Supplements and New Media

For Instructors

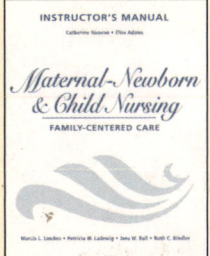

Instructor's Resource Manual
ISBN: 0130391913

This manual contains a wealth of material to help faculty plan and manage their maternity and pediatric nursing courses. It includes chapter overviews, detailed lecture suggestions and outlines, learning objectives, a complete test bank, answers to the textbook and website Thinking Critically exercises, teaching tips, and more for each chapter. The IRM also guides faculty how to assign and use the text-specific Companion Website, www.prenhall.com/london, and the Student CD-ROM that accompany the textbook.

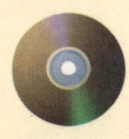

Instructor's Resource CD-ROM
ISBN: 0130391948

This cross-platform CD-ROM provides illustrations in PowerPoint from the textbook for use in classroom lectures. It also contains an electronic test bank, animations from the Student CD-ROM, and answers to the textbook and website Thinking Critically exercises, This supplement is available to faculty free upon adoption of the textbook.

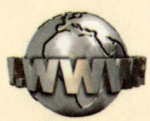

Companion Website Syllabus Manager
www.prenhall.com/london

Faculty adopting this textbook have *free* access to the online **Syllabus Manager** feature of the Companion Website, www.prenhall.com/london. It offers a whole host of features that facilitate the students' use of the Companion Website, and allows faculty to post syllabi and course information online for their students. For more information or a demonstration of Syllabus Manager, please contact your Prentice Hall Sales Representative.

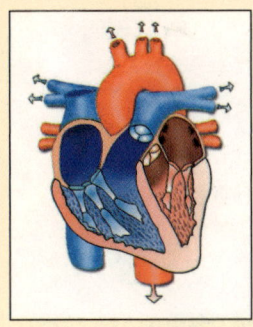

Online Course Management Systems

Also new to this package are online course companions available for schools using course management systems. The online course management solutions feature interactive modules, electronic test bank, PowerPoint images, animations and assessments. For more information about adopting an online course management system to accompany **Maternal-Newborn and Child Nursing: Family-Centered Care,** please contact your Prentice Hall Health Sales Representative or go online to www.prenhall.com/demo.

Brief Table of Contents

Maternal-Newborn & Child Nursing

FAMILY-CENTERED CARE

MARCIA L. LONDON, PhDc, RNC, NNP
Senior Clinical Instructor
Beth-El College of Nursing and Health Sciences
University of Colorado
Colorado Springs, Colorado

PATRICIA WIELAND LADEWIG, PhD, RN
Professor and Academic Dean
School for Health Care Professions
Regis University
Denver, Colorado

JANE W. BALL, DrPH, RN, CPNP
Executive Director
National Resource Center for Health Programs and Strategies
Children's National Medical Center
Washington, D.C.

RUTH C. McGILLIS BINDLER, PhD, RNC
Associate Professor
Intercollegiate College of Nursing
Washington State University
Spokane, Washington

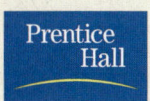
Prentice Hall

Upper Saddle River, New Jersey 07458

Library of Congress Cataloging-in-Publication Data

Maternal-newborn and child nursing: family-centered care / Marcia L. London ... [et al.].
   p. cm.
  Includes index.
  ISBN 0-13-099406-5
   1. Maternity nursing. 2. Pediatric nursing. I. London, Marcia L.

RG951 .M3145 2003
610.73'678—dc21   2002074823

Publisher: Julie Levin Alexander
Assistant to Publisher: Regina Bruno
Executive Editor: Maura Connor
Senior Managing Editor: Marilyn Meserve
Development Editor: Elena Mauceri
Assistant Editor: Yesenia Kopperman
Editorial Assistant: Sladjana Repic
Director of Production and Manufacturing: Bruce Johnson
Managing Production Editor: Patrick Walsh
Production Liaison: Danielle Newhouse
Production Editor: Lori Dalberg, Carlisle Publishers Services
Manufacturing Manager: Ilene Sanford
Design Director: Cheryl Asherman
Design Coordinator: Maria Guglielmo
Interior Designer: Lee Goldstein
Cover Designers: Lee Goldstein & Cheryl Asherman
Electronic Art Creation: Precision Graphics
Manager of Media Production: Amy Peltier
New Media Project Manager: Stephen Hartner
New Media Production: Jack Yensen, Synergy
Marketing Manager: Nicole Benson
Marketing Coordinator: Janet Ryerson
Production Information Manager: Rachele Strober
Composition: Carlisle Communications, Ltd.
Cover Printer: Lehigh Press
Printing and Binding: Von Hoffmann Press

Pearson Education, LTD.
Pearson Education Australia PTY, Limited
Pearson Education Singapore, Pte. Ltd.
Pearson Education North Asia Ltd.
Pearson Education Canada, Ltd.
Pearson Educación de Mexico, S.A. de C.V.
Pearson Education Japan
Pearson Education Malaysia, Pte. Ltd.

Permission was granted by Elsevier Science to reprint in our Nursing Care Plans the nursing intervention and outcome classifications (NIC and NOC), from McCloskey & Bulechek, *Nursing Interventions Classification* and Johnson et al., *Nursing Outcomes Classification.*

Notice: Care has been taken to confirm the accuracy of information presented in this book. The authors, editors, and the publisher, however, cannot accept any responsibility for errors or omissions or for consequences from application of the information in this book and make no warranty, express or implied, with respect to its contents.

The authors and publishers have exerted every effort to ensure that drug selections and dosages set forth in this text are in accord with current recommendations and practice at time of publication. However, in view of ongoing research, changes in government regulations, and the constant flow of information relating to drug therapy and drug reactions, the reader is urged to check the package inserts of all drugs for any change in indications of dosage and for added warnings and precautions. This is particularly important when the recommended agent is a new and/or infrequently employed drug.

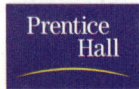
Prentice
Hall

10 9 8 7 6 5 4 3 2 1
ISBN 0-13-099406-5

Throughout the ages, nurses have made a difference—treating, healing, soothing, and caring.

And so we dedicate this book to nurses—

For their wisdom, expertise, and compassion
For their willingness to challenge the system when necessary
For their ability to remain strong during times of difficulty and stress
And for their unfailing commitment to the families they assist.

And to nursing students everywhere—

For seeking to serve others when so many have become self-serving
For committing their minds and talents to a proud profession
For accepting the challenges posed by the changes in health care
And for daring to envision a brighter tomorrow.

Then, too, as always, we honor our beloved families—

David London, Craig and Matthew
Timothy Ladewig, Ryan, his fiancée Amanda, and Erik
Ronald Ball
Julian Bindler, Dana and Ross

Contents

UNIT I
Introductory Concepts 1

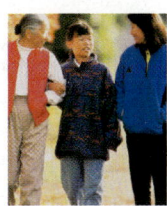

UNIT II
The Reproductive Years and Beyond 19

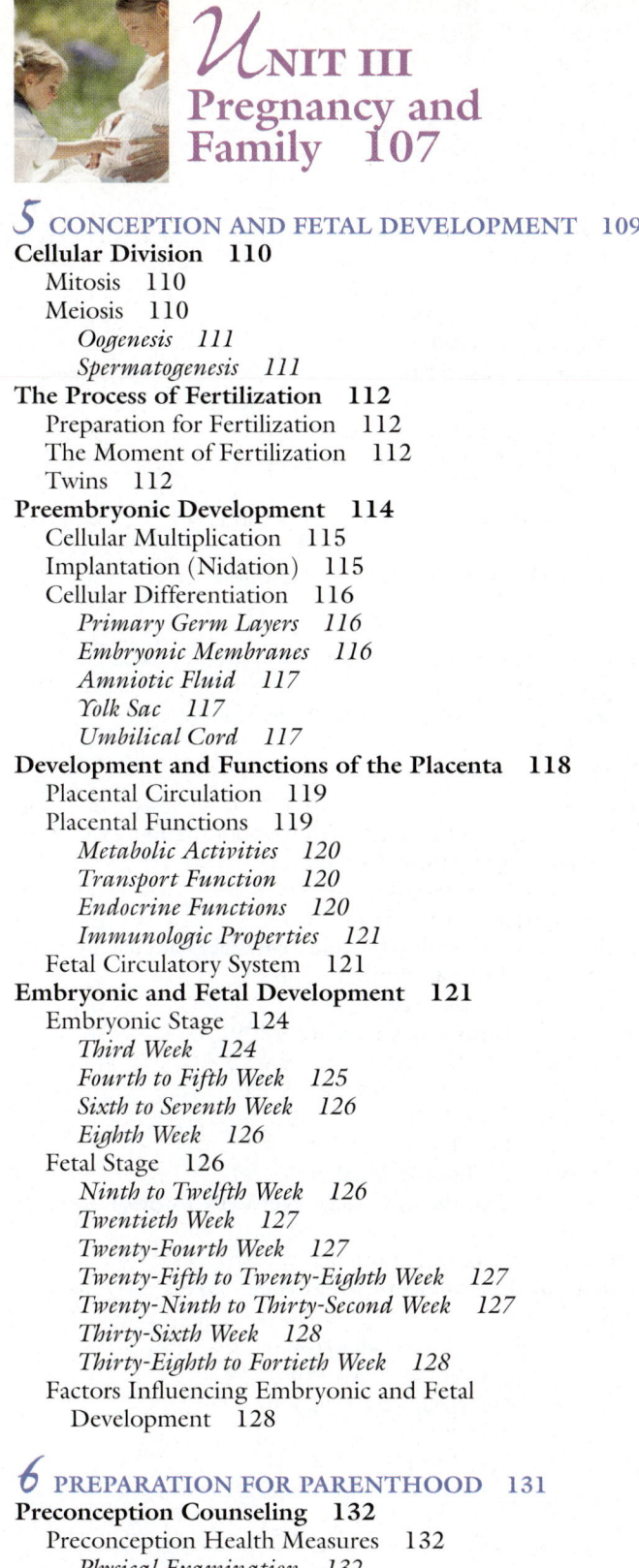

𝒰NIT V
The Postpartal Childbearing Family and Newborn 443

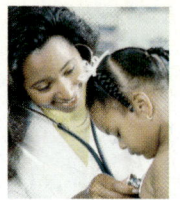

UNIT VI
Care and Needs of Children 703

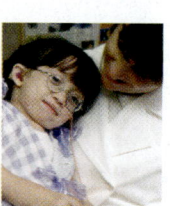

UNIT VII
Caring for Children with Alterations in Health Status 993

Preface

Today, more than ever before, nurses play a significant role in the care of families during pregnancy and the experience of birth, and then with the child's care through all stages of growth. Nurses working with childbearing and childrearing families are challenged by a variety of forces that affect the provision of nursing care. Our goal is a text that is accurate and readable, and one that helps students develop the skills and abilities they need now and in the future in an ever-changing health care environment. The underlying philosophy of *Maternal-Newborn and Child Nursing: Family-Centered Care* is that the family members are coparticipants in care, whether this is related to pregnancy and childbirth or to care of the infant or child at any stage of development.

Families experience the excitement and exhilaration of adding a healthy infant to the family, but they also experience sorrow and concern when a health problem occurs. Nurses play a pivotal role in helping families celebrate the normal life processes associated with birth and then foster the child's growth and development from infancy through adolescence. Infants and children are dependent upon their families for the care they need. Nursing care for pregnant women and children is a family-centered process. We are committed to providing a text that integrates the needs of families across the continuum from conception through adolescence.

NURSING CARE IN THE COMMUNITY

Most maternity and pediatric nursing care occurs in the community setting, especially since most pregnant women and children are healthy and have only episodic acute health conditions. Although pregnancy, birth, and the postpartal period cover a timeframe of many months, in reality most women spend only two to three days in an acute care facility. Thus, by its very nature, maternal-newborn nursing is primarily community-based nursing. Moreover, because of the changes resulting from managed care, even women with high-risk pregnancies are receiving more care in their homes and in the community and are spending less time in hospital settings.

Dramatic health care system changes have resulted in community and home care for children with serious chronic health conditions, including children needing care with advanced technology. Short-stay surgical units and short-term observation units have replaced hospitalization for many acute conditions. The nurse's role in preparing a family for their child's discharge from an acute care facility is often the transitional step to nursing care in the home and community. Information on long-term management of complex health conditions is included as these problems are especially challenging to manage in community settings. Selected ambulatory pediatric conditions are also included because students will see them in everyday life and in the hospital where these conditions are secondary to the presenting problem.

Because many graduating nurses practice in acute care facilities, this text emphasizes the information necessary to prepare students to work in that setting. Students who understand how to care for families effectively in an acute care setting can readily transfer these skills to other nursing situations and environments. However, there is a strong emphasis on helping pregnant women, parents and families care for themselves and their children in community settings.

As educators and nurses, we have organized this text to flow logically and to integrate maternity and pediatric nursing concepts carefully. For example, Chapter 1 begins with introductory concepts important for maternal, newborn, and child nursing. Later chapters focus on reproductive issues and women's health, pregnancy, birth processes, postpartum care, newborn management, and then transition into the pediatric care chapters. The pediatric chapters first address general pediatric health care concepts, and then the nursing care of children with various disorders, organized by body system. We have made efforts to reduce duplication and potentially conflicting information throughout the text.

Throughout this text, several core elements have been emphasized.

- **Assessment** is an essential and core role in the nursing process. Several chapters are dedicated to helping the student perform an assessment, at each stage along the pregnancy continuum, of the fetus and newborn, and then later of children.
- **Communication** is one of the most important skills that students need to learn. Effective communication is the very fiber of nursing practice. This book integrates communication skills in an applied manner where students can most benefit.
- We feel a strong commitment as nurses and educators to the importance of recognizing and honoring diversity and multiculturalism. The influence of the family's **culture** on health beliefs and health care practices cannot be underestimated. A brief introduction to cultural issues relevant to maternity and child nursing care is provided in Chapter 1. Content about specific cultural issues and their application to nursing care is integrated throughout the text, often made visible in **Developing Cultural Competence**

boxes. We believe this integration of issues affecting maternal-newborn and pediatric nursing care—beyond the emphasis on ethnicity alone—provides the most accessible format.

- Nursing care in **community settings** forms a dominant theme in this text. Two separate chapters, *Home Care of the Postpartal Family,* and *Nursing Considerations for the Child in the Community* provide a theoretical perspective and important tools in caring for childbearing and childrearing families in the community setting. We have also addressed this topic in focused, user-friendly features. **Nursing Care in the Community** is a special heading used throughout this text and indicated by an icon to help students recognize this content. Because we consider home care to be one form of community-based care, it often has a separate heading under Nursing Care in the Community.
- Assuring appropriate **nutrition** during pregnancy and during infancy and childhood is important to promote growth and development, as well as the health of the pregnant woman, fetus, newborn, infant, child, and adolescent. Three chapters address nutrition for the pregnant woman, the newborn, and children.
- **Pain** is now considered the fifth vital sign, and pain management is a priority in health care settings. Two chapters address pain assessment and management. Applicable pain management is discussed when appropriate in other chapters.

USE OF THE NURSING PROCESS

The nursing process is emphasized throughout the nursing care chapters. We use the heading **Nursing Management** to highlight nursing actions. Selected health issues or conditions have an expanded section on nursing management to help students understand and apply the nursing process more completely. We present sections on *Nursing Assessment and Diagnosis, Planning and Implementation,* and *Evaluation.* The health issues and conditions in this comprehensive presentation were chosen because they are seen frequently or because of their high-risk nature.

In keeping with the changing approaches to nursing care management, **Nursing Care Plans** and **Clinical Pathways** are featured throughout the text. The *nursing care plans* are designed to help students approach care from the nursing process perspective. They have integrated the new nursing diagnosis features of Nursing Intervention Classifications (NIC) and Nursing Outcome Classifications (NOC). The *clinical pathways* are designed to help students plan and manage care within normally anticipated time frames. The plans and pathways help students become familiar with these two approaches to managing care so that they are better equipped for variations in clinical settings.

Client education remains a critical element of effective nursing care, one that is emphasized and highlighted in this text. Our focus is on the teaching that nurses do at all stages of pregnancy and the childbearing process, and during the child's health visits and care for specific conditions. There is a significant emphasis on helping pregnant women, parents, and family members care for themselves and their children after leaving the hospital and also in the various community settings. A special patient education feature is integrated into many chapters of the text—**Teaching About** a special health care issue or problem includes the key teaching points for care by the family.

CRITICAL THINKING

Nurses today must be able to think critically and problem solve effectively. To support the development of critical thinking skills, **Thinking Critically** boxes provide brief scenarios that ask students to determine the appropriate response. Suggested answers to the scenarios are provided on the Student CD-ROM and the Instructor's Resource Manual so that students have feedback on their decision-making skills. Additionally, students can access a variety of critical thinking exercises and case studies on the textbook's companion website at www.prenhall.com/london.

RESEARCH AND EVIDENCE-BASED PRACTICE

Additionally, health care professionals are increasingly aware of the importance of using reliable information as the basis for planning and providing effective care. This approach, called **evidence-based practice,** draws on information from a variety of sources including nursing research. To help nurses become more comfortable integrating new knowledge into their nursing practice, we have included a brief discussion of evidence-based practice in Chapter 1. While the text uses current literature and research findings, we have chosen to present our research features on the text's website. This allows the information to be updated easily and makes it possible to provide links for further research so students can maximize their understanding of research and evidence-based practice.

NOTABLE FEATURES

Instructors and students both value in-text learning aids. We have developed a text that is easy to learn from and easy to use as a reference. In keeping with our theme of family-centered care, each chapter begins with a **Family Quote** that helps set the stage for content that follows from the family's perspective. This is followed by a list of **Key Terms.** Page numbers are included with each key term to identify the place where the term first appears in the chapter. Media related to the chapter content is highlighted in features called **MediaLink** at the beginning of each chapter. Each chapter ends with a chapter review that consists of a summary of **Chapter Highlights,** a list of **References,** and a section entitled **EXPLORE MediaLink.** This last section encourages students to use the additional chapter-specific NCLEX review, interactive exercises, and resources available on the accompanying free Student CD-ROM and the Companion Website at www.prenhall.com/london. Finally, a **Glossary** of terms commonly used in the field of maternal-newborn and child nursing can be found on the Student CD-ROM and the Companion Website, with audio pronunciations of the terms as well as printed definitions.

Students may notice a "voice" change within chapters. For example, within the more theoretical/knowledge sections of the chapters, we address the students as "the nurse". Within the nursing management sections we speak to the students directly (e.g., "Assess . . .", "Manage . . .", etc.). This way, students have a very clear understanding of their responsibilities, and can put themselves in the role of the nurse more easily. Explicit second person address ("you") is used only in boxed features.

Other features found in the text include the following:

- **Nursing Practice** features offer hands-on suggestions and clinical tips. These are placed at locations in the text that will help students apply them. They include topics such as legal and ethical considerations, nursing alerts, and home and community care considerations.
- **Developing Cultural Competence** provides information about the potential responses of different ethnic groups to health conditions or to medical or nursing care interventions.
- **Complementary Care** features present information about commonly used alternative and complementary measures to treat or provide comfort for various conditions.
- **Thinking Critically** boxes provide brief scenarios that ask students to determine the appropriate response.
- **Teaching About** is a special patient education feature that highlights a special health care issue or problem and includes the key teaching points for care by the family.
- **Drug Guides** for selected medications commonly used in maternal-newborn and child nursing are included to guide students in correctly administering the medications and evaluating their action.
- **Important lab values** are highlighted within the chapters as a tool for students to assess their patients' conditions. In addition, an appendix presents normal ranges for children by age group. The information is presented in one location because many conditions are evaluated with the same lab values.
- **Cross-reference** icons ⊂⊃ help the student to correlate related information in other chapters.
- **CD-ROM** and **Skills** icons CD SKILLS remind the student that comprehensive information related to specific skills can be found on the accompanying CD-ROM and/or the supplemental *Clinical Skills Manual*.

- **Assessment Guides,** found in the maternal-newborn chapters, assist students with diagnoses by incorporating physical assessment and normal findings, alterations and possible causes, as well as guidelines for nursing interventions.
- **Pathophysiology Illustrated** provides information about the pathophysiologic process associated with a health condition using art, graphics, and photography to enhance the student's understanding.
- **Clinical Manifestations** tables help students understand the association between the pathophysiology and the signs and symptoms of a particular condition. In some cases, these tables present several similar conditions so that students can see the differentiation between conditions. In some cases, the table includes treatment for the clinical manifestations and conditions.
- **As They Grow,** found in the pediatric-specific chapters, illustrates the anatomic and physiologic differences in infants and children from adults.
- **Growth and Development,** also found exclusively in the pediatric chapters, features provide information about the different responses of children at various ages to health conditions.

COMPREHENSIVE TEACHING AND LEARNING PACKAGE

To enhance the teaching and learning process, the following supplements have been developed in close correlation with this new textbook. The full complement of supplemental teaching materials is available to all qualified instructors from your Prentice Hall Sales Representative.

Student CD-ROM. The Student CD-ROM includes many valuable learning supplements. It is packaged free with every copy of the textbook.

- The audio glossary helps review key terms used throughout the textbook.
- Most of the nursing skills included in the supplemental *Clinical Skills Manual* for the care of the pregnant woman, newborn, and children are on the CD-ROM. The skills show the step-by-step process for performing a procedure and the rationale for specific actions.
- NCLEX-style multiple-choice questions emphasize the application of nursing care. Students can test their knowledge and gain immediate feedback through rationales for right and wrong answers.
- The CD-ROM also provides animations to help students understand and visualize difficult concepts in maternal-newborn and pediatric nursing care. CD-ROM icons CD indicate when the student should refer to the CD-ROM to view these animations.
- Students can access the answers to the Thinking Critically questions found in the textbook.
- Finally, the CD-ROM allows access to the website described later in this section.

Clinical Skills Manual. The clinical skills manual describes commonly performed maternal, newborn, women's health, and pediatric nursing skills. This colorful and highly visual manual clearly shows students the steps required to perform each skill. It is assumed that students have already had a basic skills course so the material presented focuses on techniques specific to maternal-newborn nursing and pediatrics. Both hospital-based and community-based skills are included. Margin boxes emphasize material such as clinical tips and safety considerations. The protocols for performing skills contain rationales when needed to clarify recommended actions.

Instructor's Resource Manual. This effective teaching aid guides instructors on how to use *Maternal-Newborn and Child Nursing: Family-Centered Care* for their courses. It includes lecture suggestions, objectives, test questions, answers to the textbook Thinking Critically exercises, a guide to PowerPoint images and animations on the Instructor's Resource CD-ROM, and a guide to using the Companion Website and Syllabus Manager. Finally, it includes a test bank of items that follow the NCLEX format and are classified by cognitive level, nursing process step, and client need.

Instructor's Resource CD-ROM. This practical CD-ROM provides three resources in an electronic format. First, the CD-ROM includes the complete test bank in a PC-compatible format. Second, it includes a comprehensive collection of images from the textbook in PowerPoint format, so faculty can easily import these photographs and illustrations into their own classroom lecture presentations. Finally, instructors can access the animations found on the Student CD-ROM so they can incorporate them into their lectures.

Companion Website and Syllaus Manager®. Faculty and students using this textbook may access the free Companion Website at www.prenhall.com/london. This website serves as a text-specific, interactive online workbook to *Maternal-Newborn and Child Nursing: Family-Centered Care*. The website includes modules for objectives, chapter outlines, audio glossary with definitions, discussion questions with essay responses, research activities, NCLEX review questions with automatic grading, links to other sites for student research and essay responses, additional nursing care plans and clinical pathways, and more. Instructors adopting this textbook for their courses have free access to an online Syllabus Manager with a whole host of features that facilitate the students' use of this Companion Website and allow faculty to post their syllabi online for their students. For more information or a demonstration of Syllabus Manager, please contact your Prentice Hall Sales Representative or go online to www.prenhall.com/demo.

Online Course Management Systems. Also added to this package are online course companions available for schools using Blackboard, WebCT, or Course Compass course management systems. For more information about adopting an online course management system to accompany *Maternal-Newborn and Child Nursing: Family-Centered Care,* please contact your Prentice Hall Health Sales Representative or go online to www.prenhall.com/demo.

Finally, we sense that nursing is becoming reenergized. Perhaps not surprisingly, the tragic events of September 11, 2001 have had some positive effects. People are reevaluating their lives and their goals. Many feel a strong desire to choose professions that make a difference—professions such as nursing. We, like you, know that expert nurses can have a tremendous impact on the lives of childbearing and child-rearing families. Our goal in writing this text is to help prepare nurses with the skills and knowledge to make a difference—one family at a time.

Marcia L. London
Patricia W. Ladewig
Jane W. Ball
Ruth C. Bindler

Acknowledgments

Nursing is a dynamic, exciting health care profession. As curricula develop, many nursing programs have begun to offer nursing of childbearing families and nursing of children together in a single course. This combined approach requires that faculty approach these two fields with a similar framework and philosophy, and with similar teaching methods, so that students can maximize learning. With this new text, we have sought to create a tool that will enable students to master these two critical areas of nursing—the care of childbearing families and the care of children. Creating a new, dynamic, and useful text would not be possible without the skill and dedication of a host of people.

We wish to acknowledge the contributions to the Complementary Care features in the textbook and on the Companion Website. These individuals brought their specialized knowledge to the project:

Faye Bailey, RN, BSN, C, CIMI
Carol Baldwin, PhD, RN, HNC
Karen Fontaine, RN, MSN, AASECT
Lynette Leeseberg Stamler, RN, PhD
Marilyn Joy Leeseberg, BA, MMT
Karen C. Haack, BMus.
Sylvia M. Kubsch, RN, PhD
Geralyn Jadin, RN, BSN, C
Nicette Julevics, MC, ICCE
Kathryn Landon-Malone, PNP
Sunny Pendleton Mavor, BS
John D. Mark, MD
Suzi Cekarmis Schoon, DNS, RN
Ilene Spector, DO
Maria Luisa Urdaneta, RN, PhD
Sherry Warden, PhD, RN
Beverly Yates, ND
Steven Yeomans, DC
Mark Edinger, DC

We offer our thanks to Lisa Haynie, RN, MSN, CFNP, who skillfully prepared several of our Nursing Care Plans. And we wish to express gratitude to the following individuals who contributed to the CD-ROM and Companion Website:

Ann Bianchi, MSN, RN
Calhoun Community College

Linda Cassata, MSN, RN
University of Illinois-Chicago

Bernadette Dragich, PhD, RN, FNP
Bluefield State College

Judith Halle, PhD, RN
West Virginia Wesleyan College

Pamela Hamre, MS, RN, CNM
College of St. Catherine

Tina Magers, MSN, RN
Mississippi Baptist Health Systems

Kimberly Serroha, MSN, RN
Youngstown State University

Sharon Stoffels, MSN, RNC
Boise State University

Nancy Wagner, MSN, RN
Youngstown State University

Katherine West, MPH, MSN, RN
Azusa Pacific University

We also wish to acknowledge the authors of the Instructor's Resource Manual:

Catherine Noonan, RN, MS, CPNP
Bunker Hill Community College and Boston Children's Hospital

Ellise Adams, CNM, MSN, CD (DONA), ICCE
Calhoun Community College

We would personally like to thank several people. At Prentice-Hall, Maura Connor, our editor, merits our deepest thanks. Her vision brought this project to fruition. She is a woman of energy, enthusiasm, and dedication, who gave us tremendous support and encouragement. We consider her a special friend. Our thanks also go to Julie Levin Alexander, our publisher. Julie is a woman committed to excellence and creativity. She is the driving force behind the exciting changes occurring at Prentice Hall Health and is truly a visionary in publishing. We also wish to thank Cheryl Asherman, Director of Design, for the striking design of the text and Sladjana Repic, Editorial Assistant, for helping with the myriad of details involved in preparing a manuscript of this size.

Operationally, this book exists in large part because of the tremendous dedication, patience, and skill of one woman—our developmental editor, Elena Mauceri. During the long months of hard work, Elena remained calm, focused, organized, and creative. She noted discrepancies, worked for continuity, pitched in everywhere, and earned the respect of all of us. She even ordered us massages when they were most needed! She is truly amazing and we hope to work with her on future projects.

Like Elena, Kim Wyatt, developmental editor of the Third Edition of the Ball and Bindler Pediatric Nursing textbook, helped us complete this project successfully. Kim has a thorough understanding of child health care. This understanding enabled her to suggest methods of presenting material to facilitate learning for students. She often took on extra tasks to meet deadlines and helped keep us focused on our goals.

Whitney Wood skillfully edited our chapters for writing style consistency. Her attention to making our writing clear and succinct will be valued by students and instructors.

Special thanks to the people of Carlisle Communications, especially Lori Dalberg, for coordinating production, and Joan Lyon, for her work as copyeditor. They are perceptive, organized, and skillful in all of the tasks of publishing.

Finally we all wish to thank our other co-authors. As four individuals, but two teams, we came together with our own ideas, writing styles, and vision for this book. We collaborated, argued, cajoled, and compromised. It was a challenging but rewarding process. Together we created a new and different text for maternal, newborn, and child health nursing, a book and associated learning aids that we hope will be a useful tool for legions of nursing students to come.

Marcia L. London
Patricia W. Ladewig
Jane W. Ball
Ruth C. Bindler

Reviewers

We are grateful to all the nurses, both clinicians and educators, who reviewed the manuscript of this text. Their insights, suggestions, and eye for detail helped us prepare a more relevant and useful book, one that focuses on the essential components of learning in the fields of maternal, newborn, and child health nursing.

Ann Bello, RN, MA
Illinois Valley Community College
Oglesby, IL

Ellise D. Adams, CNM, MSN
Calhoun Community College
Huntsville, AL

Deborah H. Amason, RN, MS
Floyd College
Rome, GA

Louise Aurilio, PhD, MSN, RNC, CNA
Youngstown State University
Girard, OH

Kathaleen C. Bloom, PhD, CNM
University of North Florida
Jacksonville, FL

Constance Bobik, RN, BSN, MSN
Brevard Community College
Titusville, FL

Lisa A. Broussard, MSN
University of Louisiana at Lafayette
New Iberia, LA

Judy Buzby, RN
Niagara County Community College
Sanborn, NY

Martha Craft-Rosenberg, PhD, RN, FAAN
University of Iowa
Iowa City, IA

Cheryl DeGraw, RN, MSN, CRNP
Florence Darlington Technical College
Florence, SC

Priscilla Markley Delikowski MSN, RN
Fox Valley Technical College
Appleton, WI

Shannon M. Dowdall, MSN, RN
University of Texas-Pan American
Edinburg, TX

Lynn Doyle, RN, MS, CPNP
Marian College
Fond du Lac, WI

Lori Fuhrer, RN, BSN
Brevard Community College
Titusville, FL

Lisa Haynie, RN, MSN, CFNP
University of Mississippi School of Nursing
Jackson, MS

Diane C. LaGrange, RN, MSN
University of Texas-Pan American
Edinburg, TX

Hope M. Moon, RN, MSN, CNS
Lorain County Community College
Elyria, OH

Debbie McGregor, MSN
Broward Community College
Miramar, FL

Dana Murphy-Parker, RN, BSN
Arizona Western College
Yuma, AZ

LaDonna Northington, RN, DNS
University of Mississippi School of Nursing
Jackson, MS

Roselle Partridge, RNC, MSN
Indiana University School of Nursing
Indianapolis, IN

Marlene Poe-Greskamp, RN, MSN, CFLE
Andersen University
Andersen, IN

Michelle Renaud, RN, CCRN, PhD
Pacific Lutheran University
Tacoma, WA

Lynn Rhyne, MN, RN
Coastal Georgia Community College
Brunswick, GA

Ruth Robillard, EdD, RN
University of North Florida
Jacksonville, FL

Kathy Russell, RNC, MSN
Front Range Community College
Westminster, CO

Carol Shimer, MS, RN
Pasco-Hernando Community College
New Port Richey, FL

Loretta Tharpe, RN, FNP-C
Saddleback College
Mission Viejo, CA

Sharon A. Vinten, RNC, MSN, WHNP
Indiana University School of Nursing
Indianapolis, IN

Karen Wilkinson, MN, RN, ARNP
University of Washington, School of Nursing
Seattle, WA

P. Renee Williams, RN, MSN, CCE
University of Mississippi Medical Center School of Nursing
Jackson, MS

Michele Woodbeck, MS, RN
Hudson Valley Community College
Troy, NY

STUDENT REVIEWERS

Michele Berkstresser
University of Scranton
Bridgewater, NJ

Debra Brooks
University of Scranton
Scranton, PA

Maria Delcos
Pasco-Hernando Community College
New Port Richey, FL

Mary Anne Hutchinson
Pasco-Hernando Community College
New Port Richey, FL

Tina Kunze
University of Maryland
Laurel, MD

Phyllis Thieken
Ohio University
Jackson, OH

About the Authors

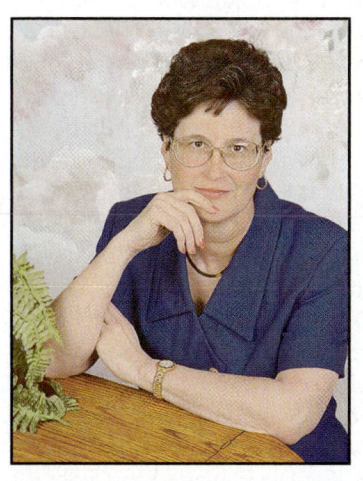

Marcia L. London

Marcia L. London has been able to combine her two greatest passions by being both a nurse caring for children and families and a teacher for almost 31 years. She received her B.S.N. and school nurse certificate from Plattsburgh State University in Plattsburgh, New York. After graduation, she began her nursing career as a pediatric nurse at St. Luke's Hospital in New York City, then moved to Pittsburgh, where she began her teaching career. Mrs. London accepted a faculty position at Pittsburgh's Children's Hospital Affiliate Program and received her M.S.N. in pediatrics as a clinical nurse specialist from the University of Pittsburgh. Mrs. London began teaching at Beth-El School of Nursing and Health Science in 1974 after opening the first intensive care nursery at Memorial Hospital of Colorado Springs. She has served in many administrative and faculty positions at Beth-El, including coordinator for nursing care of children for 28 years. Mrs. London maintains her clinical skills working in a pediatric after-hours clinic and doing undergraduate pediatric clinical supervision. She obtained her postmaster's neonatal nurse practitioner certificate in 1983 and subsequently developed the neonatal nurse practitioner (NNP) program and the master's NNP program at Beth-El. She is active nationally in neonatal nursing and was involved in the development of the *Neonatal Nurse Practitioner Educational Program Guidelines*. Mrs. London is active in nurse practitioner education in general. She is involved in the revision of the *Core Competency for Nurse Practitioners and Curriculum Guidelines for Nurse Practitioner Education*, as a member of the Education Committee of the National Organization of Nurse Practitioner Faculties. Mrs. London is currently completing her Ph.D. in higher education administration and adult studies at the University of Denver in Colorado. She feels fortunate to be involved in the education of her future colleagues. Her teaching philosophy is that, with support, students can achieve more than they may initially believe they are capable of achieving. Mrs. London and her husband have two sons and two dogs (Samantha and Betsy, daughters by proxy). Her two sons, Craig and Matthew, are studying computers and computer animation in college and are more than willing to give Mom helpful hints.

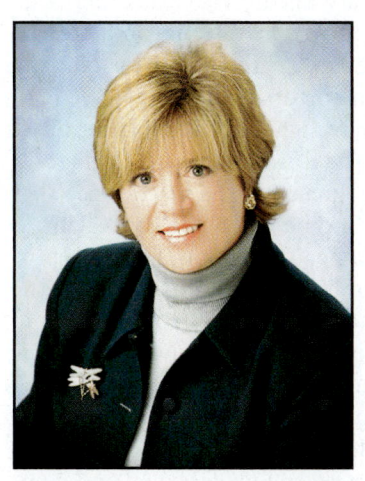

Patricia A. Wieland Ladewig

Patricia A. Wieland Ladewig received her B.S. from the College of Saint Teresa in Winona, Minnesota. After graduation, she worked as a pediatric nurse before joining the U.S. Air Force. After completing her tour of duty, Dr. Ladewig relocated at Florida, where she accepted a faculty position at Florida State University. There she embraced teaching as her calling. Over the years, she taught at several schools of nursing while earning her M.S.N. in maternal-newborn nursing from Catholic University of America in Washington, D.C., and her Ph.D. in higher education administration from the University of Denver in Colorado. In addition, she became a women's health nurse practitioner and maintained a part-time clinical practice. In 1988 Dr. Ladewig became the first director of the nursing program at Regis College in Denver and, in 1991, when the college became Regis University, she became dean of the School for Health Care Professions. Under her guidance, the Department of Nursing has added a graduate program and the School for Health Care Professions has added two departments: the Department of Physical Therapy and the Department of Health Services Administration and Management. Dr. Ladewig feels that teaching others to be excellent, caring nurses gives her the best of all worlds because it keeps her in touch with the profession she loves and enables her to help shape the future of the nursing profession. When not at work or writing textbooks, Pat and her husband, Tim, enjoy skiing, climbing Colorado's 14'ers (14,000-foot mountains, 15 of which she has climbed to date), and traveling. They are the parents of two sons, Ryan, a computer scientist who works in Denver, and Erik, a student at Regis University. Pat is especially pleased to announce that Ryan recently became engaged to a lovely young woman—Amanda—who is also a nurse!

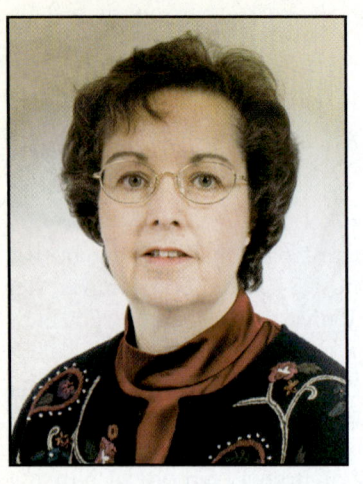

Jane W. Ball

Jane W. Ball graduated from the Johns Hopkins Hospital School of Nursing, and subsequently received a B.S. from the Johns Hopkins University. She worked in the surgical, emergency, and outpatient units of the Johns Hopkins Children's Medical and Surgical Center, first as a staff nurse and then as a pediatric nurse practitioner. This began her career as a pediatric nurse and advocate for children's health needs. Jane obtained both a master of public health and doctor of public health degree from the Johns Hopkins University Bloomberg School of Public Health with a focus on maternal and child health. After graduation she became the chief of child health services for the Commonwealth of Pennsylvania Department of Health. In this capacity she oversaw the state-funded well-child clinics and explored ways to improve education for the state's community health nurses. After relocating to Texas, she joined the faculty at the University of Texas at Arlington School of Nursing to teach community pediatrics to registered nurses returning to school for a B.S.N. During this time she became involved in writing her first textbook, *Mosby's Guide to Physical Examination,* which is currently in its fifth edition. After relocating to the Washington, D.C., area, she joined Children's National Medical Center to manage a federal project to teach instructors of emergency medical technicians from all states about the special care children need during an emergency. Exposure to the shortcomings of the emergency medical services system in the late 1980s with regard to pediatric care was a career-changing event. With federal funding, she developed educational curricula for emergency medical technicians and emergency nurses to help them provide improved care for children. A textbook entitled *Pediatric Emergencies, A Manual for Prehospital Providers* was developed from these educational ventures. For the past 10 years she has managed the federally funded Emergency Medical Services for Children National Resource Center. As executive director, Dr. Ball directs the provision of consultation and resource development for state health agencies, health professionals, families, and advocates about successful methods to improve the health care system so that children get optimal emergency care in all health care settings.

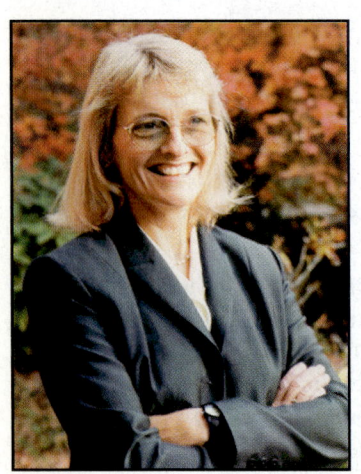

Ruth C. McGillis Bindler

Ruth Bindler received her B.S.N. from Cornell University–New York Hospital School of Nursing in New York. She worked in oncology nursing at Sloan Kettering Cancer Center in New York, and then moved to Wisconsin and became a public health nurse in Dane County, Wisconsin. Thus began her commitment to work with children as she visited children and their families at home, and served as a school nurse for several elementary, middle, and high schools. Due to this interest in child health care needs, she earned her M.S. in child development from the University of Wisconsin. A move to Washington State was accompanied by a new job as a faculty member at the Intercollegiate Center for Nursing Education in Spokane, Washington. Dr. Bindler has been fortunate to be involved for 28 years in the growth of this nursing education consortium, which is a combination of public and private universities and colleges and is now the Intercollegiate College of Nursing/Washington State University College of Nursing. Presently she teaches the theory course in child health and a course on cultural diversity and health, as well as serving as lead faculty for the theory and clinical components of child health nursing. Her first professional book, *Pediatric Medications,* was published in 1981, and she has continued to publish articles and books in the areas of pediatric medications and pediatric health. Special research interests are in the area of cardiovascular risk factors in children, a topic that was the focus of her recent Ph.D. work in human nutrition at Washington State University. Ethnic diversity has been another theme in her work. She facilitates international and other diversity experiences for students and performs research with culturally diverse children. Dr. Bindler believes that her role as a faculty member has enabled her to learn continually, to foster the development of students in nursing, and to participate fully in the profession of nursing. In addition to teaching, research, publication, and leadership, she enhances her life by service in several professional and community activities, and by activities with her family.

A GUIDE TO
*M*aternal-Newborn *M*and Child Nursing

Chapter Opening Family Quote
Each chapter begins with a Family Quote that helps set the stage for chapter content from the family's perspective.

Key Terms
Key terms introduce each chapter. Page numbers are included with each key term to identify the place where the term first appears in the chapter, in bold type.

MediaLink
MediaLink introduces each chapter of the text and lists additional specific content, animations, NCLEX Review, other interactive exercises, and tools, which appear on the accompanying Student CD-ROM and the Companion Web site.

As They Grow
Found in the pediatric chapters, As They Grow boxes illustrate the anatomic and physiologic differences between children and adults. This enhances students' knowledge in association with a specific topic and helps them to apply theoretical information in practical situations.

Cross-Referencing Icons and Media Supplements
There are three types of icons that appear regularly throughout the textbook. The link icon, ⬭ when used alone, guides students to other sections of the textbook for more information. When this link is used in combination with the CD and web icons, ⬭ WEB CD they refer students to specific animations, additional content, resources or activities contained in the media supplements accompany this textbook. The link icon used with the skills icon ⬭ SKILLS refers students to specific maternal-newborn and pediatric skills in the *Clinical Skills Manual for Maternal-Newborn and Child Nursing*. Note that many of the skills can also be found on the CD-ROM, so the CD icon is frequently used in conjunction with the skills icon.

Nursing Practice
Nursing Practice features offer hands-on suggestions and clinical tips. Placed at locations in the text that will help students apply them, they include topics such as legal and ethical considerations, nursing alerts, and home and community care considerations.

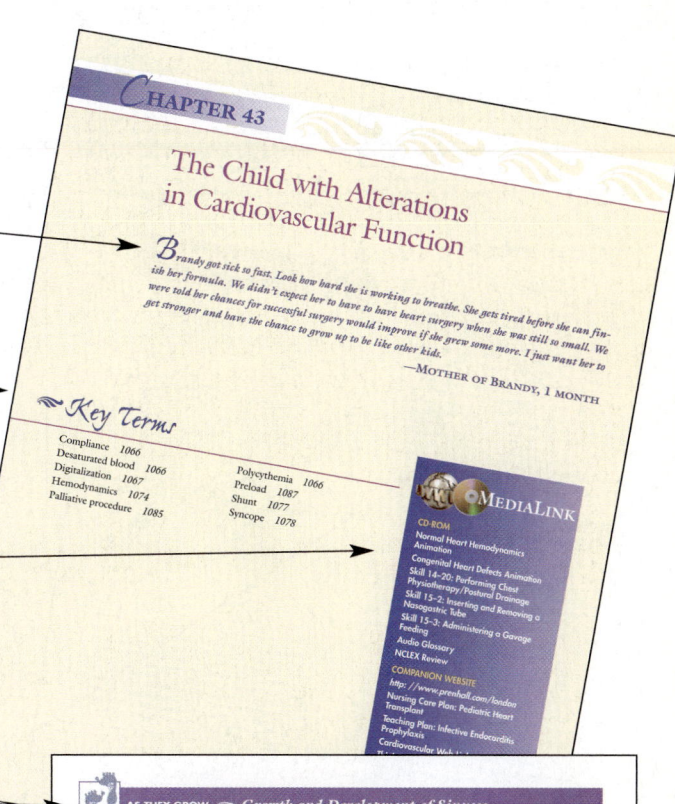

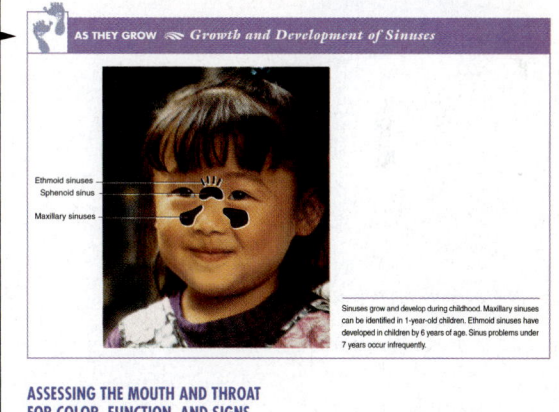

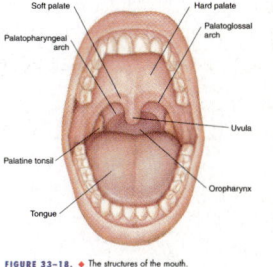

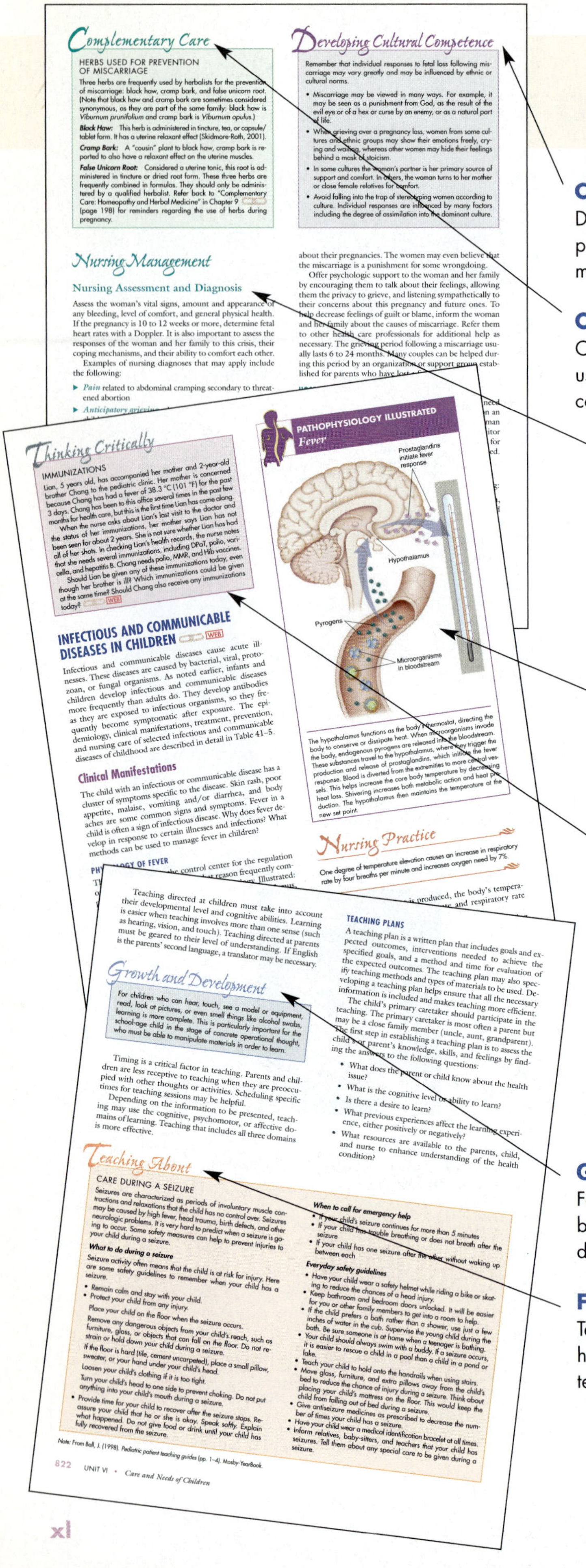

Complementary Care

HERBS USED FOR PREVENTION OF MISCARRIAGE

Three herbs are frequently used by herbalists for the prevention of miscarriage: black haw, cramp bark, and false unicorn root. (Note that black haw and cramp bark are sometimes considered synonymous, as they are part of the same family: black haw is *Viburnum prunifolium* and cramp bark is *Viburnum opulus*.)

Black Haw: This herb is administered in tincture, tea, or capsule/tablet form. It has a uterine relaxant effect (Skidmore-Roth, 2001).

Cramp Bark: A "cousin" plant to black haw, cramp bark is reported to also have a relaxant effect on the uterine muscles.

False Unicorn Root: Considered a uterine tonic, this root is administered in tincture or dried root form. These three herbs are frequently combined in formulas. They should only be administered by a qualified herbalist. Refer back to "Complementary Care: Homeopathy and Herbal Medicine" in Chapter 9 (page 198) for reminders regarding the use of herbs during pregnancy.

Developing Cultural Competence

Remember that individual responses to fetal loss following miscarriage may vary greatly and may be influenced by ethnic or cultural norms.

- Miscarriage may be viewed in many ways. For example, it may be seen as a punishment from God, as the result of the evil eye or of a hex or curse by an enemy, or as a natural part of life.
- When grieving over a pregnancy loss, women from some cultures and ethnic groups may show their emotions freely, crying and wailing, whereas other women may hide their feelings behind a mask of stoicism.
- In some cultures the woman's partner is her primary source of support and comfort. In others, the woman turns to her mother or close female relatives for comfort.
- Avoid falling into the trap of stereotyping women according to culture. Individual responses are influenced by many factors including the degree of assimilation into the dominant culture.

Nursing Management

Nursing Assessment and Diagnosis

Assess the woman's vital signs, amount and appearance of any bleeding, level of comfort, and general physical health. If the pregnancy is 10 to 12 weeks or more, determine fetal heart rates with a Doppler. It is also important to assess the responses of the woman and her family to this crisis, their coping mechanisms, and their ability to comfort each other.

Examples of nursing diagnoses that may apply include the following:

▶ *Pain* related to abdominal cramping secondary to threatened abortion

▶ *Anticipatory grieving* ...

about their pregnancies. The women may even believe that the miscarriage is a punishment for some wrongdoing.

Offer psychologic support to the woman and her family by encouraging them to talk about their feelings, allowing them the privacy to grieve, and listening sympathetically to their concerns about this pregnancy and future ones. To help decrease feelings of guilt or blame, inform the woman and her family about the causes of miscarriage. Refer them to other health care professionals for additional help as necessary. The grieving period following a miscarriage usually lasts 6 to 24 months. Many couples can be helped during this period by an organization or support group established for parents who have lost ...

PATHOPHYSIOLOGY ILLUSTRATED
Fever

Thinking Critically

IMMUNIZATIONS

Lian, 5 years old, has accompanied her mother and 2-year-old brother Chang to the pediatric clinic. Her mother is concerned because Chang has had a fever of 38.3°C (101°F) for the past 3 days. Chang has been to this office several times in the past few months for health care, but this is the first time Lian has come along.

When the nurse asks about Lian's last visit to the doctor and the status of her immunizations, her mother says Lian has not been seen for about 2 years. She is not sure whether Lian has had all of her shots. In checking Lian's health records, the nurse notes that she needs several immunizations, including DPaT, polio, varicella, and hepatitis B. Chang needs polio, MMR, and Hib vaccines.

Should Lian be given any of these immunizations today, even though her brother is ill? Which immunizations could be given at the same time? Should Chang also receive any immunizations today?

INFECTIOUS AND COMMUNICABLE DISEASES IN CHILDREN

Infectious and communicable diseases cause acute illnesses. These diseases are caused by bacterial, viral, protozoan, or fungal organisms. As noted earlier, infants and children develop infectious and communicable diseases more frequently than adults do. They develop antibodies as they are exposed to infectious organisms, so they frequently become symptomatic after exposure. The epidemiology, clinical manifestations, treatment, prevention, and nursing care of selected infectious and communicable diseases of childhood are described in detail in Table 41–5.

Clinical Manifestations

The child with an infectious or communicable disease has a cluster of symptoms specific to the disease. Skin rash, poor appetite, malaise, vomiting and/or diarrhea, and body aches are some common signs and symptoms. Fever in a child is often a sign of infectious disease. Why does fever develop in response to certain illnesses and infections? What methods can be used to manage fever in children?

PHYSIOLOGY OF FEVER

The hypothalamus functions as the body's thermostat, directing the body to conserve or dissipate heat. When microorganisms invade the body, endogenous pyrogens are released into the bloodstream. These substances travel to the hypothalamus, where they trigger the production and release of prostaglandins, which initiate the fever response. Blood is diverted from the extremities to more central vessels. This helps increase the core body temperature by decreasing heat loss. Shivering increases both metabolic action and heat production. The hypothalamus then maintains the temperature at the new set point.

Nursing Practice

One degree of temperature elevation causes an increase in respiratory rate by four breaths per minute and increases oxygen need by 7%.

Teaching directed at children must take into account their developmental level and cognitive abilities. Learning is easier when teaching involves more than one sense (such as hearing, vision, and touch). Teaching directed at parents must be geared to their level of understanding. If English is the parents' second language, a translator may be necessary.

Growth and Development

For children who can hear, touch, see a model or equipment, read, look at pictures, or even smell things like alcohol swabs, learning is more complete. This is particularly important for the school-age child in the stage of concrete operational thought, who must be able to manipulate materials in order to learn.

Timing is a critical factor in teaching. Parents and children are less receptive to teaching when they are preoccupied with other thoughts or activities. Scheduling specific times for teaching sessions may be helpful.

Depending on the information to be presented, teaching may use the cognitive, psychomotor, or affective domains of learning. Teaching that includes all three domains is more effective.

TEACHING PLANS

A teaching plan is a written plan that includes goals and expected outcomes, interventions needed to achieve the specified goals, and a method and time for evaluation of the expected outcomes. The teaching plan may also specify teaching methods and types of materials to be used. Developing a teaching plan helps ensure that all the necessary information is included and makes teaching more efficient.

The child's primary caretaker should participate in the teaching. The primary caretaker is most often a parent but may be a close family member (uncle, aunt, grandparent). The first step in establishing a teaching plan is to assess the child's or parent's knowledge, skills, and feelings by finding the answers to the following questions:

- What does the parent or child know about the health issue?
- What is the cognitive level or ability to learn?
- Is there a desire to learn?
- What previous experiences affect the learning experience, either positively or negatively?
- What resources are available to the parents, child, and nurse to enhance understanding of the health condition?

Teaching About

CARE DURING A SEIZURE

Seizures are characterized as periods of involuntary muscle contractions and relaxations that the child has no control over. Seizures may be caused by high fever, head trauma, birth defects, and other neurologic problems. It is very hard to predict when a seizure is going to occur. Some safety measures can help to prevent injuries to your child during a seizure.

What to do during a seizure

Seizure activity often means that the child is at risk for injury. Here are some safety guidelines to remember when your child has a seizure.

- Remain calm and stay with your child.
- Protect your child from any injury.

Place your child on the floor when the seizure occurs.

Remove any dangerous objects from your child's reach, such as furniture, glass, or objects that can fall on the floor. Do not restrain or hold down your child during a seizure.

If the floor is hard (tile, cement uncarpeted), place a small pillow, sweater, or your hand under your child's head.

Loosen your child's clothing if it is too tight.

Turn your child's head to one side to prevent choking. Do not put anything into your child's mouth during a seizure.

Provide time for your child to recover after the seizure stops. Reassure your child that he or she is okay. Speak softly. Explain what happened. Do not give food or drink until your child has fully recovered from the seizure.

When to call for emergency help

- If your child's seizure continues for more than 5 minutes
- If your child has trouble breathing or does not breath after the seizure
- If your child has one seizure after the other without waking up between each

Everyday safety guidelines

- Have your child wear a safety helmet while riding a bike or skating to reduce the chances of a head injury.
- Keep bathroom and bedroom doors unlocked. It will be easier for you or other family members to get into a room to help.
- If the child prefers a bath rather than a shower, use just a few inches of water in the tub. Supervise the young child during the bath. Be sure someone is at home when a teenager is bathing.
- Your child should always swim with a buddy. If a seizure occurs, it is easier to rescue a child in a pool than a child in a pond or lake.
- Teach your child to hold onto the handrails when using stairs. Move glass, furniture, and extra pillows away from the child's bed to reduce the chance of injury during a seizure. Think about placing your child's mattress on the floor. This would keep the child from falling out of bed during a seizure.
- Give antiseizure medicines as prescribed to decrease the number of times your child has a seizure.
- Have your child wear a medical identification bracelet at all times.
- Inform relatives, baby-sitters, and teachers that your child has seizures. Tell them about any special care to be given during a seizure.

Note: From Ball, J. (1998). Pediatric patient teaching guides (pp. 1–4). Mosby-YearBook.

822   UNIT VI • Care and Needs of Children

Cultural Competence
Developing Cultural Competence provides information about the potential responses of different ethnic groups to health conditions or to medical or nursing care interventions.

Complementary Care
Complementary Care features present information about commonly used alternative and complementary measures to treat or provide comfort for various conditions.

Consistent Nursing Process Coverage
The nursing process is presented in a consistent manner throughout the nursing care chapters. The heading Nursing Management highlights nursing actions, followed by sections on *Nursing Assessment and Diagnosis, Planning and Implementation,* and *Evaluation.*

Pathophysiology Illustrated
Pathophysiology Illustrated boxes visually explain the pathophysiology of certain conditions as they affect pregnant women, newborns, and children in a format that students can understand and apply.

Critical Thinking
Thinking Critically boxes provide brief scenarios that ask students to determine the appropriate response. A special icon found at the end of each Thinking Critically box refers the reader to the Companion Website students can respond to critical thinking questions about these scenarios and email responses directly to instructors.

Growth and Development
Found exclusively in the pediatric chapters, Growth and Development boxes help students focus nursing care at various stages of development.

Family and Patient Teaching
Teaching About boxes are a special patient education feature that highlights a special health care issue or problem and includes the key teaching points for care by the family.

Assessment Guides

Assessment Guides, found in the maternal-newborn chapters, assist students with diagnoses by incorporating physical assessment and normal findings, alterations and possible causes, as well as guidelines for nursing interventions.

Clinical Pathways

The Clinical Pathways are designed to help students plan and manage care within normally anticipated time frames.

Nursing Care Plans

Throughout the text, nursing care plans help students approach care from the nursing process perspective. These nursing care plans include Nursing Intervention Classifications (NIC) and Nursing Outcome Classifications (NOC). Additional Care Map activities can be found on the Companion Website.

Drug Guide

Drug Guides for selected medications commonly used in maternal-newborn and child nursing are included to guide students in correctly administering the medications and evaluating their action.

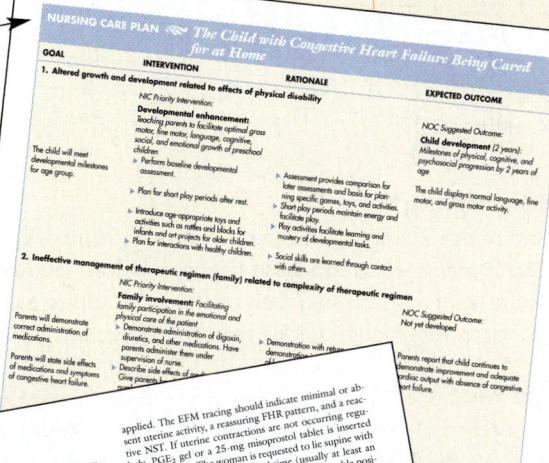

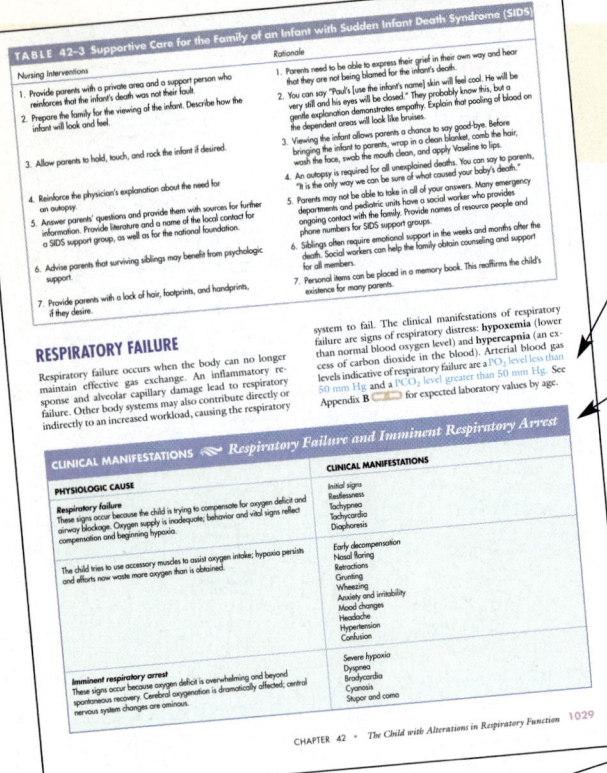

Lab Values

Important lab values are highlighted within the chapters as a tool for students to assess their patients' conditions.

Clinical Manifestations

This feature presents the etiology, clinical presentation, and clinical therapy for selected conditions.

Chapter Highlights

At the end of each chapter, students will find a summary of chapter highlights. Students who read these concepts before reading the chapter will find this helpful in focusing their attention. Chapter highlights are also an appropriate tool to quickly review the chapter content.

Explore MediaLink

Found at the end of each chapter, the EXPLORE MediaLink encourages students to use the CD-ROM and the Companion Website to apply what they have learned from the text in case studies, practice NCLEX questions, and to use additional resources.

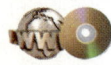 ## ADDITIONAL ONLINE RESOURCES

NCLEX Review

Both the Student CD-ROM and the Companion Website offer students numerous opportunities for practicing NCLEX questions. For each chapter, questions are graded automatically and provide complete rationales. The NCLEX review module on the Companion Website allows students to email their results directly to instructors.

Animations

The free Student CD-ROM contains many animations of difficult concepts to help students understand and visualize them.

Skills

The free Student CD-ROM includes many of the skills from the *Clinical Skills Manual*. The chapter-opening MediaLink feature specifies the skills that are related to that chapter's content, and the cross-reference and CD icons within the chapter remind the student to view these skills on the CD-ROM.

Case Studies

The case studies on the Companion Website allow students to apply concepts and principles addressed in the chapter to realistic client scenarios. Students can email their responses to critical thinking questions directly to instructors.

Care Map Activities

Interactive Care Map Activities on the Companion Website allow students to develop their own care plans based upon a specific client scenario. Students can e-mail these custom care plans to their instructors as homework assignments.

Special Features

🌀 DEVELOPING CULTURAL COMPETENCE

🌀 DRUG GUIDES

🌀 GROWTH AND DEVELOPMENT

NURSING CARE PLANS

PATHOPHYSIOLOGY ILLUSTRATED

TEACHING ABOUT

THINKING CRITICALLY

UNIT I

Introductory Concepts

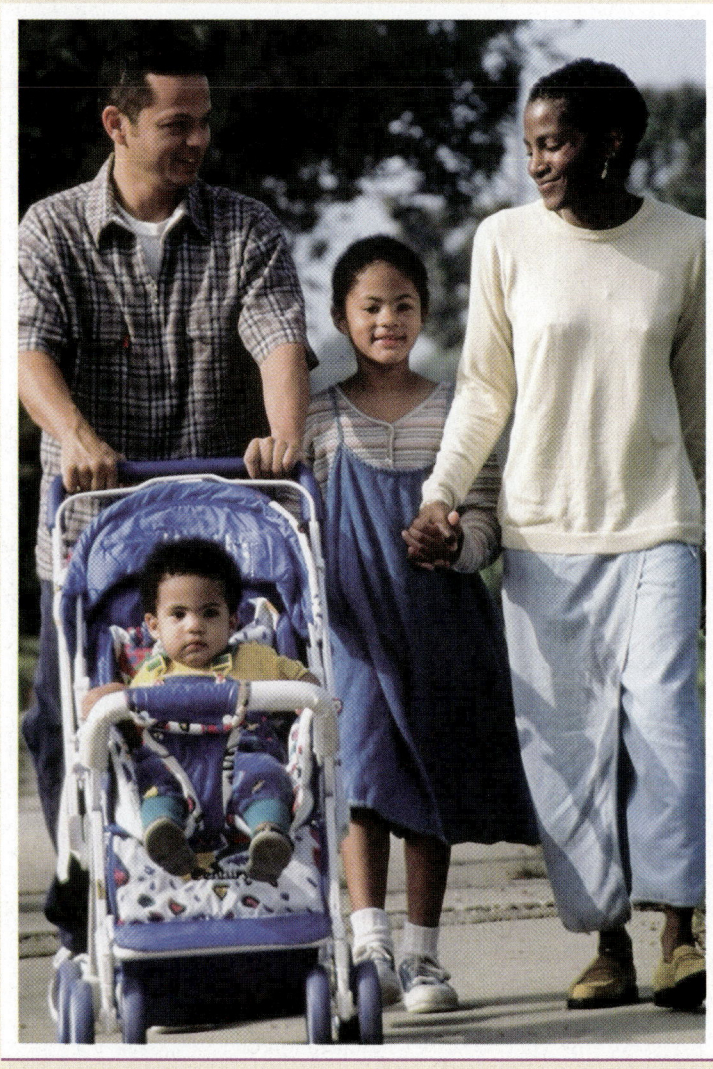

CHAPTER 1
Maternal, Newborn, and Child Health Nursing

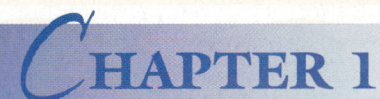

Maternal, Newborn, and Child Health Nursing

My younger son turned 21 today—officially a man now. I remember so well the night he was born in a birthing room at our local hospital. I watched my husband rock our baby and talk to him just minutes after his birth. Over the years we sought emergency health care for our son several times—when he was diagnosed with asthma as a high school freshman, when he fell skateboarding and needed surgery to put three pins in his wrist, when he fell snowboarding and dislocated his shoulder. Active kids do get their share of bumps! It is easy to take good health care for granted, but we shouldn't. It can make all the difference.

—MARJORIE, 47

Key Terms

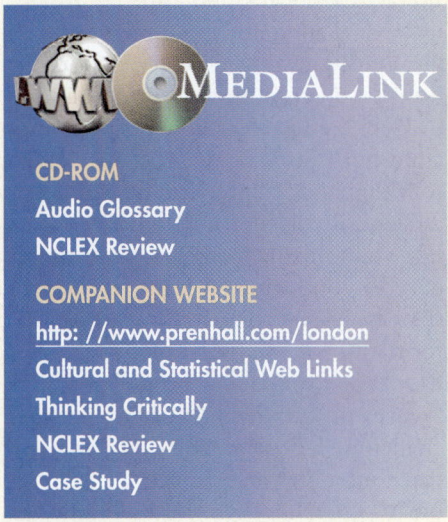

MediaLink

CD-ROM
Audio Glossary
NCLEX Review

COMPANION WEBSITE
http://www.prenhall.com/london
Cultural and Statistical Web Links
Thinking Critically
NCLEX Review
Case Study

$\mathcal{S}$killed nurses care *for* people, care *about* people, and use their expertise to help people care for themselves. Fundamentally, this is the essence of nursing. Most nurses experience special moments professionally, times in which they know that they have practiced the essence of nursing and, in doing so, have touched the lives of others. For nurses who work with childbearing families or with children and their families, the rewards that come from skilled nursing practice can be especially rich.

This chapter focuses on introductory concepts related to the nurse and childbearing families, infants, children, and adolescents.

NURSING ROLES IN MATERNAL-CHILD NURSING

Traditionally, **maternal-child nursing** refers to the care of women during pregnancy, birth, and postpartum, as well as the care of infants, children, and adolescents. However, this label is somewhat misleading because it fails to acknowledge clearly the consideration due to fathers, partners, and family members. As nurses who work with families quickly learn, a holistic, inclusive approach is crucial to effective nursing care.

The nursing process provides the framework for delivery of direct nursing care. The nurse assesses the client—whether childbearing woman, infant, child, or adolescent—and identifies the nursing diagnoses that describe the responses of the individual and family to the illness or injury. The nurse then implements and evaluates nursing care. This care is designed to meet specific physical and psychosocial needs. For children, the care is tailored to the individual developmental stage, giving the child additional responsibility for self-care with increasing age.

Nurses play a major role in minimizing the psychologic and physical distress experienced by childbearing families and by children and their families. This often involves listening to concerns, being present during stressful or emotional experiences, and implementing strategies to help the individual and family members cope. Nurses can help families by suggesting ways to support their loved one in the hospital, in community settings, and in the home.

Client education is a major component of maternal-child nursing. During pregnancy, nurses provide anticipatory guidance to prepare the woman and her partner, if he or she is involved, for the changes that each month brings. For example, the woman is taught self-care measures to relieve discomforts and learns to identify the warning signs that she should report. Similarly, both partners receive information on the psychologic changes of pregnancy that they may experience. Education for the laboring woman focuses on activities that help her deal successfully with a challenging experience—childbirth—whereas postpartum teaching addresses the needs of the woman and her newborn to prepare them for discharge.

In pediatric nursing, education is especially challenging because nurses must be prepared to work with children at various levels of understanding and to include family members in all aspects of care. As patient educators, nurses help children adapt to the hospital setting and prepare them for procedures.

When a child is ill, most hospitals encourage a parent to stay with the child and to provide much of the direct and the supportive care. Nurses teach parents to watch for important signs and responses to therapies, to increase the child's comfort, and even to provide advanced care. Taking an active role during hospitalization helps prepare the parent to assume total responsibility for care after the child leaves the hospital.

Nurses also serve as advocates, acting to safeguard and advance the interests of families. To be an effective advocate the nurse must be aware of the individual's needs, the family's needs and resources, and the health care services available in the hospital and the community. The nurse can then assist the family to make informed choices about these services and to act in their best interests. Nurses must also ensure that the policies and resources of health care agencies meet the psychosocial needs of childbearing women and of children and their families.

Collaborative practice is a comprehensive model of health care that uses a multidisciplinary team of health professionals to provide high-quality, cost-effective care. In maternal-newborn settings the team generally includes certified nurse-midwives (CNMs) (see later discussion), physicians, nurses, and other health specialists such as pharmacists, lactation consultants, or childbirth educators. Similarly, the multidisciplinary team assembled when a child has a significant health problem or handicapping condition may include physicians, nurses, social workers, physical and occupational therapists, and other specialists. Their goal is to create an interdisciplinary plan designed to meet the child's medical, nursing, developmental, educational, and psychosocial needs. Because nurses spend large amounts of time providing nursing care for the client and family, they often are better informed than other health care professionals about the family's wishes and resources. Thus, as a member of the team, the nurse serves as an advocate to ensure that the plan of care considers the family's wishes and contains appropriate services.

Case management is a process of coordinating the delivery of health care services in a manner that focuses on both quality and cost outcomes. This is often a collaborative practice with other health care providers designed to promote continuity of care. The nurse case manager has control over the use of health care resources that are considered appropriate for the client's condition and links the client and family to these services. The goal is to help the individual and family have the best health care outcome and decrease fragmentation of care, while controlling the cost of health care services. In maternal-child nursing, case management is often used for a complicated high-risk pregnancy, for the care of a hospitalized child, and for long-term care of chronic conditions.

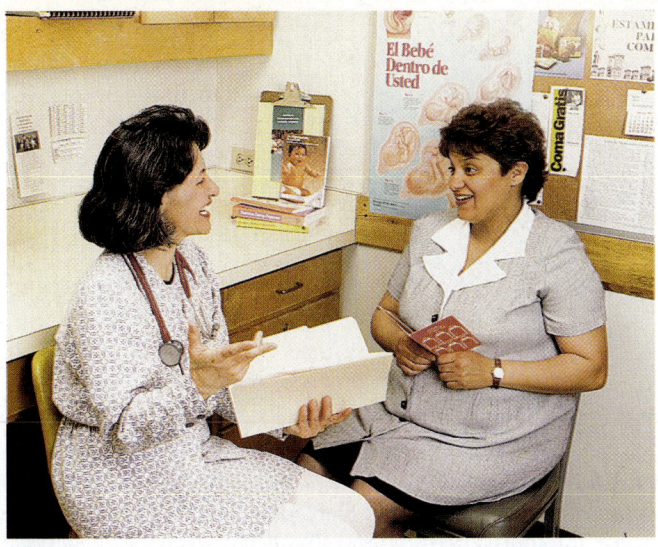

FIGURE 1–1. ◆ A certified nurse-midwife confers with her client.

Discharge planning is a form of case management. Effective discharge planning promotes a smooth, rapid, and safe transition into the community and improves the results of treatment begun in the hospital. To be a discharge planner, the nurse needs to know about community medical resources, appropriate home care agencies, educational interventions, and services reimbursed by the individual's health plan or other financial resources.

In addition, several advanced practice roles are available to maternal-child nurses with additional education. *Nurse practitioners (NPs)* who have specialized education in a master's degree program or a certificate program often provide ambulatory care services to pregnant women, neonates, children, adolescents, and families. NPs focus on physical and psychosocial assessments, including history, physical examination, and certain diagnostic tests and procedures. They make clinical judgments and begin appropriate treatments, seeking physician consultation when necessary. *Clinical nurse specialists (CNSs)* have a master's degree and specialized knowledge and competence in a specific clinical area. They often are found on mother-baby units, on pediatric units, and in intensive care units assisting staff to provide excellent, evidence-based care. The **certified nurse-midwife (CNM)** is educated in the two disciplines of nursing and midwifery and is certified by the American College of Nurse-Midwives. The CNM is prepared to manage independently the care of women at low risk for complications during pregnancy, birth, and the postpartum period, as well as the care of normal newborns (Figure 1–1 ◆).

FAMILY-CENTERED MATERNAL-CHILD CARE

Contemporary childbirth is *family centered*—that is, characterized by an emphasis on the family and the family's choices about their birth experience. Consequently, today the concept of *family-centered childbirth* is accepted and encour-

aged. Fathers and partners are active participants, not simply bystanders; siblings are encouraged to visit and meet the newest family member, and they may even attend the birth.

In addition, new definitions of family are evolving. For example, the family of a single mother may include her mother, her sister, another relative, a close friend, a lesbian partner, or the father of the child. Many cultures also recognize the importance of extended families, and several family members may provide care and support.

The family can make choices about the place of birth (hospital, birthing center, or home), the primary caregiver (physician, CNM, or even lay midwife), and birth-related experiences (position for birth, use of analgesia and anesthesia, and methods of childbirth preparation, for example).

In pediatric settings, *family-centered care* is designed to meet the emotional, social, and developmental needs of children and families seeking health care. The importance of the family in helping the child recover from illnesses and injuries is recognized. Families are often considered partners in the child's care, learning about the child's condition and participating in decisions regarding the child's care. Thus, families gain greater confidence and competence in caring for their children, which has become even more important as families play an ever-increasing role in providing care for children's health care problems. The key elements of family-centered care are provided in Table 1–1.

TABLE 1–1 Key Elements of Family-Centered Care ⬭ WEB

- Incorporating into policy and practice the recognition that the *family is the constant* in a child's life, while the service systems and support personnel within those systems fluctuate.
- Facilitating *family/professional collaboration* at all levels of hospital, home, and community care:
  - care of an individual child
  - program development, implementation, evaluation, and evolution
  - policy formation
- *Exchanging complete and unbiased information* between family members and professionals in a supportive manner at all times.
- Incorporating into policy and practice the recognition and *honoring of cultural diversity*, strengths, and individuality within and across all families, including *ethnic, racial, spiritual, social, economic, educational, and geographic diversity.*
- Recognizing and respecting *different methods of coping* and implementing comprehensive policies and programs that provide *developmental, educational, emotional, environmental, and financial supports* to meet the diverse needs of families.
- Encouraging and facilitating *family-to-family support* and networking.
- Ensuring that *hospital, home, and community service and support systems* for children needing specialized health and developmental care and their families are *flexible, accessible, and comprehensive* in responding to diverse family-identified needs.
- *Appreciating families as families* and children as children, and recognizing that they possess a wide range of strengths, concerns, emotions, and aspirations beyond their need for specialized health and developmental services and support.

Note: From Shelton, T. L., & Stepanek, J. S. (1994). *Family-centered care for children needing specialized health and developmental services.* Rockville, MD: Child Life Council, (301) 881-7090.

Contemporary Childbirth

In the early 1990s women who gave birth vaginally remained in the hospital for about 3 days. This provided time for nurses to assess the family's knowledge and skill and to complete essential teaching. Nevertheless, in the late 1990s, in an effort to control costs, discharge within 12 to 24 hours after birth became the norm. This practice did not necessarily cause problems for women with supportive families, thorough prenatal preparation, and adequate resources for necessary follow-up care. However, because early discharge severely limits the time available for client teaching, women with little knowledge, experience, or support were often inadequately prepared to care for themselves and their newborn infants. Fortunately, the negative impact of this practice gained recognition nationwide and resulted in legislation that provides for a postpartum stay of up to 48 hours following a vaginal birth and up to 96 hours following a cesarean birth at the discretion of the mother and her health care provider.

Some women choose to give birth at home. Some CNMs attend home births; other home births are attended by direct-entry midwives (lay midwives), who are not RNs. In the past, training as a lay midwife followed an apprenticeship model, with a more senior midwife teaching a younger one. Today most lay midwives complete a direct-entry midwifery education program. Currently, direct-entry midwives are working to be viewed as legitimate professionals. Their professional organization, the Midwives Alliance of North America (MANA), has adopted a statement of values and ethics and has assumed a leadership role in developing a certification process. Certification through the North American Registry of Midwives (NARM) is available for direct-entry midwives who meet established standards. The midwife who completes the process successfully can use the title **certified professional midwife (CPM)** (Myers-Ciecko, 1999).

Some provision for direct-entry midwifery exists in approximately 65% of the states in the United States; however, 60% of all direct-entry midwives practice in just four states: California, Florida, Texas, and Washington (Dower & Miller, 1999). At present, only a few managed care plans make home birth services available to their members. Time will tell whether this is an emerging trend.

Contemporary Care of Children

More than 85 million children under the age of 21 live in the United States. They account for 31.3% of the population (Figure 1–2 ◆) (U.S. Census, 2001). At one time children were valued primarily as laborers. Over the past century, however, the unique needs and qualities of children have been recognized. In today's society, children are considered to have special value; they are vulnerable and need protection.

Pediatric nursing is a specialized area of nursing that focuses on caring for today's children. Pediatric nurses

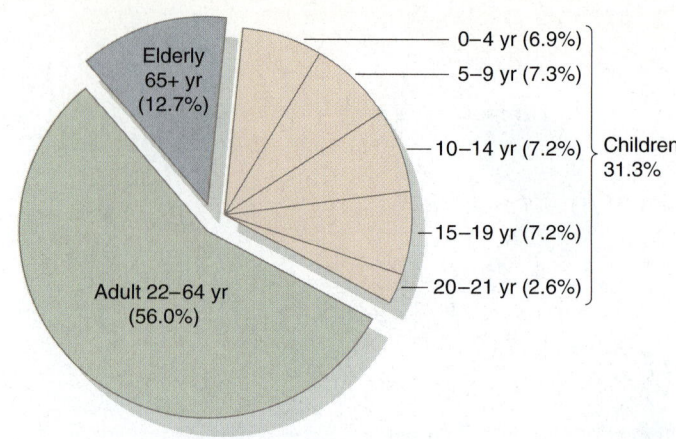

FIGURE 1–2. ◆ In 1999, children from birth to 21 years of age accounted for about one third of the population in the United States. *Note:* From U.S. Bureau of Census. (2000). *Resident population estimates of the United States by age and sex, April 1, 1990 to July 1, 1999.* Washington, DC: U.S. Government Printing Office.

function in many different settings. Within the hospital, acute care may be provided in the emergency department, observation or short-stay unit, postanesthesia unit, intensive care unit, general pediatric inpatient unit, and various outpatient clinics.

The hospital stay is now integrated into a continuum that allows children to complete therapy at home, at school, or in other community settings. Pediatric nurses assist families in making the transition from the acute hospital setting to

- The home, for a short recuperation or long-term management
- A rehabilitation center or long-term care hospital
- A nurse-managed home care or hospice program

Managing the child's transition from acute care to another setting involves planning the discharge, implementing interdisciplinary plans, helping the family to develop an emergency care plan in the event their child has an unexpected health care crisis, and collaborating with a broad range of health care professionals.

Pediatric nurses also work in several other health care settings including the following:

- In *pediatricians' offices* and health centers, nurses assess children, provide telephone counseling, and support and counsel families about growth and development and nutrition.
- In *clinic settings,* nurses assess children, assist with medical procedures, provide nursing care, and educate families to ensure the continuous management of the child's health care problem (see Figure 1–3).
- In *home health agencies,* nurses provide home care to children with acute and chronic conditions. Children may need medical treatment and nursing care for acute, self-limited, chronic, and terminal conditions.

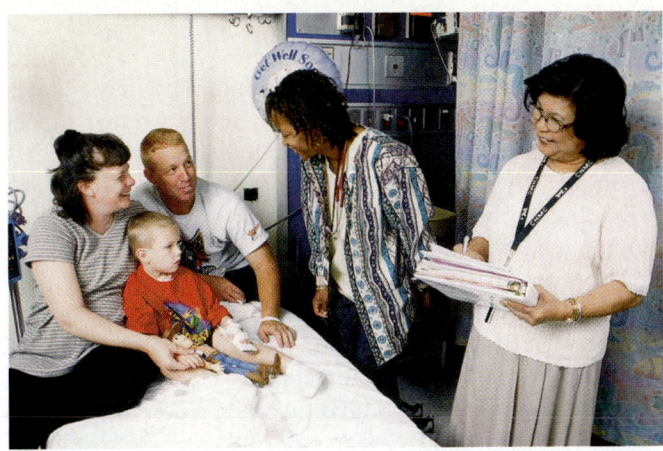

FIGURE 1–3. ◆ Children need to be involved actively in decisions regarding their care when appropriate. Here, the family and staff come together to discuss the child's care in a positive and honest manner.

Care may involve visits for specific interventions such as medication administration or "private duty" care (one-on-one nursing care).

- In *rehabilitation centers,* nurses provide inpatient and ambulatory care to help restore children to an optimal state and plan for discharge management of chronic conditions.
- In *schools,* nurses assess children, monitor their health status, and provide health education to teachers and children. Many children who are assisted by technology or have chronic conditions attend school as required by the Individuals with Disabilities Education Act (IDEA). Individual school health plans are developed, implemented, and evaluated by the school nurse.

Maternal-Child Care in the Community

Primary care is the focus of much attention as caregivers search for a new, more effective direction for health care. Primary care includes a focus on health promotion, illness prevention, and individual responsibility for one's own health. These services are best provided in community-based settings. Third-party payers and managed care organizations are beginning to recognize the importance of primary care in containing costs and maintaining health. Community-based health care systems providing primary care and some secondary care will be available in schools, workplaces, homes, churches, clinics, transitional care programs, and other ambulatory settings.

The growth and diversity of managed care plans offer both opportunities and challenges for women's and children's health care. The potential exists for managed care organizations to work with consumers to provide a model for coordinated and comprehensive well-woman and well-child care that includes improved delivery of screening and preventive services. One challenge that managed care organizations face is how to relate to essential community providers of care, such as family-planning clinics, women's health centers, and well-child centers that offer a unique service or serve groups of women and children with special needs (adolescents, women and children with disabilities, and ethnic or racial minorities).

Community-based care remains an essential element of health care for uninsured or underinsured individuals, as well as for individuals who benefit from programs such as Medicare, Medicaid, or state-sponsored health-related programs. Whereas some of these programs, such as those offered through public health departments, are broad based, others, such as parenting classes for adolescents, are geared to the needs of a specific population.

Community-based care is also part of a trend initiated by consumers, who are asking for a seamless system of family-centered, comprehensive, coordinated health care, health education, and social services. This seamless system requires coordination as clients move from primary care services to acute care facilities and then back into the community. Nurses can assume this care-management role and perform an important service for individuals and families.

Maternal-child nurses are especially sensitive to these changes in health care delivery because the vast majority of health care provided to childbearing and childrearing families takes place outside of hospitals in clinics, offices, and community-based organizations. In addition, maternal-child nurses offer specialized services such as childbirth preparation classes, sibling classes, and parenting classes.

HOME CARE

Providing health care in the home is an especially important dimension of community-based nursing care. Shorter hospital stays end in the discharge of individuals who still require support, assistance, and teaching. Home care helps fill this gap. Conversely, home care also enables infants, children, and women to remain at home with conditions that formerly would have required hospitalization.

Nurses are major providers of home care services. Home care nurses perform direct nursing care and also supervise unlicensed assistive personnel who provide less skilled levels of service. In a home setting, nurses use their skills in assessment, intervention, communication, teaching, problem solving, and organization to meet the needs of childbearing and childrearing families. They also play a major role in coordinating services from other providers, such as physical therapists or lactation consultants.

Postpartum and newborn home visits help ensure a satisfactory transition from the birthing center to the home. This trend is a positive method of meeting the needs of childbearing families and hopefully will become standard practice. Chapter 30 discusses home care and provides guidance about making a home visit. ⊂⊃ Information on home care is also provided as appropriate throughout this text.

Many children with severe chronic illnesses can be treated at home rather than by continued hospitalization. After studies in the 1980s found that home health care was substantially less expensive than hospital care (U.S. General Accounting Office, 1989), Congress amended laws to permit payment of home care services with federal funds. In 1996 nearly 600,000 children under 18 years were served by a formal home care program (National Association of Home Care, 2000). Technologic advances have resulted in the design of portable medical and infusion therapy equipment for home care. Some families have regained control over their lives by creating intensive care units in their homes. Children with conditions considered fatal 10 years ago are thriving with home care and are participating in family, community, and school life.

Complementary Therapies

Interest in complementary and alternative medicine (CAM) therapies continues to grow nationwide and will affect the care of childbearing and childrearing families. CAM includes a wide array of therapies including, for example, acupuncture, acupressure, therapeutic touch, biofeedback, massage therapy, meditation, herbal therapies, and homeopathic remedies. Information on specific therapies will be presented in boxed features entitled "Complementary Care" throughout the text, as well as on our companion website.

Research indicates that more than 42% of adults use some form of alternative practice and more than 46% have seen an alternative medicine practitioner. One third of pregnant women use CAM therapies, some of which may be potentially harmful (Ranzini, Allen, & Lai, 2001). Moreover, more than 60% of those who use complementary or alternative therapies do *not* reveal this to their regular physician (Eisenberg, Davis, Ettner, et al., 1998). The use of CAM therapies is also increasing considerably in the pediatric population. About 20% to 30% of general pediatric patients have used one or more CAM therapies; use among adolescents ranges from 50% to 75%. Rates among patients with chronic, recurrent, or incurable conditions, such as cancer, asthma, rheumatoid arthritis, and cystic fibrosis, range from 30% to 70% (Kemper, 2001). In response to this interest, the U.S. Congress established the National Center for Complementary and Alternative Medicine to evaluate alternative medical treatment, to support research and training in CAM, and to establish an information clearinghouse for the exchange of information about CAM with the public (Murphy, Kronenberg, & Wade, 1999).

It is important for nurses working with childbearing and childrearing families to become knowledgeable about complementary and alternative approaches, to become familiar with those practices that have the greatest level of documented success, and to respect and support the family's right to consider alternative approaches to traditional health care.

ACCESS TO HEALTH CARE

Not all pregnant women and children in the United States have access to health care. One in seven women (14%) lacks health care insurance (Maiese, 2001). For people living in poverty, Medicaid is the most prevalent form of insurance, covering 12.9 million people including pregnant women who fall into specified income categories.

For women who become pregnant, effective prenatal care is one of the most important approaches available to reduce adverse pregnancy outcomes. In 1998, 83% of pregnant women began prenatal care in the first trimester. However, only 74% of pregnant women received early and adequate prenatal care (Davis, Okuboye, & Ferguson, 2000). Moreover, these percentages vary significantly among groups, with black and Hispanic women less likely to receive early and adequate prenatal care (U.S. Department of Health and Human Services, 2000).

In 1998, 11.1 million children, 15.4% of those below 18 years of age, had no health insurance and 22.8% were covered by public insurance programs such as Medicaid. Of all children who lived in poverty in 1998, 26.4% had no health insurance and 57.7% were covered by public insurance (Health Resources and Services Administration, 2000). Most of these children had difficulty obtaining the most basic preventive health care, including immunizations (Figure 1–4 ◆).

Efforts to provide universal access to health care for children continue to grow. Congress passed legislation to create the Child Health Insurance Plan in 1997 to enable more children to obtain access to essential health care services. States are allocated federal funds to encourage en-

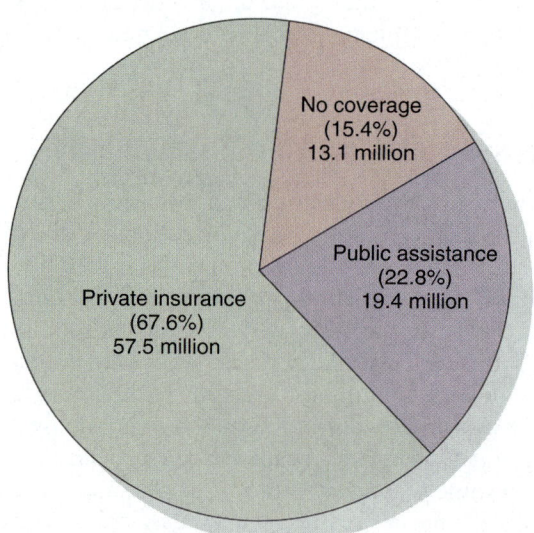

FIGURE 1–4. ◆ In the United States, who pays for children's health care? The 1998 data show that our taxes support 38% of the costs. *Note:* From Frontin, P., Employee Benefit Research Institute. (2000). *Sources of health insurance and characteristics of the uninsured: Analysis of the March 1999 current population survey* (EBRI Issue Brief No. 217). Washington, DC: EBRI.

rollment of children living with families whose income is up to 200% of the federal poverty level (Smith, Wise, Chavkin et al., 2000). Children enrolled must be provided with health benefits coverage that is substantially equal to the benefits coverage in the federal or state employee benefits plan or the plan of the largest health maintenance organization in the state. More than 3 million children were enrolled in the State Children's Health Insurance Program (SCHIP) during 2000 (Health Care Finance Administration, 2000). Many pregnant adolescents are also served in these state programs.

CULTURALLY COMPETENT CARE

The U.S. population has a varied mix of cultural groups, with ever-increasing diversity. More than 33% of all children less than 20 years of age are from families of minority populations (U.S. Census, 2001). Culture develops from socially learned beliefs, lifestyles, values, and integrated patterns of behavior that are characteristic of the family, cultural group, and community. The cultural background and values of childbearing and childrearing families are often quite different from those of the nurse.

Specific elements that contribute to a family's value system include the following:

- Religion and social beliefs
- Presence and influence of the extended family, as well as socialization within the ethnic group
- Communication patterns
- Beliefs and understanding about the concepts of health and illness
- Permissible physical contact with strangers
- Education

Specific differences in beliefs between families and health care providers are common in the following areas:

- Help-seeking behaviors
- Pregnancy and childbirth practices
- Causes of diseases or illnesses
- Death and dying
- Caretaking and caregiving
- Childrearing practices

These elements in differing degrees influence the cultural beliefs and values of an ethnic group, making the group unique. Misunderstandings may occur when the health care professional and the family come from different cultural groups. In addition, past experiences with care may have made the family angry or suspicious of providers. Nurses need to be able to recognize, respect, and respond to ethnic diversity in a way that leads to a mutually desirable outcome. The nurse must identify culturally relevant facts about the patient to provide culturally appropriate and competent care. 🔗 **WEB**

Developing Cultural Competence

Conflicts can occur within a family when traditional rituals and practices of the family's elders do not conform with current health care practices. Nurses need to be sensitive to the potential implications for the child's health care, especially after the child is discharged from the hospital. When cultural values are not part of the nursing care plan, parents may be forced to decide whether the family's beliefs should take priority over the health care professional's guidance.

When the family's cultural values are incorporated into the care plan, the family is more likely to accept and comply with the needed care, especially in the home care setting. It is important for nurses to avoid imposing personal cultural values on the families and children in their care. By learning about the values of the different ethnic groups in the community—their religious beliefs that have an impact on health care practices, their beliefs about common illnesses, and their specific healing practices—nurses can develop an individualized nursing care plan for each child and family.

STATISTICAL DATA AND MATERNAL-CHILD CARE

Health-related statistics provide an objective basis for projecting client needs, planning the use of resources, and determining the effectiveness of specific treatments. Although these statistics support no conclusions about *why* some phenomenon has occurred, they do identify certain trends and high-risk target groups. The following sections discuss descriptive statistics that are particularly important to maternal-child health care.

Birth Rate

Birth rate refers to the number of live births per 1000 people. Worldwide birth rates vary dramatically as Table 1–2 demonstrates. In the United States the birth rate increased to 14.6 in 1998, the first increase since 1990. Between 1990 and 1997 the birth rate fell 13%. The actual number of births in 1998 increased by 2% to 3,941,553. One bright spot was that the teenage birth rate declined in 1998 to 51.1 births per 1000 women between 15 and 19 years of age. This rate has decreased 18% since 1991 (Ventura, Martin, Curtin, et al., 2000).

The statistics do raise questions. For example: What is the impact of cultural differences and changing societal values on birth rates? Do birth rates change when access to information on contraception increases? What role does government policy, such as China's legislation limiting births to one child per family, play?

TABLE 1-2 Live Birth Rates and Infant Mortality Rates in Selected Countries, 1998

Country	Birth Rate	Infant Mortality Rate
Afghanistan	41.9	140.6
Argentina	19.9	18.4
Australia	13.2	5.1
Canada	11.9	5.5
China	15.1	43.3
Egypt	26.8	67.7
Ethiopia	44.3	124.6
France	11.4	5.6
Iraq	38.4	62.4
Japan	10.5	4.1
Mexico	25	24.6
United Kingdom	11.9	5.8
United States	14.3	6.3

Note: From *2000 World Almanac and Book of Facts.* (1999). Newark, NJ: World Almanac Books.

Maternal Mortality

The **maternal mortality rate** is the number of deaths from any cause during the pregnancy cycle (including the 42-day postpartal period) per 100,000 live births. In 1998 the maternal mortality rate in the United States was 7.1, a decrease from 8.4 the previous year. However, for black women in the United States the rate of death (17.1) was more than 3 times the rate for white women (5.1) (Murphy, 2000). Factors influencing the long-term decrease in maternal mortality include the increased use of hospitals and specialized health care personnel by maternity clients, the establishment of care centers for high-risk mothers and infants, the prevention and control of infection with antibiotics and improved techniques, the availability of blood products for transfusions, and the lowered rates of anesthesia-related deaths.

Infant Mortality

The **infant mortality rate** is the number of deaths of infants under 1 year of age per 1000 live births in a given population. In 1998 the U.S. infant mortality rate fell to 6.3, the lowest rate ever reported in the United States. (*Neonatal mortality* is the number of deaths of infants less than 28 days of age per 1000 live births; *perinatal mortality* includes both neonatal deaths and fetal deaths per 1000 live births; and *fetal death* is death in utero at 20 weeks or more gestation.)

The U.S. infant mortality rate continues to be an area of concern because the United States has fallen to 22nd place in infant mortality rankings among industrialized nations. Health care professionals, policy makers, and the public continue to stress the need for better prenatal care, coordination of health services, and provision of comprehen-

sive maternal-child services in the United States. In 1998 the percentage of women beginning prenatal care in the first trimester rose to 82.8%. This number has increased for 9 consecutive years (Ventura et al., 2000). In the United States, the leading causes of infant mortality vary according to the age of the infant (Figure 1–5 ◆).

The leading causes of death in neonates are congenital anomalies, low birth weight, respiratory distress syndrome, and maternal complications of pregnancy. Sudden infant death syndrome accounts for nearly 28% of infant deaths in the postneonatal period (between 1 and 12 months of age). Figure 1–5B shows the relative frequency of other major causes of death in the postneonatal period. The mortality rate for black infants is at least 2 times that for whites for the leading causes of death, except for congenital anomalies (Health Resources and Services Administration, 2000). What could account for homicide as the fifth leading cause of death in infants? (See Chapter 36.) WEB

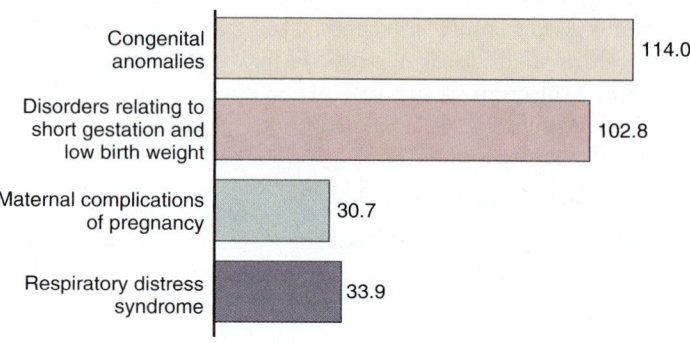

A Neonatal Mortality

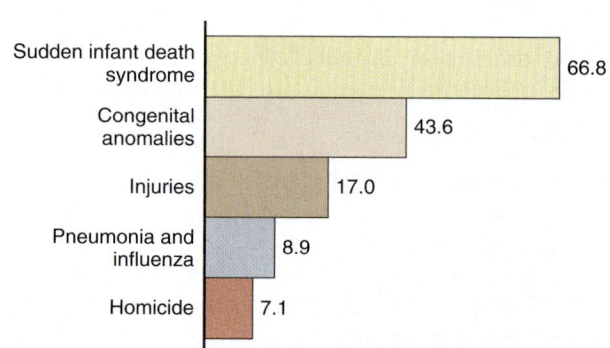

B Postneonatal Mortality

FIGURE 1-5. ◆ Leading causes of death in the United States for infants in 1998. **A,** Neonatal mortality (in infants up to 28 days old) and **B,** Postneonatal mortality (in infants between 28 days and 1 year old). In 1993 the mortality rate for sudden infant death syndrome was 109.5 per 100,000 live births. What could account for this dramatic rate reduction? (See Chapter 42 to find the answer.) *Note:* From Murphy, S. A. (2000). *Deaths: Final data for 1998. National Vital Statistics Reports, 48*(11). Hyattsville, MD: National Center for Health Statistics.

Table 1–2 identifies infant mortality rates for selected countries for 1998. As the data indicate, the range is dramatic among the countries listed. Information about birth rates and mortality rates is limited for some countries because of a lack of organized reporting mechanisms. The information raises many concerns such as access to health care during pregnancy and after birth and about standards of living, nutrition, and sociocultural factors.

Pediatric Mortality

Children have different health care problems than adults, and the problems may depend on the age and development of the child. The most common cause of death for children between 1 and 14 years of age is unintentional injury. Congenital anomalies, cancer, diseases of the heart, homicide, pneumonia/influenza, suicide, and infection with HIV/AIDS are the other major causes. ⊂⊃ [WEB] The major causes of death from unintentional injury in childhood include motor vehicle crashes (passengers and pedestrians), drowning, fires and burns, firearms, and suffocation (Health Resources and Services Administration, 2000).

Unintentional injury continues to be the leading cause of death in adolescents 15 through 19 years. Homicide, suicide, cancer, and congenital anomalies are other major causes of death. Of all deaths from unintentional and intentional injury, motor vehicle crashes are the leading cause, followed by firearms, suffocation, drowning, and poisoning. ⊂⊃ [WEB]

Pediatric Morbidity

Morbidity (an illness or injury that limits activity, requires medical attention or hospitalization, or results in a chronic condition) also varies according to the age of the child. In 1998 there were 3.4 million hospital discharges for children between 1 and 21 years of age, an average of 4.1 discharges per 100 children. See the companion website for the leading causes of hospitalization of children by age group in 1993 and 1998. ⊂⊃ [WEB] Respiratory diseases are the leading cause of hospitalization in children between 1 and 14 years of age, accounting for 31% of hospital discharges in this age group. Although injury is a leading cause of death in children 1 to 14 years, it accounted for only 9% of hospital discharges in 1998. Respiratory diseases, injury, and digestive diseases combined accounted for 45% of discharges in children 1 to 14 years. Pregnancy, childbirth, and mental disorders are among the leading causes of hospitalization in adolescents between 15 and 21 years of age (Health Resources and Services Administration, 2000).

In 1993, chronic illnesses and impairments limited the activities of more than 4.7 million children between 1 and 19 years of age. More boys than girls had activity limitations between 1 and 19 years of age (Maternal and Child Health Bureau, 1995).

Implications for Nursing Practice

Nurses can use statistics in a number of ways. For example, they can use statistical data to

- Determine populations at risk
- Assess the relationship between specific factors
- Help establish databases for specific client populations
- Determine the levels of care needed by particular client populations
- Evaluate the success of specific nursing interventions
- Determine priorities in caseloads
- Estimate staffing and equipment needs of hospital units and clinics
- Apply for funding to support health needs

Nurses who use this information are better prepared to promote the health needs of maternal-newborn clients and their families.

In the report *Healthy People 2010,* the U.S. government established updated objectives to improve pregnancy outcome and the health of women, infants, children, and young adults. These objectives focus on improving pregnancy outcomes, reducing the incidence of death and disability from the major causes of death, and so forth. Federal funding is available to health care organizations for the development of programs aimed at reducing the number of deaths from these factors in specific high-risk groups. For a complete listing of Healthy People 2010 objectives, visit our website. ⊂⊃ [WEB]

LEGAL CONSIDERATIONS IN MATERNAL-CHILD NURSING

Scope of Practice

The *scope of practice* is defined as the limits of nursing practice set forth in state statutes. Although some state practice acts continue to limit nursing practice to the traditional responsibilities of providing client care related to health maintenance and disease prevention, most state practice acts cover expanded practice roles that include collaboration with other health professionals in planning and providing care, physician-delegated diagnosis and prescriptive privilege, and the delegation of direct care tasks to other specified licensed and unlicensed personnel. A nurse must function within the scope of practice or risk being accused of practicing medicine without a license.

Standards of Nursing Care

Standards of care establish minimum criteria for competent, proficient delivery of nursing care. Such standards are designed to protect the public and are used to judge the quality of care provided. Legal interpretation of actions within standards of care is based on what a reasonably prudent nurse with similar education and experience would do in similar circumstances.

The American Nurses Association (ANA) has published standards of practice for maternal-child health. ANA and the Society of Pediatric Nurses collaborated on development of standards for pediatric clinical nursing practice. ⊂⊃ [CD] Specialty organizations, such as the Association of Women's Health, Obstetrics, and Neonatal Nurses (AWHONN), the National Association of Neonatal Nurses (NANN), and the Association of Operating Room Nurses (AORN) have also developed standards for specialty practice. ⊂⊃ [CD]

Agency policies, procedures, and protocols also provide appropriate guidelines for care standards. For example, **clinical practice guidelines** and critical pathways are comprehensive interdisciplinary care plans for a specific condition that describe the sequence and timing of interventions that should result in expected client or patient outcomes. Clinical practice guidelines or critical pathways are adopted within a health care setting to reduce variation in care management, to limit costs of care, and to evaluate the effectiveness of care (Merritt, Palmer, Bergman, et al., 1997; Melnyk, Fineout-Overholt, Stone, et al., 2000). The Joint Commission on the Accreditation of Healthcare Organizations (JCAHO), a nongovernmental agency that audits the operation of hospitals and health care facilities, has also contributed to the development of nursing standards.

Some standards carry the force of law; others, although not legally binding, carry important legal significance. Any nurse who fails to meet appropriate standards of care invites allegations of negligence or malpractice. However, any nurse who practices within the guidelines established by an agency, or follows local or national standards, is assured that clients are provided with competent nursing care, which, in turn, decreases the potential for litigation.

Informed Consent

Informed consent is a legal concept that protects a person's right to autonomy and self-determination by specifying that no action may be taken without that individual's prior understanding and freely given consent. Although this policy is usually enforced for such major procedures as surgery or regional anesthesia, it pertains to any nursing, medical, or surgical intervention. To touch a person without consent (except in an emergency) constitutes battery. Consent is not informed unless the client, or parent in the case of a child, understands the usual procedures, their rationales, and any associated risks.

The person, usually the physician, who is ultimately responsible for the treatment or procedure should provide the information necessary to obtain informed consent. In such cases the nurse's role is to witness the client's signature (or the parent's signature for a child) giving consent. The nurse may also serve as a witness if parents give verbal consent by telephone. If the nurse de-

termines that the individual does not understand the procedure or risks, the nurse must notify the physician, who must then provide additional information to ensure that the consent is informed. The nurse also responds to questions asked by adult clients or by parents and children. Anxiety, fear, pain, and medications that alter consciousness may influence an individual's ability to give informed consent. An oral consent is legal, but written consent is easier to defend in a court of law.

Children under 18 or 21 years of age, depending on state law, can legally give informed consent in the following circumstances:

- When they are minor parents of the child client
- When they are **emancipated minors** (self-supporting adolescents under 18 years of age, not subject to parental control)
- When they are adolescents between 16 and 18 years of age seeking birth control, mental health counseling, or substance abuse treatment (Dickey & Deatrick, 2000)

Mature minors (14- and 15-year-old adolescents who are able to understand treatment risks) can give consent for treatment or refuse treatment in some states.

Refusal of a treatment, medication, or procedure after appropriate information is provided also requires that the individual sign a form releasing the doctor and clinical facility from liability resulting from the effects of such a refusal. Jehovah's Witnesses' refusal of blood transfusions is an example.

Nurses are responsible for educating clients about any nursing care provided. Before each nursing intervention, the maternal-child nurse lets the individual and/or family know what to expect, thus ensuring cooperation and obtaining consent. Afterward, the nurse documents the teaching and the learning outcomes in the person's record. The importance of clear, concise, and complete nursing records cannot be overemphasized. These records are evidence that the nurse obtained consent, performed prescribed treatments, reported important observations to the appropriate staff, and adhered to acceptable standards of care.

CHILDREN AND INFORMED CONSENT

Society grants parents the responsibility and authority to give consent for their minor children. When parents are divorced, either may give informed consent. Both children and parents must understand that they have the right to refuse treatment at any time. In an emergency, consent for treatment to preserve life or limb is not required.

Parents or guardians have absolute authority to make choices about their child's health care except in specific cases:

- When the child and parents do not agree on major treatment options
- When the parents' choice of treatment does not permit lifesaving treatment for the child

- When there is a potential conflict of interest between the child and parents, such as with suspected child abuse or neglect
- When the parents are incapacitated and cannot make a decision (e.g., critically injured in the same motor vehicle crash) (Dickey & Deatrick, 2000)

In some cases the court may be requested to appoint a proxy decision maker for the child or to determine that the child is capable of making a major treatment decision.

Children should become more actively involved in decision making about treatment procedures as their reasoning skills develop. Children too young to give informed consent can be given age-appropriate information about their condition and asked about their care preferences. Their parents, however, make ultimate decisions regarding their care.

With regard to children's participation in research, federal guidelines state that children 7 years of age and older must receive information about a research project and give assent (the voluntary agreement to participate in a research project or to accept treatment) before they are enrolled. Children should be given adequate time to ask questions and be told that they have the right to refuse to participate in the study (U.S. Department of Health and Human Services, 1983; Lindeke, Hauck, & Tanner, 2000). The number of children asked to participate in research is expected to increase because of new Food and Drug Administration regulations requiring manufacturers to assess the safety and effectiveness of new drugs and biologic products in pediatric patients (Food and Drug Administration, 1998).

Right to Privacy

The *right to privacy* is the right of a person to keep his or her person and property free from public scrutiny. To protect this right for patients and families, only those responsible for their care should conduct an examination or discuss their case.

The right to privacy is protected by state constitutions, statutes, and common law. The ANA, the National League for Nursing (NLN), and JCAHO have adopted professional standards protecting the privacy of patients. Health care agencies should also have written policies dealing with patient privacy. The new Health Insurance Portability and Accountability Act of 1996, which was fully implemented in 2002, also has a provision to guarantee the security and privacy of health information.

Growth and Development

By 7 or 8 years of age, a child is able to understand concrete explanations about informed consent for research participation. By age 11, a child's abstract reasoning and logic are advanced. By age 14, an adolescent can weigh options and make decisions regarding consent as capably as an adult.

Laws, standards, and policies about privacy specify that information about clients' treatment, condition, and prognosis can be shared only by health professionals responsible for their care. Information considered vital statistics (name, age, occupation, and so on) may be revealed legally, but is often withheld because of ethical considerations. The client should be consulted as to what information may be released and to whom.

CHILDREN AND CONFIDENTIALITY

Concerns about privacy and the fear of disclosure of sensitive information to parents is a major reason why adolescents do not seek health care (Ford, Bearman, & Moody, 1999). When the child is an emancipated or mature minor, many states permit health care providers to provide birth control and treatment for sexually transmitted infections including HIV/AIDS, pregnancy, and substance abuse without informing the child's parents (Dickey & Deatrick, 2000).

If the child has a reportable disease, confidentiality may create a public health hazard. In such cases the health care professional is obligated to report the presence of the disease to the appropriate state or county agency. Suspected cases of child abuse must be reported to the appropriate agency specified by state law. In the current health care system, the complexities of treatment and the numbers of health care providers involved make it more difficult to maintain confidentiality.

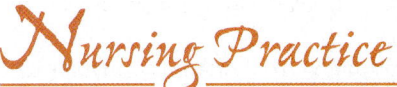

Breaching confidentiality is a potential problem for adolescents, who are just learning whom they can trust in the health care system. Make sure you openly discuss the limits of confidentiality for such things as mandatory reporting requirements with the patient and family. Inadvertent disclosure of personal information may lead to psychologic, social, or physical harm in some patients.

Patient Self-Determination Act

The federal Patient Self-Determination Act directs health care institutions to inform hospitalized patients about their rights, which include expressing a preference for treatment options and making **advance directives** (writing a living will or authorizing a durable power of attorney for health care decisions on the individual's behalf). Nurses often discuss these issues with clients and their families. Minor children and their parents should also be informed of their rights. Adolescents with serious acute or chronic conditions with a higher risk of death should be encouraged to talk with their parents about their health care wishes and to prepare advance directives jointly (Dickey & Deatrick, 2000).

Do not resuscitate (DNR) orders have become more common for children with terminal illnesses in which no further treatments are possible or desired. In many cases these children are cared for at home or in a hospice program, but some still attend school. Implementation of DNR orders for such children then becomes a community issue, to ensure that resuscitation measures are not initiated by any emergency care provider when the child has a life-threatening event. State health policies must be developed so children with these signed orders are easily identified and appropriate documentation of the orders is on file.

ETHICAL ISSUES IN MATERNAL-CHILD NURSING

Although ethical dilemmas confront nurses in all areas of practice, those related to pregnancy, birth, newborns, and children seem especially difficult to resolve.

Maternal-Fetal Conflict

Until fairly recently, the fetus was viewed legally as a nonperson. Mother and fetus were viewed as one complex client—the pregnant woman—of which the fetus was an essential part. However, advances in technology have permitted the physician to treat the fetus and monitor fetal development. The fetus is increasingly viewed as a client separate from the mother, although treatment of the fetus necessarily involves the mother. Thus, the medical emphasis has shifted from one of unity to one of duality (Hornstra, 1999).

Most women are strongly motivated to protect the health and well-being of their fetus. In some instances, however, women have refused interventions on behalf of the fetus, and forced interventions have occurred. These include forced cesarean birth, coercion of mothers who practice high-risk behaviors such as substance abuse to enter treatment, and, perhaps most controversial, mandating experimental in utero therapy or surgery in an attempt to correct a specific birth defect. These interventions infringe on the autonomy of the mother. They may also be detrimental to the baby if, as a result, maternal bonding is hindered, the mother is afraid to seek prenatal care, or the mother is herself harmed by the actions taken (Hornstra, 1999). Attempts have also been made to criminalize the behavior of women who fail to follow a physician's advice or who engage in behaviors (such as substance abuse) that are considered harmful to the fetus. This raises two thorny questions: (1) What practices should be monitored? and (2) Who will determine when the behaviors pose such a risk to the fetus that the courts should intervene?

The American College of Obstetricians and Gynecologists (ACOG) Committee on Ethics (1999) and the American Academy of Pediatrics (AAP) Committee on Bioethics (1999) both affirm the fundamental right of pregnant women to make informed, uncoerced decisions about medical interventions. ACOG and AAP also recognize that cases of maternal-fetal conflict involve two clients, both of whom deserve respect and treatment. Such cases are best resolved by using internal hospital mechanisms including counseling, the intervention of specialists, and consultation with an institutional ethics committee. Court intervention should be considered a last resort, appropriate only in extraordinary circumstances.

Abortion

Since the 1973 Supreme Court decision in *Roe v. Wade,* elective abortion has been legal in the United States. Abortion can be performed until the period of viability. After that time, abortion is permissible only when the life or health of the mother is threatened. Before viability, the rights of the mother are paramount; after viability, the rights of the fetus take precedence.

Personal beliefs, cultural norms, life experiences, and religious convictions shape people's attitudes about abortion. Ethicists have thoughtfully and thoroughly argued positions supporting both sides of the question. Nevertheless, few issues spark the intensity of response seen when the issue of abortion is raised.

At present the decision about abortion is to be made by the woman and her physician. Nurses (and other caregivers) have the right to refuse to assist with the procedure if abortion is contrary to their moral and ethical beliefs. However, if a nurse works in an institution where abortions may be performed, the nurse may be dismissed for refusing. To avoid being placed in a situation contrary to personal ethical values and beliefs, it is important to identify the practices of an institution before going to work there. A nurse who refuses to participate in an abortion because of moral or ethical beliefs has a responsibility to ensure that someone with similar qualifications is available to provide appropriate care for the client. Clients must never be abandoned, regardless of a nurse's beliefs.

Intrauterine Fetal Surgery

Intrauterine fetal surgery, an example of therapeutic research, is a therapy for anatomic lesions that can be corrected surgically and are incompatible with life if not treated. The procedure involves opening the uterus during the second trimester (before viability), performing the planned surgery, and replacing the fetus in the uterus. The risks to the fetus are substantial, and the mother is committed to cesarean births for this and subsequent pregnancies (because the upper, active segment of the uterus is entered). The parents must be informed of the experimental nature of the treatment, the risks of the surgery, the commitment to cesarean birth, and alternatives to the treatment.

As in other aspects of maternity care, caregivers must respect the pregnant woman's autonomy. The procedure involves health risks to the woman, and she retains the right to refuse any surgical procedure. Health care providers must be careful that their zeal for new technology does not lead them to focus unilaterally on the fetus at the expense of the mother.

Reproductive Assistance

Assisted reproductive technology (ART) is the term used to describe highly technologic approaches used to produce pregnancy. In vitro fertilization and embryo transfer, zygote intrafallopian transfer, gamete intrafallopian transfer, and intracytoplasmic sperm injection are examples. (See Chapter 4 for more information about these procedures.)

Some legislative efforts have been made to address consumer concerns about ART. In the United States the Federal Fertility Clinic Success Rate and Certification Act (FCSRCA) of 1992 requires standardized reporting of pregnancy success rates associated with ART programs and addresses issues related to laboratory quality. However, it does not deal with unethical practices that may occur or false reporting of success rates (Wilcox & Marks, 1996).

In Canada the Royal Commission on New Reproductive Technologies was charged with examining the range of technologies related to reproduction. Among its most important recommendations, the commission advocated legislation to prohibit several aspects of technology, such as selling human eggs, zygotes, sperm, fetuses, or fetal tissue. It also recommended that the government establish a national regulatory body to license and regulate the provision of reproductive technology services in Canada (Baird, 1996).

Surrogate childbearing is another approach to infertility. Surrogate childbearing occurs when a woman agrees to become pregnant for a childless couple. She may be artificially inseminated with the male partner's sperm or a donor's sperm or may receive a gamete transfer, depending on the infertile couple's needs. If fertilization occurs, the woman carries the fetus to term and releases the infant to the couple after birth.

These methods of resolving infertility raise ethical issues about candidate selection, responsibility for a child born with a congenital defect, and religious objections to artificial conception. Other ethical questions include the following: What should be done with surplus fertilized oocytes? To whom do frozen embryos belong? Who is liable if a woman or her offspring contracts HIV from donated sperm? Should children be told about their conception?

Embryonic Stem Cell Research

Human stem cells can be found in embryonic tissue and in the primordial germ cells of a fetus. Research has demonstrated that in tissue cultures these cells can be made to differentiate into other types of cells such as blood, nerve, or heart cells, which might then be used to treat problems such as diabetes, Parkinson and Alzheimer diseases, spinal cord injury, or metabolic disorders. The availability of specialized tissue or even organs grown from stem cells might also decrease society's dependence on donated organs for organ transplants (Ryan, 2000).

The ethical questions and dilemmas associated with embryonic stem cell research are staggering and complex. The following are two of the most pressing issues to be considered (Roche & Grodin, 2000):

- What moral status should be attached to the human embryo? How should an embryo be viewed? With full status as a person? As a cluster of undifferentiated cells with no moral status? As having status somewhere in between—that is, beyond mere cells and deserving of special respect?

- What sources of embryonic tissue are acceptable for research? Is it ever ethical to create embryos solely for stem cell research? Is there justification for using embryos remaining after fertility treatments?

Equally significant, advancements in stem cell research play a major role in the rapidly approaching convergence of reproductive and genetic technologies with all of their related ethical dilemmas, as the following discussion suggests.

The Human Genome Project

The *Human Genome Project* is an international, multidisciplinary effort to explore and map all human genetic material. (See Chapter 4 for more information.) As more genetic information becomes available, questions arise about the ethical use and protection of such information. Other emerging issues include the question of payment for genetic testing; appropriate counseling following testing; confidentiality; qualifications of individuals engaged in testing, counseling, and interventions; mandated testing; and the right to refuse to receive information about genetic findings.

Cord Blood Banking

Cord blood, taken from a newborn's umbilical cord at birth and stored or "banked," may play a role in combating leukemia, certain other cancers, and immune and blood system disorders. This is possible because cord blood, like bone marrow and embryonic tissue, contains regenerative stem cells, which can replace diseased cells in the affected individual.

Ethical issues associated with cord blood banking include the following (Smith & Thomson, 2000):

- Who owns the blood? The donor? The parents? Private blood banks? Society?

- How will informed consent be obtained and by whom?

- How will confidentiality be ensured? The family must understand that, if they choose to donate, the mother will be asked to provide a blood sample and a detailed history about her health and infectious disease status.

- How will obligations to notify the family and donor be addressed if testing of the blood reveals infectious diseases or genetic disorders?
- How will the harvested blood be allocated to ensure fairness and availability to individuals from all races, ethnic groups, and income levels?

Making Treatment Decisions for Children

Technology makes it possible to sustain the lives of children who previously would have died, thus creating many ethical issues. Problems may develop because physicians, nurses, and parents have differing opinions about treatments for an infant or child with a serious or fatal condition. Nurses often face ethical dilemmas when providing care to such a child, especially as they witness parents struggling to decide among treatment options. Ethical issues in pediatrics are often more complex because most children lack the capacity to make or to participate in medical decisions that directly affect them.

When making treatment decisions in pediatrics, health care professionals need to determine whether their responsibility is limited to the child or includes the interests of the parents. The health care institution's ethics committee often plays a role in resolving conflicts about treatment decisions. Courts should make ethical decisions only when health care professionals and parents are unable to agree about providing or withholding treatment. WEB

Terminating Life-Sustaining Treatment

Federal "Baby Doe" regulations were developed to protect the rights of infants with severe defects. Parents of such infants are usually the ultimate decision makers about the child's care. They may want to terminate treatment because of the tremendous social, emotional, and financial burden they face (Schrode, 2000). Physicians may believe treatment will help the child and improve the quality of life (sometimes defined as a meaningful existence or an ability to develop human relationships). Federal regulations require a formalized ethical decision-making process before physicians accept or reject a parent's wishes. WEB

Justifications for withholding, withdrawing, or limiting therapy include the following:

- The treatment in question has a poor rate of success.
- The burdens of the treatment outweigh the benefits, or the quality of life is poor after treatment.
- The burdens of the disease outweigh the benefits of continued survival, or the quality of life is poor before the treatment (Cassidy & Fleischman, 1996).

Each of these conditions is considered according to the individual beliefs of the members of the ethics committee and their perceptions of the value of specific interventions for an individual child. Treatment to save the infant's life is often elected if it has the potential for improving the quality of life as well. Physicians are not obligated to offer interventions that cause extreme pain and suffering when there is no potential benefit or only limited potential benefit. Treatments that only prolong life represent a misuse of expensive health care resources.

Organ Transplantation Issues

The death of a child can benefit another child through organ transplantation. WEB The National Organ Transplant Act (PL 98-507) generated laws, regulations, and guidelines for organ collection and transplantation (Frader & Thompson, 1994). For example, the transplant team cannot provide care to the potential donor. In addition, the institution has specific requirements to approach family members when brain death is suspected or confirmed to request organ donation.

Regulations are important because too few organs are available for people needing transplantation. The limited supply of organs has created numerous ethical issues.

- Which individuals on a waiting list should receive the organs available?
- Should families be permitted to pay donor families for organs?
- Should the family's ability to pay for an organ transplant give a child higher priority for an organ?
- What are the brain death and nonheartbeating criteria for children that enable organ collection to proceed?

Implications for Nursing Practice

The complex ethical issues facing maternal-child nurses have many social, cultural, legal, and professional ramifications. Ethical decisions in maternal-child nursing are often complicated by moral obligations to more than one client. Straightforward solutions to the ethical dilemmas encountered in caring for children and childbearing families are often, quite simply, not available.

Nurses must learn to anticipate ethical dilemmas, clarify their own positions related to the issues, understand the legal implications of the issues, and develop appropriate strategies for ethical decision making. To accomplish these tasks, they can read about bioethical issues, participate in discussion groups, attend courses and workshops on ethical topics pertinent to their areas of practice, and serve on ethics committees.

EVIDENCE-BASED PRACTICE IN MATERNAL-CHILD NURSING

Evidence-based practice is emerging as a force in health care. It provides a useful approach to problem solving, to clinical decision making, and to self-directed patient-centered, lifelong learning (Sackett, Straus, Richardson, et al., 2000). Of prime importance is that evidence-based practices improve the quality of care and increase the likelihood of producing the desired patient outcome. Evidence-based practice moves research findings into clinical practice. It combines several forms of scientific evidence with clinical expertise and client preferences to produce best practice. Forms of evidence may include, for example, data from clinical research studies, quality improvement measurements, and risk management measures.

As clinicians, nurses need to meet three basic competencies related to evidence-based practice. These are: (1) to recognize which clinical practices are supported by sound evidence, which practices have conflicting findings as to their effect on client outcomes, and which practices have no evidence to support their use; (2) to use data in their clinical work to evaluate outcomes of care; and (3) to appraise and integrate scientific bases into practice. Nurses need to know what data are being tracked where they work and how care practices and outcomes are improved as a result of quality improvement initiatives. However, there is more to

evidence-based practice than simply knowing what is being tracked and how the results are being used. Competent, effective nurses learn to question the very basis of their clinical work.

Special research activities related to childbearing women, children, and families can be found on the companion website. **WEB** These activities may challenge you to question the soundness and effectiveness of some of the routine care you observe in clinical practice or to confirm the scientific underpinnings of widely adopted, common practices. This may mean becoming aware that a common practice is *not* supported by empirical evidence and the practice should be changed; or it may mean becoming aware that the practice *is* supported by research, although most nurses are not cognizant of the scientific underpinning (or age of the science); or it may mean becoming aware that there is not enough scientific evidence to guide practice, in which case, more research is needed. That is the impact of evidence-based practice—it moves clinicians beyond practices of habit and opinion to practices based on high-quality, current science.

$\mathcal{C}$HAPTER HIGHLIGHTS

☙ Many nurses working with childbearing and childrearing families are expert practitioners who are able to serve as role models for nurses who have not yet attained the same level of competence.

☙ Contemporary childbirth is family centered, offers choices about birth, and recognizes the needs of siblings and other family members.

☙ Family-centered care is designed to meet the emotional, social, and developmental needs of children and families seeking health care.

☙ Case management is a process designed to coordinate the delivery of health care services in a collaborative approach that focuses on both quality and cost outcomes.

☙ The nurse who provides culturally sensitive care recognizes the importance of a family's value system, acknowledges that differences exist among people, and seeks to respect and respond to ethnic diversity in a way that leads to mutually desirable outcomes.

☙ A nurse must practice within the scope of practice or be subject to the accusation of practicing medicine without a license. The standard of care against which individual nursing practice is compared is that of a reasonably prudent nurse.

☙ Nursing standards provide information and guidelines for nurses in their own practice, in developing policies and protocols in health care settings, and in directing the development of quality nursing care.

☙ Informed consent—based on knowledge of a procedure and its benefits, risks, and alternatives—must be secured before providing treatment.

☙ Children under 18 or 21 years (depending on the state) can legally give informed consent when they are the minor parents of a child patient or when they are emancipated minors. If they are between 16 and 18 years of age, they may give consent if they are seeking birth control, mental health counseling, or substance abuse treatment.

☙ Abortion can legally be performed until the fetus reaches the age of viability. The decision to have an abortion is made by a woman in consultation with her physician.

☙ *Assisted reproductive technology* (ART) is the term used to describe highly technologic approaches used to produce pregnancy, including in vitro fertilization and embryo transfer (IVF-ET), zygote intrafallopian transfer, (ZIFT), and gamete intrafallopian transfer (GIFT).

☙ Cord blood banking provides the opportunity to have stem cells available to treat a variety of cancers and blood disorders. Its growing popularity has revealed several ethical issues.

☙ Federal "Baby Doe" regulations were developed to protect the rights of infants with severe defects.

☙ Evidence-based practice refers to clinical practice based on research findings and other available data. It increases nurses' accountability and results in better client outcomes.

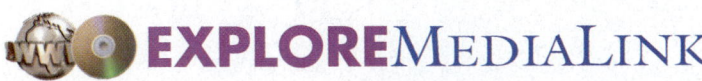 **EXPLORE**MEDIA**LINK**

NCLEX Review, Case Studies, and other interactive resources for this chapter can be found on the companion website at http://www.prenhall.com/london. Click on "Chapter 1" to select the activities for this chapter.

For animations, more NCLEX review questions, and an audio glossary, access the accompanying CD-ROM in this textbook.

REFERENCES

American Academy of Pediatrics, Committee on Bioethics. (1999). Fetal therapy—Ethical considerations (RE9817). *Pediatrics, 103*(5), 1061–1063.

American College of Obstetricians and Gynecologists, Committee on Ethics. (1999). *Patient choice and the maternal-fetal relationship* (Opinion No. 214). Washington, DC: Author.

American Nurses Association. (1998). *Standards of clinical nursing practice* (2nd ed.). Washington, DC: American Nurses Publishing.

Baird, P. A. (1996). New reproductive technologies: The Canadian perspective. *Women's Health Issues, 6*(3), 156–166.

Cassidy, R. C., & Fleischman, A. R. (1996). *Pediatric ethics—From principles to practice*. Amsterdam: Harwood Academic Publishers.

Davis, L. J., Okuboye, S., & Ferguson, S. L. (2000). Healthy people 2010: Examining a decade of maternal & infant health. *AWHONN Lifelines, 4*(3), 26–33.

Dickey, S. B., & Deatrick, J. (2000). Autonomy and decision making for health promotion in adolescence. *Pediatric Nursing, 26*(5), 461–467.

Dower, C. N., & Miller, J. E. (1999). *Taskforce on midwifery. Charting a course for the 21st century: The future of midwifery*. San Francisco: Pew Health Professions Commission and the University of California–San Francisco Center for the Health Professions.

Eisenberg, D. M., Davis, R. B., Ettner, S. L., Appel, S., Wilkey, S., VanRompey, M., & Kessler, R. C. (1998). Trends in alternative medicine use in the United States, 1990–1997. *Journal of the American Medical Association, 280*, 1569–1575.

Food and Drug Administration. (1998, December 2). Regulations requiring manufacturers to assess the safety and effectiveness of new drugs and biological products in pediatric patients. *Federal Register, 63*(231), 66631–66672. WEB

Ford, C. A., Bearman, P. S., & Moody, J. (1999). Foregone health care among adolescents. *Journal of the American Medical Association, 282*(23), 2227–2234.

Frader, J., & Thompson, A. (1994). Ethical issues in the pediatric intensive care unit. *Pediatric Clinics of North America, 41*(6), 1405–1421.

Health Care Finance Administration. (2000). *The state children's health insurance program (SCHIP)*. WEB

Health Resources and Services Administration's Maternal and Child Health Bureau. (2000). *Child health USA 2000*. Washington, DC: Government Printing Office.

Hornstra, D. (1999). A realistic approach to maternal-fetal conflict. *Neonatal Intensive Care, 12*(2), 24–31.

Kemper, K. J. (2001). Complementary and alternative medicine for children: Does it work? *Western Journal of Medicine, 174*, 272–276.

Lindeke, L. L., Hauck, M. R., & Tanner, M. (2000). Practical issues in obtaining child assent for research. *Journal of Pediatric Nursing, 15*(2), 99–104.

Maiese, D. R. (2001). Monitoring women's health through performance measures. *Title V Today, 3*(1), 6–7.

Maternal and Child Health Bureau. (1995). *Child health USA '94* (DHHS Publication No. HRSA-MCH-95-1). Washington, DC: Government Printing Office.

Melnyk, B. M., Fineout-Overholt, E., Stone, P., & Ackerman, M. (2000). Evidence-based practice: The past, the present, and recommendations for the millennium. *Pediatric Nursing, 26*(1), 77–80.

Merritt, T. A., Palmer, D., Bergman, D. A., & Shiono, P. H. (1997). Clinical practice guidelines in pediatric and newborn medicine. Implications for their use in practice. *Pediatrics, 99*(1), 100–114.

Murphy, S. L. (2000). Deaths: Final data for 1998. *National Vital Statistics Report, 48*(11), 1–106.

Murphy, P. A., Kronenberg, F., & Wade, C. (1999). Complementary and alternative medicine in women's health. *Journal of Nurse-Midwifery, 44*(3), 192–200.

Myers-Ciecko, J. A. (1999). Evolution and current status of direct-entry midwifery education, regulation, and practice in the United States, with examples from Washington state. *Journal of Nurse-Midwifery, 44*(4), 384–393.

National Association of Home Care. (2000). *Basic statistics about home care*. WEB

National Center for Human Genome Research. (2000). *Five-year research goals of the U.S. Human Genome Project*. WEB

Population Estimates Program, Population Division, U.S. Census Bureau. (2001). *Resident population estimates of the United States by age and sex: April 1, 1990 to July 1, 1999, with short-term projection to November 1, 2000*. WEB

Ranzini, A., Allen, A., & Lai, Y. (2001). Use of complementary medicine and alternative therapies among obstetric patients. *Obstetrics and Gynecology, 4*(Suppl. 1), S46.

Roche, P. A., & Grodin, M. A. (2000). The ethical challenge of stem cell research. *Women's Health Issues, 10*(3), 136–139.

Ryan, K. J. (2000). The politics and ethics of human embryo and stem cell research. *Women's Health Issues, 10*(3), 105–110.

Sackett, D. L., Straus, S. E., Richardson, W. S., Rosenberg, W., & Haynes, R. B. (2000). *Evidence-based medicine: How to practice and teach EBM*. Edinburgh Scotland: Churchill Livingstone.

Schrode, K. (2000). Baby Doe and the Baby Doe regulations. *Children's National Medical Center Pediatric Ethicscope, 11*(1), 1–4.

Smith, F. O., & Thomson, B. G. (2000). Umbilical cord blood collection, banking, and transplantation: Current status and issues relevant to perinatal caregivers. *Birth, 27*(2), 127–135.

Smith, L. A., Wise, P. H., Chavkin, W., Romero, D., & Zuckerman, B. (2000). Implications in welfare reform for child health: Emerging challenges for clinical practice and policy. *Pediatrics, 106*(5), 1117–1125.

U.S. Census. (2001). *Population estimates for children by age and race*. WEB

U.S. Department of Health and Human Services. (2000). *Healthy People 2010* (Conference Edition). Washington, DC: Author.

U.S. Department of Health and Human Services. (1983). *Protection of human subjects: Code of federal regulations* (45 CFR #46, Subpart D).

U.S. General Accounting Office. (1989). *Home care experiences of families with chronically ill children*. Washington, DC: Author.

Ventura, S. J., Martin, J. A., Curtin, S. C., Mathews, T. J., & Park, M. M. (2000). Births: Final data for 1998. *National Vital Statistics Report, 48*(3), 1–105.

Wilcox, L. S., & Marks, J. S. (1996). Regulating assisted reproductive technologies: Public health, consumer protection, and public resources. *Women's Health Issues, 6*(3), 175–180.

UNIT II

The Reproductive Years and Beyond

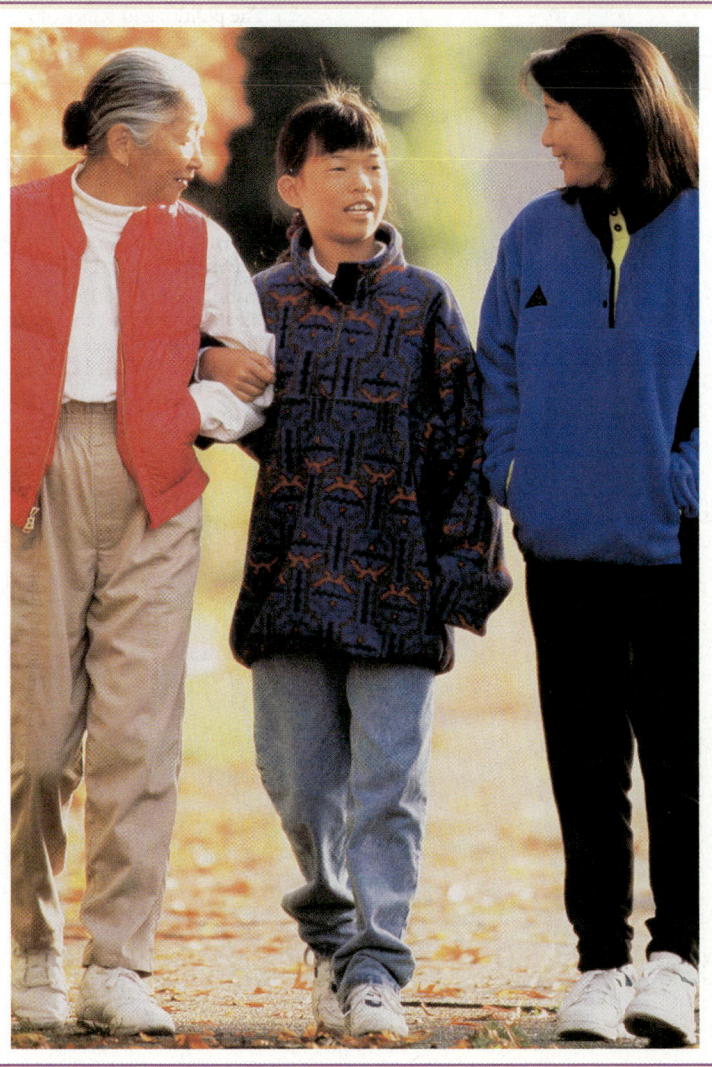

CHAPTER 2

Reproductive Anatomy and Physiology

At my last "female checkup" at the clinic, the nurse told me about their free family-planning classes. So I went to one with a friend, and I learned so much about my body and about men's bodies. I thought I knew all there was to know about that stuff—but I guess not. My boyfriend, Jontau, has been looking at the handouts they gave me, and asking me questions. I think he's completely amazed at how our bodies work. I know I am.

—SHEENA, 16

Key Terms

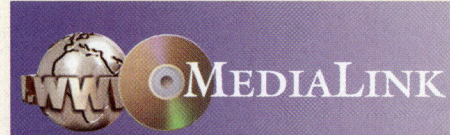

MEDIALINK

CD-ROM

Audio Glossary

NCLEX Review

Sperm Production Animation

Egg Cell Production Animation

COMPANION WEBSITE

http://www.prenhall.com/london

Reproductive Anatomy and Physiology Web Links

Thinking Critically

NCLEX Review

Case Study

$\mathcal{U}$nderstanding childbearing requires more than understanding sexual intercourse or the process by which the female and male sex cells unite. The nurse must also become familiar with the structures and functions that make childbearing possible and the phenomena that initiate it. This chapter presents the anatomic, physiologic, and sexual aspects of the female and male reproductive systems. Chapter 3 discusses the psychosocial aspects of human sexuality. ⌾

The female and male reproductive organs are *homologous*; that is, they are fundamentally similar in structure and function. The primary functions of both female and male reproductive systems are to produce sex cells and transport them to locations where their union can occur. The sex cells, called *gametes*, are produced by specialized organs called *gonads*. A series of ducts and glands within both male and female reproductive systems contributes to the production and transport of the gametes.

Although the genetic sex of an embryo is determined at fertilization, the male and female reproductive systems are undifferentiated for about the first 8 weeks of gestation. This undifferentiated period is followed by a period of rapid, dramatic changes as the reproductive organs differentiate into recognizable structures (Figure 2–1 ◆).

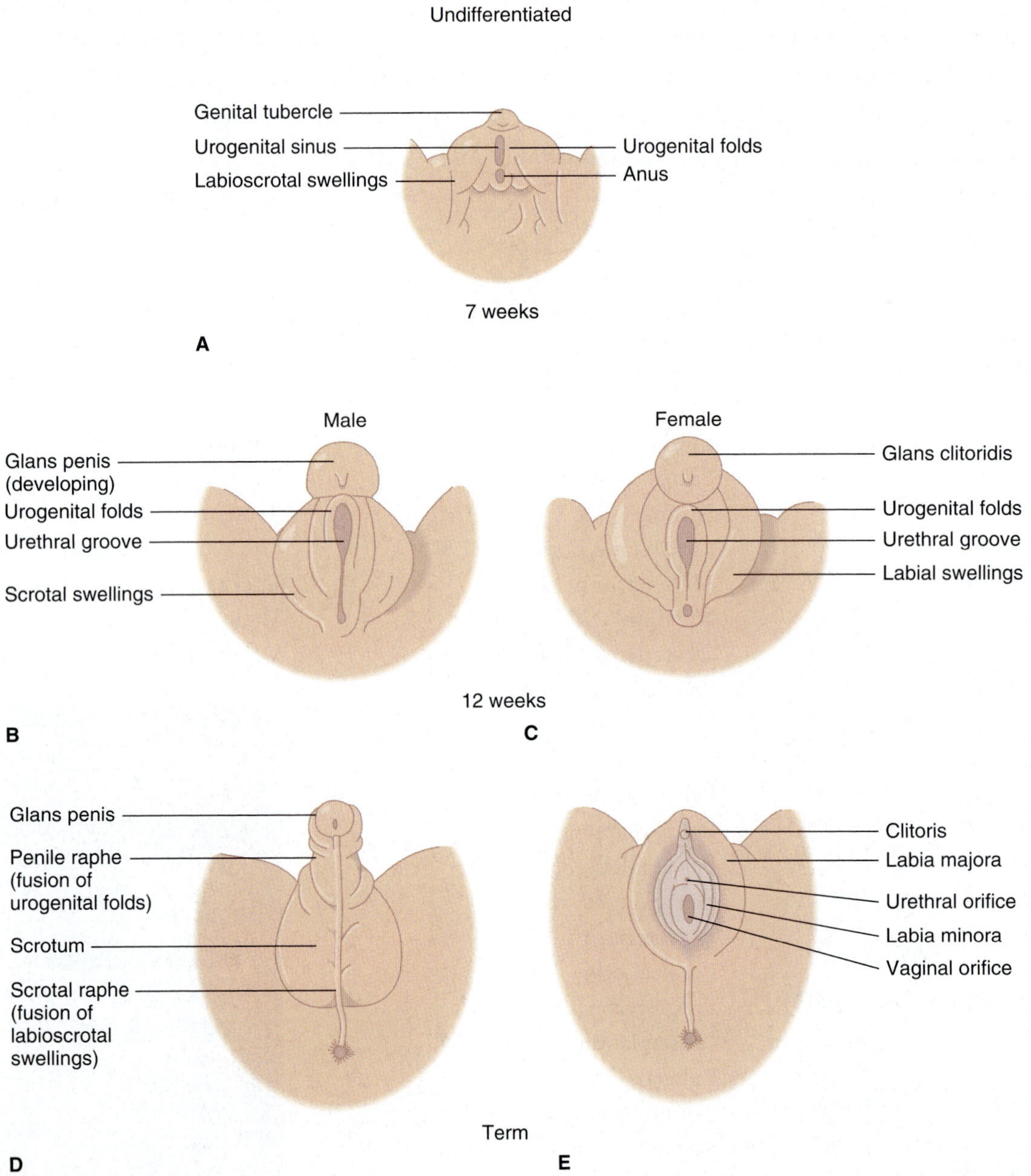

FIGURE 2–1. ◆ Sexual differentiation. **A,** At 7 weeks' gestation, male and female genitalia are identical (undifferentiated). **B** and **C,** By 12 weeks' gestation, noticeable differentiation begins to occur. **D** and **E,** Differentiation continues until birth but is almost complete at term.

PUBERTY

The term **puberty** refers to the developmental period between childhood and attainment of adult sexual characteristics and functioning. Generally, boys mature physically about 2 years later than girls. The age at onset and progress of puberty vary widely, physical changes overlap, and the sequence of events can vary from person to person. For a detailed discussion of physical changes associated with puberty see Chapters 32 and 33. ◌═◌ This diversity results from each individual's response to hormonal stimulation.

Physiology of Onset

Puberty is initiated by the maturation of the hypothalamic-pituitary-gonad complex (the *gonadostat*) and input from the central nervous system. The process, which begins during fetal life, is sequential and complex.

The central nervous system releases a neurotransmitter that stimulates the hypothalamus to synthesize and release **gonadotropin-releasing hormone (GnRH)** (Ferin, 1998). GnRH is transmitted to the anterior pituitary, where it causes the synthesis and secretion of the gonadotropins **follicle-stimulating hormone (FSH)** and **luteinizing hormone (LH)** (Figure 2–2 ◆).

Although the gonads do produce small amounts of *androgens* (male sex hormones) and *estrogens* (female sex hormones) before the onset of puberty, FSH and LH stimulate increased secretion of these hormones. Androgens and estrogens influence the development of secondary sex characteristics. FSH and LH stimulate the processes of spermatogenesis and maturation of ova.

Other hormones are involved in the onset of puberty. Although less direct, their action is essential. Abnormally high or low levels of adrenocorticotropic hormone (ACTH), thyroid hormone, or growth hormone (GH) can disrupt the onset of normal puberty (see detailed discussion in Chapter 51) ◌═◌ (Ferin, 1998).

FEMALE REPRODUCTIVE SYSTEM

The female reproductive system consists of the external and internal genitals and the accessory organs of the breasts. Because of its importance to childbearing, the bony pelvis is also discussed in this chapter.

External Genitals

All the external reproductive organs except the glandular structures can be directly inspected. The size, color, and shape of these structures vary extensively among races and individuals. The female external genitals, also referred to as the **vulva,** include the following structures (Figure 2–3 ◆):

- Mons pubis
- Labia majora
- Labia minora

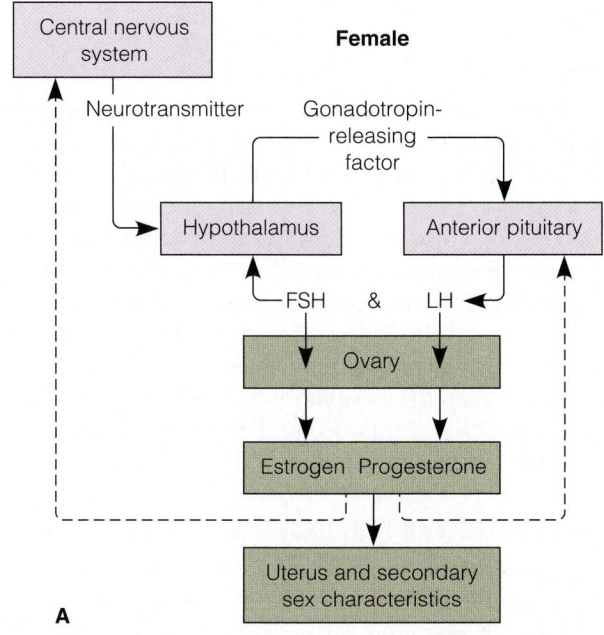
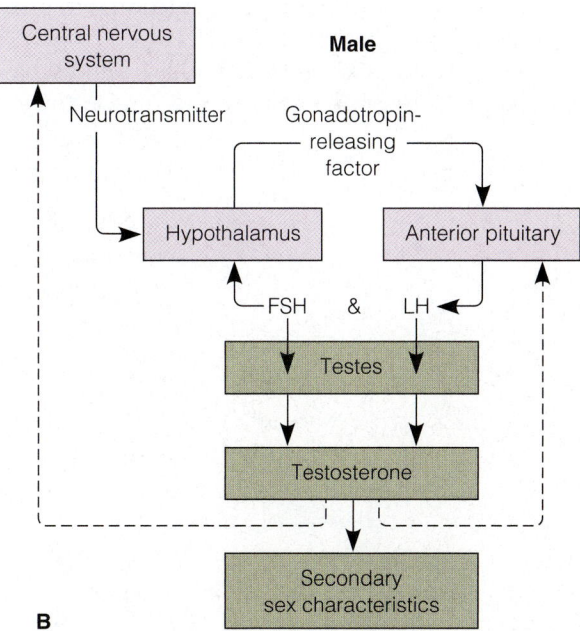

FIGURE 2–2. ◆ Physiologic changes leading to onset of puberty. **A,** In females; and **B,** in males. Solid lines illustrate stimulation of hormone production, and broken lines illustrate inhibition. Through a neurotransmitter the central nervous system stimulates the hypothalamus, which in turn produces a gonadotropin-releasing factor that causes the anterior pituitary to produce gonadotropins (FSH or LH). These hormones stimulate specific structures in the gonads to secrete steroid hormones (estrogen, progesterone, or testosterone). The rise in pituitary hormone production increases hypothalamus activity. Elevated steroid hormone levels stimulate the central nervous system and pituitary gland to inhibit hormone production.

- Clitoris
- Urethral meatus and opening of the paraurethral (Skene's) glands
- Vaginal vestibule (vaginal orifice, vulvovaginal glands, hymen, and fossa navicularis)
- Perineal body

Although they are not true parts of the female reproductive system, the urethral meatus and perineal body are considered here because of their proximity and relationship to the vulva. The vulva has a generous supply of blood and nerves. As a woman ages, estrogen secretions decrease, causing the vulvar organs to atrophy and become subject to a variety of lesions.

MONS PUBIS

The mons pubis is a softly rounded mound of subcutaneous fatty tissue beginning at the lowest portion of the anterior abdominal wall (see Figure 2–3). Also known as the mons veneris, this structure covers the front portion of the symphysis pubis. The mons pubis is covered with pubic hair, typically with the hairline forming a transverse line across the lower abdomen. The hair is short and varies from sparse and fine in Asian women to heavy, coarse, and curly in women of African descent. The mons pubis protects the pelvic bones, especially during coitus.

LABIA MAJORA

The *labia majora* are longitudinal, raised folds of pigmented skin, one on either side of the vulvar cleft. As the pair descend, they narrow and merge to form the posterior junction of the perineal skin. Their chief function is to protect the structures lying between them.

The labia majora are covered by hair follicles and sebaceous glands, with underlying adipose and muscle tissue.

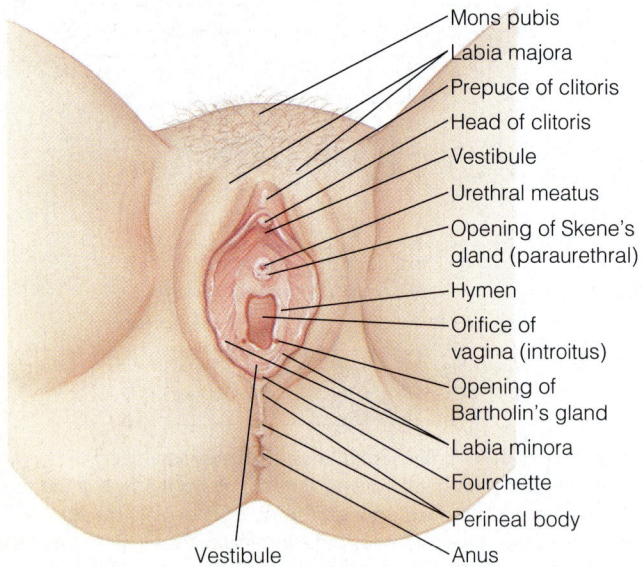

Mons pubis
Labia majora
Prepuce of clitoris
Head of clitoris
Vestibule
Urethral meatus
Opening of Skene's gland (paraurethral)
Hymen
Orifice of vagina (introitus)
Opening of Bartholin's gland
Labia minora
Fourchette
Perineal body
Anus
Vestibule

FIGURE 2–3. ◆ Female external genitals, longitudinal view.

The dartos muscle sheet is responsible for the wrinkled appearance of the labia majora as well as for their sensitivity to heat and cold. The inner surface of the labia majora in women who have not had children is moist and looks like mucous membrane, whereas after many births it is more skinlike (Cunningham, Gant, Leveno, Gilstrap, Hauth, Wenstrom, 2001). With each pregnancy, the labia majora become less prominent. Because of the extensive venous network in the labia majora, varicosities may occur during pregnancy, and obstetric or sexual trauma may cause hematomas. The labia majora share an extensive lymphatic supply with the other structures of the vulva, which can facilitate the spread of cancer in the female reproductive organs. Because of the nerves supplying the labia majora (from the first lumbar and third sacral segment of the spinal cord), certain regional anesthesia blocks will affect them and cause numbness.

LABIA MINORA

The *labia minora* are soft folds of skin within the labia majora that converge near the anus, forming the *fourchette*. Each labium minus has the appearance of shiny mucous membrane, moist and devoid of hair follicles. The labia minora are rich in sebaceous glands, which lubricate and waterproof the vulvar skin and provide bactericidal secretions. Because the sebaceous glands do not open into hair follicles but open directly onto the surface of the skin, sebaceous cysts commonly occur in this area. Vulvovaginitis in this area is very irritating because the labia minora have many tactile nerve endings. The labia minora increase in size at puberty and decrease after menopause because of changes in estrogen levels.

CLITORIS

The *clitoris,* located between the labia minora, is about 5 to 6 mm long and 6 to 8 mm across. Its tissue is essentially erectile, and it is very sensitive to touch. The glans of the clitoris is partly covered by a fold of skin called the *prepuce,* or clitoral hood. This area resembles an opening to an orifice and may be confused with the urethral meatus. Accidental attempts to insert a catheter in this area produce extreme discomfort. The clitoris has rich blood and nerve supplies and exists primarily for female sexual enjoyment. In addition, it secretes *smegma,* which along with other vulval secretions has a unique odor that may be sexually stimulating to the male.

URETHRAL MEATUS AND PARAURETHRAL GLANDS

The *urethral meatus* is located 1 to 2.5 cm beneath the clitoris in the midline of the vestibule; it often appears as a puckered, slitlike opening. At times the meatus is difficult to visualize because of the presence of blind dimples or small mucosal folds. The paraurethral glands, or *Skene's glands,* open into the posterior wall of the urethra close to its opening (see Figure 2–3). Their secretions lubricate the vaginal opening, facilitating sexual intercourse.

VAGINAL VESTIBULE

The vaginal vestibule is a boat-shaped depression enclosed by the labia majora and visible when they are separated. The vestibule contains the vaginal opening, or *introitus,* which is the border between the external and internal genitals.

The *hymen* is a thin, elastic collar or semicollar of tissue that surrounds the vaginal opening. The appearance changes during the woman's lifetime. The hymen is essentially avascular. For thousands of years, some societies have perpetuated the belief that the hymen covers the vaginal opening and is a sign of virginity. However, modern studies of female genital anatomy have revealed that the hymen does not completely cover the vaginal opening and can be torn through strenuous physical activity, masturbation, menstruation, or the use of tampons, thus dispelling old beliefs.

External to the hymen at the base of the vestibule are two small papular elevations containing the openings of the ducts of the *vulvovaginal (Bartholin's) glands.* They lie under the constrictor muscle of the vagina. These glands secrete a clear, thick, alkaline mucus that enhances the viability and motility of the sperm deposited in the vaginal vestibule. These gland ducts can harbor *Neisseria gonorrheae* and other bacteria, which can cause pus formation and abscesses in the Bartholin's glands.

PERINEAL BODY

The **perineal body** is a wedge-shaped mass of fibromuscular tissue found between the lower part of the vagina and the anus. The superficial area between the anus and the vagina is referred to as the *perineum.*

The muscles that meet at the perineal body are the external sphincter ani, both levator ani, the superficial and deep transverse perineal, and the bulbocavernosus. These muscles mingle with elastic fibers and connective tissue in an arrangement that allows a remarkable amount of stretching. During the last part of labor, the perineal body thins out until it is just a few centimeters thick. This tissue is the site of the possible episiotomy or lacerations during childbirth (see Chapter 20).

Internal Reproductive Organs

The female internal reproductive organs are the vagina, uterus, fallopian tubes, and ovaries (Figure 2–4 ◆). These are target organs for estrogenic hormones, and they play a unique part in the reproductive cycle. The internal reproductive organs can be palpated during vaginal examination and assessed with various instruments.

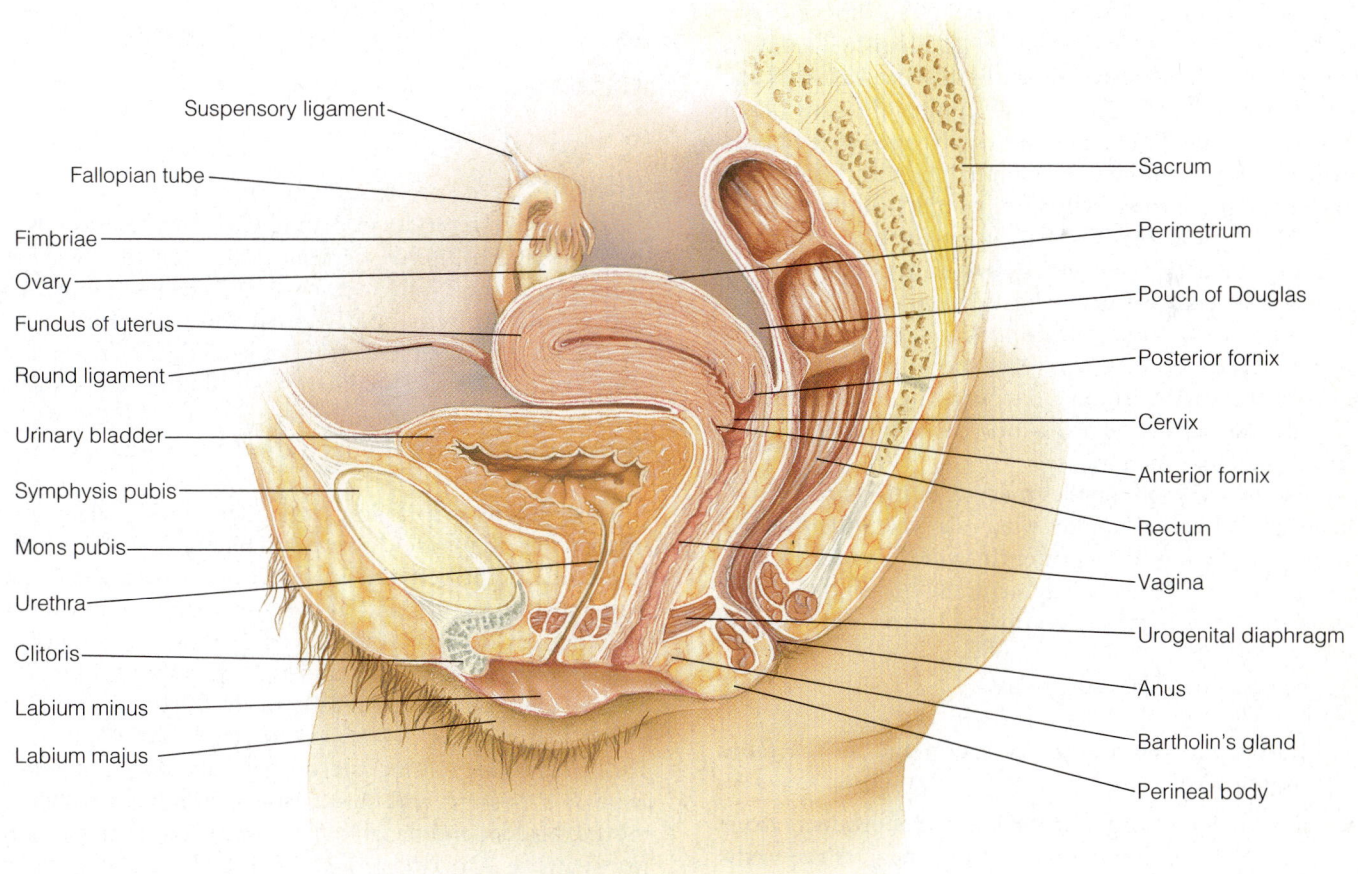

Suspensory ligament — Fallopian tube — Fimbriae — Ovary — Fundus of uterus — Round ligament — Urinary bladder — Symphysis pubis — Mons pubis — Urethra — Clitoris — Labium minus — Labium majus

Sacrum — Perimetrium — Pouch of Douglas — Posterior fornix — Cervix — Anterior fornix — Rectum — Vagina — Urogenital diaphragm — Anus — Bartholin's gland — Perineal body

FIGURE 2–4. ◆ Female internal reproductive organs.

VAGINA

The **vagina** is a muscular and membranous tube that connects the external genitals with the uterus. It extends from the vulva to the uterus. The vagina is often called the *birth canal* because it forms the lower part of the pelvis through which the fetus must pass during birth.

Because the cervix of the uterus projects into the upper part of the anterior wall of the vagina, the anterior wall is approximately 2.5 cm shorter than the posterior wall. Measurements range from 6 to 8 cm for the anterior wall and from 7 to 10 cm for the posterior wall.

In the upper part of the vagina, which is called the vaginal vault, there is a recess or hollow around the cervix. This area is called the vaginal *fornix*. Since the walls of the vaginal vault are very thin, various structures can be palpated through the walls, including the uterus, a distended bladder, the ovaries, the appendix, the cecum, the colon, and the ureters. When a woman lies on her back after intercourse, the space in the fornix permits the pooling of semen near the cervix and increases the chances of pregnancy.

The walls of the vagina are covered with ridges, or rugae, crisscrossing each other. These rugae allow the vaginal tissues to stretch enough for the fetus to pass through during childbirth.

During a woman's reproductive life, an acidic vaginal environment is normal (pH 4 to 5). The acidic environment is maintained by a symbiotic relationship between lactic acid–producing bacilli (Döderlein's bacillus or lactobacillus) and the vaginal epithelial cells. These cells contain glycogen, which is broken down by the bacilli into lactic acid. Secretion from the vaginal epithelium provides a moist environment. The amount of glycogen is regulated by the ovarian hormones. Any interruption of this process can destroy the normal self-cleaning action of the vagina. Such interruption may be caused by antibiotic therapy, douching, or use of perineal sprays or deodorants. (For discussion of comfort issues for women, see Chapter 3.) The acidic vaginal environment is normal only during the mature reproductive years and in the first days of life when maternal hormones are operating in the infant. A relatively neutral pH of 7.5 is normal from infancy until puberty and after menopause.

The vagina's blood supplies are extensive (Figure 2–5 ♦). The pudendal nerve supplies what relatively little somatic innervation there is to the lower third of the vagina. Thus, sensation during sexual excitement and coitus is reduced in this area, as is vaginal pain during the second stage of labor.

The vagina has three functions:

- To serve as the passage for sperm and for the fetus during birth

- To provide passage for the menstrual products from the uterine endometrium to the outside of the body

- To protect against trauma from sexual intercourse and infection from pathogenic organisms

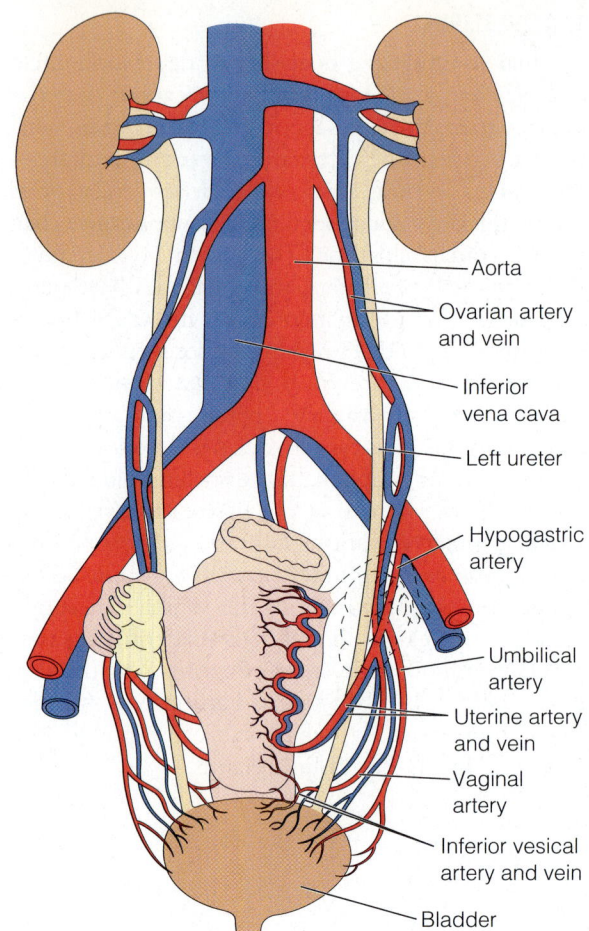

FIGURE 2–5. ♦ Pelvic blood supply.

Labels: Aorta; Ovarian artery and vein; Inferior vena cava; Left ureter; Hypogastric artery; Umbilical artery; Uterine artery and vein; Vaginal artery; Inferior vesical artery and vein; Bladder

UTERUS

As the core of reproduction and hence continuation of the human race, the uterus, or womb, has been endowed with a mystical aura. Numerous customs, taboos, mores, and values have evolved about women and their reproductive function. Although scientific knowledge has replaced much of this folklore, remnants of old ideas and superstitions persist. To provide effective care, nurses must be cognizant of their own attitudes and beliefs, as well as those of their clients.

The **uterus** is a hollow, muscular, thick-walled organ shaped like an upside-down pear (Figure 2–6 ♦). It lies in the center of the pelvic cavity between the base of the bladder and the rectum and above the vagina. The external opening of the cervix (external os) is about the level of the ischial spines. The mature uterus weighs about 50 to 70 g and is approximately 6.0–8.0 cm long, and 1 to 2.5 cm thick (Cunningham, Gant, Leveno et al., 2001).

The position of the uterus can vary depending on a woman's posture and musculature, number of children borne, bladder and rectal fullness, and even normal respiratory patterns. Only the cervix is anchored laterally. The body of the uterus can move freely forward or backward. The axis also varies. Generally, the uterus bends forward, forming a

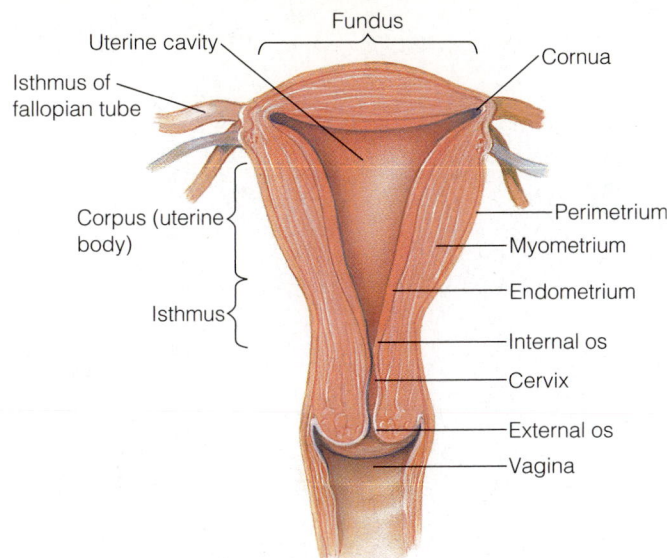

FIGURE 2–6. ◆ Structures of the uterus.

sharp angle with the vagina. There is a bend in the area of the isthmus of the uterus; from there the cervix points downward. The uterus is said to be anteverted when it is in this position. The anteverted position is considered normal.

The uterus is kept in place by three sets of supports. The upper supports are the broad and round ligaments. The middle supports are the cardinal, pubocervical, and uterosacral ligaments. The lower supports are those structures considered to make up the pelvic muscular floor.

The isthmus is a slight constriction in the uterus that divides it into two unequal parts. The upper two thirds of the uterus is the **corpus,** or uterine body, composed mainly of a smooth muscle layer (myometrium). The lower third is the cervix or neck. The rounded uppermost portion of the corpus that extends above the points of attachment of the fallopian tubes is called the **fundus.** The elongated portion of the uterus where the fallopian tubes enter is called the *cornua.*

The isthmus is about 6 mm above the uterine opening of the cervix (the internal os), and it is in this area that the uterine lining changes into the mucous membrane of the cervix; it joins the corpus to the cervix. The isthmus takes on importance in pregnancy because it becomes the lower uterine segment. With the cervix, it is a passive segment and not part of the contractile uterus. At birth this thin lower segment, situated behind the bladder, is the site for lower-segment cesarean births (see Chapter 20). 🔗

The blood and lymphatic supplies to the uterus are extensive. Innervation of the uterus is entirely by the autonomic nervous system. Even without an intact nerve supply, the uterus can contract adequately for birth; for example, hemiplegic women have adequate uterine contractions.

The function of the uterus is to provide a safe environment for fetal development. The uterine lining is cyclically prepared by steroid hormones for implantation of the embryo **(nidation).** Once the embryo is implanted, the developing fetus is protected until it is expelled.

Both the body of the uterus and the cervix are changed permanently by pregnancy. The body never returns to its prepregnant size, and the external os changes from a circular opening of about 3 mm to a transverse slit with irregular edges.

Uterine Corpus. The uterine corpus is made up of three layers. The outermost layer is the *serosal layer,* or **perimetrium,** which is composed of peritoneum. The middle layer is the *muscular uterine* layer, or **myometrium.** This muscular uterine layer is continuous with the muscle layers of the fallopian tubes and the vagina. This continuity helps these organs present a unified reaction to various stimuli—ovulation, orgasm, or the deposit of sperm in the vagina. These muscle fibers also extend into the ovarian, round, and cardinal ligaments and minimally into the uterosacral ligaments, which helps explain the vague but disturbing pelvic "aches and pains" reported by many pregnant women.

The myometrium has three distinct layers of uterine (smooth) involuntary muscles (Figure 2–7 ◆). The outer layer, found mainly over the fundus, is made up of longitudinal muscles that cause cervical effacement and expel the fetus during birth. The thick middle layer is made up of interlacing muscle fibers in figure-eight patterns. These muscle fibers surround large blood vessels, and their contraction produces a hemostatic action (a tourniquet-like action on blood vessels to stop bleeding after birth). The inner muscle layer is composed of circular fibers that form sphincters at the fallopian tube attachment sites and at the internal os. The internal os sphincter inhibits the expulsion of the uterine contents during pregnancy but stretches in labor as cervical dilatation occurs. An incompetent cervical os can be caused by a torn, weak, or absent sphincter at the internal os. The sphincters at the fallopian tubes prevent menstrual blood from flowing backward into the fallopian tubes from the uterus. Although each layer of muscle has been discussed as having a unique function, the uterine musculature actually works as a whole. The uterine contractions of labor are responsible for the dilatation of the cervix and provide the major force for the passage of the fetus through the pelvis and vaginal canal at birth.

The *mucosal* layer, or **endometrium,** of the uterine corpus is the innermost layer. This single layer is composed of columnar epithelium, glands, and stroma. From menarche to menopause, the endometrium undergoes monthly degeneration and renewal in the absence of pregnancy. As it responds to the governing hormonal cycle and prostaglandin influence, the endometrium varies in thickness from 0.5 to 5 mm. The glands of the endometrium produce a thin, watery, alkaline secretion that keeps the uterine cavity moist. This endometrial milk not only helps sperm travel to the fallopian tubes but also nourishes the developing embryo before it implants in the endometrium (see Chapter 5). 🔗

The blood supply to the endometrium is unique. Some of the blood vessels are not sensitive to cyclic hormonal control, whereas others are extremely sensitive to it. These

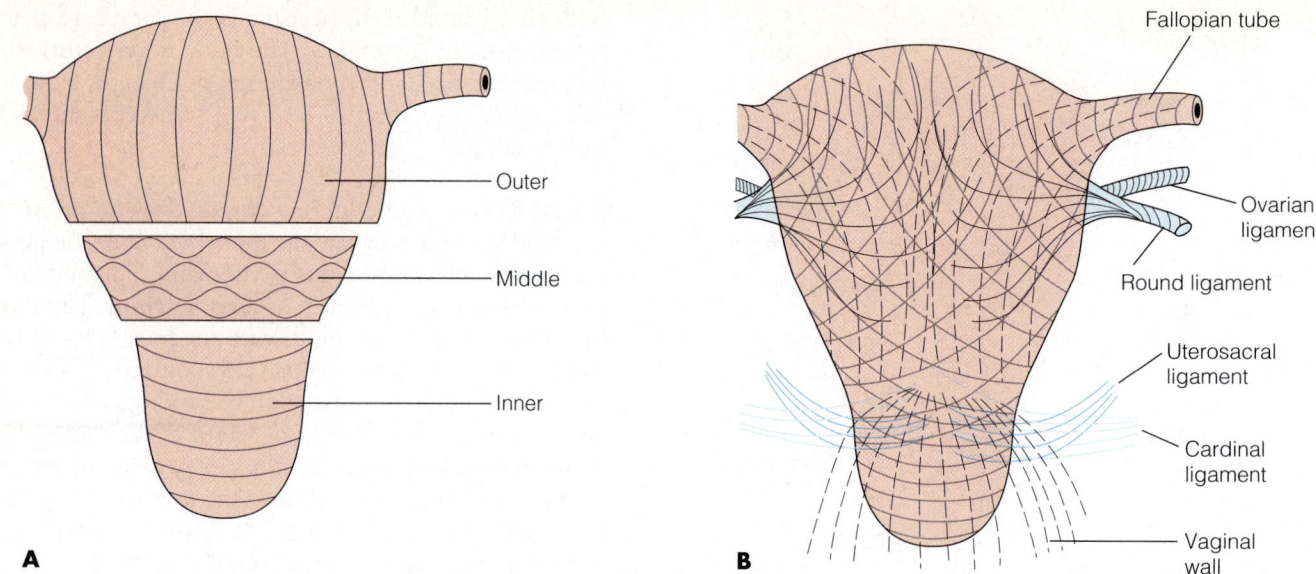

FIGURE 2–7. ◆ Uterine muscle layers. **A,** Muscle fiber placement. **B,** Interlacing of uterine muscle layers.

differing responses allow part of the endometrium to remain intact while other endometrial tissue is shed during menstruation. When pregnancy occurs and the endometrium is not shed, the reticular stromal cells surrounding the endometrial glands become the decidual cells of pregnancy. The stromal cells are highly vascular, channeling a rich blood supply to the endometrial surface.

Cervix. The narrow neck of the uterus is the **cervix.** It meets the body of the uterus at the internal os and descends about 2.5 cm to connect with the vagina at the external os (see Figure 2–6). Thus it provides a protective entrance for the body of the uterus. The cervix is divided by its line of attachment into the vaginal and supravaginal areas. The vaginal cervix projects into the vagina at an angle of from 45 to 90 degrees. The *supravaginal cervix* is surrounded by the attachments that give the uterus its main support: the uterosacral ligaments, the transverse ligaments of the cervix (Mackenrodt's ligaments), and the pubocervical ligaments.

The vaginal cervix appears pink and ends at the external os. The cervical canal appears rosy red and is lined with columnar ciliated epithelium, which contains mucus-secreting glands. Most cervical cancer begins at this *squamo-columnar junction.* The specific location of the junction varies with age and number of pregnancies. Elasticity is the chief characteristic of the cervix. Its ability to stretch is due to the high fibrous and collagenous content of the supportive tissues and also to the vast number of folds in the cervical lining.

The cervical mucus has three functions:

- To lubricate the vaginal canal
- To act as a bacteriostatic agent
- To provide an alkaline environment to shelter deposited sperm from the acidic vagina

At ovulation, cervical mucus is clearer, thinner, more profuse, and more alkaline than at other times.

Uterine Ligaments. The uterine ligaments support and stabilize the various reproductive organs. The ligaments shown in Figure 2–8 ◆ are described as follows:

1. The **broad ligament** keeps the uterus centrally placed and provides stability within the pelvic cavity. It is a double layer that is continuous with the abdominal peritoneum. The broad ligament covers the uterus anteriorly and posteriorly and extends outward from the uterus to enfold the fallopian tubes. The round and ovarian ligaments are at the upper border of the broad ligament. At its lower border, it forms the cardinal ligaments. Between the folds of the broad ligament are connective tissue, involuntary muscle, blood and lymph vessels, and nerves.

2. The **round ligaments** help the broad ligament keep the uterus in place. The round ligaments arise from the sides of the uterus near the fallopian tube insertions. They extend outward between the folds of the broad ligament, passing through the inguinal ring and canals and eventually fusing with the connective tissue of the labia majora. Made up of longitudinal muscle, the round ligaments enlarge during pregnancy. During labor the round ligaments steady the uterus, pulling downward and forward so that the presenting part of the fetus is moved into the cervix.

3. The **ovarian ligaments** anchor the lower pole of the ovary to the cornua of the uterus. They are composed of muscle fibers that allow the ligaments to contract. This contractile ability influences the position of the ovary to some extent, thus helping the fimbriae of the fallopian tubes to "catch" the ovum as it is released each month.

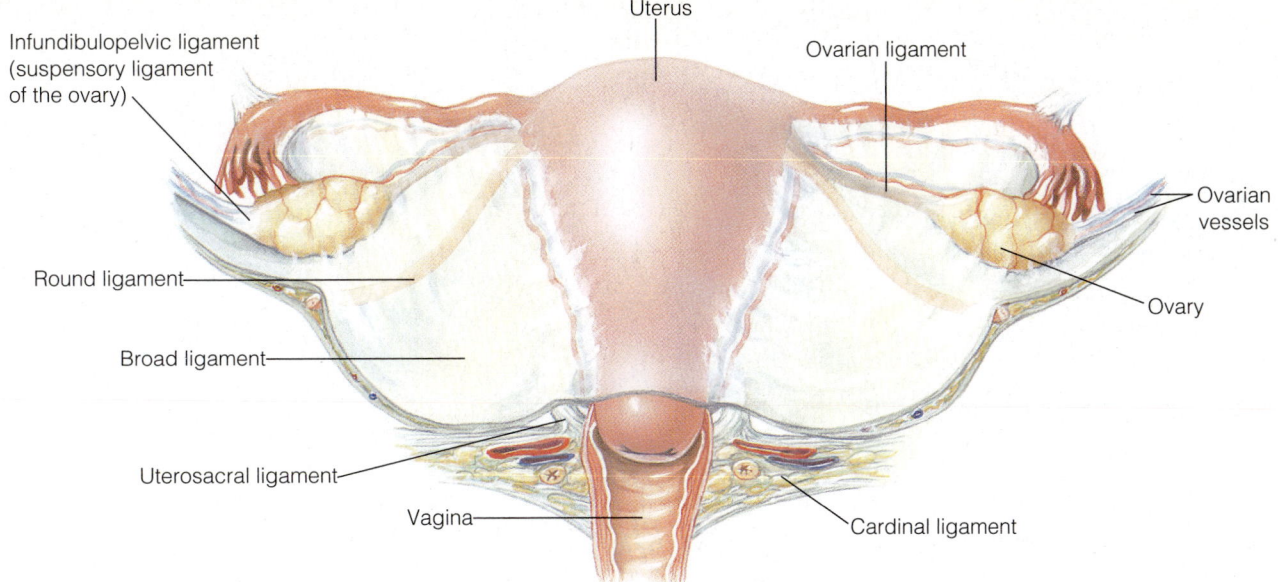

FIGURE 2–8. ◆ Uterine ligaments.

4. The **cardinal ligaments** are the chief uterine supports and suspend the uterus from the side walls of the true pelvis. These ligaments, also known as Mackenrodt's or transverse cervical ligaments, arise from the sides of the pelvic walls and attach to the cervix in the upper vagina. These ligaments prevent uterine prolapse and also support the upper vagina.

5. The **infundibulopelvic ligament** suspends and supports the ovaries. Arising from the outer third of the broad ligament, the infundibulopelvic ligament contains the ovarian vessels and nerves.

6. The **uterosacral ligaments** provide support for the uterus and cervix at the level of the ischial spines. Arising on each side of the pelvis from the posterior wall of the uterus, the uterosacral ligaments sweep back around the rectum and insert on the sides of the first and second sacral vertebrae. The uterosacral ligaments contain smooth muscle fibers, connective tissue, blood and lymph vessels, and nerves. They also contain sensory nerve fibers that contribute to dysmenorrhea (painful menstruation) (see Chapter 3).

FALLOPIAN TUBES

The two **fallopian tubes,** also known as the *oviducts* or *uterine tubes,* arise from each side of the uterus and reach almost to the sides of the pelvis, where they turn toward the ovaries (Figure 2–9 ◆). Each tube is approximately 8 to 13.5 cm long. A short section of each fallopian tube is inside the uterus; its opening into the uterus is only 1 mm in diameter. The fallopian tubes link the peritoneal cavity with the uterus and vagina. This linkage increases a woman's biologic vulnerability to disease processes.

Each fallopian tube may be divided into three parts: the isthmus, the ampulla, and the infundibulum, or fimbria.

The **isthmus** is straight and narrow, with a thick muscular wall and an opening (lumen) 2 to 3 mm in diameter. It is the site of tubal ligation, a surgical procedure to prevent pregnancy (see Chapter 3).

Next to the isthmus is the curved **ampulla,** which comprises the outer two thirds of the tube. Fertilization of the secondary oocyte by a spermatozoon usually occurs here. The ampulla ends at the fimbria, which is a funnel-shaped enlargement with many projections, called **fimbriae,** reaching out to the ovary. The longest of these, the *fimbria ovarica,* is attached to the ovary to increase the chances of intercepting the ovum as it is released.

The wall of the fallopian tube is made up of four layers: peritoneal (serous), subserous (adventitial), muscular, and mucous tissues. The peritoneum covers the tubes. The subserous layer contains the blood and nerve supply, and the muscular layer is responsible for the peristaltic movement of the tube. The mucosal layer, immediately next to the muscular layer, is composed of ciliated and nonciliated cells, with the number of ciliated cells more abundant at the fimbria. Nonciliated cells secrete a protein-rich, serous fluid that nourishes the ovum. The constantly moving tubal cilia propel the ovum toward the uterus. Because the ovum is a large cell, this ciliary action is needed to assist the tube's muscular layer peristalsis. Any malformation or malfunction of the tubes can result in infertility, ectopic pregnancy, or even sterility.

A rich blood and lymphatic supply serves each fallopian tube. Thus the tubes have an unusual ability to recover from an inflammatory process.

The fallopian tubes have three functions:

- To provide transport for the ovum from the ovary to the uterus (transport time through the fallopian tubes varies from 3 to 4 days)

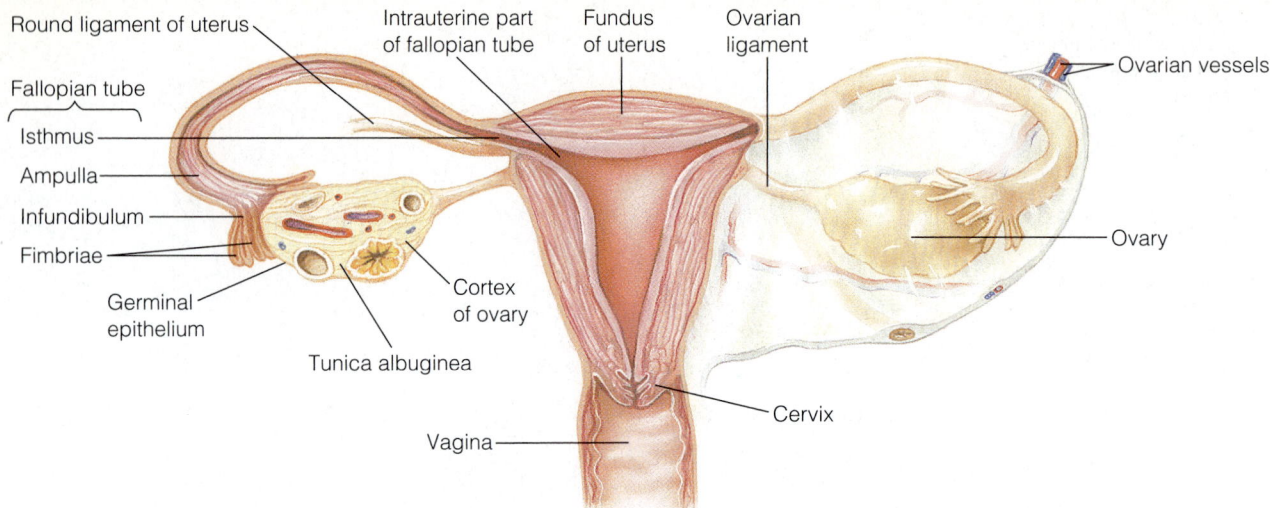

FIGURE 2–9. ◆ Fallopian tubes and ovaries.

- To provide a site for fertilization
- To serve as a warm, moist, nourishing environment for the ovum or zygote (fertilized egg) (see Chapter 5 for further discussion)

OVARIES

The **ovaries** are two almond-shaped structures just below the pelvic brim. One ovary is located on each side of the pelvic cavity. Their size varies among women and with the stage of the menstrual cycle. Each ovary weighs approximately 6 to 10 g and is 1.5 to 3 cm wide, 2 to 5 cm long, and 1 to 1.5 cm thick. The ovaries of girls are small, but they become larger after puberty. They also change in appearance from a dull white, smooth-surfaced organ to a pitted gray organ. The pitting is caused by scarring due to ovulation.

The ovaries are held in place by the broad, ovarian, and infundibulopelvic ligaments. There is no peritoneal covering for the ovaries. Although this lack of covering assists the mature ovum to erupt, it also allows easier spread of malignant cells from cancer of the ovaries. A single layer of cuboidal epithelial cells, called the germinal epithelium, covers the ovaries. The ovaries are composed of three layers: the tunica albuginea, the cortex, and the medulla. The *tunica albuginea* is dense and dull white and serves as a productive protective layer. The *cortex* is the main functional part because it contains ova, graafian follicles, corpora lutea, the degenerated corpora lutea (corpora albicantia), and degenerated follicles. The *medulla* is completely surrounded by the cortex and contains the nerves and the blood and lymphatic vessels.

The ovaries are the primary source of two important hormones: the estrogens and progesterone. Estrogens are associated with those characteristics contributing to femaleness, including breast alveolar lobule growth and duct development. The ovaries secrete large amounts of estrogen, while the adrenal cortex (extraglandular sites) produces minute amounts of estrogen in nonpregnant women.

Progesterone is often called the *hormone of pregnancy* because its effects on the uterus allow pregnancy to be maintained. The placenta is the primary source of progesterone during pregnancy. This hormone also inhibits the action of prolactin, thereby preventing lactation during pregnancy (Cunningham, Gant, Leveno, et al., 2001). The interplay between the ovarian hormones and other hormones such as FSH and LH is responsible for the cyclic changes that allow pregnancy. The hormonal and physical changes that occur during the female reproductive cycle are discussed in depth later in this chapter.

Between the ages of 45 and 55, a woman's ovaries secrete decreasing amounts of estrogen. Eventually, ovulatory activity ceases and menopause occurs.

BONY PELVIS

The female bony pelvis has two unique functions:

- To support and protect the pelvic contents
- To form the relatively fixed axis of the birth passage

Because the pelvis is so important to childbearing, its structure must be understood clearly.

BONY STRUCTURE

The pelvis is made up of four bones: two innominate bones, the sacrum, and the coccyx. The pelvis resembles a bowl or basin; its sides are the innominate bones, and its back is the sacrum and coccyx. Lined with fibrocartilage and held tightly together by ligaments (Figure 2–10 ◆), the four bones join at the symphysis pubis, the two sacroiliac joints, and the sacrococcygeal joints.

The innominate bones, popularly known as the *hip bones*, are made up of three separate bones: the ilium, ischium,

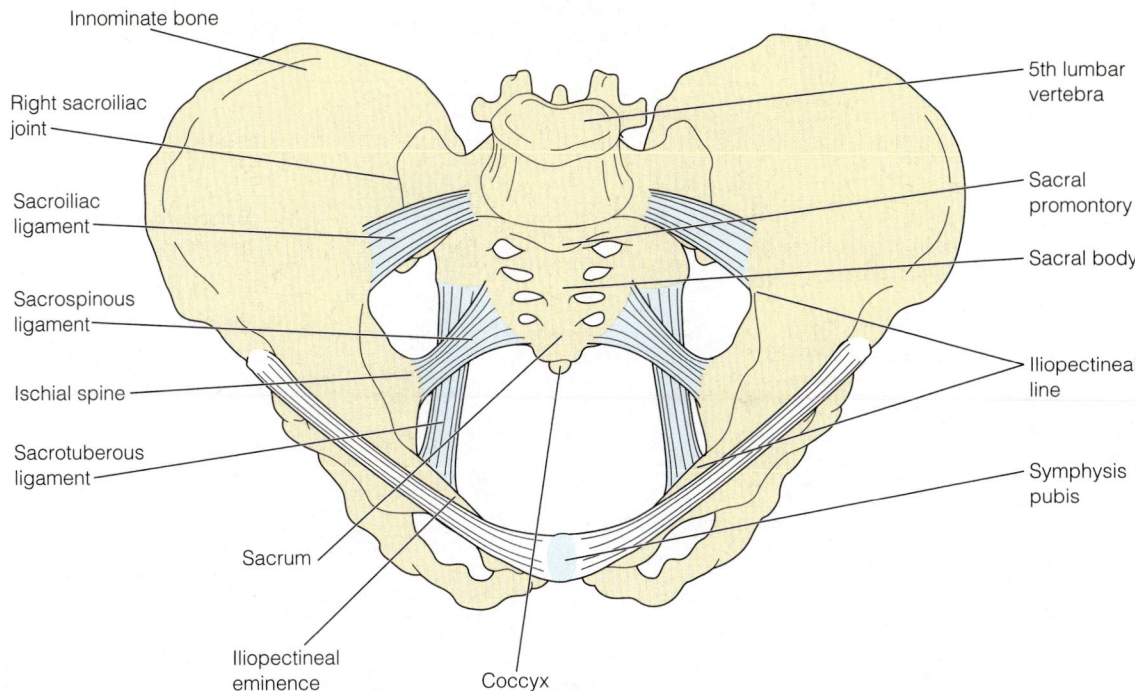

Labels on figure:
Innominate bone
Right sacroiliac joint
Sacroiliac ligament
Sacrospinous ligament
Ischial spine
Sacrotuberous ligament
Sacrum
Iliopectineal eminence
Coccyx
5th lumbar vertebra
Sacral promontory
Sacral body
Iliopectineal line
Symphysis pubis

FIGURE 2–10. ◆ Pelvic bones with supporting ligaments.

and pubis. These bones fuse to form a circular cavity, the *acetabulum,* which articulates with the femur.

The *ilium* is the broad, upper prominence of the hip. The *iliac crest* is the margin of the ilium. The **ischial spines,** the foremost projection nearest the groin, is the site of attachment for ligaments and muscles.

The *ischium,* the strongest bone, is under the ilium and below the acetabulum. The L-shaped ischium ends in a marked protuberance, the ischial tuberosity, on which the weight of a seated body rests. The ischial spines arise near the junction of the ilium and ischium and jut into the pelvic cavity. The shortest diameter of the pelvic cavity is between the ischial spines. The ischial spines serve as reference points during labor to evaluate the descent of the fetal head into the birth canal (see Chapter 15 and Figure 15–7). ⬭

The *pubis* forms the slightly bowed front portion of the innominate bone. Extending medially from the acetabulum to the midpoint of the bony pelvis, each pubis meets the other to form a joint called the **symphysis pubis.** The triangular space below this junction is known as the pubic arch. The fetal head passes under this arch during birth. The symphysis pubis is formed by heavy fibrocartilage and the superior and inferior pubic ligaments. The mobility of the inferior ligament increases during a first pregnancy and to a greater extent in subsequent pregnancies.

The sacroiliac joints also have a degree of mobility that increases near the end of pregnancy as the result of an upward, gliding movement. The pelvic outlet may be increased by 1.5 to 2 cm in the squatting, sitting, and dorsal lithotomy positions. These relaxations of the joints are induced by the hormones of pregnancy.

The *sacrum* is a wedge-shaped bone formed by the fusion of five vertebrae. On the anterior upper portion of the sacrum is a projection into the pelvic cavity known as the **sacral promontory.** This projection is another obstetric guide in determining pelvic measurements. (For a discussion of pelvic measurements, see Chapter 8.) ⬭

The small triangular bone last on the vertebral column is the *coccyx.* It articulates with the sacrum at the sacrococcygeal joint. The coccyx usually moves backward during labor to provide more room for the fetus.

PELVIC FLOOR

The muscular *pelvic floor* of the bony pelvis is designed to overcome the force of gravity exerted on the pelvic organs. It acts as a buttress to the irregularly shaped pelvic outlet, thereby providing stability and support for surrounding structures.

Deep fascia, the levator ani, and coccygeal muscles form the part of the pelvic floor known as the **pelvic diaphragm.** The components of the pelvic diaphragm function as a whole, yet they are able to move over one another. This feature provides an exceptional capacity for dilatation during birth and return to prepregnancy condition following birth. Above the pelvic diaphragm is the pelvic cavity; below and behind it is the perineum.

The levator ani muscle makes up the major portion of the pelvic diaphragm and consists of four muscles: the ileococcygeus, pubococcygeus, puborectalis, and pubovaginalis. The ileococcygeal muscle, a thin muscular sheet underlying the sacrospinous ligament, helps the levator ani support the pelvic organs. Muscles of the pelvic floor are shown in Figure 2–11 ◆ and discussed in Table 2–1.

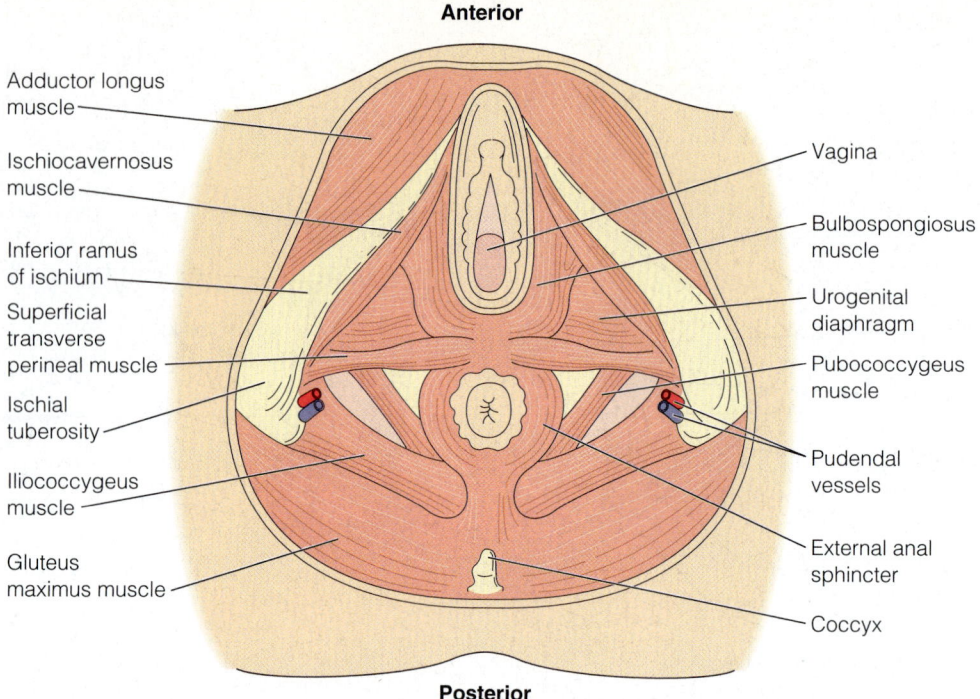

Anterior

Adductor longus muscle

Ischiocavernosus muscle

Inferior ramus of ischium

Superficial transverse perineal muscle

Ischial tuberosity

Iliococcygeus muscle

Gluteus maximus muscle

Vagina

Bulbospongiosus muscle

Urogenital diaphragm

Pubococcygeus muscle

Pudendal vessels

External anal sphincter

Coccyx

Posterior

FIGURE 2–11. ◆ Muscles of the pelvic floor. (The puborectalis, pubovaginalis, and coccygeal muscles cannot be seen from this view.)

TABLE 2–1   Muscles of the Pelvic Floor

Muscle	Origin	Insertion	Innervation	Action
Levator ani	Pubis, lateral pelvic wall, and ischial spine	Blends with organs in pelvic cavity	Inferior rectal, second and and third sacral nerves, plus anterior rami of third and fourth sacral nerves	Supports pelvic viscera; helps form pelvic diaphragm
Iliococcygeus	Pelvic surface of ischial spine and pelvic fascia	Central point of perineum, coccygeal raphe, and coccyx		Assists in supporting abdominal and pelvic viscera
Pubococcygeus	Pubis and pelvic fascia	Coccyx		
Puborectalis	Pubis	Blends with rectum; meets similar fibers from opposite side		Forms sling for rectum, just posterior to it, raises anus
Pubovaginalis	Pubis	Blends into vagina		Supports vagina
Coccygeus	Ischial spine and sacrospinous ligament	Lateral border of lower sacrum and upper coccyx	Third and fourth sacral nerves	Supports pelvic viscera; helps form pelvic diaphragm, flexes and abducts coccyx

PELVIC DIVISION

The pelvic cavity is divided into the false pelvis and the true pelvis (Figure 2–12A ◆). The **false pelvis,** the portion above the pelvic brim, or linea terminalis, serves to support the weight of the enlarged pregnant uterus and direct the presenting fetal part into the true pelvis.

The **true pelvis** is the portion that lies below the linea terminalis. The bony circumference of the true pelvis is made up of the sacrum, coccyx, and innominate bones and represents the bony limits of the birth canal. The true pelvis is of paramount importance because its size and shape must be adequate for normal fetal passage during labor and at birth.

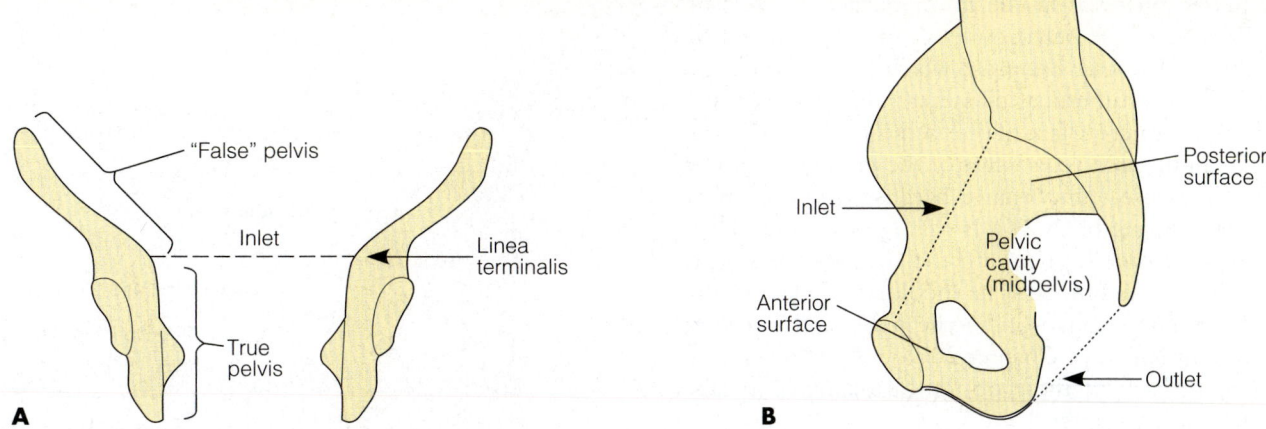

FIGURE 2–12. ◆ Female pelvis. **A,** False pelvis is shallow cavity above inlet; true pelvis is deeper portion of cavity below inlet. **B,** True pelvis consists of inlet, cavity (midpelvis), and outlet.

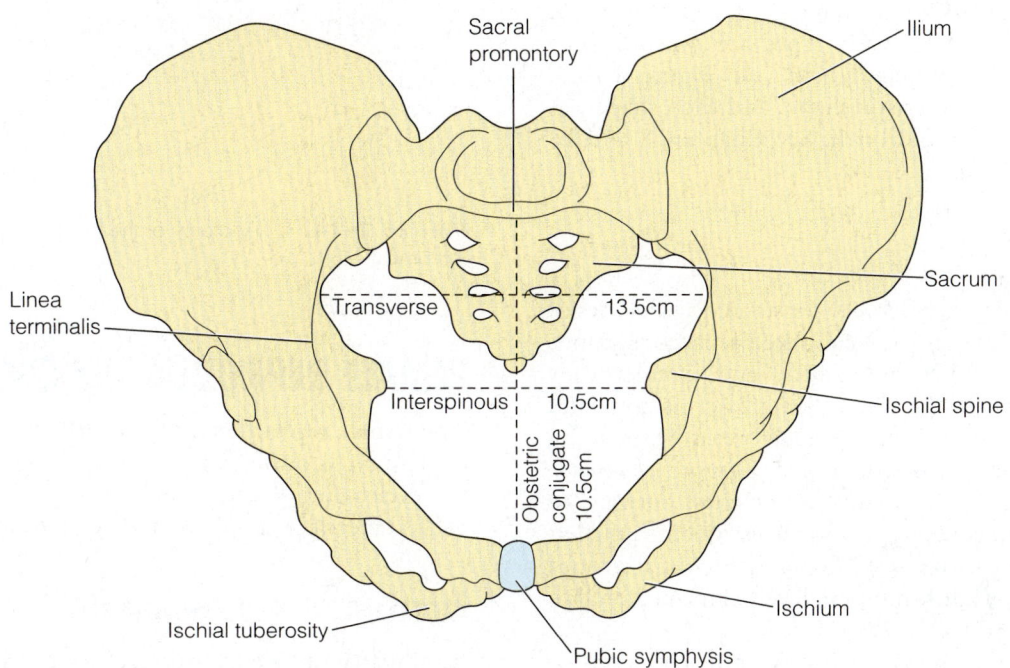

FIGURE 2–13. ◆ Pelvic planes: coronal section and diameters of the bony pelvis.

The true pelvis consists of three parts: the inlet, the pelvic cavity, and the outlet (Figure 2–12B ◆). Each part has distinct measurements that aid in evaluating the adequacy of the pelvis for childbirth. (For further discussion, see Chapter 8.) ⊂⊃

The **pelvic inlet** is the upper border of the true pelvis. The female pelvic inlet is typically rounded. Its size and shape are determined by assessing three anteroposterior diameters. The **diagonal conjugate** extends from the subpubic angle to the middle of the sacral promontory and is typically 12.5 cm. The diagonal conjugate can be measured manually during a pelvic examination. The **obstetric conjugate** extends from the middle of the sacral promontory to an area approximately 1 cm below the pubic crest. Its length is estimated by subtracting 1.5 cm from the length

of the diagonal conjugate (Figure 2–13 ◆). The fetus passes through the obstetric conjugate, and the size of this diameter determines whether the fetus can move down into the birth canal in order for engagement to occur. The true (anatomic) conjugate, or **conjugate vera,** extends from the middle of the sacral promontory to the middle of the pubic crest (superior surface of the symphysis) (Di Saia, 1999). One additional measurement, the transverse diameter, helps determine the shape of the inlet. The **transverse diameter** is the largest diameter of the inlet and is measured by using the linea terminalis as the point of reference.

The **pelvic cavity** (canal) is a curved canal with a longer posterior than anterior wall. The curvature of the lumbar spine influences the shape and tilt (inclination) of the pelvic cavity (see Figure 2–12B).

The **pelvic outlet** is at the lower border of the true pelvis. The size of the pelvic outlet can be determined by assessing the *transverse diameter,* which is also called the bi-ischial, or intertuberous, diameter. This diameter extends from the inner surface of one ischial tuberosity to the other. The pubic arch is also part of the pelvic cavity. The pubic arch has great importance because the fetus must pass under it during birth. If it is narrow, the baby's head may be pushed backward toward the coccyx, making extension of the head difficult. The shoulders of a large baby may also become wedged under the pubic arch, making birth more difficult (see Chapter 20). ⬭ The clinical assessment of each of these obstetrical diameters is discussed further in Chapter 8. ⬭

PELVIC TYPES

The Caldwell-Moloy classification of pelves is widely used to differentiate bony pelvic types (Caldwell & Moloy, 1933). The four basic types are *gynecoid, android, anthropoid,* and *platypelloid* (see Figure 15–1). Each type has a characteristic shape, and each shape has implications for labor and birth. See Chapters 8 and 15 for further discussion. ⬭

Breasts

The *breasts,* or *mammary glands,* considered accessories of the reproductive system, are specialized sebaceous glands (Figure 2–14 ◆). They are conical and symmetrically placed on the sides of the chest. The greater pectoral and anterior serratus muscles underlie each breast. Suspending the breasts are fibrous tissues, called *Cooper's ligaments,* that extend from the deep fascia in the chest outward to just under the skin covering the breast. Frequently, the left breast is larger than the right. In different racial groups breasts develop at slightly different levels in the pectoral region of the chest (Rebar, 1999).

In the center of each mature breast is the *nipple,* a protrusion about 0.5 to 1.3 cm in diameter. The nipple is composed mainly of erectile tissue, which becomes more rigid and prominent during the menstrual cycle, sexual excitement, pregnancy, and lactation. The nipple is surrounded by the heavily pigmented **areola,** which is 2.5 to 10 cm in diameter. Both the nipple and the areola are roughened by small papillae called *tubercles of Montgomery.* As an infant suckles, these tubercles secrete a fatty substance that helps lubricate and protect the breasts.

The breasts are composed of glandular, fibrous, and adipose tissue. The glandular tissue is arranged in a series of 15 to 24 lobes separated by fibrous and adipose tissue. Each lobe is made up of several lobules composed of many alveoli clustered around tiny ducts. The lining of these ducts secretes the various components of milk. The ducts from several lobules merge to form the larger *lactiferous ducts,* which open on the surface of the nipple.

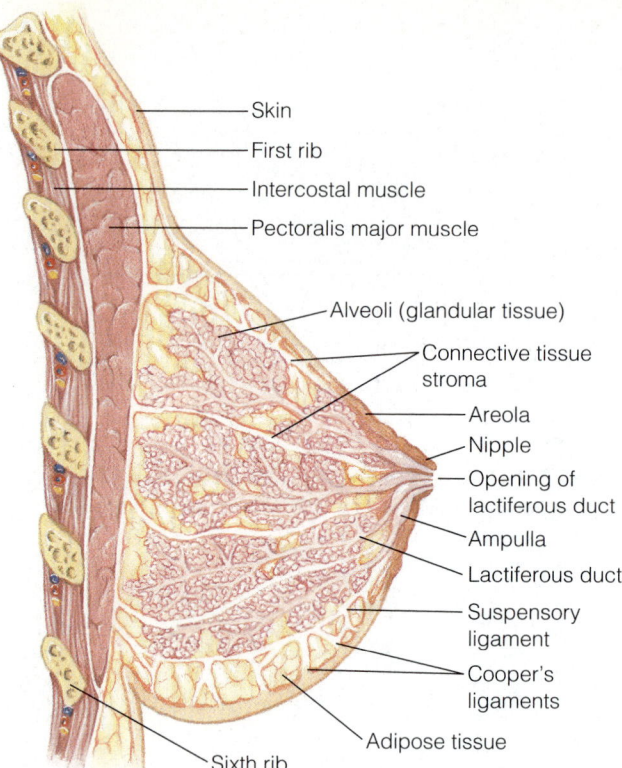

FIGURE 2–14. ◆ Anatomy of the breast: sagittal view of left breast.

Labels: Skin; First rib; Intercostal muscle; Pectoralis major muscle; Alveoli (glandular tissue); Connective tissue stroma; Areola; Nipple; Opening of lactiferous duct; Ampulla; Lactiferous duct; Suspensory ligament; Cooper's ligaments; Adipose tissue; Sixth rib

FEMALE REPRODUCTIVE CYCLE

The **female reproductive cycle (FRC)** is composed of the ovarian cycle, during which ovulation occurs, and the uterine cycle, during which menstruation occurs. These two cycles take place simultaneously (Figure 2–15 ◆).

Effects of Female Hormones

After menarche, a female undergoes a cyclic pattern of ovulation and menstruation (if pregnancy does not occur) for a period of 30 to 40 years. This cycle is an orderly process under neurohormonal control. Each month one oocyte matures, ruptures from the ovary, and enters the fallopian tube. The ovary, vagina, uterus, and fallopian tubes are major target organs for female hormones.

The ovaries produce mature gametes and secrete hormones. Ovarian hormones include the estrogens, progesterone, and testosterone. The ovary is sensitive to FSH and LH. The uterus is sensitive to estrogen and progesterone. The relative proportion of these hormones to each other controls the events of both ovarian and menstrual cycles.

ESTROGENS

Estrogens are secreted in large amounts by the ovaries in nonpregnant women. The major estrogenic effects are due primarily to three classical estrogens: estrone, β-estradiol, and estriol. The major estrogen is β-estradiol.

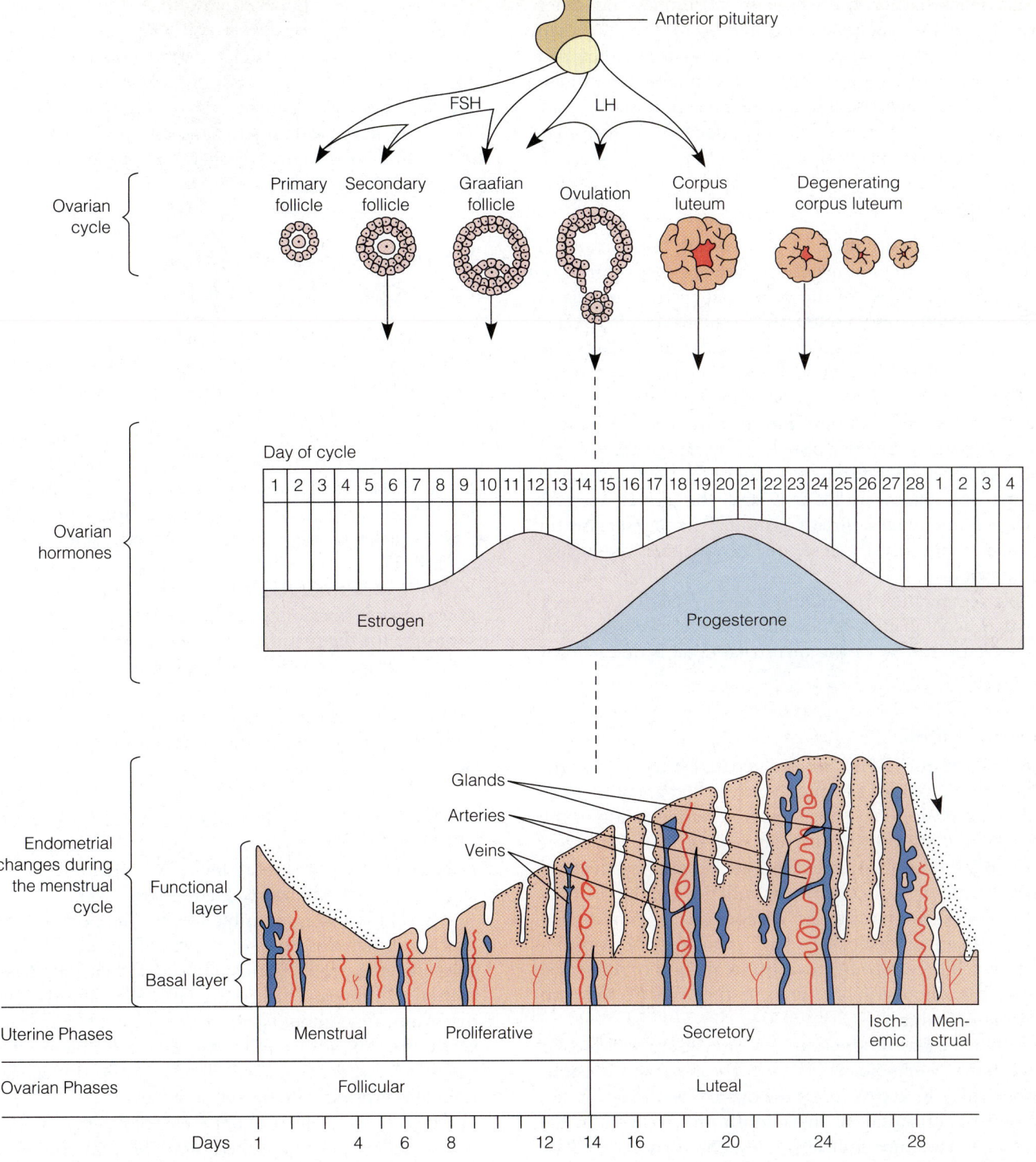

FIGURE 2–15. ◆ Female reproductive cycle: interrelationships of hormones with the four phases of the uterine cycle and the two phases of the ovarian cycle in an ideal 28-day cycle.

Estrogens control the development of the female secondary sex characteristics: breast development, widening of the hips, and deposits of tissue (fat) in the buttocks and mons pubis. Estrogens also assist in the maturation of the ovarian follicles and cause the endometrial mucosa to proliferate following menstruation. The amount of estrogens is greatest during the proliferative (follicular or estrogenic) phase of the menstrual cycle. Estrogens also cause the uterus to increase in size and weight because of increased glycogen, amino acids, electrolytes, and water. Blood supply is expanded as well. Under the influence of estrogens, myometrial contractility increases in both the uterus and the fallopian tubes, and uterine sensitivity to oxytocin increases. Estrogens inhibit FSH production and stimulate LH production.

Estrogens have effects on many hormones and other carrier proteins, such as contributing to the increased amount of protein-bound iodine in pregnant women and women who use oral contraceptives containing estrogen. Estrogens may increase libidinal feelings in humans. They decrease the excitability of the hypothalamus, which may cause an increase in sexual desire.

PROGESTERONE

Progesterone is secreted by the corpus luteum and is found in greatest amounts during the secretory (luteal or progestational) phase of the menstrual cycle. It decreases uterine motility and contractility caused by estrogens, thereby preparing the uterus for implantation after the ovum is fertilized. The endometrial mucosa is in a ready state as a result of estrogenic influence. Progesterone causes the uterine endometrium to further increase its supply of glycogen, arterial blood, secretory glands, amino acids, and water. Under the influence of progesterone, the vaginal epithelium proliferates and the cervix secretes thick, viscous mucus. Breast glandular tissue increases in size and complexity. Progesterone also prepares the breasts for lactation.

The temperature rise of about 0.3 to 0.6 °C (0.5 to 1 °F) that accompanies ovulation and persists throughout the secretory phase of the menstrual cycle is due to progesterone.

PROSTAGLANDINS

Prostaglandins (PGs) are oxygenated fatty acids produced by the cells of the endometrium and are also classified as hormones. Prostaglandins have varied action in the body depending on the different type of PGs. Generally, PGEs relax smooth muscles and are potent vasodilators; PGFs are potent vasoconstrictors and increase the contractility of muscles and arteries. Although their primary actions seem antagonistic, their basic regulatory functions in cells are achieved through an intricate pattern of reciprocal events. The discussion here sums up their role in ovulation and menstruation.

Prostaglandin production increases during follicular maturation, is dependent on gonadotropins, and is essential to ovulation. Extrusion of the ovum, resulting from the increased contractility of the smooth muscle in the theca layer of the mature follicle, is thought to be caused by $PGF_{2\alpha}$. Significant amounts of PGs are found in and around the follicle at the time of ovulation.

Although the exact mechanism by which the corpus luteum degenerates in the absence of pregnancy remains obscure, $PGF_{2\alpha}$ is thought to induce progesterone withdrawal, the lowest point of which coincides with the onset of menses.

During the late secretory phase, the level of $PGF_{2\alpha}$ is higher than that of PGE (Clark & Myatt, 1999). This event increases vasoconstriction and contractility of the myometrium, which contributes to the ischemia preceding menstruation. A high concentration of PGs may also account for the vasoconstriction of the endometrium venous lacunae, allowing for platelet aggregation at vascular rupture points and thereby preventing rapid blood loss during menstruation. The menstrual flow's high concentration of PGs may also facilitate the process of tissue digestion, which allows for an orderly shedding of the endometrium during menstruation.

Neurohumoral Basis of the Female Reproductive Cycle

The female reproductive cycle is controlled by complex interactions between the nervous and endocrine systems and their target tissues. These interactions involve the hypothalamus, anterior pituitary, and ovaries.

The hypothalamus secretes GnRH to the pituitary gland in response to signals received from the central nervous system. This releasing hormone is often called both luteinizing hormone–releasing hormone (LHRH) and follicle-stimulating hormone–releasing hormone (FSHRH).

In response to GnRH, the anterior pituitary secretes the gonadotropic hormones FSH and LH. FSH is primarily responsible for the maturation of the ovarian follicle. As the follicle matures, it secretes increasing amounts of estrogen, which enhance the development of the follicle (Ferin, 1998). (This estrogen is also responsible for the building or proliferation phase of the endometrium after it is shed during menstruation.)

Final maturation of the follicle cannot come about without the action of LH. The anterior pituitary's production of LH increases six- to tenfold as the follicle matures. The peak production of LH can precede ovulation by as much as 36 hours (Couchman & Hammond, 1999).

The LH is also responsible for the "luteinizing" of the theca and granulosa cells of the ruptured follicle. As a result, estrogen production is reduced and progesterone secretion continues. Thus, estrogen levels fall a day before ovulation; tiny amounts of progesterone are in evidence. **Ovulation** takes place following the very rapid growth of the follicle, as the sustained high level of estrogen diminishes and progesterone secretion begins.

The ruptured follicle undergoes rapid change, complete luteinization is accomplished, and the mass of cells becomes the **corpus luteum.** The lutein cells secrete large amounts of progesterone with smaller amounts of estrogen. (Concurrently, the excessive amounts of progesterone are responsible for the secretory phase of the uterine cycle.) Seven or eight days following ovulation, the corpus luteum begins to involute, losing its secretory function. The production of both progesterone and estrogen is severely diminished. The anterior pituitary responds with increasingly large amounts of FSH; a few days later LH production begins. As a result, new follicles become responsive to another ovarian cycle and begin maturing.

Ovarian Cycle

The ovarian cycle has two phases: the *follicular phase* (days 1 to 14) and the *luteal phase* (days 15 to 28 in a 28-day cycle). Figure 2–16 ◆ depicts the changes that the follicle undergoes during the ovarian cycle. In women whose menstrual cycles vary, usually only the length of the follicular phase varies, because the luteal phase is of fixed length. During the follicular phase, the immature follicle matures as a result of FSH. Within the follicle, the oocyte grows. A mature **graafian follicle** appears on about the 14th day under dual control of FSH and LH. It is a large structure, measuring about 5 to 10 mm. The mature follicle produces increasing amounts of estrogen. In the mature graafian follicle, the cells surrounding the antral cavity are granulosa cells. The oocyte is surrounded by fluid and enclosed in a thick elastic capsule called the zona pellucida.

Just before ovulation, the mature oocyte completes its first meiotic division (see Chapter 5 for a description of meiosis). As a result of this division, two cells are formed: a small cell, called a *polar body,* and a larger cell, called the *secondary oocyte.* The secondary oocyte matures into the ovum (see Figure 5–2).

As the graafian follicle matures and enlarges, it comes close to the surface of the ovary. The ovary surface forms a blisterlike protrusion 10 to 15 mm in diameter, and the follicle walls become thin. The secondary oocyte, polar body, and follicular fluid are pushed out. The ovum is discharged near the fimbria of the fallopian tube and is pulled into the tube to begin its journey toward the uterus.

Occasionally, ovulation is accompanied by midcycle pain known as *mittelschmerz.* This pain may be caused by a thick tunica albuginea or by a local peritoneal reaction to the expelling of the follicular contents. Vaginal discharge may increase during ovulation, and a small amount of blood (midcycle spotting) may be discharged as well.

The body temperature increases about 0.3 to 0.6 °C (0.5 to 1 °F) 24 to 48 hours after the time of ovulation. It remains elevated until the day before menstruation begins. There may be an accompanying sharp basal body temperature drop before the increase. These temperature changes are useful clinically to determine the approximate time ovulation occurs.

Generally, the ovum takes several minutes to travel through the ruptured follicle to the fallopian tube opening. The contractions of the tube's smooth muscle and its ciliary action propel the ovum through the tube. The ovum remains in the ampulla, where, if it is fertilized, cleavage can begin. The ovum is thought to be fertile for only 6 to 24 hours. It reaches the uterus 72 to 96 hours after its release from the ovary.

The luteal phase begins when the ovum leaves its follicle. Under the influence of LH, the corpus luteum develops from the ruptured follicle. Within 2 or 3 days, the corpus luteum becomes yellowish and spherical and increases in vascularity. If the ovum is fertilized and implants in the endometrium, the fertilized egg begins to secrete **human chorionic gonadotropin (hCG),** which is needed to maintain the corpus luteum. If fertilization does not occur, within about a week after ovulation the corpus luteum begins to degenerate, eventually becoming a connective tissue scar called the *corpus albicans.* With degeneration comes a decrease in estrogen and progesterone. This allows for an increase in LH and FSH, which trigger the hypothalamus. Approximately 14 days after ovulation (in a 28-day cycle), in the absence of pregnancy, menstruation begins.

Uterine (Menstrual) Cycle

Menstruation is cyclic uterine bleeding in response to cyclic hormonal changes. Menstruation occurs when the ovum is not fertilized and begins about 14 days after ovulation in a 28-day cycle. The menstrual discharge, also referred to as the *menses,* or *menstrual flow,* is composed of blood mixed with fluid, cervical and vaginal secretions, bacteria, mucus, leukocytes, and other cellular debris. The menstrual discharge is dark red and has a distinctive odor.

Menstrual parameters vary greatly among individuals. Generally, menstruation occurs every 28 days, plus or minus 5 to 10 days. Emotional and physical factors such as illness, excessive fatigue, stress or anxiety, and vigorous exercise programs can alter the cycle interval. Certain environmental factors such as temperature and altitude may also affect the cycle. The duration of menses is from 2 to 8 days, with the blood loss averaging 30 mL and the loss of iron averaging 0.5 to 1 mg daily.

The uterine (menstrual) cycle has four phases: menstrual, proliferative, secretory, and ischemic. Menstruation occurs during the *menstrual phase.* Some endometrial areas are shed, while others remain. Some of the remaining tips of the endometrial glands begin to regenerate. The endometrium

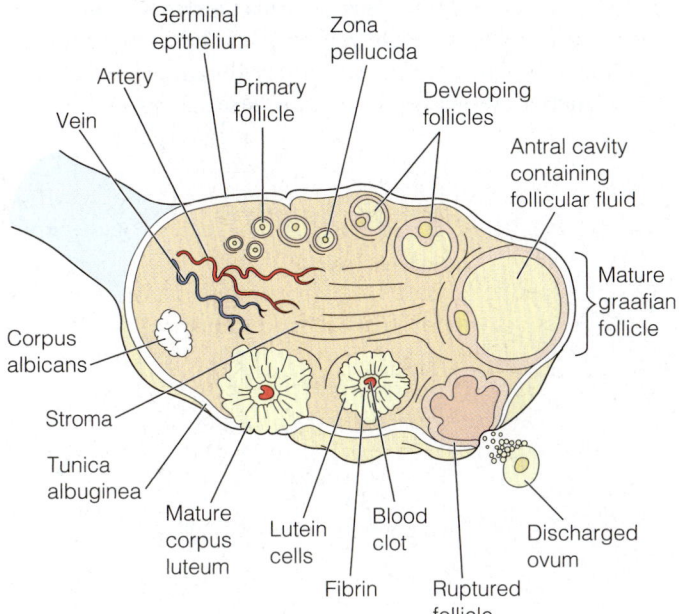

FIGURE 2–16. ◆ Various stages of development of the ovarian follicles.

Labels: Germinal epithelium; Artery; Vein; Zona pellucida; Primary follicle; Developing follicles; Antral cavity containing follicular fluid; Mature graafian follicle; Corpus albicans; Stroma; Tunica albuginea; Mature corpus luteum; Lutein cells; Fibrin; Blood clot; Ruptured follicle; Discharged ovum

is in a resting state following menstruation. Estrogen levels are low, and the endometrium is 1 to 2 mm deep. During this part of the cycle, the cervical mucosa is scanty, viscous, and opaque.

The *proliferative phase* begins when the endometrial glands enlarge, becoming twisted and longer in response to increasing amounts of estrogen. The blood vessels become prominent and dilated, and the endometrium increases in thickness six- to eightfold. This gradual process reaches its peak just before ovulation. The cervical mucosa becomes thin, clear, watery, and more alkaline, making the mucosa more favorable to spermatozoa. As ovulation nears, the cervical mucosa shows increased elasticity, called *spinnbarkheit*. At ovulation, the mucus will stretch more than 5 cm. The cervical mucosa pH increases from below 7 to 7.5 at the time of ovulation. On microscopic examination, the mucosa shows a characteristic ferning pattern (see Figure 4–3). ⬭ This fern pattern is a useful aid in assessing ovulation time.

The *secretory phase* follows ovulation. The endometrium, under estrogenic influence, undergoes slight cellular growth. Progesterone, however, causes such marked swelling and growth that the epithelium is warped into folds. The amount of tissue glycogen increases. The glandular epithelial cells begin to fill with cellular debris, become twisted, and dilate. The glands secrete small quantities of endometrial fluid in preparation for a fertilized ovum. The vascularity of the entire uterus increases greatly, providing a nourishing bed for implantation. If implantation occurs, the endometrium, under the influence of progesterone, continues to develop and become even thicker (see Chapter 5 for a discussion of implantation). ⬭

If fertilization does not occur, the *ischemic phase* begins. The corpus luteum begins to degenerate, and as a result both estrogen and progesterone levels fall. Areas of necrosis appear under the epithelial lining. Extensive vascular changes also occur. Small blood vessels rupture, and the spiral arteries constrict and retract, causing a deficiency of blood in the endometrium, which becomes pale. This is-

chemic phase is characterized by the escape of blood into the stromal cells of the uterus. The menstrual flow begins, thus beginning the menstrual cycle again. After menstruation the basal layer remains, so that the tips of the glands can regenerate the new functional endometrial layer. For further discussion, see Table 2–2.

MALE REPRODUCTIVE SYSTEM

The primary reproductive functions of the male genitals are to produce and transport sex cells (sperm) through and eventually out of the male genital tract and into the female genital tract. The external and internal genitals of the male reproductive system are shown in Figure 2–17 ◆.

TABLE 2–2 Summary of Female Reproductive Cycle		
Ovarian Cycle		
Follicular phase (days 1–14): Primordial follicle matures under influence of FSH and LH up to the time of ovulation.		
Luteal phase (days 15–28): Ovum leaves follicle; corpus luteum develops under LH influence and produces high levels of progesterone and low levels of estrogen.		
Uterine (Menstrual) Cycle		
Menstrual phase (days 1–6): Estrogen levels are low, cervical mucus is scant, viscous, and opaque.		
Proliferative phase (days 7–14): Estrogen peaks just prior to ovulation. Cervical mucus at ovulation is clear, thin, watery, alkaline, and more favorable to sperm; shows ferning pattern; and has spinnbarkheit greater than 5 cm. Just before ovulation, body temperature may drop slightly, then at ovulation body temperature rises sharply and remains elevated under influence of progesterone.		
Secretory phase (days 15–26): Estrogen drops sharply, and progesterone dominates.		
Ischemic phase (days 27–28): Both estrogen and progesterone levels drop.		

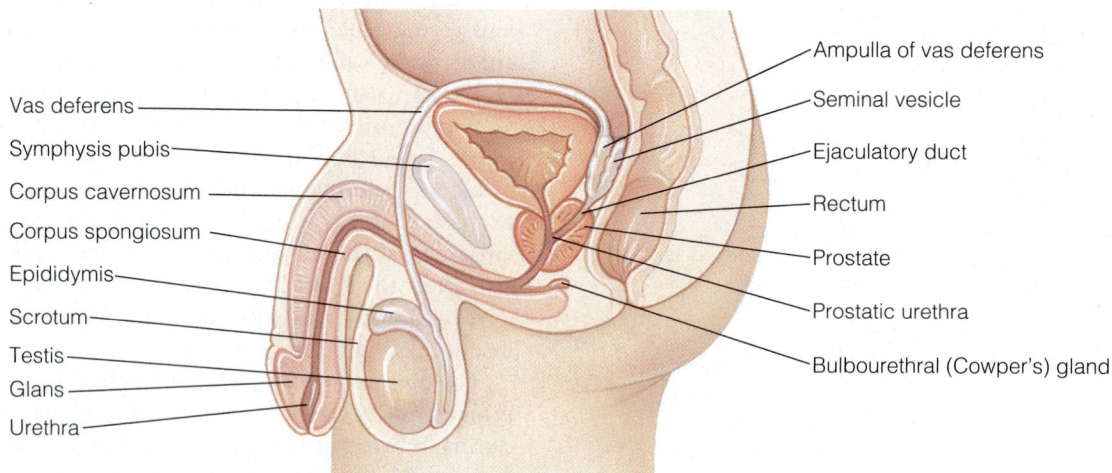

Vas deferens
Symphysis pubis
Corpus cavernosum
Corpus spongiosum
Epididymis
Scrotum
Testis
Glans
Urethra

Ampulla of vas deferens
Seminal vesicle
Ejaculatory duct
Rectum
Prostate
Prostatic urethra
Bulbourethral (Cowper's) gland

FIGURE 2–17. ◆ Male reproductive system, sagittal view.

External Genitals

The two external reproductive organs are the penis and scrotum. The *penis* is an elongated, cylindrical structure consisting of a body, called the *shaft,* and a cone-shaped end, called the *glans.* The penis lies in front of the scrotum.

The shaft of the penis is made up of three longitudinal columns of erectile tissue: the paired *corpora cavernosa* and the *corpus spongiosum.* These columns are covered by dense fibrous connective tissue and then enclosed by elastic tissue. The penis is covered by a thin outer layer of skin.

The corpus spongiosum contains the urethra and becomes the glans at the distal end of the penis. The urethra widens within the glans and ends in a slitlike opening, located in the tip of the glans, called the *urethral meatus.* A circular fold of skin arises just behind the glans and covers it. Known as the *prepuce,* or *foreskin,* it may be removed by the surgical procedure of circumcision (see Chapter 26). If the corpus spongiosum does not surround the urethra completely, the urethral meatus may occur on the ventral aspect of the penile shaft (hypospadias) or on the dorsal aspect (epispadias).

Sexual stimulation causes the penis to elongate, thicken, and stiffen, a process called *erection.* The penis becomes erect when its blood vessels become engorged, a consequence of parasympathetic nerve stimulation. If sexual stimulation is intense enough, the forceful and sudden expulsion of semen occurs through the rhythmic contractions of the penile muscles. This phenomenon is called *ejaculation.*

The penis serves both the urinary and the reproductive systems. Urine is expelled through the urethral meatus. The reproductive function of the penis is to deposit sperm in the vagina so that fertilization of the ovum can occur.

The *scrotum* is a pouchlike structure that hangs in front of the anus and behind the penis. Composed of skin and the *dartos muscle,* the scrotum shows increased pigmentation and scattered hairs. The sebaceous glands open directly onto the scrotal surface; their secretion has a distinctive odor. Contraction of the dartos and cremasteric muscles shortens the scrotum and draws it closer to the body, thus wrinkling its outer surface. The degree of wrinkling is greatest in young men and at cold temperatures and is least in older men and at warm temperatures.

Inside the scrotum are two lateral compartments. Each compartment contains a testis with its related structures. Because the left spermatic cord grows longer, the left testis and its scrotal sac hang lower than on the right. A ridge (raphe) on the external scrotal surface marks the position of the medial septum.

The function of the scrotum is to protect the testes and the sperm by maintaining a temperature lower than that of the body. Spermatogenesis cannot occur if the testes fail to descend and thus remain at body temperature. Because it is sensitive to touch, pressure, temperature, and pain, the scrotum defends against potential harm to the testes.

TABLE 2–3 Summary of Male Reproductive Organ Functions

The testes house seminiferous tubules and gonads.

- Semmiferous tubules contain sperm cells in various stages of development and undergoing meiosis.
- Sertoli's cells nourish and protect spermatocytes (phase between spermatids and spermatozoa).
- Leydig's cells are the main source of testosterone.
- Epididymides provide an area for maturation of sperm and a reservoir for mature spermatozoa.
- The vas deferens connects the epididymis with the prostate gland, then connects with ducts from the seminal vesicle to become an ejaculatory duct.
- Ejaculatory ducts provide a passageway for semen and seminal fluid into the urethra.
- Seminal vesicles secrete yellowish fluid rich in fructose, prostaglandins, and fibrinogen. This provides nutrition that increases motility and fertilizing ability of sperm. Prostaglandins also aid fertilization by making the cervical mucus more receptive to sperm.
- The prostate gland secretes thin, alkaline fluid containing calcium, citric acid, and other substances. Alkalinity counteracts acidity of ductus and seminal vesicle secretions.
- Bulbourethral (Cowper's) glands secrete alkaline, viscous fluid into semen aiding in neutralization of acidic vaginal secretions.

Internal Reproductive Organs

The male internal reproductive organs include the gonads (testes or testicles), a system of ducts (epididymides, vas deferens, ejaculatory duct, and urethra), and accessory glands (seminal vesicles, prostate gland, bulbourethral glands, and urethral glands). See Table 2–3.

TESTES

The *testes* are a pair of oval, compound glandular organs contained in the scrotum. In the sexually mature male, they are the site of spermatozoa production and the secretion of several male sex hormones.

Each testis is 4 to 6 cm long, 2 to 3 cm wide, and 3 to 4 cm thick and weighs about 10 to 15 g. Each is covered by an outer serous membrane and an inner capsule that is tough, white, and fibrous. The connective tissue sends projections inward to form septa, dividing the testis into 250 to 400 lobules. Each lobule contains one to three tightly packed, convoluted *seminiferous tubules* containing sperm cells in all stages of development.

The seminiferous tubules are surrounded by loose connective tissue that houses abundant blood and lymph vessels and *interstitial (Leydig's) cells.* The interstitial cells produce testosterone, the primary male sex hormone. The tubules also contain *Sertoli's cells,* which nourish and protect the spermatocytes. The seminiferous tubules come together to form 20 to 30 straight tubules, which in turn form an anastomotic network of thin-walled spaces, the *rete testis.* The rete testis forms 10 to 15 efferent ducts that empty into the duct of the epididymis.

Most of the cells lining the seminiferous tubules undergo **spermatogenesis,** a process of maturation in which spermatocytes become spermatozoa. (Chapter 5 further discusses the process of spermatogenesis.) Sperm production varies among and within the tubules, with cells in different areas of the same tubule undergoing different stages of spermatogenesis. The sperm are eventually released from the tubules into the epididymis, where they continue to mature. ⊐⊏ CD

Like the female reproductive cycle, the process of spermatogenesis and other functions of the testes are the result of complex neural and hormonal controls. The hypothalamus secretes releasing factors that stimulate the anterior pituitary to release the gonadotropins, FSH and LH. These hormones cause the testes to produce testosterone, which maintains spermatogenesis, increases sperm production by the seminiferous tubules, and stimulates production of seminal fluid.

Testosterone is the most prevalent and potent of the testicular hormones. It is also responsible for the development of secondary male characteristics and certain behavioral patterns. The effects of testosterone include structural and functional development of the male genital tract, emission and ejaculation of seminal fluid, distribution of body hair, promotion of growth and strength of long bones, increased muscle mass, and enlargement of the vocal cords. The action of testosterone on the central nervous system is thought to produce aggressiveness and sexual drive. The action of testosterone is constant, not cyclic like that of the female hormones. Its production is not limited to a certain number of years, but it is thought to decrease with age.

The testes have two primary functions:

- To serve as the site of spermatogenesis
- To produce testosterone

EPIDIDYMIS

The *epididymis* (plural, *epididymides*) is a duct about 5.6 m long, although it is convoluted into a compact structure about 3.75 cm long. An epididymis lies behind each testis. It arises from the top of the testis, courses downward, and then passes upward, where it becomes the vas deferens.

The epididymis provides a reservoir where maturing spermatozoa can survive for a long period. When discharged from the seminiferous tubules into the epididymis, the sperm are immotile and incapable of fertilizing an ovum. The spermatozoa remain in the epididymis for 2 to 10 days. As the sperm move along the tortuous course of the epididymis, they become both motile and fertile.

VAS DEFERENS AND EJACULATORY DUCTS

The *vas deferens,* also known as the *ductus deferens,* is about 40 cm long and connects the epididymis with the prostate. One vas deferens arises from the posterior border of each testis. It joins the spermatic cord and weaves over and between several pelvic structures until it meets the vas deferens from the opposite side. Each vas deferens terminus expands to form the *terminal ampulla.* It then unites with the seminal vesicle duct (a gland) to form the ejaculatory duct, which enters the prostate gland and ends in the prostatic urethra. The ejaculatory ducts serve as passageways for semen and fluid secreted by the seminal vesicles. The main function of the vas deferens is to rapidly squeeze the sperm from their storage sites (the epididymis and distal part of the vas deferens) into the urethra.

URETHRA

The male urethra is the passageway for both urine and semen. The urethra begins in the bladder and passes through the prostate gland, where it is called the *prostatic urethra.* The urethra emerges from the prostate gland to become the *membranous urethra.* It terminates in the penis, where it is called the *penile urethra.* In the penile urethra, goblet secretory cells are present, and smooth muscle is replaced by erectile tissue.

ACCESSORY GLANDS

The male accessory glands secrete a unique and essential component of the total seminal fluid in an ordered sequence.

The *seminal vesicles* are two glands composed of many lobes. Each vesicle is about 7.5 cm long. They are situated between the bladder and the rectum, immediately above the base of the prostate. The epithelium lining the seminal vesicles secretes an alkaline, viscid, clear fluid rich in high-energy fructose, prostaglandins, fibrinogen, and amino acids. During ejaculation, this fluid mixes with the sperm in the ejaculatory ducts. This fluid helps provide an environment favorable to sperm motility and metabolism.

The *prostate gland* encircles the upper part of the urethra and lies below the neck of the bladder. Made up of several lobes, it measures about 4 cm in diameter and weighs 20 to 30 g. The prostate is made up of both glandular and muscular tissue. It secretes a thin, milky, alkaline fluid containing high levels of zinc, calcium, citric acid, and acid phosphatase. This fluid protects the sperm from the acidic environment of the vagina and the male urethra, which could be spermicidal.

The *bulbourethral (Cowper's) glands* are a pair of small, round structures on either side of the membranous urethra. The glands secrete a clear, thick, alkaline fluid rich in mucoproteins that becomes part of the semen. This secretion also lubricates the penile urethra during sexual excitement and neutralizes the acid in the male urethra and vagina, thereby enhancing sperm motility.

The *urethral (Littre's) glands* are tiny mucus-secreting glands found throughout the membranous lining of the penile urethra. Their secretions add to those of the bulbourethral glands.

SEMEN

The male ejaculate, *semen* or *seminal fluid,* is made up of spermatozoa and the secretions of all the accessory glands. The seminal fluid transports viable and motile sperm to the female reproductive tract. Effective transportation of sperm requires adequate nutrients, an adequate pH (about 7.5), a specific concentration of sperm to fluid, and an optimal osmolarity.

A spermatozoon is made up of a *head* and a *tail.* The tail is divided into the middle piece and end piece (Figure 2–18 ◆). The head's main components are the *acrosome* and *nucleus.* The head carries the male's haploid number of chromosomes (23), and it is the part that enters the ovum at fertilization (see Chapter 5). ⬮ The tail, or flagellum, is divided into the middle and end piece and is specialized for motility.

Sperm may be stored in the male genital system for up to 42 days, depending primarily on the frequency of ejaculations. The average volume of ejaculate following abstinence for several days is 2 to 5 mL but may vary from 1 to 10 mL. Repeated ejaculation results in decreased volume. Once ejaculated, sperm can live only 2 or 3 days in the female genital tract.

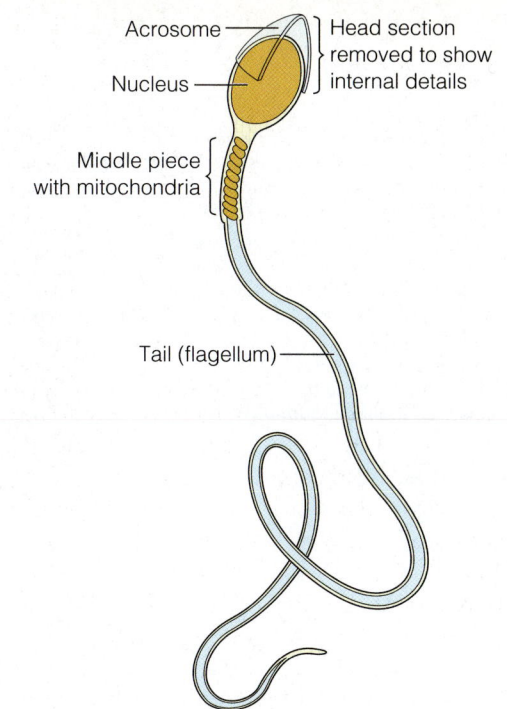

FIGURE 2–18. ◆ Schematic representation of a mature spermatozoon.

CHAPTER HIGHLIGHTS

🔁 Reproductive activities require a complex interaction between the reproductive structures, the central nervous system, and such endocrine glands as the pituitary, hypothalamus, testes, and ovaries.

🔁 The female reproductive system consists of the ovaries, where female germ cells and female sex hormones are formed; the fallopian tubes, which capture the ovum and allow transport to the uterus; the uterus, which is the implantation site for the fertilized ovum (blastocyst); the cervix, which is a protective portal for the body of the uterus and the connection between the vagina and the uterus; and the vagina, which is the passageway from the external genitals to the uterus and provides for discharge of menstrual products out of the body.

🔁 The female reproductive cycle is composed of the ovarian cycle, during which ovulation occurs, and the uterine cycle, during which menstruation occurs. These two cycles take place simultaneously and are under neurohumoral control.

🔁 The ovarian cycle has two phases: the follicular phase and the luteal phase. During the follicular phase, the primordial follicle matures under the influence of FSH and LH until ovulation occurs. The luteal phase begins when the ovum leaves the follicle and the corpus luteum develops under the influence of LH. The corpus luteum produces high levels of progesterone and low levels of estrogen.

🔁 The uterine (menstrual) cycle has four phases: menstrual, proliferative, secretory, and ischemic. Menstruation is the actual shedding of the endometrial lining, when estrogen levels are low. The proliferative phase begins when the endometrial glands begin to enlarge under the influence of estrogen and cervical mucosal changes occur; the changes peak at ovulation. The secretory phase follows ovulation, and, influenced primarily by progesterone, the uterus increases its vascularity to make ready for possible implantation. The ischemic phase is characterized by degeneration of the corpus luteum, decreases in both estrogen and progesterone levels, constriction of the spiral arteries, and escape of blood into the stromal cells of the endometrium.

🔁 The male reproductive system consists of the testes, where male germ cells and male sex hormones are formed; a series of continuous ducts through which spermatozoa are transported outside the body; accessory glands that produce secretions important to sperm nutrition, survival, and transport; and the penis, which serves as the reproductive organ of intercourse.

EXPLOREMEDIALINK

NCLEX Review, Case Studies, and other interactive resources for this chapter can be found on the companion website at http://www.prenhall.com/london. Click on "Chapter 2" to select the activities for this chapter.

For animations, more NCLEX review questions, and an audio glossary, access the accompanying CD-ROM in this textbook.

REFERENCES

Caldwell, W. E., & Moloy, H. C. (1933). Anatomical variations in the female pelvis and their effect on labor with a suggested classification [Historical article]. *American Journal of Obstetrics and Gynecology, 26,* 479–505.

Clark, K. E., & Myatt, L. (1999). Prostaglandins and the reproductive cycle. In J. J. Sciarri & T. J. Watkins (Eds.), *Gynecology and obstetrics* (Vol. 5, chap. 42, pp. 1–18). Hagerstown, MD: Harper & Row.

Couchman, G. M., & Hammond, C. B. (1999). Clinical anatomy of the female. In J. R. Scott, P. J. Di Saia, C. B. Hammond, & W. N. Spel-lacy (Eds.), *Danforth's obstetrics and gynecology* (8th ed., pp. 19–28). Philadelphia: Lippincott.

Cunningham, F. G., Gant, N. F., Leveno, K. J., Gilstrap, L. C., Hauth, J. C., & Wenstrom, K. P. (2001). *Williams obstetrics* (21st ed.). New York: McGraw-Hill.

Di Saia, P. J. (1999). Clinical anatomy of the female. In J. R. Scott, P. J. Di Saia, C. B. Hammond, & W. N. Spellacy (Eds.), *Danforth's obstetrics and gynecology* (8th ed., pp. 47–64). Philadelphia: Lippincott.

Ferin, M. (1998). The hypothalamus-hypophy-seal-ovarian axis and the menstrual cycle. In J. J. Sciarri & T. J. Watkins (Eds.), *Gynecology and obstetrics* (Vol. 5, chap. 6, pp. 1–15). Hagerstown, MD: Harper & Row.

Liu, J. H., & Rebar, R. W. (1999). Endocrinology of pregnancy. In R. K. Creasy & R. Resnik (Eds.), *Maternal-fetal medicine: Principles and practice* (4th ed., pp. 379–391). Philadelphia: Saunders.

Rebar, R. W. (1999). The breast and the physiology of lactation. In R. K. Creasy & R. Resnik (Eds.), *Maternal-fetal medicine: Principles and practice* (4th ed., pp. 106–121). Philadelphia: Saunders.

CHAPTER 3

Women's Health Care

I am 55 now, an early baby boomer. I am astonished at the changes that have occurred in women's health care in my lifetime. I remember that my mom was shocked when our family doctor taught me to do a breast exam when I turned 18. What a farsighted man. Information on sexually transmitted diseases was not as generally available. AIDS was beyond our imagination. Contraceptive options were more limited although the pill was gaining in popularity. Menopause seemed like the end of life—menopausal women were old. Today more and more of us women are becoming savvy health care consumers. We have more information, we have treatment options, we decide our own care. I think this is the most exciting change of all!

—A**LICE**

Key Terms

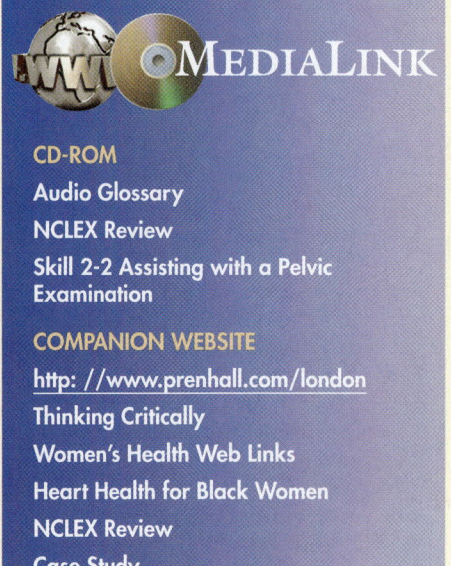

MEDIALINK

CD-ROM

Audio Glossary

NCLEX Review

Skill 2-2 Assisting with a Pelvic
Examination

COMPANION WEBSITE

http://www.prenhall.com/london

Thinking Critically

Women's Health Web Links

Heart Health for Black Women

NCLEX Review

Case Study

A woman's health care needs change throughout her lifetime. As a young girl she needs health teaching about menstruation, sexuality, and personal responsibility. As a teen she needs information about reproductive choices and safe sexual activity. During this time she should also be introduced to the importance of health care practices such as breast self-examination and regular Pap smears. The mature woman may need to be reminded of these self-care issues and prepared for physical changes that accompany childbirth and aging. By educating women about their bodies, their health care choices, and their right to be knowledgeable consumers, nurses can help women assume responsibility for the health care they receive.

The contemporary woman is likely to encounter various major or minor gynecologic or urinary problems during her lifetime. The nurse can assist a woman in this situation by providing accurate, sensitive, and supportive health education and counseling. This chapter provides information about selected aspects of women's health care with an emphasis on conditions typically addressed in a community-based setting.

NURSING CARE IN THE COMMUNITY

Women's health refers to a holistic view of women and their health-related needs within the context of their everyday lives. It is based on the awareness that a woman's physical, mental, and spiritual status are interdependent and affect her state of health or illness. The woman's view of her situation, her assessment of her needs, her values, and her beliefs are valid and important factors to be incorporated into any health care intervention.

Nurses can work with women to provide health teaching and information about self-care practices in schools, during routine examinations in a clinic or office, at senior centers, at meetings of volunteer organizations, through classes offered by local agencies or schools, or in the home. This community-based focus is the key to providing effective nursing care to women of all ages.

Developing Cultural Competence

In the course of your work as a nurse, you are bound to encounter people different from yourself. Even with the best of intentions, you may say or do something your client or the client's family finds offensive or inappropriate. If you ask someone something and get a funny look, ask what's on the person's mind. The answer may surprise you. It often leads to more honest reporting of information and a feeling of being listened to and respected. When people feel emotionally safe, cultural and other perceived differences shrink. This helps a therapeutic relationship to develop between the person you are serving and you, yourself, as the caregiver.

In reality, the vast majority of women's health care is provided outside of acute care settings. Nurses oriented to community-based care are especially effective in recognizing the autonomy of each individual and in dealing with clients holistically. This holistic approach is important in addressing not only physical problems but also major health issues such as violence against women, which may go undetected unless care providers are alert for signs of it. See "Developing Cultural Competence."

THE NURSE'S ROLE IN ADDRESSING ISSUES OF SEXUALITY

Because sexuality and its reproductive implications are such an intrinsic and emotion-laden part of life, people have many concerns, problems, and questions about sex roles, behaviors, education, inhibitions, morality, and related areas such as family planning. The reproductive implications of sexual intercourse must also be considered. Some people desire pregnancy; others wish to avoid it. Health factors are another consideration. The increase in the incidence of sexually transmitted infections, especially HIV/AIDS and herpes, has caused many people to modify their sexual practices and activities. Women frequently ask questions or voice concerns about these issues to the nurse in a clinic or ambulatory setting. Thus the nurse may need to assume the role of counselor or educator on sexual and reproductive matters.

Nurses who assume this role must recognize their own feelings, values, and attitudes about sexuality so they can be more sensitive when they encounter the values and beliefs of others. Nurses need to have accurate, up-to-date information about anatomy and physiology and about topics related to sexuality, sexual practices, and common gynecologic problems. In addition, when a woman is accompanied by her partner, it is important that the nurse be sensitive to the dynamics of the relationship between the two.

Taking a Sexual History

Nurses are often responsible for taking a woman's initial history, including her gynecologic and sexual history. To be effective, the nurse must have good communication skills and should conduct the interview in a quiet, private place free of distractions.

Opening the discussion with a brief explanation of the purpose of such questions is often helpful. For example, the nurse might say, "As your nurse I'm interested in all aspects of your well-being. Often women have concerns or questions about sexual matters, especially when they are pregnant (or starting to be sexually active). I will be asking you some questions about your sexual history as part of your general health history."

It may be helpful to use direct eye contact as much as possible unless the nurse knows it is culturally unacceptable to the woman. The nurse should do little, if any, writing during the interview, especially if the woman seems ill at ease or is discussing very personal issues. Open-ended questions are often useful in eliciting information. For example, "What, if anything, would you change about your sex life?" will elicit more information than "Are you happy with your sex life now?" The nurse needs to clarify terminology and proceed from easier topics to those that are more difficult to discuss. Throughout the interview the nurse should be alert to body language and nonverbal cues. It is important that the nurse not assume that the client is heterosexual. Some women are open about lesbian relationships; others are more reserved until they develop a sense of trust in their caregivers.

After completing the sexual history, the nurse assesses the information obtained. If there is a problem that requires further medical tests and assessments, the nurse will refer the woman to a nurse-practitioner, certified nurse-midwife, physician, or counselor as necessary. In many instances the nurse alone will be able to develop a nursing diagnosis and then plan and implement therapy. The nurse must be realistic in making assessments and planning interventions. It requires insight and skill to recognize when a woman's problem requires interventions that are beyond a nurse's preparation and ability. In such situations, it is essential that the nurse makes appropriate referrals.

MENSTRUATION

Girls today begin to learn about puberty and menstruation at a young age. Unfortunately, the source of their "education" is sometimes their peers or the media; thus the information is often incomplete, inaccurate, and sensationalized. Nurses who work with young girls and adolescents recognize this and are working hard to provide accurate health teaching and to correct misinformation about *menarche* (the onset of menses) and the menstrual cycle.

Cultural, religious, and personal attitudes about menstruation are part of the menstrual experience and often reflect negative attitudes toward women. Currently there are fewer customs associated with menstruation. In many cultures, sexual intercourse during menses is a common practice. Physiologically, it is not generally contraindicated. For most couples, the decision is one of personal preference. (The physiology of menstruation is discussed in Chapter 2.)

Counseling the Premenstrual Girl about Menarche

Many young women find it embarrassing to discuss menstruation, both because of the taboos associated with the subject and because of their immaturity. However, the most critical factor in successful adaptation to menarche is the adolescent's level of preparedness. Information should be given to premenstrual girls over time rather than all at once. This allows them to absorb information and develop questions.

The following basic information is helpful for young clients:

- *Cycle length.* Cycle length is determined from the first day of one menses to the first day of the next menses. Initially a female's cycle length is about 29 days, but the normal length may vary from 21 to 35 days. As a woman matures, cycle length often shortens to a median of 25+ days just before menopause. Cycle length often varies by a day or two from one cycle to the next, although greater normal variations may also occur.
- *Amount of flow.* The average flow is approximately 25 to 60 mL per period. Usually women characterize the amount of flow in terms of the number of pads or tampons used. Flow often is heavier at first and lighter toward the end of the period.
- *Length of menses.* Menses usually lasts from 2 to 8 days, although this may vary.

The nurse should make it clear that variations in age at menarche, length of cycle, and duration of menses are normal, because girls may worry if their experience varies from that of their peers. It also is helpful to acknowledge the negative aspects of menstruation (messiness, cramping, embarrassment) while stressing its positive role as a symbol of maturity and womanhood.

Educational Topics

PADS AND TAMPONS

Since early times women have made pads and tampons from cloth or rags, which required washing but were reusable. Commercial tampons were introduced in the 1930s.

Today adhesive-stripped minipads and maxipads and flushable tampons are readily available. However, the deodorants and increased absorbency that manufacturers have added to both sanitary napkins and tampons may prove harmful. The chemical used to deodorize can create a rash on the vulva and damage the tender mucous lining of the vagina. Excessive or inappropriate use of tampons can produce dryness or even small sores or ulcers in the vagina.

Because the use of superabsorbent tampons has been linked to the development of toxic shock syndrome (TSS) (page 68), women should avoid using them. They should use regular-absorbency tampons only for heavy menstrual flow (during the first 2 or 3 days of the period), not during the whole period, and change them every 3 to 6 hours. Because *Staphylococcus aureus,* the causative organism of TSS, is frequently found on the hands, a woman should wash her hands before inserting a fresh tampon and should avoid touching the tip of the tampon when unwrapping it or before insertion.

In the absence of a heavy menstrual flow, tampons absorb moisture, leaving the vaginal walls dry and subject to injury. The absorbency of regular tampons varies. If the tampon is hard to pull out or shreds when removed, or if the vagina becomes dry, the tampon is probably too absorbent.

A woman may want to use tampons only during the day and switch to napkins at night to avoid vaginal irritation. She should avoid using tampons on the last, spotty days of her period and should never use them for midcycle spotting or leukorrhea. If a woman experiences vaginal irritation, itching, or soreness or notices an unusual odor while using tampons, she should stop using them or change brands or absorbencies to see if that helps.

VAGINAL SPRAY, DOUCHING, AND CLEANSING

Vaginal sprays are unnecessary and can cause infections, itching, burning, vaginal discharge, rashes, and other problems. If a woman chooses to use a spray, she needs to know that these sprays are for external use only and should never be applied to irritated or itching skin or used with sanitary napkins.

Although douching is sometimes used to treat vaginal infections, douching as a hygiene practice is unnecessary, since the vagina cleanses itself. Douching washes away the natural mucus and upsets the vaginal ecology, which can make the vagina more susceptible to infection. Perfumed douches can cause allergic reactions, and too frequent use of an undiluted or strong douche solution can cause irritation or even tissue damage. Propelling water up the vagina may also erode the antibacterial cervical plug and force bacteria and germs from the vagina into the uterus. Women should avoid douching during menstruation because the cervix is dilated to permit the downward flow of menstrual fluids from the uterine lining. Douching may force tissue back up into the uterine cavity, which could contribute to endometriosis.

The mucous secretions that bathe the vagina are odor-free while they are in the vagina; odor develops only when they mingle with perspiration and are exposed to the air. Keeping one's skin clean and free of bacteria with plain soap and water is the most effective method of controlling odor. A soapy finger or soft washcloth should be used to wash gently between the vulvar folds. Bathing is as important during menses as at any other time. A long, leisurely soak in a warm tub promotes menstrual blood flow and relieves cramps by relaxing the muscles.

Keeping the vulva fresh throughout the day means keeping it dry and clean. A woman can ensure adequate ventilation by wearing cotton panties and clothes loose enough to permit the vaginal area to "breathe." After using the toilet, a woman should always wipe herself from front to back and, if necessary, follow up with a moistened paper towel or toilet paper. If an unusual odor persists despite these efforts, it may be a sign that something is awry. Certain conditions such as vaginitis produce a foul-smelling discharge.

Associated Menstrual Conditions

A variety of menstrual irregularities have been identified. An abnormally short duration of menstrual flow is termed *hypomenorrhea;* an abnormally long one is called *hyperme-* *norrhea.* Excessive, profuse flow is called *menorrhagia,* and bleeding between periods is known as *metrorrhagia.* Infrequent and too frequent menses are termed *oligomenorrhea* and *polymenorrhea,* respectively. An *anovulatory cycle* is one in which ovulation does not occur. (*Note:* Anovulatory cycles often occur during the first year after menarche and during the perimenopause, the period around the time of menopause.) Generally menstrual irregularities should be investigated to rule out disease.

AMENORRHEA

Amenorrhea, the absence of menses, is classified as primary or secondary. Primary amenorrhea exists if menstruation has not been established by 16 years of age or within 4 years of breast development. Secondary amenorrhea exists when an established menses (of longer than 3 months) ceases for at least 6 months.

Primary amenorrhea necessitates a thorough assessment of the young woman to determine its cause. Possible causes include congenital obstructions, Turner syndrome, congenital absence of the uterus, testicular feminization (external genitals appear female but uterus and ovaries are absent and testes are present), or absence or imbalance of hormones. Treatment depends on the causative factors. Some causes are not correctable.

Secondary amenorrhea is caused most frequently by pregnancy. Additional causes include lactation, hormonal imbalances, poor nutrition (anorexia nervosa, obesity, and fad dieting), ovarian lesions, strenuous exercise (associated with long-distance runners, dancers, and other athletes with low body fat ratios), debilitating systemic diseases, stress of high intensity and/or long duration, stressful life events, a change in season or climate, use of oral contraceptives, use of the phenothiazine and chlorpromazine group of tranquilizers, and syndromes such as Cushing and Sheehan. The causative factors dictate treatment. The nurse can explain that once the underlying condition has been corrected—for example, when sufficient body weight is gained—menses will resume. Athletes and women who participate in strenuous exercise routines may be advised to increase their caloric intake or reduce their exercise levels for a month or two to see whether a normal cycle ensues. If it does not, medical referral is indicated.

DYSMENORRHEA

Dysmenorrhea, or painful menstruation, occurs at, or a day before, the onset of menstruation and disappears by the end of menses. Dysmenorrhea is classified as primary or secondary. Primary dysmenorrhea is defined as cramps without underlying disease. Prostaglandins F_2 and $F_{2\alpha}$, which are produced by the uterus in higher concentrations during menses, are the primary cause. They increase uterine contractility and decrease uterine artery blood flow, causing ischemia. The end result is the painful sensation of cramps. Dysmenorrhea typically disappears after a first pregnancy and does not occur if cycles are anovulatory. Treatment of primary dysmenorrhea includes oral contraceptives (which block ovulation), prostaglandin inhibitors (such as ibuprofen, aspirin, and naproxen), and self-care measures such as regular exercise, rest, heat, and good nutrition. Biofeedback has also been used with some success.

Secondary dysmenorrhea is associated with pathology of the reproductive tract and usually appears after menstruation has been established. Conditions that most frequently cause secondary dysmenorrhea include endometriosis; residual pelvic inflammatory disease; anatomic anomalies such as cervical stenosis, imperforate hymen, and uterine displacement; ovarian cysts; and the presence of an intrauterine device. Because primary and secondary dysmenorrhea may coexist, accurate differential diagnosis is essential for appropriate treatment.

Some nutritionists suggest that vitamins B and E help relieve the discomforts associated with menstruation. Vitamin B_6 may help relieve the premenstrual bloating and irritability some women experience. Vitamin E, a mild prostaglandin inhibitor, may help decrease menstrual discomfort. Avoiding salt can decrease discomfort from fluid retention.

Heat is soothing and promotes increased blood flow. Any source of warmth, from sipping herbal tea to soaking in a hot tub or using a heating pad, may be helpful during painful periods. Massage can also soothe aching back muscles and promote relaxation and blood flow.

Regular exercise can ease menstrual discomfort and help prevent cramps and other menstrual complaints. Aerobic exercises such as jogging, cycling, swimming, and fast-paced walking are especially helpful. Persistent discomfort should be medically evaluated.

PREMENSTRUAL SYNDROME

Premenstrual syndrome (PMS) refers to a symptom complex associated with the luteal phase of the menstrual cycle (2 weeks prior to the onset of menses). The symptoms must, by definition, occur between ovulation and the onset of menses. They repeat at the same stage of each menstrual cycle and include some or all of the following:

- Psychologic: irritability, lethargy, depression, low morale, anxiety, sleep disorders, crying spells, hostility
- Neurologic: classic migraine, vertigo, syncope
- Respiratory: rhinitis, hoarseness, and occasionally asthma
- Gastrointestinal: nausea, vomiting, constipation, abdominal bloating, craving for sweets
- Urinary: retention, oliguria
- Dermatologic: acne
- Mammary: swelling and tenderness

Most women experience only some of these symptoms. The symptoms usually are most pronounced 2 or 3 days before the onset of menstruation and subside as menstrual flow begins, with or without treatment. *Premenstrual dysphoric disorder* (PMDD) is a diagnosis that may be applied to a subgroup of women with PMS whose symptoms are primarily mood related and severe (Endicott, Bardack, Grady-Weliky, et al., 2000).

The exact cause of PMS is unknown, although a variety of theories have been put forth to explain it. These include, for example, a blunted response to serotonin and imbalance of the gonadal hormones (Dell, Moskowitz, & Sondheimer, 2001).

Nursing Management

The nurse can help the woman identify specific symptoms and develop healthy behavior. After assessment, counseling for PMS may include advising the woman to restrict her intake of foods containing methylxanthines such as chocolate, cola, and coffee; restrict her intake of alcohol, nicotine, red meat, and foods containing salt and sugar; increase her intake of complex carbohydrates and protein; and increase the frequency of meals. For women whose primary symptoms are psychologic, supplementation with B-complex vitamins, especially B_6, may decrease anxiety and depression. However, treatment trials do not demonstrate a consistent effect, and megadoses of B_6 are associated with peripheral neurologic changes (Moline & Zendell, 2000). Vitamin E supplements may help reduce breast tenderness, and a program of aerobic exercise such as fast walking, jogging, and aerobic dancing is generally beneficial. In addition to vitamin supplements, pharmacologic treatments for PMS include progesterone replacement, diuretics, psychotropic drugs (such as tricyclic antidepressants and selective serotonin reuptake inhibitors), and prostaglandin inhibitors. All have been effective in some women and not in others. For women who are not planning a pregnancy, low-dose oral contraceptives, which suppress ovulation, are often helpful.

A woman benefits a great deal from an empathic relationship with a health care professional to whom she feels free to voice concerns. Encourage the woman to keep a diary to help identify life events associated with PMS. Self-care groups and self-help literature both help women feel they have control over their bodies. Some women use complementary therapies such as homeopathic remedies or herbs. Thus it is helpful to have a general familiarity with commonly used remedies. It is important that women using such alternatives seek advice from knowledgeable, experienced homeopaths or herbalists.

CONTRACEPTION

The decision to use a method of contraception may be made individually by a woman (or, in the case of vasectomy, by a man) or jointly by a couple. The decision may be motivated by a desire to avoid pregnancy, to gain control over the number of children conceived, or to determine the spacing of future children. In choosing a specific method, consistency of use outweighs the absolute reliability of the given method.

Decisions about contraception should be made voluntarily, with full knowledge of available choices, advantages, disadvantages, effectiveness, side effects, contraindications, and long-term effects. Many outside factors influence this choice, including cultural practices, religious beliefs, attitudes and personal preferences, cost, effectiveness, misinformation, practicality of method, and self-esteem. Different methods of contraception may be appropriate at different times for couples.

Fertility Awareness Methods

Fertility awareness methods, also known as *natural family planning,* are based on an understanding of the changes that occur throughout a woman's ovulatory cycle. All these methods require periods of abstinence and recording of certain events throughout the cycle; cooperation of the partners is important.

Fertility awareness methods are free, safe, and acceptable to many whose religious beliefs prohibit other methods. They provide an increased awareness of the body, involve no artificial substances or devices, encourage a couple to communicate about sexual activity and family planning, and are useful in helping a couple plan a pregnancy.

On the other hand, these methods require extensive initial counseling to be used effectively. They may interfere with sexual spontaneity; they require extensive maintenance of records for several cycles before beginning to use them; they may be difficult or impossible for women with irregular cycles to use; and, although theoretically they should be very reliable, in practice they may not be as reliable in preventing pregnancy as other methods.

The *basal body temperature (BBT)* method to detect ovulation requires that a woman take her BBT every morning upon awakening (before any activity) and record the readings on a temperature graph. To do this, she uses a BBT thermometer, which shows tenths of a degree rather than the two tenths shown on standard thermometers. She may also use tympanic thermometry (an "ear thermome-

ter"). After 3 to 4 months of recording temperatures, a woman with regular cycles should be able to predict when ovulation will occur. The method is based on the fact that the temperature sometimes drops just before ovulation and almost always rises and remains elevated for several days after. The temperature rise occurs in response to the increased progesterone levels that occur in the second half of the cycle. Figure 3–1 ◆ shows a sample BBT chart. To avoid conception, the couple abstains from intercourse on the day of the temperature rise and for 3 days after. Because the temperature rise does not occur until after ovulation, a woman who had intercourse just before the rise is at risk of pregnancy. To decrease this risk, some couples abstain from intercourse for several days before the *anticipated* time of ovulation and then for 3 days after.

The *calendar,* or *rhythm, method* is based on the assumptions that ovulation tends to occur 14 days (plus or minus 2 days) before the start of the next menstrual period, sperm are viable for 48 to 72 hours, and the ovum is viable for 24 hours. To use this method, the woman must record her menstrual cycles for 6 to 8 months to identify the shortest and longest cycles. The first day of menstruation is the first day of the cycle. The fertile phase is calculated from 18 days before the end of the shortest recorded cycle through 11 days from the end of the longest recorded cycle (Hatcher, Trussell, Stewart et al., 1998). For example, if a woman's cycle lasts from 24 to 28 days, the fertile phase would be calculated as day 6 through day 17. Once this information is obtained, the woman can identify the fertile and infertile phases of her cycle. For effective use of this method, she must abstain from intercourse during the fertile phase. The calendar method is the least reliable of the fertility awareness methods and has largely been replaced by other, more scientific approaches.

The *cervical mucus method,* sometimes called the *ovulation method* or the *Billings method,* involves the assessment of cervical mucus changes that occur during the menstrual cycle. The amount and character of cervical mucus change because of the influence of estrogen and progesterone. At

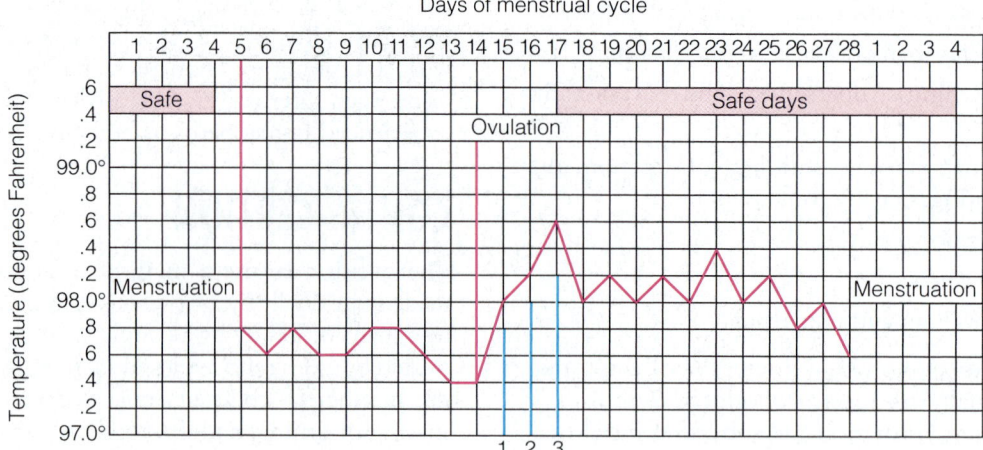

FIGURE 3–1. ◆ Sample basal body temperature chart.

the time of ovulation the mucus (estrogen-dominant mucus) is clearer, more stretchable (a quality called *spinnbarkeit*), and more permeable to sperm. It also shows a characteristic fern pattern when placed on a glass slide and allowed to dry (see Figure 4–3, page 87). During the luteal phase, the cervical mucus is thick and sticky (progesterone-dominant mucus) and forms a network that traps sperm, making their passage more difficult.

To use the cervical mucus method, the woman abstains from intercourse for the first menstrual cycle. Cervical mucus is assessed daily for amount, feeling of slipperiness or wetness, color, clearness, and spinnbarkeit, as the woman becomes familiar with varying characteristics.

The peak day of wetness and clear, stretchable mucus is assumed to be the time of ovulation. To use this method correctly, the woman should abstain from intercourse from the time she first notices that the mucus is becoming clear, more elastic, and slippery until 4 days after the last wet mucus (ovulation) day. Because this method evaluates the effects of hormonal changes, it can be used by women with irregular cycles.

The *symptothermal method* consists of various assessments made and recorded by the couple. These include information regarding cycle days, coitus, cervical mucus changes, and secondary signs such as increased libido, abdominal bloating, mittelschmerz (midcycle abdominal pain), and BBT. Through the various assessments, the couple learns to recognize signs that indicate ovulation. This combined approach tends to improve the effectiveness of fertility awareness as a method of birth control.

Situational Contraceptives

Abstinence can be considered a method of contraception, and, partly because of changing values and the increased risk of infection with intercourse, it is gaining increased acceptance.

Coitus interruptus, or *withdrawal,* is one of the oldest and least reliable methods of contraception. This method requires that the male withdraw from the female's vagina when he feels that ejaculation is impending. He then ejaculates away from the external genitalia of the woman. Failure tends to occur for two reasons: (1) this method demands great self-control on the part of the man, who must withdraw just as he feels the urge for deeper penetration with impending orgasm, and (2) some preejaculatory fluid, which can contain sperm, may escape from the penis during the excitement phase prior to ejaculation. The fact that the quantity of sperm in this preejaculatory fluid is increased after a recent ejaculation is especially significant for couples who engage in repeated episodes of intercourse within a short period of time. Couples who use this method should be aware of postcoital contraceptive options in case the man fails to withdraw in time.

Douching after intercourse is an ineffective method of contraception and is not recommended. It may actually facilitate conception by pushing sperm farther up the birth canal.

Spermicides

Spermicides, available as creams, jellies, foams, vaginal film, and suppositories, are inserted into the vagina before intercourse. They destroy sperm or neutralize vaginal secretions and thereby immobilize sperm. Spermicides that effervesce in a moist environment offer relatively rapid protection, and coitus may take place immediately after they are inserted. Suppositories may require up to 30 minutes to dissolve and will not offer protection until they do so. Instruct the woman to insert these spermicide preparations high in the vagina and maintain a supine position.

Spermicides are minimally effective when used alone, but their effectiveness increases in conjunction with a diaphragm or condom. The major advantages of spermicides are their wide availability and low toxicity. They are readily available over the counter without prescription. In addition, they provide significant protection from gonorrhea and chlamydia (Hatcher et al., 1998).

Skin irritation and allergic reactions to spermicides are the primary disadvantages. Although some studies have suggested that the use of spermicides at the time of conception or early in pregnancy may be associated with an increased risk of congenital anomalies, recent studies have shown no increased incidence (Hatcher et al., 1998).

Mechanical Contraceptives

Mechanical contraceptive methods either prevent the transport of sperm to the ovum or prevent implantation of the zygote.

MALE AND FEMALE CONDOMS

The male **condom** offers a viable means of contraception when used consistently and properly (Figure 3–2 ◆). Acceptance has been increasing as a growing number of men are assuming responsibility for regulation of fertility. The condom is applied to the erect penis, rolled from the tip to the end of the shaft, before vulvar or vaginal contact. A small space must be left at the end of the condom to allow for collection of the ejaculate, so that the condom will not break at the time of ejaculation. If the condom or vagina is dry a water-soluble lubricant, such as K-Y jelly, should be used to prevent irritation and possible condom breakage.

Care must be taken in removing the condom after intercourse. For optimal effectiveness, the man should withdraw his penis from the vagina while it is still erect and hold the condom rim to prevent spillage. If after ejaculation the penis becomes flaccid while still in the vagina, the male should hold onto the edge of the condom while withdrawing to avoid spilling the semen and to prevent the condom from slipping off.

The effectiveness of male condoms is largely determined by their use. The condom is small, disposable, and inexpensive; it has no side effects, requires no medical examination or supervision, and offers visual evidence of effectiveness. Most condoms are made of latex, although polyurethane

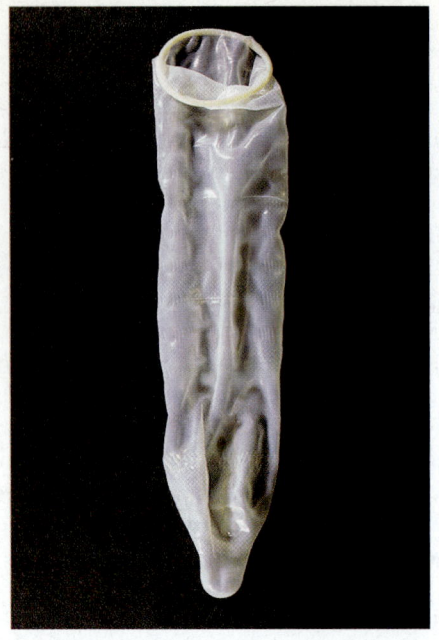

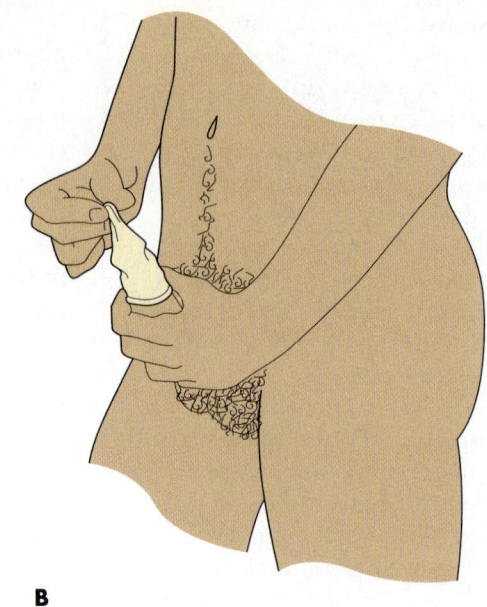

A   **B**

FIGURE 3–2. ◆ **A,** Unrolled condom with reservoir tip. **B,** Correct use of a condom.

and silicone rubber condoms are available for individuals allergic to latex. All condoms, except natural "skin" condoms, made from lamb's intestines, offer protection against both pregnancy and sexually transmitted infections (STIs). Breakage, displacement, perineal or vaginal irritation, and dulled sensation are possible disadvantages.

The male condom is becoming increasingly popular because of the protection it offers from infections. The protection condoms provide is especially useful for adolescent females because their developing cervical tissue increases their risk of contracting an STI (Jenkins & Raine, 2000). Regardless of age, however, for women, sexually transmitted infection increases the risk of pelvic inflammatory disease (PID) and resultant infertility. Many women are beginning to insist that their sexual partners use condoms, and many women carry condoms with them.

The *Reality female condom* (Figure 3–3 ◆) is a thin polyurethane sheath with a flexible ring at each end. The inner ring, at the closed end of the condom, serves as the means of insertion and fits over the cervix like a diaphragm. The second ring remains outside the vagina and covers a portion of the woman's perineum. It also covers the base of the man's penis during intercourse. Available over the counter and designed for onetime use, the condom may be inserted up to 8 hours before intercourse. The inner sheath is prelubricated but does not contain spermicide and is not designed to be used with a male condom. Data on its effectiveness against pregnancy are still limited, although the female condom has been compared favorably to other barrier methods. Because it also covers a portion of the vulva, it probably provides better protection than other methods against some pathogens.

High cost, noisiness during intercourse, and the cumbersome feel of the device make acceptability a problem for some couples.

DIAPHRAGM AND CERVICAL CAP

The **diaphragm** (Figure 3–4 ◆) is used with spermicidal cream or jelly and offers a good level of protection from conception. The woman must be fitted with a diaphragm and instructed in its use by trained personnel. The diaphragm should be rechecked for correct size after each childbirth and whenever a woman has gained or lost 15 lb or more.

The diaphragm must be inserted before intercourse, with approximately 1 teaspoonful (or 1.5 inches from the tube) of spermicidal jelly placed around its rim and in the cup. This chemical barrier supplements the mechanical barrier of the diaphragm. The diaphragm is inserted through the vagina and covers the cervix. The last step in insertion is to push the edge of the diaphragm under the symphysis pubis, which may result in a "popping" sensation. When fitted properly and correctly in place, the diaphragm should not cause discomfort to the woman or her partner. Correct placement of the diaphragm can be checked by touching the cervix with a fingertip through the cup. The cervix feels like a small, firm, rounded structure and has a consistency similar to that of the tip of the nose. The center of the diaphragm should be over the cervix. If more than 4 hours elapse between insertion of the diaphragm and intercourse, additional spermicidal cream or jelly should be used. It is necessary to leave the diaphragm in place for at least 6 hours after coitus. The diaphragm should then be removed, cleaned with mild soap

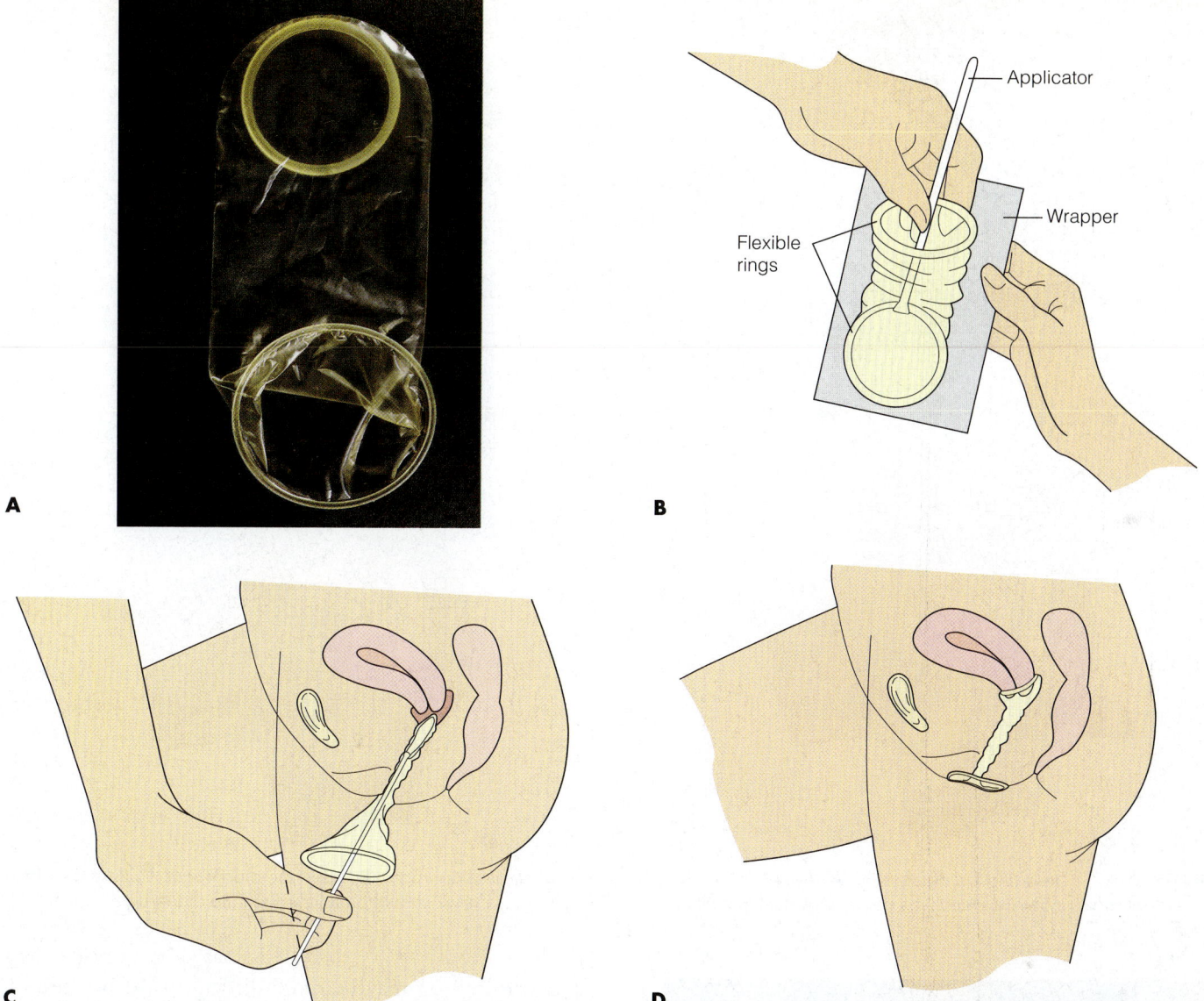

A

B

Applicator

Wrapper

Flexible
rings

C

D

FIGURE 3–3. ◆ **A,** The female condom. To insert the condom: **B,** Remove condom and applicator from wrapper by pulling up on the ring. **C,** Insert condom slowly by gently pushing the applicator toward the small of the back. **D,** When properly inserted, the outer ring should rest on the folds of skin around the vaginal opening, and the inner ring (closed end) should fit loosely against the cervix. *Note:* From Crooks, R., & Baur, K. (1993). *Our sexuality* (5th ed.). Reprinted with permission of Wadsworth, an imprint of the Wadsworth Group, a division of Thomson Learning. Fax (800) 730-2215.

and water, and allowed to air dry before it is stored in its case. If intercourse is desired again within the 6 hours, another type of contraception must be used or additional spermicidal jelly placed in the vagina with an applicator, taking care not to disturb the placement of the diaphragm. Periodically the diaphragm should be held up to the light and inspected for tears or holes.

Some couples feel that the use of a diaphragm interferes with the spontaneity of intercourse. The nurse can suggest that the partner insert the diaphragm as part of foreplay. The woman can then easily verify the placement herself.

Diaphragms are an excellent contraceptive method for women who are lactating, who cannot or do not wish to use the pill (oral contraceptives), who are smokers over age 35, or who wish to avoid the increased risk of PID associated with intrauterine devices.

Women who object to manipulating their genitals to insert the diaphragm, check its placement, and remove it may find this method unsatisfactory. It is not recommended for women with a history of urinary tract infection, because pressure from the diaphragm on the urethra may interfere with complete bladder emptying and lead to recurrent urinary tract infections. Women with a history of toxic shock syndrome should not use diaphragms or any of the barrier methods because they are left in place for prolonged periods. For the same reason, the diaphragm should not be used during a menstrual period or if a woman has abnormal vaginal discharge.

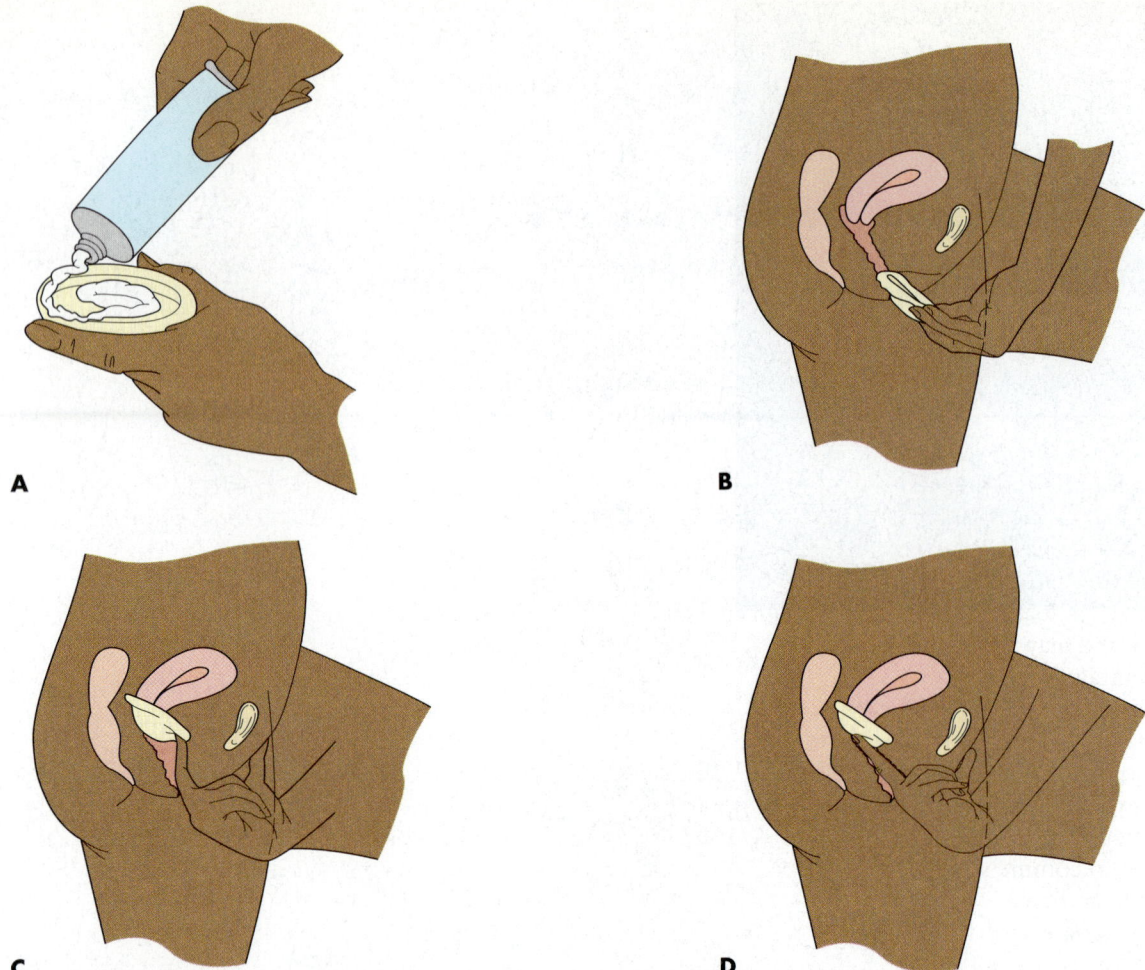

FIGURE 3–4. ◆ Inserting the diaphragm. **A,** Apply jelly to the rim and center of the diaphragm. **B,** Insert the diaphragm. **C,** Push the rim of the diaphragm under the symphysis pubis. **D,** Check placement of the diaphragm. Cervix should be felt through the diaphragm.

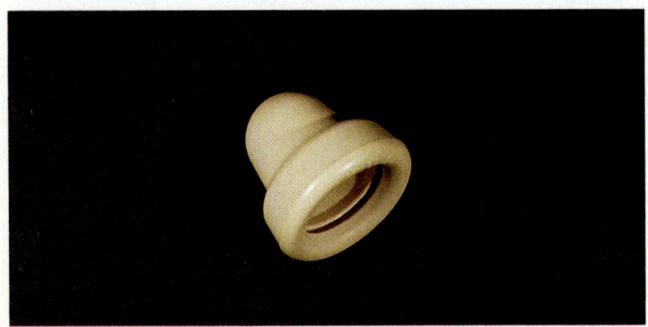

FIGURE 3–5. ◆ A cervical cap.

The **cervical cap** (Figure 3–5◆) is a cup-shaped device, used with spermicidal cream or jelly, that fits snugly over the cervix and is held in place by suction. Effectiveness rates and method of insertion are similar to those for the diaphragm. Unlike the diaphragm, however, the cap may be left in place for up to 48 hours, and it does not require additional spermicide for repeated intercourse (Hatcher et al., 1998). Advantages, disadvantages, and contraindications are similar to those associated with the diaphragm.

The cervical cap may be more difficult to fit because of limited size options. It also tends to be more difficult for women to insert and remove.

INTRAUTERINE DEVICES

The **intrauterine device (IUD)** is designed to be inserted into the uterus by a qualified health care provider and left in place for an extended period, providing continuous contraceptive protection. The exact mechanism of IUD action is not clearly understood. Current evidence on the new generation of IUDs suggests that they truly are contraceptives; they act by altering or inhibiting sperm migration and ovum transport in some way (Chez & Strathman, 1999). The IUD is also known to have local inflammatory effects on the endometrium (Hatcher et al., 1998).

Advantages of the IUD include high rate of effectiveness, continuous contraceptive protection, no coitus-related activity, and relative inexpensiveness over time. Possible adverse reactions to the IUD include discomfort to the wearer, increased bleeding during menses, PID, perforation of the uterus, intermenstrual bleeding, dysmenorrhea, and expulsion of the device.

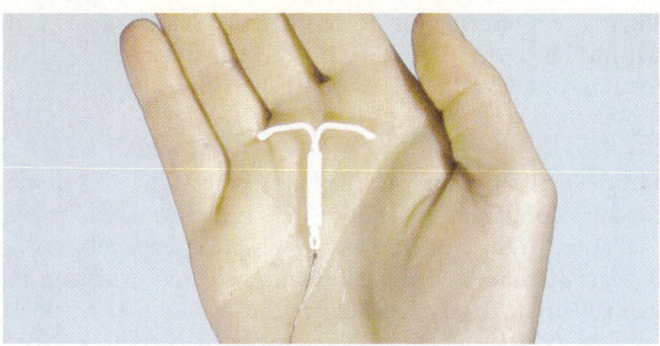

FIGURE 3–6. ◆ The Mirena Intrauterine System, which releases levonorgestrel gradually, may be left in place for up to 5 years. Note: Courtesy of Berlex Laboratories, Inc.

Two IUDs are currently available in the United States (Figure 3–6 ◆ shows the newest type, Mirena). The copper T380A (ParaGard) is highly effective and can be left in place for up to 10 years. The levonorgestrel-releasing intrauterine system (LNG-IUS) (Mirena), which releases a levonorgestrel gradually, is comparable in effectiveness to the copper T and may be left in place for up to 5 years. The primary advantage of the LNG-IUS is that it produces diminished periods or even amenorrhea (Zinger & Thomas, 2001). In fact, 14 to 20% of women have amenorrhea, which they often welcome once they are advised that the absence of menses is safe and not an indication of pregnancy (Grimes, Hanson, & Sondheimer, 2001). In general, IUDs are recommended only for women who have at least one child and are in a monogamous relationship, because these women have the lowest risk of developing a pelvic infection. It is not recommended for women with multiple sexual contacts, because they are at higher risk for sexually transmitted infections.

The IUD is inserted into the uterus with its string or tail protruding through the cervix into the vagina. It may be inserted during a menstrual period or during the 4- to 6-week postpartum check. After insertion, the clinician instructs the woman to check for the presence of the string once a week for the first month and then after each menses. She is told that she may have some cramping or bleeding intermittently for 2 to 6 weeks and that her first few menses may be irregular. Follow-up examination is suggested 4 to 8 weeks after insertion.

Women with IUDs should contact their health care providers if they are exposed to a STI or if they develop the following warning signs: late period, abnormal spotting or bleeding, pain with intercourse, abdominal pain, abnormal discharge, signs of infection (fever, chills, and malaise), or missing string. If the woman becomes pregnant with an IUD in place, the device is generally removed if the string is visible.

Hormonal Contraception

ORAL CONTRACEPTIVES

Oral contraceptives (OCs), also called *birth control pills,* are typically a combination of the hormones estrogen and progesterone. OCs work by inhibiting the release of an ovum and by maintaining cervical mucus that is hostile to sperm. Many OCs are available. The pill is taken daily for 21 days, typically beginning on the Sunday after the first day of the menstrual cycle. In most cases menses occurs 1 to 4 days after the last pill is taken. Seven days after taking her last pill, the woman restarts the pill. Thus the woman always begins the pill on the same day. Some companies offer a 28-day pack with seven "blank" pills so that the woman never stops taking a pill. The pill should be taken at approximately the same time each day—usually upon arising or before retiring in the evening.

Although they are highly effective, OCs may produce side effects ranging from breakthrough bleeding to thrombus formation. Side effects may be either progesterone or estrogen related (Table 3–1). The use of low-dose (35 μg or less estrogen) preparations has reduced many of the side effects; the newer 20-μg pills appear to provide comparable cycle control and have even fewer side effects (Rosenberg, Meyers, & Roy, 1999).

Contraindications to the use of OCs include pregnancy, previous history of thrombophlebitis or thromboembolic disease, acute or chronic liver disease of cholestatic type with abnormal function, presence of estrogen-dependent carcinomas, undiagnosed uterine bleeding, heavy smoking, hypertension, diabetes, and hyperlipidemia. In addition, women with the following conditions who use OCs need to be examined every 3 months: migraine headaches, epilepsy, depression, oligomenorrhea, and amenorrhea. Women who choose this method of contraception should be fully advised of its potential side effects.

TABLE 3–1 Side Effects Associated with Oral Contraceptives

Estrogen Effects	Progestin Effects
Alterations in lipid metabolism	Acne, oily skin
Breast tenderness, engorgement; increased breast size	Breast tenderness; increased breast size
Cerebrovascular accident	Decreased libido
Changes in carbohydrate metabolism	Decreased high-density lipoprotein (HDL) cholesterol levels
Chloasma (Melasma)	Depression
Fluid retention; cyclic weight gain	Fatigue
Headache	Hirsutism
Hepatic adenomas	Increased appetite; weight gain
Hypertension	Increased low-density lipoprotein (LDL) cholesterol levels
Leukorrhea, cervical erosion, ectopia	
Nausea	Oligomenorrhea, amenorrhea
Nervousness, irritability	Pruritus
Telangiectasia	Sebaceous cysts
Thromboembolic complications— thrombophlebitis, pulmonary embolism	

OCs also have some important noncontraceptive benefits. Many women experience relief of uncomfortable menstrual symptoms. Cramps are lessened, flow is decreased, and cycle regularity is increased. Mittelschmerz is eliminated, and the incidence of functional ovarian cysts is decreased. More important, there is a substantial reduction in the incidence of ectopic pregnancy, ovarian cancer, endometrial cancer, iron deficiency anemia, benign breast disease, and hospitalization for PID (Wallach & Grimes, 2000). In addition, OCs are considered a good solution to the physiologic problems some women experience during the perimenopause, and their use in nonsmoking women ages 40 to 45 has quadrupled since 1990 (Speroff, 1998).

The woman using OCs should contact her health care provider if she becomes depressed, becomes jaundiced, develops a breast lump, or experiences any of the following warning signs: severe abdominal pain, severe chest pain or shortness of breath, severe headaches, dizziness, changes in vision (vision loss or blurring), speech problems, or severe leg pain.

Another OC is the progesterone-only pill, also called the *minipill*. It is used primarily by women who have a contraindication to the estrogen component of the combination pills, such as history of thrombophlebitis, but are strongly motivated to use this form of contraception. The major problems with this preparation are amenorrhea or irregular spotting and bleeding patterns.

THE CONTRACEPTIVE PATCH

In late 2001 the U.S. Food and Drug Administration (FDA) approved a new hormonal contraceptive option—the contraceptive patch. The Ortho Evra Transdermal System, which releases a combination of norelgestromin and ethinyl estradiol, is being marketed as an alternative to OCs. The patch is applied to the lower abdomen, buttocks, back, or upper outer arm and is worn continuously for 1 week. This routine is followed for 3 weeks; no patch is applied for the fourth week. During the treatment-free week, the woman menstruates.

The patch is comparable to the pill in effectiveness and side effects. Research does suggest that the patch may be slightly less effective in preventing pregnancy in women who weigh more than 200 lb (90 kg) (American Society for Reproductive Medicine, 2001).

LONG-ACTING HORMONAL CONTRACEPTIVES

Subdermal implants (Norplant) consist of six silastic capsules containing levonorgestrel, a progestin, which are implanted in the woman's arm. They are effective for up to 5 years (Figure 3–7 ◆). Norplant prevents ovulation in most women. It also stimulates the production of thick cervical mucus, which inhibits sperm penetration. Norplant provides effective continuous contraception removed from the act of coitus. Possible side effects include spotting, irregular bleeding or amenorrhea, an increased incidence of ovarian cysts, weight gain, headaches, fluid retention, acne, mood changes, and depression. Women should be advised that the implant may be visible, especially in very slender users, and that it requires a minor surgical procedure to insert and remove the implants. A biodegradable form of implant, currently under development, would eliminate the need for surgical removal.

Two long-term, effective injectable contraceptives are also available: Depo-Provera and Lunelle. Both contraceptives act by suppressing ovulation and are safe, effective, convenient, private, and relatively inexpensive. They also separate birth control from the act of coitus.

Depot-medroxyprogesterone acetate (DMPA) **(Depo-Provera),** a progestin-only contraceptive, provides highly effective birth control for 3 months when given as a single injection of 150 mg. DMPA can safely be given to nursing mothers because it contains no estrogen. DMPA has been associated with decreases in bone mass density, which may be a concern for adolescents and premenopausal women because of the increased risk of osteoporosis. Side effects include menstrual irregularities, headache, weight gain, breast tenderness, and depression. Return of fertility occurs within 10 months of last injection for 50% of women but it may be delayed up to 18 months in a small percentage of women (Kaunitz, 2001).

Lunelle, a combination of medroxyprogesterone acetate and estradiol cypionate (MPA/E$_2$C), is administered

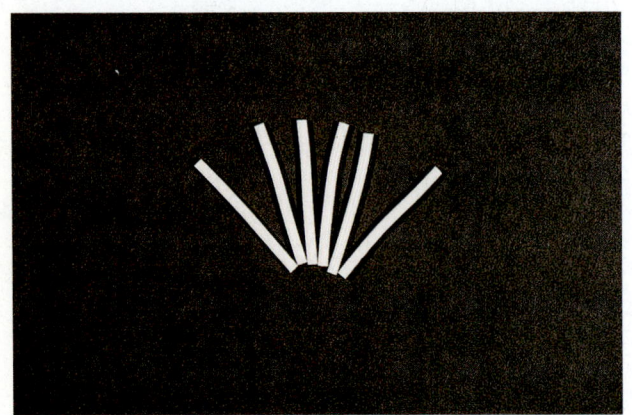

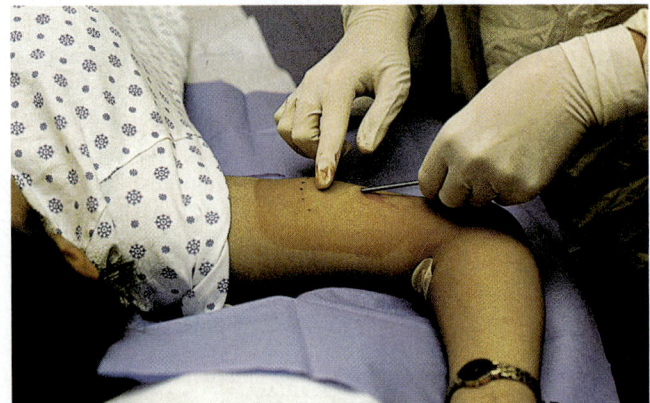

FIGURE 3–7. ◆ **A,** The Norplant system. **B,** Norplant, a long-acting progestin contraceptive, is implanted in a woman's upper arm.

monthly as an intramuscular injection. Women using Lunelle have regular menstrual bleeding patterns and rapid return to fertility when the medication is stopped. Its contraindications and side effects are the same as those of OCs.

Emergency Postcoital Contraception

Emergency contraception is indicated when a woman is worried about pregnancy because of unprotected intercourse or possible contraceptive failure (e.g., broken condom, slipped diaphragm, or too long a time between DMPA injections). Two product kits, Preven (levonorgestrel/ethinyl estradiol) and Plan B (levonorgestrel), are now FDA approved for emergency contraception. Though sometimes called the "morning-after pill," the phrase is misleading because the woman actually takes a dose (two pills with the Preven regimen and one pill with Plan B) as soon after intercourse as possible and a second dose 12 hours later. This regimen must be started within 72 hours after unprotected intercourse; the earlier the treatment is started, the greater the effectiveness. Prior to the development of these two kits, Ovral, a high-estrogen OC, was often used for emergency contraception. The Plan-B regimen is more effective than other emergency contraceptives and has a much lower incidence of associated nausea and vomiting (Grimes, Hanson, & Sondheimer, 2001).

Operative Sterilization

Before sterilization is performed on either partner, the physician provides a thorough explanation of the procedure to both. Each needs to understand that sterilization is not a decision to be taken lightly or entered into when psychologic stresses, such as separation or divorce, exist. Even though both male and female procedures are theoretically reversible, the permanency of the procedure should be stressed and understood.

Male sterilization is achieved through a relatively minor procedure called a **vasectomy.** This procedure involves surgically severing the vas deferens in both sides of the scrotum. Following vasectomy, it takes about 4 to 6 weeks and 6 to 36 ejaculations to clear the remaining sperm from the vas deferens. During that period, the couple is advised to use another method of birth control and to bring in two or three semen samples for a sperm count. The man is rechecked at 6 and 12 months to ensure that fertility has not been restored by recanalization. Side effects of a vasectomy include pain, infection, hematoma, sperm granulomas, and spontaneous reanastomosis (reconnecting).

Vasectomies can sometimes be reversed by using microsurgery techniques. Restored fertility, as measured by subsequent pregnancy, ranges from 30% to 76%, depending primarily on the length of time between vasectomy and reversal (Pollack & Barone, 2000).

Female sterilization is most frequently accomplished by **tubal ligation.** The tubes are located through a small subumbilical incision or by minilaparotomy techniques and are crushed, ligated, electrocoagulated, or banded or plugged (in the newer, reversible procedures). Tubal ligation may be done at any time. However, the postpartal period is an ideal time to perform a tubal ligation because the tubes are somewhat enlarged and easily located.

Complications of female sterilization procedures include coagulation burns on the bowel, bowel perforation, pain, infection, hemorrhage, and adverse anesthesia effects. Reversal of a tubal ligation depends on the type of procedure performed. With microsurgical techniques, a pregnancy rate of 44% to 81% is possible (DeLeon & Peters, 2000).

Male Contraception

The vasectomy and the condom, discussed previously, are currently the only forms of male contraception available in the United States. Hormonal contraception for men has yet to be developed, although studies are under way.

Nursing Management

In most cases, the nurse who provides information and guidance about contraceptive methods works with the woman partner, because most contraceptive methods are female oriented. Since a man can purchase condoms without seeing a health care provider, only with vasectomy does a man require counseling and interaction with a nurse. The nurse can play an important role in helping a woman choose a method of contraception acceptable to her and to her partner.

In addition to completing a history and assessing for any contraindications to specific methods, spend time with a woman learning about her lifestyle, personal attitudes about particular contraceptive methods, religious beliefs, personal biases, and plans for future childbearing, before helping the woman select a particular contraceptive method. Once the method is chosen, help the woman learn to use it effectively. Table 3–2 summarizes factors to consider in choosing an appropriate method of contraception.

TABLE 3–2 Factors to Consider in Choosing a Method of Contraception	
Effectiveness of method in preventing pregnancy	Personal preferences, biases
Safety of the method:	Lifestyle:
Are there inherent risks?	How frequently does client have intercourse?
Does it offer protection against STIs or other conditions?	Does she have multiple partners?
Client's age and future childbearing plans	Does she have ready access to medical care in the event of complications? Is cost a factor?
Any contraindications in client's health history	Partner's support and willingness to cooperate
Religious or moral factors influencing choice	Personal motivation to use method

USING A METHOD OF CONTRACEPTION

- Discuss factors a woman should consider in choosing a method of contraception (see Table 3–2). Note that different methods may be appropriate at different times in a woman's life.
- Review the woman's reasons for choosing a particular method and confirm any contraindications to specific methods.
- Give a step-by-step description of the correct procedure for using the method chosen. Provide opportunities for questions.
- If a technique is to be learned, such as charting BBT or inserting a diaphragm, demonstrate and then have the woman do a return demonstration as appropriate. (Note: If certain aspects are beyond your level of expertise, such as fitting a cervical cap, review the content about its use and confirm that the woman understands what she is to do.)
- Provide information on what the woman should do if unusual circumstances arise (for example, she misses a pill or forgets a morning temperature). These can be presented in a written handout as well.
- Stress warning signs that may require immediate action by the woman and explain why these signs indicate a risk. (These should also be covered in the handout.)
- Arrange to talk with the woman again soon, either by phone or at a return visit, to see if she has any questions or has encountered any problems.

Also review any possible side effects and warning signs related to the method chosen and counsel the woman about what action to take if she suspects she is pregnant. In many cases the nurse is involved in telephone counseling of women who call with questions and concerns about contraception. Thus it is vital to be knowledgeable about this topic and have resources available to find answers to less common questions.

"Teaching About: Using a Method of Contraception" provides guidelines for helping women use a method of contraception effectively.

CLINICAL INTERRUPTION OF PREGNANCY

Although abortion was legalized in the United States in 1973, the associated controversy over moral and legal issues continues. Many people are opposed to abortion for religious, ethical, or personal reasons. Others feel that access to a safe, legal abortion is every woman's right. A number of physical and psychosocial factors influence a woman's decision to seek an abortion. Some situations may involve lack of knowledge about contraceptive options, contraceptive failure, rape, or incest.

Abortion in the first trimester is technically easier and safer than abortion in the second trimester. It may be performed by dilatation and curettage (D&C), minisuction, or vacuum curettage. Second-trimester abortion may be done using dilatation and extraction (D&E), hypertonic saline, systemic prostaglandins, and intrauterine prostaglandins.

Mifepristone (Mifeprex), originally called RU-486, may be used to induce abortion medically during the first 7 weeks of pregnancy (up to 49 days following conception). Mifepristone blocks the action of progesterone, thereby altering the endometrium. After the length of the woman's gestation is confirmed, she takes a dose of mifepristone. Two days later she returns to her caregiver and takes a dose of the prostaglandin misoprostol, which induces contractions that expel the embryo/fetus. About 12 days after taking the misoprostol, the woman is seen a third time to confirm that the abortion was successful.

Nursing Management

Important aspects of nursing care for a woman who decides to have an abortion include providing information about the methods of abortion and associated risks; counseling regarding available alternatives to abortion and their implications; encouraging verbalization by the woman; providing counseling and emotional support before, during, and after the procedure; monitoring vital signs, intake, and output; providing for physical comfort and privacy throughout the procedure; and health teaching about self-care, the importance of the postabortion checkup, and contraception review.

RECOMMENDED GYNECOLOGIC SCREENING PROCEDURES

The accepted standard of care for women today involves regular screening procedures designed to detect potential problems early to permit the most effective treatment. This section focuses on some of the most commonly used screening procedures: breast self-examination and breast examination by a trained health care provider, mammography, Pap smear, and pelvic examination.

Breast Examination

Like the uterus, the breast undergoes regular cyclical changes in response to hormonal stimulation. Each month, in rhythm with the cycle of ovulation, the breasts become engorged with fluid in anticipation of pregnancy, and the woman may experience sensations of tenderness, lumpiness, or pain. If conception does not occur, the accumulated fluid drains away via the lymphatic network. *Mastodynia* (premenstrual swelling and tenderness of the breasts) is common. It usually lasts for 3 to 4 days before the onset of menses, but the symptoms may persist throughout the month.

After menopause, adipose breast tissue atrophies and is replaced by connective tissue. Elasticity is lost, and the breasts may droop and become pendulous. The recurring breast engorgement associated with ovulation ceases. If estrogen replacement therapy is used to counteract other symptoms of menopause, breast engorgement may resume.

Monthly **breast self-examination (BSE)** is the best method for detecting breast masses early. A woman who knows the texture and feel of her own breasts is far more likely to detect changes that develop. Thus it is important for a woman to develop the habit of doing routine BSE as early as possible, preferably as an adolescent. Women at high risk for breast cancer are especially encouraged to be attentive to the importance of early detection through routine BSE.

The effectiveness of BSE is determined by the woman's ability to perform the procedure correctly. She should do a BSE on a regular monthly basis about 1 week after each menstrual period, when the breasts are typically not tender or swollen. After menopause, she should perform BSE on the same day each month (as chosen by the woman). See "Teaching About: Breast Self-Examination."

Clinical breast examination by a trained health care provider, such as a physician, nurse-practitioner, or nurse-midwife, is an essential element of a routine gynecologic

Teaching About

BREAST SELF-EXAMINATION (BSE)

Begin by discussing the risk factors associated with breast cancer and the use of BSE in breast cancer detection. Then describe and demonstrate the correct procedure for BSE.

1. Timing—Instruct the woman to perform BSE on a monthly basis. Be specific based on whether she is premenopausal, pregnant, postmenopausal, or postmenopausal receiving hormone therapy.

2. Inspection—Instruct the woman to inspect her breasts by standing or sitting in front of a mirror. She should inspect them in three positions: both arms relaxed at her sides, both arms raised straight over her head, and both hands placed on her hips while she leans forward (Figure 3–8). In these positions she should do the following:

   • Note size and symmetry of the breasts. Some size difference between breasts is normal. Breasts may vary but the variations should remain constant during rest or movement—note abnormal contours.

• Note shape and direction of breasts. Breasts can be rounded or pendulous with some variation between breasts. Breasts should point slightly laterally.

• Observe for color and venous patterns. Check for redness or inflammation. A blue hue with a marked venous pattern that is focal or unilateral may indicate an area of increased blood supply due to tumor. Symmetric venous patterns are normal.

• Observe for thickening or edema. Skin edema is seen as thickened skin with enlarged pores ("orange peel"). It may indicate blocked lymph drainage due to tumor.

• Note the surface of the skin. Skin dimpling, puckering, or retraction when the hands are pressed together or against the hips suggests malignancy. Straie (stretch marks) are normal.

• Note nipple size, shape, and direction. Long-standing nipple inversion is normal, but an inverted nipple previously capable of erection is suspicious. Note any deviation, flattening, or broadening of the nipples.

• Check for rashes, ulcerations, or discharge.

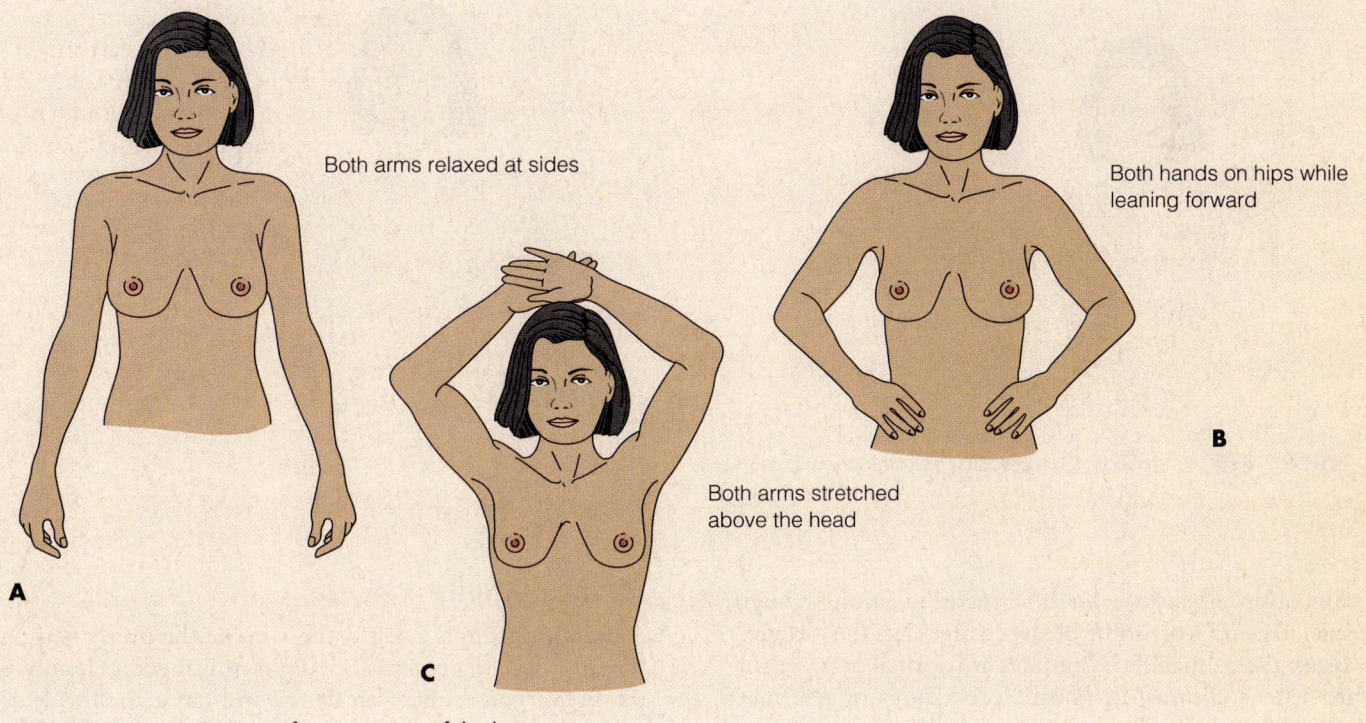

Both arms relaxed at sides

Both hands on hips while leaning forward

Both arms stretched above the head

A

C

B

FIGURE 3–8. ◆ Positions for inspection of the breasts.

(continued)

3. Palpation—Instruct the woman to palpate (feel) her breasts as follows:

- Lie down. Put one hand behind your head. With the other hand, fingers flattened, gently feel your breast. Press lightly (Figure 3–9A).

- Figure 3–9B shows you how to check each breast. Begin as you see in B and follow the arrows, feeling gently for a lump or thickening. Remember to feel all parts of each breast, including the "tail" of tissue near the armpit. Repeat the process on the second breast.

- Now repeat the same process on each breast sitting up, with your hand still behind your head (Figure 3–9C).

- Squeeze the nipple between your thumb and forefinger. Look for any discharge—clear, bloody, or milky (Figure 3–9D).

4. Take the woman's hand and help her identify her "normal bumps" (e.g., mammary ridge, ribs, nodularity in the upper, outer quadrants).

5. Determine whether she has any questions about her findings during this examination. If she has questions, palpate the area and attempt to identify whether it is normal.

6. If a breast model is available, give the woman the opportunity to palpate it and identify the lumps.

7. Provide her with a monthly reminder such as an American Cancer Society shower card.

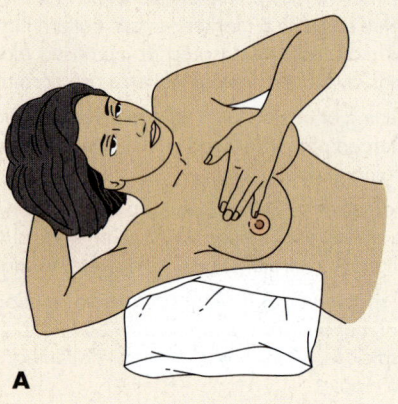

With one hand behind your head, flatten your fingers and press lightly on your breast, feeling gently for a lump or thickening.

A

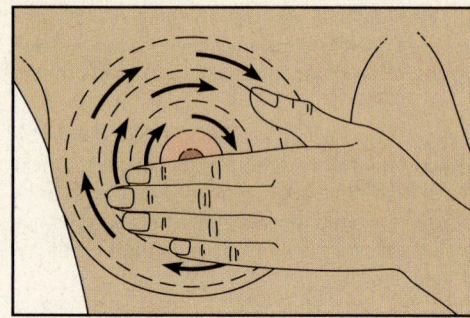

Check each breast in a circular manner, feeling all parts of the breast.

B

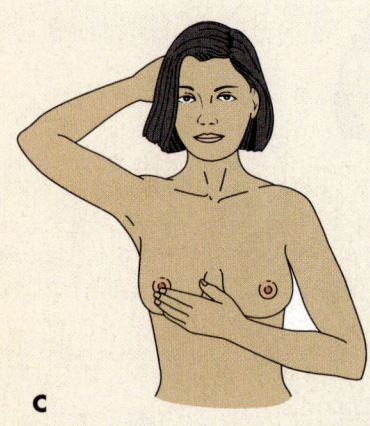

Repeat the same procedure sitting up with your hand still behind your head.

C

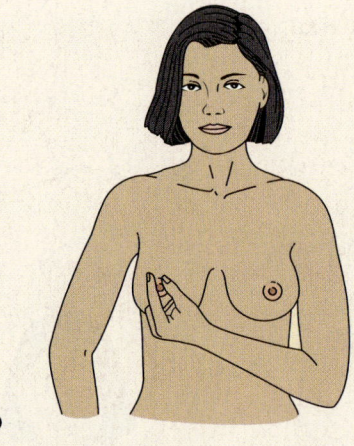

Squeeze your nipple between your thumb and forefinger; look for any clear or bloody discharge.

D

FIGURE 3–9 ◆ Procedure for breast self-examination.

examination. Experience in differentiating among benign, suspicious, and worrisome breast changes lets the caregiver reassure the woman if the findings are normal or move forward with additional diagnostic procedures or referral if the findings are suspicious or worrisome.

Mammography

A **mammogram** is a soft tissue x-ray of the breast without the injection of a contrast medium. It can detect lesions in the breast before they can be felt and has gained wide acceptance as an effective screening tool for breast cancer.

Currently the American Cancer Society recommends that all women age 40 to 49 have a mammorgram every 1 to 2 years; annually for women age 50 and over. The National Cancer Institute recommends mammograms every 1 to 2 years for women ages 40 and older.

Pap Smear and Pelvic Examination

Women who have reached the age of 18 and women, regardless of age, who are or have been sexually active should have a pelvic examination and Pap smear annually. The Papanicolaou test (*Pap smear*) has helped dramatically decrease the incidence of death from cervical cancer. Its purpose is to detect cellular abnormalities by examining a smear containing cells from the cervix and the endocervical canal. A newer test, the *ThinPrep Pap test,* is proving even more effective than the traditional Pap smear in detecting abnormalities. In this test, no slide is prepared. Instead, the cervical cells, gathered in the same way as for the Pap smear, are transferred directly to a vial of preservative fluid, thereby preserving the entire specimen.

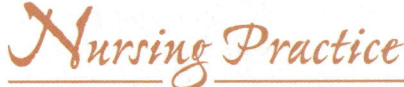

Nursing Practice

Whenever you teach about pelvic examination and Pap smear, be sure the woman understands that she should not douche for at least 24 hours beforehand. Douching can interfere with the accuracy of the Pap smear. Occasionally a caregiver will specifically request that a woman use a douche before a Pap smear; douching should only be done in this circumstance.

For best test results, also advise women to avoid intercourse and the use of other female hygiene products and spermicidal agents immediately before a specimen is obtained. Specimens should not be obtained during menstruation or when visible cervicitis exists.

The pelvic examination lets the health care provider assess a woman's vagina, uterus, ovaries, and lower abdominal area. It is often performed after the Pap smear but may also be performed without a Pap for diagnostic purposes. Women sometimes perceive the pelvic exam as uncomfortable and embarrassing. The negative feelings may cause women to delay having yearly gynecologic examinations, and this avoidance may pose a threat to life and health.

To make the pelvic examination less threatening, and thus improve health-seeking behavior, caregivers can offer the woman a mirror to watch the procedure, point out anatomic parts to her, and position and drape her to allow eye-to-eye contact with the practitioner. Caregivers encourage the woman to participate by asking questions and giving feedback.

Nurse practitioners, certified nurse-midwives, and physicians all perform pelvic examinations. Nurses assist the practitioner and the woman during the examination.

See Skill 2-2: Assisting with a Pelvic Examination in the *Clinical Skills Manual,* as well as the accompanying CD-ROM. SKILLS CD

MENOPAUSE

Menopause, the time when menses cease, is a time of transition for a woman, marking the end of her reproductive abilities. *Perimenopause* is the term applied to the period preceding menopause, usually about 2 to 8 years, when ovarian function wanes and hormonal deficiencies begin to produce syptoms. *Climacteric,* or *change of life* (often used synonymously with menopause), refers to the host of psychologic and physical alterations that occur around the time of menopause. Today the average age at menopause is 51.4 years, and the average life span of a woman in the United States is over 80 years. Thus the average woman will live one third of her life after menopause. A woman's psychologic adaptation to menopause and the climacteric is multifactorial. She is influenced by her own expectations and knowledge, physical well-being, family views, marital stability, and sociocultural expectations. As the number of women reaching menopause increases, the negative emotional connotations society once attached to menopause are diminishing, enabling menopausal women to cope more effectively and even encouraging them to view menopause as a time of personal growth.

The physical characteristics of menopause are linked to the shift from a cyclic to a noncyclic hormonal pattern. The age at onset may be influenced by nutritional, cultural, or genetic factors. The onset of menopause occurs when estrogen levels become so low that menstruation stops.

Generally, ovulation ceases 1 to 2 years before menopause, but individual variations exist. Atrophy of the ovaries occurs gradually. Follicle-stimulating hormone levels rise, and less estrogen is produced. Menopausal symptoms include atrophic changes in the vagina, vulva, and urethra and in the trigonal area of the bladder.

Many menopausal women experience a vasomotor disturbance commonly known as *hot flashes,* a feeling of heat arising from the chest and spreading to the neck and face. The hot flashes are often accompanied by sweating and sleep disturbances. These episodes may occur as often as 20 to 30 times a day and generally last 3 to 5 minutes. Some women also experience dizzy spells, palpitations, and weakness. Many women find their own most effective ways to deal with the hot flashes. Some report that using a fan or drinking a cool liquid helps relieve distress; others seek relief through hormone replacement therapy. In addition, many women use complementary therapies (see later discussion).

The uterine endometrium and myometrium atrophy, as do the cervical glands. The uterine cavity constricts. The fallopian tubes and ovaries atrophy extensively. The vaginal mucosa becomes smooth and thin, and the rugae disappear, leading to loss of elasticity. As a result, intercourse can be painful, but this problem may be overcome by using lubricating gel. Dryness of the mucous membrane can lead to burning and itching. The vaginal pH level increases as the number of Döderlein's bacilli decreases.

Postmenopausal women can still be multiorgasmic. Some women find that their sexual interest and activity improve as the need for contraception disappears and personal growth and awareness increase. Other women experience a decrease in libido at this time. Vulvar atrophy occurs late, and the pubic hair thins, turns gray or white, and may ultimately disappear. The labia shrink and lose their heightened pigmentation. Pelvic fascia and muscles atrophy, resulting in decreased pelvic support. The breasts become pendulous and decrease in size and firmness.

Long-range physical changes may include **osteoporosis,** a decrease in the bony skeletal mass. This change is thought to be associated with lowered estrogen and androgen levels, lack of physical exercise, and a chronic low intake of calcium. Moreover, the estrogen deprivation that occurs in menopausal women may significantly increase their risk of coronary heart disease. Loss of protein from the skin and supportive tissues causes wrinkling. Postmenopausal women frequently gain weight, which may be due to excessive caloric intake or to lower caloric need with the same level of intake.

Clinical Therapy

HORMONE REPLACEMENT THERAPY

Hormone replacement therapy (HRT), usually involving estrogen with or without a progestin, had been controversial for years, but currently the American College of Obstetricians and Gynecologists recommends HRT in menopause. Estrogen replacement is helpful in stopping hot flashes and night sweats and in reversing atrophic vaginal changes. Other benefits of HRT include prevention and treatment of bone loss associated with osteoporosis, improved bladder and vaginal tone, and improved quality of life. It may also offer protection against Alzheimer's disease and colon cancer (McKeon, 2002). Whether HRT increases the incidence of breast cancer is debated, but research suggests an increased risk of breast cancer in women who use HRT that includes progesterone for extended periods of time (Schairer, Lubin, Troisi, et al., 2000). Until recently HRT was thought to provide protection against cardiovascular disease, the leading cause of death in women over age 50. However, recent studies have called this into question (Manson, Shlipak, & Wenger, 2001).

When estrogen is given alone, it can produce endometrial hyperplasia and increase the risk of endometrial cancer. Thus, in women who still have a uterus, estrogen is opposed by giving a progestin, often Provera, for a portion of the cycle. HRT may be given continuously or sequentially. The continuous approach involves the daily administration of estrogen with 2.5 mg progestin. This regimen is associated with less vaginal bleeding and is sufficient to prevent endometrial hyperplasia and osteoporosis; it also retains most of estrogen's beneficial effects on the cardiovascular system (Speroff, 1999). With the sequential approach, estrogen is given the first 25 days of the month, with 5 to 10 mg progestin added during the last 12 days (days 14 to 25). Although most women prefer to take estrogen orally, some choose the transdermal estrogen skin patch. Estrogen may also be given by injection. For women experiencing decreased libido, combination estrogen-testosterone preparations are available.

A thorough history, physical examination including Pap smear, and baseline mammogram are indicated before starting HRT. An initial endometrial biopsy is indicated for women with an increased risk of endometrial cancer; biopsy is also indicated if excessive, unexpected, or prolonged vaginal bleeding occurs. Women taking estrogen should be advised to stop immediately if they develop headaches, visual changes, signs of thrombophlebitis, or chest pain.

ALTERNATIVE AND COMPLEMENTARY THERAPIES

For women who do not wish to take HRT or who have medical contraindications to it, a variety of approaches have been proposed as alternative or complementary treatment or preventive measures for the discomforts of the perimenopausal and postmenopausal years. These include diet and nutrition, specifically a high-fiber, low-fat diet with supplements of vitamins D and E. Phytoestrogens (substances with estrogen properties) can play a significant role in reducing menopausal symptoms; they are found in a number of foods, especially soy products (see "Complementary Care: Phytoestrogens"). About 10% of women have tried herbal remedies such as long quai and black cohosh, which have been used in traditional Chinese medicine for years but have not yet been well studied (Nachtigall, 2000). Weight-bearing exercises such as walking, jogging, tennis, and low-impact aerobics help increase bone mass and decrease the risk of osteoporosis. Exercise also improves cholesterol profiles and contributes to overall health. Stress management and relaxation techniques such as biofeedback, meditation, yoga, visualization, and massage may provide a sense of well-being. Some women also use homeopathic remedies and herbal treatments for symptom relief.

Complementary Care

PHYTOESTROGENS

Phytoestrogens are naturally occurring plant sterols that have an estrogen-like effect. Herbs that contain phytoestrogen include ginseng, agnus castus, beth root, black cohosh, dong quai, fenugreek, licorice, red sage, sarsaparilla, and wild Mexican yam. The phytoestrogens found in these herbs are much weaker than endogenous estrogen, but their biologic activity is equivalent to that of estradiol when the herbs are taken in large amounts (Ansbacher, 2001). Phytoestrogens are also found in soy products such as tofu. Currently, the effectiveness of the herbs and soy are receiving considerable study as more and more women elect to use alternative approaches to treat their menopausal symptoms.

PREVENTION AND TREATMENT OF OSTEOPOROSIS

Osteoporosis is more common in women who are middle-aged or older. Risk factors associated with osteoporosis include white or Asian heritage; small-boned, thin build; family history of osteoporosis; lack of regular exercise; never pregnant; early onset of menopause; consistently low intake of calcium; cigarette smoking; and moderate to heavy alcohol intake.

Pre- or postmenopausal women with four or more risk factors for osteoporosis should have their bone mass measured. Women's height should be measured at each visit, because a loss of height is often an early sign that vertebrae are being compressed because of reduced bone mass. A variety of conditions, including malabsorption syndrome, cancer, cirrhosis of the liver, chronic use of cortisone, and rheumatoid arthritis, can cause secondary arthritis, which resembles osteoporosis. If these causes have been eliminated, treatment for osteoporosis is initiated.

Prevention of osteoporosis is a primary goal of care. Women are advised to maintain an adequate calcium intake. Women over age 50 should have a daily calcium intake of 1200 mg. Most women require supplements to achieve this level. They should also have a daily vitamin D intake of 400 to 800 IU. Women are also advised to participate regularly in exercise, to consume only modest quantities of alcohol and caffeine, and to stop smoking. Alcohol and smoking have a negative effect on the rate of bone resorption.

The effectiveness of estrogen in preventing osteoporosis is well documented. Women showing evidence of bone loss are good candidates for HRT if they have no contraindications to estrogen. For women unable or unwilling to take estrogen, other medications available to treat or help prevent osteoporosis include the following (National Institutes of Health, 2000):

- Alendronate (Fosamax), etidronate (Didronel), and risedronate (Actonel): calcium regulators that act by inhibiting bone resorption and increasing bone mass
- Raloxifene (Evista): one of a new class of drugs called selective estrogen receptor modulators that preserve the beneficial effects of estrogen, including its protection against osteoporosis, but do not stimulate uterine or breast tissue
- Intranasal calcitonin: a calcium regulator that may inhibit bone loss; its value is less clear than that of the other medications listed.

Nursing Management

Most menopausal women deal well with this developmental phase of life, although some women may need counseling to adjust successfully. Nurses and other health professionals can help menopausal women achieve high-level functioning at this time in life. Of major importance is the nurse's ability to understand and provide support for the woman's views and feelings. Use an empathic approach in counseling, health teaching, and providing physical care.

Explore the question of the woman's comfort during sexual intercourse. In counseling, it may be appropriate to say, "After menopause many women notice that their vagina seems dryer and intercourse can be uncomfortable. Have you noticed any changes?" This gives the woman information and may open discussion. Then go on to explain that dryness and shrinking of the vagina can be addressed by use of a water-soluble jelly. Use of estrogen, orally or in vaginal creams, may also be indicated. Increased frequency of intercourse will maintain some elasticity in the vagina. When assessing the menopausal woman, address the question of sexual activity openly but tactfully, because the woman may have been socialized to be reticent in discussing sex.

The crucial need of women in the perimenopausal period of life is for adequate information about the changes taking place in their bodies and their lives. Supplying that information provides both a challenge and an opportunity for nurses.

VIOLENCE AGAINST WOMEN

Violence against women is a major health concern, one that costs the health care system millions of dollars and thousands of lives. Violence affects women of all ages, races, ethnic backgrounds, socioeconomic levels, educational levels, and walks of life. Two of the most common forms of violence are intimate partner abuse and rape. Even today, society not only accepts these forms of violence against women but also shifts the blame for the violence to the women themselves by asking questions such as, "How did she make him so mad?" "Why does she stay?" "What was she doing out so late?" and "Why did she dress that way?"

Female Partner Abuse

Intimate partner abuse can be defined as collective methods used to exert power and control by one individual over another in an adult domestic or intimate relationship. Gay men, heterosexual women, and lesbian women batter, but most abusers are male, and the overwhelming majority of victims are women (Gantt & Bickford, 1999). Consequently, we use the term **female partner abuse** in discussing this serious health problem.

Female partner abuse is the most common form of violence in the United States but the least reported serious crime. Research suggests that 18% to 25% of women treated in emergency departments and almost one fourth of women seeking prenatal care are victims of violence (Valente, 2000). Worldwide, as many as one in three women will be the victim of violence or sexual coercion at some point in her life (State of the World Population, 2000).

The woman may or may not be married to her abuser. She may be living with, dating, or divorced from him. Female partner abuse takes many forms, including verbal attacks, insults, intimidation, threats, emotional abuse, social isolation, economic deprivation, intellectual derision, ridicule, stalking, and physical attacks and injury. Physical battering includes slapping, kicking, shoving, punching, forms of torture, attacks with objects or weapons, and sexual assault. Women who are physically abused can also suffer psychologic and emotional abuse.

CYCLE OF VIOLENCE

In an effort to explain the experience of battered women, Walker (1984) developed the theory of the *cycle of violence.* Battering takes place in a cyclic fashion through three phases:

1. In the *tension-building phase,* the batterer demonstrates power and control. This phase is characterized by anger, arguing, blaming the woman for external problems, and possibly minor battering incidents. The woman may blame herself and believe she can prevent the escalation of the batterer's anger by her own actions.

2. The *acute battering incident* is typically triggered by some external event or internal state of the batterer. It is an episode of acute violence distinguished by lack of control, lack of predictability, and major destructiveness. The cycle of violence can be interrupted before the acute battering incident if proper interventions take place.

3. The *tranquil, loving phase* is sometimes termed the honeymoon period. This phase may be characterized by extremely kind and loving behavior on the part of the batterer as he tries to make up with the woman, or it may simply be manifested as an absence of tension and violence. Without intervention, this phase will end and the cycle of violence will continue. Over time the violence increases in severity and frequency.

CHARACTERISTICS OF BATTERED WOMEN

Battered women often hold traditional views of sex roles. Many were raised to be submissive, passive, and dependent and to seek approval from male figures. Some battered women were exposed to violence between their parents, whereas others first experienced it from their partners. Many battered women do not work outside the home. As part of the manipulation of batterers, they are isolated from family and friends and totally dependent on their partners for their financial and emotional needs.

Battered women may attribute their beatings to some personal shortcoming or inadequacy. Many believe their batterers' insults and accusations that they are bad wives or partners and negligent mothers. As these women become more isolated, they find it harder to judge who is right. Eventually they fully believe in their inadequacy, and their low self-esteem reinforces their belief that they deserve to be beaten. Battered women often feel a pervasive sense of guilt, fear, and depression. Their sense of hopelessness and helplessness reduces their problem-solving ability. Some women develop a pattern of behavior termed *learned helplessness,* in which the unknown becomes terrifying. Learned helplessness often plays a role in a woman's

decision to stay in a known, though abusive, situation rather than leave and face the unknown. Some researchers suggest that a theory of survivorship better describes the behavior of many women who experience abuse. These women actively seek help and have found creative ways to survive in a relationship when help is not forthcoming (Poirier, 1997).

CHARACTERISTICS OF BATTERERS

Batterers come from all backgrounds. They often have feelings of insecurity, socioeconomic inferiority, powerlessness, and helplessness that conflict with their assumptions of male supremacy. Emotionally immature and aggressive men have a tendency to express these overwhelming feelings of inadequacy through violence. Many batterers feel undeserving of their partners, yet they blame and punish the very women they value.

Battered women often describe their husbands or partners as lacking respect toward women in general, having come from homes where they witnessed abuse of their mothers or were themselves abused as children, and having a hidden rage that erupts occasionally. Batterers accept traditional macho values, yet when they are not angry or aggressive, they appear childlike, dependent, seductive, manipulative, and in need of nurturing. They may be well respected in the community. This dual personality of batterers reflects the conflict between their belief that they must live up to their macho image and their feelings of inadequacy in the role of husband or provider. Combined with low frustration tolerance and poor impulse control, their pervasive sense of powerlessness leads them to strike out at life's inequities by abusing women.

NURSING MANAGEMENT

Nurses often come in contact with abused women but fail to recognize them, especially if their bruises are not visible. Women at high risk for battering often have a history of alcohol or drug abuse, child abuse, or abuse in the previous or present relationship. Other possible signs of abuse include expressions of helplessness and powerlessness; low self-esteem revealed by the woman's dress, appearance, and the way she relates to health care providers; signs of depression evidenced by fatigue, hopelessness, and somatic problems such as headache, insomnia, chest pain, back pain, or pelvic pain; and possible suicide attempts. In addition, the abused woman may have a history of missed or frequently changed appointments, perhaps because she had signs of abuse that kept her from coming in or because her partner prevented it.

Because female partner abuse is so prevalent, many caregivers now advocate *universal screening of all female clients at every health encounter.* Screening should be done privately, with only the caregiver and client present, in a safe and quiet place. Specific language leads to higher disclosure rates. Possible screening questions include the following (American College of Obstetricians and Gynecologists [ACOG], 1999a):

1. Has your partner or anyone close to you ever threatened to hurt you?

2. During the past year, have you been kicked, hit, choked, or hurt physically?

3. Has your partner or anyone else ever forced you to have sex?

During the screening, assure the woman that her privacy will be respected. It is essential to remain nonjudgmental; create a warm, caring climate conducive to sharing; and demonstrate a willingness to talk about violence. A battered woman often interprets the nurse's willingness to discuss violence as permission for her to discuss it as well.

When a woman seeks care for an injury, be alert to the following cues of abuse:

- Hesitation in providing detailed information about the injury and how it occurred

- Inappropriate affect for the situation

- Delayed reporting of symptoms

- Pattern of injury consistent with abuse, including multiple injury sites involving bruises, abrasions, and contusions to the head (eyes and back of the neck), throat, chest, abdomen, or genitals

- Inappropriate explanation for the injuries

- Lack of eye contact

- Signs of increased anxiety in the presence of the possible batterer, who frequently does much of the talking

When a battered woman comes in for treatment, she needs to feel safe physically and secure in talking about her injuries and problems. If a man is with her, ask or tell him to remain in the waiting room while the woman is examined. A battered woman also needs to regain a sense of predictability by knowing what to expect and how she can interact. Provide sufficient information about what to expect in terms the woman can understand.

In providing care, let the woman work through her story, problems, and situation at her own pace. Reassure the woman that she is believed. Anticipate the woman's ambivalence (due to her fear and possible love-hate relationship with her batterer), but also respect the woman's capacity to change and grow when she is ready. The woman may need help identifying specific problems and developing realistic ideas for reducing or eliminating those problems. In all interactions, stress that no one should be abused and that the abuse is not the woman's fault.

Nursing Care in the Community.   The nurse should inform any woman suspected of being in an abusive situation of the services available in the community. A battered woman may need the following:

- Medical treatment for injuries

- Temporary shelter to provide a safe environment for her and her children

- Counseling to raise her self-esteem and help her understand the dynamics of violence

- Legal assistance for a restraining order, protection, and/or prosecution

- Financial assistance to obtain shelter, food, and clothing

- Job training or employment counseling

- An ongoing support group with counseling

If the woman returns to an abusive situation, encourage her to develop an exit plan for herself and her children, if any. As part of the plan, she should pack a change of clothing for herself and her children, including toiletries and an extra set of car and house keys. She should store these items away from the house with a friend or relative. If possible she should have money, identification papers (driver's license, social security card, and birth certificates for herself and her children), checkbook, savings account information, other financial information (such as mortgage papers, automobile papers, and pay stubs), court papers or orders, and information about the children to help her enroll them in school. She should also plan where she will go, regardless of the time of day. Ensure that the woman has a planned escape route and emergency telephone numbers she can call, including local police, a phone hotline, and a women's shelter if one is available in the community.

Working with battered women is challenging, and many health care providers feel frustrated and impotent when the women repeatedly return to their abusive situations without developing sufficient ego strength or coping abilities. On average, women leave their battering situation seven times before they stay away permanently. Nurses must realize that they cannot rescue battered women; battered women must decide on their own how to handle their situations. Effective nurses provide battered women with information that empowers them in decision making and supports their decisions, knowing that incremental assistance over the years may be the only alternative until the battered women are ready to explore other options.

Sexual Assault and Rape

Broadly, **sexual assault** is involuntary sexual contact with another person. The National Crime Victimization Survey defines **rape** as forced sexual intercourse, including both physical force as well as psychologic coercion. Forms of forced sexual intercourse include vaginal, anal, or oral penetration by the offender(s) (Rape, Abuse, and Incest National Network [RAINN], 2001). Sexual assault is one of the most underreported violent crimes in the United States. Estimates suggest that, somewhere in the United States, a woman is sexually assaulted every 2 minutes (RAINN, 2001).

Sexual assault is an act of violence expressed sexually—most commonly, a man's aggression and rage acted out against a woman. The person who commits a sexual assault may be an acquaintance, spouse, other relative, employer, or stranger. In 2000, 62% of reported rapes or assaults were committed by someone known to the victim (Rennison, 2001). No woman of any age or ethnicity is immune, but statistics indicate that young, unmarried women, women who have a low family income, and students have the highest incidence of sexual assault or attempted assault.

Assault is traumatic for any woman, regardless of her age. However, adolescent survivors of sexual assault are often reluctant to report the assault because of embarrassment, feelings of guilt, fear of retribution, lack of knowledge of their legal rights, concerns about confidentiality, lack of funds, and limited access to health care. Young adolescents may also avoid disclosing an assault to authorities because they may be worried about revealing the circumstances, especially if they involved risk-taking behaviors such as underage drinking, drug use, accepting a ride from a stranger, or socializing with older men (Holmes, 1998).

Like their victims, the assailants come from all ethnic backgrounds and walks of life. More than half are under age 25, and three out of five are married and leading "normal" sex lives. Why do men rape? Of the many theories put forth, none provides a completely satisfactory explanation. So few assailants are actually caught and convicted that a clear characteristic of the assailant has not been developed. However, rapists tend to be emotionally weak and insecure and may have difficulty maintaining interpersonal relationships. Many assailants also have trouble dealing with the stresses of daily life. Such men may become angry and overcome by feelings of powerlessness. They then commit a sexual assault as an expression of power or anger.

One type of sexual assault, *date rape* (a form of acquaintance rape), is an increasing problem on high school and college campuses. In some cases an assailant uses alcohol or other drugs to sedate his intended victim. One drug, flunitrazepam (Rohypnol) has gained notoriety as a date rape drug because it frequently produces amnesia in its victims.

RESPONSES TO SEXUAL ASSAULT

Sexual assault is a *situational crisis*. It is a traumatic event that the victim cannot be prepared to handle because it is unforeseen. Following an assault, the victim generally experiences a cluster of symptoms, described by Burgess and Holmstrom (1979) as the *rape trauma syndrome*, which last far beyond the rape itself. These phases are described in Table 3–3. Although the phases of response are listed individually, they often overlap, and individual responses and their duration may vary. A fourth phase—integration and recovery—has also been suggested (Holmes, 1998).

Research also suggests that survivors of sexual assault may exhibit high levels of posttraumatic stress disorder, the same disorder that developed in many of the veterans of the Vietnam War. Posttraumatic stress disorder is marked by varying degrees of intensity. Assault victims with this disorder often require lengthy, intensive therapy to regain a sense of trust and feeling of personal control.

CARE OF THE SEXUAL ASSAULT SURVIVOR

Survivors of sexual assault often enter the health care system by way of the emergency room. Thus the emergency room nurse is often the first person to counsel them. Because the values, attitudes, and beliefs of the caregiver necessarily affect the competence and focus of the care, it is essential that nurses clearly understand their feelings about sexual assault and assault survivors and resolve any conflicts that may exist. In many communities, specially trained sexual assault nurse examiner (SANE) nurses coordinate the care of survivors of sexual assault, gather necessary forensic evidence, and are then available as expert witnesses when assailants are tried for the crime.

The first priority in caring for a survivor of a sexual assault is to create a safe, secure milieu. Admission information is gathered in a quiet, private room. The woman should be reassured that she is safe and not alone. The nurse assesses the survivor's appearance, demeanor, and ways of communicating for the purpose of planning care. Initially, the woman is evaluated to determine the need for emergency care. Obtaining a careful, detailed history is essential. After the woman has received any necessary emergency care, a forensic chart and kit are completed.

The woman is given a thorough explanation of the procedures to be carried out and signs a consent form for the forensic examination and collection of materials. Sexual

TABLE 3–3   Phases of Recovery Following Sexual Assault

Phase	Response
Acute Phase (Disorganization)	Fear, shock, disbelief, desire for revenge, anger, anxiety, guilt, denial, embarrassment, humiliation, helplessness, dependence, self-blame, wide variety of physical reactions, lost or distorted coping mechanisms
Outward Adjustment Phase (Denial)	Survivor appears outwardly composed, denying and repressing feelings (e.g., she returns to work, buys a weapon); refuses to discuss the assault; denies need for counseling
Reorganization	Survivor makes many life adjustments, such as moving to a new residence or changing her phone number; uses emotional distancing; may engage in risky sexual behaviors; may experience sexual dysfunction, phobias, flashbacks, sleep disorders, nightmares, anxiety; has a strong urge to talk about or resolve feelings; may seek counseling or remain silent
Integration and Recovery	Time of resolution; survivor begins to feel safe and be comfortable trusting others; places blame on assailant; may become an advocate for others

assault kits contain all the necessary supplies for collecting and labeling evidence. The woman's clothing is collected and bagged, swabs of stains and secretions are taken, hair samples and any fingernail scrapings are collected, blood samples are drawn, tissue swabs are obtained, and photographs are taken. Vaginal and rectal examinations are performed, along with a complete physical examination for trauma. The woman is offered prophylactic treatment for sexually transmitted infections. The woman is also questioned about her menstrual cycle and contraceptive practices. If she could become pregnant as a result of the rape, she is offered postcoital contraceptive therapy.

Throughout the experience the nurse acts as the sexual assault survivor's advocate, providing support without usurping decision making. The nurse need not agree with all the survivor's decisions but should respect and defend her right to make them.

The family members and friends on whom the survivor calls also need nursing care. Like those of the survivor, the reactions of the family will depend on the values to which they ascribe. Many families or mates blame the survivor for the assault and feel angry with her for not having been more careful. They may also incorrectly view the assault as a sexual act rather than an act of violence. They may feel personally wronged and see the survivor as devalued or unclean. Their reactions may compound the survivor's crisis. By spending some time with family members before their first interaction with the survivor, the nurse can perhaps reduce their anxiety and absorb some of their frustrations, sparing the woman further trauma.

Sexual assault counseling, provided by qualified nurses or other counselors, is a valuable tool in helping the survivor come to terms with her assault and its impact on her life. In counseling, the woman is encouraged to explore and identify her feelings and determine appropriate actions to resolve her problems and concerns. The counselor must avoid reinforcing the prevalent myth that the assault was somehow the woman's fault. The fault lies with the assailant. The counselor also plays an important role in emphasizing that the loss of control the woman experienced during the rape was temporary and that the woman can regain a feeling of control over life.

PROSECUTION OF THE ASSAILANT

Legally, sexual assault is considered a crime against the state, and prosecution of the assailant is a community responsibility. The survivor, however, must begin the process by reporting the assault and pressing charges against her assailant. In the past, the police and the judicial system were notoriously insensitive in dealing with survivors. However, many communities now have classes designed to help officers work effectively with sexual assault survivors or have special teams to carry out this important task.

Many women who have sought to use the judicial process have had such a traumatic experience that they refer to it as a second assault. The woman may be asked repeatedly to describe the experience in intimate detail, and her reputation and testimony may be attacked by the defense attorney. In addition, publicity may intensify her feelings of humiliation, and, if her assailant is released on bail or found not guilty, she may fear retaliation.

The nurse acting as a counselor needs to be aware of the judicial sequence to anticipate rising tension and frustration in the survivor and her support system. The woman needs consistent, effective support at this crucial time.

CARE OF THE WOMAN WITH A BENIGN DISORDER OF THE BREAST

Throughout her lifetime a woman may experience a variety of breast disorders. Some, like mastitis, are acute disorders, whereas others, such as fibrocystic breast disease, are chronic. This section deals with some common breast disorders a woman may encounter. For information on breast cancer, consult a medical-surgical nursing textbook.

Fibrocystic Breast Disease

Fibrocystic breast disease, the most common of the benign breast disorders, is most prevalent in women 30 to 50 years of age. Only women whose fibrocystic breast disease is accompanied by certain histologic changes (usually found incidentally when a biopsy is done) have an increased risk of developing cancer. Fibrosis is a thickening of the normal breast tissue. Cyst formation that may accompany fibrosis is considered a later change in the condition. Fibrocystic breast disease is probably caused by an imbalance in estrogen and progesterone that distorts the normal changes of the menstrual cycle. The symptoms often increase as the woman approaches menopause and generally decrease after menopause. However, if a postmenopausal woman is treated with HRT, the cyclic breast changes may resume.

The woman often reports pain, tenderness, and swelling that occur cyclically and are most pronounced just before menses. Physical examination may reveal only mild signs of irregularity, or the breasts may feel dense, with areas of irregularity and nodularity. Women often refer to this irregularity as "lumpiness." Some women may also have expressible nipple discharge. Although unilateral discharge and serosanguineous discharge are the most worrisome findings, all breast discharge should be investigated further.

If the woman has a large, fluid-filled cyst, she may experience a localized painful area as the capsule containing the accumulated fluid distends coincident with her cycle. However, if small cysts form, the woman may experience not a solitary tender lump but a diffuse tenderness. A cyst may often be differentiated from a malignancy because a cyst is more mobile and tender and is not associated with skin retraction (pulling) in the surrounding tissue.

Mammography, sonography, palpation, and fine-needle aspiration are used to confirm fibrocystic breast disease. Often, fine-needle aspiration is the treatment as well, affording relief from the tenderness or pain. Treatment of palpable cysts is conservative; invasive procedures such as biopsy are used only if the diagnosis is questionable.

Women with mild symptoms may benefit from restricting sodium intake and taking a mild diuretic during the week before the onset of menses. This counteracts fluid retention, relieves pressure in the breast, and helps decrease the pain. In other cases, a mild analgesic is necessary. Other treatment approaches include the use of thiamine and vitamin E. In severe cases, the hormone inhibitor danazol is the drug of choice.

Some researchers suggest that methylxanthines (found in caffeine products, such as coffee, tea, colas, and chocolate, and in some medications) may contribute to the development of fibrocystic breast changes and that limiting intake of these substances will help decrease fibrocystic changes. Other research fails to demonstrate a clear association between methylxanthines and fibrocystic breast changes. Additional medical therapies that are helpful in varying degrees include OCs, progestins, and bromocriptine. All work on the principle of estrogen suppression and progesterone stimulation or augmentation.

Other Benign Breast Disorders

Fibroadenoma is a common benign tumor seen in women in their teens and early twenties. It has not been significantly associated with breast cancer. Fibroadenomas are freely movable, solid tumors that are well defined, sharply delineated, and rounded, with a rubbery texture. They are asymptomatic and nontender.

If there are any disquieting features to the appearance of a lump, fine-needle biopsy or excision of the mass may be indicated. Caution is exercised when deciding on biopsy because excision of the mass in a young girl may interfere with normal breast development. Watchful observation and possible surgical excision are the only treatments for fibroadenomas. Surgery is often deferred, but when advisable, it ends the treatment.

Intraductal papillomas, most often occurring during the menopausal years, are tumors growing in the terminal portion of a duct or, sometimes, throughout the duct system within a section of the breast. They are typically benign but have the potential to become malignant. Although relatively uncommon, they are the most frequent cause of nipple discharge in women who are not pregnant or lactating.

The majority of papillomas present as solitary nodules. These small, ball-like lesions may be detected on mammography but often are nonpalpable. A papilloma is often frightening to the woman, because her primary symptom is a discharge from the nipple that may be serosanguineous or brownish green due to old blood. The location of the papilloma within the duct system and its pattern of growth determine whether nipple discharge will be present.

If the woman reports a nipple discharge, the breast should be milked to obtain fluid. The fluid obtained is sent

for a Pap smear. The diagnosis is confirmed if papilloma cells are present. The lesion must be excised and histologically examined because of the difficulty in differentiating between a benign papilloma and a papillary carcinoma. Treatment for benign intraductal papilloma is excision with follow-up care.

Duct ectasis (comedomastitis), an inflammation of the ducts behind the nipple, commonly occurs during or near the onset of menopause and is not associated with malignancy. The condition typically occurs in women who have borne and nursed children. It is characterized by a thick, sticky nipple discharge and by burning pain, pruritus, and inflammation. Nipple retraction may also be noted, especially in postmenopausal women. Treatment is conservative, with drug therapy aimed at symptomatic relief. The major central ducts of the breast occasionally have to be excised.

Nursing Management

Nursing Assessment and Diagnosis

During the period of diagnosis of any breast disorder, the woman may be anxious about a possible change in body image or a diagnosis of cancer. Use therapeutic communication to assess the significance the woman places on her breasts; her current emotional status, coping mechanisms used during periods of stress, and knowledge and beliefs about cancer; and other variables that may influence her coping and adjustment.

Nursing diagnoses that may apply to a woman with a benign disorder of the breast include the following:

▶ *Health-seeking behaviors:* information about diagnostic procedures related to an expressed desire to understand procedures

▶ *Anxiety* related to threat to body image

Planning and Implementation

During the prediagnosis period, clarify misconceptions and encourage the woman to express her anxiety. Once a diagnosis is made, ensure that the woman understands her condition, its association to breast malignancy, and the treatment options. Also point out that frequent professional breast examinations and regular mammograms help detect any abnormalities and that the woman who practices monthly BSE, follows her caregiver's advice, and is examined regularly has taken action to protect her health.

Evaluation

Expected outcomes of nursing care include the following:

▶ The woman is able to discuss her fears, concerns, and questions during the period of diagnosis.

▶ The diagnosis is made quickly and accurately.

CARE OF THE WOMAN WITH ENDOMETRIOSIS

Endometriosis, a condition characterized by the presence of endometrial tissue outside the endometrial cavity, occurs in about 5% to 10% of premenopausal women (Esposito, Tureck, & Mastroianni, 1999). Endometriosis has been found almost everywhere in the body, including the vagina, lungs, cervix, central nervous system, and gastrointestinal tract. The most common location, however, is the pelvis. This tissue responds to the hormonal changes of the menstrual cycle and bleeds in a cyclic fashion. The bleeding results in inflammation, scarring of the peritoneum, and formation of adhesions.

Endometriosis may occur at any age after puberty, but is most common in women between ages 30 and 40. The exact cause of endometriosis is unknown. Leading theories include retrograde menstrual flow and inflammation of the endometrium, hereditary tendency, and a possible immunologic defect.

The most common symptom of endometriosis is pelvic pain, which is often dull or cramping. Usually the pain is related to menstruation and is thought to be dysmenorrhea by the affected woman. **Dyspareunia** (painful intercourse) and abnormal uterine bleeding are other common signs. The condition is often diagnosed when the woman seeks evaluation for infertility. Bimanual examination may reveal a fixed, tender, retroverted uterus and palpable nodules in the cul-de-sac. Diagnosis is confirmed by laparoscopy. However, to avoid the need for diagnostic surgery, in some cases medical therapy may be instituted based on signs and symptoms and careful pretreatment evaluation (ACOG, 1999b).

Treatment may be medical, surgical, or a combination of the two. During a laparoscopic examination to confirm the diagnosis, any visible implants of endometrial tissue are removed using excision, endocoagulation, electrocautery, or laser vaporization (ACOG, 1999b). Surgery is very effective in relieving pain symptoms, at least for a time. In women with minimal disease and symptoms, treatment includes observation, analgesics, and nonsteroidal antiinflammatory drugs. If the woman does not currently desire pregnancy, she may be started on a combined OC. OCs create a pseudopregnancy state with decreased menstrual bleeding. If OCs do not relieve symptoms, therapy with medroxyprogesterone acetate (MPA), danazol, or a gonadotropin-releasing hormone (GnRH) agonist may be indicated.

MPA causes endometrial tissue to atrophy, thereby decreasing symptoms. It may be taken orally daily or given intramuscularly every 1 to 3 months. Side effects include weight gain, bloating, acne, headaches, emotional lability, and irregular bleeding (Propst & Laufer, 1999).

Danazol is a testosterone derivative that suppresses GnRH and has high-androgen and low-estrogen effects that inhibit the growth of the endometrium. It suppresses ovulation and causes amenorrhea. Danazol has some significant side effects, however, including hirsutism, vaginal bleeding, acne, oily skin, weight gain, reduced libido, voice changes and hoarseness, clitoral enlargement, and decreased breast size.

GnRH agonists such as nafarelin acetate (given as a metered nasal spray twice daily) and leuprolide acetate (Lupron) (given once a month as an intramuscular injection) are gaining popularity because many women tolerate them better than danazol and their results in treating endometriosis are comparable. GnRH agonists suppress the menstrual cycle through estrogen antagonism. This may result in the hypoestrogen side effects of hot flashes, vaginal dryness, decreased libido, and loss of bone density (Kim & Adamson, 2000).

In more advanced cases, surgery may be done to remove endometrial implants and break up adhesions. If severe dyspareunia or dysmenorrhea are symptoms, the surgeon may perform a presacral neurectomy. In advanced cases in which childbearing is not an issue, treatment may be a hysterectomy with bilateral salpingo-oophorectomy.

Nursing Management

Nursing Assessment and Diagnosis

The nurse needs to know the symptoms of endometriosis and elicit an accurate history. If a woman is being treated for endometriosis, assess the woman's understanding of the condition, its implications, and the treatment alternatives.

Nursing diagnoses that may apply to a woman with endometriosis include the following:

▶ *Pain* related to peritoneal irritation secondary to endometriosis

▶ *Ineffective individual coping* related to depression secondary to infertility

Planning and Implementation

Be available to explain the condition, its symptoms, treatment alternatives, and prognosis. Help the woman evaluate treatment options and make appropriate choices. If medication is begun, review the dosage, schedule, possible side effects, and any warning signs. A woman with endometriosis is often advised to avoid delaying pregnancy because of the risk of infertility. The woman may wish to discuss the implications of this decision on her life choices, relationship with her partner, and personal preferences. Be a nonjudgmental listener and help the woman consider her options.

Evaluation

Expected outcomes of nursing care include the following:

▶ The woman is able to discuss her condition, its implications for fertility, and her treatment options.

▶ After considering the alternatives, the woman chooses appropriate treatment options.

CARE OF THE WOMAN WITH TOXIC SHOCK SYNDROME

Toxic shock syndrome (TSS) is primarily a disease of women at or near menses or during the postpartum period. The causative organism is *Staphylococcus aureus*. The use of superabsorbent tampons was once related to an increased incidence of TSS. That incidence has declined. Occluding the cervical os with a contraceptive device such as a diaphragm or cervical cap during menses may also increase the risk of TSS (McGregor, 2000).

Early diagnosis and treatment are important in preventing death. The most common signs of TSS include fever (often greater than 38.9 °C [102 °F]); desquamation of the skin, especially the palms and soles; rash; hypotension; and dizziness. Systemic symptoms often include vomiting, diarrhea, severe myalgia, and inflamed mucous membranes (oropharyngeal, conjunctival, or vaginal). Disorders of the central nervous system, including alterations in consciousness, disorientation, and coma, may also occur.

Women with TSS are generally hospitalized and given supportive therapy, including intravenous fluids to maintain blood pressure. Severe cases may require renal dialysis, administration of vasopressors, and intubation. Broad-spectrum antibiotic therapy (including antistaphylococcal agents) is initiated immediately until septisemia is excluded as a diagnosis; antibiotic therapy also reduces the risk of recurrence (McGregor, 2000).

Nursing Management

Nurses play a major role in helping educate women about preventing the development of TSS. It is crucial that women understand the importance of avoiding prolonged use of tampons. Women who choose to continue using tampons may reduce their risk of TSS by alternating them with napkins and avoiding overnight use of tampons. Postpartal women should avoid the use of tampons for 6 to 8 weeks after childbirth. Women who use diaphragms or cervical caps should not leave them in place for prolonged periods and should not use them during the postpartum period or when they are menstruating. Also, help make women aware of the signs and symptoms of TSS so that they will seek treatment promptly if symptoms occur.

CARE OF THE WOMAN WITH VULVOVAGINAL CANDIDIASIS

Vulvovaginal candidiasis (VVC), also called moniliasis or yeast infection, is the most common form of vaginitis affecting the vagina and vulva. *Candida albicans* is responsible for most vaginal yeast infections. Factors that contribute to VVC are the use of OCs, use of antibiotics, frequent douching, pregnancy, diabetes mellitus, and use of immunosuppressants.

The woman with VVC often complains of thick, curdy vaginal discharge, severe itching, dysuria, and dyspareunia. A male sexual partner may experience a rash or excoriation of the skin of the penis and possibly pruritus. The male may be symptomatic and the female asymptomatic.

On physical examination, the woman's labia may be swollen and excoriated if pruritus has been severe. A speculum examination reveals thick, white, tenacious cheeselike patches adhering to the vaginal mucosa. Diagnosis is confirmed by microscopic examination of the vaginal discharge; hyphae and spores are usually seen on a wet-mount preparation (Figure 3–10 ◆).

Treatment of VVC includes intravaginal insertion of miconazole, tioconazole, butoconazole, terconazole, clotrimazole, or nystatin suppositories or cream at bedtime for varying times, typically 3 to 7 nights. Some of the topical medications are available over the counter. They are indicated for women with a history of yeast infections who clearly recognize the symptoms.

VVC may also be treated with a single oral dose of fluconazole; however, fluconazole has been associated with more systemic side effects than topical agents (Sobel, 2000). Pregnant women are treated the same as nonpregnant women (Centers for Disease Control [CDC], 1998). Infection at the time of birth may cause thrush (a mouth infection) in the newborn.

Recurrent VVC (four or more symptomatic infections per year) is treated by chronic suppression including oral antifungal agents such as fluconazole (orally once a week), ketoconazole (orally each day), or itraconazole (orally every other day). As an alternative, intravaginal azole preparations may be used daily (Batteiger, 2001).

Topical miconazole usually eliminates the yeast infection from the male. However, the CDC states that treatment of the male partner is not necessary unless candidal balanitis (inflammation of the glans penis) is present or chronicity is a problem (CDC, 1998).

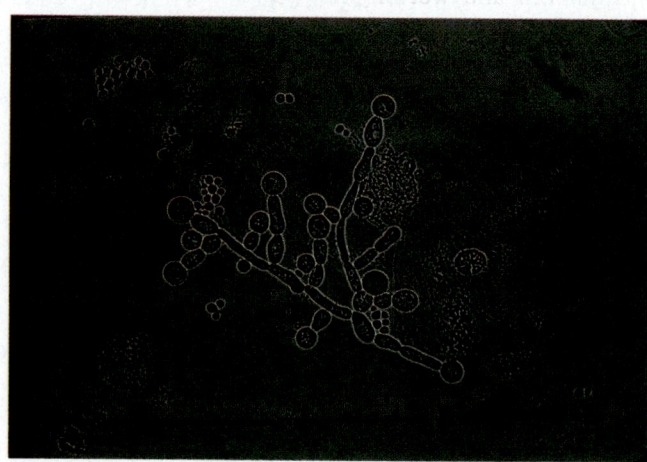

FIGURE 3–10. ◆ The hyphae and spores of *Candida albicans.* From Centers for Disease Control and Prevention.

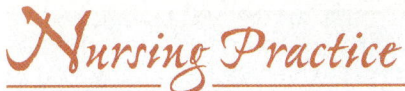

Nursing Practice

To distinguish among the common types of vaginitis and their treatments, it is useful to remember the following:

Vulvovaginal candidiasis (moniliasis)
Cause: *Candida albicans.*
Appearance of discharge: Thick, curdy, like cottage cheese
Diagnostic test: Slide of vaginal discharge (treated with potassium hydroxide) shows characteristic hyphae and spores
Treatment: Clotrimazole vaginal cream or suppositories

Bacterial vaginosis (Gardnerella vaginalis vaginitis)
Cause: *Gardnerella vaginalis*
Appearance of discharge: Gray, milky
Diagnostic test: Slide of vaginal discharge shows characteristic "clue" cells
Treatment: Metronidazole

Trichomoniasis
Cause: *Trichomonas vaginalis*
Appearance of discharge: Greenish white and frothy
Diagnostic test: Saline slide of vaginal discharge shows motile flagellated organisms
Treatment: Metronidazole

Nursing Management

Nursing Assessment and Diagnosis

The nurse should suspect VVC if a woman complains of intense vulvar itching and a curdy, white discharge. Because pregnant women with diabetes mellitus are especially susceptible to this infection, be alert for symptoms in these women. In some areas, nurses are trained to do speculum examinations and wet-mount preparations and can confirm the diagnosis themselves. In most cases, however, the nurse who suspects a vaginal infection reports it to the woman's health care provider.

Nursing diagnoses that might apply to the woman with VVC include the following:

▶ *Risk for impaired skin integrity* related to scratching secondary to discomfort of the infection

▶ *Health-seeking behaviors:* information about ways of preventing the development of VVC related to an expressed desire to learn about the infection

Planning and Implementation

If the woman is experiencing discomfort because of pruritus, recommend gentle bathing of the vulva with a weak sodium bicarbonate solution. If a topical treatment is being used, the woman will need to bathe the area before applying the medication.

Also discuss with the woman the factors that contribute to the development of VVC and suggest ways to prevent recurrences, such as wearing cotton underwear and avoiding vaginal powders or sprays that may irritate the vulva. Some women report that the addition of yogurt to the diet or the use of activated culture of plain yogurt as a vaginal douche helps prevent recurrence by maintaining high levels of lactobacilli.

Evaluation

Expected outcomes of nursing care include the following:

▶ The woman's symptoms are relieved, and the infection is cured.

▶ The woman is able to identify self-care measures to prevent further episodes of VVC.

CARE OF THE INDIVIDUAL WITH A SEXUALLY TRANSMITTED INFECTION

The occurrence of **sexually transmitted infection (STI),** or *sexually transmitted disease (STD),* has increased over the past few decades. In fact, vaginitis and STIs are the most common reasons for outpatient, community-based treatment of women.

Children and adolescents can also become infected with sexually transmitted organisms through sexual experimentation, sexual play, molestation, and sexual abuse. Adolescents are considered an at-risk population because of their inexperience and lack of knowledge about STIs. More than half of all school-age adolescents have had sexual intercourse, and 8.3% of students have had sexual intercourse before age 13 (CDC, 2000). They may disregard the importance of using barrier protection, may have multiple sexual partners, may have sex frequently, and often do not seek medical treatment until symptoms are well advanced. The adolescent who acquires an STI has a 40% chance of acquiring another STI within a year, especially if gonorrhea is the first infection (Stamm & McGregor, 2001). Of the 15 million new STI cases each year, approximately 25% occur in adolescents (CDC, 2000). The most frequently diagnosed STIs are chlamydia, genital herpes (herpes simplex type 2), gonorrhea, genital warts (human papillomavirus), trichomoniasis, and syphilis.

Additional information, including specifics as to which STIs must be reported, can be found on the companion website. **WEB** For more detailed information on the specific signs, symptoms, and treatment of males with STIs, please consult a medical-surgical nursing textbook.

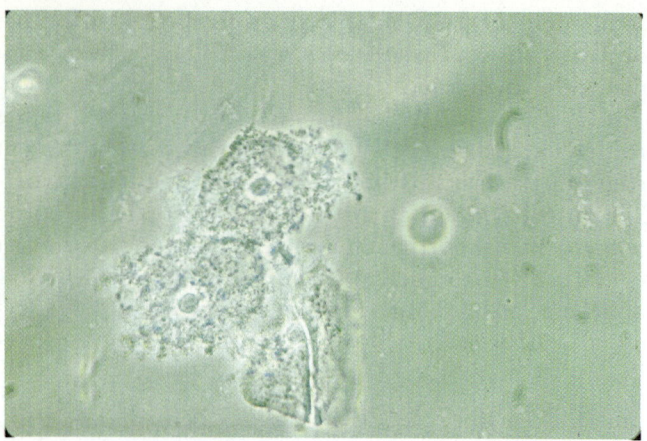

FIGURE 3–11. ◆ Depiction of the clue cells characteristically seen in bacterial vaginosis.

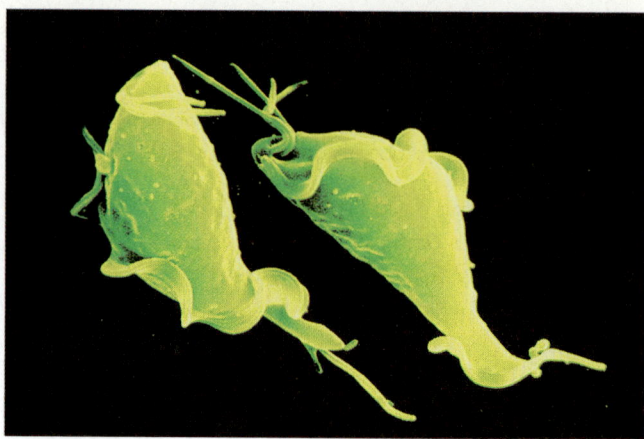

FIGURE 3–12. ◆ Microscopic appearance of *Trichomonas vaginalis.* © David Phillips/Visuals Unlimited.

Bacterial Vaginosis

Bacterial vaginosis (BV) is an alteration of normal vaginal bacterial flora that results in the loss of hydrogen peroxide–producing lactobacilli, which are normally the main vaginal flora. With the loss of this defense, bacteria such as *Gardnerella,* mycoplasmas, and anaerobes overgrow in large numbers, causing vaginitis (Thomason & Scaglione, 1999). The cause of this overgrowth is not clear, although tissue trauma and sexual intercourse may be contributing factors.

The infected woman often notices an excessive amount of thin, watery, yellow-gray vaginal discharge with a foul odor described as "fishy." The characteristic "clue" cell is seen on a wet-mount preparation (Figure 3–11 ◆). The vaginal pH is usually greater than 4.5.

The nonpregnant woman is generally treated with metronidazole (Flagyl) or clindamycin (Cleocin) orally or as a vaginal cream. Because of its potential teratogenic effects, metronidazole is avoided during the first trimester of pregnancy. During the second and third trimesters, oral metronidazole or oral clindamycin can be used (Batteiger, 2001). BV during pregnancy may be a factor in premature rupture of the membranes and preterm birth. Treatment of sexual partners is only recommended in cases of recurrent BV (Thomason & Scaglione, 1999).

Because women with BV are at increased risk for infection following a hysterectomy or surgical abortion, the CDC now recommends screening for BV prior to these procedures, whether the woman is symptomatic or not. Treatment preoperatively is indicated if BV is diagnosed (Batteiger, 2001).

Trichomoniasis

Trichomonas vaginalis is a microscopic motile protozoan that thrives in an alkaline environment. Most infections are acquired through sexual intimacy. Transmission by shared bath facilities, wet towels, or wet swimsuits may be possible (CDC, 1998). In females, symptoms of trichomoniasis include a yellow-green, frothy, odorous discharge fre-

quently accompanied by inflammation of the vagina and cervix, dysuria, and dyspareunia. Visualization of *T. vaginalis* under the microscope on a wet-mount preparation of vaginal discharge confirms the diagnosis (Figure 3–12 ◆). Most males are asymptomatic although a few may have nongonococcal urethritis (NGU).

Treatment for trichomoniasis is metronidazole (Flagyl) administered in a single 2-g dose for both male and female sexual partners; a 7-day regimen is also available (Eschenbach, 2000). Partners should avoid intercourse until both are cured (see "Nursing Practice" on page 69).

Metronidazole is contraindicated in the first trimester of pregnancy because of possible teratogenic effects on the fetus. However, no other adequate treatment exists. For women with severe symptoms after the first trimester, treatment with 2 g metronidazole in a single dose may be considered (Eschenbach, 2000). The woman and her partner should be cautioned to avoid alcohol while taking metronidazole; the combination has an effect similar to that of alcohol and disulfiram (Antabuse)—abdominal pain, flushing, and tremors.

Chlamydial Infection

Chlamydial infection, caused by *Chlamydia trachomatis,* is the most common STI in the United States. A form of chlamydia is responsible for trachoma, the world's leading cause of preventable blindness.

In males, chlamydia is a major cause of NGU. In females it can cause infections similar to those that occur with gonorrhea. It can infect the fallopian tubes, cervix, urethra, and Bartholin's glands. Pelvic inflammatory disease, infertility, and ectopic pregnancy are associated with chlamydia. The newborn of a woman with untreated chlamydia is at risk of developing ophthalmia neonatorum, which responds to erythromycin ophthalmic ointment prophylaxis at birth. The newborn may also develop chlamydia pneumonia.

Both males and females may be asymptomatic. In females, symptoms of chlamydia include a thin or purulent discharge, burning and frequency of urination, and lower abdominal pain. Diagnosis is often made after treatment of a male partner for NGU or in a symptomatic woman with a negative gonorrhea culture. Laboratory detection is now simpler because of the development of DNA amplification tests that are over 95% sensitive to *C. trachomatis*. These noninvasive tests can be done on a woman's first-voided urine of the day (Hammerschlag, 1999).

Treatment is azithromycin, doxycycline, or levofloxacin. Sexual partners are also treated; couples should abstain from intercourse for 7 days, the course of therapy. Pregnant women are treated with erythromycin ethylsuccinate or amoxicillin, although neither is highly effective (CDC, 1998). Because a prior chlamydial infection is a major risk factor for a repeat infection within the ensuing 3 to 4 months, the CDC now recommends rescreening at 3 to 4 months regardless of symptoms. Annual screening for chlamydia is recommended for sexually active teens and young women ages 20 to 25 years (Batteiger, 2001).

Gonorrhea

Gonorrhea is an infection caused by the bacteria *Neisseria gonorrhoeae*. If a nonpregnant woman contracts the disease, she is at risk of developing pelvic inflammatory disease. If a woman becomes infected after the third month of pregnancy, the mucous plug in the cervix will prevent the infection from ascending, and it will remain localized in the urethra, cervix, and Bartholin's glands until the membranes rupture. Then it can spread upward.

Often women with gonorrhea are asymptomatic. Thus it is routine to screen for this infection using a cervical culture during the initial prenatal examination. For women at high risk, the culture may be repeated during the last month of pregnancy. Cultures of the urethra, throat, and rectum may also be required for diagnosis, depending on the body orifices used for intercourse.

In females, the most common symptoms of gonorrheal infection include a purulent, greenish yellow vaginal discharge, dysuria, and urinary frequency. Some women also develop inflammation and swelling of the vulva. The cervix may appear swollen and eroded and may secrete a foul-smelling discharge in which gonococci are present. In males, urethritis, or inflammation of the urethra, is the cardinal symptom. This is marked by burning during urination and the presence of discharge from the urethra.

Treatment consists of antibiotic therapy with ceftriaxone intramuscularly and doxycycline or azithromycin administered orally. This combined approach provides dual treatment for gonorrhea and chlamydia because the two infections often occur together. Additional treatment may be required if the cultures remain positive 7 to 14 days after completion of treatment. All sexual partners must also be treated or the woman may become reinfected. Pregnant women should be treated with ceftriaxone intramuscularly or cefixime orally. This treatment is combined with erythromycin or amoxicillin to address the risk of coinfection with chlamydia (CDC, 1998).

Women should be informed of the need for reculture to verify cure and the need for abstinence or condom use until cure is confirmed. Both sexual partners should be treated if either has a positive test for gonorrhea.

Herpes Genitalis

Herpes infections are caused by the herpes simplex virus (HSV). Two types of herpes infections can occur: HSV-1 (the cold sore) typically occurs above the waist and is not sexually transmitted; HSV-2 is usually associated with genital infections. The clinical symptoms and treatment of both types are the same.

The primary episode of herpes genitalis is characterized by the development of single or multiple blisterlike vesicles. In males these usually occur on the penis or anal area. In females the vesicles occur in the genital area and sometimes affect the vaginal walls, cervix, urethra, and anus. The vesicles may appear within a few hours to 20 days after exposure and rupture spontaneously to form painful, open, ulcerated lesions. Inflammation and pain secondary to the presence of herpes lesions can cause difficult urination and urinary retention. Inguinal lymph node enlargement may be present. Flulike symptoms and genital pruritus or tingling also may be noticed. Primary episodes usually last the longest and are the most severe. Lesions heal spontaneously in 2 to 4 weeks.

After the lesions heal, the virus enters a dormant phase, residing in the nerve ganglia of the affected area. Some individuals never have a recurrence, whereas others have regular recurrences. Recurrences are usually less severe than the initial episode and seem to be triggered by emotional stress, menstruation, ovulation, pregnancy, frequent or vigorous intercourse, poor health status or a generally run-down physical condition, tight clothing, or overheating. Diagnosis is made on the basis of the clinical appearance of the lesions, Pap smear or culture of the lesions, and sometimes blood testing for antibodies.

No known cure for herpes exists. Prescriptive treatment is available to provide relief from pain and prevent complications from secondary infection. The recommended treatment of the first clinical episode of genital herpes is oral acyclovir, valacyclovir, or famciclovir. These same medications, in somewhat different dosages, are also recommended for recurrent herpes infection and for daily suppression therapy for people who have frequent recurrences (CDC, 1998). Keeping the genital area clean and dry, wearing loose clothing, and wearing cotton underwear or none at all help promote healing. If herpes is present in the genital tract of a woman during childbirth, it can have a devastating effect on the newborn. See Chapter 13. 🔗

Syphilis

Syphilis is a chronic STI caused by the spirochete *Treponema pallidum*. Syphilis is divided into early and late stages. During the early stage (primary), a chancre appears at the site where the *T. pallidum* organism entered the body. Symptoms include slight fever, loss of weight, and malaise. The chancre persists for about 4 weeks and then disappears. In 6 weeks to 6 months, secondary symptoms appear. Skin eruptions called condylomata lata, which resemble wartlike plaques and are highly infectious, may appear on the vulva. Other secondary symptoms are acute arthritis, enlargement of the liver and spleen, nontender enlarged lymph nodes, iritis, and a chronic sore throat with hoarseness.

Syphilis may also be transmitted transplacentally. When infected in utero, the newborn exhibits secondary-stage symptoms of syphilis. Transplacentally transmitted syphilis may cause intrauterine growth restriction, preterm birth, and stillbirth. As a result of the disease's impact on the fetus in utero, serologic testing of every pregnant woman is recommended; some state laws require it. Testing is done at the initial prenatal screening and repeated in the third trimester. Blood studies may be negative if blood is drawn too early in the pregnancy.

Diagnosis of syphilis is made by dark-field examination for spirochetes. Blood tests such as the venereal disease research laboratory (VDRL) test, rapid plasma reagin (RPR) test, or the more specific fluorescent treponemal antibody-absorption (FTA-ABS) test are commonly done.

For males and for females, both nonpregnant and pregnant, with syphilis of less than a year's duration, the CDC (1998) recommends 2.4 million units of benzathine penicillin G administered intramuscularly. Alternately, nonpregnant individuals may be treated with a single dose of azithromycin orally, ceftriaxone intramuscularly once daily for 10 days, or doxycycline orally twice a day for 14 days. The CDC stresses that the effectiveness of these non-penicillin-based treatments is less well documented than the traditional therapy with benzathine penicillin (Batteiger, 2001). If syphilis is of long (more than a year) duration, 2.4 million units of benzathine penicillin G is given intramuscularly once a week for 3 weeks. For men and for nonpregnant women allergic to penicillin, doxycycline can be given. The pregnant woman who is allergic to penicillin should be desensitized to penicillin (CDC, 1998). Maternal serologic testing may remain positive for 8 months, and the newborn may have a positive test for 3 months.

Condylomata Acuminata (Venereal Warts)

The infection *condylomata acuminata,* also called *venereal warts,* is a relatively common sexually transmitted condition caused by the human papillomavirus (HPV). Often an individual seeks medical care after noticing single or multiple soft, grayish pink, cauliflower-like lesions on the penis or in the genital area (Figure 3–13 ◆). In women, the moist, warm environment of the genital area is conducive to the growth of the warts, which may be present on the vulva, vagina, cervix, and anus. The incubation period following exposure is 3 weeks to 3 years.

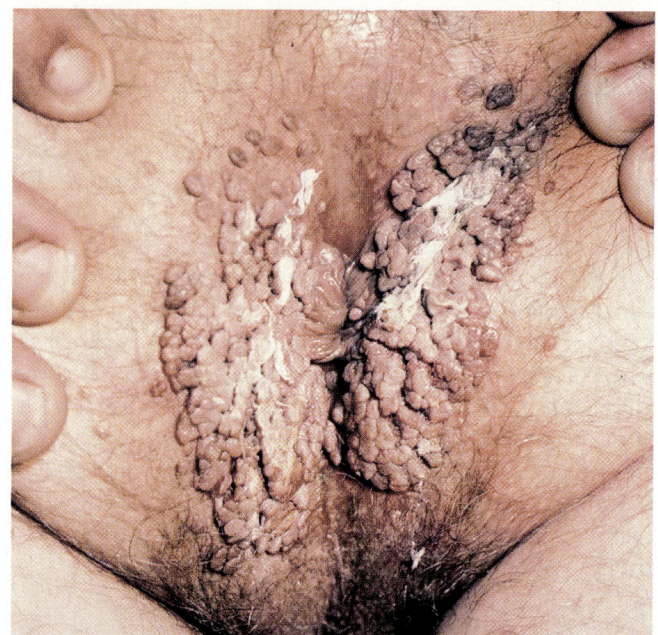

FIGURE 3–13. ◆ Condylomata acuminata on the vulva. © Ken Greer/Visuals Unlimited.

Because condylomata sometimes resemble other lesions and malignant transformation is possible, all atypical, pigmented, and persistent warts should be biopsied and treatment should be instituted promptly. The CDC does not specify a treatment of choice for genital warts but recommends that treatment be determined based on client preference, available resources, and experience of the health care provider. Client-applied therapies include podofilox solution or gel or imiquimod cream. Provider-administered therapies include cryotherapy with liquid nitrogen or cryoprobe; trichloroacetic acid (TCA); bichloroacetic acid (BCA); intralesional interferon; surgical removal by tangential scissor excision, shave excision, or curettage; or laser surgery (CDC, 1998). Topical podophyllin is no longer recommended because of its toxicity and limited effectiveness (Batteiger, 2001). Imiquimod and podofilox are not used during pregnancy because they are thought to be teratogenic and in large doses have been associated with fetal death.

Certain forms of HPV have been linked to cervical cancer. Women with HPV infections should have frequent Pap smears to monitor cervical cellular changes. Sex partners are probably infected but do not require treatment unless large lesions are present. Male or female condoms may reduce the risk of transmitting the virus to an uninfected partner.

Acquired Immunodeficiency Syndrome

Acquired immunodeficiency syndrome (AIDS) is a fatal disorder caused by the human immunodeficiency virus (HIV). Medical-surgical texts more fully describe care of people with HIV/AIDS. However, because HIV/AIDS has profound implications for a fetus if the woman is pregnant, AIDS is discussed in more detail in Chapter 12. ⊂⊐

Nursing Management

Nursing Assessment and Diagnosis

Nurses need to become adept at taking a thorough history and identifying people at risk for STIs. Risk factors include multiple sexual partners, a partner's involvement with other partners, high-risk sexual behaviors such as intercourse without barrier contraception or anal intercourse, partners with high-risk behaviors, treatment with antibiotics while taking OCs, and young age at onset of sexual activity. Be alert for signs and symptoms of STIs and be familiar with diagnostic procedures if an STI is suspected.

When children or adolescents have a possible STI, the nurse usually encounters them and their families in the emergency department, outpatient clinic, or nursing unit. Because adolescents are often afraid of the consequences of reporting symptoms, it is important to develop good assessment skills, particularly when asking questions about sexual activity, partners, and the possibility of abuse. When a child or adolescent is diagnosed with one STI, it is important to screen for others as these diseases may coexist. Adolescents who are symptomatic may postpone care because of their discomfort with examinations and cultures. Routine screening of sexually active adolescents is recommended because many have subclinical infections or are asymptomatic.

Nursing Practice

- When a child is found to have an STI, the law requires that a report be made to social services and the local health department and that an investigation take place.
- When a child younger than 10 years of age is found to have gonorrhea or another STI, consider the possibility of sexual abuse.
- Whenever anorectal symptoms are found in a child, suspect molestation.

Although each STI has certain distinctive characteristics, the following complaints warrant further investigation: presence of a sore or lesion on the penis or vulva, increased vaginal discharge, malodorous vaginal discharge, urethral discharge (males), burning with urination, dyspareunia, bleeding after intercourse, and pelvic pain. In many instances a woman is asymptomatic but may report symptoms in her partner, especially painful urination or urethral discharge. It is often helpful to ask the woman whether her partner is experiencing any symptoms.

Nursing diagnoses that may apply when an STI is diagnosed include the following:

- *Altered family processes* related to the effects of a diagnosis of STI on the couple's relationship

- *Health-seeking behaviors:* information about the long-term effects of the diagnosis on childbearing status related to an expressed request for information.

Planning and Implementation

The nurse provides the person who has an STI with information about the infection, methods of transmission, implications for pregnancy or future fertility, and the importance of thorough treatment including treatment of the partner, if indicated. The person should also understand the need to abstain from sexual activity, if necessary, during treatment.

Some STIs such as trichomoniasis or chlamydia may cause a woman concern but, once diagnosed, are rather easily treated. Other STIs may be simple to treat medically but may carry a stigma and be emotionally difficult to accept. Thus the nurse should stress prevention with all people and encourage them to require partners, especially new partners, to use condoms. See "Teaching About: Preventing STIs and Their Consequences."

Teaching About

PREVENTING STIs AND THEIR CONSEQUENCES

The risk of contracting an STI increases with the number of sexual partners. Because of the extended time between infection with HIV and evidence of infection, intercourse with an individual exposes a female or male to all the other sexual partners of that individual for the past 5 or more years. Because of this risk, it is important to take the following actions:

- Plan ahead and develop strategies to refuse sex (especially important for adolescents who may be less confident about saying "no" to casual sexual encounters), as abstinence is the best method of preventing STIs.
- Limit the number of sexual contacts and practice mutual monogamy.
- The condom is the best contraceptive method currently available (other than abstinence) for protection from STIs. Use one for every act of vaginal and anal intercourse. Other contraceptives such as the diaphragm, cervical cap, and spermicides also offer some protection against STIs.
- Plan strategies for negotiating condom use with a partner.
- Reduce high-risk behaviors. Use of recreational drugs and alcohol can increase sexual risk taking.
- Refrain from oral sex if your partner has active sores in mouth, vagina, or anus or on penis.
- Seek care as soon as you notice symptoms and make sure your partner gets treatment if indicated. Absence of symptoms or disappearance of symptoms does not mean that treatment is unnecessary if you suspect an STI. Take all prescribed medications completely.
- The presence of a genital infection may lead to an abnormal Pap smear. Women with certain infections should have more frequent Pap tests according to a schedule recommended by their caregiver. Ask your health care provider if you need more frequent Paps.

The nurse can be especially helpful in encouraging a person to explore feelings about the diagnosis. People may, for example, experience anger or feel betrayed by a partner, they may feel guilt or see their diagnosis as a form of punishment, or they may feel concern about the long-term implications for future childbearing or ongoing intimate relationships. Opportunities to discuss personal feelings in a nonjudgmental environment can be very helpful. Offer suggestions about support groups, if indicated, and assist the person in planning for future sexual activity.

More subtly, an attitude of acceptance and matter-of-factness conveys the message that the individual is an acceptable person who happens to have an infection. See "Teaching About" on page 73 for key information about STIs.

Evaluation

Expected outcomes of nursing care include the following:

▶ The infection is identified and cured, if possible; if not, supportive therapy is provided.
▶ The individual and partner can describe the infection, its method of transmission, its implications, and the therapy.
▶ The person copes successfully with the impact of the diagnosis on self-concept.

CARE OF THE WOMAN WITH PELVIC INFLAMMATORY DISEASE

Pelvic inflammatory disease (PID) occurs in approximately 1% of women between ages 15 and 39, although sexually active young women between 15 and 24 have the highest infection rate (Eschenbach, 1999). The disease is more common in women who have had multiple sexual partners, a history of PID, early onset of sexual activity, a recent gynecologic procedure, or an IUD. It usually produces a tubal infection (salpingitis) that may or may not be accompanied by a pelvic abscess. However, perhaps the greatest problem of PID is postinfection tubal damage, which is closely associated with infertility.

The organisms most frequently identified with PID are *Chlamydia trachomatis* and *Neisseria gonorrhoeae*. Symptoms of PID include bilateral sharp, cramping pain in the lower quadrants, fever, chills, purulent vaginal discharge, irregular bleeding, malaise, nausea, and vomiting. However, it is also possible to be asymptomatic and have normal laboratory values.

Diagnosis is based on examination, blood tests, gonorrhea culture, and a test for chlamydia. Physical exam usually reveals direct abdominal tenderness with palpation, adnexal tenderness, and cervical and uterine tenderness with movement (chandelier sign). A palpable mass is evaluated with ultrasound. Fluid may be aspirated via needle from the cul-de-sac of Douglas through the posterior vaginal fornix. Purulent fluid suggests an intraabdominal infection. Laparoscopy may be used to confirm the diagnosis and to enable the examiner to obtain cultures from the fallopian tubes and directly from the fluid of the cul-de-sac (Wölner-Hanssen, 1999).

Except in mild cases, the woman is hospitalized and treated with intravenous administration of cefoxitan sodium, cefotetan disodium, or clindamycin plus gentamicin. Outpatient therapy usually includes antibiotics such as cefoxitan, ceftriaxone, doxycycline, and clindamycin used singly or in combination. A new antibiotic, ofloxacin (Floxin), is now available for women with PID caused by chlamydia or gonorrhea. In addition, supportive therapy is often indicated for severe symptoms. The sexual partner should also be treated. If the woman has an IUD, it is generally removed 24 to 48 hours after antibiotic therapy is started.

Nursing Management

Nursing Assessment and Diagnosis

Be alert to factors in a woman's history that put her at risk for PID. Question the woman who has an IUD about possible symptoms, such as aching pain in the lower abdomen, foul-smelling discharge, malaise, and the like. The woman who is acutely ill will have obvious symptoms, but a low-grade infection is more difficult to detect.

Nursing diagnoses that may apply to a woman with PID include the following:

▶ *Pain* related to peritoneal irritation
▶ *Health-seeking behaviors:* information about the possible effects of PID on fertility related to a request for specific information

Planning and Implementation

The nurse plays a vital role in helping to prevent or detect PID. Accordingly, spend time discussing risk factors related to this infection. The woman who uses an IUD for contraception and has multiple sexual partners needs to understand clearly the risk she faces. Discuss signs and symptoms of PID and stress the importance of early detection.

The woman who develops PID should be counseled on the importance of completing her antibiotic treatment and of returning for follow-up evaluation. She should also understand the possibility of decreased fertility following the infection.

Evaluation

Expected outcomes of nursing care include the following:

▶ The woman describes her condition, her therapy, and the possible long-term implications of PID on her fertility.
▶ The woman completes her course of therapy and the PID is cured.

CARE OF THE WOMAN WITH AN ABNORMAL FINDING DURING PELVIC EXAMINATION

Abnormal Pap Smear Results

The Bethesda system (Table 3–4) has become the most widely used system in the United States for reporting Pap smear results. Early detection of abnormalities allows changes to be treated before cells reach the precancerous or cancerous stage. Notification of an abnormal Pap smear usually causes anxiety for a woman, so it is important that she be told in a caring way. The woman needs accurate, complete information about the meaning of the results and the next steps to be taken. She should also be given time to ask questions and express her concerns.

Diagnostic or therapeutic procedures used in cases of abnormalities include repetition of the Pap test using the ThinPrep method rather than a smear, Pap tests at shorter intervals, colposcopy and endocervical biopsy, cryotherapy, laser conizations, or large loop excision of the transformation zone (LLETZ). Management is based on the specific report.

TABLE 3–4 The Bethesda System for Classifying Pap Smears

SPECIMEN TYPE: *Indicate conventional smear (Pap smear) vs. liquid based vs. other*

SPECIMEN ADEQUACY

Satisfactory for evaluation *(describe presence or absence of endocervical/transformation zone component and any other quality indicators, e.g., partially obscuring blood inflammation etc)*

Unsatisfactory for evaluation . . . *(specify reason)*

  Specimen rejected/not processed *(specify reason)*

  Specimen processed and examined, but unsatisfactory for evaluation of epithelial abnormality because of *(specify reason)*

GENERAL CATEGORIZATION *(optional)*

Negative for intraepithelial lesion or malignancy.

Epithelial cell abnormality. See Interpretation/result *(specify 'squamous' or 'glandular' as appropriate)*

Other: See Interpretation result *(e.g., endometrial cells in a woman ≥40 years of age).*

AUTOMATED REVIEW

If case examined by automated device, specify device and result.

ANCILLARY TESTING

Provide a brief description of the test methods and report the result so that it is easily understood by the clinician.

INTERPRETATION/RESULT

  Negative for intraepithelial lesion or malignancy
  (when there is no cellular evidence of neoplasia, state this in the General Categorization above and/or in the Interpretation/Result section of the report, whether or not there are organisms or other non neoplastic findings)

    ORGANISMS:
    Trichomonas vaginalis
    Fungal organisms morphologically consistent with Candida spp.
    Shift in flora suggestive of bacterial vaginosis.
    Bacteria morphologically consistent with Actinomyces spp.
    Cellular changes associated with herpes simplex virus.

  OTHER NON-NEOPLASTIC FINDINGS *(Optional to report list not inclusive).*

    Reactive cellular changes associated with
      —inflammation (Includes typical repair)
      —radiation
      —intrauterine contraceptive device (IUD)
    Glandular cells status posthysterectomy
    Atrophy

Other

  Endometrial cells (in a woman ≥40 years of age) (Specify if negative for squamous intraepthelial lesion')

Epithelial cell abnormalities

  SQUAMOUS CELL
    Atypical squamous cells
      —of undetermined significance (ASC-US)
      —cannot exclude HSIL (ASC-H)
    Low-grade squamous intraepithelial lesion (LSIL)
      —encompassing HPV/mild dysplasia/CIN-1
    High-grade squamous intraepithelial lesion (HSIL)
      —encompassing: moderate and severe dysplasia CIS/CIN-2 and CIN-3
      —with features suspicious for invasion (*if invasion is suspected*)
    Squamous cell carcinoma
  GLANDULAR CELL
    Atypical
      —endocervical cells *(NOS or specify in comments)*
      —endometrial cells *(NOS or specify in comments)*
      —glandular cells *(NOS or specify in comments)*
    Atypical
      —endocervical cells, favor neoplastic
      —glandular cells, favor neoplastic
    Endocervical adenocarcinoma in situ
    Adenocarcinoma
      —endocervical
      —endometrial
      —extrauterine
      —not otherwise specified (NOS)
  Other malignant neoplasms *(specify)*

EDUCATIONAL NOTES AND SUGGESTIONS *(optional)*

Suggestions should be concise and consistent with clinical follow-up guidelines published by professional organizations (references to relevant publications may be included).

Courtesy of National Cancer Institute

Colposcopy has become a common second step in many cases of abnormal Pap smears. The examination, done in an office or clinic, permits more detailed visualization of the cervix in bright light, using a high-magnification microscope. The cervix can be visualized directly and again following application of acetic acid. The acetic acid causes abnormal epithelium to assume a characteristic white appearance. The colposcope can also be used to obtain a directed biopsy.

Ovarian Masses

Between 70% and 80% of ovarian masses are benign. More than 50% are functional cysts, occurring most commonly in women 20 to 40 years of age. Functional cysts are rare in women who take oral contraceptives. Ovarian cysts usually represent physiologic variations in the menstrual cycle. Dermoid cysts (cystic teratomas) and endometriomas, or "chocolate cysts," are common types of ovarian masses. No relationship exists between ovarian masses and ovarian cancer. However, ovarian cancer is the most fatal of all cancers in women because it is difficult to diagnose and often has spread throughout the pelvis before it is detected.

A woman with an ovarian mass may be asymptomatic; the mass may be noted on a routine pelvic examination. She may experience a sensation of fullness or cramping in the lower abdomen (often unilateral), dyspareunia, irregular bleeding, or delayed menstruation. Diagnosis is made on the basis of a palpable mass with or without tenderness and other related symptoms. Radiography or ultrasonography may be used to assist in the diagnosis.

The woman is often kept under observation for a month or two because most cysts resolve on their own and are harmless. Oral contraceptives may be prescribed for 1 to 2 months to suppress ovarian function. If this regimen is effective, a repeat pelvic examination should be normal. If the mass is still present after 60 days of observation and OC therapy, a diagnostic laparoscopy or laparotomy may be considered. Tubal or ovarian lesions, ectopic pregnancy, cancer, infection, or appendicitis also must be ruled before a diagnosis can be confirmed.

Surgery is not always necessary but is considered if the mass is larger than 6 to 7 cm in circumference; if the woman is over 40 years of age with an adnexal mass, a persistent mass, or continuous pain; or if the woman is taking oral contraceptives. Surgical exploration is also indicated when a palpable mass is found in an infant, a young girl, or a postmenopausal woman.

Women taking OCs should be informed of their preventive effect against ovarian masses. Women may need clear explanations about why the initial therapy is observation. A discussion of the origin and resolution of ovarian cysts may clarify this treatment plan. If a surgical treatment removes or impairs the function of one ovary, the woman needs to be assured that the remaining ovary can be expected to take over ovarian functioning and that pregnancy is still possible if desired.

Uterine Masses

Fibroid tumors, or *leiomyomas,* are among the most common benign disease entities in women and are the most common reason for gynecologic surgery. Between 20% and 50% of women develop leiomyomas by age 40. The potential for cancer is minimal. Leiomyomas are more common in women of African heritage.

Fibroid tumors vary in size from 1 to 2 cm to the size of a 10-week fetus. Frequently, the woman is asymptomatic. Lower abdominal pain, fullness or pressure, menorrhagia, metrorrhagia, or increased dysmenorrhea may occur, particularly with large tumors. Ultrasonography revealing masses or nodules can assist and confirm the diagnosis. Leiomyoma is also considered a possible diagnosis when masses or nodules involving the uterus are palpated on a pelvic examination.

The majority of these masses require no treatment and will shrink after menopause. Close observation for symptoms or an increase in size of the uterus or the masses is the only management most women need. Routine pelvic examinations every 3 to 6 months are recommended unless new symptoms appear.

If a woman notices symptoms, or pelvic examination reveals that the mass is increasing in size, surgery (myomectomy, D&C, or hysterectomy) is recommended. The choice of surgery depends on the age and reproductive status of the woman and the significance of the noted changes. Currently, two oral medications—pirfenidone and tibolone—are being tested as treatments for fibroids. These medications show promise of providing long-term relief (5 to 10 years), thereby decreasing the need for surgical intervention (Stringer, 2000).

Endometrial cancer, most commonly a disease of postmenopausal women, has a high rate of cure if detected early. The hallmark sign is vaginal bleeding in postmenopausal women not treated with HRT. Diagnosis is made by endometrial biopsy or posthysterectomy pathology examination of the uterus. The treatment is total abdominal hysterectomy and bilateral salpingo-oophorectomy. Radiation therapy may also be indicated, depending on the stage of the cancer.

NURSING MANAGEMENT

Pelvic examinations and Pap smears are not done by nurses except those with special training. In most cases, nursing assessment is directed toward an evaluation of the woman's understanding of the findings and their implications and her psychosocial response.

The woman needs accurate information on etiology, symptomatology, and treatment options. Encourage her to report symptoms and keep appointments for follow-up examination and evaluation. The woman needs realistic reassurance if her condition is benign; she may require counseling and effective emotional support if a malignancy is likely. If the management plan includes surgery, she may need the nurse's support in obtaining a second opinion and making her decision about treatment.

CARE OF THE WOMAN WITH A URINARY TRACT INFECTION

Bacteria that cause a *urinary tract infection (UTI)* usually enter the body by way of the urethra. The organisms are capable of migrating against the downward flow of urine. The shortness of the female urethra facilitates the passage of bacteria into the bladder. Other conditions associated with bacterial entry are relative incompetence of the urinary sphincter, frequent enuresis (bed-wetting) before adolescence, and urinary catheterization. Wiping from back to front after urination may transfer bacteria from the anorectal area to the urethra. Voluntarily suppressing the desire to urinate is a predisposing factor. Retention overdistends the bladder and can lead to an infection. A relationship also exists between recurring UTI and coitus. General poor health or lowered resistance to infection can increase a woman's susceptibility to UTI.

Asymptomatic bacteriuria (ASB) (bacteria in the urine actively multiplying without accompanying clinical symptoms) is a condition that becomes especially significant if the woman is pregnant. About 30% to 40% of pregnant women with untreated ASB go on to develop cystitis or pyelonephritis (Lentz, 2000). ASB is almost always caused by a single organism, typically *Escherichia coli*. Other commonly found causative organisms include *Klebsiella* and *Proteus*. A woman who has had a UTI is susceptible to recurrent infection. If a pregnant woman develops an acute UTI, especially with a high temperature, amniotic fluid infection may develop and retard the growth of the placenta.

Lower Urinary Tract Infection (Cystitis)

Because UTIs are ascending, it is important to recognize and diagnose a lower UTI early to avoid the sequelae associated with an upper UTI. Symptoms of frequency, pyuria, and dysuria without bacteriuria may indicate urethritis caused by *Chlamydia trachomatis;* it has become a common pathogen in the genitourinary system.

When cystitis develops, the initial symptom is often dysuria, specifically at the end of urination. Urgency and frequency also occur. Cystitis is usually accompanied by a low-grade fever (38.3 °C [101 °F] or lower), and hematuria is occasionally seen. Urine specimens usually contain an abnormal number of leukocytes and bacteria. Diagnosis is made with a urine culture.

Treatment depends on the causative organism. Oral trimethoprim-sulfamethoxazole, fluoroquinolones, and fomycin tromethamine are frequently used in single-dose, 3-day, and 7-day regimens. (For treatment options during pregnancy, see Table 13–4.) Phenazopyridine (Pyridium), a bladder analgesic, may also be prescribed to treat the dysuria.

Nursing Management

Nursing Assessment and Diagnosis

During each visit, note any complaints from the woman of dysuria or other urinary difficulties. If any concerns arise, obtain a clean-catch urine specimen from the woman.

Nursing diagnoses that may apply to a woman with a lower UTI include the following:

▶ *Pain* related to dysuria secondary to the UTI
▶ *Health-seeking behaviors:* information about self-care measures to prevent UTI related to an expressed desire to prevent reccurence

Planning and Implementation

Make sure the woman is aware of good hygiene practices, since most bacteria enter through the urethra after having spread from the anal area. See "Teaching About: Preventing Cystitis." Reinforce instructions or answer questions about the prescribed antibiotic, the amount of liquids to take, and the reasons for these treatments. Cystitis usually responds rapidly to treatment, but follow-up urinary cultures are important.

Evaluation

Expected outcomes of nursing care include the following:

▶ The woman implements self-care measures to help prevent cystitis.
▶ The woman can identify the signs, symptoms, therapy, and complications of cystitis.
▶ The woman's infection is cured.

Teaching About

PREVENTING CYSTITIS

Following is information for women about ways to avoid cystitis:

- If you use a diaphragm for contraception, try changing methods or using another size of diaphragm.
- Avoid bladder irritants such as alcohol, caffeine products, and carbonated beverages.
- Increase fluid intake, especially water, to a minimum of six to eight glasses per day.
- Make regular urination a habit; avoid long waits.
- Practice good genital hygiene, including wiping from front to back after urination and bowel movements.
- Be aware that vigorous or frequent sexual activity may contribute to urinary tract infection.
- Urinate before and after intercourse to empty the bladder and cleanse the urethra.
- Complete medication regimens even if symptoms decrease.
- Do not use medication left over from previous infections.
- Drink cranberry juice to acidify the urine. This has been found to relieve symptoms in some cases.

Upper Urinary Tract Infection (Pyelonephritis)

Pyelonephritis (inflammatory disease of the kidneys) is less common but more serious than cystitis and is often preceded by lower UTI. It is more common during the latter part of pregnancy or early postpartum and poses a serious threat to maternal and fetal well-being. Women with symptoms of pyelonephritis during pregnancy have an increased risk of preterm birth and of intrauterine growth restriction.

Acute pyelonephritis has a sudden onset, with chills, high temperature of 39.6 °C to 40.6 °C (103 °F to 105 °F), and flank pain (either unilateral or bilateral). The right side is almost always involved if the woman is pregnant because the large bulk of intestines to the left pushes the uterus to the right, putting pressure on the right ureter and kidney. Nausea, vomiting, and general malaise may ensue. With accompanying cystitis, the woman may experience frequency, urgency, and burning with urination.

Edema of the renal parenchyma or ureteritis with blockage and swelling of the ureter may lead to temporary suppression of urinary output. This is accompanied by severe colicky (spastic, intense) pain, vomiting, dehydration, and ileus of the large bowel. Women with acute pyelonephritis generally have increased diastolic blood pressure, positive fluorescent antibody titer (FA test), low creatinine clearance, significant bacteremia in urine culture, pyuria, and presence of white blood cell casts.

Often the woman is hospitalized and started on intravenous antibiotics. In the case of obstructive pyelonephritis, a blood culture is necessary. The woman is kept on bed rest. After the sensitivity report is received, the antibiotic is changed as necessary. If signs of urinary obstruction occur or continue, the ureter may be catheterized to establish adequate drainage.

With appropriate drug therapy, the woman's temperature should return to normal. The pain subsides and the urine shows no bacteria within 2 to 3 days. Follow-up urinary cultures are needed to determine that the infection has been eliminated completely.

Nursing Management

Nursing Assessment and Diagnosis

During a woman's visit, obtain a sexual and medical history to identify whether she is at risk for UTI. A clean-catch urine specimen is evaluated for evidence of ASB.

Nursing diagnoses that may apply to a woman with an upper UTI include the following:

▶ *Health-seeking behaviors:* information about pyelonephritis related to a request for information about treatment options.

▶ *Fear* related to the possible long-term effects of the disease

Planning and Implementation

Give the woman information to help her recognize the signs of UTI. Also discuss hygiene practices, the advantages of wearing cotton underwear, and the need to void frequently to prevent urinary stasis. Stress the importance of maintaining a good fluid intake. Drinking cranberry juice daily and taking 500 mg of vitamin C help acidify the urine and may help prevent recurrence of infection. Women with a history of UTI find it helpful to drink a glass of fluid before sexual intercourse and to void afterward.

Evaluation

Expected outcomes of nursing care include the following:

▶ The woman completes her prescribed course of antibiotic therapy.
▶ The woman's infection is cured.
▶ The woman incorporates preventive self-care measures into her daily regimen.

PELVIC RELAXATION

A *cystocele* is the downward displacement of the bladder, which appears as a bulge in the anterior vaginal wall. Genetic predisposition, childbearing, obesity, and increased age are factors that may contribute to cystocele. Symptoms of stress incontinence are most common, including loss of urine with coughing, sneezing, laughing, or sudden exertion. Vaginal fullness, a bulging out of the vaginal wall, or a dragging sensation may also be noticeable.

If pelvic relaxation is mild, Kegel exercises help restore tone. The exercises involve contraction and relaxation of the pubococcygeal muscle (see Chapter 9). Women have found these exercises helpful before and after childbirth in maintaining vaginal muscle tone. Estrogen may improve the condition of vaginal mucous membranes, especially in menopausal women. Vaginal pessaries or rings may be used if surgery is undesirable or impossible or until surgery can be scheduled. Surgery may be considered for cystoceles considered moderate to severe.

The nurse may instruct the woman in the use of Kegel exercises. Information on causes and contributing factors and discussion of possible alternative therapies greatly help the woman.

CHAPTER HIGHLIGHTS

🕊 Nurses should give girls and women information about menstrual issues, such as use of tampons; vaginal spray and douching practices; and self-care comfort measures during menstruation, such as nutrition, exercise, and use of heat and massage.

🕊 Dysmenorrhea usually begins at, or a day before, onset of menses and disappears by the end of menstruation. Therapy with hormones such as OCs or the use of nonsteroidal antiinflammatory drugs or prostaglandin inhibitors is useful. Self-care measures include improved nutrition, exercise, applications of heat, and extra rest.

🕊 Premenstrual syndrome (PMS) occurs most often in women over age 30, and symptoms occur 2 to 3 days before onset of menstruation and subside as menstruation starts, with or without treatment. Medical management usually includes progesterone agonists and prostaglandin inhibitors. Self-care measures include improved nutrition (vitamin B complex and E supplementation and avoidance of methylxanthines found in chocolate and caffeine), a program of aerobic exercise, and participation in self-care support groups.

🕊 Fertility awareness methods are natural, noninvasive methods of contraception often used by people whose religious beliefs prevent their using other methods.

🕊 Mechanical contraceptives such as the diaphragm, cervical cap, and condom act as barriers to prevent the transport of sperm. These methods are used in conjunction with a spermicide.

🕊 The intrauterine device (IUD) is a mechanical contraceptive. Research suggests it acts by immobilizing sperm or by impeding the progress of sperm from the cervix to the fallopian tubes. The IUD may also act by speeding the movement of the ovum through the fallopian tube. In addition, the IUD has a local inflammatory effect.

🕊 Oral contraceptives (OCs) are combinations of estrogen and progesterone. When taken correctly, they are the most effective of the reversible methods of fertility control.

🕊 Spermicides are far less effective in preventing pregnancy when they are not used with a barrier method.

🕊 Permanent sterilization is accomplished by tubal ligation for women and vasectomy for men. Although theoretically reversible, clients are advised that the method should be considered irreversible.

🕊 Recommendations about the frequency of screening mammograms vary somewhat. Currently the American Cancer Society recommends mammograms every 1 to 2 years for women ages 40 to 49, and annually for women ages 50 and older. The National Cancer Institute recommends mammograms every 1 to 2 years for women ages 40 and older.

🕊 Menopause is a physiologic, maturational change in a woman's life. Physiologic changes include the cessation of menses and decrease in circulating hormones. Hormonal changes sometimes bring unsettling emotional responses. The most common physiologic symptoms are hot flashes, palpitations, dizziness, and increased perspiration at night. Physical changes also include atrophy of the vagina, reduction in size and pigmentation of the labia, and myometrial atrophy. Osteoporosis becomes an increasing concern.

🕊 Current management of menopause centers around hormone replacement therapy (HRT), client health care education, and prevention of osteoporosis.

🕊 Battering occurs in a cyclic pattern called the "cycle of violence" and increases in frequency and severity over time. Nurses are in an excellent position to help battered women by recognizing their cues, diagnosing their problems appropriately, and understanding the complex dynamics of the battering family. Nurses provide information about available community resources, medical attention, and community support.

🕊 Sexual assault is an act of violence expressed sexually. Most sexual assaults are expressions of anger or power. Following sexual assault the survivor usually experiences an assortment of symptoms known as the rape trauma syndrome.

🕊 In fibrocystic breast disease, the cysts tend to be round, mobile, and well delineated. The woman generally experiences increased discomfort premenstrually. Because of their increased risk of breast cancer, women with fibrocystic breast disease should understand the importance of monthly breast self-examination.

🕊 Endometriosis is a condition in which endometrial tissue occurs outside the endometrial cavity. This tissue bleeds in a cyclic fashion in response to the menstrual cycle. The bleeding leads to inflammation, scarring, and adhesions. The primary symptoms include dysmenorrhea, dyspareunia, and infertility.

🕊 Treatment of endometriosis may be medical, surgical, or a combination. For the woman not currently desiring pregnancy, OCs are used.

🕊 Toxic shock syndrome (TSS), caused by a toxin of *Staphylococcus aureus,* is most common in women of childbearing age. There is an increased incidence in women who use tampons or barrier methods of contraception, such as the diaphragm and cervical cap.

🕊 Vulvovaginal candidiasis (VVC) (moniliasis), a vaginal infection caused by *Candida albicans,* is most common in women who use OCs, are on antibiotics, are pregnant, or have diabetes mellitus. It is generally treated with intravaginal suppositories or, in certain cases, with oral medication.

🕊 Bacterial vaginosis (BV), a common vaginal infection, is diagnosed by its characteristic fishy odor and by the presence of "clue" cells on a vaginal smear. It is treated with metronidazole unless the woman is in the first trimester of pregnancy.

🕊 Chlamydial infection is difficult to detect in a woman but may result in pelvic inflammatory disease (PID) and infertility. It is treated with antibiotic therapy.

🕊 Gonorrhea, a common sexually transmitted infection (STI), may be asymptomatic in women initially but may cause PID if not diagnosed early. The treatment of choice is penicillin.

🕊 Herpes genitalis, caused by the herpes simplex virus (HSV), is a recurrent infection with no known cure. Acyclovir (Zovirax), valacyclovir, or famciclovir may reduce the symptoms and decrease the length of viral shedding.

🕊 Syphilis, caused by *Treponema pallidum,* is an STI that is treatable if diagnosed. The characteristic lesion is the chancre. Syphilis can also be transmitted in utero to the fetus of an infected woman. The treatment of choice is penicillin.

🕊 Condylomata accuminata (venereal warts) are transmitted by the human papillomavirus (HPV). Treatment is indicated, because research suggests a possible link with abnormal cervical changes. The treatment chosen depends on the size and location of the warts.

🕊 PID may be life threatening and may lead to infertility.

🕊 Women with an abnormal finding on a pelvic examination need a careful explanation of the finding and techniques of diagnosis and emotional support during the diagnostic period.

🕊 The classic symptoms of a lower urinary tract infection (UTI) are dysuria, urgency, frequency, and sometimes hematuria.

🕊 An upper UTI is a serious infection that can permanently damage the kidneys if untreated. Generally the woman is acutely ill and requires supportive therapy as well as antibiotics.

🕊 A cystocele is a downward displacement of the bladder into the vagina. Often it is accompanied by stress incontinence. Kegel exercises may help restore tone in mild cases.

EXPLOREMediaLink

NCLEX Review, Case Studies, and other interactive resources for this chapter can be found on the companion website at http://www.prenhall.com/london. Click on "Chapter 3" to select the activities for this chapter.

For animations, more NCLEX review questions, and an audio glossary, access the accompanying CD-ROM in this textbook.

REFERENCES

American College of Obstetricians and Gynecologists. (1999a). *Domestic violence* (ACOG Educational Bulletin No. 257). Washington, DC: Author.

American College of Obstetricians and Gynecologists. (1999b). *Medical management of endometriosis* (ACOG Practice Bulletin No. 11). Washington, DC: Author.

American Society for Reproductive Medicine. (2001). Report of the 57th Annual Meeting held in Orlando Florida, October 20–25, 2001.

Ansbacher, R. (2001). Herbal medicine. *The Female Patient, 26*(1), 36–40.

Batteiger, B. (2001). STDs: Progress! Report of the International Congress of Sexually Transmitted Infections:2nd Joint Meeting of the International Society for Sexually Transmitted Diseases Research (ISSTDR) and the International Union against Sexually Transmitted Infections (IUSTI). Berlin, Germany, June 24–27, 2001.

Burgess, A. W., & Holmstrom, L. L. (1979). *Rape: Crisis and recovery.* Englewood Cliffs, NJ: Prentice-Hall.

Centers for Disease Control and Prevention. (1998). 1998 sexually transmitted disease treatment guidelines. *Mortality and Morbidity Weekly Report, 47*(RR-1), 1–116.

Centers for Disease Control and Prevention. (2000). *Tracking the hidden epidemic: Trends in STDs in the United States 2000.* Atlanta, GA: Author.

Chez, R. A., & Strathman, I. (1999). Contraception and sterilization. In J. R. Scott, P. J. Di Saia, C. B. Hammond, & W. N. Spellacy (Eds.), *Danforth's obstetrics and gynecology* (8th ed., pp. 553–566). Philadelphia: Lippincott Williams & Wilkins.

Crooks, R., & Baur, K. (1998). *Our sexuality* (7th ed.). Monterey, CA: Brooks/Cole.

Cullins, V. E., Dominguez, L., Guberski, T., Secor, R. M., & Wysocki, S. J. (1999). Treating vaginitis. *The Nurse Practitioner, 24*(10), 46–60.

DeLeon, F. D., & Peters, A. J. (2000). Reversal of female sterilization. In J. J. Sciarra (Ed.), *Gynecology and obstetrics* (Vol. 6, Chap. 46, pp. 1–6). Philadelphia: Lippincott Williams & Wilkins.

Dell, D. L., Moskowitz, D., & Sondheimer, S. J. (2001). PMS and PMDD: Identification and treatment. *Contemporary OB/GYN, 46*(4), 15–30.

Endicott, J., Bardack, L., Grady-Weliky, T. A., Ling, F. W., & Schmidt, P. J. (2000). An update on premenstrual dysphoric disorder. *The Female Patient, 25*(2), 45–56.

Eschenbach, D. A. (1999). Pelvic infections and sexually transmitted diseases. In J. R. Scott, P. J. DiSaia, C. B. Hammond, & W. N. Spellacy (Eds.), *Danforth's obstetrics and gynecology* (8th ed., pp. 579–600). Philadelphia: Lippincott Williams & Wilkins.

Eschenbach, D. A. (2000). Infectious vaginitis. In J. J. Sciarra (Ed.), *Gynecology and obstetrics* (Vol. 1, Chap. 40, pp. 1–17). Philadelphia: Lippincott Williams & Wilkins.

Esposito, M. A., Tureck, R. W., & Mastroianni, L. (1999). Understanding endometriosis. *The Female Patient, 24*(6), 79–85.

Gantt, L., & Bickford, A. (1999). Screening for domestic violence. *AWHONN Lifelines, 3*(2), 36–42.

Grimes, D. A., Hanson, V., & Sondheimer, S. (2001). New approaches to emergency contraception. *Contemporary OB/GYN, 46*(6), 89–99.

Haddix-Hill, K. (1997). The violence of rape. *Critical Care Nursing Clinics of North America, 9*(2), 167–174.

Hammerschlag, M. R. (1999). New diagnostic methods for chlamydial infection in women. *Medscape Women's Health, 4*(5), 1–7.

Hatcher, R. A., Trussell, J., Stewart, F., Cates, W., Jr., Stewart, G. K., Guest, F., et al. (1998). *Contraceptive technology* (17th ed.). New York: Ardent Media.

Holmes, M. M. (1998). The clinical management of rape in adolescents. *Contemporary OB/GYN, 43*(5), 62–78.

Jenkins, R. R., & Raine, T. (2000). Helping adolescents prevent unintended pregnancy. *Contemporary Pediatrics, 17*(5), 75–99.

Kaunitz, A. (2001). Choosing an injectable contraceptive. *Contemporary OB/GYN, 46*(6), 29–48.

Kim, A. H., & Adamson, G. D. (2000). Endometriosis. In J. J. Sciarra (Ed.), *Gynecology and obstetrics* (Vol. 1, Chap. 20, pp. 1–22). Philadelphia: Lippincott Williams & Wilkins.

Lentz, G. M. (2000). Urinary tract infections in obstetrics and gynecology. In J. J. Sciarra (Ed.), *Gynecology and obstetrics* (Vol. 2). Philadelphia: Lippincott Williams & Wilkins.

Lindsay, S. H. (1999). Menopause, naturally. *AWHONN Lifelines, 3*(5), 32–38.

Manson, J., Shlipak, M., & Wenger, N. (2001). Heart disease in older women. *Contemporary OB/GYN, 46*(8), 69–82.

McGregor, J. A. (2000). Toxic shock syndrome. In J. J. Sciarra (Ed.), *Gynecology and obstetrics* (Vol. 1, Chap. 43, pp. 1–9). Philadelphia: Lippincott Williams & Wilkins.

McKeon, V. A. (2002). Exploring HRT. *Journal of Obstetrics, Gynecologic, and Neonatal Nursing, 6*(1), 24–31.

Moline, M. L., & Zendell, S. M. (2000, March). Evaluating and managing premenstrual syndrome. *Medscape Women's Health, 5*(2), 1–3.

Nachtigall, L. E. (2000, June). Assessing alternative approaches to menopause. *Supplement to Contemporary OB/GYN,* 3–10.

National Institutes of Health. (2000, March 27–29). Osteoporosis prevention, diagnosis, and therapy. *NIH Consensus Statement Online, 17*(2), 1–34.

Poirier, L. (1997). The importance of screening for domestic violence in all women. *The Nurse Practitioner, 22*(5), 105–115.

Pollack, A. E., & Barone, M. A. (2000). Reversing vasectomy. In J. J. Sciarra (Ed.), *Gynecology and obstetrics* (Vol. 6, Chap. 48, pp. 1–5). Philadelphia: Lippincott Williams & Wilkins.

Propst, A. M., & Laufer, M. R. (1999). Diagnosing and treating adolescent endometriosis. *Contemporary OB/GYN, 44*(12), 52–59.

Rape, Abuse, and Incest National Network (RAINN). (2001). *RAINN statistics.* www.rainn.org.

Rennison, C. M. (2001). *National crime victimization survey.* Washington, DC: U.S. Department of Justice.

Rosenberg, M. J., Meyers, A., & Roy, V. (1999). Efficacy, cycle control, and side effects of low- and lower-dose oral contraceptives: A randomized trial of 20 micrograms and 35 micrograms estrogen preparations. *Contraception, 60*(6), 321–329.

Schairer, C., Lubin, J., Troisi, R., Sturgeon, S., Brinton, L., & Hoover, R. (2000). Menopausal estrogen and estrogen-progestin replacement therapy and breast cancer risk. *Journal of the American Medical Association, 283,* 485–491.

Sobol, J. (2000). Managing vulvovaginal candidiasis. *The Female Patient, 25*(5), 29–32, 45.

Speroff, L. (May 15, 1998). A quarter century of contraception: Remarkable advances, increasing success. *Contemporary OB/GYN, 43* (Special Anniversary Issue), 13–26.

Speroff, L. (1999, November). Hormone therapy and heart health in postmenopausal women. *Contemporary OB/GYN, 44* (Suppl.), 4–26.

Stamm, C. A., & McGregor, J. A. (2001). Diagnosing and treating STDs in young women. *Contemporary Pediatrics, 18*(2), 53–67.

State of the World Population. (2000). Ending violence against women and girls. *United Nations Population Trend.* New York, NY. WEB

Stringer, N. H. (2000). Pirfenidone and tibolone: Innovations in drug therapy for uterine fibroids. *The Female Patient, 25*(5), 17–25.

Thomason, J. L., & Scaglione, N. J. (1999). Bacterial vaginosis. *Contemporary OB/GYN, 44*(6), 15–24.

Valente, S. M. (2000). Evaluating and managing intimate partner violence. *The Nurse Practitioner, 25*(5), 18–33.

Walker, L. (1984). *The battered woman syndrome.* New York: Springer.

Wallach, M., & Grimes, D. A. (2000). *Modern oral contraception: Update from the Contraception Report.* Totowa, NJ: Emron.

Wölner-Hanssen, P. (1999). Pelvic inflammatory disease: Diagnosis. *Contemporary OB/GYN, 44*(8), 108–116.

Zinger, M., & Thomas, M. A. (2001). Using the levonorgestrel IUS. *Contemporary OB/GYN, 46*(5), 35–48.

CHAPTER 4

Special Reproductive Issues for Families

As we sat in the in vitro clinic waiting room, I felt great apprehension. For 4 years we had been unable to conceive. I'd been through two surgeries, dozens of blood tests, and hormone drugs that made me irrational and emotional. It was difficult at times—I blamed myself, felt out of control, and had surprisingly painful reactions to seeing mothers with babies. After many long talks we decided that if in vitro didn't work, we would adopt. Still we felt that we wanted to experience childbirth together. We were on the brink of the most expensive infertility treatment— the last resort for most infertile couples. Was this the right thing to do? Then a young nurse burst into the office, excited and out of breath. She had just come from the lab, having done a blood test, and had discovered that a client was pregnant. Watching the thrill and caring of the nurse's face helped me to decide. Yes, I was in the right place. Yes, it was worth hoping again. Even if in vitro didn't work for us, we had to try.

—Samantha, 38

Key Terms

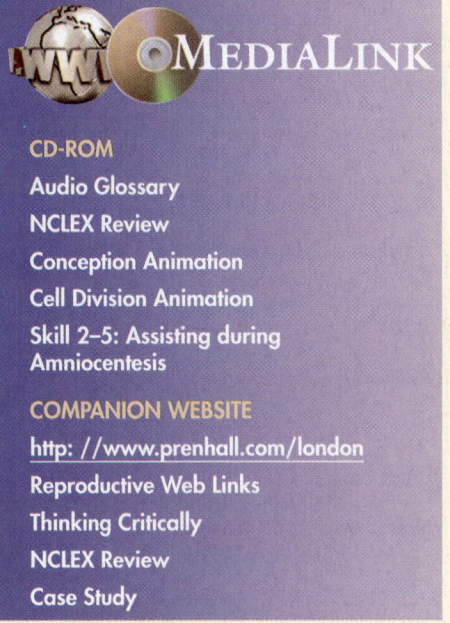

MediaLink

CD-ROM

Audio Glossary

NCLEX Review

Conception Animation

Cell Division Animation

Skill 2–5: Assisting during Amniocentesis

COMPANION WEBSITE

http://www.prenhall.com/london

Reproductive Web Links

Thinking Critically

NCLEX Review

Case Study

*P*regnancy and childbirth usually take their normal course, and a healthy baby is born without problems. But some less fortunate couples are unable to fulfill their dream of having the desired baby because of infertility or genetic problems.

This chapter explores two particularly troubling reproductive problems: the inability to conceive and the risk of bearing babies with genetic abnormalities.

INFERTILITY

Infertility is defined as lack of conception despite unprotected sexual intercourse for at least 12 months (Bopp & Seifer, 2000). Infertility has a profound emotional, psychologic, and economic impact on both the affected couples and society. Approximately 10% to 15% of couples in their reproductive years are infertile (Speroff, Glass, & Kase, 1999). *Sterility* is the term applied when there is an absolute factor preventing reproduction. **Subfertility** is used to describe a couple that has difficulty conceiving because both partners have reduced fertility (Hatcher, Stewart, Trussell, et al., 1998).

Public perception is that the incidence of infertility is increasing, but in fact there has been no significant change in the proportion of infertile couples in the United States (Speroff et al., 1999). What has changed is the composition of the infertile population; the infertility diagnosis has increased in the age group 25 to 44 because of delayed childbearing and the entry of the baby boom cohort into this age range in Western society (Bopp & Seifer, 2000).

The perception that infertility is on the rise may be related to the following factors:

- The deferring of pregnancy and then the desire to have a family within a short time frame
- The increase in assisted reproduction techniques
- The increase in availability and use of infertility services
- The increase in insurance coverage of some ethnic groups for diagnosis of and treatment for infertility
- The increased number of childless women over age 35 seeking medical attention for infertility
- The increased acceptance of infertility as a problem

Essential Components of Fertility

Understanding the elements essential for normal fertility can help the nurse identify the many factors that may cause infertility. The components necessary for normal fertility are correlated with possible causes of deviation in Table 4–1. In addition, adequate reproductive hormones must be present. With intricacies of timing and environment playing such a crucial role, it is an impressive natural phenomenon that the majority of couples in the United States are able to conceive. The remaining couples suffer infertility due to a male factor (35%), a female factor (50%), or either an unknown cause (unexplained infertility) or a problem with both partners (15%) (Speroff et al., 1999). In 35% of infertile couples, multiple causes are present. Professional intervention can help approximately 65% of infertile couples achieve pregnancy.

TABLE 4–1 Normal Fertility Components and Possible Causes of Infertility	
Necessary Norms	*Deviations from Normal*
Female	
Favorable cervical mucus	Cervicitis, cervical stenosis, use of coital lubricants, antisperm antibodies (immunologic response)
Clear passage between cervix and tubes	Myomas, adhesions, adenomyosis, polyps, endometritis, cervical stenosis, endometriosis, congenital anomalies (e.g., septate uterus, diethylstilbestrol (DES) exposure)
Patent tubes with normal motility	Pelvic inflammatory disease, peritubal adhesions, endometriosis, intrauterine device, salpingitis (e.g., chlamydia, recurrent sexually transmitted infections), neoplasm, ectopic pregnancy, tubal ligation
Ovulation and release of ova	Primary ovarian failure, polycystic ovarian disease, hypothyroidism, pituitary tumor, lactation, periovarian adhesions, endometriosis, premature ovarian failure, hyperprolactinemia, Turner syndrome
No obstruction between ovary and tubes	Adhesions, endometriosis, pelvic inflammatory disease
Endometrial preparation	Anovulation, luteal phase defect malformation, uterine infection, Asherman syndrome
Male	
Normal semen analysis	Abnormalities of sperm or semen, polyspermia, congenital defect in testicular development, mumps after adolescence, cryptorchidism, infections, gonadal exposure to x-rays, chemotherapy, smoking, alcohol abuse, malnutrition, chronic or acute metabolic disease medications (e.g., morphine, ASA, ibuprofen), cocaine, marijuana use, constrictive underclothing, heat
Unobstructed genital tract	Infections, tumors, congenital anomalies, vasectomy, strictures, trauma, varicocele
Normal genital tract secretions	Infections, autoimmunity to semen, tumors
Ejaculate deposited at the cervix	Premature ejaculation, impotence, hypospadias, retrograde ejaculation (e.g., diabetic) neurologic cord lesions, obesity (inhibiting adequate penetration)

Couples should be referred for infertility evaluation if they have been unable to conceive after at least 1 year of attempting to achieve pregnancy. If the woman is over age 35, it may be appropriate to refer the couple after only 6 to 9 months of unprotected intercourse without conception. At age 25, when couples are the most fertile, the average length of time needed to achieve conception is 5.3 months. In about 20% of cases, conception occurs within the first month of unprotected intercourse (Speroff et al., 1999).

Nurse's Role During Initial Investigation

Extensive testing for infertility is avoided until data confirm that the timing of intercourse and length of coital exposure have been adequate. The nurse provides information about the most fertile times to have intercourse during the menstrual cycle. Teaching the couple the signs and timing of ovulation and most effective times for intercourse within the cycle may solve the problem (see Table 4–2). Primary assessment, including a comprehensive history and physical examination for any obvious causes of infertility, is done before a costly, time-consuming, and emotionally trying investigation is initiated. During the first visit for the preliminary investigation, the nurse explains the basic infertility workup. The basic investigation for the couple depends on the individuals' history and usually includes assessment of ovarian function, cervical mucosal adequacy and receptivity to sperm, sperm adequacy, tubal patency, and the general condition of the pelvic organs (Bradshaw, 1998). Since about 35% of infertility is related to a male factor, a semen analysis should be one of the first diagnostic tests done before moving on to more invasive diagnostic procedures involving the woman.

The mutual desire to have children is a cornerstone of many marriages. A fertility problem is a deeply personal, emotion-laden area in a couple's life. The self-esteem of one or both partners may be threatened if the inability to conceive is perceived as a lack of virility or femininity (Leon, 2000). The nurse can provide comfort to couples by offering a sympathetic ear, a nonjudgmental approach, and appropriate information and instructions throughout the diagnostic and therapeutic process. Because counseling includes discussion of very personal matters, nurses who are comfortable with their own sexuality are able to establish rapport and elicit relevant information from couples with fertility problems.

The first interview should involve both partners and include a comprehensive history and physical examination. Table 4–3 lists the items in a complete infertility physical workup and laboratory evaluation for both partners. Figure 4–1 ◆ outlines the historical database, diagnostic tests usually performed, and health care interventions used in cases of infertility.

Tests for Infertility

Because of the high incidence of multifactorial infertility, a thorough female evaluation includes assessment of ovulatory function, as well as structure and function of the cervix, uterus, fallopian tubes, and ovaries. See Chapter 2 for an in-depth discussion of the fertility cycle. ⊂⊃ If the man's history indicates the need, he may be referred to a urologist for further testing. Evaluation of the man may include at least two semen analyses to confirm or rule out a seminal deficiency. Tests such as the hamster sperm penetration assay (SPA), acrosome reaction assay, sperm density evaluation, and semen immunobead testing for the presence of antisperm antibody (immunologic infertility) may be performed, but their usefulness is controversial.

ASSESSMENT OF THE WOMAN

Evaluation of Ovulatory Factors.
Ovulation problems account for approximately 15% of infertility causes (Speroff et al., 1999). For a review of female reproductive cycle characteristics, see Chapter 2. ⊂⊃

One basic test of ovulatory function is the **basal body temperature (BBT)** recording, which aids in identification of follicular and luteal phase abnormalities. At the initial visit, the nurse instructs the woman in the technique of recording BBT on a special form. The woman is instructed to begin a new chart on the first day of every monthly cycle. The temperature can be taken with a standard oral or rectal thermometer calibrated by tenths of a degree, making slight temperature changes readily apparent (Carcio, 1998). A special kind of thermometer (BBT) may be used to measure temperatures only between 35 °C and 37.8 °C (96 °F and 100 °F). In addition to the traditional glass and mercury thermometer, tympanic thermometry, which provides a reading in only a few seconds, may also be a valid method. In addition, computerized or digitalized BBT devices ("the Rabbit," Fertil-A-Chron) are being developed to identify the fertile period more accurately at home.

TABLE 4–2   Fertility Awareness

Avoid douching and artificial lubricants. Prevent alteration of pH of vagina and introduction of spermicidal agents.

Promote retention of sperm. The male superior position with female remaining recumbent for at least 1 hour after intercourse maximizes the number of sperm reaching the cervix.

Avoid leakage of sperm. Elevate the woman's hips with a pillow after intercourse. Avoid getting up to urinate for 1 hour after intercourse.

Maximize the potential for fertilization. Have intercourse one to three times per week at intervals no less than 48 hours.

Avoid emphasizing conception during sexual encounters to decrease anxiety and potential sexual dysfunction.

Maintain adequate nutrition and reduce stress. Using stress-reduction techniques and good nutritional habits increases sperm production.

Explore other methods to increase fertility awareness, such as home assessment of cervical mucus and basal body temperature (BBT) recordings.

Seek counsel and advice from valued friend or family member.

Consider incorporating culturally appropriate methods to enhance fertility.

TABLE 4–3 Initial Infertility Physical Workup and Laboratory Evaluation

Female	Male
PHYSICAL EXAMINATION Assessment of height, weight, blood pressure, temperature, and general health status Endocrine evaluation of thyroid for exophthalmos, lid lag, tremor, or palpable gland Optic fundi evaluation for presence of increased intracranial pressure, especially in oligomenorrheal or amenorrheal women (possible pituitary tumor) Reproductive features (including breast and external genital area) Physical ability to tolerate pregnancy	**PHYSICAL EXAMINATION** General health (assessment of height, weight, blood pressure) Endocrine evaluation (e.g., presence of gynecomastia) Visual fields evaluation for bitemporal hemianopia Abnormal hair patterns
PELVIC EXAMINATION Papanicolaou smear Culture for gonorrhea if indicated and possibly chlamydia or mycoplasma culture (opinions vary) Signs of vaginal infections Shape of escutcheon (e.g., does public hair distribution resemble that of a male?) Size of clitoris (enlargement caused by endocrine disorders) Evaluation of cervix; old lacerations, tears erosion, polyps, condition and shape of os, signs of infections, cervical mucus (evaluate for estrogen effect of spinnbarkheit and cervical ferning)	**UROLOGIC EXAMINATION** Presence or absence of phimosis Location of urethral meatus Size and consistency of each testis vas deferens and epididymis Presence of varicocele
BIMANUAL EXAMINATION Size shape, position, and motility of uterus Presence of congenital anomalies Presence of endometriosis Evaluation of adnexa ovarian size, cysts, fixations, or tumors	**RECTAL EXAMINATION** Size and consistency of prostate with microscopic evaluation of prostate fluid for signs of infection Size and consistency of seminal vesicles
RECTOVAGINAL EXAMINATION Presence of retroflexed or retroverted uterus Presence of rectouterine pouch masses Presence of possible endometriosis	**LABORATORY EXAMINATION** Complete blood count Sedimentation rate, if indicated Serology Urinalysis Rh factor and blood grouping Semen analysis If indicated testicular biopsy, buccal smear Hormonal assays, FSH, LH, prolactin
LABORATORY EXAMINATION Complete blood count Sedimentation rate, if indicated Serology Urinalysis Rh factor and blood grouping If indicated, thyroid function tests, prolactin levels, glucose tolerance test, hormonal assays including estradiol, LH, progesterone, FSH, dehydroepiandrosterone (DHEA), androstendione, testosterone, 17 α-hydroxy progesterone (17-OHP).	

The woman records daily variations on the temperature graph. The temperature graph shows a typical biphasic pattern during ovulatory cycles, whereas in anovulatory cycles it remains monophasic. The woman uses the readings on the temperature graph to detect ovulation and direct timing of intercourse (Figure 4–2 ◆).

Basal temperature for females in the preovulatory phase is usually below 36.7 °C (98 °F). As ovulation approaches, production of estrogen increases. At its peak, estrogen may cause a slight drop, then a rise, in the basal temperature. The slight drop in temperature before ovulation is often difficult to capture on the BBT chart (Carcio, 1998). Prior to ovulation, a surge of luteinizing hormone (LH) stimulates production of progesterone, causing a 0.3 °C to 0.6 °C (0.5 °F to 1 °F) rise in basal temperature. These changes in the basal temperature create the typical biphasic pattern. Figure 4–2B shows a biphasic ovulatory BBT chart. Progesterone is thermogenic (produces heat); therefore, it maintains the temperature increase during the second half of the menstrual cycle (luteal phase). Temperature elevation does not predict the day of ovulation, but it does provide supportive evidence of ovulation about a day after it has occurred. Actual release of the ovum probably occurs 24 to 36 hours before the first temperature elevation (Carcio, 1998; Speroff et al., 1999).

Based on serial BBT charts, the clinician might recommend sexual intercourse every other day beginning 3 to 4 days prior to and continuing for 2 to 3 days after the expected time of ovulation. (See "Teaching About: Methods of Determining Ovulation.")

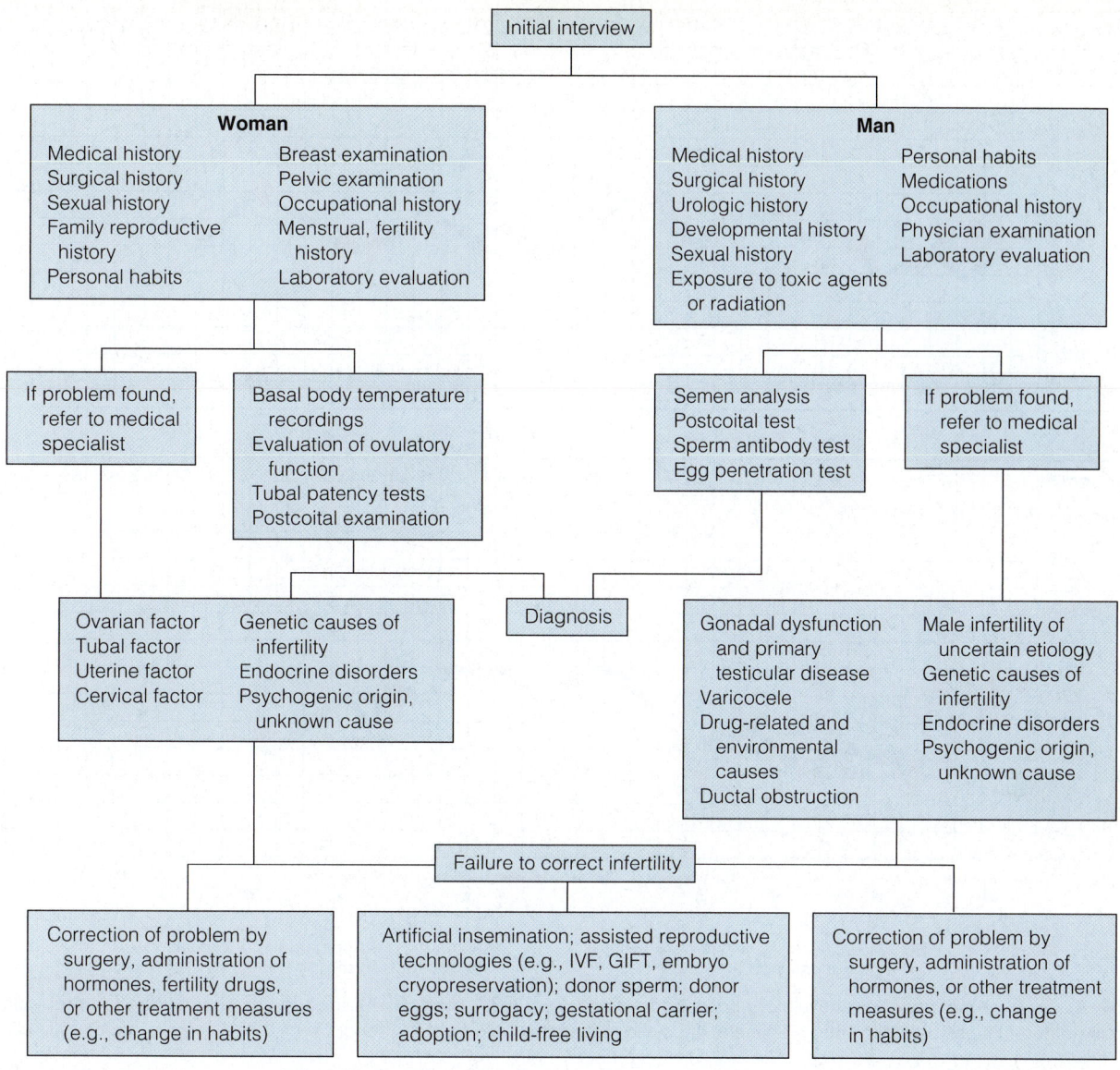

FIGURE 4–1. ◆ Flowchart for management of the infertile couple.

Hormonal assessments of ovulatory function fall into the following categories:

1. *Gonadotropin levels (FSH, LH)*. Baseline hormonal assessment of follicle-stimulating hormone (FSH) and LH provides valuable information about normal ovulatory function. Measured on cycle day 3, FSH is the single most valuable test of ovarian reserve and function. FSH should always be measured, particularly in women over age 35, to predict the potential for successful treatment with ovulation-induction treatment cycles. LH levels may be measured early in the cycle to rule out androgen excess disorders, which disrupt normal follicular development and oocyte maturation. Daily sampling of LH at midcycle can detect the LH surge. The day of the LH surge is believed to be the day of maximum fertility. Urine LH ovulation prediction kits are also available for home use to better time postcoital testing, insemination, and coitus (Moghissi, 1998).

2. *Progesterone assays*. Progesterone levels furnish the best evidence of ovulation and corpus luteum functioning. Serum levels begin to rise with the LH surge and peak about 8 days later. A level of 5 ng/mL 3 days after the LH surge confirms ovulation (Moghissi, 1998). On day 21 (7 days postovulation) a level of 10 ng/mL or higher indicates an adequate luteal phase. Hormonal assessment may also be conducted for prolactin, thyroid-stimulating hormone, and androgen (testosterone, dehydroepiandrosterone (DHEAS), and androstenedione) levels.

Endometrial biopsy provides information about the effects of progesterone produced by the corpus luteum after ovulation and endometrial receptivity. The biopsy is

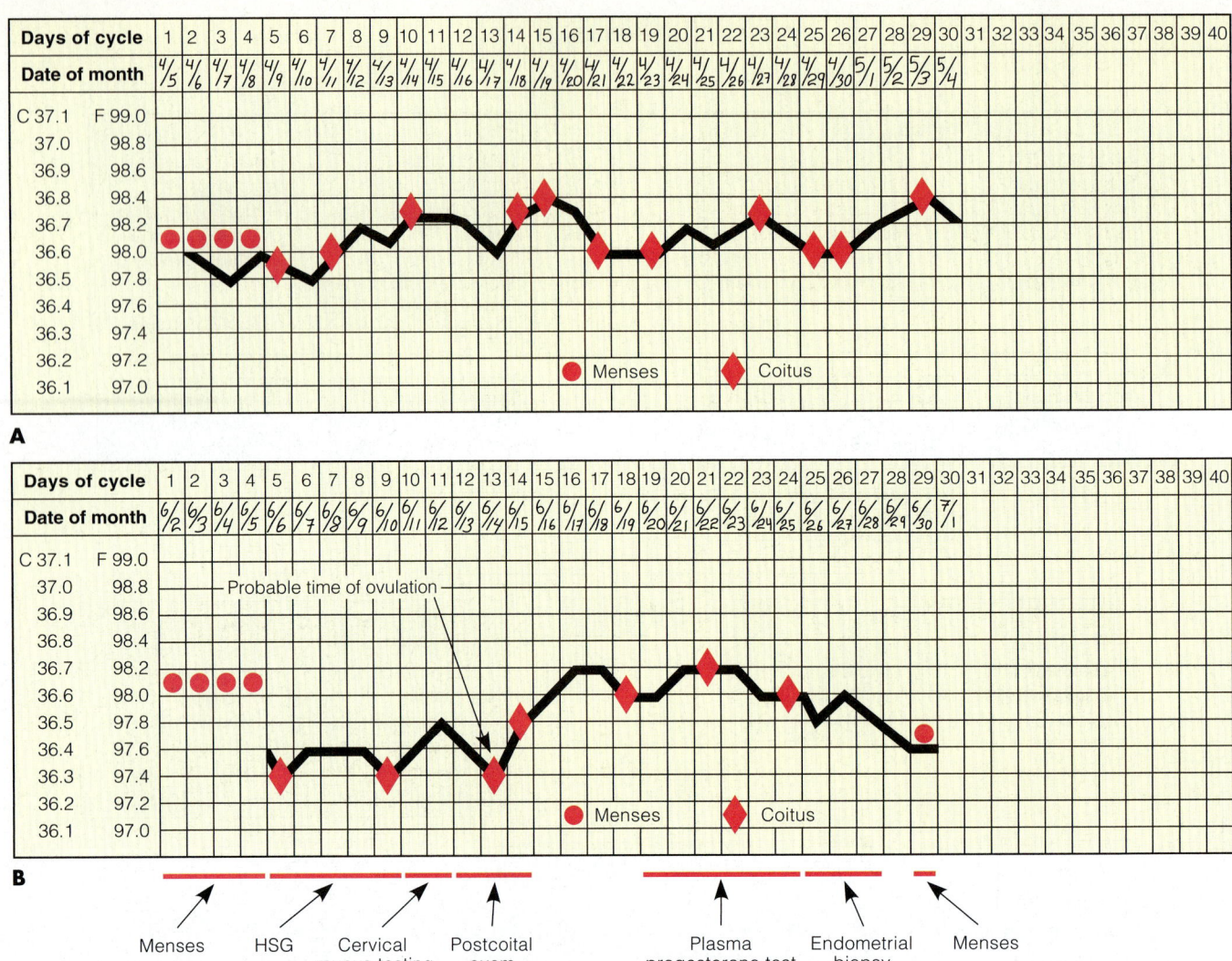

FIGURE 4–2. ◆ **A,** A monophasic, anovulatory basal body temperature (BBT) chart. **B,** A biphasic BBT chart illustrating probable time of ovulation, the different types of testing, and the time in the cycle that each would be performed.

performed not earlier than 10 to 12 days after ovulation and involves removing a sample of endometrium with a small pipette attached to suction (Speroff et al., 1999). The woman should be informed that some pelvic discomfort, cramping, and vaginal spotting are normal during and following the procedure. The onset of menses following biopsy should be disclosed for accurate interpretation of the biopsy report. A dysfunction may exist if the endometrial lining does not show the expected amount of secretory tissue for that day of the woman's menstrual cycle. Endometrial biopsies and serum progesterone assay may both be necessary to confirm luteal phase dysfunction.

Transvaginal ultrasound is an invaluable adjunct in infertility diagnosis and treatment. Transvaginal ultrasound is the method of choice for follicular monitoring of women undergoing induction cycles, for timing ovulation for insemination and intercourse, for retrieving oocytes for in vitro fertilization, and for monitoring early pregnancy. The use of a transvaginal color flow Doppler to investigate uterine blood flow may in the future help the endocrinologist

evaluate the adequacy of the developing follicle, further assess oocyte maturity and endometrial development and patterns, and improve the diagnosis of luteal phase defects (Moghissi, 1998).

Evaluation of Cervical Factors. The mucous cells of the endocervix consist predominantly of water. As ovulation approaches, the ovary increases its secretion of estrogen and produces changes in the cervical mucus. The amount of mucus increases 10-fold, and the water content rises significantly.

At ovulation, mucus elasticity (**spinnbarkheit**) increases and viscosity decreases. Excellent spinnbarkheit exists when the mucus can be stretched 8 to 10 cm or longer (Speroff et al., 1999). Mucus elasticity is determined by using two glass slides (Figure 4–3A ◆) or by grasping some mucus at the external os and stretching it through the vagina toward the introitus. (See "Teaching About: Methods of Determining Ovulation.")

The **ferning capacity** (crystallization) (Figure 4–3B ◆) of the cervical mucus also increases as ovulation approaches.

Teaching About

Ferning is caused by decreased levels of salt and water interacting with the glycoproteins in the mucus during the ovulatory period and is thus an indirect indication of estrogen production. To test for ferning, mucus is obtained from the cervical os, spread on a glass slide, allowed to air dry, and examined under the microscope. Within 24 to 48 hours postovulation, rising levels of progesterone markedly decrease the quantity of cervical mucus and increase its viscosity and cellularity. The resulting absence of spinnbarkheit and ferning capacity decreases sperm survival.

To be receptive to sperm, cervical mucus must be thin, clear, watery, profuse, alkaline, and acellular. As shown in Figure 4–4 ◆, the mazelike microscopic mucoid strands

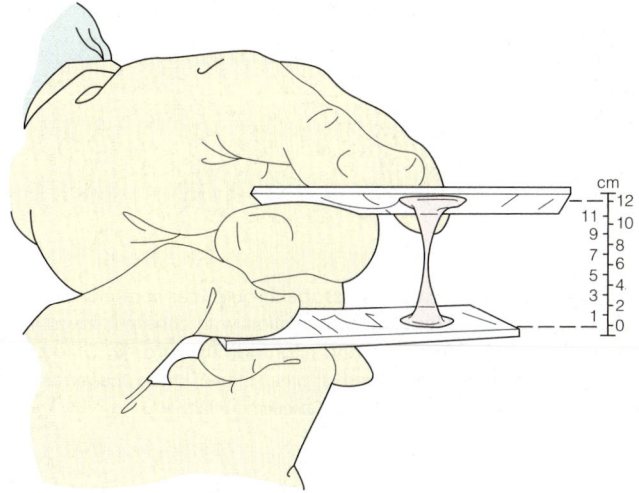

A

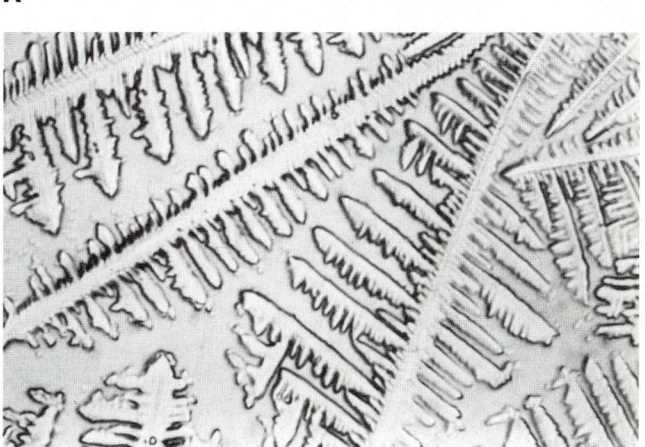

B

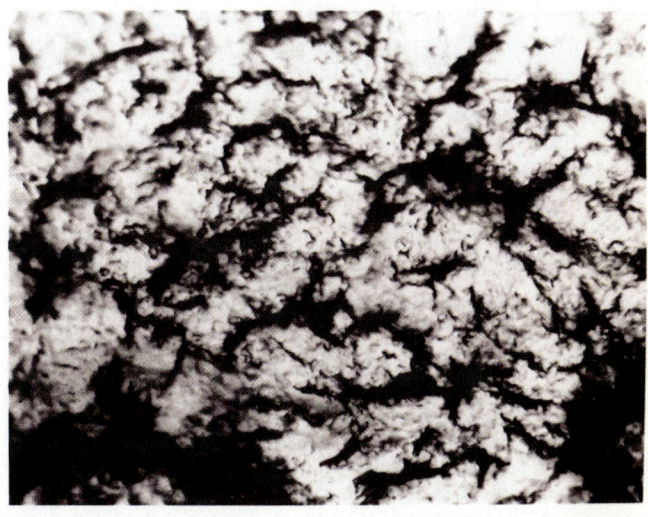

C

FIGURE 4–3. ◆ **A,** Spinnbarkheit (elasticity). **B,** Ferning pattern. **C,** Lack of ferning. *Note:* From Speroff, L., et al. (1994). *Clinical gynecologic endocrinology and infertility* (5th ed., p. 818). Baltimore: Williams & Wilkins.

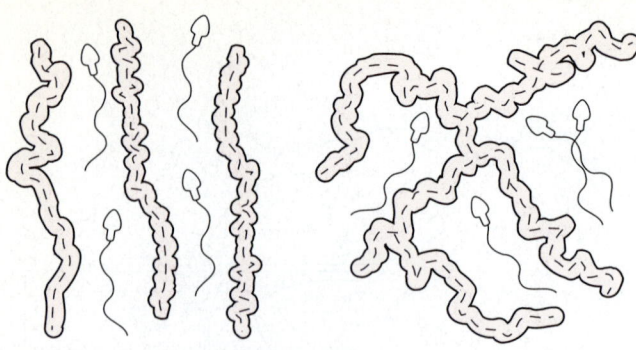

FIGURE 4–4. ◆ Sperm passage through cervical mucus. **A,** Appearance at the time of ovulation with channels favoring efficient sperm penetration and migration upward. **B,** Unfavorable mazelike configuration found at other times during the menstrual cycle. *Note:* From Corson, S. (1990). *Conquering infertility* (p. 16). New York: Prentice-Hall.

align in a parallel manner to allow for easy sperm passage. The mucus is termed *inhospitable* if these changes do not occur.

Cervical mucus inhospitable to sperm survival can have several causes, some of which are treatable. For example, estrogen secretion may be inadequate for development of receptive mucus. Cervical infection is another cause of mucosal hostility to sperm; it can be treated, depending on the type of infection. Cone biopsy, electrocautery, or cryosurgery of the cervix may remove large numbers of mucus-producing glands, creating a "dry cervix" that decreases sperm survival. Finally, treatment with clomiphene citrate may have harmful effects on cervical mucus due to its antiestrogenic properties. Therapy with supplemental estrogen for approximately 6 days before expected ovulation encourages the formation of suitable spinnbarkheit (Speroff et al., 1999). However, intrauterine insemination is more often the most appropriate therapy to overcome these obstacles. Profuse mucus is necessary for a hospitable sperm environment.

The cervix can also be the site of secretory immunologic reactions in which antisperm antibodies are produced, causing agglutination or immobilization of sperm. The most widely used serum-sperm bioassay to detect specific classes of antibodies in serum and seminal fluid is immunobead testing by radio immunoassay. The treatment for antisperm antibodies may include intrauterine insemination of the man's washed sperm to bypass the cervical factor.

The **postcoital test,** (PCT), also called the **Huhner test,** is performed 1 or 2 days before the expected date of ovulation as determined by previous BBT charts, the length of prior cycles, or a urinary LH kit. This examination evaluates the cervical mucus, sperm motility, sperm-mucus interaction, and the sperm's ability to negotiate the cervical mucus barrier (Speroff et al., 1999). The couple can have intercourse up to 12 hours before the examination. If the results are abnormal, the test should be repeated at the optimal time of 2 to 3 hours after intercourse. A small plastic catheter aspirates mucus from the internal and external os.

The mucus is measured and examined microscopically for signs of infection, spinnbarkheit, ferning, number and motility of active spermatozoa per high-power field (HPF), and number of sperm with poor or no motility. The focus of the postcoital exam on the timing of intercourse may promote sexual difficulties in some infertile couples.

Evaluation of Uterine Structures and Tubal Patency.
Tubal patency tests are usually done after BBT evaluation, semen analysis, and other less invasive tests. Tubal patency and uterine structure are usually evaluated by hysterosalpingography. Other invasive tests of tubular function are laparoscopy and hysteroscopy. Hysteroscopy may be performed earlier in the evaluation if the woman's history suggests possible tubal or adhesive disease or uterine abnormalities.

Hysterosalpingography (HSG), or hysterogram, involves an instillation of a radiopaque substance into the uterine cavity. As the substance fills the uterus and fallopian tubes and spills into the peritoneal cavity, it is viewed with x-ray techniques. This procedure can reveal tubal patency and any distortions of the uterine cavity. In addition, the oil-based dye and injection pressure used in HSG may have a therapeutic effect. This effect may be caused by the flushing of debris, breaking of adhesions, or induction of peristalsis by the instillation (Carcio, 1998). The HSG should be performed in the proliferative phase of the cycle to avoid interrupting an early pregnancy. This timing also avoids the lush secretory changes in the endometrium that occur after ovulation, which may prevent the passage of the dye through the tubes and present a false picture of cornual obstruction. HSG causes moderate discomfort. The pain is referred from the peritoneum (which is irritated by the subdiaphragmatic collection of gas) to the shoulder. The cramping may be decreased if the radiopaque dye is warmed to body temperature before instillation. Women can take an over-the-counter prostaglandin synthesis inhibitor (such as ibuprofen) 30 minutes before the procedure to decrease the pain, cramping, and discomfort. HSG can also cause recurrence of pelvic inflammatory disease, so prophylactic antibiotics are recommended to prevent infection that could be triggered by the procedure (Speroff et al., 1999). *Hysteroscopy* allows the physician to further evaluate any areas of suspicion within the uterine cavity or fallopian tubes revealed by the HSG. It is often done in conjunction with a laparoscopy, but it can be done independently and does not require general anesthesia. A fiberoptic instrument is inserted into the uterus for further evaluation of polyps, fibroids, or structural variations (Speroff et al., 1999).

Laparoscopy enables direct visualization of the pelvic organs and is usually done 6 to 8 months after the HSG unless symptoms suggest the need for earlier evaluation. Diagnostic laparoscopy is an outpatient procedure requiring the use of general anesthesia. Generally, a three-puncture approach is used; entry is made through the umbilical area, and supporting instruments are inserted in two suprapubic incisions. The peritoneal cavity is distended with carbon dioxide gas so that the pelvic organs can be directly visualized with a fiberoptic instrument. Tubular patency can be assessed by instillation of dye into the uterine cavity through the cervix. The pelvis is evaluated for endometriosis, adhesions, organ fixations, pelvic inflammatory disease, tumors, and cysts. The intraperitoneal gas is usually manually expressed at the end of the procedure. In routine preanesthesia instructions, the woman is told that she may have some discomfort from organ displacement and shoulder and chest pain caused by gas in the abdomen. She should be informed that she can resume normal activities as tolerated after 24 hours. Using postoperative pain medication and assuming a supine position may help relieve discomfort caused by any remaining gas.

ASSESSMENT OF THE MAN

A semen analysis is the single most important initial diagnostic study of the man; it should be done early in the couple's evaluation, before invasive testing of the woman. Although a postcoital test can provide information about sperm viability, it does not provide sufficient information about normal seminal parameters. To obtain adequate results, the specimen is collected after 2 to 3 days of abstinence, usually by masturbation to avoid contamination or loss of any ejaculate. If the man has difficulty producing sperm by masturbation, special medical-grade condoms are available to collect the sperm during intercourse. Neither regular nor nonlatex condoms should be used, because they contain spermicidal agents and sperm can be lost in the condom. Most lubricants also are spermicidal and should not be used unless approved by the andrology laboratory. Both seasonal and incidental variability may be seen in count and motility in successive semen analyses from the same person. Thus, a repeat semen analysis may be required to assess the man's fertility potential adequately; a minimum of two separate analyses is recommended for confirmation. In cases in which a known testicular insult has occurred (infection, high fevers, or surgery), a repeat analysis may not be done for at least 2.5 months to allow for new sperm maturation.

Sperm analysis provides information about sperm motility and morphology and a determination of the absolute number of spermatozoa present (Table 4–4). Although low numbers and motility may indicate compromised fertility, other parameters, such as morphology, motion patterns, and progression, are important prognostic indicators. Values previously thought to indicate subfertility may in fact be compatible with normal fertility when morphology, motion patterns, and progression factors are considered. An infertile specimen is one that has fewer than 20 million sperm per milliliter, less than 50% motility at 6 hours, or less than 30% normal sperm forms (Damani & Shaban, 1999). Some studies have indicated that the quality of sperm decreases with increased age (Speroff et al., 1999).

Spermatozoa have been shown to possess intrinsic antigens that can provoke male immunologic infertility. Immunologic infertility is especially apparent following vasectomy reversals or genital trauma, such as testicular torsion, in which

TABLE 4–4 Normal Semen Analysis

Factor	Value
Volume	> 2 mL
pH	7 to 8
Total sperm count	> 20 million/mL
Liquefaction	Complete in 1 hour
Motility	50% or greater forward progression
Normal forms	30% or greater
Round cells	< 5 million/mL
White cells	< 1 million/mL

Note: From World Health Organization. (1993). *The WHO laboratory manual for the examination of human semen and sperm-cervical mucus interaction* (3rd ed.). Geneva, Switzerland: Author.

autoimmunity to sperm (the man produces antibodies to his sperm) develops. Research now indicates that it is the actual presence of antibodies on the spermatozoal surface (not just the presence of antibodies in the serum) that affects sperm function and thus leads to subfertility. Treatment for antisperm antibodies is directed toward preventing the formation of antibodies or arresting the underlying mechanism that compromises sperm function. Therapies such as immunosuppression with corticosteriods have not proved effective. The treatment of choice for clinically significant antisperm antibodies is in vitro fertilization or intrauterine insemination (Damani & Shaban, 1999).

Complementary Care

COMMON TREATMENTS FOR INFERTILITY

Couples experiencing infertility may seek out alternative treatments. Some common treatments include acupuncture and herbs.

Acupuncture: Acupuncture is a therapy used in traditional Chinese medicine (TCM), and has become a very popular complementary treatment. Acupuncture involves inserting sterile needles into specific points on the body to control the flow of chi, or life energy (Gottlieb, 2000). Acupuncture treatment would focus on balancing the flow of chi in the kidneys and adrenal glands. Several clinical studies have shown acupuncture to be effective in treating infertility in both men and women (Sinclair, 2000; Siterman, Eltes, Wolfson, et al., 2000; Beal, 1999; Bartoov, Eltes, Reichart, et al., 1999; Chen, 1997; Siterman, Eltes, Wolfson, et al., 1997; Gerhard & Postneek, 1992; Stener-Victorin, Waldenstrom, Andersson, et al., 1996; Tiran & Mack, 2000).

Herbal Treatments: Herbs frequently recommended to treat infertility include ginseng and astragalus. Herbalists cite the healing and hormone-balancing effects of these herbs (Gladstar, 1993). Ginseng has historically been used in traditional chinese medicine to enhance male virility and fertility (Sinclair, 2000). Several studies also cite ginseng, as well as astralagus, in enhancing in vitro sperm motility (Chen, Xu, Chen, et al., 1999; Hong, Ku, & Wu, 1992).

The nurse should be alert for signs that the couple is pursuing complementary therapies out of desperation, and may not be using their best judgment.

Methods of Infertility Management

PHARMACOLOGICAL METHODS

If an ovulation defect is detected during the fertility testing, the treatment depends on the specific cause. If a woman has normal ovaries, a normal prolactin level, and an intact pituitary gland, *clomiphene citrate* (Clomid or Serophene) is often used (See "Drug Guide: Clomiphene Citrate"). This medication induces ovulation in 80% of women by actions at both the hypothalamic and ovarian levels; 40% of these women will become pregnant. Approximately 5% of women develop multiple-gestation pregnancies, almost exclusively twins.

The woman should be knowledgeable about side effects and call her health care provider if they occur. When visual disturbances (flashes, blurring, or spots) occur, bright lighting should be avoided. This side effect disappears within a few days or weeks after discontinuation of therapy

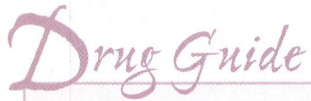

CLOMIPHENE CITRATE (CLOMID, SEROPHENE)

Overview of Action

Clomid stimulates follicular growth by stimulating the release of FSH and LH. Ovulation is expected to occur 5 to 9 days after last dose. Used when anovulation is caused by hypothalamic dysfunction luteal phase dysfunction or oligo-ovulation and for in vitro fertilization protocols.

Route, Dosage, Frequency

Administered orally. Fifty mg/day to 150 mg/day for 5 days beginning from day 3 to day 5 of the menstrual cycle. Usually start with 50 mg/day and increase dose 50 mg to a maximum of 200–250 mg (Leibowitz & Hoffman, 2000). May need to give estrogen simultaneously if decrease in cervical mucus occurs.

Contraindications

Presence of ovarian enlargement ovarian cysts hyperstimulation syndrome, liver disease, visual problems, pregnancy.

Side Effects

Antiestrogenic effects may cause decrease in cervical mucus production and endometrial lining development. Other side effects include vasomotor flushes; abdominal distention and ovarian enlargement secondary to follicular growth (bloating) and multiple corpus luteum formation; pain, soreness, breast discomfort; nausea and vomiting, visual symptoms (spots, flashes); headaches; dryness or loss of hair; multiple pregnancies.

Nursing Considerations

Determine if couple has been advised to have sexual intercourse every other day for 1 week beginning 5 days after the last day of medications.

Instruct couple on use of BBT chart to assess whether ovulation has occurred or instruct on the use of urinary LH kits to predict the onset of LH surge. Also inform couple that ultrasound, plasma progesterone, and postcoital test may be done. Remind couples that if the woman doesn't have a period she must be checked for the possibility of pregnancy before another trial of Clomid is started.

(Speroff et al., 1999). Hot flashes may be due to the antiestrogenic properties of clomiphene citrate. The woman can obtain some relief by increasing intake of fluids and using fans. Therapy using *human menopausal gonadotropins (hMG),* which include *menotropins* (Pergonal®, Hemegon™, and Repronex) and *urofollitropin* (Fertinex), is indicated as a first line of therapy for anovulatory infertile women with low to normal levels of gonadotropins (FSH and LH) and as a second line of therapy in women who fail to ovulate or conceive with clomiphene citrate therapy and in women undergoing assisted reproduction to induce superovulation. Menotropin is a combination of FSH and LH obtained from postmenopausal women's urine. Urofollitropin (FSH only) is indicated for women who have excessive androgen production, such as those with *polycystic ovary disease (PCO).* Clients with polycystic ovary disease have high endrogenous LH levels. Urofollitropin, which is predominantly FSH, is used to equalize the hormonal ratio and induce ovulation.

Gonadotropin therapy requires close observation by use of serum estradiol levels and ultrasound. Monitoring of follicle development is necessary to minimize the risk of multiple pregnancy and to avoid hyperstimulation syndrome. The daily dose of medication given is titrated based on serum estradiol and ultrasound findings. When follicle maturation has occurred, human chorionic gonadotropin (hCG) may be administered by intramuscular injection to stimulate ovulation. The couple is advised to have intercourse 24 to 36 hours after hCG administration and for the next 2 days. Women who elect to have hMG medication usually have passed through all other forms of management without conceiving. Strong emotional support and thorough education are needed because of the numerous office visits and injections. Often the male partner is instructed, with return demonstration, to administer the daily injections (Leibowitz & Hoffman, 2000). High prolactin levels may impair the glandular production of FSH and LH or block their action on the ovaries. When hyperprolactinemia accompanies anovulation, the infertility may be treated with *bromocriptine* (Parlodel). This medication acts directly on the prolactin-secreting cells in the anterior pituitary. It inhibits the pituitary's secretion of prolactin, thus preventing suppression of the pulsatile secretion of FSH and LH. Thus, normal menstrual cycles are restored and ovulation is induced by allowing FSH and LH production. If treatment is successful, the tests of ovulatory function will indicate that ovulation is occurring with a normal luteal phase. Bromocriptine should be discontinued if pregnancy is suspected or at the anticipated time of ovulation because of its possible teratogenic effects. Side effects include nausea, diarrhea, dizziness, headache, and fatigue. To minimize side effects for women who are extremely sensitive, treatment may be initiated with a dose of 1.25 mg, slowly building tolerance toward the usual dose of 2.5 mg given twice daily. An intravaginal preparation may also be used to decrease the occurrence of side effects (Carcio, 1998).

When endometriosis is determined to be the cause of infertility, *danazol* (Danocrine®) may be given to suppress ovulation and menstruation and to effect atrophy of the ectopic endometrial tissue. Temporary suppression has been shown to result in healing of the endometriosis. The treatment regimen may last for 6 to 12 months or longer, depending on the severity of the disease. Other pharmacologic treatments involve use of oral contraceptives or oral medroxyprogesterone acetate and gonadotropin-releasing hormone (GnRH) agonists (Leibowitz & Hoffman, 2000; Yuen, 1999). The management and care of endometriosis is further discussed in Chapter 3.

Treatment of luteal phase defects may include the use of progesterone to augment luteal phase progesterone levels. Ovulation-induction agents, such as clomiphene citrate or menotropins, may be used to augment proliferative phase FSH production in the developing follicle. It is also common to use progesterone supplementation in conjunction with these ovulation-induction agents if the drug alone does not correct the luteal phase. Occasionally, hCG therapy may be used in the luteal phase to stimulate corpus luteum production of progesterone.

THERAPEUTIC INSEMINATION

Therapeutic insemination has replaced the previously used term *artificial insemination* and involves depositing semen at the cervical os or in the uterus by mechanical means. *Therapeutic donor insemination (TDI)* is the current term for use of donor semen, and *therapeutic husband insemination (THI)* is the current term for use of the husband's semen. THI is used in cases of inadequate volumes of sperm, decreased motility, and anatomic defects accompanied by inadequate deposition or penetration of semen, or retrograde ejaculation (Sigman, 1999). It is also indicated in cases of unexplained infertility and some cases of female factor infertility, such as scant or inhospitable mucus, persistent cervicitis, or cervical stenosis. Because the seminal fluid contains high levels of prostaglandins, intrauterine insemination prevents the violent reaction of nausea, severe cramps, abdominal pain, and diarrhea that can result from the absorption of prostaglandins by the uterine lining (Sigman, 1999). Sperm preparation for intrauterine insemination involves washing sperm from the seminal plasma.

TDI is considered in cases of azoospermia (absence of sperm), inherited male sex-linked disorders, and autosomal dominant disorders. Some states have specified the parental rights of single women and donors, but most are silent on this issue (Speroff et al., 1999).

TDI has become more complicated and expensive in the past decade because of the need for strict screening and processing procedures. Guidelines established by the American Fertility Society (1994) include mandatory medical (genetic) and infectious disease screening of both donor and recipient, the need for informed consent from all parties, the need to limit the number of pregnancies per donor, and the need for accurate means of record keeping.

Finally, because of the risk of transmitting infectious diseases, donated sperm must be frozen and quarantined for 6 months from the time of acquisition, and the donor must be retested before sperm can be released for use.

Numerous factors need to be evaluated before TDI is performed. Has every possible effort been made to diagnose and treat the cause of the male infertility? Do tests indicate normal fertility and sperm-ovum transport in the woman? Has the couple had an opportunity to discuss this option with an infertility counselor to explore the issues of secrecy, disclosure, and potential feelings of loss the couple (particularly the male partner) may feel about not having a genetic child? Are there any religious constraints? After making the decision, the couple should allow themselves time to further assess their concerns and explore their feelings individually and together to ensure that this option is acceptable to both.

Intrauterine insemination, with or without ovulation-induction therapy, is an option for many couples before more aggressive treatments such as in vitro fertilization and gamete intrafallopian transfer are employed.

IN VITRO FERTILIZATION

The **in vitro fertilization (IVF)** procedure is selectively used in cases in which infertility has resulted from tubal factors, mucus abnormalities, male infertility, unexplained infertility, male and female immunologic infertility, and cervical factors. In IVF a woman's eggs are collected from her ovaries, fertilized in the laboratory, and placed into her uterus after normal embryo development has begun. If the procedure is successful, the embryo continues to develop in the uterus, and pregnancy proceeds naturally.

The potential for a successful pregnancy with IVF is maximized when three to four embryos (rather than one) are placed in the uterus. For this reason, fertility drugs are used to induce ovulation prior to the process. Follicular development and oocyte maturity are monitored frequently with ultrasound and hormonal assays. Monitoring usually begins around cycle day 5, and medications are titrated according to individual response. When follicles appear mature, hCG is given to stimulate final egg maturation and control the induction of ovulation. Egg retrieval is performed approximately 35 hours later. Once the eggs are fertilized and progress to the embryo stage, the embryos are placed in the uterus. After the procedure, the woman is advised to engage in only minimal activity for 12 to 24 hours, and progesterone supplementation is prescribed. Success with IVF depends on many factors, but especially the woman's age and the specific indication. Women have a good chance of achieving pregnancy with an average of three cycles of IVF. Many couples find the emotional, physical, and financial costs of going beyond three cycles too great (Speroff et al., 1999). Clinical delivery rates reported by the Society of Assisted Reproductive Technology (SART) in 1997 were 28.7% per embryo transfer for women regardless of age or indication (American Society for Reproductive Medicine, 2000). The increase in maternal and neonatal morbidity associated with IVF because of the rates of multiple gestation remains an issue. Differences in successful IVF may exist between various ethnic groups (Sharara & McClamrock, 2000).

OTHER ASSISTED REPRODUCTIVE TECHNIQUES

Gamete intrafallopian transfer (GIFT) involves the retrieval of oocytes by laparoscopy; immediate placement of the oocytes in a catheter with washed, motile sperm; and placement of the gametes into the fimbriated end of the fallopian tube. Fertilization occurs in the fallopian tube as with normal conception (in vivo) [CD] rather than in the laboratory (in vitro). From the GIFT technology evolved procedures such as *zygote intrafallopian transfer (ZIFT) and* **tubal embryo transfer (TET).** In these procedures eggs are retrieved and incubated with the man's sperm. However, the eggs are transferred back to the woman's body at a much earlier stage of cell division [CD] than in IVF and, as in GIFT, are placed in the fallopian tube or tubes and not the uterus. In tubal embryo transfer the placement is done at the embryo stage. These procedures allow fertilization to be documented, which is not possible with GIFT, and the pregnancy rate is theoretically increased when the fertilized ovum is placed in the fallopian tube. IVF success rates approximate those that have been achieved with the GIFT procedure, and IVF is a much less invasive and costly procedure. For these reasons, GIFT and other tubal procedures have lost some acceptance and IVF techniques are more often used. However, GIFT may be more acceptable to adherents of some religions, since fertilization does not occur outside the woman's body. Other technologies involve oocyte donation and cryopreservation of the embryo (Kingsberg, Applegarth, & Janata, 2000).

Several new reproductive technologies can help families with genetic problems or infertile women who are unable to carry a pregnancy. The diagnosis of genetic disorders via blastomere analysis before implantation gives couples the option of forgoing the attempt to establish a pregnancy and thereby avoiding a difficult decision about terminating an affected pregnancy (Verp, 1999a). Assisted embryo hatching is a micromanipulation procedure that has proved to be an effective adjunct therapy in IVF. IVF using a gestational carrier allows infertile women who are genetically sound but unable to carry a pregnancy to exercise the option of having their own biologic child (Pergament & Fiddler, 2000).

Nursing Care in the Community

Infertility therapy taxes a couple's financial, physical, and emotional resources. Treatment can be costly, and often insurance coverage is limited. Years of effort and numerous evaluations and examinations may take place before conception occurs, if it occurs at all. In a society that values children and considers them to be the natural result of marriage, infertile couples face a myriad of tensions and

discrimination. Clinic nurses need to be constantly aware of the emotional needs of the couple confronting infertility evaluation and treatment. Often an intact marriage will become stressed with intrusive infertility procedures and treatments. Constant attention to temperature charts and instructions about their sex life from a person outside the relationship naturally affect the spontaneity of a couple's interactions. Tests and treatments may heighten feelings of frustration or anger between partners. The need to share this intimate area of a relationship, especially when one or the other is identified as "the cause" of infertility, may precipitate feelings of guilt or shame. Infertility often becomes a central focus for role identity, especially for women (Greil, 1997). The couples may experience feelings of loss of control, feelings of reduced competency and defectiveness, loss of status and ambiguity as a couple, a sense of social stigma, stress on the marital and sexual relationship, and strained relationships with health care providers. The nurse's role can be summarized as that of counselor, educator, and advocate. Throughout the evaluation process, nurses play a key role in lessening the stress these couples must endure by providing resources and accurate information about what is entailed in treatment and what physical, emotional, and financial demands the couple can anticipate throughout the process (Glover, Hunter, Richards, et al., 2000).

The nurse's ability to assess and respond to emotional and educational needs is essential to give infertile couples a sense of control (Carcio, 1998; Klock & Greenfeld, 2000). An assessment tool such as an infertility questionnaire (Table 4–5) may be helpful. Extensive and repeated explanations and written instruction may be necessary because the couple's anxiety often overwhelms their ability to retain all the information given. It is important to use a nursing framework that recognizes the multidimensional needs of the infertile individual or couple within physical, social, psychologic, spiritual, and environmental contexts.

Infertility may be perceived as a loss by one or both partners. Affected individuals have described this loss as loss of their relationship with spouse, family, or friends; their health; their status or prestige; their self-esteem and self-confidence; their security; and the potential child. One such loss alone may lead to depression, but in many cases the crisis of infertility evokes feelings of all these losses (Bradshaw, 1998). Each couple passes through several stages of feelings, not unlike those identified by Kübler-Ross: surprise, denial, anger, isolation, guilt, grief, and resolution. The impact of these feelings on the couple and how fast they move into resolution, if ever, may depend on the cause and on the duration of treatment. Each partner may progress through the stages at different rates (Sandelowski, 1994). Nonjudgmental acceptance and a professional, caring attitude on the nurse's part can go far in dissipating the negative emotions the couple may experience while going through these stages.

This is also a time when the nurse may assess the couple's relationship: Are they able and willing to communicate verbally and share feelings? Are they mutually supportive?

TABLE 4–5 Infertility Questionnaire

Self-Image

1. I feel bad about my body because of our inability to have a child.
2. Since our infertility, I feel I can do anything as well as I used to.
3. I feel as attractive as before our infertility.
4. I feel less masculine/feminine because of our inability to have a child.
5. Compared with others, I feel I am a worthwhile person.
6. Lately, I feel I am sexually attractive to my wife/husband.
7. I feel I will be incomplete as a man/woman if we cannot have a child.
8. Having an infertility problem makes me feel physically incompetent.

Guilt/Blame

1. I feel guilty about somehow causing our infertility.
2. I wonder if our infertility problem is due to something I did in the past.
3. My spouse makes me feel guilty about our problem.
4. There are times when I blame my spouse for our infertility.
5. I feel I am being punished because of our infertility.

Sexuality

1. Lately I feel I am able to respond to my spouse sexually.
2. I feel sex is a duty, not a pleasure.
3. Since our infertility problem, I enjoy sexual relations with my spouse.
4. We have sexual relations for the purpose of trying to conceive.
5. Sometimes I feel like a "sex machine," programmed to have sex during the fertile period.
6. Impaired fertility has helped our sexual relationship.
7. Our inability to have a child has increased my desire for sexual relations.
8. Our inability to have a child has decreased my desire for sexual relations.

Note: The questionnaire is scored on a Likert scale, with responses ranging from "strongly agree" to "strongly disagree." Each question is scored separately, and the mean score is determined for each section (Self-Image, Guilt/Blame, and Sexuality) The total mean score is then divided by 3. A final mean score of greater than 3 indicates distress. *Note:* From Bernstein, J., Potts, N,. & Mattox, J. H. (1985). Assessment of psychological dysfunction associated with infertility. *Journal of Obstetric, Gynecologic, and Neonatal Nursing, 14* (Suppl.), 64S, Table 1.

The answers to such questions may help the nurse to identify areas of strength and weakness and to construct an appropriate plan of care. Referral to mental health professionals is helpful when the emotional issues become too disruptive in the couple's relationship or life. The couple should be aware of infertility support and education organizations such as RESOLVE, which may help meet some of their needs and validate their feelings. Finally, individual or group counseling with other infertile couples may help the couple resolve feelings brought about by their own difficult situation.

ADOPTION

Infertile couples consider various alternatives for resolving their infertility; adoption is one option that will be considered at several points during the treatment process. The adoption of an infant can be a difficult and frustrating experience for everyone involved. As couples begin to consider adoption, an important aspect of this exploration is the reading of magazines and informational books on adoption, attending adoption support groups and conferences, and meeting with adoptive parents to discuss their experiences with adoption (Carcio, 1998). Some couples seek international adoption or consider adopting older children, children with handicaps, or children of mixed parentage because the adoption process in such cases is quicker and more children are available. Nurses in the community can assist couples considering adoption by providing information on community resources for adoption and support through the adoption process. Couples also need support if they choose to remain childless.

PREGNANCY AFTER INFERTILITY

The feeling of being infertile does not necessarily disappear with pregnancy. Although there may be initial ecstasy, couples may face a whole new arena of fear and anxiety, and the parents-to-be often do not know where they "fit in." They may feel a great sense of isolation because those who have had no trouble conceiving cannot relate to the physical and emotional pain they endured to achieve the pregnancy. Contact with their past support system composed of other infertile couples may vanish when peers learn they have resolved their infertility problems. Although the desperation to become pregnant may have superseded the couple's ability to acknowledge their concerns about undergoing various treatments or procedures, questions about the repeated cycle of fertility drugs or the achievement of pregnancy through IVF technology or cryopreservation may now arise. The expectant couple may be very concerned about the potential of these treatments to adversely affect the fetus (Buitendijk, 1999). Couples may need reassurance throughout the pregnancy to allay these anxieties. The nurse can assist couples who conceive after infertility by acknowledging their past experiences of infertility treatment; validating their fears and anxieties as they face childbirth classes, birth, and parenting issues; and providing support and education about what to anticipate physically and emotionally throughout the pregnancy.

GENETIC DISORDERS

Even when conception has been achieved, families can have special reproductive concerns. The desired and expected outcome of any pregnancy is the birth of a healthy, "perfect" baby. Parents experience grief, fear, and anger when they discover that their baby has been born with a defect or a genetic disease. Such an abnormality may be evident at birth or may not appear for some time. The baby may have inherited a disorder from one parent, or both, creating guilt and strife within the family.

Regardless of the type or scope of the problem, parents will have many questions: "What did I do?" "What caused it?" "Will it happen again?" The nurse must anticipate the couple's questions and concerns and guide, direct, and support the family. To do so, the nurse must have a basic knowledge of genetics and genetic counseling. Many congenital malformations and diseases are genetic or have a strong genetic component. Others are not genetic at all. Professional nurses can help expedite this questioning process if they understand the principles involved and can direct the family to the appropriate resources to help them cope with the questions and fears surrounding birth defects.

Chromosomes and Chromosomal Analysis

All hereditary material is carried on tightly coiled strands of DNA known as **chromosomes.** Chromosomes carry the genes, the smallest units of inheritance. The *Human Genome Project,* which began in 1988, has made remarkable advances toward determining the exact DNA sequence of every human gene. ⬭ [WEB]

All *somatic (body) cells* contain 46 chromosomes, which is the *diploid* number; the sperm and egg contain 23 chromosomes, or the *haploid* number ⬭ (see Chapter 5). There are 23 pairs of homologous chromosomes (a matched pair of chromosomes, one inherited from each parent); 22 of the pairs are **autosomes** (nonsex chromosomes), and one pair is made up of the sex chromosomes, X and Y. A normal female has a 46,XX chromosome constitution; a normal male has a 46,XY chromosome constitution (Figures 4–5 ◆ and 4–6 ◆). The **karyotype,** or pictorial analysis of these chromosomes, is usually obtained from specially treated and stained peripheral blood lymphocytes. Placental tissue taken from a site near the insertion of the cord and deep enough to include chorion can also be sent for karyotyping.

Chromosomal abnormalities can occur in either the autosomes or the sex chromosomes and can be divided into two categories: abnormalities of number and abnormalities of structure. Even small alterations in chromosomes can cause problems, especially those associated with delayed growth and development. The child need not have obvious major congenital malformations to be affected. Some of these abnormalities can be passed on to other offspring. Thus, in some cases, chromosomal analysis is appropriate even if clinical manifestations are mild. Whatever the case, too much or too little genetic material usually produces adverse effects on a child's growth and development. The Human Genome Project has already led to the identification of the gene associated with certain abnormalities such as fragile X and cystic fibrosis (Williams, 2000).

Autosomal Abnormalities

Abnormalities of chromosome number are most commonly seen as trisomies, monosomies, and mosaicism. In all three cases, the abnormality is most often caused by nondisjunction. Nondisjunction occurs when paired chromosomes fail to separate during cell division. If nondisjunction occurs in either the sperm or the egg before fertilization, the

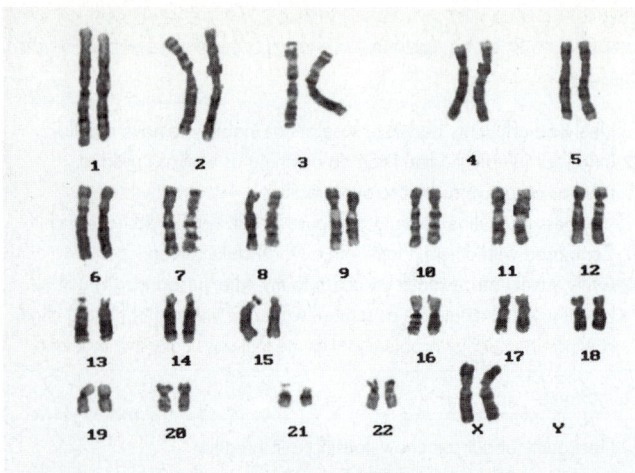

FIGURE 4–5. ◆ Normal female karyotype. Courtesy of David Peakman. Reproductive Genetics Center, Denver, CO.

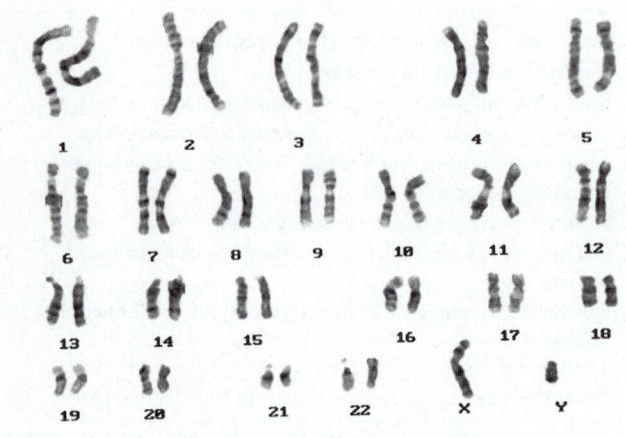

FIGURE 4–6. ◆ Normal male karyotype. Courtesy of David Peakman, Reproductive Genetics Center, Denver, CO.

resulting zygote (fertilized egg) will have an abnormal chromosome makeup in all of the cells (trisomy or monosomy). If nondisjunction occurs after fertilization, the developing zygote will have cells with two or more different chromosome makeups, evolving into two or more different cell lines (mosaicism).

Trisomies are the product of the union of a normal gamete (egg or sperm) with a gamete that contains an extra chromosome. The individual will have 47 chromosomes and is trisomic (has three copies of the same chromosome) for whichever chromosome is extra (Table 4–6). Down syndrome (formerly called mongolism) is the most common trisomy abnormality seen in children (Figure 4–7 ◆). The presence of the extra chromosome 21 produces distinctive clinical features (Figure 4–8 ◆). With the advent of modern surgical techniques and antibiotics, children with Down syndrome are now living into their fifth and sixth decades.

Two other common trisomies are trisomy 18 and trisomy 13 (see Table 4–6 and Figures 4–9 ◆ and 4–10 ◆).

TABLE 4–6 Chromosomal Syndromes

Altered Chromosome: 21	Characteristics
Genetic defect: trisomy 21 (Down syndrome) (secondary nondisjunction or 14/21 unbalanced translocation) Incidence: average 1 in 700 live births, incidence variable with age of woman (Figure 4–8)	CNS: mental retardation; hypotonia at birth Head: flattened occiput; depressed nasal bridge; mongoloid slant of eyes; epicanthal folds; white specking of the iris (Brushfield spots); protrusion of the tongue; high, arched palate; low-set ears Hands: broad, short fingers; abnormalities of finger and foot; dermal ridge patterns (dermatoglyphics); transverse palmar crease (simian line) Other: congenital heart disease

Altered Chromosome: 18	Characteristics
Genetic defect: trisomy 18 Incidence: 1 in 3,000 live births (Figure 4–9)	CNS: mental retardation; severe hypotonia Head: prominent occiput; low-set ears; corneal opacities; ptosis (drooping eyelids) Hands: third and fourth fingers overlapped by second and fifth fingers; abnormal dermatoglyphics; syndactyly (webbing of fingers) Other: congenital heart defects; renal abnormalities; single umbilical artery; gastrointestinal tract abnormalities; rocker-bottom feet; cryptorchidism; various malformations of other organs

Altered Chromosome: 13	Characteristics
Genetic defect: trisomy 13 Incidence: 1 in 5,000 live births (Figure 4–10)	CNS: mental retardation; severe hypotonia; seizures Head: microcephaly; microphthalmia and/or coloboma (keyhole-shaped pupil); malformed ears; aplasia of external auditory canal; micrognathia (abnormally small lower jaw); cleft lip and palate Hands: polydactyly (extra digits); abnormal posturing of fingers; abnormal dermatoglyphics Other: congenital heart defects; hemangiomas; gastrointestinal tract defects; various malformations of other organs

Altered Chromosome: 5P	Characteristics
Genetic defect deletion of short arm of chromosome 5 (cri du chat, or cat cry syndrome) Incidence: 1 in 20,000 live births	CNS: severe mental retardation; a catlike cry in infancy Head: microcephaly; hypertelorism (widely spaced eyes); epicanthal folds; low-set ears Other: failure to thrive; various organ malformations

Altered Chromosome: XO (Sex Chromosome)	Characteristics
Genetic defect: only one X chromosome in female (Turner syndrome) Incidence: 1 in 300–7,000 live female births (Figure 4–11)	CNS: no intellectual impairment; some perceptual difficulties Head: low hairline; webbed neck Trunk: short stature; cubitus valgus (increased carrying angle of arm); excessive nevi (congenital discoloration of skin due to pigmentation); broad, shieldlike chest with widely spaced nipples; puffy feet; no toenails Other: fibrous streaks in ovaries; underdeveloped secondary sex characteristics; primary amenorrhea; usually infertile; renal anomalies; coarctation of the aorta

Altered Chromosome: XXY (Sex Chromosome)	Characteristics
Genetic defect: extra X chromosome in male (Klinefelter syndrome) Incidence: 1 in 1,000 live male births, approximately 1%–2% of institutionalized males	CNS: mild mental retardation Trunk: occasional gynecomastia (abnormally large male breasts); eunuchoid body proportions (lack of male muscular and sexual development) Other: small, soft testes; underdeveloped secondary sex characteristics: usually sterile

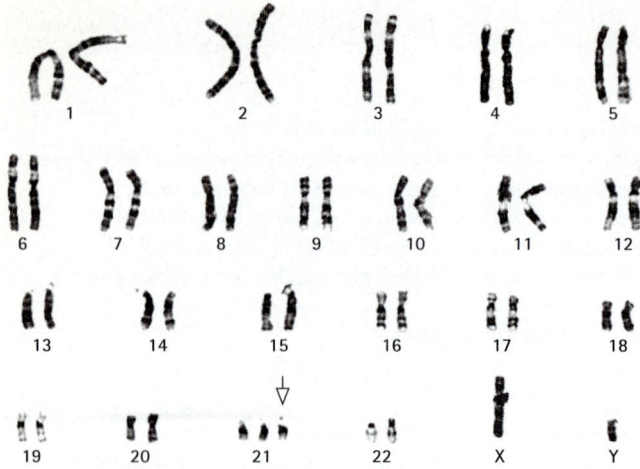

FIGURE 4–7. ◆ Karyotype of a male who has trisomy 21, Down syndrome. *Note:* the extra 21 chromosome. Courtesy of David Peakman, Reproduction Genetics Center, Denver, CO.

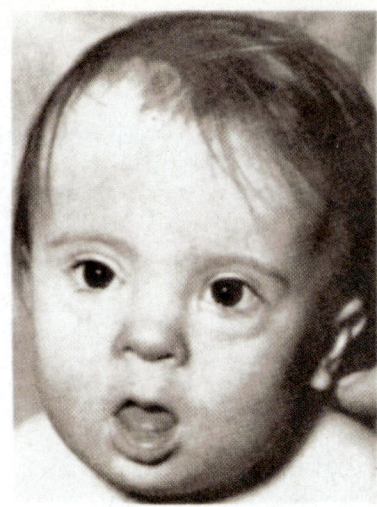

FIGURE 4–8. ◆ A child with Down syndrome. *Note:* From Jones, K. L. (1988). *Smith's recognizable patterns of human malformations* (4th ed.). Philadelphia: Saunders.

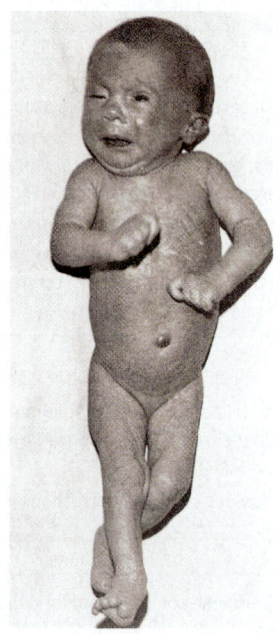

FIGURE 4–9. ◆ Infant with trisomy 18. *Note:* From Jones, K. L. (1988). *Smith's recognizable patterns of human malformations* (4th ed.). Philadelphia: Saunders.

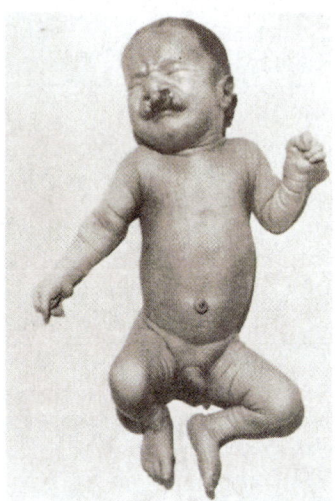

FIGURE 4–10. ◆ Infant with trisomy 13. *Note:* From Jones, K. L. (1988). *Smith's recognizable patterns of human malformations* (4th ed.). Philadelphia: Saunders.

The prognosis for both trisomy 13 and 18 is extremely poor. Most children (70%) die within the first 3 months of life secondary to complications related to respiratory and cardiac abnormalities. However, 10% survive the first year of life; therefore, the family needs to plan for the possibility of long-term care of a severely affected infant and for family support.

Monosomies occur when a normal gamete unites with a gamete that is missing a chromosome. In this case the individual has only 45 chromosomes and is said to be monosomic. Monosomy of an entire autosomal chromosome is incompatible with life.

Mosaicism occurs after fertilization and results in an individual who has two different cell lines, each with a different chromosomal number. Mosaicism tends to be more common in the sex chromosomes than in the autosomes; when it occurs in the autosomes it is most common in those with Down syndrome. A person with many classic signs of Down syndrome but with normal or near-normal intelligence should be investigated for the possibility of mosaicism.

Abnormalities of chromosome structure involve only parts of the chromosome and occur in two forms: translocation and deletions or additions. Some children born with Down syndrome have an abnormal rearrangement of chromosomal material known as a *translocation.* Clinically, the two types of Down syndrome are indistinguishable. What is of major importance to the family is that the two different types have significantly different risks of recurrence. The only way to distinguish the two types of Down syndrome is to do a chromosome analysis. Risk of trisomy is 1 in 700 live births; in contrast, the risk is 1 in 1,500 live births with a balanced translocation. The translocation occurs when the carrier parent has 45 chromosomes, usually with one chromosome fused to another. A common translocation is one in which the parent has one normal 14, one normal 21, and one 14/21 chromosome. Since all the chromosomal material is present and functioning normally, the parent is clinically normal. This individual is known as a *balanced translocation carrier.* When a person who is a balanced translocation carrier has a child with a partner who has a structurally normal chromosome constitution, the child can have a normal number of chromosomes, be a carrier, or have an extra chromosome 21. A child with an extra chromosome 21 has an *unbalanced translocation* and has Down syndrome.

Structure abnormality is also caused by *additions* or *deletions* of chromosomal material. Any portion of a chromosome may be lost or added, generally leading to some adverse effect. Depending on how much chromosomal material is involved, the clinical effects may be mild or severe. Many types of additions and deletions have been described, such as the deletion of the short arm of chromosome 5 (cri du chat, or cat cry, syndrome) or the deletion of the long arm of chromosome 18 (see Table 4–6).

Sex Chromosome Abnormalities

To better understand abnormalities of the **sex chromosomes,** the nurse should know that in a female, at an early embryonic stage, one of the two normal X chromosomes becomes inactive. The inactive X chromosome forms a dark staining area known as the *Barr body.* The normal female has one Barr body, since one of her two X chromosomes has been inactivated. The normal male has no Barr bodies because he has only one X chromosome.

The most common sex chromosome abnormalities are Turner syndrome in females (45, XO with no Barr bodies present; see Figure 4–11 ◆) and Klinefelter syndrome in males (47, XXY with one Barr body present). See Table 4–6 for clinical descriptions of these abnormalities and Chapter 51 for nursing management. 🔗

Modes of Inheritance

Many inherited diseases are produced by an abnormality in a single gene or pair of genes. In such instances, the chromosomes are grossly normal. The defect is at the gene level. Some of these gene defects can be detected by technologies such as DNA and biochemical assays. The two major categories of inheritance are **mendelian (single-gene) inheritance** and **nonmendelian (multifactorial) inheritance.** Each single-gene trait is determined by a pair of genes working together. These genes are responsible for the observable expression of the traits (e.g., blue eyes, fair skin), referred to as the **phenotype.** The total genetic makeup of an individual is referred to as the **genotype** (pattern of the genes on the chromosomes).

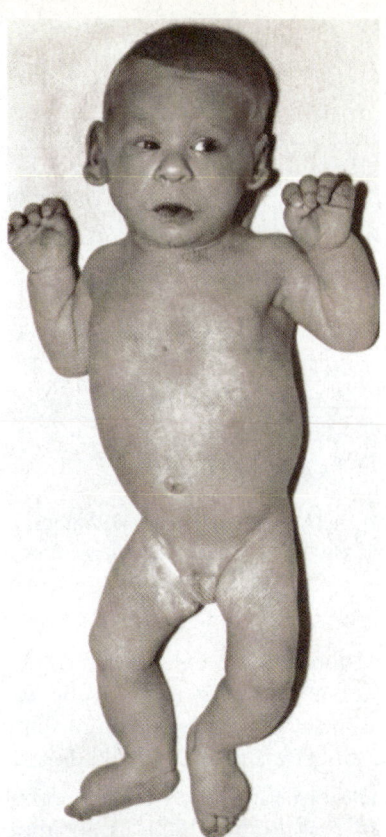

FIGURE 4–11. ◆ Infant with Turner syndrome at 1 month of age. Note prominent ears. *Note:* From Lemli, L., & Smith, D. W. (1963). The XO syndrome: A study of the differentiated phenotype in 25 patients. *Journal of Pediatrics, 63,* 577.

One of the genes for a trait is inherited from the mother, the other from the father. A person who has two identical genes at a given locus is *homozygous* for that trait. A person is *heterozygous* for a particular trait when he or she has two different *alleles* (alternate forms of the same gene) at a given locus on a pair of homologous chromosomes.

The best-known modes of single-gene inheritance are autosomal dominant, autosomal recessive, X-linked (sex-linked) recessive, and X-linked dominant mode of inheritance, which is less common.

AUTOSOMAL DOMINANT INHERITANCE

A person is said to have an autosomal dominantly inherited disorder if the disease trait is heterozygous; that is, the abnormal gene overshadows the normal gene of the pair to produce the trait. It is essential to remember that in autosomal dominant inheritance

1. An affected person generally has an affected parent. Thus the family **pedigree** (graphic representation of a family tree) usually shows multiple generations with the disorder.
2. An affected person has a 50% chance of passing on the abnormal gene to each of his or her children (Figure 4–12 ◆).

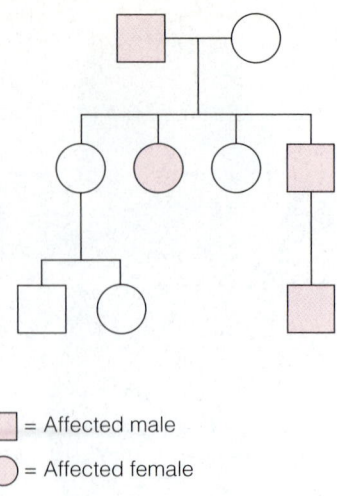

■ = Affected male

● = Affected female

FIGURE 4–12. ◆ Autosomal dominant pedigree. One parent is affected. Statistically, 50% of offspring will be affected, regardless of sex.

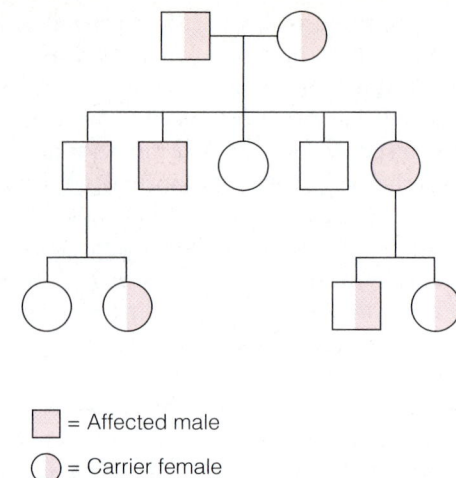

■ = Affected male

◗ = Carrier female

FIGURE 4–13. ◆ Autosomal recessive pedigree. Both parents are carriers. Statistically, 25% of offspring are affected, regardless of sex.

3. Males and females are equally affected, and a father can pass the abnormal gene on to his son. This is an important principle when distinguishing autosomal dominant disorders from X-linked disorders.

4. Autosomal dominant inherited disorders have varying degrees of presentation. This is an important factor when counseling families concerning autosomal dominant disorders. A parent with a mild form of the disease may have a child with a more severe form.

Some common autosomal dominant inherited disorders are Huntington disease, polycystic kidney disease, neurofibromatosis (von Recklinghausen disease), and achondroplastic dwarfism.

AUTOSOMAL RECESSIVE INHERITANCE

In an autosomal recessive inherited disorder, the person must have two abnormal genes to be affected. The notion of a *carrier state* is appropriate here. A carrier is heterozygous for the abnormal gene and clinically normal. It is not until two people mate and pass on the same abnormal gene that affected children may appear. It is essential to remember that in autosomal recessive inheritance

1. An affected person may have clinically normal parents, but both parents are carriers of the abnormal gene (Figure 4–13 ◆).

2. With two carrier parents there is a 25% chance that the abnormal gene will be passed on to any of their offspring. Each pregnancy has a 25% chance of resulting in an affected child.

3. If a child of two carrier parents is clinically normal, there is a 50% chance that he or she is a carrier of the gene.

4. Both males and females are equally affected.

5. There is an increased history of consanguineous matings (mating of close relatives).

Some common autosomal recessive inherited disorders are cystic fibrosis, phenylketonuria, (PKU), galactosemia, sickle-cell anemia, Tay-Sachs disease, and most metabolic disorders.

X-LINKED RECESSIVE INHERITANCE

X-linked, or sex-linked, disorders are those for which the abnormal gene is carried on the X chromosome. Thus, an X-linked disorder is manifested in a male who carries the abnormal gene on his X chromosome. His mother is considered to be a carrier when the normal gene on one X chromosome overshadows the abnormal gene on the other X chromosome. It is essential to remember that in X-linked recessive inheritance

1. There is no male-to-male transmission. Affected males are related through the female line (see Figure 4–14 ◆).

2. There is a 50% chance that a carrier mother will pass the abnormal gene to each of her sons, who will thus be affected. There is a 50% chance that a carrier mother will pass the normal gene to each of her sons, who will thus be unaffected. Finally, there is a 50% chance that a carrier mother will pass the abnormal gene to each of her daughters, who will become carriers.

3. Fathers affected with an X-linked disorder cannot pass the disorder to their sons, but all their daughters become carriers of the disorder.

Common X-linked recessive disorders are hemophilia, Duchenne muscular dystrophy, and color blindness.

X-LINKED DOMINANT INHERITANCE

X-linked dominant disorders are rare, the most common being vitamin D–resistant rickets and now the recognized fragile X syndrome. When X-linked dominant inheritance does occur, the pattern is similar to that of X-linked recessive inheritance except that heterozygous females are

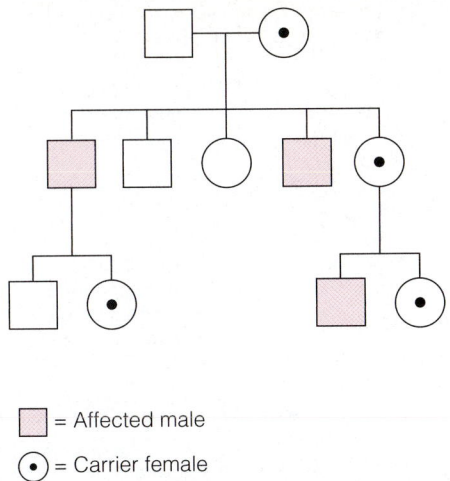

■ = Affected male

◉ = Carrier female

FIGURE 4–14. ◆ X-linked recessive pedigree. The mother is the carrier. Statistically, 50% of male offspring are affected, and 50% of female offspring are carriers.

affected. It is essential to remember that in X-linked dominant inheritance there is no male-to-male transmission. Affected fathers will have affected daughters but no affected sons.

FRAGILE X SYNDROME

Fragile X syndrome is a common inherited form of mental retardation second only to Down syndrome among all causes of moderate mental retardation in males (Hogge & Lanasa, 1999). Fragile X syndrome is a central nervous system disorder linked to a "fragile" site on the X chromosome. It is characterized by moderate mental retardation, large protuberant ears, and large testes after puberty. The carrier females do not have the abnormal features, but about one third are mildly mentally retarded. See Chapter 51 for management and nursing care discussion. ⊂⊃

MULTIFACTORIAL INHERITANCE

Many common congenital malformations, such as cleft palate, heart defects, spina bifida, dislocated hips, clubfoot, and pyloric stenosis, are caused by an interaction of many genes and environmental factors. They are, therefore, multifactorial in origin. It is essential to remember that in multifactorial inheritance

1. The malformations may vary from mild to severe. For example, spina bifida may range in severity from mild (spina bifida occulta) to more severe (myelomeningocele). It is believed that the more severe the defect, the greater the number of genes present for that defect.

2. There is often a sex bias. For example, pyloric stenosis is more common in males, whereas cleft palate is more common among females. When a member of the less commonly affected sex shows the condition, a greater number of genes must usually be present to cause the defect.

3. In the presence of environmental influences (such as seasonal changes, altitude, irradiation, chemicals in the environment, or exposure to toxic substances), fewer genes are needed to manifest the disease in the offspring.

4. In contrast to single-gene disorders, there is an additive effect in multifactorial inheritance. The more family members who have the defect, the greater the risk that the next pregnancy will also be affected.

Although most congenital malformations are multifactorial traits, a careful family history should always be taken, since cleft lip and palate, certain congenital heart defects, and other malformations occasionally can be inherited as autosomal dominant or recessive traits. Other disorders thought to be within the multifactorial inheritance group are diabetes, hypertension, some heart diseases, and mental illness.

Prenatal Diagnostic Tests

Parent-child and family-planning counseling have become a major responsibility of professional nurses. To be effective counselors, nurses must have the most up-to-date information about prenatal diagnosis. It is essential that couples be completely informed about the known and potential risks of each of the genetic diagnostic procedures. Nurses must recognize the emotional impact on the family of a decision to have or not have a genetic diagnostic procedure. The ability to diagnose certain genetic diseases has enormous implications for the practice of preventive health care. Several methods are available for prenatal diagnosis, although some are still experimental.

GENETIC ULTRASOUND

Ultrasound may be used to assess the fetus for genetic or congenital problems. With ultrasound, one can visualize the fetal head for abnormalities in size, shape, and structure (for a detailed discussion of ultrasound technology, see Chapter 14). ⊂⊃ Craniospinal defects (anencephaly, microcephaly, hydrocephalus), thoracic malformations (diaphragmatic hernia), gastrointestinal malformations (omphalocele, gastroschisis), renal malformations (dysplasia or obstruction), and skeletal malformations (caudal regression, conjoined twins) are only some of the disorders that have been diagnosed in utero by ultrasound. Screening by ultrasound for congenital anomalies is best done at 18 to 20 weeks, when fetal structures have developed completely. There is no information documenting harm to the fetus or long-term effects from exposure to ultrasound. However, complete safety is not guaranteed; therefore, the practitioner and the parents must evaluate the risks against the benefits on an individual basis.

GENETIC AMNIOCENTESIS

The major method of prenatal diagnosis is genetic amniocentesis (Figure 4–15 ◆ and Skill 2–5). ⊂⊃ SKILLS CD

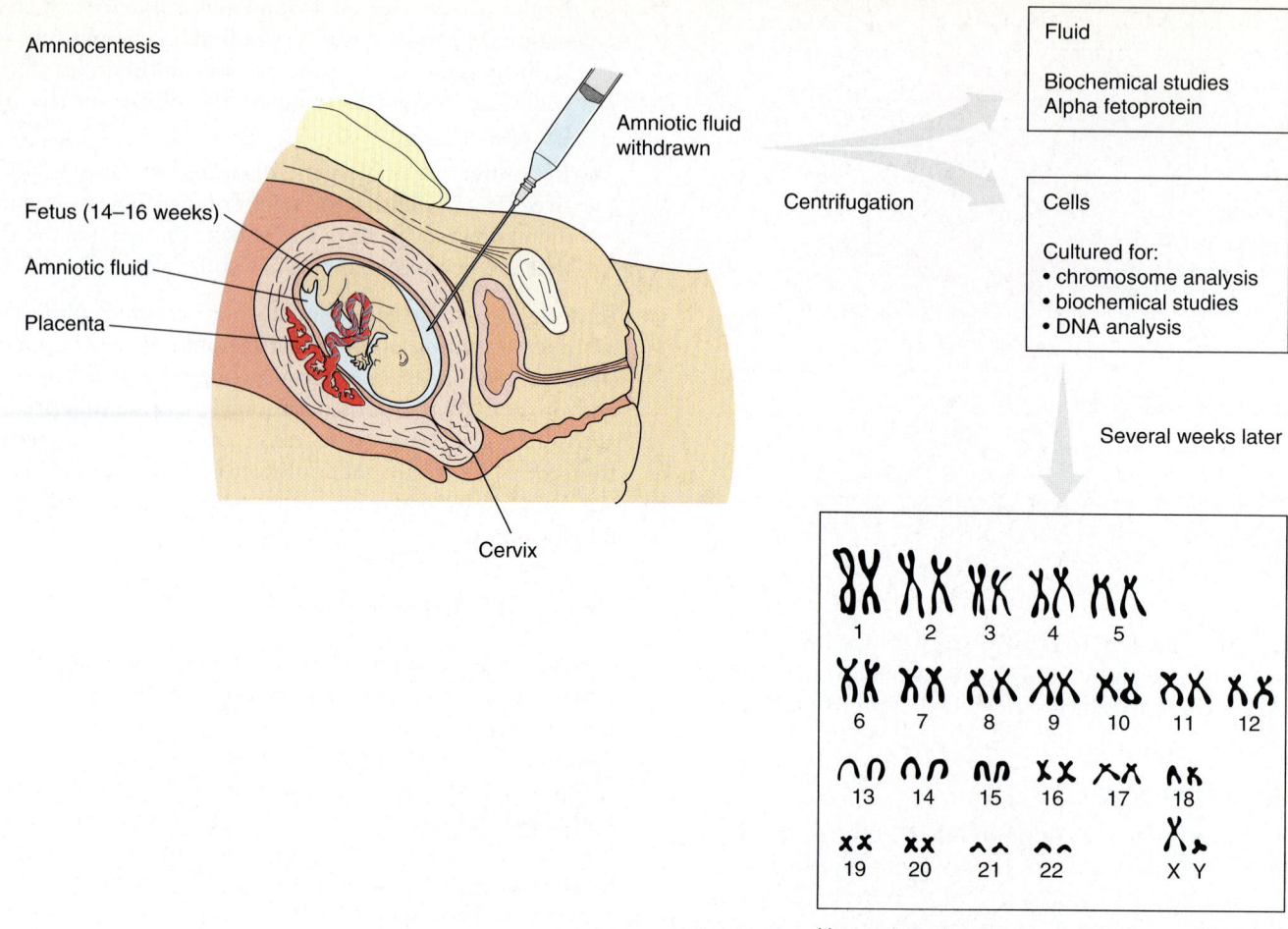

Amniocentesis

Amniotic fluid withdrawn

Fetus (14–16 weeks)

Amniotic fluid

Placenta

Cervix

Centrifugation

Fluid

Biochemical studies
Alpha fetoprotein

Cells

Cultured for:
• chromosome analysis
• biochemical studies
• DNA analysis

Several weeks later

Human karyotype

FIGURE 4–15. ◆ Genetic amniocentesis for prenatal diagnosis is done at 14 to 16 weeks' gestation.

The indications for genetic amniocentesis include the following:

1. *Maternal age 35 or older at the time of birth.* Women age 35 or older are at greater risk for having children with chromosomal abnormalities (see Chapter 10 for further discussion). Chromosomal abnormalities due to maternal age include trisomy 21, trisomy 13, trisomy 18, XXX, or XXY. The risk of having a live-born infant with a chromosome problem is 1 in 200 for a 35-year-old woman; the risk for trisomy 21 is 1 in 365 (Newberger, 2000). At age 45, the risks are 1 in 20 and 1 in 40, respectively.

2. *Previous child born with a chromosomal abnormality.* Young couples who have had a child with a trisomy 21, 18, or 13 have an approximately 1% to 2% risk of a future child having a chromosomal abnormality.

3. *Parent with balanced translocation (chromosomal abnormality).* A woman who carries a balanced 14/21 translocation has a risk of approximately 10% to 15% that her children will be affected with the unbalanced translocation of Down syndrome; if the father is the carrier, there is a 2% to 5% risk.

4. *Family history of known or suspected mendelian genetic disorder.* In families in which the woman is a known or possible carrier of an X-linked disorder such as hemophilia A or B, or Duchenne muscular dystrophy, genetic amniocentesis, chorionic villus sampling (CVS), or percutaneous umbilical blood sampling (PUBS) may be options. For a known female carrier, the risk of an affected male fetus is 50%. Now DNA testing may make it possible to distinguish affected males from nonaffected males in some disorders. In disorders in which female carriers can be distinguished from non-carriers, only the carrier females would be offered prenatal diagnosis. When both parents are carriers of an autosomal recessive disease, there is a 25% risk *for each pregnancy* that the fetus will be affected. Diagnosis is made by testing the cultured amniotic fluid cells (enzyme level, substrate level, product level, or DNA) or the fluid itself. Autosomal recessive diseases identified by amniocentesis are hemoglobinopathies such as sickle-cell anemia, thalassemia, and cystic fibrosis.

5. *Parents carrying an inborn error of metabolism that can be diagnosed in utero.* Metabolic disorders detectable in utero include argininosuccinicaciduria,

cystinosis, Fabry disease, galactosemia, Gaucher disease, homocystinuria, Hunter syndrome, Hurler syndrome, Krabbe disease, Lesch-Nyhan syndrome, maple syrup urine disease, metachromatic leukodystrophy, methylmalonic aciduria, Niemann-Pick disease, Pompe disease, Sanfilippo syndrome, and Tay-Sachs disease.

6. *Family history of neural tube defects.* Genetic amniocentesis is available to couples who have had a child with neural tube defects or who have a family history of these conditions, which include anencephaly, spina bifida, and myelomeningocele. Neural tube defects are usually multifactorial traits.

PERCUTANEOUS UMBILICAL BLOOD SAMPLING AND CHORIONIC VILLUS SAMPLING

Percutaneous umbilical blood sampling is a technique used for obtaining blood that allows for rapid chromosome diagnosis, genetic studies, or transfusion for Rh isoimmunization or hydrops. Chorionic villus sampling is used in selected regional centers, and its diagnostic capability is similar to that of amniocentesis. Its advantages are that diagnostic information is available at 8 to 10 weeks' gestation and that products of conception are tested directly. For further discussion, see Chapter 14.

ALPHA-FETOPROTEIN (AFP)

The maternal circulation or amniotic fluid is tested for alpha-fetoprotein (AFP). The maternal serum AFP (MSAFP) level is elevated in cases of infants with open neural tube defects, anencephaly, omphalocele, and gastroschisis; fetal death; vaginal bleeding; or multiple gestations (Rose & Mennuti, 2000). A woman with a family history of neural tube defects should consult her prenatal care provider for recommended folic acid dosages. Low MSAFP level has been associated with Down syndrome. MSAFP testing is done at 15 to 22 weeks' gestation (Scioscia, 1999). Ultrasound and amniocentesis are offered to patients with low or high MSAFP levels. Inaccurate dating is the most common cause for abnormal AFP; therefore, ultrasound dating is very important (Rose & Mennuti, 2000). With high MSAFP levels, normal amniotic fluid AFP, and normal ultrasound, there is an increased risk for preterm labor, perinatal death, and intrauterine growth retardation.

IMPLICATIONS OF PRENATAL DIAGNOSTIC TESTING

It is imperative that counseling precede any procedure for prenatal diagnosis. Many questions and points must be considered if the family is to reach a satisfactory decision. See Table 4–7 and "Developing Cultural Competence: Genetic Screening Recommendations for Various Ethnic and Age Groups." With the advent of diagnostic techniques such as amniocentesis and chorionic villus sampling, couples at risk who would not otherwise have additional children can decide to conceive. Following prenatal diagnosis, a couple can decide not to have a child with a genetic

TABLE 4–7 Couples Who May Benefit from Prenatal Diagnosis

Women age 35 or over at time of birth

Couples with a balanced translocation (chromosomal abnormality)

Family history of known or suspected mendelian genetic disorder (e.g., cystic fibrosis, hemophilia A & B, Duchenne muscular dystrophy)

Couples with a previous child with chromosomal abnormality

Couples in which either partner or a previous child is affected with, or in which both partners are carriers for, a diagnosable metabolic disorder

Family history of birth defects and/or mental retardation (e.g., neural tube defects, congenital heart disease, cleft lip and/or palate)

Ethnic groups at increased risk for specific disorders (see "Developing Cultural Competence")

Couples with history of two or more first-trimester spontaneous abortions

Women with an abnormal maternal serum alpha-fetoprotein (MSAFP or AFP3) test

Women with a teratogenic risk secondary to an exposure or maternal health condition (e.g., diabetes)

disease. For many couples, prenatal diagnosis is not a solution, however, since the only method of preventing a genetic disease is preventing the birth by terminating the pregnancy. The decision about whether to use prenatal diagnosis can only be made by the family. Even when termination is not an option, prenatal diagnosis can give parents an opportunity to prepare for the birth of a child with special needs, contact the families of children with similar problems, or access support services before the birth.

Every pregnancy has a 3% to 4% risk of resulting in an infant with a birth defect. When an abnormality is detected or suspected before birth, an attempt is made to determine the diagnosis by assessing the family health history (via the pedigree) and the pregnancy history and by evaluating the fetal anomaly or anomalies via ultrasound. Health care professionals can then present the parents with options. A family with a baby who has a lethal anomaly, such as trisomy 13 or 18, may wish to consider nonaggressive intervention. Many disorders can be diagnosed prenatally; the list has grown and continues to grow almost daily. Nurses should consult experts on a specific disorder before giving information to couples or discussing options. Treatment of prenatally diagnosed disorders may begin during the pregnancy, thus possibly preventing irreversible damage. For example, a mother carrying a fetus with galactosemia may follow a galactose-free diet. In light of the philosophy of preventive health care, information that can be obtained prenatally should be made available to all couples who are expecting a baby or who are contemplating pregnancy.

POSTNATAL DIAGNOSIS

Questions about genetic disorders (cause, treatment, and prognosis) are most often first discussed in the newborn nursery or during the infant's first few months of life. When a child is born with anomalies, has a stormy newborn period, or does not progress as expected, a genetic

Developing Cultural Competence

GENETIC SCREENING RECOMMENDATIONS FOR VARIOUS ETHNIC AND AGE GROUPS

Background of Population at Risk	Disorder	Screening Test	Definitive Test
Ashkenazic Jewish	Tay-Sachs disease	Decreased serum hexosaminidase-A	CVS* or amniocentesis for hexosaminidase-A assay
African; Hispanic from Caribbean, Central America, or South America,	Sickle-cell anemia	Presence of sickle-cell hemoglobin; confirmatory hemoglobin electrophoresis	CVS or amniocentesis for genotype determination; direct molecular studies
Greek, Italian	beta-thalassemia	Mean corpuscular volume < 80%; confirmatory hemoglobin electrophoresis	CVS or amniocentesis for genotype determination (direct molecular studies or indirect RFLP† analysis)
Southeast Asian (Vietnamese, Loatian, Cambodian), Filipino	alpha-thalassemia	Mean corpuscular volume < 80%; confirmatory hemoglobin electrophoresis	CVS or amniocentesis for genotype determination (direct molecular studies)
Women over age 35 (all ethnic groups)	Chromosomal trisomies	None	CVS or amniocentesis for cytogenetic analysis
Women of any age (all ethnic groups; particularly suggested for women from British Isles, Ireland)	Neural tube defects and selected other anomalies	Maternal serum alpha-fetoprotein (MSAFP)	Amniocentesis for amniotic fluid, alpha-fetoprotein, and acetylcholinesterase assays

*Chorionic villus sampling.
†Restriction fragment length polymorphism.

---

evaluation may be warranted. An accurate diagnosis and an optimal treatment plan incorporate the following:

- Complete and detailed history to determine whether the problem is prenatal (congenital), postnatal, or familial in origin
- Thorough physical examination, including dermatoglyphics analysis (Figure 4–16 ◆)
- Laboratory analysis, which includes chromosome analysis; enzyme assay for inborn errors of metabolism; DNA studies (both direct and by linkage); and antibody titers for infectious teratogens, such as toxoplasmosis, rubella, cytomegalovirus, and herpesvirus (TORCH syndrome) (see Chapter 13 for further discussion of these tests) ⬭
- Counsel and support for the family

To make an accurate diagnosis, the geneticist consults with other specialists and reviews the current literature. This permits the geneticist to evaluate all the available information before arriving at a diagnosis and plan of action. The Human Genome Project will have significant implications for the identification and management of inherited disorders. Once genes have been identified, it will be possible to detect their presence in carriers and lead to better genetic counseling. New genetic material might be inserted into cells to provide important missing information (gene transfer) as may be possible in cystic fibrosis, or medications can be specifically designed to target the disease on a molecular level (Jaffe, Bush, Gedes, et al., 1999; Tolstoi & Smith, 1999).

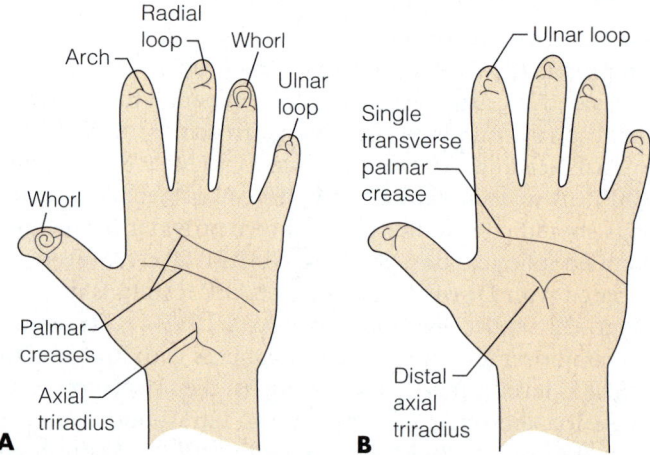

FIGURE 4–16. ◆ Dermatoglyphic patterns of the hands in **A,** a normal individual, and **B,** a child with Down syndrome. Note the single transverse palmar crease, distally placed axial triradius, and increased number of ulnar loops.

However, concerns have been voiced about ethical considerations with genetic research. What guidelines are needed to protect children and families so that genetic testing does not lead to discrimination in future employment or health insurance? Who should be tested for genetic diseases, and who should have access to the results? Since children cannot yet give informed consent for genetic testing (see Chapter 1 for discussion of informed consent), ⬭ it is recommended that children and adolescents should have genetic testing *only* when medical treatment could help if the disease is identified, or when another family member might benefit from the knowledge for their own health and the child will not be harmed by the testing (American Academy of Pediatrics, Committee on Genetics, 2000). Whenever genetic testing is performed, counseling about the results must be made available. Some nurses are choosing special educational programs to enable them to work in the growing field of genetics and health care.

Nursing Practice

The explosion in knowledge and clinical therapy related to genetics will offer challenges to those in health care. Just because a genetic test for a disease exists, should it be done on all newborns? What might be the potential harmful uses of information obtained about someone's genetic information? What forms of disadvantage and discrimination might occur if someone was known to carry a gene for breast cancer, a neurologic disease, or Alzheimer disease? The rapidly advancing technology demands a focus on the ethical aspects of use of genetic tests and information. The Ethical, Legal, and Social Implications (ELSI) Program of the National Human Genome Research Institute has been established to explore these issues (American Academy of Pediatrics, 2000; Giarelli & Jacobs, 2000). WEB

Nursing Care in the Community

Genetic counseling is a communication process in which a genetic counselor gives a family the most complete and accurate information about the occurrence or the risk of recurrence of a genetic disease in that family (Verp, 1999b).

In retrospective genetic counseling, time is a crucial factor. One cannot expect a couple who has just learned that their child has a birth defect or Down syndrome to take in any information concerning future risks. However, the couple should never be "put off" from genetic counseling for so long that they conceive another affected child because of lack of information. The perinatal nursing team nurse frequently has the first contact with the parents who have a newborn with a congenital abnormality. At the birth of an affected child, the nurse can inform the parents that genetic counseling is available before they attempt to have another child. Genetic counseling is an appropriate course of action for any family wondering, "Will it happen again?" The family nurse practitioner, neonatal nurse practitioner, or family-planning nurse is in an excellent position to reach at-risk families before the birth of another baby with a congenital problem. Genetic counseling referral is advised for any of the following categories:

1. *Congenital abnormalities, including developmental delay.* Any couple who has a child or a relative with a congenital malformation may be at increased risk and should be so informed. If developmental delay of

unidentified cause has occurred in a family, there may be an increased risk of recurrence. In many cases the genetic counselor will identify the cause of a malformation as a teratogen (see Chapter 9). The family should be aware of teratogenic substances so they can avoid exposure during any subsequent pregnancy.

2. *Familial disorders.* Families should be told that certain diseases may have a genetic component and that the risk of their occurrence in a particular family may be higher than that in the general population. Such disorders as diabetes, heart disease, cancer, and mental illness fall into this category.

3. *Known inherited diseases.* Families may know that a disease is inherited but not know the mechanism or the specific risk for them. An important point to remember is that family members who are not at risk for passing on a disorder should be as well informed as family members who are at risk.

4. *Metabolic disorders.* Any family at risk for having a child with a metabolic disorder or biochemical defect should be referred. Because most inborn errors of metabolism are inherited in an autosomal recessive manner, a family may not be identified as being at risk until the birth of an affected child. Carriers of the sickle-cell trait can be identified before they conceive a child, and the risk of having an affected child can be determined. Prenatal diagnosis of an affected fetus is only available experimentally.

5. *Chromosomal abnormalities.* As discussed previously, any couple who has had a child with a chromosomal abnormality may be at increased risk of having another child similarly affected. This group includes families in which there is concern about a possible translocation. After a couple has been referred to the genetics clinic, they are sent a form requesting information on the health status of various family members. At this time, the nurse can help by discussing the form with the couple or clarifying the information needed to complete it.

A pedigree and history facilitate identification of other family members who might also be at risk for the same disorder (Figure 4–17 ◆). The couple being counseled may wish to notify relatives at risk so that they, too, can begin genetic counseling. When done correctly, the family history and pedigree can be powerful tools for determining a family's risk.

The counselor gathers additional information about the pregnancy, the affected child's growth and development, and the family's understanding of the problem. Generally, the child undergoes a physical examination. Other family members may also be examined. If laboratory tests such as chromosomal analyses, metabolic studies, or viral titers are indicated, they are performed at this time. The genetic counselor may then give the parents some preliminary information based on the data at hand.

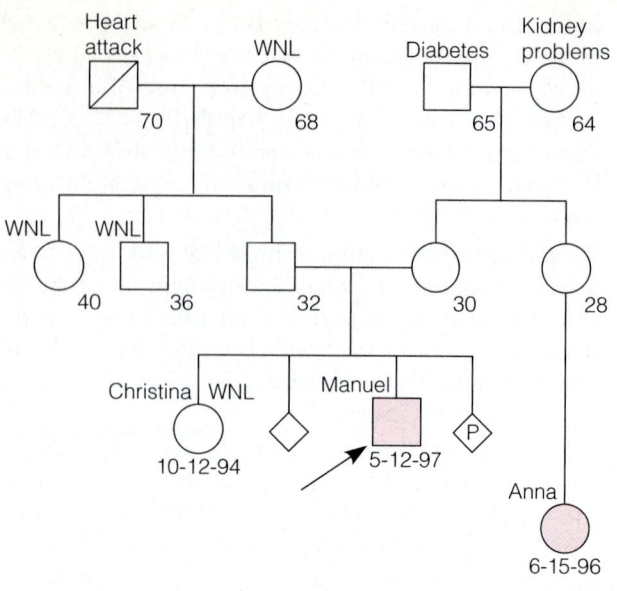

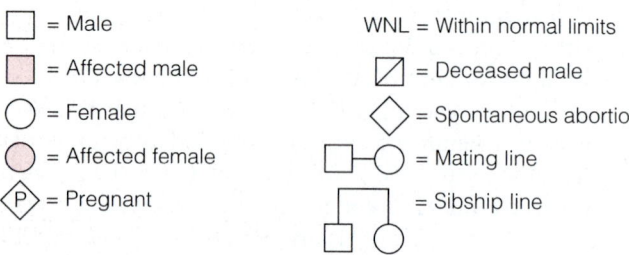

FIGURE 4–17. ◆ Screening pedigree. Arrow indicates the nearest family member affected with the disorder being investigated. Basic data have been recorded. Numbers refer to the ages of the family members.

Finally, the nurse elicits information concerning ethnic background, family origin, and religion. Many genetic disorders are more common among certain ethnic groups or more commonly found in particular geographic areas. For example, compared with individuals of other ethnic backgrounds, families from the British Isles are at higher risk for neural tube defects, Ashkenazic Jews (from eastern Europe) are at higher risk for Tay-Sachs disease, people of African descent are at higher risk for sickle-cell anemia, and people of Mediterranean heritage are at higher risk for thalassemias.

FOLLOW-UP COUNSELING

When all the data have been carefully examined and analyzed, the couple returns for a follow-up visit. At this time, the genetic counselor gives the parents all the information available, including the medical facts, diagnosis, probable course of the disorder, and any available management; the inheritance pattern for this particular family and the risk of recurrence; and the options or alternatives for dealing with the risk of recurrence. The remainder of the counseling session is spent discussing the course of action that seems appropriate to the family in view of the risk and family goals. Among the options or alternatives are prenatal diagnosis,

early detection and treatment, and, in some cases, adoption, artificial insemination, and delayed childbearing. The couple may consider therapeutic donor insemination, discussed earlier in this chapter. This alternative is appropriate, for example, if the male partner has an autosomal dominant disorder; TDI would decrease to zero the risk of having an affected child (if the sperm donor is not at risk) because the child would not inherit any genes from the affected parent. If the man has an X-linked disorder and does not wish to continue the gene in the family (all his daughters would be carriers), TDI is an alternative to terminating all pregnancies with a female fetus. If the man is a carrier for a balanced translocation and if termination of pregnancy is against family ethics, TDI is the most appropriate alternative. If both parents are carriers of an autosomal recessive disorder, TDI lowers the risk to a very low level or to zero if a carrier test is available. Finally, TDI may be appropriate if the couple is at high risk for a multifactorial disorder.

Couples who are young and at risk may decide to delay childbearing for a few years. These couples may find in a few years that prenatal diagnosis is available or that a disease can be detected and treated early to prevent irreversible damage.

The family may return to the genetic counselor a number of times to ask questions and express concerns. It is most desirable for the nurse working with the family to attend many or all of these counseling sessions. Because the nurse has already established a rapport with the couple, she or he can act as a liaison between the family and the genetic counselor. Hearing directly what the genetic counselor says helps the nurse clarify the issues for the family, which in turn helps them formulate questions.

When the parents have completed the counseling sessions, the counselor sends them and their certified nurse-midwife or physician a letter detailing the contents of the sessions. The parents keep this document for reference. See Table 4–8.

A nurse with the appropriate knowledge of genetics is in an ideal position to help couples review what has been discussed during the counseling sessions and to answer any additional questions they might have. As families return to daily living, the nurse can provide helpful information on

TABLE 4–8 Nursing Responsibilities in Genetic Counseling

Identify families at risk for genetic problems.
Determine how the genetic problem is perceived and what information is desired before proceeding.
Assist families in acquiring accurate information about the specific problem.
Act as liaison between family and genetic counselor.
Assist the family in understanding and dealing with information received.
Provide information on support groups.
Aid families in coping with this crisis.
Provide information about known genetic factors.
Assure continuity of nursing care to the family.

the day-to-day aspects of caring for a child, answer questions as they arise, support parents in their decisions, and refer families to other health and community agencies (Lewis, 2001). If the couple is considering having more children, or if siblings want information about their affected brother or sister, the nurse should recommend that the family return for another follow-up visit with the genetic counselor. Appropriate options can again be defined and discussed, and any new information can be given to the family. Many genetic centers have found the public health nurse to be the ideal health professional to provide such follow-up care.

Nurses must be careful not to assume a diagnosis, determine carrier status or recurrence risks, or provide genetic counseling without adequate information and training. Inadequate, inappropriate, or inaccurate information may be misleading or harmful. Health care professionals need to learn the appropriate referral systems and options for care in their region.

CHAPTER HIGHLIGHTS

- A couple is considered infertile when they do not conceive after 1 year of unprotected coitus.

- A thorough history and physical exam of both partners are essential as a basis for infertility investigation.

- General fertility investigations include evaluation of ovarian function, cervical mucus adequacy and receptivity to sperm, sperm number and function, tubal patency, general condition of the pelvic organs, and certain laboratory tests.

- Among cases of infertility, 35% involve male factors, 50% involve female factors, and 15% have no identifiable cause; 35% have multifactorial causes.

- Medications may be prescribed to induce ovulation, facilitate cervical mucus formation, reduce antibody concentration, increase sperm count and motility, and suppress endometriosis.

- The emotional aspects of infertility may be even more difficult for the couple than the testing and therapy.

- The nurse needs to be prepared to dispel myths and provide accurate information about infertility.

- The nurse assesses coping responses and initiates counseling referrals as indicated.

- In autosomal dominant inherited disorders, an affected parent has a 50% chance of having an affected child. Such disorders equally affect males and females. Some of the common autosomal dominant inherited disorders are Huntington disease, polycystic kidney disease, and neurofibromatosis (von Recklinghausen disease).

- Autosomal recessive inherited disorders are characterized by both parents being carriers; each offspring having a 25% chance of having the disease, a 25% chance of not being affected, and a 50% chance of being a carrier; and males and females being equally affected. Some common autosomal recessive inherited disorders are cystic fibrosis, phenylketonuria, galactosemia, sickle-cell anemia, Tay-Sachs disease, and most metabolic disorders.

- X-linked recessive disorders are characterized by no male-to-male transmission, effects limited to males, a 50% chance that a carrier mother will pass the abnormal gene to her son, a 50% chance that a carrier mother will not transmit the abnormal gene to her son, a 50% chance that the daughter of a carrier mother will be a carrier, and a 100% chance that daughters of affected fathers will be carriers. Common X-linked recessive disorders are hemophilia, color blindness, and Duchenne muscular dystrophy.

- Multifactorial inheritance disorders include cleft lip and palate, spina bifida, dislocated hips, clubfoot, and pyloric stenosis.

- Some genetic conditions that can currently be diagnosed prenatally are craniospinal defects, renal malformations, hemophilia, fragile X syndrome, thalassemia, cystic fibrosis, many inborn errors of metabolism such as Tay-Sachs disease, and neural tube defects. This list expands daily as new technology allows for the detection of more conditions.

- The chief tools of prenatal diagnosis are ultrasound, serum alpha-fetoprotein testing, amniocentesis, chorionic villus sampling, and percutaneous umbilical blood sampling.

- Based on sound knowledge about common genetic problems, the nurse should prepare the family for counseling and act as a resource person during and after the counseling sessions.

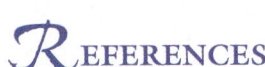

EXPLOREMediaLink

NCLEX Review, Case Studies, and other interactive resources for this chapter can be found on the companion website at http://www.prenhall.com/london. Click on "Chapter 4" to select the activities for this chapter.

For animations, more NCLEX review questions, and an audio glossary, access the accompanying CD-ROM in this textbook.

REFERENCES

American Academy of Pediatrics, Committee on Genetics. (2000). Molecular genetic testing in pediatric practice: A subject review. *Pediatrics, 106*, 1494–1497.

American Fertility Society. (1994). *Infertility: Questions and answers.* Washington, DC: Author.

American Society for Reproductive Medicine. (2000). Assisted reproductive technology in the United States: 1997 results generated from the American Society for Reproductive

Medicine/Society for Assisted Reproductive Technology Registry. *Fertility and Sterility, 74*(4), 641–655.

Bartoov, B., Eltes, F., Reichart, M., Langzam, J., Lederman, H., & Zabludovsky, N. (1999). Quantitative ultramorphological analysis of human sperm: Fifteen years of experience in the diagnosis and management of male factor infertility. *Archives of Andrology, 43*(1), 13–25.

Beal, M. W. (1999). Acupuncture and acupressure. Applications to women's reproductive health care. *Journal of Nurse Midwifery, 44*(3), 217–230.

Bernstein, J. (1985). Assessment of psychological dysfunction associated with infertility. *Journal of Obstetric, Gynecologic, and Neonatal Nursing, 14*(Suppl.), 63.

Bopp, B. L., & Seifer, D. B. (2000). Age and reproduction. In J. J. Sciarri & T. J. Watkins (Eds.), *Gynecology and obstetrics* (Vol. 5, chap. 72, pp. 1–26). Philadelphia: Lippincott Williams & Wilkins.

Bradshaw, K. D. (1998). Evaluation and management of the infertile couple. In J. J. Sciarri & T. J. Watkins (Eds.), *Gynecology and obstetrics* (Vol. 5, chap. 50, pp. 1–15). Hagerstown, MD: Harper & Row.

Buitendijk, S. E. (1999). Children after in vitro fertilization. *International Journal of Technology Assessment in Health Care, 15*(1), 52–65.

Carcio, H. A. (1998). *Management of the infertile woman.* Philadelphia: Lippincott-Raven.

Chen, B. Y. (1997). Acupuncture normalizes dysfunction of hypothalamic-pituitary-ovarian axis. *Acupuncture and Electro-therapeutics Research, 22*(2), 97–108.

Chen, J. C., Xu, M. X., Chen, L. D., Chen, Y. N., Chiu, T. H. (1999). Effect of Panax notoginseng extracts on inferior sperm motility in vitro. *The American Journal of Chinese Medicine, 27,* 123–128.

Damani, M. N., & Shaban, S. F. (1999). Medical treatment of male infertility. In J. J. Sciarri & T. J. Watkins (Eds.), *Gynecology and obstetrics* (Vol. 5, chap. 65, pp. 1–20). Hagerstown, MD: Harper & Row.

Gerhard, I., & Postneek, F. (1992). Auricular acupuncture in the treatment of female infertility. *Gynecological Endocrinology, 6*(3), 171–181.

Giarelli, E., & Jacobs, L. A. (2000). Issues related to the use of genetic material and information. *Oncology Nursing Forum, 27,* 459–467.

Gladstar, R. (1993). *Herbal healing for women.* New York, New York: Simon & Schuster.

Glover, L., Hunter, M., Richards, J. M., Katz, M., & Abel, P. D. (2000). Development of the fertility adjustment scale. *Fertility and Sterility, 72*(4), 623–628.

Gottlieb, B. (2000). *Alternative cures: The most effective natural home remedies for 160 health problems.* Emmaus, PA: Rodale Press.

Greil, A. L. (1997). Infertility and psychological distress: A critical review of the literature. *Social Science & Medicine, 54*(11), 679–704.

Hatcher, R. A., Stewart, F., Trussell, J., Kowal, D., Guest, F., Stewart, G. K., et al. (1998).

Contraceptive technology (17th ed.). New York: Ardent Media.

Hogge, W. A., & Lanasa, M. C. (1999). *Molecular and mendelian disorders.* In J. J. Sciarri & T. J. Watkins (Eds.), *Gynecology and obstetrics* (Vol. 5, chap. 115, pp. 1–13). Hagerstown, MD: Harper & Row.

Hong, C. Y., Ku, J., & Wu, P. (1992). Astnagalus membranaceus stimulates human sperm motility in vitro. *The American Journal of Chinese Medicine, 20,* 289–294.

Jaffe, A., Bush, A., Gedes, D. M., & Alton, E. W. (1999). Prospects for gene therapy in cystic fibrosis. *Archives of Diseases in Children, 80,* 286–289.

Kingsberg, S. A., Applegarth, L. D., & Janata, J. W. (2000). Embryo donation programs and policies in North America: Survey results and implications for health and mental health professionals. *Fertility and Sterility, 73*(2), 215–220.

Klock, S. C., & Greenfeld, D. A. (2000). Psychological status of in vitro fertilization patients during pregnancy: A longitudinal study. *Fertility and Sterility, 73*(6), 1159–1164.

Leibowitz, D., & Hoffman, D. (2000). Fertility drug therapies: Past, present, and future. *Journal of Obstetric, Gynecologic, and Neonatal Nursing, 29*(2), 201–210.

Leon, I. G. (2000). Psychology of reproduction: Pregnancy, parenthood, and parental ties. In J. J. Sciarri & T. J. Watkins (Eds.), *Gynecology and obstetrics* (Vol. 6, chap. 62, pp. 1–29). Philadelphia: Lippincott Williams & Wilkins.

Lewis, J. A. (2001). Understanding genetics: Shaping the foundation for future nursing practice. *Lifelines, 5*(2), 50–56.

Mackta, J., & Weiss, J. O. (1994). The role of genetic support groups. *Journal of Obstetric, Gynecologic, and Neonatal Nursing, 23*(6), 519–523.

Miller, P. B., & Soules, M. R. (1998). Luteal phase deficiency: Pathophysiology, diagnosis, and treatment. In J. J. Sciarri & T. J. Watkins (Eds.), *Gynecology and obstetrics* (Vol. 5, chap. 56, pp. 1–29). Hagerstown, MD: Harper & Row.

Moghissi, K. S. (1998). How to document ovulation. In J. J. Sciarri & T. J. Watkins (Eds.), *Gynecology and obstetrics* (Vol. 5, chap. 54, pp. 1–14). Hagerstown, MD: Harper & Row.

Newberger, D. S. (2000). Down syndrome: Prenatal risk assessment and diagnosis. *American Family Physician, 62*(4), 825–832, 837–838.

Pergament, E., & Fiddler, M. (2000). Indications and patient selection for preimplantation-related chromosome abnormalities. In J. J. Sciarri & T. J. Watkins (Eds.), *Gynecology and obstetrics* (Vol. 5, chap. 107, pp. 1–7). Philadelphia: Lippincott Williams & Wilkins.

Rose, N. C., & Mennuti, M. T. (2000). Alpha-fetoprotein and neural tube defects. In J. J. Sciarri & T. J. Watkins (Eds.), *Gynecology and obstetrics* (Vol. 3, chap. 116, pp. 1–14). Philadelphia: Lippincott Williams & Wilkins.

Sandelowski, M. (1994). On infertility. *Journal of Obstetric, Gynecologic, and Neonatal Nursing, 23*(9), 749–752.

Scioscia, A. L. (1999). Prenatal genetic diagnosis. In R. K. Creasy & R. Resnik (Eds.), *Maternal-fetal medicine* (4th ed., pp. 40–62). Philadelphia: Saunders.

Sharara, F. I., & McClamrock, H. D. (2000). Differences in in vitro fertilization (IVF) outcome between white and black women in an inner-city, university-based IVF program. *Fertility and Sterility, 73*(6), 1170–1173.

Sigman, M. (1999). Therapeutic insemination. In J. J. Sciarri & T. J. Watkins (Eds.), *Gynecology and obstetrics* (Vol. 5, chap. 67, pp. 1–21). Hagerstown, MD: Harper & Row.

Sinclair, S. (2000). Male infertility: Nutritional and environmental considerations. *Alternative Medicine Review, 5*(1), 28–38.

Siterman, S., Eltes, F., Wolfson, V., Lederman, H., & Bartoov, B. (2000). Does acupuncture treatment affect sperm density in males with very low sperm count? A pilot study. *Andrologia, 32*(1), 31–39.

Siterman, S., Eltes, F., Wolfson, V., Zabludovsky, N., Bartoov, B. (1997). Effect of acupuncture on sperm parameters of males suffering from subfertility related to low sperm quality. *Archives of Andrology, 39,* 155–161.

Speroff, L., Glass, R. H., & Kase, N. G. (1999). *Clinical gynecologic endocrinology and infertility* (6th ed.). Philadelphia: Lippincott Williams & Wilkins.

Stener-Victorin, E., Waldenstrom, U., Andersson, S. A., & Wikland, M. (1996). Reduction of blood flow impedance in the uterine arteries of infertile women with electro-acupuncture. *Human Reproduction, 11*(6), 1314–1317.

Tiran, D., & Mack, S. (2000). *Complementary therapies for pregnancy and childbirth* (2nd ed.). Philadelphia: Harcourt Publishers Limited.

Tolstoi, L. G., & Smith, C. L. (1999). Human genome project and cystic fibrosis—A symbiotic relationship. *Journal of the American Dietetic Association, 99,* 1421–1427.

Verp, M. S. (1999a). Antenatal diagnosis of chromosomal abnormalities. In J. J. Sciarri & T. J. Watkins (Eds.), *Gynecology and obstetrics* (Vol. 3, chap. 113, pp. 1–17). Hagerstown, MD: Harper & Row.

Verp, M. S. (1999b). Genetic counseling. In J. J. Sciarri & T. J. Watkins (Eds.), *Gynecology and obstetrics* (Vol. 3, chap. 111, pp. 1–13). Hagerstown, MD: Harper & Row.

Williams, J. K. (2000). Impact of genome research on children and their families. *Journal of Pediatric Nursing, 15*(4), 207–211.

World Health Organization. (1992). *WHO manual for the examination of human semen and sperm–cervical mucus interaction.* Cambridge, UK: Cambridge University Press.

Yuen, B. H. (1999). New methods for induction of ovulation. In J. J. Sciarri & T. J. Watkins (Eds.), *Gynecology and obstetrics* (Vol. 5, chap. 70, pp. 1–13). Hagerstown, MD: Harper & Row.

UNIT III

Pregnancy and Family

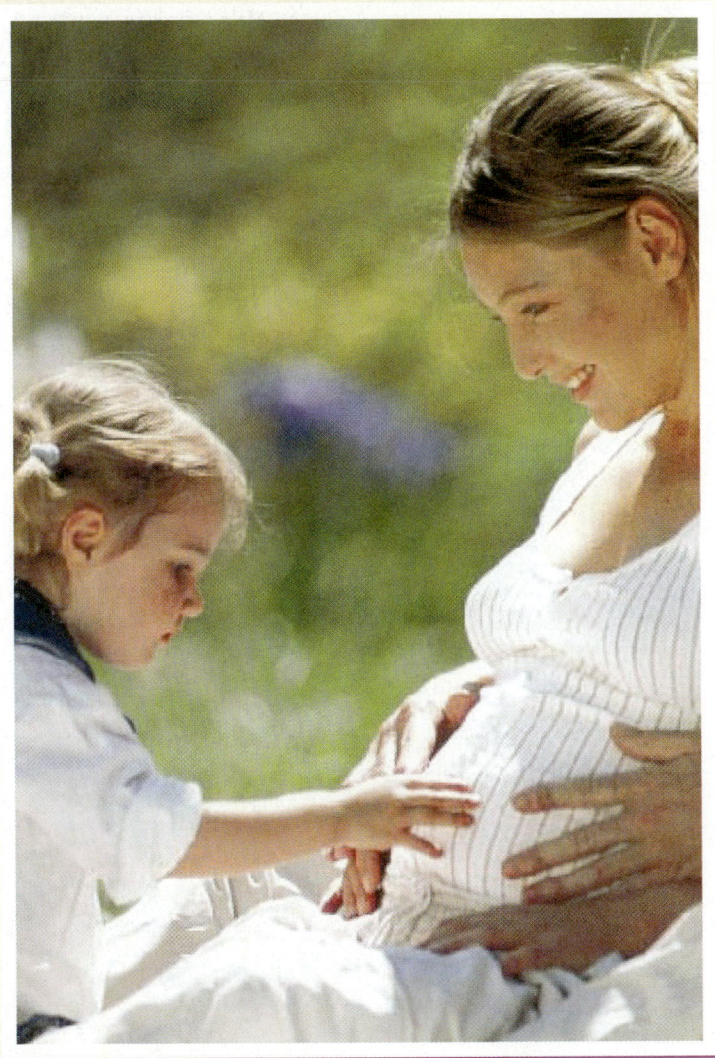

CHAPTER 5

Conception and Fetal Development

$\mathcal{M}$y friends tease me when I say this, but I know the moment my son was conceived. My husband and I had both been so busy at work, but finally we planned a getaway weekend. It was wonderful. We got back some of the magic as we took long walks and talked. Until that weekend, whenever we discussed having children it was always "maybe someday."

On the second night, we decided to skip the diaphragm for the first time. Our lovemaking seemed so special and magic—a true reflection of the emotional closeness we had recaptured. We are convinced that Michael is the result of that night together.

—MICHELLE, 29

Key Terms

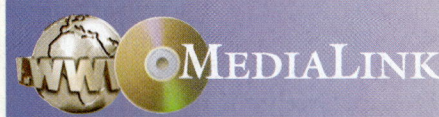

WWW MediaLink

CD-ROM

Conception Animation

Cell Division Animation

Egg Cell Animation

Sperm Cell Animation

Placenta Formation Animation

Fetal Heart Formation and Circulation
Animation

Audio Glossary

NCLEX Review

COMPANION WEBSITE

http://www.prenhall.com/london

Conception and Fetal Development
Web Links

Thinking Critically

NCLEX Review

Case Study

$\mathcal{O}$ur bodies are very similar, in both structure and function. Even our chromosomes are made of the same biochemical substances. What, then, makes each of us unique? The answer lies in the physiologic mechanisms of heredity, the processes of cellular division, and the environmental factors that influence our development from the moment we are conceived. This chapter explores the processes involved in conception and fetal development—the basis of human uniqueness.

CELLULAR DIVISION

Each human begins life as a single cell (fertilized ovum or zygote). This single cell reproduces itself, and in turn each resulting cell also reproduces itself in a continuing process. The new cells are similar to the cells from which they came. Cells are reproduced by either mitosis or meiosis, two different but related processes. **Mitosis** produces exact copies of the original cell, making growth and development possible, and in mature individuals it is the process by which our body cells continue to divide and replace themselves. **Meiosis** is a process of cell division leading to the development of eggs and sperm needed to produce a new organism.

Mitosis

During mitosis, the cell undergoes several changes ending in cell division. As the last phase of cell division nears completion, a furrow develops in the cell cytoplasm, which divides it into two *daughter cells,* each with its own nucleus. Daughter cells have the same **diploid number of chromosomes** (46) and same genetic makeup as the cell from which they came. After a cell with 46 chromosomes goes through mitosis, the result is two identical cells, each with 46 chromosomes.

Meiosis

Meiosis is a special type of cell division by which diploid cells give rise to sperm and ova. Meiosis consists of two successive cell divisions. In the first division, the chromosomes replicate, doubling the structure of each of the 46 chromosomes. Next, a pairing takes place between homologous chromosomes (Sadler, 2000). Instead of separating immediately, as in mitosis, the chromosomes become closely intertwined. At each point of contact, there is a physical exchange of genetic material between the chromatids (the arms of the chromosomes). New combinations are provided by the newly formed chromosomes; these combinations account for the wide variation of traits in people (e.g., hair or eye color). The chromosome pairs then separate, and the members of the pair move to opposite sides of the cell. The cell divides, forming two daughter cells, each with 23 double-structured chromosomes—the same amount of deoxyribonucleic acid (DNA) as a normal somatic cell

(Moore, Persaud & Shiota, 2000). In the second division, the chromatids of each chromosome separate and move to opposite poles of each of the daughter cells. Cell division occurs, resulting in the formation of four cells, each containing 23 single chromosomes (the **haploid number of chromosomes**). These daughter cells contain only half the DNA of a normal somatic cell (See Table 5–1).

Mutations may occur during the second meiotic division, if two of the chromatids do not move apart rapidly enough when the cell divides. When this happens, the still-paired chromatids are carried into one of the daughter cells and eventually form an extra chromosome. This condition, *autosomal nondisjunction* (chromosomal mutation), is harmful to the offspring if fertilization occurs.

Another type of chromosomal mutation can occur if chromosomes break during meiosis. If the broken segment is lost, the result is a shorter chromosome; this situation is known as *deletion*. If the broken segment becomes attached to another chromosome, a harmful mutation called a *translocation* is the result. The effects of translocation and autosomal nondisjunction are described in Chapter 4. 🔗

Meiosis occurs during *gametogenesis,* the process by which germ cells, or **gametes,** are produced. The gametes must have a haploid number (23) of chromosomes so that when the female gamete (egg or ovum) and the male gamete (sperm or spermatozoon) unite to form the *zygote* (fertilized ovum), the normal human diploid number of chromosomes (46) is reestablished.

TABLE 5–1 Comparison of Meiosis and Mitosis
Meiosis
Purpose
Produce reproductive cells (gametes). Reduction of chromosome number by half (from diploid [46] to haploid [23]), so that when fertilization occurs the normal diploid number is restored. Introduces genetic variability.
Cell division
Two-stage reduction.
Number of daughter cells
Four daughter cells, each containing one half the number of chromosomes as the mother cell, or 23 chromosomes. Nonidentical to original cell.
Mitosis
Purpose
Produce cells for growth and tissue repair. Cell division characteristic of all somatic cells.
Cell division
One-stage cell division.
Number of daughter cells
Two daughter cells identical to the mother cell, each with the diploid number (46 chromosomes).

OOGENESIS

Oogenesis is the process by which the female gametes, or ova, are produced. The ovaries begin to develop early in the fetal life of the female. All the ova that the female will produce are formed by the sixth month of fetal life. The ovary gives rise to oogonial cells, which develop into *oocytes*. Meiosis begins in all oocytes before the female fetus is born but stops before the first division is complete and remains in this arrested phase until puberty. During puberty, the mature primary oocyte proceeds (by oogenesis) through the first meiotic division in the graafian follicle of the ovary.

The first meiotic division produces two cells of unequal size with different amounts of cytoplasm but with the same number of chromosomes. These two cells are the *secondary oocyte* and a minute *polar body*. Both the secondary oocyte and the polar body contain 22 double-structured autosomal chromosomes and one double-structured sex chromosome (X). At the time of ovulation, a second meiotic division begins immediately and proceeds as the oocyte moves down the fallopian tube. Division is again not equal, and the secondary oocyte moves into the metaphase stage of cell division, where its meiotic division is arrested.

When the secondary oocyte completes the second meiotic division after fertilization, the result is a mature ovum with the haploid number of chromosomes and virtually all the cytoplasm. In addition, the second polar body (also haploid) forms at this time. The first polar body has also divided in two, producing two additional polar bodies. Thus, at the completion of meiosis, four haploid cells have been produced: the three polar bodies, which eventually disintegrate, and one ovum (Sadler, 2000) (Figure 5–1 ◆). [CD]

SPERMATOGENESIS

During puberty, the germinal epithelium in the seminiferous tubules of the testes begins the process of spermatogenesis, which produces the male gamete (sperm) [CD]. The diploid spermatogonium replicates before it enters the first meiotic division, during which it is called the primary spermatocyte. During this first meiotic division, the spermatogonium forms two cells called secondary spermatocytes, each of which contains 22 double-structured autosomal chromosomes and either a double-structured X sex chromosome or a double-structured Y sex chromosome. During the second meiotic division, they divide to form four spermatids, each with the haploid number of chromosomes. The spermatids undergo a series of changes during which they lose most of their cytoplasm and become sperm (spermatozoa) (see Figure 5–1).

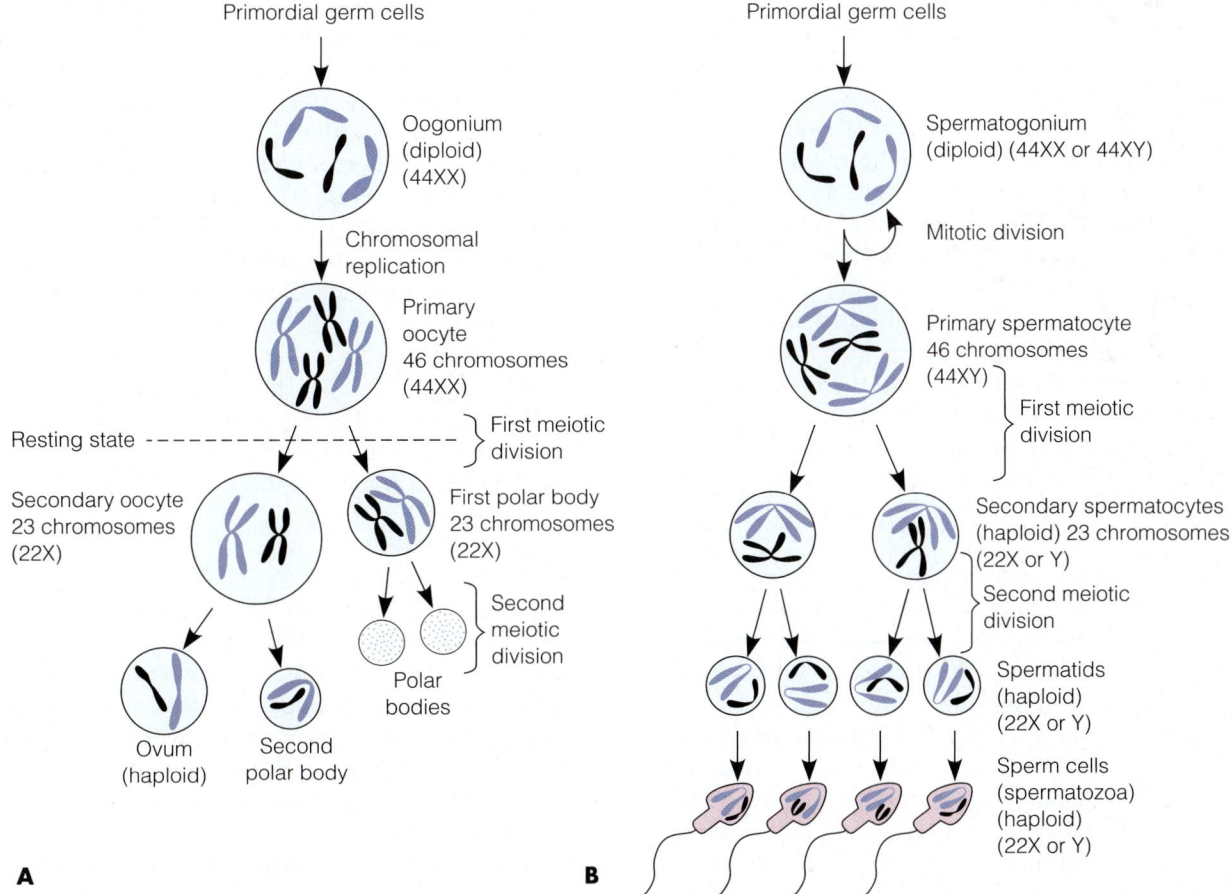

FIGURE 5–1. ◆ Gametogenesis involves meiosis within the ovary and testis. **A,** During meiosis, each oogonium produces a single haploid ovum once some cytoplasm moves into the polar bodies. **B,** Each spermatogonium produces four haploid spermatozoa.

THE PROCESS OF FERTILIZATION

Fertilization is the process by which a sperm fuses with an ovum to form a new diploid cell, or zygote. Following are the events that lead to fertilization. ⬭ CD

Preparation for Fertilization

The process of fertilization takes place in the ampulla (outer third) of the fallopian tube. During ovulation, high estrogen levels increase peristalsis within the fallopian tubes, which helps move the ovum through the tube toward the uterus. The ovum has no inherent power of movement. The high estrogen levels also cause a thinning of the cervical mucus, facilitating movement of the sperm through the cervix, into the uterus, and up the fallopian tube.

The ovum's cell membrane is surrounded by two layers of tissue. The layer closest to the cell membrane is called the *zona pellucida.* It is a clear, noncellular layer whose thickness influences the fertilization rate. Surrounding the zona pellucida is a ring of elongated cells, called the *corona radiata* because they radiate from the ovum like the gaseous corona around the sun. These cells are held together by hyaluronic acid.

The mature ovum and spermatozoa have only a brief time to unite. Ova are considered fertile for about 12 to 24 hours after ovulation. Sperm can survive in the female reproductive tract for 48 to 72 hours but are believed to be healthy and highly fertile for only about 24 hours (De Jonge, 2000).

In a single ejaculation, the male deposits approximately 200 to 500 million spermatozoa in the vagina, of which only hundreds of sperm actually reach the ampulla. (Brannigan & Lipshultz, 2000). The spermatozoa propel themselves up the female tract by the flagellar movement of their tails. Transit time from the cervix into the fallopian tube can be as short as 5 minutes but usually takes an average of 4 to 6 hours (Cunningham, Gant, Leveno, Gilstrap, Hauth & Wenstrom, 2001). Prostaglandins in the semen may increase uterine smooth muscle contractions, which help transport the sperm. The fallopian tubes have a dual ciliary action that facilitates movement of the ovum toward the uterus and movement of the sperm from the uterus toward the ovary.

The sperm's nucleus, which contains its genetic material, is compacted into the head of the sperm and covered by a protective cap called an *acrosome,* which is in turn covered by a plasma membrane. The sperm must undergo two processes before fertilization can occur: capacitation and the acrosomal reaction. **Capacitation** is the removal of the plasma membrane overlying the spermatozoa's acrosomal area and the loss of seminal plasma lipids, proteins, and the glycoprotein coat. If the sperm plasma membrane is not removed, the sperm will not be able to fertilize the ovum (Brannigan & Lipshultz, 2000). Capacitation occurs in the female reproductive tract (aided by uterine enzymes) and is thought to take about 7 hours.

The **acrosomal reaction** follows capacitation. The acrosomes of the sperms surrounding the ovum release their enzymes (hyaluronidase, a protease called acrosin, and corona-dispersing enzymes) and thus break down the hyaluronic acid in the ovum's corona radiata (Brannigan & Lipshultz, 2000). Hundreds of acrosomes must rupture before enough hyaluronic acid is cleared for a single sperm to penetrate the ovum's zona pellucida successfully. At the moment of penetration, a cellular change in the ovum renders it impenetrable by other sperm (Figure 5–2 ◆).

The Moment of Fertilization

After the sperm enters the ovum, a chemical signal prompts the secondary oocyte to complete the second meiotic division, forming the nucleus of the ovum and ejecting the second polar body. Then the nuclei of the ovum and sperm swell and approach each other. The true moment of fertilization occurs as the nuclei unite. Their individual nuclear membranes disappear, and their chromosomes pair up to produce the diploid **zygote.** Since each nucleus contains a haploid number of chromosomes (23), this union restores the diploid number (46). The zygote contains a new combination of genetic material that results in an individual different from either parent and anyone else.

It is also at the moment of fertilization that the sex of the zygote is determined. The two chromosomes (the sex chromosomes) of the 23rd pair—either XX or XY—determine the sex of an individual. X chromosomes are larger and bear more genes than Y chromosomes. Females have two X chromosomes, and males have an X and a Y chromosome. Whereas the mature ovum produced by oogenesis can have only one type of sex chromosome—an X—spermatogenesis produces two sperm with an X chromosome and two sperm with a Y chromosome. When each gamete contributes an X chromosome, the resulting zygote is female. When the ovum contributes an X and the sperm contributes a Y chromosome, the resulting zygote is male. As discussed in Chapter 4, certain traits are termed *sex-linked* because they are controlled by the genes on the X sex chromosome. Two examples of sex-linked traits are color blindness and hemophilia. ⬭

Twins

Twins occur in approximately 1 in 80 pregnancies, and triplets occur in 1 in 8,000 pregnancies (Spellacy, 1999). Twins have been reported to occur more often among black women than among white women and more often among white women than among women of Asian origin (Benirschke, 1999a). Among all groups, as parity (having given birth to a viable infant) increases, so does the chance for multiple births.

Twins may be either fraternal or identical. If they are fraternal, they are dizygotic, which means they arise from two separate ova fertilized by two separate spermatozoa (Figure 5–3 ◆). There are two placentas, two chorions,

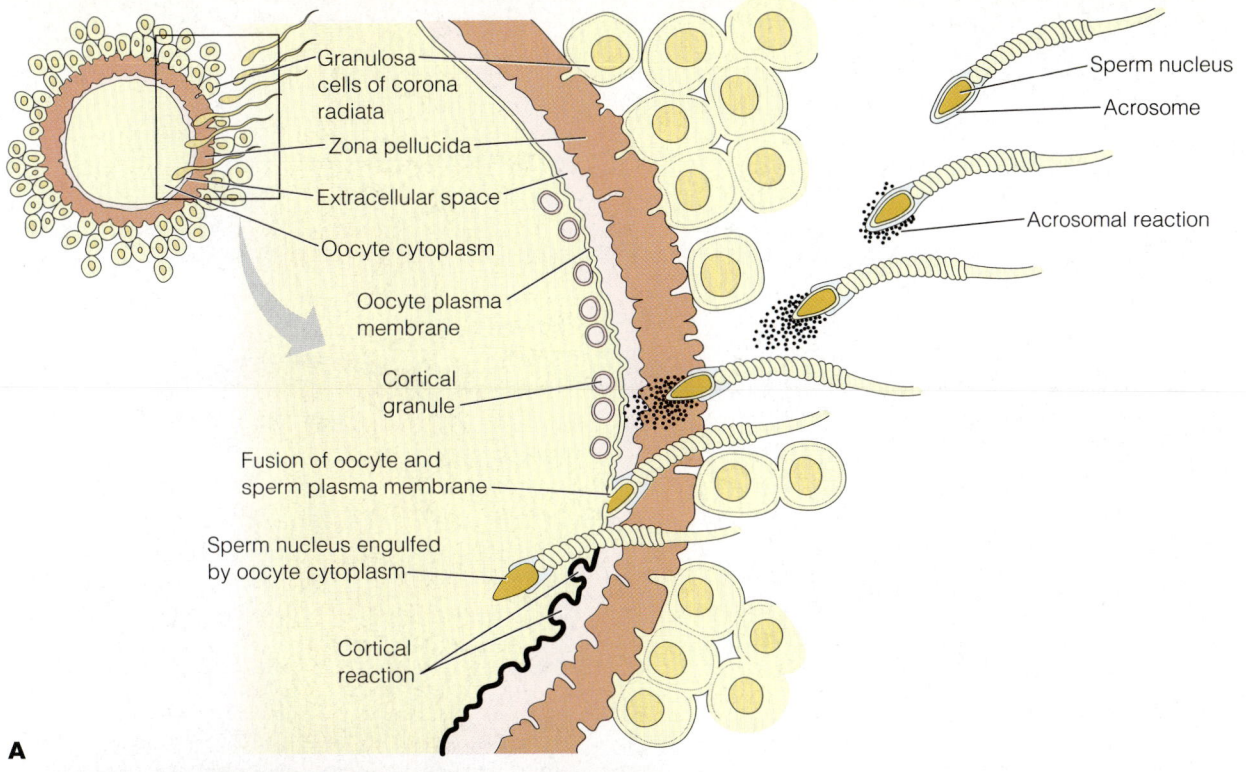

A

- Granulosa cells of corona radiata
- Zona pellucida
- Extracellular space
- Oocyte cytoplasm
- Oocyte plasma membrane
- Cortical granule
- Fusion of oocyte and sperm plasma membrane
- Sperm nucleus engulfed by oocyte cytoplasm
- Cortical reaction
- Sperm nucleus
- Acrosome
- Acrosomal reaction

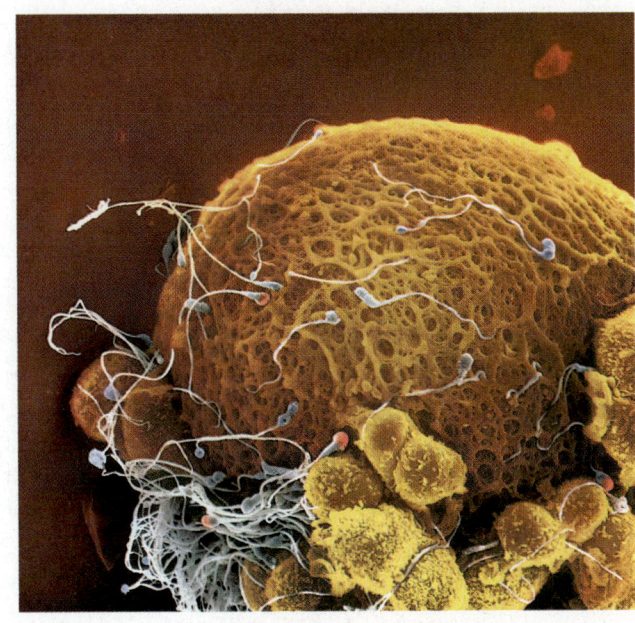

B

FIGURE 5–2. ◆ Sperm penetration of an ovum. **A,** The sequential steps of oocyte penetration by a sperm are depicted moving from top to bottom. **B,** Scanning electron micrograph of a human sperm surrounding a human ovum (750×). The smaller spherical cells are granulosa cells of the corona radiata. *Note:* Scanning electron micrograph from Nilsson, L. (1990). *A child is born.* New York: Dell Publishing.

and two amnions; however, the placentas sometimes fuse and appear to be one. Despite their birth relationship, fraternal twins are no more similar to each other than they would be to siblings born singly. They may be of the same or different sex.

The likelihood of dizygotic twinning increases with maternal age up to about age 35 and then decreases abruptly. The chance of dizygotic twins increases with parity, in conceptions that occur in the first 3 months of marriage, and also with coital frequency. The chance of dizygotic twinning decreases during periods of malnutrition and during winter and spring for women living in the northern hemisphere. Studies indicate that dizygotic twins occur in certain families, perhaps because of genetic factors that result in elevated serum gonadotropin levels and thus double ovulation (Spellacy, 1999).

Identical, or monozygotic, twins develop from a single fertilized ovum. They are of the same sex and have the same genotype (appearance). Identical twins usually have a common placenta (see Figure 5–3). Monozygosity is not affected by environment, race, physical characteristics, or fertility.

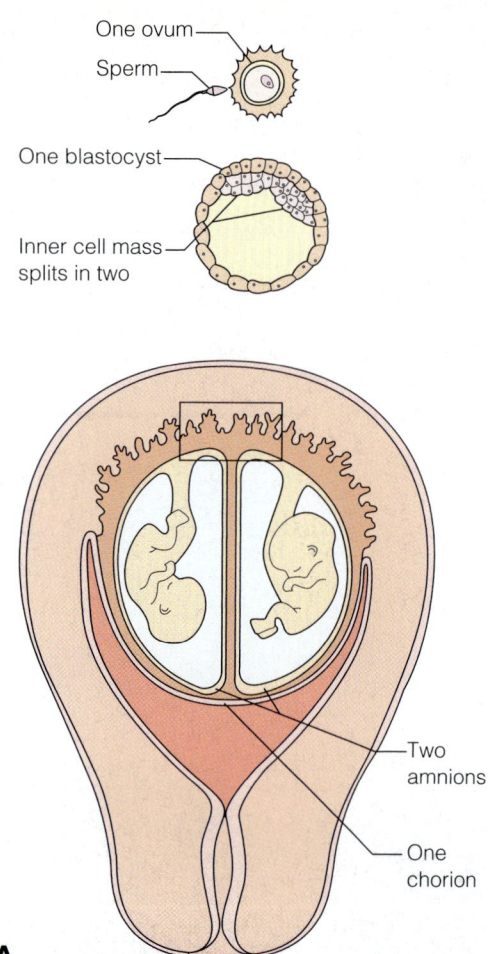

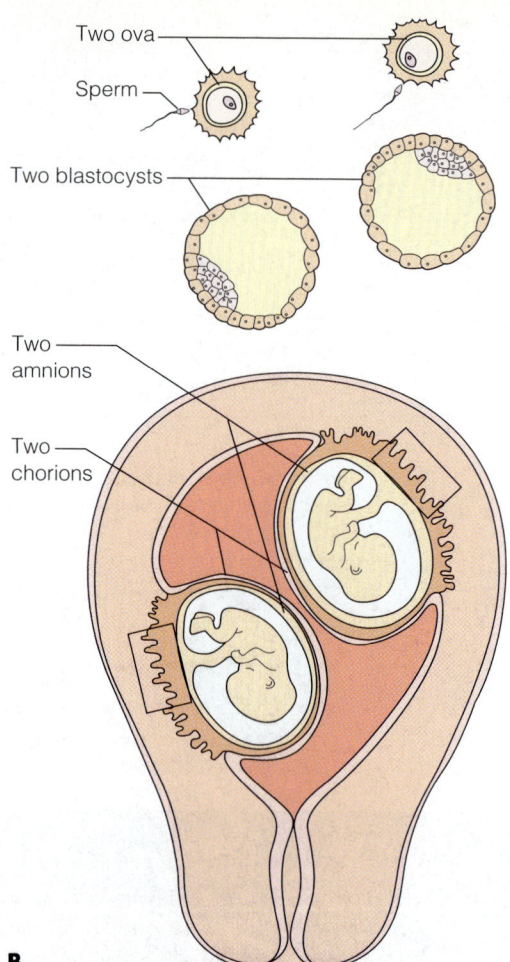

FIGURE 5–3. ◆ **A,** Formation of identical twins. **B,** Formation of fraternal twins. (Note separate placentas.)

Monozygotic twins originate from division of the fertilized ovum at different stages of early development, after the zygote consists of thousands of cells. Complete separation of the cellular mass into two parts is necessary for twin formation. The number of amnions and chorions present depends on the timing of the division:

1. If division occurs within 3 days of fertilization (before the inner cell mass and chorion are formed), two embryos, two amnions, and two chorions will develop. This dichorionic-diamniotic situation occurs about 20% to 30% of the time, and there may be two distinct placentas or a single fused placenta.

2. If division occurs about 5 days after fertilization (when the inner cell mass is formed and the chorion cells have differentiated but those of the amnion have not), two embryos develop with separate amniotic sacs. These sacs will eventually be covered by a common chorion; thus there will be a monochorionic-diamniotic placenta.

3. If the amnion has already developed, approximately 7 to 13 days after fertilization, division results in two embryos with a common amniotic sac and a common chorion (a monochorionic-monoamniotic placenta). This type occurs about 1% of the time (Spellacy, 1999).

Monozygotic twinning is considered a random event and occurs in approximately 3.5 per 1,000 live births (Spellacy, 1999). The survival rate of monozygotic twins is 10% lower than that of dizygotic twins, and congenital anomalies are more prevalent. Both twins may have the same malformation.

PREEMBRYONIC DEVELOPMENT

The first 14 days of development, starting the day the ovum is fertilized (conception), are called the preembryonic stage, or the stage of the ovum (Craven & Ward, 1999). Development after fertilization can be divided into two phases: cellular multiplication and cellular (embryonic membrane) differentiation. This stage is characterized by rapid cellular multiplication and differentiation and the establishment of the embryonic membranes and primary germ layers. These phases and the process of implantation (nidation), which occurs between them, are discussed next.

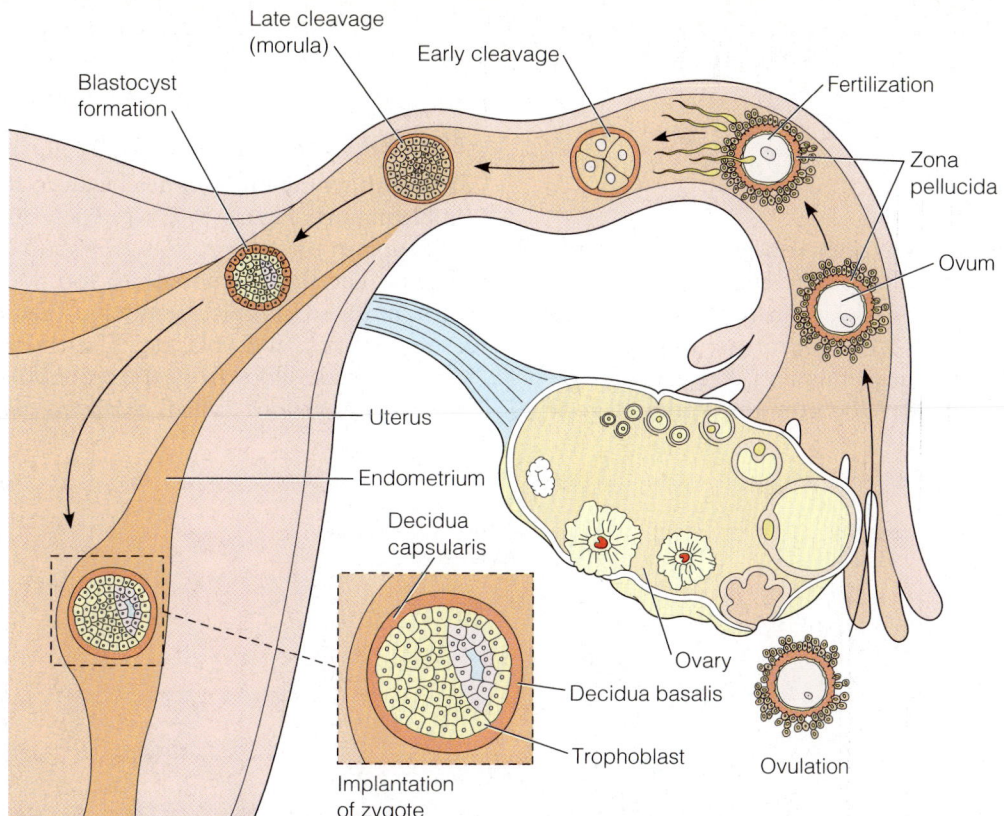

FIGURE 5–4. ◆ During ovulation, the ovum leaves the ovary and enters the fallopian tube. Fertilization generally occurs in the outer third of the fallopian tube. Subsequent changes in the fertilized ovum from conception to implantation are depicted.

Cellular Multiplication

Cellular multiplication begins as the zygote moves through the fallopian tube toward the cavity of the uterus. This transport takes 3 days or more and is accomplished mainly by a very weak fluid current in the fallopian tube resulting from the beating action of the ciliated epithelium that lines the tube.

The zygote now enters a period of rapid mitotic divisions called **cleavage,** during which it divides into two cells, four cells, eight cells, and so on. These cells, called *blastomeres,* are so small that the developing cell mass is only slightly larger than the original zygote. The blastomeres are held together by the zona pellucida, which is under the corona radiata. The blastomeres eventually form a solid ball of 12 to 16 cells called the **morula.** As the morula enters the uterus, its intracellular fluid increases, and a cavity begins to form within it. The inner solid mass of cells is called the **blastocyst.** The outer layer of cells that surrounds the cavity and replaces the zona pellucida is the **trophoblast.** Eventually, the trophoblast develops into one of the embryonic membranes, the chorion. The blastocyst develops into a double layer of cells called the embryonic disc, from which the embryo and the other embryonic membrane (the amnion) will develop. The journey of the fertilized ovum to its destination in the uterus is illustrated in Figure 5–4 ◆. 🔖 CD

Implantation (Nidation)

While floating in the uterine cavity, the blastocyst is nourished by the uterine glands, which secrete a mixture of lipids, mucopolysaccharides, and glycogen. The trophoblast attaches itself to the surface of the endometrium for further nourishment. The most frequent site of attachment is the upper part of the posterior uterine wall. Between days 7 and 10 after fertilization, the zona pellucida disappears and the blastocyst implants itself by burrowing into the uterine lining. It penetrates down toward the maternal capillaries until it is completely covered (Ahokas & McKinney, 2000). The lining of the uterus thickens below the implanted blastocyst, and the cells of the trophoblast grow down into the thickened lining, forming processes called *villi.*

Under the influence of progesterone, the endometrium increases in thickness and vascularity in preparation for implantation and nutrition of the ovum. After implantation, the endometrium is called the *decidua.* The portion of the decidua that covers the blastocyst is called the **decidua capsularis,** the portion directly under the implanted blastocyst is the **decidua basalis,** and the portion that lines the rest of the uterine cavity is the **decidua vera (parietalis)** (Ahokas & McKinney, 2000). The maternal part of the placenta develops from the decidua basalis, which contains large numbers of blood vessels (see magnified insert in

Figure 5–4). The chorionic villi in contact with the decidua basalis will form the fetal portion of the placenta.

Cellular Differentiation

PRIMARY GERM LAYERS

About the 10th to 14th day after conception, the homogeneous mass of blastocyst cells differentiates into the primary germ layers (Figure 5–5 ◆). These three layers, the **ectoderm, mesoderm,** and **endoderm,** are formed at the same time as the embryonic membranes, and all tissues, organs, and organ systems develop from these primary germ

cell layers (see Table 5–2). For example, differentiation of the endoderm results in the formation of the epithelium lining the respiratory and digestive tracts (Figure 5–6 ◆).

EMBRYONIC MEMBRANES

The **embryonic membranes** begin to form at the time of implantation (Figure 5–7 ◆). These membranes protect and support the embryo as it grows and develops inside the uterus. The first membrane to form is the **chorion,** the outermost embryonic membrane that encloses the amnion, embryo, and yolk sac. The chorion, a thick membrane that develops from the trophoblast, has many fingerlike projections called *chorionic villi* on its surface.

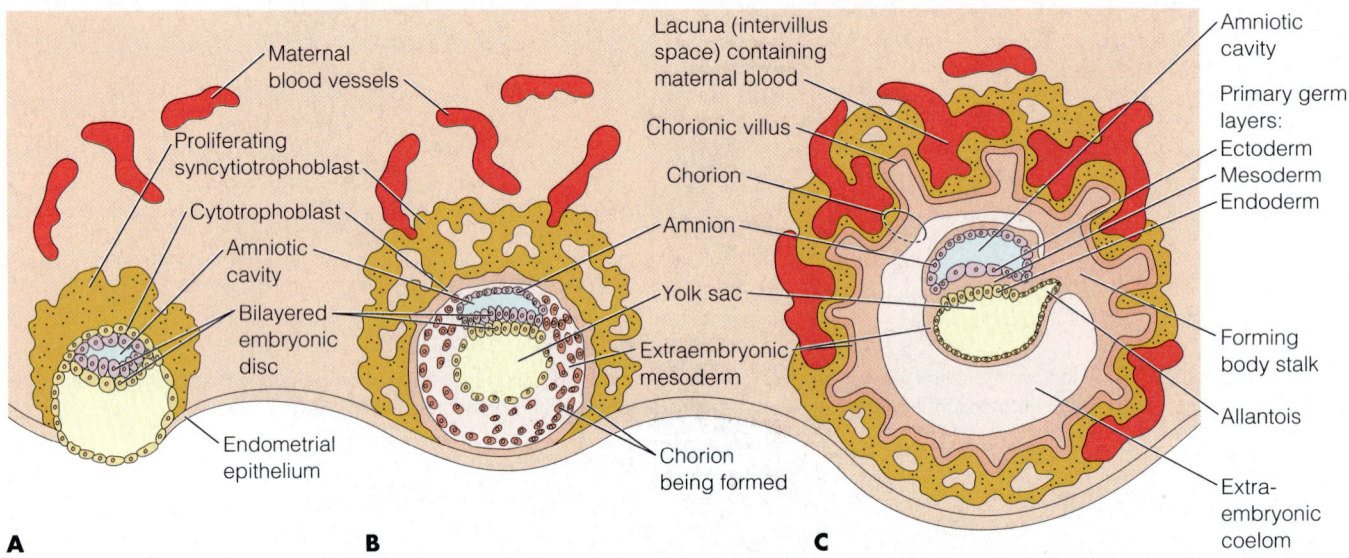

FIGURE 5–5. ◆ Formation of primary germ layers. **A,** Implantation of a 7 1/2-day blastocyst in which the cells of the embryonic disc are separated from the amnion by a fluid-filled space. The erosion of the endometrium by the syncytiotrophoblast is ongoing. **B,** Implantation is completed by day 9, and extraembryonic mesoderm is beginning to form a discrete layer beneath the cytotrophoblast. **C,** By day 16 the embryo shows all three germ layers, a yolk sac, and an allantois (an outpouching of the yolk sac that forms the structural basis of the body stalk, or umbilical cord). The cytotrophoblast and associated mesoderm have become the chorion, and chorionic villi are developing.

TABLE 5–2 Derivation of Body Structures from Primary Cell Layers

Ectoderm	Mesoderm	Endoderm
Epidermis	Dermis	Respiratory tract epithelium
Sweat glands	Wall of digestive tract	Epithelium (except nasal), including pharynx,
Sebaceous glands	Kidneys and ureter (suprarenal cortex)	tongue, tonsils, thyroid, parathyroid, thymus,
Nails	Reproductive organs (gonads, genital ducts)	and tympanic cavity
Hair follicles	Connective tissue (cartilage, bone, joint cavities)	Lining of digestive tract
Lens of eye	Skeleton	Primary tissue of liver and pancreas
Sensory epithelium of internal and external	Muscles (all types)	Urethra and associated glands
ear, nasal cavity, sinuses, mouth, and	Cardiovascular system (heart, arteries, veins,	Urinary bladder (except trigone)
anal canal	blood, bone marrow)	Vagina (parts)
Central and peripheral nervous systems	Pleura	
Nasal cavity	Lymphatic tissue and cells	
Oral glands and tooth enamel	Spleen	
Pituitary gland		
Mammary glands		

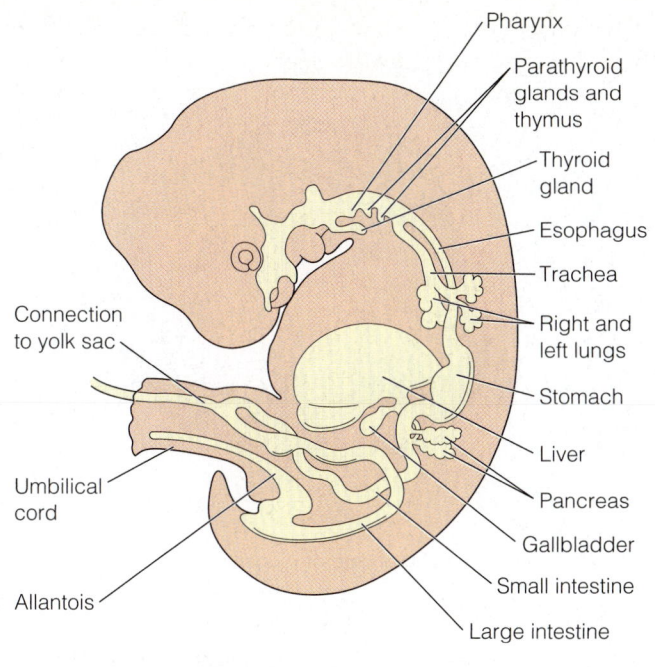

5-week embryo

FIGURE 5–6. ◆ Endoderm differentiates to form the epithelial lining of the digestive and respiratory tracts and associated glands.

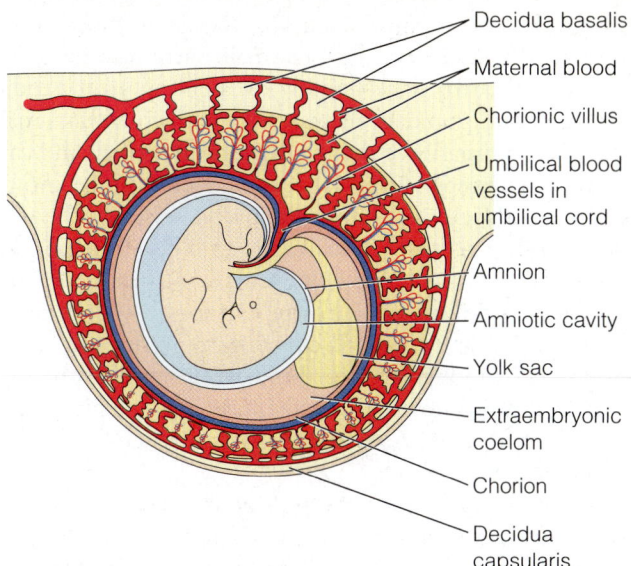

FIGURE 5–7. ◆ Early development of primary embryonic membranes. At 4 1/2 weeks, the decidua capsularis (placental portion enclosing the embryo on the uterine surface) and decidua basalis (placental portion encompassing the elaborate chorionic villi and maternal endometrium) are well formed. The chorionic villi lie in blood-filled intervillous spaces within the endometrium. The amnion and yolk sac are well developed.

These chorionic villi can be used for early genetic testing of the embryo at 8 to 10 weeks' gestation by chorionic villi sampling (see Chapter 14). The villi degenerate, except for those just under the embryo, which grow and branch into depressions in the uterine wall, forming the fetal portion of the placenta. By the fourth month of pregnancy, the surface of the chorion is smooth except at the place of attachment to the uterine wall.

The second membrane, the **amnion,** originates from the ectoderm, a primary germ layer, during the early stages of embryonic development. The amnion is a thin protective membrane that contains amniotic fluid. The space between the membrane and the embryo is the amniotic cavity. This cavity surrounds the embryo and yolk sac, except where the developing embryo (germ-layer disc) attaches to the trophoblast via the umbilical cord. As the embryo grows, the amnion expands until it comes in contact with the chorion. These two slightly adherent fetal membranes form the fluid-filled amniotic sac, or **bag of waters,** that protects the floating embryo.

AMNIOTIC FLUID

Amniotic fluid functions as a cushion to protect against mechanical injury. It also helps control the embryo's temperature, permits symmetrical external growth of the embryo, prevents adherence of the amnion, and allows freedom of movement so that the embryo-fetus can change position, thus aiding in musculoskeletal development. The amount of amniotic fluid at 10 weeks is about 30 mL, and it increases to 350 mL at 20 weeks. After 20 weeks, the

volume ranges from 700 to 1,000 mL. The amniotic fluid volume is constantly changing as the fluid moves back and forth across the placental membrane. As the pregnancy continues, the fetus contributes to the volume of amniotic fluid by excreting urine. The fetus swallows up to 600 mL every 24 hours, and about 400 mL of amniotic fluid flows out of the fetal lungs each day (Gilbert & Brace, 1993). See Chapter 19 for an in-depth discussion of alterations in amniotic fluid volume.

Amniotic fluid is slightly alkaline and contains albumin, uric acid, creatinine, lecithin, sphingomyelin, bilirubin, vernix, leukocytes, epithelial cells, enzymes, and fine hair called lanugo.

YOLK SAC

In humans, the yolk sac is small and functions early in embryonic life. It develops as a second cavity in the blastocyst on about day 8 or 9 after conception. It forms primitive red blood cells during the first 6 weeks of development, until the embryo's liver takes over the process. As the embryo develops, the yolk sac is incorporated into the umbilical cord, where it can be seen as a degenerated structure after birth.

UMBILICAL CORD

The **umbilical cord** is formed from the amnion. The *body stalk,* which attaches the embryo to the yolk sac, contains blood vessels that extend into the chorionic villi. The body stalk fuses with the embryonic portion of the placenta to provide a circulatory pathway from the chorionic villi to the embryo (see Figure 5–10). As the body stalk elongates to become the umbilical cord, the vessels in the cord decrease to one large vein and two smaller arteries. About 1% of umbilical cords have only two vessels, an artery and a vein; this condition may be associated with congenital malformations primarily of the renal, gastrointestinal, and cardiovascular systems. A specialized connective tissue known as **Wharton's jelly** surrounds the blood vessels in the umbilical cord. This tissue, plus the high blood volume pulsating through the vessels, prevents compression of the umbilical cord in utero. At term (38 to 42 weeks' gestation), the average cord is 2 cm (0.8 in) across and about 55 cm (22 in) long. The cord can attach itself to the placenta in various sites. Central insertion into the placenta is considered normal. (See Chapter 19 for a discussion of the various attachment sites. ⬭)

Umbilical cords appear twisted or spiraled. This is most likely caused by fetal movement (Benirschke, 1999b). A true knot in the umbilical cord rarely occurs; if it does, the cord is usually long. More common are so-called false knots, caused by the folding of cord vessels. A nuchal cord is said to exist when the umbilical cord encircles the fetal neck.

DEVELOPMENT AND FUNCTIONS OF THE PLACENTA

The **placenta** is the means of metabolic and nutrient exchange between the embryonic and maternal circulations. Placental development and circulation do not begin until the third week of embryonic development. ⬭ [CD] The placenta develops at the site where the embryo attaches to the uterine wall. Expansion of the placenta continues until about the 20th week, when it covers approximately one half of the internal surface of the uterus. After 20 weeks' gestation, the placenta becomes thicker but not wider. At 40 weeks' gestation, the placenta is about 15 to 20 cm (5.9 to 7.9 in) in diameter and 2.5 to 3 cm (1 to 1.2 in) in thickness. At that time, it weighs about 400 to 600 g (14 to 21 oz).

The placenta has two parts: the maternal and fetal portions. The maternal portion consists of the decidua basalis and its circulation. Its surface is red and fleshlike. The fetal portion consists of the chorionic villi and their circulation. The fetal surface of the placenta is covered by the amnion, which gives it a shiny, gray appearance (Figures 5–8 ◆ and 5–9 ◆).

Development of the placenta begins with the chorionic villi. The trophoblastic cells of the chorionic villi form spaces in the tissue of the decidua basalis. These spaces fill with maternal blood, and the chorionic villi grow into them. As the chorionic villi differentiate, two trophoblastic layers appear: an outer layer, called the *syncytium* (consisting of syncytiotrophoblasts), and an inner layer, known as the *cytotrophoblast* (see Figure 5–5). The cytotrophoblast thins out and disappears about the fifth month, leaving only a single layer of syncytium covering the chori-

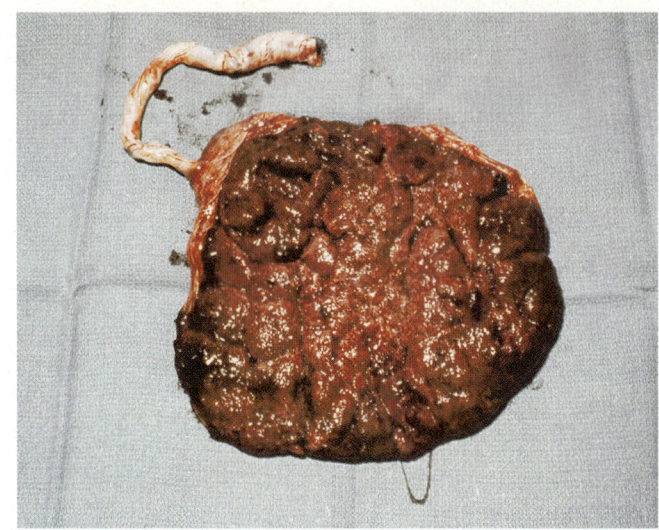

FIGURE 5–8. ◆ Maternal side of placenta.

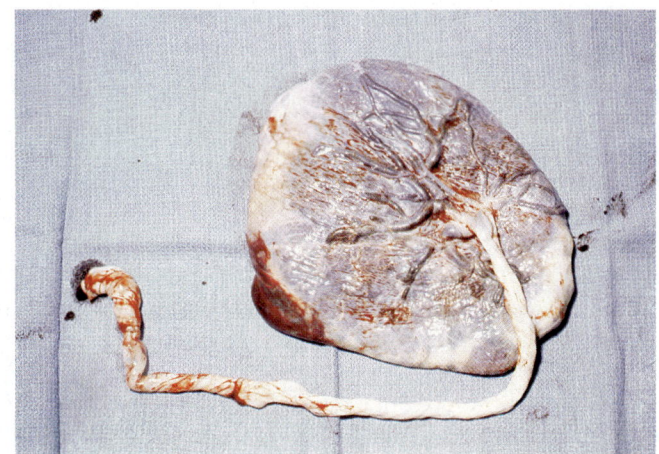

FIGURE 5–9. ◆ Fetal side of placenta.

onic villi. The syncytium is in direct contact with the maternal blood in the intervillous spaces. It is the functional layer of the placenta and secretes the placental hormones of pregnancy.

A third, inner layer of connective mesoderm develops in the chorionic villi, forming *anchoring villi*. These anchoring villi eventually form the septa (partitions) of the placenta. The septa divide the mature placenta into 15 to 20 segments called **cotyledons** (subdivisions of the placenta made up of anchoring villi and decidual tissue). In each cotyledon, the *branching villi* form a highly complex vascular system that allows compartmentalization of the utero placental circulation. The exchange of gases and nutrients takes place across these vascular systems.

Exchange of substances across the placenta is minimal during the first 3 to 5 months of development because of limited permeability. The villous membrane is initially too thick. As the villous membrane thins, placental permeability increases until about the last month of pregnancy, when permeability begins to decrease as the placenta ages.

In the fully developed placenta, fetal blood in the villi and maternal blood in the intervillous spaces are separated by three to four thin layers of tissue.

Placental Circulation

After implantation of the blastocyst, the cells distinguish themselves into fetal cells and trophoblastic cells. The proliferating trophoblast successfully invades the decidua basalis of the endometrium, first opening the uterine capillaries and later opening the larger uterine vessels. The chorionic villi are an outgrowth of the blastocystic tissue. As these villi continue to grow and divide, the fetal vessels begin to form. The intervillous spaces in the decidua basalis develop as the endometrial spiral arteries are opened.

By the fourth week, the placenta has begun to function as a means of metabolic exchange between embryo and mother. The completion of the maternal-placental-fetal circulation occurs about 17 days after conception, when the embryonic heart begins functioning (Benirschke, 1999b). By 14 weeks, the placenta is a discrete organ. It has grown in thickness as a result of growth in the length and size of the chorionic villi and accompanying expansion of the intervillous space.

In the fully developed placenta's umbilical cord, fetal blood flows through the two umbilical arteries to the capillaries of the villi, becomes oxygen enriched, and then flows back through the umbilical vein into the fetus (Figure 5–10 ◆). Late in pregnancy, a soft blowing sound (*funic souffle*) can be heard over the area of the umbilical cord.

The sound is synchronous with the fetal heartbeat and fetal blood flow through the umbilical arteries.

Maternal blood, rich in oxygen and nutrients, spurts from the spiral uterine arteries into the intervillous spaces. These spurts are produced by the maternal blood pressure. The blood is directed toward the chorionic plate, and as the spurt loses pressure, it becomes lateral (spreads out). Fresh blood enters continuously and exerts pressure on the contents of the intervillous spaces, pushing blood toward the exits in the basal plate. The blood then drains through the uterine and other pelvic veins. A *uterine souffle,* timed precisely with the mother's pulse, is also heard just above the mother's symphysis pubis during the last months of pregnancy. This souffle is caused by the augmented blood flow entering the dilated uterine arteries.

Braxton Hicks contractions (see Chapter 15) ⬭ are believed to facilitate placental circulation by enhancing the movement of blood from the center of the cotyledon through the intervillous space. Placental blood flow is enhanced when the woman is lying on her left side because the vena cava is not compromised.

Placental Functions

Placental exchange functions occur only in those fetal vessels in intimate contact with the covering syncytial membrane. The syncytium villi have brush borders containing many microvilli, which greatly increase the exchange rate between maternal and fetal circulation (Sadler, 2000).

The placental functions, many of which begin soon after implantation, include fetal respiration, nutrition, and

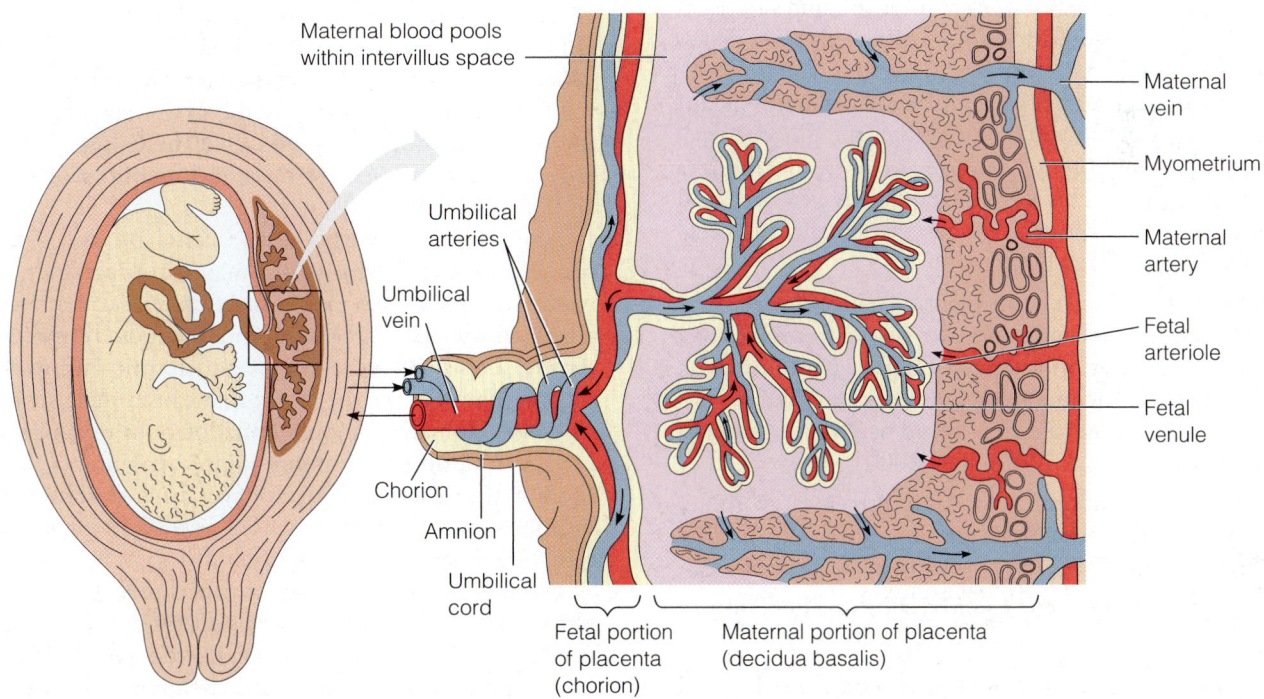

FIGURE 5–10. ◆ Vascular arrangement of the placenta. Arrows indicate the direction of blood flow. Maternal blood flows through the uterine arteries to the intervillous spaces of the placenta and returns through the uterine veins to maternal circulation. Fetal blood flows through the umbilical arteries into the villous capillaries of the placenta and returns through the umbilical vein to the fetal circulation.

excretion. To carry out these functions, the placenta is involved in metabolic and transfer activities. In addition, it has endocrine functions and special immunologic properties.

METABOLIC ACTIVITIES

The placenta continuously produces glycogen, cholesterol, and fatty acids for fetal use and hormone production. The placenta also produces numerous enzymes required for fetoplacental transfer, breaks down certain substances such as epinephrine and histamine, and stores glycogen and iron.

TRANSPORT FUNCTION

The placental membranes actively control the transfer of a wide range of substances by five major mechanisms:

1. *Simple diffusion* moves substances from an area of higher concentration to an area of lower concentration. Substances that move across the placenta by simple diffusion include water, oxygen, carbon dioxide, electrolytes (sodium and chloride), anesthetic gases, and drugs. Insulin and steroid hormones originating from the adrenals and thyroid hormones also cross the placenta, but at a very slow rate. The rate of oxygen transfer across the placental membrane is greater than that allowed by simple diffusion, indicating that oxygen is also transferred by some type of facilitated diffusion transport. Unfortunately, many substances of abuse, such as cocaine, cross the placenta via simple diffusion.

2. *Facilitated transport* involves a carrier system to move molecules from an area of greater concentration to an area of lower concentration at a more rapid rate than by simple diffusion. Molecules such as glucose, galactose, and some oxygen are transported by this method. The glucose level in the fetal blood ordinarily is approximately 20% to 30% lower than the glucose level in the maternal blood, because the fetus metabolizes glucose rapidly. This lower level, in turn, causes rapid transport of additional glucose from the maternal blood into the fetal blood.

3. *Active transport* can work against a concentration gradient and allows molecules to move from areas of lower concentration to areas of higher concentration. Amino acids, calcium, iron, iodine, water-soluble vitamins, and glucose are transferred across the placenta this way (Ahokas & McKinney, 2000).

4. *Pinocytosis* is important for transferring large molecules such as albumin and gamma globulin. Ameba-like cells engulf materials, forming plasma droplets.

5. *Hydrostatic* and *osmotic pressures* allow the bulk flow of water and some solutes.

Other modes of transfer also exist. For example, fetal red blood cells pass into the maternal circulation through breaks in the placental membrane, particularly during labor and birth. Certain cells, such as maternal leukocytes, and

microorganisms, such as viruses (e.g., HIV, which causes AIDS) and the bacterium *Treponema pallidum,* which causes syphilis, can also cross the placental membrane under their own power (Moore, Persaud, & Shiota, 2000). Some bacteria and protozoa infect the placenta by causing lesions and then entering the fetal blood system.

Reduction of the placental surface area, as with abruptio placentae (partial or complete premature separation of an abnormally implanted placenta), lessens the area that is functional for exchange. Placental diffusion distance also affects exchange. In conditions such as diabetes and placental infection, edema of the villi increases the diffusion distance, thus increasing the distance the substance has to be transferred. Blood flow alteration changes the transfer rate of substances. Decreased blood flow in the intervillous space is seen in labor and with certain maternal diseases such as hypertension. Mild fetal hypoxia increases the umbilical blood flow, but severe hypoxia results in decreased blood flow.

As the maternal blood picks up fetal waste products and carbon dioxide, it drains back into the maternal circulation through the veins in the basal plate. Fetal blood is hypoxic by comparison; it therefore attracts oxygen from the mother's blood. Affinity for oxygen increases as the fetal blood gives up its carbon dioxide, which also decreases its acidity.

ENDOCRINE FUNCTIONS

The placenta produces hormones vital to the survival of the fetus. These include human chorionic gonadotropin (hCG); human placental lactogen (hPL); and two steroid hormones, estrogen and progesterone.

The hormone hCG is similar to luteinizing hormone (LH) and prevents the normal involution of the corpus luteum at the end of the menstrual cycle. If the corpus luteum stops functioning before the 11th week of pregnancy, spontaneous abortion occurs. The hCG also causes the corpus luteum to secrete increased amounts of estrogen and progesterone.

After the 11th week, the placenta produces enough progesterone and estrogen to maintain pregnancy. In the male fetus, hCG also exerts an interstitial cell-stimulating effect on the testes, resulting in the production of testosterone. This small secretion of testosterone during embryonic development is the factor that causes male sex organs to grow. Human chorionic gonadotropin may play a role in the trophoblast's immunologic capabilities (ability to exempt the placenta and embryo from rejection by the mother's system), and it is used as a basis for pregnancy tests (see Chapter 7).

Human chorionic gonadotropin is present in maternal blood serum as early as 10 days after fertilization, just as soon as implantation has occurred, and is detectable in maternal urine at the time of missed menses. It reaches its maximum level at 45 to 60 days' gestation and then begins to decrease as placental hormone production increases (Ahokas & McKinney, 2000).

Progesterone is a hormone essential for pregnancy. It increases the secretions of the fallopian tubes and uterus to provide appropriate nutritive matter for the developing morula and blastocyst. It also appears to aid in ovum transport through the fallopian tube (Ahokas & McKinney, 2000). Progesterone causes decidual cells to develop in the uterine endometrium, and it must be present in high levels for implantation to occur. Progesterone also decreases the contractility of the uterus, thus preventing uterine contractions from causing spontaneous abortion.

Prior to stimulation by hCG, the production of progesterone by the corpus luteum reaches a peak about 7 to 10 days after ovulation. Implantation occurs at about the same time as this peak. At 16 days after ovulation, progesterone reaches a level between 25 and 50 mg/day and continues to rise slowly in subsequent weeks (Cunningham, Gant & Leveno, et al., 2001). After 10 weeks, the placenta (specifically, the syncytiotrophoblast) takes over the production of progesterone and secretes it in tremendous quantities late in pregnancy.

By 7 weeks, the placenta produces more than 50% of the estrogens in the maternal circulation. *Estrogens* serve mainly a proliferative function, causing enlargement of the uterus, breasts, and breast glandular tissue. Estrogens also have a significant role in increasing vascularity and vasodilation, particularly in the villous capillaries toward the end of pregnancy. Placental estrogens increase markedly toward the end of pregnancy, to as much as 30 times the daily production in the middle of a normal monthly menstrual cycle. The primary estrogen secreted by the placenta is different from that secreted by the ovaries. The placenta secretes mainly *estriol*, whereas the ovaries secrete primarily *estradiol*. The placenta cannot synthesize estriol by itself. The fetal adrenal glands provide essential precursors that are transported to the placenta for the final conversion to estriol.

The hormone *human placental lactogen (hPL)*, also called human chorionic somatomammotropin (hCS), is similar to human pituitary growth hormone; hPL stimulates certain changes in the mother's metabolic processes. These changes ensure that more protein, glucose, and minerals are available for the fetus. Secretion of hPL can be detected by about 4 weeks after conception.

IMMUNOLOGIC PROPERTIES

The placenta and embryo are transplants of living tissue within the same species and are therefore considered *homografts.* Unlike other homografts, the placenta and embryo appear exempt from immunologic reaction by the host. Most recent data suggest that the placental hormones (progesterone and hCG) suppress cellular immunity during pregnancy. One theory suggests that trophoblastic tissue is immunologically inert. It may contain a cell coating that masks transplantation antigens, repels sensitized lymphocytes, and protects against antibody formation.

Fetal Circulatory System

The circulatory system of the fetus has several unique features that, by maintaining the blood flow to the placenta, provide the fetus with oxygen and nutrients while removing carbon dioxide and other waste products.

Most of the blood supply bypasses the fetal lungs, since they do not carry out respiratory gas exchange. The placenta assumes the function of the fetal lungs by supplying oxygen and allowing the fetus to excrete carbon dioxide into the maternal bloodstream. Figure 5–11 ◆ shows the fetal circulatory system. The blood from the placenta flows through the umbilical vein, which enters the abdominal wall of the fetus at the site that, after birth, is the umbilicus (belly button). It divides into two branches, one of which circulates a small amount of blood through the fetal liver and empties into the inferior vena cava through the hepatic vein. The second and larger branch, called the **ductus venosus,** empties directly into the fetal vena cava. This blood then enters the right atrium, passes through the **foramen ovale** into the left atrium, and pours into the left ventricle, which pumps it into the aorta. Some blood returning from the head and upper extremities by way of the superior vena cava is emptied into the right atrium and passes through the tricuspid valve into the right ventricle. This blood is pumped into the pulmonary artery, and a small amount passes to the lungs for nourishment only. The larger portion of blood passes from the pulmonary artery through the **ductus arteriosus** into the descending aorta, bypassing the lungs. Finally, blood returns to the placenta through the two umbilical arteries, and the process is repeated. ⌾ CD

The fetus obtains oxygen via diffusion from the maternal circulation because of the gradient difference of PO_2 of 50 mm Hg in maternal blood in the placenta to 30 mm Hg PO_2 in the fetus. At term the fetus receives oxygen from the mother's circulation at a rate of 20 to 30 mL per minute (Sadler, 2000). Fetal hemoglobin facilitates obtaining oxygen from the maternal circulation, because it carries as much as 20% to 30% more oxygen than adult hemoglobin. For further discussion, see Chapter 21. ⌾

Fetal circulation delivers the highest available oxygen concentration to the head, neck, brain, and heart (coronary circulation) and a lesser amount of oxygenated blood to the abdominal organs and the lower body. This circulatory pattern leads to cephalocaudal (head-to-tail) development in the fetus.

EMBRYONIC AND FETAL DEVELOPMENT

Pregnancy is calculated to last an *average* of 10 lunar months: 40 weeks, or 280 days. This period of 280 days is calculated from the onset of the last normal menstrual period to the time of birth. Estimated date of birth (EDB) is usually calculated by this method. The postfertilization age, or postconception age, of the fetus is calculated to be *about* 2 weeks less, or 266 days (38 weeks) after estimated time of fertilization. This latter measurement is more

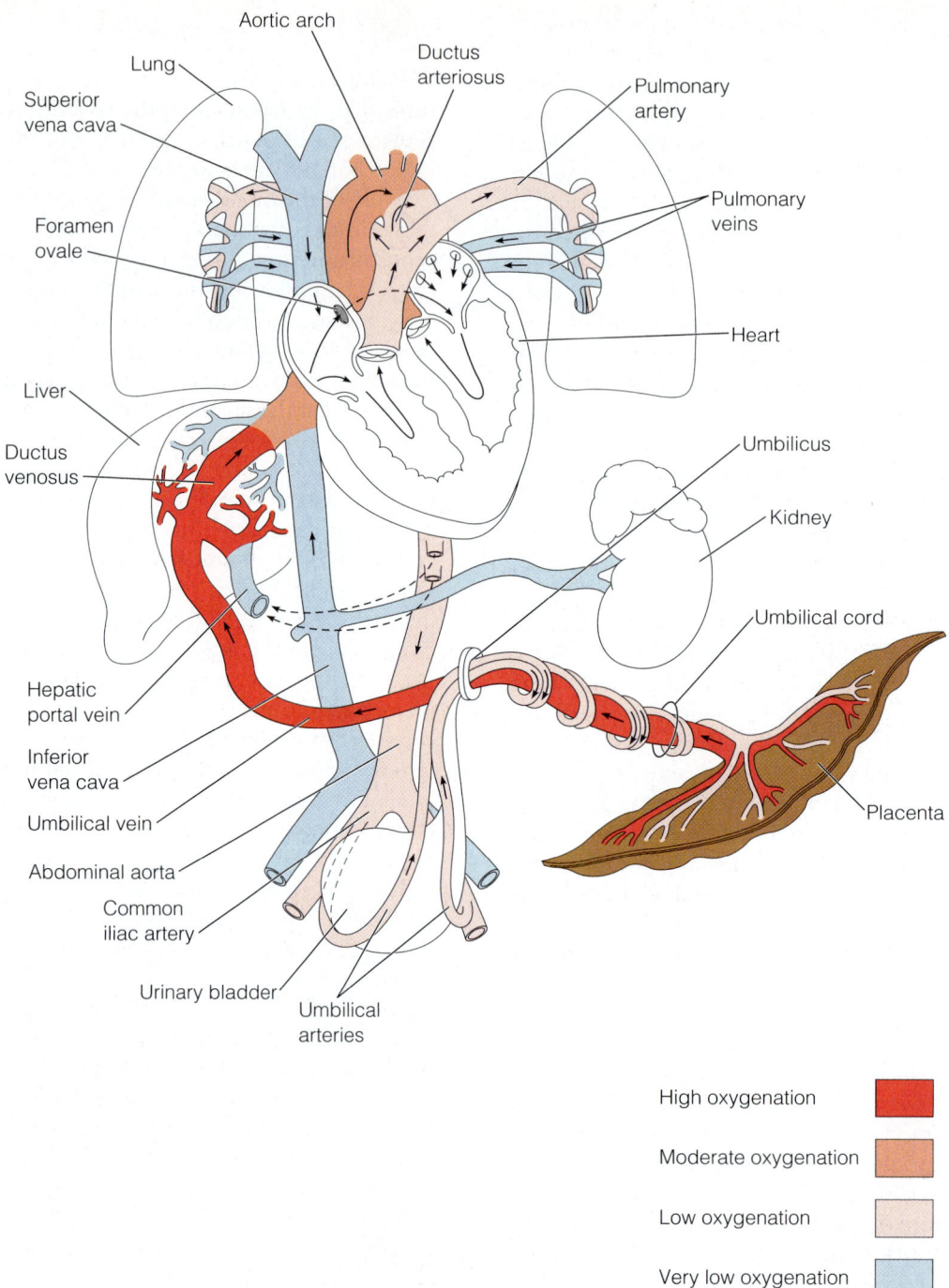

Aortic arch
Ductus arteriosus
Lung
Pulmonary artery
Superior vena cava
Pulmonary veins
Foramen ovale
Heart
Liver
Umbilicus
Ductus venosus
Kidney
Umbilical cord
Hepatic portal vein
Inferior vena cava
Umbilical vein
Abdominal aorta
Placenta
Common iliac artery
Urinary bladder
Umbilical arteries

High oxygenation

Moderate oxygenation

Low oxygenation

Very low oxygenation

FIGURE 5–11. ◆ Fetal circulation. Blood leaves the placenta and enters the fetus through the umbilical vein. After circulating through the fetus, the blood returns to the placenta through the umbilical arteries. The ductus venosus, the foramen ovale, and the ductus arteriosus allow the blood to bypass the fetal liver and lungs.

accurate because it measures time from the fertilization of the ovum, or conception. The basic events of organ development in the embryo and fetus are outlined in Table 5–3. The time periods in the table are postfertilization or **postconception age periods.** For detailed discussion of the development of each body system, see Chapter 21. ⌒

Human development follows three stages. The preembryonic stage, as we have seen, consists of the first 14 days of development after the ovum is fertilized; the embryonic stage covers the period from day 15 until approximately the end of the eighth week; and the fetal stage extends from the end of the eighth week until birth.

TABLE 5-3 **Summary of Organ System Development**

AGE: 2-3 WEEKS

Length: 2 mm C–R (crown to rump)

Nervous system: Groove forms along middle back as cells thicken; neural tube forms from closure to neural groove.

Cardiovascular system: Beginning of blood circulation; tubular heart begins to form during third week.

Gastrointestinal system: Liver begins to function.

Genitourinary system: Formation of kidneys beginning.

Respiratory system: Nasal pits forming.

Endocrine system: Thyroid tissue appears.

Eyes: Optic cup and lens pit have formed; pigment in eyes.

Ear: Auditory pit is now enclosed structure.

AGE: 4 WEEKS

Length: 4–6 mm C–R

Weight: 0.4 g

Nervous system: Anterior portion of neural tube closes to form brain; closure of posterior end forms spinal cord.

Musculoskeletal system: Noticeable limb buds.

Cardiovascular system: Tubular heart beats at 28 days, and primitive red blood cells circulate through fetus and chorionic villi.

Gastrointestinal system: Mouth: formation of oral cavity; primitive jaws present; esophagotracheal septum begins division of esophagus and trachea. Digestive tract: stomach forms; esophagus and intestine become tubular; ducts of pancreas and liver forming.

AGE: 5 WEEKS

Length: 8 mm C–R

Weight: Only 0.5% of total body weight is fat (to 20 weeks).

Nervous system: Brain has differentiated and cranial nerves are present.

Musculoskeletal system: Developing muscles have innervation.

Cardiovascular system: Atrial division has occurred.

AGE: 6 WEEKS

Length: 12 mm C–R

Musculoskeletal system: Bone rudiments present; primitive skeletal shape forming; muscle mass begins to develop; ossification of skull and jaws begins.

Cardiovascular system: Chambers present in heart; groups of blood cells can be identified.

Gastrointestinal system: Oral and nasal cavities and upper lip formed; liver begins to form red blood cells.

Respiratory system: Trachea, bronchi, and lung buds present.

Ear: Formation of external, middle, and inner ear continues.

Sexual development: Embryonic sex glands appear.

AGE: 7 WEEKS

Length: 18 mm C–R

Cardiovascular system: Fetal heartbeats can be detected.

Gastrointestinal system: Mouth: tongue separates; palate folds. Digestive tract: stomach attains final form.

Genitourinary system: Separation of bladder and urethra from rectum.

Respiratory system: Diaphragm separates abdominal and thoracic cavities.

Eyes: Optic nerve formed; eyelids appear, thickening of lens.

Sexual development: Differentiation of sex glands into ovaries and testes begins.

AGE: 8 WEEKS

Length: 2.5–3 cm C–R

Weight: 2 g

Musculoskeletal system: Digits formed; further differentiation of cells in primitive skeleton; cartilaginous bones show first signs of ossification development of muscles in trunk, limbs, and head; some movement of fetus now possible.

Cardiovascular system: Development of heart essentially complete; fetal circulation follows two circuits—four extraembryonic and two intraembryonic.

Gastrointestinal system: Mouth: completion of lip fusion. Digestive tract: rotation in midgut; anal membrane has perforated.

Ear: External, middle, and inner ear assuming final forms.

Sexual development: Male and female external genitals appear similar until end of ninth week.

AGE: 10 WEEKS

Length: 5–6 cm C–H (crown to heel)

Weight: 14 g

Nervous system: Neurons appear at caudal end of spinal cord; basic divisions of brain present.

Musculoskeletal system: Fingers and toes begin nail growth.

Gastrointestinal system: Mouth: separation of lips from jaw; fusion of palate folds. Digestive tract: developing intestines enclosed in abdomen.

Genitourinary system: Bladder sac formed.

Endocrine system: Islets of Langerhans differentiated.

Eyes: Eyelids fused closed; development of lacrimal duct.

Sexual development: Males: production of testosterone and physical characteristics between 8 and 12 weeks.

AGE: 12 WEEKS

Length: 8 cm C–R; 11.5 cm C–H

Weight: 45 g

Musculoskeletal system: Clear outlining of miniature bones (12–20 weeks), process of ossification is established throughout fetal body; appearance of involuntary muscles in viscera.

Gastrointestinal system: Mouth: completion of palate. Digestive tract: appearance of muscles in gut; bile secretion begins; liver is major producer of red blood cells.

Respiratory system: Lungs acquire definitive shape.

Skin: Pink and delicate.

Endocrine system: Hormonal secretion from thyroid; insulin present in pancreas.

Immunologic system: Appearance of lymphoid tissue in fetal thymus gland.

AGE: 16 WEEKS

Length: 13.5 cm C–R; 15 cm C–H

Weight: 200 g

Musculoskeletal system: Teeth beginning to form hard tissue that will become central incisors.

Gastrointestinal system: Mouth: differentiation of hard and soft palate. Digestive tract: development of gastric and intestinal glands; intestines begin to collect meconium.

Genitourinary system: Kidneys assume typical shape and organization.

Skin: Appearance of scalp hair; lanugo present on body; transparent skin with visible blood vessels; sweat glands developing.

Eye, ear, and nose: Formed.

Sexual development: Sex determination possible.

(continued)

TABLE 5-3 • Summary of Organ System Development—continued

AGE: 18 WEEKS

Musculoskeletal system: Teeth beginning to form hard tissue (enamel and dentine) that will become lateral incisors.

Cardiovascular system: Fetal heart tones audible with fetoscope at 16–20 weeks.

AGE: 20 WEEKS

Length: 19 cm C–R; 25 cm C–H

Weight: 435 g (6% of total body weight is fat)

Nervous system: Myelination of spinal cord begins.

Musculoskeletal system: Teeth beginning to form hard tissue that will become canine and first molar. Lower limbs are of final relative proportions.

Gastrointestinal system: Fetus actively sucks and swallows amniotic fluid; peristaltic movements begin.

Skin: Lanugo covers entire body; brown fat begins to form; vernix caseosa begins to form.

Immunologic system: Detectable levels of fetal antibodies (IgG type).

Blood formation: Iron is stored and bone marrow is increasingly important.

AGE: 24 WEEKS

Length: 23 cm C–R; 28 cm C–H

Weight: 780 g

Nervous system: Brain looks like mature brain.

Musculoskeletal system: Teeth are beginning to form hard tissue that will become the second molars.

Respiratory system: Respiratory movements may occur (24–40 weeks). Nostrils reopen. Alveoli appear in lungs and begin production of surfactant; gas exchange possible.

Skin: Reddish and wrinkled, vernix caseosa present.

Immunologic system: IgG levels reach maternal levels.

Eyes: Structurally complete.

AGE: 28 WEEKS

Length: 27 cm C–R; 35 C–H

Weight: 1,200–1,250 g

Nervous system: Begins regulation of some body functions.

Skin: Adipose tissue accumulates rapidly; nails appear; eyebrows and eyelashes present.

Eyes: Eyelids open (28–32 weeks).

Sexual development: Males: testes descend into inguinal canal and upper scrotum.

AGE: 32 WEEKS

Length: 31 cm C–R; 38–43 cm C–H

Weight: 2,000 g

Nervous system: More reflexes present.

AGE: 36 WEEKS

Length: 35 cm C–R; 42–48 cm C–H

Weight: 2,500–2,750 g

Musculoskeletal system: Distal femoral ossification centers present.

Skin: Pale; body rounded, lanugo disappearing, hair fuzzy or woolly; few sole creases; sebaceous glands active and helping to produce vernix caseosa (36–40 weeks).

Ears: Earlobes soft with little cartilage.

Sexual development: Males: scrotum small and few rugae present; descent of testes into upper scrotum to stay (36–40 weeks). Females: labia majora and minora equally prominent.

AGE: 38–40 WEEKS

Length: 40 cm C–R; 48–52 C–H

Weight: 3,200+ g (16% of total body weight is fat)

Respiratory system: At 38 weeks, lecithin-sphingomyelin (L/S) ratio approaches 2:1 (indicates decreased risk of respiratory distress from inadequate surfactant production if born now).

Skin: Smooth and pink; vernix present in skin folds; moderate to profuse silky hair; lanugo on shoulders and upper back; nails extend over tips or digits; creases cover sole.

Ears: Earlobes firmer due to increased cartilage.

Sexual development: Males: rugous scrotum. Females: labia majora well developed and minora small or completely covered.

Note: Age refers to postfertilization or postconception age.

Note: From Sadler, T. W. (1985). *Langman's medical embryology* (7th ed.). Baltimore: Williams & Wilkins; and Moore, K. L., & Persand, T. V. N. (1998). *The developing human: Clinically oriented embryology* (6th ed.). Philadelphia: Saunders.

Embryonic Stage

The stage of the **embryo** starts on day 15 (the beginning of the third week after conception) and continues until approximately the eighth week, or until the embryo reaches a *crown-to-rump (C–R)* length of 3 cm (1.2 in). This length is usually reached about 56 days after fertilization (the end of the eighth gestational week). During the embryonic stage, tissues differentiate into essential organs and the main external features develop (Figure 5–12 ◆). The embryo is the most vulnerable to teratogens during this period.

THIRD WEEK

In the third week, the embryonic disc becomes elongated and pear shaped, with a broad cephalic end and a narrow caudal end. The ectoderm has formed a long cylindrical tube for brain and spinal cord development. The gastrointestinal tract, created from the endoderm, appears as another tubelike structure communicating with the yolk sac. The most advanced organ is the heart. At 3 weeks, a single tubular heart forms just outside the body cavity of the embryo.

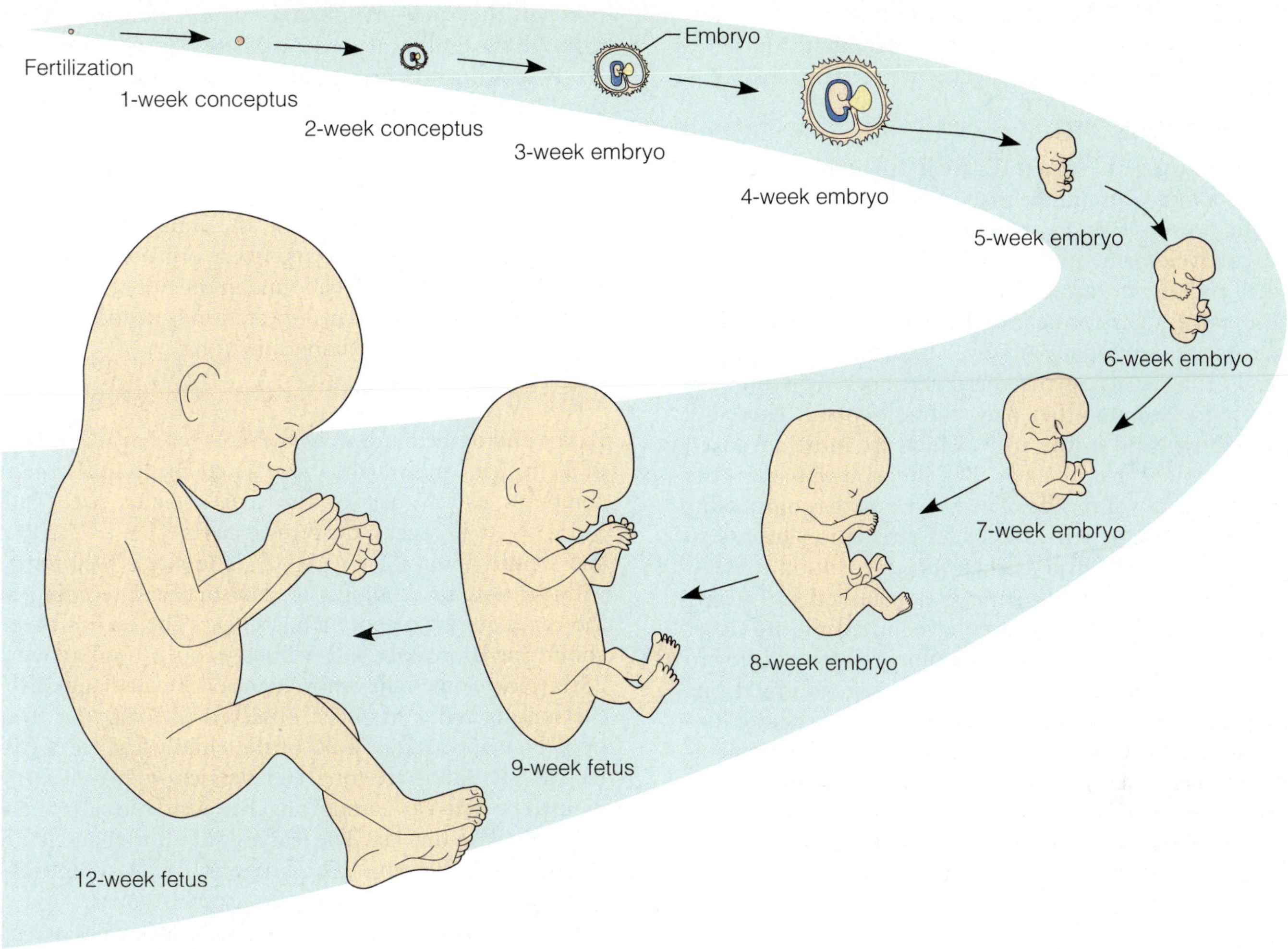

Fertilization

1-week conceptus

2-week conceptus

3-week embryo

Embryo

4-week embryo

5-week embryo

6-week embryo

7-week embryo

8-week embryo

9-week fetus

12-week fetus

FIGURE 5–12. ◆ The actual size of a human conceptus from fertilization to the early fetal stage. The embryonic stage begins in the third week after fertilization; the fetal stage begins in the ninth week.

FOURTH TO FIFTH WEEK

During days 21 to 32, *somites* (a series of mesodermal blocks) form on either side of the embryo's midline. The vertebrae that form the spinal column will develop from these somites. Prior to 28 days, arm and leg buds are not visible, but the tail bud is present. The pharyngeal arches—which will form the lower jaw, hyoid bone, and larynx—develop at this time. The pharyngeal pouches appear now; these pouches will form the eustachian tube and cavity of the middle ear, the tonsils, and the parathyroid and thymus glands. The primordia of the ear and eye are also present. By the end of 28 days, the tubular heart is beating at a regular rhythm and pushing its own primitive blood cells through the main blood vessels.

During the fifth week, the optic cups and lens vessels of the eye form and the nasal pits develop. Partitioning in the heart occurs with the dividing of the atrium. The embryo has a marked C-shaped body, accentuated by the rudimentary tail and the large head folded over a protuberant trunk (Figure 5–13 ◆). By day 35, the arm and leg buds are well developed, with paddle-shaped hand and foot plates. The

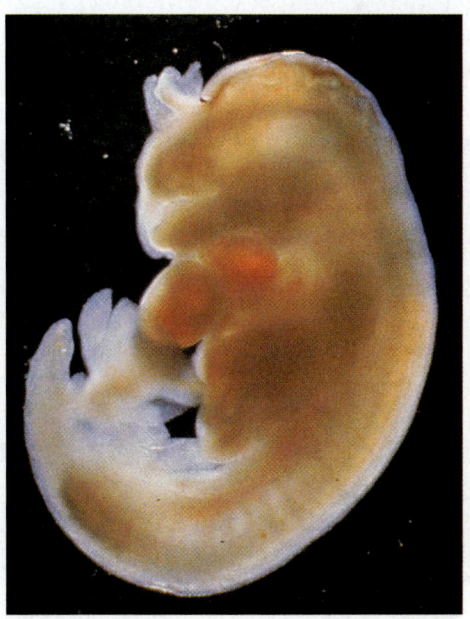

FIGURE 5–13. ◆ The embryo at 5 weeks. The embryo has a marked C-shaped body and a rudimentary tail.

heart, circulatory system, and brain show the most advanced development. The brain has differentiated into five areas, and 10 pairs of cranial nerves are recognizable.

SIXTH TO SEVENTH WEEK

At 6 weeks the head structures are more highly developed and the trunk is straighter than in earlier stages. The upper and lower jaws are recognizable, and the external nares are well formed. The trachea has developed, and its caudal end is bifurcated for beginning lung formation. The upper lip has formed, and the palate is developing. The ears are developing rapidly. The arms have begun to extend ventrally across the chest, and both arms and legs have digits, although they may still be webbed. There is a slight elbow bend in the arms, which are more advanced in development than the legs. Beginning at this stage, the prominent tail will recede. The heart now has most of its definitive characteristics, and fetal circulation begins to be established. The liver starts to produce blood cells. At 7 weeks the head of the embryo is rounded and nearly erect (Figure 5–14 ◆). The eyes have shifted and are closer together, and the eyelids are beginning to form. Prior to this time the rectal and urogenital passages formed one tube that ended in a blind pouch; they now separate into two tubular structures. The intestines enter the extraembryonic coelom in the area of the umbilical cord (called umbilical herniation) (Moore et al., 2000). At this point the beginnings of all essential external and internal structures are present.

EIGHTH WEEK

At 8 weeks the embryo is approximately 3 cm (1.2 in) long C–R and clearly resembles a human being. Facial features continue to develop. The eyelids begin to fuse. Auricles of the external ears begin to assume their final shape, but they are still set low (Moore et al., 2000). External genitals appear, but the embryo's sex is not clearly discernible, and the rectal passage opens with the perfora-

tion of the anal membrane. The circulatory system through the umbilical cord is well established. Long bones are beginning to form, and the large muscles are now capable of contracting.

Fetal Stage

By the end of the eighth week, the embryo is sufficiently developed to be called a **fetus.** Every organ system and external structure that will be found in the full-term newborn is present. The remainder of gestation is devoted to refining structures and perfecting function.

NINTH TO TWELFTH WEEK

By the end of the ninth week the fetus reaches a C–R length of 5 cm (2 in) and weighs about 14 g. The head is large and comprises almost half of the fetus's entire size (Figure 5–15 ◆). At 12 weeks, the fetus reaches 8 cm (3.2 in) C–R and weighs about 45 g (1.6 oz). The face is well formed, with the nose protruding, the chin small and receding, and the ear acquiring a more adult shape. The eyelids close at about the 10th week and will not reopen until about the 28th week. Some reflex movement of the lips suggestive of the sucking reflex has been observed at 3 months. Tooth buds now appear for all 20 of the child's first teeth (baby teeth). The limbs are long and slender, with well-formed digits. The fetus can curl the fingers toward the palm and begins to make a tiny fist. The legs are still shorter and less developed than the arms. The urogenital tract completes its development, well-differentiated genitals appear, and the kidneys begin to produce urine. Red blood cells are produced primarily by the liver. Fetal heart rates can be ascertained by electronic devices between 8 and 12 weeks. The rate is 120 to 160 beats per minute.

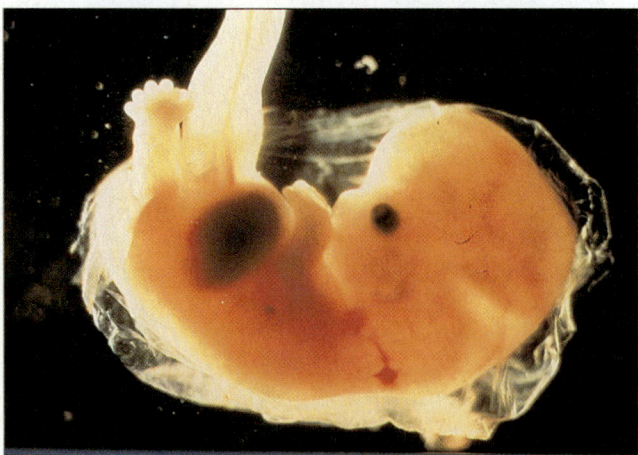

FIGURE 5–14. ◆ The embryo at 7 weeks. The head is rounded and nearly erect. The eyes have shifted forward and closer together, and the eyelids begin to form.

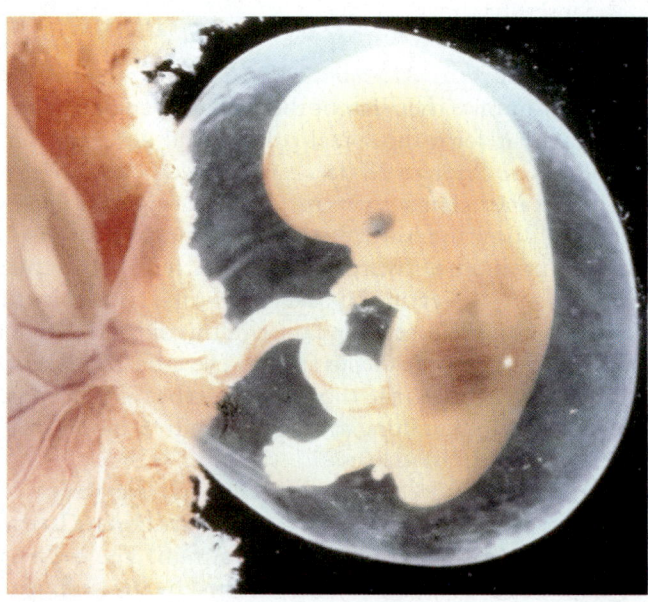

FIGURE 5–15. ◆ The fetus at 9 weeks. Every organ system and external structure is present. *Note:* From Nilsson, L. (1990). *A child is born.* New York: Dell Publishing.

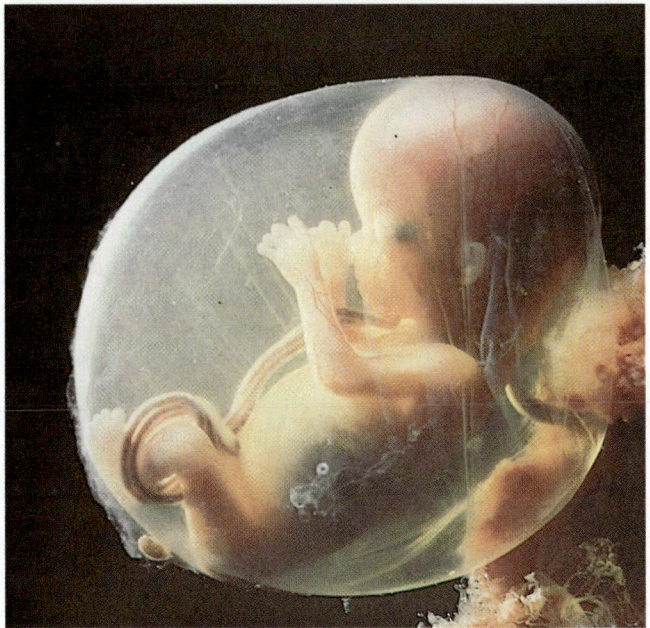

FIGURE 5–16. ◆ The fetus at 14 weeks. During this period of rapid growth the skin is so transparent that blood vessels are visible beneath it. More muscle tissue and body skeleton have developed, and they hold the fetus more erect. *Note:* From Nilsson, L. (1990). *A child is born.* New York: Dell Publishing.

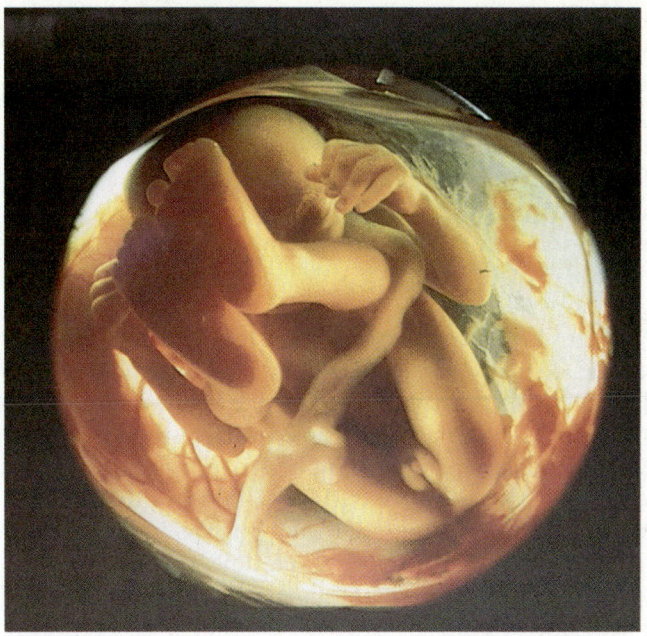

FIGURE 5–17. ◆ The fetus at 20 weeks. The fetus now weighs 435 to 465 g and measures about 19 cm. Subcutaneous deposits of brown fat make the skin a little less transparent. "Woolly" hair covers the head, and nails have developed on the fingers and toes. *Note:* From Nilsson, L. (1990). *A child is born.* New York: Dell Publishing.

Between 13 and 16 weeks is a period of rapid growth. **Lanugo,** or fine hair, begins to develop, especially on the head. The skin is so transparent that blood vessels are clearly visible beneath it. More muscle tissue and body skeleton have developed and hold the fetus more erect (Figure 5–16 ◆). Active movements are present; the fetus stretches and exercises its arms and legs. It makes sucking motions, swallows amniotic fluid, and produces meconium in the intestinal tract.

TWENTIETH WEEK

The fetus doubles its C–R length and now measures 19 cm (8 in) long. Fetal weight is between 435 and 465 g (15.2 and 16.3 oz). Lanugo covers the entire body and is especially prominent on the shoulders. Subcutaneous deposits of brown fat, which has a rich blood supply, make the skin less transparent. Nipples now appear over the mammary glands. The head is covered with fine, woolly hair, and the eyebrows and eyelashes are beginning to form. Nails are present on both fingers and toes. Muscles are well developed, and the fetus is active (Figure 5–17 ◆). The mother feels fetal movement known as quickening. The fetal heartbeat is audible through a fetoscope. Quickening and fetal heartbeat can help in validating the estimated date of birth.

TWENTY-FOURTH WEEK

The fetus at 24 weeks reaches a crown-to-heel (C–H) length of 28 cm (11.2 in). It weighs about 780 g (1 lb, 10 oz). The hair on the head is growing long, and eyebrows and eyelashes have formed. The eye is structurally complete and will soon open. The fetus has a reflex hand grip (grasp reflex) and, by the end of 6 months, a startle reflex. Skin covering the body is reddish and wrinkled, with little subcutaneous fat. Skin on the hands and feet has thickened, with skin ridges on palms and soles forming distinct foot- and fingerprints. The skin over the entire body is covered with **vernix caseosa,** a protective cheeselike, fatty substance secreted by the sebaceous glands. The alveoli in the lungs are just beginning to form.

TWENTY-FIFTH TO TWENTY-EIGHTH WEEK

At 6 months the fetal skin is still red, wrinkled, and covered with vernix caseosa. During this time the brain is developing rapidly, and the nervous system is complete enough to provide some degree of regulation of body functions. The eyelids open and close under neural control. In the male fetus, the testes begin to descend into the scrotal sac. Respiratory and circulatory systems have developed; even though the lungs are still physiologically immature, they are sufficiently developed to provide gas exchange. A fetus born at this time will require immediate and prolonged intensive care to survive and then to decrease the risk of major handicap. The fetus at 28 weeks is about 35 to 38 cm (14 to 15 in) long C–H and weighs 1,200 to 1,250 g (2 lb, 10.5 oz to 2 lb, 12 oz).

TWENTY-NINTH TO THIRTY-SECOND WEEK

At 30 weeks the pupillary light reflex is present (Moore et al., 2000). The fetus is gaining weight from an increase in body muscle and fat and weighs about 2,000 g (4 lb,

6.5 oz), with a length of about 38 to 43 cm (15 to 17 in), by 32 weeks of age. The central nervous system has matured enough to direct rhythmic breathing movements and partially control body temperature. However, the lungs are not yet fully mature. Bones are fully developed but soft and flexible. The fetus begins storing iron, calcium, and phosphorus. In males the testicles may be located in the scrotal sac but are often still high in the inguinal canals.

THIRTY-SIXTH WEEK

The fetus begins to get plump, and less wrinkled skin covers the deposits of subcutaneous fat. Lanugo begins to disappear, and the nails reach the edge of the fingertips. By 35 weeks of age the fetus has a firm grasp and exhibits spontaneous orientation to light. By 36 weeks of age the weight is usually 2,500 to 2,750 g (5 lb, 12 oz to 6 lb, 11.5 oz), and the C–H length of the fetus is about 42 to 48 cm (16 to 19 in). An infant born at this time has a good chance of surviving but may require some special care, especially if there is intrauterine growth retardation.

THIRTY-EIGHTH TO FORTIETH WEEK

The fetus is considered full term 38–40 weeks after conception. The C–H length varies from 48 to 52 cm (19 to 21 in), with males usually longer than females. Generally, males also weigh more than females. The weight at term is about 3,000 to 3,600 g (6 lb, 10 oz to 7 lb, 15 oz). The skin is pink and has a smooth, polished look. The only lanugo left is on the upper arms and shoulders. The hair on the head is no longer woolly but is coarse and about 1 inch long. Vernix caseosa is present, with heavier deposits remaining in the creases and folds of the skin. The body and extremities are plump, with good skin turgor, and the fingernails extend beyond the fingertips. The chest is prominent but still a little smaller than the head, and mammary glands protrude in both sexes. The testes are in the scrotum or palpable in the inguinal canals.

As the fetus enlarges, amniotic fluid diminishes to about 500 mL or less, and the fetal body mass fills the uterine cavity. The fetus assumes what is called its position of comfort, or lie. The head is generally pointed downward, following the shape of the uterus (and possibly because the head is heavier than the feet). The extremities, and often the head, are well flexed. After 5 months, feeding patterns, sleeping patterns, and activity patterns become established, so at term the fetus has its own body rhythms and individual style of response. Table 5–4 summarizes some important developmental milestones.

Factors Influencing Embryonic and Fetal Development

Factors that may affect embryonic development include the quality of the sperm or ovum from which the zygote was formed, the genetic code established at fertilization, and the adequacy of the intrauterine environment. If the

TABLE 5–4 Fetal Development: What Parents Want to Know

4 weeks:	The fetal heart begins to beat.
8 weeks:	All body organs are formed.
8–12 weeks:	Fetal heart rate can be heard by ultrasound Doppler device.
16 weeks:	Baby's sex can be seen.
	Although thin, the fetus looks like a baby.
20 weeks:	Heartbeat can be heard with fetoscope.
	Mother feels movement (quickening).
	Baby develops a regular schedule of sleeping, sucking, and kicking.
	Hands can grasp.
	Baby assumes a favorite position in utero.
	Vernix (lanolin-like covering) protects the body, and lanugo (fine hair) keeps oil on skin.
	Head hair, eyebrows, and eyelashes present.
24 weeks:	Weighs 1 lb, 10 oz.
	Activity is increasing.
	Fetal respiratory movements begin.
28 weeks:	Eyes begin to open and close.
	Baby can breathe at this time.
	Surfactant needed for breathing at birth is formed.
	Baby is two thirds its final size.
32 weeks:	Baby has fingernails and toenails.
	Subcutaneous fat is being laid down.
	Baby appears less red and wrinkled.
38–40 weeks:	Baby fills total uterus.
	Baby gets antibodies from mother.

environment is unsuitable before cellular differentiation occurs, all the cells of the zygote are affected. The cells may die, which causes spontaneous abortion, or growth may be slowed, depending on the severity of the situation. When differentiation is complete and the fetal membranes have formed, an injurious agent has the greatest effect on those cells undergoing the most rapid growth. Thus the time of injury is critical in the development of anomalies.

Because organs are formed primarily during embryonic development, the growing organism is considered most vulnerable to noxious agents during the first months of pregnancy; therefore, it is important to know the gestational age of the embryo or fetus to determine the potential effects of teratogens. Any agent, such as a drug, virus, or radiation, that can cause development of abnormal structures in an embryo is called a *teratogen*. Chapter 7 discusses the effects of specific teratogenic agents on the developing fetus.

Adequacy of the maternal environment is also important during the periods of rapid embryonic and fetal development. Maternal nutrition can affect brain development. The period of maximum brain growth and myelination begins with the fifth lunar month before birth and continues during the first 6 months after birth, when there is a twofold increase in myelination (Volpe, 2000).

Amino acids, glucose, and fatty acids are considered to be the primary dietary factors in brain growth. A subtle type of damage that affects the associative capacity of the brain, possibly leading to learning disabilities, may be caused by nutritional deficiency at this stage. Maternal nutrition may also predispose offspring to the development of adult coronary heart disease, hypertension, and diabetes in babies who were small or disproportionate at birth. (Maternal nutrition is discussed in depth in Chapter 11.) ⬭

Maternal hyperthermia during the first trimester has raised concern about possible central nervous system defects and failure of neural tube closure. Maternal substance abuse also affects the intrauterine environment and is discussed in Chapters 12 and 13. ⬭

CHAPTER HIGHLIGHTS

🐚 Humans have 46 chromosomes, which are divided into 23 pairs—22 pairs of autosomes and 1 pair of sex chromosomes.

🐚 Mitosis is the process by which additional somatic (body) cells are formed. It provides growth and development of the organisms and replacement of body cells.

🐚 Meiosis is the process by which new organisms are formed. It occurs during gametogenesis (oogenesis and spermatogenesis) and consists of two successive cell divisions (reduction division), which produce a gamete with 23 chromosomes (22 autosomal chromosomes and 1 sex chromosome), the haploid number of chromosomes.

🐚 Gametes must have a haploid number of chromosomes (23) so that when the female gamete (ovum) and the male gamete (spermatozoon) unite (fertilization) to form the zygote, the normal human diploid number of chromosomes (46) is reestablished.

🐚 An ovum is considered fertile for about 24 hours after ovulation, and the sperm is capable of fertilizing the ovum for only about 24 hours after it is deposited in the female reproductive tract.

🐚 Fertilization usually takes place in the ampulla (outer third) of the fallopian tube.

🐚 Both capacitation and acrosomal reaction must occur for the sperm to fertilize the ovum. Capacitation is the removal of the plasma membrane, which exposes the acrosomal covering of the sperm head. Acrosomal reaction is the deposit of hyaluronidase in the corona radiata, which allows the sperm head to penetrate the ovum.

🐚 Females have two X chromosomes, and males have an X and a Y chromosome (carried by the sperm). To produce a male child, the mother contributes an X chromosome and the father contributes a Y chromosome.

🐚 Twins are either monozygotic (identical) or dizygotic (fraternal). Dizygotic twins arise from two separate ova fertilized by two separate spermatozoa. Monozygotic twins develop from a single ovum fertilized by a single spermatozoon.

🐚 Preembryonic development first proceeds via cellular multiplication in which the zygote undergoes rapid mitotic division called cleavage. As a result of cleavage, the zygote divides and multiplies into cell groupings called blastomeres, which are held together by the zona pellucida. The blastomeres eventually become a solid ball of cells called the morula. When a cavity forms in the morula cell mass, the inner solid cell mass is called the blastocyst.

🐚 Implantation usually occurs in the upper part of the posterior uterine wall when the blastocyst burrows into the uterine lining.

🐚 After implantation, the endometrium is called the decidua. Decidua capsularis is the portion that covers the blastocyst. Decidua basalis is the portion that is directly under the blastocyst. Decidua vera is the portion that lines the rest of the uterine cavity.

🐚 Primary germ layers give rise to all tissues, organs, and organ systems. The three primary germ cell layers are ectoderm, endoderm, and mesoderm.

🐚 Embryonic membranes are called the amnion and the chorion. The amnion is formed from the ectoderm and is a thin protective membrane that contains the amniotic fluid and the embryo. The chorion is a thick membrane that develops from the trophoblast and encloses the amnion, embryo, and yolk sac.

🐚 Amniotic fluid cushions the fetus against mechanical injury, controls the embryo's temperature, allows symmetrical external growth, prevents adherence to the amnion, and permits freedom of movement.

🐚 The umbilical cord contains two umbilical arteries, which carry deoxygenated blood from the fetus to the placenta, and one umbilical vein, which carries oxygenated blood from the placenta to the fetus. The umbilical cord normally has a central insertion into the placenta. Wharton's jelly, a specialized connective tissue, helps prevent compression of the umbilical cord in utero.

🐚 The placenta develops from the chorionic villi and decidua basalis and has two parts: The maternal portion, consisting of the decidua basalis, is red and fresh looking; the fetal portion, consisting of chorionic villi, is covered by the amnion and appears shiny and gray. The placenta is made up of 15 to 20 segments called cotyledons.

🐚 The placenta serves metabolic functions, endocrine (production of hPL, hCG, estrogen, and progesterone), and immunologic functions. It acts as the fetus's respiratory organ, is an organ of excretion, and aids in the exchange of nutrients.

🐚 Stages of fetal development include the preembryonic stage (the first 14 days of human development starting at the time of fertilization), the embryonic stage (from day 15 after fertilization, or the beginning of the third week, until approximately 8 weeks), and the fetal stage (from 8 weeks until birth, at approximately 40 weeks after the last normal menstrual period).

🐚 Significant events that occur during the embryonic stage include the fetal heart beginning to beat at 4 weeks and the establishment of fetal circulation at 6 weeks.

🐚 The fetal stage is devoted to refining structures and perfecting function. Some significant developments during the fetal stage are as follows:
- At 8 to 12 weeks, all organ systems are formed and simply require maturation.
- At 16 weeks, the sex can be determined visually.
- At 20 weeks, the fetal heartbeat can be auscultated by a fetoscope, and the mother can feel movement (quickening).
- At 24 weeks, vernix caseosa covers the entire body.

- At 26 to 28 weeks, the eyes reopen.
- At 32 weeks, skin appears less wrinkled and red, since subcutaneous fat has been laid down.
- At 36 weeks, fingernails reach the ends of fingers.

- At 40 weeks, vernix caseosa is apparent only in the creases and folds of the skin, and lanugo remains on upper arms and shoulders only.

🐦 The embryo is particularly vulnerable to teratogenesis during the first 8 weeks of cell differentiation and organ system development.

EXPLOREMediaLink

NCLEX Review, Case Studies, and other interactive resources for this chapter can be found on the companion website at http://www.prenhall.com/london. Click on "Chapter 5" to select the activities for this chapter.

For animations, more NCLEX review questions, and an audio glossary, access the accompanying CD-ROM in this textbook.

REFERENCES

Ahokas, R. A., & McKinney, E. T. (2000). Development and physiology of the placenta and membranes. In J. J. Sciarra & T. J. Watkins (Eds.), *Gynecology and obstetrics* (Vol. 2, chap. 11, pp. 1–21). Philadelphia: Lippincott Williams & Wilkins.

Benirschke, K. (1999a). Multiple gestation: Incidence, etiology, and inheritance. In R. K. Creasy & R. Resnik (Eds.), *Maternal-fetal medicine* (4th ed., pp. 585–597). Philadelphia: Saunders.

Benirschke, K. (1999b). Normal development. In R. K. Creasy & R. Resnik (Eds.), *Maternal-fetal medicine* (4th ed., pp. 63–71). Philadelphia: Saunders.

Brannigan, R. E., & Lipshultz, L. I. (2000). Sperm transport and capacitation. In J. J. Sciarra & T. J. Watkins (Eds.), *Gynecology and obstetrics* (Vol. 5, chap. 45, pp. 1–9). Philadelphia: Lippincott Williams & Wilkins.

Craven, C., & Ward, K. (1999). Embryology, fetus, and placenta: Normal and abnormal. In J. R. Scott, P. J. Di Saia, C. B. Hammond, & W. N. Spellacy (Eds.), *Danforth's obstetrics and gynecology* (8th ed., pp. 29–46). Philadelphia: Lippincott Williams & Wilkins.

Cunningham, F. G., Gant, N. G., Leveno, K. J., Gilstrap III, L. C., Hauth, J. C. & Wenstrom, K. O. (2001). *Williams Obstetrics* (21st. ed.) New York: McGraw-Hill.

De Jonge, C. J. (2000). Egg transport and fertilization. In J. J. Sciarra & T. J. Watkins (Eds.), *Gynecology and obstetrics* (Vol. 5, chap. 46, pp. 1–7). Philadelphia: Lippincott Williams & Wilkins.

Gilbert, W. M., & Brace, R. A. (1993). Amniotic fluid volume and normal flows to and from the amniotic cavity. *Seminars in Perinatology, 17*(3), 150–157.

Moore, K. L., Persaud, T. V. N., & Shiota, K. (2000). *Color atlas of clinical embryology* (2nd ed.). Philadelphia: Saunders.

Sadler, T. W. (2000). *Langman's medical embryology* (8th ed.). Philadelphia: Lippincott, Williams & Wilkins.

Spellacy, W. N. (1999). Multiple pregnancies. In J. R. Scott, P. J. Di Saia, C. B. Hammond, & W. N. Spellacy (Eds.), *Danforth's obstetrics and gynecology* (8th ed., pp. 293–300). Philadelphia: Lippincott Williams & Wilkins.

Volpe, J. J. (2000). *Neurology of the newborn* (4th ed.). Philadelphia: Saunders.

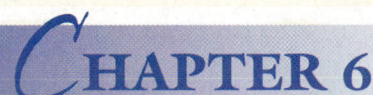

CHAPTER 6

Preparation for Parenthood

We took our childbirth education classes with seven other couples. Our instructor, who was a nurse, was great—warm and funny but very knowledgeable. After we all had given birth she had everyone over to her house for a "reunion." We lined the babies up together on the sofa and took a picture. They leaned against each other, topsy-turvy. It was hilarious. My son is now 23 but I still love that picture of him. What memories it triggers of such a very special time!

—TRISH, 45

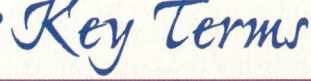

Key Terms

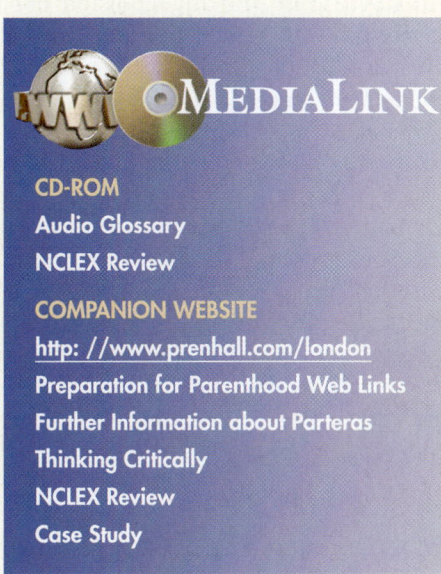

MEDIALINK

CD-ROM
Audio Glossary
NCLEX Review

COMPANION WEBSITE
http://www.prenhall.com/london
Preparation for Parenthood Web Links
Further Information about Parteras
Thinking Critically
NCLEX Review
Case Study

As pregnancy progresses, expectant parents begin to look forward to their birth experience and the challenges of parenthood. This is a time for plans and decisions. Where will the birth be? Who do they wish to be present? How will they prepare themselves for this experience?

Today's professional nurse can assist a pregnant woman or expectant couple, if the partner is involved, to make the choices that are part of pregnancy and birth. For first-time parents, the decisions may seem numerous and complicated, and the nurse has a unique opportunity to help them establish a pattern of decision making that will serve them well in their years as parents.

PRECONCEPTION COUNSELING

One of the first questions a couple should ask themselves is whether they wish to have children. This decision involves consideration of each person's goals, expectations of the relationship, and desire to be a parent. Sometimes one person wishes to have a child, but the other does not. In such situations, an open discussion is essential to reach a mutually acceptable decision.

Couples who wish to have children need to decide about the timing of pregnancy. When do they believe it would be best to become parents? For couples who have religious beliefs that do not support contraception or who feel that fertility planning is unnatural, planning the timing of the pregnancy is unacceptable and irrelevant. These couples can still take steps to ensure that they are in the best possible physical and mental health when pregnancy occurs.

Preconception Health Measures

The nurse begins by teaching the couple about known or suspected health risks. The nurse advises the woman who smokes to cease smoking if possible or to limit her cigarette intake to less than half a pack per day. Because of the hazards of secondhand smoke, it is helpful if her partner refrains from smoking around her. Although the effects of caffeine are less clearly understood, the woman is advised to avoid or limit her intake of caffeine. Alcohol, social drugs, and street drugs pose a real threat to the fetus. A woman who uses any prescription or over-the-counter medications needs to discuss the implications of their use with her health care provider. It is best to avoid using any medication if possible. Because of the possible teratogenic effects of environmental hazards, the nurse urges the couple contemplating pregnancy to determine whether they are exposed to any environmental hazards at work or in their community.

PHYSICAL EXAMINATION

It is wise for both partners to have a physical examination to identify any health problems so that they can be corrected if possible. These problems might include medical

Complementary Care

AYURVEDA AND PRECONCEPTION LIFESTYLE

Ayurveda is an ancient system of natural and medical healing that originated in India. *Ayur* means "life" and *veda* means "science." It includes a wide range of modalities, including the use of diet, herbs, massage, exercise, music therapy, aromatherapy, meditation, and yoga, among others. Ayurvedic practitioners believe that these modalities should be practiced not only during pregnancy, but also prior to conception for optimal maternal and fetal health.

Ayurvedic practitioners would recommend that both the mother *and* father take part in a healthy lifestyle prior to conception. Some of the preconception lifestyle recommendations would include:

- Avoiding stress and overwork
- Avoiding alcohol, tobacco, and drugs
- Avoiding meat and dairy products, and eating primarily a vegetarian diet
- Striving for a positive emotional relationship between the man and woman

In Chapter 41, see "Complementary Care: Ayurvedic Treatment of the Common Cold" for more information.

conditions such as high blood pressure or obesity; problems that threaten fertility, such as certain sexually transmitted infections; or conditions that keep the individual from achieving optimal health, such as anemia or colitis. If the family history indicates previous genetic disorders, or if the couple is planning pregnancy when the woman is over age 35, the health care provider may suggest that the couple consider genetic counseling. In addition to the history and physical exam, the woman may have a variety of laboratory tests. (See "Assessment Guide: Initial Prenatal Assessment" in Chapter 8.) The woman is advised to have a dental examination and any necessary dental work done prior to conception to avoid exposure to x-rays and the risk of infection while she is pregnant.

NUTRITION

Prior to conception it is advisable for the woman to be at an average weight for her body build and height. The woman is advised to follow a nutritious diet that contains ample quantities of all the essential nutrients. Some nutritionists advocate emphasizing the following nutrients: calcium, protein, iron, B-complex vitamins, vitamin C, folic acid, and magnesium. Intake of certain vitamins in megadoses can cause severe fetal problems and should be avoided.

Neural tube defects such as spina bifida and meningomyelocele in the newborn have been associated with low maternal folate. To decrease this risk, women of childbearing age are advised to consume 0.4 mg folate daily. This quantity is typically found in a multivitamin tablet (American Academy of Pediatrics, 1999). (See Chapter 11 for further discussion of nutrition.)

EXERCISE

A woman is advised to continue her present pattern of exercise or to establish a regular exercise plan beginning at least 3 months before she attempts to become pregnant. An exercise routine that she enjoys and maintains will provide the best results. Exercise that includes some aerobic conditioning and some general muscle toning improves the woman's circulation and general health. Once an exercise program is well established, the woman is generally encouraged to continue it during pregnancy.

CONTRACEPTION

A woman who takes oral contraceptives is advised to stop taking the pill and have two or three normal menses before attempting to conceive. This waiting period allows the natural hormonal cycle to return and facilitates dating the subsequent pregnancy. A woman using an intrauterine device is advised to have it removed and to wait 1 month before attempting to conceive. During the waiting period, she can use barrier methods of contraception (condoms, diaphragm, or cervical cap with spermicides).

CONCEPTION

Most preconception recommendations focus on helping the couple attain their best possible health state so that they do not enter pregnancy with unnecessary risks. Conception is a personal and emotional experience, and even if a couple is prepared, they may feel some ambivalence. Ambivalence is a normal response, but they may need reassurance that the feeling will pass. A couple may get so caught up in preparation and in their efforts to "do things right" that they lose sight of the pleasure they derive from each other and their lives together and cease to value the joy of spontaneity in their relationship. It is often helpful for the health care provider to remind an overly zealous couple to take pleasure in the present moment.

CHILDBEARING DECISIONS

Once the couple has conceived, they should begin exploring their options for a health care provider and birth setting, as well as labor support and sibling preparation, if appropriate. These decisions are influenced by a variety of factors.

Care Provider

One of the first decisions facing expectant parents is the selection of a health care provider. The nurse assists them by explaining the various options and outlining what can be expected from each. A thorough understanding of the differences of educational preparation, skill level, general philosophy, and characteristics of practice of certified nurse-midwives, obstetricians, family practice physicians, and lay midwives is essential. The nurse can encourage expectant parents to investigate the care provider's credentials, edu-

Developing Cultural Competence

Sometimes nurses make the mistake of assuming that a pregnant woman will make the same decisions about the birth experience as the nurse would have. However, the choices a woman and her family make are influenced by many factors, including ethnic background, culture, and religious beliefs. These factors may profoundly influence decisions such as care provider (male or female), birth setting, labor support person(s), use of medications for analgesia, position during birth, saving the placenta, dietary practices immediately postpartum, and a host of other issues. There is no one right way to give birth.

cation and training, philosophy of childbirth, fee schedule or insurance plans accepted, and availability to new clients; they can often get this information by telephoning the provider's office. The nurse can help the expectant parents develop a list of questions for their first visit to a care provider to help determine compatibility. These questions might include the following:

- Who is in practice with you, or who covers for you when you are unavailable?

- How do your partners' philosophies compare with yours?

- How do you feel about my partner, other support person, or other children coming to the prenatal visits?

- What are your feelings about _____ (fill in special desires for the birth event, such as different positions assumed during labor, episiotomy, induction of labor, other people present during the birth, breastfeeding immediately after the birth, no separation of infant and parents following birth, and so on)?

- If a cesarean birth is necessary, could my partner be present?

- Are you familiar with _____ (fill in complementary or alternative forms of health care that may be used currently if applicable)? How will this practice impact my plan of care?

Choosing a care provider is just one of the decisions pregnant women and couples make. A method that has helped many couples make these choices is a **birth preference plan.** By writing down preferences, prospective parents identify aspects of the childbearing experience that are most important to them. (A sample birth preference sheet is presented in Figure 6–1 ◆). Used as a tool for communication among the expectant parents, the health care provider, and the health care professionals at the birth setting, the written plan identifies options that are available as well as those that are not.

The preference sheet or plan also helps pregnant women and couples set priorities. Using the plan, they identify areas that they want to incorporate into their own birth

Choice	I would like to have		Available	
	Yes	No	Yes	No
Care provider:				
Certified nurse-midwife	___	___	___	___
Obstetrician	___	___	___	___
Lay midwife	___	___	___	___
Birth setting	___	___	___	___
Hospital:				
Birthing room	___	___	___	___
Delivery room	___	___	___	___
Birth center	___	___	___	___
Home	___	___	___	___
Partner present	___	___	___	___
Doula present	___	___	___	___
During labor and birth	___	___	___	___
During cesarean	___	___	___	___
During whole postpartum period	___	___	___	___
During labor:				
Ambulate as desired	___	___	___	___
Shower if desired	___	___	___	___
Wear own clothes	___	___	___	___
Use whirlpool	___	___	___	___
Use rocking chair	___	___	___	___
Have enema	___	___	___	___
Water birth	___	___	___	___
Intermittent electronic fetal monitor	___	___	___	___
Membranes:				
Rupture naturally	___	___	___	___
Amniotomy if needed	___	___	___	___
Labor stimulation if needed	___	___	___	___
Medication:				
Identify type desired	___	___	___	___
Food and fluids or ice as desired	___	___	___	___
Music during labor and birth	___	___	___	___
Massage	___	___	___	___
Therapeutic touch	___	___	___	___
Position during birth:				
On side	___	___	___	___
Hands and knees	___	___	___	___
Kneeling	___	___	___	___
Squatting	___	___	___	___
Birthing chair	___	___	___	___
Birthing bed	___	___	___	___
Other:	___	___	___	___
Family present (sibs)	___	___	___	___
Filming of birth/videotaping	___	___	___	___
Leboyer	___	___	___	___
Episiotomy	___	___	___	___
Partner to cut umbilical cord	___	___	___	___
Hold baby immediately after birth	___	___	___	___
Breastfeed immediately after birth	___	___	___	___
No separation after birth	___	___	___	___
Save the placenta	___	___	___	___
Collect cord blood	___	___	___	___
Newborn care:				
Eye treatment for the baby	___	___	___	___
Vitamin K injection	___	___	___	___
Breastfeeding	___	___	___	___
Formula feeding	___	___	___	___
Glucose water	___	___	___	___
Circumcision	___	___	___	___
Postpartum care:				
Rooming-in	___	___	___	___
Short stay (48° after vaginal birth)	___	___	___	___
Sibling visitation	___	___	___	___
Infant care classes	___	___	___	___
Self-care classes	___	___	___	___
Home visits following discharge	___	___	___	___
Home doula	___	___	___	___
Other:	___	___	___	___

FIGURE 6–1. ◆ Birth preference sheet. The column on the left lists various choices that the couple may consider during their childbirth experience. Once the couple has considered each of the choices, they may mark the "yes" or "no" space in the middle columns. The right columns are used to note the availability of some of the choices. For instance, the couple may want to use hydrotherapy (whirlpool) during labor, but the birthing settings in their community do not have whirlpool tubs available. All choices need to be made in the context of what is available in the couple's community.

experience. They can then discuss the document at a visit with their certified nurse-midwife or other care provider and use it to compare their wishes with the philosophy and beliefs of the provider.

Expectant parents also need to consider the qualities they want in a care provider for the newborn. They may want to visit several before the birth to select someone who will meet their needs and those of their child.

Pregnant women and couples will make many more choices, all with associated benefits and risks. Some are explored in Table 6–1. Although many birth experiences are very close to the desired experience, at times expectations cannot be met. This may be because of the unavailability of some choices in the community, limitations set by insurance providers, or unexpected problems during pregnancy or birth. It is important for the nurse to help expectant parents keep sight of what is realistic for their situation while also acting as an advocate for them.

Birth Setting

The nurse can help expectant parents choose a birth setting by suggesting they tour facilities and talk with nurses there as well as with friends or acquaintances who are recent parents. However, the choice of health care provider may largely determine the birth setting. Questions that expectant parents might ask of new parents include the following:

- What kind of care and support did you receive during labor?
- If the setting has both labor and delivery rooms and birthing rooms, was a birthing room available when you wanted it?
- Were you encouraged to be mobile during labor or do what you wanted to do (walking, sitting in a rocking chair, sitting in a whirlpool bath, standing in a shower, and so on)? If not, were there reasonable circumstances that prevented you from doing so?
- Were you encouraged to be involved in your plan of care and kept well informed of progress or proposed changes?
- Was your labor partner or coach treated well?
- Were your birth preferences respected? Did you share them with the facility before the birth? If something did not work, why do you think there were problems?

TABLE 6–1 Benefits and Risks of Some Consumer Decisions During Pregnancy, Labor, and Birth

Issue	Benefits	Risks
Breastfeeding	No additional expense Contains maternal antibodies Decreases incidence of infant otitis media, vomiting, and diarrhea Easier to digest than formula Immediately after birth, promotes uterine contractions and decreases incidence of postpartum hemorrhage	Transmission of pollutants to newborn Irregular ovulation and menses can cause false sense of security and nonuse of contraceptives Increased nutritional requirement in mother
Enema	May facilitate labor Increases space for infant in pelvis May increase strength of contractions May prevent contamination of sterile field	Increases discomfort and anxiety

Ambulation during labor	Comfort for laboring woman
	May assist in labor progression by
	  a. Stimulating contractions
	  b. Allowing gravity to help descent of fetus
	  c. Giving sense of independence and control
		Cord prolapse will rupture membranes unless engagement has occurred
		Birth of infant in undesirable situations

Electronic fetal monitoring	Helps evaluate fetal well-being Helps identify fetal stress Useful in diagnostic testing Helps evaluate labor progress	Supine postural hypotension Intrauterine perforation (with internal uterine pressure device) Infection (with internal monitoring) Decreases personal interaction with mother because of attention paid to the machine Mother is unable to ambulate or change her position freely
Whirlpool (jet hydrotherapy)	Increased relaxation Decreased anxiety Stimulation of labor Nonmedicated pain relief Slight decrease in blood pressure Increased diuresis	May slow contractions if used before active labor is established Possible risk of infection if membranes are ruptured Slight increase in maternal temperature and heart rate and fetal heart rate during whirlpool and/or in first 30 minutes after being in tub
Analgesia	Maternal relaxation facilitates labor	All drugs reach the fetus in varying degrees and with varying effects
Episiotomy	May facilitate birth in emergency situations	Increased pain after birth and for 3 months following birth Infection Increased frequency of third- and fourth-degree lacerations (Wolcott & Conry, 2000)

- During labor, did the nurse offer or suggest a variety of comfort measures?
- How were medications handled during labor? Were you comfortable with this arrangement?
- Were siblings welcomed in the birth setting? After the birth?
- Was the nursing staff helpful after the baby was born? Did you receive self-care and infant care information? Did you have a choice about what information was provided?

Labor Support

Another important choice the expectant family faces is how active a support role the father or partner wants to take during labor and birth. Although many partners are comfortable acting as the primary physical and emotional support for the laboring woman, some partners are not. Studies have found that many men are discouraged when the comfort measures they learned in childbirth classes do not seem to work in labor, and they are left with a negative feeling about the experience (Chapman, 2000). In lieu of the partner, other options for labor support include asking a friend or family member to attend the birth and help with comfort needs, contacting a local childbirth advocate group for a volunteer referral, or hiring a specialized childbirth support person, known as a **doula.**

The role of the doula is to attend to the needs of the childbearing family. Specially trained to assist with births and provide support to new parents and family members, the doula is an adjunct to the health care team. In a managed care environment in which nursing staff are often stretched thinly, a doula can be an asset to the nurse by attending to the many comfort needs of the laboring mother and her family (England & Horowitz, 1998; Simkin, 1999). Another labor support person that is more culturally specific is a partera. Women of Mexican descent, in particular, may choose to employ these direct-entry midwives (see "Developing Cultural Competence" on parteras for further information).

$\mathcal{D}$eveloping Cultural Competence

The increasing numbers of Mexican Americans living in the United States make it important for nurses to become familiar with the use of *parteras* by many members of this population. Parteras are one of several types of **curanderos** (traditional healers) found in Latino communities. Parteras or direct-entry midwives—not to be confused with certified nurse-midwives—are usually women in their 40s or older who are themselves mothers or grandmothers. They have learned their skills from their mothers or other respected elder women.

Traditionally, it is a cultural preference that a pregnant woman be attended by a partera and give birth at home or in a birthing center. The partera stays with the expectant mother all through active labor. Parteras are trained to do perineal massage and manual stretching of muscles and soft tissues of the birth canal, instead of episiotomies. They do not conduct vaginal exams. The partera uses no medicines, no forceps, no episiotomy, no stitches, no oxytocins, and no breaking of the amniotic membrane to hasten birth. Parteras acknowledge the body/mind/soul and spiritual connection of the client (Arizága, 1999).

Not all women wishing to have their babies at home assisted by a partera are able to do so. U.S. midwifery laws prohibit the partera from accepting as clients women who are severely overweight, diabetic, hypertensive, or anemic, or who have been told by a physician that they have a medical problem that would make home birth unsafe. 🔗 WEB

Sibling Participation in the Birth

Some expectant parents may wish to have their other children present at the birth. Children who will attend a birth can be prepared through books, audiovisual materials, use of models, discussion, and sibling classes. Nurses can assist parents with sibling preparation by helping them understand the stresses a child may experience. For example, the child may become frightened if the laboring mom is irritable and visibly showing discomfort, feel left out when there is a new child to love, or feel disappointed if a brother is born when a sister was expected.

During the birth it is important that a sibling have his or her own support person whose sole responsibility is tending to the child's needs. The support person needs to be familiar to the child; warm, sensitive, and flexible; knowledgeable about the birth process; and comfortable with sexuality and birth. This person must be prepared to interpret what is happening for the child and to intervene when necessary. For example, the support person needs to be prepared to remove the child from the birthing room at the child's request or if the situation warrants that action.

Siblings should be allowed to react to the birth in whatever manner they choose, as long as it is not disruptive. They should understand that they can stay or leave the room as they choose. They should also feel free to ask questions and express feelings.

In general, siblings who are present at birth tend to have feelings of interest and the desire to nurture "our" baby, as opposed to jealousy and rivalry directed at "Mom's" baby. The mother does not disappear mysteriously into the hospital and return with a demanding outsider. Instead, the family attending the birth together finds a new opportunity for closeness and growth by sharing in the birth of a new member.

CLASSES FOR FAMILY MEMBERS DURING PREGNANCY

Prenatal education programs provide important opportunities to share information about pregnancy and childbirth and to enhance the parents' decision-making skills. The content of each class is generally directed by the overall goals of the program. The nurse who knows the types of prenatal programs available in the community can direct expectant parents to programs that meet their special needs and learning goals.

From the expectant parents' point of view, class content is best presented in chronology with the pregnancy. Thus, prenatal classes are often divided into early and late classes (Table 6–2).

Early Classes: First Trimester

Early prenatal classes often include prepregnant women and couples as well as those in early pregnancy. The classes cover early gestational changes; self-care during pregnancy; fetal development and environmental dangers for the fetus; sexuality in pregnancy; birth settings and types of care providers; nutrition, rest, and exercise suggestions; common discomforts of pregnancy and relief measures; psychologic changes in pregnancy for the woman and man; methods of coping with stress; and the benefits of following a healthful lifestyle. Early classes provide information about factors that place the woman at risk for preterm labor and about how to recognize symptoms of preterm labor. Early classes should also present information about breastfeeding and bottle-feeding. Most women (50% to 80%) have made their infant feeding decision before the sixth month of pregnancy.

Later Classes: Second and Third Trimesters

The later classes focus on preparation for the birth, including birth choices (episiotomy, medications, fetal monitoring, epidural, and so forth), postpartum self-care, infant care and feeding, and newborn safety issues. Since many expectant parents purchase a car seat before the birth of their child, later classes should also include information about the importance of car seats, how they work, and how to select an approved car seat.

Childbirth preparation classes are an ideal time to incorporate infant stimulation concepts. These concepts help develop parenting skills and enhance prenatal and neonatal bonding. Tactile, vestibular, and auditory stimulation

TABLE 6–2 Possible Content of Classes for Childbirth Preparation

Early Classes (First Trimester)

Early gestational changes
Self-care during pregnancy
Fetal development, environmental dangers for the fetus
Sexuality in pregnancy
Birth settings and types of care providers
Nutrition, rest, and exercise suggestions
Relief measures for common discomforts of pregnancy
Psychologic changes in pregnancy
Information for getting pregnancy off to a good start

Later Classes (Second and Third Trimesters)

Preparation for birth process
Postpartum self-care
Birth choices (e.g., episiotomy, medications, fetal monitoring, enema)
Relaxation techniques
Breathing techniques
Infant stimulation or infant massage
Newborn safety issues, such as car seats

Adolescent Preparation Classes

How to be a good parent
Newborn care
Health dangers for the baby
Healthy diet during pregnancy
How to recognize when baby is ill
Baby care: physical and emotional

Breastfeeding Programs

Advantages and disadvantages
Techniques of breastfeeding
Methods of breast milk storage
Involvement of fathers in feeding process

can be explained. As the uterine wall thins during the pregnancy, the mother and father are better able to feel the baby, and the fetus can sense the parents' stroking and patting through the abdominal wall. Abdominal effleurage (a light stroking movement made over the abdominal wall with the fingertips) can provide tactile stimulation to the fetus.

The pelvic-tilt exercise provides vestibular stimulation through movement of the fetus. Rocking in a rocking chair is also a comfortable way to provide both relaxation for the expectant woman and vestibular stimulation for the fetus. Playing music can provide auditory stimulation. Classical music is found to stimulate the fetus.

Adolescent Parenting Classes

Adolescents have special learning needs during pregnancy. Areas of concern for teens focus on how to be a good par-

ent, how to care for a new baby, health dangers to the baby, and healthful foods to eat during pregnancy. Teens also need to learn how to recognize when the baby is sick, protect the baby from accidents, and make the baby feel happy and loved. Expectant teens are often eager to hear more about the birth process (especially ways to cope with pain during the birth process), the personal health of the mother, the discomforts and life changes that accompany pregnancy, and sexuality.

Breastfeeding Programs

Programs offering information on breastfeeding are increasing. For many years, a primary source of information has been **La Leche League,** a nonprofit organization that promotes breastfeeding. Certified lactation educators; clinical lactation consultants; and nurses at birthing centers, hospitals, and health clinics can also provide information. Expectant parents learn positioning and techniques of breastfeeding, advantages and disadvantages, and methods of breast pumping and milk storage. The father's support and encouragement of the mother is vital, so it is important to include him in the educational programs and decision making. Some fathers may feel ambivalent or resentful about breastfeeding and need opportunities in the prenatal period to discuss and share feelings and experiences.

Sibling Preparation: Adjustment to a Newborn

The birth of a new sibling is a significant event in a child's life. Attendance at sibling preparation classes can enhance positive adjustment (Figure 6–2 ◆). The classes usually focus on reducing the child's anxiety, giving the child opportunities to express feelings and concerns, and encouraging realistic expectations of the newborn. Parents learn strategies to prepare the child for the birth and help the child cope with a new family member.

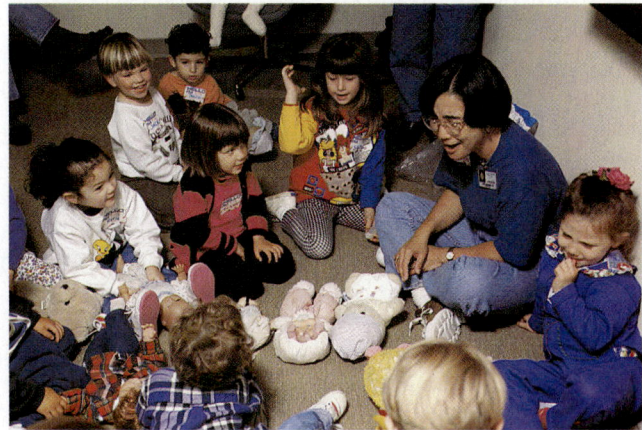

FIGURE 6–2. ◆ It is especially important that siblings be well prepared when they are going to be present for the birth. However, all siblings can benefit from information about birth and the new baby ahead of time.

Sibling preparation can be addressed through a formal class or in a less formal way by providing a booklet for parents that addresses issues affecting both parents and children.

Classes for Grandparents

Grandparents are an important source of support and information for prospective and new parents. They are now often included in the birthing process. Prenatal programs for grandparents can be an important source of information about current beliefs and practices in childbearing. The most useful content may include changes in birthing and parenting practices and helpful tips for being a supportive grandparent. Grandparents who will be integral members of the labor and birth team need information about that role.

EDUCATION OF THE FAMILY HAVING CESAREAN BIRTH

Cesarean birth is an alternative method of birth. However, because the need for a cesarean birth is rarely known in advance, specific classes covering this alternative are uncommon. Since one out of every four or five births is by cesarean, preparation for this possibility should be an integral part of every childbirth education curriculum.

Cesarean birth class content should cover what the parents can expect to happen during a cesarean birth, what they might feel, and what choices are available. All pregnant women and couples should be encouraged to discuss with their certified nurse-midwife or physician the progression of events if a cesarean birth becomes necessary.

Preparation for Repeat Cesarean Birth

When expectant parents are anticipating a repeat cesarean birth, they have time to plan and prepare. Many birthing units provide preparation classes for repeat cesarean birth. Parents who have had previous negative experiences need an opportunity to describe what contributed to their feelings. They should be encouraged to identify what they would like to change and to list interventions that would make the experience more positive. Those who have had positive experiences require reassurance that their needs and desires will be met in a similar manner. In addition, all parents are encouraged to air any fears or anxieties.

A specific concern of the woman facing a repeat cesarean is anticipation of pain. She needs reassurance that subsequent cesarean births are often less painful than the first. In addition, planned cesarean births involve less fatigue than unplanned procedures because they are not preceded by a long, strenuous labor. Providing this information will help the woman cope more effectively with stressful stimuli, including pain.

Preparation for Parents Desiring Vaginal Birth after Cesarean Birth (VBAC)

Parents who have had a cesarean birth and are now anticipating a vaginal birth have unique needs. Because they may have unresolved questions and concerns about the last birth, it is helpful to begin the series of classes with an informational session. The nurse can supply information about the criteria necessary to attempt a trial of labor and identify decisions to be made regarding the birth experience. Some childbirth educators suggest that parents prepare two birth preference plans: one for vaginal birth and one for cesarean birth. Preparation of the birth plans seems to give parents some sense of control over the birth experience and tends to increase the positive aspects of the experience.

CHILDBIRTH PREPARATION METHODS

Childbirth preparation classes are usually taught by *certified childbirth educators.* Various types of childbirth preparation are available. Vital to each method is the educational component, which helps alleviate fear. The classes vary in coverage of subjects related to the maternity cycle, but all teach relaxation and coping techniques, as well as what to expect during labor and birth. Most classes also feature exercises to relax and condition muscles and breathing exercises for use in labor. The greatest differences among the methods lie in the theories of why they work and in the specific comfort techniques and breathing patterns they teach.

Childbirth preparation offers several advantages. Most important is that judicious use of analgesics and anesthetics optimizes the baby's health. Another advantage is the satisfaction of the parents, for whom childbirth becomes a shared and profound emotional experience. In addition, each method has been shown to shorten labor. All nurses should know how these techniques differ, so that they can support each birth experience effectively.

Programs for Preparation

Some antepartal classes, specifically oriented to preparation for labor and birth, have a name associated with a theory of pain reduction in childbirth. The most common methods of this type are the Lamaze (psychoprophylactic), Kitzinger (sensory-memory), and Bradley (partner-coached childbirth). Each of these programs is designed to provide the woman or couple with self-help measures so that the pregnancy and birth are healthy and happy events (Haire, 1999). Table 6–3 identifies differentiating characteristics of each method.

The psychoprophylactic method is the childbirth preparation method generally called **Lamaze** classes. Psychoprophylactic means "mind prevention." Dr. Fernand Lamaze, a French obstetrician, introduced this method of childbirth preparation to the Western world. In 1960, pro-

TABLE 6-3 Summary of Selected Childbirth Preparation Methods

Method	Characteristics	Breathing Technique
Lamaze	See narrative discussion in text.	
Bradley	Frequently referred to as partner- or husband-coached natural childbirth. Uses various exercises and slow, controlled abdominal breathing to accomplish relaxation.	Uses primarily abdominal breathing.
Kitzinger	Uses sensory memory to help the woman understand and work with her body in preparation for birth. Incorporates the Stanislavsky method of acting as a way to teach relaxation.	Uses chest breathing in conjunction with abdominal relaxation.

ponents of the method formed a nonprofit group called the American Society for Psychoprophylaxis in Obstetrics (ASPO). This organization offers a standardized training and certification for childbirth educators, and has helped establish many programs throughout the United States. Lamaze has become one of the most familiar types of childbirth education.

Another prominent organization that provides educational resources and certification for educators is the International Childbirth Education Association (ICEA). Also formed in 1960, this organization does not advocate a particular method of childbirth preparation but rather promotes a philosophy of "freedom of choice based on knowledge of alternatives" (International Childbirth Education Association, 2000). Many expectant parents find this approach consistent with their own desires to experience birth as informed health care consumers. ICEA educators often teach a combination of techniques designed to meet individual needs.

Body-Conditioning Exercises

Some body-conditioning exercises, such as the pelvic tilt, pelvic rock, and Kegel exercises, are taught in childbirth preparation classes. Other exercises strengthen the abdominal muscles for the expulsive phase of labor. (See Chapter 8 for a description of recommended exercises.)

Relaxation Exercises

Relaxation during labor allows the woman to conserve energy and the uterine muscles to work more efficiently. Without practice it is difficult to relax the whole body in the midst of intense uterine contractions. Progressive relaxation exercises such as those taught to induce sleep can be helpful during labor. "Teaching About: Touch Relaxation" provides information on one approach, which is based on interaction between the woman and her partner.

Teaching About

TOUCH RELAXATION

Touch relaxation technique often combines patterned abdominal breathing with focused relaxation. It may be used to achieve relaxation of specific body parts or for general body relaxation.

Goals

The woman learns to release tension in the areas that her partner touches. The partner learns to watch his or her partner carefully and becomes attuned to tense, tightened muscles.

Technique

- The partner gently touches the woman's brow.
- The woman uses abdominal breathing. As she breathes in through her nose, her abdomen rises, and as she breathes out through her mouth, her abdomen falls. As each breath is released, she lets all tightness and tension flow out with the breath.
- The partner continues to lightly touch her brow until relaxation is felt. The partner may want to provide quiet encouragement such as, "You are doing fine, you are releasing the tension in your forehead." After at least five breaths, the partner may now touch the woman's shoulders and repeat the pattern described earlier.
- The partner moves on to the arms, chest, abdomen, thighs, and calves. The last aspect is to breathe in, let the whole body relax and go limp, and slowly release the breath. It will be helpful at the end of each labor contraction to let the body go limp and release all tension.
- As the couple practices, it is important for the woman to relax each part of her body. When she is in labor it will not be possible to go through the whole body; however, the woman can indicate what would be most helpful (e.g., touch her shoulder during each contraction). The partner can also be alert for signs of muscle tension and tightening. As the partner and woman practice touch relaxation, they may want to make the situation more realistic. They could decide that uterine contractions are occurring every 5 minutes and are lasting for 30 seconds. A clock will help the partner keep track of time. The partner can indicate that a contraction is beginning and suggest the woman begin her breathing. To help her focus, the partner may touch her shoulder or hand. In some instances, it is helpful for the partner to breathe along with the woman. Each couple can determine what works best for them.

An additional exercise specific to Lamaze is *disassociation relaxation*. The woman is taught to become familiar with the sensation of contracting and relaxing the voluntary muscle groups throughout her body. She then learns to contract a specific muscle group and relax the rest of her body. The exercise conditions the woman to relax uninvolved muscles while the uterus contracts, creating an active relaxation pattern.

The relaxation techniques described are most effective if the woman practices them daily both alone and with her support person. During a practice session, the partner begins by checking the woman's neck, shoulders, arms, and legs for relaxation. As tense areas are found, the helper encourages the woman to relax those body parts. By gentle touch and verbal cues the woman learns to respond to her own perceptions of tense muscles and also to the suggestion from others.

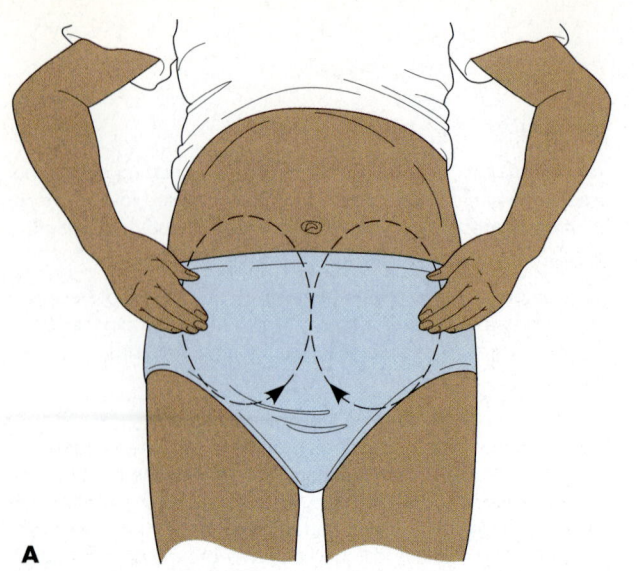
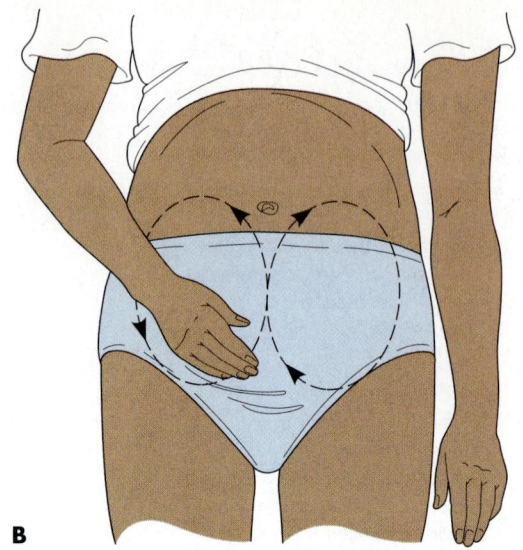

A

B

FIGURE 6–3. ◆ Effleurage is light stroking of the abdomen with the fingertips. **A,** Starting at the symphysis, the woman lightly moves her fingertips up and around in a circular pattern. **B,** An alternative approach involves using one hand in a figure-eight pattern. This light stroking can also be done by the support person.

Relaxation may also be promoted by cutaneous stimulation. One type commonly used prior to the transitional phase of labor is known as **abdominal effleurage** (Figure 6–3 ◆). This light abdominal stroking can relieve mild to moderate pain but not intense pain.

Breathing Techniques

Breathing techniques are a key element of most childbirth preparation programs. They help keep the mother and her unborn baby adequately oxygenated and help the mother relax and focus her attention appropriately. Breathing techniques are best taught during the final trimester of pregnancy. The nurse then supports the mother's use of breathing techniques during labor. Breathing techniques are described in Chapter 17. ⬭

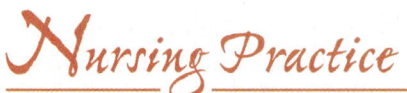

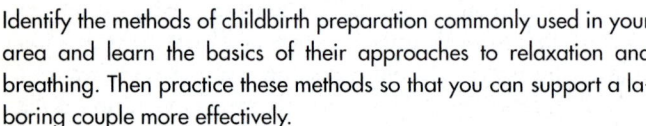

Identify the methods of childbirth preparation commonly used in your area and learn the basics of their approaches to relaxation and breathing. Then practice these methods so that you can support a laboring couple more effectively.

PREPARATION FOR CHILDBIRTH THAT SUPPORTS INDIVIDUALITY

Childbirth educators stress the value of individuality when providing information to expectant parents about childbirth. The goal is to encourage women to incorporate their own natural responses into coping with the pain of labor and birth. Self-care activities that may be used include vocalization or "sounding" to relieve tension in pregnancy and labor, massage (light touch) to facilitate relaxation, use of warm water for showers or bathing during labor, visualization (imagery), relaxing music, and subdued lighting.

Nurses need to encourage expectant mothers and couples to make the birth a personal experience. A woman might choose to bring items from home that help create a more personal birthing space. These items might include warm socks, extra pillows, bath powder, lotion, or a favorite blanket. She may wish to bring photos of special people or places. Many expectant parents enjoy listening to tapes of favorite music or watching favorite home videos. Such personalization of the birth experience may give expectant parents feelings of increased serenity and empowerment (England & Horowitz, 1998).

CHAPTER HIGHLIGHTS

🪶 Preconception counseling may help couples make decisions regarding childbearing.

🪶 Prenatal classes may be offered early and late in the pregnancy. Expectant parents tend to want information in chronological sequence with the pregnancy.

🪶 Pregnant adolescents have special learning needs related to pregnancy, the birthing process, and newborn care.

🪶 Siblings are often included in the birthing process, and special classes are available for them.

🪶 Information regarding cesarean birth is beneficial in prenatal classes.

🪶 Prenatal education programs vary in their goals, content, and method of teaching, but all seek to enhance knowledge and decrease anxiety.

🪶 Lamaze is a psychoprophylactic method of preparing for labor and birth. The classes include information on toning exercises, relaxation exercises and techniques, and breathing methods for labor.

🪶 Childbirth education groups, such as ICEA and ASPO, provide consumer health information and certification for teaching prenatal classes.

🪶 Childbirth classes must meet the individual needs of families and their members.

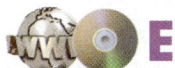 **EXPLORE**MediaLink

NCLEX Review, Case Studies, and other interactive resources for this chapter can be found on the companion website at http://www.prenhall.com/london. Click on "Chapter 6" to select the activities for this chapter.

For animations, more NCLEX review questions, and an audio glossary, access the accompanying CD-ROM in this textbook.

REFERENCES

American Academy of Pediatrics. (1999). Folic acid for the prevention of neural tube defects. *Pediatrics, 104*(2), 325–327.

Arizága, G. (1999). Curanderismo as holistic medicine. In G. Cajeta (Ed.), *A people's ecology: explorations in sustainable living,* (pp. 210–233). Santa Fe, NM: Clear Light Publishers.

Chapman, L. L. (2000). Expectant fathers and labor epidurals. *American Journal of Maternal-Child Nursing, 25*(3), 133–138.

England, P., & Horowitz, R. (1998). *Birthing from within.* Albuquesque, NM: Pantera Press.

Haire, D. (1999). The history of childbirth education. *International Journal of Childbirth Education, 14*(4), 26.

International Childbirth Education Association. (2000). ICEA philosophy statement. *International Journal of Childbirth Education, 15*(1).

Simkin, P. (1999). Labor support: Where has it been and where is it going? *International Journal of Childbirth Education, 14*(4), 22.

Wolcott, H. D., & Conry, J. A. (2000). Normal labor. In A. T. Evans & K. R. Niswander (Eds.), *Manual of obstetrics* (6th ed., pp. 392–424). Philadelphia: Lippincott, Williams & White.

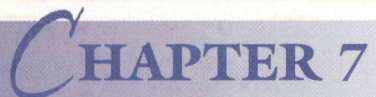

CHAPTER 7

Physical and Psychologic Changes of Pregnancy

Our son and his wife just told us they are pregnant. I am going to be a grandfather! I have tried to be a good father, to give my boy love, to teach him to respect others, to show him what it means to be a real man, someone a family can count on. Guess time will tell if the lessons took—I'm betting they have.

—PATRICK, 52

Key Terms

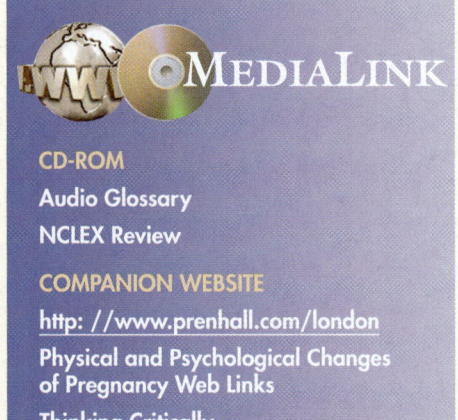

MediaLink

CD-ROM

Audio Glossary

NCLEX Review

COMPANION WEBSITE

http://www.prenhall.com/london

Physical and Psychological Changes of Pregnancy Web Links

Thinking Critically

NCLEX Review

Case Study

*P*regnancy is divided into three trimesters, each a 3-month period. Each trimester brings predictable changes for both the mother and fetus. How does pregnancy affect the woman physically and psychologically? How does it affect her family, including siblings, partners, and the grandparents, like Patrick? This chapter describes the physical and psychologic changes caused by pregnancy, and the responses of the entire family to pregnancy. It also presents the various cultural factors that can affect a pregnant woman's well-being. Subsequent chapters build on this information in describing effective approaches to planning and providing care.

ANATOMY AND PHYSIOLOGY OF PREGNANCY

Reproductive System

UTERUS

Before pregnancy, the uterus is a small, almost solid, pear-shaped organ measuring approximately 7.5 × 5 × 2.5 cm and weighing about 60 g (2 oz). At the end of pregnancy it measures about 28 × 24 × 21 cm and weighs approximately 1100 g; its capacity has also increased from about 10 mL to 5000 mL (5 L) or more (Cunningham, Gant, Leveno et al., 2001). The change is primarily due to the enlargement (hypertrophy) of the preexisting myometrial cells as a result of the stimulating influence of estrogen and the distention caused by the growing fetus. Only a limited increase in cell number (hyperplasia) occurs. The fibrous tissue between the muscle bands increases markedly, which adds to the strength and elasticity of the muscle wall. The enlarging uterus, developing placenta, and growing fetus require additional blood flow to the uterus. ⊂⊃ CD By the end of pregnancy, one sixth of the total maternal blood volume is contained within the vascular system of the uterus.

Braxton Hicks contractions, which are irregular, generally painless contractions of the uterus, occur intermittently throughout pregnancy. They may be felt through the abdominal wall beginning about the fourth month of pregnancy. In later months, these contractions become uncomfortable and may be confused with true labor contractions.

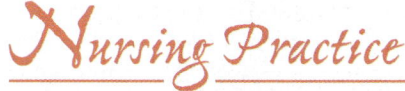

Nursing Practice

Beginning early in pregnancy, have the woman feel her uterus periodically so that she becomes familiar with the size and the way it feels. As her pregnancy progresses, she then will be more likely to identify Braxton Hicks contractions and preterm labor, if it occurs.

CERVIX

Estrogen stimulates the glandular tissue of the cervix, which increases in cell number and becomes hyperactive. The endocervical glands secrete a thick, sticky mucus that accumulates and forms the **mucus plug**, which seals the endocervical canal and prevents the ascent of organisms into the uterus. This mucus plug is expelled when cervical dilatation begins. The hyperactivity of the glandular tissue also increases the normal physiologic mucorrhea, at times resulting in profuse discharge. Increased cervical vascularity also causes both the softening of the cervix (**Goodell's sign**) and its bluish discoloration (**Chadwick's sign**).

OVARIES

The ovaries stop producing ova during pregnancy, but the corpus luteum continues to produce hormones until about weeks 6 to 8. The progesterone the corpus luteum secretes until about the seventh week of pregnancy maintains the endometrium until the placenta assumes the task. The corpus luteum then begins to regress and is almost completely obliterated by the middle of pregnancy.

VAGINA

Estrogen causes a thickening of the vaginal mucosa, a loosening of the connective tissue, and an increase in vaginal secretions. These secretions are thick, white, and acidic (pH 3.5 to 6.0). The acid pH helps prevent bacterial infection but favors the growth of yeast organisms. Thus the pregnant woman is more susceptible to monilial infection than usual.

The supportive connective tissue of the vagina loosens throughout pregnancy. By the end of pregnancy, the vagina and perineal body are sufficiently relaxed to permit passage of the infant. Because blood flow to the vagina is increased, the vagina may show the same blue-purple color (Chadwick's sign) as the cervix.

BREASTS

Estrogen and progesterone cause many changes in the mammary glands. The breasts enlarge and become more nodular as the glands increase in size and number in preparation for lactation. Superficial veins become more prominent, the nipples become more erectile, and the areolas darken. Montgomery's follicles (sebaceous glands) enlarge, and **striae** (reddish stretch marks that slowly turn silver after childbirth) may develop.

Colostrum, an antibody-rich yellow secretion, may leak or be expressed from the breasts during the last trimester. Colostrum gradually converts to mature milk during the first few days after childbirth.

Respiratory System

Many respiratory changes occur to meet the increased oxygen requirements of a pregnant woman. The volume of air breathed each minute increases 30% to 40%. In addition, progesterone decreases airway resistance, permitting a 15%

to 20% increase in oxygen consumption, as well as increases in carbon dioxide production and in the respiratory functional reserve.

As the uterus enlarges, it presses upward and elevates the diaphragm. The subcostal angle increases, so that the rib cage flares. The anteroposterior diameter increases, and the chest circumference expands by as much as 6 cm; as a result, there is no significant loss of intrathoracic volume. Breathing changes from abdominal to thoracic as pregnancy progresses, and descent of the diaphragm on inspiration becomes less possible. Some hyperventilation and difficulty in breathing may occur.

Nasal stuffiness and epistaxis (nosebleeds) may also occur because of estrogen-induced edema and vascular congestion of the nasal mucosa.

Cardiovascular System

Blood volume progressively increases beginning in the first trimester, increases rapidly in the second trimester, and slows in the third. It peaks near term, at about 40 to 45% above nonpregnant levels. This increase is due to increases in both erythrocytes and plasma.

During pregnancy, blood flow increases to organ systems with an increased workload. Thus, blood flow increases to the uterus and kidneys, while hepatic and cerebral flow remains unchanged. Cardiac output begins to increase early in pregnancy and remains elevated throughout gestation.

The pulse may increase by as many as 10 to 15 beats per minute at term. The blood pressure decreases slightly, reaching its lowest point during the second trimester. It gradually increases to near prepregnant levels by the end of the third trimester.

The enlarging uterus puts pressure on pelvic and femoral vessels, interfering with returning blood flow and causing stasis of blood in the lower extremities. This condition may lead to dependent edema and varicosity of the veins in the legs, vulva, and rectum (hemorrhoids) in late pregnancy. This increased blood volume in the lower legs may also make the pregnant woman prone to postural hypotension.

When the pregnant woman lies supine, the enlarging uterus may press on the vena cava, thus reducing blood flow to the right atrium, lowering blood pressure, and causing dizziness, pallor, and clamminess. The enlarging uterus may also press on the aorta and its collateral circulation (Cunningham et al., 2001). This condition is called **supine hypotensive syndrome.** It may also be referred to as **vena caval syndrome** or **aortocaval compression** (Figure 7–1◆). It can be corrected by having the woman lie on her side or by placing a pillow or wedge under her right hip.

The total erythrocyte (red blood cell) volume increases by about 30% in women who receive iron supplementation but only about 18% without iron supplementation. This increase in erythrocytes is necessary to transport the additional oxygen required during pregnancy. However, the increase in plasma volume during pregnancy averages about

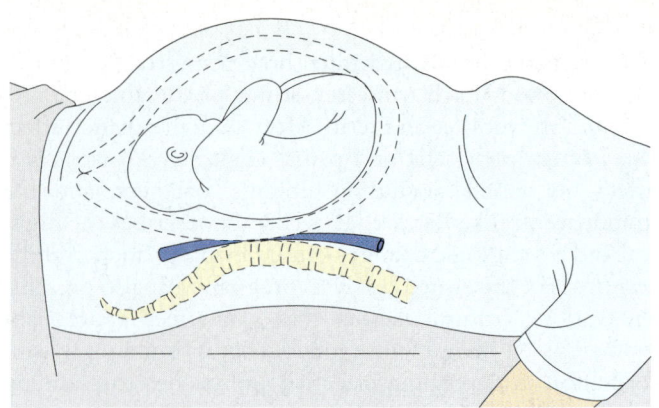

FIGURE 7–1. ◆ Vena caval syndrome. The gravid uterus compresses the vena cava when the woman is supine. This reduces the blood flow returning to the heart and may cause maternal hypotension.

50%. Because the plasma volume increase (50%) is greater than the erythrocyte increase (30%), the hematocrit, which measures the concentration of red blood cells in the plasma, decreases by an average of about 7% during pregnancy. This decrease is referred to as the **physiologic anemia of pregnancy** (pseudoanemia).

Iron is necessary for hemoglobin formation, and hemoglobin is the oxygen-carrying component of erythrocytes. Thus the increase in erythrocyte levels results in an increased need for iron by the pregnant woman. Even though the gastrointestinal absorption of iron is moderately increased during pregnancy, it is usually necessary to add supplemental iron to the diet to meet the expanded red blood cell and fetal needs.

Leukocyte production increases slightly to an average of 5,000 to 12,000/mm^3. During labor and early postpartum, these levels may reach 25,000/mm^3 or higher (Cunningham et al., 2001).

Both fibrin and plasma fibrinogen levels increase during pregnancy. Although the blood-clotting time of the pregnant woman does not differ significantly from that of the nonpregnant woman, clotting factors VII, VIII, IX, and X increase; thus pregnancy is a somewhat hypercoagulable state. These changes, coupled with venous stasis in late pregnancy, increase the pregnant woman's risk of developing venous thrombosis.

Gastrointestinal System

Nausea and vomiting are common during the first trimester because of elevated human chorionic gonadotropin levels and changed carbohydrate metabolism. Gum tissue may soften and bleed easily. The secretion of saliva may increase and even become excessive (ptyalism).

Elevated progesterone levels cause smooth muscle relaxation, resulting in delayed gastric emptying and decreased peristalsis. As a result, the pregnant woman may complain of bloating and constipation. These symptoms are aggravated as the enlarging uterus displaces the stomach upward and the intestines laterally and posteriorly. The cardiac sphincter also relaxes, and heartburn (pyrosis) may occur due to reflux of acidic secretions into the lower esophagus. Hemorrhoids frequently develop in late pregnancy from constipation and from pressure on vessels below the level of the uterus.

The emptying time of the gallbladder is prolonged during pregnancy as a result of smooth muscle relaxation from progesterone. This, coupled with the elevated levels of cholesterol in the bile, can predispose the woman to gallstone formation.

Urinary Tract

During the first trimester, the enlarging uterus is still a pelvic organ and presses against the bladder, producing urinary frequency. This symptom decreases during the second trimester, when the uterus becomes an abdominal organ and pressure against the bladder lessens. Frequency reappears during the third trimester, when the presenting part descends into the pelvis and again presses on the bladder, reducing bladder capacity, contributing to hyperemia, and irritating the bladder.

The ureters (especially the right ureter) elongate and dilate above the pelvic brim. The glomerular filtration rate rises by as much as 50% beginning in the second trimester and remains elevated until birth. To compensate for this increase, renal tubular reabsorption also increases. However, glycosuria is sometimes seen during pregnancy because of the kidneys' inability to reabsorb all the glucose filtered by the glomeruli. Glycosuria may be normal or may indicate gestational diabetes, so it always warrants further testing.

Skin and Hair

Changes in skin pigmentation commonly occur during pregnancy. They are thought to be stimulated by increased estrogen, progesterone, and α-melanocytic-stimulating hormone levels. Pigmentation of the skin increases primarily in areas that are already hyperpigmented: the areola, the nipples, the vulva, and the perianal area. The skin in the middle of the abdomen may develop a pigmented line, the **linea nigra,** which usually extends from the umbilicus or above to the pubic area (Figure 7–2◆). Facial **chloasma** or **melasma gravidarum** (also known as the "mask of pregnancy"), a darkening of the skin over the forehead and around the eyes, may develop. Melasma is more prominent in dark-haired women and is aggravated by exposure to the sun. Fortunately, it fades or becomes less prominent soon after childbirth when the hormonal influence of pregnancy subsides. In addition, the sweat and sebaceous glands are often hyperactive during pregnancy. Striae, or stretch marks, are reddish, wavy streaks that may appear on the abdomen, thighs, buttocks, and breasts. They result from reduced connective tissue strength due to elevated adrenal steroid levels.

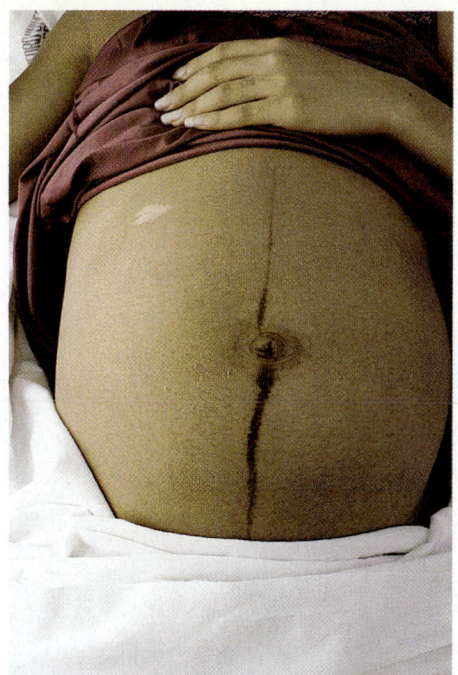

FIGURE 7–2. ◆ Linea nigra.

Vascular spider nevi, small, bright-red elevations of the skin radiating from a central body, may develop on the chest, neck, face, arms, and legs. They may be caused by increased subcutaneous blood flow in response to elevated estrogen levels.

The rate of hair growth may decrease during pregnancy; the number of hair follicles in the resting or dormant phase also decreases. After birth, the number of hair follicles in the resting phase increases sharply and the woman may notice increased hair shedding for 1 to 4 months. Practically all hair is replaced within 6 to 12 months, however (Cunningham et al., 2001).

Musculoskeletal System

No demonstrable changes occur in the teeth of pregnant women. The dental caries that sometimes accompany pregnancy are probably caused by inadequate oral hygiene and dental care, especially if the woman has problems with bleeding gums or nausea and vomiting.

The joints of the pelvis relax somewhat because of hormonal influences. The result is often a waddling gait. As the pregnant woman's center of gravity gradually changes, the lumbar spinal curve becomes accentuated, and her posture changes (Figure 7–3◆). This posture change compensates for the increased weight of the uterus anteriorly and frequently results in low backache.

Pressure of the enlarging uterus on the abdominal muscles may cause the rectus abdominis muscle to separate, producing **diastasis recti.** If the separation is severe and muscle tone is not regained postpartally, subsequent pregnancies will not have adequate support and the woman's abdomen may appear pendulous.

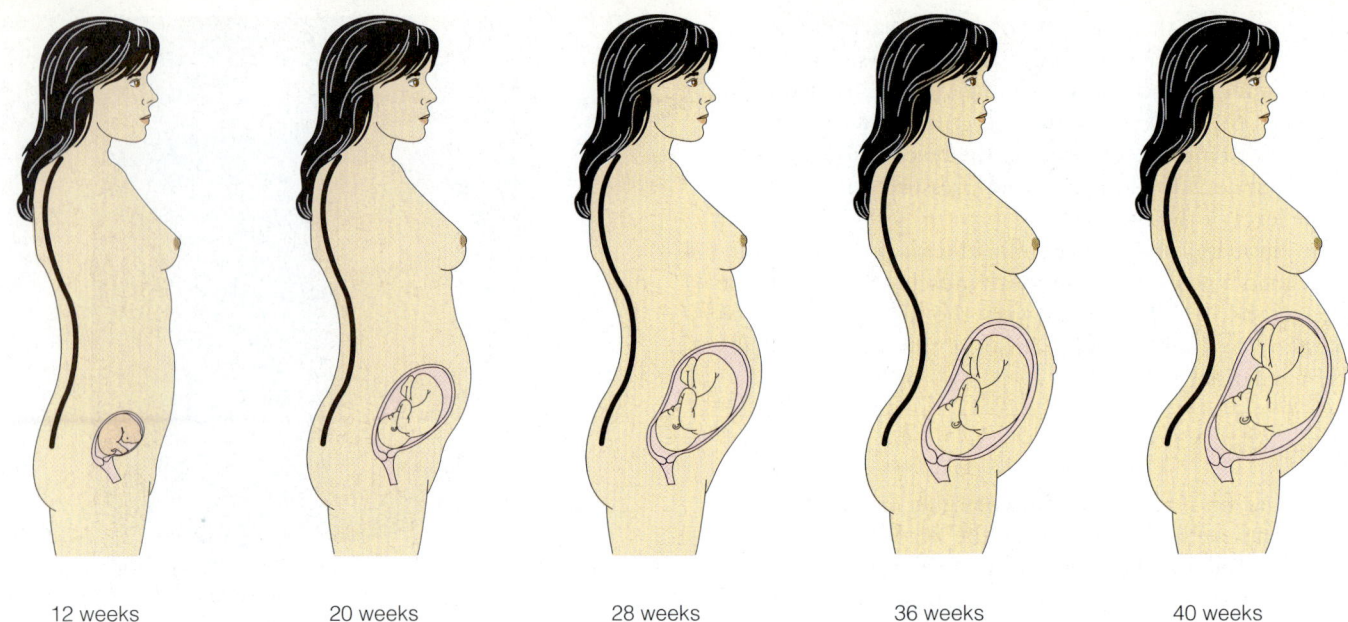

| 12 weeks | 20 weeks | 28 weeks | 36 weeks | 40 weeks |

FIGURE 7–3. ◆ Postural changes during pregnancy. Note the increasing lordosis of the lumbosacral spine and the increasing curvature of the thoracic area.

Metabolism

Most metabolic functions increase during pregnancy because of the increased demands of the growing fetus and its support system. For a detailed discussion of nutrient, vitamin, and mineral metabolism, see Chapter 11. ⬭

WEIGHT GAIN

The recommended weight gain for women of normal weight before pregnancy is 25 to 35 lb (11.4 to 15.9 kg); for women who were overweight, the recommended gain is 15 to 25 lb (6.8 to 11.4 kg). Underweight women are advised to gain the weight needed to reach their ideal weight plus 25 to 35 lb (11.4 to 15.9 kg) (Mattson & Smith, 2000). The average pattern of weight gain is 3.5 to 5 lb (1.6 to 2.3 kg) during the first trimester and 12 to 15 lb (5.5 to 6.8 kg) during each of the last two trimesters. Adequate nutrition and weight gain are important during pregnancy (see discussion in Chapter 11). ⬭

WATER METABOLISM

Increased water retention, a basic alteration of pregnancy, is caused by several interrelated factors. The increased level of steroid sex hormones affects sodium and fluid retention. The lowered serum protein also influences fluid balance, as do increased intracapillary pressure and permeability. The extra water is needed for the fetus, placenta, and amniotic fluid and the mother's increased blood volume, interstitial fluids, and enlarged organs.

NUTRIENT METABOLISM

The fetus makes its greatest protein and fat demands during the second half of pregnancy, doubling in weight during the last 6 to 8 weeks. Protein (contributing nitrogen) must be stored during pregnancy to maintain a constant level within the breast milk and to avoid depletion of maternal tissues. Carbohydrate needs also increase, especially during the second and third trimesters. Fats are more completely absorbed during pregnancy, and the level of free fatty acids increases in response to human placental lactogen. The levels of lipoproteins and cholesterol also increase. Because of these changes, increased levels of dietary fat or reduced carbohydrate production may lead to ketonuria in the pregnant woman.

Endocrine System

THYROID

The thyroid gland often enlarges slightly during pregnancy because of increased vascularity and hyperplasia of glandular tissue. Estrogen increases its capacity to bind thyroxine, resulting in an increase in serum protein-bound iodine. The basal metabolic rate increases by as much as 25% during pregnancy. However, within a few weeks after birth all thyroid function returns to normal limits.

PITUITARY

Pregnancy is made possible by the hypothalamic stimulation of the anterior pituitary gland, which in turn produces follicle-stimulating hormone (FSH), which stimulates ovum growth, and luteinizing hormone (LH), which brings about ovulation. Stimulation of the pituitary also prolongs the ovary's corpus luteal phase, which maintains the endometrium in case conception occurs. Prolactin, another anterior pituitary hormone, is responsible for initial lactation.

The posterior portion of the pituitary secretes vasopressin (antidiuretic hormone) and oxytocin. Vasopressin causes vasoconstriction, which results in increased blood pressure; it also helps regulate water balance. Oxytocin promotes uterine contractility and stimulates ejection of milk from the breasts (the letdown reflex) in the postpartum period.

ADRENALS

During pregnancy, circulating cortisol, which regulates carbohydrate and protein metabolism, increases in response to increased estrogen levels. Cortisol blood levels return to normal within 1 to 6 weeks postpartum. In addition, the adrenals secrete increased levels of aldosterone by the early part of the second trimester. This increase in aldosterone in a normal pregnancy may be the body's protective response to the increased sodium excretion associated with progesterone (Cunningham et al., 2001).

PANCREAS

The pregnant woman has increased insulin needs, and the pancreatic islets of Langerhans, which secrete insulin, are stressed to meet this increased demand. Any marginal pancreatic function quickly becomes apparent, and the woman may show signs of gestational diabetes.

HORMONES IN PREGNANCY

Human Chorionic Gonadotropin. The trophoblast secretes human chorionic gonadotropin (hCG) in early pregnancy. This hormone stimulates progesterone and estrogen production by the corpus luteum to maintain the pregnancy until the placenta is developed sufficiently to assume that function.

Human Placental Lactogen. Also called human chorionic somatomammotropin, human placental lactogen (hPL) is produced by the syncytiotrophoblast. Human placental lactogen is an antagonist of insulin; it increases the amount of circulating free fatty acids for maternal metabolic needs and decreases maternal metabolism of glucose to favor fetal growth.

Estrogen. Estrogen, secreted originally by the corpus luteum, is produced primarily by the placenta as early as the seventh week of pregnancy. Estrogen stimulates uterine development to provide a suitable environment for the fetus. It also helps develop the ductal system of the breasts in preparation for lactation.

Progesterone. Progesterone, also produced initially by the corpus luteum and then by the placenta, plays the greatest role in maintaining pregnancy. It maintains the endometrium and inhibits spontaneous uterine contractility, preventing early spontaneous abortion. Progesterone also helps develop the acini and lobules of the breasts in preparation for lactation.

Relaxin. Relaxin is detectable in the serum of a pregnant woman by the time of the first missed menstrual period. Relaxin inhibits uterine activity, diminishes the strength of uterine contractions, aids in the softening of the cervix, and has the long-term effect of remodeling collagen. Its primary source is the corpus luteum, but small amounts are believed to be produced by the placenta and uterine decidua.

PROSTAGLANDINS IN PREGNANCY

Prostaglandins are lipid substances that can arise from most body tissues but occur in high concentrations in the female reproductive tract and are present in the decidua during pregnancy. The exact functions of prostaglandins during pregnancy are still unknown, although it has been proposed that they are responsible for maintaining reduced placental vascular resistance. Decreased prostaglandin levels may contribute to preeclampsia-eclampsia. Prostaglandins are also believed to play a role in the complex biochemistry that initiates labor.

SIGNS OF PREGNANCY

Many of the changes women experience during pregnancy are used to diagnose the pregnancy itself. They are called the subjective, or presumptive, changes; the objective, or probable, changes; and the diagnostic, or positive, changes of pregnancy.

Subjective (Presumptive) Changes

The subjective changes of pregnancy are the symptoms the woman experiences and reports. Because they can be caused by other conditions, they cannot be considered proof of pregnancy (Table 7–1). The following subjective signs can be diagnostic clues when other signs and symptoms of pregnancy are also present.

Amenorrhea, or the absence of menses, is the earliest symptom of pregnancy. Missing more than one menstrual period, especially in a woman whose cycle is ordinarily regular, is an especially useful diagnostic clue.

Nausea and vomiting in pregnancy (NVP) occur frequently during the first trimester. Because these symptoms often occur in the early part of the day, they are commonly referred to as **morning sickness.** In reality, the symptoms may occur at any time and can range from a mere distaste for food to severe vomiting. Women who experience NVP tend to have a decreased incidence of spontaneous abortion and perinatal mortality.

Excessive fatigue may be noted within a few weeks after the first missed menstrual period and may persist throughout the first trimester.

Urinary frequency is experienced during the first trimester as the enlarging uterus presses on the bladder.

Changes in the breasts are frequently noted in early pregnancy. These changes include tenderness and tingling

TABLE 7–1 Differential Diagnosis of Pregnancy: Subjective Changes

Subjective Changes	Possible Alternative Causes
Amenorrhea	Endocrine factors; early menopause; lactation; thyroid, pituitary, adrenal, ovarian dysfunction
	Metabolic factors; malnutrition, anemia, climatic changes, diabetes mellitus, degenerative disorders, long-distance running
	Psychologic factors: emotional shock, fear of pregnancy or sexually transmitted infection, intense desire for pregnancy (pseudocyesis), stress
	Obliteration of endometrial cavity by infection or curettage
	Systemic disease (acute or chronic), such as tuberculosis or malignancy
Nausea and vomiting	Gastrointestinal disorders
	Acute infections such as encephalitis
	Emotional disorders such as pseudocyesis or anorexia nervosa
Urinary frequency	Urinary tract infection
	Cystocele
	Pelvic tumors
	Urethral diverticula
	Emotional tension
Breast tenderness	Premenstrual tension
	Chronic cystic mastitis
	Pseudocyesis
	Hyperestrinism
Quickening	Increased peristalsis
	Flatus ("gas")
	Abdominal muscle contractions
	Shifting of abdominal contents

TABLE 7–2 Differential Diagnosis of Pregnancy: Objective Changes

Objective Changes	Possible Alternative Causes
Changes in pelvic organs	Increased vascular congestion
Goodell's sign	Estrogen-progestin oral contraceptives
Chadwick's sign	Vulvar, vaginal, cervical hyperemia
Hegar's sign	Excessively soft walls of nonpregnant uterus
Uterine enlargement	Uterine tumors
Enlargement of abdomen	Obesity, ascites, pelvic tumors
Braxton Hicks contractions	Hematometra, pedunculated, submucous, and soft myomas
Uterine souffle	Large uterine myomas, large ovarian tumors, or any condition with greatly increased uterine blood flow
Pigmentation of skin	Estrogen-progestin oral contraceptives
Chloasma	Melanocyte hormonal stimulation
Linea nigra	
Nipples and areola	
Abdominal striae	Obesity, pelvic tumor
Ballottement	Uterine tumors or polyps, ascites
Pregnancy tests	Increased pituitary gonadotropins at menopause, choriocarcinoma, hydatidiform mole
Palpation for fetal outline	Uterine myomas

sensations, increased pigmentation of the areola and nipple, and changes in Montgomery's glands. The veins also become more visible and form a bluish pattern beneath the skin.

Quickening, or the mother's perception of fetal movement, occurs about 18 to 20 weeks after the last menstrual period in a woman pregnant for the first time but may occur as early as 16 weeks in a woman who has been pregnant before. Quickening is a fluttering sensation in the abdomen that gradually increases in intensity and frequency.

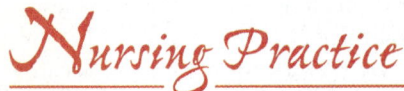

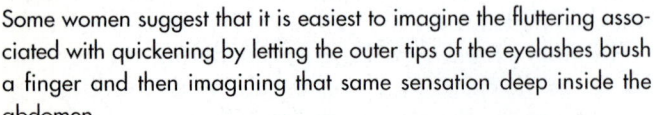

Some women suggest that it is easiest to imagine the fluttering associated with quickening by letting the outer tips of the eyelashes brush a finger and then imagining that same sensation deep inside the abdomen.

Objective (Probable) Changes

An examiner can perceive the objective changes that occur in pregnancy. Since these changes can also have other causes, they do not confirm pregnancy (Table 7–2).

Changes in the pelvic organs—the only physical changes detectable during the first 3 months of pregnancy—are caused by increased vascular congestion. These changes are noted on pelvic examination. There is a softening of the cervix called Goodell's sign. Chadwick's sign is a bluish, purple, or deep-red discoloration of the mucous membranes of the cervix, vagina, and vulva (some sources consider this a presumptive sign). **Hegar's sign** is a softening of the isthmus of the uterus, the area between the cervix and the body of the uterus (Figure 7–4◆). **McDonald's sign** is an ease in flexing the body of the uterus against the cervix.

General enlargement and softening of the body of the uterus can be noted after the eighth week of pregnancy. The fundus of the uterus is palpable just above the symphysis pubis at about 10 to 12 weeks' gestation and at the level of the umbilicus at 20 to 22 weeks' gestation (Figure 7–5◆).

Enlargement of the abdomen during the childbearing years is usually regarded as evidence of pregnancy, especially if it is continuous and accompanied by amenorrhea.

Braxton Hicks contractions can be palpated most commonly after the 28th week. As the woman approaches the end of pregnancy, these contractions may become uncomfortable. They are then often called *false labor.*

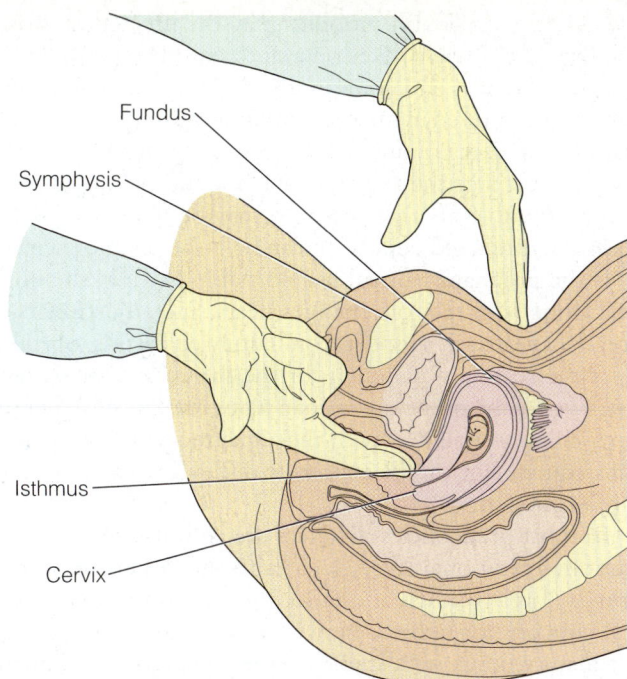

FIGURE 7–4. ◆ Hegar's sign, a softening of the isthmus of the uterus, can be determined by the examiner during a vaginal examination.

Fundus
Symphysis
Isthmus
Cervix

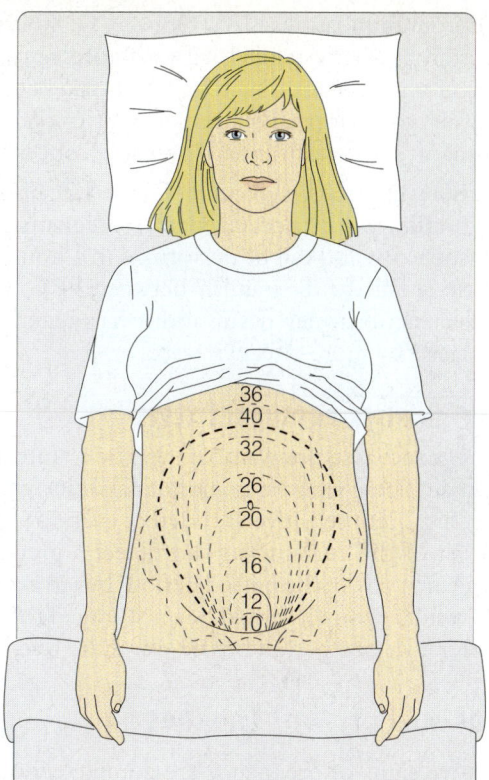

FIGURE 7–5. ◆ Approximate height of the fundus at various weeks of pregnancy.

Uterine souffle may be heard when the examiner auscultates the abdomen over the uterus. It is a soft, blowing sound that occurs at the same rate as the maternal pulse and is caused by the increased uterine blood flow and blood pulsating through the placenta. It is sometimes confused with the *funic souffle*, a soft, blowing sound of blood pulsating through the umbilical cord. The funic souffle occurs at the same rate as the fetal heart rate.

Changes in pigmentation of the skin are common in pregnancy. The nipples and areola may darken, and the linea nigra may develop. Facial *melasma* (chloasma) may become noticeable, and striae may appear.

The *fetal outline* may be identified by palpation in many pregnant women after 24 weeks' gestation. **Ballottement** is the passive fetal movement elicited when the examiner inserts two gloved fingers into the vagina and pushes against the cervix. This action pushes the fetal body up, and, as it falls back, the examiner feels a rebound.

Pregnancy tests detect the presence of hCG in the maternal blood or urine. These are not considered a positive sign of pregnancy because other conditions can cause elevated hCG levels.

CLINICAL PREGNANCY TESTS

A variety of assay techniques are available to detect hCG during early pregnancy.

- Hemagglutination-inhibition test (Pregnosticon R), an immunoassay, is based on the fact that no clumping of cells occurs when the urine of a pregnant woman is added to the hCG-sensitized red blood cells of sheep.

- Latex agglutination test (Gravindex and Pregnosticon Slide tests), also an immunoassay, is based on the fact that latex particle agglutination is inhibited in the presence of urine containing hCG.

The two tests just described are done on the first early morning urine specimen of the woman because it is adequately concentrated. The tests become positive within 10 to 14 days after the first missed period.

Several pregnancy tests are done on maternal serum, including the following:

- β-subunit radioimmunoassay (RIA) uses an antiserum with specificity for the β-subunit of hCG in maternal blood. This very accurate pregnancy test becomes positive a few days after presumed implantation, thereby permitting early diagnosis of pregnancy.

- Immunoradiometric assay (IRMA) (Neocept, Pregnosis) uses a radioactive antibody to identify the presence of hCG in the serum. This test can detect very low concentrations of hCG and requires only about 30 minutes to perform.

- Enzyme-linked immunosorbent assay (ELISA)(Model Sensichrome, Quest Confidot) does not use radioisotopes but a substance that results in a color change after binding. The test is sensitive, quick, and can detect hCG levels as early as 7 to 9 days after ovulation and conception, which is 5 days before the first missed period (Buster & Carson, 1996).

- Fluoroimmunoassay (FIA) (Opus hCG, Stratus hCG) uses an antibody tagged with a fluorescent label to detect serum hCG. The test, which takes about 2 to 3 hours to perform, is extremely sensitive and is used primarily to identify and follow hCG concentrations.
- Radioreceptor assay (Biocept-G) uses the principle of high-affinity receptors to detect pregnancy. It is a sensitive test and can be performed in 1 hour, but because it fails to distinguish between hCG and LH, cross reactions may occur and it has generally been replaced by more effective tests.

OVER-THE-COUNTER PREGNANCY TESTS

Home pregnancy tests are available over the counter at a reasonable cost. These enzyme immunoassay tests, performed on urine, are quite sensitive and detect even low levels of hCG. Most of the current kits can detect a pregnancy as early as the first day of the missed period, but to avoid false-negative results, women should be encouraged to wait 6 to 9 days after a missed period before using the test.

Diagnostic (Positive) Changes

The positive signs of pregnancy are completely objective, cannot be confused with a pathologic state, and offer conclusive proof of pregnancy.

The *fetal heartbeat* can be detected with an electronic Doppler device as early as weeks 10 to 12 of pregnancy.

Fetal movement is actively palpable by a trained examiner after about the 20th week of pregnancy.

Visualization of the fetus by ultrasound examination confirms a pregnancy. The gestational sac can be observed by 4 to 5 weeks' gestation (2 to 3 weeks after conception). Fetal parts and fetal movement can be seen as early as 8 weeks' gestation. Transvaginal ultrasound has been used to detect a gestational sac as early as 10 days after implantation (Cunningham et al., 2001).

PSYCHOLOGIC RESPONSE OF THE EXPECTANT FAMILY TO PREGNANCY

Pregnancy is a turning point in a family's life, and thus it is accompanied by stress and anxiety, whether the pregnancy is desired or not. For beginning families, pregnancy is the transition period from childlessness to parenthood. If the pregnancy results in the birth of a child, the couple enters a new, irreversible stage of their life together. **WEB**
The expectant couple may be unaware of the physical, emotional, and cognitive changes of pregnancy and may anticipate no problems from such a normal event. Thus they may be confused and distressed by new feelings and behaviors that are essentially normal.

If the expectant woman is married or has a stable partner, she no longer is only a mate but must also assume the role of mother. Her partner will experience a role change,

too. Career goals and mobility may be affected, and the couple's relationship takes on a different meaning to them and their families and community. Routines and family dynamics are altered with each pregnancy, requiring readjustment and realignment. As pregnancy progresses, the couple must face the anxieties of labor and birth and must also deal with fears that the baby may be ill or disfigured. Classes in prepared childbirth can help the couple prepare.

If the pregnant woman has no stable partner, she must deal alone with the role changes, fears, and adjustments of pregnancy or seek support from family or friends. She also faces the reality of planning for the future as a single parent. Even if the pregnant woman plans to relinquish her infant, she must still deal with the adjustments of pregnancy. This adjustment can be especially difficult without a good support system.

In most pregnancies, finances are an important consideration. Traditional lore relegates to the father the role of primary breadwinner, and indeed finances are often a very real concern for fathers. However, in today's society even pregnant women with stable partners recognize the financial impact of a child and may feel concern about financial issues. For the single mother, finances may be a major source of concern.

Decisions about financial matters need to be made at this time. Will the woman work during her pregnancy and return to work after her child is born? If so, who will provide child care? Couples may also need to decide about the division of domestic tasks. Any differences of opinion must be discussed openly and resolved so that the family can meet the needs of its members.

Pregnancy can be viewed as a developmental stage with its own distinct developmental tasks. For a couple, it can be a time of support or conflict, depending on the amount of adjustment each is willing to make to maintain the family's equilibrium. Most pregnant women turn to their partners as their primary source of social support. In particular, a woman needs support from her partner that affirms that she is valued and that her baby will be welcomed and accepted (Logsdon, 2000–2001).

During a first pregnancy, the couple plans together for the child's arrival, collecting information on how to be parents. At the same time, each continues to participate in some separate activities with friends or family members. The availability of a social support network is an important factor in psychosocial well-being during pregnancy. The social network is often a major source of advice for the pregnant woman. However, both sound and unsound information may be conveyed.

During pregnancy, the expectant mother and father both face significant changes and must deal with major psychosocial adjustments (Table 7–3). Other family members, especially other children of the woman or couple and the grandparents-to-be, must also adjust to the pregnancy.

For some, pregnancy is more than a developmental stage; it is a *crisis*. Crisis can be defined as a disturbance or conflict in which the individual cannot maintain a state of

TABLE 7–3 Parental Reactions to Pregnancy

First Trimester	Second Trimester	Third Trimester
MOTHER'S REACTIONS Informs father secretively or openly Feels ambivalent toward pregnancy, anxious about labor and responsibility of child Is aware of physical changes, daydreams of possible miscarriage Develops special feelings for and renewed interest in her own mother, with formation of a personal identity	**MOTHER'S REACTIONS** Remains regressive and introspective, projects all problems with authority figures onto partner, may become angry as if lack of interest is sign of weakness in him Continues to deal with feelings as a mother and looks for furniture as something concrete May have other extreme of anxiety and wait until ninth month to look for furniture and clothes for baby Feels movement and is aware of fetus and incorporates it into herself Dreams that partner will be killed, telephones him often for reassurance Experiences more distinct physical changes; sexual desires may increase or decrease	**MOTHER'S REACTIONS** Experiences more anxiety and tension, with physical awkwardness Feels much discomfort and insomnia from physical condition Prepares for birth, assembles layette, picks out names Dreams often about misplacing baby or not being able to give birth, fears birth of deformed baby Feels ecstasy and excitement, has spurt of energy during last month
FATHER'S REACTIONS Differ according to age, parity, desire for child, economic stability Acceptance of pregnant woman's attitude or complete rejection and lack of communication Is aware of his own sexual feelings, may develop more or less sexual arousal Accepts, rejects, or resents mother-in-law May develop new hobby outside of family as sign of stress	**FATHER'S REACTIONS** If he can cope, will give her extra attention she needs; if he cannot cope, will develop a new time-consuming interest outside of home May develop a creative feeling and a "closeness to nature" May become involved in pregnancy and buy or make furniture Feels for movement of baby, listens to heartbeat, or remains aloof, with no physical contact May have fears and fantasies about himself being pregnant, may become uneasy with this feminine aspect in himself May react negatively if partner is too demanding, may become jealous of physician and of physician's importance to partner and her pregnancy	**FATHER'S REACTIONS** Adapts to alternative methods of sexual contact Becomes concerned over financial responsibility May show new sense of tenderness and concern, treats partner like doll Daydreams about child as if older and not newborn, dreams of losing partner Renewed sexual attraction to partner Feels he is ultimately responsible for whatever happens

equilibrium. Pregnancy can be considered a *maturational crisis*, since it is a common event in the normal growth and development of the family. During such a crisis, the individual or family is in disequilibrium. Egos weaken, usual defense mechanisms are not effective, unresolved material from the past reappears, and relationships shift. If the crisis is not resolved, it will result in maladaptive behaviors in one or more family members and possible disintegration of the family. Families that are able to resolve a maturational crisis will return successfully to normal functioning and can even strengthen the bonds in the family relationship.

The Mother

Pregnancy alters body image and also necessitates a re-ordering of social relationships and changes in roles of family members. The way each woman meets the stresses of pregnancy is influenced by her emotional makeup, her sociologic and cultural background, and her acceptance or rejection of the pregnancy. However, many women manifest similar psychologic and emotional responses during pregnancy, including ambivalence, acceptance, introversion, mood swings, and changes in body image.

A woman's attitude toward her pregnancy can be a significant factor in its outcome. Even if the pregnancy is planned, there is an element of surprise at first. Many women commonly experience feelings of *ambivalence* during early pregnancy. This ambivalence may be related to feelings that the timing is somehow wrong; worries about the need to modify existing relationships or career plans; fears about assuming a new role; unresolved emotional conflicts with the woman's own mother; and fears about pregnancy, labor, and birth. These feelings may be more pronounced if the pregnancy is unplanned or unwanted. Indirect expressions of ambivalence include complaints about considerable physical discomfort, prolonged or frequent depression, significant dissatisfaction with changing body shape, excessive mood swings, and difficulty in accepting the life changes resulting from the pregnancy (Lederman, 1996).

Women who view their pregnancy as unwanted are more likely to delay prenatal care and to experience complications. The support and opinion of the woman's current partner, even if he is not the father of the child, has a major impact on pregnancy wantedness. Financial and emotional support from the partner are essential to the woman's positive attitude (Kroelinger & Oths, 2000). Involving the partner in the prenatal care may help promote a supportive attitude.

Conflicts about adapting to pregnancy are no more pronounced for older pregnant women (age 35 and over) than for younger ones. Moreover, older pregnant women tend to be less concerned about the normal physical changes of pregnancy and are confident about handling issues that arise during pregnancy and parenting. This difference may result because mature pregnant women have more experience with problem solving. However, mature pregnant women may have fewer pregnant peers and thus may have fewer people with whom to share concerns and expectations (Stark, 1997).

Pregnancy produces marked changes in a woman's body within a relatively short period of time. Pregnant women experience changes in body image because of physical alterations and may feel a loss of control over their bodies during pregnancy and later during childbirth. These perceptions are related to a certain extent to personality factors, social network responses, and attitudes toward pregnancy. Although changes in body image are normal, they can be very stressful for the woman. Explanation and discussion of the changes may help both the woman and her partner deal with the stress associated with this aspect of pregnancy.

Fantasies about the unborn child are common among pregnant women. However, the themes of the fantasies (baby's appearance, gender, traits, impact on parents, and so forth) vary by trimester and also differ between women pregnant for the first time and women who already have children (Sorenson & Schuelke, 1999).

FIRST TRIMESTER

During the first trimester, feelings of disbelief and ambivalence are paramount. The woman's baby does not seem real, and she focuses on herself and her pregnancy. She may experience one or more of the early symptoms of pregnancy, such as breast tenderness or morning sickness, which are unsettling and at times unpleasant.

During this time, the expectant mother begins to exhibit some characteristic behavioral changes. She may become increasingly introspective and passive. She may be emotionally labile, with characteristic mood swings from joy to despair. She may fantasize about a miscarriage and feel guilt because of these fantasies. She may worry that these thoughts will harm the baby in some way.

SECOND TRIMESTER

During the second trimester, quickening occurs. This perception of fetal movement helps the woman think of her baby as a separate person, and she generally becomes excited about the pregnancy even if earlier she was not. The woman becomes increasingly introspective as she evaluates her life, her plans, and her child's future. This introspection helps the woman prepare for her new mothering role. Emotional lability, which may be unsettling to her partner, persists. In some instances, the partner may react by withdrawing. This withdrawal is especially distressing to the woman, because she needs increased love and affection. Once the couple understands that these behaviors are characteristic of pregnancy, they are easier to accept; however, they may be sources of stress to some extent throughout pregnancy.

As pregnancy becomes more noticeable, the woman's body image changes. She may feel great pride, embarrassment, or concern. Generally women feel best during the second trimester, which is a relatively tranquil time.

THIRD TRIMESTER

In the third trimester, the woman feels pride about her pregnancy and anxiety about labor and birth. Physical discomforts increase, and the woman is eager for the pregnancy to end. She experiences increased fatigue, her body movements are awkward, and her interest in sexual activity may decrease. The woman tends to be concerned about the health and safety of her unborn child and may worry that she will not cope well during childbirth. Toward the end of this period, there is often a surge of energy as the woman prepares a "nest" for the infant. Many women report bursts of energy, during which they vigorously clean and organize their homes.

PSYCHOLOGICAL TASKS OF THE MOTHER

Rubin (1984) has identified four major tasks that the pregnant woman undertakes to maintain her intactness and that of her family and at the same time incorporate her new child into the family system. These tasks form the foundation for a mutually gratifying relationship with her infant.

1. *Ensuring safe passage through pregnancy, labor, and birth.* The pregnant woman feels concern for both her unborn child and herself. She looks for competent maternity care to provide a sense of control. She may seek information from literature, observation of other pregnant women and new mothers, and discussion with others. She often engages in self-care activities related to diet, exercise, alcohol consumption, and so forth. In the third trimester she becomes more aware of external threats in the environment—a toy on the stairs, the awkwardness of an escalator—that pose a threat to her well-being. Sleep becomes more difficult and she longs for birth even though it, too, is frightening.

2. *Seeking acceptance of this child by others.* The birth of a child alters a woman's primary support group (her family) and her secondary affiliative groups. The woman slowly and subtly alters her network to meet the needs of her pregnancy. In this adjustment the woman's partner is the most important figure. The partner's

support and acceptance help form a maternal identity. If there are other children in the home, the mother also works to ensure their acceptance of the coming child. The woman without a partner looks to others such as a family member or friend for this support.

3. *Seeking commitment and acceptance of herself as mother to the infant (binding-in).* During the first trimester the child remains a rather abstract concept. With quickening, however, the child begins to become a real person, and the mother begins to develop bonds of attachment. The mother experiences the movement of the child within her in an intimate, exclusive way, and out of this experience bonds of love form. The mother develops a fantasy image of her ideal child. This binding-in process, characterized by its strong emotional component, motivates the pregnant woman to become competent in her role and provides satisfaction for her in the role of mother (Mercer, 1995).

4. *Learning to give of oneself on behalf of one's child.* Childbirth involves many acts of giving. The man "gives" a child to the woman; she in turn "gives" a child to him. Life is given to an infant; a sibling is given to older children of the family. The woman begins to develop a capacity for self-denial and learns to delay immediate personal gratification to meet the needs of another. Baby showers and gifts are acts of giving that increase the mother's self-esteem and help her recognize the separateness and needs of the coming baby.

Accomplishment of these tasks helps the expectant woman develop her self-concept as mother. The expectant woman who was well nurtured by her own mother may view her mother as a role model and emulate her; the woman who views her mother as a "poor mother" may worry that she will make similar mistakes (Lederman, 1996). A woman's self-concept as a mother expands with actual experience and continues to grow through subsequent childbearing and child rearing.

The Father

For the expectant father, pregnancy is a psychologically stressful time because he, too, must make the transition from nonparent to parent or from parent of one or more to parent of two or more. Expectant fathers who have more self-actualizing behaviors, exercise regularly, use more stress management techniques, and have good interpersonal support tend to find pregnancy less stressful and feel more confident about parenting (Walker, Fleschler, & Heaman, 1998).

Initially, expectant fathers may feel pride in their virility, which pregnancy confirms, but also have many of the same ambivalent feelings expectant mothers have. The extent of ambivalence depends on many factors, including the father's relationship with his partner, his previous experience with pregnancy, his age, his economic stability, and whether the pregnancy was planned.

In adjusting to his role, the expectant father must first deal with the reality of the pregnancy and then gain recognition as a parent from his partner, family, friends, coworkers, and society—and from his baby as well. The expectant mother can help her partner adjust if she has a definite sense of the experience as their pregnancy and their infant and not her pregnancy and her infant.

The expectant father must establish a fatherhood role, just as the woman develops a motherhood role. Fathers who are most successful at this task generally like children, are excited about the prospect of fatherhood, are eager to nurture a child, and have confidence in their ability to be a parent. They also share the experiences of pregnancy and birth with their partners (Lederman, 1996). (See Table 7–3.)

FIRST TRIMESTER

After the initial excitement attending the announcement of the pregnancy, an expectant father may begin to feel left out. He may be confused by his partner's mood changes. He might resent the attention she receives and her need to modify their relationship as she experiences fatigue and possibly a decreased interest in sex. In addition, he might be concerned about what kind of father he will be. During this time, his child is a "potential" baby. Fathers often picture interacting with a child of 5 or 6 years, not a newborn. The pregnancy itself may seem unreal until the woman shows more physical signs.

SECOND TRIMESTER

The father's role in the pregnancy is still vague in the second trimester, but his involvement may increase as he watches and feels fetal movement and listens to the fetal heartbeat during a prenatal visit. Like expectant mothers, expectant fathers need to confront and resolve some of their conflicts about the parenting they received. A father needs to sort out which behaviors of his own father he wants to imitate and which he wants to avoid.

Evidence suggests that the father-to-be's anxiety is lessened if both parents agree on the paternal role the man is to assume. For example, if both see his role as that of breadwinner, the man's stress is low. However, if the man views his role as that of breadwinner and the woman expects him to be actively involved in child care, his stress increases. Thus the ability of the couple to negotiate a mutually agreeable role for the man may provide a significant coping mechanism for expectant fathers (Diemer, 1997).

As the woman's appearance begins to change, her partner may have several reactions. Her appearance may decrease his sexual interest, or it may have the opposite effect. Because of the variety of emotions both partners may feel, communication and acceptance remain important.

THIRD TRIMESTER

If the couple's relationship has grown through effective communication of their concerns and feelings, the third trimester is often a rewarding time. They may attend childbirth classes and make concrete preparations for the arrival of the baby. If the father has developed a detached attitude about the pregnancy, however, it is unlikely he will become a willing participant, even though his role becomes more obvious.

Concerns and fears may recur. The father may worry about hurting the unborn baby during intercourse or become concerned about labor and birth. Also, he may wonder what kind of parents he and his partner will be.

COUVADE

Couvade has traditionally referred to the observance of certain rituals and taboos by the male to signify the transition to fatherhood. This observance affirms his psychosocial and biophysical relationship to the woman and child. More recently, the term has been used to describe the unintentional development of physical symptoms such as fatigue, increased appetite, difficulty sleeping, depression, headache, or backache by the partner of a pregnant woman. Men who demonstrate couvade syndrome may tend to have a higher degree of paternal role preparation and be involved in more activities related to this preparation.

Siblings

Bringing a new baby home often marks the beginning of sibling rivalry. The siblings view the baby as a threat to the security of their relationships with their parents. Parents who recognize this potential problem early in pregnancy and begin constructive actions can minimize the problem of sibling rivalry.

Preparation of the young child begins several weeks before the anticipated birth. Because they do not have a clear concept of time, young children should not be told too early about the pregnancy. From the toddler's point of view, several weeks is an extremely long time. The mother may let the child feel the baby moving in her uterus, explaining that the uterus is "a special place where babies grow." The child can help the parents put the baby clothes in drawers or prepare the baby's room.

Consistency is important in dealing with young children. They need reassurance that certain people, special things, and familiar places will continue to exist after the new baby arrives. The crib is often an important though transient object in a child's life. If it is to be given to the new baby, the parents should thoughtfully help the older child adjust to this change. Any move from crib to bed or from one room to another should precede the baby's birth by several weeks or more. If the new baby will share a room with siblings, the parents must also discuss this situation with the older child or children.

If the child is ready, toilet training is most effective several months before or after the baby's arrival. It is not unusual for an older, toilet-trained child to regress to wetting or soiling because of the attention the newborn gets for such behavior. The older, weaned child may want to nurse or drink from the bottle again after the baby arrives. If the

new mother anticipates these behaviors, they will be less frustrating during her early postpartum days.

Pregnant women may find it helpful to bring their children on a prenatal visit to the certified nurse-midwife or physician to give them an opportunity to listen to the fetal heartbeat. Such a visit helps make the baby seem more real to the children.

If siblings are school-age children, pregnancy should be viewed as a family affair. Teaching should be suitable to the child's level of understanding and may be supplemented with appropriate books. Taking part in family discussions, attending sibling preparation classes, feeling fetal movement, and listening to the fetal heartbeat help the school-age child take part in the experience of pregnancy and not feel like an outsider.

Older children or adolescents may appear to have sophisticated knowledge but may have many misconceptions about pregnancy and birth. The parents should make opportunities to discuss their concerns and involve the children in preparations for the new baby.

Even after birth, siblings need to feel that they are taking part. Having siblings visit their mother and the new baby at the hospital or birthing center will help. After the baby comes home, siblings can share in "showing off" the new baby.

Sibling preparation is essential, but other factors are equally important. These factors include how much parental attention the new arrival receives, how much attention the older child receives after the baby comes home, and how well the parents handle regressive or aggressive behavior.

Grandparents

The first relatives told about a pregnancy are usually the grandparents. Often, the expectant grandparents become increasingly supportive of the couple, even if conflicts previously existed. But it can be difficult for even sensitive grandparents to know how deeply to become involved in the childrearing process.

Because grandparenting can occur over a wide expanse of years, people's response to this role can vary considerably. Younger grandparents leading active lives may not demonstrate as much interest as the young couple would like. In other cases, expectant grandparents may give advice and gifts unsparingly. For grandparents, conflict may be related to the expectant couple's need to feel in control of their lives, or it may stem from events signaling changing roles in the grandparents' own lives (e.g., retirement, financial concerns, menopause, or death of a friend). Some parents of expectant couples may already be grandparents with a developed style of grandparenting. This influences their response to the pregnancy.

Because childbearing and childrearing practices have changed, family cohesiveness is promoted by effective communication and frank discussion between young couples and interested grandparents about the changes and the reasons for them. Classes for grandparents may provide information about changes in birth and parenting practices. These classes help familiarize grandparents with new parents' needs and may offer suggestions for ways in which the grandparents can support the childbearing couple.

CULTURAL VALUES AND REPRODUCTIVE BEHAVIOR

Cultures have a universal tendency to create ceremonial rituals or rites around important life events. The rituals and customs of a group are a reflection of the group's values. Thus the identification of cultural values is useful in predicting reactions to pregnancy. An understanding of male and female roles, family lifestyles, religious values, or the meaning of children in a culture may explain reactions of joy or shame.

Health values and beliefs are also important in understanding reactions and behavior. Certain behaviors can be expected if a culture views pregnancy as a sickness, whereas other behaviors can be expected if the culture views pregnancy as a natural occurrence. Prenatal care may not be a priority for women who view pregnancy as a natural phenomenon or for women challenged by financial constraints.

Generalization about cultural characteristics or values is difficult because not every individual in a culture may display these characteristics. Just as variations are seen between cultures, variations are also seen within cultures. For example, because of their exposure to the American culture, a third-generation Cambodian-American family might have very different values and beliefs from those of a Cambodian family that has recently immigrated to America. For this reason, the nurse needs to supplement a general knowledge of cultural values and practices with a complete assessment of the individual's values and practices.

The meaning assigned to childbearing may vary from culture to culture. For example, most Native-American groups generally view pregnancy as a natural condition, and children are desired. In some cultures, a woman who gives birth, especially to a son, achieves higher status. This is true in traditional Chinese families, for example. Similarly, in the western United States, people of the Mormon faith view motherhood as the most important aspect of a woman's life, comparable to the male role of priesthood. In traditional Mexican-American families, having children may be seen as proving the male's manliness, or machismo, a desired trait among many Mexican-American men.

Health Beliefs

Although many cultures view pregnancy as a natural occurrence, it may also be seen as a time of increased vulnerability. In Orthodox Judaism, for example, it is a man's responsibility to procreate, but it is a woman's right, not her obligation, to do so. This is because, according to Orthodox Jewish law, the health of the mother, both physically and mentally, is of primary concern, and she should never be obliged to do something that threatens her life (Bodo & Gibson, 1999a).

Individuals of many cultures take certain protective precautions based on their beliefs. In Mexican-American culture, the concept of *mal aire*, or bad air, is sometimes related to evil spirits. It is thought that air, especially night air, may enter the body and cause harm. For many Vietnamese women, lifting the arms above the head is believed to increase the risk of preterm birth. Vietnamese women also are discouraged from sitting or lying down for lengthy periods because doing so might permit the baby to become too large (Bodo & Gibson, 1999b).

Most taboos stemming from the belief in evil spirits are grounded in fear of injuring the unborn child. Taboos also arise from the belief that a pregnant woman has evil powers. As a result, pregnant women are sometimes prohibited from taking part in certain community activities.

The equilibrium model of health is based on the concept of balance between light and dark, heat and cold. Some Eastern philosophies focus on the notion of *yin* and *yang*. Yin represents the female, passive principle—darkness, cold, and wetness—whereas yang is the masculine, active principle—light, heat, and dryness. When the two are combined, they are all that can be. The hot-cold classification is seen in cultures in Latin America, the Near East, and Asia.

Mexican Americans may consider illness to be an excess of either hot or cold. To restore health, imbalances are often corrected by the proper use of foods, medications, or herbs also classified as hot or cold. For example, an illness attributed to an excess of cold will be treated with hot foods or medications. The classification of foods is not always consistent, but it conforms to a general structure of traditional knowledge. Certain foods, spices, herbs, and medications are perceived to cool or heat the body. These perceptions do not necessarily correspond to the actual temperature; some hot dishes are said to have a cooling quality.

Complementary Care

HERBS DURING PREGNANCY

Pharmaceutical companies continue to refuse to include children and babies in their studies of drug safety, claiming excessive costs and other research problems. As a result, very few over-the-counter or prescription drugs can claim to be safe for pregnant women and nursing mothers. The same can be said for herbal medicines. Although herbs have been researched extensively in Europe and Asia, there has been little clinical research done in the United States on the use of herbs in pregnancy. Every pregnant or nursing woman must be extremely cautious about everything she ingests—foods, liquids, medications, and herbs. If a problem warrants intervention, she and her primary health care provider should discuss the benefits and risks of all treatments, synthetic and natural.

More information regarding the use of herbs in pregnancy can be found in Chapter 9.

Southeast Asians believe it is important to keep the woman "warm" after birth, because blood, which is considered "hot," has been lost, and the woman is at risk of becoming "cold." Therefore, they avoid cold drinks and foods following birth (Mattson, 1995). In contrast, many women in India consider pregnancy a "hot" period and eat "cool" foods to balance the hot state (Choudhry, 1997).

Health Practices

Health care practices during pregnancy are influenced by numerous factors, such as the prevalence of traditional home remedies and folk beliefs, the importance of indigenous healers, and the influence of professional health care workers. In an urban setting, the age, length of time in the city, marital status, and strength of the family may affect these patterns. Socioeconomic status is also important, since modern medical services are more accessible to those who can afford them.

An awareness of alternative health sources is crucial for health professionals, since these practices affect health outcomes. For example, in traditional Mexican-American culture, mothers are often influenced by *familism*, a close-knit, interdependent network of nuclear and extended family members who are connected for the good of the family. Familism is also reflected in a high regard for parental roles, and young mothers seek and follow the advice of their mothers or older women in the childbearing period (Lederman & Miller, 1998).

Indigenous healers are also important to specific cultures. In the Mexican-American culture, the healer is called a *curandero* or *curandera* (see Developing Cultural Competence on page 136). In some Native-American tribes, the medicine man or woman may fulfill the healing role. Herbalists are often found in Asian cultures, and faith healers, root doctors, and spiritualists are sometimes consulted by members of some African cultures.

Cultural Factors and Nursing Care

Health care providers are often unaware of the cultural characteristics they themselves demonstrate. Without cultural awareness, caregivers tend to project their own cultural responses onto foreign-born clients; clients from different socioeconomic, religious, or educational groups; or clients from different regions of the country. This projection leads caregivers to assume that the clients are demonstrating a specific behavior for the same reason that they themselves would. Moreover, health care providers often fail to realize that medicine has its own culture, which has been dominated historically by traditional middle-class values and beliefs (American College of Obstetricians and Gynecologists, 1998).

Ethnocentrism is the conviction that the values and beliefs of one's own cultural group are the best or only acceptable ones. It is characterized by an inability to understand the beliefs and worldview of another culture. To a certain extent, all of us are guilty of ethnocentrism, at least some of the time. Thus the nurse who values stoicism during labor may be uncomfortable with the more vocal response of some Latin American women. Another nurse may be disconcerted by a Southeast Asian woman who believes that pain is something to be endured rather than alleviated and who is intent on maintaining self-control in labor (Mattson, 1995).

Health care providers sometimes believe that if members of other cultures do not share Western values and beliefs, they should adopt them. For example, a nurse who believes strongly in equality of the sexes may find it difficult to remain silent if a woman from a Middle Eastern culture defers to her husband in decision making. It is important to remember that pressure to defy cultural values and beliefs can be stressful and anxiety provoking for women.

To address issues of cultural diversity in the provision of health care, emphasis is being placed on developing cultural competence—that is, the skills and knowledge necessary to appreciate, respect, and work with individuals from different cultures. Cultural competence requires self-awareness, awareness and understanding of cultural differences, and the ability to adapt clinical skills and practices as needed (Beckman & Dysart, 2000). It begins with the recognition that culture is the essence of a person's being; that it is more than ethnic, racial, or linguistic differences; and that many kinds of "cultures" exist. These other cultures—for example, women who have been abused, women who have experienced perinatal loss, or women who have undergone ritual circumcision—may be less visible, but they reflect significant life experiences and shape people's responses to experiences (Callister, 2001).

Cultural assessment is an important aspect of prenatal care. The nurse needs to identify the prospective parents' main beliefs, values, and behaviors about pregnancy and childbearing. This includes information about ethnic background, amount of affiliation with the ethnic group, patterns of decision making, religious preference, language, communication style, and common etiquette practices.

In planning care, the nurse considers the extent to which the woman's personal values, beliefs, and customs are in accord with the values, beliefs, and customs of the woman's identified cultural group, the nurse providing care, and the health care agency. If discrepancies exist, the nurse then considers whether the woman's system is supportive, neutral, or harmful in relation to possible interventions. If the woman's system is supportive or neutral, it should be incorporated into the plan. For example, individual food practices or methods of pain expression may differ from those of the nurse or agency but would not necessarily pose a risk to the woman. On the other hand, certain cultural practices might pose a threat to her health. For example, some Filipinas will not take any medication during pregnancy. The health care provider may consider a certain medication essential to the woman's well-being. In this case, the woman's cultural belief may be detrimental to her own health. The nurse and client must carefully discuss the reasons for her refusal. After discussing and understanding the reasons, the nurse faces three possible outcomes: (1) identifying ways to persuade the woman to accept the proposed medication, (2) accepting the woman's decision to refuse the medication, or (3) explaining alter-

nate therapies that might be acceptable to the woman in light of her cultural beliefs.

"Developing Cultural Competence: Providing Effective Prenatal Care to Families of Different Cultures" summarizes the key actions a nurse can take to become more culturally aware.

Developing Cultural Competence

Nurses who are interacting with expectant families from a different culture or ethnic group can provide more effective, culturally sensitive nursing care by

- Critically examining their own cultural beliefs
- Identifying personal biases, attitudes, stereotypes, and prejudices
- Making a conscious commitment to respect the values and beliefs of others
- Using sensitive, current language when describing others' cultures
- Learning the rituals, customs, and practices of the major cultural and ethnic groups with whom they have contact
- Including cultural assessment and assessment of the family's expectations of the health care system as a routine part of prenatal nursing care

- Incorporating the family's cultural practices into prenatal care as much as possible
- Fostering an attitude of respect for and cooperation with alternative healers and caregivers whenever possible
- Providing for the services of an interpreter if language barriers exist
- Learning the language (or at least several key phrases) of at least one of the cultural groups with whom they interact
- Recognizing that ultimately it is the woman's right to make her own health care choices
- Evaluating whether the client's health care beliefs have any potential negative consequences for her health

CHAPTER HIGHLIGHTS

🕊 Virtually all systems of a woman's body are altered in some way during pregnancy.

🕊 Blood pressure decreases slightly during pregnancy. It reaches its lowest point in the second trimester and gradually increases to near normal levels in the third trimester.

🕊 The enlarging uterus may cause pressure on the vena cava when the woman lies supine, causing supine hypotensive syndrome.

🕊 A physiologic anemia may occur during pregnancy because the total plasma volume increases more than the total number of erythrocytes. This difference produces a drop in the hematocrit.

🕊 The glomerular filtration rate increases somewhat during pregnancy. Glycosuria may be caused by the body's inability to reabsorb all the glucose filtered by the glomeruli.

🕊 Changes in the skin include the development of chloasma; linea nigra; darkened nipples, areola, and vulva; striae; and spider nevi.

🕊 Insulin needs increase during pregnancy. A woman with a latent deficiency state may respond to the increased stress on the islets of Langerhans by developing gestational diabetes.

🕊 The subjective (presumptive) signs of pregnancy are symptoms experienced and reported by the woman, such as amenorrhea, nausea and vomiting, fatigue, urinary frequency, breast changes, and quickening.

🕊 The objective (probable) signs of pregnancy can be perceived by the examiner but may be caused by conditions other than pregnancy.

🕊 The diagnostic (positive) signs of pregnancy can be perceived by the examiner and can be caused only by pregnancy.

🕊 During pregnancy, the expectant mother may experience ambivalence, acceptance, introversion, emotional lability, and changes in body image.

🕊 Rubin (1984) has identified four developmental tasks for the pregnant woman: (1) ensuring safe passage through pregnancy, labor, and birth; (2) seeking acceptance of this child by others; (3) seeking commitment and acceptance of herself as mother to the infant; and (4) learning to give of herself on behalf of her child.

🕊 The father faces a series of adjustments as he accepts his new role. The father must deal with the reality of pregnancy, gain recognition as a parent, and confront and resolve any personal conflicts about the fathering he himself received.

🕊 Siblings of all ages require assistance in dealing with the birth of a new baby.

🕊 Cultural values, beliefs, and behaviors influence a family's response to childbearing and the health care system.

🕊 Ethnocentrism is the belief that one's own cultural beliefs, values, and practices are the best ones—indeed, the only ones worth considering. To combat ethnocentrism, health care providers need to develop cultural competency.

🕊 A cultural assessment does not have to be exhaustive, but it should focus on factors that will influence the practices of the childbearing family with regard to health needs.

EXPLORE MediaLink

NCLEX Review, Case Studies, and other interactive resources for this chapter can be found on the companion website at http://www.prenhall.com/london. Click on "Chapter 7" to select the activities for this chapter.

For animations, more NCLEX review questions, and an audio glossary, access the accompanying CD-ROM in this textbook.

REFERENCES

American College of Obstetricians and Gynecologists. (1998). *Cultural competency in health care* (Opinion No. 201). Washington, DC: Author.

Beckman, C. R. B., & Dysart, D. (2000). The challenge of multicultural medical care. *Contemporary OB/GYN, 45*(12), 12–33.

Bodo, K., & Gibson, N. (1999a). Childbirth customs in Orthodox Jewish traditions. *Canadian Family Physician, 45,* 682–686.

Bodo, K., & Gibson, N. (1999b). Childbirth customs in Vietnamese traditions. *Canadian Family Physician, 45,* 690–697.

Buster, J. E., & Carson, S. A. (1996). Endocrinology and diagnosis of pregnancy. In S. G. Gabbe, J. R. Niebyl, & J. L. Simpson (Eds.), *Obstetrics: Normal and problem pregnancies* (3rd ed.). New York: Churchill-Livingstone.

Callister, L. C. (2001). Culturally competent care of women and newborns: Knowledge, attitude, and skills. *Journal of Obstetric, Gynecologic, and Neonatal Nursing, 30*(2), 209–215.

Choudhry, U. K. (1997). Traditional practices of women from India: Pregnancy, childbirth, and newborn care. *Journal of Obstetric, Gynecologic, and Neonatal Nursing, 26*(5), 533–539.

Cruikshank, D. P., Wigton, T. R., & Hays, P. M. (1996). Maternal physiology in pregnancy. In S. G. Gabbe, J. R. Niebyl, & J. L. Simpson (Eds.), *Obstetrics: Normal and problem pregnancies* (3rd ed.). New York: Churchill-Livingstone.

Cunningham, F. G., Gant, N. F., Leveno, K. J., Gilstrap, L. C., III, Hauth, J. C., & Wenstrom, K. D. (2001). *Williams obstetrics* (21st ed.). New York: McGraw-Hill.

Diemer, G. A. (1997). Expectant fathers: Influence of perinatal education on stress, coping, and spousal relations. *Research in Nursing and Health, 20*(4), 281–293.

Kroelinger, C. D., & Oths, K. S. (2000). Partner support and pregnancy wantedness. *Birth, 27*(2), 112–119.

Lederman, R. P. (1996). *Psychosocial adaptation in pregnancy* (2nd ed.). New York: Springer.

Lederman, R., & Miller, D. S. (1998). Adaptations to pregnancy in three different ethnic groups: Latin-American, African-American, and Anglo-American. *Canadian Journal of Nursing Research, 30*(3), 37–51.

Logsdon, M. C. (2000–2001). Helping hands: Exploring the cultural implications of social support during pregnancy. *AWHONN Lifelines, 4*(6), 29–32.

Mattson, S. (1995). Culturally sensitive perinatal care for Southeast Asians. *Journal of Obstetric, Gynecologic, and Neonatal Nursing, 24*(4), 335–341.

Mattson, S., & Smith, J. E. (2000). *Core curriculum for maternal-newborn nursing* (2nd ed.). Philadelphia: Saunders.

Mercer, R. T. (1995). *Becoming a mother.* New York: Springer.

Rubin, R. (1984). *Maternal identity and the maternal experience.* New York: Springer.

Sorenson, D. S., & Schuelke, P. (1999). Fantasies of the unborn among pregnant women. *Maternal-Child Nursing, 24*(2), 92–97.

Stark, M. A. (1997). Psychosocial adjustment during pregnancy: The experience of mature gravidas. *Journal of Obstetric, Gynecologic, and Neonatal Nursing, 26*(2), 206–211.

Walker, L. O., Fleschler, R. G., & Heaman, M. (1998). Is a healthy lifestyle related to stress, parenting confidence, and health symptoms among new fathers? *Canadian Journal of Nursing Research, 30*(3), 21–36.

CHAPTER 8

Antepartal Nursing Assessment

I'm 16—just got my license—so it was weird telling my friends that my mom is pregnant. I was embarrassed (and a little jealous) at first but now I kind of like the idea of having a baby sister. Mom had an amniocentesis because she is 37, so we know it's a girl. My mom has been great about including me and telling me what is going on. I've gone to a couple of her prenatal appointments so I got to hear the heartbeat and I saw the baby moving on ultrasound. I'm surprised by how interesting I am finding everything. Don't laugh, but I think I might like to be a nurse-midwife someday.

—KRISTA, 16

Key Terms

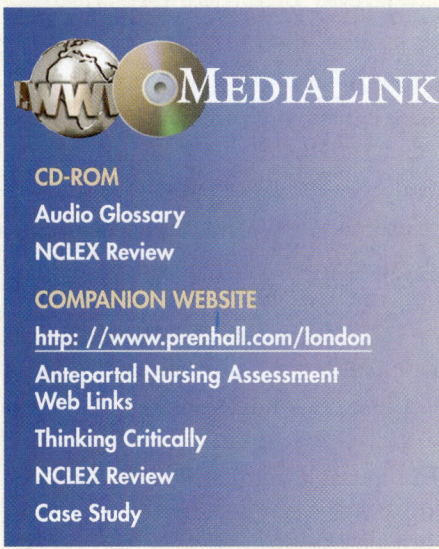

MediaLink

CD-ROM
Audio Glossary
NCLEX Review

COMPANION WEBSITE
http://www.prenhall.com/london
Anteparial Nursing Assessment
Web Links
Thinking Critically
NCLEX Review
Case Study

*H*ow can the registered nurse (RN) caring for a pregnant woman establish an environment of comfort and open communication with each antepartal visit? Including the family in the prenatal visits, such as inviting Krista to listen to the fetal heartbeat, is one way. The RN may complete many areas of prenatal assessment. Advanced practice nurses such as certified nurse-midwives (CNMs) are able to perform complete antepartal assessments. This chapter focuses on the prenatal assessments completed initially and at subsequent visits to provide optimum care for the childbearing family.

INITIAL CLIENT HISTORY

The course of a pregnancy depends on a number of factors, including the woman's prepregnancy health, presence of disease states, emotional status, and past health care. A thorough history helps determine the status of a woman's prepregnancy health.

Definition of Terms

The following terms are used in recording the history of maternity clients:

Gestation: the number of weeks since the first day of the last menstrual period.

Abortion: birth that occurs before the end of 20 weeks' gestation.

Term: the normal duration of pregnancy (38 to 42 weeks' gestation).

Antepartum: time between conception and the onset of labor; usually used to describe the period during which a woman is pregnant; used interchangeably with *prenatal*.

Intrapartum: time from the onset of true labor until the birth of the infant and placenta.

Postpartum: time from birth until the woman's body returns to a nonpregnant condition.

Preterm or premature labor: labor that occurs after 20 weeks' but before completion of 37 weeks' gestation.

Postterm labor: labor that occurs after 42 weeks' gestation.

Gravida: any pregnancy, regardless of duration, including present pregnancy.

Nulligravida: a woman who has never been pregnant.

Primigravida: a woman who is pregnant for the first time.

Multigravida: a woman who is in her second or any subsequent pregnancy.

Para: birth after 20 weeks' gestation regardless of whether the infant is born alive or dead.

Nullipara: a woman who has had no births at more than 20 weeks' gestation.

Primipara: a woman who has had one birth at more than 20 weeks' gestation, regardless of whether the infant was born alive or dead.

Multipara: a woman who has had two or more births at more than 20 weeks' gestation.

Stillbirth: an infant born dead after 20 weeks' gestation.

The terms *gravida* and *para* are used in relation to pregnancies, not to the number of fetuses. Thus twins, triplets, and so forth count as one pregnancy and one birth.

The following examples illustrate how these terms are applied in clinical situations:

1. Jean Sanchez has one child born at 38 weeks' gestation and is pregnant for the second time. At her initial prenatal visit, the nurse indicates her obstetric history "gravida 2 para 1 ab 0." Jean Sanchez's present pregnancy terminates at 16 weeks' gestation. She is now "gravida 2 para 1 ab 1."

2. Liz Buehl is pregnant for the fourth time. At home she has a child born at 35 weeks' gestation. One pregnancy ended at 10 weeks' gestation, and she gave birth to another infant stillborn at term. At her antepartal assessment, the nurse records her obstetric history as "gravida 4 para 2 ab 1."

To provide more comprehensive data, a more detailed approach is used in some settings. Using the detailed system, *gravida* keeps the same meaning, but the meaning of *para* changes because the detailed system counts each infant born rather than the number of pregnancies carried to viability (Cunningham, Gant, Leveno et al, 2001; Varney, 1997). Thus, for example, twins count as one pregnancy but two babies.

A useful acronym for remembering the system is TPAL:

T: number of *term* infants born—that is, the number of infants born after 37 weeks' gestation or more

P: number of *preterm* infants born—that is, the number of infants born after 20 weeks' but before the completion of 37 weeks' gestation

A: number of pregnancies ending in either spontaneous or therapeutic *abortion*

L: number of currently *living children*

Using this approach, the nurse would have initially described Jean Sanchez (see the first example) as "gravida 2 para 1001." Following Jean's spontaneous abortion, she would be "gravida 2 para 1011." Liz Buehl would be described as "gravida 4 para 1111" (See Figure 8–1 ◆).

Name	Gravida	**T**erm	**P**reterm	**A**bort	**L**iving Child
Jean Sanchez	2	1	0	0	1
Liz Buehl	4	1	1	1	1

FIGURE 8–1 ◆ The TPAL approach provides detailed information about the woman's pregnancy history.

Client Profile

The history is essentially a screening tool to identify factors that may place the mother or fetus at risk during the pregnancy. The following information is obtained for each pregnant woman at the first prenatal assessment:

1. Current pregnancy
   - First day of last normal menstrual period (LMP)
   - Presence of cramping, bleeding, or spotting since LMP
   - Woman's opinion about the time when conception occurred and when infant is due
   - Woman's attitude toward pregnancy (Is this pregnancy planned? Wanted?)
   - Results of pregnancy tests, if completed
   - Any discomforts since LMP such as nausea, vomiting, urinary frequency, fatigue, or breast tenderness

2. Past pregnancies
   - Number of pregnancies
   - Number of abortions, spontaneous or induced
   - Number of living children
   - History of previous pregnancies, length of pregnancy, length of labor and birth, type of birth (vaginal, forceps or vacuum-assisted birth, or cesarean), type of anesthesia used (if any), woman's perception of the experience, and complications (antepartal, intrapartal, and postpartal)
   - Neonatal status of previous children: Apgar scores, birth weights, general development, complications, and feeding patterns
   - Loss of a child (miscarriage, elective or medically indicated abortion, stillbirth, neonatal death, relinquishment, or death after the neonatal period) What was the experience like for her? What coping skills helped? How did her partner, if involved, respond?
   - If Rh negative, was medication received after birth to prevent sensitization?
   - Prenatal education classes and resources (books)

3. Gynecologic history
   - Date of last Pap smear; any history of abnormal Pap smear
   - Previous infections: vaginal, cervical, or sexually transmitted
   - Previous surgery
   - Age at menarche
   - Regularity, frequency, and duration of menstrual flow
   - History of dysmenorrhea
   - Sexual history
   - Contraceptive history (If birth control pills were used, did pregnancy occur immediately following cessation of pills? If not, how long after?)

4. Current medical history
   - Weight
   - Blood type and Rh factor, if known
   - General health including nutrition, normal dietary practices, and regular exercise program (type, frequency, and duration)
   - Any medications presently being taken (including prescription, nonprescription, homeopathic, or herbal medications) or taken since the onset of pregnancy
   - Previous or present use of alcohol, tobacco, or caffeine (Ask specifically about the amounts of alcohol, cigarettes, and caffeine [specify coffee, tea, colas, or chocolate] consumed each day.)
   - Illicit drug use or abuse (Ask about specific drugs such as cocaine, crack, and marijuana.)
   - Drug allergies and other allergies
   - Potential teratogenic insults to this pregnancy such as viral infections, medications, x-ray examinations, surgery, or cats in the home (possible source of toxoplasmosis)
   - Presence of disease conditions such as diabetes, hypertension, cardiovascular disease, renal problems, or thyroid disorder
   - Record of immunizations (especially rubella)
   - Presence of any abnormal symptoms

5. Past medical history
   - Childhood diseases
   - Past treatment for any disease condition (Any hospitalizations? History of hepatitis? Rheumatic fever? Pyelonephritis?)
   - Surgical procedures
   - Presence of bleeding disorders or tendencies (Has she received blood transfusions?)

6. Family medical history
   - Presence of diabetes, cardiovascular disease, cancer, hypertension, hematologic disorders, tuberculosis, or preeclampsia-eclampsia
   - Occurrence of multiple births
   - History of congenital diseases or deformities
   - Occurrence of cesarean births and cause, if known

7. Religious, spiritual, and cultural history
   - Does the woman wish to specify a religious preference on her chart? Does she have any religious beliefs or practices that might influence her health care or that of her child, such as prohibition against receiving blood products, dietary considerations, or circumcision rites?
   - What practices are important to maintain her spiritual well-being?
   - Might practices in her culture or that of her partner influence her care or that of her child?

8. Occupational history
   - Occupation
   - Physical demands (Does she stand all day, or are there opportunities to sit and elevate her legs? Any heavy lifting?)
   - Exposure to chemicals or other harmful substances
   - Opportunity for regular meals and breaks for nutritious snacks
   - Provision for maternity or family leave
9. Partner's history
   - Presence of genetic conditions or diseases
   - Age
   - Significant health problems
   - Previous or present alcohol intake, drug use, or tobacco use
   - Blood type and Rh factor
   - Occupation
   - Educational level; methods by which he learns best
   - Attitude toward the pregnancy
10. Personal information about the woman
    - Age
    - Educational level; methods by which she learns best
    - Race or ethnic group (to identify need for prenatal genetic screening and racially or ethnically related risk factors)
    - Housing; stability of living conditions
    - Economic level
    - Acceptance of pregnancy
    - Any history of emotional or physical deprivation or abuse of herself or children or any abuse in her current relationship (Ask specifically whether she has been hit, slapped, kicked, or hurt within the past year or since she has been pregnant. Ask whether she is afraid of her partner or anyone else. If yes, of whom is she afraid? [Ask only when she is alone.])
    - History of emotional problems
    - Support systems available to her
    - Personal preferences about the birth (expectations of both the woman and her partner, presence of others, and so on) (See Chapter 6. 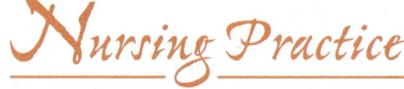)
    - Plans for care of child following birth
    - Feeding preference for the baby (breast or bottle?)

Obtaining Data

A questionnaire is used in many instances to obtain information. The woman should complete the questionnaire in a quiet place with a minimum of distractions. The nurse can get further information in an interview, which allows the pregnant woman to clarify her responses to questions and gives the nurse and client the opportunity to begin developing rapport.

The partner can be encouraged to attend the prenatal examinations. The partner is often able to contribute to the history and may use the opportunity to ask questions or express concerns.

High-Risk Screening

Risk factors are any findings that suggest the pregnancy may have a negative outcome, for either the woman or her unborn child. Screening for risk factors is an important part of the prenatal assessment. Many risk factors can be identified during the initial assessment; others may be detected during subsequent prenatal visits. It is important to identify high-risk pregnancies early so that appropriate interventions can be started promptly. Not all risk factors threaten a pregnancy equally; thus, many agencies use a scoring sheet to determine the degree of risk. Information must be updated throughout pregnancy as necessary. Any pregnancy may begin as low risk and change to high risk because of complications.

Table 8–1 identifies the major risk factors currently recognized. The table also identifies maternal and fetal or newborn implications if the risk is present in the pregnancy.

INITIAL PRENATAL ASSESSMENT

The prenatal assessment focuses on the woman holistically by considering physical, cultural, and psychosocial factors that influence her health. The establishment of the nurse-client relationship is a chance to begin developing an atmosphere conducive to interviewing, support, and education. Because many women are excited and anxious at the first antepartal visit, the initial psychosocial-cultural assessment is general.

As part of the initial psychosocial-cultural assessment, discuss with the woman any religious or spiritual, cultural, or socioeconomic factors that influence the woman's expectations of the childbearing experience. It is especially helpful to be familiar with common practices of the members of various religious and cultural groups who reside in the community.

After obtaining the history, prepare the woman for the physical examination. The physical examination begins with assessment of vital signs; then the woman's body is examined. The pelvic examination is performed last.

Before the examination, the woman should provide a clean urine specimen. When her bladder is empty, the woman

Nursing Practice

In a clinic or office setting, gowns and goggles for the health care provider are usually not necessary because splashing of body fluids is unlikely. Gloves are worn for procedures that involve contact with body fluids such as drawing blood for lab work, handling urine specimens, and conducting pelvic examinations.

TABLE 8-1　Prenatal High-Risk Factors

Factor	Maternal Implications	Fetal or Neonatal Implications
SOCIAL AND PERSONAL		
Low income level and/or low educational level	Poor antenatal care Poor nutrition ↑ risk preecalmpsia	Low birth weight Intrauterine growth restriction (IUGR)
Poor diet	Inadequate nutrition ↑ risk anemia ↑ risk of preeclampsia	Fetal malnutrition Prematurity
Living at high altitude	↑ hemoglobin	Prematurity IUGR ↑ hemoglobin (polycythemia)
Multiparity >3	↑ risk antepartum or postpartum hemorrhage	Anemia Fetal death
Weight <45.5 kg (100 lb)	Poor nutrition Cephalopelvic disproportion Prolonged labor	IUGR Hypoxia associated with difficult labor and birth
Weight >91 kg (200 lb)	↑ risk hypertension ↑ risk cephalopelvic disproportion ↑ risk diabetes	↓ fetal nutrition ↑ risk macrosomia
Age < 16	Poor nutrition Poor antenatal care ↑ risk preeclampsia ↑ risk cephalopelvic disproportion	Low birth weight ↑ fetal demise
Age > 35	↑ risk preeclampsia ↑ risk cesarean birth	↑ risk congenital anomalies ↑ chromosomal aberrations
Smoking one pack/day or more	↑ risk hypertension ↑ risk cancer	↓ placental perfusion →↓ O$_2$ and nutrients available Low birth weight IUGR Preterm birth
Use of addicting drugs	↑ risk poor nutrition ↑ risk of infection with IV drugs ↑ risk HIV, hepatitis C	↑ risk congenital anomalies ↑ risk low birth weight Neonatal withdrawal Lower serum bilirubin
Excessive alcohol consumption	↑ risk poor nutrition Possible hepatic effects with long-term consumption	↑ risk fetal alcohol syndrome
PREEXISTING MEDICAL DISORDERS		
Diabetes mellitus	↑ risk preeclampsia, hypertension Episodes of hypoglycemia and hyperglycemia ↑ risk cesarean birth	Low birth weight Macrosomia Neonatal hypoglycemia ↑ risk congenital anomalies ↑ risk respiratory distress syndrome
Cardiac disease	Cardiac decompensation Further strain on mother's body ↑ maternal death rate	↑ risk fetal demise ↑ prenatal mortality
Anemia: hemoglobin <9 g/dL (white) <29% hematocrit (white) <8.2 g/dL hemoglobin (black) <26% hematocrit (black)	Iron-deficiency anemia Low energy level Decreased oxygen-carrying capacity	Fetal death Prematurity Low birth weight
Hypertension	↑ vasospasm ↑ risk central nervous system irritability → convulsions ↑ risk cerebrovascular accident ↑ risk renal damage	↓ placental perfusion → low birth weight Preterm birth

TABLE 8–1 Prenatal High-Risk Factors—continued

Factor	Maternal Implications	Fetal or Neonatal Implications
PREEXISTING MEDICAL DISORDERS *continued*		
Thyroid disorder	↑ infertility	↑ spontaneous abortion
Hypothyroidism	↓ basal metabolic rate, goiter, myxedema	↑ risk congenital goiter
Hyperthyroidism	↑ risk postpartum hemorrhage ↑ risk preeclampsia Danger of thyroid storm	Mental retardation → cretinism ↑ incidence congenital anomalies ↑ incidence preterm birth ↑ tendency to thyrotoxicosis
Renal disease (moderate to severe)	↑ risk renal failure	↑ risk IUGR ↑ risk preterm birth
Diethylstilbestrol (DES) exposure	↑ infertility, spontaneous abortion ↑ cervical incompetence	↑ spontaneous abortion ↑ risk preterm birth
OBSTETRIC CONSIDERATIONS		
Previous Pregnancy		
Stillborn	↑ emotional or psychologic distress	↑ risk IUGR ↑ risk preterm birth
Habitual abortion	↑ emotional or psychologic distress ↑ possibility diagnostic workup	↑ risk abortion
Cesarean birth	↑ possibility repeat cesarean birth	↑ risk preterm birth ↑ risk respiratory distress
Rh or blood group sensitization	↑ financial expenditure for testing	Hydrops fetalis Icterus gravis Neonatal anemia Kernicterus Hypoglycemia
Large baby	↑ risk cesarean birth ↑ risk gestational diabetes	Birth injury Hypoglycemia
Current Pregnancy		
Rubella (first trimester)		Congenital heart disease Cataracts Nerve deafness Bone lesions Prolonged virus shedding
Rubella (second trimester)		Hepatitis Thrombocytopenia
Cytomegalovirus		IUGR Encephalopathy
Herpesvirus type 2	Severe discomfort Concern about possibility of cesarean birth, fetal infection	Neonatal herpesvirus type 2 2% hepatitis with jaundice Neurologic abnormalities
Syphilis	↑ incidence abortion	↑ fetal demise Congenital syphilis
Abruptio placenta and placenta previa	↑ risk hemorrhage Bed rest Extended hospitalization	Fetal or neonatal anemia Intrauterine hemorrhage ↑ fetal demise
Preeclampsia or eclampsia	See hypertension	↓ placental perfusion → low birth weight
Multiple gestation	↑ risk postpartum hemorrhage ↑ risk preterm labor	↑ risk preterm birth ↑ risk fetal demise
Elevated hematocrit >41% (white) >38% (black)	Increased viscosity of blood	Fetal death rate 5 times normal rate
Spontaneous premature rupture of membranes	↑ uterine infection	↑ risk preterm birth ↑ fetal demise

is more comfortable during the pelvic examination and the examiner can palpate the pelvic organs more easily. After the woman empties her bladder, ask her to disrobe and give her a gown and sheet or some other protective covering.

Increasing numbers of nurses, such as CNMs and other nurses in advanced practice, are prepared to perform complete physical examinations. The nurse who is not an advanced practitioner assesses the woman's vital signs, explains the procedures to allay apprehension, positions her for examination, and assists the examiner as necessary.

Thoroughness and a systematic procedure are the most important considerations when performing the physical portion of an antepartal examination. See "Assessment Guide: Initial Prenatal Assessment," starting below. To promote completeness, the assessment guide is organized in three columns that address the areas to be assessed (and normal findings), the variations or alterations that may be observed, and nursing responses to the data. Be aware that certain organs and systems are assessed concurrently with others during the physical portion of the examination.
Text continues on page 172.

ASSESSMENT GUIDE ≈ *Initial Prenatal Assessment*

Physical Assessment/Normal Findings	Alterations and Possible Causes*	Nursing Responses to Data†
VITAL SIGNS		
Blood pressure (BP): 90;—140/60—90 mm Hg	High BP (essential hypertension; renal disease; pregestational hypertension; apprehension or anxiety associated with pregnancy diagnosis, exam, or other crises; preeclampsia if initial assessment not done until after 20 weeks' gestation)	BP > 140/90 requires immediate consideration; establish women's BP; refer to physician if necessary. Assess women's knowledge about high BP; counsel on self-care and medical management.
Pulse: 60—90 beats/min. rate may increase 10 beats/min during pregnancy	Increased pulse rate (excitement or anxiety, cardiac disorders)	Count for 1 full minute; note irregularities.
Respirations: 16–24 breaths/min (or pulse rate divided by four); pregnancy may induce a degree of hyperventilation; thoracic breathing predominant	Marked tachypnea or abnormal patterns	Assess for respiratory disease.
Temperature: 36.2–37.6°C (98–99.6°F)	Elevated temperature (infection)	Assess for infection process or disease state if temperature is elevated; refer to physician or CNM.
WEIGHT		
Depends on body build	Weight < 45 kg (100 lb) or > 91 kg (200 lb); rapid, sudden weight gain (preeclampsia)	Evaluate need for nutritional counseling; obtain information on eating habits, cooking practices, foods regularly eaten, income limitations, need for food supplements, pica and other abnormal food habits. Note initial weight to establish baseline for weight gain throughout pregnancy.
SKIN		
Color: Consistent with racial background; pink nail beds	Pallor (anemia); bronze, yellow (hepatic disease; other causes of jaundice)	The following tests should be performed: complete blood count (CBC), bilirubin level, urinalysis, and blood urea nitrogen (BUN).
	Bluish, reddish, mottled; dusky appearance or pallor of palms and nail beds in dark-skinned women (anemia)	If abnormal, refer to physician.
Condition: Absence of edema (slight edema of lower extremities is normal during pregnancy)	Edema (preeclampsia); rashes, dermatitis (allergic response)	Counsel on relief measures for slight edema. Initiate preeclampsia assessment; refer to physician.
Lesions: Absence of lesions	Ulceration (varicose veins, decreased circulation)	Further assess circulatory status; refer to physician if lesion is severe.
Spider nevi common in pregnancy	Petechiae, multiple bruises, ecchymosis (hemorrhagic disorders; abuse)	Evaluate for bleeding or clotting disorder. Provide opportunities to discuss abuse if suspected.
Moles	Change in size or color (carcinoma)	Refer to physician.
Pigmentation: Pigmentation changes of pregnancy include linea nigra, striae gravidarum, melasma		Assure woman that these are normal manifestations of pregnancy and explain the physiologic basis for the changes.
Café-au-lait spots	Six or more (Albright syndrome or neurofibromatosis)	Consult with physician.
	***Possible causes of alterations were placed in parentheses.**	**†This column provides guidelines for further assessment and initial nursing intervention.**

(continued)

Physical Assessment/Normal Findings	Alterations and Possible Causes*	Nursing Responses to Data†
NOSE		
Character of mucosa: Redder than oral mucosa; in pregnancy nasal mucosa is edematous in response to increased estrogen, resulting in nasal stuffiness (rhinitis of pregnancy) and nosebleeds	Olfactory loss (first cranial nerve deficit)	Counsel woman about possible relief measures for nasal stuffiness and nosebleeds (epistaxis); refer to physician for olfactory loss.
MOUTH		
May note hypertrophy of gingival tissue because of estrogen	Edema, inflammation (infection); pale in color (anemia)	Assess hematocrit for anemia; counsel regarding dental hygiene habits. Refer to physician or dentist if necessary. Routine dental care appropriate during pregnancy (no x-ray studies, no nitrous anesthesia).
NECK		
Nodes: Small, mobile, nontender nodes	Tender, hard, fixed, or prominent nodes (infection, carcinoma)	Examine for local infection; refer to physician.
Thyroid: Small, smooth, lateral lobes palpable on either side of trachea; slight hyperplasia by third month of pregnancy	Enlargement or nodule tenderness (hyperthyroidism)	Listen over thyroid for bruits, which may indicate hyperthyroidism. Question woman about dietary habits (iodine intake). Ascertain history of thyroid problems; refer to physician.
CHEST AND LUNGS		
Chest: Symmetric, elliptic, smaller anteroposterior (A-P) than transverse diameter	Increased A-P diameter, funnel chest, pigeon chest (emphysema, asthma, chronic obstructive pulmonary disease [COPD])	Evaluate for emphysema, asthma, pulmonary disease (COPD).
Ribs: Slope downward from nipple line	More horizontal (COPD) Angular bumps Rachitic rosary (vitamin C deficiency)	Evaluate for COPD. Evaluate for fractures. Consult physician. Consult nutritionist.
Inspection and palpation: No retraction or bulging of intercostal spaces (ICS) during inspiration or expiration; symmetric expansion	ICS retractions with inspiration, bulging with expiration; unequal expansion (respiratory disease)	Do thorough initial assessment. Refer to physician.
Tactile fremitus	Tachypnea, hyperpnea, Cheyne-Stokes respirations (respiratory disease)	Refer to physician.
Percussion: Bilateral symmetry in tone	Flatness of percussion, which may be affected by chest wall thickness	Evaluate for pleural effusions; consolidations, or tumor.
Low-pitched resonance of moderate intensity	High diaphragm (atelectasis or paralysis), pleural effusion	Refer to physician.
Auscultation: Upper lobes—bronchovesicular sounds above sternum and scapulas; equal expiratory and inspiratory phases.	Abnormal if heard over any other area of chest	Refer to physician.
Remainder of chest: vesicular breath sounds heard; inspiratory phase longer (3:1)	Rales, rhonchi, wheezes; pleural friction rub; absence of breath sounds; bronchophony, egophony, whispered pectoriloquy	Refer to physician.
	*Possible causes of alterations were placed in parentheses.	†This column provides guidelines for further assessment and initial nursing intervention.

Physical Assessment/Normal Findings	Alterations and Possible Causes*	Nursing Responses to Data†
BREASTS Supple; symmetric in size and contour; darker pigmentation of nipple and areola; may have supernumerary nipples, usually 5–6 cm below normal nipple line	"Pigskin" or orange-peel appearance, nipple retractions, swelling, hardness (carcinoma); redness, heat, tenderness, cracked or fissured nipple (infection)	Encourage monthly self-examination; instruct woman how to examine own breasts.
Axillary nodes unpalpable or pellet sized	Tenderness, enlargement, hard node (carcinoma); may be visible bump (infection)	Refer to physician if evidence of inflammation.
Pregnancy changes: 1. Size increase noted primarily in first 20 weeks. 2. Become nodular. 3. Tingling sensation may be felt during first and third trimester; woman may report feeling of heaviness. 4. Pigmentation of nipples and areolas darkens. 5. Superficial veins dilate and become more prominent. 6. Striae seen in multiparas. 7. Tubercles of Montgomery enlarge. 8. Colostrum may be present after 12th week. 9. Secondary areola appears at 20 weeks, characterized by series of washed-out spots surrounding primary areola. 10. Breasts less firm, old striae may be present in multiparas.		Discuss normalcy of changes and their meaning with the woman. Teach and/or institute appropriate relief measures. Encourage use of supportive, well-fitting brassiere.
HEART Normal rate, rhythm, and heart sounds *Pregnancy changes:* 1. Palpitations may occur due to sympathetic nervous system disturbance. 2. Short systolic murmurs that increase in held expiration are normal due to increased volume.	Enlargement, thrills, thrusts, gross irregularity or skipped beats, gallop rhythm or extra sounds (cardiac disease)	Complete an initial assessment. Explain normalcy of pregnancy-induced changes. Refer to physician if indicated.
ABDOMEN Normal appearance, skin texture, and hair distribution; liver nonpalpable; abdomen nontender. *Pregnancy changes:* 1. Purple striae may be present (or silver striae on a multipara) as well as finea nigra. 2. Diastasis of the rectus muscles late in pregnancy.	Muscle guarding (anxiety, acute tenderness); tenderness, mass (ectopic pregnancy, inflammation, carcinoma)	Assure woman of normalcy of diastasis. Provide initial information about appropriate prenatal and postpartum exercises. Evaluate woman's anxiety level. Refer to physician if indicated.
3. Size; Flat or rotund abdomen; progressive enlargement of uterus due to pregnancy. 10–12 weeks; Fundus slightly above symphysis pubis. 16 weeks: Fundus halfway between symphysis and umbilicus. 20–22 weeks: Fundus at umbilicus. 28 weeks: Fundus three finger breadths above umbilicus 36 weeks: Fundus just below ensiform cartilage.	Size of uterus inconsistent with length of gestation (intrauterine growth restriction [UGR], multiple pregnancy, fetal demise, hydatidiform mole)	Reassess menstrual history regarding pregnancy dating. Evaluate increase in size using McDonald's method. Use ultrasound to establish diagnosis.
	*Possible causes of alterations were placed in parentheses.	†This column provides guidelines for further assessment and initial nursing intervention.

(continued)

Physical Assessment/Normal Findings	Alterations and Possible Causes*	Nursing Responses to Data†
ABDOMEN *continued*		
4. Fetal heartbeats: 120–160 beats/min may be heard with Doppler at 10–12 weeks' gestation; may be heard with fetoscope at 17–20 weeks.	Failure to hear fetal heartbeat with Doppler (fetal demise, hydatidiform mole)	Refer to physician. Administer pregnancy tests. Use ultrasound to establish diagnosis.
5. Fetal movement palpable by a trained examiner after the 18th week.	Failure to feel fetal movements after 20 weeks' gestation (fetal demise, hydatidiform mole)	Refer to physician for evaluation of fetal status.
6. Ballottement: During fourth to fifth month fetus rises and then rebounds to original position when uterus is tapped sharply.	No ballottement (oligohydramnios)	Refer to physician for evaluation of fetal status.
EXTREMITIES		
Skin warm, pulses palpable, full range of motion; may be some edema of hands and ankles in late pregnancy; varicose veins may become more pronounced; palmar erythema may be present	Unpalpable or diminished pulses (arterial insufficiency); marked edema (preeclampsia)	Evaluate for other symptoms of heart disease; initiate follow-up if woman mentions that her rings feel tight. Discuss prevention and self-treatment measures for varicose veins; refer to physician if indicated.
SPINE		
Normal spinal curves: Concave cervical, convex thoracic, concave lumbar	Abnormal spinal curves; flatness, kyphosis, lordosis	Refer to physician for assessment of cephalopelvic disproportion (CPD).
In pregnancy, lumbar spinal curve may be accentuated	Backache	May have implications for administration of spinal anesthetics; see Chapter 9 for relief measures.
Shoulders and iliac crests should be even	Uneven shoulders and iliac crests (scoliosis)	Refer very young women to a physician; discuss back-stretching exercises with older women.
REFLEXES		
Normal and symmetric	Hyperactivity, clonus (preeclampsia)	Evaluate for other symptoms of preeclampsia.
PELVIC AREA		
External female genitals: Normally formed with female hair distribution; in multiparas, labia majora loose and pigmented; urinary and vaginal orifices visible and appropriately located	Lesions, hematomas, varicosities, inflammation of Bartholin's glands; clitoral hypertrophy (masculinization)	Explain pelvic examination procedure (see Skill 2–2). SKILLS Encourage woman to minimize her discomfort by relaxing her hips. Provide privacy.
Vagina: Pink or dark pink, vaginal discharge odorless, nonirritating; in multiparas, vaginal folds smooth and flattened; may have episiotomy scar	Abnormal discharge associated with vaginal infections	Obtain vaginal smear. Provide understandable verbal and written instructions about treatment for woman and partner, if indicated.
Cervix: Pink color; os closed except in multiparas, in whom os admits fingertip	Eversion, reddish erosion, nabothian or retention cysts, cervical polyp; granular area that bleeds (carcinoma of cervix); lesions (herpes, human papillomavirus [HPV] Presence of string or plastic tip from cervix (intrauterine device [IUD] in uterus)	Provide woman with a hand mirror and identify genital structures for her; encourage her to view her cervix if she wishes. Refer to physician if indicated. Advise woman of potential serious risks of leaving an IUD in place during pregnancy; refer to physician for removal.
*Possible causes of alterations were placed in parentheses.	†This column provides guidelines for further assessment and initial nursing intervention.	

Physical Assessment/Normal Findings	Alterations and Possible Causes*	Nursing Responses to Data†
PELVIC AREA *continued*		
Pregnancy changes:	Absence of Goodell's sign (inflammatory conditions, carcinoma)	Refer to physician.
1–4 weeks' gestation: Enlargement in anteroposterior diameter		
4–6 weeks' gestation: Softening of cervix (Goodell's sign), softening of isthmus of uterus (Hegar's signs); cervix takes on bluish coloring (Chadwick's sign)		
8–12 weeks' gestation: Vagina and cervix appear bluish violet in color (Chadwick's sign)		
Uterus: Pear shaped, mobile; smooth surface	Fixed (pelvic inflammatory disease [PID]); nodular surface (fibromas)	Refer to physician.
Ovaries: Small, walnut shaped, nontender (ovaries and fallopian tubes are located in the adnexal areas)	Pain or movement of cervix (PID); enlarged or nodular ovaries (cyst, tumor, tubal pregnancy, corpus luteum of pregnancy)	Evaluate adnexal areas; refer to physician.
PELVIC MEASUREMENTS		
Internal measurements:	Measurement below normal	Vaginal birth may not be possible if deviations are present.
1. Diagonal conjugate at least 11.5 cm (Figure 8–5)		
2. Obstetric conjugate estimated by subtracting 1.5–2 cm from diagonal conjugate	Disproportion of pubic arch	
3. Inclination of sacrum	Abnormal curvature of sacrum	
4. Motility of coccyx; external intertuberosity diameter > 8 cm	Fixed or malposition of coccyx	
ANUS AND RECTUM		
No lumps, rashes, excoriation, tenderness; cervix may be felt through rectal wall	Hemorrhoids, rectal prolapse; nodular lesion (carcinoma)	Counsel about appropriate prevention and relief measures; refer to physician for further evaluation.
LABORATORY EVALUATION		
Hemoglobin: 12–16 g/dL; women residing in areas of high altitude may have higher levels of hemoglobin	< 12 g/dL (anemia)	Note: Wear gloves when drawing blood. Hemoglobin < 12 g/dL requires nutritional counseling; < 11 g/dL requires iron supplementation.
ABO and Rh typing: Normal distribution of blood types	Rh negative	If Rh negative, check for presence of anti-Rh antibodies. Check partner's blood type; if partner is Rh positive, discuss with woman the need for antibody titers during pregnancy, management during the intrapartal period, and possible candidacy for RhIgG. (See Chapter 13).
Complete blood count (CBC)		
Hematocrit: 38%–47% physiologic anemia (pseudoanemia) may occur	Marked anemia or blood dyscrasias	Perform CBC and Schilling differential cell count.
Red blood cells (RBC): 4.2–5.4 million/μL		
	*Possible causes of alterations were placed in parentheses.	†This column provides guidelines for further assessment and initial nursing intervention.

(continued)

Physical Assessment/Normal Findings	Alterations and Possible Causes*	Nursing Responses to Data†
LABORATORY EVALUATION *continued*		
White blood cells (WBC): 5,000– 12,000/μL	Presence of infection; may be elevated in pregnancy and with labor	Evaluate for other signs of infection.
Differential Neutrophils: 40%–60% Bands: up to 5% Eosinophils: 1%–3% Basophils: up to 1% Lymphocytes: 20%–40% Monocytes: 4%–8%		
Syphilis tests: Serologic tests for syphilis (STS), complement fixation test, veneral disease research laboratory (VDRL) test—nonreactive	Positive reaction STS—tests may have 25%–45% incidence of biologic false-positive results; false results may occur in individuals who have acute viral or bacterial infections, hypersensitivity reactions, recent vaccinations, collagen disease, malaria, or tuberculosis	Positive results may be confirmed with the fluorescent treponemal antibody-absorption (FTA-ABS) tests; all tests for syphilis give positive results in the secondary stage of the disease; antibiotic tests may cause negative test results.
Gonorrhea culture: Negative	Positive	Refer for treatment.
Urinalysis (u/a); Normal color, specific gravity; pH 4.6–8	Abnormal color (porphyria, hemaglobinuria, bilirubinemia); alkaline urine (metabolic alkalemia, *Proteus* infection, old specimen)	Repeat u/a; refer to physician.
Negative for protein, red blood cells, white blood cells, casts	Positive findings (contaminated specimen, kidney disease)	Repeat u/a; refer to physician.
Glucose: Negative (small degree of glycosuria may occur in pregnancy)	Glycosuria (low renal threshold for glucose diabetes mellitus)	Assess blood glucose level; test urine for ketones.
Rubella titer: Hemagglutination-inhibition (HAI) test—1:10 indicates woman is immune	HAI titer < 1:10	Immunization will be given on postpartum or within 6 weeks after childbirth. Instruct woman whose titers are > 1:10 to avoid children who have rubella.
Hepatitis B screen for hepatitis B surface antigen (HbsAg); negative	Positive	If negative, consider referral for hepatitis B vaccine. If positive, refer to physician. Infants born to women who test positive are given hepatitis B immune globulin soon after birth followed by first dose of hepatitis B vaccine.
HIV screen: Offered to all women; encouraged for those at risk; negative	Positive	Refer to physician.
Illicit drug screen: Offered to all women; negative	Positive	Refer to physician.
Sickle cell screen for clients of African descent: Negative	Positive; test results would include a description of cells	Refer to physician.
Pap smear: Negative	Test results that show atypical cells	Refer to physician. Discuss with the woman the meaning of the findings and the importance of follow-up.

Cultural Assessment	Variations to Consider*	Nursing Responses to Data†
Determine the woman's fluency in English.	Woman may be fluent in a language other than English.	Work with a knowledgable translater to provide information and answer questions.
Ask the woman how she prefers to be addressed.	Some women prefer informality; other prefer to use titles.	Address the woman according to her preference. Maintain formality in introducing oneself if that seems preferred.
	*Possible causes of alterations were placed in parentheses.	†This column provides guidelines for further assessment and initial nursing intervention.

Cultural Assessment	Variations to Consider*	Nursing Responses to Data†
Determine customs and practices regarding prenatal care:	Practices are influenced by individual preference, cultural expectations, or religious beliefs.	Honor a woman's practices and provide for specific preferences unless they are contraindicated because of safety.
• Ask the woman if there are certain practices she expects to follow when she is pregnant.	Some women believe that they should perform certain acts related to sleep, activity, or clothing.	Have information printed in the language of different cultural groups that live in the area.
• Ask the woman if there are any activities she cannot do while she is pregnant.	Some women have restrictions or taboos they follow related to work, activity, sexual, environmental, or emotional factors.	
• Ask the woman whether there are certain foods she is expected to eat or avoid while she is pregnant. Determine whether she has lactose intolerance.	Foods are an important cultural factor. Some women may have certain foods they must eat or avoid; many women have lactose intolerance and have difficulty consuming sufficient calcium.	Respect the woman's food preferences, help her plan an adequate prenatal diet within the framework of her preferences, and refer to a dietitian if necessary.
• Ask the woman whether the gender of her caregiver is of concern.	Some women are comfortable only with a female caregiver.	Arrange for a female caregiver if it is the woman's preference.
• Ask the woman about the degree of involvement in her pregnancy that she expects or wants from her support person, mother, and other significant people.	A woman may not want her partner involved in the pregnancy. For some the role falls to the woman's mother or a female relative or friend.	Respect the woman's preferences about her partner or husband's involvement; avoid imposing personal values or expectations.
• Ask the woman about her sources of support and counseling during pregnancy.	Some women seek advice from a family member, *curandera*, tribal healer, and so forth.	Respect and honor the woman's sources of support.
PSYCHOLOGIC STATUS		
Excitement and/or apprehension, ambivalence	Marked anxiety (fear of pregnancy diagnosis, fear of medical facility)	Establish lines of communication. Active listening is useful. Establish trusting relationship. Encourage woman to take active part in her care.
	Apathy; display of anger with pregnancy diagnosis	Establish communication and begin counseling. Use active listening techniques.
EDUCATIONAL NEEDS		
May have questions about pregnancy or may need time to adjust to reality of pregnancy		Establish educational, supporting environment that can be expanded throughout pregnancy.
SUPPORT SYSTEMS		
Can identify at least two or three individuals with whom woman is emotionally intimate (partner, parent, sibling, friend)	Isolated (no telephone, unlisted number); cannot name a neighbor or friend whom she can call upon in an emergency; does not perceive parents as part of her support system	Institute support system through community groups. Help woman to develop trusting relationship with health care professionals.
FAMILY FUNCTIONING		
Emotionally supportive Communications adequate Mutually satisfying Cohesiveness in times of trouble	Long-term problems or specific problems related to this pregnancy, potential stressors within the family, pessimistic attitudes, unilateral decision making, unrealistic expectations of this pregnancy or child	Help identify the problems and stressors, encourage communication, and discuss role changes and adaptations.
ECONOMIC STATUS		
Source of income is stable and sufficient to meet basic needs of daily living and medical needs	Limited prenatal care; poor physical health; limited use of health care system; unstable economic status	Discuss available resources for health maintenance and the birth. Institute appropriate referral for meeting expanding family's needs—food stamps and so forth.
STABILITY OF LIVING CONDITIONS		
Adequate, stable housing for expanding family's needs	Crowded living conditions; questionable supportive environment for newborn	Refer to appropriate community agency. Work with family on self-help ways to improve situation.
	*Possible causes of alterations were placed in parentheses.	†This column provides guidelines for further assessment and initial nursing intervention.

Nursing interventions based on assessment of the normal physical and psychosocial changes of pregnancy, evaluation of the cultural influences associated with pregnancy, and mutually defined client teaching and counseling needs are discussed further in Chapter 9.

Determination of Due Date

Childbearing families generally want to know the "due date," or the date around which childbirth will occur. Historically the due date has been called the estimated date of confinement (EDC). The concept of confinement is, however, rather negative, and there is a trend in the literature to avoid it by referring to the due date as the EDD or estimated date of delivery. Childbirth educators often stress that babies are not "delivered" like a package; they are born. In keeping with a view that emphasizes the normalcy of the process, this text refers to the due date as the **estimated date of birth (EDB)**.

To calculate the EDB it is helpful to know the date of the LMP. However, some women have episodes of irregular bleeding or fail to keep track of menstrual cycles. Thus, other techniques also help to determine how far along a woman is in her pregnancy—that is, at how many weeks' gestation she is. Techniques include evaluating uterine size, determining when quickening occurs, and auscultating fetal heart rate with a Doppler device or ultrasound.

Nägele's Rule

The most common method of determining the EDB is **Nägele's rule.** To use this method, begin with the first day of the LMP, subtract 3 months, and add 7 days. For example,

First day of LMP	November 21
Subtract 3 months	− 3 months
	August 21
Add 7 days	+ 7 days
EDB	August 28

It is simpler to change the months to numeric terms:

November 21 becomes	11-21
Subtract 3 months	− 3
	8-21
Add 7 days	+ 7
EDB	August 28

A gestation calculator or wheel lets the caregiver calculate the EDB even more quickly (Figure 8–2 ◆).

If a woman with a history of menses every 28 days remembers her LMP and was not taking oral contraceptives before becoming pregnant, Nägele's rule may be a fairly accurate determiner of the EDB. However, ovulation usually occurs 14 days before the onset of the next menses, not 14 days after the previous menses. Consequently, if her cycle is irregular, or 35 to 40 days long, the time of ovulation

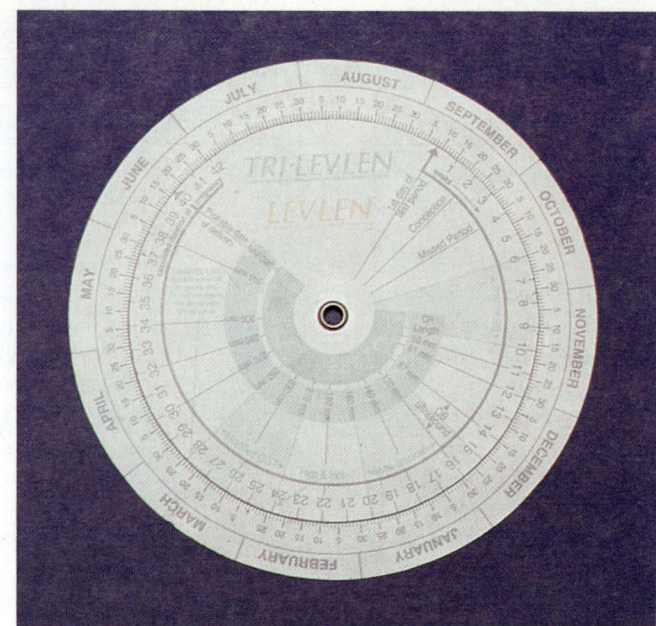

FIGURE 8–2 ◆ The EDB wheel can be used to calculate the due date. To use it, place the "last menses began" arrow on the date of the woman's LMP. Then read the EDB at the arrow labeled 40. In this case the LMP is September 8 and the EDB is June 17.

may be delayed by several days. If she has been using oral contraceptives, ovulation may be delayed several weeks following her last menses. Then, too, a postpartum woman who is breastfeeding may resume ovulating but be amenorrheic for a time, making calculation impossible. Thus Nägele's rule, although helpful, is not foolproof.

Uterine Assessment

PHYSICAL EXAMINATION

When a woman is examined in the first 10 to 12 weeks of her pregnancy and her uterine size is compatible with her menstrual history, uterine size may be the single most important clinical method for dating her pregnancy. In many cases, however, women do not seek maternity care until well into their second trimester, when it becomes much more difficult to evaluate specific uterine size. In obese women it is difficult to determine uterine size early in a pregnancy because the uterus is more difficult to palpate.

Fundal Height

Fundal height may be used as an indicator of uterine size, although this method is less accurate late in pregnancy. A centimeter tape measure is used to measure the distance abdominally from the top of the symphysis pubis to the top of the uterine fundus (McDonald's method) (Figure 8–3 ◆). Fundal height in centimeters correlates well with weeks of gestation between 22 to 24 weeks and 34 weeks. Thus, at 26 weeks' gestation, fundal height is probably about 26 cm. If the woman is very tall or very short, fundal height will differ. To be most accurate, fundal height should be

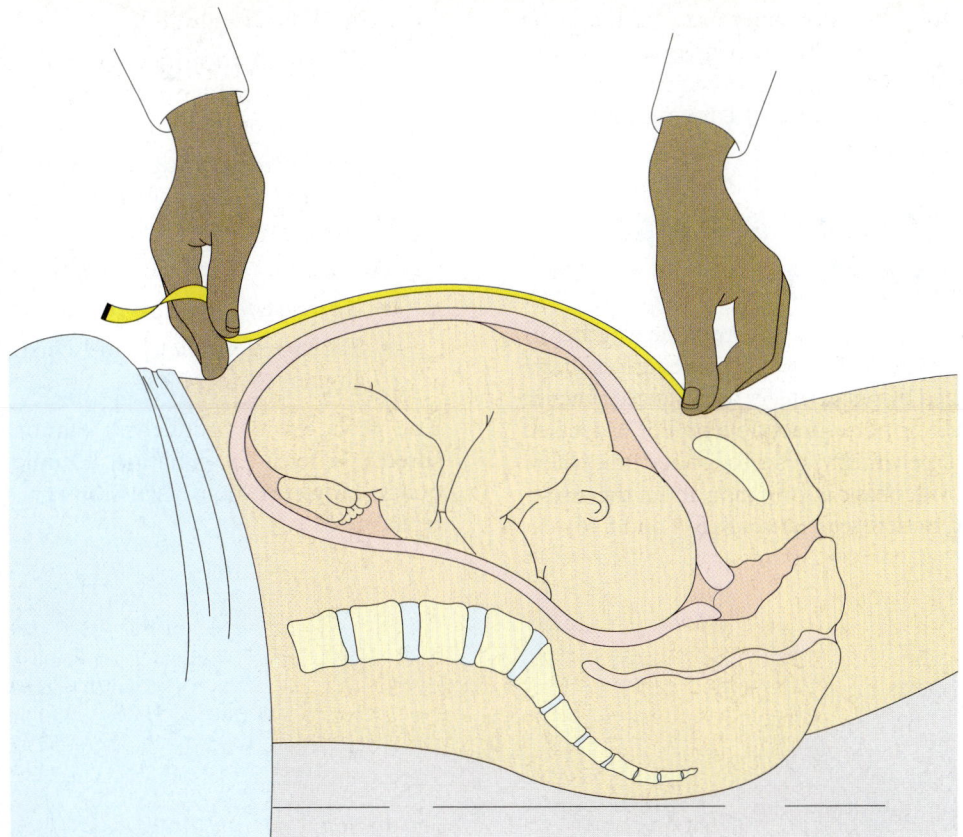

FIGURE 8-3 ◆ A cross-sectional view of fetal position when McDonald's method is used to assess fundal height.

measured by the same examiner each time. The woman should have voided within 1/2 hour of the exam and should lie in the same position each time. In the third trimester, variations in fetal weight decrease the accuracy of fundal height measurements.

A lag in progression of measurements of fundal height from month to month and week to week may signal intrauterine growth restriction (IUGR). A sudden increase in fundal height may indicate twins or hydramnios (excessive amount of amniotic fluid).

Fetal Development

QUICKENING

Fetal movements felt by the mother, called quickening, may indicate that the fetus is nearing 20 weeks' gestation. However, quickening may be experienced between 16 and 22 weeks' gestation, so this method is not completely accurate.

FETAL HEARTBEAT

The ultrasonic Doppler device (Figure 8–4 ◆) is the primary tool for assessing fetal heartbeat. It can detect fetal heartbeat, on average, at 8 to 12 weeks' gestation. If an ultrasonic Doppler is not available, a fetoscope may be used, although in current practice it is seldom necessary. The fetal heartbeat can be detected by fetoscope as early as week 16 and almost always by 19 or 20 weeks' gestation.

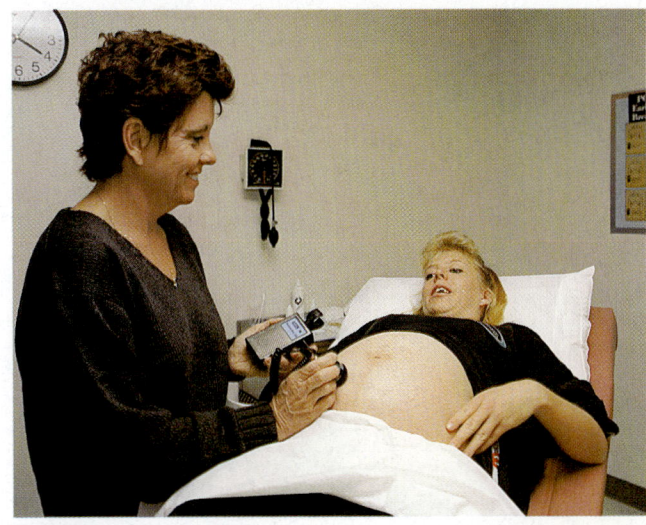

FIGURE 8-4 ◆ Listening to the fetal heartbeat with a Doppler device.

ULTRASOUND

In the first trimester, ultrasound scanning can detect a gestational sac as early as 5 to 6 weeks after the LMP, fetal heart activity by 6 to 7 weeks, and fetal breathing movement by 10 to 11 weeks of pregnancy. Crown-to-rump measurements can be made to assess fetal age until the fetal head can be visualized clearly. Biparietal diameter (BPD) can then be used. BPD measurements can be made by approximately 12 to 13 weeks and are most accurate between 20 and 30 weeks, when rapid growth in the biparietal diameter occurs. (See Chapter 14 for discussion of fetal ultrasound scanning.) 🔗

ASSESSMENT OF PELVIC ADEQUACY (CLINICAL PELVIMETRY)

The pelvis can be assessed vaginally to determine whether its size is adequate for a vaginal birth. This procedure, *clinical pelvimetry*, is performed by physicians or by advanced practice nurses such as CNMs or nurse-practitioners. For a detailed description of clinical pelvimetry, refer to a nurse-midwifery text. This section provides basic information about the assessment of the inlet and outlet (see Figures 8–5 ◆ and 8–6 ◆).

1. Pelvic inlet (Figure 8–5)
   - **Diagonal conjugate** (the distance from the lower posterior border of the symphysis pubis to the sacral promontory) at least 11.5 cm
   - **Obstetric conjugate** (a measurement approximately 1.5 cm smaller than the diagonal conjugate) 10 cm or more
2. Pelvic outlet (Figures 8–5 and 8–6)
   - *Anteroposterior diameter*, 9.5 to 11.5 cm
   - *Transverse diameter* (bi-ischial or intertuberous diameter), 8 to 10 cm

The pelvic cavity (midpelvis) cannot be accurately measured by clinical examination. Examiners estimate its adequacy. However, that discussion is also beyond the scope of this text.

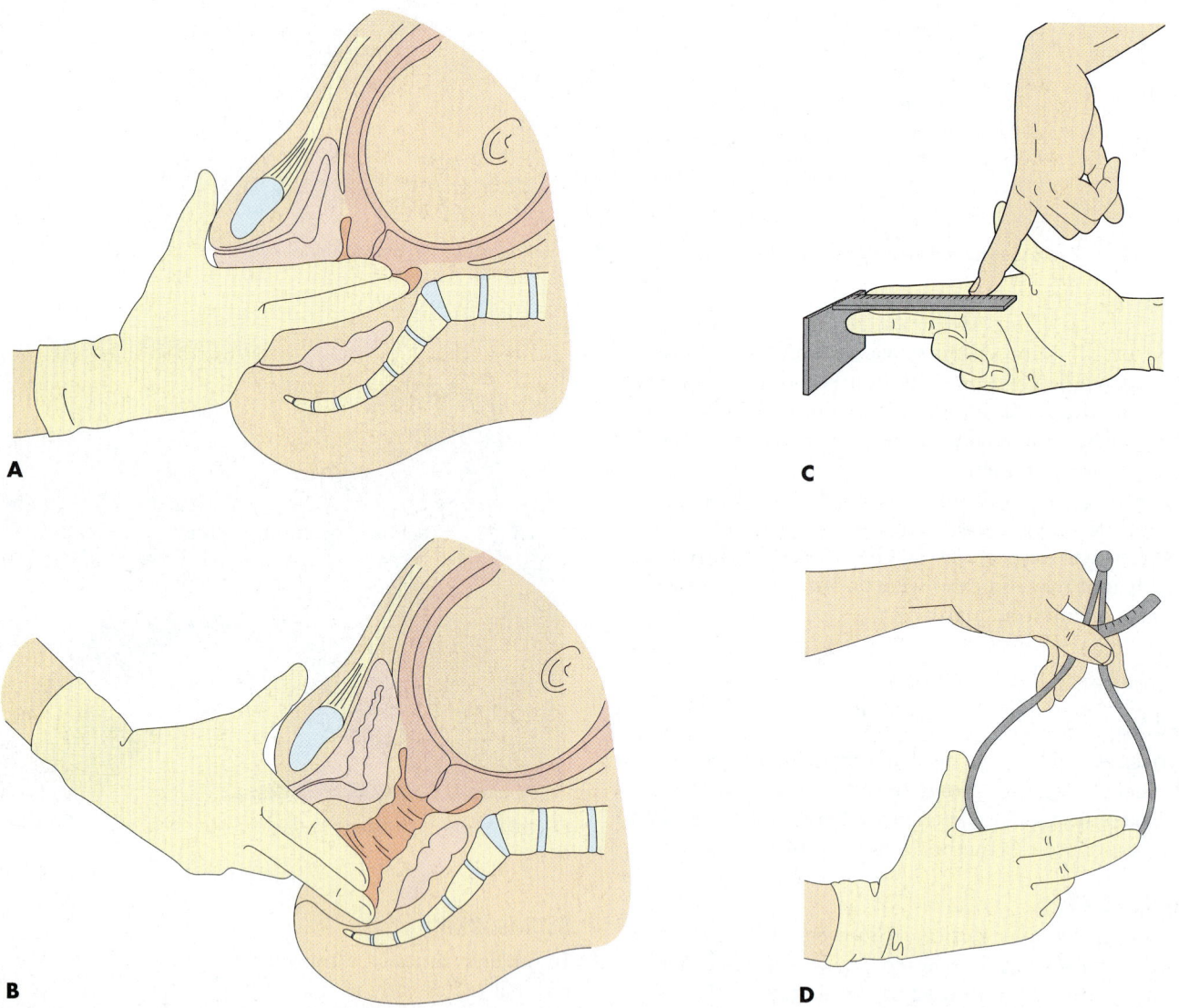

A

B

C

D

FIGURE 8–5 ◆ Manual measurement of inlet and outlet. **A,** Estimation of the diagonal conjugate, which extends from the lower border of the symphysis pubis to the sacral promontory. **B,** Estimation of the anteroposterior diameter of the outlet, which extends from the lower border of the symphysis pubis to the tip of the sacrum. **C,** and **D,** Methods that may be used to check the manual estimation of anteroposterior measurements.

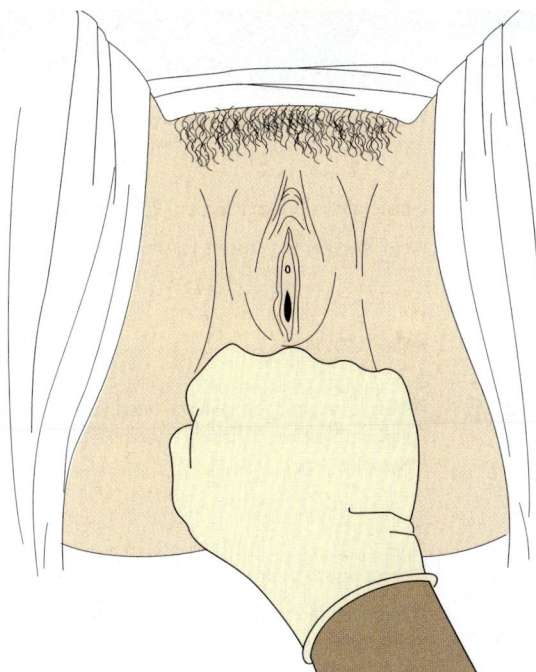

FIGURE 8–6 ◆ Use of a closed fist to measure the outlet. Most examiners know the distance between their first and last proximal knuckles. If they do not, they can use a measuring device.

SUBSEQUENT CLIENT HISTORY

At subsequent prenatal visits, continue to gather data about the course of the pregnancy to date and the woman's responses to it. Also ask about the adjustment of the support person and of other children, if any, in the family. As pregnancy progresses, inquire about the preparations the family has made for the new baby.

Ask specifically whether the woman has experienced any discomfort, especially the kinds of discomfort that are often seen at specific times during a pregnancy. Inquire about physical changes that relate directly to the pregnancy, such as fetal movement. Also ask about the danger signs of pregnancy (see Table 8–2).

Other pertinent information includes any exposure to contagious illnesses, medical treatment and therapy prescribed for nonpregnancy problems since the last visit, and any prescription or over-the-counter medications that were not prescribed as part of the woman's prenatal care.

Periodic prenatal examinations offer a chance to assess the childbearing woman's psychologic needs and emotional status. If the woman's partner attends the antepartal visits, they can also be a time to identify the partner's needs and concerns. The woman should have sufficient time to ask questions and air concerns. If a nurse provides the time and demonstrates genuine interest, the woman will be more at ease bringing up questions that she may believe are silly or has been afraid to verbalize.

Be sensitive to religious or spiritual, cultural, and socioeconomic factors that may influence a family's response to pregnancy, as well as to the woman's expectations of the health care

TABLE 8–2 Danger Signs in Pregnancy	
The woman should report the following danger signs in pregnancy immediately:	
Danger Sign	*Possible Cause*
Sudden gush of fluid from from vagina	Premature rupture of membranes
Vaginal bleeding	Abruptio placentae, placenta previa
	Lesions of cervix or vagina "Bloody show"
Abdominal pain	Premature labor, abruptio placentae
Temperature above 38.3°C (101°F) and chills	Infection
Dizziness, blurring of vision, double vision, spots before eyes	Hypertension, preeclampsia
Persistent vomiting	Hyperemesis gravidarum
Severe headache	Hypertension, preeclampsia
Edema of hands, face, legs, and feet	Preeclampsia
Muscular irritability, convulsions	Preeclampsia, eclampsia
Epigastric pain	Preeclampsia, ischemia in major abdominal vessel
Oliguria	Renal impairment, decreased fluid intake
Dysuria	Urinary tract infection
Absence of fetal movement	Maternal medication, obesity, fetal death

system. Avoid stereotyping clients simply by asking each woman about her expectations for the antepartal period. Although many women's responses may reflect what are thought to be traditional norms, other women will have decidedly different views or expectations that represent a blending of beliefs or cultures. During the antepartal period, it is also essential to begin assessing the readiness of the woman and her partner (if possible) to assume their responsibilities as parents successfully.

SUBSEQUENT PRENATAL ASSESSMENT

The "Assessment Guide: Subsequent Prenatal Assessment" provides a systematic approach to the regular physical examinations the pregnant woman should undergo for optimal antepartal care and also provides a model for evaluating both the pregnant woman and the expectant father, if he is involved in the pregnancy.

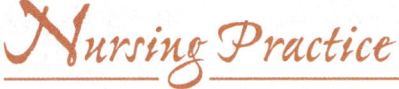

When assessing blood pressure, have the pregnant woman sit up with her arm resting on a table so that her arm is at the level of her heart. Expect a decrease in blood pressure from baseline during the second trimester because of typical physiologic changes. If the decrease does not occur, evaluate further for signs of preeclampsia.

Physical Assessment/Normal Findings	Alterations and Possible Causes*	Nursing Responses to Data†
VITAL SIGNS		
Temperature: 36.2–37.6 °C (98–99.6 °F)	Elevated temperature (infection)	Evaluate for signs of infection. Refer to physician.
Pulse: 60–90/min Rate may increase 10 beats/min during pregnancy	Increase pulse rate (anxiety, cardiac disorders)	Note irregularities. Assess for anxiety and stress.
Respiration: 16–24/min.	Marked tachypnea or abnormal patterns (respiratory disease)	Refer to physician.
Blood pressure: 90–140/60–90 (falls in second trimester)	>140/90 or increase of 30 mm systolic and 15 mm diastolic (PIH)	Assess for edema, proteinuria, and hyperreflexia. Refer to physician. Schedule appointments more frequently.
WEIGHT GAIN		
First trimester: 1.6–2.3 kg (3.5–5 lb) *Second trimester:* 5.5–6.8 kg (12–15 lb) *Third trimester:* 5.5–6.8 kg (12–15 lb)	Inadequate weight gain (poor nutrition, nausea, IUGR) Excessive weight gain (excessive caloric intake, edema, preeclampsia)	Discuss appropriate weight gain. Provide nutritional counseling. Assess for presence of edema or anemia.
EDEMA		
Small amount of dependent edema, especially in last weeks of pregnancy	Edema in hands, face, legs, and feet (preeclampsia)	Identify any correlation between edema and activities, blood pressure, or proteinuria. Refer to physician if indicated.
UTERINE SIZE		
See Assessment Guide: Initial Prenatal Assessment for normal changes during pregnancy	Unusually rapid growth (multiple gestation, hydatidiform mole, hydramnios, miscalculation of EDB)	Evaluate fetal status. Determine height of fundus (page 172). Use diagnostic ultrasound.
FETAL HEARTBEAT		
120–160/min Funic souffle	Absence of fetal heartbeat after 20 weeks' gestation (maternal obesity, fetal demise)	Evaluate fetal status.
LABORATORY EVALUATION		
Hemoglobin: 12–16 g/dL Pseudoanemia of pregnancy	<12 g/dL (anemia)	Provide nutritional counseling. Hemoglobin is repeated at 7 months' gestation. Women of Mediterranean heritage need a close check on hemoglobin because of possibility of thalassemia.
Triple screen (also called multiple marker screening [MMS]) serum test done at 16–18 weeks' gestation. Evaluates three factors—maternal serum alpha-fetoprotein (MSAFP), estriol, and hCG: normal levels	Evaluated MSAFP (neural tube defect, underestimated gestational age, multiple gestation, Rh disease). Low level (trisomy 21 [Down syndrome], trisomy 18). Elevated hCG combined with lower than normal estriol and MSAFP (Down syndrome) (ACOG, 2000)	Refer to physician.
Indirect Coombs test done on Rh—women: Negative (done at 28 weeks' gestation)	Rh antibodies present (maternal sensitization has occurred)	If Rh—and unsensitized, RhIgG prophylaxis given (see Chapter 13). If Rh antibodies present, RhIgG *not* given; fetus monitored closely for isoimmune hemolytic disease.
	*Possible causes of alterations are placed in parentheses.	†This column provides guidelines for further assessment and initial nursing intervention.

Physical Assessment/Normal Findings	Alterations and Possible Causes*	Nursing Responses to Data†
LABORATORY EVALUATION		
50-g 1-hour glucose screen (done between 24 and 28 weeks' gestation)	Plasma glucose level > 140 mg/dL (gestational diabetes mellitus [GDM]) *Note:* Some facilities use level > 130 mg/dL, which identifies 90% of women with GDM (American Diabetes Association, 2000)	Discuss implications of GDM. Refer for a diagnostic 100-g oral glucose tolerance test.
Urinalysis: See Assessment Guide: Initial Prenatal Assessment for normal findings	See Assessment Guide: Initial Prenatal Assessment for deviations	Repeat urinalysis at 7 months' gestation. Repeat dipstick test at each visit.
Protein: Negative	Proteinuria, albuminuria (contamination by vaginal discharge, urinary tract infection, preeclampsia)	Obtain dipstick urine sample. Refer to physician if deviations are present.
Glucose: Negative *Note:* Glycosuria may be present due to physiologic alterations in glomerular filtrations rate and renal threshold	Persistent glycosuria (diabetes mellitus)	Refer to physician.
Screening for Group B streptococcal disease (GBS) (Rectal and vaginal cultures obtained at 35–37 weeks' gestation)	GBS disease in mother increases risk of GBS in the newborn.	Refer to CNM or physician. If results positive, woman is offered antibiotic therapy in the intrapartal period. Therapy must be administered at least 4 hours before childbirth for maximum effectiveness (Mead, 1999).

Cultural Assessment	Variations to Consider*	Nursing Responses to Data†
Determine the mother's (and family's) attitudes about the sex of the unborn child.	Some women have no preference about the sex of the child; others do. In many cultures, boys are especially valued as firstborn children.	Provide opportunities to discuss preferences and expectations; avoid a judgmental attitude to the response.
Ask about the woman's expectations of childbirth. Will she want someone with her for the birth? Whom does she choose? What is the role of her partner?	Some women want their partner present for labor and birth; others prefer a female relative or friend. Some women expect to be separated from their partner once cervical dilatation has occurred (Andrews & Boyle, 1998).	Provide information on birth options but accept the woman's decision about who will attend. Explore reasons for not preparing for the baby. Support the mother's preferences and provide information about possible sources of assistance if the decision is related to a lack of resources.
Ask about preparations for the baby. Determine what is customary for the woman.	Some women may have a fully prepared nursery; others may not have a separate room for the baby.	

Psychosocial Assessment	Variations to Consider*	Nursing Responses to Data †
EXPECTANT MOTHER		
Psychologic status *First trimester:* Incorporates idea of pregnancy; may feel ambivalent, especially if she must give up desired role; usually looks for signs of verification of pregnancy, such as increase in abdominal size or fetal movement	Increased stress and anxiety Inability to establish communication; inability to accept pregnancy; inappropriate response or actions; denial of pregnancy; inability to cope	Encourage woman to take an active part in her care. Establish lines of communication. Establish a trusting relationship. Counsel as necessary. Refer to appropriate professional as needed.
Second trimester: Baby becomes more real to woman as abdominal size increases and she feels movement; she begins to turn inward, becoming more introspective		
Third trimester: Begins to think of baby as separate being; may feel restless and may feel that time of labor will never come; remains self-centered and concentrates on preparing place for baby		
	*Possible causes of alterations are placed in parentheses.	†This column provides guidelines for further assessment and initial nursing intervention.

(continued)

Physical Assessment/Normal Findings	Alterations and Possible Causes*	Nursing Responses to Data†
EXPECTANT MOTHER *continued*		
Educational Needs	Inadequate information	Provide information and counseling.
Self-care measures and knowledge about the following:		
Health promotion		
Breast care		
Hygiene		
Rest		
Exercise		
Nutrition		
Relief measures for common discomforts of pregnancy		
Danger signs in pregnancy (Table 8–2, page 175)		
Sexual activity: Woman knows how pregnancy affects sexual activity	Lack of information about effects of pregnancy and/or alternative positions during sexual intercourse	Provide counseling.
Preparation for parenting: Appropriate preparation	Lack of preparation (denial, failure to adjust to baby, unwanted child)	Counsel. If lack of preparation is due to inadequacy of information, provide information (Chapter 9). 🔗
Preparatin for Childbirth *Client aware of the following:*		If couple chooses particular technique, refer to classes (see Chapter 6 for description of childbirth preparation techniques). 🔗
1. Prepared childbirth techniques		Encourage prenatal class attendance.
2. Normal processes and changes during childbirth.		Educate woman during visits based on current physical status. Provide reading list for more specific information.
3. Problems that may occur as a result of drug and alcohol use and of smoking	Continued abuse of drugs and alcohol; denial of possible effect on self and baby	Review danger signs that were presented on initial visit.
Woman has met other physician or nurse-midwife who may be attending her birth in the absence of primary caregiver	Introduction of new individual at birth may increase stress and anxiety for woman and partner	Introduce woman to all members of group practice.
	***Possible causes of alterations are placed in parentheses.**	**†This column provides guidelines for further assessment and initial nursing intervention.**

The recommended frequency of antepartal visits in an uncomplicated pregnancy is as follows:

- Every 4 weeks for the first 28 weeks' gestation
- Every 2 weeks until 36 weeks' gestation
- After week 36, every week until childbirth

During the subsequent antepartal assessments, most women demonstrate ongoing psychologic adjustment to pregnancy. However, some women may exhibit signs of possible psychologic problems such as the following:

- Increasing anxiety
- Inability to establish communication
- Inappropriate responses or actions
- Denial of pregnancy
- Inability to cope with stress
- Intense preoccupation with the sex of the baby
- Failure to acknowledge quickening
- Failure to plan and prepare for the baby (e.g., living arrangements, clothing, and feeding methods)
- Indications of substance abuse

If the woman's behavior indicates possible psychologic problems, the nurse can provide ongoing support and counseling and also refer the woman to appropriate professionals.

Physical Assessment/Normal Findings	Alterations and Possible Causes*	Nursing Responses to Data†
EXPECTANT FATHER		
Impending Labor	Lack of information	Provide appropriate teaching, stressing importance of seeking appropriate medical assistance.
Client knows signs of impending labor:		
1. Uterine contractions that increase in frequency, duration, and intensity		
2. Bloody show		
3. Expulsion of mucous plug		
4. Rupture of membranes		
EXPECTANT FATHER		
Psychologic Status		
First trimester: May express excitement over confirmation of pregnancy and of his virility; concerns move toward providing for financial needs; energetic, may identify with some discomfortsof pregnancy and may even exhibit symptoms	Increasing stress and anxiety; inability to establish communication; inability to accept pregnancy diagnosis; withdrawal of support; abandonment of the mother	Encourage expectant father to come to prenatal visits. Establish lines of communication. Establish trusting relationship.
Second trimester: May feel more confident and be less concerned with financial matters; may have concerns about wife's changing size and shape, her increasing introspection		Counsel. Let expectant father know that it is normal for him to experience these feelings.
Third trimester: May have feelings of rivalry with fetus, especially during sexual activity; may make changes in his physical appearance and exhibit more interest in himself; may become more energetic; fantasizes about child but usually imagines older child; fears mutilation and death of woman and child		Include expectant father in pregnancy activities as he desires. Provide education, information, and support. Increasing numbers of expectant fathers are demonstrating desire to be involved in many or all aspects of prenatal care, education, and preparation.
	*Possible causes of alterations are placed in parentheses.	†This column provides guidelines for further assessment and initial nursing intervention.

CHAPTER HIGHLIGHTS

〰 A complete history forms the basis of prenatal care and is reevaluated and updated as necessary throughout the pregnancy.

〰 The initial prenatal assessment is a careful and thorough physical examination and cultural and psychosocial assessment designed to identify variations and potential risk factors.

〰 Laboratory tests completed at the initial visit, such as a complete blood count, ABO and Rh blood typing, hepatitis B screen, urinalysis, Pap smear, gonorrhea culture, rubella titer, and various blood screens, provide information about the woman's health during early pregnancy and also help detect potential problems.

〰 The estimated date of birth (EDB) can be calculated by using Nägele's rule. Using this approach, one begins with the first day of the last menstrual period (LMP), subtracts 3 months, and adds 7 days. A gestational calculator or "wheel" may also be used to calculate the EDB.

〰 Accuracy of the EDB may be evaluated by physical exam to assess uterine size, measurement of fundal height, and ultrasound. Perception of quickening and auscultation of fetal heartbeat are also helpful in confirming the gestation of a pregnancy.

〰 The diagonal conjugate is the distance from the lower posterior border of the symphysis pubis to the sacral promontory. The obstetric conjugate is estimated by subtracting 1.5 cm from the length of the diagonal conjugate.

〰 The nurse begins evaluating the woman psychosocially during the initial prenatal assessment. This assessment continues and is modified throughout the pregnancy.

〰 Religious, cultural, and ethnic beliefs may strongly influence the woman's attitudes and apparent cooperation with care during pregnancy.

EXPLOREMediaLink

NCLEX Review, Case Studies, and other interactive resources for this chapter can be found on the companion website at http://www.prenhall.com/london. Click on "Chapter 8" to select the activities for this chapter.

For animations, more NCLEX review questions, and an audio glossary, access the accompanying CD-ROM in this textbook.

REFERENCES

American College of Obstetricians and Gynecologists (ACOG). (2000). *Planning your pregnancy and birth* (3rd ed.). Washington, DC: Author.

American Diabetes Association. (2000). Position statement: Gestational diabetes mellitus. *Diabetes Care, 23*(Suppl. 1), 1–6.

Andrews, M. M., & Boyle, J. S. (1998). *Transcultural concepts in nursing care* (2nd ed.). Glenview, IL: Scott, Foresman/Little, Brown.

Cunningham, F. G., Grant, N. F., Leveno, K. J., Gilstrap, L. C., III, Hauth, J. C., & Wenstrom, K. D. (2001). *Williams Obstetrics* (21st ed.) New York: McGraw-Hill.

Mead, P. B. (1999). Perinatal GBS: Guidelines worth following. *Contemporary Pediatrics, 16*(1), 67–79.

Varney, H. (1997). *Varney's midwifery* (3rd ed.). Sudbury, MA: Jones and Bartlett.

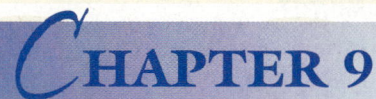

CHAPTER 9

The Expectant Family: Needs and Care

We have what I guess you would call a blended family. I have two college-age sons from my first marriage, and my wife has a 12-year-old boy. She is expecting our first child now. Because she is 38, she had an amniocentesis done and we know that this baby is a girl. How excited we all are! I don't think anything could have done more to unite us as a new family. Now if we can just agree on a name.

—RICARDO, 46

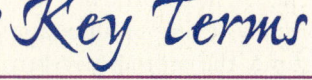
Key Terms

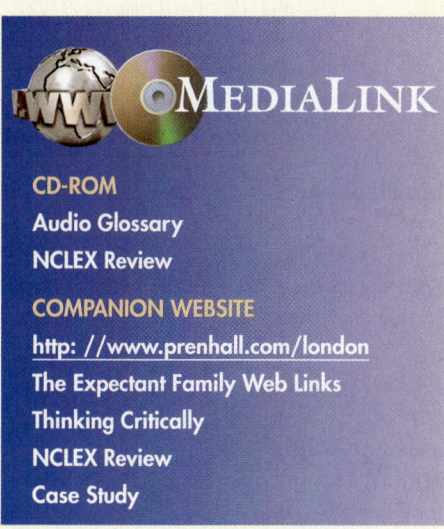

MediaLink

CD-ROM
Audio Glossary
NCLEX Review

COMPANION WEBSITE
http://www.prenhall.com/london
The Expectant Family Web Links
Thinking Critically
NCLEX Review
Case Study

$\mathscr{F}$rom the moment a woman finds out she is pregnant, she faces a future marked by dramatic changes—changes in her appearance, in her relationships, and in her psychologic state. In coping with these changes, she and her loved ones need to make adjustments in their daily lives.

Nurses caring for pregnant women need an up-to-date understanding of pregnancy to be effective in implementing the nursing process as they plan and provide care. With this in mind, Chapter 7 provided a database for the nurse by presenting material related to the normal physical, social, cultural, and psychologic changes of pregnancy. Chapter 8 then used that database to begin discussing nursing care management by focusing on assessment. This chapter further addresses nursing care management as it relates to the needs of the expectant woman and her loved ones.

Nursing Management

Nursing Diagnosis During Pregnancy

The nurse may see a pregnant woman only once every 3 to 4 weeks during the first several months of her pregnancy. Therefore a written care plan or critical path that incorporates the database, nursing diagnoses, and client goals is essential to ensure continuity of care.

The nurse can anticipate that, for many women with a low-risk pregnancy, certain nursing diagnoses will be made more frequently than others. The diagnoses will, of course, vary from woman to woman and according to the time in the pregnancy. After formulating an appropriate diagnosis, the nurse and woman establish related goals to guide the nursing plan and interventions.

Planning and Implementation During Pregnancy

Once nursing diagnoses have been identified, the next step is to establish priorities of nursing care. Sometimes priorities of care are based on the most immediate needs or concerns expressed by the woman. For example, during the first trimester, when she is experiencing nausea or is concerned about sexual intimacy with her partner, the woman is not likely to want to hear about labor and birth. At other times, priorities may develop from findings during a prenatal examination. For example, a woman who is showing signs of preeclampsia (a pregnancy complication discussed in Chapter 13) may feel physically well and find it hard to accept the nurse's emphasis on the need for frequent rest periods. It then becomes the responsibility of medical and nursing professionals to help the woman and her family to understand the significance of a problem and to plan interventions to deal with it.

NURSING CARE IN THE COMMUNITY

Prenatal care, especially for women with low-risk pregnancies, is community based, typically in a clinic or a private office. The health care community recognizes the value of providing a primary care nurse in these settings to coordinate holistic care for each childbearing family. The nurse in a clinic or health maintenance organization may be the only source of continuity for the woman, who may see a different physician or certified nurse-midwife at each visit. The nurse can be extremely effective in working with the expectant family by answering their questions; providing complete information about pregnancy, prenatal health care activities, and community resources; and supporting the health care activities of the woman and her family. Communities often have a wealth of services and educational opportunities available for pregnant women and their families, and the knowledgeable nurse can help expectant mothers to assess and access these services.

Throughout the prenatal period, the nurse shares information with the family, both verbally and through written materials. The nurse also provides anticipatory guidance to help the family plan for changes that will occur after childbirth. The nurse encourages the expectant couple to identify and discuss issues that could be sources of postpartal stress. Issues to be addressed beforehand may include the sharing of infant and household chores, help in the first few days after childbirth, options for baby-sitting to allow the mother (and couple) some free time, the mother's return to work after the baby's birth, and sibling rivalry. Couples resolve these issues in different ways, but postpartal adjustment tends to be easier for couples who agree on the issues beforehand than for couples who do not confront and resolve these issues.

HOME CARE

Home care can be of benefit to any pregnant woman, but it is especially effective in removing barriers for women who have difficulty accessing health care. These barriers may include lack of locally available health care facilities, problems with transportation to the facility, or schedule conflicts with available appointment times because of employment hours or family responsibilities.

In-home nursing assessments vary according to the experience and preparation of the nurse and include current history, vital signs, weight, urine screen, physical activity, dietary intake, reflexes, tests of fetal well-being, and cervical examinations, if indicated. Once the assessments are completed, the nurse can determine the level of follow-up home care or telephone contact needed. See Chapter 29 for further discussion of home care of the childbearing family.

Currently, home care is most often used for women with prenatal complications that can be managed without hospitalization if effective nursing assessment and care are provided in the home (see Chapters 12 and 13).

CARE OF THE EXPECTANT FATHER AND SIBLINGS

The well-being of the pregnant woman is intertwined with the well-being of those to whom she is closest. Thus, the nurse also addresses the needs of the woman's family. Although the expectant father is often involved in the pregnancy, his presence cannot be assumed. If he is not part of the family structure, it is important to assess the woman's support system to determine which significant people in her life will play a major role during this childbearing experience.

Anticipatory guidance of the expectant father, if he is involved in the pregnancy, is a necessary part of any plan of care. He may need information about the anatomic, physiologic, and emotional changes that occur for both the expectant mother and father during and after pregnancy, the couple's sexuality and sexual response, and the reactions that he is experiencing. He may wish to express his feelings about the sex of the child, his ability to parent, and other topics.

If it is culturally acceptable to the couple and personally acceptable to the expectant father, refer the couple to expectant parents' classes. These classes provide valuable information about pregnancy and childbirth, using a variety of teaching strategies such as discussion, films, demonstrations with educational models, and written handouts. Some classes even give the father the opportunity to get a "feel" for pregnancy by wearing a pregnancy simulator (Figure 9–1 ◆). Such classes also offer the couple an opportunity to gain support from other couples.

The nurse assesses the father's intended degree of participation during labor and birth and his knowledge of what to expect. If the couple prefers that his participation

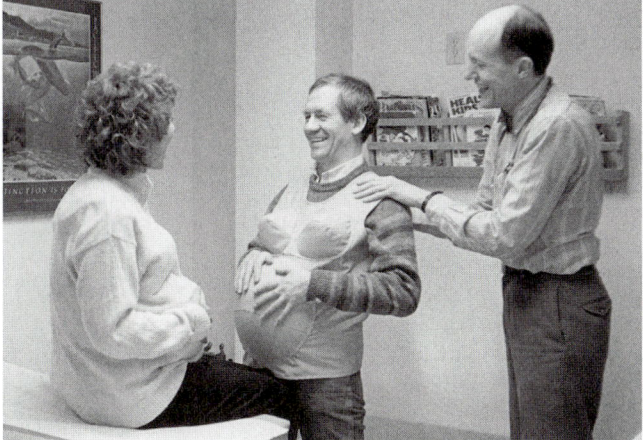

FIGURE 9–1. ◆ The Empathy Belly® is a pregnancy simulator that allows males and females to experience some of the symptoms of pregnancy. The "belly," which weighs 33 lb, produces symptoms such as shortness of breath, bladder pressure, shift in the center of gravity with resulting waddling gait, increased lordosis and backache, and fatigue. It also can simulate fetal kicking movements. *Note:* From Birthways Childbirth Resource Center.

be minimal or restricted, support the decision. With this type of consideration and collaboration, the father is less apt to develop feelings of alienation, helplessness, and guilt during the pregnancy. As the couple's relationship is strengthened and the father's self-esteem raised, he is better able to provide physical and emotional support to his partner during labor and birth.

In the plan for prenatal care, the nurse also incorporates a discussion about the negative feelings older children may develop. Parents may be distressed to see an older child become aggressive toward the newborn. Parents who are unprepared for the older child's feelings of anger, jealousy, and rejection may respond inappropriately in their confusion and surprise. The nurse emphasizes that open communication between parents and children (or acting out feelings with a doll if the child is too young to verbalize) helps children master their feelings. Children may feel less neglected and more secure if they know that their parents are willing to help with their anger and aggressiveness.

COMMON DISCOMFORTS OF PREGNANCY

The common discomforts of pregnancy result from physiologic and anatomic changes and are fairly specific to each of the three trimesters. Table 9–1 identifies the common discomforts of pregnancy, their possible causes, and self-care measures that often help relieve the discomfort.

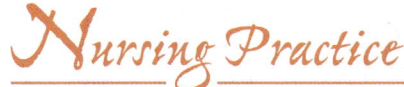

At each prenatal visit, focus your teaching on changes or possible discomforts the woman might encounter during the coming month and the next trimester. If the pregnancy is progressing normally, spend a few minutes describing her baby at this stage of development.

First Trimester

NAUSEA AND VOMITING

Nausea and vomiting are early, very common symptoms in pregnancy. These symptoms appear sometime after the first missed menstrual period and usually cease by the fourth missed menstrual period. Some women develop an aversion to specific foods, many experience nausea when they get up in the morning, and others experience nausea throughout the day or in the evening.

The exact cause of nausea and vomiting of pregnancy is unknown, but it is thought to be multifactorial. An elevated human chorionic gonadotropin (hCG) level is believed to be a major factor, but changes in carbohydrate metabolism, fatigue, and emotional factors may also play a role.

TABLE 9-1   Self-Care Measures for Common Discomforts of Pregnancy

Discomfort	Influencing Factors	Self-Care Measures
FIRST TRIMESTER		
Nausea and vomiting	Increased levels of human chorionic gonadotropin Changes in carbohydrate metabolism Emotional factors Fatigue	Avoid odors or causative factors. Eat dry crackers or toast before arising in morning. Have small but frequent meals. Avoid greasy or highly seasoned foods. Take dry meals with fluids between meals. Drink carbonated beverages.
Urinary frequency	Pressure of uterus on bladder in both first and third trimesters	Void when urge is felt. Increase fluid intake during the day. Decrease fluid intake *only* in the evening to decrease nocturia.
Fatigue	Specific causative factors unknown May be aggravated by nocturia due to urinary frequency	Plan time for a nap or rest period daily. Go to bed earlier. Seek family support and assistance with responsibilities so that more time is available to rest.
Breast tenderness	Increased levels of estrogen and progesterone	Wear well-fitting, supportive bra.
Increased vaginal discharge	Hyperplasia of vaginal mucosa and increased production of mucus by the endocervical glands due to the increase in estrogen levels	Promote cleanliness by daily bathing. Avoid douching, nylon underpants, and pantynose; cotton underpants are more absorbent; powder can be used to maintain dryness if not allowed to cake.
Nasal stuffiness and nosebleed (epistaxis)	Elevated estrogen levels	May be unresponsive, but cool-air vaporizer may help; avoid use of nasal sprays and decongestants.
Ptyalism (excessive, often bitter salivation)	Specific causative factors unknown	Use astringent mouthwashes, chew gum, or stuck hard candy.
SECOND AND THIRD TRIMESTERS		
Heartburn (pyrosis)	Increased production of progesterone, decreasing gastrointestinal motility and increasing relaxation of cardiac sphincter, displacement of stomach by enlarging uterus, thus regurgitation of acidic gastric contents into the esophagus	Eat small and more frequent meals. Use low-sodium antacids. Avoid overeating, fatty and fried foods, lying down after eating, and sodium bicarbonate.
Ankle edema	Prolonged standing or sitting Increased levels of sodium due to hormonal influences Circulatory congestion of lower extremities Increased capillary permeability Varicose veins	Practice frequent dorsiflexion of feet when prolonged sitting or standing is necessary. Elevate legs when sitting or resting. Avoid tight garters or restrictive bands around legs.
Varicose veins	Venous congestion in the lower veins that increases with pregnancy Hereditary factors (weakening of walls of veins, faulty valves) Increased age and weight gain	Elevate legs frequently. Wear supportive hose. Avoid crossing legs at the knees, standing for long periods, garters, and hosiery with constrictive bands.

In addition to common self-care measures (see "Complementary Care: Ginger and Acupressure for Morning Sickness"), some women find 25 mg of pyridoxine (vitamin B$_6$) taken three times a day helpful in reducing symptoms; if B$_6$ is not effective, caregivers often recommend doxylamine (Unisom), an over-the-counter antihistamine (Chez & Niebyl, 2000). Advise a woman to contact her health care provider if she vomits more than once a day or shows signs of dehydration such as dry mouth and concentrated urine. In such cases, the physician/certified nurse-midwife might order an antiemetic. However, antiemetics should be avoided if possible during this time because of possible harmful effects on embryo development.

URINARY FREQUENCY

Urinary frequency, a common discomfort of pregnancy, occurs early in pregnancy and again during the third trimester because the enlarging uterus puts pressure on the bladder. Although frequency is considered normal during the first and third trimesters, advise the woman to tell her health care provider about signs of bladder infection such as pain, burning with voiding, or blood in the urine. Fluid

Discomfort	Influencing Factors	Self-Care Measures
SECOND AND THIRD TRIMESTERS		
Hemorrhoids	Constipation (see following discussion) Increased pressure from gravid uterus on hemorrhoidal veins	Avoid constipation. Apply ice packs, topical ointments, anesthetic agents, warm soaks, or sitz baths; gently reinsert into rectum as necessary.
Constipation	Increased levels of progesterone, which cause general bowel sluggishness Pressure of enlarging uterus on intestine Iron supplements Diet, lack of exercise, and decreased fluids	Increase fluid intake, fiber in the diet, and exercise. Develop regular bowel habits. Use stool softeners as recommended by physician.
Backache	Increased curvature of the lumbosacral vertebrae as the uterus enlarges Increased levels of hormones, which cause softening of cartilage in body joints Fatigue Poor body mechanics	Use proper body mechanics. Practice the pelvic—tilt exercise. Avoid uncomfortable working heights, high-heeled shoes, lifting heavy loads, and fatigue.
Leg cramps	Imbalance of calcium/phosphorous ratio Increased pressure of uterus on nerves Fatigue Poor circulation to lower extremities Pointing the toes	Practice dorsiflexion of feet to stretch affected muscle. Evaluate diet. Apply heat to affected muscles. Arise slowly from resting position.
Faintness	Postural hypotension Sudden change of position causing venous pooling in dependent veins Standing for long periods in warm area Anemia	Avoid prolonged standing in warm or stuffy environments. Evaluate hematocrit and hemoglobin.
Dyspnea	Decreased vital capacity from pressure of enlarging uterus on the diaphragm	Use proper posture when sitting and standing. Sleep propped up with pillows for relief if problem occurs at night.
Flatulence	Decrease gastrointestinal motility leading to delayed emptying time Pressure of growing uterus on large intestine Air swallowing	Avoid gas-forming foods. Chew food thoroughly. Get regular daily exercise. Maintain normal bowel habits.
Carpal tunnel syndrome	Compression of median nerve in carpal tunnel of wrist Aggravated by repetitive hand movements	Avoid aggravating hand movements. Use splint as prescribed. Elevate affected arm.

Complementary Care

GINGER AND ACUPRESSURE FOR MORNING SICKNESS

Ginger and acupressure are among the most frequently used alternative therapies for the nausea and vomiting of morning sickness.

Ginger: Ginger is widely used in traditional Chinese medicine but without contraindications in pregnancy (Blumenthal et al., 2000). Many clinical trials have confirmed the effectiveness and safety of ginger (Aikins Murphy, 1998; Fulder & Tenne, 1996; Jewell & Young, 2000; Vutyavanich, Kraisarin, & Ruangsri, 2001; Weidner & Sigwart, 2001); yet Skidmore-Roth (2001) cites that it is an abortifacient (abortion-inducing) when used in large doses. Although no specific clinical studies are cited in this latter source, ginger should be used with caution during pregnancy, and the dosage should not exceed 1 g of dried root daily (Hardy,

2000). Ginger is available in many forms, including capsules, candied, or as a tea. See "Complementary and Alternative Therapies" later in this chapter for more information on the use of herbs during pregnancy. Also, refer to Table 9–3.

Acupressure: Acupressure, like acupuncture, is a therapy based on the ancient philosophy of traditional Chinese medicine. Acupressure involves the application of pressure using fingers or thumbs to stimulate and balance the body's healing energy known by the Chinese as chi. A specific acupressure point that relieves nausea is located on the forearm, three fingerwidths above the wrist closest to the palm, toward the elbow. The point is pressed firmly for 30 seconds every couple of minutes (Gottlieb, 2000). A motion sickness wristband (brand names include Sea-Band and Acuband) can be purchased that puts gentle pressure on this acupressure point (Steele, French, Gatherer-Boyles, et al., 2001).

intake should never be decreased to prevent frequency. The woman needs to maintain an adequate fluid intake—at least, 2,000 mL (8 to 10 8-oz glasses) per day. Also, encourage her to empty her bladder frequently (about every 2 hours while awake).

FATIGUE

Marked fatigue is so common in early pregnancy that it is considered a presumptive sign of pregnancy. It is aggravated if the woman cannot sleep through the night because of urinary frequency. Typically it resolves after the end of the first trimester.

BREAST TENDERNESS

Sensitivity of the breasts occurs early and continues throughout the pregnancy. Increased levels of estrogen and progesterone contribute to soreness and tingling of the breasts and increased sensitivity of the nipples.

INCREASED VAGINAL DISCHARGE

Increased whitish vaginal discharge, called **leukorrhea,** is common in pregnancy. It occurs as a result of hyperplasia of the vaginal mucosa and increased mucus production by the endocervical glands. The increased acidity of the secretions encourages the growth of *Candida albicans,* so the woman is more susceptible to monilial vaginitis.

NASAL STUFFINESS AND EPISTAXIS

Once pregnancy has progressed somewhat, elevated estrogen levels may produce edema of the nasal mucosa, which results in nasal stuffiness, nasal discharge, and obstruction. Epistaxis (nosebleeds) may also result. Cool air vaporizers and normal saline nasal sprays may help, but the problem is often unresponsive to treatment. Women experiencing these problems find it difficult to sleep and may resort to using medicated nasal sprays and decongestants. Such interventions may provide initial relief but can actually increase nasal stuffiness over time. Pregnant women should avoid using any medications, if possible.

PTYALISM

Ptyalism is a rare discomfort of pregnancy in which excessive, often bitter saliva is produced. The cause is unknown, and effective treatments are limited.

Second and Third Trimesters

The discomforts discussed in this section usually do not appear until the third trimester in primigravidas but may occur earlier with each succeeding pregnancy.

HEARTBURN (PYROSIS)

Heartburn is the regurgitation of acidic gastric contents into the esophagus. It creates a burning sensation in the esophagus and sometimes leaves a bad taste in the mouth. Heartburn during pregnancy appears to be primarily a result of the displacement of the stomach by the enlarging

Complementary Care

MEADOWSWEET FOR HEARTBURN

Meadowsweet has traditionally been used as a pain reliever (the analgesic substance *salicin* was first isolated from meadowsweet leaves in 1827); it also provides relief for heartburn (Blumenthal, 2000). However, because it contains salicylates, a woman with a sensitivity to aspirin should not take meadowsweet. See "Complementary and Alternative Therapies" later in this chapter for more information on the use of herbs during pregnancy.

uterus. The increased production of progesterone in pregnancy, decreases in gastrointestinal motility, and relaxation of the cardiac (esophageal) sphincter also contribute to heartburn.

Liquid forms of low-sodium antacids are often most effective in providing relief. Advise women that antacids containing aluminum may cause constipation, and antacids containing magnesium can cause diarrhea. Let women know that they should avoid sodium bicarbonate (baking soda) and Alka-Seltzer because they may lead to electrolyte imbalance.

If maternal heartburn is severe, not relieved by antacids, and accompanied by gastrointestinal reflux, an antisecretory agent (H_2-blocker) such as ranitidine (Zantac), cimetidine (Tagamet), or omeprazole (Losec) may be helpful. Research has not linked them with an excessive risk of birth defects, preterm birth, or intrauterine growth restriction, and up to 85% of pregnant women use at least one of these medications to control acid reflux ("Good News for Pregnant Women," 1999).

ANKLE EDEMA

Most women experience ankle edema in the last part of pregnancy because of the increasing difficulty of venous return from the lower extremities. Prolonged standing or sitting and warm weather increase the edema. It is also associated with varicose veins. Ankle edema becomes a concern only when accompanied by hypertension or proteinuria or when the edema is not postural in origin.

VARICOSE VEINS

Varicose veins are a result of weakening of the walls of veins or faulty functioning of the valves. Poor circulation in the lower extremities predisposes people to varicose veins in the legs and thighs, as does prolonged standing or sitting. The pregnant uterus puts pressure on the pelvic veins, preventing good venous return, so it may aggravate existing problems or contribute to obvious changes in the veins of the legs (Figure 9–2 ◆).

Surgical correction of varicose veins is not generally recommended during pregnancy. Advise the woman that treatment may be needed after she gives birth because the problem will be aggravated by a succeeding pregnancy.

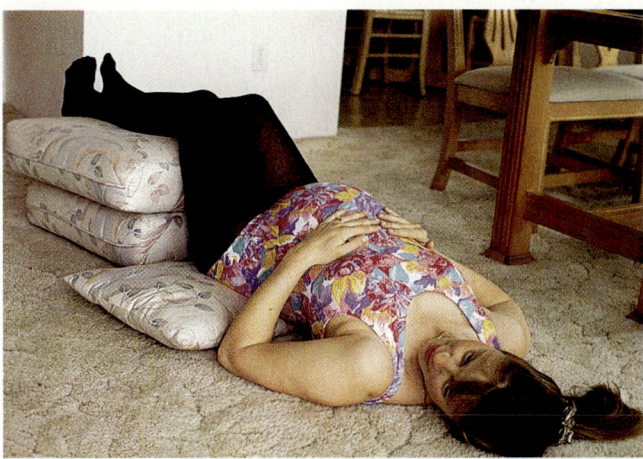

FIGURE 9–2. ◆ Swelling and discomfort from varicosities can be decreased by lying down with the legs and one hip elevated (to avoid compression of the vena cava).

Complementary Care

HORSE CHESTNUT FOR VARICOSE VEINS

Horse chestnut seed extract may be helpful in preventing or reducing varicose veins (Blumenthal, 2000; Gottlieb, 2000). It is available in oral form (capsules, tincture, etc.), as well as topical (gel) form. It is reported to combine well with other herbs that improve peripheral circulation, such as ginkgo leaf and bilberry fruit (Morgan & Bone, 1998). See "Complementary and Alternative Therapies" later in this chapter for more information on the use of herbs during pregnancy. See also Table 9–3.

Although less common, varicosities in the vulva and perineum may also develop. They produce aching and a sense of heaviness. Wearing two sanitary pads inside the underpants sometimes provides support for vulvar varicosities. A woman may relieve uterine pressure on the pelvic veins by resting on her side. Blocks placed under the foot of her bed to elevate it slightly may also help.

FLATULENCE

Flatulence results from decreased gastrointestinal motility, leading to delayed emptying, and from pressure on the large intestine by the growing uterus. Air swallowing may also contribute to the problem.

HEMORRHOIDS

Hemorrhoids are varicosities of the veins in the lower rectum and the anus. During pregnancy, the gravid uterus presses on the veins and interferes with venous circulation. In addition, the straining that accompanies constipation is frequently a contributing cause of hemorrhoids.

Some women may not be bothered by hemorrhoids until the second stage of labor, when the hemorrhoids appear as they push. These hemorrhoids usually become asymptomatic a few days after childbirth. Symptoms of hemor-

rhoids include itching, swelling, pain, and bleeding. Women who have had hemorrhoids before pregnancy will probably experience difficulties with them during pregnancy.

Some women find relief by gently reinserting the hemorrhoid. The woman lies on her side, places some lubricant on her finger, and presses against the hemorrhoids, pushing them inside. She holds them in place for 1 to 2 minutes and then gently withdraws her finger. The anal sphincter should then hold them inside the rectum. The woman will find it especially helpful if she can maintain a side-lying (Sims') position for a time, so this method is best done before bed or prior to a daily rest period.

CONSTIPATION

Conditions that predispose the pregnant woman to constipation include general bowel sluggishness caused by increased progesterone and steroid metabolism; displacement of the intestines, which increases with the growth of the fetus; and the oral iron supplements most pregnant women need. In severe or preexisting cases of constipation, the woman may need stool softeners, mild laxatives, or suppositories as recommended by her caregiver.

BACKACHE

Many pregnant women experience backache, due primarily to exaggeration of the lumbosacral curve that occurs as the uterus enlarges and becomes heavier. Maintaining good posture and using proper body mechanics throughout pregnancy can help prevent backache. Advise the pregnant woman to avoid bending over at the waist to pick up objects and to bend from the knees instead (Figure 9–3 ◆). She should place her feet 12 to 18 inches apart to maintain body balance. If the woman uses work surfaces that require her to bend, advise her to adjust the height of the surfaces.

LEG CRAMPS

Leg cramps are painful muscle spasms in the gastrocnemius muscles. They occur most often after the woman has gone to bed at night but may occur at other times. Extension of the foot can often cause leg cramps. Warn the pregnant woman not to extend the foot during childbirth preparation exercises or during rest periods. The exact cause of leg cramps is not known, but pressure of the enlarged uterus on pelvic nerves or blood vessels leading to the legs may be a contributing factor (Varney, 1997), especially during the third trimester.

Stretching provides immediate relief of the muscle spasm. With the woman lying on her back, another person presses the woman's knee down to straighten her leg while pushing her foot toward her leg. The woman may also stand and put her foot flat on the floor. Massage and warm packs can alleviate the discomfort of leg cramps (Figure 9–4 ◆). Also, a diet that includes daily portions of both calcium and phosphorus may help prevent leg cramps (Varney, 1997).

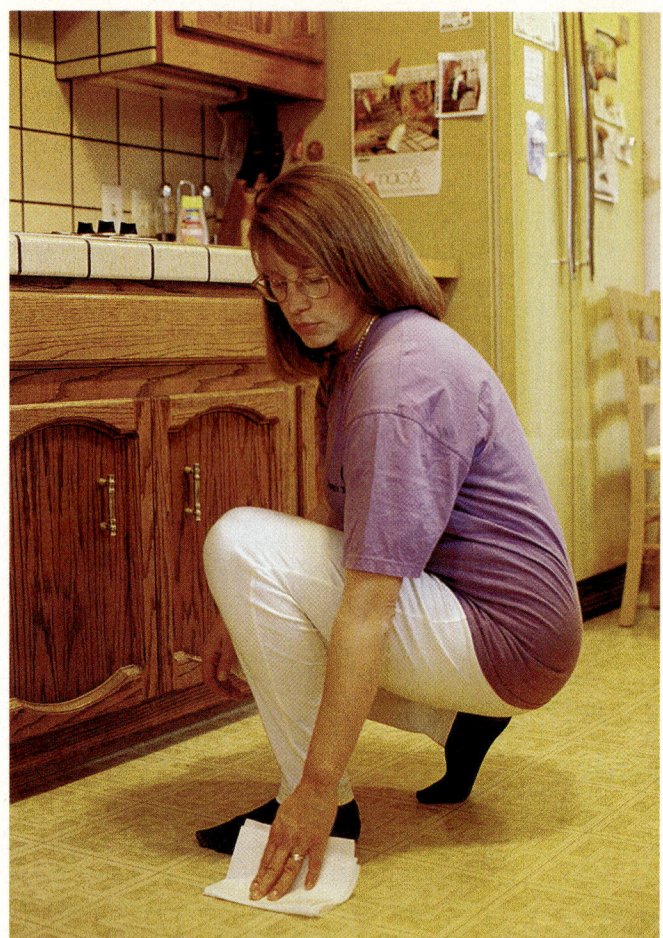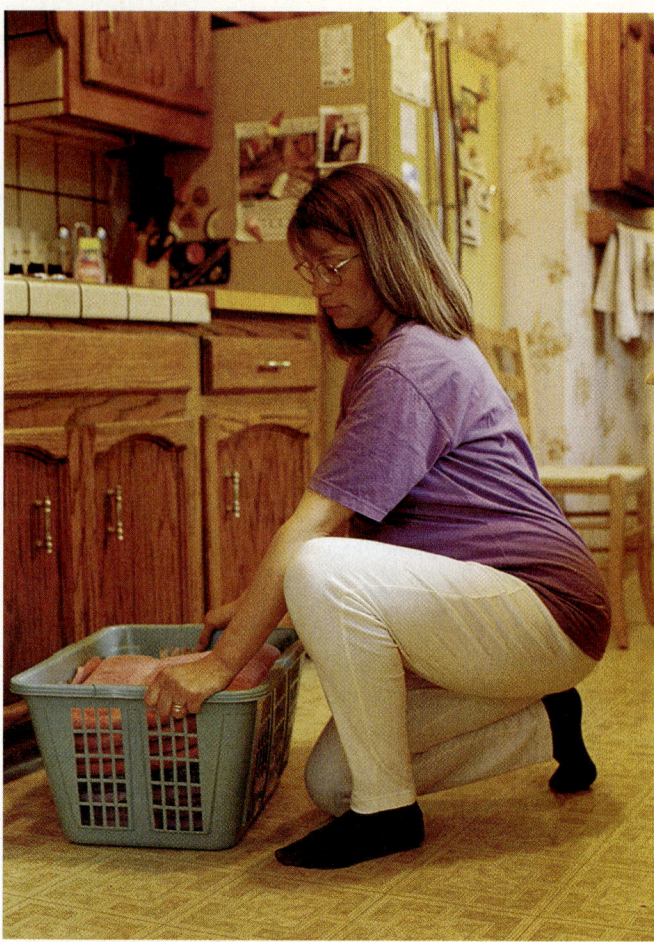

FIGURE 9–3. ◆ When picking up objects from floor level or lifting objects, the pregnant woman must use proper body mechanics.

Complementary Care

PHYSICAL MODALITIES FOR RELIEF OF BACKACHE AND OTHER PREGNANCY-RELATED MUSCULAR PAIN

Massage Therapy for Low Back Pain: Massage often helps relieve the low back pain associated with pregnancy. During the first 4 months of pregnancy, the body should be massaged with a gentle, soft touch. The best position for lumbar massage is with the woman sitting on a stool, resting her arms on a table, and leaning her forehead against her arms. The person doing the massage kneels on the floor behind her, which enhances the ability to apply an effective amount of pressure to the back muscles. 🔗 **WEB**

Yoga: Many women find that the regular practice of yoga builds and tones muscles, increases flexibility, improves endurance, and promotes a state of relaxation. One of the many applications of yoga is in pregnancy and childbirth. In fact, many of the techniques taught in childbirth classes, such as focus, relaxation, and systematic breathing, have their roots in yoga. The gentle stretching of the poses helps ease the muscle aches of pregnancy and strengthens the muscles that will be used during childbirth. The breathing techniques may lessen the shortness of breath that often accompanies advanced pregnancy.

Yoga practiced while pregnant is slightly different from regular yoga in that some poses are contraindicated. These poses are the extreme stretching positions and any position that puts pressure on the uterus. Full forward bends will probably be uncomfortable for both woman and baby. A woman's center of balance has shifted completely, and thus she must be careful with balance poses. Pregnant women should never lie on the stomach for any pose. If any pose feels uncomfortable, the woman should stop at once. If she experiences dizziness, sudden swelling, extreme shortness of breath, or vaginal bleeding, she should see her midwife or doctor immediately.

Reflexology for Sciatica: Reflexology is a field of therapy that uses specific touch techniques to stimulate "reflex points and areas" on the feet, hands, and ears. Reflexologists believe that each of these points corresponds to a specific part of the body. The growing baby can put pressure on the large sciatic nerve. The pressure inflames the nerve, causing severe lower back pain that radiates into the legs. Reflexology may help this condition. The reflex points for the sciatic nerve are on the heel. A woman in her second or third trimester can press gently and release with her thumbs to stimulate first one whole heel, then the other. Each heel can be worked for a minute or two twice a day until the pain is gone.

Women who are in the first trimester of pregnancy should not have reflexology that stimulates the uterine points on the hands, feet, or ears. In general, it's best for pregnant women to receive reflexology that uses light, gentle pressure (Gottlieb, 2000).

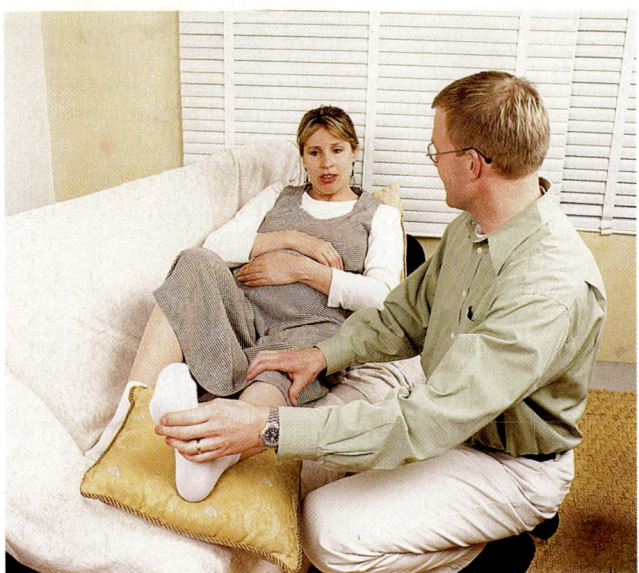

FIGURE 9–4. ◆ The expectant father can help relieve the woman's painful leg cramps by flexing her foot and straightening her leg.

FAINTNESS

Many pregnant women occasionally feel faint, especially in warm, crowded areas. Faintness is caused by a combination of changes in the blood volume and postural hypotension due to pooling of blood in the dependent veins. Sudden change of position or standing for prolonged periods can also cause this sensation, and the woman may faint.

If a woman begins to feel faint from prolonged standing or from being in a stuffy room, she should sit down and lower her head between her knees. If this procedure does not help, she should ask someone to help her to an area where she can lie down and get fresh air. Advise the woman that when getting up from a resting position, it is important to move slowly. Women whose jobs require standing in one place for long periods should march in place regularly to increase venous return from the legs.

SHORTNESS OF BREATH (DYSPNEA)

Shortness of breath occurs as the uterus rises into the abdomen and causes pressure on the diaphragm. This problem worsens in the last trimester because the enlarged uterus presses directly on the diaphragm, decreasing vital capacity. The primigravida experiences considerable relief from shortness of breath in the last few weeks of pregnancy, when **lightening** occurs, and the fetus and uterus move down in the pelvis. Because the multigravida does not usually experience lightening until labor, she tends to feel short of breath throughout the latter part of her pregnancy.

DIFFICULTY SLEEPING

Many physical factors in late pregnancy may make sleeping difficult. The enlarged uterus may make it difficult to find a comfortable position for sleep, and an active fetus may aggravate the problem. Other discomforts of pregnancy such as urinary frequency, shortness of breath, and leg cramps may also make it hard to sleep.

ROUND LIGAMENT PAIN

As the uterus enlarges during pregnancy, the round ligaments stretch and hypertrophy as the uterus rises up in the abdomen, causing pain. The woman may feel concern when she first experiences round ligament pain, because it is often intense and causes a "grabbing" sensation in the lower abdomen and inguinal area. Warn the pregnant woman of this possible discomfort. Once it has been determined that the cause of the pain is not a medical complication such as appendicitis, the woman may find that applying a heating pad to the abdomen brings relief.

CARPAL TUNNEL SYNDROME

Carpal tunnel syndrome, characterized by numbness and tingling of the hand near the thumb, occurs in about one-fourth of pregnant women (Cunningham, Gant, Leveno et al., 2001). It is caused by compression of the median nerve in the carpal tunnel of the wrist. The syndrome is aggravated by repetitive hand movements such as typing and may disappear following childbirth. Treatment usually involves splinting and avoiding aggravating movements, but surgery may be needed in severe cases if more conservative approaches are not effective.

PROMOTION OF SELF-CARE DURING PREGNANCY

Cultural Considerations in Pregnancy

As discussed in Chapter 8, actions during pregnancy are often determined by cultural beliefs. Table 9–2 presents activities encouraged or forbidden by some specific cultures. The table is not meant to be all-inclusive, nor is it meant to imply that all members of a given culture hold these beliefs. Rather, it offers a few examples of cultural activities that may be important to some clients during the prenatal period.

In working with clients of other cultures, health professionals should be open to and respectful of other beliefs. Culturally competent nurses recognize that each childbearing family, shaped by culture and life experience, has expectations of both its members and the health care system during pregnancy and birth.

Language barriers often pose a challenge in providing effective prenatal nursing care. Whenever possible it is important to have an interpreter—family member, friend, or staff person—present at prenatal visits so it is possible to provide basic information about pregnancy and prenatal care. Also give the woman chances to ask questions or express concerns. It is essential to have printed material available in the woman's language.

TABLE 9-2 Cultural Beliefs and Practices during Pregnancy

Here are a few examples of cultural beliefs and practices related to pregnancy. It is important not to make assumptions about a client's beliefs, because cultural norms vary greatly within a culture and from generation to generation. The nurse should observe the client carefully and take the time to ask questions. Clients will benefit greatly from the nurse's increased awareness of their cultural beliefs and practices.

Belief or Practice	Nursing Consideration
HOME REMEDIES Pregnant women of Native-American background may use herbal remedies. An example is the dandelion, which contains a milky juice in its stem believed to increase breast milk flow in mothers who choose to breastfeed (Spector, 2000). Clients of Chinese descent may drink ginseng tea for faintness after childbirth or as a sedative when mixed with bamboo leaves. Some people of African heritage may use self-medication for pregnancy discomforts—for example, laxatives to prevent or treat constipation (Spector, 2000).	Find out what medications and home remedies your client is using and counsel your client regarding overall effects. It is common for individuals to avoid telling health care workers about home remedies; the client may feel her use of home remedies will be judged unfavorably. Phrase your questions in a sensitive, accepting way.
NUTRITION Some women of Italian background may believe that it is necessary to satisfy desires for certain foods in order to prevent congenital anomalies. Also, they may believe that they must eat food that they smell, or else the fetus will move "inside," which will result in a miscarriage. Pregnant women of African descent may continue the tradition of eating clay, dirt, or starch, which they believe will benefit the mother and fetus (Spector, 2000). To practice *Tae Kyo,* a set of rules for safe childbirth, pregnant women of Korean descent may practice food taboos by eating particular high-quality foods and avoiding other foods believed to cause an unhealthy fetus (Choi, 1995).	Discuss the client's beliefs and practices in regard to nutrition during pregnancy. Obtain a diet history from the client. Discuss the importance of a well-balanced diet during pregnancy, with consideration of the client's cultural beliefs and practices. In some cases, you might want to suggest remedies that may be more effective—for example, eating high-fiber foods to reduce constipation. If the home remedy is not harmful, there is no reason to ask a client to discontinue this practice.
ALTERNATIVE HEALTH CARE PROVIDERS Pregnant women of Mexican background may choose to seek out the care of a *partera* (midwife) for prenatal and intrapartal care. A *partera* speaks their language, shares a similar culture, and can deliver pregnant women at home or in a birthing center instead of a hospital. Some people in Hispanic-American communities may use the *curandero,* the folk healer. The *curandero* frequently uses herbs, massage, and religious artifacts for treatment (Spector, 2000).	Discuss the variety of choices of health care providers available to the pregnant woman. Contrast the benefits and risks of different settings for prenatal care and birth. Provide reassurance that the goal of health care during pregnancy and birth is a healthy outcome for mother and baby, with respect for the specific cultural beliefs and practices of the client.
EXERCISE Pregnant women of Italian descent may fear changing their body position in certain ways because they believe doing so may cause the fetus to develop abnormally (Spector, 2000). Some people of Southeast Asian background believe that inactivity during pregnancy will result in a difficult labor (Mattson, 1995). Some people of European, African, and Mexican descent believe that reaching over the head during pregnancy can harm the baby.	Ask your client whether there are any activities she is afraid to do because of the pregnancy. Assure her that reaching over her head will not harm the baby and evaluate other activities related to their effect on the pregnancy.
SPIRITUALITY Native Americans of the Navajo tribe may meet with the medicine man 2 months prior to birth, feeling that the prayers will ensure a safe birth and healthy baby. Some people of European background may tend to pay more attention to spirituality in their life to alleviate fears and ensure a safe birth.	Encourage the use of support systems and spiritual aids that provide comfort for the mother.

In caring for pregnant women of Native-American descent, it is helpful to consider the following general points (Cesario, 2001):

➡ Because there are more than 500 federally recognized tribes in the United States, it is difficult to summarize common cultural characteristics of Native Americans.

➡ Many Native-American tribes are matrilineal. Women are respected and heeded in decision making and the children belong to the clan of their mother.

➡ Three-generation extended families are common and the grandparents and aunts and uncles often assume primary responsibility for discipline and education of the children. Thus it is important to learn whether a new mother will be the primary caregiver for her infant.

➡ Many tribes are "present-oriented," viewing events such as childbearing as part of the rhythms of life. Thus, during pregnancy a Native-American woman is often focused on the pregnancy itself and not on issues that will follow such as contraception or childrearing practices. This has implications for the focus of the teaching a nurse offers.

Fetal Activity Monitoring

Many caregivers encourage pregnant women to monitor their unborn child's well-being by regularly assessing fetal activity beginning at 28 weeks' gestation. Vigorous activity generally provides reassurance of fetal well-being, but a marked decrease in activity or cessation of movement may indicate a problem that needs immediate evaluation. Fetal activity is affected by fetal sleep, sound, time of day, blood glucose levels, cigarette smoking, and some illicit drugs such as crack and cocaine. At times a healthy fetus may be minimally active or inactive. A variety of methods for tracking fetal activity have been developed. They focus on having the woman keep a **fetal movement record** (FMR) using a technique such as the Cardiff Count-to-Ten method. An FMR is noninvasive and lets the pregnant woman monitor and record movements easily and without expense. See "Teaching About: Assessing Fetal Activity."

Breast Care

Whether the pregnant woman plans to bottle- or breast-feed her infant, support of the breasts is important to promote comfort, retain breast shape, and prevent back strain, particularly if the breasts become large and pendulous. The sensitivity of the breasts in pregnancy is often relieved by good support.

A well-fitting, supportive brassiere has the following qualities:

- The straps are wide and do not stretch (elastic straps soon lose their tautness with the weight of the breasts and frequent washing).

ASSESSING FETAL ACTIVITY

- Explain that fetal movements are first felt around 18 weeks' gestation. From that time the fetal movements get stronger and easier to detect. A slowing or stopping of fetal movement may be an indication that the fetus needs some attention and evaluation.

- Explain procedure for Cardiff Count-to-Ten method or for the daily fetal movement record. For both methods, advise the woman to
  - Beginning at about 27 weeks' gestation, keep a daily record of fetal movement.
  - Try to begin counting at about the same time each day, about 1 hour after a meal if possible.
  - Lie quietly in a side-lying position.

- Using the Cardiff card, have the woman place an X for each fetal movement until she has recorded 10. Movement varies considerably, but most women feel fetal movement at least 10 times in 3 hours (see Figure 9–5 ◆).

- Using the daily fetal movement record, have the woman count three times a day for 20 to 30 minutes each session. If there are fewer than three movements in a session, have the woman count for 1 hour or more.

- Explain when to contact the care provider:
  - If there are fewer than 10 movements in 3 hours
  - If overall the fetus's movements are slowing, and it takes much longer each day to note 10 movements
  - If there are no movements in the morning
  - If there are fewer than 3 movements in 8 hours

- Evaluate learning by having the woman explain the method and by asking the woman to fill the card in using a fictitious situation. At each prenatal visit the expectant woman's record is reviewed, and this provides another opportunity for evaluation of learning. Review of the record provides opportunities for questions and clarification.

- Describe procedures and demonstrate how to assess fetal movement. Sit beside the woman and show her how to place her hand on the fundus to feel fetal movement.

- Provide a written teaching sheet for the woman's use at home.

- Demonstrate how to record fetal movements on the Cardiff Count-to-Ten scoring card or on the daily fetal movement record.

- Watch the woman fill out the record as examples are provided. Encourage her to complete the record each day and bring it with her to each prenatal visit. Assure her that the record will be discussed at each prenatal visit, and questions may be addressed at that time if desired.

- Provide the woman with a name and phone number in case she has further questions.

- The cups hold all breast tissue comfortably.

- The brassiere has tucks or other devices that allow it to expand and accommodate the enlarging chest circumference.

- The brassiere supports the nipple line approximately midway between the elbow and shoulder but is not pulled up in the back by the weight of the breasts.

FIGURE 9–5. ◆ Fetal movement assessment method: The Cardiff Count-to-Ten scoring card (adaptation).

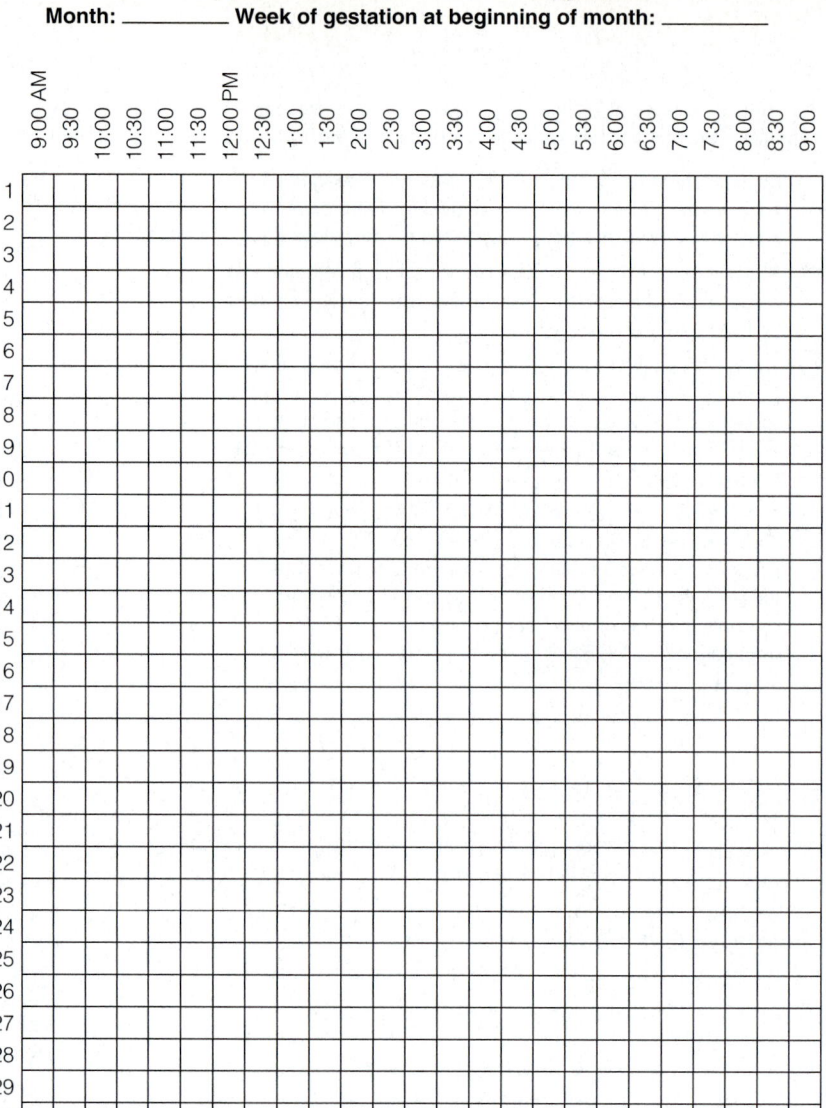

Sample Cardiff–Count–to–Ten scoring card

Month: _____ Week of gestation at beginning of month: _____

Cleanliness of the breasts is important, especially as the woman begins producing colostrum. Colostrum that crusts on the nipples can be removed with warm water. Advise the woman planning to breastfeed not to use soap on her nipples because of its drying effect.

Nipple preparation, generally begun during the third trimester, helps prevent soreness during the first few days of breastfeeding. Nipple preparation promotes the distribution of the natural lubricants produced by Montgomery's tubercles and helps develop the protective layer of skin over the nipple. Women who are planning to nurse can begin by going braless when possible and by exposing their nipples to sunlight and air. Rubbing the nipples removes protective oils and is best avoided, but rolling the nipple—grasping it between thumb and forefinger and gently rolling it for a short time each day—helps prepare for breastfeeding. However, advise women with a history of preterm labor not to use this

technique because nipple stimulation triggers the release of oxytocin. See Chapter 14 for further discussion of the effects of nipple stimulation on contractions. ⊂⊃

Nipple rolling is more difficult for women with flat or inverted nipples, but it can still be useful in preparing for breastfeeding. Breast shields designed to correct inverted nipples can be worn during pregnancy. The shields appear to be the only available measure that offers help to some women with inverted nipples (Figure 9–6 ◆). Other women gain no benefit from them (Chey & Friedman, 2000). For further discussion of inverted nipples, see Chapter 24. ⊂⊃

Oral stimulation of the nipple by the woman's partner during sex play is also an excellent technique for toughening the nipple in preparation for breastfeeding. The nurse should encourage couples who enjoy this stimulation to continue it throughout the pregnancy, except when the woman has a history of preterm labor, as discussed earlier.

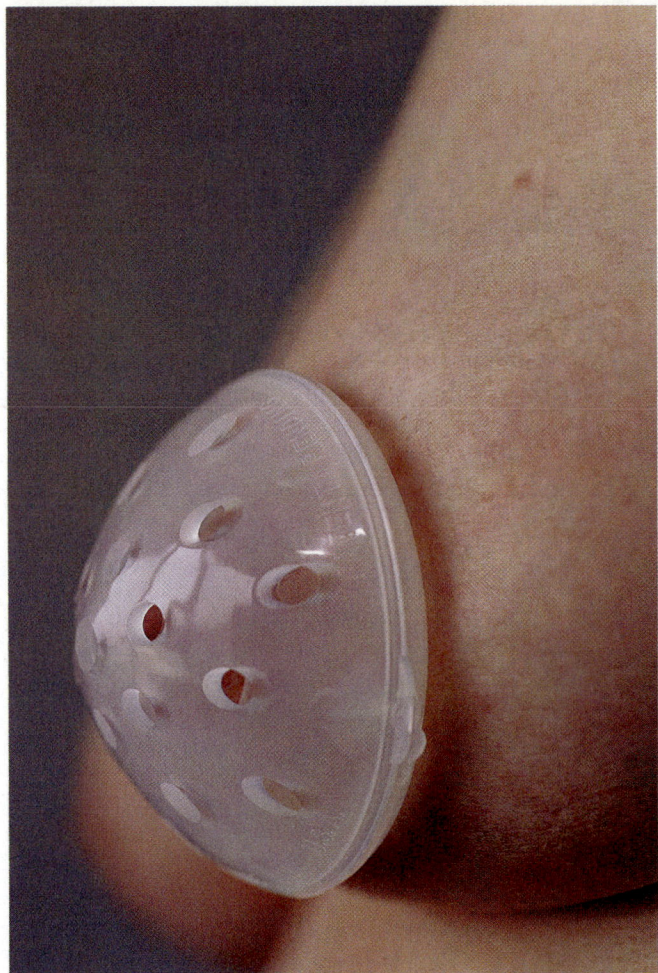

FIGURE 9-6. ◆ This breast shield is designed to increase the protractility of inverted nipples. Worn the last 3 to 4 months of pregnancy, it exerts gentle pulling pressure at the edge of the areola, gradually forcing the nipple through the center of the shield. It may be used after childbirth if still necessary.

Clothing

Clothing in pregnancy is generally an important factor in the woman's feelings about herself and her appearance. Clothes should be loose and nonconstricting. Maternity clothing can be expensive and is worn for a relatively short time, so women may economize by wearing regular clothing, sharing clothes with friends, sewing their own garments, or buying used maternity clothes.

High-heeled shoes tend to aggravate back discomfort by increasing the curvature of the lower back. Women who experience backache or have problems with balance do best to avoid them. Shoes should fit properly and feel comfortable.

Bathing

Perspiration and mucoid vaginal discharge increase during pregnancy. Keep in mind that cultural norms often influence bathing and cleansing practices. A pregnant woman may choose to cleanse only some portions of her body regularly or may elect to take showers or tub baths. Advise women to be careful in the tub because balance becomes a problem in late pregnancy. Rubber mats and hand grips are important safety devices. Also, vasodilation due to warm water may cause the woman to feel faint when she gets out of the tub, so she may need assistance, especially during the last trimester.

Employment

In general, women with low risk pregnancies can continue working until the start of labor. However, studies of women employed outside the home during pregnancy and those who do not work show distinct differences. Pregnant women whose jobs require prolonged standing have a higher incidence of preterm birth. Women with physically demanding jobs have an increased incidence of preterm birth, hypertension, and fetal growth restriction (Cunningham et al., 2001).

Overfatigue, excessive physical strain, fetotoxic hazards in the environment, and medical or obstetric complications are the major deterrents to certain types of employment during pregnancy. In the last half of pregnancy, women whose occupations involve balance should make adjustments as needed.

Fetotoxic hazards are always a concern to the expectant couple. The pregnant woman (or the woman contemplating pregnancy) who works in industry should contact her company physician or nurse about possible hazards in her work environment and should do her own reading and research on environmental hazards as well. Her partner can also find out how hazards in his workplace might affect his sperm.

Travel

Pregnant women without complications can travel as usual. Pregnant women should avoid travel if they have a history of bleeding or preeclampsia or if multiple births are anticipated.

Travel by automobile can be tiring, aggravating many of the discomforts of pregnancy. The pregnant woman needs frequent opportunities to get out of the car and walk. (A good pattern is to stop every 2 hours and walk around for about 10 minutes.) She should wear both lap and shoulder belts; the lap belt should fit snugly and be positioned under the abdomen and across the upper thighs. Seat belts help save the lives of expectant mothers and fetuses (Cunningham et al., 2001). Fetal death in car accidents is sometimes caused by placental separation (abruptio placentae) as a result of uterine distortion. Shoulder belts decrease the risk of traumatic flexion of the woman's body, making placental separation less likely.

As pregnancy progresses, long-distance trips are best taken by plane or train. Remind near-term women who travel to think about the availability of medical care at the destination.

Activity and Rest

Exercise during pregnancy helps maintain maternal fitness and muscle tone, leads to improved self-image, promotes regular bowel function, increases energy, improves sleep, relieves tension, helps control weight gain, and is associated with improved postpartum recovery. A woman with an uncomplicated pregnancy can and should continue normal participation in exercise. The woman can check with her certified nurse-midwife or physician about strenuous sports such as skiing and horseback riding. The skilled sportswoman should not usually be discouraged from participating in these activities if her pregnancy is uncomplicated. However, pregnancy is not the appropriate time to learn a new or strenuous sport.

Certain conditions contraindicate exercise. These conditions include rupture of the membranes, preeclampsia, incompetent cervix or cerclage placement, persistent vaginal bleeding, risk factors for preterm labor, evidence of intrauterine growth restriction, and chronic medical conditions that might be negatively impacted by vigorous exercise (Dickerson & Chez, 1999).

The American College of Obstetricians and Gynecologists (ACOG) has developed the following guidelines about exercise during pregnancy (ACOG, 1994):

- Even mild to moderate exercise is beneficial during pregnancy. Regular exercise, which occurs at least three times a week, is preferred.

- After the first trimester, women should avoid exercising in the supine position. In most pregnant women, the supine position is associated with decreased cardiac output. Since uterine blood flow is reduced during exercise as blood is shunted from the visceral organs to the muscles, the remaining cardiac output is further decreased. Similarly, women should also avoid standing motionless for prolonged periods.

- Because decreased oxygen is available for aerobic exercise during pregnancy, women should modify the intensity of their exercise based on their symptoms, should stop when they become fatigued, and should avoid exercising to the point of exhaustion. Non-weight-bearing exercises such as swimming and cycling are recommended because they decrease the risk of injury and provide fitness with comfort.

- As pregnancy progresses and the center of gravity changes, especially in the third trimester, women should avoid exercises in which the loss of balance could pose a risk to mother or fetus. Similarly, women should avoid any type of exercise that might result in even mild abdominal trauma.

Research shows that the ACOG guidelines are safe for sedentary women who want to begin exercising during pregnancy. A woman who had exercised regularly before becoming pregnant can continue a weight-bearing exercise routine of moderate intensity for up to 60 minutes 5 days per week throughout her pregnancy (Clapp, 2001). The following guidelines apply to all pregnant women:

- A normal pregnancy requires an additional 300 kcal per day. Women who exercise regularly during pregnancy should be careful to ensure that their diet is adequate.

- To avoid overheating, especially during the first trimester, pregnant women who exercise should wear clothing that is comfortable and loose, drink plenty of fluids, and avoid the prolonged overheating that can come from vigorous exercise in hot, humid weather. Hyperthermia may have teratogenic effects on the fetus (Heffernan, 2000). For the same reason, pregnant women are advised to avoid hot tubs and saunas.

- Women should avoid reaching their maximum physical effort during pregnancy. As a general rule, their pulse rates should not exceed 140 beats per minute (Shrock, 2000).

The woman should wear a supportive bra and appropriate shoes when exercising. She should also warm up and stretch to help prepare the joints for activity and cool down with a period of mild activity to help restore circulation and avoid pooling of blood. A moderate, rhythmic exercise routine involving large muscle groups such as swimming, cycling, or brisk walking is best. Jogging or running is acceptable for women already conditioned to these activities as long as they avoid exercising at maximum effort and overheating.

Exercising pregnant women should be alert for warning signs such as pain of any kind, nausea or vomiting, swelling, back pain, decreased or absent fetal movement, difficulty walking, dizziness, blurred vision, palpitations, pubic pain, shortness of breath, tachycardia, uterine contractions, vaginal bleeding, or fluid loss (Heffernan, 2000). The woman should stop exercising if these symptoms occur and

Thinking Critically

COUNSELING REGARDING STRENUOUS PHYSICAL ACTIVITY

Constance Petrowski, a 24-year-old, G1P0, world-class marathon runner, is 11 weeks pregnant when she sees you, the nurse-midwife, for her first prenatal exam. Because of her low body fat, her menses have always been irregular, and it had not occurred to Constance that she might be pregnant. Constance tells you that she has just begun serious training for a marathon that is to take place when she is about 22 weeks pregnant. Constance says she has been told that it is fine to continue any physical activity at which one is proficient and says that she would like to compete in the marathon because she believes she has a chance to come in as one of the top three women runners. What should you tell Constance about competing in the marathon? WEB

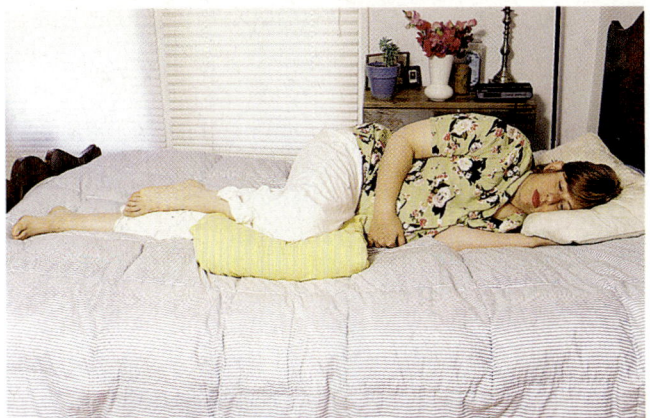

FIGURE 9–7. ◆ Position for relaxation and rest as pregnancy progresses.

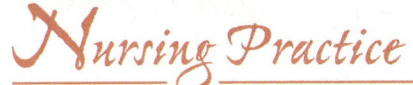 

Doing the pelvic rock on hands and knees may aggravate back strain. Teach women with a history of minor back problems to do the pelvic rock only in the standing position.

ABDOMINAL EXERCISES

A basic exercise to increase abdominal muscle tone is tightening abdominal muscles with each breath. It can be done in any position, but it is best learned while lying supine. With knees flexed and feet flat on the floor, the woman expands her abdomen and slowly takes a deep breath. Exhaling slowly, she gradually pulls in her abdominal muscles until they are fully contracted. She relaxes for a few seconds and then repeats the exercise.

Partial sit-ups strengthen abdominal muscle tone and are done according to individual comfort levels. A partial sit-up must be done with the knees flexed and the feet flat on the floor to avoid strain on the lower back. The woman stretches her arms toward her knees as she slowly pulls her head and shoulders off the floor to a comfortable level (if she has poor abdominal muscle tone, she may not be able to pull up very far). She then slowly returns to the starting position, takes a deep breath, and repeats the exercise. To strengthen the oblique abdominal muscles, she repeats the process but stretches the left arm to the side of her right knee, returns to the floor, takes a deep breath, and then reaches with the right arm to the left knee.

Women can do these exercises approximately five times in a sequence, and repeat the sequence at other times during the day as desired. It is important to do the exercises slowly to prevent muscle strain and overtiring.

PERINEAL EXERCISES

Perineal muscle tightening, also called **Kegel exercises,** strengthens the pubococcygeus muscle and increases its elasticity (Figure 9–9 ◆). The woman can feel the specific muscle group to be exercised by stopping urination midstream. Doing Kegel exercises while urinating is discouraged, however, because this practice has been associated with urinary stasis and urinary tract infection.

Childbirth educators sometimes use the following technique to teach Kegel exercises. They tell the woman to think of her perineal muscles as an elevator. When she relaxes, the elevator is on the first floor. To do the exercises, she contracts, bringing the elevator to the second, third, and fourth floors. She keeps the elevator on the fourth floor for a few seconds, and then gradually relaxes the area. If the exercise is properly done, the woman does not contract the muscles of the buttocks and thighs. Kegel exercises can be done at almost any time. Some women use ordinary events—for instance, stopping at a red light or talking on the telephone—as a cue to remember to do the exercise.

modify her exercise program. If the symptoms persist, the woman should contact her caregiver.

During pregnancy, adequate rest is important for both physical and emotional health. Women need more sleep, particularly in the first and last trimesters, when they tire easily. Without enough rest, pregnant women have less resilience. Finding time to rest during the day may be difficult for women who work outside the home or who have small children. The nurse can help the expectant mother examine her daily schedule to develop a realistic plan for short periods of rest and relaxation.

Sleeping becomes more difficult during the last trimester because of the enlarged abdomen, increased frequency of urination, and greater activity of the fetus. Finding a comfortable position becomes difficult. Figure 9–7 ◆ shows a position most pregnant women find comfortable. Women can also prepare for sleep with progressive relaxation techniques similar to those taught in prepared childbirth classes.

Exercises to Prepare for Childbirth

Certain exercises help strengthen muscle tone in preparation for birth and promote more rapid restoration of muscle tone after birth. A few of the more common body-conditioning exercises for pregnancy are discussed here.

The **pelvic tilt,** or pelvic rocking, helps prevent or reduce back strain as it strengthens abdominal muscles. To do the pelvic tilt, the pregnant woman lies on her back and puts her feet flat on the floor. This flexes the knees and helps prevent strain or discomfort. She decreases the curvature in her back by pressing her spine toward the floor. With her back pressed to the floor, the woman tightens her abdominal muscles as she tightens and tucks in her buttocks. The woman can also do the pelvic tilt on her hands and knees (Figure 9–8 ◆), while sitting in a chair, or while standing with her back against a wall. The woman should maintain the body alignment that results when the pelvic tilt is done correctly as much as possible throughout the day.

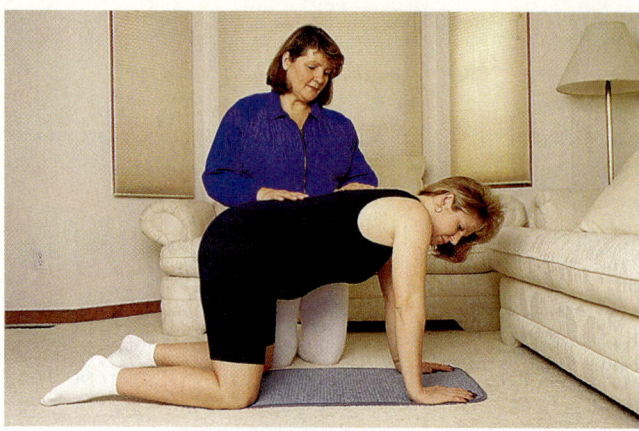

A

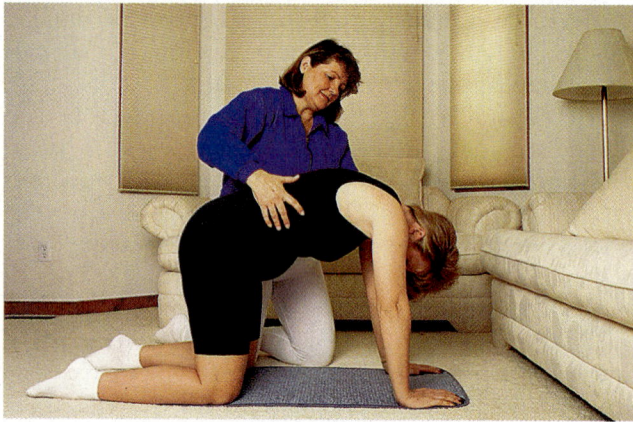

B

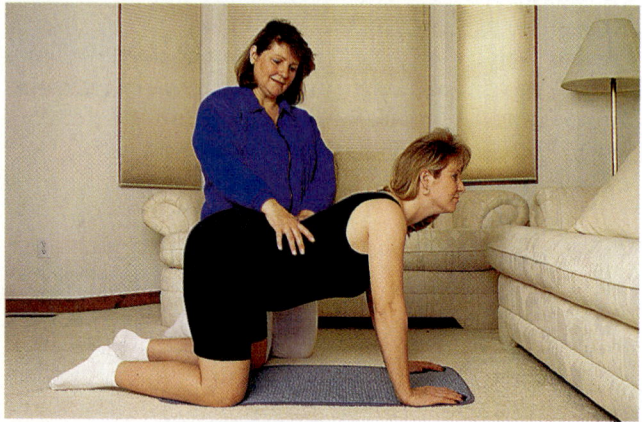

C

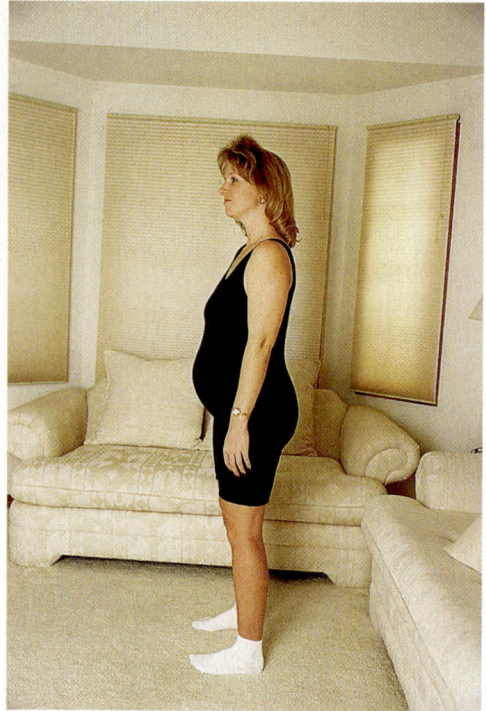

D

FIGURE 9–8. ◆ **A,** Starting position when the pelvic tilt is done on hands and knees. The back is flat and parallel to the floor, the hands are below the head, and the knees are directly below the buttocks. **B,** A prenatal yoga instructor offers pointers for proper positioning for the first part of the tilt: head up, neck long and separated from the shoulders, buttocks up, and pelvis thrust back, allowing the back to drop and release on an inhaled breath. **C,** The instructor helps the woman assume the correct position for the next part of the tilt. It is done on a long exhalation, allowing the pregnant woman to arch her back, drop her head loosely, push away from her hands, and draw in the muscles of her abdomen to strengthen them. Note that in this position the pelvis and buttocks are tucked under, and the buttock muscles are tightened. **D,** Proper posture. The knees are slightly bent but not locked, and the pelvis and buttocks are tucked under, thereby lengthening the spine and helping support the weighty abdomen. With her chin tucked in, this woman's neck, shoulders, hips, knees, and feet are all in a straight line perpendicular to the floor. Her feet are parallel. This is also the starting position for doing the pelvic tilt while standing.

INNER THIGH EXERCISES

The nurse can advise the pregnant woman to assume a cross-legged sitting position whenever possible. This "tailor sit" stretches the muscles of the inner thighs in preparation for labor and birth.

Sexual Activity

Because of the physiologic, anatomic, and emotional changes of pregnancy, couples usually have many questions and concerns about sexual activity during pregnancy. Often, these questions are about possible injury to the baby or the woman during intercourse and about changes in the desire each partner feels for the other.

In the past, couples were often warned to avoid sexual intercourse during the last 6 to 8 weeks of pregnancy to prevent complications such as infection or premature rupture of the membranes. However, these fears seem to be unfounded. In a healthy pregnancy, there is no medical reason to limit sexual activity. Intercourse is contraindicated for medical reasons such as multiple pregnancy, threatened abortion, incompetent cervix, a partner with

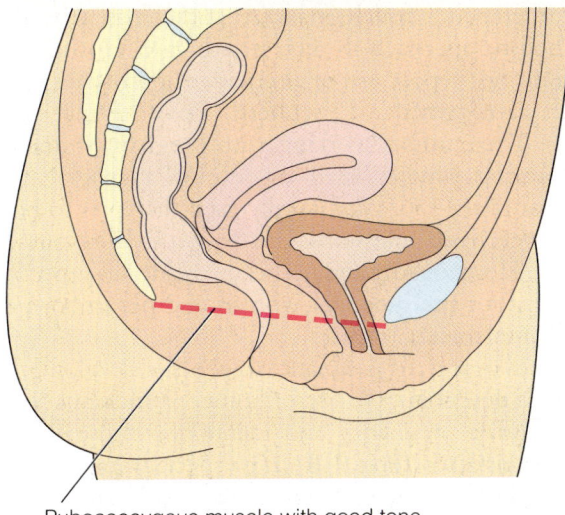

Pubococcygeus muscle with good tone

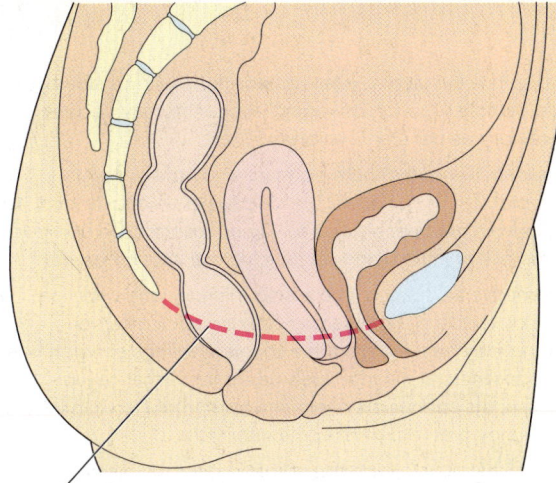

Pubococcygeus muscle with poor tone

FIGURE 9–9. ◆ Kegel exercises. The woman learns to tighten the pubococcygeus muscle, which improves support to the pelvic organs.

sexually transmitted infection, or a maternal history of miscarriage following orgasm (Shrock, 2000). Most caregivers also advise against intercourse when the membranes are ruptured and in women with a history of preterm labor.

The expectant mother may experience changes in sexual desire and response. Often, these changes are related to the various discomforts that occur throughout pregnancy. For instance, during the first trimester, fatigue or nausea and vomiting may decrease sexual desire. During the second trimester, many of these discomforts are lessened and sexual satisfaction increases. During the third trimester, interest in sex may again decrease as the woman becomes more uncomfortable and tired. Shortness of breath, urinary frequency, leg cramps, and decreased mobility may also lessen sexual desire and activity. If they are not already doing so, the couple should consider coital positions other than male superior, such as side-by-side, female superior, and vaginal rear entry.

Sexual activity does not have to include intercourse. Many of the nurturing and sexual needs of the pregnant woman can be satisfied by cuddling, kissing, and being held. The warm, sensual feelings that accompany these activities can be an end in themselves. Her partner, however, may choose to masturbate more frequently than before.

Many factors in pregnancy also affect the sexual desires of men. The man's previous relationship with the partner, acceptance of the pregnancy, attitudes toward the partner's change of appearance, and concern about hurting the expectant mother or baby can all play a role. Some men find it difficult to view their partners as sexually appealing while they are adjusting to the concept of them as mothers. Other men find their partners' pregnancies arousing and experience feelings of increased happiness, intimacy, and closeness.

The expectant couple should be aware of their changing sexual desires, the normality of these changes, and the importance of communicating these changes to each other so that they can make nurturing adaptations. It is important that the couple feel free to express concerns about sexual activity. Use a relaxed manner when responding to questions and giving anticipatory guidance. See "Teaching About: Sexual Activity During Pregnancy."

Teaching About

SEXUAL ACTIVITY DURING PREGNANCY

In starting a discussion about sexual activity during pregnancy, universal statements that give permission, such as "Many couples experience changes in sexual desire during pregnancy. What kind of changes have you experienced?" are often effective.

In your teaching, explain the following points to the woman and her partner:

- The pregnant woman may experience changes in desire during the course of pregnancy. During the first trimester, discomforts such as nausea, fatigue, and breast tenderness may make intercourse less desirable for many women. In the second trimester, as symptoms decrease, desire may increase. In the third trimester, discomfort and fatigue may lead to decreased desire in the woman.

- Men may notice changes in their level of desire, too. This may be related to feelings about their partner's changing appearance, their belief about the acceptability of sexual activity with a pregnant woman, or concern about hurting the woman or fetus. Some men find the changes of pregnancy erotic; others must adjust to the notion of their partners as mothers.

- The woman may notice that orgasms are much more intense during the last weeks of pregnancy and may be followed by cramping.

- Because of the pressure of the enlarging uterus on the vena cava, the woman should not lie flat on her back for intercourse after about the fourth month. If the couple prefer that position, a pillow should be placed under her right hip

(continued)

to displace the uterus. Alternate positions such as side-by-side, female superior, or vaginal rear entry may become necessary as her uterus enlarges.

- Sexual activities that both partners enjoy are generally acceptable. It is not advisable for couples who favor anal sex to go from anal penetration to vaginal penetration because of the risk of introducing *Escherichia coli* into the vagina.

- Alternative methods of expressing intimacy and affection such as cuddling, holding and stroking each other, and kissing may help maintain the couple's feelings of warmth and closeness. If the man feels desire for further sexual release, his partner may help him masturbate to ejaculation, or he may prefer to masturbate in private.

- Sexual intercourse is contraindicated once the membranes are ruptured or if bleeding is present. Women with a history of preterm labor may be advised to avoid intercourse because the oxytocin that is released with orgasm stimulates uterine contractions and may trigger preterm labor. Because oxytocin is also released with nipple stimulation, fondling the breasts may also be contraindicated in those cases.

- Stress the importance of open communication so that the couple feel comfortable expressing their feelings, preferences, and concerns.

- Deal with any specific questions about the physical and psychologic changes that the couple may have.

Dental Care

Proper dental hygiene is important in pregnancy. In fact, research suggests a link between periodontal disease in pregnant women and preterm birth and low-birth-weight infants (Carl, Roux, & Matacale, 2000). In spite of such discomforts as nausea and vomiting, gum hypertrophy, and heartburn, it is important for pregnant women to maintain regular oral hygiene.

Encourage the pregnant woman to have a dental checkup early in her pregnancy. General dental repair and extractions can be done during pregnancy, preferably in the second trimester and under local anesthetic (Carl et al., 2000). The woman should inform her dentist of her pregnancy so that she is not exposed to teratogenic substances. Dental x-ray examinations and extensive dental work need to be delayed until after the birth when possible.

Immunizations

Immunizations with attenuated live viruses, such as rubella vaccine, should not be given in pregnancy because of the teratogenic effect of the live viruses on the developing embryo. Vaccinations using killed viruses may be used, however.

Complementary and Alternative Therapies

As discussed in Chapter 1 ⬭, many women use complementary and alternative medicine such as homeopathy, herbal medicine, acupressure and acupuncture, biofeed-

back, therapeutic touch, massage, and chiropractic as part of a holistic approach to their health care. However, they often do not report use of alternative approaches to their health care provider (Eisenberg, Davis, Ettner, et al., 1998). Thus, nurses working with pregnant women and childbearing families need to develop a general understanding of the more commonly used therapies to be able to answer basic questions and to provide resources as needed. Homeopathy and herbal medicine have special implications for the pregnant woman and her unborn child (see Complementary Care).

Nurses caring for pregnant women can develop printed materials describing the use of homeopathic remedies and herbs during pregnancy and identifying those that may present a risk (see Table 9–3). It is especially important that women choosing these complementary approaches consult

Complementary Care

HOMEOPATHY AND HERBAL MEDICINE

Homeopathy: Homeopathy means "like suffering." Homeopathic medicine is based on the theory that a miniscule amount of a substance can cure symptoms in a sick person that are similar to the symptoms the substance causes in healthy people. Thus, for example, ipecac, which induces vomiting, may be used to treat a person who is vomiting, such as a pregnant woman with severe nausea and vomiting (Brennan, 1999). Currently homeopathic practitioners use about 2000 plant, animal, and mineral substances.

Homeopathic therapies are available for pregnancy-related symptoms such as musculoskeletal disorders, anemia, nausea, ptyalism, pica, threatened miscarriage, and preterm labor. According to homeopathic theory, homeopathic remedies either help an individual or have no effect. However, a healing crisis or aggravation of symptoms can occur if the remedy is given in too high a potency or repeated too frequently (Brennan, 1999). More information about homeopathy can be found on our companion website. ⬭ [WEB]

Herbal Medicine: Herbal medicine uses therapies derived from plants. Many have been used for centuries in different parts of the world and are well recognized. In fact, countries such as Germany, Canada, England, and France recognize the benefits of scores of herbs and include information about their use as part of formal educational programs for physicians and pharmacists.

In the United States, herbs are categorized as dietary supplements rather than drugs and are often used by pregnant women. It is best to advise pregnant women interested in using herbs to follow three basic principles: (1) if at all possible, avoid the use of herbs, even tonic herbs, during the first trimester (with the exception of ginger in amounts less than 1 g daily); (2) avoid standardized or highly concentrated extracts because the risk of side effects tends to be higher than with whole plant extracts; and (3) do not take essential oils internally (Belew, 1999). In addition, pregnant women need to avoid certain categories of herbs such as abortifacient (abortion-inducing) herbs, herbs that induce menstruation, nervous system stimulants, stimulant laxatives, and so forth. Lists identifying common herbs that women are advised to avoid or use with caution during pregnancy and lactation are available; an example is shown in Table 9–3.

TABLE 9–3 Common Herbs to Avoid in Pregnancy

Aloe spp.	Kava kava
Black cohosh	Licorice
Buckthorn	Ma huang
Cascara sagrada	Pennyroyal
Chamomile, Roman	Rue
Chaste tree berry	Sage
Dong quai	Senna
Feverfew	St. John's Wort
Goldenseal	Stinging nettle
Gotu kola	Tansy
Guggul	Wormwood
Horehound	Yarrow
Horseradish (fresh)	

Use with caution:
Garlic
Ginger
Turmeric

*Avoid excessive consumption relative to usual and customary food use.

Note: From Hardy, M. (2000). Herbs of special interest to women. *Journal of the American Pharmaceutical Association, 40*(2), 234–242.

someone who is knowledgeable, well trained, and experienced in the specific therapy and that they buy their herbs or homeopathic remedies from reputable manufacturers.

Teratogenic Substances

Substances that adversely affect the normal growth and development of the fetus are called teratogens (see Chapter 3). 🔗 Many substances are known or suspected teratogens, including, for example, certain medications, psychotropic drugs, and alcohol. The harmful effects of others, such as some pesticides or exposure to x-rays in the first trimester of pregnancy, have also been documented. It is essential to provide pregnant women with information about recognized teratogens and environmental risks.

Medications

The use of medications during pregnancy, including prescriptions, over-the-counter drugs, and herbal remedies, is of great concern. Many pregnant women need medication to treat infections, allergies, or other pathologic processes. In these situations, the problem can be very complex. Care providers do not prescribe known teratogenic agents and can usually replace them with safer medications. However, even when a woman is highly motivated to avoid taking any medications, she may have taken potentially teratogenic medications before her pregnancy was confirmed, especially if she has an irregular menstrual cycle.

The fetus is at highest risk for gross abnormalities during the first trimester of pregnancy, when fetal organs are first developing. The classic period of teratogenesis in a woman with a 28-day cycle extends from day 31 after the last menstrual period (17 days after fertilization) to day 71 (54 days after fertilization) (Niebyl, 1999). Many factors influence teratogenic effects, including the type of teratogen and the dose, the stage of embryo development, and the genetic sensitivity of the mother and fetus (ACOG, 1997b). For example, the commonly prescribed acne medication isotretinoin (Accutane) is associated with a high incidence of spontaneous abortion and congenital malformations if taken early in pregnancy.

To provide information for caregivers and clients, the U.S. Food and Drug Administration has developed the following classification system for medications administered during pregnancy:

Category A: Controlled studies in women have demonstrated no associated fetal risk. Few drugs fall into this category.

Category B: Animal studies show no risk, but there are no controlled studies in women, or animal studies indicate a risk, but controlled human studies fail to demonstrate a risk. The penicillins fall into this category.

Category C: Either (1) no adequate animal or human studies are available or (2) animal studies show teratogenic effects, but no controlled studies in women are available. Many drugs fall into this category, which, because of the lack of information, is a problematic one for caregivers. Epinephrine, beta-blockers, and zidovudine (a drug used to decrease perinatal transmission of HIV) fall into this category.

Category D: Evidence of human fetal risk exists, but the benefits of the drug in certain situations are thought to outweigh the risks. Examples of drugs in this category include tetracycline, vincristine, lithium, and hydrochlorothiazide.

Category X: The demonstrated fetal risks clearly outweigh any possible benefit. Examples of drugs in this category include isotretinoin (Accutane), the acne medication, which can cause multiple central nervous system, facial, and cardiovascular anomalies.

If a woman has taken a drug in category D or X, she should be informed of the risks associated with that drug and of her alternatives. Similarly, a woman who has taken a drug in the safer categories can be reassured (Cunningham et al., 2001).

Although the first trimester is the critical period for teratogenesis, some medications are known to have a teratogenic effect when taken in the second and third trimesters. For example, tetracycline taken in late pregnancy is commonly associated with staining of teeth in children and has been shown to depress skeletal growth, especially in premature infants. Sulfonamides taken in the last few weeks of pregnancy are known to compete with bilirubin attachment of protein-binding sites, increasing the risk of jaundice in the newborn (Niebyl, 1999).

Pregnant women need to avoid all medication—prescribed, homeopathic, or over-the-counter—if possible. If no alternative exists, it is wisest to select a well-known medication rather than a newer drug whose potential teratogenic effects may not be known. When possible, the oral form of a drug should be used, and it should be prescribed in the lowest possible therapeutic dose for the shortest time possible. Caution is the watchword for nurses caring for pregnant women who have been taking medications. It is essential that pregnant women check with their certified nurse-midwives or physicians about any herbs or medications they were taking when pregnancy began and about any nonprescription drugs they are thinking of using. The advantage of using a particular medication must outweigh the risks. Any medication with possible teratogenic effects is best avoided.

TOBACCO

Infants of mothers who smoke during pregnancy have a higher incidence of low birth weight than infants of mothers who do not smoke. For women with a twin pregnancy, this effect is even more pronounced (Pollack, Lantz, & Frohna, 2000). Smoking during pregnancy has also been associated with preterm birth, premature rupture of the membranes, placenta previa, abruptio placentae, sudden infant death syndrome, higher morbidity, and lower IQ (Todd, LaSala, & Neil-Urban, 2001). The risk is related to the number of cigarettes smoked. Smoking has also been linked to an increased risk of cleft lip and palate in the newborn (Chung, Kowalski, Kim, et al., 2000). The specific mechanism of smoking's effect on the fetus is not known. However, the main ingredients in cigarette smoke that account for adverse effects in the fetus are carbon monoxide and nicotine, because they decrease the availability of oxygen to maternal and fetal tissues.

Currently about 12.9% of women smoke during pregnancy. This rate has declined steadily since 1989—a positive trend. Unfortunately, tobacco use by pregnant teens continues to increase (Ventura, Martin, Curtin, et al., 2000). Women who smoke tend to stop smoking or at least reduce their intake once pregnancy is confirmed. Unfortunately, a majority of women who quit smoking during pregnancy resume following childbirth, although this percentage is lower for women who quit early in pregnancy. Any decrease in smoking during pregnancy most likely improves fetal outcome, and researchers continue to explore approaches designed to help women quit smoking. Pregnancy may be a difficult time for a woman to stop smoking, but the nurse should encourage her to reduce the number of cigarettes she smokes daily. The perceived need to protect her unborn child may increase her motivation.

ALCOHOL

Fetuses of women who drink heavily are at increased risk of developing **fetal alcohol syndrome** (Chapter 25). This syndrome, which is characterized by growth restric-

tion, facial anomalies, and central nervous system dysfunction of varying severity, is the major cause of mental retardation in the Western world (Brennan, 1999).

The effects of moderate drinking during pregnancy are unclear. Research indicates an increased incidence of lowered birth weight and some neurologic effects, such as attention deficit disorder. Evidence suggests that the risk of teratogenic effects increases proportionately with increased average daily intake of alcohol. Although an occasional drink during pregnancy does not carry any known risk, no safe level of drinking during pregnancy has been identified (Niebyl, 1999). Caregivers recommend that pregnant women abstain from all alcohol during pregnancy. In most cases, once a woman becomes aware of her pregnancy, she decreases her consumption of alcohol. However, the alcohol consumed after conception and before pregnancy is diagnosed remains a cause for concern.

Assessment of alcohol intake is a major part of every woman's medical history. Ask questions in a direct, nonjudgmental manner. All women need to be counseled about the role of alcohol in pregnancy. If heavy consumption is involved, refer the pregnant woman immediately to an alcoholic treatment program. Counselors in these programs need to know about a woman's pregnancy before drug therapy is suggested, since certain drugs may be harmful to the developing fetus. For example, the drug disulfiram (Antabuse), often used in conjunction with alcohol treatment, is suspected to be a teratogenic agent.

CAFFEINE

Current research offers no evidence that caffeine has teratogenic effects in humans. However, maternal coffee consumption decreases iron absorption and may increase the risk of anemia (Niebyl, 1999). Until more definitive data are available, nurses can advise women about common sources of caffeine, including coffee, tea, colas, and chocolate, and suggest that they moderate their daily caffeine intake.

MARIJUANA

The prevalence of marijuana use in our society raises many concerns about its effect on the fetus, but no teratogenic effects of marijuana use during pregnancy have yet been documented (Niebyl, 1999). Research on marijuana use in pregnancy is difficult, however, because it is an illegal drug. Unreliability of reporting, lack of a representative population, inability to determine strength or composition of the marijuana used (including the presence of herbicides), and use of other drugs at the same time all complicate the research being done.

COCAINE

A woman who uses cocaine during pregnancy is at increased risk for acute myocardial infarction, cardiac arrhythmias, ruptured ascending aorta, seizures, cerebrovascular accidents, hyperthermia, bowel ischemia, and sudden death (Cunningham et al., 1997). Cocaine use during pregnancy has been related to abruptio placentae, preterm birth, fetal distress, low birth weight, neonatal withdrawal, sudden infant death syndrome (SIDS), and spontaneous pneumothorax (Chan, Pham, & Reece, 1997). Several congenital anomalies have also been linked to maternal cocaine use, including, for example, genitourinary anomalies, congenital heart defects, limb reduction defects, and central nervous system anomalies (Cunningham et al., 2001) (see also Chapter 12). ⬭

As the number of women of childbearing age using cocaine increases, health care providers need to become more alert to early signs of cocaine use. It is often difficult for a nurse or physician to face the fact that a client is using cocaine, but ongoing alertness and an open, nonjudgmental approach are important in early detection. Urine screening for cocaine is valuable, but because cocaine is metabolized rapidly, the drug screen is negative within 24 to 48 hours after cocaine use. Thus it is probable that many expectant mothers who use cocaine are not identified.

Evaluation

Throughout the antepartal period, evaluation is an ongoing and essential part of effective nursing care. In evaluating the effectiveness of the interactions, try creative solutions that are logical and carefully thought out. Creative solutions are especially important in dealing with families from other cultures. If a practice is important to a woman and not harmful, the culturally competent nurse will not discourage it.

In completing an evaluation, be alert for situations that require referral for further evaluation. For example, a woman who has gained 4 lb in a single week does not require counseling about nutrition; she needs further assessment for preeclampsia. The nurse who has a sound knowledge of theory will recognize this need and act immediately.

Throughout the course of pregnancy, certain criteria determine the quality of care. In essence, nursing care has been effective if:

- The common discomforts of pregnancy are quickly identified and are relieved or lessened effectively.
- The woman is able to discuss the physiologic and psychologic changes of pregnancy.
- The woman uses self-care measures, if needed, during pregnancy.
- The woman avoids substances and situations that pose a risk to her or her child's well-being.
- The woman seeks regular prenatal care.

CARE OF THE EXPECTANT COUPLE OVER AGE 35

Today an increasing number of women are choosing to have their first baby after age 35 (Table 9–4). In fact, in the United States the rate of first births to women between the

TABLE 9–4 Pregnancy in Women over Age 35

- Couples who choose pregnancy at a later age are usually financially secure and have made a thoughtful, planned choice.
- If the woman has no existing health problems, her risk during pregnancy is not appreciably higher than that of the general population.
- The decreased fertility of women over age 35 may make conception more difficult.
- The incidence of Down syndrome increases somewhat in women over age 35 and significantly in those over age 40.
- The couple may choose to have amniocentesis or chorionic villus sampling to gain information about the health of their fetus.

ages of 35 and 39 has nearly doubled since 1978, from 19 per 1000 women to 37.4. For women between the ages of 40 and 44, the birth rate increased by over 90% during the same period (Ventura et al., 2000). Many factors have contributed to this trend, including the following:

- The availability of effective birth control methods
- The expanded roles and career options available for women
- The increased number of women getting advanced education, pursuing careers, and delaying parenthood until they are established professionally
- The increased incidence of later marriage and second marriage
- The high cost of living, which causes some young couples to delay childbearing until they are more secure financially
- The increased number of women in this older reproductive age group due to the baby boom between 1946 and 1964
- The increased availability of specialized fertilization procedures, which may help women previously considered infertile

There are advantages to having a first baby after age 35. Single women or couples who delay childbearing until they are older tend to be well educated and financially secure. Usually their decision to have a baby was deliberately and thoughtfully made (Figure 9–10 ◆). Compared with younger women, women over age 35 tend to be more emotionally stable and more likely to get early prenatal care and demonstrate healthful behaviors during their pregnancy. Because of their greater life experiences, they also are more aware of the realities of having a child and what it means to have a baby at their age (Windridge & Berryman, 1999). Many of the women have experienced fulfillment in their careers and feel secure enough to take on the added responsibility of a child. Some women are ready to make a change in their lives, wanting to stay home with a new baby. Those who plan to continue working typically can afford good child care.

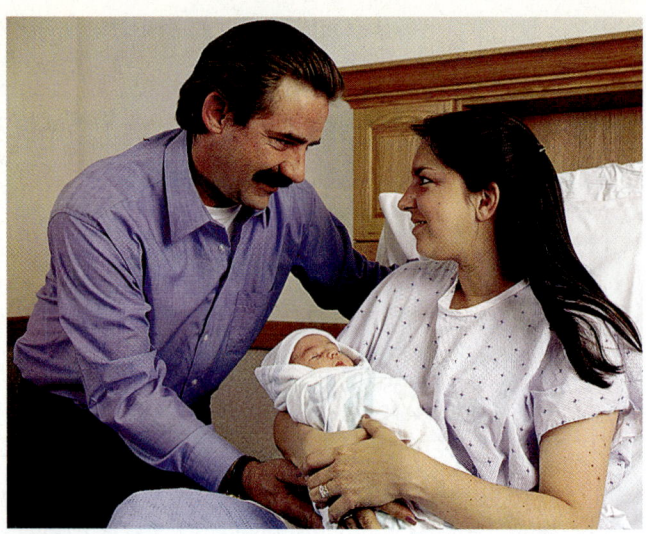

FIGURE 9–10 ♦ For many older couples, the decision to have a child may be very rewarding.

Medical Risks

In the United States, the risk of fetal death has declined dramatically over the past 30 years for women of all ages. However, the risk for fetal death remains highest among teenagers and among women age 40 and older (National Center for Health Statistics, 1999). In addition, women who give birth to a first child after age 40 have a higher risk of preterm birth, preeclampsia, and perinatal mortality (Scholz, Haas, & Petru, 1999), as well as a higher incidence of low-birth-weight infants and infants with congenital malformations (Gilbert, Nesbitt, & Danielson, 1999). In both the United States and Canada, the risk of maternal mortality, though low, increases with maternal age. For women age 40 or older, the risk of dying from a pregnancy-related or pregnancy-aggravated cause is 5 times higher than the risk for women ages 20 to 24 years (Hoyert, Danel, & Tully, 2000).

Women over age 35, and, even more, women over age 40, are more likely to have chronic medical conditions that can complicate a pregnancy. Preexisting medical conditions such as hypertension or diabetes probably play a more significant role than age in maternal well-being and the outcome of pregnancy (Cunningham et al., 2001). The cesarean birth rate is also increased in pregnant women over age 35. This may be related both to pregnancy complications and to increased concern by the woman and her physician about the pregnancy outcome (Windridge & Berryman, 1999).

The risk of conceiving a child with Down syndrome increases with age, especially over age 35. Amniocentesis is routinely offered to all women over age 35 to permit the early detection of several chromosomal abnormalities, including Down syndrome. Genetic testing is not routinely offered to couples in whom there is only advanced pater-

nal age, because there is not enough evidence to determine a paternal age at which to start genetic testing. However, advanced paternal age affects autosomal dominant inherited diseases, such as neurofibromatosis, achondroplasia, and Marfan syndrome (ACOG, 1997a).

A triple screening blood test, also called *multiple marker screen (MMS)*, detects levels of specific serum markers—namely, maternal serum alpha-fetoprotein (MSAFP), hCG, and unconjugated estriol. The test, offered to all pregnant women at about 16 to 18 weeks gestation, is especially important for women over age 35 because of the increased risk of Down syndrome. If a fetus has Down syndrome, hCG levels tend to be higher than normal, while estriol and MSAFP levels tend to be lower than normal. If the levels indicate high risk, further assessments are warranted (ACOG, 2000). Although these tests are not as definite as amniocentesis or chorionic villus sampling in detecting abnormalities, they are safer and less expensive.

Special Concerns of the Expectant Couple over Age 35

No matter what their age, most expectant couples have concerns about the well-being of the fetus and their ability to parent. Expectant parents over age 35 often have additional concerns about their age, especially the closer they are to age 40. Some couples are concerned about whether they will have enough energy to care for a new baby. Of greater concern is their ability to deal with the needs of the child as they age.

The financial concerns of the older couple are usually different from those of the younger couple. The older couple is generally more financially secure, but when their "baby" is ready for college, the older couple may be close to retirement and might not have the means to provide for their child. The older couple may also be forced to face their own mortality. Certainly the realization of one's mortality is not uncommon in midlife, but instead of confronting this issue at 40 to 45 years of age or later, the older expectant couple may confront the issue earlier as they consider what will happen as their child grows.

Older couples facing pregnancy in a late or second marriage or after therapy for infertility may find themselves somewhat isolated socially. They may feel different because they are often the only couple in their peer group expecting their first baby. In fact, many of their peers are likely to be parents of adolescents or young adults and may be grandparents as well.

Older couples who already have children may respond quite differently to learning that the woman is pregnant, depending on whether the pregnancy was planned or unexpected. Other factors influencing their response include their children's, family's, and friends' attitudes toward the pregnancy; the impact on their lifestyle; and the financial implications of having another child. Sometimes couples who had previously been married to other mates will choose to have a child together. *Blended families* are formed when "her" children, "his" children, and "their" children come together as a new family group.

Health care professionals may treat the older expectant couple differently than they would a younger couple. They may offer older women more medical procedures, such as amniocentesis and ultrasound, than younger women. They may also discourage an older woman from using a birthing room or birthing center even if she is healthy because her age is considered to put her at risk.

The woman who has delayed pregnancy may be concerned about the limited amount of time that she has to bear children. When pregnancy does not occur as quickly as she had hoped, the older woman may become increasingly anxious as time slips away on her "biological clock." When an older woman becomes pregnant but has a spontaneous abortion, her grief for the loss of her unborn child is exacerbated by her anxiety about her ability to conceive again in the time remaining to her.

Nursing Management

Nursing Assessment and Diagnosis

In working with a woman in her late 30s or 40s who is pregnant, make the same assessments as are indicated in caring for any woman who is pregnant. Assess physical status, the woman's understanding of pregnancy and its changes, the couple's attitudes about the pregnancy and their expectations of the impact a baby will have on their lives, their health teaching needs, the degree of support the woman has, and her knowledge of infant care.

The nursing diagnoses applicable to pregnant women in general apply to pregnant women over age 35. Examples of other nursing diagnoses that may apply include the following:

▶ *Decisional conflict* related to unexpected pregnancy
▶ *Moderate anxiety* related to uncertainty about fetal well-being

Planning and Implementation

Once an older couple has made the decision to have a child, respect and support the couple in this decision. As with any client, discuss risks, identify concerns, and promote strengths. Do not make the woman's age an issue. It is helpful in promoting a sense of well-being to treat the pregnancy as normal unless the woman has specific health risks.

As the pregnancy continues, identify and discuss concerns the woman may have related to her age or to specific health problems. The older woman who has made a conscious decision to become pregnant often has carefully thought through potential problems and may actually have fewer concerns than a younger woman or one with an unplanned pregnancy.

Childbirth education classes are important in promoting adaptation to the event of childbirth for expectant couples of any age. However, older expectant couples, who are still in the minority, often feel uncomfortable in classes in which most of the participants are much younger. Consequently, classes for expectant parents over age 35 are now available in many communities.

Women who are over age 35 and having their first baby tend to be better educated than other health care consumers. These clients frequently know the kind of care and services they want and may be assertive in their interactions with the health care system. Do not be intimidated by these individuals and do not assume that anticipatory guidance and support are not needed. Instead, support the couple's strengths and be sensitive to their individual needs.

In working with older expectant couples or an older single woman, be sensitive to special needs. A particularly difficult issue these couples face is the possibility of bearing an unhealthy child or a child with a genetic disorder. As discussed previously, a triple screening test, also called multiple marker screen (MMS), is useful in assessing for Down syndrome. Because of the risk of Down syndrome in these families, amniocentesis is often suggested.

For couples who agree to amniocentesis, the first few months of pregnancy are a difficult time. Amniocentesis cannot be done until week 14 of pregnancy, and the chromosomal studies take roughly 2 weeks to complete. Their fear that the fetus is at risk may delay the successful completion of the psychologic tasks of early pregnancy.

Support couples who decide to have amniocentesis by providing information and answering questions about the procedure and by providing comfort and emotional support during the amniocentesis. If the results indicate that the fetus has Down syndrome or another genetic abnormality, ensure that the couple has complete information about the condition, its range of possible manifestations, and its developmental implications.

Evaluation

Expected outcomes of nursing care include the following:

▶ The woman and her partner are knowledgeable about the pregnancy and express confidence in their ability to make appropriate health care choices.

▶ The expectant couple (and their children) are able to cope with the pregnancy and its implications for the future.

▶ The woman receives effective health care throughout her pregnancy and during birth and the postpartum period.

▶ The woman and her partner develop skills in child care and parenting.

CHAPTER HIGHLIGHTS

◈ Provision of anticipatory guidance about childbirth, the postpartum period, and childrearing is a primary responsibility of the nurse caring for women in an antepartal setting.

◈ The nurse assesses the expectant father's knowledge level and intended degree of participation and then works with the couple to help ensure a satisfying experience.

◈ Culturally based practices and proscribed activities may have an impact on the childbearing family.

◈ The common discomforts of pregnancy occur as a result of physiologic and anatomic changes. The nurse provides the woman with information about self-care activities aimed at reducing or relieving discomfort.

◈ To make self-care choices and acquire desired healthful habits, a pregnant woman requires accurate information about a range of subjects, from exercise to sexual activity and from bathing to immunization.

◈ Teratogenic substances are substances that adversely affect the normal growth and development of the fetus.

◈ A pregnant woman should avoid taking prescribed medications or using over-the-counter preparations during pregnancy.

◈ Evidence exists that smoking, consuming alcohol, or using "social" drugs such as marijuana or cocaine during pregnancy may be harmful to the fetus.

◈ Maternal assessment of fetal activity keeps the woman "in touch" with her fetus and provides ongoing assessment of fetal status.

◈ Childbirth among women over age 35 is becoming increasingly common. It poses fewer health risks than previously believed and seems to offer advantages for the woman or couple who make the choice.

◈ A major risk for the older expectant couple relates to the increased incidence of Down syndrome in children born to women over age 35 or 40. Amniocentesis can provide information as to whether the fetus has Down syndrome. The couple can then decide whether they wish to continue the pregnancy.

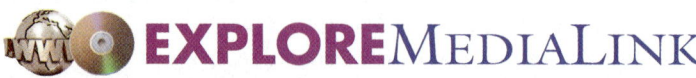 **EXPLORE**MediaLink

NCLEX Review, Case Studies, and other interactive resources for this chapter can be found on the companion website at http://www.prenhall.com/london. Click on "Chapter 9" to select the activities for this chapter.

For animations, more NCLEX review questions, and an audio glossary, access the accompanying CD-ROM in this textbook.

REFERENCES

Aikins Murphy, P. (1998). Alternative therapies for nausea and vomiting of pregnancy. *Obstetrics and Gynecology, 91*(1), 149–155.

American College of Obstetricians and Gynecologists. (1994). *Exercise during pregnancy and the postpartum period* (ACOG Technical Bulletin No. 189). Washington, DC: Author.

American College of Obstetricians and Gynecologists. (1997a). *Advanced paternal age* (ACOG Committee Opinion No. 189). Washington, DC: Author.

American College of Obstetricians and Gynecologists. (1997b). *Teratology* (ACOG Educational Bulletin No. 236). Washington, DC: Author.

American College of Obstetricians and Gynecologists. (2000). *Planning your pregnancy and birth* (3rd ed.). Washington, DC: Author.

Belew, C. (1999). Herbs and the childbearing woman: Guidelines for midwives. *Journal of Nurse-Midwifery, 44*(3), 231–246.

Blumenthal, M. (2000). *Herbal medicine: Expanded Commission E Monographs.* Austin, TX: American Botanical Council.

Brennan, P. (1999). Homeopathic remedies in prenatal care. *Journal of Nurse-Midwifery, 44*(3), 291–299.

Carl, D. L., Roux, G., & Matacale, R. (2000). Exploring dental hygiene and perinatal outcomes. *AWHONN Lifelines, 4*(1), 22–27.

Cesario, S. K. (2001). Care of the Native American woman: Strategies for practice, education, and research. *Journal of Obstetric, Gynecologic, and Neonatal Nursing, 30*(1), 13–19.

Chan, L., Pham, H., & Reece, E. A. (1997). Pneumothorax in pregnancy associated with cocaine use. *American Journal of Perinatology, 14*(7), 385–388.

Chez, R. A., & Friedmann, A. K. (2000). Offering effective breastfeeding advice. *Contemporary OB/GYN, 45*(8), 32–50.

Chez, R. A., & Niebyl, J. (2000). Management of nausea and vomiting in pregnancy: Traditional therapies. *Contemporary OB/GYN, 45*(3), 130–136.

Choi, E. C. (1995). A contrast of mothering behaviors in women from Korea and the United States. *Journal of Obstetric, Gynecologic, and Neonatal Nursing, 24*(4), 363–369.

Chung, K. C., Kowalski, C. P., Kim, H. M., & Buchman, S. R. (2000). Maternal cigarette smoking during pregnancy and the risk of having a child with cleft lip/palate. *Plastic and Reconstructive Surgery, 105*(2), 485–491.

Clapp, J. F., III. (2001). Recommending exercise during pregnancy. *Contemporary OB/GYN, 46*(1), 30–40.

Collins, C. (1998). Yoga: Intuition, preventive medicine, and treatment. *Journal of Obstetric, Gynecologic, and Neonatel Nursing. 27*(5), 563–568.

Cunningham, F. G., Gant, N. F., Leveno, K. J., Gilstrap, L. C., III, Hauth, J. C., & Wenstrom, K. D. (2001). *Williams obstetrics* (21st ed.). New York: McGraw-Hill.

Dickerson, V. M., & Chez, R. A. (1999). Normal pregnancy and prenatal care. In J. R. Scott, P. J. DiSaia, C. B. Hammond, & W. N. Spellacy (Eds.), *Danforth's obstetrics and gynecology* (8th ed., pp. 65–90). Philadelphia: Lippincott Williams & Wilkins.

Eisenberg, D. M., Davis, R. B., Ettner, S. L., Appel, S., Wilkey, S., Van Rompey, M., et al. (1998). Trends in alternative medicine use in the United States, 1990–1997. *Journal of the American Medical Association, 280*, 1569–1575.

Fontaine, K. L. (2000). *Healing practices: Alternative therapies for nursing.* Upper Saddle River, NJ: Prentice Hall.

Fulder, S., & Tenne, M. (1996). Ginger as an anti-nausea remedy in pregnancy: The issue of safety. *HerbalGram, 38,* 47–50.

Gilbert, W. M., Nesbitt, T. S., & Danielson, B. (1999). Childbearing beyond age 40: Pregnancy outcome in 24,032 cases. *Obstetrics and Gynecology, 93*(1), 9–14.

Good news for pregnant women with heartburn. (1999). *Contemporary OB/GYN, 44*(12), 50.

Gottlieb, B. (2000). *Alternative cures.* Emmaus PA: Rodale Press.

Hardy, M. (2000). Herbs of special interest to women. *Journal of the American Pharmaceutical Association, 40*(2), 234–242.

Heffernan, A. E. (2000). Exercise and pregnancy in primary care. *Nurse Practitioner, 25*(3), 42–60.

Hoyert, D. L., Danel, I., & Tully, P. (2000). Maternal mortality, United States and Canada, 1982–97. *Birth, 27*(1), 4–11.

Jackson, E. A. (2001). Is ginger root effective for decreasing the severity of nausea and vomiting in early pregnancy? *Journal of Family Practice, 50*(8), 720.

Jewell, D., & Young, G. (2000). Interventions for nausea and vomiting in early pregnancy. *Cochrane Database Systems Review,* (2), CD000145.

Marti, J. (1998). *The alternative health and medicine encyclopedia* (2nd ed.). Detroit, MI: Visible Ink Press.

Mattson, S. (1995). Culturally sensitive perinatal care for Southeast Asians. *Journal of Obstetric, Gynecologic, and Neonatal Nursing, 24*(4), 335–341.

Morgan, M., & Bone, K. (1998). *Professional review: Horsechestnut. Medicinal Herb, 65,* 1–4.

National Center for Health Statistics. (1999, December 15). *Infant mortality rates vary by race and ethnicity* [News release]. Hyattsville, MD: Author.

Niebyl, J. R. (1999). Teratology and drugs in pregnancy. In J. R. Scott, P. J. DiSaia, C. B. Hammond, & W. N. Spellacy (Eds.), *Danforth's obstetrics and gynecology* (8th ed., pp. 197–212). Philadelphia: Lippincott Williams & Wilkins.

Pollack, H., Lantz, P. M., & Frohna, J. G. (2000). Maternal smoking and adverse birth outcomes among singletons and twins. *American Journal of Public Health, 90*(3), 395–400.

Pugh, L. C., Milligan, R., Parks, P. L., Lenz, E. R., & Kitzman, H. (1999). Clinical approaches in the assessment of childbearing fatigue. *Journal of Obstetric, Gynecologic, and Neonatal Nursing, 28*(1), 74–80.

Scholz, H. S., Haas, J., & Petru, E. (1999). Do primiparas aged 40 years or older carry an increased obstetric risk? *Preventive Medicine, 29*(4), 263–266.

Shrock, P. (2000). Exercise and physical activity during pregnancy. In J. J. Sciarra (Ed.), *Gynecology and obstetrics* (Vol. 2, Chap. 8, pp. 1–17). Philadelphia: Lippincott Williams & Wilkins.

Skidmore-Roth, L. (2001). *Mosby's handbook of herbs & natural supplements.* St. Louis, MO: Mosby.

Spector, R. E. (2000). *Cultural diversity in health and illness* (5th ed.). Upper Saddle River, NJ: Prentice-Hall Health.

Steele, N. M., French, J., Gatherer-Boyles, J., Newman, S., & Leclaire, S. (2001). Effect of acupressure by sea-bands on nausea and vomiting of pregnancy. *Journal of Obstetric, Gynecologic, and Neonatal Nursing, 30*(1), 61–70.

Todd, S., LaSala, K. B., & Neil-Urban, S. (2001). An integrated approach to prenatal smoking cessation. *American Journal of Maternal-Child Nursing, 26*(4), 185–190.

Varney, H. (1997). *Varney's midwifery* (3rd ed.). Sudbury, MA: Jones and Bartlett.

Ventura, S. J., Martin, J. A., Curtin, S. A., Mathews, T. J., & Parks, M. M. (2000). Births: Final data for 1998. *National Vital Statistics Reports, 48*(3), 1–105.

Vutyavanich, T., Kraisarin, T., & Ruangsri, R. (2001). Ginger for nausea and vomiting in pregnancy: Randomized, double-masked, placebo-controlled trial. *Obstetrics and Gynecology, 97*(4), 577–582.

Weidner, M. S., & Sigwart, K. (2001). Investigation of the teratogenic potential of a *Zingiber officinale* extract in the rat. *Reproductive Toxicology, 15*(1), 75–80.

Windridge, K. C., & Berryman, J. C. (1999). Women's experiences of giving birth after 35. *Birth, 26*(1), 16–23.

Adolescent Pregnancy

I was a child when I had my daughter—just 16—and so afraid. I was one of the lucky ones though. My parents were wonderfully supportive and I went to a special teen clinic for my pregnancy. The nurses really taught me a lot about my body and about taking care of my baby. With help and encouragement from Mom and Dad, I got by. Last spring, at age 28 I graduated with a degree in nursing. I wanted a job with real security and opportunity, but more important, I want to give something back, to give others a little of the support I received.

—JOANNA, 29

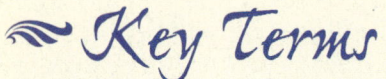

Key Terms

Early adolescence   *207*   Late adolescence   *207*
Emancipated minors   *213*   Middle adolescence   *207*

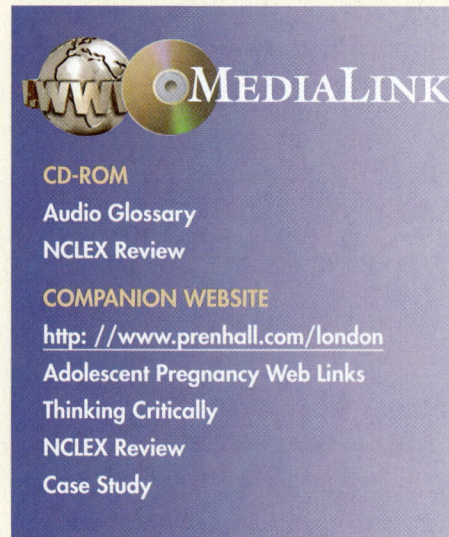

MediaLink

CD-ROM
Audio Glossary
NCLEX Review

COMPANION WEBSITE
http://www.prenhall.com/london
Adolescent Pregnancy Web Links
Thinking Critically
NCLEX Review
Case Study

$\mathcal{P}$regnancy is an especially challenging time if the expectant mother is an adolescent. In the United States each year almost 1 million teenage girls become pregnant; 78% of these pregnancies are unintended. Of these pregnancies, nearly two fifths are terminated by therapeutic abortion, and about 14% end in miscarriage (Alan Guttmacher Institute, 1999). More than half the teens who become pregnant give birth and keep their babies.

The U.S. birth rate (number of births per 1000 women) for adolescents age 15 to 19 dropped from 62.1 per 1000 in 1991 to 48.5 per 1000 in 2000, a 22% decline. Nevertheless, the United States continues to have one of the highest levels of adolescent childbearing among industrialized nations (National Campaign to Prevent Teen Pregnancy, 2002). The incidence of sexual activity among teens in many other countries is as high as it is in the United States. Researchers suggest that these countries may have lower adolescent pregnancy rates because of family influences, a greater openness about sexuality, better access to contraceptives, and a more comprehensive approach to sex education.

This chapter explores the issue of adolescent pregnancy and the role of the nurse in meeting the special needs and concerns of pregnant adolescents and their families. It concludes with a discussion of efforts to prevent adolescent pregnancy.

OVERVIEW OF THE ADOLESCENT PERIOD

Physical Changes

Puberty—that period during which an individual becomes capable of reproduction—is a maturational process that can last from 1.5 to 6 years. The major physical changes of puberty include a growth spurt, weight change, and the appearance of secondary sexual characteristics. Menarche, or the time of the first menstrual period, usually occurs in the last half of this maturational process, with the average age between 12 and 13. The initial menstrual cycles are usually irregular and often anovulatory, although they are not always so. Thus contraception is important for all sexually active adolescents.

Psychosocial Development

Many writers have described the developmental tasks of adolescence, based on a variety of classic theories. The following are major developmental tasks of this period (Steinberg, 1999):

- Developing a sense of identity
- Gaining autonomy and independence

- Developing truly intimate relationships—that is, relationships characterized by honesty, openness, trust, and self-disclosure
- Developing comfort with one's own sexuality
- Developing a sense of achievement

Resolution of these tasks is a developmental process that occurs over time. Although average ages for the completion of tasks have been identified, these ages are somewhat arbitrary and are affected by many factors, including culture, religion, and socioeconomic status.

In **early adolescence** (age 14 and under) the teen still sees authority in the parents. However, he or she begins the process of gaining independence from the family by spending more time with friends. Conformity to peer group standards is important. The adolescent in this phase is very egocentric and is a concrete thinker, with only minimal ability to see him- or herself in the future or foresee the consequences of his or her behavior. Teens perceive their locus of control as external; that is, their destinies are controlled by others such as parents and school authorities.

Middle adolescence (ages 15 to 17 years) is the time for challenging; experimenting with drugs, alcohol, and sex is a common avenue for rebellion. Middle adolescents seek independence and turn increasingly to their peer groups. They begin to move from concrete thinking to formal operational thought but are not yet able to anticipate the long-term implications of all their actions. These years are often a time of great turmoil for the family as the adolescent struggles for independence and challenges the family's values and expectations.

In **late adolescence** (ages 18 to 19 years) teens are more at ease with their individuality and decision-making ability. They can think abstractly and anticipate consequences. Late adolescents are capable of formal operational thought. They learn to solve problems, to conceptualize, and to make decisions. These abilities help them see themselves as having control, which leads to the ability to understand and accept the consequences of their behavior.

FACTORS CONTRIBUTING TO ADOLESCENT PREGNANCY

Among adolescents there is great peer pressure to become sexually active during the teen years. Premarital sexual activity is commonplace, and teenage pregnancy is more socially acceptable today than it was in the past. Sexual innuendo permeates every aspect of the popular media, but issues of sexual responsibility are commonly ignored. Figure 10–1 ◆ identifies reasons teens cite for having sex.

Pregnancy risk taking (sexual activity without use of pregnancy prevention measures) stems from a variety of factors. Many adolescents do not consciously decide to be sexually active—they do not plan or expect to have sex. Pregnancy risk taking has also been linked to a lack of knowledge about contraception or delay in seeking con-

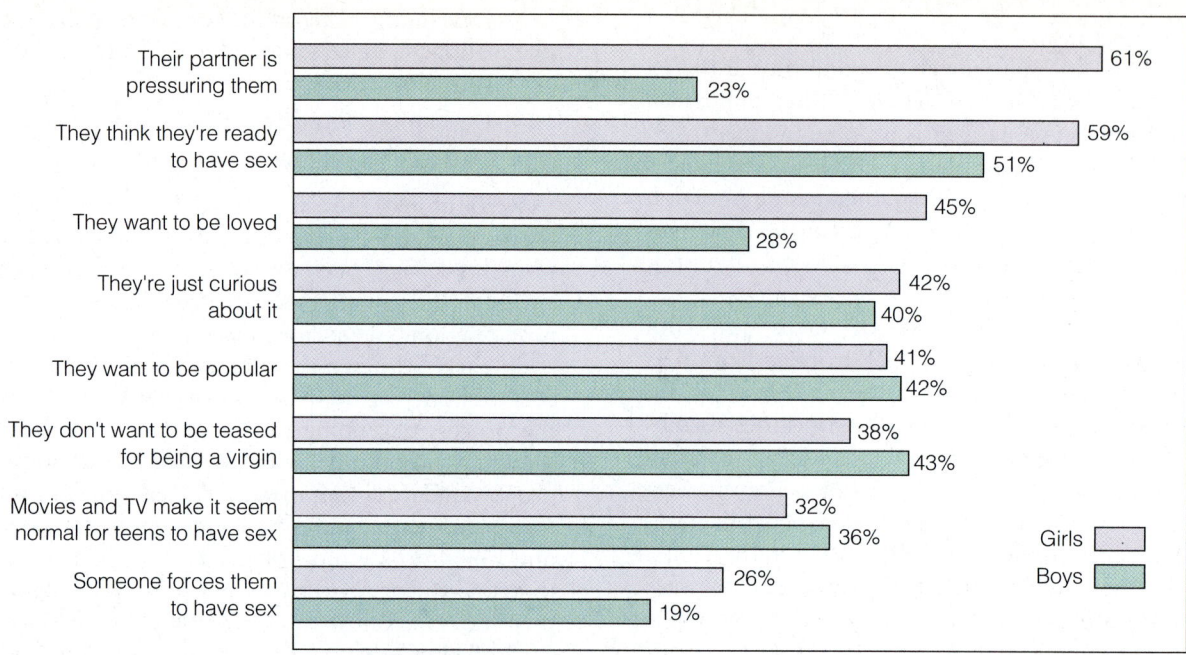

FIGURE 10–1. ◆ Why teens have sex. *Note:* From *The Kaiser Family Foundation Survey on Teens and Sex: What They Say. Teens Today Need to Know, and Who They Listen To.* June 1996. Menlo Park, CA: The Henry J. Kaiser Family Foundation.

traception. Delay may be attributed to the adolescent's worry that parents will find out, fear of the physical examination, the belief that contraception is dangerous, and ambivalence (Kendig & Omvig, 2001).

Some young teenagers may deliberately plan to get pregnant. The adolescent girl may use pregnancy for various subconscious or conscious reasons: to punish her father and/or mother, to escape from an undesirable home situation, to gain attention, or to feel that she has someone to love and to love her. Pregnancy may also be a young woman's form of acting out.

About three fourths of adolescents use some form of contraception (often a condom) the first time they have sexual intercourse, and 9 out of 10 sexually active adolescent girls and their partners use contraception, although not always correctly or consistently (Graydanus, Patel, & Rimsza, 2001). Compared with other teens, teens with future goals (that is, college or job) tend to use birth control more consistently; if they become pregnant, they are also more likely to have abortions. Adolescents who do not have access to middle-class opportunities tend to maintain their pregnancies, because they see pregnancy as their only option for adult status; 83% of births to unmarried teens occur to those from poor or low-income families (Alan Guttmacher Institute, 1999).

The younger the teen when she first gets pregnant, the more likely she is to have another pregnancy in her teens (East & Felice, 1996). Moreover, the likelihood of repeat pregnancies increases when the teen is living with her sexual partner and has dropped out of school. Daughters of women who had a baby in their early teens are at higher risk for teen pregnancy themselves.

Social and Cultural Factors

In the United States, the adolescent birth rate is higher among black and Latino teens than among white teens. However, pregnancy rates in these two groups are decreasing steadily (Santelli, 2000). To some degree, the discrepancy probably reflects the impact of poverty—a disproportionately higher number of black and Latino youths live in poverty—and the influence of ethnic or cultural norms.

Internationally, adolescent women are more likely to welcome a pregnancy in a country in which Islam is the predominant religion, where large families are desired, where social change is slow in coming, and where most childbearing occurs within marriage. Early pregnancy is less desired in countries in which the reverse is true.

Abuse as a Factor

More teens who become pregnant were sexually abused as children. In fact, maltreatment of any kind is a high-risk contributor to early teen pregnancy (Stock, Bell, Boyer, et al., 1997). Teenage pregnancy can result from an incestuous relationship. In the very young adolescent, incest or sexual abuse should be suspected as a possible cause of

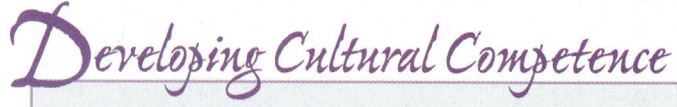

Developing Cultural Competence

Throughout the world, the higher a woman's educational level, the more likely she is to delay marriage and childbirth.

pregnancy. Teenage pregnancy could also be caused by other nonvoluntary sexual experiences such as acquaintance rape.

RISKS TO THE ADOLESCENT MOTHER

Physiologic Risks

Adolescents over age 15 who receive early, thorough prenatal care are at no greater risk during pregnancy than women over age 20. Unfortunately, many adolescents fail to seek early prenatal care and fail to cooperate with the recommendations they receive. Thus, risks for pregnant adolescents include preterm births, low-birth-weight infants, cephalopelvic disproportion, iron deficiency anemia, and preeclampsia and its sequelae. In the adolescent age group, prenatal care is the critical factor that most influences pregnancy outcome.

Teenagers ages 15 to 19 have a high incidence of sexually transmitted infections (STIs), including herpesvirus, syphilis, and gonorrhea. The incidence of chlamydial infection is also increased in this age group. The presence of such infections during a pregnancy greatly increases the risk to the fetus (Chapter 13 ⬭). Other problems seen in adolescents are cigarette smoking and drug use. By the time pregnancy is confirmed, the fetus may already have been harmed by these substances.

Psychologic Risks

The major psychologic risk to the pregnant adolescent is the interruption of her developmental tasks. Adding the tasks of pregnancy to her developmental tasks creates a huge amount of psychologic work, the completion of which will affect the adolescent's and her newborn's futures. Table 10–1 suggests typical behaviors of the adolescent when she becomes aware of her pregnancy. In reviewing these behaviors, the nurse should realize that other factors may influence individual response.

Sociologic Risks

Being forced into adult roles before completing adolescent developmental tasks causes a series of events that may result in prolonged dependence on parents, lack of stable relationships with the opposite sex, and lack of economic and

TABLE 10–1 Initial Reaction to Awareness of Pregnancy

Age	Adolescent Behavior	Nursing Implications
Early adolescent (14 and under)	Fears rejection by family and peers. Enters health care system with an adult, most likely mother (parents still seen as locus of control). Value system still closely reflects that of parents, so still turns to parents for decision or approval of decision. Pregnancy probably not result of intimate relationship. Is self-conscious about normal adolescent changes in body. Self-consciousness and low self-esteem likely to increase with rapid breast enlargement and abdominal enlargement of pregnancy.	Be nonjudgmental in approach to care. Focus on needs and concerns of adolescent, but if parent accompanies daughter, include parent in plan of care. Encourage both to express concerns and feelings regarding pregnancy and options: abortion, maintaining pregnancy, and adoption. Be realistic and concrete in discussion implications of each option. During physical exam of adolescent, respect increased sense of modesty. Explain in simple and concrete terms physical changes that are produced by pregnancy versus puberty. Explain each step of physical exam in simple and concrete terms.
Middle adolescent (15–17 years)	Fears rejection by peers and parents. Unsure in whom to confide. May seek confirmation of pregnancy on own with increased awareness of options and services, such as over-the-counter pregnancy kits and Planned Parenthood. If in an ongoing, caring relationship with partner (peer), may choose him as confidant. Economic dependence on parents may determine if and when parents are told. Future educational plans and perception of parental support or lack of support are significant factors in decision regarding termination or maintenance of the pregnancy. Possible conflict in parental and own developing value system.	Be nonjudgmental in approach to care. Reassure adolescent that confidentiality will be maintained. Help adolescent identify significant individuals in whom she can confide to help make a decision about the pregnancy. Be aware of state laws regarding requirement of parental notification if abortion intended. Also be aware of state laws regarding requirements for marriage: usually, minimum age for both parties is 18; 16- and 17-year-olds are, in most states, allowed to marry only with consent of parents. Encourage adolescent to be realistic about parental response to pregnancy.
Older adolescent (18–19 years)	Most likely to confirm pregnancy on own and at an earlier date due to increased acceptance and awareness of consequences of behavior. Likely to use pregnancy kit for confirmation. Relationship with father of baby, future educational plans, and own value system are among significant determinants of decision about pregnancy.	Be nonjudgmental in approach to care. Reassure adolescent that confidentiality will be maintained. Encourage adolescent to identify significant individuals in whom she can confide. Refer to counseling as appropriate. Encourage adolescent to be realistic about parental response to pregnancy.

social stability. Many teenage mothers drop out of school during their pregnancy. Many never complete their education. Lack of education reduces the quality of jobs available to them. Childbearing at an early age is a strong predictor of need for public assistance, especially in lower socioeconomic groups and when the pregnant teen's family does not support her (National Campaign to Prevent Teen Pregnancy, 1997).

Adolescent mothers frequently fail to establish a stable family, especially if they have a second child while still in their teens. Their family structure tends to be single-parent and matriarchal, often the same type in which the adolescents themselves were raised. Some pregnant adolescents choose to marry the father of the baby, who may be a teenager. Unfortunately, the majority of adolescent marriages end in divorce (Roye & Balk, 1996). This fact should not be surprising because pregnancy and marriage interrupt the adolescents' childhood and basic education. Lack of maturity in dealing with an intimate relationship also contributes to marital breakdown.

The increased incidence of maternal complications, preterm birth, and low-birth-weight babies among teen mothers also impacts society because many of these mothers are on welfare. The need for increased financial support for good prenatal care and nutritional programs remains critical.

Table 10–2 identifies the early adolescent's response to the developmental tasks of pregnancy. Middle and older adolescents respond differently, reflecting their progression through developmental tasks. In addition to her maturational level, the amount of nurturing the pregnant adolescent receives is a critical factor in the way she handles pregnancy and motherhood.

Risks for Her Child

Children of adolescent parents are at a disadvantage in many ways because teens are not developmentally or economically prepared to be parents. In general, children of teenage mothers are found to be at a developmental disadvantage compared with children whose mothers were older at the time of their birth. Many factors contribute to these differences, especially the adverse social and economic conditions many teenage mothers face. These factors result in high rates of family instability, disadvantaged neighborhoods, and high rates of behavior problems. In addition,

---

TABLE 10–2   The Early Adolescent's Response to the Developmental Tasks of Pregnancy

Stage	Developmental Tasks of Pregnancy	Early Adolescent's Response to Pregnancy	Nursing Implications
First trimester	Pregnancy confirmation. Seeking early prenatal care as a confirmation tool. Begins to evaluate her diet and general health habits. Initial ambivalence common. Usually supportive partner.	May delay confirmation of pregnancy until late part of first trimester or later. Reasons for delay may include lack of awareness that she is pregnant, fear of confiding in anyone, and denial. Rapid enlargement and sensitivity of breasts are embarrassing and frightening to early adolescent—may be perceived as changes of puberty. If confiding in mother, may be experiencing family turmoil in response to pregnancy.	Explain physiologic changes of pregnancy versus those associated with puberty. Explain that ambivalence is normal with any pregnancy, but recognize it as a much greater concern with adolescent pregnancy. Emphasize need for good nutrition as important for her well-being as much as infant's (prevention of PIH and anemia). Use simple explanations and lots of audiovisual aids. Have adolescent listen to fetal heart rate with Doppler.
Second trimester	Changes in physical appearance begin, and fetal movement is experienced, causing pregnancy to be experienced as a reality. Begins wearing maternity clothes to accommodate the physical changes. As a result of quickening she perceives her fetus as a real baby and begins preparing for the maternal role and new relationships with her partner and members of her family.	Some teenagers may delay validation of pregnancy until now, with family turmoil occurring at this time. Abdominal enlargement and quickening may be perceived as loss of control over body image. May try to maintain prepregnant weight and wear restrictive clothing to control and conceal changing body. Becomes dependent on her own mother for support. Egocentric; unable to develop a maternal role at this time.	Continue to discuss importance of good nutrition and adequate weight gain as noted above. Discuss ways of utilizing common teenage clothing (large sweatshirts, blouses) to promote comfort but preserve adolescent image to some degree. Discuss plans being made for baby, continued educational plans, and role of teen's parents.
Third trimester	At end of second trimester begins to view fetus as separate from self. Buys baby clothes and supplies. Prepares a place for the baby. Realistic about what baby is like. Prepares to give birth to infant. Anxiety increases as labor and birth approach and has concerns about well-being of fetus.	May focus on "wanting it to be over." May have trouble individuating fetus. May have fantasies, dreams, or nightmares about childbirth. Natural fears of labor and birth greater than with older primigravida. Probably has not been in a hospital, and may associate this with negative experiences.	Assess whether adolescent is preparing for baby by buying supplies and preparing a place in the home. Childbirth education is important. Provide hospital tour. Assess for discomforts of pregnancy, such as heartburn and constipation. Adolescent may be uncomfortable mentioning these and other problems.

these children do not do as well in school and are less likely to complete high school. Children born to adolescent mothers also have higher rates of abuse and neglect, resulting in significantly higher rates of foster care placement (National Campaign to Prevent Teen Pregnancy, 1997).

PARTNERS OF ADOLESCENT MOTHERS

Almost half of the fathers of infants of adolescent mothers are not teens but are 20 years of age or older (East & Felice, 1996). Of these men, approximately one fifth are 6 or more years older than the adolescent mother (Taylor, Chavez, Chabra, et al., 1999). The poorer the man's education, the greater the risk that he will father the child of an adolescent, possibly because he is seeking an intellectual and emotional equal in his sex partner. Often the older partners of pregnant adolescents are similar to adolescent fathers socioeconomically. They have experienced early school failure, are unemployed, and are no more likely than adolescent fathers to support the mother (Roye & Balk, 1996). Adult paternity also tends to be higher when the teenage mother was born outside the United States. This difference may reflect cultural norms (Taylor et al., 1997).

Adolescent males tend to become sexually active at an earlier age than females, and they have more sexual partners in their teenage years. When the father is an adolescent, he, too, has uncompleted developmental tasks for his age group and is no better prepared psychologically than his female counterpart to deal with the consequences of pregnancy. Consequently, the adolescent who attempts to assume his responsibility as a father faces many of the same psychologic and sociologic risks as the adolescent mother. The mother and father are generally from similar socioeconomic backgrounds and have similar educational levels.

Adolescent fathers tend to achieve less formal education than older fathers, and they enter the workforce earlier. They tend to pursue less prestigious careers and have less job satisfaction. They often marry at a younger age than older fathers and have more children.

Although they may not be married, many adolescent couples have meaningful relationships. The male partners may be very involved in the pregnancy and may be present for the birth. Research suggests that a teen who has a close, satisfying relationship with her baby's father is more likely to demonstrate maternal role behaviors during pregnancy and positive maternal attachment after birth (Bloom, 1998). Unfortunately, research also indicates that the father has decreasing contact with the mother and infant over time, even when he is involved in the birth (Taylor et al., 1999).

The role of the parents of the adolescent father has not been well studied. Some research indicates that sons are more involved with their babies when they believe that their own mothers expect it. Similarly, the mothers of teen fathers seem to influence the parenting behaviors their sons demonstrate. Adolescent fathers' need for continued parenting and their young age are the main barriers to their ability to perform the parental role (Dallas & Chen, 1999).

Some adolescent fathers face negative reactions from people, including their own families and the families of their young partners. They may experience others' anger, shame, and disappointment. Their relationships with their peers may be altered as well.

The lack of responsibility shown by some unmarried fathers has caused a shift in cultural and community attitudes. Fathers are included on birth certificates far more frequently today than in the past. This inclusion helps ensure the fathers' rights and encourages them to meet their responsibilities to their children. In addition, legal paternity gives children access to military and social security benefits and to medical information about their fathers.

In some situations the pregnant adolescent female may not want to identify or contact the father of the baby, and the male may not readily acknowledge paternity. Those situations include rape, exploitative sexual relations, incest, and casual sexual relations. If health care providers suspect any of the first three causes, further investigation into the situation is important for the well-being of the pregnant adolescent, and referral to other resources should be made as appropriate.

Health care providers should support the adolescent father in his decision to assume responsibility. It is important, however, that the pregnant adolescent have the chance to decide whether she wants the father to participate in her health care. If the adolescents perceive that they have a caring relationship, the adolescent father may want to be supportive and protective but probably does not understand the physical and psychologic changes his female partner is experiencing. The young man needs education about pregnancy, childbirth, child care, and parenting.

Although the adolescent father may have been included in the health care of the young woman throughout the pregnancy, it is not unusual for her to want her mother as her primary support person during labor and birth. Younger adolescents are especially likely to choose their mothers for this role. It is important both to support the pregnant adolescent's wishes and to acknowledge and support the adolescent father's wishes as appropriate.

As a part of counseling, the nurse should assess the young man's stressors, his support systems, his plans for involvement in the pregnancy and childbearing, and his future plans. He should be referred to social services for counseling about his educational and vocational future. When the father is involved in the pregnancy, the young mother feels less deserted, more confident in her decision making, and better able to discuss her future.

REACTIONS OF FAMILY AND SOCIAL NETWORK TO ADOLESCENT PREGNANCY

The reactions of families and support groups to adolescent pregnancy vary widely. In families that foster children's educational and career goals, adolescent pregnancy is often a shock. Anger, shame, and sorrow are common reactions. The majority of pregnant adolescents from these families are likely to choose abortion, with the exception of teens whose cultural and religious beliefs prevent them from seeking abortions.

In populations in which adolescent pregnancy is more prevalent and more socially acceptable, family and friends may be more supportive of the adolescent parents. In many cases, the teen's friends and mother are present at the birth. The expectant couple may also have friends who are already teen parents. Some male partners of these adolescent mothers see pregnancy and the birth of a baby as signs of adult status and increased sexual prowess—a source of pride.

The mother of the pregnant adolescent is usually among the first to be told about the pregnancy. She typically becomes involved with decision making, especially with the young adolescent, about issues such as maintaining the pregnancy, abortion, and dealing with the father-to-be and his family.

Once the pregnant adolescent decides how to proceed, it is often her mother who helps the teen access health care and accompanies her to her first prenatal visit. If the pregnancy is maintained, the mother may participate in prenatal care and classes and can be an excellent source of support for her daughter. She should be encouraged to participate if the mother-daughter relationship is positive. If the baby's father is involved in the pregnancy, he and the pregnant adolescent's mother may be able to work together to support the teenage mother. The pregnant adolescent's mother should be updated on childbearing practices to clarify any misconceptions she might have. During labor and birth, the mother may be a key figure for her daughter, offering reassurance and instilling confidence in the teen.

It is commonly believed that the adolescent and her infant will fare better if they live in the same household as the teen's mother, now the grandmother. However, research suggests that the best outcomes for the adolescent and her infant occur when there is regular assistance from the grandmother but they do not live together (Spieker & Bensley, 1994). The wise grandmother gently encourages a balance between helping her daughter to be a parent and allowing her to complete the tasks of adolescence and become more independent.

Nursing Management

Nursing Assessment and Diagnosis

Establish a knowledge base to plan interventions for the adolescent mother-to-be and family. Areas of assessment include history of family and personal physical health, developmental level and impact of pregnancy, and emotional and financial support. Also assess the family and social support network and the father's degree of involvement in the pregnancy.

As with all pregnant women, it is important to have information on general physical health. This may be the first time the adolescent has ever provided a health history. Consequently, it may be helpful to ask very specific questions and give examples if the young woman appears confused about a question. The teen's mother may be best able to answer questions about family history because the adolescent is often unaware of this information.

Assess the following areas: family and personal health history, medical history, menstrual history, obstetric and gynecologic history, and substance abuse history. It is also important to assess the maturational level of each person. The adolescent's development level and the impact of pregnancy are reflected in the degree of recognition of the realities and responsibilities involved in teenage pregnancy and parenting. Also assess the mother's self-concept (including body image), her relationship with the significant adults in her life, her attitude toward her pregnancy, and her coping methods in the situation, as well as the teen's knowledge of, attitude toward, and anticipated ability to care for the coming baby.

The socioeconomic status of the pregnant adolescent often places the baby at risk throughout life, beginning with conception. It is essential to assess family and social support systems, as well as the extent of financial support available.

The nursing diagnoses applicable to pregnant women in general apply to the pregnant adolescent. Other nursing diagnoses are influenced by the adolescent's age, support systems, socioeconomic situation, health, and maturity. Examples of nursing diagnoses specific to the pregnant adolescent may include the following:

▶ *Health-seeking behaviors:* information about child care related to expressed desire to parent effectively

▶ *Altered nutrition:* less than body requirements related to poor eating habits

▶ *Self-esteem disturbance* related to unanticipated pregnancy

Planning and Implementation

NURSING CARE IN THE COMMUNITY

Early, thorough prenatal care is the most critical factor in reducing risk for the adolescent mother and her newborn. Many innovative community programs have evolved to provide care for high-risk clients during the childbearing experience and beyond. Research suggests that a planned, multidimensional approach that includes preparation for motherhood classes, a series of focused prenatal home visits, and monthly visits for the first year after birth results in a reduced rate of preterm births and fewer days of infant hospitalization (Koniak-Griffin, Mathenge, Anderson, et al., 1999). Nurses in community-based agencies can help adolescents access the health care system as well as social services and other support services (e.g., food banks and the Women, Infants, and Children Program [WIC]). These nurses are also involved extensively in counseling and client teaching.

Issue of Confidentiality

Most states in the United States have passed legislation that confirms the right of some minors to assume the rights of adults; they are then called **emancipated minors.** An adolescent may be considered emancipated if he or she is self-supporting and living away from home, married, pregnant, a parent, or in the military service. The pregnant adolescent, even if very young, is generally considered emancipated and has the right and responsibility to consent to health care for herself and, later, for her child. If she is considered emancipated, she is entitled to confidentiality in her dealings with health care providers. Only with her agreement can other adults, including her parents, be included in communication.

Development of a Trusting Relationship with the Pregnant Adolescent

The first visit to the clinic or caregiver's office may make the young woman feel anxious and vulnerable. Making this first experience as positive as possible for the young woman will encourage the adolescent to return for follow-up care and to cooperate with her caregivers and will help her recognize the importance of health care for her and her baby. Developing a trusting relationship with the pregnant adolescent is essential. Honesty, respect, and a caring attitude promote self-esteem.

Depending on the adolescent's age, this may be her first pelvic examination, an anxiety-provoking experience for any woman. Provide explanations during the procedure. A gentle and thoughtful examination technique will help the young woman to relax.

Nursing Practice

During the initial pelvic examination, with the consent of the examiner, offer the teen a hand held mirror. A mirror is helpful in enabling the young woman to see her cervix, thus educating her about her anatomy. It also gives her an active role in the exam if she so desires.

Promotion of Self-Esteem and Problem-Solving Skills

Assist the adolescent in her decision-making and problem-solving skills so that she can proceed with her developmental tasks and begin to assume responsibility for her life and that of her newborn. Many adolescents are not aware of the legally available options to deal with an unplanned pregnancy. In an open, nonjudgmental way, without imposing personal values, educate the teen about her alternatives: terminating the pregnancy, maintaining the pregnancy and parenting the infant, or relinquishing the infant for adoption. The nurse can also provide information about community resources available to help with each alternative. Once the teen has decided on a course of action,

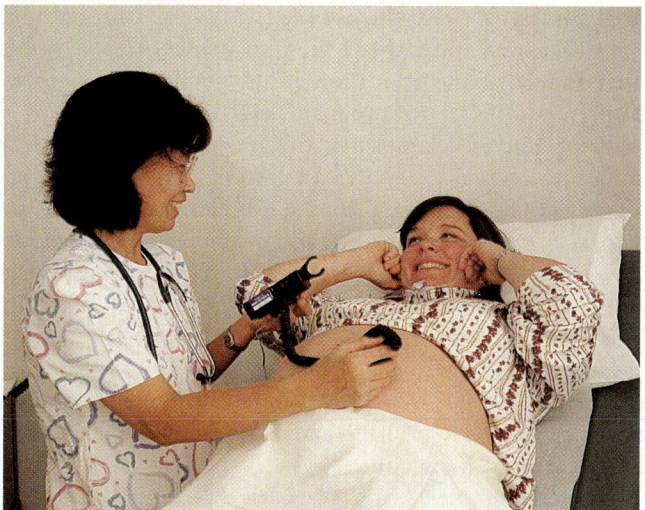

FIGURE 10–2. ◆ The nurse gives this young mother an opportunity to listen to her baby's heartbeat.

caregivers should respect her decision and support her efforts to achieve her goals.

If the adolescent chooses to continue her pregnancy, the nurse describes what she can expect over the prenatal period and provides an explanation and rationale for each procedure as it occurs. This overview fosters the adolescent's understanding and gives her some control (Figure 10–2 ◆).

Early adolescents tend to be egocentric and oriented to the present. They may not think it is important that their health and habits affect the fetus. Thus, it is often helpful to emphasize how these practices affect the teens themselves. Early adolescents also need help in problem solving and in visualizing the future so they can plan effectively.

Middle adolescents are developing the ability to think abstractly and can recognize that actions may have long-term consequences. They may not yet have acquired assertive communication skills, however, and may be reluctant to ask questions. Therefore, ask teens directly if they have questions. Middle adolescents can absorb more detailed health teaching and apply it.

Late adolescents can think abstractly, plan for the future, and function in a manner comparable to older pregnant women. They can also handle complex information and apply it.

Promotion of Physical Well-Being

Baseline weight and blood pressure measurements are valuable in assessing weight gain and predisposition to preeclampsia. Encourage the adolescent to take part in her care by measuring and recording her own weight. Use this time as an opportunity for assisting the young woman in problem solving and encourage her to ask herself the following questions: "Have I gained too much or too little weight?" "What influence does my diet have on my weight?" "How can I change my eating habits?"

Also introduce the subject of nutrition during measurement of baseline and subsequent hemoglobin and hematocrit values. Because the adolescent is at risk for anemia, she needs education about the importance of iron in her diet. Indeed, basic education about nutrition is a critical component of care for pregnant teens.

Preeclampsia-eclampsia is the most prevalent medical complication of pregnant adolescents. Blood pressure readings of 140/90 mm Hg are not acceptable as the determinant of preeclampsia in adolescents. Women ages 14 to 20 years without evidence of high blood pressure usually have diastolic readings between 50 and 66 mm Hg. Gradual increases from the prepregnant diastolic readings, along with excessive weight gain, must be evaluated as precursors to preeclampsia. Establishment of baseline readings is one reason early prenatal care is vital to management of the pregnant adolescent.

Adolescents have an increased incidence of STIs. The initial prenatal examination should include gonococcal and chlamydial cultures; wet-mount prep for *Candida, Trichomonas,* and *Gardnerella;* and tests for syphilis. Although today's teens are knowledgeable about HIV/AIDS, they know much less about other STIs, especially with regard to symptoms and risk reduction, so education is important. If the adolescent's history indicates that she is at increased risk for HIV, she should be given information about it and offered HIV screening.

Discuss substance abuse with the adolescent. It is important to review the risks associated with the use of tobacco, caffeine, drugs, and alcohol. The young woman should be aware of how these substances affect both her and her fetus's development.

Ongoing care should include the same assessments that an older pregnant woman receives. Pay special attention to evaluating fetal growth by determining when quickening occurs and by measuring fundal height, fetal heart rate, and fetal movement. If there is a question of size-date discrepancy by 2 cm either way when assessing fundal height, an ultrasound is warranted to establish fetal age so that instances of intrauterine growth restriction can be detected early.

Thinking Critically

EVALUATING AN ADOLESCENT'S NUTRITIONAL NEEDS

Cindy Lenz, a 15-year-old Gr1P0, is 16 weeks pregnant when she arrives for her second prenatal visit. She is drinking diet soda and eating potato chips as she waits for her appointment. Her 18-year-old boyfriend is with her. While reviewing her history, you remember that Cindy had tried to get pregnant for several months. Her boyfriend, a high school dropout, has a part-time job. Cindy is still living at home, although she does not get along with her mother or sister. She plans to stay in school until her baby is born because she has two other friends at school who are also pregnant. As you weigh Cindy, you ask a few questions about her nutritional habits and find that she eats a lot of junk food and very few vegetables or fruits. How should you discuss Cindy's nutritional needs with her? WEB

Promotion of Family Adaptation

Assess the family situation during the first prenatal visit and find out the level of involvement the adolescent wants from each of her family members and the father of the child, as well as her perception of their present support. If the mother and daughter agree, the mother should be included in the client's care. Also help the teen's mother assess and meet her daughter's needs. Some adolescents become more dependent during pregnancy, and some become more independent. The mother can ease and encourage her daughter's self-growth by understanding how best to respond to and support the adolescent.

The adolescent's relationship with her father is also affected by her pregnancy. Provide information to the father and encourage his involvement to whatever degree is acceptable to both daughter and father.

Finally, the father of the adolescent's infant should not be forgotten in promoting the family's adaptation to the pregnancy. He should be included in prenatal visits, classes, health teaching, and in the birth itself to the extent that he wishes and that is acceptable to the teenage mother. He should also have the opportunity to express his feelings and concerns and to have his questions answered.

Facilitation of Prenatal Education

School systems attempt to meet prenatal education needs in many ways. The most effective method appears to be mainstreaming the pregnant adolescent in academic classes with her peers and adding classes appropriate to her needs during pregnancy and postpartum. Classes about growth and development beginning with the newborn and early infancy periods can help teenage parents to develop realistic expectations of their infants and may help decrease child abuse. Mainstreaming is an ideal way to help teens complete their education while learning the skills they need to cope. Vocational guidance in this setting is also beneficial as they plan for their futures.

Most childbirth educators believe that prenatal classes with other teens are best, even though they can be challenging to teach (Figure 10–3 ◆). The pregnant teen may be accompanied by her mother, her boyfriend, or her girlfriends. Those who bring girlfriends may bring a different one each time, and giggling and side conversations may occur. Such activity reflects the short attention span of the teen and is fairly typical. Thus, to keep the attention of the participants, it is important to use a variety of teaching strategies including audiovisual aids, demonstrations, and games.

Goals for prenatal classes may include the following:

▶ Providing anticipatory guidance about pregnancy
▶ Preparing participants for labor and birth
▶ Helping participants identify the problems and conflicts of teenage pregnancy and parenting
▶ Promoting increased self-esteem
▶ Providing information about available community resources
▶ Helping participants develop adaptive coping skills

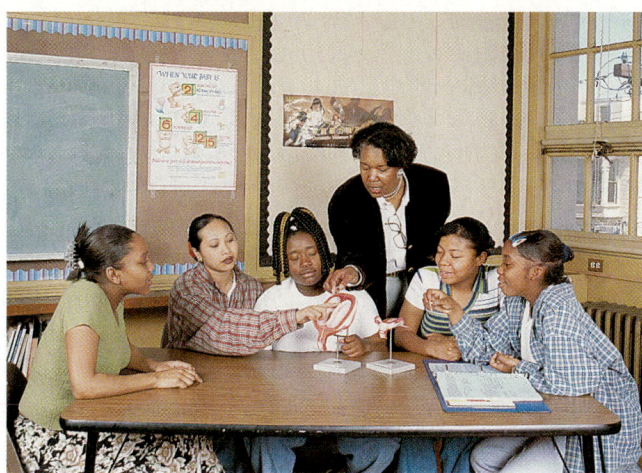

FIGURE 10–3. ◆ Young adolescents may benefit from prenatal classes designed for them.

Although parenting topics are sometimes included in prenatal classes for adolescents, teens may not retain the information because they tend to be present-oriented. Parenting skills are crucial, but adolescents generally are not ready to learn about these skills until birth makes the newborn—and thus parenting—a reality.

HOSPITAL-BASED NURSING CARE

The adolescent's mother is often present during the teen's labor and birth. The father of the baby may also be involved. Close girlfriends may arrive soon after the teen is admitted. At admission, ask the teen who will be her primary support person in labor and who she wants involved in the labor and birth. This information may also be included on her prenatal record.

The adolescent in labor has the same care needs as any pregnant woman. However, she may require more sustained care. Be readily available and answer questions simply and honestly, using lay terminology. Also help the adolescent's support people understand their roles in assisting the teen. If the father of the baby is involved, encourage him, at his own level of comfort, to play an active role in all phases of the birth process, perhaps by supporting the teen's relaxation techniques, feeding her ice chips, timing her contractions, and coaching her with her breathing. Recommend hand-holding, back rubs, and supportive touching.

During the postpartum period, most teens do not foresee that they will become sexually active in the near future and are often adamant that they will not become pregnant again for a long time. However, the statistics demonstrate a different reality. Consequently, predischarge teaching should include information about the resumption of ovulation and the importance of contraception. It is especially helpful to provide this information to both the adolescent mother and her sexual partner. Encourage the couple to use condoms and spermicide until they choose another method of birth control.

As part of discharge planning, ensure that the teen is aware of community resources available to assist her and her family. Postpartum classes, especially with peers, can be particularly beneficial. Such classes address a variety of topics including postpartum adaptation, infant and child development, parenting skills, and the like.

Evaluation

Expected outcomes of nursing care include the following:

▶ A trusting relationship is established with the pregnant adolescent.

▶ The adolescent is able to use her problem-solving abilities to make appropriate choices.

▶ The adolescent follows the recommendations of the health care team and receives effective health care throughout her pregnancy, the birth, and the postpartum period.

▶ The adolescent, her partner (if he is involved), and their families are able to cope successfully with the effects of the pregnancy.

▶ The adolescent is able to discuss pregnancy, prenatal care, and childbirth.

▶ The adolescent develops skill in child care and parenting.

PREVENTION OF ADOLESCENT PREGNANCY

In 1996 the National Campaign to Prevent Teen Pregnancy was founded. The group's purpose is to reduce teenage pregnancy one third by 2005 (National Campaign to Prevent Teen Pregnancy, 2000). The National Campaign is a private, nonprofit organization made up of a broad spectrum of religious, political, social, human services, health, and academic organizations. Not surprisingly, the National Campaign has found that adolescent pregnancy is a multifaceted problem with no easy answers. The best approach is local and is based on strong, community-wide involvement with a variety of programs directed at the multiple causes of the problem (Kirby, 1997).

One of the major problems in local communities continues to be intense conflict among different groups about how to approach adolescent pregnancy prevention. Some groups believe that abstinence is the only answer, whereas others believe that abstinence programs do not work with the many teens who are already sexually active. The latter groups believe that sex education and easy availability of contraception are the answers. Ironically, a comprehensive review of research suggests that neither of the proposed solutions, individually or together, is as effective in reducing the teen pregnancy rate as many believe. The risk factors most closely associated with teen birth rates **WEB** appear to be poverty, low educational achievement, poor self-esteem, family dysfunction, and high-risk behaviors in general. Thus research suggests that programs to address these societal problems and give teens hope for a different future are more effective than programs narrowly focused on teen sexual activity (Moore & Sugland, 1996; Stevens-Simon, Kelly, Singer, et al., 1996). In teen populations with job accessibility and education, easy, confidential access to sex education and contraception is also important in reducing teen pregnancy rates (Table 10–3).

The cause or motivation for pregnancy varies from one community to another. In inner-city areas, where there are high rates of poverty, low self-esteem, school failure, early behavioral problems, and delinquent behaviors, programs that promote self-esteem, deal with these social ills, and provide hope for these youth are critical. However, the National Campaign has identified similar characteristics in successful programs, regardless of the type of offering or community. Some of the critical characteristics of effective adolescent pregnancy prevention programs include the following:

- Involvement of adolescents in the planning of programs
- Good role models from the same cultural and racial backgrounds
- Long-term and intensive programs
- Sufficient focus on the adolescent male population

TABLE 10–3 Community Approaches to Preventing Adolescent Pregnancy

I. PLANNING

- Involve all sectors of the community (e.g., business groups, religious groups, civic organizations, health and human service providers, schools, media).
- Commit to adequate, long-term funding.
- Include teens in planning effective programs.
- Target high-risk populations within the community.
- Target males as well as females.
- Plan programs that are culturally appropriate and age appropriate as well as locally relevant.

II. SAMPLE COMPONENTS OF A COMMUNITY PROGRAM

- Youth development activities, such as tutoring, mentoring, after-school activities, community volunteer work.
- Community-based adolescent health clinics.
- School dropout prevention.
- Opportunities for career counseling and job training.
- Comprehensive sexuality education, which not only includes accurate information about sexually transmitted infections and contraception but also teaches adolescents skills to avoid peer pressure and promote responsible relationships.

- Educational programs for teachers and religious leaders who teach sexuality education.
- Educational programs for parents on communication skills and increasing knowledge.
- Peer training to act as educators and to give support.

III. EVALUATION

- Evaluation of the process is essential and should include reports about services that are being delivered plus basic demographics (i.e., who attends the program over time).
- Knowledge, attitudes, and intent should also be evaluated; however, these factors have not been found to be significantly related to the adolescents' actual behaviors (Philliber & Namerow, 1995).
- Evaluation of the impact of specific programs may be too expensive for most communities because it involves experimental research that is difficult to implement (i.e., large sample size, control groups, random assignment into groups, and long-term follow-up).
- Pregnancy rates and birth rates are not likely to change rapidly (Kirby, 1997; Moore & Sugland, 1996).

---

*C*HAPTER HIGHLIGHTS

∽ Although the U.S. birth rate (number of births per 1000 women) for adolescents dropped from 62 per 1,000 in 1991 to 51 per 1000 in 1998, the United States continues to have one of the highest levels of adolescent childbearing among industrialized nations.

∽ Many factors contribute to the high teenage pregnancy rate, including earlier age at first experience with sexual intercourse, lack of knowledge about conception, lack of easy access to contraception, lessened stigma associated with adolescent pregnancy in some populations, poverty, early school failure, and early childhood sexual abuse.

∽ Physical risks of adolescent pregnancy include preterm births, low-birth-weight infants, cephalopelvic disproportion, iron-deficiency anemia, and preeclampsia and its sequelae.

∽ In the adolescent age group, prenatal care is the critical factor that most influences pregnancy outcome.

∽ The major psychologic risk the pregnant adolescent faces is the interruption of her own developmental tasks.

∽ In general, the children of teenage mothers are found to be at a developmental disadvantage compared with children whose mothers were older at the time of their birth.

∽ Almost half of the fathers of infants of adolescent mothers are age 20 or older but are often similar to adolescent fathers psychosocially and no more likely to be able to support the mother.

Factors affecting an adolescent's response to pregnancy include her degree of achievement of the developmental tasks of adolescence (which can be closely associated with age), as well as cultural, religious, and socioeconomic factors.

Often the adolescent has little understanding of pregnancy, childbirth, or parenting. Consequently, education is a primary responsibility of the nurse.

Adolescent pregnancy prevention programs should be multifaceted, target males as well as females, and involve community-wide approaches.

EXPLOREMEDIALINK

NCLEX Review, Case Studies, and other interactive resources for this chapter can be found on the companion website at http://www.prenhall.com/london. Click on "Chapter 10" to select the activities for this chapter.

For animations, more NCLEX review questions, and an audio glossary, access the accompanying CD-ROM in this textbook.

REFERENCES

Alan Guttmacher Institute. (1996). *Issues in brief: Risks and realities of early childbearing.* Washington, DC: Author.

Alan Guttmacher Institute. (1999). *Issues in brief: Teen sex and pregnancy, 1999.* Washington, DC: Author.

Bloom, K. C. (1998). Perceived relationship with the father of the baby and maternal attachment in adolescents. *Journal of Obstetric, Gynecologic, and Neonatal Nursing, 27*(4), 420–430.

Clark, L. R., Cohall, A. T., & Joffe, A. (1998). Beyond the birds and the bees: Talking to teens about sex. *Contemporary OB/GYN, 43*(4), 35–61.

Cockey, C. D. (1997). Preventing teen pregnancy: It's time to stop kidding around. *AWHONN Lifelines, 1*(3), 32–40.

Dallas, C. M., & Chen, S. C. (1999). Perspectives of women whose sons become adolescent fathers. *American Journal of Maternal-Child Nursing, 24*(5), 247–251.

East, P. L., & Felice, M. E. (1996). *Adolescent pregnancy and parenting: Findings from a racially diverse sample.* Hillsdale, NJ: Erlbaum.

Graydanus, D., Patel, D., & Rimsza, M. (2001). Contraception in the adolescent: An update. *Pediatrics, 107*(3), 526–73.

Kendig, S., & Omvig, K. J. (2001, Spring/Summer). Why are teens still getting pregnant despite contraceptive options? *Contemporary Nurse Practitioner*, 10–20.

Kirby, D. (1997). *No easy answers: Research findings on programs to reduce teen pregnancy (summary).* Washington, DC: National Campaign to Prevent Teen Pregnancy.

Koniak-Griffin, D., Mathenge, C., Anderson, N. L. R., & Verzemnieks, I. (1999). An early intervention program for adolescent mothers: A nursing demonstration project. *Journal of Obstetric, Gynecologic, and Neonatal Nursing, 28*(1), 51–59.

Moore, K., & Sugland, B. (1996). *Next steps and best bets: Approaches to preventing adolescent childbearing.* Washington, DC: Child Trends.

National Campaign to Prevent Teen Pregnancy. (2000). Fact sheet report.

National Campaign to Prevent Teen Pregnancy. (2002). United States birth rates for teens, 15–19. www.teenpregnancy.org

Philliber, S., & Namerow, P. (1995, December). *Trying to maximize the odds: Using what we know to prevent teen pregnancy.* Paper presented at technical assistance workshop to support the Teen Pregnancy Prevention Program. Division of Reproductive Health, Centers for Disease Control and Prevention, Atlanta, GA.

Roye, C. F., & Balk, S. J. (1996). The relationship of partner support to outcomes for teenage mothers and their children: A review. *Journal of Adolescent Health, 19*(2), 86–93.

Santelli, J., Linburg, L., Abma, J., & McNeely, C. (2000). Adolescent sexual behaviors. Estimates and trends from four nationally representative surveys. *Family Planning Perspectives, 32*(4), 156–165, 194.

Singh, S., & Darroch, J. E. (2000). Adolescent pregnancy and childbearing: Levels and trends in developed countries. *Family Planning Perspectives, 32*(1), 14–23.

Spieker, S. J., & Bensley, L. (1994). Roles of living arrangements and grandmother social support in adolescent mothering and infant attachment. *Developmental Psychology, 30*(1), 102–111.

Steinberg, L. (1999). *Adolescence* (5th ed.). Boston: McGraw-Hill.

Stevens-Simon, C., Kelly, L., Singer, D., & Cox, A. (1996). Why pregnant adolescents say they did not use contraceptives prior to conception. *Journal of Adolescent Health, 19*(1), 48–53.

Stock, J. L., Bell, M. A., Boyer, D. K., & Connell, F. A. (1997). Adolescent pregnancy and sexual risk-taking among sexually abused girls. *Family Planning Perspectives, 29*(5), 200–203, 227.

Taylor, D., Chavez, G., Adams, E., Chabra, A., & Shah, R. (1999). Demographic characteristics in adult paternity for first births to adolescents under 15 years of age. *Journal of Adolescent Health 24*(4), 251–58.

Taylor, D., Chavez, G., Chabra, A., & Boggess, J. (1997). Risk factors for adult paternity in births to adolescents. *Obstetrics and Gynecology, 89*(2), 199–205.

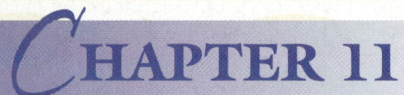
Maternal Nutrition

When I was young I thought nutrition was boring. Now that I am pregnant I find it endlessly fascinating. I realize how important good nutrition is for me, for my husband, and for the well-being of our child. My mother just laughs and reminds me about the times I resisted her efforts to help me develop better eating habits. Oh well, it is just another example of how smart our parents get as we get older!

—MARIA, 26

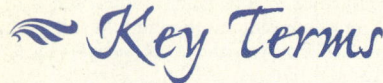

Key Terms

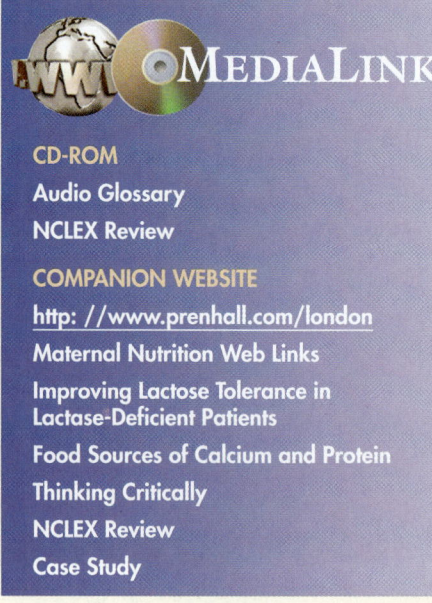

MEDIALINK

CD-ROM

Audio Glossary

NCLEX Review

COMPANION WEBSITE

http: //www.prenhall.com/london

Maternal Nutrition Web Links

Improving Lactose Tolerance in Lactase-Deficient Patients

Food Sources of Calcium and Protein

Thinking Critically

NCLEX Review

Case Study

woman's nutritional status before and during pregnancy can significantly influence her health and that of her fetus. In most prenatal clinics and offices, nurses offer nutritional counseling directly or work closely with the nutritionist in providing nutritional assessment and teaching.

This chapter focuses on the nutritional needs of a normal pregnant woman. Special sections consider the nutritional needs of the pregnant adolescent and the woman after giving birth.

Fetal growth occurs in three overlapping stages: (1) growth by increase in cell number, (2) growth by increases in cell number and cell size, and (3) growth by increase in cell size alone. Nutritional problems that interfere with cell division may have permanent consequences. If the nutritional deficit occurs when cells are mainly enlarging, the changes are usually reversible when normal nutrition resumes.

Growing fetal and maternal tissues require increased quantities of essential dietary components. These are listed in the **dietary reference intakes (DRIs)** as either *recommended dietary allowances* (RDA) or *adequate intake* (AI). `WEB` `CD` Women can get most of the recommended nutrients by eating a well-balanced diet each day. The basic food groups and recommended amounts during pregnancy and lactation are presented in Table 11–1.

MATERNAL WEIGHT GAIN

Maternal weight gain is an important factor in fetal growth and infant birth weight. Optimal weight gain depends on the woman's weight for height (body mass index) and her prepregnant nutritional state. An adequate weight gain indicates an adequate caloric intake. However, it does not ensure that the woman has a good diet nutritionally. The pregnant woman must maintain the nutritional quality of her diet as her weight gain progresses.

The Institute of Medicine (1992) recommends optimum ranges of weight gain, as follows:

- Underweight woman: 28 to 40 lb (12.5 to 18 kg)
- Normal-weight woman: 25 to 35 lb (11.5 to 16 kg)
- Overweight woman: 15 to 25 lb (7 to 11.5 kg)
- Obese woman: ≤15 lb (≤7 kg)

The average maternal weight gain is distributed as follows:

11 lb (5 kg)	Fetus, placenta, amniotic fluid
2 lb (0.9 kg)	Uterus
4 lb (1.8 kg)	Increased blood volume
3 lb (1.4 kg)	Breast tissue
5 to 10 lb (2.3 to 4.5 kg)	Maternal stores

For a normal-weight woman the ideal pattern of weight gain during pregnancy is a gain of 3.5 to 5 lb (1.6 to 2.3 kg) during the first trimester, followed by a gain of about 1 lb (0.5 kg) per week during the second and third trimesters. A normal-weight woman who is expecting twins should gain about 1.5 lb per week during the second and third trimesters of her pregnancy (Brown & Carlson, 2000).

The pattern of weight gain is important. A woman should generally gain 10 to 13 lb (4.5 to 6 kg) by 20 weeks' gestation. If she has not, the nurse should offer further nutritional evaluation and counseling. Sudden, sharp increases (weight gains of 3 to 5 lb [1.4 to 2.3 kg] in 1 week) may indicate excessive fluid retention related to preeclampsia-eclampsia and needs to be evaluated. Inadequate gains (less than 2.2 lb [1 kg] per month during the second and third trimesters) or excessive gains (more than 6.6 lb [3 kg] per month) should be assessed and the need for nutritional counseling considered.

Pregnancy is not a time for dieting, and severe dieting during pregnancy can result in maternal ketosis, a threat to fetal well-being. Counseling the pregnant woman to eat according to the Food Guide Pyramid (Figure 11–1 ◆) places less emphasis on the amount of her weight gain and more on the quality of her diet.

Women 10% or more below their recommended weight before conception have an increased risk of giving birth to a low-birth-weight infant and have an increased risk of developing preeclampsia (Institute of Medicine, 1990). Underweight women are generally advised to increase their caloric intake by 500 kilocalories (kcal) above the nonpregnant RDA, as opposed to the 300-kcal increase. They should also consume 20 g additional protein. This is often difficult for underweight women, especially if they have a small appetite, and they will need support and encouragement from family and health care providers.

NUTRITIONAL REQUIREMENTS

The RDA for almost all nutrients increases during pregnancy, although the amount of increase varies with each nutrient. These increases reflect the additional requirements of both the mother and the developing fetus (see Table 11–1).

Folic acid and iron are the only nutritional supplements generally recommended during pregnancy. An adequate diet can usually meet the increased need for other vitamins and minerals. To avoid possible deficiencies, however, many health care professionals still recommend a daily vitamin supplement.

Calories

The term **calorie** (cal) designates the amount of heat required to raise the temperature of 1 g of water 1 °C. The **kilocalorie** (kcal) is equivalent to 1,000 cal and is the unit used to express the energy value of food.

The RDA for calories during pregnancy is as follows: no increase during the first trimester but an increase of

TABLE 11-1 Daily Food Plan for Pregnancy and Lactation

Food Group	Nutrients Provided	Food Source	Recommended Daily Amount During Pregnancy	Recommended Daily Amount During Lactation
Dairy products	Protein; riboflavin; vitamins A, D, and others; calcium; phosphorus; zinc, magnesium	Milk—whole, 2%, skim, dry, buttermilk Cheeses—hard, semisoft, cottage Yogurt—plain, low-fat Soybean milk—canned, dry	Four (8-oz) cups (five for teenagers) used plain or with flavoring, in shakes, soups, puddings, custards, cocoa Calcium in 1 cup milk equivalent to 1 1/2 cups cottage cheese, 1 1/2 oz hard or semisoft cheese, 1 cup yogurt, 1 1/2 cups ice cream (high in fat and sugar)	Four (8-oz) cups (five for teenagers); equivalent amount of cheese, yogurt, and so forth
Meat and meat alternatives	Protein; iron; thiamine; niacin, and other vitamins; minerals	Beef, pork, veal, lamb, poultry, animal organ meats, fish, eggs; legumes; nuts, seeds, peanut butter, grains in proper vegetarian combination (vitamin B_{12} supplement needed)	Three servings (one serving = 2 oz), combination in amounts necessary for same nutrient equivalent (varies greatly)	Four servings
Grain products, whole grain or enriched	B vitamins; iron; whole grain also has zinc, magnesium, and other trace elements; provides fiber	Breads and bread products such as cornbread, muffins, waffles, hotcakes, biscuits, dumplings, cereals, pastas, rice	Six to eleven servings daily: one serving = one slice bread, 3/4 cup or 1 oz dry cereal, 1/2 cup rice or pasta	Same as for pregnancy
Fruits and fruit juices	Vitamins A and C; minerals; raw fruits for roughage	Citrus fruits and juices, melons, berries, all other fruits and juices	Two to four servings (one serving for vitamin C): one serving = one medium fruit, 1/2–1 cup fruit, 4 oz orange or grapefruit juice	Same as for pregnancy
Vegetables and vegetable juices	Vitamins A and C; minerals; provides roughage	Leafy green vegetables; deep yellow or orange vegetables such as carrots, sweet potatoes, squash, tomatoes; green vegetables such as peas, green beans, broccoli; other vegetables such as beets, cabbage, potatoes, corn, lima beans	Three to five servings (one serving of dark green or deep yellow vegetable for vitamin A): one serving = 1/2–1 cup vegetable, two tomatoes, one medium potato	Same as for pregnancy
Fats	Vitamins A and D; linoleic acid	Butter, cream cheese, fortified table spreads; cream, whipped cream, whipped toppings; avocado, mayonnaise, oil, nuts	As desired in moderation (high in calories): one serving = 1 tbsp butter or enriched margarine	Same as for pregnancy
Sugar and sweets		Sugar, brown sugar, honey, molasses	Occasionally, if desired	Same as for pregnancy
Desserts		Nutritious desserts such as puddings, custards, fruit whips, and crisps; other rich, sweet desserts and pastries	Occasionally, if desired	Same as for pregnancy
Beverages		Coffee, decaffeinated beverages, tea, bouillon, carbonated drinks	As desired, in moderation	Same as for pregnancy
Miscellaneous		Iodized salt, herbs, spices, condiments	As desired	Same as for pregnancy

Note: The pregnant woman should eat regularly, three meals a day, with nutritious snacks of fruit, cheese, milk, or other foods between meals if desired. (More frequent but smaller meals are also recommended. Four to six (8-oz) glasses of water and a total of 8 to 10 (8-oz) cups total fluid intake should be consumed daily. Water is an essential nutrient.

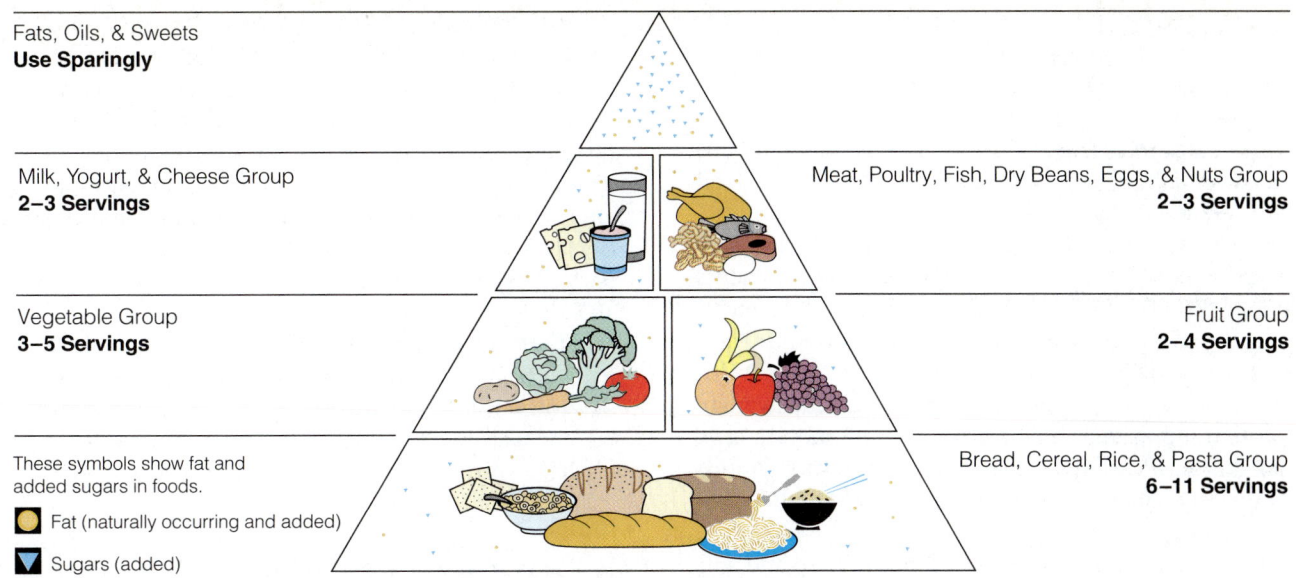

Fats, Oils, & Sweets
Use Sparingly

Milk, Yogurt, & Cheese Group
2–3 Servings

Meat, Poultry, Fish, Dry Beans, Eggs, & Nuts Group
2–3 Servings

Vegetable Group
3–5 Servings

Fruit Group
2–4 Servings

These symbols show fat and
added sugars in foods.

Fat (naturally occurring and added)

Sugars (added)

Bread, Cereal, Rice, & Pasta Group
6–11 Servings

FIGURE 11–1. ◆ The Food Guide Pyramid provides a quick reference for people interested in healthful eating. The largest portion of the pyramid is devoted to grains, rice, bread, and pasta, and the smallest portion of the pyramid is devoted to fats, oils, and sweets, which should be used sparingly. *Note:* From U.S. Department of Agriculture; U.S. Department of Health and Human Services.

Teaching About

300 kcal/day during the second and third trimesters. Prepregnant weight, height, maternal age, health status, and activity level all influence caloric needs, and weight should be monitored regularly during the pregnancy. See "Teaching About: Adding 300 kcal During Pregnancy."

Carbohydrates

Carbohydrates provide the body's main source of energy as well as the fiber necessary for proper bowel functioning.

If the total caloric intake is not adequate, the body uses protein for energy. Protein then becomes unavailable for growth needs. In addition, protein breakdown leads to ketosis.

The carbohydrate and caloric needs of the pregnant woman increase, especially during the last two trimesters. Carbohydrate intake promotes weight gain and growth of the fetus, placenta, and other maternal tissues. Dairy products, fruits, vegetables, and whole-grain cereals and breads all contain carbohydrates and other important nutrients.

Protein

Protein supplies the amino acids required for the growth and development of maternal tissues, such as the uterus and breasts, and to meet fetal needs. This is especially important during the last half of pregnancy, when fetal growth is greatest.

The protein requirement for a pregnant woman is 60 g/day, an increase of 20% over prepregnancy requirements (Reifsnider & Gill, 2000). Animal products such as meat, fish, poultry, and eggs provide high-quality protein. Dairy products are also important protein sources. A quart of milk supplies 32 g of protein, more than half the average daily protein requirement. A woman can incorporate milk into her diet in a variety of dishes, including soups, puddings, custards, sauces, and yogurt. Beverages such as hot chocolate and milk-and-fruit drinks can also be included, but they are high in calories. Various kinds of hard and soft cheeses and cottage cheese are excellent protein sources, although cream cheese is considered a fat source only. Women who have allergies to milk, are lactose intolerant, or practice vegetarianism may find soy milk acceptable. It can be used in cooked dishes or as a beverage. Tofu, or soybean curd, can replace cottage cheese. ⊂⊃ WEB

If the woman consumes little or no protein from animal sources, it is necessary to combine foods of plant origin to get the amino acids necessary for a complete protein. Examples of combined proteins are beans and rice, peanut butter on whole-grain bread, and whole-grain cereal and milk. Except in unusual medical situations, the pregnant woman should get protein through natural foods and avoid using protein and amino acid supplements.

Fat

Fats are valuable sources of energy for the body. Fats are more completely absorbed during pregnancy, resulting in a marked increase in serum lipids, lipoproteins, and cholesterol and decreased elimination of fat through the bowel. Fat deposits in the fetus increase from about 2% at midpregnancy to almost 12% at term. The RDA for fat is less than 30% of daily caloric intake, of which less than 10% should be saturated fat.

Minerals

CALCIUM AND PHOSPHORUS

Calcium and phosphorus are involved in the mineralization of fetal bones and teeth, energy and cell production, and acid-base buffering. The body absorbs and uses calcium more efficiently during pregnancy. Some calcium and phosphorus are required early in pregnancy, but most fetal bone calcification occurs during the last 2 to 3 months. Teeth begin to form at about 8 weeks' gestation and are formed by birth. The 6-year molars begin to calcify just before birth.

The recommended (AI) intake for calcium for the pregnant or lactating woman, age 19 or older, is 1000 mg/day. It is 1300 mg/day for pregnant women under age 19. If calcium intake is low, fetal needs will be met at the mother's expense by demineralization of bone.

A diet that includes 4 cups of milk or an equivalent dairy alternative will provide sufficient calcium. Smaller amounts of calcium are supplied by legumes, nuts, dried fruits, and dark green leafy vegetables (such as kale, cabbage, collards, and turnip greens). ⊂⊃ WEB

The RDA for phosphorus is 700 mg/day for the pregnant or lactating woman age 19 and older. It is 1250 mg/day for women under 19 years. Because phosphorus is so widely available in foods, the daily requirement is readily supplied through calcium- and protein-rich foods.

IODINE

Iodine is an essential part of the thyroid hormone thyroxine. The thyroid gland may become enlarged if iodine is not replaced by adequate dietary intake or an additional supplement. Moreover, cretinism may occur in the infant if the mother has a severe iodine deficiency. Pregnant women can meet the iodine allowance of 220 μg/day by using iodized salt. When salt is restricted, the physician may prescribe an iodine supplement.

SODIUM

Sodium is essential for proper metabolism and the regulation of fluid balance. Sodium intake in the form of salt is never entirely restricted during pregnancy, even when hypertension is present. The pregnant woman may season food to taste during cooking but should avoid using extra salt at the table. She can avoid excessive intake by eliminating salty foods such as potato chips, ham, sausages, and sodium-based seasonings.

ZINC

Zinc is needed for protein metabolism and the synthesis of DNA and RNA. It is essential for normal fetal growth and development as well as milk production during lactation. The RDA during pregnancy is 11 mg/day for women age 19 and older. Sources include meats, shellfish, poultry, whole grains, and legumes.

MAGNESIUM

Magnesium is essential for cellular metabolism and structural growth. The RDA for pregnancy is 350 mg/day for women age 19 to 30. Good sources include milk, whole grains, dark green vegetables, nuts, and legumes.

IRON

Iron requirements increase during pregnancy because of the growth of the fetus and placenta and the increased maternal blood volume. Anemia in pregnancy is mainly caused by low iron stores, although it may also be caused by inadequate intake of other nutrients, such as vitamins B_6 and B_{12}, folic acid, ascorbic acid, copper, and zinc. *Iron de-*

ficiency anemia is generally defined as a decrease in the oxygen-carrying capacity of the blood. Anemia leads to a significant reduction in hemoglobin in the volume of packed red cells per deciliter of blood (hematocrit) or in the number of erythrocytes. Iron deficiency anemia may be associated with preterm birth and higher maternal morbidity (Wenstrom & Malee, 1999).

Fetal demands for iron further contribute to symptoms of anemia in the pregnant woman. The fetal liver stores iron, especially during the third trimester. The infant needs this stored iron during the first 4 months of life to compensate for the normally inadequate levels of iron in breast milk and non-iron-fortified formulas.

To prevent anemia, the woman must balance iron requirements and intake. Adequate iron intake is a problem for nonpregnant women and a greater one for pregnant women. By carefully choosing foods high in iron, the woman can increase her daily iron intake considerably. Lean meats, dark green leafy vegetables, eggs, and wholegrain and enriched breads and cereals are the usual food sources of iron. Other iron sources include dried fruits, legumes, shellfish, and molasses.

Iron absorption is usually higher for animal products than for vegetable products. However, the woman can increase absorption of iron from nonmeat sources by combining them with meat or a food rich in vitamin C. The RDA for iron during pregnancy is 27 mg/day, but this intake is almost impossible to achieve through diet alone. Thus the pregnant woman should take a supplement of simple iron salt, such as ferrous gluconate, ferrous fumarate, or ferrous sulfate. The Centers for Disease Control and Prevention (CDC) recommend a daily supplement of 30 mg elemental iron beginning at the first prenatal visit (CDC, 1998). Unfortunately iron supplements often cause gastrointestinal discomfort, especially if taken on an empty stomach. Taking the iron supplement after a meal may help reduce this discomfort. Iron supplements may also cause constipation, so an adequate fluid intake is important in pregnancy.

Vitamins

Vitamins are organic substances needed for life and growth. They are found in small amounts in specific foods and generally cannot be synthesized by the body in adequate amounts.

Vitamins are grouped according to solubility. Vitamins A, D, E, and K dissolve in fat; vitamin C and the B-complex vitamins dissolve in water. An adequate intake of all vitamins is essential during pregnancy; however, several are required in larger amounts to fulfill specific needs.

FAT-SOLUBLE VITAMINS

The fat-soluble vitamins, A, D, E, and K, are stored in the liver and thus are available if the dietary intake becomes inadequate. The major complication related to these vitamins is not deficiency but toxicity due to overdose. Unlike water-soluble vitamins, excess amounts of vitamins A, D, E, and K are not excreted in the urine. Symptoms of vita-

min toxicity include nausea, gastrointestinal upset, dryness and cracking of the skin, and loss of hair.

Vitamin A is involved in the growth of epithelial cells, which line the entire gastrointestinal tract and make up the skin. It also plays a role in the metabolism of carbohydrates and fats. Without vitamin A, the body cannot synthesize glycogen, and the body's ability to handle cholesterol is also affected. In addition, the protective layer of tissue surrounding nerve fibers does not form properly if vitamin A is lacking.

Probably the best known function of vitamin A is its effect on vision in dim light. A person's ability to see in the dark depends on the eye's supply of retinol, a form of vitamin A. Adequate vitamin A prevents night blindness. Vitamin A is associated with the formation and development of healthy eyes in the fetus. The RDA for vitamin A is 770 µg/day for pregnant women ages 19 and older.

Although routine supplementation with vitamin A is not recommended, supplementation with 5000 IU is indicated for women whose dietary intake may be inadequate, such as strict vegetarians and recent emigrants from countries where deficiency of vitamin A is endemic (American College of Obstetricians and Gynecologists [ACOG], 1998). Excessive intake of preformed vitamin A is toxic to both children and adults. Some evidence indicates that excessive intake of vitamin A in the fetus can cause birth defects.

Rich plant sources of vitamin A include deep green, deep orange, and yellow vegetables; animal sources include egg yolk, cream, butter, and fortified margarine and milk. Liver has long been identified as a source of vitamin A. However, because of today's animal feeding practices, animal liver now contains exceptionally high doses of vitamin A; in fact, a single serving may contain twice the recommended daily allowance. Thus, to avoid toxicity, researchers recommend that women who are pregnant or trying to conceive avoid eating liver and liver products, including liver sausage and pâté (Doyle, 1998).

Vitamin D is best known for its role in the absorption and use of calcium and phosphorus in skeletal development. To supply the needs of the developing fetus, the pregnant woman should have a vitamin D intake of 5 µg/day.

Main food sources of vitamin D include fortified milk, margarine, butter, and egg yolks. Drinking a quart of milk daily provides the vitamin D needed during pregnancy.

Excessive intake of vitamin D usually comes from high-potency vitamin preparations, not from the diet. Overdoses during pregnancy can cause hypercalcemia, or high blood calcium levels, due to withdrawal of calcium from the skeletal tissue. Symptoms of toxicity include excessive thirst, loss of appetite, vomiting, weight loss, irritability, and high blood calcium levels.

The major function of vitamin E, or tocopherol, is antioxidation. Vitamin E takes on oxygen, thus preventing another substance from undergoing chemical change. For example, vitamin E helps spare vitamin A by preventing its oxidation in the intestinal tract and in the tissues. It decreases the oxidation of polyunsaturated fats, thus helping to retain the flexibility and health of the cell membrane. For this reason, vitamin E affects the health of all cells in the body.

Vitamin E is also involved in certain enzymatic and metabolic reactions. It is essential for the synthesis of nucleic acids required in the formation of red blood cells in the bone marrow. Vitamin E is useful in treating certain types of muscular pain and intermittent claudication, in surface healing of wounds and burns, and in protecting lung tissue from the damaging effects of smog. These functions may help explain the abundant claims and cures attributed to vitamin E, many of which have not been scientifically proved.

The recommended intake of vitamin E for pregnant women is unchanged at 15 mg/day. The vitamin E requirement varies with the polyunsaturated fat content of the diet. Vitamin E is widely distributed in foodstuffs, especially vegetable fats and oils, whole grains, greens, and eggs. Excessive intake of vitamin E has been associated with abnormal coagulation in the newborn.

Vitamin K, or menadione (as used synthetically in medicine), is essential for the synthesis of prothrombin, so its function is related to normal blood clotting. It is synthesized in the intestinal tract by the *Escherichia coli* bacteria normally found in the large intestine. However, the body's need for vitamin K is not totally met by synthesis. Green leafy vegetables are excellent sources. The RDI for vitamin K does not increase during pregnancy. It is an AI of 90 μg/day.

Intake of vitamin K is usually adequate in a well-balanced prenatal diet. Problems may arise if an illness is present that results in malabsorption of fats or if antibiotics are used for an extended period, which would inhibit vitamin K synthesis by destroying intestinal *E. coli*.

WATER-SOLUBLE VITAMINS

Water-soluble vitamins are excreted in the urine. Since only small amounts are stored, adequate amounts must be consumed daily. During pregnancy, the concentration of water-soluble vitamins in the maternal serum falls, whereas high concentrations are found in the fetus.

The RDA for vitamin C (ascorbic acid) increases in pregnancy from 75 to 85 mg. Vitamin C's major function is to aid in the formation and development of connective tissue and the vascular system. Ascorbic acid is essential to the formation of collagen, which binds cells together. If the collagen begins to disintegrate because of a lack of ascorbic acid, cell functioning is disturbed and cell structure breaks down, resulting in muscular weakness, capillary hemorrhage, and eventual death. These are symptoms of scurvy, the disease caused by vitamin C deficiency. Infants fed mainly cow's milk become deficient in vitamin C, and they are the main group that develops these symptoms. Surprisingly, newborns of women who have taken megadoses of vitamin C may have a rebound form of scurvy.

Maternal plasma levels of vitamin C progressively decrease during pregnancy, with values at term being about half those found at midpregnancy. It appears that ascorbic acid concentrates in the placenta; levels in the fetus are 50% or more above maternal levels.

A nutritious diet should meet the pregnant woman's needs for vitamin C without additional supplementation. Common food sources of vitamin C include citrus fruit, tomatoes, cantaloupe, strawberries, potatoes, broccoli, and other leafy greens. Ascorbic acid is readily destroyed by water and oxidation. Therefore, foods containing vitamin C must be stored and cooked properly.

The B vitamins include thiamine (B_1), riboflavin (B_2), niacin, folic acid, pantothenic acid, vitamin B_6, and vitamin B_{12}. These vitamins serve as vital coenzyme factors in many reactions such as cell respiration, glucose oxidation, and energy metabolism. The quantities needed increase as caloric intake increases to meet the metabolic and growth needs of the pregnant woman.

The thiamine requirement increases from the prepregnant level of 1.1 mg/day to 1.4 mg/day. Sources include pork, milk, potatoes, and enriched breads and cereals.

Riboflavin deficiency is manifested by *cheilosis* (fissures and cracks of the lips and corners of the mouth) and other skin lesions. During pregnancy, women may excrete less riboflavin and still require more because of increased energy and protein needs. An additional 0.3 mg/day is recommended. Sources include milk, eggs, enriched breads, and cereals.

Niacin intake should increase 4 mg/day during pregnancy for pregnant women ages 19 and older. Sources of niacin include meat, fish, poultry, whole grains, enriched breads, cereals, and peanuts.

Folic acid, or folate, is required for normal growth, reproduction, and lactation. It prevents the macrocytic, megaloblastic anemia of pregnancy. Megaloblastic anemia due to folate deficiency is rarely found in the United States, but it does occur. The RDA increases to 600 μg during pregnancy.

More importantly, an inadequate intake of folic acid has been associated with neural tube defects (NTDs) (spina bifida, meningomyelocele) in the fetus or newborn. Because the average daily intake of folic acid from dietary sources is only about half the RDA for nonpregnant women (400 μg), the CDC, the March of Dimes Birth Defects Foundation, and the National Council on Folic Acid have worked to educate women about the importance of consuming folic acid daily. Specifically, the U.S. Public Health Service recommends that all women of childbearing age (15 to 45 years) consume 0.4 mg of folic acid daily from supplements, because half of all U.S. pregnancies are unplanned and NTDs occur very early in pregnancy (3 to 4 weeks after conception), before most women realize they are pregnant (Mersereau, 2000). The CDC estimates that 50% to 70% of NTDs could be prevented if this recommendation was followed, especially before conception and during early pregnancy (first trimester) (CDC, 2000). Large dose supplementation (4.0 mg/day) is recommended for women who have had a previous NTD-affected pregnancy and are planning another pregnancy (ACOG, 1996).

The best food sources of folates are fresh green leafy vegetables, peanuts, and whole-grain breads and cereals. Folic acid can be made inactive by oxidation, ultraviolet light, and heating. It can easily be lost during improper storage and cooking. To prevent unnecessary loss, foods should be stored covered to protect them from light, cooked with only a small amount of water, and not overcooked.

No allowance has been set for pantothenic acid in pregnancy, but 5 mg/day is considered a safe, adequate intake. Sources include meats, egg yolk, legumes, and whole-grain cereals and breads.

Vitamin B_6 (pyridoxine) is associated with amino acid metabolism; thus a higher-than-average protein intake requires increased pyridoxine intake. The RDA for vitamin B_6 during pregnancy is 2.6 mg, an increase of 0.2 mg over the allowance for nonpregnant women. Generally, the slightly increased need can be supplied by dietary sources, which include wheat germ, yeast, fish, liver, pork, potatoes, and lentils.

Vitamin B_{12}, or cobalamin, is the cobalt-containing vitamin found only in animal sources. Women of reproductive age rarely have a B_{12} deficiency. Vegans (see later discussion on vegetarian diets) can develop a deficiency, however, so it is essential that their dietary intake be supplemented with this vitamin. The RDA during pregnancy is 2.6 mg/day. A deficiency may be due to a congenital inability to absorb vitamin B_{12}, resulting in pernicious anemia. Infertility is a complication of this type of anemia.

Fluid

Water is essential for life, and it is found in all body tissues. It is necessary for many biochemical reactions. It also serves as a lubricant, as a medium of transport for carrying substances in and out of the body, and as an aid in temperature control. A pregnant woman should consume at least 8 to 10 (8-oz) glasses of fluid each day, of which 4 to 6 glasses should be water. Because of their sodium content, diet sodas should be consumed in moderation. Caffeinated beverages have a diuretic effect, which is counterproductive to increasing fluid intake.

VEGETARIANISM

Vegetarianism is the dietary choice of many people for religious, health, or ethical reasons. There are several types of vegetarians. **Lacto-ovovegetarians** include milk, dairy products, and eggs in their diet. **Lactovegetarians** include dairy products but no eggs in their diets. **Vegans** are "pure" vegetarians who will not eat any food from animal sources.

The expectant woman who is vegetarian must eat the proper combination of foods to obtain adequate nutrients. If her diet allows, a woman can obtain ample and complete proteins from dairy products and eggs. An adequate, pure vegan diet contains protein from unrefined grains (brown rice, whole wheat), legumes (beans, split peas, lentils), nuts in large quantities, and a variety of cooked and fresh vegetables and fruits. Seeds may provide adequate protein in the vegetarian diet if the quantity is large enough. If the vegetarian woman's diet contains sufficient calories, it will also contain sufficient protein if she follows the recommendations for complementing proteins. Figure 11–2 ◆ depicts the vegetarian food pyramid.

A daily supplement of 4 mg of vitamin B_{12} is necessary because vegans use no animal products. If the woman uses soy milk, only partial supplementation may be needed. If she uses no soy milk, she needs daily supplements of 1200 mg of calcium and 10 mg of vitamin D.

Because the best sources of iron and zinc are animal products, vegan diets may also be low in these minerals. In addition, a high fiber intake may reduce mineral (calcium, iron, and zinc) bioavailability. Nurses need to emphasize the use of foods containing these nutrients. A vegetarian food group guide appears in Table 11–2.

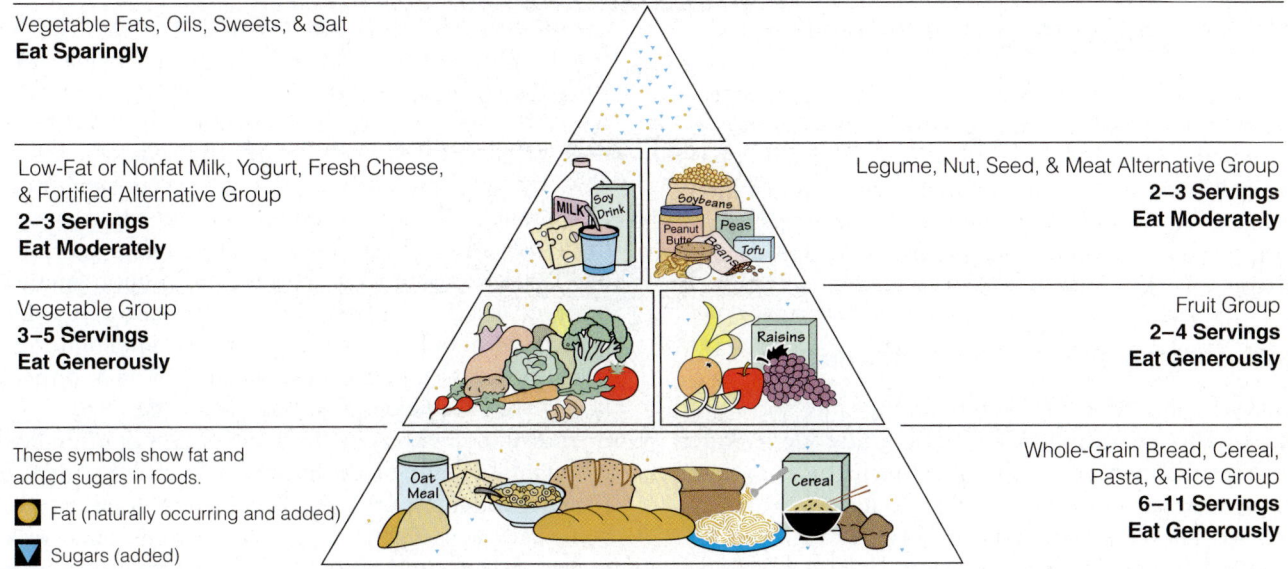

FIGURE 11–2. ◆ The vegetarian food pyramid. *Note:* From the Health Connection, 55 West Oak Ridge Drive, Hagerstown, MD 21740-7390. Adapted.

TABLE 11–2	Vegetarian Food Groups			
Food Group	Mixed Diet	Lacto-ovovegetarian	Lactovegetarian	Vegan
Grain	Bread, cereal, rice, pasta	Bread, cereal, rice, pasta	Bread, cereal, rice, pasta	Bread, cereal, rice, pasta
Fruit	Fruit, fruit juices	Fruit, fruit juices	Fruit, fruit juices	Fruit, fruit juices
Vegetable	Vegetables, vegetable juices	Vegetables, vegetable juices	Vegetables, vegetable juices	Vegetables, vegetable juices
Dairy and dairy alternatives	Milk, yogurt, cheese	Milk, yogurt, cheese	Milk, yogurt, cheese	Fortified soy milk, rice milk
Meat and meat alternatives	Meat, fish, poultry, eggs, legumes, tofu, nuts, nut butters	Eggs, legumes, tofu, nuts, nut butters	Legumes, tofu, nuts, nut butters	Legumes, tofu, nuts, nut butters

Complementary Care

NUTRITIONAL CONTENT OF HERBS

Several herbs are good sources of various vitamins and minerals. Like other "whole" foods, herbs contain all the necessary nutrients and enzymes to increase bioavailability versus isolated substances (such as in vitamin and mineral supplements).

Dandelion root and herb: Contains high concentrations of vitamins A and C, beta carotene, and potassium (Blumenthal, 2000; Kemper, 1999).

Oat straw: Rich in calcium and magnesium, plus iron, manganese, and zinc (Blumenthal, 2000; Skidmore-Roth, 2001). Note that this is the same plant from which we derive oatmeal.

Raspberry leaf: Contains vitamin C and naturally chelated iron (Skidmore-Roth, 2001).

It is best to advise pregnant women interested in using herbs to follow three basic principles: (1) if at all possible, avoid the use of herbs, even tonic herbs, during the first trimester (with the exception of ginger in amounts less than 1 g daily); (2) avoid standardized or highly concentrated extracts because the risk of side effects tends to be higher than with whole plant extracts; and (3) do not take essential oils internally (Belew, 1999).

FACTORS INFLUENCING NUTRITION

It is important to consider the many factors that affect a client's nutrition. What are the age, lifestyle, and culture of the pregnant woman? What food beliefs and habits does she have? What a person eats is determined by availability, economics, and symbolism. These factors and others influence the expectant mother's acceptance of dietary recommendations.

Lactase Deficiency (Lactose Intolerance)

Some individuals have difficulty digesting milk and milk products. This condition, known as **lactase deficiency (lactose intolerance),** results from an inadequate amount of the enzyme lactase, which breaks down the milk sugar lactose into smaller digestible substances.

Lactase deficiency is found in many people of African, Mexican, Native-American, Ashkenazic Jewish, and Asian descent. People of northern European heritage are usually not affected. WEB Symptoms include abdominal distention, discomfort, nausea, vomiting, loose stools, and cramps.

In counseling pregnant women who might be intolerant of milk and milk products, be aware that even one glass of milk can produce symptoms. Milk in cooked form, such as custards, is sometimes tolerated, as are cultured or fermented dairy products such as buttermilk, some cheeses, and yogurt. In some instances, the enzyme lactase may be taken to alleviate this problem. It is available as a chewable tablet to be taken before ingesting milk products or as a liquid to add to milk itself. Lactase-treated milk is also available commercially in some grocery stores.

Eating Disorders

In any given client population, it is probable that about 3% will have an eating disorder (Herrin, 1999). Two serious eating disorders, anorexia nervosa and bulimia nervosa, develop most commonly in adolescent girls but often continue into adulthood. Both conditions are psychologic disorders that can have a major impact on physiologic well-being.

Anorexia nervosa is characterized by an extreme fear of weight gain and fat. People with this problem have distorted body images and perceive themselves as fat even when they are extremely underweight. Their dietary intake is very restrictive in both variety and quantity. They may also engage in excessive exercise to prevent weight gain.

Bulimia is characterized by bingeing (secretly consuming large amounts of food in a short time) and purging. Self-induced vomiting is the most common method of purging; laxatives and/or diuretics may also be used. Individuals with bulimia nervosa often maintain normal or near-normal weight for their height, so it is difficult to know whether bingeing and purging occur.

Individuals with anorexia nervosa do not often become pregnant because of the physiologic changes that affect their reproductive systems. Women with bulimia can become pregnant. Their self-induced vomiting may produce many of the same complications as hyperemesis gravidarum (see Chapter 13). In both anorexia nervosa and bulimia, a multidisciplinary approach to treatment, involving medical, nursing, psychiatric, and dietetic practitioners, is indicated. Pregnant women with eating disorders need to be closely monitored and supported throughout their pregnancies.

Pica

Pica is the persistent eating of substances such as dirt, clay, starch, freezer frost, burned matches, or ashes that are not ordinarily considered edible or nutritionally valuable. Most women who practice pica in pregnancy eat such substances only during that time.

Iron deficiency anemia is the most common concern in pica. Eating laundry starch or certain types of clay may contribute to iron deficiency because they interfere with iron absorption. The ingestion of large quantities of clay could fill the intestine and cause fecal impaction; eating starch may be associated with excessive weight gain.

Assessment for pica is an important part of a nutritional history. However, a woman may be embarrassed about her cravings or reluctant to discuss them for fear of criticism. Using a nonjudgmental approach, give the woman information that can help her decrease or eliminate this practice.

Common Discomforts of Pregnancy

Gastrointestinal functioning can be altered at times during pregnancy, resulting in discomforts such as nausea, vomiting, heartburn, and constipation. Although these changes can be uncomfortable for the woman, they are seldom a major problem. These discomforts and dietary modifications that may provide relief are discussed in Chapter 9.

Cultural, Ethnic, and Religious Influences

Cultural, ethnic, and religious backgrounds determine people's experiences with food and influence food preferences and habits (Figure 11–3 ◆). People of different nationalities are accustomed to eating different foods because of the kinds of foodstuffs available in their countries of origin. The way food is prepared varies, depending on the customs and traditions of the ethnic and cultural group. In addition, the laws of certain religions forbid the use of some foods and direct the preparation and serving of meals. (See "Developing Cultural Competence.")

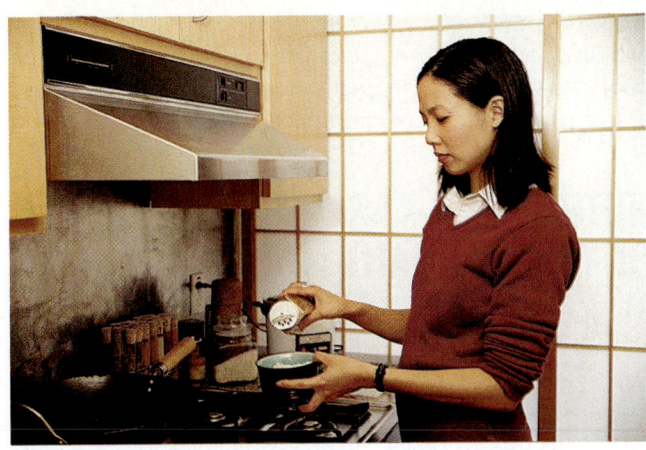

FIGURE 11–3. ◆ Food preferences and habits are affected by cultural factors.

In each culture, certain foods have symbolic meaning. Generally these symbolic foods are related to major life experiences such as birth, death, or developmental milestones. Although generalizations have been made about the food practices of ethnic and religious groups, there are many variations. The extent to which people continue to eat traditional ethnic foods and follow food-related ethnic customs is affected by their exposure to other cultures and the availability, quality, and cost of traditional foods.

It is common for health care providers to give dietary advice from their own cultural context. When working with pregnant women from any ethnic background, it is important to understand the impact of the woman's cultural beliefs on her eating habits and to identify any beliefs she may have about food and pregnancy. Talking with the client can help determine the level of influence that traditional food customs exert. It is then possible to give dietary advice in a way that is meaningful to the woman and her family.

Psychosocial Factors

Various psychosocial factors may influence a woman's food choices. The sharing of food has long been a symbol of friendliness, warmth, and social acceptance in many cultures. Some foods and food practices are associated with status. Some foods are prepared "just for company"; others are served only on special occasions or holidays.

Socioeconomic level may be a determinant of nutritional status. Poverty-level families cannot afford the same foods that higher income families can. Thus pregnant women with low incomes are frequently at risk for poor nutrition.

Knowledge about the basic components of a balanced diet is essential. Often educational level is related to economic status, but even people on very limited incomes can prepare well-balanced meals if they know enough about nutrition.

The expectant woman's attitudes and feelings about her pregnancy influence her nutritional status. For example, foods may be used as a substitute for the expression of

Developing Cultural Competence

The kosher diet followed by many Jewish people forbids the eating of pig products and shellfish. Certain cuts of meat from sheep and cattle are allowed as are fish with fins and scales. In addition, many Jews believe that meat and milk should not be mixed and eaten at the same meal.

emotions, such as anger or frustration, or as a way of expressing feelings of joy. The woman who is depressed or does not wish to be pregnant may manifest these feelings in loss of appetite or overindulgence in certain foods.

NUTRITIONAL CARE OF THE PREGNANT ADOLESCENT

Nutritional care of the pregnant adolescent is of particular concern to health care professionals. Many adolescents are nutritionally at risk because of a variety of complex emotional, social, and economic factors. Important nutrition-related factors to assess in pregnant adolescents include low prepregnant weight, low weight gain during pregnancy, young age at menarche, smoking, excessive prepregnant weight, anemia, unhealthy lifestyle (drugs or alcohol use), chronic disease, and history of an eating disorder.

The nutritional needs of adolescents are generally estimated by using the RDA for nonpregnant teenagers (ages 9 to 13 or 14 to 18) and adding nutrient amounts recommended for all women. If she is mature (more than 4 years since menarche), the pregnant adolescent's nutritional needs approach those reported for pregnant adults. However, adolescents who become pregnant less than 4 years after menarche are at risk due to their physiologic and anatomic immaturity. They are more likely than older adolescents to still be growing, which can impact the fetus's development. Thus young adolescents (age 14 and under) need to gain more weight than older adolescents (18 years and older) to produce babies of equal size.

In determining the optimal weight gain for the pregnant adolescent, add the recommended weight gain for an adult pregnancy to that expected during the postmenarcheal year in which the pregnancy occurs. If the teenager is underweight, additional weight gain is recommended to bring her to a normal weight for her height.

Specific Nutrient Concerns

Caloric needs of pregnant adolescents vary widely. Major factors in determining caloric needs include whether growth has been completed and the physical activity level of the individual. Figures as high as 50 kcal/kg have been suggested for young, growing teens who are very active physically. A satisfactory weight gain usually confirms an adequate caloric intake.

An inadequate iron intake is a major concern with the adolescent diet. Iron needs are high for the pregnant teen due to the requirement for iron by the enlarging maternal muscle mass and blood volume. Iron supplements are definitely indicated.

Calcium is another important nutrient for pregnant adolescents. Inadequate intake of calcium is often a problem in this age group. An intake of 1200 mg/day of calcium is recommended to promote bone mineralization in the adolescent and support fetal skeletal growth. This is

400 mg/day more than the recommended amount for nonpregnant adults over age 24. An extra serving of dairy products is usually suggested for teenagers. Calcium supplementation is indicated for teens who dislike milk, unless they consume enough other dairy products or significant calcium sources.

Because folic acid plays a role in cell reproduction, it is also an important nutrient for pregnant teens. As previously indicated, a supplement is usually recommended for all pregnant females, whether adult or teenaged.

Other nutrients and vitamins must be considered when evaluating the overall nutritional quality of the teenager's diet. Nutrients that have frequently been found to be deficient in this age group include zinc and vitamins A, D, and B_6. Eating a wide variety of foods—especially fresh and lightly processed foods—helps the teen get adequate amounts of trace minerals, fiber, and other vitamins.

Dietary Patterns

Healthy adolescents often have irregular eating patterns. Many skip breakfast, and most tend to be frequent snackers. Teens rarely follow the traditional three-meals-a-day pattern. Their day-to-day intake often varies drastically, and they eat food combinations that may seem bizarre to adults. Despite these practices, adolescents usually achieve a better nutritional balance than most adults would expect.

A variety of factors influence adolescent food choices, including hunger, food cravings, time and convenience, appeal of food, food availability, parental influence (including family religion and culture), food benefits, mood, body image, habit, media, cost, vegetarian beliefs, and situation-specific factors. Barriers adolescents cite to increased consumption of vegetables, fruits, and dairy products and decreased consumption of high-fat foods include taste preferences for other foods, a lack of a sense of urgency about personal health, and the cost of more healthful foods. In addition, the places adolescents typically eat when away from home—school and fast-food restaurants—do not offer these foods or they fail to make them appealing (Neumark-Sztainer, Story, Perry, et al., 1999).

In assessing the diet of the pregnant adolescent, it is important to consider the eating pattern over time, not simply a single day's intake. Once the pattern is identified, direct counseling toward correcting deficiencies.

Counseling Issues

Counseling about nutrition and healthy eating practices is an important element of care for pregnant teenagers that nurses can effectively provide in a community setting. This counseling may be individualized, involve other teens, or provide a combination of both approaches. If an adolescent's family member does most of the meal preparation, it may be useful to include that person in the discussion if the adolescent agrees. Clinics and schools often offer classes and focused activities designed to address this topic.

The pregnant teenager will soon become a parent, and her understanding of nutrition will influence not only her well-being but also that of her child. However, teens tend to live in the present, and counseling that stresses long-term changes may be less effective than more concrete approaches. In many cases, group classes are effective, especially those with other teens.

POSTPARTUM NUTRITION

Nutritional needs change following childbirth. Nutrient requirements vary depending on whether the mother decides to breastfeed. An assessment of postpartal nutritional status is necessary before nutritional guidance is given.

Postpartal Nutritional Status

Postpartal nutritional status is determined based on the new mother's weight, hemoglobin and hematocrit levels, clinical signs, and dietary history. As mentioned previously, an ideal weight gain during pregnancy is 25 to 35 lb (11.5 to 16 kg). After birth there is a weight loss of approximately 10 to 12 lb. Additional weight loss is most rapid during the next few weeks as the body adjusts to the end of pregnancy. The mother's weight then begins to stabilize. This weight stabilization may take 6 months or longer.

The increased weight gain now recommended during pregnancy may have important implications for women postpartally unless they receive adequate counseling. Women who gain between 25 and 35 lb while pregnant have a net gain of about 3.5 lb (1.6 kg) 6 months after childbirth. Furthermore, multiparous women tend to lose less weight postpartally than primiparas; women who return to work outside the home tend to lose more weight than those who do not. The mother's weight should be considered in terms of ideal weight, prepregnancy weight, and weight gain during pregnancy. Refer women who want information about weight reduction to a dietitian.

Hemoglobin and erythrocyte levels should return to normal within 2 to 6 weeks after childbirth. Iron supplements are generally continued for 2 to 3 months following childbirth to build stores depleted by pregnancy.

Constipation is a common problem following birth. To prevent it, the woman should maintain a high fluid intake, which helps keep the stool soft. Dietary sources of fiber, such as whole grains, fruits, and vegetables, also help prevent constipation.

Get specific information on dietary intake and eating habits directly from the woman. Visiting the mother during mealtimes provides an opportunity for unobtrusive nutritional assessment. Which foods has the woman selected? Is her diet nutritionally sound? A comment focusing on a positive aspect of her meal selection may initiate a discussion of nutrition.

Notify the dietitian about any woman whose cultural or religious beliefs require specific foods so that appropriate meals can be prepared for her. Also consider referring women with unusual eating habits or numerous questions about good nutrition to the dietitian. In addition, provide literature on nutrition so that the woman will have a source of information at home.

Nutritional Care of Nonnursing Mothers

After birth, the nonnursing mother's dietary requirements return to prepregnancy levels. If the mother has a good understanding of nutritional principles, it is sufficient to advise her to reduce her daily caloric intake by about 300 kcal and to return to prepregnancy levels for other nutrients.

If the mother has a limited understanding of nutrition, now is the time to teach her the basic principles and the importance of a well-balanced diet. Her eating habits and dietary practices will eventually be reflected in the diet of her child.

If the mother has gained excessive weight during pregnancy (or perhaps was overweight before pregnancy) and wishes to lose weight, a referral to the dietitian is appropriate. The dietitian can design weight-reduction diets to meet nutritional needs and food preferences. Weight loss goals of 1 to 2 lb/week are usually suggested.

In addition to meeting her own nutritional needs, the new mother is usually interested in learning how to provide for her infant's nutritional needs. A discussion of infant feeding that includes topics such as selecting infant formulas, formula preparation, and vitamin and mineral supplementation is appropriate and generally well received.

Nutritional Care of Nursing Mothers

A breastfeeding woman needs increased nutrients. Table 11–1 provides a sample daily food guide for lactating women. It is especially important for the nursing mother to consume sufficient calories, because inadequate caloric intake can reduce milk volume. However, milk quality generally remains unaffected. The nursing mother should increase her calories by about 200 kcal over her pregnancy requirement, or 500 kcal over her prepregnancy requirement. In the woman who breastfeeds exclusively, caloric requirements usually peak at 6 months postpartum because after that time infants generally begin to eat supplemental foods (Reifsnider & Gill, 2000).

Because protein is an important ingredient in breast milk, an adequate intake while breastfeeding is essential. An intake of 65 g/day during the first 6 months of breastfeeding and 62 g/day during the second 6 months is recommended. As in pregnancy, it is important to consume adequate nonprotein calories to prevent the use of protein as an energy source.

Calcium is an important ingredient in milk production. Requirements during lactation return to prepregnancy levels for women ages 19–50—an AI of 1000 mg/day. If the intake of calcium from food sources is not adequate, calcium supplements are recommended.

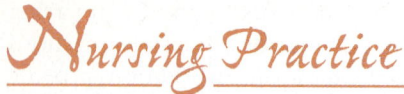

Nursing Practice

Explain to breastfeeding mothers that liquids are especially important during lactation, because inadequate fluid intake may decrease milk volume. Encourage them to drink at least 8 to 10 (8-oz) glasses of fluid daily, including water, juice, milk, and soups.

Iron is not a principal mineral component of milk; thus the needs of lactating women are not substantially different from those of nonpregnant women. However, supplementation for 2 to 3 months after childbirth is advisable to replenish maternal stores depleted by pregnancy.

In addition to counseling nursing mothers on how to meet their increased nutrient needs during breastfeeding, discuss a few issues related to infant feeding. For example, many mothers are concerned about how specific foods they eat will affect their babies during breastfeeding. Generally the nursing mother need not avoid any foods except those to which she might be allergic. Occasionally, however, some nursing mothers find that their babies are affected by certain foods. Onions, turnips, cabbage, chocolate, spices, and seasonings are commonly listed as offenders. The best advice to give the nursing mother is to avoid those foods she suspects cause distress in her infant. For the most part, however, she should be able to eat any nourishing food she wants without fear that her baby will be affected. For further discussion of successful infant feeding, see Chapter 27.

Nursing Management

Nursing Assessment and Diagnosis

In order to plan an optimal diet with each woman, it is essential to assess nutritional status. The woman's chart and a client interview provide information about (1) the woman's height and weight, as well as her weight gain during pregnancy; (2) pertinent laboratory values, especially hemoglobin and hematocrit; (3) clinical signs that have possible nutritional implications, such as constipation, anorexia, or heartburn; and (4) dietary history to evaluate the woman's views on nutrition as well as her specific nutrient intake.

While gathering data, seek information about psychologic, cultural, and socioeconomic factors that may influence food intake. Also use the opportunity to discuss important aspects of nutrition within the context of the family's needs and lifestyle. A nutritional questionnaire is often useful in gathering and recording important facts. This information can be used to develop an intervention plan to fit the woman's individual needs. The sample questionnaire shown in Figure 11–4 ♦ has been filled in to demonstrate this process.

Once information is obtained, begin to analyze the information, formulate appropriate nursing diagnoses, and, with the woman, develop goals and desired outcomes. For a woman during the first trimester, for example, the diagnosis may be "altered nutrition: less than body requirements related to nausea and vomiting." In other cases, the woman may have excessive weight gain. In such situations the diagnosis might be "altered nutrition: more than body requirements related to excessive caloric intake." Be specific in addressing issues such as inadequate intake of nutrients including iron, calcium, or folic acid; problems with nutrition because of a limited food budget; problems related to physiologic alterations including anorexia, heartburn, or nausea; and behavioral problems related to excessive dieting, binge eating, and so on. At other times the diagnosis "health-seeking behaviors" may seem most appropriate, especially if the woman asks for information about nutrition.

Planning and Implementation

After determining the nursing diagnosis, plan an approach to address any nutritional deficiencies or improve the overall quality of the diet. To be truly effective, this plan must be made in cooperation with the woman. The following example demonstrates ways to plan with the woman based on the nursing diagnosis.

▶ *Diagnosis:* Altered nutrition: less than body requirements related to low intake of calcium.

▶ *Client goal:* The woman will increase her daily intake of calcium to the minimum RDA levels.

▶ Implementation:

1. Plan with the woman how to add more milk or dairy products to the diet (specify amounts).
2. Encourage the use of other calcium sources such as leafy greens and legumes.
3. Plan for the addition of powdered milk in cooking and baking.
4. If none of the preceding options are realistic or acceptable, consider the use of calcium supplements.

Most families can benefit from guidance about food purchasing and preparation. Advise women to plan food purchases thoughtfully by preparing general menus and a list before shopping. It is also helpful to monitor sales, compare brands, and be cautious when purchasing "convenience" foods, which tend to be expensive. Other techniques for keeping food costs down without jeopardizing quality include buying food in season, using bulk foods when appropriate, using whole-grain or enriched products, buying lower grade eggs (grading has no relation to the egg's nutritional value but indicates color of the shell, delicacy of flavor, and so forth), and avoiding foods from specialty shops and foods in elaborate packaging.

NUTRITIONAL QUESTIONNAIRE

Name __Susan Longmont__ Date __7-22-02__

Age __20__

Ethnic group __Caucasian__

Religion __Protestant__

Gravida __1__ Para __0__ EDB __3-24-03__

Age of youngest child? __NA__

Birth weights of previous children? __NA__

Usual nonpregnant weight __115__ Present weight __125__

Weight gain during last pregnancy? __NA__

Vitamin supplements? __none__

Current medications? __aspirin for headache__

Do you smoke? __yes__ How much per day? __1-1½ packs__

Eating patterns:

1. How many meals per day? __2__ when __12:30 pm 6:30 pm__

2. How many snacks per day? __3__ when __10:30 am 4:00 pm 10:00 pm__

3. What other foods are important to your usual diet? __chocolate and candy bars__

4. Amount per day __4 bars/week__

5. Do you have any different food preferences now? __no__

6. Do you eat nonfoods such as:

		Amount
laundry starch	no	NA
ice	yes	10 cubes/day
other (name)	no	NA

7. What foods do you dislike or do not eat? __spinach and dried beans__

8. For added information complete a typical daily intake (24 hour recall is suggested).

Do you have special problems in food preparation such as:

1. Physical disability __yes__ __no ✔__ Explain ____

2. Cooking appliances __yes__ __no ✔__ Explain ____

3. Refrigeration of food __yes__ __no ✔__ Explain ____

Who does the meal planning? __I do.__ shopping? __We both do.__

cooking? __I do most of the time but my husband likes to help.__

Are there transportation problems? __We have only one car but we go in the evening.__

Financial situation: __My husband is working and going to school.__

__I am not working.__ Food Stamps __yes__ WIC __no__

Do you have any previous nutritional problems? __No. I have never paid much attention__

__to food before, but now I have lots of questions.__

Are there any problems with this pregnancy? Nausea __Yes, in the morning.__

Constipation __No__ Other __NA__

Assessment by the nurse following the completion of the questionnaire.

Basic estimated nutrient and caloric value of typical daily intake.

Please circle one of the following:

Protein intake was	low	(adequate)	high
Caloric intake was	low	adequate	(high)
Calcium intake was	(low)	adequate	high
Iron intake was	(low)	adequate	high
Vitamin C intake was	low	(adequate)	high

FIGURE 11-4. ◆ Sample nutritional questionnaire used in nursing management of a pregnant woman.

NURSING CARE IN THE COMMUNITY

Food is a significant portion of a family's budget, and meeting nutritional needs may be a challenge for families on limited incomes. Community-based services offered through clinics, local agencies, schools, and volunteer organizations address these needs. Increasingly nurses play an important role in managing such community-based services, especially services focusing on client education. In addition, most communities offer special assistance to qualifying families to meet their nutritional needs. The Food Stamp Program provides stamps or coupons for participating households whose net monthly income is below a specified level. These stamps can be used to purchase food for the household each month.

The Special Supplemental Food Program for Women, Infants, and Children (WIC) is designed to assist pregnant or breastfeeding women with low incomes and their children under 5 years of age. The program provides food assistance, nutrition education, and referrals to health care providers. The food distributed, including dried beans and peas, peanut butter, eggs, cheese, milk, fortified adult and infant cereals, juice, and iron-fortified formula, is designed to provide good sources of iron, protein, and certain vitamins for people with an inadequate diet. Research indicates that participation in the WIC program during pregnancy and infancy is associated with a reduced risk of infant death (Moss & Carver, 1998).

Evaluation

Once a plan has been developed and implemented, work with the woman to identify ways of evaluating its effectiveness. This may involve keeping a food journal, writing out weekly menus, returning for weekly weigh-ins, and the

like. If anemia is a special problem, periodic hematocrit assessments are also indicated. Refer women with serious nutritional deficiencies to a dietitian.

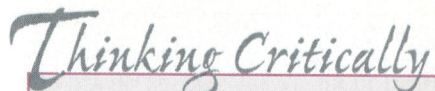

Thinking Critically

EVALUATING A PREGNANT WOMAN'S DIET

Jane is 14 weeks pregnant. The rate and total amount of her weight gain during the first trimester have been consistent with recommendations. She has gained an average of 0.5 kg (1 lb) per week during both of the past 2 weeks. Her appetite is good, and she consumes three meals per day and snacks between meals on occasion.

Jane has altered her diet because she is concerned about excessive weight gain. She told you that she has decreased her intake from the bread and dairy groups in order to limit her calorie intake. Because she has omitted most dairy products, she has increased her consumption of salads and broccoli to provide calcium sources.

A diet history revealed the following:

➡ Grain: 3 to 4 servings, mainly cereal and rice

➡ Fruit: 2 to 4 servings, fresh fruit

➡ Vegetables: 3 to 5 servings, salads, peas, corn, broccoli

➡ Meat: 4 to 5 servings, beef, pork, chicken

➡ Dairy: occasionally cheese, ice cream, pudding

➡ Fats, oils, occasionally salad dressings, sweets, margarine, desserts

➡ Beverages: 8 to 10 servings, soda, juices, water

After assessing her diet history, what is your evaluation of Jane's diet? How could you counsel her? **WEB**

CHAPTER HIGHLIGHTS

≈ Maternal weight gains averaging 25 to 35 lb (11.5 to 16 kg) for a normal-weight woman are associated with the best reproductive outcomes.

≈ If the diet is adequate, folic acid and iron are the only supplements generally recommended during pregnancy.

≈ Because of the risk of NTDs, a national campaign is under way to encourage all women of childbearing age to take a 0.4-mg supplement of folic acid daily.

≈ Women should not restrict calories to reduce weight during pregnancy.

≈ It is most healthful for pregnant women to eat regularly and choose a wide variety of foods, especially fresh and lightly processed foods.

≈ Taking megadoses of vitamins during pregnancy is unnecessary and potentially dangerous.

≈ In vegetarian diets, special emphasis is placed on obtaining ample protein, calories, calcium, iron, vitamin D, vitamin B_{12}, and zinc through food sources or supplementation if necessary.

≈ Evaluation of physical, psychosocial, and cultural factors that affect food intake is essential before the nurse can determine nutritional status and plan nutritional counseling.

≈ Adolescents who become pregnant less than 4 years after menarche have higher nutritional needs than older pregnant adolescents and are considered to be at high biologic risk.

≈ Weight gains during adolescent pregnancy need to accommodate recommended gains for a normal pregnancy plus necessary gains due to maternal growth.

≈ After giving birth, the nonnursing mother's dietary requirements return to prepregnancy levels.

≈ Nursing mothers need an adequate calorie and fluid intake to maintain ample milk volume.

EXPLOREMediaLink

NCLEX Review, Case Studies, and other interactive resources for this chapter can be found on the companion website at http://www.prenhall.com/london. Click on "Chapter 11" to select the activities for this chapter.

For animations, more NCLEX review questions, and an audio glossary, access the accompanying CD-ROM in this textbook.

REFERENCES

American College of Obstetricians and Gynecologists. (1996). *Nutrition and women* (ACOG Educational Bulletin No. 229). Washington, DC: Author.

American College of Obstetricians and Gynecologists. (1998). *Vitamin A supplementation during pregnancy* (ACOG Committee Opinion No. 196). Washington, DC: Author.

Belew, C. (1999). Herbs and the childbearing woman: Guidelines for midwives. *Journal of Nurse-Midwifery, 44*(3), 231–246.

Blumenthal, M. (2000). *Herbal medicine: Expanded Commission E Monographs.* Austin, TX: American Botanical Council.

Brown, J. E., & Carlson, M. (2000). Nutrition and multifetal pregnancy. *Journal of the American Dietetic Association, 100*(3), 343–348.

Centers for Disease Control and Prevention (CDC). (1998). Recommendations to prevent and control iron deficiency in the United States. *Morbidity and Mortality Weekly Reports, 47*(RR-3), 1–36.

Centers for Disease Control and Prevention (CDC). (2000). *Folic acid now.* Birth Defects and Pediatric Genetics Branch, National Center for Environmental Health. Atlanta, GA: Author.

Doyle, W. (1998). Nutrition and pregnancy. *Nursing Times, 94*(Suppl. 16), 22–28.

Herrin, M. (1999). Balancing the scales: Nutritional counseling for women with eating disorders. *AWHONN Lifelines, 3*(4), 26–34.

Institute of Medicine, Subcommittee for a Clinical Application Guide. (1992). *Nutrition during pregnancy and lactation: An implementation guide.* Washington, DC: National Academy Press.

Institute of Medicine, Subcommittee on Dietary Intake and Nutrient Supplements During Pregnancy, Committee on Nutrition Status During Pregnancy and Lactation, Food and Nutrition Board. (1990). *Nutrition during pregnancy: Weight gain and nutrient supplements.* Washington, DC: National Academy Press.

Kemper, K. J. (1999, November). Longwood Herbal Task Force and the Center for Holistic Pediatric Education and Research: Monograph on Dandelion *(Taraxacum offinalis).*

Mersereau, P. W. (2000). Preventing neural tube birth defects: A national campaign. *Small Talk, 12*(2), 1–5.

Moss, N., & Carver, K. (1998). The effect of WIC and Medicaid on infant mortality in the United States. *American Journal of Public Health, 88*(9), 1354–1361.

National Research Council, Food and Nutrition Board. (1989). *Recommended dietary allowances* (10th ed.). Washington, DC: National Academy Press.

Neumark-Sztainer, D., Story, M., Perry, C., & Casey, M. A. (1999). Factors influencing food choices of adolescents: Findings from focus-group discussions with adolescents. *Journal of the American Dietetic Association, 99*(8), 929–938.

Reifsnider, E., & Gill, S. L. (2000). Nutrition for the childbearing years. *Journal of Obstetric, Gynecologic, and Neonatal Nursing, 29*(1), 43–55.

Simpson, M., Parsons, M., Greenwood, J., & Wade, K. (2001). Raspberry leaf in pregnancy: Its safety and efficacy. *Journal of Midwifery and Women's Health, 46*(2), 51–59.

Skidmore-Roth, L. (2001). *Mosby's handbook of herbs & natural supplements.* St. Louis, MO: Mosby.

Wenstrom, K. D., & Malee, D. W. (1999). Medical and surgical complications of pregnancy. In J. R. Scott, P. J. DiSaia, C. B. Hammond, & W. N. Spellacy (Eds.), *Danforth's obstetrics and gynecology* (8th ed., pp. 327–362). Philadelphia: Lippincott Williams & Wilkins.

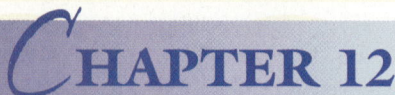

CHAPTER 12

Pregnancy at Risk: Pregestational Problems

When I learned I had gestational diabetes I felt panicky. My grandmother died of diabetes and it has always scared me. However, by taking each day as it came, cooperating with my care-givers, and watching my diet I did fine and gave birth to a beautiful 7 pound 10 ounce daughter. One good thing has come of the experience—I'm no longer so terrified of developing diabetes. I have become far more careful about taking care of myself and I now think of diabetes as a chronic disease to be controlled.

—SUEANN, 34

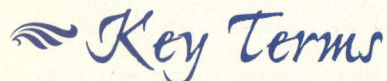

Key Terms

Acquired immunodeficiency syndrome (AIDS) *248*

Gestational diabetes mellitus (GDM) *239*

Human immunodeficiency virus (HIV) *248*

Macrosomia *240*

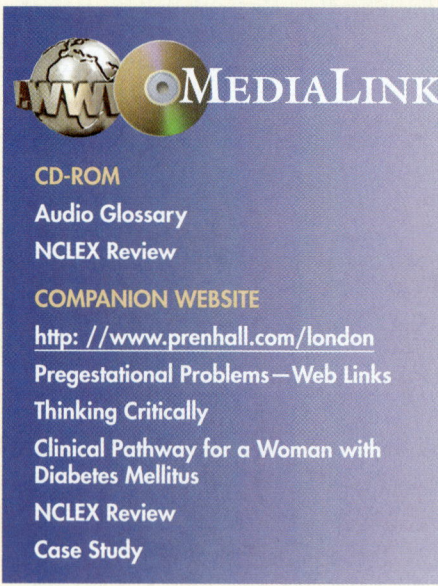

MEDIALINK

CD-ROM
Audio Glossary
NCLEX Review

COMPANION WEBSITE
http://www.prenhall.com/london
Pregestational Problems—Web Links
Thinking Critically
Clinical Pathway for a Woman with Diabetes Mellitus
NCLEX Review
Case Study

_F_or some women, pregnancy may become a life-threatening event because of potential or existing complications. These complications can be the result of factors such as age, parity, blood type, socioeconomic status, psychologic health, or pre-existing chronic illnesses. This chapter focuses on women with pregestational medical disorders and their possible effects on the pregnancy.

CARE OF THE WOMAN WITH SUBSTANCE ABUSE PROBLEMS

Substance abuse occurs when a person experiences difficulties with work, family, social relations, and health as a result of alcohol or drug use. Research suggests that more than 5% of all pregnant women use illegal drugs during pregnancy, with even higher rates in certain subgroups

(Howell, Heiser, & Harrington, 1999). Drugs that are commonly misused include alcohol, cocaine, marijuana, amphetamines, barbiturates, hallucinogens, heroin, and other narcotics. Table 12–1 identifies some addictive drugs and their effects on the fetus or newborn.

Drug use during pregnancy, particularly in the first trimester, may have a negative effect on the health of the woman and the growth and development of the fetus. Unfortunately, prenatal drug use may be the most frequently missed diagnosis in all of maternity care. Physicians and nurses may fail to ask women about drug and alcohol use because of their own lack of knowledge, discomfort, or biases. Often substance-abusing women wait until late in pregnancy to seek health care. Moreover, the substance-abusing woman who seeks early prenatal care may not voluntarily reveal her addiction, so caregivers should be alert for a history or physical signs that might indicate substance abuse.

TABLE 12–1   Possible Effects of Selected Drugs of Abuse or Addiction on Fetus and Neonate

Maternal Drug	Effect on Fetus and Neonate
DEPRESSANTS	
Alcohol	Mental retardation, microcephaly, midfacial hypoplasia, cardiac anomalies, intrauterine growth restriction (IUGR), potential teratogenic effects, fetal alcohol syndrome (FAS), fetal alcohol effects (FAE)
Narcotics	
Heroin	Withdrawal symptoms, convulsions, death, IUGR, respiratory alkalosis, hyperbilirubinemia
Methadone	Fetal distress, meconium aspiration; with abrupt termination of the drug, severe withdrawal symptoms, neonatal death
Barbiturates	Neonatal depression, increased anomalies; teratogenic effect (?); withdrawal symptoms, convulsions, hyperactivity, hyperreflexia, vasomotor instability
Phenobarbital	Bleeding (with excessive doses)
"T's and Blues" (combination of the following)	
Talwin (narcotic)	Safe for use in pregnancy; depresses respiration if taken close to time of birth
Amytal (barbiturate)	See barbiturates
Tranquilizers	
Phenothiazine derivatives	Withdrawal, extrapyramidal dysfunction, delayed respiratory onset, hyperbilirubinemia, hypotonia or hyperactivity, decreased platelet count
Diazepam (Valium)	Hypotonia, hypothermia, low Apgar score, respiratory depression, poor sucking reflex, possible cleft lip
Antianxiety drugs	
Lithium	Congenital anomalies, especially Ebstein anomaly; lethargy and cyanosis in the newborn
STIMULANTS	
Amphetamines	
Amphetamine sulfate (Benzedrine)	Generalized arthritis, learning disabilities, poor motor coordination, transposition of the great vessels, cleft palate
Dextroamphetamine sulfate (Dexedrine)	Congenital heart defects, hyperbilirubinemia
Cocaine	Cerebral infarctions, microcephaly, learning disabilities, poor state organization, decreased interactive behavior, central nervous system (CNS) anomalies, cardiac anomalies, genitourinary anomalies, sudden infant death syndrome (SIDS)
Caffeine (more than 600 mg/day)	Spontaneous abortion, IUGR, increased incidence of cleft palate, other anomalies suspected
Nicotine (half to one pack cigarettes/day)	Increased rate of spontaneous abortion, increased incidence of placental abruption, small for gestational age (SGA), small head circumference, decreased length, SIDS
PSYCHOTROPICS	
PCP ("angel dust")	Flaccid appearance, poor head control, impaired neurologic development
LSD	Chromosomal breakage?
Marijuana	IUGR, potential impaired immunologic mechanisms

Nursing Practice

Keep in mind that at least 1 of 10 women in the United States, regardless of socioeconomic status or ethnic background, is currently abusing a substance. If you consider that possibility with every woman, you will ask the important questions about drug use and be alert for signs of substance abuse.

Providing effective prenatal care to chemically dependent women is often challenging for clinicians. However, pregnancy is a time when most women are receptive to caring interventions. See "Nursing Practice."

Substances Commonly Abused During Pregnancy

ALCOHOL

Alcohol is a central nervous system (CNS) depressant and a potent teratogen. In fact, the use of alcohol during pregnancy has been described as the leading preventable cause of mental retardation (Andres, 1999). The incidence of alcohol abuse is highest among women ages 20 to 40 years although alcoholism is also seen in teenagers. Chronic abuse of alcohol can undermine maternal health by causing malnutrition (especially folic acid and thiamine deficiencies), bone marrow suppression, increased incidence of infections, and liver disease.

Alcohol is toxic to the fetus, although its exact effects on the fetus are only partly understood. The ethanol of alcohol may interfere with protein synthesis and placental transfer of glucose and amino acids; it may also contribute to vasoconstriction and a resulting hypoxemia in the fetus (Andres, 1999).

The effects of alcohol on the fetus may result in a group of signs known as *fetal alcohol syndrome (FAS)*. The syndrome has characteristic physical and mental abnormalities that vary in severity. (See discussion in Chapter 25.)
There is no final answer to how much alcohol a woman can safely drink during pregnancy. The expectant woman should avoid alcohol completely during the early weeks of pregnancy, when organ formation (organogenesis) is occurring. During the remainder of pregnancy, an occasional drink carries no currently known risk; however, no alcohol at all is safest (Niebyl, 1999).

As a result of alcohol dependence, a woman may have withdrawal seizures in the intrapartal period as early as 12 to 48 hours after she stops drinking. Delirium tremens may occur in the postpartal period, and the newborn may suffer a withdrawal syndrome. Nurses in the maternal-newborn unit must be aware of the manifestations of alcohol abuse so they can prepare for the woman's special needs. Care includes sedation to decrease irritability and tremors, seizure precautions, intravenous (IV) fluid therapy for hydration, and preparation for an addicted newborn. Although high doses of sedatives and analgesics may be necessary for the woman, caution is advised because these medications can cause fetal depression.

Breastfeeding generally is not contraindicated, although alcohol is excreted in breast milk. Excessive alcohol consumption may intoxicate the infant and inhibit the maternal letdown reflex. Discharge planning for the alcohol-addicted mother and newborn needs to be correlated with the social service department of the hospital.

COCAINE AND CRACK

Approximately 1 in 10 pregnant women is believed to use cocaine, with even higher rates reported in urban areas (Kenner & D'Apolito, 1997). Cocaine acts at the nerve terminals to prevent the reuptake of dopamine and norepinephrine, which in turn results in vasoconstriction, tachycardia, and hypertension. Placental vasoconstriction decreases blood flow to the fetus. The onset of cocaine effects occurs rapidly, but the euphoria lasts only about 30 minutes. Euphoria and excitement are usually followed by irritability, depression, pessimism, fatigue, and a strong desire for more cocaine. This pattern often leads the user to take repeated doses to sustain the effect. Cocaine metabolites may be present in the urine of a pregnant woman for as long as 4 to 7 days after use.

Cocaine can be taken by IV injection or by snorting the powdered form. *Crack*, a form of freebase cocaine that is made up of baking soda, water, and cocaine mixed into a paste and microwaved to form a rock, can be smoked. Smoking crack leads to a quicker, more intense high because the drug is absorbed through the large surface area of the lungs.

The cocaine user is difficult to identify prenatally. Because cocaine is illegal, many women are reluctant to admit that they use it. The nurse may recognize subtle signs of cocaine use, including mood swings and appetite changes, and withdrawal symptoms such as depression, irritability, nausea, lack of motivation, and psychomotor changes.

Major adverse maternal effects of cocaine use include seizures and hallucinations, pulmonary edema, cerebral hemorrhage, respiratory failure, and heart problems. Women who use cocaine have an increased incidence of spontaneous abortion, abruptio placentae, preterm birth, and stillbirth.

Fetal exposure to cocaine increases the risk of intrauterine growth restriction (IUGR), small head circumference, shorter body length, malformations of the genitourinary tract, and lower Apgar scores. Newborns exposed to cocaine in utero may have neurobehavioral disturbances, marked irritability, an exaggerated startle reflex, labile emotions, and an increased risk of sudden infant death syndrome (SIDS). (See Chapter 25 for further discussion.)
Cocaine crosses into breast milk and may cause symptoms in the breastfeeding infant, including extreme irritability, vomiting, diarrhea, dilated pupils, and apnea. Thus

women who continue to use cocaine after childbirth should avoid nursing.

MARIJUANA

Estimates of marijuana use during pregnancy vary widely and range from 3% (based on self-report) to 35% (based on urine screen) (Andres, 1999). To date, there is no strong evidence that marijuana has teratogenic effects on the fetus (Niebyl, 1999). However, the impact of heavy marijuana use on pregnancy is difficult to evaluate because of the variety of social factors that influence the results.

HEROIN

Heroin is an illicit CNS depressant narcotic that alters perception and produces euphoria. It is an addictive drug that is generally administered IV, although a snortable form of heroin called Karachi is available. Pregnancy in women who use heroin is considered high risk because of the increased incidence in these women of poor nutrition, iron deficiency anemia, and preeclampsia. Women addicted to heroin also have a higher incidence of sexually transmitted infections because many rely on prostitution to support their drug habit.

The fetus of a heroin-addicted woman is at increased risk for IUGR, meconium aspiration, and hypoxia. The newborn frequently shows signs of heroin addiction such as restlessness; shrill, high-pitched cry; irritability; fist sucking; vomiting; and seizures. Signs of withdrawal usually appear within 72 hours and may last for several days. (See discussion in Chapter 25.)

METHADONE

Methadone is the most commonly used therapy for women dependent on opioids such as heroin. Methadone blocks withdrawal symptoms and reduces or eliminates the craving for narcotics. Dosage should be individualized at the lowest possible therapeutic level. Methadone crosses the placenta and has been associated with preeclampsia, placental problems, and abnormal fetal presentation (Kearney, 1997).

Prenatal exposure to methadone may result in reduced head circumference and lower birth weight. The newborn may experience withdrawal symptoms that are often more severe and longer lasting than those associated with heroin, possibly because of the longer half-life of methadone (Wang, 1999).

Clinical Therapy

A team approach to the care of the pregnant woman with substance abuse problems ensures the management necessary to provide safe labor and birth for the woman and her child.

The management of drug addiction may include hospitalization if necessary to start detoxification. "Cold turkey" withdrawal is not advisable during pregnancy because of the possible risk to the fetus. Maintenance and support therapy are given during weekly prenatal visits. Urine screening is also done regularly throughout pregnancy if the woman has a known or suspected substance abuse problem. This testing helps to identify the type and amount of drug being abused.

Nursing Management

Nursing Assessment and Diagnosis

Because of the prevalence of substance abuse, it is important to screen all pregnant women for substance abuse during the health history. Several simple screening tools are available. In addition, be alert for clues in the history or appearance of the woman that suggest substance abuse. If abuse is suspected, ask direct questions, beginning with less threatening questions about use of tobacco, caffeine, and over-the-counter medications. Then progress to questions about alcohol intake and finally to questions focusing on past and current use of illegal drugs. A matter-of-fact, nonjudgmental approach is more likely to elicit honest responses.

When assessing a woman with a known substance abuse problem, focus on the woman's general health status, with specific attention to nutritional status, susceptibility to infections, and evaluation of all body systems. Also assess the woman's understanding of the impact of substance abuse on herself and on her pregnancy.

Nursing diagnoses that may apply to a woman at risk because of substance abuse include the following:

▶ *Altered nutrition:* less than body requirements related to inadequate food intake secondary to substance abuse

▶ *Risk for infection* related to use of inadequately cleaned syringes and needles secondary to IV drug use

▶ *Knowledge deficit* related to a lack of information about the impact of substance abuse on the fetus

Planning and Implementation

Prevention of substance abuse during pregnancy is the ideal nursing goal and is best accomplished through education. Unfortunately, many women who abuse substances do not receive regular health care and may not seek care until they are far along in pregnancy.

Thus it is important to focus on ongoing assessment and client teaching. Consider providing information about the relationship between substance abuse and existing health problems and the implications for the woman's unborn child. Establishing a relationship of trust and support helps ensure the woman's cooperation. If possible, discuss strategies to help the woman quit (addiction treatment programs, 12-step programs, individual counseling) and suggest a referral for more in-depth assessment by a specialist.

Preparation for labor and birth should be part of prenatal planning. Nonnarcotic psychologic support and careful explanation of the labor process may help relieve the woman's fear, tension, and discomfort. If pain medication is necessary, it should not be withheld; the notion that it will contribute to further addiction is mistaken. Preferred methods of pain relief include the use of psychoprophylaxis and regional blocks such as epidurals or local anesthetics such as pudendal block and local infiltration. Immediate intensive care should be available for the newborn, who is often depressed, small for gestational age (SGA), and premature. (For care of the addicted newborn, see Chapter 25.)

Evaluation

Expected outcomes of nursing care include the following:

▶ The woman is able to describe the impact of her substance abuse on herself and her unborn child.

▶ The woman gives birth to a healthy infant.

▶ The woman accepts a referral to social services (or another appropriate community agency) for follow-up care after discharge.

CARE OF THE WOMAN WITH DIABETES MELLITUS

Diabetes mellitus (DM) is an endocrine disorder of carbohydrate metabolism resulting from inadequate production or use of insulin. It occurs in about 1% to 14% of all pregnancies, depending on the population served (American Diabetes Association [ADA], 2000a). Insulin, produced by the β-cells of the islets of Langerhans in the pancreas, lowers blood glucose levels by enabling glucose to move from the blood into muscle and adipose tissue cells.

Carbohydrate Metabolism in Normal Pregnancy

In early pregnancy the rise in serum levels of estrogen, progesterone, and other hormones stimulates increased insulin production by the maternal pancreas and increased tissue response to insulin. Thus an anabolic (building-up) state exists during the first half of pregnancy, with storage of glycogen in the liver and other tissues.

In the second half of pregnancy, placental secretion of human placental lactogen (hPL) and prolactin (from the decidua), as well as elevated cortisol and glycogen levels, cause increased resistance to insulin and decreased glucose tolerance. This decreased effectiveness of insulin results in a catabolic (destructive) state during fasting periods, such as during the night or after meal absorption. Because increasing amounts of circulating maternal glucose and amino acids are diverted to the fetus, maternal fat is metabolized much more readily during fasting periods than in a nonpregnant woman. As a result of this lipolysis (maternal metabolism of fat), ketones may be present in the urine.

The delicate system of checks and balances between glucose production and glucose use is stressed by the growing fetus, who derives energy from glucose taken solely from maternal stores. This stress is known as the *diabetogenic effect of pregnancy*. Thus any preexisting disruption in carbohydrate metabolism is augmented by pregnancy, and any diabetic potential may precipitate gestational diabetes mellitus.

Pathophysiology of Diabetes Mellitus

In DM, the pancreas does not produce enough insulin to allow necessary carbohydrate metabolism. Without adequate insulin, glucose does not enter the cells and they become energy depleted. Blood glucose levels remain high (hyperglycemia), and the cells break down their stores of fats and protein for energy. Protein breakdown results in a negative nitrogen balance; fat metabolism causes ketosis.

These pathologic developments cause the four cardinal signs and symptoms of DM: polyuria, polydipsia, polyphagia, and weight loss. Polyuria (frequent urination) results because water is not reabsorbed by the renal tubules due to the osmotic activity of glucose. Polydipsia (excessive thirst) is caused by dehydration from polyuria. Polyphagia (excessive hunger) is caused by tissue loss and a state of starvation, which results from the inability of the cells to use the blood glucose. Weight loss (seen with marked hyperglycemia) is due to the use of fat and muscle tissue for energy.

Classification

Diabetes has been classified in several ways. Table 12–2 shows the classification of DM proposed in 1999, which is based on its cause. This classification contains four main categories: type 1 diabetes, type 2 diabetes, other specific types, and gestational diabetes mellitus (GDM). The former classification, developed by the National Diabetes Data Group in 1979, is based to a degree on the type of pharmacologic treatment used. Thus it included type I (insulin-dependent diabetes mellitus [IDDM]) and type II

TABLE 12–2 Etiologic Classification of Diabetes Mellitus

I. Type 1 diabetes* (β-cell destruction, usually leading to absolute insulin deficiency)
   A. Immune mediated
   B. Idiopathic
II. Type 2 diabetes* (may range from predominantly insulin resistance with relative insulin deficiency to a predominantly secretory defect with insulin resistance)
III. Other specific types†
IV. Gestational diabetes mellitus

*Patients with any form of diabetes may require insulin treatment at some stage of their disease. Such use of insulin does not classify the patient.
†The more detailed classification, which can be found in medical-surgical texts and the original source, provides eight subcategories of type.
Note: From the 1999 Report of the Expert Committee on the Diagnosis and Classification of Diabetes Mellitus. *Diabetes Care,* Suppl. 5. Adapted.

TABLE 12-3 White's Classification of Diabetes in Pregnancy

Class	Criterion
A	Chemical diabetes
B	Maturity onset (age over 20 years), duration under 10 years, no vascular lesions
C_1	Age 10 to 19 years at onset
C_2	10 to 19 years' duration
D_1	Under 10 years at onset
D_2	Over 20 years' duration
D_3	Benign retinopathy
D_4	Calcified vessels of legs
D_5	Hypertension
E	No longer sought
F	Nephropathy
G	Many failures
H	Cardiopathy
R	Proliferating retinopathy
T	Renal transplant (added by Tagatz and colleagues of the University of Minnesota)

Note: From White, P. (1978). Classification of obstetric diabetes. *American Journal of Obstetrics and Gynecology, 130,* 228. Used with permission.

(non-insulin-dependent diabetes mellitus [NIDDM]) as well as the broad categories impaired glucose tolerance and gestational diabetes mellitus. As health care moves to adopt the newer, etiology-based system, the older terms, IDDM and NIDDM, are still being used in many facilities.

Table 12–3 shows White's classification of diabetes in pregnancy. This classification is useful for describing the extent of the disease.

Gestational diabetes mellitus (GDM) is defined as any degree of glucose intolerance that has its onset or is first diagnosed during pregnancy. The woman may remain asymptomatic or may have a mild form of the disease. Diagnosis of GDM is very important, however, because even mild diabetes causes increased risk for perinatal morbidity and mortality. Furthermore, with time, many women with GDM progress to overt type 1 or type 2 diabetes mellitus.

Influence of Pregnancy on Diabetes

Pregnancy can affect diabetes significantly because the physiologic changes of pregnancy can drastically alter insulin requirements. Pregnancy may also alter the progress of vascular disease secondary to DM. Pregnancy can affect diabetes in the following ways:

- DM may be difficult to control because insulin requirements are changeable.
  - During the first trimester, the need for insulin frequently decreases. Levels of hPL, an insulin antagonist, are low; fetal needs are minimal; and the woman may consume less food because of nausea and vomiting.

- Nausea and vomiting may cause dietary fluctuations and increase the risk of hypoglycemia, formerly called insulin shock.
  - Insulin requirements begin to rise in the second trimester as glucose use and glucose storage by the woman and fetus increase. Insulin requirements may double or quadruple by the end of pregnancy as a result of placental maturation and hPL production.
  - Increased energy needs during labor may require increased insulin to balance IV glucose.
  - Usually an abrupt decrease in insulin requirement occurs after the passage of the placenta and the resulting loss of hPL in maternal circulation.
- A decreased renal threshold for glucose leads to a higher incidence of glycosuria.
- The risk of ketoacidosis, which may occur at lower serum glucose levels in the pregnant woman with DM than in the nonpregnant diabetic, increases.
- The vascular disease that accompanies DM may progress during pregnancy.
  - Hypertension may occur, contributing to vascular changes.
  - Nephropathy may result from renal impairment, and retinopathy may develop.

Influence of Diabetes on Pregnancy Outcome

The pregnancy of a woman who has diabetes carries a higher risk of complications, especially perinatal mortality and congenital anomalies. Tight metabolic control (glucose between 70 and 120 mg/dL) reduces this risk. New techniques for monitoring blood glucose level, delivering insulin, and monitoring the fetus also help reduce perinatal mortality.

MATERNAL RISKS

The prognosis for the pregnant woman with gestational, type 1, or type 2 diabetes without significant vascular damage is positive. However, diabetic pregnancy still carries a higher risk of complications than normal pregnancy.

Hydramnios, or an increase in the volume of amniotic fluid, occurs in 10% to 20% of pregnant diabetic women. It is thought to be a result of excessive fetal urination because of fetal hyperglycemia (Spellacy, 1999). Premature rupture of membranes and onset of labor may occasionally be a problem with hydramnios.

Preeclampsia and eclampsia occur more often in diabetic pregnancies than in normal pregnancies, especially when vascular changes already exist (Moore, 1999).

Hyperglycemia can lead to ketoacidosis as a result of the increase in ketone bodies (which are acidic) released in the blood from the metabolism of fatty acids. Decreased gastric motility and the anti-insulin effects of hPL also predispose the woman to ketoacidosis. Ketoacidosis usually develops slowly but, if untreated, can lead to coma and death for mother and fetus.

The pregnant woman with diabetes is also at increased risk for monilial vaginitis and urinary tract infections because of increased glycosuria, which contributes to a favorable environment for bacterial growth.

FETAL-NEONATAL RISKS

Many of the problems of the neonate result directly from high maternal plasma glucose levels. In the presence of untreated maternal ketoacidosis, the risk of fetal death increases to 50% (Spellacy, 1999).

For the general population, the risk of giving birth to a child with a major congenital anomaly is 1% to 2%. For diabetic mothers this risk increases threefold (Spellacy, 1999). This increased incidence of congenital anomalies is probably related to high glucose levels in early pregnancy (Moore, 1999). Most anomalies involve the heart, central nervous system, and skeletal system. One anomaly, *sacral agenesis,* appears almost exclusively in infants of diabetic mothers. In sacral agenesis, the sacrum and lumbar spine fail to develop and the lower extremities develop incompletely. Preconception counseling and strict diabetes control before conception help reduce the incidence of congenital anomalies.

Characteristically, infants of diabetic mothers on insulin therapy (or White's classes A, B, and C; see Table 12–3) are large for gestational age (LGA) as a result of the high maternal levels of blood glucose, from which the fetus derives its glucose. These elevated levels continually stimulate the fetal islets of Langerhans to produce insulin. This hyperinsulin state causes the fetus to use the available glucose, which leads to excessive growth (known as **macrosomia**) and fat deposits. If born vaginally, the macrosomic infant is at increased risk for shoulder dystocia and traumatic birth injuries and may be at increased risk for impaired glucose tolerance in later childhood (Moore, 1999).

Once the umbilical cord is cut after birth, the generous maternal blood glucose supply stops. However, continued islet cell hyperactivity leads to high insulin levels and depleted blood glucose (hypoglycemia) in 2 to 4 hours. Macrosomia can be significantly reduced by tight maternal blood glucose control.

Infants of mothers with advanced diabetes (vascular involvement) may demonstrate IUGR. IUGR occurs because vascular changes in the diabetic woman decrease the efficiency of placental perfusion and the fetus is not as well sustained.

Respiratory distress syndrome appears to result from high levels of fetal insulin, which inhibit some fetal enzymes necessary for surfactant production. Polycythemia (excessive number of red blood cells) in the newborn is mainly due to the diminished ability of glycosylated hemoglobin in the mother's blood to release oxygen. Hyperbilirubinemia is a direct result of the inability of immature liver enzymes to metabolize the increased bilirubin resulting from the polycythemia.

Thinking Critically

COUNSELING REGARDING THE GLUCOSE TOLERANCE TEST

Patti Chang is a 35-year-old, gravida 3 para 2, well-educated, active Chinese-American woman with no history of glucose intolerance. Her two children were born healthy at 36 weeks' gestation. She receives the usual 50-g glucose tolerance test at 26 weeks' gestation, and her plasma level is 160 mg/dL. She seems irritated and frustrated when her obstetrician tells her that it would be best to perform a 3-hour fasting glucose tolerance test. After the physician leaves the room, Patti asks you the following questions: "Will the glucose hurt my baby? What will the treatment be?" How will you answer the questions? Why does Patti seem so upset? ⚬—⚬ WEB

Clinical Therapy

Until recently, all pregnant women were given a 1-hour oral glucose tolerance test (GTT) between 24 and 28 weeks' gestation to screen for GDM. The American Diabetes Association no longer recommends universal screening. Rather, the ADA now recommends that women who are at average risk be screened at 24 to 28 weeks using the 1-hour GTT. Women at average risk include the following (ADA, 2000a):

- Age 25 or older
- Obese women of any age
- Family history of DM in a first-degree relative
- Member of an ethnic group with a high prevalence of diabetes (Hispanic, black, Native American, Asian American)
- History of abnormal glucose tolerance
- History of poor obstetric outcome

To do the 1-hour GTT, the woman drinks a 50-g oral glucose solution at any time during the day and provides a blood sample one hour later. If the plasma glucose level exceeds 130 mg/dL, a 3-hour oral GTT is necessary (ADA, 2000a).

During pregnancy, GDM is diagnosed by using a 3-hour, 100-g oral GTT. To do this test, the woman eats a high-carbohydrate (greater than 200 g carbohydrate daily) diet for 3 days before her scheduled test. She then drinks a 100-g oral glucose solution in the morning after an overnight fast of between 8 and 14 hours. Plasma glucose levels are determined fasting and at 1, 2, and 3 hours. Gestational diabetes is diagnosed if two or more of the following values are equaled or exceeded:

Fasting	95 mg/dL
1 hour	180 mg/dL
2 hours	155 mg/dL
3 hours	140 mg/dL

Pregnant women considered at high risk for DM should have a blood glucose screening as soon as possible. A fasting plasma glucose level > 126 mg/dL or a casual (any time of the day) plasma glucose level > 200 mg/dL is diagnostic of GDM if confirmed on a subsequent day. If not confirmed, the 3-hour GTT is indicated. Women at high risk for GDM but with negative initial findings should be retested at 24 to 28 weeks (ADA, 2000a).

LABORATORY ASSESSMENT OF LONG-TERM GLUCOSE CONTROL

Measurement of glycosylated hemoglobin levels provides information about the long-term (previous 4 to 8 weeks) control of hyperglycemia. The test measures the percentage of glycohemoglobin in the blood. Glycohemoglobin, or HbA_{1c}, is the hemoglobin to which a glucose molecule is attached. Because glycosylation is a rather slow and essentially irreversible process, the test is not reliable for screening for gestational diabetes or for close daily control. Women with abnormal HbA_{1c} values of 9.2% to 11.1% have a 23% risk of having an infant with a malformation (Moore, 1999).

Antepartal Management of Diabetes Mellitus

To ensure an optimally healthy mother and newborn, good prenatal care using a team approach must be a top priority. The woman with gestational diabetes may find the diagnosis shocking and upsetting. She needs clear explanations and teaching to gain her cooperation in ensuring a good outcome. The nurse educator plays a major role in this counseling. The woman with pregestational diabetes needs to understand what changes she can expect during pregnancy; she should receive such teaching in preconception counseling.

DIETARY REGULATION

The pregnant woman with diabetes needs to increase her caloric intake by about 300 kcal/day. During the first trimester, she generally requires about 30 kcal/kg of ideal body weight. During the second and third trimesters, she needs about 35 kcal/kg of ideal body weight (Spellacy, 1999). Approximately 40% to 50% of the calories should come from complex carbohydrates, 15% to 20% from protein, and 30% from fats (Curet, 2000). The food is divided among three meals and three snacks. The bedtime snack is the most important and should include both protein and complex carbohydrates to prevent nighttime hypoglycemia. A nutritionist should work out meal plans with the woman based on the woman's lifestyle, culture, and food preferences. The woman needs to be familiar with the use of food exchanges so she can plan her own meals.

GLUCOSE MONITORING

Glucose monitoring is essential to determine the need for insulin and to assess glucose control. Many physicians have the woman come in for weekly assessment of her fasting glucose levels and one or two postprandial levels. In addition, frequent self-monitoring of glucose levels is paramount in maintaining good glucose control. Self-monitoring is discussed on page 246.

INSULIN ADMINISTRATION

Many women with gestational diabetes need insulin to maintain normal glucose levels. Those with pregestational diabetes typically are already on insulin. In either case, human insulin should be used because it is the least likely to cause an allergic reaction. Insulin is given either in multiple injections or by continuous subcutaneous infusion. Multiple injections are more common and generally produce excellent results. Most women receive a combination of intermediate and regular insulin. Recently, some clinicians have moved away from the use of regular human insulin, replacing it with a fast-acting human analogue called lispro. Lispro is associated with better glucose control (Jovanovic, 2000). Often a four-dose approach is used, with regular insulin or lispro taken before each meal and NPH or Lente insulin added at bedtime (Curet, 2000). Other clinicians vary the NPH and regular insulin patterns slightly but still prefer a four-dose approach.

Oral hypoglycemics are never used during pregnancy because their use has been associated with prolonged fetal hypoglycemia and they may be teratogenic (Spellacy, 1999).

EVALUATION OF FETAL STATUS

Information about the well-being, size, and maturation of the fetus is important for planning the course of pregnancy and the timing of birth. In pregnancies complicated by diabetes, the fetus is at increased risk of neural tube defects such as spina bifida, so maternal serum alpha-fetoprotein (MSAFP) screening is done at 16 to 20 weeks' gestation (see Chapter 14).

Ultrasound is done at 18 weeks to determine gestational age and detect anomalies. It is then repeated at 28 weeks to monitor fetal growth for IUGR or macrosomia. Some agencies do fetal biophysical profiles (ultrasound evaluations of fetal well-being that assess fetal breathing movements, fetal activity, reactivity, muscle tone, and amniotic fluid volume) as part of an ongoing evaluation of fetal status.

Daily maternal evaluation of fetal activity is begun at about 28 weeks. Twice weekly nonstress testing (NST) using a fetal monitor is begun at 32 weeks for women with preexisting DM and for women with GDM who require insulin. Nonstress tests may be delayed until closer to term in women with GDM (Landon, 2000). If the NST is nonreactive, a fetal biophysical profile or contraction stress test is performed. (For an explanation of these tests, see Chapter 14.)

Intrapartal Management of Diabetes Mellitus

During the intrapartal period, medical therapy focuses on the following:

- *Timing of birth.* Most pregnant women with diabetes, regardless of the type, are allowed to go to term, with elective induction of labor and vaginal birth planned at 38 to 40 weeks' gestation. Cesarean birth may be indicated if signs of fetal distress exist. Birth before term may be indicated for diabetic women with vascular changes and worsening hypertension or if evidence of IUGR exists (Landon, 2000). To determine fetal lung maturity, amniotic fluid (obtained by amniocentesis) is evaluated for lecithin/sphingomyelin (L/S) ratio and the presence of phosphatidylglycerol (see Chapter 14). ⊂⊃ Preterm induced birth, often by cesarean, is considered if prenatal testing indicates that the fetus is deteriorating.

- *Labor management*. Frequently maternal insulin requirements decrease dramatically during labor. Consequently maternal glucose levels are measured hourly to determine insulin need. The primary goal in controlling maternal glucose levels intrapartally is to prevent neonatal hypoglycemia (Curet, 2000). Often two IV lines are used, one with a 5% dextrose solution and one with a saline solution. The saline solution is then available for piggybacking insulin or if a bolus is needed. Because insulin clings to plastic IV bags and tubing, the tubing should be flushed with insulin before the prescribed amount is added. During the second stage of labor and the immediate postpartal period, the woman may not need additional insulin. The IV insulin is discontinued at the end of the third stage of labor.

Postpartal Management of Diabetes Mellitus

Generally maternal insulin requirements fall significantly during the postpartal period because, with placental separation, hormone levels fall and the anti-insulin effect ceases. For the first 24 hours postpartum, women with pre-existing diabetes typically require very little insulin. They are usually managed with a sliding scale. Afterward, a more regular insulin dosage pattern can be reestablished. Women with mild diabetes not requiring insulin often have sufficient glucose control and do not require any therapy while they are hospitalized. Antihyperglycemics are contraindicated during breastfeeding. Consequently a nursing woman with diabetes that is not controlled by diet alone may need insulin for a time (Kjos, 2000).

Women with GDM who did not require insulin during pregnancy generally do not need it during the postpartum period. Clinicians routinely discontinue insulin for women with GDM following childbirth and then monitor blood glucose levels. If elevated glucose levels develop, oral antihyperglycemic agents may be tried if the woman is not breastfeeding (Curet, 2000). The woman should be reassessed 6 weeks postpartum to determine whether her glucose levels are normal. If the levels are normal, she should be reassessed at a minimum of 3-year intervals (ADA, 2000a).

The establishment of parent-child relationships is a high priority during the postpartum period. Therefore if the newborn requires a special-care nursery, the parents need ongoing information, support, and encouragement to visit and be involved in the newborn's care.

Encourage breastfeeding as beneficial to both mother and baby. Evidence suggests that breastfed infants have a lower risk of developing diabetes than infants who are bottle-fed (Moore, 1999). Calorie needs increase during lactation to 500 to 800 kcal above prepregnant requirements, and insulin must be adjusted accordingly. Home blood glucose monitoring should continue for the insulin-dependent diabetic.

The woman and her partner, if he is involved, should also receive information on family planning. Barrier methods of contraception (diaphragm, cervical cap, condom) used with a spermicide are safe, effective, economical, and the method of choice for insulin-dependent diabetic women. The use of oral contraceptives by diabetic women is somewhat controversial. Many physicians who prescribe low-dose oral contraceptives to women with diabetes restrict them to women who have no vascular disease and do not smoke. The progesterone-only pill has a higher failure rate but is otherwise safer. Many couples who have completed their families choose elective sterilization.

Nursing Management

The "Nursing Care Plan" for a woman with diabetes mellitus, on pages 243–245, summarizes nursing management during the antepartum, intrapartum, and postpartum periods.

Nursing Assessment and Diagnosis

Whether diabetes has been diagnosed before pregnancy occurs or the diagnosis is made during pregnancy (GDM), careful assessment of the disease process and the woman's understanding of diabetes is important. Thorough physical examination—including assessment for vascular complications of the disease, any signs of infectious conditions, and urine and blood testing for glucose—is essential on the first prenatal visit. Follow-up visits are usually scheduled twice a month during the first two trimesters and once a week during the last trimester.

Assessment provides information about the woman's ability to cope with the combined stress of pregnancy and diabetes and to follow a recommended regimen of care. Determine the woman's knowledge about diabetes and self-care before developing a teaching plan.

Nursing diagnoses that may apply to the pregnant woman with diabetes include the following:

▶ *Risk for altered nutrition:* more than body requirements related to imbalance between intake and available insulin

▶ *Risk for injury* related to possible complications secondary to hypoglycemia or hyperglycemia

▶ *Altered family processes* related to the need for hospitalization secondary to DM

GOAL	INTERVENTION	RATIONALE	EXPECTED OUTCOME
1. Risk for altered nutrition: Less than body requirements related to poor carbohydrate metabolism			
	NIC Intervention:		NOC Outcome:
	Nutrition management: *Assistance with or provision of a balanced dietary intake of foods and fluids*		**Nutritional status:** *Extent to which nutrients are available to meet metabolic needs*
Client will maintain adequate nutrition throughout pregnancy.	▶ Emphasize importance of regular prenatal visits for assessment of weight gain, blood sugar levels, fetal heart tones, urine ketones, and fundal height measurement.	▶ Regular follow-up and assessment of weight, blood sugar levels, fetal heart tones, urine ketones, and fundal height will promote a healthy pregnancy and outcome, as well as allow for modifications in the treatment regimen if necessary.	The client will maintain adequate nutrition as evidenced by adequate weight gain, controlled blood sugar levels, verbalization of understanding of personal treatment regimen, and appropriate fetal growth and development during pregnancy.
	▶ Coordinate care with a dietitian to assist client in meal planning and educate client on the daily caloric needs of pregnancy.	▶ A daily intake of high-quality foods promotes fetal growth and controls maternal glucose levels.	
	▶ Instruct client on signs and symptoms of hyperglycemia: polyphagia, nausea, hot flushes, polydipsia, polyuria, fruity breath, abdominal cramps, rapid deep breathing, headache, weakness, drowsiness, and general malaise. Instruct client on signs and symptoms of hypoglycemia: hunger, clammy skin, irritability, slurred speech, seizures, tachycardia, headache, pallor, sweating, disorientation, shakiness, blurred vision, and, if untreated, coma or convulsions.	▶ Maintaining a euglycemic state throughout pregnancy aids in preventing diabetic complications and promotes a positive pregnancy outcome.	
	▶ Instruct client on management of hyperglycemia and hypoglycemia.		
	▶ Include family members in meal planning.	▶ Gives the family member a sense of involvement and an understanding of the importance of adequate nutrition in pregnancy.	Client will recognize signs and intervene appropriately.
2. Risk for fetal injury related to possible complications associated with altered tissue perfusion secondary to maternal diagnosis of diabetes mellitus			
	NIC Intervention:		NOC Outcome:
	High-risk pregnancy care: *Identification and management of a high-risk pregnancy to promote healthy outcomes for mother and baby*		**Risk control:** *Actions to eliminate or reduce actual, personal, and modifiable health threats*
Uncomplicated birth of a healthy newborn.	▶ Assess fetal heart tones for reassuring variability and accelerations.	▶ Reassuring fetal heart rate variability and accelerations are interpreted as adequate placental oxygenation.	The fetus will not exhibit signs and symptoms of altered tissue perfusion as evidenced by positive fetal activity, reassuring fetal heart rate patterns, a biophysical profile score between 8 and 10, negative CST, L/S ratio indicating fetal lung maturity, and a reactive nonstress test.
	▶ Instruct mother on how to lie in a left recumbent position after eating and record how many fetal movements she feels in an hour.	▶ More than five fetal kicks in an hour are indicative of fetal well-being.	
	▶ **Collaborative:** Perform oxytocin challenge test (OCT)/contraction stress test (CST) and nonstress tests as determined by physician.	▶ Fetal surveillance testing assesses fetal well-being and adequate placental perfusion.	

(continued)

GOAL	INTERVENTION	RATIONALE	EXPECTED OUTCOME
	▶ Prepare client for frequent ultrasound assessments.	▶ Ultrasonography is indicated at 8, 12, 18, 28, and 36–38 weeks per physician's orders to confirm gestational age and fetal well-being.	
	▶ Prepare client for amniocentesis procedure.	▶ A sample of amniotic fluid contains two phospholipids (lecithin/sphingomyelin) that can be used to detect fetal lung maturity and enables medical personnel to prepare for a potential preterm birth.	
	▶ Assist physician with biophysical profile assessment.	▶ Helps assure fetal well-being and a positive fetal outcome.	

3. Health-seeking behaviors related to lack of information about the effects of blood sugar on pregnancy

GOAL	INTERVENTION	RATIONALE	EXPECTED OUTCOME
	NIC Intervention: **Health education:** *Developing and providing instruction and learning experiences to facilitate voluntary adaptation of behavior conducive to health in individuals, families, groups, or communities*		NOC Outcome: **Health-seeking behavior:** *Actions to promote optimal wellness, recovery, and rehabilitation*
The client and her family will verbalize the importance of maintaining blood sugar within prescribed ranges during pregnancy.	▶ Assess the client and family's cognitive level and develop a teaching strategy that will facilitate learning at that level.	▶ Behavior changes occur when teaching strategies are appropriate for the client and family's cognitive level.	The client and family members will verbalize understanding of the effects of blood sugar fluctuations on pregnancy as evidenced by asking questions and seeking health information when necessary. The client adheres to personal treatment regimen throughout pregnancy.
	▶ Teach blood glucose monitoring, insulin administration, and predicted insulin needs throughout pregnancy, and then have client and family members repeat the discussion.	▶ Basic understanding of the relationship between blood sugar levels and how insulin needs change throughout pregnancy will foster compliance with prescribed regimen.	
	▶ Emphasize the importance of maintaining a healthy diet and exercise program during pregnancy. Encourage client and family to develop a sample diabetic diet and exercise regimen that is appropriate for pregnancy while present in the clinic or hospital and evaluate for appropriateness.	▶ Involves the client and her family members in her care and the evaluation method promotes positive reinforcement and a time for modifications of regimen if necessary.	
	▶ Emphasize the importance of prenatal care for the purpose of maternal and fetal surveillance.	▶ Frequent prenatal visits allow for modifications in regimen and promote a healthy pregnancy outcome.	

4. Risk for infection related to increased levels of glucose in urine

GOAL	INTERVENTION	RATIONALE	EXPECTED OUTCOME
	NIC Intervention: **Infection control:** *Minimizing the acquisition and transmission of infectious agents*		NOC Outcome: **Knowledge: Infection control:** *Extent of understanding conveyed about prevention and control of infection*
The client will have no urinary tract infections (UTIs) during pregnancy.	▶ Encourage client to utilize preventive measures to prevent UTIs: increasing intake of water and cranberry juice, wearing cotton underwear, wiping perineum from front to back, voiding frequently, and voiding before and immediately after sexual intercourse.	▶ Utilizing preventive measures decreases the likelihood of patient acquiring a UTI.	Client will remain free of UTIs during pregnancy as evidenced by verbalizing and complying with appropriate preventive measures, increasing fluid intake, and negative urine samples during prenatal visits.

GOAL	INTERVENTION	RATIONALE	EXPECTED OUTCOME
	▶ Instruct client on the signs and symptoms of UTIs: urinary frequency, dysuria, cloudy urine, hematuria, lower back pain, and foul-smelling urine. **Collaborative:** ▶ Instruct client on how to obtain a clean-catch urine sample and send to lab for culture and sensitivity per physician's orders. ▶ Administer prescribed antibiotic therapy and teach client about medication, adverse effects, and appropriate dosage. ▶ Encourage client to drink 8–10 glasses of water each day.	▶ Client will be aware of signs and symptoms of UTIs and report to physician for immediate intervention. ▶ A clean-catch urine sample will contain bacteria if a UTI is present. ▶ Antibiotic therapy is the appropriate treatment for a UTI. Compliance increases when a client fully understands medication regimen. ▶ Increased fluid intake assists in flushing bacteria out of the urinary tract system.	
5. Anxiety related to unfamiliarity with diagnosis			
	NIC Intervention: **Anxiety reduction:** *Minimizing apprehension, dread, foreboding, or uneasiness related to an unidentified source of anticipated danger*		NOC Outcome: **Anxiety control:** *Ability to eliminate or reduce feelings of apprehension and tension from an unidentifiable source*
The client expresses less anxiety	▶ Assess client's level of anxiety (mild-1, moderate-2, or severe-3) and have client verbalize causes of anxiety. ▶ Share information on diabetes such as nutrition, exercise, and glucose control in a clear and concise manner. ▶ Instruct client on anxiety-reducing techniques such as imagery, breathing exercises, and massage used in pregnancy. ▶ Refer client to a diabetes support group.	▶ Verbalization of anxiety provokers encourages expression of feelings and questions. ▶ Accurate information gives the client a sense of control and comfort. ▶ Gives client the tools necessary for decreasing anxiety. ▶ A support group allows clients with similar problems to express concerns and share information with each other.	The client demonstrates appropriate coping strategies as evidenced by utilizing resources efficiently and verbalizing feelings of anxiety and the ways to deal with them.

Planning and Implementation

For the woman with preexisting diabetes, a nurse and a physician may provide prepregnancy counseling using a team approach. Ideally they see the couple before pregnancy so that the DM can be evaluated. The outlook for pregnancy is good if the diabetes is of recent onset without vascular complications, provided that glucose levels can be controlled.

For women with GDM, nursing care focuses heavily on client education about the condition, its implications, and its management.

NURSING CARE IN THE COMMUNITY

In many cases, women with gestational diabetes mellitus are stabilized in the hospital and necessary teaching for self-care is begun. Women with preexisting diabetes may also require hospitalization for stabilization of their dia-

betes. In either case, the majority of ongoing teaching and supervision of pregnant women with diabetes is then carried out by nurses in clinics, community agencies, and the women's homes.

Effective Insulin Use

Ensure that the woman and her partner understand the purpose of insulin, the types of insulin to be used, and the correct procedure for administering it. Instruct the woman's partner about insulin administration in case it becomes necessary for the partner to give it. For some highly motivated women whose glucose levels are not well controlled with multiple injections, the continuous infusion pump may improve glucose control.

Teach the woman how and when to monitor her blood glucose level, the desired range of blood glucose levels, and the importance of good control (Figure 12–1 ◆). Most women use a glucose meter to monitor blood sugar level

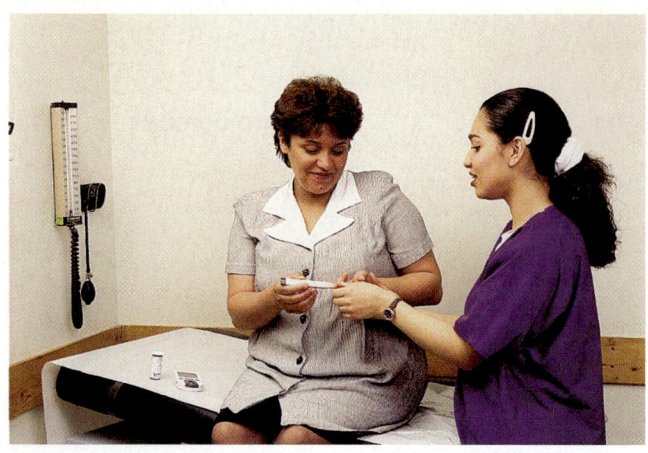

FIGURE 12–1. ◆ The nurse teaches the pregnant woman with gestational diabetes mellitus how to do home glucose monitoring.

because the meter is more accurate, but some women use a visual method of monitoring. With either method, teach the woman to follow the manufacturer's directions exactly; to wash her hands thoroughly before puncturing her finger; to touch the blood droplet, not her finger, to the test pad on the strip; and to store the test strips as directed and discard them after the expiration date. Diabetic clients need to keep a record of each blood sugar reading. Specific record sheets are available for this purpose.

Planned Exercise Program

Regardless of the type of diabetes, unless otherwise medically contraindicated, exercise is important for the woman's overall well-being. If she is used to a regular exercise program, encourage her to continue. Advise the woman to exercise after meals when blood sugar levels are high, to wear diabetic identification, to carry a simple sugar such as hard candy (because of the possibility of exercise-induced hypoglycemia), to monitor her blood glucose levels regularly, and to avoid injecting insulin into an extremity that will soon be used during exercise.

If the woman has not been following a regular exercise plan, encourage her to begin gradually. Due to alterations in metabolism with exercise, the woman's blood glucose should be well controlled before she begins an exercise program.

Teaching for Self-Care

Using the information gained during the nursing assessment of the pregnant woman with diabetes, provide appropriate teaching to the woman and her family so that the woman can meet her own health care needs as much as possible.

▶ *Glucose monitoring.* Home monitoring of blood glucose levels is the most accurate and convenient method to determine insulin dose and assess control. Women learn self-monitoring techniques that they perform four to six times a day according to a specified schedule. They then regulate their insulin dosage based on blood glucose

values and anticipated activity level. Women are encouraged to maintain blood glucose levels in normal ranges as follows: before meals, 70 to 100 mg/dL; 2 hours after a meal, <120 mg/dL (ADA, 2000b).

▶ *Symptoms of hypoglycemia and ketoacidosis.* The pregnant diabetic woman must recognize symptoms of changing glucose levels and take appropriate action by immediately checking her capillary blood glucose level. If it is less than 60 mg/dL, she should take 20 g of carbohydrate, wait 20 minutes, and then retest her glucose level. The necessary carbohydrate can be obtained by drinking about a cup and a half (12 oz) of whole milk, orange or apple juice, or cola. Many people overtreat their symptoms by continuing to eat, but doing so can cause rebound hyperglycemia. The woman should carry a snack at all times and should have other fast sources of glucose (simple carbohydrates) at hand to treat an insulin reaction when milk or juice is not available. Family members also learn how to inject glucagon in case food does not work or is not feasible (e.g., in the presence of severe morning sickness).

▶ *Smoking.* Smoking has harmful effects on both the maternal vascular system and the developing fetus and is contraindicated for both pregnancy and diabetes.

▶ *Travel.* Insulin can be kept at room temperature while traveling. Insulin supplies should be kept with the traveler and not packed in the baggage. Special meals can be arranged by notifying most airlines a few days before departure. The woman should wear a diabetic identification bracelet or necklace and should check with her physician for any instructions or advice before traveling.

▶ *Support groups.* Many communities have diabetes support groups or education classes that are helpful to women with newly diagnosed diabetes.

▶ *Cesarean birth.* Chances for a cesarean birth increase if the pregnant woman is diabetic. The possibility should be anticipated; caregivers may suggest enrollment in cesarean birth preparation classes. The couple may prefer simply to discuss cesarean birth with the nurse and their obstetrician and read some books on the topic.

HOSPITAL-BASED NURSING CARE

Hospitalization may become necessary during the pregnancy to evaluate blood glucose levels and adjust insulin dosages. In such cases, monitor the woman's status and provide teaching so that she is knowledgeable about her condition and its management. See the Clinical Pathway for a woman with diabetes mellitus on the companion website. 🔗 **WEB**

During the intrapartal period, continue to monitor the woman's status, maintain her IV fluids, remain alert for signs of hypoglycemia, and provide the care indicated for any woman in labor. If a cesarean birth becomes necessary, provide appropriate care, as described in Chapter 17. 🔗

Evaluation

Expected outcomes of nursing care include the following:

▶ The woman is able to discuss her condition and its possible impact on her pregnancy, labor and birth, and postpartal period.

▶ The woman participates in developing a health care regimen to meet her needs and follows it throughout her pregnancy.

▶ The woman avoids developing hypoglycemia or hyperglycemia.

▶ The woman gives birth to a healthy newborn.

▶ The woman is able to care for her newborn.

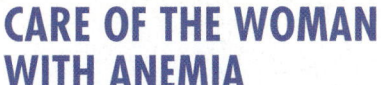

CARE OF THE WOMAN WITH ANEMIA

Anemia indicates inadequate levels of hemoglobin (Hb) in the blood. During pregnancy, anemia is defined as hemoglobin less than 10 g/dL (Wenstrom & Malee, 1999). The common anemias of pregnancy are due either to insufficient hemoglobin production related to nutritional deficiency in iron or folic acid during pregnancy or to hemoglobin destruction in an inherited disorder such as sickle cell anemia. Table 12–4 describes these common anemias.

TABLE 12–4 Anemia and Pregnancy			
Condition	*Brief Description*	*Maternal Implications*	*Fetal/Neonatal Implications*
Iron deficiency anemia	Condition caused by inadequate iron intake resulting in hemoglobin levels below 11g/dL. To prevent this, most women are advised to take supplemental iron during pregnancy.	Pregnant woman with this anemia tires easily, is more susceptible to infection, has increased chance of PIH and postpartal hemorrhage, and cannot tolerate even minimal blood loss during birth.	Risk of low birth weight, prematurity, stillbirth, and neonatal death increases in women with severe iron-deficiency anemia (maternal Hb less than 6 g/dL). Fetus may be hypoxic during labor due to impaired uteroplacental oxygenation.
Sickle cell anemia	Recessive autosomal disease present in about 1 in 600 African Americans in the United States (the sickle cell trait is carried by 8%) (Scioscia, 1999). The disease is characterized by sickling of the RBCs in the presence of decreased oxygenation. Condition may be marked by crisis with profound anemia, jaundice, high temperature, infarction, and acute pain. Crisis is treated by partial exchange transfusion, rehydration with IV fluids, antibiotics, and analgesics. The fetus is monitored throughout.	Pregnancy may aggravate anemia and bring on more crises. Risk of developing preeclampsia increases. Risk of urinary tract infection, pneumonia, congestive heart failure, and pulmonary infarction also increases. The goal of treatment is to reduce the anemia and maintain good health. Oxygen supplementation should be used continuously during labor. Additional blood should be available if transfusion is necessary following birth.	Abortion, fetal death, and prematurity may occur. IUGR is also a characteristic finding in newborns of women with sickle cell anemia.
Folic acid deficiency anemia	Folic acid deficiency is the most common cause of megaloblastic anemia. In the absence of folic acid, immature RBCs fail to divide, become enlarged (megaloblastic), and are fewer in number. Increased folic acid metabolism during pregnancy and lactation can result in deficiency. Because the condition is difficult to diagnose, the best approach is prevention. All women who could become pregnant should take a multivitamin containing 400 μg (0.4 mg) daily (generally found in prenatal vitamins) before conception and through at least the first trimester of pregnancy (Mersereau, 2000). Some authorities recommend increasing the amount of synthetic folate to 0.6 mg daily once pregnancy is confirmed (Institute of Medicine, 1998). The condition is treated with 1 mg folate daily (see Chapter 11).	Folate deficiency is the second most common cause of anemia in pregnancy. Severe deficiency increases the risk that the mother may need a blood transfusion following birth due to anemia. She also has an increased risk of hemorrhage due to thrombocytopenia and is more susceptible to infection. Folic acid is readily available in foods such as fresh leafy green vegetables, red meat, fish, poultry, and legumes, but it is easily destroyed by overcooking or cooking with large quantities of water.	Maternal folic acid deficiency has been associated with an increased risk of neural tube defects (NTDs) such as spina bifida, meningomyelocele, and anencephaly in the newborn. Adequate folic acid intake can reduce the incidence of NTDs by 50% to 70% (CDC, 1999). Folic acid may also help prevent other birth defects, including cleft lip and cleft palate (March of Dimes [MOD], 1999). Women who have already had one baby with an NTD are generally advised to take a larger dose of folic acid daily—typically 4 mg (MOD, 1999).

CARE OF THE WOMAN WITH HIV INFECTION

Human immunodeficiency virus (HIV) infection is one of today's major health concerns. It leads to a progressive disease that ultimately results in **acquired immunodeficiency syndrome (AIDS).** From 1996 to the present, the incidence of AIDS has been decreasing, although the rate of decrease has slowed; concurrently the number of people living with AIDS has increased. These changes have been attributed to the effect of new treatment options (Centers for Disease Control and Prevention [CDC], 2000). Homosexual and bisexual men still make up the largest group of infected people. Women account for 17% of cases. Cases of perinatal AIDS have also decreased significantly in the past several years primarily because of the use of zidovudine (ZDV) therapy in pregnant women with HIV (Levine, 2001). (See "Developing Cultural Competence.")

Pathophysiology of HIV and AIDS

HIV, which causes AIDS, typically enters the body through blood, blood products, or other body fluids such as semen, vaginal fluid, and breast milk. HIV affects specific T cells, thereby decreasing the body's immune responses. This makes the affected person susceptible to opportunistic infections such as *Pneumocystis carinii*, which causes a severe pneumonia, candidiasis, cytomegalovirus, tuberculosis, and toxoplasmosis.

Once infected with the virus, the person develops antibodies that can be detected with the enzyme-linked immunosorbent assay (ELISA) and confirmed with the Western blot test. Antibodies usually develop within 6 to 12 weeks after exposure, although in some people this latent period is longer. An asymptomatic period of approximately 5 to 11 years follows seroconversion (Minkoff, 1999). The majority of pregnant women fall into this category.

The diagnosis of AIDS is made when a person is HIV positive and has one of several specific opportunistic infections.

Maternal Risks

AIDS-defining diseases that are more common in women than in men include wasting syndrome, esophageal candidiasis, and herpes simplex virus disease.

Non-AIDS-defining gynecologic disorders, such as candidiasis or cervical pathology, are prevalent among women in all stages of HIV.

Many women who are HIV positive choose to avoid pregnancy because of the risk of infecting the fetus and the likelihood of dying before the child is raised. Women who become pregnant should be advised that pregnancy is not believed to accelerate the progression of HIV/AIDS, that the use of ZDV during pregnancy significantly reduces the risk of transmitting the HIV to the fetus, and that most medications used to treat HIV can be taken during the pregnancy (Minkoff, 1999).

Fetal-Neonatal Risks

AIDS may develop in infants whose mothers are seropositive, usually due to perinatal transmission. Perinatal transmission occurs transplacentally, at birth when the infant is exposed to maternal blood and vaginal secretions, and via breast milk. The risk to infants born to mothers who are HIV positive is estimated to be about 25%. When the pregnant woman receives ZDV therapy, that risk decreases to 5% to 8%. When ZDV therapy is combined with a scheduled cesarean birth, the risk is further reduced to about 2% (American College of Obstetricians and Gynecologists [ACOG], 1999).

Often infants have a positive antibody titer for up to 15 months due to the passive transfer of maternal antibodies. For further discussion of the infant who is HIV positive, see Chapter 25.

Clinical Therapy

All women who are pregnant or planning a pregnancy should be offered HIV testing using ELISA. If the results are positive, the Western blot test is used to confirm the diagnosis. Women who test positive should be counseled about the implications of the diagnosis for themselves and their fetus to ensure an informed reproductive choice. The care of the woman who chooses to continue her pregnancy focuses on stabilizing the disease, preventing opportunistic infections and the transmission of the virus from mother to fetus, and providing psychosocial and educational support. ZDV therapy should be recommended to all infected pregnant women to reduce the rate of perinatal transmission. This therapy involves administration of ZDV during pregnancy and labor and to the newborn for the first 6 weeks of life (Mofenson, 1999).

The woman infected with HIV should be evaluated and treated for other sexually transmitted infections and for conditions occurring more commonly in women with HIV, such as tuberculosis, cytomegalovirus, toxoplasmosis, and cervical dysplasia. If there is no history of hepatitis B, she should receive the hepatitis vaccine, as well as the pneumococcal vaccine and an annual flu shot. In addition to routine prenatal laboratory tests, a platelet count and a complete blood count with differential should be obtained at the first prenatal visit and repeated each trimester to identify anemia, thrombocytopenia, and leukopenia, which are associated with both HIV infection and antiviral therapy.

At each prenatal visit, asymptomatic, HIV-infected women are monitored for early signs of complications, such as weight loss in the second or third trimesters or fever. The clinician inspects the mouth for signs of infections such as thrush (candidiasis) or hairy leukoplakia; the lungs are auscultated for signs of pneumonia; and the lymph nodes, the liver, and the spleen are palpated for signs of enlargement. Each trimester the woman should have a visual examination and examination of the retina to detect such complications as toxoplasmosis.

In addition to routine prenatal testing, the woman who is HIV positive should be assessed regularly for serologic changes indicating that HIV/AIDS is progressing. This assessment includes the absolute CD4 lymphocyte count, which provides the number of helper T4 cells. When the CD4 count reaches a level of $200/mm^3$ or lower, opportunistic infections are more likely to develop.

A pregnancy complicated by HIV infection, even if asymptomatic, is considered high risk, and the fetus is monitored closely. Weekly nonstress testing is begun at 32 weeks' gestation, and serial ultrasounds are done to detect IUGR. Biophysical profiles are also indicated (see Chapter 14). Invasive procedures such as amniocentesis are avoided when possible to prevent the contamination of a noninfected infant.

Because cesarean birth further reduces the risk of transmission of HIV vertically from mother to baby, ACOG recommends that birth by scheduled cesarean be offered to all HIV-infected women. To decrease the risk of rupture of the membranes before the onset of labor, the cesarean is best done at 38 completed weeks of gestation. Intravenous ZDV prophylaxis should be given before surgery (ACOG, 1999).

HIV-positive women are at increased risk for complications such as intrapartal or postpartal hemorrhage, postpartal infection, poor wound healing, and infections of the genitourinary tract. Thus they need careful monitoring and appropriate therapy as indicated. Research suggests that breastfeeding increases the risk of HIV transmission to the newborn. Consequently, the HIV-positive woman should be cautioned against breastfeeding her infant.

Because of the profound implications of HIV infection for the woman, her family, the child, and her health care providers, screening is recommended for women who are at increased risk, including the following: IV drug users; prostitutes; women whose current or previous sexual partners have been bisexual, have abused IV drugs, have hemophilia, or have tested positive for HIV; and women from countries where heterosexual transmission is common. In addition, clinical facilities in areas with a large population of people who test positive for HIV may require routine HIV screening of all prenatal clients.

Nursing Management

Nursing Assessment and Diagnosis

A woman who tests positive for HIV may be asymptomatic or may present with any of the following signs or symptoms: fatigue, anemia, malaise, progressive weight loss, lymphadenopathy, diarrhea, fever, neurologic dysfunction, cell-mediated immunodeficiency, or evidence of Kaposi's sarcoma (purplish, reddish brown lesions either externally or internally). If a woman tests positive for HIV or is involved in a relationship that places her at high risk, assess the woman's knowledge level about the disease, its implications for her and her fetus, and self-care measures the woman can take.

Examples of nursing diagnoses that might apply for a pregnant woman who tests positive for HIV include the following:

▶ *Knowledge deficit* related to lack of information about HIV/AIDS and its long-term implications for the woman and her unborn child

▶ *Risk for infection* related to altered immunity secondary to HIV infection

▶ *Ineffective family coping* related to the implications of a positive HIV test in one of the family members

Nursing Plan and Implementation

NURSING CARE IN THE COMMUNITY

Women need to understand that HIV/AIDS is a fatal disease. HIV infection can be avoided if women practice safe sex, including insisting that their partners wear a latex condom for each act of intercourse and avoiding sharing IV drug needles. Women at high risk for HIV/AIDS should be offered premarital and prepregnancy screening for HIV antibodies (ACOG, 1997).

In monitoring the asymptomatic pregnant woman who is HIV positive, be alert for nonspecific symptoms such as fever, weight loss, fatigue, persistent candidiasis, diarrhea, cough, skin lesions, and behavior changes. These may be signs of developing symptomatic HIV infection. Laboratory findings such as decreased hemoglobin, hematocrit, and CD4 lymphocytes; elevated erythrocyte sedimentation rate (ESR); and abnormal complete blood count, differential, and platelets may indicate complications such as infection or progression of the disease.

Education about optimal nutrition and maintenance of wellness is important; review the information frequently with the woman. Give her information about her ZDV prophylaxis and the importance of following the established regimen for herself during pregnancy and for her newborn after birth.

HOSPITAL-BASED NURSING CARE

The "Clinical Pathway for a Woman with HIV/AIDS" beginning on page 250 summarizes essential nursing management during the antepartum, intrapartum, and postpartum periods.

CLINICAL PATHWAY ❧ *For A Woman With HIV/AIDS*

Category	Antepartal Management	Intrapartal Management*	Postpartal Management*
Referral	• Perinatologist • Internist • Social worker • Psych clinical nurse practitioner • Dietary/nutritionist • Infectious disease consult	• Obtain prenatal record	• Home nursing referral if indicated **Expected Outcomes** Appropriate resources identified and utilized

Assessments	• Obtain course of present pregnancy
	• Assess estimated gestational age
	• Assess any sensitivity to medications
	• Obtain history of any infections
	• Obtain complete physical examination to include:
	  • Fetal size, fetal status (FHR), and fetal maturity
	  • Signs of fatigue, weakness, recurrent diarrhea, pallor, night sweats
	  • Lymphadenopathy
	  • Present weight and amount of weight gain or weight loss
	  • Presence of nonproductive cough, fever, sore throat, chills, shortness of breath (*Pneumocystis carinii* pneumonia)
	  • Dark purplish marks or lesions, especially on the lower extremities (Kaposi's sarcoma)
	  • Oral, gingival lesions
	• Obtain diagnostic studies:
	  • Ultrasound
	  • Fetal maturity studies (L/S ratio, PG creatinine)
	  • Hemoglobin and hematocrit
	  • WBC
	  • HIV-I
	  • CD4+ T lymphocyte count
	  • ESR
	  • Differential
	  • Platelet count
		• Assess for signs of infection	• Monitor daily Hct
			• Continue normal postpartum assessment q8h
			• Feeding technique with newborn: should be progressing
			• TPR assessment: q8h; all WNL; report temperature >38°C (100.4°F)
			• Continue assessment of comfort level
			Expected Outcomes
			Potential/actual health problems and complications identified and minimized

Teaching/ psychosocial	• Room orientation
	• Explain signs and symptoms of worsening disease and importance of notifying RN
	• Explain s/sx of labor
	• Increase pt awareness of fetal monitoring
	• Evaluation of client teaching
		• Tour of ICN
		• Discuss with woman:
		  a. Mode of childbirth
		  b. Postpartum expectation
			• Implement normal postpartum teaching and psychosocial support
			Expected Outcomes
			Client verbalizes/demonstrates understanding and incorporation of teaching

Nursing care management and reports	• Assess emotional response so that support and teaching can be planned accordingly • Weigh woman • Obtain food history • Establish rapport • Provide opportunities to talk without interruption • Monitor for signs of infection • Maintain appropriate isolation precautions	• Ongoing monitoring of blood pressure • Electronic fetal monitoring in place • Try to have same nurses caring for woman during her hospitalization • Maintain appropriate BSI precautions • Monitor for signs of infection Provide supportive care	• Continue sitz baths prn • May shower if ambulating without difficulty • DC buffalo cap (heparin lock) if present • Maintain appropriate isolation precautions • Monitor for signs of infection **Expected Outcomes** Maternal and fetal well-being maximized Active involvement of client in plan of care to include physical, emotional, and spiritual needs

Category	Antepartal Management	Intrapartal Management*	Postpartal Management*
Activity	• Decreased stimulation in room • Limit visitors	Encourage position change and activity as tolerated	• Up ad lib **Expected Outcome** Level of activity has not exacerbated condition
Comfort	• Assess for discomfort • Provide comfort measures as needed	• Assess for discomfort • Provide comfort measures as needed	• Continue with pain management techniques **Expected Outcome** Optimal comfort maintained
Nutrition	• Plan high-protein, high-calorie diet	• Ice chips; popsicles	• Continue diet and fluids **Expected Outcome** Nutritional needs met with emphasis on appetite enhancement and reduction of deficiencies
Elimination			**Expected Outcome** Intake and output WNL
Medications		• Continuous IV infusion	• May take own prenatal vitamins • Rh immune globulin (RhoGAM) administered if indicated • Rubella vaccine administered if indicated **Expected Outcomes** Perfusion and hydration supported Ongoing treatments maintained

Discharge planning/ home care Family	• Assess home care needs
	• If the client is asymptomatic, the primary nursing activity is client teaching regarding
	  • Disease process
	  • Screening and health care for sex partners as appropriate
	  • Impact of disease on pregnancy
	  • Methods of HIV transmission
	  • Precautions to take in preventing the spread of infection
	  • Options in regard to pregnancy
	  • Available community resources
	  • Signs and symptoms to report to health care provider including common discomforts of pregnancy such as nausea and fatigue and complications such as premature rupture of membranes, vaginal bleeding, and preterm labor
	  • Importance of regular prenatal visits
	• Provide teaching regarding nutritional needs
	• Refer to community resources
	• Discuss disease process, impact on pregnancy, and pregnancy options
	• Provide support and counseling
			• Review discharge instruction sheet and checklist
			• Describe postpartum warning signs and when to call CNM/physician
			• Provide prescriptions and gift pack
			• Arrangements made for baby pictures
			• Postpartum visit scheduled
			• Newborn check schedule
			• Discuss the implications of breastfeeding (current information suggests that the virus may be spread in breast milk)
			• Provide information on transmission of HIV and measures to prevent infection. Discuss household safety issues (eg, it is acceptable to use same dishes, safe to sleep in same bed, safe to use same bathroom, can hold and hug children, should avoid sharing razors and toothbrushes and should wear gloves and use 10% bleach solution to clean spills of body fluids or disinfect bathroom). Inform the woman that sexual abstinence is safest; otherwise latex condoms should be used.
			Expected Outcomes
			Discharge teaching completed with emphasis on follow-up continuing health care needs, adequate support network

Involvement	• Assess woman's major concerns regarding losing fetus, relationship with other children, relationship with partner • Assess support systems	• Encourage family member to stay with the woman as long as possible throughout labor and childbirth	• Family members urged to visit • Continue to involve support persons in teaching • Shows parental bonding behaviors • Plans made for providing support to mother following discharge. Support persons verbalize understanding of need for woman to rest, eat nutritionally, recover. **Expected Outcomes** Family demonstrates resource utilization, integration of newborn into family, helpful coping skills
Date			

*Interventions for a woman with a normal labor and birth and during the early postpartum period may be found in those appropriate clinical pathways.
BSI, body substance isolation; ESR, erythrocyte sedimentation rate; FHR, fetal heart rate; hct, hematocrit; ICN, intensive care nursery; IV, intravenous; L/S ratio, Lecithin/sphingomyelin ratio; PG, phosphotidyl glycerol; Q8h, every 8 hours; s/sx, signs/symptoms; WBC, white blood count; WNL, within normal limits.

Nurses who deal with childbearing families are exposed frequently to blood and body fluids and need to pay careful attention to the universal precautions addressed in introductory nursing courses as a preparation for clinical practice (see "Nursing Practice"). Protocols have been established for postexposure treatment of a caregiver who experiences a needlestick or exposure to body fluids of a person with positive or unknown HIV status. The effectiveness of the therapy, usually a combined drug approach, depends on starting rapidly (Catanzarite, Piacquadio, Stanco, et al., 1999). Thus, such exposure should be reported immediately.

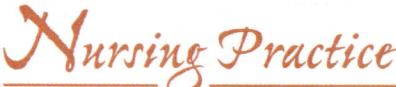

Nursing Practice

Universal precautions were developed in 1987 in response to the increasing prevalence of HIV/AIDS. They provide specific information about practices designed to reduce your exposure to infection. In particular, always follow the cardinal rule in caring for pregnant women: *if it's wet and it's not yours, use protection when handling it!*

TEACHING FOR SELF-CARE

The psychologic implications of HIV/AIDS for the childbearing family are staggering. The woman is faced with the knowledge that she and her newborn, if infected, have a decreased life expectancy. If her infant is not infected, she must face the probability that others will raise her child. The couple must deal with the impact of the illness on the partner, who may or may not be infected, and on other children. The woman and her family may feel fearful, helpless, angry, and isolated.

It is important to preserve confidentiality and the woman's right to privacy. Help ensure that the woman receives complete, accurate information about her condition and ways she might cope. Teach about transmission prevention using language the woman and her partner understand. In addition, ensure that the woman is referred to a comprehensive program that includes social services, psychologic support, and appropriate health care (Sinclair, 1999–2000).

Evaluation

Expected outcomes of nursing care include the following:

► The woman discusses the implications of her HIV infection (or diagnosis of AIDS), its implications for her unborn child and for herself, the method of transmission, and the treatment options.

► The woman uses information about social services (or other agency referral) for follow-up assistance and counseling.

► The woman begins to verbalize her feelings about her condition and its implications for her and her family.

CARE OF THE WOMAN WITH HEART DISEASE

Pregnancy results in increased cardiac output, heart rate, and blood volume. The normal heart is able to adapt to these changes without difficulty. The woman with heart disease, however, has decreased cardiac reserve, making it more difficult for her heart to handle the higher workload of pregnancy.

Approximately 4% of pregnant women of childbearing age have preexisting heart disease (Wenstrom & Malee, 1999). The pathology found in a pregnant woman with heart disease varies with the type of disorder. The more common conditions are discussed briefly here.

Congenital heart defects account for most cases of heart disease in women of childbearing age (Wenstrom & Malee, 1999). Those most commonly seen in pregnant women include atrial septal defect, ventricular septal defect, patent ductus arteriosus, coarctation of the aorta, and tetralogy of Fallot.

For women with congenital heart disease, the impact of pregnancy depends on the specific defect. If the heart defect has been surgically repaired and no evidence of heart disease remains, the woman may undertake pregnancy with confidence. Because of the risk of subacute bacterial endocarditis, even in cases where the defect was corrected surgically, antibiotic prophylaxis is often recommended at the time of birth. Women with congenital heart disease who experience cyanosis should be counseled to avoid pregnancy because the risk to mother and fetus is high.

Rheumatic fever, which may develop in untreated group A β-hemolytic streptococcal infections, is an inflammatory connective tissue disease that can involve the heart, joints, central nervous system, skin, and subcutaneous tissue. Once it occurs, rheumatic fever can recur; it is serious primarily because of the permanent damage it can do to the heart— rheumatic heart disease. Fortunately, rheumatic heart disease has declined rapidly in the past four decades, primarily because of the availability of antibiotics for treatment.

Rheumatic heart disease results when recurrent inflammation from bouts of rheumatic fever causes scar tissue to form on the valves. The scarring results in stenosis (failure of the valve to open completely), regurgitation due to failure of the valve to close completely, or a combination of both, thereby increasing the workload of the heart. Although mitral valve stenosis is most common, the aortic and tricuspid valves may also be affected.

The increased blood volume of pregnancy, coupled with the pregnant woman's need for increased cardiac output, stresses the heart of a woman with mitral stenosis and increases her risk of developing congestive heart failure. Even the woman who has no symptoms at the onset of her pregnancy is at risk.

Mitral valve prolapse (MVP) is usually asymptomatic and commonly found in women of childbearing age. The condition is more common in women than in men and seems to run in families. In MVP, the mitral valve leaflets tend to prolapse into the left atrium during ventricular systole because the chordae tendineae that support them are long, stretched, and thin. This produces a characteristic systolic click on auscultation. In more pronounced cases of MVP, mitral valve regurgitation occurs, producing a systolic murmur.

Women with MVP usually tolerate pregnancy well. Most women require assurance that they can continue with normal activities. A few women experience symptoms—primarily palpitations, chest pain, and dyspnea—which are often due to arrhythmias. They are usually treated with propranolol hydrochloride (Inderal). Limiting caffeine intake also helps decrease palpitations. Prophylactic antibiotics at the time of birth to prevent bacterial endocarditis are not usually necessary for women whose only sign of MVP is a systolic click. Antibiotics are recommended, however, for women with a systolic murmur (Shabetai, 1999).

Peripartum cardiomyopathy is a dysfunction of the left ventricle that occurs in the last month of pregnancy or the first 5 months postpartum in a woman with no previous history of heart disease. The cause is unknown, but the mortality rate is as high as 25% to 50% (Sheffield & Cunningham, 1999). The symptoms are similar to those of congestive heart failure: dyspnea, orthopnea, fatigue, cough, chest pain, palpitations, and edema. The woman may have an enlarged heart, tachycardia, rales, and a third heart sound. Treatment includes digoxin, diuretics, vasodilators as necessary, anticoagulants, and strict bed rest (Wenstrom & Malee, 1999). The condition may resolve with bed rest as the heart gradually returns to normal size. Subsequent pregnancy is strongly discouraged because the disease tends to recur during pregnancy.

Clinical Therapy

The primary goal of clinical therapy is early diagnosis and ongoing management of the woman with cardiac disease. Echocardiogram, chest x-ray, auscultation of heart sounds, and sometimes cardiac catheterization are essential for establishing the type and severity of the heart disease. The severity of the disease can also be determined by the individual's ability to perform ordinary physical activity. The following classification of functional capacity has been standardized by the Criteria Committee of the New York Heart Association (1979):

- *Class I.* Asymptomatic. No limitation of physical activity.
- *Class II.* Slight limitation of physical activity. Asymptomatic at rest; symptoms occur with heavy physical activity.
- *Class III.* Moderate to marked limitation of physical activity. Symptomatic during less-than-ordinary physical activity.
- *Class IV.* Inability to carry on any physical activity without discomfort. Even at rest the person experiences symptoms of cardiac insufficiency or anginal pain.

Women in classes I and II usually experience a normal pregnancy and have few complications, whereas those in classes III and IV are at risk for more severe complications. Because anemia increases the work of the heart, it should be diagnosed early and treated if present. Infections, even if minor, also increase cardiac workload and should be treated.

DRUG THERAPY

The pregnant woman with heart disease may need drug therapy in addition to the iron and vitamin supplements ordinarily prescribed to maintain health during pregnancy. Antibiotics, usually penicillin if not contraindicated by allergy, are used during pregnancy to prevent recurrent bouts of rheumatic fever and subsequent heart valve damage. Antibiotics are also recommended during labor and the early postpartum period to prevent bacterial endocarditis in women with either acquired or congenital disease. If the woman develops coagulation problems, the anticoagulant heparin may be used. Heparin is safest for the fetus because it does not cross the placenta. The thiazide diuretics and furosemide (Lasix) may be used to treat congestive heart failure if it develops. Digitalis glycosides and common antiarrhythmic drugs may be used to treat cardiac failure and arrhythmias. These agents cross the placenta but have no reported teratogenic effect.

Labor and Birth

Spontaneous natural labor with adequate pain relief is usually recommended for women in classes I and II. Special attention should be given to the prompt recognition and treatment of any signs of heart failure. Those in classes III and IV may have labor induced and may need to be hospitalized before the onset of labor for cardiac stabilization. They also require invasive cardiac monitoring during labor.

Use of low forceps provides the safest method of birth, with lumbar epidural anesthesia to reduce the stress of pushing. Cesarean birth is used only if fetal or maternal indications exist, not on the basis of heart disease alone.

Nursing Management

Nursing Assessment and Diagnosis

Assess the stress of pregnancy on the heart's functioning during every antepartal visit. Note the category of functional capacity assigned to the woman; take the woman's pulse, respirations, and blood pressure; and compare the findings with the normal values expected during pregnancy. Then determine the woman's activity level, including rest, and any changes in the pulse and respirations since previous visits. At every prenatal visit, ask the woman about any increased fatigue with activity because fatigue is an early sign of decompensation. Identify and evaluate other factors that would increase strain on the heart. These factors might include anemia, infection, anxiety, lack of a support system, and household and career demands.

The following signs and symptoms, if they are progressive, indicate congestive heart failure:

▶ Cough (frequent, with or without blood-stained sputum [hemoptysis])

▶ Dyspnea (progressive, on exertion)

▶ Edema (progressive, generalized, including extremities, face, eyelids)

▶ Heart murmurs (heard on auscultation)

▶ Palpitations

▶ Rales (auscultated in lung bases)

▶ Weight gain (related to fluid retention)

Progressiveness of the cycle is the critical factor because some of these same signs and symptoms are seen to a minor degree in a pregnancy without cardiac problems.

Nursing diagnoses that might apply to the pregnant woman with heart disease include the following:

▶ *Decreased cardiac output:* easy fatigability

▶ *Impaired gas exchange* related to pulmonary edema secondary to cardiac decompensation

▶ *Fear* related to the effects of the maternal cardiac condition on fetal well-being

Planning and Implementation

Nursing care is directed toward maintaining a balance between cardiac reserve and cardiac workload.

NURSING CARE IN THE COMMUNITY

Antepartal Nursing Care

The priority of nursing action varies based on the severity of the disease process and the individual needs of the woman determined by the nursing assessment. Ensure that the woman and her family thoroughly understand her condition and its management and that they recognize signs of potential complications; this level of understanding will decrease their anxiety. Providing thorough explanations, using printed material, and giving frequent opportunities to ask questions and discuss concerns lets the woman better meet her own health care needs and seek assistance appropriately.

As part of health teaching, explain the purposes of the required dietary and activity changes. A diet high in iron, protein, and essential nutrients but low in sodium, with adequate calories to ensure normal weight gain best meets the nutrition needs of the woman with cardiac disease. To help preserve her cardiac reserves, the woman may need to restrict her activities. In addition, 8 to 10 hours of sleep, with frequent daily rest periods, are essential. Because upper respiratory infections may tax the heart and lead to decompensation, the woman must avoid contact with sources of infection.

During the first half of pregnancy, the woman is seen approximately every 2 weeks to assess cardiac status. During the second half of pregnancy, the woman is seen weekly. These assessments are especially important between weeks 28 and 30, when the blood volume reaches its maximum. If symptoms of cardiac decompensation occur, prompt medical intervention is indicated to correct the cardiac problem.

HOSPITAL-BASED NURSING CARE

Intrapartum Period

Labor and birth exert tremendous stress on the woman and her fetus. This stress could be fatal to the fetus of a woman with cardiac disease, because the fetus may be receiving a decreased oxygen and blood supply. Thus the intrapartal care of a woman with cardiac disease is aimed at reducing physical exertion and the accompanying fatigue.

Evaluate maternal vital signs frequently to determine the woman's response to labor. A pulse rate greater than 100 beats per minute or respirations greater than 25 per minute may indicate the onset of cardiac decompensation and require further evaluation. Also auscultate the woman's lungs frequently for evidence of rales and carefully observe for other signs that she is developing decompensation.

To ensure cardiac emptying and adequate oxygenation, encourage the laboring woman to assume either a semi-Fowler's or side-lying position, with her head and shoulders elevated. Oxygen by mask, diuretics to reduce fluid retention, sedatives and analgesics, prophylactic antibiotics, and digitalis may also be used as indicated by the woman's status. Remain with the woman to support her. It is essential to keep the woman and her family informed of labor progress and management plans, collaborating with them to fulfill their wishes for the birth experience as much as possible. Maintain an atmosphere of calm to lessen the anxiety of the woman and her family.

Continuous electronic fetal monitoring provides ongoing assessment of the fetal response to labor. To prevent overexertion and the accompanying fatigue, encourage the woman to sleep and relax between contractions and give her emotional support and encouragement. Epidural anesthesia is often used to decrease exertion. During pushing, encourage the woman to use shorter, more moderate open-glottis pushing, with complete relaxation between pushes. Forceps or vacuum extraction may be used if pushing is too difficult. Monitor vital signs closely during the second stage.

Postpartum Period

The postpartum period is a significant time for the woman with cardiac disease. As extravascular fluid returns to the bloodstream for excretion, cardiac output and blood volume increase. This physiologic adaptation places great strain on the heart and may lead to decompensation, especially in the first 48 hours after birth.

To detect any possible problems, the woman remains in the hospital for about a week to rest and recover. Monitor her vital signs frequently, and assess for signs of decompensation. She stays in the semi-Fowler's or side-lying position, with her head and shoulders elevated, and begins a gradual, progressive activity program. Appropriate diet and stool softeners facilitate bowel movement without undue strain.

Give the woman opportunities to discuss her birth experience and help her deal with any feelings or concerns that distress her. Encourage maternal-infant attachment by providing frequent opportunities for the mother to interact with her child.

No evidence exists that breastfeeding stresses the heart. Thus the only concern about breastfeeding for women with cardiovascular disease is related to medications the mother may be taking (Friedman & Polifka, 1996). These should be evaluated for the likelihood of passing into the milk or affecting lactation. Assist the breastfeeding mother to a comfortable side-lying position, with her head moderately elevated, or to a semi-Fowler's position. To conserve the mother's energy, position the newborn at the breast and be available to burp the baby and reposition him or her at the other breast.

In addition to providing the normal postpartum discharge teaching, ensure that the woman and her family understand the signs of possible problems from her heart disease or other postpartal complications. Work with the woman and her family to plan an activity schedule. Visiting nurse referrals may be necessary, depending on the woman's health status.

Evaluation

Expected outcomes of nursing care include the following:

▶ The woman participates in developing an appropriate health care regimen and follows it throughout her pregnancy.

▶ The woman gives birth to a healthy infant.

▶ The woman avoids congestive heart failure, thromboembolism, and infection.

▶ The woman is able to identify signs and symptoms of possible postpartum complications.

▶ The woman is able to care effectively for her newborn infant.

OTHER MEDICAL CONDITIONS AND PREGNANCY

A woman with a preexisting medical condition needs to be aware of the possible impact of pregnancy on her condition, as well as the impact of her condition on the successful outcome of her pregnancy. Table 12–5 discusses some less common medical conditions in relation to pregnancy.

TABLE 12–5 Less Common Medical Conditions and Pregnancy			
Condition	Brief Description	Maternal Implications	Fetal/Neonatal Implications
Rheumatoid arthritis	Chronic inflammatory disease believed to be caused by a genetically influenced antigen-antibody reaction. Symptoms include fatigue, low-grade fever, pain and swelling of joints, morning stiffness, pain on movement. Treated with salicylates, physical therapy, and rest. Corticosteroids used cautiously if not responsive to above.	Usually there is remission of rheumatoid arthritis symptoms during pregnancy, often with a relapse postpartum. Anemia may be present due to blood loss from salicylate therapy. Mother needs extra rest, particularly to relieve weight-bearing joints, but needs to continue range-of-motion exercises. If in remission, may stop medication during pregnancy.	Possibility of prolonged gestation and longer labor with heavy salicylate use. Possible teratogenic effects of salicylates.
Epilepsy	Chronic disorder characterized by seizures; may be idiopathic or secondary to other conditions, such as head injury, metabolic and nutritional disorders such as phenylketonuria (PKU) or vitamin B_6 deficiency, encephalitis, neoplasms, or circulatory interferences. Treated with anticonvulsants.	Vast majority of pregnancies in women with seizure disorders are uneventful and have an excellent outcome. Women with more frequent seizures before pregnancy may have exacerbations during pregnancy, but this may be related to lack of cooperation with drug regimen or sleep deprivation. During pregnancy the woman should continue to be treated with the medication that best controls her seizures. Folic acid therapy should be started prior to conception if possible. Folic acid and vitamin D are indicated throughout pregnancy (Samuels, 1996b).	There is an increased incidence of stillbirth in women with epilepsy. Also, anticonvulsant medications are associated with an increased incidence of congenital anomalies, especially cleft lip and heart defects, although the incidence has decreased in recent years. This may be due to the fact that the current ability to determine blood levels of medications has led to more accurate dosages and the resultant use of a single medication; consequently multiple medications are used less often (Samuels, 1996b).

(continued)

TABLE 12–5 Less Common Medical Conditions and Pregnancy—continued

Condition	Brief Description	Maternal Implications	Fetal/Neonatal Implications
Hepatitis B	Hepatitis B, caused by the hepatitis B virus (HBV), is a major, growing health problem. Groups at risk include those from areas with a high incidence (primarily developing countries), illegal intravenous (IV) drug users, prostitutes, homosexuals, those with multiple sex partners, or occupational exposure to blood, although many infected people have no identifiable source of infection. HBV transmission is blood borne, primarily sexually and perinatally transmitted. Because of the dramatic increase and the difficulty of vaccinating high-risk individuals before they become infected, the CDC now recommend (1) testing all pregnant women for the presence of hepatitis B surface antigen (HBsAg), (2) routine vaccination of all newborns, (3) vaccination of older children at high risk for hepatitis B, (4) vaccination of children ages 11–12 years who have not previously received the vaccine, and (5) vaccination of adolescents and adults at high risk for infection (CDC, 1998).	Hepatitis B does not usually affect the course of pregnancy. However, chronic HBV carriers have a great potential for infecting others when exposure to blood and body fluids occurs. In addition, chronic carriers may develop long-term sequelae, such as chronic liver disease and liver cancer. Approximately 4,000 to 5,000 deaths are caused annually by liver disease associated with chronic HBV infection. It is now recommended that all pregnant women be tested for the presence of HBsAg. A woman who tests negative may be given the hepatitis vaccine.	Perinatal transmission most often occurs at or near the time of childbirth. Infants infected perinatally have a 90% risk of becoming chronically infected if not treated (CDC, 1998). Recommendations now include routine vaccination of all neonates born to HBsAg-negative women and immunoprophylaxis to all newborns of HBsAg-positive women.
Hyperthyroidism (thyrotoxicosis)	Enlarged, overactive thyroid gland; increased T4: thyroid-binding globulin (TBG) ratio and increased basal metabolic rate (BMR). Symptoms include muscle wasting, tachycardia, excessive sweating, and exophthalmos. Treatment by antithyroid drug propylthiouracil (PTU) while monitoring free T4 levels. Surgery used only if drug intolerance exists.	Mild hyperthyroidism is not dangerous. Increased incidence of PIH and postpartum hemorrhage if not well controlled. Serious risk related to thyroid storm characterized by high fever, tachycardia, sweating, and congestive heart failure. Now occurs rarely. When diagnosed during pregnancy, may be transient or permanent.	Neonatal thyrotoxicosis is rare. Even low doses of antithyroid drug in mother may produce a mild fetal/neonatal hypothyroidism; higher dose may produce a goiter or mental deficiencies. Fetal loss not increased in euthyroid women. If untreated, rates of abortion, intrauterine death, and stillbirth increase. Breastfeeding contraindicated for women on antithyroid medication because it is excreted in the milk (may be tried by woman on low dose if neonatal T4 levels are monitored).
Hypothyroidism	Characterized by inadequate thyroid secretions (decreased T4:TBG ratio), elevated thyroid-stimulating hormone, lowered BMR, and enlarged thyroid gland (goiter). Symptoms include lack of energy, excessive weight gain, cold intolerance, dry skin, and constipation. Treated by thyroxine replacement therapy.	Long-term replacement therapy usually continues at same dosage during pregnancy as before. Weekly nonstress test (NST) after 35 weeks' gestation.	If mother untreated, fetal loss 50%; high risk of congenital goiter or true cretinism. Therefore newborns are screened for T4 level. Children of mothers with even mild deficiency may show evidence of negative impact on neuropsychologic development (Haddow, Palomaki, Allan, et al., 1999).
Maternal phenylketonuria (PKU) (hyperphenylalaninemia)	Inherited recessive single gene anomaly causing a deficiency of the liver enzyme needed to convert the amino acid phenylalanine to tyrosine, resulting in high serum levels of phenylalanine. Brain damage and mental retardation occur if not treated early.	Low phenylalanine diet is mandatory before conception and during pregnancy. The woman should be counseled that her children will either inherit the disease or be carriers, depending on the zygosity of the father for the disease. Treatment at a PKU center is recommended.	Risk to fetus if maternal treatment is not begun preconception. In untreated women increased incidence of fetal mental retardation, microcephaly, congenital heart defects, and growth retardation. Fetal phenylalanine levels are approximately 50% higher than maternal levels.
Multiple sclerosis	Neurologic disorder characterized by destruction of the myelin sheath of nerve fibers. The condition occurs primarily in young adults, more commonly in females, and is marked by periods of remission; progresses to marked physical disability in 10 to 20 years.	Associated with remission during pregnancy but with slightly increased relapse rate postpartum (Confavreux, Hutchinson, Hours, et al., 1998). Rest is important; help with child care should be planned. Uterine contraction strength is not diminished, but because sensation is frequently lessened, labor may be almost painless.	Increased evidence of a genetic predisposition. Therefore, reproductive counseling is recommended.

TABLE 12-5 Less Common Medical Conditions and Pregnancy—continued

Condition	Brief Description	Maternal Implications	Fetal/Neonatal Implications
Systemic lupus erythematosus (SLE)	Chronic autoimmune collagen disease, characterized by exacerbations and remissions; symptoms range from characteristic rash to inflammation and pain in joints, fever, nephritis, depression, cranial nerve disorders, and peripheral neuropathies.	Women are generally advised that SLE should be in remission for at least 5–7 months before conceiving. Pregnancy does not appear to alter the long-term prognosis of women with SLE, but maternal morbidity and mortality increase. They also face an increased risk of permanent renal or central nervous system (CNS) deterioration after pregnancy (Classen, Paulson, & Zacharias, 1998). Most maternal deaths occur in the postpartal period and are caused by pulmonary hemorrhage or lupus pneumonitis (Samuels, 1996a).	Increased incidence of spontaneous abortion, stillbirth, prematurity, and IUGR. Infants born to women with SLE may have characteristic skin rash, which usually disappears after 6 months. Infants are at increased risk for complete congenital heart block, a condition that can be diagnosed prenatally. Women with SLE and certain antibodies are at risk. A fetal echocardiogram is done between 18 and 24 weeks of gestation and treatment is started if necessary (Reichlin, 1998).
Tuberculosis (TB)	Infection caused by *Mycobacterium tuberculosis;* inflammatory process causes destruction of lung tissue, increased sputum, and coughing. Associated primarily with poverty, crowded living spaces, and malnutrition and may be found among refugees from countries where TB is prevalent. Pregnant women with active TB are treated with triple therapy: isoniazid, rifampin, and ethambutol; breastfeeding women receive the three drugs plus pyrazinamide in a four-agent therapy (Newton, 2000).	The incidence of TB has begun to increase significantly since the late 1980s, and it is increasingly associated with HIV infection (Newton, 2000). If TB is inactive due to prior treatment, relapse rate is no greater than for nonpregnant women. When isoniazid is used during pregnancy, the woman should take supplemental pyridoxine (vitamin B_6). Extra rest and limited contact with others is required until disease becomes inactive.	If maternal TB is inactive, mother may breastfeed and care for her infant. If TB is active and mother is *not* receiving treatment at the time of birth, both mother and infant are treated. Some physicians advocate separating mother and infant for first week of therapy. Others feel the benefits do not outweigh the hardship of separation (Newton, 2000). Isoniazid crosses the placenta, but most studies show no teratogenic effects. Rifampin crosses the placenta; possibility of harmful effects are still being studied.

CHAPTER HIGHLIGHTS

∾ Almost any health problem that a person can have when not pregnant can coexist with pregnancy. Some problems, such as anemias, may be exacerbated by pregnancy. Others, such as collagen disease, may go into temporary remission with pregnancy. Regardless of the health problem, careful health care is needed throughout pregnancy to improve the outcome for mother and fetus.

∾ The diagnosis of high-risk pregnancy can shock an expectant couple. Providing emotional support, teaching about the condition and prognosis, and educating for self-care are important nursing measures that help clients cope.

∾ Substance abuse (either drugs or alcohol) not only is detrimental to the mother's health but also may have profound, lasting effects on the fetus. Nurses need to be alert to signs of substance abuse and nonjudgmental in their care of women with substance abuse problems.

∾ The key point in the care of the pregnant diabetic is scrupulous maternal plasma glucose control. This is best achieved by home blood glucose monitoring, multiple daily insulin injections, and a careful diet.

∾ To reduce the incidence of congenital anomalies and other problems in the newborn, the woman should maintain a normal blood glucose level before conception and throughout the pregnancy. Diabetics more than most other clients need to be educated about their condition and involved with their own care.

∾ HIV infection, which is transmitted via blood and body fluids, may also be transmitted vertically from the mother to the fetus. Currently there is no definitive treatment for HIV/AIDS.

∾ The risk of vertical transmission of HIV infection is reduced dramatically with the administration of ZDV to the mother prenatally and during labor and to the newborn. The risk can be reduced even further by scheduled cesarean birth before the onset of labor or rupture of the membranes.

∾ Nurses should use blood and body fluid precautions (universal precautions) in caring for all women to avoid potential spread of infection.

∾ Cardiac disease during pregnancy requires careful assessment, limitation of activity, and knowing and reporting signs of impending cardiac decompensation by both client and nurse.

EXPLOREMEDIALINK

NCLEX Review, Case Studies, and other interactive resources for this chapter can be found on the companion website at http://www.prenhall.com/london. Click on "Chapter 12" to select the activities for this chapter.

For animations, more NCLEX review questions, and an audio glossary, access the accompanying CD-ROM in this textbook.

REFERENCES

American College of Obstetricians and Gynecologists. (1997). *Human immunodeficiency virus infections in pregnancy* (ACOG Technical Bulletin No. 232). Washington, DC: Author.

American College of Obstetricians and Gynecologists. (1999). *Scheduled cesarean delivery and the prevention of vertical transmission of HIV infection* (ACOG Committee Opinion No. 219). Washington, DC: Author.

American Diabetes Association. (2000a). Position statement: Gestational diabetes mellitus. *Diabetes Care, 23* (Suppl. 1), S77–S79.

American Diabetes Association. (2000b). Position statement: Preconception care of women with diabetes. *Diabetes Care, 23* (Suppl. 1), S65–S68.

Andres, R. L. (1999). Social and illicit drug use in pregnancy. In R. K. Creasy & R. Resnik (Eds.), *Maternal-fetal medicine* (4th ed., pp. 145–164). Philadelphia: Saunders.

Catanzarite, V. A., Piacquadio, K. M., Stanco, L. M., Kollisch, N., Chinn, R., & Gardner, S. (1999). Preventing transmission of AIDS and hepatitis to obstetric-care workers. *Contemporary OB/GYN, 44*(8), 39–55.

Centers for Disease Control and Prevention. (1998). 1998 guidelines for the treatment of sexually transmitted disease. *Morbidity and Mortality Weekly Report, 47* (RR-1).

Centers for Disease Control and Prevention. (1999). *National Folic Acid Program of the National Center for Environmental Health* (NCEH Publication No. 99–0082). Atlanta, GA: Author.

Centers for Disease Control and Prevention. (2000). *HIV/AIDS Surveillance Report, 12*(1), 1–18.

Classen, S. R., Paulson, P. R., & Zacharias, S. R. (1998). Systemic lupus erythematosis: Perinatal and neonatal implications. *Journal of Obstetric, Gynecologic, and Neonatal Nursing, 27*(5), 493–500.

Confavreux, C., Hutchinson, M., Hours, M. M., Cortinovis-Tourniaire, P., & Moreau, T. (1998). Rate of pregnancy-related relapse in multiple sclerosis. *New England Journal of Medicine, 339*(5), 339–340.

Criteria Committee of the New York Heart Association. (1979). *Nomenclature and criteria for diagnosis of diseases of the heart and great vessels* (8th ed.). New York: New York Heart Association.

Curet, L. B. (2000). Obstetric management of diabetes mellitus in pregnancy. In J. J. Sciarra, (Ed.), *Maternal and fetal medicine* (Vol. 3, chap. 14, pp. 1–10).

Friedman, J. M., & Polifka, J. E. (1996). *The effects of drugs on the fetus and nursing infant.* Baltimore: Johns Hopkins University Press.

Haddow, J. E., Palomaki, G. E., Allan, W. C., Williams, J. R., Knight, G. J., Gagnon, J., et al.

(1999). Maternal thyroid deficiency during pregnancy and subsequent neuropsychological development of the child. *New England Journal of Medicine, 341*(8), 549–555, 601–602.

Hoffman-Terry, M. L. (1999, October). *Defining the epidemic in American women.* 1999 National Conference on Women and HIV/AIDS: Navigating into the New Millennium through Collaboration, Los Angeles.

Howell, E. M., Heiser, N., & Harrington, M. (1999). A review of recent findings on substance abuse treatment for pregnant women. *Journal of Substance Abuse Treatment, 16*(3), 195–219.

Institute of Medicine, Standing Committee on the Scientific Evaluation of Dietary Reference Intakes, Food and Nutrition Board. (1998, April 7). *Dietary reference intakes: Folate, other B vitamins, and choline.* Washington, DC: National Academy Press.

Jovanovic, L. (2000). Role of diet and insulin treatment of diabetes in pregnancy. *Clinical Obstetrics and Gynecology, 43*(1), 46–55.

Kearney, M. H. (1997). Drug treatment for women: Traditional models and new directions. *Journal of Obstetric, Gynecologic, and Neonatal Nursing, 26*(4), 459–468.

Kenner, C., & D'Apolito, K. (1997). Outcomes for children exposed to drugs in utero. *Journal of Obstetric, Gynecologic, and Neonatal Nursing, 26*(5), 595–603.

Kjos, S. L. (2000). Postpartum care of the woman with diabetes. *Clinical Obstetrics and Gynecology, 43*(1), 75–82.

Landon, M. B. (2000). Obstetric management of pregnancies complicated by diabetes mellitus. *Clinical Obstetrics and Gynecology, 43*(1), 65–74.

Levine, A. M. (2001, July). *Management of HIV-infected women and mother-to-child HIV transmission.* Paper presented at the First IAS Conference on HIV Pathogenesis and Treatment, Buenos Aires, Argentina.

Mandeville, L. K. (1992). Diabetes mellitus in pregnancy. In L. K. Mandeville & N. H. Troiano (Eds.), *High-risk intrapartum nursing.* (pp. 165–186). Philadelphia: Lippincott.

March of Dimes. (1999). *Folic acid.* Wilkes-Barre, PA: Author.

Mersereau, P. W. (2000). Preventing neural tube defects: A national campaign. *Small Talk, 12*(2), 1–5.

Minkoff, H. L. (1999). Human immunodeficiency virus and other perinatal infections. In J. R. Scott et al. (Eds.), *Danforth's obstetrics and gynecology* (8th ed., pp. 393–406). Philadelphia: Lippincott Williams & Wilkins.

Mofenson, L. M. (1999). Can perinatal HIV infection be eliminated in the United States? *Journal of the American Medical Association, 282*(6), 577–579.

Moore, T. R. (1999). Diabetes in pregnancy. In R. K. Creasy & R. Resnik (Eds.), *Maternal-fetal medicine* (4th ed., pp. 964–995). Philadelphia: Saunders.

Newton, E. R. (2000). Tuberculosis and pregnancy. In J. J. Sciarra (Ed.), *Maternal and fetal medicine* (Vol. 3, chap. 49, pp. 1–15).

Niebyl, J. R. (1999). Teratology and drugs in pregnancy. In J. R. Scott, P. J. DiSaia, C. B. Hammond, & W. N. Spellacy (Eds.), *Danforth's obstetrics and gynecology* (8th ed., pp. 197–212). Philadelphia: Lippincott Williams & Wilkins.

Reichlin, M. (1998). Systemic lupus erythematosis and pregnancy. *Journal of Reproductive Medicine, 43*(4), 355–360.

Samuels, P. (1996a). Collagen vascular diseases. In S. G. Gabbe, J. R. Niebyl, & J. L. Simpson (Eds.), *Obstetrics: Normal and problem pregnancies* (3rd ed., pp. 1101–1118). New York: Churchill-Livingstone.

Samuels, P. (1996b). Neurologic disorders. In S. G. Gabbe, J. R. Niebyl, & J. L. Simpson (Eds.), *Obstetrics: Normal and problem pregnancies* (3rd ed., pp. 1135–1154). New York: Churchill-Livingstone.

Scioscia, A. L. (1999). Prenatal genetic diagnosis. In R. K. Creasy & R. Resnik (Eds.), *Maternal-fetal medicine* (4th ed., pp. 918–926). Philadelphia: Saunders.

Shabetai, R. (1999). Cardiac diseases. In R. K. Creasy & R. Resnik (Eds.), *Maternal-fetal medicine* (4th ed., pp. 927–941). Philadelphia: Saunders.

Sheffield, J. S., & Cunningham, F. G. (1999). Diagnosing and managing cardiomyopathy. *Contemporary OB/GYN, 44,* 74–78.

Sinclair, B. P. (1999–2000). HIV and women: Understand your responsibilities; reduce your risk. *AWHONN Lifelines, 3*(6), 35–38.

Spellacy, W. N. (1999). Diabetes mellitus and pregnancy. In J. R. Scott, P. J. DiSaia, C. B. Hammond, & W. N. Spellacy (Eds.), *Danforth's obstetrics and gynecology* (8th ed., pp. 301–308). Philadelphia: Lippincott Williams & Wilkins.

Wang, E. C. (1999). Methadone treatment during pregnancy. *Journal of Obstetric, Gynecologic, and Neonatal Nursing, 28*(6), 615–622.

Wenstrom, K. D., & Malee, M. P. (1999). Medical and surgical complications of pregnancy. In J. R. Scott, P. J. DiSaia, C. B. Hammond, & W. N. Spellacy (Eds.), *Danforth's obstetrics and gynecology* (8th ed., pp. 327–362). Philadelphia: Lippincott Williams & Wilkins.

CHAPTER 13

Pregnancy at Risk: Gestational Onset

When we decided to have children we were so excited, so ready. I never expected that I would have two miscarriages. I can't tell you how hard that was to handle. Even today, with two healthy children, I remember the pain, the loss, the sense of failure, and I grieve for the children we will never know.

—JASMINE, 36

Key Terms

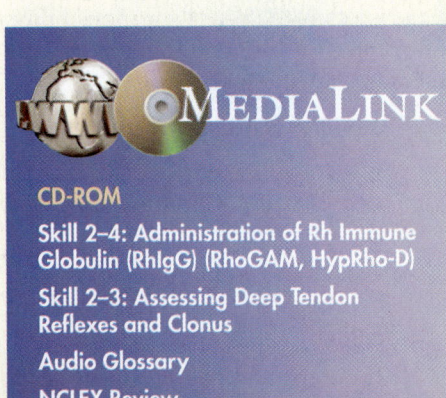

MediaLink

CD-ROM

Skill 2–4: Administration of Rh Immune Globulin (RhIgG) (RhoGAM, HypRho-D)

Skill 2–3: Assessing Deep Tendon Reflexes and Clonus

Audio Glossary

NCLEX Review

COMPANION WEBSITE

http://www.prenhall.com/london

Pregestational Problems—Web Links

Thinking Critically

NCLEX Review

Case Study

*I*n some pregnancies, problems arise that place the woman and her unborn child at risk. Regular prenatal care helps detect these complications quickly so that effective care can be provided. This chapter focuses on problems that develop during pregnancy, those with a gestational onset.

CARE OF THE WOMAN WITH A BLEEDING DISORDER

During the first and second trimesters, the major cause of bleeding is **abortion.** This is the expulsion of the fetus prior to viability, which is considered to be 20 weeks' gestation or weight of less than 500 g (Cunningham, Gant, Leveno et al., 2001). Abortions are either *spontaneous* (occurring naturally) or *induced* (occurring as a result of medical or surgical means). Because the term *abortion* may have a negative connotation, spontaneous abortion is often called **miscarriage.**

Other complications that can cause bleeding in the first half of pregnancy are ectopic pregnancy and gestational trophoblastic disease, discussed shortly. In the second half of pregnancy, particularly in the third trimester, the two major causes of bleeding are placenta previa and abruptio placentae. (See Chapter 19.) 🔗 Regardless of the cause of bleeding, the nurse has certain general responsibilities in providing nursing care.

General Principles of Nursing Intervention

Spotting is relatively common during pregnancy and usually occurs following sexual intercourse or exercise because of trauma to the highly vascular cervix. However, the woman is advised to have an evaluation of any spotting or bleeding that occurs during pregnancy.

It is often the nurse's responsibility to make the initial assessment of bleeding. In general, the following nursing measures are indicated:

- Monitor blood pressure and pulse frequently.
- Observe the woman for behaviors indicative of shock, such as pallor, clammy skin, perspiration, dyspnea, or restlessness.
- Count and weigh pads to assess amount of bleeding over a given time period; save any tissue or clots expelled.
- If pregnancy is of 12 weeks' gestation or beyond, assess fetal heart tones with a Doppler.
- Prepare for intravenous (IV) therapy. There may be standing orders to begin IV therapy on bleeding clients.
- Prepare equipment for examination and have oxygen available.
- Collect and organize all data, including antepartal history, onset of bleeding episode, and laboratory studies (hemoglobin, hematocrit, hormonal assays) for analysis.
- Notify other members of the health care team including the physician or nurse-midwife, operating room staff if a surgical procedure is planned, and so forth.
- Obtain an order to type and crossmatch for blood if evidence of significant blood loss exists.
- Assess coping mechanisms of the woman in crisis. Give emotional support to enhance her coping abilities by continuous, sustained presence; by clear explanation of procedures; and by communicating her status to her family. Prepare the woman for possible fetal loss. Assess her expressions of anger, denial, silence, guilt, depression, or self-blame.

CARE OF THE WOMAN HAVING A MISCARRIAGE (SPONTANEOUS ABORTION)

Many pregnancies end in the first trimester because of spontaneous abortion. The incidence is about 20% for clinically recognized pregnancies but may be much higher (Lyon, 2000). A woman may assume she is having a heavy period when she is really having an early miscarriage.

A majority of early miscarriages are related to chromosomal abnormalities. Other causes include teratogenic drugs, faulty implantation due to abnormalities of the female reproductive tract, a weakened cervix, placental abnormalities, chronic maternal diseases, endocrine imbalances, and maternal infections. Research does not support the belief that accidents and psychic trauma are primary causes of spontaneous abortion.

Spontaneous abortion can be extremely distressing to the couple desiring a child. Chances for carrying the next pregnancy to term after one miscarriage are as good as they are for the general population. Thereafter, however, chances of successful pregnancy decrease with each succeeding miscarriage.

Classification

Spontaneous abortions, or miscarriages, are subdivided into the following categories:

- *Threatened abortion.* The embryo or fetus is jeopardized by unexplained bleeding, cramping, and backache. The cervix is closed. Bleeding may persist for days. It may be followed by partial or complete expulsion of the embryo or fetus, placenta, and membranes (sometimes called the "products of conception") (Figure 13–1 ◆).
- *Imminent abortion.* Bleeding and cramping increase. The internal cervical os dilates. Membranes may rupture. The term *inevitable abortion* also applies.

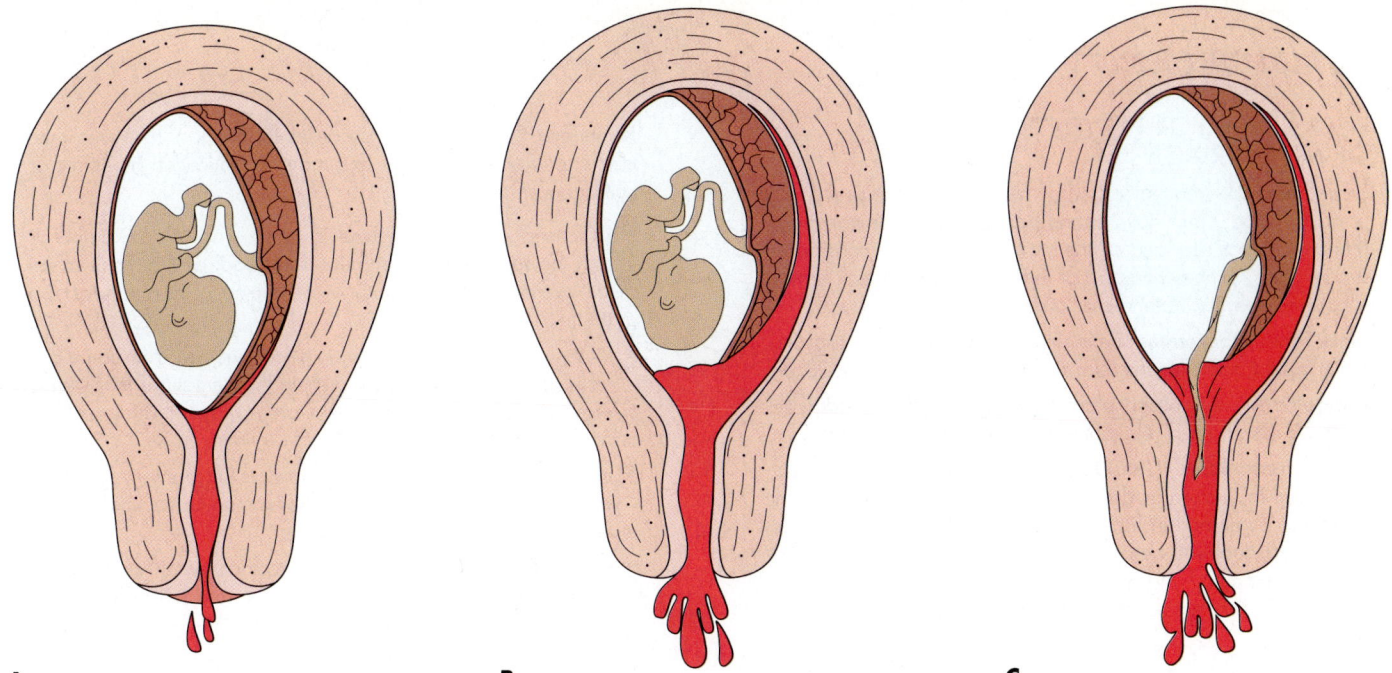

FIGURE 13–1. ◆ Types of spontaneous abortion. **A,** Threatened. The cervix is not dilated, and the placenta is still attached to the uterine wall, but some bleeding occurs. **B,** Imminent. The placenta has separated from the uterine wall, the cervix has dilated, and the amount of bleeding has increased. **C,** Incomplete. The embryo or fetus has passed out of the uterus, but the placenta remains.

- *Complete abortion.* All the products of conception are expelled.
- *Incomplete abortion.* Some of the products of conception are retained, most often the placenta. The internal cervical os is dilated slightly.
- *Missed abortion.* The fetus dies in utero but is not expelled. Uterine growth ceases, breast changes regress, and the woman may report a brownish vaginal discharge. The cervix is closed. If the fetus is retained beyond 6 weeks, the breakdown of fetal tissues results in the release of thromboplastin, and disseminated intravascular coagulation (DIC) may develop.
- *Recurrent (habitual) abortion.* Abortion occurs consecutively in three or more pregnancies.
- *Septic abortion.* Infection is present. It may occur with prolonged, unrecognized rupture of the membranes, pregnancy with an intrauterine device (IUD) in place, or attempts by unqualified individuals to end a pregnancy.

Clinical Therapy

One of the more reliable indicators of potential spontaneous abortion is the presence of pelvic cramping and backache. These symptoms are usually absent in bleeding caused by polyps, ruptured cervical blood vessels, or cervical erosion. Ultrasound scanning may be used to detect the presence of a gestational sac or fetal heartbeat if the cause of bleeding is unclear. Results of human chorionic go-

nadotropin (hCG) levels are not particularly helpful because hCG levels fall slowly after fetal death and therefore cannot confirm a live embryo or fetus. Hemoglobin and hematocrit are obtained to assess blood loss. Blood is typed and crossmatched for possible replacement needs.

The therapy prescribed for the pregnant woman with bleeding is bed rest, abstinence from sex, and perhaps sedation. If bleeding persists and abortion is imminent or incomplete, the woman may be hospitalized, IV therapy or blood transfusions may be started to replace fluid, and dilatation and curettage (D&C) or suction evacuation is performed to remove the remainder of the products of conception. If the woman is Rh negative and not sensitized, Rh immune globulin (RhoGAM) is given within 72 hours (see discussion on Rh sensitization later in this chapter).

In missed abortions, the products of conception usually are expelled spontaneously, usually within about 2 weeks. Diagnosis is based on history, pelvic examination, and a negative pregnancy test and may be confirmed by ultrasound if necessary. Because of the psychologic stress of carrying a dead fetus and the risk of DIC, treatment is indicated once the diagnosis is made (Cunningham, et al., 2001). A D & C or suction evacuation is done if the pregnancy is in the first trimester. In the second trimester, labor is induced or dilatation and evacuation (D&E) may be used.

For recurrent miscarriage, the American College of Obstetricians and Gynecologists (ACOG) recommends testing the woman for certain antibodies that can cause her body to reject a pregnancy and testing the couple for genetic abnormalities (ACOG, 2001).

Nursing Management

Nursing Assessment and Diagnosis

Assess the woman's vital signs, amount and appearance of any bleeding, level of comfort, and general physical health. If the pregnancy is 10 to 12 weeks or more, determine fetal heart rates with a Doppler. It is also important to assess the responses of the woman and her family to this crisis, their coping mechanisms, and their ability to comfort each other.

Examples of nursing diagnoses that may apply include the following:

▶ *Pain* related to abdominal cramping secondary to threatened abortion

▶ *Anticipatory grieving* related to expected loss of unborn child

Planning and Implementation

NURSING CARE IN THE COMMUNITY

If a woman in her first trimester of pregnancy begins cramping or spotting, she is often evaluated on an outpatient basis. Provide analgesics for pain relief if the woman's cramps are severe, and explain what is occurring throughout the process.

Feelings of shock or disbelief are normal. Couples who approached the pregnancy with joy and excitement now feel grief, sadness, and possibly anger. Because many women, even with planned pregnancies, feel some ambivalence initially, guilt is also a common emotion. These feelings may be even stronger for women who were negative about their pregnancies. The women may even believe that the miscarriage is a punishment for some wrongdoing.

Offer psychologic support to the woman and her family by encouraging them to talk about their feelings, allowing them the privacy to grieve, and listening sympathetically to their concerns about this pregnancy and future ones. To help decrease feelings of guilt or blame, inform the woman and her family about the causes of miscarriage. Refer them to other health care professionals for additional help as necessary. The grieving period following a miscarriage usually lasts 6 to 24 months. Many couples can be helped during this period by an organization or support group established for parents who have lost a fetus or newborn.

HOSPITAL-BASED NURSING CARE

A woman with an incomplete or missed abortion may need a D&C or other procedure, which is typically done on an outpatient basis. Barring any complications, the woman can return home a few hours after the procedure. Monitor the woman's condition closely and provide instruction for self-care. Administer Rh immune globulin if it is indicated.

Evaluation

Expected outcomes of nursing care include the following:

▶ The woman is able to explain spontaneous abortion, the treatment measures employed in her care, and long-term implications for future pregnancies.

▶ The woman suffers no complications.

▶ The woman and her partner begin verbalizing their grief and acknowledge that the grieving process lasts several months.

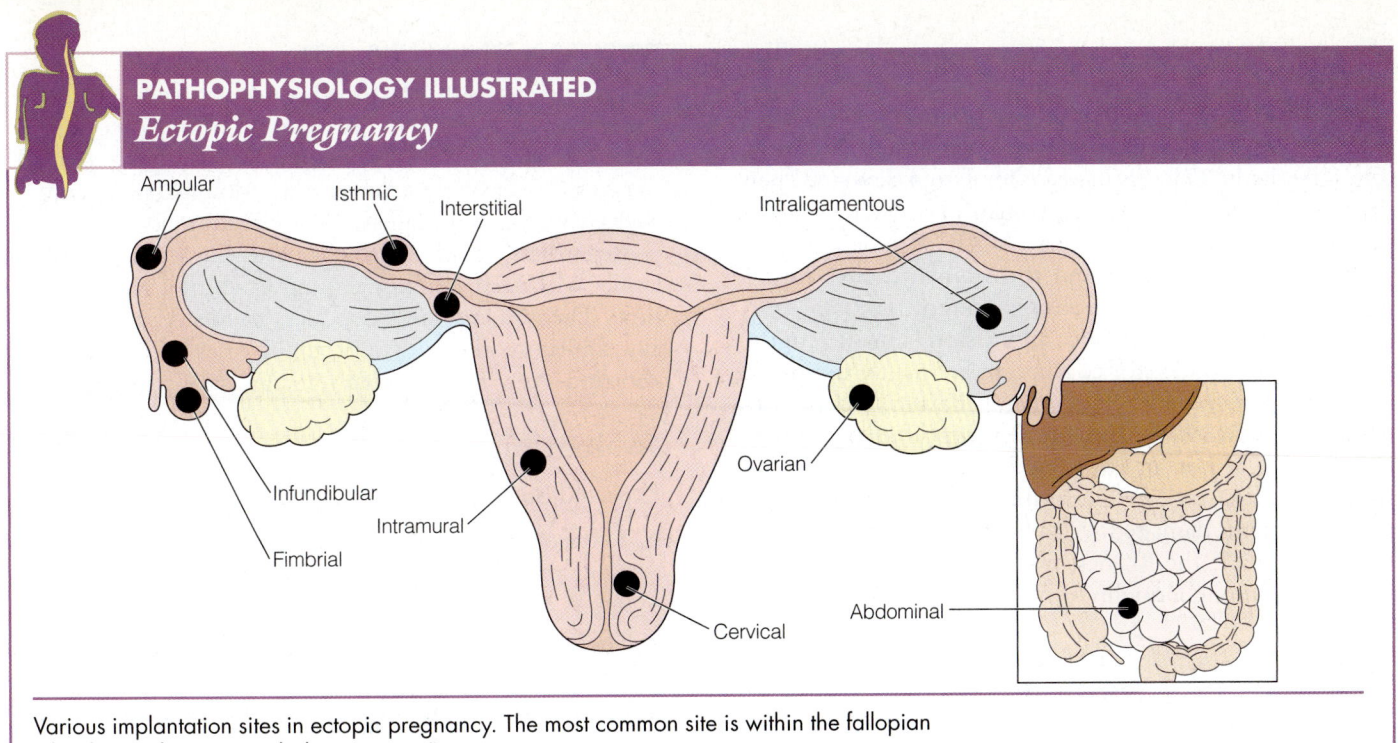

PATHOPHYSIOLOGY ILLUSTRATED
Ectopic Pregnancy

Various implantation sites in ectopic pregnancy. The most common site is within the fallopian tube, hence the name "tubal pregnancy."

CARE OF THE WOMAN WITH AN ECTOPIC PREGNANCY

Ectopic pregnancy (EP) is the implantation of the fertilized ovum in a site other than the endometrial lining of the uterus. It has many causes including tubal damage from pelvic inflammatory disease (PID), previous tubal surgery, congenital anomalies of the tube, endometriosis, previous EP, presence of an IUD, and in utero exposure to diethylstilbestrol (DES).

The incidence of EP has increased in the past several years. Currently 1% to 2% of all pregnancies are ectopic (Lyon, 2000). EP occurs when the fertilized ovum is prevented or slowed in its passage through the tube and thus implants before it reaches the uterus. The most common location for implantation is the ampulla of the fallopian tube. "Pathophysiology Illustrated: Ectopic Pregnancy" identifies other implantation sites.

Initially symptoms of pregnancy may be present, including amenorrhea, breast tenderness, and nausea. The hormone hCG is present in the blood and urine. As the pregnancy progresses, the chorionic villi grow into the wall of the tube or site of implantation and a blood supply is established. When the embryo outgrows this space, the tube ruptures and there is bleeding into the abdominal cavity. This bleeding irritates the peritoneum, causing the characteristic symptoms of sharp, one-sided pain, syncope, and referred shoulder pain. The woman may also have lower abdominal pain. Vaginal bleeding occurs when the embryo dies and the decidua begins to slough.

Physical examination usually reveals adnexal tenderness. (The *adnexae* are the areas of the lower abdomen located over each ovary and fallopian tube.) An adnexal mass is palpable about half the time. Bleeding tends to be slow and chronic, and the abdomen gradually becomes rigid and very tender. With bleeding into the abdominal cavity, pelvic examination is very painful, and a mass of blood may be palpated in the lower abdomen. Laboratory tests may reveal low hemoglobin and hematocrit levels and rising leukocyte levels. The hCG titers are lower than in regular pregnancy.

Clinical Therapy

Diagnosis of EP begins with an assessment of menstrual history, including the date of the last menstrual period, followed by a pelvic exam to identify any pelvic masses and tenderness. Serum β-hCG levels are drawn and reassessed in 48 hours if necessary. A woman with EP tends to have abnormally low hCG levels. Moreover, in normal pregnancy, hCG levels double every 48 to 72 hours. Nondoubling hCG levels occur in EP. If the β-hCG levels are above 1500 IU/L, transvaginal ultrasound is used to check for a uterine pregnancy or an adnexal mass. Confirming a uterine pregnancy nearly eliminates the diagnosis of EP (Tulandi, 1999).

Treatment may be medical or surgical. Methotrexate is used for the woman who desires future pregnancy if her ectopic pregnancy is unruptured and of 3.5 cm size or less and if her condition is stable. In addition, there must be no fetal heart motion and the woman must have no evidence of a blood disorder or kidney or liver disease. The methotrexate is given intramuscularly (IM). As an outpatient, the woman is monitored for increasing abdominal pain. Serum β-hCG titers are also monitored regularly. Typically the hCG levels increase for 1 to 4 days and then decrease. If they do not, the woman may need a second dose of methotrexate or surgery (ACOG, 1998a).

If surgery is indicated and the woman desires future pregnancies, treatment involves salpingostomy via a laparoscope. With this method, an incision is made lengthwise and the products of conception are gently removed. The surgical incision is left open and allowed to close naturally (Tulandi, 1999). If the tube is ruptured or if future childbearing is not an issue, laparoscopic salpingectomy (removal of the tube) is performed, leaving the ovary in place unless it is damaged. With both medical and surgical therapies for EP, the Rh-negative nonsensitized woman is given Rh immune globulin to prevent sensitization.

Nursing Management

Nursing Assessment and Diagnosis

When the woman with a suspected ectopic pregnancy is admitted to the hospital, it is important to assess the appearance and amount of vaginal bleeding and to monitor vital signs for signs of developing shock. Assess the woman's emotional state and coping abilities and determine the couple's informational needs. The woman may experience marked abdominal discomfort, so determine her level of pain. If surgery is necessary, complete the appropriate ongoing assessments postoperatively.

Nursing diagnoses that may apply for a woman with EP include the following:

▶ *Pain* related to abdominal bleeding secondary to tubal rupture

▶ *Health-seeking behaviors:* request for information about treatment of ectopic pregnancy and its long-term implications related to stated unfamiliarity with the condition

Planning and Implementation

NURSING CARE IN THE COMMUNITY

Women with EP are often seen initially in a clinic or office setting. Be alert to the possibility of EP if a woman presents with complaints of abdominal pain and lack of menses for 1 to 2 months. If a woman is to receive medical treatment using methotrexate, she is followed as an outpatient. Advise the woman that some abdominal pain is common following the injection, but generally it is mild and lasts only 24 to 48 hours. More severe pain might indicate treatment failure and should be evaluated. The woman should also report heavy vaginal bleeding, dizziness, or tachycardia (ACOG, 1998a). Stress the need to return for follow-up hCG testing.

HOSPITAL-BASED NURSING CARE

Once a diagnosis of EP is made and surgery is scheduled, the nurse starts an IV as ordered and begins preoperative teaching. Immediately report signs of developing shock. If the woman is experiencing severe abdominal pain, administer analgesics and evaluate their effectiveness.

Regardless of the treatment used, the woman and her family will need emotional support during this difficult time. Their feelings and responses to this crisis are generally similar to those that occur in cases of spontaneous abortion. As a result, similar nursing actions are required.

Evaluation

Expected outcomes of nursing care include the following:

▶ The woman is able to explain ectopic pregnancy, treatment alternatives, and implications for future childbearing.

▶ The woman and her caregivers detect possible complications early and manage them successfully.

▶ The woman and her partner are able to begin verbalizing their loss.

CARE OF THE WOMAN WITH GESTATIONAL TROPHOBLASTIC DISEASE

Gestational trophoblastic disease (GTD) includes hydatidiform mole, invasive mole (chorioadenoma destruens), and choriocarcinoma, a form of cancer.

Hydatidiform mole (molar pregnancy) is a disease in which (1) abnormal development of the placenta occurs, resulting in a fluid-filled, grapelike cluster; and (2) the trophoblastic tissue proliferates. The disease results in the loss of the pregnancy and the possibility, though remote, of developing choriocarcinoma, a form of cancer, from the trophoblastic tissue.

Hydatidiform mole is found in about 1 in 1000 pregnancies (Cunningham et al., 2001). Molar pregnancies are classified into two types, complete and partial, both of which meet the previously mentioned criteria. A complete mole develops from an ovum containing no maternal genetic material, an "empty egg," which is fertilized by a normal sperm. The embryo dies very early, no circulation is established, the hydropic vesicles are avascular, and no embryonic tissue is found. Choriocarcinoma seems to be associated exclusively with the complete mole.

The partial mole usually has a triploid karyotype (69 chromosomes), generally because of failure of either the ovum or sperm to undergo the first meiotic division. There may be a fetal sac or even a fetus with a heartbeat. The fetus has multiple anomalies and little chance for survival. Often partial moles are recognized only after miscarriage, and they may go unnoticed even then.

Invasive mole (chorioadenoma destruens) is similar to a complete mole, but it involves the uterine myometrium. Treatment is the same as for complete mole.

Clinical Therapy

Initially the clinical picture is similar to that of pregnancy. However, classic signs soon appear. Vaginal bleeding occurs almost universally. It is often brownish (like prune juice) due to liquefaction of the uterine clot, but it may be bright red. Uterine enlargement greater than expected for gestational age is a classic sign, present in about 50% of cases. In the remainder of cases, the uterus is appropriate or small for the gestational age. Hydropic vesicles may be passed; if so, they are diagnostic. With a partial mole the vesicles are often smaller and may not be noticed. In addition, because serum hCG levels are higher with molar pregnancy than with normal pregnancy, the woman may experience hyperemesis gravidarum. Anemia occurs frequently due to blood loss and poor nutrition secondary to hyperemesis. Symptoms of preeclampsia prior to 24 weeks' gestation strongly suggest a molar pregnancy. No fetal heart tones are heard, and no fetal movement is palpated. Transvaginal ultrasound is used for diagnosis.

Therapy begins with suction evacuation of the mole and curettage of the uterus to remove all fragments of the placenta. Early evacuation decreases the possibility of other complications. If the woman is older and has completed her childbearing, or if there is excessive bleeding, hysterectomy may be the treatment of choice to reduce the risk of choriocarcinoma.

Because of the risk of choriocarcinoma, the woman treated for hydatidiform mole should receive extensive follow-up therapy, typically for a year. Follow-up care includes baseline chest x-ray exam to detect metastasis, physical exam including pelvic exam, and regular measurements of hCG levels. The woman should avoid pregnancy during that time because the elevated hCG levels associated with pregnancy would cause confusion about whether cancer had developed.

Continued high or rising hCG titers are abnormal. If they occur, a D&C is performed, and the tissue is examined. If cancer cells are found, treatment at a center specializing in GTD is advised. Chemotherapy is started using methotrexate alone or with other chemotherapy agents. If, after a year of monitoring, the hCG serum titers are within normal limits, a couple may be assured that a normal pregnancy can be anticipated, with a low risk of recurring hydatidiform mole.

Nursing Management

Nursing Assessment and Diagnosis

It is important to observe for symptoms of hydatidiform mole at each antepartal visit. The classic symptoms are found more frequently with the complete mole. Before evacuation, the partial mole may be difficult to distinguish from a missed abortion. If a molar pregnancy is diagnosed, assess the woman's (or the couple's) understanding of the condition and its implications.

Nursing diagnoses that may apply include the following:

▶ *Fear* related to the possible development of choriocarcinoma

▶ *Anticipatory grieving* related to the loss of the pregnancy secondary to GTD

Planning and Implementation

NURSING CARE IN THE COMMUNITY

When a molar pregnancy is suspected, the woman needs emotional support. Answer questions about the condition and explain what ultrasound and other diagnostic procedures will entail. If a molar pregnancy is diagnosed, support the parents as they deal with their grief about the lost pregnancy. Health care counselors, a member of the clergy, or a professional counselor may also be of help.

HOSPITAL-BASED NURSING CARE

When the woman is hospitalized for removal of the mole, monitor vital signs and vaginal bleeding for signs of hemorrhage. Also determine whether abdominal pain is present and evaluate the woman's emotional state and coping ability. Have typed and crossmatched blood available for surgery. Administer oxytocin as ordered to keep the uterus contracted and to prevent hemorrhage. If the woman is Rh negative and not sensitized, give Rh immune globulin to prevent antibody formation.

Help ensure that the woman understands the importance of the follow-up visits. She is advised to delay becoming pregnant again until after the follow-up program is completed.

Evaluation

Expected outcomes of nursing care include the following:

▶ The woman has a smooth recovery following successful evacuation of the mole.

▶ The woman is able to explain GTD and its treatment, follow-up, and long-term implications for pregnancy.

▶ The woman and her partner are able to begin talking about their grief at the loss of their anticipated child.

▶ The woman can discuss the importance of follow-up care and indicates her willingness to cooperate with the regimen.

CARE OF THE WOMAN WITH AN INCOMPETENT CERVIX

Incompetent cervix refers to the premature dilatation of the cervix, usually in the fourth or fifth month of pregnancy. It is associated with repeated second trimester abortions.

Possible causes include cervical trauma, infection, congenital cervical or uterine anomalies, or increased uterine volume (as with a multiple gestation).

Diagnosis is based on a positive history of repeated, relatively painless and bloodless second trimester abortions. Serial pelvic exams early in the second trimester reveal progressive effacement and dilatation of the cervix and bulging of the membranes through the cervical os. If incompetent cervix is suspected, serial ultrasound provides information on dilatation of the internal cervical os before a dilated external os is detected.

Incompetent cervix is managed surgically with a Shirodkar procedure (cerclage)—or a modification of it by McDonald—which reinforces the weakened cervix by encircling it at the level of the internal os with suture material. A purse-string suture is placed in the cervix in the first trimester or early in the second trimester. Once the suture is in place, a cesarean birth may be planned (to prevent repeating the procedure in subsequent pregnancies), or the suture may be cut at term and vaginal birth permitted. The woman must understand the importance of contacting her physician immediately if her membranes rupture or labor begins. The physician can remove the suture to prevent possible complications.

CARE OF THE WOMAN WITH HYPEREMESIS GRAVIDARUM

Hyperemesis gravidarum, a relatively rare condition, is excessive vomiting during pregnancy. It may be mild at first, but true hyperemesis may progress to a point at which the woman not only vomits everything she swallows but also retches between meals.

Although the exact cause of hyperemesis is unclear, increased levels of hCG may play a role. Other variables under investigation include a possible dysfunction of the pituitary-adrenal axis, an increase in thyroid function, and psychologic factors (Wenstrom & Malee, 1999).

In severe cases, hyperemesis causes dehydration, which leads to fluid-electrolyte imbalance and alkalosis from loss of hydrochloric acid. Hypovolemia, hypotension, tachycardia, increased hematocrit and blood urea nitrogen (BUN), and decreased urine output can also occur. If untreated, metabolic acidosis may develop. Severe potassium loss may disrupt cardiac functioning. Starvation causes muscle wasting and severe protein and vitamin deficiencies. Fetal or embryonic death may result, and the woman may suffer irreversible metabolic changes or death.

Clinical Therapy

The goals of treatment include control of vomiting and dehydration, restoration of electrolyte balance, and maintenance of adequate nutrition. Some women require hospitalization. For the first 24 to 48 hours, the woman is given nothing by mouth, and IV fluids are administered.

Potassium chloride is often added to the IV to prevent hypokalemia. The nausea and vomiting are treated with drugs such as the phenothiazines (prochlorperazine, chlorpromazine, promethazine) and antihistamines such as meclizine and dimenhydrinate. If her condition does not improve, total parenteral nutrition may be needed. She then begins controlled oral feedings.

Nursing Management

Nursing Assessment and Diagnosis

When a woman is hospitalized for control of vomiting, assess the amount and character of any emesis, intake and output, fetal heart rate, signs of jaundice or bleeding, and her emotional state.

Nursing diagnoses that may apply include the following:

▶ *Altered nutrition: less than body requirements* related to persistent vomiting secondary to hyperemesis

▶ *Fear* related to the effects of hyperemesis on fetal well-being

Planning and Implementation

NURSING CARE IN THE COMMUNITY

Parenteral therapy provided at home in collaboration with a physician and a registered dietitian is sometimes used to enable the woman to remain in her home. This therapy also gives an opportunity to observe family interactions and evaluate the home environment. This assessment helps determine the pregnant woman's level of support, any significant stressors in her life, and her understanding of nutrition and self-care measures.

HOSPITAL-BASED NURSING CARE

Nursing care is supportive and directed at maintaining a relaxed, quiet environment away from food odors or offensive smells. Once oral feedings resume, food needs to be attractively served. Oral hygiene is important because the mouth is dry and may be irritated from vomitus. Monitor weight regularly. Because emotional factors have been found to play a major role in this condition, psychotherapy may be recommended. With proper treatment, prognosis is favorable.

Evaluation

Expected outcomes of nursing care include the following:

▶ The woman is able to explain hyperemesis gravidarum, its therapy, and its possible effects on her pregnancy.

▶ The woman's condition is corrected and complications are avoided.

CARE OF THE WOMAN WITH PREMATURE RUPTURE OF MEMBRANES

Premature rupture of membranes (PROM) is spontaneous rupture of the membranes and leakage of amniotic fluid prior to the onset of labor. Preterm PROM (pPROM) is the rupture of membranes that occurs before 37 weeks' gestation and is found in 1% to 2% of pregnancies (Weitz, 2001). PROM is associated with infection, previous history of PROM, hydramnios, multiple pregnancy, urinary tract infection, amniocentesis, placenta previa, abruptio placentae, trauma, incompetent cervix, bleeding during pregnancy, and maternal genital tract anomalies.

Maternal risk of infection is increased as is the risk of cesarean birth. Fetal-newborn implications include risk of respiratory distress syndrome (with pPROM), fetal sepsis due to ascending pathogens, malpresentation, prolapse of the umbilical cord, and increased perinatal morbidity and mortality.

Clinical Therapy

A sterile speculum examination is done to detect the presence of amniotic fluid in the vagina. If fluid is not obviously pooling, the diagnosis can be confirmed with nitrazine paper (which turns deep blue) and a microscopic examination (ferning test). Digital examination increases the risk of infection and is not recommended unless prompt birth is expected (ACOG, 1998c).

Fetal well-being is assessed through a fetal heart rate tracing or biophysical profile. In addition, the gestational age of the fetus is calculated. The gestational age of the fetus and the presence or absence of infection determine the direction of treatment for PROM. If maternal signs of infection are evident, antibiotic therapy (usually by IV infusion) is started immediately, and the fetus is born vaginally or by cesarean regardless of the gestational age. Prophylactic antibiotics are often administered for the first 48 hours while awaiting culture results. Upon admission to the nursery, the newborn is assessed for sepsis and placed on antibiotics. (Chapter 26 provides further information about the newborn with sepsis.) ⊂⊃

Management of PROM in the absence of infection and gestation of less than 37 weeks is usually conservative. The woman is hospitalized on bed rest. On admission, complete blood cell count (CBC), C-reactive protein, and urinalysis are obtained. Continuous electronic fetal monitoring may be ordered at the beginning of treatment but usually is discontinued after a few hours, unless the fetus is estimated to be very low birth weight. Regular nonstress tests (NSTs) or biophysical profiles are used to monitor fetal well-being. (These tests are discussed in Chapter 14. ⊂⊃) Maternal blood pressure, pulse, and temperature and fetal heart rate (FHR) are assessed every 4 hours. Regular laboratory evaluations are done to detect maternal infection. Vaginal exams are avoided to decrease the chance

of infection. As the gestation approaches 34 weeks, fetal lung maturity studies are indicated (American Academy of Pediatrics & ACOG, 1997).

Although controversial, after initial treatment and observation, if leaking of fluid ceases, some women (typically those with sufficient amniotic fluid, no infection, and cervical dilatation less than 4 cm) may be followed at home. The woman is advised to continue bed rest (with bathroom privileges), monitor her temperature and pulse four times a day, keep a fetal movement chart, and have regular NSTs (Parsons & Spellacy, 1999a).

Corticosteroid administration to promote fetal lung maturity and prevent respiratory distress syndrome remains controversial because of possible harmful effects on the fetus and mother. Currently a single course of corticosteroid treatment (typically 12 mg betamethasone IM every 24 hours for two doses or 6 mg dexamethasone IM every 12 hours for four doses [Weitz, 2001]) is recommended for women with PROM between 24 and 34 weeks of gestation, if there is no intra-amniotic infection. At this point, however, experts have determined that there is not sufficient evidence to recommend the routine use of repeat courses of antenatal corticosteroids (Cerrato, 2001). (See "Drug Guide: Betamethasone".)

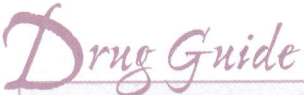

Drug Guide

BETAMETHASONE (CELESTONE SOLUSPAN)
Pregnancy Risk Category: C

Overview of Maternal-Fetal Action
Studies have provided ample evidence that glucocorticoids such as betamethasone are capable of inducing pulmonary maturation and decreasing the incidence of respiratory distress syndrome in preterm infants. The mechanism by which corticosteroids accelerate fetal lung maturity is unclear, but it is related to the stimulation of enzyme activity by the drug. The enzyme is required for biosynthesis of surfactant by the type II pneumocytes. Surfactant is essential to the proper functioning of the lung in that it decreases the surface tension of the alveoli. Glucocorticoids also increase the rate of glycogen depletion, which leads to thinning of the interalveolar septa and increases the size of the alveoli. The thinning of the epithelium brings the capillaries into closer proximity with the air spaces and improves oxygen exchange.

Route, Dosage, Frequency
Prenatal maternal IM injections of 12 mg of betamethasone are given once a day for 2 days. Dexamethasone may also be given in doses of 6 mg every 6 hours for four doses (Guinn & Lee, 2000). To obtain maximum results, birth should be delayed for at least 24 hours after completing the first round of treatment. The effect of corticosteroids may be transient. Currently, it is suggested by some that the treatment regimen be repeated every week up to 34 weeks' gestation for the undelivered fetus with an immature lung profile, but this approach is controversial (Guinn & Lee, 2000).

(continued)

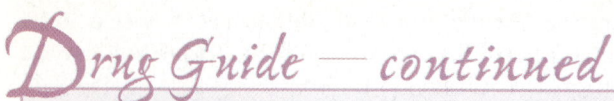

Drug Guide — continued

Contraindications

Inability to delay birth

Adequate lecithin-sphingomyelin (L/S) ratio

Presence of a condition that necessitates immediate birth (e.g., maternal bleeding)

Presence of maternal infection, diabetes mellitus, hypertension

Gestational age greater than 34 completed weeks

Maternal Side Effects

Increased risk for infection has not been supported in large studies. There may, however, be some increase in the incidence of infection in women with premature rupture of the membranes. Maternal hyperglycemia may occur during corticosteroid administration. Insulin-dependent diabetics may require insulin infusions for several days to prevent ketoacidosis. Corticosteroids may increase the risk of pulmonary edema, especially when used concurrently with tocolytics (Iams, 1996a; National Institutes of Health, 1994).

Effects on Fetus or Neonate

Lowered cortisol levels at birth, but rebound occurs by 2 hours of age

Hypoglycemia

Increased risk of neonatal sepsis

Animal studies have shown serious fetal side effects such as reduced head circumference, reduced weight of the fetal adrenal and thymus glands, and decreased placental weight. Human studies have not shown these effects, however.

Nursing Considerations

Assess for presence of contraindications.

Provide education regarding possible side effects.

Administer betamethasone deep into gluteal muscle, avoiding injection into deltoid (high incidence of local atrophy). (Dexamethasone may be administered IM or IV.)

Periodically evaluate blood pressure, pulse, weight, and edema.

Assess lab data for electrolytes and blood glucose level.

Although concomitant use of betamethasone and tocolytic agents has been implicated in increased risk of pulmonary edema, the betamethasone has little mineral corticoid activity; therefore, it probably does not add significantly to the salt and water retention effects of β-adrenergic agonists. Other causes of noncardiogenic pulmonary edema should also be investigated if pulmonary edema develops during administration of betamethasone to a woman in preterm labor.

Nursing Management

Nursing Assessment and Diagnosis

Determining the length of time the membranes have been ruptured is a major part of the intrapartal assessment. Ask the woman when her membranes ruptured and when labor began, because the risk of infection may be directly related to the time involved. Observe the mother for signs and symptoms of infection by reviewing her white blood cell count, temperature, pulse rate, and the character of her amniotic fluid. Check her hydration status. When a preterm or cesarean birth is anticipated, evaluate the childbirth preparation and coping abilities of the woman and her partner.

Nursing diagnoses that may apply to a woman with PROM include the following:

- ▶ *Risk for infection* related to premature rupture of membranes
- ▶ *Impaired gas exchange* in the fetus related to compression of the umbilical cord secondary to prolapse of the cord
- ▶ *Risk for ineffective individual coping* related to unknown outcome of the pregnancy

Planning and Implementation

Nursing actions should focus on the woman, her partner, and the fetus. Report signs of infection to the certified nurse-midwife or physician. Evaluate uterine activity and fetal response to the labor but do not do vaginal exams unless absolutely necessary. Encourage the woman to rest on her left side to promote optimal uteroplacental perfusion. Use comfort measures to help her rest and relax. Ensure that the woman is well hydrated, particularly if her temperature is elevated.

Education is another important aspect of nursing care. The woman and her partner, if he is involved, need to understand the implications of PROM and all treatment methods. It is important to address side effects and alternative treatments. The couple needs to know that although the membranes are ruptured, amniotic fluid continues to be produced.

Providing psychologic support for the couple is critical. Listen empathetically, relay accurate information, and provide explanations as needed. Preparing the couple for a cesarean birth, a preterm newborn, and the possibility of fetal or newborn demise may be necessary.

Evaluation

Expected outcomes of nursing care include the following:

- ▶ The woman's risk of infection and cord prolapse decrease.
- ▶ The couple is able to discuss the implications of PROM and all treatments and alternative treatments.
- ▶ The pregnancy is maintained without trauma to the mother or fetus.

CARE OF THE WOMAN AT RISK DUE TO PRETERM LABOR

Labor that occurs between 20 and 37 completed weeks of pregnancy is called **preterm labor.** Prematurity continues to be the number one perinatal and neonatal problem in the United States, with 11% of all live births occurring prematurely (Creasy & Iams, 1999). Often preterm labor is related to multiple risk factors. Risk factors can be classified as follows (Aerts & Iams, 1999):

- *Nonrecurrent risk factors:* placenta previa, abruptio placentae, hydramnios, second-trimester bleeding, fetal anomaly or death
- *Recurrent or treatable factors in the mother:* genital tract infection, incompetent cervix, uterine malformations, uterine fibroids, low socioeconomic status, limited prenatal care, poor nutritional status, low prepregnancy weight, tobacco or drug use, occupation or work requirement, sexual activity, anemia
- *Recurrent but not treatable:* history of preterm birth, race, DES exposure

Maternal implications of preterm labor include psychologic stress related to the baby's condition and physiologic stress related to medical treatment for preterm labor. Fetal-neonatal implications include increased morbidity and mortality, especially due to respiratory distress syndrome, increased risk of trauma during birth, and maturational deficiencies (fat storage, heat regulation, immaturity of organ systems).

Clinical Therapy

Women at risk for preterm labor are taught to recognize the symptoms associated with it and, if any symptoms are present, to notify their certified nurse-midwife or physician immediately. Prompt diagnosis is necessary to stop preterm labor before it progresses to the point at which intervention will be ineffective.

Three tests are useful both in screening high-risk women and in helping confirm a diagnosis of preterm labor:

- *Fetal fibronectin (fFN).* Fetal fibronectin is a protein normally found in the fetal membranes and decidua. It is found in the cervicovaginal fluid in early pregnancy but is not usually present in significant quantities between 18 and 36 weeks' gestation. A positive fFN test (fFN found in the cervicovaginal fluid) during this time puts the woman at increased risk for preterm birth. Conversely, a negative test is over 99% accurate for predicting no preterm birth within 7 days. The procedure for collecting a sample is similar to that of the Pap smear; results can be available within 1 hour (Chez, 1999).
- *Salivary estriol.* Research indicates that maternal estriol levels rise about 3 weeks before birth, either preterm or term. Estriol can be measured in the maternal blood or saliva, although saliva is preferred because it is a stable method and no venipuncture is necessary. Salivary estriol levels are most reliable in predicting preterm birth after 30 weeks' gestation. The saliva sample should be collected during the day (estriol levels are elevated at night) but not within 30 minutes of eating (Chez, 1999).

- *Transvaginal ultrasound (sonography).* The length of the cervix can be measured fairly reliably after 16 weeks' gestation using an ultrasound probe inserted into the vagina. A cervix that is shorter than expected may be useful in assisting a physician to identify the need for a cerclage to prevent preterm birth because of incompetent cervix. In general, cervical length less than 25 mm prior to term is abnormal (Aerts & Iams, 1999).

Diagnosis of preterm labor is confirmed if the pregnancy is between 20 and 37 weeks, and if there are documented uterine contractions (four in 20 minutes or six to eight in 1 hour), documented cervical change of 1 cm or more, cervical dilatation of more than 2 cm, or a positive fFN level (Creasy & Iams, 1999).

The goal of clinical therapy is to prevent the preterm birth of a compromised infant. Attempts to prevent labor are *not* indicated if one or more of the following conditions are present: severe preeclampsia or eclampsia, chorioamnionitis, hemorrhage, maternal cardiac disease, poorly controlled diabetes mellitus or thyrotoxicosis, severe abruptio placentae, fetal anomalies incompatible with life, fetal death, acute fetal distress, or fetal maturity.

The initial management of preterm labor is directed toward maintaining good uterine blood flow, detecting uterine contractions, and quieting the fetus. The mother is asked to lie on her side to increase profusion, and an IV infusion is started to promote maternal hydration.

Tocolysis is the use of medications in an attempt to stop labor. Drugs currently used as tocolytics include the β-adrenergic agonists (also called β-mimetics), magnesium sulfate ($MgSO_4$), prostaglandin synthetase inhibitors, and calcium channel blockers. The β-mimetics (ritodrine [Yutopar] and terbutaline sulfate [Brethine]) and $MgSO_4$ are the most widely used tocolytics. Ritodrine is approved by the U.S. Food and Drug Administration (FDA) for tocolysis; however, it is much less frequently used than terbutaline, which is not approved by the FDA for this use.

Although tocolytic drugs suppress uterine contractions and allow pregnancy to continue, they may cause maternal side effects; the most serious is maternal pulmonary edema. Reducing the dose and duration of therapy sometimes reduces the side effects.

Because it is effective and has fewer side effects than the β-mimetics, $MgSO_4$ administered IV is often the initial drug of choice for therapy. Therapy with $MgSO_4$ is indicated in women with cardiopulmonary disease, diabetes, or infection. In all other cases, the selection of $MgSO_4$ or β-mimetics depends on the experience of the health care providers. Oral tocolytics are not effective in preventing preterm labor (Cunningham et al., 2001).

For $MgSO_4$, the recommended loading dose is 4 to 6 g IV using an infusion pump over 20 minutes, followed by a maintenance dose of 1 to 4 g/hr titrated to response and side effects (Creasy & Iams, 1999). The therapy is continued for 12 to 24 hours at the lowest rate that maintains cessation of contractions.

Side effects with the loading dose may include flushing, a feeling of warmth, headache, nystagmus, nausea, and dizziness. Other side effects include lethargy, sluggishness, and pulmonary edema (see "Drug Guide: Magnesium Sulfate"). Fetal side effects may include hypotonia and lethargy that persists for 1 or 2 days following birth.

One calcium channel blocker, nifedipine, is becoming increasingly popular as a tocolytic because it is easily administered orally or sublingually and has few serious maternal side effects. It decreases smooth muscle contractions by blocking the slow calcium channels at the cell surface. The most common side effects are related to arterial vasodi-

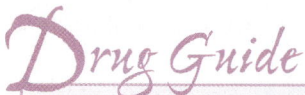

Drug Guide

MAGNESIUM SULFATE (MgSO₄)
Pregnancy Risk Category: B

Overview of Obstetric Action

$MgSO_4$ acts as a central nervous system depressant by decreasing the quantity of acetylcholine released by motor nerve impulses and thereby blocking neuromuscular transmission. This action reduces the possibility of convulsion, which is why $MgSO_4$ is used in the treatment of preeclampsia. Because magnesium sulfate secondarily relaxes smooth muscle, it may decrease the blood pressure, although it is not considered an antihypertensive. $MgSO_4$ may also decrease the frequency and intensity of uterine contractions; as a result it is also used as a tocolytic in the treatment of preterm labor.

Route, Dosage, Frequency

$MgSO_4$ is generally given IV to control dosage more accurately and prevent overdosage. An occasional physician still prescribes IM administration. However, it is painful and irritating to the tissues and does not permit the close control that IV administration does. The IV route allows for immediate onset of action. It must be given by infusion pump for accurate dosage.

For Treatment of Preterm Labor

Loading dose: 4 to 6 g $MgSO_4$ in 250-mL solution administered over a 20-minute period

Maintenance dose: 1 to 4 g/hr via infusion pump (Creasy & Iams, 1999)

For Treatment of Preeclampsia

Loading dose: 2 to 4 g $MgSO_4$ administered over a 5-minute period

Maintenance dose: 1 g/hr via infusion pump (Roberts, 1999)

Note: $MgSO_4$ is excreted via the kidneys. Because women in preterm labor typically have normal renal function, they generally require higher levels of magnesium to achieve a therapeutic range than women who have preeclampsia and may have compromised renal function. Maintenance dose may need to be adjusted based on serum magnesium levels.

Maternal Contraindications

Diagnosed maternal myasthenia gravis is the only absolute contraindication to the administration of $MgSO_4$. A history of myocardial damage or heart block is a relative contraindication to use of the drug because of the effects on nerve transmission and muscle contractility. Extreme care is necessary in administration to women with impaired renal function because the drug is eliminated by the kidneys, and toxic magnesium levels may develop quickly.

Maternal Side Effects

Most maternal side effects are dose related. Lethargy and weakness related to neuromuscular blockade are common. Sweating, a feeling of warmth, flushing, and nasal congestion may be related to peripheral vasodilation. Other common side effects include nausea and vomiting, constipation, visual blurring, headache, and slurred speech. Signs of developing toxicity include depression or absence of reflexes, oliguria, confusion, respiratory depression, circulatory collapse, and respiratory paralysis. Rapid administration of large doses may cause cardiac arrest.

Effects on Fetus or Neonate

The drug readily crosses the placenta. Some authorities suggest that transient decrease in fetal heart rate variability may occur; others report that no change occurred. In general, $MgSO_4$ therapy does not pose a risk to the fetus. Occasionally, the newborn may demonstrate neurologic depression or respiratory depression, loss of reflexes, and muscle weakness. Ill effects in the newborn may actually be related to fetal growth retardation, prematurity, or perinatal asphyxia.

Nursing Considerations

1. Monitor the blood pressure closely during administration.
2. Monitor maternal serum magnesium levels as ordered (usually every 6 to 8 hours). Therapeutic levels are in the range of 4.8 to 9.6 mg/dL. Reflexes often disappear at serum magnesium levels of 8 to 12 mg/dL; respiratory depression occurs at levels of 15 to 17 mg/dL; cardiac arrest occurs at levels above 30 mg/dL (Sibai, 1996; Silver, 1996).
3. Monitor respirations closely. If the rate is less than 12/min, magnesium toxicity may be developing, and further assessments are indicated. Many protocols require stopping the medication if the respiratory rate falls below 12/min.
4. Assess knee jerk (patellar tendon reflex) for evidence of diminished or absent reflexes. Loss of reflexes is often the first sign of developing toxicity. Also note marked lethargy or decreased level of consciousness and hypotension.
5. Determine urinary output. Output less than 30 mL/hr may result in the accumulation of toxic levels of magnesium.
6. If the respirations or urinary output fall below specified levels or if the reflexes are diminished or absent, no further magnesium should be administered until these factors return to normal.
7. The antagonist of $MgSO_4$ is calcium. Consequently, an ampule of calcium gluconate should be available at the bedside. The usual dose is 1 g given IV over a period of about 3 minutes.
8. Monitor fetal heart tones continuously with IV administration.
9. Continue $MgSO_4$ infusion for approximately 24 hours after birth as prophylaxis against postpartum seizures if given for preeclampsia-eclampsia.
10. If the mother has received $MgSO_4$ close to birth, the newborn should be closely observed for signs of magnesium toxicity for 24 to 48 hours.

Note: Protocols for $MgSO_4$ administration may vary somewhat according to agency policy. Consequently, individuals are referred to their own agency protocols for specific guidelines.

lation and include hypotension, tachycardia, facial flushing, and headache. Nifedipine may be coadministered with the β-mimetics. However, it should not be used with magnesium because both drugs block calcium, and simultaneous administration has been implicated in serious maternal side effects related to low calcium levels.

Prostaglandin synthesis inhibitors such as indomethacin (Indocin) are being used for tocolysis in selected instances. However, potential fetal side effects, such as constriction of the ductus arteriosus, have been reported, especially in pregnancies at 32 weeks' gestation and beyond. Consequently, indomethacin use is limited to pregnancies < 32 weeks' gestation; the duration of therapy should be < 72 hours, if possible (Vermillion & Scardo, 2000).

As in the treatment of pPROM, in treating preterm labor, a single course of antenatal corticosteroids using betamethasone or dexamethasone appears to help fetal lung maturation. However, the routine use of repeated courses of antenatal corticosteroids is not recommended (Cerrato, 2001). (See "Drug Guide: Betamethasone.")

Nursing Management

Nursing Assessment and Diagnosis

During the antepartal period, identify the woman at risk for preterm labor by noting the presence of predisposing factors. During the intrapartal period, assess the progress of labor and the physiologic impact of labor on the mother and fetus.

Nursing diagnoses that may apply to the woman with preterm labor include the following:

▶ *Fear* related to risk of early labor and birth
▶ *Ineffective individual coping* related to need for constant attention to pregnancy

Planning and Implementation

NURSING CARE IN THE COMMUNITY

Once the woman at risk for preterm labor has been identified, she needs to be taught about the importance of recognizing the onset of labor (see "Teaching About: Preterm Labor").

Periodic home visits by a home care nurse are an important part of care. During these visits the nurse completes physical assessments similar to those done in the hospital and assesses the woman's emotional state. The nurse can also provide information about support groups and other community resources for women at risk for preterm birth.

Increasing the woman's awareness of the subtle symptoms of preterm labor is an important teaching objective. The signs and symptoms of preterm labor include the following:

▶ Uterine contractions that occur every 10 minutes or less, with or without pain
▶ Mild menstrual-like cramps felt low in the abdomen

Teaching About

PRETERM LABOR
- Describe the dangers of preterm labor, especially the risk of prematurity in the infant, and all the potential problems.
- Explain that many of the early symptoms of labor, such as backache and increased bloody show, may be subtle initially.
- Summarize self-care measures (see Table 13–1) the woman can take to prevent preterm labor.
- Teach the woman how to palpate for uterine contractions. Demonstrate and ask for a return demonstration.

▶ Pelvic pressure that feels like the baby pressing down
▶ Rupture of membranes
▶ Constant or intermittent low, dull backache
▶ A change in the vaginal discharge (an increase in amount, a change to more clear and watery, or a pinkish tinge)
▶ Abdominal cramping with or without diarrhea

Also teach the woman to evaluate contraction activity once or twice a day. She does so by lying down tilted to one side with a pillow behind her back for support. The woman places her fingertips on the fundus of the uterus, which is above the umbilicus (navel). She checks for contractions (hardening or tightening in the uterus) for about 1 hour. It is important for the pregnant woman to know that uterine contractions occur occasionally throughout the pregnancy. If they occur every 10 minutes for 1 hour, however, the cervix could begin to dilate, and labor could begin.

Ensure that the woman knows when to report signs and symptoms. If contractions occur every 10 minutes (or more frequently) for 1 hour, if any of the other signs and symptoms are present for 1 hour, or if clear fluid begins leaking from the vagina, the woman should telephone her physician or certified nurse-midwife and make arrangements to be checked for ongoing labor. When a woman is at risk for preterm labor, she may have many episodes of contractions and other signs or symptoms. Thus the woman's call must be taken seriously. If she is treated positively, she will feel freer to report problems as they arise.

Preventive self-care measures are also very important. They are described in Table 13–1.

HOSPITAL-BASED NURSING CARE

Supportive nursing care is important to the woman in preterm labor during hospitalization. It is important to promote bed rest, monitor vital signs, measure intake and output, monitor the fetal heart rate continuously, and monitor uterine contractions. Having the woman lie on her left side facilitates maternal-fetal circulation. Keep vaginal examinations to a minimum. If tocolytic agents are being administered, monitor the mother and fetus closely for any adverse effects.

TABLE 13–1 Self-Care Measures to Prevent Preterm Labor

Rest two or three times a day lying on your left side.

Drink 2 to 3 quarts of water or fruit juice each day. Avoid caffeine drinks. Filling a quart container and drinking from it will eliminate the need to keep track of numerous glasses of fluid.

Empty your bladder at least every 2 hours during waking hours.

Avoid lifting heavy objects. If small children are in the home, work out alternatives for picking them up, such as sitting on a chair and having them climb onto your lap.

Contact your healthcare provider if you experience menstrual-like cramping, unusual low back pain, unusual vaginal discharge, increased pelvic pressure, or more than 5 uterine contractions in 1 hour (whether painful or not).

Pace necessary activities to avoid overexertion.

Sexual activity may need to be modified or avoided.

Try to focus on 1 day or 1 week at a time rather than on longer periods of time.

If on bed rest, get dressed each day and rest on a couch rather than becoming isolated in the bedroom.

Find pleasurable ways to help compensate for limitations of activities and boost the spirits.

Note: Prepared in consultation with Adele Grant, RN, Coordinator of the Prematurity Prevention Program, University of Washington Medical Center.

Whether preterm labor is arrested or proceeds, the woman and her partner, if he is involved, experience intense psychologic stress. Provide emotional support to help decrease the anxiety associated with the risk of a preterm newborn. Also recognize the stress of prolonged bed rest and of lack of sexual contact and help the couple find satisfactory ways of dealing with those stresses. With empathetic communication, it is possible to assist the couple to express their feelings, which commonly include guilt and anxiety, and identify and implement coping mechanisms. Keep the couple informed about the labor progress, the treatment regimen, and the status of the fetus. In the event of imminent vaginal or cesarean birth, offer the couple brief but ongoing explanations to prepare them for the actual birth process and the events following the birth.

Evaluation

Expected outcomes of nursing care include the following:

▶ The woman is able to discuss the cause, identification, and treatment of preterm labor.

▶ The woman states that she feels comfortable in her ability to cope with her situation and has resources to call on.

▶ The woman can describe appropriate self-care measures and can identify characteristics that need to be reported to her caregiver.

▶ The woman successfully gives birth to a healthy infant.

CARE OF THE WOMAN WITH A HYPERTENSIVE DISORDER

A number of hypertensive disorders can occur during pregnancy. Hypertension is defined as a blood pressure of 140/90 or greater. The working group of the National High Blood Pressure Education Program (2000) recommends the following classification of hypertensive disorders:

- Gestational hypertension
- Preeclampsia
- Eclampsia
- Chronic hypertension
- Preeclampsia superimposed on chronic hypertension

Preeclampsia and Eclampsia

Preeclampsia, the most common hypertensive disorder in pregnancy, typically occurs after 20 weeks' gestation. At a minimum, it is characterized by the development of hypertension and proteinuria ≥ 0.3 g protein in a 24-hour specimen or $\geq 1 +$ dipstick. The higher the blood pressure or proteinuria, the more certain the diagnosis (Cunningham et al., 2001). Previously, edema was listed as a cardinal sign of preeclampsia but is no longer included because it is such a common finding in pregnancy.

Preeclampsia, typically categorized as mild or severe, is a progressive disorder. In its most severe form, **eclampsia,** generalized seizures or coma develop. If a woman has a seizure, she is considered eclamptic. Most often preeclampsia is seen in the last 10 weeks of gestation, during labor, or in the first 48 hours after childbirth. Although birth of the fetus is the only known cure for preeclampsia, it can be controlled with early diagnosis and careful management. Preeclampsia is seen more often in teenagers and in women over age 35, especially if they are primigravidas. Other risk factors include obesity, history of hypertension, black ethnicity, and multiple gestation (Cunningham et al., 2001).

Developing Cultural Competence

- The incidence of ectopic pregnancy is higher for nonwhite women than for whites in every age category.
- The incidence of preeclampsia is also related to genetic predisposition. Women of African-American descent are at higher risk.
- Until recently, researchers thought that the incidence of GTD was significantly higher in women of Asian ancestry. However, population-based studies show that the incidence of GTD in most of the world is similar to that found in the United States—about 1 in 1000 pregnancies (Cunningham et al., 2001)

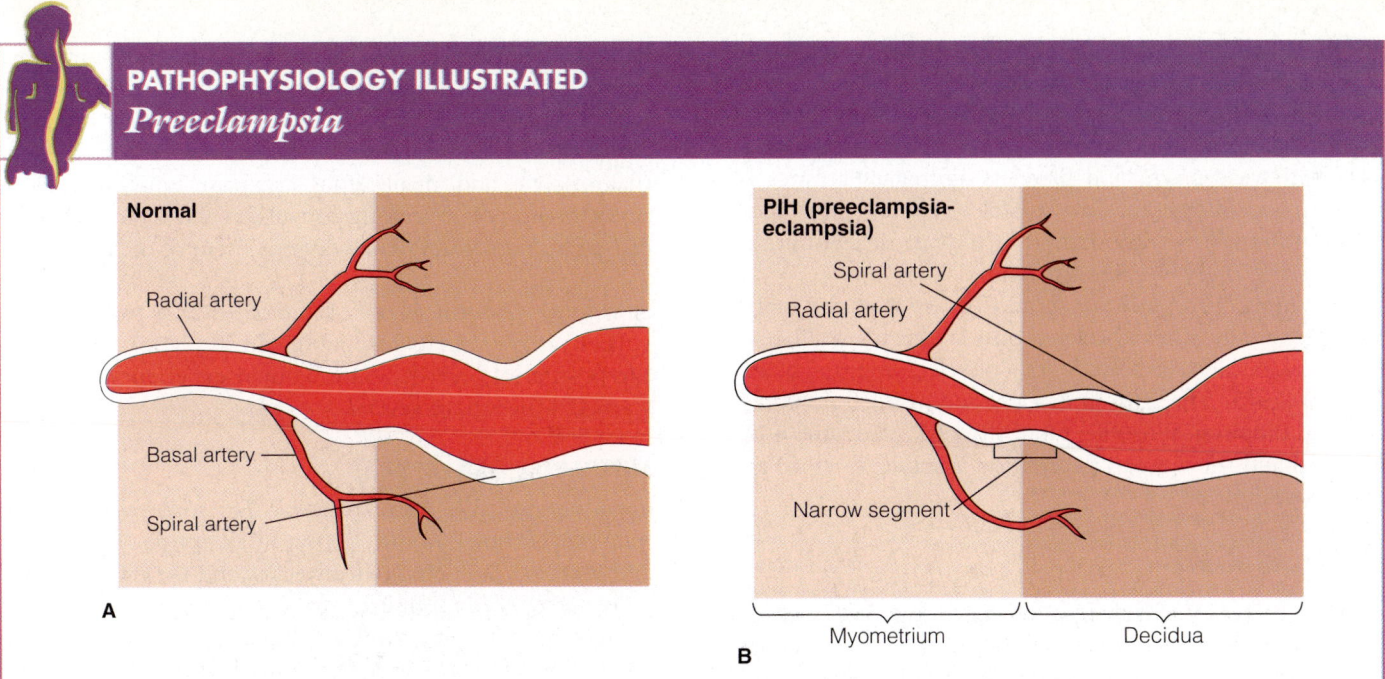

PATHOPHYSIOLOGY ILLUSTRATED
Preeclampsia

A, In a normal pregnancy, the passive quality of the spiral arteries permits increased blood flow to the placenta.
B, In preeclampsia vasoconstriction of the myometrial segment of the spiral arteries occurs.

PATHOPHYSIOLOGY OF PREECLAMPSIA

The cause of preeclampsia-eclampsia remains unknown, despite decades of research. Preeclampsia affects all the major systems of the body. The following pathophysiologic changes are associated with the disease:

- In normal pregnancy, the lowered peripheral vascular resistance and the increased maternal resistance to the pressor effects of angiotensin II result in lowered blood pressure. In preeclampsia, blood pressure begins to rise after 20 weeks' gestation, probably due to a gradual loss of resistance to angiotensin II. This response has been linked to the ratio between the prostaglandins prostacyclin and thromboxane. Prostacyclin is a potent vasodilator. It is decreased in preeclampsia, often several weeks before symptoms develop. This changes the ratio between the two prostaglandins, allowing the potent vasoconstriction and platelet-aggregating effects of thromboxane to dominate. This effect is intensified in the later weeks of preeclamptic pregnancy when levels of thromboxane increase (Mills, DerSimonian, Raymond, et al., 1999).

- In addition, nitric oxide, a potent vasodilator, plays a role in the pregnant woman's resistance to vasopressors. Decreased nitric oxide production in women with preeclampsia may contribute to the development of hypertension (Branch & Porter, 1999).

- The loss of normal vasodilation of uterine arterioles and the concurrent maternal vasospasm result in decreased placental perfusion (see "Pathophysiology Illustrated: Preeclampsia"). The effect on the fetus may be growth restriction, decrease in fetal movement, and chronic hypoxia or fetal distress.

- In preeclampsia, normal renal perfusion is decreased. With a reduction of the glomerular filtration rate, serum levels of creatinine, BUN, and uric acid begin to rise from normal pregnant levels, while urine output decreases. Sodium is retained in increased amounts, which results in increased extracellular volume, increased sensitivity to angiotensin II, and edema. Stretching of the capillary walls of the glomerular endothelial cells allows the large protein molecules, primarily albumin, to escape in the urine, decreasing serum albumin levels. The decreased serum albumin concentration causes decreased plasma colloid osmotic pressure. This lowered pressure results in a further movement of fluid to the extracellular spaces, which also contributes to the development of edema.

- The decreased intravascular volume causes increased viscosity of the blood and a corresponding rise in hematocrit.

HELLP syndrome (**h**emolysis, **e**levated **l**iver enzymes, and **l**ow **p**latelet count) is sometimes associated with severe preeclampsia. Women who experience this multiple-organ-failure syndrome have high morbidity and mortality rates, as do their offspring.

The hemolysis that occurs is termed *microangiopathic hemolytic anemia*. It is thought that red blood cells are fragmented during passage through small, damaged blood vessels. Elevated liver enzymes occur from blood flow that is obstructed by fibrin deposits. Hyperbilirubinemia and jaundice may also be seen. Liver distention causes epigastric pain. Thrombocytopenia (low platelet count) is a frequent finding in preeclampsia. Vascular damage is associated with vasospasm, and platelets aggregate at sites of damage, resulting in low platelet count (less than $100,000/mm^3$). Symptoms may include nausea, vomiting, flulike symptoms, or epigastric pain.

The mother's condition should be assessed and stabilized, especially if her platelet counts are very low. Platelet transfusions are indicated for platelet counts below $20,000/mm^3$. The fetus is also assessed, using a nonstress test and biophysical profile. Once HELLP syndrome is diagnosed and the woman's condition is stable, birth of the child is indicated.

Maternal Risks

Central nervous system changes associated with preeclampsia-eclampsia are hyperreflexia, headache, and seizures. Hyperreflexia may be due to increased intracellular sodium and decreased intracellular potassium levels. Cerebral vasospasm causes headaches, and cerebral edema and vasoconstriction are responsible for seizures. There is also increased risk for renal failure, abruptio placentae, DIC, ruptured liver, and pulmonary embolism.

Fetal-Neonatal Risks

Infants of women with hypertension during pregnancy have an increased risk for morbidity and mortality. They also tend to be small for gestational age. The cause is related specifically to maternal vasospasm and hypovolemia, which result in fetal hypoxia and malnutrition. In addition, the neonate may be premature because of the necessity for early birth. At birth, the newborn may be oversedated because of medications given to the mother. The newborn may also have hypermagnesemia due to treatment of the woman with large doses of $MgSO_4$.

Clinical Therapy

CLINICAL MANIFESTATIONS AND DIAGNOSIS

Mild Preeclampsia. Women with mild preeclampsia may exhibit few if any symptoms. The blood pressure is elevated to 140/90 mm Hg or higher, 1 + proteinuria may occur, and liver enzymes may be elevated minimally. Although it is no longer considered a diagnostic sign of preeclampsia, edema may be present.

Severe Preeclampsia. Severe preeclampsia may develop suddenly. Signs include a diastolic blood pressure of 110 mm Hg or higher; persistent dipstick albumin measures of 2 + or more or 24-hour urine protein level of 2 g or more; and elevated hematocrit, serum creatinine, uric acid, and liver enzymes. Other characteristic symptoms are frontal headaches, blurred vision, scotomata (spots before the eyes), nausea, vomiting, irritability, hyperreflexia, cerebral distur-

bances, oliguria (≤ 500 mL of urine in 24 hours), pulmonary edema with moist breath sounds and dyspnea, cyanosis, retinal edema (retinas appear wet and glistening), narrowed segments on the retinal arterioles when examined with an ophthalmoscope, and, finally, epigastric pain. Epigastric pain is often the sign of impending convulsion and is thought to be caused by increased vascular engorgement of the liver.

Eclampsia. Eclampsia, characterized by a grand mal convulsion, may occur before labor, during labor, or early in the postpartal period. Some women experience only one seizure; others have several.

ANTEPARTAL MANAGEMENT

Home Care of Mild Preeclampsia. For some women with mild preeclampsia, home care is now an option. The mother and fetus are evaluated twice weekly, and the mother is encouraged to set aside at least two 2- to 3-hour blocks of time for rest in a side-lying position. It is extremely important to advise the woman to report to the doctor if she develops signs of worsening preeclampsia (Branch & Porter, 1999).

Hospital Care of Mild Preeclampsia. The woman is placed on bed rest, primarily on her left side, to decrease pressure on the vena cava, thereby increasing venous return, circu-

Complementary Care

HERBS AND SUPPLEMENTS USED TO TREAT HYPERTENSION

There are several herbs and supplements that are used by herbalists to help reduce hypertension: burdock, dandelion, hawthorn, and the supplement coenzyme Q10.

Burdock (Seeds): Burdock seeds (not the root) are used for their hypotensive and diuretic properties. It is administered in extract, tincture, and tea form. Note that the chemical constituents in the root appear to be stronger than in the seeds, and may be a uterine stimulant—so pregnant women should be advised against using this portion of the burdock plant.

Dandelion: Dandelion root is used as an antihypertensive. It is also used as a diuretic, thereby reducing the effects of hypertension. It is administered in extract, tincture, capsule, and tea form.

Hawthorn (Leaf and Flower): The hawthorn leaf and flower are frequently used in cardiac disorders, including hypertension. It is administered in extract, tincture, capsule, and tea form. Note that potential uteroactivity has been found in the use of hawthorn berries, so the pregnant woman should be advised against using this part of the hawthorn plant (Blumenthal, 2000).

These herbs should only be administered by a qualified herbalist. Refer back to "Complementary Care: Homeopathy and Herbal Medicine" in Chapter 9 (page 198) for reminders regarding the use of herbs during pregnancy.

Coenzyme Q10: Coenzyme Q10 is a fat-soluble vitamin-like compound known as ubiquinone (Skidmore-Roth, 2001). It is used to treat a variety of cardiac disorders, including hypertension.

Note: Licorice in any form should be avoided, as it has a hypertensive effect.

latory volume, and placental and renal perfusion. Her diet should be well balanced and moderate to high in protein (80 to 100 g/day, or 1.5 g/kg/day) to replace protein lost in the urine. Sodium intake should be moderate, not to exceed 6 g/day. Excessively salty foods should be avoided, but sodium restriction and diuretics are no longer used in treating preeclampsia.

To achieve a safe outcome for the fetus, tests to evaluate fetal status are done more frequently as preeclampsia progresses. The following tests are used:

- Fetal movement record
- Nonstress test (NST)
- Ultrasonography every 3 or 4 weeks for serial determination of growth
- Biophysical profile
- Serum creatinine determinations
- Amniocentesis to determine fetal lung maturity
- Doppler velocimetry beginning at 30 to 32 weeks to screen for fetal compromise

Severe Preeclampsia. In severe cases, birth may be the treatment of choice for both mother and fetus, even if the fetus is immature. Other medical therapies for severe preeclampsia include the following:

- *Bed rest.* Bed rest must be complete. Stimuli that may bring on a seizure should be reduced.
- *Diet.* A high-protein, moderate-sodium diet is given as long as the woman is alert and has no nausea or indication of impending seizure.
- *Anticonvulsants.* MgSO$_4$ is the treatment of choice for convulsions. Its depressant action on the central nervous system reduces the possibility of seizure (see "Drug Guide: Magnesium Sulfate").
- *Fluid and electrolyte replacement.* The goal of fluid intake is to achieve a balance between correcting hypovolemia and preventing circulatory overload. Fluid intake may be oral or supplemented with IV therapy. IV fluids may be started "to keep lines open" in case they are needed for drug therapy even when oral intake is adequate. Electrolytes are replaced as indicated by daily serum electrolyte levels.
- *Sedative.* A sedative such as diazepam (Valium) or phenobarbital is sometimes given to encourage quiet bed rest.
- *Antihypertensives.* Hydralazine (Apresoline), labetalol (Normodyne), and nifedipine (Procardia) are the antihypertensive medications most commonly used (Kurdas, 2001). In general, antihypertensive therapy is given for diastolic blood pressures of 110 mm Hg or above only in cases where the gestational age of the fetus is critical (25 to 30 weeks). Otherwise, for women beyond 30 weeks, childbirth is induced (Roberts, 1999).

Eclampsia. An eclamptic seizure requires immediate, effective treatment. A bolus of 4 to 6 g MgSO$_4$ is given IV over 5 minutes to control convulsions. A sedative such as diazepam or amobarbitol is used only if the seizures are not controlled by MgSO$_4$. Dilantin may be used for seizure prevention. The lungs are auscultated for pulmonary edema. The woman is observed for circulatory and renal failure and signs of cerebral hemorrhage. Furosemide (Lasix) may be given for pulmonary edema; digitalis may be given for circulatory failure. Intake and output are monitored hourly.

The woman is observed for signs of labor. She is also checked every 15 minutes for evidence of vaginal bleeding and abdominal rigidity, which might indicate abruptio placentae. While she is comatose, she is positioned on her side with the side rails up.

Because of the severity of her condition, the woman is often cared for in an intensive care unit. Invasive hemodynamic monitoring of either central venous pressure or pulmonary artery wedge pressure may be started using a Swan-Ganz catheter. When the condition of the woman and the fetus are stabilized, induction of labor is considered, because birth is the only known cure for preeclampsia-eclampsia. The woman and her partner should be given a careful explanation about her status and that of her unborn child and the treatment they are receiving. Plans for further treatment and for birth must be discussed with them.

INTRAPARTAL MANAGEMENT

Labor may be induced by IV oxytocin when there is evidence of fetal maturity and cervical readiness. In very severe cases, cesarean birth may be necessary even if the fetus is immature. The woman may receive IV oxytocin and MgSO$_4$ simultaneously. Infusion pumps should be used, and bags and tubing must be carefully labeled.

Analgesics may be used to decrease discomfort or the woman may have an epidural block. Birth in the Sims' or semisitting position should be considered. If the lithotomy position is used, a wedge should be placed under the right buttock to displace the uterus. The wedge should also be used if birth is by cesarean. Oxygen is administered to the woman during labor if the need is indicated by fetal response to the contractions.

A pediatrician or neonatal nurse practitioner must be available to care for the newborn at birth. This caregiver must be informed of all amounts and times of medication the woman has received during labor.

POSTPARTUM MANAGEMENT

The woman with preeclampsia usually improves rapidly after giving birth, although seizures can still occur during the first 48 hours postpartum. When the hypertension is severe, the woman may continue to receive antihypertensives or MgSO$_4$ postpartally.

Nursing Management

See "Clinical Pathway for a Woman with Preeclampsia-Eclampsia" for a detailed summary of nursing care management.

CLINICAL PATHWAY 〜 *For a Woman with Preeclampsia-Eclampsia*

Category	Antepartal Management	Intrapartal Management*	Postpartal Management*
Referral	• Perinatologist • Internist • Social worker • Psych clinical nurse practitioner • Dietary/nutritionist	• Obtain prenatal record	• Home nursing referral if indicated **Expected Outcomes** Appropriate resources identified and utilized
Assessments	• Electronic fetal monitoring (EFM) ____ q4h ____ q8h ____ Continuous • NST ____ qd • Ultrasound as indicated • Assess for headache, visual disturbances, epigastric pain, edema, DTRs, clonus, and protein in urine	• Assess prenatal BP readings and compare to baseline reading • Assess for headache, visual disturbances, epigastric pain, edema, DTRs, clonus, and protein in urine	• BP q4h for first 48h then q8h until discharge • Monitor daily hematocrit • Continue normal postpartum assessment q8h • Feeding technique with newborn: should be progressing • TPR assessment; q8h; all WNL: report temperature >38°C (100.4°F) • Continue assessment of comfort level • Assess for headache, visual disturbances, epigastric pain, edema, DTRs, clonus, and protein in urine **Expected Outcomes** Findings indicate hypertension reduced or stabilized Unstable or escalating hypertension identified in timely manner

Teaching/ psychosocial	• Room orientation
	• Explain signs and symptoms of worsening disease and importance of notifying RN
	• Explain s/sx of labor
	• Increase pt awareness of fetal monitoring, importance of bed rest and lying on left side
	• Evaluation of client teaching
		• Tour of ICN
		• Discuss with woman:
		  a. Mode of childbirth
		  b. Progression of disease and possible use of MgSO$_4$ prior to birth
		  c. Postpartum expectation
			• Implement normal postpartum teaching and psychosocial support (see Chapter 22)
			Expected Outcomes
			Verbalizes or otherwise demonstrates understanding of teaching
			Incorporates teaching of BP management into self-care

Nursing care management and reports	• CBC daily
	• Biochemical profile
	• U/A dipstick for protein and ketones with each void as well as specific gravity
	• 24-hour urine for total protein and creatinine clearance
	• VS q4h or more frequently if indicated
	• I&O q8h; fluid restriction ____ mL as ordered
	• DTRs and clonus q4h; report 3+ or 4+ results
	• Daily weight
	• Seizure precautions
	  • Headache, visual distress, epigastric pain: report abnormal findings
	  • Edema (ongoing)
	  • Auscultate lungs for moist respirations and report
	  • Assess hourly for vaginal bleeding and/or uterine irritability or contractions
	• Observe for alertness, mood changes, and signs of impending convulsion or coma
	• Assess emotional response so that support and teaching can be planned accordingly
		• Ongoing monitoring of blood pressure
		• Ongoing monitoring of edema
		• Assess urine for proteinuria every shift
		• Electronic fetal monitoring in place
		• Assess woman for worsening signs of PIH (placental separation, pulmonary edema, renal failure, and fetal distress)
		• Try to have same nurses caring for woman during her hospitalization
			• Continue sitz bath prn
			• May shower if ambulating without difficulty
			• DC buffalo cap (heparin lock) if present
			• Continue to monitor VS, breath sounds, edema, epigastric pain, DTRs, clonus, and protein in urine until return to normal limits
			Expected Outcomes
			Hypertension reduced or controlled
			Maternal-fetal complications quickly identified and minimized
			Feels safe in environment and remains injury free

Category	Antepartal Management	Intrapartal Management*	Postpartal Management*
Comfort	• Assess for discomfort • Provide comfort measures as needed	• Assess for discomfort • Provide comfort measures as needed	• Continue with pain management techniques **Expected Outcomes** Comfort level is maintained
Activity	• BP with BRP • Decreased stimulation in room • Limit visitors • Encourage left lateral recumbent position	• Positioned on side • Encouraged to push while lying on side • Birth is in a side-lying position if possible	• Up ad lib when VS have stabilized **Expected Outcomes** Level of activity has not exacerbated condition
Nutrition	• Regular diet	• Ice chips	• Continue diet and fluids **Expected Outcomes** Nutritional needs met
Elimination	• Report urine output <30 mL/hr or urine specific gravity >1.040	• Monitor urine output	• Monitor urine output • I/O recorded for 48h after birth **Expected Outcomes** Intake and output WNL

Medications	• Heparin lock or IV
	• If gestational age indicates:
	  • Celestone Soluspan
	  • TRH
	• MgSO$_4$ per infusion pump if indicated
	• Assess home care needs
		• Continuous IV infusion
		• MgSO$_4$ infusion pump if indicated
			• Continue MgSO$_4$ as indicated
			• May take own prenatal vitamins
			• Rh immune globulin and rubella vaccine administered if indicated
			Expected Outcomes
			Hypertensive crisis prevented
			Pain level controlled
			Perfusion of tissues supported

Discharge planning/ home care			• Review discharge instruction and checklist • Describe postpartum warning signs and when to call CNM/physician • Provide prescriptions; gift pack given to woman • Arrangements made for baby pictures if desired • Postpartum visit scheduled • Newborn check scheduled **Expected Outcomes** Discharged with plan for follow-up health care and blood pressure monitoring Support network identified
Family involvement	• Assess woman's major concerns (e.g., fear for fetus, relationship with other children, relationship with partner)	• Encourage family members to stay with the woman as long as possible throughout labor and childbirth	• Family members urged to visit • Continue to involve support persons in teaching • Evidence of parental bonding behaviors apparent • Plans being made for providing support to mother following discharge; support persons verbalize understanding of need for woman to rest, eat nutritionally, recover **Expected Outcomes** Family able to participate as desired
Date			

*Interventions for a woman with a normal labor and birth and during the early postpartum period may be found in those appropriate clinical pathways.

BP, blood pressure; BRP, bathroom privileges; CBC, complete blood count; CNM/physician, certified nurse-midwife/physician; DTRs, deep tendon reflexes; Hct, hematocrit; Heparin lock, intravenous catheter that allows intermittent access; ICN, intensive care nursery; I&O, intake and output; IV, intravenous; NST, nonstress test; PRN, as needed or as desired; s/sx, signs and symptoms; TPR, temperature, pulse, respiration; VS, vital signs; WNL, within normal limits.

Nursing Assessment and Diagnosis

Take and record the blood pressure during each antepartal visit. If the blood pressure rises, or if the normal decrease in blood pressure expected between 8 and 28 weeks of pregnancy does not occur, the woman should be followed closely. Also check the woman's urine for proteinuria at each visit.

If hospitalization becomes necessary, assess the following:

► *Blood pressure*. Assess every 1 to 4 hours, or more frequently if indicated by medication or other changes in the woman's status.

► *Temperature*. Take every 4 hours, or every 2 hours if elevated.

► *Pulse and respirations*. Determine pulse rate and respirations along with blood pressure.

► *Fetal heart rate*. Check the fetal heart rate with the blood pressure or monitor continuously with the electronic fetal monitor if the situation indicates.

► *Urinary output*. Measure every voiding. The woman frequently has an indwelling catheter. In this case, urine output can be assessed hourly. Output should be 700 mL or greater in 24 hours, or at least 30 mL/hr.

► *Urine protein*. Evaluate urinary protein hourly if an indwelling catheter is in place or with each voiding. Readings of 3+ or 4+ indicate loss of 5 g or more of protein in 24 hours.

► *Urine specific gravity*. Check specific gravity of the urine hourly or with each voiding. Readings over 1.040 correlate with oliguria and proteinuria.

► *Weight*. Weigh the woman daily at the same time, wearing the same robe or gown and slippers. Weighing may be omitted if the woman is to maintain strict bed rest.

► *Pulmonary edema*. Observe the woman for coughing. Auscultate the lungs for moist respirations.

► *Deep tendon reflexes*. Assess the woman for evidence of hyperreflexia in the brachial, wrist, patellar, or Achilles' tendons (Table 13–2). The patellar reflex is the easiest to assess (see Skills manual). Clonus is assessed by vigorously dorsiflexing the foot while the knee is held in a fixed position (Figure 13–2 ◆). Normally no clonus is present. If it is present, it is measured as beats and recorded as such. See Skill 2–3 in the *Clinical Skills Manual*, as well as the CD-ROM that accompanies this text. ⌬ SKILLS CD

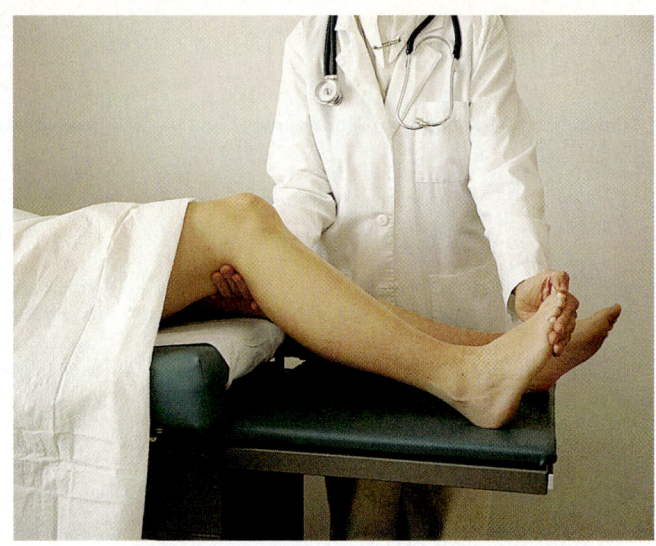

FIGURE 13–2. ◆ To elicit clonus, with the knee flexed and the leg supported, sharply dorsiflex the foot, hold it momentarily and then release it. Normally the foot returns to its usual position of plantar flexion. Clonus is present if the foot "jerks" or taps against the examiner's hand. If so, the number of taps or beats of clonus is recorded.

► *Placental separation*. Assess hourly for vaginal bleeding and/or uterine rigidity.

► *Headache*. Ask about the existence and location of any headache.

► *Visual disturbance*. Ask about any visual blurring or changes or scotomata. The results of the daily fundoscopic exam should be recorded on the chart.

► *Epigastric pain*. Ask about any epigastric pain. It is important to differentiate it from simple heartburn, which tends to be familiar and less intense.

► *Laboratory blood tests*. Daily tests of hematocrit to measure hemoconcentration; BUN, creatinine, and uric acid levels to assess kidney function; clotting studies for signs of thrombocytopenia or DIC; liver enzymes; and electrolyte levels are all indicated.

► *Level of consciousness*. Observe the woman for alertness, mood changes, and any signs of impending convulsion.

► *Emotional response and level of understanding*. Carefully assess the woman's emotional response so that support and teaching can be planned accordingly.

In addition, assess the effects of any medications administered. It is important to be familiar with the more commonly used medications and their purpose, implications, and associated untoward or toxic effects.

Examples of nursing diagnoses that might apply include the following:

► *Fluid volume deficit* related to fluid shift from intravascular to extravascular space secondary to vasospasm

► *Risk for injury* related to the possibility of seizure secondary to cerebral vasospasm or edema

TABLE 13–2 Deep Tendon Reflex Rating Scale	
Rating	Assessment
4+	Hyperactive; very brisk, jerky, or clonic response; abnormal
3+	Brisker than average; may not be abnormal
2+	Average response; normal
1+	Diminished response; low normal
0	No response; abnormal

Planning and Implementation

NURSING CARE IN THE COMMUNITY

A woman with preeclampsia may fear losing her fetus, may worry about her personal relationship with her other children and her personal and sexual relationship with her partner, may be concerned about finances, and may also feel bored and a little resentful if she faces prolonged bed rest. If she has small children, she may have trouble providing for their care. Help the couple identify and discuss these concerns. Offer information and explanations if certain aspects of therapy cause difficulty. Refer the woman and her family to community resources such as support groups or homemaker services as appropriate.

The woman needs to know which symptoms are significant and should be reported at once. Usually the woman with mild preeclampsia is seen once or twice weekly, but she may need to come in earlier than her next appointment if symptoms indicate that her condition is progressing.

HOSPITAL-BASED NURSING CARE

The development of severe preeclampsia is a cause for increased concern about the prognosis for the woman and her fetus. Explain medical therapy and its purpose and offer honest, hopeful information. Keep the couple informed of fetal status and discuss other concerns the couple may express. Provide as much information as possible and seek other sources of information or aid for the family as needed. Offer to contact a member of the clergy or hospital chaplain for additional support if the couple so chooses.

Maintain a quiet, low-stimulus environment for the woman. She should be in a private room in a quiet location where she can be watched closely. Visitors are limited to close family members or main support persons. The woman should maintain the left lateral recumbent position most of the time, with side rails up for her protection. Unlimited phone calls are avoided because the phone ringing unexpectedly may be too jarring. To avoid a sense of isolation, however, some women find it preferable to limit calls to a certain time of day. Bright lights and sudden loud noises may precipitate seizures in the woman with severe preeclampsia.

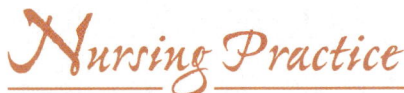

When caring for a woman with preeclampsia who is receiving IV MgSO₄, it is imperative that you follow protocols for monitoring blood levels of magnesium. You are probably already aware of the common signs of increasing magnesium levels, such as diminished reflexes and decreased respiratory rate. However, you can also watch for some subtle clues that may suggest either the therapeutic or toxic range. When a woman's magnesium level is in the therapeutic range, she usually has some slurring of speech, awkwardness of movement, and decreased appetite. If the woman begins to have difficulty swallowing and begins to drool, she may be approaching the toxic range.

Monitor the effectiveness of medications administered. Be alert for signs of untoward effects or developing toxic levels.

The occurrence of a convulsion is frightening to any family members who may be present, although the woman will not be able to recall it when she becomes conscious. Therefore, it is essential to offer explanations to the family members and the woman herself later.

A grand mal seizure has both a tonic phase, marked by pronounced muscular contraction and rigidity, and a clonic phase, marked by alternate contraction and relaxation of the muscles, which causes the woman to thrash about wildly. When the tonic phase of the contraction begins, turn the woman to her side (if she is not already in that position) to aid circulation to the placenta. Turn her head face down to allow saliva to drain from her mouth. Attempting to insert a padded tongue blade is no longer advocated in many facilities; in others, it is used if it can be inserted without force because it may prevent injury to the woman's mouth. The side rails should be padded or a pillow put between the woman and each side rail.

After 15 to 20 seconds the clonic phase starts. When the thrashing subsides, intensive monitoring and therapy begin. An oral airway is inserted, the woman's nasopharynx is suctioned, and oxygen is administered by nasal catheter. Fetal heart tones are monitored continuously. Maternal vital signs are monitored every 5 minutes until they are stable, then every 15 minutes.

Nursing Management During Labor and Birth

The woman is kept positioned on her left side as much as possible. Both the woman and the fetus are monitored carefully throughout labor. Note the progress of labor and remain alert for signs of worsening preeclampsia or its complications.

During the second stage of labor, encourage the woman to push in the side-lying position if possible. If she is unable to do so comfortably or effectively, she can be helped to a semisitting position for pushing and can then resume the lateral position between contractions. Birth is in the side-lying position or in the lithotomy position with a wedge placed under the woman's right hip. Encourage a family member or other support person to stay with the woman as much as possible. Keep the woman and her support person informed of the progress and plan of care. Whenever possible, respect their wishes concerning the birth experience.

Nursing Management During the Postpartal Period

Because the woman with preeclampsia is hypovolemic, even normal blood loss can be serious. Assess the amount of vaginal bleeding and observe the woman for signs of shock. Monitor blood pressure and pulse every 4 hours for 48 hours. Check hematocrit daily. Assess the woman for any further signs of preeclampsia. Measure intake and output. Normal postpartum diuresis helps eliminate edema and is a favorable sign.

Postpartal depression can develop after such a difficult pregnancy. To help prevent it, provide opportunities for frequent maternal-infant contact and encourage family members to visit. The couple may have many questions, so be available for discussion. Give the couple family-planning information. Oral contraceptives may be used if the woman's blood pressure has returned to normal by the time they are prescribed (usually 4 to 6 weeks after birth).

Evaluation

Expected outcomes of nursing care include the following:

▶ The woman is able to explain preeclampsia-eclampsia, its implications for her pregnancy, the treatment regimen, and possible complications.

▶ The woman suffers no eclamptic seizures.

▶ The woman and her caregivers detect early evidence of increasing severity of the preeclampsia or possible complications so that treatment measures can be instituted.

▶ The woman gives birth to a healthy newborn.

Chronic Hypertensive Disease

Chronic hypertension exists when the blood pressure is 140/90 mm Hg or higher before pregnancy or before the 20th week of gestation or when hypertension persists for more than 12 weeks following childbirth (National High Blood Pressure Education Program, 2000). The cause of chronic hypertension has not been determined. In most women, the disease is mild.

The goals of care are to prevent the development of preeclampsia and to ensure normal growth of the fetus. The woman is seen regularly for prenatal care (every 2 weeks until 28 weeks and then weekly until birth). The woman is taught the importance of daily rest periods in the left lateral recumbent position and also learns to monitor her blood pressure at home. Sodium is limited to about 2 g/day.

Antihypertensive medication is continued throughout pregnancy in women with severe chronic hypertension (blood pressure over 160/100 mm Hg). The drug of choice is methyldopa (Aldomet). Serial measurement of hematocrit, serum creatinine, serum uric acid, creatinine clearance, and 24-hour output of urine protein may be necessary (Branch & Porter, 1999).

Nursing care is directed at providing information so that the woman can meet her health care needs. Provide information about her diet, the need for regular rest, her medications, the need for blood pressure control, and any procedures used to monitor the well-being of her fetus.

Chronic Hypertension with Superimposed Preeclampsia

Preeclampsia may develop in a woman previously found to have chronic hypertension. Close monitoring and careful management are indicated if the following signs develop: (1) new-onset proteinuria in a hypertensive woman with no proteinuria before 20 weeks' gestation; or (2) sudden increase in blood pressure or proteinuria or a platelet count $< 100,000/mm^3$ in a woman with hypertension and proteinuria before 20 weeks of gestation (Cunningham et al., 2001). A woman with chronic hypertension who develops superimposed preeclampsia often progresses quickly to eclampsia, sometimes before 30 weeks of pregnancy.

Gestational Hypertension

Gestational hypertension is characterized by hypertension occurring for the first time during pregnancy but not accompanied by proteinuria. It is called *transient hypertension* if preeclampsia does not develop and if the blood pressure returns to normal within 12 weeks following childbirth (Kurdas, 2001).

CARE OF THE WOMAN AT RISK FOR RH SENSITIZATION

The Rh blood group is present on the surface of erythrocytes of most of the population. When it is present, a person is said to be Rh positive. Those without the factor are Rh negative. If an Rh-negative individual is exposed to Rh-positive blood, an antigen-antibody response occurs, and the person forms anti-Rh agglutinin and is said to be sensitized. Subsequent exposure to Rh-positive blood can then cause a serious reaction that results in agglutination and hemolysis of red blood cells. Sensitization most often occurs when an Rh-negative woman carries an Rh-positive fetus, either to term or to termination by miscarriage or induced abortion. It can also occur if an Rh-negative nonpregnant woman receives an Rh-positive blood transfusion.

The red blood cells from the fetus invade the maternal circulation, thereby stimulating the production of Rh antibodies. Because this transfer of RBCs usually occurs at birth, the first child is not affected. In a subsequent pregnancy, however, Rh antibodies cross the placenta and enter the fetal circulation, causing severe hemolysis. The destruction of fetal red blood cells causes anemia in the fetus (Figure 13–3).

Fetal-Neonatal Risks

Although maternal sensitization can now be prevented by administration of **Rh immune globulin** (**RhoGAM,** or RhIgG), infants still die of Rh hemolytic disease. If treatment is not initiated, the anemia resulting from this disorder can cause marked fetal edema, called **hydrops fetalis.** Congestive heart failure may result; marked jaundice (called *icterus gravis*), which can lead to neurologic damage (kernicterus), is also possible. This severe hemolytic syndrome is known as **erythroblastosis fetalis.**

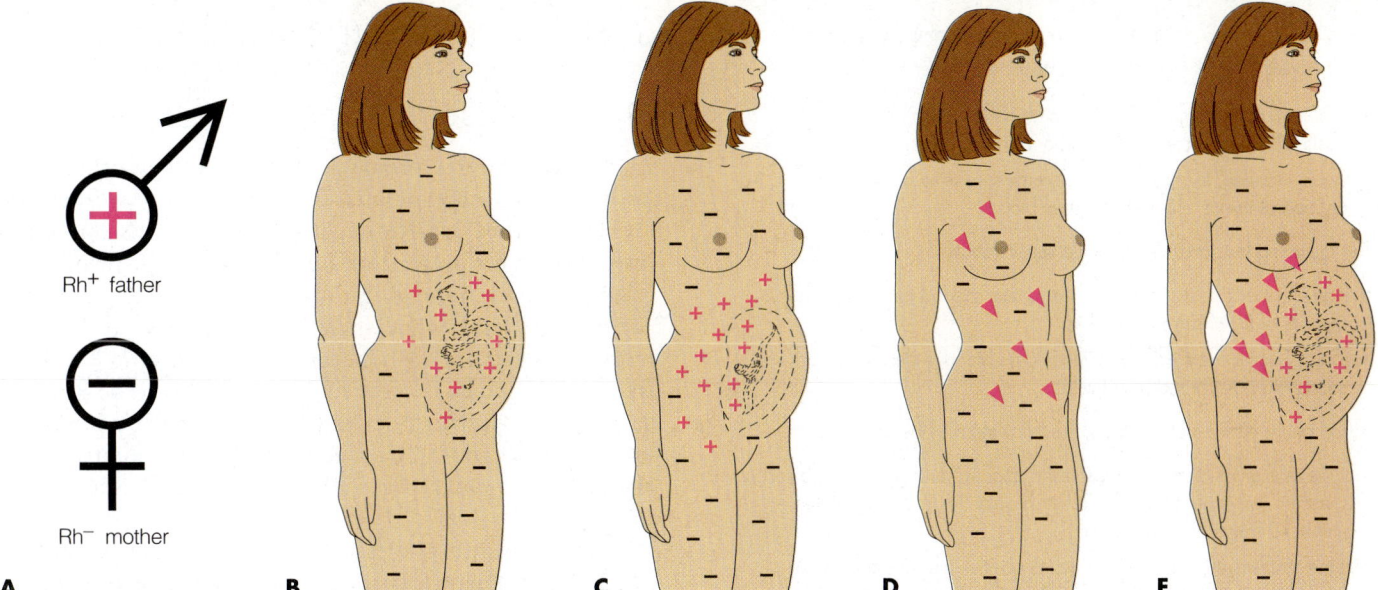

FIGURE 13–3. ◆ Rh isoimmunization sequence. **A,** Rh-positive father and Rh-negative mother. **B,** Pregnancy with Rh-positive fetus. Some Rh-positive blood enters the mother's bloodstream. **C,** As the placenta separates, the mother is further exposed to the Rh-positive blood. **D,** Anti-Rh-positive antibodies (triangles) are formed. **E,** In subsequent pregnancies with an Rh-positive fetus, Rh-positive red blood cells are attacked by the anti-Rh-positive maternal antibodies, causing hemolysis of the red blood cells in the fetus.

Screening for Rh Incompatibility and Sensitization

At the first prenatal visit, caregivers (1) take a history of previous sensitization, abortions, blood transfusions, or children who developed jaundice or anemia during the newborn period; (2) determine maternal blood type (ABO) and Rh factor and do a routine Rh antibody screen; and (3) identify other medical complications such as diabetes, infections, or hypertension. When assessment identifies an Rh-negative woman who may be pregnant with an Rh-positive fetus, an antibody screen (indirect Coombs' test) is done to determine if the woman is sensitized (has developed isoimmunity) to the Rh antigen. The indirect Coombs' test measures the number of antibodies in the maternal blood.

Negative antibody titers and a negative indirect Coombs' test can identify the fetus not at risk. However, the titers cannot reliably point out the fetus in danger, since titer level does not correlate with the severity of the disease. Antibody titers are determined periodically throughout the pregnancy. If the maternal antibody titer is 1:16 or greater, an optical density (ΔOD) analysis of the amniotic fluid is performed. This ΔOD analysis measures the amount of pigment from the breakdown of red blood cells and can determine the severity of the hemolytic process.

Ultrasound should be done at 14 to 16 weeks to determine gestational age. Then serial ultrasounds and amniotic fluid analysis can be used to follow fetal progress. Ascites and subcutaneous edema are signs of severe fetal involvement. Other indicators of the fetal condition include an increase in fetal heart size and hydramnios.

Clinical Therapy

The goals of clinical management are the early identification and treatment of maternal conditions that predispose to hemolytic disease, evaluation of the Rh-sensitized woman, treatment for the affected newborn, and prevention of Rh sensitization if none is present.

ANTEPARTAL MANAGEMENT

Prevention of Isoimmunization. Since transplacental hemorrhage is possible during pregnancy, an antibody screen is performed on an Rh-negative woman at 28 weeks' gestation. If she has no antibody titer, she is given an IM injection of 300 μg Rh immune globulin (RhoGAM, HypRho-D). The Rh immune globulin provides passive antibody protection against Rh antigens. This "tricks" the body, which does not then produce antibodies of its own (active immunity). As discussed later, Rh immune globulin is also given postpartally.

When the woman is Rh negative and not sensitized and the father is Rh positive or unknown, Rh immune globulin is also given after each abortion (whether spontaneous or induced), ectopic pregnancy, amniocentesis, or stillbirth. If abortion or ectopic pregnancy occurs in the first trimester, a smaller (50 μg) dose of Rh immune globulin (MICRhoGAM or Mini-Gamulin Rh) is used. A full dose is used following second-trimester amniocentesis or the birth of a stillborn infant (Scott & Branch, 1999).

Rh immune globulin is not given to the newborn or the father. It should not be given to a previously sensitized woman. However, sometimes after birth or an abortion the results of the blood test do not clearly show whether

TABLE 13-3 Rh Sensitization

When trying to work through Rh problems, remember the following:

- A potential problem exists when an Rh-negative mother and an Rh-positive father conceive a child who is Rh-negative.
- In this situation, the mother may become sensitized or produce antibodies to her fetus's Rh-negative blood.

The following tests are used to detect sensitization:

- Indirect Coombs' test—done on the mother's blood to measure the number of Rh-positive antibodies.
- Direct Coombs' test—done on the infant's blood to detect antibody-coated Rh-positive red blood cells.

Based on the results of these tests, the following may be done:

- If the mother's indirect Coombs' test is negative and the infant's direct Coombs' test is negative, the mother is given Rh immune globulin within 72 hours of birth.
- If the mother's indirect Coombs' test is positive and her Rh-positive infant has a positive direct Coombs' test, Rh immune globulin is not given; in this case the infant is carefully monitored for hemolytic disease.
- It is recommended that Rh immune globulin be given at 28 weeks antenatally to decrease possible transplacental bleeding concerns.

Rh immune globulin is also administered after each abortion (spontaneous or therapeutic), ectopic pregnancy, or amniocentesis.

---

the mother is already sensitized to the Rh antigen. In such cases, the Rh immune globulin is given; it will cause no harm (see Table 13–3). (The treatment of the newborn is discussed in Chapter 25.)

Care of the Sensitized Fetus. Two primary interventions can help the fetus whose blood cells are being destroyed by maternal antibodies: early birth and intrauterine transfusion. Both carry risks. Ideally, birth should be delayed until fetal maturity is confirmed at about 36 to 37 weeks.

If ΔOD indicates severe anemia or when fetal hydrops is present, percutaneous umbilical blood sampling (PUBS) (see Chapter 14) is performed to determine fetal hematocrit. If the hematocrit is low (generally below 30%), the fetus is given an intrauterine blood transfusion (Cunningham et al., 2001). Severely sensitized fetuses may require birth at 32 to 34 weeks.

POSTPARTAL MANAGEMENT

The Rh-negative mother who has no antibody titer (indirect Coombs' test negative, nonsensitized) and has given birth to an Rh-positive fetus (direct Coombs' test negative) is given an injection of Rh immune globulin within 72 hours of childbirth so she does not have time to produce antibodies to fetal cells that entered her bloodstream when the placenta separated. Rh immune globulin provides her with temporary passive immunity, which prevents the development of permanent active immunity (antibody formation).

Nursing Management

Nursing Assessment and Diagnosis

As part of the initial prenatal history, ask the mother if she knows her blood type and Rh factor. Many women are aware that they are Rh negative and that this status has implications for pregnancy. Ask the woman if she has ever received Rh immune globulin, if she has had any previous pregnancies and what their outcome was, and if she knows her partner's Rh factor. If the partner is Rh negative, there is no risk to the fetus, who will also be Rh negative. If the woman does not know what Rh type she is, intervention cannot begin until the initial laboratory data are obtained. Once that is done, plan care based on the findings.

If the woman becomes sensitized during her pregnancy, nursing assessment focuses on the knowledge and coping skills of the woman and her family. After birth, review data about the Rh type of the fetus. If the newborn is Rh positive, the mother is Rh negative, and no sensitization has occurred, it is necessary to administer Rh immune globulin.

Nursing diagnoses that might apply include the following:

▸ *Health-seeking behaviors:* information about Rh immune globulin related to an expressed need to understand the implications of being Rh negative and pregnant

▸ *Ineffective individual coping* related to depression secondary to the development of indications of the need for fetal exchange transfusion

Planning and Implementation

During the antepartal period, explain the mechanisms involved in isoimmunization and answer any questions the woman and her partner have. It is imperative that the woman understand the importance of receiving Rh immune globulin after every miscarriage, abortion, or ectopic pregnancy. In addition, explain the purpose of the Rh immune globulin administered at 28 weeks' gestation if the woman is not sensitized.

If the woman is sensitized to the Rh factor, it poses a threat to any Rh-positive fetus she carries. Provide emotional support to the family to help the members deal with their concern and any feelings of guilt about the infant's condition. If an intrauterine transfusion becomes necessary, provide support while also assuming responsibility as part of the health care team.

During labor, when caring for an Rh-negative woman who has not been sensitized, ensure that the woman's blood is assessed for any antibodies and also has been cross-matched for Rh immune globulin. The postpartum nurse is usually responsible for administering the Rh immune globulin IM if the newborn is Rh positive. See Skill 2–4 in the *Clinical Skills Manual*, as well as the CD-ROM that accompanies this text. CD SKILLS

Evaluation

Expected outcomes of nursing care include the following:

▶ The woman is able to explain the process of Rh sensitization and its implications for her unborn child and for subsequent pregnancies.

▶ If the woman has not been sensitized, she is able to discuss the importance of receiving Rh immune globulin when necessary and cooperates with the recommended dosage schedule.

▶ The woman gives birth to a healthy newborn.

▶ If complications develop for the fetus or newborn, they are detected quickly and therapy is instituted.

CARE OF THE WOMAN AT RISK DUE TO ABO INCOMPATIBILITY

ABO incompatibility occurs in about 20% to 25% of pregnancies, but it rarely causes significant hemolysis (Scott & Branch, 1999). In most cases, ABO incompatibility is limited to type O mothers with a type A or B fetus. Group O infants, because they have no antigenic sites on the red blood cells, are never affected regardless of the mother's blood type. The incompatibility occurs as a result of the interaction of antibodies present in maternal serum and the antigen sites on the fetal red blood cells.

Anti-A and anti-B antibodies are naturally occurring; that is, women are naturally exposed to the A and B antigens through the foods they eat and through exposure to infection by gram-negative bacteria. As a result, some women have high serum anti-A and anti-B titers before they become pregnant. Once they become pregnant, the maternal serum anti-A and anti-B antibodies cross the placenta and produce hemolysis of the fetal red blood cells. With ABO incompatibility, the first infant is often involved, and no relationship exists between the appearance of the disease and repeated sensitization from one pregnancy to the next.

Unlike Rh incompatibility, antepartal treatment is never warranted. As part of the initial assessment, however, note whether the potential for an ABO incompatibility exists (type O mother and type A or B father). This alerts caregivers so that, following birth, the newborn can be assessed carefully for the development of hyperbilirubinemia (see Chapter 26).

CARE OF THE WOMAN REQUIRING SURGERY DURING PREGNANCY

Elective surgery should be delayed until the postpartum, but essential surgery can generally be done during pregnancy. Surgery poses some risks, however. The incidence of miscarriage is increased for women who have surgery in the first trimester. There is also an increased incidence of fetal mortality and of low-birth-weight (less than 2500 g) infants. Finally, when surgery is necessary, the incidence of preterm labor and intrauterine growth restriction increases.

Although general preoperative and postoperative care is similar for pregnant and nonpregnant women, special considerations must be kept in mind whenever the surgical client is pregnant. The early second trimester is the best time to operate because there is less risk of miscarriage or early labor, and the uterus is not so large as to block the surgical site.

To prevent uterine compression of major blood vessels while the woman is supine, the caregiver must place a wedge under the woman's right hip to tilt the uterus during both surgery and recovery. The decreased intestinal motility and delayed gastric emptying that occur in pregnancy increase the risk of vomiting when anesthetics are given and during the postoperative period. Thus a nasogastric tube is usually inserted before a pregnant woman has major surgery. An indwelling urinary catheter prevents bladder distention, decreases risk of injury to the bladder, and permits monitoring of output.

Pregnancy causes increased secretions of the respiratory tract and engorgement of the nasal mucous membrane, often making breathing through the nose difficult. Consequently, pregnant women often need an endotracheal tube to maintain an airway during surgery. Caregivers must guard against maternal hypoxia. During surgery, uterine circulation decreases, and fetal oxygenation may be reduced quickly. Fetal heart rate must be monitored electronically during and after surgery. Blood loss is also monitored throughout the procedure and following it.

Postoperatively, encourage the woman to turn, breathe deeply, and cough regularly and to use any ventilation therapy, such as incentive spirometry, to avoid developing pneumonia. The pregnant woman is at increased risk for thrombophlebitis, so apply antiembolism stockings, encourage leg exercises while the woman is in bed, and have her ambulate as soon as possible.

Discharge teaching is very important. The woman and her family should understand what to expect regarding activity level, discomfort, diet, medications, and any special considerations. In addition, they should know the warning signs they need to report to the physician immediately.

CARE OF THE WOMAN SUFFERING TRAUMA FROM AN ACCIDENT

Trauma complicates about 1 in 12 pregnancies; motor vehicle accidents are the most common cause of trauma, accounting for two thirds of injuries. Falls and direct assaults account for most of the remaining cases. (Domestic violence, which may be the cause of trauma, is discussed next.) Most accidents produce non-life-threatening injuries and result in pregnancy loss 1% to 5% of the time. Abruptio placentae is a complication in 40% to 50% of women who sustain severe trauma (ACOG, 1998b).

Late in pregnancy, when balance and coordination are affected, the woman may fall. Her protruding abdomen is vulnerable to a variety of minor injuries. The fetus is usually well protected by the amniotic fluid, which distributes the force of a blow equally in all directions, and by the muscle layers of the uterus and abdominal wall. In early pregnancy, while the uterus is still in the pelvis, it is shielded from blows by the surrounding pelvic organs, muscles, and bones.

Trauma that causes concern includes blunt trauma (from an automobile accident, for example); penetrating abdominal injuries, such as knife and gunshot wounds; and the complications of maternal shock, premature labor, and spontaneous abortion. Maternal mortality most often occurs from head trauma or hemorrhage. Uterine rupture is a rare but life-threatening complication of trauma. It may result from strong deceleration forces in an automobile accident, with or without seat belts. Traumatic separation of the placenta can occur; it causes a high rate of fetal mortality. Premature labor, often following rupture of membranes during an accident, is another serious hazard to the fetus. Premature labor can begin even if the woman is not injured. To help prevent trauma from automobile accidents, all pregnant women should wear both lap seat belts and shoulder harnesses (ACOG, 1998b).

Treatment of major injuries during pregnancy focuses initially on life-saving measures for the woman. Such measures include establishing an airway, controlling external bleeding, and administering IV fluid to alleviate shock. The woman must be kept on her left side to prevent further hypotension. Fetal heart rate is monitored. Exploratory surgery may be necessary following abdominal trauma to determine the extent of injuries. If the fetus is near term and the uterus has been damaged, cesarean birth is indicated. If the fetus is still immature, the uterus can often be repaired, and the pregnancy continues until term.

In cases of trauma in which the mother's life is not directly threatened, fetal monitoring for 4 hours should be sufficient if there are no contractions, vaginal bleeding, uterine tenderness, or leaking amniotic fluid. Abruptio placentae may occur following a blow to the abdomen. Increased uterine irritability in the first few hours after trauma helps identify women who may be at risk for this potentially catastrophic complication.

CARE OF THE BATTERED PREGNANT WOMAN

Female partner abuse, the intentional injury of a woman by her partner, often begins or increases during pregnancy. The incidence of abuse during pregnancy ranges from 4% to 8% (ACOG, 1999a). Physical abuse may result in loss of pregnancy, preterm labor, low-birth-weight infants, and fetal death. Abused women have higher rates of complications such as anemia, infection, low weight gain, and first- and second-trimester bleeding (McFarlane, Parker, Soeken, et al., 1999).

The first step toward helping the battered woman is to identify her. Asking every woman about abuse at various times during pregnancy is crucial because a woman may not disclose abuse until she knows her caregivers better. ACOG (1999a) recommends screening for abuse at the first prenatal visit, at least once each trimester, and then again during the postpartum period.

Chronic psychosomatic symptoms can also be an indicator of abuse. The woman may have nonspecific or vague complaints. It is important to assess old scars around the head, chest, arms, abdomen, and genitalia. Any bruising or evidence of pain is also evaluated. Be especially alert for signs of bruising or injury to the woman's breasts, abdomen, or genitalia because these areas are common targets of violence during pregnancy. Other indicators include a decrease in eye contact; silence when the partner is in the room; and a history of nervousness, insomnia, drug overdose, or alcohol problems. Frequent visits to the emergency room and a history of accidents without understandable causes are possible indicators of abuse.

The goals of treatment are to identify the woman at risk, to increase her decision-making abilities to decrease the risk for further abuse, and to provide a safe environment for the woman and her unborn child. An environment that is private, accepting, and nonjudgmental is necessary so the woman can express her concerns. She needs to be aware of community resources available to her, such as emergency shelters; police, legal, and social services; and counseling. Ultimately, it is the woman's decision to either seek assistance or return to old patterns.

Because abuse often begins during pregnancy, it may be a new, unexpected experience for the woman, one she believes is an isolated incident. She needs to know that battering may continue after childbirth and may extend to the child as well. This is an important time to provide information and establish a trusted link for the woman with a health professional. (For further discussion see Chapter 3).

CARE OF THE WOMAN WITH A TORCH INFECTION

The TORCH group of infectious diseases are those identified as causing serious harm to the embryo-fetus: **t**oxoplasmosis, **r**ubella, **c**ytomegalovirus, and **h**erpes simplex virus type 2. (Some sources identify the O as "other infections.") Exposure of the woman during the first 12 weeks of gestation may cause developmental anomalies in the fetus.

Toxoplasmosis

Toxoplasmosis is caused by the protozoan *Toxoplasma gondii*. It is barely noticeable in adults, but, when contracted in pregnancy, it can profoundly affect the fetus. The pregnant woman may contract the organism by eating raw or undercooked meat or by contact with the feces of infected cats, either through the cat litter box or by gardening in areas frequented by cats.

FETAL-NEONATAL RISKS

The likelihood of fetal infection increases with each trimester of pregnancy, but the risk of serious impact on the fetus decreases. Thus maternal infection contracted during the first trimester is associated with the lowest incidence of fetal infection but the highest risk of severe fetal disease or death. Maternal infection that occurs before conception is rarely associated with congenital effects (Lopez, Dietz, Wilson, et al., 2000). Most infants born with congenital toxoplasmosis are asymptomatic at birth but develop symptoms later. The infection may vary from mild to severe. In mild cases, retinochoroiditis (inflammation of the retina and choroid of the eye) may be the only recognizable damage, and it and other manifestations may not appear until adolescence or young adulthood. Severe neonatal disorders associated with congenital infection include convulsions, coma, microcephaly, and hydrocephalus. The infant with a severe infection may die soon after birth. Survivors are often blind, deaf, and severely retarded.

CLINICAL THERAPY

Diagnosis can be made by serologic testing of antibody titers, specifically *Toxoplasma*-specific antibodies IgG and IgM using the indirect fluorescent antibody (IFA) test. Titers become positive within 1 to 2 weeks after infection and may persist for months or years (Minkoff, 1999).

Prenatal diagnosis is possible using a culture of amniotic fluid or a sample of fetal blood, which is then tested for *Toxoplasma*-specific IgM. If diagnosis can be established by physical findings, history, and blood tests, the woman may be treated with sulfadiazine, pyrimethamine, and spiramycin. Treatment of the mother can reduce the incidence of fetal infection significantly. If toxoplasmosis is diagnosed before 20 weeks' gestation, pyrimethamine should be avoided unless a therapeutic abortion is planned because the drug can have teratogenic effects.

Nursing Management

Nursing Assessment and Diagnosis

The incubation period for the disease is 10 days. The woman with acute toxoplasmosis may be asymptomatic, or she may develop myalgia, malaise, rash, splenomegaly, and enlarged posterior cervical lymph nodes. Symptoms usually disappear in a few days or weeks.

Nursing diagnoses that might apply include the following:

▶ *Risk for altered health maintenance* related to lack of knowledge about ways in which a pregnant woman can contract toxoplasmosis

▶ *Anticipatory grieving* related to potential effects on infant of maternal toxoplasmosis

Planning and Implementation

During the antepartal period, discuss methods of preventing toxoplasmosis. The woman must understand the importance of avoiding poorly cooked or raw meat, especially pork, beef, lamb, and, in the Arctic region, caribou. Fruits and vegetables should be washed. She should avoid contact with the cat litter box and have someone else clean it frequently, since it takes approximately 48 hours for a cat's feces to become infectious. Stress the importance of wearing gloves when gardening and of avoiding garden areas frequented by cats.

Evaluation

Expected outcomes of nursing care include the following:

▶ The woman is able to discuss toxoplasmosis, its methods of transmission, the implications for her fetus, and measures she can take to avoid contracting it.

▶ The woman implements health measures to avoid contracting toxoplasmosis.

▶ The woman gives birth to a healthy newborn.

Rubella

The effects of rubella (German measles) on the fetus and newborn are great because rubella causes a chronic infection that begins in the first trimester of pregnancy and may persist for months after birth.

FETAL-NEONATAL RISKS

The period of greatest risk for the effects of rubella on the fetus is the first trimester. Clinical signs of congenital infection include congenital heart disease, intrauterine growth restriction, and cataracts. Cataracts may be unilateral or bilateral and may be present at birth or develop in the newborn period. A petechial rash is present in some infants, and hepatosplenomegaly and hyperbilirubinemia are frequently seen. Other abnormalities, such as mental retardation or cerebral palsy, may become evident in infancy. Diagnosis in the newborn can be made in the presence of these conditions and with an elevated rubella IgM antibody titer at birth. Infants born with congenital rubella syndrome are infectious and should be isolated.

The expanded rubella syndrome relates to effects that may develop for years after the infection. These include an increased incidence of insulin-dependent diabetes mellitus; sudden hearing loss; glaucoma; and a slow, progressive form of encephalitis.

CLINICAL THERAPY

The best therapy for rubella is prevention. Live attenuated vaccine is available and should be given to all children. Women of childbearing age should be tested for immunity and vaccinated if susceptible once it is established that they are not pregnant.

As part of the prenatal laboratory screen, the woman is evaluated for rubella using hemagglutination inhibition (HAI), a serology test. The presence of a 1:16 titer or greater is evidence of immunity. A titer less than 1:8 indicates susceptibility to rubella. Because the vaccine is made with attenuated virus, pregnant women are not vaccinated. However, it is considered safe for newly vaccinated children to have contact with pregnant women.

If a woman becomes infected during the first trimester, therapeutic abortion is a legally available alternative.

Nursing Management

Nursing Assessment and Diagnosis

A woman who develops rubella during pregnancy may be asymptomatic or may show signs of a mild infection including a maculopapular rash, lymphadenopathy, muscular achiness, and joint pain. The presence of IgM antirubella antibody is diagnostic of a recent infection. These titers remain elevated for approximately 1 month after infection.

Nursing diagnoses that may apply to the woman who develops rubella early in her pregnancy include the following:

▶ *Ineffective family coping* due to an inability to accept the possibility of fetal anomalies secondary to maternal rubella exposure

▶ *Risk for altered health maintenance* related to lack of knowledge about the importance of rubella immunization before becoming pregnant

Planning and Implementation

Support is vital for the couple considering abortion due to a diagnosis of rubella. Such a decision may trigger a crisis for the couple. The parents need objective data to understand the possible effects on their unborn fetus and the long-term prognosis.

Evaluation

Expected outcomes of nursing care include the following:

▶ The woman is able to describe the implications of rubella exposure during the first trimester of pregnancy.

▶ If exposure occurs in a woman who is not immune, she is able to identify her options and make a decision about continuing her pregnancy that is acceptable to her and her partner.

▶ The nonimmune woman receives the rubella vaccine during the early postpartal period.

▶ The woman gives birth to a healthy infant.

Cytomegalovirus

Cytomegalovirus (CMV) causes both congenital and acquired infections referred to as cytomegalic inclusion disease (CID). This virus can be transmitted by asymptomatic pregnant women across the placenta to the fetus or by the cervical route during birth.

CMV is the most common congenital infection in the United States (ACOG, 2000). Nearly half of adults have antibodies for the virus. The virus can be found in virtually all body fluids. It can be passed between humans by any close contact, such as kissing, breastfeeding, and sexual intercourse. Asymptomatic CMV infection is particularly common in children and gravid women. It is a chronic, persistent infection in that the individual may shed the virus continually over many years. The cervix can harbor the virus, and an ascending infection can develop after birth. Although the virus is usually innocuous in adults and children, it may be fatal to the fetus.

Accurate diagnosis in the pregnant woman depends on the presence of CMV in the urine, a rise in IgM levels, and identification of the CMV antibodies within the serum IgM fraction. At present, no treatment exists for maternal CMV or for the congenital disease in the neonate.

Congenital CMV infection afflicts 1% to 2% of all newborns born in the United States. Of these, about 10% have signs of the disease at birth, and 5% to 15% more go on to develop problems (Oshiro, 1999). The mortality rate for severely affected newborns is 30% (ACOG, 2000). Subclinical infections in the newborn may produce mental retardation and hearing loss, sometimes not recognized for several months, or learning disabilities not seen until childhood.

For the fetus, this infection can result in extensive tissue damage that leads to fetal death; in survival with microcephaly, hydrocephaly, cerebral palsy, or mental retardation; or in survival with no damage at all. The infected newborn is often small for gestational age. The principal tissues and organs affected are the blood, brain, and liver. However, virtually all organs are potentially at risk.

Herpes Simplex Virus

Herpes simplex virus (HSV-1 or HSV-2) infection can cause painful lesions in the genital area. Lesions may also develop on the cervix. This condition and its implications for nonpregnant women are discussed in Chapter 3. Herpes infection as it relates to a pregnant woman is discussed here as part of the TORCH complex of infections.

FETAL-NEONATAL RISKS

Primary infection poses the greatest risk to both the mother and her infant. Primary infection has been associated with spontaneous abortion, low birth weight, and preterm birth. Transmission to the fetus almost always occurs after the membranes rupture and the virus ascends or during birth through an infected birth canal. Transplacental infection is rare. Approximately 50% of all infants born vaginally to a mother experiencing a primary genital HSV infection develop some form of herpes infection. Of these infants, about 60% will die in the neonatal period; of the survivors, about half will develop severe problems such as microcephaly, mental retardation, seizures, retinal dysplasia, apnea, and coma (Minkoff, 1999).

The infected infant is often asymptomatic at birth but develops symptoms of fever (or hypothermia), jaundice, seizures, and poor feeding after an incubation period of 2 to 12 days. Approximately half of infected infants develop the characteristic vesicular skin lesions. Vidarabine has been useful in decreasing serious effects from neonatal herpes, but no definitive treatment exists as yet. Some experts treat asymptomatic infants who were exposed to HSV during birth with acyclovir. Positive herpes cultures taken 24 to 48 hours after birth should be obtained before treatment (Centers for Disease Control and Prevention, 1998).

CLINICAL THERAPY

The vesicular lesions of herpes have a characteristic appearance, and they rupture easily. Definitive diagnosis is made by culturing active lesions.

ACOG (1999b) recommends antiviral therapy for women with primary HSV infection during pregnancy to decrease viral shedding and promote healing. Women with recurrent infection may also benefit from antiviral therapy. Three medications are available for that purpose: acyclovir, valaclovir, and famciclovir. Acyclovir has been shown to be effective and safe during pregnancy, but it is not as well absorbed as the other two drugs.

If there is no evidence of genital infection, vaginal birth is preferred. However, if the woman has any signs of active genital lesions or prodromal symptoms of infection such as vulvar pain or burning, cesarean birth is indicated. The woman with active HSV infection and ruptured membranes should also give birth by cesarean as soon as the necessary caregivers and equipment can be assembled (ACOG, 1999b).

HSV has not been found in breast milk. Present experience shows that breastfeeding is acceptable if there are no herpes lesions on the mother's breasts and if she washes her hands well to prevent any direct transfer of the virus.

Nursing Management

Nursing Assessment and Diagnosis

During the initial prenatal visit it is important to learn whether the woman or her partner have had previous herpes infections. If so, ongoing assessment is indicated as pregnancy progresses.

Nursing diagnoses that may apply include the following:

▶ *Sexual dysfunction* related to unwillingness to engage in sexual intercourse secondary to the presence of active herpes lesions

▶ *Ineffective individual coping* related to depression secondary to the risk to the fetus if herpes lesions are present at birth

Planning and Implementation

Client education about this fast-spreading disease is crucial. Women should be informed of the association of HSV infection with spontaneous abortion, newborn mortality and morbidity, and the possibility of cesarean birth. A woman needs to inform all health care providers of her infection. She should also know of the possible association of genital herpes with cervical cancer and the importance of a yearly Pap smear.

The woman who acquired HSV infection as an adolescent may be devastated as a mature adult who wants to have a family. She may be helped by counseling that allows her to express the negative feelings she may have about the infection. Literature may also be helpful and is available from Planned Parenthood and public health agencies. The American Social Health Association has established the HELP program to provide information on genital herpes. The association has a quarterly journal, *The Helper,* for clients with HSV infection.

Evaluation

Expected outcomes of nursing care include the following:

▶ The woman is able to describe her infection with regard to its method of spread, therapy and comfort measures, implications for her pregnancy, and long-term implications.

▶ The woman gives birth to a healthy infant.

OTHER INFECTIONS IN PREGNANCY

In addition to the TORCH infections, other infections contribute to risk during pregnancy. Spontaneous abortion is frequently the result of a severe maternal infection. Some evidence links infection and prematurity. In addition, if the pregnancy is carried to term in the presence of infection, the risk of maternal and fetal morbidity and mortality increases. Thus it is essential to maternal and fetal health that infection be diagnosed and treated promptly.

Table 13–4 provides a summary of other major infections and their implications for pregnancy. Urinary tract, vaginal, and sexually transmitted infections are also discussed in Chapter 3.

TABLE 13–4   Infections that Put Pregnancy at Risk

Condition and Causative Organism	Signs and Symptoms	Treatment	Implications for Pregnancy
GENERAL INFECTION			
Group B streptococcal disease (GBS): *Streptococcus agalactiae*	GBS is commonly found in the vagina and rectum of asymptomatic pregnant women. GBS causes urinary tract infection and has been linked to PROM, preterm labor, amnionitis, and postpartum infection (Cunningham et al., 2001). Inrapartum transmission from mother to fetus can cause serious infection in the newborn.	To prevent transmission to the newborn during birth, IV penicillin or ampicillin is administered to the mother during labor. Two screening options are recommended to detect maternal GBS: Screening approach: Collect vaginal and rectal swabs for GBS from all pregnant women at 35–37 weeks' gestation. If positive, give intrapartum antibiotics. Risk factor approach: Use intrapartum prophylaxis for women with risk factors (previous infant with GBS disease, less than 37 weeks' gestation, membranes ruptured $\geq$18 hr, temperature $\geq$ 100.4°F [38°C]) (CDC, 1996).	In the United States, GBS is the leading bacterial infection associated with newborn morbidity and mortality. In infants the most common signs of early infection are pneumonia, meningitis, and septicemia. Most infection can be prevented by intrapartum antibiotic therapy (Parks, Yetman, Moyer, et al., 2000).
URINARY TRACT INFECTIONS (UTI)			
Asymptomatic bacteriuria (ASB): *Escherichia, Klebsiella, Proteus* most common	Bacteria present in urine on culture with no accompanying symptoms.	Oral sulfonamides early in pregnancy, ampicillin and nitrofurantoin (Furadantin) in late pregnancy.	Women with ASB in early pregnancy may go on to develop cystitis or acute pyelonephritis by third trimester if not treated. Oral sulfonamides taken in the last few weeks of pregnancy may lead to neonatal hyperbilirubinemia and kernicterus.
Cystitis (lower UTI): Causative organisms same as for ASB	Dysuria, urgency, frequency; low-grade fever and hematuria may occur. Urine culture (clean catch) shows $\uparrow$ leukocytes. Presence of 10^5 (100,000) or more colonies bacteria per mL urine.	Same	If not treated, infection may ascend and lead to acute pyelonephritis.
Acute pyelonephritis: Causative organisms same as for ASB	Sudden onset. Chills, high fever, flank pain. Nausea, vomiting, malaise. May have decreased urine output, severe colicky pain, dehydration. Increased diastolic BP, positive fluorescent antibody (FA) test, low creatinine clearance. Marked bacteremia in urine culture, pyuria, WBC casts.	Hospitalization; IV antibiotic therapy. Other antibiotics safe during pregnancy include carbenicillin, methenamine, cephalosporins. Catheterization if output is $\downarrow$. Supportive therapy for comfort. Follow-up urine cultures are necessary.	Increased risk of premature birth and intrauterine growth restriction (IUGR). These antibiotics interfere with urinary estriol levels and can cause false interpretations of estriol levels during pregnancy.
VAGINAL INFECTIONS			
Vulvovaginal candidiasis (yeast infections): *Candida albicans*	Often thick, white, curdy discharge, severe itching, dysuria, dyspareunia. Diagnosis based on presence of hyphae and spores in a wet-mount preparation of vaginal secretions.	Intravaginal insertion of miconazole or clotrimazole suppositories at bedtime for 1 week. Cream may be prescribed for topical application to the vulva if necessary.	If the infection is present at birth and the fetus is born vaginally, the fetus may contract thrush.
Bacterial vaginosis: *Gardnerella vaginalis*	Thin, watery, yellow-gray discharge with foul odor often described as "fishy." Wet-mount preparation reveals "clue cells." Application of potassium hydroxide (KOH) to a specimen of vaginal secretions produces a pronounced fishy odor.	Nonpregnant women treated with oral metronidazole (Flagyl). In second and third trimesters, oral metronidazole administered in a lower dose; clindamycin orally and metronidazole vaginal gel are alternatives (CDC, 1998).	Metronidazole has potential teratogenic effects when used in the first trimester. Possible $\uparrow$ risk of PROM and preterm birth. Confirmatory studies needed (CDC, 1998).

TABLE 13–4 **Infections that Put Pregnancy at Risk—continued**

Condition and Causative Organism	Signs and Symptoms	Treatment	Implications for Pregnancy
VAGINAL INFECTIONS (CONTINUED)			
Trichomoniasis: *Trichomonas vaginalis*	Occasionally asymptomatic. May have frothy greenish gray vaginal discharge, pruritus, urinary symptoms. Strawberry patches may be visible on vaginal walls or cervix. Wet-mount preparation of vaginal secretions shows motile flagellated trichomonads.	During early pregnancy, symptoms may be controlled with clotrimazole vaginal suppositories. Both partners are treated, but no adequate treatment exists. After first trimester, a single 2-g dose of metronidazole may be used (CDC, 1998).	Metronidazole has potential teratogenic effects. Associated with ↑ risk of PROM and preterm birth (CDC, 1998).
SEXUALLY TRANSMITTED INFECTIONS			
Chlamydial infection: *Chlamydia trachomatis*	Women are often asymptomatic. Symptoms may include thin or purulent discharge, urinary burning and frequency, or lower abdominal pain. Lab test available to detect monoclonal antibodies specific for *Chlamydia*.	Although nonpregnant women are treated with tetracycline, it may permanently discolor fetal teeth. Thus, pregnant women are treated with erythromycin ethyl succinate.	Infant of woman with untreated chlamydial infection may develop newborn conjunctivitis, which can be treated with erythromycin eye ointment (but not silver nitrate). Infant may also develop chlamydial pneumonia. May be responsible for premature labor and fetal death.
Syphilis: *Treponema pallidum*, a spirochete	Primary stage: chancre, slight fever, malaise. Chancre lasts about 4 weeks, then disappears. Secondary stage: occurs 6 weeks to 6 months after infection. Skin eruptions (condyloma lata); also symptoms of acute arthritis, liver enlargement, iritis, chronic sore throat with hoarseness. Diagnosed by blood tests such as VDRL, RPR, FTA, ABS. Dark-field examination or spirochetes may also be done.	For syphilis less than 1 year in duration: 2.4 million U benzathine penicillin G IM. For syphilis of more than 1 year's duration: 2.4 million U benzathine penicillin G once a week for 3 weeks. Sexual partners should also be screened and treated.	Syphilis can be passed transplacentally to the fetus. If untreated, one of the following can occur: second-trimester abortion, stillborn infant at term, congenitally infected infant, uninfected live infant.
Gonorrhea: *Neisseria gonorrhoeae*	Majority of women asymptomatic; disease often diagnosed during routine prenatal cervical culture. If symptoms are present they may include purulent vaginal discharge, dysuria, urinary frequency, inflammation and swelling of the vulva. Cervix may appear eroded.	Nonpregnant women are treated with cefixime orally or ceftriaxone IM plus doxycycline. Pregnant woman are treated with ceftriaxone plus erythromycin (CDC, 1998). If the woman is allergic to ceftriaxone, spectinomycin is used. All sexual partners are also treated.	Infection at time of birth may cause ophthalmia neonatorum in the newborn.
Condyloma acuminata: caused by a papovavirus	Soft, grayish pink lesions on the vulva, vagina, cervix, or anus.	Podophyllin not used during pregnancy. Trichloroacetic acid, liquid nitrogen, or cryotherapy CO_2 laser therapy done under colposcopy is also successful (CDC, 1998).	Possible teratogenic effect of podophyllin. Large doses have been associated with fetal death.

CHAPTER HIGHLIGHTS

≫ Several health problems associated with bleeding arise from pregnancy, such as spontaneous abortion, ectopic pregnancy (EP), and gestational trophoblastic disease (GTD). The nurse needs to be alert to early signs of these situations, to guard the woman against heavy bleeding and shock, to facilitate the medical treatment, and to provide educational and emotional support.

≫ EP is the implantation of a fertilized ovum in a site other than the uterus. Treatment may be medical, using IM methotrexate, or surgical.

≫ Incompetent cervix, the premature dilatation of the cervix, is the most common cause of second-trimester abortion. It is treated surgically with a Shirodkar-Barter operation (cerclage), which involves placing a purse-string suture in the cervix to keep it closed.

≫ Hyperemesis gravidarum, excessive vomiting during pregnancy, may cause fluid and electrolyte imbalance, dehydration, and signs of starvation in the mother and, if severe enough, death of the fetus. Treatment is aimed at controlling the vomiting, correcting fluid and electrolyte imbalance, correcting dehydration, and improving nutritional status.

≫ Both premature rupture of the membranes and preterm labor place the fetus at risk. Women with PROM and no signs of infection are managed conservatively with bed rest and careful monitoring of fetal well-being. Women with a history of preterm labor are often placed on home fetal-monitoring programs. If preterm labor develops, tocolytics are often effective in stopping labor, but they have associated side effects.

≫ Hypertension may exist before pregnancy or may develop during pregnancy. Preeclampsia can lead to growth retardation for the fetus, and if untreated it may lead to convulsions (eclampsia) and even death for the mother and fetus. A woman's understanding of the disease process helps motivate her to maintain the required rest periods in the left lateral recumbent position. Antihypertensive or anticonvulsive drugs may be part of the therapy.

≫ Rh incompatibility can exist when an Rh-negative woman and an Rh-positive partner conceive a child who is Rh positive. The use of Rh immune globulin has greatly decreased the incidence of severe sequelae due to Rh because the drug "tricks" the body into thinking antibodies have been produced in response to the Rh antigen.

≫ The impact of surgery, trauma, or battering on the pregnant woman and her fetus is related to the seriousness, the timing in the pregnancy, and to other factors influencing the situation.

≫ Physical violence often begins or continues during pregnancy. The nurse needs to be alert for signs of abuse, including bruising or injury to the breasts, abdomen, or genitalia. The woman should be given information about female partner abuse and about community resources available to assist her.

≫ TORCH is an acronym standing for toxoplasmosis, rubella, cytomegalovirus, and herpes, all of which pose a grave threat to the fetus.

≫ Sexually transmitted infections pose less of a threat to the fetus if detected early and treated quickly.

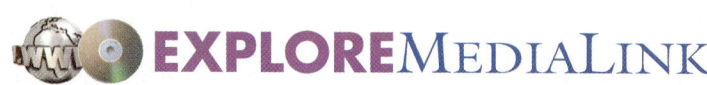

EXPLOREMediaLink

NCLEX Review, Case Studies, and other interactive resources for this chapter can be found on the companion website at http://www.prenhall.com/london. Click on "Chapter 13" to select the activities for this chapter.

For animations, more NCLEX review questions, and an audio glossary, access the accompanying CD-ROM in this textbook.

REFERENCES

Aerts, M., & Iams, J. D. (1999). Prevention of spontaneous preterm birth. *Contemporary OB/GYN, 44*(5), 128–136.

American Academy of Pediatrics and American College of Obstetricians and Gynecologists. (1997). Obstetric complications. In *Guidelines for prenatal care* (4th ed., pp. 127–146). Elk Grove Village, IL: Author.

American College of Obstetricians and Gynecologists. (1996). *Home uterine activity monitoring* (ACOG Committee Opinion No. 172). Washington, DC: Author.

American College of Obstetricians and Gynecologists. (1998a). *Medical management of tubal pregnancy* (ACOG Practice Bulletin No. 3). Washington, DC: Author.

American College of Obstetricians and Gynecologists. (1998b). *Obstetric aspects of trauma management* (ACOG Educational Bulletin No. 251). Washington, DC: Author.

American College of Obstetricians and Gynecologists. (1998c). *Premature rupture of membranes* (ACOG Practice Bulletin No. 1). Washington, DC: Author.

American College of Obstetricians and Gynecologists. (1999a). *Domestic violence* (ACOG Educational Bulletin No. 257). Washington, DC: Author.

American College of Obstetricians and Gynecologists. (1999b). *Management of herpes in pregnancy* (ACOG Practice Bulletin No. 8). Washington, DC: Author.

American College of Obstetricians and Gynecologists. (2000). *Perinatal viral and parasitic infections* (ACOG Practice Bulletin No. 20). Washington, DC: Author.

American College of Obstetricians and Gynecologists. (2001). *Management of early pregnancy loss* (ACOG Practice Bulletin). Washington, DC: Author.

Blumenthal, M. (2000). *Herbal medicine: Expanded Commission E Monographs.* Austin, TX: American Botanical Council.

Branch, D. W., & Porter, T. F. (1999). Hypertensive disorders of pregnancy. In J. R. Scott, P. J. DiSaia, C. B. Hammond, & W. N. Spellacy (Eds.), *Danforth's obstetrics and gynecology* (8th ed., pp. 309–326). Philadelphia: Lippincott Williams & Wilkins.

Centers for Disease Control and Prevention. (1996). Prevention of perinatal group B streptococcal disease: A public health perspective. *Morbidity and Mortality Weekly Report, 45*(RR-7), 1–25.

Centers for Disease Control and Prevention. (1998). 1998 sexually transmitted disease treatment guidelines. *Morbidity and Mortality Weekly Report, 47*(RR-1), 1–116.

Cerrato, P. L. (2001). An authoritative voice on antenatal corticosteroids. *Contemporary OB/GYN, 46*(3), 125–131.

Chez, R. A. (1999). Prevention of preterm birth: Putting three new tools into practice. *Contemporary OB/GYN, 44*(6), 53–78.

Creasy, R. K., & Iams, J. D. (1999). Preterm labor and delivery. In R. K. Creasy & R. Resnik (Eds.), *Maternal-fetal medicine* (4th ed., pp. 498–531). Philadelphia: Saunders.

Cunningham, F. G., Gant, N. F., Leveno, K. J., Gilstrap, L. C., III, Hauth, J. C., & Wenstrom, K. D. (2001). *Williams obstetrics* (21st ed.). New York: McGraw-Hill.

Guinn, D., & Lee, M. J. (2000). Multiple courses of antenatal corticosteroids: New concerns. *Contemporary OB/GYN, 45*(2), 63–69.

Iams, J. (1996a). Preterm birth. In S. G. Gabbe, J. R. Niebyl, & J. L. Simpson (Eds.), *Obstetrics: Normal and problem pregnancies* (3rd ed., pp. 743–820). New York: Churchill-Livingstone.

Iams, J. (1996b). Tocolysis. In J. T. Queenan & J. C. Hobbins (Eds.), *Protocols for high risk pregnancies* (pp. 539–546). Cambridge, MA: Blackwell.

Kurdas, C. (2001). New guidelines for detecting and managing hypertension in pregnancy. *Contemporary OB/GYN, 46*(2): 15–25.

Lopez, A., Dietz, V. J., Wilson, M., Navin, T. R., & Jones, J. L. (2000). Preventing congenital toxoplasmosis. *Morbidity and Mortality Weekly Report, 49*(RR-2), 57–75.

Lyon, D. S. (2000). First-trimester bleeding and pain. *The Female Patient, 25*(12), 80–84.

Martin, J. N., & Magann, E. F. (1999). High-dose dexamethasone: A promising therapeutic option for HELLP. *Contemporary OB/GYN, 44*(11), 55–64.

McFarlane, J., Parker, B., Soeken, K., Silva, C., & Reed, S. (1999). Severity of abuse before and during pregnancy for African American, Hispanic, and Anglo women. *Journal of Nurse-Midwifery, 44*(2), 139–144.

Mills, J. L., DerSimonian, R., Raymond, E., Morrow, J. D., Roberts, L. J., II, Clemens, J. D., et al. (1999). Prostacyclin and thromboxane changes predating clinical onset of preeclampsia. *Journal of the American Medical Association, 282*(4), 356–362.

Minkoff, L. (1999). Human immunodeficiency virus and other perinatal infections. In J. R. Scott, P. J. DiSaia, C. B. Hammond, & W. N. Spellacy (Eds.), *Danforth's obstetrics and gynecology* (8th ed., pp. 393–406). Philadelphia: Lippincott Williams & Wilkins.

National High Blood Pressure Education Program, (2000). Working group report on high blood pressure in pregnancy. *American Journal of Obstetrics and Gynecology, 83*, 51–54.

National Institutes of Health. (1994, February 28-March 2). *Effect of Corticosteroids for fetal maturation on perinatal outcomes.* National Institutes of Health Consensus Development Conference Statement.

Oshiro, B. T. (1999). Cytomegalovirus infection in pregnancy. *Contemporary OB/GYN, 44*(11), 16–24.

Parks, D. K., Yetman, R. J., Moyer, V., & Kennedy, K. (2000). Early-onset neonatal group B streptococcal infection: Implications for practice. *Journal of Pediatric Health Care, 14*(6), 264–269.

Parsons, M. T., & Spellacy, W. N. (1999a). Premature rupture of membranes. In J. R. Scott, P. J. DiSaia, C. B. Hammond, & W. N. Spellacy (Eds.), *Danforth's obstetrics and gynecology* (8th ed., pp. 269–278). Philadelphia: Lippincott Williams & Wilkins.

Parsons, M. T., & Spellacy, W. N. (1999b). Preterm labor. In J. R. Scott, P. J. DiSaia, C. B. Hammond, & W. N. Spellacy (Eds.), *Danforth's obstetrics and gynecology* (8th ed., pp. 257–268). Philadelphia: Lippincott Williams & Wilkins.

Roberts, J. M. (1999). Pregnancy-related hypertension. In R. K. Creasy & R. Resnik (Eds.), *Maternal-fetal medicine* (4th ed., pp. 833–872). Philadelphia: Saunders.

Scott, J. R. (1999). Early pregnancy loss. In J. R. Scott, P. J. DiSaia, C. B. Hammond, & W. N. Spellacy (Eds.), *Danforth's obstetrics and gynecology* (8th ed., pp. 143–154). Philadelphia: Lippincott Williams & Wilkins.

Scott, J. R., & Branch, D. W. (1999). Immunologic disorders in pregnancy. In J. R. Scott, P. J. DiSaia, C. B. Hammond, & W. N. Spellacy (Eds.), *Danforth's obstetrics and gynecology* (8th ed., pp. 363–392). Philadelphia: Lippincott Williams & Wilkins.

Skidmore-Roth, L. (2001). *Mosby's handbook of herbs and natural supplements.* St. Louis, MO: Mosby.

Sibai, B. M. (1996). Hypertension in pregnancy. In S. G. Gabbe, J. R. Niebyl, & J. L. Simpson (Eds.), *Obstetrics: Normal and problem pregnancies* (3rd ed., pp. 935–996). New York: Churchill Livingstone.

Silver, H. (1996). Hypertensive disorders. In K. R. Niswander & A. T. Evans (Eds.), *Manual of obstetrics* (pp. 283–295). Boston: Little, Brown.

Simon, E. P., & Schwartz, J. (1999). Medical hypnosis for hyperemesis gravidarum. *Birth, 26*(4), 248–253.

Tulandi, T. (1999). New protocols for ectopic pregnancy. *Contemporary OB/GYN, 44*(10), 42–55.

Vermillion, S. T., & Scardo, J. A. (2000). Using indomethacin as a tocolytic. *Contemporary OB/GYN, 45*(7), 102–108.

Weitz, B. W. (2001). Premature rupture of the fetal membranes: an update for advanced practice nurses. *American journal of maternal-child nursing 26*(2), 86–92.

Wenstrom, K. D., & Malee, M. P. (1999). Medical and surgical complications of pregnancy. In J. R. Scott, P. J. DiSaia, C. B. Hammond, & W. N. Spellacy (Eds.), *Danforth's obstetrics and gynecology* (8th ed., pp. 327–362). Philadelphia: Lippincott Williams & Wilkins.

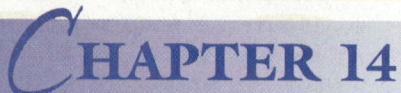

CHAPTER 14

Assessment of Fetal Status

My first pregnancy was so tenuous that I didn't know from one moment to the next how it would end. I hoped for our baby's safety, but in the end the baby died. When I became pregnant the next time, I was very nervous. Being able to see the baby on ultrasound helped me so much. I knew then that our baby was alive and growing.

—SHARON, 29

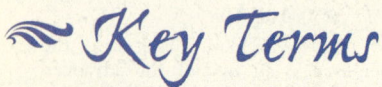 **Key Terms**

Amniocentesis *302*
Chorionic villus sampling
  (CVS) *304*
Biophysical profile (BPP) *299*
Contraction stress test (CST) *300*
Lecithin/sphingomyelin (L/S)
  ratio *303*
Nonstress test (NST) *297*

Percutaneous umbilical blood
  sampling (PUBS) *304*
Phosphatidylglycerol (PG) *303*
Surfactant *303*
Ultrasound *294*
Triple test *303*

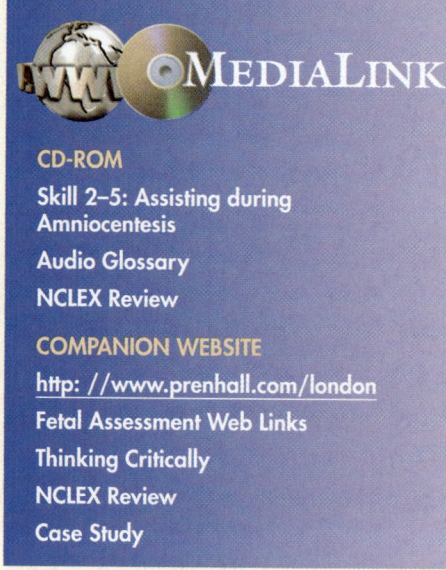

MediaLink

CD-ROM
Skill 2–5: Assisting during Amniocentesis
Audio Glossary
NCLEX Review

COMPANION WEBSITE
http://www.prenhall.com/london
Fetal Assessment Web Links
Thinking Critically
NCLEX Review
Case Study

The past few decades have produced a notable increase in the number of techniques used to assess fetal well-being. From the relatively simple maternal assessment of fetal movement to more complex diagnostic tests guided by ultrasound, each technique is used to obtain accurate and helpful data about the growing fetus. For example, specialized diagnostic tests can provide information about the normal growth of the fetus, the presence of congenital anomalies, the location of the placenta, and fetal lung maturity (Table 14–1). At times just one test is done, and in other circumstances a combination of testing is needed.

Some of these diagnostic techniques pose risks to the fetus and possibly to the pregnant woman, and the risk to both should be considered before the decision to perform the test is made. The health care provider must be certain that the advantages outweigh the potential risks and added expense. In addition, the diagnostic accuracy and applicability of these tests may vary. Certainly not all high-risk pregnancies require the same tests. Conditions that indicate a pregnancy at risk include the following:

- Maternal age less than 16 or more than 35 years
- Chronic maternal hypertension, preeclampsia, diabetes mellitus, or heart disease
- Presence of Rh isoimmunization
- A maternal history of unexplained stillbirth
- Suspected intrauterine growth restriction
- Pregnancy prolonged past 42 weeks' gestation
- Multiple gestation

See Chapter 7 for further discussion of prenatal at-risk factors and Chapters 12 and 13 for descriptions of various conditions that may threaten the successful completion of pregnancy.

Nursing care for the woman who is undergoing diagnostic testing focuses on outcomes to ensure that she understands the reasons for the test, understands the test results, and has had support during the test (see Table 14–2). In addition, other objectives include completing the tests without complication and ensuring that the safety of the mother and her unborn child has been maintained.

TABLE 14–1 Summary of Screening and Diagnostic Tests

Goal	Test	Timing
To validate the pregnancy	Ultrasound: gestational sac volume	5 and 6 weeks after last menstrual period by endovaginal ultrasound
To determine how advanced the pregnancy is	Ultrasound: crown–rump length	6 to 10 weeks' gestation
	Ultrasound: biparietal diameter, femur length, abdomen circumference	13 to 40 weeks' gestation
To identify normal growth of the fetus	Ultrasound: biparietal diameter	Most useful from 20 to 30 weeks' gestation
	Ultrasound: head/abdomen ratio	13 to 40 weeks' gestation
	Ultrasound: estimated fetal weight	About 24 to 40 weeks' gestation
To detect congenital anomalies and problems	Ultrasound	18 to 40 weeks' gestation
	Chorionic villus sampling	8 to 12 weeks' gestation
	Amniocentesis	16 to 18 weeks' gestation
	Fetoscopy	18 weeks' gestation
	Percutaneous blood sampling	Second and third trimesters
	Triple test or quadruple test	About 10 weeks' gestation
To localize the placenta	Ultrasound	Usually in third trimester or before amniocentesis
To assess fetal status	Biophysical profile	Approximately 28 weeks to birth
	Maternal assessment of fetal activity	About 28 weeks to birth
	Nonstress test	Approximately 28 weeks to birth
	Contraction stress test	After 28 weeks
To diagnose cardiac problems	Fetal echocardiography	Second and third trimesters
To assess fetal lung maturity	Amniocentesis	33 to 40 weeks
	L/S ratio	33 weeks to birth
	Phosphatidylglycerol	33 weeks to birth
	Phosphatidylcholine	33 weeks to birth
To obtain more information about breech presentation	Ultrasound	Just before labor is anticipated or during labor

TABLE 14-2 Sample Nursing Approaches to Pretest Teaching
Assess whether the woman knows the reason the screening or diagnostic test is being recommended.
Examples:
"Has your doctor or nurse-midwife told you why this test is necessary?"
"Sometimes tests are done for many different reasons. Can you tell me why you are having this test?"
"What is your understanding about what the test will show?"
Provide an opportunity for questions.
Examples:
"Do you have any questions about the test?"
"Is there anything that is not clear to you?"
Explain the test procedure, paying particular attention to any preparation the woman needs prior to the test.
Example:
"The test that has been ordered for you is designed to . . ." (Add specific information about the particular test. Give the explanation in simple language.)
Validate the woman's understanding of the preparation.
Example:
"Tell me what you will have to do to get ready for this test."
Give permission for the woman to continue to ask questions if needed.
Example:
"I'll be with you during the test. If you have any questions at any time, please don't hesitate to ask."

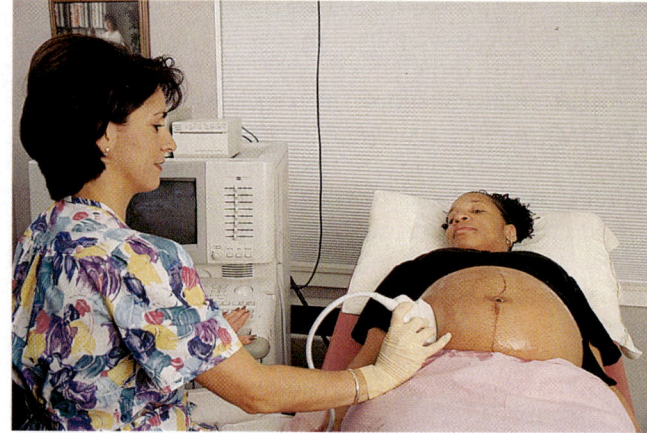

FIGURE 14–1. ◆ Ultrasound scanning permits visualization of the fetus in utero.

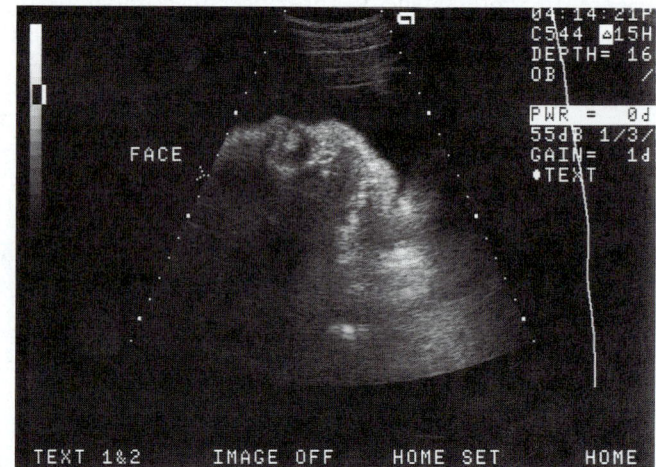

FIGURE 14–2. ◆ Ultrasound of fetal face.

MATERNAL ASSESSMENT OF FETAL ACTIVITY

Clinicians now generally agree that vigorous fetal activity provides reassurance of fetal well-being and that marked decrease in activity or cessation of movement may indicate possible fetal compromise (or even death) requiring immediate follow-up (Cunningham, Gant, Leveno, et al., 2001). Although there is considerable variation among individuals, the number of daily movements during the third trimester is a maximum of 575 until 32 weeks' gestation and then decreases to an average of 280 (12 to 15 gross fetal body movements per hour) (Jasper, 2000). In women with a multiple gestation, daily fetal movements are significantly higher. During the last few weeks of gestation the fetus spends 60% to 70% of its time in an active sleep state (Jasper, 2000).

Fetal activity is affected by many factors, including time of day, sleep states of the fetus, sound, blood glucose levels, cigarette smoking, and drugs. The expectant mother's perception of fetal movements and her commitment to completing a fetal movement record may vary. When a woman understands the purpose of the assessment, how to complete the form, whom to call with questions, and what to report—and has the opportunity for follow-up during each visit—she generally sees completing the fetal activity record as an important activity. The nurse is available to answer questions and clarify areas of concern. (See further discussion and "Teaching About: Assessing Fetal Activity" in Chapter 9.)

ULTRASOUND

Valuable information about the fetus may be obtained from **ultrasound** testing. Intermittent ultrasonic waves (high-frequency sound waves) are transmitted by an alternating current to a transducer, which is applied to the woman's abdomen. The ultrasonic waves deflect off tissues within the woman's abdomen, showing structures of varying densities (Figures 14–1 ◆ and 14–2 ◆). Diagnostic ultrasound has several advantages. It is noninvasive, painless, and nonradiating to both the woman and the fetus, and it has no known harmful effects to either. Serial studies (several ultrasound tests done over a span of time) may be done for assessment and comparison. Soft tissue masses (such as tumors) can be differentiated, the fetus can be visualized, fetal growth can be followed (especially in the presence of multiple gestation), and a number of potential problems can be averted (Barnhart, Simhan, & Kamelle, 1999). In addition, the ultrasonographer or physician obtains results immediately.

Future research in fetal well-being will be generated and enhanced by the use of the three-dimensional ultrasound. It is believed that this new technology will produce more accurate fetal growth and weight assessments (Zelop, 2000).

Procedures

The two most common methods of ultrasound scanning are transabdominal and endovaginal.

TRANSABDOMINAL ULTRASOUND

In the transabdominal approach, the examiner moves a transducer across the woman's abdomen. The woman is often scanned with a full bladder; when the bladder is full, the examiner can assess other structures, especially the vagina and cervix, in relation to the bladder. The ability to see the lower portion of the uterus and cervix is particularly important when vaginal bleeding is noted and placenta previa is the suspected cause. The woman is advised to drink 1 to 1.5 quarts of water approximately 2 hours before the examination, and she is asked to refrain from emptying her bladder. If the bladder is not sufficiently filled, she is asked to drink three to four (8-oz) glasses of water and is rescanned 30 to 45 minutes later. Mineral oil or a transmission gel is generously spread over the woman's abdomen, and the sonographer slowly moves a transducer over the abdomen to obtain a picture of the contents of the uterus. Ultrasound testing takes 20 to 30 minutes. The woman may feel discomfort due to pressure applied over a full bladder. In addition, if the woman lies on her back during the test, shortness of breath can develop. This may be relieved by elevating her upper body during the test.

ENDOVAGINAL ULTRASOUND

The endovaginal approach uses a probe inserted into the vagina. Once inserted, the endovaginal probe is close to the structures being imaged and so produces a clearer, more defined image. The improved images obtained by endovaginal ultrasound have enabled sonographers to identify structures and fetal characteristics earlier in pregnancy (Owen, Neely, & Northen, 1999). Internal visualization can also be used as a predictor for preterm birth in high-risk cases (Berghella, Daly, Tolosa, et al., 1999). Use of the ultrasound to detect shortened cervical length or funneling (a cone-shaped indentation in the cervical os) is helpful in predicting preterm labor, especially in women who have a history of preterm birth (Andrews, Copper, Hauth, et al., 2000).

After the procedure is fully explained to the woman, she is prepared in the same manner as for a pelvic examination: in the lithotomy position, with appropriate drapes to pro-vide privacy, and a female attendant in the room. It is important that her buttocks are at the end of the table so that, once inserted, the probe can be moved in various directions. A small, lightweight vaginal transducer is covered with a specially fitted sterile sheath, a condom, or one finger of a glove. Ultrasound coupling gel is then applied to the covering, making insertion into the vagina easier and providing a medium for enhancing the ultrasound image. The endovaginal procedure can be accomplished with an empty bladder, and most women do not feel discomfort during the exam. The probe is smaller than a speculum, so insertion is usually completed with ease. The woman may feel the movement of the probe during the exam as various structures are imaged. Some women may want to insert the probe themselves to enhance their comfort, whereas others would feel embarrassed even to be asked. The certified nurse-midwife, physician, or ultrasonographer offers the choice based on the rapport she or he has with the woman.

Clinical Applications

Ultrasound testing can be of benefit in the following ways (Barnhart et al., 1999; Berghella et al., 1999):

- Early identification of pregnancy. (Pregnancy may be detected as early as the fifth or sixth week after the last menstrual period [LMP].)
- Observation of fetal heartbeat and fetal breathing movements. Fetal breathing movements have been observed as early as the 11th week of gestation.
- Identification of more than one embryo or fetus.
- Measurement of the biparietal diameter of the fetal head or the fetal femur length. These measurements help determine the gestational age of the fetus and identify intrauterine growth restriction.
- Clinical estimations of birth weight. This assessment helps to identify macrosomia (infants greater than 4,000 g at birth). Macrosomia has been identified as a predictor of birth-related trauma (O'Reilly-Green & Divon, 2000).
- Detection of fetal anomalies such as anencephaly and hydrocephalus.
- Examination of fetal cardiac structures (*echocardiography*).
- Identification of *amniotic fluid index (AFI)*. The maternal abdomen is divided into quadrants. The umbilicus is used to divide the upper and lower sections, and the linea nigra divides the right and left sections. The vertical diameter of the largest amniotic fluid pocket in each quadrant is measured. All measurements are totaled to obtain the AFI in centimeters. Women with an AFI of more than 20 cm are considered to have hydramnios, and women with less than 5 cm at term are considered to have oligohydramnios. Both hydramnios and oligohydramnios

are associated with increased risk to the fetus (Wolfe & Moore, 2002).

- Location of the placenta. The placenta is located before amniocentesis to avoid puncturing the placenta. Ultrasound is also used to determine the presence of placenta previa.
- Placental grading. As the fetus matures, the placenta calcifies. These changes can be detected by ultrasound and graded according to the degree of calcification (Jasper, 2000).
- Detection of fetal death. Inability to visualize the fetal heart beating and the separation of the bones in the fetal head are signs of fetal death.
- Determination of fetal position and presentation.
- Accompanying procedures such as amniocentesis, periumbilical blood sampling, intrauterine procedures, and other procedures to be discussed shortly.

Risks of Ultrasound

Ultrasound has been used clinically for over 40 years, and to date no clinical studies verify harmful effects to the mother or the fetus or newborn. The use of ultrasound in pregnancy has spanned nearly three generations. Many pregnant patients themselves received diagnostic ultrasound in utero with no adverse effect (Manning, 1999).

Nursing Management

It is important for the nurse to ascertain whether the woman understands why the ultrasound is being suggested. Provide an opportunity for the woman to ask questions, and act as an advocate if there are questions or concerns that need to be addressed before the ultrasound examination. Explain the preparation needed and ensure that it is done. After the test is completed, help clarify or interpret test results for the woman and her partner, if necessary.

DOPPLER BLOOD FLOW STUDIES (UMBILICAL VELOCIMETRY)

Umbilical velocimetry, a noninvasive ultrasound test, assesses placental function by measuring blood flow changes that occur in maternal and fetal circulation. An ultrasound beam, like that provided by the pocket Doppler (a handheld ultrasound device), is directed at the umbilical artery (in some cases a maternal vessel such as the arcuate can also be used). The signal is reflected off the red blood cells moving within the vessels and creates a "picture" (waveform) that looks like a series of waves (Figures 14–3 ◆ and 14–4 ◆). The highest velocity peak of the waves is the systolic measurement, and the lowest point is the diastolic velocity. To interpret the waveforms, the systolic (S) peak is divided by the end-diastolic (D) component. This calculation is called

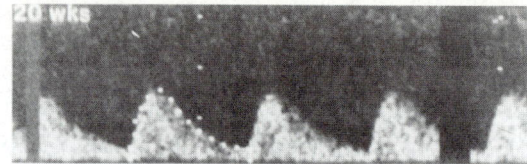
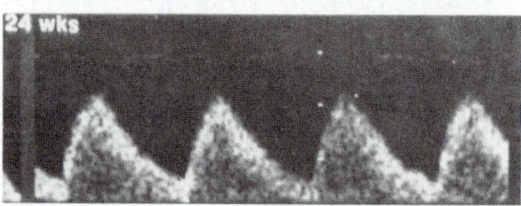
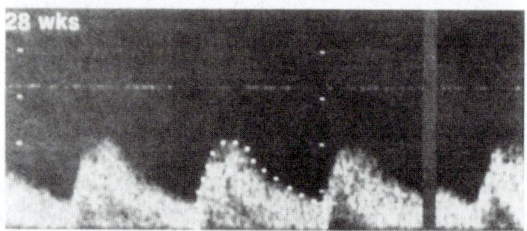
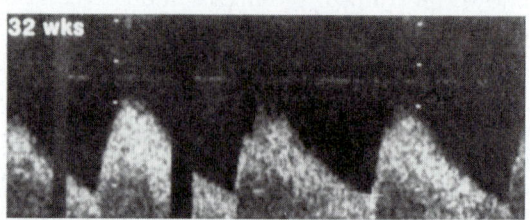
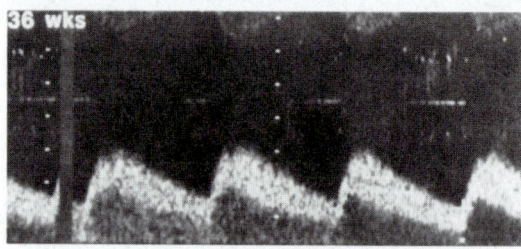
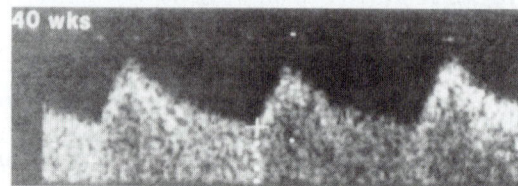

FIGURE 14–3. ◆ Serial studies of the umbilical artery velocity waveforms in a normal pregnancy from one client. *Note:* From Cundiff, J. L., Haubrich, K. L., & Hinzman, N. G. (1990). Umbilical artery Doppler flow studies during pregnancy. *Journal of Obstetric, Gynecologic, and Neonatal Nursing, 19*(6), 475, Figure 3.

the S/D ratio. The normal S/D ratio is below 2.6 by 26 weeks' gestation and below 3 at term. When uteroplacental perfusion decreases (because of narrowing of the vessels), it causes an increase in placental bed resistance and a decrease in diastolic flow, resulting in an elevated S/D ratio. Abnormal elevations are considered to be 3 and above (Jasper, 2000). Doppler blood flow studies are helpful in assessing

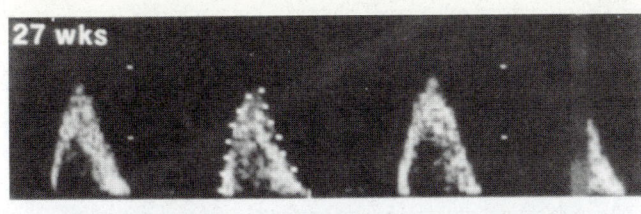

FIGURE 14–4. ◆ Two examples of abnormal umbilical artery velocity waveforms taken from a client with intrauterine growth restriction. *Note:* From Cundiff, J. L., Haubrich, K. L., & Hinzman, N. G. (1990). Umbilical artery Doppler flow studies during pregnancy. *Journal of Obstetric, Gynecologic, and Neonatal Nursing, 19*(6), 475, Figure 4.

and managing pregnancies with suspected uteroplacental insufficiency before asphyxia occurs (American College of Obstetricians and Gynecologists, 2000).

Doppler blood flow studies are relatively easy to obtain. The woman lies supine with a wedge under the left hip (to promote uteroplacental perfusion). Warmed transducer gel is applied to the abdomen, and a pulsed-wave Doppler device is used to ascertain the blood flow. The Doppler flow study takes about 15 to 20 minutes. Doppler flow studies can be initiated at 16 to 18 weeks' gestation and are then scheduled at regular intervals for women at risk.

NONSTRESS TEST

The **nonstress test (NST),** a widely used method of evaluating fetal status, may be used alone or as part of a more comprehensive diagnostic assessment called a biophysical profile (see discussion later in this chapter). The NST is based on the knowledge that when the fetus has adequate oxygenation and an intact central nervous system, there are accelerations of the fetal heart rate (FHR) with fetal movement. An NST requires an electronic fetal monitor to observe and record these fetal heart rate accelerations (see discussion of acceleration in Chapter 16). A nonreactive NST is fairly consistent in identifying at-risk fetuses. The advantages of the NST are as follows:

- It is quick to perform, permits easy interpretation, and is inexpensive.
- It can be done in an office or clinic setting.
- There are no known side effects.

The disadvantages of the NST include the following:

- It is sometimes difficult to obtain a suitable tracing.
- The woman has to remain relatively still for at least 20 minutes.

Procedure for NST

The test can be done with the woman in a reclining chair or in bed in a semi-Fowler's or side-lying position. Research has shown that the semi-Fowler's position may shorten the time needed to conduct the NST (Nathan, Haberman, Burgess, et al., 2000). An electronic fetal monitor is used to obtain a tracing of the FHR and fetal movement. The examiner puts two elastic belts on the woman's abdomen. One belt holds a device that detects uterine or fetal movement; the other belt holds a device that detects the FHR. As the NST is done, each fetal movement is documented, so that associated or simultaneous FHR changes can be evaluated. Women with a high-risk factor will probably begin having NSTs at 30 to 32 weeks' gestation and at frequent intervals for the remainder of the pregnancy.

Interpretation of NST Results

The results of the NST are interpreted as follows:

- *Reactive test.* A reactive NST shows at least two accelerations of FHR with fetal movements of 15 beats per minute, lasting 15 seconds or more, over 20 minutes (Figure 14–5 ◆). This is the desired result (Table 14–3).
- *Nonreactive test.* In a nonreactive test, the reactive criteria are not met. For example, the accelerations are not as much as 15 beats per minute or do not last 15 seconds (Figure 14–6 ◆).
- *Unsatisfactory test.* An NST is unsatisfactory if the data cannot be interpreted or there was inadequate fetal activity.

It is important that anyone who performs the NST understand the significance of any decelerations of the FHR during testing. If decelerations are noted, the certified nurse-midwife or physician should be notified for further evaluation of fetal status. (See Chapter 16 for further discussion of FHR decelerations.)

Clinical Management

The clinical management of potential fetal stress or distress may vary somewhat among clinicians depending on the clinical judgment of the care provider. One commonly used protocol is as follows: If the NST is reactive in less than 30 minutes, the test is concluded and rescheduled as indicated by the high-risk condition that is present; if it is nonreactive, the test time is extended for 30 minutes at a time until the results are reactive, and then the test is rescheduled as indicated. If the FHR remains nonreactive, additional testing (such as diagnostic ultrasound and biophysical profile) or immediate birth is considered; if the NST is nonreactive and spontaneous decelerations of the FHR are present, diagnostic ultrasound and biophysical profile are performed and birth is recommended (Figure 14–7 ◆).

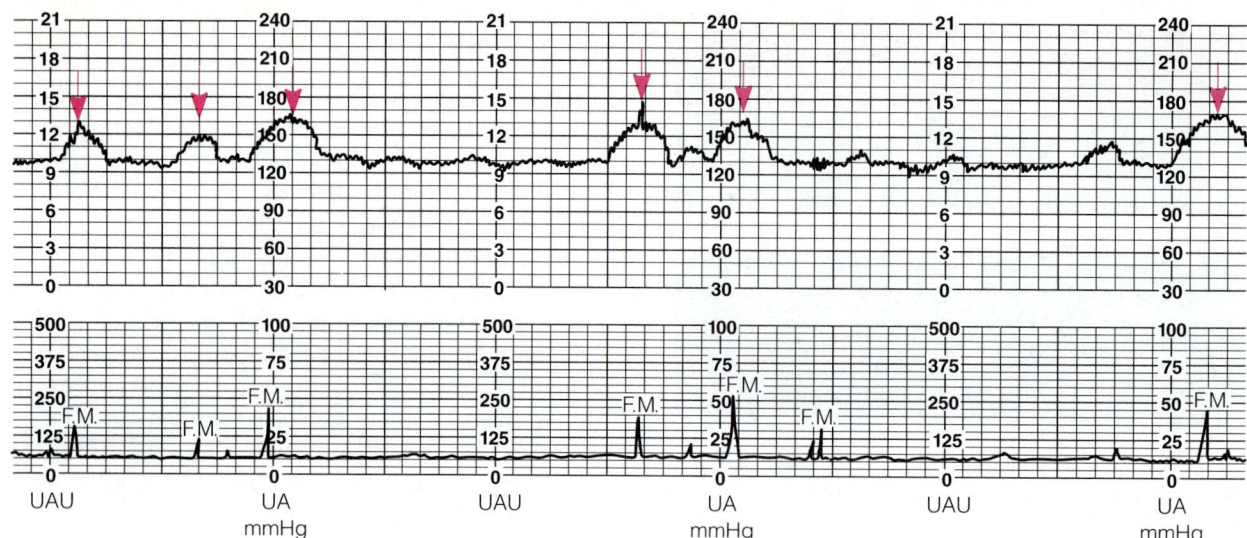

FIGURE 14–5. ◆ Example of a reactive nonstress test (NST). Accelerations of 15 bpm lasting 15 seconds with each fetal movement (FM). Top of strip shows FHR; bottom of strip shows uterine activity tracing. Note that FHR increases (above the baseline) at least 15 beats and remains at that rate for at least 15 seconds before returning to the former baseline.

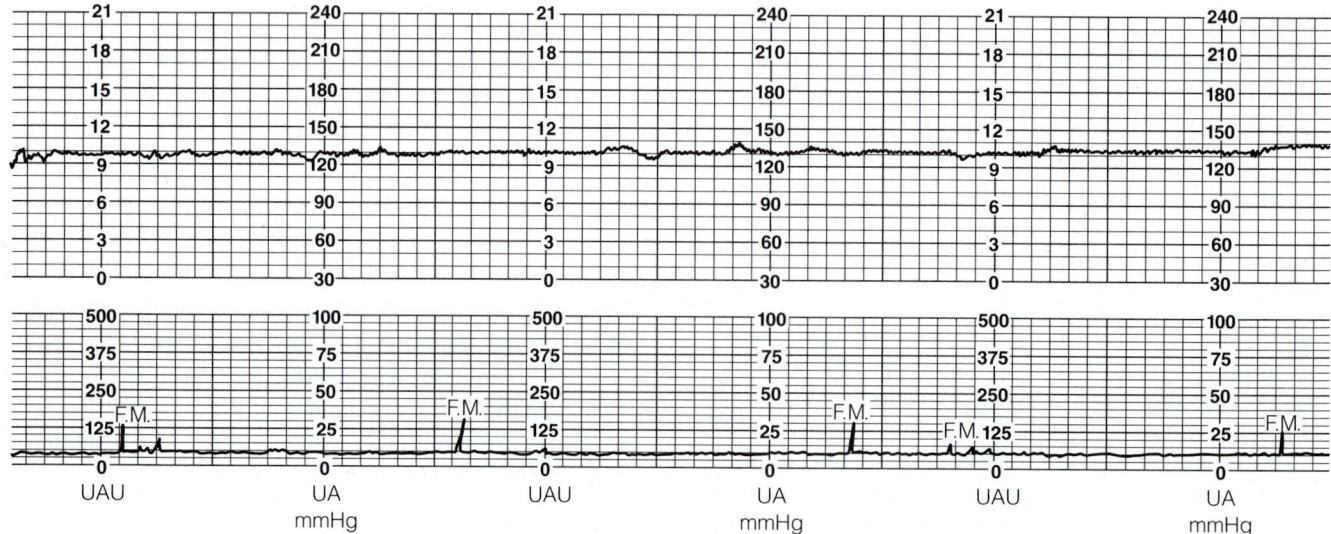

FIGURE 14–6. ◆ Example of a nonreactive NST. There are no accelerations of FHR with FM. Baseline FHR is 130 bpm. The tracing of uterine activity is on the bottom of the strip.

TABLE 14-3	Nonstress Test
Diagnostic Value	*Results*
Demonstrates fetus's ability to respond to its environment by acceleration of FHR with movement.	• Reactive test: Accelerations of 15 beats/min above the baseline, lasting 15 sec in a 20-min window, are present, indicating fetal well-being. • Nonreactive test: Accelerations are not present, indicating that the fetus is sick or asleep.

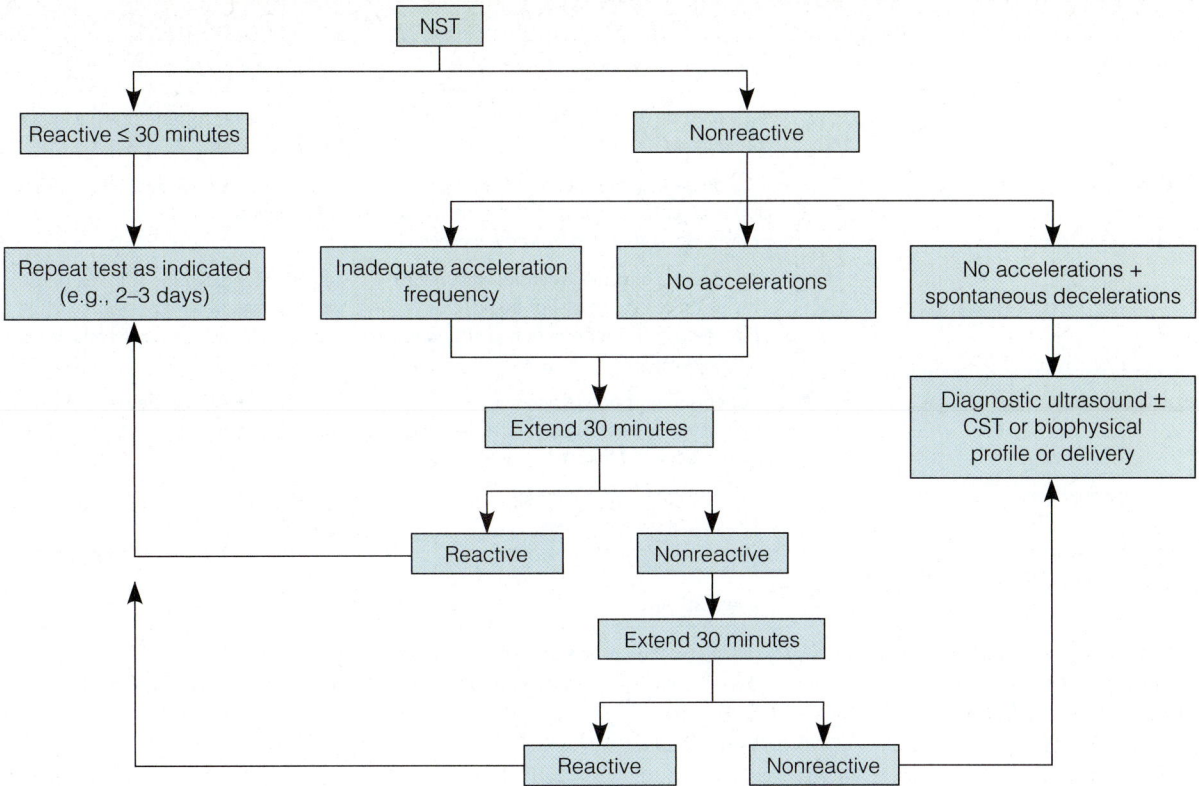

FIGURE 14–7. ◆ NST management scheme. *Note:* From Devoe, L. D. (1989). Nonstress and contraction stress testing. In R. Depp, D. A. Eschenbach, & J. J. Sciarri (Eds.), *Gynecology and obstetrics* (Vol. 3, p. 9, Figure 5). Philadelphia: Lippincott.

Many testing guidelines vary in frequency, recommending a retest either once or twice a week, depending upon the at-risk condition that exists. In some situations, such as preterm premature rupture of membranes, testing may be done daily (Jasper, 2000; Parer, 1999).

Nursing Management

Evaluate the woman's understanding of the NST and the possible results. Review the reasons for the NST and the procedure before beginning the test. Administer the NST, interpret the results, and report the findings to the certified nurse-midwife or physician and the expectant woman.

FETAL ACOUSTIC STIMULATION TEST (FAST) AND VIBROACOUSTIC STIMULATION TEST (VST)

Acoustic (sound) and vibroacoustic (vibration and sound) stimulation of the fetus can be used as an adjunct to the NST. A handheld, battery-operated device is applied to the woman's abdomen over the area of the fetal head. This device generates a low-frequency vibration and a buzzing sound that are intended to induce movement and associated accelerations of FHR in fetuses with a nonreactive NST and in fetuses with decreased variability of FHR during labor. (See discussion of variability in Chapter 16.) The sound stimulus lasts for 1 to 2 seconds; if no accelerations occur, it can be repeated up to three times for up to 3 seconds (Cunningham et al., 2001). Whether the fetus responds more to the vibration or to the sound is not known. Two FHR accelerations of 15 beats per minute, lasting 15 seconds, in a 10-minute period, indicate a reactive test (Jasper, 2000; Schmidt, 2000). Advantages of the fetal acoustic stimulation test and the vibroacoustic stimulation test are

* Both are noninvasive and easy to perform.
* Results are rapidly available.
* Time for the NST is shortened.

BIOPHYSICAL PROFILE

The **biophysical profile (BPP)** is a comprehensive assessment of five biophysical variables: fetal breathing movement, fetal movements of body or limbs, fetal tone (extension and flexion of extremities), amniotic fluid volume (visualized as pockets of fluid around the fetus), and reactive FHR with activity (reactive NST). The first four variables are assessed by ultrasound scanning; FHR reactivity is assessed with the NST. By combining these five assessments, the BPP helps to identify the compromised fetus and to confirm the healthy fetus. A score of 2 is assigned to each normal find-

TABLE 14-4 Biophysical Profile Scoring: Technique and Interpretation

Biophysical Variable	Normal (Score = 2)	Abnormal (Score = 0)
Fetal breathing movements	≥1 episode of ≥30 seconds in 30 minutes	Absent or no episode of ≥30 seconds in 30 minutes
Gross body movements	≥3 discrete body or limb movements in 30 minutes (Episodes of active continuous movement considered as single movement.)	≤2 episodes of body or limb movements in 30 minutes
Fetal tone	≥1 episode of active extension with return to flexion of fetal limb(s) or trunk (Opening and closing of hand considered normal tone.)	Either slow extension with return to partial flexion or movement of limb in full extension or absent fetal movement
Reactive fetal heart rate	≥2 episodes of acceleration of ≥ 15 bpm and of ≥ 15 seconds associated with fetal movement in 20 minutes	<2 episodes of acceleration of fetal heart rate or acceleration of <15 bpm in 20 minutes
Qualitative amniotic fluid volume	≥1 pocket of fluid measuring ≥1 cm in two perpendicular planes	Either no pockets or a pocket <1 cm in two perpendicular planes

Management Based on Biophysical Profile Score Attained Score	Intervention
10 of 10 or 8 of 10, with normal amniotic fluid volume	No intervention is needed; normal finding.
8 of 10 with abnormal amniotic fluid volume	If fetal renal function is normal and membranes are intact, delivery is indicated.
6 of 10 with normal amniotic fluid volume	Equivocal
4 of 10, 2 of 10, or 0 of 10	Deliver fetus.

Note: From Manning, F. (1999). Fetal assessment by evaluation of biophysical variables. In R. K. Creasy & R. Resnik (Eds.), *Maternal-fetal medicine* (4th ed., pp. 319–330). Philadelphia: Saunders.

ing, and 0 to each abnormal one, for a maximum score of 10. The absence of a specific activity is difficult to interpret, since it may be indicative of central nervous system depression or simply the resting state of a healthy fetus. Scores of 8 (with normal amniotic fluid) and 10 are considered normal. Such scores have the least chance of being associated with a compromised fetus unless a decrease in the amount of amniotic fluid is noted, in which case the infant's birth may be indicated (Jasper, 2000). A management protocol regarding BPP is outlined in Table 14–4.

The BPP is indicated when there is risk of placental insufficiency or fetal compromise because of the following:

- Intrauterine growth restriction
- Maternal diabetes mellitus
- Maternal heart disease
- Maternal chronic hypertension
- Maternal preeclampsia or eclampsia (pregnancy-induced hypertension)
- Maternal sickle cell anemia
- Suspected fetal postmaturity (more than 42 weeks' gestation)
- History of previous stillbirths
- Rh sensitization
- Abnormal estriol excretion
- Hyperthyroidism

- Renal disease
- Nonreactive NST

CONTRACTION STRESS TEST

The **contraction stress test (CST)** evaluates the respiratory function (oxygen and carbon dioxide exchange) of the placenta. It lets the health care team identify the fetus at risk for intrauterine asphyxia by observing how the FHR responds to the stress of uterine contractions (spontaneous or induced). During contractions, intrauterine pressure increases. Blood flow to the intervillous space of the placenta is reduced momentarily, thereby decreasing oxygen transport to the fetus. A healthy fetus usually tolerates this reduction well and maintains a steady heart rate. If the placental reserve is insufficient, fetal hypoxia, depression of the myocardium, and a decrease in FHR occur.

Although the CST is not used as frequently as in the past, it is still used when the availability of other technology is reduced (such as during night shifts) or where it is limited (such as at small community hospitals or birthing centers). It may also be used as an adjunct to other forms of fetal assessment. In many areas, however, the CST has given way to the BPP.

The CST is contraindicated if there is third-trimester bleeding from placenta previa or marginal abruptio placentae, previous cesarean with classical incision (vertical incision in the fundus of the uterus), premature rupture of the membranes, incompetent cervix, or multiple gestation.

Procedure

The critical component of the CST is the presence of uterine contractions. They may occur spontaneously (which is unusual prior to the onset of labor), or they may be induced (stimulated) with oxytocin (Pitocin) administered intravenously. Another method of obtaining oxytocin is through the use of breast stimulation during a breast self-stimulation test (also called nipple self-stimulation); the posterior pituitary produces oxytocin in response to stimulation of the breasts or nipples.

An electronic fetal monitor is used to provide continuous data about the FHR and uterine contractions. After a 15-minute baseline recording of uterine activity and FHR, the tracing is evaluated for evidence of spontaneous contractions. If three spontaneous contractions of good quality and lasting 40 to 60 seconds occur in a 10-minute window, the results are evaluated, and the test is concluded. If no contractions occur or they are insufficient for interpretation, oxytocin is administered intravenously, or breast self-stimulation is done to produce contractions of good quality. (See Chapter 20 for more information on nursing care management of oxytocin induction.)

Interpretation of CST Results

The CST is classified as follows:

- *Negative.* A negative CST shows three contractions of good quality lasting 40 or more seconds in 10 minutes without evidence of late decelerations. This is the desired result. It implies that the fetus can handle the hypoxic stress of uterine contractions.

- *Positive.* A positive CST shows repetitive persistent late decelerations with more than 50% of the contractions (even if the contraction frequency is fewer than three in 10 minutes) (American College of Obstetricians and Gynecologists, 1999). This is not a desired result. The hypoxic stress of the uterine contraction causes a slowing of the FHR. The pattern will not improve and will most likely get worse with additional contractions (Figure 14–8 ◆).

- *Equivocal or suspicious.* An equivocal or suspicious test has nonpersistent late decelerations or decelerations associated with hyperstimulation (contraction frequency of < 2 minutes or duration of > 90 seconds). When this test result occurs, more information is needed.

Clinical Application

A negative CST implies that the placenta is functioning normally, fetal oxygenation is adequate, and the fetus will be able to withstand the stress of labor, if it occurs within the ensuing week. A positive CST with a nonreactive NST presents evidence that the fetus will not likely withstand the stress of labor. Although a negative CST is reliable in predicting fetal status, a positive result needs to be verified. As many as 50% of fetuses with positive CSTs may tolerate labor without any further signs of fetal stress (a false-positive result) (Parer, 1999). See Table 14–5.

Nursing Management

Ascertain the woman's understanding of the CST, the reasons for the test, and the possible results before the test begins. Written consent is required in some settings. In this case, the certified nurse-midwife or physician is responsible

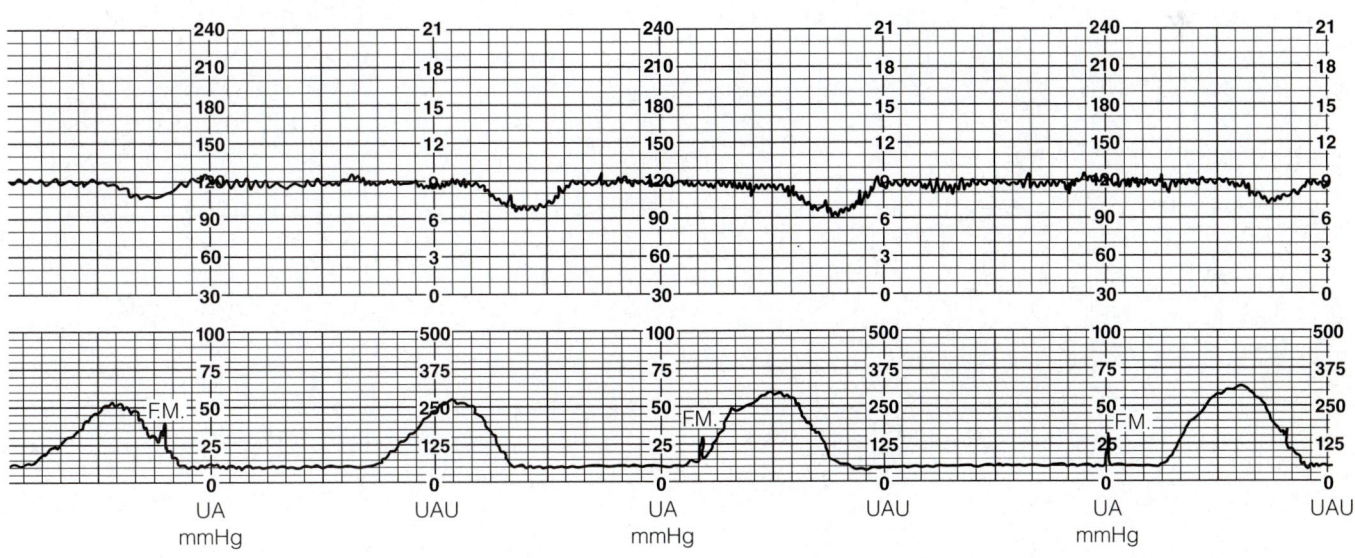

FIGURE 14–8. ◆ Example of a positive contraction stress test (CST). Repetitive late decelerations occur with each contraction. Note that there are no accelerations of FHR with three fetal movements (FM). The baseline FHR is 120 bpm. Uterine contractions (bottom half of strip) occurred four times in 12 minutes.

TABLE 14–5	Contraction Stress Test
Diagnostic Value	Results
Demonstrates reaction of FHR to stress of uterine contraction.	• Negative test: Stress of uterine contraction does not cause a late deceleration of the FHR. • Positive test: Stress of uterine contraction is associated with a late deceleration of the FHR.

for fully informing the woman about the test. Administer the CST, interpret the results, and report the findings to the certified nurse-midwife or physician and the expectant woman. Throughout the procedure, perform critical assessments and provide continual reassurance to the woman and her support person.

AMNIOTIC FLUID ANALYSIS

Amniocentesis is a procedure used to obtain amniotic fluid for testing. The amniotic fluid is withdrawn by a needle inserted through the abdominal wall into the uterus (Figure 14–9 ◆). The analysis of amniotic fluid provides valuable information about fetal status. Amniocentesis is a fairly simple procedure, although complications do occur

rarely (less than 1% of cases). See Skill 2–5 in the *Clinical Skills Manual,* as well as the CD-ROM that accompanies this text, for more information. ⊂▭ CD SKILLS

Nursing Management

Assist the physician during the amniocentesis and support the woman undergoing the procedure. Although the physician has explained the procedure in advance so that the woman can give informed consent, the woman is likely to be apprehensive both about the amniocentesis itself and about the information it may reveal. She may become anxious during the procedure and need additional emotional support. Provide support by further clarifying the physician's instructions or explanations, by relieving the woman's physical discomfort when possible, and by responding verbally and physically to the woman's need for reassurance.

Obtain maternal blood pressure, temperature, pulse, respirations, and FHR baseline data prior to the procedure and then monitor these parameters every 15 minutes during the procedure. Assist with the real-time ultrasound in order to assess needle position during the amniocentesis. Real-time ultrasound is used to identify fetal parts and locate pockets of amniotic fluid.

Following the amniocentesis, reiterate explanations given by the physician and provide opportunities for questions.

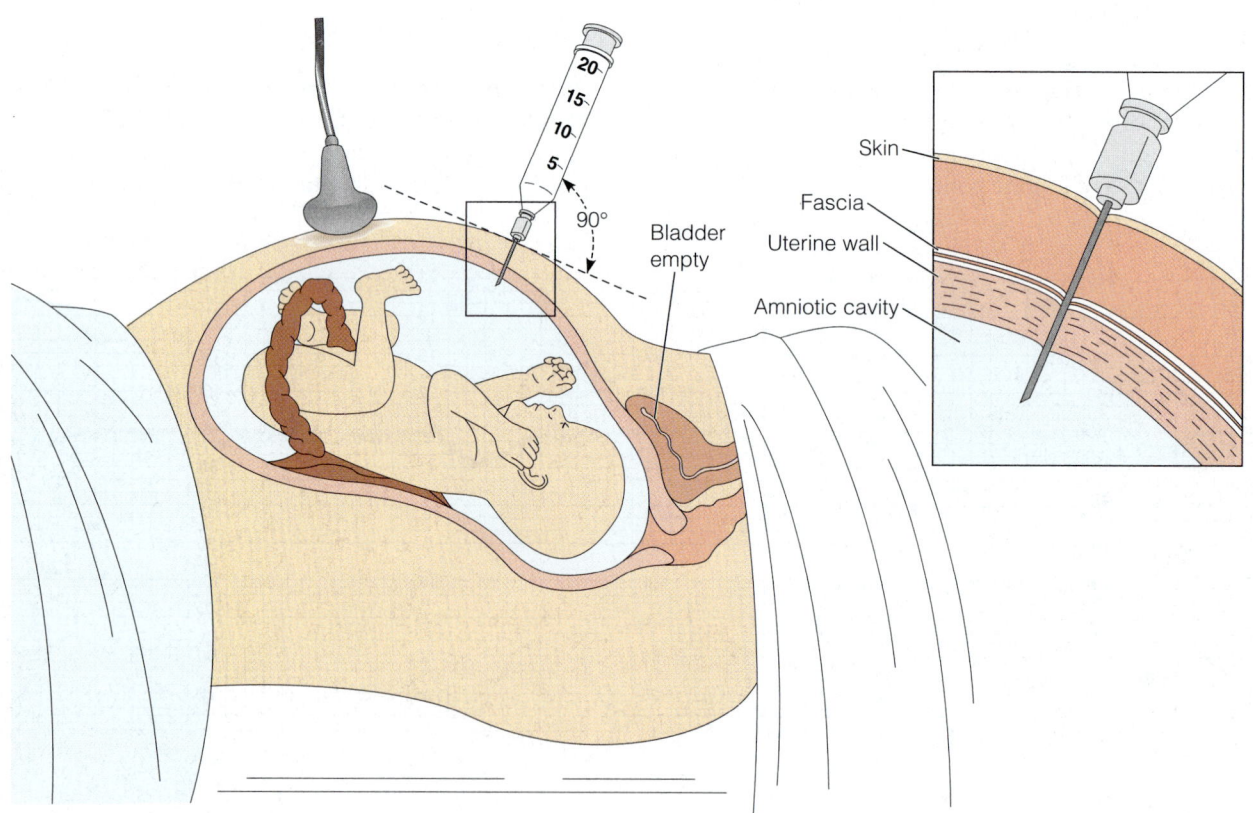

FIGURE 14–9. ◆ Amniocentesis. The woman is scanned by ultrasound to determine the placental site and to locate a pocket of amniotic fluid. Then the needle is inserted into the uterine cavity to withdraw amniotic fluid.

Review the experience with the woman and explain self-care measures. Monitor the woman's blood pressure, pulse, respirations, and the FHR. The woman's fundus is monitored with an external fetal heart monitor for 20 to 30 minutes after the amniocentesis. If the woman develops supine hypotension, initiate a treatment plan to increase venous return and cardiac output such as lying on her left side. The women's blood type and need for Rh immune globulin is determined. Prior to discharge, the woman should understand the side effects that are to be reported to her primary care provider.

Reportable side effects of an amniocentesis include:

- Unusual fetal hyperactivity or lack of movement
- Vaginal discharge—clear drainage or bleeding
- Uterine contractions or abdominal pain
- Fever or chills

The woman is encouraged to engage in only light activity for 24 hours after amniocentesis to decrease uterine irritability. She is also encouraged to increase her fluid intake to increase uteroplacental circulation and thereby replace the amniotic fluid.

Diagnostic Uses of Amniocentesis

A number of studies can be performed on amniotic fluid following amniocentesis. These tests can provide information about genetic disorders (see Chapter 4), ⌘ fetal health, and fetal lung maturity. The remainder of this section describes the amniotic fluid studies. Concentrations of certain substances in amniotic fluid provide information about the health status of the fetus. For example, the **triple test** assesses for appropriate levels of alpha fetoprotein, human chorionic gonadotrophin, and unconjugated estriol. The triple test is the current standard used to screen for Down syndrome (trisomy 21), trisomy 18, and neural tube defect. A more sensitive and accurate detector of trisomy 21, the quadruple screen (adds measurement of the substance Diameric Inhibin-A), will replace the triple screen as the standard in the near future (McColgin, 1999).

When managing a high-risk pregnancy, the caregiver is faced with the possibility of naturally occurring preterm labor or the need to terminate the pregnancy by induction of labor or cesarean birth. Indications for early termination of pregnancy include premature rupture of membranes and developing amnionitis (infection of the amnion), severe preeclampsia or eclampsia, bleeding problems (HELLP syndrome, placenta previa, abruptio placenta, and disseminated intravascular coagulation), worsening Rh sensitization, and placental insufficiency. When an infant is born before the lungs are mature, the risk of complications such as respiratory distress syndrome is high.

EVALUATION OF FETAL MATURITY

Because gestational age, birth weight, and the rate of development of organ systems do not necessarily correspond, amniotic fluid may also be analyzed to determine the maturity of the fetal lungs.

Lecithin/Sphingomyelin (L/S) Ratio. The alveoli of the lungs are lined with a substance called **surfactant,** which is composed of phospholipids. Surfactant lowers the surface tension of the alveoli when the newborn exhales. When a newborn with mature pulmonary function takes its first breath, a tremendously high pressure is needed to open the lungs. By lowering the alveolar surface tension, surfactant stabilizes the alveoli, and a certain amount of air always remains in the alveoli during expiration. Thus, when the infant exhales, the lungs do not collapse. An infant born before synthesis of surfactant is complete is unable to maintain lung stability. Each breath requires the same effort as the first. This results in underinflation of the lungs and the development of respiratory distress syndrome (RDS).

Fetal lung maturity can be ascertained by determining the **lecithin/sphingomyelin (L/S) ratio;** lecithin and sphingomyelin are two components of surfactant. Early in pregnancy, the sphingomyelin concentration in amniotic fluid is greater than the concentration of lecithin, and so the L/S ratio is low (lecithin levels are low and sphingomyelin levels are high). At about 32 weeks' gestation, sphingomyelin levels begin to fall and the amount of lecithin begins to increase. By 35 weeks' gestation, an L/S ratio of 2:1 (also reported as 2.0) is usually achieved in the normal fetus. A 2:1 L/S ratio indicates that the risk of respiratory distress syndrome is very low (Jobe, 1999). Under certain conditions of stress (a physiologic problem in the mother, placenta, and/or fetus), the fetal lungs mature more rapidly.

Phosphatidylglycerol. Phosphatidylglycerol (PG) is another phospholipid in surfactant. PG is not present in the fetal lung fluid early in gestation. It appears when fetal lung maturity has been attained, at about 35 weeks' gestation. Since the presence of PG is associated with fetal lung maturity, when it is present the risk of respiratory distress syndrome is low. PG determination is also useful in blood-contaminated specimens. Since PG is not present in blood or vaginal fluids, its presence reliably predicts lung maturity (Jobe, 1999). See Table 14–6.

TABLE 14–6	L/S Ratio and PG
Diagnostic Value	Results
Provides information to help determine fetal lung maturity.	• L/S ratio of 2:1 and presence of PG correlate with 35 weeks' gestation. • An L/S ratio lower than 2:1 and/or an absence of PG may indicate underinflation of lungs and an increased risk for development of respiratory distress syndrome.

OTHER FETAL DIAGNOSTIC TESTING

Chorionic villus sampling (CVS) involves obtaining a small sample of chorionic villi from the developing placenta. CVS is performed in some medical centers for first-trimester diagnosis of genetic, metabolic, and DNA studies. The advantages of this procedure are early diagnosis and short waiting time for results. Whereas amniocentesis is not done until at least 16 weeks' gestation, CVS is performed between weeks 8 and 12 (Scioscia, 1999).

Percutaneous umbilical blood sampling is used to obtain a fetal blood sample for a variety of blood disorders, chromosome abnormalities, and certain diseases, as well as fetal karyotyping. This procedure uses ultrasound-guided imaging to locate the fetal umbilical cord. A needle is introduced through the maternal abdomen into the umbilical cord and a blood sample is aspirated.

CHAPTER HIGHLIGHTS

☞ Maternal assessment of fetal activity can be used as a screening tool to provide information about fetal well-being.

☞ Ultrasound offers a valuable way to assess intrauterine fetal growth because the growth can be followed over a period of time. It is noninvasive and painless, allows the certified nurse-midwife or physician to study the gestation serially, is nonradiating to both the woman and her fetus, and has no known harmful effects.

☞ Doppler blood flow studies are used to assess placental function and sufficiency.

☞ An NST is based on the knowledge that the FHR normally increases in response to fetal activity and to sound stimulation. The desired result is a reactive test.

☞ A fetal BPP includes five variables (fetal breathing movement, fetal body movement, fetal tone, amniotic fluid volume, and FHR reactivity) to assess the fetus at risk for intrauterine compromise.

☞ A CST provides a way to observe the response of the FHR to the stress of uterine contractions. The desired result is a negative test.

☞ Amniocentesis can be used to obtain amniotic fluid for a variety of tests, including the L/S ratio and PG.

☞ The L/S ratio can be used to assess fetal lung maturity. The presence of PG also provides information about fetal lung maturity.

☞ The triple test (and quadruple screen) measures substances contained in the amniotic fluid that provide information regarding the presence of fetal anomalies, such as neural tube defects and Down syndrome.

EXPLORE MediaLink

NCLEX Review, Case Studies, and other interactive resources for this chapter can be found on the companion website at http://www.prenhall.com/london. Click on "Chapter 14" to select the activities for this chapter.

For animations, more NCLEX review questions, and an audio glossary, access the accompanying CD-ROM in this textbook.

REFERENCES

American College of Obstetricians and Gynecologists. (1999). *Antepartum fetal surveillance* (Practice Bulletin No. 9). Washington, DC: Author.

American College of Obstetricians and Gynecologists. (2000). *Intrauterine growth restriction* (Practice Bulletin No. 12). Washington, DC: Author.

Andrews, W. W., Copper, R., Hauth, J. C., Goldenberg, R. L., Neely, C., & Dubard, M. (2000). Second-trimester cervical ultrasound associations with increased risk of recurrent early spontaneous delivery. *Obstetrics and Gynecology, 95*(2), 222–226.

Barnhart, K. T., Simhan, H., & Kamelle, S. A. (1999). Diagnostic accuracy of ultrasound above and below the beta-hCG discriminatory zone. *Obstetrics and Gynecology. 94,* 583–586.

Berghella, V., Daly, S. F., Tolosa, J. E., DiVito, M., Chalmers, R., Garg, N., et al. (1999). Prediction of preterm delivery with transvaginal ultrasound of the cervix in patients with high-risk pregnancies: Does cerclage prevent prematurity? *American Journal of Obstetrics and Gynecology, 181,* 809–810.

Cunningham, F. G., Gant, N. F., Leveno, K. J., Gilstrap, L. C., Hauth, J. C., & Wenstrom, K. D. (2001). *Williams obstetrics* (21st ed.). New York: McGraw-Hill.

Jasper, M. L. (2000). Antepartum fetal assessment. In S. Mattson & J. E. Smith (Eds.), *AWHONN: Maternal newborn nursing* (2nd ed., pp. 127–160). Philadelphia: Saunders.

Jobe, A. H. (1999). Fetal lung development: Tests for maturation, induction of maturation, and treatment. In R. K. Creasy & R. Resnik (Eds.), *Maternal-fetal medicine* (4th ed., pp. 270–299). Philadelphia: Saunders.

Manning, F. (1999). General principles and applications of ultrasound. In R. K. Creasy & R. Resnik (Eds.), *Maternal-fetal medicine.* (4th ed., pp. 169–206). Philadelphia: Saunders.

McColgin, S. W. (1999, November). *Multiple marker screening revisited.* Paper presented at the Memorial Hospitals 3rd Annual Obstetrics Conference, *Update in OB/GYN.* Colorado Springs, CO.

Nathan, E. B., Haberman, S., Burgess, T., & Minkoff, H. (2000). The relationship of maternal position to the results of brief nonstress tests: A randomized clinical trial. *American Journal of Obstetrics and Gynecology, 182*(5), 1070–1072.

O'Reilly-Green, C., & Divon, M. (2000). Sonographic and clinical methods of diagnosis of macrosomia. *Clinical Obstetrics and Gynecology, 44,* 309–320.

Owen, J., Neely, C., & Northen, A. (1999). Transperineal versus endovaginal ultrasonography examination of the cervix in the midtrimester: A blended comparison. *American Journal of Obstetrics and Gynecology, 181,* 780.

Parer, J. T. (1999). Fetal heart rate. In R. K. Creasy & R. Resnik (Eds.), *Maternal-fetal medicine* (4th ed., pp. 270–299). Philadelphia: Saunders.

Schmidt, J. (2000). Intrapartum fetal assessment. In S. Mattson & J. E. Smith (Eds.), *AWHONN: Maternal newborn nursing* (2nd ed., pp. 272–299). Philadelphia: Saunders.

Scioscia, A. L. (1999). Prenatal genetic diagnosis. In R. K. Creasy & R. Resnik (Eds.), *Maternal-fetal medicine* (4th ed., pp. 40–62). Philadelphia: Saunders.

Wolfe, R. B. & Moore, T. R. (2002). Amniotic fluid and nonimmune hydrops fetalis. In A. A. Fanaroff & R. J. Martin (Eds.). *Neonatal-Perinatal Medicine: Diseases of the fetus and infant* (7th ed. pp. 351–370). St. Louis: Mosby.

Zelop, C. M. (2000). Prediction of fetal weight with the use of three-dimensional ultrasound. *Clinical Obstetrics and Gynecology, 44,* 321–325.

UNIT IV

Birth and the Family

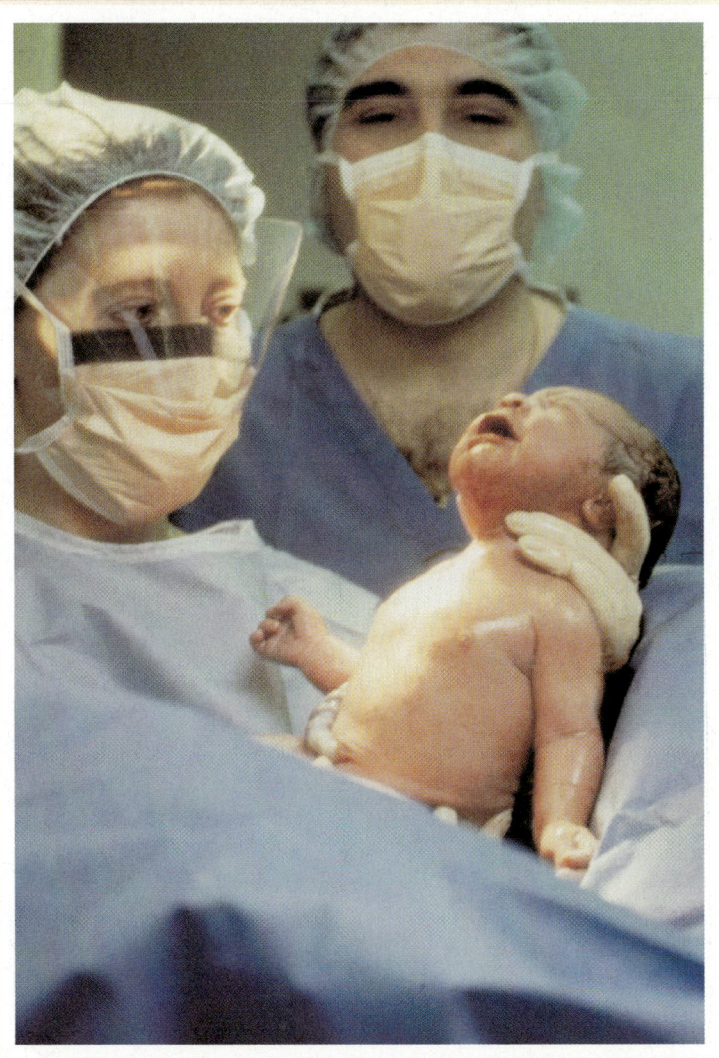

CHAPTER 15

Processes and Stages of Labor and Birth

I think experts refer to us as a blended family. I have two sons, ages 12 and 9, from a previous marriage. They live part-time with us and part-time with their father. My husband has a 15-year-old daughter who lives with her mother. Here I am, 6 months pregnant with our first child together. It has been quite the time, getting used to the idea of a baby and trying to include our children in the pregnancy. They have all heard the heartbeat and felt the baby move. My sons are pretty blasé about it. I didn't know how Jack's daughter would respond but she has been great. Maybe this new baby will help us all grow closer together. I sure hope so.

—LETETIA, 34

Key Terms

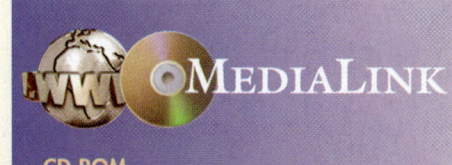

MEDIALINK

CD-ROM

Audio Glossary

NCLEX Review

Rupturing Membranes Animation

Vaginal Delivery Animation

Placenta Delivery Animation

COMPANION WEBSITE

http://www.prenhall.com/london

Labor and Birth Web Links

Thinking Critically

NCLEX Review

Case Study

Complementary Care: Additional Information on Visualization

*I*n the final weeks of pregnancy, both mother and baby begin to prepare for birth. The onset of labor begins a remarkable change in the relationship between the woman and her baby. In those hours and moments the birth process may seem to carry all the power in the universe. The mother-to-be and her partner may feel stretched beyond their normal limits of concentration, purpose, endurance, and pain as they work to bring forth a precious new life.

This chapter focuses on the processes and stages of labor. Subsequent chapters describe intrapartum assessment and nursing care.

CRITICAL FACTORS IN LABOR

Five factors are important in the process of labor and birth: the passage, the fetus, the relationship between the passage and the fetus, the forces of labor, and the psychosocial con-

siderations. Abnormalities that affect any component of these critical forces can alter the outcome of labor and jeopardize both the expectant woman and her baby. These factors are described in this section and summarized in Table 15–1. (Complications are discussed in Chapter 19.)

The Birth Passage

The true pelvis, which forms the bony canal through which the fetus must pass, is divided into three sections: the inlet, the pelvic cavity (midpelvis), and the outlet. (See Chapter 2 for discussion of the pelvis and Chapter 8 for assessment techniques.)

The Caldwell-Moloy classification of pelvises is widely used to differentiate bony pelvis types. The four classic types of pelvis are *gynecoid, android, anthropoid,* and *platypelloid* (Caldwell & Moloy, 1933) (Figure 15–1 ◆). The gynecoid, or female, pelvis is most common. All diameters of the gy-

---

TABLE 15–1 Critical Forces in Labor

The birth passage
- Size of the pelvis (diameters of the pelvic inlet, midpelvis or pelvic cavity, and outlet)
- Type of pelvis (gynecoid, android, anthropoid, platypelloid, or a combination)
- Ability of the cervix to dilate and efface and ability of the vaginal canal and the external opening of the vagina (the introitus) to distend

The fetus
- Fetal head (size and presence of molding)
- Fetal attitude (flexion or extension of the fetal body and extremities)
- Fetal lie
- Fetal presentation (the part of the fetal body entering the pelvis first in a single- or multiple-gestation pregnancy)
- Placenta (implantation site)

The relationship between the passage and the fetus
- Engagement of fetal presenting part
- Station (location of fetal presenting part within the maternal pelvis)
- Fetal position (relationship of the presenting part to one of the four quadrants of the maternal pelvis)

Primary forces of labor
- Frequency, duration, and intensity of uterine contractions as the fetus moves through the birth passage
- Effectiveness of the maternal pushing effort
- Duration of labor

Psychosocial considerations
- Physical preparation for childbirth
- Sociocultural values and beliefs
- Previous childbirth experience
- Support from significant others
- Emotional status

TABLE 15–2 Implications of Pelvic Type for Labor and Birth

Pelvic Type	Pertinent Characteristics	Implications for Birth
Gynecoid	Inlet rounded with all inlet diameters adequate Midpelvis diameters adequate with parallel side walls Outlet adequate	Favorable for vaginal birth
Android	Inlet heart-shaped, with short posterior sagittal diameter Midpelvis diameters reduced Outlet capacity reduced	Not favorable for vaginal birth Descent into pelvis is slow Fetal head enters pelvis in transverse or posterior position, with arrest of labor frequent
Anthropoid	Inlet oval in shape, with long anteroposterior diameter Midpelvis diameters adequate Outlet adequate	Favorable for vaginal birth
Platypelloid	Inlet oval in shape, with long transverse diameters Midpelvis diameters reduced Outlet capacity inadequate	Not favorable for vaginal birth Fetal head engages in transverse position Difficult descent through midpelvis Frequent delay of progress at outlet of pelvis

Note: Description of pelvic shape is exaggerated for easier comprehension.

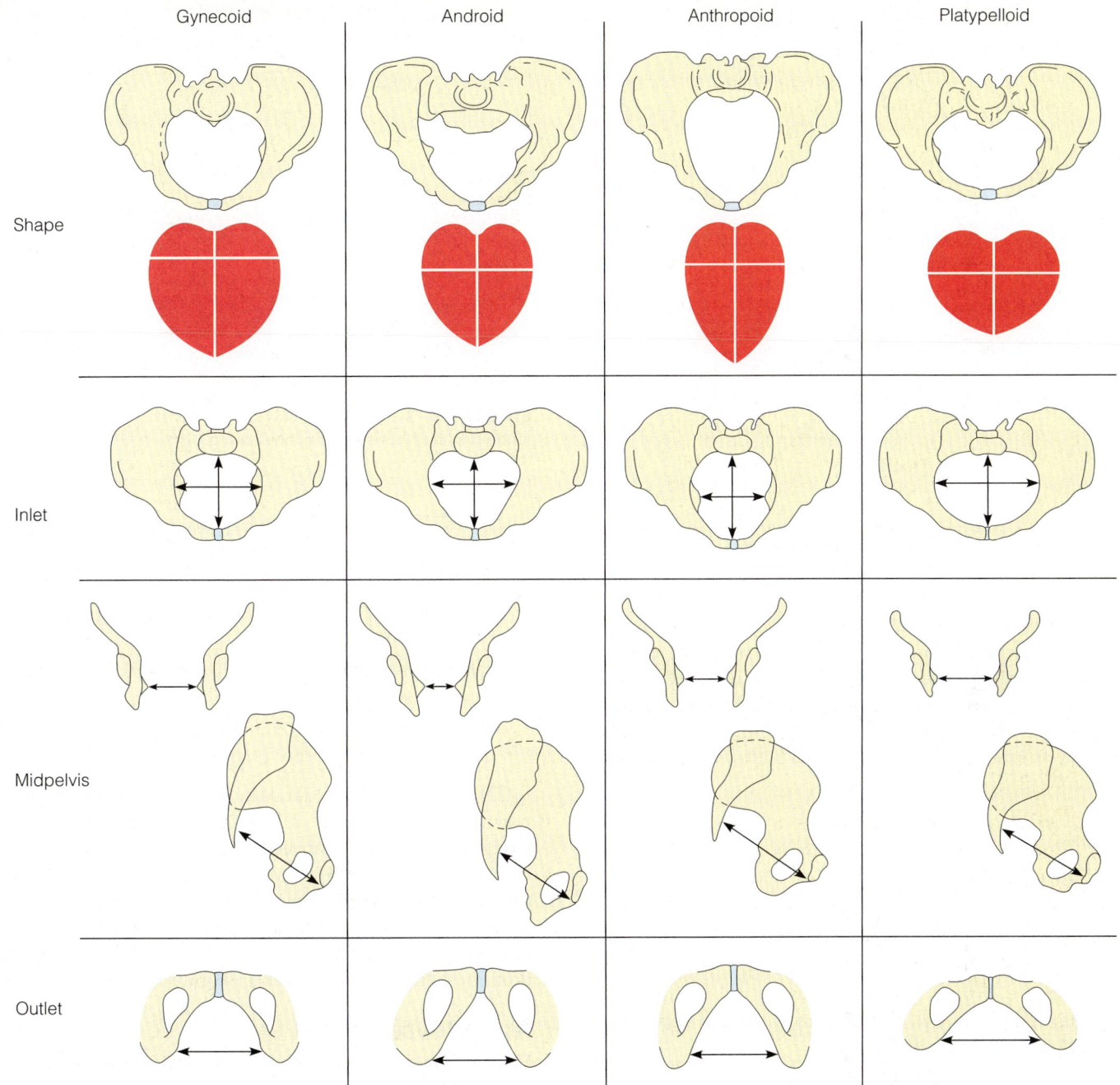

	Gynecoid	Android	Anthropoid	Platypelloid
Shape				
Inlet				
Midpelvis				
Outlet				

FIGURE 15–1. ◆ Comparison of Caldwell-Moloy pelvic types.

necoid are adequate for childbirth. Implications of each type of pelvis for childbirth are summarized in Table 15–2.

The Fetus

FETAL HEAD

The fetal skull (cranium) has three major parts: the face, the base of the skull, and the vault of the cranium (roof). The bones of the face and cranial base are well fused and essentially fixed. The base of the cranium is composed of the two temporal bones, each with a sphenoid and eth-moid bone. The bones composing the vault are the two frontal bones, the two parietal bones, and the occipital bone (Figure 15–2 ◆). These bones are not fused, so this portion of the head can adjust in shape as the presenting part passes through the narrow portions of the pelvis. The cranial bones overlap under pressure of the powers of labor and the demands of the unyielding pelvis. This overlapping is called **molding.** Once the head (the least compressible and largest part of the fetus) has been born, the birth of the rest of the body is rarely delayed.

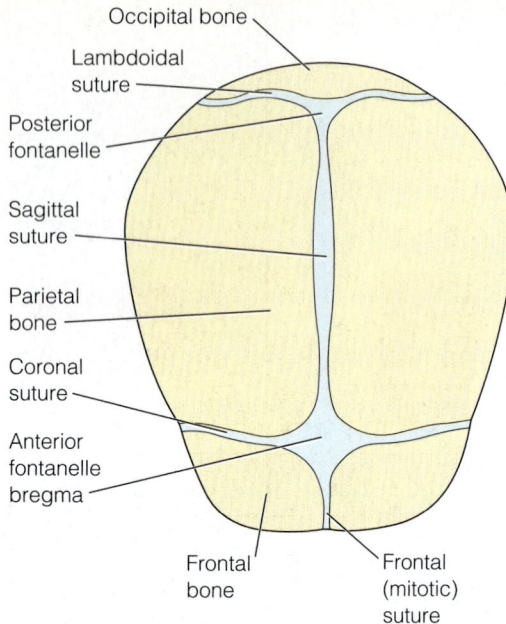

FIGURE 15–2. ◆ Superior view of the fetal skull.

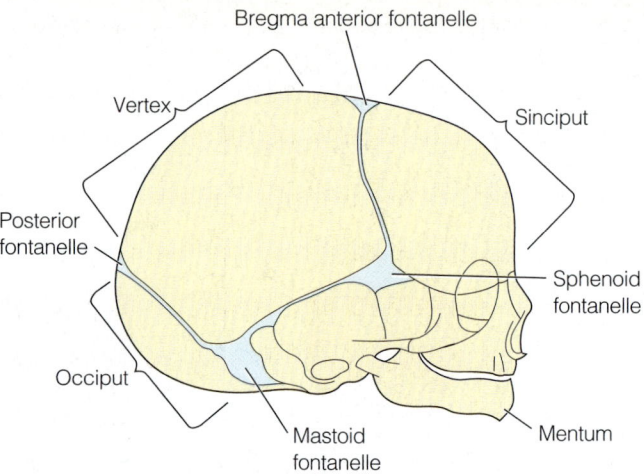

FIGURE 15–3. ◆ Lateral view of the fetal skull identifying the landmarks that have significance during birth.

The **sutures** of the fetal skull are membranous spaces between the cranial bones. The intersections of the cranial sutures are called **fontanelles.** These sutures allow for molding of the fetal head and help the clinician to identify the position of the fetal head during vaginal examination. The impor-tant sutures of the cranium are as follows (see Figure 15–2):

- *Frontal (mitotic) suture:* located between the two frontal bones; becomes the anterior continuation of the sagittal suture
- *Sagittal suture:* located between the parietal bones; divides the skull into left and right halves; runs an-teroposteriorly, connecting the two fontanelles
- *Coronal sutures:* located between the frontal and parietal bones; extend transversely left and right from the anterior fontanelle
- *Lambdoidal suture:* located between the two parietal bones and the occipital bone; extends transversely left and right from the posterior fontanelle

The anterior and posterior fontanelles are clinically use-ful (along with the sutures) in identifying the position of the fetal head in the pelvis and in assessing the status of the newborn after birth. The anterior fontanelle is diamond shaped and measures about 2 by 3 cm. It permits growth of the brain by remaining unossified for as long as 18 months. The posterior fontanelle is much smaller and closes within 8 to 12 weeks after birth. It is shaped like a small triangle and marks the meeting point of the sagittal suture and the lambdoidal suture.

Following are several important landmarks of the fetal skull (Figure 15–3 ◆):

- *Mentum:* fetal chin
- *Sinciput:* anterior area known as the brow
- *Bregma:* large diamond-shaped anterior fontanelle
- *Vertex:* area between the anterior and posterior fontanelles
- *Posterior fontanelle:* intersection between posterior cranial sutures
- *Occiput:* area of the fetal skull occupied by the occip-ital bone, beneath the posterior fontanelle

The diameters of the fetal skull vary considerably within normal limits. Some diameters shorten and others lengthen as the head is molded during labor. Fetal head di-ameters are measured between the various landmarks on the skull. For example, the suboccipitobregmatic diameter is the distance from the undersurface of the occiput to the center of the bregma, or anterior fontanelle. Typical fetal skull measurements are given in Figure 15–4 ◆.

FETAL ATTITUDE AND FETAL LIE

Fetal attitude refers to the relation of the fetal parts to one another. The normal attitude of the fetus is one of moderate flexion of the head, flexion of the arms onto the chest, and flexion of the legs onto the abdomen (Figure 15–5 ◆).

Fetal lie refers to the relationship of the cephalocaudal axis (spinal column) of the fetus to the cephalocaudal axis of the woman. The fetus may assume either a longitudinal or a transverse lie. A *longitudinal lie* occurs when the cephalocaudal axis of the fetus is parallel to the woman's spine. A *transverse lie* occurs when the cephalocaudal axis of the fetus is at a right angle to the woman's spine.

FETAL PRESENTATION

Fetal presentation is determined by fetal lie and by the body part of the fetus that enters the pelvic passage first.

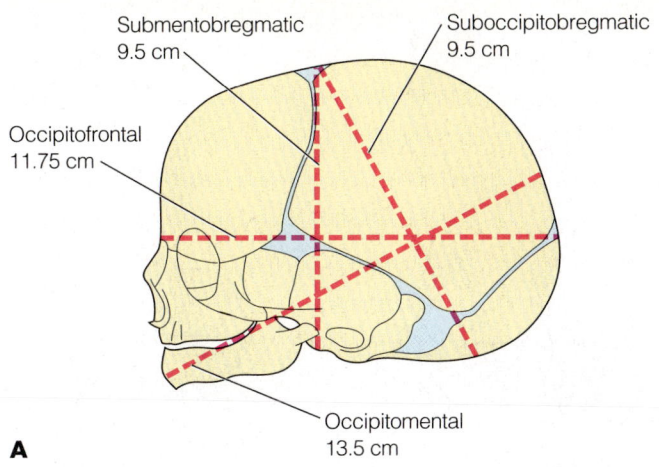

A

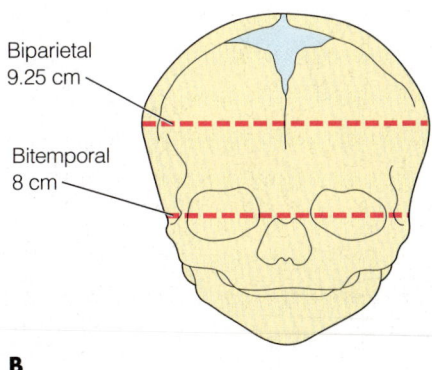

B

FIGURE 15–4. ◆ **A,** Typical anteroposterior diameters of the fetal skull. When the vertex of the fetus presents and the fetal head is flexed with the chin on the chest, the smallest anteroposterior diameter (suboccipitobregmatic) enters the birth canal. **B,** Transverse diameters of the fetal skull.

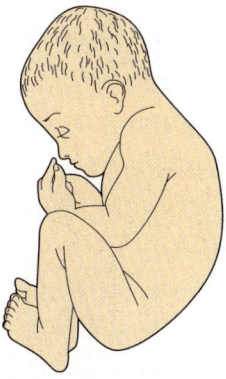

FIGURE 15–5. ◆ Fetal attitude. The attitude (or relationship of body parts) of this fetus is normal. The head is flexed forward, with the chin almost resting on the chest. The arms and legs are flexed.

This portion of the fetus is referred to as the **presenting part.** Fetal presentation may be cephalic, breech, or shoulder. Cephalic presentation, in which the fetal head presents itself to the passage, occurs in approximately 97% of term births. When this presentation occurs, labor and birth are likely to proceed normally. Breech and shoulder presentations are associated with difficulties during labor, and labor does not proceed as expected; therefore, they are called **malpresentations** (see Chapter 19 for discussion). 🔗

The cephalic presentation can be further classified according to the degree of flexion or extension of the fetal head (attitude).

- In *vertex presentation*, the most common presentation, the fetal head is completely flexed onto the chest, and the smallest diameter of the fetal head (suboccipitobregmatic) presents to the maternal pelvis (Figure 15–6A ◆). The occiput is the presenting part.

- In *military presentation*, the fetal head is neither flexed nor extended. The occipitofrontal diameter presents to the maternal pelvis (Figure 15–6B ◆); the top of the head is the presenting part.

- In *brow presentation*, the fetal head is partially extended. The occipitomental diameter, the largest anteroposterior diameter, is presented to the maternal pelvis (see Figure 15–6C ◆); the sinciput is the presenting part (see Figure 15–3).

- In *face presentation*, the fetal head is completely extended. The submentobregmatic diameter presents to the maternal pelvis (Figure 15–6D ◆); the face is the presenting part.

Breech presentations occur in 3% of term births. These presentations are classified according to the attitude of the fetus's hips and knees. In all variations of the breech presentation, the sacrum is the landmark to be noted.

- In *complete breech*, the fetal knees and hips are both flexed; the thighs are on the abdomen, and the calves are on the posterior aspect of the thighs. The buttocks and feet of the fetus present to the maternal pelvis. (Refer to Chapter 19, Figure 19–7.) 🔗

- In *frank breech*, the fetal hips are flexed, and the knees are extended. The buttocks of the fetus present to the maternal pelvis.

- In *footling breech*, the fetal hips and legs are extended, and the feet of the fetus present to the maternal pelvis. In a single footling, one foot presents; in a double footling, both feet present.

A shoulder presentation is also called a *transverse lie.* Most frequently, the shoulder is the presenting part and the acromion process of the scapula is the landmark to be noted. However, the fetal arm, back, abdomen, or side may present in a transverse lie. (See Chapter 19.) 🔗

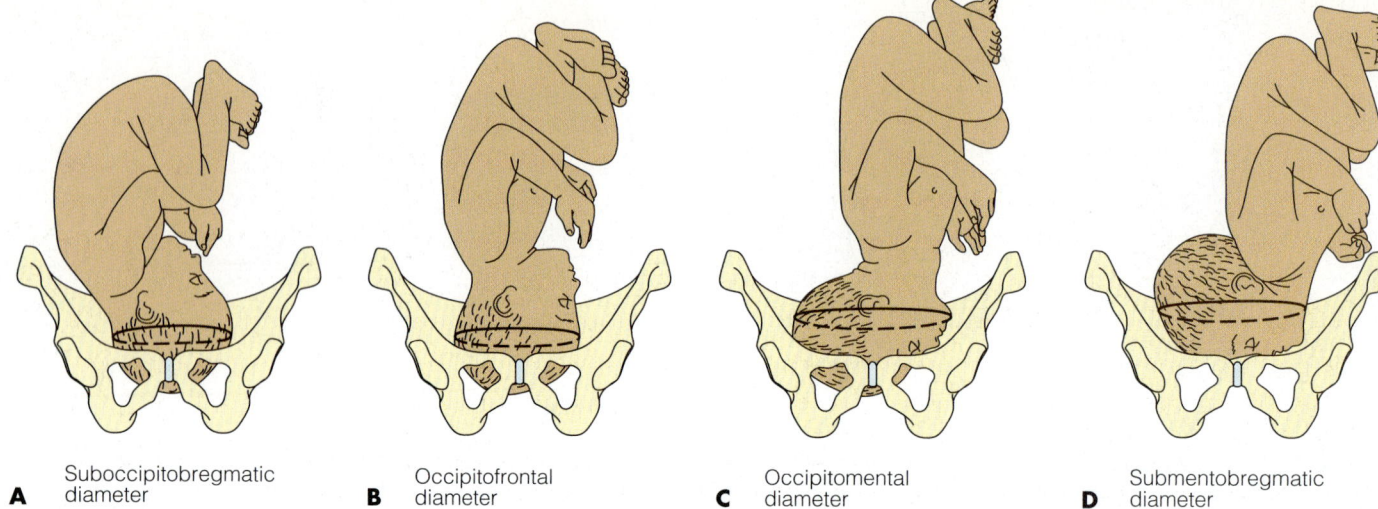

| **A** Suboccipitobregmatic diameter | **B** Occipitofrontal diameter | **C** Occipitomental diameter | **D** Submentobregmatic diameter |

FIGURE 15–6. ◆ Cephalic presentation. **A,** Vertex presentation. Complete flexion of the head allows the suboccipitobregmatic diameter to present to the pelvis. **B,** Military (median vertex) presentation with no flexion or extension. The occipitofrontal diameter presents to the pelvis. **C,** Brow presentation. The fetal head is in partial (halfway) extension. The occipitomental diameter, which is the largest diameter of the fetal head, presents to the pelvis. **D,** Face presentation. The fetal head is in complete extension, and the submentobregmatic diameter presents to the pelvis.

Level of spines (station 0)

BPD

BPD

BPD

Inlet

Inlet

Inlet

A

B

C

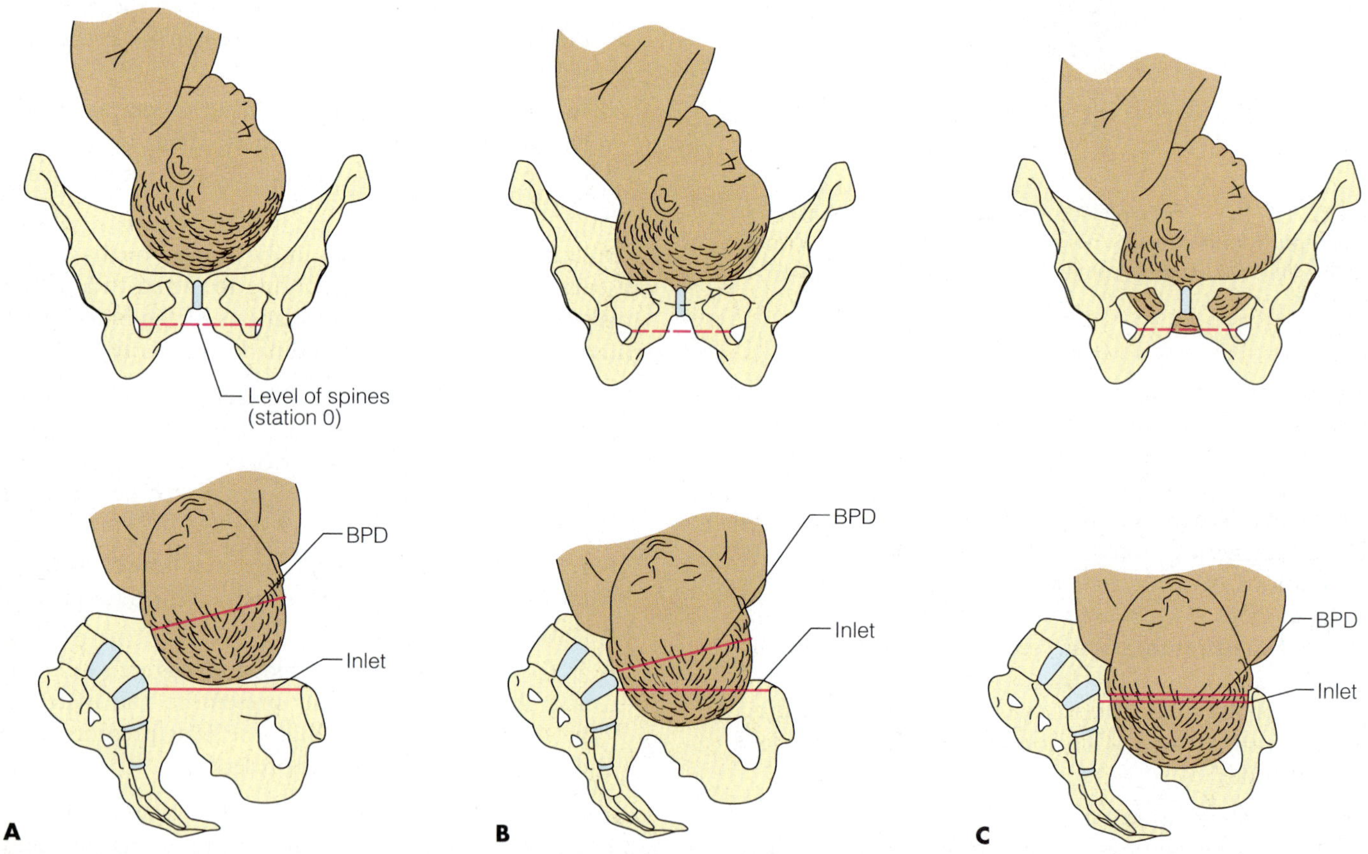

FIGURE 15–7. ◆ Process of engagement in cephalic presentation. **A,** Floating. The fetal head is directed down toward the pelvis but can still easily move away from the inlet. **B,** Dipping. The fetal head dips into the inlet but can be moved away by exerting pressure on the fetus. **C,** Engaged. The biparietal diameter (BPD) of the fetal head is in the inlet of the pelvis. In most instances the presenting part (occiput) is at the level of the ischial spines (zero station).

Functional Relationships of Presenting Part and Passage

ENGAGEMENT

Engagement of the presenting part occurs when the largest diameter of the presenting part reaches or passes through the pelvic inlet (Figure 15–7 ◆). Engagement can be determined by vaginal examination. In primigravidas, engagement occurs approximately 2 weeks before term. Multiparas, however, may experience engagement several weeks before the onset of labor or during the process of labor. Engagement confirms the adequacy of the pelvic inlet. Engagement does not, however, indicate whether the midpelvis and outlet are also adequate.

STATION

Station refers to the relationship of the presenting part to an imaginary line drawn between the ischial spines of the maternal pelvis. In a normal pelvis, the ischial spines mark the narrowest diameter through which the fetus must pass. These spines are not sharp protrusions that harm the fetus but blunted prominences at the midpelvis. The ischial spines as a landmark have been designated as zero station (Figure 15–8 ◆). If the presenting part is higher than the ischial spines, a negative number is as-

signed, noting centimeters above zero station. Positive numbers indicate that the presenting part has passed the ischial spines. Station −5 is at the pelvic inlet, and station + 4 is at the outlet. If the presenting part can be seen at the woman's perineum, birth is imminent. During labor, the presenting part should move progressively from the negative stations to the midpelvis at zero station and into the positive stations. If the presenting part fails to descend in the presence of strong contractions, there may be disproportion between the maternal pelvis and fetal presenting part.

FETAL POSITION

Fetal position refers to the relationship of a designated landmark on the presenting fetal part to the front, sides, or back of the maternal pelvis. The landmark on the fetal presenting part is related to four imaginary quadrants of the pelvis: left anterior, right anterior, left posterior, and right posterior. These quadrants designate whether the presenting part is directed toward the front, back, left, or right of the passage. The landmark chosen for vertex presentations is the occiput, and the landmark for face presentations is the mentum. In breech presentations, the sacrum is the designated landmark, and the acromion process on the scapula is the landmark in shoulder presentations. If the landmark is directed toward the side of the pelvis, fetal position is designated as *transverse,* rather than anterior or posterior. Three notations are used to describe the fetal position:

1. Right (R) or left (L) side of the maternal pelvis
2. The landmark of the fetal presenting part: occiput (O), mentum (M), sacrum (S), or acromion process (A)
3. Anterior (A), posterior (P), or transverse (T), depending on whether the landmark is in the front, back, or side of the pelvis

The abbreviations of these notations help the health care team communicate the fetal position. Thus, when the fetal occiput is directed toward the back and to the left of the birth passage, the abbreviation used is LOP (left occiput-posterior). The term *dorsal* (D) is used when denoting the fetal position in a transverse lie; it refers to the fetal back. Thus, RADA indicates that the acromion process of the scapula is directed toward the woman's right and the fetus's back is anterior. The most common occurring positions are illustrated in Figure 15–9 ◆. The most common fetal position is occiput anterior. When this position occurs, labor and birth are likely to proceed normally. Positions other than occiput anterior are more frequently associated with problems during labor; therefore they are called *malpositions.* (See Chapter 19.) 🔗

Assessment techniques to determine fetal position include inspection and palpation of the maternal abdomen and vaginal examination. They are discussed in Chapter 16. 🔗

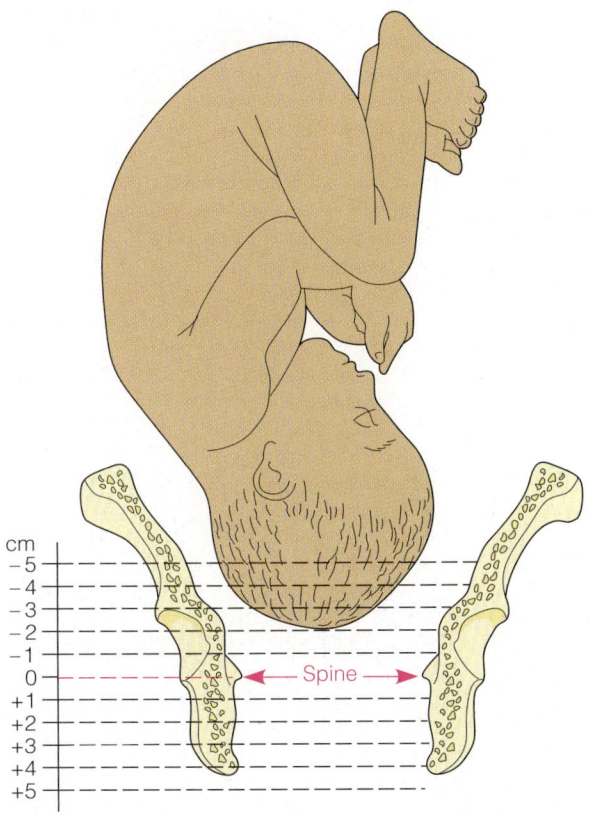

FIGURE 15–8. ◆ Measuring the station of the fetal head while it is descending. In this view the station is −2/−3.

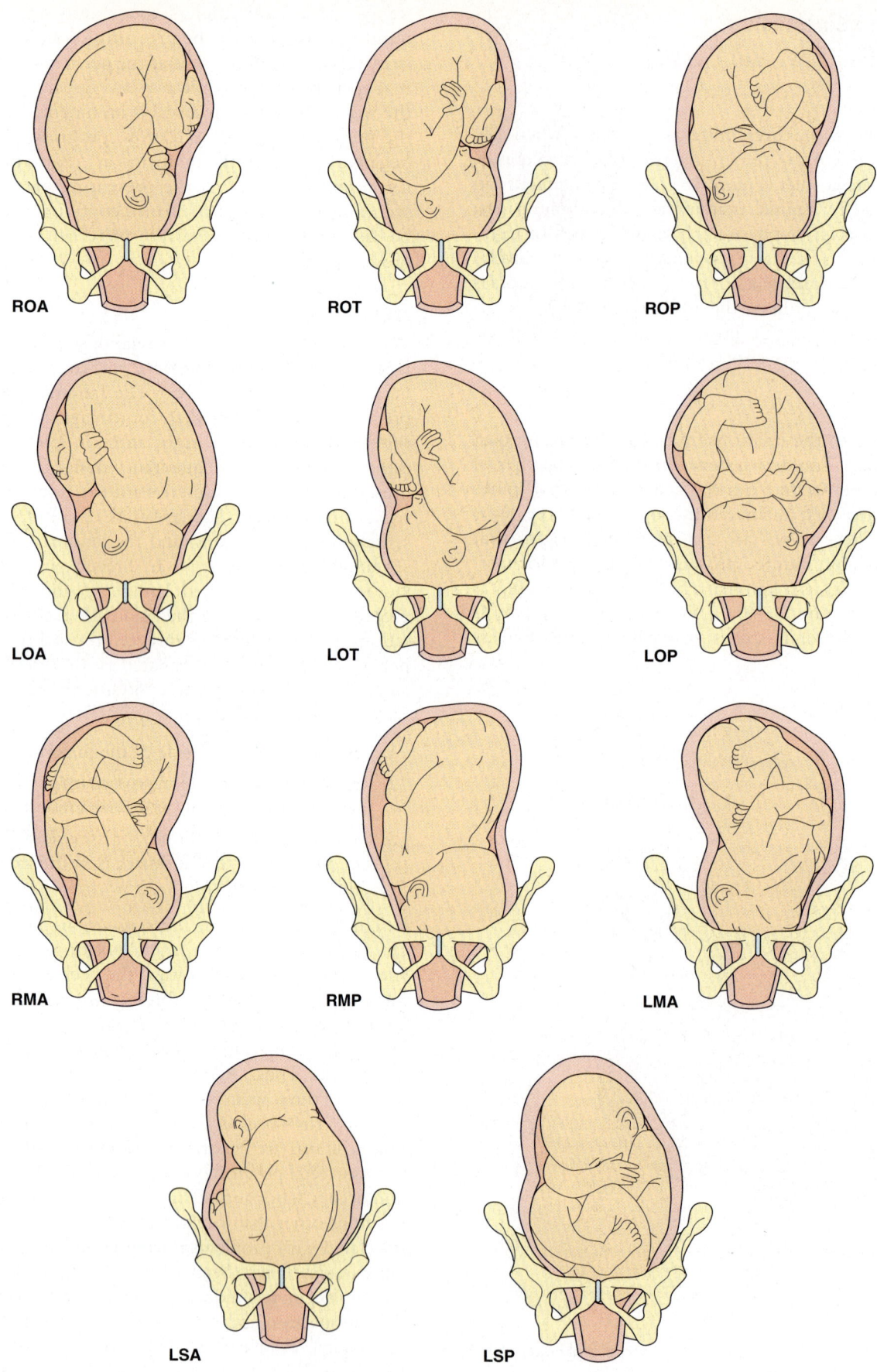

ROA **ROT** **ROP**

LOA **LOT** **LOP**

RMA **RMP** **LMA**

LSA **LSP**

FIGURE 15–9. ◆ Categories of presentation.

The Forces of Labor

Primary and secondary forces work together to achieve birth of the fetus, the fetal membranes, and the placenta. The *primary force* is uterine muscular contractions, which cause the complete effacement and dilatation of the cervix. The *secondary force* is the use of abdominal muscles to push during the second stage of labor. The pushing adds to the primary force after full dilatation.

In labor, uterine contractions are rhythmic but intermittent. Between contractions a period of relaxation occurs. This allows uterine muscles to rest and provides relief for the laboring woman. It also restores uteroplacental circulation, which is important to fetal oxygenation and adequate circulation in the uterine blood vessels.

Each contraction has three phases: (1) *increment*, the building up of the contraction (the longest phase); (2) *acme*, or the peak of the contraction; and (3) *decrement*, or the letting up of the contraction. The terms *frequency*, *duration*, and *intensity* are used to describe uterine contractions during labor. **Frequency** refers to the time between the beginning of one contraction and the beginning of the next contraction. **Duration** is measured from the beginning of a contraction to the completion of that same contraction (Figure 15–10 ◆). **Intensity** refers to the strength of the contraction during acme. In most instances, intensity is estimated by palpating the uterine fundus during a contraction, but it may be measured directly with an intrauterine catheter. When estimating intensity by palpation, the nurse determines whether it is mild, moderate, or strong by judging the amount of indentability of the uterine wall during the acme of a contraction. If the uterine wall can be indented easily, the contraction is considered mild. Strong intensity exists when the uterine wall cannot be indented. Moderate intensity falls somewhere between. When intensity is measured with an intrauterine catheter, the normal resting pressure in the uterus (between contractions) averages 10 to 12 mm Hg. During acme the intensity ranges from 25 to 40 mm Hg in early labor, 50 to 70 mm Hg in active labor, 70 to 90 mm Hg during transition, and 70 to 100 mm Hg while the woman is pushing in the second stage (Varney, 1997). (See Chapter 16 for further discussion of assessment techniques.)

At the beginning of labor, contractions are usually mild, last about 30 seconds, and occur about every 5 to 7 minutes. As labor progresses, duration of contractions increases to about 60 seconds, intensity increases, and frequency is every 2 to 3 minutes. Contractions are involuntary; the laboring woman cannot control their duration, frequency, or intensity.

Psychosocial Considerations

Similar psychosocial factors affect the mother and the father. Both are making a transition to a new role, and both have expectations of themselves during the labor and birth experience.

Although many expectant mothers and fathers attend childbirth preparation classes, they still tend to be concerned about what labor will be like, whether they will be able to perform the way they expect, whether the discomfort and pain will be more than the mother expects or can cope with, and whether the father can provide helpful support (Mauger, 2000). A common fear expressed in childbirth preparation classes is of "losing it," which often means loss of control or loss of a preconceived image of the "right" way to give birth. It is helpful for the prospective parents to be assured that there is no definitively correct way to approach labor and birth.

Every woman is uncertain about what her labor will be like. A woman approaching her first labor faces a totally new experience, whereas the woman who has given birth before knows that each labor is unique and different. Every woman wonders if she will live up to her expectations for herself, whether she will be injured through laceration, episiotomy, or cesarean incision, and whether loved ones will be as supportive as she hopes. The woman faces an irrevocable event—childbirth—and, with it, changes in lifestyle, relationships, and self-image. The woman must also deal with concerns about her loss of control of body functions, emotional responses to an unfamiliar situation, and reactions to the pain associated with labor.

Various factors influence a woman's reaction to the physical and emotional challenge of labor (Table 15–3). Her accomplishment of the tasks of pregnancy, usual coping mechanisms in response to stressful life events, support

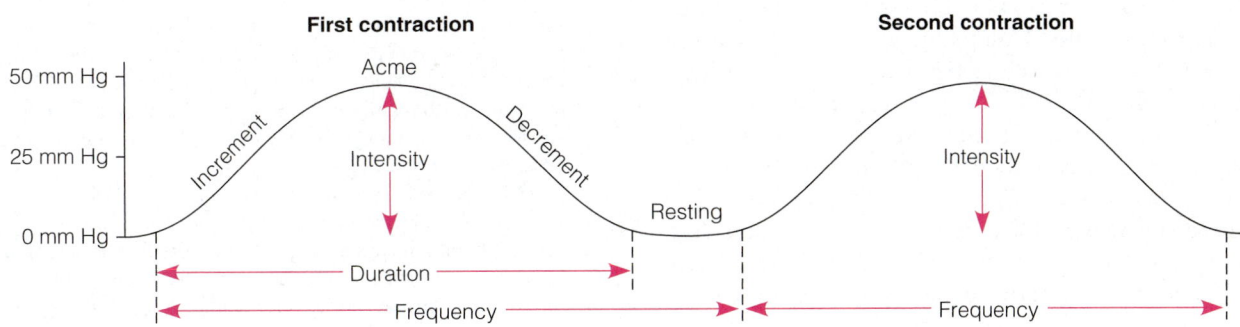

FIGURE 15–10. ◆ Characteristics of uterine contractions.

TABLE 15–3 Factors Associated with a Positive Birth Experience

Motivation for the pregnancy

Attendance at childbirth education classes

A sense of competence or mastery

Self-confidence and self-esteem

Positive relationship with mate

Maintaining control during labor

Support from mate or other person during labor

Not being left alone in labor

Trust in the medical and nursing staff

Having personal control of breathing patterns, comfort measures

Choosing a physician or certified nurse-midwife who has a similar philosophy of care

Receiving clear information regarding procedures

system, preparation for childbirth, and cultural influences are all significant factors.

Expectant women mentally prepare for labor through meaningful actions and imaginary rehearsal. The actions frequently consist of "nesting behavior" (housecleaning, decorating the nursery) and a "psyching up" for the labor, which varies depending on the woman's self-confidence, self-esteem, and previous experiences with stress. Specific actions to prepare for labor may focus on becoming better informed and prepared. In addition, just as a woman tries on the maternal role during pregnancy, fantasizing about labor seems to help her understand and become better prepared for it. Fantasies about the excitement of the baby's birth and the sharing of the experience are positive forms of preparation (Mullaly, 2000).

Many women fear the pain of contractions. They not only see the pain as threatening but also associate it with a loss of control over their bodies and emotions. It is important to realize that the discomfort and stresses of labor are an expected part of the process. Assurances that labor is progressing normally can go a long way toward reducing anxiety and thereby reducing pain. A wide variety of coping techniques may help both the laboring woman and her partner, including, for example, relaxation exercises, massage, and controlled breathing. Women are likely to feel empowered and better able to cope with labor if they recognize that maintaining control is not important or perhaps even possible. (See "Complementary Care: Music During Childbirth" and "Complementary Care: Visualization for Childbirth," as well as the feature on aromatherapy in Chapter 16.) ⬭

The laboring woman's support system may also influence the course of labor and birth. Although some women prefer not to have a support person or family member with them, for many women, the presence of the father and other significant persons (especially the nurse) tends to have a positive effect. A labor partner's presence at the bedside provides a means to enhance communication and to

Complementary Care

MUSIC DURING CHILDBIRTH

The therapeutic use of music to help with pain management is becoming increasingly popular. Browning (2001) conducted a study with a group of primiparas to determine the value of music as a tool in reducing the pain of labor and birth. During their pregnancy, study participants chose preferred music and listened to it daily. They also received information about focused listening. During labor all the women used the music to help distract themselves from the pain or from their current situation and all of them found that the music assisted with relaxation.

The following suggestions are useful in using music in labor (Browning, 2001):

1. Have the woman select the music herself, preferably during pregnancy.

2. Have her listen to it daily when she is in a relaxed state. That way she will begin associating the music with a pleasant activity and will develop a conditioned response to it in labor.

3. Several different tapes should be made to provide variety and avoid boredom during labor.

4. Make a special tape of music that has particular significance for the couple and use it during the birth. Consider having lullabies on the other side of the tape. These can be played for the newborn after birth.

5. Let the mother's response to the music be the guide to its use.

Complementary Care

VISUALIZATION FOR CHILDBIRTH

Visualization uses the power of the mind to influence psychologic and physiologic states. Guided imagery is a specific form of visualization that uses a leader or audiotape to paint a picture in the mind of a pleasant scene that stimulates natural healing responses, alleviates anxiety, promotes relaxation, and/or brings about changes in attitude and behavior. For example, visualization can prepare a pregnant woman to handle the different stages of labor and birth. During pregnancy a woman can imagine her unborn baby, sleeping and floating inside of her. During the early stage of labor a woman can imagine her labor contractions as hugs to the baby or waves in the ocean crashing to shore (Kilson, 2001). The calm in between waves can be used as analogies of rest for the laboring woman and unborn baby. In the second stage of labor, images of a rose bud blossoming into a flower can be used to assist cervical dilatation. Images of a playground slide can help in bringing the baby down, crowning, and the actual birth itself. The third stage of labor is also receptive to visualization techniques that help the mother deliver the placenta while relaxing and regaining control.

Many benefits of visualization are a direct result of decreased stress. Deep relaxation counters the effects of stress by arousing the parasympathetic nervous system, resulting in decreases in heart rate, respiratory rate, oxygen consumption, blood pressure, muscle tension, and gastric acidity. ⬭ **WEB**

demonstrate feelings of love. Communication needs may include talking and the use of affectionate and understanding words from the partner. Showing love may take the form of holding hands, hugging, or touching.

How the woman views the birth experience in hindsight may have implications for mothering behaviors. It appears that any activities by the expectant woman or by health care providers that enhance the birth experience are beneficial to the mother-baby connection. The father's experience of childbirth and his opportunities for bonding may have important implications for fathering as well.

THE PHYSIOLOGY OF LABOR
Possible Causes of Labor Onset

The process of labor usually begins between the 38th and the 42nd week of gestation, when the fetus is mature and ready for birth. The exact cause of labor onset is not clearly understood. However, some important aspects have been identified: progesterone relaxes smooth muscle tissue, estrogen stimulates uterine muscle contractions, and connective tissue loosens to permit the softening, thinning, and eventual opening of the cervix (Smith, 1999). Currently, researchers are focusing on several promising areas of research about labor onset.

PROGESTERONE WITHDRAWAL HYPOTHESIS

Progesterone, produced by the placenta, relaxes uterine smooth muscle by interfering with the conduction of impulses from one cell to the next. During pregnancy, progesterone exerts a quieting effect and the uterus generally does not have coordinated contractions. Toward the end of gestation, biochemical changes decrease the availability of progesterone to myometrial cells and may be associated with an antiprogestin that inhibits the relaxant effect but allows other progesterone actions such as lactogenesis (Liggins, 1997). With the decreased availability of progesterone, estrogen is better able to stimulate contractions (Challis, 1999).

PROSTAGLANDIN HYPOTHESIS

Although the exact relationship between prostaglandin and the onset of labor is not yet known, the effect is clinically demonstrated by the successful induction of labor after vaginal application of prostaglandin E. In addition, preterm labor may be stopped by using an inhibitor of prostaglandin synthesis (Challis, 1999; Liggins, 1997).

The amnion and decidua are the focus of research on the source of prostaglandins. Once prostaglandin is produced, stimuli for its synthesis may include rising levels of estrogen, decreased availability of progesterone, and increased levels of oxytocin, platelet-activating factor, and endothelin-1 (Challis, 1999; Liggins, 1997).

CORTICOTROPHIN-RELEASING HORMONE

Corticotrophin-releasing hormone (CRH) has a possible role in labor onset. It increases during pregnancy, with a sharp increase at term. Also, plasma CRH increases prior to preterm labor, and CRH levels are elevated in multiple gestation. Finally, CRH is known to stimulate the synthesis of prostaglandin F and prostaglandin E by amnion cells (Smith, 1999).

Myometrial Activity

In true labor, the muscles of the upper uterine segment shorten and exert a longitudinal pull on the cervix with each contraction, causing effacement. **Effacement** is the drawing up of the internal os and the cervical canal into the side walls of the uterus. The cervix changes progressively from a long, thick structure to one that is tissue-paper thin (Figure 15–11 ◆). In primigravidas, effacement usually occurs before dilatation.

The uterus elongates with each contraction, decreasing the horizontal diameter. This elongation causes a straightening of the fetal body, pressing the upper portion against the fundus and thrusting the presenting part down toward the lower uterine segment and the cervix. The pressure exerted by the fetus is called the fetal axis pressure. As the uterus elongates, the longitudinal muscle fibers are pulled upward over the presenting part. This action and the hydrostatic pressure of the fetal membranes cause cervical dilatation. The cervical os and cervical canal widen from less than 1 cm to approximately 10 cm, allowing birth of the fetus. When the cervix is completely dilated and retracted up into the lower uterine segment, it can no longer be palpated. At the same time the round ligament pulls the fundus forward, aligning the fetus with the bony pelvis.

Intra-abdominal Pressure

After the cervix is completely dilated, the maternal abdominal muscles contract as the woman pushes. This pushing action (called bearing down) aids in expulsion of the fetus and placenta. If the cervix is not completely dilated, however, bearing down can cause cervical edema (which retards dilatation), possible tearing and bruising of the cervix, and maternal exhaustion.

Musculature Changes in the Pelvic Floor

The levator ani muscle and fascia of the pelvic floor draw the rectum and vagina upward and forward with each contraction, along the curve of the pelvic floor. As the fetal head descends to the pelvic floor, the pressure of the presenting part causes the perineal structure, which was once 5 cm in thickness, to thin to less than 1 cm. The anus everts, exposing the interior rectal wall as the fetal head descends forward (Cunningham, Gant, Leveno et al., 2001).

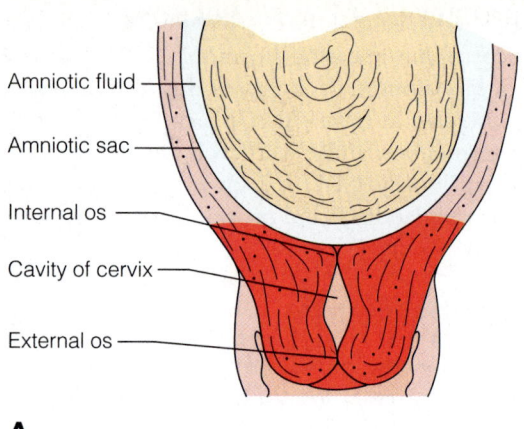

Amniotic fluid
Amniotic sac
Internal os
Cavity of cervix
External os

A

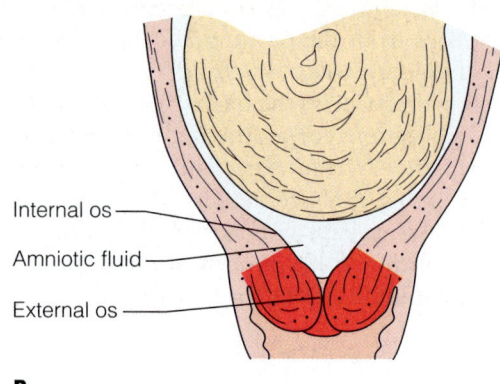

Internal os
Amniotic fluid
External os

B

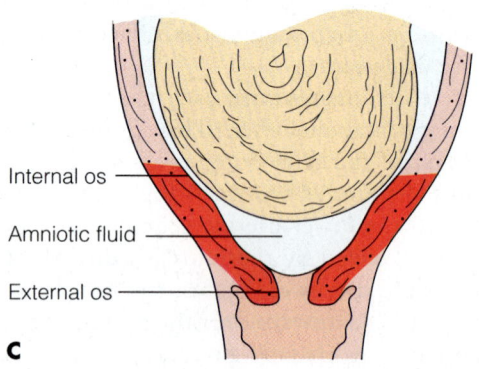

Internal os
Amniotic fluid
External os

C

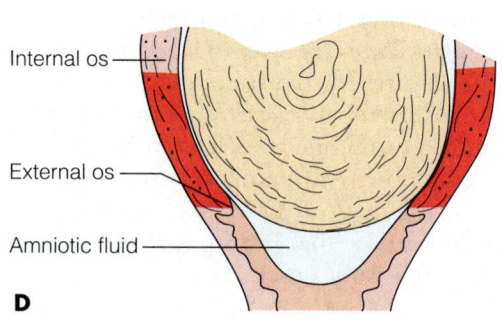

Internal os
External os
Amniotic fluid

D

FIGURE 15–11. ◆ Effacement of the cervix in the primigravida. **A,** Beginning of labor. There is no cervical effacement or dilatation. The fetal head is cushioned by amniotic fluid. **B,** Beginning cervical effacement. As the cervix begins to efface, more amniotic fluid collects below the fetal head. **C,** Cervix about one half effaced and slightly dilated. The increasing amount of amniotic fluid exerts hydrostatic pressure. **D,** Complete effacement and dilatation.

Premonitory Signs of Labor

Most primigravidas and many multiparas experience the following signs and symptoms of impending labor.

LIGHTENING

Lightening describes the effects that occur when the fetus begins to settle into the pelvic inlet (engagement). With fetal descent, the uterus moves downward, and the fundus no longer presses on the diaphragm, which allows breathing to become easier. However, with increased downward pressure of the presenting part, the woman may notice the following:

- Leg cramps or pains due to pressure on the nerves that pass through the obturator foramen in the pelvis
- Increased pelvic pressure
- Increased venous stasis, leading to edema in the lower extremities
- Increased vaginal secretions resulting from congestion of the vaginal mucous membranes

BRAXTON HICKS CONTRACTIONS

Before the onset of labor, **Braxton Hicks contractions** (the irregular, intermittent contractions that have been occurring throughout the pregnancy) may become uncomfortable. The pain seems to be focused in the abdomen and groin but may feel like the "drawing" sensations experienced by some women with dysmenorrhea. When these contractions are strong enough for the woman to believe she is in labor, she is said to be in *false labor*. False labor is uncomfortable and may be exhausting. Since the contractions can be fairly regular, the woman has no way of knowing if they are true labor (see later discussion).

CERVICAL CHANGES

Considerable change occurs in the cervix during the prenatal and intrapartal period. At the beginning of pregnancy the cervix is rigid and firm, and it must soften so it can stretch and dilate to allow the fetus passage. This softening of the cervix is called *ripening*.

As term approaches, collagen fibers in the cervix are broken down by certain enzymes. As the fibers change, their ability to bind together decreases, while the water content of the cervix increases. All these changes result in a weakening and softening of the cervix.

BLOODY SHOW

During pregnancy, cervical secretions accumulate in the cervical canal to form a barrier called a *mucus plug*. With softening and effacement of the cervix, the mucus plug is often expelled, resulting in a small amount of blood loss from the exposed cervical capillaries. The resulting pink-tinged secretions are called **bloody show.** Bloody show is considered a sign that labor will begin within 24 to 48 hours. Vaginal examination that includes manipulation of the cervix may also result in a blood-tinged discharge, which may be confused with bloody show.

RUPTURE OF MEMBRANES ⬭ CD

In about 12% of women at term, the amniotic membranes rupture before the onset of labor. This is called *rupture of membranes* (ROM). After the membranes rupture, 80% of these women experience onset of labor within 24 hours. If membranes rupture and labor does not begin spontaneously within 12 to 24 hours, labor may be induced to decrease the risk of infection. Labor is induced only if the pregnancy is near term (Varney, 1997).

When the membranes rupture, the amniotic fluid may be expelled in large amounts. If engagement has not occurred, there is danger of the umbilical cord washing out with the fluid (prolapsed cord). In addition, the open pathway into the uterus increases the risk of infection. Because of these risks, when the membranes rupture, the woman is advised to call her certified nurse-midwife or physician and proceed to the hospital or birthing center. In some instances, the fluid is expelled in small amounts and may be confused with episodes of urinary incontinence associated with urinary urgency, coughing, or sneezing. The discharge should be checked to determine its source and the appropriate action. (See Chapter 16 for assessment techniques.) ⬭

SUDDEN BURST OF ENERGY

Some women report a sudden burst of energy approximately 24 to 48 hours before labor. The cause of the energy spurt is unknown. In prenatal teaching, warn prospective mothers not to overexert themselves during this energy burst to avoid being overtired when labor begins.

OTHER SIGNS

Additional premonitory signs include the following:

- Weight loss of 1 to 3 lb resulting from fluid loss and electrolyte shifts produced by changes in estrogen and progesterone levels
- Diarrhea, indigestion, or nausea and vomiting just before onset of labor

The causes of these signs are unknown.

Differences Between True and False Labor

The contractions of true labor produce progressive dilatation and effacement of the cervix. They occur regularly and increase in frequency, duration, and intensity. The discomfort of true labor contractions usually starts in the back and radiates around to the abdomen. The pain is not relieved by ambulation (in fact, walking may intensify the pain).

The contractions of false labor do not produce progressive cervical effacement and dilatation. Classically, they are irregular and do not increase in frequency, duration, and intensity. The contractions may be perceived as a hardening or "balling up" without discomfort, or discomfort may occur mainly in the lower abdomen and groin. The discomfort may be relieved by ambulation, changes of position, or a hot shower (Lieberman & Holt, 2000). Many times the only way to differentiate accurately between true and false labor is to assess dilatation. The woman must feel free to come in for accurate assessment of labor and should be counseled not to feel foolish if the labor is false. Reassure the woman that false labor is common and that it often cannot be distinguished from true labor except by vaginal examination (Table 15–4).

STAGES OF LABOR AND BIRTH

The labor process is divided into phases and stages of labor. These represent theoretical separations in the process. A laboring woman does not usually experience distinct differences from one to the other.

The *first stage* begins with the onset of true labor and ends when the cervix is completely dilated to 10 cm. The *second stage* begins with complete dilatation and ends with the birth of the baby. The *third stage* begins with the birth of the baby and ends with the delivery of the placenta.

Some clinicians identify a *fourth stage*. During this stage, which lasts 1 to 4 hours after delivery of the placenta, the

TABLE 15–4 Comparison of True and False Labor	
True Labor	*False Labor*
Contractions occur at regular intervals.	Contractions are irregular.
Interval between contractions gradually shortens.	Usually no change.
Contractions increase in duration and intensity.	Usually no change.
Discomfort begins in back and radiates around to abdomen.	Discomfort is usually in abdomen.
Intensity usually increases with walking.	Walking has no effect on or lessens contractions.
Cervical dilatation and effacement are progressive.	No change.

uterus contracts to control bleeding at the placental site (Cunningham et al., 2001). (The care of the laboring woman is discussed in Chapter 17.) ⚭

First Stage

The first stage of labor is divided into the *latent, active,* and *transition* phases. Each phase of labor is characterized by physical and psychologic changes.

LATENT PHASE

The latent phase starts with the beginning of regular contractions, which are usually mild. The woman feels able to cope with the discomfort. She may be relieved that labor has finally started. Although she may be anxious, she is able to recognize and express those feelings of anxiety. The woman is often talkative and smiling and is eager to talk about herself and answer questions. Excitement is high, and her partner or other support person is often as elated as she is.

Uterine contractions become established during the latent phase and increase in frequency, duration, and intensity. They may start as mild contractions lasting 15 to 20 seconds with a frequency of 10 to 20 minutes and progress to moderate ones lasting 30 to 40 seconds with a frequency of 5 to 7 minutes. As the cervix begins to dilate, it also effaces, although little or no fetal descent is evident. For a woman in her first labor (nullipara), the latent (or early) phase of the first stage of labor averages 8.6 hours but should not exceed 20 hours. The latent phase in multiparas averages 5.3 hours but should not exceed 14 hours.

At the beginning of labor, the amniotic membranes bulge through the cervix in the shape of a cone. **Spontaneous rupture of membranes (SROM)** generally occurs at the height of an intense contraction with a gush of fluid out of the vagina. ⚭ **CD** In many instances, the membranes are ruptured by the certified nurse-midwife or physician, using an instrument called an *amnihook*. This procedure is called *amniotomy,* or **artificial rupture of membranes (AROM).**

ACTIVE PHASE

When a woman enters the early active phase, her anxiety tends to increase as she senses the intensification of contractions and pain. She begins to fear a loss of control and may use a variety of coping mechanisms. Some women show decreased ability to cope and a sense of helplessness. Women who have support people and family available may feel greater satisfaction and less anxiety than those without support. During this phase, the cervix dilates from about 3 to 4 cm, to 8 cm. Fetal descent is progressive. Cervical dilatation averages 1.2 cm/hr in nulliparas and 1.5 cm/hr in multiparas.

TRANSITION PHASE

The transition phase is the last part of the first stage of labor. When the woman enters transition, she may show sig-

nificant anxiety. She becomes acutely aware of the increasing force and intensity of the contractions. She may become restless, frequently changing position. By the time the woman enters the transition phase, she is inner directed and often tired. She may fear being left alone at the same time the support person may be feeling the need for a break. Reassure the woman that she will not be left alone. Be available as relief support at this time and keep the woman informed about where her labor support people are, if they leave the room.

During the active and transition phases, contractions become more frequent and longer in duration, and they increase in intensity. By the end of the active phase, contractions have a frequency of 2 to 3 minutes, a duration of 60 seconds, and strong intensity. During transition, contractions have a frequency of about every 2 minutes, a duration of 60 to 90 seconds, and strong intensity. Cervical dilatation slows as it progresses from 8 to 10 cm and the rate of fetal descent dramatically increases. The average rate of descent is 1.6 cm/hr and at least 1 cm/hr in nulliparas and 5.4 cm/hr and at least 2.1 cm/hr in multiparas. The transition phase does not usually last longer than 3 hours for nulliparas or longer than 1 hour for multiparas.

As dilatation approaches 10 cm, the woman may feel increased rectal pressure and an uncontrollable desire to bear down, the amount of bloody show may increase, and the membranes may rupture (if it has not already occurred). The woman may also fear that she will be "torn open" or "split apart" by the force of the contractions. With the peak of a contraction, she may experience a sensation of pressure so great that it seems to her that her abdomen will burst open with the force. Inform the woman that what she is feeling is normal. The woman may doubt her ability to cope with labor and may become apprehensive, irritable, and withdrawn. She may be terrified of being left alone, though she does not want anyone to talk to or touch her. However, with the next contraction she may ask for verbal and physical support. Other characteristics of this phase may include the following:

- Hyperventilation, as the woman increases her breathing rate
- Generalized discomfort, including low backache, shaking and cramping in legs, and increased sensitivity to touch
- Increased need for partner's and/or nurse's presence and support
- Restlessness
- Increased apprehension and irritability
- Difficulty understanding directions
- A sense of bewilderment, frustration, and anger at the contractions
- Requests for medication
- Hiccuping, belching, nausea, or vomiting
- Beads of perspiration on the upper lip or brow

The woman in this phase may be amnesic and sleep between her now frequent contractions. Her support persons may start to feel helpless and may turn to the nurse for increased help as their efforts to alleviate her discomfort seem less effective.

Second Stage ⊂⊃ CD

The second stage of labor begins with complete cervical dilatation and ends with birth of the infant. The second stage is usually completed within 2 hours after the cervix becomes fully dilated for primigravidas; the stage averages 15 minutes for multiparas. Contractions continue with a frequency of about every 2 minutes, a duration of 60 to 90 seconds, and strong intensity. Descent of the fetal presenting part continues until it reaches the perineal floor.

As the fetal head descends, the woman usually has the urge to push because of pressure of the fetal head on the sacral and obturator nerves. As she pushes, contraction of the maternal abdominal muscles exerts intra-abdominal pressure. As the fetal head continues its descent, the perineum begins to bulge, flatten, and move anteriorly. The amount of bloody show may increase. The labia begin to part with each contraction. Between contractions the fetal head appears to recede. With succeeding contractions and maternal pushing effort, the fetal head descends farther. **Crowning** occurs when the fetal head is encircled by the external opening of the vagina (introitus), and it means birth is imminent.

A childbirth-prepared woman may feel some relief that the acute pain she felt during the transition phase is over (see Table 15–5). She may also be relieved that the birth is near and she can push. Some women feel a sense of purpose now that they can be actively involved. Others, particularly those without childbirth preparation, may become frightened and fight each contraction. Such behavior may be disconcerting to the woman's support persons. The woman may feel she has lost her ability to cope and become embarrassed, or she may demonstrate extreme irritability toward the staff or her supporters as she attempts to regain control over forces against which she feels helpless. Most women feel acute, increasingly severe pain and a burning sensation as the perineum distends.

SPONTANEOUS BIRTH (VERTEX PRESENTATION)

As the fetal head distends the vulva with each contraction, the perineum becomes extremely thin and the anus stretches and protrudes. With time, the head extends under the symphysis pubis and is born. When the anterior shoulder meets the underside of the symphysis pubis, a gentle push by the mother aids in the birth of the shoulders. The body then follows (Figure 15–12 ◆). (Birth of a fetus in other than a vertex presentation is discussed in Chapter 19.) ⊂⊃

POSITIONAL CHANGES OF THE FETUS

For the fetus to pass through the birth canal, the fetal head and body must adjust to the passage by certain positional changes. These changes, called **cardinal movements** or mechanisms of labor, are described in the order in which they occur (Figure 15–13 ◆).

Descent.   Descent occurs because of four forces: (1) pressure of the amniotic fluid, (2) direct pressure of the uterine fundus on the breech, (3) contraction of the abdominal muscles, and (4) extension and straightening of the fetal body. The head enters the inlet in the occiput transverse or oblique position because the pelvic inlet is widest from side to side. The sagittal suture is an equal distance from the maternal symphysis pubis and sacral promontory.

Flexion.   Flexion occurs as the fetal head descends and meets resistance from the soft tissues of the pelvis, the muscles of the pelvic floor, and the cervix. As a result of the resistance, the fetal chin flexes downward onto the chest.

Internal Rotation.   The fetal head must rotate to fit the diameter of the pelvic cavity, which is widest in the anteroposterior diameter. As the occiput of the fetal head

TABLE 15–5 Characteristics of Labor

	First Stage			Second Stage
	Latent Phase	Active Phase	Transition Phase	
Nullipara	8.6 hr	4.6 hr	3.6 hr	Up to 3 hr
Multipara	5.3 hr	2.4 hr	Variable	0–30 min
Cervical dilatation	0–3 cm	4–7 cm	8–10 cm	
Contractions				
Frequency	Every 3–30 min	Every 2–3 min	Every 1½–2 min	Every 1½–2 min
Duration	20–40 sec	40–60 sec	60–90 sec	60–90 sec
Intensity	Begin as mild and progress to moderate; 25–40 mm Hg by intrauterine pressure catheter (IUPC)	Begin as moderate and progress to strong; 50–70 mm Hg by IUPC	Strong by palpation; 70–90 mm Hg by IUPC	Strong by palpation; 70–100 mm Hg by IUPC

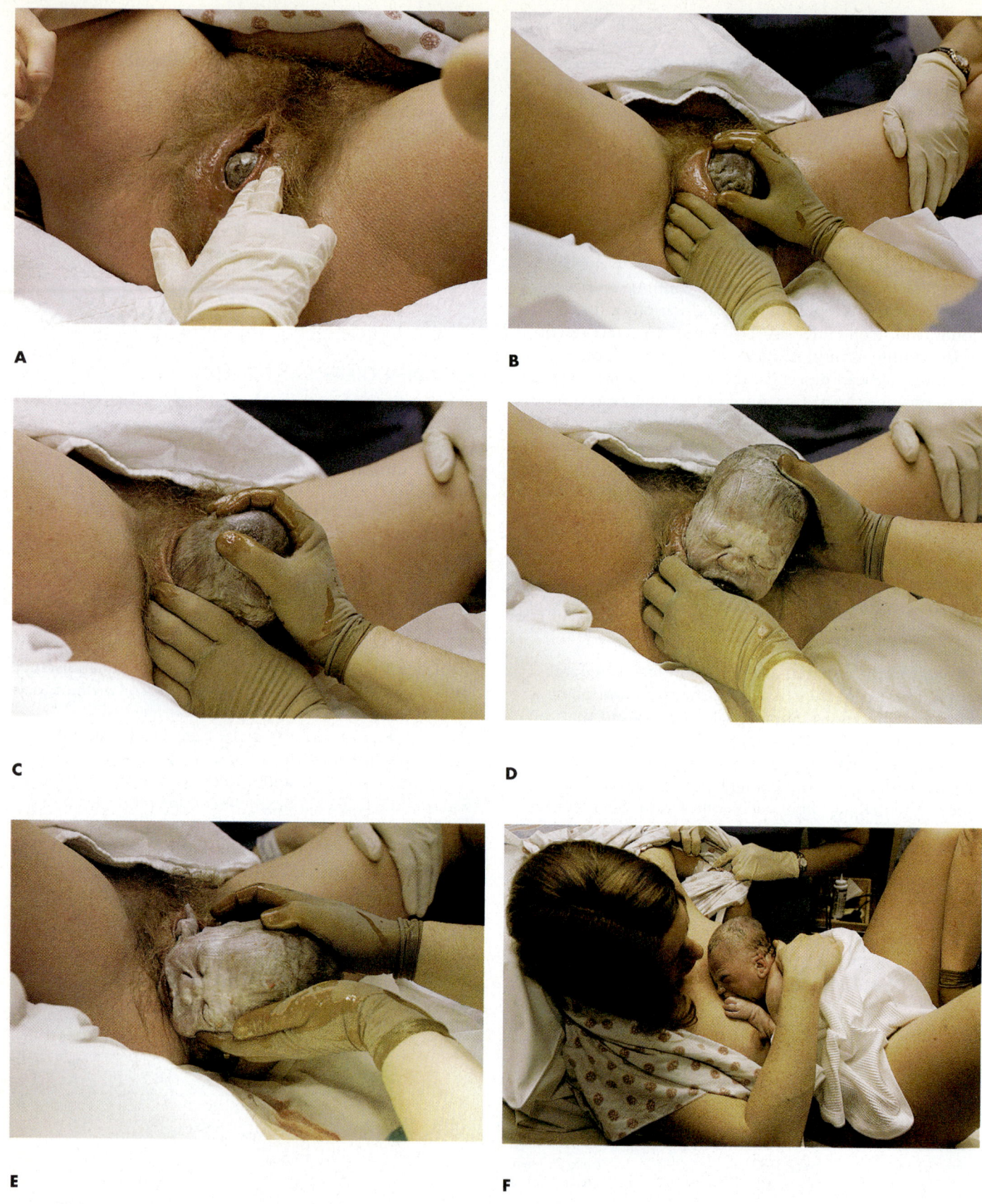

A

B

C

D

E

F

FIGURE 15–12. ◆ The birth sequence.

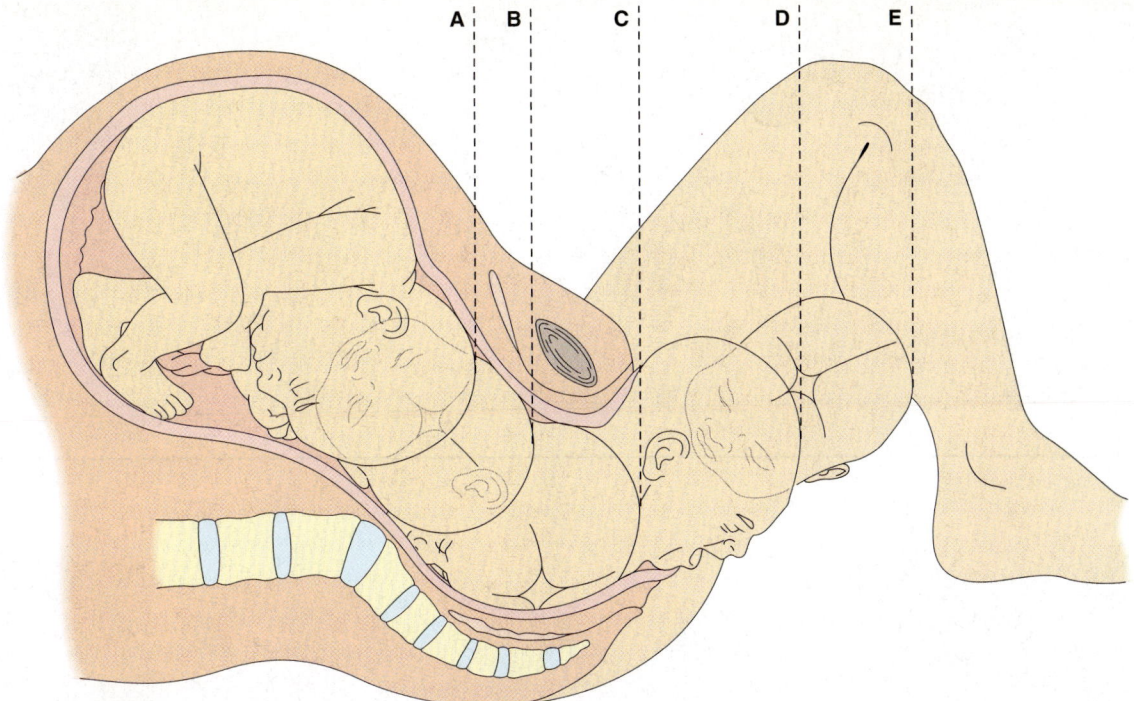

FIGURE 15–13. ◆ Mechanisms of labor. **A, B,** Descent. **C,** Internal rotation. **D,** Extension. **E,** External rotation.

meets resistance from the levator ani muscles and their fascia, the occiput rotates—usually from left to right—and the sagittal suture aligns in the anteroposterior pelvic diameter.

Extension. The resistance of the pelvic floor and the mechanical movement of the vulva opening anteriorly and forward assist with extension of the fetal head as it passes under the symphysis pubis. With this positional change, the occiput, then brow and face, emerge from the vagina.

Restitution. The shoulders of the fetus enter the pelvic inlet obliquely and remain oblique when the head rotates to the anteroposterior diameter through internal rotation. Because of this rotation, the neck becomes twisted. Once the head is born and is free of pelvic resistance, the neck untwists, turning the head to one side (restitution), and aligns with the position of the back in the birth canal.

External Rotation. As the shoulders rotate to the anteroposterior position in the pelvis, the head turns farther to one side (external rotation).

Expulsion. After the external rotation, and through the pushing efforts of the laboring woman, the anterior shoulder meets the undersurface of the symphysis pubis and slips under it. As lateral flexion of the shoulder and head occurs, the anterior shoulder is born before the posterior shoulder. The body follows quickly.

Third Stage

PLACENTAL SEPARATION

After the infant is born, the uterus contracts firmly, decreasing its capacity and the surface area of placental attachment. The placenta begins to separate because of this decreased surface area. As separation occurs, bleeding results in the formation of a hematoma between the placental tissue and the remaining decidua. This hematoma speeds the separation process. The membranes are the last to separate. They are peeled off the uterine wall as the placenta descends into the vagina. Signs of placental separation usually appear about 5 minutes after the birth of the newborn. These signs are (1) a globular-shaped uterus, (2) a rise of the fundus in the abdomen, (3) a sudden gush or trickle of blood, and (4) further protrusion of the umbilical cord out of the vagina.

PLACENTAL DELIVERY 🔗 CD

When the signs of placental separation appear, the woman may bear down to aid in placental expulsion. If this fails and the certified nurse-midwife or physician has ascertained that the fundus is firm, gentle traction may be applied to the cord while pressure is exerted on the fundus. The weight of the placenta as it is guided into the placental collection pan aids in the removal of the membranes from the uterine wall. A placenta is considered to be retained if 30 minutes have elapsed from completion of the second stage of labor.

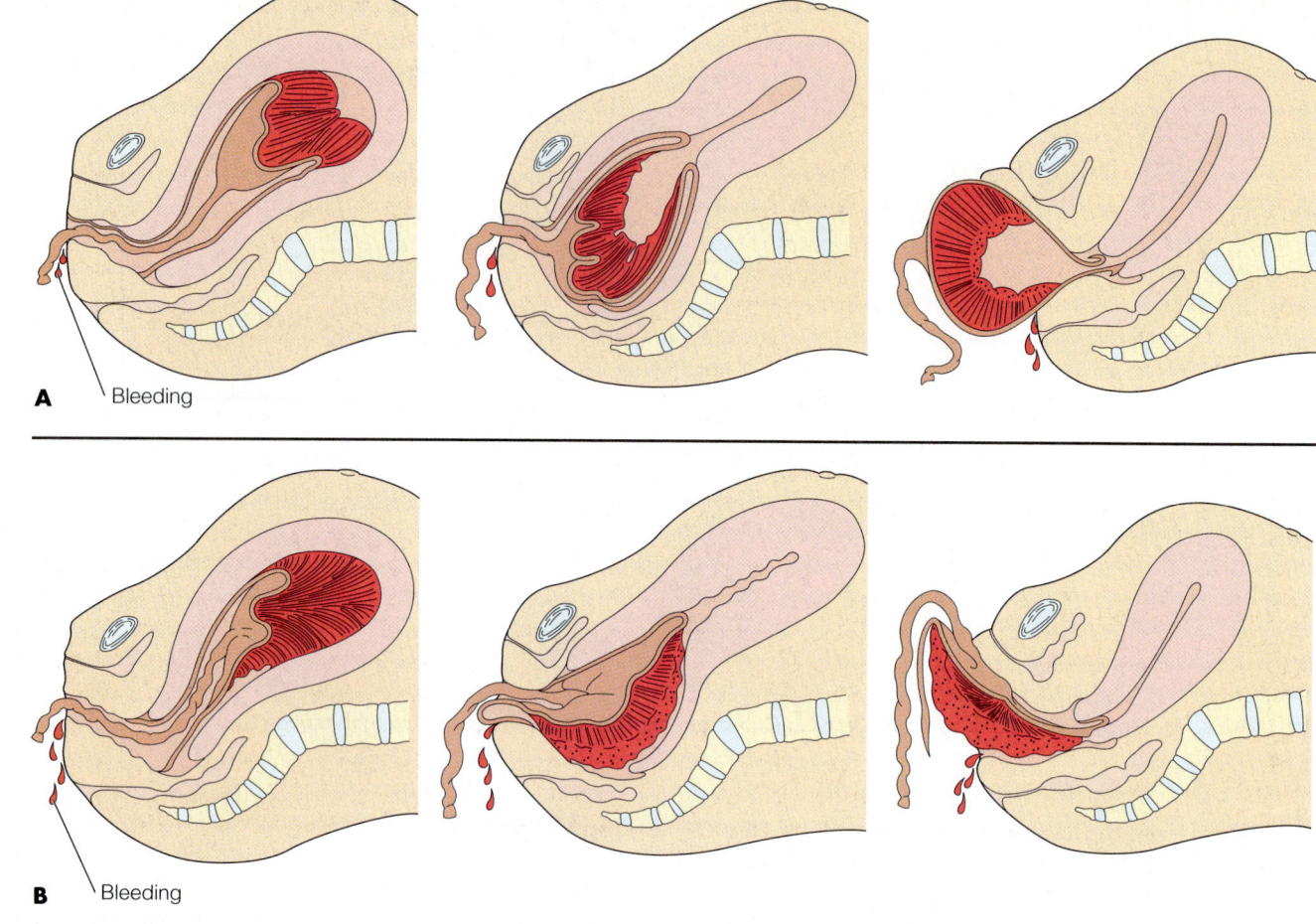

FIGURE 15–14. ◆ Placental separation and expulsion. **A,** Schultze mechanism. **B,** Duncan mechanism.

If the placenta separates from the inside to the outer margins, it is delivered with the fetal (shiny) side presenting (Figure 15–14 ◆). This is known as the Schultze mechanism of placental delivery or, more commonly, "shiny Schultze." If the placenta separates from the outer margins inward, it rolls up and presents sideways with the maternal surface delivering first. This is known as the Duncan mechanism and is commonly called "dirty Duncan" because the placental surface is rough. (Interventions for the third stage are discussed in Chapter 17.)

Fourth Stage

The fourth stage of labor is the time, from 1 to 4 hours after birth, during which physiologic readjustment of the mother's body begins. With the birth, hemodynamic changes occur. Blood loss ranges from 250 to 500 mL. With this blood loss and removal of the weight of the pregnant uterus from the surrounding vessels, blood is redistributed into venous beds. This results in a moderate drop in both systolic and diastolic blood pressure, increased pulse pressure, and moderate tachycardia (Cunningham et al., 2001).

The uterus remains contracted in the midline of the abdomen. The fundus is usually midway between the symphysis pubis and umbilicus. Its contracted state constricts the vessels at the site of placental implantation. Immediately after birth of the placenta, the cervix is widely spread and thick.

Nausea and vomiting usually cease. The woman may be thirsty and hungry. She may experience a shaking chill, which is thought to be associated with the ending of the physical exertion of labor. The bladder is often hypotonic due to trauma during the second stage and/or the administration of anesthetics that decrease sensations. Hypotonic bladder can lead to urinary retention. (Nursing care during this stage is discussed in Chapter 17.)

MATERNAL SYSTEMIC RESPONSE TO LABOR

Cardiovascular System

Uterine contractions and the pain, anxiety, and apprehension a laboring woman experiences stress her cardiovascular system. With each contraction, 300 to 500 mL of blood volume is forced back into the maternal circulation, which results in an increase in cardiac output of as much as 31% (Monga, 1999). Cardiac output increases more as the laboring woman experiences pain with uterine contractions and her anxiety and apprehension increase.

Maternal position also affects cardiac output. In the supine position, cardiac output lowers, heart rate increases, and stroke volume decreases. When the woman turns to a lateral (side-lying) position, cardiac output increases by as much as 25% to 30% (Monga, 1999).

Blood Pressure

As a result of increased cardiac output, blood pressure rises during uterine contractions. In the first stage, systolic pressure increases by 35 mm Hg and diastolic pressure increases by about 25 mm Hg. There may be further increases in the second stage during pushing (Monga, 1999).

Respiratory System

Oxygen demand and consumption increase when labor begins because of the presence of uterine contractions. As anxiety and pain from contractions increase, hyperventilation frequently occurs. With hyperventilation there is a fall in $PaCO_2$, and respiratory alkalosis results (Smith, 2000).

By the end of the first stage, most women have developed a mild metabolic acidosis compensated by respiratory alkalosis. As they push in the second stage of labor, the women's $PaCO_2$ levels may rise along with blood lactate levels (due to muscular activity), and mild respiratory acidosis occurs. By the time the baby is born (end of second stage), the woman has metabolic acidosis uncompensated for by respiratory alkalosis. The changes in acid-base status that occur in labor are quickly reversed in the fourth stage because of changes in women's respiratory rates. Acid-base levels return to pregnancy levels by 24 hours after birth, and to nonpregnant values a few weeks after birth (Blackburn & Loper, 1992).

Renal System

During labor there is an increase in maternal renin, plasma renin activity, and angiotensinogen. This elevation is thought to be important in the control of uteroplacental blood flow during birth and the early postpartal period. Structurally, the base of the bladder is pushed forward and upward when engagement occurs. The pressure from the presenting part may impair blood and lymph drainage from the base of the bladder, leading to edema (Cunningham et al., 2001).

Gastrointestinal System

During labor, gastric motility and absorption of solid food are reduced. Gastric emptying time is prolonged, and gastric volume (amount of contents that remain in the stomach) remains increased, regardless of the time the last meal was taken. Some narcotics also delay gastric emptying time and add to the risk of aspiration if general anesthesia is used.

Immune System and Other Blood Values

The white blood cell count (WBC) increases to 25,000 to 30,000/mm^3 during labor and the early postpartum. The change in WBC is mostly due to increased neutrophils resulting from a physiologic response to stress. The increased WBC makes it difficult to identify an infection. Maternal blood glucose levels decrease because the body uses glucose as an energy source during contractions. Decreased blood glucose levels lead to a decrease in insulin requirements.

Pain

According to the gate-control theory, pain results from activity in several interacting specialized neural systems. The gate-control theory proposes that a mechanism in the dorsal horn of the spinal column serves as a valve, or gate, that increases or decreases the flow of nerve impulses from the periphery to the central nervous system (CNS). The size of the transmitting fibers and the nerve impulses that descend from the brain influence the gate mechanism. Psychologic processes such as past experiences, attention, and emotion may influence pain perception and response by activating the gate mechanism. The gates may be opened or closed by CNS activities, such as anxiety or excitement, or selective localized activity.

The gate-control theory has two important implications for childbirth. Pain can be reduced by tactile stimulation and may be modified by activities controlled by the CNS. Tactile stimulation includes back rub, sacral pressure, and effleurage, while CNS-controlled activities include suggestion, distraction, and conditioning.

CAUSES OF PAIN DURING LABOR

The pain associated with the first stage of labor is unique in that it accompanies a normal physiologic process. Even though perception of the pain of childbirth varies among women, there is a physiologic basis for discomfort during labor. Pain during the first stage of labor arises from (1) dilatation of the cervix, which is the primary source of pain; (2) stretching of the lower uterine segment; (3) pressure on adjacent structures; and (4) hypoxia of the uterine muscle cells during contraction (Wesson, 2000). The areas of pain include the lower abdominal wall and the areas over the lower lumbar region and the upper sacrum.

During the second stage of labor, discomfort is due to (1) hypoxia of the contracting uterine muscle cells, (2) distention of the vagina and perineum, and (3) pressure on adjacent structures. The area of pain increases as shown in Figures 15–15 ◆ and 15–16 ◆.

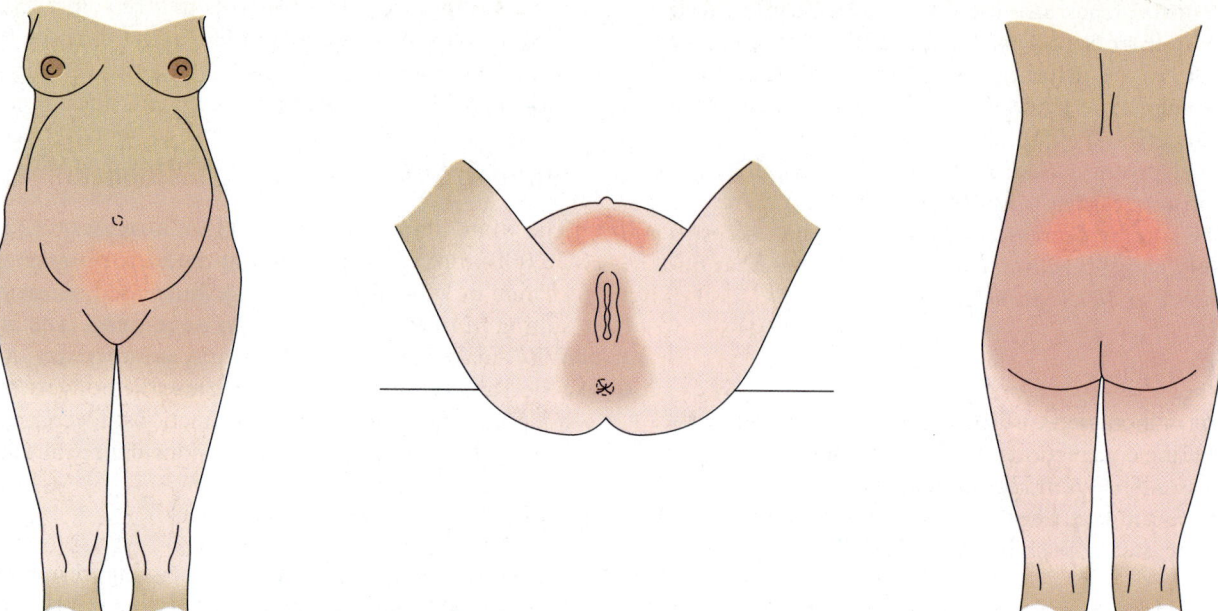

FIGURE 15–15. ◆ Distribution of labor pain during the later phase of the first stage and early phase of the second stage. The darkest colored areas indicate the location of the most intense pain, moderate color indicates moderate pain, and lighter color indicates mild pain. The uterine contractions, which at this stage are very strong, produce intense pain. *Note:* From Bonica, J. J. (1972). *Principles and practice of obstetric analgesia and anesthesia* (p. 109). Philadelphia: Davis.

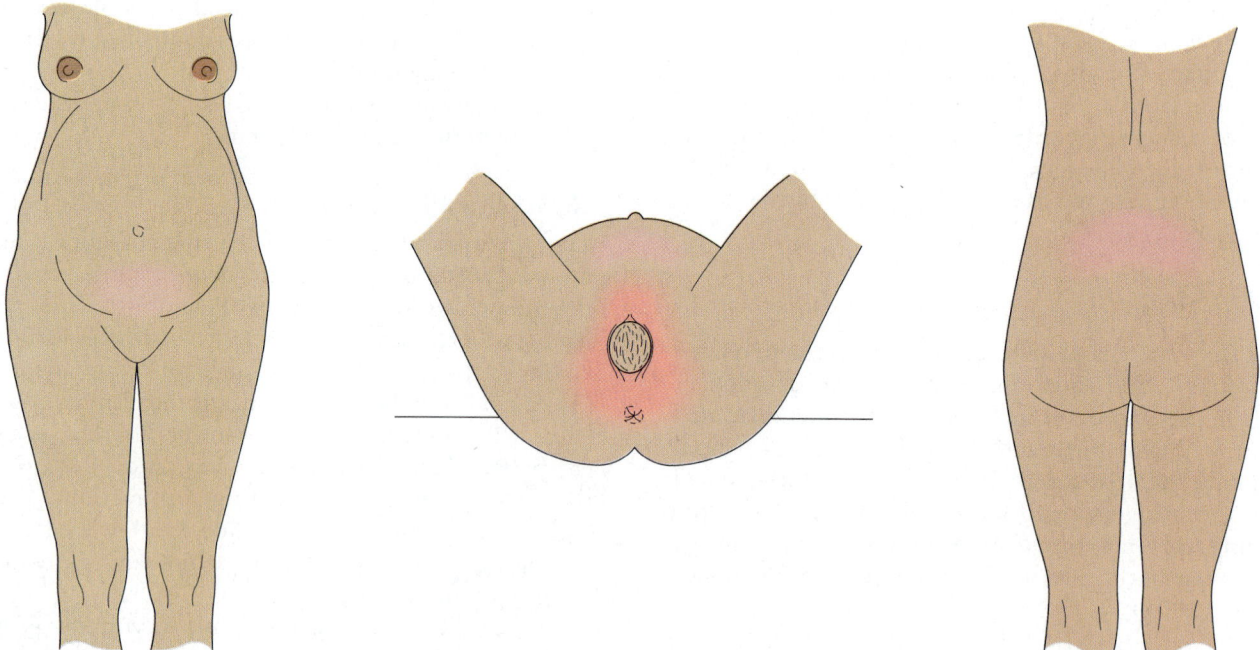

FIGURE 15–16. ◆ Distribution of labor pain during the later phase of the second stage and actual birth. The perineal component is the primary cause of discomfort. Uterine contractions contribute much less to the level of pain. *Note:* From Bonica, J. J. (1972). *Principles and practice of obstetric analgesia and anesthesia* (p. 109). Philadelphia: Davis.

Pain during the third stage results from uterine contractions and cervical dilatation as the placenta is expelled. This stage of labor is short, and after it anesthesia is needed primarily for episiotomy repair.

FACTORS AFFECTING RESPONSE TO PAIN

Many factors affect the individual's perception and response to pain. For example, preparation for childbirth classes may reduce the need for analgesia during labor. In addition, people tend to respond to painful stimuli in the way that is acceptable in their culture. In some cultures, it is natural to communicate pain, no matter how mild, whereas members of other cultures stoically accept pain. Fatigue and sleep deprivation may also influence response to pain. The tired woman has less energy and ability to use such strategies as distraction or imagination to deal with pain. As a result, she may lose her ability to cope with labor and choose analgesics or other medications to relieve the discomfort.

The woman's previous experience with pain and her anxiety level also affect her ability to manage current and future pain. Those who have had experience with pain seem more sensitive to painful stimuli than those who have not. Unfamiliar surroundings and events can increase anxiety, as does separation from family and loved ones. Anticipation of discomfort and questions about whether she can cope with the contractions may also increase anxiety.

Both attention and distraction influence the perception of pain. When pain sensation is the focus of attention, the perceived intensity is greater. A sensory stimulus such as a back rub can be a distraction that focuses the woman's attention on the stimulus rather than the pain.

FETAL RESPONSE TO LABOR

When the fetus is healthy, the mechanical and hemodynamic changes of normal labor have no adverse effects. Certain physiologic responses do occur, however.

- *Heart rate changes.* Early fetal heart rate decelerations can occur with intracranial pressures of 40 to 55 mm Hg, as the head pushes against the cervix. This early deceleration is believed to be due to hypoxic depression of the central nervous system, which is under vagal control. The absence of head compression decelerations in some fetuses during labor is explained by the existence of a threshold reached more gradually in the presence of intact membranes and lack of maternal resistance. These early decelerations are harmless in a normal fetus. Blood flow is decreased to the fetus at the peak of each contraction, which leads to a slow decrease in pH. During the second stage of labor, as uterine contractions become longer and stronger and the woman holds her breath to push, the fetal pH decreases more rapidly. The base deficit increases, and fetal oxygen saturation drops about 10% (Manning, 1999).

- *Hemodynamic changes.* The adequate exchange of nutrients and gases in the fetal capillaries and intervillous spaces depends in part on the fetal blood pressure. Fetal blood pressure protects the normal fetus during the anoxic periods caused by the contracting uterus during labor. The fetal and placental reserve is usually enough to see the fetus through these anoxic periods unharmed (Meschia, 1999).

- *Fetal sensation.* Beginning at about 37 or 38 weeks' gestation, the fetus is able to experience sensations of light, sound, and touch. The full-term fetus is able to hear music and the maternal voice. Even in utero, the fetus is sensitive to light and will move away from a bright light source. Additionally, the term baby is aware of pressure sensations during labor such as the touch of the caregiver during a vaginal exam or pressure on the head as a contraction occurs. Although the fetus may not be able to process this input, as the woman labors the fetus is experiencing the labor as well.

CHAPTER HIGHLIGHTS

- Five factors continuously interact during the process of labor and birth: the birth passage, the fetus, the relationship between the passage and the fetus, the forces of labor (contractions and pushing efforts), and the emotional components the woman brings to the birth setting (psychosocial status).
- The fetal head contains bones that are not fused. This allows for some overlapping and for a change in the shape of the head called molding to facilitate birth.
- Fetal attitude refers to the relation of the fetal parts to one another. The head is usually moderately flexed at midline, and the extremities are flexed close to the body.

- Fetal lie refers to the relationship of the cephalocaudal axis of the fetus to the maternal spine. The fetal lie is either longitudinal or transverse.
- Fetal presentation is determined by the body part lying closest to the maternal pelvis. Fetal presentation can be cephalic (head down), breech (buttocks or one or both feet), or shoulder.
- Fetal position is the relationship of the landmark on the presenting fetal part to the front, sides, or back of the maternal pelvis.
- Engagement of the presenting part takes place when the largest diameter of the presenting part reaches or passes through the pelvic inlet.

- Station refers to the relationship of the presenting part to an imaginary line between the ischial spines of the maternal pelvis. Negative numbers (−5 through −1) are above the pelvic inlet and ischial spines, and the fetus is not engaged. Zero (0) station is at the pelvic inlet, and positive numbers (+1 through +4) indicate descent below the ischial spines.

- Each uterine contraction has an increment, acme, and decrement.

- Contraction frequency is the time from the beginning of one contraction to the beginning of the next contraction. Contraction duration is the time from the beginning to the end of one contraction, while intensity is the strength of the contraction during acme. Intensity is termed mild, moderate, or strong.

- The woman's response to labor pain can be affected by education, culture, fatigue, personal meaning of pain, previous experience, anxiety, and availability of coping techniques and support.

- Possible causes of labor include progesterone withdrawal, prostaglandin release, or increased concentrations of CRH.

- Premonitory signs of labor include lightening, Braxton Hicks contractions, cervical softening and effacement, bloody show, sudden burst of energy, weight loss, and sometimes rupture of membranes.

- True labor contractions occur regularly, with an increase in frequency, duration, and intensity over time. The contractions usually start in the back and radiate around the abdomen. The discomfort is not relieved by ambulation or rest. False labor contractions do not produce progressive cervical effacement and dilatation. They are usually irregular and do not increase in intensity. The discomfort may be relieved by changes in activity.

- There are four stages of labor and birth: the first stage extends from the beginning of true labor to complete dilatation of the cervix; the second stage extends from complete dilatation of the cervix to birth; the third stage extends from birth to expulsion of the placenta; and the fourth stage extends from expulsion of the placenta to a period of 1 to 4 hours after.

- The fetus accommodates itself to the maternal pelvis in a series of movements called the cardinal movements of labor, which include descent, flexion, internal rotation, extension, external rotation, expulsion, and restitution.

- Placental separation is indicated by lengthening of the umbilical cord, a small spurt of blood, change in uterine shape, and a rise of the fundus in the abdomen.

EXPLORE MediaLink

NCLEX Review, Case Studies, and other interactive resources for this chapter can be found on the companion website at http://www.prenhall.com/london. Click on "Chapter 15" to select the activities for this chapter.

For animations, more NCLEX review questions, and an audio glossary, access the accompanying CD-ROM in this textbook.

REFERENCES

Blackburn, S. T., & Loper, D. L. (1992). *Maternal, fetal, and neonatal physiology*. Philadelphia: Saunders.

Browning, C. A. (2001). Using music during childbirth. *Birth, 27*(4), 272–276.

Caldwell, W. E., & Moloy, H. C. (1933). Anatomical variations in the female pelvis and their effect on labor with a suggested classification. *American Journal of Obstetrics and Gynecology, 26*, 479.

Challis, J. R. G. (1999). Characteristics of parturition. In R. K. Creasy & R. R. Resnik (Eds.), *Maternal-fetal medicine* (4th ed., pp. 484–497). Philadelphia: Saunders.

Cunningham, F. G., Gant, N. F., Leveno, K. J., Gilstrap, L. C., Hauth, J. C., & Wenstrom, K. D. (2001). *Williams obstetrics* (21st ed.). New York: McGraw-Hill.

Kilson, K. (2001). *Beach imagery*. BC Media Group. WEB

Lieberman, A. B., & Holt, L. H. (2000). *Nine months and a day*. Boston: Harvard Common Press.

Liggins, G. C. (1997). Biology of parturition. In R. K. Creasy (Ed.), *Management of labor and delivery*. Malden, MA: Blackwell.

Manning, F. (1999). Fetal assessment by evaluation of biophysical variables. In R. K. Creasy & R. R. Resnik (Eds.), *Maternal-fetal medicine* (4th ed., pp. 319–330). Philadelphia: Saunders.

Mauger, B. (2000). *Reclaiming the spirituality of birth: Healing for mothers and babies*. Rochester, VT: Healing Arts Press.

Meschia, G. (1999). Placental respiratory gas exchange and fetal oxygenation. In R. K. Creasy & R. R. Resnik (Eds.), *Maternal-fetal medicine* (4th ed., pp. 260–269). Philadelphia: Saunders.

Monga, M. (1999). Maternal cardiovascular and renal adaptation to pregnancy. In R. K. Creasy & R. R. Resnik (Eds.), *Maternal-fetal medicine* (4th ed., pp. 783–796). Philadelphia: Saunders.

Mullaly, L. M. (2000). Psychology of pregnancy. In S. Mattson & J. E. Smith (Eds.), *AWHONN: Maternal newborn nursing* (2nd ed., pp. 101–114). Philadelphia: Saunders.

Smith, K. (2000). Normal childbirth. In S. Mattson & J. E. Smith (Eds.), *AWHONN: Maternal newborn nursing* (2nd ed., pp. 241–270). Philadelphia: Saunders.

Smith, R. (1999). Corticotrophin-releasing hormone and the fetoplacental clock: An Australian perspective. *American Journal of Obstetrics and Gynecology, 180*, S269–S271.

Stern, D. N., & Bruschweiler-Stern, N. (1998). *The birth of a mother*. New York: Perseus Books.

Varney, H. (1997). *Nurse-midwifery* (3rd ed.). Boston: Blackwell.

Wesson, N. (2000). *Labor pain: A natural approach to easing delivery*. Rochester, VT: Healing Arts Press.

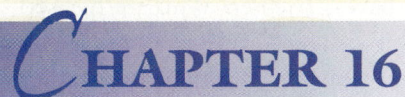

CHAPTER 16

Intrapartal Nursing Assessment

It was strange. After months of waiting for my baby's birth, labor took me by surprise. I wasn't quite ready to move from being pregnant to being a mother. Not that I had any choice!

—TAMMY, 23

Key Terms

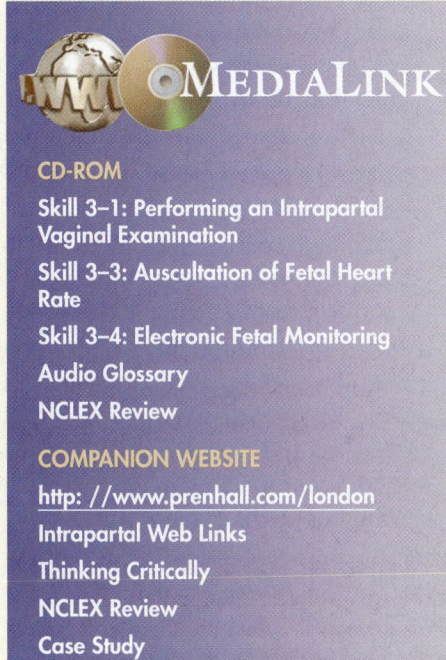

MEDIALINK

CD-ROM

Skill 3–1: Performing an Intrapartal Vaginal Examination

Skill 3–3: Auscultation of Fetal Heart Rate

Skill 3–4: Electronic Fetal Monitoring

Audio Glossary

NCLEX Review

COMPANION WEBSITE

http://www.prenhall.com/london

Intrapartal Web Links

Thinking Critically

NCLEX Review

Case Study

The physiologic events during labor call for many adaptations by the mother and the fetus. Thus, frequent and accurate assessments are crucial. The woman's partner or chosen support person is also an integral part of the childbirth experience. In nursing practice, the traditional assessment techniques of observation, palpation, and auscultation are augmented by the judicious use of technology such as ultrasound and electronic monitoring. These tools may provide more detailed information for assessment; however, it is important for the nurse to remember that the technology only provides data; it is the nurse who monitors the mother and her baby.

MATERNAL ASSESSMENT

History

Obtain a brief oral history when the woman is admitted to the birthing area. Each agency has its own admission forms, but they usually include the following information:

- Woman's name and age
- Attending physician or certified nurse-midwife
- Personal data: blood type; Rh factor; results of serology testing; prepregnant and present weight; allergies to medications, foods, or other substances; prescribed and over-the-counter medications taken during pregnancy; and history of drug and alcohol use and smoking during the pregnancy
- History of previous illness, such as tuberculosis, heart disease, diabetes, and so forth
- Problems in the prenatal period, such as elevated blood pressure, bleeding problems, recurrent urinary tract infections, other infections
- Pregnancy data: gravida, para, abortions, and perinatal deaths
- The method chosen for infant feeding
- Type of prenatal education classes (childbirth education classes)
- Woman's preferences about labor and birth, such as no episiotomy, no analgesics or anesthetics, or the presence of the father or others at the birth
- Pediatrician or family practice physician
- Additional data: history of special tests such as nonstress test (NST), biophysical profile (BPP), or ultrasound; history of any preterm labor; onset of labor; amniotic fluid membrane status; and brief description of previous labor and birth

The psychosocial history is a critical component of intrapartal nursing assessment. Begin the assessment when the woman is admitted to the birthing area by obtaining information such as the following:

- Does the woman have a partner? Who are her support people?
- Is she safe in her relationship with the baby's father? Was there any physical or emotional abuse before or during the pregnancy? If so, what interventions were made?

In questioning the woman about safety and abuse issues, be aware that abuse affects as many as one in five pregnant women. The following screening questions should be asked universally when the woman is alone so that she can answer freely (American College of Obstetricians and Gynecologists, 1999):

1. Has anyone close to you ever threatened to harm you?
2. Have you ever been hit, slapped, kicked, choked, or otherwise physically hurt by someone? If yes, by whom? Total number of times?
3. Has anyone, including your partner, ever forced you to have sex?
4. Are you afraid of your partner or anyone you mentioned?

- Has the woman experienced rape or sexual assault? Note: Given the prevalence of sexual violence against women in our society (the reported incidence is one in three women, regardless of age) it is essential to consider that the woman may have experienced sexual violence at some point in her life. In this case, she may be anxious about the labor process, or may become anxious during labor.
- Has she had difficulty or problems with previous pregnancies, labors, or births that would increase her anxiety now?
- Have emotional problems been present during the past few months? What interventions have occurred?

It is important to obtain the history in a setting that promotes trust and the establishment of a relationship. Some questions are straightforward, but others require care and privacy (the nurse and the woman alone together) to ensure that the woman has a safe environment in which to respond.

Nursing Practice

Many nurses have difficulty asking questions about domestic violence, sexual abuse, and drug or alcohol use during pregnancy. However, this information is necessary to provide the best nursing care possible. To create a relationship of trust in which the client feels safe answering uncomfortable questions, the following tips may be helpful:

▸ Explore your own beliefs and values.
▸ Use open-ended questions.
▸ Be receptive to the answers.
▸ Be accepting of others' life experiences.

Intrapartal High-Risk Screening

Screening for intrapartal high-risk factors is an integral part of assessing the normal laboring woman. As the history is obtained, note the presence of any factors that may be associated with a high-risk condition. For example, the woman who reports a physical symptom such as intermittent bleeding needs further assessment to rule out abruptio placentae or placenta previa before the admission process continues. It is also important to recognize the implications of a high-risk condition for the laboring woman and her fetus. For example, if there is an abnormal fetal presentation, labor may be prolonged, prolapse of the umbilical cord is more likely, and the possibility of a cesarean birth is increased.

Although physical conditions are major factors that increase risk in the intrapartal period, sociocultural variables such as poverty, nutrition, the amount of prenatal care, cultural beliefs about pregnancy, and communication patterns may also precipitate a high-risk situation. In addition, women who suffer from posttraumatic stress disorder may be at increased risk for some pregnancy complications (Seng, Oakley, Samselle, et al., 2001).

Begin gathering data about sociocultural factors as the woman enters the birthing area. Observe the communication pattern between the woman and her support person or people and their responses to admission questions and initial teaching. If the woman and those supporting her do not speak English and translators are not available among the birthing unit staff, the course of labor and the ability of caregivers to interact and provide support and education are affected. The couple must receive information in their primary language to make informed decisions. Communication may also be affected by cultural practices such as beliefs about when to speak, who should ask questions, or whether it is acceptable to let others know about discomfort (Austin et al., 1999).

A partial list of intrapartal risk factors appears in Table 16–1. Keep these factors in mind during the intrapartal assessment.

TABLE 16–1 Intrapartal High-Risk Factors

Factor	Maternal Implications	Fetal-Neonatal Implications
Abnormal presentation	↑ Incidence of cesarean birth ↑ Incidence of prolonged labor	↑ Incidence of placenta previa Prematurity ↑ Risk of congenital abnormality Neonatal physical trauma ↑ Risk of intrauterine growth restriction (IUGR)
Multiple gestation	↑ Uterine distention → ↑ risk of postpartum hemorrhage ↑ Risk of cesarean birth ↑ Risk of preterm labor	Low birth weight Prematurity ↑ Risk of congenital anomalies Feto-fetal transfusion
Hydramnios	↑ Discomfort ↑ Dyspnea ↑ Risk of preterm labor Edema of lower extremities	↑ Risk of esophageal or other high-alimentary-tract atresias ↑ Risk of CNS anomalies (myelocele)
Oligohydramnios	Maternal fear of "dry birth"	↑ Incidence of congenital anomalies ↑ Incidence of renal lesions ↑ Risk of IUGR ↑ Risk of fetal acidosis ↑ Risk of cord compression Postmaturity
Meconium staining of amniotic fluid	↑ Psychologic stress due to fear for baby	↑ Risk of fetal asphyxia ↑ Risk of meconium aspiration ↑ Risk of pneumonia due to aspiration of meconium
Premature rupture of membranes	↑ Risk of infection (chorioamnionitis) ↑ Risk of preterm labor ↑ Anxiety Fear for the baby Prolonged hospitalization ↑ Incidence of tocolytic therapy	↑ Perinatal morbidity Prematurity ↑ Birth weight ↑ Risk of respiratory distress syndrome Prolonged hospitalization

(continued)

TABLE 16-1   Intrapartal High-Risk Factors—continued

Factor	Maternal Implications	Fetal-Neonatal Implications
Induction of labor	↑ Risk of hypercontractility of uterus ↑ Risk of uterine rupture Length of labor if cervix not ready ↑ Anxiety	Prematurity if gestational age not assessed correctly Hypoxia if hyperstimulation occurs
Abruptio placentae/placenta previa	Hemorrhage Uterine atony ↑ Incidence of cesarean birth	Fetal hypoxia/acidosis Fetal exsanguination ↑ Perinatal mortality
Failure to progress in labor	Maternal exhaustion ↑ Incidence of augmentation of labor ↑ Incidence of cesarean birth	Fetal hypoxia/acidosis Intracranial birth injury
Precipitous labor (<3 hours)	Perineal, vaginal, cervical lacerations ↑ Risk of postpartum hemorrhage	Tentorial tears
Prolapse of umbilical cord	↑ Fear for baby Cesarean birth	Acute fetal hypoxia/acidosis
Fetal heart aberrations	↑ Fear for baby ↑ Risk of cesarean birth, forceps, vacuum Continuous electronic monitoring and intervention in labor	Tachycardia, chronic asphyxic insult, bradycardia, acute asphyxic insult Chronic hypoxia Congenital heart block
Uterine rupture	Hemorrhage Cesarean birth for hysterectomy ↑ Risk of death	Fetal anoxia Fetal hemorrhage ↑ Neonatal morbidity and mortality
Postdates (>42 weeks)	↑ Anxiety ↑ Incidence of induction of labor ↑ Incidence of cesarean birth ↑ Use of technology to monitor fetus ↑ Risk of shoulder dystocia	Postmaturity syndrome ↑ Risk of fetal-neonatal mortality and morbidity ↑ Risk of antepartum fetal death ↑ Incidence or risk of large baby
Diabetes	↑ Risk of hydramnios ↑ Risk of hypoglycemia or hyperglycemia ↑ Risk of preeclampsia-eclampsia	↑ Risk of malpresentation ↑ Risk of macrosomia ↑ Risk of IUGR ↑ Risk of respiratory distress syndrome ↑ Risk of congenital anomalies
Pregnancy-induced hypertension	↑ Risk of seizures ↑ Risk of stroke ↑ Risk of HELLP	↑ Risk of small-for-gestational-age baby ↑ Risk of preterm birth ↑ Risk of mortality
AIDS/STD	↑ Risk of additional infections	↑ Risk of transplacental transmission

Intrapartal Physical and Psychosociocultural Assessment

A physical examination is part of the admission procedure and part of the ongoing care of the woman. Although the intrapartal physical assessment is not as complete and thorough as the initial prenatal physical examination (Chapter 8), ⚭ it does involve assessment of some body systems and the actual labor process. See "Assessment Guide: Intrapartal—First Stage of Labor" for a framework to use when examining the laboring woman.

The physical assessment portion includes assessments performed immediately on admission as well as ongoing assessments. When labor is progressing very quickly, there may not be time for a complete nursing assessment. In that case, the critical physical assessments include maternal vital signs, labor status, fetal status, and laboratory findings.

The cultural assessment portion provides a starting point for this increasingly important aspect of assessment. Individualized nursing care can best be planned and implemented when the values and beliefs of the laboring woman are known and honored (Callister, 2001). It is sometimes challenging to achieve a balance between cultural awareness and the risk of stereotyping because cultural responses are influenced by so many factors. Nurses are most effective when they combine an awareness of the major cultural values and beliefs of a specific group with the recognition that individual differences have an impact.

Physical Assessment/Normal Findings	Alterations and Possible Causes*	Nursing Responses to Data†
VITAL SIGNS		
Blood pressure (BP): <130 systolic and <85 diastolic in adult 18 years of age or older or no more than 15–20 mm Hg rise in systolic pressure over baseline BP during early pregnancy	High BP (essential hypertension, preeclampsia, renal disease, apprehension or anxiety) Low BP (supine hypotension)	Evaluate history of preexisting disorders and check for presence of other signs of preeclampsia. Do not assess during contractions; implement measures to decrease anxiety and reassess. Turn woman on her side and recheck BP. Provide quiet environment. Have O₂ available.
Pulse: 60–90 beats per minute (bpm)	Increased pulse rate (excitement or anxiety, cardiac disorders, early shock)	Evaluate cause, reassess to see if rate continues; report to physician.
Respirations: 14–22/minute (or pulse rate divided by 4)	Marked tachypnea (respiratory disease), hyperventilation in transition phase	Assess between contractions; if marked tachypnea continues, assess for signs of respiratory disease.
Pulse oxygen 95% or greater	Hyperventilation (anxiety)	Encourage slow breaths if woman is hyperventilating.
Temperature: 36.2–37.6 °C (98–99.6 °F)	>90%; hypoxia, hypotension, hemorrhage	Apply O₂; notify physician
	Elevated temperature (infection, dehydration, prolonged rupture of membranes, epidural regional block)	Assess for other signs of infection or dehydration.
WEIGHT		
25–30 lb greater than prepregnant weight	Weight gain >30 lb (fluid retention, obesity, large infant, diabetes mellitus, preeclampsia), weight gain <15 lb (SGA).	Assess for signs of edema. Evaluate pattern from prenatal record.
LUNGS		
Normal breath sounds, clear and equal	Rales, rhonchi, friction rub (infection), pulmonary edema, asthma	Reassess; refer to physician.
FUNDUS		
At 40 weeks' gestation located just below xiphoid process	Uterine size not compatible with estimated date of birth (SGA, large for gestational age [LGA], hydramnios, multiple pregnancy)	Reevaluate history regarding pregnancy dating. Refer to physician for additional assessment.
EDEMA		
Slight amount of dependent edema	Pitting edema of face, hands, legs, abdomen, sacral area (preeclampsia)	Check deep tendon reflexes for hyperactivity; check for clonus; refer to physician.
HYDRATION		
Normal skin turgor, elastic	Poor skin turgor (dehydration)	Assess skin turgor; refer to physician for deviations.
PERINEUM		
Tissues smooth, pink color (see Prenatal Initial Physical Assessment Guide, Chapter 8) 🔗	Varicose veins of vulva, herpes lesions	Exercise care while doing a perineal prep; note on client record need for follow-up in postpartal period; reassess after birth; refer to physician.
Clear mucus; may be blood tinged with earthy or human odor	Profuse, purulent, foul-smelling drainage	Suspected gonorrhea or chorioamnionitis; report to physician; initiate care to newborn's eyes; notify neonatal nursing staff and pediatrician.
	*Possible causes of alterations are placed in parentheses.	†This column provides guidelines for further assessment and initial nursing intervention.

(continued)

Physical Assessment/Normal Findings	Alterations and Possible Causes*	Nursing Responses to Data†
PERINEUM— *continued*		
Presence of small amount of bloody show that gradually increases with further cervical dilatation	Hemorrhage	Assess BP and pulse, pallor, diaphoresis; report any marked changes. (*Note:* Gaping of vagina or anus and bulging of perineum are signs that suggest the onset of the second stage of labor.) Follow universal precautions.
LABOR STATUS		
Uterine contractions: regular pattern	Failure to establish a regular pattern, prolonged latent phase Hypertonicity Hypotonicity	Evaluate whether woman is in true labor; ambulate if in early labor. Evaluate client status and contractile pattern. Obtain a 20-minute EFM strip. Notify physician or CNM.
Cervical dilatation: progressive cervical dilatation from size of fingertip to 10 cm (see Skill 3–1 in the Clinical Skills Manual, as well as the CD-ROM that accompanies this text) ⊂⊃ SKILLS CD	Rigidity of cervix (frequent cervical infections, scar tissue, failure of presenting part to descend)	Evaluate contractions, fetal engagement, position, and cervical dilatation. Inform client of progress.
Cervical effacement: progressive thinning of cervix (see Skill 3–1) ⊂⊃ SKILLS CD	Failure to efface (rigidity of cervix, failure of presenting part to engage); cervical edema (pushing effort by woman before cervix is fully dilated and effaced, trapped cervix)	Evaluate contractions, fetal engagement, and position. Notify physician or CNM if cervix is becoming edematous; work with woman to prevent pushing until cervix is completely dilated. Keep vaginal exams to a minimum.
Fetal descent: progressive descent of fetal presenting part from station −5 to +4 (see Skill 3–1 Procedure 16–1) ⊂⊃ SKILLS CD	Failure of descent (abnormal fetal position or presentation, macrosomic fetus, inadequate pelvic measurement)	Evaluate fetal position, presentation, and size. Evaluate maternal pelvic measurements.
Membranes: may rupture before or during labor	Rupture of membranes more than 12–24 hours before initiation of labor	Assess for ruptured membranes using Nitrazine test tape before doing vaginal exam. Follow body substance isolation (BSI) precautions. Instruct woman with ruptured membranes to remain on bed rest if presenting part is not engaged and firmly down against the cervix. Keep vaginal exams to a minimum to prevent infection. When membranes rupture in the birth setting, **immediately assess FHR** to detect changes associated with prolapse of umbilical cord (FHR slows).

Findings on Nitrazine test tape:
Membranes probably intact
 	
  Yellow   pH 5.0
  Olive   pH 5.5
  Olive green pH 6.0
	False-positive results may be obtained if large amount of bloody show is present, previous vaginal examination has been done using lubricant, or tape is touched by nurse's fingers.	Assess fluid for consistency, amount, odor, assess FHR frequently. Assess fluid at regular intervals for presence of meconium staining.
		Follow BSI precautions while assessing amniotic fluid.

Membranes probably ruptured
 	
  Blue-green   pH 6.5
  Blue-gray   pH 7.0
  Deep blue   pH 7.5
		Teach woman that amniotic fluid is continually produced (to allay fear of "dry birth").
		Teach woman that she may feel amniotic fluid trickle or gush with contractions.
		Change chux pads often.

Amniotic fluid clear, with earthy or human odor, no foul-smelling odor	Greenish amniotic fluid (fetal stress)	Assess FHR; do vaginal exam to evaluate for prolapsed cord; apply fetal monitor for continuous data; report to physician.
	Strong or foul odor (amnionitis)	Take woman's temperature and report to physician.
	***Possible causes of alterations are placed in parentheses.**	**†This column provides guidelines for further assessment and initial nursing intervention.**

Physical Assessment/Normal Findings	Alterations and Possible Causes*	Nursing Responses to Data†
FETAL STATUS		
FHR: 120–160 bpm	<120 or >160 bpm (fetal stress); abnormal patterns on fetal monitor: decreased variability, late decelerations, variable decelerations, absence of accelerations with fetal movement	Initiate interventions based on particular FHR pattern.
Presentation: Cephalic, 97% Breech, 3%	Face, brow, breech, or shoulder presentation	Report to physician; after presentation is confirmed as face, brow, breech, or shoulder, woman may be prepared for cesarean birth.
Position: left-occiput-anterior (LOA) most common	Persistent occipital-posterior (OP) position; transverse arrest	Carefully monitor maternal and fetal status.
Activity: fetal movement	Hyperactivity (may precede fetal hypoxia)	Carefully evaluate FHR; apply fetal monitor.
	Complete lack of movement (fetal distress or fetal demise)	Carefully evaluate FHR; apply fetal monitor. Report to physician or CNM.
LABORATORY EVALUATION		
Hematologic tests Hemoglobin: 12–16 g/dL	<12 g/dL (anemia, hemorrhage)	Evaluate woman for problems due to decreased oxygen-carrying capacity caused by lowered hemoglobin.
Complete blood count (CBC) Hematocrit: 38%–47% Red blood cell count (RBC): 4.2–5.4 million/mm³ White blood cell count (WBC): 4,500–11,000/mm³, although leukocytosis to 20,000/mm³ is not unusual Platelets: 150,000–400,000/mm³	Presence of infection or blood dyscrasias, loss of blood (hemorrhage, disseminated intravascular coagulation [DIC])	Evaluate for other signs of infection or for petechiae, bruising, or unusual bleeding.
Serologic testing Serologic test for syphilis (STS) or venereal disease research laboratory (VDRL) test: nonreactive	Positive reaction (Chapter 8, Initial Prenatal Physical Assessment Guide) 🔗	For reactive test, notify newborn nursery and pediatrician.
Rh factor	Rh-positive fetus in Rh-negative woman	Assess prenatal record for titer levels during pregnancy. Obtain cord blood for direct Coombs' at birth.
Urinalysis Glucose: negative	Glycosuria (low renal threshold for glucose, diabetes mellitus)	Assess blood glucose level; test urine for ketones; ketonuria and glycosuria require further assessment of blood sugar levels.‡
Ketones: negative	Ketonuria (starvation ketosis)	
Proteins: negative	Proteinuria (urine specimen contaminated with vaginal secretions, fever, kidney disease); proteinuria of 2+ or greater found in uncontaminated urine may be a sign of ensuing preeclampsia	Instruct woman in collection technique; incidence of contamination from vaginal discharge is common.
Red blood cells: negative	Blood in urine (calculi, cystitis, glomerulonephritis, neoplasm)	Assess collection technique (may be bloody show).
White blood cells: negative	Presence of white blood cells (infection in genitourinary tract)	Assess for signs of urinary tract infection.
Casts: none	Presence of casts (nephrotic syndrome)	

†This column provides guidelines for further assessment and initial nursing intervention.

‡Glycosuria should not be discounted. The presence of glycosuria necessitates follow-up.

*Possible causes of alterations are placed in parentheses.

(continued)

Cultural Assessment[§]	Variations to Consider	Nursing Responses to Data[†]
Cultural influences determine customs and practices regarding intrapartal care	Individual preferences may vary.	
Ask the following questions: Who would you like to remain with you during your labor and birth?	She may prefer only her coach to remain or may also want family and/or friends.	Provide support for her wishes by encouraging desired people to stay. Provide information to others (with the woman's permission) who are not in the room.
What would you like to wear during labor?	She may be more comfortable in her own clothes.	Offer supportive materials such as chux pad if needed to protect her own clothing. Avoid subtle signals to the woman that she should not have chosen to remain in her own clothes. Have other clothing available if the woman desires. If her clothing becomes contaminated, it will be simple to place it in a plastic bag. The nurse can soak soiled clothing in cool water. The nurse needs to remember to wear disposable gloves and a plastic apron if splashing is anticipated.
What activity would you like during labor?	She may want to ambulate most of the time, stand in the shower, sit in the Jacuzzi (see "Complementary Care: Hydrotherapy" in Chapter 17), sit in a chair or on a stool, remain on the bed, and so forth.	Support the woman's wishes; provide encouragement and complete assessments in a manner so her activity and positional wishes are disturbed as little as possible.
What position would you like for the birth?	She may feel more comfortable in lithotomy with stirrups and her upper body elevated, or side-lying or sitting in birthing bed, or standing, or squatting, or on hands and knees.	Collect any supplies and equipment needed to support her in her chosen birthing position. Provide information to the coach regarding any changes that may be needed based on the chosen position.
Is there anything special you would like?	She may want the room darkened or to have curtains and windows open, music playing (see "Complementary Care: Music During Childbirth" in Chapter 15), a Leboyer birth, certain scents (see "Complementary Care: Aromatherapy in Childbirth" in this chapter), her coach to cut the umbilical cord, to save a portion of the umbilical cord, to save the placenta, to videotape the birth, and so forth.	Support requests and communicate requests to any other nursing or medical personnel (so requests can continue to be supported and not questioned). If another nurse or physician does not honor the request, act as advocate for the woman by continuing to support her unless her desire is truly unsafe.
Ask the woman if she would like fluids and ask what temperature she prefers.	She may prefer clear fluids other than water (tea, clear juice). She may prefer iced, room-temperature, or warmed fluids.	Provide fluids as desired.
Observe the woman's response when privacy is difficult to maintain and her body is exposed.	Some women do not seem to mind being exposed during an exam or procedure; others feel acute discomfort.	Maintain privacy and respect the woman's sense of privacy. If the woman is unable to provide specific information, the nurse may draw from general information regarding cultural variation: a Southeast Asian woman may not want any family member in the room during exam or procedures. Her partner may not be involved with coaching activities during labor or birth. Saudi women may need to remain covered during the labor and birth and avoid exposure of any body part. The husband may need to be in the room but remain behind a curtain or screen so he does not view his wife at this time.
If the woman is to breastfeed, ask if she would like to feed her baby immediately after birth.	She may want to feed her baby right away or may want to wait a little while.	

§These are only a few suggestions. We do not mean to imply that this is a comprehensive cultural assessment; rather, it is a tool to encourage cultural sensitivity.

†This column provides guidelines for further assessment and initial nursing intervention.

Cultural Assessment[§]	Variations to Consider	Nursing Responses to Data[†]
PREPARATION FOR CHILDBIRTH		
Woman has some information regarding process of normal labor and birth.	Some women do not have any information regarding childbirth.	Add to present information base.
Woman has breathing and/or relaxation techniques to use during labor.	Some women do not have any method of relaxation or breathing to use, and some do not desire them.	Support breathing and relaxation techniques that client is using; provide information if needed.
RESPONSE TO LABOR		
Latent phase: relaxed, excited, anxious for labor to be well established	May feel unable to cope with contractions because of fear, anxiety, or lack of information	Provide support and encouragement; establish trusting relationship.
Active phase: becomes more intense, begins to tire Transitional phase: feels tired, may feel unable to cope, needs frequent coaching to maintain breathing patterns	May remain quiet and without any sign of discomfort or anxiety, may insist that she is unable to continue with the birthing process	Provide support and coaching if needed.
Coping mechanisms: ability to cope with labor through utilization of support system, breathing, relaxation techniques	May feel marked anxiety and apprehension, may not have coping mechanisms that can be brought into this experience, or may be unable to use them at this time.	Support coping mechanisms if they are working for the woman; provide information and support if she exhibits anxiety or needs alternative to present coping methods.
	Survivors of sexual abuse may demonstrate fear of IVs or needles, may recoil when touched, may insist on a female caregiver, may be very sensitive to body fluids and cleanliness, and may be unable to labor lying down (Burrian, 1995).	Encourage participation of coach or significant other if a supportive relationship seems apparent. Establish rapport and a trusting relationship. Provide information that is true and offer your presence.
ANXIETY		
Some anxiety and apprehension is within normal limits	May show anxiety through rapid breathing, nervous tremors, frowning, grimacing, clenching of teeth, thrashing movements, crying, increased pulse and blood pressure.	Provide support, encouragement, and information. Teach relaxation techniques; support controlled breathing efforts. May need to provide a paper bag to breathe into if woman says her lips are tingling. Note FHR.
SOUNDS DURING LABOR		
	Some women are very quiet; others moan or make a variety of noises.	Provide a supportive environment. Encourage woman to do what is right for her.
SUPPORT SYSTEM		
Physical intimacy between mother and father (or mother and support person); caretaking activities such as soothing conversation, touching	Some women would prefer no contact; others may show clinging behaviors.	Encourage caretaking activities that appear to comfort the woman; encourage support to the woman; if support is limited, the nurse may take a more active role.
Support person stays in close proximity	Limited interaction may come from a desire for quiet.	Encourage support person to stay close (if this seems appropriate).
Relationship between mother and father (or support person): involved interaction	The support person may seem to be detached and maintain little support, attention, or conversation.	Support interactions; if interaction is limited, the nurse may provide more information and support.
		Ensure that coach or significant other has short breaks, especially prior to transition.

[§]These are only a few suggestions. We do not mean to imply that this is a comprehensive cultural assessment; rather, it is a tool to encourage cultural sensitivity.

[†]This column provides guidelines for further assessment and initial nursing intervention.

Developing Cultural Competence

The following list provides a few examples of the beliefs and taboos of some Native-American women related to childbirth (Cesario, 2001):

- If a pregnant woman eats the feet of animals, her infant will be born feet first.
- If a pregnant woman eats an animal's tail, her infant will get stuck in the birth canal.
- Weaving or tying knots during pregnancy will cause umbilical cord complications.
- If the woman naps during labor it may cause a change in the desired sex of her infant.
- A lengthy labor may result if a woman is exposed to cold during pregnancy because cold causes the woman's bag of waters to freeze, thereby holding the infant back.
- When the infant's cord is being cut following birth the mother should bite on a white pebble. This ensures that the infant's teeth will be white and strong.

TABLE 16–2 Contraction and Labor Progress Characteristics

Contraction Characteristics

Latent phase:	Every 10–30 min × 20–40 sec; mild, progressing to Every 5–7 min × 30–40 sec; moderate
Active phase:	Every 2–3 min × 40–60 sec; moderate to strong
Transition phase:	Every 1 1/2–2 min × 60–90 sec; strong

Labor Progress Characteristics

Primipara:	1.2 cm/hr dilatation 1 cm/hr descent < 2 hr in second stage
Multipara:	1.5 cm/hr dilatation < 2 cm/hr descent < 1 hr in second stage

"Developing Cultural Competence" provides examples of selected beliefs of some Native-American women.

The final section of the assessment guide addresses psychosocial factors. The laboring woman's psychosocial status is an important part of the total assessment. The woman has previous ideas, knowledge, and fears about childbearing. By assessing her psychosocial status, the nurse can meet the woman's needs for information and support.

While performing the intrapartal assessment, it is crucial to follow the Centers for Disease Control and Prevention (CDC) guidelines to prevent exposure to body substances. Provide information about the precautions in a factual manner.

Methods of Evaluating Labor Progress

CONTRACTION ASSESSMENT

Uterine contractions may be assessed by palpation or continuous electronic monitoring.

Palpation. Assess contractions for frequency, duration, and intensity by placing one hand on the uterine fundus. Keep the hand relatively still because excessive movement may stimulate contractions or cause discomfort. Determine the frequency of the contractions by noting the time from the beginning of one contraction to the beginning of the next. If contractions begin at 7:00, 7:04, and 7:08, for example, their frequency is every 4 minutes. To determine contraction duration, note the time when tensing of the fundus is first felt (beginning of contraction) and again as relaxation occurs (end of contraction). During the acme of the contraction, intensity can be evaluated by estimating the indentability of the fundus. Assess at least three successive contractions to provide enough data to determine the contraction pattern. See Table 16–2 for a review of characteristics in different phases of labor.

Complementary Care

AROMATHERAPY IN CHILDBIRTH

Aromatherapy is the use of aromas for physical, mental, and emotional healing. The primary sources of healing aromas are essential oils distilled from herbs and flowers. Essential oils are volatile, which means that their molecules quickly evaporate into the environment. When you inhale an essential oil molecule, its active components react with the olfactory membrane in your nose, which is directly linked to the limbic system and hypothalamus in the brain. These two areas play a crucial role in regulating your emotions, mind, and body (Gottlieb, 2000).

Essential oils can also be applied directly to the skin. Because the oil is not only inhaled but also absorbed into the bloodstream, the effect can be doubled (Gottlieb, 2000). Essential oils are quite potent and can irritate the skin, so they should be diluted with a carrier oil such as sesame or sweet almond oil before being used on the skin. The fragrance of the essential oil in the carrier oil does not have to be intense to be effective. In fact, the more intense the odor, the less pleasant it becomes.

For a few days before the expected due date and during labor, jasmine or lavender oil can be massaged into the abdomen and lower back using long, smooth movement and fairly firm pressure. The woman may find small circular movements of the lower back to be soothing. Both jasmine and lavender strengthen contractions and provide some analgesia. If the woman complains of feeling hot during labor, a few drops of lavender can be added to cool water, which is then used to sponge her face and body.

Note that women should not use essential oils during the first 3 months of pregnancy, since many oils contain thujone, a chemical that has been shown to have an abortive effect (Gottlieb, 2000).

This is also a good time to assess the laboring woman's perception of pain. For example, how does she describe the pain? What is her affect? Is this contraction more uncomfortable than the last one? Note and chart the woman's affect and response to the contractions.

Electronic Monitoring of Contractions   Electronic monitoring of uterine contractions provides continuous data. In many birth settings, electronic monitoring is routine for high-risk clients and women having oxytocin-induced labor; other facilities monitor all laboring women.

Electronic monitoring may be done externally, with a device placed against the maternal abdomen, or internally, with an **intrauterine pressure catheter.** When monitoring by external means, the portion of the monitoring equipment called a tocodynamometer, or "toco," is positioned against the fundus of the uterus and held in place with an elastic belt (see Figure 16–1 ◆). The toco contains a flexible disk that responds to pressure. When the uterus contracts, the fundus tightens and the change in pressure against the toco is amplified and transmitted to the electronic fetal monitor. The monitor displays the uterine contraction as a pattern on graph paper.

External monitoring provides a continuous recording of the frequency and duration of uterine contractions and is noninvasive. However, it does not accurately record the intensity of the uterine contraction, and it is difficult to obtain an accurate fetal heart rate (FHR) in some women, such as those who are very obese, those who have hydramnios (an abnormally large amount of amniotic fluid), or those whose fetus is very active. In addition, the belt may bother the woman if it requires frequent readjustment when she changes position.

Internal intrauterine monitoring provides the same data and also provides accurate measurement of uterine contraction intensity (the strength of the contraction and the actual pressure within the uterus). After membranes have ruptured, the certified nurse-midwife or physician inserts the intrauterine pressure catheter into the uterine cavity and connects it by a cable to the electronic fetal monitor. A small micropressure device located in the tip of the catheter measures the pressure within the uterus in the resting state and during each contraction. Internal electronic monitoring is used when it is imperative to have accurate intrauterine pressure readings to evaluate the stress on the uterus.

In addition, it is important to evaluate the woman's labor status by palpating the intensity and resting tone of the uterine fundus during contractions.

CERVICAL ASSESSMENT

Cervical dilatation and effacement are evaluated directly by vaginal examination (see Skill 3–1 in the *Clinical Skills Manual,* as well as the CD-ROM that accompanies this text). ▭ CD SKILLS The vaginal examination can also provide information about membrane status, characteristics of amniotic fluid, fetal position, and station. See Figures 16–2 ◆, 16–3 ◆, and 16–4 ◆.

FETAL ASSESSMENT

Fetal Position and Presentation

Fetal position and presentation are determined by inspecting the woman's abdomen, palpating it, performing a vaginal examination, and auscultating FHR. Ultrasound may also be used.

INSPECTION

Observe the woman's abdomen for size and shape. Assess the lie of the fetus by noting whether the uterus projects up and down (longitudinal lie) or left to right (transverse lie).

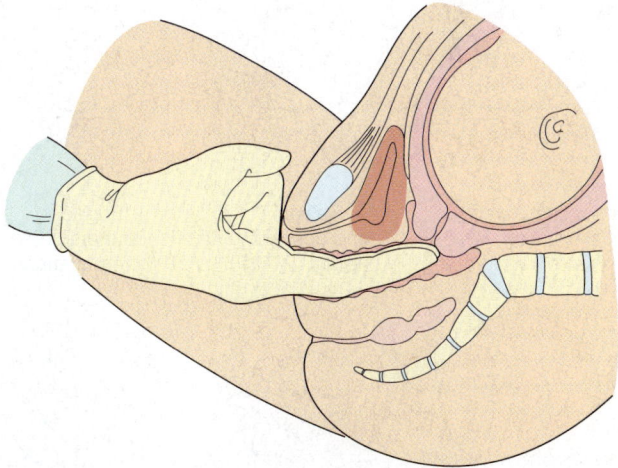

FIGURE 16–2. ◆ To gauge cervical dilatation, the nurse place the index and middle fingers against the cervix and determines the size of the opening. Before labor begins, the cervix is long (approximately 2.5 cm), the sides feel thick, and the cervical canal is closed, so an examining finger cannot be inserted. During labor, the cervix begins to dilate, and the size of the opening progresses from 1 cm to 10 cm in diameter.

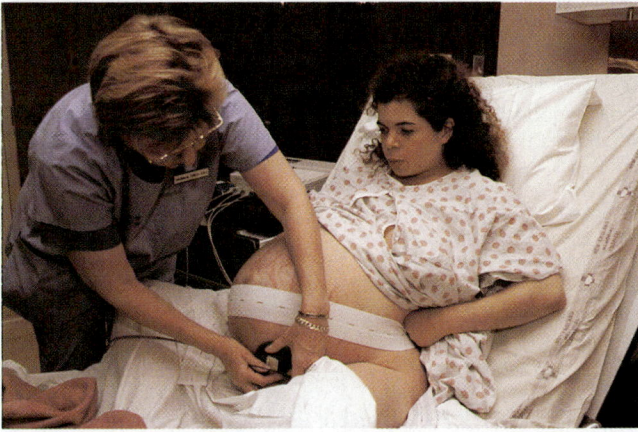

FIGURE 16–1. ◆ Woman in labor with external monitor applied. The tocodynamometer placed on the uterine fundus is recording uterine contractions. The lower belt holds the ultrasonic device that monitors the fetal heart rate. The belts can be adjusted for comfort.

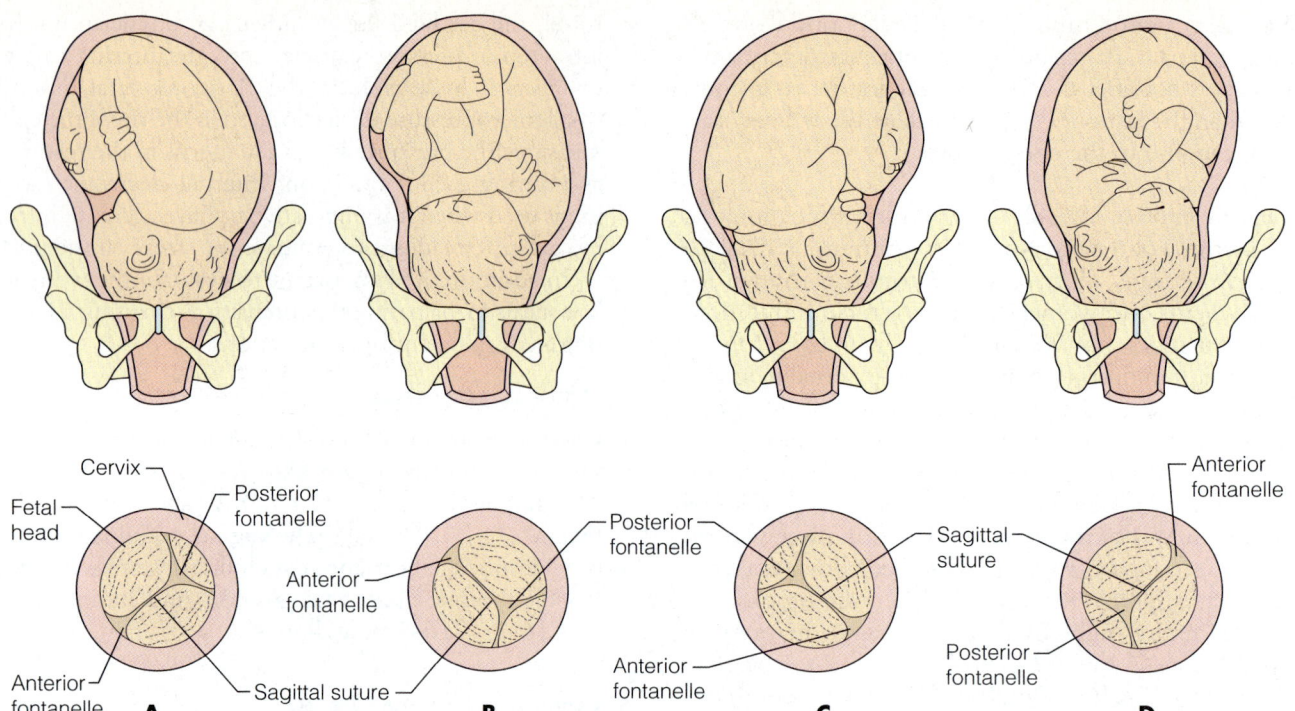

FIGURE 16-3. ◆ Palpating the presenting part (portion of the fetus that enters the pelvis first). **A,** Left occiput anterior (LOA). The occiput (area over the occipital bone on the posterior part of the fetal head) is in the left anterior quadrant of the woman's pelvis. When the fetus is LOA, the posterior fontanelle (located just above the occipital bone and triangular in shape) is in the upper left quadrant of the maternal pelvis. **B,** Left occiput posterior (LOP). The posterior fontanelle is in the lower left quadrant of the maternal pelvis. **C,** Right occiput anterior (ROA). The posterior fontanelle is in the upper right quadrant of the maternal pelvis. **D,** Right occiput posterior (ROP). The posterior fontanelle is in the lower right quadrant of the maternal pelvis. *Note:* The anterior fontanelle is diamond shaped. Because of the roundness of the fetal head, only a portion of the anterior fontanelle can be seen in each of the views, so it appears to be triangular in shape.

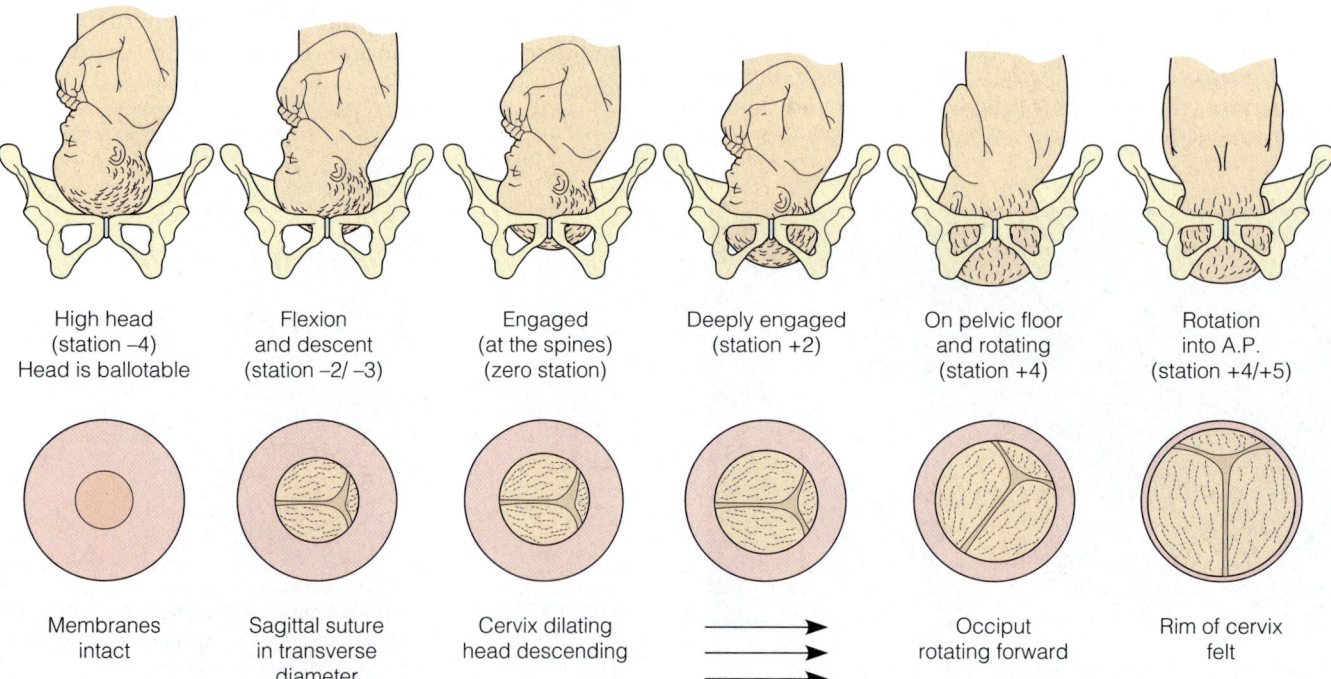

FIGURE 16-4. ◆ **Top:** The fetal head progressing through the pelvis. **Bottom:** The changes the nurse will detect on palpation of the occiput through the cervix while doing a vaginal examination. *Note:* Reprinted from Myles, M. F. (1975). *Textbook for midwives* (p. 246), by permission of the publisher: Churchill-Livingstone.

342   UNIT IV • *Birth and the Family*

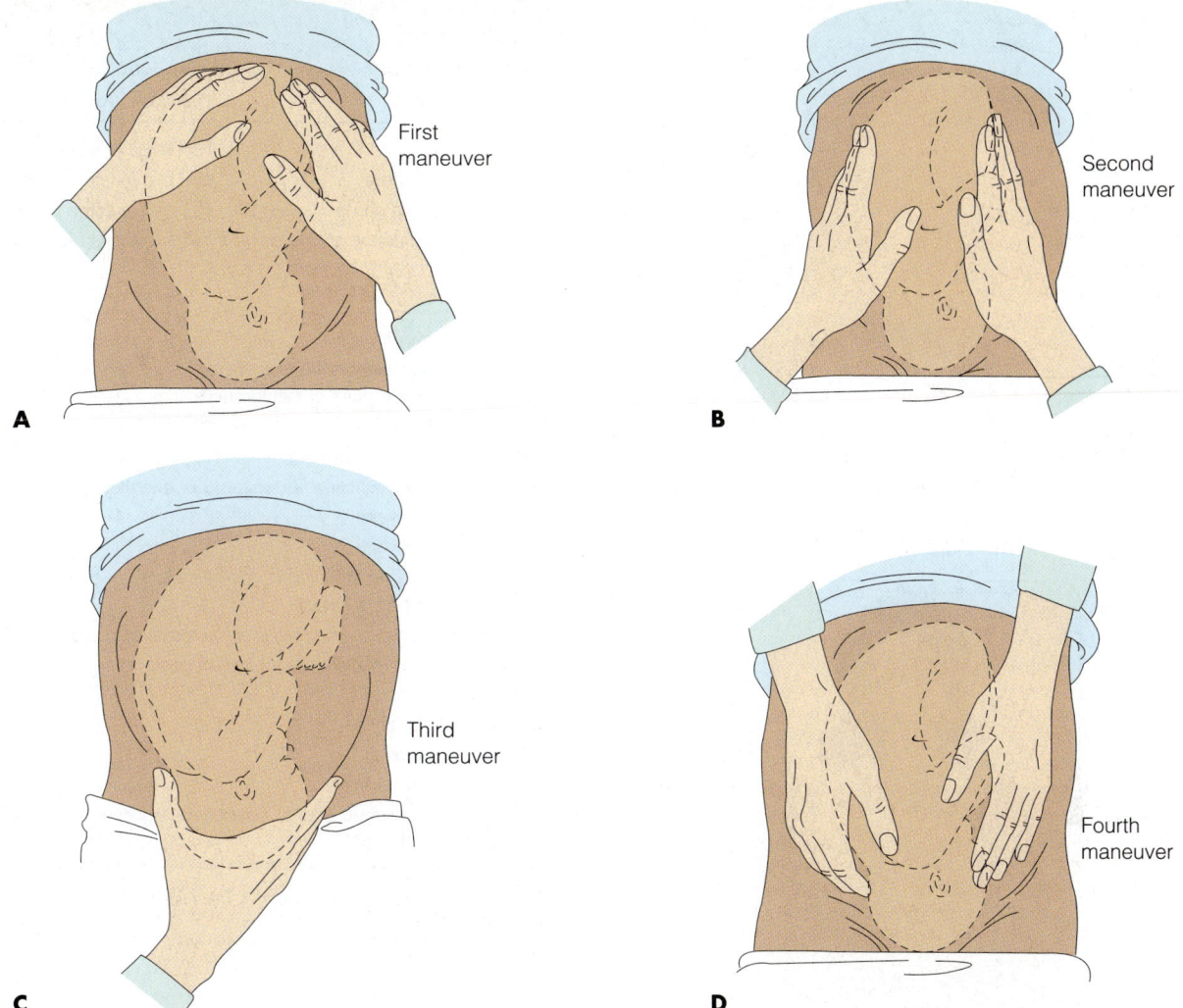

FIGURE 16–5. ◆ Leopold's maneuvers for determining fetal position and presentation. **A,** First maneuver: Facing the woman, palpate the upper abdomen with both hands. Note the shape, consistency, and mobility of the palpated part. The fetal head is firm and round and moves independently of the trunk. The buttock feels softer, and it moves with the trunk. **B,** Second maneuver: Moving the hands on the pelvis, palpate the abdomen with gentle but deep pressure. The fetal back, on one side of the abdomen, feels smooth, and the fetal extremities on the other side feel knobby. **C,** Third maneuver: Place one hand just above the symphysis. Note whether the part palpated feels like the fetal head or the breech and whether it is engaged. **D,** Fourth maneuver: Facing the woman's feet, place both hands on the lower abdomen and move hands gently down the sides of the uterus toward the pubis. Note the cephalic prominence or brow.

PALPATION: LEOPOLD'S MANEUVERS

Leopold's maneuvers are a systematic way to evaluate the maternal abdomen. Frequent practice increases the examiner's skill in determining fetal position by palpation. Leopold's maneuvers may be difficult to perform on an obese woman or on a woman who has excessive amniotic fluid (hydramnios). Before performing Leopold's maneuvers have the woman (1) empty her bladder and (2) lie on her back with her feet on the bed and her knees bent. (See Figure 16–5 ◆ for technique.)

VAGINAL EXAMINATION AND ULTRASOUND

During a vaginal examination, the examiner can palpate the presenting part if the cervix is dilated. The exam also provides information about the position of the fetus and the degree of flexion of its head (in cephalic presentations). Visualization by ultrasound is used when the fetal position cannot be determined by abdominal palpation (see Chapter 14). ⊂▭⊃

Auscultation of Fetal Heart Rate

The handheld Doppler ultrasound or the fetoscope is used to auscultate the FHR between, during, and immediately after uterine contractions. Instead of listening haphazardly over the woman's abdomen for the FHR, it is useful to perform Leopold's maneuvers first. Leopold's maneuvers not only indicate the probable location of the FHR but also help determine the presence of multiple fetuses, fetal lie, and fetal presentation. The FHR is heard most clearly at

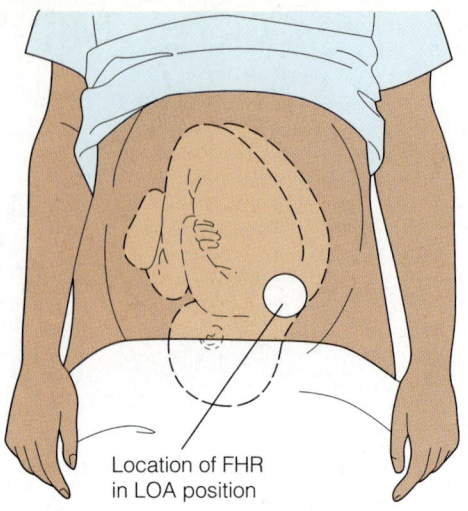

Location of FHR
in LOA position

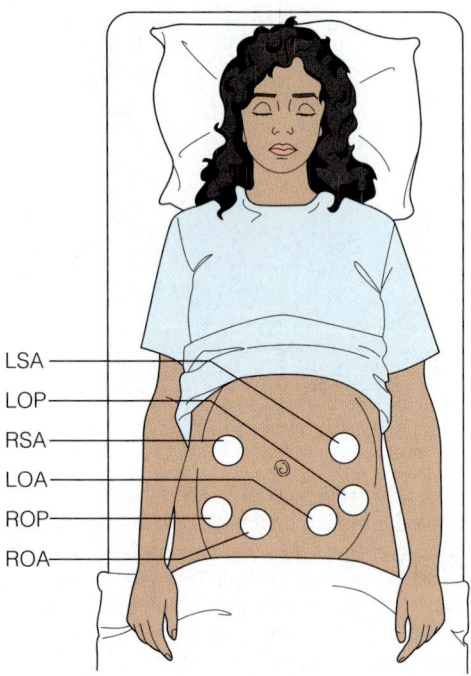

LSA
LOP
RSA
LOA
ROP
ROA

FIGURE 16–6. ◆ Location of FHR in relation to the more commonly seen fetal positions.

the fetal back (see Figure 16–6 ◆). Thus, in a cephalic presentation, the FHR is best heard in the lower quadrant of the maternal abdomen. In a breech presentation, it is heard at or above the level of the maternal umbilicus. In a transverse lie, FHR may be heard best just above or just below the umbilicus. As the presenting part descends and rotates through the pelvic structure during labor, the location of the FHR tends to descend and move toward the midline.

After the FHR is located, it is usually counted for 30 seconds and multiplied by 2 to obtain the number of beats per minute (bpm). Check the woman's pulse against the

fetal sounds. If the rates are the same, readjust the Doppler or fetoscope. Occasionally listen for a full minute, through and just after a contraction, to detect any abnormal heart rate, especially if the FHR is over 160 bpm (tachycardia), under 120 bpm (bradycardia), or irregular. If the FHR is irregular or has changed markedly from the last assessment, listen for a full minute through and immediately after a contraction (see Skill 3–3 in the *Clinical Skills Manual*, as well as the CD-ROM that accompanies this text CD SKILLS and Table 16–3 for guidelines about how often to auscultate the FHR).

It is important to note that intermittent auscultation has been found to be as effective as the electronic method for fetal surveillance. A growing number of health care professionals, doctors and nurses alike, are beginning to question the widespread use of a technology that has not proven its overall worth (Feinstein, 2000; Parer & King, 2000).

Electronic Monitoring of Fetal Heart Rate

Electronic fetal monitoring produces a continuous tracing of the FHR, which allows visual assessment of many characteristics of the FHR (see Skill 3–4 in the *Clinical Skills Manual*, as well as the CD-ROM that accompanies this text). CD SKILLS

INDICATIONS FOR ELECTRONIC MONITORING

If one or more of the following factors are present, the FHR and contractions are monitored by electronic fetal monitoring:

- Previous history of a stillborn (fetus dies in the uterus) at 38 or more weeks' gestation
- Presence of a complication of pregnancy (e.g., pregnancy-induced hypertension, placenta previa, abruptio placentae, multiple gestation, prolonged or premature rupture of membranes)
- Induction of labor (labor that is begun as a result of some type of intervention such as an intravenous infusion of oxytocin [Pitocin])
- Preterm labor (gestation less than 37 completed weeks)
- Decreased fetal movement
- Fetal stress or distress
- Meconium staining of amniotic fluid (meconium has been released into the amniotic fluid by the fetus, which may indicate a problem)

METHODS OF ELECTRONIC MONITORING OF FHR

External monitoring of the fetus is usually accomplished by ultrasound. A transducer, which emits continuous sound waves, is placed on the maternal abdomen. When placed correctly, the sound waves bounce off the fetal heart and are picked up by the electronic monitor. The actual moment-by-moment FHR is displayed graphically on a screen (Figure 16–7 ◆). In some instances, the monitor may track the maternal heart rate instead of the fetal heart rate. Avoid this error by comparing the maternal pulse to the FHR.

Recent advances in technology have led to the development of new ambulatory methods of external monitoring. Using a telemetry system, a small, battery-operated transducer transmits signals to a receiver connected to the monitor. This system, held in place with a shoulder strap, allows the woman to ambulate, helping her to feel more comfortable and less confined during labor. In contrast, the system depicted in Figure 16–7 requires the woman to remain close to the electrical power source for the monitor.

Internal monitoring requires an internal spiral electrode. To place the spiral electrode on the fetal occiput, the amniotic membranes must be ruptured, the cervix must be dilated at least 2 cm, the presenting part must be down against the cervix, and the presenting part must be known (that is, the examiner must be able to detect the actual part of the fetus that is down against the cervix). If all these factors are present, the labor and birth nurse, the physician, or the certified nurse-midwife inserts a sterile internal spiral electrode into the vagina and places it against the fetal presenting part. The spiral electrode is rotated clockwise until it is attached to the presenting part. Wires that extend from the spiral electrode are attached to a leg plate (which

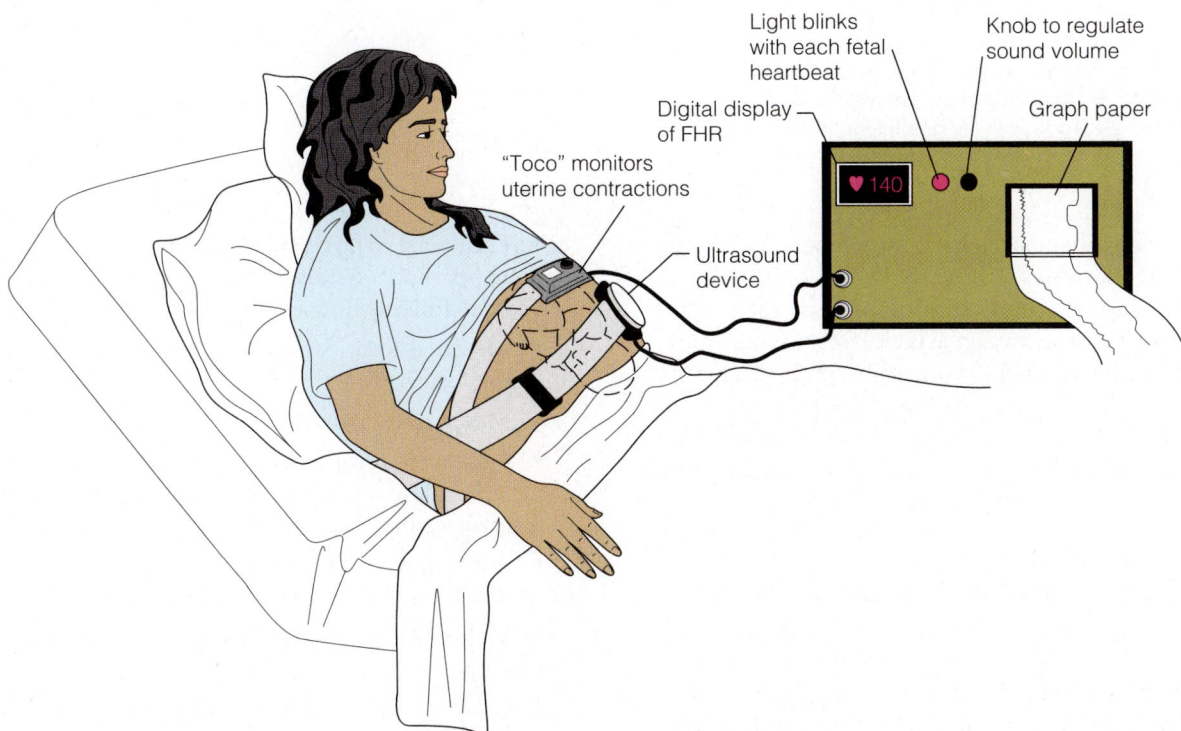

FIGURE 16–7. ◆ Electronic fetal monitoring by external technique. The tocodynamometer ("toco") is placed over the uterine fundus. The toco provides information that can be used to monitor uterine contractions. The ultrasound device is placed over the area of the fetal back. This device transmits information about the FHR. Information from both the toco and the ultrasound device is transmitted to the electronic fetal monitor. The FHR is displayed in a digital display (as a blinking light), on the special monitor paper, and audibly (by adjusting a button on the monitor). The uterine contractions are displayed on the special monitor paper as well.

Labels in figure:
- Light blinks with each fetal heartbeat
- Knob to regulate sound volume
- Digital display of FHR
- Graph paper
- "Toco" monitors uterine contractions
- Ultrasound device
- ♥ 140

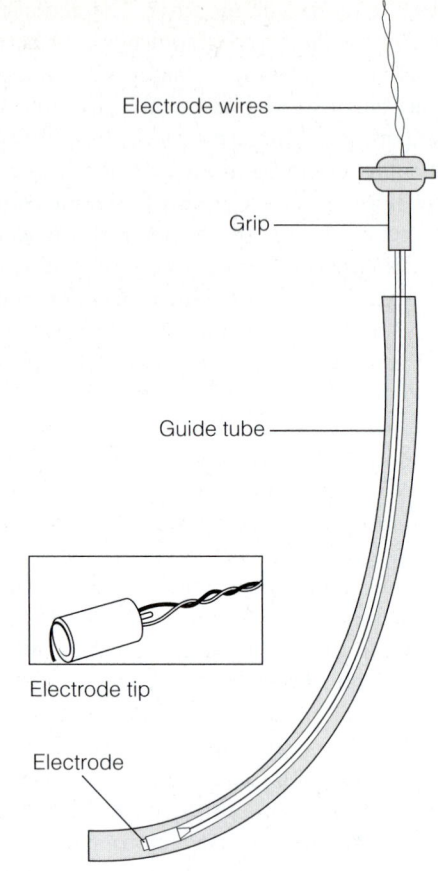

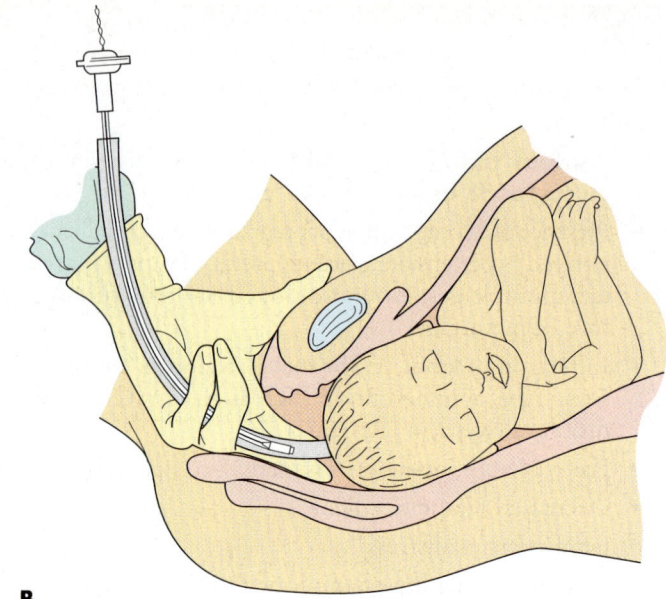

FIGURE 16–8. ◆ Technique for internal, direct fetal monitoring.
A, Spiral electrode. **B,** Attaching the spiral electrode to the scalp.
C, Attached spiral electrode with the guide tube removed.

is placed on the woman's thigh) and then attached to the electronic fetal monitor. This method of monitoring the FHR provides more accurate continuous data than external monitoring, because the signal is clearer and movement of the fetus or the woman does not interrupt it (Figure 16–8 ◆). The FHR tracing at the top of Figure 16–9 ◆ was obtained by internal monitoring with a spiral electrode; the uterine contraction tracing at the bottom of the figure was obtained by external monitoring with a toco.

BASELINE FETAL HEART RATE

The **baseline rate** refers to the average FHR observed during a 10-minute period of monitoring. Normal FHR (baseline rate) ranges from 120 to 160 bpm. There are two abnormal variations of the baseline rate—those above 160 bpm (tachycardia) and those below 120 bpm (bradycardia). Another change affecting the baseline is called variability, a change in FHR over a few seconds to a few minutes.

Fetal tachycardia is a sustained rate of 161 bpm or above. Marked tachycardia is 180 bpm or above. Causes of tachycardia include the following (Parer, 1999):

- Early fetal hypoxia, which leads to stimulation of the sympathetic system as the fetus compensates for reduced blood flow
- Maternal fever, which accelerates the metabolism of the fetus
- Maternal dehydration
- Beta-sympathomimetic drugs such as ritodrine, terbutaline, atropine, and isoxsuprine, which have a cardiac stimulant effect
- Amnionitis (fetal tachycardia may be the first sign of developing intrauterine infection)
- Maternal hyperthyroidism (thyroid-stimulating hormones may cross the placenta and stimulate FHR)
- Fetal anemia (the heart rate is increased to improve tissue perfusion)

Tachycardia is considered an ominous sign if it is accompanied by late decelerations, severe variable decelerations, or decreased variability. If tachycardia is associated with maternal fever, treatment may include antipyretics and/or antibiotics.

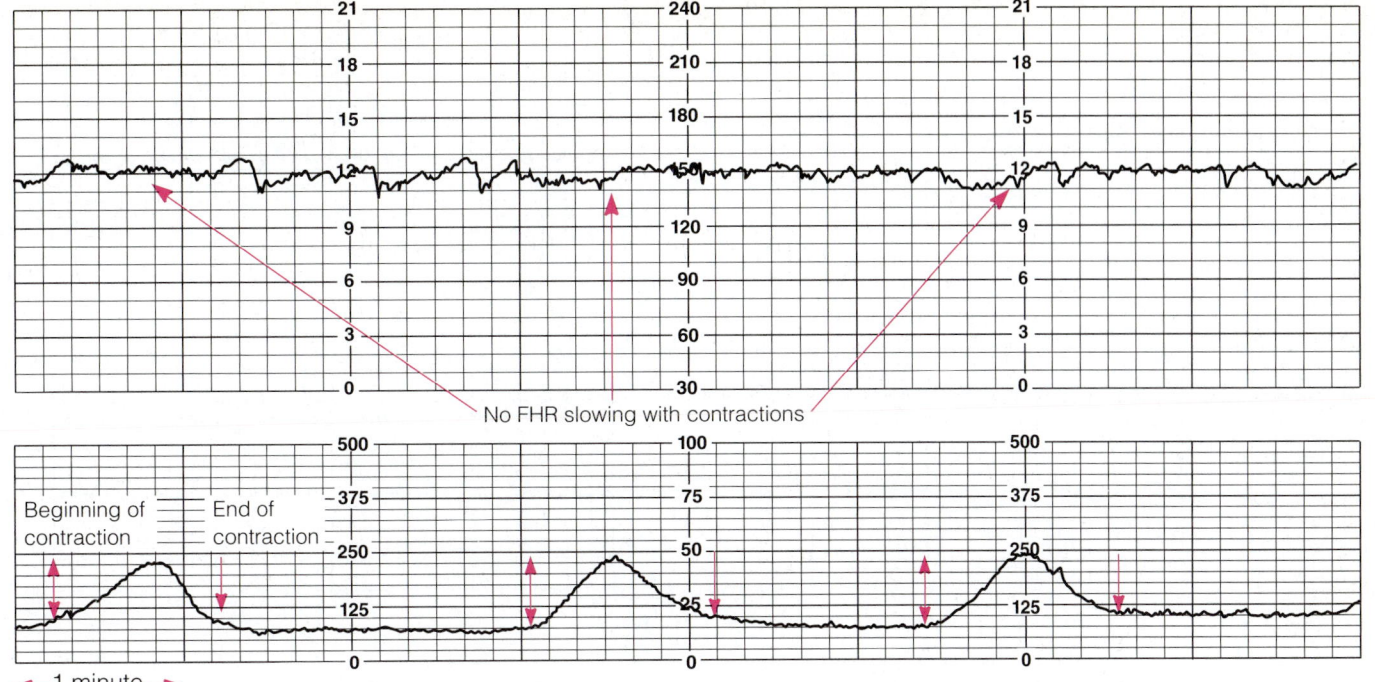

FIGURE 16–9. ◆ Normal FHR pattern obtained by internal monitoring. Note normal FHR, 140 to 158 bpm, presence of long- and short-term variability, and absence of deceleration with adequate contractions. Arrows on the bottom of tracing indicate beginnings of uterine contractions.

Fetal bradycardia is a rate less than 110 to 120 bpm during a 10-minute period or longer. Causes of fetal brady-cardia include the following (Parer, 1999; Schmidt, 2000):

- Late (profound) fetal hypoxia (depression of my-ocardial activity)
- Maternal hypotension, which results in decreased blood flow to the fetus
- Prolonged umbilical cord compression; fetal baro-ceptors are activated by cord compression and this produces vagal stimulation, which results in de-creased FHR
- Fetal arrhythmia, which is associated with complete heart block in the fetus

Bradycardia may be a benign or an ominous sign. If av-erage long-term variability exists, the bradycardia is con-sidered benign. When bradycardia is accompanied by de-creased long-term variability and late decelerations, it is considered a sign of advanced fetal distress (Parer, 1999).

VARIABILITY

Baseline variability is a measure of the interplay (the push-pull effect) between the sympathetic and parasym-pathetic nervous systems. There are two types of fetal heart variability. **Short-term variability (STV)** is the beat-to-beat change in FHR. It represents fluctuations of the baseline. STV can only be measured via internal (scalp electrode) means and is classified as either present or ab-sent. **Long-term variability (LTV)** is the waviness or rhythmic fluctuations (called cycles) of the FHR tracing, which occur three to five times per minute. LTV can be classified as absent, decreased, average, increased, or marked (see Figure 16–10 ◆). The most important aspect of LTV is that even in the presence of abnormal or ques-tionable FHR patterns, if the variability is normal, the fe-tus is not suffering from cerebral asphyxia.

Causes of decreased variability include the following (Parer, 1999):

- Hypoxia and acidosis (decreased blood flow to the fetus)
- Administration of drugs such as meperidine hy-drochloride (Demerol), diazepam (Valium), or hy-droxyzine (Vistaril), which depress the fetal central nervous system
- Fetal sleep cycle (during fetal sleep, LTV is de-creased; fetal sleep cycles usually last for 20 to 30 minutes)
- Fetus of less than 32 weeks' gestation (fetal neuro-logic control of heart rate is immature)

Causes of increased variability include the following (Parer, 1999):

- Early mild hypoxia (variability increases as a result of compensatory mechanism)
- Fetal stimulation (stimulation of autonomic nervous system because of abdominal palpation, maternal vaginal examination, application of spiral electrode on fetal head, or acoustic stimulation)

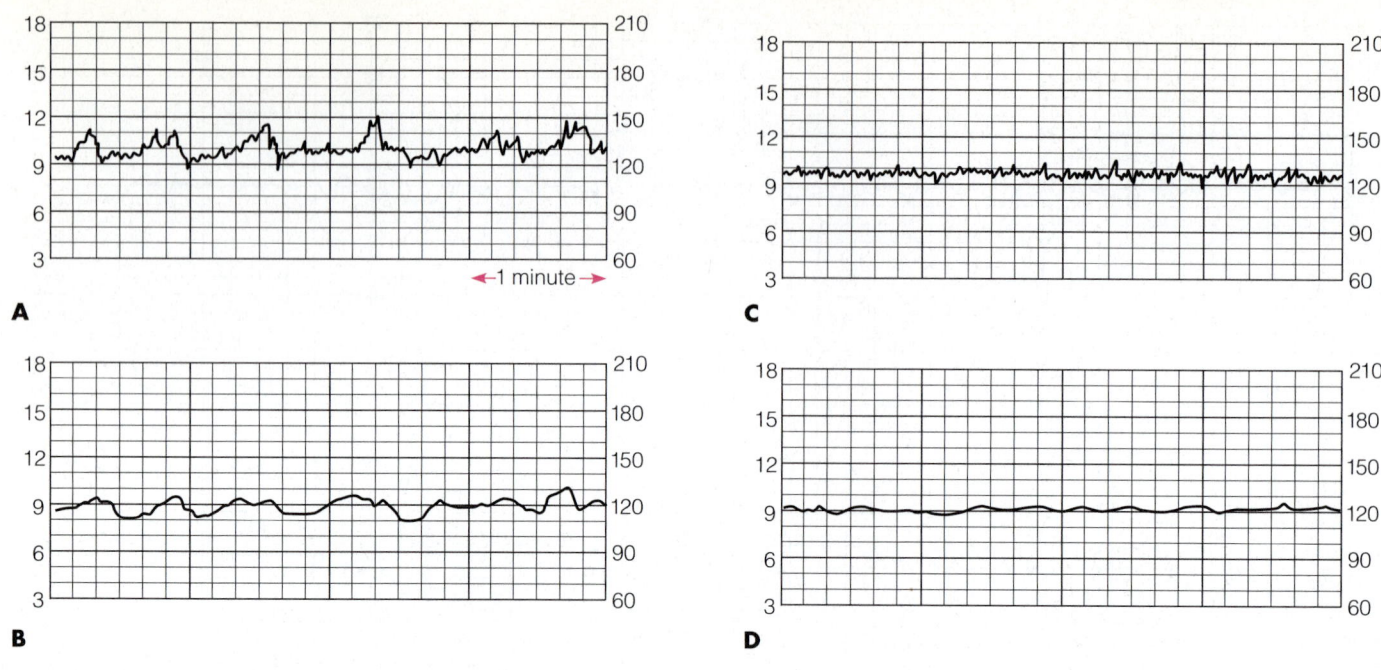

FIGURE 16–10. ◆ Short- and long-term variability. **A,** Increased LTV; STV present. **B,** Average LTV; STV absent. **C,** Absent LTV; STV present. **D,** Absent LTV; STV absent.

Decreasing variability that does not appear to be associated with a fetal sleep cycle or the administration of drugs is a warning sign of fetal distress. It is especially ominous if decreased variability is accompanied by late decelerations, explained shortly.

External electronic fetal monitoring is not an adequate method to assess STV. If decreased variability is noted on monitoring, application of a spiral electrode should be considered to obtain more accurate information.

ACCELERATIONS

Accelerations are transient increases in the FHR normally caused by fetal movement. When the fetus moves, the heart rate increases, just as the heart rates of adults increase during exercise. Often, accelerations accompany uterine contractions, usually due to fetal movement in response to the pressure of the contractions. Accelerations of this type are thought to be a sign of fetal well-being and adequate oxygen reserve. The accelerations with fetal movement form the basis for nonstress tests (see Chapter 14). ⌾

DECELERATIONS

Decelerations are periodic decreases in FHR from the normal baseline. They are categorized as early, late, and variable according to the time of their occurrence in the contraction cycle and their waveform (Figure 16–11 ◆). When the fetal head is compressed, cerebral blood flow is decreased, which leads to central vagal stimulation and results in early deceleration. The onset of early deceleration occurs before the onset of the uterine contraction. This type of deceleration is of uniform shape, is usually considered benign, and does not require intervention.

Late deceleration is caused by uteroplacental insufficiency resulting from decreased blood flow and oxygen transfer to the fetus through the intervillous spaces during uterine contractions. The onset of the deceleration occurs after the onset of a uterine contraction and is of a uniform shape that tends to reflect associated uterine contractions. The late deceleration pattern is considered a nonreassuring sign but does not necessarily require immediate childbirth.

Variable decelerations occur if the umbilical cord becomes compressed, thus reducing blood flow between the placenta and fetus. The resulting increase in peripheral resistance in the fetal circulation causes fetal hypertension. The fetal hypertension stimulates the baroreceptors in the aortic arch and carotid sinuses, which slow the FHR. The onset of variable decelerations varies in timing with the onset of the contraction, and the decelerations are variable in shape. This pattern requires further assessment. Nursing interventions for late and variable decelerations in FHR are presented in Table 16–4.

A *sinusoidal pattern* appears similar to a waveform. The characteristics of this pattern include presence of LTV, absence of STV, and accelerations with fetal movement. This pattern is associated with Rh isoimmunization, fetal anemia, and a chronic fetal bleed. It may also occur with the administration of medications such as meperidine (Demerol) or butorphanol tartrate (Stadol). When it appears in association with medication, the pattern is usually temporary (Kang & Boehm, 1999).

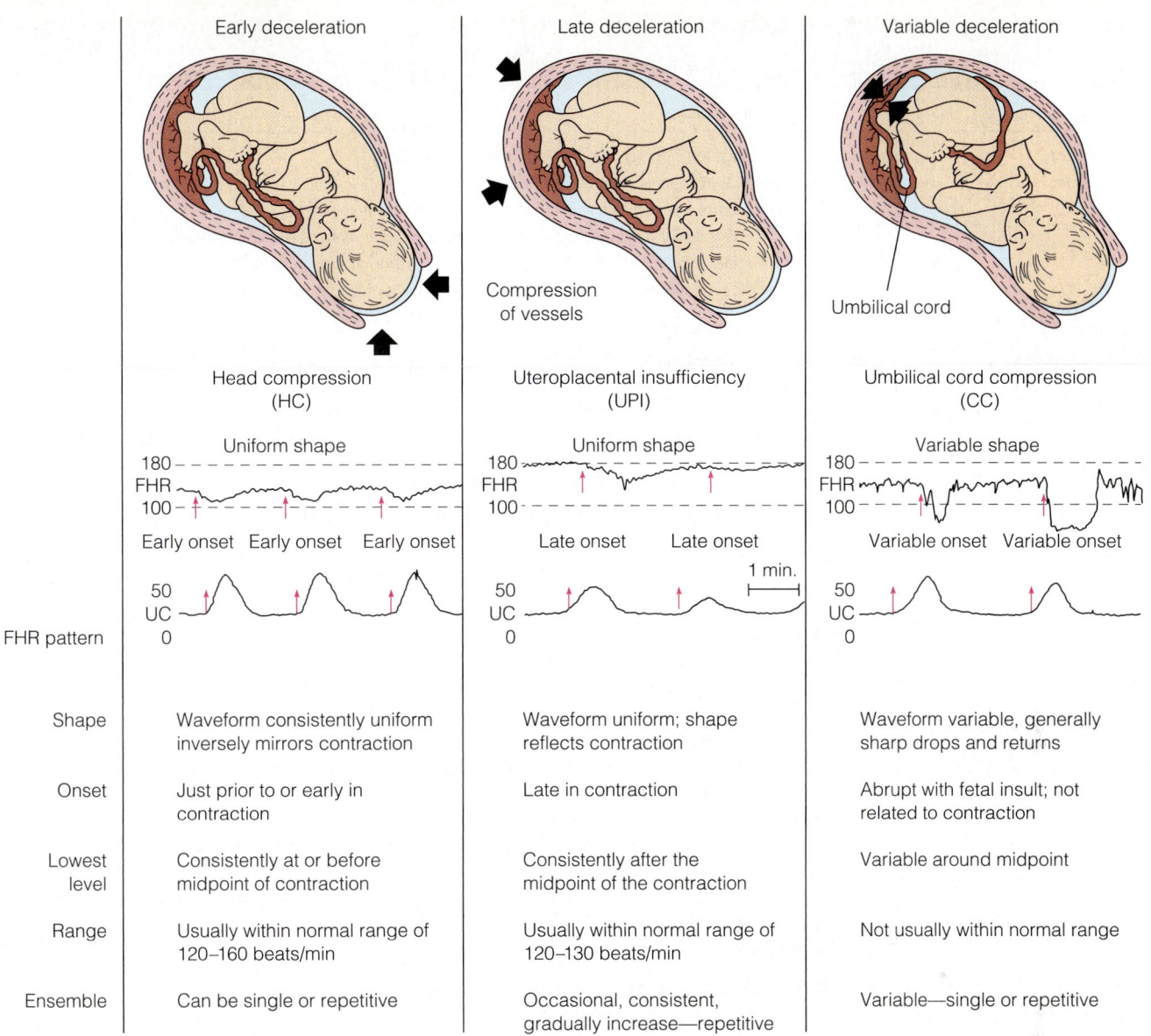

	Early deceleration	Late deceleration	Variable deceleration
	Head compression (HC)	Uteroplacental insufficiency (UPI)	Umbilical cord compression (CC)
FHR pattern	Uniform shape — Early onset	Uniform shape — Late onset	Variable shape — Variable onset
Shape	Waveform consistently uniform inversely mirrors contraction	Waveform uniform; shape reflects contraction	Waveform variable, generally sharp drops and returns
Onset	Just prior to or early in contraction	Late in contraction	Abrupt with fetal insult; not related to contraction
Lowest level	Consistently at or before midpoint of contraction	Consistently after the midpoint of the contraction	Variable around midpoint
Range	Usually within normal range of 120–160 beats/min	Usually within normal range of 120–130 beats/min	Not usually within normal range
Ensemble	Can be single or repetitive	Occasional, consistent, gradually increase—repetitive	Variable—single or repetitive

FIGURE 16–11. ◆ Types and characteristics of early, late, and variable decelerations. *Note:* From Hon, E. (1976). *An introduction to fetal heart rate monitoring* (2nd ed., p. 29). Los Angeles: University of Southern California School of Medicine.

PSYCHOLOGIC REACTIONS TO ELECTRONIC MONITORING

Responses to electronic fetal monitoring can be varied and complex. Many women have little knowledge of monitoring unless they have attended a prenatal class that dealt with this subject. Some women react to electronic monitoring positively, viewing it as a reassurance that "the baby is OK." They may also feel that the monitor helps identify problems that develop in labor. Other women may have ambivalent or even negative feelings about the monitor. They may think that the monitor is interfering with a natural process, and they do not want the intrusion. Some women may find that the equipment, wires, and sounds increase their anxiety. The discomfort of lying in one position and fear of injury to the baby are other objections.

NURSING RESPONSIBILITIES

A key strength of technology is its ability to explain and possibly predict health patterns or problems with precision. However, this advantage has the potential to dehumanize the nurse-client relationship. Therefore, it is important to recognize that every encounter with the childbearing family offers an opportunity to provide education and empowerment to the laboring woman and her partner. Helping to provide information when needed, answering questions, and encouraging the woman to make decisions establish a trusting nurse-client relationship.

Technology has been advancing at a rapid rate in the labor and birthing arena, and each new development challenges nurses to understand, include, and balance technology

TABLE 16-4 Guidelines for Management of Variable, Late, and Prolonged Deceleration Patterns

Pattern	Nursing Interventions
Variable decelerations Isolated or occasional Moderate	Report findings to physician or CNM and document in chart. Provide explanation to woman and partner. Change maternal position to one in which FHR pattern is most improved. Discontinue oxytocin if it is being administered and other interventions are unsuccessful. Perform vaginal examination to assess for prolapsed cord or change in labor progress. Monitor FHR continuously to assess current status and for further changes in FHR pattern.
Variable decelerations Severe and uncorrectable	Give oxygen if indicated. Report findings to physician or CNM and document in chart. Provide explanation to woman and partner. Prepare for probable cesarean birth. Follow interventions listed above. Prepare for vaginal birth unless baseline variability is decreasing or FHR is progressively rising—then cesarean, forceps, or vacuum birth is indicated. Assist physician with fetal scalp sampling if ordered. Prepare for cesarean birth if scalp pH shows acidosis or downward trend.
Late decelerations	Give oxygen if indicated. Report findings to physician or CNM and document in chart. Provide explanation to woman and partner. Monitor for further FHR changes. Maintain maternal position on left side. Maintain good hydration with IV fluids (normal saline or lactated Ringer's). Discontinue oxytocin if it is being administered and late decelerations persist despite other interventions. Administer oxygen by face mask at 7 to 10 L/min. Monitor maternal blood pressure and pulse for signs of hypotension; possibly increase flow rate of IV fluids to treat hypotension. Follow physician's orders for treatment for hypotension if present. Increase IV fluids to maintain volume and hydration (normal saline or lactated Ringer's). Assess labor progress (dilatation and station). Assist physician with fetal blood sampling: If pH stays above 7.25, physician will continue monitoring and resample; if pH shows downward trend (between 7.25 and 7.2) or is below 7.2, prepare for birth by most expeditious means.
Late decelerations with tachycardia or decreasing variability	Report findings to physician or CNM and document in chart. Maintain maternal position on left side. Administer oxygen by face mask at 7 to 10 L/min. Discontinue oxytocin if it is being administered. Assess maternal blood pressure and pulse. Increase IV fluids (normal saline or lactated Ringer's). Assess labor progress (dilatation and station). Prepare for immediate cesarean birth. Explain plan of treatment to woman and partner. Assist physician with fetal blood sampling (if ordered).
Prolonged decelerations	Perform vaginal examination to rule out prolapsed cord or to determine progress in labor status. Change maternal position as needed to try to alleviate decelerations. Discontinue oxytocin if it is being administered. Notify physician or CNM of findings and initial interventions and document in chart. Provide explanation to woman and partner. Increase IV fluids (normal saline or lactated Ringer's). Administer tocolytic if hypertonus noted and ordered by physician or CNM. Anticipate normal FHR recovery following deceleration if FHR previously normal. Anticipate intervention if FHR previously abnormal or deceleration lasts >3 minutes.

with holistic nursing practice. Before using the electronic fetal monitor, explain the reason for its use and the information that it can provide. After applying the monitor, record basic information on the monitor strip. These data should include the date, client's name, physician or certified nurse-midwife's name, hospital number, age, gravida, para, estimated date of birth, membrane status, and maternal vital signs. As the monitor strip runs and care is provided, occurrences during labor should be recorded not only in the medical record but also on the monitor strip. This information helps the health care team assess current status and evaluate the tracing.

Note the following information on the tracing (American Academy of Pediatrics & American College of Obstetricians and Gynecologists, 1997):

- Vaginal examination (dilatation, effacement, station, position)
- Amniotomy or spontaneous rupture of membranes, color of amniotic fluid
- Maternal vital signs
- Maternal position in bed and changes of position
- Application of spiral electrode or intrauterine pressure catheter
- Medications given
- Oxygen administration
- Maternal behaviors (emesis, coughing, hiccups)
- Fetal scalp stimulation or fetal scalp blood sampling
- Vomiting
- Pushing
- Administration of anesthesia blocks

In addition, if the monitor does not automatically add the time on the strip at specific intervals, include the time when recording any information on the strip. If more than one nurse is adding information to the monitor strip, it is essential to initial each note. The tracing is considered a legal part of the woman's medical record and is submissible as evidence in court.

It is important for the laboring woman to feel that what is happening to her is the central focus. Acknowledge this need by always speaking to and looking at the woman when entering the room, before looking at the monitor.

EVALUATION OF FHR TRACINGS

It is important to use a systematic approach in evaluating FHR tracings. Evaluation of the electronic monitor tracing begins by looking at the uterine contraction pattern:

- Determine the uterine resting tone.
- Assess the contractions: What is the frequency? What is the duration? What is the intensity (if internal monitoring)?

The next step is to evaluate the FHR tracing:

- Determine the baseline: Is the baseline within the normal range? Is there evidence of tachycardia? Is there evidence of bradycardia?
- Determine FHR variability: Is STV present or absent? Is LTV average? Minimal? Absent? Moderate? Marked?
- Determine if a sinusoidal pattern is present.
- Determine if there are periodic changes: Are accelerations present? Do they meet the criteria for a reactive nonstress test? Are decelerations present? Are they uniform in shape? If so, determine if they are early or late decelerations. Are they nonuniform in shape? If so, determine whether they are variable decelerations.

After evaluating the FHR tracing for the factors just listed, classify the tracing as reassuring (normal) or nonreassuring (worrisome). Reassuring patterns contain normal parameters and do not require additional treatment or intervention.

Characteristics of reassuring FHR patterns include the following:

- Baseline rate is 120 to 160 bpm.
- STV is present.
- LTV ranges from three to five cycles per minute. Periodic patterns consist of accelerations with fetal movement, and early decelerations may be present.

Nonreassuring patterns may indicate that the fetus is becoming stressed and intervention is needed. Characteristics of nonreassuring patterns include the following:

- Severe variable decelerations (FHR drops below 70 bpm for longer than 30 to 45 seconds and is accompanied by rising baseline or decreasing variability or slow return to baseline)
- Late decelerations of any magnitude
- Absence of variability (no STV or LTV present)
- Prolonged deceleration (a deceleration that lasts 60 to 90 seconds or more)
- Severe (marked) bradycardia (FHR baseline of 70 bpm or less)

Nonreassuring patterns may require continuous monitoring and more involved treatment and intervention (see Table 16–4).

It is vital to provide information to the laboring woman about the FHR pattern and the interventions, if necessary, that will help her fetus. Most women are aware that something is happening. Sharing information with them provides reassurance that a potential or actual problem is identified and that they are active participants in the interventions. Occasionally a problem arises that requires immediate intervention. In that case, it may be helpful to say something like "It is important for you to turn on your left side right now because the baby is having a little difficulty. I'll explain what is happening in just a few moments." This type of response lets the woman know that although an action needs to be accomplished rapidly, information will soon be provided. In the haste to act quickly, nurses and other caregivers must not forget that it is the woman's body and her baby.

Scalp Stimulation Test

When there is a question regarding fetal status, a scalp stimulation test can be used before the more invasive fetal blood sampling. In this test, the examiner applies pressure to the fetal scalp while doing a vaginal examination. The fetus who is not in any stress or distress responds with an acceleration of the FHR (Cunningham, Gant, Leveno, et al., 2001).

Fetal Scalp Blood Sampling

When nonreassuring or confusing FHR patterns are noted, additional information about the acid-base status of the fetus is needed. This information may be obtained by **fetal blood sampling.** The physician usually draws the blood sample from the fetal scalp but may obtain it from the fetal buttocks if the fetus is in the breech position (Gilstrap, 1999).

Before fetal blood can be sampled, the membranes must be ruptured, the cervix must be dilated at least 2 to 3 cm, and the presenting part must not be above −2 station. Sampling is not done when FHR patterns are ominous. It is contraindicated in acute emergencies and in cases of vaginal bleeding. In these instances, birth by the most expeditious means is indicated.

Normal fetal pH values during labor are above 7.25; 7.2 to 7.25 is considered borderline, warranting further sampling. Values below 7.2 are nonreassuring and necessitate birth without delay (Gilstrap, 1999).

The more information that is available from FHR monitoring, the less need there is for fetal blood sampling. This adjunctive procedure is indicated only when FHR patterns are not interpretable, are worsening, or are suggestive of high risk. Fetal blood sampling may prevent unnecessary cesarean birth.

CHAPTER HIGHLIGHTS

↝ Intrapartal assessment includes attention to both the physical and psychosociocultural parameters of the laboring woman, assessment of the fetus, and ongoing assessment for conditions that place the woman and her fetus at increased risk.

↝ A vaginal examination determines the status of fetal membranes; cervical dilatation and effacement; and fetal presentation, position, and station.

↝ Fetal presentation and position may be assessed by palpation using Leopold's maneuvers, vaginal examination, or ultrasound.

↝ Electronic fetal monitoring is accomplished by indirect ultrasound or by direct methods that require the placement of a spiral electrode on the fetal presenting part. The normal range of FHR is 120 to 160 bpm.

↝ Short-term variability of the FHR can only be assessed by direct electronic monitoring.

↝ Baseline changes of the FHR include tachycardia (160 bpm or more for a 10-minute period), bradycardia (less than 120 bpm for a 10-minute period), and variability.

↝ Periodic changes are transient decelerations or accelerations of the FHR from the baseline. Accelerations are normally caused by fetal movement; decelerations may be early, late, variable, or sinusoidal.

↝ Early decelerations are due to compression of the fetal head during contractions and are considered reassuring. Late decelerations are associated with uteroplacental insufficiency and are considered ominous. Variable decelerations are associated with compression of the umbilical cord and require further assessment. Sinusoidal patterns are characterized by an undulant sine wave.

↝ Birthing room nurses have responsibilities in recognizing and interpreting fetal monitoring patterns, notifying the physician or certified nurse-midwife of problems, and initiating corrective and supportive measures when needed.

↝ Fetal scalp stimulation can be used when fetal status is in question.

↝ Fetal acid-base status may be assessed by fetal blood sampling.

EXPLOREMediaLink

NCLEX Review, Case Studies, and other interactive resources for this chapter can be found on the companion website at http://www.prenhall.com/london. Click on "Chapter 16" to select the activities for this chapter.

For animations, more NCLEX review questions, and an audio glossary, access the accompanying CD-ROM in this textbook.

REFERENCES

American Academy of Pediatrics & American College of Obstetricians and Gynecologists. (1997). *Guidelines for perinatal care* (4th ed.).Washington, DC: Author.

American College of Obstetricians and Gynecologists. (1999). *Domestic violence* (ACOG Educational Bulletin No. 257). Washington, DC: Author.

Association of Women's Health, Obstetric, and Neonatal Nurses. (1998). *Standards for professional nursing practice in the care of women and newborns* (5th ed.). Washington, DC: Author.

Austin, G., Gallop, R., McCay, E., Peternelj-Taylor, C., & Bayer, M. (1999). Culturally competent care for psychiatric clients who have a history of sexual abuse. *Clinical Nursing Research, 8,* 5–25.

Burrian, J. (1995). Helping survivors of sexual abuse through labor. *Maternal-Child Nursing Journal, 20*(5), 252–255.

Callister, L. C. (2001). Culturally competent care of women and newborns: Knowledge, attitude, and skills. *Journal of Obstetric, Gynecologic, and Neonatal Nursing, 30*(2), 209–215.

Cesario, S. K. (2001). Care of the Native American woman: Strategies for practice, education, and research. *Journal of Obstetric, Gynecologic, and Neonatal Nursing, 30*(1), 13–18.

Cunningham, F. G., Gant, F. G., Leveno, K. L., Gilstrap, L. C., Hauth, J. C., & Wenstrom, K. D. (2001). *Williams obstetrics* (21st ed.). New York: McGraw-Hill.

Feinstein, N. (2000). Fetal heart rate auscultation: Current and future practice. *Journal of Obstetric and Gynecological Nurses, 29*(3), 306–314.

Fontaine, K. L. (2000). *Healing practices: Alternative therapies for nursing.* Upper Saddle River, NJ: Prentice Hall.

Gilstrap, L. (1999). Fetal acid-base balance. In R. K. Creasy & R. Resnik (Eds.), *Maternal-fetal medicine* (4th ed., pp. 331–340). Philadelphia: Saunders.

Gottlieb, B. (2000). *Alternative cures.* Emmaus, PA: Rodale Books.

Kang, A. H., & Boehm, F. H. (1999). The clinical significance of intermittent sinusoidal fetal heart rate. *American Journal of Obstetrics and Gynecology, 180,* 151–152.

Parer, J. (1999). Fetal heart rate. In R. K. Creasy & R. Resnik (Eds.), *Maternal-fetal medicine* (4th ed., pp. 270–299). Philadelphia: Saunders.

Parer, J., & King, T. (2000). Fetal heart rate monitoring: Is it salvageable? *American Journal of Obstetrics and Gynecology, 182*(4), 982–987.

Schmidt, J. (2000). Intrapartal fetal assessment. In S. Mattson & J. E. Smith (Eds.), *Maternal-newborn nursing* (2nd ed., pp. 271–299). Philadelphia: Saunders.

Schnaubelt, K. 1999. *Medical aromatherapy.* Berkeley, CA: Frog, LTD.

Seng, J. S., Oakley, D. J., Samselle, C. M., Killion, C., Graham-Bermann, S., & Liberzon, I. (2001). Posttraumatic stress disorder and pregnancy complications. *Obstetrics & Gynecology, 97*(1), 17–22.

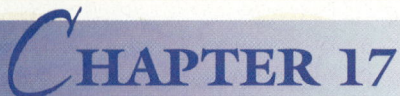

CHAPTER 17

The Family in Childbirth: Needs and Care

For as long as I can remember, I have been fascinated with birth. Currently, I am a labor and delivery nurse at our town's only hospital. I'm still fascinated with birth but a little nervous, too. You see, I was just admitted in early labor with my first child. Before I got here I worried that I would be a "bad" patient or that I would lose my cool. How silly I was. All that matters is that my baby is healthy and that I am able to take care of him effectively. (Yes. We know it is a boy!)

—AMANDA, 31

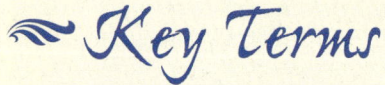
Key Terms

Apgar scoring system   *374*
Birthing room   *355*
Precipitous birth   *378*

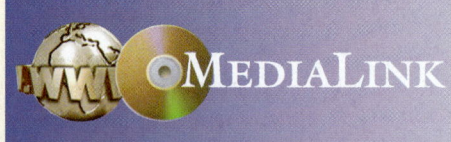
⊙MediaLink

CD-ROM

Skill 4–2: Performing Nasal Pharyngeal Suctioning

Skill 5–1: Evaluating Lochia

Vaginal Delivery Animation

Audio Glossary

NCLEX Review

COMPANION WEBSITE

http://www.prenhall.com/london

Family in Childbirth Web Links

Complementary Care: Doula Information

Thinking Critically

NCLEX Review

Case Study

can obtain essential information about the woman and her pregnancy within a few minutes after admission, initiate any immediate interventions needed, and establish individualized priorities.

The woman may be facing a number of unfamiliar procedures that seem routine for health care providers. It is important to remember that all women have the right to determine what happens to their bodies. The woman's informed consent should be obtained prior to any procedure that involves touching her.

If indicated, assist the woman into bed. A side-lying or semi-Fowler's position rather than a supine position is most comfortable and avoids supine hypotensive syndrome (vena caval syndrome). After obtaining the essential information from the woman and her records, begin the intrapartal assessment. (Chapter 16 considers intrapartal maternal assessment in depth.) ⬭ Once the assessment is complete, it is possible to make effective nursing decisions about intrapartal care, such as the following:

- Should ambulation or bed rest be encouraged?
- Is more frequent monitoring needed?
- What does the woman want during her labor and birth?
- Is a support person available?
- What special needs do this woman and her partner have?

Auscultate the fetal heart rate (FHR). (See Chapter 16.) ⬭ Determine the woman's blood pressure, pulse, respirations, and oral temperature and assess contraction frequency, duration, and intensity (possibly while gathering other data). Before the vaginal examination, inform the woman about the procedure and its purpose; afterward, report the findings. If there are signs of advanced labor (frequent contractions, an urge to bear down, and so on), a vaginal examination must be done quickly. If there are signs of excessive bleeding or if the woman reports episodes of painless bleeding in the last trimester, suspect placenta previa and do not do a vaginal examination.

Results of FHR assessment, uterine contraction evaluation, and the vaginal examination help determine whether the rest of the admission process can proceed at a leisurely pace or whether additional interventions are required. For example, a FHR of 110 beats per minute on auscultation indicates that a fetal monitor should be applied immediately to obtain additional data. The woman's vital signs can be assessed once the monitor is in place.

After obtaining admission data, collect a clean voided midstream urine specimen. The woman with intact membranes may collect her specimen in the bathroom. If the membranes are ruptured and the presenting part is not engaged, the woman generally remains in bed to avoid prolapse of the umbilical cord. Views vary about the wisdom of ambulation once the membranes are ruptured. The decision is generally based on physical findings, clinician orders, the woman's desires, agency policy, and safety concerns.

Use a dipstick to test the woman's urine for the presence of protein, ketones, and glucose before sending the sample to the laboratory. This procedure is especially important if edema or elevated blood pressure is noted on admission. Proteinuria of 1+ or more may be a sign of impending preeclampsia. Glycosuria (sugar in the urine) is found frequently in pregnant women because of the increased glomerular filtration rate in the proximal tubules and the inability of these tubules to increase reabsorption of glucose. However, it may also be associated with gestational diabetes, so do not discount it. While the woman is collecting the urine specimen, gather the equipment needed for any procedures ordered by the certified nurse-midwife (CNM) or physician. In the past, complete or partial shaving of the pubic area (called a *prep*) was standard. This practice is becoming increasingly rare because the benefit to the woman is questionable (Varney, 1997).

Laboratory tests are done during early admission. Hemoglobin and hematocrit values help determine the oxygen-carrying capacity of the circulatory system and the woman's ability to withstand blood loss at birth. Elevation of the hematocrit may reveal hemoconcentration of blood, which occurs with edema or dehydration. A low hemoglobin, in the absence of other evidence of bleeding, suggests anemia. Blood may be typed and crossmatched if the woman is in a high-risk category. Additional serologic testing may be performed as indicated.

In many hospitals, the admission process also includes signing an informed consent for treatment and providing information about advanced directives. In all cases an identification bracelet is attached to the expectant woman's wrist.

Depending on how rapidly labor is progressing, the nurse notifies the CNM or physician before or after completing the admission procedures. The report should include the following information: parity, cervical dilatation and effacement, station, presenting part, status of the membranes, contraction pattern, FHR, vital signs that are not in the normal range, any significant prenatal history, the woman's birth preferences, and her reaction to labor.

Enter a nursing admission note into the computer or the charting system. The admission note should include the reason for admission, the date and time of the woman's arrival and notification of the CNM or physician, the condition of the woman and her baby, and labor and membrane status (American Academy of Pediatrics & American College of Obstetricians and Gynecologists, 1997).

NURSING MANAGEMENT DURING THE FIRST STAGE OF LABOR

After completing the nursing assessment and diagnosis steps, create a plan of care to achieve identified nursing goals. For instance, if the woman and her support person did not have the opportunity to attend preparation for childbirth classes, the nursing goal would be to provide desired information. To accomplish this goal, the nurse would assess the current level of the couple's understanding and then plan to provide brief explanations as labor progresses.

Integration of Family Expectations

Families come into the birth setting with basic expectations that they will not be harmed and that the labor and birth will be safe for the mother and baby. In addition, women look for the following from their nurses:

- Emotional support, which includes sustained presence of the nurse, praise, encouragement, reassurance, and companionship.
- Comfort measures such as the use of touch, provision of ice chips and fluids, massage, assistance with care, and a bath or shower.
- Information and advice, which includes offering information about procedures, interventions as they occur, and reports of labor progress.
- Advocacy to help the woman and her partner achieve their goals, hopes, and dreams for their labor and birth experience.
- Support of the partner including encouragement, praise for his or her efforts, an opportunity for rest breaks, and role modeling.

Integration of Cultural Beliefs

Knowledge of values, customs, and practices of different cultures is as important during labor as it is in the prenatal period. Without this knowledge, a nurse is less likely to understand a family's behavior and may attempt to impose personal values and beliefs on them. As cultural sensitivity increases, so does the likelihood of providing high-quality care.

The following sections briefly present a few possible cultural responses to labor. It is difficult to present even such a limited discussion in a clear, nonjudgmental way, because once a statement is made it may appear stereotypic, and of course no statement of a specific behavior can accurately reflect the preference of all people in a group. Always remain aware that an individual example of a birthing practice will never be pertinent to all women in a given group. General information about any culture or belief system needs to be viewed as background to help caregivers meet each individual's needs and desires.

MODESTY

Modesty is an important consideration for women regardless of culture. However, some women may be more uncomfortable than others with the degree of exposure needed for certain procedures during labor and the birth process. Some women may be particularly uncomfortable when men are present and feel more comfortable with women; others may be uncomfortable with exposure of

personal body parts regardless of the gender of the caregivers. Be alert to the woman's responses to examinations and procedures and provide the draping and privacy the woman needs. It is more prudent to assume that embarrassment will occur with exposure and take measures to provide privacy than to assume that it will not matter to the woman if she is exposed during procedures. For example, some Asian women are not accustomed to male physicians and attendants. Modesty is of great concern, and exposure of as little of the woman's body as possible is strongly recommended.

PAIN EXPRESSION

The manner in which a woman chooses to deal with the discomfort of labor varies widely. Some women seem to turn inward and remain very quiet during the whole process. They speak only to ask others to leave the room or cease conversation. Others may be very vocal, with behaviors such as counting out loud, moaning quietly, crying, or use of loud vocalization. They may also turn from side to side or change positions frequently.

In Asian cultures it is important for individuals to act in a way that will not bring shame on the family. Therefore, the Korean woman may not express pain outwardly for fear of shaming herself or her family, and Filipina women say it is best to lie quietly (Lauderdale, 1999; Wesson, 2000). Silence is valued in Chinese society, so a woman of that heritage is usually quiet and stoic in order to avoid dishonoring herself or her family (Wesson, 2000). Hispanic women are encouraged to be patient and not to cry out or the "uterus will rise up" (Lauderdale, 1999). South or Central American women may view pain during labor as a symbol of love toward the baby: the more intense the pain, the more intense the love (Scott-Ramos, 1996). It is important to support a woman's individual expression, whatever it may be (as long as harm is not done to another), in order to enhance the birthing experience for mother, baby, and family.

CULTURAL BELIEFS: SOME EXAMPLES

Hmong women from Laos report that squatting during childbirth is common in their culture (Lauderdale, 1999). During labor they may want to be active and move about. The husband is frequently present and actively involved in providing comfort. Traditionally, the woman prefers that the amniotic membranes not be ruptured until just before birth. It is thought that the escape of fluid at this time makes the birth easier. During labor the woman usually prefers only "hot" foods and warm water to drink (Lauderdale, 1999). As soon as the baby is born, a soft-boiled egg must be given to the mother to restore her energy.

Vietnamese women usually maintain self-control and may even smile throughout labor. They may prefer to walk about during labor and to give birth in a squatting position. The woman may avoid drinking cold water and prefer fluids at room temperature. The newborn is protected from praise to prevent jealousy (Calhoun, 1986).

Latina women have identified expectations of their partners during labor and birth such as wanting their partners to stay with them and to reassure them that everything will be all right. As they labor, the women want their partners to show their love and to speak using affectionate words (Khazoyan & Anderson, 1994).

Muslim women may have their husband, a female friend or relative, or a male relative with them during childbirth. Family support may be particularly important but does not preclude the importance of the nurse's presence. The woman may want to retain her head covering *(khimar),* and may prefer to wear two long-sleeved gowns to enhance modesty. It is important for a female nurse, physician, or CNM to perform examinations whenever possible. If a male physician or nurse is involved, the woman may want her husband to remain in the room.

Maternity nurses can provide culturally sensitive care by first becoming acquainted with the beliefs and practices of the various subcultures in their communities. In the birthing situation, the truly effective nurse supports the family's cultural practices as long as it is safe to do so.

Support of the Adolescent During Birth

As with all women, each adolescent in labor is different. Assess what each teen brings to the experience by considering the following:

- Has the young woman received prenatal care?
- What are her attitudes and feelings about the pregnancy?
- Who will attend the birth and what is the person's relationship to her?
- What preparation has she had for the experience?
- What are her expectations and fears regarding labor and birth?
- How has her culture influenced her?
- What are her usual coping mechanisms?
- Does she plan to keep the newborn?

Adolescent women are at highest risk for pregnancy and labor complications and must be assessed carefully. Fetal well-being is established by fetal monitoring. Be especially alert for any physiologic complications of labor. The young woman's prenatal record is carefully reviewed for risks, and she is screened for preeclampsia, cephalopelvic disproportion, anemia, drugs ingested during pregnancy, sexually transmitted infections, and size-date discrepancies.

The support role of the nurse depends on the young woman's support system during labor. The adolescent may not be accompanied by someone who will stay with her during childbirth, or she may have her mother, the father of the baby, or a close friend as her labor partner. Regardless of whether the teen has a support person, it is important to establish a trusting relationship with her. In this way, it is possible to help the teen understand what is happening to her. Establishing rapport without recrimination for possible inappropriate behavior is essential. The adolescent given positive reinforcement for "work well done" will leave the experience with increased self-esteem, despite the emotional problems that may accompany her situation.

If a support person accompanies the adolescent, that person also needs encouragement and support. Explain changes in the young woman's behavior and describe ways the support person can be of help.

The adolescent who has taken childbirth education classes is generally better prepared for labor than the adolescent who has not. However, keep in mind that the younger the adolescent, the less she may be able to participate actively in the process, even if she has taken prenatal classes.

The very young adolescent (age 14 and under) has fewer coping mechanisms and less experience to draw on than her older counterparts. Because her cognitive development is incomplete, the younger adolescent may have fewer problem-solving capabilities. She may be more threatened by the experience, and she may be more vulnerable to stress and discomfort.

The very young adolescent needs someone to rely on at all times during labor. She may be more childlike and dependent than older teens. Be sure instructions and explanations are simple and concrete. During the transition phase, the young teenager may become withdrawn and unable to express her need to be nurtured. Touch, soothing encouragement, and measures to provide comfort help her maintain control and meet her needs for dependence. During the second stage of labor, the young adolescent may feel as if she is losing control and may reach out to those around her. Remain calm and give clear, simple directions to help the teen cope with feelings of helplessness.

The middle adolescent (age 15 to 17 years) often attempts to remain calm and unflinching during labor. Nevertheless, a caring attitude still helps the young woman. Many older adolescents believe that they "know it all," but they may be no more prepared for childbirth than their younger counterparts. Positive reinforcement and a nonjudgmental manner will help them save face. If the adolescent has not taken childbirth preparation classes, she may require preparation and explanations. The older teenager's (age 18 to 19) response to the stresses of labor, however, is similar to that of the adult woman.

Even if the adolescent is planning to relinquish her newborn, she should be given the option of seeing and holding the infant. She may be reluctant to do this at first, but the mother's grieving process is facilitated if she sees the infant. However, seeing or holding the newborn should be the young woman's choice. (See Chapter 22 for further discussion of the relinquishing mother and the adolescent parent.) ⌖

Promotion of Comfort in the First Stage

The first step in planning care is to talk with the woman and her partner, if present, to identify their goals. Usually the couple is concerned with discomfort, so it is helpful to identify factors that may contribute to discomfort. These factors include uncomfortable positions, diaphoresis, continual leaking of amniotic fluid, a full bladder, a dry mouth, anxiety, and fear. Nursing interventions can minimize the effects of these factors. These interventions are described later in this section.

There are many responses to pain. As the intensity of the contraction increases with the progress of labor, the woman becomes less aware of the environment and may have difficulty hearing and understanding verbal instructions. The pattern of coping with labor contractions varies from the use of highly structured breathing techniques to turning inward. Low moaning that begins deep in the throat, rocking or swaying, facial grimacing, and using loud vocalizations are all effective means of dealing with the power of labor and birth (England & Horowitz, 1998). Some women feel that making sounds helps them cope and do the work of labor, whereas others make loud sounds only as they lose their perception of control.

The most frequent physiologic manifestations of pain are increased pulse and respiratory rates, dilated pupils, increased blood pressure, and muscle tension. In labor, these reactions are transitory because the pain is intermittent. Increased muscle tension is most significant because it may impede the progress of labor. Women in labor often tighten skeletal muscles voluntarily during a contraction and remain motionless. This method of dealing with the contractions may actually increase the level of discomfort because of muscular tension, but the women may believe it is the only acceptable way to cope with the pain.

A woman generally wants touching, massage, effleurage (see Chapter 6), ⌖ and other forms of physical contact during the first part of labor, but when she moves into the transition phase, she may rebuff all efforts and pull away. Women may provide verbal and nonverbal signs such as crying, moaning, and beseeching the coach or nurse to hold their hand or rub their back. They may reach out and grasp the support person or indicate their anxiety or fear through eye contact. However, some women are uncomfortable with being touched at all, regardless of the phase of labor. It is important to confirm the woman's preferences and to meet each family on its own terms, always keeping in mind that this is their experience.

Many nurses like to incorporate touch into their nursing care, and they readily respond to the woman's needs. As the nurse and woman or couple work together to increase comfort during contractions, a ritual of supportive

measures begins to develop. The nurse watches for cues and nonverbal behaviors and asks for feedback from the woman. As labor progresses, the nurse and couple use their prior experience and growing rapport to change comfort measures as needed.

A decrease in the intensity of discomfort is one of the goals of nursing support during labor. Nursing measures used to decrease pain include the following:

- Ensuring general comfort
- Providing information to decrease anxiety
- Using specific supportive relaxation techniques
- Encouraging controlled breathing
- Administering pharmacologic agents as ordered by the physician or CNM

GENERAL COMFORT

General comfort measures are of great importance during labor. By relieving minor discomforts, the nurse helps the woman optimize her ability to cope with pain.

Encourage the woman to ambulate as long as there are no contraindications, such as vaginal bleeding or rupture of membranes before the fetus is engaged in the pelvis. Even if the woman prefers not to walk around, upright positions such as sitting in a rocker or leaning against a wall or bed can enhance comfort. If she stays in bed, encourage the woman to assume positions that she finds comfortable. A side-lying position is generally the most advantageous for the laboring woman, although frequent position changes seem to achieve more efficient contractions. Take care to support all body parts, with the joints kept slightly flexed. For instance, when the woman is in a side-lying position, pillows may be placed against her chest and under the uppermost arm. Place a pillow or folded bath blanket between her knees to support the uppermost leg and relieve tension or muscle strain. A pillow placed at the woman's midback also helps provide support. If the woman is more comfortable on her back, elevate the head of the bed to relieve the pressure of the uterus on the vena cava. Pillows may be placed under each arm and under the knees to provide further support. Because a pregnant woman is at increased risk for thrombophlebitis, excessive pressure behind the knee and calf should be avoided. Assess pressure points frequently.

Back rubs and frequent changes of position contribute to comfort and relaxation (see Figure 17–1 ◆). Wearing socks or slippers may alleviate cold feet, just as adjusting the room's thermostat can offset excessive warmth. Attention to such details allows the woman to focus on the more important issues of giving birth.

Diaphoresis and the constant leaking of amniotic fluid can dampen the woman's gown and bed linen. Fresh, smooth, dry bed linen promotes comfort. To avoid having to change the bottom sheet following rupture of the membranes, replace chux pads at frequent intervals (following body substance isolation precautions). Keep the woman's

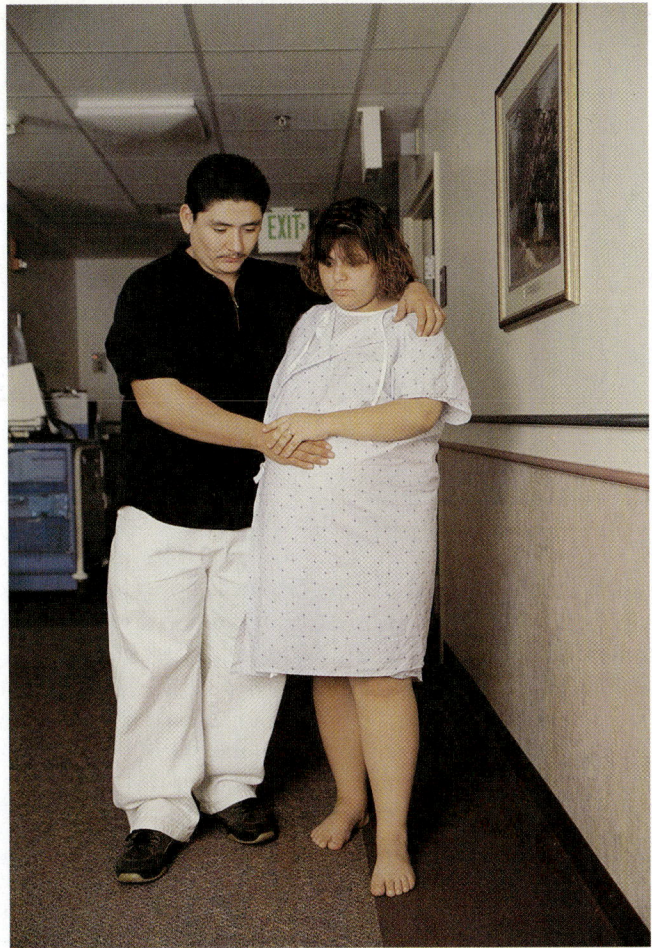

FIGURE 17–1. ◆ Woman and her partner walking in the hospital during labor.

perineal area as clean and dry as possible to promote comfort and to prevent infection.

A full bladder adds to the discomfort during a contraction and may prolong labor by interfering with the descent of the fetus. The bladder should be kept as empty as possible. Even if the woman is voiding, urine may be retained because of the pressure of the fetal presenting part. To detect a full bladder, palpate directly over the symphysis pubis. Some regional analgesia procedures contribute to the inability to void, and catheterization may be necessary. Encourage the woman to empty her bladder every 1 to 2 hours.

Family members also need to be encouraged to maintain their own comfort. Because they are paying attention to the laboring woman, they may forget their own needs. It may be necessary to encourage them to take breaks, to eat and drink, and to rest.

HANDLING ANXIETY

A woman's anxiety as she begins labor is related to a combination of factors inherent to the process. A moderate amount of anxiety about the pain enhances the woman's ability to deal with it. In contrast, an excessive degree of anxiety decreases her ability to cope. Women in the latent

phase of labor who have increased anxiety about safety and their ability to cope are much more likely to describe their pain as unbearable. They are also more likely to have FHR decelerations in labor, a slow second stage, and/or a cesarean birth, and they are more likely to need pediatric assistance for neonatal resuscitation at birth (Varney, 1997).

To decrease anxiety not related to pain, give information (which eases fear of the unknown), establish rapport with the couple (which helps them preserve their personal integrity), and express confidence in the couple's ability to work with the labor process. It is important to demonstrate genuine concern for the laboring woman. Remaining with the woman as much as possible conveys a caring attitude and dispels fears of abandonment. Praise for breathing, relaxation, and pushing efforts not only encourages repetition of the behavior but also decreases anxiety about the ability to cope with labor.

CLIENT TEACHING

Providing truthful information about the nature of the discomfort that will occur during labor is important. Stressing the intermittent nature and maximum duration of the contractions can be most helpful. The woman can cope with pain better when she knows that a period of relief will follow. Describing the type of discomfort and specific sensations that will occur as labor progresses helps the woman recognize these sensations as normal and expected when she does experience them.

Descriptions of sensations are best accompanied by information on specific comfort measures. Some women experience the urge to push during transition, when the cervix is not fully dilated and effaced. Panting can control this sensation (it is difficult to pant and bear down at the same time). If time permits, explain the purpose of panting and have the woman practice before the technique is needed.

Thorough orientation and explanation of surroundings, procedures, and equipment being used also decrease anxiety, thereby reducing pain. Being attached to an electronic monitor can produce fear because equipment of this type is associated with critically ill people. Explain beeps, clicks, and other strange noises and give a simplified explanation of the monitor strip. Emphasize that the use of the fetal monitor provides a way to assess the well-being of the fetus during labor. In addition, show the woman and her partner or support person how the monitor can help them identify the beginnings of contractions. At the onset of each contraction, encourage the woman to begin her breathing technique to lessen her perception of pain.

Labor and childbirth may be a critical time for the woman with a history of childhood sexual abuse. Thus, all women entering the health care arena need to be evaluated for a history of sexual abuse. However, a woman who has been abused may or may not be able to address this issue with the nurse, because sharing such personal information with a stranger is difficult. It is therefore especially important to be alert for nonverbal cues, such as unexplained anxiety, unrelenting pain, and/or fear during vaginal exams, and to be prepared to offer additional teaching and relaxation support to help offset the woman's anxiety.

SUPPORTIVE RELAXATION TECHNIQUES

Tense muscles increase resistance to the descent of the fetus and contribute to maternal fatigue. This fatigue increases pain perception and decreases the woman's ability to cope with the pain. Comfort measures, massage, water therapy (see "Complementary Care: Water Therapy During Labor"), techniques for decreasing anxiety, and client teaching can contribute to relaxation. Adequate sleep and rest are also important. Encourage the laboring woman to use the periods between contractions for rest and relaxation. A prolonged prodromal phase of labor may have kept her awake. Moreover, a woman beginning labor is naturally excited, making it difficult for her to sleep even if her contractions are mild and infrequent.

Distraction helps increase relaxation and ability to cope with discomfort. During early labor, conversation or activities such as light reading or playing cards or other games serve as distractions. It may be helpful to have the woman concentrate on a pleasant experience she has had in the past. Other techniques include the use of a specific visual or mental focal point, patterns of breathing and the accompanied sounds, or visualization (England & Horowitz, 1998). (See the "Complementary Care" features on the use of music and visualization during labor and birth in Chapter 15. More information can also be found on our website. ⬭⬭ WEB)

Touch is another type of distraction (Figure 17–2◆). Although some women regard touching as an invasion of privacy or threat to their independence, many want to

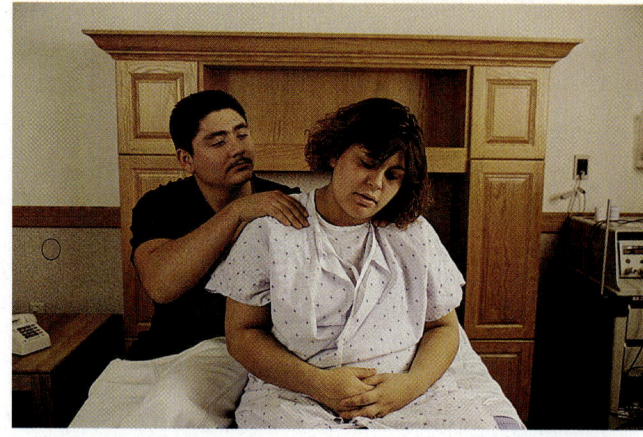

FIGURE 17–2. ◆ The woman's partner provides support and encouragement during labor.

touch and be touched during a painful experience. Nurses can make themselves available to the woman who desires touch. Place a hand on the side of the bed within the woman's reach. The person who needs touch will reach out for contact. (See "Complementary Care: Intuitive Touch".) Mild to moderate abdominal discomfort during contractions may be relieved or lessened by effleurage. Firm pressure on the lower back or sacral area may relieve back pain associated with labor. To apply firm pressure, place a hand or a rolled, warmed towel or blanket in the small of the woman's back. In addition to the measures just described, enhance the woman's relaxation by providing encouragement and support for her controlled breathing techniques.

Complementary Care

WATER THERAPY DURING LABOR

Centuries old, water immersion in hot springs, and more recently in Jacuzzis and spas, is used all over the world to promote relaxation. Current evidence supports hydrotherapy in labor as an effective method for pain management (Teschendorf & Evans, 2000). A study reported in Perez (1995) and conducted by Guyette found that women who labored in water felt better, were more relaxed, and had less pain. Compared to women who did not labor in water, they were significantly less afraid, cleaner, freer, more peaceful, and more in control.

Water immersion offers both psychologic and physiologic benefits. Physiologically, water provides the right counterpressure and support for the stretching tissues. However, several studies have reported adverse neonatal and maternal effects of water births, such as neonatal and maternal sepsis due to contaminated water. In addition, infants may require more resuscitation measures in water births (Eckert, Turnbull, & MacLennan, 2001). A sanitized tub is extremely important. Some women may choose to labor *and* give birth in a water environment; only women with low-risk pregnancies should consider this option, and they should be made aware of the possible risks.

Complementary Care

INTUITIVE TOUCH

Intuitive touch is the nurse's intentional use of physical contact with the woman with the intent of helping to slow down and regulate the breathing pattern. This type of touch has also been referred to as purposeful, affective, comforting, or empathetic touch (Bottorff, 1993; Snyder & Nojima, 1998).

Evidence suggests that touch induces the relaxation response, which is mediated through the neuroendocrine and sympathetic nervous systems. Deep relaxation results in decreased heart rate, respiratory rate and volume, oxygen consumption, blood pressure, skeletal muscle tension, and gastric acidity and motility, and it increases peripheral blood flow and the activity of natural killer cells.

A variety of techniques can be used. These include handholding; stroking or patting of a woman's arm, face, or legs; placing one hand on her shoulder; putting an arm around her shoulders; and hugging. To implement intuitive touch, use long, slow, up-and-down strokes on the woman's limbs. You do not need special training to use this intervention; all that is needed is the intention to help regulate the breathing pattern and the willingness to use a little time to achieve this goal.

BREATHING TECHNIQUES

Breathing techniques may help the laboring woman. Used correctly, they increase the woman's pain threshold, permit relaxation, enhance the woman's ability to cope with the uterine contractions, and allow the uterus to function more efficiently.

Many women learn patterned-paced breathing during prenatal education classes. This type of controlled breathing often has three levels. The woman tends to begin with the first level and then proceed to the next when she feels the need. Regardless of the level of breathing used, a cleansing breath begins and ends each pattern. A cleansing breath involves only the chest. It consists of inhaling through the nose and exhaling through pursed lips (Table 17–1).

First Pattern. The first pattern may also be called slow, deep breathing or slow-paced breathing. During the breathing movements only the chest moves. The woman inhales

---

TABLE 17–1 Nursing Support of Patterned-Paced Breathing

Determine which breathing method the woman (couple) has learned.
Provide encouragement as needed in maintaining breathing pattern.
Provide support to the labor coach and assist as needed.

LAMAZE BREATHING PATTERN LEVELS

First level (slow paced)

Pattern begins and ends with a cleansing breath (in through the nose and out through pursed lips as if cooling a spoonful of hot food). While inhaling through the nose and exhaling through pursed lips, slow breaths are taken, moving only the chest. The rate should be approximately 6–9/minute or 2 breaths/15 seconds. The coach or nurse may assist by reminding the woman to take a cleansing breath, and then the breaths could be counted out if needed to maintain pacing. The woman inhales as someone counts "one one thousand, two one thousand, three one thousand, four one thousand." Exhalation begins and continues through the same count.

First level for use during uterine contractions (The level begins and ends with a cleansing breath [CB].)

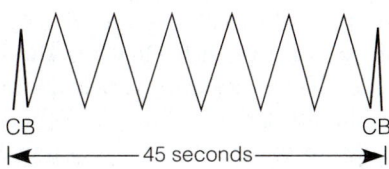

Second level (modified paced)

Pattern begins and ends with a cleansing breath. Breaths are then taken in and out silently through the mouth at approximately 4 breaths/5 seconds. The jaw and entire body need to be relaxed. The rate can be accelerated to 2–2 1/2 breaths/second. The rhythm for the breaths can be counted out as "one and two and one and two and. . ." with the woman exhaling on the numbers and inhaling on "and."

Second level

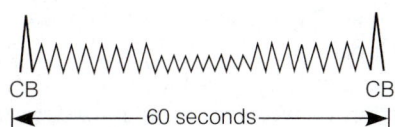

Third level (pattern paced)

Pattern begins and ends with a cleansing breath. All breaths are rhythmic, in and out through the mouth. Exhalations are accompanied by a "hee" or "hoo" sound in a varying pattern, 2:1, which begins as 3:1 (hee hee hee hoo) and can change to 2:1 (hee hee hoo) or 1:1 (hee hoo) as the intensity of the contraction changes. The rate should not be more rapid than 2–2 1/2 breaths/second. The rhythm of the breaths would match a "one and two and . . ." count.

Third level (Darkened spike represents "hoo.")

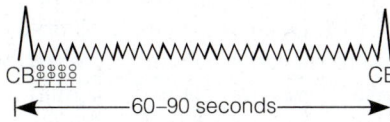

ABDOMINAL BREATHING PATTERN CUES

The abdomen moves outward during inhalation and downward during exhalation.
The rate remains slow, with approximately 6–9 breaths/minute.

Breathing sequence for abdominal breathing.

QUICK METHOD

When the woman has not learned a particular method and is in the active phase of labor, the nurse may teach her a combination of two patterns. Abdominal breathing may be used until labor is more advanced. Then a more rapid pattern consisting of two short blows from the mouth followed by a longer blow can be used. (This pattern is called "pant-pant-blow" even though all exhalations are a blowing motion.)

Pant-pant-blow breathing pattern

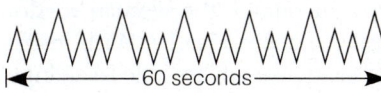

---

slowly through her nose. She moves her chest up and out during the inhalation. She exhales through pursed lips. The breathing rate is 6 to 9 breaths a minute.

Second Pattern. The second pattern is also called shallow or modified-paced breathing. The woman begins with a cleansing breath and at the end of the cleansing breath pushes out a short breath. She then inhales and exhales through the mouth at a rate of about 4 breaths every 5 seconds. This pattern can be altered into a more rapid rate that does not exceed 2 to 2 1/2 breaths every second.

Third Pattern. The third pattern is also called pant-blow or patterned-paced breathing. It is similar to modified-paced breathing except the breathing is punctuated every few breaths by a forceful exhalation through pursed lips. A pattern of 4 breaths may be used to begin. All breaths are kept equal and rhythmic. As the contraction becomes more intense, the woman may adjust the pattern as needed to 3:1, 2:1, and finally 1:1.

If the woman has not learned a controlled breathing technique, teaching her may be difficult when she is admitted in active labor. In this instance, teach abdominal and pant-pant-blow breathing (see Table 17–1). In abdominal breathing, the woman moves the abdominal wall upward as she inhales and downward as she exhales. This method tends to lift the abdominal wall off the contracting uterus and thus may provide some pain relief. The breathing is deep and rhythmic. As transition approaches, the woman may feel the need to breathe more rapidly. To avoid breathing too rapidly, the woman can use the pant-pant-blow breathing pattern.

As the woman uses her breathing technique, assess and support the interaction between the woman and her support person or partner. In the absence of a partner, or when the partner wants a less active role in the support of the laboring woman, an additional care provider, often called a *doula*, may be present. The doula enhances the comfort and decreases the anxiety of the expectant family. A doula can be a valuable advocate to the laboring woman, as well as an asset to the labor nurse. For example, the doula might support the woman by helping identify the beginning of each contraction and encouraging her as she breathes through it (see "Complementary Care: The Doula").

Hyperventilation is the result of an imbalance of oxygen and carbon dioxide (i.e., too much carbon dioxide is exhaled, and too much oxygen remains in the body). Hyperventilation may occur when a woman breathes very rapidly over a prolonged period. The signs and symptoms of hyperventilation are tingling or numbness in the tip of the nose, lips, fingers, or toes; dizziness; spots before the eyes; or spasms of the hands or feet (carpal-pedal spasms). If hyperventilation occurs, encourage the woman to slow her breathing rate and take shallow breaths. With instruction and encouragement, many women are able to change their breathing to correct the problem. It may also help to count out loud for the woman so she can pace her breathing dur-

ing contractions. If the signs and symptoms continue or become more severe (they progress from numbness to spasms), the woman can breathe into a paper surgical mask or a paper bag until symptoms go away. Breathing into a mask or bag causes rebreathing of carbon dioxide. During this time, remain with the woman to reassure her.

In some instances, analgesics or regional anesthetic blocks may be used to increase comfort and relaxation during labor. (See Chapter 18.) Table 17–2 summarizes labor progress, possible responses of the laboring woman, and support measures.

Special Assessments and Care Throughout the First Stage of Labor

LATENT PHASE

As discussed in Chapter 16, it is important to assess the physical well-being of the woman and her fetus. Monitor maternal temperature every 4 hours unless the temperature is over 37.5 °C (99.6 °F); in such cases take it every hour. Monitor blood pressure, pulse, and respirations every hour. If the woman's blood pressure is over 140/90 mm Hg or her pulse is more than 100, notify the CNM or physician and reevaluate the blood pressure and pulse more frequently. Palpate uterine contractions for frequency, intensity, and duration and auscultate the FHR every 60 minutes for low-risk women and every 30 minutes for high-risk women. Auscultate the FHR throughout one contraction and for about 15 seconds after the contraction to ensure that there are no decelerations. If the FHR baseline is not in the 120 to 160 range

TABLE 17–2 Normal Progress, Psychologic Characteristics, and Nursing Support During the First and Second Stages of Labor

Phase	Cervical Dilatation	Uterine Contractions	Woman's Response	Support Measures
STAGE 1 Latent phase	1–4 cm	Every 10–20 minutes, 15–20 seconds' duration Mild intensity *progressing to* Every 5–7 minutes, 30–40 seconds' duration Moderate intensity	Usually happy, talkative, and eager to be in labor Exhibits need for independence by taking care of own bodily needs and seeking information	Establish rapport on admission and continue to build during care. Assess information base and learning needs. Be available to consult regarding breathing technique if needed; teach breathing technique if needed and in early labor. Orient family to room, equipment, monitors, and procedures. Encourage woman and partner to participate in care as desired. Provide needed information. Assist woman into position of comfort; encourage frequent change of position; encourage ambulation during early labor. Offer fluids or ice chips. Keep couple informed of progress. Encourage woman to void every 1 to 2 hours. Assess need for an interest in using visualization to enhance relaxation and teach if appropriate.
Active phase	4–7 cm	Every 2–3 minutes, 40–60 seconds' duration Moderate to strong intensity	May experience feelings of helplessness Exhibits increased fatigue and may begin to feel restless and anxious as contractions become stronger Expresses fear of abandonment Becomes more dependent because she is less able to meet her needs	Encourage woman to maintain breathing patterns. Provide quiet environment to reduce external stimuli. Provide reassurance, encouragement, support; keep couple informed of progress. Promote comfort by giving back rubs, sacral pressure, cool cloth on forehead, assistance with position changes, support with pillows, effleurage. Provide ice chips, ointment for dry mouth and lips. Encourage to void every 1 to 2 hours. Offer shower, whirlpool, or warm bath if available.
Transition phase	8–10 cm	Every 2 minutes, 60–75 seconds' duration Strong intensity	Tires and may exhibit increased restlessness and irritability May feel she cannot keep up with labor process and is out of control Physical discomforts Fear of being left alone May fear tearing open or splitting apart with contractions	Encourage woman to rest between contractions. If she sleeps between contractions, wake her at beginning of contraction so she can begin breathing pattern (increases feeling of control). Provide support, encouragement, and praise for efforts. Keep couple informed of progress; encourage continued participation of support persons. Promote comfort as listed earlier but recognize that many women do not want to be touched when in transition. Provide privacy. Provide ice chips, ointment for lips. Encourage to void every 1 to 2 hours.
STAGE 2	Complete	Every 2 minutes	May feel out of control, helpless, panicky	Assist woman in pushing efforts. Encourage woman to assume position of comfort. Provide encouragement and praise her efforts. Keep couple informed of progress. Provide ice chips. Maintain privacy as woman desires.

or if decelerations are heard, continuous electronic monitoring is recommended (Table 17–3).

Offer fluids in the form of clear liquids or ice chips frequently, unless complications exist that may result in a cesarean birth. Some certified childbirth educators advise the woman to bring lollipops to help combat the dryness that occurs with some of the labor breathing patterns. Because gastric emptying time is prolonged during labor, solid foods are usually avoided. However, fasting during labor is a controversial practice. Some providers believe that eating and

drinking during labor should be an option. Based on the current literature, many nurse-midwifery practices now encourage mothers to eat and drink as tolerated (Varney, 1997).

ACTIVE PHASE

During the active phase, contractions have a frequency of 2 to 3 minutes, a duration of 50 to 60 seconds, and a moderate intensity. Palpate contractions every 15 to 30 minutes. As the contractions become more frequent and intense, vaginal exams assess cervical dilatation and effacement

TABLE 17–3   Nursing Assessments in the First Stage

Phase	Mother	Fetus
Latent	Blood pressure, respirations each hour if in normal range	Fetal heart rate (FHR) every 60 minutes for low-risk women and every 30 minutes for high-risk women if normal characteristics present (average variability, baseline in the 120–160 beats per minute range, without late or variable decelerations) (AWHONN, 1998).
	Temperature every 4 hours unless over 37.5 °C (99.6 °F) or membranes ruptured, then every hour	Note fetal activity.
	Uterine contractions every 30 minutes	If electronic fetal monitor in place, assess for reactive nonstress test (NST).
Active	Blood pressure, pulse, respirations every hour if in normal range	FHR every 30 minutes for low-risk women and every 15 minutes for high-risk women if normal characteristics are present (AWHONN, 1998).
	Uterine contractions every 30 minutes	
Transition	Blood pressure, pulse, respirations every 30 minutes	FHR every 30 minutes for low-risk women and every 15 minutes for high-risk women if normal characteristics are present (AWHONN, 1998).

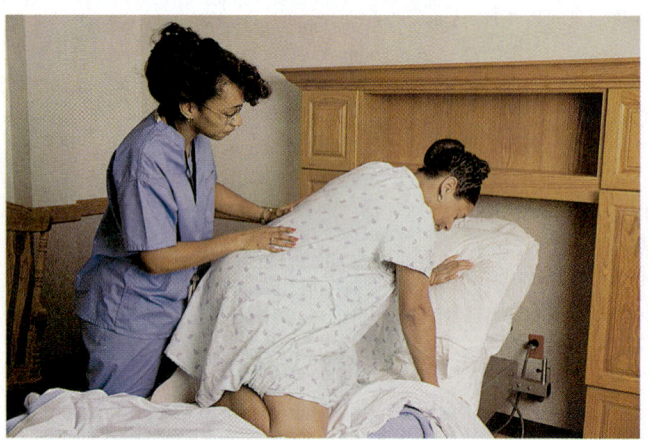

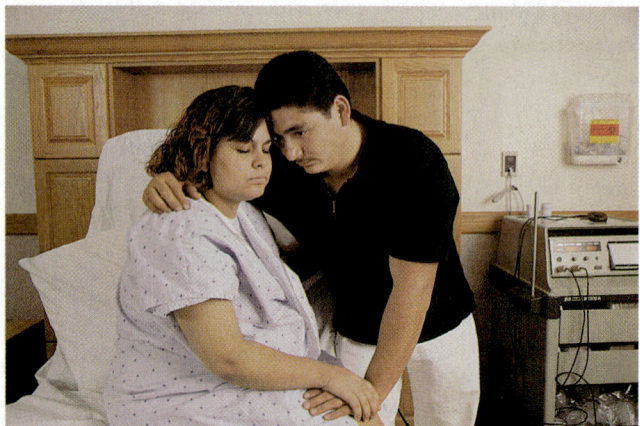

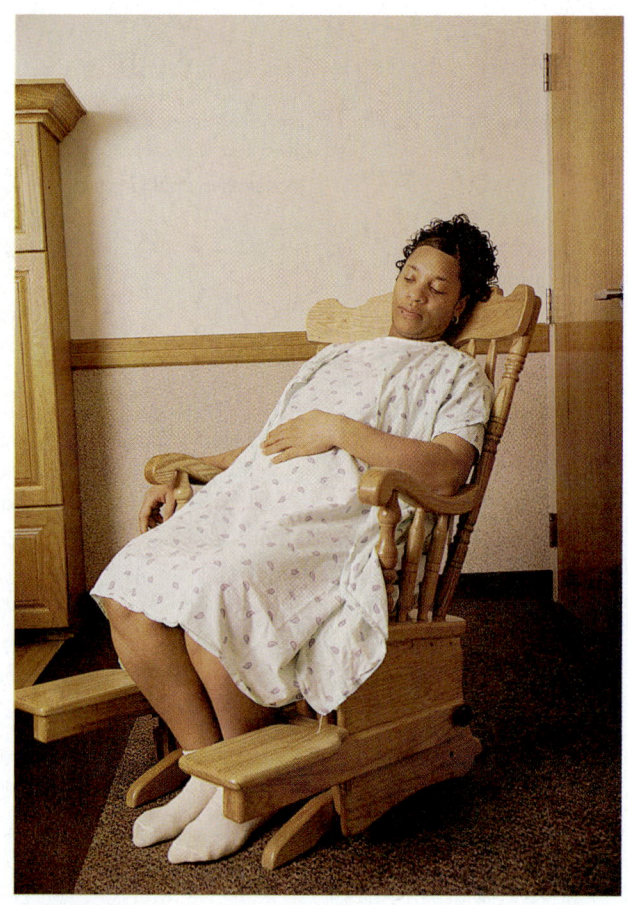

FIGURE 17–3. ◆ The laboring woman is encouraged to choose a comfortable position. The nurse modifies assessments and intervention as necessary.

and fetal station and position. During the active phase, the cervix dilates from 4 to 7 cm, and vaginal discharge and bloody show increase. Monitor maternal blood pressure, pulse, and respirations every hour for low-risk women (unless elevated, as previously noted) and every 30 minutes for high-risk women. Auscultate the FHR every 30 minutes for low-risk women and every 15 minutes for high-risk women

(Association of Women's Health, Obstetric, and Neonatal Nurses [AWHONN], 1999).

A woman who has been ambulatory up to this point may now wish to sit in a chair or on a bed (Figure 17–3 ◆). If the woman wants to lie on the bed, encourage her to assume a side-lying position. Help her into a comfortable position and place pillows to support her body. To increase

TABLE 17-4 Deviations from Normal Labor Process Requiring Immediate Intervention

Problem	Immediate Action
Woman admitted with vaginal bleeding or history of painless vaginal bleeding	Do not perform vaginal examination. Assess fetal heart rate (FHR). Evaluate amount of blood loss. Evaluate labor pattern. Notify physician or certified nurse-midwife (CNM) immediately.
Presence of greenish or brownish amniotic fluid	Continuously monitor FHR. Evaluate dilatation of cervix and determine if umbilical cord is prolapsed. Evaluate presentation (vertex or breech). Maintain woman on complete bed rest on left side. Notify physician or CNM immediately.
Absence of FHR and fetal movement	Notify physician or CNM. Provide truthful information and emotional support to laboring couple. Remain with the couple.
Prolapse of umbilical cord	Relieve pressure on cord manually. Continuously monitor FHR; watch for changes in FHR pattern. Notify physician or CNM. Assist woman into knee-chest position. Administer oxygen.
Woman admitted in advanced labor; birth imminent	Prepare for immediate birth. Obtain critical information: Estimated date of birth (EDB) History of bleeding problems History of medical or obstetric problems Past and/or present use or abuse of prescription, over-the-counter (OTC), or illicit drugs Problems with this pregnancy FHR and maternal vital signs Whether membranes are ruptured and how long since rupture Blood type and Rh Direct another person to contact physician or CNM. Do not leave woman alone. Provide support to couple. Put on gloves.

comfort, offer a back rub or effleurage or place a cool cloth on the woman's forehead or across her neck. Because vaginal discharge increases, change the chux pad frequently. Washing the perineum with warm soap and water removes secretions and increases comfort. During such procedures, wear disposable gloves to avoid exposure to vaginal discharge.

If the amniotic membranes have not ruptured previously, they may do so during this phase. When the membranes rupture, note the color, odor, and consistency of the amniotic fluid and the time of rupture and immediately auscultate the FHR. The fluid should be clear, with no odor. Fetal stress leads to intestinal and anal sphincter relaxation, and meconium may be released into the amniotic fluid, which turns the fluid greenish brown. Whenever meconium-stained fluid is present, apply an electronic monitor to assess the FHR continuously. Note the time of rupture because medical practice suggests that birth should occur within 24 hours of rupture of membranes.

Prolapse of the umbilical cord is a possible risk when membranes rupture and the fetus is not engaged because the amniotic fluid coming through the cervix might wash the umbilical cord out through the cervix. With each contraction the cord would then become trapped between the presenting part and the maternal pelvis. The FHR is auscultated because a drop in the rate might indicate an undetected prolapsed cord. Immediate intervention is necessary to remove pressure on a prolapsed umbilical cord (see Chapter 19). (See Table 17–4 for other deviations from normal.)

TRANSITION

During transition, the contraction frequency is every 2 to 3 minutes, duration is 60 to 90 seconds, and intensity is strong. Cervical dilatation increases from 8 to 10 cm, effacement is complete (100%), and there is usually a heavy amount of bloody show. Palpate contractions at least every 15 minutes. Sterile vaginal examinations may be done more frequently because this stage of labor usually is accompanied by rapid change. Take the maternal blood pressure, pulse, and respirations at least every 30 minutes, and auscultate FHR every 15 minutes.

Comfort measures are important in this phase of labor, but continual assessment is required to intervene appropriately. The woman may rapidly change from wanting a back rub and other hands-on care to wanting to be left completely alone. The support person and the nurse need to follow her cues and change interventions as needed. Because the woman is breathing more rapidly, increase her comfort by offering small spoons of ice chips to moisten her mouth or offer petroleum jelly for her dry lips. Encourage the woman to rest between contractions. If analgesics have been administered, a quiet environment enhances the quality of rest between contractions. Awaken the woman just before a contraction begins so that she can begin patterned breathing.

Some women have difficulty coping during this time and need help with their breathing. Either the support person or the nurse can breathe along with the woman during each contraction to help her maintain her pattern. It is helpful to encourage the woman and to assure her that she is doing a good job. The woman will begin to feel increased rectal pressure as the fetal presenting part moves down the birth canal. To help prevent cervical edema, encourage the woman to refrain from pushing until the cervix is completely dilated.

The end of transition and the beginning of the second stage may be indicated by a change in the woman's voice or the sounds she is making. As the fetus moves down and she feels increased pressure and a bearing-down sensation, her voice tends to deepen. A moan during a contraction takes on a more guttural quality.

NURSING MANAGEMENT DURING THE SECOND STAGE OF LABOR

The second stage is reached when the cervix is fully dilated (10 cm). The contractions continue as in the transition phase. Assess maternal pulse and blood pressure and FHR every 5 to 15 minutes.

As the woman pushes during the second stage, she may make a variety of sounds. A low-pitched, grunting sound ("uhhh") usually indicates that the woman is working with the pushing. The nurse who feels comfortable with maternal sounds and stays sensitive to changes in the sounds may be able to detect if the woman is losing her ability to cope. For instance, if the woman feels afraid of the sensations produced by her pushing effort, her sound may change to a high-pitched cry or whimper, and the nurse can then provide extra support (Wesson, 2000). Some nurses and physicians may encourage the woman to push harder and not let any breath out. The belief is that making noise decreases the pushing effort, although research disputes this.

During the second stage, the woman may interpret rectal pressure as a need to move her bowels. The instinctive response is to resist and to tighten muscles rather than bear down (push). A sensation of splitting apart also occurs in the latter part of the second stage, and the woman may fear the urge to push. The woman who expects these sensations and understands that bearing down contributes to progress at this stage is more likely to do so effectively.

When the urge to bear down becomes uncontrollable and pushing begins, the nurse can help by encouraging the woman and by assisting with positioning (Figure 17–4 ◆). The woman may want to be supported with pillows in a semireclining position, be side-lying, position herself on her hands and knees, or use a squatting bar. Most women spontaneously push very effectively in response to messages from their body. However, in some settings sustained, forceful pushing is believed to be necessary. In that case, when the contraction begins, the woman is told to take a cleansing breath or two, then to take a third large breath and hold it while pushing down with her abdominal muscles (called the *Valsalva maneuver*). Studies have shown that when the woman uses the more natural approach to pushing, the second stage of labor is either the same length or shorter than that of women using the Valsalva maneuver (Varney, 1997).

A nullipara is usually prepared for birth when perineal bulging is noted. A multipara usually progresses far more quickly, so she may be prepared for the birth when the cervix is dilated 7 to 8 cm. As the birth approaches, the woman's partner or support person also prepares for the birth.

Monitor the woman's blood pressure and the FHR between contractions, and palpate the contractions until the birth. Continue to assist the woman in her pushing efforts, keep both the woman and the coach informed of procedures and progress, and support them both throughout the birth.

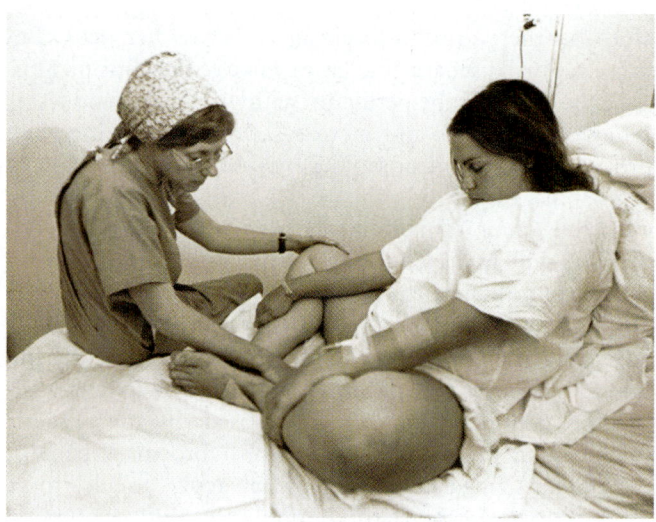

FIGURE 17–4. ◆ The nurse provides support during pushing efforts.

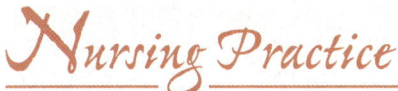
In addition to assisting the woman and her partner, the nurse also assists the physician or certified nurse-midwife (CNM) in preparing for the birth. The physician or CNM dons a sterile gown and gloves and may place sterile drapes over the woman's abdomen and legs. An episiotomy may be done just before the actual birth if needed. (See the discussion of episiotomy in Chapter 20.)

Promotion of Comfort in the Second Stage

Most of the comfort measures used during the first stage remain appropriate at this time. Applying cool cloths to the face and forehead may help cool the woman involved in the intense physical exertion of pushing. The woman may feel hot and want to remove some covers. Care still needs to be taken to provide privacy even though covers are removed. Encourage the woman to rest and relax all muscles during the periods between contractions. With the support person(s), help the woman into a pushing position with each contraction. Sips of fluids or ice chips may relieve dry mouth.

Assisting During Birth

Shortly before the birth, the birthing room or delivery room is prepared with the equipment and materials that may be needed. Family members do not need to change into other clothing if the birth occurs in a birthing room; they don a disposable scrub suit if the birth is to occur in a delivery room or surgery suite. Good handwashing is required of the nurses and CNM or physician. Nurses who will be in direct contact with the mother at the time of birth need to wear protective clothing such as an apron or gown with a splash apron, disposable gloves, and eye covering. The CNM or physician also needs to wear a plastic apron or a gown with a splash apron, eye covering, and sterile gloves.

If for any reason the laboring woman is to give birth in a location other than the birthing room (such as in the case of a cesarean birth), she is moved on her bed or a cart shortly before birth. To ensure safety, the side rails should be raised into a locked position. It is important that the woman move from one bed to another between contractions. During the contraction, the woman feels increased discomfort and may be involved in pushing efforts. Take care to preserve her privacy during the transfer. The labor bed or transfer cart must be carefully braced against the delivery table to ensure the woman's safety during the transfer.

Even though there are differences in the delivery room setting, the family can still be together during the birth. Encourage family members to participate, because the delivery room environment may seem intimidating. The family member may hesitate to continue providing support because of fear of interfering or being in the way.

MATERNAL BIRTHING POSITIONS

Until modern times the upright posture for birth was considered normal in most societies. Women chose to squat, kneel, stand, or sit for birth. The recumbent position (lithotomy) became more usual in the Western world because of the convenience it offers in applying technology. The lithotomy position has thus become the conventional manner in which North American women give birth in hospitals. In seeking alternative positions, consumers and professionals alike are refocusing on the comfort of the laboring woman rather than on the convenience of the CNM or physician (Figures 17–5 ◆ and 17–6 ◆ and Table 17–5).

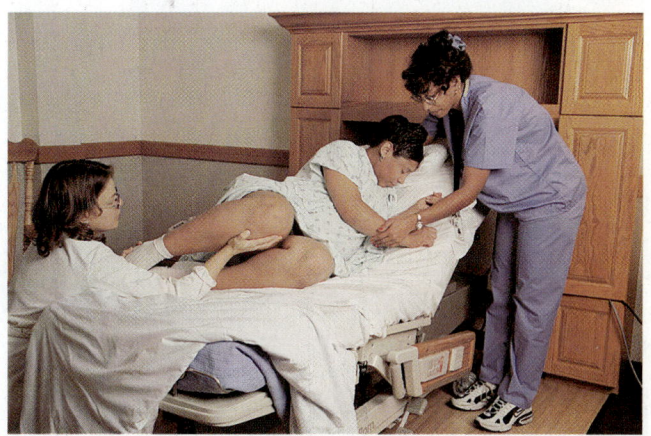

A

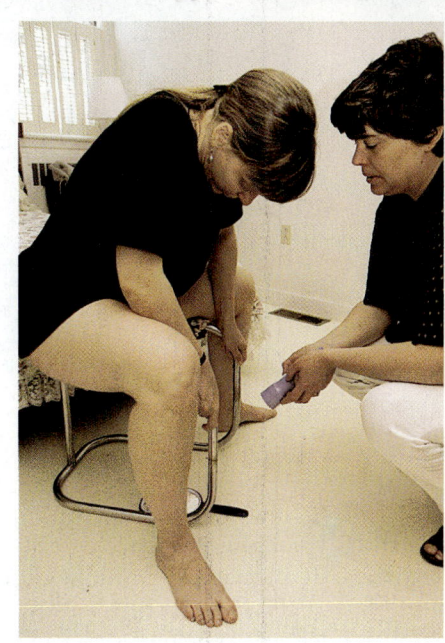

B

FIGURE 17–5. ◆ Birthing positions. **A,** Side-lying position. **B,** Using a birthing stool.

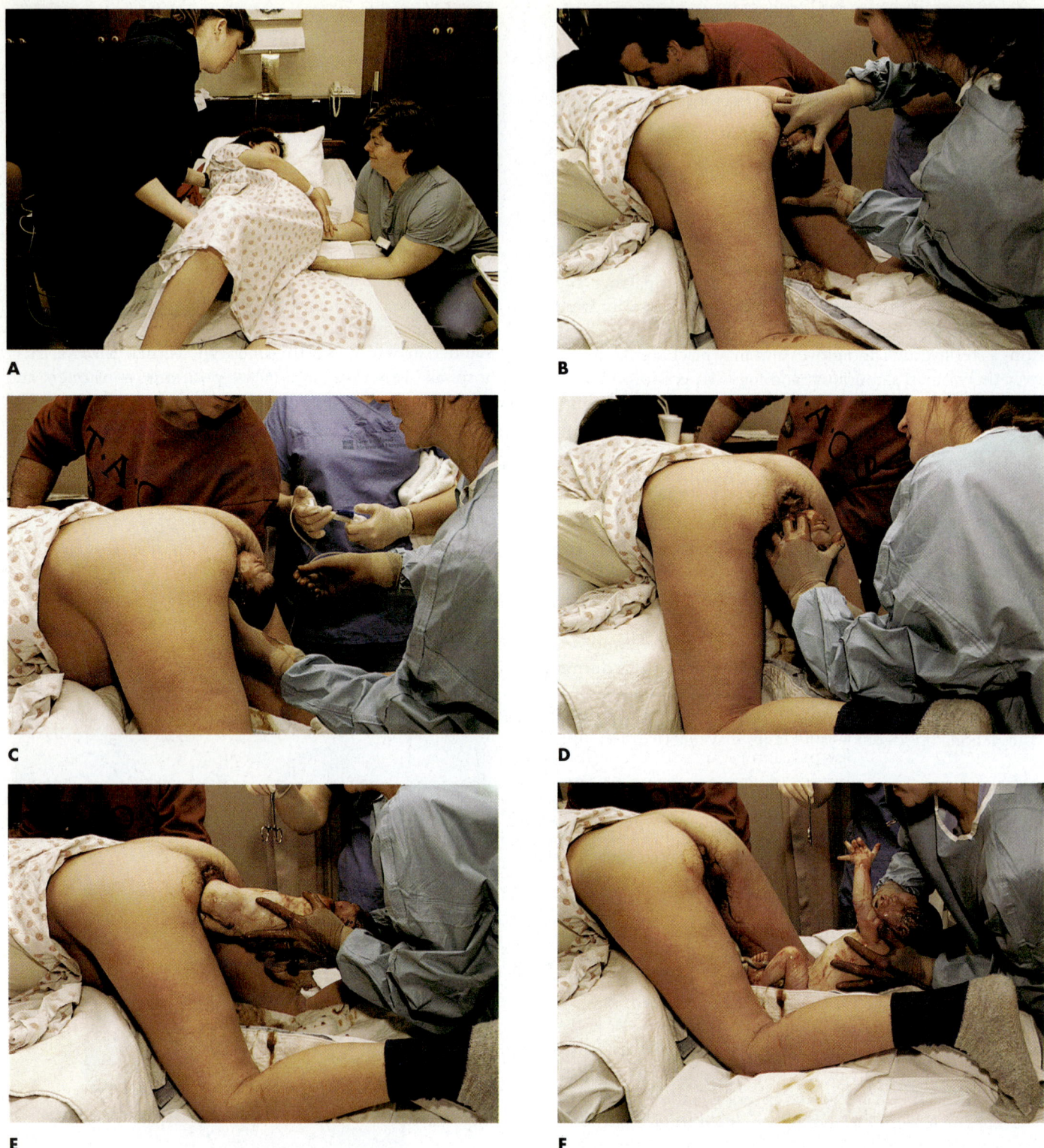

FIGURE 17–6. ◆ A birthing sequence.

The woman is typically positioned for birth on a bed with leg supports, in a squatting position, or perhaps on her hands and knees. If a birthing bed is used, the back is elevated 30 to 60 degrees to help the woman bear down. Stirrups, if needed and used, are padded to avoid pressure. If helping the woman place her legs in the stirrups, lift both legs simultaneously to avoid strain on abdominal, back, and perineal muscles. Adjust the stirrups to fit the woman's legs. The feet are supported in the stirrup holders. The height and angle of the stirrups are adjusted so there is no pressure on the backs of the knees or the calves, which might cause discomfort and postpartal vascular problems.

TABLE 17–5 Comparison of Birthing Positions

Position	Advantages	Disadvantages	Nursing Actions
Sitting on birthing stool	Gravity aids descent and expulsion of infant. Does not compromise venous return from lower extremities. Woman can view birth process.	It is difficult to provide support for the woman's back.	Encourage woman to sit in a position that increases her comfort.
Semi-Fowler's	Does not compromise venous return from lower extremities. Woman can view birth process.	If legs are positioned wide apart, relaxation of perineal tissues is decreased.	Assess that upper torso is evenly supported. Increase support of body by changing position of bed or using pillows as props.
Left lateral Sims'	Does not compromise venous return from lower extremities. Increases perineal relaxation and decreases need for episiotomy. Appears to prevent rapid descent.	It is difficult for the woman to see the birth.	Adjust position so that the upper leg lies on the bed (scissor fashion) or is supported by the partner or on pillows.
Squatting	Size of pelvic outlet is increased. Gravity aids descent and expulsion of newborn. Second stage may be shortened.	It may be difficult to maintain balance while squatting.	Help woman maintain balance. Use a birthing bar if available.
Sitting in birthing bed	Gravity aids descent and expulsion of the fetus. Does not compromise venous return from lower extremities. Woman can view the birth process. Leg position may be changed at will.		Ensure that legs and feet have adequate support.
Hands and knees	Increases perineal relaxation and decreases need for episiotomy. Increases placental and umbilical blood flow and decreases fetal distress. Improves fetal rotation. Nurse is better able to assess perineum. Nurse has better access to fetal nose and mouth for suctioning at birth. Facilitates birth of infant with shoulder dystocia.	Woman cannot view birth. There is decreased contact with birth attendant. Caregivers cannot use instruments. There may be increased maternal fatigue.	Adjust birthing bed by dropping the foot down. Supply extra pillows for increased support.

CLEANSING THE PERINEUM

After the woman has been positioned for the birth, her vulvar and perineal areas are cleansed to increase her comfort and to remove any bloody discharge. Depending on agency protocol or on physician or CNM orders, perineal cleansing methods range from use of soapy water to aseptic technique. Once the cleansing is completed, the woman returns to the desired birthing position.

CONTINUED LABOR SUPPORT

Both the woman's partner and the nurse who has been with the woman during the labor continue to provide support during contractions. The woman is encouraged to push with each contraction and, as the fetal head emerges, is asked to take shallow breaths or to pant to prevent pushing. While supporting the head, the physician or certified nurse-midwife assesses whether the umbilical cord is around the fetal neck and removes it if it is, then suctions the mouth and nose with a bulb syringe. The mouth is suctioned first to prevent reflex inhalation of mucus when the nostrils are touched with the bulb syringe tip. The woman is encouraged to push again as the rest of the newborn's body is born. Figure 17–6 depicts a birthing experience.

NURSING MANAGEMENT DURING THE THIRD AND FOURTH STAGES OF LABOR

Initial Care of the Newborn

The CNM or physician places the newborn on the mother's abdomen or in the radiant-heated unit. The newborn is maintained in a modified Trendelenburg position. In this position, gravity aids drainage of mucus from the nasopharynx and trachea. Dry the newborn immediately. Help keep the infant warm by placing warmed blankets over the newborn or by placing the newborn in skin-to-skin contact with the mother. If the newborn is in a radiant-heated unit, he or she is dried, placed on a dry blanket, and left uncovered. Because radiant heat warms the outer surface of objects, a newborn wrapped in blankets will receive no benefit from the unit.

Suction the newborn's nose and mouth with a bulb syringe as needed. Most immediate care of the newborn can be done while the newborn is in the parent's arms or in the radiant-heated unit.

APGAR SCORING SYSTEM

The **Apgar scoring system** (Table 17–6) evaluates the physical condition of the newborn at birth. The newborn is rated 1 minute after birth and again at 5 minutes and receives a total score (Apgar score) ranging from 0 to 10 based on the following assessments:

1. *Heart rate* is auscultated or palpated at the junction of the umbilical cord and skin. This is the most important assessment. A newborn heart rate of less than 100 beats per minute indicates the need for immediate resuscitation.

2. *Respiratory effort* is the second most important Apgar assessment. Complete absence of respirations is termed *apnea*. A vigorous cry indicates adequate respirations.

3. *Muscle tone* is determined by evaluating the degree of flexion and resistance to straightening of the extremities. A normal newborn's elbows and hips are flexed, with the knees positioned up toward the abdomen.

4. *Reflex irritability* is evaluated by stroking the baby's back along the spine or by flicking the soles of the feet. A cry merits a full score of 2. A grimace is 1 point, and no response is 0.

5. *Skin color* is inspected for cyanosis and pallor. Generally, newborns have blue extremities, with a pink body, which merits a score of 1. This condition is termed *acrocyanosis* and is present in many normal newborns at 1 minute after birth. A totally pink newborn scores a 2, and a totally cyanotic, pale infant scores 0. Newborns with darker skin are not pink in color. Their skin color is assessed for pallor and acrocyanosis.

A score of 8 to 10 indicates a newborn in good condition who requires only nasopharyngeal suctioning and perhaps some oxygen near the face (called "blow-by" oxygen). If the Apgar score is below 8, resuscitative measures may be needed. (See the discussion in Chapter 25. 🔗)

CARE OF UMBILICAL CORD

If the clinician has not placed some type of cord clamp on the newborn's umbilical cord, the nurse does so. Before

TABLE 17-6   The Apgar Scoring System

Sign	Score		
	0	*1*	*2*
Heart rate	Absent	Slow—below 100	Above 100
Respiratory effort	Absent	Slow—irregular	Good crying
Muscle tone	Flaccid	Some flexion of extremities	Active motion
Reflex irritability	None	Grimace	Vigorous cry
Color	Pale blue	Body pink, blue extremities	Completely pink

Note: From Apgar V: The newborn (Apgar) scoring system, reflections and advice. (1968, August). *Pediatric Clinics of North America, 13,* 645.

applying the cord clamp, examine the cut end of the cord for the presence of two arteries and one vein. The umbilical vein is the largest vessel, and the arteries are seen as smaller vessels. Record the number of vessels on the birth and newborn records. The cord is clamped approximately 1/2 to 1 inch from the abdomen to allow room between the abdomen and clamp as the cord dries. Abdominal skin must not be clamped, because this will cause necrosis of the tissue. The most common type of cord clamp is the plastic Hollister cord clamp (Figure 17–7 ◆). The Hollister clamp is removed in the nursery about 24 hours after the cord has dried.

CORD BLOOD COLLECTION FOR BANKING

A growing number of parents are arranging for cord blood banking (see discussion in Chapter 1 🔗). Immediately after the newborn's umbilical cord is clamped and cut and the placenta is expelled, the CNM or physician withdraws blood from the remaining umbilical cord and the placenta. The blood is placed in a special container that parents receive from the Cord Blood Registry and bring with them for the birth. The parents should have any special directions that are required for storage and care of the container.

PHYSICAL ASSESSMENT OF THE NEWBORN

The nurse performs an abbreviated systematic physical assessment in the birthing area to detect any abnormalities (Table 17–7). First, note the size of the newborn and the contour and size of the head in relationship to the rest of the body. The newborn's posture and movements indicate tone and neurologic functioning.

Inspect the skin for discoloration, presence of vernix caseosa and lanugo, and signs of trauma and *desquamation* (peeling of skin). *Vernix caseosa* is a white, cheesy substance found normally on newborns. It is absorbed within 24 hours after birth. Vernix is abundant on preterm infants and absent on postterm newborns. Fine hair *(lanugo)* is often seen on preterm newborns on their shoulders, foreheads, backs, and cheeks. Desquamation is seen in postterm newborns.

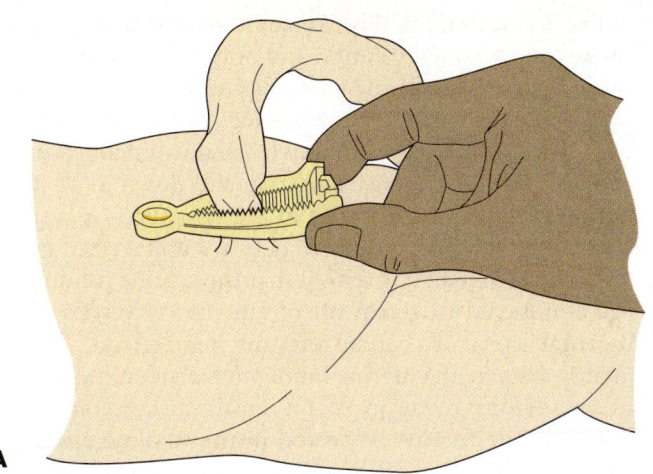

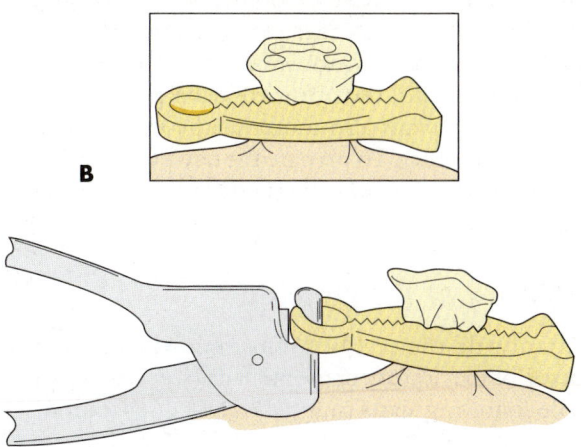

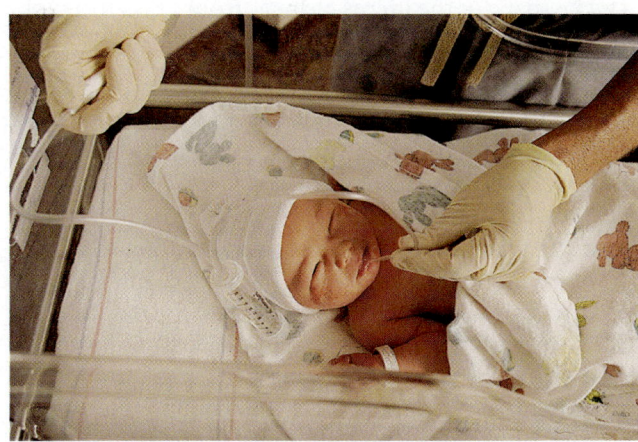

FIGURE 17–7. ◆ Hollister cord clamp. **A,** Clamp is positioned 1/2 to 1 inch from the abdomen and then secured. **B,** Cut cord. The one vein and two arteries can be seen. **C,** Plastic device for removing clamp after cord has dried. After the cord is cut, the nurse grasps the Hollister clamp on either side of the cut area and gently separates it.

TABLE 17–7	Initial Newborn Evaluation
Assess	*Normal Findings*
Respirations	Rate 36–60, irregular
	No retractions, no grunting
Apical pulse	Rate 120–160 and somewhat irregular
Temperature	Skin temp above 36.5 °C (97.8 °F)
Skin color	Body pink with bluish extremities
Umbilical cord	Two arteries and one vein
Gestational age	Should be 38–42 weeks to remain with parents for extended time
Sole creases	Sole creases that involve the heel

In general, expect scant amount of vernix on upper back, axilla, groin; lanugo only on upper back; ears with incurving of upper 2/3 of pinnae and thin cartilage that springs back from folding; male genitals—testes palpated in upper or lower scrotum; female genitals—labia majora larger, clitoris nearly covered

In the following situations, newborns should generally be stabilized rather than remaining with parents in the birth area for an extended period of time:

Apgar less than 8 at 1 minute and less than 9 at 5 minutes or baby requires resuscitation measures (other than whiffs of oxygen)

Respirations below 30 or above 60, with retractions and/or grunting

Apical pulse below 120 or above 160 with marked irregularities

Skin temperature below 36.5 °C (97.8 °F)

Skin color pale blue or circumoral pallor

Baby less than 38 or more than 42 weeks' gestation

Baby very small or very large for gestational age

Congenital anomalies involving open areas in the skin (meningomyelocele)

FIGURE 17–8. ◆ To clear secretions from the newborn's nose or oropharynx, a DeLee mucus trap (shown here) or other suction device is used. One end of the suction tubing is connected to low suction, the other end of the tubing is inserted 3 to 5 inches into the newborn's nose or mouth. Suction is applied as the tubing is pulled out. Repeat the process for as long as fluid is aspirated.

Observe the nares (nostrils) for flaring and, as the newborn cries, inspect the palate for cleft palate. Look for mucus in the nose and mouth; remove it with a bulb syringe as needed. Inspect the chest for respiratory rate and the presence of retractions. If retractions are present, assess the newborn for grunting or stridor. A normal respiratory rate is 30 to 60 per minute. Auscultate the lungs bilaterally for breath sounds. Absence of breath sounds on one side could mean pneumothorax. Rales may be heard immediately after birth because a small amount of fluid may remain in the lungs; this fluid will be absorbed. Rhonchi indicate aspiration of oral secretions. If there is excessive mucus or respiratory distress, suction the newborn with a mucus trap. (See Figure 17–8 ◆, as well as Skill 5–1 in the *Clinical Skills Manual* and the CD-ROM that accompanies this text.) ◻ CD SKILLS Note and record elimination of urine or meconium on the newborn record.

NEWBORN IDENTIFICATION

Place two ID bands on the newborn—one on the wrist and one on the ankle. The bands must fit snugly so they will not be lost. To ensure correct identification, while still in the birthing or delivery room give the mother and her partner each a band that matches that of the baby. The bands allow access to the infant care areas and should not be removed until the infant is discharged.

Many hospitals also footprint the newborn and fingerprint the mother. To prepare the newborn for footprinting, wipe the soles of both the newborn's feet to remove any vernix caseosa.

Delivery of the Placenta

After birth, the certified nurse-midwife or physician prepares for the delivery of the placenta (see Chapter 15). The following signs suggest placental separation:

1. The uterus rises upward in the abdomen.
2. As the placenta moves downward, the umbilical cord lengthens.
3. A sudden trickle or spurt of blood appears.
4. The shape of the uterus changes from a disk to a globe.

While waiting for these signs, palpate the uterus to check for ballooning caused by uterine relaxation and subsequent bleeding into the uterine cavity. After the placenta has separated, the woman may be asked to bear down to aid delivery of the placenta.

Oxytocics are frequently given at the time of the delivery of the placenta, so the uterus will contract and bleeding will be minimized. Oxytocin (Pitocin), 10 units, may be added to an intravenous (IV) infusion or given intramuscularly or by slow IV push. Some physicians order methylergonovine maleate (Methergine), 0.2 mg, administered intramuscularly, or carboprost tromethamine (Hemabate), 250 μg/mL, administered intramuscularly. In addition to administering the ordered medications, assess and record maternal blood pressure before and after administration of oxytocics. For further information, refer to "Drug Guide: Oxytocin" (in Chapter 20) and "Drug Guide: Methylergonovine Maleate" (in Chapter 28).

After the delivery of the placenta, the CNM or physician inspects the placental membranes to make sure they are intact and that all cotyledons are present. If there is a defect or a part missing from the placenta, a manual uterine examination is done. On the birth record, note the time of delivery of the placenta.

After the placenta is expelled, the physician or CNM inspects the vagina and cervix for lacerations and makes any necessary repairs. The episiotomy may be repaired now if it has not been done previously (see Chapter 20).

Special Assessments and Care of the New Mother

The period of 1 to 4 hours immediately following the expulsion of the placenta, during which the mother's condition stabilizes, is often referred to as the fourth stage of labor and birth. This is actually the initial recovery period.

The nurse washes the woman's perineum with gauze squares and warmed solution and dries the area well with a towel before placing the maternity pad. If stirrups have been used, remove the woman's legs from the stirrups at the same time to avoid muscle strain. Encourage the woman to move her legs gently up and down in a bicycle motion. The woman remains in the same bed or is transferred to a recovery room bed; help her don a clean gown.

After childbirth, it is critical that the uterine fundus stay well contracted to clamp off uterine blood vessels at the placental site and thereby prevent hemorrhage. Consequently, palpate the uterine fundus at frequent intervals for the first 4 hours to ensure that it remains firmly contracted. Normally the fundus is located in the midline and at or below the umbilicus. Palpate the fundus (Figure 17–9 ◆) but do not massage it unless it is soft (boggy). When a uterus becomes boggy, pooling of blood occurs within it, causing clots. Anything left in the uterus prevents it from contracting effectively. Thus, if it becomes boggy or appears to rise in the abdomen, massage the fundus until firm; then with one hand supporting the uterus at the symphysis pubis, use the other hand to exert steady pressure on the fundus to express retained clots. The uterus is very tender at this time so do all palpation and massage as gently as possible.

In some women the uterus becomes so relaxed that it cannot be found when palpation is attempted. In this case,

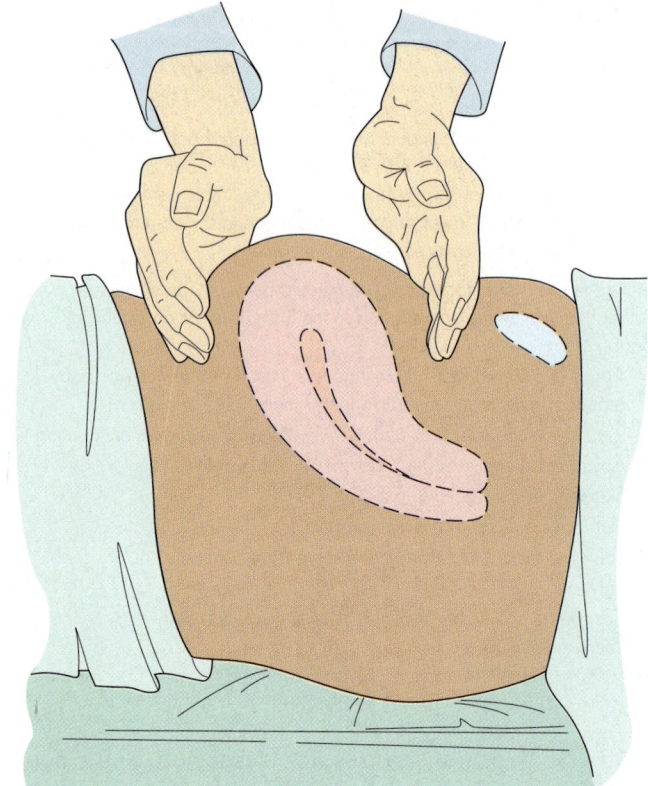

FIGURE 17–9. ◆ Suggested method of palpating the fundus of the uterus during the fourth stage. The left hand is placed just above the symphysis pubis, and gentle downward pressure is exerted. The right hand is cupped around the uterine fundus.

place one hand in the midline of the abdomen at about the level of the umbilicus and begin to make kneading motions. This motion generally stimulates the uterus to contract and it then feels like a firm, hard object.

During the recovery period it is essential to monitor maternal vital signs closely. Check the maternal blood pressure at 5- to 15-minute intervals to detect any changes. Blood pressure should return to the prelabor level due to an increased volume of blood returning to the maternal circulation from the uteroplacental shunt. Pulse rate should be slightly lower than it was during labor. Baroreceptors cause a vagal response, which slows the pulse. A rise in blood pressure may be a response to oxytocic drugs or may be caused by preeclampsia. A lowered blood pressure and a rising pulse rate may reflect blood loss (Table 17–8).

Also monitor the woman's temperature. Frequently women have tremors in the immediate postpartum period, possibly caused by a difference in internal and external body temperatures (higher temperature inside the body than outside). Another theory is that the woman is reacting to the fetal cells that have entered the maternal circulation at the placental site. A heated bath blanket placed next to the woman is helpful and can be replaced as often as the mother desires.

Inspect the bloody vaginal discharge for amount and chart it as minimal, moderate, or heavy and with or without clots. This discharge, lochia rubra, should be bright red. A soaked perineal pad contains approximately 100 mL of blood. If the perineal pad becomes soaked in a 15-minute period or if blood pools under the buttocks, continuous observation is necessary (see Skill 4–2 in the *Clinical Skills Manual*, as well as in the CD-ROM that accompanies this text). ⊂⊃ [CD] [SKILLS] When the fundus is firm, a continuous trickle of blood may signal

laceration of the vagina or cervix or an unligated vessel in the episiotomy.

If the fundus rises and displaces to the right, it is important to consider two factors:

1. As the uterus rises, the uterine contractions become less effective and increased bleeding may occur.

2. The most common cause of uterine displacement is bladder distention.

Palpate the bladder to determine whether it is distended. The bladder fills rapidly with the extra fluid volume returned from the uteroplacental circulation (and with any fluid received intravenously during labor and birth). The postpartal woman may not realize that her bladder is full because trauma to the bladder and urethra during childbirth and the use of regional anesthesia decrease bladder tone and the urge to void.

Use a variety of measures to help the mother to void. Place a warm towel across the lower abdomen or pour warm water over the perineum to relax the urinary sphincter and facilitate voiding. If the woman is unable to void, catheterization is necessary.

The perineum is inspected for edema and hematoma formation. An ice pack often reduces the swelling and alleviates the discomfort of an episiotomy.

The couple may be tired, hungry, and thirsty. Some agencies serve the couple a meal. The tired mother will probably drift off into a welcome sleep. The partner can also be encouraged to rest, since the supporting role is physically and mentally tiring. If the mother is not in a birthing room, she is usually transferred from the birthing unit to the postpartal or mother-baby area after 2 hours or more, depending on agency policy and whether the following criteria are met:

- Stable vital signs
- No bleeding
- Undistended bladder
- Firm fundus
- Sensations fully recovered from any anesthetic agent received during birth

Enhancing Attachment

Dramatic evidence indicates that the first few hours and even minutes after birth are an important period for the attachment of mother and infant. If this period of contact can occur during the first hour after birth, the newborn will be in the quiet state and able to interact with parents by looking at them. Newborns also turn their heads in response to a spoken voice. (See Chapter 21 for further discussion of newborn states.) ⊂⊃

The first parent-newborn contact may be brief (a few minutes), to be followed by a more extended contact after uncomfortable procedures (delivery of the placenta and

TABLE 17–8 Maternal Adaptations Following Birth	
Characteristic	*Normal Finding*
Blood pressure	Returns to prelabor level
Pulse	Slightly lower than in labor
Uterine fundus	In the midline at the umbilicus or one to two finger breadths below the umbilicus
Lochia	Red (rubra), small to moderate amount (from spotting on pads to 1/4–1/2 of pad covered in 15 minutes)
	Does not exceed saturation of one pad in first hour
Bladder	Nonpalpable
Perineum	Smooth, pink, without bruising or edema
Emotional state	Wide variation, including excited, exhilarated, smiling, crying, fatigued, verbal, quiet, pensive, and sleepy

suturing of the episiotomy) are completed. When the newborn is returned to the mother, help her begin breastfeeding if she so desires. The baby may seek out the mother's breast, and early contact between the two can greatly affect breastfeeding success. Even if the newborn does not actively nurse, he or she can lick, taste, and smell the mother's skin. This activity by the newborn stimulates the maternal release of prolactin, which promotes the onset of lactation.

Darkening the birthing room by turning out most of the lights causes newborns to open their eyes and gaze around. This in turn enhances eye-to-eye contact with the parents. (Note: If the physician or CNM needs a light source, the spotlight can be left on.) Treatment of the newborn's eyes may also be delayed. Many parents who establish eye contact with the newborn are content to quietly gaze at their infant. Others may show more active involvement by touching or inspecting the newborn. Some mothers talk to their babies in a high-pitched voice, which seems to be soothing to newborns. Some couples verbally express amazement and pride when they see they have produced a beautiful, healthy baby. Their verbalization enhances feelings of accomplishment and ecstasy. Figure 17–10 ◆ shows a new parent establishing bonds with his newborn son.

Both parents need to be encouraged to do whatever they feel most comfortable doing. Some parents prefer only limited contact with the newborn immediately after birth and instead want private time together in a quiet en-vironment. In spite of the current zeal for providing immediate attachment opportunities, nursing personnel need to be aware of parents' wishes. The desire to delay interaction with the newborn does not necessarily imply a decreased ability of the parents to bond with their newborn. (See Chapter 26 for further discussion of parent-newborn attachment.) ⬭

NURSING MANAGEMENT DURING NURSE-ATTENDED BIRTH

Occasionally labor progresses so rapidly that the maternity nurse is faced with the task of assisting in the actual birth of the baby. This is called a **precipitous birth.** The attending maternity nurse has the primary responsibility for providing a physically and psychologically safe experience for the woman and her baby. A woman whose certified nurse-midwife or physician is not present may feel disappointed, frightened, abandoned, angry, and cheated. She may fear what is going to happen and feel that everything is out of her control. In working with the woman, the nurse provides support by keeping her informed about the labor progress and assuring her that the nurse will stay with her.

If birth is imminent, the nurse must not leave the mother alone. The nurse can direct auxiliary personnel to contact the CNM or physician and retrieve the emergency birth pack ("precip pack"). An emergency birth pack should be readily accessible to birthing rooms. A typical pack contains the following items:

1. A small drape that can be placed under the woman's buttocks to provide a sterile field
2. A bulb syringe to clear mucus from the newborn's mouth
3. Two sterile clamps (Kelly or Rochester) to clamp the umbilical cord before applying a cord clamp
4. Sterile scissors to cut the umbilical cord
5. A sterile umbilical cord clamp, either Hesseltine or Hollister
6. A baby blanket to wrap the newborn in after birth
7. A package of sterile gloves

As the materials are being gathered, the nurse must remain calm; the woman is reassured by the composure of the nurse and feels that the nurse is competent. At all times during the birth, the nurse provides suggestions such as when to maintain a controlled breathing pattern and when to push, supports the woman's efforts, and provides reassurance.

The nurse assists in the precipitous birth as follows: The woman is encouraged to assume a comfortable position. If time permits, the nurse scrubs his or her hands with soap and water and puts on sterile gloves. Sterile drapes are

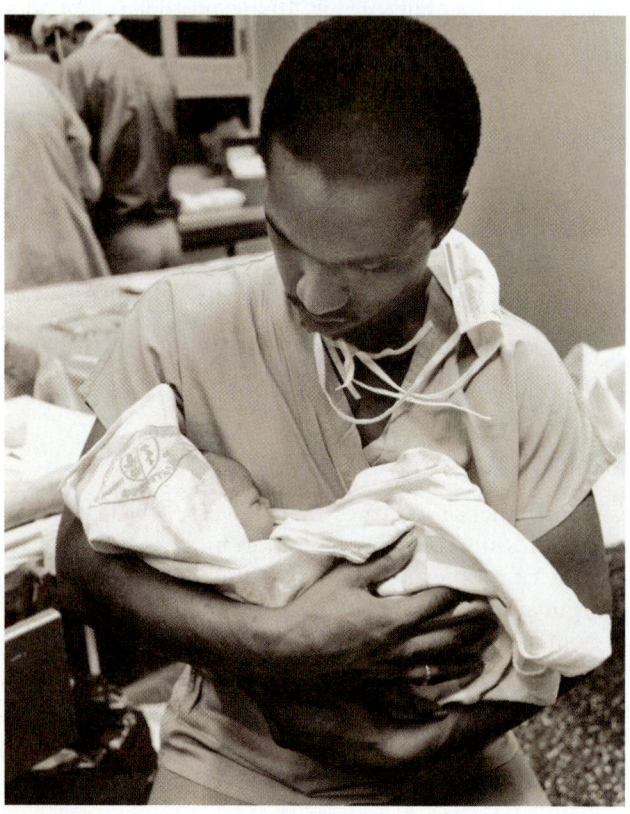

FIGURE 17–10. ◆ A father holds his newborn.

placed under the woman's buttocks. The nurse may place an index finger inside the lower portion of the vagina and the thumb on the outer portion of the perineum and gently massage the area to help stretch perineal tissues and prevent perineal lacerations. This procedure is called "ironing the perineum."

When the infant's head crowns, the nurse instructs the woman to pant, which decreases her urge to push. The nurse checks whether the amniotic sac is intact. If it is, the nurse tears the sac so the newborn will not breathe in amniotic fluid with the first breath.

With one hand, the nurse applies gentle pressure against the fetal head to prevent it from popping out rapidly. The nurse does not hold the head back forcibly. Rapid birth of the head may result in tears in the woman's perineal tissues. In the fetus, the rapid change in pressure within the fetal head may cause subdural or dural tears. The nurse supports the perineum with the other hand and allows the head to be born between contractions.

As the woman continues to pant, the nurse inserts one or two fingers along the back of the fetal head to check for the umbilical cord. If there is a nuchal cord (umbilical cord around the neck), the nurse bends his or her fingers like a fish hook, grasps the cord, and pulls it over the baby's head. It is important to check that the cord is not wrapped around the neck more than one time. If the cord is tightly looped and cannot be slipped over the baby's head, two clamps are placed on the cord, the cord is cut between the clamps, and the cord is unwound.

Immediately after birth of the head, the nurse suctions the baby's mouth, throat, and nasal passages. The nurse then places one hand on each side of the head and exerts gentle downward traction until the anterior shoulder passes under the symphysis pubis. Then gentle upward traction aids the birth of the posterior shoulder. The nurse then instructs the woman to push gently so that the rest of the body can be born quickly. The newborn must be supported as he or she emerges.

The newborn is held at the level of the uterus to facilitate blood flow through the umbilical cord. The combination of amniotic fluid and vernix makes the newborn very slippery, so the nurse must be careful to avoid dropping the baby. The nose and mouth of the newborn are suctioned again, using a bulb syringe. The nurse then dries the newborn to prevent heat loss.

As soon as the nurse determines that the newborn's respirations are adequate, the infant can be placed on the mother's abdomen. The newborn's head should be slightly lower than the body to aid drainage of fluid and mucus. The weight of the newborn on the mother's abdomen stimulates uterine contractions, which aid in placental separation. The umbilical cord should not be pulled.

The nurse is alert for signs of placental separation (slight gush of dark blood from the vagina, lengthening of the cord, or a change in uterine shape from discoid to globular). When these signs are present, the nurse tells the mother to push so that the placenta can be delivered. The nurse inspects the placenta to determine whether it is intact.

The nurse checks the firmness of the uterus. The fundus may be gently massaged to stimulate contractions and decrease bleeding. Putting the newborn to breast also stimulates uterine contractions through release of oxytocin from the pituitary gland.

The umbilical cord may now be cut. The nurse places two sterile Kelly clamps approximately 1 to 3 inches from the newborn's abdomen. The cord is cut between the Kelly clamps with sterile scissors. The nurse places a sterile umbilical cord clamp adjacent to the clamp on the newborn's cord, between the clamp and the newborn's abdomen. The clamp must not be placed snugly against the abdomen, because the cord will dry and shrink.

The nurse cleanses the area under the mother's buttocks and inspects her perineum for lacerations. Bleeding from lacerations may be controlled by pressing a clean perineal pad against the perineum and instructing the woman to keep her thighs together.

If the CNM or physician's arrival is delayed or if the newborn is having respiratory distress, the newborn should be transported immediately to the nursery. The newborn must be properly identified before he or she leaves the birth area. The nurse notes and places on a birth record the following information:

1. Position of fetus at birth
2. Presence of cord around neck or shoulder (nuchal cord)
3. Time of birth
4. Apgar scores at 1 and 5 minutes after birth
5. Gender of newborn
6. Time of expulsion of placenta
7. Method of placental expulsion
8. Appearance and intactness of placenta
9. Mother's condition
10. Any medications given to mother or newborn (per agency protocol)

EVALUATION

Evaluation determines the effectiveness of nursing care. As a result of comprehensive nursing care during the intrapartal period, the following outcomes may be anticipated:

- The mother's physical and psychologic well-being has been maintained and supported.
- The baby's physical and psychologic well-being has been protected and supported.
- The couple have had input into the birth process and have participated as much as they desired.
- The mother and her baby have had a safe birth.

CHAPTER HIGHLIGHTS

☞ During labor, before procedures are begun, it is important to explain what will be done, the reasons, potential benefits and risks, and possible alternatives. These explanations help the woman determine what happens to her body.

☞ Behavioral responses to labor vary with the phase of labor, the preparation the woman has had, and her previous experience, cultural beliefs, and developmental level.

☞ The childbearing family may have a variety of expectations of the nurse during labor and birth. Some families want to make all decisions themselves with limited nursing contact, others want a moderate amount of contact and see the relationship as a cooperative venture, and some families want a lot of involvement and look to the nurse to instill confidence in them that everything will be all right.

☞ Each woman's cultural beliefs affect her needs for privacy, expression of discomfort, and expectations for the birth and the role she wishes the father to play in the birth event.

☞ The adolescent mother has special needs in the birth setting. Her developmental needs require specialized nursing care.

☞ The laboring woman's comfort may be increased by general comfort measures, supportive relaxation techniques, methods of handling anxiety, controlled breathing, and support by a caring person.

☞ Maternal birthing positions include a wide variety of possibilities, from side-lying to sitting, squatting, and semi-Fowler's.

☞ Immediate assessments of the newborn include evaluation of the Apgar score and an abbreviated physical assessment. These early assessments help determine the need for resuscitation and whether the newborn's adaptation to extrauterine life is progressing normally. The newborn who is not experiencing problems may remain with the parents for an extended period after birth.

☞ Immediate care of the newborn also includes maintenance of respirations, promotion of warmth, prevention of infection, and accurate identification.

☞ The placenta separates from the uterine wall and is expelled with either the maternal or fetal side emerging from the vagina. The maternal side contains the cotyledons and appears rough in texture; this presentation may be associated with retention of placental fragments.

☞ The fourth stage includes the first 1 to 4 hours following birth. Many physiologic and psychologic changes occur during this period.

☞ At times a baby is born rapidly without the physician or CNM present. This event is referred to as a precipitous birth. The nurse in the birthing area remains with the woman and attends her during the birth until a CNM or physician can be present.

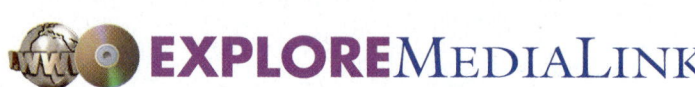 **EXPLORE**MediaLink

NCLEX Review, Case Studies, and other interactive resources for this chapter can be found on the companion website at http://www.prenhall.com/london. Click on "Chapter 17" to select the activities for this chapter.

For animations, more NCLEX review questions, and an audio glossary, access the accompanying CD-ROM in this textbook.

REFERENCES

American Academy of Pediatrics & American College of Obstetricians and Gynecologists. (1997). *Guidelines for perinatal care* (4th ed.). Washington, DC: Author.

Association of Women's Health, Obstetric, and Neonatal Nurses. (1998). *Standards for professional nursing practice in the care of women and newborns* (5th ed). Washington, DC: Author.

Association of Women's Health, Obstetric, and Neonatal Nurses. (1999). Guidelines for fetal monitoring. In L. K. Mandeville & N. H. Troiano (Eds.), *High-risk & critical care intrapartum nursing*. Philadelphia: Lippincott.

Bottorff, J. (1993). The use and meaning of touch caring for patients with cancer. *Oncology Nursing Forum, 20,* 531–538.

Calhoun, M. A. (1986). The Vietnamese woman: Health/illness attitudes and behaviors. In P. N. Stearn (Ed.), *Women, health, and culture*. Washington, DC: Hemisphere.

Drake, P. (1996). Addressing developmental needs of pregnant adolescents. *Journal of Obstetric, Gynecologic, and Neonatal Nursing, 25,* 518.

Eckert, K., Turnbull, D., & MacLennan, A. (2001). Immersion in water in the first stage of labor: A randomized clinical trial. *Birth, 28*(2), 84–93.

England, P., & Horowitz, R. (1998). *Birthing from within*. Albuquerque, NM: Partera Press.

Guyette, L. *Laboring in water*. Denver: University of Colorado Health Sciences Center. (1995, November). In P. Perez, *Pushing through the 90s: Changing times, changing roles*. Conference proceedings. Green Bay, WI: St. Vincent Hospital.

Hodnett, E. (1996). Nursing support of the laboring woman. *Journal of Obstetric, Gynecologic, and Neonatal Nursing, 25,* 257.

Hutchinson, M. K., & Baqi-Aziz, M. (1994). Nursing care of the childbearing Muslim family. *Journal of Obstetric, Gynecologic, and Neonatal Nursing, 23*(9), 767.

Khazoyan, C. M., & Anderson, N. L. R. (1994). Latinas' expectations for their partners during childbirth. *Maternal-Child Nursing Journal, 19,* 226.

Lauderdale, J. (1999). Childbearing and transcultural nursing care issues. In M. M. Andrews & J. S. Boyle (Eds.), *Transcultural concepts in nursing care* (3rd ed., pp. 81–106). Philadelphia: Lippincott.

Lipson, J. G., Dibble, S. L., & Minarik, P. A. (1996). *Culture and nursing care: A pocket guide*. San Francisco: University of California at San Francisco Nursing Press.

Perez, P. (1995, November). *Pushing through the 90s: Changing times, changing roles*. Conference proceedings. Green Bay, WI: St. Vincent Hospital.

Scott-Ramos, I. (1996). Culturally sensitive care giving for the Latino woman. *Journal of Obstetric, Gynecologic, and Neonatal Nursing, 25,* 67.

Snyder, M., & Nojima, Y. (1998). Purposeful touch. In M. Snyder & R. Lindquist, *Complementary/alternative therapies in nursing* (3rd ed., pp. 149–158). New York: Springer Publishing.

Stern, D. N., & Bruschweiler-Stern, N. (1998). *The birth of a mother*. New York: Basic Books.

Teschendorf, M. E., & Evans, C. P. (2000). Hydrotherapy during labor: An example of developing a practice policy. *American Journal of Maternal-Child Nursing, 25*(4), 198–203.

Varney, H. (1997). *Varney's midwifery* (3rd ed.). Sudbury, MA: Jones & Bartlett.

Waymire, V. (1997). A triggering time: Childbirth may recall sexual abuse memories. *Association of Women's Health, Obstetric, and Neonatal Nursing–Lifelines, 23,* 47–50.

Wesson, N. (2000). *Labor pain: A natural approach to easing delivery*. Rochester, NY: Healing Arts Press.

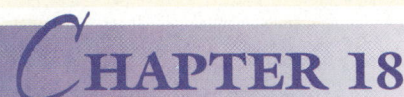

CHAPTER 18

Pain Relief Therapies During Birth

We had attended our classes and practiced through the last few weeks, but I was not ready for the amount of discomfort that I felt during my labor. I've always been able to handle pain much better, but this pain was very different. I had hoped to go through all of labor and birth without medications, but we had talked about it and I knew that if I felt I needed something, it would be all right. My nurse was also helpful and supportive of my decision. She helped me feel that I was making a good decision and that I wasn't failing somehow.

—KYUNG-AIE, 36

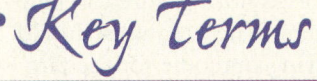

Key Terms

Epidural block   *386*

General anesthesia   *391*

Local anesthesia   *390*

Pudendal block   *390*

Regional analgesia   *384*

Regional anesthesia   *384*

Spinal block   *389*

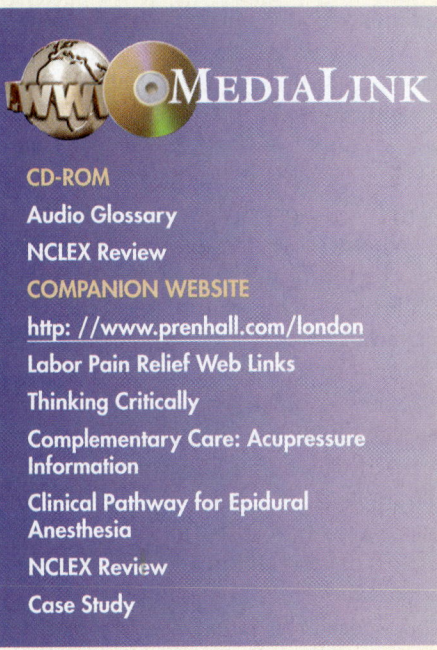

MediaLink

CD-ROM

Audio Glossary

NCLEX Review

COMPANION WEBSITE

http://www.prenhall.com/london

Labor Pain Relief Web Links

Thinking Critically

Complementary Care: Acupressure Information

Clinical Pathway for Epidural Anesthesia

NCLEX Review

Case Study

Like Kyung-aie, the childbearing woman experiences many demanding sensations and discomforts during labor and birth. What comfort measures can the nurse provide to help her have a positive childbirth experience? Nursing interventions directed toward pain relief begin with non-pharmacologic measures such as providing information, support, and physical comfort. The perinatal nurse should develop experience in a variety of pain management strategies. Measures to promote comfort include back rubs, hydrotherapy (bath, shower), the application of cool cloths to her forehead, and encouragement. Some laboring women need no further interventions. For other women, the progression of labor brings increasing discomfort that interferes with their ability to perform breathing techniques and maintain a sense of comfort. Pharmacologic agents such as systemic drugs, epidural analgesics, intrathecal narcotics, and regional nerve blocks may be used to decrease discomfort, increase relaxation, and reestablish the woman's sense of balance and control. The methods are not all mutually exclusive, and any of them may be used in combination with other comfort measures. See Chapter 17 for application of comfort measures during the various stages of labor and birth.

Developing Cultural Competence

A woman's cultural background may influence her responses to pain. Following are generalizations of how some cultures perceive pain and pain responses:

- Mexican-American women may moan rhythmically and massage their thighs and abdomen when in pain.
- Haitian women may prefer massage, movement, and position changes to increase comfort.
- Filipino women may lie quietly because they believe that noise and activity increase labor pain.
- Black, Puerto Rican, and Middle Eastern women are often verbally expressive of pain.
- Native-American women may be viewed as stoic, using meditation, self-control, and traditional herbs.
- Thailand women's silent but restless behavior can reflect high levels of pain.
- Japanese, Chinese, Vietnamese, Laotian, and other women of Asian descent may feel that crying out during labor is shameful.
- Samoan women may believe no verbal response is allowed.

CULTURAL INFLUENCES ON EXPRESSION OF CHILDBIRTH PAIN

Labor is painful for most women; only a few experience a natural painless birth. However, how each woman copes with the pain depends on factors which might include cultural attitudes toward normalcy and conduct of birth, perceptions of childbirth pain, expectations of how a woman should act in labor (pain behaviors), the degree and quality of social support, and the physiologic processes involved (Lauderdale, 1999; Squire, 2000; York, Bhuttarowas, & Brown, 1999).

Although systemic analgesics and regional local anesthetic blocks may affect the fetus, so does the pain and stress experienced by the laboring woman. During labor, maternal respirations and oxygen consumption increase, which decreases the amount of oxygen available to the fetus. In addition, the pain and stress can lead to metabolic acidosis and the release of catecholamine, which causes maternal blood vessels to constrict, lessening oxygen and nutrient supply to the fetus (Creehan, 2000).

Many couples who have had childbirth education approach childbirth confident that the techniques they have learned will enable them to cope with the discomforts of labor. There is a good deal of peer pressure on expectant parents to have the "ideal" birth experience. They may plan a natural childbirth, and the need for analgesia may make them feel inadequate and guilty. The nurse has a very special role in helping a woman and her partner to accept alterations in their original plan and to recognize the

unique qualities of their birth experience. Reassurance that accepting analgesia for discomfort is not a failure can help maintain the woman's self-esteem. The emphasis should be on achieving a healthy, satisfying outcome for the family. Ultimately, it is essential to listen and honor the request of the laboring woman about the effectiveness of non-pharmacologic techniques during her labor. There will always be laboring women who need or desire pharmacologic agents. In the absence of any medical contraindications, a woman's request is sufficient medical justification for providing pharmacologic pain relief during labor (American College of Obstetricians and Gynecologists [ACOG] 2000).

PHARMACOLOGIC ANALGESIA

The goal of pharmacologic analgesia during labor is to provide maximum pain relief at minimum risk for the mother and fetus. To reach this goal, clinicians must consider a number of factors, including the following:

- All systemic drugs used for pain relief during labor cross the placental barrier by simple diffusion, but some drugs cross more readily than others.
- Drug action in the body depends on the rate at which the substance is metabolized by liver enzymes and excreted by the kidneys.
- High drug doses may remain in the fetus for long periods because fetal liver enzymes and kidney excretion are inadequate for metabolizing analgesic agents.

Nursing Management

Analgesic drugs provide pain relief for the laboring woman but also affect the fetus and the labor process. Analgesia given too early may prolong labor and depress the fetus; if given too late it is of minimal use to the woman and may cause neonatal respiratory depression. Assess the mother and fetus and evaluate the contraction pattern before administering prescribed systemic medications.

Maternal assessment parameters include:

- The woman is willing to receive medication after being advised about it.
- Vital signs are stable.

Fetal assessment parameters include:

- The fetal heart rate (FHR) baseline is between 120 and 160 beats per minute, and no late decelerations or nonreassuring FHR patterns are present.
- Short-term variability is present, and long-term variability is average.
- The fetus exhibits normal movement, and accelerations are present with fetal movement.
- The fetus is at term.

Assessment of labor includes:

- Contraction pattern is well established.
- The cervix is dilated at least 4 to 5 cm in nulliparas and 3 to 4 cm in multiparas.
- The fetal presenting part is engaged.
- There is progressive descent of the fetal presenting part. No complications that would preclude administrating an analgesic agent are present.

If normal parameters are absent, further assessments in collaboration with the physician/certified nurse-midwife may be needed.

Before administering the medication, once again ascertain whether the woman has a history of any drug reactions or allergies and provide information about the medication (see Table 18–1). After giving the medication, record the drug name, dose, route, and site, and the woman's blood pressure and pulse, on the FHR monitor strip and on the woman's records. If the woman is alone, raise side rails to provide safety. Assess the FHR for possible adverse effects of the medication.

When an analgesic medication is administered by intramuscular (IM) or subcutaneous route, it takes a few minutes for the effect to be felt. Continue with other supportive measures to enhance comfort, such as ensuring a quiet environment, providing a back rub or cool cloth, assisting with relaxation and visualization exercises, or providing therapeutic touch until the woman feels the effect of the medication. When the medication begins to take effect, the woman may sleep between contractions. This short period of rest helps her relax and can restore her energy. When an intravenous (IV) route is ordered by the certified nurse-midwife/physician, the effect of the drug will be felt within a few minutes, so if any change of position is necessary or if the woman needs to void, suggest that these activities be completed before the drug administration. Some women may be so uncomfortable that they do not want anything except the medication. In this case, administering the medication first would be more helpful for the woman.

Narcotic Analgesic: Butorphanol Tartrate (Stadol)

Butorphanol tartrate (Stadol) is a synthetic parenteral analgesic agent that can be given by the IM or IV route. Its onset of action is rapid after IV injection, peak analgesia occurs in 30 to 60 minutes, and the duration is from 3 to 4 hours (Wilson, Shannon, & Strang, 2001). The recommended initial dose is 2 mg administered IM every 3 to 4 hours. If it is given IV, the dosage is reduced. Respiratory depression of both the mother and fetus or neonate can occur. The effects of butorphanol can be reversed with naloxone (Narcan). Butorphanol should not be used for women with a known opiate dependency and should be used with caution if drug dependence is suspected because it may precipitate withdrawal (Wilson et al., 2001).

Urinary retention following administration of butorphanol is not common but does occur. Therefore, be alert

---

TABLE 18–1 What Women Need to Know about Pain Relief Medications

Before receiving medications, the woman should understand the following:

- Type of medication administered
- Route of administration
- Expected effects of medication
- Implications for fetus or neonate
- Safety measures needed (e.g., remain in bed with side rails up)

Complementary Care

ACUPRESSURE FOR LABOR PAIN

The acupressure point for labor and delivery is found in the webbing between the thumb and index finger. This point should never be stimulated during pregnancy since it stimulates uterine contractions. The mother places her right thumb on the back of her left hand and her right index finger on the front of the left hand at the acupressure point. She can rub the point to stimulate labor and squeeze the point to decrease labor pain. Another acupressure point is found between the inner anklebone and the Achilles' tendon. Squeezing for 1 minute on each ankle reduces labor pain. See our companion website for more information on acupressure, including an interview with a labor and delivery nurse on her use of acupressure to relieve labor pain. [WEB]

for bladder distention when a woman has received butor-phanol for analgesia during labor, has IV fluids infusing, and receives regional anesthesia for the birth. Butorphanol needs to be protected from light and stored at room temperature (Wilson et al., 2001).

Opiate Antagonist: Naloxone (Narcan)

Since naloxone is an antagonist with little or no agonistic effect, it exhibits little pharmacologic activity in the absence of narcotics. Naloxone can be used to reverse the mild respiratory depression that follows administration of small doses of opiates. The drug is useful for respiratory depression caused by fentanyl, morphine, and meperidine, as well as butorphanol and nalbuphine hydrochloride. Naloxone is the drug of choice when the depressant is unknown because it will cause no further depression (Wilson et al., 2001). An initial dose of 0.4 to 2 mg may be administered IV to the laboring woman. Naloxone may be given to the newborn if needed after birth. (See "Drug Guide: Naloxone Hydrochloride: Narcan" 🔗 in Chapter 29.)

Thinking Critically

COUNSELING THE WOMAN ON USE OF ANALGESIA

Luisa Silva, a 33-year-old G1 P O, is 32 weeks' pregnant. She is trying to decide whether she should accept any analgesia during her labor. She has finished childbirth education classes and wants an unmedicated labor and birth. She says, "I want to do this on my own, but I'm afraid it may be too much. Will it be OK if I need to take something?" What will you tell her? 🔗 **WEB**

REGIONAL ANESTHESIA AND ANALGESIA

Regional anesthesia is the temporary loss of sensation produced by injecting an anesthetic agent (called a local) into direct contact with nervous tissue. Loss of sensation happens because the local agents stabilize the cell membrane, which prevents initiation and transmission of nerve impulses. The regional anesthetic blocks most commonly used in childbirth include the epidural, spinal, and combined epidural-spinal blocks. Epidural blocks may be used for analgesia during labor and vaginal birth and for anesthesia during cesarean birth.

An epidural relieves pain associated with the first stage of labor by blocking the sensory nerves supplying the uterus. Pain associated with the second stage of labor and with birth can be alleviated with epidural, combined epidural-spinal, and pudendal blocks (see Figure 18–1 ◆).

Until fairly recently, the same anesthetic agents used for regional epidurals were also used to produce **regional anal-**

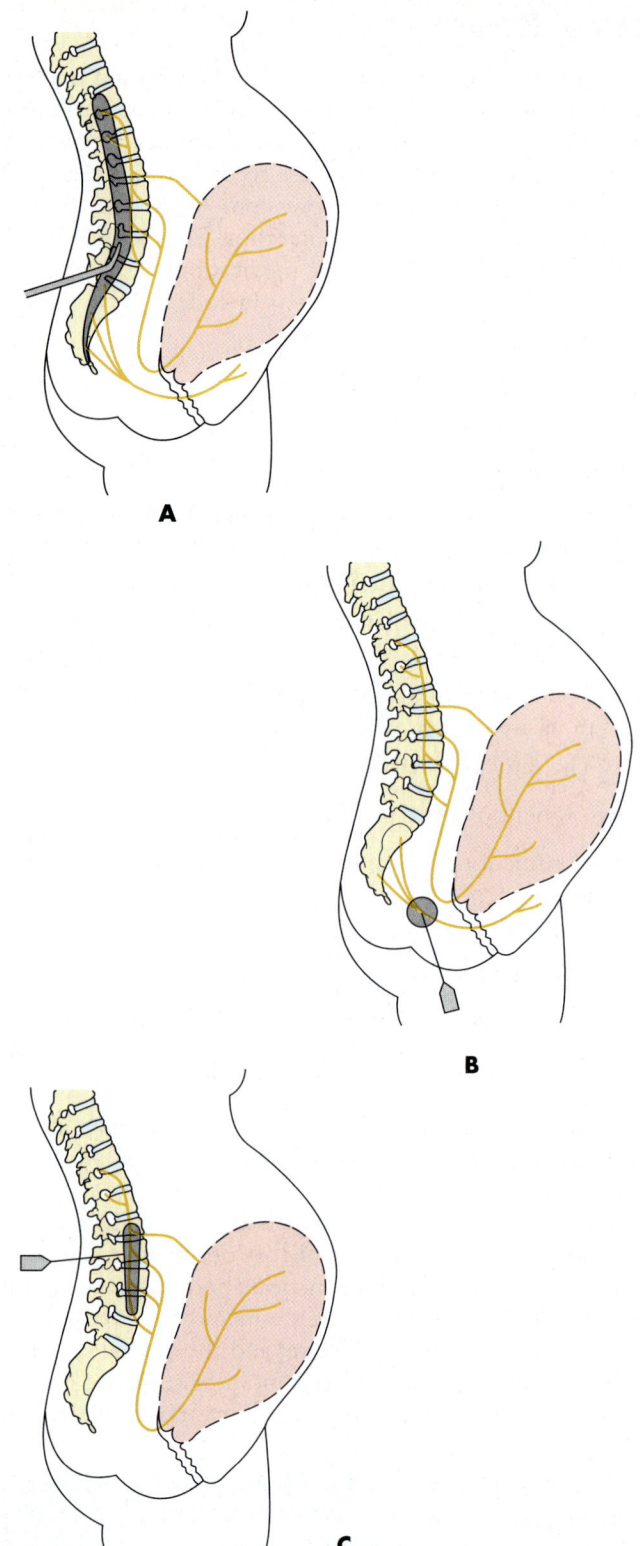

FIGURE 18–1. ◆ Schematic diagram showing pain pathways and sites of interruption. **A,** Lumbar epidural block: the dark area demonstrates peridural (epidural) space and nerves affected, and the gray tube represents a continuous plastic catheter. **B,** Pudendal block: relief of perineal pain. **C,** Lumbar sympathetic (spinal) block: relief of uterine pain only. *Note:* From Bonica, J. J. (1972). *Principles and practice of obstetric analgesia and anesthesia* (pp. 492, 512, 521, 614). Philadelphia: Davis.

gesia (pain relief) during labor. This practice was problematic because the anesthetic agents used alter the transmission of impulses to the bladder, making voiding difficult. The agents also interfere with blood pressure stability and leg movement. In addition, the descent of the fetus may be slowed because of the woman's decreased ability to push during the second stage of labor (Wong, 2001). To address these difficulties, regional analgesia is now obtained by injecting a narcotic such as fentanyl along with only a small amount of local anesthetic agent. This approach relieves the woman's pain while minimizing side effects.

The intrathecal injection of narcotics results in another type of regional analgesia. In this case, the narcotic is injected into the subarachnoid space. Fentanyl citrate and preservative-free morphine are the most commonly used drugs. The woman's pain is usually relieved, but she may experience urinary retention, pruritus, nausea, and vomiting (Karch, 2001; Wong, 2001).

Nursing care during administration of regional analgesia is directed toward helping the woman void prior to the injection, assisting her with positioning during and after the procedure, monitoring and assessing vital signs and respiratory status, monitoring analgesic effect, and determining fetal well-being. Additional measures may be needed to address pruritus, nausea and vomiting, and urinary retention.

As with other procedures, the woman needs to know how the block is given, the expected effect on her and the fetus, advantages and disadvantages, and possible complications (Creehan, 2000). Many women discuss possible anesthetic blocks with their care provider at some point in the pregnancy. If they have not, it is important to give them an opportunity to ask questions and obtain information before receiving the block while in labor.

Anesthetic Agents for Regional Blocks

Local anesthetic agents block the conduction of nerve impulses from the periphery to the central nervous system by preventing the propagation of an action potential from the source of pain (Wong, 2001). The types of nerve fibers are differentially sensitive to the various anesthetic agents. In general, the smaller the fiber, the more sensitive it is to local agents. For example, it is possible to block the small C and A delta fibers, which transmit pain and temperature, without blocking the larger A alpha, A beta, and A gamma fibers, which continue to maintain a sense of pressure, muscle tone, position sense, and motor function.

Absorption of local anesthetics depends primarily on the vascularity of the area of injection. The agents themselves contribute to increased blood flow by causing vasodilation. High concentrations of drugs cause greater vasodilation. Good maternal physical condition or a high metabolic rate aids absorption. Malnutrition, dehydration, electrolyte imbalance, and cardiovascular and pulmonary problems increase the potential for toxic effects. The pH of tissues affects the rate of absorption, which has implications for fetal complications such as acidosis. The addition of vaso-

constrictors such as epinephrine delays absorption and prolongs the anesthetic effect. Epinephrine decreases uteroplacental blood flow, making it an undesirable additive in many situations. The breakdown of local anesthetics in the body is accomplished by the liver and plasma esterase, and the resulting substance is eliminated by the kidneys. It is important to use the weakest concentration and the smallest amount necessary to produce the desired results.

Types of Local Anesthetic Agents

Three types of local anesthetic agents are currently available: esters, amides, and opiates. The ester type includes procaine hydrochloride (Novocain), chloroprocaine hydrochloride (Nesacaine), and tetracaine hydrochloride (Pontocaine). Esters are rapidly metabolized; therefore, toxic maternal levels are not as likely to be reached, and placental transfer to the fetus is prevented. Amide types include lidocaine hydrochloride (Xylocaine), mepivacaine hydrochloride (Carbocaine), and bupivacaine hydrochloride (Marcaine). Amide types are more powerful and longer acting agents. They readily cross the placenta, can be measured in the fetal circulation, and affect the fetus for a prolonged period.

Opioids are used with epidural blocks for labor. Some of the agents used include morphine, fentanyl, butorphanol, and meperidine (Faucher & Brucker, 2000). When only opioids are used epidurally, rather than in combination with another type of agent, the amount of pain relief is not as effective, especially toward the end of labor; therefore, a combination of opioids and a low dose of local are given (Wong, 2001).

Adverse Maternal Reactions to Anesthetic Agents

Reactions to local anesthetic agents range from mild symptoms to cardiovascular collapse. Mild reactions include palpitations, tinnitus, apprehension, confusion, and a metallic taste in the mouth. Moderate reactions include more severe degrees of mild symptoms plus nausea and vomiting, hypotension, and muscle twitching, which may progress to convulsions. Severe reactions are sudden loss of consciousness, coma, severe hypotension, bradycardia, respiratory depression, and cardiac arrest. Anesthetic agents should not be used unless an IV line is in place.

The preferred treatment for a mild toxic reaction is administration of oxygen and IV injection of a short-acting barbiturate to diminish anxiety.

Neonatal Neurobehavioral Effects of Anesthesia and Analgesia

Many studies have focused on the neurobehavioral effects on the newborn of pharmacologic agents used during labor and birth. Although analgesic and anesthetic agents may alter the behavioral and adaptive function of the newborn, physiologic factors such as hunger, degree of

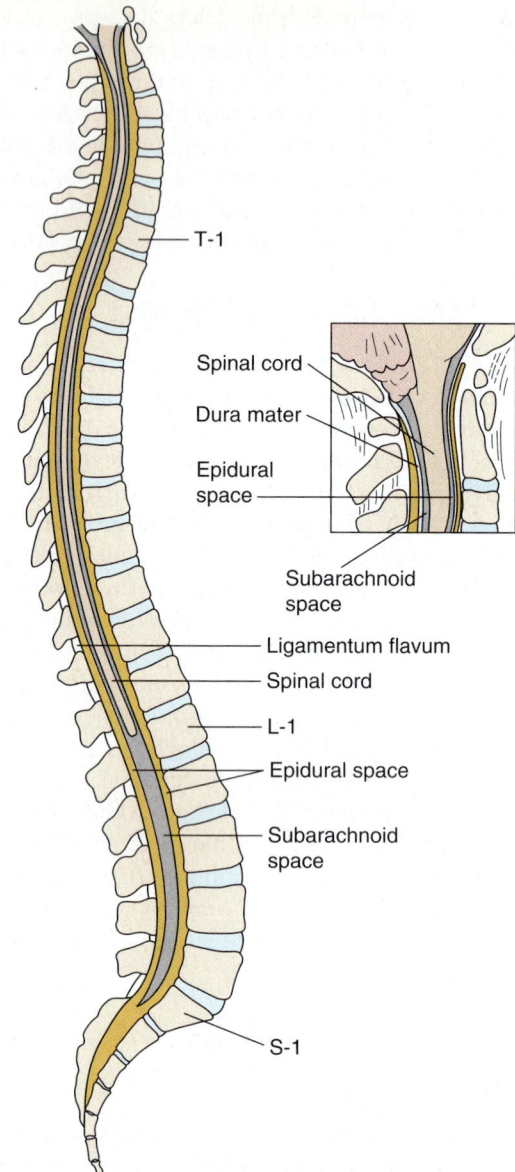

FIGURE 18–2. ◆ The epidural space is between the dura mater and the ligamentum flavum, extending from the base of the skull to the end of the sacral canal.

hydration, and time within the sleep-wake cycle may also exert an influence.

Epidural Block

A lumbar **epidural block** involves injection of an anesthetic agent into the epidural space to provide pain relief throughout labor. The epidural space, a potential space between the dura mater and the ligamentum flavum, is accessed through the lumbar area (Figure 18–2 ◆). The epidural is most frequently used as a continuous block to provide analgesia and anesthesia from active labor through episiotomy repair (Figure 18–3 ◆).

Epidurals have become a relatively common method of analgesia and anesthesia during labor and birth in the

United States. An epidural can be given as soon as active labor is established (Holt, Diehl, & Wright, 1999). Insurance providers have limited some women's access to epidural anesthesia; however, ACOG (2000) believes that a woman's request is sufficient justification for providing an epidural.

ADVANTAGES

The epidural block relieves discomfort during labor and birth, and the woman is fully awake and a part of the birth process. The continuous epidural allows different blocking for each stage of labor, so that the fetus is able to descend and rotate in the maternal pelvis; many times the woman's urge to bear down is preserved.

DISADVANTAGES

The most common complication of an epidural block is maternal hypotension, which is generally prevented by IV fluid administration, left uterine displacement, and maternal positioning on her side. In some instances, labor progress and fetal descent may be slowed, pushing efforts in the second stage may be less effective, and the use of forceps or a vacuum extractor is more common (Main, Main, & Moore, 2000). Delay in return of bladder sensation may result in the need for catheterization during labor and in the fourth stage.

CONTRAINDICATIONS

The absolute contraindications for epidural block are client refusal, infection at the site of the needle puncture, maternal problems with blood coagulation (coagulopathies), specific drug allergy to the agent being used, and hypovolemic shock (Wong, 2001).

NURSING MANAGEMENT

Assessment of the woman's knowledge level about an epidural block is essential. Before providing information, determine the woman's current knowledge and evaluate factors related to learning, such as primary language spoken, ability to hear and interpret information, and the presence of anxiety. If the woman is not able to understand because of a language barrier or inability to hear, locate and provide an interpreter. Although the nurse is an integral person in providing information, the anesthesiologist is the essential person to provide information to obtain written informed consent.

In preparation for the epidural, encourage the woman to empty her bladder, because the block may interfere with her ability to void. Assess maternal blood pressure, pulse, and respirations and FHR to determine that normal parameters are present and to establish a baseline. Continuous electronic fetal monitoring to assess fetal status and frequent monitoring of maternal blood pressure and pulse for hypotension are essential. An IV infusion is usually begun with an 18-gauge plastic indwelling catheter. A large-gauge catheter is used so that IV fluids can be administered quickly if hypotension occurs. A bolus of 500 to 1,000 mL of IV fluid (lactated Ringer's or normal saline) over 15 to 30 min-

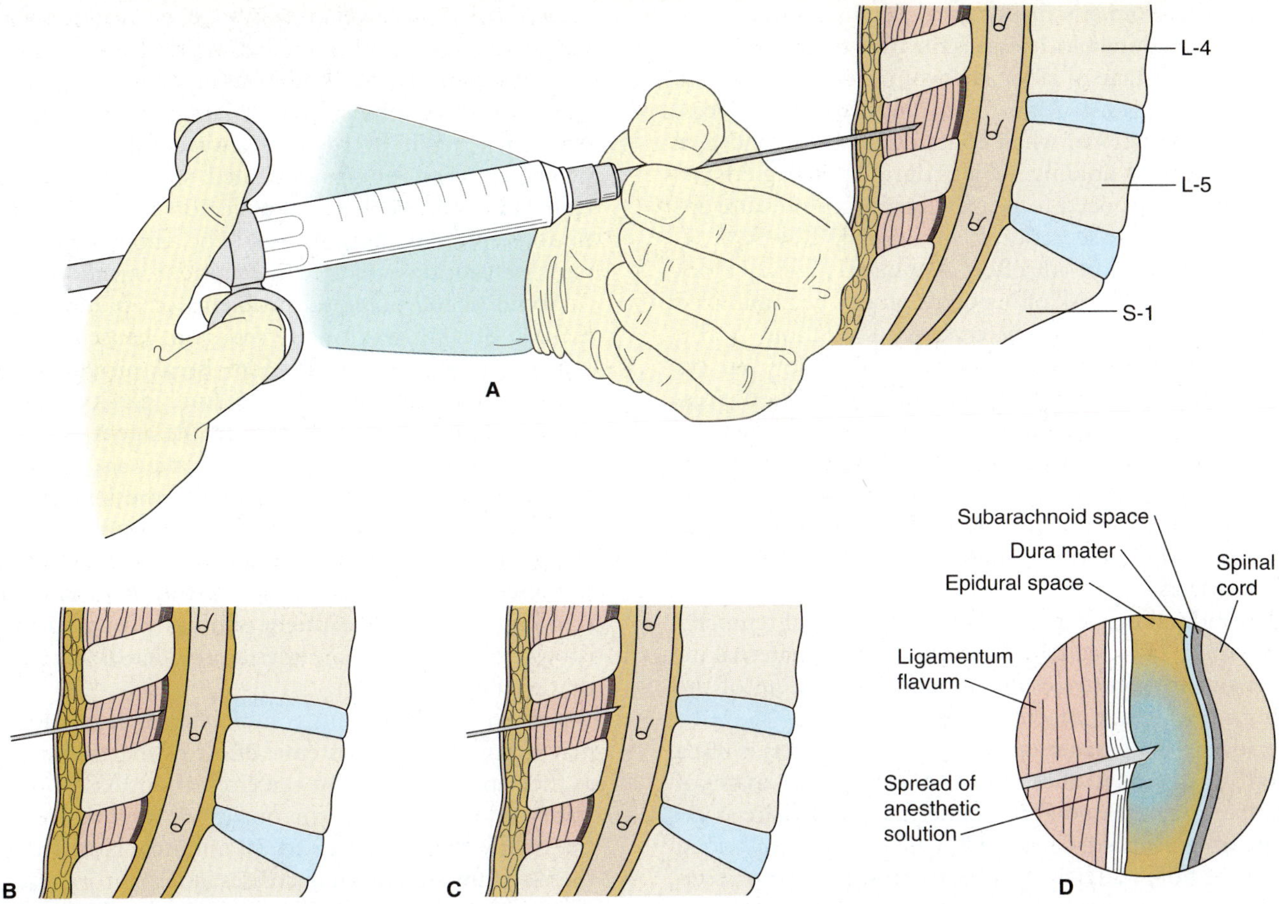

FIGURE 18-3. ◆ Technique for lumbar epidural block. **A,** Proper position of insertion. **B,** Needle in the ligamentum flavum. **C,** Tip of needle in epidural space. **D,** Force of injection pushing dura away from tip of needle. *Note: From Bonica, J. J. (1972). Principles and practice of obstetric analgesia and anesthesia (p. 631). Philadelphia: Davis.*

utes is given before beginning the epidural block. IV fluids with dextrose are avoided because they can cause increased fetal insulin production and hypoglycemia after birth.

Help the woman into a side-lying position at the edge of the bed, where the mattress is firmer and provides more support. Support the woman's head with a small pillow so it remains in alignment with the spine. A pillow may also be placed in front of her chest to provide support for her upper arm. Her back needs to remain straight, with the shoulders square. Her legs are bent and her knees kept together so that the upper hip does not roll forward and cause the spine to twist. Proper positioning is essential to avoid severe spinal flexion because it can decrease the epidural space and increase the possibility of puncturing the dura. The block may also be given with the woman in a sitting position, with her back arched and her feet supported on a stool. After positioning, continue to provide support and try to ensure that the woman does not move during the procedure. After the block is administered, assess maternal vital signs frequently per protocol until the block wears off. The blood pressure can be monitored by a mechanical blood pressure device or by the nurse directly. The vital signs are recorded on the fetal monitor strip and/or on the client record. Encourage the woman to

maintain a side-lying position (preferably left lateral tilt) to maximize uteroplacental blood flow; change her position (from side to side) frequently to increase circulation, promote comfort, and avoid a one-sided block. Assess the woman's ability to lift her legs and her level of sensation every 30 minutes to monitor the effects of the nerve block.

Nursing Practice

An important assessment following the administration of regional blocks, such as the epidural, is the location and degree of lost sensation. Landmarks (called dermatomes) can be used to measure and document where these sensory levels begin and end. Some useful tips include the following:

- ▶ Use dermatome level charts.
- ▶ Use a cool alcohol prep pad to check for areas and levels of sensation.
- ▶ Assess dermatome levels approximately every 30 minutes.
- ▶ Evaluate the level of anesthesia. The anesthesia level is too high if the patient reports numbness in her chest, face, or tongue or any difficulty breathing. Be alert for statements such as "I feel like I can't take a full breath" or "My tongue feels funny."

Assess the woman's bladder for distention frequently because the epidural block lessens the urge to urinate. During the second stage of labor, the woman with an epidural block may need assistance with pushing. It may be necessary to tell the woman when contractions begin and give extra assistance by holding her legs during pushing efforts. The woman's legs need to be protected from pressure applied to them while sensation is diminished.

The most common side effect of epidural regional block is hypotension. The risk of hypotension can be minimized by a preload fluid bolus of crystalloid solution (Yerby, 2000). If hypotension occurs, increase the IV flow rate (to increase intravascular volume and raise the blood pressure), ensure or verify left uterine displacement (to increase circulation), and administer oxygen (to improve oxygenation). If blood pressure is not restored in 1 to 2 minutes, administer ephedrine, 3 to 6 mg IV, per physician order (Creehan, 2000). Also continuously assess FHR to monitor fetal effects.

The epidural may cause elevation of maternal temperature (pyrexia). Pyrexia may be confused with maternal infection and frequently results in additional testing of the newborn to rule out infection (Yerby, 2000).

Headache (which may occur with spinal blocks) is not a side effect of epidural anesthesia because the dura mater of the spinal canal has not been penetrated and there is no leakage of spinal fluid. Therefore, lying flat for a prescribed number of hours after birth is not necessary. Motor control of the legs is weak but not totally absent after birth. Return of complete sensation and the ability to control the legs are essential before ambulation is attempted. Recovery may take several hours, depending on the anesthetic agent and the dose given.

To assess sensation, touch various parts of the woman's legs and abdomen bilaterally to determine if the touch can be felt. Evaluate motor control by asking the woman to raise her knees, to lift her feet (one at a time) off the bed, or to dorsiflex her foot. Even though assessments may indicate that sensation and motor control have returned, be ready to support the woman's weight as she stands and quickly return her to bed if motor control is inadequate. In addition, blood pressure assessments help determine the safety of ambulation. Assess blood pressure while the woman is lying down, then sitting in the bed. As long as blood pressure values remain stable (no evidence of orthostatic hypotension), assess a standing blood pressure. It is advisable to have additional assistance when the woman stands for the first time, to maintain safety. See the companion website for "Clinical Pathway for Epidural Anesthesia." ⊂▭⊃ WEB

Continuous Epidural Infusion

Epidural anesthesia may be given with a continuous infusion pump. Some of the benefits include good to excellent analgesia, infrequent nausea, minimal sedation, decreased anxiety, earlier mobilization, retained cough reflex, de-creased risk of deep vein thrombosis, decreased myocardial oxygen demand, and ease of administration.

Obviously, ease of administration does not imply lack of need for close observation. Malfunctioning equipment with subsequent overdose is always a possibility. Fortunately, infusion pumps designed specifically for use in epidural anesthesia have safety factors incorporated. Continuous epidural infusions should be administered with the same precautions used for intermittent injections.

Some of the potential problems of epidural infusions include breakthrough pain, sedation, nausea and vomiting, pruritus, and hypotension. Breakthrough pain may occur at any time during the epidural infusion but usually occurs when the infusion rate of the agent is below the recommended therapeutic rate. It may also occur when the infusion pump rate is altered or the integrity of the epidural line is broken. When breakthrough pain occurs, check the integrity of the epidural infusion line and notify the anesthesiologist or nurse anesthetist. There may be standing orders for treatment of breakthrough pain, but it is best to inform the anesthesia provider of any problems that occur.

General sedation and resulting respiratory depression may occur from the systemic effect of the epidural agents as they are absorbed into the circulation. Assess the respiratory rate, along with the quality of respirations, no less frequently than every 15 to 30 minutes. Notify the anesthetist of any significant decreases in respiratory rate or respiratory pattern change. If respiratory rate decreases below 19 respirations per minute, naloxone may be given to counteract the effect of the anesthetic agent; typically respirations then return to a normal rate.

Nausea and vomiting can occur at any time during or after epidural infusion. Give an antiemetic if one is ordered and notify the anesthesiologist. The nausea and vomiting can make the woman very uncomfortable, and the infusion rate of the epidural may need to be decreased or terminated to alleviate this discomfort.

Pruritus (itching and rash) may occur at any time during the epidural infusion. It usually appears first on the face, neck, or torso and is usually the result of the agent in the epidural infusion. Pruritus is most often seen with the administration of epidural morphine (Creehan, 2000). Treatment generally involves administration of diphenhydramine hydrochloride (Benadryl). If no standing order exists, notify the anesthetist and identify the problem. The epidural infusion may need to be decreased or terminated.

Hypotension may occur from hypovolemia or from the effect of the epidural. Treatment involves administering oxygen by mask, administering a bolus of crystalloid fluid, and notifying the anesthetist. Usually standing orders for treatment of hypotension are graded in terms of the degree of hypotension. The epidural infusion may have to be terminated and the woman placed in the Trendelenburg position. See "Clinical Pathway for Epidural Anesthesia" on our companion website for further nursing assessment and interventions. ⊂▭⊃ WEB

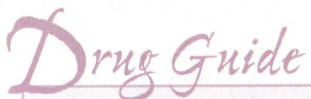

Drug Guide

POSTBIRTH EPIDURAL MORPHINE

Overview of Action

Epidural morphine is used to provide relief of pain associated with cesarean birth, extensive episiotomies (mediolaterals), or third- and fourth-degree lacerations. Epidural morphine pain relief results directly from its effect on the opiate receptors in the spinal cord (it depresses pain impulse transmission). Morphine binds opiate receptors, thereby altering both the perception of and the emotional response to pain. Women experience little or no discomfort or pain during recovery and for up to 24 hours afterward. There is no motor or sympathetic block or associated hypotension. Onset of analgesia is slower, but duration is longer.

Dosage, Route

Five to 10 mg of morphine is injected through a catheter into the epidural space, providing relief for about 24 hours (Wilson et al., 2001).

Maternal Contraindications

Hypersensitivity to opiates

Narcotic addiction

Chronic debilitating respiratory disease

Reduced blood volume

Maternal Side Effects

Late-onset respiratory depression (rare but may occur 8 to 12 hours after administration)

Nausea and vomiting (occurring between 4 and 7 hours after injection)

Itching (begins within 3 hours and lasts up to 10 hours)

Urinary retention

Somnolence (rarely)

Side effects can be managed with naloxone.

Effect on Fetus or Neonate

No adverse effects since medication is injected after birth of baby

Nursing Considerations

Assess client's sensitivity to narcotics on admission.

Monitor and evaluate analgesic effect. Ask client about comfort level and notify anesthesiologist of inadequate pain relief.

If present, check epidural catheter for obvious knots, breaks, and leakage at insertion site and catheter hub.

Assess for pruritus (scratching and rubbing, especially around the face and neck).

Administer comfort measures for narcotic-induced pruritus, such as lotion, back rubs, cool or warm packs, or diversional activities. If the itching can be tolerated, naloxone should be avoided, especially because it counteracts the pain relief.

If allergic reaction (urticaria, edema, or respiratory difficulties) occurs, administer naloxone or diphenhydramine per physician order.

Provide comfort measures for nausea or vomiting, such as frequent oral hygiene or gradual increase in activity; administration of naloxone, trimethobenzamide, or metoclopramide HCl per physician order.

Assess postural blood pressure and heart rate before ambulation.

Assist the woman with her first ambulation and then as needed.

Assess respiratory function frequently for the first 24 hours, then every 2 to 8 hours as needed. Also assess level of consciousness and mucous membrane color. May need to monitor client via apnea monitor for 24 hours and use continuous pulse oximetry.

Monitor urinary output and assess bladder for distention. Assist client to void.

Epidural Narcotic Analgesia after Birth

To provide analgesia for approximately 24 hours after the birth, the anesthesiologist may inject an opioid, such as morphine sulfate (Duramorph), into the epidural space immediately after the birth. The analgesic effect begins approximately 30 to 60 minutes after the injection. The side effects include pruritus, nausea and vomiting, and urinary retention. The onset seems to occur early, and it resolves within 14 to 16 hours after the birth. (See "Drug Guide: Postbirth Epidural Morphine.")

Spinal Block

In a **spinal block,** a local anesthetic agent is injected directly into the spinal fluid in the spinal canal to provide anesthesia for cesarean birth and occasionally for vaginal birth. The technique of administration varies depending on whether the spinal block is being given for a cesarean or vaginal birth.

ADVANTAGES

The advantages of spinal block are immediate onset of anesthesia, relative ease of administration, a need for smaller drug volume, and maternal compartmentalization of the drug.

DISADVANTAGES

The primary disadvantage of spinal block is blockade of sympathetic nerve fibers, resulting in a high incidence of hypotension; maternal hypotension may lead to fetal hypoxia. In addition, uterine tone is maintained, which makes intrauterine manipulation difficult. The level of spinal block is less predictable in laboring women.

CONTRAINDICATIONS

Contraindications for spinal block include severe hypovolemia, regardless of the cause; central nervous system disease; infection over the puncture site; allergy to local anesthetic agents; coagulation problems; and client refusal (Creehan, 2000).

NURSING MANAGEMENT

If an IV infusion is not already in place, it is started with a 16- to 18-gauge plastic catheter, and a bolus of 500 to 1,000 mL is infused rapidly. Assess maternal vital signs and the FHR to establish a baseline and then position the woman in a sitting position (or a side-lying position). The woman sits on the side of the bed or operating room table and places her feet on a stool. The woman places her arms between her knees or up around the nurse's shoulders, bows her head, and arches her back to widen the intervertebral spaces. Support the woman in this position and palpate the uterus to identify the beginning of uterine contractions (if labor is present). The physician injects the anesthetic agent between contractions. If the anesthetic agent is injected during a contraction, the level of anesthesia obtained is higher and may compromise respirations.

The woman remains in a sitting position for 30 seconds and then returns to a lying position, with a rolled towel or blanket under her right hip to displace the uterus from the vena cava. Monitor maternal blood pressure and pulse frequently per protocol or physician's order. Also reassess the blood pressure when the woman is moved after birth, because movement may lower blood pressure.

If the spinal block is being used during vaginal birth, monitor uterine contractions and instruct the woman to bear down during a contraction. The block usually reduces the woman's ability to push, and the birth may be assisted with forceps or vacuum extractor (see Chapter 20).

After birth, the temporary motor paralysis of the woman's legs continues. Use caution when moving the woman from the birthing bed (or operating room table) to protect her from injury. The woman remains flat in bed for 6 to 12 hours following the block; she may not regain sensation and control of her bladder for 8 to 12 hours and may need to be catheterized. An indwelling bladder catheter is usually inserted before surgery for women undergoing cesarean birth.

Combined Spinal-Epidural Block

Spinal anesthesia may be combined with an epidural block. The combined spinal-epidural (CSE) block can be used for labor analgesia and for cesarean birth. The anesthetic and analgesic agents used differ according to the purpose of the CSE block. A CSE is accomplished by inserting an epidural needle into the epidural space. A narrow-gauge atraumatic (24- to 27-gauge pencil point) needle is inserted through the epidural needle, through the dura, and into the cerebral spinal fluid. A small amount of local anesthetic agent, opioid, or both is injected, and the atraumatic needle is withdrawn. An epidural catheter is then threaded through the epidural needle and into the epidural space. The epidural needle is removed, and the epidural catheter is secured.

An advantage of CSE block is that the spinal (intrathecal) anesthetic and/or analgesic agent has a faster onset than medications that are injected into the epidural space. Most drugs are used in low dose, so spinal analgesia may be given in early labor to assist in alleviating labor pain

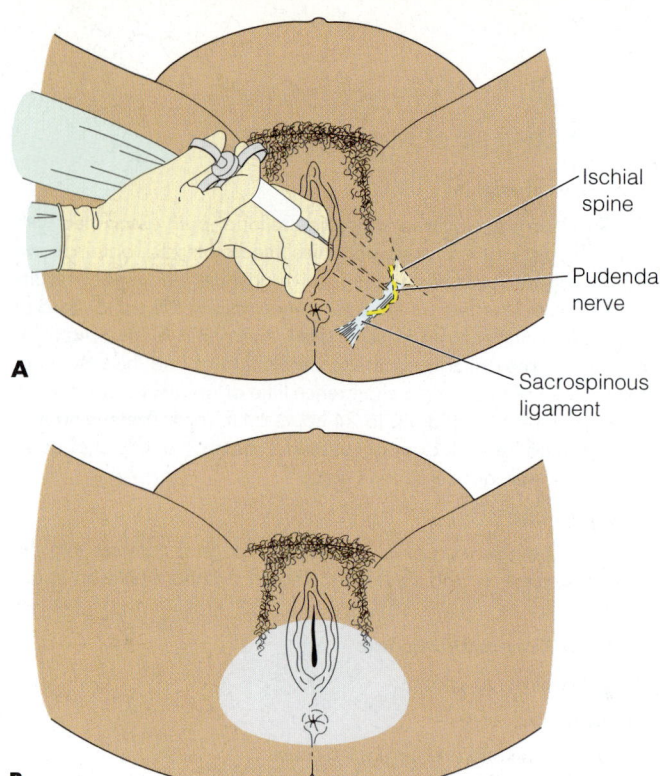

FIGURE 18-4. ◆ **A,** Pudendal block by the transvaginal approach. **B,** Area of perineum affected by pudendal block.

without motor block. The epidural is activated when active labor begins (Wong, 2001).

Pudendal Block

A **pudendal block,** administered by a transvaginal method, intercepts signals to the pudendal nerve. The pudendal block provides perineal anesthesia for the latter part of the first stage of labor, the second stage, birth, and episiotomy repair. The pudendal block relieves the pain of perineal distention but not the discomfort of uterine contractions (Figure 18-4 ◆).

Advantages of the pudendal block are ease of administration and absence of maternal hypotension. It also may be used to decrease the discomfort of low forceps or vacuum-assisted birth. Because a pudendal block does not alter maternal vital signs or FHR, additional assessments are not necessary. Explain the procedure and answer any questions.

The disadvantages of the pudendal block include possible broad ligament hematoma, perforation of the rectum, and trauma to the sciatic nerve. A moderate dose of anesthetic agent has minimal ill effects on the course of labor, but the urge to push may decrease.

Local Infiltration Anesthesia

Local anesthesia is accomplished by injecting an anesthetic agent into the intracutaneous, subcutaneous, and intramuscular areas of the perineum (Figure 18-5 ◆). It is

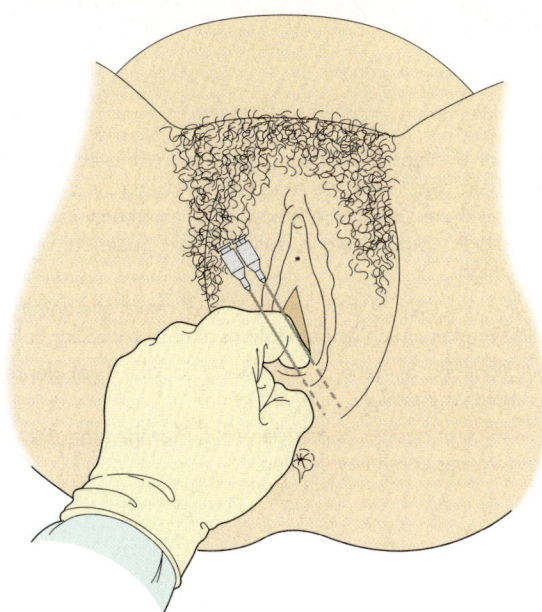

FIGURE 18–5. ◆ Technique of local infiltration for episiotomy and repair. *Note:* From Bonica, J. J. (1972). *Principles and practice of obstetric analgesia and anesthesia* (p. 505). Philadelphia: Davis.

generally used at the time of birth, both in preparation for an episiotomy if one is needed and for the episiotomy repair. Women who have followed some type of prepared childbirth method and want minimal analgesia and anesthesia usually do not object to local anesthesia for the episiotomy. The administration procedure is technically uncomplicated and is practically free from complications.

A disadvantage of local infiltration is that large amounts of local anesthetic must be used to infuse the tissues. Although any local anesthetic may be used, chloroprocaine hydrochloride (Nesacaine), lidocaine hydrochloride (Xylocaine), and mepivacaine hydrochloride (Carbocaine) are the agents of choice because of their capacity for diffusion. Because local anesthetic agents have no effect on maternal vital signs or FHR, additional assessments are unnecessary.

GENERAL ANESTHESIA

Occasionally, **general anesthesia** (induced unconsciousness) may be needed for cesarean birth and for surgical intervention with some complications. The method used to achieve general anesthesia is usually a combination of IV injection and inhalation of anesthetic agents.

Complications of General Anesthesia

A primary danger of general anesthesia is fetal depression. Most general anesthetic agents reach the fetus in about 2 minutes. The depression in the fetus is directly proportional to the depth and duration of the anesthesia. The poor fetal metabolism of general anesthetic agents is similar to that of analgesic agents administered during labor. General anesthesia is not advocated when the fetus is considered to be at high risk, particularly in preterm birth.

The majority of general anesthetic agents cause some degree of uterine relaxation. They may also cause vomiting and aspiration. Since pregnancy results in decreased gastric motility, and the onset of labor halts the process almost entirely, food eaten hours earlier may remain undigested in the stomach. Find out when the laboring woman last ate and record this information on the client's chart and on her anesthesia record. Even when food and fluids have been withheld, the gastric juice produced during fasting is highly acidic and can cause chemical pneumonitis if aspirated.

Nursing Care During General Anesthesia

Prophylactic antacid therapy to reduce the acidic content of the stomach before general anesthesia is common practice. A nonparticulate antacid (such as Bicitra) is often used. Cimetidine (Tagamet) has also been suggested by some anesthesiologists.

Before induction of anesthesia, place a wedge under the woman's right hip to displace the uterus and prevent vena caval compression in the supine position. The woman should also be preoxygenated with 3 to 5 minutes of 100% oxygen. Start IV fluids so that access to the intravascular system is immediately available.

During the process of rapid induction of anesthesia, apply cricoid pressure to occlude the esophagus and prevent possible aspiration; the esophagus is occluded by depressing the cricoid cartilage 2 to 3 cm posteriorly. Maintain cricoid pressure until the anesthesiologist has placed the endotracheal tube and indicates that the pressure can be released. Figure 18–6 ◆ shows the appropriate technique.

It should be noted that this discussion of obstetric analgesia and anesthesia applies only to a healthy woman and fetus. Pain relief during labor and birth for women with high-risk conditions, such as preterm labor, pregnancy-induced hypertension, diabetes mellitus, or bleeding complications, requires skilled decision making, close observation, and awareness of all the potential threats to both the woman and her baby.

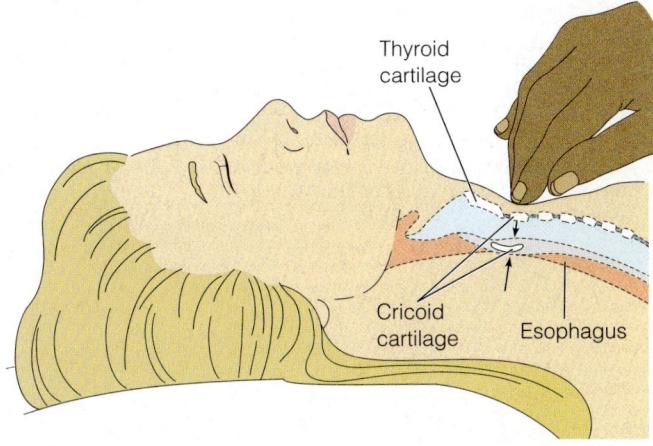

FIGURE 18–6. ◆ Proper position for fingers in applying cricoid pressure until a cuffed endotracheal tube is placed by the anesthesiologist or nurse anesthetist. The cricoid cartilage is depressed 2 to 3 cm posteriorly so that the esophagus is occluded.

CHAPTER HIGHLIGHTS

≋ Pain relief during labor may be enhanced by childbirth preparation methods and by the administration of analgesics and/or regional anesthesia blocks.

≋ The goal of pharmacologic pain relief during labor is to provide maximum pain relief with minimal risk for the mother and fetus.

≋ The best time for administering analgesia is determined after a complete assessment. An analgesic agent is generally administered to nulliparas when the cervix has dilated 4 to 5 cm and to multiparas when the cervix has dilated 3 to 4 cm.

≋ Analgesic agents include a variety of drugs, such as butorphanol tartrate (Stadol) and nalbuphine hydrochloride (Nubain).

≋ Narcotic antagonists (such as naloxone) counteract the respiratory depressant effect of the opiate narcotics by acting at specific receptor sites in the central nervous system.

≋ Regional analgesia and anesthesia are achieved by injecting local anesthetic agents into an area that will bring the agent into direct contact with nerve tissue. Methods most commonly used in childbearing include epidural block, spinal block, pudendal block, and local infiltration.

≋ Adverse reactions of the woman to local anesthetic agents range from mild symptoms such as palpitations to cardiovascular collapse.

≋ Complications of general anesthesia include fetal depression, uterine relaxation, vomiting, and aspiration.

≋ The choice of analgesia and anesthesia for the high-risk woman and fetus requires careful evaluation.

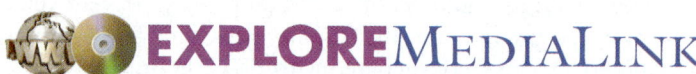

EXPLORE MediaLink

NCLEX Review, Case Studies, and other interactive resources for this chapter can be found on the companion website at http://www.prenhall.com/london. Click on "Chapter 18" to select the activities for this chapter.

For animations, more NCLEX review questions, and an audio glossary, access the accompanying CD-ROM in this textbook.

REFERENCES

American College of Obstetricians and Gynecologists. (2000). *Pain relief during labor* (Committee Opinion No. 231). Washington, DC: Author.

Cook, A., & Wilcox, G. (1997). Pressuring pain. Alternative therapies for labor pain management. *AWHONN Lifelines, 1*(2), 36–41.

Creehan, P. A. (2000). Pain relief and comfort measures during labor. In K. R. Simpson & P. A. Creehan (Eds.), *AWHONN perinatal nursing* (chap. 11, pp. 417–444). Philadelphia: Lippincott, Williams & Wilkins.

Faucher, M. A., & Brucker, M. C. (2000). Intrapartum pain: Pharmacologic management. *Journal of Obstetric, Gynecologic, and Neonatal Nursing, 29*(2), 169–180.

Holt, R. O., Diehl, S. J., & Wright, J. (1999). Station and cervical dilation at epidural placement in predicting cesarean risk. *Obstetrics and Gynecology, 93,* 281–284.

Karch, A. M. (2001). *Lippincott's nursing drug guide*. Philadelphia: Lippincott Williams & Wilkins.

Lauderdale, J. (1999). Childbearing and transcultural nursing care issues. In M. M. Andrews & J. S. Boyle (Eds.), *Transcultural concepts in nursing care* (3rd ed.). Philadelphia: Lippincott.

Main, D. M., Main, E. K., & Moore, D. H. (2000). The relationship between maternal care and uterine dysfunction: A continuous effect throughout reproductive life. *American Journal of Obstetrics and Gynecology, 182*(6), 1312–1317.

PDR nurse's handbook. (2001). Montvale, NJ: Demar Publishers.

Squire, C. (2000). Sociocultural aspects of pain. In M. Yerby (Ed.), *Pain in childbearing: Key issues in management*. London: Harcourt Publishers Limited.

Wilson, B. A., Shannon, M. T., & Strang, C. L. (Eds.), (2001). *Nursing drug guide: 2001*. Upper Saddle River, NJ: Prentice-Hall.

Wong, C. A. (2001). Analgesia and anesthesia for labor and delivery. In J. J. Sciarri & T. J. Watkins (Eds.), *Gynecology and obstetrics* (Vol. 3, chap. 90, pp 1–35). Philadelphia: Lippincott Williams & Wilkins.

Yerby, M. (2000). Pharmacological methods of pain relief. In M. Yerby (Ed.), *Pain in childbearing: Key issues in management*. London: Harcourt Publishers Limited.

York, R., Bhuttarowas, P., & Brown, L. P. (1999). Nursing in Thailand and its relationship to childbearing practices. *American Journal of Maternal Child Nursing, 24*(3), 145–150.

CHAPTER 19

Childbirth at Risk

We arrived at the birthing unit with such wonderful plans for the birth of our first baby. I was able to do my breathing and work through the labor pains with the assistance of my husband and the nurse until transition started. Then suddenly my baby's heart rate dropped— it changed its rhythm. The change lasted for about 20 seconds but it felt like a lifetime. The nurse helped me to my side, took my hand, and just stayed with my husband and me while we waited and watched the fetal monitor. There were no further problems, but I will never forget that moment.

—YOLANDA, 26

Key Terms

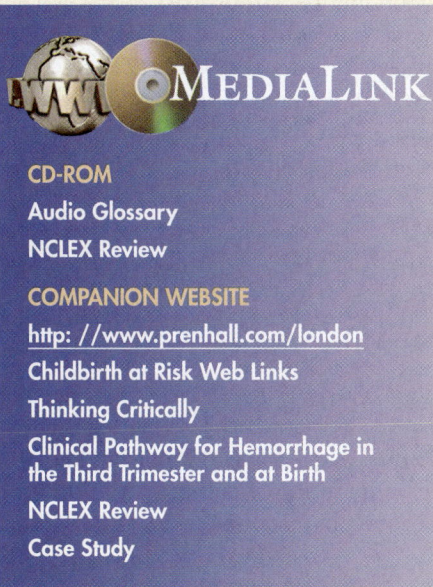

MEDIALINK

CD-ROM
Audio Glossary
NCLEX Review

COMPANION WEBSITE
http://www.prenhall.com/london
Childbirth at Risk Web Links
Thinking Critically
Clinical Pathway for Hemorrhage in the Third Trimester and at Birth
NCLEX Review
Case Study

Successful labor requires the harmonious functioning of five components: emotional factors, contractile forces, fetus, pelvis, and relationship between the fetus and the pelvis. (These components are described in depth in Chapter 15.) ⌐⊐ Disruptions in any of the five components may affect the others and cause dystocia (abnormal or difficult labor). The most common of these disruptions are discussed in this chapter.

CARE OF THE WOMAN AT RISK DUE TO ANXIETY AND FEAR

Anxiety and fear have an enormous effect on labor, especially when unexpected complications may jeopardize the life or health of the mother and/or fetus. A childbirth experience that was initially approached with expectation and confidence may become fraught with anxiety and uncertainty. In labor, anxiety and fear may exacerbate pain. The resulting increase in catecholamine release in turn increases physical distress and results in myometrial dysfunction and possibly ineffectual labor.

A frequent outcome of increased levels of fear, anxiety, and loss of control in childbirth is the development of posttraumatic stress disorder. Women who experience unexpectedly high levels of labor intervention and who feel unsatisfied with their health care are much more likely to exhibit long-term symptoms of posttraumatic stress disorder, such as episodes of intense fear, persistent reexperiencing of the traumatic event(s), and recurring feelings of helplessness and horror (Creedy, Shochet, & Horsfall, 2000).

Clinical Therapy

The goal of clinical therapy is to provide strategies that will help decrease the anxiety of the woman and her partner. Research suggests that childbirth experience is enhanced if caregivers give the laboring woman opportunities to talk about concerns and make choices about her care, even when complications exist (Berg & Dahlberg, 1998). The nurse can use therapeutic communication and sharing of information to allay anxiety for both the woman and her support person. When needed, pharmacologic measures such as sedatives and analgesics may be ordered to help the woman feel calmer.

Nursing Management

Nursing Assessment and Diagnosis

Unless birth is imminent or severe complications exist, begin the assessment by reviewing the woman's background. Factors such as age, marital and socioeconomic status, culture, methods of coping, and understanding of the labor process all contribute to the woman's psychologic response to labor. In addition, if the woman has other children, she may have unresolved concerns or fears related to a previous childbirth experience. As labor progresses, stay alert to the woman's verbal and nonverbal behavioral responses to the pain and anxiety of labor. The woman who is agitated and seems uncooperative or is too quiet and compliant may require further appraisal for posttraumatic stress symptoms (Saito, Ylikorkala, & Halmesmaki, 1999). Verbal cues such as "Is everything okay?" "I'm really nervous," or "What's going on?" usually indicate some degree of anxiety and concern. Other women may be irritable, require frequent explanations, or repeat questions. Also observe for nonverbal cues, including a tense posture, clenched hands, or pain out of proportion to the stage of labor (Roberts, Reardon, & Rosenfeld, 1999). Recognizing the impact of fatigue on pain and anxiety is another important nursing function.

Nursing diagnoses that may apply to the woman with excessive fear or anxiety include the following:

▶ *Anxiety* related to stress of the labor process

▶ *Fear* related to unknown outcome of labor

▶ *Pain* related to increased anxiety and stress

Planning and Implementation

The primary nursing interventions center on providing support to the laboring woman and her partner or family. Families that have attended prenatal classes may benefit from encouragement as they use some of the coping techniques they have learned (see Chapter 6). ⌐⊐ When something unexpected happens (such as fetal stress or distress), the woman may lose confidence in her ability to handle her pain and to maintain a level of control in the situation. Help the woman regain some balance by providing information and including her in any decision making (see Chapters 17 and 18). ⌐⊐

Unprepared couples can be taught a great deal at the time of admission, especially if active labor has not yet begun. To relieve some apprehension and fear, give clear but succinct information about the labor process, medical procedures, the environment, simple breathing exercises, and relaxation techniques. Even a woman in active labor who has had no prior preparation can relax a great deal in response to physical comfort measures, touch, frequent attention, therapeutic interaction, and possibly analgesics.

The nurse's ability to help the woman and her partner cope with the stress of labor is directly related to the rapport they have established. A calm, caring, confident, nonjudgmental approach not only acknowledges the anxiety but may also identify the source of the distress. Once the causative factors are known, implement appropriate interventions such as offering information, comfort measures, touch, or therapeutic communication. At times a woman (or couple) experiencing increased anxiety presents so many challenges that the nurse feels reluctant about being in the labor room for prolonged periods. However, the nurse's presence is the single most important factor that women identify as helping them during labor (Dahlberg, Berg, & Lundgren, 1999).

Evaluation

Expected outcomes of nursing care include the following:

▶ The woman experiences decreased physiologic signs of stress and increased physical and psychologic comfort.

▶ The fear experienced by the woman and her family decreases.

▶ The woman is able to verbalize feelings about her labor.

CARE OF THE WOMAN WITH DYSTOCIA RELATED TO DYSFUNCTIONAL UTERINE CONTRACTIONS

Dystocia, or difficult labor, may be due to a wide variety of problems, the most common of which is dysfunctional (or uncoordinated) uterine contractions. These uncoordinated contractions result in a prolonged labor (Bowes, 1999). Contractions that result in a more normal progression of labor tend to be moderate to strong when palpated and occur regularly (two to four contractions in 10 minutes in early labor and four to five per 10 minutes in later phases). Dysfunctional contractions are typically irregular in strength, timing, or both. These irregular uterine contractions often arrest cervical dilatation.

Hypertonic Labor Patterns

In hypertonic labor patterns, ineffectual uterine contractions of poor quality occur in the latent phase of labor, and the resting tone of the myometrium increases. Contractions usually become more frequent, but their intensity may decrease. The contractions are painful but ineffective in dilating and effacing the cervix, and a prolonged latent phase may result.

Maternal risks of hypertonic labor include

• Increased discomfort due to uterine muscle cell anoxia

• Fatigue as the pattern continues and no labor progress results

• Stress on coping abilities

• Dehydration and increased incidence of infection if labor is prolonged

Fetal-neonatal risks include

• Fetal distress because contractions and increased resting tone interfere with the uteroplacental exchange

• Prolonged pressure on the fetal head, which may result in cephalhematoma, caput succedaneum, or excessive molding (Figure 19–1 ◆)

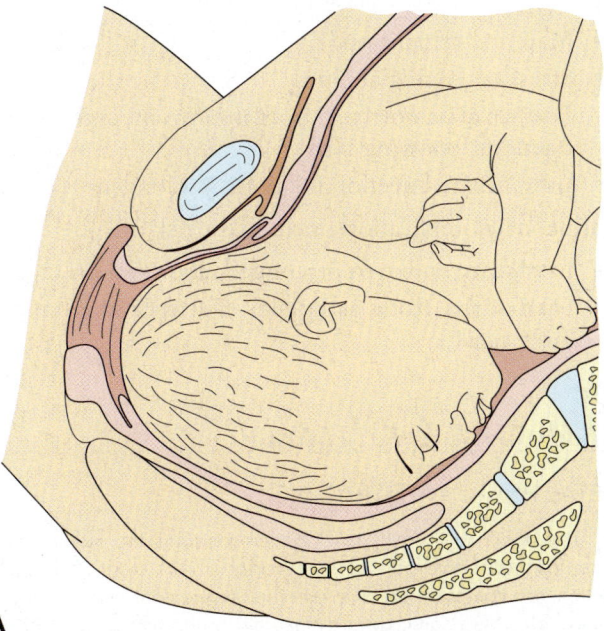

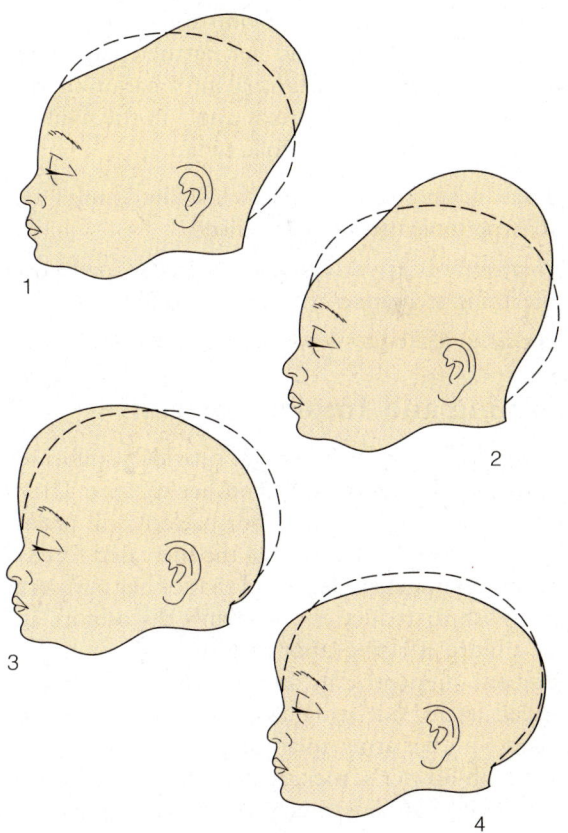

FIGURE 19–1. ◆ Effects of labor on the fetal head. **A,** Caput succedaneum formation. The presenting portion of the scalp area is encircled by the cervix during labor, causing swelling of the soft tissue. **B,** Molding of the fetal head in cephalic presentations: (1) occiput anterior, (2) occiput posterior, (3) brow, (4) face.

CLINICAL THERAPY

Management of hypertonic labor may include bed rest and sedation to promote relaxation and reduce pain. If the hypertonic pattern continues and develops into a prolonged latent phase, oxytocin infusion or amniotomy may be considered (see Chapter 20). These methods are instituted only after **cephalopelvic disproportion (CPD)** and fetal malpresentation have been ruled out. When an oxytocin infusion is used to stimulate uterine contractions, the physician or certified nurse-midwife (CNM) needs to assess whether vaginal birth is possible (i.e., whether the maternal pelvis is large enough for the fetus to pass through). If the maternal pelvic diameters are less than average, or if the fetus is particularly large or is in a malpresentation or malposition, CPD is said to be present. In the presence of true CPD, labor is not stimulated because vaginal birth is not possible.

Nursing Management

Nursing Assessment and Diagnosis

As part of the labor assessment, evaluate the relationship between the intensity of the pain being experienced and the degree to which the cervix is dilating and effacing. Also note whether anxiety is negatively affecting labor progress. Evidence of increasing frustration and discouragement on the part of the mother and her partner may indicate the need to provide some additional information or assurance.

Nursing diagnoses that may apply to the woman in hypertonic labor include the following:

▶ *Pain* related to the woman's inability to relax secondary to hypertonic uterine contractions

▶ *Ineffective individual coping* related to ineffectiveness of breathing techniques to relieve discomfort

▶ *Anxiety* related to slow labor progress

Planning and Implementation

A key nursing responsibility is to provide comfort and support to the laboring woman and her partner. The woman experiencing a hypertonic labor pattern will probably be very uncomfortable because of the increased force of contractions. Her anxiety level and that of her partner may be high. Work to reduce the woman's discomfort and promote a more effective labor pattern.

Suggest supportive measures such as a change of position: left lateral side-lying, high Fowler's, on her knees in the bed with her arms up around the top of the bed while it is in high Fowler's, rocking in a rocking chair, sitting up, and walking. Soothing measures, such as a warm shower, a Jacuzzi, a quiet environment, music the woman finds soothing, a back rub, therapeutic touch, and visualization, and comfort measures, such as mouth care, change of linens, effleurage, and relaxation exercises, may also be helpful. If sedation is ordered, ensure that the environment is conducive to relaxation. The labor partner may also need assistance in helping the woman cope. A calm, understanding approach offers the woman and her partner further support. Providing information about the cause of the hypertonic labor pattern and assuring the woman that she is not overreacting to the situation are important nursing actions.

Client education is key for the woman experiencing hypertonic labor. She needs information about the dysfunctional labor pattern and the possible implications for her and her baby. Information will help relieve anxiety and thereby increase relaxation and comfort. Explain treatment options and offer opportunities to ask questions.

Evaluation

Expected outcomes of nursing care include the following:

▶ The woman has increased comfort and decreased anxiety.

▶ The woman and her partner are able to cope with the labor.

▶ The woman experiences a more effective labor pattern.

Hypotonic Labor Patterns

A hypotonic labor pattern usually develops in the active phase of labor, after labor has been well established. Hypotonic labor is characterized by fewer than two to three contractions in a 10-minute period (Figure 19–2 ◆). Hypotonic labor may occur when the uterus is overstretched from a twin gestation, or in the presence of a large fetus, hydramnios, or grand multiparity. Bladder or bowel distention and CPD may also be associated with this pattern. Maternal implications of hypotonic labor patterns include the risk of

• Maternal exhaustion

• Stress on coping abilities

• Postpartal hemorrhage from insufficient uterine contractions following birth

• Intrauterine infection if labor is prolonged

Fetal-neonatal implications include the risk of

• Fetal distress due to prolonged labor pattern

• Fetal sepsis from pathogens that ascend from the birth canal

Thinking Critically

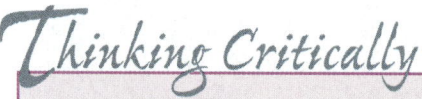

FETAL HEART RATE TRACING

A fetal heart rate (FHR) tracing demonstrates the following: baseline heart rate of 140 with variability of 6 to 10 bpm. When you compare the FHR with the uterine contractions, you note that there is a slowing of the FHR at the time of the contraction and that the FHR tracing looks like the contraction curve, but it is upside down. Based on this tracing, what would you do? **WEB**

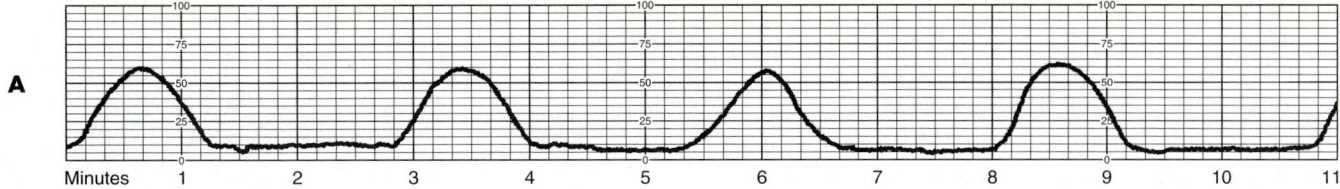

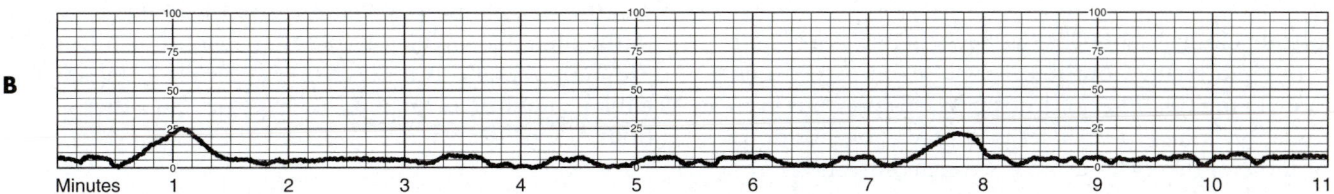

FIGURE 19–2. ◆ Comparison of labor patterns. **A,** Normal uterine contraction pattern. In this example, contraction frequency is every 3 minutes; duration is 60 seconds. The baseline resting tone is below 10 mm Hg. **B,** Hypotonic uterine contraction pattern. In this example, the contraction frequency is every 7 minutes (with some uterine activity between contractions), duration is 50 seconds, and intensity increases approximately 25 mm Hg during contractions.

CLINICAL THERAPY

Improving the quality of the uterine contractions while ensuring a safe outcome for the woman and her baby are the goals of therapy. Before beginning treatment for hypotonic labor, the physician or CNM makes sure pelvic measurements are adequate and establishes gestational age if fetal maturity is in question. After CPD, fetal malpresentation, and fetal immaturity have been ruled out, oxytocin (Pitocin) may be given intravenously (IV) via an infusion pump to improve the quality of uterine contractions. IV fluid maintains adequate hydration and prevents maternal exhaustion. Amniotomy may be used to stimulate the labor process.

Some physicians support **active management of labor (AMOL),** a process whereby labor is managed from the beginning with amniotomy, timed cervical exams are performed, and augmentation of labor with IV administration of oxytocin is begun if a specified level of progress is not met. Supporters of active management of labor contend that it is a preventative treatment that reduces the chance for protracted labor (Simpson & Poole, 1998).

Noticeable progress in the labor process demonstrates an improvement in the quality of uterine contractions. If the labor pattern does not become effective or if other complications develop, further interventions, including cesarean birth, may be necessary.

Nursing Management

Nursing Assessment and Diagnosis

Assessment of contractions (for frequency and intensity), maternal vital signs, and fetal heart rate (FHR) provides data to evaluate maternal-fetal status. Also be alert for signs and symptoms of infection and dehydration. Because of the stress associated with a prolonged labor, observing the woman and her partner's success in implementing coping mechanisms is important.

Nursing diagnoses that may apply to the woman in hypotonic labor include the following:

▶ *Pain* related to uterine contractions secondary to dysfunctional labor

▶ *Health-seeking behaviors* related to lack of information about dysfunctional labor

Planning and Implementation

Nursing measures to promote maternal-fetal physical well-being include frequent monitoring of contractions, maternal vital signs, and FHR. If amniotic membranes are ruptured, assess the amniotic fluid for meconium (dark green or black fetal stool). If there is meconium in the amniotic fluid, close observation of fetal status is more critical because it often indicates that the fetus is experiencing some form of stress. An intake and output record provides a way of determining maternal hydration or dehydration. Encourage the woman to void every 2 hours, and check her bladder for distention. Because labor may be prolonged, continue to monitor the woman for signs of infection (elevated temperature, chills, foul-smelling amniotic fluid). Vaginal examinations should be kept to a minimum to decrease the risk of introducing an infection. (The nursing implications of oxytocin infusion are presented in Chapter 20.)

Clients experiencing a hypotonic labor pattern require emotional support. Help the woman and her partner cope with the frustration of a lengthy labor process. Combine a warm, caring approach with techniques to reduce anxiety and discomfort.

The teaching plan must include information regarding the dysfunctional labor process and implications for the mother and baby. Disadvantages of and alternatives to treatment also need to be discussed and understood.

Evaluation

Expected outcomes of nursing care include the following:

▶ The woman maintains comfort during labor.

▶ The woman understands the type of labor pattern that is occurring and the treatment plan.

Precipitous Labor and Birth

Precipitous labor is labor that lasts less than 3 hours and results in rapid birth. Contributing factors in precipitous labor are (1) multiparity, (2) large pelvis, (3) previous precipitous labor, and (4) a small fetus in a favorable position. One or more of these factors, plus strong contractions, result in a rapid descent of the infant through the birth canal.

Precipitous labor and precipitous birth are not the same. A precipitous birth is an unexpected, sudden, and often unattended birth. (See Chapter 17 for discussion of emergency birth.)

Maternal risks of precipitous labor include

- Loss of coping abilities
- Lacerations of the cervix, vagina, and perineum due to rapid descent and birth of the fetus
- Postpartal hemorrhage due to undetected lacerations or inadequate uterine contractions after birth

Fetal-neonatal implications include

- Fetal distress or hypoxia from decreased uteroplacental circulation due to intense uterine contractions
- Cerebral trauma from rapid descent through the birth canal

CLINICAL THERAPY

Any woman with a history of precipitous labor requires close monitoring in the last few weeks of pregnancy. If the cervix softens and begins to dilate, the woman may be scheduled for immediate induction of labor.

NURSING MANAGEMENT

During the intrapartal nursing assessment, identify a woman at increased risk of precipitous labor because of a previous history of precipitous or short labor, for example. During labor the presence of one or both of the following factors may indicate potential problems:

- Accelerated cervical dilatation (>2 cm/hr in multigravidas and >1.2 cm/hr in primigravidas) and fetal descent
- Intense uterine contractions with little uterine relaxation between contractions

If the woman has a history of precipitous labor, she is closely monitored, and an emergency birth pack is kept at hand. Stay in constant attendance if possible and promote comfort and rest by assisting the woman to a comfortable position, providing a quiet environment, and administer-

ing sedatives as needed. Give information and support before and after the birth.

To avoid possible precipitous labor and hyperstimulation of the uterus during oxytocin administration, be alert to the dangers of oxytocin overdosage (see "Drug Guide: Oxytocin" in Chapter 20). ⊂⊃ If the woman receiving oxytocin develops an accelerated labor pattern, the oxytocin is discontinued immediately, and the woman is turned on her left side to improve uterine perfusion. Oxygen may be administered to increase the available oxygen in the maternal circulating blood, which in turn increases the amount available for exchange at the placental site. The fetus is monitored for signs of hypoxia and other indications of fetal distress.

CARE OF THE WOMAN WITH POSTTERM PREGNANCY

A **postterm pregnancy** is one that extends more than 294 days or 42 weeks past the first day of the last menstrual period. It is important to distinguish between the terms *postdate*, which means that the pregnancy has gone beyond the estimated date of birth, and *postterm*, which indicates that the pregnancy has gone at least 1 day beyond 42 complete weeks from the last menstrual period (Martin, 2000). The actual incidence of post-term pregnancies is small, approximately 3% to 7%. The cause of true postterm pregnancy is unknown, but it seems to occur more frequently in primigravidas and women over age 35 (Berkowitz & Garite, 2001).

Maternal risks associated with postterm pregnancy include the following (Martin, 2000):

- Probable labor induction
- Increased risk for large-for-gestational-age (LGA) infant
- Increased incidence of forceps-assisted, vacuum-assisted, or cesarean birth
- Increased psychologic stress as the due date passes and concern for the baby increases

Fetal risks include the following (Martin, 2000):

- Decreased perfusion from the placenta
- Oligohydramnios (decreased amount of amniotic fluid), which increases the risk of cord compression
- Meconium aspiration (aspiration of meconium-stained amniotic fluid by the fetus at the time of birth), which is more likely if oligohydramnios and thick meconium are present

Some fetuses continue to grow beyond the 42nd week of pregnancy and can be excessively large at birth (macrosomia). In other cases, the intrauterine environment becomes unfavorable for growth, and at birth the infant has lost muscle mass and subcutaneous fat. The macrosomic fetus is at risk for birth trauma, while the small-for-gestational-age

(SGA) fetus is at risk for fetal distress during labor because there is often associated oligohydramnios (Martin, 2000).

Clinical Therapy

When the 40th week of gestation is completed and birth has not occurred, most obstetricians begin using the non-stress test (NST) and biophysical profile (BPP) (especially the amniotic fluid volume portion of the BPP) as assessment tools. These tests may be done two to three times a week to help evaluate fetal well-being (Berkowitz & Garite, 2001). If the fetal assessment tests indicate a problem, the clinician intervenes to accomplish the birth.

Nursing Management

Nursing Assessment and Diagnosis

When the woman is admitted into the birthing area, ongoing assessments of fetal well-being begin as soon as the postterm condition has been verified. Identify reassuring FHR characteristics and assess for nonreassuring patterns, such as nonperiodic variable decelerations (which may indicate cord compression), so that corrective actions can be taken. When the amniotic membranes rupture, assess the fluid for meconium. In addition, assess the woman's knowledge about the condition, implications for her baby, risks, and possible interventions.

Nursing diagnoses that may apply to the woman with postterm pregnancy include the following:

▶ *Health-seeking behaviors* related to lack of information about postterm pregnancy

▶ *Fear* related to the unknown outcome for the baby

▶ *Ineffective individual coping* related to anxiety about the status of the baby

Planning and Implementation

NURSING CARE IN THE COMMUNITY

If the woman has not been assessing fetal movement every day, teach her how to do so. It is vital to stress the importance of identifying inadequate fetal movement and immediately contacting her health care provider. (See Chapter 9 for further discussion of techniques to detect fetal movement.)

Client education about the postterm pregnancy is another important nursing responsibility. Address the implications and associated risks for the baby, as well as possible treatment plans. The woman and her partner need opportunities to ask questions and clarify information.

HOSPITAL-BASED NURSING CARE

Promoting fetal well-being requires careful assessment of the response of the fetus during labor. If oligohydramnios exists, a continuous FHR tracing is obtained and evaluated

frequently. The decreased amount of fluid may allow compression of the umbilical cord, resulting in variable decelerations. If the fetus is macrosomic, careful assessment of labor progress (contraction characteristics, progressive cervical dilatation, fetal descent) is also needed.

Emotional support is a key nursing intervention for women with pregnancies that extend past the due date. Women experiencing postterm pregnancy frequently feel increased stress and anxiety and have difficulty coping. Encouragement, support, and recognition of the woman's anxiety are helpful.

Evaluation

Expected outcomes of nursing care include the following:

▶ The woman has knowledge about the postterm pregnancy.

▶ The woman and her partner feel supported and able to cope with the postterm pregnancy.

▶ Fetal status is maintained, any abnormalities are quickly identified, and supportive measures are initiated.

CARE OF THE WOMAN AND FETUS AT RISK DUE TO FETAL MALPOSITION

The occiput-posterior (OP) position is the most common fetal malposition. When the fetus is OP, the occiput of the fetal head is directed toward the back of the maternal pelvis. During labor, 87% of OP fetuses rotate to an occiput-anterior (OA) position (Rivlin, 2000).

A variation of OP called the **persistent occiput-posterior (POP) position** occurs in 5% of labors. In this case the fetus enters and travels the birth canal in the OP position, and is born that way. POP is associated with android and anthropoid pelvic shapes. Labor may be prolonged; however, most POP fetuses are born without the aid of forceps (Rivlin, 2000).

Maternal risks related to the POP position include

• Risk of third- or fourth-degree perineal lacerations during birth

• Risk of extension of a midline episiotomy

Fetal implications do not include an increased mortality risk unless labor is prolonged or additional interventions such as forceps-assisted, vacuum-assisted, or cesarean birth are required.

Clinical Therapy

Clinical treatment focuses on close monitoring of maternal and fetal status and labor progress to determine whether vaginal or cesarean birth is the safer method. A cesarean birth is chosen if maternal or fetal problems make a vaginal birth unwise or if CPD is present. Although most POP fetuses are born vaginally, in some cases forceps-assisted birth may be necessary. The forceps can be used to deliver the fetus while it is still in the OP position or to rotate the occiput to an anterior position (Scanzoni's maneuver). A vacuum-assistance device may also accomplish rotation from left occiput-posterior (LOP) or right occiput-posterior (ROP) to an anterior position. (See Chapter 20 for further discussion of forceps and vacuum extraction.)

Nursing Management

Nursing Assessment and Diagnosis

Signs and symptoms of a POP position include complaints of intense back pain by the laboring woman, a dysfunctional labor pattern, hypotonic labor (the fetal head does not put adequate pressure on the cervix), arrest of dilatation, or arrest of fetal descent. The back pain is caused by the fetal occiput compressing the sacral nerves. Further assessment may reveal a depression in the maternal abdomen above the symphysis. FHR is typically heard far laterally on the abdomen, and on vaginal examination the CNM/physician finds the wide, diamond-shaped anterior fontanelle in the anterior portion of the pelvis. This fontanelle may be difficult to feel because of molding of the fetal head.

Nursing diagnoses that may apply to women with POP include the following:

▶ *Pain* related to back discomfort secondary to the OP position

▶ *Ineffective individual coping* related to unanticipated discomfort and slow progress in labor

Planning and Implementation

Changing maternal posture has been used for many years to enhance rotation of OP or occiput-transverse (OT) to OA. A number of position changes may be tried. For instance, the woman may be asked to lie on one side and then asked to move to the other side as the fetus begins to rotate. This side-lying position may promote rotation; it also enables the support person to apply counterpressure on the sacral area to decrease discomfort. A knee-chest position provides a downward slant to the vaginal canal, directing the fetal head downward on descent. A hands-and-knees position is often effective in rotating the fetus. In addition to maintaining a hands-and-knees position on the bed, the woman may try pelvic rocking, and the support person may firmly stroke the abdomen. The stroking begins over the fetal back and swings around to the other side of the abdomen. After the fetus has rotated, the woman lies in a Sims' position on the side opposite the fetal back.

Evaluation

Expected outcomes of nursing care include the following:

▶ The woman's discomfort is decreased.

▶ The coping abilities of the woman and her partner are strengthened.

CARE OF THE WOMAN AND FETUS AT RISK DUE TO FETAL MALPRESENTATION

In a normal presentation, the occiput is the presenting part (Figure 19–3A ◆). Fetal malpresentations include brow, face, breech, shoulder (transverse lie), and compound presentation.

Brow Presentation

In a brow presentation, the forehead of the fetus becomes the presenting part. The fetal head is between flexion and extension (military position, Figure 19–3B ◆), and the fetal head enters the birth canal with the widest diameter of the head (occipitomental—14 cm) foremost (Figure 19–3C ◆).

The brow presentation occurs more often in multiparas than in nulliparas and is thought to be due to lax abdominal and pelvic musculature. Many brow presentations spontaneously convert to face or occipital presentations (Bowes, 1999).

Maternal implications of brow presentation include increased risk of

• Longer labor due to ineffective contractions and slow or arrested fetal descent

• Cesarean birth if brow presentation persists

Fetal-neonatal risks include increased mortality because of cerebral and neck compression and damage to the trachea and larynx (Rivlin, 2000). In addition, the newborn may have facial edema and exaggerated molding of the head.

CLINICAL THERAPY

If a brow presentation fails to convert to occipital or face presentation, cesarean birth is indicated, in most cases (Rivlin, 2000). If a vaginal birth is attempted, the woman is closely monitored for CPD and will probably need an episiotomy. Right mediolateral (RML) or left mediolateral (LML) episiotomy is preferable, because the more common midline episiotomy has the risk of extending into the anus and rectum (fourth-degree laceration).

Nursing Management

Nursing Assessment and Diagnosis

A brow presentation can be detected on vaginal examination (with ultrasound or x-ray confirmation) by palpation

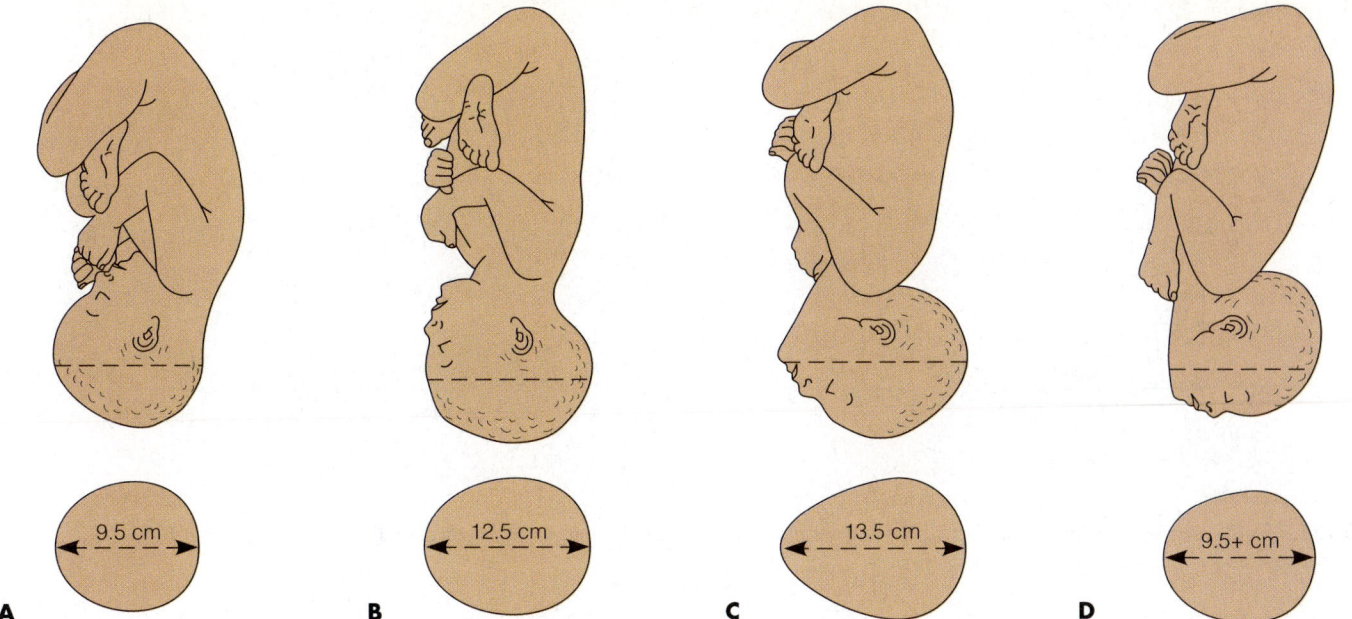

FIGURE 19–3. ◆ Types of cephalic presentations. **A,** The occiput is the presenting part because the head is flexed and the fetal chin is against the chest. The largest anteroposterior (AP) diameter that presents and passes through the pelvis is approximately 9.5 cm. **B,** Military presentation. The head is neither flexed nor extended. The presenting AP diameter is approximately 12.5 cm. **C,** Brow presentation. The largest diameter of the fetal head (approximately 13.5 cm) presents in this situation. **D,** Face presentation. The AP diameter is 9.5 cm.
Note: From Danforth, D. N., & Scott, J. R. (Eds.). (1990). *Obstetrics and gynecology* (5th ed., p. 170, Figure 8–9). New York: Lippincott.

of the diamond-shaped anterior fontanelle on one side and orbital ridges and root of the nose on the other side (Rivlin, 2000).

Nursing diagnoses that may apply to a woman with a brow presentation include the following:

▶ *Health-seeking behaviors* related to lack of information about the possible maternal-fetal effects of brow presentation

▶ *Risk for injury to the fetus* related to pressure on fetal structures secondary to brow presentation

Planning and Implementation

Closely observe the woman for labor problems and the fetus for signs of stress or distress. Observe the fetus closely during labor for signs of hypoxia, as evidenced by late decelerations and bradycardia.

Also provide emotional support to the family. Explain the fetal position to the woman and her support person or interpret what the CNM or physician has told them. Stay close at hand to reassure the couple, inform them of any changes, and assist them with labor-coping techniques. In face and brow presentations, the newborn's face may be edematous. The couple may need help in beginning the attachment process because of the newborn's facial appearance. After the infant is inspected for any abnormalities, the pediatrician and nurse can assure the couple that the facial edema is only temporary and will subside in 3 or 4 days and that the molding will be much less visible in a few days (even though completion of the process takes several weeks).

Evaluation

Expected outcomes of nursing care include the following:

▶ The woman and her partner understand the implications and associated problems of brow presentation.

▶ The mother and her baby have a safe labor and birth.

Face Presentation

In a face presentation, the face of the fetus is the presenting part (Figure 19–4 ◆; also see Figure 19–3D). The fetal head is hyperextended even more than in the brow presentation. Face presentation occurs most frequently in multiparas, in preterm birth, and in the presence of anencephaly. The incidence of face presentation is about 1 in 500 births (Bowes, 1999).

Maternal risks related to face presentation include

• Increased risk of CPD and prolongation of labor

• Increased risk of infection (with prolonged labor)

• Cesarean birth if fetal chin is posterior (mentum posterior)

Fetal-neonatal risks include

• Cephalhematoma of the face

• Edema of the face and throat if the fetal chin is anterior (mentum anterior) and a vaginal birth occurs (may also occur during fetal descent)

• Pronounced molding of the head

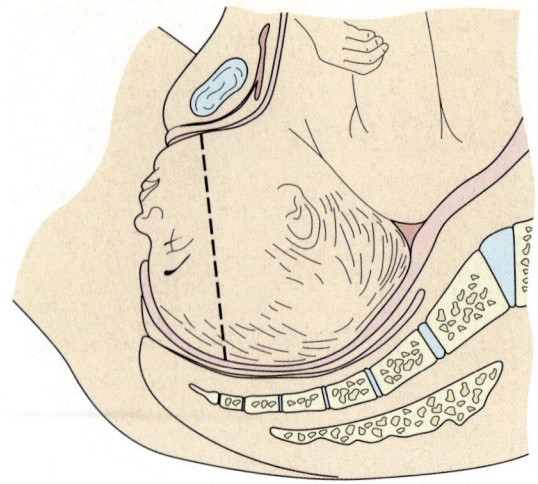

A

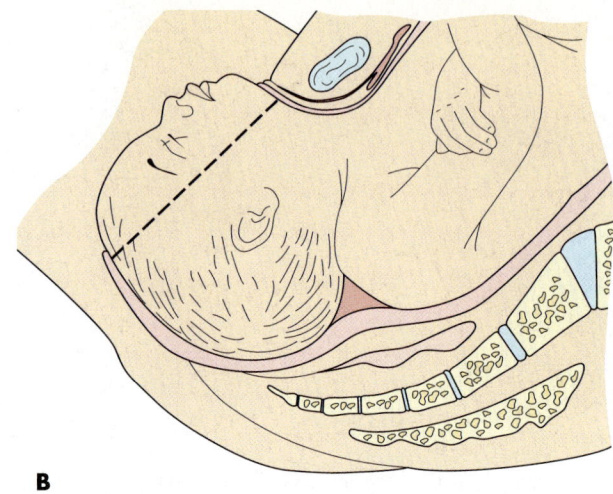

B

FIGURE 19–4. ◆ Mechanism of birth in face (mentoanterior) position. **A,** The submentobregmatic diameter at the outlet. **B,** The fetal head is born by the movement of flexion.

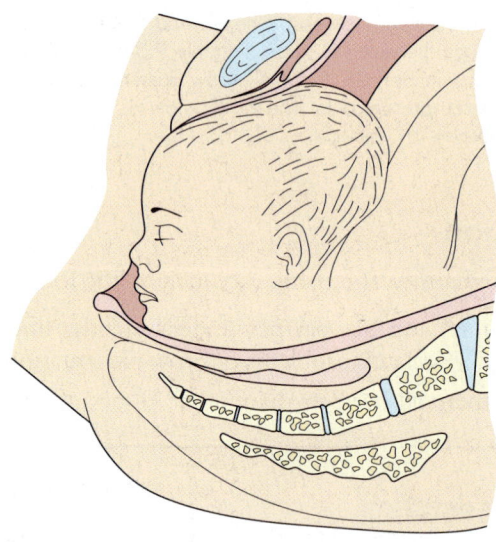

FIGURE 19–5. ◆ Face presentation. Mechanism of birth in mentoposterior position. Fetal head is unable to extend farther. The face becomes impacted.

CLINICAL THERAPY

A vaginal birth may be anticipated if no CPD is present, the chin (mentum) is anterior, the labor pattern is effective, and no fetal stress or distress is present. If the mentum is posterior, a vaginal birth is not possible and a cesarean birth is necessary (Figure 19–5 ◆).

Nursing Management

Nursing Assessment and Diagnosis

When performing Leopold's maneuvers, the back of the fetus is difficult to outline, and a deep furrow can be pal-

pated between the hard occiput and the fetal back (Figure 19–6 ◆). Fetal heart tones are audible on the side where the fetal feet are palpated. It may be difficult to determine by vaginal examination whether a breech or face is presenting, especially if facial edema is already present. During the vaginal examination, try to palpate the saddle of the nose and the gums. When assessing engagement, remember that the face has to be deep within the pelvis before the biparietal diameters have entered the inlet.

Nursing diagnoses that may apply to the woman with a fetus in face presentation include the following:

▶ *Fear* related to unknown outcome of the labor
▶ *Risk for injury to the newborn's face* related to edema secondary to the birth process

Planning and Implementation

Nursing interventions are the same as those indicated for the brow presentation.

Evaluation

Expected outcomes of nursing care include the following:

▶ The woman and her partner understand the implications and associated problems of face presentation.
▶ The mother and her baby have a safe labor and birth.

Breech Presentation

The exact cause of breech presentation (Figure 19–7 ◆) is unknown. This malpresentation occurs in about 3% to 4% of labors and is frequently associated with preterm birth, placenta previa, hydramnios, multiple gestation, uterine anomalies (such as bicornuate uterus), and fetal anomalies (especially anencephaly and hydrocephaly) (Bofill, 2000).

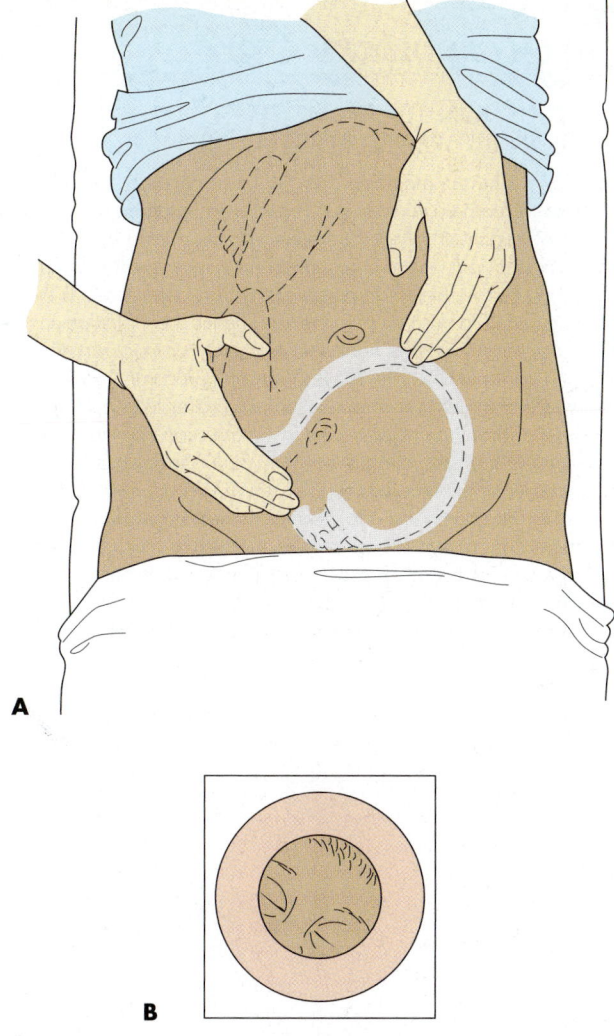

FIGURE 19–6. ◆ Face presentation. **A,** Palpation of the maternal abdomen with the fetus in right mentum posterior (rmp) position. **B,** Vaginal examination may permit palpation of facial features of the fetus.

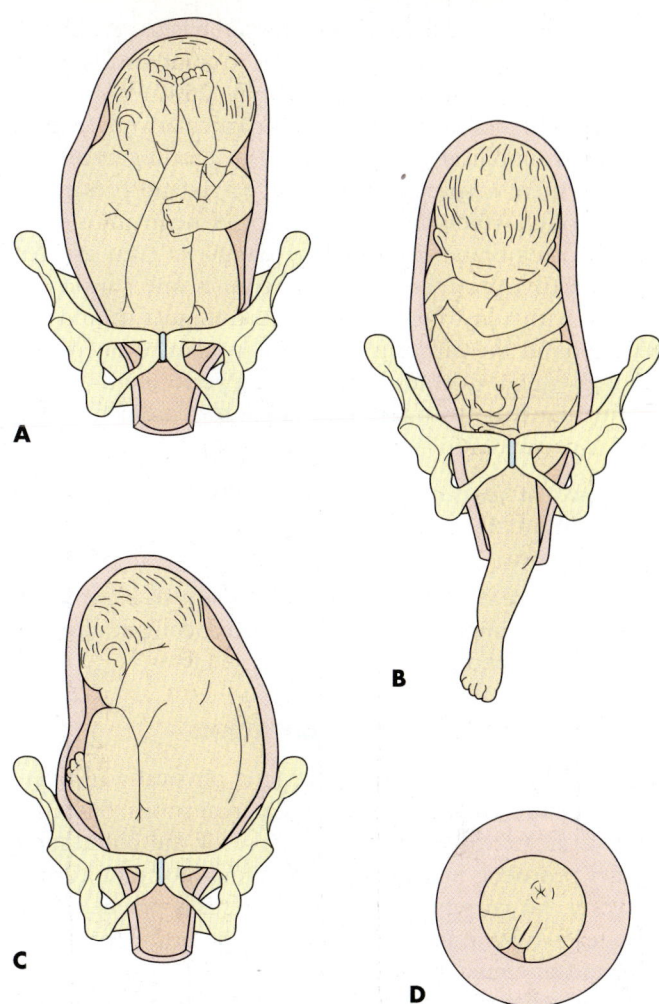

FIGURE 19–7. ◆ Breech presentation. **A,** Frank breech. **B,** Incomplete (footling) breech. **C,** Complete breech in left sacral anterior (lsa) position. **D,** On vaginal examination the nurse may feel the anal sphincter. The tissue of the fetal buttocks feels soft.

The maternal implication of breech presentation is a likelihood of cesarean birth. Fetal-neonatal implications include the following (Gimovsky, 2000):

- Higher perinatal morbidity and mortality rates
- Increased risk of prolapsed cord, especially in incomplete breeches, because space is available between the cervix and presenting part
- Increased risk of cervical cord injuries due to hyperextension of the fetal head during vaginal birth
- Increased risk of birth trauma (especially of the head) during either vaginal or cesarean breech birth

CLINICAL THERAPY

Current clinical therapy is directed toward converting the breech presentation to a cephalic presentation prior to the beginning of labor. Therefore, an external cephalic version (ECV) may be attempted at 36 to 38 weeks' gestation as long as the woman is not in labor (Bofill, 2000; Gimovsky, 2000). (See Chapter 20 ⬚ for discussion of external version.) Opinions differ about the best method of birth for the fetus in a breech presentation. When the fetus is still in breech presentation and labor occurs, the method of birth varies depending on gestational age, estimated fetal weight, type of breech, and physician preference.

Nursing Management

Nursing Assessment and Diagnosis

Frequently, it is the nurse who first recognizes a breech presentation. On palpation the nurse feels the firm fetal head in the uterine fundus and the wider sacrum in the lower part of the abdomen. If the sacrum has not descended, ballottement causes the entire fetal body to move. Furthermore,

FHR is usually auscultated above the umbilicus. Passage of meconium into the amniotic fluid due to compression of the fetus's intestinal tract is common (Bofill, 2000).

If membranes are ruptured, be particularly alert for a prolapsed umbilical cord, especially in footling breeches, because there is space between the cervix and presenting part through which the cord can slip. If the infant is small and the membranes rupture, the danger is even greater. The risk of a prolapsed umbilical cord is one reason any woman with a history of ruptured membranes should not walk around the birthing area until a full assessment, including vaginal examination, has been performed.

Nursing diagnoses that may apply to a woman with a breech presentation include the following:

▶ *Impaired gas exchange in the fetus* related to interruption in umbilical blood flow secondary to compression of the cord

▶ *Health-seeking behaviors* related to lack of information about the implications and associated complications of breech presentation for the mother and fetus

Planning and Implementation

During labor, promote maternal-fetal physical well-being by frequently assessing fetal and maternal status. Since the fetus is at increased risk for prolapse of the cord, some agency protocols may call for continuous fetal monitoring; however, no current research supports this practice. Provide teaching and information about the breech presentation and the nursing care needed.

Although as many as 90% of infants in breech presentations are born by cesarean birth, a few are born vaginally (Bofill, 2000). Assist with the vaginal birth by including Piper forceps (used to guide the after-coming fetal head) in the birth table setup. Assist the physician if forceps are needed for the birth. If the family and CNM or physician decide on a cesarean birth, intervene as with any cesarean birth.

Evaluation

Expected outcomes of nursing care include the following:

▶ The woman and her partner understand the implications and associated problems of breech presentation.

▶ Major complications are recognized early and corrective measures are instituted.

▶ The mother and baby have a safe labor and birth.

Transverse Lie (Shoulder Presentation) of a Single Fetus

A transverse lie occurs in approximately 1 in 300 term births (Bowes, 1999). Maternal conditions associated with a transverse lie are grand multiparity with relaxed uterine muscles and placenta previa (Figure 19–8 ◆).

Complementary Care

MOXIBUSTION TO PROMOTE VERSION IN BREECH PRESENTATIONS

Traditional Chinese medicine uses the herb mugwort in the form of moxa to promote version in a breech presentation. Moxa is a system of treatment, often combined with acupuncture, in which an herb is dried, rolled into cones (like incense cones), and placed on certain meridian points of the body. The moxa is then lit and allowed to burn close to the skin, hence the—*bustion* component of the name. The heat and pungency of mugwort stimulates the point, and energy moves through (Gladstar, 1993). It is believed that the effect of moxibustion increases fetal activity.

The meridian point that is used in moxibustion to promote version in breech presentation is acupoint BL 67, located beside the outer corner of the fifth toenail (Cardini & Weixin, 1998). Treatment may take from 7 days to 2 weeks. In two recent clinical studies, moxibustion was found to be an effective modality in the management of breech presentation (Cardini & Weixin, 1998; Kanakura, Kometani, Nagata, et al., 2001).

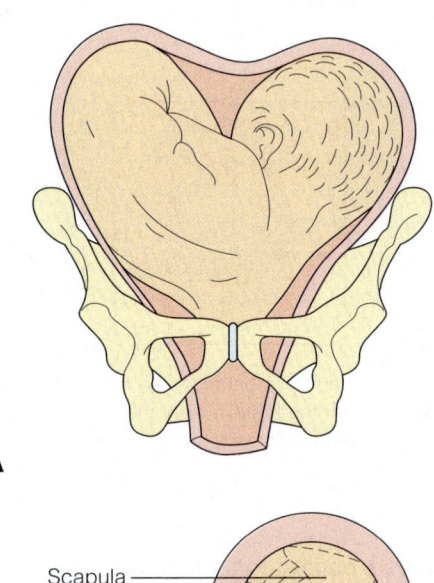

A

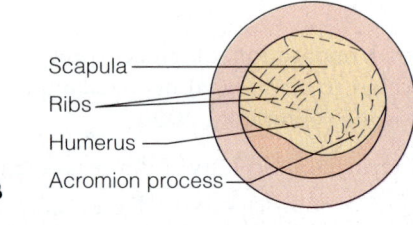

Scapula
Ribs
Humerus
Acromion process

B

FIGURE 19–8. ◆ Transverse lie. **A,** Shoulder presentation. **B,** On vaginal examination the nurse may feel the acromion process as the fetal presenting part.

CLINICAL THERAPY

The management of shoulder presentation depends on the gestational age. If discovered before term, the management is expectant (watchful), because some fetuses may change presentation without any intervention. When a shoulder presentation is still evident at 37 completed weeks of gestation, an external cephalic version attempt (followed, if successful, by induction of labor) is recommended, because the associated risk of prolapsed cord is significant. Intrapartum external cephalic version is often successful, reducing the need for cesarean birth by as much as 50% (Rivlin, 2000).

NURSING MANAGEMENT

The nurse can identify a transverse lie by inspection and palpation of the abdomen, by auscultation of FHR, and by vaginal examination. On inspection the woman's abdomen appears widest from side to side as a result of the long axis of the infant's body lying parallel to the ground and across the mother's uterus.

On palpation no fetal part is felt in the fundal portion of the uterus or above the symphysis. The head may be palpated on one side and the breech on the other. FHR is usually auscultated just below the midline of the umbilicus. On vaginal examination, if a presenting part is palpated, it is the ridged thorax or possibly an arm compressed against the chest.

Assist in the interpretation of the fetal presentation and provide information and support to the couple. Also assess maternal and fetal status frequently and prepare the woman for a cesarean birth. (See Chapter 20 for further information about teaching related to cesarean birth.)

Compound Presentation

A compound presentation is one in which there are two presenting parts, such as the occiput and fetal hand or the complete breech and fetal hand. Most compound presentations resolve themselves spontaneously, but others require additional manipulation at birth.

CARE OF THE WOMAN AND FETUS AT RISK DUE TO MACROSOMIA

Fetal **macrosomia** is defined as a newborn weight of more than 4,000 g at birth. Some sources suggest that the fetus not be considered macrosomic unless it weighs 4,500 g or more and that considerations of ethnic grouping be incorporated as well (Hogg & Kimberlin, 2000). The condition is more common among offspring of large parents and diabetic women and in cases of grand multiparity and post-term gestation (Gherman & Gonik, 2001).

Maternal implications of macrosomia include increased risk of

- CPD
- Dysfunctional labor
- Soft tissue laceration during vaginal birth
- Postpartal hemorrhage

Fetal-neonatal implications include increased risk of

- Meconium aspiration
- Asphyxia

- Shoulder dystocia, in which, after birth of the head, the anterior shoulder fails to deliver either spontaneously or with gentle traction (Gherman & Gonik, 2001)
- Upper brachial plexus injury and fractured clavicles

Clinical Therapy

The occurrence of maternal and fetal problems associated with excessively large infants may be lessened somewhat by identifying macrosomia before the onset of labor. If a large fetus is suspected, the maternal pelvis should be evaluated carefully. Fetal size can be estimated by palpating the crown-to-rump length of the fetus in utero and by ultrasound or x-ray pelvimetry. Clinical studies have demonstrated that palpation and ultrasound are equally effective assessments of fetal weight; both provide accurate estimates in about 65% of cases (O'Reilly-Green & Divon, 2000). Whenever the uterus appears excessively large, hydramnios, an oversized fetus, or multiple pregnancies must be considered as the possible cause.

When fetal weight is estimated to be 4,500 g or more, a cesarean birth is usually planned. The best method of birth for an estimated fetal weight of 4,000 to 4,500 g is debated. The discussion centers primarily on the incidence of shoulder dystocia during vaginal birth and the difficulty in accurately estimating the fetal weight. Unexpected shoulder dystocia during vaginal birth can be a grave problem. As an emergency measure the CNM or physician may ask the nurse to assist the woman into the McRoberts maneuver (sharp flexion of the thighs toward the hips and abdomen) or to apply gentle suprapubic pressure in an attempt to aid in the delivery of the fetal shoulders (Gherman & Gonik, 2001).

Nursing Management

Assist in identifying women at risk for carrying a large fetus and those who exhibit signs of macrosomia. Because these women are prime candidates for dystocia and its complications, assess the FHR frequently for indications of fetal stress and evaluate the rates of cervical dilatation and fetal descent.

The fetal monitor is applied for continuous fetal evaluation. Early decelerations (caused by fetal head compression) could mean size disproportion at the bony inlet. Report any sign of labor dysfunction or fetal distress to the physician or CNM immediately.

Support the laboring woman and her partner and give them information about the implications of macrosomia and possible associated problems. During the birth, continue to provide support and encouragement to the couple.

Inspect macrosomic newborns after birth for cephalhematoma and Erb's palsy and inform the nursery staff of any problems so that they will observe the newborn closely for cerebral, neurologic, and motor problems. The presence of a macrosomic fetus means that the uterus has been stretched farther than it would have been with an average-sized fetus. The overstretching may lead to contractile problems during labor or after birth. After birth the over-stretched uterus may not contract well (uterine atony) and will feel boggy (soft). In this case, uterine hemorrhage is likely. Massage the fundus of the uterus to stimulate contraction; IV oxytocin may be needed. Closely monitor maternal vital signs for deviation suggestive of shock.

CARE OF THE WOMAN WITH MULTIPLE GESTATION

In part due to advances in infertility treatments, the incidence of twins in the United States is approximately 1 in 45 pregnancies, and the overall multifetal birth rate has more than doubled since 1991 (Miller, Ransom, Shalhoub, et al., 2000). Spontaneous twin and other multiple-gestation pregnancies can develop either from the fertilization of two (or more) separate ova or from the division of one fertilized ovum. Twins from two separate ova are called dizygotic and may be of the same or different sexes. In this type of twinning, there are two amnions (diamniotic) and two chorions (dichorionic). In multiple-gestation pregnancies, each fetus usually has its own amniotic sac. The incidence of spontaneous twins varies but is highest in African Americans, women of greater age and parity, and women who are tall and tend to be heavier. The incidence is low in the Asian population (Benirschke, 1999; Miller et al., 2000).

Twins from one fertilized ovum are called monozygotic and are always of the same sex. If the fertilized ovum (zygote) divides within the first 72 hours after fertilization, the siblings will be dichorionic (trichorionic and so on) and diamniotic (triamniotic and so on). The most common monozygotic twins result from division that occurs from the fourth to the eighth day after fertilization; the embryos develop one chorion (monochorionic) and separate amnions (diamniotic or multiamniotic). The relationship of membranes among triplets and other high-order gestations generally follows the same principles as for twins, except that monochorionic and dichorionic amniotic sacs may coexist (Benirschke, 1999; W. E. Roberts, 2000). The terminology is important because the perinatal morbidity and mortality rates differ greatly among different types of multiple-gestation pregnancies (Keith, Papiernik, & Oleszczuk, 1998).

During the prenatal period, visualization of two gestational sacs at 5 to 6 weeks, fundal height greater than expected for the length of gestation, and auscultation of heart rates that differ by at least 10 beats per minute are the most likely clues to multiple-gestation pregnancies. In addition, the alpha-fetoprotein level is usually elevated in twin or multiple-gestation pregnancies and many women experience severe nausea and vomiting (due to elevated levels of the human chorionic gonadotropin [hCG] hormone) (Malone & D'Alton, 1999).

Maternal Implications

During her pregnancy, the woman may experience physical discomfort such as shortness of breath, dyspnea on exertion, backaches, and pedal edema. Other associated problems include urinary tract infections, pregnancy-induced hypertension (PIH), preterm labor, and placenta previa (Malone & D'Alton, 1999). Complications during labor include abnormal fetal presentations, uterine dysfunction, prolapsed cord, and hemorrhage at birth or shortly after (W. E. Roberts, 2000).

Fetal-Neonatal Implications

The perinatal mortality rate is approximately 10 times greater for twins than for a single fetus (W. E. Roberts, 2000). The perinatal mortality rate for monoamniotic siblings has been estimated to be as high as 50% to 60% (Benirschke, 1999). Fetal problems include decreased intrauterine growth rate for each fetus, increased incidence of fetal anomalies, increased risk of prematurity and its associated problems, and abnormal presentations (W. E. Roberts, 2000).

Clinical Therapy

Once the presence of twins has been detected, preventing and treating problems that infringe on the development and birth of normal fetuses is the most significant clinical goal. Prenatal visits are more frequent for women with twins than for those with one fetus. Women with multiple-gestation pregnancies need to understand the nutritional implications of multiple fetuses, the assessment of fetal activity, the signs of preterm labor, and the danger signs of pregnancy.

Serial ultrasounds assess the growth of each fetus and provide early recognition of intrauterine growth restriction (IUGR). Some physicians believe that bed rest in the lateral position enhances utero-placental-fetal blood flow and decreases the risk of preterm labor. Others question the value of bed rest for the prevention of periodic uterine contractions, which seem to precede preterm labor (W. E. Roberts, 2000). More recent strategies include work leave and lifestyle modifications (Papiernik, Keith, Oleszcuzuk, et al., 1998).

Testing usually begins at 30 to 34 weeks' gestation and may include NST, BPP, and Doppler ultrasound to assess umbilical blood waveforms (Rodis, Arky, Egan, et al., 1999). A reactive NST is associated with good fetal outcome if birth occurs within 1 week of the testing. The NST is done every 3 to 7 days until birth or until results become nonreactive. The BPP is also accurate in assessing fetal status with twin pregnancies. A BPP of 8 or better for each fetus is considered reassuring, and weekly or biweekly BPPs and NSTs continue until birth.

Intrapartal management requires careful attention to maternal and fetal status. The mother should have an IV with a large-bore needle in place. Anesthesia and cross-

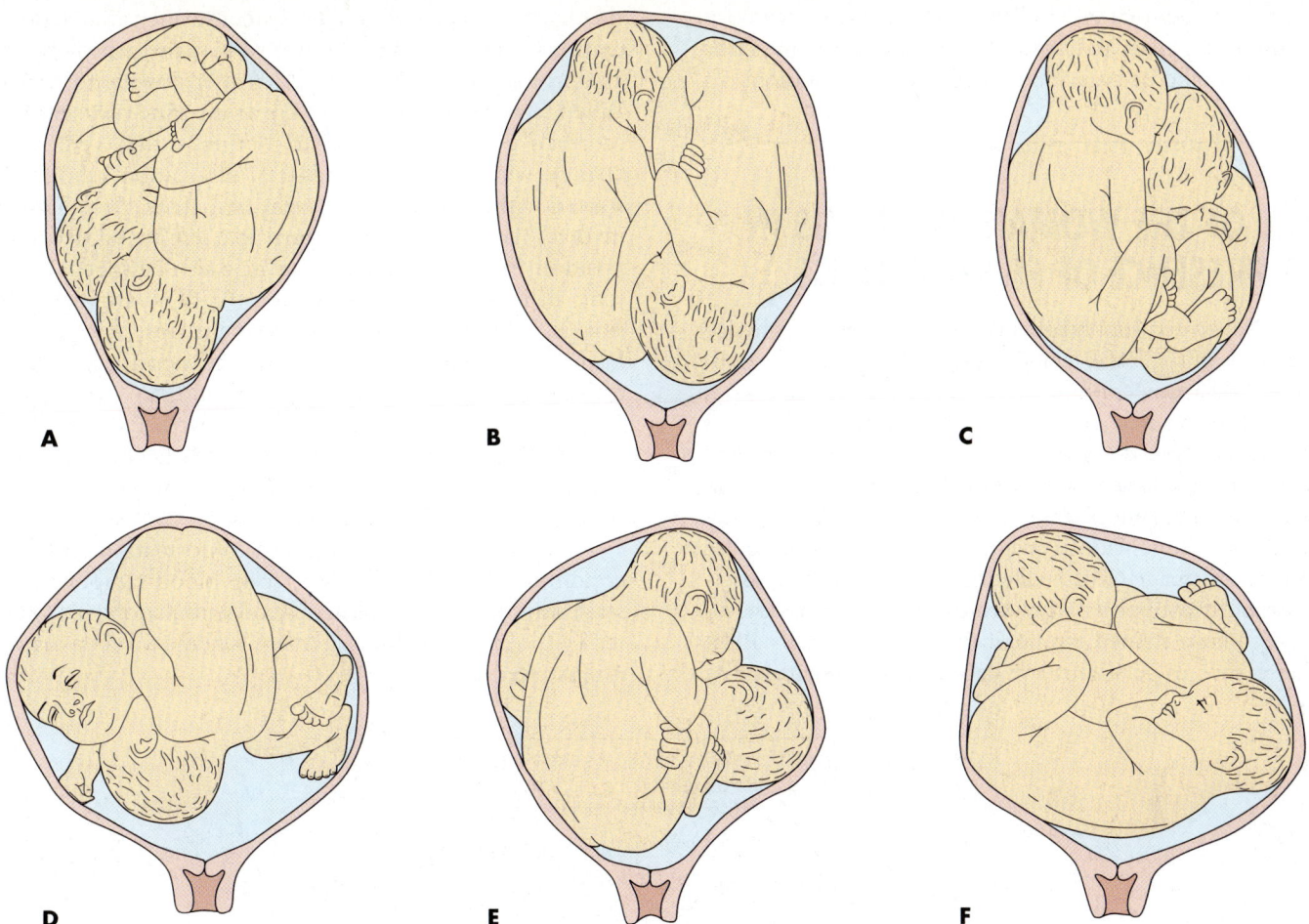

FIGURE 19–9. ◆ Twins may be in any of these presentations while in utero.

matched blood should be readily available. The twins are monitored by dual electronic fetal monitoring.

The decision about method of birth, which depends on a variety of factors, may not be made until labor occurs. The presence of maternal complications such as placenta previa, abruptio placentae, or severe PIH usually indicates the need for cesarean birth. Fetal factors such as severe IUGR, preterm birth, fetal anomalies, fetal distress, and unfavorable fetal position or presentation also require cesarean birth.

Any combination of presentations and positions can occur with multiple births. Figure 19–9 ◆ shows some possible presentations of twins. When the presenting fetus is in a nonvertex position, cesarean birth is usually indicated (Malone & D'Alton, 1999).

Nursing Management

NURSING CARE IN THE COMMUNITY

During pregnancy the woman may need counseling about diet and daily activities. Help her plan meals to meet her increased needs. A daily intake of 4,000 kcal (minimum) and 135 g of protein is recommended for optimal weight gain and fetal growth. A prenatal vitamin and 1 mg of folic acid should also be taken daily. A weight gain of 40 to 50 lb, with a 15- to 20-lb weight gain by 20 weeks, has been recommended for women with multiple-gestation pregnancy (Papiernik et al., 1998).

Counseling about daily activities may include encouraging the woman to plan frequent rest periods during the day. The rest period is most effective if the woman rests in a side-lying position (which increases uteroplacental blood flow) and elevates her lower legs and feet to reduce edema. Back discomfort may be relieved by pelvic rocking, maintaining good posture, and using good body mechanics when lifting objects and moving about.

HOSPITAL-BASED NURSING CARE

During labor, the FHRs of the siblings are monitored continuously by electronic fetal monitor (EFM). Electronic monitoring equipment now makes it possible to monitor the fetuses simultaneously, whether by external or internal means. They are monitored throughout labor and vaginal birth or up to the time of abdominal incision if a cesarean is done.

After birth, prepare to receive two or more newborns instead of one. This means duplicating everything, including resuscitation equipment, radiant warmers, and newborn identification papers and bracelets. Two or more physicians or nurses should be available for newborn resuscitation.

CARE OF THE WOMAN AND FETUS IN THE PRESENCE OF FETAL DISTRESS

When the oxygen supply is insufficient to meet the physiologic needs of the fetus, fetal distress may result. The condition may be acute, chronic, or a combination of the two. A variety of factors may contribute to fetal distress. The most common are cord compression and uteroplacental insufficiency, possibly caused by preexisting maternal or fetal disease or placental abnormalities. If the resulting hypoxia persists and metabolic acidosis occurs, the situation could cause permanent damage to or be life threatening for the fetus.

The most common early warning signs of fetal distress are meconium-stained amniotic fluid and ominous FHR patterns such as persistent late decelerations (regardless of

the depth of deceleration), persistent severe variable decelerations (especially if the return to baseline is prolonged), and prolonged decelerations (Uckan & Townsend, 1999). When fetal distress is indicated, **intrauterine resuscitation** (corrective measures used to optimize the oxygen exchange within the maternal-fetal circulation) should be started without delay. Treatment of maternal hypotension involves having the woman turn to a left lateral decubitus position (right lateral decubitus may also be tried), beginning an IV infusion or increasing the flow rate if an infusion is already in place, or, if cord prolapse is suspected, having the woman assume a knee-chest position. Uterine activity can be decreased by discontinuing IV oxytocin administration or administering a tocolytic agent (such as terbutaline) to decrease contraction frequency and intensity. Oxygen is also administered to the woman via facial mask (Uckan & Townsend, 1999).

Caregivers can obtain additional information about the condition of the fetus by fetal scalp blood sampling, fetal scalp stimulation, or fetal acoustical stimulation (see Chapter 14). The management scheme for fetal distress is illustrated in Figure 19–10 ◆.

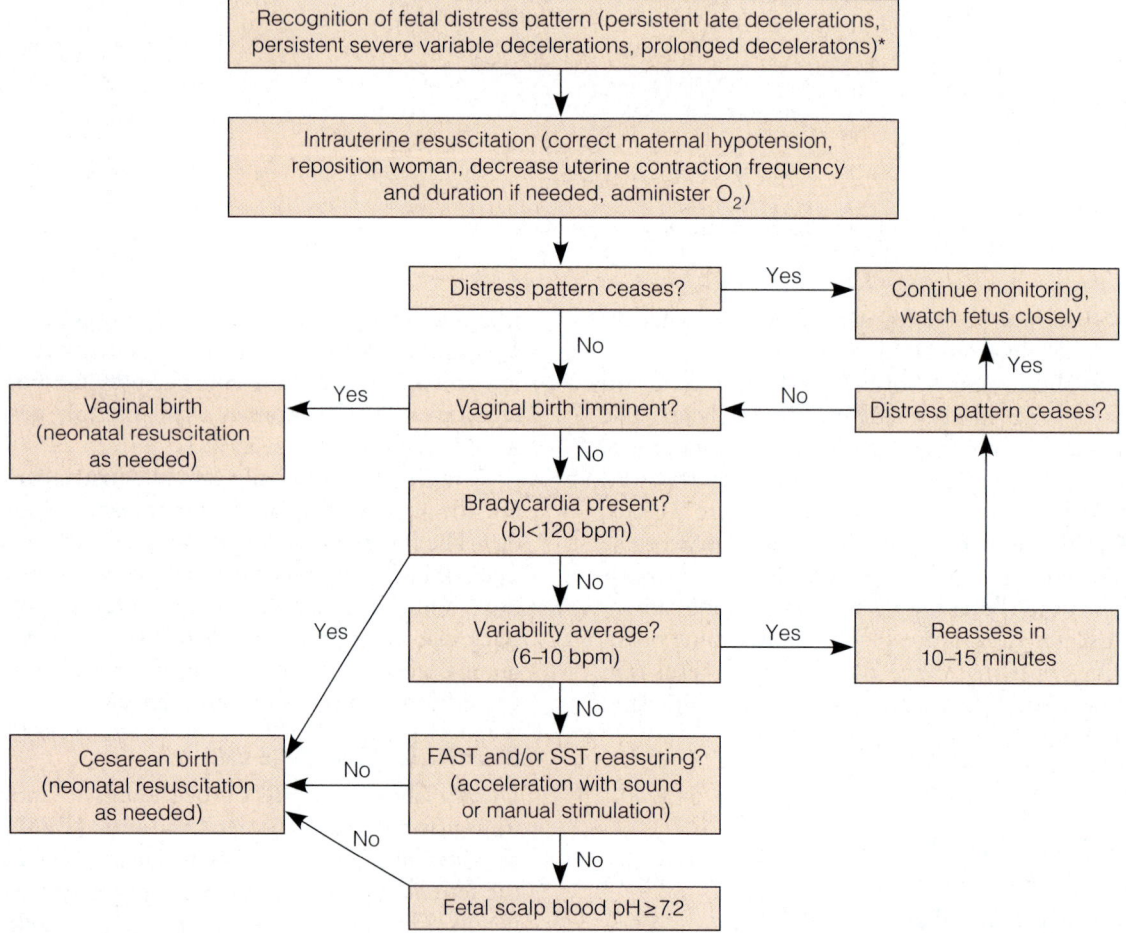

FIGURE 19–10. ◆ Intrapartum management of fetal distress. Note: bl = baseline; FAST = fetal acoustic stimulation test; SST = scalp stimulation test. *Note:* From Strong, T. H. (1990). Fetal distress in the intrapartum period. In E. J. Quilligan & F. P. Zuspan (Eds.), *Current therapy in obstetrics and gynecology* (3rd ed.). Philadelphia: Saunders. *Huddleston, J. F., & Freeman, R. K. (1992). Estimation of fetal well-being. In A. A. Fanaroff & R. S. Martin (Eds.), *Neonatal-perinatal medicine: Diseases of the fetus and newborn* (5th ed.). St. Louis, MO: Mosby-Year Book.

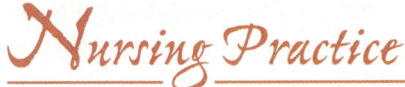

To determine whether the FHR is reassuring, look for the following (Schmidt, 2000):

- Baseline heart rate is between 120 and 160 bpm.
- Long-term variability is average.
- Short-term variability (can only be assessed with an internal EFM device) is present.
- Accelerations are spontaneous.
- Decelerations are absent or limited to early or occasional variables (see Chapter 14).

Maternal Implications

Indications of fetal distress greatly increase the psychologic stress of a laboring woman. Professional staff members may become so involved in assessing fetal status and initiating corrective measures that they fail to provide the woman and her partner with explanations and emotional support. It is imperative to offer both. In many instances, if birth is not imminent, the woman must undergo cesarean birth. This method of birth may be a source of fear and of frustration, too, if the couple prepared for a shared vaginal birth experience.

CLINICAL THERAPY

When evidence of possible fetal distress exists, treatment centers on improving the blood flow to the fetus by correcting maternal hypotension, decreasing the intensity and frequency of contractions if present, providing IV fluids to the woman as needed, administering oxygen, and gathering further information about fetal status. Fetal response to intrauterine resuscitation measures dictates subsequent actions.

NURSING MANAGEMENT

Review the woman's prenatal history and note the presence of any conditions (such as PIH, diabetes, renal disease, intrauterine growth restriction (IUGR) that may be associated with decreased uteroplacental-fetal blood flow. When the membranes rupture, assess the FHR immediately and note the characteristics of the amniotic fluid. As labor progresses, be especially alert to suspicious changes in the FHR. At all times, encourage and support maternal positioning that maximizes utero-placental-fetal blood flow.

CARE OF THE FAMILY AT RISK DUE TO INTRAUTERINE FETAL DEATH

Intrauterine fetal death (IUFD), often referred to as fetal demise, accounts for one half of perinatal mortality after 20 weeks' gestation. Fetal death results from unknown causes or from a number of physiologic maladaptations including preeclampsia or eclampsia, abruptio placentae, placenta previa, diabetes, infection, congenital anomalies, and isoimmune disease.

Prolonged retention of the dead fetus may lead to the development of disseminated intravascular coagulation (DIC), also called consumption coagulopathy, in the mother. After the release of thromboplastin from the degenerating fetal tissues into the maternal bloodstream, the extrinsic clotting system is activated, triggering the formation of multiple tiny blood clots. Fibrinogen and factors V and VII are subsequently depleted, and the woman begins to display symptoms of DIC. Fibrinogen levels begin a linear descent 3 to 4 weeks after the death of the fetus and continue to decrease in the absence of appropriate medical intervention.

Clinical Therapy

When fetal death has occurred, abdominal x-ray examination may reveal Spalding's sign, an overriding of the fetal cranial bones. In addition, maternal estriol levels fall. Diagnosis of intrauterine fetal death is confirmed by absence of heart action on ultrasound. Most women have spontaneous labor within 2 weeks of fetal death. If other complications are not present, some physicians wait for labor to begin spontaneously (Anderson, 2000). In the absence of spontaneous labor, induction measures are begun.

Nursing Management

Nursing Assessment and Diagnosis

Cessation of fetal movement reported by the mother to the nurse is frequently the first indication of fetal death. It is followed by a gradual decrease in the signs and symptoms of pregnancy. Fetal heart tones are absent, and fetal movement is no longer palpable. Once fetal demise is established, assess the family members' ability to adapt to their loss. Open communication between the mother, her partner, and the health team members contributes to a realistic understanding of the medical condition and its associated treatments. It may be helpful to discuss prior experiences the family has had with stress and what they feel were their perceived coping abilities at that time. Identifying the family's social supports and resources is also important.

Nursing diagnoses that may apply include the following:

- *Grief* related to death of the fetus
- *Ineffective individual and family coping* related to depression secondary to loss of a child
- *Ineffective family coping* related to death of a child

Planning and Implementation

The parents of a stillborn infant suffer a devastating experience that precipitates an intense emotional trauma. During the pregnancy, the couple has already begun the attachment process, which now must be terminated through the grieving process. Although enough similarity among individuals exists to identify some common phases in the course of grief, the process is "more fluid than an ordering of discrete phases would seem to imply" (Kay, Roman, & Schulte, 1997, p. 8). Therefore, it is important to recognize and honor the individual, using the three phases of grief that follow as general guidelines (Kay et al., 1997).

1. Often the first phase is protest of the death of the fetus. This is likely to result in immediate shock and numbness, followed by disbelief and denial. In most cases this inability to grasp the reality of the loss is short lived and is followed by distress. When the caregiver first suspects fetal demise, the mother or parents may initially attempt to dismiss the possibility because the loss is too difficult to consider. When the death is confirmed, there may be a brief period during which the family refuses to believe it, followed by development of visible signs of loss such as weeping.

2. The second phase is disorganization, which involves developing awareness of the finality of the loss. Feelings of profound sadness and a deep yearning for the lost baby develop. Isolation, loneliness, and meaninglessness manifest into withdrawal from everyone and everything. The most common characteristic of disorganization is preoccupation with painful thoughts and visions of the lost infant.

3. Reorganization is the third and final phase. This step in the mourning process is the most individual of all, as the bereaved parents slowly begin to reengage with the world. The time frame varies greatly, but eventually painful memories become less frequent and new activities are begun. However, this phase may be accompanied by transitory feelings of guilt for enjoying life again in spite of the loss.

Nursing Practice

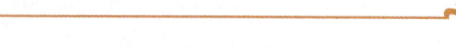

No matter who you are, or how much nursing experience you have, when an expectant family is in pain because of their loss, you will probably feel that you do not have the right thing to say. "I'm sorry and I don't know what to say" is a start.

Some facilities use a checklist to ensure that caregivers address important aspects of working with the parents. The checklist becomes a communication tool as staff members share information particular to the couple. Such a checklist might include the following items:

▶ When fetal death has been confirmed before admission, inform the staff so they can avoid making inappropriate remarks.

▶ Allow the woman and her partner to remain together as much as they wish. Provide privacy and a supportive environment.

▶ Stay with the couple; do not leave them alone and isolated.

▶ As much as possible, have the same nurse provide care to increase the support for the couple. Develop a care plan to provide for continuity of care.

▶ Have the most experienced labor and birth nurse auscultate for fetal heart tones to avoid the searching that a more inexperienced nurse might feel compelled to do. Avoid the temptation to listen again "to make sure."

▶ Listen to the couple; do not offer explanations. They require solace without minimizing the situation.

▶ Facilitate active participation of the woman and her partner in the labor and birth process. Help them to make decisions about who is present and what rituals will occur during the birth process. Allow the woman to make the decision regarding anesthesia and analgesia during labor and birth.

▶ Give parents accurate information about plans for labor and birth.

▶ Provide ongoing opportunities for the couple to ask questions.

▶ Arrange for the woman to be assigned to a room that is away from new mothers and babies. If early discharge is an option, allow the family to make that decision.

▶ Encourage the couple to experience the grief that they feel. A couple may have intense feelings that they are unable to share with each other. Encourage them to talk and allow their emotions to show freely. Help them understand that they may each experience different feelings.

▶ Give the couple an opportunity to see and hold the stillborn infant in a private, quiet location. (Advocates of seeing the stillborn believe that viewing assists in dispelling denial and enables the couple to progress to the next step in the grieving process.) If they choose to see their stillborn infant, prepare the couple for what they will see by saying "the baby is cold," "the baby is blue," "the baby is bruised," or other appropriate statements.

▶ Some families may elect to bathe or dress their stillborn; support them in their choice.

▶ Take a photograph of the infant and let the family know it is available if they want it now or some time in the future.

▶ Offer a card with footprints, crib card, identification band, and possibly a lock of hair to the parents. These items may be kept with the photo if the parents do not want them at this time.

▶ Prepare the couple to return home. If there are siblings, each will usually progress through age-appropriate grieving. Provide the parents with information about normal mourning reactions, both psychologic and physiologic.

- Give the mother educational materials that discuss the changes she will experience in returning to a nonpregnant state.
- Provide information about community support groups, including group name, contact person (if possible), and phone number. Use materials such as the book *When Hello Means Goodbye* by Schwiebert and Kirk (1985).
- Contact religious support systems if the parents desire.

The nurse experiences many of the same grief reactions as the parents of a stillborn infant. It is important to have support persons and colleagues available for counseling and support.

Evaluation

Expected outcomes of nursing care include the following:

- Family members express their feelings about the death of their baby.
- Family members participate in the decision of whether to see their baby and other decisions about the baby.
- The family has resources available for continued support.
- Family members know the community resources available and have names and phone numbers to use if they choose.
- The family is moving into and through the grieving process.

CARE OF THE WOMAN AND FETUS AT RISK DUE TO PLACENTAL PROBLEMS

The most common types of placental problems are abruptio placentae, placenta previa, and abnormalities in placental formation and structure. Because the placenta is very vascular, problems are usually associated with maternal and possibly fetal hemorrhage. Abruptio placentae is a major emergency in labor and birth and requires rapid, effective interventions. Although placenta previa is primarily an antepartal problem, it is presented here for the sake of comparison. Causes and sources of hemorrhage are highlighted in Table 19–1.

Abruptio Placentae

Abruptio placentae is the premature separation of a normally implanted placenta from the uterine wall. Premature separation is considered a catastrophic event because of the severity of the resulting hemorrhage. The incidence of abruptio placentae is approximately 1 in 100 births and occurs more frequently in pregnancies complicated by hypertension and cocaine abuse. The risk of recurrence is much higher than for the general population (Yeo, Ananth, & Vintzileos, 2001).

TABLE 19-1 Causes and Sources of Hemorrhage

Causes and Sources	Signs and Symptoms
Antepartal Period	
Abortion	Vaginal bleeding
	Intermittent uterine contractions
	Rupture of membranes
Placenta previa	Painless vaginal bleeding after seventh month
Abruptio placentae	
Partial	Vaginal bleeding: no increase in uterine pain
Severe	Vaginal bleeding may or may not be present
	Extreme tenderness of abdominal area
	Rigid, boardlike abdomen
	Increase in size of abdomen
Intrapartal Period	
Placenta previa	Bright-red vaginal bleeding
Abruptio placentae	Same signs and symptoms listed earlier
Uterine atony in stage 3	Bright-red vaginal bleeding
	Ineffectual contractility
Postpartal Period	
Uterine atony	Boggy uterus
	Dark vaginal bleeding
	Presence of clots
Retained placental fragments	Boggy uterus
	Dark vaginal bleeding
	Presence of clots
Lacerations of cervix or vagina	Firm uterus
	Bright-red blood

The cause of abruptio placentae is largely unknown. Theories have been proposed relating its occurrence to decreased blood flow to the placenta through the sinuses during the last trimester. Excessive intrauterine pressure caused by hydramnios or multiple-gestation pregnancy, maternal hypertension, cigarette smoking, alcohol ingestion, increased maternal age and parity, trauma, and sudden changes in intrauterine pressure (as with amniotomy) have been suggested as contributing factors (Yeo et al., 2001).

Abruptio placentae is subdivided into three types (Figure 19–11):

- *Marginal*. In this case the placenta separates at its edges, the blood passes between the fetal membranes and the uterine wall, and the blood escapes vaginally (also called marginal sinus rupture).

- *Central*. In this situation, the placenta separates centrally, and the blood is trapped between the placenta and the uterine wall. Entrapment of the blood results in concealed bleeding.

- *Complete*. Massive vaginal bleeding is seen in the presence of total separation.

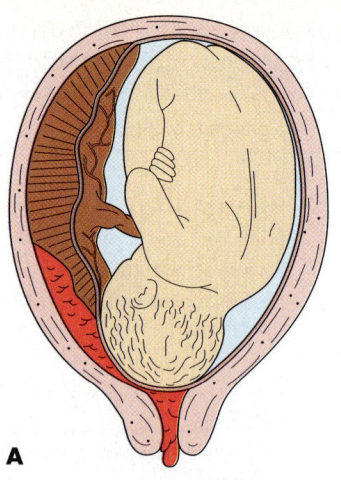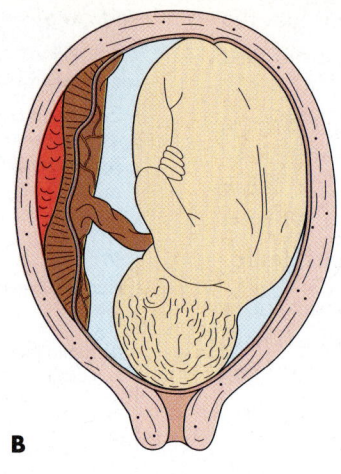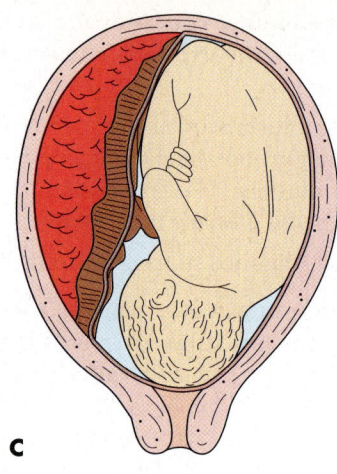

FIGURE 19–11. ◆ Abruptio placentae. **A,** Marginal abruption with external hemorrhage. **B,** Central abruption with concealed hemorrhage. **C,** Complete separation.

TABLE 19–2	Differential Signs and Symptoms of Placenta Previa and Abruptio Placentae	
	Placenta Previa	*Abruptio Placentae*
Onset	Quiet and sneaky	Sudden and stormy
Bleeding	External	External or concealed
Color of blood	Bright red	Dark venous
Anemia	= Blood loss	> Apparent blood loss
Shock	= Blood loss	> Apparent blood loss
Toxemia	Absent	May be present
Pain	Only during labor	Severe and steady
Uterine tenderness	Absent	Present
Uterine tone	Soft and relaxed	Firm to stony hard
Uterine contour	Normal	May enlarge and change shape
Fetal heart tones	Usually present	Present or absent
Engagement	Absent	May be present
Presentation	May be abnormal	No relationship

Note: From Oxom, H. (1986). *Human labor and birth* (5th ed., p. 507). Reproduced with permission from the McGraw-Hill Companies.

The signs and symptoms of these three types of placental abruption are listed in Table 19–2. In severe cases of central abruptio placentae, the blood invades the myometrial tissues between the muscle fibers. This occurrence accounts for the uterine irritability that is a significant sign of abruptio placentae. If hemorrhage continues, eventually the uterus turns entirely blue because the muscle fibers are filled with blood. After birth the uterus contracts poorly. This condition is known as Couvelaire uterus and frequently necessitates hysterectomy.

As a result of the damage to the uterine wall and the retroplacental clotting with central abruption, large amounts of thromboplastin are released into the maternal blood supply. This thromboplastin in turn triggers the development of DIC and resultant hypofibrinogenemia. Fibrinogen levels, ordinarily elevated in pregnancy, may drop in minutes to the point at which blood will no longer coagulate (Yeo, et al., 2001).

MATERNAL IMPLICATIONS

Postpartal problems depend in large part on the severity of the intrapartal bleeding, coagulation defects (DIC), hypofibrinogenemia, and time between separation and birth. Moderate to severe hemorrhage results in hemorrhagic shock, which may prove fatal to the mother if it is not rapidly reversed. In the postpartal period, women with this disorder are at risk for hemorrhage and renal failure due to shock, vascular spasm, intravascular clotting, or a combination of these factors.

FETAL-NEONATAL IMPLICATIONS

Perinatal mortality associated with abruptio placentae ranges from 20% to 40% (Yeo et al., 2001). In severe cases, in which most of the placenta has separated, the infant mortality rate is 100%. In less severe separation, fetal outcome depends on the level of maturity. The most serious complications in the newborn arise from preterm labor, anemia, and hypoxia. If fetal hypoxia progresses unchecked, irreversible brain damage or fetal demise may result. Thorough assessment and prompt action on the part of the health team can improve both fetal and maternal outcomes.

CLINICAL THERAPY

Because of the risk of DIC, evaluating the results of coagulation tests is imperative. In DIC, fibrinogen levels and platelet counts usually decrease; prothrombin times and partial thromboplastin times are normal to prolonged. If the values are not markedly abnormal, serial testing may be helpful in establishing an abnormal trend indicative of coagulopathy. Another test determines levels of fibrin-degradation products; these values rise with DIC.

After establishing the diagnosis, emphasis is placed on maintaining the cardiovascular status of the mother and developing a plan for effecting the birth of the fetus. The birth method selected depends on the condition of the woman and fetus; in many circumstances, cesarean birth may be the safest option.

If the separation is mild and the pregnancy is near term, labor may be induced and the fetus born vaginally with as little trauma as possible. If rupture of membranes and oxytocin infusion by pump do not initiate labor, a cesarean birth is required. A long delay would raise the risk of increased hemorrhage, with resulting hypofibrinogenemia.

Specific tests for coagulation failure are:

- Partial thromboplastin time (normal = 35 to 45 s)
- Prothrombin time (normal = 10 to 14 s)
- Thrombin time (normal = 10 to 15 s)
- Fibrinogen levels (normal = 2.5 to 4 g/L)
- Fibrin degradation products
- Whole blood screen and platelet count

Supportive actions to decrease the risk of DIC include typing and crossmatching for blood transfusions (at least four units), evaluating the clotting mechanism, and providing IV fluids (Perry, 2000a).

In cases of moderate to severe placental separation, a cesarean birth is done concurrently with treatment of hypofibrinogenemia by IV infusion of coagulation factors or plasma. Vaginal birth is impossible with a Couvelaire uterus, because the uterus would not contract properly in labor. Severe hemorrhage necessitates cesarean birth to allow an immediate hysterectomy to save both the woman and the fetus.

The hypovolemia that accompanies severe abruptio placentae is life threatening and requires the administration of whole blood. If the fetus is alive but in distress, emergency cesarean birth is the method of choice. With a stillborn fetus, vaginal birth is preferable unless maternal shock from hemorrhage is uncontrollable (Perry, 2000a). Central venous pressure (CVP) monitoring may be needed to evaluate IV fluid replacement. A normal CVP of 10 cm H_2O is the goal. Elevations of CVP may indicate fluid overload

and pulmonary edema. Laboratory testing provides ongoing data about hemoglobin, hematocrit, and coagulation status. The hematocrit is maintained through the administration of packed red blood cells or whole blood (Perry, 2000a). Measures are taken to stimulate labor to prevent DIC. An amniotomy may be performed, and oxytocin is given to hasten delivery. Progressive dilatation and effacement usually occur (Perry, 2000a).

NURSING MANAGEMENT

Electronic monitoring of the uterine contractions and resting tone between contractions provides information about the labor pattern and effectiveness of the oxytocin induction. Since uterine resting tone is frequently increased with abruptio placentae, it must be evaluated frequently for further increase. Abdominal girth measurements may be ordered hourly and are obtained by placing a tape measure around the maternal abdomen at the level of the umbilicus. Another method of evaluating uterine size, which increases as more bleeding occurs at the site of abruption, involves placing a mark at the top of the uterine fundus; the distance from the symphysis pubis to the mark may be measured hourly. Begin continuous fetal monitoring immediately to monitor for fetal distress.

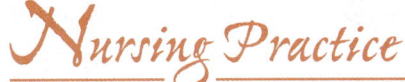 

The amount of bleeding per vagina is no guide to the degree of placental separation.

Placenta Previa

In **placenta previa,** the placenta is implanted in the lower uterine segment rather than the upper portion of the uterus. This implantation may be on a portion of the lower segment or over the internal cervical os. As the lower uterine segment contracts and dilates in the later weeks of pregnancy, the placental villi are torn from the uterine wall, thus exposing the uterine sinuses at the placental site. Bleeding begins, but because its amount depends on the number of sinuses exposed, initially it may be either scanty or profuse (Figure 19–12 ♦).

The cause of placenta previa is unknown. Statistically it occurs in about 1 in every 200 births. Women with a previous history of placenta previa have a recurrence rate as high as 10% to 15%. Other factors associated with placenta previa are multiparity, increasing age, placenta accreta, defective development of blood vessels in the decidua, and a large placenta (Perry, 2000b).

FETAL-NEONATAL IMPLICATIONS

The prognosis for the fetus depends on the extent of placenta previa. Changes in the FHR and meconium staining of the amniotic fluid may be apparent. In a profuse bleeding

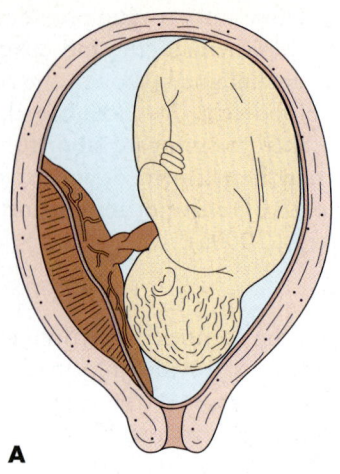
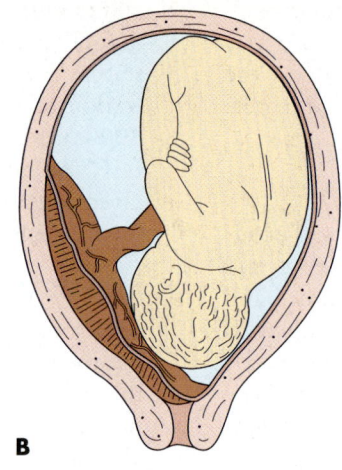
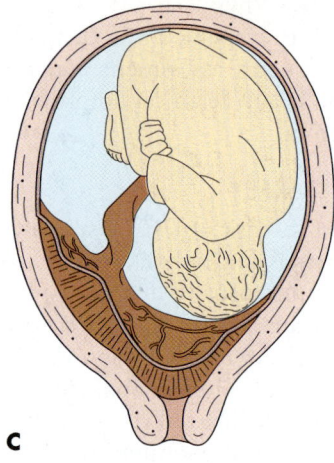

A **B** **C**

FIGURE 19–12. ◆ Placenta previa. **A,** Low placental implantation. **B,** Partial placenta previa. **C,** Total placenta previa.

episode, the fetus is compromised and suffers some hypoxia. FHR monitoring is imperative when the woman is admitted, particularly if a vaginal birth is anticipated, because the presenting part of the fetus may obstruct the flow of blood from the placenta or umbilical cord. If fetal distress occurs, cesarean birth is indicated. After birth, blood sampling should be done to determine whether the intrauterine bleeding episodes of the woman have caused anemia in the newborn.

CLINICAL THERAPY

The goal of medical care is to identify the cause of bleeding and to provide treatment that will ensure birth of a mature newborn. Indirect diagnosis is made by localizing the placenta through tests that require no vaginal examination. The most common diagnostic test is the ultrasound scan (Figure 19–13◆). If placenta previa is ruled out, a vaginal examination can be performed with a speculum to determine the cause of bleeding (such as cervical lesions).

The differential diagnosis of placental or cervical bleeding takes careful consideration. Partial separation of the placenta may also present with painless bleeding, and true placenta previa may not demonstrate overt bleeding until labor begins, thus confusing the diagnosis.

Care of the woman with painless late-gestational bleeding depends on (1) the week of gestation during which the first bleeding episode occurs and (2) the amount of bleeding (Figure 19–14◆). If the pregnancy is less than 37 weeks' gestation, expectant management is used to delay birth until about 37 weeks' gestation to allow the fetus to mature. Expectant management involves stringent regulation of the following:

1. Bed rest with bathroom privileges as long as the woman is not bleeding
2. No vaginal exams
3. Monitoring blood loss, pain, and uterine contractility
4. Evaluating FHR with an external fetal monitor

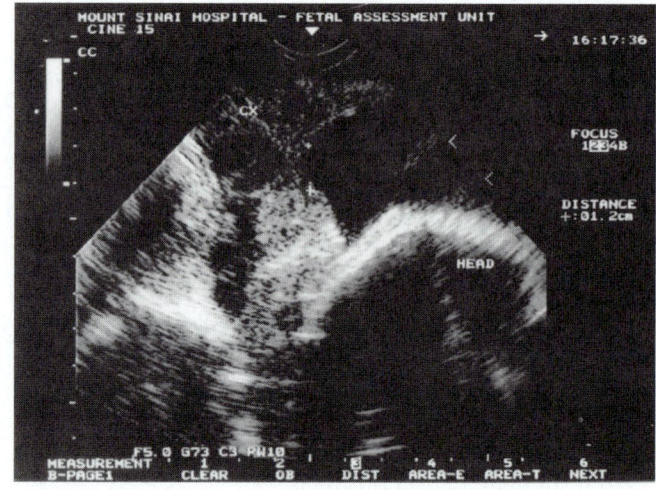

FIGURE 19–13. ◆ Ultrasound of placenta previa.

5. Monitoring maternal vital signs
6. Complete laboratory evaluation: hemoglobin, hematocrit, Rh factor, and urinalysis
7. Intravenous fluid (lactated Ringer's solution)
8. Two units of crossmatched blood available for transfusion

If frequent, recurrent, or profuse bleeding persists, or if fetal well-being appears threatened, a cesarean birth may be performed.

Nursing Management

Nursing Assessment and Diagnosis

Assessment of the woman with placenta previa must be ongoing to prevent or treat complications that are potentially

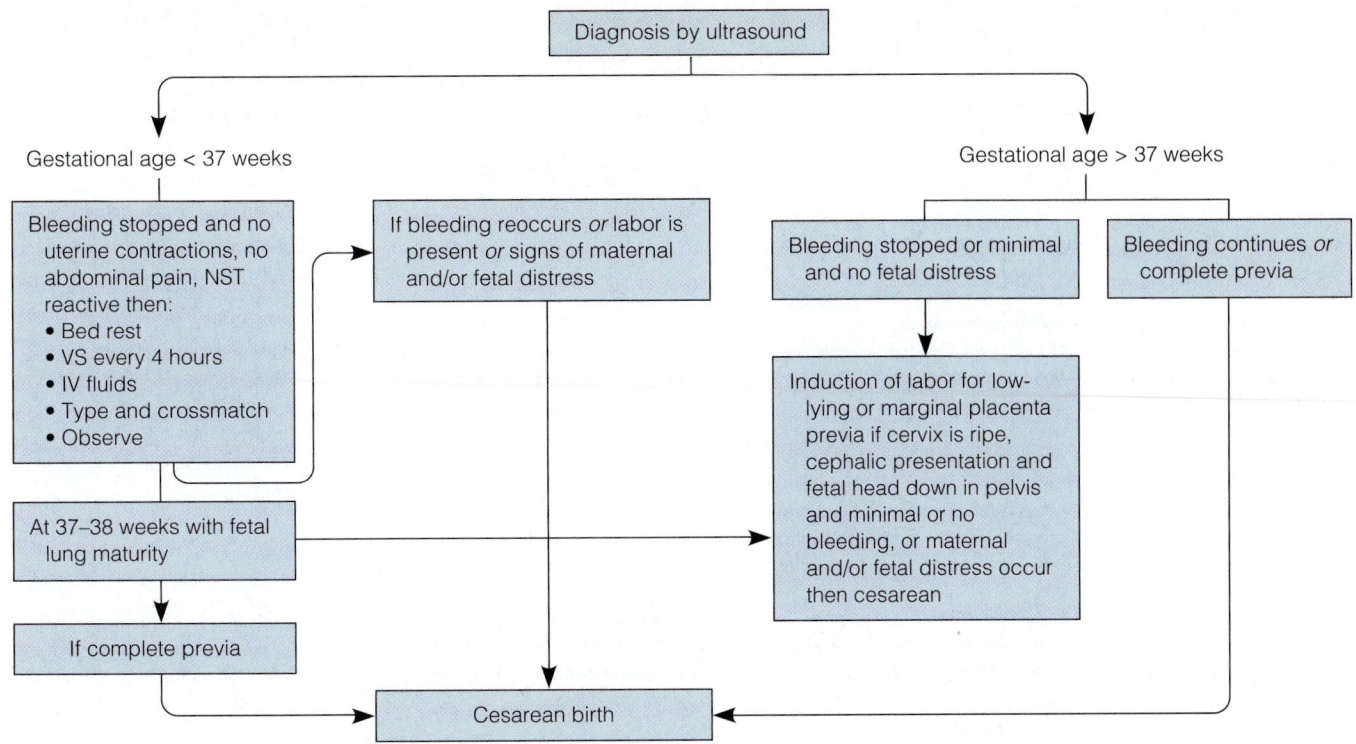

FIGURE 19–14. ◆ Management of placenta previa. *Note:* From Barker, R. K., Fields, D. H., & Kaufman, S. A. (1990). *Quick reference to OB-GYN procedures* (3rd ed.). New York: Lippincott/Harper & Row.

lethal to the mother and fetus. Painless, bright-red vaginal bleeding is the most accurate diagnostic sign of placenta previa. If this sign develops during the last 3 months of pregnancy, placenta previa should always be considered until ruled out by examination. The first bleeding episode is generally scanty. If no vaginal examinations are performed, it often subsides spontaneously. However, each subsequent hemorrhage is more profuse.

The uterus remains soft, and if labor begins, it relaxes fully between contractions. The FHR usually remains stable unless profuse hemorrhage and maternal shock occur. As a result of the placement of the placenta, the fetal presenting part is often unengaged, and transverse lie is common.

Assess blood loss, pain, and uterine contractility both subjectively and objectively. Maternal vital signs and the results of blood and urine tests provide additional data about the woman's condition. Evaluate the FHR with continuous external fetal monitoring. Another pressing nursing responsibility is to observe and verify the family's ability to cope with the anxiety associated with an unknown outcome.

Nursing diagnoses that may apply include the following:

▶ *Fluid volume deficit* related to hypovolemia secondary to excessive blood loss

▶ *Risk for impaired fetal gas exchange* related to decreased blood volume and maternal hypotension

▶ *Anxiety* related to concern for own personal status and the baby's safety

Planning and Implementation

Monitor the woman and her fetus to determine the status of the bleeding and the responses of the mother and baby. Vital signs, intake and output, and other pertinent assessments must be made frequently. Use the electronic monitor tracing to evaluate fetal status. Have a whole-blood setup ready for IV infusion and establish a patent IV line before caregivers undertake any intrusive procedures. Monitor maternal vital signs every 15 minutes in the absence of hemorrhage and every 5 minutes with active hemorrhage. Connect the external tocodynamometer to the maternal abdomen to monitor uterine activity continuously.

Providing emotional support for the family is an important nursing care goal. During active bleeding, direct the assessments and management toward physical support. However, emotional aspects need to be addressed simultaneously. Explain the assessments and treatment measures needed. Make time for questions, and act as an advocate in obtaining information for the family. Offer emotional support by staying with the family and using touch.

Promoting neonatal physiologic adaptation is another important nursing responsibility. Check the newborn's hemoglobin, cell volume, and erythrocyte count immediately and then monitor them closely. The newborn may require oxygen, administration of blood, and admission into a special care nursery. See "Nursing Care Plan: Hemorrhage in the Third Trimester" and Clinical Pathway.

GOAL	INTERVENTION	RATIONALE	EXPECTED OUTCOME

1. High risk for fluid volume deficit related to excessive vascular loss during pregnancy.

	NIC Intervention:		*NOC Outcome:*
	Fluid management: *Promotion of fluid balance and prevention of complications resulting from abnormal or undesired fluid levels*		**Fluid balance:** *Balance of water in the intracellular and extracellular compartments of the body*
Patient will not experience significant fluid volume deficit during the third trimester of pregnancy.	▶ Monitor vital signs (i.e., temperature—normal range is 96.8–100.4, pulse—normal is 60–80, respirations—normal is 12–20, blood pressure—normal range is 110/70 to 138/88, central venous pressure—normal range is 5–10 mm H_2O). Compare present blood pressure with woman's baseline blood pressure. Note pulse pressure.	▶ Any deviations in a patient's baseline vital signs could indicate intravascular fluctuations.	The patient will show signs of adequate fluid volume during pregnancy as evidenced by vital signs within normal limits, capillary refill < 3 seconds, adequate sensorium, and urine output > 30 mL/hr.
	▶ Instruct patient on initiating pad counts. Teach patient how to weigh pads and chux with each gram = to approximately 1 mL of blood loss.	▶ The combination of weighing and counting pads and chux assists medical personnel in determining patient blood loss.	
	▶ Report amount of blood loss within a specific period of time (e.g., 50 mL of bright red blood on pad in 20 minutes).		
	▶ Monitor urinary output hourly and measure urine specific gravity (normal: 1.010–1.025).	▶ A decrease in urinary output (30 cc/hr) and an increase in specific gravity suggest dehydration and a need for an increase in fluid intake.	
	▶ Palpate bilateral peripheral pulses (normal: equal and strong) and note capillary refill (normal: < 3 seconds). Also, assess skin color and temperature (normal: pink, warm, dry, and intact).	▶ Helps determine signs of circulatory loss or hypovolemic shock that include weak pulses, capillary refill > 3 seconds, skin color that is cyanotic or pallor, and skin temperature that is cool and clammy.	
	▶ Assess mental status at frequent intervals.	▶ Excessive blood loss can lead to changes in mentation.	
	▶ Assess patient for signs and symptoms of disseminated intravascular coagulation.	▶ Provides vital information on maternal status.	
	▶ Instruct patient on importance of strict bed rest and avoidance of any sexual activity that may lead to orgasm.	▶ Bleeding may cease with limited activity. Pressure on the abdomen and orgasm can stimulate uterine activity, thereby causing bleeding.	
	▶ Monitor fetal status and uterine activity by continuous fetal monitoring.	▶ May determine origin of bleeding and fetal well-being.	
	Collaborative: Collect and review blood work: CBC, type and crossmatch, Rh titer, fibrinogen levels, platelet count, APTT, PT, and hCG levels.	▶ Determines blood loss and need for intervention if blood work is abnormal.	
	▶ Administer appropriate isotonic IV solutions and blood products (e.g., plasma expanders, whole blood, serum albumin, or packed red blood cells) as ordered by physician.	▶ Reverses shock symptoms by increasing blood volume.	
	▶ Insert Foley catheter.	▶ Close monitoring of urinary output will aid in determining adequate renal perfusion.	

GOAL	INTERVENTION	RATIONALE	EXPECTED OUTCOME

2. Risk for altered tissue perfusion (uteroplacental) related to hypovolemia secondary to excessive maternal blood loss.

	NIC Intervention:		NOC Outcome:
	Electronic fetal monitoring: *Electronic evaluation of fetal heart rate response to movement, external stimuli, or uterine contractions during antepartal testing*		**Circulation status:** *Extent to which blood flows unobstructed, unidirectionally, and at an appropriate pressure through large vessels of the systemic and pulmonary circuits*
The fetus will have no evidence of hypoxia during pregnancy.	▸ Assess maternal vital signs.	▸ Closely monitoring maternal physiologic status and circulatory status will assist in determining if an episode of bleeding has occurred and allow for interventions to protect maternal and fetal well-being.	
	▸ Monitor fetal heart tones continuously, assessing for variability, accelerations, and decelerations, and record.	▸ Continuous electronic fetal monitoring will aid in detecting signs of fetal hypoxia and allow time for appropriate intervention.	Fetus will demonstrate adequate tissue perfusion as evidenced by fetal heart tones that remain within 120–160 bpm, long-term variability and short-term variability present, positive periodic changes (no variable or late decelerations), and fetal scalp blood pH > 7.25.
	▸ Encourage patient to adhere to a strict lateral lying bed rest regimen.	▸ Promotes good placental/fetal oxygen exchange because pressure on the inferior vena cava is relieved.	
	▸ Assess fundal height.	▸ Determines an approximate gestational age.	
	▸ Assess labor progression by determining cervical dilatation and effacement if contractions are present.	▸ Provides information on maternal labor status.	
	Collaborative:		
	▸ Perform scalp stimulation to assess fetal accelerations.	▸ An FHR acceleration is considered 15 beats above the baseline lasting for 15 seconds and is indicative of fetal well-being.	
	▸ Assess amniotic fluid for meconium.	▸ Impaired gas exchange relaxes fetal intestinal motility causing expulsion of meconium into amniotic fluid.	
	▸ Assist physician during ultrasonography and amniocentesis (L/S ratio sample).	▸ Determines viability and alerts appropriate medical personnel of fetal age if delivery is imminent.	

3. Fear/anxiety related to personal and fetal well-being secndary to third-trimester hemorrhage.

	NIC Intervention:		NOC Outcome:
	Anxiety reduction: *Minimizing apprehension, dread, foreboding, or uneasiness related to an unidentified source of anticipated danger*		**Fear control:** *Ability to eliminate or reduce disabling feelings of alarm aroused by an identifiable source*
The patient will verbalize a decrease in fear and anxiety.	▸ Maintain frequent contact with patient and family members.	▸ Establishes trust with patient and family members and the patient will not feel alone or abandoned.	The patient will actively seek infor-mation about diagnosis and prognosis.
	▸ Provide patient with accurate, reliable information concerning diagnosis and prognosis.	▸ Fear and anxiety will lessen when patient is informed of health status and is allowed to make decisions based on present situation.	The patient and family members develop appropriate coping strategies that decrease fear and anxiety.
	▸ Allow patient and family members to verbalize origination of fears.	▸ Recognizing the origination of fear gives the patient and family the appropriate tool to begin the process of developing coping strategies for dealing with the fears.	
	▸ Explain all procedures in an easy-to-understand, nonthreatening manner, and allow patient and family members to ask questions.	▸ Accurate information prepares patient and family members of the impending procedures, thereby reducing fear of the unknown.	

Evaluation

Expected outcomes of nursing care include the following:

▶ The cause of hemorrhage is recognized promptly and corrective measures are taken.

▶ The woman's vital signs remain in the normal range.

▶ Any other complications are recognized and treated early.

▶ The family understands what has happened and the implications and associated problems of placenta previa.

▶ The woman and her baby have a safe labor and birth.

Other Placental Problems

Other problems of the placenta are presented in Table 19–3.

CARE OF THE WOMAN AND FETUS WITH A PROLAPSED UMBILICAL CORD

A **prolapsed umbilical cord** results when the umbilical cord precedes the fetal presenting part. When this occurs, pressure is placed on the umbilical cord as it is trapped between the presenting part and the maternal pelvis. Consequently, the vessels carrying blood to and from the fetus are compressed (Figure 19–15). Prolapse of the cord

TABLE 19–3   Placental and Umbilical Cord Variations

Placental Variation	Maternal Implications	Fetal-Neonatal Implications	
SUCCENTURIATE PLACENTA One or more accessory lobes of fetal villi will develop on the placenta.	Postpartal hemorrhage from retained lobe	None, as long as all parts of the placenta remain attached until after birth of the fetus	
CIRCUMVALLATE PLACENTA A double fold of chorion and amnion form a ring around the umbilical cord, on the fetal side of the placenta.	Increased incidence of late abortion, antepartal hemorrhage, and preterm labor	Intrauterine growth restriction, prematurity, fetal death	
BATTLEDORE PLACENTA The umbilical cord is inserted at or near the placental margin.	Increased incidence of preterm labor and bleeding	Prematurity, fetal distress	
VELAMENTOUS INSERTION OF THE UMBILICAL CORD The vessels of the umbilical cord divide some distance from the placenta in the placental membranes.	Hemorrhage if one of the vessels is torn	Fetal distress, hemorrhage	

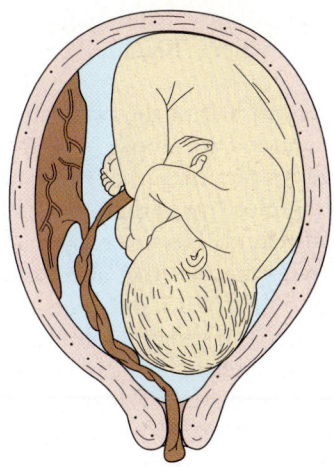

FIGURE 19–15. ◆ Prolapse of the umbilical cord.

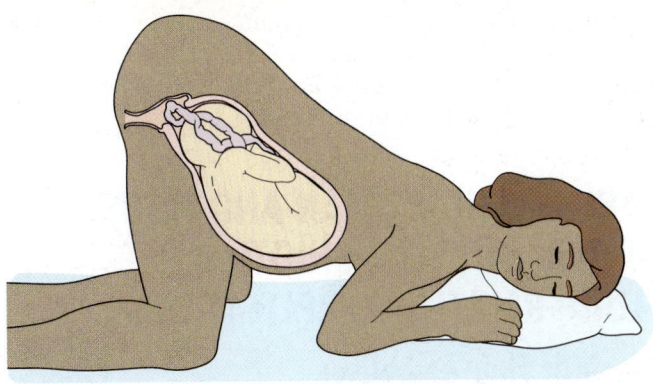

FIGURE 19–16. ◆ Knee-chest position is used to relieve cord compression during cord prolapse emergency.

may occur with rupture of the membranes if the presenting part is not well engaged in the pelvis.

Maternal Implications

Although a prolapsed cord does not directly precipitate physical alterations in the woman, her immediate concern for the baby creates enormous stress. The woman may need to deal with some unusual interventions, a cesarean birth, and, in some circumstances, the death of her baby.

Fetal-Neonatal Implications

Compression of the cord results in decreased blood flow and leads to fetal distress. If labor is under way, the cord is compressed further with each contraction. If the pressure on the cord is not relieved, the fetus will die.

Clinical Therapy

Preventing the occurrence of prolapse of the cord is the preferred medical approach. A laboring woman with a confirmed rupture of membranes will be kept horizontal, usually in bed, until the fetal head is well engaged and the risk of a prolapse is significantly decreased. If a prolapse occurs, relieving the compression on the cord is critical to fetal outcome. The medical and nursing team must work together to facilitate birth.

Bed rest is indicated for all laboring women with a history of ruptured membranes, until engagement with no cord prolapse has been documented. Furthermore, with spontaneous rupture of membranes or amniotomy, the FHR should be auscultated for at least a full minute and at the beginning and end of contractions for several contractions. If fetal bradycardia is detected on auscultation, a vaginal exam is performed to rule out cord prolapse. In the presence of cord prolapse, electronic monitor tracings show severe, moderate, or prolonged variable decelerations with baseline bradycardia. If these patterns are found, the woman is examined vaginally.

If a loop of cord is discovered, the examiner's gloved fingers must remain in the vagina to provide firm pressure on the fetal head (to relieve compression) until the physician or CNM arrives. This is a lifesaving measure. The mother is given oxygen via face mask, and the FHR is monitored to determine whether the cord compression is adequately relieved.

The force of gravity can be employed to relieve umbilical cord compression. The woman assumes the knee-chest position or the bed is adjusted to the Trendelenburg position, and the woman is transported to the delivery or operating room in this position (see Figure 19–16 ◆). The nurse must remember that the cord may be occultly prolapsed with an actual loop extending into the vagina or lying alongside the presenting part. It may be pulsating strongly or so weakly that it is difficult to determine upon palpation of the cord whether the fetus is alive.

Nursing Management

Because there are few outward signs of cord prolapse, each pregnant woman is advised to call her physician or CNM when the membranes rupture and to go to the office, clinic, or birthing facility. A sterile vaginal examination determines if there is danger of cord prolapse. If the presenting part is well engaged, the risk of cord prolapse is minimal, and the woman may ambulate as desired. If the presenting part is not well engaged, bed rest is recommended to prevent cord prolapse.

Because cord prolapse can be associated with fetal death, some physicians and CNMs insist that bed rest be maintained after rupture of membranes regardless of fetal engagement. This can lead to conflict if the laboring woman and her partner do not hold the same opinions. Ease this situation by helping the physician or CNM and the couple communicate.

During labor, any alteration of the FHR or the presence of meconium in the amniotic fluid indicates the need to assess for cord prolapse. Vaginal birth is possible with prolapsed cord if the cervix is completely dilated and pelvic measurements are adequate.

If these conditions are not present, cesarean birth is the method of choice. The woman is taken to the surgical delivery room, and the examiner continues to relieve the pressure on the cord until the infant is born.

CARE OF THE WOMAN AND FETUS AT RISK DUE TO AMNIOTIC FLUID–RELATED COMPLICATIONS

Amniotic Fluid Embolism

In the presence of a small tear in the amnion or chorion high in the uterus, a small amount of amniotic fluid may leak into the chorionic plate and enter the maternal system as an **amniotic fluid embolism.** The fluid can also enter at areas of placental separation or cervical tears. Under pressure from the contracting uterus, the fluid is driven into the maternal circulation and then the maternal lungs. The more debris in the amniotic fluid (such as meconium), the greater the maternal problems. This condition frequently occurs during or after the birth when the woman has had a difficult, rapid labor. Suddenly she experiences respiratory distress, circulatory collapse, acute hemorrhage, and cor pulmonale as the embolism blocks the vessels of the lungs. The woman exhibits a sudden onset of dyspnea, cyanosis, cardiovascular collapse, shock, and coma. Birth must be facilitated immediately to obtain a live fetus.

CLINICAL THERAPY

Any woman exhibiting chest pain, dyspnea, cyanosis, frothy sputum, tachycardia, hypotension, and massive hemorrhage requires the cooperation of every member of the health team if her life is to be saved. Medical interventions are supportive. Recovery is contingent on return of the mother's cardiovascular and respiratory stability. If necessary, the birth is assisted to enhance the health of the newborn.

NURSING MANAGEMENT

In the absence of the physician or CNM, administer oxygen under positive pressure until medical help arrives. Establish an IV line quickly. If respiratory and cardiac arrest occurs, initiate cardiopulmonary resuscitation immediately.

Prepare the equipment necessary for blood transfusion and for the insertion of the CVP line. As the blood volume is replaced, using fresh whole blood to provide clotting factors, monitor the CVP frequently. In the presence of cor pulmonale, fluid overload could easily occur.

Hydramnios

Hydramnios (also called polyhydramnios) occurs when there is more than 2,000 mL of amniotic fluid. The exact cause of hydramnios is unknown; however, in about 20% of cases it is associated with major congenital anomalies (Rosemond, 2000). In addition to the fetal implications,

the maternal implications include significantly increased incidence of cesarean birth (Biggio, Wenstrom, Dubarb, et al., 1999).

During the second half of the pregnancy, the fetus begins to swallow and inspire amniotic fluid and to urinate, which contributes to the amount of amniotic fluid present. In cases of hydramnios, no pathology has been found in the amniotic epithelium. However, hydramnios is associated with fetal malformations that affect the fetal swallowing mechanism and neurologic disorders in which the fetal meninges are exposed in the amniotic cavity. This condition is also found in cases of anencephaly, in which the fetus is thought to urinate excessively due to overstimulation of the cerebrospinal centers. When monozygotic twins manifest hydramnios, it is because the twin with the increased blood volume urinates excessively. The weight of the placenta has been found to be increased in some cases of hydramnios, indicating that increased functioning of the placental tissue may be a factor.

There are two types of hydramnios: chronic and acute. In the chronic type, the fluid volume gradually increases and is a problem of the third trimester. Most cases are of this variety. In acute cases, the volume increases rapidly over a period of a few days. The acute type is usually diagnosed between 20 and 24 weeks' gestation.

MATERNAL IMPLICATIONS

When the amount of amniotic fluid is 3,000 mL or more, the woman experiences shortness of breath and edema in the lower extremities from compression of the vena cava. Milder forms of hydramnios occur more frequently and are associated with minimal symptoms. Hydramnios is associated with maternal disorders such as diabetes and Rh sensitization and with multiple-gestation pregnancies.

If the amniotic fluid is removed rapidly before birth, abruptio placentae can result from too sudden a change in the size of the uterus. Because of overdistention of uterine muscles, uterine dysfunction can occur in the intrapartal period, and the incidence of postpartal hemorrhage increases.

FETAL-NEONATAL IMPLICATIONS

Fetal malformations and preterm birth are common with hydramnios; thus the perinatal mortality rate is fairly high. Prolapsed cord can occur when the membranes rupture, a further complication for the fetus. The incidence of malpresentations also increases.

CLINICAL THERAPY

Hydramnios is managed with supportive treatment unless the intensity of the woman's distress and symptoms dictates otherwise. If the accumulation of amniotic fluid is severe enough to cause maternal dyspnea and pain, hospitalization and removal of the excessive fluid are required. Fluid can be removed vaginally or by amniocentesis. The dangers of performing the technique vaginally are prolapsed cord and the inability to remove the fluid slowly. If amniocentesis is performed, it should be done with the aid of sonography to prevent inadvertent damage to the fetus and placenta. The fluid should be removed slowly to prevent abruption (Rosemond, 2000).

NURSING MANAGEMENT

Hydramnios should be suspected when the fundal height increases out of proportion to the gestational age. As the amount of fluid increases, it may be difficult to palpate the fetus and auscultate the FHR. In more severe cases, the maternal abdomen appears extremely tense and tight on inspection. On sonography, large spaces can be seen between the fetus and the uterine wall.

When amniocentesis is performed, it is vital to maintain sterile technique to prevent infection. Offer support to the couple by explaining the procedure to them.

If the fetus has been diagnosed with a congenital defect in utero or is born with the defect, psychologic support is needed to assist the family. Often the nurse collaborates with social services to offer the family this additional help.

Oligohydramnios

Oligohydramnios, in which the amount of amniotic fluid is severely reduced and concentrated, is a rare maternal finding. The exact cause of this condition is unknown. It is found in cases of postmaturity, with IUGR secondary to placental insufficiency, and in fetal conditions associated with major renal malformations, including renal aplasia with dysplastic kidneys and obstructive lesions of the lower urinary tract (Rosemond, 2000). If oligohydramnios occurs in the first part of pregnancy, there is a danger of fetal adhesions (one part of the fetus may adhere to another part).

MATERNAL IMPLICATIONS

Labor can be dysfunctional, and progress is slow.

FETAL-NEONATAL IMPLICATIONS

During the gestational period, fetal skin and skeletal abnormalities may occur because fetal movement is impaired as a result of reduced amniotic fluid volume. Because there is less fluid available for the fetus to use during fetal breathing movements, pulmonary hypoplasia may develop. During the labor and birth, the lessened amounts of fluid reduce the cushioning effect for the umbilical cord, and cord compression is more likely to occur. Decreased amniotic fluid also contributes to fetal head compression.

CLINICAL THERAPY

During the antepartum period, oligohydramnios may be suspected when the uterus does not increase in size according to the dates, the fetus is easily palpated and outlined by the examiner, and the fetus is not ballotable. The fetus can be assessed by BPPs, NSTs, and serial ultrasound. During labor, the fetus is monitored by continuous EFM to detect cord compression, which is indicated by variable decelerations. Some clinicians advocate the use of an amnioinfusion

(a transcervical instillation of 500 mL of warmed sterile saline, followed by a continuous infusion rate of 100 to 200 mL/hr) after membranes have ruptured to decrease the frequency and severity of variable decelerations in the FHR during labor (Rosemond, 2000). The infusion of saline provides more fluid for the umbilical cord to float in and thereby lessens or prevents cord compression.

NURSING MANAGEMENT

Continuous EFM is an important part of the assessment during the labor and birth. Evaluate the EFM tracing for the presence of variable decelerations or other nonreassuring signs (such as increasing or decreasing baseline, decreased variability, or presence of late decelerations). If variable decelerations are noted, change the woman's position (to relieve pressure on the umbilical cord), and notify the CNM or physician. After the birth, evaluate the newborn for signs of congenital anomalies, pulmonary hypoplasia, and postmaturity.

CARE OF THE WOMAN WITH CEPHALOPELVIC DISPROPORTION (CPD)

The birth passage includes the maternal bony pelvis, beginning at the pelvic inlet and ending at the pelvic outlet, and the maternal soft tissues within these anatomic areas. A contracture (narrowed diameter) in any of the described areas can result in CPD if the fetus is larger than the pelvic diameters. Abnormal fetal presentations and positions occur in CPD as the fetus moves to accommodate its passage through the maternal pelvis.

The gynecoid and anthropoid pelvic types are usually adequate for vertex birth, but the android and platypelloid types are predisposed to CPD. Certain combinations of types also can result in pelvic diameters inadequate for vertex birth. (See Chapter 15 for a description of pelvic types and their implications for childbirth.)

Types of Contractures

The pelvic inlet is contracted if the shortest anterior-posterior diameter is less than 10 cm or the greatest transverse diameter is less than 12 cm. The anterior-posterior diameter may be approximated by measuring the diagonal conjugate, which in the contracted inlet is less than 11.5 cm. Clinical and x-ray pelvimetry determine the smallest anterior-posterior diameter through which the fetal head must pass.

The treatment goal is to allow the natural forces of labor to push the biparietal diameter of the fetal head beyond the potential interspinous obstruction. Although forceps may be used, they cause difficulty because pulling on the head destroys flexion, and the space is further diminished. A bulging perineum and crowning indicate that the obstruction has been passed.

An interischial tuberous diameter of less than 8 cm constitutes an outlet contracture. Outlet and midpelvic contractures frequently occur simultaneously. Whether vaginal birth can occur depends on the woman's interischial tuberous diameters and the fetal posterosagittal diameter.

Maternal Implications

Labor is prolonged in the presence of CPD. Membrane rupture can result from the force of the unequally distributed contractions being exerted on the fetal membranes. In obstructed labor, in which the fetus cannot descend, uterine rupture can occur. With delayed descent, necrosis of maternal soft tissues can result from pressure exerted by the fetal head. Eventually, necrosis can cause fistulas from the vagina to other nearby structures. Difficult, forceps-assisted births can also result in damage to maternal soft tissue.

Fetal-Neonatal Implications

If the membranes rupture and the fetal head has not entered the inlet, there is a danger of cord prolapse. Excessive molding of the fetal head can result. Traumatic, forceps-assisted birth can damage the fetal skull and central nervous system.

Clinical Therapy

Fetopelvic relationships can be assessed by comparing pelvic measurements obtained by a manual exam before labor and by computed tomography (CT) with estimated weight of the fetus as obtained by ultrasound measurements.

When the pelvic diameters are borderline or questionable, a trial of labor (TOL) may be advised. In this process, the woman continues to labor, and the care team makes careful, frequent assessments of cervical dilatation and fetal descent. As long as there is continued progress, the trial of labor continues. If progress ceases, the decision for a cesarean birth is made.

Nursing Management

The adequacy of the maternal pelvis for a vaginal birth should be assessed both during and before labor. During the intrapartal assessment, the size of the fetus and its presentation, position, and lie must also be considered. (See Chapter 16 for intrapartal assessment techniques.)

Suspect CPD when labor is prolonged, cervical dilatation and effacement are slow, and engagement of the presenting part is delayed. The couple may need support in coping with the stresses of this complicated labor. Keep the couple informed of what is happening and explain the procedures being used. This knowledge reassures the couple that measures are being taken to resolve the problem.

Nursing actions during the trial of labor are similar to care during any labor except that cervical dilatation and fetal descent are assessed more frequently. Monitor both contractions and the fetus continuously. Any signs of fetal distress are reported to the CNM or physician immediately.

The mother may be positioned in a variety of ways to increase the pelvic diameters. Sitting or squatting increases the outlet diameters and may be effective when there is failure of or slow fetal descent. Changing from one side to the other or maintaining a hands-and-knees position may assist the fetus in the OP position to change to an OA position. The mother may instinctively want to assume one of these positions. If not, encourage a change of position.

CARE OF THE WOMAN AT RISK DUE TO COMPLICATIONS OF THE THIRD AND FOURTH STAGES OF LABOR

Lacerations

Lacerations of the cervix or vagina may be indicated when bright-red vaginal bleeding persists in the presence of a well-contracted uterus. The incidence of lacerations is higher when the childbearing woman is young or a nullipara, has an epidural, has forceps-assisted birth and an episiotomy, and has not done perineal massage or preparation during pregnancy. Vaginal and perineal lacerations are often categorized in terms of degree, as follows:

- First-degree laceration is limited to the fourchette, perineal skin, and vaginal mucous membrane.
- Second-degree laceration involves the perineal skin, vaginal mucous membrane, underlying fascia, and muscles of the perineal body; it may extend upward on one or both sides of the vagina.
- Third-degree laceration extends through the perineal skin, vaginal mucous membranes, and perineal body and involves the anal sphincter; it may extend up the anterior wall of the rectum.
- Fourth-degree laceration is the same as third-degree but extends through the rectal mucosa to the lumen of the rectum; it may be called a third-degree laceration with a rectal wall extension.

Placenta Accreta

The chorionic villi attach directly to the myometrium of the uterus in placenta accreta. Two other types of placental adherence are placenta increta, in which the myometrium is invaded, and placenta percreta, in which the myometrium is penetrated. The adherence itself may be total, partial, or focal, depending on the amount of placental involvement. The incidence of placenta accreta is 1 in 2,500. Placenta accreta is the most common type and accounts for 80% of adherent placentas.

The primary complication with placenta accreta is maternal hemorrhage and failure of the placenta to separate following birth of the infant. An abdominal hysterectomy may be necessary, depending on the amount and depth of involvement.

CHAPTER HIGHLIGHTS

✍ Anxiety and fear have a profound effect on labor, particularly when complications that might jeopardize the mother or fetus occur.

✍ A hypertonic labor pattern is characterized by painful contractions that are not effective in effacing and dilating the cervix. It usually leads to a prolonged latent phase.

✍ Hypotonic labor patterns begin normally and then progress to infrequent, less intense contractions.

✍ Precipitous labor is extremely rapid labor and birth that lasts less than 3 hours. It is associated with an increased risk to the mother and newborn infant.

✍ Postterm pregnancy is one that extends more than 294 days, or 42 weeks, past the first day of the last menstrual period.

✍ The OP position of the fetus during labor prolongs the labor process, causes severe back discomfort in the laboring woman, and predisposes her to vaginal and perineal trauma and lacerations during birth.

✍ The types of fetal malpresentations include face, brow, breech, and shoulder.

✍ A fetus or newborn weighing more than 4,000 g is termed *macrosomic*. Problems may occur during labor, birth, and the early neonatal period.

✍ Preventing and treating problems that infringe on the development and birth of normal fetuses are significant medical-nursing activities once the presence of twins or multiple-gestation pregnancies has been detected.

✍ Fetal distress is indicated by persistent late decelerations, persistent severe variable decelerations, and prolonged decelerations. If fetal distress is recognized and treated appropriately, the fetus may be spared any permanent damage.

✍ Intrauterine fetal death poses a major nursing challenge to provide support and care for the parents.

✍ Abruptio placentae is the separation of the placenta from the side of the uterus prior to birth of the infant. Abruptio placentae may be central, marginal, or complete.

✍ Placenta previa occurs when the placenta implants low in the uterus near or over the cervix. A low-lying or marginal placenta is one that lies near the cervix. In partial placenta previa, part of the placenta lies over the cervix; in complete placenta previa, the cervix is completely covered.

✍ Prolapsed umbilical cord results when the umbilical cord precedes the fetal presenting part. This places pressure on the umbilical cord and diminishes blood flow to the fetus.

✍ Amniotic fluid embolism occurs when a bolus of amniotic fluid enters the maternal circulation and then the maternal lungs. The maternal mortality rate is very high with this complication.

✍ Hydramnios (also called polyhydramnios) occurs when there is more than 2,000 mL of amniotic fluid within the amniotic membranes. Hydramnios is associated with fetal malformations that affect fetal swallowing and with maternal diabetes mellitus, Rh sensitization, and multiple-gestation pregnancies.

✍ Oligohydramnios is present when there is a severely reduced volume of amniotic fluid. Oligohydramnios is associated with IUGR, with postmaturity, and with fetal renal or urinary malfunctions. The fetus is more likely to experience variable decelerations because the amniotic fluid is insufficient to keep pressure off the umbilical cord.

✍ CPD occurs when there is a narrowed diameter in the maternal pelvis. The narrowed diameter is called a contracture and may occur in the pelvic inlet, the midpelvis, or the outlet. If pelvic measurements are borderline, a trial of labor may be attempted. Failure of cervical dilatation or fetal descent necessitates a cesarean birth.

✍ Third- and fourth-stage complications usually involve hemorrhage. The causes of hemorrhage include lacerations of the birth canal or cervix and placenta accreta.

EXPLORE MediaLink

NCLEX Review, Case Studies, and other interactive resources for this chapter can be found on the companion website at http://www.prenhall.com/london. Click on "Chapter 19" to select the activities for this chapter.

For animations, more NCLEX review questions, and an audio glossary, access the accompanying CD-ROM in this textbook.

REFERENCES

Anderson, G. D. (2000). Fetal demise. In M. E. Rivlin & R. W. Martin (Eds.), *Manual of clinical problems in obstetrics and gynecology* (5th ed., pp. 122–126). Philadelphia: Lippincott.

Benirschke, K. (1999). Multiple gestation: Incidence, etiology, and inheritance. In R. K. Creasy & R. Resnik (Eds.), *Maternal-fetal medicine* (4th ed., pp. 585–597). Philadelphia: Saunders.

Berg, M., & Dahlberg, K. (1998). A phenomenological study of women's experiences of complicated childbirth. *Midwifery, 14,* 23–29.

Berkowitz, K. M., & Garite, T. J. (2001). Postdatism. In J. J. Sciarri & T. J. Watkins (Eds.), *Gynecology and obstetrics* (Vol. 2, chap. 54, pp. 1–9). Philadelphia: Lippincott Williams & Wilkins.

Biggio, J. R., Wenstrom, K. D., Dubarb, M. B., & Cliver, S. P. (1999). Hydramnios: Prediction of adverse perinatal outcomes. *Obstetrics and Gynecology, 94*(5), 762–773.

Bofill, J. A. (2000). Breech presentation. In M. E. Rivlin & R. W. Martin (Eds.), *Manual of clinical problems in obstetrics and gynecology* (5th ed., pp. 143–146). Philadelphia: Lippincott.

Bowes, W. A. (1999). Clinical aspects of normal and abnormal labor. In R. K. Creasy & R. Resnik (Eds.), *Maternal-fetal medicine* (4th ed., pp. 541–568). Philadelphia: Saunders.

Cardini, F., & Weixin, H. (1998). Moxibustion for correction of breech presentation: A randomized controlled trial. *Journal of the American Medical Association, 280*(18), 1580–1584.

Creedy, D. K., Shochet, I. M., & Horsfall, J. (2000). Childbirth and the development of acute traumatic symptoms: Incidence and contributing factors. *Birth, 27*(2), 104–111.

Dahlberg, K., Berg, M., & Lundgren, I. (1999). Commentary: Studying maternal experiences of childbirth. *Birth, 26*(4), 215–217.

Gherman, R. B., & Gonik, B. (2001). Shoulder dystocia. In J. J. Sciarri & T. J. Watkins (Eds.), *Gynecology and obstetrics* (Vol. 2, chap. 79, pp. 1–7). Philadelphia: Lippincott Williams & Wilkins.

Gladstar, R. (1993). Herbal healing for women. New York: Simon & Schuster

Gimovsky, M. L. (2000). Abnormal fetal lie and presentation. In J. J. Sciarri & T. J. Watkins (Eds.), *Gynecology and obstetrics* (Vol. 2, chap. 76, pp. 1–15). Philadelphia: Lippincott Williams & Wilkins.

Hogg, B. B., & Kimberlin, D. F. (2000). Delivery of the small and large infant. In M. E. Rivlin & R. W. Martin (Eds.), *Manual of clinical problems in obstetrics and gynecology* (5th ed., pp. 179–182). Philadelphia: Lippincott.

Kanakura, Y., Kometani, K., Nagata, T., Niwa, K., Kamatsuki, H., & Shinzato, Y., et al. (2001). Moxibustion treatment of breech presentation. *American Journal of Chinese Medicine, 29*(1), 37–45.

Kay, J., Roman, B., & Schulte, H. M. (1997). Pregnancy loss and the grief process. In J. R. Woods & J. L. Esposito (Eds.), *Loss during pregnancy or in the newborn period: Principles of care with clinical cases and analyses* (pp. 5–36). Pittman, NJ: Jannetti Publications.

Keith, L., Papiernik, E., & Oleszcuzuk, J. J. (1998). How should the efficacy of prenatal care be tested in twin gestation? *Clinical Obstetrics and Gynecology, 41,* 85–93.

Malone, F. D., & D'Alton, M. E. (1999). Multiple gestation: Clinical characteristics and management. In R. K. Creasy & R. Resnik (Eds.), *Maternal-fetal medicine* (4th ed., pp. 598–615). Philadelphia: Saunders.

Martin, J. N. (2000). Postterm pregnancy. In M. E. Rivlin & R. W. Martin (Eds.), *Manual of clinical problems in obstetrics and gynecology* (5th ed., pp. 105–108). Philadelphia: Lippincott.

Miller, V. L., Ransom, S. B., Shalhoub, A., Sokol, R. J., & Evans, M. I. (2000). Multifetal pregnancy reduction: Perinatal and fiscal outcomes. *American Journal of Obstetrics and Gynecology, 182*(6), 1575–1579.

O'Reilly-Green, C., & Divon, M. (2000). Sonographic and clinical methods in diagnosis of macrosomia. *Clinical Obstetrics and Gynecology, 43*(2) 309–325.

Papiernik, E., Keith, L., Oleszcuzuk, J. J., & Cervantes, A. (1998). What interventions are useful in reducing the rate of preterm delivery in twins? *Clinical Obstetrics and Gynecology, 41,* 13–23.

Perry, K. G., Jr. (2000a). Abruptio placentae. In M. E. Rivlin & R. W. Martin (Eds.), *Manual of clinical problems in obstetrics and gynecology* (5th ed., pp. 21–23). Philadelphia: Lippincott.

Perry, K. G., Jr. (2000b). Placenta previa. In M. E. Rivlin & R. W. Martin (Eds.), *Manual of clinical problems in obstetrics and gynecology* (5th ed., pp. 18–20). Philadelphia: Lippincott.

Rivlin, M. E. (2000). Nonbreech abnormal presentations, positions, and lies. In M. E. Rivlin & R. W. Martin (Eds.), *Manual of clinical problems in obstetrics and gynecology* (5th ed., pp. 146–149). Philadelphia: Lippincott.

Roberts, S. J., Reardon, K. M., & Rosenfeld, S. (1999). Childbirth sexual abuse: Surveying its impact on primary care. *AWHONN Lifelines, 3,* 39–45.

Roberts, W. E. (2000). Multifetal gestation. In M. E. Rivlin & R. W. Martin (Eds.), *Manual of clinical problems in obstetrics and gynecology* (5th ed., pp. 95–100). Philadelphia: Lippincott.

Rodis, J. F., Arky, L., Egan, J. F. X., Borgida, A. F., Leo, M. V., & Campbell, W. A. (1999).

Comprehensive fetal ultrasonography measurements in triplet gestation. *American Journal of Obstetrics and Gynecology, 181*(5), 1128–1132.

Rosemond, R. L. (2000). Hydramnios and oligohydramnios. In M. E. Rivlin & R. W. Martin (Eds.), *Manual of clinical problems in obstetrics and gynecology* (5th ed., pp. 149–152). Philadelphia: Lippincott.

Saito, T., Ylikorkala, O., & Halmesmaki, E. (1999). Factors associated with fear of delivery in second pregnancies. *Obstetrics and Gynecology, 94*(5), 679–682.

Schmidt, J. (2000). Intrapartum fetal assessment. In S. Mattson & J. E. Smiths (Eds.), *AWHONN: Maternal newborn nursing* (4th ed., pp. 272–299). Philadelphia: Saunders.

Schwiebert, P., & Kirk, P. (1985). *When hello means goodbye.* Eugene, OR: Health Sciences University.

Scott, J. R. (1999). Placenta previa and abruption. In J. R. Scott, P. J. DiSaia, C. B. Hammond, & W. N. Spellacy (Eds.), *Danforth's obstetrics and gynecology* (8th ed., pp. 407–418). Philadelphia: Lippincott.

Simpson, K. R., & Poole, J. H. (1998). *Cervical ripening, and induction and augmentation of labor* (AWHONN Symposium). Washington, DC: Association of Women's Health, Obstetric and Neonatal Nurses.

Uckan, E. M., & Townsend, N. S. (1999). Fetal adaptation. In L. K. Mandeville & N. H. Troiano (Eds.), *AWHONN: High-risk and critical care intrapartum nursing* (2nd ed., pp. 32–50). Philadelphia: Lippincott.

Yeo, L., Ananth, C. V., & Vintzileos, A. M. (2001). Placental abruption. In J. J. Sciarri & T. J. Watkins (Eds.), *Gynecology and obstetrics* (Vol. 2, chap. 50, pp. 1–25). Philadelphia: Lippincott Williams & Wilkins.

CHAPTER 20

Birth-Related Procedures

With our first baby, all of a sudden I had to have a cesarean. Everything happened so fast but our son was OK, and that's all that mattered. With our second baby, I wanted to try a vaginal birth. Even though I wanted to, I was afraid. I don't know what I would have done without my nurse. She stayed with me the whole time and kept giving me support. She explained what was happening and gave encouragement. I felt safe. I had a beautiful baby girl after 8 hours of labor.

—MARIANNE, 22

Key Terms

Amnioinfusion (AI) *434*

Amniotomy *427*

Cervical ripening *427*

Episiotomy *434*

External cephalic version (ECV) *426*

Forceps *436*

Internal version *426*

Labor augmentation *429*

Labor induction *428*

Vacuum-assisted birth *438*

Vaginal birth after cesarean (VBAC) *441*

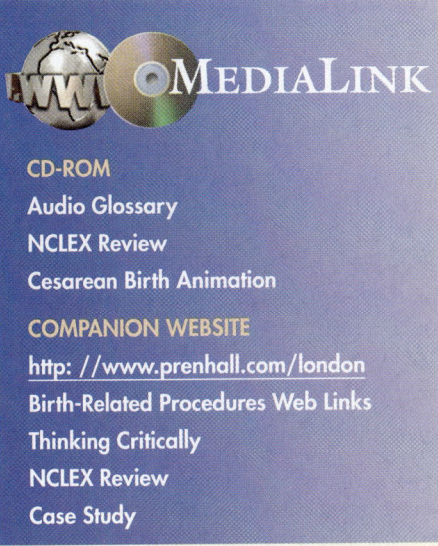

MEDIALINK

CD-ROM
Audio Glossary
NCLEX Review
Cesarean Birth Animation

COMPANION WEBSITE
http://www.prenhall.com/london
Birth-Related Procedures Web Links
Thinking Critically
NCLEX Review
Case Study

Most births occur without the need for operative obstetric intervention. In some instances, however, procedures are necessary to maintain safety for the woman and the fetus. The most common are amniotomy, induction of labor, episiotomy, cesarean birth, and vaginal birth following a previous cesarean birth.

Generally, women know they may need an obstetric procedure during their labor and birth. However, some women expect to have a "natural" experience and do not anticipate the need for medical intervention. This conflict between expectation and the need for intervention presents a challenge to maternity nurses. The nurse provides information about any procedure to help the woman and her partner understand what is proposed, the anticipated benefits and possible risks, and any alternatives.

CARE OF THE WOMAN DURING VERSION

Version, or turning the fetus, is a procedure used to change the fetal presentation by abdominal or intrauterine manipulation. The most common type of version is **external cephalic version (ECV),** in which the fetus is changed from a breech to a cephalic presentation by external manipulation of the maternal abdomen (Figure 20–1 ◆). A

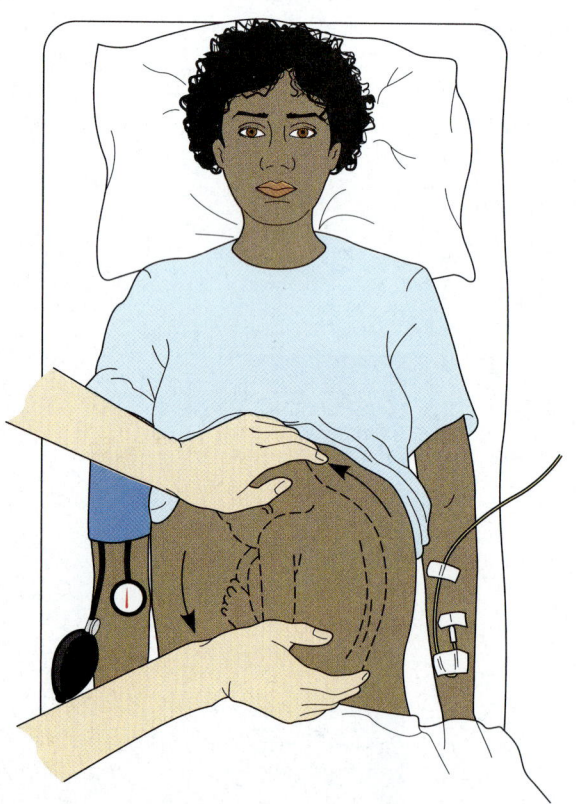

FIGURE 20–1. ◆ External (or cephalic) version of the fetus. A new technique involves pressure on the fetal head and buttocks so that the fetus completes a "backward flip" or "forward roll."

less common type, called **internal version** (or podalic version), is used only with the second fetus during a vaginal twin birth and only if the twin does not descend readily or shows signs of distress. In an internal version, medication is used to relax the uterus and the obstetrician places a hand inside the uterus, grabs the fetus's feet, and draws them down through the cervix.

External Version

If breech or shoulder presentation (transverse lie) is detected in the later weeks of pregnancy, an external version may be attempted. Before the external version is begun, an ultrasound is used to locate the placenta and to confirm fetal presentation.

The following criteria should be met prior to performing external version:

- The pregnancy is 36 or more weeks' gestation. A version may result in complications that require immediate birth by cesarean (Cruikshank, 1999).
- A nonstress test (NST) done immediately before the version is reactive. A reactive NST indicates fetal well-being.
- The fetal breech is not engaged. Once the presenting part is engaged it is difficult, if not impossible, to do a version.

Contraindications include the following (Bowes, 1999):

- Maternal problems, such as uterine anomalies, pregnancy-induced hypertension (PIH), or third-trimester bleeding
- Complications of pregnancy, such as rupture of membranes, oligohydramnios, hydramnios, or placenta previa
- Previous cesarean birth or other significant uterine surgery
- Multiple gestation
- Nonreassuring fetal heart rate (FHR) or other evidence of uteroplacental insufficiency
- Fetal abnormalities, such as intrauterine growth restriction or nuchal cord

Before the external version begins, an intravenous (IV) line is established to administer medications in case of difficulty. The woman receives terbutaline to relax the uterus. The version is discontinued in the presence of severe maternal pain or significant FHR bradycardia or decelerations.

Nursing Management

On admission, begin a thorough assessment by verifying that there are no contraindications to the version procedure. Obtain maternal vital signs and a reactive NST. This initial assessment period provides an ideal time for educating the woman and her partner and for addressing their concerns. Encourage them to express their understanding and expectations of the procedure. At the same time, discuss the possibility of failure of the external cephalic version and slight risk of cesarean birth if the fetus becomes distressed. Explaining what will happen in either of these circumstances will better prepare the woman and her partner in case intervention becomes necessary.

Throughout the procedure, continue to monitor maternal blood pressure, pulse, and comfort level frequently (because the mother may experience pain during the procedure). Ascertain fetal well-being before, intermittently during, and for (at least) 30 minutes after the procedure, using electronic fetal monitoring (EFM), ultrasound, or both. Also assess maternal-fetal response to the tocolytic. Provide aftercare instructions, which may include maternal monitoring for contractions and fetal movement (fetal kick counts).

CARE OF THE WOMAN DURING AMNIOTOMY

Amniotomy is the artificial rupture of the amniotic membranes (AROM). It is probably the most common operative procedure in obstetrics. Because the amniotomy requires that an instrument, called an amnihook, be inserted through the cervix, at least 2 cm of cervical dilatation is required. The amniotomy may be performed in hope of starting labor (inducing) or at any time during the first stage to augment labor (accelerate the progress). An amniotomy done after 3 cm of cervical dilatation will probably shorten the length of labor (Wolcott & Conry, 2000). Amniotomy may also be done during labor to apply an internal fetal heart monitoring electrode to the scalp, to insert an intrauterine pressure catheter, or to obtain a fetal scalp blood sample for acid-base determination and fetal pH monitoring. In addition, amniotomy allows assessment of the color and composition of amniotic fluid.

AROM Procedure

While performing a vaginal examination, the physician or certified nurse-midwife (CNM) introduces an amnihook into the vagina and makes a small tear in the amniotic membrane, which allows amniotic fluid to escape.

Nursing Management

Explain the AROM procedure to the woman and then assess fetal presentation, position, and station, because amniotomy is usually delayed until engagement has occurred. Ask the woman to assume a semireclining position and drape her for privacy. Assess the FHR just before and immediately after the amniotomy, and compare the two FHR assessments. If there are marked changes, check for prolapse of the cord (see Chapter 19). Inspect the amniotic fluid for amount, color, odor, and the presence of meconium or blood. While wearing disposable gloves,

cleanse and dry the perineal area and change the underpads. Because there is now an open pathway for organisms to ascend into the uterus, the number of vaginal exams must be kept to a minimum to reduce the chance of introducing an infection. In addition, monitor the woman's temperature at least every 2 hours. Provide information about the expected effects of the amniotomy. It is important for the woman to know that amniotic fluid is constantly produced, because some may worry that they will experience a "dry birth."

CARE OF THE WOMAN DURING CERVICAL RIPENING

Prostaglandin E$_2$

Prostaglandin E$_2$ (PGE$_2$) gel or tablets for **cervical ripening** (softening and effacing the cervix) may be used for the pregnant woman at or near term when there is a medical or obstetric indication for induction of labor. Two commonly used products are Prepidil and Cervidil. These preparations have been demonstrated to cause cervical ripening and shorter labor and to lower requirements for oxytocin during labor induction. Vaginal birth is achieved within 24 hours for most women (Oei, Lidewijde, & Mol, 2000).

Prostaglandin cervical ripening preparations are best used only in a hospital birthing unit, and it is recommended that an obstetrician be readily available in case an emergency cesarean birth is needed (Cunningham, Gant, Leveno et al., 2001). See "Drug Guide: Dinoprostone (Cervidil) Vaginal Insert" for additional information.

Misoprostol (Cytotec)

Misoprostol (Cytotec) is a synthetic PGE$_1$ analogue that may also be used to ripen the cervix and induce labor. It is available in tablet form. Some contraindications for the use of misoprostol include the following (ACOG, 1999b):

- Presence of uterine contractions three times in 10 minutes
- Significant maternal asthma
- History of previous uterine scar or bleeding during the pregnancy
- Presence of placenta previa
- Nonreassuring FHR tracing

Nursing Management

Physicians, CNMs, and birthing room nurses who have had special education and training may administer PGE$_2$ products and misoprostol. The woman and her support person(s) are provided information about the procedure, and any questions are answered. Maternal vital signs are assessed for baseline, and an electronic fetal monitor is

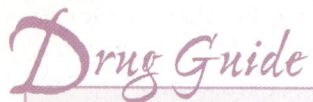
Drug Guide

applied. The EFM tracing should indicate minimal or absent uterine activity, a reassuring FHR pattern, and a reactive NST. If uterine contractions are not occurring regularly, PGE₂ gel or a 25-mg misoprostol tablet is inserted into the vagina. The woman is requested to lie supine with a right hip wedge for a specified time (usually at least an hour). The woman can then assume any comfortable position. Monitor the woman for uterine hyperstimulation and FHR abnormalities (changes in baseline rate, variability, presence of decelerations) for at least 2 hours following insertion (Schmidt, 1999).

During administration of PGE₂, if nausea and vomiting are present or contractions occur more frequently than every 2 minutes (and/or last >75 seconds) the gel is removed.

CARE OF THE WOMAN DURING LABOR INDUCTION

ACOG defines **labor induction** as the stimulation of uterine contractions before the spontaneous onset of labor, with or without ruptured fetal membranes, for the purpose of accomplishing birth. Induction may be indicated in the presence of the following (ACOG, 1999a):

- Diabetes mellitus
- Renal disease
- Pregnancy-induced hypertension or preeclampsia
- Premature rupture of membranes (PROM)
- History of rapid labor (precipitous labor and birth)
- Chorioamnionitis
- Postterm gestation
- Mild abruptio placentae with no fetal distress
- Intrauterine fetal demise
- Intrauterine fetal growth restriction
- Isoimmunization

All contraindications to spontaneous labor and vaginal birth are contraindications to the induction of labor. Relative maternal contraindications include but are not limited to the following (Cunningham, et al., 2001):

- Client refusal
- Placenta previa or vasa previa
- Transverse fetal lie
- Prior classic uterine incision (vertical incision in the upper portion of the uterus)
- Active genital herpes infection
- Some instances of positive maternal HIV status

Before induction is attempted, appropriate assessment must indicate that both the woman and fetus are ready for the onset of labor. This includes evaluation of fetal maturity and cervical readiness.

Labor Readiness

FETAL MATURITY

The gestational age of the fetus is best evaluated by accurate menstrual dating and serial ultrasounds. Amniotic fluid studies also provide valuable information in assessing fetal lung maturity (see Chapter 14).

CERVICAL READINESS

A vaginal examination helps determine whether cervical changes favorable for induction have occurred. Bishop (1964) developed a prelabor scoring system that is helpful in predicting the potential success of induction (Table 20–1). Components evaluated are cervical dilatation, effacement, consistency, and position, as well as the station of the fetal presenting part. The examiner gives a score of 0, 1, 2, or 3 to each assessed characteristic. The higher the total score for all the criteria, the more likely that labor will occur. The lower the total score, the higher the failure rate. A favorable cervix is the most important criterion for a successful induction (Cunningham et al., 2001). A cervix that is anterior, soft, 50% effaced, and dilated at least 2 cm, with the fetal head at 21 to 11 station or lower (Bishop score of 9) is favorable for successful induction. If the cervix is unfavorable, a method of cervical ripening may be tried.

Fetal fibronectin (fFN) assay has been suggested as a biochemical marker for impending term labor and successful labor induction (Rozenberg, Goffinet, & Hessabi, 2000). The presence of fetal fibronectin in the cervicovaginal secretions has correlated with successful induction of labor (Kiss, Ahner, Hohlagschwandtner, et al., 2000). Currently, the high cost of fFN testing limits its clinical use.

Induction by Oxytocin Infusion

Oxytocin initiates uterine contractions to induce labor and may also be used to enhance ineffective contractions (**labor augmentation**). A primary line of 1,000 mL of electrolyte solution (e.g., lactated Ringer's solution) is started IV. Ten units of oxytocin (Pitocin) are added to a secondary line of IV fluid so the resulting mixture will contain 10 mU/mL of oxytocin (1 mU/min, or 6 mL/h), and the prescribed dose can be calculated easily. After the primary infusion is started, the oxytocin solution is piggybacked into the primary tubing port closest to the catheter insertion. The infusion is then administered using an infusion pump to control the flow rate precisely. The rate of infusion is based on physician or CNM protocol and careful assessment of the contraction pattern. The goal for induction is to achieve stable contractions every 2 to 3 minutes that last 40 to 60 seconds. The uterus should relax to full baseline resting tone between each contraction. Progress is determined by changes in the effacement and dilatation of the cervix and station of the presenting part.

Oxytocin induction is not without some associated risks, including hyperstimulation of the uterus, resulting in uterine contractions that are too frequent or too intense, with an increased resting tone. Hypertonic contractions may lead to decreased placenta perfusion and fetal distress. Other risks include uterine rupture and water intoxication (Wilson, Shannon, & Strang, 2001).

Induction by Misoprostol

During misoprostol induction, an IV is started to ensure access if needed later, and a 25-mg misoprostol tablet is inserted into the posterior vaginal fornix. The dose may be repeated every 3 to 4 hours until there are at least three uterine contractions in 10 minutes (ACOG, 1999b).

Nursing Management

During client teaching about induction of labor, discuss the purpose, the procedure itself, nursing care that will be provided, assessments, comfort measures, and a review of breathing techniques that may be used during labor. Regardless of the induction method used, close observation and accurate, ongoing assessments are mandatory to provide safe, optimal care for both woman and fetus. A qualified obstetrician should be readily accessible to manage any complications that may occur. As contractions are established, perform vaginal examinations to evaluate cervical dilatation, effacement, and station. The frequency of

---

TABLE 20-1   Prelabor Status Evaluation Scoring System

Factor	Assigned Value			
	0	1	2	3
Cervical dilatation	Closed	1–2 cm	3–4 cm	5 cm or more
Cervical effacement	0%–30%	40%–50%	60%–70%	80% or more
Fetal station	−3	−2	−1,0	+1, or lower
Cervical consistency	Firm	Moderate	Soft	
Cervical position	Posterior	Midposition	Anterior	

Reprinted with permission from the American College of Obstetricians and Gynecologists. (*Obstetrics and Gynecology*, 1964, 24, 266.)

vaginal examinations primarily depends on the woman's parity, comfort level, and strength of her contractions. If evaluating the need for analgesia, perform a vaginal examination to avoid giving the medication too early and increasing the risk of prolonging labor and to identify advanced dilatation and imminent birth.

Although the use of misoprostol (Cytotec) for labor induction has been studied since 1993, universal protocols have not been established. One proposed protocol (Wilson, 2000) recommends the following:

- Obtain baseline vital signs, then repeat blood pressure, pulse, and respiration every 30 minutes (×2), then lengthen time to 4-hour intervals (temperature every 2 hours if membranes are ruptured) after each administration of Cytotec

- Perform vaginal exam to determine cervical status and fetal presentation

- Apply fetal monitor and obtain NST

- Monitor uterine activity and FHR continuously for 2 hours; if reassuring, the woman may be permitted to ambulate until the next scheduled dose

- Obtain IV access and administer IV fluids as ordered

- Delay administration of additional doses for 2 hours (and monitor uterine activity) if membranes rupture

- Oxytocin may be given 2 hours after last dose of misoprostol

Oxytocin induction protocols recommend obtaining baseline data (maternal temperature, pulse, respirations, blood pressure), a 20- to 30-minute EFM recording demonstrating a reassuring FHR, a reactive NST, and the contraction status before the induction is started. The fetal monitor provides continuous data.

Before each increase of the oxytocin infusion rate the nurse assesses the following:

- Maternal blood pressure and pulse

- Contraction status including frequency, duration, intensity, and resting tone

- FHR baseline, variability, and reactivity, noting the presence of accelerations, any decelerations, or bradycardia

For additional information about nursing interventions during use of oxytocin, see "Drug Guide: Oxytocin (Pitocin)" and "Clinical Pathway for Induction of Labor."

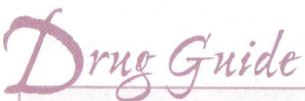
Drug Guide

OXYTOCIN (PITOCIN)

Overview of Obstetric Action

Oxytocin (Pitocin) exerts a selective stimulatory effect on the smooth muscle of the uterus and blood vessels. It affects the myometrial cells of the uterus by increasing the excitability of the muscle cell, increasing the strength of the muscle contraction, and supporting propagation of the contraction (movement of the contraction from one myometrial cell to the next). Its effect on the uterine contraction depends on the dosage used and on the excitability of the myometrial cells. During the first half of gestation, there is little excitability of the myometrium, and the uterus is fairly resistant to the effects of oxytocin. However, from midgestation on, the uterus responds increasingly to exogenous IV oxytocin. Cautious use of diluted oxytocin administered IV at term results in a slow rise of uterine activity.

The circulatory half-life of oxytocin is 3 to 5 minutes. It takes approximately 40 minutes for a particular dose of oxytocin to reach a steady-state plasma concentration.

The effects of oxytocin on the cardiovascular system can be pronounced. Blood pressure initially may decrease but after prolonged administration increase by 30% above the baseline. Cardiac output and stroke volume increase. With doses of 20 mU/min or above, oxytocin exerts an antidiuretic effect, decreasing free water exchange in the kidney and markedly decreasing urine output.

Oxytocin is used to induce labor at term and to augment uterine contractions in the first and second stages of labor. It may also be used immediately after birth to stimulate uterine contraction and thereby control uterine atony.

Route, Dosage, Frequency

For induction of labor: Add 10 units of Pitocin (1 mL) to 1,000 mL of IV solution. (The resulting concentration is 10 mU oxytocin per 1 mL of IV fluid.) Using an infusion pump, administer IV, starting at 0.5 to 1 mU/min and increasing by 1 to 2 mU/min every 40 to 60 minutes. Alternatively, start at 1 to 2 mU/min and increase by 1 mU/min every 15 minutes until a good contraction pattern (every 2 to 3 minutes and lasting 40 to 60 seconds) is achieved.

Maternal Contraindications

- Severe preeclampsia or eclampsia (pregnancy-induced hypertension)

- Predisposition to uterine rupture (in nullipara over 35 years of age, multigravida 4 or more, overdistention of the uterus, previous major surgery of the cervix or uterus)

- Cephalopelvic disproportion

- Malpresentation or malposition of the fetus, cord prolapse

- Preterm infant

- Rigid, unripe cervix; total placenta previa

- Presence of fetal distress

Maternal Side Effects

Hyperstimulation of the uterus results in hypercontractility, which in turn may cause the following:

- Abruptio placentae

- Impaired uterine blood flow, leading to fetal hypoxia

- Rapid labor, leading to cervical lacerations

- Rapid labor and birth, leading to lacerations of cervix, vagina, or perineum; uterine atony; fetal trauma

- Uterine rupture

- Water intoxication (nausea, vomiting, hypotension, tachycardia, cardiac arrhythmia) if oxytocin is given in electrolyte-free solution or at a rate exceeding 20 mU/min; hypotension with rapid IV bolus administration postpartum

Effect on Fetus or Neonate

- Primarily associated with the presence of hypercontractility of the maternal uterus, which decreases the oxygen supply to the fetus and is reflected by irregularities or decrease in FHR

- Hyperbilirubinemia

- Trauma from rapid birth

Nursing Considerations

- Explain induction or augmentation procedure to client.

- Apply fetal monitor and obtain 15- to 20-minute tracing and NST to assess FHR before starting IV oxytocin.

- For induction or augmentation of labor, start with primary IV and piggyback secondary IV with oxytocin and infusion pump.

- Ensure continuous monitoring of the fetus and uterine contractions.

- The maximum rate is 40 mU/min (ACOG, 1999a). Not all protocols recommend a maximum dose. When indicated, the maximum dose is generally between 16 and 40 mU/min. Decrease oxytocin by similar increments once labor has progressed to 5 or 6 cm dilatation. Protocols may vary from one agency to another.

    0.5 mU/min = 3 mL/hr

    1 mU/min = 6 mL/hr

    1.5 mU/min = 9 mL/hr

    2 mU/min = 12 mL/hr

    4 mU/min = 24 mL/hr

    6 mU/min = 36 mL/hr

    8 mU/min = 48 mL/hr

    10 mU/min = 60 mL/hr

    12 mU/min = 72 mL/hr

    15 mU/min = 90 mL/hr

    18 mU/min = 108 mL/hr

    20 mU/min = 120 mL/hr

- Assess FHR, maternal blood pressure, pulse, frequency and duration of uterine contractions, and uterine resting tone before each increase in the oxytocin infusion rate.

- Record all assessments and IV rate on monitor strip and on client's chart.

- Record oxytocin infusion rate in milliunits per minute and milliliters per hour (e.g., 0.5 mU/min [3 mL/hr]).

- Assess cervical dilatation as needed.

- Provide nursing comfort measures.

- Discontinue IV oxytocin infusion and infuse primary solution when (1) fetal distress is noted (bradycardia, late or variable decelerations), (2) uterine contractions are more frequent than every 2 minutes, (3) duration of contractions exceeds more than 60 seconds, or (4) insufficient relaxation of the uterus between contractions or a steady increase in resting tone is noted (ACOG, 1999a). In addition to discontinuing IV oxytocin infusion, turn client to side, and if fetal distress is present, administer oxygen by tight face mask at 7 to 10 L/min; notify physician.

- Maintain intake and output record.

For augmentation of labor:

Prepare and administer IV Pitocin as for labor induction. Increase rate until labor contractions are of good quality. The flow rate is gradually increased at no less than every 30 minutes to a maximum of 10 mU/min. In some settings or in a situation when limited fluids may be administered, a more concentrated solution may be used. When 10 U Pitocin are added to 500 mL IV solution, the resulting concentration is 1 mU/min = 3 mL/hr. If 10 U Pitocin are added to 250 mL IV solution, the concentration is 1 mU/min = 1.5 mL/hr.

For administration after delivery of placenta:

- One dose of 10 U Pitocin (1 mL) is given intramuscularly or added to IV fluids for continuous infusion.

- Assess FHR, maternal blood pressure, pulse, frequency and duration of uterine contractions, and uterine resting tone before each increase in oxytocin infusion rate.

- Record all assessments and IV rate on monitor strip and on client's chart. Record oxytocin infusion rate in milliunits per minute and milliliters per hour (e.g., 0.5 mU/min [3 mL/hr]).

- Record on monitor strip all client activities (such as change of position, vomiting), procedures done (amniotomy, sterile vaginal examination), and administration of analgesic agents to allow for interpretation and evaluation of tracing.

- Assess cervical dilatation as needed.

- Provide nursing comfort measures.

- Discontinue IV oxytocin infusion and infuse primary solution when (1) fetal stress or distress is noted (tachycardia or bradycardia, late or variable decelerations), (2) uterine contractions are more frequent than every 2 minutes, (3) duration of contractions exceeds 60 seconds, or (4) insufficient relaxation of the uterus between contractions or a steady increase in resting tone is noted (ACOG, 1999a). In addition to discontinuing IV oxytocin infusion, turn client to side, and if fetal distress is present, administer oxygen by tight face mask at 7 to 10 L/min; notify physician.

- Maintain intake and output record. Assess intake and output every hour.

Category	Immediate Care	Outcomes
Referral	Review prenatal record Advise certified nurse-midwife (CNM) or physician of admission Anesthesia	**Expected Outcomes** Appropriate resources identified and utilized
Assessments	Previous pregnancies, present pregnancy, and childbirth preparation Estimated gestational age of the fetus Assess woman's feelings regarding induction as well as knowledge base regarding the induction process Assess knowledge of breathing techniques; if woman does not have a method to use, teach breathing techniques before starting oxytocin infusion	**Expected Outcomes** Potential and actual complications identified
Teaching/ psychosocial	Provide emotional support through teaching and answering all questions	**Expected Outcomes** Woman verbalizes or demonstrates understanding of information given
Nursing care management and reports	Examination of pregnant uterus (Leopold's maneuvers to determine fetal size and position) Vaginal examination to evaluate cervical readiness: • Ripe cervix feels soft to the examining finger, is located in a medial to anterior position, is more than 50% effaced, and is 2–3 cm dilated • Unripe cervix feels firm to the examining finger, is long and thick, is perhaps in a posterior position, and is dilated little or not at all Presence of contractions Membranes intact or ruptured Maternal vital signs and a 20-minute baseline fetal monitoring strip prior to induction to determine fetal well-being Diagnostic studies: • Fetal maturity tests (lecithin/sphingomyelin [L/S] ratio, creatinine concentrations, ultrasonography), NST, CST, BPP • Maternal blood studies (complete blood count [CBC], hemoglobin, hematocrit, blood type, Rh factor) • Urinalysis Monitor for nausea, vomiting, hypotension, tachycardia, cardiac arrhythmias, headache, mental confusion, decreased urinary output Monitor FHR by continuous electronic fetal monitoring; do not start infusion or advance rate (if induction has already begun) if FHR is not in range of 120–160 bpm, if decelerations are present, or if variability decreases Evaluate and document maternal BP and pulse before beginning induction and then before each increase in infusion rate; do not advance infusion rate in presence of maternal hypertension or hypotension or radical changes in pulse rate If the woman becomes hypotensive: • Keep her on her side; may change to other side • Discontinue oxytocin infusion • Increase rate of primary IV line • Monitor FHR • Notify physician • Assess for cause of hypotension Evaluate and document contraction frequency, duration, and intensity prior to each increase in infusion rate Discontinue oxytocin infusion if: • Contractions are more frequent than every 2 minutes • Contraction duration exceeds 90 seconds • Uterus does not relax between contractions	**Expected Outcomes** Progression of labor and birth without difficulty Potential and actual complications minimized

BP, blood pressure; bpm, beats per minute; BPP, biophysical profile; CBC, complete blood count; CST, contraction stress test; FHR, fetal heart rate; I&O, intake and output; IV, intravenous; NST, nonstress test; Prn, as needed; WNL, within normal limits

Category	Immediate Care	Outcomes
Nursing care management and reports *continued*	Increase oxytocin IV infusion rate every 20 minutes until adequate contractions are achieved. Do not exceed an infusion rate of 20–40 mL/min. (*Note:* Protocols directing how often oxytocin is increased may vary from 15 to 60 minutes. See ACOG, 1999a, for guidelines and refer to institutional protocols.) Check infusion pump to ensure oxytocin is infusing. Check whether pump is on, chamber refills and empties, level of fluid in IV bottle becomes lower. If problem is found, correct and restart infusion at beginning dose. Check main IV site frequently. Check piggyback connection to primary tubing to ensure solution is not leaking. Evaluate cervical dilatation by vaginal examination as indicated. Monitor FHR continuously (normal range is 120–160 bpm). In episodes of bradycardia (<120 bpm) lasting for more than 30 seconds, administer oxygen by face mask at 7–10 L/min. Stop oxytocin infusion. Position woman on left side if quick recovery of FHR does not occur. Carefully evaluate fetal tachycardia (>160 bpm). Sustained tachycardia may necessitate discontinuation of oxytocin infusion. Assess for presence of meconium staining. Notify physician.	
Activity	Ambulate until 5–10 cm, dilated, then bed Position woman in left lateral or semi-Fowler's position Encourage her to avoid supine position	**Expected Outcomes** Activity individualized for woman
Comfort	Provide support to woman as she uses breathing techniques Encourage use of effleurage, back rub, and other supportive measures Assess need for analgesia or anesthesia	**Expected Outcomes** Optimal comfort level maintained
Nutrition	IV or lactated Ringer's solution Ice chips, clear fluids	**Expected Outcomes** Nutritional and hydration needs met
Elimination	Encourage voiding every 2 hours; monitor and record intake and output	**Expected Outcomes** Intake and output WNL
Medications	Start primary IV as ordered Administer oxytocin in electrolyte solution (piggyback oxytocin onto primary IV at closest site to IV needle insertion) Pain medications prn	**Expected Outcomes** Induction or augmentation of labor occurs within expected parameters
Discharge planning/home care	Photo packet Birth certificate worksheet Sibling visitation Car seat	**Expected Outcomes** Individualized discharge teaching completed
Family involvement	Family visitation policy per institutional protocol Encourage significant other to stay close and assist with breathing of woman	**Expected Outcomes** Family or support person involvement maximized
Date		

Complementary Care

HOLISTIC METHODS FOR CERVICAL RIPENING AND INDUCTION

In addition to the medical (allopathic) cervical ripening and induction methods previously discussed, a variety of more natural, noninvasive methods may also be used. These methods include sexual intercourse; self or partner nipple or breast stimulation; the use of herbs, castor oil, or enemas; acupuncture; stripping or sweeping the amniotic membranes; and mechanical dilatation of the cervix with balloon catheters (Summers, 1997). The cautions and contraindications are the same as those for medical induction of labor.

Although not frequently presented in medical (allopathic) or nursing texts, the natural methods are very effective (Summers, 1997). Many CNMs and their clients desire a less medical approach to birth and want to use natural methods whenever possible. It is important for basic nursing students, nurses, and consumers to be aware of all aspects of pregnancy care.

Sexual intercourse is a logical method of inducing cervical ripening and uterine contractions; female orgasm stimulates contractions, and male ejaculate contains a rich source of prostaglandins. In addition, breast and nipple stimulation, which are often part of lovemaking, cause the production of endogenous oxytocin, which in turn stimulates the uterus to contract (Summers, 1997).

Herbal preparations and other homeopathic solutions have not been scientifically studied to the same extent as other natural methods. The caregiver needs a thorough personal knowledge or ongoing consultation with a homeopathic physician to safely recommend the use of these approaches during late pregnancy (McFarlin, Gibson, O'Rear, et al., 1999).

Castor oil has been used for many years but has not been frequently studied as a method of labor induction. The mechanism by which castor oil stimulates uterine contractions is not understood. Some practitioners consider it to be an old-fashioned, nonuseful substance, whereas others have noted that it is especially effective for primigravidas (Summers, 1997).

CARE OF THE WOMAN DURING AMNIOINFUSION

Amnioinfusion (AI) is a technique by which warmed, sterile normal saline or Ringer's lactate solution is introduced into the uterus through an intrauterine pressure catheter (IUPC). Amnioinfusion can be used intrapartally to increase the volume of fluid in cases of oligohydramnios, in which cord compression causes FHR deceleration and fetal distress. It provides an extra cushion of fluid that relieves pressure on the umbilical cord and promotes increased perfusion to the fetus. Amnioinfusion is also used to dilute moderate to heavy meconium released in utero by a stressed fetus; when used for meconium dilution, amnioinfusion has resulted in a significant decrease of meconium below the cords after birth and a decrease in meconium aspiration. At birth, if the infant inhales any meconium present in the amniotic fluid, serious breathing problems and pneumonia may result (Pierce, Gaudier, & Sanches-Ramos, 2000). Amnioinfusion may also be indicated for preterm labor with premature rupture of membranes.

Nursing Management

The nurse is often the first person to detect changes in FHR associated with cord compression or to observe meconium-stained amniotic fluid. When cord compression is suspected, the immediate intervention is to assist the laboring woman to another position. If this intervention is not successful in restoring the FHR, an amnioinfusion may be considered.

Explain the amnioinfusion procedure and indications to the woman and her support person before initiation. Amnioinfusions are usually lactated Ringer's solution or normal saline. During the bolus infusion, monitoring is essential to avoid iatrogenic polyhydramnios (Tucker, 2000). Calculate the amount of fluid returned. If 250 mL has been infused with no return, discontinue the amnioinfusion until the fluid has returned.

Help administer the amnioinfusion, assess the woman's vital signs and contraction status, and monitor the FHR by continuous EFM. It is important to provide ongoing information to the laboring woman and her partner and to answer questions as they arise. Comfort measures and positioning are vital because the woman is now on bed rest. Frequently change disposable underpads and provide perineal care because fluid leaks constantly from the vagina.

CARE OF THE WOMAN DURING AN EPISIOTOMY

An **episiotomy** is a surgical incision of the perineal body to enlarge the outlet. The second most common procedure in maternal-child care, the episiotomy has long been thought to minimize the risk of lacerations of the perineum and the overstretching of perineal tissues (Peleg, Kennedy, Merrill, et al., 1999). Though very common, the routine use of episiotomy is being seriously questioned. In clinical practice, research has shown that major perineal trauma (extension to or through the anal sphincter) is four times more likely with a midline episiotomy (Maier & Maloni, 1997) and that a repeat of the trauma is likely to occur with subsequent births. Other complications associated with episiotomy are blood loss, infection, pain, and perineal discomfort that may continue for days or weeks past birth, including painful intercourse (Eason & Feldman, 2000). Personal beliefs, education, and experience of the practitioner appear to influence the decision to perform an episiotomy (Low, Seng, Murtland, et al., 2000).

Factors That Predispose Women to Episiotomy

Overall factors that place a woman at increased risk for episiotomy are primigravida, large or macrosomic fetus, occiput-posterior position, use of forceps or vacuum extractor, and shoulder dystocia (Maier & Maloni, 1997).

Preventative Measures

Following are some general tips that may help reduce the incidence of routine episiotomies:

- Kegel exercises throughout pregnancy to improve vaginal tone

- Perineal massage during pregnancy (Labrecque, Eason, & Marcoux, 2000)
- Natural gentle pushing that coincides with the woman's natural urges during labor
- Assuming an upright position and avoiding the lithotomy position or pulling back on legs (which tightens the perineum)
- Open-glottis breathing during pushing in second-stage labor

Episiotomy Procedure

There are two types of episiotomy in current practice: midline and mediolateral (Figure 20–2 ◆). Just before birth, when approximately 3 to 4 cm of the fetal head is visible during a contraction, the episiotomy is performed using sharp scissors with rounded points. The incision begins at the bottom center of the perineal body and extends either straight down the midline or at a 45-degree angle in either mediolateral direction.

The episiotomy is usually performed with regional or local anesthesia but may be done without anesthesia in emergency situations. It is generally proposed that as crowning occurs, the distention of the tissues causes numbing. Repair of the episiotomy (episiorrhaphy) and any lacerations is completed either during the period between birth of the neonate and before expulsion of the placenta or after expulsion of the placenta. Adequate anesthesia must be given for the repair.

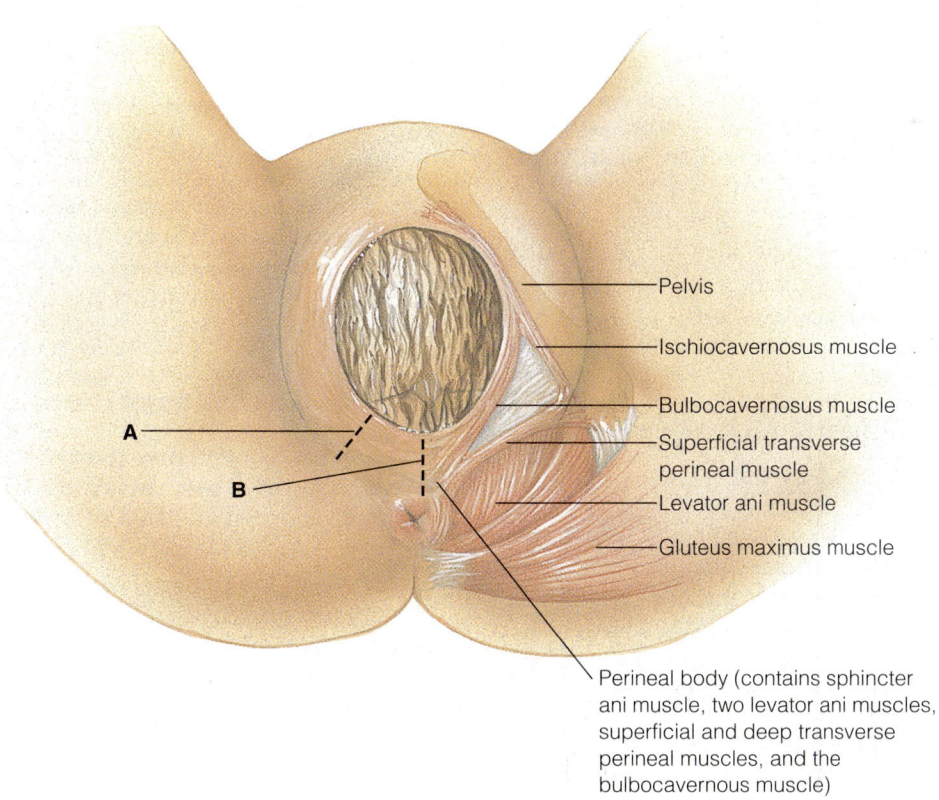

Pelvis
Ischiocavernosus muscle
Bulbocavernosus muscle
Superficial transverse perineal muscle
Levator ani muscle
Gluteus maximus muscle

Perineal body (contains sphincter ani muscle, two levator ani muscles, superficial and deep transverse perineal muscles, and the bulbocavernous muscle)

FIGURE 20–2. ◆ The two most common types of episiotomy are midline and mediolateral. **A,** Right mediolateral. **B,** Midline.

Nursing Management

The woman needs nursing support during the episiotomy and the repair because she may feel some pressure sensations. Without adequate anesthesia she may feel pain. Placing a hand on her shoulder and talking with her can provide comfort and distraction from the repair process. If the woman is having more discomfort than she can comfortably handle, act as an advocate in communicating the woman's needs to the physician or CNM. At all times the woman needs to be the one who decides whether the amount of discomfort she is experiencing is tolerable. She should never be told, "This doesn't hurt." She is the person experiencing the discomfort, and her evaluation needs to be respected.

The type of episiotomy is recorded on the birth record. This information should also be included in a report to subsequent caregivers so that they can make adequate assessments and institute relief measures.

Comfort measures may begin immediately after birth with the application of an ice pack to the perineum. For optimal effect the ice pack should be applied for 20 to 30 minutes and removed for at least 20 minutes before being reapplied. Assess the perineal tissues frequently to prevent injury from the ice pack. Inspect the episiotomy site every 15 minutes during the first hour after the birth for redness, swelling, tenderness, and hematomas. As part of postpartum care, instruct the mother in perineal hygiene care and comfort measures.

It is important for nurses to recognize that perineal pain continues for a period of time. Many women experience significant pain for a week after the birth; some continue to have pain at 8 weeks postpartum, or may have pain for a much longer period. Do not discount this pain: Women who experience prolonged pain tend to have problems with breastfeeding and depression and are reluctant to reestablish sexual activity.

Nursing advocacy is needed to promote selective rather than routine episiotomy. It is imperative that each nurse stay current regarding new information and research in order to maintain current practice standards.

CARE OF THE WOMAN DURING FORCEPS-ASSISTED BIRTH

Forceps are surgical instruments designed to assist in the birth of a fetus by providing either traction or the means to rotate the fetal head to an occiput-anterior position. In medical literature and practice, forceps-assisted birth is also known as *instrumental delivery* or *operative vaginal delivery*. The three categories of forceps application are:

1. *Outlet forceps* are applied when the fetal skull has reached the perineum, the fetal scalp is visible, and the sagittal suture is in the anteroposterior diameter or right or left occiput anterior or posterior position. Rotation is not more than 45 degrees.

2. *Low forceps* are applied when the leading edge (presenting part) of the fetal skull is at a station of $\geq +2$ cm and not on the pelvic floor.

3. *Midforceps* are applied when the fetal head is engaged.

Forceps may be indicated in the presence of any condition that threatens the mother or fetus and can be relieved by birth. Conditions that put the woman at risk include heart or pulmonary disease, maternal exhaustion, or high level of regional analgesia that diminishes the woman's expulsive efforts. Fetal conditions include premature placental separation and fetal distress (ACOG, 2000b). Forceps may be used electively to shorten the second stage of labor and assist the woman's pushing effort.

Before forceps are used, the following conditions must be met (Charles, 1999):

- The cervix must be completely dilated and the exact position and station of the fetal head known.
- Membranes must be ruptured to allow a firm grasp on the fetal head, which must be engaged and in vertex or face presentation.
- The type of pelvis should be known, because certain pelvic types do not permit rotation.
- The maternal bladder should be empty and adequate anesthesia given.
- No degree of cephalopelvic disproportion can be present.

Neonatal and Maternal Risks

Some neonates may develop a small area of ecchymosis and/or edema along the sides of the face as a result of forceps application. Caput succedaneum or cephalhematoma (with subsequent hyperbilirubinemia) may occur, as may transient facial paralysis (ACOG, 2000b).

Maternal risks include possible lacerations of the birth canal, extensions of a median episiotomy into the anus, increased bleeding, bruising, and perineal edema.

Nursing Management

Ongoing assessment may allow the nurse to note the variables associated with an increased rate of instrument-assisted or operative birth. Nursing care measures could then be directed toward variables that may reduce the incidence of these factors. For example, labor dystocia may be corrected by changing maternal position, ambulation, and frequent bladder emptying. FHR abnormalities may be improved by position changes, increased fluid intake, and/or adequate oxygen exchange.

If a forceps-assisted birth is required, explain the procedure to the woman. Assess maternal comfort level before the application of forceps. With adequate regional anes-

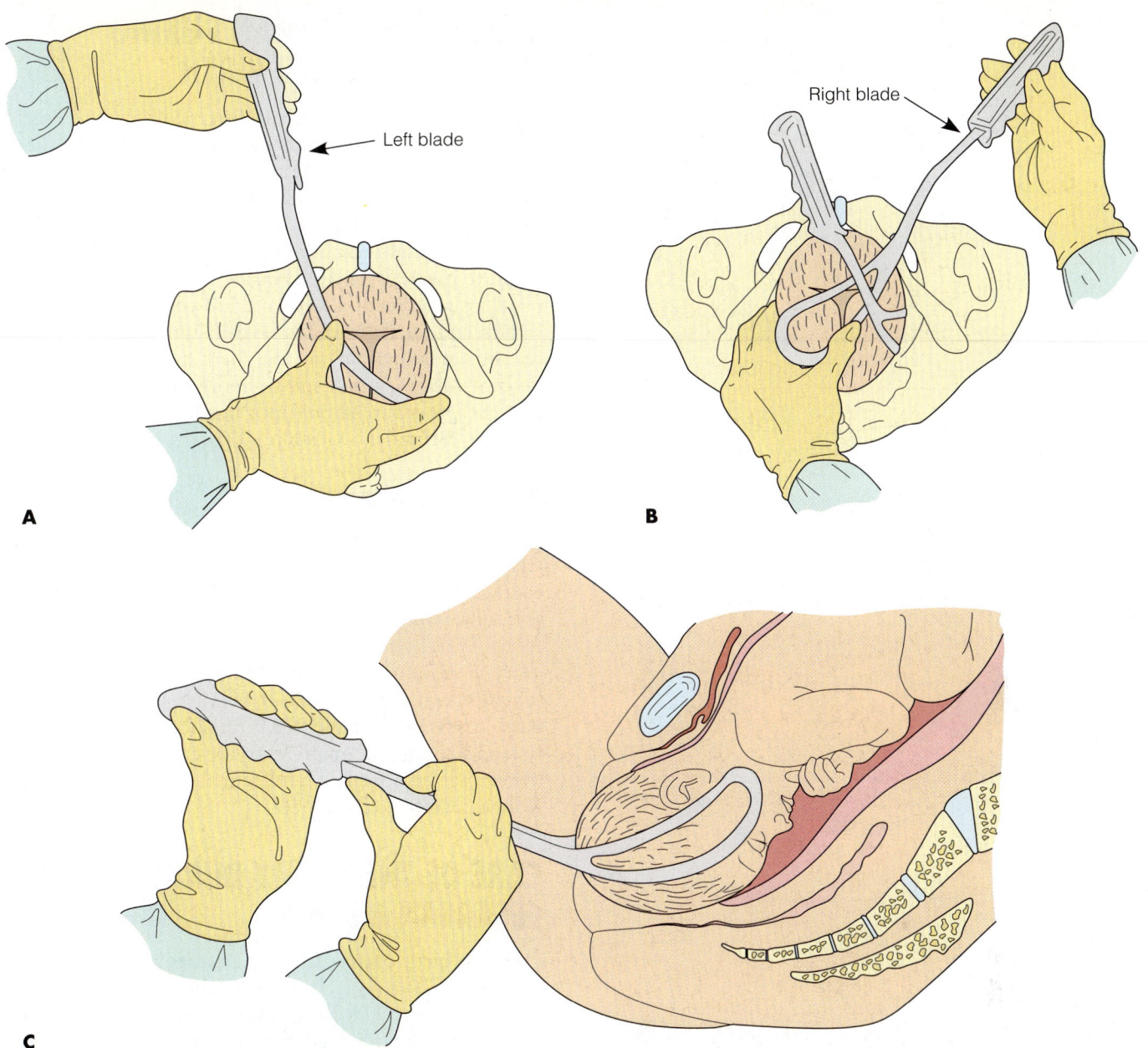

FIGURE 20–3. ◆ Application of forceps in occiput-anterior (OA) position. **A,** The left blade is inserted along the left side wall of the pelvis over the parietal bone. **B,** The right blade is inserted along the right side wall of the pelvis over the parietal bone. **C,** With correct placement of the blades, the handles lock easily. During uterine contractions, traction is applied to the forceps in a downward and outward direction to follow the birth canal.

thesia the woman should feel some pressure during the procedure but no pain. Encourage the woman to use breathing techniques that help prevent her from pushing during application of the forceps (Figure 20–3 ◆). Monitor contractions and advise the physician when one is present because traction is only applied with a contraction. With each contraction the physician provides traction on the forceps as the woman pushes. It is not uncommon to observe mild fetal bradycardia as traction is being applied to the forceps. This bradycardia results from head compression and is transient.

Immediately following birth, assess the newborn for facial edema, bruising, caput succedaneum, cephalhematoma, and any sign of cerebral edema. Prepare parents and show them any forcep marks; provide reassurance that they usually disappear in a few days. In the fourth stage, assess the woman for perineal swelling, bruising, hematoma, excessive bleeding, and hemorrhage. In the postpartum period it is important to assess for signs of infection if lacerations occurred during the procedure. Give the woman a chance to ask questions and reiterate explanations. Also discuss nursing assessments of the woman and her newborn.

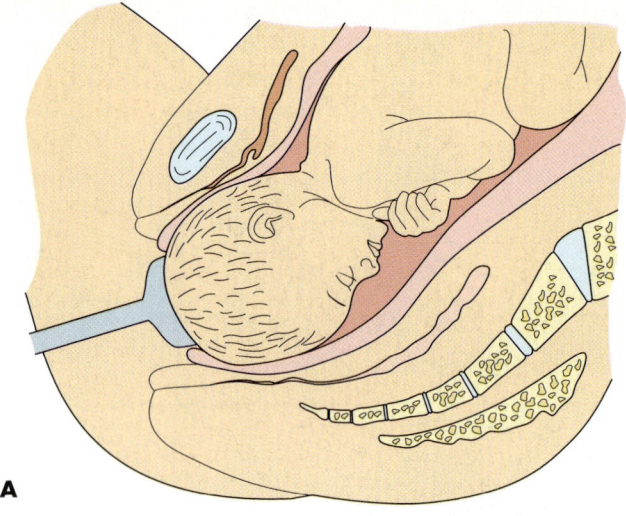

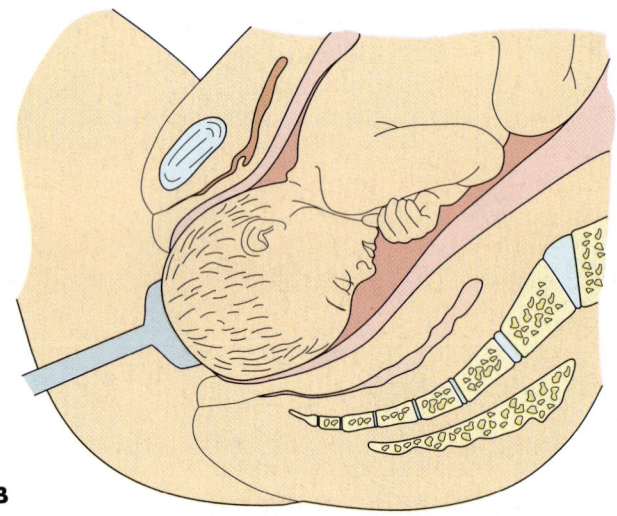

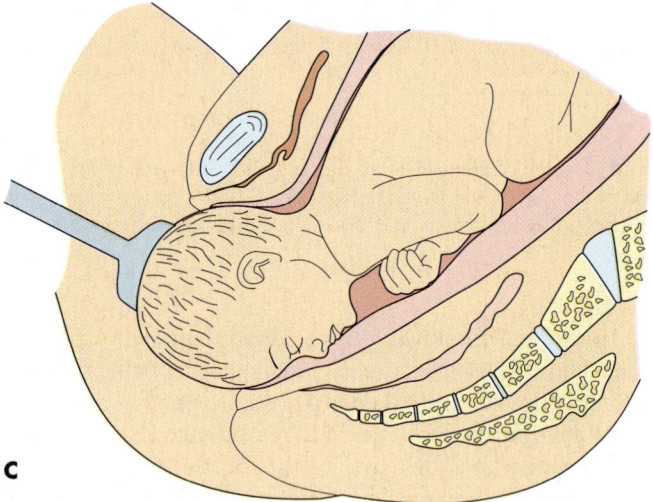

FIGURE 20–4. ◆ Vacuum extractor traction. **A,** The cup is placed on the fetal occiput and suction is created. Traction is applied in a downward and outward direction. **B,** Traction continues in a downward direction as the fetal head begins to emerge from the vagina. **C,** Traction is maintained to lift the fetal head out of the vagina.

CARE OF THE WOMAN DURING VACUUM-ASSISTED BIRTH

Vacuum-assisted birth is an obstetric procedure used to facilitate the birth of a fetus by applying suction to the fetal head. The vacuum extractor is composed of a soft suction cup attached to a suction bottle (pump) by tubing. The suction cup, which comes in various sizes, is placed against the fetal occiput, and the pump is used to create negative pressure (suction) inside the cup. Traction is applied in coordination with uterine contractions, descent occurs, and the fetal head is born (Figure 20–4 ◆). General recommendations include that there should be progressive descent with each pull and no more than three pulls; and that the procedure should not last longer than 20 to 30 minutes (Brumfield, Gilstrap, O'Grady, et al., 1999).

Nursing Management

The nurse is responsible for keeping the woman and her partner informed about what is happening during the procedure. If adequate regional anesthesia has been administered, the woman feels only pressure during the procedure. Assess FHR by continuous EFM or by auscultation at least every 5 minutes. Reassure the parents that the caput (chignon) on the baby's head will disappear within 2 to 3 days. Assessment of the newborn should include inspection and continued observation for cephalhematomas, intracerebral hemorrhage, and retinal hemorrhages (Sachs, Kobelin, Castro, et al., 1999).

CARE OF THE FAMILY DURING CESAREAN BIRTH

Cesarean birth occurs through an abdominal and uterine incision. ⬭⬭ 🆒 It is one of the oldest surgical procedures known. Until the 20th century, cesarean procedures were primarily used in an attempt to save the fetus of a dying woman. As the maternal and perinatal morbidity and mortality rates associated with cesarean birth steadily decreased throughout the 20th century, the proportion of cesarean births increased. Following the 1970's dramatic rise in surgical births, a steady decline began in 1989, primarily due to efforts to contain health care costs. In 1996 the total cesarean rate had decreased to 20.6% (Curtin & Mathews, 2000). However, in recent years the total percentage of cesarean births has again begun to rise and at the end of 1999 the rate was 22% (Cockey, 2000).

In an effort to generate and analyze data that can be used to appropriately decrease the rising cesarean birth rate, ACOG (2000a) developed the *Evaluation of Cesarean Delivery* document. This resource is aimed at obtaining accurate statistics for clinicians and institutions using case mix adjusted data for two groups who have had cesareans: nulliparous women with a single, full-term fetus in vertex presentation (first-time cesareans) and multiparous women who have had one prior low-transverse cesarean birth for a single full-term fetus in a vertex presentation (repeat cesareans). These two groups were chosen because together they comprise two thirds of cesarean births in the United States but represent the greatest variation in cesarean rates. ACOG recommends that physicians and hospitals monitor their cesarean rates for these two groups and then compare their rates with benchmark rates (Cockey, 2000). Other factors, such as the continuous presence of a nurse or trained support person, may also help lower cesarean birth rates and warrant further consideration (Sams, 2000).

Indications

Cesarean births are performed in the presence of a variety of maternal and fetal conditions. Commonly accepted indications include complete placenta previa, cephalopelvic disproportion, placental abruption, active genital herpes, umbilical cord prolapse, failure to progress in labor, proven fetal distress, benign and malignant tumors that obstruct the birth canal, and cervical cerclage (Keane, 1997). More controversial indications include breech presentation, previous cesarean birth, major congenital anomalies, and severe Rh isoimmunization. It should be noted that cesarean births have a higher maternal mortality rate than vaginal births and the morbidity factors associated with a surgical delivery are infection, reactions to anesthetic agents, blood clots, and bleeding (Bowes, 1999).

Skin Incisions

The skin incision for a cesarean birth is either transverse (Pfannenstiel) or vertical and is not indicative of the type of incision made into the uterus. The transverse incision is made across the lowest and narrowest part of the abdomen. Since the incision is made just below the pubic hairline, it is almost invisible after healing. The limitation of this type of skin incision is that it does not allow for extension of the incision if needed. This incision is used when time is not of the essence (e.g., with failure to progress and no fetal or maternal distress), because it usually requires more time to make and repair.

The vertical incision is made between the navel and the symphysis pubis. This type of incision is quicker and is therefore preferred in cases of fetal distress when rapid birth is indicated, with preterm or macrosomic infants, or when the woman is significantly obese. Time factors, client preference, or physician preference determine the type of skin incision.

Uterine Incisions

The type of uterine incision depends on the need for the cesarean. The choice of incision affects the woman's opportunity for a subsequent vaginal birth and her risks of a ruptured uterine scar with a subsequent pregnancy. The two major types of uterine incisions are in the lower uterine segment and in the upper segment of the uterine corpus. The lower uterine segment incision most commonly used is a transverse incision, although a vertical incision may also be used (Figure 20–5 ◆).

Nursing Management

PREPARATION FOR CESAREAN BIRTH

Because one of every five births is a cesarean, make preparation for this possibility an integral part of all prenatal education. Encourage pregnant women and their partners to discuss the possibility of a cesarean birth with their

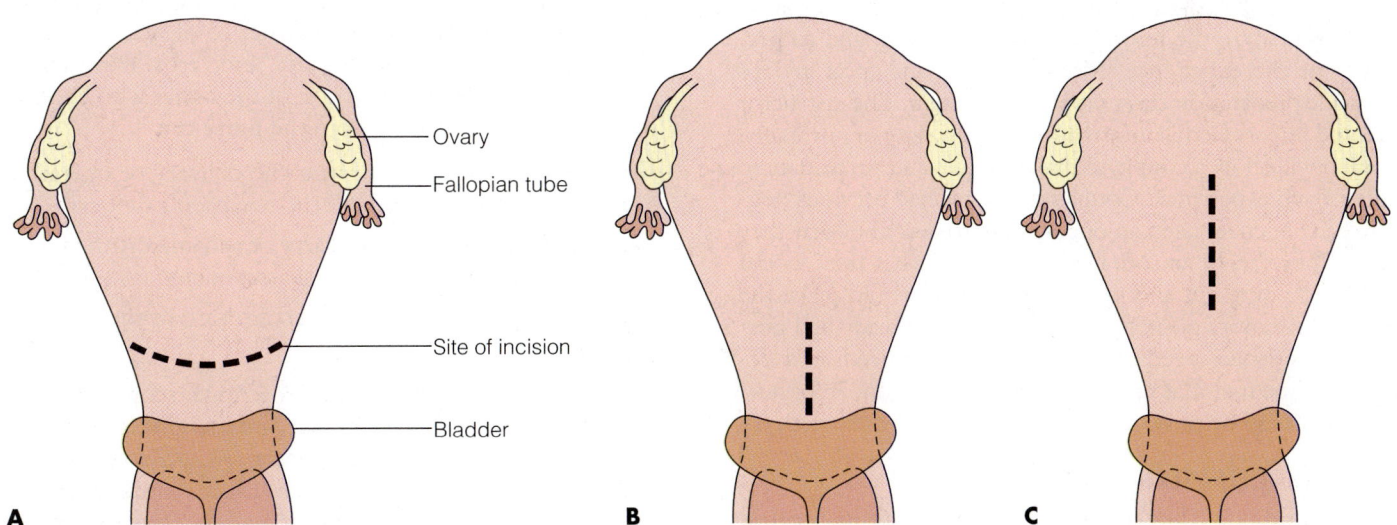

FIGURE 20–5. ◆ Uterine incisions for a cesarean birth. **A,** This transverse incision in the lower uterine segment is called a Kerr incision. **B,** The Sellheim incision is a vertical incision in the lower uterine segment. **C,** This view illustrates the classic uterine incision that is done in the body (corpus) of the uterus. The classic incision was commonly used in the past but is associated with increased risk of uterine rupture in subsequent pregnancies and labor.

obstetrician or CNM and at the same time discuss their specific needs and desires under those circumstances. Their preferences may include the following:

- Participating in the choice of anesthetic
- Father (or significant other) being present during the procedures and/or birth
- Father (or significant other) being present in the recovery or postpartum room
- Audio recording and/or taking pictures of the birth
- Delayed instillation of eye drops to promote eye contact between parent and infant in the first hours after birth
- Physical contact or holding the infant while in the operating and/or recovery room (by the father if the mother cannot hold the newborn)
- Breastfeeding immediately after birth or in the recovery area

Information that couples need about cesarean birth includes the following:

- What preparatory procedures to expect
- Description or viewing of the delivery room
- Types of anesthesia for birth and analgesia available postpartum
- Sensations that may be experienced
- Roles of significant others
- Interaction with newborn
- Immediate recovery phase
- Postpartum phase

Relay this information in a birth-oriented context rather than a surgery-oriented one.

REPEAT CESAREAN BIRTH

When a couple is anticipating a cesarean birth, they have time to analyze the information they are given and to prepare for the experience. Many hospitals and local groups provide preparation classes for cesarean birth. The instructor should impart factual information and a feeling of normality, which will allow a couple to make choices and participate in their birth experience. Couples who have had previous negative experiences need an opportunity to describe what they felt. They can be encouraged to identify what they would like to be different and to list options that would make the experience more positive. Those who have already had positive experiences need reassurance that their needs and desires will be met in a similar manner. In addition, an opportunity should be provided to discuss any fears or anxieties.

EMERGENCY CESAREAN BIRTH

The period preceding surgery must be used to its greatest advantage. It is imperative that caregivers use their most effective communication skills in supporting the couple. The nurse describes what the couple may anticipate during the next few hours. Asking the couple "What questions or concerns do you have about the decision?" gives them an opportunity for clarification. The nurse can prepare the woman in stages, giving her information and the rationale for interventions before beginning any procedure. It is essential to tell the woman (1) what is going to happen, (2) why it is being done, and (3) what sensations she may experience. This allows the woman to be informed and to consent to the procedure, which gives her a sense of control and reduces her feelings of helplessness.

To reduce the likelihood of serious pulmonary damage if gastric contents are aspirated, antacids may be administered within 30 minutes of surgery. If epidural anesthesia is used, the nurse may assist with the procedure, monitor the woman's blood pressure and response, and continue EFM. An abdominal and perineal prep is done, and an indwelling catheter is inserted to prevent bladder distention. An IV line is started with a large-bore needle to permit blood administration if it becomes necessary. Preoperative medication may be ordered. The pediatrician should be notified and preparation made to receive the new baby. The nurse ensures that the infant warmer is working and that resuscitation equipment is available.

The nurse assists in positioning the woman on the operating table. Fetal heart rate is assessed before surgery and during preparation because fetal hypoxia can result from the supine position. A hip wedge (folded blanket or towels) is placed under the right hip to tip the uterus slightly and reduce compression of blood vessels A last-minute check is done to ensure that the fetal scalp electrode has been removed if the fetus was internally monitored.

Birth

Every effort should be made to include the father or partner in the birth experience. When attending the cesarean birth, the partner wears protective coverings similar to those worn by others in the operating suite. A stool beside the woman's head allows the partner to sit nearby to provide physical touch, visual contact, and verbal reassurance.

To promote the participation of the father who chooses not to be in the delivery room the nurse can

1. Allow the father to be near the delivery or operating room, where he can hear the newborn's first cry
2. Encourage the father to carry or accompany the infant to the nursery for the initial assessment
3. Involve the father in postpartum care in the recovery room

After birth the nurse assesses the Apgar score and completes the same initial assessment and identification procedures used for vaginal births. Make every effort to assist the parents in bonding with their infant. If the mother is awake, free one of her arms so that she can touch and stroke the infant. Place the newborn on the mother's chest or hold it in an en face position. If physical contact is not possible, provide a running narrative so the mother knows what is happening with her baby. Help the anesthesiologist or nurse anesthetist raise the mother's head so she can see her infant immediately after birth. Encourage the parents to talk to the baby, and let the father hold the baby until he or she is taken to the nursery.

Analgesia and Anesthesia

There is no perfect anesthesia for cesarean birth. Each has its advantages, disadvantages, possible risks, and side effects. Goals for analgesia and anesthesia administration include safety, comfort, and emotional satisfaction for the client (see Chapter 18). 🔗

Immediate Postpartal Recovery Period

The nurse caring for the postpartum woman assesses the mother's vital signs every 5 minutes until they are stable, then every 15 minutes for an hour, then every 30 minutes until she is discharged to the postpartum unit. Remain with the woman until she is stable.

Evaluate the dressing and perineal pad every 15 minutes for at least an hour. Gently palpate the fundus to determine whether it is remaining firm; it may be palpated by placing a hand to support the incision. IV oxytocin is usually administered to promote the contractility of the uterine musculature. If the woman has been under general anesthesia, she should be positioned on her side to facilitate drainage of secretions, turned, and assisted with coughing and deep breathing every 2 hours for at least 24 hours. If she has received a spinal or epidural anesthetic, check the level of anesthesia every 15 minutes until full sensation has returned. It is important to monitor intake and output and to observe the urine for bloody tinge, which could mean surgical trauma to the bladder. The physician prescribes medication to relieve the mother's pain and nausea, and it is administered as needed.

CARE OF THE WOMAN UNDERGOING VAGINAL BIRTH AFTER CESAREAN (VBAC)

There is an increasing trend to have a trial of labor and **vaginal birth after cesarean (VBAC)** in cases of nonre-curring indications (such as umbilical cord accident, placenta previa, or fetal distress). This trend has been influenced by consumer demand and studies that support VBAC as a viable alternative to repeat cesarean.

The ACOG (1999c) guidelines state that the following aspects need to be considered for VBAC:

- A woman with one or two prior low transverse uterine incisions may be counseled and encouraged to attempt VBAC.
- There should be a clinically adequate pelvis and no other uterine scars or previous rupture.
- A prior classic or T-shaped uterine incision or other transfundal uterine surgery is a contraindication to VBAC.
- Anesthesia and surgical team are available for emergent cesarean birth.
- A physician is immediately available throughout active labor capable of monitoring labor and performing an emergent cesarean birth.

The most common risks associated with VBAC are hemorrhage and a less than 1% occurrence of uterine scar separation or rupture (ACOG, 1999c).

Nursing Management

The nursing care of a woman undergoing VBAC varies according to institutional protocols. Generally, if the woman is at very low risk, a heplock is inserted for IV access if needed, continuous EFM is used, and clear fluids may be taken. A woman at higher risk may require additional precautionary measures. Take care to ensure that the woman and her partner feel safe but not unduly restricted by the VBAC status.

Supportive and comfort measures are very important. The woman may be excited about this opportunity to experience labor and vaginal birth, or she may be hesitant and frightened about the possibility of complications. The presence of the nurse is important in providing information and encouragement for the laboring woman and her partner.

CHAPTER HIGHLIGHTS

🖎 An external (or cephalic) version may be done after 36 weeks' gestation to change a breech presentation to a cephalic presentation. The benefits of the version are that a lower risk vaginal birth may be anticipated. The version is accomplished with the use of tocolytics to relax the uterus.

🖎 Amniotomy (AROM) is performed to hasten labor. The risks are prolapse of the umbilical cord and infection.

🖎 Prostaglandin E$_2$ may be used before an induction of labor to soften the cervix (called cervical ripening).

🖎 Labor is induced for many reasons. The medical (allopathic) methods include amniotomy and IV oxytocin infusion. Nursing responsibilities are heightened during an induced labor.

🖎 An episiotomy may be done just before birth of the fetus. Although very prevalent in the United States, its routine use is being questioned.

- Forceps-assisted birth can be accomplished using outlet, low, or midforceps.

- A vacuum extractor is a soft, pliable cup attached to suction that can be applied to the fetal head and used in much the same way as forceps.

- At least one in five births is now accomplished by cesarean. The nurse has a vital role in providing information, support, and encouragement to the couple participating in a cesarean birth.

- Vaginal birth after cesarean (VBAC) is occurring more frequently now than in the past.

EXPLOREMediaLink

NCLEX Review, Case Studies, and other interactive resources for this chapter can be found on the companion website at http://www.prenhall.com/london. Click on "Chapter 20" to select the activities for this chapter.

For animations, more NCLEX review questions, and an audio glossary, access the accompanying CD-ROM in this textbook.

REFERENCES

American College of Obstetricians and Gynecologists. (1999a). *Induction of labor* (Practical Bulletin No. 10). Washington, DC: Author.

American College of Obstetricians and Gynecologists Committee on Practice. (1999b). *Induction of labor with misoprostol*. Washington, DC: Author.

American College of Obstetricians and Gynecologists Committee. (1999c). *Vaginal birth after previous cesarean delivery* (Practice Bulletin No. 5). Washington, DC: Author.

American College of Obstetricians and Gynecologists (2000a). *Evaluation of cesarean delivery*. Washington, DC: Author.

American College of Obstetricians and Gynecologists (2000b). *Operative vaginal delivery* (Practice Bulletin No. 17). Washington, DC: Author.

Bishop, E. H. (1964). Pelvic scoring for elective inductions. *Obstetrics and Gynecology, 24,* 266.

Bowes, W. A., Jr. (1999). Clinical aspects of normal and abnormal labor. In R. K. Creasy & R. Resnik (Eds.), *Maternal-fetal medicine* (4th ed., pp. 541–568). Philadelphia: Saunders.

Brumfield, C., Gilstrap, L. C., O'Grady, J. P., Ross, M. G., & Schifrin, B. S. (1999). Cutting your legal risks with vacuum-assisted deliveries. *OBG Management, 3,* 2–6.

Charles, A. G. (1999). Forceps delivery and vacuum extraction. In P. V. Dilts & J. J. Sciarri (Eds.), *Gynecology and obstetrics* (Vol. 2). Philadelphia: Lippincott.

Cockey, C. D. (2000). Curbing cesarean rates: ACOG releases new comprehensive recommendations. *AWHONN: Lifelines, 4*(5), 17.

Cruikshank, D. P. (1999). Malpresentations and umbilical cord complications. In J. R. Scott, P. J. DiSaia, C. B. Hammond, & W. N. Spellacy (Eds.), *Danforth's obstetrics and gynecology* (8th ed., pp. 419–436). Philadelphia: Lippincott Williams & Wilkins.

Cunningham, F. G., Gant, N. F., Leveno, K. J., Gilstrap, L. C., Hauth, J. C., & K. D. Wenstrom. Induction and augmentation of labor. *Williams obstetrics,* New York: McGraw-Hill. (21st ed. pp. 469–481).

Curtin, S. C., & Mathews, T. J. (2000). U.S. obstetric procedures, 1998. *Birth, 27*(2), 136–140.

Eason, E., & Feldman, P. (2000). Much ado about a little cut: Is episiotomy worthwhile? *Obstetrics and Gynecology, 95*(4), 616–618.

Forrest Pharmaceuticals, Inc. (1995). *Cervidil Dinoprostone 10 mg. Vaginal insert.* St. Louis, MO: UAB Laboratories.

Keane, D. P. (1997). Operative procedures. In R. K. Creasy (Ed.), *Management of labor and delivery* (pp. 414–457). Malden, MA: Blackwell Science.

Kiss, H., Ahner, R., Hohlagschwandtner, M., Leitch, H., & Huslein, P. (2000). Fetal fibronectin as a predictor of term labor: A literature review. *Acta Obstetricia et Gynecologica Scandinavica, 79*(1), 3–7.

Labrecque, M., Eason, E., & Marcoux, S. (2000). Randomized controlled trial of perineal massage during pregnancy: Perineal symptoms three months after delivery. *American Journal of Obstetrics and Gynecology, 182*(1, Pt.1), 76–80.

Low, L. K., Seng, J. S., Murtland, T. L., & Oakley, D. (2000). Clinician-specific episiotomy rates: Impacts on perineal outcomes. *Journal of Nurse-Midwifery and Women's Health, 45*(2), 87–93.

Maier, J. S., & Maloni, J. A. (1997). Nurse advocacy for selective versus routine episiotomy. *Journal of Obstetric, Gynecologic, and Neonatal Nursing, 26,* 155–161.

McFarlin, B. L., Gibson, M. H., O'Rear, J., & Harman, P. (1999). A national survey of herbal preparation use by nurse-midwives for labor stimulation: Review of the literature and recommendations for practice. *Journal of Nurse-Midwifery, 44,* 205–216.

Oei, S. G., Lidewijde, J., & Mol, B. W. J. (2000). Randomized trial of administration of prostaglandin E₂ gel for induction of labor in the morning or the evening. *Journal of Perinatal Medicine, 28,* 20–25.

Peleg, D., Kennedy, C. M., Merrill, D., & Zlatnik, F. J. (1999). Risk of repetitions of a severe perineal laceration. *Obstetrics and Gynecology, 93,* 1021–1024.

Pierce, J., Gaudier, F. L., & Sanches-Ramos, L. (2000). Intrapartum amniofusion for meconium-stained fluid: Meta-analysis of prospective clinical trials. *Obstetrics and Gynecology, 95*(6, Pt. 2), 1051–1056.

Rozenberg, P., Goffinet, F., & Hessabi, M. (2000). Comparison of the Bishop score, ultrasonographically measured cervical length, and fetal fibronectin assay in predicting time until delivery and type of delivery at term. *American Journal of Obstetrics and Gynecology, 182*(1, Pt.1), 108–113.

Sachs, B. P., Kobelin, C., Castro, M. A., & Frigoletto, F. (1999). Sounding: The risks of lowering the cesarean-delivery rate. *New England Journal of Medicine, 340,* 54–57.

Sams, L. (2000). Evaluating cesarean deliveries: Exploring ACOG's recommendations to improve outcomes. *AWHONN: Lifelines, 4*(5), 15.

Schmidt, J. (1999). Prolonged pregnancy. In L. K. Mandeville & N. H. Troiano (Eds.), *AWHONN: High risk and critical care intrapartum nursing* (2nd ed., pp. 123–138). Philadelphia: Lippincott.

Summers, L. (1997). Methods of cervical ripening and labor induction. *Journal of Nurse-Midwifery, 42,* 71–82.

Tucker, S. M. (2000). *Pocket guide to fetal monitoring and assessment* (4th ed.). St. Louis, MO: Mosby.

Wilson, B. A., Shannon, M. T., & Strang, C. L. (Eds.). (2001). *Nursing drug guide: 2001.* Upper Saddle River, NJ: Prentice-Hall.

Wilson, C. (2000). The nurse's role in misoprostol induction: A proposed protocol. *Journal of Obstetric, Gynecologic, and Neonatal Nursing, 28*(6), 574–583.

Wolcott, H. D., & Conry, J. A. (2000). Normal labor. In A. T. Evans & K. R. Niswander (Eds.), *Manual of obstetrics* (6th ed., pp. 392–424). Philadelphia: Lippincott Williams & Wilkins.

UNIT V

The Postpartal Childbearing Family and Newborn

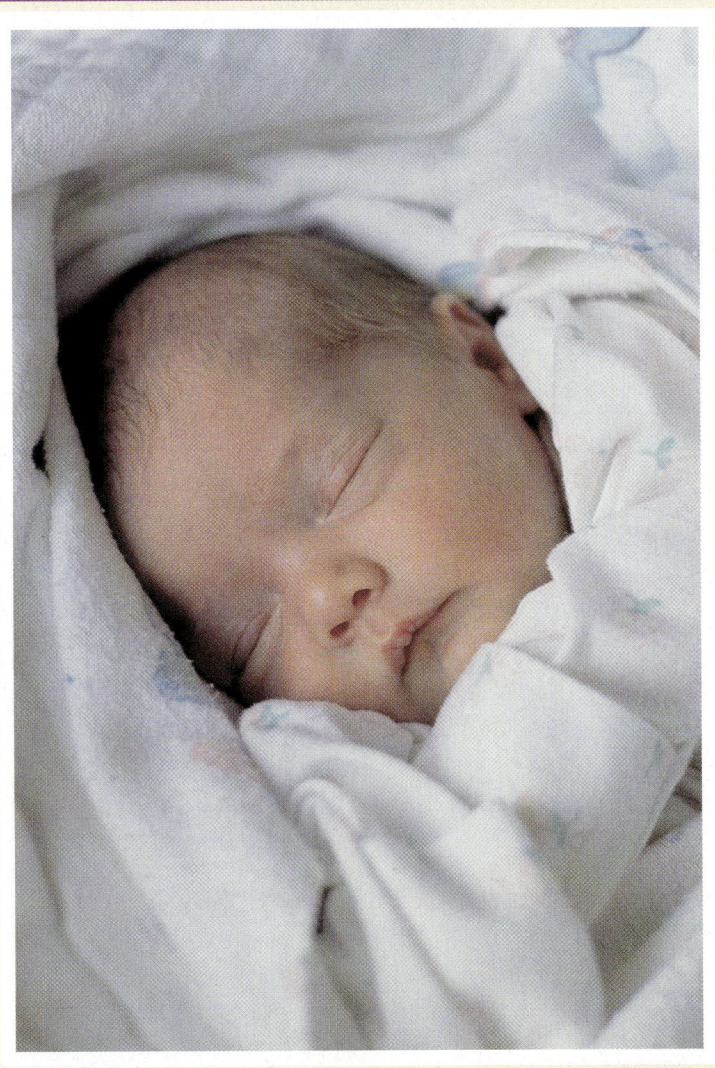

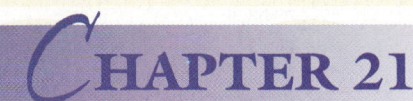

Postpartal Adaptation and Nursing Assessment

I acutely felt the fatigue and sense of loss of the relationship with my baby that I had during pregnancy. But then the wonderful part happened with the reuniting with my new daughter. Holding her, having her latch on to my breast to get nourishment and her looking into my eyes to say "hello Mom."

—SUSAN, 34

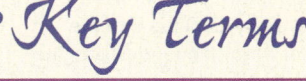 Key Terms

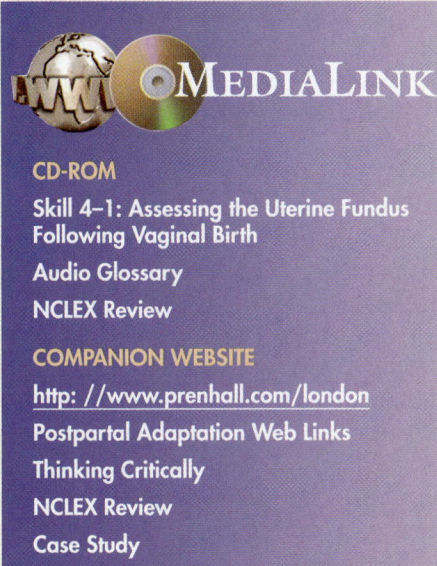

MEDIALINK

CD-ROM
Skill 4–1: Assessing the Uterine Fundus Following Vaginal Birth
Audio Glossary
NCLEX Review

COMPANION WEBSITE
http://www.prenhall.com/london
Postpartal Adaptation Web Links
Thinking Critically
NCLEX Review
Case Study

*T*he **puerperium,** or postpartal period, is when the woman adjusts, physically and psychologically, to the process of childbirth. It begins immediately after birth and continues for approximately 6 weeks, or until the body has returned to a near prepregnant state. This chapter describes the physiologic and psychologic changes that occur postpartally and the basic aspects of a thorough postpartal assessment. How can the nurse help the woman adjust to these changes?

POSTPARTAL PHYSICAL ADAPTATIONS

Comprehensive nursing assessment is based on a sound understanding of the normal anatomic and physiologic processes of the puerperium. These processes involve the reproductive organs and other major body systems.

Reproductive System

INVOLUTION OF THE UTERUS

The term **involution** is used to describe the rapid reduction in size and the return of the uterus to a nonpregnant state. Following separation of the placenta, the decidua of the uterus is irregular, jagged, and varied in thickness. The spongy layer of the decidua is cast off as lochia, while the inner layer forms the basis for the development of new endometrium. Except at the placenta attachment site, this process takes about 3 weeks. Bleeding from the larger uterine vessels of the placenta site is controlled by compression of the retracted uterine muscle fibers. The clotted blood is gradually absorbed by the body. Some of these vessels are eventually obliterated and replaced by new vessels with smaller lumens.

Rather than forming a fibrous scar in the decidua, the placenta site heals by a process of exfoliation. In this process, the site is undermined by the growth of the endometrial tissue both from the margins of the site and from the fundi of the endometrial glands left in the basal layer of the site. The infarcted superficial tissue then becomes necrotic and is sloughed off (Cunningham, Gant, Leveno, et al., 2001). Exfoliation is a very important aspect of involution. If healing of the placenta site left a fibrous scar, the area available for future implantation would be limited, as would the number of possible pregnancies.

The uterus gradually decreases in size as the cells grow smaller and the hyperplasia of pregnancy reverses. Protein material in the uterine wall is broken down and absorbed. Factors that slow uterine involution include prolonged labor, anesthesia or excessive analgesia, difficult birth, grand multiparity, a full bladder, and incomplete expulsion of all of the placenta or fragments of the membranes. Factors that enhance involution include an uncomplicated labor and birth, complete expulsion of the placenta or membranes, breastfeeding, and early ambulation.

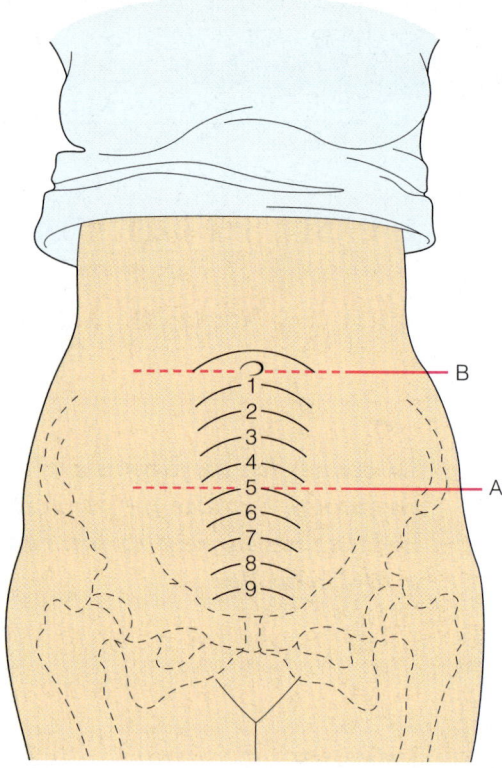

FIGURE 21–1. ◆ Involution of the uterus. **A,** Immediately after delivery of the placenta, the top of the fundus is in the midline and approximately halfway between the symphysis pubis and the umbilicus. **B,** About 6 to 12 hours after birth, the fundus is at the level of the umbilicus. The height of the fundus then decreases about one finger breadth (approximately 1 cm) each day.

CHANGES IN FUNDAL POSITION

Immediately following the birth of the placenta, the uterus contracts to the size of a large grapefruit. The **fundus,** or top portion of the uterus, is situated in the midline midway between the symphysis pubis and the umbilicus (Figure 21–1 ◆). The walls of the contracted uterus are in close proximity, and the uterine blood vessels are firmly compressed by the myometrium. Within 6 to 12 hours after birth, the fundus of the uterus rises to the level of the umbilicus. A fundus that is above the umbilicus and is boggy (feels soft and spongy rather than firm and well contracted) is associated with excessive uterine bleeding. A **boggy uterus** results from collected blood and clot formation causing the fundus to rise and the interruption of uterine contractions. When the fundus is higher than expected on palpation and is not in the midline (usually deviated to the right), distention of the bladder should be suspected.

After birth the top of the fundus remains at the level of the umbilicus for about half a day. On the first postpartum day, the top of the fundus is located about 1 cm below the umbilicus. The top of the fundus descends approximately one finger breadth per day until it descends into the pelvis within 2 weeks on average (Cunningham et al., 2001).

If the mother is breastfeeding, endogenous oxytocin released by the posterior pituitary in response to suckling hastens this process. Barring complications, the uterus approaches its prepregnant size and location by 5 to 6 weeks.

LOCHIA

The uterus rids itself of the debris remaining after birth through a discharge called **lochia,** which is classified according to its appearance and contents. **Lochia rubra** is dark red. It occurs for the first 3 to 4 days and contains epithelial cells, erythrocytes, leukocytes, shreds of decidua, and occasionally fetal meconium, lanugo, and vernix caseosa. Lochia should not contain large (plum-sized) clots; if it does the cause should be investigated without delay. **Lochia serosa** is a pinkish color. It follows from about the 4th until the 10th day. Lochia serosa is composed of serous exudate (hence the name), shreds of degenerating decidua, erythrocytes, leukocytes, cervical mucus, and numerous microorganisms (Cunningham et al., 2001). Gradually the red blood cell component decreases, and **lochia alba,** a creamy or yellowish discharge, persists for an additional week or two. This final discharge is composed primarily of leukocytes, decidual cells, epithelial cells, fat, cervical mucus, cholesterol crystals, and bacteria. When the lochia flow stops, the cervix is considered closed, and chances of infection ascending from the vagina to the uterus decrease. Like menstrual discharge, lochia flow has a musty, stale odor that is not offensive. Foul-smelling lochia suggests infection and should be assessed promptly.

The total volume of lochia is about 240 to 270 mL, and the amount gradually declines with each passing day (Scoggin, 2000). The amount of discharge is greater in the morning due to pooling in the vagina and uterus while the mother lies sleeping. The amount of lochia may also be increased by exertion or breastfeeding.

Evaluation of lochia is necessary not only to determine the presence of hemorrhage but also to assess uterine involution. The type, amount, and consistency of lochia determine the stage of healing of the placenta site, and a progressive change from bright red at birth to dark red to pink to white or clear discharge should occur. Persistent discharge of lochia rubra or a return to lochia rubra indicates subinvolution or late postpartal hemorrhage (see Chapter 23).

CERVICAL CHANGES

Following birth the cervix is flabby and formless and may appear bruised. The external os is markedly irregular and closes slowly. It admits two fingers for a few days following birth, but by the end of the first week it admits only a fingertip.

The shape of the external os is permanently changed by the first childbearing. The characteristic dimplelike os of the nullipara changes to the lateral slit (fish-mouth) os of the multipara. After significant cervical laceration or several lacerations, the cervix may appear lopsided.

VAGINAL CHANGES

Following birth the vagina appears edematous and may be bruised. Small superficial lacerations may be evident, and the rugae are obliterated. The apparent bruising is due to pelvic congestion and will quickly disappear. The hymen, torn and jagged, heals irregularly, leaving small tags called the carunculae myrtiformes.

The size of the vagina decreases and rugae return within 3 weeks, facilitating the gradual return to smaller, although not nulliparous, dimensions (Harrison, 2000). By 6 weeks the nonlactating woman's vagina usually appears normal. The lactating woman is in a hypoestrogenic state because of ovarian suppression, and her vaginal mucosa may be pale and without rugae; the effects of the lowered estrogen level may lead to dyspareunia (painful intercourse). Tone and contractility of the vaginal orifice may be improved by perineal tightening exercises such as Kegel's (see Chapter 9). The labia majora and labia minora are more flaccid in the woman who has borne a child than in the nullipara.

PERINEAL CHANGES

During the early postpartal period the soft tissue in and around the perineum may appear edematous, with some bruising (Figure 21–2 ◆). If an episiotomy is present, the edges should be drawn together. Occasionally ecchymosis occurs, which may delay healing.

RECURRENCE OF OVULATION AND MENSTRUATION

The return of ovulation and menstruation varies for each postpartal woman. Menstruation generally returns in 40% to 45% of nonnursing mothers between 6 and 8 weeks after birth; 50% of the first cycles are anovulatory (Cunningham et al., 2001). Overall, 75% of nonnursing mothers resume menstruation by 12 weeks and the remaining 25% within 6 months following birth (Scoggin, 2000).

The return of ovulation and menstruation in nursing mothers is usually prolonged. It is associated with the length

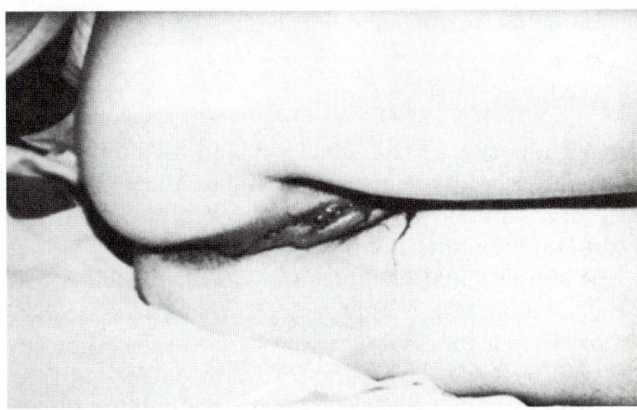

FIGURE 21–2. ◆ Bruising and edema of the vulva and perineum in a primipara 3 days after a forceps delivery. *Note:* From Bennett, V. R., & Brown, L. K. (1989). *Myles textbook for midwives* (11th ed. p. 235). By permission of the publisher Churchill Livingstone.

of time the woman breastfeeds and whether formula supplements are used. If a nursing mother breastfeeds for less than 1 month, the return of menstruation and ovulation is similar to that of the nonnursing mother. In women who exclusively breastfeed, menstruation is usually delayed for at least 3 months. However, since ovulation precedes menstruation, breastfeeding is not a reliable means of contraception, especially after the first 3 weeks postpartum (American College of Obstetricians and Gynecologists, 2000).

Abdomen

Following birth the stretched abdominal wall appears loose and flabby, but it responds to exercise within 2 to 3 months. In the grand multipara, in the woman in whom overdistention of the abdomen has occurred, or in the woman with poor muscle tone before pregnancy, the abdomen may fail to regain good tone and will remain flabby. **Diastasis recti abdominis,** a separation of the abdominal muscle, may occur with pregnancy, especially in women with poor abdominal muscle tone. If diastasis occurs, part of the abdominal wall has no muscular support but is formed only by skin, subcutaneous fat, fascia, and peritoneum. If rectus muscle tone is not regained, support may be inadequate during future pregnancies. Inadequate support may result in a pendulous abdomen and increased maternal backache. Fortunately, diastasis responds well to exercise, and abdominal muscle tone can improve significantly.

Striae (stretch marks), caused by stretching and rupture of the elastic fibers of the skin, are red to purple at the time of birth. These marks gradually fade after a time but remain visible.

Lactation

During pregnancy, breast development in preparation for lactation results from the influence of both estrogen and progesterone. After birth, the interplay of maternal hormones leads to milk production. (For further details, see the section on breastfeeding in Chapter 27.) ⊙⊙

Gastrointestinal System

Hunger following birth is common, and the mother may enjoy a light meal. She may also be quite thirsty and may drink large amounts of fluid. This helps replace fluids lost in labor, in the urine, and through perspiration.

The bowels tend to be sluggish following birth because of the lingering effects of progesterone and decreased abdominal muscle tone. Women who have had an episiotomy may tend to delay elimination for fear of increasing their pain or in the belief that their stitches will be torn if they bear down. In refusing or delaying the bowel movement, the woman may cause increased constipation and more pain when bowel elimination finally occurs.

The woman with a cesarean birth may receive clear liquids shortly after surgery; once bowel sounds are present,

her diet is quickly advanced to solid food. The woman may experience some initial discomfort from flatulence; it is relieved by early ambulation and antiflatulent medications. It may take a few days for the bowel to regain its tone, especially if general anesthesia was used. The woman who has had a cesarean or a difficult birth may benefit from stool softeners.

Urinary Tract

The postpartal woman has an increased bladder capacity, swelling and bruising of the tissue around the urethra, decreased sensitivity to fluid pressure, and a decreased sensation of bladder filling. Consequently, she is at risk for overdistention, incomplete bladder emptying, and a buildup of residual urine. Women who have had an anesthetic block have inhibited neural functioning of the bladder and are more susceptible to bladder distention, difficulty voiding, and bladder infections.

Puerperal diuresis causes rapid filling of the bladder. Thus, adequate bladder elimination is an immediate concern. Urinary stasis increases the chances that a urinary tract infection will develop. A full bladder may also increase the tendency toward uterine relaxation by displacing the uterus and interfering with contractility, all of which may lead to hemorrhage. In the absence of infection, the dilated ureters and renal pelves return to prepregnant size by the end of the sixth week.

Vital Signs

A maternal temperature of up to 38 °C (100.4 °F) may occur after childbirth as a result of the exertion and dehydration of labor. After the first 24 hours, the woman should be afebrile, and a temperature of 38 °C (100.4 °F) or greater suggests infection. (See discussion in Chapter 23.) ⊙⊙

Blood pressure readings should remain stable after childbirth. A decrease may indicate physiologic readjustment to decreased intrapelvic pressure, or it may be related to uterine hemorrhage. Blood pressure elevations, especially when accompanied by headache, suggest pregnancy-induced hypertension, and the woman should be evaluated further. Puerperal bradycardia with rates of 50 to 70 beats per minute commonly occurs during the first 6 to 10 days of the postpartal period. It may be related to decreased cardiac effort, the decreased blood volume following placental separation and contraction of the uterus, and increased stroke volume. Tachycardia occurs less frequently and is related to increased blood loss or difficult, prolonged labor and birth.

Blood Values

Blood values should return to the prepregnant state by the end of the postpartal period. Pregnancy-associated activation of coagulation factors may continue for variable amounts of time after birth. This condition, in conjunction with trauma, immobility, or sepsis, predisposes the woman to thromboembolism.

Nursing Practice

During the first few hours after birth, the woman may have some orthostatic hypotension; it will cause her to have a lower blood pressure reading in a sitting position. For the most accurate reading, measure her blood pressure with her in the same position each time, preferably lying on her back with her arm at her side.

Nonpathologic leukocytosis often occurs, with white blood cell counts of 25,000 to 30,000/µL, with the increase predominantly consisting of granulocytes (Cunningham et al., 2001). Hemoglobin and hematocrit levels may be difficult to interpret in the first 2 days after birth because of the changing blood volume. In general, a decrease of two percentage points from the hematocrit at admission to the birthing unit indicates a blood loss of 500 mL (Varney, 1997). Hemoglobin and hematocrit values should approximate or exceed prelabor values within 2 to 6 weeks as normal concentrations are reached. As extracellular fluid is excreted, hemoconcentration coincides with a rise in hematocrit.

Weight Loss

An initial weight loss of about 10 to 12 lb occurs as a result of the birth of the infant, placenta, and amniotic fluid. Puerperal diuresis accounts for the loss of an additional 5 lb during the early puerperium. By the sixth to eighth week after birth, many women have returned to approximately prepregnant weight if they gained the average 25 to 30 lb. For others, a return to prepregnant weight may take longer. A woman who is physically active prior, during, and after pregnancy completion loses more weight (8.6 lb) than a comparable, but less active counterpart (3 lb) (Sampselle, Seng, Yeo, et al., 1999).

Postpartal Chill

Frequently the mother experiences a shaking chill immediately after birth, related to a nervous response or to vasomotor changes. If not followed by fever, this chill is of no clinical concern, but it is uncomfortable for the woman. Increase the woman's comfort by covering her with a warmed blanket and encouraging her to relax. Some women may also find a warm drink helpful. Later in the puerperium, chill and fever indicate infection and require further evaluation.

Postpartal Diaphoresis

The woman experiences greatly increased perspiration as the body eliminates excess fluid and waste products via the skin during the puerperium. Diaphoretic (sweating) episodes frequently occur at night, and the woman may awaken drenched with perspiration. This perspiration is not significant clinically, but the mother should be protected from chilling.

Afterpains

Afterpains, caused by intermittent uterine contractions, are more common in multiparas than in primiparas. Although the uterus of the primipara usually remains consistently contracted, the lost tone of the multiparous uterus results in alternate contraction and relaxation. This phenomenon also occurs if the uterus has been markedly distended, as with a multiple-gestation pregnancy or hydramnios, or if clots or placental fragments were retained. These afterpains may cause the mother severe discomfort for 2 to 3 days after birth. The administration of oxytocic agents stimulates uterine contraction and increases the discomfort of the afterpains. Because endogenous oxytocin is released when the infant suckles, breastfeeding also increases the frequency and severity of the afterpains. The nursing mother may find it helpful to take a mild analgesic approximately 1 hour before feeding her infant. The nurse can assure the nursing mother that the prescribed analgesics are not harmful to the newborn and help improve the quality of the breastfeeding experience. An analgesic is also helpful at bedtime if the afterpains interfere with the mother's rest.

POSTPARTAL PSYCHOLOGIC ADAPTATIONS

Maternal Role

The postpartal period is a time of readjustment and adaptation for the entire childbearing family, but especially for the mother. The woman experiences a variety of responses as she adjusts to a new family member, postpartum discomforts, changes in her body image, and the reality that she is no longer pregnant. During the first day or two after birth, the woman tends to be passive and somewhat dependent. She follows suggestions, hesitates to make decisions, and is still rather preoccupied with her needs. She may have a great need to talk about her perceptions of her labor and birth. Talking helps her work through the process, sort out the reality from her fantasized experience, and clarify anything that she did not understand. Food and sleep are major needs. In her early work, Rubin (1961) labeled this the *taking-in* period.

By the second or third day after birth, the new mother is ready to resume control over her life. She may be concerned about controlling her body functions such as elimination. If she is breastfeeding, she may worry about the quality of her milk and her ability to nurse her baby. If her baby spits up after a feeding, she may view it as a personal failure. She may also feel that the nurse handles her baby more proficiently than she does. She requires assurance that she is doing well as a mother. Rubin labeled this the *taking-hold* period (1961). Today's mothers seem to be more independent and adjust more rapidly, exhibiting behaviors of "taking in" and "taking hold" in shorter time periods than those previously identified.

Postpartally the woman must adjust to a changed body image. Women often express dissatisfaction about their appearance and concern about the return of their weight and figure to normal. Multiparas tend to be more positive than primiparas. This difference may result because the multipara's previous experience has prepared her for the fact that the body does not immediately return to a prepregnant state.

The psychologic outcomes of the postpartal period are far more positive when the parents have access to a support network. Women and their partners may find that family relationships become increasingly important, but the increased family interaction can be a source of stress. The new parents may also have increasing contact with other parents of small children while contact with coworkers declines. Of great concern are women and their partners who have no family or friends to form a social network. Isolation at a time when the woman feels an increased need for support can result in tremendous stress and is often a contributing factor in situations of child neglect or abuse.

Maternal role attainment is the process by which a woman learns mothering behaviors and becomes comfortable with her identity as a mother. Formation of a maternal identity occurs with each child a woman bears. As the mother grows to know this child and forms a relationship, the mother's maternal identity gradually, systematically evolves and she "binds in" to the infant (Rubin, 1984).

Maternal role attainment often occurs in four stages (Mercer, 1995):

1. The anticipatory stage occurs during pregnancy. The woman looks to role models, especially her own mother, for examples of how to mother.

2. The formal stage begins when the child is born. The woman is still influenced by the guidance of others and tries to act as she believes others expect her to act.

3. The informal stage begins when the mother begins to make her own choices about mothering. The woman begins to develop her own style of mothering and finds ways of functioning that work well for her.

4. The personal stage is the final stage of maternal role attainment. When the woman reaches this stage, she is comfortable with the notion of herself as mother.

In most cases, maternal role attainment occurs within 3 to 10 months after birth. Social support, the woman's age and personality traits, the temperament of her infant, and the family's socioeconomic status all influence the woman's success in attaining the maternal role.

The postpartum woman faces a number of challenges as she adjusts to her new role:

- For many women, finding time for themselves is one of the greatest challenges. It is often difficult for the new mother to find time to read a book, talk to her partner, or even eat a meal without interruption.

- Women also report feelings of incompetence because they have not mastered all aspects of the mothering role. Often they are unsure of what to do in a given situation (Nicolson, 1999).

- The next greatest challenge involves fatigue resulting from sleep deprivation. The demands of nighttime care are tremendously draining, especially if the woman has other children.

- Another challenge faced by the new mother involves the feeling of responsibility that having a child brings. Women experience a sense of lost freedom, an awareness that they will never again be quite as carefree as they were before becoming mothers.

- Mothers sometimes cite the infant's behavior as a challenge, especially when the child is about 8 months old. Stranger anxiety develops, the infant begins crawling and getting into things, teething may cause fussiness, and the baby's tendency to put everything in his or her mouth requires constant vigilance by the parent.

All too often postpartum nurses are unaware of the long-term adjustments and stresses that the childbearing family faces as its members adjust to new and different roles. Nurses can help by providing anticipatory guidance about the realities of being a mother. Agencies should have literature available for reference at home. Ongoing parenting groups give parents an opportunity to discuss problems and become comfortable in new roles.

Postpartum Blues

The **postpartum blues** consist of a transient period of depression that often occurs during the first few days of the puerperium. It may be manifested by tearfulness, anorexia, difficulty in sleeping, and a feeling of letdown. This depression frequently occurs while the woman is still hospitalized, but it may occur at home as well. Psychologic adjustments and hormonal factors are thought to be the main cause, although fatigue, discomfort, and overstimulation may play a part. The postpartum blues usually resolve naturally, but if persistent or worsening symptoms develop, the woman may need evaluation for postpartum depression (see Chapter 23). ⬭

DEVELOPMENT OF PARENT-INFANT ATTACHMENT

A mother's first interaction with her infant is influenced by many factors, including her involvement with her family of origin, her relationships, the stability of her home environment, the communication patterns she developed, and the degree of nurturing she received as a child. These factors have shaped the person she has become. Certain personal characteristics are also important:

- *Level of trust.* What level of trust has this mother developed in response to her life experiences? What is her philosophy of child rearing? Will she be able to treat her infant as a unique individual with changing needs that should be met as much as possible?
- *Level of self-esteem.* How much does she value herself as a woman and as a mother? Does she feel generally able to cope with the adjustments of life?
- *Capacity for enjoying herself.* Is the mother able to find pleasure in everyday activities and human relationships?
- *Interest in and adequacy of knowledge about childbearing and child rearing.* What beliefs about the course of pregnancy, the capacities of newborns, and the nature of her emotions influence her behavior at first contact with her infant and later?
- *Prevailing mood or usual feeling tone.* Is the woman predominantly content, angry, depressed, or anxious? Is she sensitive to her own feelings and those of others? Will she be able to accept her own needs and to obtain support in meeting them?
- *Reactions to the present pregnancy.* Was the pregnancy planned? Did it go smoothly? Were there ongoing life events that enhanced her pregnancy or depleted her reserves of energy?

By the time of birth, each mother has developed an emotional orientation of some kind to the baby based on these factors.

Initial Attachment Behavior

New mothers demonstrate a fairly regular pattern of maternal behaviors at first contact with a normal newborn. In a progression of touching activities, the mother proceeds from fingertip exploration of the newborn's extremities toward palmar contact with larger body areas and finally to enfolding the infant with the whole hand and arms. The time taken to accomplish these steps varies from minutes to days. The mother increases the proportion of time spent in the **en face** position (Figure 21–3 ◆). She arranges herself or the newborn so that she has direct face-to-face and eye-to-eye contact. There is an intense interest in having the infant's eyes open. When the infant's eyes are open, the mother characteristically greets the newborn and talks in high-pitched tones to him or her.

In most instances the mother relies heavily on her senses of sight, touch, and hearing in getting to know what her baby is really like. She tends also to respond verbally to any sounds emitted by the newborn, such as cries, coughs, sneezes, and grunts. The sense of smell may be involved as well.

In addition to interacting with the newborn, the mother is undergoing her own emotional reactions to the whole

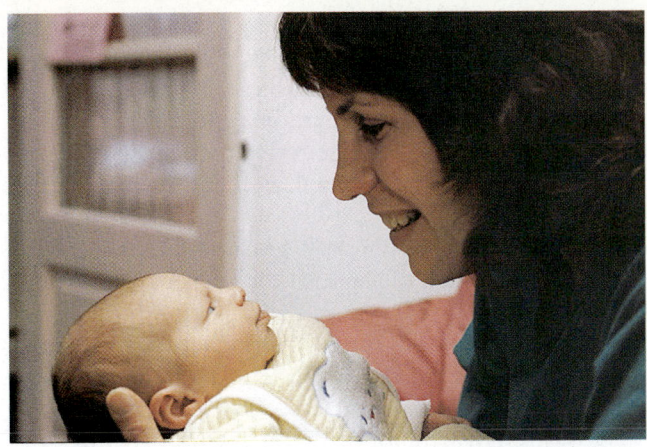

FIGURE 21–3. ◆ The mother has direct face-to-face and eye-to-eye contact in the en face position.

experience and, more specifically, to the baby as she perceives him or her. The frequency of the "I can't believe" reaction leads to speculation that human gains as well as losses may initially be met with a degree of shock, disbelief, and denial. A feeling of emotional distance from the newborn is quite common: "I feel like he is a stranger." On the other hand, feelings of connectedness between the newborn and the rest of the family can be expressed in positive or negative terms: "She's got your cute nose, Daddy" or "Oh, no! He looks just like the first one, and he was an impossible baby." A mother's facial expressions or the frequency and content of her questions may demonstrate concerns about the infant's general condition or normality, especially if her pregnancy was complicated or if a previously delivered baby was not healthy.

What are the characteristic behaviors of a newborn? Unless care is taken to effect a gentle birth, a number of harsh stimuli assault the senses of the newborn at birth. The newborn is probably suctioned, held with his or her head somewhat downward, exposed to bright lights and cool air, and in some way cleaned. The infant usually responds by crying. In fact, caregivers typically stimulate the newborn to cry to reassure themselves that the baby is well and normal. When newborns no longer need to concentrate most of their energy on physical and physiologic responses to the immediate crisis of birth, they are able to lie quietly with their eyes open, looking about, moving their limbs occasionally, making sucking motions, and possibly attempting to get their hands to their mouths. Placed in proximity to the mother, the newborn appears to focus briefly on her face and attend to her voice in the first moments of life.

During the first few days after her child's birth, the new mother applies herself to the task of getting to know her baby. This is termed the acquaintance phase. If the infant gives clear behavioral cues about needs, the infant's responses to mothering will be predictable, which will make the mother feel effective and competent. Other behaviors that make an infant more attractive to caretakers are smiling, grasping a finger, nursing eagerly, and being easy to console. During this time the newborn is also becoming acquainted. Within a few days after birth, infants show signs of recognizing recurrent situations and responding to changes in routine. To the extent that their mother is their world, it can be said that they are actively acquainting themselves with her.

During the phase of mutual regulation, mother and infant seek to deal with the issue of the degree of control to be exerted by each partner in their relationship. In this phase of adjustment, a balance is sought between the needs of the mother and the needs of the infant. The most important consideration is that each should obtain a good measure of enjoyment from the interaction. During the mutual adjustment phase, negative maternal feelings are likely to surface or intensify. Because "everyone knows that mothers love their babies," these negative feelings often go unexpressed and are allowed to build up. If they are expressed, the response of friends, relatives, or health care personnel is often to deny the feelings to the mother: "You don't mean that." Some negative feelings are normal in the first few days after birth, and the nurse should be supportive when the mother vocalizes these feelings.

When mutual regulation arrives at the point where both mother and infant primarily enjoy each other's company, reciprocity has been achieved. **Reciprocity** is an interactional cycle that occurs simultaneously between mother and infant. It involves mutual cuing behaviors, expectancy, rhythmicity, and synchrony. The mother develops a new relationship with an individual who has a unique character and evokes a response entirely different from the fantasy response of pregnancy. When reciprocity is synchronous, the interaction between mother and infant is mutually gratifying and is sought and initiated by both partners. They find pleasure and delight in each other's company and grow in mutual love. The new mother who feels comfortable and competent in her role provides a stimulating and nurturing environment and facilitates her infant's development (Fowles, 1998).

FATHER-INFANT INTERACTIONS

Traditionally in Western cultures the primary role of the expectant father has been one of support for the pregnant woman. However, commitment to family-centered maternity care has fostered interest in understanding the feelings and experiences of the new father. Evidence suggests that the father has a strong attraction to his newborn and that the feelings he experiences are similar to the mother's feelings of attachment (Figure 21–4 ◆). The characteristic sense of absorption, preoccupation, and interest in the infant demonstrated by fathers during early contact is termed **engrossment.**

SIBLINGS AND OTHERS

Infants are capable of maintaining a number of strong attachments without loss of quality. These attachments may

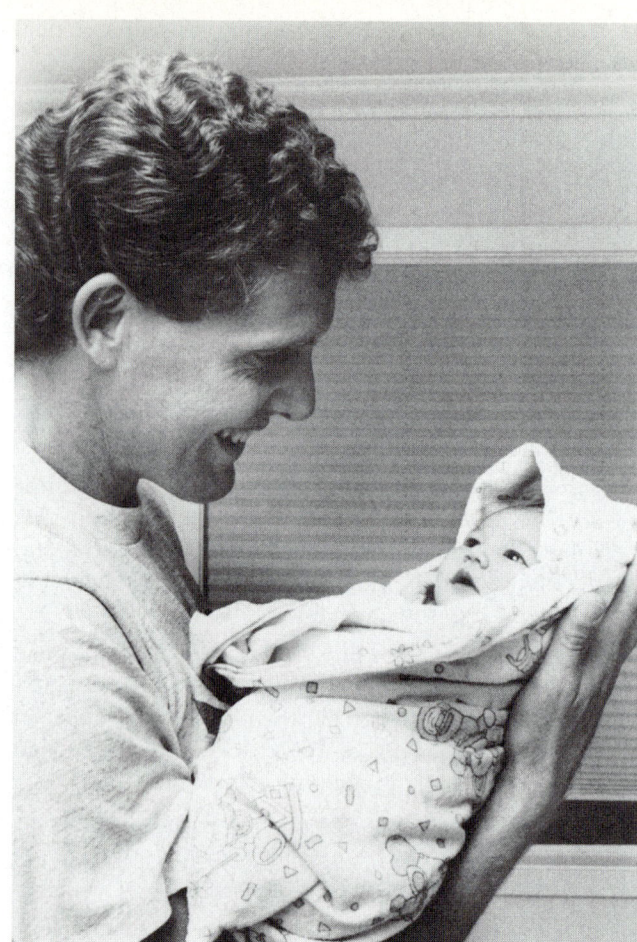

FIGURE 21–4. ◆ The father experiences strong feelings of attraction during engrossment.

include siblings, grandparents, aunts, and uncles. The social setting and personality of the individual seem to be significant factors in the development of multiple attachments. The advent of open visiting hours and rooming-in permits siblings and grandparents to participate in the attachment process.

Cultural Influences in the Postpartal Period

Western culture places primary emphasis on the events of birth. Many cultures place greater emphasis on the postpartum period. Proscription may exist against contact with others, contact with food or objects, and avoidance of sexual relationships. These practices may serve to reduce the risks of infection, and promote healing, lactation, and attachment (Andrews & Boyle, 1999). The new mother's culture and personal values also influence her beliefs about her postpartal care. Her expectations about food, fluids, rest, hygiene, medications and relief measures, support and counsel, and other aspects of her life are influenced by the beliefs and values of her family and cultural group. Sometimes, a new mother's wishes differ from what the physician or nurse expects.

Nurses belong to a particular personal culture and are also part of the health care cultural group. As part of the health care cultural group, nurses may take on some practices that support the general beliefs of that group, such as offering food in the recovery period after birth, providing iced fluids, expecting the woman to ambulate as soon as possible, and assuming the woman will want to shower and perhaps wash her hair soon after giving birth. It is important for nurses to recognize that they are approaching their client's care from their own perspective and that, to individualize care for each mother, they need to offer and support individual choices. Although describing particular practices of differing cultural groups always involves some generalization, it is helpful for nurses to understand some of the possible differences in beliefs and practices (Mayberry, Affonso, Shibuya, et al., 1999). The woman of European heritage may expect to eat a full meal and have large amounts of iced fluids after the birth, in the belief that the food restores energy and the fluids help replace fluid lost during the labor. She may want to ambulate shortly after the birth and shower, wash her hair, and put on a fresh gown. She may expect a short stay in the hospital and may or may not be interested in educational classes. Many cultures emphasize certain postpartal routines or rituals for mother and baby that are designed to restore the harmony, or the hot-cold balance, of the body (Howard & Berbiglia, 1997). Some women of Mexican, African, and Asian cultures may avoid cold after birth. This prohibition includes cold air, wind, and all water (even if heated). On the other hand, some traditional Mexican women may avoid eating "hot" foods such as pork just after the birth of a baby (considered a "hot" experience). It is important to note that individuals may define hot and cold conditions and foods differently. The nurse should ask each woman what she can eat and what foods she thinks would be helpful for healing (Chondhey, 1997). The nurse may encourage family members to bring preferred food and drink.

In many cultures, such as the Native Americans, the extended family plays an essential role during the puerperium. The grandmother is often the primary helper to the mother and newborn. She brings wisdom and experience, allowing the new mother time to rest and giving her ready access to someone who can help with problems and concerns as they arise. It is important to ensure access of all family members during the postpartal period. Visiting rules may be broadened to allow family members access to the mother and newborn. These practices show respect and foster a blending of old and new behaviors to meet the goals of all concerned (Cesario, 2001). African-American mothers model their mothering skills after their older female relatives. In addition, these same older female relatives usually provide childcare if the mother is unable to fulfill her responsibilities (Gichia, 2000).

POSTPARTAL NURSING ASSESSMENT

Comprehensive care is based on a thorough assessment that identifies individual needs or potential problems. See "Assessment Guide: Postpartal—First 24 Hours after Birth."

Risk Factors

Ongoing assessment and client education during the puerperium are designed to meet the needs of the childbearing family and to detect and treat possible complications. Table 21–1 identifies factors that may place the new mother at risk during the postpartal period. Use this knowledge during the assessment and be particularly alert for possible complications associated with identified risk factors.

TABLE 21–1	Postpartal High-Risk Factors
Factor	Maternal Implication
PIH	↑ Blood pressure ↑ CNS irritability ↑ Need for bed rest → ↑ risk thrombophlebitis
Diabetes	Need for insulin regulation Episodes of hypoglycemia or hyperglycemia ↓ Healing
Cardiac disease	↑ Maternal exhaustion
Cesarean birth	↑ Healing needs ↑ Pain from incision ↑ Risk of infection ↑ Length of hospitalization
Overdistention of uterus (multiple gestation, hydramnios)	↑ Risk of hemorrhage ↑ Risk of anemia ↑ Stretching of abdominal muscles ↑ Incidence and severity of afterpains
Abruptio placentae, placenta previa	Hemorrhage → anemia ↓ Uterine contractility after birth → ↑ infection risk
Precipitous labor (<3 hours)	↑ Risk of lacerations to birth canal → hemorrhage
Prolonged labor (>24 hours)	Exhaustion ↑ Risk of hemorrhage Nutritional and fluid depletion ↑ Bladder atony and/or trauma
Difficult birth	Exhaustion ↑ Risk of perineal lacerations ↑ Risk of hematomas ↑ Risk of hemorrhage → anemia
Extended period of time in stirrups at birth	↑ Risk of thrombophlebitis
Retained placenta	↑ Risk of hemorrhage ↑ Risk of infection

Physical Assessment/Normal Findings	Alterations and Possible Causes*	Nursing Responses to Data†
VITAL SIGNS		
Blood pressure (BP): Should remain consistent with baseline BP during pregnancy.	High BP (PIH, essential hypertension, renal disease, anxiety).	Evaluate history of preexisting disorders and check for other signs of PIH (edema, proteinuria).
	Drop in BP (may be normal; uterine hemorrhage).	Assess for other signs of hemorrhage (↑ pulse, cool clammy skin).
Pulse: 50–90 beats/minute.	Tachycardia (difficult labor and birth, hemorrhage).	Evaluate for other signs of hemorrhage (↓ BP, cool clammy skin).
May be bradycardia of 50–70 beats/minute.		
Respirations: 16–24/minute.	Marked tachypnea (respiratory disease).	Assess for other signs of respiratory disease.
Temperature: 36.2–38 °C (98–100.4 °F)	After first 24 hours temperature of 28 °C (100.4 °F) or above suggests infection.	Assess for other signs of infection; notify physician or certified nurse-midwife.
BREASTS		
General appearance: Smooth, even pigmentation, changes of pregnancy still apparent; one may appear larger.	Reddened area (mastitis).	Assess further for signs of infection.
Palpation: Depending on postpartal day, may be soft, filling, full, or engorged.	Palpable mass (caked breast, mastitis).	Assess for other signs of infection: If blocked duct, consider heat, massage, position change for breastfeeding.
	Engorgement (venous stasis).	
	Tenderness, heat, edema (engorgement, caked breast, mastitis).	Assess for further signs.
		Report mastitis to physician or certified nurse-midwife.
Nipples: Supple, pigmented, intact; become erect when stimulated.	Fissures, cracks, soreness (problems with breastfeeding), not erectile with stimulation (inverted nipples).	Reassess technique; recommend appropriate interventions.
ABDOMEN		
Musculature: Abdomen may be soft, have a "doughy" texture; rectus muscle intact.	Separation in musculature (diastasis recti abdominis).	Evaluate size of diastasis; teach appropriate exercises for decreasing the separation.
Fundus: Firm, midline; following expected process of involution.	Boggy (full bladder, uterine bleeding).	Massage until firm; assess bladder and have woman void if needed; attempt to express clots when firm. If bogginess remains or recurs, report to physician or certified nurse-midwife.
May be tender when palpated.	Constant tenderness (infection).	Assess for evidence of endometritis.
LOCHIA		
Scant to moderate amount, earthy odor; no clots.	Large amount, clots (hemorrhage).	Assess for firmness, express additional clots; begin peripad count.
	Foul-smelling lochia (infection).	Assess for other signs of infection; report to physician or certified nurse-midwife.
Normal progression: First 1–3 days: rubra. Following rubra	Failure to progress normally or return to rubra from serosa (subinvolution).	Report to physician or certified nurse-midwife.
Days 3–10: serosa (alba seldom seen in hospital).		
PERINEUM		
Slight edema and bruising in intact perineum.	Marked fullness, bruising, pain (vulvar hematoma).	Assess size; apply ice glove or ice pack; report to physician or certified nurse-midwife.
Episiotomy: No redness, edema, ecchymosis, or discharge, edges well approximated.	Redness, edema, ecchymosis, discharge, or gaping stitches (infection).	Encourage sitz baths; review perineal care, appropriate wiping techniques.
Hemorrhoids: None present, if present, should be small and nontender.	Full, tender, inflamed hemorrhoids.	Encourage sitz baths, side-lying position; Tucks pads, anesthetic ointments, manual replacement of hemorrhoids, stool softeners, increased fluid intake.
COSTOVERTEBRAL ANGLE (CVA) TENDERNESS		
None.	Present (kidney infection).	Assess for other symptoms of urinary tract infection (UTI); obtain clean-catch urine sample; report to physician or certified nurse-midwife.

*Possible causes of alterations are placed in parentheses.

†This column provides guidelines for further assessment and initial nursing actions.

Physical Assessment/Normal Findings	Alterations and Possible Causes*	Nursing Responses to Data†
LOWER EXTREMITIES No pain with palpation; negative Homans' sign.	Positive findings (thrombophlebitis).	Report to physician or certified nurse-midwife.
ELIMINATION Urinary output: Voiding in sufficient quantities at least every 4–6 hours; bladder not palpable.	Inability to void (urinary retention). Symptoms of urgency, frequency, dysuria (UTI).	Employ nursing interventions to promote voiding; if not successful, obtain order for catheterization. Report symptoms of UTI to physician or certified nurse-midwife.
Bowel elimination: Should have normal bowel movement by second or third day after birth.	Inability to pass feces (constipation due to fear of pain from episiotomy, hemorrhoids, perineal trauma).	Encourage fluids, ambulation, roughage in diet; sitz baths to promote healing of perineum; obtain order for stool softener.

Cultural Assessment‡	Variations to Consider	Nursing Responses to Data†
Determine customs and practices regarding postpartum care. Ask the mother whether she would like fluids and ask what temperature she prefers. Ask the mother what foods or fluids she would like. Ask the mother whether she would prefer to be alone during breastfeeding.	Individual preference may include • Room-temperature or warmed fluids rather than iced drinks. • Special foods or fluids to hasten healing after childbirth. Some women may be hesitant to have someone with them when their breast is exposed.	Provide for specific request if possible. If woman is unable to provide specific information, the nurse may draw from general information regarding cultural variation. Mexican women may want food and fluids that restore hot-cold balance to the body. Women of European background may ask for iced fluids. Provide privacy as desired by mother.

Psychosocial Assessment/ Normal Findings	Variations to Consider	Nursing Responses to Data†
PSYCHOLOGIC ADAPTATION During first 24 hours: Passive; preoccupied with own needs; may talk about her labor and birth experience; may be talkative, elated, or very quiet. By 12 hours: Beginning to assume responsibility; some women eager to learn; easily feels overwhelmed.	Very quiet and passive; sleeps frequently (fatigue from long labor; feelings of disappointment about some aspect of the experience; may be following cultural expectation). Excessive weepiness, mood swings, pronounced irritability (postpartum blues; feelings of inadequacy; culturally prescribed behavior).	Provide opportunities for adequate rest; provide nutritious meals and snacks that are consistent with what the woman desires to eat and drink; provide opportunities to discuss birth experience in nonjudgmental atmosphere if the woman desires to do so. Explain postpartum blues; provide supportive atmosphere; determine support available for mother; consider referral for evidence of profound depression.
ATTACHMENT *En face* position; holds baby close; cuddles and soothes; calls by name; identifies characteristics of family members in infant; may be awkward in providing care. Initially may express disappointment over sex or appearance of infant but within 1–2 days demonstrates attachment behaviors.	Continued expressions of disappointment in sex, appearance of infant; refusal to care for infant; derogatory comments; lack of bonding behaviors (difficulty in attachment, following expectations of cultural/ethnic group).	Provide reinforcement and support for infant caretaking behaviors; maintain nonjudgmental approach and gather more information if caretaking behaviors are not evident.
CLIENT EDUCATION Has basic understanding of self-care activities and infant care needs; can identify signs of complications that should be reported.	Unable to demonstrate basic self-care and infant care activities (knowledge deficit; postpartum blues; following prescribed cultural behavior and will be cared for by grandmother or other family member).	Determine whether woman understands English and provide interpreter if needed; provide reinforcement of information through conversation and through written material (remember that some women and their families may not be able to understand written materials because of language difficulties or inability to read); provide information regarding infant care skills that are culturally consistent; give woman opportunity to express her feelings; consider social service home referral for women who have no family or other support, are unable to take in information about self-care and infant care, and demonstrate no caretaking activities.

‡These are only a few suggestions. It is not our intent to imply this is a comprehensive cultural assessment.

*Possible causes of alterations are placed in parentheses.

†This column provides guidelines for further assessment and initial nursing actions.

Physical Assessment

Remember several principles in preparing for and completing the assessment of the postpartal woman:

- Select a time that will provide the most accurate data. Palpating the fundus when the woman has a full bladder, for example, may give false information about the progress of involution.
- Record the findings as clearly as possible.
- Perform the procedures as gently as possible to avoid unnecessary discomfort.
- Explain the purpose of regular assessment.

While performing the physical assessment, the nurse should also be teaching the woman. For example, when assessing the breasts of a nursing woman, discuss breast milk production, the letdown reflex, and breast self-examination. A new mother may be very receptive to instruction on postpartal abdominal tightening exercises when the nurse assesses the woman's fundal height and diastasis. The assessment is also an excellent time to provide information about the body's postpartal physical and anatomic changes as well as danger signs to report (see Table 21–2). Because the time new mothers spend in the postpartum unit is often limited, use every available opportunity for client education about self-care. One of the best opportunities comes during the normal postpartal assessment. To assist nurses in recognizing these opportunities, examples of client teaching during the assessment are provided throughout the following discussion.

VITAL SIGNS

The nurse may choose to organize the physical assessment in a variety of ways. Many nurses begin by assessing vital signs because the findings are more accurate when they are obtained with the woman at rest. In addition, establishing whether the vital signs are within the expected normal range will help determine if other assessments are needed.

For instance, if the temperature is elevated, consider the time since birth and gather information to determine whether the woman is dehydrated or an infection is present.

Temperature elevations (less than 38 °C [100.4 °F]) due to normal processes should last for only 24 hours. Evaluate any elevation of temperature in light of associated signs and symptoms and carefully review the woman's history to identify other factors, such as premature rupture of membranes or prolonged labor, which might increase the incidence of infection in the genital tract.

Alterations in vital signs may indicate complications; assess them at regular intervals. The blood pressure should remain stable, but the pulse often shows a characteristic slowness that is no cause for alarm. Pulse rates return to prepregnant norms very quickly unless complications arise.

Inform the woman of the results of the vital signs assessment and provide information about the normal changes in blood pressure and pulse. This may be an opportunity to determine whether the mother knows how to assess her own and her infant's temperature and how to read a thermometer.

AUSCULTATION OF LUNGS

The breath sounds should be clear. Women who have been treated for preterm labor or pregnancy-induced hypertension are at higher risk for pulmonary edema (see Chapter 13 for further discussion). 🔗

BREASTS

The nurse can first assess the fit and support provided by the bra and offer information about how to select a supportive bra. A properly fitting bra supports the breasts and helps maintain breast shape by limiting stretching of supporting ligaments and connective tissue. If the mother is breastfeeding, the straps of the bra should be cloth, not elastic, and easily adjustable. The back should be wide and have at least three rows of hooks to adjust for fit. Traditional nursing bras have a fixed inner cup and a separate half cup that can be unhooked for breastfeeding while the cup continues to support the breast. Purchasing a nursing bra one size too large during pregnancy will usually result in a good fit because the breasts increase in size with milk production.

Then ask the woman to remove her bra so the breasts can be examined. Note the size and shape of the breasts and any abnormalities, reddened areas, or engorgement. Lightly palpate the breasts for softness, slight firmness associated with filling, firmness associated with engorgement, warmth, and tenderness. Assess the nipples for fissures, cracks, soreness, and inversion. Teach the woman the characteristics of the breast and explain how to recognize problems such as fissures and cracks.

Assess the nonnursing mother for evidence of breast discomfort, and institute relief measures if necessary. (See discussion of lactation suppression in the nonnursing mother in Chapter 22.) 🔗 Breast assessment findings for a nursing woman may be recorded as follows: breasts soft, filling, no evidence of nipple tenderness or cracking.

TABLE 21–2	Common Postpartal Concerns

Several postpartal occurrences cause special concern for mothers. The nurse will frequently be asked about the following events:

Source of Concern	Explanation
Gush of blood that sometimes occurs when she first arises	Due to normal pooling of blood in vagina when the woman lies down to rest or sleep; gravity causes blood to flow out when she stands
Night sweats	Normal physiologic occurrence that results as body attempts to eliminate excess fluids that were present during pregnancy; may be aggravated by plastic mattress pad
Afterpains	More common in multiparas; due to contractions

ABDOMEN AND FUNDUS

Before examination of the abdomen, the woman should void. This practice ensures that a full bladder is not displacing the uterus or causing any uterine atony; if atony is present, other causes must be investigated.

The nurse determines the relationship of the fundus to the umbilicus and also assesses the firmness of the fundus. Measure the top of the fundus in finger breadths above, below, or at the umbilicus (Figure 21–5 ◆). See Skill 4-1 in the *Clinical Skills Manual,* as well as the accompanying CD-ROM, for more information. **CD SKILLS**

Note whether the fundus is in the midline or displaced to either side of the abdomen. If not midline, the uterus position should be located. Because the most common cause of displacement is a full bladder, this finding requires further assessment. Measure urine output for the next few hours until normal elimination status is established. Record the results of the assessment. Fundal height is recorded in finger breadths (e.g., "2 FB ⇓ U; 1 FB ⇑ U"). Determine whether the fundus is firm. If it is not firm, massage the abdomen lightly until the fundus is firm. If massage was necessary, record the intervention as " Uterus Boggy → firm with light massage." While completing the assessment, teach the woman about fundal position. The mother can be assisted in gently massaging her fundus to determine firmness. The nurse correlates the position and firmness of the fundus with lochial flow.

In the woman who has had a cesarean birth, the abdominal incision is exquisitely tender. Therefore, palpate the fundus with extreme care. Also inspect the abdominal incision for any signs of infection, including drainage, foul odor, or redness. During the assessment, teach the woman about her incision. Characteristics of normal healing may be reviewed and signs of infection discussed.

LOCHIA

The nurse then evaluates the lochia, including character, amount, odor, and the presence of clots. Disposable gloves must be worn when assessing the perineum and lochia. Nurses may put on the gloves before beginning the assessment, just before assessing the abdomen and fundus, or when they are ready to assess the perineum and lochia. During the first 1 to 3 days the lochia should be rubra. A few small clots are normal and occur as a result of blood pooling in the vagina. However, the passage of numerous or large clots is abnormal, and the cause should be investigated immediately. After 3 to 4 days, the lochia flow becomes serosa.

Lochia should never exceed a moderate amount, such as four to eight partially saturated perineal pads daily, with an average of six. However, because this number is influenced by an individual woman's pad-changing practices, as well as the absorbency of the pad, ask about the length of time the current pad has been in use, whether the amount is normal, and whether any clots were passed before this examination, such as during voiding. If heavy bleeding is reported but not seen, ask the woman to put on a clean perineal pad and then reassess the woman's pad in 1 hour (Figure 21–6 ◆). When a more accurate assessment of blood loss is needed, the perineal pads can be weighed,

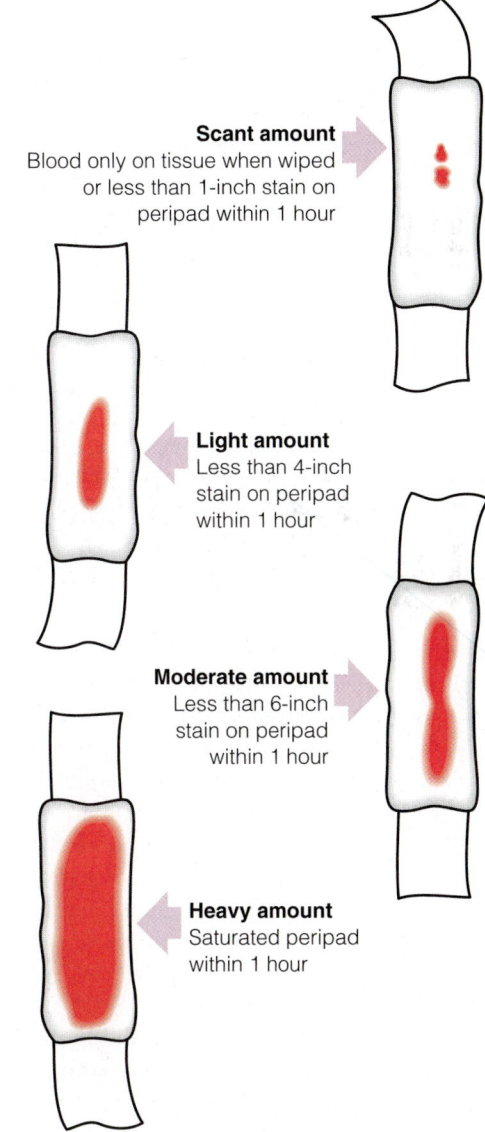

Scant amount
Blood only on tissue when wiped or less than 1-inch stain on peripad within 1 hour

Light amount
Less than 4-inch stain on peripad within 1 hour

Moderate amount
Less than 6-inch stain on peripad within 1 hour

Heavy amount
Saturated peripad within 1 hour

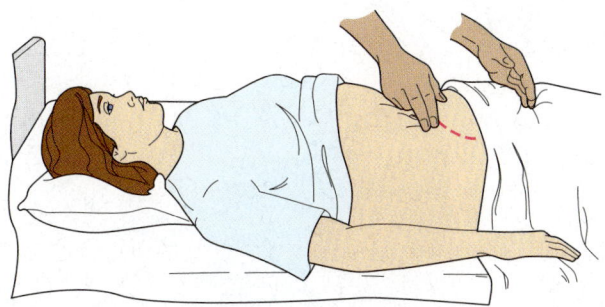

FIGURE 21–5. ◆ Measurement of descent of fundus for the woman with vaginal birth. The fundus is located two finger breadths below the umbilicus.

FIGURE 21–6. ◆ Suggested guideline for assessing lochia volume. *Note:* From Jacobson, H. (1985, May–June). A standard for assessing lochia volume. *Maternal-Child Nursing.*

with 1 g considered the approximate equivalent of 1 mL of blood. Clots and heavy bleeding may be caused by uterine relaxation (atony) or retained placental fragments and may require further assessment. Because of the evacuation of the uterine cavity during cesarean birth, women with such surgery usually have less lochia after the first 24 hours than mothers who give birth vaginally. If the woman is at increased risk for bleeding, or is actually experiencing heavy flow of lochia rubra, the physician may also order methylergonovine maleate (Methergine). See "Drug Guide: Methylergonovine Maleate (Methergine)," Chapter 22.

The odor of the lochia is nonoffensive and never foul. If a foul odor is present, so is an infection. The amount of lochia is charted first, followed by character. For example:

- Lochia: moderate rubra
- Lochia: small rubra/serosa

Client teaching during assessment of the lochia may center on normal changes that can be expected in the amount and color of the flow. Review hygienic measures if appropriate. Approach the teaching of hygienic practices delicately and with the goals of promoting comfort, enhancing tissue healing, and preventing infection. Avoid value-laden statements about the need for cleanliness or control of body odor.

Thinking Critically

ASSESSING LOCHIA

You have completed your assessment of Patty Clark, a 24-year-old gravida 2 para 2, who is 24 hours past childbirth. The fundus is just above the umbilicus and slightly to the right. Lochia rubra is present, and a pad is soaked every 2 hours. What would you do? **WEB**

PERINEUM

Inspect the perineum with the woman lying in a Sims' position. Lift the buttock to expose the perineum and anus.

If an episiotomy was done or a laceration required suturing, assess the wound and evaluate the state of healing by observing for ecchymosis and approximation. After 24 hours some edema may still be present, but the skin edges should be "glued" together (well approximated) so that gentle pressure does not separate them. Gentle palpation should elicit minimal tenderness, and there should be no hard areas suggesting infection. Ecchymosis interferes with normal healing, as does infection.

Foul odors associated with drainage indicate infection. Also observe the incision for warmth, redness, tenderness, edema, and separation. Next assess whether hemorrhoids are present around the anus. If present, they are assessed for size, number, and pain or tenderness. During the assessment, talk with the woman to determine the effectiveness of comfort measures that have been used. Provide

teaching about the episiotomy. Some women do not thoroughly understand what and where an episiotomy is, and they may believe that the stitches must be removed as with other types of surgery. Frequently, when women fear that the stitches must be removed manually, they are afraid to ask about them. While explaining the findings of the assessment, provide information about the episiotomy, its location, and the signs that are being assessed. In addition, casually add that the sutures are special and will dissolve slowly over the next few weeks as the tissues heal. By the time the sutures are dissolved the tissues are strong and the incision edges will not separate. This is also an opportunity to teach comfort measures (see Chapter 30).

An example of charting a perineal assessment might be: Midline episiotomy; no edema, tenderness, or ecchymosis present. Skin edges well approximated. Woman reports pain relief measures are controlling discomfort.

LOWER EXTREMITIES

If thrombophlebitis occurs, the most likely site is in the woman's legs. To assess for it, her legs should be stretched out straight and relaxed with the knees flexed. Grasp the woman's foot and sharply dorsiflex it. No discomfort or pain should be present. The second leg is assessed in the same way. If pain is elicited, notify the certified nurse-midwife or physician that the woman has a positive Homans' sign (Figure 21–7 ◆). The pain is caused by inflammation of the vessel. Also evaluate the legs for edema by comparing both legs, since usually only one leg is involved. Any areas of redness, tenderness, and increased skin temperature are also noted.

Early ambulation is an important aspect in the prevention of thrombophlebitis. Most women are able to be up shortly after birth. The cesarean birth client requires range of motion exercises until she is ambulating more freely.

Client teaching associated with assessment of the lower extremities focuses on the signs and symptoms of thrombophlebitis. In addition, review self-care measures to promote circulation and measures to prevent thrombophlebitis,

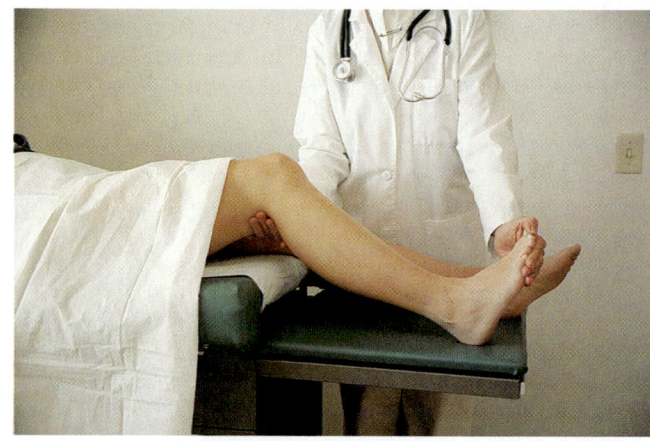

FIGURE 21–7. ◆ Homans' sign: With the woman's knee flexed, the nurse dorsiflexes the foot. Pain in the foot or leg is a positive Homans' sign.

such as ambulation and avoiding pressure behind the knees, using the knee gatch on the bed, and crossing the legs.

ELIMINATION

During the hours after birth, carefully monitor a new mother's bladder status. A boggy uterus, a displaced uterus, or a palpable bladder are signs of bladder distention and require nursing intervention. Following birth the woman should void within 4 hours (Cunningham et al., 2001). Encourage her to void every 4 to 6 hours. Assess the bladder for distention until the woman demonstrates complete emptying of the bladder with each voiding. The nurse may employ techniques to facilitate voiding, such as helping the woman out of bed to void or pouring warm water on the perineum. Catheterization is required when the bladder is distended and the woman cannot void or when no voiding has occurred in 8 hours. The cesarean birth mother may have an indwelling catheter inserted prophylactically. Make the same assessments in evaluating bladder emptying once the catheter is removed.

During the physical assessment, ask the woman about the adequacy of her fluid intake, whether she feels she is emptying her bladder completely when she voids, and any signs of urinary tract infection she may be experiencing.

Also ask about the new mother's intestinal elimination and any concerns she may have about it. Many mothers fear that the first bowel movement will be painful and possibly even damaging if an episiotomy has been done. Stool softeners may be ordered to increase bulk and moisture in the fecal material and to allow more comfortable and complete evacuation. Constipation is avoided to prevent pressure on sutures, which may increase discomfort. To enhance bowel elimination and help the woman reestablish her normal bowel pattern, encourage ambulation, increased fluid intake (up to 2,000 mL/day or more), and additional fresh fruits and roughage in her diet.

During the assessment, provide information about postpartum diuresis and explain why the woman may be emptying her bladder so frequently. The need for additional fluid intake with suggestions of specific amounts may be helpful. The woman should drink at least eight 8-oz glasses of water or juice per day in addition to other fluids. Discuss signs of urinary retention and overflow voiding and review symptoms of urinary tract infection if it seems an appropriate moment for teaching. Also review methods of assisting bowel elimination and provide opportunities for the woman to ask questions.

REST AND SLEEP STATUS

As part of the postpartal assessment, evaluate the amount of rest a new mother is getting. If the woman reports difficulty sleeping at night, try to determine the cause. If it is simply the strange environment, a warm drink and back rub may prove helpful. Appropriate nursing measures are indicated if the woman is bothered by normal postpartal discomforts such as afterpains, diaphoresis, or episiotomy or hemorrhoidal pain.

Encourage a daily rest period and schedule hospital activities to allow time for napping. Also provide information about the fatigue new mothers experience and the impact it can have on a woman's emotions and sense of control.

NUTRITIONAL STATUS

Determination of postpartal nutritional status is based primarily on information provided by the mother and on direct assessment. During pregnancy the daily recommended dietary allowances call for increases in calories, protein, and most vitamins and minerals. After birth, the nonnursing mother's dietary requirements return to prepregnancy levels.

Visiting the mother during mealtime provides an opportunity for unobtrusive nutritional assessment and counseling. Advise the nonnursing mother about the need to reduce her caloric intake by about 300 kcal and to return to prepregnancy levels for other nutrients. The nursing mother, on the other hand, should increase her caloric intake by about 200 kcal over the pregnancy requirements, or a total of 500 kcal over the nonpregnant requirement. Basic discussion often proves helpful, followed by referral as needed. In all cases, literature on nutrition should be provided, so that the woman will have a source of information after discharge.

Inform the dietitian of any mother who is a vegetarian or whose cultural or religious beliefs require specific foods. Appropriate meals can then be prepared for her. Many women, especially those who gained excessive weight, are interested in losing weight after birth. The dietitian can design weight-reduction diets to meet nutritional needs and food preferences. The nurse may also refer women with unusual eating habits or numerous questions about good nutrition to the dietitian.

New mothers are advised that it is common practice to prescribe iron supplements for 3 months after birth. The hematocrit is then checked at the postpartal visit to detect any anemia (Cunningham et al., 2001).

Psychologic Assessment

Adequate assessment of the mother's psychologic adjustment is an integral part of postpartal evaluation. This assessment focuses on the mother's general attitude, feelings of competence, available support systems, and caregiving skills. It also evaluates her fatigue level, sense of satisfaction, and ability to accomplish her developmental tasks.

Fatigue is often a highly significant factor in a new mother's apparent disinterest in her newborn (Troy, 1999). Frequently the woman is so tired from a long labor and birth that everything seems to be an effort. To avoid inadvertently classifying a very tired mother as one with a potential attachment problem, the nurse should do a psychologic assessment on more than one occasion. After a nap the new mother is often far more receptive to her baby and her surroundings.

Some new mothers have little or no experience with newborns and may feel totally overwhelmed. They may show these feelings by asking questions and reading all available material or by becoming passive and quiet because they simply cannot deal with their feelings of inadequacy. Unless a nurse questions the woman about her plans and previous experience in a supportive, nonjudgmental way, the nurse might conclude that the woman is disinterested, withdrawn, or depressed.

Problem clues might include excessive continued fatigue, marked depression, excessive preoccupation with physical status or discomfort, evidence of low self-esteem, lack of support systems, marital problems, inability to care for or nurture the newborn, and current family crises (illness, unemployment, and so on). These characteristics frequently indicate a potential for maladaptive parenting, which may lead to child abuse or neglect (physical, emotional, intellectual) and cannot be ignored. Referrals to public health nurses or other available community resources may provide greatly needed assistance and alleviate potentially dangerous situations.

Assessment of Early Attachment

A nurse in any of the various postpartal settings can periodically observe and note progress toward attachment. The following questions can be addressed in the course of nurse-client interaction:

- Is the mother attracted to her newborn? To what extent does she seek face-to-face contact and eye contact? Has she progressed from fingertip touch, to palmar contact, to enfolding the infant close to her own body? Is attraction increasing or decreasing? If the mother does not exhibit increasing attraction, why not? Do the reasons lie primarily within her, in the baby, or in the environment?

- Is the mother inclined to nurture her infant? Is she progressing in her interactions with her infant?

- Does the mother act consistently? If not, is the source of unpredictability within her or her infant?

- Is her mothering consistently carried out? Does she seek information and evaluate it objectively? Does she develop solutions based on adequate knowledge of valid data? Does she evaluate the effectiveness of her maternal care and adjust appropriately?

- Is she sensitive to the newborn's needs as they arise? How quickly does she interpret her infant's behavior and react to cues? Does she seem happy and satisfied with the infant's responses to her efforts? Is she pleased with feeding behaviors? How much of this ability and willingness to respond is related to the baby's nature and how much to her own?

- Does she seem pleased with her baby's appearance and sex? Is she experiencing pleasure in interaction with her infant? What interferes with the enjoyment? Does she speak to the baby frequently and affectionately? Does she call him or her by name? Does she

point out family traits or characteristics she sees in the newborn?

- Are there any cultural factors that might modify the mother's response? For instance, is it customary for the grandmother to assume most of the child care responsibilities while the mother recovers from childbirth?

When the nurse has addressed these questions and assembled the facts, the nurse's intuition and knowledge should combine to answer three more questions: Is there a problem in attachment? What is the problem? What is its source? Then devise a creative approach to the problem as it presents itself in the context of a unique, developing mother-infant relationship.

ASSESSMENT OF PHYSICAL AND DEVELOPMENTAL TASKS

During the first several postpartal weeks, the woman must accomplish certain physical and developmental tasks:

- Restoring physical condition
- Developing competence in caring for and meeting the needs of her infant
- Establishing a relationship with her new child
- Adapting to altered lifestyles and family structure resulting from the addition of a new member

The new mother may have an inadequate or incorrect understanding of what to expect during the early postpartal weeks. She may be concerned with restoring her figure and be surprised by continuing physical discomfort from sore breasts, episiotomy, or hemorrhoids. Fatigue is perhaps her greatest yet most underestimated problem during the early weeks. It may be aggravated if she has no extended family support or there are other young children at home. Developing skill and confidence in caring for an infant may be especially anxiety provoking for a new mother. As she struggles to establish a mutually acceptable pattern with her baby, small unanticipated concerns may seem monumental. The woman may begin to feel inadequate and, if she lacks support systems, isolated.

Nurses have been in the forefront of health care providers in attempting to improve the care currently provided during the postpartal period. Many obstetricians and nurse practitioners now routinely see all postpartal women 1 to 2 weeks after birth in addition to the routine 6-week checkup. This extra visit provides an opportunity for physical assessment as well as evaluation of the mother's psychologic and informational needs.

Postdischarge Care

Postdischarge care for the postpartal woman may be accomplished by home visits or follow-up phone calls. A home visit 1 to 3 days after discharge provides opportunities for further assessment and teaching. (See discussion of postpartum home care in Chapter 30.) 🔗

The follow-up telephone call is usually made by a nurse from the postpartal unit of the agency where the mother gave birth. It is made soon after discharge and is designed to provide assessment and care if necessary, to reinforce knowledge and provide additional teaching, and to make referrals if indicated (Stark, 2000).

Paternal satisfaction with the birth experience and its associated stresses influences marital happiness and family life (Rogers & White, 1998). A family approach involving the father, infant, other siblings, and grandparents permits a total evaluation and provides an opportunity for all family members to ask questions and express concerns. Such an approach also promotes diagnosis and treatment of disturbed family patterns to prevent future problems of neglect or abuse.

CHAPTER HIGHLIGHTS

🐚 The uterus involutes rapidly, primarily through a reduction in cell size.

🐚 Involution is assessed by measuring fundal height. The fundus is at the level of the umbilicus within a few hours after childbirth and should decrease by approximately one finger breadth per day.

🐚 The placental site heals by a process of exfoliation, so no scar formation occurs.

🐚 Lochia flow progresses from rubra to serosa to alba and is assessed in terms of type, quantity, and characteristics.

🐚 The abdomen may be flabby initially. Diastasis recti should be measured.

🐚 Constipation may develop postpartally because of decreased tone, limited diet, and denial of the urge to defecate due to fear of pain.

🐚 Decreased bladder sensitivity, increased capacity, and postpartal diuresis may lead to problems with bladder elimination. A fundus that is boggy but does not respond to massage, is higher than expected, or deviates to the side usually indicates a full bladder.

🐚 Postpartally a healthy woman should be normotensive and afebrile. Bradycardia is common. The white blood cell count is often elevated. Activation of clotting factors predisposes the woman to thrombus formation.

🐚 Psychologic adaptations include maternal role attainment and attachment to the newborn.

🐚 In consideration of the client's background, the nurse should recognize and respect cultural variations and individual preferences.

🐚 Postpartal assessment should be completed in a systematic way, usually cephalocaudally. It provides a tremendous opportunity for informal teaching.

🐚 In the weeks following birth, the woman's physical condition returns to a nonpregnant state and she gains competence and confidence in herself as a parent.

EXPLOREMEDIALINK

NCLEX Review, Case Studies, and other interactive resources for this chapter can be found on the companion website at http://www.prenhall.com/london. Click on "Chapter 21" to select the activities for this chapter.

For animations, more NCLEX review questions, and an audio glossary, access the accompanying CD-ROM in this textbook.

REFERENCES

American College of Obstetricians and Gynecologists. (2000). *Breast feeding: Maternal and infant aspects* (Education Bulletin No. 258). Washington, DC: Author.

Andrews, M. M., & Boyle, J. S. (1999). *Transcultural concepts in nursing care* (3rd ed.). Philadelphia: J. B. Lippincott.

Cesario, S. K. (2001). Care of the Native American woman: Strategies for practice, education, and research. *Journal of Obstetric, Gynecologic and Neonatal Nursing, 30*(1), 13–18.

Chondhey, U. K. (1997). Traditional practices of women from India: Pregnancy, childbirth, and newborn care. *Journal of Obstetric, Gynecologic, and Neonatal Nursing, 26*(5), 533–539.

Cunningham, F. G., Gant, N. F., Leveno, K. J., Gilstrap, L. C., Hauth, J. C., & Wenstrom, K. D. (2001). *Williams obstetrics* (21st ed.). Whitby, Ontario, Canada: McGraw-Hill Ryerson.

Fowles, E. R. (1998). The relationship between maternal role attainment and postpartum depression. *Health Care for Women International, 19,* 83–94.

Gichia, J. E. U. (2000). Mothers and others: African-American women's preparation for motherhood. *American Journal of Maternal Child Nursing, 25*(2), 86–91.

Harrison, J. M. (2000). Physiological changes of the puerperium. *British Journal of Midwifery, 8*(8), 483–488.

Howard, J. Y., & Berbiglia, V. A. (1997). Caring for childbearing Korean women. *Journal of Obstetric, Gynecologic, and Neonatal Nursing, 26*(6), 665–671.

Mayberry, L. J., Affonso, D. D., Shibuya, J., & Clemmens, D. (1999). Integrating cultural values, beliefs, and customs into pregnancy and postpartum care: Lessons learned from a Hawaiian public health nursing project. *Journal of Perinatal and Neonatal Nursing, 13*(1), 15–26.

Mercer, R. T. (1995). *Becoming a mother.* New York: Springer.

Nicolson, P. (1999). *Post-natal depression: Psychology, science, and the transition to motherhood.* New York: Routledge.

Rogers, S. J., & White, L. K. (1998). Satisfaction with parenting: The role of marital happiness, family structure, and parents' gender. *Journal of Marriage and the Family, 60,* 293–308.

Rubin, R. (1961). Puerperal change. *Nursing Outlook, 9,* 753.

Rubin, R. (1984). *Maternal identity and the maternal experience.* New York: Springer.

Sampselle, C. M., Seng, J., Yeo, S., Killion, C., & Oakley, D. (1999). Physical activity and postpartum well being. *Journal of Obstetric, Gynecologic, and Neonatal Nursing, 28*(1), 41–49.

Scoggin, J. (2000). Physical and psychological changes. In S. Mattson & J. Smith (Eds.), *AWHONN: Core curriculum for maternal-newborn nursing* (2nd ed., pp. 302–316). Philadelphia: Saunders.

Stark, M. A. (2000). Is it difficult to concentrate during the third trimester and postpartum? *Journal of Obstetric, Gynecologic, and Neonatal Nursing, 29*(4), 378–389.

Troy, N. W. (1999). A comparison of fatigue and energy levels at 6 weeks and 14 to 19 months postpartum. *Clinical Nursing Research, 8*(2), 135–152.

Varney, H. (1997). *Varney's midwifery* (3rd ed.). Sudbury, MA: Jones & Bartlett.

NURSING CARE IN THE COMMUNITY

Various services are available to meet the needs of the childbearing family during the postpartum and beyond. These services range from educational, such as classes on nutrition, infant care, and parenting, to specific health care programs, such as well-baby checks, family-planning services, and the like. Some are offered by private caregivers, others by city, county, state, or federal agencies. In all cases, the goal is to help ensure that the mother, infant, and all family members have the opportunity to meet their health care needs, regardless of their resources.

Home Health Care

Home health care is one of the most important forms of community-based nursing care offered to postpartum families. Home care visits and phone contacts help ensure that new parents have the necessary skills and resources to adequately care for their new infant and any other family members. (Home care is discussed in depth in Chapter 30.)

NURSING MANAGEMENT DURING THE EARLY POSTPARTUM PERIOD

Nursing Diagnosis

For most postpartal women, physical recovery goes smoothly. Consequently, caregivers too often assume that the woman and her family have no real needs and that no care plan is needed. Nothing could be further from the truth. Every member of the family has needs, although the needs may not be obvious, especially if they are psychologic or educational in nature.

The postpartum family's needs, which should be identified during assessment, are the basis for developing nursing diagnoses. Many nurses have suggested that nursing diagnoses are difficult to make in a wellness setting because of their emphasis on "problems." Nurses involved in the effort to formulate standardized diagnoses recognize this difficulty and continue working to develop nursing diagnoses more congruent with wellness settings.

Many agencies that use nursing diagnoses prefer to use only the NANDA list. Consequently, physiologic alterations form the basis of many postpartum diagnoses. Examples of such diagnoses include

- Constipation related to fear of tearing stitches or pain
- Pain related to perineal edema or episiotomy from birth

Fortunately, diagnoses have now been developed that focus on the positive aspects of childbirth and parenting. Examples of these diagnoses include

- Health-seeking behaviors: information about infant care related to an expressed desire to improve parenting skills

- Family coping: potential for growth related to successful adjustment to new baby

After completing the assessment and diagnosis steps of the nursing process, the nurse identifies expected outcomes and selects nursing interventions that will help the family meet the expected outcomes.

Planning and Implementation

Nursing management is individualized to meet the needs of each woman and her newborn. The plan of care needs to consider the baby's schedule, as well as the physical and psychologic well-being of each family member. An important component of nursing care is client teaching, which must be individualized to the learning ability and readiness of the parent(s). As part of the teaching role, the nurse discusses desired outcomes and goals with the mother and family members. Interventions can then be designed to achieve optimal health promotion.

Promotion of Maternal Physical Well-Being

The nurse can promote and restore maternal physical well-being by monitoring uterine status, vital signs, cardiovascular status, elimination patterns, nutritional needs, sleep and rest, and support and educational needs. In addition, the postpartum woman may need medications to promote comfort, treat anemia, provide immunity to rubella, and prevent development of antigens (in the nonsensitized Rh-negative woman).

MONITORING UTERINE STATUS

Complete an assessment of the uterus as discussed in Chapter 21. The assessment interval is usually every 15 minutes for the first hour after childbirth, every 30 minutes for the next hour, and then hourly for approximately 2 hours. After that, monitor uterine status every 8 hours or more frequently if problems arise such as bogginess, positioning out of midline, heavy lochia flow, or the presence of clots (Table 22–1). Occasionally a woman needs medications to promote uterine contractions. See "Drug Guide: Oxytocin (Pitocin)" in Chapter 20 and "Drug Guide: Methylergonovine Maleate (Methergine)" in this chapter. Monitor amount, consistency, color, and odor of the lochia on an ongoing basis (Table 22–2).

TABLE 22–1 Position of the Uterine Fundus Following Birth

Immediately after birth: The top of the fundus is in the midline about midway between the symphysis pubis and umbilicus.

Six to twelve hours after birth: The top of the fundus is in the midline and at the level of the umbilicus.

One day after birth: The top of the fundus is in the midline and one finger breadth below the umbilicus.

Second day after birth and thereafter: The top of the fundus remains in the midline and descends about one finger breadth per day.

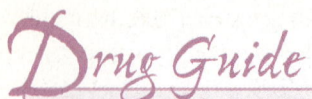
Drug Guide

METHYLERGONOVINE MALEATE (METHERGINE)

Overview of Action

Methylergonovine maleate (Methergine) is an ergot alkaloid that stimulates smooth muscle tissue. Because the uterus is especially sensitive to this drug, it is used postpartally to stimulate the uterus to contract in order to decrease blood loss by clamping off uterine blood vessels and to promote involution. In addition, the drug has a vasoconstrictive effect on all blood vessels, especially the larger arteries. This may result in hypertension, particularly in a woman whose blood pressure is already elevated.

Route, Dosage, Frequency

Methergine has a rapid onset of action and may be given orally or intramuscularly.

Usual IM dose: 0.2 mg following delivery of the placenta. The dose may be repeated every 2 to 4 hours if necessary.

Usual oral dose: 0.2 mg every 4 hours (six doses).

Maternal Contraindications

Pregnancy, hepatic or renal disease, cardiac disease, and hypertension or pregnancy-induced hypertension contraindicate use of this drug. Methylergonovine maleate must be used with caution during lactation (Karch, 2001).

Maternal Side Effects

Hypertension, nausea, vomiting, headache, bradycardia, dizziness, tinnitus, abdominal cramps, palpitations, dyspnea, chest pain, and allergic reactions may be noted.

Effects on Fetus or Neonate

Because Methergine has a long duration (3 hours [Karch, 2001]) and action and can thus produce tetanic contractions, it should never be used during pregnancy or in labor, when it may result in a sustained uterine contraction that may cause amniotic fluid embolism (increased pressure in uterus may allow entry of amniotic fluid under the edge of the placenta and thus entry into the maternal venous system), uterine rupture, cervical and perineal lacerations (resulting from tetanic contractions and rapid birth of the baby), and hypoxia and intracranial hemorrhage in the baby (because of tetanic contractions, which severely decrease the maternal-placental-fetal blood flow, or uterine rupture, which causes cessation of blood flow to the unborn baby) (*PDR Nurse's Handbook,* 2001).

Nursing Considerations

- Monitor fundal height and consistency and the amount and character of the lochia.

- Assess the blood pressure before and routinely throughout drug administration.

- Observe for adverse effects or symptoms of ergot toxicity (ergotism) such as nausea and vomiting, headache, muscle pain, cold or numb fingers and toes, chest pain, and general weakness (*PDR Nurse's Handbook,* 2001).

- Provide client and family teaching about the importance of not smoking during Methergine administration (nicotine from cigarettes leads to constricted vessels and may lead to hypertension) and about signs of toxicity.

TABLE 22–2 Changes in Lochia That Cause Concern		
Change	Possible Problem	Nursing Action
Presence of clots	Inadequate uterine contractions that allow bleeding from vessels at the placental site.	Assess location and firmness of fundus. Assess voiding pattern. Record and report findings.
Persistent lochia rubra	Inadequate uterine contractions; retained placental fragments; infection	Assess location and firmness of fundus. Assess activity pattern. Assess for signs of infection. Record and report findings.

Promotion of Comfort and Relief of Pain

Potential sources of postpartum discomfort include an edematous perineum; an episiotomy, perineal laceration, or extension; vaginal hematoma; engorged hemorrhoids; or engorged breasts with sore nipples.

RELIEF OF PERINEAL DISCOMFORT

Before selecting a method to help relieve perineal discomfort, assess the perineum to determine the degree of edema and so on. It is also important to ask the woman if she believes any special measures will be particularly effective and to offer her choices when possible. Wear disposable gloves while applying all relief measures and complete handwashing before and after using the gloves. At all times it is essential to remember good hygiene practices, such as moving from the front (area of the symphysis pubis) to the back (area around the anus) of the perineum. Avoiding contamination between the anal area and the urethral/vaginal area is vital to prevent infection.

Ice Pack. If an episiotomy is done at the time of birth, an ice pack is generally applied to the perineum to reduce edema and provide numbing of the tissues, which promotes comfort. In some agencies, chemical ice bags are used. Folding both ends toward the middle usually activates these ice bags. To make an inexpensive ice bag, fill a disposable glove with ice chips or crushed ice and then tape the top of the glove to close it. To protect the perineum from burns caused by contact with such an ice pack, rinse the glove under running water to remove any powder and then wrap it in an absorbent towel or washcloth before placing it against the perineum. For best results, follow a pattern of applying the ice pack for approximately 20 minutes and then removing it for about 10 minutes. Usually ice packs are needed for the first 24 hours. Provide information about the purpose of the ice pack, as well as anticipated effects, benefits, and possible problems, and explain how to make an ice pack for home use if edema is present and early discharge is planned.

Nursing Practice

You may be surprised by how quickly the postpartum woman shows signs of bladder distention, possibly as soon as 1 to 2 hours after childbirth. It results because of normal postpartum diuresis. You can help prevent overdistention by palpating the woman's bladder frequently and encouraging her to void. When attempting to void for the first time after vaginal birth, some mothers may feel the urge to urinate but be unable to begin the flow of urine. Possible interventions include letting her hear running water by turning water on in the sink or tub, running warm water in the sink and having her place one hand in the water, and/or placing her feet in a basin of warm water.

Sitz Bath. The warmth of the water in the sitz bath provides comfort, decreases pain, and promotes circulation to the tissues. This promotes healing and reduces the incidence of infection. Sitz baths may be ordered three times a day (tid) and as needed (prn). Prepare the sitz bath by cleaning the sitz bath equipment and adding water at 102 to 105 °F. Encourage the woman to remain in the sitz bath for about 20 minutes. It is important for the woman to have a clean, unused towel to pat dry her perineum after the sitz bath and to have a clean perineal pad to apply. Be alert during the first sitz bath because the warm, moist heat and warm environment may cause the woman to faint. Place a call bell well within reach and check on the woman frequently to maintain safety. Signs that she may feel faint include expressed feelings of dizziness, a floaty or spacy feeling, or difficulty hearing.

Cool sitz baths have gained popularity because they are effective in reducing perineal edema. Until research supports one temperature (warm or cold) as more effective, it may be best to offer the woman a choice. Provide information about the purpose and use of the sitz bath; anticipated effects, benefits, and possible problems; and safety measures to prevent injury from fainting, slipping, or excessive water temperature. Home use of sitz baths may be recommended for the woman with an extensive episiotomy, and the woman may use a portable sitz bath or her bathtub. It is important to emphasize that in using a bathtub, the woman draws only 4 to 6 inches of water, assesses the temperature, and uses the water only for the sitz and not for bathing. If the woman takes a tub bath, she should release the water, have a helper clean the tub, and draw new water prior to the sitz bath to prevent infection.

Topical Agents. Topical anesthetics such as Dermoplast aerosol spray and Americaine spray may be used to relieve perineal pain. Advise the woman to apply the anesthetic after a sitz bath or perineal care. Witch hazel compresses may be used to relieve perineal pain and edema. Nupercainal ointment or Tucks pads may be ordered for relief of hem-

orrhoidal pain. Provide information about the spray or topical agent. The woman needs to understand the purpose, use, anticipated effects and benefits, and possible problems associated with the product. It is important to emphasize the need for the woman to wash her hands before and after using the topical treatments.

Perineal Care. Perineal care after each elimination cleanses the perineum and helps promote comfort. Many agencies provide "peri-bottles" that the woman can use to squirt warm tap water over her perineum following elimination. To cleanse her perineum, the woman should use moist antiseptic towelettes or toilet paper in a blotting (patting) motion and should be taught to start at the front (area just under the symphysis pubis) and proceed toward the back (area around the anus), to prevent contamination from the anal area. Similarly, she should apply the perineal pad from front to back (place the front portion against the perineum first).

Demonstrate how to cleanse the perineum and assist the woman as necessary. Many women have never used perineal pads and will need help in using them during the postpartum period. The pad needs to be placed snugly against the perineum but should not produce pressure. If the pad is worn too loosely, it may rub back and forth, irritating perineal tissues and causing contamination between the anal and vaginal areas (for information regarding the care of the perineum following an episiotomy see "Teaching About: Episiotomy Care").

Teaching About

EPISIOTOMY CARE

Describe the process of wound healing. Discuss the risks of contamination of the episiotomy by bacteria from the anal area.

Describe techniques that are used to keep the episiotomy clean and promote healing:

- Sitz bath
- Use of peri-bottle following each voiding or defecation
- Pad change following each elimination and at regular intervals

Describe comfort measures:

- Ice pack or ice-filled glove to perineum immediately following childbirth
- Sitz bath
- Judicious use of analgesics or topical anesthetics
- Tightening buttocks before sitting

Identify signs of episiotomy infection (redness, edema, drainage, poor approximation of the edges).

Advise the woman to contact her caregiver if signs of infection develop.

RELIEF OF HEMORRHOIDAL DISCOMFORT

Some mothers experience hemorrhoidal pain after giving birth. Relief measures include sitz baths, topical anesthetic ointments, rectal suppositories, or witch hazel pads applied directly to the anal area. The woman may be taught to replace external hemorrhoids digitally in her rectum. She may also find it helpful to maintain a side-lying position when possible and to avoid prolonged sitting. Encourage the woman to maintain an adequate fluid intake, and administer stool softeners to ensure greater comfort with bowel movements. The hemorrhoids usually disappear a few weeks after birth if the woman did not have them before her pregnancy.

RELIEF OF AFTERPAINS

Afterpains are the result of intermittent uterine contractions. A primipara may not have afterpains because her uterus is able to maintain a contracted state. Multiparous women and those who have had a multiple gestation preg-

nancy or hydramnios frequently have discomfort from afterpains as the uterus contracts intermittently. Breastfeeding women are also more likely to have afterpains than bottle-feeding women because of the release of oxytocin when the infant suckles. For relief the woman can lie prone, with a small pillow under her lower abdomen. The discomfort may feel intensified for about 5 minutes but then diminishes greatly if not completely. The prone position applies pressure to the uterus and thus stimulates contractions. When the uterus maintains a constant contraction, the afterpains cease. Additional nursing interventions include a sitz bath (for warmth), ambulation, or administration of an analgesic. For breastfeeding mothers, an analgesic administered an hour before nursing helps promote comfort and enhances maternal-infant interaction (Table 22–3).

Provide information about the cause of afterpains and methods to decrease discomfort. Explain any medications that are ordered, including their expected effect, benefits, and possible side effects, and any special considerations

---

TABLE 22–3 Essential Information for Common Postpartum Drugs

EMPIRIN #3 (325 MG ASPIRIN AND 30 MG CODEINE)

Drug class: Narcotic analgesic.

Dose/Route: Usual adult dose: 1–2 tablets PO every 4 hours prn.

Indication: For relief of mild to moderate pain.

Adverse Effects: Aspirin: Nausea, dyspepsia, epigastric discomfort, dizziness.

Codeine: Respiratory depression, apnea, light-headedness, dizziness, nausea, sweating, dry mouth, constipation, facial flushing, suppression of cough reflex, ureteral spasm, urinary retention, pruritus.

Nursing Implications: Determine whether woman is sensitive to aspirin or codeine; has history of impaired hepatic or renal function. Monitor bowel sounds, respiration, urine output.

Administer with food or after meals if GI upset occurs; encourage woman to drink one full glass (240 mL) with the tablet to reduce the risk of the tablet lodging in the esophagus.

Client Teaching: Inform client about name of drug, expected action, possible side effects, that it is secreted in breast milk (*Note:* Some physicians and certified nurse-midwives may avoid ordering this medication for nursing mothers), and review safety measures (assess for dizziness, use side rails, call for assistance when getting out of bed and ambulating, report to nurse any signs of adverse effects); ask if she has any questions.

Nursing Diagnosis Related to Drug Therapy: *Knowledge deficit* related to lack of information about the drug therapy.

Risk for injury related to dizziness secondary to effect of drug.

PERCOCET (325 MG ACETAMINOPHEN AND 5 MG OXYCODONE)

Drug Class: Narcotic analgesic

Drug/Route: 1–2 tablets PO every 4 hours prn.

Indication: For moderate to moderately severe pain. Can be used in aspirin-sensitive women.

Adverse Effects: Acetaminophen: Hepatotoxicity, headache, rash, hypoglycemia.

Oxycodone: Respiratory depression, apnea, circulatory depression, euphoria, facial flushing, constipation, suppression of cough reflex, ureteral spasm, urinary retention.

Nursing Implications: Determine whether woman is sensitive to acetaminophen or codeine; has bronchial asthma, respiratory depression, convulsive disorder.

Observe woman carefully for respiratory depression if given with barbiturates or sedative/hypnotics. Consider that women who have undergone cesarean birth may have depressed cough reflex, so teaching and encouragement to deep breathe and cough are needed.

Monitor bowel sounds, urine and bowel elimination.

Client Teaching: Teaching should include name of drug, expected effect, possible adverse effects, that drug is secreted in the breast milk, encouragement to report any signs of adverse effects immediately.

Nursing Diagnoses Related to Drug Therapy: *Ineffective breathing pattern* related to respiratory depression.

Constipation related to slowed gastrointestinal activity.

---

such as the possibility of dizziness or sleepiness with particular medications.

RELIEF OF DISCOMFORT FROM IMMOBILITY

Discomfort may be caused by immobility. The woman who has been in stirrups for any length of time may experience muscular aches from such positioning. Moreover, depending on the effort they exerted in pushing during labor, women often experience joint pains and muscular pain in both arms and legs.

Early ambulation helps reduce the incidence of complications such as constipation and thrombophlebitis. It also helps promote a feeling of general well-being. Provide information about ambulation and the importance of monitoring signs of dizziness or weakness.

Assist the woman the first few times she gets up during the postpartum period. Fatigue, effects of medications, loss of blood, and lack of food intake may cause feelings of dizziness or faintness when she stands up. Because this may be a problem during the woman's first shower, remain in the room, check the woman frequently, and have a chair close by in case she becomes faint. During this first shower, explain use of the emergency call button in the bathroom. Tell the woman that if she becomes faint during a future shower, she should sit down and call for help.

TABLE 22–3 Essential Information for Common Postpartum Drugs—continued

RUBELLA VIRUS VACCINE, LIVE (MERUVAX 2)

Dose/Route: Single dose vial, inject subcutaneously in outer aspect of the upper arm.

Indication: Stimulate active immunity against rubella virus.

Adverse Effects: Burning or stinging at the injection site; about 2–4 weeks later may have rash, malaise, sore throat, or headache.

Nursing Implications: Determine whether woman has sensitivity to neomycin (vaccine contains neomycin); is immunosuppressed, or has received blood transfusions (not to be administered within 3 months of blood transfusion, plasma transfusion, or serum immune globulin).
Note: If a woman is to receive both RhoGAM and rubella, there is a possibility that the formation of antibodies to rubella may be suppressed by the RhoGAM injection. Most physicians will go ahead and order both injections and retest for maternal rubella immune status in about 3 months (Varney, 1997).

Client Teaching: Name of drug, expected effect, possible adverse effects, possible comfort measures to use if adverse effects occur, rubella titer will be assessed in about 3 months. Instruct woman to *avoid pregnancy for 3 months* following vaccination. Provide information regarding contraceptives and their use.

Nursing Diagnosis Related to Drug Therapy: Health-Seeking Behavior: information about contraception related to an expressed desire to avoid pregnancy following rubella vaccination.

Pain related to rash and malaise.

RHOGAM (RH IMMUNE GLOBULIN SPECIFIC FOR D ANTIGEN)

Dose/Route: Postpartum: One vial IM within 72 hours of birth. Antepartal: One vial microdose RhoGAM IM at 28 weeks in Rh-negative women; after amniocentesis, spontaneous or therapeutic abortion, or ectopic pregnancy.

Indication: Prevention of sensitization to the Rh factor in Rh-negative women and to prevent hemolytic disease in the newborn in subsequent pregnancies. Mother must be Rh negative, not previously sensitized to Rh factor. Infant must be Rh positive, direct antiglobulin negative.

Adverse Effects: Soreness at injection site.

Nursing Implications: Confirm that criteria for administration are present. Ensure correct vial is used for the client (each vial is crossmatched to the specific woman and must be carefully checked).

Inject entire contents of vial.

Client Teaching: Name of drug, expected action, possible side effects; report soreness at injection site to nurse; woman should carry information regarding Rh status and dates of RhoGAM injections with her at all times; explain use of RhoGAM with subsequent pregnancies.

Nursing Diagnoses Related to Drug Therapy: *Knowledge deficit* related to lack of information about the need for the RhoGAM and future implications.

Pain related to soreness at injection site.

SECONAL SODIUM (SECOBARBITAL SODIUM)

Drug Class: Sedative, short-acting barbiturate

Dose/Route: 100 mg PO at bedtime.

Indication: Promote sleep.

Adverse Effects: Somnolence, confusion, ataxia, vertigo, nightmares, hypoventilation, bradycardia, hypotension, nausea, vomiting, rashes.

Nursing Implications: Determine whether woman has sensitivity to barbiturates, or respiratory distress. Monitor respirations, blood pressure, pulse. Modify environment to increase relaxation and promote sleep. Monitor for drug interaction if woman also is taking tranquilizers or TACE.

Client Teaching: Name of drug, expected effect, possible adverse effects, safety measures (side rails, use call bell, ask for assistance when out of bed); medication is secreted in breast milk.

Nursing Diagnoses Related to Drug Therapy: *Risk for injury* related to possible ataxia or vertigo.

Altered thought processes related to drug-induced confusion.

Knowledge deficit related to lack of information about drug therapy.

RELIEF OF POSTPARTUM DIAPHORESIS

Postpartum diaphoresis (excessive perspiration) may cause discomfort for new mothers. Offer a fresh, dry gown and change the bed linens to enhance comfort. Some women may feel refreshed by a shower. It is important to consider cultural practices and realize that some women of Hispanic or Asian cultural background may prefer not to shower in the first few days following birth. Because diaphoresis may also increase thirst, offer fluids regularly. Again, consider cultural practices. Women of western European background may prefer iced water, whereas Asian women may prefer water at room temperature. It is important to ascertain the woman's wishes rather than operate solely from personal values. Provide information about the normalcy of diaphoresis and methods to increase comfort.

Suppression of Lactation in the Nonnursing Mother

For the woman who chooses not to breastfeed, lactation may be suppressed by mechanical inhibition. Although signs of engorgement do not usually appear until the second or third postpartum day, prevention of engorgement is best accomplished when the woman begins mechanical inhibition of lactation as soon as possible after birth. Ideally prevention involves having the woman begin wearing a supportive, well-fitting bra within 6 hours after birth. She wears the bra continuously until lactation is suppressed (usually about 5 to 7 days) and removes it only for showers. The bra provides support and eases the discomfort that can occur with tension on the breasts because of fullness. Ice packs should be applied over the axillary area of each breast for 20 minutes four times daily. This practice, too, should begin soon after birth. Ice is also useful in relieving discomfort if engorgement occurs.

Advise the woman to avoid any stimulation of her breasts by her baby, herself, breast pumps, or her partner until the sensation of fullness has passed (usually about 5 to 7 days). Such stimulation increases milk production and delays suppression. Heat is avoided for the same reason. Encourage the mother to let shower water flow over her back rather than her breasts.

Promotion of Rest and Graded Activity

Following childbirth, some women feel exhausted and in need of rest. Other women may be euphoric and full of energy, ready to relive and recount the experience of birth repeatedly. Provide a period for airing of feelings and then encourage a period of rest.

Physical fatigue often affects other adjustments and functions of the new mother. For example, fatigue can reduce milk flow, thereby increasing problems with establishing breastfeeding. Energy is also needed to adjust to a new infant and to assume new roles. Encourage rest by organizing care activities to avoid frequent interruptions for the woman. It is helpful for the new mother to know that fatigue may persist for several weeks or even months. Persistent fatigue is compounded by physical, psychologic, situational, and environmental factors (Parks, Lenz, Milligan, et al., 1999).

Although most mothers feel tired, if they consider pregnancy and birth as a natural process, they tend to see themselves as healthy and well. However, some mothers view the postpartum as a time of sickness. For instance, some Korean women and their families view the new mother as sick and in need of care by the mother-in-law and the baby's father. A Korean mother may do some things, but for the most part it will be activities such as picking up the baby from the nursery rather than activity directed toward herself (Schneiderman, 1996).

POSTPARTUM EXERCISES

Postpartum exercise is associated with positive views of the childbirth experience (Sampselle, Seng, Yeo, et al., 1999). Encourage the woman to begin simple exercises while in the birthing unit and to continue them at home. Inform her that increased lochia or pain means she should reevaluate her activity and make necessary alterations. Most agencies provide a booklet describing suggested postpartum activities. (Exercise routines vary for women undergoing cesarean birth or tubal ligation after childbirth.) (See Figure 22–1 ◆ for a description of some commonly used exercises.)

FIGURE 22–1. ◆ Postpartum exercises. Begin with 5 repetitions two or three times daily and gradually increase to 10 repetitions. First day: **A,** Abdominal breathing. Lying supine, inhale deeply using the abdominal muscles. The abdomen should expand. Then exhale slowly through pursed lips, tightening the abdominal muscles. **B,** Pelvic rocking. Lying supine with arms at sides, knees bent, and feet flat, tighten abdomen and buttocks and attempt to flatten back onto floor. Hold for a count of 10, then arch the back, causing the pelvis to "rock." On second day add the following: **C,** Chin to chest. Lying supine with no pillow, legs straight, raise head and attempt to touch chin to chest. Slowly lower head. **D,** Arm raises. Lying supine, arms extended perpendicular to the body, raise arms until hands touch. Lower slowly. On fourth day add the following: **E,** Knee rolls. Lying supine with knees bent, feet flat, arms extended to the side, roll knees slowly to one side, keeping shoulders flat. Return to original position and roll to opposite side. **F,** Buttocks lift. Lying supine, arms at sides, knees bent, feet flat, slowly raise the buttocks and arch the back. Return slowly to starting position. On sixth day add the following: **G,** Abdominal tighteners. Lying supine, knees bent, feet flat, slowly raise the head toward the knees. Arms should extend along either side of the legs. Return slowly to original position. **H,** Knee to abdomen. Lying supine, arms at sides, bend one knee and thigh until foot touches buttocks. Straighten leg and lower it slowly. Repeat with other leg. After 2 to 3 weeks, more strenuous exercises such as side leg raises may be added as tolerated. Kegel exercises, begun antepartally, should be done many times daily during postpartum to restore vaginal and perineal tone.

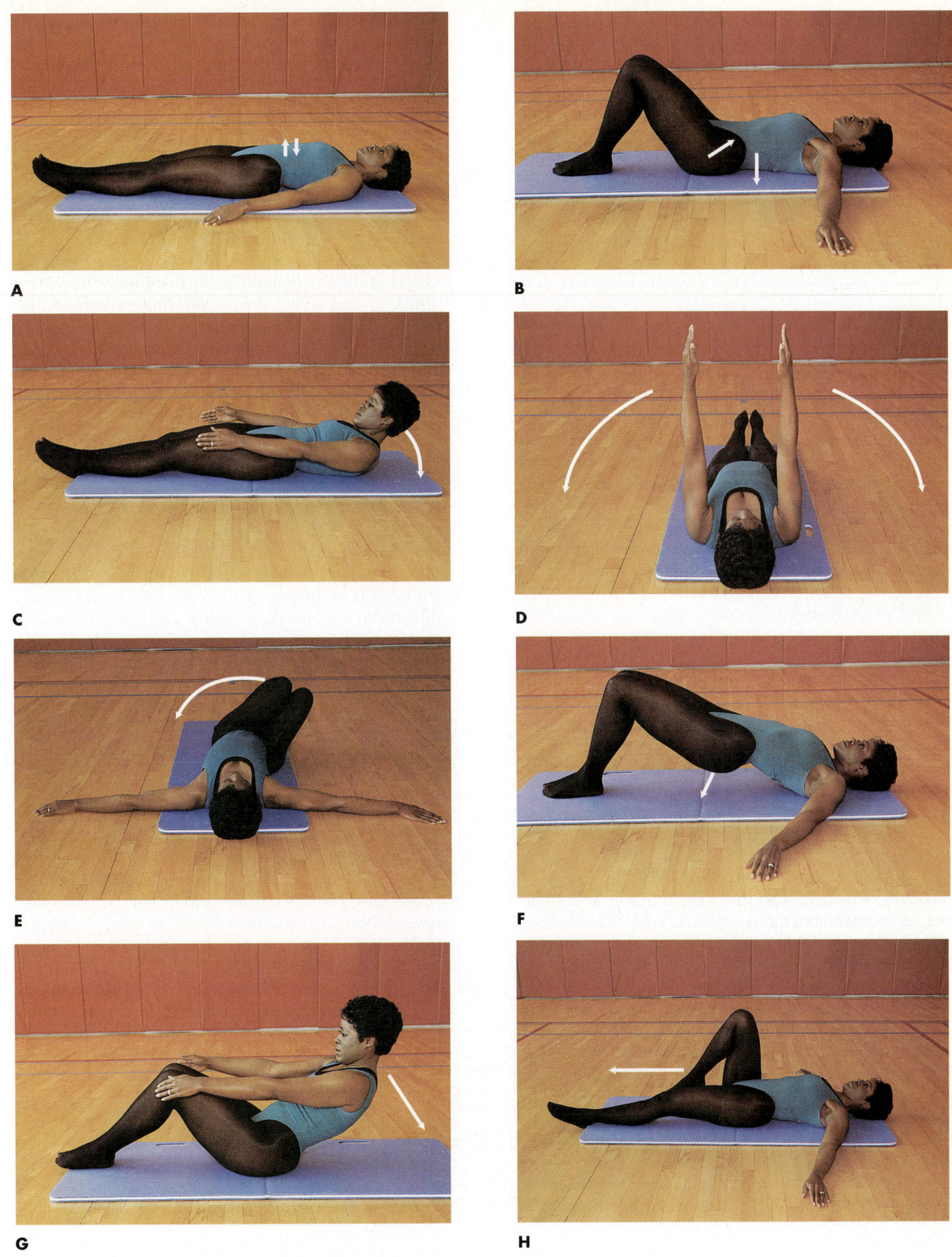

A

B

C

D

E

F

G

H

RESUMPTION OF ACTIVITIES

Ambulation and activity may gradually increase after birth. The new mother should avoid heavy lifting, excessive stair climbing, and strenuous activity. One or two daily naps are essential and are most easily achieved if the mother sleeps when her baby does.

By the second week at home, the woman may resume light housekeeping. Although it is customary to delay returning to work for 6 weeks, most women are physically able to resume practically all activities by 4 to 5 weeks. Delaying the return to work until after the final postpartum examination minimizes the possibility of problems.

Pharmacologic Interventions

RUBELLA VACCINE

Women who have a rubella titer of less than 1:10, or test antibody negative on the enzyme-linked immunosorbent assay (ELISA), are usually given rubella vaccine in the postpartum period (Cunningham, Gant, Leveno, et al., 2001) (see Table 22–3). Ensure that the woman understands the purpose of the vaccine and the need to avoid becoming pregnant in the next 3 months. To ensure that the woman understands, obtain an informed consent before giving the vaccine. Because avoiding pregnancy is so important, counseling about contraception is suggested.

RH IMMUNE GLOBULIN

All Rh-negative women who meet specific criteria should receive Rh immune globulin (RhoGAM) within 72 hours after childbirth to prevent sensitization from the fetomaternal transfusion of Rh-positive fetal red blood cells. (See Chapter 13.) The Rh-negative woman needs to understand the implications of her Rh-negative status in future pregnancies. Provide opportunities for her and her partner to ask questions.

Promotion of Maternal Psychologic Well-Being

The birth of a child, with the changes in role and the increased responsibilities it produces, is a time of emotional stress for the new mother. During the early postpartum period the mother may be emotionally labile, and mood swings and tearfulness are common. Initially the mother may repeatedly discuss her experiences of labor and birth. This allows the mother to integrate her experiences (Banks-Wallace, 1999). If she believes that she did not cope well with labor, she may have feelings of inadequacy and may benefit from reassurance that she did well. Some women feel that they did not have any perception of time during the labor and birth and want to know how long it really lasted, or they may not remember the entire experience. In this case, it is helpful to talk with the woman and provide the information that she is missing and wants.

During this time the new mother must also adjust to the loss of her fantasized child and accept the child she has borne. This task may be more difficult if the child is not of the desired sex or if he or she has birth defects (see Chapter 29).

Immediately after the birth (the taking-in period) the mother is focused on bodily concerns and may not be fully ready to learn about personal and infant care. Following this initial dependent period, the mother typically becomes concerned about her ability to be a successful parent (the taking-hold period). During this time the mother needs reassurance that she is effective. She also tends to be receptive to teaching and demonstration designed to help her in mothering successfully. The depression, weepiness, and "let-down feeling" that characterize the postpartum blues are often a surprise for the new mother. Provide reassurance that these feelings are normal, an explanation about why they occur, and a supportive environment so that she can cry if she wishes without feeling guilty.

Promotion of Effective Parent Education

Meeting the educational needs of the new mother and her family is an important nursing responsibility. Each woman's educational needs vary based on her age, background, experience, and expectations. In addition, because the mother is in the postpartum area for a brief period, it is difficult to address all individual characteristics and informational needs.

Assess the learning needs of the new mother through observation and tactfully phrased questions. For example, "What plans have you made for handling things when you get home?" may elicit a response of several words and may provide the opportunity for some information sharing and guidance. Some agencies also use checklists of common concerns for new mothers. The woman can check the concerns that are of interest to her.

Plan and implement teaching in a logical, nonthreatening way based on knowledge and respect of the family's cultural values and beliefs. Unless an activity would be harmful, most cultural customs can be supported and encouraged. Postpartum units use a variety of approaches to teaching, including handouts, formal classes, videotapes, and individual interaction.

Regardless of the teaching technique, timing is important. The new mother becomes more receptive to teaching after the first 24 to 48 hours, when she is ready to assume responsibility for her own care and that of her newborn (Lamp & Howard, 1999). Unfortunately, many women are discharged during the first 48 hours after birth. Consequently, many units provide printed material for new mothers to consult if questions arise at home. Timing is also important for new fathers, who are more likely to attend teaching sessions if they are scheduled in the late afternoon or early evening.

Thinking Critically

READY TO GO HOME?

You walk in and find Dana Sullivan, a 29-year-old G2P2, crying 48 hours after a repeat cesarean birth. She states, "I'm not ready to go home. With my first baby they made me go home after 2 days. Can they make me again?" How would you respond? **WEB**

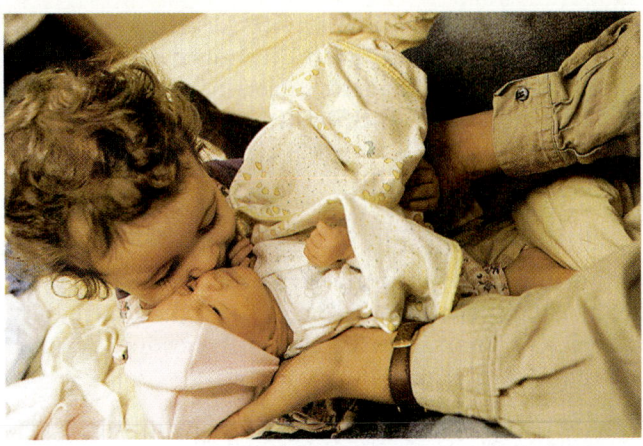

FIGURE 22–2. ◆ The sister of this newborn becomes acquainted with the new family member during a nursing assessment.

Teaching should include information on role change and psychologic adjustments as well as skills. Anticipatory guidance can help prepare new parents for the many changes they will experience with a new family member.

Information is also essential for women with specialized educational needs such as the mother who has had a cesarean birth, the parents of twins, the parents of an infant with congenital anomalies, and so on (Koniak-Griffin, Mathenge, Anderson, et al., 1999). Nurses who are attuned to these individual problems can begin providing guidance as soon as possible. Evaluation may take several forms: return demonstrations, question-and-answer sessions, and even formal evaluation tools. Follow-up phone calls after discharge provide additional evaluative information and continue the helping process for the family.

Promotion of Family Wellness

The promotion of family wellness involves several considerations, including a satisfactory maternity experience, the need for follow-up care for mother and infant, and birth control. The new or expanding family may also need information about adjustment of siblings and resuming sexual relations.

Today most facilities support family-centered care called **mother-baby care** or **couplet care.** It provides increased opportunities for parent-child interaction because the newborn shares the mother's unit and they are cared for together. Mother-baby care enables the mother to have time to bond with her baby and learn to care for him or her in a supportive environment. It is especially conducive to a hunger-demand feeding schedule for both breast- and bottle-feeding babies. It also allows the father, siblings, and friends to help with the care of the new baby.

Mother-baby unit policies must be flexible enough to permit the mother to return the baby to the nursery if she finds it necessary because of fatigue or physical discomfort. Some mother-baby units also return the newborns to a central nursery at night so the mothers can get more rest. Mother-baby care provides excellent opportunities for family bonds to grow because the father, mother, newborn, and often siblings can begin functioning as a family unit immediately.

REACTIONS OF SIBLINGS

Sibling visits help meet the needs of both the siblings and their mother. A visit to the mother-baby unit reassures children that their mother is well and still loves them. It also provides an opportunity for the children to become familiar with the new baby. For the mother the pangs of separation are lessened as she interacts with her children and introduces them to the newest family member (Figure 22–2 ◆).

Although the parents have prepared their children for the presence of a new brother or sister, the actual arrival of the baby in the home requires some adjustments. If small children are waiting at home, it is helpful if the father carries the infant inside so that the mother's arms are free to hug her older children. Many mothers bring a doll home with them for an older child. Caring for the doll alongside the mother or father helps the child to identify with the parents. This identification helps decrease anger and the need to regress for attention.

Parents may also provide supervised times when older children can hold the new baby and perhaps even help with a bottle-feeding. The older children feel a sense of accomplishment and learn tenderness and caring—qualities appropriate for both males and females. The nurse can help the parents come up with ways to show the other children that they, too, are valued and have their own places in the family.

SEXUAL ACTIVITY AND CONTRACEPTION

Previously, couples were discouraged from engaging in sexual intercourse until 6 weeks postpartum. Currently, couples are advised to abstain from intercourse until the episiotomy has healed and the lochial flow has stopped (usually by the end of the third week). (For a more detailed discussion on resumption of sexual activity see Chapter 30.)

Because many couples resume sexual activity before the scheduled postpartum exam, family-planning information should be made available before discharge (Barrett, Pendry, Peacock, et al., 2000). Unfortunately, because of in-hospital time restraints, this subject is often overlooked. (Specific contraceptive methods are discussed in detail in Chapter 3.) 🔗

Promotion of Parent-Infant Attachment

Nursing interventions to enhance the quality of parent-infant attachment should be designed to promote feelings of well-being, comfort, and satisfaction. Following are some suggestions for ways of promoting this:

- Determine the childbearing and childrearing goals of the infant's mother and father and support them wherever possible in planning care for the family. This includes giving the parents choices about their labor and birth and their initial time with their new infant.

- Postpone eye prophylaxis for 1 hour after birth to facilitate eye contact between parents and their newborn (eye ointment clouds the newborn's vision and makes eye contact difficult for the baby).

- Provide time in the first hour after birth for the new family to become acquainted, with as much privacy as possible.

- Arrange the health care setting so that the individual nurse-client relationship can be developed. A primary nurse can develop rapport and assess the mother's strengths and needs.

- Encourage the parents to involve the siblings in integrating the infant into the family by bringing them to the birthing center for visits.

- Use anticipatory guidance from conception through the postpartum period to prepare the parents for expected problems of adjustment.

- Include parents in any nursing intervention, planning, and evaluation. Give choices whenever possible.

- Initiate and support measures to alleviate fatigue in the parents.

- Help parents identify, understand, and accept both positive and negative feelings related to the overall parenting experience.

- Support and assist parents in determining the personality and unique needs of their infant.

Whenever possible, mother-baby care should be available. This practice gives the mother a chance to learn her newborn's normal patterns and develop confidence in caring for him or her. It also allows the father more uninterrupted time with his infant in the first days of life. If mother and baby are doing well, if help is available for the mother at home, and if the family and certified nurse-midwife or physician agree, early discharge may be advantageous.

The beginnings of parent-newborn attachment may be observed in the first few hours after birth. Continued assessments may occur in home visits after discharge. In assessing attachment, it is important to remember that cultural values, beliefs, and practices will direct child care activities and self-care practices. For example, some Mexican-American women treat the umbilical stump by placing a coin or belly band over it. People in many countries, for example, Greece, Iran, Italy, and Malaysia, often place amulets on the baby or in the crib for protection (Spector, 2000). (See Table 22–4 for behaviors related to infant attachment.)

TABLE 22–4	Parent Attachment Behaviors	
Assessment Area	*Attachment*	*Behavior Requiring Assessment and Information*
Caretaking	Talks with baby	Does not refer to baby
	Demonstrates and seeks eye-to-eye contact	Completes activities without addressing the baby or looking at the baby
	Touches and holds baby	Lack of interaction
	Changes diapers when needed	Does not recognize need for or demonstrate concern for baby's comfort
	Baby is clean	Feeding occurs intermittently
	Clothing is appropriate for room temperature	Baby does not gain weight
	Feeds baby as needed and baby is gaining weight	Waits for baby to cry and then hesitates to respond
	Positions baby comfortably and checks on baby	
Perception of the baby	Has knowledge of expected child development	Has unrealistic expectations of the baby's abilities and behaviors
	Understands that the baby is dependent and cannot meet parent's needs	Expects love and interaction from the baby
		Believes that the baby will fulfill parent's needs
	Accepts sex and characteristics of child	Is strongly distressed over sex of baby or feels that some aspect of the baby is unacceptable
Support	Has friends who are available for support	Is alone or isolated
	Seems to be comfortable with being a parent	Is on edge, tense, anxious, and hesitant with the baby
	Has realistic beliefs of parent role	Demonstrates difficulty incorporating parenting with own wants and needs

Please note: These are a few of the behaviors that may be associated with attachment. It is vitally important for the nurse to observe the parents on more than one occasion and to take into consideration individual characteristics, values, beliefs, and customs.

Developing Cultural Competence

The following information applies to many women from Southeast Asia during the postpartum period:

- Childbirth gives the woman increased status in her community.
- The female support system of relatives, especially the mother, mother-in-law, and sisters, is of special importance during postpartum for information on self-care and activities to avoid as well as assistance with household chores.
- The postpartum is viewed as a time for rest, often bed rest, for a month or more. During that time the woman is expected to do little except breastfeed (Davis, 2001).
- The newborn should be shielded from compliments because they may attract the attention of evil spirits (Spector, 2000).
- Because of the blood loss associated with childbirth, the body is in a "cold" state afterward. To regain balance, the woman should have "hot" drinks and foods (warm water, rice, boiled chicken, and so forth). She should also avoid baths and showers, which cool the body (Davis, 2001).

NURSING MANAGEMENT AFTER CESAREAN BIRTH

After a cesarean birth the new mother has postpartum needs similar to those of women who have given birth vaginally. Because she has undergone major abdominal surgery, the woman's nursing care needs are also similar to those of other surgical clients.

Promotion of Maternal Physical Well-Being

The chances of pulmonary infection are increased because of immobility after the use of narcotics and sedatives and because of the altered immune response in postoperative clients. Therefore, encourage the woman to cough and deep breathe every 2 to 4 hours while awake until she is ambulating frequently. In addition, encourage leg exercises every 2 hours until the woman is ambulating. These exercises increase circulation, help prevent thrombophlebitis, and also aid intestinal motility by tightening abdominal muscles.

Monitor and manage the woman's pain during the postpartum period. Sources of pain include incisional pain, gas pain, referred shoulder pain, periodic uterine contractions (afterbirth pains), and pain from voiding, defecation, or constipation. Nursing interventions are oriented toward preventing or alleviating pain or helping the woman cope with pain. Implement the following measures:

- Administer analgesics as needed, especially during the first 24 to 72 hours after childbirth. Use of analgesics relieves the woman's pain and enables her to be more mobile and active.
- Promote comfort through proper positioning, back rubs, oral care, and the reduction of noxious stimuli such as noise and unpleasant odors.

- Encourage visits by significant others, including the newborn. These visits distract the woman from the painful sensations and help reduce her fear and anxiety.
- Encourage the use of breathing, relaxation, and distraction (e.g., stimulation of cutaneous tissue) techniques taught in childbirth preparation class.

Epidural analgesia administered just after the cesarean birth is an effective method of pain relief for most women in the first 24 hours following birth (see "Drug Guide: Postpartum Epidural Morphine").

The physician may order **patient-controlled analgesia** (PCA). With this approach, the woman is given a bolus of

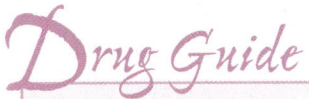

Drug Guide

POSTPARTUM EPIDURAL MORPHINE

Overview of Obstetric Action

Epidural morphine is used to provide relief of pain associated with cesarean birth, extensive episiotomies (mediolaterals), or third- and fourth-degree lacerations. Pain relief results directly from its effect on the opiate receptors in the spinal cord (it depresses pain impulse transmission). Morphine binds opiate receptors, thereby altering both the perception of and emotional response to pain. Women experience little or no discomfort during recovery and for up to 24 hours afterward. There is no motor or sympathetic block or associated hypotension. Onset of analgesia is slower, but duration is longer.

Route, Dosage, Frequency

Morphine (5 to 7.5 mg) is injected through a catheter into the epidural space, providing pain relief for about 24 hours (Karch, 2001).

Maternal Contraindications

Allergy to morphine, narcotic addiction, chronic debilitating respiratory disease, infection at the injection site, or administration of parenteral corticosteroids in past 14 days.

Maternal Side Effects

Late-onset respiratory depression (rare but may occur 8 to 12 hours after administration), nausea and vomiting (occurring between 4 and 7 hours after injection), itching (begins within 3 hours and lasts up to 10 hours), urinary retention, and, rarely, somnolence. Side effects can be managed with naloxone.

Neonatal Effects

No adverse effects since it is injected after birth of the baby.

Nursing Considerations

- Obtain history: sensitivity (allergy) to morphine, presence of any contraindications.
- Assess orientation, reflexes, skin color, texture, breath sounds, presence of lesions or infection over area of lumbar spine, voiding pattern, urinary output within normal limits (Karch, 2001).
- Monitor and evaluate analgesic effect. Ask client about comfort level and notify anesthesiologist of inadequate pain relief.

(continued)

- Check catheter for obvious knots, breaks, and leakage at insertion site and catheter hub.
- Assess for pruritus (scratching and rubbing, especially around face and neck).
- Administer comfort measures for narcotic-induced pruritus, such as lotion, back rubs, cool/warm packs, or diversional activities. If the itching can be tolerated, naloxone should be avoided, especially since it counteracts the pain relief.
- If allergic reaction (urticaria, edema, or respiratory difficulties) occurs, administer naloxone or diphenhydramine per physician order.
- Provide comfort measures for nausea and vomiting, such as frequent oral hygiene or gradual increase of activity; administer naloxone, trimethobenzamide (Tigan), or metoclopramide HCl per physician order.
- Assess postural blood pressure and heart rate before ambulation.
- Assist client with her first ambulation and then as needed.
- Assess respiratory function every hour for 24 hours, then q2-8 h as needed. Also assess level of consciousness and mucous membrane color. May need to monitor client via apnea monitor for 24 hours.
- Monitor urinary output and assess bladder for distention. Assist client to void.

analgesia, usually morphine or meperidine, at the beginning of therapy. Using a special intravenous (IV) pump system, the woman presses a button to self-administer small doses of the medication as needed. For safety, the pump is preset with a time lockout so that the woman cannot deliver another dose until a specified period of time has elapsed. The use of a PCA helps women feel a greater sense of control and less dependence on nursing staff. The frequent, smaller doses help the woman experience rapid pain relief without grogginess and a drugged feeling and also avoid the discomfort associated with injections.

If a general anesthetic was used, abdominal distention may produce marked discomfort for the woman during the first few postpartum days. Measures to prevent or minimize abdominal distention include leg exercises, abdominal tightening, ambulation, avoiding carbonated or very hot or cold beverages, avoiding the use of straws, and providing a high-protein, liquid diet for the first 24 to 48 hours, until bowel sounds return. Medical intervention for gas pain includes using rectal suppositories and enemas to stimulate passage of flatus and stool and encouraging the woman to lie on her left side. Lying on the left side allows the gas to rise from the descending colon to the sigmoid colon so that it can be expelled more readily.

Nurses can minimize discomfort and promote satisfaction as the mother assumes the activities of her new role. Assistance in assuming comfortable positions when holding or breastfeeding the infant will do much to increase the mother's sense of competence and comfort.

The cesarean birth mother usually does extremely well postoperatively. Most women are ambulating by the day after the surgery. Usually by the second postpartum day the incision can be covered with plastic wrap so the woman can shower, which seems to provide a mental as well as physical lift. Most women are discharged by the third day after birth.

Promotion of Parent-Infant Interaction after Cesarean Birth

Many factors associated with cesarean birth may hinder successful maternal-infant interaction. These factors include the physical condition of the mother and newborn and maternal reactions to stress, anesthesia, and medications. The mother and her infant may be separated after birth because of birthing unit routines, prematurity, or neonatal complications. A healthy infant born by uncomplicated cesarean is no more fragile than one born vaginally. However, some agencies automatically place cesarean birth infants in the high-risk nursery for a time. This practice may cause anxiety for the parents and interfere with early parent-infant interaction.

Signs of depression, anger, or withdrawal may indicate a grief response to the loss of the fantasized birth experience. Fathers as well as mothers may experience feelings of "missing out," guilt, or even jealousy toward another couple who had a vaginal birth. The cesarean birth couple may need the opportunity to tell their story repeatedly to work through these feelings. Thus, it is important to provide factual information about the situation and support the couple's effective coping behaviors.

By the second or third day the cesarean birth mother moves into the "taking-hold period" and is usually receptive to learning how to care for herself and her infant. Emphasize home management. Encourage the mother to let others assume responsibility for housekeeping and cooking. Fatigue not only prolongs recovery but also interferes with breastfeeding and mother-infant interaction.

The presence of the father or significant other during the birth process positively influences the woman's perception of the birth event. His or her presence reduces the woman's fears, enhances her sense of control, and enables the couple to share feelings and respond to one another with touch and eye contact. Later, they have the opportunity to relive the experience and fill in any gaps or missing pieces. The presence of the father or significant other is especially valuable if the mother has had general anesthesia. He or she can take pictures, hold the baby, and foster the discovery process by directing the mother's attention to the details of the newborn.

The reactions to a cesarean birth depend on how the woman defines that experience. Her reality is what she perceives it to be. If the woman's attitude is more positive than negative, successful resolution of subsequent stressful events is more likely. Often the mothering role is perceived as an extension of the childbearing role. Inability to fulfill expected childbearing behavior (vaginal birth) may lead to parental feelings of role failure and frustration. It is important to help families alter their negative definitions of cesarean birth and to encourage positive perceptions.

NURSING MANAGEMENT FOR THE POSTPARTUM ADOLESCENT

The adolescent mother has special postpartum needs, depending on her level of maturity, support system, and cultural background. The nurse needs to assess maternal-infant interaction, roles of support people, plans for discharge, knowledge of childrearing, and plans for follow-up care. It is important that a community health service contact the adolescent shortly after discharge.

Contraception counseling is an essential part of teaching. The incidence of repeat pregnancies during adolescence is high. The younger the adolescent, the more likely she is to become pregnant again. (See Chapter 10 on adolescent pregnancy.)

The nurse has many opportunities to teach the teen about her newborn in the postpartum unit. As a role model, the manner in which the nurse handles the newborn greatly influences the young mother. The father should be included in as much of the teaching as possible.

A newborn examination done at the bedside gives the teen information about her baby's health and shows her possible positions for holding a baby. The nurse can also use this time to provide information about newborn and infant behavior. Parents who have some idea of what to expect from their infant are less frustrated with the newborn's behavior.

The adolescent mother appreciates positive feedback about her newborn and her developing maternal responses. Praise and encouragement increase her confidence and self-esteem. Group classes for adolescent mothers should include information about infant care skills, taking the baby's temperature, clearing the nose and mouth, growth and development, infant feeding, well-baby care, and danger signals in the ill newborn.

Ideally, teenage mothers should visit adolescent clinics, for assessment of the mother and newborn, for several years after birth. In this way, the adolescent's enrollment in classes on parenting, need for vocational guidance, and school attendance can be supported and followed closely. School systems offering classes for young mothers are an excellent way of helping adolescents finish school and learn how to parent at the same time.

NURSING MANAGEMENT FOR THE WOMAN WHO IS RELINQUISHING HER BABY

Sometimes a woman is unable to parent her baby. The woman may be single, an adolescent, or economically restricted, or the pregnancy may be the result of incest or rape. She may feel that she is not emotionally ready for the responsibilities of parenthood. Her partner may strongly disapprove of the pregnancy. These and many other reasons may cause the woman to continue to reject her pregnancy. An emotional crisis arises as she attempts to resolve the problem. She may choose to have an abortion, to carry the fetus to term and parent the baby, or to have the baby and relinquish it for adoption.

A mother's decision to relinquish her infant is an extremely difficult one. There are social pressures against giving up one's child. Some women may want to prove to themselves that they can manage on their own by keeping their baby. The mother who chooses to let her child be adopted usually experiences intense ambivalence. These feelings may heighten just before birth and upon seeing her baby. After childbirth, the mother needs to complete a grieving process to work through her loss.

The mother who decides to relinquish the child has usually made considerable adjustments in her lifestyle to give birth to this child. She may not have told friends and relatives about the pregnancy and so she may lack an extended support system. During the prenatal period, the nurse can help the woman by encouraging her and providing opportunities to express her grief, loneliness, guilt, and other feelings.

When the relinquishing mother is admitted to the birthing unit, the nurse should be informed about the mother's decision to relinquish the baby. The nurse needs to respect any special requests for the birth and encourage the woman to express her emotions. After the birth the mother should have access to the baby; she will decide whether she wants to see the newborn. Seeing the newborn often aids the grieving process. When the mother sees her baby, she may feel strong attachment and love. The nurse needs to assure the woman that these feelings do not mean that her decision to relinquish the child is a wrong one; relinquishment is often a painful act of love (Arms, 1990). Postpartum nursing care also includes arranging ongoing care for the relinquishing mother.

If a woman decides to parent an unwanted child, the nurse should be aware of the potential for parenting problems. Families with unwanted children are more crisis prone than others, although in many cases, parents grow to love their child after attachment occurs. The nurse should be ready to initiate crisis strategies or make appropriate referrals as the need arises.

DISCHARGE INFORMATION

Ideally, preparation for discharge begins the moment a woman enters the birthing unit to give birth. Nursing efforts should be directed toward assessing the parents' knowledge, expectations, and beliefs and then providing anticipatory guidance and teaching accordingly. Since teaching is one of the primary responsibilities of the postpartum nurse, many agencies have elaborate teaching programs and videos. Before the actual discharge, spend time with the parents to determine if they have any last-minute questions. In general, discharge teaching includes at least the following information:

- The signs of possible complications (Table 22–5) and encouragement for the woman to contact her caregiver if she develops any of them.

- Review of literature the woman has received explaining recommended postpartum exercises, the need for adequate rest, the need to avoid overexertion initially, and the recommendation to abstain from sexual intercourse until lochia has ceased. The woman may take either a tub bath or shower and may continue sitz baths at home. If the family desires information about birth control methods, the nurse can provide such information at this time.

- The phone number of the mother-baby unit and encouragement to call if she has any questions or concerns.

- Information on local agencies and/or support groups, such as La Leche League and Mothers of Twins, that might be of particular assistance to the new mother.

- Information geared to the specific nutritional needs of breastfeeding or bottle-feeding mothers. If the mother has been receiving vitamins and/or iron supplements, the nurse encourages her to continue until the first postpartum examination.

- When to schedule the first appointment for her postpartum examination and for her newborn's first well-baby examination.

- The procedure for obtaining copies of her infant's birth certificate.

TABLE 22–5 Signs of Postpartum Complications
After discharge, a woman should contact her physician or certified nurse-midwife if any of the following develop:
• Sudden, persistent or spiking fever
• Change in the character of the lochia—foul smell, return to bright-red bleeding, excessive amount, passage of large clots
• Evidence of mastitis, such as breast tenderness, reddened areas, malaise
• Evidence of thrombophlebitis, such as calf pain, tenderness, redness
• Evidence of urinary tract infection, such as urgency, frequency, burning on urination
• Continued severe or incapacitating postpartum depression

- How to provide basic care for the infant; when to anticipate that the cord will fall off; when the infant can have a tub bath; when the infant will need his or her first immunizations; and so on. Parents should also be comfortable feeding and handling the baby, and should be aware of basic safety considerations, including the need to use a car seat whenever the infant is in a car.

- The signs and symptoms that indicate possible problems in the infant and who the parents should contact about them.

- Plans for home care visits so that the parents know when to expect the visit and what it entails (see Chapter 30).

Use this final opportunity to reassure the couple of their ability to be successful parents. Stress the infant's need to feel loved and secure and urge parents to talk to each other and work together to solve any problems that arise.

The ideal teaching situation is a family approach involving the mother, the father, the infant, and possibly other siblings. This approach permits a total evaluation and provides opportunities for all family members to ask questions and express concerns. It also promotes diagnosis and treatment of disturbed family patterns to prevent future problems of neglect or abuse. A sample postpartal teaching checklist is found on the web site. WEB

Evaluation

Anticipated outcomes of nursing care of the postpartum family include the following:

- The mother is reasonably comfortable and has learned pain relief measures.

- The mother is rested and understands how to add activity over the next few days and weeks.

- The mother's physiologic and psychologic well-being have been supported.

- The mother verbalizes her understanding of self-care measures.

- The new parents demonstrate how to care for their baby.

- The new parents have had opportunities to form attachment with their baby.

- The cesarean birth mother has been supported and has received safe care.

CHAPTER HIGHLIGHTS

🐚 Postpartum discomfort may be due to a variety of factors, including engorged breasts, an edematous perineum, an episiotomy or extension, engorged hemorrhoids, or hematoma formation. Various self-care approaches are helpful in promoting comfort.

🐚 Lactation suppression may be accomplished by mechanical techniques.

🐚 The new mother requires opportunities to discuss her childbirth experience with an empathetic listener.

🐚 In the first day or two after birth, maternal behaviors are dependent and comfort oriented. Then the woman becomes more independent and ready to assume responsibility.

🐚 Mother-baby care provides the childbearing family with opportunities to interact with their new member during the first hours and days of life. It enables the family to develop some confidence and skill in a safe environment.

🐚 Sexual intercourse may resume once the episiotomy has healed and lochia has ceased.

🐚 After a cesarean birth, the woman has the nursing care needs of an abdominal surgical client in addition to her needs as a postpartum client. She may also require assistance in working through her feelings if the cesarean birth was unexpected.

🐚 Postpartally the nurse evaluates the adolescent mother in terms of her level of maturity, available support systems, cultural background, and existing knowledge, then plans care accordingly.

🐚 The mother who decides to relinquish her baby needs emotional support. She should be able to decide whether to see and hold her baby, and any special requests regarding the birth should be honored.

🐚 Prior to discharge the couple should be given any information necessary for the woman to provide appropriate self-care. Parents should have a basic skill in caring for their newborn and should be familiar with warning signs of possible complications for mother or baby. Printed information is valuable in helping couples deal with questions that may arise at home.

🐚 Because of the trend toward early discharge, follow-up care is more important than ever. Many approaches are used, especially home visits and telephone follow-up.

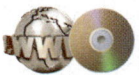 **EXPLORE**MediaLink

NCLEX Review, Case Studies, and other interactive resources for this chapter can be found on the companion website at http://www.prenhall.com/london. Click on "Chapter 22" to select the activities for this chapter.

For animations, more NCLEX review questions, and an audio glossary, access the accompanying CD-ROM in this textbook.

REFERENCES

Arms, S. (1990). *Adoption: A handbook of hope*. Berkeley, CA: Celestial Arts.

Banks-Wallace, J. (1999). Storytelling as a tool for providing holistic care to women. *American Journal of Maternal-Child Nursing, 24,* 20–24.

Barrett, G., Pendry, E., Peacock, J., Victor, C., Thakar, R., & Manyonda, I. (2000). Women's sexual health after childbirth. *British Journal of Obstetrics and Gynecology, 107*(20), 186–195.

Cunningham, F. G., Gant, N. F., Leveno, K. J., Gilstrap, L. C., III, Hauth, J. C., & Wenstrom, K. D. (2001). *Williams obstetrics* (21st ed.). New York: McGraw-Hill.

Davis, R. E. (2001). The postpartum experience for Southeast Asian women in the United States. *American Journal of Maternal-Child Nursing, 26*(4), 208–213.

Karch, A. M. (2001). *Lippincott's nursing drug guide*. Philadelphia, PA: Lippincott.

Koniak-Griffin, D., Mathenge, C., Anderson, N. L., & Verzemnieks, I. (1999). An early intervention program for adolescent mothers: A nursing demonstration project. *Journal of Obstetric, Gynecologic, and Neonatal Nursing, 28,* 51–59.

Lamp, J. M., & Howard, P. A. (1999). Guiding parents' use of the Internet for newborn education. *American Journal of Maternal-Child Nursing, 24,* 33–36.

Parks, P. L., Lenz, E. R., Milligan, R. A., & Han, H. R. (1999). What happens when fatigue lingers for 18 months after delivery? *Journal of Obstetric, Gynecologic, and Neonatal Nursing, 28,* 87–93.

PDR nurse's handbook. (2001). Montvale, NJ: Demar Publishers.

Sampselle, C. M., Seng, J., Yeo, S., Killian, C., & Oakley, D. (1999). Physical activity and postpartum wellbeing. *Journal of Obstetric, Gynecologic, and Neonatal Nursing, 28,* 41–49.

Schneiderman, J. U. (1996). Postpartum nursing for Korean mothers. *American Journal of Maternal-Child Nursing, 21*(3), 155–158.

Spector, R. E. (2000). *Cultural diversity in health & illness* (5th ed.). Upper Saddle River, NJ: Prentice Hall Health.

Varney, H. (1997). *Varney's midwifery* (3rd ed.). Sudbury, MA: Jones and Bartlett.

CHAPTER 23

The Postpartal Family at Risk

We are surviving. Maybe just. I was told that babies ate at six-ten-two-six-ten-two, but no one said that he would eat at five-seven-nine-eleven or so it seems. I am either getting ready to feed him or just finished feeding and changing him. But I love him without bounds. I feel a need to protect him from ever being hurt or wounded. During that first week, when I was tired and recovering from the emergency cesarean, I was afraid that I would not be able to shelter and help this young son grow up.

—KATE, 34

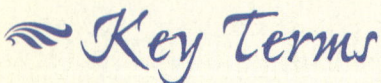

Key Terms

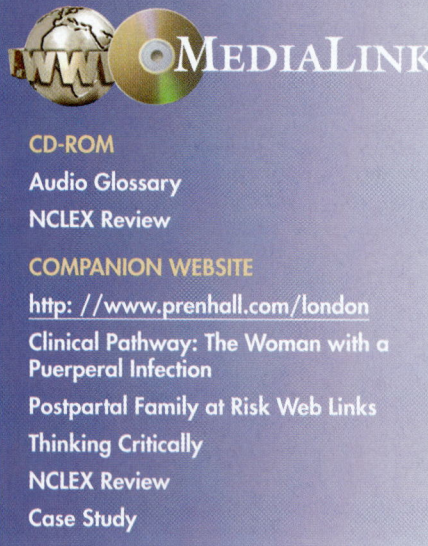

MediaLink

CD-ROM
Audio Glossary
NCLEX Review

COMPANION WEBSITE
http://www.prenhall.com/london
Clinical Pathway: The Woman with a Puerperal Infection
Postpartal Family at Risk Web Links
Thinking Critically
NCLEX Review
Case Study

The postpartal period is typically viewed as a smooth, uneventful transition time—and it usually is. However, the nurse must be aware of problems that may develop postpartally and their implications for the childbearing family.

NURSING MANAGEMENT OF THE POSTPARTAL FAMILY AT RISK

Hospital-Based Care

Ongoing comprehensive nursing assessment of postpartal clients is an important aspect of care. Systematic data collection allows the nurse to note the normality of findings and identify early signs of complications that might necessitate a longer hospital stay. Data collected before hospital discharge provide baseline findings against which subsequent data, collected by telephone or home visits, can be evaluated.

Signs and symptoms of many postpartal complications (late hemorrhage, mastitis, thromboembolic disease, major depression) typically occur only after the woman has returned home; they may appear even though she met criteria for early discharge. Consequently, it is critical that predischarge teaching for the woman and her partner (or her support person) include signs of postpartal complications; findings to report to her physician or certified nurse-midwife; and preventive measures, if available. Written instructions to supplement any discussion are of great value in the early weeks at home with a newborn, when life can be chaotic and instructions may be forgotten. Be sure the family has telephone numbers for postpartum follow-up services and other resources to answer questions. Communicating an attitude of willingness to answer questions and listen to concerns makes the parents more comfortable calling later for what they might otherwise perceive as issues too trivial to bother someone about.

Nursing Care in the Community

Telephone or home visit follow-up may recognize complications and, therefore, treat them more quickly than might otherwise be possible. (See Chapter 30 for a more detailed discussion of home care for the postpartum family.)

CARE OF THE WOMAN WITH POSTPARTAL HEMORRHAGE

Hemorrhage in the postpartal period is described as either early (immediate) or late (delayed) postpartal hemorrhage. **Early postpartal hemorrhage** occurs in the first 24 hours after childbirth. **Late postpartal hemorrhage** occurs from 24 hours to 6 weeks after birth. The traditional definition of postpartal hemorrhage has been a loss of more than 500 mL of blood following childbirth. That definition is currently being questioned, however, because careful quantification indicates that the average blood loss in a vaginal birth is actually greater than 500 mL, and the average blood loss after cesarean childbirth exceeds 1000 mL (Cunningham, Gant, Leveno, et al., 2001). Some clinicians think postpartal hemorrhage can be objectively and reliably defined as either a decrease in the hematocrit of 10 points between the time of admission and the time postbirth or the need for fluid replacement following childbirth (American College of Obstetricians and Gynecologists [ACOG], 1998). Clinical estimation of blood loss at childbirth is difficult because blood mixes with amniotic fluid and is obscured as it oozes onto sterile drapes or is sponged away; without vigilance, it may be difficult over the next hours to appreciate the significance of slow, steady blood loss.

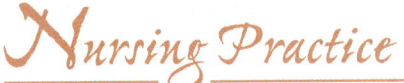

Women who are natural redheads tend to experience heavier bleeding after childbirth.

Early Postpartal Hemorrhage

The normal mechanism for hemostasis after delivery of the placenta is contraction of the interlacing uterine muscles to occlude the open sinuses that previously brought blood into the placenta. Uterine atony, the absence of prompt and sustained uterine contractions, can result in significant blood loss. Other causes of postpartal hemorrhage include laceration of the genital tract; episiotomy; retained placental fragments; vulvar, vaginal, or subperitoneal hematomas; uterine inversion; and coagulation disorders.

Uterine Atony

Uterine atony (relaxation of the uterus) is a common cause of early postpartal hemorrhage (Cunningham et al., 2001). Although uterine atony can occur after any childbirth, its contributing factors include the following:

- Overdistention of the uterus due to multiple gestation, hydramnios, or a large infant (macrosomia)
- Rapid or prolonged labor, which indicates that the uterus is contracting abnormally
- Oxytocin augmentation or induction of labor
- Grand multiparity, because stretched uterine musculature contracts less vigorously
- Use of anesthesia or other drugs, such as magnesium sulfate and terbutaline, that cause the uterus to relax
- Intra-amniotic infection
- Pregnancy-induced hypertension (PIH)
- Operative delivery

- Retained placental fragments
- Placenta previa
- Asian or Hispanic heritage

Hemorrhage from uterine atony may be slow and steady rather than sudden and massive. The blood may escape the vagina or collect in the uterus, evident as large clots. Because of the increased blood volume associated with pregnancy, changes in maternal blood pressure and pulse may not occur until blood loss has been significant. The woman with PIH is an exception because she does not have the normal hypervolemia of pregnancy and cannot tolerate even normal postchildbirth blood loss.

Ideally, postpartal hemorrhage is prevented, beginning with adequate prenatal care, good nutrition, avoidance of traumatic procedures, risk assessment, early recognition, and management of complications as they arise. Any woman at risk should be typed and crossmatched for blood and have intravenous lines in place with needles suitable for blood transfusion (18-gauge minimum).

After expulsion of the placenta, the fundus is palpated to ensure that it is firmly contracted. If it is not firm (if it is boggy), fundal massage is performed until the uterus contracts. Fundal massage is painful for the woman who has not received regional anesthesia; consequently, she will need explanation for why this uncomfortable procedure is necessary and support as massage is initiated. If bleeding is excessive, the clinician will likely order intravenous oxytocin at a rapid infusion rate and may elect to do a bimanual massage (Figure 23–1A ◆). Other uterine stimulants may be necessary to manage postpartal uterine atony. Table 23–1 summarizes critical nursing information about the use of uterine stimulants. The clinician uses hemoglobin and hematocrit results to determine the need for intravenous fluid replacement and blood transfusion. Vessel

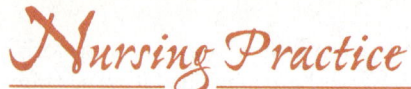

Nursing Practice

As you know, bogginess indicates that the uterus is not contracting well, which results in increased uterine bleeding. This blood may remain in the uterus and form clots or may result in increased flow. In assessing the amount of blood loss, you must first massage the uterus until it is firm and then express clots. Do not be misled by the firmness of a woman's uterus. Significant bleeding can have causes other than uterine atony. To accurately determine the amount of blood loss, it is not sufficient to assess only the perineal pad. You should also ask the woman to turn on her side so you can assess underneath her for pooling of blood.

ligation may be used to slow blood loss and allow normal clotting mechanisms to occur (ACOG, 1998; Bowes, 1999). Arterial embolization may be used when the bleeding is not immediately life threatening. In severe, uncontrolled hemorrhage, surgical management may be the only alternative.

Lacerations of the Reproductive Tract

Early postpartum hemorrhage is associated with lacerations of the perineum, vagina, or cervix. Several factors predispose women to higher risk of reproductive tract lacerations:

- Nulliparity
- Epidural anesthesia
- Precipitous childbirth
- Forceps- or vacuum-assisted birth
- Macrosomia

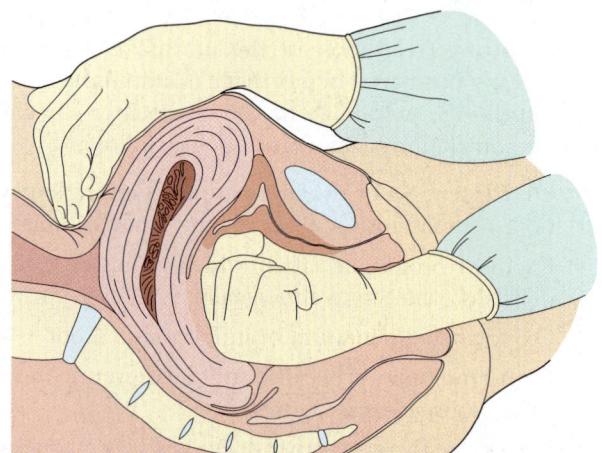

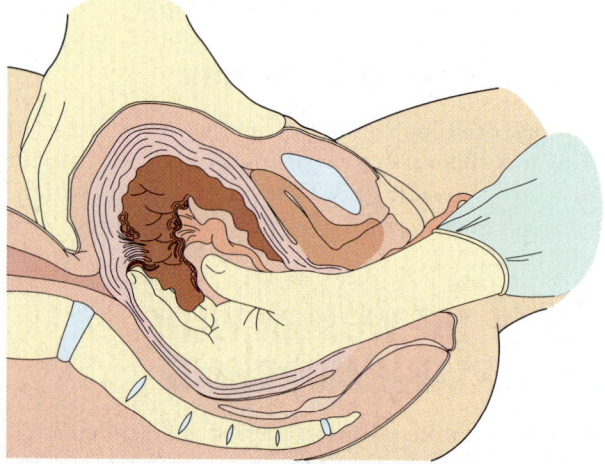

FIGURE 23–1. ◆ **A,** Manual compression of the uterus and massage with the abdominal hand usually will effectively control hemorrhage from uterine atony. **B,** Manual removal of placenta. The fingers are alternately abducted, adducted, and advanced until the placenta is completely detached. Both procedures are performed only by the medical clinician. *Note:* From Cunningham, F. G., MacDonald, P. C., & Gant, N. F. (Eds.). (1989). *Williams obstetrics* (18th ed., pp. 417–418). New York: McGraw-Hill, Inc. Adapted.

"stitches." If the hematoma is in the posterior vaginal area, rectal pressure may also be a presenting complaint. Hematomas in the upper vagina may cause difficulty voiding because of pressure against the urinary meatus or urethra. Rather than automatically attributing complaints of perineal pain to an episiotomy, examine the perineal area for signs of hematomas: ecchymosis; edema; tenseness of tissue overlying the hematomas; fluctuant, bulging mass at the introitus; and extreme tenderness to palpation. Estimate the size of the hematoma on first assessment of the perineum so that it is easier to identify increases in size and the potential blood loss. Notify the physician or certified nurse-midwife if a hematoma is suspected.

Nursing diagnoses that may apply to a woman experiencing postpartal hemorrhage include:

▶ *Health-seeking behaviors* related to lack of information about signs of delayed postpartal hemorrhage

▶ *Fluid volume deficit* related to blood loss secondary to uterine atony, lacerations, or retained placental fragments

Planning and Implementation

If the uterus is soft and boggy, massage it until firm. If the uterus is not contracting well and appears larger than anticipated, clots may be expressed during fundal massage. Once clots are removed, the uterus tends to contract more effectively.

If the woman seems to have a slow, steady, free flow of blood, begin to weigh the perineal pads (500 mL fluid weighs approximately 1 lb [454 g]) and monitor the woman's vital signs every 15 minutes, or more frequently if indicated. If the fundus is displaced upward or to one side because of a full bladder, encourage the woman to empty her bladder—or catheterize her if she is unable to void—to allow for efficient uterine contractions.

During the initial postpartum period, maintain the vascular access started during labor in case additional fluid or blood is necessary. When physicians and certified nurse-midwives write orders that specify "discontinue IV after present bottle," the astute postpartum nurse assesses the consistency of the fundus and the presence of normal versus excessive lochia before discontinuing the infusion. If the assessments are not reassuring, the nurse continues the intravenous (IV) infusion and notifies the physician or certified nurse-midwife.

Assess the woman for signs of anemia, such as fatigue, pallor, headache, thirst, and orthostatic changes in pulse or blood pressure and review the results of all hematocrit determinations. Monitor all medical interventions, intravenous infusions, blood transfusions, oxygen therapy, and medications such as uterine stimulants as necessary and evaluate them for effectiveness. Also monitor urinary output to determine adequacy of fluid replacement and renal perfusion and report amounts less than 30 mL/h to the physician. Help the woman plan activities so that she can rest adequately.

The woman experiencing anemia and fatigue related to hemorrhage may need assistance with self-care and progressive ambulation for several days. When she is able to be out of bed to shower, a shower chair permits independence while providing a measure of safety in case the woman feels weak or dizzy. The emergency call light should be easily accessible.

The mother may find it difficult to care for her baby because of the fatigue associated with blood loss. It is often possible to find ways to promote maternal-infant attachment while accommodating the health needs of the mother. The mother may need extra help caring for her infant. Work with the woman's partner and family to find ways to help the mother cope. Decrease the risk of vulvar or vaginal hematoma by applying an ice pack to the woman's perineum during the first hour after birth and intermittently thereafter for the next 8 to 12 hours. If a hematoma develops despite preventive measures, a sitz bath after the first 12 hours aids fluid absorption once the bleeding has stopped and promotes comfort, as does the judicious use of analgesics.

The woman and her family or other support persons should receive clear, preferably written, explanations of the normal postpartum course, including changes in the lochia and fundus and signs of abnormal bleeding. Instructions for preventing bleeding should include fundal massage, ways to assess the fundal height and consistency, and inspection of any episiotomy and lacerations, if possible. Advise the woman and her family to contact her caregiver if any signs of postpartal hemorrhage occur (Table 23–2). If iron supplementation is ordered, provide instructions for proper dosage to enhance absorption and avoid constipation and nausea.

NURSING CARE IN THE COMMUNITY

The woman may continue to need help with self-care for a time. Advise her to rise slowly to minimize the likelihood of orthostatic hypotension. Until she regains strength, she should be seated when holding the newborn.

The support person who assumes responsibility for grocery shopping and meal preparation needs advice about the importance of including foods high in iron in the daily menus. Having the woman indicate her preferences from a

TABLE 23-2 Signs of Postpartal Hemorrhage
Excessive or bright-red bleeding
A boggy fundus that does not respond to massage
Abnormal clots
Any unusual pelvic discomfort or backache
Persistent bleeding in the presence of a firmly contracted uterus
Rise in the level of the fundus of the uterus
Increased pulse or decreased BP
Hematoma formation or bulging/shiny skin in the perineal area
Decreased level of consciousness

list of such foods will promote cooperation with the diet. Explain the rationale for continuing medications containing iron.

The woman should continue to count perineal pads for several days so that she can recognize any recurring problems with excessive blood loss. The debilitated condition and anemia associated with hemorrhage increase the woman's risk of puerperal infection. She and her caregivers should use good handwashing and minimize exposure to infection in the home. Give the woman's caregiver a list of the signs of infection and ensure that he or she understands the importance of alerting the physician immediately if signs occur.

A sense of emergency often accompanies late postpartal hemorrhage. Because it commonly occurs 1 to 2 weeks after birth, the couple is generally at home, involved in the day-to-day activities demanded by their new roles, when the unexpected, excessive bleeding begins. Quick decisions about child care arrangements must often be made so that the mother can return to the hospital. Both mother and father are likely to be alarmed by the excessive bleeding and concerned about her prognosis. There may be additional worries about separation from the newborn, especially when the mother is breastfeeding. The father may find himself torn between the needs of the mother and those of the newborn. Ideally, arrangements can be made to minimize separation of the family members.

Evaluation

Expected outcomes of nursing care include the following:

▶ Signs of postpartal hemorrhage are detected quickly and managed effectively.

▶ Maternal-infant attachment is maintained successfully.

▶ The woman can identify abnormal changes that might occur following discharge and understands the importance of notifying her caregiver if they develop.

CARE OF THE WOMAN WITH A REPRODUCTIVE TRACT INFECTION OR WOUND INFECTION

Puerperal infection affects the reproductive tract; it is associated with childbirth and occurs any time up to 6 weeks postpartum. The most common infection is metritis (endometritis), which is limited to the uterus. However, infection can spread by way of the lymphatic system to become a progressive disease resulting in parametrial cellulitis and peritonitis.

The standard definition of **puerperal morbidity,** established in the 1930s by the Joint Committee on Maternal Welfare, is a temperature of 38 °C (100.4 °F) or higher, with the temperature occurring on any 2 of the first 10 postpartum days, exclusive of the first 24 hours, and when taken by mouth by standard technique at least four times a day. However, serious infections can occur in the first 24 hours or may cause only persistent low-grade temperatures. Therefore, careful assessment of all postpartum women with elevated temperatures is essential. Antibiotic therapy is only one cause of the decrease in postpartal morbidity and mortality seen today. Aseptic technique, fewer traumatic operative births, a better understanding of labor dystocia, improved surgical intervention, and a population generally at less risk from malnutrition and chronic debilitative disease have also contributed to this reduction.

The vagina and cervix of approximately 70% of all healthy pregnant women contain pathogenic bacteria that, alone or in combination, are sufficiently virulent to cause excessive infection. However, other factors must be present for infection to occur. Uterine infections are relatively uncommon following uncomplicated vaginal births, but they continue to be a major source of morbidity for women who give birth by cesarean. See "Nursing Care Plan for the Woman with a Puerperal Infection."

Postpartal Uterine Infection

Postpartal uterine infection is known variously as metritis, endometritis, endomyometritis, and endoparametritis. Risk factors for postpartal uterine infection include the following:

- Cesarean birth, which is the single most significant risk

- Prolonged rupture of the amniotic membranes

- Multiple vaginal examinations during labor

- Compromised health status (due to low socioeconomic status, anemia, obesity, cigarette smoking, use of illicit drugs or alcohol)

- Use of fetal scalp electrode or intrauterine pressure catheter for internal monitoring during labor

- Obstetric trauma (including episiotomy and lacerations of perineum, vagina, or cervix)

- Chorioamnionitis

- Preexisting bacterial vaginosis or *Chlamydia trachomatis* infection

- Instrument-assisted childbirth (vacuum or forceps)

- Manual removal of the placenta

- Lapses in aseptic technique by surgical staff

Endometritis (Metritis)

Endometritis or **metritis,** an inflammation of the endometrium, occurs postpartally in 2% to 5% of women delivered vaginally and 15% to 20% of those delivered by cesarean (Quilligan & Zuspan, 2000). After expulsion of the placenta, the placental site provides an excellent culture medium for bacterial growth. The rest of the decidua is

GOAL	INTERVENTION	RATIONALE	EXPECTED OUTCOME
1. Risk for spread of infection related to traumatized tissues			
	NIC Intervention:		*NOC Outcome:*
	Infection control: *Minimizing the acquisition and transmission of infectious agents*		**Risk control:** *Actions to eliminate or reduce actual, personal, and modifiable health threats*
The patient will be free of complications associated with infection.	▶ Encourage patient, staff, and family members to adhere to a strict handwashing policy	▶ Handwashing kills bacteria and prevents cross-contamination.	The patient will be free of complications associated with infection as evidenced by practicing behaviors that prevent the spread of infection and promote timely wound healing.
	▶ Review the patient's prenatal, intrapartal, and postpartal records for underlying problems that could contribute to poor wound healing or increase risk for spread of infection.	▶ Identifying underlying problems gives the caregiver an opportunity to initiate preventive measures that will promote healthy wound healing and stop the spread of infection.	
	▶ Monitor blood pressure, pulse, respiration, and temperature.	▶ Obtain baseline data; signs and symptoms of septic shock produce a ↓ in blood pressure and an ↑ in respirations.	
	▶ Instruct patient on proper perineal care including: wiping perineum front to back after voiding, perineal washes after voiding and defecating, and changing peri-pads frequently.	▶ Proper perineal care techniques enhance good hygiene and assist in removing urine and fecal contaminants from perineum. Changing peri-pads frequently decreases skin contact with a moist medium that favors bacteria growth.	
	▶ Encourage patient to consume 2000 mL of fluid a day.	▶ Maintains hydration and increases circulating volume.	
	▶ Encourage use of the sitz bath, surgigator, or the perineal light two to four times a day for at least 10–15 minutes.	▶ Moist or dry heat to the perineum increases blood flow and promotes healing.	
	▶ Encourage early ambulation.	▶ Enhances circulation and drainage of lochia.	
	▶ Assess and report signs and symptoms of infection in perineum including: erythema, edema, discharge, pain, and approximation of wound edges (REEDA).	▶ Identifying signs and symptoms of infection early allows for prompt treatment and healing.	
	Collaborative: Obtain lab work as ordered by physician including: culture and sensitivity, CBC with differential, and WBC count.	▶ Identifies abnormal lab values for early intervention. In addition, identifies infection and its causative organism for appropriate antibiotic treatment.	
	▶ Administer antibiotic therapy as ordered by the physician.	▶ Fights present infection and helps prevent the spread of further infection.	
	▶ Promote wound drainage by assisting physician in opening wound if necessary. Also, if wound is greater than 2–3 cm, pack with iodoform gauze.	▶ Iodoform gauze is used to maintain patency of wound opening. This promotes drainage and prevents abscesses from developing.	
	▶ Report signs and symptoms of severe infections: foul-smelling lochia, uterine subinvolution, uterine tenderness, severe lower abdominal pain, elevated temperature, elevated WBC count, general malaise, chills, lethargy, tachycardia, nausea and vomiting, and abdominal rigidity.	▶ Reporting signs and symptoms of severe infections early allows for initiation of appropriate therapy by physician and prevents further spread of the invading pathogen.	

(continued)

GOAL	INTERVENTION	RATIONALE	EXPECTED OUTCOME
2. Pain related to the infection process			
	NIC Intervention:		*NOC Outcome:*
	Pain management: *Alleviation of pain or a reduction in pain to a level of comfort that is acceptable to the patient*		**Pain level:** *Amount of reported or demonstrated pain.*
The patient will be free of pain.	▶ Assess pain location and intensity, have patient describe on a scale from 1 (mild) –10 (severe). Assess nonverbal signs of pain, including facial grimacing and agitation.	▶ Assesses the need for pain management and evaluates interventions already implemented.	Patient is free of pain as evidenced by verbalization of pain relief and the exhibition of a relaxed demeanor.
	▶ Encourage patient to discuss anxiety and fears.	▶ Reduces anxiety/fear and may decrease the patient's perception of pain.	
	▶ Encourage frequent rest periods and decrease disturbing environmental stimuli.	▶ Frequent rest periods will conserve client's energy. Increasing environmental stimuli may increase client's pain perception.	
	▶ Promote relaxation by encouraging diversional activities and the use of exercises including: radio/television, reading, guided imagery, deep breathing techniques, massage, visualization, and meditation.	▶ Promotes relaxation and refocuses patient's attention away from the intensity of pain.	
	Collaborative: Administer analgesics as ordered by the physician.	▶ Relieves pain and reduces anxiety.	
3. Risk for altered parent/infant attachment related to pain secondary to maternal infection			
	NIC Intervention:		*NOC Outcome:*
	Attachment promotion: *Facilitation of the development of the parent-infant relationship*		**Parent-infant attachment:** *Behaviors that demonstrate an enduring affectionate bond between a parent and infant*
Mother will have no problems bonding with infant and assuming responsibility for the care of the infant.	▶ Provide quality time for mother and infant contact.	▶ Aids in the bonding process.	Mother will bond with infant as evidenced by exhibiting appropriate attachment behaviors when interacting with infant, providing care to self and infant, and verbalization of understanding of the parenting role.
	▶ Encourage partner or family members to give patient videos and pictures of the infant if the mother's condition requires separation from the infant.	▶ Promotes bonding and gives the mother reassurance that the infant is being cared for.	
	▶ Encourage partner and family members to become involved with the care of the infant and verbalize interaction to the mother.	▶ Allows mother to feel as though she is involved in the care of the infant.	
	▶ Encourage mother to feed (breast or bottle) infant if her condition is stable. If mother is unable to breastfeed, encourage and assist her in pumping her breasts to maintain milk production.	▶ Hands-on participation in the infant's care gives mother a positive outlook.	
	▶ Assess maternal support systems.	▶ As mother is recovering, she will need assistance in household organization and personal care.	
	Collaborative: Offer referrals to home health services, doula services, and/or support groups.	▶ Assures patient's well-being, and identifies problems that may require intervention.	

also susceptible to pathogenic bacteria because of its thinness (approximately 2 mm) and its large blood supply. The cervix may also be a bacterial breeding ground because of the multiple small lacerations attending normal labor and spontaneous birth. Both aerobic and anaerobic organisms cause postpartal uterine infections. Late-onset postpartal endometritis or metritis is most commonly associated with genital mycoplasmas, *Gardnerella vaginalis,* and *Chlamydia trachomatis. C. trachomatis* has a longer replication time and latency period than other bacteria and is not consistently eradicated by antibiotics used for early postpartal infections.

In mild cases of endometritis the woman generally has discharge that is either scant or profuse, bloody, and foul smelling. In more severe cases, she also has uterine tenderness; sawtooth temperature spikes, usually between 38.3 and 40 °C (101 and 104 °F); tachycardia; and chills. Foul-smelling lochia is cited as a classic sign of endometritis, but in the case of infection with β-hemolytic streptococcus, the lochia may be scant and odorless (Cunningham et al., 2001).

Pelvic Cellulitis (Parametritis) and Peritonitis

Pelvic cellulitis (parametritis) is infection involving the connective tissue of the broad ligament or, in more severe forms, the connective tissue of all the pelvic structures. The infection generally ascends upward in the pelvis by way of the lymphatics in the uterine wall but this may also occur if pathogenic organisms invade a cervical laceration that extends upward into the connective tissue of the broad ligament—a direct pathway into the pelvis.

A pelvic abscess may form in postpartal **peritonitis** (infection involving the peritoneal cavity) and is most commonly found in the uterine ligaments, the cul-de-sac of Douglas, and the subdiaphragmatic space. Pelvic cellulitis may be a secondary result of pelvic vein thrombophlebitis. This condition occurs when the clot, usually in the right ovarian vein, becomes infected and the wall of the vein breaks down from necrosis, spilling the infection into the connective tissues of the pelvis.

A woman with parametritis may have a variety of symptoms, including marked high temperature (38.9 to 40 °C [102 to 104 °F]) chills, malaise, lethargy, abdominal pain, subinvolution of the uterus, tachycardia, and local and referred rebound tenderness. If peritonitis develops, the woman becomes acutely ill, with severe pain, marked anxiety, high fever, rapid and shallow respirations, pronounced tachycardia, excessive thirst, abdominal distention, nausea, and vomiting.

Perineal Wound Infections

Given the degree of bacterial contamination that occurs with normal vaginal birth, it is surprising that more women do not have infections of the episiotomy or repaired lacerations of the perineum, vagina, or vulva. When perineal wound infection occurs, it is recognized by the classic signs: redness, warmth, edema, purulent drainage, and, later, gaping of the previously well-approximated wound. Local pain may be severe. Infected perineal wounds, like other infected wounds, are treated by draining purulent material. Sutures are removed, and the wound is left open. A regimen of broad-spectrum antibiotics is used. When the surface of the wound is free of infectious exudate and tissue granulation is evident, the mother returns for secondary closure of the wound under regional anesthesia (Cunningham et al., 2001).

Cesarean Wound Infection

The infection rate following cesarean births is 4% to 12%, with the highest rate occurring after emergency cesarean because there is more traumatization of the tissue (Gibbs & Sweet, 1999). Signs of an abdominal wound infection, which may not be evident until after discharge, include erythema; warmth; skin discoloration; edema; tenderness; purulent drainage, sometimes mixed with sanguineous liquid; and gaping of the wound edges. Fever, pain, malodorous lochia, and other systemic signs are also common. Culture of the wound drainage commonly reveals mixed pathogens.

Clinical Therapy

The infection site and causative organism are diagnosed by careful history and complete physical examination, blood tests, aerobic and anaerobic endometrial cultures (which may be of limited value because multiple organisms are usually present), and urinalysis to rule out urinary tract infection. When a localized infection develops, it is treated with antibiotics, sitz baths, and analgesics as necessary. If an abscess has developed or a stitch site is infected, the suture is removed and the area is allowed to drain. Packing the wound with saline gauze twice to three times daily, using aseptic technique, allows removal of necrotic debris when packing is removed. Broad-spectrum antibiotic coverage treats postpartal wound infections (Gibbs & Sweet, 1999). Endometritis (metritis) is treated aggressively with intravenous antibiotics. With appropriate antibiotic coverage, improvement should occur within a few days. Antibiotics are generally continued until the woman is afebrile for 24 to 48 hours. The severity of the infection determines the route and dosage. Careful monitoring is also necessary to prevent the development of a more serious infection.

Parametritis and peritonitis are treated with intravenous antibiotics. Treatment begins with broad-spectrum antibiotics effective against the most commonly occurring causative organisms, until the results of culture and sensitivity reports are available. If multiple organisms are present, the approach to antibiotic therapy is continued unless no improvement is observed; then the antibiotic is changed.

An abscess is frequently manifested by the development of a palpable mass and may be confirmed with ultrasound.

It usually requires incision and drainage to prevent rupture into the peritoneal cavity and the possible development of peritonitis. After drainage, the cavity may be packed with iodoform gauze to promote drainage and facilitate healing.

The woman with a severe systemic infection is acutely ill and may require care in an intensive care unit. Supportive therapy includes maintenance of adequate hydration with intravenous fluids, analgesic medications, ongoing assessment of the infection, and possibly continuous nasogastric suctioning if paralytic ileus develops.

Nursing Management

Nursing Assessment and Diagnosis

Inspect the woman's perineum every 8 to 12 hours for signs of early infection. The REEDA scale is a reminder to consider redness, edema, ecchymosis, discharge, and approximation. Immediately report any degree of induration (hardening) to the clinician. Note and report fever, malaise, abdominal pain, foul-smelling lochia, tachycardia, and other signs of infection so that treatment can begin.

Nursing diagnoses that may apply to the woman with a puerperal infection include the following:

- ► *Risk for injury* related to the spread of infection
- ► *Pain* related to the presence of infection
- ► *Risk for altered parenting* related to delayed parent-infant attachment secondary to woman's malaise and other symptoms of infection

Planning and Implementation

HOSPITAL-BASED NURSING CARE

The nurse caring for a woman during the postpartal period is responsible for teaching the woman self-care measures that are helpful in preventing infection. The woman should understand the importance of perineal care, good hygiene practices to prevent contamination of the perineum (including wiping from front to back, changing perineal pads after voiding), and thorough handwashing. Once edema and perineal pain are under control, encourage sitz baths, which are cleansing and promote healing. Adequate fluid intake and a diet high in protein and vitamin C, which are necessary for wound healing, also help prevent infection.

If the woman is seriously ill, ongoing assessment of urine specific gravity and intake and output is necessary. Carefully administer antibiotics as ordered and regulate the intravenous fluid rate. Ongoing assessment of the woman's condition is vital to detect subtle changes in her health status. Keep the woman comfortable by providing hygiene, positioning, oral hygiene, and pain relief.

Promoting maternal-infant attachment can be difficult with the acutely ill woman. It may help to provide pictures of the infant and keep the mother informed of the infant's

well-being. See "Clinical Pathway: The Woman with a Puerperal Infection" on our website for specific nursing care measures.

NURSING CARE IN THE COMMUNITY

The woman with a puerperal infection needs assistance when she is discharged from the hospital. If the family cannot provide it, a referral to home care services is needed. Home care services should be contacted as soon as puerperal infection is diagnosed so that the nurse can meet with the woman for a family and home assessment and development of a home care plan. The family needs instruction in the care of a newborn, including feeding, bathing, cord care, immunizations, and significant observations that should be reported. A well-baby appointment should be scheduled. Breastfeeding mothers receiving antibiotics should be instructed to inspect the infant's mouth for signs of thrush and to report the finding to their physician.

Teach the mother about activity, rest, medications, diet, and signs and symptoms of complications, and schedule a return medical visit. She needs to know the importance of taking the entire course of prescribed antibiotics even though she may begin to feel better before the bottle is empty. She also needs to know the importance of pelvic rest; that is, she should not use tampons or douches or have intercourse until she has been examined by the physician and told it is safe to resume those activities.

Evaluation

Expected outcomes of nursing care include the following:

- ► The infection is quickly identified and treated successfully, without further complications.
- ► The woman understands the infection and the purpose of therapy; she cooperates with ongoing antibiotic therapy after discharge.
- ► Maternal-infant attachment is maintained.

CARE OF THE WOMAN WITH A URINARY TRACT INFECTION

The postpartal woman is at increased risk for urinary tract problems due to the normal postpartal diuresis, increased bladder capacity, decreased bladder sensitivity from stretching or trauma, and possible inhibited neural control of the bladder after general or regional anesthesia and contamination from catheterization.

Emptying the bladder is vital. Women who have not sufficiently recovered from the effects of anesthesia cannot void spontaneously, and catheterization is necessary. Retention of residual urine, bacteria introduced at the time of catheterization, and a bladder traumatized by birth combine to provide an excellent environment for the development of cystitis.

Overdistention of the Bladder

Overdistention occurs postpartally when the woman is unable to empty her bladder as a result of the predisposing factors previously identified. After the effects of regional anesthesia have worn off, postpartal urinary retention is highly indicative of urinary tract infection (UTI).

Clinical Therapy

Overdistention in the early postpartal period is often managed by draining the bladder with a straight catheter as a onetime measure. If the overdistention recurs or is diagnosed later in the postpartal period, an indwelling catheter is generally ordered for 24 hours.

Nursing Management

Nursing Assessment and Diagnosis

The overdistended bladder appears as a large mass, reaching sometimes to the umbilicus and displacing the uterine fundus upward. Increased vaginal bleeding occurs, the fundus is boggy, and the woman may complain of cramping as the uterus attempts to contract. Some women also experience backache and restlessness.

Nursing diagnoses that may apply when a woman has difficulties with overdistention of the bladder include the following:

▶ *Risk for infection* related to urinary stasis secondary to overdistention

▶ *Urinary retention* related to decreased bladder sensitivity and normal postpartal diuresis

Planning and Implementation

Diligent monitoring of the bladder during the recovery period and preventive health measures greatly reduce the chances for overdistention of the bladder. Encouraging the mother to void spontaneously and helping her use the toilet, if possible, or the bedpan, if she has received conductive anesthesia, prevents overdistention in most cases. Help the woman to a normal position for voiding (i.e., sitting with the legs and feet lower than the trunk) and provide privacy to encourage voiding. The woman should receive medication for whatever pain she may be having before she attempts to void because pain may cause a reflex spasm of the urethra. Applying perineal ice packs after childbirth helps minimize edema, which may interfere with voiding. Pouring warm water over the perineum or having the woman void in the sitz bath may also be effective.

If catheterization becomes necessary, use careful, meticulous aseptic technique. The vagina and vulva are traumatized to some degree by vaginal birth, and edema is common. Because this edema may obscure the urinary meatus, be extremely careful cleansing the vulva and inserting the catheter. It is imperative to discard a catheter that has inadvertently been introduced into the vagina and thus contaminated. Because postpartal trauma and edema make catheterization uncomfortable, be careful and gentle not only in inserting the catheter but also in handling and cleaning the perineal area.

Clamp the catheter after draining the desired amount of urine and tape it firmly to the woman's leg. Take the woman's vital signs before and after the procedure and note the woman's responses. Then carefully document the procedure and assessment findings. After an hour, the catheter may be unclamped and placed on gravity drainage. This technique protects the bladder and prevents rapid intra-abdominal decompression. When the indwelling catheter is removed, a urine specimen is often sent to the laboratory. The tip of the catheter may also be removed and sent for culture.

Evaluation

Expected outcomes of nursing care include the following:

▶ The woman voids adequately.

▶ The woman does not develop infection due to stasis of urine.

▶ The woman uses self-care measures to decrease bladder overdistention.

CYSTITIS (LOWER URINARY TRACT INFECTION)

Escherichia coli has been demonstrated to be the causative agent in most cases of postpartal cystitis and pyelonephritis (in both lower and upper UTI). Generally, the infection ascends the urinary tract from the urethra to the bladder and then to the kidneys because vesiculoureteral reflux (backward flow of urine) forces contaminated urine into the renal pelvis.

Clinical Therapy

When cystitis is suspected, a clean-catch midstream urine sample is obtained for microscopic examination, culture, and sensitivity tests. The specimen may require collection by the nurse with the woman on a bedpan because few postpartal women can collect a true midstream, clean-catch specimen without contaminating the specimen with lochia. A catheterized specimen is avoided when possible because of the increased risk of infection. When the bacterial concentration is greater than 100,000 colonies of the same organism per milliliter of fresh urine, infection is generally present. Counts between 10,000 and 100,000 suggest infection, particularly if clinical symptoms are noted.

In the clinical setting, antibiotic therapy is often begun before culture and sensitivity reports are available. Frequently used antibiotics include a preparation of trimethoprim and sulfamethoxazole (Bactrim, Septra), one of the short-acting sulfonamides, nitrofurantoin (Macrodantin), and, in the case of sulfa allergy, ampicillin. The antibiotic is changed later if indicated by the results of the sensitivity report. Antispasmodics or urinary analgesic agents, such as phenazopyridine hydrochloride (Pyridium), may be given to relieve discomfort.

Nursing Management

Nursing Assessment and Diagnosis

Symptoms of cystitis often appear 2 to 3 days after childbirth. The initial symptoms of cystitis may include frequency, urgency, dysuria, and nocturia. Hematuria and suprapubic pain may also be present. A slightly elevated temperature may occur, but systemic symptoms are often absent. When a UTI progresses to pyelonephritis, systemic symptoms usually occur, and the woman becomes acutely ill. Symptoms include chills, high fever, flank pain (unilateral or bilateral), nausea, and vomiting, in addition to all the signs of lower UTI. Costovertebral angle tenderness on palpation and pain may or may not be present. Get a urine culture so that sensitivity can identify the causative organism.

Nursing diagnoses that may apply if a woman develops a UTI postpartally include the following:

▶ *Pain* with voiding related to dysuria secondary to infection

▶ *Health-seeking behaviors* related to lack of information about self-care measures to prevent UTI

Planning and Implementation

Screening for asymptomatic bacteriuria in pregnancy should be routine. Encourage frequent emptying of the bladder during labor and postpartum to prevent overdistention and trauma to the bladder. Catheterization technique and nursing actions to prevent overdistention (previously discussed) also apply. Be sure the woman with pyelonephritis understands the importance of follow-up care after discharge to prevent recurrence or further complications.

Advise the postpartal woman to continue good perineal hygiene after discharge, to maintain a good fluid intake (at least 8 to 10 8-oz glasses daily), especially of water, and to empty her bladder whenever she feels the urge to void, but at least every 2 to 4 hours while awake. Once sexual intercourse is resumed, the new mother should void before (to prevent bladder trauma) and after intercourse (to wash contaminants from the vicinity of the urinary meatus). Wearing underwear with a cotton crotch to facilitate air circulation also reduces the risk of UTI. Acidification of the urine is thought to aid in preventing and managing UTI. Therefore, advise the woman to avoid carbonated beverages, which increase the alkalinity of urine, and to drink unsweetened cranberry, plum, apricot, and prune juices, which increase the acidity of urine.

Evaluation

Expected outcomes of nursing care include the following:

▶ Signs of UTI are detected quickly and the condition is treated successfully.

▶ The woman uses self-care measures to prevent the recurrence of UTI as part of her personal hygiene routine.

▶ The woman cooperates with any long-term therapy or follow-up.

▶ Maternal-infant attachment is maintained and the woman can care for her newborn effectively.

CARE OF THE WOMAN WITH MASTITIS

Mastitis is an infection of the breast connective tissue that occurs primarily in lactating women. The usual causative organisms are *Staphylococcus aureus, Haemophilus parainfluenzae, H. influenzae,* and *Streptococcus* species. Because symptoms seldom occur before the second to fourth week postpartum, birthing unit nurses often are not fully aware of how uncomfortable and acutely ill the woman can be; they must ensure that all breastfeeding women are taught preventive techniques and ways of recognizing this condition if it develops.

The infection usually begins when bacteria invade the breast tissue. Often the tissue has been traumatized in some way (fissured or cracked nipples, overdistention, manipulation, milk stasis) and is especially susceptible to pathogenic invasion. The most common sources of these organisms are the infant's nose and throat, but other sources include the hands of the mother or birthing unit personnel and the woman's circulating blood.

Poor drainage of milk, lowered maternal defenses due to fatigue or stress, and poor hygiene practices make the woman susceptible to mastitis (Lauwers & Shinskie, 2000). Tight clothing, missed feedings, poor support of pendulous breasts, lack of regular breast pumping when away from the baby, and a baby who suddenly begins to sleep through the night can result in milk stasis, which is a milder inflammatory condition.

Infectious mastitis is a more serious infection, with fever, headache, flulike symptoms, and a warm, reddened, painful area of the breast, often wedge shaped because of the connective tissue septal divisions of the breast (Figure 23–2 ◆).

In some cases *Candida albicans* is the causative organism of mastitis, entering the breast through a small fissure or abrasion on the nipple. Signs include late-onset nipple pain, followed by shooting pain during and between feedings. Eventually, the skin of the affected breast becomes pink, flaking, and pruritic.

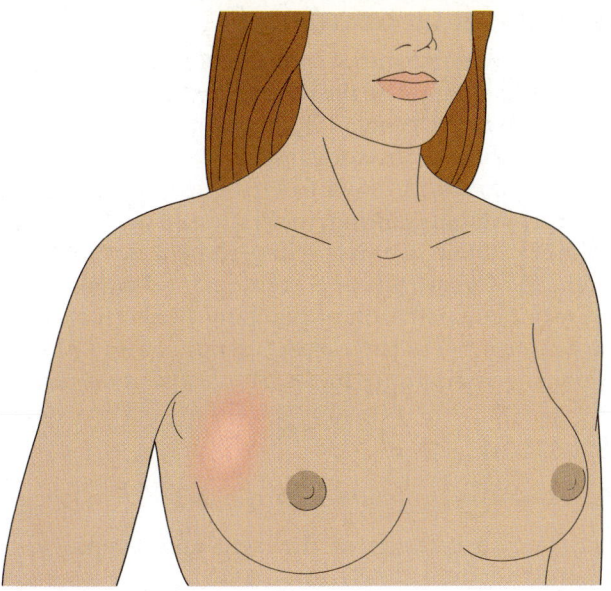

FIGURE 23–2. ◆ Mastitis. Erythema and swelling are present in the upper outer quadrant of the breast. Axillary lymph nodes are often enlarged and tender. The segmental anatomy of the breast accounts for the demarcated, often v-shaped wedge of inflammation.

Complementary Care

PROBIOTICS

Probiotics are a category of dietary supplements consisting of beneficial microorganisms (*pro* means "for," and *biotic* means "life" versus *antibiotics*, which literally means "against life"). Probiotics compete with disease-causing microorganisms in the gastrointestinal tract. When antibiotics are taken, they kill many of the beneficial bacteria that exist naturally in the digestive tract. Supplementing with probiotics after a course of antibiotics is frequently prescribed by nutritionists and complementary practitioners. Commonly used probiotics include *Lactobacillus acidophilus* and *Bifidobacterium bifidum;* there are other species of *Lactobacillus and Bifidobacterium* that have been shown to be effective in such conditions as diarrhea and vaginal infections (Elmer, 2001). *Bifidobacterium* also competes against *Candida albicans.* Probiotics can be taken in the form of powder, capsules, and suppositories, or in fermented milk products such as yogurt or *kefir.*

Clinical Therapy

Diagnosis is usually based on history and physical examination; a culture and sensitivity may be done. A culture and sensitivity assessment of breast milk allows susceptibility-directed antibiotic therapy; a leukocyte count of 1 million/mL and bacterial colony count of greater than 10,000/mL is diagnostic (Gibbs & Sweet, 1999). Treatment involves bed rest (may be needed for the first several days), use of a supportive bra, frequent breastfeeding, local application of warm, moist-heat compresses, and analgesics (such as acetaminophen) as needed. Nonsteroidal anti-inflammatory agents are recommended to treat both fever and inflammation. Also, a 10-day course of antibiotics (usually a penicillinase-resistant penicillin) is completed (Johnson & Riddick, 2000). Continued emptying of the breast by nursing or pumping improves the outcome, decreases the duration of symptoms, and decreases the incidence of breast abscess. Thus, continued breastfeeding is recommended in the presence of mastitis. The woman should be contacted within 24 hours of initiation of treatment to ensure that symptoms are subsiding (Lauwers & Shinskie, 2000). Early treatment may prevent the progression of milk stasis and noninfectious inflammation to mastitis; 10% of all mastitis cases result in abscess formation requiring aspiration (if small) or, more commonly but still rare, incision and drainage (Cunningham et al., 2001).

Nursing Management

Nursing Assessment and Diagnosis

Each day, assess breast consistency, skin color, surface temperature, nipple condition, and presence of pain to detect early signs of problems that may predispose a woman to mastitis. Watch the mother nursing her baby to ensure proper technique.

If an infection develops, assess for contributing factors such as cracked nipples, poor hygiene, engorgement, supplemental feedings, change in routine or infant feeding pattern, abrupt weaning, and lack of proper breast support so that these factors can be corrected as part of the treatment plan.

Nursing diagnoses that may apply to the woman with mastitis include the following:

▶ *Health-seeking behaviors* related to lack of information about appropriate breastfeeding practices

▶ *Ineffective breastfeeding* related to pain secondary to development of mastitis

Planning and Implementation

Preventing mastitis is far simpler than treating it. Ideally, mothers learn proper breastfeeding technique prenatally. The nurse helps the mother breastfeed soon after childbirth and reviews correct technique. Comanagement of breastfeeding between the nurse and a certified lactation specialist is often possible. Encourage new mothers, even those not breastfeeding, to wear a good supportive bra at all times to prevent milk stasis, especially in the lower lobes.

Meticulous handwashing by the breastfeeding mother and all personnel is the primary measure in preventing epidemic nursery infections and subsequent maternal mastitis. Prompt attention to mothers who have blocked milk ducts eliminates stagnant milk as a growth medium for bacteria. If the mother finds that one area of her breast feels distended, she can rotate the position of her infant for nursing, manually express milk remaining in the breast after nursing (usually necessary only if the infant is not sucking well), or massage the caked area toward the nipple as the infant nurses. Mothers who develop mastitis can apply warm, moist compresses to the affected area before and during breastfeeding. Encourage the mother to breastfeed frequently, starting with the unaffected breast until letdown occurs in the affected breast, then feeding from the affected breast until it is emptied completely (Lauwers & Shinskie, 2000). While feeding on the affected breast, the baby's chin is pointed toward the inflamed area. After nursing, the mother can leave a small amount of milk on each nipple to prevent cracking and allow nipples to air dry. Early identification of and intervention for sore nipples are also essential.

DISCHARGE PLANNING AND HOME CARE TEACHING

Stress to the breastfeeding woman the importance of adequate breast and nipple care to prevent the development of cracks and fissures, a common portal for bacterial entry. (For a detailed discussion of breastfeeding, see Chapter 27.)

The woman should be aware of the importance of regular, complete emptying of the breasts to prevent engorgement and stasis. She should also understand the role of letdown in successful breastfeeding, correct positioning of the infant on the nipple, proper latch-on, and the principle of supply and demand. If the mother is taking antibiotics, she needs to understand the importance of completing the full course of antibiotics, even if the infection seems to clear quickly. Breastfeeding mothers returning to work outside the home need information on how to do so successfully. Because mastitis tends to develop after discharge, it is important to include information about signs and symptoms in the discharge teaching and printed materials (Table 23–3). All flulike symptoms should be considered a sign of mastitis until proven otherwise. If symptoms develop, the woman should contact her caregiver immediately because prompt treatment helps to prevent abscess formation.

NURSING CARE IN THE COMMUNITY

The home care nurse who suspects mastitis on the basis of assessment findings refers the woman to the physician. The nurse may be asked to obtain a sample of breast milk to be cultured for the causative organism.

If the mother feels too ill to breastfeed or develops an abscess that prevents nursing, the home care nurse can help the mother obtain a breast pump to help her maintain lactation and can provide opportunities for demonstration and return demonstration of pumping. Referral to a lactation consultant or to La Leche League can be invaluable to the woman's physical and emotional adjustment to mastitis.

Evaluation

Expected outcomes of nursing care include the following:

▶ The woman is aware of the signs and symptoms of mastitis.

▶ The woman's mastitis is detected early and treated successfully.

▶ The woman can continue breastfeeding if she chooses.

▶ The woman understands self-care measures she can employ to prevent the recurrence of the mastitis.

CARE OF THE WOMAN WITH POSTPARTAL THROMBOEMBOLIC DISEASE

Thromboembolic disease may occur antepartally, but it is generally considered a postpartal complication. Venous thrombosis refers to thrombus formation in a superficial or deep vein, with the accompanying risk that a portion of the clot might break off and result in pulmonary embolism. When the thrombus is formed in response to inflammation in the vein wall, it is termed **thrombophlebitis.** In this type of thrombosis, the clot tends to be more firmly attached and therefore is less likely to result in embolism. In noninflammatory venous thrombosis (also called phle-

TABLE 23–3	Comparison of Findings of Engorgement, Plugged Duct, and Mastitis		
Characteristics	Engorgement	Plugged Duct	Mastitis
Onset	Gradual, immediately postpartum	Gradual, after feedings	Sudden, after 10 days
Site	Bilateral	Unilateral	Usually unilateral
Swelling and heat	Generalized	May shift, little or no heat	Localized, red, hot, and swollen
Pain	Generalized	Mild but localized	Intense but localized
Body temperature	<38.4 °C (101.1 °F)	<38.4 °C (101.1 °F)	>38.4 °C (101.1 °F)
Systemic symptoms	Feels well	Feels well	Flulike symptoms

Note: From Lawrence, R. A. (1994). *Breastfeeding: A guide for the medical profession* (p. 261). St. Louis, MO: Mosby.

bothrombosis) the clot, caused by venous stasis, tends to be more loosely attached and the risk of embolism is greater.

Factors contributing directly to the development of thromboembolic disease postpartally include (1) increased amounts of certain blood-clotting factors; (2) postpartal thrombocytosis (increased quantity of circulating platelets and their increased adhesiveness); (3) release of thromboplastin substances from the tissue of the decidua, placenta, and fetal membranes; and (4) increased amounts of fibrinolysis inhibitors. Predisposing factors include (1) obesity, increased maternal age, and high parity; (2) anesthesia and surgery, with possible vessel trauma and venous stasis due to prolonged inactivity; (3) previous history of venous thrombosis; (4) maternal anemia, hypothermia, or heart disease; (5) endometritis (metritis); and (6) varicosities. Thromboembolic disease is more likely to occur after cesarean birth than after vaginal birth (Laros, 1999).

Superficial Vein Leg Disease

Superficial thrombophlebitis is far more common postpartally than during pregnancy. Often the clot involves one of the saphenous veins. This disorder is more common in women with preexisting varices (enlarged veins), although it is not limited to these women. Symptoms—including tenderness in a portion of the vein, some local heat and redness, normal temperature or low-grade fever, and occasionally slight elevation of the pulse—usually become apparent about the third or fourth postpartal day. Treatment involves application of local heat, elevation of the affected limb, bed rest, analgesics, and the use of elastic support hose. Anticoagulants are usually not necessary unless complications develop. Pulmonary embolism is extremely rare. Occasionally the involved veins have incompetent valves, and, as a result, the problem may spread to the deeper leg veins, such as the femoral vein.

Deep Vein Thrombosis

Deep vein thrombosis (DVT) is more frequently seen in women with a history of thrombosis. Certain obstetric complications, such as hydramnios, PIH, and operative birth, are associated with an increased incidence. After a clinical diagnosis of DVT, a woman's risk in subsequent pregnancy is as high as 20% (Clarke-Pearson, 2000).

Clinical manifestations may include edema of the ankle and leg and an initial low-grade fever often followed by high temperature and chills. Depending on the vein involved, the woman may complain of pain in the popliteal and lateral tibial areas (popliteal vein), pain in the entire lower leg and foot (anterior and posterior tibial veins), inguinal tenderness (femoral vein), or pain in the lower abdomen (iliofemoral vein). The Homans' sign (refer to Figure 21–7) 🔗 may or may not be positive, but pain often results from calf pressure. Because of reflex arterial spasm, sometimes the limb is pale and cool to the touch—

the so-called *milk leg* or *phlegmasia alba dolens*—and peripheral pulses may be decreased.

Septic Pelvic Thrombophlebitis

Septic pelvic thrombophlebitis is a complication that develops in conjunction with infections of the reproductive tract and is more common in women who have had a cesarean birth. The diagnosis is suspected when infection is unresponsive to antibiotics. Abdominal pain, flank pain, or both, sometimes accompanied by guarding, occurs on the second or third day postpartum, along with fever and tachycardia. Bimanual examination may reveal a parametrial mass. On occasion, paralytic ileus develops. Treatment consists of anticoagulation and antibiotic therapy. Although most women show significant clinical improvement with antibiotics, a sawtooth fever spike and chills may persist (Laros, 1999).

Clinical Therapy

Because cases of thromboembolic disease are seldom clear-cut, diagnosis involves a variety of approaches, such as client history and physical examination, real-time ultrasonography with color, Doppler ultrasonography, and contrast venography (increased circumference of affected extremity). In questionable cases, venography provides the most accurate diagnosis of DVT; unfortunately, however, it is not practical for multiple examinations or prospective screening and may itself induce phlebitis (Cunningham et al., 2001).

Treatment involves intravenous heparin, using an infusion pump to permit continuous, accurate infusion of medication. Strict bed rest and elevation of the leg are required; analgesics are given as necessary. If fever is present, deep thrombophlebitis is suspected, and the woman is also given antibiotics. In most cases, thrombectomy (surgical removal of the clot) is not necessary.

Once the symptoms have subsided (usually in several days), the woman may begin ambulation while wearing elastic support stockings. Intravenous heparin is continued until prothrombin time reaches 1.5 to 1.7, and treatment with sodium warfarin (Coumadin) is begun. The woman continues taking Coumadin for 2 to 6 months at home. While taking warfarin, prothrombin times are assessed periodically to maintain correct dosage levels.

Thinking Critically

ASSESSING POSTPARTAL LEG PAIN

Lei Chang, G1P1, had a cesarean birth after a prolonged labor and failure to progress. As she is walking in the hallway with her husband, you notice that Lei is limping slightly, and you comment on that observation. Lei responds that she is having pain in her right lower leg. She says, "Maybe I pulled a muscle during labor." What would you do? 🔗 [WEB]

Nursing Management

Nursing Assessment and Diagnosis

Carefully assess the woman's history for factors predisposing her to development of thrombosis or thrombophlebitis. In addition, be alert to any complaints of pain in the legs, inguinal area, or lower abdomen because such pain may indicate DVT. Also assess the woman's legs for edema, temperature change, or pain with palpation.

Nursing diagnoses that may apply to a postpartal woman with a thrombolic disease include the following:

▶ *Altered tissue perfusion in periphery* related to obstructed venous return

▶ *Pain* related to tissue hypoxia and edema secondary to vascular obstruction

▶ *Risk for altered parenting* related to decreased maternal-infant interaction secondary to bed rest and intravenous lines

Planning and Implementation

Evaluate the need for support hose for women with varicosities during labor and the postpartum period. Adequate fluid intake is necessary during labor to prevent dehydration. Because trauma is often a factor in the development of thrombophlebitis, avoid keeping the woman's legs elevated in stirrups for prolonged periods. If stirrups are used, they should be comfortably padded and adjusted to provide correct support and prevent pressure on popliteal vessels. In addition, encourage early ambulation after birth; the knee gatch on the bed should be avoided. Encourage women confined to bed after a cesarean birth to perform regular leg exercises to promote venous return.

Once DVT is diagnosed, maintain the heparin therapy, provide appropriate comfort measures, and monitor the woman closely for signs of pulmonary embolism. Also assess for evidence of bleeding related to heparin and keep the antagonist for heparin, protamine sulfate, readily available.

Tell the woman to avoid prolonged standing or sitting because these positions contribute to venous stasis. Advise the woman to avoid crossing her legs because of the pressure it causes. Recommend that the woman take frequent breaks during car trips and while working if she sits most of the day. Walking is acceptable because it promotes venous return. Remind the woman to mention her history of thrombosis or thrombophlebitis to her physician during subsequent pregnancies so that preventive measures can be instituted early.

Women discharged while taking warfarin must understand the purpose of the medication and be alert for signs of bleeding such as bleeding gums, epistaxis, petechiae or ecchymosis, and evidence of blood in the urine or stool. Because careful monitoring is important, the woman should clearly understand the need to keep scheduled appointments for prothrombin time assessment. Certain medications such as aspirin and other nonsteroidal anti-inflammatory drugs increase anticoagulant activity and should be avoided; when she is taking warfarin the woman should check for possible medication interaction before taking any other medication. Encourage the woman to carry a MedicAlert card in case of emergency, inform all health care providers—including dentists—that she is taking anticoagulants, and have vitamin K available in case of bleeding (Shaver, 1999).

Warfarin is excreted in the breast milk but is not considered hazardous to the nursing infant (Nadeau, Alpert, Constantino, et al., 2000). (See "Clinical Pathway: The Woman with Thromboembolic Disease" for specific nursing care measures.)

NURSING CARE IN THE COMMUNITY

Because the mother with postpartal thromboembolic disease will depend on others for much of her initial home care, it is helpful for the father of the newborn to be involved in preparations for discharge. Allow ample time to answer questions and clarify instructions, verbally and in writing. Evaluate how well both the mother and father have understood instructions about the plan of care. It is especially important to assess the couple's plans to ensure complete bed rest for the mother. They might explore ways for her to maintain bed rest and still spend quality time with her newborn and any other children. For example, young children can sit on the bed for storytelling or play quiet games, and the newborn's crib can be placed next to the mother's bed. Many concerns will not surface until the couple actually returns home and fully comprehends the reality of their situation. For that reason, it is valuable to provide them with an accessible resource person and to plan telephone or home visit follow-up care.

Signs of postpartum thrombophlebitis may not occur until after discharge from the birthing unit. Therefore, teach all couples to recognize its signs and symptoms and appreciate the importance of reporting them immediately and of not massaging the affected leg. If signs and symptoms occur after discharge, a short readmission may be required. In that case every effort is made to allow mother, father, and newborn to remain together.

Evaluation

Expected outcomes of nursing care include the following:

▶ If thrombophlebitis develops, it is detected quickly and managed successfully, without further complications.

▶ At discharge the woman can explain the purpose, dosage regimen, and necessary precautions of any prescribed medications such as anticoagulants.

▶ The woman can discuss the self-care measures and ongoing therapies (such as the use of elastic stockings) indicated.

▶ The woman has bonded successfully with her newborn and is able to care for her baby effectively.

Category	Antepartal Management	Intrapartal Management	Postpartal Management
Referral	Perinatologist Internist Social worker Psychiatric clinical nurse practitioner Dietary/nutritionist Infectious disease consult	Obtain prenatal record	Home nursing referral if indicated **Expected Outcomes** Appropriate resources identified and utilized
Assessment	Obtain hx of present pregnancy Assess estimated gestational age Assess any sensitivity to medications Obtain complete physical examination to include • Fetal size, fetal status (FHR), and fetal maturity • Signs of fatigue, weakness, recurrent diarrhea, pallor, night sweats • Present weight and amount of weight gain or weight loss Obtain diagnostic studies: • Ultrasound • Fetal maturity studies (L/S ratio, PG, creatinine) • Hemoglobin, hematocrit, platelet count • WBC and differential • HIV • CD4+ T lymphocyte count • ESR		Monitor daily Hct Continue normal postpartum assessment q8h Feeding technique with newborn: should be good or improving TPR assessment: q8h; all WNL; report temperature > 38 °C (100.4 °F) Continue assessment of comfort level Assess for superficial thrombophlebitis: • Tenderness along involved vein • Areas of palpable thrombosis • Warmth and redness in the involved area Deep venous thrombosis (DVT): • Positive Homans' sign (pain occurs when foot is dorsiflexed while leg is extended) • Tenderness and pain in affected area • Fever (initially low, followed by high fever and chills) • Edema in affected extremity • Pallor and coolness in affected limb • Diminished peripheral pulses • Increased potential for pulmonary embolus Immediately report any signs of pulmonary embolism, including the following: • Sudden onset of severe chest pain, often located substernally • Apprehension and sense of impending catastrophe • Cough (may be accompanied by hemoptysis) • Tachycardia • Fever • Hypotension • Diaphoresis, pallor, weakness • Shortness of breath • Neck engorgement • Friction rub and evidence of atelectasis upon auscultation **Expected Outcomes** Findings indicate complications of thrombosis minimized, and condition stable or improved
Comfort			Continue with pain management techniques No aspirin or ibuprofen; acetaminophen may be ordered Provide supportive nursing comfort measures such as back rubs, provision of quiet time for sleep, diversional activities Maintain warm, moist soaks as ordered, with legs elevated

*All of the interventions for a normal labor and birth and postpartal client may be found in those appropriate clinical pathways.

(continued)

Category	Antepartal Management	Intrapartal Management	Postpartal Management
Teaching/ psychosocial	Room orientation Explain s/s of labor Increase client awareness of fetal monitoring Evaluation of client teaching	*Tour of NICU* Discuss with woman: • Mode of childbirth • Postpartum expectation	Implement normal postpartum teaching and psychosocial support (see Chapter 22) 🔗 Maintain mother-infant attachment; when mother is on bed rest provide frequent contacts for mother and infant; modified rooming-in is possible if the crib is placed close to the mother's bed and nurse checks often to help mother lift or move infant **Expected Outcomes** Woman demonstrates/verbalizes understanding of plan of care and teaching Infant-maternal bonding unimpaired
Nursing care management and reports	Assess emotional response so that support and teaching can be planned accordingly Weigh woman Obtain food history Establish rapport Provide opportunities to talk without interruption Monitor for signs of infection Maintain appropriate isolation precautions	Ongoing monitoring of blood pressure Electronic fetal monitoring in place Try to have same nurses caring for woman during her hospitalization Monitor for signs of infections **Expected Outcomes** Maternal/fetal circulation optimized	Continue sitz baths prn May shower if ambulating without difficulty DC buffalo cap (heparin lock) if present Monitor for signs of infection For DVT obtain prothrombin time (PT) and review prior to beginning warfarin; repeat periodically per physician order **Expected Outcomes** Thromboembolic disease treated successfully, without related complications
Activity and comfort	Decreased stimulation in room including visitors		Maintain bed rest and limb in elevated position Initiate progressive ambulation following the acute phase; provide properly fitting elastic stockings prior to ambulation for management of superficial thrombophlebitis and DVT **Expected Outcomes** Activity initiated as appropriate Optimal comfort maintained
Nutrition	Plan high-protein, high-calorie diet		Continue diet and fluids **Expected Outcomes** Nutritional needs met
Elimination			
Medications		Continuous IV infusion	May take own prenatal vitamins RhoGAM administered if indicated Rubella vaccine administered if indicated For DVT, administer intravenous heparin as ordered by continuous intravenous drip, heparin lock, or subcutaneously, including • Monitor IV or heparin lock site for signs of infiltration • Obtain Lee-White clotting times or partial thromboplastin time (PTT) per physician order and review prior to administering heparin • Observe for signs of anticoagulant overdose with resultant bleeding, including the following: hematuria, epistaxis, ecchymosis, and bleeding gums • Provide protamine sulfate per physician order to combat bleeding problems related to heparin overdose **Expected Outcomes** Thrombosis resolved and control of related bleeding problems achieved Minimized complications and side effects

Category	Antepartal Management	Intrapartal Management	Postpartal Management
Discharge planning/home care	Assess home care needs Provide support and counseling		Discuss ways to avoid circulatory stasis such as avoiding prolonged standing, sitting, and crossing legs Review need to wear support stockings and to plan for rest periods with legs elevated In the presence of DVT, discuss the following: • The use of warfarin, its side effects, possible interactions with other medications, and need to have dosage assessed through periodic checks of the prothrombin time • Signs of bleeding, which may be associated with warfarin sodium and which need to be reported immediately, including the following: hematuria, epistaxis, ecchymosis, bleeding gums, and rectal bleeding • Monitor menstrual flow: bleeding may be heavier • Review need for woman to eat a consistent amount of leafy green vegetables (lettuce, cabbage, brussels sprouts, broccoli) every day (high in vitamin K, also affects dose of warfarin and PT balance) • Tell the woman to report any bleeding that continues more than 10 minutes Instruct the woman to do the following: • Routinely inspect the body for bruising • Carry MedicAlert card indicating she is on anticoagulant therapy • Use electric razor to avoid scratching skin • Use soft-bristle toothbrush • Avoid alcohol intake or keep intake at a minimum • Avoid taking any other drugs without checking with the physician • Be aware that stools may change color to pink, red, or black as result of anticoagulant use • Advise all health providers, including dentists, that she is taking anticoagulants Review discharge instructions and checklist Provide list or make appropriate referrals to available community resources Describe postpartum warning signs and when to call CNM or physician Provide prescriptions; gift pack given to woman Make arrangements for baby pictures if desired Schedule postpartum visit Schedule newborn checkup **Expected Outcomes** Client discharge teaching done with emphasis on follow-up care, continued therapy needs, and precautions Support network identified

Category	Antepartal Management	Intrapartal Management	Postpartal Management
Family involvement	Assess support systems	Encourage family member to stay with the woman as long as possible throughout labor and childbirth	Involve support persons in teaching Plans made for providing support to mother following discharge; support persons verbalize understanding of need for woman to rest, eat nutritionally, recover Encourage woman to express her concerns to her partner; assist couple in planning ways to manage while woman is hospitalized and after her discharge Encourage partner or support person to bring other children to hospital to visit mother and meet new sibling Encourage partner or support person to bring in family pictures; encourage phone calls Contact social services if indicated to obtain additional assistance for family if needed **Expected Outcomes** Family demonstrates resource availability and utilization Family bonding and development unimpaired
Date			

CNM, certified nurse-midwife; DC, discharge; Hct, hematocrit; NICU, neonatal intensive care unit; IV, intravenous; heparin lock, intravenous catheter that allows intermittent access; hx, history; prn, as needed; s/s, signs and symptoms; TPR, temperature, pulse, and respiration; WNL, within normal limits.

CARE OF THE WOMAN WITH A POSTPARTUM PSYCHIATRIC DISORDER

Many types of psychiatric problems may occur in the postpartum period. The classification of postpartum psychiatric disorders is a subject of some controversy. The *Diagnostic and Statistical Manual of Mental Disorders,* 4th edition *(DSM-IV)* (American Psychiatric Association, 1994), has added a postpartum onset specifier to the mood disorder diagnostic category of psychiatric disorders. It is proposed that postpartum psychiatric disorders be considered one diagnosable syndrome with three subclasses: (1) adjustment reaction with depressed mood, (2) postpartum psychosis, and (3) postpartum major mood disorder. The incidence, etiology, symptoms, treatment, and prognosis vary with each subclass.

Adjustment reaction with depressed mood is also known as postpartum, maternal, or "baby blues." It is characterized by mild depression interspersed with happier feelings. Postpartum blues typically occur within a few days after the baby's birth and are self-limiting, lasting from a few hours to several days (O'Hara, 1999). The depression is more severe in primiparas than in multiparas and seems related to the rapid alteration of estrogen, progesterone, and prolactin levels after birth. New mothers experiencing postpartum blues commonly report feeling overwhelmed, unable to cope, fatigued, anxious, irritable, and oversensitive. A key feature is episodic tearfulness, often without an identifiable reason.

Validating the existence of this phenomenon, labeling it as a real but normal adjustment reaction, and providing reassurance can offer a measure of relief. Assistance with self- and infant care, information, and family support aids recovery. The partner should be encouraged to watch for and report signs that the new mother is not returning to a more normal mood but slipping into a deeper depression.

Postpartum psychosis, which has an incidence of 1 to 2 per 1000, usually becomes evident within the first 3 months postpartum. Symptoms include agitation, hyperactivity, insomnia, mood lability, confusion, irrationality, difficulty remembering or concentrating, poor judgment, delusions, and hallucinations. Improvement is seen in 95% of women in 2 to 3 months (O'Hara, 1999). Treatment may include hospitalization, antipsychotics, sedatives, electroconvulsive therapy, removal of the infant, social support, and psychotherapy.

Postpartum major mood disorder, also known as postpartum depression, develops in about 7% to 16% of all postpartum women in North America (O'Hara, 1999). Although it may occur at any time during the first postpartum year, the periods of greatest risk occur around the fourth week, just before the initiation of menses, and upon weaning. Surprisingly, it is not associated with depression during pregnancy.

Risk factors for postpartum depression include the following:

- Primiparity
- Ambivalence about maintaining the pregnancy
- History of postpartum depression or bipolar illness
- Lack of social support
- Lack of a stable and supportive relationship with parents or partner
- The woman's dissatisfaction with herself, including body image problems and eating disorders

Clinical Therapy

Medication, individual or group psychotherapy, and practical assistance with child care and other demands of daily life are common treatment measures. Support groups have proved to be successful adjuncts to such treatment. Within a support group of postpartal women and their partners, a couple may feel consolation that they are not alone in their experience. Moreover, the group provides a forum for exchanging information about postpartum depression, learning stress-reduction measures, and experiencing renewed self-esteem and support. If a support group is not available locally, the woman and her family may be encouraged to contact Depression after Delivery (DAD), a national support network that provides literature and volunteers (P.O. Box 1282, Morrisville, PA 19067, or 800-944-4773).

Nursing Management

Nursing Assessment and Diagnosis

Assessment for factors predisposing a client to postpartal depression or psychosis should begin prenatally. Questions designed to detect problems can be included as part of the routine prenatal history interview or questionnaire. Beck (1995) developed a practical and simple screening checklist to use during routine care with all postpartum women to identify those who might be experiencing postpartum depression so that early management might be initiated (Table 23–4). Willingness to listen as the mother shares her experiences of postpartum depression not only enables the nurse to recognize symptoms and initiate timely management but also conveys to the mother a sense of caring (Beck, 1999). Be aware that depressive symptomatology frequently occurs among first-time mothers of low socioeconomic status. Chronic stressors and inadequate social support are significant factors associated with postpartum depression (Seguin, Potvin, St-Denis, et al., 1999).

In providing daily care, observe the woman for objective signs of depression—anxiety, irritability, poor concentration, forgetfulness, sleep difficulties, appetite change, fatigue, and tearfulness—and listen for statements indicating feelings of failure and self-accusation. Note severity and duration of symptoms. Behavior and verbalizations that are bizarre or seem to indicate a potential for violence against herself or others, including the infant, are reported as soon as possible for further evaluation.

Be aware that many normal physiologic changes of the puerperium are similar to symptoms of depression (lack of sexual interest, appetite change, fatigue). It is essential that observations be as specific and as objective as possible and that they be carefully documented.

Possible nursing diagnoses that may apply to a woman with a postpartum psychiatric disorder include the following:

▶ *Ineffective individual coping* related to postpartum depression
▶ *Risk for altered parenting* related to postpartal mental illness

Planning and Implementation

Nurses working in antepartal settings or teaching childbirth classes play indispensable roles in helping prospective parents appreciate the lifestyle changes and role demands of parenthood. Offering realistic information and anticipatory guidance and debunking myths about the perfect mother or perfect newborn may help prevent postpartum depression. Social support teaching guides are available for nurses to help postpartum women explore their needs for postpartum support (Logsdon, Birkimer, & Usui, 2000). Alert the mother, spouse, and other family members to the possibility of postpartum blues in the early days after birth and reassure them of the short-term nature of the condition. Describe symptoms of postpartum depression and encourage the mother to call her health care provider if symptoms become severe, if they fail to subside quickly, or if at any time she feels she is unable to function. Encouraging the mother to plan how she will manage at home and providing concrete suggestions on how to cope aid in her adjustment to motherhood.

NURSING CARE IN THE COMMUNITY

Home visits, especially for early-discharge families, are essential to fostering positive adjustments for the new family constellation. Telephone follow-up at 3 weeks postpartum to ask whether the mother is experiencing difficulties is also helpful.

Women with a history of depression or postpartum psychosis should be referred to a mental health professional for counseling and biweekly visits between the second and sixth week postpartum for evaluation of depression. Medication, social support, and assistance with child care may also be necessary.

In all women the presence of three symptoms or one symptom of depression for 3 days may signal serious depression and requires immediate referral to a mental health professional. Also make an immediate referral if the mother

TABLE 23-4   Suggested Questions to Elicit Responses from the Postpartum Depression Checklist (PDC)*

LACK OF CONCENTRATION
Are you experiencing difficulty concentrating?
Does your mind seem to be filled with cobwebs?
Does it seem at times like fogginess sets in?

LOSS OF INTERESTS
Do you feel your life is empty of your previous interests and goals?
Have you lost interest in your hobbies that used to bring you pleasure and enjoyment?

LONELINESS
Are you experiencing feelings of loneliness?
Do you feel as though no one really understands what you are experiencing?
Do you feel uncomfortable around other people?
Have you been isolating yourself from other people?

INSECURITY
Have you been feeling insecure, fragile, or vulnerable?
Does the responsibility of motherhood seem overwhelming?

OBSESSIVE THINKING
Is your mind constantly filled with obsessive thinking such as, "What's wrong with me?" "Am I going crazy?" "Why can't I enjoy being with my baby?"
When trying to fall asleep at night, is your mind still racing with repetitive thoughts?

LACK OF POSITIVE EMOTIONS
Are you experiencing feelings of emptiness?
Do you feel like a robot just going through the motions?
When caring for your infant/child, do you feel any joy or love?

LOSS OF SELF
Do you feel as though you are not the same person you used to be?
Are you afraid that your life will never be normal again?

ANXIETY ATTACKS
Are you experiencing uncontrollable anxiety attacks?
Are you experiencing periods of palpitations, chest pains, sweating, or tingling hands?
When going through an anxiety attack, do you feel as though you're losing your mind?

LOSS OF CONTROL
Do you feel you are in control of your emotions and thoughts?
Are you experiencing loss of control in any aspects of your life?

GUILT
Are you feeling guilty because you believe you are not giving your infant/child the love and attention he/she needs?
Are you experiencing guilt over thoughts of harming your infant/child?
Do you feel you are a good mother?

CONTEMPLATING DEATH
Have you experienced thoughts of harming yourself?
Have you been feeling so low that the thought of leaving this world was appealing to you?

*Bold print reflects areas of concern expressed by depressed women in Beck's qualitative studies. Questions answered "Yes" by women during screening with this checklist can be followed with further dialogue between nurse and client.

Note: From Beck, C. T. (1995). Screening methods for postpartum depression. *Journal of Obstetric, Gynecologic, and Neonatal Nursing, 24*(4), 311, Table 2. Used with permission of Lippincott-Raven Publishers.

has rejected the infant or threatened or been aggressive against the infant. In such cases the newborn is never left unattended with the mother. A diagnosis of postpartum depression or other psychiatric disorder poses major problems for the family, especially the father (Meighan, Davis, Thomas, et al., 1999). The symptoms of these disorders are difficult to witness and may be harder to understand than physical problems such as hemorrhage and infection. The father may feel hurt by his partner's hostility, worry that she is becoming insane, or be baffled by her mood swings and lack of concern about herself, the newborn, or household responsibilities. Very real practical matters—running the household; managing the children, including the totally dependent newborn; and caring for the mother—may be added to his usual routines and work responsibilities.

Information, emotional support, and assistance in providing or obtaining care for the infant may be needed.

Help family members by identifying community resources and making referrals to public health nursing services and social services. Postpartum follow-up and visits from a psychiatric home health nurse are especially important.

Evaluation

Expected outcomes of nursing care include the following:

▶ Signs of potential postpartal disorders are detected quickly and therapy is implemented.

▶ The newborn is cared for effectively by the father or another support person until the mother is able to do her share.

CHAPTER HIGHLIGHTS

☞ The main causes of early postpartal hemorrhage are uterine atony, lacerations of the vagina and cervix, and retained placental fragments.

☞ The most common postpartal infection is endometritis, which is limited to the uterine cavity.

☞ A postpartal woman is at increased risk for developing urinary tract problems due to normal postpartal diuresis, increased bladder capacity, decreased bladder sensitivity from stretching or trauma, and, possibly, inhibited neural control of the bladder following the use of anesthetic agents.

☞ Mastitis is an inflammation of the breast caused by a variety of organisms and is primarily seen in breastfeeding women. Symptoms seldom occur before the second to fourth week after birth.

☞ Thromboembolic disease originating in the veins of the leg, thigh, or pelvis may occur in the antepartum or postpartum periods and may create a pulmonary embolus.

☞ Although many different types of psychiatric problems may be encountered in the postpartal period, depression is the most common. Episodes occur frequently in the week after childbirth and are typically transient.

☞ Telephone calls and home visits are effective measures for extending comprehensive care into the home setting of the postpartum family at risk.

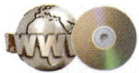 EXPLOREMediaLink

NCLEX Review, Case Studies, and other interactive resources for this chapter can be found on the companion website at http://www.prenhall.com/london. Click on "Chapter 23" to select the activities for this chapter.

For animations, more NCLEX review questions, and an audio glossary, access the accompanying CD-ROM in this textbook.

REFERENCES

American College of Obstetricians and Gynecologists. (1998). *Postpartum hemorrhage* (ACOG Educational Bulletin No. 243). Washington, DC: Author.

American Psychiatric Association. (1994). *Diagnostic and statistical manual of mental disorders: DSM-IV* (4th ed.). Washington, DC: Author.

Beck, C. T. (1995). Perceptions of nurses' caring by mothers experiencing postpartum depression. *Journal of Obstetric, Gynecologic, and Neonatal Nursing, 24*(9), 819–825.

Beck, C. T. (1999). Maternal depression and child behaviour problems: A meta-analysis. *Journal of Advanced Nursing, 29*(3), 623–629.

Bowes, W. (1999). Clinical aspects of normal and abnormal labor. In R. K. Creasy & R. Resnik (Eds.), *Maternal-fetal medicine* (4th ed., pp. 541–568). Philadelphia: Saunders.

Cash, J. C., & Glass, C. A. (2000). *Family practice guidelines.* Philadelphia: Lippincott.

Clarke-Pearson, D. L. (2000). Venous thromboembolic disease in pregnancy. In E. J. Quilligan & F. P. Zuspan (Eds.), *Current therapy in obstetrics and gynecology* (5th ed., pp. 368–371). Philadelphia: W. B. Saunders.

Cunningham, F. G., Gant, N. F., Leveno, K. J., Gilstrap, L. C., III, Hauth, J. C., & Wenstrom, K. D. (2001). *Williams obstetrics* (21st ed.). New York: McGraw-Hill.

Elmer, G. W. (2001). Probiotics: "Living drugs." *American Journal of Health System Pharmacy, 58*(12), 1101–1109.

Gibbs, R. S., & Sweet, R. L. (1999). Maternal and fetal infectious disorders. In R. K. Creasy & R. Resnik (Eds.), *Maternal-fetal medicine* (4th ed., pp. 659–724). Philadelphia: Saunders.

Johnson, J. V., & Riddick, D. H. (2000). The nonlactating human breast. In J. J. Sciarri & T. J. Watkins (Eds.), *Gynecology and obstetrics* (Vol. 5, pp. 1–19). Philadelphia, PA: Lippincott Williams & Wilkins.

Laros, R. K. (1999). Thromboembolic disease. In R. K. Creasy & R. Resnik (Eds.), *Maternal-fetal medicine* (4th ed., pp. 821–832). Philadelphia: Saunders.

Lauwers, J., & Shinskie, D. (2000). *Counseling the nursing mother: The lactation consultant's reference* (3rd ed.). Boston: Jones & Bartlett.

Logsdon, M. C., Birkimer, J. C., & Usui, W. M. (2000). The link of social support and postpartum depressive symptoms in African-American women with low incomes. *Journal of Maternal-Child Nursing, 25*(5), 262–266.

Meighan, M., Davis, M. W., Thomas, S. P., & Droppleman, P. G. (1999). Living with postpartum depression: The father's experience. *Journal of Maternal-Child Nursing, 24*(4), 202–208.

Nadeau, C., Alpert, B., Constantino, T., McGinn, R., Coyne, M., Ahern, K., et al. (2000). The challenges of oral anticoagulation. *Patient Care for the Nurse Practitioner, 3*(12), 12–25.

O'Hara, M. W. (1999). Postpartum mental disorders. In J. J. Sciarri & T. J. Watkins (Eds.), *Gynecology and obstetrics* (Vol. 6, pp. 1–19). Philadelphia: Lippincott Williams & Wilkins.

Quilligan, E. J., & Zuspan, F. P. (2000). *Current therapy in obstetrics and gynecology* (5th ed.). Philadelphia: W. B. Saunders.

Seguin, L., Potvin, L., St-Denis, M., & Loiselle, J. (1999). Depressive symptoms in the late postpartum among low socioeconomic status women. *Birth, 26*(3), 157–163.

Shaver, D. C. (1999). Thromboembolic disease. In J. J. Sciarri & T. J. Watkins (Eds.), *Gynecology and obstetrics* (Vol. 2, pp. 1–11). Philadelphia: Lippincott Williams & Wilkins.

CHAPTER 24

The Physiologic Responses of the Newborn to Birth

I remember clearly when they held him up for us to see and my husband and I cried and laughed and it was so amazing. He was 9 1/2 pounds and was so beautiful. Even though my labor was long, his Apgars were high, and he didn't even cry—not until we dressed him, anyway.

—CRYSTAL, 26

❧ Key Terms

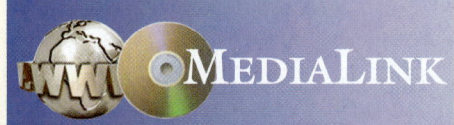

MediaLink

CD-ROM

Skill 5–1: Performing Nasal Pharyngeal Suctioning

Fetal Heart Formation and Circulation Animation

Audio Glossary

NCLEX Review

COMPANION WEBSITE

http://www.prenhall.com/london

Physiologic Responses of the Newborn to Birth—Web Links

Thinking Critically

NCLEX Review

Case Study

The newborn period includes the time from birth through the 28th day of life. During this period, the newborn adjusts from intrauterine to extrauterine life. The nurse needs to be knowledgeable about a newborn's normal physiologic and behavioral adaptations and to be able to recognize alterations from normal.

To begin life as a separate being, the baby must immediately establish respiratory gas exchange in conjunction with marked circulatory changes. These radical and rapid changes are crucial to the maintenance of extrauterine life. The first few hours of life, in which the newborn stabilizes respiratory and circulatory functions, are called **neonatal transition.** All other newborn body systems change their level of functioning and become established over a longer period of time during the neonatal period.

RESPIRATORY ADAPTATIONS

Although significant respiratory events occur at birth, certain intrauterine factors also enhance the newborn's ability to breathe.

Intrauterine Factors Supporting Respiratory Function

FETAL LUNG DEVELOPMENT

The respiratory system is in an ongoing state of development during fetal life, and lung development continues into early childhood. During the first 20 weeks' gestation, development is limited to the differentiation of pulmonary, vascular, and lymphatic structures.

At 20 to 24 weeks, alveolar ducts begin to appear, followed by primitive alveoli at 24 to 28 weeks. During this time, the alveolar epithelial cells begin to differentiate into type I cells (structures necessary for gas exchange) and type II cells (structures that provide for the synthesis and storage of surfactant). **Surfactant** is a mixture of surface-active phospholipids that reduces the surface tension of pulmonary fluids and contributes critically to the elasticity of pulmonary tissue.

At 28 to 32 weeks' gestation, the number of type II cells increases further, and surfactant is produced by a choline pathway within them. Surfactant production by this pathway peaks at about 35 weeks' gestation and remains high until term, paralleling late fetal lung development. At this time, the lungs are structurally developed enough to permit maintenance of lung expansion and adequate exchange of gases.

Clinically, the peak production of lecithin corresponds closely with a marked decrease in the incidence of respiratory distress syndrome for babies born after 35 weeks' gestation. Production of sphingomyelin (another component of surfactant) remains constant throughout gestation. The newborn born before the lecithin/sphingomyelin (L/S)

ratio is 2:1 will have varying degrees of respiratory distress. (See discussion of L/S ratio in Chapter 29).

FETAL BREATHING MOVEMENTS

The newborn's ability to breathe air immediately when exposed to the extrauterine environment appears to be the consequence of weeks of intrauterine practice. In this respect, breathing can be seen as a continuation of an intrauterine process; the lungs convert from a fluid-filled to a gas-filled organ. Fetal breathing movements (FBMs) occur as early as 11 weeks' gestation (see Chapter 14 for discussion). They develop the chest wall muscles and the diaphragm and, to a lesser extent, regulate lung fluid volume and resultant lung growth.

Initiation of Breathing

To maintain life, the lungs must function immediately after birth. Two radical changes must take place:

1. Pulmonary ventilation must be established through lung expansion following birth.
2. A marked increase in the pulmonary circulation must occur.

The first breath of life—the gasp in response to mechanical, chemical, thermal, and sensory changes associated with birth—starts the serial opening of the alveoli. So begins the transition from a fluid-filled environment to an air-breathing, independent, extrauterine life. Figure 24–1 ◆ summarizes the initiation of respiration.

MECHANICAL EVENTS

During the latter half of gestation, the fetal lungs continuously produce fluid. This fluid expands the lungs almost completely, filling the air spaces. Some lung fluid moves up into the trachea and into the amniotic fluid and is then swallowed by the fetus.

Production of lung fluid diminishes 2 to 4 days before the onset of labor. However, approximately 80 to 110 mL of fluid remains in the respiratory passages of a normal full-term fetus at birth. It must be removed from the lungs to permit adequate movement of air. The primary mechanical events that initiate respiration involve the removal of fluid from the lungs as the fetus passes through the birth canal. During birth the fetal chest is compressed, increasing intrathoracic pressure, and approximately one third of the fluid is squeezed out of the lungs. After the birth of the newborn's trunk, the chest wall recoils. This chest recoil creates a negative intrathoracic pressure, which is thought to produce a small, passive inspiration of air that replaces the fluid that is squeezed out.

After this first inspiration, the newborn exhales, with crying, against a partially closed glottis, creating positive intrathoracic pressure. The high positive intrathoracic pressure distributes the inspired air throughout the alveoli and begins to establish functional residual capacity (FRC), the air left in the lungs at the end of a normal expiration.

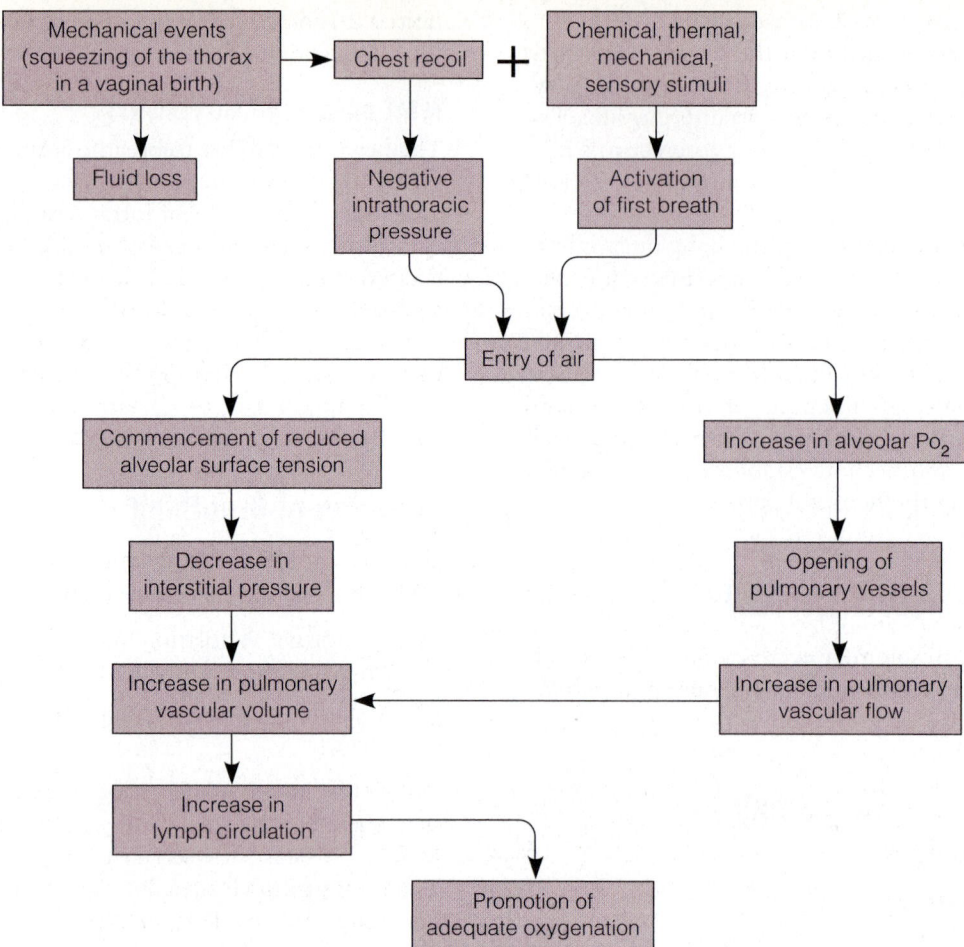

FIGURE 24–1. ◆ Initiation of respiration in the newborn.

The higher intrathoracic pressure also increases absorption of fluid via the capillaries and lymphatic system. The negative intrathoracic pressure created when the diaphragm moves down with inspiration causes lung fluid to flow from the alveoli across the alveolar membranes into the pulmonary interstitial tissue.

With each succeeding breath, the lungs expand. Because the protein concentration is higher in the pulmonary capillaries than in the interstitial tissue, oncotic pressure draws the interstitial fluid into the capillaries and lymphatic tissue. Lung expansion helps the remaining lung fluid move into the interstitial tissue. As pulmonary vascular resistance decreases, pulmonary blood flow increases, and more fluid is absorbed into the bloodstream. In the healthy term newborn, lung fluid moves rapidly into the interstitial tissue but may take several hours to move into the lymph and blood vessels. About 80% of the fluid is reabsorbed within 2 hours after birth, and it is completely absorbed within 12 to 24 hours after birth.

Although the initial chest compression and recoil generally clear the airways of accumulated fluid and permit further inspiration, some clinicians believe mucus and fluid should be suctioned from the newborn's mouth and oropharynx. They use a mucus trap attached to suction as soon as the newborn's head and shoulders are born and again as the newborn adapts to extrauterine life and stabilizes (see Skill 5–1). ⊂⊃ SKILLS CD A variety of factors may cause problems with lung fluid clearance and the start of respiration. The lymphatic system may be underdeveloped, decreasing the rate at which the fluid is absorbed from the lungs. Prenatal or intrapartal complications can interfere with adequate lung expansion and cause failure to decrease pulmonary vascular resistance, resulting in decreased pulmonary blood flow. These complications include inadequate compression of the chest wall in a very small newborn, the absence of chest wall compression in a newborn born by cesarean birth, respiratory depression due to maternal anesthesia, or aspiration of amniotic fluid or meconium.

CHEMICAL STIMULI

An important chemical stimulator that contributes to the onset of breathing is transitory asphyxia of the fetus and newborn. The first breath is an inspiratory gasp triggered by elevation in PCO_2 and decrease in pH and PO_2, the natural result of a normal vaginal birth with cessation of placental gas exchange when the cord is clamped. These changes, present in all newborns to some degree, stimulate the aortic and carotid chemoreceptors, initiating impulses that trigger the medulla's respiratory center. Although this brief asphyxia is a significant stimulator, prolonged asphyxia is abnormal and acts as a central nervous system (CNS) respiratory depressant.

THERMAL STIMULI

A significant decrease in environmental temperature after birth, 37 °C to 21–23.9 °C (98.6 °F to 70–75 °F), also helps newborns begin breathing. The cold stimulates skin nerve endings, and the newborn responds with rhythmic respirations. Normal temperature changes at birth are apparently within acceptable physiologic limits. However, excessive cooling may cause profound depression and evidence of cold stress (see Chapter 29 for discussion of cold stress).

SENSORY STIMULI

As the fetus moves from a familiar, comfortable, quiet environment to one of sensory abundance, a number of physical and sensory influences help respiration begin. They include the numerous tactile, auditory, and visual stimuli of birth.

During intrauterine life, the fetus is in a dark, sound-dampened, fluid-filled environment and is nearly weightless. After birth the newborn experiences light, sounds, and the effects of gravity for the first time. Historically, clinicians provided vigorous stimulation by slapping the buttocks or heels of the newborn, but the emphasis today is on gentle physical contact. Thoroughly drying the newborn and placing it in skin-to-skin contact with the mother's chest and abdomen provide ample stimulation in a far more comforting way and also decrease heat loss.

Factors Opposing the First Breath

Three major factors may oppose the initiation of respiratory activity: (1) alveolar surface tension, (2) viscosity of lung fluid within the respiratory tract, and (3) degree of lung compliance.

The contracting force between the moist surfaces of the alveoli is called *alveolar surface tension*. This tension, required for healthy respiratory function, would nevertheless cause the small airways and alveoli to collapse between each inspiration if surfactant were not present. By reducing the attracting force between alveoli, surfactant prevents the alveoli from completely collapsing with each expiration and thus promotes lung expansion. Similarly, surfactant promotes lung compliance, the ability of the lung to fill with air easily. When surfactant decreases, compliance also decreases, and the pressure needed to expand the alveoli with air increases. Resistive forces of the fluid-filled lung, combined with the small radii of the airways, mean that 30 to 40 cm of water pressure are needed to open the lung initially (Thureen, Deacon, O'Neill, et al., 1999). The first breath usually establishes FRC that is 30% to 40% of the fully expanded lung volume. This FRC allows alveolar sacs to remain partially expanded on expiration, decreasing the need for continuous high pressures for each of the following breaths. Subsequent breaths require only 6 to 8 cm H_2O pressure to open alveoli during inspiration. Therefore, the first breath of life is usually the most difficult.

Cardiopulmonary Physiology

The onset of respiration stimulates cardiovascular system changes necessary for successful transition to extrauterine life, hence the term **cardiopulmonary adaptation.** As air enters the lungs, PO_2 rises in the alveoli, relaxing the pulmonary arteries and triggering a decrease in pulmonary vascular resistance. As pulmonary vascular resistance decreases, the vascular flow in the lung increases to 100% 24 hours after birth. The greater blood volume in the lungs contributes to the conversion from fetal circulation to newborn circulation. After pulmonary circulation is established, blood is distributed throughout the lung, although the alveoli may or may not be fully open. For adequate oxygenation to occur, the heart must deliver sufficient blood to functional, open alveoli. Shunting of blood is common in the early newborn period. Bidirectional blood flow, or right-to-left shunting through the ductus arteriosus, may divert a significant amount of blood away from the lungs, depending on the pressure changes of respiration, crying, and the cardiac cycle. This shunting in the newborn period is also responsible for the unstable transitional period in cardiopulmonary function.

Oxygen Transport

The transportation of oxygen to the peripheral tissues depends on the type of hemoglobin in the red blood cells. In the fetus and newborn, a variety of hemoglobins exist, the most significant being fetal hemoglobin (Hb F) and adult hemoglobin (Hb A). Approximately 70% to 90% of the hemoglobin in the fetus and newborn is of the fetal variety.

Since Hb F has a greater affinity for oxygen than does Hb A, the oxygen saturation in the newborn's blood is greater than in the adult's, but the amount of oxygen available to the tissues is less. This situation is beneficial prenatally, because the fetus must maintain adequate oxygen uptake in the presence of very low oxygen tension (umbilical venous PO_2 cannot exceed the uterine venous PO_2). This high concentration of oxygen in the blood makes hypoxia in the newborn particularly difficult to recognize. Clinical manifestations of cyanosis do not appear until blood levels of oxygen are low. In addition, alkalosis (increased pH) and hypothermia can result in less oxygen being available to the body tissues, whereas acidosis, hypercarbia, and hyperthermia can result in less oxygen being bound to hemoglobin and more oxygen being released to the body tissues.

Maintaining Respiratory Function

The lung's ability to maintain oxygenation and ventilation (the exchange of oxygen and carbon dioxide) is influenced by such factors as lung compliance and airway resistance. Anatomic differences in the newborn reduce elastic recoil of the lung tissue and thereby decrease lung compliance. The newborn has a relatively large heart and mediastinal structures that reduce available lung space. Also, the newborn chest is equipped with weak intercostal muscles and a rigid rib cage with horizontal ribs and a high diaphragm, which restricts the space available for lung expansion. The large abdomen further encroaches on the high diaphragm to decrease lung space. Another factor that limits ventilation is airway resistance, which depends on the radii, length, and number of airways and are also reduced in the newborn when compared to the adult.

Characteristics of Newborn Respiration

The normal newborn respiratory rate is 30 to 60 breaths per minute. Initial respirations may be largely diaphragmatic and shallow and irregular in depth and rhythm. The abdomen's movements are synchronous with the chest movements. When the breathing pattern includes pauses lasting 5 to 15 seconds, **periodic breathing** is occurring. Periodic breathing is rarely associated with differences in skin color or heart rate changes, and it has no prognostic significance. Tactile or other sensory stimulation increases the inspired oxygen and converts periodic breathing patterns to normal breathing patterns during neonatal transition. With deep sleep, the pattern is reasonably regular. Periodic breathing occurs with rapid-eye-movement (REM) sleep, and grossly irregular breathing is evident with motor activity, sucking, and crying. Cessation of breathing lasting more than 20 seconds is defined as *apnea* and is abnormal in term newborns. Apnea may or may not be associated with changes in skin color or heart rate (drop below 100 beats per minute). Apnea always needs to be further evaluated.

The newborn must breath through the nose, and any obstruction will cause respiratory distress, so it is important to keep the nose and throat clear. Immediately after birth, and for about the next 2 hours after birth, respiratory rates of 60 to 70 breaths per minute are normal. Some cyanosis and acrocyanosis are normal for several hours; after that the infant's color improves steadily. If respirations drop below 30 or exceed 60 per minute when the infant is at rest, or if retractions, cyanosis, or nasal flaring and expiratory grunting occur, the clinician should be notified. Any increased use of the intercostal muscles (retractions) may indicate respiratory distress. (See Chapter 29 and Table 29–1 for signs of respiratory distress).

CARDIOVASCULAR ADAPTATIONS

As described earlier, the onset of respiration triggers increased blood flow to the lungs after birth. This greater blood volume contributes to the conversion from fetal circulation to neonatal circulation.

TABLE 24-1 Fetal and Neonatal Circulation

System	Fetal	Neonatal
Pulmonary blood vessels	Constricted, with very little blood flow; lungs not expanded	Vasodilation and increased blood flow; lungs expanded; increased oxygen stimulates vasodilation.
Systemic blood vessels	Dilated, with low resistance; blood mostly in placenta	Arterial pressure rises due to loss of placenta; increased systemic blood volume and resistance.
Ductus arteriosus	Large, with no tone; blood flow from pulmonary artery to aorta	Reversal of blood flow; now from aorta to pulmonary artery because of increased left atrial pressure. Ductus is sensitive to increased oxygen and body chemicals and begins to constrict.
Foramen ovale	Patent, with increased blood flow from right atrium to left atrium	Increased pressure in left atrium attempts to reverse blood flow and shuts one-way valve.

Fetal-Newborn Transitional Physiology

During fetal life, blood with a higher oxygen content is diverted to the heart and brain. Blood in the descending aorta is less oxygenated and supplies the kidney and intestinal tract before it is returned to the placenta. Limited amounts of blood, pumped from the right ventricle toward the lungs, enter the pulmonary vessels. In the fetus, increased pulmonary resistance forces most of this blood through the ductus arteriosus into the descending aorta (see Table 24–1). See fetal heart animation on the CD-ROM. **CD**

Marked cardiovascular system changes occur at birth. Expansion of the lungs with the first breath decreases pulmonary vascular resistance and increases pulmonary blood flow. Pressure in the left atrium increases as blood returns from the pulmonary veins. Pressure in the right atrium drops, and systematic vascular resistance increases as umbilical venous blood flow is halted when the cord is clamped. These physiologic mechanisms mark the transition from fetal to neonatal circulation and show the interplay of cardiovascular and respiratory systems (Figure 24–2 ◆).

Five major areas of change occur in cardiopulmonary adaptation (Figure 24–3 ◆):

1. *Increased aortic pressure and decreased venous pressure.* Clamping of the umbilical cord eliminates the placental vascular bed and reduces the intravascular space. Consequently, aortic (systemic) blood pressure increases. At the same time, blood return via the inferior vena cava decreases, resulting in a decreased right atrial pressure and a small decrease in pressure in the venous circulation.

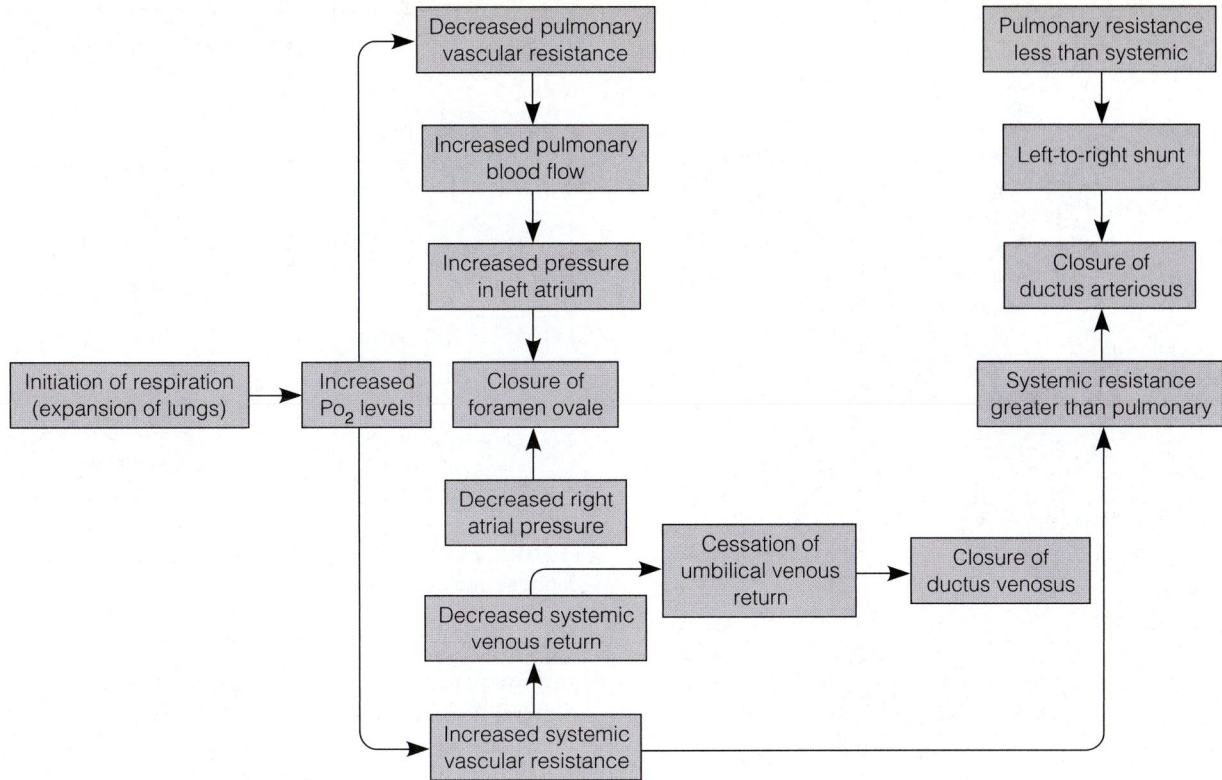

FIGURE 24-2. ◆ Transitional circulation: conversion from fetal to neonatal circulation.

2. *Increased systemic pressure and decreased pulmonary artery pressure.* With the loss of the low-resistance placenta, systemic resistance pressure increases, resulting in greater systemic pressure. At the same time, lung expansion increases pulmonary blood flow, and the increased blood PO_2 associated with initiation of respirations dilates pulmonary blood vessels. The combination of vasodilation and increased pulmonary blood flow decreases pulmonary artery resistance. As the pulmonary vascular beds open, the systemic vascular pressure increases, enhancing perfusion of the other body systems.

3. *Closure of the foramen ovale.* Closure of the foramen ovale is a function of changing atrial pressures. In utero, pressure is greater in the right atrium, and the foramen ovale is open after birth. Decreased pulmonary resistance and increased pulmonary blood flow increase the pulmonary venous return into the left atrium, raising left atrial pressure slightly. The decreased pulmonary vascular resistance and the decreased umbilical venous return to the right atrium also lower right atrial pressure. The pressure gradients across the atria are now reversed, left atrial pressure is greater, and the foramen ovale is functionally closed 1 to 2 hours after birth. However, a slight right-to-left shunting may occur in the early newborn period. Any increase in pulmonary resistance or right atrial pressure, such as occurs with crying, acidosis, or cold

stress, may cause the foramen ovale to reopen, resulting in a right-to-left shunt. Permanent closure occurs within 6 months.

4. *Closure of the ductus arteriosus.* Initial elevation of the systemic vascular pressure above the pulmonary vascular pressure increases pulmonary blood flow by reversing the flow through the ductus arteriosus. Blood now flows from the aorta into the pulmonary artery. Furthermore, although oxygen causes the pulmonary arterioles to dilate, an increase in blood PO_2 triggers the opposite response in the ductus arteriosus—it constricts.

In utero, the placenta provides prostaglandin E_2 (PGE_2), which causes ductus vasodilation. With the loss of the placenta and increased pulmonary blood flow, PGE_2 levels drop, leaving the active constriction by PO_2 unopposed. If the lungs fail to expand or if PO_2 levels drop, the ductus remains patent. Fibrosis of the ductus occurs within 3 weeks after birth, but functional closure happens within 15 hours after birth (Nelson, 1999).

5. *Closure of the ductus venosus.* Although the mechanism initiating closure of the ductus venosus is not known, it appears to be related to mechanical pressure changes after severing of the cord, redistribution of blood, and cardiac output. Closure of the bypass forces perfusion of the liver. Fibrosis of the ductus venosus occurs within 2 months.

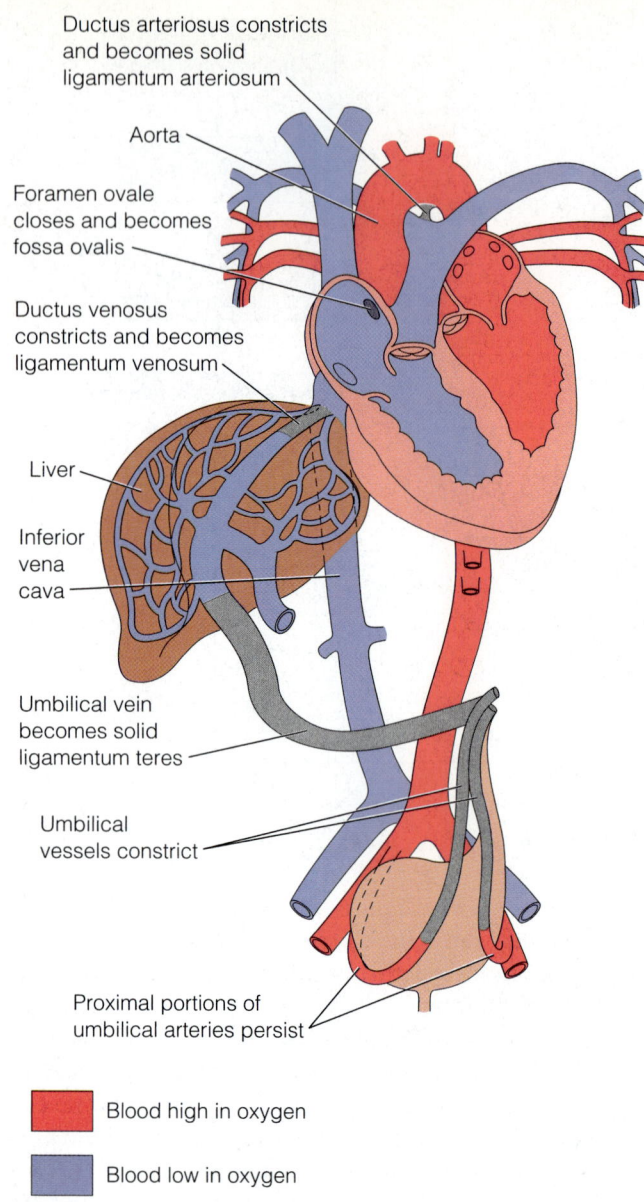

Ductus arteriosus constricts
and becomes solid
ligamentum arteriosum

Aorta

Foramen ovale
closes and becomes
fossa ovalis

Ductus venosus
constricts and becomes
ligamentum venosum

Liver

Inferior
vena
cava

Umbilical vein
becomes solid
ligamentum teres

Umbilical
vessels constrict

Proximal portions of
umbilical arteries persist

■ Blood high in oxygen

■ Blood low in oxygen

FIGURE 24–3. ◆ Major changes that occur in the newborn's circulatory system. *Note:* From Hole, J. W. (1993). *Human anatomy and physiology* (6th ed.). Dubuque, IA: W. C. Brown. All rights reserved. Reprinted by permission.

Characteristics of Cardiac Function

HEART RATE

Shortly after the first cry and the start of changes in cardiopulmonary circulation, the newborn heart rate accelerates to 175 to 180 beats per minute. The average resting heart rate in the first week of life is 110 to 150 beats per minute in a quiet, healthy, full-term newborn, but may vary significantly during deep sleep or active awake states (Lissauer, 2002). In the full-term newborn, the heart rate may drop to a low of 85 beats per minute during sleep. Apical pulse rates should be obtained by auscultation for a full minute, preferably when the newborn is asleep. Peripheral pulses of all extremities should also be evaluated to detect

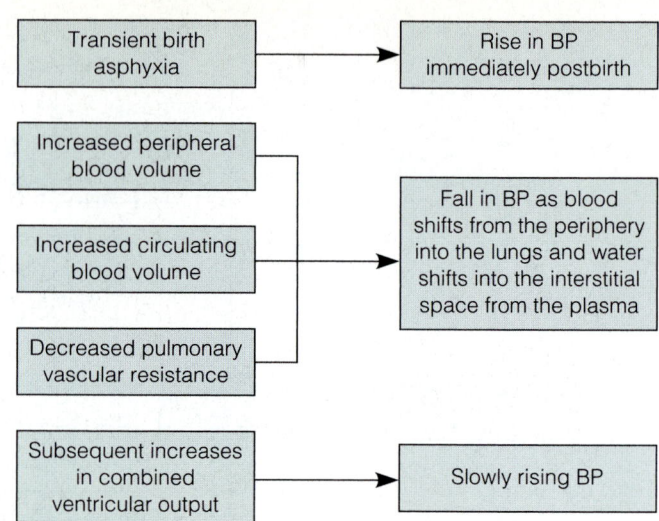

| Transient birth asphyxia | → | Rise in BP immediately postbirth |

Increased peripheral blood volume		
Increased circulating blood volume	→	Fall in BP as blood shifts from the periphery into the lungs and water shifts into the interstitial space from the plasma
Decreased pulmonary vascular resistance		

| Subsequent increases in combined ventricular output | → | Slowly rising BP |

FIGURE 24–4. ◆ Response of blood pressure (BP) to neonatal changes in blood volume.

any inequalities or unusual characteristics. However, peripheral radial pulses are difficult to palpate in the newborn. They can be assessed when blood pressure is measured if blood pressure readings are taken on all four extremities.

BLOOD PRESSURE

The blood pressure tends to be highest immediately after birth and then descends to its lowest level about 3 hours later. By days 4 to 6, the blood pressure rises and plateaus at a level approximately the same as the initial level. Blood pressure is sensitive to the changes in blood volume that occur in the transition to newborn circulation (Figure 24–4 ◆). Peripheral perfusion pressure is a particularly sensitive indicator of the newborn's ability to compensate for alterations in blood volume prior to changes in blood pressure. Capillary refill should be less than 2 to 3 seconds when the skin is blanched.

Blood pressure during the first 12 hours of life varies with the birth weight. Crying may cause an elevation of 20 mm Hg in both the systolic and diastolic blood pressure. An accurate blood pressure is best obtained with the Doppler technique or a 1- to 2-in cuff and a stethoscope over the brachial artery.

HEART MURMURS

Murmurs are produced by turbulent blood flow. They may be heard when blood flows across an abnormal valve or across a stenosed valve, when there is an atrial or ventricular septal defect, or when there is increased flow across a normal valve. In newborns, 90% of all murmurs are transient and not associated with anomalies. Because of the current practice of early discharge, murmurs associated with ventricular septal defect and patent ductus arteriosus are not often picked up until the first well-baby checkup at 4 to 6 weeks of age. Murmurs are sometimes absent even in seriously malformed hearts (Zahka & Lane, 2002).

CARDIAC WORKLOAD

Before birth the right ventricle does approximately two thirds of the cardiac work, resulting in increased size and thickness of the right ventricle at birth. After birth the left ventricle must assume a larger share of the cardiac workload, and it progressively increases in size and thickness. This may explain why right-sided heart defects are better tolerated than left-sided ones and why left-sided heart defects rapidly become symptomatic after birth.

HEMATOPOIETIC SYSTEM

Fetal erythrocytes are large but few in number. After birth, the red blood cell (RBC) count gradually increases as cell size decreases. Neonatal RBCs have a life span of 80 to 100 days, approximately two thirds the life span of adult RBCs. In the first days of life, hematocrit may rise 1 to 2 g/dL above fetal levels as a result of placental transfusion, low oral fluid intake, and diminished extracellular fluid volume. By 1 week postnatally, peripheral hemoglobin is comparable to fetal blood counts. The hemoglobin level declines progressively over the first 2 to 3 months of life (Polin & Fox, 1998). This initial decline in hemoglobin creates a phenomenon known as **physiologic anemia of infancy.**

Leukocytosis is a normal finding, because the stress of birth stimulates increased production of neutrophils during the first few days of life. Neutrophils then decrease to 35% of the total leukocyte count by 2 weeks of age. Eventually, lymphocytes become the predominant type of leukocyte and the total white blood cell count falls.

Blood volume of the term infant is estimated to be 80 to 85 mL/kg of body weight. For example, an 8-lb (3.6-kg) newborn has a blood volume of 290 to 309 mL. Blood volume varies with the amount of placental transfusion during the delivery of the placenta, as well as other factors, including the following:

1. *Delayed cord clamping and the normal shift of plasma to the extravascular spaces.* Newborn hemoglobin and hematocrit values are higher when a placental transfusion occurs after birth. Placental vessels contain about 100 mL of blood at term, most of which can be transfused into the newborn by holding the newborn below the level of the placenta and delaying cord clamping. Blood volume increases by 50% with delayed cord clamping (Polin & Fox, 1998). The increase is reflected by a rise in hemoglobin level and an increase in the hematocrit to about 65% after birth (compared with 48% when the cord is clamped immediately). Although not a routine practice, for greatest accuracy, the initial hemoglobin and hematocrit levels should be measured in the cord blood.

2. *Gestational age.* There appears to be a positive association between gestational age, RBC numbers, and hemoglobin concentration.

TABLE 24–2 Normal Term Newborn Cord Blood Values	
Laboratory Data	*Normal Range*
Hemoglobin	14–20 g/dl
Hematocrit	43–63%
WBC	10,000–30,000/mm³
Neutrophils	40%–80%
Platelets	150,000–350,000/mm³
Reticulocytes	3%–7%
Blood volume	82.3 mL/kg (third day after early cord clamping)
	92.6 mL/kg (third day after delayed cord clamping)
Sodium	126–166 mEq/L
Potassium	5.6–12.0 mEq/L
Chloride	98–110 mEq/L
Calcium	8.2–11.1 mg/dL
Glucose	45–96 mg/dL

3. *Prenatal and/or perinatal hemorrhage.* Significant prenatal or perinatal bleeding decreases the hematocrit level and causes hypovolemia.

4. *The site of the blood sample.* Hemoglobin and hematocrit levels are significantly higher in capillary blood than in venous blood. Sluggish peripheral blood flow creates RBC stasis, increasing RBC concentration in the capillaries. Consequently, blood samples from venous blood sites are more accurate than those from capillary sites.

The concentration of serum electrolytes in the blood indicates the fluid and electrolyte status of the newborn. See Table 24–2 for normal term newborn electrolyte and blood values.

TEMPERATURE REGULATION

Temperature regulation is the maintenance of thermal balance by losing heat to the environment at a rate equal to heat production. Newborns are homeothermic; they attempt to stabilize their internal (core) body temperatures within a range in spite of significant temperature variations in their environment.

Thermoregulation in the newborn can be closely related to the rate of metabolism and oxygen consumption. Within a specific environmental temperature range, called the **neutral thermal environment (NTE),** the rates of oxygen consumption and metabolism are minimal, and internal body temperature is maintained because of thermal balance (LeBlanc, 2002). Thus the normal newborn requires higher environmental temperatures to maintain a thermoneutral environment. Several newborn characteristics affect the establishment of a thermal stability:

- The newborn has decreased subcutaneous fat and a thin epidermis.
- Blood vessels are closer to the skin than in an adult. Therefore, changes in environmental temperature influence the circulating blood, and in turn influence the hypothalamic temperature-regulating center.
- The flexed posture of the term newborn decreases the surface area exposed to the environment, thereby reducing heat loss.

Size and age may also affect the establishment of an NTE. For example, the preterm or small-for-gestational-age (SGA) newborn has less adipose tissue and is hypoflexed and therefore requires higher environmental temperatures to achieve a thermal neutral environment. Larger, well-insulated newborns may be able to cope with lower environmental temperatures. If the environmental temperature falls below the lower limits of the NTE, the newborn responds with increased oxygen consumption and metabolism, which results in greater heat production. Prolonged exposure to the cold may result in depleted glycogen stores and acidosis. Oxygen consumption also increases if the environmental temperature is above the NTE.

Heat Loss

A newborn is at a distinct disadvantage in maintaining a normal temperature. With a large body surface in relation to mass and a limited amount of insulating subcutaneous fat, the full-term newborn loses about four times the heat an adult does. The newborn's poor thermal stability is primarily due to excessive heat loss rather than impaired heat production. Because of the risk of hypothermia and possible cold stress, minimizing heat loss in the newborn after birth is essential (see Chapters 17 and 26 for nursing measures).

Two major routes of heat loss are from the internal core of the body to the body surface and from the external surface to the environment. Usually the core temperature is higher than the skin temperature, resulting in continuous transfer of heat to the surface (LeBlanc, 2002). The greater the difference in temperature between core and skin, the more rapid the transfer. The transfer is accomplished through an increase in oxygen consumption, depletion of glycogen stores, and metabolizing of brown fat. Heat loss from the body surface to the environment takes place in four ways—by convection, radiation, evaporation, and conduction (Figure 24–5 ◆).

- **Convection** is the loss of heat from the warm body surface to the cooler air currents. Air-conditioned rooms, air currents with a temperature below the infant's skin temperature, oxygen by mask, and removal from an incubator for procedures increase convective heat loss in the newborn.

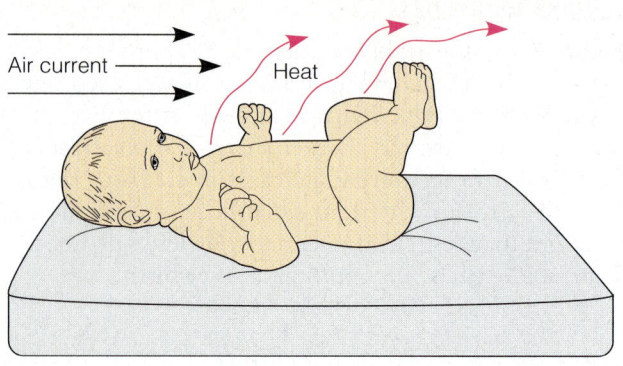

A Convection

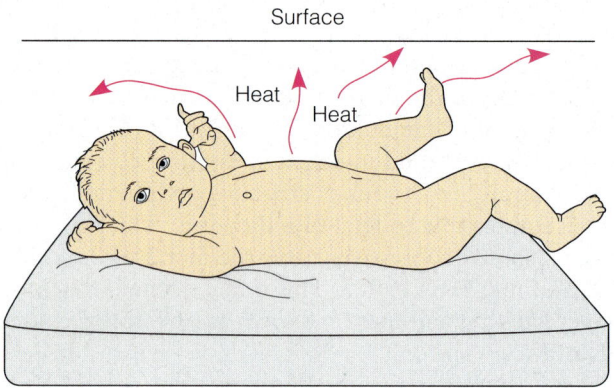

B Radiation

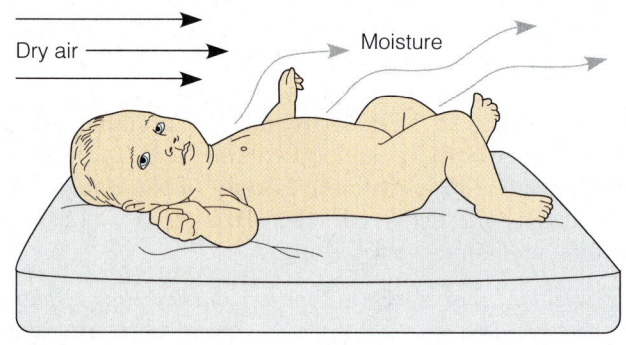

C Evaporation

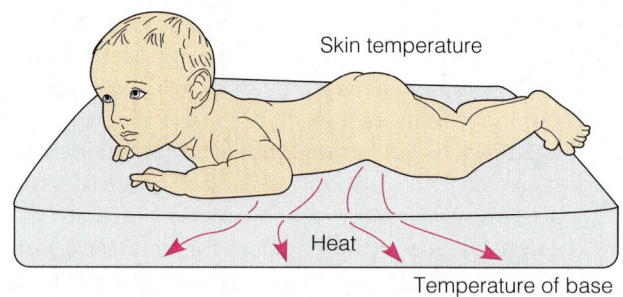

D Conduction

FIGURE 24–5. ◆ Methods of heat loss. **A,** Convection. **B,** Radiation. **C,** Evaporation. **D,** Conduction.

- **Radiation** losses occur when heat transfers from the heated body surface to cooler surfaces and objects not in direct contact with the body. The walls of a room or of an incubator are potential causes of heat loss by radiation, even if the ambient temperature of the incubator is within the thermal neutral range for that infant. Placing cold objects (such as ice for blood gases) onto the incubator or near the infant in the radiant warmer will increase radiant losses.

- **Evaporation** is the loss of heat incurred when water is converted to a vapor. The newborn is particularly prone to lose heat by evaporation immediately after birth (when wet with amniotic fluid), and during baths; therefore, drying the newborn is critical.

- **Conduction** is the loss of heat to a cooler surface by direct skin contact. Chilled hands, cool scales, cold examination tables, and cold stethoscopes can cause loss of heat by conduction. Even if objects are warmed to the incubator temperature, the temperature difference between the infant's core temperature and the ambient temperature may be significant. This difference results in heat transfer.

Once the infant has been dried after birth, the greatest losses of heat generally result from radiation and convection, because of the newborn's large body surface compared with weight, and from thermal conduction, because of the marked difference between core temperature and skin temperature. The newborn can respond to the cooler environmental temperature with adequate peripheral vasoconstriction, but this mechanism is not entirely effective because of the minimal amount of fat insulation present, the large body surface, and ongoing thermal conduction. Therefore, minimizing the baby's heat loss and preventing hypothermia are imperative. (See Chapter 29 for nursing measures to prevent hypothermia and cold stress.)

Heat Production (Thermogenesis)

When exposed to a cool environment, the newborn requires additional heat. The newborn has several physiologic mechanisms that increase heat production, or thermogenesis. They include increased basal metabolic rate, muscular activity, and chemical thermogenesis (also called nonshivering thermogenesis [NST]) (Baumgart, Harrsch, & Touch, 1999).

NST, an important mechanism of heat production unique to the newborn, occurs when skin receptors perceive a drop in the environmental temperature and, in response, transmit sensations to stimulate the sympathetic nervous system. NST uses the infant's stores of **brown adipose tissue (BAT)** (also called brown fat) to provide heat in the cold-stressed newborn. It first appears in the fetus at about 26 to 30 weeks' gestation and continues to increase until 2 to 5 weeks after the birth of a term infant, unless the fat is depleted by cold stress. BAT is deposited in the midscapular area, around the neck, and in the axil-

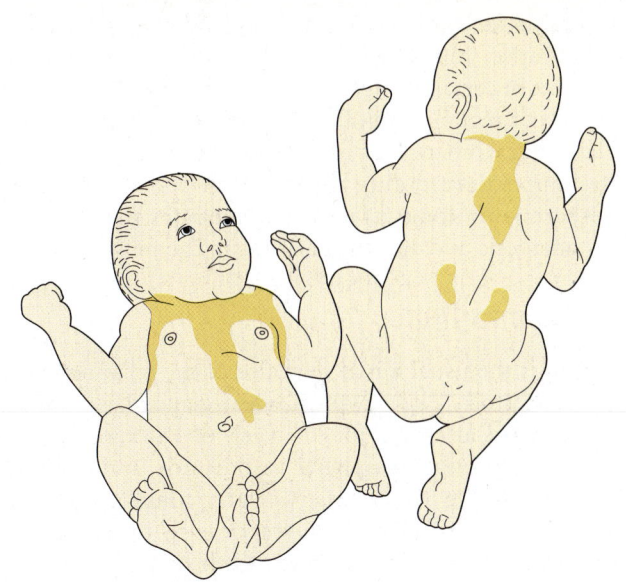

FIGURE 24–6. ◆ The distribution of brown adipose tissue (brown fat) in the newborn. Note: From Davis, V. (1980, November–December). The structure and function of brown adipose tissue in the neonate. *Journal of Obstetric, Gynecologic, and Neonatal Nursing, 9,* 369. Adapted.

las, with deeper placement around the trachea, esophagus, abdominal aorta, kidneys, and adrenal glands (Figure 24–6 ◆). BAT constitutes 2% to 6% of the newborn's total body weight. Brown fat receives its name from the dark color caused by its enriched blood supply, dense cellular content, and abundant nerve endings. The large numbers of brown fat cells increase the speed with which triglycerides are metabolized to produce heat. These characteristics promote rapid metabolism, heat generation, and heat transfer to the peripheral circulation.

A newborn rarely shivers. If he or she does, it means the metabolic rate has already doubled. The extra muscular activity does little to produce needed heat.

Thermographic studies of newborns exposed to cold show an increase in the skin heat produced over the newborn's brown fat deposits between 1 and 14 days of age. However, if the brown fat supply has been depleted, the metabolic response to cold is limited or lacking. The resulting hypothermia causes an increase in basal metabolism and an increase in oxygen consumption. A decrease in the environmental temperature of 2 °C, from 33 to 31 °C, is sufficient to double the oxygen consumption of a term newborn. Keeping the normal newborn warm promotes normal oxygen requirements, whereas chilling can cause the newborn to show signs of respiratory distress.

When exposed to cold, the normal term newborn is usually able to cope with the increase in oxygen requirements, but the preterm newborn may be unable to increase ventilation to the necessary level of oxygen consumption. (See Chapter 29 for discussion of cold stress.) Because oxidation of fatty acids depends on the availability of oxygen, glucose, and adenosine triphosphate (ATP), the newborn's ability to generate heat can be altered by pathologic events such as hypoxia, acidosis, and hypoglycemia or by medication that blocks the release of norepinephrine. The effect of certain drugs, such as meperidine (Demerol), may prevent metabolism of brown fat. Meperidine given to the laboring woman leads to a greater fall in the newborn's body temperature during the neonatal period. Newborn hypothermia prolongs as well as potentiates the effects of many analgesic and anesthetic drugs in the newborn.

Response to Heat

Sweating is the usual initial response of the term newborn to hyperthermia. The newborn sweat glands have limited function until after the fourth week of extrauterine life; heat is lost through peripheral vasodilation and evaporation of insensible water loss. Oxygen consumption and metabolic rate also increase in response to hyperthermia. Severe hyperthermia can lead to death or to gross brain damage if the baby survives.

HEPATIC ADAPTATIONS

In the newborn, the liver is frequently palpable 2 to 3 cm below the right costal margin. It is relatively large and occupies about 40% of the abdominal cavity. The newborn liver plays a significant role in iron storage, carbohydrate metabolism, conjugation of bilirubin, and coagulation.

Iron Storage and RBC Production

As RBCs are destroyed after birth, the iron is stored in the liver until needed for new RBC production. Newborn iron stores are determined by total body hemoglobin content and length of gestation. The term newborn has about 270 mg of iron at birth, and about 140 to 170 mg of this amount is in the hemoglobin. If the mother's iron intake has been adequate, enough iron will be stored to last until the infant is about 5 months of age. After about 6 months of age, foods containing iron or iron supplements must be given to prevent anemia.

Carbohydrate Metabolism

At term, the newborn's cord blood glucose level is 70% to 80% of the maternal blood glucose level (Cornblath, Hawdon, Williams, et al., 2000). Newborn carbohydrate reserves are relatively low. One third of this reserve is in the form of liver glycogen. Newborn glycogen stores are twice those of the adult. The newborn enters an energy crunch at the time of birth, with the removal of the maternal glucose supply and the increased energy expenditure associated with the birth process and extrauterine life. Newborns consume fuel sources at a faster rate because of the work of breathing, loss of heat when exposed to cold, activity, and activation of muscle tone.

Glucose is the main source of energy in the first 4 to 6 hours after birth. During the first 2 hours of life, the serum blood glucose level declines, then rises, and finally reaches a steady state 2 to 3 hours after birth (Cornblath, et al., 2000). Using a Chemstrip, the nurse assesses the glucose level on admission to the newborn nursery and again 4 hours later. As stores of liver and muscle glycogen and blood glucose decrease, the newborn compensates by changing from a predominantly carbohydrate metabolism to fat metabolism. Energy can be derived from fat and protein, as well as from carbohydrates. The amount and availability of each of these "fuel substrates" depend on the ability of immature metabolic pathways (which lack specific enzymes or hormones) to function in the first few days of life.

Conjugation of Bilirubin

Conjugation of bilirubin is the conversion of yellow lipid-soluble pigment into water-soluble pigment. Unconjugated (indirect) bilirubin is a breakdown product derived from hemoglobin released primarily from destroyed RBCs. Unconjugated bilirubin is not in excretable form and is a potential toxin. **Total serum bilirubin** is the sum of conjugated (direct) and unconjugated (indirect) bilirubin.

Fetal unconjugated bilirubin crosses the placenta to be excreted, so the fetus does not need to conjugate bilirubin. Total bilirubin at birth is usually less than 3 mg/dL unless an abnormal hemolytic process has been present in utero. After birth the newborn's liver must begin to conjugate bilirubin by itself. This produces a rise in serum bilirubin levels in the first few days of life.

The bilirubin formed after RBCs are destroyed is transported in the blood bound to albumin. The bilirubin is transferred into the hepatocytes and bound to two intracellular binding proteins. These two proteins determine the amount of bilirubin held in a liver cell for processing and consequently determine the amount of bilirubin uptake into the liver. The activity of glucuronyl transferase attaches unconjugated bilirubin to glucuronic acid (product of liver glycogen), producing conjugated (direct) bilirubin. Direct bilirubin is excreted into the common duct and duodenum. The conjugated (direct) bilirubin then progresses down the intestines, where bacteria transform it into urobilinogen. This product is not reabsorbed but is excreted as a yellow-brown pigment in the stools.

Even after the bilirubin has been conjugated and bound, it can be changed back to unconjugated bilirubin via the enterohepatic circulation. In the intestines, β-glucuronidase enzyme acts to split off (deconjugate) the bilirubin from glucuronic acid if gut bacteria have not first acted on it to produce urobilinogen; the free bilirubin is reabsorbed through the intestinal wall and brought back to the liver via portal vein circulation. This recycling of the bilirubin and decreased ability to clear bilirubin from the system are prevalent in babies with very high β-glucuronidase activity levels and in those with delayed bacterial colonization of the gut (such as those receiving antibiotics) and further increase the newborn's susceptibility to jaundice (Figure 24–7 ◆).

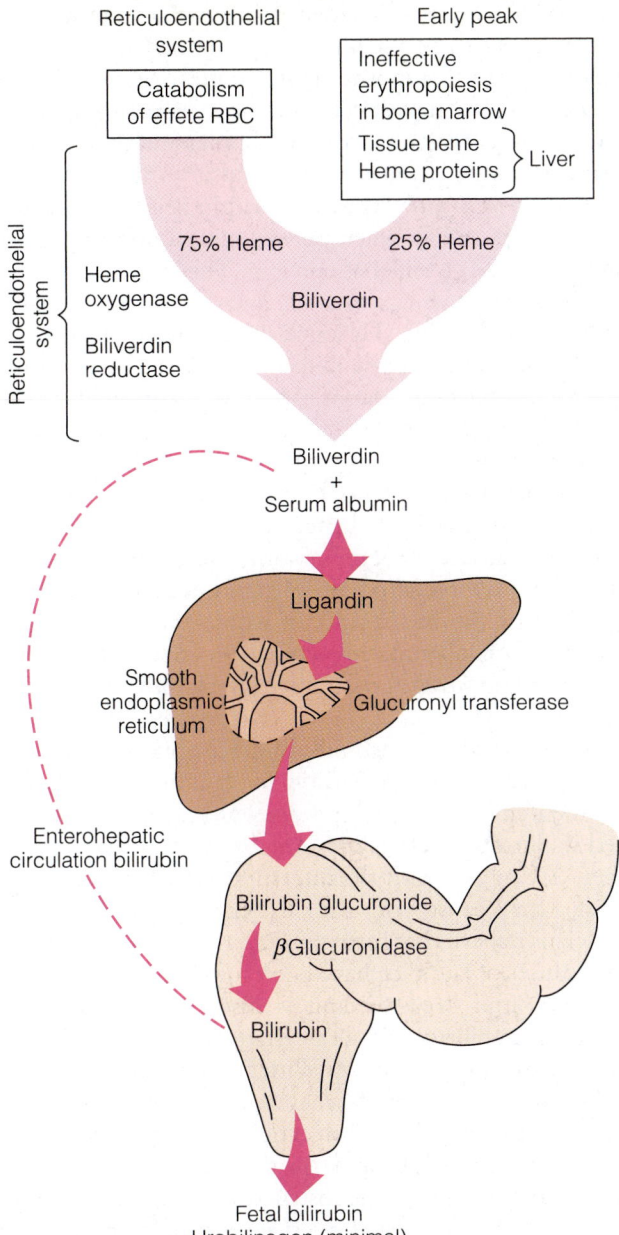

FIGURE 24–7. ◆ Conjugation of bilirubin in the newborn.
Note: From Avery, G. B., Fletcher, M. A., & MacDonald, M. G. (1994). *Neonatology: Pathophysiology and management of the newborn* (4th ed., p. 635). Philadelphia: Lippincott.

The newborn liver has relatively less glucuronyl transferase activity in the first few weeks of life than an adult liver. This lower hepatic activity, along with a relatively large bilirubin load, decreases the liver's ability to conjugate bilirubin and increases susceptibility to jaundice.

Physiologic Jaundice

Physiologic jaundice is caused by accelerated destruction of fetal RBCs, impaired conjugation of bilirubin, and increased bilirubin reabsorption from the intestinal tract.

This condition is not pathologic, but a normal biologic response of the newborn.

Maisels (1999) describes four factors that may interact to create physiologic jaundice:

1. *Increased amounts of bilirubin delivered to the liver.* The increased blood volume due to delayed cord clamping combined with faster RBC destruction in the newborn raises the bilirubin level in the blood. A proportionately larger amount of nonerythrocyte bilirubin forms in the newborn. Therefore, newborns have two to three times greater production or breakdown of bilirubin than do adults. Forceps, which sometimes cause facial bruising or cephalhematoma (entrapped hemorrhage), can increase the amount of bilirubin to be handled by the liver. Decreased oxygen supplies to the liver associated with neonatal hypoxia or congenital heart disease increase the bilirubin level. Reduced bowel motility, intestinal obstruction, or delayed passage of meconium increases the circulation of bilirubin in the enterohepatic pathway, resulting in higher bilirubin values.

2. *Defective hepatic uptake of bilirubin from the plasma.* If the newborn does not ingest adequate calories, the formation of hepatic binding proteins diminishes, resulting in higher bilirubin levels.

3. *Defective conjugation of the bilirubin.* Decreased glucuronyl transferase activity, as in hypothyroidism, and inadequate caloric intake cause the intracellular binding proteins to remain saturated and result in greater unconjugated bilirubin levels in the blood. The fatty acids in breast milk are thought to compete with bilirubin for albumin-binding sites and therefore impede bilirubin processing.

4. *Defect in bilirubin excretion.* A congenital infection may cause impaired excretion. Delay in introduction of bacterial flora and decreased intestinal motility can also delay excretion and increase enterohepatic circulation of bilirubin.

About 50% of term and 80% of preterm newborns exhibit physiologic jaundice on about the second or third day after birth. The characteristic yellow color results from increased levels of unconjugated (indirect) bilirubin, which are a normal product of RBC breakdown and reflect the body's temporary inability to eliminate bilirubin. Serum levels of bilirubin are about 4 to 6 mg/dL before the yellow coloration of the skin and sclera appear. The signs of physiologic jaundice appear after the first 24 hours postnatally. This time frame differentiates physiologic jaundice from pathologic jaundice (see Chapter 26), ⊂⊃ seen at birth or within the first 24 hours of postnatal life.

In the past it was thought that during the first week, unconjugated bilirubin levels in physiologic jaundice should not exceed 13 mg/dL in the term or preterm newborn. Peak bilirubin levels are reached between days 3 and 5 in the term infant and between days 5 and 7 in the preterm infant. But these values are established for European and American Caucasian newborns. Chinese, Japanese, Korean, and Native-American newborns have considerably higher bilirubin levels that are not as apparent and that persist for longer periods with no apparent ill effects (Halamek & Stevenson, 2002).

The nursery or postpartum room environment, including lighting, may hinder the early detection of the degree and type of jaundice. Pink walls and artificial lights mask the beginning of jaundice in newborns. Daylight helps the observer recognize jaundice early.

If jaundice is suspected, quickly assess the newborn's coloring by pressing the skin, generally on the forehead or nose, with a finger. As blanching occurs, observe the icterus (yellow coloring). Several newborn care procedures decrease the probability of high bilirubin levels; specifically, the nurse can:

- Maintain the newborn's skin temperature at 36.5 °C (97.8 °F) or above, because cold stress results in acidosis. Acidosis in turn decreases available serum albumin–binding sites, weakens albumin-binding powers, and causes elevated unconjugated bilirubin levels.

- Monitor stool for amount and characteristics. Bilirubin is eliminated in the feces; inadequate stooling may result in reabsorption and recycling of bilirubin. Encourage early breastfeeding because the laxative effect of colostrum increases excretion of stool.

- Encourage early feedings to promote intestinal elimination and bacterial colonization and to provide the calories needed to form hepatic binding proteins.

If jaundice becomes apparent, nursing care is directed toward keeping the newborn well hydrated and promoting intestinal elimination. (For specific nursing management and therapies, see "Clinical Pathway for the Newborn with Hyperbilirubinemia" in Chapter 29.)

Physiologic jaundice may be very upsetting to parents; they require emotional support and thorough explanation of the condition. If the baby is placed under phototherapy, additional days of hospitalization may be required, which may also be disturbing to parents. They can be encouraged to provide for the emotional needs of their newborn by continuing to feed, hold, and caress the infant. If the mother is discharged, the parents are encouraged to return for feedings and feel free to telephone or visit whenever possible. In many instances, the mother, especially if she is breastfeeding, may elect to remain hospitalized with her newborn; support this decision. Alternatively, the newborn may be treated with home phototherapy.

Breastfeeding and Breast Milk Jaundice

Breastfeeding is implicated in jaundice in some newborns. *Breastfeeding jaundice* occurs in the first days of life in breastfed newborns. Breastfeeding jaundice appears to be associated with poor feeding practices and not with any change in milk composition. Prevention of early breastfeeding jaundice includes encouraging frequent (every 2 to 3 hours) breastfeeding, avoiding supplementation, and accessing maternal lactation counseling.

In *breast milk jaundice*, the bilirubin begins to rise after the first week of life, when physiologic jaundice is waning after the mother's milk has come in. The level peaks at 5 to 10 mg/dL at 2 to 3 weeks of age and declines over the first several months of life (Halamek & Stevenson, 2002).

Some women's breast milk may contain several times the normal concentration of certain free fatty acids. These free fatty acids may compete with bilirubin for binding sites on albumin and inhibit the conjugation of bilirubin or increase lipase activity, disrupting the RBC membrane. Increased lipase activity enhances absorption of bile across the gastrointestinal tract membrane, thereby increasing the enterohepatic circulation of bilirubin. In the past it was thought that the breast milk of women whose newborns have breast milk jaundice contained an enzyme that inhibited glucuronyl transferase, but this hypothesis has been discounted.

Newborns with breast milk jaundice appear well, and at present kernicterus with this type of jaundice has not been documented. Temporary cessation of nursing may be advised if bilirubin reaches presumed toxic levels of approximately 20 mg/dL or if the interruption is necessary to establish the cause of the hyperbilirubinemia. Most physicians believe that breastfeeding may be resumed once other causes of jaundice have been ruled out. Within 24 to 36 hours after breastfeeding is discontinued, the newborn's serum bilirubin levels begin to fall dramatically (Halamek & Stevenson, 2002). With resumption of nursing, the bilirubin concentration may have a slight rise of 2 to 3 mg/dL with a subsequent decline. Nursing mothers need encouragement and support in their desire to breastfeed their infants, assistance and instruction about pumping and expressing milk during the interrupted nursing period, and reassurance that nothing is wrong with their milk or mothering abilities (see Table 24–3).

TABLE 24-3 **Jaundice**	
Physiologic Jaundice	*Breast Milk Jaundice*
Physiologic jaundice occurs after the first 24 hours of life.	Bilirubin levels begin to rise after first week of life after mature breast milk comes in.
During the first week of life, bilirubin should not exceed 13 mg/dL. Some pediatricians allow levels up to 15 mg/dL.	Peak of 5–10 mg/dL is reached at 2 to 3 weeks of age.
Bilirubin levels peak at 3 to 5 days in term infants.	It may be necessary to interrupt nursing for a short period when bilirubin reaches 20 mg/dL.

Coagulation

The liver plays an important part in blood coagulation during fetal life and continues this function to some degree during the first few months after birth. Coagulation factors II, VII, IX, and X (synthesized in the liver) are activated under the influence of vitamin K and therefore are considered vitamin K dependent. The absence of normal flora needed to synthesize vitamin K in the newborn gut results in low levels of vitamin K and creates a transient change in blood coagulation between the second and fifth day of life. From a low point at about 2 to 3 days after birth, these coagulation factors rise slowly, but they do not approach adult levels until 9 months of age or later. Other coagulation factors with low umbilical cord blood levels are XI, XII, and XIII. Fibrinogen and factors V and VII are near adult ranges.

Although newborn bleeding problems are rare, an injection of vitamin K (AquaMEPHYTON) is given prophylactically on the day of birth to combat potential clinical bleeding problems. (Chapter 26 discusses hemorrhagic disease of the newborn in greater depth.) ⫘

Platelet counts at birth are in the same range as for older children, but newborns may have mild transient difficulty in platelet aggregation functioning. Phototherapy accentuates this platelet problem.

Prenatal maternal therapy with phenytoin sodium (Dilantin) or phenobarbital also causes abnormal clotting studies and newborn bleeding in the first 24 hours after birth. Infants born to mothers receiving warfarin sodium (Coumadin) may bleed, because these agents cross the placenta and accentuate existing deficiencies in vitamin K–dependent factor.

GASTROINTESTINAL ADAPTATIONS

By 36 to 38 weeks' gestation, the gastrointestinal system is adequately mature, with enzymatic activity and the ability to transport nutrients. The full-term newborn has enough intestinal and pancreatic enzymes to digest most simple carbohydrates, proteins, and fats.

The carbohydrates newborns must digest are usually disaccharides (lactose, maltose, sucrose). Lactose is the primary carbohydrate in the breastfeeding newborn and is generally easily digested and well absorbed. The only enzyme lacking is pancreatic amylase, which remains relatively deficient during the first few months of life. Newborns have trouble digesting starches (changing more complex carbohydrates into maltose), so they should not eat them until after the first few months of life.

Although proteins require more digestion than carbohydrates, they are well digested and absorbed from the newborn intestine. The newborn digests and absorbs fats less efficiently because of the minimal activity of the pancreatic enzyme lipase. The newborn excretes about 10% to 20% of the dietary fat intake, compared with 10% for the adult. The newborn absorbs the fat in breast milk more completely than the fat in cows' milk, because breast milk consists of more medium-chain triglycerides and contains lipase. (See Chapter 27 for further discussion of infant nutrition.) ⫘

By birth, the newborn has experienced swallowing, gastric emptying, and intestinal propulsion. In utero, fetal swallowing is accompanied by gastric emptying and peristalsis of the fetal intestinal tract. By the end of gestation, peristalsis becomes much more active in preparation for extrauterine life. Fetal peristalsis is also stimulated by anoxia, causing the expulsion of meconium into the amniotic fluid in more mature fetuses.

Air enters the stomach immediately after birth. The small intestine is filled with air within 2 to 12 hours and the large bowel within 24 hours. The salivary glands are immature at birth, and the newborn produces little saliva until about age 3 months. The newborn's stomach has a capacity of about 50 to 60 mL. It empties intermittently, starting within a few minutes of the beginning of a feeding and ending 2 to 4 hours after feeding. The newborn's gastric pH becomes less acidic about a week after birth and remains less acidic than that of adults for the next 2 to 3 months. The cardiac sphincter is immature, as is neural control of the stomach, so some regurgitation may happen in the newborn period. Regurgitation of the first few feedings during the first day or two of life can usually be lessened by avoiding overfeeding and by burping the newborn well during and after the feeding.

When no other signs and symptoms are evident, vomiting is limited and ceases within the first few days of life. Continuous vomiting or regurgitation should be observed closely. If the newborn has swallowed bloody or purulent amniotic fluid, lavage of the stomach may be indicated in the term newborn to relieve the problem. Bilious vomiting is abnormal and must be evaluated thoroughly because it might represent a condition that warrants prompt surgical intervention.

Adequate digestion and absorption are essential for newborn growth and development. If optimal nutritional support is available, postnatal growth should parallel intrauterine growth; that is, after 30 weeks' gestation, the fetus gains 30 g/day and adds 1.2 cm to body length daily. To gain weight at the intrauterine rate, the term newborn requires 120 cal/kg/day. After birth, caloric intake is often insufficient for weight gain until the newborn is 5 to 10 days old. During this time, term newborns may lose 5% to 10% of their weight. A shift of intracellular water to extracellular space and insensible water loss account for the 5% to 10% weight loss; thus, failure to lose weight when caloric intake is inadequate may indicate fluid retention.

Term newborns usually pass meconium within 8 to 24 hours of life and almost always within 48 hours. **Meconium** is formed in utero from the amniotic fluid and its constituents, intestinal secretions, and shed mucosal cells. It is recognized by its thick, tarry black or dark-green appearance. Transitional (thin brown to green) stools con-

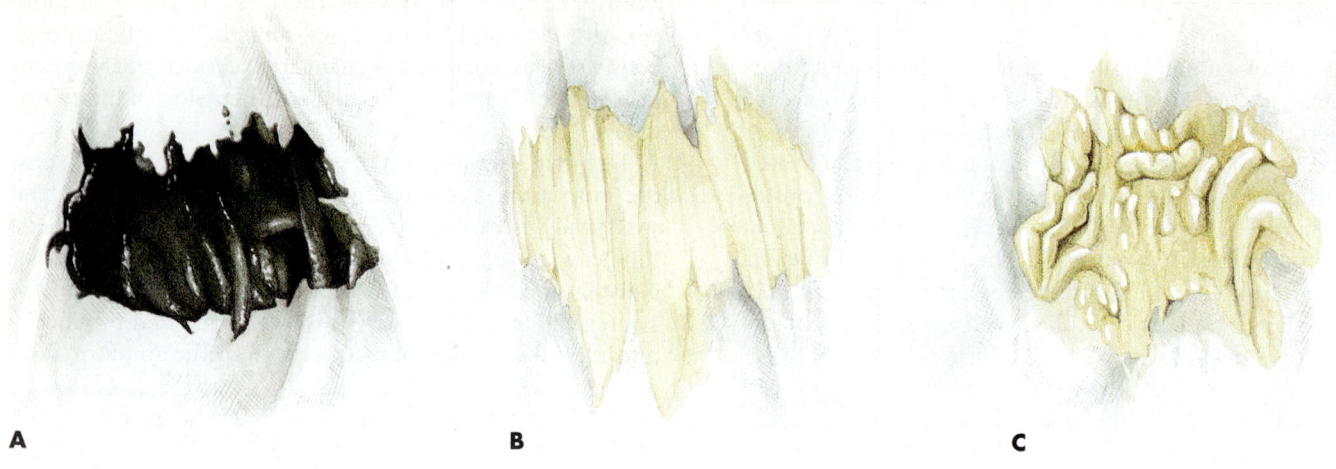

FIGURE 24–8. ◆ Newborn stool samples. **A,** Meconium stool. **B,** Breast milk stool. **C,** Cow's milk stool.

Table 24–4 Physiologic Adaptations to Extrauterine Life	
Respiratory, Skin Temperature, and Blood Glucose	*Stools (progress from):*
Periodic breathing may be present	Meconium (thick, tarry, black)
Desired skin temperature 36–36.5 °C (96.8–97.7 °F) stabilizes 4 to 6 hours after birth.	Transitional stools (thin, brown to green)
Desired blood glucose level reaches 60–70 mg/dL by third postnatal day.	Breastfed infants (yellow-gold, soft, or mushy) Bottle-fed infants (pale yellow, formed, and pasty)

sisting of part meconium and part fecal material are passed for the next day or two, and then the stools become entirely fecal. Generally the stools of a breastfed newborn are pale yellow (but may be pasty green); they are more liquid and more frequent than those of formula-fed newborns, whose stools are paler (Figure 24–8 ◆). Frequency of bowel movement varies but ranges from one every 2 to 3 days to as many as 10 daily. Totally breastfed infants often progress to stools that occur every 5 to 7 days. Mothers should be counseled that the newborn is not constipated as long as the bowel movement remains soft (see Table 24–4).

URINARY ADAPTATIONS

Kidney Development and Function

Certain physiologic features of the newborn's kidneys influence the newborn's ability to handle body fluids and excrete urine:

1. The term newborn's kidneys have a full complement of functioning nephrons by 34 to 36 weeks' gestation.

2. The glomerular filtration rate of the newborn's kidney is low compared with the adult rate. Because of this physiologic inefficiency, the newborn's kidney is unable to dispose of water rapidly when necessary because the kidney favors reabsorption of sodium.

3. The juxtamedullary portion of the nephron has limited capacity to reabsorb HCO_3^- and H^- and concentrate urine. The limitation of tubular reabsorption can lead to inappropriate loss of substances in the glomerular filtrate, such as amino acids, bicarbonate, glucose, and sodium. Full-term newborns are less able than adults to concentrate urine (reabsorb water back into the blood) because the tubules are short and narrow. They have a greater capacity for glomerular filtration than for tubular reabsorption and secretion. Also the reduced ability to concentrate urine is due to the limited excretion of solutes (principally sodium, potassium, chloride, bicarbonate, urea, and phosphate) in the growing newborn. Babies gain the ability to concentrate urine fully by 3 months of age.

Because the newborn has difficulty concentrating urine, the effect of excessive insensible water loss or restricted fluid intake is unpredictable. The newborn kidney is also limited in its dilutional capabilities. Concentrating and dilutional limitations of renal function are important considerations in monitoring fluid therapy to prevent dehydration or overhydration.

Characteristics of Newborn Urinary Function

Many newborns void immediately after birth, and the voiding frequently goes unnoticed. Among normal newborns, 93% void by 24 hours after birth and 98% void by 48 hours after birth (Thureen, et al., 1999). A newborn who has not voided by 48 hours should be assessed for adequacy of fluid intake, bladder distention, restlessness, and symptoms of pain. The appropriate clinical personnel should be notified if indicated.

TABLE 24–5 Newborn Urinalysis Values

Protein < 5–10 mg/dL	Casts 0
WBC < 2–3	Bacteria 0
RBC 0	Color pale yellow

The initial bladder volume is 6 to 44 mL of urine. Unless edema is present, normal urinary output is often limited, and the voidings are scanty until fluid intake increases. The fluid of edema is eliminated by the kidneys, so newborns with edema have a much higher urinary output. The first 2 days postnatally, the newborn voids two to six times daily, with a urine output of 15 mL/day. The newborn subsequently voids 5 to 25 times every 24 hours, with a volume of 25 mL/kg per day.

Following the first voiding, the newborn's urine frequently appears cloudy (due to mucus content) and has a high specific gravity, which decreases as fluid intake increases. Occasionally, pink stains ("brick dust spots") appear on the diaper. These are caused by urates and are innocuous. Blood may occasionally be observed on the diapers of female newborns. This pseudomenstruation is related to the withdrawal of maternal hormones. Males may have bloody spotting from a circumcision if performed. In the absence of apparent causes for bleeding, the clinician should be notified. Normal urine during early infancy is straw colored and almost odorless, although odor occurs when certain drugs are given, metabolic disorders exist, or infection is present. Table 24–5 contains urinalysis values for the normal newborn.

IMMUNOLOGIC ADAPTATIONS

The newborn's immune system is not fully activated until sometime after birth. The limitations in the newborn's inflammatory response result in failure to recognize, localize, and destroy invasive bacteria. Thus the signs and symptoms of infection are often subtle and nonspecific in the newborn. The newborn also has a poor hypothalamic response to pyrogens; therefore, fever is not a reliable indicator of infection. In the neonatal period, hypothermia is a more reliable sign of infection.

The most common class of immune cells are immunoglobulins, a type of antibody secreted by lymphocytes and plasma cells into body fluids. Of the three major types of immunoglobulins primarily involved in immunity—IgG, IgA, and IgM—only IgG crosses the placenta. The pregnant woman forms antibodies in response to illness or immunization, in a process called **active acquired immunity.** The transfer of IgG antibodies to the fetus in utero results in **passive acquired immunity,** since the fetus does not produce the antibodies itself. IgG immunoglobulins are very active against bacterial toxins.

Because the maternal IgG is transferred primarily during the third trimester, preterm newborns (especially those born prior to 34 weeks' gestation) may be more susceptible to infection. In general, newborns have immunity to tetanus, diphtheria, smallpox, measles, mumps, poliomyelitis, and a variety of other bacterial and viral diseases. The period of resistance varies. Immunity against common viral infections such as measles may last 4 to 8 months, whereas immunity to certain bacteria may disappear within 4 to 8 weeks.

The normal newborn produces antibodies in response to an antigen but not as effectively as an older child does. Immunization usually begins at 2 months of age; then the infant can develop active acquired immunity.

IgM immunoglobulins are produced in response to blood group antigens, gram-negative enteric organisms, and some viruses in the expectant mother. Because IgM does not normally cross the placenta, most or all is produced by the fetus beginning at 10 to 15 weeks' gestation. Elevated levels of IgM at birth may indicate placental leaks or, more commonly, antigenic stimulation in utero. Consequently, elevations suggest that the newborn was exposed to an intrauterine infection such as syphilis or TORCH syndrome (toxoplasmosis, rubella, cytomegalovirus, herpesvirus hominis type 2 infection). (For further discussion, see Chapter 13.) The lack of available maternal IgM in the newborn also accounts for the susceptibility to gram-negative enteric organisms such as *Escherichia coli.*

The functions of IgA immunoglobulins are not fully understood. IgA appears to provide protection mainly on secreting surfaces such as the respiratory tract, gastrointestinal tract, and eyes. Serum IgA does not cross the placenta and is not normally produced by the fetus in utero. Unlike the other immunoglobulins, IgA is not affected by gastric action. Colostrum, the forerunner of breast milk, is very high in the secretory form of IgA. It may provide some passive immunity to the infant of a breastfeeding mother. Newborns begin to produce secretory IgA in their intestinal mucosa about 4 weeks after birth.

NEUROLOGIC AND SENSORY-PERCEPTUAL FUNCTIONING

The newborn's brain is about one fourth the size of an adult's, and myelination of nerve fibers is incomplete. Unlike the cardiovascular and respiratory systems, which undergo tremendous changes at birth, the nervous system is minimally influenced by the actual birth process. Because many biochemical and histologic changes have yet to occur in the newborn's brain, the postnatal period is considered a risky time for brain and nervous system development. For neurologic development—including development of intellect—to proceed, the brain and other nervous system structures must mature in an orderly, unhampered fashion. (For discussion of cranial nerves, see Chapter 25.)

Intrauterine Factors Influencing Newborn Behavior

Newborns respond to and interact with the environment in a predictable pattern of behavior that is somewhat shaped by their intrauterine experience. Intrinsic factors such as maternal nutrition and external factors such as the mother's physical environment affect this intrauterine experience. Depending on the newborn's intrauterine experience, neonatal behavioral responses to various stresses vary from dealing quietly with the stimulation, to becoming overreactive and tense, to a combination of the two.

Factors such as exposure to intense auditory stimuli in utero can eventually be manifested in the behavior of the newborn. For example, the fetal heart rate (FHR) initially increases when the pregnant woman is exposed to auditory stimuli, but repetition of the stimuli leads to decreased FHR. Thus the newborn who was exposed to intense noise during fetal life is significantly less reactive to loud sounds postnatally.

Characteristics of Newborn Neurologic Function

The normal newborn's usual position involves partially flexed extremities with the legs near the abdomen. When awake, the newborn's extremities may exhibit purposeless, uncoordinated bilateral movements.

The organization and quality of the newborn's motor activity are influenced by a number of factors, including the following (Brazelton, 1984):

- Sleep-alert states
- Environmental stimuli, such as heat, light, cold, and noise
- Conditions causing a chemical imbalance, such as hypoglycemia
- Hydration status
- State of health
- Recovery from the stress of labor and birth

Eye movements can be seen during the first few days of life. An alert newborn is able to fixate on faces and geometric objects or patterns such as black-and-white stripes. A bright light shining in the newborn's eyes elicits the blinking reflex.

The cry of the newborn should be lusty and vigorous. High-pitched cries, weak cries, and no cries are all causes for concern.

The newborn's body grows in a cephalocaudal (head-to-toe), proximal-distal fashion. The newborn is somewhat hypertonic; that is, there is resistance to extending the elbow and knee joints. Muscle tone should be symmetric. Diminished muscle tone and flaccidity may indicate neurologic dysfunction.

Specific symmetric deep tendon reflexes can be elicited in the newborn. Plantar flexion is present. The knee jerk is brisk; a normal ankle clonus may involve three to four beats. Other reflexes, including the Moro, grasping, Babinski, rooting, and sucking reflexes, are characteristic of neurologic integrity (see Chapter 25).

Complex behavioral patterns reflect the newborn's neurologic maturation and integration. Newborns who can bring a hand to their mouth may be demonstrating motor coordination as well as a self-quieting technique, thus increasing the complexity of the behavioral response. Newborns also possess complex, organized defensive motor patterns; for example, they can remove an obstruction, such as a cloth across the face.

Periods of Reactivity

The baby usually shows a predictable pattern of behavior during the first several hours after birth, characterized by two **periods of reactivity** separated by a sleep phase.

FIRST PERIOD OF REACTIVITY

The first period of reactivity lasts approximately 30 minutes after birth. During this period the newborn is awake and active and may appear hungry and have a strong sucking reflex. This is a natural opportunity to initiate breastfeeding if the mother has chosen it. Bursts of random, diffuse movements alternating with relative immobility may occur. Respirations are rapid, as high as 80 breaths per minute, and there may be retraction of the chest, transient flaring of the nares, and grunting. The heart rate is rapid, and the rhythm may be irregular. Bowel sounds are usually absent.

PERIOD OF INACTIVITY TO SLEEP PHASE

After approximately half an hour the newborn's activity gradually diminishes, and the heart rate and respirations decrease as the newborn enters the sleep phase. The sleep phase may last from a few minutes to 2 to 4 hours. During this period, the newborn will be difficult to awaken and will show no interest in sucking. Bowel sounds become audible, and cardiac and respiratory rates return to baseline values.

SECOND PERIOD OF REACTIVITY

During the second period of reactivity, the newborn is again awake and alert. This period lasts 4 to 6 hours in the normal newborn. Physiologic responses are variable during this stage. The heart and respiratory rates increase; however, be alert for apneic periods, which may cause a drop in the heart rate. The newborn is stimulated to continue breathing during such times. The newborn may change color rapidly and become mildly cyanotic or mottled during these fluctuations. Production of respiratory and gastric mucus increases, and the newborn responds by gagging, choking, and regurgitating.

Continued close observation and intervention may be required to maintain a clear airway during this period of reactivity. The gastrointestinal tract becomes more active. The newborn often passes the first meconium stool during this second active stage, and may also have an initial voiding. The newborn shows he or she is ready to be fed by such behaviors as sucking, rooting, and swallowing. If feeding was not begun in the first period of reactivity, it is done at this time. (See Chapters 26 and 27 for further discussion of this first feeding.)

Behavioral States of the Newborn

The behavior of the newborn can be divided into two categories, the sleep state and the alert state (Brazelton, 1999). These postnatal behavioral states are similar to those that have been identified during pregnancy. Subcategories are identified under each major category.

SLEEP STATES

The sleep states are as follows:

1. *Deep or quiet sleep.* The baby has closed eyes with no eye movements; regular, even breathing; and jerky motions or startles at regular intervals. Behavioral responses to external stimuli are likely to be delayed. Startles are rapidly suppressed, and changes in state are not likely. Heart rate may range from 100 to 120 beats per minute.

2. *Active rapid eye movement (REM).* The baby has irregular respirations; closed eyes, with rapid eye movements visible through the lids; irregular sucking motions; minimal activity; and irregular but smooth movement of the extremities. Environmental and internal stimuli may initiate a startle reaction and a change of state.

Newborn sleep cycles have been recognized and defined according to duration. The length of the cycle depends on the age of the newborn. At term, REM active sleep and quiet sleep occur in intervals of 45 to 50 minutes. About 45% to 50% of the total sleep of the newborn is active sleep, 35% to 45% is quiet sleep, and 10% is transitional between these two periods. It is hypothesized that REM sleep stimulates the growth of the neural system. Over time, the newborn's sleep-wake patterns become diurnal; that is, the newborn sleeps at night and stays awake during the day. (See Chapter 25 for a short discussion of Brazelton's assessment of newborn states.)

ALERT STATES

In the first 30 to 60 minutes after birth, many newborns display a quiet alert state, characteristic of the first period of reactivity (Figure 24–9 ◆). Nurses should use these alert states to encourage bonding and breastfeeding. These periods of alertness tend to be short the first 2 days after birth to allow the baby to recover from the birth process. Subsequent alert states are of choice or of necessity (Brazelton,

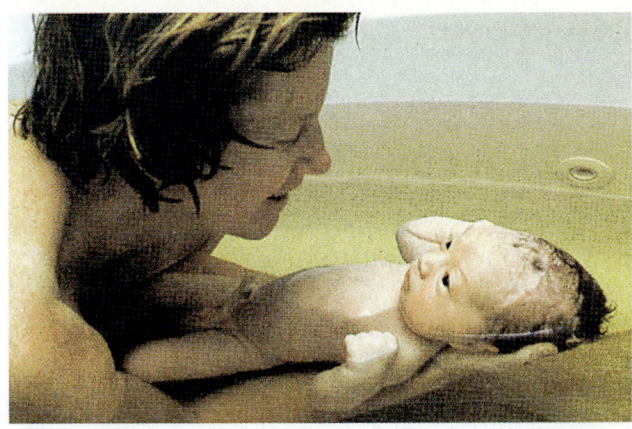

FIGURE 24–9. ◆ Mother and newborn gaze at each other. This quiet, alert state is the optimum state for interaction between baby and parents.

1999). The newborn's increasing choice of wakefulness indicates a maturing capacity to achieve and maintain consciousness. Heat, cold, and hunger are but a few of the stimuli that can cause wakefulness by necessity. Once the disturbing stimuli are removed, the baby tends to fall back asleep.

The following are subcategories of the alert state (Brazelton, 1999):

1. *Drowsy or semidozing.* The behaviors common to the drowsy state are open or closed eyes; fluttering eyelids; semidozing appearance; and slow, regular movements of the extremities. Mild startles may be noted from time to time. Although reaction to a sensory stimulus is delayed, it often causes a change of state.

2. *Wide awake.* In the wide-awake state, the newborn is alert and follows and fixates on attractive objects, faces, or auditory stimuli. Motor activity is minimal, and the response to external stimuli is delayed.

3. *Active awake.* In the active-awake state the newborn's eyes are open and motor activity is quite intense, with thrusting movements of the extremities. Environmental stimuli increase startles or motor activity, but individual reactions are difficult to distinguish because of the generally high activity level.

4. *Crying.* Intense crying is accompanied by jerky motor movements. Crying serves several purposes for the newborn. It may be a distraction from disturbing stimuli such as hunger and pain. Fussiness often allows the newborn to discharge energy and reorganize behavior. Most important, crying elicits an appropriate response of help from the parents.

Behavioral-Sensory Capacities of the Newborn

Habituation is the newborn's ability to process and respond to visual and auditory stimulation. For example,

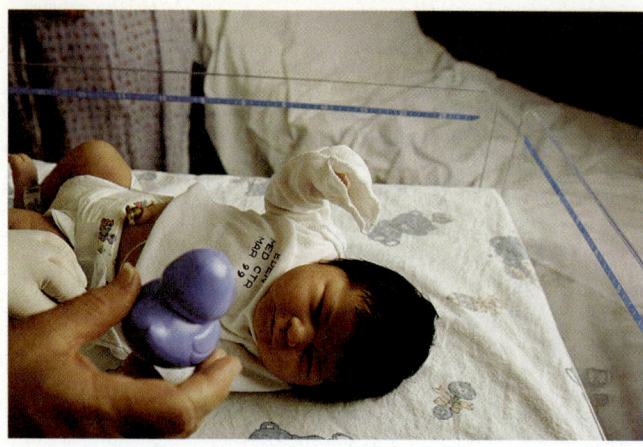

FIGURE 24–10. ◆ Head turning to follow movement.

when a bright light is flashed into the newborn's eyes, the initial response is blinking, constriction of the pupil, and perhaps a slight startle reaction. However, with repeated stimulation, the newborn's response repertoire gradually diminishes and disappears. The capacity to ignore repetitious disturbing stimuli is a newborn defense mechanism readily apparent in the noisy, well-lit nursery.

Orientation is the newborn's ability to be alert to, follow, and fixate on complex visual stimuli that are appealing and attractive. The newborn prefers the human face and eyes and bright shiny objects. As the face or object comes into the line of vision, the newborn responds with bright, wide eyes, still limbs, and fixed staring. This intense visual involvement may last several minutes, during which time the newborn can follow the stimulus from side to side. Figure 24–10 ◆ illustrates this response. The newborn uses this sensory capacity to become familiar with family, friends, and surroundings.

Self-quieting ability refers to newborns' ability to quiet and comfort themselves. Their repertoire includes hand-to-mouth movements, sucking on a fist or tongue, and attending to external stimuli. Neurologically impaired newborns cannot use self-quieting activities and require more frequent comforting from caregivers when stimulated. For example, drug-positive newborns often exhibit abnormal sleep and feeding patterns and irritability.

AUDITORY CAPACITY

The newborn responds to auditory stimulation with a definite, organized behavior repertoire. The stimulus used to assess auditory response should match the state of the newborn. A rattle is appropriate for light sleep, a voice for an awake state, and a clap for deep sleep. As the newborn hears the sound, the cardiac rate rises, and may have a minimal startle reflex. If the sound is appealing, the newborn will become alert and search for its source.

OLFACTORY CAPACITY

Newborns can apparently select people by smell. In one study, newborns could distinguish their mothers' breast pads from those of other mothers at just 5 days of age (Brazelton, 1999).

TASTE AND SUCKING

The newborn responds differently to varying tastes. Sugar, for example, increases sucking. Newborns fed with a rubber nipple versus the breast also show sucking pattern variations. When breastfeeding, the newborn sucks in bursts, with frequent regular pauses. The bottle-fed newborn tends to suck at a regular rate, with infrequent pauses.

When awake and hungry, the newborn makes rapid searching motions in response to the rooting reflex. Once feeding begins, the newborn establishes a sucking pattern according to the method of feeding. Finger sucking happens not only postnatally but also in utero. The newborn often uses nonnutritive sucking as a self-quieting activity, which helps develop self-regulation. For bottle-fed infants, there is no reason to discourage nonnutritive sucking with a pacifier. For breastfed infants, pacifiers should be offered only after breastfeeding is well established. If the pacifier is offered too soon, the breastfed infant may develop "nipple confusion," and have difficulty learning to suck from the breast (see Chapter 27). 🔗

TACTILE CAPACITY

The newborn is very sensitive to being touched, cuddled, and held. Often a mother's first response to an upset or crying newborn is touching or holding. Swaddling, placing a hand on the abdomen, or holding the arms to prevent a startle reflex are other ways to sooth the newborn. The settled newborn can then attend to and interact with the environment.

CHAPTER HIGHLIGHTS

☙ Newborn respiration is initiated primarily by chemical and mechanical events, in association with thermal and sensory stimulation.

☙ Surfactant is crucial to keeping the lungs expanded during expiration by reducing alveolar surface tension.

☙ The newborn is an obligatory nose breather. Respirations change from being primarily shallow, irregular, and diaphragmatic to synchronous abdominal and chest breathing. Normal respiratory rate is 30 to 60 beats per minute.

- Periodic breathing is normal, and newborn sleep states affect breathing patterns.

- The status of the cardiopulmonary system may be measured by evaluating the heart rate, blood pressure, and presence or absence of murmurs. The normal heart rate is 120 to 160 beats per minute.

- Blood values in the newborn are modified by several factors, such as site of the blood sample, gestational age, prenatal and/or perinatal hemorrhage, and the timing of the clamping of the umbilical cord.

- Blood glucose levels should reach a steady state by 4 hours of age.

- The newborn is considered to have established thermoregulation when oxygen consumption and metabolic activity are minimal.

- Evaporation is the primary heat loss mechanism in newborns who are wet from amniotic fluid or a bath. In addition, excessive heat loss occurs from radiation and convection, because of the newborn's larger surface area compared with weight, and from thermal conduction, because of the marked difference between core temperature and skin temperature.

- The primary source of heat in the cold-stressed newborn is brown adipose tissue.

- The normal newborn can digest and absorb nutrients necessary for newborn growth and development.

- The newborn's liver plays a crucial role in iron storage, carbohydrate metabolism, conjugation of bilirubin, and coagulation.

- Physiologic jaundice may be seen between 3 and 5 days of life in term infants.

- The newborn's stools change from meconium (thick, tarry, dark green) to transitional stools (thin, brown-to-green) and then to the distinct forms for either breastfed newborns (yellow-gold, soft, or mushy) or bottle-fed newborns (pale yellow, formed, and pasty). Most newborns pass their first stool within 24 hours of birth.

- The newborn's kidneys have decreased rate of glomerular flow, limited tubular reabsorption, limited excretion of solutes, and limited ability to concentrate urine. Most newborns void within 24 hours of birth.

- The immune system in the newborn is not fully activated until sometime after birth, but the newborn possesses some immunologic abilities.

- Neurologic and sensory-perceptual functioning in the newborn are evident from the newborn's interaction with the environment, synchronized motor activity, and well-developed sensory capacities.

- The first period of reactivity lasts for 30 minutes after birth. The newborn is alert and hungry at this time, making this a natural opportunity to promote attachment.

- The second period of reactivity requires close monitoring by the nurse because apnea, decreased heart rate, gagging, choking, and regurgitation are likely to occur and require nursing intervention.

- The behavioral states in the newborn can be divided into sleep states and alert states.

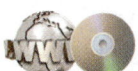 **EXPLOREMEDIALINK**

NCLEX Review, Case Studies, and other interactive resources for this chapter can be found on the companion website at http://www.prenhall.com/london. Click on "Chapter 24" to select the activities for this chapter.

For animations, more NCLEX review questions, and an audio glossary, access the accompanying CD-ROM in this textbook.

REFERENCES

Baumgart, S., Harrsch, S. C., & Touch, S. M. (1999). Thermoregulation. In G. B. Avery, M. A. Fletcher, & M. G. MacDonald (Eds.), *Neonatology: Pathophysiology and management of the newborn* (5th ed., pp. 395–408). Philadelphia: Lippincott.

Brazelton, T. B. (1984). *Neonatal behavioral assessment scale* (2nd ed.). London: Heineman.

Brazelton, T. B. (1999). Behavioral competence. In G. B. Avery, M. A. Fletcher, & M. G. MacDonald (Eds.), *Neonatology: Pathophysiology and management of the newborn* (5th ed., pp. 321–332). Philadelphia: Lippincott.

Cornblath, M., Hawdon, J. M., Williams, A. F., Aynsley-Green, A., Ward-Platt, M. P., Schwartz, R., et al. (2000). Controversies regarding definition of neonatal hypoglycemia: Suggested operational thresholds. *Pediatrics, 105*(5), 1141–1145.

Halamek, L. P., & Stevenson, D. K. (2002). Neonatal jaundice and liver disease. In A. A. Fanaroff & R. J. Martin (Eds.), *Neonatal-perinatal medicine* (7th ed., pp. 1309–1350). St. Louis, MO: Mosby.

Johnston, P. G. B. (1998). *The newborn child* (8th ed.). New York: Churchill.

LeBlanc, M. H. (2002). The physical environment. In A. A. Fanaroff & R. J. Martin (Eds.), *Neonatal-perinatal medicine* (7th ed., pp. 512–530). St. Louis, MO: Mosby.

Lissauer, T. (2002). Physical examination of the newborn. In A. A. Fanaroff & R. J. Martin (Eds.), *Neonatal-perinatal medicine* (7th ed., pp. 441–450). St. Louis, MO: Mosby.

Maisels, M. J. (1999). Jaundice. In G. B. Avery, M. A. Fletcher, & M. G. MacDonald (Eds.), *Neonatology: Pathophysiology and manage-*

ment of the newborn (5th ed., pp. 765–819). Philadelphia: Lippincott.

Nelson, N. M. (1999). The onset of respiration. In G. B. Avery, M. A. Fletcher, & M. G. MacDonald (Eds.), *Neonatology: Pathophysiology and management of the newborn* (5th ed., pp. 257–278). Philadelphia: Lippincott.

Polin, R. A., & Fox, W. W. (1998). *Fetal and neonatal physiology* (2nd ed.). Philadelphia: Saunders.

Thureen, P. J., Deacon, J., O'Neill, P., & Hernandez, J. (1999). *Assessment and care of the well newborn*. Philadelphia: Saunders.

Zahka, K. G., & Lane, J. R. (2002). Approach to the neonate with cardiovascular disease. In A. A. Fanaroff & R. J. Martin (Eds.), *Neonatal-perinatal medicine* (7th ed., pp. 1112–1120). St. Louis, MO: Mosby.

CHAPTER 25

Nursing Assessment of the Newborn

ike most parents, when I held my son for the first time, I checked that all his fingers and toes were present. Then he looked at me with wide, bright, serious eyes and began my introduction to his unique personality.

—LEAH, 23

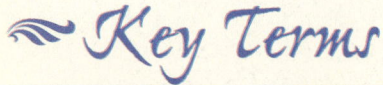 Key Terms

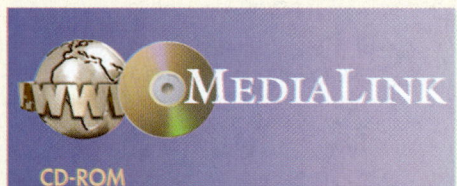

MediaLink

CD-ROM

Clinical Estimation of Gestational Age

Audio Glossary

NCLEX Review

COMPANION WEBSITE

http://www.prenhall.com/london

Techniques for Assessing Selected Primitive Reflexes, with Normal Findings and Their Expected Age of Occurrence

Nursing Assessment of the Newborn Web Links

Thinking Critically

NCLEX Review

Case Study

Unlike the adult, the newborn communicates needs primarily by behavior. Because the nurse is the most consistent observer of the newborn, he or she can translate this behavior into information about the newborn's condition and respond with appropriate nursing interventions. This chapter focuses on the assessment of the newborn and the interpretation of the findings. Newborn assessment is a continuous process designed to evaluate development and adjustments to extrauterine life. In the birth setting, the Apgar scoring procedure (see Chapter 17 ⊂⊃ for discussion) and careful observation form the basis of assessment and are correlated with information such as the following:

- Maternal prenatal care history
- Birthing history
- Maternal analgesia and anesthesia
- Complications of labor or birth
- Treatment instituted immediately after birth, in conjunction with determination of clinical gestational age
- Consideration of the classification of newborns by weight and gestational age and by neonatal mortality risk
- Physical examination of the newborn

The nurse incorporates data from these sources with the assessment findings during the first 1 to 4 hours after birth to formulate a plan for nursing intervention. The various newborn assessments and the data obtained from them are only valuable to the degree to which they are shared with the parents. The parents must be included in the assessment process from the moment of their child's birth. The Apgar score and its meaning should be explained immediately to the family. As soon as possible, the parents should take part in the physical and behavioral assessments as well.

Encourage the parents to identify their newborn's unique behavioral characteristics. Promote attachment by giving parents a chance to explore their newborn in private and identify individual physical and behavioral characteristics. The nurse's supportive responses to parents' questions and observations are essential throughout the assessment process. The newborn physical examination therefore is the beginning of newborn health surveillance and health education for the newborn's family that continues into the community setting.

TIMING OF NEWBORN ASSESSMENTS

During the first 24 hours of life, the newborn makes the critical transition from intrauterine to extrauterine life. The risk of mortality and morbidity is statistically high during this period. Assessment of the newborn is essential to en-

sure that the transition is proceeding successfully (Rinehart, Terrone, & Magann, 2000).

There are three major time frames for assessments of newborns while they are in the birth facility:

- The first assessment is done in the birthing area immediately after birth to determine the need for resuscitation or other interventions. The stable newborn can stay with the family after birth to initiate early attachment. The newborn with complications is usually taken to the nursery for further evaluation and intervention.
- A second assessment is done within the first 4 hours after birth as part of routine admission procedures. During this assessment, the nurse carries out a brief physical examination to estimate gestational age ⊂⊃ CD WEB and evaluate the newborn's adaptation to extrauterine life. No later than 2 hours after birth, the admitting nursery nurse should evaluate the newborn's status and any problems that place the newborn at risk (American Academy of Pediatrics [AAP] & American College of Obstetricians and Gynecologists [ACOG], 1997).
- Before discharge, a certified nurse-midwife, physician, or nurse practitioner carries out a behavioral assessment and a complete physical examination to detect any emerging or potential problems. A general assessment is also done at this time.

This chapter presents the procedures for estimating gestational age and performing the complete physical examination and behavioral assessment (see Table 25–1). (Chapter 17 discusses the immediate postbirth assessment.) ⊂⊃

TABLE 25–1 Timing and Types of Newborn Assessments

Assess immediately after birth
- Need for resuscitation
- If newborn is stable and can be placed with parents to initiate early attachment and bonding

Assessments within 1 to 4 hours after birth
- Progress of newborn's adaptation to extrauterine life
- Determination of gestational age
- Ongoing assessment for high-risk problems

Assessment procedures within first 24 hours or prior to discharge
- Complete physical examination (Depending on agency protocol, the nurse may complete some components independently, with the certified nurse-midwife, physician, or nurse practitioner completing the exam prior to discharge.)
- Nutritional status and ability to bottle-feed or breastfeed satisfactorily
- Behavioral state organization abilities

ESTIMATION OF GESTATIONAL AGE

Establish the newborn's gestational age in the first 4 hours after birth so that careful attention can be given to age-related problems. Traditionally a newborn's gestational age was determined from the date of the pregnant woman's last menstrual period, but this method was accurate only 75% to 85% of the time. Because of the problems that develop with the preterm newborn or the newborn whose weight is inappropriate for gestational age, a more accurate system was developed to postnatally evaluate the newborn. Once learned, the procedure can be done in a few minutes. *It is essential to wear gloves when assessing the newborn in these early hours after birth and before the first bath.*

Clinical **gestational age assessment tools** have two components: external physical characteristics and neurologic or neuromuscular development. Physical characteristics generally include sole creases, amount of breast tissue, amount of lanugo, cartilaginous development of the ear, and testicular descent and scrotal rugae or labial development. These objective clinical criteria are not influenced by labor and birth and do not change significantly within the first 24 hours after birth. The optimal accuracy of gestational age estimates are most accurate when done within 12 hours of birth.

Neurologic examination facilitates assessment of functional or physiologic maturation in addition to physical development. However, the newborn's nervous system is unstable during the first 24 hours of life; neurologic findings based on reflexes or assessments dependent on the higher brain centers may not be reliable. If the neurologic findings drastically deviate from the gestational age derived by evaluation of external characteristics, a second assessment is done in 24 hours.

The neurologic assessment components (excluding reflexes) can aid in assessing the gestational age of newborns of less than 34 weeks' gestation. Between 26 and 34 weeks, neurologic changes are significant, whereas significant physical changes are less evident. One significant neurologic change is that extensor tone is replaced by flexor tone in a caudocephalad (tail-to-head) progression.

Ballard, Khoury, Wedig, et al. (1991) developed the *estimation of gestational age by maturity rating,* a simplified version of the well-researched Dubowitz tool. Ballard's tool gives each physical and neuromuscular finding a value, and the total score is matched to a gestational age (Figure 25–1 ◆). The maximum score on Ballard's tool is 50, which corresponds to a gestational age of 44 weeks.

For example, after completing a gestational assessment of a 1-hour-old newborn, the nurse gives a score of 3 to all the physical characteristics, for a total of 18, and gives a score of 3 to all neuromuscular assessments, for a total of 18. The physical characteristics score of 18 is added to the neurologic score of 18 for a total score of 36, which correlates with 38+ weeks' gestation. Because all newborns have slightly varied development of physical characteristics and maturation of neurologic function, scores usually differ instead of all being 3, as in this example.

Postnatal gestational age assessment tools can overestimate preterm gestational age and underestimate postterm gestational age. The tools have been shown to lose accuracy for newborns of fewer than 28 weeks' or more than 43 weeks' gestation. Also the assessments should be made within 12 hours of birth to optimize accuracy, especially in infants of less than 26 weeks' gestational age (Ballard et al., 1991). Current research still suggests that gestational age scoring scales need to be refined so they can better help determine the care given extremely premature infants (Donovan, Tyson, Ehrenkranz, et al., 1999).

In carrying out gestational age assessments, keep in mind that some maternal conditions, such as pregnancy-induced hypertension (PIH), diabetes, and maternal analgesia and anesthesia, may affect certain gestational assessment components and warrant further study. Maternal diabetes, although it appears to accelerate fetal physical growth, seems to retard maturation. Maternal hypertensive states, which retard fetal physical growth, seem to speed maturation.

Newborns of women with PIH have a poor correlation with the criteria involving active muscle tone and edema. Maternal analgesia and anesthesia may cause respiratory depression in the baby. Babies with respiratory distress syndrome (RDS) tend to be flaccid and edematous and to assume a "froglike" posture. These characteristics affect the scoring of the neuromuscular components of the assessment tool.

Assessment of Physical Characteristics

First, evaluate observable characteristics without disturbing the baby (Rinehart et al., 2000). Selected physical characteristics common to all gestational assessment tools are presented here in the order in which they can be evaluated most effectively:

1. *Resting posture,* although a neuromuscular component, should be assessed as the baby lies undisturbed on a flat surface (Figure 25–2 ◆).

2. *Skin* in the preterm newborn appears thin and transparent, with veins prominent over the abdomen early in gestation. As term approaches, the skin appears opaque because of increased subcutaneous tissue. Disappearance of the protective vernix caseosa promotes skin desquamation and is commonly seen in postmature infants (infants of more than 42 weeks' gestational age and showing signs of placental insufficiency; see Chapter 28). ⬭

3. *Lanugo,* a fine hair covering, decreases as gestational age increases. The amount of lanugo is greatest at 28 to 30 weeks and then disappears, first from the face and then from the trunk and extremities.

NEWBORN MATURITY RATING & CLASSIFICATION

ESTIMATION OF GESTATIONAL AGE BY MATURITY RATING
Symbols: X - 1st Exam O - 2nd Exam

NEUROMUSCULAR MATURITY

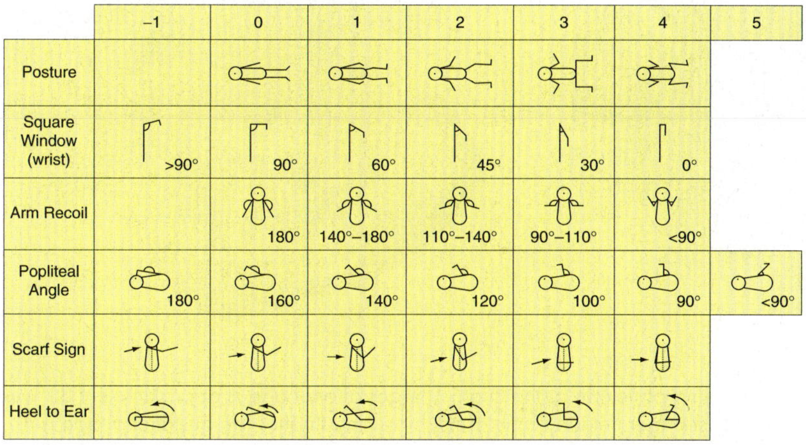

	–1	0	1	2	3	4	5
Posture							
Square Window (wrist)	>90°	90°	60°	45°	30°	0°	
Arm Recoil		180°	140°–180°	110°–140°	90°–110°	<90°	
Popliteal Angle	180°	160°	140°	120°	100°	90°	<90°
Scarf Sign							
Heel to Ear							

PHYSICAL MATURITY

Skin	sticky friable transparent	gelatinous red, translucent	smooth pink, visible veins	superficial peeling &/or rash, few veins	cracking pale areas rare veins	parchment deep cracking no vessels	leathery cracked wrinkled
Lanugo	none	sparse	abundant	thinning	bald areas	mostly bald	
Plantar Surface	heel-toe 40–50mm:–1 <40mm:–2	>50mm no crease	faint red marks	anterior transverse crease only	creases ant. 2/3	creases over entire sole	
Breast	imperceptible	barely perceptible	flat areola no bud	stippled areola 1–2mm bud	raised areola 3–4mm bud	full areola 5–10mm bud	
Eye/Ear	lids fused loosely:–1 tightly:–2	lids open pinna flat stays folded	sl. curved pinna; soft; slow recoil	well curved pinna; soft but ready recoil	formed & firm instant recoil	thick cartilage ear stiff	
Genitals male	scrotum flat, smooth	scrotum empty faint rugae	testes in upper canal rare rugae	testes descending few rugae	testes down good rugae	testes pendulous deep rugae	
Genitals female	clitoris prominent labia flat	prominent clitoris small labia minora	prominent clitoris enlarging minora	majora & minora equally prominent	majora large minora small	majora cover clitoris & minora	

Gestation by Dates _____ wks

Birth Date _____ Hour _____ am/pm

APGAR _____ 1 min _____ 5 min

MATURITY RATING

score	weeks
–10	20
–5	22
0	24
5	26
10	28
15	30
20	32
25	34
30	36
35	38
40	40
45	42
50	44

SCORING SECTION

	1st Exam = X	2nd Exam = O
Estimating Gest Age by Maturity Rating	_____Weeks	_____Weeks
Time of Exam	Date _____ Hour_____ am/pm	Date _____ Hour_____ am/pm
Age at Exam	_____ Hours	_____ Hours
Signature of Examiner	_____ M.D.	_____ M.D.

FIGURE 25–1. ◆ Newborn maturity rating and classification. If a 1-hour-old newborn is given a score of 3 for each of the physical characteristics and neuromuscular assessments, the newborn's total score would be 36. A total score of 36 correlates with 38+ weeks' gestation. *Note:* From Ballard, J. L., Khoury, J. C., Wedig, K., Wang, L., Eilers-Walsmann, B. L., & Lipp, R. (1991). New Ballard score, expanded to include extremely premature infants. *Journal of Pediatrics, 119,* 417.

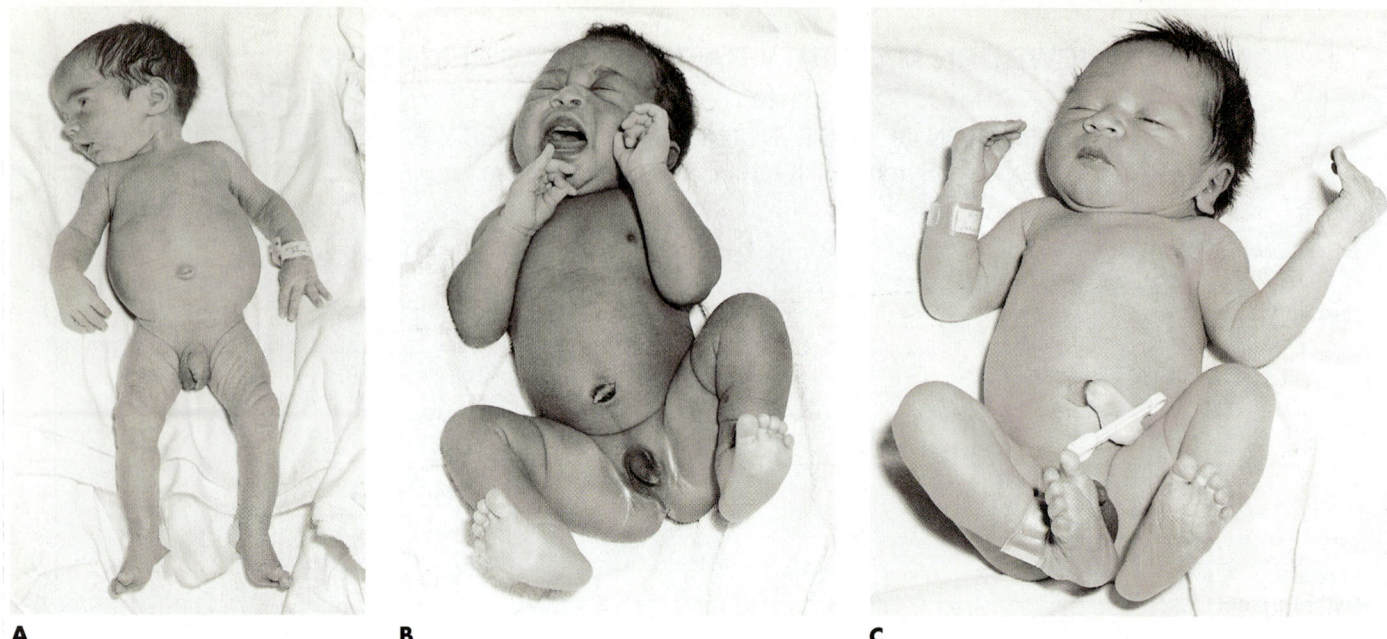

FIGURE 25–2. ◆ Resting posture. **A,** Newborn exhibits beginning of flexion of the thigh. The gestational age is approximately 31 weeks. Note the extension of the upper extremities. **B,** Newborn exhibits stronger flexion of the arms, hips, and thighs. The gestational age is approximately 35 weeks. **C,** The full-term newborn exhibits hypertonic flexion of all extremities. *Note:* Reprinted by permission of V. Dubowitz, MD, Hammersmith Hospital, London, England.

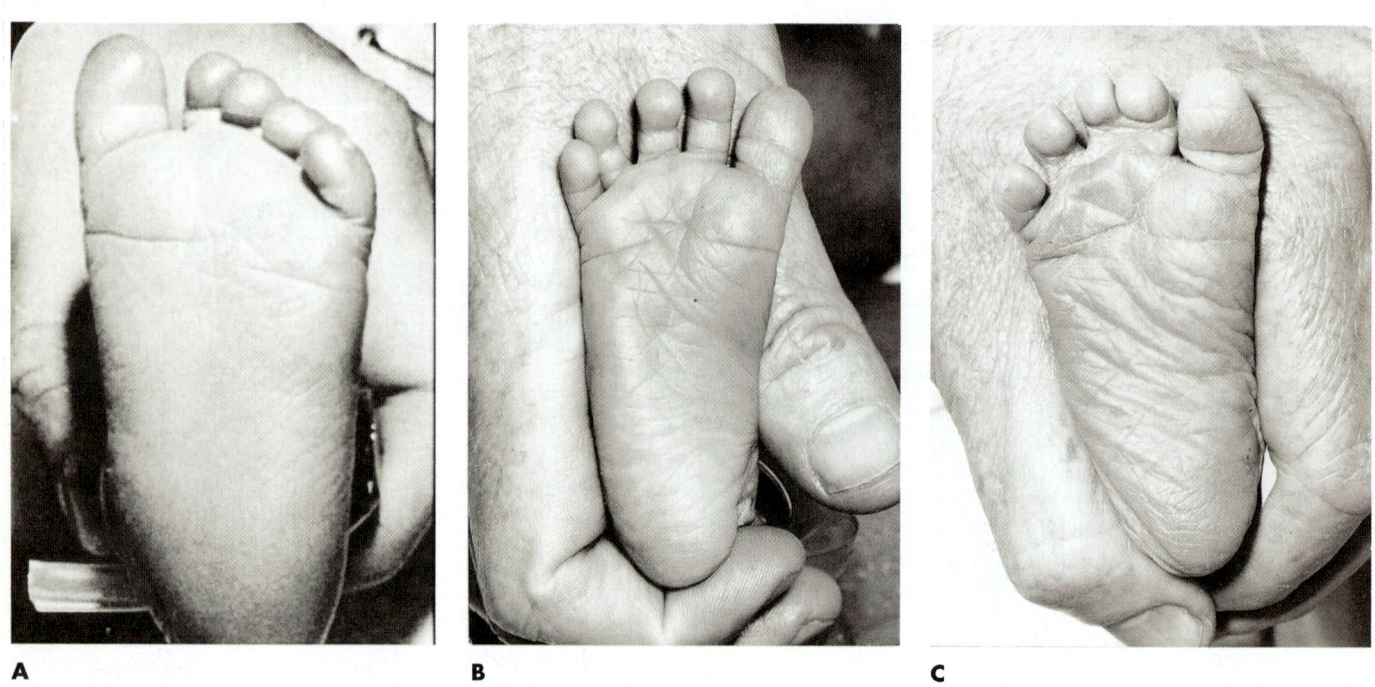

FIGURE 25–3. ◆ Sole creases. **A,** Newborn has a few sole creases on the anterior portion of the foot. Note the slick heel. The gestational age is approximately 35 weeks. **B,** Newborn has a deeper network of sole creases on the anterior two thirds of the sole. Note the slick heel. The gestational age is approximately 37 weeks. **C,** The term newborn has deep sole creases down to and including the heel as the skin loses fluid and dries after birth. Sole (plantar) creases can be seen even in preterm newborns. *Note:* **B** and **C** reprinted by permission of V. Dubowitz, MD, Hammersmith Hospital, London, England.

4. *Sole (plantar) creases* reliably indicate gestational age in the first 12 hours of life. After this, the skin of the foot begins drying, and superficial creases appear. Development of sole creases begins at the top (anterior) portion of the sole and, as gestation progresses, proceeds to the heel (Figure 25–3 ◆). Peeling may also occur. Plantar creases vary with race. In newborns of African descent, sole creases may be less developed at term.

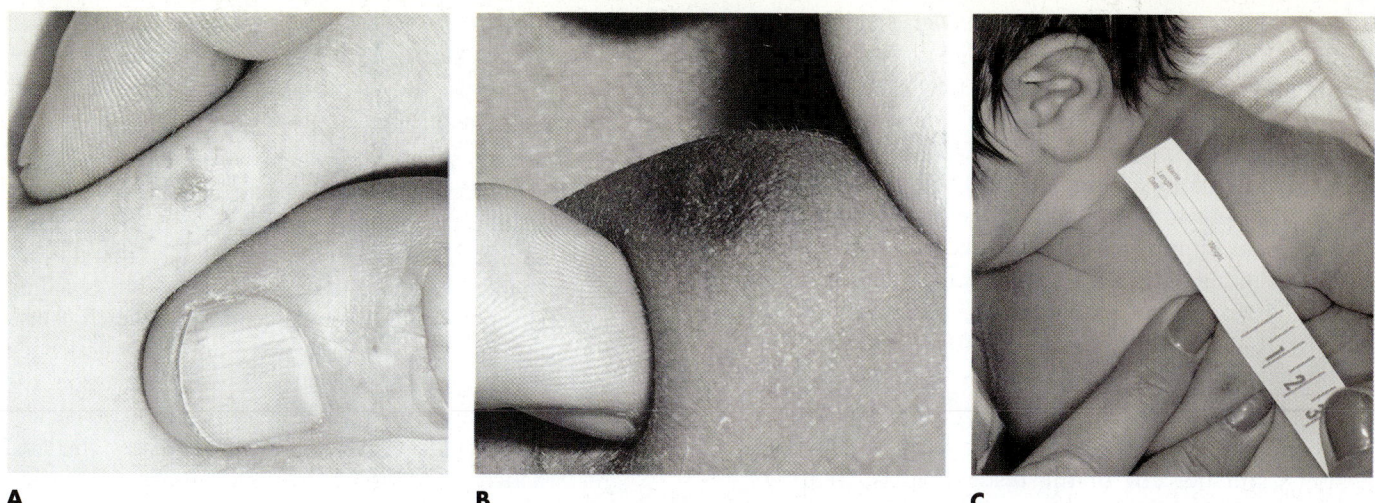

FIGURE 25–4. ◆ Breast tissue. **A,** Newborn has a visible raised area. On palpation the area is 4 mm. The gestational age is 38 weeks. **B,** Newborn has 10 mm breast tissue area. The gestational age is 40 to 44 weeks. **C,** Gently compress the tissue between the middle and index fingers and measure the tissue in centimeters or millimeters. Absence of or decreased breast tissue often indicates premature or small-for-gestational-age newborn. *Note:* **A** and **B** reprinted by permission of V. Dubowitz, MD, Hammersmith Hospital, London, England.

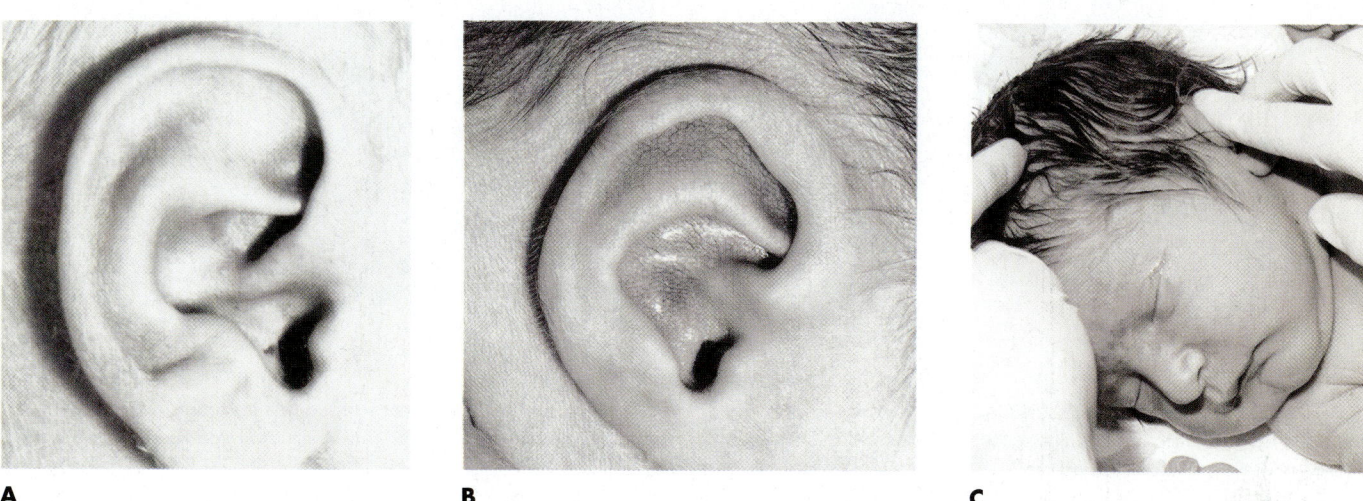

FIGURE 25–5. ◆ Ear form and cartilage. **A,** The ear of the infant at approximately 36 weeks' gestation shows incurving of the upper two thirds of the pinna. **B,** Infant at term shows well-defined incurving of the entire pinna. **C,** If the auricle stays in the position in which it is pressed or returns slowly to its original position, it usually means the gestational age is less than 38 weeks. *Note:* **A** and **B** reprinted by permission of V. Dubowitz, MD, Hammersmith Hospital, London, England.

5. The *areola* and breast tissue are assessed for size. At term gestation, the tissue measures between 0.5 and 1 cm (5 and 10 mm). As gestation progresses, the breast tissue mass and areola enlarge. To assess size, gently palpate the *breast bud tissue* by applying the forefinger and middle finger to the breast area and measuring the tissue between them in centimeters or millimeters (Figure 25–4 ◆). During the assessment, never grasp the nipple, because skin and subcutaneous tissue will prevent accurate estimation of size. Do this procedure gently to avoid causing trauma to the breast tissue. A large breast tissue mass can occur as a result of specific conditions other than advanced gestational age or the effects of maternal hormones on the baby. The newborn of a diabetic mother tends to be large for gestational age (LGA), and the accelerated development of breast tissue reflects subcutaneous fat deposits. Small-for-gestational-age (SGA) term or postterm newborns may have used subcutaneous fat (which would have been deposited as breast tissue) to survive in utero; as a result, their lack of breast tissue may indicate a gestational age of 34 to 35 weeks, even though other factors indicate a term or postterm newborn.

6. *Ear form and cartilage distribution* develop with gestational age. The cartilage gives the ear its shape and substance (Figure 25–5◆). In a newborn of less than

34 weeks' gestation, the ear is relatively shapeless and flat; it has little cartilage, so the ear folds over on itself and remains folded. By approximately 36 weeks' gestation, some cartilage and slight incurving of the upper pinna are present, and the pinna springs back slowly when folded. (Test this response by holding the top and bottom of the pinna together with the forefinger and thumb and then releasing them or by folding the pinna of the ear forward against the side of the head, releasing it, and observing the response.) By term, the newborn's pinna is firm, stands away from the head, and springs back quickly from the folding.

7. *Male genitals* are evaluated for size of the scrotal sac, presence of rugae (wrinkles and ridges in the scrotum), and descent of the testes (Figure 25–6 ◆). Prior to 36 weeks, the scrotum has few rugae, and the testes are palpable in the inguinal canal. By 36 to 38 weeks, the testes are in the upper scrotum, and rugae have developed over the anterior portion of the scrotum. By term, the testes are generally in the lower scrotum, which is pendulous and covered with rugae.

8. The appearance of the *female genitals* depends in part on subcutaneous fat deposition and therefore relates to fetal nutritional status (Figure 25–7 ◆). The clitoris varies in size, and occasionally is so swollen that it is difficult to identify the sex of the newborn. This swelling may be due to adrenogenital syndrome, which causes the adrenals to secrete excessive amounts of androgen and other hormones. At 30 to 32 weeks' gestation, the clitoris is prominent, and the labia majora are small and widely separated. As gestational age increases, the labia majora increase in size. At 36 to 40 weeks, they nearly cover the clitoris. At 40 weeks and beyond, the labia majora cover the labia minora and clitoris.

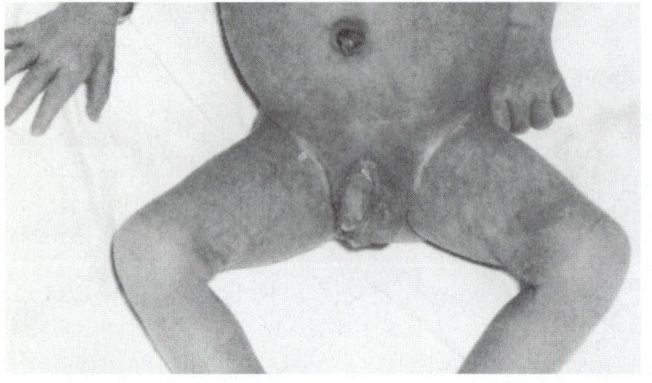

A

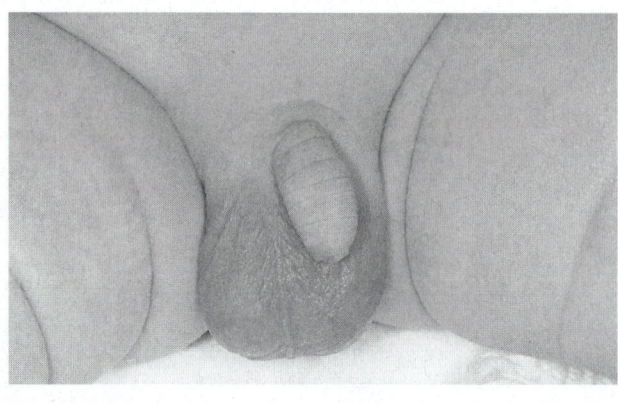

B

FIGURE 25–6. ◆ Male genitals. **A,** Preterm newborn's testes are not within the scrotum. The scrotal surface has few rugae. **B,** Term newborn's testes are generally fully descended. The entire surface of the scrotum is covered by rugae. *Note:* **A** reprinted by permission of V. Dubowitz, MD, Hammersmith Hospital, London, England.

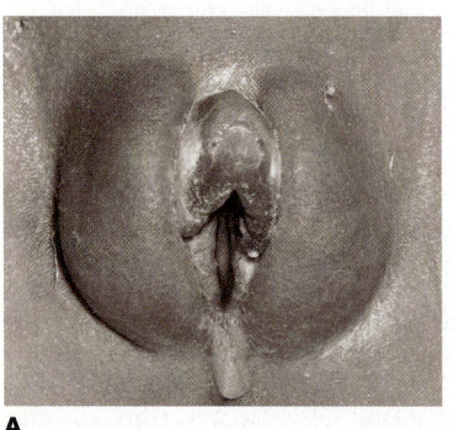

A

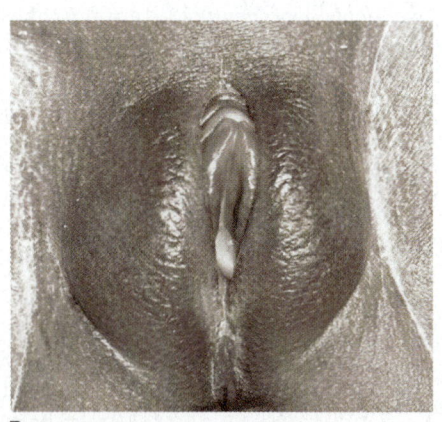

B

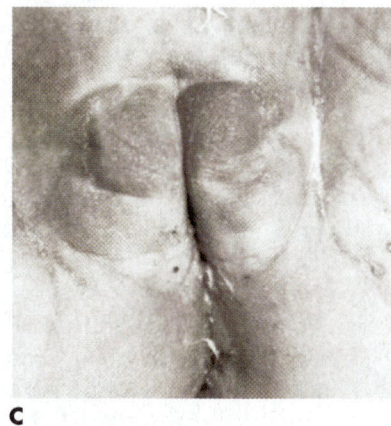

C

FIGURE 25–7. ◆ Female genitals. **A,** Newborn has a prominent clitoris. The labia majora are widely separated, and the labia minora, viewed laterally, would protrude beyond the labia majora. The gestational age is 30 to 36 weeks. **B,** The clitoris is still visible. The labia minora are now covered by the larger labia majora. The gestational age is 36 to 40 weeks. **C,** The term newborn has well-developed, large labia majora that cover both clitoris and labia minora. *Note:* Reprinted by permission of V. Dubowitz, MD, Hammersmith Hospital, London, England.

Other physical characteristics assessed by some gestational age scoring tools include the following:

1. *Vernix* covers the preterm newborn. The postterm newborn has little vernix. After noting vernix distribution, the birthing area nurse (wearing gloves) dries the newborn to prevent evaporative heat loss, thus disturbing the vernix and potentially altering this gestational age criterion. The birthing area nurse must communicate to the newborn nurse the amount of vernix and the areas of vernix coverage.

2. *Hair* of the preterm newborn has the consistency of matted wool or fur and lies in bunches rather than in the silky, single strands of the term newborn's hair.

3. *Skull firmness* increases as the fetus matures. In a term newborn the bones are hard, and the sutures are not easily displaced. Do not attempt to displace the sutures forcibly.

4. *Nails* appear and cover the nail bed at about 20 weeks' gestation. Nails extending beyond the fingertips may indicate a posttermnewborn.

Assessment of Neuromuscular Maturity Characteristics

The central nervous system of the fetus matures at a fairly constant rate. Tests have been designed to evaluate neurologic status as manifested by neuromuscular tone development and correlated with gestational ages. In the fetus, neuromuscular tone develops from the lower to the upper extremities.

The neuromuscular evaluation requires more manipulation and disturbances than the physical evaluation of the newborn. The neuromuscular evaluation (see Figure 25–1) is best performed when the baby's condition has stabilized. Evaluate the following characteristics:

1. The *square window sign* is elicited by gently flexing the newborn's hand toward the ventral forearm until resistance is felt. The angle formed at the wrist is measured (Figure 25–8 ◆).

2. *Recoil* is a test of flexion development. Because flexion first develops in the lower extremities, test recoil in the legs first. Place the newborn on its back on a flat surface. With a hand on the newborn's knees, place the baby's legs in flexion, then extend them parallel to each other and flat on the surface. The response to this maneuver is recoil of the newborn's legs. According to gestational age, they may not move or they may return slowly or quickly to the flexed position. Preterm infants have less muscle tone than term infants, so preterm infants have less recoil. Test arm recoil by flexion at the elbow and extension of the arms at the newborn's side. While the baby is in the supine position, completely flex both elbows, hold them in this position for 5 seconds, extend the arms at the baby's side, and release them. On release, the elbows of a full-term newborn form an angle of less than 90 degrees and rapidly recoil back to a flexed position. The elbows of a preterm newborn have slower recoil time and form an angle greater than 90 degrees. Arm recoil is also slower in healthy but fatigued newborns after birth; therefore, arm recoil is best elicited after the first hour of birth, when the baby has had time to recover from the stress of the birth. Deep sleep state also decreases the arm recoil response. Assess arm recoil bilaterally to rule out brachial palsy.

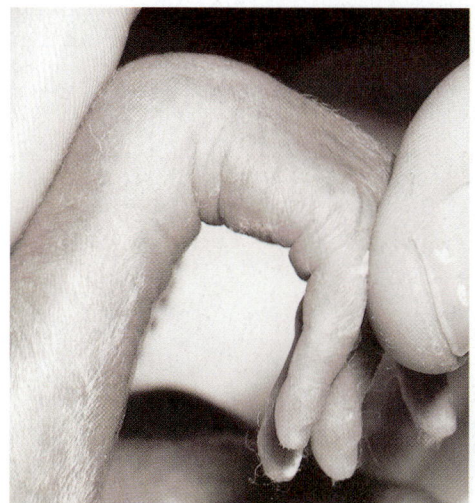
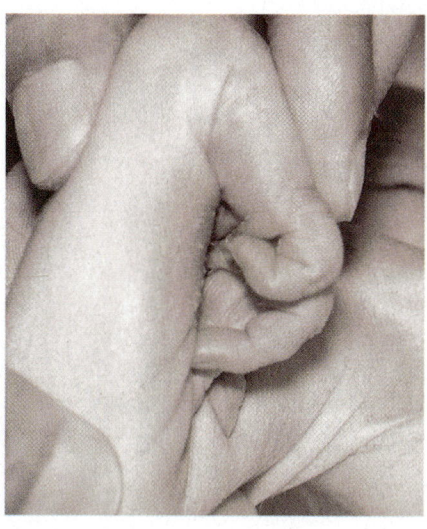
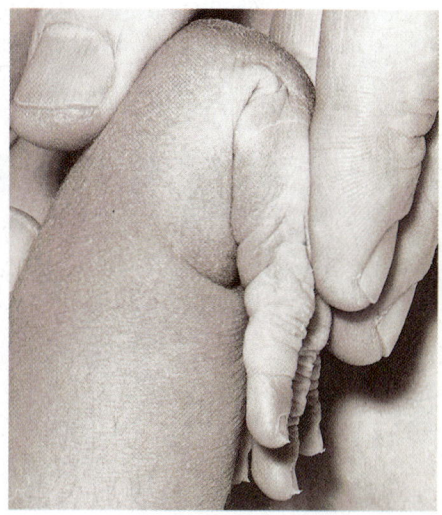

A **B** **C**

FIGURE 25–8. ◆ Square window sign. **A,** This angle is 90 degrees and suggests an immature newborn of 28 to 32 weeks' gestation. **B,** A 30-degree angle is commonly found from 39 to 40 weeks' gestation. **C,** A 0-degree angle can occur from 40 to 42 weeks. *Note:* Reprinted by permission of V. Dubowitz, MD, Hammersmith Hospital, London, England.

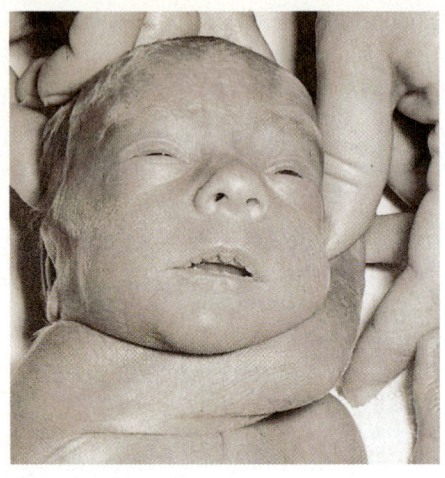
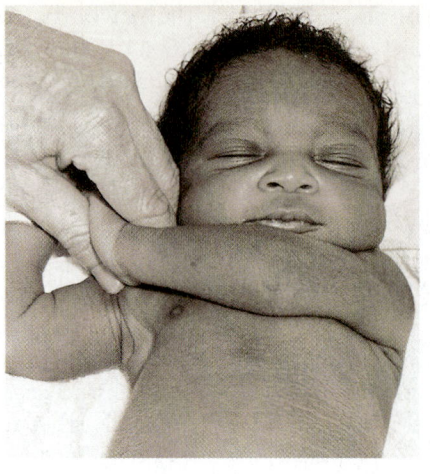
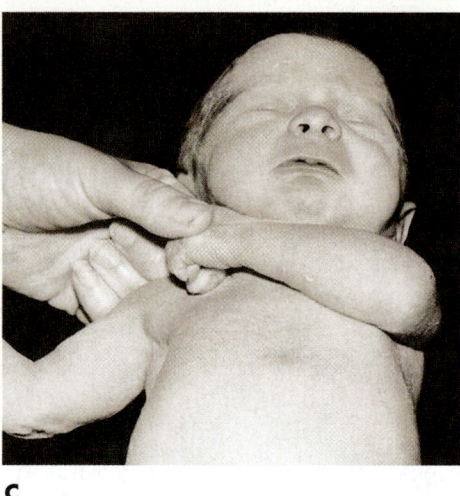

A   **B**   **C**

FIGURE 25–9. ◆ Scarf sign. **A,** No resistance is noted until after 30 weeks' gestation. The elbow moves readily past the midline. **B,** The elbow is at midline at 36 to 40 weeks' gestation. **C,** Beyond 40 weeks' gestation the elbow will not reach the midline. *Note:* Reprinted by permission of V. Dubowitz, MD, Hammersmith Hospital, London, England.

3. The *popliteal angle* (degree of knee flexion) is determined with the newborn flat on its back. Flex the thigh on the abdomen and chest, and place the index finger of the other hand behind the newborn's ankle to extend the lower leg until resistance is met. Measure the angle formed. Results vary from no resistance in the very immature newborn to an 80-degree angle in the term newborn.

4. The *scarf sign* is elicited by placing the newborn supine and drawing an arm across the chest toward the newborn's opposite shoulder until resistance is met. Note the location of the elbow in relation to the midline of the chest (Figure 25–9 ◆).

5. The *heel-to-ear extension* is performed by placing the newborn in a supine position and then gently drawing the foot toward the ear on the same side until resis-

tance is felt. Allow the knee to bend during the test. It is important to hold the buttocks down to keep from rolling the baby. Assess both the proximity of foot to ear and the degree of knee extension. The leg of a preterm, immature newborn remains straight and the foot goes to the ear or beyond. With advancing gestational age the newborn demonstrates increasing resistance to this maneuver. Delay maneuvers involving the lower extremities of newborns who had frank breech presentation to allow leg positioning to be resolved.

6. *Ankle dorsiflexion* is determined by flexing the ankle on the shin. Use a thumb to push on the sole of the newborn's foot while the fingers support the back of the leg. Then measure the angle formed by the foot and the interior leg (Figure 25–10 ◆). Intrauterine position and congenital deformities can influence this sign.

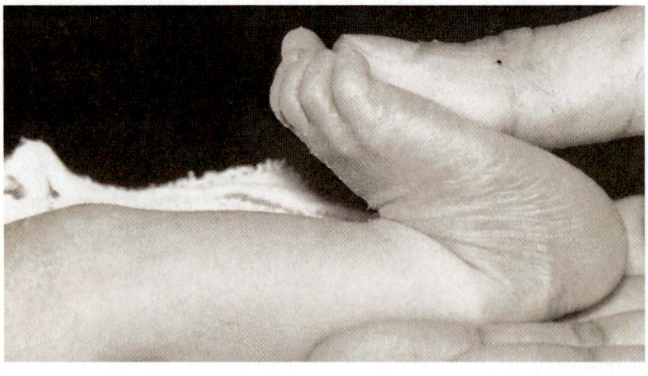
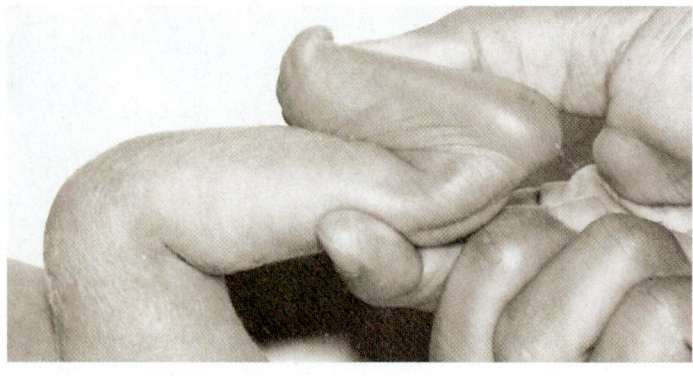

A   **B**

FIGURE 25–10. ◆ Ankle dorsiflexion. **A,** A 45-degree angle indicates 32 to 36 weeks' gestation. A 20-degree angle indicates 36 to 40 weeks' gestation. **B,** A 0-degree angle is common at 40 weeks' or more gestational age. *Note:* Reprinted by permission of V. Dubowitz, MD, Hammersmith Hospital, London, England.

7. *Head lag* (neck flexor) is measured by pulling the newborn to a sitting position and noting the degree of head lag. Total lag is common in newborns up to 34 weeks' gestation, whereas postterm newborns (42+ weeks) hold their heads in front of their body lines. Full-term newborns can support their heads momentarily.

8. *Ventral suspension* (horizontal position) is evaluated by holding the newborn prone on the hand. Note the position of the head and back and the degree of flexion in the arms and legs. Some flexion of arms and legs indicates 36 to 38 weeks' gestation; fully flexed extremities, with head and back even, are characteristic of a term newborn.

9. *Major reflexes* such as sucking, rooting, grasping, Moro, tonic neck, Babinski, and others are evaluated during the newborn exam. See discussion of reflexes on pages 551–552.

When the gestational age determination and birth weight are considered together, the newborn can be identified as *one whose growth is below the 10th percentile, or small for gestational age (SGA); appropriate for gestational age (AGA); or above the 90th percentile, or large for gestational age (LGA)* (Figure 25–11 ◆). This determination enables the nurse to anticipate possible physiologic problems and, in conjunction with a complete physical examination, to establish a plan of care appropriate for the individual newborn. For example, an SGA newborn often requires frequent glucose monitoring and early feedings. (See Chapter 28 for more complete discussion of these categories and the potential problems associated with them.)

Plot the gestational age against the newborn's length, head circumference, and weight on the appropriate growth chart to determine if these measurements fall

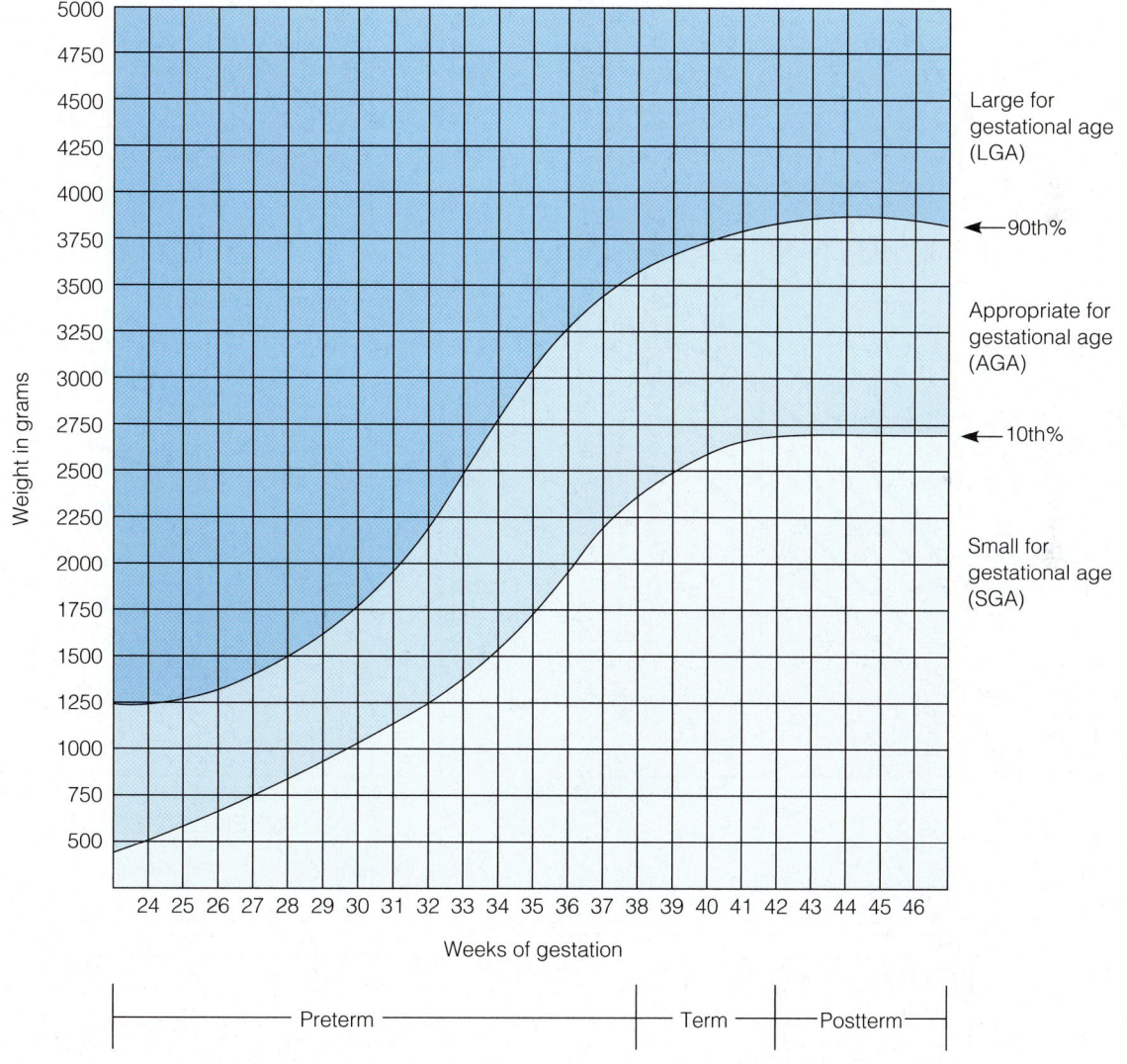

FIGURE 25–11. ◆ Classification of newborns by birth weight and gestational age. The nurse places the newborn's birth weight and gestational age on the graph and classifies the newborn as large for gestational age (LGA), appropriate for gestational age (AGA), or small for gestational age (SGA). *Note:* From Battaglia, F. C., & Lubchenco, L. O. (1967). A practical classification of newborn infants by weight and gestational age. *Journal of Pediatrics, 71,* 161.

CLASSIFICATION OF NEWBORNS—
BASED ON MATURITY AND INTRAUTERINE GROWTH

Symbols: X-1st Exam   O-2nd Exam

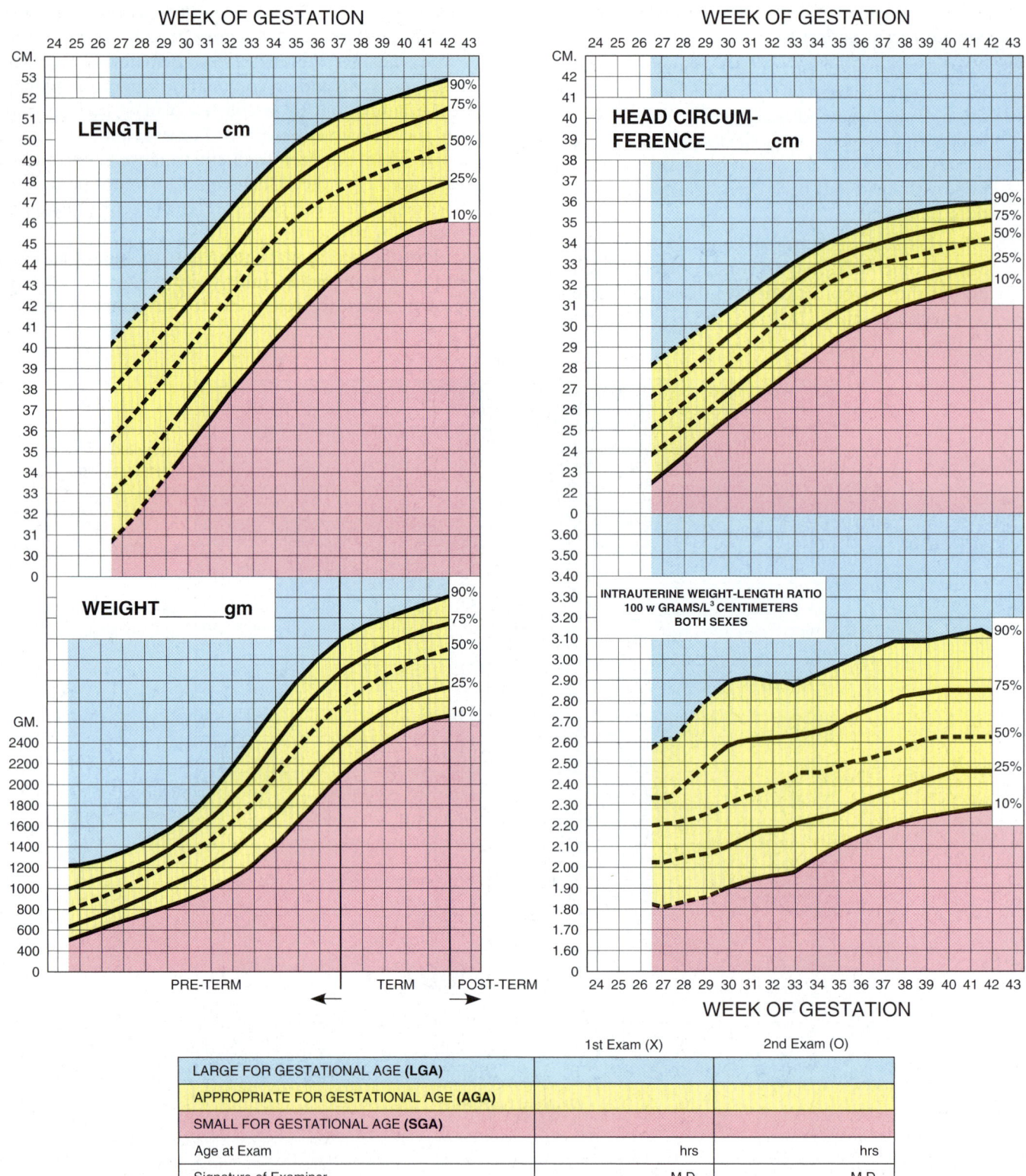

FIGURE 25–12. ◆ Classification of newborns based on maturity and intrauterine growth. *Note:* From Lubchenco, L. O., Hansman, C., & Boyd, E. (1966). Intrauterine growth in length and head circumference as estimated from live births at gestational ages from 26 to 42 weeks. *Pediatrics, 37,* 403–408; and Battaglia, F. C., & Lubchenco, L. O. (1967). A practical classification of newborn infants by weight and gestational age. *Journal of Pediatrics, 71,* 159. Adapted.

within the average range—the 10th to 90th percentile for the corresponding gestational age Figure 25–12 ◆). These correlations further document the level of maturity and appropriate category for the newborn. The comparison of the infant's weight-length ratio further helps identify SGA infants as having symmetric or asymmetric growth restriction. (See Chapter 28 for further discussion.) ⬭

PHYSICAL ASSESSMENT

After the initial determination of gestational age and related potential problems, carry out a more extensive physical assessment. Choose a warm, well-lit area that is free of drafts. Completing the physical assessment in the presence of the parents gives a chance to acquaint them with their unique newborn. Perform the examination in a systematic, head-to-toe manner, and record all findings. When assessing the physical and neurologic status of the newborn, first consider general appearance and then proceed to specific areas.

A guide for systematically assessing the newborn appears on pages 553–563. Normal findings, alterations, and related causes are presented and correlated with suggested nursing responses. The findings are typical for a full-term newborn.

General Appearance

The newborn's head is disproportionately large for its body. The center of the baby's body is the umbilicus rather than the symphysis pubis as in the adult. The body appears long and the extremities short. The flexed position that the newborn maintains contributes to the short appearance of the extremities. The hands are tightly clenched. The neck looks short because the chin rests on the chest. Newborns have a prominent abdomen, sloping shoulders, narrow hips, and rounded chests. They tend to stay in a flexed position similar to the one maintained in utero and will offer resistance when the extremities are straightened. After a breech birth, the feet are usually dorsiflexed, and it may take several weeks for the newborn to assume the typical newborn posture.

Weight and Measurements

The normal full-term white newborn has an average birth weight of 3405 g (7 lb, 8 oz). Newborns of African-, Asian-, or Mexican-American descent are usually somewhat smaller at term (Overpeck, Hediger, Zhang, et al., 1999; Wu & Daniel, 2001). Other factors that influence weight are age and size of parents, health of mother (smoking and malnutrition decrease birth weight), and the interval between pregnancies (short intervals, such as every year, result in lower birth weight) (Basso, Olsen, Knudsen, et al., 1998). After the first week, and for the first 6 months, the newborn's weight increases about 198 g (7 oz) weekly.

Approximately 70% to 75% of the newborn's body weight is water. During the initial newborn period (the first 3 or 4 days), term newborns have a physiologic weight loss of about 5% to 10% because of fluid shifts. This weight loss may reach 15% for preterm newborns. Large babies also tend to lose more weight because of greater fluid loss in proportion to birth weight. If weight loss is greater than 10%, clinical reappraisal is indicated. Factors contributing to weight loss include small fluid intake resulting from delayed breastfeeding or a slow adjustment to the formula, increased volume of meconium excreted, and urination. Weight loss may be marked in the presence of temperature elevation (because of associated dehydration) or consistent chilling (because of nonshivering thermogenesis).

The length of the normal newborn is difficult to measure because the legs are flexed and tensed. To measure length, place babies flat on their backs with their legs extended as much as possible (Figure 25–13 ◆). The average length is 50 cm (20 in), and the range is 48 to 52 cm (18 to 22 in). The newborn will grow approximately 1 inch a month for the next 6 months. This is the period of most rapid growth.

At birth the newborn's head is one third the size of an adult's head. The circumference (biparietal diameter) of the newborn's head is 32 to 37 cm (12.5 to 14.5 in). For accurate measurement, place the tape over the most prominent part of the occiput, just above the eyebrows (Figure 25–14A ◆). The circumference of the newborn's head is approximately 2 cm greater than the circumference of the newborn's chest at birth, and the two parts remain in this proportion for the next few months. (For factors that alter this measurement, see "Head" later in this chapter.) It is best to take another head circumference on the second day if the newborn experienced significant head molding or developed a caput from the birth process.

At birth the average circumference of the chest is 32 cm (12.5 in) and ranges from 30 to 35 cm (12 to 14 in). Take chest measurements with the tape measure placed at the lower edge of the scapulas and brought around anteriorly,

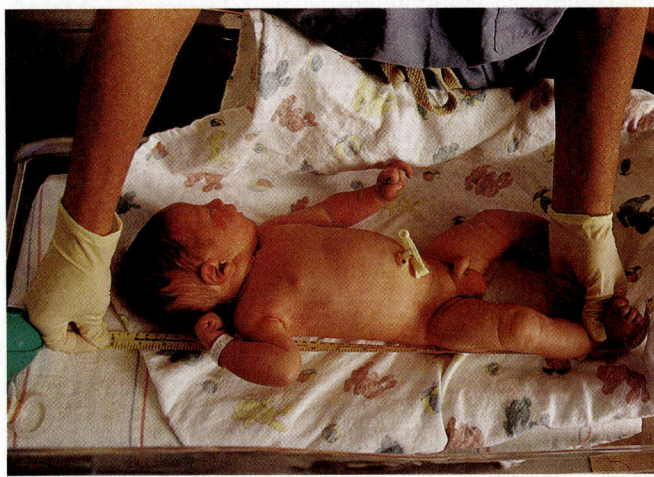

FIGURE 25–13. ◆ Measuring the length of the newborn.

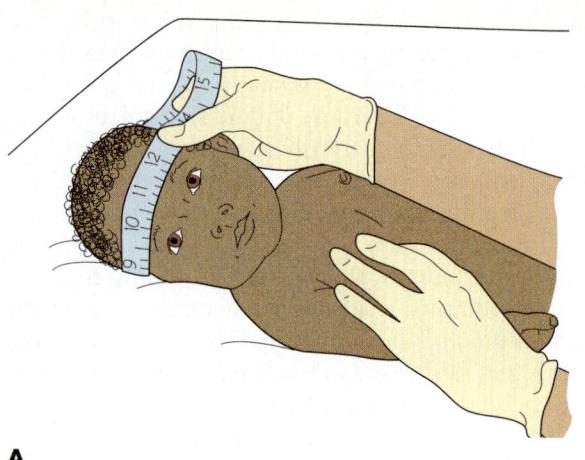

A

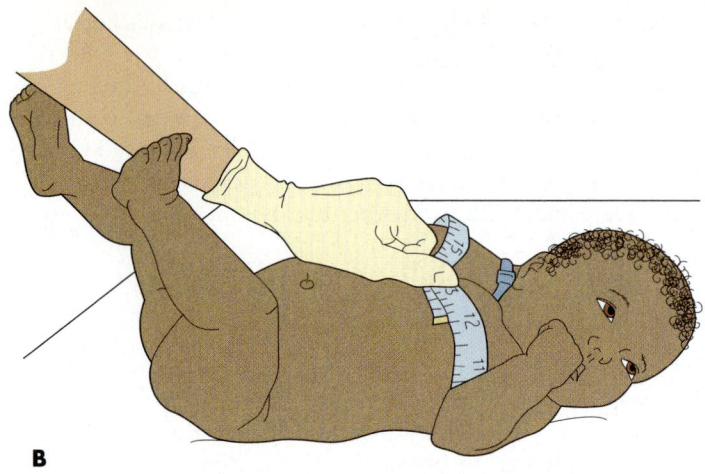

B

FIGURE 25–14. ◆ **A,** Measuring the head circumference of the newborn. **B,** Measuring the chest circumference of the newborn.

TABLE 25-2 Newborn Measurements

Weight
- Average: 3405 g (7 lb, 8 oz)
- Range: 2500–4000 g (5 lb, 8 oz–8 lb, 13 oz)
- Weight is influenced by racial origin and maternal age and size.
- Physiologic weight loss: 5%–10% for term newborns, up to 15% for preterm newborns
- Growth: 198 g (7 oz) per week for first 6 months

Length
- Average: 50 cm (20 in)
- Range: 48–52 cm (18–22 in)
- Growth: 2.5 cm (1 in) per month for first 6 months

Head Circumference
- 32–37 cm (12.5–14.5 in)
- Approximately 2 cm larger than chest circumference

Chest Circumference
- Average: 32 cm (12.5 in)
- Range: 30–35 cm (12–14 in)

directly over the nipple line (Figure 25–14B ◆). The abdominal circumference, or girth, may also be measured at this time, by placing the tape around the newborn's abdomen at the level of the umbilicus, with the bottom edge of the tape at the top edge of the umbilicus (see Table 25–2).

Temperature

Initial assessment of the newborn's temperature is critical. In utero, the temperature of the fetus is about the same as, or slightly higher than, the expectant mother's. When babies enter the outside world, their temperature can suddenly drop as a result of exposure to cold drafts and the skin's heat loss mechanisms.

If no heat conservation measures are started, the normal term newborn's deep body temperature falls 0.1 °C (0.2 °F) per minute; skin temperature drops 0.3 °C (0.5 °F) per minute. Skin temperature markedly decreases within 10 minutes after exposure to room air. The temperature should stabilize within 8 to 12 hours. Temperature is monitored when the newborn is admitted to the nursery and at least every 30 minutes until the newborn's status has remained stable for 2 hours. After that, assess temperature at least once every 8 hours, or according to institutional policy (AAP & ACOG, 1997). (See Chapter 24 for a discussion of the physiology of temperature regulation.)

Temperature can be assessed by the axillary skin method, a continuous skin probe, the rectal route, or a tympanic thermometer. Axillary temperature reflects body (core) temperature and the body's compensatory response to the thermal environment. Axillary temperatures are the preferred method and are considered to be a close estimation of the rectal temperature. In preterm and term newborns, there is less than 0.1 °C (0.2 °F) difference between the two sites. With the axillary method, the thermometer must remain in place at least 3 minutes unless an electronic thermometer is used (Figure 25–15 ◆). Axillary temperature ranges from 36.5 to 37 °C (97.7 to 98.6 °F). Keep in mind that axillary temperatures can be misleading, because the friction caused by apposition of the inner arm skin and

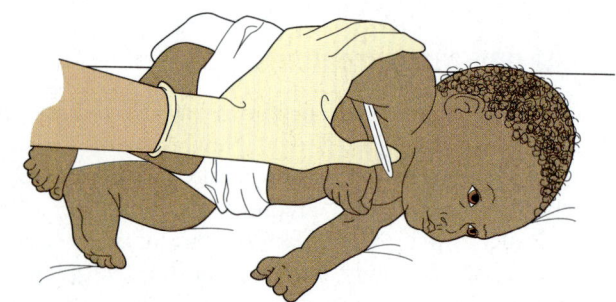

FIGURE 25–15. ◆ Axillary temperature measurement. The thermometer should remain in place for 3 minutes. The nurse presses the newborn's arm tightly but gently against the thermometer and the newborn's side, as illustrated.

upper chest wall and the nearness of brown fat to the probe may elevate the temperature.

Skin temperature is measured most accurately by continuous skin probe, especially for small newborns or newborns maintained in incubators or under radiant warmers. Normal skin temperature is 36 to 36.5 °C (96.8 to 97.7 °F). Continuous skin temperature assessment allows time to begin interventions before a more serious fall in core temperature occurs (Figure 25–16 ◆).

Rectal temperature is assumed to be the closest approximation to core temperature, but the accuracy of this method depends on the depth to which the thermometer is inserted. Normal rectal temperature is 36.6 to 37.2 °C (97.8 to 99 °F). The rectal route is not recommended as a routine method, because it may irritate the rectal mucosa and increase chances of perforation.

Many institutions use tympanic thermometers, portable sensor probes with disposable covers that are placed in the auditory canal. The probe uses infrared technology to measure the temperature of the internal carotid artery blood flow within several seconds. Research suggests that tympanic and digital thermometer axillary temperatures are accurate estimations of body temperature in the *healthy* newborn (Sganga, Wallace, Kiehl, et al., 2000). Current research still questions the accuracy of tympanic thermometer readings from sick or potentially ill newborns (Sganga et al., 2000).

Temperature instability, a deviation of more than 1 °C (2 °F) from one reading to the next, or a subnormal temperature may indicate an infection. In contrast to an elevated temperature in older children, an increased temperature in a newborn may indicate reactions to too much covering, too hot a room, or dehydration. Dehydration, which tends to increase body temperature, occurs in newborns whose feedings have been delayed for any reason. Newborns may respond to overheating (a temperature greater than 37.5 °C [99.5 °F]) by increased restlessness and eventually by perspiration. The perspiration appears initially on the head and face and then on the chest. Many newborns initially cannot perspire, so they increase their respiratory and heart rates, which increases oxygen consumption.

Skin Characteristics

Although the newborn's skin color varies with genetic background, all healthy newborns have a pink tinge to their skin. The ruddy hue results from increased red blood cell concentrations in the blood vessels and limited subcutaneous fat deposits.

Skin pigmentation is slight in the newborn period, so color changes may be seen even in darker-skinned babies. A newborn who is cyanotic at rest and pink only with crying may have choanal atresia (congenital blockage of the passageway between the nose and pharynx). If crying increases the cyanosis, heart or lung problems may be suspected. Very pale newborns may be anemic or have hypovolemia (low BP) and should be evaluated for these problems.

Acrocyanosis (bluish discoloration of the hands and feet) may be present in the first 2 to 6 hours after birth (Figure 25–17 ◆). This condition is caused by poor peripheral circulation, which results in vasomotor instability and capillary stasis, especially when the baby is exposed to cold. If the central circulation is adequate, the blood supply should return quickly when the skin is blanched with a finger. Blue hands and nails are a poor indicator of oxygenation in a newborn. Assess the face and mucous membranes for pinkness reflecting adequate oxygenation.

Mottling (lacy pattern of dilated blood vessels under the skin) occurs as a result of general circulation fluctuations. It may last several hours to several weeks or may come and go periodically. Mottling may be related to chilling or prolonged apnea.

Harlequin sign (clown) color change is occasionally noted: A deep red color develops over one side of the new-

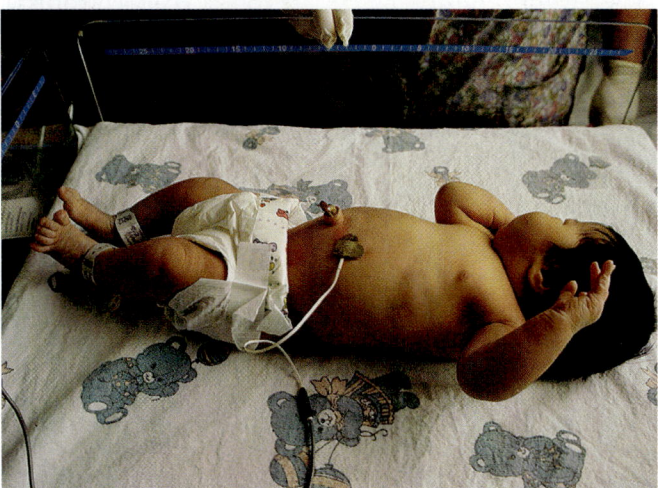

FIGURE 25–16. ◆ Temperature monitoring for the newborn. A skin thermal sensor is placed on the newborn's abdomen, upper thigh, or arm and secured with porous tape or a foil-covered foam pad.

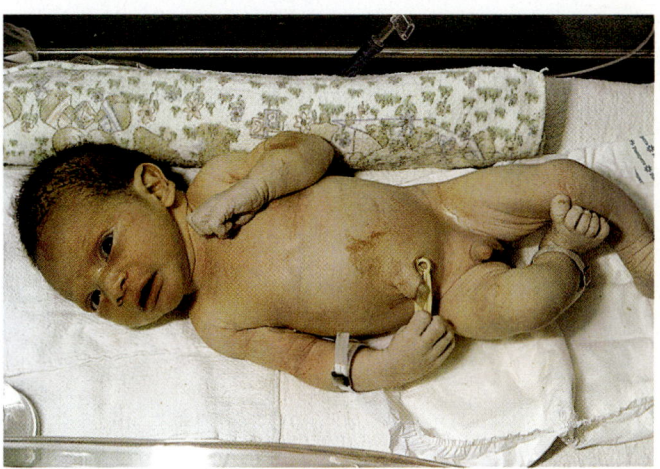

FIGURE 25–17. ◆ Acrocyanosis.

born's body while the other side remains pale, so that the skin resembles a clown's suit. This color change results from a vasomotor disturbance in which blood vessels on one side dilate while the vessels on the other side constrict. It usually lasts from 1 to 20 minutes. Affected newborns may have single or multiple episodes, but they are transient and clinically significant.

Jaundice is first detectable on the face (where skin overlies cartilage) and the mucous membranes of the mouth and has a head-to-toe progression (Moyer, Ahn, & Sneed, 2000). Evaluate it by blanching the tip of the nose, the forehead, the sternum, or the gum line. This procedure must be done in appropriate lighting. If jaundice is present, the area will appear yellowish immediately after blanching. Another area to assess for jaundice is the sclera. Evaluation and determination of the cause of jaundice must begin immediately to prevent possibly serious sequelae. The jaundice may be related to breastfeeding (in a few cases), hematomas, immature liver function, or bruises from forceps, or it may be caused by blood incompatibility, oxytocin (Pitocin) augmentation or induction, or severe hemolysis process. Report any jaundice noted before a newborn is 24 hours of age to the physician or nurse practitioner. (For detailed discussion of causes and assessment of jaundice, see Chapter 29.)

Erythema toxicum is a perifollicular eruption of lesions that are firm, vary in size from 1 to 3 mm, and consist of a white or pale yellow papule or pustule with an erythematous base. It is often called "newborn rash" or "flea bite" dermatitis. The rash may appear suddenly, usually over the trunk and diaper area, and is frequently widespread (Figure 25–18 ◆). The lesions do not appear on the palms of the hands or the soles of the feet. The peak incidence is at 24 to 48 hours of life. The condition rarely presents at birth or after 5 days of life. The cause is unknown, and no treatment is necessary. Some clinicians believe it may be caused by irritation from clothing. The lesions disappear in a few hours or days. If a maculopapular rash appears, a smear of the aspirated papule will show numerous eosinophils on staining; no bacteria will be cultured.

Milia, which are exposed sebaceous glands, appear as raised white spots on the face, especially across the nose (Figure 25–19 ◆). No treatment is necessary, because they will clear up spontaneously within the first month. Infants of African heritage have a similar condition called transient neonatal pustular melanosis.

Skin turgor is assessed to determine hydration status, the need for early feedings, and the presence of any infectious processes. The usual place to assess skin turgor is over the abdomen or the thigh. Skin should be elastic and return to its original shape.

Vernix caseosa, a whitish, cheeselike substance, covers the fetus while in utero and lubricates the skin of the newborn. The skin of the term or postterm newborn has less vernix and is frequently dry; peeling is common, especially on the hands and feet.

Forceps marks may be present after a difficult forceps birth. The newborn may have reddened areas over the cheeks and jaws. It is important to reassure the parents that these marks will disappear, usually within 1 or 2 days. Transient facial paralysis resulting from the forceps pressure is a rare complication. Vacuum extractor suction marks on the vertex of the scalp are often seen when vacuum extractors are used to assist with the birth. These marks are benign and do not indicate any underlying brain lesions.

Birthmarks

Telangiectatic nevi (stork bites) appear as pale pink or red spots and are frequently found on the eyelids, nose, lower occipital bone, and nape of the neck (Figure 25–20 ◆). These lesions are common in newborns with light complexions and are more noticeable during periods of crying. These areas have no clinical significance and usually fade by the second birthday.

Mongolian spots are macular areas of bluish black or gray-blue pigmentation on the dorsal area and the buttocks (Figure 25–21 ◆). They are common in newborns of Asian and African descent and other dark-skinned races. They gradually fade during the first or second year of life.

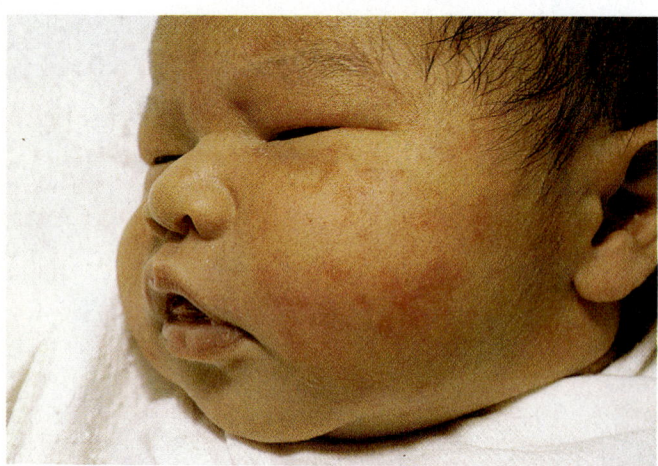

FIGURE 25–18. ◆ Erythema toxicum.

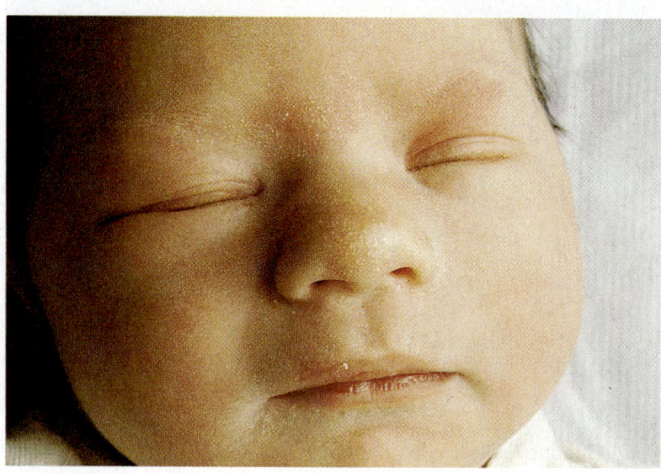

FIGURE 25–19. ◆ Facial milia.

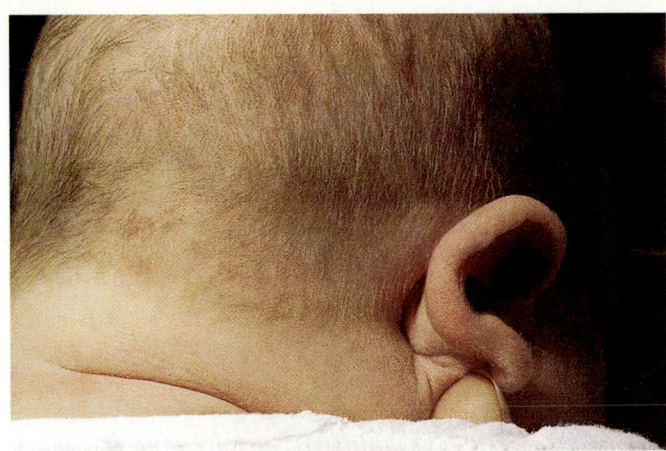

FIGURE 25–20. ◆ Stork bites.

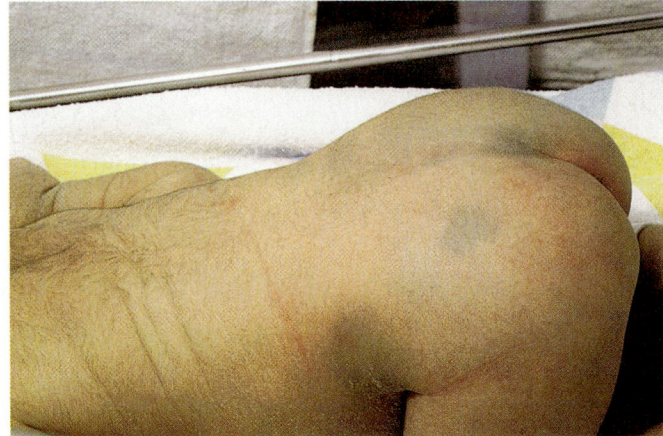

FIGURE 25–21. ◆ Mongolian spots.

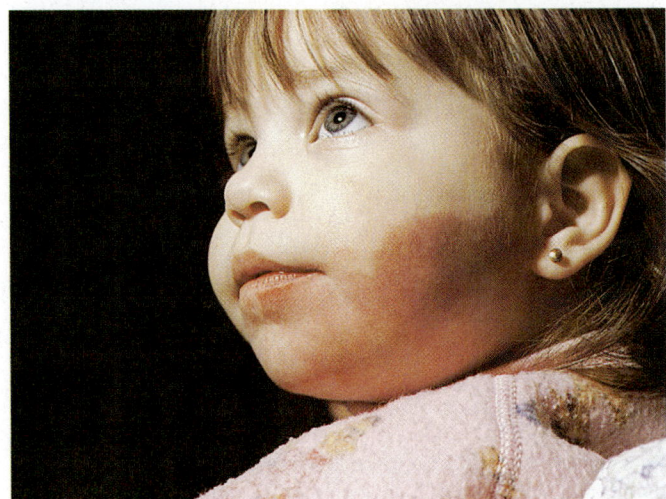

FIGURE 25–22. ◆ Port-wine stain.

They may be mistaken for bruises and should be documented in the newborn's chart.

Nevus flammeus (port-wine stain), a capillary angioma directly below the epidermis, is a nonelevated, sharply demarcated, red-to-purple area of dense capillaries (Figure 25–22 ◆). In infants of African descent, it may appear as a purple-black stain. The size and shape vary, but it commonly appears on the face. It does not grow in size, does not fade with time, and does not blanch as a rule. The birthmark may be concealed by using an opaque cosmetic cream. If convulsions and other neurologic problems accompany the nevus flammeus, the clinical picture suggests Sturge-Weber syndrome, with involvement of the fifth cranial nerve (the ophthalmic branch of the trigeminal nerve).

Nevus vasculosus (strawberry mark), a capillary hemangioma, consists of newly formed and enlarged capillaries in the dermal and subdermal layers. It is a raised, clearly delineated, dark-red, rough-surfaced birthmark commonly found in the head region. Such marks usually grow (often rapidly) starting during the second or third week of life and may not reach their fullest size for 1 to 3 months (Rinehart et al., 2000). They begin to shrink and start to resolve spontaneously several weeks to months after they reach peak growth. Tell parents that a pale purple or gray spot on the surface of the hemangioma signals the start of resolution. The best cosmetic effect is achieved when the lesions are allowed to resolve spontaneously.

Birthmarks frequently worry parents. The mother may be especially anxious, fearing that she is to blame ("Is my baby 'marked' because of something I did?"). Guilt is common when parents have misconceptions about the cause. Identify and explain them to the parents. Providing appropriate information about the cause and course of birthmarks often relieves the fears and anxieties of the family. Note any bruises, abrasions, or birthmarks seen on admission to the nursery.

Head

GENERAL APPEARANCE

The newborn's head is large (approximately one fourth of the body size), with soft, pliable skull bones. The head may appear asymmetric in the newborn of a vertex birth. This asymmetry, called **molding,** is caused by overriding of the cranial bones during labor and birth (Figure 25–23 ◆). The degree of molding varies with the amount and length of pressure exerted on the head. Within a few days after birth, the overriding usually diminishes and the suture lines become palpable. Because head measurements are affected by molding, a second measurement is indicated a few days after birth. The heads of breech-born newborns and those born by elective cesarean are characteristically round and well shaped because no pressure was exerted on them during birth. Any extreme differences in head size may indicate microcephaly or hydrocephalus. Variations in the shape, size, or appearance of the head measurements may be due to *craniostenosis* (premature closure of the cranial sutures), which needs to be corrected through surgery to allow brain growth, and *plagiocephaly* (asymmetry caused by pressure on the fetal head during gestation).

Two *fontanelles* ("soft spots") may be palpated on the newborn's head. Fontanelles, openings at the juncture of the cranial bones, can be measured with the fingers. Accurate measurement requires the examiner's finger to be measured in centimeters. Carry out the assessment with the newborn in a sitting position and not crying. The diamond-shaped *anterior fontanelle* is approximately 3 to 4 cm long by 2 to 3 cm wide. It is located at the juncture of the frontal and parietal bones. The *posterior fontanelle*, smaller and triangular, is formed by the parietal bones and the occipital bone and is 0.5 by 1 cm. The fontanelles are smaller immediately after birth than several days later because of molding. The anterior fontanelle closes within 18 months, whereas the posterior fontanelle closes within 8 to 12 weeks.

The fontanelles are a useful indicator of the newborn's condition. The anterior fontanelle may swell when the newborn cries or passes a stool or may pulsate with the heartbeat, which is normal. A bulging fontanelle usually signifies increased intracranial pressure, and a depressed fontanelle indicates dehydration. Palpate the sutures between the cranial bones for amount of overlapping. In newborns whose growth has been restricted the sutures may be wider than normal, and the fontanelles may also be larger due to impaired growth of the cranial bones. In addition to inspecting the newborn's head for degree of molding and size, evaluate it for soft tissue edema and bruising.

CEPHALHEMATOMA

Cephalhematoma is a collection of blood resulting from ruptured blood vessels between the surface of a cranial bone (usually parietal) and the periosteal membrane (Figure 25–24 ◆). The scalp in these areas feels loose and slightly edematous. These areas emerge as defined hematomas between the first and second day. Although external pressure may cause the mass to fluctuate, it does not in-

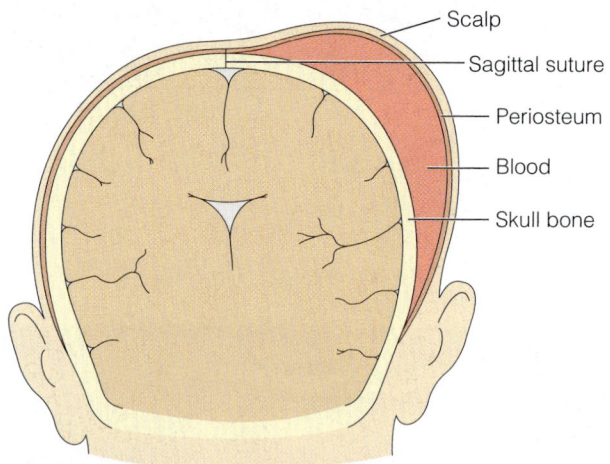

Scalp

Sagittal suture

Periosteum

Blood

Skull bone

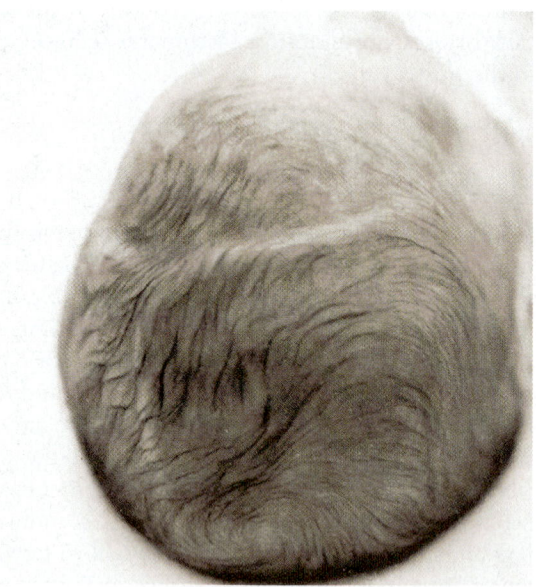

FIGURE 25–23. ◆ Overlapped cranial bones produce a visible ridge in a small, premature newborn. Easily visible overlapping does not occur often in term infants. *Note:* From Korones, S. B. (1986). *High-risk newborn infants* (4th ed.). St. Louis, MO: Mosby.

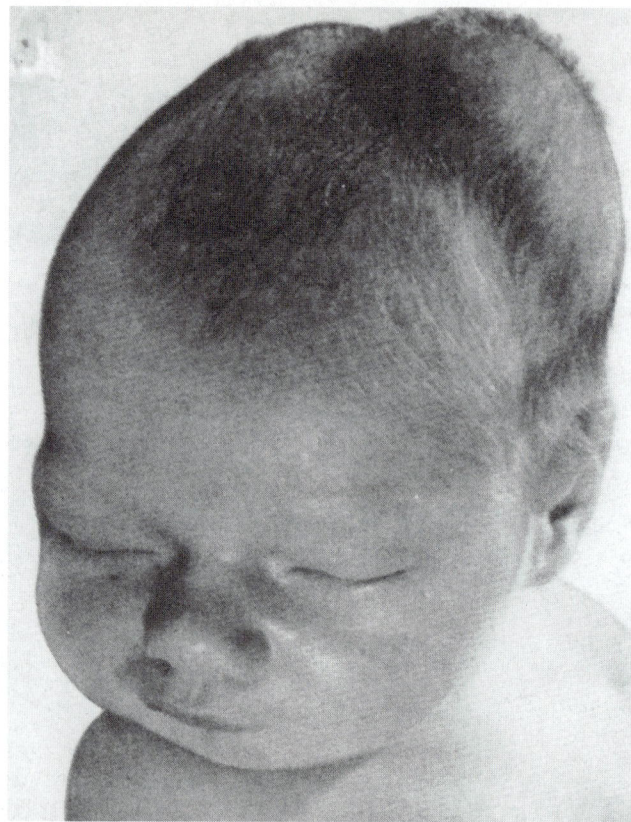

FIGURE 25–24. ◆ Cephalhematoma is a collection of blood between the surface of a cranial bone and the periosteal membrane. This is a cephalhematoma over the left parietal bone. *Note:* From Potter, E. L., & Craig, J. M. (1975). *Pathology of the fetus and infant* (3rd ed.). St. Louis: Mosby–Yearbook Medical Publishers. Reproduced with permission.

crease in size when the newborn cries. Cephalhematomas may be unilateral or bilateral and do not cross suture lines. They are relatively common in vertex births and may disappear within 2 to 3 weeks or very slowly over subsequent months. They may be associated with physiologic jaundice, because extra red blood cells are destroyed within the cephalhematoma.

CAPUT SUCCEDANEUM

Caput succedaneum is a localized, easily identifiable, soft area of the scalp, generally resulting from a long and difficult labor or vacuum extraction. The sustained pressure of the presenting part against the cervix results in compression of local blood vessels, and venous return is slowed. Slowed venous return in turn causes an increase in tissue fluids, an edematous swelling, and occasional bleeding under the periosteum. The caput may vary from a small area to a severely elongated head. The fluid in the caput is reabsorbed within 12 hours to a few days after birth. Caputs resulting from vacuum extractors are sharply outlined, circular areas up to 2 cm thick. They disappear more slowly than naturally occurring edema. It is possible to distinguish between a cephalhematoma and a caput because the caput overrides suture lines (Figure 25–25 ◆), whereas the cephalhematoma, because of its location, never crosses a suture line (Table 25–3). Also, caput succedaneum is present at birth, whereas cephalhematoma is not.

Face

The newborn's face is well designed to help the newborn suckle. Sucking (fat) pads are located in the cheeks, and a labial tubercle (sucking callus) is frequently found in the center of the upper lip. The chin is recessed, and the nose is flattened. The lips are sensitive to touch, and the sucking reflex is easily initiated.

Evaluate symmetry of the eyes, nose, and ears. See "Newborn Physical Assessment Guide" on pages 553–563 for deviations in symmetry and variations in size, shape, and spacing of facial features.

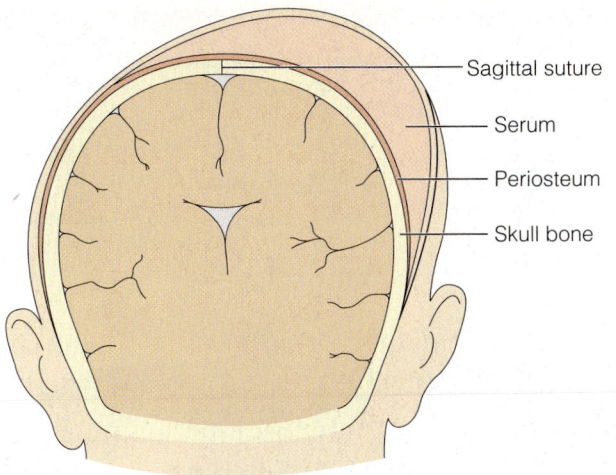

Sagittal suture

Serum

Periosteum

Skull bone

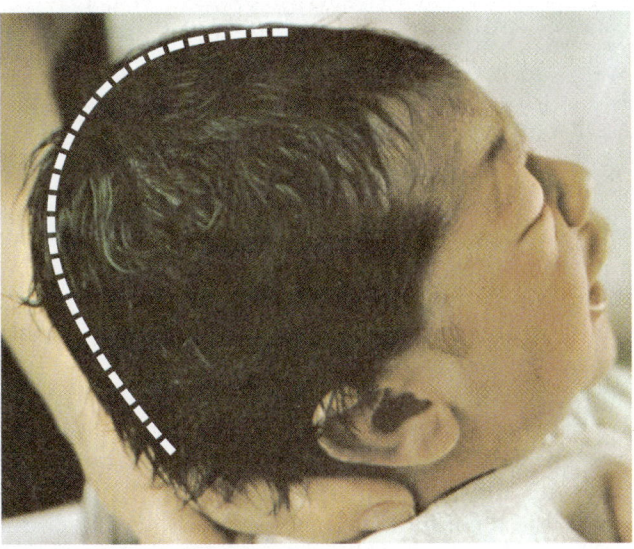

FIGURE 25–25. ◆ Caput succedaneum is a collection of fluid (serum) under the scalp. Courtesy of Mead Johnson Nutritionals, Evansville, IN.

Assess facial movement symmetry to determine the presence of facial palsy. Facial paralysis appears when the newborn cries; the affected side is immobile, and the palpebral (eyelid) fissure widens (Figure 25–26 ◆). Paralysis may result from forceps-assisted birth or pressure on the facial nerve from the maternal pelvis during birth. Facial paralysis usually disappears within a few days to 3 weeks, although in some cases it may be permanent.

Eyes

The eyes of the newborn of northern European descent are a blue-gray or slate–blue-gray color. The sclera tends to be bluish white because of its relative thinness. A blue sclera is associated with osteogenesis imperfecta. The infant's eye color is usually established at approximately 3 months, although it may change any time up to 1 year. Dark-skinned newborns tend to have dark eyes at birth.

TABLE 25–3 Comparison of Cephalhematoma and Caput Succedaneum

CEPHALHEMATOMA
- Collection of blood between cranial (usually parietal) bone and periosteal membrane
- Does not cross suture lines
- Does not increase in size with crying
- Appears on first and second day
- Disappears after 2 to 3 weeks or may take months

CAPUT SUCCEDANEUM
- Collection of fluid, edematous swelling of the scalp
- Crosses suture lines
- Present at birth or shortly thereafter
- Reabsorbed within 12 hours or a few days after birth

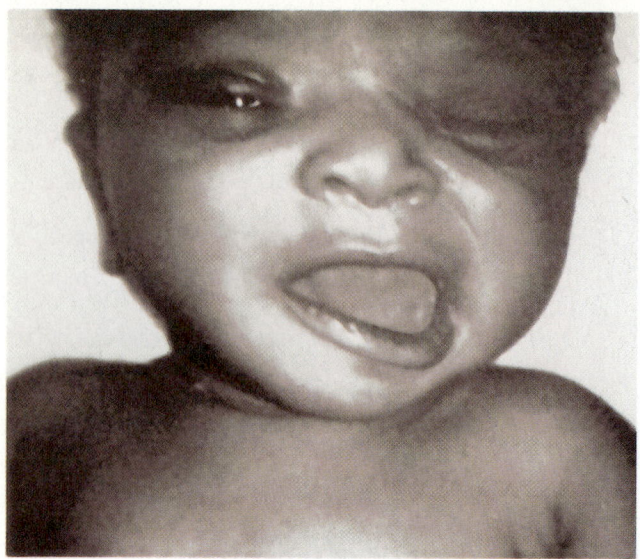

FIGURE 25–26. ◆ Facial paralysis. Paralysis of the right side of the face from injury to right facial nerve. *Note:* From Potter, E. L., & Craig, J. M. (1975). *Pathology of the fetus and infant* (3rd ed.). St. Louis: Mosby–Yearbook Medical Publishers. Courtesy of Dr. Ralph Platow.

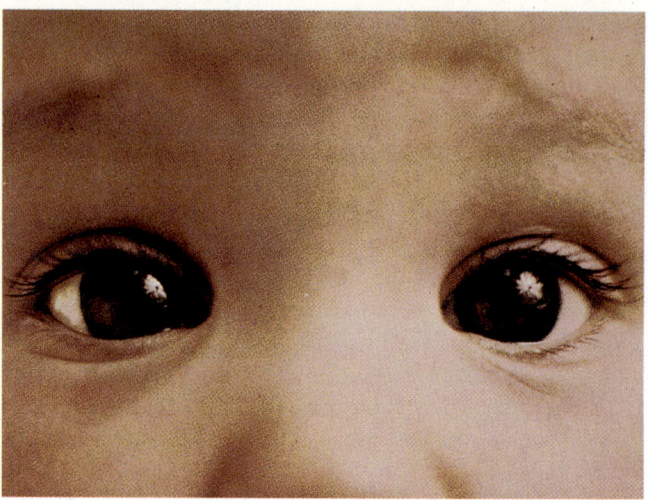

FIGURE 25–27. ◆ Transient strabismus may be present in the newborn due to poor neuromuscular control. Courtesy of Mead Johnson Nutritionals, Evansville, IN.

Check the eyes for size, equality of pupil size, reaction of pupils to light, blink reflex to light, and edema and inflammation of the eyelids. The eyelids are usually edematous during the first few days of life because of the pressure associated with birth.

Erythromycin and tetracycline are now frequently used prophylactically instead of silver nitrate and usually do not cause chemical irritation of the eye. The instillation of silver nitrate drops in the newborn's eyes may cause edema, and **chemical conjunctivitis** may appear a few hours after instillation, but it disappears in 1 to 2 days. If infectious conjunctivitis exists, the newborn has the same purulent (greenish yellow) discharge exudate as in chemical conjunctivitis, but it is caused by gonococcus, *Chlamydia,* staphylococci, or a variety of gram-negative bacteria and requires treatment with ophthalmic antibiotics. Onset is usually after the second day. Edema of the orbits or eyelids may persist for several days, until the newborn's kidneys can eliminate the fluid.

Small **subconjunctival hemorrhages** appear in about 10% of newborns and are commonly found on the sclera. These hemorrhages are caused by the changes in vascular tension or ocular pressure during birth. They will remain for a few weeks and are of no pathologic significance. Parents need reassurance that the newborn is not bleeding from within the eye and that vision will not be impaired.

The newborn may demonstrate transient strabismus caused by poor neuromuscular control of eye muscles (Figure 25–27 ◆). It gradually regresses in 3 to 4 months. The "doll's eye" phenomenon is also present for about 10 days after birth. As the newborn's head position is changed to the left and then to the right, the eyes move to the opposite direction. This results from underdeveloped integration of head-eye coordination.

Observe the newborn's pupils for opacities or whiteness and for the absence of a normal red retinal reflex. Red retinal reflex is a red-orange flash of color observed when an ophthalmoscope light reflects off the retina. In a newborn with dark skin color, the retina may appear paler or more grayish. Absence of red reflex occurs with cataracts. Congenital cataracts should be suspected in newborns of mothers with a history of rubella, cytomegalic inclusion disease, or syphilis.

The newborn's cry is commonly tearless because the lacrimal structures are immature at birth and are not usually fully functional until the second month of life. However, some newborns produce tears. Poor oculomotor coordination and absence of accommodation limit visual abilities, but newborns have peripheral vision, can fixate on objects near (10 to 20 in) their face for short periods, can accommodate to large objects (3 in tall by 3 in wide), and can seek out high-contrast geometric shapes. Newborns can perceive faces, shapes, and colors and begin to show visual preferences early. Newborns generally blink in response to bright lights, to a tap on the bridge of the nose (glabellar reflex), or to a light touch on the eyelids. Pupillary light reflex is also present. Examination of the eye is best accomplished by rocking the newborn from an upright position to the horizontal a few times or by other methods, such as diminishing overhead lights, which elicit an opened-eye response.

Nose

The newborn's nose is small and narrow. Infants are characteristically nose breathers for the first few months of life and generally remove obstructions by sneezing. The nose is patent if the newborn breathes easily with the mouth closed. If respiratory difficulty occurs, check for choanal atresia.

The newborn can smell after the nasal passages are cleared of amniotic fluid and mucus. They demonstrate this ability by searching for milk. Newborns turn their heads toward a milk source, whether bottle or breast. They react to strong odors, such as alcohol, by turning their heads away or blinking.

Mouth

The lips of the newborn should be pink, and a touch on the lips should produce sucking motions. Saliva is normally scant. The taste buds develop before birth, and the newborn can easily discriminate between sweet and bitter flavors.

The easiest way to examine the mouth completely is to stimulate infants gently to cry by depressing their tongue, thereby causing them to open the mouth fully. It is extremely important to examine the entire mouth to check for a cleft palate, which can be present even in the absence of a cleft lip (Thurdeen, Deacon, O'Neill, et al., 1999) (Figure 25–28 ◆). Always remove glove powder before examining the newborn's mouth.

Occasionally, an examination of the gums will reveal *precocious teeth* over the area where the lower central incisor will erupt. If they appear loose, they should be removed to prevent aspiration. Gray-white lesions (inclusion cysts) on the gums may be confused with teeth. On the hard palate and gum margins, **Epstein's pearls,** small glistening white specks (keratin-containing cysts) that feel hard to the touch, are often present. They usually disappear in a few weeks and are of no significance. **Thrush** may appear as white patches that look like milk curds adhering to the mucous membranes and cause bleeding when removed. Thrush is caused by *Candida albicans,* often acquired from an infected vaginal tract during birth or if the mother uses poor handwashing when handling her newborn. Thrush is treated with a preparation of nystatin (Mycostatin).

A newborn who is tongue-tied has a ridge of frenulum tissue attached to the underside of the tongue at varying lengths from its base, causing a heart shape at the tip of the tongue. "Clipping the tongue," or cutting the ridge of tissue, is not recommended. This ridge does not affect speech or eating, but cutting creates an entry for infection.

Transient nerve paralysis resulting from birth trauma may be manifested by asymmetric mouth movements when the newborn cries or by difficulty with sucking and feeding.

Ears

The ears of the newborn should be soft and pliable and should recoil readily when folded and released. In the normal newborn, the top of the ear (pinna) should be parallel to the outer and inner canthus of the eye. Inspect the ears for shape, size, position, and firmness of cartilage. *Low-set ears* are characteristic of many syndromes and may indicate chromosomal abnormalities (especially trisomy 13 and 18), mental retardation, and internal organ abnormalities, especially bilateral renal agenesis as a result of embryologic developmental deviations (Figure 25–29 ◆). *Preauricular skin tags* may be present just in front of the ear.

After the first cry, the newborn's hearing becomes acute as mucus from the middle ear is absorbed, the eustachian tube becomes aerated, and the tympanic membrane becomes visible. Evaluate the newborn's hearing by noting the baby's response to loud or moderately loud noises unaccompanied by vibrations. The sleeping newborn should stir or awaken in response to nearby sounds. (This is not a very accurate test, but it may alert the examiner to a possible problem.) The AAP endorses universal newborn hearing screening (UNHS) in birthing units (AAP, 1999). The newborn can discriminate the individual characteristics of the human voice and is especially sensitive to sound levels within the normal conversational range (Sininger, Doyle, & Moore, 1999). The newborn in a noisy nursery may habituate to the sounds and not stir unless the sound is sudden or much louder than usual.

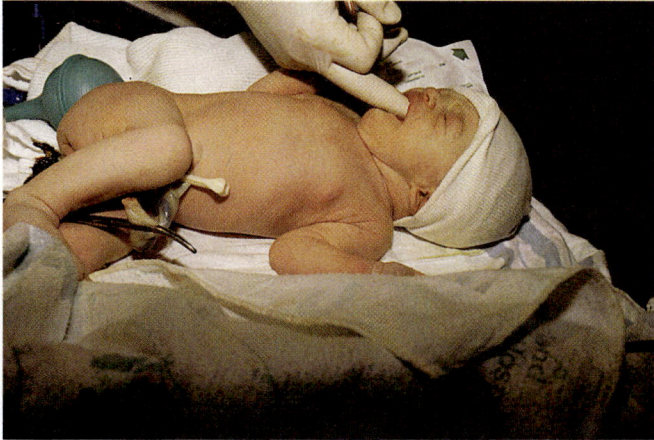

FIGURE 25–28. ◆ The nurse inserts a gloved index finger into the newborn's mouth and feels for any openings along the hard and soft palates. *Note:* Gloves or a finger cot are always worn to examine the palate.

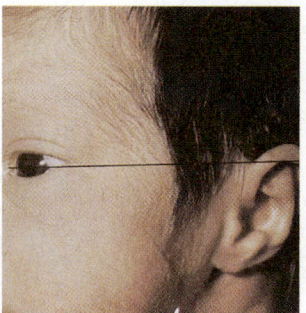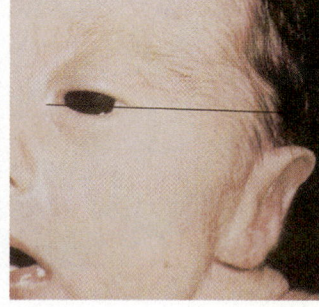

FIGURE 25–29. ◆ The position of the external ear may be assessed by drawing a line across the inner and outer canthus of the eye to the insertion of the ear. **A,** Normal position. **B,** True low-set position. Courtesy of Mead Johnson Nutritionals, Evansville, IN.

Neck

A short neck, creased with skin folds, is normal. Because muscle tone is not well developed, the neck cannot support the full weight of the head, which rotates freely. The head lags considerably when the newborn is pulled from a supine to a sitting position, but the prone newborn is able to raise the head slightly. Palpate the neck for masses and lymph nodes and inspect it for webbing. Determine adequacy of range of motion and neck muscle function by fully extending the head in all directions. Consider injury to the sternocleidomastoid muscle (congenital torticollis) if the neck is rigid.

Evaluate the clavicles for evidence of fractures, which occasionally occur during difficult births or in newborns with broad shoulders. The normal clavicle is straight. If fractured, a lump and a grating sensation (crepitus) during movements may be palpated along the course of the side of the break. Elicit Moro reflex (page 551) to evaluate bilateral equal movement of the arms. If the clavicle is fractured, the response will be demonstrated only on the unaffected side.

Chest

The thorax is cylindrical at birth, and the ribs are flexible. Assess the general appearance of the chest. A protrusion at the lower end of the sternum, called the *xiphoid cartilage,* is frequently seen. It is under the skin and will become less apparent after several weeks as adipose tissue accumulates.

Engorged breasts occur frequently in both male and female newborns. This condition, which occurs by the third day, is a result of maternal hormonal influences and may last up to 2 weeks (Figure 25–30 ◆). A whitish secretion from the nipples may also be noted. The newborn's breast should not be massaged or squeezed, because this may cause a breast abscess. Extra nipples, or *supernumerary nipples,* are occasionally noted below and medial to the true nipples. These harmless pink or brown (in darker-skinned newborns) spots vary in size and do not contain glandular tissue. Differentiate accessory nipples from a pigmented nevi (mole) by placing the fingertips alongside the accessory nipple and pulling the adjacent tissue laterally. The accessory nipple will appear dimpled. At puberty the accessory nipple may darken.

Cry

The newborn's cry should be strong, lusty, and of medium pitch. A high-pitched, shrill cry is abnormal and may indicate neurologic disorders or hypoglycemia. Periods of crying usually vary in length after consoling measures are used. Babies' cries are an important method of communication and alert caregivers to changes in the baby's condition and needs.

Respiration

Normal breathing for a term newborn is 30 to 60 respirations per minute and is predominantly diaphragmatic, with associated rising and falling of the abdomen during inspiration and expiration. Note any signs of respiratory distress, nasal flaring, intercostal or xiphoid retraction, expiratory grunt or sigh, seesaw respirations, or tachypnea (greater than 60 breaths per minute or sustained). Also note hyperexpansion (chest appears high) or hypoexpansion (chest appears low) of the anteroposterior diameter of the chest. Both the anterior and posterior chest are auscultated. Some breath sounds are heard better when the newborn is crying, but localizing and identifying breath sounds are difficult in the newborn. Upper airway noises and bowel sounds may also be heard over the chest wall and make auscultation difficult. Because sounds may be transmitted from the unaffected lung to the affected lung, the absence of breath sounds may not be diagnosed. Air entry may be noisy in the first couple of hours until lung fluid resolves, especially after cesarean births. Brief periods of apnea (episodic breathing) occur, but no color or heart rate changes occur in healthy, term newborns.

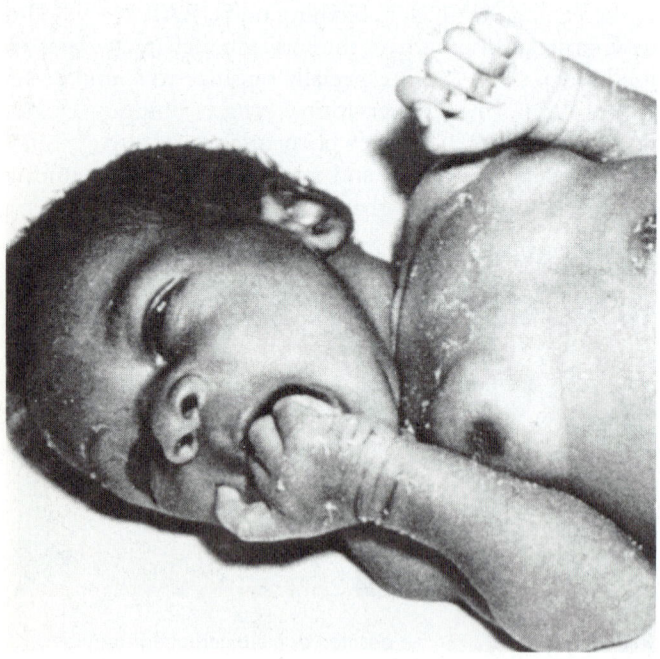

FIGURE 25–30. ◆ Breast hypertrophy. *Note:* From Korones, S. B. (1986). *High-risk newborn infants* (4th ed.). St. Louis, MO: Mosby.

Nursing Practice

Vital sign assessments are most accurate if the newborn is at rest, so measure pulse and respirations first if the baby is quiet. To soothe a crying baby, try placing your moistened gloved finger in the baby's mouth and then complete your assessment while the baby suckles.

Heart

Heart rates can be as rapid as 180 beats per minute in newborns and fluctuate a great deal, especially if the baby moves or is startled. The normal range is 120 to 160 beats per minute. The heart is examined for rate and rhythm, position of the apical impulse, and heart sound intensity. The physician should reassess dysrhythmias.

The pulse rate is variable and is influenced by physical activity, crying, state of wakefulness, and body temperature. The examiner auscultates over the entire heart region (precordium), below the left axilla, and below the scapula. Apical pulse rates are obtained by auscultation for a full minute, preferably when the newborn is asleep.

The placement of the heart in the chest should be determined when the newborn is in a quiet state. The heart is relatively large at birth and is located high in the chest, with its apex somewhere between the fourth and fifth intercostal space. A shift of heart tones in the mediastinal area to either side may indicate pneumothorax, dextrocardia (heart placement on the right side of the chest), or a diaphragmatic hernia. The experienced nurse can diagnose these and many other problems early with a stethoscope.

Normally, the heart beat has a "toc tic" sound. A slur or slushing sound (usually after the first sound) may indicate a murmur. Although 90% of all murmurs are transient and are considered normal, a physician should monitor them closely. Many murmurs are related to a patent ductus arteriosus, which closes in about 1 to 2 days. In newborns, a low-pitched, musical murmur heard just to the right of the apex of the heart is fairly common. Occasionally, significant murmurs are heard, including the murmur of a patent ductus arteriosus, aortic or pulmonary stenosis, or small ventricular septal defect. (See Chapter 28 for a discussion of congenital heart defects.)

Also evaluate peripheral pulses (brachial, femoral, pedal) to detect any lags or unusual characteristics. Palpate brachial pulses bilaterally for equality and compare them with the femoral pulses. Palpate femoral pulses by applying gentle pressure with the middle finger over the femoral canal (Figure 25–31 ◆). Decreased or absent femoral pulses indicate coarctation of the aorta and require additional investigation. A wide difference in blood pressure between the upper and lower extremities also indicates coarctation.

The measurement of blood pressure is best accomplished by using the Doppler technique or a 1- to 2-inch cuff and a stethoscope over the brachial artery (Figure 25–32 ◆). If a Doppler device is used, the newborn's extremities must be immobilized during the assessment, and the cuff should cover two thirds of the upper arm or upper leg. Movement, crying, and inappropriate cuff size can give inaccurate measurements of the blood pressure.

Blood pressure may not be measured routinely on healthy newborns, but it is essential for newborns who are having distress, are premature, or are suspected of cardiac anomaly (Thureen et al., 1999). Infants who have birth asphyxia and are on ventilators have significantly lower sys-

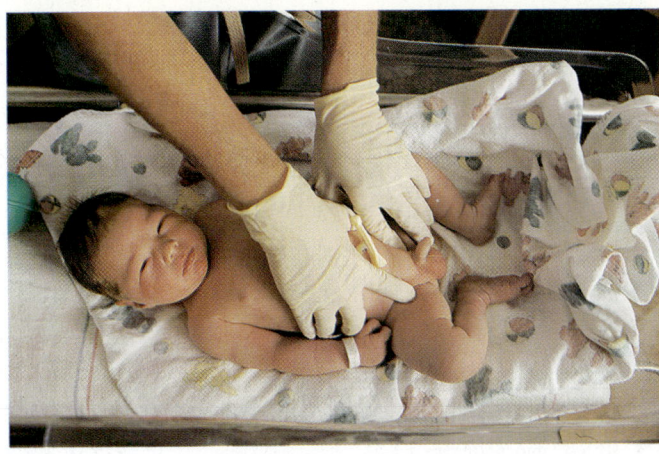

A

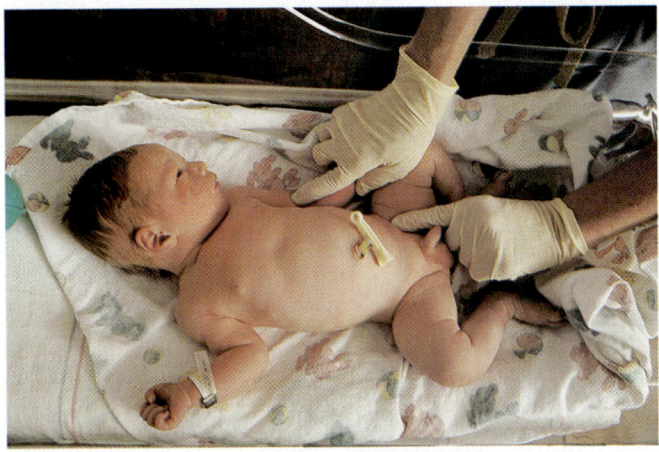

B

FIGURE 25–31. ◆ **A,** Bilaterally palpate the femoral arteries for rate and intensity of the pulses. Press fingertip gently at the groin as shown. **B,** Compare the femoral pulses to the brachial pulses by palpating the pulses simultaneously for comparison of rate and intensity.

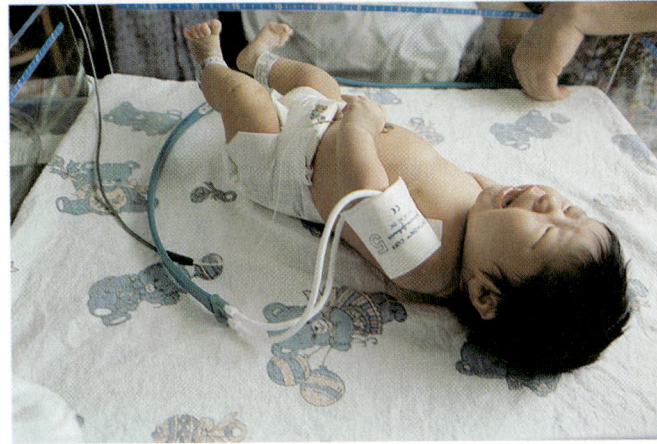

FIGURE 25–32. ◆ Blood pressure measurement using a Doppler device. The cuff can be applied to the upper arm or thigh.

TABLE 25–4 Newborn Vital Signs

Pulse
- 120–160 bpm
- During sleep as low as 100 bpm; if crying, up to 180 bpm
- Apical pulse counted for 1 full minute

Respirations
- 30–60 respirations/minute
- Predominantly diaphragmatic but synchronous with abdominal movements
- Respirations are counted for 1 full minute

Blood Pressure
- 80–60/45–40 mm Hg at birth
- 100/50 mm Hg at day 10

Temperature
- Normal range: 36.5–37.5 °C (97.7–99.4 °F)
- Axillary: 36.4–37.2 °C (97.5–99 °F)
- Skin: 36–36.5 °C (96.8–97.7 °F)
- Rectal: 36.6–37.2 °C (97.8–99 °F)

tolic and diastolic blood pressures than healthy infants. If cardiac anomaly is suspected, blood pressure is measured in all four extremities (Table 25–4).

Abdomen

The nurse can learn a great deal about the newborn's abdomen without disturbing the infant. The abdomen should be cylindrical and protrude slightly. A certain amount of laxness of the abdominal muscles is normal. A scaphoid (hollow-shaped) appearance suggests the absence of abdominal contents. No cyanosis should be present, and few if any blood vessels should be apparent to the eye. There should be no gross distention or bulging. The more distended the abdomen, the tighter the skin becomes, with engorged vessels appearing. Distention is the first sign of many of the abnormalities found in the gastrointestinal tract.

Before palpating the abdomen, auscultate for bowel sounds in all four quadrants. Bowel sounds may be present by 1 hour after birth. Palpation can cause a transient decrease in intensity of the bowel sounds.

Abdominal palpation should be done systematically. Palpate each of the four abdominal quadrants and move in a clockwise direction until all four quadrants have been palpated for softness, tenderness, and the presence of masses.

Umbilical Cord

Initially the umbilical cord is white and gelatinous in appearance, with the two umbilical arteries and one umbilical vein readily apparent. Because a single umbilical artery is frequently associated with congenital anomalies, count the vessels during the newborn assessment. The cord begins drying within 1 or 2 hours of birth and is shriveled and blackened by the second or third day. Within 7 to 10 days

it sloughs off, although a granulating area may remain for a few days longer.

Cord bleeding is abnormal and may result because the cord was inadvertently pulled or the cord clamp was loosened. Foul-smelling drainage is also abnormal and is generally caused by infection, which requires immediate treatment to prevent septicemia. If the newborn has a patent urachus (abnormal connection between the umbilicus and bladder), moistness or draining urine may be apparent at the base of the cord.

Serous or serosanguineous drainage that continues after the cord falls off may indicate a granuloma. It appears as a small red button deep in the umbilicus. A physician cauterizes it with a silver nitrate stick (O'Donnell, Glick, & Cory, 1998).

Genitals

FEMALE INFANTS

Examine the labia majora, labia minora, and clitoris and note the size of each as appropriate for gestational age. A vaginal tag or hymenal tag is often evident and usually disappears in a few weeks. During the first week of life, the newborn may have a vaginal discharge composed of thick, whitish mucus. This discharge, which can become tinged with blood, is called **pseudomenstruation** and is caused by the withdrawal of maternal hormones. Smegma, a white, cheeselike substance, is often present between the labia. Removing it may traumatize tender tissue.

MALE INFANTS

Inspect the penis to determine whether the urinary orifice is correctly positioned. *Hypospadias* occurs when the urinary meatus is located on the ventral surface of the penis. It occurs most commonly among people of western European descent. *Phimosis* is a condition in which the opening of the foreskin (prepuce) is small and the foreskin cannot be pulled back over the glans at all. This condition may interfere with urination, so the adequacy of the urinary stream should be evaluated.

Inspect the scrotum for size and symmetry, palpating to verify the presence of both testes and to rule out *cryptorchidism* (failure of testes to descend). Palpate the testes separately between the thumb and forefinger, with the thumb and forefinger of the other hand placed together over the inguinal canal. Scrotal edema and discoloration are common in breech births. *Hydrocele* (a collection of fluid surrounding the testes in the scrotum) is common in newborns and should be identified. It usually resolves without intervention. A discolored or dusky scrotum and solid testis should raise the suspicion of testicular torsion (Juretschke, 2000).

Anus

Inspect the anal area to verify that it is patent and has no fissure. Imperforate anus and rectal atresia may be ruled out by observation. Digital examination, if necessary, is done by a physician or nurse practitioner. The nurse also notes the passage of the first meconium stool. Atresia of the gastrointestinal tract or meconium ileus with resultant obstruction must be considered if the newborn does not pass meconium in the first 24 hours of life.

Extremities

Examine extremities for gross deformities, extra digits or webbing, clubfoot, and range of motion. Normal newborn extremities appear short, are generally flexible, and move symmetrically.

ARMS AND HANDS

Nails extend beyond the fingertips in term newborns. Count fingers and toes. *Polydactyly* is the presence of extra digits on either the hands or the feet. *Syndactyly* refers to fusion (webbing) of fingers or toes. Inspect the hands for normal palmar creases. A single palmar crease, called *simian line* (see Figure 4–16), is frequently present in children with Down syndrome.

Brachial palsy, paralysis of portions of the arm, results from trauma to the brachial plexus during a difficult birth. It occurs commonly when strong traction is exerted on the head of the newborn in an attempt to deliver a shoulder lodged behind the symphysis pubis in the presence of shoulder dystocia. Brachial palsy may also occur during a breech birth if an arm becomes trapped over the head and traction is exerted.

The portion of the arm affected is determined by the nerves damaged. **Erb-Duchenne paralysis (Erb's palsy)** involves damage to the upper arm (fifth and sixth cervical nerves) and is the most common type. Injury to the eighth cervical and first thoracic nerve roots and the lower portion of the plexus produces the relatively rare *lower arm injury*. The *whole-arm type* results from damage to the entire plexus.

With Erb-Duchenne paralysis the newborn's arm lies limply at the side. The elbow is held in extension, with the forearm pronated. The newborn is unable to elevate the arm, and the Moro reflex cannot be elicited on the affected side (Figure 25–33 ◆). Lower arm injury causes paralysis of the hand and wrist; complete paralysis of the limb occurs with the whole-arm type.

Carefully instruct the parents in the correct method of performing passive range of motion exercises (to prevent muscle contractures and restore function) and arrange supervised practice sessions. In more severe cases, splinting of the arm is indicated until the edema decreases. The arm is held in a position of abduction and external rotation with the elbow flexed 90 degrees.

Complete recovery occurs within a few months with minimal trauma (amount of nerve damage resulting from trauma and hemorrhage within the nerve sheath). Routine orthopedic follow-up should occur in all cases, because growth plate problems can occur years later. Moderate trauma may result in partial paralysis. Recovery is unlikely with severe trauma, and muscle wasting may develop.

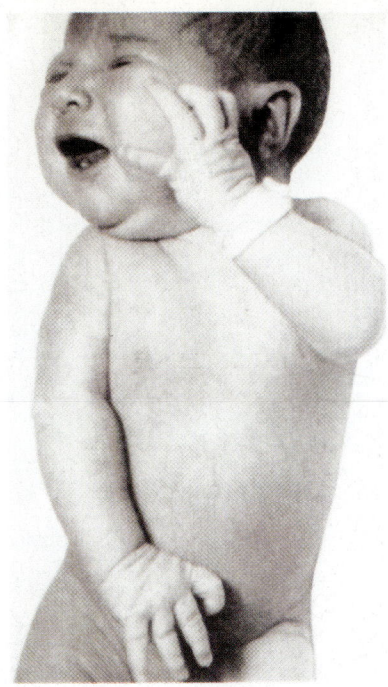

FIGURE 25–33. ◆ Right Erb's palsy resulting from injury to the fifth and sixth cervical roots of the brachial plexus. *Note:* From Potter, E. L., & Craig, J. M. (1975). *Pathology of the fetus and infant* (3rd ed.). St. Louis: Mosby–Yearbook Medical Publishers. Reproduced with permission.

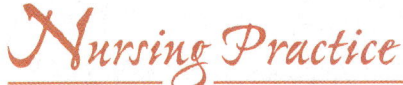

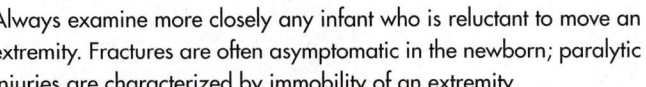

Always examine more closely any infant who is reluctant to move an extremity. Fractures are often asymptomatic in the newborn; paralytic injuries are characterized by immobility of an extremity.

LEGS AND FEET

The newborn's legs should be of equal length, with symmetric skin folds. However, they may assume a "fetal posture" secondary to position in utero, and it may take several days for the legs to relax into a normal position. Perform **Ortolani's maneuver** to rule out the possibility of congenital hip dysplasia (hip dislocation). With the newborn relaxed and quiet on a firm surface, with hips and knees flexed at a 90-degree angle, grasp the infant's thigh with the middle finger over the greater trochanter and lift the thigh to bring the femoral head from its posterior position toward the acetabulum. With gentle abduction of the thigh, the femoral head is returned to the acetabulum. The examiner feels a sense of reduction or a "clunk" as the femoral head returns. This reduction is audible. To perform **Barlow's maneuver,** grasp and adduct the infant's thigh and apply gentle downward pressure. Dislocation is felt as the femoral head is then returned to the acetabulum using Ortolani's maneuver, confirming the diagnosis of an unstable or dislocated hip (Figure 25–34 ◆).

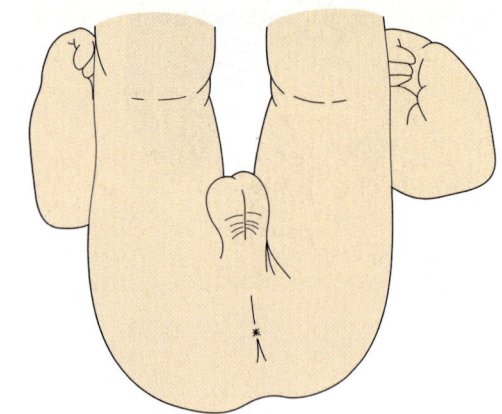

A

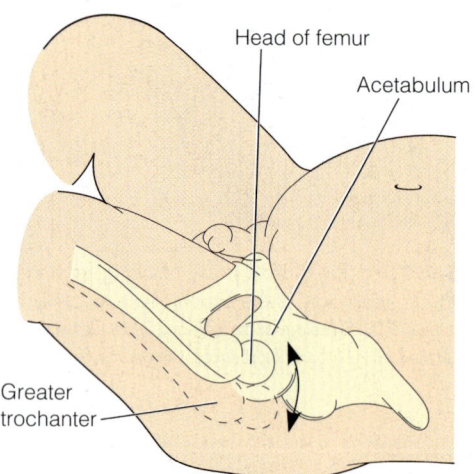

Head of femur

Acetabulum

Greater
trochanter

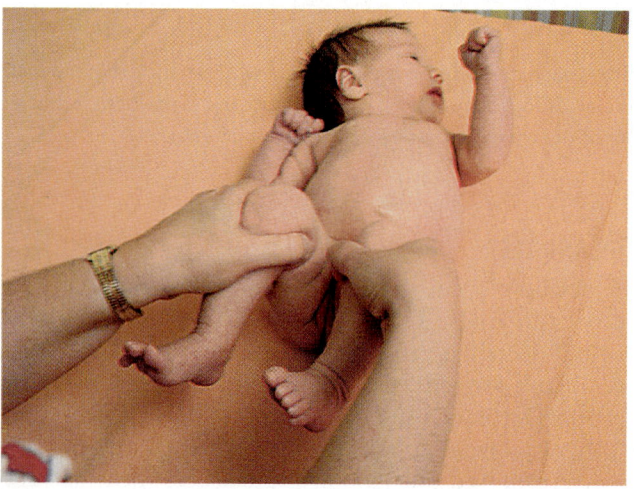

B

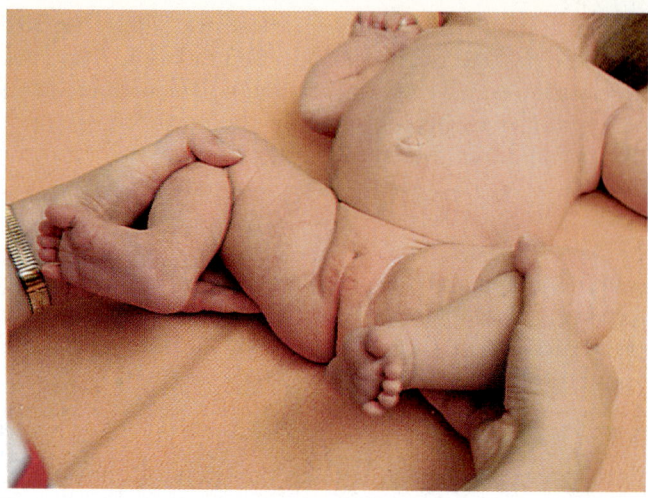

D

FIGURE 25–34. ◆ A, Congenitally dislocated right hip in a young infant as seen on gross inspection. **B,** Barlow's (dislocation) maneuver. Baby's thigh is grasped and adducted (placed together) with gentle downward pressure. Dislocation is palpable as femoral head slips out of acetabulum. **C,** Ortolani's maneuver puts downward pressure on the hip and then inward rotation. If the hip is dislocated, this maneuver forces the femoral head over the acetabular rim with a noticeable "clunk."

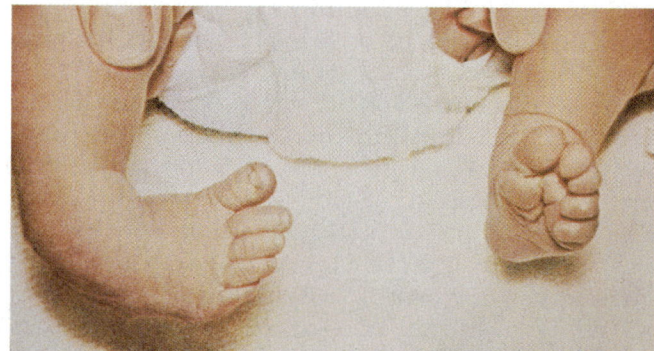

A

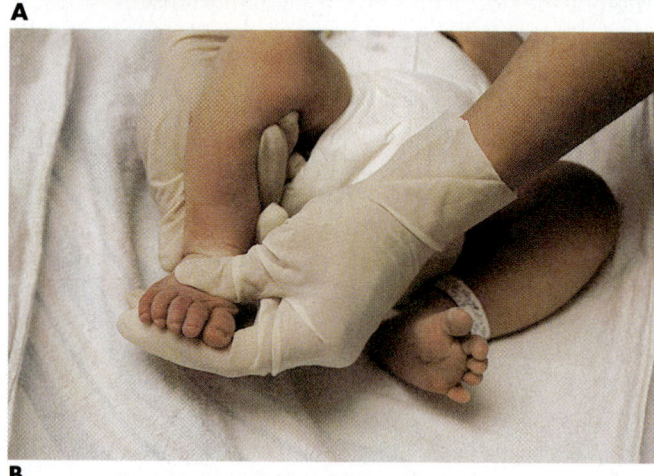

B

FIGURE 25–35. ◆ A, Unilateral talipes equinovarus (clubfoot). **B,** To determine the presence of clubfoot, the nurse moves the foot to the midline. Resistance indicates true clubfoot.
Reprinted with permission of Mead Johnson Nutritionals.

Examine the feet for evidence of clubfoot. Intrauterine position frequently causes the feet to appear to turn inward (Figure 25–35 ◆). This finding is termed a "positional" clubfoot. If the feet can easily be returned to the midline by manipulation, no treatment is indicated; teach range of motion exercises to the family. Further investigation is indicated when the foot will not turn to a midline position or align readily. This condition is a severe "true clubfoot," or talipes equinovarus.

Back

With the newborn prone, examine the back. The spine should appear straight and flat, since the lumbar and sacral curves do not develop until the newborn begins to sit. Examine the base of the spine for a dermal sinus. A nevus pilosus ("hairy nerve") is only occasionally found at the base of the spine in newborns, but it is significant because it is often associated with spina bifida. A pilonidal dimple should be examined to ascertain that there is no connection to the spinal canal.

Assessment of Neurologic Status

The neurologic examination should begin with a period of observation, noting the general physical characteristics and behaviors of the newborn. Important behaviors to assess are the *state of alertness, resting posture, cry,* and *quality of muscle tone and motor activity.*

The usual position of the newborn is with partially flexed extremities, with the legs abducted to the abdomen. When awake, the newborn may exhibit purposeless, uncoordinated bilateral movements of the extremities. If these movements are absent, minimal, or obviously asymmetric, neurologic dysfunction should be suspected. Eye movements are observable during the first few days of life. An alert newborn is able to fixate on faces and brightly colored objects. A bright light shining in the newborn's eyes elicits the blinking response.

Evaluate muscle tone by moving various parts of the body while the head of the newborn is in a neutral position. The newborn is somewhat hypertonic; that is, there should be resistance to extending the elbow and knee joints. Muscle tone should be symmetric. Diminished muscle tone and flaccidity require further evaluation.

Tremors are common in the full-term newborn and must be evaluated to differentiate them from convulsions. A fine jumping of the muscle is likely to be a central nervous system (CNS) disorder and requires further evaluation. Tremors may also be related to hypoglycemia or hypocalcemia. Newborn seizures may consist of no more than chewing or swallowing movements, deviations of the eyes, rigidity, or flaccidity because of CNS immaturity.

It is possible to elicit specific deep tendon reflexes, but they have limited value unless they are obviously asymmetric. The knee jerk is typically brisk; a normal ankle clonus may involve three or four beats. Plantar flexion is present.

The immature CNS of the newborn is characterized by a variety of reflexes. Because the newborn's movements are uncoordinated, methods of communication are limited, and control of body functions is drastically limited, the reflexes serve a variety of purposes. Some are protective (blink, gag, sneeze), some aid in feeding (rooting, sucking) and may not be very active if the infant has eaten recently, and some stimulate human interaction (grasping). Carefully assess newborn reflex and general neurologic activity (Pressler & Hepworth, 1997).

The most common reflexes found in the normal newborn are the following:

- The **tonic neck reflex** (fencer position) is elicited when the newborn is supine and the head is turned to one side. In response, the extremities on the same side straighten, whereas on the opposite side they flex (Figure 25–36 ◆). This reflex may not be seen during the early newborn period, but once it appears it persists until about the third month.
- The **Moro reflex** is elicited when the newborn is startled by a loud noise or lifted slightly above the crib and then suddenly lowered. In response, the newborn straightens arms and hands outward while the knees flex. Slowly the arms return to the chest, as in an embrace. The fingers spread, forming a C, and the newborn may cry (Figure 25–37 ◆). This reflex may persist until about 6 months of age.
- The **grasping reflex** is elicited by stimulating the newborn's palm with a finger or object; the newborn grasps and holds the object or finger firmly enough to be lifted momentarily from the crib (Figure 25–38 ◆).
- The **rooting reflex** is elicited when the side of the newborn's mouth or cheek is touched. In response, the newborn turns toward that side and opens the lips to suck (if not fed recently) (Figure 25–39 ◆).

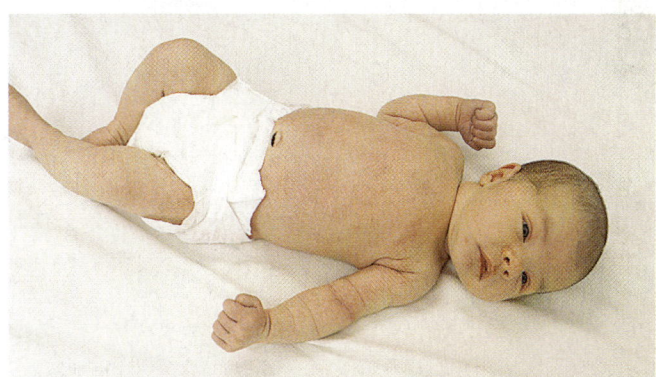

FIGURE 25–36. ◆ Tonic neck reflex.

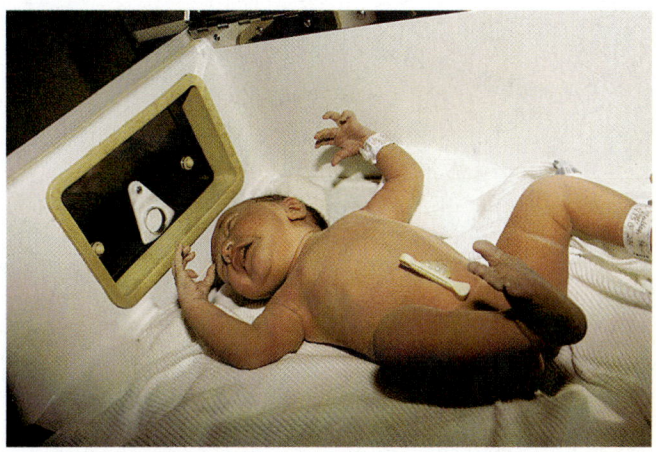

FIGURE 25–37. ◆ Moro reflex.

- The **sucking reflex** is elicited when an object is placed in the newborn's mouth or anything touches the lips. Newborns suck even while sleeping; this is called *nonnutritive sucking,* and it can have a quieting effect on the baby.

- The **Babinski reflex (plantar reflex),** or fanning and hyperextension of all toes, occurs when the lateral aspect of the sole is stroked from the heel upward across the ball of the foot (see Figure 25–40 ◆). In adults, the toes flex.

- **Trunk incurvation (Galant reflex)** is seen when the newborn is prone. Stroking the spine causes the pelvis to turn to the stimulated side.

In addition to these reflexes, newborns can *blink, yawn, cough, sneeze,* and draw back from pain (protective reflexes). They can even move a little on their own. When placed on their stomachs, they push up and try to crawl (prone crawl). When held upright with one foot touching a flat surface, the newborn puts one foot in front of the other and "walks" *(stepping reflex)* (Figure 25–41 ◆). This reflex is more pronounced at birth and is lost in 4 to 8 weeks.

Use the following steps to assess CNS integration:

1. Insert a gloved finger into the newborn's mouth to elicit a sucking reflex.
2. As soon as the newborn is sucking vigorously, assess hearing and vision responses by noting changes in sucking in the presence of a light, a rattle, and a voice.
3. The newborn should respond to such stimuli with a brief cessation of sucking, followed by continuous sucking with repetitious stimulation.

This examination demonstrates auditory and visual integrity as well as the capability of complex behavioral interactions. Refer to "Newborn Physical Assessment Guide" for a summary of the stimulus for, and response of, the common newborn reflexes.

Newborn Physical Assessment Guide

Following is a guide for systematically assessing the newborn (pages 553–563). Normal findings, alterations, and related causes are presented and correlated with suggested nursing responses. The findings are typical for a full-term newborn.

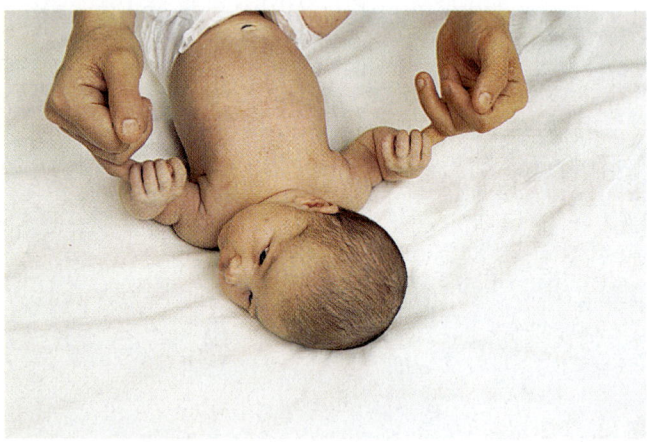

FIGURE 25–38. ◆ Grasping reflex.

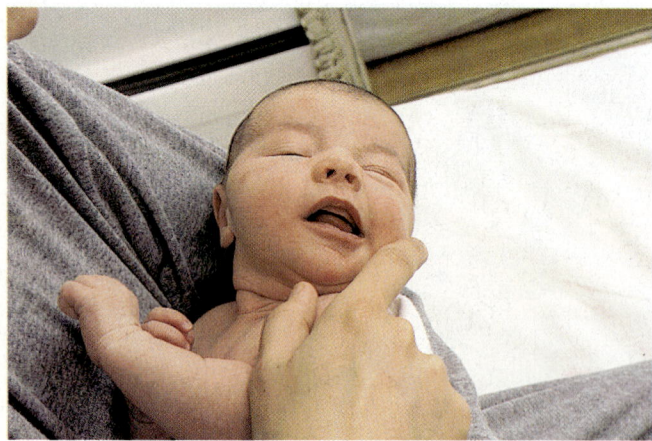

FIGURE 25–39. ◆ Rooting reflex.

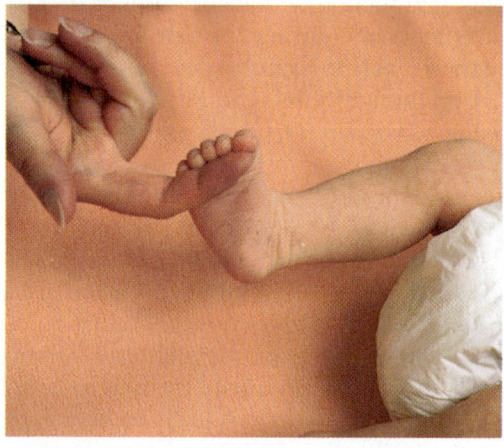

FIGURE 25–40. ◆ The Babinski (or plantar) reflex.

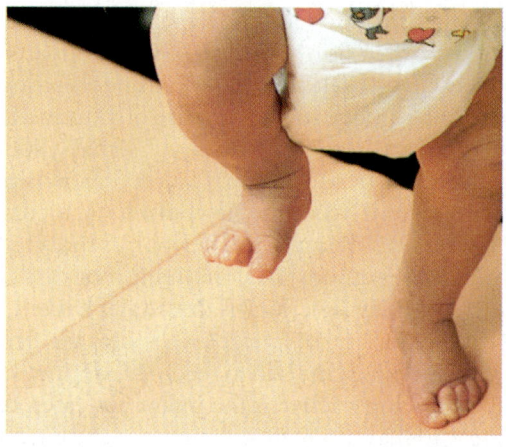

FIGURE 25–41. ◆ The stepping reflex disappears between 4 and 8 weeks of age.

Physical Assessment/Normal Findings	Alterations and Possible Causes*	Nursing Responses to Data†
VITAL SIGNS		
Blood pressure (BP) At birth: 80–60/45–40 mm Hg Day 10: 100/50 mm Hg (may be unable to measure diastolic pressure with standard sphygmomanometer)	Low BP (hypovolemia, shock)	Monitor BP in all cases of distress, prematurity, or suspected anomaly. Low BP: Refer to physician immediately so measures to improve circulation are begun.
Pulse 120–160 bpm (if asleep, 100 bpm; if crying, up to 180 bpm)	Weak pulse (decreased cardiac output) Bradycardia (severe asphyxia, arrhythmia) Tachycardia (over 160 bpm at rest) (infection, central nervous system problems, arrhythmia)	Assess skin perfusion by blanching (capillary refill test). Correlate finding with BP assessments; refer to physician. Carry out neurologic and thermoregulation assessments.
Respirations 30–60 breaths/minute Synchronization of chest and abdominal movements Diaphragmatic and abdominal breathing Transient tachypnea	Tachypnea (pneumonia, respiratory distress syndrome [RDS]) Rapid, shallow breathing (hypermagnesemia due to large doses given to mothers with PIH) Respirations below 30 breaths/minute (maternal anesthesia or analgesia) Expiratory grunting; subcostal and substernal retractions; flaring of nares (respiratory distress); apnea (cold stress, respiratory disorder)	Identify sleep-wake state; correlate with respiratory pattern. Evaluate for all signs of respiratory distress; report findings to physician. Evaluate for cold stress. Report findings to physician or nurse practitioner.
Crying Strong and lusty Moderate tone and pitch Cries vary in length from 3 to 7 minutes after consoling measures are used	High pitched, shrill (neurologic disorder, hypoglycemia) Weak or absent (CNS disorder, laryngeal problem)	Discuss newborn's use of cry for communication. Assess and record abnormal cries. Reduce environmental noises.
Temperature Axilla 36.4–37.2 °C (97.5–99 °F) Rectal 36.6–37.2 °C (97.8–99 °F); 36.8 °C (98.8 °F) desired Heavier neonates tend to have higher body temperatures	Elevated temperature (room too warm, too much clothing or covers, dehydration, sepsis, brain damage) Subnormal temperature (brain stem involvement, cold, sepsis) Swings of more than 2 °F from one reading to next or subnormal temperature (infection)	Notify physician of elevation or drop. Counsel parents on possible causes of elevated or low temperatures, appropriate home care measures, when to call physician. Teach parents how to take rectal and/or axillary temperature; assess parents' information regarding use of thermometer; provide teaching as needed.
Weight 2500–4000 g (5 lb, 8 oz–8 lb, 13 oz)	<2748 g (<6 lb) = SGA or preterm infant >4050 g (>9 lb) = LGA or infants of diabetic mothers	Plot weight and gestational age on growth chart to identify high-risk infants. Ascertain body build of parents. Counsel parents regarding appropriate caloric intake.
Within first 3 to 4 days, normal weight loss of 5%–10% Large babies tend to lose more due to greater fluid loss in proportion to birth weight except infants of diabetic mothers	Loss greater than 15% (small fluid intake, loss of meconium and urine, feeding difficulties)	Notify physician of net losses or gains. Calculate fluid intake and losses from all sources (insensible water loss, radiant warmers, phototherapy lights).
Length 48–52 cm (18–22 in) Grows 10 cm (3 in) during first 3 months	Less than 45 cm (congenital dwarf) Short/long bones proximally (achondroplasia) Short/long bones distally (Ellis-van Creveld syndrome)	Assess for other signs of dwarfism. Determine other signs of skeletal system adequacy. Plot progress at subsequent well-baby visits.
	*Possible causes of alterations are placed in parentheses.	**†This column provides guidelines for further assessment and initial nursing interventions.**

(continued)

Physical Assessment/Normal Findings	Alterations and Possible Causes*	Nursing Responses to Data†
POSTURE		
Body usually flexed, hands may be tightly clenched, neck appears short because chin rests on chest	Only extension noted, inability to move from midline (trauma, hypoxia, immaturity)	Record spontaneity of motor activity and symmetry of movements.
In breech births, feet are usually dorsiflexed	Constant motion (maternal caffeine intake)	If parents express concern about newborn's movement patterns, reassure and further evaluate if appropriate.
SKIN		
Color		
Color consistent with genetic background	Pallor of face conjunctiva (anemia, hypothermia, anoxia)	Discuss with parents common skin color variations to allay fears.
Newborns of European descent: pink-tinged or ruddy color over face, trunk, extremities	Beefy red (hypoglycemia, immature vasomotor reflexes, polycythemia)	Document extent and time of occurrence of color change.
Newborns of African or Native-American descent; pale pink with yellow or red tinge		
Newborns of Asian descent: pink or rosy red to yellow tinge		
Common variations: acrocyanosis, circumoral cyanosis, or harlequin color change	Meconium staining (fetal distress)	Obtain Hb and hematocrit values; obtain bilirubin levels.
	Jaundice (hemolytic reaction from blood incompatibility within first 24 hours, sepsis)	Assess for respiratory difficulty.
		Differentiate between physiologic and pathologic jaundice.
Mottled when undressed	Cyanosis (choanal atresia, CNS damage or trauma, respiratory or cardiac problem, cold stress)	Assess degree of (central or peripheral) cyanosis and possible causes; refer to physician.
Minor bruising over buttocks in breech presentation and over eyes and forehead in facial presentations		Discuss with parents cause and course of minor bruising related to labor and birth.
Texture		
Smooth, soft, flexible; may have dry, peeling hands and feet	Generalized cracked or peeling skin (SGA or postterm; blood incompatibility; metabolic, kidney dysfunction)	Report to physician.
		Instruct parents to shampoo the scalp and anterior fontanelle areas daily with soap; rinse well; avoid use of oil.
	Seborrheic-dermatitis (cradle cap)	
	Absence of vernix (postmature)	
	Yellow vernix (bilirubin staining)	
Turgor		
Elastic, returns to normal shape after pinching	Maintains tent shape (dehydration)	Assess for other signs and symptoms of dehydration.
Pigmentation		
Clear; milia across bridge of nose, forehead, or chin will disappear within a few weeks		Advise parents not to pinch or prick these pimplelike areas.
Café-au-lait spots (one or two)	Six or more (neurologic disorder such as von Recklinghausen disease, cutaneous neurofibromatosis)	If there are six or more café-au-lait spots, refer for genetic and neurologic consult.
Mongolian spots common over dorsal area and buttocks in dark-skinned infants		Assure parents of normalcy of this pigmentation; it will fade in first year or two.
Erythema toxicum	Impetigo (group A β-hemolytic streptococcus or *Staphylococcus aureus* infection)	If impetigo occurs, instruct parents about hand-washing and linen precautions during home care.
	Hemangiomas:	Collaborate with physician.
Telangiectatic nevi	Nevus flammeus (port-wine stain)	Counsel parents about birthmark's progression to allay misconceptions.
	Nevus vasculosus (strawberry hemangioma)	
	Cavernous hemangiomas	Record size and shape of hemangiomas.
		Refer for follow-up at well-baby clinic.
	Rashes (infection)	Assess location and type of rash (macular, papular, vesicular).
Rashes		Obtain history of onset, prenatal history, and related signs and symptoms.
	Generalized petechiae (clotting abnormalities)	
Petechiae of head or neck (breech presentation, cord around neck)		Determine cause; advise parents if further health care is needed.

Physical Assessment/Normal Findings	Alterations and Possible Causes*	Nursing Responses to Data†
HEAD		
General appearance, size, movement Round, symmetric, and moves easily from left to right and up and down; soft and pliable	Asymmetric, flattened occiput on either side of the head (plagiocephaly) Head held at angle (torticollis)	Instruct parents to change infant's sleeping positions frequently.
	Unable to move head side to side (neurologic trauma)	Determine adequacy of all neurologic signs.
Circumference: 32–37 cm (12.5–14.5 in); 2 cm greater than chest circumference Head one fourth of body size	Extreme differences in size may be due to microencephaly (Cornelia de Lange syndrome, cytomegalic inclusion disease [CID]), rubella, toxoplasmosis, chromosome abnormalities), hydrocephalus (meningomyelocele, achondroplasia), anencephaly (neural tube defect) Head is 3 cm or more larger than chest circumference (preterm, hydrocephalus)	Measure circumference from occiput to frontal area using metal or paper tape. Measure chest circumference using metal or paper tape and compare to head circumference. Record measurements on growth chart. Reevaluate at well-baby visits.
Common variations Molding Breech and cesarean newborns' heads are round and well shaped	Cephalhematoma (trauma during birth, persists up to 3 weeks) Caput succedaneum (long labor and birth; disappears in 1 week)	Evaluate neurologic response. Observe for hyperbilirubinemia. Reassure parents regarding common manifestations due to birth process and when they should disappear.
Fontanelles Palpation of juncture of cranial bones Anterior fontanelle: 3–4 cm long by 2–3 cm wide, diamond shaped Posterior fontanelle: 1–2 cm at birth, triangle shaped Slight pulsation Moderate bulging noted with crying, stooling; pulsations with heartbeat	Overlapping of anterior fontanelle (malnourished or preterm newborn) Premature closure of sutures (craniostenosis) Late closure (hydrocephalus) Moderate to severe pulsation (vascular problems) Bulging (increased intracranial pressure, meningitis) Sunken (dehydration)	Discuss normal closure times with parents and care of "soft spots" to allay misconceptions. Refer to physician. Observe for signs and symptoms of hydrocephalus. Refer to physician. Report to physician. Evaluate neurologic status. Evaluate hydration status.
HAIR		
Texture Smooth with fine texture variations (*Note:* Variations depend on ethnic background.)	Coarse, brittle, dry hair (hypothyroidism) White forelock (Waardenburg syndrome)	Instruct parents regarding routine care of hair and scalp.
Distribution Scalp hair high over eyebrows (Spanish-Mexican hairline begins midforehead and extends down back of neck.)	Low forehead and posterior hairlines may indicate chromosomal disorders.	Assess for other signs of chromosomal aberrations. Refer to physician.
FACE		
Symmetric movement of all facial features, normal hairline, eyebrows and eyelashes present		Assess and record symmetry of all parts, shape, regularity of features, sameness or differences in features.
Spacing of features Eyes at same level, nostrils equal size, cheeks full, and sucking pads present	Eyes wide apart—ocular hypertelorism (Apert syndrome, cri-du-chat, Turner syndrome)	Observe for other signs and symptoms indicative of disease states or chromosomal aberrations.
Lips equal on both sides of midline	Abnormal face (Down syndrome, cretinism, gargoylism)	
Chin recedes when compared to other bones of face	Abnormally small jaw—micrognathia (Pierre Robin syndrome, Treacher Collins syndrome)	Maintain airway; do not position supine. Initiate surgical consultation and referral.
Movement Makes facial grimaces	Inability to suck, grimace, and close eyelids (cranial nerve injury)	Initiate neurologic assessment and consultation.
Symmetric when resting and crying	Asymmetry (paralysis of facial cranial nerve)	Assess and record symmetry of all parts, shape, regularity of features, and sameness or differences in features.
	*Possible causes of alterations are placed in parentheses.	**†This column provides guidelines for further assessment and initial nursing interventions.**

(continued)

Physical Assessment/Normal Findings	Alterations and Possible Causes*	Nursing Responses to Data†
EYES		
General placement and appearance		
Bright and clear; even placement; slight nystagmus (involuntary cyclical eye movements)	Gross nystagmus (damage to third, fourth, and sixth cranial nerves)	
Concomitant strabismus	Constant and fixed strabismus	Reassure parents that strabismus is considered normal up to 6 months.
Move in all directions		
Blue- or slate-blue gray	Lack of pigmentation (albinism)	Discuss with parents any necessary eye precautions.
	Brushfield spots may indicate Down syndrome (a light or white speckling of the outer two thirds of the iris)	Assess for other signs of Down syndrome.
Brown color at birth in dark-skinned infants		Discuss with parents that permanent eye color is usually established by 3 months of age.
Eyelids		
Position: above pupils but within iris, no drooping	Elevation or retraction of upper lid (hyperthyroidism)	Assess for signs of hydrocephalus and hyperthyroidism.
	"Sunset sign" lid retraction and downward gaze (hydrocephalus), ptosis (congenital or paralysis of oculomotor muscle)	Evaluate interference with vision in subsequent well-baby visits.
Eyes on parallel plane	Upward slant in non-Asians (Down syndrome)	Assess for other signs of Down syndrome.
Epicanthal folds in Asian and 20% of newborns of northern European descent	Epicanthal folds (Down syndrome, cri-du-chat syndrome)	
Movement		
Blink reflex in response to light stimulus	Blink absent (CNS injury)	Evaluate neurologic status.
Eyes open wide in dimly lit room		Refer to physician.
Inspection		
Edematous for first few days of life, resulting from birth and instillation of silver nitrate (chemical conjunctivitis); no lumps or redness	Purulent drainage (infection); infectious conjunctivitis (gonococcus, chlamydia, staphylococcus, or gram-negative organisms)	Initiate good handwashing. Refer to physician.
	Marginal blepharitis (lid edges red, crusted, scaly)	Evaluate infant for seborrheic dermatitis; scales can be removed easily.
Cornea		
Clear	Ulceration (herpes infection); large cornea or corneas of unequal size (congenital glaucoma)	Refer to ophthalmologist.
Corneal reflex present	Clouding, opacity of lens (cataract)	Assess for other manifestations of congenital herpes; institute nursing care measures.
Sclera		
May appear bluish in newborn, then white; slightly brownish color frequent in newborns of African descent	True blue sclera (osteogenesis imperfecta)	Refer to physician.
Pupils		
Pupils equal in size, round, and react to light by accommodation	Anisocoria—unequal pupils (CNS damage)	Refer for neurologic examination.
	Dilation or constriction (intracranial damage, retinoblastoma, glaucoma)	
	Pupils nonreactive to light or accommodation (brain injury)	
Slight nystagmus in newborn who has not learned to focus	Nystagmus (labyrinthine disturbance, CNS disorder)	
Pupil light reflex demonstrated at birth or by 3 weeks of age		
Conjunctiva		
Chemical conjunctivitis	Pale color (anemia)	Obtain hematocrit and hemoglobin.
Subconjunctival hemorrhage		Reassure parents that chemical conjunctivitis will subside in 1 to 2 days and subconjunctival hemorrhage disappears in a few weeks.
Palpebral conjunctiva (red but not hyperemic)	Inflammation or edema (infection, blocked tear duct)	

Physical Assessment/Normal Findings	Alterations and Possible Causes*	Nursing Responses to Data†
EYES— *continued*		
Vision		
20/150	Cataracts (congenital infection)	Record any questions about visual acuity and initiate follow-up evaluation at first well-baby checkup.
Tracks moving object to midline		
Fixed focus on objects at a distance of about 10–20 in; may be difficult to evaluate in newborn		
Prefers faces, geometric designs, and black and white to colors		
Lashes and lacrimal glands		
Presence of lashes (lashes may be absent in preterm newborns)	No lashes on inner two thirds of lid (Treacher Collins syndrome); bushy lashes (Hurler syndrome); long lashes (Cornelia de Lange syndrome)	
Cry commonly tearless	Excessive tearing (plugged lacrimal duct, natal narcotic withdrawal), glaucoma	Demonstrate to parents how to milk blocked tear duct.
		Refer to ophthalmologist if tearing is excessive before third month of life.
NOSE		
Appearance of external nasal aspects		
May appear flattened as a result of birth process	Continued flat or broad bridge of nose (Down syndrome)	Arrange consultation with specialist.
Small and narrow in midline, even placement in relationship to eyes and mouth	Low bridge of nose, beaklike nose (Apert syndrome, Treacher Collins syndrome)	Initiate evaluation of chromosomal abnormalities.
	Upturned (Cornelia de Lange syndrome)	
Patent nares bilaterally (nose breathers)	Blockage of nares (mucus and/or secretions), choanal atresia	Inspect for obstruction of nares.
Sneezing common to clear nasal passages	Flaring nares (respiratory distress)	Maintain oral airway until surgical correction is made.
Responds to odors, may smell breast milk	No response to stimulating odors	Inspect for obstruction of nares.
MOUTH		
Function of facial, hypoglossal, glossopharyngeal, and vagus nerves		
Symmetry of movement and strength	Mouth draws to one side (transient seventh cranial nerve paralysis due to pressure in utero or trauma during birth, congenital paralysis)	Initiate neurologic consultation.
		Administer eye care if eye on affected side of face is unable to close.
	Fishlike shape (Treacher Collins syndrome)	
Presence of gag, swallowing, coordinated with sucking reflexes	Suppressed or absent reflexes	Evaluate other neurologic functions of these nerves.
Adequate salivation		
Palate (soft and hard)		
Hard palate dome shaped	High-steepled palate (Treacher Collins syndrome), bifid uvula (congenital anomaly)	Assess for other congenital anomalies.
Uvula midline with symmetric movement of soft palate		
Palate intact, sucks well when stimulated	Clefts in either hard or soft palate (polygenic disorder)	Initiate a surgical consultation referral.
Epithelial (Epstein's) pearls appear on mucosa		Assure parents that these are normal and will disappear at 2 or 3 months of age.
Esophagus patent, some drooling common in newborn	Excessive drooling or bubbling (esophageal atresia)	Test for patency of esophagus.
	*Possible causes of alterations are placed in parentheses.	**†This column provides guidelines for further assessment and initial nursing interventions.**

(continued)

Physical Assessment/Normal Findings	Alterations and Possible Causes*	Nursing Responses to Data†
MOUTH—continued		
Tongue		
Free moving in all directions, midline	Lack of movement or asymmetric movement (neurologic damage)	Further assess neurologic functions.
	Tongue-tied	Test reflex elevation of tongue when depressed with tongue blade.
	Deviations from midline (cranial nerve damage)	Check for signs of weakness or deviation.
Pink color, smooth to rough texture, noncoated	White cheesy coating (thrush)	Differentiate between thrush and milk curds.
	Tongue has deep ridges	Reassure parents that tongue pattern may change from day to day.
Tongue proportional to mouth	Large tongue with short frenulum (cretinism, Down syndrome, other syndromes)	Evaluate in well-baby clinic to assess development delays.
		Initiate referrals.
EARS		
External ear		
Without lesions, cysts, or nodules	Nodules, cysts, or sinus tracts in front of ear	Evaluate characteristics of lesions.
	Adherent earlobes	Counsel parents to clean external ear with washcloth only; discourage use of cotton-tip applicators.
	Low set	
	Preauricular skin tags	Refer to physician for ligation.
Hearing		
Eustachian tubes are cleared with first cry		
Absence of all risk factors	Presence of one or more risk factors	Assess history of risk factors for hearing loss.
Attends to sounds; sudden or loud noise elicits Moro reflex	No response to sound stimuli (deafness)	Test for Moro reflex.
NECK		
Appearance		
Short, straight, creased with skin folds	Abnormally short neck (Turner syndrome)	Report findings to physician.
	Arching or inability to flex neck (meningitis, congenital anomaly)	
Posterior neck lacks loose extra folds of skin	Webbing of neck (Turner syndrome, Down syndrome, trisomy 18)	Assess for other signs of the syndromes.
Clavicles		
Straight and intact	Knot or lump on clavicle (fracture during difficult birth)	Obtain detailed labor and birth history; apply figure-eight bandage.
Moro reflex elicitable	Unilateral Moro reflex response on unaffected side (fracture of clavicle, brachial palsy, Erb-Duchenne paralysis)	Collaborate with physician.
Symmetric shoulders	Hypoplasia	
CHEST		
Appearance and size		
Circumference: 32.5 cm, 1–2 cm less than head		Measure at level of nipples after exhalation.
Wider than it is long		
Normal shape without depressed or prominent sternum	Funnel chest (congenital or associated with Marfan syndrome)	Determine adequacy of other respiratory and circulatory signs.
Lower end of sternum (xiphoid cartilage) may be protruding; less aparent after several weeks	Continued protrusion of xiphoid cartilage (Marfan syndrome, "pigeon chest")	Assess for other signs and symptoms of various syndromes.
Sternum 8 cm long	Barrel chest	
Expansion and retraction		
Bilateral expansion	Unequal chest expansion (pneumonia, pneumothorax, respiratory distress)	Assess respiratory effort regularity, flaring of nares, difficulty on both inspiration and expiration.
No intercostal, subcostal, or supracostal retractions	Retractions (respiratory distress)	Record and consult physician.
	See-saw respirations (respiratory distress)	

Physical Assessment/Normal Findings	Alterations and Possible Causes*	Nursing Responses to Data†
CHEST—*continued*		
Auscultation		
Breath sounds are louder in infants	Decreased breath sounds (decreased respiratory activity, atelectasis, pneumothorax)	Perform assessment and report to physician any positive findings.
Chest and axilla clear on crying	Increased breath sounds (resolving pneumonia or in cesarean births)	
Bronchial breath sounds (heard where trachea and bronchi closest to chest wall, above sternum and between scapulae):		
Bronchial sounds bilaterally	Adventitious or abnormal sounds (respiratory disease or distress)	Evaluate color for pallor or cyanosis.
Air entry clear		Report to physician.
Rales may indicate normal newborn atelectasis		
Cough reflex absent at birth, appears in 2 or more days		
Breasts		
Flat with symmetric nipples	Lack of breast tissue (preterm or SGA)	
Breast tissue diameter 5 cm or more at term	Discharge	Evaluate for infection
Distance between nipples 8 cm	Breast abscesses	.
Breast engorgement occurs on third day of life; liquid discharge may be expressed in term newborns	Enlargement	Reassure parents of normality of breast engorgement.
Nipples	Supernumerary nipples	No intervention is necessary.
	Dark-colored nipples	
HEART		
Auscultation		
Location: lies horizontally, with left border extending to left of midclavicle		
Regular rhythm and rate	Arrhythmia (anoxia), tachycardia, bradycardia	Refer all arrhythmia and gallop rhythms.
Determination of point of maximal impulse (PMI)	Malpositioning (enlargement, abnormal placement, pneumothorax, dextrocardia, diaphragmatic hernia)	Initiate cardiac evaluation.
Usually lateral to midclavicular line at third or fourth intercostal space		
Functional murmurs	Location of murmurs (possible congenital cardiac anomaly)	Evaluate murmur: location, timing, and duration; observe for accompanying cardiac pathology symptoms; ascertain family history.
No thrills		
Horizontal groove at diaphragm shows flaring of rib cage to mild degree	Marked rib flaring (vitamin D deficiency)	Initiate cardiopulmonary evaluation; assess pulses and blood pressures in all four extremities for equality and quality.
	Inadequacy of respiratory movement	
ABDOMEN		
Appearance		
Cylindrical, with some protrusion; appears large in relation to pelvis; some laxness of abdominal muscles	Distention, shiny abdomen with engorged vessels (gastrointestinal abnormalities, infection, congenital megacolon)	Examine abdomen thoroughly for mass or organomegaly.
No cyanosis, few vessels seen	Scaphoid abdominal appearance (diaphragmatic hernia)	Measure abdominal girth. Report deviations of abdominal size.
Diastasis recti—common in infants of African descent	Increased or decreased peristalsis (duodenal stenosis, small bowel obstruction)	Assess other signs and symptoms of obstruction.
	Localized flank bulging (enlarged kidneys, ascites, absent abdominal muscles)	Refer to physician

*Possible causes of alterations are placed in parentheses.

†This column provides guidelines for further assessment and initial nursing interventions.

(continued)

Physical Assessment/Normal Findings	Alterations and Possible Causes*	Nursing Responses to Data†
ABDOMEN— *continued*		
Umbilicus		
No protrusion of umbilicus (protrusion of umbilicus common in infants of African descent)	Umbilical hernia Patent urachus (congenital malformation)	Measure umbilical hernia by palpating the opening and record; it should close by 1 year of age; if not, refer to physician.
Bluish white color	Omphalocele	
Cutis navel (umbilical cord projects), granulation tissue present in navel	Gastroschisis Redness or exudate around cord (infection) Yellow discoloration (hemolytic disease, meconium staining)	Cover omphalocele with sterile, moist dressing. Instruct parents on cord care and hygiene.
Two arteries and one vein apparent	Single umbilical artery (congenital anomalies)	Refer anomalies to physician.
Begins drying 1 to 2 hours after birth No bleeding	Discharge or oozing of blood from the cord	
Auscultation and percussion	Bowel sounds in chest (diaphragmatic hernia)	Collaborate with physician.
Soft bowel sounds heard shortly after birth every 10–30 seconds	Absence of bowel sounds Hyperperistalsis (intestinal obstruction)	Assess for other signs of dehydration and/or infection.
Femoral pulses		
Palpable, equal, bilateral	Absent or diminished femoral pulses (coarctation of aorta)	Monitor blood pressure in upper and lower extremities.
Inguinal area		
No bulges along inguinal area No inguinal lymph nodes felt	Inguinal hernia	Initiate referral. Continue follow-up in well-baby clinic.
Bladder		
Percusses 1–4 cm above symphysis	Failure to void within 24–48 hours after birth	Check whether baby voided at birth.
Emptied about 3 hours after birth; if not, at time of birth	Exposure of bladder mucosa (exstrophy of bladder)	Consult with clinician.
Urine—inoffensive, mild odor	Foul odor (infection)	Obtain urine specimen if infection is suspected.
GENITALS		
Gender clearly delineated	Ambiguous genitals	Refer for genetic consultation.
MALE		
Penis		
Slender in appearance, about 2.5 cm long, 1 cm wide at birth	Micropenis (congenital anomaly) Meatal atresia	Observe and record first vioding.
Normal urinary orifice, urethral meatus at tip of penis	Hypospadias, epispadias	Collaborate with physician in presence of abnormality. Delay circumcision.
Noninflamed urethral opening	Urethritis (infection)	Palpate for enlarged inguinal lymph nodes and record painful urination.
Foreskin adheres to glans	Ulceration of meatal opening (infection, inflammation)	Evaluate whether ulcer is due to diaper rash; counsel regarding care.
Uncircumcised foreskin tight for 2 to 3 months	Phimosis—if still tight after 3 months	Instruct parents on how to care for uncircumcised penis.
Circumcised Erectile tissue present		Teach parents how to care for circumcision.
Scrotum		
Skin loose and hanging or tight and small; extensive rugae and normal size	Large scrotum containing fluid (hydrocele) Red, shiny scrotal skin (orchitis)	Shine a light through scrotum (transilluminate) to verify diagnosis.
Normal skin color	Minimal rugae, small scrotum	Assess for prematurity.
Scrotal discoloration common in breech		
Testes		
Descended by birth; not consistently found in scrotum	Undescended testes (cryptorchidism)	If testes cannot be felt in scrotum, gently palpate femoral, inguinal, perineal, and abdominal areas for presence.
Testes size 1.5–2 cm at birth	Enlarged testes (tumor) Small testes (Klinefelter syndrome or adrenal hyperplasia)	Refer to and collaborate with physician for further diagnostic studies.

Physical Assessment/Normal Findings	Alterations and Possible Causes*	Nursing Responses to Data†
FEMALE		
Mons		
Normal skin color, area pigmented in dark-skinned infants		
Labia majora cover labia minora in term and postterm newborns; symmetric size appropriate for gestational age	Hematoma, lesions (trauma) Labia minora prominent	Evaluate for recent trauma. Assess for prematurity.
Clitoris		
Normally large in newborn Edema and bruising in breech birth	Hypertrophy (hermaphroditism)	Refer to genetic workup.
Vagina		
Urinary meatus and vaginal orifice visible (0.5 cm circumference) Vaginal tag or hymenal tag disappears in a few weeks	Inflammation; erythema and discharge (urethritis) Congenital absence of vagina	Collect urine specimen for laboratory examination. Refer to physician.
Discharge; smegma under labia	Foul-smelling discharge (infection)	Collect data and further evaluate reason for discharge.
Bloody or mucoid discharge	Excessive vaginal bleeding (blood coagulation defect)	
BUTTOCKS AND ANUS		
Buttocks symmetric	Pilonidal dimple	Examine for possible sinus. Instruct parents about cleansing this area.
Anus patent and passage of meconium within 24–48 hours after birth	Imperforate anus, rectal atresia (congenital gastrointestinal defect)	Evaluate extent of problems. Initiate surgical consultation. Perform digital examination to ascertain patency if patency uncertain.
No fissures, tears, or skin tags	Fissures	
EXTREMITIES AND TRUNK		
Short and generally flexed; extremities move symmetrically through range of motion but lack full extension	Unilateral or absence of movement (spinal cord involvement) Fetal position continued or limp (anoxia, CNS problems, hypoglycemia)	Review birth record to assess possible cause.
All joints move spontaneously; good muscle tone, of flexor type, birth to 2 months	Spasticity when infant begins using extensors (cerebral palsy, lack of muscle tone, "floppy baby" syndrome) Hypotonia (Down syndrome)	Collaborate with physician.
Arms		
Equal in length Bilateral movement Flexed when quiet	Brachial palsy (difficult birth) Erb-Duchenne paralysis Muscle weakness, fractured clavicle Absence of limb or change of size (phocomelia, amelia)	Report to clinician.
Hands		
Normal number of fingers	Polydactyly (Ellis-van Creveld syndrome) Syndactyly—one limb (developmental anomaly) Syndactyly—both limbs (genetic component)	Report to clinician.
Normal palmar crease	Simian line on palm (Down syndrome)	Refer for genetic workup.
Normal-sized hands	Short fingers and broad hand (Hurler syndrome)	
Nails present and extend beyond fingertips in term newborn.	Cyanosis and clubbing (cardiac anomalies) Nails long or yellow stained (postterm)	Evaluate for history of distress in utero.
	***Possible causes of alterations are placed in parentheses.**	**†This column provides guidelines for further assessment and initial nursing interventions.**

(continued)

Physical Assessment/Normal Findings	Alterations and Possible Causes*	Nursing Responses to Data†
EXTREMITIES AND TRUNK—continued		
Spine		
C-shaped spine	Spina bifida occulta (nevus pilosus)	Evaluate extent of neurologic damage; initiate care of spinal opening.
Flat and straight when prone	Dermal sinus	
Slight lumbar lordosis	Myelomeningocele	
Easily flexed and intact when palpated	Head lag, limp, floppy trunk (neurologic problems)	
At least half of back devoid of lanugo		
Full-term infant in ventral suspension should hold head at 45-degree angle, back straight		
Hips		
No sign of instability	Sensation of abnormal movement, jerk, or snap of hip dislocation	Examine all newborn infants for dislocated hip prior to discharge from birthing center.
Hips abduct to more than 60 degrees		If this is suspected, refer to orthopedist for further evaluation.
		Reassess at well-baby visits.
Inguinal and buttock skin creases		
Symmetric inguinal and buttock creases	Asymmetry (dislocated hips)	Refer to orthopedist for evaluation.
		Counsel parents regarding symptoms of concern and discuss therapy.
Legs		
Legs equal in length	Shortened leg (dislocated hips)	Refer to orthopedist for evaluation.
Legs shorter than arms at birth	Lack of leg movement (fractures, spinal defects)	Counsel parents regarding symptoms of concern and discuss therapy.
Feet		
Foot is in straight line	Talipes equinovarus (true clubfoot)	Discuss differences between positional and true clubfoot with parents.
Positional clubfoot—based on position in utero		Teach parents passive manipulation of foot.
Fat pads and creases on soles of feet	Incomplete sole creases in first 24 hours of life (premature)	Refer to orthopedist if not corrected by 3 months of age.
Talipes planus (flat feet) normal under 3 years of age		Reassure parents that flat feet are normal in infants.
NEUROMUSCULAR		
Motor function		
Symmetric movement and strength in all extremities	Limp, flaccid, or hypertonic (CNS disorders, infection, dehydration, fracture)	Appraise newborn's posture and motor functions by observing activities and motor characteristics.
May be jerky or have brief twitchings	Tremors (hypoglycemia, hypocalcemia, infection, neurologic damage)	Evaluate electrolyte imbalance, hypoglycemia, and neurologic functioning.
Head lag not over 45 degrees	Delayed or abnormal development (preterm, neurologic involvement)	
Neck control adequate to maintain head erect briefly	Asymmetry of tone or strength (neurologic damage)	Refer for genetic evaluation.
REFLEXES		
Blink		
Stimulated by flash of light; response is closure of eyelids	Lack of blink response (damage to cranial nerve, CNS injury)	Assess neurologic status.
Pupillary reflex		
Stimulated by flash of light; response is constriction of pupil	Lack of reflex (damage to cranial nerve, CNS injury)	
Moro		
Response to sudden movement or loud noise should be one of symmetric extension and abduction of arms with fingers extended; then return to normal relaxed flexion	Asymmetry of body response (fractured clavicle, injury to brachial plexus)	Discuss normality of this reflex in response to loud noises and/or sudden movements.
Infant lying on back: slightly raised head suddenly released; infant held horizontally, lowered quickly about 6 in, and stopped abruptly	Consistent absence (brain damage)	Absence of reflex requires neurologic evaluation.
Fingers form a C		
Present at birth; disappears by 6 months of age		

Physical Assessment/Normal Findings	Alterations and Possible Causes*	Nursing Responses to Data†
REFLEXES—*continued*		
Rooting and sucking Turns in direction of stimulus to cheek or mouth; opens mouth and begins to suck rhythmically when finger or nipple is inserted into mouth; difficult to elicit after feeding; disappears by 4 to 7 months of age Sucking is adequate for nutritional intake and meeting oral stimulation needs; disappears by 12 months	Poor sucking or easily fatigable (preterm, breastfed infants of barbiturate-addicted mothers, possible cardiac problem) Absence of response (preterm, neurologic involvement, depressed newborns)	Evaluate strength and coordination of sucking. Observe newborn during feeding and counsel parents about mutuality of feeding experience and newborn's responses.
Palmar grasp Fingers grasp adult finger when palm is stimulated and held momentarily; lessens at 3 to 4 months of age	Asymmetry of response (neurologic problems)	Evaluate other reflexes and general neurologic functioning.
Plantar grasp Toes curl downward when sole of foot is stimulated; lessens by 8 months	Absent (defects of lower spinal column)	Assess for other lower extremity neurologic problems.
Stepping When held upright and one foot touching a flat surface, will step alternately; disappears at 4 to 8 weeks of age	Asymmetry of stepping (neurologic abnormality)	Evaluate muscle tone and function on each side of body. Refer to specialist.
Babinski Fanning and extension of all toes when one side of sole is stroked from heel upward across ball of foot; disappears at about 12 months	Absence of response (low spinal cord defects)	Refer for further neurologic evaluation.
Tonic neck Fencer position—when head is turned to one side, extremities on same side extend and on opposite side flex; this reflex may not be evident during early neonatal period; disappears at 3 to 4 months of age Response often more dominant in leg than in arm	Absent after 1 month of age or persistent asymmetry (cerebral lesion)	Assess neurologic functioning.
Prone crawl While on abdomen, neonate pushes up and tries to crawl	Absence or variance of response (preterm, weak, or depressed newborns)	Evaluate motor functioning. Refer to specialist.
Trunk incurvation (Galant) In prone position, stroking of spine causes pelvis to turn to stimulated side	Failure to rotate to stimulated side (neurologic damage)	
	*Possible causes of alterations are placed in parentheses.	**†This column provides guidelines for further assessment and initial nursing interventions.**

Newborn Behavioral Assessment

Two conflicting forces influence parents' perceptions of their newborn. One is their preconceptions, based on hopes and fears, of what their newborn will be like. The other is their initial reaction to the baby's temperament, behaviors, and physical appearance. Nurses can help parents identify their baby's specific behaviors.

The **Brazelton Neonatal Behavioral Assessment Scale** provides valuable guidelines for assessing the newborn's state changes, temperament, and individual behavior patterns. It provides a way for the health care provider, in conjunction with the parents (primary caregivers), to identify and understand the individual newborn's states and capabilities. Families learn which responses, interventions, or activities best meet the special needs of their newborn, and this understanding fosters positive attachment experiences.

Thinking Critically

ASSESSING NEWBORN BEHAVIOR

Maria Reyes, a 19-year-old G2 now P2 mother, delivered a 40-week-old female neonate 24 hours ago. The newborn exam was normal. Mrs. Reyes asks about the newborn's exam. She says she has noticed that the baby cries more than her first child did and seems to require holding for longer periods of time after feeding before "quieting down." She is concerned that she is doing something wrong and wants to know when her newborn will start to act like her first baby. What should you discuss with her about newborn behavior? 🔗 WEB

The assessment tool identifies the newborn's repertoire of behavioral responses to the environment and also documents the newborn's neurologic adequacy and capabilities. The examination usually takes 20 to 30 minutes and involves about 30 tests. Some items are scored according to the newborn's response to specific stimuli. Others, such as consolability and alertness, are scored as a result of continuous behavioral observations throughout the assessment. (For a complete discussion of all test items and maneuvers, see Brazelton & Nugent, 1995.)

Assess the newborn initially in a quiet, softly lit room, if possible. First determine the newborn's state of consciousness, because scoring and introduction of the test items are correlated with the sleep or waking state. The newborn's state depends on physiologic variables, such as the amount of time from the last feeding, positioning, environmental temperature, and health status; presence of such external stimuli as noises and bright lights; and the wake-sleep cycle of the newborn. An important characteristic of the newborn period is the pattern of states, as well as the transitions from one state to another. The pattern of states predicts the newborn's receptivity and ability to respond to stimuli in a cognitive manner. Babies learn best in a quiet, alert state and in a supportive, protective environment that provides appropriate stimuli.

Observe the newborn's sleep-wake patterns (as discussed in Chapter 24), 🔗 including the rapidity with which the newborn moves from one state to another, ability to be consoled, and ability to diminish the impact of disturbing stimuli. The following questions may provide a framework for assessment:

- Does the newborn's response style and ability to adapt to stimuli indicate a need for parental interventions that will alert the newborn to the environment so that he or she can grow socially and cognitively?

- Are parental interventions necessary to lessen the outside stimuli, as in the case of the baby who responds to sensory input with intensity?

- Can the baby control the amount of sensory input that he or she must deal with?

The behaviors, and the sleep-wake states in which they are assessed, are categorized as follows:

1. *Habituation.* Assess the newborn's ability to diminish or shut down innate responses to specific repeated stimuli, such as a rattle, bell, light, or pinprick to heel.

2. *Orientation to inanimate and animate visual and auditory assessment stimuli.* Observe how often and where the newborn attends to auditory and visual stimuli. Orientation to the environment is determined by an ability to respond to clues given by others and by a natural ability to fix on and follow a visual object horizontally and vertically. This capacity and parental appreciation of it are important for positive communication between infant and parents; the parents' visual (en face) and auditory (soft, continuous voice) presence stimulates their newborn to orient to them. Inability or lack of response may indicate visual or auditory problems. It is important for parents to know that their newborn can turn to voices soon after birth or by 3 days of age and can become alert at different times with a varying degree of intensity in response to sounds.

3. *Motor activity.* Evaluate several components. Assess motor tone of the newborn in the most characteristic state of responsiveness. This summary assessment includes overall use of tone as the newborn responds to being handled—whether during spontaneous activity, prone placement, or horizontal holding—and overall assessment of body tone as the newborn reacts to all stimuli.

4. *Variations.* Assess frequency of alert states, state changes, color changes (throughout all states as examination progresses), activity, and peaks of excitement.

5. *Self-quieting activity.* This assessment is based on how often, how quickly, and how effectively newborns can use their resources to quiet and console themselves when upset or distressed. Considered in this assessment are such self-consoling activities as putting hand to mouth, sucking on a fist or the tongue, and attuning to an object or sound. Also consider the newborn's need for outside consolation (e.g., seeing a face; being rocked, held, or dressed; using a pacifier; being swaddled).

6. *Cuddliness or social behaviors.* This area encompasses the newborn's need for, and response to, being held. Also consider how often the newborn smiles. These behaviors influence the couple's self-esteem and feelings of acceptance or rejection. Cuddling also appears to be an indicator of personality. Cuddlers appear to enjoy, accept, and seek physical contact; are easier to placate; sleep more; and form earlier and more intense attachments. Noncuddlers are active and restless, have accelerated motor development, and are intolerant of physical restraint. Smiling, even as a grimace reflex, greatly influences parent-newborn feedback. Parents identify this response as positive.

CHAPTER HIGHLIGHTS

❧ A perinatal history, determination of gestational age, physical examination, and behavior assessment form the basis for a complete newborn assessment.

❧ The common physical characteristics included in the gestational age assessment are skin, lanugo, sole (plantar) creases, breast tissue and size, ear form and cartilage, and genitalia.

❧ The neuromuscular components of gestational age scoring tools are usually posture, square window sign, popliteal angle, arm recoil, heel-to-ear extension, and scarf sign.

❧ After determining the gestational age and gestational classification of the baby (SGA, AGA, LGA), the nurse can assess how the newborn will make the transition to extrauterine life and anticipate potential physiologic problems.

❧ Normal ranges for vital signs assessed in the newborn are as follows: heart rate, 120 to 160 beats per minute; respirations, 30 to 60 respirations per minute; axillary temperature, 36.4 to 37.2 °C (97.5 to 99 °F); skin temperature, 36 to 36.5 °C (96.8 to 97.7 °F); rectal temperature, 36.6 to 37.2 °C (97.8 to 99 °F); and blood pressure at birth, 80–60/45–40 mm Hg.

❧ Normal newborn measurements are as follows: weight range, 2500 to 4000 g (5 lb, 8 oz, to 8 lb, 13 oz), with weight dependent on maternal size and age; length range, 45 to 52 cm (18 to 22 in); and head circumference range, 32 to 37 cm (12.5 to 14.5 in)—approximately 2 cm larger than the chest circumference.

❧ Commonly elicited newborn reflexes are tonic neck, Moro, grasp, rooting, sucking, and blink.

❧ Newborn behavioral abilities include habituation, orientation to visual and auditory stimuli, motor activity, cuddliness, and self-quieting activity.

❧ An important role of the nurse during the physical and behavioral assessments of the newborn is to teach parents about their newborn and involve them in their baby's care. This involvement facilitates the parents' identification of their newborn's uniqueness and allays their concerns.

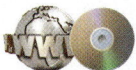

EXPLOREMediaLink

NCLEX Review, Case Studies, and other interactive resources for this chapter can be found on the companion website at http://www.prenhall.com/london. Click on "Chapter 25" to select the activities for this chapter.

For animations, more NCLEX review questions, and an audio glossary, access the accompanying CD-ROM in this textbook.

REFERENCES

American Academy of Pediatrics. (1999). Newborn and infant hearing loss: Detection and intervention. *Pediatrics, 103*(2), 527–530.

American Academy of Pediatrics, Committee on Fetus and Newborn, & American College of Obstetricians and Gynecologists, Committee on Obstetrics. (1997). *Guidelines for perinatal care* (4th ed.). Evanston, IL: Author.

Ballard, J. L., Khoury, J. C., Wedig, K., Wang, L., Eilers-Walsmann, B. L., & Lipp, R. (1991). New Ballard score, expanded to include extremely premature infants. *Journal of Pediatrics, 119*(3), 417–423.

Basso, O., Olsen, J., Knudsen, L. B., & Christensen, K. (1998). Low birth weight and preterm birth after short interpregnancy intervals. *American Journal of Obstetrics and Gynecology, 178*(2), 259–263.

Brazelton, T. B., & Nugent, J. K. (1995). *The neonatal behavioral assessment scale* (3rd ed.). London: MacKeith.

Donovan, E. F., Tyson, J. E., Ehrenkranz, R. A., Verter, J., Wright, L. L., Korones, S. B., et al. (1999, August). Inaccuracy of Ballard scores before 28 weeks' gestation. *Journal of Pediatrics, 135*, 147–152.

Juretschke, L. J. (2000). Unilateral neonatal testicular torsion. *Journal of Obstetrics, Gynecologic, and Neonatal Nursing, 29*(5), 451–456.

Moyer, V. A., Ahn, C., & Sneed, S. (2000, April). Accuracy of clinical judgment in neonatal jaundice. *Archives of Pediatric and Adolescent Medicine, 154*, 391–394.

O'Donnell, K. A., Glick, P. L., & Cory, M. G. (1998). Pediatric umbilical problems. *Pediatric Clinics of North America, 45*(4), 791–799.

Overpeck, M. D., Hediger, M. L., Zhang, J., Trumble, A. C., & Klebanoff, M. A. (1999). Birth weight for gestational age of Mexican American infants born in the United States. *Obstetrics and Gynecology, 93*(6), 943–947.

Pressler, J. L., & Hepworth, J. T. (1997). Newborn neurologic screening using NBAS reflexes. *Neonatal Network, 16*(6), 33–46.

Rinehart, T. T., Terrone, D. A., & Magann, E. (2000). The normal neonate: Assessment of early physical findings. In J. J. Sciarri & T. J. Watkins (Eds.), *Gynecology and obstetrics* (Vol. 2, chap. 97, pp. 1–15). Philadelphia: Lippincott, Williams & Wilkins.

Sganga, A., Wallace, R., Kiehl, E., Irving, T., & Witter, L. (2000). A comparison of four methods of normal newborn temperature measurements. *American Journal of Maternal Child Nursing, 25*(2), 76–79.

Sininger, Y. S., Doyle, K. J., & Moore, J. K. (1999). The case for early identification of hearing loss in children. *Pediatric Clinics of North America, 46*(1), 1–14.

Thurdeen, P. J., Deacon, J., O'Neill, P., & Hernandez, J. (1999). *Assessment and care of the well newborn*. Philadelphia: Saunders.

Wu, Tsu-Yin, & Daniel, L. (2001). Growth of immigrant Chinese infants in the first year of life. *American Journal of Maternal/Child Nursing, 26*(4), 202–207.

CHAPTER 26

Normal Newborn: Needs and Care

*W*hen our daughter was laid in my arms right after birth she was so delicate. I had not dared to hope that we would be blessed with a girl because there were so few girls in my husband's family. Our 2-year-old niece was the first girl in 107 years, so I had pretty much decided that another boy would be just fine. But here she was, right here in my arms.

—CATHERINE, 32

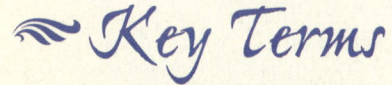 Key Terms

Circumcision   *575*
Newborn screening tests   *582*
Parent-newborn attachment   *577*

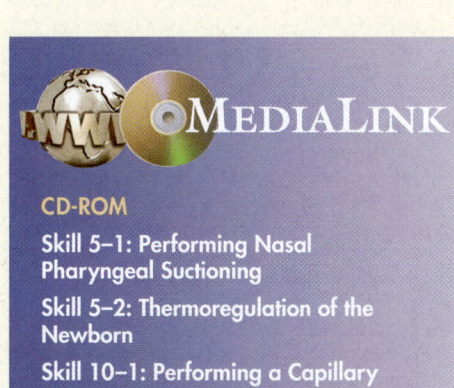

MediaLink

CD-ROM

Skill 5–1: Performing Nasal Pharyngeal Suctioning

Skill 5–2: Thermoregulation of the Newborn

Skill 10–1: Performing a Capillary Puncture

Audio Glossary

NCLEX Review

COMPANION WEBSITE

http://www.prenhall.com/london

Newborn Needs and Care Web Links

Thinking Critically

NCLEX Review

Case Study

In the absence of any newborn distress, continue with the admission by taking the newborn's vital signs. The initial temperature is taken by the axillary method; a normal axillary temperature range is 36.5 to 37 °C (97.7 to 98.6 °F).

Once the initial temperature is taken, monitor the core temperature either by obtaining axillary temperatures at intervals or by placing a skin sensor on the newborn for continuous reading. The usual skin sensor placement site is the newborn's abdomen, but placement on the upper thigh or arm can give a reading closely correlated with the mean body temperature. Monitor the vital signs for a healthy term newborn at least every 30 minutes until the newborn's condition has remained stable for 2 hours (AAP, 1997). The newborn's respirations may be irregular yet still be normal. Brief periods of apnea, lasting only 5 to 10 seconds with no color or heart rate changes, are considered normal. The normal pulse range is 120 to 160 beats per minute, and the normal respiratory range is 30 to 60 respirations per minute.

MAINTENANCE OF A NEUTRAL THERMAL ENVIRONMENT

A neutral thermal environment is essential to minimize the newborn's need for increased oxygen consumption and use of calories to maintain body heat in the optimal range of 36.4 to 37.2 °C (97.5 to 99 °F). If the newborn becomes hypothermic, the body's response can lead to metabolic acidosis, hypoxia, and shock.

A neutral thermal environment is best achieved by performing the newborn assessment and interventions with the newborn unclothed and under a radiant warmer. The radiant warmer thermostat is controlled by a thermal skin sensor taped to the newborn's abdomen, upper thigh, or arm. The sensor indicates when the newborn's temperature exceeds or falls below the acceptable temperature range. Be aware that leaning over the newborn may block the radiant heat waves from reaching the newborn.

It is common practice in some institutions to cover the newborn's head with a cap made of wool lined with gauze and cotton, Thinsulate, or cotton and polyester fill terry cloth to prevent further heat loss, in addition to placing the baby under a radiant warmer ("Neonatal Thermoregulation," 1997).

When the newborn's temperature is normal and vital signs are stable (about 2 to 4 hours after birth), the baby may be given a sponge bath. However, this admission bath may be postponed for some hours if the newborn's condition dictates or the parents wish to give the first bath. In light of early discharge practices (12 to 48 hours), healthy term infants can be safely bathed immediately after the admission assessment is completed (Varda & Behnke, 2000). The baby is bathed while still under the radiant warmer; the bathing may be done in the parents' room. Bathing the newborn offers an excellent opportunity for teaching and welcoming parents' involvement in the care of their baby. 🔗 WEB

Recheck the baby's temperature after the bath and, if it is stable, dress the newborn in a shirt, diaper, and cap; wrap the baby; and place the newborn in an open crib at room temperature or in the mother's arms. If the baby's axillary temperature is below 36.4 °C (97.5 °F), the baby returns to the radiant warmer for gradual rewarming and to prevent hypothermia. Once the newborn is rewarmed, take steps to prevent further heat loss, such as keeping the newborn away from cool surfaces or instruments, drafts, open windows or doors, and air conditioners. Blankets and clothing are stored in a warm place. (See "Temperature Regulation" in Chapter 24, plus Skill 5–2). 🔗 SKILLS CD

Nursing Practice

A cap can be fashioned from a piece of stockinette to help reduce heat loss from the head.

Drug Guide

VITAMIN K₁ PHYTONADIONE (AQUAMEPHYTON)

Overview of Neonatal Action

Phytonadione is used in prophylaxis and treatment of hemorrhagic disease of the newborn. It promotes liver formation of the clotting factors, II, VII, IX, and X. At birth, the neonate does not have the bacteria in the colon that are necessary for synthesizing fat-soluble vitamin K_1. Therefore, the newborn may have decreased levels of prothrombin during the first 5 to 8 days of life, reflected by a prolongation of prothrombin time.

Route, Dosage, Frequency

Intramuscular injection is given in the vastus lateralis thigh muscle. A one-time-only prophylactic dose of 0.5 to 1 mg is given intramuscularly in the birthing area or within 1 hour of birth (Zenk et al., 2000).

If the mother received anticoagulants during pregnancy, an additional dose may be ordered by the physician and is given at 6 to 8 hours after the first injection. IM/SC concentration: 1 mg/0.5 mL (neonatal strength); can use 10 mg/mL concentration to minimize volume injected.

Neonatal Side Effects

Pain and edema may occur at injection site. Allergic reactions, such as rash and urticaria, may also occur.

Nursing Considerations

- Protect drug from light.
- Give vitamin K_1 before circumcision procedure.
- Observe for signs of local inflammation.
- Observe for jaundice and severe hemolytic anemia, especially in preterm infants.
- Observe for bleeding (usually occurs on second or third day). Bleeding may be seen as generalized ecchymoses or bleeding from umbilical cord, circumcision site, nose, or gastrointestinal tract. Results of serial prothrombin time (PT) and partial thromboplastin time (PTT) should be assessed.

PREVENTION OF COMPLICATIONS
OF HEMORRHAGIC DISEASE OF NEWBORN

A prophylactic injection of vitamin K$_1$ (AquaMEPHYTON) is given to prevent hemorrhage, which can occur due to low prothrombin levels in the first few days of life. See "Drug Guide: Vitamin K$_1$ Phytonadione (AquaMEPHYTON)." The potential for hemorrhage is thought to result from the absence of gut bacterial flora, which influences the production of vitamin K$_1$ in the newborn (see Chapter 29 for further discussion). 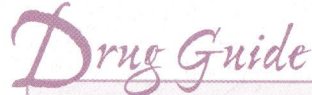 Newborns receive a single dose of 0.5 to 1 mg of natural vitamin K$_1$ (phytonadione) parenterally (preferred) or subcutaneously within 1 hour of birth (Zenk, Sills, & Koeppel, 2000).

The vitamin K$_1$ injection is given intramuscularly in the middle third of the vastus lateralis muscle, in the lateral aspect of the thigh (Figure 26–2 ◆). An alternate site is the rectus femoris muscle in the anterior aspect of the thigh. However, this site is near the sciatic nerve and femoral artery and should be used with caution (Figure 26–3 ◆).

Parents may request that vitamin K be given by mouth. Oral vitamin K has not been shown to be as effective as parenteral administration and is not currently recommended for use in the United States (AAP, 1997).

PREVENTION OF EYE INFECTION

The nurse is also responsible for giving the legally required prophylactic eye treatment for *Neisseria gonorrhoeae*, which may have infected the newborn of an infected mother during the birth process. A variety of topical agents appear to be equally effective. Ophthalmic ointments that are used include 1% silver nitrate, 0.5% erythromycin (Ilotycin Ophthalmic) (see "Drug Guide: Erythromycin Ophthalmic Ointment [Ilotycin Ophthalmic]"), and 1% tetracycline. Erythromycin is also effective against chlamydia, which has a higher incidence rate than gonorrhea.

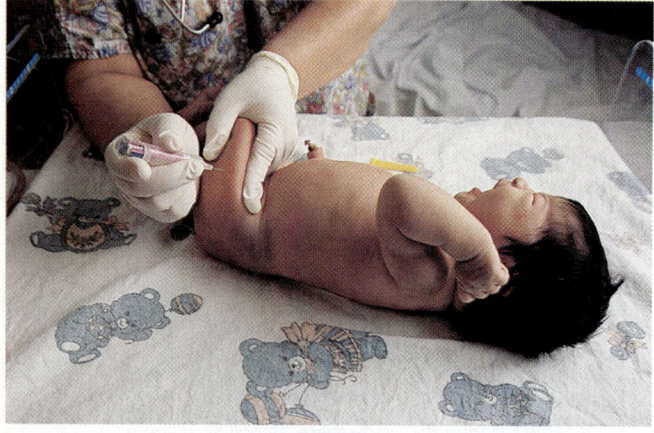

FIGURE 26–2. ◆ Procedure for vitamin K injection. Cleanse area thoroughly with alcohol swab and allow skin to dry. Bunch the tissue of the upper outer thigh (vastus lateralis muscle) and quickly insert a 25-gauge 5/8-in needle at a 90-degree angle to the thigh. Aspirate, then slowly inject the solution to distribute the medication evenly and minimize the baby's discomfort. Remove the needle and gently massage the site with an alcohol swab.

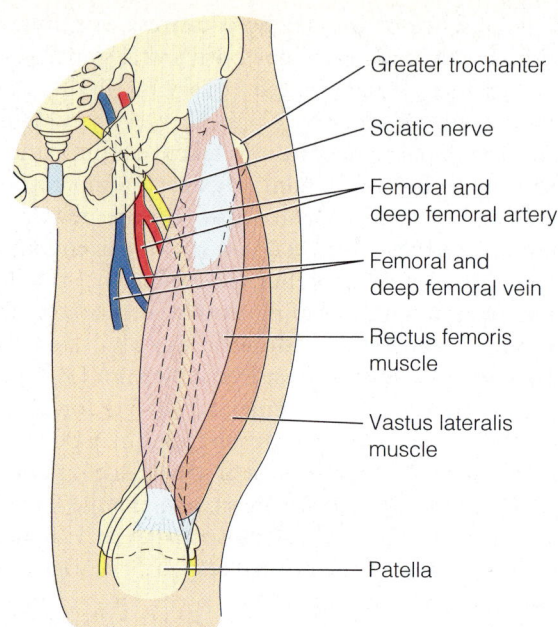

- Greater trochanter
- Sciatic nerve
- Femoral and deep femoral artery
- Femoral and deep femoral vein
- Rectus femoris muscle
- Vastus lateralis muscle
- Patella

FIGURE 26–3. ◆ Injection sites. The middle third of the vastus lateralis muscle is the preferred site for intramuscular injection in the newborn. The middle third of the rectus femoris is an alternate site, but its proximity to major vessels and the sciatic nerve requires caution in using this site for injection.

Drug Guide

ERYTHROMYCIN OPHTHALMIC OINTMENT (ILOTYCIN OPHTHALMIC)

Overview of Neonatal Action

Erythromycin (Ilotycin Ophthalmic) is used as prophylactic treatment of ophthalmia neonatorum, which is caused by the bacteria *Neisseria gonorrhoeae*. Preventive treatment of gonorrhea in the newborn is required by law. Erythromycin is also effective treatment against ophthalmic chlamydial infections. It is either bacteriostatic or bactericidal, depending on the organisms involved and the concentration of drug.

Pregnancy risk category: C
Route, Dosage, Frequency

Ophthalmic ointment (0.5%) is instilled as a narrow ribbon or strand, 1/4 inch long, along the lower conjunctival surface of each eye, starting at the inner canthus. It is instilled only once in each eye. The ointment may be administered in the birthing area or, alternatively, later in the nursery so that eye contact between infant and parent is facilitated and the bonding process immediately after birth is not interrupted.

Neonatal Side Effects

Sensitivity reaction, such as edema, inflammation, or drainage, may interfere with ability to focus and may cause edema and inflammation. Side effects usually disappear in 24 to 48 hours.

(continued)

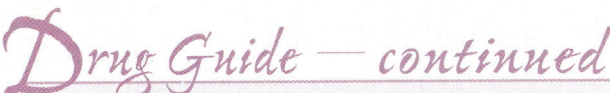

Drug Guide — continued

Nursing Considerations

- Wash hands immediately prior to instillation to prevent introduction of bacteria.
- Clean the newborn's eyes to remove any drainage.
- Use new tube or single-use container for ophthalmic ointment administration shortly after birth.
- Massage eyelids gently to distribute the ointment (Zenk et al., 2000).
- May wipe away excess after 1 minute (AAP, 1997).
- Do not irrigate the eyes after instillation.
- Observe for hypersensitivity.
- Teach parents about need for eye prophylaxis. Educate them regarding side effects and signs that need to be reported to the health care provider.

TABLE 26–2 Signs of Newborn Distress
Increased respiratory rate (more than 60/minute) or difficult respirations
Sternal retractions
Nasal flaring
Grunting
Excessive mucus
Facial grimacing
Cyanosis (central: skin, lips, tongue)
Abdominal distention or mass
Vomiting of bile-stained material
Absence of meconium elimination within 48 hours of birth
Absence of urine elimination within 48 hours of birth
Jaundice of the skin within 24 hours of birth or due to hemolytic process
Temperature instability (hypothermia or hyperthermia)
Jitteriness or blood glucose < 40 mg%

Note: From Tappero, E. P., & Honeyfield, M. E. (1996). *Physical assessment of the newborn* (2nd ed.). Petaluma, CA: NICU Ink. Adapted.

Successful eye prophylaxis requires that the medication be instilled into the lower conjunctival sac of each eye (Figure 26–4 ◆). Massage the eyelid gently to distribute the ointment. Instillation may be delayed up to 1 hour after birth to allow eye contact during parent-newborn bonding.

Eye prophylaxis medications can cause chemical conjunctivitis, which gives the newborn some discomfort and may interfere with the ability to focus on the parents' faces. The resulting edema, inflammation, and discharge may worry parents if they have not been told that the side effects will clear in 24 to 48 hours.

EARLY ASSESSMENT OF NEONATAL DISTRESS

During the first 24 hours of life, be constantly alert for signs of distress in the newborn. If the newborn is with the parents during this period, take extra care to teach them how to maintain their newborn's temperature, recognize the hallmarks of newborn distress, and respond immediately to signs of respiratory problems. Teach the parents to observe the newborn for changes in color or activity, rapid breathing with chest retractions, or facial grimacing. Their interventions include nasal and oral suctioning with a bulb syringe, positioning, and vigorous fingertip stroking of the newborn's spine to stimulate respiratory activity if necessary. Be immediately available in case the newborn develops distress (Table 26–2).

A common cause of neonatal distress is early-onset group B streptococcal (GBS) disease. Infected mothers transmit GBS infection to their infants during labor and birth; thus it is recommended that at-risk mothers receive intrapartum antimicrobial prophylaxis (IAP) for GBS disease. Assess and observe all infants of mothers identified as at risk for signs and symptoms of sepsis (bacteremia, pneumonia, or meningitis).

INITIATION OF FIRST FEEDING

The timing of the first feeding varies depending on whether the newborn is to be breastfed or bottle-fed and whether there were any complications during pregnancy or birth, such as maternal diabetes, intrauterine growth restriction (IUGR), and so forth. Mothers who choose to breastfeed their newborns may seek to put their baby to the breast while in the birthing area. Encourage this practice because successful, long-term breastfeeding during infancy appears to be related to beginning breastfeedings in the first few hours of life. Sleep-wake states affect feeding

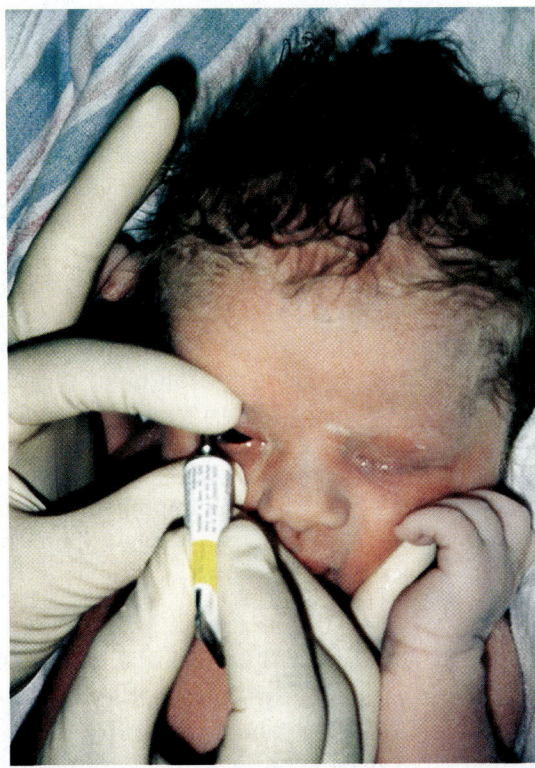

FIGURE 26–4. ◆ Ophthalmic ointment. Retract lower eyelid outward to instill 1/4-in-long strand of ointment from a single-dose tube along the lower conjunctival surface.

behavior and need to be considered when evaluating the newborn's sucking ability (MacMullen & Dulski, 2000). Formula-fed newborns usually begin the first feedings by 5 hours of age, during the second period of reactivity when they awaken and appear hungry. Signs indicating newborn readiness for the first feeding are active bowel sounds, absence of abdominal distention, and a lusty cry that quiets with rooting and sucking behaviors when a stimulus is placed near the lips.

FACILITATION OF PARENT-NEWBORN ATTACHMENT

Eye-to-eye contact between the parents and their newborn is extremely important during the early hours after birth, when the newborn is in the first period of reactivity. The newborn is alert during this time, the eyes are wide open, and the baby often makes direct eye contact with human faces within optimal range for visual acuity (7 to 8 in). It is theorized that this eye contact is an important foundation in establishing attachment in human relationships (Klaus & Klaus, 1985). Consequently, administration of the prophylactic eye medication is often delayed for the first hour after birth to provide an opportunity for a period of eye contact between parents and their newborn. An interactive bath can also facilitate attachment. During the interactive bath experience, the newborn becomes an active participant and parents are drawn into an interaction with their newborn. Interpret the infant's behavior, model ways to respond to the behavior, and support parental strategies for doing so (Karl, 1999).

NURSING MANAGEMENT FOR NEWBORN CARE DURING STAY IN BIRTHING UNIT

The following section discusses nursing care management for newborn care during stay in birthing unit.

Nursing Diagnosis

Examples of nursing diagnoses that may apply during daily care of the newborn include the following:

- *Altered nutrition: Less than body requirements* related to limited nutritional and fluid intake and increased caloric expenditure
- *Altered urinary elimination* related to meatal edema secondary to circumcision
- *Risk for infection* related to umbilical cord healing, circumcision site, or immature immune system
- *Health-seeking behaviors* related to care needs of circumcised and uncircumcised newborns or pros and cons of breastfeeding and bottle-feeding
- *Altered family processes* related to integration of newborn into family unit or demands of newborn feeding schedule

Planning and Implementation

MAINTENANCE OF CARDIOPULMONARY FUNCTION

Assess vital signs every 6 to 8 hours or more, depending on the newborn's status. The newborn should always be in a propped, side-lying position when left unattended to prevent aspiration and facilitate drainage of mucus. Keep a bulb syringe within easy reach, and teach parents to do so, in case the baby needs oral-nasal suctioning. If the newborn has respiratory difficulty, clear the airway. Vigorous fingertip stroking of the baby's spine will frequently stimulate respiratory activity. A cardiorespiratory monitor can be used on newborns who are not being observed at all times and are at risk for decreased respiratory or cardiac function. Indicators of risk are pallor, cyanosis, ruddy color, apnea, and other signs of instability. Changes in skin color may indicate the need for closer assessment of temperature, cardiopulmonary status, and hematocrit and bilirubin levels.

Thinking Critically

A NEWBORN WITH RESPIRATORY DIFFICULTY

A mother calls you to her room. She sounds frightened and says her baby cannot breathe. You find the mother cradling her infant in her arms. The infant is mildly cyanotic, waving her arms, and has mucus coming from her nose and mouth. What would you do? **WEB**

MAINTENANCE OF NEUTRAL THERMAL ENVIRONMENT

Make every effort to maintain the newborn's temperature within the normal range. Make certain the newborn is dressed and exposed to the air as little as possible. Use a head covering for the small newborn, who has less subcutaneous fat to act as insulation in maintaining body heat. Routinely monitor the ambient temperature of the room where the newborn is kept and carry out all nursing care activities as quickly as possible. A newborn whose temperature falls below optimal levels uses calories to maintain body heat rather than for growth. Chilling also decreases the affinity of serum albumin for bilirubin, thereby increasing the likelihood of newborn jaundice. In addition, it increases oxygen use and may cause respiratory distress.

On the other hand, an overheated newborn increases activity and respiratory rate in an attempt to cool the body. Both measures deplete caloric reserves, and the increased respiratory rate leads to increased insensible fluid loss ("Neonatal Thermoregulation," 1997).

PROMOTION OF ADEQUATE HYDRATION AND NUTRITION

Newborn nutrition is addressed in depth in Chapter 27. Record caloric and fluid intake and enhance adequate hydration by maintaining a neutral thermal environment and offering early and frequent feedings. Early feedings promote gastric emptying and increase peristalsis, thereby decreasing the potential for hyperbilirubinemia by decreasing the amount of time fecal material is in contact with beta glucuronidase in the small intestine. This enzyme frees the bilirubin from the feces, allowing it to be reabsorbed into the vascular system. Record voiding and stooling patterns. The first voiding should occur within 24 hours and the first passage of stool within 48 hours. When they do not occur, continue the normal observation routine while assessing for abdominal distention, bowel sounds, hydration, fluid intake, and temperature stability.

Weigh the newborn at the same time each day for accurate comparisons. A weight loss of up to 10% for term newborns is considered normal during the first week of life. This weight loss is the result of limited intake, loss of excess extracellular fluid, and passage of meconium. Tell parents about the expected weight loss, the reason for it, and the expectations for regaining the birth weight. Birth weight is usually regained by 2 weeks if feedings are adequate.

Excessive handling can cause an increase in the newborn's metabolic rate and caloric use. Be alert to the newborn's subtle cues of fatigue, including a decrease in muscle tension and activity in the extremities and neck, as well as loss of eye contact, which may be manifested by fluttering or closure of the eyelids. Quickly cease stimulation when signs of fatigue appear and demonstrate to parents the need to be aware of newborn cues and to wait for periods of alertness for contact and stimulation. Assess the woman's comfort and latching-on techniques, if breastfeeding, or bottle-feeding techniques.

PROMOTION OF SKIN INTEGRITY

Newborn skin care, including bathing, is important for the health and appearance of the individual newborn and for infection control within the nursery. Ongoing skin care involves cleansing the buttock and perianal areas with fresh water and cotton or a mild soap and water with diaper changes. Assess the umbilical cord for signs of bleeding or infection, such as oozing and foul smell. Antimicrobial agents (triple-dye or bacitracin) may be applied to the normal newborn's cord if the baby is in a hospital nursery (World Health Organization [WHO], 1999). The nursery nurse is responsible for cord care per agency policy, which may be after the cord is cut only, once a day for the first 3 days of life, or each time the diaper is changed. In 24-hour rooming-in systems, in which the mother is the primary caregiver and clean cord care is practiced, application of an antiseptic to the stump is probably not needed because the risk of contaminating the cord is low (WHO, 1999). Clean cord care includes washing hands with clean water and soap before and after care. Alcohol is probably not effective in preventing microbial colonization of the cord and omphalitis and can delay drying of the cord.

PROMOTION OF SAFETY AND PREVENTION OF COMPLICATIONS

Safety of the newborn is paramount. It is essential that the nurse and other caregivers verify the identity of the newborn by comparing the numbers and names on the identi-

fication bracelets of mother and newborn before giving a baby to a parent. Another form of identification band has a built-in sensor unit that sounds an alarm if the baby is transported beyond set birthing unit boundaries. Individual birthing units should practice safety measures to prevent infant abduction and provide information to parents regarding their role in this area (Carroll, 2000). Parental measures to prevent abduction include the following:

- Checking that identification bands are in place as they care for their infant and, if not, have them replaced immediately
- Allowing only people with proper birthing unit identification to remove their baby from the parent's room
- Returning baby to nursery or having baby accompany the parent when leaving the room
- Reporting presence of any suspicious people on the birthing unit

Infection in the nursery is best prevented by requiring that all personnel who have direct contact with newborns scrub for 2 to 3 minutes from the fingertips to and including the elbows at the beginning of each shift. The hands must also be washed with soap and rubbed vigorously for 15 seconds ("Neonatal Skin Care," 1997) before and after contact with every newborn and after touching any soiled surface such as the floor or one's hair or face. Parents are often instructed to use an antiseptic hand cleaner before touching the baby. Anyone with an infection should refrain from working with newborns until the infection has cleared. A few agencies ask family members to wear gowns (preferably disposable) over their street clothes. Parents need to be taught that everyone handling the baby should always wash their hands before doing so, even after the baby is home.

Newborns are at continued risk for the complications of hemorrhage, late-onset cardiac symptoms, and infection. Pallor may be an early sign of hemorrhage and must be reported to the physician. The newborn is placed on a cardiorespiratory monitor to permit continuous assessment. Several newborn conditions put newborns at risk for hemorrhage. Cyanosis that is not relieved by oxygen administration requires emergency intervention, may indicate a congenital cardiac condition or shock, and requires ongoing assessment. Assess the circumcision for signs of hemorrhage and infection. The first voiding after a circumcision is also a significant assessment in evaluating for possible urinary obstruction due to trauma and edema. Apply petroleum jelly gauze to the circumcision site to prevent bleeding. The gauze is removed and replaced if it gets soiled.

CIRCUMCISION

Circumcision is a surgical procedure in which the prepuce, an epithelial layer covering the penis, is separated from the glans penis and excised. This procedure supposedly permits exposure of the glans for easier cleaning.

The parents make the decision about circumcision for their newborn male child. In most cases the choice is based on cultural, social, and family tradition. Circumcision was originally a religious rite practiced by Jews and Muslims. The practice gained widespread cultural acceptance in the United States but is much less common in Europe. Many parents choose circumcision because they want their male child to have a physical appearance similar to that of his father or the majority of other children. Other parents feel that it is expected by society. Another commonly cited reason for circumcising newborn males is to prevent the need for anesthesia, hospitalization, pain, and trauma if the procedure is needed later in life (Kauffman, Clark & Castro, 2001). During the prenatal period, ensure that parents have clear and current information regarding the risks and benefits of circumcision.

Current Recommendations. As in the past, recommendations regarding circumcision vary. The 1999 AAP policy statement does not recommend routine circumcision but acknowledges that medical indications for circumcision still exist. The organization recommends that analgesia (e.g., EMLA cream, dorsal penile nerve block [DPNB], subcutaneous ring block) be used during circumcision to decrease procedural pain (Kaufman, Clark & Castro, 2001). If a circumcision is to be performed, it should be done using the least painful method.

Circumcision should not be performed if the newborn is premature or compromised, has a known bleeding problem, or is born with a genitourinary defect such as hypospadias or epispadias, because the foreskin may be needed in future surgical repairs.

Nurse's Role. The nurse plays an essential role in providing parents with current information about circumcision. Nurses can facilitate parental informed consent because of their knowledge of the medical, social, and psychologic aspects of newborn circumcision. A well-informed nurse can allay parents' anxiety by sharing information and allowing them to express their concerns. Parents must be informed about potential risks and benefits of circumcision. Hemorrhage, infection, difficulty in voiding, separation of the edges of the circumcision, discomfort, and restlessness are early potential problems. Later there is a risk that the glans and urethral meatus may become irritated and inflamed from contact with the ammonia in urine. Adhesions and/or progressive stenosis, entrapment of the penis, and damage to the urethra are all potential complications that could require surgical correction (Kaufman et al., 2001). Potential benefits include reduction in the risk of urinary tract infections (UTIs), sexually transmitted infections, and penile cancer.

Be sure the parents of an uncircumcised male infant have information about hygienic practices. Tell them that the foreskin and glans are two similar layers of cells that separate from each other. The separation process begins prenatally and is normally completed between 3 to 5 years

of age. In the process of separation, sterile sloughed cells build up between the layers. This buildup looks similar to the smegma secreted after puberty, and it is harmless. Occasionally during the daily bath, the parent can gently test for retraction. If retraction has occurred, daily gentle washing of the glans with soap and water is sufficient to maintain adequate cleanliness. The parents should teach the child to incorporate this practice into his daily self-care activities. If circumcision is desired, the procedure is performed when the newborn is well stabilized and has received his initial physical examination by a health care provider. The parents may also choose to have the circumcision done after discharge. However, they need to be advised that if the baby is older than 1 month, the current practice is to hospitalize him for the procedure. Prior to a circumcision, ensure that the physician has explained the procedure and determines whether anesthesia is to be used, whether the parents have any further questions about the procedure, and that the circumcision permit is signed. Gather the equipment and prepare the newborn by removing the diaper and placing him on a circumcision board or some other type of restraint, but restraining only the legs. In Jewish circumcision ceremonies, the infant is held by the father or godfather and given wine before the procedure.

A variety of techniques may be used for circumcision (Figures 26–5 ◆ and 26–6 ◆), and it is an almost bloodless procedure. However, make special note of infants with a family history of bleeding disorders or with mothers who took anticoagulants, including aspirin, prenatally. During the procedure, assess the newborn's response. One consideration is pain being experienced by the newborn. A DPNB using 1% lidocaine without epinephrine significantly

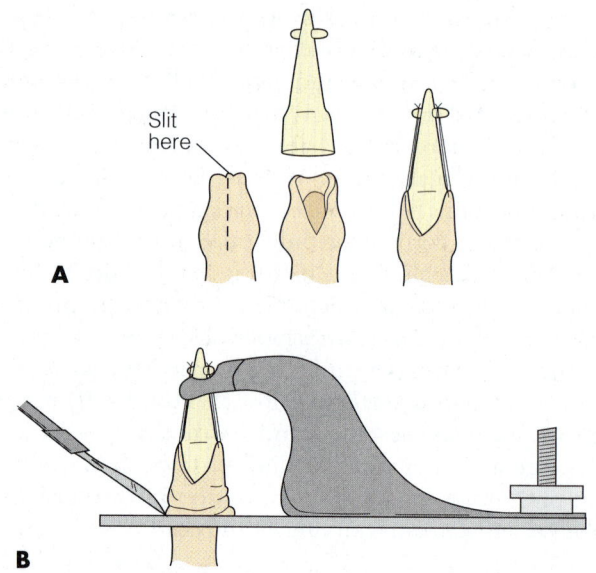

FIGURE 26–5. ◆ Circumcision using a circumcision clamp. **A,** The prepuce is drawn over the cone and **B,** the clamp is applied. Pressure is maintained for 3 to 4 minutes, and then excess prepuce is cut away.

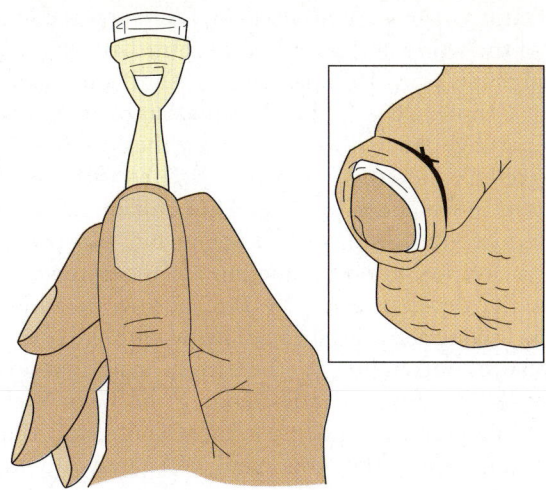

FIGURE 26–6. ◆ Circumcision using the Plastibell. The bell is fitted over the glans. A suture is tied around the bell's rim and the excess prepuce is cut away. The plastic rim remains in place for 3 to 4 days until healing occurs. The bell may be allowed to fall off; it is removed if still in place after 8 days.

minimizes the pain and the shifts in behavioral patterns associated with circumcision, such as crying, irritability, and erratic sleep cycles. Other studies are investigating the use of topical anesthetic applied 60 to 90 minutes before prepuce removal, acetaminophen, and cryoanalgesia (Kaufman et al., 2001; Taddio, Pollock, Gilbert-MacLeod, et al., 2000). Provide comfort measures such as lightly stroking the baby's head, providing a pacifier, and talking to him.

Following the circumcision, the infant should be held and comforted by a family member or the nurse. Be alert to any cues that these measures are overstimulating the newborn instead of comforting him. Such cues include turning away of the head, increased generalized body movement, skin color changes, hyperalertness, and hiccuping. Assess the infant every hour for the first 12 hours or per agency protocol for any abnormal bleeding and apply gentle pressure as needed. A and D ointment, petroleum jelly, or antibiotic ointment is placed on the penis to keep the diaper from adhering to the site in all procedures except those using the Plastibell. New ointment is applied with each diaper change, or at least four to five times a day for 24 to 48 hours. Check that the newborn voids and for adequacy of the urine stream and presence of blood. The newborn may cry when he voids after circumcision because of the ammonia in the urine. He should be positioned on his back or side with the diaper fastened loosely to prevent undue pressure. He may remain fussy for several hours and be less interested in feedings than before the procedure.

Before discharge, show the parents the appearance of a normal circumcised penis. Initially the glans penis is dark red and then becomes covered with whitish yellow exudate. Explain that the whitish yellow exudate around the glans is normal granulation tissue and not indicative of an infection. The exudate may be noted for about 2 or 3 days and should not be removed. Instruct parents to squeeze warm water gently over the penis to remove urine and feces and pat it dry after each diaper change. They should use soap only after the circumcision is healed. They should also fasten the diaper loosely for 2 to 3 days, because the glans remains tender. Parents need to provide extra holding, feeding, and nonnutritive sucking opportunities for a day or two. Instruct the family to look at the penis for bleeding or possible signs of infection (greenish discharge, swelling, redness). If bleeding occurs, they should apply light pressure intermittently to the site with a sterile gauze pad and notify the health care provider.

If the Plastibell is used, inform parents that it may remain in place for up to 8 days and then fall off. If it is still in place after 8 days, it may require manual removal by the clinician.

ENHANCEMENT OF PARENT-INFANT ATTACHMENT AND PARENTAL KNOWLEDGE OF NEWBORN CARE

The nurse encourages **parent-newborn attachment** by involving both parents with the new family member. (For specific interventions, see Chapters 17 and 22 and "Teaching About: What Parents Need to Know About Enhancing Attachment.")

Teaching About

WHAT PARENTS NEED TO KNOW ABOUT ENHANCING ATTACHMENT

- Information on the periods of reactivity and expected newborn responses (see Chapter 24).
- The gradual developmental nature of the bonding process and the reciprocal interactive nature of the process.
- The infant's capabilities for interaction such as nonverbal communication abilities. Nonverbal communications include movement, gaze, touch, facial expressions, and vocalizations—including crying. Eye contact is considered one of the cardinal factors in developing infant-parent attachment and will be integrated with touching and vocal behaviors.
- Touching, including stroking, patting, massaging, and kissing, will progress to interactive touch between parent and infant; parents need to assimilate these behaviors into daily routine with their baby.
- Parents need to incorporate comforting techniques, including use of sound, swaddling, rocking, stroking, and massage, into their daily baby care routines.
- The infant's behaviors will change as the infant matures and it is important for parents to be consistent in response to their infant's cues and needs.
- Information about available pamphlets, videos, and support groups in the community.

A Letter From Your Baby

Dear Parents:

I come to you a small, immature being with my own style and personality. I am yours for only a short time; enjoy me.

1. Please take time to find out who I am, how I differ from you and how much I can bring you joy.

2. Please feed me when I am hungry. I never knew hunger in the womb, and clocks and time mean little to me.

3. Please hold, cuddle, kiss, touch, stroke, and croon to me. I was always held closely in the womb and was never alone before.

4. Please don't be disappointed when I am not the perfect baby that you expected, nor disappointed with yourselves that you are not the perfect parents.

5. Please don't expect too much from me as your newborn baby, or too much from yourself as a parent. Give us both six weeks as a birthday present—six weeks for me to grow, develop, mature and become more stable and predictable, and six weeks for you to rest and relax and allow your body to get back to normal.

6. Please forgive me if I cry a lot. Bear with me and in a short time, as I mature, I will spend less and less time crying and more time socializing.

7. Please watch me carefully and I can tell you the things that soothe, console and please me. I am not a tyrant who was sent to make your life miserable, but the only way I can tell you that I am not happy is with my cry.

8. Please remember that I am resilient and can withstand the many natural mistakes you will make with me. As long as you make them with love, you cannot ruin me.

9. Please take care of yourself and eat a balanced diet, rest and exercise so that when we are together, you have the health and strength to take care of me.

10. Please take care of your relationship with others. Relationships that are good for you, support both you and me.

Although I may have turned your life upside down, please realize that things will be back to normal before long.

Thank you,

Your Loving Child

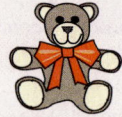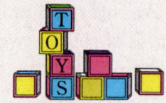

FIGURE 26–7. ◆ A Letter from your baby.

Infant massage is a common child care practice in many parts of the world and has recently gained attention in the United States (see "Complementary Care" on infant massage in Chapter 28). Parents can be taught to use infant massage as a method to facilitate the bonding process and to reduce the stress and pain associated with colic, constipation, inoculations, and teething. Infant massage not only induces relaxation for the infant but also provides a calming and feel-good interaction for the parents, which fosters the development of warm, positive relationships. Discuss waking activities such as talking with the baby while making eye contact, holding the baby in an upright position (sitting or standing), gently bending the baby back and forth while grasping under the knees and supporting the head and back with the other hand, and gently rubbing the baby's hands and feet. Quieting activities may include swaddling or bundling the baby to increase a sense of security; using slow, calming movements; and talking softly, singing, or humming to the baby. Also be aware of cultural variations in newborn care such as timing of naming the newborn, giving compliments about the baby, and needing good luck charms. The nurse plays a vital role in fostering parent-infant attachment (Figure 26–7 ◆).

Planning and Implementation in Preparation for Discharge

PARENT TEACHING

The nurse who is responsible for the care of the mother and newborn should assume the primary responsibility for education. Nearly every contact with the parents presents an opportunity for sharing information that can facilitate their sense of competence in newborn care. Recognize and respect the many ways of providing safe care. Unless harmful to the newborn, the parents' methods of giving care should be reinforced rather than contradicted. In addition, be sensitive to the cultural beliefs and values of the family (See "Developing Cultural Competence").

The information that follows is provided to increase the nurse's knowledge of newborn care and can also be used to meet parents' needs for information. Parents may be familiar with handling and caring for infants, or this may be their first time to interact with a newborn. If they are new parents, the sensitive nurse gently teaches them by example and provides instructions geared to their needs and previous knowledge about the various aspects of newborn care.

The length of stay in the birthing unit for mother and baby after birth is often 48 hours or less. The challenge for the nurse is to use every opportunity to teach, guide, and support individual parents, fostering their capabilities and confidence in caring for their newborn. Including mother-baby care and home care instruction on the night shift assists with education needs for early-discharge parents.

Observe how parents interact with their newborn during feeding and caregiving activities. Even during a short stay, there are opportunities to provide information and

Developing Cultural Competence

Following are examples of cultural beliefs and practices regarding baby care:*

Umbilical Cord

People of Latin American or Filipino cultural background may use an abdominal binder or bellyband to protect against dirt, injury, and umbilical hernia. They may also apply oils to the stump of the cord or tape metal to the umbilicus to ward off evil spirits.

People of northern European ancestry may expect a sterile cutting of the cord at birth. They may allow the stump to air dry and discard the cord once it falls off.

Some Latin American cultures cauterize the stump with a hot flame, hot coal, or the like (WHO, 1999).

In Kenya, women may express colostrum to the cord stump (WHO, 1999).

In Ecuador, the cord is left long in girls to prevent a small uterus and problems with childbirth (WHO, 1999).

Parent-Infant Contact

People of Asian ancestry may pick up the baby as soon as it cries, or they may carry the baby at all times.

Some Native Americans, notably the Navajos, may use cradle boards.

Korean mothers may be reluctant to pick up or touch their infant, deferring infant care to the paternal grandmother (Schneiderman, 1996).

The Muslim father traditionally calls praise to Allah in the newborn's right ear and cleans the infant after birth (Hutchinson & Baqi-Aziz, 1994).

Feeding

Some people of Asian heritage may breastfeed their babies for the first 1 to 2 years of life. Many Cambodian refugees practice breastfeeding on demand without restriction, or, if bottle-feeding, provide a "comfort bottle" in between feedings (Rasbridge & Kulig, 1995). People of Iranian heritage may breastfeed female babies longer than male babies. Some people of African ancestry may wean their babies after they begin to walk. Most Korean mothers resist breastfeeding in the hospital, contending that they do not have "milk," and state that they will begin breastfeeding at home (Schneiderman, 1996). Some Asians, Hispanics, Eastern Europeans, and Native Americans may delay breastfeeding because they believe colostrum is "bad" (Lipson, Dibble, & Minarik, 1996).

Circumcision

People of Muslim and Jewish ancestry practice circumcision as a religious ritual (Hutchinson & Baqi-Aziz, 1994).

Many natives of Africa and Australia practice circumcision as a puberty rite.

Native Americans and people of Asian and Latin American cultures rarely perform circumcision.

Only 15% of the world's male population is circumcised.

Health and Illness

Some people from Latin American cultural backgrounds may believe that touching the face or head of an infant when admiring it will ward off the "evil eye." They may also neglect to cut the baby's nails to avoid nearsightedness and instead put mittens on the baby's hands to prevent scratching. They also may believe that fat babies are healthy.

Some people of Asian heritage may not allow anyone to touch the baby's head without asking permission.

Some Orthodox Jews believe that saying the baby's name before the formal naming ceremony will harm the baby.

Some Asians and Haitians delay naming their infants (Geissler, 1998).

Some people of Vietnamese ancestry believe that cutting a baby's hair or nails will cause illness.

*The information is meant only to provide examples of some of the behaviors that may be found within certain cultures. Not all members of a culture practice the behaviors described.
Note: Adapted from Andrews, M. M. (1999). Transcultural perspectives in the nursing care of children and adolescents. In M. M. Andrews & J. S. Boyle (Eds.), *Transcultural concepts in nursing care* (3rd ed.). Philadelphia: Lippincott; Riordan, J., & Auerbach, K. G. (1999). *Breastfeeding and human lactation* (2nd ed.). Boston: Jones & Bartlett; World Health Organization. (1999). *Care of the umbilical cord: A review of the evidence* [On-line]. Available: www.who.int/rht/documents/MSM98-4

observe whether the parents are comfortable with changing the diapers of, wrapping, handling, and feeding their newborn. Do both parents get involved in the newborn's care? Is the mother depending on someone else to help her at home? Does the mother give reasons (e.g., "I'm too tired," "My stitches hurt," or "I'll learn later") for not wanting to be involved in her newborn's care? As the family provides care, enhance parental confidence by giving them positive feedback. If the parents encounter problems, express confidence in their abilities to master the new skill or information, suggest alternatives, and serve as a role model. All these factors need to be considered when evaluating the educational needs of the parents (Ruchala, 2000).

Several methods may be used to teach families about newborn care. Daily newborn care videos or classes are a nonthreatening way to convey general information. Individual instruction is helpful to answer specific questions or to clarify something that may have been confusing in class (Figure 26–8 ◆). Currently, many birthing centers have 24-hour educational video channels or videos to be viewed in the mother's room on a variety of postpartum and newborn care issues. With shorter stays, most teaching unfortunately tends to focus on infant feeding and immediate physical care needs of the mothers, with limited anticipatory guidance provided in other areas (Cavendish & Jackson, 1999). One-to-one teaching while the nurse is in the mother's room is the most effective educational method. Both first-time and experienced postpartum mothers rated individual teaching as the most effective method of instruction. For the hearing-impaired parent, videotapes with the information in both spoken and signed formats will be most helpful. Birthing centers should have handouts available for families who do not speak English and either interpreters or language interpreter phones.

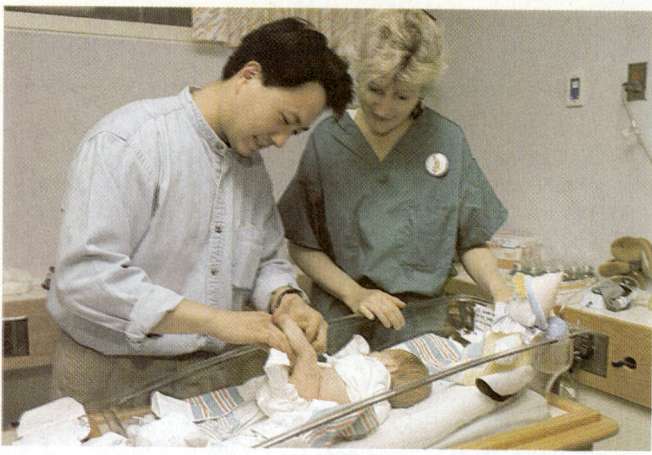

FIGURE 26–8. ◆ Individualizing family education. Father returns demonstration of diapering his son.

Nursing Practice

Remember that left-handed people tend to hold the baby over their right shoulder, and right-handed people do the opposite. This keeps the dominant hand free. However, most health personnel wear their name tags on the left side. To avoid scratching the baby's face, wear your name tag on the same side as your dominant hand.

GENERAL INSTRUCTIONS FOR NEWBORN CARE

Picking up a newborn is one of the first concerns of both student nurses and parents who have not had the experience. The newborn is easily picked up by sliding one hand under the neck and shoulders and the other hand under the buttocks or between the legs and then gently lifting the newborn. This technique provides security and support for the head (which the newborn is unable to support until 3 or 4 months of age).

The AAP (1997) recommends that healthy term infants be placed on their back or side to decrease the risk of sudden infant death syndrome. The nurse should demonstrate the proper positioning of the newborn and correct use of the bulb syringe. He or she can be an excellent role model for families in the area of safety. The baby should never be left alone anywhere but in the crib. Remind the mother that while she and the newborn are together in the birthing unit, she should never leave the baby alone for security reasons and because newborns spit up frequently the first day or two after birth.

Information on newborn bathing, cord care, and temperature assessment is provided to the parents prior to discharge. Current evidence does not support the routine application of topical antimicrobials to the drying umbilical cord (Dore, Buchan, Coulas, et al., 1998; WHO, 1999). Parents need to know the normal changes in the cord and

possible problems that may occur such as bright-red bleeding or greenish yellow drainage from the cord stump. If bleeding or drainage occurs, advise the parents to call their health care provider. (See "Teaching About: What to Tell Parents about Infant Care.")

Teaching About

WHAT TO TELL PARENTS ABOUT INFANT CARE

Immediate Safety Measures for the Newborn

Watch for excessive mucus: use bulb syringe to remove mucus. Have baby sleep on his or her back in crib or in someone's arms.

Voiding and Stool Characteristics and Patterns

Urine is straw to amber color without foul smell.

At least 6 to 10 wet diapers a day.

Normal progression of stool changes: (1) meconium (thick, tarry, dark green); (2) transitional stools (thin, brown to green); (3a) breastfed infant: yellow-gold, soft or mushy stools; (3b) bottle-fed infant: pale yellow, formed and pasty stools.

Only 1 to 2 stools a day for formula-fed baby.

Six to 10 small, loose yellow stools per day or only one stool every few days after breastfeeding is well established (after about 1 month).

Cord Care

Wash hands with clean water and soap before and after care. Keep the cord dry and exposed to air or loosely covered with clean clothes. (If cultural custom demands binding of the abdomen, a sanitary method such as the use of a clean piece of gauze can be recommended.)

Clean cord and skin around base with a cotton swab or cotton ball. Clean two to three times a day or with each diaper change. Touching the cord, applying unclean substances to it, and applying bandages should be avoided. Do not give tub baths until cord falls off in 7 to 14 days.

Fold diapers below umbilical cord to air-dry the cord (contact with wet or soiled diapers slows the drying process and increases the possibility of infection).

Check cord each day for any odor, oozing of greenish yellow material, or reddened areas around the cord. Expect tenderness around the cord and darkening and shriveling of cord. Report to health care provider any signs of infection.

Normal changes in cord: Cord should look dark and dry up before falling off. A small drop of blood may present when cord falls off.

Never pull the cord or attempt to loosen it.

Care Required for Circumcision and Uncircumcised Infants
Circumcision Care:

Squeeze soapy water over circumcision site once a day.

Rinse area off with warm water and pat dry.

Apply small amount of petroleum jelly (unless a Plastibell is in place) with each diaper change.

Fasten diaper loosely over penis.

Since the glans is sensitive, avoid placing baby on his stomach.

(continued)

Teaching About

Check for any foul-smelling drainage or bleeding at least once a day.

Let Plastibell fall off by itself (about 8 days after circumcision).

Plastibell should not be pulled off.

Light, sticky, yellow drainage (part of healing process) may form over head of penis.

Uncircumcised Care:

Clean uncircumcised penis with water during diaper changes and with bath.

Do not force foreskin back over the penis; foreskin will retract normally over time (may take 3 to 5 years).

Techniques for Waking and Quieting Newborns

Techniques for Waking Baby:

Loosen clothing, change diaper.

Hand-express milk onto baby's lips.

Talk with baby while making eye contact.

Hold baby in upright position (sitting or standing).

Have baby do sit-ups (gently and rhythmically bend baby back and forth while grasping the baby under his or her knees and supporting baby's head and back with your other hand).

Play patty-cake with baby.

Stimulate rooting reflex (brush one cheek with hand or nipple).

Increase skin contact (gently rub hands and feet).

Techniques for Quieting Baby:

Check for soiled diaper.

Swaddle or bundle baby (bring arms and legs into midline, which increases sense of security).

Use slow, calming movements with baby.

Softly talk, sing, or hum to baby.

Signs of Illness and Use of Thermometer

See Table 26–3, page 584.

Review with the family how to take axillary or tympanic temperatures and discuss the different types of thermometers. It is important that families understand the differences and know how to select a thermometer. The newborn's temperature needs to be taken only when signs of illness are present. Advise parents to call their physician or pediatric nurse practitioner immediately if they observe any signs of illness.

Thinking Critically

SIGNS OF ILLNESS?

You are caring for a new mother who had her first child, a daughter, about 4 hours ago. She appears visibly upset when changing her infant's diaper and says she thinks something is wrong because her daughter has tissue protruding from her vagina and some blood in her diaper. What would you do? 🔗 **WEB**

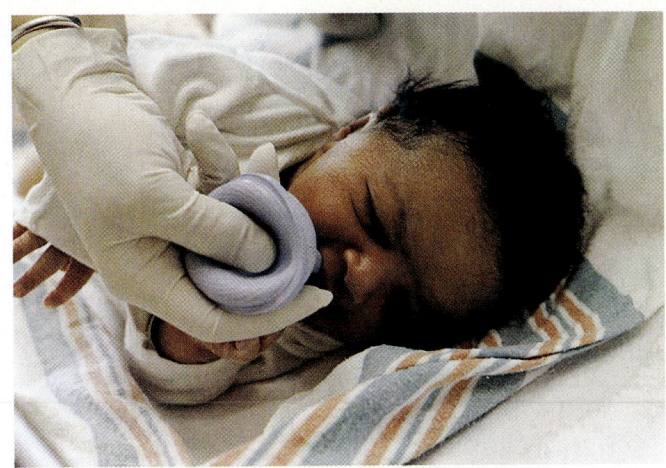

FIGURE 26–9. ◆ Nasal and oral suctioning. The bulb is compressed, the tip is placed in either the mouth or the nose, and the bulb is released.

NASAL AND ORAL SUCTIONING

Most newborns are obligatory nose breathers for the first months of life. They generally maintain air passage patency by coughing or sneezing. During the first few days of life, however, the newborn has increased mucus, and gentle suctioning with a bulb syringe may be indicated. Demonstrate the use of the bulb syringe in the mouth and nose and have the parents do a return demonstration. The parents should repeat this demonstration of suctioning and cleansing the bulb before discharge so they feel confident in performing the procedure. Care should be taken to apply only gentle suction to prevent nasal bleeding.

To suction the newborn, compress the bulb syringe before placing the tip in the nostril. The nurse or parent must take care not to occlude the passageway. Let the bulb re-expand slowly by releasing the compression on the bulb (Figure 26–9 ◆). Remove the bulb syringe from the nostril, and compress the drainage out of the bulb and onto a tissue. The bulb syringe may also be used in the mouth if the newborn is spitting up and unable to handle the excess secretions. Once the bulb is compressed, place the tip of the bulb syringe about 1 inch to one side of the newborn's mouth, and release the compression. The resulting suction draws up the excess secretions. Repeat the procedure on the other side of the mouth. Avoid the roof of the mouth and back of the throat because suction in these areas might stimulate the gag reflex. The bulb syringe should be washed in warm, soapy water and rinsed in warm water daily and as needed after use. A bulb syringe should always be kept near the newborn. New parents and nurses who are inexperienced with newborns may fear that the baby will choke and are relieved to know how to take action if such an event occurs. They should be advised to turn the newborn's head to the side or down as soon as there is any indication of gagging or vomiting and to use the bulb syringe as needed.

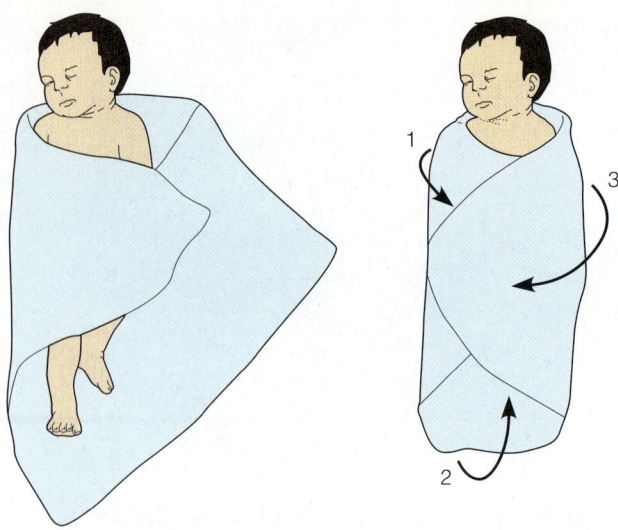

FIGURE 26–10. ◆ One method of swaddling a baby.

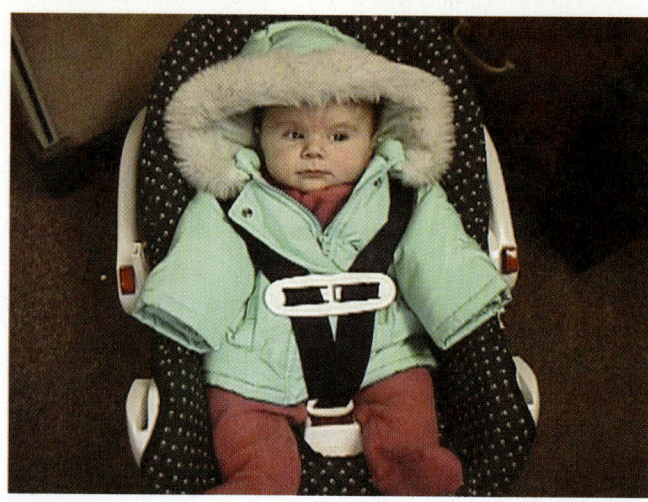

FIGURE 26–11. ◆ Infant car restraint for use from birth to about 12 months of age.

SWADDLING THE NEWBORN

Swaddling (wrapping) helps the newborn maintain body temperature, provides a feeling of closeness and security, and may be effective in quieting a crying baby. Place a blanket on the crib (or secure surface) in the shape of a diamond. Fold down the top corner of the blanket slightly, and place the newborn with the head at the upper edge of the blanket. Wrap the right corner of the blanket around the newborn and tuck it under the left side (not too tightly—the newborn needs a little room to move). Pull the bottom corner up to the chest, and wrap the left corner around the newborn's right side (Figure 26–10 ◆). The nurse can show this wrapping technique to a new mother so she will feel more skilled in handling her baby.

SLEEP AND ACTIVITY

Perhaps nothing is more individual to each newborn than the sleep-activity cycle. It is important to recognize the individual variations of each newborn and to assist parents as they develop sensitivity to their newborn's communication signals and rhythms of activity and sleep. (See Chapter 24 for a more detailed discussion of sleep-wake activity). ⊂⊃

CAR SAFETY CONSIDERATIONS

Half the children killed or injured in automobile accidents could have been protected by federally approved car seats. Newborns should go home from the birthing unit in a car seat adapted to fit newborns (Figure 26–11 ◆). Ensure that all parents understand the benefits of child safety seat use and proper installation (AAP Committee on Injury and Poison Prevention, 1999). For more detail, see Chapter 32. ⊂⊃

NEWBORN SCREENING AND IMMUNIZATION PROGRAM

Before the newborn and mother are discharged from the birthing unit, inform the parents about the normal **new-born screening tests** and tell them when to return to the birthing center or clinic if further tests are needed. The disorders that can be identified from a drop of blood obtained by a heel stick are cystic fibrosis, galactosemia, homocystinuria, hypothyroidism, maple syrup urine disease, phenylketonuria (PKU), and hemoglobinopathies. See Chapters 44 and 51 for detailed discussion of management. ⊂⊃ Early discharge puts infants at risk for delayed or even missed diagnosis of PKU and congenital hypothyroidism because of decreased sensitivity of screening; infants should be retested by 2 weeks of age if the first test was done prior to 24 hours after birth. The accuracy of the test for PKU is directly related to the newborn's age. The likelihood of detecting PKU increases as the infant grows older, so the infant needs to be at least 24 hours old for a valid test (Wallman, 1998).

The Centers for Disease Control and Prevention (CDC) and the AAP recommend universal hepatitis B immunization programs during newborn and early infancy (Selekman, 2000). The current recommendation is that newborns receive the first vaccine dose within 12 hours of birth (0.5 mL of either vaccine preparation). Infants born to HBsAg-positive mothers should receive hepatitis B vaccine and 0.5 mL hepatitis B immune globulin (HBIG) within 12 hours of birth at separate injection sites. (See "Drug Guide: Hepatitis B Vaccine," on page 584.) Parents need to be advised if the birthing center provides newborn hepatitis vaccinations so that an appropriate follow-up program can be set in motion.

Teach the family all necessary caregiving methods before discharge. A checklist may be helpful to determine whether the teaching has been completed and to verify the parents' knowledge on leaving the birthing unit (Figure 26–12 ◆). Review all areas with the mother and father, without rushing, and take time to answer all queries. Note any concerns of the parents or nurse.

NURSERY TEACHING CHECKLIST

Please read the *Mother/Baby* information booklet given to you after delivery. After reading it, please go through the following list and check whether you understand each topic or need to know more.

		I know this already	Doesn't apply to me	I need to know more	Taught/ reviewed/ demonstrated
Baby Care	What to do if baby is choking or gagging				
	Safety				
	How to do skin care/cord care				
	How to take care of the circumcision or genital area				
	How to know if my baby is sick and what to do				
	What is jaundice and how to detect it				
	Use of thermometer				
	Use of bulb syringe				
	How and when to burp baby				
	Newborn behavior: crying/comforting				
	How to position baby after feeding				
	What does demand scheduling mean				
Breastfeeding	How to position baby for feeding				
	How to get baby to latch on to my nipple properly				
	When and how long to nurse				
	Removal of baby from my nipple				
	What is the supply and demand concept				
	What is the letdown reflex				
	When does breast milk come in				
	Supplementing				
	Proper diet for breastfeeding mothers				
	Prevention and comfort measures for sore nipples				
	Prevention and comfort measures for engorgement				
	When and how to use a breast pump				
	How to express milk by hand				
	How to go back to work and continue to breastfeed				
Bottle Feeding	How to feed my baby a bottle				
	Reasons for NOT propping bottles				
	How to clean nipple/bottle				
	How to mix formula				
	What formula should my baby drink				
Safety	**Use of infant car seat**				
	Back to Sleep				
	Shaken Baby Syndrome				

Other information:

_____

_____

_____

_____

I have received and understand the instructions given on the above topics.

_____ _____
MOTHER'S SIGNATURE DATE

Videos reviewed/ Literature given:

_____

Language Spoken by Mother:

☐English ☐Spanish ☐Other _____

Interpreter Used? ☐Yes ☐No ☐Family Interprets

Nurse's Signature(s):

_____

_____

_____

FIGURE 26–12. ◆ Infant teaching checklist is completed by the time of discharge. *Note:* From Presbyterian/St. Luke's Medical Center, Denver, CO. Adapted.

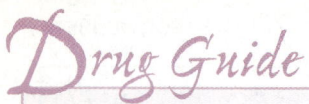

Drug Guide

HEPATITIS B VACCINE (ENGERIX-B, RECOMBIVAX HB)

Overview of Neonatal Action

Hepatitis B vaccine is used as a prophylactic treatment against all subtypes of hepatitis B virus. It provides passive immunization for newborns of HBsAg-negative and HBsAg-positive mothers. Hepatitis B can be transmitted across the placenta but most newborns are infected during birth.

The vaccine is produced from baker's yeast and plasmid containing HBsAg gene.

Hepatitis B (thimerosal free) vaccine contains more than 95% HBsAg protein and is an inactivated (noninfective) product. Universal immunization is recommended.

Infants of HBsAg-positive mothers should concurrently receive 0.5 mL of HBIG prophylaxis at separate injection sites.

Route, Dosage, Frequency

First dose of 0.5 mL (10 mcg) is given intramuscularly into the anterolateral thigh within 12 hours of birth for infants born to HBsAg-positive mothers. The second dose of vaccine is given at 1 month of age and is followed by a final dose at 6 months of age.

Infants born to HBsAg-negative mothers receive their first dose of vaccine at birth, the second dose at 1 to 2 months of age, and the third dose at 6 to 18 months (Zenk et al., 2000).

Infants whose mother's HBsAg status is unknown receive the same doses of vaccine as infants born to HBsAg-positive mothers.

Neonatal Side Effects

The only common side effect is soreness at the injection site. Occasional side effects include erythema, swelling, warmth and induration at the injection site, irritability, or low-grade fever (37.7 °C [99.8 °F]).

Nursing Considerations

Delay administration during active infection; the vaccine will not prevent infection during the incubation period.

The vaccine should be used as supplied. Do not dilute. Shake well.

Store in refrigerator at 2 to 8 °C. Do not freeze.

Do not inject intravenously or interdermally.

Monitor for adverse reactions. Monitor temperature closely.

Have epinephrine available to treat possible allergic reactions.

Responsiveness to the vaccine is age dependent. Preterm infants weighing less than 1000 g have lower seroconversion rates. Consider delaying the first dose until infant is term PCA (postconceptual age) or use a 4-dose schedule.

NURSING CARE IN THE COMMUNITY

By discussing with parents ways to meet their newborn's needs, ensure safety, and appreciate the newborn's unique characteristics and behaviors, and by assisting parents in establishing links with their community-based health care provider, the nurse can get the new family off to a good start. To assist parents in caring for their newborn at home, some physicians encourage pediatric prenatal visits so that this contact is established before birth. Public health nurses have long been involved in newborn care and parent education. In some programs the birthing unit staff nurses visit new families in their homes within a few hours or days of discharge to bridge the gap between early discharge and routine health care checkups (AAP Council on Child and Adolescent Health, 1998; Lieu, Braverman, Escobar, et al., 2000). Parents need to know the signs of illness, how to reach the pediatrician or after-hours clinic, and the importance of follow-up after discharge (Table 26–3). Parents should also check with their clinician for advice about over-the-counter medications to be kept in the medicine cabinet.

Education is a wonderful aspect of family-centered maternity care. The nurse who takes the time to get the family off to a good start can feel the satisfaction of providing optimal care.

Evaluation

Expected outcomes of nursing care include the following:

- The newborn's adaptation to extrauterine life is completed successfully.
- The newborn feeding pattern is satisfactorily established.
- The parents demonstrate safe techniques in caring for their newborn.
- The parents express understanding of the bonding process and display attachment behaviors.
- Parents verbalize developmentally appropriate behavioral expectations of their newborn and knowledge of community-based newborn follow-up care.

TABLE 26–3 When Parents Should Call Their Health Care Provider

Temperature above 38.4 °C (101 °F) rectally or 38 °C (100.4 °F) axillary or below 36.1 °C (97 °F) rectally or 36.6 °C (97.8 °F) axillary

Continual rise in temperature

More than one episode of forceful vomiting or frequent vomiting (over 6 hours)

Refusal of two feedings in a row

Lethargy (listlessness), difficulty in awakening baby

Inconsolable infant (quieting techniques are not effective) or continuous high-pitched cry

Cyanosis (bluish discoloration of skin) with or without a feeding

Absence of breathing longer than 15 seconds

Reddened umbilical cord

Abdominal distention, crying when trying to pass stools, or absence of stools after stool pattern is established

Two consecutive green or black watery stools or increased frequency of stools

No wet diapers for 18 to 24 hours or fewer than six wet diapers per day after 4 days of age

Increasing jaundice (yellow tone) of the skin and jaundice over abdomen and extremities

Pustules, rashes, or blisters other than normal, newborn rash

Development of eye drainage

The overall goal of newborn nursing care is to provide comprehensive care while promoting the establishment of the new family unit.

In the period immediately after birth, during which adaptation to extrauterine life occurs, the newborn requires close monitoring to ensure normal transition.

Nursing goals during the first 4 hours after birth (admission period) are to maintain a clear airway, maintain a neutral thermal environment, initiate oral feedings, facilitate attachment, and prevent hemorrhage and infection.

The newborn is routinely given prophylactic vitamin K to prevent possible hemorrhagic disease of the newborn.

Prophylactic eye treatment for *Neisseria gonorrhoeae* is legally required for all newborns.

Nursing goals for ongoing newborn care include maintenance of cardiopulmonary function, maintenance of neutral thermal environment and skin integrity, promotion of adequate hydration and nutrition, promotion of safety, enhancement of attachment and family knowledge of child care, and prevention of complications.

Following a circumcision, the newborn must be observed closely for signs of pain, bleeding, inability to void, and infection.

Prior to discharge, the nurse provides parent teaching on nasal and oral suctioning, wrapping the newborn, sleep and activity, and safety considerations.

Newborn screening for cystic fibrosis, galactosemia, homocystinuria, hypothyroidism, maple syrup urine disease, phenylketonuria, and hemoglobinopathies is done on all newborns in the first 1 to 3 days after birth.

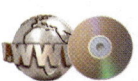

EXPLOREMediaLink

NCLEX Review, Case Studies, and other interactive resources for this chapter can be found on the companion website at http://www.prenhall.com/london. Click on "Chapter 26" to select the activities for this chapter.

For animations, more NCLEX review questions, and an audio glossary, access the accompanying CD-ROM in this textbook.

REFERENCES

American Academy of Pediatrics. (1997): *Guidelines for perinatal care* (4th ed.). Chicago: Author.

American Academy of Pediatrics, Council on Child and Adolescent Health. (1998). The role of home-visitation programs in improving health outcomes for children and families. *Pediatrics, 101*(3), 486–489.

American Academy of Pediatrics, Committee on Injury and Poison Prevention. (1999). Safe transportation of newborns at hospital discharge. *Pediatrics, 104*(4), 986–987.

Andrews, M. M. (1999). Transcultural perspectives in the nursing care of children and adolescents. In M. M. Andrews & J. S. Boyle (Eds.), *Transcultural concepts in nursing care* (3rd ed., pp. 107–159). Philadelphia: Lippincott.

Carroll, V. (2000). Infant abduction: Lowering the risk. *AWHONN Lifelines, 3*(6), 25–27.

Cavendish, R., & Jackson, L. (1999). *Early discharge of the term newborn: Guideline for practice.* Des Plaines, IL: National Association of Neonatal Nurses.

Dore, S., Buchan, D., Coulas, S., Hamber, L., Stewart, M., Cowan, D., et al., (1998). Alcohol versus natural drying for the newborn cord care. *Journal of Obstetric, Gynecologic, and Neonatal Nursing, 27*(6), 621–628.

Geissler, E. M. (1998). *Pocket guide to cultural assessment* (2nd ed.). St. Louis, MO: Mosby.

Hutchinson, M. K., & Baqi-Aziz, M. (1994). Nursing care of the childbearing Muslim family. *Journal of Obstetric, Gynecologic, and Neonatal Nursing, 23*(9), 767–771.

Karl, D. J. (1999). The newborn bath: Using infant neurobehavior to connect parents and newborns. *American Journal of Maternal Child Nursing, 24*(6), 280–286.

Kaufman, M. W., Clark, J. Y. & Castro, C. L. (2001). Neonatal circumcision: Benefits, risks, and family teaching. *American Journal of Maternal Child Nursing, 26*(4), 197–201.

Klaus, M., & Klaus, P. (1985). *The amazing newborn.* Menlo Park, CA: Addison-Wesley.

Lieu, T. A., Braverman, P. A., Escobar, G. J., Fischer, A. F., Jensvold, N. G., & Capra, A. M. (2000). A randomized comparison of home and clinic follow-up visits after early postpartum hospital discharge. *Pediatrics, 105*(5), 1058–1065.

Lipson, J. G., Dibble, S. L., & Minarik, P. A. (1996). *Culture and nursing care: A pocket guide.* San Francisco: University of California at San Francisco Nursing Press.

MacMullen, N. J., & Dulski, L. A. (2000). Factors related to sucking ability in healthy newborns. *Journal of Obstetric, Gynecologic, and Neonatal Nursing, 29*(4), 390–396.

Neonatal Skin Care. (1997). *NANN guidelines for practice.* Petaluma, CA: National Association of Neonatal Nurses.

Neonatal Thermoregulation. (1997). *NANN guidelines for practice.* Petaluma, CA: National Association of Neonatal Nurses.

Rasbridge, L. A., & Kulig, J. C. (1995). Infant feeding among Cambodian refugees. *American Journal of Maternal Child Nursing, 20*(4), 213–218.

Riordan, J., & Auerbach, K. G. (1999). *Breastfeeding and human lactation* (2nd ed.). Boston: Jones & Bartlett.

Ruchala, P. L. (2000). Teaching new mothers: Priorities of nurses and postpartum women. *Journal of Obstetric, Gynecologic, and Neonatal Nursing, 29*(3), 265–273.

Schneiderman, J. U. (1996). Postpartum nursing for Korean mothers. *American Journal of Maternal Child Nursing, 21*(3), 155–158.

Selekman, J. (2000). Immunization schedule 2000. *Pediatric Nursing, 26*(2), 209–210.

Taddio, A., Pollock, N., Gilbert-MacLeod, C., & Ohlsson, K. (2000). Combined analgesia and local anesthesia to minimize pain during circumcision. *Archives of Pediatric and Adolescent Medicine, 154*, 620–623.

Varda, K. E., & Behnke, R. S. (2000). The effect of timing of initial bath on newborn's temperature. *Journal of Obstetric, Gynecologic, and Neonatal Nursing, 29*(1), 27–32.

Wallman, C. M. (1998). Newborn genetic screening. *Neonatal Network, 17*(3), 55–60.

World Health Organization. (1999). *Care of the umbilical cord: A review of the evidence* [On-line]. Available: www.who.int/rht/documents/MSM98-4

Zenk, K. E., Sills, J. H., & Koeppel, R. M. (2000). *Neonatal medications and nutrition: A comprehensive guide* (2nd ed.). Santa Rosa, CA: NICU Ink.

CHAPTER 27

Newborn Nutrition

I had been told that most babies ate every 3 to 4 hours and slept the rest of the time. But not my son! He wanted to nurse every 2 hours, and sometimes more often than that. I wanted to meet his needs but felt consumed by them. It was hard to adjust to the fact that I could not get done what I usually accomplished. Once I accepted this fact, I felt free to enjoy the time I was spending with my son.

—RYAN'S MOTHER, 30

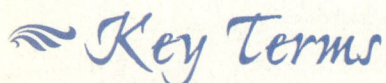

Key Terms

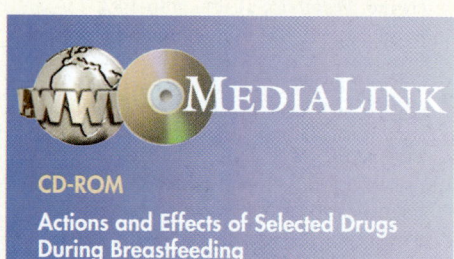

MediaLink

CD-ROM

Actions and Effects of Selected Drugs During Breastfeeding

Audio Glossary

NCLEX Review

COMPANION WEBSITE

http://www.prenhall.com/london

Newborn Nutrition Web Links

Thinking Critically

NCLEX Review

Case Study

*F*eeding their newborn is an exciting, satisfying, but often worrisome task for parents. Meeting this essential need of their new child helps parents strengthen their attachment to their child and fosters their self-images as nurturers and providers, yet carries great responsibility. Whether a woman chooses to breastfeed or formula feed, she can be reassured that she can adequately meet her infant's needs. As questions about feeding arise, the nurse works with the woman to help her develop skill in her chosen method. In every interaction, it is the nurse's responsibility to support the parents and promote the family's sense of confidence.

NUTRITIONAL NEEDS OF THE NEWBORN

The newborn's diet must supply nutrients to meet the rapid rate of physical growth and development. A neonatal diet should include protein, carbohydrate, fat, water, vitamins, and minerals. The recommended dietary allowances (RDAs) for birth through the first 6 months have been established. The calories (105 to 108 kcal/kg/day or 50 to 55 kcal/lb/day) in the newborn's diet are divided among protein, carbohydrate, and fat. Protein is needed for rapid cellular growth and maintenance. Carbohydrates provide energy. Fat provides calories, regulates fluid and electrolyte balance, and develops the newborn brain and neurologic system. Fluid requirements are high (140 to 160 mL/kg/day or 64 to 73 mL/lb/day) because the newborn cannot concentrate urine. Fluid needs increase further during illness or hot weather.

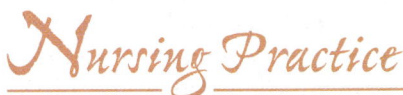
Nursing Practice

Following are newborn caloric and fluid needs:

▶ Caloric intake: 50 to 55 kcal/lb/day or 105 to 108 kcal/kg/day
▶ Fluid requirements: 64 to 73 mL/lb/day or 140 to 160 mL/kg/day
▶ Weight gain: First 6 months—1 oz/day Second 6 months—0.5 oz/day

The infant's iron needs are affected by accumulation of iron stores during fetal life and the mother's iron and other food intake if she is breastfeeding. Ascorbic acid (usually in the form of fruit juices) and meat, poultry, and fish enhance iron absorption in the mother, just as they do later in the infant. The newborn needs adequate minerals and vitamins to prevent deficiency states such as scurvy, cheilosis, and pellagra.

Formula-fed babies gain weight faster than breastfed babies because of the higher protein in commercially prepared formula and the larger volumes of formula needed to obtain the necessary nutrients. (Because breast milk is digested more easily than formula, the nutrients are more readily available.) Formula-fed infants tend to regain their birth weight by 10 days after birth and may gain 30 g (1 oz) or more per day, up to 6 months of age. Healthy breastfed babies tend to regain their birth weight about 14 days after birth and gain approximately 15 g (0.5 oz) per day in the first 6 months of life. Formula-fed infants generally double their weight within 3.5 to 4 months, whereas nursing infants double their weight at about 5 months of age.

Breast Milk Feeding

The composition of human milk varies with the stage of lactation, the time of the day, the time during the feeding, maternal nutrition, and gestational age of the newborn at birth. During the establishment of lactation there are three stages of human milk: colostrum, transitional milk, and mature milk.

Colostrum is a yellowish or creamy-appearing fluid that is thicker than the mature milk and contains more protein, fat-soluble vitamins, and minerals (American College of Obstetricians and Gynecologists [ACOG], 2000). It also contains high levels of immunoglobulins (antibodies such as IgA) and can be a source of passive immunity for the newborn. Colostrum production begins early in pregnancy and may last for several days after birth. Usually colostrum is replaced by transitional milk within 2 to 4 days after birth.

Transitional milk is produced from the end of colostrum production until approximately 2 weeks postpartum. This milk contains lactose, water-soluble vitamins, elevated levels of fat, and more calories than colostrum.

The final milk produced, **mature milk,** contains about 10% solids (carbohydrates, proteins, fats) for energy and growth; the rest is water, which is vital for maintaining hydration. The composition of mature milk varies according to the time during the feeding. **Foremilk** is the milk obtained at the beginning of the feeding. It is high in water content and contains vitamins and protein. **Hindmilk** is released after the initial letdown, or release of milk, and has a higher fat concentration. Although mature milk appears similar to skim milk (watery and somewhat bluish in color) and may cause mothers to question whether their milk is "rich enough," mature breast milk provides 20 kcal/oz, as do most prepared formulas. However, the percentage of calories derived from protein is lower in breast milk than in formulas, and a greater percentage of calories is derived from fat. In breastfed babies, protein metabolism produces less nitrogen waste, which has a positive effect on the infant's immature renal system.

ACOG (2000) recommends breast milk as the optimal food for the first 6 to 12 months of life. It is believed that breastfeeding provides newborns and infants with immunologic, nutritional, and psychosocial advantages.

IMMUNOLOGIC ADVANTAGES
Immunologic advantages of breastfeeding include varying degrees of protection from respiratory and gastrointestinal infections, otitis media, meningitis, sepsis, and allergies

(ACOG, 2000). This protection of the breastfed baby extends from the neonatal period through age 18 months, when the baby's own immunoglobulins become active. Secretory IgA, an immunoglobulin in colostrum and breast milk, has antiviral, antibacterial, and antigenic-inhibiting properties. Secretory IgA plays a role in decreasing the permeability of the small intestine to antigenic macromolecules (Johnson & Riddick, 2000). Other properties in colostrum and breast milk that inhibit the growth of bacteria and viruses are *Lactobacillus bifidus,* lysozymes, lactoperoxidase, lactoferrin, transferrin, and various immunoglobulins. Immunoglobulins to the poliomyelitis virus are also present in the breast milk of mothers who have immunity to this virus. Because these immunoglobulins may inhibit the desired intestinal infection and immune response of the infant, some clinics suggest that breastfeeding be withheld for 30 to 60 minutes following the administration of the Sabin oral polio vaccine. In addition to its immunologic properties, breast milk is non-allergenic.

NUTRITIONAL ADVANTAGES

Breast milk is composed of lactose, lipids, polyunsaturated fatty acids, and amino acids, especially taurine, and has a whey-to-casein protein ratio that facilitates its digestion, absorption, and full use compared to formulas (Johnson & Riddick, 2000). Some researchers believe that the high concentration of cholesterol and the balance of amino acids in breast milk make it the best food for myelination and neurologic development (Johnson & Riddick, 2000). High cholesterol levels in breast milk may stimulate the production of enzymes that lead to efficient metabolism of cholesterol, thereby reducing its harmful long-term effects on the cardiovascular system. Breast milk provides newborns with minerals in more appropriate doses than formulas do (Lawrence & Lawrence, 1999). Although the concentration of iron in breast milk is much lower than that in prepared formulas, it is much more readily and fully absorbed and appears sufficient to meet the infant's iron needs for the first 4 to 6 months. The AAP and ACOG (1997) state that breastfed newborns generally do not need supplemental iron before the age of 4 to 6 months. Furthermore, supplemental iron may decrease the ability of breast milk to protect the newborn by interfering with lactoferrin, an iron-binding protein that enhances the absorption of iron and has anti-infective properties.

Another advantage of breast milk is that all its components are delivered to the infant in an unchanged form, and vitamins are not lost through processing and heating. If the breastfeeding mother is taking daily multivitamins, her diet is adequate, and the baby is exposed to sunlight for 30 minutes a week if wearing a diaper or 2 hours a week if fully clothed, vitamin D supplements are not necessary for the exclusively breastfed infant (Lauwers & Shinskie, 2000). If the mother's diet or vitamin intake is inadequate or questionable, caregivers may choose to prescribe additional vitamins for the infant.

PSYCHOSOCIAL ADVANTAGES

The psychosocial advantages of breastfeeding are primarily those associated with maternal-infant attachment. The mother's level of oxytocin generally increases with breastfeeding, and studies indicate that this hormonal change coincides with more even mood responses and increased feelings of maternal well-being. Breastfeeding enhances attachment by providing the opportunity for frequent, direct skin contact between the newborn and the mother. The newborn's sense of touch is highly developed at birth and is a primary means of communication. The tactile stimulation associated with breastfeeding can communicate warmth, closeness, and comfort. The increased closeness lets both newborn and mother learn each other's behavioral cues and needs. The mother's sense of accomplishment in being able to satisfy her baby's needs for nourishment and comfort is enhanced when the newborn sucks vigorously and is satiated and calmed by the breastfeeding. Some mothers prefer breastfeeding as a way to extend the close, unique, nourishing relationship between mother and baby that existed before the baby's birth.

Breastfeeding twins not only is possible but can enhance the mother's individualization and attachment to each newborn. The fantasy of a single baby is replaced more readily with the reality of two individual babies when the mother has close and frequent contact with each. Fathers are encouraged to be a part of the feeding experience by offering fresh pumped or thawed (frozen) breast milk to the baby at one or more feedings daily.

CONTRAINDICATIONS AND DISADVANTAGES

There are some medical contraindications to breastfeeding. A mother with a diagnosis of breast cancer should not breastfeed so that she can begin treatment immediately. Women with HIV or AIDS are counseled against breastfeeding except in countries where the risk of neonatal death from diarrhea and other disease (excluding AIDS) is high. Breastfeeding is also contraindicated for the infant suffering from galactosemia (Calamaro, 2000). Maternal medications may preclude breastfeeding, as discussed in Chapters 12 and 28. ⬭ Medications such as metronidazole (Flagyl), used to treat trichomoniasis, pass into breast milk and may be harmful to the infant (Johnson & Riddick, 2000). Management of newborn jaundice may include a brief suspension of breastfeeding (see Chapter 29). ⬭

In the dominant Western culture, in which women actively pursue activities outside the home, being "tied down" to an infant for 9 to 12 feedings every day may be considered inconvenient and stressful. Another often-cited disadvantage of breastfeeding is the exclusion of the father from the nurturing involved in feeding the infant. However, nurturing encompasses more than just feeding, and the father can comfort and attend to the baby in many other ways (Figure 27–1 ◆).

Opinions vary on the advisability of continuing breastfeeding if the mother becomes pregnant with another

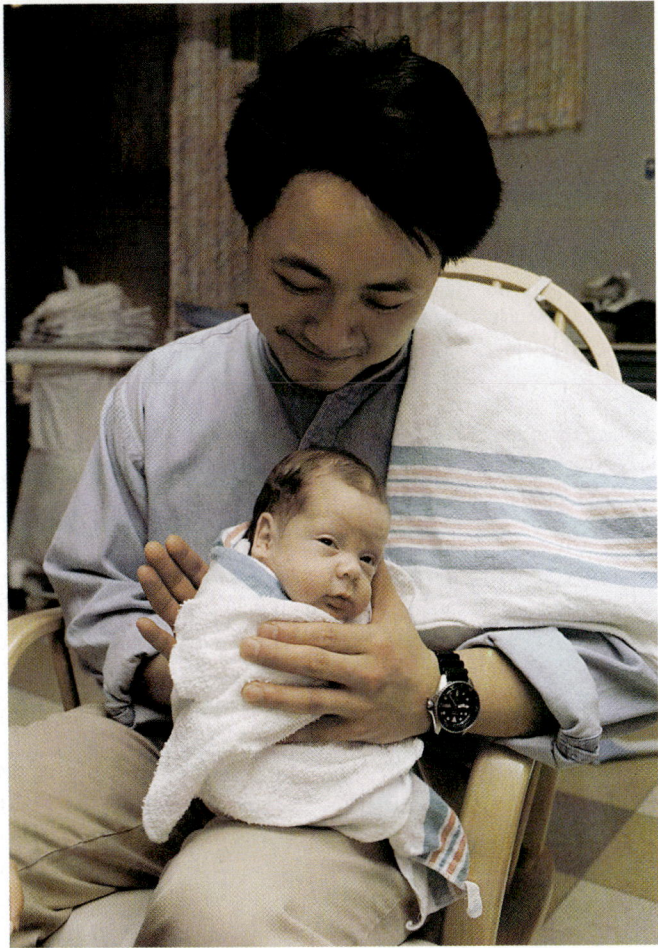

FIGURE 27-1. ◆ A father can nurture his baby in many ways.

child. Some believe the nutritional demands on the pregnant mother are too great and advocate gradual weaning. Others suggest that with adequate rest, a proper diet, and strong emotional support, continued breastfeeding during pregnancy is a valid choice. The practice of nursing one infant throughout pregnancy and then breastfeeding both infants after birth is called tandem nursing. When pregnancy occurs, the decision is best made individually after considering maternal health and motivation and the age of the first child.

Although many mothers learn about breastfeeding from written sources, family and friends, and **La Leche League** (an international lay support and information group), the nurse needs to be a ready source of information, encouragement, and support as well. The nurse can be helpful when parents are deciding whether to breastfeed, after the birth process when breastfeeding is just being established, and after the family returns home.

Formula Feeding

Although breastfeeding is increasing in popularity, formula feeding is a viable and nurturing choice, particularly in developed countries, and meets the goal of successful growth of the baby. The closeness and warmth that can occur during breastfeeding is also an integral part of bottle-feeding. An advantage of bottle-feeding is that parents can share equally in this nurturing, caring experience with their baby. Numerous types of commercially prepared lactose formulas meet the nutritional needs of the infant. These formulas contain more tyrosine and phenylalanine and less taurine than breast milk does. Because many commercial formulas use a cow's milk base, they tend to have a high renal solute load, high protein and casein content, high proportion of saturated fats, low amounts of linoleic acid, poor mineral bioavailability, and increased risk for allergies to cow's milk proteins (Walker & Creehan, 2001).

Many companies make enriched formulas that are similar to breast milk. These formulas have sufficient levels of carbohydrate, protein, fat, vitamins, and minerals to meet the newborn's nutritional needs. Commercial formulas have been developed to minimize the harmful components of cow's milk. The formulas are enriched with carnitine and/or taurine and vitamins, particularly vitamin D; some of them are also enriched with long-chain polyunsaturated fatty acids. The three categories of infant formulas are formulas with cow's milk base, soy protein–based formulas, and specialized or therapeutic formulas. Soy protein–based formulas substitute soy protein supplemented with methionine for cow's milk protein and are used for primary lactase deficiency or galactosemia conditions. Specialized formulas such as casein-hydrolysated formulas (e.g., Nutramigen, Pregestimil, Alimentum) are used when an infant has an allergy or intolerance to cow's milk protein. The AAP recommends hydrolysated formulas for infants with allergy or intolerance to cow's milk protein to avoid risk of concomitant allergy to soy protein (AAP Committee on Nutrition, 2000). Whey-hydrolysated formulas, such as Carnation Good Start, can also be used for infants with cow's milk allergy, but not if the child has an IgE-mediated allergy to cow's milk.

POTENTIAL CONTRAINDICATIONS

If formula is prepared improperly (such as by adding too much powder), the excess salts (i.e., sodium) may harm the newborn's kidneys and may lead to thirst in the formula-fed infant, causing overfeeding. If formula is overdiluted, the infant will not receive adequate nutrients. Another potential problem with formulas is an allergic reaction in the newborn. The infant's small intestine is permeable to macromolecules such as those found in cow's milk–based formulas. A formula's foreign protein can cause an allergic reaction, with such signs as vomiting, colic, diarrhea, colitis, reluctance to feed, and eczema (see Table 27–1).

Clinicians recommend that parents who bottle-feed use iron-fortified formulas or supplements to avoid iron-deficiency anemia (AAP Committee on Nutrition, 1999). The RDA for iron is 6 mg/day from birth to 6 months. However, too much iron in the form of iron-fortified cereal may interfere with the infant's natural ability to defend against disease. Parents also need to be informed about the con-

TABLE 27-1   Comparison of Breastfeeding and Formula Feeding

Breastfeeding	Iron-Enriched Formula Feeding
Nutrition	
Breast milk is species specific (i.e., perfect balance of proteins, carbohydrates, fats, vitamins, and minerals for human infants).	Formula is as close to human milk as possible, but nutrients are not as efficiently utilized.
Breast milk contains higher levels of lactose, cystine, and cholesterol, which are necessary for brain and nerve growth.	Nutritional adequacy depends on proper preparation (overdilution results in decreased nutrients delivered to infant).
Proteins are easily digested and fats are well absorbed.	Some babies cannot tolerate the fats or carbohydrates found in regular formula. Companies offer alternative formulas.
Composition varies according to gestational age and stage of lactation, thereby meeting the changing nutritional requirements of individual infants as they grow.	
Infants determine the volume of milk consumed.	Pediatrician or caregiver determines the volume consumed. Overfeeding may occur if caregiver is determined that baby empty bottle.
Frequency of feeding is determined by infant cues.	Feeding is determined by infant's cues.
Anti-infective and Antiallergic Properties	
Breast milk contains immunoglobulins, enzymes, and leukocytes that protect against pathogens.	Formula is linked to an increased number of GI and respiratory infections.
Bacteriostatic properties permit storage at room temperature up to 6 hours, in refrigerator for 24 hours, and freezing for 6 months.	Potential for bacterial contamination exists during preparation and storage.
Breast milk decreases the incidence of allergy by eliminating exposure to potential antigens (cow and soy protein).	Some babies are allergic to cow or soy protein. Formula companies are offering alternative formulas suitable for babies who develop allergies.
Psychosocial Aspects	
Skin-to-skin contact enhances closeness.	Formula feeding provides an opportunity for positive parent-infant interaction.
Hormones of lactation promote maternal feelings and sense of well-being.	
The value system of an industrial society can create barriers to successful breastfeeding: Mother may feel ashamed or embarrassed. Breastfeeding after return to work may be difficult.	
Father is not able to breastfeed, but he can feed expressed breast milk from a bottle and nurture the infant in ways other than feeding.	Father can feed the baby.
Cost	
Healthy diet for mother.	Formula is an expense.
Optional, but recommended, items include nursing pads, nursing bras.	Bottles or disposable nursers with plastic liners, nipples, and nipple caps must be purchased.
A breast pump may be needed.	
Refrigeration is necessary for storing expressed milk.	
Convenience	
The milk is always the perfect temperature.	A refrigeration system is necessary if mixing formula for more than one feeding at a time or using large containers or ready-to-feed formula.
No preparation time is needed.	Varying amounts of time are involved in formula preparation.
The mother must be available to feed or provide expressed milk to be given in her absence.	Anyone can feed the baby.
If she misses a feeding, the mother must express milk to maintain lactation.	
The mother may experience slight discomfort in the early days of lactation.	
Maternal medication may interrupt breastfeeding.	

stipation that sometimes results from iron-enriched formula and about various methods of alleviating it.

The AAP and ACOG (1997) recommended that infants be given breast milk or iron-fortified formula rather than whole milk until 1 year of age. Neither unmodified cow's milk (i.e., whole milk) nor skim milk is an acceptable alternative for infant feeding. The level of protein in unmodified cow's milk is much higher (50% to 75% greater) than in human milk, is poorly digested, and may cause bleeding of the gastrointestinal tract. It is also has higher levels of calcium, phosphorus, sodium, and potassium, which increase renal solute load and result in greater obligatory water loss. Skim milk lacks adequate calories, fat content, and essential fatty acids necessary for proper development of the infant's neurologic system. Nutritionists advise against giving cow's milk with decreased fat content (2% milk) or skim milk to children under 2 years of age.

NEWBORN FEEDING

Initial Feeding

The physiologic and behavioral cues of the newborn determine the time of the first feeding. The nurse should assess for active bowel sounds, absence of abdominal distention, and a lusty cry that quiets and is replaced with rooting and sucking behaviors when a stimulus is placed near the lips. These signs indicate that the newborn is hungry and physically ready to tolerate the feeding. The first feeding provides an opportunity for the nurse to assess the effectiveness of the newborn's suck, swallow, and gag reflexes. Encourage the mother who plans to breastfeed to nurse her newborn immediately after birth and allow the baby to nurse to satiety. Because colostrum is not irritating if aspirated (which may occur because of the newborn's initial uncoordinated sucking and swallowing abilities) and is readily absorbed by the respiratory system, breastfeeding can usually begin immediately after birth. Contraindications to immediate nursing include heavy sedation of the mother and physical compromise of either mother or baby. Offer bottle-feeding newborns formula as soon as they show an interest.

Early breastfeeding benefits both mother and newborn because oxytocin helps expel the placenta and prevent excessive maternal blood loss, lactation is accelerated, and the infant receives the immunologic protection of colostrum. For both breastfed and formula-fed infants, early feeding stimulates peristalsis, helping to eliminate the by-products of bilirubin conjugation (which decreases the risk of jaundice), and enhances maternal-infant attachment.

Throughout the first 2 hours after birth, especially during the first 20 to 30 minutes, the infant is usually alert and ready to nurse. However, newborn suckling patterns vary, and although many babies are eager to suckle at this time, some simply lick or nuzzle the nipple. This behavior is beneficial because the licking stimulates the release of oxytocin, which aids uterine involution and lactation (letdown). Assure the mother that this is a positive breastfeeding interaction (Riordan & Auerbach, 1999). Within minutes after birth the newborn shows early odor-based recognition of the mother's breasts. Maternal breast odors elicit preferential head orientation, which helps guide the newborn to the nipple (Porter & Winberg, 1999).

Assessment of the newborn's physiologic status is of primary and ongoing concern to the nurse throughout the first feeding. Extreme fatigue coupled with rapid respiration, circumoral cyanosis, and diaphoresis of the head and face may indicate cardiovascular complications and should be assessed further. The initial feeding also requires assessment of the infant for the rare congenital anomalies such as tracheoesophageal fistula and esophageal atresia (see Chapter 28). ⊂⊃ Findings associated with esophageal anomalies include maternal polyhydramnios and increased oral mucus in the infant. In cases of esophageal atresia, the newborn takes the feeding well initially, but, as the esophageal pouch fills, the feeding is quickly regurgitated unchanged. If a fistula is present, the infant gags, chokes, regurgitates mucus, and may become cyanotic as fluid passes through the fistula and into the lungs.

It is not unusual for the newborn to regurgitate some mucus and water following a feeding, even if it was taken without difficulty. Consequently, observe the newborn closely and position the baby on the right side after a feeding to aid drainage and facilitate gastric emptying.

Establishing a Feeding Pattern

An "on-demand" feeding program facilitates each baby's own rhythm and helps a new mother establish lactation. The newborn rapidly digests breast milk and may want to nurse 8 to 10 times in a 24-hour period. After the initial period of alertness and eagerness to suckle, the infant progresses to light sleep, then deep sleep, followed by increased wakefulness and interest in nursing. As wakefulness and interest in nursing increase, the infant will often cluster 5 to 10 feeding episodes over 2 to 3 hours, followed by a 4- to 5-hour deep sleep. After this cluster of minifeeds and deep sleep, the infant will feed frequently but at more regular intervals. Maternal medications received during labor may affect newborn feeding behavior by delaying early cluster feedings. Delays in the normal feeding patterns depend on the specific drug and its half-life. ⊂⊃ CD WEB

Some newborns whose mothers received epidural analgesia have been noted to be irritable and demonstrate reduced motor organization, poor self-quieting skills, and decreased visual skills and alertness (Riordan & Auerbach, 1999).

Couplet care permits the mother to learn about and respond to her infant's early feeding cues. Early cues that indicate a newborn is interested in feeding include hand-to-mouth or hand-passing-mouth motion, whimpering, sucking, and rooting (Mulford, 1992). Satiety behaviors can include withdrawal of head from nipple, falling asleep, relaxation of hands, and relief of body tension. When couplet care is not available, a supportive nursing staff and flexible nursery policies allow the mother to feed her infant on cue. It is very frustrating to a new mother to attempt to feed a newborn who is sound asleep because he or she is either not hungry or exhausted from crying. Parents can identify their baby's hunger cues that may include crying (a late sign of hunger), hand fisting, and body tenseness.

Although people often accept crying as normal and healthy behavior for newborns, it may actually delay the transition to extrauterine life. Crying involves a Valsalva maneuver that increases pulmonary vascular pressure, which may cause unoxygenated blood to be shunted into systemic circulation through the foramen ovale and ductus arteriosus. Therefore, it may be advantageous for the baby to be in the room with the mother; she will respond to the baby's needs more quickly than the nursery staff may be able to, resulting in less infant crying.

Formula-fed newborns may awaken for feedings every 2 to 5 hours but are frequently satisfied with feedings every 3 to 4 hours. Because formula is digested more slowly, the bottle-fed infant may go longer between feedings but should not go longer than 4 hours. Babies may begin skipping the night feeding about 8 to 12 weeks after birth (Riordan & Auerbach, 1999). The need for a night feeding is individual and depends on the size and development of the infant.

Both breastfed and bottle-fed infants experience growth spurts at certain times and require increased feeding. The breastfeeding mother may meet these increased demands by nursing more frequently to increase her milk supply. It takes about 24 hours for the milk supply to increase adequately to meet the new demand (Lawrence & Lawrence, 1999). A slight increase in feedings meets the formula-fed infant's needs.

NURSING CARE IN THE COMMUNITY

Nourishing her newborn is a major concern of the new mother. Her feelings of success or failure may influence her self-concept as she assumes her maternal role. With proper instruction, support, and encouragement from professionals, feeding becomes a source of pleasure and satisfaction to both the parents and infant.

Promotion of Successful Infant Feeding

Parents may see feeding their baby as the center of their relationship with this new family member. Whether the mother has chosen to formula-feed or breastfeed, the nurse can be instrumental in the mother's success while in the birthing unit and during the early days at home. Feeding and caring for newborns may be routine tasks for the nurse, but the mother's success or failure during the first few times may determine whether she sees herself as an adequate mother. The newborn's response to caring is an expression of personality but often has great significance for parents. A parent may interpret the newborn's behavior as rejection, which may alter the progress of parent-child relationships. A parent may also interpret the sleepy infant's refusal to suck or inability to retain formula as evidence of parental incompetence. The breastfeeding mother may deduce that the newborn does not like her if he or she fails to take her nipple readily. Conversely, infants pick up messages from the muscular tension of those holding them.

A nurse who is sensitive to the needs of the mother can form a relationship with her that permits teaching about techniques and emotions connected with the feeding. Breastfeeding women frequently express disappointment in the help birthing unit nurses give them; they say they would like more encouragement, support, and practical information about feeding their newborn, especially with early discharge. Nonnursing mothers express similar concerns. Consistency in teaching by nurses is essential. A new mother becomes very frustrated if she is shown a number of different methods of feeding her newborn. With the technologic advances in formula production and the availability of knowledge about breastfeeding techniques, the mother should be confident that the choice she makes will promote normal growth and development of her newborn.

The mother usually decides to breastfeed or formula feed by the sixth month of pregnancy and often even before conception. However, she may not make her final decision until admission to the birth center. The decision is often influenced by relatives, especially the baby's father and maternal grandmother (Susin, Giugliani, Kummer, et al., 1999), by friends, and by social customs rather than being based on knowledge about the nutritional and psychologic needs of the mother and her newborn.

The goals of Healthy People 2010 continue to be 75% of infants breastfeeding in the early postpartal period and 50% taking in at least some human milk until age 6 months (Davis, Okuboye, & Ferguson, 2000). It is the health care provider's responsibility to provide the parents with accurate information about the distinct advantages of breastfeeding to the mother and infant. In times of short stays, the Baby-Friendly Hospital Initiative program promotes breastfeeding by designating hospitals as centers for breastfeeding education (Dodgson, Allard-Hale, Bramscher, et al., 1999). Unfortunately, as of 1998, only 17 hospitals in the United States had implemented the program (Davis, et al., 2000). Parents have a right to hear about the data so they can make their own informed choices. ACOG (2000) supports the following "Ten Hospital Practices to Encourage and Support Breastfeeding":

- Maintain a written breastfeeding policy that is communicated to all health care staff.
- Train all pertinent health care staff in skills needed to implement this policy.
- Inform all pregnant women about the benefits of breastfeeding.
- Offer all mothers the chance to begin breastfeeding within 1 hour of birth.
- Show breastfeeding mothers how to breastfeed and how to maintain lactation even if they are separated from their infants.
- Give breastfeeding infants only breast milk unless medically indicated.
- Facilitate rooming-in; encourage all mothers and infants to remain together during their hospital stay.
- Encourage unrestricted breastfeeding when baby exhibits hunger cues or signals or on the mother's request.
- Encourage exclusive suckling at the breast by avoiding pacifiers or artificial nipples.
- Refer mothers to established breastfeeding and mother's support groups and services, and foster the establishment of those services when they are not available.

The 1994 report of the Healthy Babies National Coalition Expert Work Group recommended that the UNICEF-WHO Baby-Friendly Hospital Initiative be adapted to use in the United States as the United States Breastfeeding Health Initiative, using the adapted 10 steps just listed.

Once the parents have made an informed choice of feeding method, the nurse's primary responsibilities are to support the family's decision and to help the family achieve a positive result. No woman should be made to feel either inadequate or superior because of her choice in feeding. There are advantages and disadvantages to breastfeeding and bottle-feeding, but positive bonds in parent-child relationships can be developed with either method.

Before a feeding, make the mother as comfortable as possible. Preparations may include voiding, washing her hands, and assuming a comfortable position. The woman who has had a cesarean birth needs support so that the infant does not rest on her abdomen for long periods. When breastfeeding, she may be more comfortable lying on her side with a pillow behind her back and one between her legs. Position the newborn next to the woman's breast and place a rolled towel or small pillow behind the infant for support. At first the mother will need assistance in turning from side to side and burping the newborn. She may prefer to breastfeed sitting up with a pillow on her lap and the infant resting on the pillow rather than directly on her abdomen. It may be helpful to place a rolled pillow under the arm supporting the infant's head. The football hold, an alternative position, prevents pressure on the incision while allowing the mother a clear view of the infant's face. See Figure 27–2 ◆ for a variety of breastfeeding positions.

Mothers who have undergone cesarean birth frequently use the sitting position to bottle-feed. If incisional pain makes this position difficult, she may want to assume the side-lying position. The infant can be moved to a semisitting position against a pillow close to the mother. Depending on the newborn's level of hunger, the parents may want to use the time before feeding to get acquainted with their infant. The presence of the nurse during part of this time to answer questions and provide reinforcement of parenting skills will be helpful for the family. For the sleepy baby, a period of playful activity—such as gently rubbing the feet and hands or adjusting clothing and loosening coverings to expose the infant to room air—may increase alertness so that, when the feeding is initiated, the infant is ready and sucks eagerly. If an infant is overly hungry and upset, talking quietly and rocking gently may help the baby calm down so that he or she can find and grasp the nipple effectively. After the feeding, when the infant is satisfied and asleep, parents may explore their newborn's unique characteristics. Routines must be flexible enough to allow this time for the family. Couplet care offers spontaneous, frequent encounters for the family and provides opportunities to practice handling skills, thereby increasing confidence in care after discharge. It also encourages feeding in response to the baby's cues rather than feeding by a fixed schedule. However, understand and support the mother's choice to have her newborn cared for in the nursery so she can rest. This rest time is especially important if she must care for herself, the newborn, and other children without adult help at home.

Nursing Practice

As you help new mothers with breastfeeding, it is important to create a relaxed environment and approach to breastfeeding. Encourage the mom to get into a comfortable position, well supported with pillows. Remind her to bring the baby to her breast rather than leaning forward to the baby.

Cultural Considerations in Infant Feeding

It is important to understand how culture and society influence infant feeding. Motherhood itself changes the woman's lifestyle. Perceptions of the mother's role and of breastfeeding as a biologic act also influence the mother's comfort with breastfeeding. Some mothers identify shame, modesty, and embarrassment as reasons they chose not to breastfeed. The amount of body contact considered acceptable also influences parental behaviors. North American and European societies sometimes consider it indecent to expose the breast, believe that too much handling spoils children, and regard weaning as a sign of infant development (Lawrence & Lawrence, 1999).

Also understand the impact of culture on the idiosyncrasies of specific feeding practices. How soon women want to begin breastfeeding after birth is culturally determined. For example, in many cultures (Mexican-American, Navajo, Filipino, and Vietnamese) and in some countries (Guinea, Pakistan) colostrum is not offered to the newborn (Geissler, 1998; Riordan & Auerbach, 1999). Breastfeeding begins only after the milk flow is established. In many Asian cultures, the newborn is given boiled water until the mother's milk flows. The newborn is fed on demand, and cries are responded to immediately. If the crying continues, evil spirits may be blamed and a priest's blessing may be sought. Although many of the Hmong women of Laos combine breastfeeding with some bottle-feeding, they usually find expressing their milk or pumping their breasts unacceptable. Suggest other methods of providing relief if breast engorgement develops. Most Muslim mothers breastfeed because the Qur'an (Koran) encourages it until the child is 2 years old (Hutchinson & Baqi-Aziz, 1994). Japanese women are returning to breastfeeding as the method of feeding for the baby's first year (Riordan & Auerbach, 1999).

The African American culture tends to emphasize plentiful feeding. Solid foods are introduced early and may even be added to the infant's formula. African American

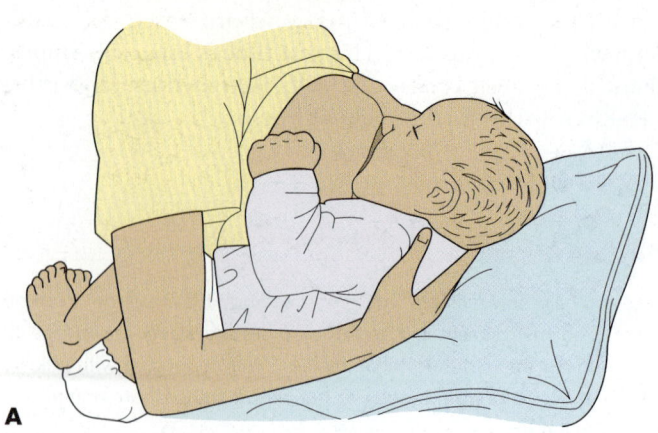

A

- Hold the baby's back and shoulders in the palm of your hand.
- Tuck the baby up under the arm, keeping the baby's ear, shoulder and hip in a straight line.
- Support the breast to touch baby's lips., Once the baby's mouth is open wide, pull the baby quickly to you.
- Hold your breast until the baby nurses easily.

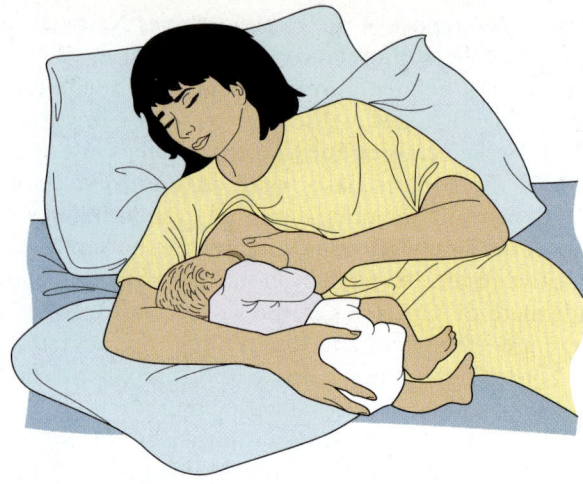

B

- Lie on your side with a pillow at your vack and lay the baby so you are facing each other.
- To start, prop yourself up; on your elbow and support your breast with that hand.
- Pull the baby close to you, lining up the baby's mouth with your nipple.
- Hold you breast with the opposite hand. Once the baby is nursing well, lie back down.

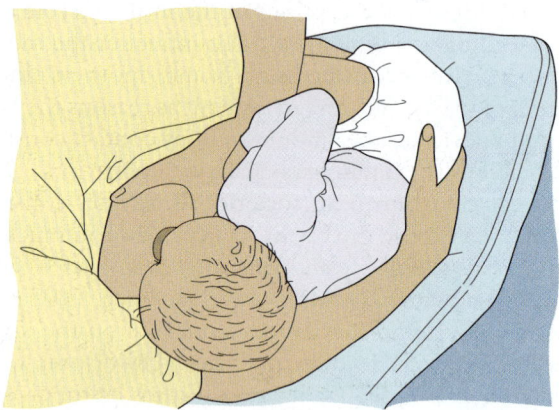

C

- Cradle the baby in the arm closest to the breast, with the baby's head in the crook of the arm.
- Have the baby's body facing you, tummy-to-tummy.
- Use your opposite hand to support the breast.

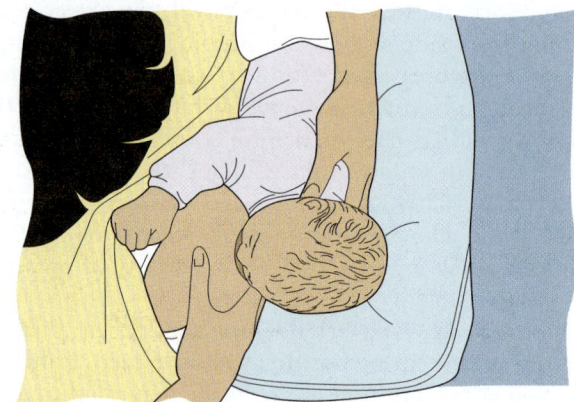

D

- Lay your baby on pillows across your lap.
- Turn the baby to face you.
- Reach across your lap to support the baby's back and shoulders with the palm of your hand.
- Support your breast from underneath. Once the baby's mouth is open wide, pull your baby quickly onto your breast.

FIGURE 27–2. ◆ Four common breastfeeding positions. **A,** Football hold. **B,** Lying down. **C,** Cradling. **D,** Across the lap.
Note: From *Breastfeeding: A special relationship.* Breastfeeding Education Resources, 1-800-869-7892, Raleigh, NC. Copyright Lactation Consultants of NC.

mothers view frequent feeding as an expression of hardiness and a positive behavioral characteristic for their children for the future (Vezeau, 1991). For the traditional Mexican, a fat baby is considered healthy and infants are fed on demand. "Spoiling" is encouraged.

These are but a few of the cultural practices related to feeding. When faced with an infant care practice different from the ones to which they are accustomed, nurses need to evaluate the effect of the practice. Different practices are not necessarily inferior. Intervene only if the practice is actually harmful to the mother and baby.

Physiology of the Breasts and Lactation

The female breast is divided into 15 to 24 lobes separated from one another by fat and connective tissue. These lobes are subdivided into lobules, composed of small units called alveoli, where milk is synthesized by the alveolar secretory epithelium. The lobules have a system of lactiferous ductiles that join larger ducts and eventually open onto the nipple surface. During pregnancy, increased levels of estrogen stimulate breast development in preparation for lactation. Birth results in a rapid drop in estrogen and progesterone with a concomitant increase in the secretion of **prolactin.** This hormone promotes milk production by stimulating the alveolar cells of the breast. Prolactin levels rise in response to the infant suckling. The newborn's suckling also stimulates the release of oxytocin from the posterior pituitary. This hormone increases the contractility of the myoepithelial cells lining the walls of the mammary ducts, and a flow of milk results. This is called the **letdown reflex,** or milk ejection reflex. Mothers have described the letdown reflex as a prickling or tingling sensation during which they feel the milk coming down. Other signs of letdown include increased uterine cramps and increased lochia (during the early postpartum period), milk leaking from the other breast, and a feeling of relaxation. It is not unusual for the breasts to leak some milk before feeding.

The letdown reflex can be stimulated by the newborn's sucking, presence, or cry, or even by maternal thoughts about her baby. It may also occur during sexual orgasm because oxytocin is released. Conversely, the mother's lack of self-confidence, fear of embarrassment, or pain connected with breastfeeding may prevent the milk from being ejected into the duct system. Milk production decreases with repeated inhibition of the milk ejection reflex. Failure to empty the breasts frequently and completely also decreases production. As milk accumulates and is not withdrawn, the buildup of pressure in the alveoli suppresses secretion. Once lactation is established, prolactin production decreases. Oxytocin and sucking continue to facilitate milk production.

Client Education for Breastfeeding Self-Care

The nurse caring for the breastfeeding mother should help the woman achieve independence and success in her feeding efforts (Figure 27–3 ◆). Prepared with a knowledge of the anatomy and physiology of the breast and lactation, the components and positive effects of breast milk, and techniques of breastfeeding, the nurse can help the woman and her family use their own resources to achieve a successful experience.

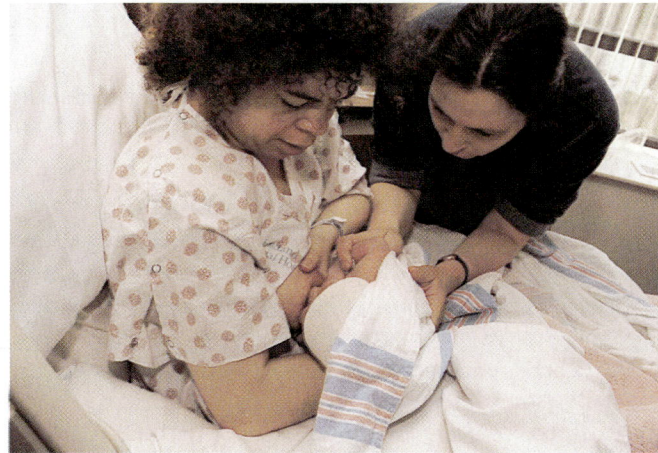

FIGURE 27–3. ◆ For many mothers, the nurse's support and knowledge are instrumental in establishing successful breastfeeding.

BREASTFEEDING PROCESS

The objectives involved in breastfeeding are (1) to provide adequate nutrition, (2) to facilitate maternal-infant attachment, and (3) to prevent trauma to the nipples. Direct information and support toward these goals. When assisting the mother with breastfeeding, use disposable gloves because breast milk and newborn saliva are body substances

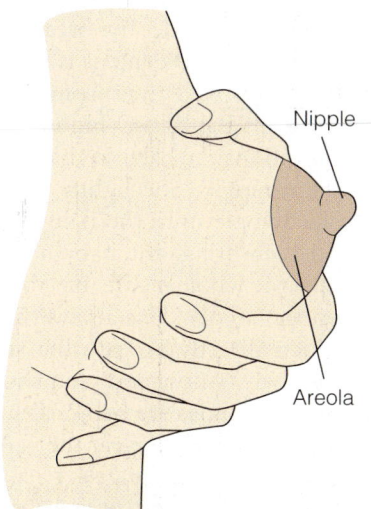

Nipple

Areola

A

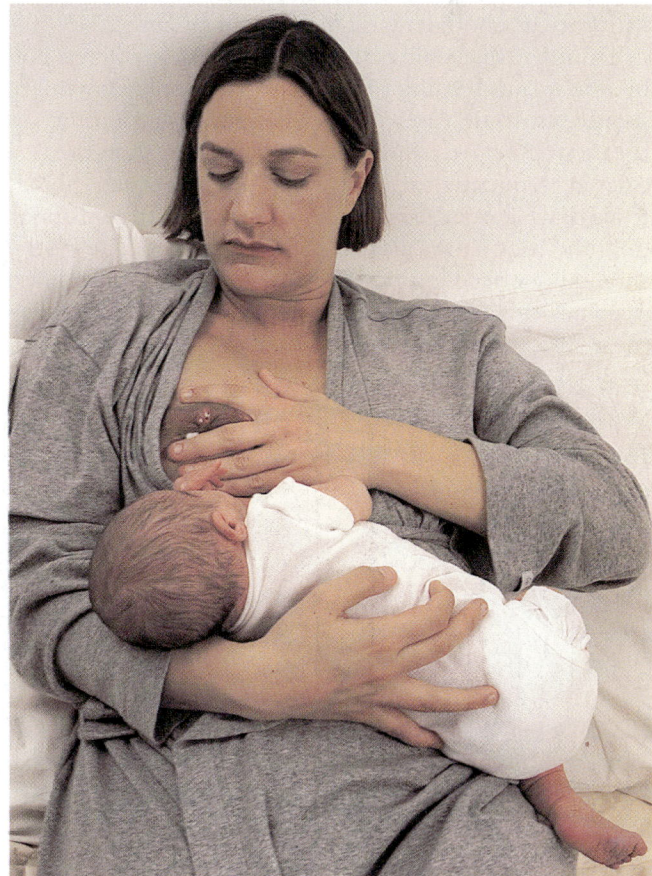

B

FIGURE 27–4. ◆ **A,** C-hold. **B,** Scissors hold.
Note: **A** courtesy of The WRS Group, Waco, TX.

that call for standard precautions. To facilitate successful breastfeeding, arrange for privacy, help the mother find a comfortable position, and position the baby comfortably close to the mother. The mother should support her breast with her hand, using the C-hold or the scissors hold. In the C-hold the mother places her thumb well above the areola and the rest of her fingers below the areola and under the breast. The mother may also use the scissors hold, placing her index finger above the areola and her other three fingers below the areola and under the breast. Either method of presenting the breast to the infant is acceptable as long as the mother's hand is well away from the nipple so the baby can "latch on" to the breast (Figure 27–4 ◆).

The mother positions the baby so that her or his nose is at the level of the nipple. She lightly tickles the baby's lower lip with her nipple until the baby opens her or his mouth wide and then brings the baby to the breast. The baby needs to take the whole nipple into the mouth so that the gums are on the areola. This allows the jaws to compress the milk ducts directly beneath the areola when the baby suckles. The baby's nose and chin should touch the breast. If the breast occludes the baby's airway, simply lifting up on the breast will usually clear the nares. The baby's lips should be relaxed and flanged outward, with the tongue over the lower gum. At this point the baby should be facing the mother (tummy to tummy or chest to chest), with the ear, shoulder, and hip aligned (Figure 27–5 ◆).

During early feedings the infant should be offered both breasts at each feeding to stimulate the supply-demand response. In some cases the newborn will suckle only one breast well before falling asleep. As long as each breast is offered frequently (at least every 2 hours), single-breast feeds of whatever duration the baby wishes are appropriate until the baby shows a desire for both breasts. The mother should breastfeed until she becomes relaxed to the point of sleepiness—a delightful side effect of oxytocin secretion—

or until she notes cues from the infant suggesting satiety (suckling activity ceases or the baby falls asleep). The length of the feedings is up to the mother; she need not watch a clock. Literature suggests that imposing time limits for breastfeeding does not prevent nipple soreness and in fact interferes with successful feeding. For example, the length of nursing time necessary to stimulate the milk ejection reflex varies with the individual. If the mother feeds according to the clock and disengages the baby before letdown, the baby will not get the hindmilk. Because the

Teaching About

BREASTFEEDING

Following is information that is helpful to nursing mothers:

Basics of Milk Production

Milk produced according to demand

Milk stored in sinuses under areola

Adequate maternal fluid intake required

Milk supply established by frequent nursing (every 1½ to 3 hours)

Letdown reflex: flow of milk initiated by newborn's sucking, presence, or cry; by mother's thoughts; or during maternal orgasm

Positioning Baby at the Breast

Turn baby's entire body toward mother with mouth adjacent to nipple and the ear; shoulder and hip are in direct alignment

Mother should assume a comfortable position with arms supported

Direct nipple straight into baby's mouth so that during sucking, jaw compresses ducts directly beneath areola

Lightly brush infant's mouth with breast to stimulate rooting reflex (but avoid touching both cheeks)

Procedure for Feeding

Avoid arbitrary time limits (since letdown reflex may take up to 3 minutes)

Allow baby to nurse at first breast until breast is emptied

Insert finger in baby's mouth near nipple to break suction

Burp baby before changing breast

Burp baby again at end of feeding

To prevent skin breakdown, wash nipple with warm water and dry thoroughly

Helpful Hints

Be certain baby is well awake before attempting feeding

Alternate breast at which baby begins feeding (use safety pin as reminder)

Lift breast slightly or press lightly on breast above nose if mother's breast occludes infant's nares

Rotate baby's position at breast to avoid undue trauma to nipples and improve emptying of ducts

Avoid supplementary formula feedings until lactation is established

Check with caregiver before taking any medication while breastfeeding (because medications may cross into breast milk)

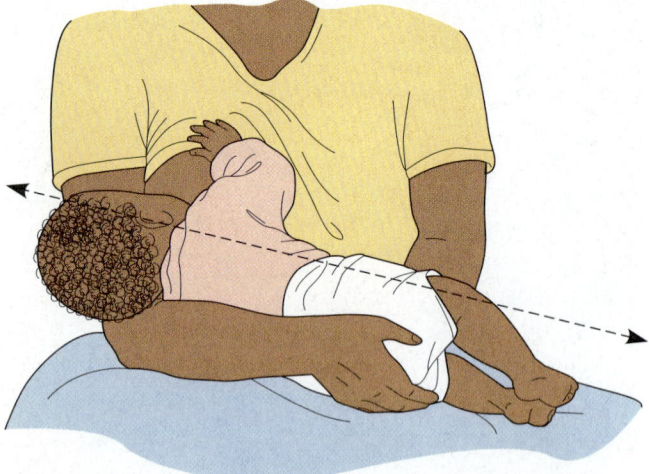

FIGURE 27–5. ◆ Infant in good breastfeeding position: tummy-to-tummy, with ear, shoulder, and hip aligned. *Note:* from Riordan, J., & Auerbach, K. (1993). *Breastfeeding and lactation* (p. 248). Sudbury, MA: Jones & Bartlett Publishers. Adapted.

hindmilk is higher in fat and calories than the foremilk, the baby will be less satisfied, will need to nurse again sooner, and will gain less weight. The mother should learn to feed in response to her baby's cues and her body, not an arbitrary time schedule. If the mother wishes to end the feeding before the infant falls asleep or detaches himself or herself, she should break the suction by gently inserting her fingers between the baby's gums. Burping between feedings on each breast and at the end of the feeding continues to be necessary. If the infant has been crying, it is also advisable to burp before beginning feeding.

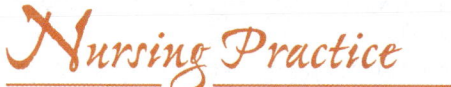

Nursing Practice

To encourage a sleepy baby to breastfeed, unwrap the baby and provide for lots of skin-to-skin contact between the mother and baby; have the mother rest with the baby near her breast so the baby can feel and smell the breast. Encourage the mother to watch for feeding cues, such as hand-to-mouth activity, fluttering eyelids, vocalization but not necessarily crying, and mouthing activities.

BREASTFEEDING ASSESSMENT

During the birthing unit stay, carefully monitor the progress of the breastfeeding mother and child. A system-

atic assessment of several breastfeeding episodes gives a chance to teach the new mother about lactation and the breastfeeding process, provide anticipatory guidance, and evaluate the need for follow-up care after discharge. Criteria for evaluating a breastfeeding session include maternal and infant cues, latch-on, position, letdown, nipple condition, infant response, and maternal response. The literature provides various tools to guide the assessment and documentation of the breastfeeding efforts. The LATCH scoring table is one example (Figure 27–6 ◆).

LEAKING

Initially more milk is produced than the infant requires. During the first few weeks, infant needs and maternal responses are not yet well attuned, daily variabilities of feeding frequency and duration are greatest, and most women experience breast leaking. Stimuli that result in letdown or leaking breast milk include hearing a baby cry and even thinking about the baby. Forewarn the mother about this possibility and recommend that she place breast pads in her bra to absorb the secretions. Caution the woman to remove wet pads frequently to prevent irritation to the nipples and infection. (Breast pads with plastic liners interfere with air circulation; the plastic should be removed before using them.) Once breastfeeding is well established—usually after the first month—the mother may also be taught to apply direct pressure to the breast with her hand or forearm when leaking occurs.

	0	1	2
L Latch	Too sleepy or reluctant No latch achieved	Repeated attempts Hold nipple in mouth Stimulate to suck	Grasps breast Tongue down Lips flanged Rhythmic sucking
A Audible swallowing	None	A few with stimulation	Spontaneous and intermittent <24 hours old Spontaneous and frequent >24 hours old
T Type of nipple	Inverted	Flat	Everted (after stimulation)
C Comfort (breast/nipple)	Engorged Cracked, bleeding, large blisters or bruises Severe discomfort	Filling Reddened/small blisters or bruises Mild/moderate discomfort	Soft Nontender
H Hold (positioning)	Full assist (staff holds infant at breast)	Minimal assist (i.e., elevate head of bed, place pillows for support) Teach one side; mother does other Staff holds and then mother takes over	No assist from staff Mother able to position and hold infant

FIGURE 27–6. ◆ LATCH: a breastfeeding charting and documentation tool. LATCH was created to provide a systematic method for breastfeeding assessment and charting. It can be used to assist the mother in establishing breastfeeding and define areas of needed intervention. *Note:* From Jensen , D., Wallace, S., & Kelsay, P. (1994). LATCH: A breastfeeding charting system and documentation tool. *Journal of Obstetric, Gynecologic, and Neonatal Nursing, 23*(1), 29, 24(1), 13 & 1994, 1995. Association of Women's Health, Obstetric, and Neonatal Nurses. All rights reserved.

If the baby is pulling the tongue back, humping the tongue, or thrusting the tongue, you can use digital suck training to bring the tongue down and forward. Place a finger in the baby's mouth, pad side up. When the baby starts sucking well, turn your finger so that the pad is down. If the baby is sucking correctly, the tongue will come forward and cup the finger, and the baby will continue to suckle. Performing this technique before feedings encourages the baby to use the tongue correctly.

SUPPLEMENTARY BOTTLE-FEEDING

Supplementary bottle-feedings for the breastfeeding infant may weaken or confuse the sucking reflex or decrease the infant's interest in nursing. The newborn has to open her or his mouth wider to grasp the mother's nipple than to grasp a bottle nipple. The shape of the mouth and lips and the sucking mechanism are also different for sucking the breast and the bottle nipple. While suckling at the breast, the infant's tongue moves front to back, squeezing the milk from the nipple. While sucking on a rubber nipple, the tongue pushes forward against the nipple to control the milk flow. Some breastfeeding babies who are given supplementary bottles cannot adjust to these different techniques and push the mother's nipple out of their mouth in subsequent breastfeeding attempts. This can be frustrating for both mother and baby. Breastfeeding mothers should avoid introducing bottles until breastfeeding is well established. Parents are often concerned because they have no visual assurance about the amount of breast milk consumed. Teach the mother the signs of milk transfer to the infant (i.e., audible swallowing, milk appearing in the baby's mouth, her breast feeling soft after feeding, milk leaking from the opposite breast) (Mulford, 1992). In addition, if the infant gains weight and has six or more wet diapers per day without supplementary feedings of water or formula, he or she is receiving adequate amounts of milk. Parents should know that because breast milk is more easily digested than formula, the breastfed infant becomes hungry sooner. Thus the frequency of breastfeeding is greater than that of bottle-feeding. The parents may also expect the infant to demand more frequent nursing during growth spurts, such as ages 10 days to 2 weeks, 5 to 6 weeks, and 2.5 to 3 months.

EXPRESSION OF MILK

If the mother who wants to breastfeed is unable to nurse for medical or workplace reasons, she needs information about other means of stimulating milk production and storing the breast milk. The choice of method (manual or with breast pump) may depend on the mother's physiologic capabilities to produce the desired amount of milk and her personal

Babies are probably getting enough milk if

▶ They are nursing at least eight times in 24 hours.
▶ In a quiet room, their mothers can hear them swallow while nursing.
▶ Their mothers' breasts appear to soften after nursing.
▶ The number of wet diapers increases by the fourth or fifth day after birth, or there are at least six to eight wet diapers every 24 hours after day 5.
▶ The baby's stools are yellow or are beginning to lighten in color by the fourth or fifth day after birth.
▶ Offering a supplemental bottle is not a reliable indicator; most babies will take a few ounces even if they are getting enough breast milk.

preference. During the early postpartum period, if the baby cannot nurse at the breast (as in the case of some preterm or sick infants), the mother needs frequent breast stimulation to establish and increase her milk supply to prepare for later breastfeeding. She should use an electric breast pump at least eight times in each 24-hour period (Riordan & Auerbach, 1999). Research has shown that a pulsatile electric pump and double setup (allowing both breasts to be stimulated simultaneously) results in higher prolactin levels and a greater volume of milk than does manual expression (Lauwers & Shinskie, 2000). After lactation is established, the mother may express the breast milk by the method that she finds most effective and convenient.

To express her milk manually, the woman washes her hands, then massages her breast to stimulate letdown. To massage her breast, the woman grasps the breast with both hands at the base of the breast near the chest wall. Using her palms, she firmly slides her hands toward her nipple. She repeats this process several times. Then she is ready to begin hand expression. The woman generally uses her left hand for her right breast and her right hand for her left breast. However, some women prefer to use the hand on the same side as the breast. Encourage the woman to use the method she finds most effective. The woman grasps the areola with her thumb on the top and her first two fingers on the lower portion (Figure 27–7). Without allowing her fingers to slide on her skin, she pushes inward toward the chest and then squeezes her fingers together while pulling forward on the areola. She can use a container to catch any fluid that is squeezed out. She rotates her hand slightly so that she can repeat the process. She continues to reposition her hand and repeat the process to empty all the milk sinuses.

Breast pumps use suction to express milk. Some have collection systems to conveniently store the milk. Hand pumps are portable and inexpensive. Battery-operated

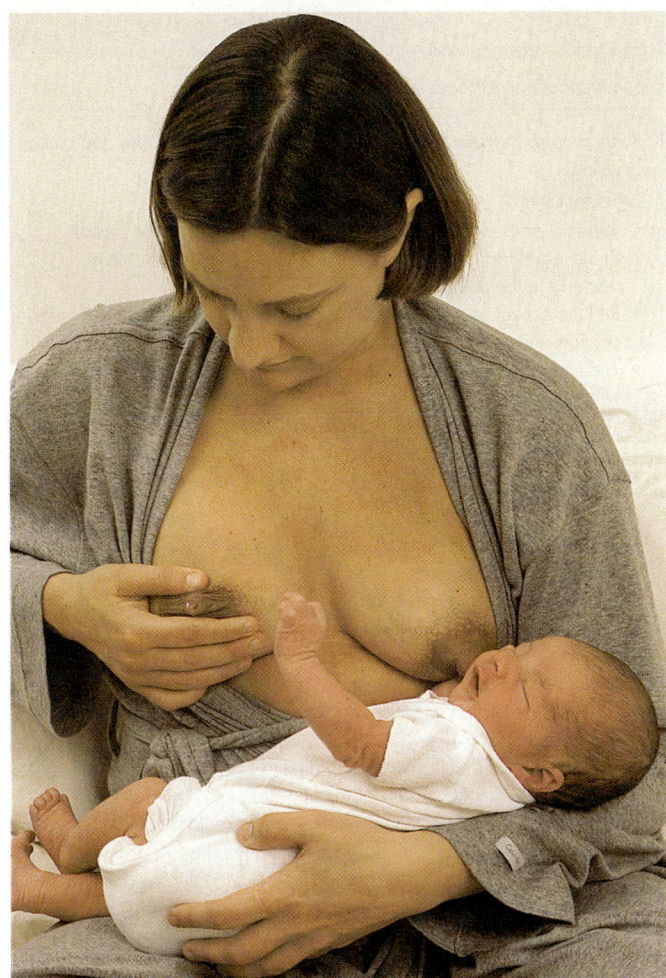

FIGURE 27–7. ◆ Hand position for manual expression of milk.

pumps are more efficient than hand pumps but are also more expensive. Electric pumps are more efficient but are bulky and expensive; however, they can be rented in many areas. Many agencies have a variety of pumps available and provide instruction on correct use (Table 27–2). Videotapes and photographs are also useful in demonstrating the process to new mothers.

STORING BREAST MILK

Breast milk has bacteriostatic qualities because of its IgA and IgG antibodies, which retard bacterial growth. It is recommended that refrigerated milk be used within 2 days. If breast milk is to be refrigerated and then fed to the infant, it should be stored in clean plastic containers; the white blood cells will adhere to glass, and their protective effect will be lost. Breast milk can be frozen in either glass or plastic; freezing destroys the white blood cells anyway. Breast milk can be stored in a freezer compartment inside the refrigerator for up to 2 weeks, in a self-contained freezer unit of a refrigerator for up to 3 to 4 months, and in a separate deep freeze unit at 0 °F or less for up to 6 months. Frozen breast milk can be thawed by initially running cool water over the container, then gradually adding warm water until the milk is thawed. The container should then be gently shaken to return to suspension the fat molecules that separate during freezing. Breast milk should not be defrosted under hot running water or in boiling water. Breast milk should never be microwaved. Uneven heating patterns may alter the composition of the milk and can create hot spots that can burn the baby's mouth.

EXTERNAL SUPPORTS

Nurses, dietitians, childbirth educators, certified nurse-midwives, lactation consultants, mother-to-mother support groups, and physicians must collaborate to provide consistent, timely information and support and to attend to the new mother's special needs. Breastfeeding mothers who work outside the home and are supported in their decision tend to breastfeed their infants for longer periods.

La Leche League International is an organized group of volunteers who provide education about breastfeeding and assistance to women who are breastfeeding infants. Through its small, neighborhood-based groups, it sponsors activities, provides printed materials, rents electric breast pumps, offers one-to-one counseling to mothers with questions or problems, and provides group support to breastfeeding mothers. Lactation consultants offer a variety of services through private practice and health care facilities.

Numerous books, pamphlets, and educational videos are also available to help the breastfeeding mother. The mother needs the support of all family members, her physician or certified nurse-midwife, pediatrician or certified nurse practitioner, and all nursing personnel, because often the attitudes of these people ultimately lead the woman to success or failure.

DRUGS AND BREASTFEEDING

It has long been recognized that certain medications taken by the mother may affect her infant. It should be noted that (1) most drugs pass into breast milk, (2) almost all medications appear in only small amounts in human milk (usually less than 1% of the maternal dosage), and (3) very few drugs are contraindicated for breastfeeding women.

The properties of a drug influence its passage into breast milk, as does the amount of the drug taken, the frequency and route of administration, and the timing of the dose in relationship to infant feeding. The drug's effects are influenced by the infant's age, the feeding frequency, the volume of milk taken, and the degree of absorption through the gastrointestinal tract. Four adjustments should be made when administering drugs to a nursing mother to decrease the effects on the infant (Auerbach, 1999):

1. Long-acting forms of drugs should be avoided. The infant may have difficulty metabolizing and excreting them, and accumulation may be a problem.

2. Absorption rates and peak blood levels should be considered in scheduling the administration of the drugs.

TABLE 27–2 Recommendations for the Nursing Mother Who Uses a Pump

General Pumping Recommendations	Recommendations for Specific Types of Pumps
1. Read the instructions on the use and cleaning of a pump before expressing milk. 2. Wash hands before each pumping session. 3. Frequency: For occasional pumping, pump during, after, or between feedings, whichever gives the best results. Most mothers tend to express more milk in the morning. Working mothers should use the pump on a regular basis for the number of nursings that are missed. For premature or ill babies who are not at breast, the number of pumpings should total eight or more in 24 hours. Initiation of pumping should be delayed no longer than 6 hours following birth unless medically indicated. This ensures appropriate development and sensitivity of prolactin receptors. More frequent pumping avoids the buildup of excessive back pressure of milk during engorgement. 4. Duration: With single-sided pumping, optimal duration is 10 to 15 minutes with an electric pump and 10 to 20 minutes with a manual pump. If double pumping with an electric or two battery-operated pumps, 8 to 10 minutes is optimal. Encourage mothers to tailor these times to their own situation. 5. Technique: • Elicit the milk ejection reflex before using any pump. • Use only as much suction as is needed to maintain milk flow. • Massage the breast in quadrants during pumping to increase intramammary pressure. • Allow enough time for pumping to avoid anxiety. • Use inserts or different flanges if needed to obtain the best fit between pump and breast. • Avoid long periods of uninterrupted vacuum. • Stop pumping when the milk flow is minimal or has ceased.	1. Avoid pumps that use rubber bulbs to generate vacuum; they can cause bruising. 2. Cylinder pumps: • When 0-rings are used, they must be in place for proper suction. • Remove gaskets after each use for cleaning to avoid harboring bacteria in the pump. • Roll the gasket on the inner cylinder back and forth to restore it to its original shape. • The pump stroke may need to be shortened as the outer cylinder fills with milk. • The user may need to empty the outer cylinder once or twice during pumping. • Hand position should be palm up with the elbow held close to the body. 3. Battery-operated pumps: • Use alkaline batteries. • Replace batteries when cycles per minute decrease. • Interrupt vacuum frequently to avoid nipple pain and damage. • Use an AC adapter when possible, especially if the pump generates fewer than six cycles per minute. • Consider renting an electric pump for pumping that will continue for longer than 1 or 2 months. • Use two pumps simultaneously if pumping time is limited or to increase the quantity of milk obtained. • Choose a pump in which the vacuum can be regulated. • Massage the breast by quadrants during pumping. 4. Semiautomatic pumps: • Vacuum may be easier to control if the mother does not lift her finger completely off the hole but rolls it back and forth rhythmically so that the vacuum is efficient but not painful. 5. Automatic electric pumps: • Use the lowest pressure setting that is efficient. • Use a double setup (simultaneous pumping) when time is limited to increase the milk supply and for prematurity, maternal or infant illness, or other special situations.

Note: From Riordan, J., & Auerbach, K. (1999). *Breastfeeding and human lactation* (2nd ed., p. 283). Sudbury, MA: Jones & Bartlett Publishers. Reprinted with permission.

Less of the drug crosses into the milk if the medication is given immediately after the woman has nursed her baby.

3. The infant should be closely observed for any signs of drug reaction, including rash, fussiness, lethargy, or changes in sleeping or feeding patterns.

4. Whenever alternatives are available, the drug that shows the least tendency to pass into breast milk should be selected.

The mother should be informed about the potential of most drugs to cross into breast milk. She should also be advised to tell any physician who prescribes medications for her that she is breastfeeding. CD WEB

In counseling the nursing mother, the health care provider needs to weigh the benefits of the medication against the possible risk to the infant and its possible effect on breastfeeding. The potential risk to the infant must also be weighed against the effect of interrupting breastfeeding.

POTENTIAL PROBLEMS IN BREASTFEEDING

Because mothers are discharged from the birthing unit before breastfeeding is well established, they are frequently alone when they encounter changes in the breastfeeding process. Many women stop nursing if the situations they encounter seem problematic. Offer anticipatory guidance regarding common breastfeeding phenomena and give the woman resources to use after discharge. (See Chapter 30 for a detailed discussion of self-care measures the nurse can suggest to a woman with a breastfeeding problem after discharge from the birthing unit.)

Complementary Care

HERBS, HOMEOPATHY, AND ESSENTIAL OILS FOR BREASTFEEDING

Herbs: Herbs thought to increase milk supply include alfalfa, dandelion, fennel, horsetail, red raspberry, caraway, and anise. The mother may drink caraway tea to reduce colic in the breastfeeding infant. Caraway tea also may be given directly to infants to treat colic (Skidmore-Roth, 2001). Chaste tree (also known as vitex) may also be helpful in cases of insufficient lactation (Blumenthal, 2000). The following herbs may decrease milk supply, so they should be avoided until a woman is no longer breastfeeding: black walnut, sage, parsley, and yarrow (Balch & Balch, 2001; Gladstar, 1993). Black cohosh, blessed thistle, cascara sagrada, horseradish, garlic, cinnamon bark, kava kava, and senna are also contraindicated during lactation (Blumenthal, 2000).

Homeopathy: Pulsatilla, a homeopathic remedy, is used to improve a deficient flow of milk or dry up the milk if the mother is weaning the child.

Essential Oils: Cracked nipples often respond to calendula cream or ointment, found in health food stores. The nursing mother should wash her nipples off very well before feeding her child. Oil of peppermint, as a cold compress, may relieve breast engorgement or assist in the process of weaning. Place four to five drops of peppermint oil in ice cold water. Although essential oils feel like water, chemically they are oils and as such do not mix with the water. Dip a piece of clean fabric into the water so that the cloth picks up the essential oil on the surface. Wring out the fabric and place it on the breasts. Again, the breast should be washed completely before feeding. Women who are allergic to ragweed may find they are also allergic to calendula.

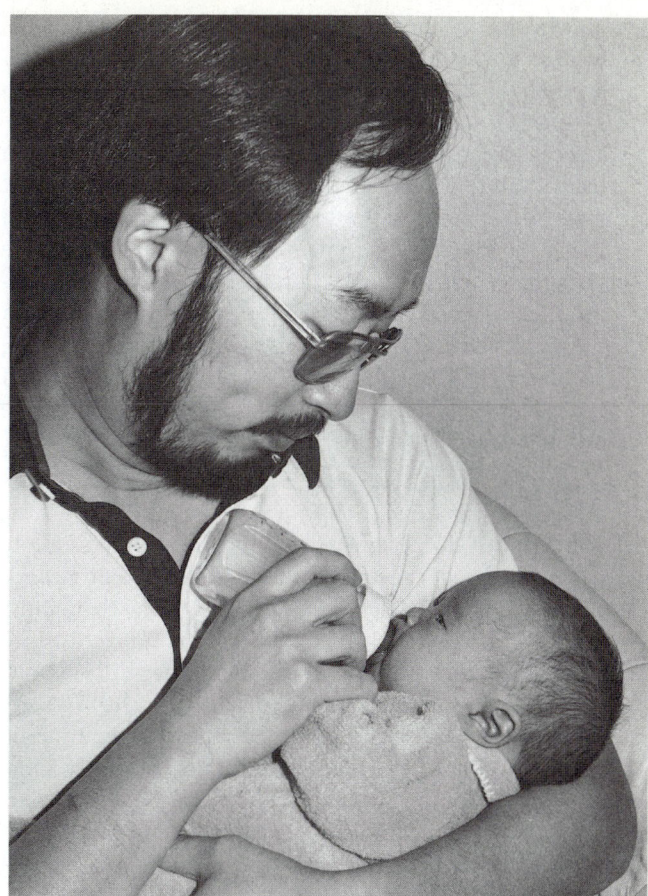

FIGURE 27–8. ◆ An infant is supported comfortably during bottle-feeding.

Client Education for Formula Feeding

With the great emphasis placed on successful breastfeeding, the teaching needs of the formula-feeding new mother may be overlooked. Encourage the mother who has chosen to bottle-feed her infant to assume a comfortable position with adequate arm support so that she can easily hold her infant. Most women cradle their infants in the crook of the arm close to the body, which provides the intimacy and cuddling so essential to an infant and offers the same benefits of closeness as breastfeeding. If the mother has had only limited experience in feeding infants, she may need some guidelines to feed her newborn successfully. The following information helps parents facilitate adequate nutrition and foster attachment:

1. Always hold bottles; never prop them. Positional otitis media may develop if the infant is fed horizontally, because milk and nasal mucus may block the eustachian tube. Holding the infant provides social and close physical contact for the baby and an opportunity for parent-child interaction and bonding (Figure 27–8 ◆).

2. The nipple should have a hole big enough to allow milk to flow in drops when the bottle is inverted. Too large an opening may cause overfeeding or regurgita-

tion because of rapid feeding. If feeding is too fast, change the nipple and help the infant eat more slowly by stopping the feeding frequently for burping and cuddling.

3. Point the nipple directly into the mouth, not toward the palate or tongue, and place it on top of the tongue. The nipple should be full of liquid at all times to prevent ingestion of extra air, which decreases the amount of feeding and increases discomfort. Nipples vary in shape, amount of energy needed to obtain the formula, and rate of formula flow.

4. Burp the infant at intervals, preferably at the middle and end of the feeding. An infant who seems to swallow a great deal of air while sucking may need more frequent burping. If the infant has cried before being fed, he or she may have swallowed air; in such cases, burp the infant before beginning to feed or after taking just enough to calm down. Burp the infant by holding him or her upright on the shoulder or in a sitting position on the lap with the infant's chin and chest supported on one hand. Then gently pat or stroke the infant's back with the other hand. Too-frequent burping may confuse a newborn attempting to coordinate sucking, swallowing, and breathing simultaneously.

5. Newborns frequently regurgitate small amounts of feedings. The amount may look large to the inexperienced parent, but it is normal. Initially it may be due to excessive mucus and gastric irritation from foreign substances such as aspirated blood in the stomach from birth. Later, regurgitation may result when the infant feeds too rapidly and swallows air. It may also happen when the infant is overfed and the cardiac sphincter allows the excess to be regurgitated. Because this is common, experienced mothers and nurses generally keep a burp cloth available. Although regurgitation is normal, vomiting or a forceful expulsion of fluid is not. When forceful expulsion occurs, further evaluation may be indicated, especially if other symptoms are present.

6. A fat baby is not necessarily a healthy one. Avoid overfeeding or feeding infants every time they cry. Encourage but do not force the infant to feed and allow the infant to set the pace once feedings are established. Parents sometimes set artificial goals—"the baby must take all 5 oz"—and keep feeding the child until those goals are met, even though the infant may not be hungry. Overfeeding results in infant obesity. During early feedings, however, the infant may need simple tactile stimulation—such as gently rubbing feet and hands, adjusting clothing, and loosening coverings—to maintain adequate sucking long enough to complete a full feeding. The desirable amount and frequency of formula feeding vary with the infant's postnatal age. From birth to 2 months of age, the baby takes six to eight feedings of approximately 2 to 4 oz of formula at each feeding within a 24-hour period.

The forms of formula are ready-to-feed, liquid concentrate, and powdered (Table 27–3). See Chapter 31 for discussion of the advantages and disadvantages of formula preparation and Teaching About Newborn Bottle-feeding.

The nurse is responsible for discussing formula preparation and sterilization techniques with families. Cleanliness is essential, but sterilization is necessary only if the water

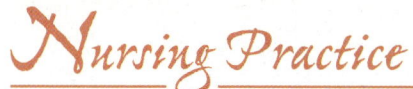

When you help a mother bottle-feed her baby for the first time, you can help her avoid many potential frustrations. The first is often "flying arms" as the baby waves his or her arms in the air. The second is the "chin plunge," as the baby's head falls forward in the mother's tentative hold. To avoid the latter, help the mother with positioning. A third frustration may arise when she tries to correctly place the nipple in the mouth. To ensure correct placement, put your index finger on the baby's chin and gently pull downward while quickly sliding the nipple in over the tongue.

source is questionable. Bottles may be effectively prepared in the dishwasher or washed thoroughly in warm, soapy water and rinsed well. The temperature of dishwashers may weaken nipples, so they should be washed thoroughly by hand and rinsed well. Tap water, if from an uncontaminated source, may be used to mix powdered formulas, which are less expensive than the concentrated or ready-to-use formulas. Honey should not be used as a sugar source because of the danger of infant botulism.

Bottles may be prepared individually, or up to one day's supply of formula may be prepared at one time. Extra bottles can be stored in the refrigerator and warmed slightly before feeding. Ready-to-use disposable bottles of formula are convenient but expensive. Formula left in bottles after a feeding should be discarded. The Special Supplemental Food Program for Women, Infants, and Children (WIC) provides 8 lb of powdered formula or 403 oz of concentrated liquid formula per month. Individual states make provisions about when WIC nutritionists may distribute soy formulas and whether prescriptions are needed for special or therapeutic formulas.

Nutritional assessment of the infant includes nutritional history from the parents, weight gain, growth chart percentiles, and physical examination. See Chapter 31 for more in-depth discussion of infant nutrition.

TABLE 27–3 Formula Preparation		
Ready to Feed	Formula Concentrate	Powdered Formula
(20 kcal/oz; available in 32-oz cans or 4-oz bottles)	(available in 13-oz cans)	(52 scoops per can) Mix one unpacked level scoop of powdered formula with each 60 mL (2 oz) of warm water.
Use within 30 minutes to 1 hour once opened.	Mix equal amounts of concentrate and water from uncontaminated source. This provides a 20 kcal/30 mL (1 oz) dilution.	Always pour water into bottle first; then add powder and stir well.
Do not dilute. Use directly from can, no mixing required.	For example, for a 4-oz feeding mix 2 oz of formula concentrate with 2 oz water.	Make sure the powder and water are well mixed to ensure the formula composition is 20 kcal/30 mL (1 oz).
Just add clean nipple to bottle.	Wash punch-type can opener and top of formula can before opening.	After opening, keep can tightly covered and use contents within 1 month to ensure freshness.
Most expensive type of formula preparation.	Prepare a single feeding by measuring water and liquid directly into nursing bottle.	Least expensive type.
	Cover opened concentrate formula cans with foil or plastic wrap and refrigerate until next bottle is made up.	

Teaching About

NEWBORN BOTTLE-FEEDING

Following is information that is helpful for bottle-feeding families:

Types of Formula

Ready-to-feed: use directly from the can.

Concentrate: dilute with water before feeding.

Powder: add water and mix well for proper concentration.

Amount of Formula

Start with 3 oz in each bottle (since a newborn usually takes 1 to 3 oz every 2 1/2 to 4 hours).

Expect increases in baby's appetite with demand feeding (as baby needs more he or she will start finishing each bottle).

Don't feed the baby a partially used bottle after 1 hour at room temperature.

Don't feed the baby a partially used bottle after 4 hours in refrigerator.

Prepare a fresh bottle for each feeding; don't add new formula to old.

Refrigerate bottles made in advance.

Don't feed the baby an opened, refrigerated can of concentrated or ready-to-feed formula after 48 hours.

Temperature of Formula

Mother or family member can try a bottle directly from the refrigerator, but most babies prefer warm formula, close in temperature to breast milk.

Warm bottle under hot tap water, in bottle warmer, or in pan of heated water.

Always test temperature of formula by sprinkling a few drops on wrist.

BE VERY CAREFUL if using a microwave oven to warm formula, as milk is superheated and plastic bottle bags may burst; use "defrost" setting on microwave oven and carefully check temperature of formula before feeding.

Positioning the Baby for Feeding

Hold baby close, establishing eye contact as in breastfeeding.

Hold baby's bottom or foot firmly, keeping his or her back straight to aid digestion and provide a sense of security.

Quiet baby before feeding.

Alternate the side baby is fed from to give baby two-sided stimulation.

Avoid feeding while baby is on his or her back.

Don't prop the bottle.

Procedure for Feeding

Nipple hole should allow only drops of milk to flow.

Keep nipple full with milk to decrease air ingestion.

How to Burp a Baby

Position baby so his or her head rests on mother's shoulder or face down on lap, or sit baby on lap with baby's chin and chest supported.

Gently pat or stroke baby's back.

Burp baby halfway through feeding and at end of feeding.

Learn baby's preferred burping position and whether baby is a slow or quick burper.

Regurgitation of small amounts of formula is common.

Have "burp cloth" available.

CHAPTER HIGHLIGHTS

🙠 The RDA for calories for the newborn is 105 to 108 kcal/kg/day (50 to 55 kcal/lb/day).

🙠 The nurse must monitor the first feeding because this is when the newborn may initially show signs of cardiac complications or anomalies of the upper gastrointestinal tract.

🙠 Breast milk has immunologic and nutritional properties that make it the optimal food for the first year of life.

🙠 Signs indicating newborn readiness for the first feeding are active bowel sounds, absence of abdominal distention, and a lusty cry that quiets with rooting and sucking behaviors when a stimulus is placed near the lips.

🙠 Mature breast milk and commercially prepared formulas (unless otherwise noted) provide 20 kcal/oz.

🙠 Breastfed infants need supplements of iron after 6 months of age.

🙠 Nurses must recognize that cultural values influence infant feeding practices, be sensitive to ethnic backgrounds of minority populations, and understand that the dominant culture in any society defines "normal" maternal-infant feeding interactions.

🙠 Breastfed infants are getting adequate nutrition if they are gaining weight and have at least six wet diapers a day when they are not receiving additional water supplements.

🙠 Breastfeeding mothers should be encouraged to ensure that the infant is correctly positioned at the breast, with a large portion of the areola in the infant's mouth. The mother is advised to rotate positions to ensure that all ducts are emptied.

🙠 Most maternal medications are transmitted through breast milk. The effects on the infant and lactation depend on a variety of factors, including route of administration, timing of the dose with respect to feeding time, and multiple properties of the medication.

🙠 Formula-fed infants regain their birth weight by 10 days of age and gain 1 oz/day for the first 6 months and 0.5 oz/day for the second 6 months; birth weight is doubled at 3.5 to 4 months of age.

Healthy breastfed babies gain approximately 0.5 oz/day in the first 6 months of life, regain their birth weight by about 14 days of age, and double their birth weight at approximately 5 months of age.

🙾 Formula-fed infants need no vitamin or mineral supplements other than iron, if it is not already in the formula, and fluoride, if it is not obtained in the water system.

🙾 The bottle-feeding mother may need help feeding and burping her infant. She will also benefit from information about feeding schedules and types of formula.

🙾 The use of skim milk or cow's milk with lowered fat content is not recommended for children under 2 years of age.

EXPLOREMEDIALINK

NCLEX Review, Case Studies, and other interactive resources for this chapter can be found on the companion website at http://www.prenhall.com/london. Click on "Chapter 27" to select the activities for this chapter.

For animations, more NCLEX review questions, and an audio glossary, access the accompanying CD-ROM in this textbook.

REFERENCES

American Academy of Pediatrics, Committee on Nutrition. (1999). Iron fortification of infant formulas. *Pediatrics, 104*(1), 119–123.

American Academy of Pediatrics, Committee on Nutrition. (2000). Hypoallergenic infant formulas. *Pediatrics, 106*(2), 346–349.

American Academy of Pediatrics & American College of Obstetricians and Gynecologists. (1997). *Guidelines for perinatal care* (4th ed.). Washington, DC: Author.

American College of Obstetricians and Gynecologists. (2000). *Breastfeeding: Maternal and infant aspects* (ACOG Educational Bulletin No. 258). Washington, DC: Author.

Auerbach, K. G. (1999). Breastfeeding and maternal medication use. *Journal of Obstetric, Gynecologic, and Neonatal Nursing, 28*(5), 554–562.

Balch, J. F, & Balch, P. A. (2001). *Prescription for nutritional healing* (3rd ed.). Garden City, NY: Avery Publishing Group.

Blumenthal, M. (2000). *Herbal medicine: Expanded Commission E Monographs.* Austin, TX: American Botanical Council.

Calamaro, C. J. (2000). Infant nutrition in the first year of life: Tradition or science? *Pediatric Nursing, 26*(2), 211–215.

Davis, L. J., Okuboye, S., & Ferguson, S. L. (2000). Healthy People 2010: Examining a decade of maternal and infant health. *AWHONN Lifelines, 4*(3), 26–33.

Dodgson, J. E., Allard-Hale, C. J., Bramscher, A., Brown, F., & Duckett, L. (1999). Adherence to the ten steps of the Baby-Friendly Hospital Initiative in Minnesota hospitals. *Birth, 26*(4), 239–246.

Fontaine, K. L. (2000). *Healing practices: Alternative therapies for nursing.* Upper Saddle River, NJ: Prentice Hall.

Geissler, E. M. (1998). *Pocket guide to cultural assessment* (2nd ed.). St. Louis, MO: Mosby.

Gladstar, R. (1993). *Herbal healing for women.* New York: Simon & Schuster.

Hershoff, A. (2000). *Homeopathic remedies.* Garden City Park, NY: Avery Publishing.

Hutchinson, M. K., & Baqi-Aziz, M. (1994). Nursing care of the childbearing Muslim family. *Journal of Obstetric, Gynecologic, and Neonatal Nursing, 23*(9), 767–771.

Johnson, J. V., & Riddick, D. H. (2000). The breast during pregnancy and lactation. In J. J. Sciarra & T. J. Watkins (Eds.), *Gynecology and obstetrics* (Vol. 5, chap. 31, pp. 1–12). Philadelphia, PA: Lippincott Williams & Wilkins.

Lauwers, J., & Shinskie, D. (2000). *Counseling the nursing mother: A lactation consultant's guide* (3rd ed.). Sudbury, MA: Jones & Bartlett.

Lawrence, R. A., & Lawrence, R. M. (1999). *Breastfeeding: A guide for the medical profession* (5th ed.). St Louis, MO: Mosby.

Mulford, C. (1992). The mother-baby assessment (MBA): An "Apgar score" for breastfeeding. *Journal of Human Lactation, 8*(2), 79–82.

Porter, R. H., & Winberg, J. (1999). Unique salience of maternal breast odors for newborn infants. *Neuroscience and Biochemical Reviews, 23,* 439–449.

Riordan, J., & Auerbach, K. (1999). *Breastfeeding and human lactation* (2nd ed.). Boston: Jones & Bartlett.

Skidmore-Roth, L. (2001). *Mosby's handbook of herbs and natural supplements.* St. Louis, MO: Mosby.

Susin, L. R. O., Giugliani, E. R. J., Kummer, S. C., Maciel, M., Simon, C., & da Silveira, L. C. (1999). Does parental breastfeeding knowledge increase breastfeeding rates? *Birth, 26*(3), 149–156.

Vezeau, T. M. (1991). Investigating "greedy." *American Journal of Maternal Child Nursing, 16*(6), 337–338.

Walker, M., & Creehan, P. (2001). Newborn nutrition. In K. R. Simpson & P. A. Creehan (Eds.), *AWHONN perinatal nursing* (2nd ed., pp. 568–571). Philadelphia, PA: Lippincott Williams & Wilkins.

Weil, A. (2000). *Eating well for optimal health.* New York: Alfred A. Knopf.

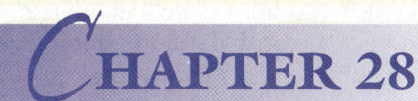
The Newborn at Risk: Conditions Present at Birth

There is an initial flurry of activity when my baby is taken into the NICU. Now my entire universe, everything that I am, constricts down to focus on our little one. She hardly dents this world, a withery face that shows a kind of infinitely pained acceptance, breath and heartbeat almost nothing, and a pose that moves to rest, resisting nothing. I look at my small daughter with eyes naked with amazement and unsure joy.

—JONTELLE, 42

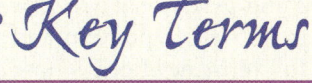
Key Terms

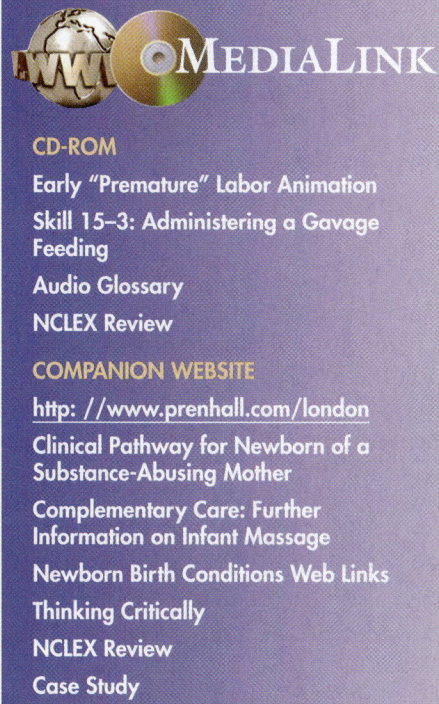

MEDIALINK

CD-ROM

Early "Premature" Labor Animation

Skill 15–3: Administering a Gavage
Feeding

Audio Glossary

NCLEX Review

COMPANION WEBSITE

http://www.prenhall.com/london

Clinical Pathway for Newborn of a
Substance-Abusing Mother

Complementary Care: Further
Information on Infant Massage

Newborn Birth Conditions Web Links

Thinking Critically

NCLEX Review

Case Study

Within the past 30 years, the field of neonatology has expanded greatly. Many levels of nursery care have evolved in response to increasing knowledge about at-risk newborns: special care, intensive care, and convalescent or transitional care. As part of the multidisciplinary health care team, the nurse is a competent professional who provides the holistic care necessary in the often high-tech perinatal environment.

In addition to the availability of a high level of newborn care, various other factors influence the outcome of these at-risk infants, including:

- Birth weight
- Gestational age
- Type and length of newborn illness
- Environmental factors
- Maternal factors
- Maternal-infant separation

IDENTIFICATION OF AT-RISK NEWBORNS

An at-risk newborn is one susceptible to illness (morbidity) or even death because of dysmaturity, immaturity, physical disorders, or complications of birth. In most cases, the pregnancy has involved one or more predictable risk factors, such as:

- Low socioeconomic level of the mother and limited access to health care
- Exposure to environmental dangers such as toxic chemicals and illicit drugs
- Preexisting maternal conditions such as heart disease, diabetes, hypertension, and renal disease
- Maternal factors such as age and parity
- Medical conditions related to pregnancy and their associated complications
- Pregnancy complications such as abruptio placentae

Various risk factors and their specific effects on the pregnancy outcome are listed in Table 8–1, in Chapter 8. Knowing these factors and the risks they bring allows the health care team to anticipate the birth of at-risk newborns. The pregnancy can be closely monitored, treatment can be started as necessary, and arrangements can be made for birth to occur at a facility with appropriate resources to care for both mother and baby.

Most at-risk infants can be identified before the onset of labor, so prenatal assessment and care are crucial. However, because the course of labor and birth and the infant's ability to withstand the stress of labor cannot be predicted, the nurse's use of electronic fetal heart monitoring or fetal heart rate auscultation by Doppler plays a significant role in de-

tecting stress or distress in the fetus. Immediately after birth the Apgar score helps identify the at-risk newborn, but it is not the only indicator of possible long-term outcome.

The newborn classification and neonatal mortality risk chart is another useful tool for identifying newborns at risk. Before this classification tool was developed, birth weight of less than 2500 g was the sole criterion for determining immaturity. Clinicians then recognized that a newborn could weigh more than 2500 g and still be immature. Conversely, an infant weighing less than 2500 g might be functionally at term or beyond. Thus, birth weight and gestational age together are now the criteria used to assess neonatal maturity and mortality risk.

According to the newborn classification and neonatal mortality risk chart, gestation is divided as follows:

- Preterm: less than 37 (completed) weeks
- Term: 38 to 41 (completed) weeks
- Postterm: greater than 42 weeks

As shown in Figure 28–1 ◆, large-for-gestational-age (LGA) newborns are those above the 90th percentile curve. Appropriate-for-gestational-age (AGA) newborns are those between the 10th percentile and 90th percentile curves. Small-for-gestational-age (SGA) newborns are those below the 10th percentile curve on the Denver intrauterine growth curves. A newborn is assigned to a category depending on birth weight and gestational age. For example, a newborn classified as Pr SGA is preterm and small for gestational age. The full-term newborn whose weight is appropriate for gestational age is classified F AGA. The assigned newborn classification may vary according to the intrauterine growth curve chart used; therefore, the chart used should correlate with the characteristics of the client population. It is also important to remember that intrauterine growth curve charts are influenced by altitude and the ethnicity of the newborn population used to create the chart.

Neonatal mortality risk is the chance of death during the newborn period—that is, the first 28 days of life. The neonatal mortality risk decreases as both gestational age and birth weight increase. Infants who are preterm and SGA have the highest neonatal mortality risk. The previously high mortality rates for LGA newborns have decreased at most perinatal centers because of improved management of diabetes in pregnancy and increased recognition of potential problems of LGA newborns.

Newborn morbidity can be anticipated based on birth weight and gestational age. In Figure 28–2 ◆ the infant's birth weight is located on the vertical axis, and the gestational age in weeks is found along the horizontal axis. The area where the two meet on the graph identifies common problems. This tool helps determine the needs of particular infants for special observation and care. For example, an infant of 2000 g at 40 weeks' gestation should be carefully assessed for evidence of neonatal distress, hypoglycemia, congenital anomalies, congenital infection, and polycythemia.

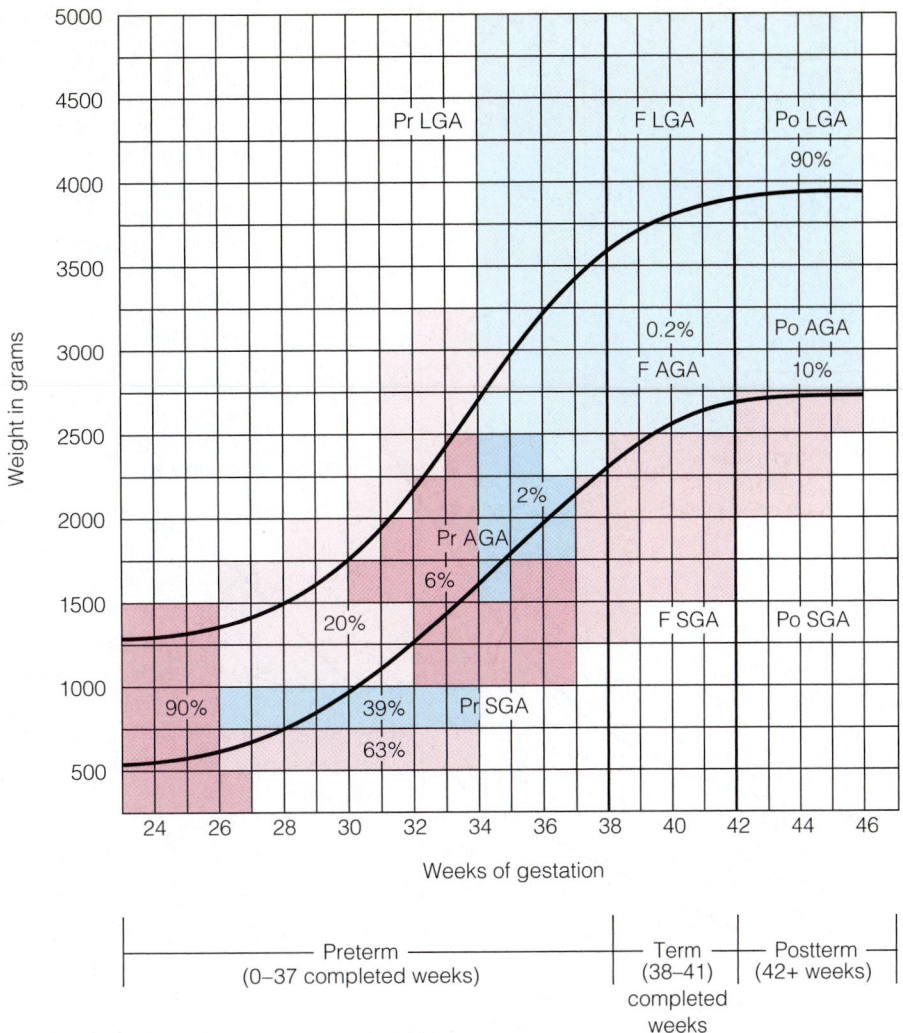

FIGURE 28–1. ◆ Newborn classification and neonatal mortality risk chart. Infants are classified according to weight as small for gestational age (SGA), appropriate for gestational age (AGA), or large for gestational age (LGA) and by weeks of newborn as preterm (Pr), term (F), or postterm (Po). Corresponding neonatal mortality risks are indicated by the percentage in the various colored regions.
Note: From Koops, B. L., Morgan, L. P., & Battaglia, F. C. (1982). Neonatal mortality risk in relationship to birth weight and gestational age. *Journal of Pediatrics, 101*(6), 969.

Identifying the nursing care needs of the at-risk newborn depends on minute-to-minute observations of the changes in the newborn's physiologic status. Direct nursing care toward the following:

- Decreasing physiologically stressful situations
- Constantly observing for subtle signs of change in clinical condition
- Interpreting laboratory data and coordinating interventions
- Conserving the infant's energy for healing and growth
- Providing for developmental stimulation and maintenance of sleep cycle
- Helping the family develop attachment behaviors
- Involving the family in planning and providing care

CARE OF THE NEWBORN WITH IUGR/SGA

Infants are considered **small for gestational age (SGA)** when they are less than two standard deviations or at less than the third percentile (10th for Denver curves because of the lower birth weight at higher altitudes) (Figure 28–3 ◆). When possible, the birth weight charts used to assign the SGA classification to a newborn should be based on the local population into which the newborn is born (Kliegman & Das, 2002). An SGA newborn may be preterm, term, or postterm. An undergrown newborn may also be said to have **intrauterine growth restriction (IUGR),** which describes pregnancy circumstances resulting in limited fetal growth. The terms SGA and IUGR are not necessarily interchangeable.

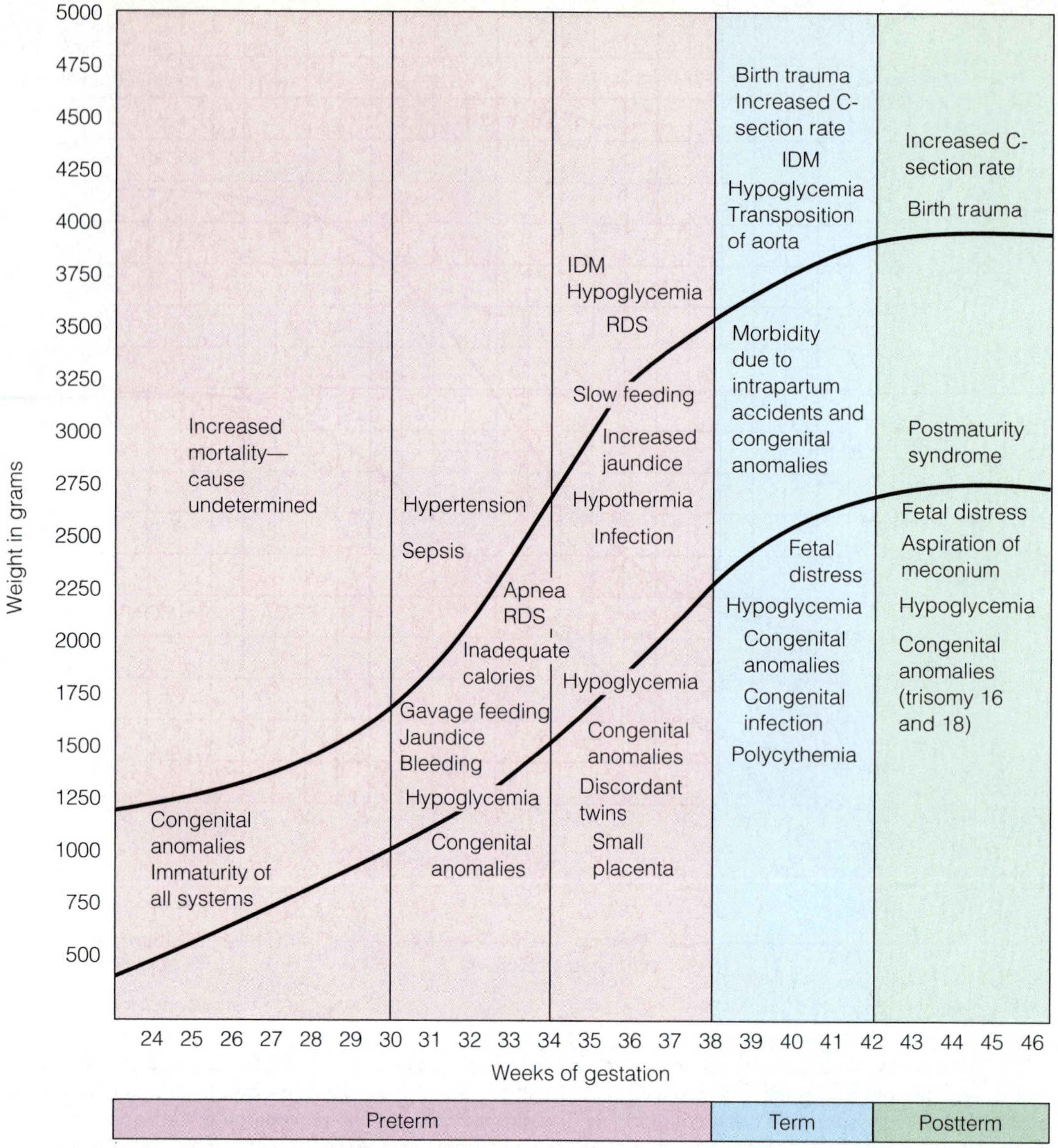

FIGURE 28–2.

Chart: Weight in grams (y-axis, 500 to 5000) vs. Weeks of gestation (x-axis, 24 to 46)

24–30 weeks region:
- Increased mortality—cause undetermined
- Congenital anomalies Immaturity of all systems

30–34 weeks region:
- Hypertension
- Sepsis
- Apnea RDS
- Inadequate calories
- Gavage feeding Jaundice Bleeding
- Hypoglycemia
- Congenital anomalies

34–38 weeks region:
- IDM Hypoglycemia RDS
- Slow feeding
- Increased jaundice
- Hypothermia
- Infection
- Hypoglycemia
- Congenital anomalies
- Discordant twins
- Small placenta

38–42 weeks region:
- Birth trauma Increased C-section rate IDM Hypoglycemia Transposition of aorta
- Morbidity due to intrapartum accidents and congenital anomalies
- Fetal distress
- Hypoglycemia
- Congenital anomalies
- Congenital infection
- Polycythemia

42–46 weeks region:
- Increased C-section rate
- Birth trauma
- Postmaturity syndrome
- Fetal distress
- Aspiration of meconium
- Hypoglycemia
- Congenital anomalies (trisomy 16 and 18)

Bottom bar: Preterm | Term | Postterm

FIGURE 28–2. ◆ Neonatal morbidity by birth weight and gestational age. *Note:* From Lubchenco, L. O. (1976). The high-risk infant (p. 122). Philadelphia: Saunders.

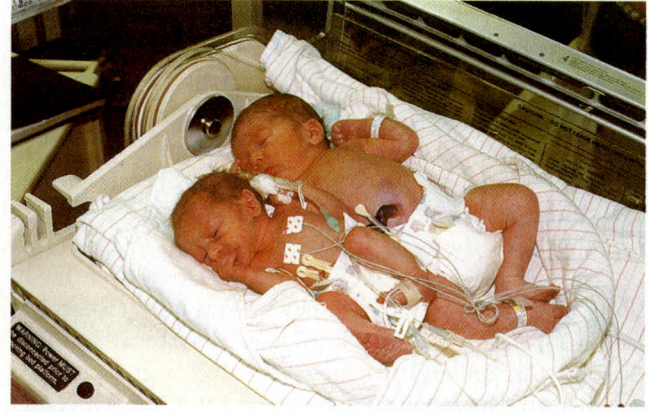

FIGURE 28–3. ◆ Thirty-five-week gestational age twins. Twin B (on left) is SGA and weighs 1260 g and twin A (on right) is AGA and weighs 2605 g. Courtesy of Carol Harrigan, RNC, MSN, NNP.

SGA infants have an increased incidence of perinatal asphyxia and perinatal mortality compared to AGA infants (Cunningham, MacDonald, Gant, et al., 2001). The incidence of polycythemia and hypoglycemia is also higher in this group of infants. See Chapter 44 for a discussion of polycythemia and Chapter 29 for a discussion of hypoglycemia. ⊝⊃

Factors Contributing to IUGR

IUGR may be caused by maternal, placental, or fetal factors and may not be apparent antenatally. In the normal pregnancy, intrauterine growth is linear from approximately 28 to 38 weeks' gestation. After 38 weeks, growth is variable, depending on the growth potential of the fetus and placental function. The most common causes of growth restriction are:

- *Maternal factors.* Primiparity, grand multiparity, multiple-gestation pregnancy (twins, triplets, and so on), smoking, lack of prenatal care, age extremes (< 16 years or > 40 years), and low socioeconomic status (which can result in inadequate health care, inadequate education, and inadequate living conditions) affect IUGR (Cunningham et al., 2001). Before the third trimester, the nutritional supply to the fetus far exceeds its needs. Only in the third trimester does maternal malnutrition limit fetal growth.

- *Maternal disease.* Maternal heart disease, substance abuse (drugs, alcohol, smoking), sickle cell anemia, phenylketonuria (PKU), and asymptomatic pyelonephritis are associated with SGA. Complications associated with pregnancy-induced hypertension (PIH), chronic hypertensive vascular disease, and advanced diabetes mellitus cause diminished blood flow to the uterus.

- *Environmental factors.* High altitude, exposure to x-rays, excessive exercise, work-related exposure to toxins, hyperthermia, and maternal use of teratogenic drugs (such as nicotine, alcohol, antimetabolites, anticonvulsants, narcotics, and cocaine) affect fetal growth (Cunningham et al., 2001).

- *Placental factors.* Placental conditions such as small placenta, infarcted areas, abnormal cord insertions, placenta previa, and thrombosis may affect circulation to the fetus; the circulation becomes more deficient with increasing gestational age.

- *Fetal factors.* Congenital infections (rubella, toxoplasmosis, syphilis, cytomegalic inclusion disease), congenital malformations, discordant twins (see Chapter 5), sex of the fetus (females tend to be smaller), chromosomal syndromes, and inborn errors of metabolism can predispose a fetus to fetal growth disturbances.

Identifying fetuses with IUGR is the first step in detecting common disorders associated with affected newborns. The perinatal history of maternal conditions, early dating of pregnancy by first-trimester ultrasound measurements, antepartal testing (nonstress test, contraction stress test, biophysical profile [see Chapter 14]), Doppler velocimetry, gestational age assessment, and the physical and neurologic assessment of the newborn are also important (Cunningham et al., 2001).

Patterns of IUGR

Intrauterine growth occurs by an increase in both cell number and cell size. If insult occurs early during the critical period of organ development in the fetus, fewer new cells are formed, organs are small, and organ weight is subnormal. In contrast, growth failure that begins later in pregnancy does not affect the total number of cells, only their size. The organs are normal, but their size is diminished. There are two clinical pictures of newborns:

- *Symmetric (proportional) IUGR* is caused by long-term maternal conditions (such as chronic hypertension, severe malnutrition, chronic intrauterine infection, substance abuse, anemia) or fetal genetic abnormalities (Kliegman & Das, 2002). Symmetric IUGR can be noted by ultrasound in the first half of the second trimester. In symmetric IUGR there is chronic, prolonged retardation of growth in the size of organs, weight, length, and, in severe cases, head circumference.

- *Asymmetric (disproportional) IUGR* is associated with an acute compromise of uteroplacental blood flow. Some causes are placental infarcts, PIH, and poor weight gain in pregnancy. The growth restriction may not be evident before the third trimester because, although weight is decreased, length and head circumference remain appropriate for that gestational age. Birth weight is below the 10th percentile, whereas head circumference and/or length may be between the 10th and 90th percentiles. Asymmetric IUGR newborns are particularly at risk for perinatal asphyxia, pulmonary hemorrhage, hypocalcemia, and hypoglycemia in the newborn period.

Despite growth restriction, physiologic maturity develops according to gestational age. Therefore, the SGA newborn may be more physiologically mature than the preterm AGA newborn and less predisposed to complications of prematurity such as respiratory distress syndrome and hyperbilirubinemia. The SGA newborn's chances for survival are better than those of the preterm AGA newborn because of organ maturity, although this newborn still faces many other potential difficulties.

Common Complications of the SGA Newborn

The complications occurring most frequently in the SGA newborn include:

- *Asphyxia.* The SGA newborn suffers chronic hypoxia in utero, which leaves little reserve to withstand the demands of normal labor and birth. Thus, fetal hypoxia and its potential systemic problems can occur. Cesarean birth may be necessary.

- *Aspiration syndrome.* In utero, hypoxia can cause the fetus to gasp during birth, aspirating amniotic fluid into the lower airways. It can also lead to relaxation of the anal sphincter and passage of meconium. This can result in aspiration of the meconium with the first breaths after birth.

- *Temperature instability.* Diminished subcutaneous fat (used for survival in utero), depletion of brown fat in utero, and a large surface area decrease the IUGR newborn's ability to conserve heat. The flexed position assumed by the term SGA newborn diminishes the effect of surface area somewhat.

- *Hypoglycemia.* An increase in metabolic rate in response to heat loss and poor hepatic glycogen stores causes hypoglycemia. In addition, the newborn is compromised by inadequate supplies of enzymes to activate gluconeogenesis (conversion of nonglucogen sources such as fatty acids and proteins to glucose).

- *Polycythemia.* The increased number of red blood cells in the SGA newborn is considered a physiologic response to in utero chronic hypoxic stress.

Newborns with significant IUGR tend to have a poor prognosis, especially when born before 37 weeks' gestation. Factors contributing to poor outcome include:

- *Congenital malformations.* Congenital malformations occur 10 to 20 times more frequently in SGA infants than in AGA infants (Kliegman & Das, 2002). The more severe the IUGR, the greater the chance for malformation as a result of impaired mitotic activity and cellular hypoplasia.

- *Intrauterine infections.* Fetuses exposed to intrauterine infections such as rubella and cytomegalovirus are profoundly affected by the offending virus's direct invasion of the brain and other vital organs, resulting in IUGR.

- *Continued growth difficulties.* SGA newborns tend to be shorter than newborns of the same gestational age. Asymmetric IUGR infants can be expected to catch up in weight and approach their inherited growth potential when given an optimal environment. Symmetric SGA infants reportedly have varied growth potential but tend not to catch up to their peers (Kliegman & Das, 2002).

- *Learning difficulties.* Often, SGA newborns can exhibit subsequent learning disabilities. The disabilities are characterized by hyperactivity, short attention span, and poor fine motor coordination (reading, writing, drawing). Some hearing loss and speech defects also occur.

Clinical Therapy

The goal of clinical therapy is early recognition and implementation of the medical management of potential problems.

Nursing Management

Nursing Assessment and Diagnosis

The nurse assesses gestational age and identifies signs of potential complications associated with SGA infants. All body parts of the symmetric IUGR infant are in proportion, but they are below normal size for the baby's gestational age.

Therefore, the head does not appear overly large or the length excessive in relation to the other body parts. These newborns are generally vigorous. The asymmetric IUGR infant appears long, thin, and emaciated, with loss of subcutaneous fat and muscle mass. The baby may have loose skin folds; dry, desquamating skin; and a thin and often meconium-stained cord. The head appears relatively large (although it approaches normal size) because the chest size and abdominal girth are decreased. The baby may have a vigorous cry and appear alert and wide eyed.

Nursing diagnoses that may apply to the SGA newborn include the following:

- ▶ *Impaired gas exchange* related to aspiration of meconium

- ▶ *Hypothermia* related to decreased subcutaneous fat

- ▶ *Risk for injury to tissues* related to decreased glycogen stores and impaired gluconeogenesis

- ▶ *Risk for altered tissue perfusion* related to increased blood viscosity

Planning and Implementation

HOSPITAL-BASED NURSING CARE

Hypoglycemia, the most common metabolic complication of IUGR, produces such sequelae as CNS abnormalities and mental retardation. Conditions such as asphyxia, hyperviscosity, and cold stress may also affect the baby's outcome. Pay meticulous attention to physiologic parameters for immediate nursing management and reduction of long-term disorders. (See "Clinical Pathway for Small-for-Gestational-Age Newborns," pages 611–612.)

NURSING CARE IN THE COMMUNITY

The long-term needs of the SGA newborn include careful follow-up evaluation of patterns of growth and possible disabilities that may later interfere with learning or motor functioning. Long-term follow-up care is essential for infants with congenital malformations, congenital infections, and obvious sequelae from physiologic problems. In addition, the parents of the IUGR newborn need support, because a positive environment can enhance the baby's growth and the child's ultimate outcome.

Evaluation

Anticipated outcomes of nursing care include the following:

- ▶ The SGA newborn is free from respiratory compromise.

- ▶ The SGA newborn maintains a stable temperature and glucose homeostasis.

- ▶ The SGA newborn gains weight and takes nipple feedings without developing physiologic distress or fatigue.

- ▶ The parents verbalize their concerns about their baby's health problems and understand the rationale behind management of their newborn.

Category	Day of Birth—First 4 Hours	Remaining Day of Birth
Referral	Report from L&D, neonatal nurse practitioner Check ID bands Prn consults: high-risk peds, genetics	Check ID bands q shift As parents desire, obtain circumcision permit after their discussion with MD Lactation consult prn
Assessments	(Refer to "Newborn Clinical Pathway," Chap. 26) • Complete set of VS • Admission wt, length, HC • Assess skin color • Gestational age assessment • Assess for s/s hypoglycemia. Chemstrip ASAP after birth, then follow SGA policy and procedure for blood glucose monitoring • Assess for polycythemia: follow policy for treatment prn	Vital signs: T/P/R q4h and prn, BP prn Newborn assessment q shift (See "Newborn Clinical Pathway," Chap. 26). Continue hypoglycemia assessments, chemstrips per SGA protocol Assess mother-baby interaction
Teaching/psychosocial	(See "Newborn Clinical Pathway," Chap. 26) Admission activities performed at mother's bedside if possible, orient to nursery, handwashing, assess teaching needs Teach parents rationale for SGA protocol	(See "Newborn Clinical Pathway," Chap. 26) Reinforce previous teaching Teach parent/guardian feeding methods, burping, diapering, calming techniques, s/s of stress, elimination norms
Nursing care management and reports	Diagnostic tests: blood type, Rh, Coombs' on cord blood when applicable, chemstrip within 1 h of birth and q1–2h until feedings initiated per protocol Check chemstrip before at least two feedings or until condition stabilizes (chemstrip > 40 mg/dL × 2)	Femoral pulse or BP all four extremities if early DC Hct per policy Hearing screen Cord care per policy Bathe per policy
Activity and comfort	Place under radiant warmer, attach skin probe to maintain NTE Soothe baby as needed with voice, touch, nesting in warmer	Leave in radiant warmer until stable, then swaddle in open crib Incubator if temp instability; adjust incubator for infant size and gestation to maintain NTE
Nutrition	Initiate breast- or bottle-feeding as soon as mother and baby conditions allow Lavage and gavage prn Supplement breast when medically indicated or ordered by MD per policy Feed SGA infants q3–4h Monitor feeding tolerance, suck	Continue feeding schedule: small frequent feedings, high-calorie formula, nutritional fortifiers
Elimination	Note first void and stool if not at birth	Note all voids, amount and color of stools q4h
Medication	AquaMEPHYTON IM, dosage according to infant wt per MD orders, Ilotycin ophth ointment OU	Hep B vaccine as ordered by MD after consent signed by parent
Discharge planning/ home care	Hep B consent reviewed with parents Plan DC with parent/guardian in 1–3 days Evaluate for social services/home care/discharge planning needs	Hep B consent signed by parents Birth certificate instructions/worksheet Car seat for DC
Family involvement	Evaluate psychosocial needs Evaluate parent teaching Access community resources prn, i.e., Teen "Healthy Starts"	Assess parents' knowledge of newborn behavior and reflexes Encourage family involvement in infant's care as possible and as infant tolerates
Date		

ASAP, as soon as possible; C/S birth, cesarean birth; ID, identification; DC, discharge; HC, head circumference; Hct, hematocrit; LD, labor and delivery; NTE, neutral thermal environment; ophth, ophthalmic; OU, both eyes; q, every; SGA, small for gestational age; s/s, signs and symptoms; vag, vaginal; VS, vital signs; wt, weight; WNL, within normal limits.

Category	Day 1	Day 2/3 (if applicable)
Referral	Check ID bands q shift	Check ID bands q shift **Expected Outcomes** Mother/baby ID bands correlate at time of discharge Consults completed prn
Assessments	Assess thermoregulation Assess for potential complications: perinatal asphyxia, aspiration syndrome, hypoglycemia, hypocalcemia, polycythemia Assess mother-baby interaction	Assess color for jaundice Assess for apnea Assess mother-baby interaction **Expected Outcomes** Physical assessments, VS WNL; no complications of SGA noted
Teaching/psychosocial	(See "Newborn Clinical Pathway," Chap. 26) Reinforce previous teaching Parent teaching: bathing, cord care, skin/nail care, use of thermometer, activity, sleep patterns, soothing activities, reflexes, jaundice, growth/feeding patterns	Final discharge teaching (see "Newborn Clinical Pathway," Chap. 26) Review infant safety, s/s of illness, and when to call health care provider with parents **Expected Outcomes** Mother verbalizes comprehension of instructions, demonstrates care capabilities
Nursing care management and reports	Scalp treatment BID Daily wt Newborn assessment q shift Check circumcision site q diaper change Unclamp cord clamp Cord care per policy Total bilirubin level prn	Newborn assessment q shift Daily wt Check circumcision site Cord care per policy Note hearing test results Femoral pulse or BP all four extremities **Expected Outcomes** Physical assessments WNL; cord unclamped and dry without s/s of infection; circ site unremarkable; gaining wt or wt stabilized to not > 10% loss, labs WNL
Activity and comfort	Swaddled in open crib Incubator if temp instability; adjust incubator for infant size and gestation to maintain NTE	**Expected Outcomes** Maintains temp WNL swaddled in open crib
Nutrition	Continue enhanced feeding schedule, gavage prn per MD orders Supplement breast only when medically indicated/policy or ordered by MD/NP Encourage on-demand feeds, minimally q3–4h, breast or bottle	Continue enhanced feeding schedule, gavage prn per MD/NP orders **Expected Outcomes** Infant tolerates feedings, feeds on demand, breastfeeds without supplement, nipples without problems; regaining lost wt or wt stabilized
Elimination	Evaluate all voids and stool color q8h **Expected Outcomes** Voids and stools without difficulty	Note all voids and stool color q shift **Expected Outcomes** Voids qs, stools without difficulty and WNL
Medication	Hep B vaccine before discharge	**Expected Outcomes** Infant has received ophth ointment OU and AquaMEPHYTON injection; received first Hep B vaccine if ordered and parental consent given
Discharge planning/ home care	Newborn photographs Complete birth certificate packet If vag birth, complete DC teaching	If C/S birth, complete DC instructions (see "Newborn Clinical Pathway," Chap. 26) **Expected Outcomes** Infant DC home with mother; mother verbalizes follow-up appointment time/date
Family involvement	Bath, newborn care, and feeding classes Newborn channel as available Assess mother-baby bonding and interaction Incorporate significant others and siblings in care Support positive parenting behaviors Evaluate mother/parent teaching	Assess mother-baby bonding and interaction Identify community referral needs and refer to community agencies **Expected Outcomes** Demonstrates caring and family incorporation of infant
Date		

CARE OF THE LARGE-FOR-GESTATIONAL-AGE (LGA) NEWBORN

A newborn whose birth weight is at or above the 90th percentile on the intrauterine growth curve (at any week of gestation) is considered **large for gestational age (LGA).** Some AGA newborns have been incorrectly categorized as LGA because of miscalculation of the date of conception due to postconceptual bleeding. Careful gestational age assessment is essential to identify the potential needs and problems of such infants.

The most well-known condition associated with excessive fetal growth is maternal diabetes (White's classes A–C; see Table 12–3 in Chapter 12); however, only a minority of large newborns are born to diabetic mothers. The cause of the majority of cases of LGA newborns is unclear, but certain factors or situations have been found to correlate with their birth (Langer, 2000):

- Genetic predisposition is correlated proportionately to the mother's prepregnancy weight and to weight gain during pregnancy. Large parents tend to have large infants.

- Multiparous women have two to three times the number of LGA infants as primigravidas.

- Male infants are typically larger than female infants.

- Infants with erythroblastosis fetalis, Beckwith-Wiedemann syndrome (a genetic condition associated with omphalocele and neonatal hypoglycemia and hyperinsulinemia), or transposition of the great vessels are usually large.

The increase in the LGA infant's body size is characteristically proportional, although head circumference and body length are in the upper limits of intrauterine growth. The exception to this rule is the infant of the diabetic mother, whose body weight increases while length and head circumference may remain in the normal range. Macrosomic infants have poor motor skills and have difficulty in regulating behavioral states. LGA infants tend to be more difficult to arouse to a quiet alert state and may have feeding difficulties.

Common Complications of the LGA Newborn

Disorders of the LGA newborn can include the following:

- *Birth trauma due to cephalopelvic disproportion (CPD).* Often, LGA newborns have a biparietal diameter greater than 10 cm (4 in) or are associated with a maternal fundal height measurement greater than 42 cm (16 in) without hydramnios. Because of their excessive size, there are more breech presentations and shoulder dystocias. These complications may result in asphyxia, fractured clavicles, brachial palsy, facial paralysis, phrenic nerve palsy, depressed skull fractures, hematomas, and bleeding due to birth trauma.

- *Increased incidence of cesarean births due to fetal size.* Mothers and infants have all the risk factors associated with cesarean births (Chatfield, 2001).

- *Hypoglycemia, polycythemia, and hyperviscosity.* These disorders are most often seen in infants with diabetic mothers, erythroblastosis fetalis, and Beckwith-Wiedemann syndrome.

NURSING MANAGEMENT

The perinatal history, in conjunction with ultrasonic measurement of fetal skull and gestational age testing, is important in identifying an at-risk LGA newborn. Direct essential nursing care toward monitoring vital signs, screening for hypoglycemia and polycythemia, and observing for signs and symptoms related to birth trauma. Address parental concerns about the visual signs of birth trauma and the potential for continuation of the overweight pattern. Help parents learn to arouse and console their newborn and facilitate attachment behaviors. Mothers of LGA infants with facial or head bruising may be reluctant to interact with their newborns because they fear hurting their infant. The nursing care for complications associated with LGA newborns is similar to the care needed by the infant of a diabetic mother and will be discussed in the next section.

CARE OF THE INFANT OF A DIABETIC MOTHER (IDM)

Infants of diabetic mothers (IDMs) are considered at risk and require close observation the first few hours to the first few days of life. Mothers with severe diabetes or diabetes of long duration (type 1, or White's classes D–F, associated with vascular complications) may give birth to SGA infants. The typical IDM (type 1 when the diabetes is poorly controlled, or White's classes A–C), however, is LGA. The infant is macrosomic, ruddy in color, and has excessive adipose tissue (Figure 28–4 ◆). The umbilical cord and placenta are large. There is a higher incidence of

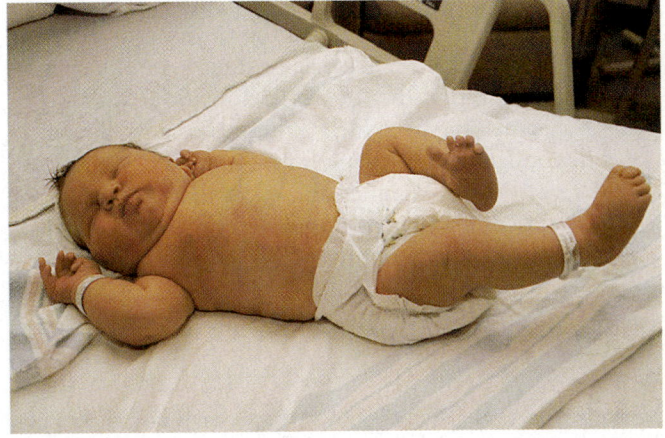

FIGURE 28–4. ◆ Macrosomic infant of diabetic mother. X-ray exam of this infant may reveal caudal regression of the spine.

macrosomic infants born to certain ethnic groups (Native Americans, Mexican Americans, African Americans, Pacific Islanders).

IDMs have decreased total body water, particularly in the extracellular spaces, and are therefore not edematous. Their excessive weight is due to increased weight of the visceral organs, cardiomegaly (hypertrophy), and increased body fat. The only organ not affected is the brain.

The excessive fetal growth of the IDM is caused by exposure to high levels of maternal glucose, which readily crosses the placenta. The fetus responds to these high glucose levels with increased insulin production and hyperplasia of the pancreatic beta cells. The insulin's main action is to help glucose enter muscle and fat cells. Once in the cells, glucose is converted to glycogen and stored. Insulin also inhibits the breakdown of fat to free fatty acids, thereby maintaining lipid synthesis, increasing the uptake of amino acids, and promoting protein synthesis. Insulin is an important regulator of fetal metabolism and has a "growth hormone" effect that increases linear growth. IDMs may be obese as children (Uvena-Celebrezze & Catalano, 2000).

Common Complications of the IDM

Although IDMs are usually large, they are immature in physiologic functions and exhibit many of the problems of the preterm (premature) infant. The complications most often seen in an IDM are:

- *Hypoglycemia.* Even without the high-glucose maternal blood supply, this newborn continues to produce high levels of insulin, which deplete the blood glucose within hours after birth. IDMs also have less ability to release glucagon and catecholamines, which normally stimulate glucagon breakdown and glucose release. The incidence of hypoglycemia in IDMs varies from 30% to 50% (Uvena-Celebrezze & Catalano, 2000), according to the degree of success in controlling the maternal diabetes, the maternal blood sugar level at birth, the length of labor, the class of maternal diabetes, and early versus late feedings of the newborn.

- *Hypocalcemia.* Tremors are the obvious clinical sign of hypocalcemia. They may be due to the IDM's prematurity and to the stresses of difficult pregnancy, labor, and birth, which predispose any infant to hypocalcemia. Diabetic women tend to have decreased serum magnesium levels at term because of increased urinary calcium excretion, which causes secondary hypoparathyroidism in their infants.

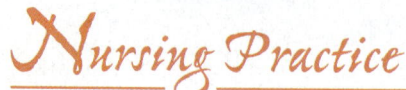

When beginning fluids on an IDM, it is sometimes best to start at a higher concentration of dextrose to avoid hypoglycemia episodes.

- *Hyperbilirubinemia.* This condition may be seen at 48 to 72 hours after birth. It may be caused by slightly decreased extracellular fluid volume, which increases the hematocrit level, and hepatic immaturity. Enclosed hemorrhages resulting from complicated vaginal birth may also cause hyperbilirubinemia. Infants with polycythemia may also have an increased rate of bilirubin production.

- *Birth trauma.* Since most IDMs are LGA, trauma may occur during labor and birth.

- *Polycythemia.* An IDM's decreased extracellular volume may cause this condition. Fetal hyperglycemia and hyperinsulinism result in increased oxygen consumption, leading to fetal hypoxia (Uvena-Celebrezze & Catalano, 2000). Hemoglobin A_{1c} binds oxygen, decreasing the oxygen available to the fetal tissues. This tissue hypoxia stimulates increased erythropoietin production, which increases both the hematocrit level and the potential for hyperbilirubinemia. See Chapter 12 for discussion of hemoglobin A_{1c}.

- *Respiratory distress syndrome (RDS).* This complication occurs especially in newborns of diabetic mothers in White's classes A–C. Insulin antagonizes the cortisol-induced stimulation of lecithin synthesis that is necessary for lung maturation. Therefore, IDMs may have less mature lungs than expected for their gestational age. There is also a decrease in the phospholipid phosphatidylglycerol (PG), which stabilizes surfactant. The insufficiency of PG increases the incidence of RDS. RDS does not appear to be a problem for infants born of diabetic mothers in White's classes D–F; instead, the stresses of poor uterine blood supply may lead to increased production of steroids, which accelerates lung maturation. IDMs may also have a delay in closure of the ductus arteriosus and decreases in postnatal pulmonary artery pressure (Uvena-Celebrezze & Catalano, 2000).

- *Congenital birth defects.* These may include transposition of the great vessels, ventricular septal defect, patent ductus arteriosus, small left colon syndrome, and sacral agenesis (caudal regression) (Uvena-Celebrezze & Catalano, 2000). Early close control of maternal glucose levels before and during pregnancy decreases the risk of birth defects.

Clinical Therapy

Prenatal management is directed toward controlling maternal glucose levels, which minimizes the common complications of IDMs. Because the onset of hypoglycemia occurs between 1 and 3 hours after birth in IDMs (with a spontaneous rise to normal levels by 4 to 6 hours), blood glucose determinations should be done initially on cord blood, hourly during the first 4 hours after birth, and at 4-hour intervals until the risk period (about 24 hours) has passed or per agency protocol.

IDMs whose serum glucose level falls below 40 mg/dL should have early feedings with formula or breast milk (colostrum). A lethargic infant may need to be gavage fed. If oral feedings cannot maintain normal glucose levels or if seizures occur, an intravenous infusion of glucose is necessary. Once the blood glucose level has been stable for 24 hours, the infusion rate can be decreased as oral feedings are increased. The newborn's blood glucose levels must be carefully monitored. Dextrose (25% to 50%) as a rapid infusion is contraindicated because it may lead to severe rebound hypoglycemia after an initial brief increase in glucose level.

Nursing Management

Nursing Assessment and Diagnosis

Do not be lulled into thinking that a big baby is a mature baby. In almost every case, because of the infant's large size, the IDM will appear older than gestational age scoring indicates. Consider both the gestational age and whether the baby is AGA or LGA in planning and providing safe care. In caring for the IDM, assess for signs of respiratory distress, hyperbilirubinemia, birth trauma, and congenital anomalies.

Nursing diagnoses that may apply to IDMs include:

- ▶ *Altered nutrition: less than body requirements* related to increased glucose metabolism secondary to hyperinsulinemia
- ▶ *Impaired gas exchange* related to respiratory distress secondary to impaired production of surfactant
- ▶ *Ineffective family coping: compromise* related to the illness of the baby

Planning and Implementation

Nursing care of the IDM is directed toward early detection and ongoing monitoring of hypoglycemia (with glucose tests) and polycythemia (with central hematocrits), RDS, and hyperbilirubinemia. (These conditions are presented in Chapter 29.) Also assess for signs of birth trauma and congenital anomalies.

Parent teaching is directed toward preventing macrosomia and the resulting fetal-neonatal problems with early and ongoing diabetic control. Advise parents that with early identification and care most IDMs' neonatal problems have no significant sequelae.

Evaluation

Expected outcomes of nursing care include the following:

- ▶ The IDM's respiratory distress and metabolic problems are minimized.
- ▶ The parents understand the effects of maternal diabetes on the baby and the preventive steps they can initiate to decrease its impact on subsequent fetuses.

- ▶ The parents verbalize their concerns about their baby's health problems and understand the rationale behind management of their newborn.

CARE OF THE POSTTERM NEWBORN

The **postterm newborn** is any newborn born after 42 weeks' gestation. The term *postmature* applies only to the infant who is born after 42 completed weeks of gestation **and** who also demonstrates characteristics of the *postmaturity syndrome*.

Postterm, or prolonged, pregnancy occurs in approximately 4% to 14% of all pregnancies (Cunningham et al., 2001). The cause of postterm pregnancy is not completely understood, but there are several associated factors. (See Chapter 19 for discussion of maternal factors.) Many pregnancies classified as prolonged are thought to be a result of inaccurate estimates of date of birth (EDB). Posterm pregnancy is more common in Australian, Greek, and Italian ethnic groups. Most babies born after prolonged pregnancy are of normal size and health; some keep on growing and are over 4000 g at birth, which supports the contention that the postterm fetus can remain well nourished. Potential intrapartal problems for these healthy but large fetuses are CPD and shoulder dystocia. See Chapter 19 for discussion of the necessary assessments and interventions for CPD and shoulder dystocia.

Only about 5% of postterm newborns show signs of postmaturity syndrome. Most of the following discussion addresses the fetus who is not tolerating the prolonged pregnancy, is hypoxic because of compromised uteroplacental blood flow, and is considered to have postmaturity syndrome.

Common Complications of the Newborn with Postmaturity Syndrome

The truly postmature newborn is at high risk for morbidity and has a mortality rate two to three times greater than that of term infants. Although today the percentages are extremely low, most postmature fetal deaths occur during labor, because the fetus uses up necessary body reserves. Decreased placental function impairs oxygenation and nutrition transport, leaving the fetus prone to hypoglycemia and asphyxia when the stresses of labor begin. The following are common disorders of the postmature newborn:

- *Hypoglycemia,* from nutritional deprivation and depleted glycogen stores.
- *Meconium aspiration* in response to in utero hypoxia. Oligohydramnios increases the danger of aspirating thick meconium. Severe meconium aspiration syndrome increases the baby's chance of developing persistent pulmonary hypertension, pneumothorax, and pneumonia.

- *Polycythemia* due to increased production of red blood cells (RBCs) in response to hypoxia.
- *Congenital anomalies* of unknown cause.
- *Seizure* activity because of hypoxic insult.
- *Cold stress* because of loss or poor development of subcutaneous fat.

The long-term effects of postmaturity syndrome are unclear. At present, studies do not agree on how postmaturity syndrome affects weight gain and IQ scores (Resnik & Calder, 1999). Prolonged pregnancy itself is not solely responsible for the postmaturity syndrome. The characteristics of postmature newborns are primarily caused by a combination of advanced gestational age, placental aging and subsequent insufficiency, and continued exposure to amniotic fluid.

Clinical Therapy

The aim of antenatal management is to differentiate the fetus who has postmaturity syndrome from the fetus who is large, well nourished, alert, and tolerating the prolonged (postterm) pregnancy. (Antenatal and intrapartal tests to evaluate fetal status and determine obstetric management are discussed in more depth in Chapters 14 and 19.) If the amniotic fluid is meconium stained, an amnioinfusion may be done during labor. This procedure dilutes the meconium, decreasing the risk of meconium aspiration syndrome. (For detailed discussion of clinical management and care of the newborn at risk for meconium aspiration, see Chapter 29.) Hypoglycemia is monitored by serial glucose determinations per agency protocols. If not in respiratory distress, the baby may be given glucose infusions or early feedings, but these measures must be instituted with caution because of the possibility of asphyxia.

As with SGA infants, peripheral and central hematocrits are tested to diagnose polycythemia. Fluid resuscitation can be initiated, and in extreme cases a partial exchange transfusion may be necessary to prevent polycythemia and adverse sequelae such as hyperviscosity. Oxygen is provided for respiratory distress. In addition, decreased liver glycogen stores can cause temperature instability and excessive loss of heat. (See Chapter 29 for thermoregulation techniques.)

Nursing Management

Nursing Assessment and Diagnosis

Assess the newborn for signs of postmaturity syndrome. The newborn with postmaturity syndrome appears alert; this wide-eyed, alert appearance is not necessarily a positive sign because it may indicate chronic intrauterine hypoxia. Postmature newborns are often voracious eaters.

The infant typically has dry, cracking, parchmentlike skin without vernix or lanugo (Figure 28–5 ◆). Fingernails

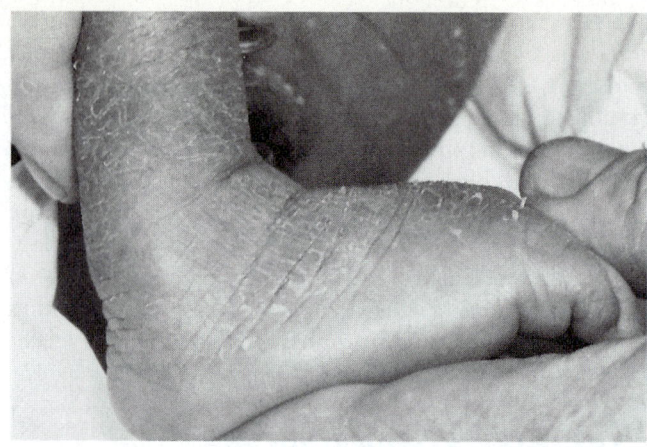

FIGURE 28–5. ◆ Postterm infant demonstrates deep cracking and peeling of skin. *Note:* Reprinted by permission of V. Dubowitz, MD, Hammersmith Hospital, London, England.

are long, and scalp hair is profuse. The infant's body appears long and thin. The wasting involves depletion of previously stored subcutaneous tissue, causing the skin to be loose. Fat layers are almost nonexistent.

Postmature newborns frequently have meconium staining, which colors the nails, skin, and umbilical cord. The varying shades (yellow to green) of meconium staining can give some clue as to whether the expulsion of meconium in utero was a recent or chronic problem. Green coloring indicates a more recent event.

Nursing diagnoses that may apply to the postmature newborn include the following:

▶ *Hypothermia* related to decreased liver glycogen and brown fat stores

▶ *Altered nutrition: less than body requirements* related to increased use of glucose secondary to in utero stress and decreased placenta perfusion

▶ *Impaired gas exchange in the lungs and at the cellular level* related to airway obstruction from meconium aspiration

Planning and Implementation

HOSPITAL-BASED NURSING CARE

Nursing interventions are primarily supportive. The nurse needs to:

▶ Monitor cardiopulmonary status, because the stresses of labor are poorly tolerated and can result in hypoxemia in utero and possible asphyxia at birth.

▶ Provide warmth to counterbalance the infant's poor response to cold stress and decreased liver glycogen and brown fat stores.

▶ Frequently monitor blood glucose and initiate early feeding (at 1 or 2 hours of age) or intravenous glucose per physician order.

- Obtain a central line hematocrit to determine accurately the presence of polycythemia.

Encourage parents to express their feelings and fears about the newborn's condition and potential long-term problems. Give careful explanations of procedures, include the parents in the development of care plans for their baby, and encourage follow-up care as needed.

Evaluation

Expected outcomes of nursing care include the following:

- The postterm newborn establishes effective respiratory function.

- The postmature baby is free of metabolic alterations (hypoglycemia) and maintains a stable temperature.

CARE OF THE PRETERM (PREMATURE) NEWBORN

With the help of modern technology, infants are surviving at younger gestational ages, but not without significant morbidity. The incidence of preterm births in the United States is approximately 8%. In socioeconomically deprived populations, it is 15% (American Academy of Pediatrics [AAP] & American College of Obstetricians and Gynecologists [ACOG], 1997). Prematurity and low birth weight are common in single and young mothers. (See Chapter 13 for a discussion of preterm labor.)

A **preterm infant** is any infant born before the completion of 37 weeks' gestation. The length of gestation and thus the level of maturity vary even in the "premature" population. Figure 28–6 ◆ shows a preterm newborn.

The major problem of the preterm newborn is the variable immaturity of all systems, which depends on the length of gestation. The preterm newborn must traverse

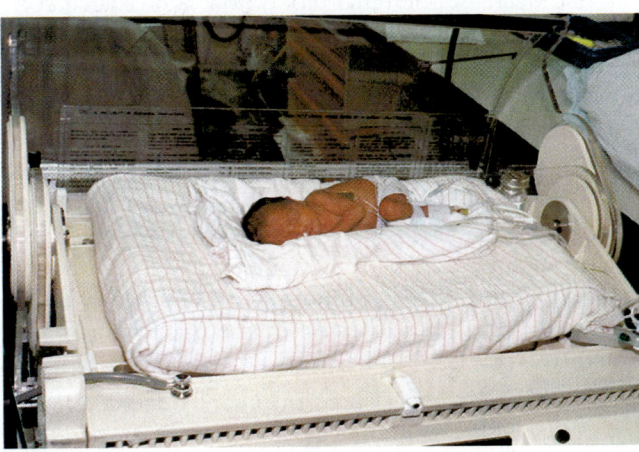

FIGURE 28–6. ◆ A 6-day-old, 28-week gestational age, 960-g preterm infant. Courtesy of Carol Harrigan, RNC, MSN, NNP.

the same complex, interconnected pathways from intrauterine to extrauterine life as the term newborn. Immaturity means the premature newborn is ill equipped to make this transition smoothly. Maintenance of the preterm newborn falls within narrow physiologic parameters.

Alteration in Respiratory and Cardiac Physiology

The preterm newborn is at risk for respiratory problems because the lungs are not fully mature and not fully ready to take over the process of oxygen and carbon dioxide exchange without assistance until 37 to 38 weeks' gestation. Critical factors in the development of respiratory distress include:

1. The preterm infant is unable to produce adequate amounts of surfactant. (See Chapter 24 for discussion of respiratory adaptation and development.) Inadequate surfactant lessens compliance (ability of the lung to fill with air easily), so the inspiratory pressure needed to expand the lungs with air is higher. The collapsed (or atelectatic) alveoli will not exchange oxygen and carbon dioxide. As a result, the infant becomes hypoxic, pulmonary blood flow is inefficient, and the preterm newborn's available energy is depleted.

2. The muscular coat of pulmonary blood vessels is incompletely developed. Consequently, the pulmonary arterioles do not constrict as well in response to decreased oxygen levels. Lower pulmonary vascular resistance leads to left-to-right shunting of blood through the ductus arteriosus back into the lungs.

3. The ductus arteriosus usually responds to increasing oxygen levels and prostaglandin E levels by vasoconstriction; in the preterm infant, who is more susceptible to hypoxia, the ductus may remain open. A patent ductus increases the blood volume to the lungs, causing pulmonary congestion, increased respiratory effort, carbon dioxide retention, and bounding femoral pulses. The common complications of the cardiopulmonary system in preterm infants are discussed later in this chapter and in Chapter 29.

Alteration in Thermoregulation

Heat loss is a major problem in preterm newborns that the nurse can do much to prevent. Two factors limiting heat production, however, are the availability of glycogen in the liver and the amount of brown fat available for metabolism. Both of these limiting factors appear in the third trimester. If the baby is chilled after birth, both glycogen and brown fat stores are metabolized rapidly for heat production, leaving the newborn with no reserves in the event of future stress. Since preterm infants have small muscle mass and cannot shiver, little heat is produced.

Five physiologic and anatomic factors cause heat loss:

1. The preterm baby has a higher ratio of body surface to body weight. This means that the baby's ability to produce heat (based on body weight) is much less than the potential for losing heat (based on surface area). Heat loss in a preterm infant weighing 1500 g is five times greater per unit of body weight than in an adult.

2. The preterm baby has very little subcutaneous fat, which is the human body's insulation. Without adequate insulation, heat is easily conducted from the core of the body (warmer temperature) to the surface of the body (cooler temperature). The body loses heat as the blood vessels, which lie close to the skin surface in the preterm infant, transport blood from the body core to the subcutaneous tissues.

3. The preterm baby has thinner, more permeable skin than the term infant, contributing to a greater insensible water loss as well as to heat loss.

4. The posture of the preterm baby is another important factor influencing heat loss. Flexion of the extremities decreases the amount of surface area exposed to the environment. Extension increases the surface area exposed to the environment and thus increases heat loss. The gestational age of the infant influences the amount of flexion, from completely hypotonic and extended at 28 weeks to strong flexion displayed by 36 weeks.

5. The preterm baby has a decreased ability to vasoconstrict superficial blood vessels and conserve heat in the body core.

In summary, gestational age is directly proportional to the ability to maintain thermoregulation; thus the more preterm the newborn, the less able the infant is to maintain heat balance. Preventing heat loss with a neutral thermal environment is one of the most important considerations in nursing management of the preterm infant. Cold stress, with its accompanying severe complications, can be prevented (see Chapter 29).

Alteration in Gastrointestinal Physiology

The basic structure of the gastrointestinal (GI) tract is formed early in gestation. Maturation of the digestive and absorptive process is more variable, however, and occurs later in gestation. As a result of GI immaturity, the preterm newborn has the following ingestion, digestive, and absorption problems:

- A marked danger of aspiration and its complications due to the infant's poorly developed gag reflex, incompetent esophageal cardiac sphincter, and poor sucking and swallowing reflex.
- Difficulty in meeting high caloric and fluid needs for growth due to small stomach capacity.

- Limited ability to convert certain essential amino acids to nonessential amino acids. Certain amino acids, such as histidine, taurine, and cysteine, are essential to the preterm infant but not to the term infant.
- Inability to handle the increased osmolarity of formula protein due to kidney immaturity. The preterm infant requires a higher concentration of whey protein than of casein.
- Difficulty absorbing saturated fats because of decreased bile salts and pancreatic lipase. Severe illness may also prevent intake of adequate nutrients.
- Difficulty with lactose digestion initially because processes may not be fully functional during the first few days of a preterm infant's life. The preterm newborn can digest and absorb most simple sugars.
- Rickets and significant bone demineralization due to deficiency of calcium and phosphorus, which are deposited primarily in the last trimester.
- Increased basal metabolic rate and increased oxygen requirements due to fatigue associated with sucking.
- Feeding intolerance and necrotizing enterocolitis (NEC) as a result of diminished blood flow and tissue perfusion to the intestinal tract due to prolonged hypoxia and hypoxemia at birth.

Alteration in Renal Physiology

The kidneys of the preterm infant are immature compared with those of the term infant. This situation poses clinical problems in the management of fluid and electrolyte balance. Specific characteristics of the preterm infant include:

- The glomerular filtration rate (GFR) is lower because of decreased renal blood flow. The GFR is directly related to lower gestational age, so the more preterm the newborn, the lower the GFR. The GFR is also decreased in the presence of diseases or conditions that decrease the renal blood flow and oxygen content, such as severe respiratory distress and perinatal asphyxia. The preterm infant may have anuria and oliguria after severe asphyxia with associated hypotension.
- The preterm infant's kidneys have a limited ability to concentrate urine or to excrete excess amounts of fluid. This means that if excess fluid is administered, the infant is at risk for fluid retention and overhydration. If too little is administered, the infant will become dehydrated because of the inability to retain adequate fluid.
- The kidneys of the preterm infant begin excreting glucose (glycosuria) at a lower serum glucose level than those of the term infant. Therefore, glycosuria with hyperglycemia is common.

- The kidney's buffering capacity is reduced, predisposing the infant to metabolic acidosis. Bicarbonate is excreted at a lower serum level, and acid is excreted more slowly. Therefore, after periods of hypoxia or insult, the preterm infants' kidneys need a longer time to excrete the accumulated lactic acid. Sodium bicarbonate is frequently required to treat the metabolic acidosis.

- The immaturity of the renal system affects the preterm infant's ability to excrete drugs. Because excretion time is longer, many drugs are given over longer intervals in the preterm infant (i.e., every 12 hours instead of every 8 hours). Urine output must be carefully monitored when the infant is receiving nephrotoxic drugs such as gentamicin, nafcillin, and others. If urine output is poor, drugs can become toxic in the infant much more quickly than in the adult.

Alteration in Reactivity Periods and Behavioral States

The newborn infant's response to extrauterine life is characterized by two periods of reactivity (see Chapter 21). The preterm infant's periods of reactivity are delayed. In the very ill infant, these periods of reactivity may not be observed at all because the infant may be hypotonic and unreactive for several days after birth.

As the preterm newborn grows and the condition stabilizes, identifying behavioral states and traits unique to each infant becomes increasingly possible. In general, stable preterm infants do not demonstrate the same behavioral states as term infants. Preterm infants tend to be more disorganized in their sleep-wake cycles and are unable to attend as well to the human face and objects in the environment. Neurologically, their responses (sucking, muscle tone, states of arousal) are weaker than full-term infants' responses.

Management of Nutrition and Fluid Requirements

Early feedings are extremely valuable in maintaining normal metabolism and lowering the possibility of such complications as hypoglycemia, hyperbilirubinemia, hyperkalemia, and azotemia. However, the preterm infant is at risk for complications that may develop because of immaturity of the digestive system.

The oral (enteral) caloric intake necessary for growth in an uncompromised healthy preterm newborn is 110 to 130 kcal/kg/day. In addition to these relatively high caloric needs, the preterm newborn requires more protein, 3 to 3.5 g/kg/day, as opposed to 2 to 2.5 g/kg/day for the full-term infant (Merenstein & Gardner, 1998). To meet these needs, many institutions use breast milk or special preterm formulas. Whether breast milk or formula is used, feeding regimens are established based on the in-

fant's weight and estimated stomach capacity. Initial formula feedings are gradually increased as the infant tolerates them. It may be necessary to supplement oral feedings with parenteral fluids to maintain adequate hydration and caloric intake until the baby is on full oral feedings.

In addition to a higher calorie and protein formula, preterm infants should receive supplemental multivitamins, including vitamin E and trace minerals. A diet high in polyunsaturated fats (which preterm infants tolerate best) increases the requirement for vitamin E. Preterm infants fed iron-fortified formulas have higher red cell hemolysis and lower vitamin E concentrations and thus require additional vitamin E. Preterm formulas also need to contain medium-chain triglycerides (MCTs) and additional amino acids such as cysteine, as well as calcium, phosphorus, and vitamin D supplements to increase mineralization of bones. Rickets and significant bone demineralization have been documented in very-low-birth-weight infants and otherwise healthy preterm infants.

Nutritional intake is considered adequate when the infant consistently gains 20 to 30 g/day. At first the baby may not gain weight for several days, but total weight loss should not exceed 15% of the total birth weight or more than 1% to 2% per day. Some institutions add the criteria of head circumference growth and increase in body length of 1 cm per week, once the newborn is stable.

Fluid requirement calculations take into account the infant's weight and postnatal age. Recommendations for fluid therapy in the preterm infant are approximately 80 to 100 mL/kg/day for day 1, 100 to 120 mL/kg/day for day 2, and 120 to 150 mL/kg/day by day 3 of life. These amounts may be increased up to 200 mL/kg/day if the infant is very small, receiving phototherapy, or under a radiant warmer because of increased insensible water losses. Fluid losses can be minimized through the use of heat shields and humidity, or "swamping."

Common Complications of Preterm Newborns

The goals of medical and nursing care are to anticipate and manage the complications associated with prematurity and meet the preterm infant's growth and development needs. The most common of these complications are:

1. *Apnea.* Apnea of prematurity refers to cessation of breathing for 20 seconds or longer or for less than 20 seconds when associated with cyanosis and bradycardia. Apnea is a common problem in the preterm infant (less than 37 weeks' gestation) and is thought to be primarily a result of neuronal immaturity, which contributes to the preterm infant's irregular breathing patterns. Factors that adversely affect brain nerve cells include hypoxia, acidosis, edema, intracranial bleeding, hyperbilirubinemia, hypoglycemia, hypocalcemia, and sepsis. Gastroesophageal reflux (GER) has been implicated in apnea. It is believed that GER causes laryngospasm, which leads to bradycardia and apnea.

2. *Patent ductus arteriosus (PDA)*. The ductus arteriosus fails to close because of decreased pulmonary arteriole musculature and hypoxemia. Symptomatic PDA is often seen around the time when premature infants are recovering from RDS. Patent ductus arteriosus often prolongs the course of illness in a preterm newborn and leads to chronic pulmonary dysfunction.

3. *Respiratory distress syndrome (RDS)*. Respiratory distress results from inadequate surfactant production.

4. *Intraventricular hemorrhage (IVH)*. Intraventricular hemorrhage is the most common type of intracranial hemorrhage in small preterm infants, especially those weighing less than 1500 g or of less than 34 weeks' gestation. Up to 35 weeks' gestation the preterm's brain ventricles are lined by the germinal matrix, which is highly susceptible to hypoxic events such as respiratory distress, birth trauma, and birth asphyxia. The germinal matrix is very vascular, and its blood vessels rupture in the presence of hypoxia.

5. *Anemia of prematurity*. The preterm infant is at risk for anemia because of the rapid rate of growth required, shorter RBC life, excessive blood sampling, decreased iron stores, and deficiency of vitamin E.

Other common problems of preterm infants such as hypocalcemia and NEC are discussed earlier in the physiologic sections. (For an in-depth discussion of RDS, hyperbilirubinemia, hypoglycemia, and sepsis see Chapter 29.)

Long-Term Needs and Outcome

The care of preterm infants and their families continues after they leave the nursery. Follow-up care is extremely important because many developmental problems are not noted until an infant is older and begins to demonstrate motor delays or sensory disability.

Within the first year of life, low-birth-weight preterm infants face higher mortality rates than term infants. Causes of death include sudden infant death syndrome (SIDS)—which occurs about five times more frequently in the preterm infant—respiratory infections, and neurologic defects. Morbidity is also much higher among preterm infants, with those weighing less than 1500 g at highest risk for long-term complications.

The most common long-term needs observed in preterm infants include the following:

- *Retinopathy of prematurity (ROP)*. Premature newborns are particularly susceptible to characteristic retinal changes, known as ROP, which can impair vision. The disease is now viewed as multifactorial in origin. Increased survival of very-low-birth-weight (VLBW) infants may be the most important factor in the increased incidence of ROP.

- *Bronchopulmonary dysplasia (BPD)*. Long-term lung disease results when positive pressure respirator therapy and high oxygen concentration damage the alveolar epithelium. Infants with BPD have long-term dependence on oxygen therapy and an increased incidence of respiratory infection during their first few years of life. For further discussion see Chapter 42.

- *Speech defects*. The most common speech defects involve delayed development of receptive and expressive ability that may persist into the school-age years.

- *Neurologic defects*. The most common neurologic defects include cerebral palsy, hydrocephalus, seizure disorders, lower IQ, and learning disabilities. However, the socioeconomic climate and family support systems are extremely important influences on the child's ultimate school performance when there are no major neurologic defects. Families can be reminded that risk does not equal injury, injury does not equal damage, and description of damage does not allow a precise prediction about recovery or outcome.

- *Auditory defects*. Preterm infants have a 1% to 4% incidence of moderate to profound hearing loss and should have a formal audiologic exam before discharge and at 3 to 6 months (corrected age). The test currently used to measure newborn hearing functions is the evoked otoacoustic emissions (EOAE) test. Any infant with repeated abnormal results should be referred to speech-and-language specialists.

When evaluating the infant's abilities and disabilities, it is important for parents to understand that developmental progress must be assessed from the expected date of birth, not from the actual date of birth. Developmental level cannot be evaluated based on chronologic age. In addition, the parents need the consistent support of health care professionals in the long-term management of their infant to promote the highest quality of life possible.

Nursing Management

Nursing Assessment and Diagnosis

Assess the physical characteristics and gestational age of the preterm newborn accurately to anticipate the special needs and problems of the baby. Physical characteristics vary greatly depending on gestational age, but these characteristics are common:

▶ Color is usually pink or ruddy but may be acrocyanotic. (Cyanosis, jaundice, and pallor are abnormal and should be noted.)

▶ Skin is reddened and translucent, blood vessels are readily apparent, there is little subcutaneous fat.

▶ Lanugo is plentiful and widely distributed.

▶ Head size appears large in relation to body.

▶ Skull bones are pliable; fontanelle is smooth and flat.

- Ears have minimal cartilage and are pliable, folded over.
- Nails are soft, short.
- Genitals are small; testes may not be descended.
- Resting position is flaccid, froglike.
- Cry is weak, feeble.
- Reflexes (sucking, swallowing, gag) are poor.
- Activity consists of jerky, generalized movements. (Seizure activity is abnormal.)

Determination of gestational age in preterm newborns requires knowledge and experience in administering gestational assessment tools. The tool used should be specific, reliable, and valid. (For a discussion of gestational age assessment tools, see Chapter 25.) ⬭ Nursing diagnoses that may apply to the preterm newborn include:

- *Impaired gas exchange* related to immature pulmonary vasculature and inadequate surfactant production
- *Altered nutrition: less than body requirements* related to weak suck and swallow reflexes and decreased ability to absorb nutrients
- *Ineffective thermoregulation* related to hypothermia secondary to decreased glycogen and brown fat stores
- *Ineffective family coping* related to anger or guilt at having delivered a premature baby

Planning and Implementation

MAINTENANCE OF RESPIRATORY FUNCTION

Preterm newborns have increased danger of respiratory obstruction. Their bronchi and trachea are so narrow that mucus can obstruct the airway. Maintain patency through judicious suctioning, but only suction as needed.

Positioning can also affect respiratory function, especially in the preterm newborn. If the baby is in the supine position, slightly elevate the infant's head to maintain the airway, being careful to avoid hyperextension of the neck because the trachea will collapse. Also, because the newborn has weak neck muscles and cannot control head movement, maintain this head position by placing a small roll under the shoulders. Because the prone position splints the chest wall and decreases the amount of respiratory effort used to move the chest wall, it facilitates chest expansion and improves air entry and oxygenation. Weak or absent cough or gag reflexes increase the premature newborn's chance of aspiration. Ensure that the infant's position facilitates drainage of mucus or regurgitated formula.

Monitor heart and respiratory rates with cardiorespiratory monitors and observe the newborn for alterations in cardiopulmonary status. Signs of respiratory distress include:

- Cyanosis (serious sign when generalized)
- Tachypnea (sustained respiratory rate greater than 60/minute after first 4 hours of life)
- Retractions
- Expiratory grunting
- Flaring nostrils
- Apneic episodes
- Presence of rales or rhonchi on auscultation
- Diminished air entry

If respiratory distress occurs, administer oxygen per physician or nurse practitioner order to relieve hypoxemia. If hypoxemia is not treated immediately, it may result in patent ductus arteriosus or metabolic acidosis. When administering oxygen to the newborn, monitor the oxygen concentration with devices such as the transcutaneous oxygen monitor ($tcPO_2$) or the pulse oximeter. Monitoring of oxygen concentration in the baby's blood is essential since hyperoxemia may lead to ROP.

Consider respiratory function during feeding. To prevent aspiration and increased energy expenditure and oxygen consumption, ensure that the infant's gag and suck reflexes are intact before starting oral feedings.

MAINTENANCE OF NEUTRAL THERMAL ENVIRONMENT

Providing a neutral thermal environment minimizes the oxygen consumption required to maintain a normal core temperature; it also prevents cold stress and facilitates growth by decreasing the calories needed to maintain body temperature. The preterm infant's immature central nervous system provides poor temperature control, and stores of brown fat are decreased. A small infant (< 1200 g) can lose 80 kcal/kg/day through radiation of body heat.

Use all the usual thermoregulation measures discussed in Chapter 26. ⬭ In addition, to minimize heat loss and temperature instability effects:

1. Warm and humidify oxygen to minimize evaporative heat loss and decrease oxygen consumption.
2. Place the baby in a double-walled incubator or use a Plexiglas heat shield over small preterm infants in single-walled incubators to avoid radiative heat losses. Some institutions use radiant warmers and plastic wrap over the baby and pipe in humidity (swamping). Do not use Plexiglas shields on radiant warmer beds because they block the infrared heat.
3. Avoid placing the baby on cold surfaces such as metal treatment tables and cold x-ray plates; pad cold surfaces with diapers and use radiant warmers during procedures, place infant on prewarmed mattresses, and warm hands before handling the baby to prevent heat transfer via conduction.
4. Use warmed ambient humidity.
5. Keep the skin dry and place a cap on the baby's head to prevent heat loss via evaporation. (The head makes up 25% of the total body size.)
6. Keep radiant warmers, incubators, and cribs away from windows and cold external walls and out of drafts to prevent heat loss by radiation.

7. Use a skin probe to monitor the baby's skin temperature. Correlate ambient temperatures with the skin probe in the incubator using the servocontrol rather than the manual mode. The temperature should be 36 to 37 °C (96.8 to 97.7 °F). Temperature fluctuations indicate hypothermia or hyperthermia. Be careful not to place skin temperature probes over bony prominences, areas of brown fat, poorly vasoreactive areas such as extremities, or excoriated areas ("Neonatal Thermoregulation," 1997).

8. Warm formula or stored breast milk before feeding.

9. Use reflector patch over the skin temperature probe when using a radiant warmer bed so that the probe does not sense the higher infrared temperature as the baby's skin temperature and therefore decrease the heater output.

Once preterm infants are medically stable, they can be clothed with a double-thickness cap, cotton shirt, and diaper and, if possible, swaddled in a blanket. Begin the process of weaning to a crib when the premature infant is medically stable, does not require assisted ventilation, weighs approximately 1500 g, has 5 days of consistent weight gain, and is taking oral feedings and when apnea and bradycardia episodes have stabilized. Be familiar with the institution's protocol for weaning to a crib.

MAINTENANCE OF FLUID AND ELECTROLYTE STATUS

Keep the newborn hydrated by providing adequate intake based on weight, gestational age, chronologic age, and volume of sensible and insensible water losses. Adequate fluid intake should compensate for increased insensible losses and the amount needed for renal excretion of metabolic products. Minimize insensible water losses by providing high ambient humidity, humidifying oxygen, using heat shields, covering the skin with plastic wrap, and placing the infant in a double-walled incubator.

Evaluate the baby's hydration status by assessing and recording signs of dehydration. Early signs of dehydration include loss of weight, dry oral mucous membranes, decreased urine output and increased specific gravity (>1.013), and then depressed fontanelle and poor skin turgor (skin returns to normal position slowly when squeezed gently). Also identify signs of overhydration by observing the newborn for edema or excessive weight gain and by comparing urine output with fluid intake.

Weigh the preterm infant at least once daily at the same time each day. *Weight change is one of the most sensitive indicators of fluid balance.* Weighing diapers is also important for accurate input and output measurement (1 mL = 1 g). A comparison of intake and output measurements over an 8- or 24-hour period provides important information about renal function and fluid balance. Assessment of patterns and whether they show a net gain or loss over several days is also essential to fluid management. In addition, monitor blood serum levels and pH to evaluate for electrolyte imbalances. Periodically obtain urine specific grav-

ity and pH. Urine osmolality provides an indication of hydration, although this factor must be correlated with other assessments (e.g., serum sodium). Hydration is considered adequate when the urine output is 1 to 3 mL/kg/hr.

Accurate hourly intake calculations when administering intravenous fluids are essential to prevent overload. Ensure accuracy by using neonatal or pediatric infusion pumps. To prevent electrolyte imbalance and dehydration, take care to give the correct intravenous (IV) solutions and volumes and concentrations of formulas.

PROVISION OF ADEQUATE NUTRITION AND PREVENTION OF FATIGUE DURING FEEDING

The preterm infant is fed by various methods depending on the infant's gestational age, health and physical condition, and neurologic status. The three most common oral feeding methods are bottle, breast, and gavage (discussed later in this section). Preterm infants who cannot tolerate any oral (enteral) feedings may be nourished by total parenteral nutrition (TPN). TPN uses hyperalimentation to provide calories, vitamins, minerals, protein, and glucose and intralipids to provide essential fatty acids.

Bottle-Feeding

Preterm infants who have a coordinated suck and swallow reflex are usually at least 34 weeks' gestation; those continually gaining weight (20 to 30 g/day) may be fed by bottle. To avoid excessive expenditure of energy, a soft, smaller nipple may be used. The infant is fed in a semisitting position and burped gently after each 1/2 to 1 oz. The feeding should take no longer than 15 to 20 minutes. Preterm infants often progress from parenteral feedings to complete oral or nipple feedings in five or six phases. Babies who are progressing from gavage feedings to bottle-feeding should start with one session of bottle-feeding a day and slowly increase the number of times a day a bottle is given until the baby tolerates all feedings from a bottle.

Also assess the infant's ability to suck. Sucking may be affected by age, asphyxia, sepsis, intraventricular hemorrhage, or other neurologic insult. Before initiating bottle-feeding, observe for signs of stress, such as tachypnea (more than 60 respirations per minute), respiratory distress, or hypothermia, which may increase the risk of aspiration. During the feeding, observe the infant for signs of feeding difficulty (tachypnea, cyanosis, bradycardia, lethargy, uncoordinated suck and swallow).

Breastfeeding

Mothers who wish to breastfeed their preterm infants are given the opportunity to put the infant to the breast as soon as the infant has demonstrated a coordinated suck and swallow reflex, is showing consistent weight gain, and can control body temperature outside of the incubator, regardless of weight. Preterm infants tolerate breastfeeding with higher transcutaneous oxygen pressures and better maintenance of body temperature than during bottle-feeding. In addition to breast milk's many benefits for the

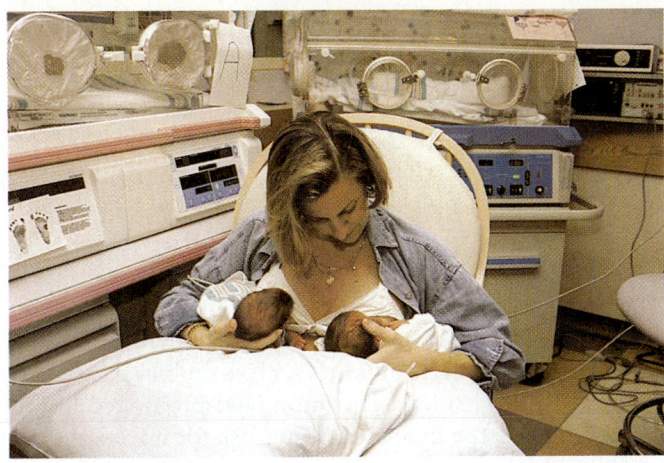

FIGURE 28–7. ◆ Mother visits intensive care unit to breastfeed her preterm twin infants.

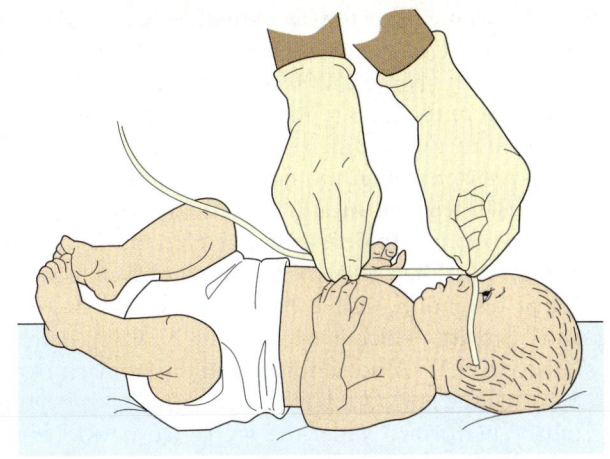

FIGURE 28–8. ◆ Measuring gavage tube length.

infant, breastfeeding allows the mother to contribute actively to the infant's well-being (Figure 28–7 ◆). Encourage mothers to breastfeed because of the numerous benefits if they choose to do so. It is important to be aware of the advantages of breastfeeding, as well as the possible disadvantages of breast milk as the sole source of food for the preterm infant (see Chapter 27). ⊂⊃

The football hold is often a convenient position for breastfeeding preterm babies. Feeding may take up to 45 minutes, and babies should be burped as they alternate breasts. Monitor the length of feeding time so that the preterm infant does not burn too many calories. Coordinate a flexible feeding schedule so babies can nurse during alert times and be allowed to set their own pace. Feedings should be on demand, but a maximum number of hours between feedings should be set. By initiating skin-to-skin holding of low-birth-weight infants in the early intensive care phase, mothers can significantly increase milk volume and thereby overcome lactation problems (Moran, Radzyminski, Higgins, et al., 1999). Even if the infant cannot be put to the breast, mothers can pump their breasts, and the breast milk can be given via gavage. A double pumping system produces higher levels of prolactin than sequential pumping of the breasts.

When progressing from gavage to breastfeeding, the mother begins with one feeding at the breast and then gradually increases the number of times during the day that the baby breastfeeds. When breastfeeding is not possible because the infant is too small or too weak to suck at the breast, the mother may express her breast milk into a cup. The milk touches the infant's lips and is lapped by the protruding motions of the tongue.

Gavage Feeding

The gavage feeding method is used with preterm infants (less than 34 weeks' gestation) who lack or have a poorly coordinated suck and swallow reflex or are ill and ventilator dependent. Gavage feeding may be used as an adjunct to nipple feeding if the infant tires easily or as an alterna-

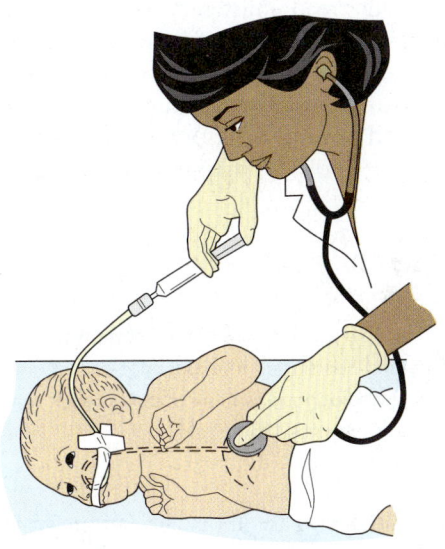

FIGURE 28–9. ◆ Auscultation for placement of gavage tube.

tive if an infant is losing weight because of the energy expenditure required for nippling (see Skill 15–3). ⊂⊃ [SKILLS] [CD] Gavage feedings are administered by either the nasogastric or orogastric route and by intermittent bolus or continuous drip method (see Figures 28–8 ◆ and 28–9 ◆).

Slow Progression to Full Enteral Feeds to Prevent Fatigue

Both nipple and gavage methods are initially supplemented with IV therapy until oral intake is sufficient to support growth (110 to 130 kcal/kg/day). Early, small-volume enteral feedings (0.1 to 0.5 mL/hr), called hypocaloric or trophic feedings, have proved to benefit the very-low-birth-weight infant. Gastrointestinal priming with these small-volume enteral feedings is not intended to contribute to the total nutritional intake but rather to enhance gut metabolism. Trophic feedings may also help encourage earlier advancement to full feedings, thereby decreasing the development of NEC and the complications of parenteral nutrition (Newell, 2000). Formula or breast milk (with or without fortifiers to increase caloric content) is incorporated into the feedings slowly. Initially, the feeding may be at quarter strength, then half strength, and so on.

Before each feeding, measure abdominal girth and auscultate the abdomen to determine the presence and quality of bowel sounds. Such assessments permit early detection of abdominal distention, visible bowel loops, and decreased peristaltic activity, which may indicate NEC or paralytic ileus. Also check for residual formula in the stomach before feeding when the newborn is fed by gavage. This procedure also can be performed when the nipple-fed newborn presents with abdominal distention. The presence of increasing residual formula indicates intolerance to the type or amount of feeding or the increase in amount of feeding. Residual formula is usually readministered (because digestive processes have already been initiated) and subtracted from the amount to be given at that feeding. Carefully watch for other signs of feeding intolerance including guaiac-positive stools (occult blood in stools), lactose in the stools (reducing substance in the stools), vomiting, and diarrhea.

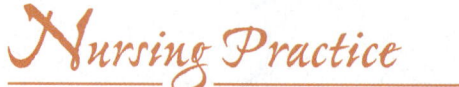

For an otherwise healthy, growing premature infant who is receiving total enteral intake and has started to experience apnea and bradycardia, one differential diagnosis to think about is reflux rather than sepsis, although sepsis may need to be ruled out.

Preterm newborns who are ill or who fatigue easily with nipple-feedings are usually fed by gavage. The infant is essentially passive with these methods, thus conserving energy and calories. As the baby matures, gavage feedings are replaced with breast- or bottle-feedings to help strengthen the sucking reflex and meet oral and emotional needs. Signs that indicate readiness for oral feedings are a strong gag reflex, nonnutritive sucking, rooting behavior, gestational age of 34 weeks or more, and weight over 1500 g. Both low-birth-weight and preterm infants nipple-feed more effectively in a quiet state. Establish a gradual nipple-feeding program, such as one nipple-feeding per day, then one nipple-feeding per shift, and then a nipple-feeding every other feeding. Monitor daily weights because often there is a small weight loss when nipple-feedings are started. After feedings, place the baby on the right side (with support to maintain this position) to enhance gastric emptying and decrease the chance of aspiration if regurgitation occurs. Gastroesophageal reflux is not uncommon in preterm newborns.

Involve the parents in feeding their preterm baby. This involvement is essential to the development of attachment between parents and infant. In addition, it teaches parents about the care of their infant and helps them cope with the situation.

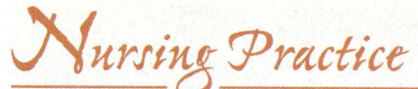

Residual feeding may indicate early NEC and should be called to the attention of the clinician.

PREVENTION OF INFECTION

The preterm newborn is susceptible to infection because of an immature immune system and thin and permeable skin. Invasive procedures, techniques such as umbilical catheterization and mechanical ventilation, and prolonged hospitalization place the infant at greater risk for infection.

Strict handwashing, reverse isolation, and use of equipment for only one infant help minimize the preterm newborn's exposure to infectious agents. In addition, most nurseries have adopted the standard precautions recommended by the Centers for Disease Control and Prevention (CDC) of isolating every baby. Staff members are required to complete a 2- to 3-minute scrub using iodine-containing antibacterial solutions, which inhibit growth of gram-positive cocci and gram-negative rod organisms. Other specific nursing interventions include limiting visitors; requiring visitors to wash their hands; and maintaining strict aseptic practices when changing IV tubing and solutions (IV solutions and tubing should be changed every 24 hours), administering parenteral fluids, and assisting with sterile procedures. Incubators and radiant warmers should be changed weekly. Prevent pressure-area breakdown by changing the baby's position regularly, doing range of motion exercises, and using a sheepskin (covered with a blanket or diapered beneath the infant's head) or a water bed. To avoid skin tears, a protective transparent covering can be applied over vulnerable joints but is used very sparingly (Siegfried, 1998). Chemical skin preps and tape may cause skin trauma and should be avoided as much as possible.

If infection (sepsis) occurs in the preterm newborn, the nurse may be the first to identify its subtle clinical signs. Inform the clinician of the findings immediately and implement the treatment plan per clinician orders. (For specific nursing care required for the newborn with an infection, see Chapter 29.)

PROMOTION OF PARENT-INFANT ATTACHMENT

Nurses need to take measures to promote positive parental feelings toward the preterm newborn. For example, give photographs of the baby to parents to take home or to the mother if she is in a different hospital or too ill to come to the nursery and visit. Place the infant's first name on the incubator as soon as it is known to help the parents feel that their infant is a unique and special person. Provide a weekly card with the baby's footprint, weight, and length to promote bonding. Give parents the telephone number of the nursery or intensive care unit and the names of staff members so that they have access to information about their

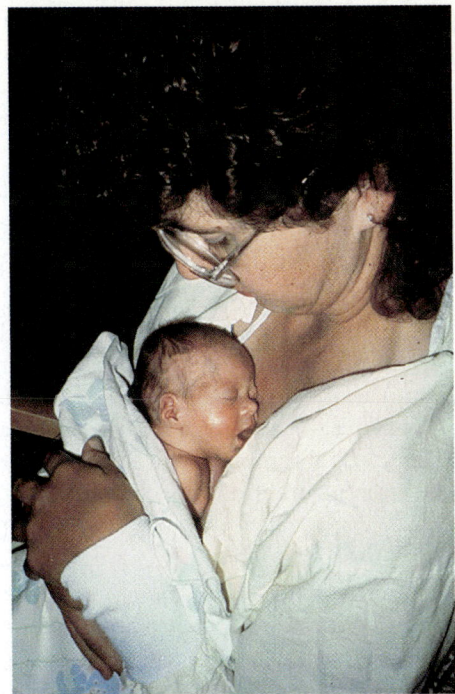

FIGURE 28–10. ◆ Kangaroo (skin-to-skin) care facilitates closeness and attachment between parents and their premature infant. Courtesy of Kadlac Medical Center Kangaroo Care Study and Carol Thompson, RNC, MSN, NNP.

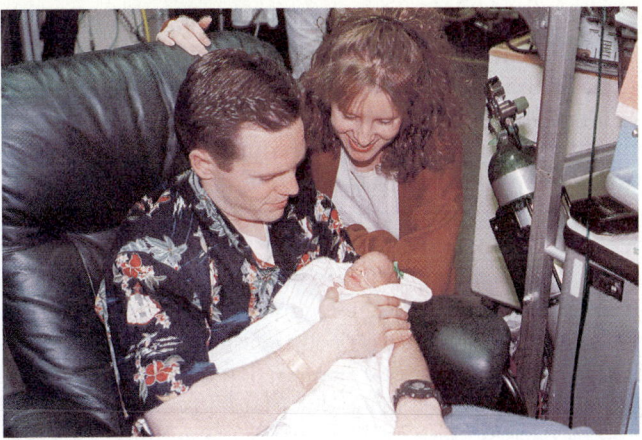

FIGURE 28–11. ◆ Family bonding occurs when parents have opportunities to spend time with their infant. Courtesy of Carol Harrigan, RNC, MSN, NNP.

baby at any time of the day or night. Encourage visits from siblings and grandparents to foster attachment.

Early parental involvement in the care of and decisions about their baby gives the parents more realistic expectations for the future. The unique combination of personality characteristics of the infant and of the parents influences the bonding and interactive process for the family. By observing each infant's patterns of behavior and responses, especially sleep-wake states, the nurse can teach parents optimal times for interacting with their infant. The parents and nurse can plan nursing care around the times when the infant is alert and best able to attend. In addition, the more knowledge parents have about the meaning of their infant's responses, behaviors, and cues for interaction, the better prepared they will be to meet their newborn's needs and form a positive attachment with their child. Parents need education to develop caregiving skills. Encourage their daily participation (if possible), as well as early and frequent visits. Give parents opportunities to touch, hold, talk to, and care for the baby. Skin-to-skin contact (kangaroo care) helps parents feel close to their small infants (Figure 28–10 ◆). Kangaroo care improves sleep periods and parents' perception of their caregiving ability (Moran et al., 1999). Parental involvement in difficult care decisions is essential and discussed in greater detail in Chapter 29. ⊂⊃

Some parents progress easily to touching and cuddling their infant; others do not. Parents need to know that their feelings are normal and that the progression of acquain-

tanceship is slow. Rooming-in can provide another opportunity for the stable preterm infant and family to get acquainted; it offers both privacy and readily available help (Figure 28–11 ◆).

PROMOTION OF DEVELOPMENTALLY SUPPORTIVE CARE

Prolonged separation and the neonatal intensive care unit (NICU) environment necessitate individualized baby sensory stimulation programs. The nurse plays a key role in determining the appropriate type and amount of visual, tactile, and auditory stimulation (Horns, 1998).

Some preterm infants are not developmentally able to deal with more than one sensory input at a time. The Assessment of Preterm Infant Behavior (APIB) scale (Als, Lester, Tronick, et al., 1982) identifies individual preterm newborn behaviors according to five areas of development. The preterm baby's behavioral reactions to stimulation are observed, and developmental interventions are then based

Complementary Care

INFANT MASSAGE

Infant massage has been practiced for many centuries. Practitioners report such physiologic benefits as stimulating blood and lymphatic flow, promoting weight gain in premature infants, and regulating sleep patterns. Many emotional and behavior benefits are also cited by practitioners. Classes are also available to teach parents how to perform massage on their infants. Massage demonstrates compassion while increasing the parent's empathy and understanding of the baby. It helps parents learn to interpret their baby's behavioral cues such as facial expression, various crying patterns, and other body language. At the same time it helps the infant to learn about his or her various body parts and feel how they integrate into the whole. For more detailed information, including an interview with a certified infant massage instructor (CIMI), see our website. ⊂⊃ **WEB**

on reducing detrimental environmental stimuli to the lowest possible level and providing appropriate opportunities for development (Als, 1998).

The NICU environment contains many detrimental stimuli that the nurse can help reduce. Noise levels can be lowered by replacing alarms with lights or silencing them quickly and keeping conversations away from the baby's bedside. Dimmer switches should be used to shield the baby's eyes from bright lights, and blankets may be placed over the top portion of the incubator. Dimming the lights may encourage infants to open their eyes and be more responsive to their parents. Plan nursing care to decrease the number of times the baby is disturbed. Place signs (such as, "Quiet Please") near the bedside to allow the baby some periods of uninterrupted sleep (Blackburn, 1998). Some other suggested developmentally supportive interventions include:

▶ Use containment measures when turning or moving the infant or doing procedures such as suctioning. Use the hands to hold the infant's arms and legs, flexed, close to the midline of the body. Containment measures help stabilize the infant's motor and physiologic subsystems during stressful activities.

▶ Touch the infant gently and avoid sudden postural changes.

▶ Promote self-consoling and soothing activities, such as placing blanket rolls or approved manufactured devices next to the infant's sides and against the feet to provide "nesting." Swaddle the infant with the extremities in a flexed position and ensure that the hands can reach the face for hand-to-mouth activities, which can be consoling (Figure 28–12 ◆).

▶ Simulate the kinesthetic advantages (decreased motor activity, improved sleep, fewer behavior state changes) of the intrauterine environment by using sheepskin or approved water beds.

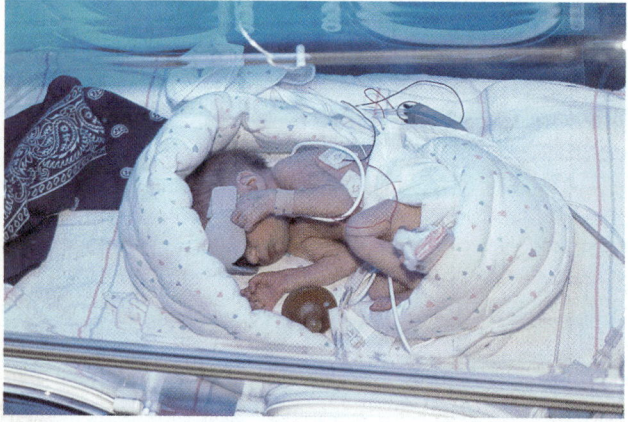

FIGURE 28–12. ◆ Infant is "nested." Hand-to-mouth behavior facilitates self-consoling and soothing activities. Courtesy of Theresa Kledzik, RN, Developmental Nurse, Memorial Hospital, Colorado Springs, Colorado.

▶ Provide opportunities for nonnutritive sucking with a pacifier. Nonnutritive sucking improves oxygen saturation; decreases body movements; improves sleep, especially after feedings; and increases weight gain (Engebretson & Wardell, 1997).

▶ Provide objects for the infant to grasp (e.g., a piece of blanket, oxygen tubing, a finger) during caregiving. Grasping may comfort the baby.

Teaching the parents to read behavioral cues will help them move at their infant's own pace when providing stimulation. Parents are ideally equipped to meet the baby's need for stimulation. Stroking, rocking, cuddling, quiet singing, and talking to the baby can all be integral parts of the baby's care. Visual stimulation in the form of *en face* interaction with caregivers and mobiles is also important.

PREPARATION FOR HOME CARE

Parents are often anxious when their premature infant is transferred out of the NICU or is discharged home. Parents of preterm babies should receive the same postpartal teaching as any parent taking a new infant home. In preparing for discharge, encourage the parents to spend time caring directly for their baby. Direct caregiving familiarizes them with their baby's behavior patterns and helps them establish realistic expectations about the infant. Some NICUs have a special room near the nursery where parents can spend the night with their baby before discharge. Discharge instruction includes breast- and bottle-feeding techniques, formula preparation, and vitamin administration. If the mother wishes to breastfeed, teach her to pump her breasts to keep the milk flowing and provide milk even before discharge. Give information on bathing, diapering, hygiene, and normal elimination patterns and prepare the parents to expect changes in the color of the baby's stool, number of bowel movements, and timing of elimination when the infant is switched from bottle- to breastfeeding. This information can prevent unnecessary concern by the parents. Also discuss normal growth and development patterns, reflexes, and activity for preterm infants. In these discussions, emphasize ways to promote bonding behaviors and deal with newborn crying. Care of the preterm infant with complications, preventing infections, recognizing signs of a sick baby, and the need for continued medical follow-up are other key issues.

Families with preterm infants usually do not need to be referred to community agencies, such as visiting nurse assistance. However, referral may be necessary if the infant has severe congenital abnormalities, feeding problems, or complications with infections or respiratory problems or if the parents seem unable to cope with an at-risk baby. Parents of preterm infants can benefit from meeting with others in a similar situation to share common experiences and concerns. Refer parents to support groups and make connections for parents with early education intervention centers.

Evaluation

Expected outcomes of nursing care include:

▶ The preterm newborn is free of respiratory distress and establishes effective respiratory function.

▶ The preterm newborn gains weight and shows no signs of fatigue or aspiration during feedings.

▶ The parents verbalize their anger and guilt feelings about the birth of a preterm baby and show attachment behavior such as frequent visits and growing confidence in their caregiving activities.

CARE OF THE NEWBORN WITH CONGENITAL ANOMALIES

The birth of a baby with a congenital defect places both newborn and family at risk. Many congenital anomalies can be life threatening if not corrected within hours after birth; others are very visible and cause the families emotional distress. When one congenital anomaly is found, health care providers should look for other ones, particularly in body systems that develop at the same time during gestation. Table 28–1 identifies some common anomalies and their early management and nursing care in the neonatal period. More detailed discussions of these congenital anomalies are found in the appropriate system alterations chapters later in the text.

CARE OF THE NEWBORN WITH CONGENITAL HEART DEFECTS

Congenital heart defects occur in 4 to 5 per 1000 live births. They account for one third of the deaths caused by congenital defects in the first year of life. Because accurate diagnosis and surgical treatment are now available, many such deaths can be prevented. Corrective cardiac surgery is being done at earlier ages; for example, more than half the children undergoing surgery are less than 1 year of age, and one fourth are less than 1 month old. It is crucial for the nurse to have comprehensive knowledge of congenital heart disease to detect deviations from normal and initiate interventions.

Factors that can contribute to congenital heart malformation can be classified as environmental or genetic; environmental factors are quite varied. For example, infections of the pregnant woman, such as rubella, cytomegalovirus, coxsackie B, and influenza, have been implicated. Steroids, alcohol, lithium, and some anticonvulsants have been shown to cause malformations of the heart. Seasonal spraying of pesticides has also been linked to an increase in congenital heart defects.

Clinicians are also beginning to see cardiac defects in infants of mothers with PKU who do not follow their diets.

Chromosomal factors may include Down syndrome and trisomy 13/15 and 16/18. Increased incidence and risk of recurrence of specific defects occur in families.

The most common cardiac defects seen in the first 6 days of life are left ventricular outflow obstructions (mitral stenosis, aortic stenosis or atresia), hypoplastic left heart, coarctation of the aorta, PDA (the most common defect, especially in premature infants), transposition of the great vessels, tetralogy of Fallot, and large ventricular septal defect or atrial septal defects. Many cardiac defects may not manifest themselves until after discharge from the birthing unit.

Nursing Management

The neonatal nurse's primary goal is to identify cardiac defects early and notify the physician. The three most common manifestations of cardiac defect are cyanosis, detectable heart murmur, and congestive heart failure signs (tachycardia, tachypnea, diaphoresis, hepatomegaly, cardiomegaly). "Pathophysiology Illustrated: Cardiac Defects of the Early Newborn Period" on page 631 shows the pathophysiology as well as the clinical manifestations and medical-surgical management of selected cardiac defects.

Initial repair of heart defects in the newborn period is becoming more commonplace. The staff of the NICUs are involved in both the preoperative and postoperative care of newborns. The benefits for the infant of being cared for by NICU staff include the staff's knowledge of neonatal anatomy and physiology, experience in supporting the family, and an awareness of the developmental needs of the newborn.

After the baby is stabilized, decisions are made about ongoing care. The parents need careful and complete explanations and the chance to take part in decision making. They also require ongoing emotional support. Families with any baby born with a congenital anomaly also need genetic counseling about future conception. Parents need opportunities to verbalize their concerns about their baby's health. Be sure they understand the rationale for follow-up care.

CARE OF THE NEWBORN OF A SUBSTANCE-ABUSING MOTHER

An **infant of a substance-abusing mother (ISAM)** was formerly called an infant of an addicted mother. This terminology changed because abuse without addiction can provoke the same outcomes for the newborn. The newborn of an alcoholic or drug-addicted woman may also be alcohol or drug dependent. After birth, when an infant's connection with the maternal blood supply is severed, the newborn may suffer withdrawal. In addition, the drugs ingested by the mother may be teratogenic, resulting in congenital anomalies.

Congenital Anomaly	Nursing Assessments	Nursing Goals and Interventions
Congenital hydrocephalus	Enlarged head Enlarged or full fontanelles Split or widened sutures "Setting sun" eyes	Assess presence of hydrocephalus; Measure and plot occipital-frontal baseline measurements; then measure head circumference once a day. Check fontanelle for bulging and sutures for widening. Assist with head ultrasound and transillumination. Maintain skin integrity. Change position frequently. Clean skin creases after feeding or vomiting. Use sheepskin pillow under head. Postoperatively, position head off operative site. Watch for signs of infection.
Choanal atresia	Occlusion of posterior nares Cyanosis and retractions at rest Snorting respirations Difficulty breathing during feeding Obstruction by thick mucus	Assess patency of nares: Listen for breath sounds while holding baby's mouth closed and alternately compressing each nostril. Assist with passing feeding tube to confirm diagnosis. Maintain respiratory function: Assist with taping airway in mouth to prevent respiratory distress. Position with head elevated to improve air exchange.
Cleft lip	Unilateral or bilateral visible defect May involve external nares, nasal cartilage, nasal septum, and alveolar process Flattening or depression of midfacial contour 	Provide nutrition: Feed with special nipple. Burp frequently (increased tendency to swallow air and reflex vomiting). Clean cleft with sterile water (to prevent crusting on cleft prior to repair). Support parental coping: Assist parents with grief over loss of idealized baby. Encourage verbalization of their feelings about visible defect. Provide role model in interacting with infant. (Parents internalize others' responses to their newborn.) (At left) Unilateral cleft lip with cleft abnormally involving both hard and soft palates.
Cleft palate	Fissure connecting oral and nasal cavity May involve uvula and soft palate May extend forward to nostril involving hard palate and maxillary aveolar ridge Difficulty in sucking Expulsion of formula through nose	Prevent aspiration/infection: Place prone or in side-lying position to facilitate drainage. Suction nasopharyngeal cavity (to prevent aspiration or airway obstruction). During newborn period, feed in upright position with head and chest tilted slightly backward (to aid swallowing and discourage aspiration). Provide nutrition: Feed with special nipple that fills cleft and allows sucking. Also decreases chance of aspiration through nasal cavity. Clean mouth with water after feedings. Burp after each ounce (tend to swallow large amounts of air). Thicken formula to provide extra calories. Plot weight gain patterns to assess adequacy of diet. Provide parental support: Refer parents to community agencies and support groups. Encourage verbalization of frustrations because feeding process is long and frustrating. Praise all parental efforts. Encourage parents to seek prompt treatment for upper respiratory infection (URI) and teach them ways to decrease URI.

(continued)

Congenital Anomaly	Nursing Assessments	Nursing Goals and Interventions
Tracheoesophageal fistula (type 3)	History of maternal hydramnios Excessive mucous secretions Constant drooling Abdominal distention beginning soon after birth Periodic choking and cyanotic episodes Immediate regurgitation of feeding Clinical symptoms of aspiration pneumonia (tachypnea, retractions, rhonchi, decreased breath sounds, cyanotic spells) Failure to pass nasogastric tube	Maintain respiratory status and prevent aspiration: Withhold feeding until esophageal patency is determined. Quickly assess patency before putting to breast in birth area. Place on low intermittent suction to control saliva and mucus (to prevent aspiration pneumonia). Place in warmed, humidified incubator (liquefies secretions, facilitating removal). Elevate head of bed 20–40 degrees (to prevent reflux of gastric juices). Keep quiet (crying causes air to pass through fistula and to distend intestines, causing respiratory embarrassment). Maintain fluid and electrolyte balance. Give fluids to replace esophageal drainage and maintain hydration. Provide parent education: Explain staged repair—provision of gastrostomy and ligation of fistula, then repair of atresia. Keep parents informed; clarify and reinforce physician's explanations regarding malformation, surgical repair, pre- and postoperative care, and prognosis (knowledge is ego strengthening). Involve parents in care of infant and in planning for future; facilitate touch and eye contact (to dispel feelings of inadequacy, increase self-esteem and self-worth, and promote incorporation of infant into family).

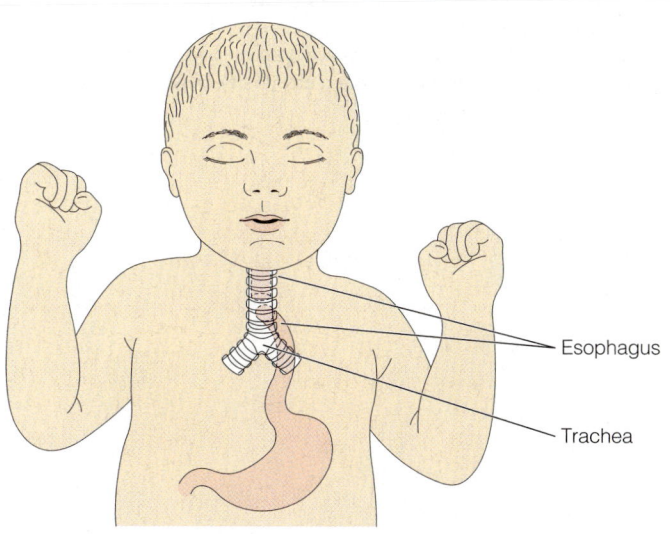

Esophagus

Trachea

(At left) The most frequently seen type of congenital tracheoesophageal fistula and esophageal atresia.

Diaphragmatic hernia	Difficulty initiating respirations Gasping respirations with nasal flaring and chest retraction Barrel chest and scaphoid abdomen Asymmetric chest expansion Breath sounds may be absent, usually on left side Heart sounds displaced to right Spasmodic attacks of cyanosis and difficulty in feeding Bowel sounds may be heard in thoracic cavity	Nurse should never ventilate with bag and mask O_2 because the stomach will inflate, further compressing the lungs. Maintain respiratory status: Immediately administer oxygen. Initiate gastric decompression. Place in high semi-Fowler's position (to use gravity to keep abdominal organs' pressure off diaphragm). Turn to affected side to allow unaffected lung expansion. Carry out interventions to alleviate respiratory and metabolic acidosis. Assess for increased secretions around suction tube (denotes possible obstruction). Aspirate and irrigate tube with air or sterile water.

Lung

Esophagus

Segment of small intestine

Diaphragm

Stomach

Liver

(At left) Diaphragmatic hernia. Note compression of the lung by the intestine on the affected side.

(continued)

Congenital Anomaly	Nursing Assessments	Nursing Goals and Interventions
Myelomeningocele	Saclike cyst containing meninges, spinal cord, and nerve roots in thoracic and/or lumbar area Myelomeningocele directly connects to subarachnoid space so hydrocephalus often associated No response or varying response to sensation below level of sac May have constant dribbling of urine Incontinence or retention of stool Anal opening may be flaccid	Prevent trauma and infection. Position on abdomen or on side and restrain (to prevent pressure and trauma to sac). Meticulously clean buttocks and genitals after each voiding and defecation (to prevent contamination of sac and decrease possibility of infection). May put protective covering over sac (to prevent rupture and drying). Observe sac for oozing of fluid or pus. Credé bladder (apply downward pressure on bladder with thumbs, moving urine toward the urethra) as ordered to prevent urinary stasis. Assess amount of sensation and movement below defect. Observe for complications. Obtain occipital-frontal circumference baseline measurements; then measure head circumference once a day (to detect hydrocephalus). Check fontanelle for bulging.

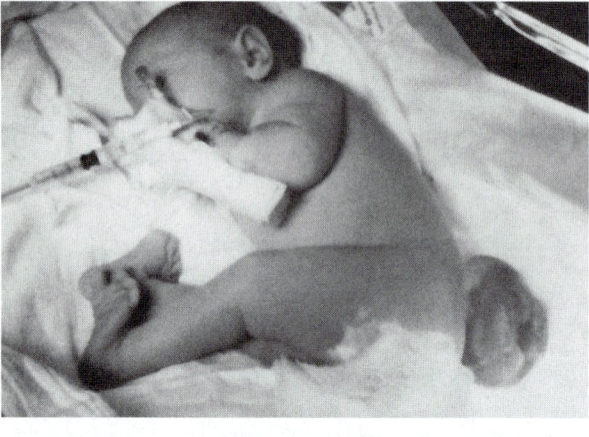

(At left) Newborn with lumbar myelomeningocele.
Source: Courtesy of Dr. Paul Winchester.

Omphalocele	Herniation of abdominal contents into base of umbilical cord May have an enclosed transparent sac covering	Maintain hydration and temperature: Provide D_5LR and albumin for hypovolemia. Place infant in sterile bag up to and covering defect. Cover sac with moistened sterile gauze, and place plastic wrap over dressing (to prevent rupture of sac and infection). Initiate gastric decompression by insertion of nasogastric tube attached to low suction (to prevent distention of lower bowel and impairment of blood flow). Prevent infection and trauma to defect. Position to prevent trauma to defect. Administer broad-spectrum antibiotics.
Imperforate anus, congenital dislocated hip, and clubfoot	See discussion in Chapter 25, Anus and Extremities	Identify defect and initiate appropriate referral early.

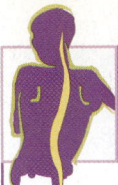

Congenital Heart Defect	*Clinical Findings*	*Medical-Surgical Management*
ACYANOTIC **Patent ductus arteriosus (PDA)** ↑ in females, maternal rubella, RDS, <1500 g preterm newborns, high-altitude births	Harsh grade 2–3 machinery murmur upper left sternal border (LSB) just beneath clavicle ↑ difference between systolic and diastolic pulse pressure Can lead to right heart failure and pulmonary congestion ↑ left atrial (LA) and left ventricular (LV) enlargement, dilated ascending aorta ↑ pulmonary vascularity	Indomethacin—0.2 mg/kg orally (prostaglandin inhibitor) Surgical ligation, occlusive coil Use of O₂ therapy and blood transfusion to improve tissue oxygenation and perfusion Fluid restriction and diuretics

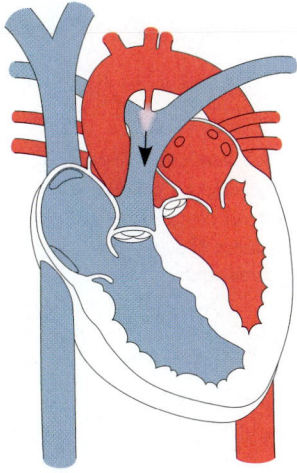

The patent ductus arteriosus is a vascular connection that, during fetal life, short-circuits the pulmonary vascular bed and directs blood from the pulmonary artery to the aorta. Postnatally, blood shunts through the ductus from the aorta to the pulmonary artery.

Atrial septal defect (ASD) ↑ in females and Down syndrome	Initially frequently asymptomatic Systolic murmur second left intercostal space (LICS) With large ASD, diastolic rumbling murmur lower left sternal (LLS) border Failure to thrive, upper respiratory infection (URI), poor exercise tolerance	Surgical closure with patch or suture
Ventricular septal defect (VSD) ↑ in males	Initially asymptomatic until end of first month or large enough to cause pulmonary edema Loud, blowing systolic murmur at third to fourth intercostal space (ICS). Inc. pulmonary blood flow Right ventricular hypertrophy Rapid respirations, growth failure, feeding difficulties CHF at 6 weeks to 2 months of age	Follow medically—some spontaneously close Use of lanoxin and diuretics in right congestive heart failure (CHF) Surgical closure with Dacron patch
Coarctation of aorta Can be preductal or postductal	Absent or diminished femoral pulses Increased brachial pulses Late systolic murmur left intrascapular area Systolic BP in lower extremities Enlarged left ventricle Can present in CHF at 7–21 days of life	Surgical resection of narrowed portion of aorta Prostaglandin E₁ to maintain peripheral perfusion No afterload reducer drugs

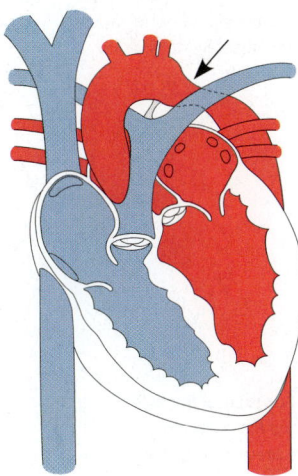

Coarctation of the aorta is characterized by a narrowed aortic lumen. The lesion produces an obstruction to the flow of blood through the aorta, causing an increased left ventricular pressure and workload.

(continued)

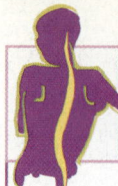
Congenital Heart Defect	Clinical Findings	Medical-Surgical Management
Hypoplastic left heart syndrome	Normal at birth—cyanosis and shocklike congestive heart failure develop within a few hours to days	PGE_1 until decision made
	Soft systolic murmur just left of the sternum	Transplant
	Diminished pulses	Currently no effective corrective treatment
	Aortic and/or mitral atresia	
	Tiny, thick-walled left ventricle	
	Large, dilated, hypertrophied right ventricle	
	X-ray, cardiac enlargement and pulmonary venous congestion	
CYANOTIC **Tetralogy of Fallot** (Most common cyanotic heart defect) Pulmonary stenosis Overriding aorta Right ventricular hypertrophy Ventricular septal defect (VSD)	May be cyanotic at birth or within first few months of life	Prevention of dehydration, intercurrent infections
	Harsh systolic murmur LSB	Alleviation of paroxysmal dyspneic attacks
	Crying or feeding increases cyanosis and respiratory distress	Palliative surgery to increase blood flow to the lungs
	X-ray boot-shaped appearance secondary to small pulmonary artery	Corrective surgery—resection of pulmonic stenosis, closure of VSD with Dacron patch
	Right ventricular enlargement	

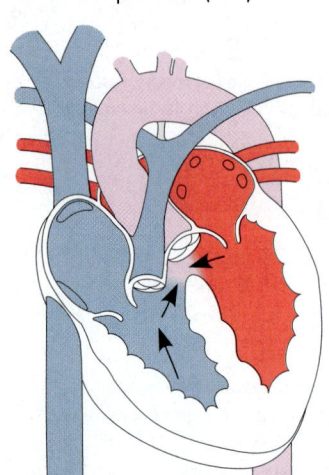

In tetralogy of Fallot, the severity of symptoms depends on the degree of pulmonary stenosis, the size of the ventricular septal defect, and the degree to which the aorta overrides the septal defect.

Transposition of great vessels (TGA) (↑ females, IDMs, LGAs)	Cyanosis at birth or within 3 days	Prostaglandin E to vasodilate ductus to keep it open
	Possible pulmonic stenosis murmur	Inotropic support
	Right ventricular hypertrophy	Initial surgery to create opening between right and left side of heart if none exists
	Polycythemia	Total surgical repair—usually the arterial switch procedure—done within first few days of life
	"Egg on its side" x-ray	

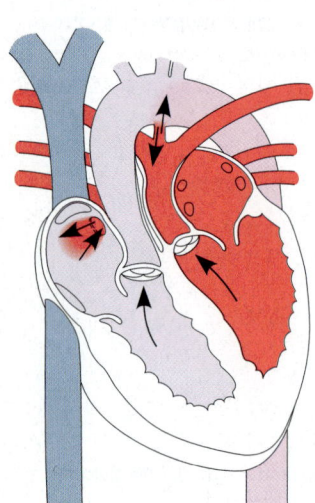

Complete transposition of great vessels is an embryonic defect caused by a straight division of the bulbar trunk without normal spiraling. As a result, the aorta originates from the right ventricle, and the pulmonary artery from the left ventricle. An abnormal communication between the two circulations must be present to sustain life.

Alcohol Dependence

The **fetal alcohol syndrome (FAS)** includes a series of malformations frequently found in infants exposed to alcohol in utero. It has been estimated that the complete FAS syndrome occurs in 5.2 live births per 10,000 (AAP Committee on Substance Abuse and Committee on Children with Disabilities, 2000). FAS rates are higher among Native Americans, Alaska natives, blacks, and those of low socioeconomic status. Fetal alcohol effects (FAE), or **alcohol-related birth defects (ARBD),** are usually determined only by a positive maternal drinking history and cognitive difficulties (Gardner, 2000). The new diagnostic categories for FAS take into consideration the various clinical manifestations of FAS, the social and family environment, and, if available, the maternal alcohol history (Hess & Kenner, 1998).

Although it is known that ethanol freely crosses the placenta to the fetus, it is still not known whether the alcohol alone or the breakdown products of alcohol cause the damage. (Chapter 12 ⬭ discusses alcohol abuse in pregnancy. The effects of other substances often combined with alcohol, such as nicotine, diazepam (Valium), marijuana, and caffeine, as well as poor diet, enhance the likelihood of FAS.

LONG-TERM COMPLICATIONS FOR THE INFANT WITH FAS

The long-term prognosis for the FAS newborn is less than favorable. Many FAS infants are evaluated for organic and inorganic failure to thrive. These infants have a delay in oral feeding development but have a normal progression of oral motor function. Many FAS infants nurse poorly and have persistent vomiting until 6 to 7 months of age. They have difficulty adjusting to solid foods and show little spontaneous interest in food.

Central nervous system dysfunctions are the most common and serious problem associated with FAS. Hypotonicity and increased placidity are seen in these infants. They also have a decreased ability to block out repetitive stimuli. Children exhibiting FAS can be severely mentally retarded or have normal intelligence. Generally the more abnormal the facial features, the lower the IQ scores. Often there is little improvement in intelligence (as measured by IQ) despite positive environmental and educational factors (Hess & Kenner, 1998). These children show impulsivity, cognitive impairment, and speech and language abnormalities indicative of CNS involvement (Ostrea, Posecion, & Villanueva, 1999).

Nursing Management

Nursing Assessment and Diagnosis

The nurse assesses the newborn for the following characteristics typical of FAS:

▶ Abnormal structural development and CNS dysfunction, including mental retardation, microcephaly, and hyperactivity.

▶ Growth deficiencies. Infants with FAS are often growth retarded; weight, length, and head circumference are affected. These infants show a persistent postnatal growth deficiency, with head circumference and linear growth most affected.

▶ Distinctive facial abnormalities. These include short palpebral fissures; epicanthal folds; broad nasal bridge; flattened midfacies; short, upturned, or beaklike nose; micrognathia (abnormally small lower jaw); hypoplastic maxilla; thin upper lip or vermilion border; and smooth philtrum (groove on upper lip) (Malanga & Kosofsky, 1999).

▶ Associated anomalies. Abnormalities affecting cardiac (primarily septal and valvular defects), ocular, renal, and skeletal (especially involving joints, such as congenital dislocated hips) systems are often noted.

In the first week of life, an alcohol-exposed newborn may show symptoms that include sleeplessness, excessive arousal states, unconsolable crying, abnormal reflexes, hyperactivity with little ability to maintain alertness and attentiveness to environment, jitteriness, abdominal distention, and exaggerated mouthing behaviors such as hyperactive rooting and increased nonnutritive sucking. These symptoms commonly persist throughout the first month of life but may continue longer (Ostrea et al., 1999). The infant's alcohol dependence is physiologic, not psychologic. Signs and symptoms of withdrawal often appear within 6 to 12 hours and at least within the first 3 days of life. Seizures after the neonatal period are rare.

Planning and Implementation

HOSPITAL-BASED NURSING CARE

Awareness of the signs and symptoms of FAS is important in planning and delivering nursing care. Nursing care of the FAS newborn is aimed at avoiding heat loss, providing adequate nutrition, and reducing environmental stimuli. The FAS baby is most comfortable in a quiet, dimly lit environment. Because of their feeding problems, these infants require extra time and patience during feedings. It is important to provide consistency in the staff working with the baby and parents and to keep personnel and visitors to a minimum at any one time.

Tell the alcohol-dependent mother that breastfeeding is not contraindicated but that excessive alcohol consumption may intoxicate the newborn and inhibit the letdown reflex. Monitor the newborn's vital signs closely and observe for evidence of seizure activity and respiratory distress.

NURSING CARE IN THE COMMUNITY

Infants affected by maternal alcohol abuse are also at risk psychologically. Restlessness, sleeplessness, agitation, resistance to cuddling or holding, and frequent crying can be frustrating to parents because their efforts to relieve the distress are unrewarded. Feeding difficulties can also result in frustrations for the caregiver and digestive upsets for the infant. Frustration may cause the parents to punish the baby or result in the unconscious desire to stay away from the infant. Either outcome may create an unstable family environment and result in failure to thrive.

Focus on providing support for the parents and reinforcing positive parenting activity. Prior to discharge, give parents opportunities to provide baby care so that they can feel confident about interpreting their baby's cues and meeting the baby's needs. Referring the family to social services and visiting nurse or public health nurse associations is essential for the well-being of the infant. Follow-up care and teaching can strengthen the parents' skill and coping abilities and help them create a stable, healthy environment for their family. The infant with FAS or ARBD should be involved in intervention programs that monitor the child's developmental progress, health, and home environment.

Evaluation

Expected outcomes of nursing care include the following:

▶ The FAS newborn is able to tolerate feedings and gain weight.

▶ The FAS infant's hyperirritability or seizures are controlled, and the baby has suffered no physical injuries.

▶ The parents are able to identify the special needs of their newborn and accept outside assistance as needed.

Drug Dependency

Drugs abused by the pregnant woman can include the following legal and illegal substances, used alone or in combination: tobacco, cocaine, phencyclidine (PCP), methamphetamines, inhalants, marijuana, heroin, and methadone.

Drug-dependent infants are predisposed to a number of problems. Since almost all drugs cross the placenta and enter the fetal circulation, the fetus can develop problems in utero or soon after birth.

The greatest risks to the fetus of the drug-abusing mother are as follows:

- *Intrauterine asphyxia.* Asphyxia is often a direct result of fetal withdrawal secondary to maternal withdrawal. Fetal withdrawal is accompanied by hyperactivity, with increased oxygen consumption. Insufficiency of oxygen can lead to fetal asphyxia. Moreover, women addicted to narcotics tend to have a higher incidence of PIH, abruptio placentae, and placenta previa, resulting in placental insufficiency and fetal asphyxia.

- *Intrauterine infection.* Sexually transmitted infection, HIV infection, and hepatitis are often connected with the pregnant addict's lifestyle. Such infections can involve the fetus.

- *Alterations in birth weight.* These alterations may depend on the type of drug the mother uses. Women who smoke or use heroin have infants of lower birth weight who are SGA. Women maintained on methadone have higher-birth-weight infants, some of whom are LGA.

- *Low Apgar scores.* These low scores may be related to the intrauterine asphyxia or the medication the woman received during labor. The use of a narcotic antagonist (nalorphine or naloxone) to reverse respiratory depression is contraindicated because it may precipitate acute withdrawal in the infant.

Patterns of abuse of alcohol, nicotine, marijuana, and heroin in childbearing women have changed very little, but the incidence of cocaine (especially crack) use has risen dramatically (see Chapter 12 for more discussion of maternal substance abuse). Marijuana, alcohol, and nicotine are sometimes used in conjunction with cocaine.

COMMON COMPLICATIONS OF THE DRUG-DEPENDENT NEWBORN

The newborn of a woman who abused drugs during her pregnancy is predisposed to the following problems:

- *Respiratory distress.* The heroin-addicted newborn frequently suffers respiratory stress, mainly meconium-aspiration pneumonia and transient tachypnea. Meconium aspiration is usually secondary to increased oxygen consumption and activity experienced by the fetus during intrauterine withdrawal. Transient tachypnea may develop because narcotics inhibit the reflex responsible for clearing the lungs. Respiratory distress syndrome, however, occurs less often in heroin-addicted newborns, even in those who are premature, because they have tissue-oxygen-unloading capabilities comparable to those of a 6-week-old term infant. In addition, heroin stimulates production of glucocorticoids via the anterior pituitary gland.

- *Jaundice.* Newborns of methadone-addicted women may develop jaundice due to prematurity. By contrast, infants of mothers addicted to heroin or cocaine have a lower incidence of hyperbilirubinemia because these substances contribute to early maturity of the liver.

- *Congenital anomalies and growth retardation.* Anomalies of the genitourinary and cardiovascular systems are slightly more common in infants of heroin- and cocaine-addicted mothers. Infants of cocaine-addicted mothers exhibit congenital malformations involving bony skull defects, such as microencephaly, and symmetric intrauterine growth retardation, cardiac defects, and genitourinary defects. Congenital anomalies, however, are rare (Bauer, 1999).

- *Behavioral abnormalities.* Babies exposed to cocaine have poor state organization. They exhibit decreased interactive behaviors when tested with the Brazelton Neonatal Behavioral Assessment Scale (Bauer, 1999). These infants also have difficulty moving through the various sleep and awake states and have problems attending to and actively engaging in auditory and visual stimuli.

- *Withdrawal.* The most significant postnatal problem of the drug-exposed newborn is opiate withdrawal (usually from heroin or methadone). Withdrawal manifestations often begin after discharge, especially with short birthing unit stays. See "Clinical Manifestations" for a discussion of withdrawal symptoms.

LONG-TERM EFFECTS

During the first 2 years of life, many cocaine-exposed infants demonstrate behavior lability and are unable to express strong feelings such as pleasure, anger, or distress, or even a strong reaction to being separated from their parents. Cocaine-exposed infants are at higher risk for motor development problems, delays in expressive language skills, and feeding difficulties because of swallowing problems (Eyler & Behnke, 1999).

Infants of drug-addicted mothers often have a higher incidence of gastrointestinal and respiratory illnesses. These illnesses can be related not to drug exposure but to the mother's lack of education regarding proper infant care, feeding, and hygiene.

Another important long-term complication is the high rate (15 to 20 per 1000 births) of SIDS in heroin- or methadone-exposed infants. After birth the infant born to a drug-dependent mother may also be neglected, abused, or both (Ostrea et al., 1999).

CLINICAL THERAPY

For optimal fetal and neonatal outcome, the opiate-addicted woman should receive complete prenatal care as early as possible (Chapter 12) and pharmacologic management of neonatal withdrawal. She should be started on a methadone program, with the aim of preventing heroin use (Buchi, 1998). The maintenance dose of methadone should be sufficient to ensure this goal (Kandall, Doberczak, Jantunen, et al., 1999). It is not recommended that the woman be withdrawn completely from narcotics while pregnant because it induces fetal withdrawal with poor newborn outcomes.

Newborn treatment may include management of newborn complications; serologic tests for syphilis, HIV, and hepatitis B; urine or hair drug screen and/or meconium analysis; and social service referral (Smeriglio & Wilcox, 1999). Drugs used to control withdrawal symptoms vary and may be regionally based. They include phenobarbital, paregoric, oral morphine sulfate solution, Donnatal elixir, and simethicone (Mylicon) drops. Nutritional support is important in light of the increase in energy expenditure that withdrawal may entail.

Nursing Management

Nursing Assessment and Diagnosis

Early identification of the newborn needing medical or pharmacologic interventions because of maternal substance abuse decreases the incidence of neonatal mortality and morbidity. During the newborn period, nursing assessment focuses on:

▶ Discovering the mother's last drug intake and dosage level through the perinatal history and laboratory tests. Women may be reluctant to disclose this information; therefore, a nonjudgmental interview technique is essential (Smeriglio & Wilcox, 1999).

▶ Assessing for congenital malformations and the complications related to intrauterine withdrawal such as SGA, intrauterine asphyxia, meconium aspiration, and prematurity.

▶ Identifying the signs and symptoms of newborn withdrawal or neonatal abstinence syndrome.

Clinical manifestations of newborn withdrawal can be classified in five groups.

Although many signs and symptoms of drug withdrawal are similar to those seen with hypoglycemia and hypocalcemia, drug addicted babies have normal glucose and calcium values. Assess the severity of withdrawal with a scoring system based on clinical manifestations. The system evaluates the infant on potentially life-threatening signs such as vomiting, diarrhea, weight loss, irritability, tremors, and tachypnea (Table 28–2).

Nursing diagnoses that may apply to drug-dependent newborns include:

▶ *Altered nutrition: less than body requirements* related to vomiting and diarrhea, uncoordinated suck and swallow reflex, and hypertonia secondary to withdrawal

▶ *Sleep pattern disturbance* related to CNS excitation secondary to drug withdrawal

▶ *Altered parenting* related to hyperirritable behavior of the infant

▶ *Ineffective family coping: disabling* related to drug abuse, poverty, and lack of education

Planning and Implementation

HOSPITAL-BASED NURSING CARE

Care of the drug-dependent newborn is based on reducing withdrawal symptoms and promoting adequate respiration, temperature, and nutrition. See "Clinical Pathway for Newborn of a Substance-Abusing Mother" on the companion website and "Nursing Care Plan for the Newborn of a Substance-Abusing Mother" on pages 637–638 for specific nursing measures. **WEB** General nursery care measures include the following:

▶ Temperature regulation

Central nervous system signs
- Hyperactivity
- Hyperirritability (persistent shrill cry)
- Increased muscle tone
- Exaggerated reflexes
- Tremors and myoclonic jerks
- Sneezing, hiccups, yawning
- Short, unquiet sleep
- Fever (accompanies the increased neuromuscular activities)

Respiratory signs
- Tachypnea (> 60 breaths per minute when quiet)
- Excessive secretions

Gastrointestinal signs
- Disorganized, vigorous suck
- Vomiting
- Drooling
- Sensitive gag reflex
- Hyperphagia
- Diarrhea
- Abdominal cramping
- Poor feeding (< 15 mL on first day of life; takes longer than 30 minutes per feeding)

Vasomotor signs
- Stuffy nose, yawning, sneezing
- Flushing
- Sweating
- Sudden, circumoral pallor

Cutaneous signs
- Excoriated buttocks, knees, elbows
- Facial scratches
- Pressure-point abrasions

▶ Careful monitoring of pulse and respirations every 15 minutes until stable; stimulation if apnea occurs

▶ Small, frequent feedings, especially if the infant has vomiting, regurgitation, and diarrhea

▶ IV therapy as needed

▶ Medications as ordered, such as phenobarbital and paregoric (but not methadone because of possible neonatal addiction to it); use of paregoric is controversial because it contains alcohol and camphor (AAP Committee on Drugs, 1998)

▶ Positioning on the right side to avoid possible aspiration of vomitus or secretions

▶ Monitoring frequency of diarrhea and vomiting and weighing infant every 8 hours during withdrawal

▶ Observation for problems of SGA or LGA newborns

▶ Swaddling with hands near mouth to minimize injury and help achieve more organized behavioral state; gentle, vertical rocking can calm an infant who is out of control

▶ Placing newborn in quiet, dimly lit area of nursery

NURSING CARE IN THE COMMUNITY

Parents need assistance to prepare for what they can expect for the first few months at home. At the time of discharge, tell the mother to anticipate mild jitteriness and irritability in the newborn, which may persist from 8 to 16 weeks, depending on the initial severity of the withdrawal. Infants with neonatal abstinence syndrome are at a significantly higher risk for SIDS when the mother used heroin or cocaine. The infant should sleep supine and home apnea monitoring should be implemented (Blatt, Mequid, & Church, 2000). Help the mother learn feeding techniques, comforting measures, how to recognize newborn cues, and appropriate parenting responses (French, Pituch, Brandt, et al., 1998). Counsel parents about available resources, such as support groups, and when to seek further care. Ongoing evaluation is necessary because of the potential for long-term problems. Follow-up on missed appointments can bring parents back into the health care system, thereby improving parent and infant outcomes and promoting a positive, interactive environment after birth.

TABLE 28-2   Assessment of the Clinical Severity of Neonatal Narcotic Withdrawal

Symptom	Mild	Moderate	Severe
Vomiting	Spitting up	Extensive vomiting for three successive feedings	Vomiting associated with imbalance of serum electrolytes
Diarrhea	Watery stools < four times per day	Watery stools five to six times per day for 3 days; no electrolyte imbalance	Diarrhea associated with imbalance of serum electrolytes
Weight loss	< 10% of birth weight	10%–15% of birth weight	> 15%
Irritability	Minimal	Marked but relieved by cuddling or feeding	Unrelieved by cuddling or feeding
Tremors or twitching	Mild tremors when stimulated	Marked tremors or twitching when stimulated	Convulsions
Tachypnea	60–80 breaths/minute	80–100 breaths/minute	>100 breaths/minute; associated with respiratory alkalosis

Source: Ostrea, E. M., Chavez, C. J., & Stryker, J. S. (1978). *The care of the drug dependent woman and her infant* (p. 33), Lansing, MI, Michigan Department of Public Health.

GOAL	INTERVENTION	RATIONALE	EXPECTED OUTCOME

1. High risk for infant CNS injury related to perinatal substance abuse

GOAL	INTERVENTION	RATIONALE	EXPECTED OUTCOME
The newborn will be free of signs and symptoms of CNS injury.	*NIC Intervention:* **Newborn monitoring:** *Measurement and interpretation of physiologic status of the neonate the first 24 hours after delivery* ▶ Obtain prenatal records and question patient about history of drug addiction. Include duration, type of drug or drugs used, time and amount of last dose taken prior to delivery. ▶ Assess newborn for signs and symptoms of withdrawal (i.e., high-pitched shrill cry, sneezing, vomiting, diarrhea, hypertonicity, restlessness, and wakefulness). ▶ Provide a quiet and calm environment. Swaddle infant tightly and place in a side-lying or prone position. ▶ Carefully plan tests and/or treatments to avoid excessive stimuli. ▶ Use soothing techniques such as, rocking, cuddling, soft music, and soft tones when speaking. ▶ Administer appropriate medications as ordered by physician. Monitor efficacy and side effects of these medications that may include: paregoric and phenobarbital.	▶ Noting the mother's last drug ingestion will provide the medical staff with an approximate time frame to expect the infant to exhibit withdrawal symptoms. ▶ The average symptoms of withdrawal occur 72 hours after birth; however, symptoms may appear as early as 6–24 hours after birth. ▶ Providing a quiet environment decreases stimuli; therefore, reducing CNS symptoms. ▶ Planning care promotes rest and reduces external stimuli. ▶ These activities promote comfort, security, and infant bonding. ▶ These medications aid patient in alleviating symptoms related to withdrawal.	*NOC Outcome:* **Neurologic status:** *Extent to which the peripheral and central nervous systems receive, process, and respond to internal and external stimuli* Infant will have no signs and symptoms of CNS injury as evidenced by reduced hyperactivity, irritability, normal sleep-wake pattern, no jitteriness, and no seizure activity.

2. Risk for ineffective airway clearance related to suppression of respiratory system

GOAL	INTERVENTION	RATIONALE	EXPECTED OUTCOME
Infant will be free of signs and symptoms of respiratory distress after birth.	*NIC Intervention:* **Respiratory monitoring:** *Collection and analysis of patient data to ensure airway patency and adequate gas exchange* ▶ Obtain maternal prenatal, labor, and delivery records. ▶ Assess infant's respiratory rate and effort, skin color, heart rate, presence or absence of cough reflex, and symptoms of respiratory distress. ▶ Position infant in a side-lying or semi-Fowler's position. ▶ Monitor infant for temperature elevation. **Collaboration:** *Obtain arterial blood gases as ordered by physician.* ▶ Monitor infant's cardiac status and pulmonary status using EKG and pulse oximetry.	▶ Provides information of fetal stress that may have occurred during the prenatal or intrapartal period. In addition, the delivery record will provide information concerning infant's respiratory status at birth; for example, the Apgar score. ▶ Maternal narcotic consumption may depress the cough reflex and respiratory center of the infant after birth. Symptoms such as cyanosis, tachycardia, grunting, retractions, and nasal flaring may indicate hypoxia. ▶ Prevents aspiration. ▶ Temperature elevation may cause metabolic rate and oxygen needs to increase when associated with CNS stimulation. ▶ Oxygen demands increase with drug withdrawal. Obtaining ABGs will provide medical personnel baseline information of infant's respiratory status and effective medical interventions can be initiated. ▶ Provides medical personnel with cardiac and pulmonary status.	*NOC Outcome:* **Respiratory status: Gas exchange:** *Alveolar exchange of CO_2 or O_2 to maintain arterial blood gas concentrations*

(continued)

GOAL	INTERVENTION	RATIONALE	EXPECTED OUTCOME
3. Altered nutrition: less than body requirements related to poor sucking and swallowing			
	NIC Intervention:		*NOC Outcome:*
	Nutrition therapy: *Administration of food and fluids to support metabolic processes of a patient who is malnourished or at high risk for becoming malnourished*		**Nutritional status:** *Extent to which nutrients are available to meet metabolic needs*
The infant will gain or maintain weight.	▶ Review gestational age assessment.		The infant will tolerate feedings, maintain weight, or gain weight as evidenced by no regurgitation or aspiration of feedings, adequate weight gain according to weight graph.
	▶ Assess infant's sucking and swallowing reflexes.	▶ Oral feeding may be difficult due to CNS hyperactivity and GI hypermobility	
	▶ Monitor regurgitation, vomiting, diarrhea.	▶ GI hypermobility, irritation, and CNS stimulation can increase nutritional needs.	
	▶ Use bulb syringe before feedings if having problems with nasal stuffiness and congestion.	▶ Allows infant to breathe easier by ridding the nasal passages of excessive mucous.	
	▶ Initiate appropriate feedings per physician's orders (i.e., oral, gavage, or IV feedings).	▶ Facilitates nutritional intake because SGA infants require 110–120 kcal/kg/day for adequate nutrition.	
	▶ Provide small frequent feedings of a high calorie formula.		
	▶ Position infant on right side after feedings.	▶ Prevents regurgitation and promotes gastric emptying.	
	▶ Monitor infant's weight and document on graph.	▶ Identifies abnormalities in weight gain/loss and allows for early intervention when necessary.	
4. Risk for altered parenting related to lack of knowledge of infant care			*NOC Outcome:*
	NIC Intervention:		**Parenting:** *Provision of an environment that promotes optimum growth and development of dependent children*
	Teaching: Infant care: *Instruction on nurturing and physical care needed during the first year of life*		The patient will demonstrate ability to perform basic infant care tasks as evidenced by exhibiting appropriate attachment behaviors (i.e., talking and holding infant), feeding infant, and bathing infant.
The patient will demonstrate ability to independently provide infant care.	▶ Assess mother's desire to learn infant care tasks as well as evaluate her present physical and emotional stability.	▶ Will provide knowledge of mother's ability to care for infant.	
	▶ Instruct mother on coping strategies (i.e., exercise, listening to music, and discussing concerns openly) to manage stressful situations.	▶ Will give mother the tools to handle stress, thereby decreasing the chances of exhibiting abusive behavior.	
	▶ Assess mother's insight into her own chemical dependency.	▶ Assistance in enrollment into a chemical dependency program may be necessary before mother can independently care for infant.	
	▶ Instruct mother on signs and symptoms of withdrawal and treatment interventions.	▶ Assists the mother in understanding infant's behaviors and gives her the tools to intervene without feeling anxious.	
	▶ Encourage mother and family members to perform basic infant care tasks.	▶ Facilitates attachment and increases parenting competence.	

Evaluation

Expected outcomes of nursing care include the following:

▶ The newborn tolerates feedings, gains weight, and has a decreased number of stools.

▶ The parents learn ways to comfort their newborn.

▶ The parents cope with their frustrations and begin to use outside resources as needed.

CARE OF THE NEWBORN AT RISK FOR HIV/AIDS

An increasing number of newborns are born infected with HIV or at risk for acquiring it in the newborn period or early infancy. Perinatal and neonatal transmission can occur across the placenta or through breast milk or contaminated blood. Maternal-to-newborn vertical transmission rates are about 25% to 30% in the United States; most infants born to infected mothers remain uninfected (Freij & Sever, 1999). The risk of vertical transmission can be decreased by two thirds in mothers taking zidovudine during gestation. (For discussion of maternal and fetal HIV/AIDS see Chapter 12 and for the infant with HIV/AIDS see Chapter 40.) ◯▭

CARE OF THE NEWBORN WITH INBORN ERRORS OF METABOLISM

Inborn errors of metabolism are a group of hereditary disorders transmitted by mutant genes. Most are transmitted by an autosomal recessive gene, requiring two heterozygous parents to produce a homozygous infant with the disorder. Carriers of some disorders can be identified by special tests, and some inborn errors of metabolism can be detected in utero. Some of the inborn errors of metabolism (especially those associated with mental retardation) are now detected neonatally through newborn screening programs (see Chapter 26). ◯▭ For more extensive discussion of inborn errors of metabolism see Chapter 51. ◯▭

$\mathcal{C}$HAPTER HIGHLIGHTS

☞ Early identification of potential high-risk fetuses through assessment of prepregnant, prenatal, and intrapartal factors helps nurses strategically time their observations and interventions.

☞ High-risk newborns, whether premature, SGA, LGA, postterm, IDM, or ISAM, have many similar problems, although their problems are based on different physiologic processes.

☞ SGA newborns are at risk for perinatal asphyxia and resulting aspiration syndrome, hypothermia, hypoglycemia, hypocalcemia, polycythemia, congenital anomalies, and intrauterine infections. Long-term problems include continued growth and learning difficulties.

☞ LGA newborns are at risk for birth trauma as a result of CPD, hypoglycemia, polycythemia, and hyperviscosity.

☞ IDMs are at risk for hypoglycemia, hypocalcemia, hyperbilirubinemia, polycythemia, and respiratory distress due to delayed maturation of their lungs.

☞ Postterm newborns often have the following problems: CPD (shoulder dystocia) and birth traumas, hypoglycemia, polycythemia, meconium aspiration, cold stress, and possible seizure activity. Long-term complications may involve poor weight gain and low IQ scores.

☞ The common problems of the preterm newborn are a result of the baby's immature body systems. Potential problems include RDS, patent ductus arteriosus, hypothermia and cold stress, feeding difficulties and NEC, marked insensible water loss and loss of buffering agents through the kidneys, infection, anemia of prematurity, apnea and intraventricular hemorrhage, retinopathy of prematurity, and behavioral state disorganization. Long-term needs and problems include bronchopulmonary dysplasia, speech defects, sensorineural hearing loss, and neurologic defects.

☞ Newborns of alcohol-dependent mothers are at risk for physical characteristic alterations and the long-term complications of feeding problems; CNS dysfunction, including low IQ, hyperactivity, and language abnormalities; and congenital anomalies.

☞ Newborns born to drug-dependent mothers experience drug withdrawal as well as respiratory distress, jaundice, congenital anomalies, and behavioral abnormalities. Early recognition and intervention can help avoid or minimize the potential long-term physiologic and emotional consequences of these difficulties.

☞ Newborns exposed to HIV/AIDS require early recognition and treatment to lessen the severity of the physiologic and emotional consequences and to implement CDC guidelines.

☞ Cardiac defects are a significant cause of morbidity and mortality in the newborn period. Early identification and nursing and medical care of newborns with cardiac defects are essential to improve the outcome of these infants. Care is directed toward lessening the workload of the heart and decreasing oxygen and energy consumption.

☞ Inborn errors of metabolism such as galactosemia, PKU, and MSUD are often included in a newborn screening program designed to prevent mental retardation through dietary management and medication.

☞ The nursing care of the newborn with special problems involves understanding normal physiology, the pathophysiology of the disease process, clinical manifestations, supportive or corrective therapies, and rationale behind nursing interventions. Only with this theoretic background can the nurse make appropriate observations about responses to therapy and development of complications.

☞ Parents of the at-risk newborn need support from nurses and health care providers to understand the special needs of their baby and feel confident in their ability to care for their children at home.

🌐💿 EXPLORE MediaLink

NCLEX Review, Case Studies, and other interactive resources for this chapter can be found on the companion website at http://www.prenhall.com/london. Click on "Chapter 28" to select the activities for this chapter.

For animations, more NCLEX review questions, and an audio glossary, access the accompanying CD-ROM in this textbook.

REFERENCES

Als, H. (1998). Developmental care in the newborn intensive care unit. *Current Opinion in Pediatrics, 10,* 138–142.

Als, H., Lester, B. M., Tronick, E., & Brazelton, T. B. (1982). Assessment of preterm infant behavior (APIB). In B. M. Fitzgerald Lester & M. W. Yogman (Eds.), *Theory and research in behavioral pediatrics* (Vol. 1, pp. 35–82). New York: Plenum.

American Academy of Pediatrics, Committee on Drugs. (1998). Neonatal drug withdrawal. *Pediatrics, 101*(6), 1079–1088.

American Academy of Pediatrics, Committee on Substance Abuse and Committee on Children with Disabilities. (2000). Fetal alcohol syndrome and alcohol-related neurodevelopmental disorders. *Pediatrics, 106*(2), 358–361.

American Academy of Pediatrics & American College of Obstetricians and Gynecologists. (1997). *Guidelines for perinatal care* (4th ed.). Elk Grove Village, IL: Author.

Anderson, M. S., & Hay, W. W. (1999). Intrauterine growth restriction and the small-for-gestational-age infant. In G. B. Avery, M. A. Fletcher, & M. G. MacDonald (Eds.), *Neonatology: Pathophysiology and management of the newborn* (5th ed., pp. 411–444). Philadelphia: Lippincott Williams & Wilkins.

Bauer, C. R. (1999). Perinatal effects of prenatal drug exposure. *Clinics in Perinatology, 26*(1), 87–106.

Blackburn, S. (1998). Environmental impact of the NICU on developmental outcomes. *Journal of Pediatric Nursing, 13*(5), 279–289.

Blatt, S. D., Mequid, V., & Church, C. C. (2000). Prenatal cocaine: What's known about outcomes? *Contemporary Pediatrics, 17*(5), 43–57.

Buchi, K. F. (1998). The drug-exposed infant in the well-baby nursery. *Clinics in Perinatology, 25*(2), 335–350.

Chatfield, J. (2001). ACOG issues guidelines on fetal macrosomia. *American Family Physician, 64*(1), 169–170.

Cunningham, F. G., MacDonald, P. C., Gant, N. F., Leveno, K. J., Gilstrap, L. C., Hauth, J. C., et al. (2001). *Williams obstetrics* (21st ed.). New York: McGraw-Hill.

Engebretson, J. C., & Wardell, D. W. (1997). Developing of a pacifier for low-birth-weight infants' nonnutritive sucking. *Journal of Obstetric, Gynecologic, and Neonatal Nursing, 26*(6), 660–664.

Eyler, F. D., & Behnke, M. (1999). Early development of infants exposed to drugs prenatally. *Clinics in Perinatology, 26*(1), 107–150.

Freij, B. J., & Sever, J. L. (1999). Chronic infections. In G. B. Avery, M. A. Fletcher, & M. G. MacDonald (Eds.), *Neonatology: Pathophysiology and management of the newborn* (5th ed., pp. 1123–1188). Philadelphia: Lippincott Williams & Wilkins.

French, E. D., Pituch, M., Brandt, J., & Pohorecki, S. (1998). Improving interactions between substance-abusing mothers and their substance-exposed newborns. *Journal of Obstetric, Gynecologic, and Neonatal Nursing, 27*(3), 262–269.

Gardner, J. (2000). Fetal alcohol syndrome. *American Journal of Maternal Child Nursing, 25*(5), 252–257.

Hess, D. J., & Kenner, C. (1998). Families caring for children with fetal alcohol syndrome: The nurse's role in early identification and intervention. *Holistic Nursing Practice, 12*(3), 47–54.

Horns, K. M. (1998). Being-in-tune caregiving. *Journal of Perinatal Neonatal Nursing, 12*(3), 38–49.

Kandall, S. R., Doberczak, T. M., Jantunen, M., & Stein, J. (1999). The methadone-maintained pregnancy. *Clinics in Perinatology, 26*(1), 173–183.

Kliegman, R. M., & Das, Utpala G. (2002). Intrauterine growth retardation. In A. A. Fanaroff & R. J. Martin (Eds.), *Neonatal-perinatal medicine: Diseases of the fetus and infant* (7th ed., pp. 228–262). St. Louis, MO: Mosby.

Langer, O. (2000). Fetal macrosomia: Etiologic factors. *Clinical Obstetrics and Gynecology, 43*(2), 283–297.

Malanga, C. J., & Kosofsky, B. E. (1999). Mechanisms of action of drugs of abuse on the developing fetal brain. *Clinics in Perinatology, 26*(1), 17–37.

Merenstein, G. B., & Gardner, S. L. (1998). *Handbook of neonatal intensive care* (4th ed.). St. Louis, MO: Mosby.

Moran, M., Radzyminski, S. G., Higgins, K. R., Dowling, D. A., Miller, M. J., & Cranston Anderson, G. (1999). Maternal kangaroo (skin-to-skin) care in the NICU beginning 4 hours postbirth. *Journal of Maternal Child Nursing, 24*(2), 74–79.

Neonatal thermoregulation. (1997). In *NANN guidelines for practice.* (pp. 1–15) Petaluma, CA: National Association of Neonatal Nurses.

Newell, S. J. (2000). Enteral feeding of the micropremie. *Clinics in Perinatology, 27*(1), 221–234.

Ostrea, E. M., Posecion, E. C., & Villanueva, M. E. T. (1999). The infant of the drug-dependent mother. In G. B. Avery, M. A. Fletcher, & M. G. MacDonald (Eds.), *Neonatology: Pathophysiology and management of the newborn* (5th ed., pp. 1407–1446). Philadelphia: Lippincott Williams & Wilkins.

Resnik, R., & Calder, A. (1999). Post-term pregnancy. In R. K. Creasy & R. Resnik (Eds.), *Maternal-fetal medicine* (4th ed., pp. 532–540). Philadelphia: Saunders.

Siegfried, E. C. (1998). Neonatal skin and skin care. *Dermatologic Clinics, 16*(3), 437–446.

Smeriglio, V. L., & Wilcox, H. C. (1999). Prenatal drug exposure and child outcome: Past, present, future. *Clinics in Perinatology, 26*(1), 1–16.

Uvena-Celebrezze, J., & Catalano, P. M. (2000). The infant of the woman with gestational diabetes mellitus. *Clinical Obstetrics and Gynecology, 43*(1), 127–139.

CHAPTER 29

The Newborn at Risk: Birth-Related Stressors

We watched him breathe every precious breath. He was covered with wires and tubes. The rhythmic tides of his sleeping and feeding spaciously measured his days and nights. We kept watch. He was special to us and we would say over and over, "Daddy and mommy are here and we love you."

—ALAN AND CLAUDIA, PARENTS OF A BABY WITH RDS

Key Terms

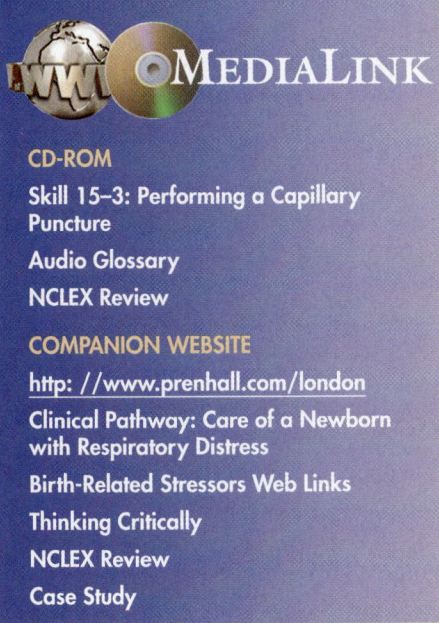

MediaLink

CD-ROM

Skill 15–3: Performing a Capillary Puncture

Audio Glossary

NCLEX Review

COMPANION WEBSITE

http://www.prenhall.com/london

Clinical Pathway: Care of a Newborn with Respiratory Distress

Birth-Related Stressors Web Links

Thinking Critically

NCLEX Review

Case Study

$\mathcal{M}$arked homeostatic changes happen during the transition from fetal to neonatal life. The most rapid anatomic and physiologic changes of this period occur in the cardiopulmonary system, so the newborn's major problems are usually related to this system. These problems include asphyxia, respiratory distress, cold stress, jaundice, hemolytic disease, and anemia. Ideally, problems are anticipated and identified prenatally, and appropriate intervention measures are begun at or immediately after birth.

CARE OF THE NEWBORN AT RISK DUE TO ASPHYXIA

Neonatal asphyxia results in circulatory, respiratory, and biochemical changes. Circulatory patterns that accompany asphyxia indicate the newborn's inability to make the transition to extrauterine circulation—in effect, a return to fetal circulatory patterns. Failure of lung expansion and establishment of respiration rapidly produces hypoxia (decreased PaO_2), acidosis (decreased pH), and hypercarbia (increased PCO_2). These biochemical changes cause pulmonary vasoconstriction, with retention of high pulmonary vascular resistance, hypoperfusion of the lungs, and a large right-to-left shunt through the ductus arteriosus. The foramen ovale opens (as right atrial pressure exceeds left atrial pressure), and blood flows from right to left. (See Chapter 24 for a review of normal newborn cardiopulmonary adaptation.)

Biochemical changes that occur in asphyxia contribute to these circulatory changes. The most serious biochemical abnormality is a change from aerobic to anaerobic metabolism in the presence of hypoxia. This change results in the accumulation of lactate and the development of metabolic acidosis. Simultaneous respiratory acidosis may also occur due to a rapid increase in PCO_2 during asphyxia. In response to hypoxia and anaerobic metabolism, the amounts of free fatty acids (FFAs) and glycerol in the blood increase. Glycogen stores are also mobilized to provide a continuous glucose source for the brain. Hepatic and cardiac stores of glycogen may be used up rapidly during an asphyxial attack.

The newborn has several protective mechanisms against hypoxic insults. These include a relatively immature brain and a resting metabolic rate lower than that of adults, an ability to mobilize substances within the body for anaerobic metabolism and to use energy more efficiently, and an intact circulatory system able to redistribute lactate and hydrogen ions in tissues still being perfused. Unfortunately, severe, prolonged hypoxia overcomes these protective mechanisms, resulting in brain damage or death of the newborn.

The newborn who is apneic at birth requires immediate resuscitative efforts. The need for resuscitation can be anticipated if specific risk factors are present during the pregnancy or labor and birth.

Risk Factors Predisposing to Asphyxia

The need for resuscitation may be anticipated if the mother demonstrates the antepartal and intrapartal risk factors described in Tables 7–1 and 16–1. Neonatal risk factors for resuscitation are as follows:

- Nonreassuring fetal heart rate pattern
- Difficult birth
- Fetal blood loss
- Apneic episode unresponsive to tactile stimulation
- Inadequate ventilation
- Prematurity
- Structural lung abnormality (congenital diaphragmatic hernia, lung hypoplasia)
- Cardiac arrest

Risk factors are not always apparent prenatally. Particular attention must be paid to all at-risk pregnancies during the intrapartal period. Certain aspects of labor and birth challenge the oxygen supply to the fetus, and often the at-risk fetus has less tolerance for the stress of labor and birth.

Clinical Therapy

The initial goal of medical management is to identify the fetus at risk for asphyxia, so that resuscitative efforts can begin at birth. Fetal biophysical assessment (see Chapter 14), combined with monitoring of fetal pH, fetal heart rates during the intrapartal period, and fetal oximetry if available, may help identify fetal distress. If the fetus is in distress, appropriate measures can be taken to deliver the fetus immediately, before major damage occurs, and to treat the asphyxiated newborn.

In addition to the fetal biophysical profile, fetal scalp blood sampling may indicate asphyxic insult and the degree of fetal acidosis, when considered in relation to the stage of labor, uterine contractions, and the presence of nonreassuring fetal heart rate (FHR) patterns. The stress of labor causes an intermittent decrease in exchange of gases in the placental intervillous space, which causes the fall in pH and fetal acidosis. The acidosis is primarily metabolic.

During labor, a fetal pH of 7.2 or higher is considered normal. A pH value of 7.2 or less is considered an ominous sign. However, low fetal pH without associated hypoxia can be caused by maternal acidosis secondary to prolonged labor, dehydration, and maternal lactate production. The treatment of fetal or newborn asphyxia is resuscitation. The goals of resuscitation are to provide an adequate airway with expansion of the lungs, to decrease the PCO_2 and increase the PO_2, to support adequate cardiac output, and to minimize oxygen consumption by reducing heat loss.

Resuscitation Management

Initial resuscitative management of the newborn is extremely important. Caregivers should keep the infant in a head-down position before the first gasp to avoid aspiration of the oropharyngeal secretions and must suction the oropharynx and nasopharynx immediately. Clearing the nasal and oral passages of obstructive fluid establishes a patent airway. Suctioning is always performed before resuscitation so that mucus, blood, or meconium is not aspirated into the lungs. After the first few breaths, the nurse places the newborn in a level position under a radiant heat source and dries the baby quickly with towels to maintain skin temperature at about 36.5 °C (97.7 °F). The newborn may be placed on the mother's chest or abdomen "skin-to-skin" as another heat source. Drying is also a good stimulation to breathing. Heat loss through evaporation is tremendous during the first few minutes of life. The temperature of a wet, 1500-g baby in a cold (16 °C [62 °F]) birthing room can drop 1 °C every 3 minutes. Hypothermia increases oxygen consumption. In an asphyxiated infant, it increases the hypoxic insult and may lead to severe acidosis and respiratory distress.

Assessment of the newborn's need for resuscitation begins at birth. The nurse should note the time of the first gasp, first cry, and onset of sustained respirations in the order of occurrence. The Apgar score (see Chapter 17) may help determine the severity of the neonatal depression and predict neonatal survival. However, all neonates should be fully resuscitated and interventions should never be delayed pending the 1-minute Apgar score (Baskett, 2000; Casey, McIntire, & Leveno, 2001; Patel, Piotrowski, Nelson, et al., 2001).

Breathing is established with the simplest form of resuscitative measures first, progressing to more complicated methods as required:

1. Simple stimulation is provided by rubbing the newborn's back or flicking the feet.

2. If respirations have not been initiated or are inadequate (gasping or occasional respirations), the lungs must be inflated with positive pressure. The mask is positioned securely on the face (over nose and mouth, avoiding the eyes), with the infant's head in a "sniffing" or neutral position (Figure 29–1 ◆). Hyperextension of the infant's neck obstructs the trachea. An airtight connection is made between the baby's face and the mask (thus allowing the bag to inflate). The lungs are inflated rhythmically by squeezing the bag. Oxygen can be delivered at 100% with an anesthesia bag with manometer or modified self-inflating bag and adequate liter flow of at least 5 L/min. The self-inflating (Ambu or Hope) bag delivers only 40% oxygen unless it has been adapted with an attached oxygen reservoir. In addition, it may not be possible to maintain adequate inspiratory pressure. In a crisis

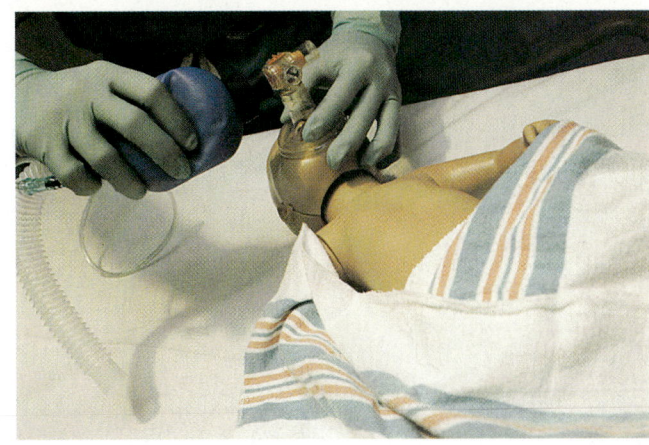

FIGURE 29–1. ◆ Demonstration of resuscitation of an infant with bag and mask. Note that the mask covers the nose and mouth, and the head is in a neutral position. The resuscitating bag is placed to the side of the baby so that chest movement can be seen.

situation, it is crucial that 100% oxygen be delivered with adequate pressure.

3. The rise and fall of the chest are observed for proper ventilation. Air entry and heart rate are checked by auscultation. Manual resuscitation is coordinated with any voluntary efforts. The rate of ventilation should be between 40 and 60 breaths per minute. Pressure should be adequate to move the chest wall. The pressure gauge (manometer) must be in place to avoid overdistention of the newborn's lungs and other problems such as pneumothorax or abdominal distention. In newborns with normal lungs, 15 to 25 cm H_2O may be adequate. If the newborn has lung disease, 20 to 40 cm H_2O may be necessary. If the newborn has not taken a first breath after birth, pressures of > 30 cm H_2O may be transiently required to expand collapsed alveoli. If ventilation is adequate, the chest moves with each inspiration, bilateral breath sounds are audible, and the lips and mucous membranes become pink. Distention of the stomach is controlled by inserting a nasogastric tube for decompression.

4. Endotracheal intubation may be needed. However, most newborns, except for very-low-birth-weight (VLBW) infants (< 1500 g), can be resuscitated by bag and mask ventilation. With preterm neonates, positive end expiratory pressure (PEEP) is required to help prevent alveolar collapse (Wong & Stenson, 2001). If the baby is intubated and the color and heart rate fail to respond to ventilatory efforts, poor or improper placement of an endotracheal tube may be the cause. If the baby is intubated properly, suspect pneumothorax, diaphragmatic hernia, or hypoplastic lungs (Potter's association).

Once breathing has been established, the heart rate should increase to over 100 beats per minute. If the heart

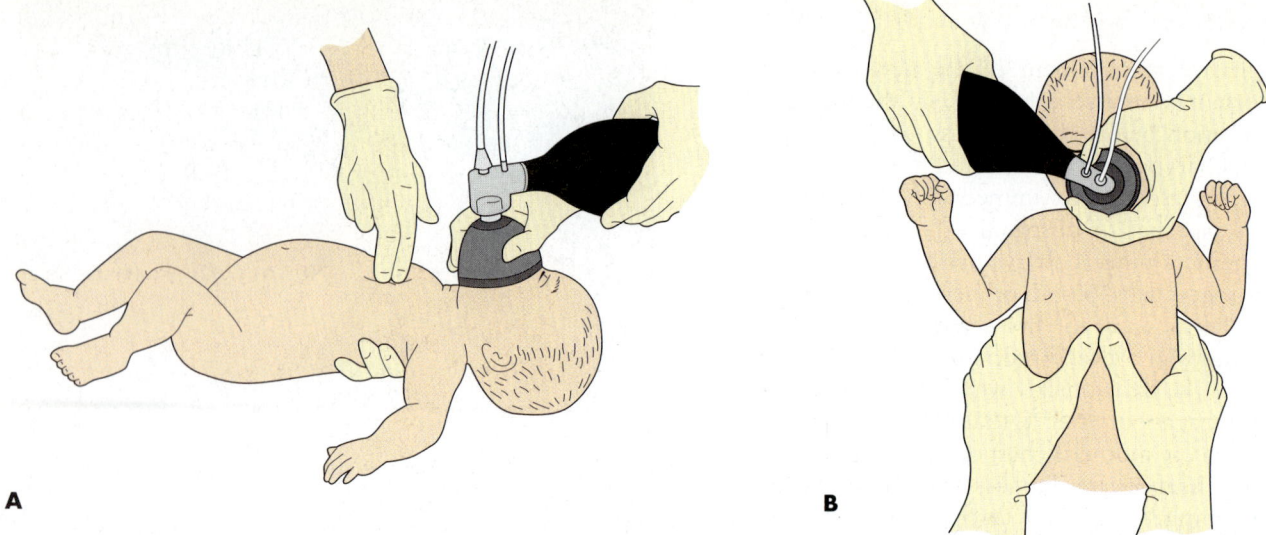

FIGURE 29–2. ◆ External cardiac massage. The lower third of the sternum is compressed with two fingertips or thumbs at a rate of 90 compressions per minute. **A,** The two-fingers method uses the tips of two fingers of one hand to compress the sternum and the other hand or a firm surface to support the infant's back. **B,** The thumb method uses the fingers to support the infant's back and uses both thumbs to compress the sternum and is the *preferred method.*

rate is absent or if it remains less than 60 beats per minute after 30 seconds of adequate assisted ventilation with 100% oxygen, external cardiac massage (chest compression) is begun. Chest compressions are started immediately if there is no detectable heartbeat. The procedure for performing chest compressions is:

1. The infant is positioned properly on a firm surface.
2. The resuscitator may (Figure 29–2 ◆) stand at the foot of the infant and place both thumbs over the lower third of the sternum (just below an imaginary line drawn between the nipples), with the fingers wrapped around and supporting the back, or use the two-finger method. The two-thumb method is preferred because it may provide better coronary perfusion pressure; however, it makes access to the umbilical cord for medication administration more difficult (Klaus & Fanaroff, 2001).
3. The sternum is depressed to sufficient depth to generate a palpable pulse or approximately one third of the anterior-posterior depth of the chest at a rate of 90 compressions per minute (American Academy of Pediatrics [AAP] & American Heart Association [AHA], 2000). Use a 3:1 ratio of heartbeat to assisted ventilation.

Drugs that should be available in the birthing area include those needed in the treatment of shock, cardiac arrest, and narcosis.

If, after 30 seconds of ventilation and cardiac compression, the newborn has not responded with spontaneous respirations and a heart rate above 60 beats per minute, resuscitative medications are necessary (AAP & AHA, 2000). The most accessible route for administering medications is the umbilical vein. If bradycardia is present, epinephrine (0.1 to 0.3 mL/kg of a 1:10,000 solution) is given through the umbilical vein catheter or the peripheral IV setup. When epinephrine is administered by endotracheal tube (if an IV has not yet been started), two to three times the IV dose of epinephrine is given, followed immediately by 1 mL of normal saline (Young & Mangum, 2001). Sodium bicarbonate is rarely given in the delivery room. It is given only in the case of a severely asphyxiated newborn to correct metabolic acidosis and only after effective ventilation is established. Dextrose is given to prevent progression of hypoglycemia. A 10% dextrose in water intravenous solution is usually sufficient to prevent or treat hypoglycemia in the birthing area. Naloxone hydrochloride (0.1 mg/kg), a narcotic antagonist, is used to reverse narcotic depression (Young & Mangum, 2001). See "Drug Guide: Naloxone Hydrochloride (Narcan)."

If shock develops (low blood pressure or poor peripheral perfusion), the baby may be given a volume expander such as 5% albumin, normal saline, or lactated Ringer's solution in a dose of 10 mL/kg. Whole blood (O negative crossmatched against the mother), fresh frozen plasma, plasminate, and packed red blood cells can also be used for volume expansion and treatment of shock (Niermeyer, Kattwinkel, Van Reempts, et al., 2000). In some instances of prolonged resuscitation associated with shock and poor response to resuscitation, dopamine (5 mg/kg/min) may be necessary.

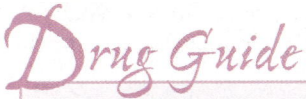

NALOXONE HYDROCHLORIDE (NARCAN)

Overview of Neonatal Action

Naloxone hydrochloride (Narcan) is used to reverse respiratory depression due to acute narcotic toxicity. It displaces morphine-like drugs from receptor sites on the neurons; therefore, the narcotics can no longer exert their depressive effects. Naloxone reverses narcotic-induced respiratory depression, analgesia, sedation, hypotension, and pupillary constriction.

Route, Dosage, Frequency

Intravenous dose is 0.1 to 0.2 mg/kg (0.25 to 0.5 mL/kg of 0.4 mg/mL preparation) concentration at birth, including premature infants. This drug is usually given through the umbilical vein or endotracheal tube, although naloxone can be given intramuscularly or subcutaneously. The use of "neonatal" naloxone (Narcan 0.02 mg/mL) is discouraged because of the extremely large fluid volumes needed.

Reversal of drug depression occurs within 1 to 2 minutes after IV administration. The duration of action is variable (minutes to hours) and depends on the amount of the drug present and the rate of excretion. Dose may be repeated in 3 to 5 minutes. If there is no improvement after two or three doses, discontinue naloxone administration. If initial reversal occurs, repeat dose as needed.

Neonatal Contraindications

Naloxone should not be administered to infants of narcotic-addicted mothers because it may precipitate acute withdrawal syndrome (increased HR and BP, vomiting, tremors).

Respiratory depression may result from nonmorphine drugs, such as sedatives, hypnotics, anesthetics, or other nonnarcotic CNS depressants.

Neonatal Side Effects

Excessive doses may result in irritability, increased crying, and possible prolongation of partial thromboplastin time (PTT).

Tachycardia may occur.

Nursing Considerations

- Monitor respirations closely—rate and depth.
- Assess for return of respiratory depression when naloxone effects wear off and effects of longer acting narcotics reappear.
- Have resuscitative equipment, O_2, and ventilatory equipment available.
- Monitor bleeding studies.
- Note that naloxone is incompatible with alkaline solutions.
- Store at room temperature and protect from light.
- Compatible with heparin.

Nursing Management

Nursing Assessment and Diagnosis

Communication between the obstetric office or clinic and the birthing area nurse helps identify newborns who may need resuscitation. When the woman arrives in the birthing area, the nurse should have the antepartal record and should note any contributory perinatal history factors and assess present fetal status. As labor progresses, nursing assessments include ongoing monitoring of fetal heartbeat and its response to contractions, assisting with fetal scalp blood sampling, and observing for the presence of meconium in the amniotic fluid to assess for fetal asphyxia. In addition, alert the resuscitation team and the practitioner responsible for the newborn's care of any potential high-risk laboring women.

Nursing diagnoses that may apply to the newborn with asphyxia include the following:

▶ *Ineffective breathing pattern* related to lack of spontaneous respirations at birth secondary to in utero asphyxia

▶ *Decreased cardiac output* related to impaired oxygenation

▶ *Ineffective family coping* related to baby's lack of spontaneous respirations at birth and fear of losing their newborn

Planning and Implementation

HOSPITAL-BASED NURSING CARE

After identifying possible high-risk situations, the next step in effective resuscitation is to assemble the necessary equipment and ensure proper functioning. Provide for pH and blood gas determination as well. Necessary equipment includes a radiant warmer that provides an overhead radiant heat source (a thermostatic mechanism taped to the infant's abdomen triggers the radiant warmer to turn on or off to maintain a level of thermoneutrality) and an open bed for easy access to the newborn. It is essential to keep the newborn warm. Dry the newborn quickly with warmed towels or blankets to prevent evaporative heat loss and place him or her under the radiant warmer with the servo-control set at 36.5 °C (97.7 °F).

Resuscitative equipment in the birthing room must be sterilized after each use. In the high-risk nursery, resuscitation may be needed at any time. Equipment reliability must be maintained at all times. Inspect all equipment—bag and mask, oxygen and flow meter, laryngoscope, and suction machine—for damaged or nonfunctioning parts before a birth or when setting up an admission bed. A systematic check of the emergency cart and equipment is a routine responsibility of each shift.

Training and knowledge about resuscitation are vital to personnel in the birth setting for both normal and at-risk births. Since resuscitation must be a two-person effort for high-risk newborns, call for additional support as needed. One member must have the skill to perform airway management and ventilation. Record resuscitative efforts on the newborn's chart so that all members of the health care team have access to the information.

Birthing room resuscitation is particularly distressing for parents. If the need for resuscitation is anticipated, reassure the parents that a team will be present at the birth to care specifically for their newborn. As soon as the infant's condition has stabilized, a member of the interdisciplinary team needs to discuss the newborn's condition with the parents. The parents may have many fears about the reasons for resuscitation and the condition of their baby after resuscitation.

Evaluation

Expected outcomes of nursing care include the following:

▶ The risk of asphyxia is promptly identified, and intervention is started early.

▶ The newborn's metabolic and physiologic processes are stabilized, and recovery is proceeding without complications.

▶ The parents can verbalize the reason for resuscitation and what was done to resuscitate their newborn.

▶ The parents can verbalize their fears about the resuscitation process and potential implications for their baby's future.

CARE OF THE NEWBORN WITH RESPIRATORY DISTRESS

One of the most severe conditions to which the newborn may fall victim is respiratory distress—an inappropriate respiratory adaptation to extrauterine life. The nurse caring for a baby with respiratory distress needs to understand the normal pulmonary and circulatory physiology (Chapter 24), the pathophysiology of the disease process, clinical manifestations, and supportive and corrective therapies. Only with this knowledge can the nurse make appropriate observations about responses to therapy and development of complications. Unlike the verbalizing adult client, the newborn communicates needs only by behavior. The neonatal nurse interprets this behavior as clues about the baby's condition.

Respiratory distress syndrome (RDS), also called hyaline membrane disease (HMD), is the result of a primary absence, deficiency, or alteration in the production of pulmonary surfactant. It is a complex disease that affects approximately 20,000 to 30,000 infants a year in the United States, most of whom are preterm infants. Nearly 50% of these infants are born at gestational ages of 26 to 28 weeks (Whitsett, Pryhuber, Rice, et al., 1999). The syndrome occurs more frequently in premature white infants than in black infants and almost twice as often in males as in females.

Not all the factors precipitating the pathologic changes of RDS have been determined, but two main factors are associated with its development:

1. *Prematurity.* All preterm newborns—whether AGA, SGA, or LGA—and especially IDMs are at risk for RDS. The incidence of RDS increases with the degree of prematurity, and most deaths occur in newborns weighing less than 1500 g. The maternal and fetal factors resulting in preterm labor and birth, complications of pregnancy, cesarean birth (and its indications), and familial tendency are all associated with RDS.

2. *Surfactant deficiency disease.* Normal pulmonary adaptation requires adequate surfactant, a lipoprotein that coats the inner surfaces of the alveoli. Surfactant provides alveolar stability by decreasing the alveoli's surface tension and tendency to collapse. Surfactant is produced by type II alveolar cells starting at about 24 weeks' gestation. In the normal or mature newborn lung, it is continuously synthesized, oxidized during breathing, and replenished. Adequate surfactant levels lead to better lung compliance and permit breathing with less work. RDS is due to alterations in surfactant quantity, composition, function, or production.

Nursing Practice

An alveolus can be thought of as a small balloon filled with water and no air. When the balloon is emptied, the water droplets that remain inside the balloon increase the surface tension. As a result, the sides of the balloon stick together. The increased surface tension makes reinflation very difficult.

Development of RDS indicates a failure to synthesize surfactant, which is required to maintain alveolar stability (see Chapter 24). On expiration this instability increases atelectasis, which causes hypoxia and acidosis because of the lack of gas exchange. These conditions further inhibit surfactant production and cause pulmonary vasoconstriction. The resulting lung instability causes the biochemical problems of hypoxemia (decreased P_{O_2}), hypercarbia (increased P_{CO_2}), and acidemia (decreased pH) which further increases pulmonary vasoconstriction and hypoperfusion. The cycle of events of RDS leading to eventual respiratory failure is diagrammed in "Pathophysiology Illustrated: Respiratory Distress Syndrome (RDS)."

Because of these pathophysiologic conditions, the newborn must expend increasing amounts of energy to reopen the collapsed alveoli with every breath, so that each breath becomes as difficult as the first. The progressive expiratory atelectasis upsets the physiologic homeostasis of the pulmonary and cardiovascular systems and prevents adequate gas exchange. Lung compliance decreases, which accounts

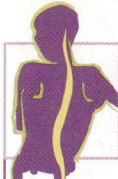
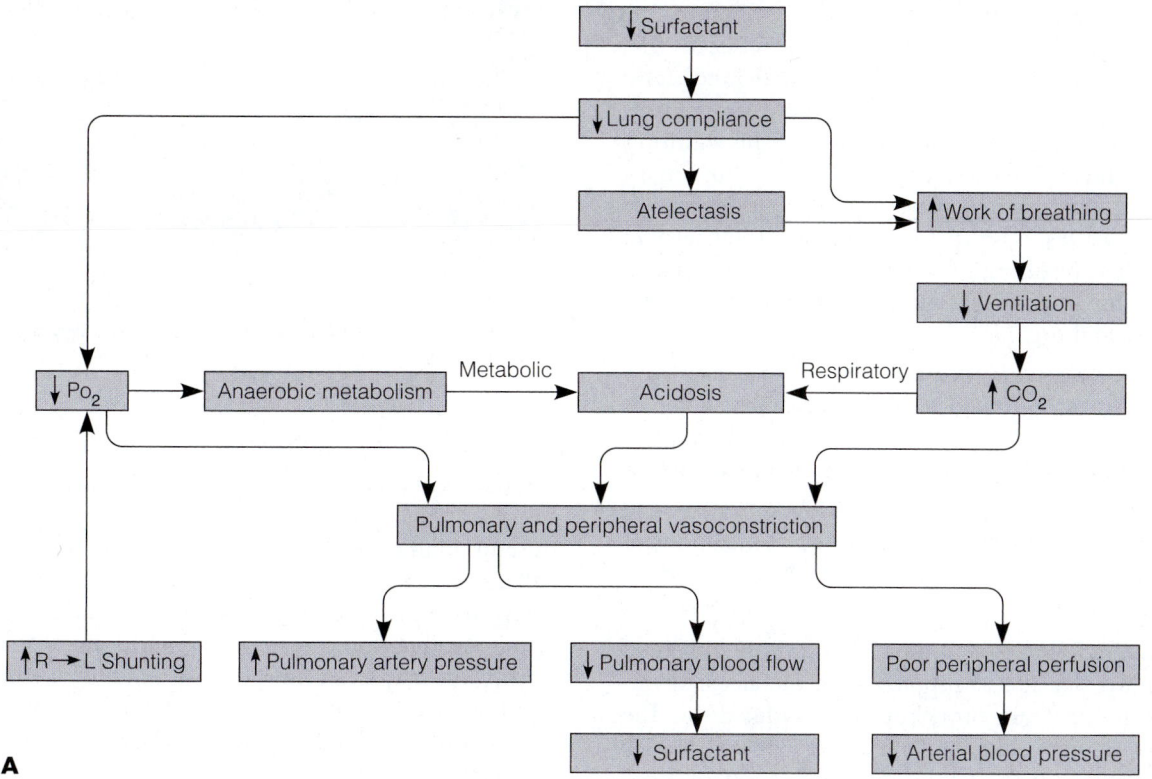

A

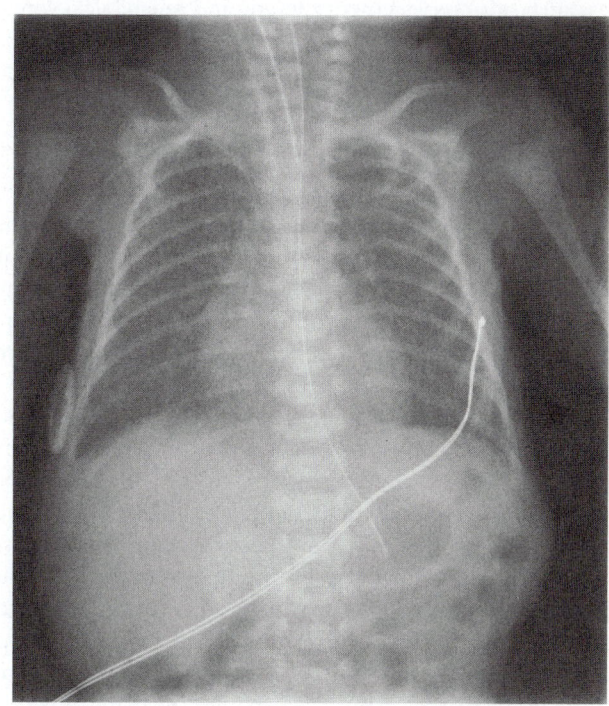

B

A, Cycle of events of RDS leading to eventual respiratory failure. *Note:* From Gluck, L., & Kulovich, M. V. (1973). Fetal lung development. *Pediatric Clinics of North America, 20,* 375. Modified. **B,** RDS chest x-ray. chest radiograph of respiratory distress syndrome characterized by a reticulogranular pattern with areas of microatelectasis of uniform opacity and air bronchograms. Courtesy of Carol Harrigan, RNC, MSN, NNP.

for the difficulty of inflation, labored respirations, and increased work of breathing.

The physiologic alterations of RDS produce the following complications:

1. *Hypoxia.* As a result of hypoxia, the pulmonary vasculature constricts, pulmonary vascular resistance increases, and pulmonary blood flow is reduced. Increased pulmonary vascular resistance may precipitate a return to fetal circulation as the ductus opens and blood flow is shunted around the lungs. This shunting increases the hypoxia and further decreases pulmonary perfusion. Hypoxia also causes impairment or absence of metabolic response to cold; reversion to anaerobic metabolism, resulting in lactate accumulation (acidosis); and impaired cardiac output, which decreases perfusion to vital organs.

2. *Respiratory acidosis.* Increased PCO_2 and decreased pH are results of alveolar hypoventilation, whereas persistently rising PCO_2 and decreases in pH are poor prognostic signs of pulmonary function and adequacy.

3. *Metabolic acidosis.* Because the cells lack oxygen, the newborn begins an anaerobic pathway of metabolism, with resulting base deficit (loss of bicarbonate) and increasing acidemia.

The classic radiologic picture of RDS is diffuse bilateral reticulogranular density, with portions of the air-filled tracheobronchial tree (air bronchogram) outlined by the opaque ("white-out") lungs and widespread atelectasis. (see "Pathophysiology Illustrated"). The progression of x-ray findings parallels the pattern of resolution, which usually occurs in 7 to 10 days, and the time of surfactant reappearance, unless surfactant replacement therapy and mechanical ventilation has been used (Newman, 1999). Echocardiography is a valuable tool in diagnosing vascular shunts that move blood either away from or toward the lungs.

Clinical Therapy

Antenatally, respiratory distress due to preterm labor is treated with therapies to enhance fetal lung development (see Chapter 13). ⊂⊃ The goals of postnatal therapy are to maintain adequate oxygenation and ventilation, correct acid-base imbalance, and provide the supportive care required to maintain homeostasis.

Supportive medical management consists of ventilation therapy, transcutaneous oxygen and carbon dioxide monitoring, blood gas monitoring, correction of acid-base imbalance, environmental temperature regulation, adequate nutrition, and protection from infection. Ventilation therapy is directed toward preventing hypoventilation and hypoxia. Mild cases of RDS may require only increased humidified oxygen concentrations. Moderately afflicted infants may need continuous positive airway pressure (CPAP). Babies with severe RDS require mechanical ventilatory assistance from a respirator (Figure 29–3 ◆). High-

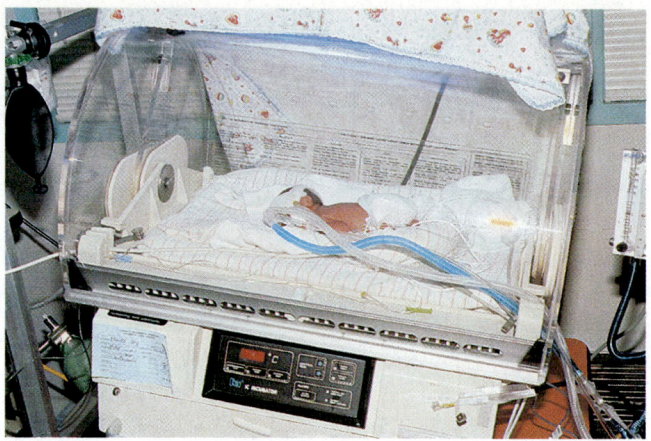

FIGURE 29–3. ◆ One-day-old, 29 weeks' gestational age, 1450-g baby on respirator and in isolette. Courtesy of Carol Harrigan, RNC, MSN, NNP.

frequency or jet ventilation has been tried when conventional ventilator therapy has not been successful (Whitsett et al., 1999). Nitric oxide inhalation therapy may also be a useful adjunctive therapy for infants with RDS (Lemons, Blackmon, Kanto, et al., 2000). Short-term and long-term steroids and bronchodilators are also used to improve respiratory function. Infants who have air leak respiratory problems may need morphine or fentanyl for pain control and sedation. Concurrent use of the ventilator and pancuronium (Pavulon) for muscle relaxation is controversial.

Surfactant replacement therapy decreases the severity of RDS in low-birth-weight newborns. Surfactant replacement therapy is delivered through an endotracheal tube and may be given in either the birthing room or the nursery, as indicated by the severity of RDS. Repeat doses are often required. The most frequent reported response to treatment is rapidly improved oxygenation and decreased need for ventilatory support (AAP Committee on Fetus and Newborn, 1999).

Nursing Management

Nursing Assessment and Diagnosis

Look for characteristics of RDS such as increasing cyanosis, tachypnea (> 60 respirations/min.), grunting respirations, nasal flaring, significant retractions, and apnea. Table 29–1 reviews clinical findings associated with respiratory distress in general. The Silverman-Andersen index (Figure 29–4 ◆) may be helpful in evaluating the signs of respiratory distress in the birthing area.

Nursing diagnoses that may apply to the newborn with RDS include the following:

▶ *Impaired gas exchange* related to inadequate lung surfactant

TABLE 29–1 Clinical Assessments Associated with Respiratory Distress

Clinical Picture	Significance
SKIN COLOR	
Pallor or mottling	These represent poor peripheral circulation due to systemic hypotension and vasoconstriction and pooling of independent areas (usually in conjunction with severe hypoxia).
Cyanosis (bluish tint)	Depending on hemoglobin concentration, peripheral circulation, intensity and quality of viewing light, and acuity of observer's color vision, this is frankly visible in advanced hypoxia. Central cyanosis is most easily detected by examination of mucous membranes and tongue.
Jaundice (yellow discoloration of skin and mucous membranes due to presence of unconjugated [indirect] bilirubin)	Metabolic alterations (acidosis, hypercarbia, asphyxia) of respiratory distress mean the newborn is predisposed to having bilirubin dissociate from albumin-binding sites and be deposited in the skin and central nervous system.
Edema (presents as slick, shiny skin)	This is characteristic of preterm infants because their total protein concentration is low, with a decrease in colloidal osmotic pressure and transudation of fluid. Edema of hands and feet is frequently seen within first 24 hours and resolved by fifth day in infants with severe RDS.
RESPIRATORY SYSTEM	
Tachypnea (normal respiratory rate 30–60/minute, elevated respiratory rate 60+/minute)	Increased respiratory rate is the most frequent and easily detectable sign of respiratory distress after birth. This compensatory mechanism attempts to increase respiratory dead space to maintain alveolar ventilation and gas exchange in the face of an increase in mechanical resistance. As a decompensatory mechanism it increases workload and energy output by increasing respiratory rate, which causes increased metabolic demand for oxygen and thus increases alveolar ventilation on an already overstressed system. Shallow, rapid respirations increase dead space ventilation, thus decreasing alveolar ventilation.
Apnea (episode of nonbreathing for more than 20 seconds; periodic breathing, a common "normal" occurrence in preterm infants, is defined as apnea of 5–10 seconds alternating with 10–15 seconds of ventilation)	This poor prognostic sign indicates cardiorespiratory disease, CNS disease, metabolic alterations, intracranial hemorrhage, sepsis, or immaturity. Physiologic alterations include decreased oxygen saturation, respiratory acidosis, and bradycardia.
Chest	Inspection of the thoracic cage includes shape, size, and symmetry of movement. Respiratory movements should be symmetric and diaphragmatic; asymmetry reflects pathology (pneumothorax, diaphragmatic hernia). Increased anteroposterior diameter indicates air trapping (meconium aspiration syndrome).
Labored respirations (Silverman-Anderson index in Figure 29–4 indicates severity of retractions, grunting, and nasal flaring, which are signs of labored respirations)	Indicates marked increase in the work of breathing.
Retractions (inward pulling of soft parts of the chest cage— suprasternal, substernal, intercostal, subcostal—at inspiration)	These reflect the significant increase in negative intrathoracic pressure necessary to inflate stiff, noncompliant lungs. Infants try to increase lung compliance by using accessory muscles. Lung expansion markedly decreases. Seesaw respirations are seen when the chest flattens with inspiration and the abdomen bulges. Retractions increase the work of breathing and oxygen need so that assisted ventilation may be necessary due to exhaustion.
Flaring nares (inspiratory dilation of nostrils)	This compensatory mechanism attempts to lessen the resistance of the narrow nasal passage.
Expiratory grunt (Valsalva maneuver in which the infant exhales against a closed glottis, thus producing an audible moan)	This increases transpulmonary pressure, which decreases or prevents atelectasis, thus improving oxygenation and alveolar ventilation. Intubation should not be tried unless the infant's condition is rapidly deteriorating, because it prevents this maneuver and allows the alveoli to collapse.
Rhythmic body movement with labored respirations (chin tug, head bobbing, retractions of anal area)	This is a result of using abdominal and other respiratory accessory muscles during prolonged forced respirations.
Auscultation of chest reveals decreased air exchange, with harsh breath sounds or fine inspiratory rales; rhonchi may be present	Decrease in breath sounds and distant quality may indicate interstitial or intrapleural air or fluid.

(continued)

Clinical Picture	Significance
CARDIOVASCULAR SYSTEM	
Continuous systolic murmur may be audible	Patent ductus arteriosus is common with hypoxia, pulmonary vasoconstriction, right-to-left shunting, and congestive heart failure.
Heart rate usually within normal limits (fixed heart rate may occur with a rate of 110–120/minute)	A fixed heart rate indicates a decrease in vagal control.
Point of maximal impulse usually located at fourth to fifth intercostal space, left sternal border	Displacement may reflect dextrocardia, pneumothorax, or diaphragmatic hernia.
HYPOTHERMIA	This is inadequate functioning of metabolic processes that require oxygen to produce necessary body heat.
MUSCLE TONE	
Flaccid, hypotonic, unresponsive to stimuli	These may indicate deterioration in the newborn's condition and possible CNS damage due to hypoxia, acidemia, or hemorrhage.
Hypertonia and/or seizure activity	

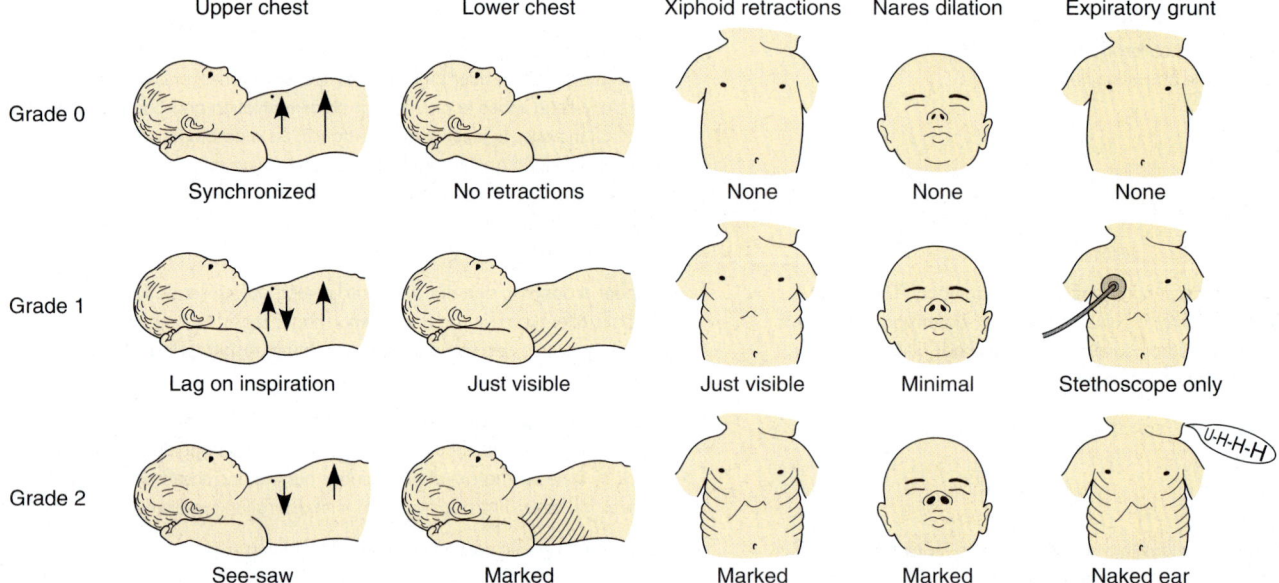

FIGURE 29–4. ◆ Evaluation of respiratory status using the Silverman-Andersen index. The baby's respiratory status is assessed. A grade of 0, 1, or 2 is determined for each area, and a total score is charted in the baby's record or on a copy of this tool and placed in the chart. *Note:* From Ross Laboratories, Nursing Aid No. 2. Columbus, OH; Silverman, W. A., & Andersen, D. H. (1956). *Pediatrics, 17,* 1–10. Copyright 1956, American Academy of Pediatrics.

▶ *Altered nutrition: less than body requirements* related to increased metabolic needs of the stressed infant

▶ *Risk for infection* related to invasive procedures

Planning and Implementation

HOSPITAL-BASED NURSING CARE

Based on clinical parameters, the neonatal nurse implements therapeutic approaches to maintain physiologic homeostasis and provides supportive care to the newborn with RDS. (See "Nursing Care Plan for the Newborn with Respiratory Distress Syndrome." See also "Clinical Pathway: Care of a Newborn with Respiratory Distress" on the companion website) ⊂▭⊃ **WEB**

Nursing interventions and criteria for instituting mechanical ventilation depend on institutional protocol. Methods of oxygen monitoring and nursing interventions are included in Table 29–2. The nursing care of infants on ventilators or with umbilical artery catheters is not discussed here. These infants have severe respiratory distress and are cared for in neonatal intensive care units by nurses with advanced knowledge and training. The parents of a baby with respiratory distress should be provided with a very supportive environment.

GOAL	INTERVENTION	RATIONALE	EXPECTED OUTCOME

1. Risk for ineffective breathing pattern related to immature lung development

	NIC Priority Intervention: **Respiratory monitoring:** *Collection and analysis of patient data to ensure airway patency and adequate gas exchange*		NOC Suggested Outcome: **Respiratory status: Ventilation:** *Movement of air in and out of the lungs*
The infant will maintain an effective breathing pattern.	▶ Review maternal delivery records noting medications given to mother prior to birth and the infant's condition at birth such as Apgar scores and resuscitative measures.	▶ Several drugs suppress respiratory function in the newborn.	The infant will maintain an effective breathing pattern as evidenced by: respirations are 30–60 breaths/ minute, arterial blood gases are within a normal range, infant is free of signs of retractions or nasal flaring, and blood pH is 7.35–7.45.
	▶ Initiate cardiac and respiratory monitoring and calibrate these monitors every 8 hours.	▶ Close monitoring detects periodic apneic spells and allows for medical intervention if necessary.	
	▶ Monitor infant's respiratory rate and rhythm, pulse, blood pressure and activity	▶ Increases in respiratory rate and pulse, alteration in rhythm, and blood pressure may indicate respiratory distress.	
	▶ Assess skin color; note signs of cyanosis, duskiness, and pallor.	▶ Any changes in the normal skin color may indicate a physiologic change occurring.	
	▶ Clear infant's airway by suctioning PRN.	▶ Opens airway by clearing mucus and allows maximum respiratory effort.	
	▶ Administer warmed, humidified oxygen by oxygen hood and monitor the oxygen concentrations every 30 minutes.	▶ Prevents mucosal dryness and maintains an even level of oxygen administration.	
	▶ Do not allow oxyhood to touch infant's face; maintain a stable oxygen concentration by increasing and decreasing oxygen by 5%–10% increments.	▶ Allowing oxyhood to touch infant's face may cause apnea by stimulating the facial nerve.	
	Collaborative: Obtain arterial blood gases per physician orders.	▶ Obtaining arterial blood gases is essential in managing an infant receiving oxygen. Suctioning may cause a discrepancy in ABG readings and should be avoided.	
	a. Maintain constant O_2 concentration for 15–30 minutes before sample is obtained.		
	b. Avoid stimulating infant 15 minutes prior to obtaining sample.		
	c. Avoid suctioning infant prior to obtaining sample.		
	d. Obtain sample in heparinized tuberculin syringe and maintain the temperature of the sample.		
	e. Assess the patency of the IV line to prevent clot formation, then replace blood used to clear line.		
	f. Flush line with 3 cc heparinized solution before restarting flow of IV fluids.		
	g. Monitor transcutaneous pulse oximeter continuously or hourly and record. Rotate sensor site every 3–4 hours.		
	▶ Assess infant's need for mechanical ventilation: apnea present, hypoxia ($PaO_2 < 50$ mm Hg), hypercapnia ($PaCO_2 > 60$ mm Hg), respiratory acidosis (pH < 7.2)	▶ Mechanical ventilation improves oxygenation and ventilation resulting in rise in PaO_2 and decrease in $PaCO_2$.	
	▶ Administer mechanical ventilation per hospital protocol.	▶ CPAP or PEEP can be administered by nasal prongs, nasopharyngeal or oral intubation.	

(continued)

GOAL	INTERVENTION	RATIONALE	EXPECTED OUTCOME

2. Ineffective thermoregulation related to increased respiratory effort

	NIC Priority Intervention:		*NOC Suggested Outcome:*
	Temperature regulation: *Attaining and/or maintaining body temperature within a normal range*		**Thermoregulation: Neonate:** *Balance among heat production, heat gain, and heat loss during the neonatal period*
The infant will exhibit no signs of hypothermia.	▶ Review maternal prenatal and intra-partum records. Note any medications mother received during these times.	▶ Medications such as Demerol and magnesium sulfate used by the mother during the prenatal or intrapartum periods significantly interfere with the infant's ability to retain heat.	The infant will not exhibit signs and symptoms of hypothermia as evidenced by temperature maintenance of 97.7–99.1 °F and no signs and symptoms of respiratory distress.
	▶ Assess infant's temperature frequently.	▶ Hypothermia leads to pulmonary vasoconstriction because of the increase in oxygen consumption.	
	▶ Observe for signs of increased oxygen consumption and metabolic acidosis.	▶ Cold stress leads to increased oxygen needs; thereby, brown fat is utilized to maintain body temperature.	
	▶ Warm all inspired gases and record temperature of delivered gases.	▶ Hypoxia and acidoses further depresses surfactant production.	Cold air/oxygen blown in face of newborn is stimulus for consumption of oxygen and glucose and increased metabolic rate.
	▶ Utilize radiant warmers or isolettes with servocontrols, incubators, and open cribs with appropriate clothing.	▶ Maintains neutral thermal environment.	
	▶ Note signs and symptoms of respiratory distress, including tachypnea, apnea, cyanosis, acrocyanosis, bradycardia, lethargy, weak cry, and hypotonia.	▶ These signs can predispose the infant to metabolic acidosis.	

3. Altered nutrition: less than body requirements related to increase metabolic needs in the infant

	NIC Priority Intervention:		*NOC Suggested Outcome:*
	Newborn monitoring: *Measurement and interpretation of physiologic status of the neonate the first 24 hours*		**Nutritional status: Food and fluid intake:** *Amount of food and fluid taken into the body over a 24-hour period*
Infant will gain weight in a normal curve.	▶ Assess suck, swallow, gag, and cough reflexes.	▶ Prevents feeding problems and assists in determining the best method of feeding for infant.	The infant will maintain steady weight gain as evidenced by < 2%/day weight loss, tolerates oral feedings, and urine output is 1–3 mL/kg/hour.
	▶ Assess respiratory status of infant. If problems are noted, notify physician.	▶ In the presence of respiratory distress, avoid oral fluids and initiate parenteral nutrition per physician's orders.	
	▶ Monitor IV rates per infusion pump (60–80 mL/kg/day) as ordered by physician.	▶ Allows for close monitoring of fluid intake.	
	▶ Record hourly intake and output and daily weights.	▶ IV fluids are administered to replace sensible and insensible water loss, as well as evaporative water loss secondary to infant respiratory distress. Monitoring I&O will prevent circulatory system overload that can lead to pulmonary edema and cardiac problems.	
	▶ Provide total parenteral nutrition (TPN) when indicated.	▶ TPN is used as nutritional alternative if bowel sounds are not present and infant remains in acute distress.	
	▶ Advance, based on tolerance, from intravenous to gastrointestinal feedings. Gavage or nipple feedings are used, and IV is used as supplement (discontinued when oral intake is sufficient).	▶ If IV discontinued before oral intake is established, baby will not receive adequate calories.	
		▶ Formula or breast milk stimulate GI hormones necessary for a functional absorptive GI tract.	
		▶ Avoid complications associated with nutrition by IV route only.	
	▶ Provide adequate caloric intake: consider amount of intake, type of formula, route of administration, and need for supplementation of intake by other routes.	▶ Calories are essential to prevent catabolism of body proteins, and metabolic acidosis due to starvation or inadequate caloric intake.	
	▶ Assess infusion site for signs and symptoms of infection including: erythema, edema, and drainage with a foul odor.	▶ Appropriate intervention can be initiated when signs and symptoms of infection are detected early. Treatment may avoid infection and sepsis in the infant.	

GOAL	INTERVENTION	RATIONALE	EXPECTED OUTCOME
4. Risk for fluid volume deficit related to increased insensible water losses			
The infant will not exhibit signs of dehydration and will display appropriate weight gain.	**NIC Priority Intervention:** **Fluid monitoring:** *Collection and analysis of patient data to regulate fluid balance* ▶ Observe for weight fluctuations by obtaining daily weights. ▶ Document cumulative balances of intake (IV fluid administration and feedings) and output (urine collection bags, weighing or counting diapers) hourly. ▶ Obtain urinalysis, monitor closely specific gravity and nitrites. ▶ Monitor vital signs including blood pressure, pulse, temperature, and mean arterial pressure. ▶ Assess client for signs of dehydration (i.e., poor skin turgor, pale mucous membranes, and sunken anterior fontanel). ▶ Assess IV site for signs of infection (erythema and edema) and infiltration. **Collaborative:** Obtain labs for Hct, serum calcium, serum magnesium, serum potassium, blood urea nitrogen (BUN), creatinine, and uric acid levels. ▶ Administer fluids, blood products, and electrolytes as ordered by physician.	▶ Fluctuations in weight may indicate water imbalance or inadequate caloric intake. ▶ Balanced fluid intake and output suggest homeostasis. ▶ Specific gravity > 1.013 and nitrites present in the urine are indicative of not enough fluid intake. ▶ A MAP of less than 25 mm Hg may indicate hypotension. ▶ Detecting signs and symptoms of dehydration early in the infant are important because early intervention is vital to prevent further damage. ▶ If signs and symptoms of infection are noted, intervention is necessary and IV site should be changed. ▶ Determines necessity for TPN administration. ▶ Replaces low nutrient stores and treats anemia if present.	**NOC Suggested Outcome:** **Fluid balance:** *Balance of water in the intracellular and extracellular compartments of the body* The infant will be free of signs and symptoms of dehydration as evidenced by intake equaling output, urine specific gravity in normal range, and a weight gain of at least 20–30 grams/day.

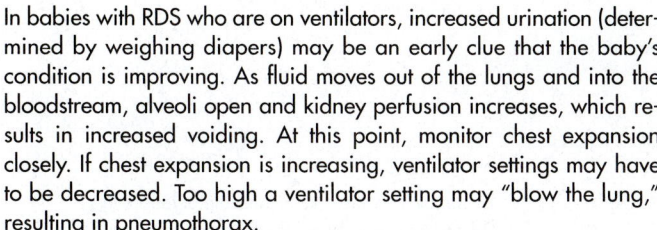

Nursing Practice

In babies with RDS who are on ventilators, increased urination (determined by weighing diapers) may be an early clue that the baby's condition is improving. As fluid moves out of the lungs and into the bloodstream, alveoli open and kidney perfusion increases, which results in increased voiding. At this point, monitor chest expansion closely. If chest expansion is increasing, ventilator settings may have to be decreased. Too high a ventilator setting may "blow the lung," resulting in pneumothorax.

Evaluation

Expected outcomes of nursing care include the following:

▶ The risk of RDS is promptly identified and early intervention is initiated.

▶ The newborn is free of respiratory distress and metabolic alterations.

▶ The parents verbalize their concerns about their baby's health problem and survival and understand the rationale behind the management of their newborn.

Transient Tachypnea of the Newborn

Some AGA preterm and near-term infants may develop progressive respiratory distress that can resemble classic RDS. They may have had intrauterine or intrapartal asphyxia due to maternal oversedation, maternal bleeding, prolapsed cord, breech birth, or maternal diabetes. The newborn then fails to clear the airway of lung fluid, mucus, and other debris or has an excess of fluid in the lungs due to aspiration of amniotic or tracheal fluid. Transient tachypnea is also more prevalent in cesarean birth newborns who have not had the thoracic squeeze that occurs during vaginal birth and removes some of the lung fluid.

Usually the newborn experiences little or no difficulty at the onset of breathing. However, shortly after birth, expiratory grunting, flaring of the nares, and mild cyanosis may be noted in the newborn breathing room air. Tachypnea is usually present by 6 hours of age, with respiratory rates as high as 100 to 140 breaths per minute.

CLINICAL THERAPY

Initial x-ray findings may be identical to those showing RDS within the first 3 hours. However, radiographs of infants with transient tachypnea usually reveal a generalized overexpansion of the lungs (hyperaeration of alveoli),

TABLE 29–2 Oxygen Monitors

Type	Function and Rationale	Nursing Interventions
PULSE OXIMETRY—SPO$_2$ Estimates beat-to-beat arterial oxygen saturation. Microprocessor measures saturation by the absorption of red and infrared light as it passes through tissue. Changes in absorption related to blood pulsation through vessel determine saturation and pulse rate (Merenstein & Gardner, 1998).	Calibration is automatic. Less dependent on perfusion than TcP$_{O_2}$ and TcPCO$_2$; however, functions poorly if peripheral perfusion is decreased due to low cardiac output. Much more rapid response time than TcPO$_2$—offers real-time readings. Can be located on extremity, digit, or palm of hand, leaving chest free; not affected by skin characteristics. Requires understanding of oxyhemoglobin dissociation curve. Pulse oximeter reading of 85% to 95% reflects clinically safe range of saturation. Extreme sensitivity to movement; decreases if average of 7th or 14th beat is selected rather than beat to beat. Poor correlation with extreme hyperoxia.	Understand and use oxyhemoglobin dissociation curve. Monitor trends over time and correlate with arterial blood gases (Merenstein & Gardner, 1998). Check disposable sensor at least q8h. Use disposable cuffs (reusable cuffs allow too much ambient light to enter, and readings may be inaccurate).
TRANSCUTANEOUS OXYGEN MONITOR—TcP$_{O_2}$ Measures oxygen diffusion across the skin. Clark electrode is heated to 43 °C (preterm) or 44 °C (term) to warm the skin beneath the electrode and promote diffusion of oxygen across the skin surface. P$_{O_2}$ is measured when oxygen diffuses across the capillary membrane, skin, and electrode membrane (Merenstein & Gardner, 1998).	When transcutaneous monitors are properly calibrated and electrodes are appropriately positioned, they provide reliable, continuous, noninvasive measurements of P$_{O_2}$, PCO$_2$, and oxygen saturation. Readings vary when skin perfusion is decreased. Reliable as trend monitor. Frequent calibration necessary to overcome mechanical drift. Following membrane change, machine must "warm up" 1 hour prior to initial calibration; otherwise, after turning it on, it must equilibrate for 30 minutes prior to calibration. When placed on infant, values will be low until skin is heated; approximately 15 minutes required to stabilize. Second-degree burns are rare but possible if electrodes remain in place too long. Decreased correlations noted with older infants (related to skin thickness), with infants with low cardiac output (decreased skin perfusion), and with hyperoxic infants. The adhesive that attaches the electrode may abrade the fragile skin of the preterm infant. May be used for both preductal and postductal monitoring of oxygenation for observations of shunting.	Use TcP$_{O_2}$ to monitor trends of oxygenation with routine nursing care procedures. Clean electrode surface to remove electrolyte deposits; change solution and membrane once a week. Allow machine to stabilize before drawing arterial gases; note reading when gases are drawn and use values to correlate. Ensure airtight seal between skin surface and electrode; place electrodes on clean, dry skin on upper chest, abdomen, or inner aspect of thigh; avoid bony prominences. Change skin site and recalibrate at least every 4 hours; inspect skin for burns; if burns occur, use lowest temperature setting and change position of electrode more frequently. Adhesive disks may be cut to a smaller size, or skin prep may be used under the adhesive circle only; allow membrane to touch skin surface at center.

which is identified principally by flattened contours of the diaphragm. Dense streaks (increased vascularity) radiate from the hilar region and represent engorgement of the lymphatic vessels, which clear alveolar fluid when air breathing begins. Within 48 to 72 hours, the chest x-ray examination is normal (Newman, 1999).

Thinking Critically

TRANSIENT TACHYPNEA OF THE NEWBORN

You are caring for baby girl Linn, who is a 39-week, AGA female born by repeat cesarean birth to a 34-year-old G3 now P3 mother. Baby Linn's Apgar scores were 7 and 9 at 1 and 5 minutes. At 2 hours of age, an elevated respiratory rate of 70 to 80 and mild cyanosis were noted. She is now receiving 30% oxygen and has a respiratory rate of 100 to 120. The baby's clinical course, chest x-ray examination, and lab work are all consistent with transient tachypnea of the newborn. Her mother calls you to ask about her baby. She tells you that her last child was born at 30 weeks' gestation, had respiratory distress syndrome requiring ventilator support, and was hospitalized for 6 weeks. She asks you, "Is this the same respiratory distress?" What will you tell her? **WEB**

Ambient oxygen concentrations of 30% to 50%, usually under an oxyhood, may be required to correct the hypoxemia (Figure 29–5 ◆). Fluid and electrolyte requirements should be met with intravenous fluids during the acute phase of the disease. Oral feedings are contraindicated because of rapid respiratory rates. The infant should be improving by 8 to 24 hours. The clinical course of transient tachypnea lasts approximately 72 hours. Mild respiratory and metabolic acidosis may be present at 2 to 6 hours.

When hypoxemia is severe and tachypnea continues, persistent pulmonary hypertension must be considered and treatment measures initiated. If pneumonia is suspected initially, antibiotics may be administered prophylactically.

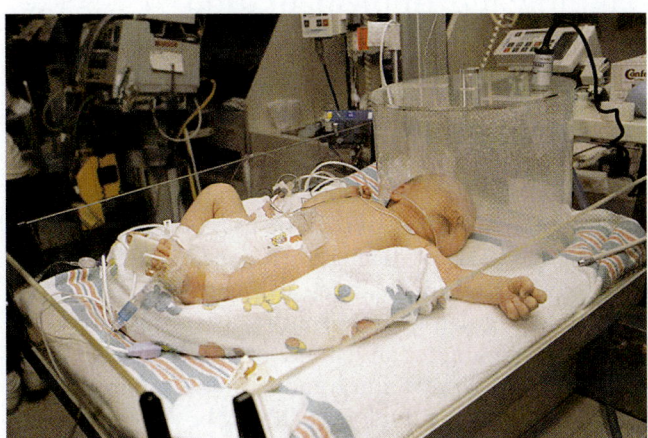

FIGURE 29–5. ◆ An infant under an oxyhood.

NURSING MANAGEMENT

For nursing actions, see "Nursing Care Plan for the: Newborn with Respiratory Distress Syndrome" as well as "Clinical Pathway: Care of a Newborn with Respiratory Distress" on the companion website. **WEB**

CARE OF THE NEWBORN WITH MECONIUM ASPIRATION SYNDROME

Meconium in the amniotic fluid indicates an asphyxial insult to the fetus before or during labor. The physiologic response to asphyxia is increased intestinal peristalsis, relaxation of the anal sphincter, and passage of meconium into the amniotic fluid. However, passage of meconium in a breech position does not necessarily indicate asphyxia.

Approximately 13% of live-born infants are born through meconium-stained amniotic fluid (MSAF). Of the newborns born through MSAF, 5% to 12% develop **meconium aspiration syndrome (MAS)** (Wiswell, Gannon, Jacob, et al., 2000). This fluid may be aspirated into the tracheobronchial tree in utero or during the first few breaths taken by the newborn. This syndrome primarily affects term, SGA, and postterm newborns and those who have experienced a long labor.

Meconium in the lungs produces a ball-valve action (air is allowed in but not exhaled), so that alveoli overdistend and rupture, resulting in pulmonary air leaks such as pneumomediastinum or pneumothorax . The meconium also triggers a chemical pneumonitis in the lung, with oxygen and carbon dioxide trapping and hyperinflation. Secondary bacterial pneumonia can occur. Clinical manifestations of MAS include (1) fetal hypoxia in utero a few days or a few minutes before birth, indicated by a sudden increase in fetal activity followed by diminished activity, slowing of FHR or weak and irregular heartbeat, loss of beat-to-beat variability, and meconium staining of amniotic fluid; and (2) signs of distress at birth, such as pallor, cyanosis, apnea, slow heartbeat, and low Apgar scores (below 6) at 1 and 5 minutes. As the victims of intrauterine asphyxia, meconium-stained newborns, or newborns that have aspirated meconium, are depressed at birth and require resuscitation to establish adequate respiratory effort.

After the initial resuscitation, the severity of clinical symptoms depends on the extent of aspiration. Many infants need mechanical ventilation at birth because of immediate signs of distress (generalized cyanosis, tachypnea, and severe retractions). An overdistended, barrel-shaped chest with increased anteroposterior diameter is common. Auscultation reveals diminished air movement, with prominent rales and rhonchi. Abdominal palpation may reveal a displaced liver caused by diaphragmatic depression resulting from the overexpansion of the lungs. The skin, nails, and umbilical cord usually have yellowish staining.

The chest x-ray film reveals nonuniform, coarse, patchy densities and hyperinflation (9 to 11 rib expansion). Evidence of pulmonary air leak is frequently present. Extreme hypoxia is also caused by the cardiopulmonary shunting and resultant failure to oxygenate and can lead to persistent pulmonary hypertension of the newborn (PPHN). See Chapter 42 for discussion of PPHN. 🔗

Clinical Therapy

The maternity and pediatric teams must work together to prevent MAS. The most effective form of preventive management is as follows:

1. After the head of the newborn is born and while the shoulders and chest are still in the birth canal, the baby's oropharynx and then nasopharynx are suctioned. (This is also done with a cesarean birth.) To decrease the possibility of HIV transmission, low-pressure wall suction is used.

2. If the infant has absent or depressed respirations, heart rate < 100 beats per minute, or poor muscle tone, direct tracheal suctioning is recommended. The glottis is visualized with a laryngoscope and the trachea suctioned (Wiswell et al., 2000).

If the newborn's head is not adequately suctioned on the perineum (when the head is born but the shoulder and chest are still in the vagina), respiratory or resuscitative efforts will push meconium into the airway and into the lungs. Stimulation of the newborn should be avoided to minimize respiratory movements. Further resuscitative efforts are undertaken as indicated, following the same principles of clinical therapy used for asphyxia (discussed earlier in this chapter). Resuscitated newborns should be transferred immediately to the nursery for closer observation. An umbilical arterial line may be used for direct monitoring of arterial blood pressures; blood sampling for pH and blood gases; and infusion of intravenous fluids, blood, or medications. Treatment usually involves delivering high levels of oxygen and pressure ventilation. Ventilation with low positive end-expiratory pressure (PEEP) is preferred to avoid pulmonary air leaks. Unfortunately, high pressures may be needed to cause sufficient expiratory expansion of obstructed airways or to stabilize airways weakened by inflammation so that the most distal atelectatic alveoli are ventilated.

Surfactant replacement therapy is most effective when used prophylactically. It improves oxygenation and decreases the incidence of air leaks. Systemic blood pressure and pulmonary blood flow must be maintained; this may be accomplished using medications and/or volume expanders.

Full-term newborns over 3.17 kg (7 lb) with respiratory failure who are not responding to ventilator therapy may need treatment with high-frequency ventilation and/or nitric oxide therapy or extracorporeal membrane oxygenation (ECMO). ECMO treatment, a form of heart-lung by-pass, has proved successful for newborns with meconium aspiration, pneumonia, and PPHN who are not responding to traditional treatments.

Treatment includes chest physiotherapy (chest percussion, vibration, and drainage) to remove debris. Prophylactic intravenous antibiotics are frequently given. Bicarbonate (to correct metabolic acidosis) may be necessary for several days for severely ill newborns. Mortality in term or postterm infants is very high, because the cycle of hypoxemia and acidemia is difficult to break.

Nursing Management

Nursing Assessment and Diagnosis

During the intrapartal period, observe for signs of fetal hypoxia and meconium staining of amniotic fluid. At birth, assess the newborn for signs of distress. Carefully observe for complications such as pulmonary air leaks; anoxic cerebral injury manifested by convulsions; myocardial injury evidenced by congestive heart failure or cardiomegaly; disseminated intravascular coagulation (DIC) resulting from hypoxic hepatic damage that depresses liver-dependent clotting factors; anoxic renal damage demonstrated by hematuria, oliguria, or anuria; fluid overload; sepsis secondary to bacterial pneumonia; and any signs of intestinal necrosis from ischemia, including gastrointestinal obstruction or hemorrhage.

Nursing diagnoses that may apply to the newborn with MAS and the infants' parents include:

▶ *Ineffective gas exchange* related to aspiration of meconium and amniotic fluid during birth

▶ *Altered nutrition: less than body requirements* related to respiratory distress and increased energy requirements

▶ *Ineffective family coping: compromised* related to life-threatening illness in term newborn

Planning and Implementation

HOSPITAL-BASED NURSING CARE

Initial interventions are aimed at preventing aspiration by helping remove the meconium from the infant's oropharynx and nasopharynx before the first extrauterine breath. When significant aspiration occurs, the primary goals of therapy are to maintain appropriate gas exchange and minimize complications. Nursing interventions after resuscitation should include maintaining adequate oxygenation and ventilation, regulating temperature, performing glucose testing by glucometer at 2 hours of age to check for hypoglycemia, observing intravenous fluids administration, calculating necessary fluids (which may be restricted in the first 48 to 72 hours due to cerebral edema), providing caloric requirements, and monitoring intravenous antibiotic therapy.

Evaluation

Expected outcomes of nursing care include the following:

▶ The risk of MAS is promptly identified and early intervention is initiated.

▶ The newborn is free of respiratory distress and metabolic alterations.

▶ The parents verbalize their concerns about their baby's health problem and survival and understand the rationale behind the management of their newborn.

CARE OF THE NEWBORN WITH COLD STRESS

Cold stress is excessive heat loss that requires a newborn to use compensatory mechanisms (such as increased respirations and nonshivering thermogenesis) to maintain core body temperature. Newborns experience heat loss that results in cold stress through the mechanisms of evaporation, convection, conduction, and radiation. (See Chapter 24 for types of thermoregulation.) Heat loss at birth that leads to cold stress can play a significant role in the severity of RDS and the ultimate outcome for the infant.

The amount of heat an infant loses depends largely on the actions of the nurse or caregiver. Both preterm and SGA newborns are at risk for cold stress because they have decreased adipose tissue, brown fat stores, and glycogen available for metabolism.

As discussed in Chapter 24, the newborn infant's major source of heat production in nonshivering thermogenesis (NST) is brown fat metabolism. The infant's ability to respond to cold stress by NST is impaired in the presence of several conditions:

- Hypoxemia (PO_2 less than 50 torr)
- Intracranial hemorrhage or any CNS abnormality
- Hypoglycemia (blood glucose level < 40 mg/dL)

When these conditions occur, the infant's temperature should be monitored closely and the neutral thermal environment conscientiously maintained. The nurse must recognize these conditions and treat them as soon as possible. The metabolic consequences of cold stress can be devastating and potentially fatal to an infant. Oxygen requirements rise, glucose use increases, acids are released into the bloodstream, and surfactant production decreases. The effects are graphically depicted in Figure 29–6 ◆.

Nursing Management

Observe the baby for signs of cold stress, including increased movement and respirations, decreased skin temperature and peripheral perfusion, development of hypoglycemia, and possibly development of metabolic acidosis.

Assess skin temperature because vasoconstriction, which decreases skin temperature, is the initial response to cold stress. Therefore, monitoring rectal temperature is not satisfactory. A decrease in rectal temperature means that the infant has long-standing cold stress, with decompensation in the newborn's ability to maintain core body temperature.

If skin temperature decreases, determine whether hypoglycemia is present. Hypoglycemia is a result of the metabolic effects of cold stress and is suggested by glucometer values below 45 mg/dL, tremors, irritability or lethargy, apnea, or seizure activity.

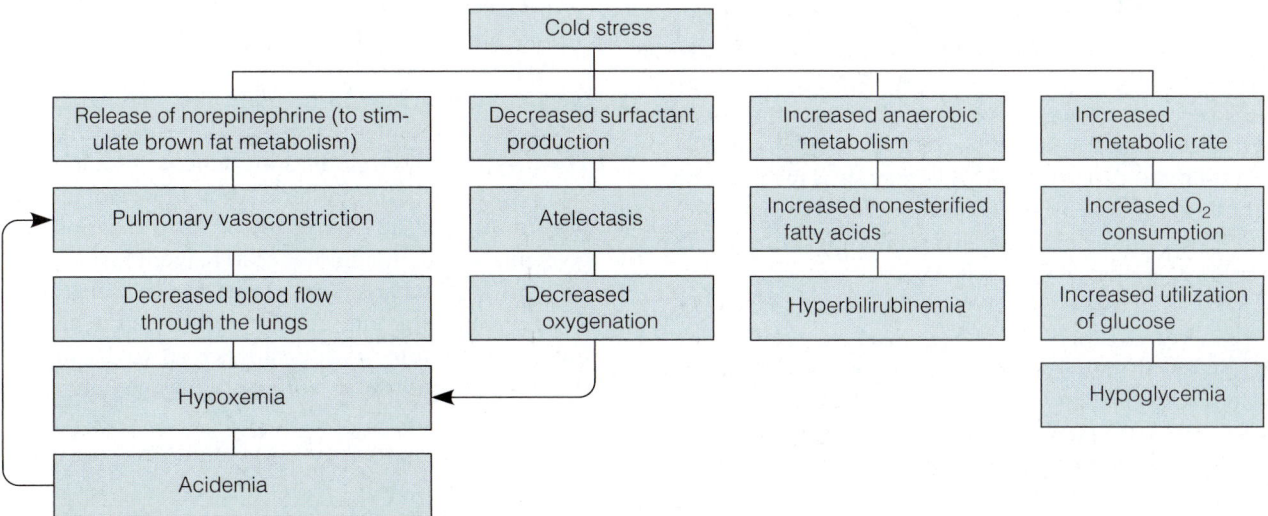

FIGURE 29–6. ◆ Cold stress chain of events. The hypothermic, or cold-stressed, newborn attempts to compensate by conserving heat and increasing heat production. These physiologic compensatory mechanisms initiate a series of metabolic events that result in hypoxemia and altered surfactant production, metabolic acidosis, hypoglycemia, and hyperbilirubinemia.

If the baby becomes hypothermic, initiate the following care plan ("Neonatal Thermoregulation," 1997):

- Keep the ambient air temperature 1 to 1.5 °C higher than the infant's temperature.
- Warm the newborn slowly because rapid temperature elevation may cause hypotension and apnea.
- Increase the air temperature in hourly increments of 1 °C until infant's temperature is stable.
- Monitor skin temperature every 15 to 30 minutes to determine if the newborn's temperature is increasing.
- Remove plastic wrap, caps, and heat shields while rewarming the infant so that cool air is not trapped along with the warm air.
- Warm intravenous fluids prior to infusion.
- Block heat loss by evaporation, radiation, convection, and conduction and maintain the newborn in a neutral thermal environment.

Assess for anaerobic metabolism and treat the resulting metabolic acidosis. Burning brown fat increases oxygen consumption, lactic acid levels, and metabolic acidosis. Hypoglycemia may be reversed by adequate glucose intake, as described in the following section.

CARE OF THE NEWBORN WITH HYPOGLYCEMIA

A widely used cutoff point or threshold for intervention in newborn hypoglycemia is a plasma glucose concentration of 40 mg/dL (Cornblath, Hawdon, Williams, et al., 2000). Plasma glucose values < 20 to 25 mg/dL should be treated with parenteral glucose, regardless of the age or gestation. **Hypoglycemia** is the most common metabolic disorder in IDMs, SGA infants, and preterm AGA infants. The pathophysiology of hypoglycemia differs for each classification.

AGA preterm infants have not been in utero long enough to store glycogen and fat. As a result, they have decreased ability to carry out gluconeogenesis. This situation is further aggravated by the tissues' increased use of glucose (especially in the brain and heart) during stress and illness (chilling, asphyxia, sepsis, RDS).

Infants of White's classes A–C or type 1 diabetic mothers have increased stores of glycogen and fat (see Chapter 28) and higher circulating insulin and insulin responsiveness levels than other newborns. Because the high in utero glucose loads stop at birth, the newborn experiences rapid, profound hypoglycemia. The SGA infant has used up glycogen and fat stores because of intrauterine malnutrition and has a blunted hepatic enzymatic response with which to produce and use glucose. Any newborn stressed at birth (from asphyxia or cold) also quickly uses up available glucose stores and becomes hypoglycemic. In addition, epidural anesthesia may alter maternal-fetal glucose homeostasis, resulting in hypoglycemia (Kalhan & Parimi, 2002).

Clinical Therapy

The goal of management includes early identification of hypoglycemia through observation and screening of newborns at risk. The newborn may be asymptomatic, or any of the following may occur:

- Lethargy, jitteriness
- Poor feeding
- Vomiting
- Pallor
- Apnea, irregular respirations, respiratory distress, cyanosis
- Hypotonia, possible loss of swallowing reflex
- Tremors, jerkiness, seizure activity
- High-pitched cry

Differential diagnosis of a newborn with nonspecific hypoglycemic symptoms includes determining if the newborn has any of the following:

- CNS disease
- Sepsis
- Metabolic aberrations
- Polycythemia
- Congenital heart disease
- Drug withdrawal
- Temperature instability
- Hypocalcemia

Aggressive treatment is recommended after a single low blood glucose value if the infant shows any of these symptoms. In at-risk infants, routine screening should be done frequently during the first 4 hours of life and then whenever any of the noted clinical manifestations appear or at 4-hour intervals until the risk period has passed.

Hypoglycemia may also be defined as a glucose oxidase reagent strip below 45 mg/dL, but only when corroborated with laboratory plasma glucose testing (see Skill 10–3. **SKILLS** Bedside glucose oxidase strip tests can screen for hypoglycemia, but laboratory determinations must confirm the results before a diagnosis of hypoglycemia can be made. Glucose reagent strips should not be used by themselves to screen for and diagnose hypoglycemia, because their results depend on the baby's hematocrit and there is a wide variance (5 to 15 mg/dL) between their results and laboratory plasma determinations.

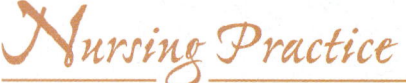

Nursing Practice

Wrapping the foot in a warm washcloth or disposable diaper is a simple way to create adequate vasodilation for taking a blood specimen.

Blood glucose sampling techniques can significantly affect the accuracy of the blood glucose value. Common bedside methods use whole blood, an enzymatic reagent strip, and a reflectance meter or color chart. It is important to note that whole blood glucose concentrations are 10% to 15% lower than plasma glucose concentrations (Kalhan & Parimi, 2002). The higher the hematocrit, the greater the difference between whole blood and plasma values. Also, venous blood glucose concentrations are approximately 15% to 19% lower than arterial blood glucose concentrations because the tissues extract some glucose before the blood enters the venous system ("Neonatal Hypoglycemia," 2000). Newer techniques, such as using a glucose oxidase analyzer or an optical bedside glucose analyzer, are more reliable for bedside screening but must also be validated with laboratory chemical analysis.

Nursing Practice

Blood samples for the laboratory should be placed on ice and analyzed within 30 minutes of drawing to prevent the red blood cells from continuing to metabolize glucose.

Adequate caloric intake is important. Early formula feeding or breastfeeding is a major preventive approach. If early feeding meets the infant's fluid and caloric needs, the blood glucose concentration is likely to remain above the hypoglycemic level. During the first hours after birth, asymptomatic newborns may also be given oral glucose. Another plasma glucose measurement is then obtained 30 to 60 minutes after feeding. For at-risk newborns who are feeding, blood sampling should be done before feeding.

Intravenous infusions of a dextrose solution (5% to 10%) begun immediately after birth also should prevent hypoglycemia. Plasma glucose levels are obtained when the parenteral infusion is started. However, in the very small AGA infant, infusions of 10% dextrose solution may cause hyperglycemia to develop, requiring an alteration in the glucose concentration. Infants require 6 to 8 mg/kg/min of glucose to maintain normal glucose concentrations. Therefore, an intravenous glucose solution should be calculated based on the infant's body weight, with blood glucose tests to determine adequacy of the infusion treatment.

A rapid infusion of 25% to 50% dextrose is contraindicated because it may lead to profound rebound hypoglycemia following an initial brief increase. In prolonged hypoglycemic periods, corticosteroids may be administered. It is thought that steroids enhance gluconeogenesis from noncarbohydrate protein sources (Kalhan & Parimi, 2002). The untreated hypoglycemia may result in permanent, untreatable CNS damage or death.

Nursing Management

Nursing Assessment and Diagnosis

The objectives of nursing assessment are to identify newborns at risk and to screen symptomatic infants. For newborns diagnosed with hypoglycemia, assessment is ongoing and includes careful monitoring of glucose values. In addition, urine dipstick and urine volume tests (monitor only if above 1 to 3 mL/kg/hr) may be evaluated frequently for osmotic diuresis and glycosuria.

Nursing diagnoses that may apply to the newborn with hypoglycemia include:

▶ *Altered nutrition: less than body requirements* related to increased glucose use secondary to physiologic stress

▶ *Ineffective breathing pattern* related to tachypnea and apnea

▶ *Pain* related to frequent heel sticks secondary to glucose monitoring

Planning and Implementation

Monitor infants in at-risk groups no later than 2 hours after birth and before feedings or whenever there are abnormal signs (Cornblath et al., 2000). Monitor the IDM within 30 minutes of birth. Once an at-risk infant's blood sugar level is stable, glucose testing every 2 to 4 hours (or per agency protocol), or prior to feedings, adequately monitors glucose levels. The infant's lateral heel is the preferred site for the glucose sample, so that the posterior tibial nerve and artery and the important longitudinally oriented fat pad of the heel will not be damaged (Figures 29–7 ◆ and 29–8 ◆).

Calculate glucose requirements and maintain intravenous glucose for any symptomatic infant with low serum

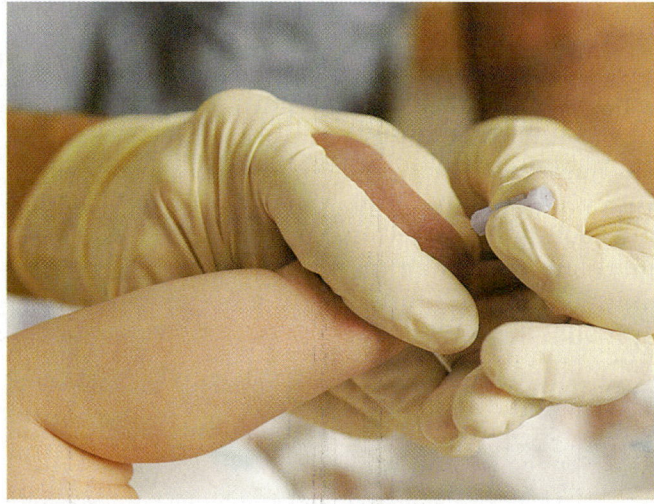

FIGURE 29–7. ◆ Heel sticks. With a quick, piercing motion, puncture the lateral heel with a microlance. Be careful not to puncture too deeply.

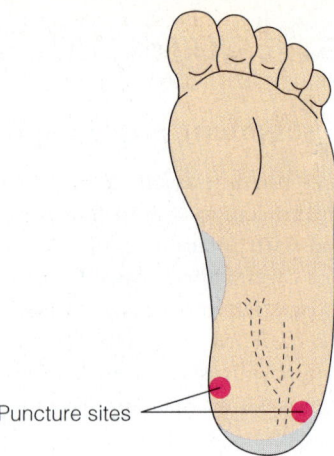

FIGURE 29–8. ◆ Potential sites for heel sticks. Avoid shaded areas to prevent injury to arteries and nerves in the foot and the important longitudinally oriented fat pad of the heel, which in later years could impede walking.

glucose levels. Careful attention to glucose monitoring is again required during the transition from intravenous to oral feedings. Titration of intravenous glucose may be required until the infant can take adequate amounts of formula or breast milk to maintain a normal blood sugar level. Titrate by decreasing the concentration of parenteral glucose gradually to 5%, then reducing the rate of infusion to 6 mg/kg/min, then to 4 mg/kg/min, and slowly discontinuing it over 4 to 6 hours.

The feeding method greatly influences glucose and energy requirements. In addition, the therapeutic nursing measure of nonnutritive sucking during gavage feedings has been reported to increase the baby's daily weight gain and lead to earlier bottle-feeding or breastfeeding and discharge. Nonnutritive sucking may also lower activity levels, which allows newborns to conserve their energy stores. Activity can increase energy requirements; crying alone can double the baby's metabolic rate. Establishing and maintaining a neutral thermal environment have a potent influence on the newborn's metabolism. Pay careful attention to environmental conditions, physical activity, and organization of care and integrate these factors into nursing care. Identify any discrepancies between the baby's caloric requirements and intake and weigh the newborn daily at consistent times, preferably before a feeding. Only then can findings of unusual losses or gains, as well as the pattern of weight gain, be considered reliable.

Evaluation

Expected outcomes of nursing care include the following:

▶ The risk of hypoglycemia is promptly identified, and intervention is started early.

▶ The newborn's metabolic and physiologic processes are stabilized, and recovery is proceeding without sequelae.

CARE OF THE NEWBORN WITH JAUNDICE

The most common abnormal physical finding in newborns is jaundice. **Jaundice** is a yellowish coloration of the skin and sclera of the eyes that develops from deposit of the yellow pigment bilirubin in lipid tissues. Normally, the placenta clears fetal unconjugated (indirect) bilirubin in utero, so total bilirubin at birth is usually less than 3 mg/dL unless an abnormal hemolytic process has been present. Postnatally, the infant must conjugate bilirubin (convert a lipid-soluble pigment into a water-soluble pigment) in the liver.

The rate and amount of conjugation of bilirubin depend on the rate of hemolysis, the bilirubin load, the maturity of the liver, and the presence of albumin-binding sites. (See Chapter 24 ⚭ for discussion of conjugation of bilirubin.) The liver of a normal, healthy term infant is usually mature enough and producing enough glucuronyl transferase that the total serum bilirubin does not reach a pathologic level. However, physiologic jaundice remains a common problem for the term newborn and may require phototherapy. Physiologic jaundice is due to the newborn's shorter red cell life span, slower uptake by the liver, lack of intestinal bacteria, and poorly established hydration.

Pathophysiology

Serum albumin-binding sites can usually meet the normal demands of the newborn. However, certain conditions tend to decrease the sites available. Fetal or neonatal asphyxia and neonatal drugs such as indomethacin decrease the binding affinity of bilirubin to albumin, because acidosis impairs albumin's capacity to hold bilirubin. Hypothermia and hypoglycemia release free fatty acids that dislocate bilirubin from albumin. Also, premature infants have less albumin available. Maternal use of sulfa drugs or salicylates interferes with conjugation or with serum albumin-binding sites by competing with bilirubin for these sites.

Although the exact mechanism of bilirubin-produced neuronal injury is uncertain, high concentrations of total bilirubin can be neurotoxic. Unconjugated bilirubin has a high affinity for extravascular tissue, such as fatty tissue (subcutaneous tissue) and the brain. Bilirubin not bound to albumin can cross the blood-brain barrier, damage cells of the CNS, and produce kernicterus or bilirubin encephalopathy. **Kernicterus** (meaning "yellow nucleus") refers to deposits of indirect or unconjugated bilirubin in the basal ganglia of the brain and to the permanent neurologic sequelae of untreated hyperbilirubinemia. The classic bilirubin encephalopathy of kernicterus most commonly found with Rh and ABO blood group incompatibility is less common today due to aggressive treatment with phototherapy and exchange transfusions. But cases of kernicterus are reappearing as a result of early discharge and the increased incidence of dehydration (as a result of discharge before the mother's milk is established).

Causes of Hyperbilirubinemia

The most common type of **hyperbilirubinemia** (elevation of bilirubin level) seen in newborns is physiologic jaundice; see Chapter 24 for more detailed discussion. A primary cause of pathologic hyperbilirubinemia is **hemolytic disease of the newborn** secondary to Rh incompatibility. All pregnant women who are Rh negative or who have blood type O (possible ABO blood incompatibility) should be asked about outcomes of any previous pregnancies and history of blood transfusion. Prenatal amniocentesis with spectrophotographic examination may be indicated. Cord blood from newborns is evaluated for bilirubin level, which should not exceed 5 mg/dL. Newborns of Rh-negative and O blood type mothers are carefully assessed for jaundice and levels of serum bilirubin.

Isoimmune hemolytic disease, also known as **erythroblastosis fetalis,** occurs when an Rh-negative mother is pregnant with an Rh-positive fetus and maternal antibodies cross the placenta. Maternal antibodies enter the fetal circulation, then attach to and destroy the fetal red blood cells (RBCs). The fetal system responds by increasing RBC production. Jaundice, anemia, and compensatory erythropoiesis result. A marked increase in immature RBCs (erythroblasts) also occurs, hence the designation erythroblastosis fetalis. With the use of RhoGAM, the incidence of erythroblastosis fetalis has dropped dramatically.

Hydrops fetalis, the most severe form of erythroblastosis fetalis, occurs when maternal antibodies attach to the Rh site on the fetal RBCs, making them susceptible to destruction; severe anemia and multiorgan system failure result. Cardiomegaly with severe cardiac decompensation and hepatosplenomegaly occurs. Severe generalized massive edema (anasarca) and generalized fluid effusion into the pleural cavity (hydrothorax), pericardial sac, and peritoneal cavity (ascites) develop. Jaundice is not present initially because the bilirubin pigments are excreted through the placenta into the maternal circulation. The hydropic hemolytic disease process is also characterized by hyperplasia of the pancreatic islets, which predisposes the infant to neonatal hypoglycemia similar to that of IDMs. In addition, the associated thrombocytopenia and hypoxic damage to the capillaries means these infants have increased bleeding tendencies. Hydrops is a frequent cause of intrauterine death among infants with Rh disease.

ABO incompatibility (the mother is blood type O and the baby is blood type A or B) may result in jaundice, although it rarely results in hemolytic disease severe enough to be clinically diagnosed and treated. Newborns with ABO incompatibility occasionally have hepatosplenomegaly, but hydrops fetalis and stillbirth are rare.

Certain prenatal and perinatal factors predispose the newborn to hyperbilirubinemia. During pregnancy, predisposing maternal conditions include hereditary spherocytosis, diabetes, intrauterine infections, and gram-negative bacilli infections that stimulate production of maternal isoimmune antibodies, drug ingestion (such as sulfas, salicylates, novobiocin, diazepam), and oxytocin.

In addition to Rh or ABO incompatibility, other conditions predispose the newborn to hyperbilirubinemia: polycythemia (central hematocrit 65% or more), pyloric stenosis, obstruction or atresia of the biliary duct or of the lower bowel, low-grade urinary tract infection, sepsis, hypothyroidism, enclosed hemorrhage (cephalhematoma, large bruises), asphyxia neonatorum, hypothermia, acidemia, and hypoglycemia. Neonatal hepatitis, atresia of the bile ducts, and gastrointestinal atresia all can alter bilirubin metabolism and excretion.

The prognosis for a newborn with hyperbilirubinemia depends on the extent of the hemolytic process and the underlying cause. Severe hemolytic disease results in fetal and early neonatal death from the effects of severe anemia—cardiac decompensation, edema, ascites, and hydrothorax. Hyperbilirubinemia may lead to kernicterus if not aggressively treated. The resulting neurologic damage may cause death, cerebral palsy, possible mental retardation, or hearing loss or, to a lesser degree, perceptual impairment, delayed speech development, hyperactivity, muscle incoordination, or learning difficulties.

Clinical Therapy

Early prenatal identification of the fetus at risk for Rh or ABO incompatibility allows prompt treatment. (See Chapter 13 for discussion of in utero management of this condition.) When one or more predisposing factors for jaundice is present, the maternal and neonatal blood types should be tested in the laboratory for Rh or ABO incompatibility. Other needed laboratory evaluations are Coombs' test, serum bilirubin levels (direct and total), hemoglobin, reticulocyte percentage, white cell count, and positive smear for cellular morphology.

Neonatal hyperbilirubinemia must be considered pathologic if any of the following criteria are met (Augustine, 1999):

1. Clinically evident jaundice in the first 24 hours of life
2. Serum bilirubin concentration rising by more than 5 mg/dL/day
3. Total serum bilirubin concentrations exceeding 15 mg/dL in term infants or 10 mg/dL in premature babies
4. Conjugated bilirubin concentrations greater than 1 mg/dL
5. Persistence of clinical jaundice beyond 10 days in term infants or beyond 21 days in preterm infants; mild jaundice in breastfed newborns after 2 weeks of age

Initial diagnostic procedures are aimed at differentiating jaundice resulting from increased bilirubin production, impaired conjugation or excretion, increased intestinal reabsorption, or a combination of these factors. The Coombs' test determines whether jaundice is due to Rh or ABO incompatibility.

If the hemolytic process is due to Rh sensitization, laboratory findings reveal the following: (1) an Rh-positive neonate with a positive Coombs' test; (2) increased erythropoiesis with many immature circulating red blood cells (nucleated blastocysts); (3) anemia, in most cases; (4) elevated levels (5 mg/dL or more) of bilirubin in cord blood; and (5) a reduction in albumin-binding capacity. Maternal data may include an elevated anti-Rh titer and spectrophotometric evidence of a fetal hemolytic process.

The indirect Coombs' test measures the amount of Rh-positive antibodies in the mother's blood. Rh-positive RBCs are added to the maternal blood sample. If the mother's serum contains antibodies, the Rh-positive RBCs agglutinate (clump) when rabbit immune antiglobulin is added, which is a positive test result.

The direct Coombs' test reveals antibody-coated (sensitized) Rh-positive RBCs in the newborn. Rabbit immune antiglobulin is added to the specimen of neonatal blood cells. If the neonatal RBCs agglutinate, they have been coated with maternal antibodies, a positive result.

If the hemolytic process is due to ABO incompatibility, laboratory findings reveal an increase in reticulocytes. The resulting anemia is usually not significant during the newborn period and is rare later on. The direct Coombs' test may be negative or mildly positive, whereas the indirect Coombs' test may be strongly positive. Infants with a positive direct Coombs' test have increased incidence of jaundice, with bilirubin levels above 10 mg/dL. Increased numbers of spherocytes (spherical, plump, mature erythrocytes) are seen on a peripheral blood smear. Increased numbers of spherocytes are not seen on blood smears from infants with Rh disease.

Whatever the cause of hyperbilirubinemia, treatment is directed toward preventing bilirubin toxic effects. Although kernicterus is rare, there is evidence that healthy term infants are at risk. Early discharge of newborns from birthing centers has significantly influenced the diagnosis and management of neonatal jaundice, increasing the emphasis on outpatient and home care management. A health care practitioner should follow up on all infants discharged before 48 hours after birth within 2 to 3 days of discharge for assessment of jaundice (AAP Provisional Committee for Quality Improvement and Subcommittee on Hyperbilirubinemia, 1994).

Therapeutic management of hyperbilirubinemia includes phototherapy, exchange transfusion, infusion of albumin, and drug therapy. Hemolytic disease may be treated with phototherapy, exchange transfusion, and drug therapy. When determining the appropriate management of hyperbilirubinemia due to hemolytic disease, the three relevant variables are the newborn's (1) serum bilirubin level, (2) birth weight, and (3) age in hours. If a newborn has hemolysis with an unconjugated bilirubin level of 14 mg/dL, weighs less than 2500 g (birth weight), and is 24 hours old or less, an exchange transfusion may be the best management. However, if that same newborn is over 24 hours of age, which is past the time when an increase in bilirubin would be due to pathologic causes, phototherapy may be the treatment of choice to prevent the possible complication of kernicterus.

PHOTOTHERAPY

Phototherapy is the exposure of the newborn to high-intensity light. It may be used alone or in conjunction with exchange transfusion to reduce serum bilirubin levels. The light exposure (using a bank of fluorescent lightbulbs or bulbs in the blue-light spectrum) decreases serum bilirubin levels in the skin by facilitating biliary excretion of unconjugated bilirubin. When the tissue absorbs the light, unconjugated bilirubin is converted into two isomers, called photobilirubin. The photobilirubin moves from the tissues to the blood by diffusion. In the blood it is bound to albumin and transported to the liver. It moves into the bile and is excreted into the duodenum for removal with feces without requiring conjugation by the liver. In addition, the photodegradation products formed when light oxidizes bilirubin can be excreted in the urine.

Phototherapy plays an important role in preventing a rise in bilirubin levels but does not alter the underlying cause of jaundice, and hemolysis may continue to produce anemia. It is generally accepted that phototherapy should be started at 4 to 5 mg/dL below the calculated exchange level for each infant (see Table 29–3). Sick newborns of less than 1000 g should have phototherapy instituted at a bilirubin concentration of 5 mg/dL. Many authors have recommended "prophylactic" phototherapy in the first 24 hours of life in high-risk, very-low-birth-weight infants (Cashore, 2000). Sick preterm infants who are at least 1500 g should begin phototherapy when the bilirubin level is 10 mg/dL. Any term newborn older than 24 to 48 hours of age with a bilirubin level of 20 mg/dL or above and illness or associated conditions may need an exchange transfusion (Maisels, 1999).

Phototherapy can be provided by banks of phototherapy lights, by a fiberoptic blanket attached to a halogen light source around the trunk of the newborn, or by a combination of both delivery methods (AAP Provisional Committee for Quality Improvement and Subcommittee on Hyperbilirubinemia, 1994).

With the fiberoptic blanket, the light stays on at all times, and the newborn is accessible for care, feeding, and diaper changes. The eyes are not covered. The babies do not get overheated, and fluid and weight loss are not complications of this system. Furthermore, the infant is accessible to the parents and the blanket is less alarming than standard phototherapy (Thureen, Deacon, O'Neill, et al., 1999). Many institutions and pediatricians use fiberoptic blankets for home care. A combination of a fiberoptic light source in the mattress under the baby and a standard light source above has also been recommended (MacMahon, Stevenson, & Oski, 1998).

TABLE 29–3 American Academy of Pediatrics Guidelines for the Management of Hyperbilirubinemia in the Healthy Term Newborn

Age (hours)	Total Serum Bilirubin Level, mg/dL (μmol/L)			
	Consider Phototherapy*	Phototherapy	Exchange Transfusion if Intensive Phototherapy Fails†	Exchange Transfusion and Intensive Phototherapy
25–48‡	≥12 (210)	≥15 (260)	≥20 (340)	≥25 (430)
49–72	≥15 (260)	≥18 (310)	≥25 (430)	≥30 (510)
>72	≥17 (290)	≥20 (340)	≥25 (430)	≥30 (510)

*Phototherapy at these total serum bilirubin (TSB) levels is a clinical option, meaning that the intervention is available and may be used on the basis of individual clinical judgment.
†Intensive phototherapy should produce a decline of TSB of 1 to 2 mg/dL within 4 to 6 hours, and the TSB level should continue to decline and remain below the threshold level for exchange transfusion. If this does not happen, phototherapy has failed.
‡Term infants who are clinically jaundiced at 24 hours old are not considered healthy and require further evaluation.
Note: Used with permission of the American Academy of Pediatrics. (1994). Practice parameter: Management of hyperbilirubinemia in the healthy term newborn. Pediatrics, 94, 560.

EXCHANGE TRANSFUSION

Exchange transfusion is the withdrawal and replacement of the newborn's blood with donor blood. It is used to treat anemia with RBCs that are susceptible to maternal antibodies, remove sensitized RBCs that would be lysed soon, remove serum bilirubin, and provide bilirubin-free albumin to increase the binding sites for bilirubin. Concerns about exchange transfusion are related to the use of blood products, which include the potential for HIV and hepatitis infection.

Nursing Management

Nursing Assessment and Diagnosis

Assessment is aimed at identifying prenatal and perinatal factors that predispose the newborn to the development of jaundice and at recognizing the jaundice as soon as it is apparent. Clinically, ABO incompatibility presents as jaundice and occasionally as hepatosplenomegaly. Fetal hydrops or erythroblastosis is rare (see Chapter 13). Suspect hemolytic disease of the newborn if the placenta is enlarged; if the newborn is edematous, with pleural and pericardial effusion plus ascites; if pallor or jaundice is noted during the first 24 to 36 hours; if hemolytic anemia is diagnosed; or if the spleen and liver are enlarged. Carefully note changes in behavior and observe for evidence of bleeding. If laboratory tests indicate elevated bilirubin levels, check the newborn for jaundice about every 2 hours and record observations.

To check for jaundice in lighter-skinned babies, blanch the skin over a bony prominence (forehead, nose, sternum) by pressing firmly with the thumb. After pressure is released, if jaundice is present, the area appears yellow before normal color returns. Check oral mucosa and the posterior portion of the hard palate and conjunctival sacs for yellow pigmentation in darker-skinned babies. Assessment

in daylight gives the best results, because pink walls and surroundings may mask yellowish tints, and yellow light makes differentiation of jaundice difficult. Record and report the time at onset of jaundice. If jaundice appears, careful observation of the increase in depth of color and of the newborn's behavior is mandatory.

Assess the newborn's behavior for neurologic signs associated with hyperbilirubinemia, which are rare but may include hypotonia, diminished reflexes, lethargy, or seizures.

Nursing diagnoses that may apply to care of a newborn with jaundice include:

▶ *Fluid volume deficit* related to increased insensible water loss and frequent loose stools

▶ *Sensory-perceptual alterations* related to neurologic damage secondary to kernicterus

▶ *Risk for altered parenting* related to parenting a newborn with jaundice

Planning and Implementation

HOSPITAL-BASED NURSING CARE

Hospital-based care is described in "Clinical Pathway: Care of a Newborn with Hyperbilirubinemia." If phototherapy lights are used, expose the newborn's entire skin surface to the light. Minimal covering may be applied over the genitals and buttocks to expose maximum skin surface while still protecting the bedding from soiling. Measure phototherapy success every 12 hours or with daily serum bilirubin levels. Turn lights off while blood is drawn to ensure accurate serum bilirubin levels. Because it is not known if phototherapy injures the delicate eye structures, particularly the retina, apply eye patches over the newborn's closed eyes during exposure to banks of phototherapy lights (see Figure 29–9 ◆). Stop phototherapy and remove the eye patches at least once per shift to assess the eyes for conjunctivitis. Also remove patches to allow eye contact during feeding (social stimulation) or when parents are visiting (to promote parental attachment).

Category	Day 1	Day 2/Discharge
Referral	Refer to lactation consultant	**Expected Outcomes** Consults completed
Assessments	Lab work (CBC, Rh, Coombs' direct, retic count, bilirubin level, both direct and indirect) Hearing test if bilirubin > 18 Obtain maternal/paternal history Obtain birth and newborn history Assess sclera and skin color for jaundice; assess mucous membranes for jaundice with dark pigmented skin Continue routine newborn assessments (see "Newborn Clinical Pathway," Chap. 26)	Bilirubin levels as ordered BID Assess for s/s dehydration Assess sclera and skin color for progression of jaundice **Expected Outcomes** Physical assessments, VS WNL; skin/mucous membranes pink, sclera clear of jaundice color; laboratory work WNL, total bilirubin level stabilized or decreasing
Teaching/psychosocial	Evaluate additional psychosocial needs of parents/family Orient family to nursery, equipment, patient room if rooming-in Instruct parents on s/s of hyperbilirubinemia (slight lethargy, irritability) Discuss possible side effects of phototherapy (stool character changes, increased fluid loss, temp changes, rash, altered sleep-wake patterns) Instruct parents on care and treatment of hyperbilirubinemia: • Phototherapy rationale, indications, and precautions • Placement of bili mask over closed eyes • Lab draws: rationale, frequency • Accurate intake and output to monitor for s/s dehydration Review cord care, skin care, care of genitalia (circumcision care as applicable) Review role of pumping breasts if necessary and offering formula for limited period of time	Teach/encourage parents to provide cuddling, tactile stimulation, and eye contact during diaper changes and feedings, talk to baby frequently Reinforce previous teaching; evaluate parental comprehension Provide opportunities for parents to express concerns/feelings **Expected Outcomes** Parents verbalize comprehension of care of infant with hyperbilirubinemia and potential sequelae of no treatment; parents verbalize comprehension of the risks/benefits of phototherapy as treatment; parents demonstrate developmentally appropriate care for infant during diaper changes and feedings; parents verbalize concerns, ask appropriate questions prn
Nursing care management and reports	Vital signs q4h with axillary temps Monitor thermoregulation Daily wt Initiate phototherapy as indicated and ordered • Maintain bili mask over eyes • Keep genitalia covered per policy • Check eyes for discharge, excessive pressure, corneal abrasions • Expose as much skin surface as possible to bili lights • Bilimeter reading q shift • No lotion or ointment on infant skin • Turn bili lights off during lab draws Continue infant assessments including • Note and document skin color q shift • Thorough skin care with diaper changes; note s/s breakdown, rash • Assess neuro status for s/s abnormality q interaction (hypotonia, lethargy, poor sucking reflex)	VS q4h with axillary temps Monitor thermoregulation, maintain NTE Daily wt Continue phototherapy as indicated • Maintain bili mask over eyes • Cover genitalia per policy • Check eyes for discharge, conjunctivitis, corneal abrasions • Expose as much skin surface as possible to bili lights • Bilimeter reading q shift • No lotion or ointment on infant skin • Turn bili lights off during lab draws Continue infant assessments as per day 1 **Expected Outcomes** VS WNL; wt stabilized or gaining wt; no s/s kernicterus; skin integrity intact; skin and mucous membranes pink; eyes without drainage, sclera clear; labs WNL, with stabilized or decreasing bilirubin level
Activity and comfort	Nest in open crib if infant able to maintain temp beneath bili lights Isolette if infant unable to maintain temp beneath bili lights Reposition q2–4h Remove bili mask, swaddle, and cuddle during feedings Cluster care procedures, remove from lights for feedings	Nest in open crib if infant's temp stable beneath bili lights Isolette if infant unable to maintain temp beneath bili lights **Expected Outcomes** Infant's temp WNL; infant able to rest with nested boundaries; infant cuddled, has eye contact with caregiver during care procedures and feedings

bili, bilirubin; CPR, cardiopulmonary resuscitation; DC, discharge; info, information; IV, intravenous; lab draws, laboratory blood withdrawal; MD/NP, medical doctor/nurse practitioner; NSY, nursery; NTE, neutral thermal environment; prn, as needed; s/s, signs and symptoms; VS, vital signs; WNL, within normal limits; wt, weight.

Category	Day 1	Day 2/Discharge
Nutrition	Breast- or bottle-feed q2–4h Monitor for dehydration, supplement with oral/IV fluid as indicated Remove newborn from bili lights, remove mask for feedings	Continue to feed q2–4h, monitor for dehydration, cuddle for feeding **Expected Outcomes** Infant tolerating feedings q2–4h without sequelae
Elimination	Record urine color and frequency Specific gravity each void Record quantity and characteristics each stool Strict intake and output (weigh diapers before discarding)	Continue noting urine and stool quantity and characteristics **Expected Outcomes** Voids qs, stools qs without difficulty, stool characteristics WNL for resolving hyperbilirubinemia; specific gravity WNL, no s/s dehydration
Medication	Evaluate routine meds Evaluate need for IV fluids	**Expected Outcomes** Routine meds given; IV fluids administered prn, IV fluids tapered as oral intake adequate to prevent dehydration
Discharge planning/ home care	Evaluate social services/visiting nurse/DC planning needs Possible home phototherapy Schedule follow-up bili levels as outpatient; follow-up with MD/NP	Offer info on CPR classes and/or film, give CPR booklet **Expected Outcomes** Infant DC home with parent(s); mother verbalizes follow-up appointments
Family involvement	Evaluate additional psychosocial needs Orient family to NSY, equipment, room Discuss rationale for treatment and possible side effects of phototherapy with family (stool changes, increased fluid loss, possible temp instability, slight lethargy, rash, altered sleep-wake patterns) Instruct family on infant's care while undergoing phototherapy: • Safety precautions—bili mask, isolette door closed and latched, covering genitalia per policy • Skin care, cord care, circ care as appropriate • Lab draws, rationale for intake and output As necessary, review role of pumping breasts and offering formula for limited time Encourage parent/significant other/sibling involvement in infant care as possible Evaluate family's understanding of information	Encourage parents to provide tactile stimulation during feeding and diaper changes Encourage cuddling and eye contact during feedings Offer suggestions to comfort restless infant: • Nesting beneath bili lights • Talking softly/singing quietly to infant • Taped music or tape recording of evening activities from home • Rhythmic patting of infant's buttocks • Firm, nonstroking touch, assisting with control of extremities • Pacifier for nonnutritive sucking Encourage family/friend support of mother/parents (i.e., meals, rest, child care for siblings, allow expression of concerns/feelings) **Expected Outcomes** Parents verbalize understanding of rationale and possible side effects of phototherapy; parents/family demonstrate safety precautions when caring for infant; parents getting meals, rest, verbalize support given
Date		

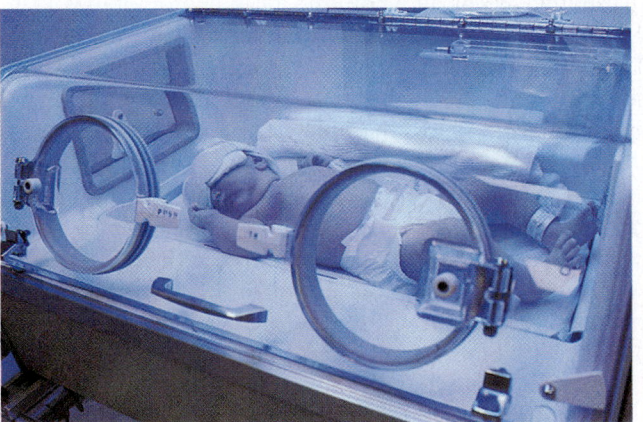

FIGURE 29–9. ◆ Infant receiving phototherapy. The phototherapy light is positioned over the incubator. Bilateral eye patches are always used to protect the baby's eyes during phototherapy.

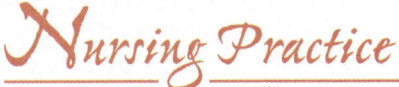 *Nursing Practice*

If the area of jaundice around the eyes begins to disappear, then the eye patches are allowing light to enter and better eye protection is needed.

Most phototherapy units provide the desired level of irradiance with the infant 45 to 50 cm below the lamps. Use a photometer to measure and maintain desired irradiance levels. Disadvantages of lights are that they create a difficult work environment and can distort an infant's color.

Monitor the newborn's temperature to prevent hyperthermia and hypothermia. The newborn needs additional fluids to compensate for the increased water lost through the skin and loose stools. Loose stools and increased urine output result from increased bilirubin excretion. Observe the infant for signs of dehydration and perianal excoriation.

A benign transient bronze discoloration of the skin may occur with phototherapy when the infant has elevated direct serum bilirubin levels or liver disease. As a side effect of phototherapy, some newborns develop a maculopapular rash. In addition to assessing the newborn's skin color for jaundice and bronzing, examine the skin for developing pressure areas. Reposition the newborn at least every 2 hours to permit the light to reach all skin surfaces, to prevent pressure areas, and to vary the stimulation to the infant. Keep track of the number of hours each lamp is used so that it can be replaced before its effectiveness is lost. Be careful about using ointment under bilirubin lights because this combination may cause burns.

The terms *jaundice, hyperbilirubinemia, exchange transfusion,* and *phototherapy* may sound frightening and threatening. Some parents may feel guilty about their baby's condition and think they have caused the problem. Under stress, parents may not be able to understand the physician's first explanations. Anticipate that the parents will need explanations repeated and clarified and that they may need help voicing their questions and fears. Encourage eye and tactile contact with the newborn. Coach parents when they visit with the baby. After the mother's discharge, keep parents informed of their infant's condition and encourage them to return to the hospital or call at any time so that they can be fully involved in the care of their infant. Tell parents that they can expect a rebound of 1 to 2 mg/dL after discontinuation of phototherapy and a follow-up bilirubin test may be done.

While the mother is still hospitalized, phototherapy can also be carried out in the parents' room if the only problem is hyperbilirubinemia. The parents must be willing to keep the baby in the room for 24 hours a day, be able to take emergency action (e.g., for choking) if necessary, and complete instruction checklists. Some institutions require that parents sign a consent form. Instruct the parents but also continue to monitor the infant's temperature, activity, intake and output, and positioning of eye patches at regular intervals (Table 29–4).

TABLE 29–4 Instructional Checklist for In-Room Phototherapy

Explain and demonstrate the placement of eye patches and explain that they must be in place when the infant is under the lights.

Explain the clothing to be worn (diaper under lights, dress and wrap when away from the lights).

Explain the importance of taking the infant's temperature regularly.

Explain the importance of adequate fluid intake.

Explain the charting flow sheet (intake, output, eyes covered).

Explain how to position the lights at a proper distance.

Explain the need to keep the infant under phototherapy except during feeding and diaper changes.

NURSING CARE IN THE COMMUNITY

If the baby is to receive phototherapy at home, teach the parents to record the infant's temperature, weight, fluid intake and output, stools, and feedings and to use the phototherapy equipment. In addition, if phototherapy lights are being used, parents must agree that the baby will be exposed to the lights for long periods of time; that they will hold the baby for only short periods for feeding, comforting, and cleansing of the perineal area; and that the room temperature will be regulated to minimize heat loss. Fiberoptic phototherapy blankets eliminate the need for eye patches, decrease heat loss because the baby is clothed, and provide more chances for baby-parent interaction. The best method of home phototherapy depends on the cause of the hyperbilirubinemia and the rate of progression of the jaundice.

Evaluation

Expected outcomes of nursing care include the following:

▶ The risks for development of hyperbilirubinemia are identified, and action is taken to minimize the potential impact of hyperbilirubinemia.

▶ The baby does not have any corneal irritation or drainage, skin breakdown, or major fluctuations in temperature.

▶ Parents understand the rationale for, goal of, and expected outcome of therapy.

▶ Parents verbalize their concerns about their baby's condition and identify how they can facilitate their baby's improvement.

CARE OF THE NEWBORN WITH ANEMIA

Neonatal anemia is often difficult to recognize by clinical evaluation alone. The hemoglobin concentration in a term newborn is 15 to 20 g/dL, slightly higher than that in premature newborns, in whom the mean hemoglobin is 14 to 18 g/dL. (Infants with hemoglobin values of less than 14 g/dL [term] and 13 g/dL [preterm] are usually considered anemic.) The most common causes of neonatal anemia are blood loss, hemolysis, and impaired RBC production.

Blood loss (hypovolemia) occurs in utero from placental bleeding (placenta previa or abruptio placentae). Intrapartal blood loss may be fetomaternal, fetofetal, or the result of umbilical cord bleeding. Birth trauma to abdominal organs or the cranium may produce significant blood loss, and cerebral bleeding may occur because of hypoxia.

Excessive hemolysis of RBCs is usually a result of blood group incompatibilities but may be due to infections. The most common cause of impaired RBC production is a genetically transmitted deficiency in G6PD. Anemia and jaundice are the presenting signs. A condition known as

physiologic anemia results from the normal gradual drop in hemoglobin for the first 6 to 12 weeks of life. Theoretically, the bone marrow stops production of RBCs as a response to the elevated oxygenation of extrauterine respirations. When the amount of hemoglobin decreases, reaching levels of 10 to 11 g/dL at about 8 to 12 weeks of age in term newborns, the bone marrow begins production of RBCs again, and the anemia disappears.

Anemia in preterm newborns is seen earlier than in term newborns, and increased production of RBCs does not start until hemoglobin is 7 to 10 g/dL. The preterm baby's hemoglobin reaches a low sooner (by 6 weeks after birth) than does a term newborn's (8 to 12 weeks) because a preterm infant's RBC survival time is shorter than that of a term newborn (Doyle, Schmidt, & Zipursky, 1999). This difference is due to several factors: the preterm infant's rapid growth rate, decreased iron stores, and an inadequate production of erythropoietin (EPO) (Juul, 1999).

Clinical Therapy

Hematologic problems can be anticipated based on the pregnancy history and clinical manifestations. The age at which anemia is first noted is also of diagnostic value. Clinically, light-skinned anemic infants are very pale when they do not have other symptoms of shock and usually have abnormally low RBC counts. In acute blood loss, symptoms of shock, such as pallor, low arterial blood pressure, and a decreasing hematocrit value, may be present. The initial laboratory workup should include hemoglobin and hematocrit measurements, reticulocyte count, ferritin concentrations, examination of peripheral blood smear, bilirubin determinations, direct Coombs' test of infant's blood, and examination of maternal blood smear for fetal erythrocytes (Kleihauer-Betke test). Clinical management depends on the severity of the anemia and on whether blood loss is acute or chronic. The baby should be placed on constant cardiac and respiratory monitoring. Mild or slow chronic anemia may be treated adequately with iron supplements alone or with iron-fortified formulas. Frequent determinations of hemoglobin, hematocrit, and bilirubin levels (in hemolytic disease) are essential. In severe cases of anemia, transfusions are the treatment of choice. Management of anemia of prematurity includes recombinant human erythropoietin (rEPO) and supplemental iron. Blood transfusions (dedicated units of blood) are kept to a minimum (Juul, 1999).

Nursing Management

Assess the newborn for symptoms of anemia (pallor). If the blood loss is acute, the baby may show signs of shock (a capillary filling time greater than 3 seconds, decreased pulses, tachycardia, low blood pressure). Continued observation identifies physiologic anemia as the preterm newborn grows. Signs of compromise include poor weight gain, tachycardia, tachypnea, and apneic episodes. Promptly report any symptoms indicating anemia or shock. Record the amount of blood drawn for all laboratory tests so that total blood removed can be assessed and replaced by transfusion when necessary. For long-term management see Chapter 44.

CARE OF THE NEWBORN WITH POLYCYTHEMIA

Polycythemia, a condition in which blood volume and hematocrit values are increased, is more common in SGA and full-term infants with delayed cord clamping, maternal-fetal and twin-to-twin transfusions, or chronic intrauterine hypoxia than in other newborns (Doyle et al., 1999). An infant is considered polycythemic when the central venous hematocrit value is greater than 65% to 70% or the venous hemoglobin level is greater than 22 g/dL during the first week of life. Other conditions that present with polycythemia are chromosomal anomalies such as trisomy 21, 18, and 13; endocrine disorders such as hypoglycemia and hypocalcemia; and births at altitudes over 5000 feet.

Clinical Therapy

The goal of therapy is to reduce the central venous hematocrit value to a range of 55% to 60% in symptomatic infants (Doyle et al., 1999). To decrease the RBC mass, the symptomatic infant receives a partial exchange transfusion in which blood is removed from the infant and replaced millimeter for millimeter with fresh frozen plasma or 5% albumin. The infant needs supportive treatment of presenting symptoms until the condition is resolved; this usually happens spontaneously after the partial exchange transfusion.

Nursing Management

Assess for, record, and report symptoms of polycythemia. Also do an initial screening of the newborn's hematocrit value on admission to the nursery. If a capillary hematocrit is done, warming the heel prior to obtaining the blood helps to decrease falsely high values. Peripheral venous hematocrit samples are usually obtained from the antecubital fossa.

Many infants are asymptomatic, but as symptoms develop, they are related to the increased blood volume, hyperviscosity (thickness) of the blood, and decreased deformability of RBCs, all of which result in poor perfusion of tissues. The infants have a characteristic plethoric (ruddy) appearance. The most common symptoms include:

- Tachycardia and congestive heart failure due to the increased blood volume
- Respiratory distress with grunting, tachypnea, and cyanosis; increased oxygen need; or respiratory hemorrhage due to pulmonary venous congestion, edema, and hypoxia

- Hyperbilirubinemia due to increased numbers of RBCs breaking down
- Decrease in peripheral pulses, discoloration of extremities, alteration in activity or neurologic depression, renal vein thrombosis with decreased urine output, hematuria, or proteinuria due to thromboembolism
- Jitteriness, decreased activity and tone, and seizures due to decreased perfusion of the brain and increased vascular resistance secondary to sluggish blood flow, which can result in neurologic or developmental problems
- Gastrointestinal-feeding difficulties, necrotizing enterocolitis (NEC)
- Metabolic-hypoglycemia, hypocalcemia

Observe closely for the signs of distress or change in vital signs during the partial exchange. Assess carefully for partial exchange transfusion complications such as transfusion overload (which may result in congestive heart failure), irregular cardiac rhythm, bacterial infection, hypovolemia, and anemia. Reunite the newborn with the parents as soon as the baby's status permits.

CARE OF THE NEWBORN WITH INFECTION

Newborns up to 1 month of age are particularly susceptible to an infection, referred to as **sepsis neonatorum,** caused by organisms that do not cause significant disease in older children. Once any infection occurs in the newborn, it can spread rapidly through the bloodstream, regardless of its primary site. The incidence of primary neonatal sepsis is 1 to 5 per 1000 live births (0.1% to .5%) (Edwards, 2002). Nosocomial infection frequency are less in the normal newborn infants and increase for infants in the neonatal intensive care unit (NICU).

One predisposing factor is prematurity. Prematurity and low birth weight are associated with nosocomial infection rates up to 15 times higher than average. The general debilitation and underlying illnesses often associated with prematurity mean that newborns need invasive procedures such as umbilical catheterization, intubation, resuscitation, ventilator support, monitoring, parenteral alimentation (especially lipid emulsions), and prior broad-spectrum antibiotic therapy. However, even full-term infants are susceptible, because their immunologic systems are immature. They lack the complex factors involved in effective phagocytosis and the ability to localize infection or to respond with a well-defined, recognizable inflammatory response. In addition, newborns lack the IgM immunoglobin necessary to protect against bacteria, because it does not cross the placenta (refer to Chapter 24 ⬭ for immunologic adaptations in the newborn period).

Most nosocomial infections in the NICU present as bacteremia or sepsis, urinary tract infections, meningitis, or pneumonia. Maternal antepartal infections such as rubella, toxoplasmosis, cytomegalic inclusion disease, and herpes may cause congenital infections and resulting disorders in the newborn. Intrapartal maternal infections, such as amnionitis and those resulting from premature rupture of membranes and precipitous birth, are sources of neonatal infection (see Chapter 13 ⬭ for more detailed information). Passage through the birth canal and contact with the vaginal flora (β-hemolytic streptococci, herpes, listeria, gonococci) expose the infant to infection (Table 29–5). When the fetus or newborn has an infection anywhere, the adjacent tissues or organs are very easily penetrated. The blood-brain barrier is ineffective. Septicemia is more common in males, except for infections caused by group B β-hemolytic streptococcus.

Gram-negative organisms (especially *Escherichia coli, Enterobacter, Proteus,* and *Klebsiella*) and the gram-positive organism β-hemolytic streptococcus are the most common causative agents. *Pseudomonas* is a common fomite contaminant of ventilator support and oxygen therapy equipment. Gram-positive bacteria, especially coagulase-negative staphylococci, are common pathogens in nosocomial bacteremias, pneumonias, and urinary tract infections. Other gram-positive bacteria that commonly cause infection are enterococci and *Staphylococcus aureus* (Edwards, 2002).

Protection of the newborn from infections starts prenatally and continues throughout pregnancy and birth. Prenatal prevention should include maternal screening for sexually transmitted infections and monitoring of rubella titers in women who test negative. Intrapartally, sterile technique is essential. Smears from genital lesions are taken, and placenta and amniotic fluid cultures are obtained if amnionitis is suspected. If genital herpes is present toward term, cesarean birth may be indicated. All newborns' eyes should be treated with silver nitrate or an antibiotic ophthalmic ointment to prevent damage from gonococcal infection. Prophylactic antibiotic therapy, for asymptomatic (group B streptococcus) GBS-culture-positive women during the intrapartum period, helps prevent early-onset sepsis (Schuchat, 1998).

Clinical Therapy

Cultures should be taken as soon after birth as possible for infants with a history of possible exposure to infection in utero (e.g., premature rupture of membranes [PROM] more than 24 hours before birth or questionable maternal history of infection). They are obtained before antibiotic therapy is begun.

1. Two blood cultures are obtained from different peripheral sites. They are taken from a peripheral rather than an umbilical vessel, because catheters may yield false-positive results due to contamination. The skin is prepared by cleaning with an antiseptic solution, such as one containing iodine, and allowed to dry; the specimen is obtained with a sterile needle and syringe.

2. Spinal fluid culture is done following a spinal tap.

TABLE 29–5   Maternally Transmitted Newborn Infections

Infection	Nursing Assessment	Nursing Plan and Implementation
GROUP B STREPTOCOCCUS 1%–2% colonized, with 1 in 10 developing disease Early onset—usually within hours of birth or within first week Late onset—1 week to 3 months	Severe respiratory distress (grunting and cyanosis) May become apneic or demonstrate symptoms of shock Meconium-stained amniotic fluid seen at birth	Early assessment of clinical signs necessary. Assist with x-ray examination—shows aspiration pneumonia or hyaline membrane disease. Immediately obtain blood, gastric aspirate, external ear canal, and nasopharynx cultures. Administer antibiotics, usually aqueous penicillin or ampicillin combined with gentamicin, as soon as cultures are obtained. Early assessment and intervention are essential to survival.

SYPHILIS
Spirochetes cross placenta after 16th–18th week of gestation
	Check perinatal history for positive maternal serology
	Assess infant for
	    Elevated cord serum IgM and FTA-ABS IgM
	    Rhinitis (snuffles)
	    Fissures on mouth corners and excoriated upper lip
	    Red rash around mouth and anus
	    Copper-colored rash over face, palms, and soles
	    Irritability
	    Generalized edema, particularly over joints; bone lesions; painful extremities
	    Hepatosplenomegaly, jaundice
	    Congenital cataracts
	    SGA and failure to thrive
		Refer to evaluate for blindness, deafness, learning or behavioral problems.
		Use isolation techniques until infants have been on antibiotics for 48 hours.
		Administer penicillin.
		Provide emotional support for parents because of their feelings about mode of transmission and potential long-term sequelae.

GONORRHEA
Approximately 30%–35% of newborns born vaginally to infected mothers acquire the infection
	Assess for
	    Ophthalmia neonatorum (conjunctivitis)
	    Purulent discharge and corneal ulcerations
	    Neonatal sepsis with temperature instability, poor feeding response, and/or hypotonia, jaundice
		Administer 1% silver nitrate solution or ophthalmic antibiotic ointment (see "Drug Guide: Erythromycin [Ilotycin] Ophthalmic Ointment" in Chapter 26) or, in lieu of silver nitrate, penicillin.
		Make a follow-up referral to evaluate any loss of vision.

HERPES TYPE 2 1 in 7500 births Usually transmitted during vaginal birth; a few cases of in utero transmission have been reported	Small cluster vesicular skin lesions over all the body Check perinatal history for active herpes genital lesions Disseminated form—DIC, pneumonia, hepatitis with jaundice, hepatosplenomegaly, and neurologic abnormalities. Without skin lesions, assess for fever or subnormal temperature, respiratory congestion, tachypnea, and tachycardia	Carry out careful handwashing and gown and glove isolation with linen precautions. Administer intravenous vidarabine (Vira A) or acyclovir (Zovirax). Make a follow-up referral to evaluate potential sequelae of microcephaly, spasticity, seizures, deafness, or blindness. Encourage parental rooming-in and touching of their newborn. Show parents appropriate handwashing procedures and precautions to be used at home if mother's lesions are active. Obtain throat, conjunctiva, cerebral spinal fluid (CSF), blood, urine, and lesion cultures to identify herpesvirus type 2 antibiotics in serum IgM fraction. Cultures positive in 24–48 hours.
ORAL CANDIDAL INFECTION (THRUSH) Acquired during passage through birth canal	Assess newborn's buccal mucosa, tongue, gums, and inside the cheeks for white plaques (seen 5 to 7 days of age) Check diaper area for bright-red, well-demarcated eruptions Assess for thrush periodically when newborn is on long-term antibiotic therapy	Differentiate white plaque areas from milk curds by using cotton tip applicator (if it is thrush, removal of white areas causes raw, bleeding areas). Maintain cleanliness of hands, linen, clothing, diapers, and feeding apparatus. Instruct breastfeeding mothers on treating their nipples with nystatin. Administer gentian violet (1%–2%) swabbed on oral lesions 1 hour after feeding or nystatin instilled in baby's oral cavity and on mucosa. Swab skin lesions with topical nystatin. Discuss with parents that gentian violet stains mouth and clothing. Avoid placing gentian violet on normal mucosa; it causes irritation.
CHLAMYDIA TRACHOMATIS Acquired during passage through birth canal	Assess for perinatal history of preterm birth Symptomatic newborns present with pneumonia—conjunctivitis after 3–4 days Chronic follicular conjunctivitis (corneal neovascularization and conjunctival scarring)	Instill ophthalmic erythromycin (see "Drug Guide: Erythromycin [Ilotycin] Ophthalmic Ointment" in Chapter 26). Make a follow-up referral for eye complications and late development of pneumonia at 4–11 weeks postnatally.

3. The specimen for urine culture is best obtained by a suprapubic bladder aspiration.

4. Skin cultures are taken of any lesions or drainage from lesions or reddened areas.

5. Nasopharyngeal, rectal, ear canal, and gastric aspirate cultures may be obtained.

Other laboratory investigations include a complete blood count, chest x-ray examination, serology, and gram stains of cerebrospinal fluid, urine, skin exudate, and umbilicus. White blood cell (WBC) count with differential may indicate the presence or absence of sepsis. A level of 30,000 WBCs may be normal in the first 24 hours of life, and a low WBC count may indicate sepsis. A low neutrophil count and a high band (immature WBCs) count indicate an infection. Stomach aspirate should be sent for culture and smear if a gonococcal infection or amnionitis is suspected. The C-reactive protein level may or may not be elevated. Serum IgM levels are elevated (normal level less than 20 mg/dL) in response to transplacental infections. If available, counterimmunoelectrophoresis tests for specific bacterial antigens are performed.

Evidence of congenital infections may be seen on skull x-ray films (cerebral calcifications such as in cytomegalovirus, toxoplasmosis), on bone x-ray films (syphilis, cytomegalovirus), and in serum-specific IgM levels (rubella). Cytomegalovirus infection is best diagnosed by urine culture.

Because neonatal infection causes high mortality, therapy begins before results of the septic workup are obtained. A combination of two broad-spectrum antibiotics, such as ampicillin and gentamicin, is given in large doses until a culture with sensitivities is obtained.

After the pathogen and its sensitivities are determined, appropriate specific antibiotic therapy is begun. Combinations of penicillin or ampicillin and kanamycin have been used in the past, but new kanamycin-resistant enterobacteria and penicillin-resistant staphylococcus mean gentamicin must increasingly be used.

Rotating aminoglycosides has been suggested to prevent development of resistance. Use of cephalosporins and, in particular, cefotaxime has emerged as an alternative to aminoglycoside therapy in the treatment of neonatal infections. Duration of therapy varies from 7 to 14 days (Table 29–6). If cultures are negative and symptoms subside, antibiotics may be discontinued after 3 days. Supportive physiologic care may be required to maintain respiratory, hemodynamic, nutritional, and metabolic homeostasis.

Nursing Management

Nursing Assessment and Diagnosis

The nurse most often notices symptoms of infection during daily care of the newborn. The infant may deteriorate rapidly in the first 12 to 24 hours after birth if β-hemolytic streptococcal infection is present, with signs and symptoms mimicking RDS. In other cases, the onset of sepsis may be gradual, with more subtle signs and symptoms. The most common signs include:

1. Subtle behavioral changes; the infant "is not doing well" and is often lethargic or irritable (especially after the first 24 hours) and hypotonic; color changes may include pallor, duskiness, cyanosis, or a "shocky" appearance; skin is cool and clammy

2. Temperature instability, manifested by either hypothermia (recognized by a decrease in skin temperature) or, rarely in newborns, hyperthermia (elevation of skin temperature) necessitating a corresponding increase or decrease in incubator temperature to maintain a neutral thermal environment

3. Feeding intolerance, as evidenced by a decrease in total intake, abdominal distention, vomiting, poor sucking, lack of interest in feeding, and diarrhea

4. Hyperbilirubinemia

5. Tachycardia initially, followed by spells of apnea or bradycardia

Signs and symptoms may suggest CNS disease (jitteriness, tremors, seizure activity), respiratory system disease (tachypnea, labored respirations, apnea, cyanosis), hematologic disease (jaundice, petechial hemorrhages, hepatosplenomegaly), or gastrointestinal disease (diarrhea, vomiting, bile-stained aspirate, hepatomegaly). A differential diagnosis is necessary because symptoms are similar to those of other more specific conditions.

Nursing diagnoses that may apply to the infant with sepsis neonatorum and the family include:

▸ *Risk for infection* related to immature immunologic system

▸ *Fluid volume deficit* related to feeding intolerance

▸ *Ineffective family coping* related to present illness resulting in prolonged hospital stay for the newborn

Planning and Implementation

In the nursery, environmental control and prevention of acquired infection are the responsibilities of the neonatal nurse. Promote strict handwashing technique for all who enter the nursery, including nursing colleagues; physicians; laboratory, x-ray, and respiratory therapists; and parents. Be prepared to assist in the aseptic collection of specimens for laboratory investigations. Scrupulous equipment care—changing and cleaning of incubators at least every 7 days, removing and sterilizing wet equipment every 24 hours, preventing cross use of linen and equipment, cleaning sink-side equipment such as soap containers periodically, and taking special care with the open radiant warmers (access without prior handwashing is much more likely than with the closed incubator)—prevents fomite contamination or contamination through improper handwashing. An infected newborn can be effectively

TABLE 29-6 Neonatal Sepsis Antibiotic Therapy

Drug	Dose (mg/kg) Total Daily Dose	Schedule for Divided Doses	Route	Comments
Ampicillin	50–100 mg/kg	Every 12 hours* Every 8 hours†	IM or IV	Effective against gram-positive microorganisms, *Haemophilus influenzae*, and most *Escherichia coli* strains. Higher doses indicated for meningitis. Used with aminoglycoside for synergy.
Cefotaxime	50 mg/kg 100–150 mg/kg/day	Every 12 hours* Every 8 hours†	IM or IV	Active against most major pathogens in infants; effective against aminoglycoside-resistant organisms; achieves CSF bactericidal activity; lack of ototoxicity and nephrotoxicity; wide therapeutic index (levels not required); resistant organisms can develop rapidly if used extensively; ineffective against *Pseudomonas, Listeria*.
Gentamicin	2.5–3 mg/kg 5–7.5 mg/kg/day	Every 12–24 hours*‡ Every 8–24 hours†	IM or IV	Effective against gram-negative rods and staphylococci; may be used instead of kanamycin against penicillin-resistant staphylococci and *E. coli* strains and *Pseudomonas aeruginosa*. May cause ototoxicity and nephrotoxicity. Need to follow serum levels. Must never be given as IV push. Must be given over at least 30–60 minutes. In presence of oliguria or anuria, dose must be decreased or discontinued. In infants less than 1000 g or 29 weeks, lower dosage 2.5–3 mg/kg/day. Monitor serum levels before administration of second dose. Peak 5–10 µg/mL Trough 1–2 µg/mL
Methicillin	25–50 mg/dose 50–100 mg/kg/day	Every 12 hours* Every 6–8 hours†	IM or IV	Effective against penicillinase-resistant staphylococci. Monitor CBC and UA. Slow IV push.
Nafcillin	25–50 mg/kg 50–100 mg/kg/day	Every 8–12 hours* Every 6–8 hours†	IM or IV	Effective against penicillinase-resistant staphylococci. Caution in presence of jaundice.
Penicillin G (aqueous crystalline)	25,000–50,000 IU/kg 50,000–125,000 IU/kg/day	Every 12 hours* Every 8 hours†	IM or IV	Initial sepsis therapy effective against most gram-positive micro-organisms except resistant staphylococci; can cause heart block in infants.
Vancomycin	10–20 mg/kg 30 mg/kg/day	Every 12–24 hours*‡ Every 8 hours†	IV	Effective for methicillin-resistant strains (*Staphylococcus epidermidis*); must be administered by slow intravenous infusion to avoid prolonged cutaneous eruption. For smaller infants, < 1200 g, < 29 weeks, smaller dosages and longer intervals between doses. Nephrotoxic, especially in combination with aminoglycosides. Slow IV infusion over at least 60 minutes. Peak 25–40 µg/mL Trough 5–10 µg/mL

*Up to 7 days of age. †Greater than 7 days of age. ‡Dependent on GA.

isolated in an incubator and receive close observation. Discourage visits to the nursery area by unnecessary personnel.

Administer antibiotics as ordered by the nurse practitioner or physician. In addition to the five rights of drug administration, be knowledgeable about the following:

▶ The proper dose to be administered, based on the weight of the newborn and desired peak and trough levels

▶ The appropriate route of administration, because some antibiotics cannot be given intravenously

▶ Admixture incompatibilities, because some antibiotics are precipitated by intravenous solutions or by other antibiotics

▶ Side effects and toxicity

In term infants being treated for infections, neonatal home infusion of antibiotics should be considered as a viable alternative to continued hospitalization. The infusion of antibiotics at home by skilled RNs facilitates parent-infant bonding while meeting the infant's ongoing health care needs (Anastasi, 1998).

In addition to antibiotic therapy, physiologic supportive care is essential in caring for a septic infant. Responsibilities of the nurse include:

▶ Observe for resolution of symptoms or development of other symptoms of sepsis.

▶ Maintain neutral thermal environment with accurate regulation of humidity and oxygen administration.

▶ Provide respiratory support: administer oxygen and observe and monitor respiratory effort.

▶ Provide cardiovascular support: observe and monitor pulse and blood pressure; observe for hyperbilirubinemia, anemia, and hemorrhagic symptoms.

▶ Provide adequate calories; oral feedings may be discontinued due to increased mucus, abdominal distention, vomiting, and aspiration.

▶ Provide fluids and electrolytes to maintain homeostasis; monitor weight changes, urine output, and urine specific gravity.

▶ Observe for the development of hypoglycemia, hyperglycemia, acidosis, hyponatremia, and hypocalcemia.

Restricting parental visits has not been shown to have any effect on the rate of infection and may be harmful for the newborn's psychologic development. With instruction and guidance, both parents should be allowed to handle the baby and participate in daily care. Support of the parents is crucial. They need to be informed of the newborn's prognosis as treatment continues and to be involved in care as much as possible (Figure 29–10 ◆). They also need to understand how infection is transmitted.

Evaluation

Expected outcomes of nursing care include the following:

▶ The risks for development of sepsis are identified early, and immediate action is taken to minimize the development of the illness.

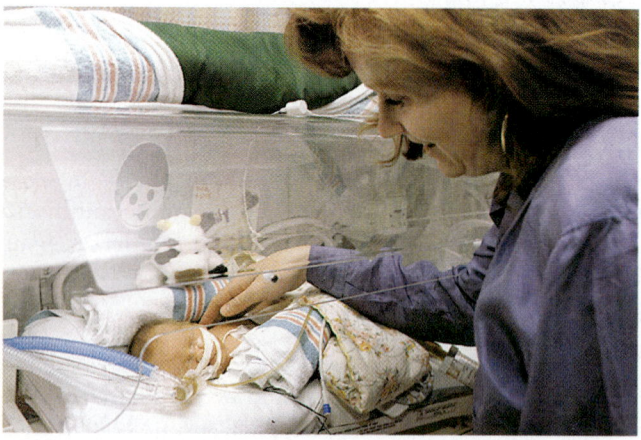

FIGURE 29–10. ◆ When parents participate in their baby's care, they tend to develop realistic expectations about the child's long-term developmental needs.

▶ Appropriate use of aseptic technique protects the newborn from further exposure to illness.

▶ The baby's symptoms are relieved, and the infection is treated.

▶ The parents verbalize their concerns about their baby's illness and understand the rationale behind the management of their newborn.

CARE OF FAMILY WITH BIRTH OF AN AT-RISK NEWBORN

The birth of a preterm or ill infant or an infant with a congenital anomaly is a serious crisis for a family. Family members have acute grief reactions to the loss of the idealized baby they have envisioned. In a preterm birth, the mother is denied the last few weeks of pregnancy that seem to prepare her psychologically for the stress of birth and the attachment process. Attachment at this time is fragile, and interruption of the process by separation can affect the future mother-child relationship. Feelings of guilt and failure often plague mothers of preterm newborns. They may question themselves: "Why did labor start?" or "What did I do [or not do]?" A woman may have guilt fantasies and wonder: "Was it because I had sexual intercourse with my husband [a week, 3 days, a day] ago?" "Was it because I carried three loads of wash up from the basement?" or "Am I being punished for something done in the past—even in childhood?"

The birth of the newborn with an illness or congenital abnormalities also engenders feelings of guilt and failure. As in the birth of a preterm infant, the woman may entertain ideas of personal guilt: "What did I do [or not do] to cause this?" or "Am I being punished for something?"

The birth of an at-risk newborn alters parental reactions and steps of attachment. Parents must recognize and deal with a variety of new feelings, reactions, and stresses before they can establish a healthy parent-infant relationship.

Although reactions and steps of attachment are altered by the birth of these infants, a healthy parent-child relationship can occur. Kaplan and Mason (1974) have identified four psychologic tasks as essential for coping with the stress of an at-risk newborn and for providing a basis for the maternal-infant relationship:

1. Anticipatory grief as a psychologic preparation for possible loss of the child while still hoping for his or her survival

2. Acknowledgment of maternal failure to produce a term or perfect newborn expressed as anticipatory grief and depression and lasting until the chances of survival seem secure

3. Resumption of the process of relating to the infant, which was interrupted by the threat of nonsurvival; continuous threat of death or abnormality may impair this task, and the mother may be slow in her response of hope for the infant's survival

4. Understanding of the special needs and growth patterns of the at-risk newborn, which are temporary and yield to normal patterns

Most authorities agree that the birth of a preterm infant or an infant with a problem requires major adjustments as the parents are forced to surrender the image they had nurtured for so long of their ideal child. *Grief work*, the emotional reaction to a significant loss, must occur before adequate attachment to the actual child is possible. Parental detachment precedes parental attachment.

Solnit and Stark (1961) postulate that grief and mourning over the loss of the loved object—the idealized child—mark parental reactions to a child with abnormalities. Simultaneously, they must adopt the imperfect child as the new love object. Parental responses to a child with health problems may be viewed as a five-stage process (Klaus & Kennell, 1982):

1. *Shock* is felt at the reality of the birth of this child. This stage may be characterized by forgetfulness, amnesia about the situation, and a feeling of desperation.

2. There is disbelief *(denial)* of the reality of the situation, characterized by a refusal to believe the child has a problem . This stage is exemplified by assertions that "It didn't really happen!" or "There has been a mistake; it's someone else's baby."

3. *Depression* over the reality of the situation and a corresponding grief reaction follows acceptance of the situation. This stage is characterized by much crying and sadness. Anger may also emerge at this stage. A projection of blame on others or on self and feelings of "not me" are characteristic of this stage.

4. *Equilibrium and acceptance* are characteristic of a decrease in the emotional reactions of the parents. This stage is variable and may be prolonged by a continuing threat to the infant's survival. Some parents feel chronic sorrow in relation to their child.

5. *Reorganization* of the family is necessary to deal with the child's problems. Mutual support of the parents facilitates this process, but the crisis of the situation may precipitate alienation between the mother and father.

Nursing Management

Nursing Assessment and Diagnosis

A positive nurse-family relationship helps information gathering in areas of concern. A concurrent illness of the mother or other family members or other concurrent stress (lack of hospitalization insurance, loss of job, age of parents) may change the family response to the baby. Feelings of apprehension, guilt, failure, and grief expressed verbally or nonverbally are important aspects of the nursing history. These observations enable all professionals to be aware of the parental state, coping behaviors, and readiness for attachment, bonding, and caretaking. Appropriate nursing observations during interviewing and relating to the family include the nurse's assessment of:

1. *Level of understanding:* observations concerning the ability to assimilate the information given and to ask appropriate questions; the need for constant repetition of information

2. *Behavioral responses:* appropriateness of behavior in relation to information given; lack of response; flat affect

3. *Difficulties with communication:* deafness (reads lips only); blindness; dysphagia; understanding only of foreign language

4. *Paternal and maternal education level:* parents unable to read or write; parents with eighth-grade-level education; parents with a graduate-level degree or health care background

Documenting such information, gathered through continuing contact and development of a therapeutic relationship with the family, lets all professionals understand and use the nursing history to provide continuous individual care.

Visiting and caregiving patterns indicate the level or lack of parental attachment. A record of visits, caretaking procedures, affect (in relating to the newborn), and telephone calls is essential. It is important to note serial observations rather than just isolated observations that cause concern. Grant (1978) has developed a conceptual framework depicting adaptive and maladaptive responses to parenting of an infant with an actual or potential problem (Figure 29–11 ◆).

If a pattern of distancing behaviors evolves, intervene appropriately. Follow-up studies have found that a statistically significant number of preterm, sick, and congenitally defective infants suffer from failure to thrive, battering, or other parenting disorders. Early detection and intervention prevents these aberrations in parenting behaviors from leading to irreparable damage or death.

Nursing diagnoses that may apply to the family of a newborn at risk include:

▶ *Dysfunctional grieving* related to loss of idealized newborn

▶ *Fear* related to emotional involvement with an at-risk newborn

▶ *Altered parenting* related to impaired bonding secondary to feelings of inadequacy about caretaking activities

Planning and Implementation

HOSPITAL-BASED NURSING CARE

Support of Parents for Initial Visit to the Newborn

Before parents see their child, prepare them for the visit. Maintain a positive, realistic attitude about the infant. An

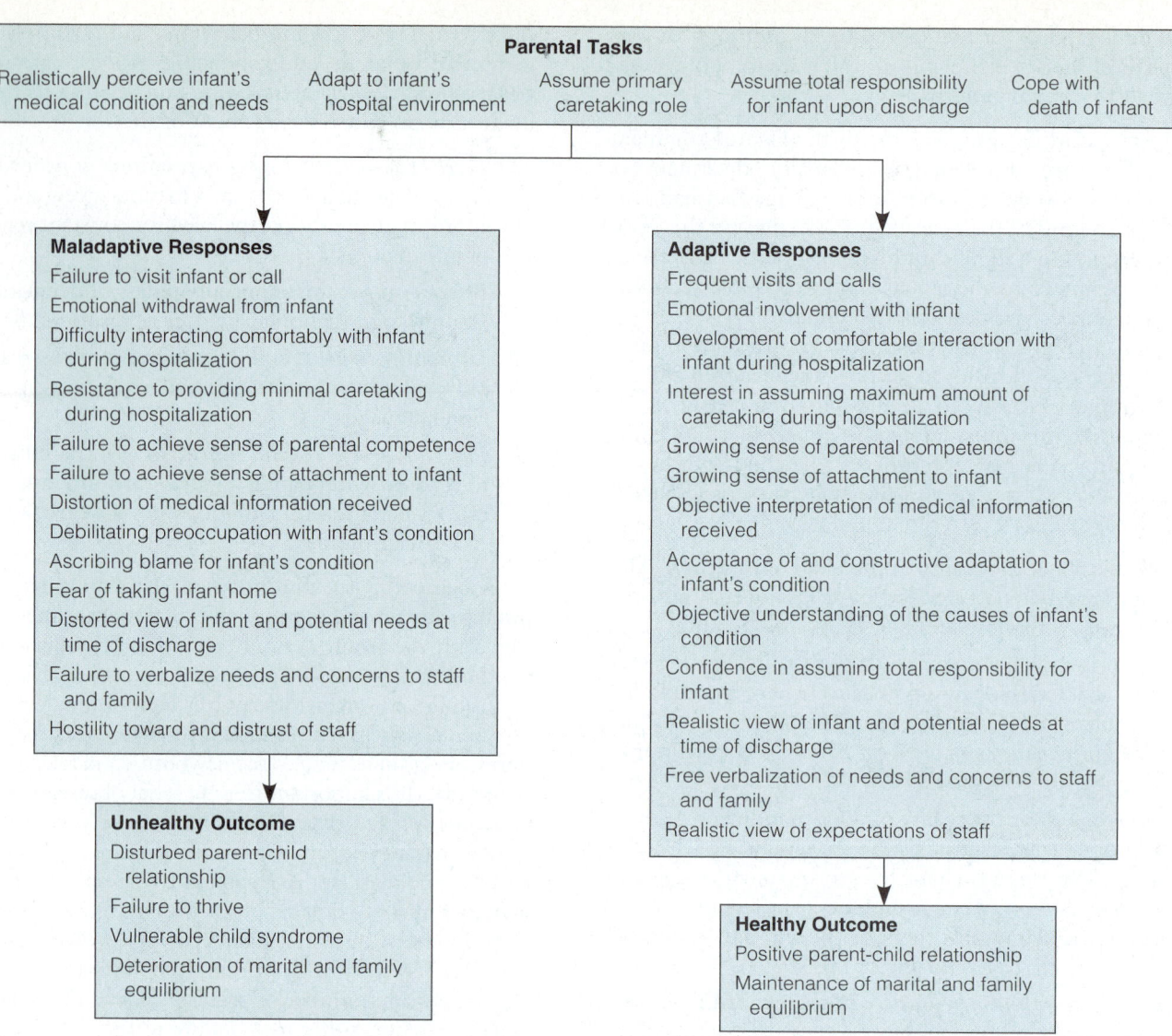

Parental Tasks

| Realistically perceive infant's medical condition and needs | Adapt to infant's hospital environment | Assume primary caretaking role | Assume total responsibility for infant upon discharge | Cope with death of infant |

Maladaptive Responses

Failure to visit infant or call

Emotional withdrawal from infant

Difficulty interacting comfortably with infant during hospitalization

Resistance to providing minimal caretaking during hospitalization

Failure to achieve sense of parental competence

Failure to achieve sense of attachment to infant

Distortion of medical information received

Debilitating preoccupation with infant's condition

Ascribing blame for infant's condition

Fear of taking infant home

Distorted view of infant and potential needs at time of discharge

Failure to verbalize needs and concerns to staff and family

Hostility toward and distrust of staff

Adaptive Responses

Frequent visits and calls

Emotional involvement with infant

Development of comfortable interaction with infant during hospitalization

Interest in assuming maximum amount of caretaking during hospitalization

Growing sense of parental competence

Growing sense of attachment to infant

Objective interpretation of medical information received

Acceptance of and constructive adaptation to infant's condition

Objective understanding of the causes of infant's condition

Confidence in assuming total responsibility for infant

Realistic view of infant and potential needs at time of discharge

Free verbalization of needs and concerns to staff and family

Realistic view of expectations of staff

Unhealthy Outcome

Disturbed parent-child relationship

Failure to thrive

Vulnerable child syndrome

Deterioration of marital and family equilibrium

Healthy Outcome

Positive parent-child relationship

Maintenance of marital and family equilibrium

FIGURE 29–11. ◆ Maladaptive and adaptive parental responses during crisis period, showing unhealthy and healthy outcomes.
Note: From Grant, P. (1978). Psychological needs of families of high-risk infants. *Family and Community Health, 1*(3), 93; with permission of Aspen Publishers, Inc., © 1978.

overly negative, fatalistic attitude further alienates the parents from their infant and retards attachment behaviors. Instead of beginning to bond with their child, the parents will anticipate their loss and begin the process of grieving. Once started, the grieving process is difficult to reverse.

Before preparing parents for the first view of their infant, observe the baby. All infants exhibit strengths as well as deficiencies; prepare the parents to see both the deviations and the normal aspects of their infant. The nurse may say, "Your baby is small, about the length of my two hands. She weighs 2 lb, 3 oz, but is very active and cries when we disturb her. She is having some difficulty breathing but is breathing without assistance and in only 35% oxygen."

Describe the equipment being used for the at-risk newborn and its purpose before the parents enter the intensive care unit. Many NICUs have booklets for parents to read before entering the units. Explanations and pictures make

the parents better prepared to deal with the feelings they may experience when they see their infant for the first time.

Upon entering the unit, parents may be overwhelmed by the sounds of monitors, alarms, and respirators, as well as by the unfamiliar language and "foreign" atmosphere. Preparing the parents by having the same health care professionals accompany them to the unit can be reassuring. The primary nurse and physician caring for the newborn need to be with the parents when they first visit their baby. Parental reactions vary, but initially there is usually an element of shock. Help them by providing chairs and time to regain composure. Slow, complete, and simple explanations— first about the infant and then about the equipment—allay fear and anxiety.

As parents attempt to deal with the initial stages of shock and grief, they may fail to grasp new information. They may need repeated explanations to accept the reality of the situation, procedures, equipment, and the infant's condition on subsequent visits.

Misconceptions about equipment and its placement on the infant and about its potential harm are common. Such questions as "Does the fluid go into the brain?" "Does the white wire on the abdomen go into the stomach?" and "Does the monitor make the baby's heart beat?" reveal fear for the infant's safety and misconception about the machines. Alleviate these worries by simple explanations of all equipment being used.

Concern about the infant's physical appearance is common yet may remain unvoiced. Parents may express such concerns as "He looks so small and red—like a drowned rat," "Why do her genitals look so abnormal?" and "Will that awful-looking mouth [cleft lip and palate] ever be normal?" Anticipate and address such questions. Use of pictures, such as of an infant after cleft lip repair, may be reassuring to doubting parents. Knowledge of the development of a "normal" preterm infant allows the nurse to make reassuring statements such as "The baby's labia may look very abnormal to you, but they are normal for her level of maturity. As she grows, the outer lips of the labia will become larger and the clitoris will be covered, and the genitals will then look as you expect them to. She is normal for her level of maturity."

The nursing staff set the tone of the NICU. Nurses foster the development of a safe, trusting environment by viewing the parents as essential caregivers, not as visitors or nuisances in the unit. Providing privacy when needed and offering easy access to staff and facilities are important in developing an open, comfortable environment. An uncrowded and welcoming atmosphere lets parents know they are welcome there. However, even in crowded physical surroundings, the nurses can convey an attitude of openness and trust.

A trusting relationship is essential for collaborative efforts in caring for the infant. Therapeutically use personal responses to relate to the parents on a one-to-one basis. Each person has different needs, different ways of adapting to crisis, and different means of support. Use techniques that feel real and spontaneous and avoid words or actions that feel foreign. Gauge interventions so that they match the parents' pace and needs.

Facilitation of Attachment if Neonatal Transport Occurs

Transport to a regional referral center that may be some distance from the parents' community may be necessary. It is essential that the mother see and touch her infant before the infant is transported. Bring the mother to the nursery or take the infant in a warmed transport incubator to the mother's bedside to let her see the infant before transportation to the center. When the infant reaches the referral center, a staff member should call the parents with information about the infant's condition during transport, safe arrival at the center, and present condition.

Occasionally the mother may be unable to see the infant before transport (e.g., if she is still under general anesthesia or experiencing complications such as shock, hemorrhage, or seizures). In these cases, before the infant is transported, take a photograph of the infant to give to the mother, and provide an explanation of the infant's condition and problems and a detailed description of the infant's characteristics. An additional photograph is also helpful for the father to share with siblings or extended family. With the increased attention on improved fetal outcome, prenatal maternal transports, rather than neonatal transports, are occurring more frequently. This practice gives the mother of an at-risk infant the opportunity to visit and care for her infant during the early postpartal period.

Promotion of Touching and Parental Caretaking

Parents visiting a small or sick infant may need several visits to become comfortable and confident in their ability to touch the infant without injuring him or her. Barriers such as incubators, incisions, monitor electrodes, and tubes may delay the mother's development of comfort in touching the newborn. Knowledge of this normal delay in touching behavior will help the nurse understand parental behavior.

Klaus and Kennell (1982) have demonstrated a significant difference in the amount of eye contact and touching behaviors of mothers of normal newborns and mothers of preterm infants. Whereas mothers of normal newborns progress within minutes to palm contact of the infant's trunk, mothers of preterm infants are slower to progress from fingertip to palm contact and from the extremities to the trunk. Mothers may need several visits to the nursery to progress to palm contact with the infant's trunk.

Use support, reassurance, and encouragement to help the mother develop positive feelings about her parenting abilities and her importance to her infant. Touching facilitates familiarity with the infant and thus establishes a bond between mother and infant. Touching and seeing the infant help the mother realize the normal aspects and potential of her baby (Figure 29–12 ◆).

Encourage parents to meet their newborn's need for stimulation. Stroking, rocking, cuddling, singing, and talking should be an integral part of the parents' caretaking responsibilities. Promote bonding by encouraging parents to visit and become involved in their baby's care (Figure 29–13 ◆). When visiting is impossible, the parents should feel free to phone whenever they wish to receive information about their baby. A warm, receptive attitude provides support. Facilitate parenting by personalizing a baby to the parents, by referring to the infant by name or by relating personal behavioral characteristics. Remarks such as "Jenny loves her pacifier" help make the infant seem individual and unique.

Caretaking may be delayed for the mother of a preterm, at-risk, or sick infant. The variety of equipment needed for life support is hardly conducive to anxiety-free caretaking by the parents. However, parents may care for even the

STAGE I: Touching

Uses fingertips

Uses whole hand

Strokes child

Holds and studies child "*en face*"

Spontaneously lowers crib rails to fondle, hold, or talk to child

↓

STAGE II: Caretaking

Provides clean clothing, toys, grooming aids

Performs activities of daily living (bathing, diapering, feeding, dressing)

Performs caretaking tasks with proficiency and expresses pleasure in meeting infant's needs

Able to comfort child when distressed or crying

Able to meet child's special health needs (suctioning, cleaning stoma sites, treatments)

↓

STAGE III: Identity

Brings linens from home

Takes photographs

Brings individualized toys

Can make personalized observations about child

Offers suggestions and makes demands for personalized care

Demonstrates "advocacy" behavior

Feels he or she can care for child better than anyone else

Demonstrates consistent visiting and/or calling pattern

Questions focus on total child, not only physiologic parameters

FIGURE 29–12. ◆ Stages of parenting behavior toward infants in intensive care. *Note:* From work of Rubin, Schaeffer, Jay, and Schraeder by Schraeder, B. D. (1980). Attachment and parenting despite lengthy intensive care. *American Journal of Maternal Child Nursing 5,* 38. Reprinted with permission from the American Journal of Nursing Company, 1980. Adapted.

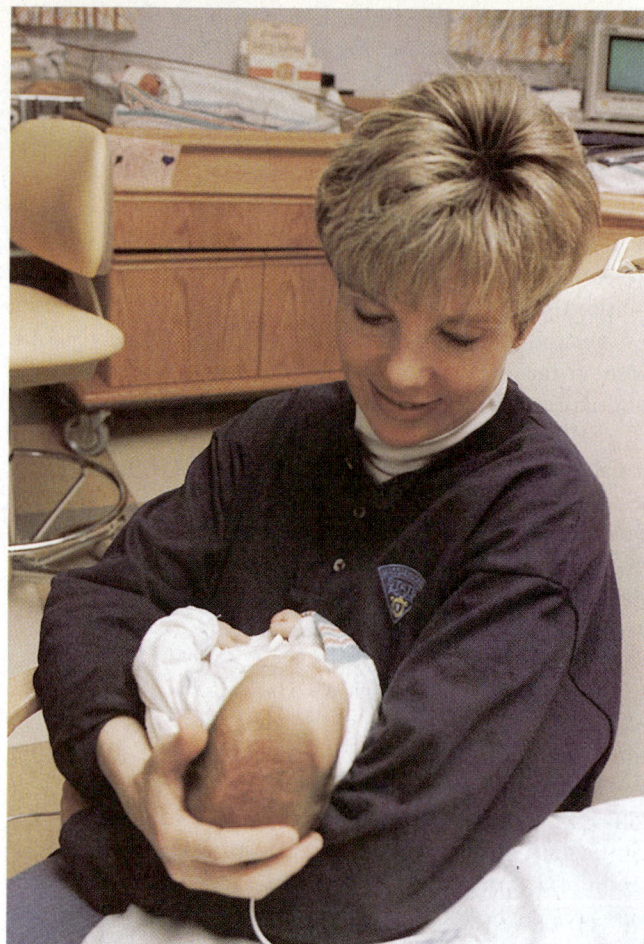

FIGURE 29–13. ◆ It is important that the parents of high-risk infants be given the opportunity to get acquainted with their children. Physical contact is extremely important in the bonding process and should be encouraged whenever possible.

sickest infant, if only in a small way. Promote the parents' success by facilitating parental caretaking. Demonstration and explanation, followed by support of the parents in initial caretaking behaviors, positively reinforce this behavior. Changing their infant's diaper, providing skin or oral care, or helping turn the infant may at first provoke anxiety, but the parents will become more comfortable and confident in caretaking and feel satisfied by the baby's reactions and their ability "to do something." Complimenting the parents' competence in caretaking also increases their self-esteem, which may have been damaged by feelings of guilt and failure. It is vitally important to never give the parents a task that they might not be able to accomplish.

Often parents of high-risk infants have ambivalent feelings toward the nurse. As they watch the nurse competently perform caretaking tasks, they may feel both grateful for the nurse's abilities and expertise and jealous of the nurse's ability to care for their infant. These feelings may take the form of criticism of the care of the infant, manipulation of staff, or personal guilt. Instead of fostering (by silence) these inferiority feelings of parents, recognize that such feelings are needed to intervene appropriately to enhance parent-infant attachment. For example, avoid making unfavorable comparisons between the baby's responses to parental and nursing caretaking. During a quiet time it may help to encourage the parents to talk about their hopes and fears and to facilitate their involvement in parent groups (Raines, 1998). Parents are also often anxious when their baby is transferred from the NICU to the "regular nursery." They may feel that their infant is not being cared for as proficiently because the nurses are not at the infant's bedside as often as they were in the NICU.

Nurses who are understanding and secure are able to support the parents' egos instead of collecting rewards for themselves. To reinforce positive parenting behaviors, professionals must first believe in the importance of the parents. The nurse can hardly convince doubting parents of their importance to the infant if he or she does not really believe it. Convey by both attitudes and words that they are good parents and have an important contribution to make in the care of their infant. Unless as much care is taken in facilitating parental attachment as in providing physiologic care, the outcome may not be a healthy family.

Verbalizations that improve parental self-esteem are essential and easily shared. For example, point out that, in addition to physiologic use, breast milk is important because of the emotional investment of the mother. Pumping, storing, labeling, and delivering quantities of breast milk is a time-consuming labor of love for mothers. Positive remarks about breast milk reinforce the maternal behavior of caretaking and providing for her infant: "Breast milk is something that only you can give your baby," "You really have brought a lot of milk today," "Look how rich this breast milk is," or "Even small amounts of milk are important, and look how rich it is." If the infant begins to gain weight while being fed breast milk, it is important to point this correlation out to the mother. Advise the parents that initial weight loss with beginning nipple-feedings is common because of the increased energy expended when the infant begins active rather than passive nutritional intake.

Provision of care by the parents is appropriate even for very sick infants with lethal anomalies who are likely to die. Detachment is easier after attachment, because the parents are comforted by the knowledge that they did all they could for their child while he or she was alive.

Facilitation of Family Adjustment

During crisis, it is difficult to maintain interpersonal relationships. Yet in a newborn intensive care area, the parents are expected to relate to many different care providers. It is important that parents have as few professionals as possible relaying information to them. A primary nurse should coordinate care and provide continuity for parents. Care providers are individuals and thus will use different terms, inflections, and attitudes. These subtle differences are monumental to parents and may confuse, confound, and produce anxiety. The transfer of the baby from NICU to a step-down unit or transport back to the home hospital provokes parental anxiety because they must now deal with new health care professionals. The nurse not only functions as a liaison between the parents and the various professionals interacting with the infant and parents but also offers clarification, explanation, interpretation of information, and support to the parents.

Encourage parents to deal with the crisis with help from their support system. The support system attempts to meet the emotional needs and to provide support for the family members in crisis and stress situations. Biologic kinship is not the only valid criterion for a support system; an emotional kinship is the most important factor. In our mobile society of isolated nuclear families, the support system may be a next-door neighbor, a best friend, or perhaps a schoolmate. Search out the significant others in the lives of the parents and help them understand the problems so that they can support the parents.

The impact of the crisis on the family is individual and varied. Find out about the family's ability to adapt to the situation through interaction with the family. To institute appropriate interventions, view the birth of the infant (normal newborn, preterm infant, infant with congenital anomaly) as it is defined by the family.

It is important to encourage open intrafamily communication. Discourage the family from keeping secrets from one another, especially between spouses, because secrets undermine the trust of relationships. Well-meaning rationales such as "I want to protect her," "I don't want him to worry about it," and so on can be destructive to open communication and to the basic element of a relationship—trust.

Open communication is especially important when the mother is hospitalized apart from the infant. The first person to visit the infant relays information regarding the infant's care and condition to the mother and family. In this situation, the mother has had minimal contact, if any, with her infant. Because of her anxiety and isolation, she may mistrust all those who provide information (the father, nurse, physician, or extended family) until she sees the infant for herself. This can put tremendous stress on the relationship between spouses. The parents (and family) should be given information together. This practice helps overcome misunderstandings and misinterpretations and promotes cooperative working through of problems.

Encourage the entire family—siblings as well as other relatives—to visit and obtain information about the baby. Interventions that help the family cope with the situation include providing support, confronting the crisis, and understanding the reality. Support, explanations, and the helping role must extend to the kin network, as well as to the nuclear family, to aid the extended family in communication and support ties with the nuclear family.

Do not overlook the needs of siblings. Siblings have been looking forward to the new baby, and they, too, suffer a degree of loss. Young children may react with hostility and older ones with shame at the birth of an infant with an anomaly. Both reactions may make them feel guilty. Parents, who may be preoccupied with working through their own feelings, often cannot give the other children the attention and support they need. Sometimes another child becomes the focus of family tension. Anxiety thus directed can take the form of finding fault or of overconcern. This is a form of denial; the parents cannot face the real worry—the infant at risk. After assessing the situation, the observant nurse can ensure that another family member or friend steps in to support the siblings of the affected baby.

Respect and seek to meet the desires and needs of the people involved and understand that differences can exist side by side. It is often possible to elicit the parents' feelings about the experience by asking "How are you doing?" The emphasis is on the word *you*, and the interest must be sincere.

Families with children in the NICU may become friends and support one another. To encourage the development of these friendships and to provide support, many units have established parent groups. The core of the groups consists of parents whose infants were once in the intensive care unit. Most groups make contact with families within a day or two of the infant's admission to the unit, through either phone calls or visits to the hospital. Early one-on-one parent contacts are more effective than discussion groups in helping families work through their feelings. This personalized method gives the grieving parents a chance to express personal feelings about the pregnancy, labor, and birth and their different-than-expected infant with others who have experienced the same feelings and with whom they can identify.

NURSING CARE IN THE COMMUNITY

Predischarge planning begins once the infant's condition becomes stable and it seems likely the newborn will survive (AAP Committee on Fetus and Newborn, 1998). Adequate predischarge teaching helps parents transform any feelings of inadequacy they may have into feelings of self-assurance and attachment. From the beginning, teach the parents about their infant's special needs and growth patterns (Bracht, Ardal, Bot, et al., 1998). This teaching and involvement are best facilitated by a nurse who is familiar with the infant and his or her family over a period of time and who has developed a comfortable and supportive relationship with them.

Provide home care instructions in an optimal environment for parental learning. Learning should take place over time, to avoid bombarding the parents with instructions in the day or hour before discharge. Parents often enjoy performing minimal caretaking tasks, with gradual expansion of their role. Many NICUs provide facilities for parents to room-in with their infants for a few days before discharge. This practice allows parents a degree of independence in the care of their infant with the security of nursing help nearby. It is particularly helpful for anxious parents, parents who have not had the opportunity to spend extended time with their infant, or parents who will be giving complex physical care at home, such as tracheostomy care (Costello & Chapman, 1998; Dracup, Doering, Moser, et al., 1998).

In addressing the basic elements of home care instruction be sure to do the following:

1. Teach the parents routine well-baby care, such as bathing, taking a temperature, preparing formula, and breastfeeding.

2. Help parents learn to do special procedures as needed by the newborn, such as gavage or gastrostomy feedings, tracheostomy or enterostomy care, medication administration, cardiopulmonary resuscitation (CPR), and operation of the apnea monitor. Before discharge, the parents should be as comfortable as possible with these tasks and should demonstrate independence. Written instructions are useful for parents to refer to once they are home with the infant, but they should not replace actual participation in the infant's care.

3. Refer parents to community health and support organizations. The Visiting Nurses' Association, public health nurses, or social services can assist the parents in the stressful transition from hospital to home by providing the necessary home teaching and support. Some NICUs have their own parent support groups to help bridge the gap between hospital and home care. Parents can also find support from a variety of community organizations, such as mothers-of-twins groups, trisomy 13 clubs, the March of Dimes Birth Defects Foundation, handicapped children services, and teen mother and child programs. Each community has numerous agencies capable of assisting the family in adapting emotionally, physically, and financially to the chronically ill infant. Be familiar with community resources and help the parents identify which agencies may benefit them.

4. Help parents recognize the growth and development needs of their infant. A development program begun in the hospital can be continued at home, or refer parents to an infant development program in the community.

5. Arrange medical follow-up care before discharge. A family pediatrician, a well-baby clinic, or a specialty clinic may provide follow-up care for the infant. The first appointment should be made before the infant is discharged from the hospital (Hussey-Gardner, Wachtel, & Viscardi, 1998).

6. Evaluate the need for special equipment for infant care (such as a respirator, oxygen, apnea monitor) in the home. Any equipment or supplies should be in the home before the infant's discharge.

Further evaluation after the infant has gone home is useful in determining whether the crisis has been resolved satisfactorily. The parents are usually given the intensive care nursery's telephone number to call for support and advice. It is a good idea for staff to follow up with each family with visits or telephone calls at intervals for several weeks to assess and evaluate the infant's (and parents') progress.

Evaluation

Expected outcomes of nursing care include the following:

▶ The parents can verbalize their feelings of grief and loss.

- The parents verbalize their concerns about their baby's health problems, care needs, and potential outcome.

- The parents participate in their infant's care and show attachment behaviors.

Considerations for the Nurse Who Works with At-Risk Newborns

The birth of a baby with a problem is a traumatic event with the potential for either disruption or growth of the involved family. Throughout the pregnancy, both parents, together and separately, have felt excitement, experienced thoughts of acceptance, and pictured what their baby would look like. Both parents have wished for a perfect baby and feared an unhealthy one. Each parent and family member must accept and adjust when the fantasized fears become reality.

The period of waiting between suspicion and confirmation of abnormality or dysfunction is a very anxious one for parents because it is difficult, if not impossible, to begin attachment to the infant if the newborn's future is questionable. During the waiting period parents need support and acknowledgment that this is an anxious time and they must be kept informed about efforts to gather additional data and to maintain the infant's viability. It is helpful to tell both parents about the problem at the same time, with the baby present. An honest discussion of the problem and anticipatory management at the earliest possible time by health professionals help the parents (1) maintain trust in the physician and nurse, (2) appreciate the reality of the situation by dispelling fantasy and misconception, (3) begin the grieving process, and (4) mobilize internal and external support.

In their sensitive and vulnerable state, parents are acutely perceptive of others' responses and reactions (particularly nonverbal) to the child. Parents are likely to identify with the responses of others. Therefore, it is imperative that medical and nursing staff be fully aware of and come to terms with their feelings so they are comfortable and at ease with the baby and grieving family.

Nurses may feel uncomfortable, may not know what to say to parents, or may fear confronting their own feelings as well as those of the parents. Each nurse must work out personal reactions with instructors, peers, clergy, parents, or significant others. It is helpful to have a stockpile of therapeutic questions and statements to initiate meaningful dialogue with parents. Opening statements might include the following: "You must be wondering what could have caused this," "Are you thinking that you [or someone else] may have done something?" "How can I help?" and "Are you wondering how you are going to manage?" Avoid statements such as "It could have been worse," "It's God's will," "You have other children," "You are still young and can have more," and "I understand how you feel." This child is important now. The entire multidisciplinary team may need to pool its resources and expertise to help the parents of children born with problems or disorders so that both parents and children thrive.

Nurses cannot provide support unless they themselves are supported. Working in an emotional environment of life-and-death situations takes its toll on staff. NICUs are among the most stressful areas in health care for patients, families, and nurses. Nurses bear most of the stress and largely determine the atmosphere of the NICU. The nurse's ability to cope with stress is the key to creating an emotionally healthy environment and a positive working atmosphere. The emotional needs and feelings of the staff must be recognized and dealt with so that staff can support the parents. An environment of openness to feelings and support in dealing with their human needs and emotions is essential for personnel. As caregivers, nurses may be unaware of their need to grieve for their own losses in the NICU. Nurses must also go through the grief work that parents experience. Techniques such as group meetings, individual support, and primary care nursing may help maintain staff mental health. The staff NICU nurses may never see the long-term results of the specialized, sensitive care they give to parents and their newborns. Their only immediate evidence of effective care may be the beginning of resolution of parental grief, discharge of a recovered, thriving infant to the care of happy parents, and the beginning of reintegration of family life.

CHAPTER HIGHLIGHTS

- The sick newborn—whether preterm, term, or postterm—must be managed within narrow physiologic parameters.

- These parameters (respiratory and thermal regulation) maintain physiologic homeostasis and prevent iatrogenic stress to the already stressed infant.

- The nursing care of the newborn with special problems involves understanding normal physiology, the pathophysiology of the disease process, clinical manifestations, and supportive or corrective thera-

pies. Only with this theoretical background can the nurse caring for newborns make appropriate observations about responses to therapy and development of complications.

- Asphyxia results in significant circulatory, respiratory, and biochemical changes in the newborn that make the successful transition to extrauterine life difficult. Asphyxia requires early identification and resuscitative management.

- Newborn conditions that commonly present with respiratory distress and require oxygen and ventilator assistance are respiratory distress syndrome, meconium aspiration syndrome, and transient tachypnea of the newborn.

~ Cold stress sets up the chain of physiologic events of hypoglycemia, pulmonary vasoconstriction, hyperbilirubinemia, respiratory distress, and metabolic acidosis. Nurses are responsible for early detection and initiation of treatment for hypoglycemia.

~ Differentiation between pathologic and physiologic jaundice is the key to early and successful intervention.

~ Anemia (decreased red blood cell volume) and polycythemia (increased volume) place the newborn at risk for alterations in blood flow and the oxygen-carrying capacity of the blood.

~ Nursing assessment of the septic newborn involves identification of very subtle clinical signs that are also seen in other clinical disease states.

~ The nurse facilitates interdisciplinary communication with the parents and identifies their understanding of their infant's care and their needs for emotional support.

~ Parents of at-risk newborns need support from nurses and health care providers to understand the special needs of their baby and to feel comfortable in an overwhelming and often unfamiliar environment.

EXPLOREMEDIALINK

NCLEX Review, Case Studies, and other interactive resources for this chapter can be found on the companion website at http://www.prenhall.com/london. Click on "Chapter 29" to select the activities for this chapter.

For animations, more NCLEX review questions, and an audio glossary, access the accompanying CD-ROM in this textbook.

REFERENCES

American Academy of Pediatrics & American Heart Association. (2000). *Textbook of neonatal resuscitation* (4th ed.). (J. Kattwinkel & J. Short, Eds.). Elk Grove Village, IL: Author.

American Academy of Pediatrics Committee on Fetus and Newborn. (1998). Hospital discharge of the high-risk neonate—proposed guidelines. *Pediatrics, 102*(2), 411–417.

American Academy of Pediatrics Committee on Fetus and Newborn. (1999). Surfactant replacement therapy for respiratory distress syndrome. *Pediatrics, 103*(3), 684–685.

American Academy of Pediatrics Provisional Committee for Quality Improvement and Subcommittee on Hyperbilirubinemia. (1994). Practice parameter: Management of hyperbilirubinemia in the healthy term newborn. *Pediatrics, 94*(4, Pt. 1), 558–565. (Published erratum appears in 1995 *Pediatrics, 95*[3], 458–461.)

Anastasi, J. M. (1998). Innovations in care: Neonatal home antibiotic infusion therapy. *Neonatal Network, 17*(4), 33–38.

Augustine, M. C. (1999). Hyperbilirubinemia in the healthy term newborn. *Nurse Practitioner, 24*(4), 24–41.

Baskett, T. F. (2000). The resuscitation greats: Virginia Apgar and the newborn Apgar score. *Resuscitation, 47*, 215–217.

Bracht, M., Ardal, F., Bot, A., & Cheng, C. M. (1998). Initiation and maintenance of a hospital-based parent group for parents of premature infants: Key factors for success. *Neonatal Network, 17*(3), 33–37.

Casey, B. M., McIntire, D. D., & Leveno, K. J. (2001). The continuing value of the Apgar score for the assessment of newborn infants. *New England Journal of Medicine, 344*(7), 467–471.

Cashore, W. J. (2000). Bilirubin and jaundice in the micropremie. *Clinics in Perinatology, 27*(1), 171–178.

Cornblath, M., Hawdon, J. M., Williams, A. F., Aynsley-Green, A., Ward-Platt, M. P., Schwartz, R., et al. (2000). Controversies regarding definition of neonatal hypoglycemia: Suggested operational thresholds. *Pediatrics, 105*(5), 1141–1145.

Costello, A., & Chapman, J. (1998). Mother's perception of the care-by-parent program prior to hospital discharge of their preterm infants. *Neonatal Network, 17*(4), 37–42.

Doyle, J. J., Schmidt, V., & Zipursky, A. (1999). Hematology. In G. B. Avery, M. A. Fletcher, & M. G. MacDonald (Eds.), *Neonatology: Pathophysiology and management of the newborn* (5th ed., pp. 1045–1092). Philadelphia: Lippincott Williams & Wilkins.

Dracup, K., Doering, L. V., Moser, D. K., & Evangelista, L. (1998). Retention and use of cardiopulmonary resuscitation skills in parents of infants at risk for cardiopulmonary arrest. *Pediatric Nursing, 24*(3), 219–225.

Edwards, M. S. (2002). Postnatal bacterial infections. In A. A. Fanaroff & R. J. Martin (Eds.), *Neonatal-perinatal medicine: Diseases of the fetus and infant* (7th ed.), Vol 2. pp. 706–735. St. Louis: Mosby.

Gaynes, R. P., Edwards, J. R., Jarvis, W. R., Culver, D. H., Tolson, J. S., & Martone, W. J. (1996). Nosocomial infections among neonates in high risk nurseries in the United States. National Nosocomial Infections Surveillance System. *Pediatrics, 98*(3, Pt. 1), 357–361.

Gomez, M., Hansen, T., & Corbet, A. (1998). Therapies for intractable respiratory failure. In H. W. Taeusch & R. A. Ballard (Eds.), *Avery's diseases of the newborn* (7th ed., pp. 576–594). Philadelphia: Saunders.

Grant, P. (1978). Psychological needs of families of high-risk infants. *Families and Community Health, 1*(3), 93–97.

Hansen, T. N., Cooper, T. R., & Weisman, L. E. (1998). *Contemporary diagnosis and management of neonatal respiratory diseases* (2nd ed.). Newton, PA: Handbooks in Health Care.

Hussey-Gardner, B. T., Wachtel, R. C., & Viscardi, R. M. (1998). Parent perceptions of an NICU follow-up clinic. *Neonatal Network, 17*(1), 33–39.

Juul, S. E. (1999). Erythropoietin in the neonate. *Current Problems in Pediatrics, 29*, 133–149.

Kalhan, S. C., & Parimi, P. S. (2002). Metabolic and endrocrine disorders. In A. A. Fanaroff & R. J. Martin (Eds.), *Neonatal-perinatal medicine: Diseases of the fetus and infant* (7th ed., Vol. 2, pp. 1351–1376). St. Louis, MO: Mosby.

Kaplan, D. M., & Mason, E. A. (1974). Maternal reactions to premature birth viewed as an acute emotional disorder. In H. J. Parad (Ed.), *Crisis intervention* (pp. 118–128). New York: Family Services Association of America.

Klaus, M. H., & Fanaroff, A. A. (2001). *Care of the high-risk neonate* (5th ed.). Philadelphia: Saunders.

Klaus, M. H., & Kennell, J. H. (1982). *Maternal-infant bonding* (2nd ed.). St. Louis, MO: Mosby.

Lemons, J. A., Blackmon, L. R., Kanto, W. P., MacDonald, H. M., Miller, C. A., Rosenfeld, W., et al. (2000). Use of inhaled nitric oxide. *Pediatrics, 106*(2), 344–345.

MacMahon, J. R., Stevenson, D. K., & Oski, F. A. (1998). Management of neonatal hyperbilirubinemia. In H. W. Taeusch & R. R. Ballard (Eds.), *Avery's diseases of the newborn* (7th ed., pp. 995–1002). Philadelphia: Saunders.

Maisels, M. J. (1999). Jaundice. In G. B. Avery, M. A. Fletcher, & M. G. MacDonald (Eds.), *Neonatology: Pathophysiology and management of the newborn* (5th ed., pp. 765–820). Philadelphia: Lippincott Williams & Wilkins.

Merenstein, G. B., & Gardner, S. L. (1998). *Handbook of neonatal intensive care* (4th ed.). St. Louis, MO: Mosby.

Neonatal hypoglycemia. (2000). *NANN guidelines for practice* (pp. 1–16). Des Plaines, IL: National Association of Neonatal Nurses.

Neonatal thermoregulation. (1997). *NANN guidelines for practice* (pp. 1–15). Petaluma, CA: NICU Ink.

Newman, B. (1999). Imaging of medical disease of the newborn lung. *Radiologic Clinics of North America, 37*(6), 1049–1065.

Niermeyer, S., Kattwinkel, J., Van Reempts, P., Nadkarni, V., Phillips, B., Ziderman, D., et al. (2000). International guidelines for neonatal resuscitation: An excerpt from the guidelines 2000 for cardiopulmonary resuscitation and emergency cardiovascular care: International consensus on science. *Pediatrics, 106*(3), E29.

Patel, D., Piotrowski, Z. H., Nelson, M. R., & Sabich, R. (2001). Effect of statewide neonatal resuscitation training program on Apgar scores among high-risk neonates in Illinois. *Pediatrics, 107*(4), 648–655.

Raines, D. A. (1998). Values of mothers of low birth weight infants in the NICU. *Neonatal Network, 17*(4), 41–46.

Schuchat, A. (1998). Epidemiology of group B streptococcal disease in the United States: Shifting paradigms. *Clinical Microbiology Reviews, 11*(3), 497–513.

Solnit, A., & Stark, M. (1961). Mourning and the birth of a defective child. *Psychoanalytic Study of the Child, 16,* 505.

Thureen, P. J., Deacon, J., O'Neill, P., & Hernandez, J. (1999). *Assessment and care of the well newborn*. Philadelphia: Saunders.

Whitsett, J. A., Pryhuber, G. S., Rice, W. R., Warner, B. B., & Wert, S. E. (1999). Acute respiratory disorders. In G. B. Avery, M. A. Fletcher, & M. G. MacDonald (Eds.), *Neonatology: Pathophysiology and management of the newborn* (5th ed., pp. 485–508). Philadelphia: Lippincott Williams & Wilkins.

Wiswell, T. E., Gannon, C. M., Jacob, J., Goldsmith, L., Szyld, E., Weiss, K., et al. (2000). Delivery room management of the apparently vigorous meconium-stained neonate: Results of the multicenter, international collaborative trial. *Pediatrics, 105*(1), 1–7.

Wong, C. M., & Stenson, B. J. (2001). Resuscitation of the preterm neonate. *Current Paediatrics, 11,* 172–176.

Young, T. E., & Mangum, O. B. (2001). *Neofax®: A manual of drugs used in neonatal care* (13th ed.). Raleigh, NC: Acorn Publishing.

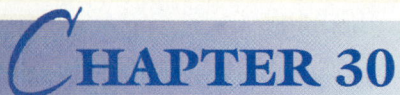

CHAPTER 30

Home Care of the Postpartum Family

I remember how terrified I was when we brought our first child home from the hospital. Neither of our mothers could come to stay and I was absolutely terrified. I survived but it was hard. My daughter is expecting her first child next month and she wants me to come out to help her. Thank God. I don't want to be a "buttinski" mother but I really want to be there for her... and I guess for me, too!

—LOIS, 53

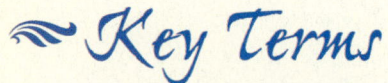

Key Terms

Active awake state   *690*

Crying state   *690*

Quiet alert state   *690*

Quiet sleep   *690*

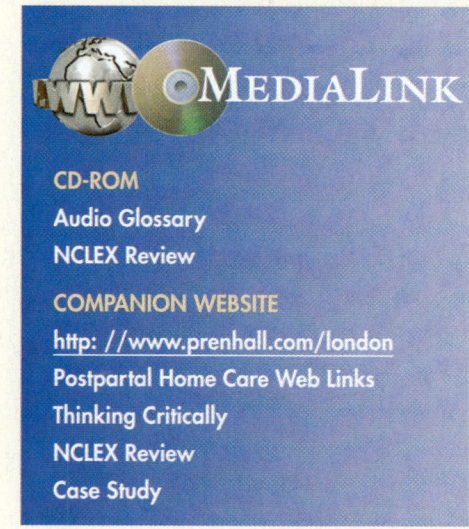

MEDIALINK

CD-ROM
Audio Glossary
NCLEX Review

COMPANION WEBSITE
http://www.prenhall.com/london
Postpartal Home Care Web Links
Thinking Critically
NCLEX Review
Case Study

$\mathcal{H}$ome care has become essential because the length of stay in the birth setting has steadily decreased over the past few years. The length of time in the hospital or birthing center after birth has been referred to as *short stay*.

As the length of stay has declined, a number of new issues have been identified. New mothers discharged in 48 hours or less after childbirth must adjust to motherhood without the benefit of the assessment and teaching that are possible with a longer stay (Fishbein & Burggraf, 1998). The shortened stay (less than 48 hours) raises issues for the newborn because many conditions, such as jaundice, ductal-dependent cardiac lesions, and gastrointestinal obstructions, may take longer than 2 days to develop, and identification of these problems depends on a skilled, experienced professional (AAP Committee on Fetus and Newborn, 1995). However, research suggests that there is no increase in neonatal readmission when early discharge is combined with a structured program of postpartum home visits (Bragg, Rosenn, Khoury, et al., 1997).

Short stays also have implications for the mother. They may compromise the stability of her health, availability of support systems, and opportunities to become comfortable with her new baby, and less than 48 hours is too little time to establish breastfeeding (AAP Committee on Fetus and Newborn, 1995). Furthermore, in the first 24 hours after childbirth, the mother is in the taking-in phase, which is not conducive to learning. The AAP Committee on Fetus and Newborn (1995) has developed minimum criteria to guide the timing of early discharge to enhance excellence in maternal-newborn care (Table 30–1).

In 1998 the U.S. federal government passed legislation that guaranteed a minimum stay of up to 48 hours following vaginal birth and up to 96 hours following cesarean birth at the discretion of the mother and her care provider. It does not require follow-up visits for women who leave earlier than the mandated time. Currently more than half the states have passed legislation strengthening the federal legislation by mandating coverage for home care follow-up (Carpenter, 1998).

As the length of stay decreases, nurses in the birthing center are pressed to complete essential assessments, ensure holistic care, and provide education about maternal self-care and newborn care. The new family, eager to learn about important aspects of care, also needs to rest and spend time with the newborn. The needs of the family and the goals of the health care provider can be addressed by providing postpartum home care.

Home care for the postpartum family is focused more on assessment, teaching, and counseling than on physical care. Postpartum home care gives nurses a chance to enhance information and self- and infant care techniques initially presented in the birth setting. In addition, the home setting lets the nurse and family interact in a more relaxed environment in which the family has control of

TABLE 30–1 Minimal Criteria for Discharge of Newborns

1. Uncomplicated prenatal, intrapartal, and postpartal course and vaginal birth.
2. A single baby who is term, 38–42 weeks, and average weight for gestational age (AGA).
3. The newborn's vital signs are within normal limits and have been stable for the 12 hours preceding discharge (respirations <60/min; apical pulse 100–160 beats per minute; axillary temperature of 36.1–37 °C in an open crib with appropriate clothing).
4. The newborn has passed at least one stool and has urinated.
5. At least two feedings have been successfully completed, and the baby's ability to coordinate sucking, swallowing, and breathing has been observed and documented.
6. No physical abnormalities have been found that require continued hospitalization.
7. If a circumcision has been done, no excessive bleeding has been evident for at least 2 hours before discharge.
8. There has been no significant jaundice in the first 24 hours of life.
9. The mother has received education about breast- or bottle-feeding; the newborn's expected stool and urinary patterns; care of circumcision; cord, skin, and genital care; ways to recognize signs of illness or distress and common infant problems; signs of jaundice and who to contact if develops; infant safety, including positioning of baby after feeding and for sleep; and use of a car seat.
10. Review of pertinent laboratory data including maternal syphilis and hepatitis B surface antigen status; cord or infant blood type.
11. Completion of screening tests (e.g., PKU).
12. First hepatitis B vaccine has been administered or appointment for administration has been scheduled within the first week.
13. Method and schedule for continuing care has been ascertained and planned, and the family is aware of the plan.
14. Family assessment has been completed for social and environmental risk factors such as history of previous child abuse or neglect; spousal or partner abuse either preceding or beginning during the pregnancy; parental substance abuse; lack of support within the family or community; lack of funds, shelter, or food; mental illness of one of the parents that impairs ability to care for self and newborn; single first-time mother without social support.

Source: Committee on Fetus and Newborn. (1995). Hospital stay for healthy term newborns. *Pediatrics, 96*(4), 788. Adapted.

the setting. In some instances, the challenges of assessing and enhancing self-care and infant care may be unique in the home, and the nurse has many opportunities to exercise critical thinking to develop creative options with the family.

THE HOME VISIT

In planning a home visit, the nurse should clearly understand the purpose of the visit and the content to be addressed. Other important considerations include ways of creating and fostering relationships with families, techniques for preplanning and executing the visit while maintaining safety, documentation of the visit, and telephone follow-up.

The postpartum home visit differs from community health visits in that only one or two home visits are typically planned, and long-term follow-up by the postpartum nurse is not anticipated. Although the postpartum home visit is comprehensive, it focuses specifically on the postpartum family's needs and care.

The established guidelines for discharge of the mother and baby mean the nurse can expect certain levels of health and wellness. However, because the status of the mother and newborn can change, the nurse should stay alert for deviations from the norm.

Purposes of the Home Visit

The postpartum home visit usually occurs within 24 to 48 hours of discharge and is conducted by a registered nurse who is experienced in postpartum maternal and newborn care. Before the home visit, the nurse prepares by identifying the purpose of the home visit and gathering anticipated materials and equipment. A personal contact while the woman is still in the birth setting or a previsit telephone call is used to arrange the appointment with the woman and her family. During the previsit contact, it is important for the nurse to identify clearly the purpose and goals of the visit and to begin establishing rapport.

The postpartum home visit has many purposes. It provides an opportunity to assess the status of the mother and infant after birth for signs of any complications, to complete follow-up blood work if needed, and to ascertain current informational needs. The home visit also provides time to cover additional information in a more relaxed setting. In addition, the nurse assesses adaptation of the family to the new baby and adjustment of any siblings and addresses the need for referrals.

Fostering a Caring Relationship with the Family

It is important to recognize that the dynamics of the home visit are different from those of the hospital or birthing center. In the home, the family members have control of their environment and the nurse is an invited visitor. The nurse can rely on the same characteristics of a caring relationship that have been integral to hospital-based practice—regard, genuineness, empathy, trust, and rapport—but the relationship may take on new elements as the nurse moves into the home setting for the first time.

Maintaining Safety

In the past, nurses were perceived as a mainstay of communities and could move in most settings without fear or concern for safety. However, today some communities are not safe for visiting nurses. It is important to follow some basic safety rules when making a home visit. Specifically, know the address and ask for directions during the previsit contact. If the area is not familiar, trace out the route on a map before leaving for the visit and take the map along. It is also wise to wear a name tag and sensible shoes. Avoid wearing expensive jewelry or pins of a religious or political nature that might be seen as offensive. A cellular phone or pager is advisable for any community visitor, as is a working flashlight, especially for night visits. In addition, carry sufficient change to call from a pay phone if necessary. Notify a supervisor when leaving for a visit and check in as soon as the visit is done.

Many agencies that provide home care services have established violence prevention programs to help ensure safety. Nurses in the community need to be aware of their environment and alert to environmental cues, whether overt or subtle. In addition, the following recommendations are important (Durkin & Wilson, 1999):

- Drive around a neighborhood before making a visit to identify potential cues to violence. Avoid walking through a crowd or staying in an elevator with others if it makes you uneasy.
- Lock personal belongings in the trunk of the car, out of sight.
- Pay attention to the body language of anyone present, not just the client. Be alert for signs that a person is becoming angry (reddened neck and face, clenched fists, pacing).
- Be aware of personal body language and how it might be interpreted. (For example, avoid crossing arms or shoving hands in pockets, which may suggest hostility; remain calm and convey a sense of respect at all times.)
- Leave the home immediately if a gun is visible and the client or family member refuses to put it away.
- If a situation arises that feels unsafe, end the visit.

If the visit is in an area that seems very unsafe, it may be wise for two nurses to go together. Avoid entering areas where violence is in progress. In such cases, return to the car and call 911.

It is always important to be aware of one's surroundings and the people who are nearby. First home visits may feel uncomfortable because they are unfamiliar, but experience increases comfort (Figure 30–1 ◆).

Carrying Out the Home Visit

When the client or family answers the door, the nurse introduces himself or herself and confirms that the location is correct. If a place to sit is not indicated, ask "Where is the best place to sit so that we can talk for a while?" In some homes, the mother or family may offer refreshments, and this may be an important aspect of welcoming a visitor. In this case, it is helpful to accept the refreshment graciously.

Complete planned assessments, provide direct care as necessary, carry out family and client teaching, make necessary referrals to community agencies, and schedule additional home visits or telephone contact. Report significant medical concerns to the certified nurse-midwife or physician immediately and plan for appropriate follow-up (Carpenter, 1998). The aspects assessed and addressed during the home visit are discussed in the following sections.

HOME CARE: THE NEWBORN

Positioning and Handling

If the mother or other family members seem unsure about handling or positioning the baby, show them how to position and handle the newborn as needed. As the family members provide care, instill confidence by giving them positive feedback. If a family member encounters problems, suggest alternatives and serve as a role model.

When the newborn is out of the crib, one of the following holds can be used (Figure 30–2 ◆). The *cradle hold* is frequently used during feeding. It provides a sense of warmth and closeness, permits eye contact, frees one of the adult's hands, and provides security because the cradling protects the newborn's body. Gripping the baby's thigh with the hand while the arm supports the newborn's body provides extra security. The *upright position* provides security and a sense of closeness and is ideal for burping. One hand should support the neck and shoulders, while the other hand holds the buttocks or is placed between the newborn's legs. The newborn may also be held upright in a cloth sling carrier that gently holds the baby against the parent's chest and frees the hands for other tasks. The *football hold* frees one of the caregiver's hands and permits eye

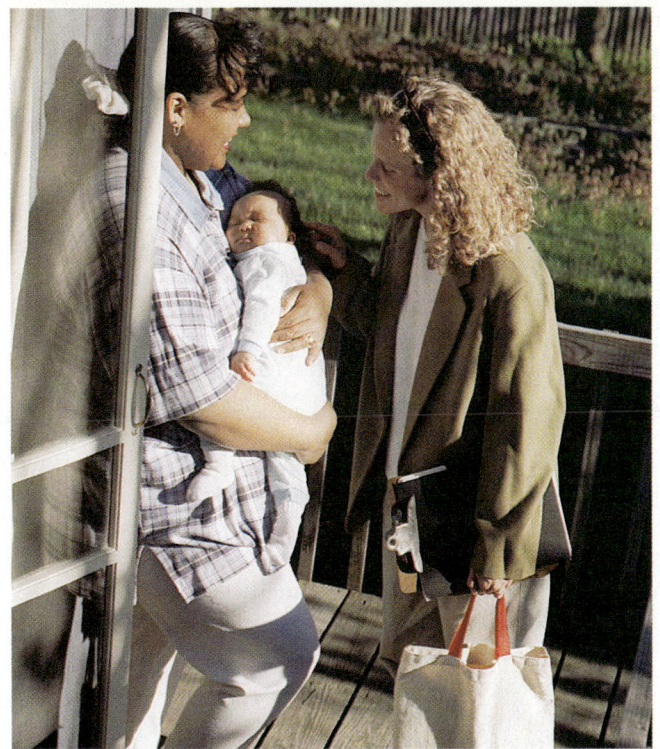

FIGURE 30–1. ◆ Nurse arriving for a home visit.

Developing Cultural Competence

During a home visit, be sensitive to culture cues. In most cultures there is a designated family caretaker—possibly a mother, aunt, or grandmother. Seek her cooperation and support for any interventions. Your client is more likely to agree to your suggestion if the designated caregiver approves (Mattson, 2000).

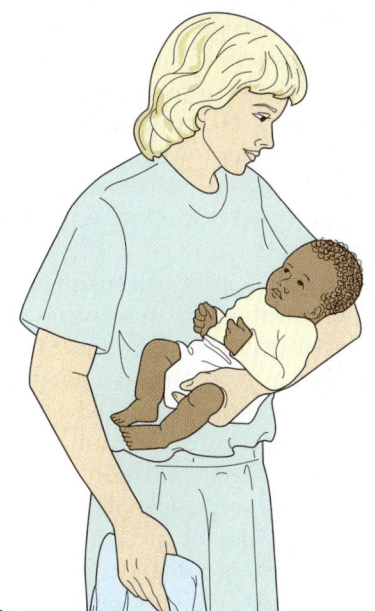
A

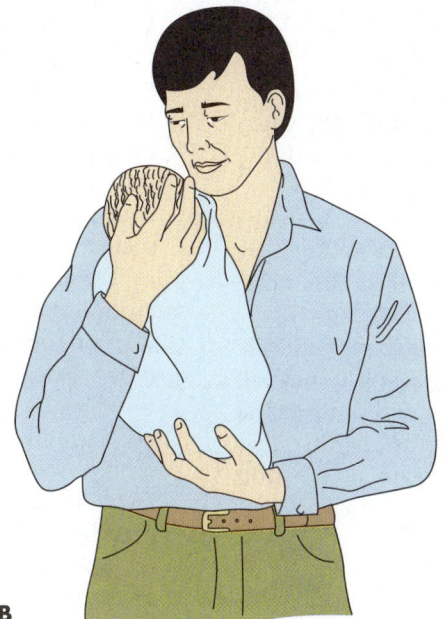
B

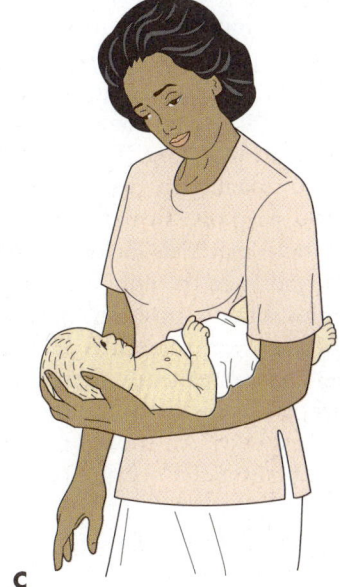
C

FIGURE 30–2. ◆ Various positions for holding an infant. **A,** Cradle hold. **B,** Upright position. **C,** Football hold.

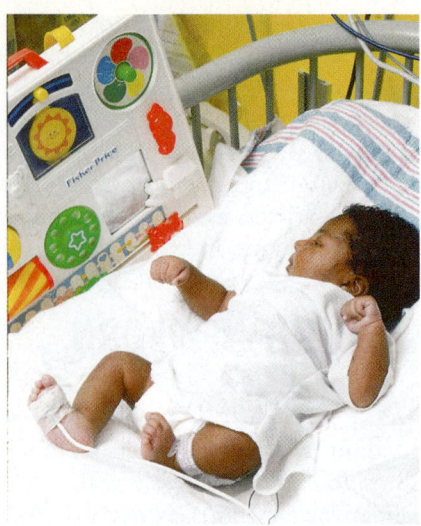

FIGURE 30–3. ◆ Babies should be placed on their backs to sleep.

contact. This hold is ideal for shampooing, carrying, or breastfeeding. It frees the caregiver to talk on the telephone or do the myriad tasks that await attention at this busy time.

Because of the increased incidence of sudden infant death syndrome (SIDS) in babies who sleep on their stomachs, experts now recommend that babies be placed on their backs to sleep (Figure 30–3 ◆). Although some parents worry about the possibility of aspiration in babies who sleep on their backs, research indicates that there is no increased risk of choking or regurgitation in healthy babies who sleep on their backs. Certain infants may need to be placed on their stomachs, including premature infants with respiratory distress (severe breathing problems), infants with symptoms of gastroesophageal reflux (severe spitting up), and infants with certain upper airway abnormalities. There may be other valid reasons for infants to be placed on their stomachs for sleep. Parents should discuss their individual circumstances with their care provider.

To help infants improve their neck and shoulder strength, they can be positioned on their stomachs when they are awake and someone is in the same room with the infant and watching. This is called "tummy time."

Additionally, to decrease the risk of SIDS, the baby should sleep on a firm, flat mattress without pillows. Fluffy and loose materials including toys and blankets should be removed from the crib.

The infant's position should be changed periodically during the early months of life, because skull bones are soft, and permanently flattened areas may develop if the newborn consistently lies in one position. In the first days of life, a newborn should not be left in a supine position when unattended because of the danger of aspiration.

Newborn Feeding

Newborn feeding is discussed in detail in Chapter 27. ⬭ Problems a breastfeeding mother may face at home

are discussed later in this chapter. Regardless of feeding method, it is important to assess the newborn's fluid and nutritional intake. Weigh the newborn while nude as part of the physical assessment. If the weight loss since birth is 10% or more, assess the baby for signs of dehydration such as loose skin with decreased turgor, dry mucous membranes, sunken anterior fontanel, and decreased frequency and amount of voiding and stooling. Newborns who are postterm, small for gestational age, and one of a multiple gestation are at high risk for breastfeeding difficulty (Locklin & Jansson, 1999).

Bathing

If the parents are not comfortable about bathing their newborn, a bath demonstration is a straightforward way to provide information to them. Because excess bathing and the use of soap remove natural skin oils and dry out the newborn's sensitive skin, bathing should be done every other day or twice a week. Sponge baths are recommended for the first 2 weeks or until the umbilical cord completely falls off and the umbilicus has healed. Some agencies use a tub bath for the bath demonstration.

At home, the family may want to use a small plastic tub, a clean kitchen or bathroom sink, or a large bowl as the baby's tub. Expensive baby tubs are not necessary, but some prefer to purchase them. Before starting, if no one else is at home, the parent may want to take the phone off the hook and put a sign on the door to prevent being disturbed. Having someone home during the first few baths will be helpful, because that person can get forgotten items, attend to interruptions, and provide moral support. The room should be warm and free of drafts.

SPONGE BATHS

After the supplies are gathered, the tub is filled with water that is warm to the touch. Even though the newborn will not be placed in the tub, the bath giver carefully tests the water temperature with an elbow or forearm. An unperfumed, mild soap such as Castile or Neutrogena should be used and kept on a soap dish or paper towel, not added to the water. The newborn should be wrapped in a blanket, with a T-shirt and diaper on, to keep her or him warm and secure.

To start the bath, the adult wraps a washcloth once around the index finger and wets it with water. Soap is not used on the face. The bath giver gently wipes each eye from inner to outer corner. This direction prevents the potential for clogging the tear duct at the inner corner, where the eye naturally drains. A different portion of the washcloth is used for each eye to prevent cross-contamination. Cotton balls can also be used for this purpose, a new one for each eye. Some swelling and drainage may be present the first few days after birth because of eye prophylaxis. The bath giver washes the ears next by wrapping the washcloth once around an index finger and gently cleaning the external ear and behind the ear. Cotton swabs are never used in the ear canal because it is possible to put the swab too far into the ear and damage the ear drum. In addition, the swab may push any discharge farther down into the ear canal. The caregiver then wipes the remainder of the baby's face. Many babies start to cry at this point. The face should be washed every day and the mouth and chin wiped off after each feeding.

The neck is washed thoroughly with the washcloth. Soap may now be used. Formula or breast milk and lint collect in the skin folds of the neck, so it may be helpful to sit the newborn up, supporting the neck and shoulders with one hand while washing the neck with the other hand.

Next the bath giver unwraps the blanket, removes the T-shirt, and wets the chest, back, and arms with the washcloth. The bath giver may then lather the hands with soap and wash the baby's chest, back, and arms. Wetting the cord is avoided, if possible, because it delays drying. Soap is rinsed off with the wet washcloth, and the upper part of the body is dried with a towel or blanket. The newborn's upper body is then wrapped with a clean, dry blanket to prevent a chill. The bath giver then unwraps the newborn's legs, wets them with the washcloth, and lathers, rinses, and dries them well. If the newborn has dry skin, a small amount of unscented lotion or ointment (petroleum jelly or A + D ointment) may be used. Ointments are thought to be better than lotions for dry, cracked feet and hands. Baby oil is not recommended, because it clogs skin pores. Powders are not currently recommended. Families should be warned that baby powder can cause serious respiratory problems if inhaled. If parents want to use powder, they should be advised to use one that is talc free. They should also shake the powder into the hand and then pat it on the newborn rather than shaking it directly onto the baby.

The genital area should be cleansed with soap and water daily and with water after each wet or dirty diaper. Females should be washed from the front of the genitalia toward the rectum to prevent fecal contamination of the urethra and thus the bladder. Newborn girls often have a thick, white mucus discharge or a slight bloody discharge from the vaginal area. This discharge is normal for the first 1 to 2 weeks after birth and should be wiped off with a damp cloth during diaper changes.

Parents of uncircumcised males should cleanse the penis daily. Even minimal retraction of the foreskin is not advised (see in-depth discussion of care of uncircumcised male babies in Chapter 26). Males who have been circumcised also need daily gentle cleansing. The bath giver rubs a very wet washcloth over a bar of soap, then squeezes the washcloth above the baby's penis, letting the soapy water run over the circumcision site. The area is rinsed off with plain warm water and lightly patted dry. A small amount of petroleum jelly, A + D ointment, or bactericidal ointment may be put on the circumcised area, but excessive amounts may block the meatus and should be avoided. It is important to avoid using ointments if a Plastibell is in place because use of ointments may cause the Plastibell ring to slip off the penis too early. The Plastibell usually falls off

within 5 to 8 days. If it does not, the family needs to call the health care provider.

The diaper area is cleansed with each diaper change to prevent diaper rash. Despite routine cleansing, a diaper rash may still occur. Baby powder or cornstarch is not recommended for diaper rash. Baby powder may cake with urine and irritate the perineal area; cornstarch may promote fungal infection. Ointments that provide a barrier, such as zinc oxide, A + D ointment, and petroleum jelly, are more effective. If the ointment does not help the rash, families using disposable diapers should try another brand. If they use cloth diapers, a different detergent or fabric softener, more thorough rinsing, and hanging them in the sun to dry may solve the problem. If the rash persists, parents should discuss the problem with their nurse practitioner or physician, because it may be due to a yeast or fungal infection.

The umbilical cord should be kept clean and dry. The presence of the umbilical vessels in the cord makes it a common entry area for infection. The cord stump generally falls off in 7 to 14 days. The diaper should be folded down to allow air to circulate around the cord. The parents should consult their health care provider if redness, bright-red bleeding, or puslike drainage with foul odor appears around the umbilicus or if the area remains unhealed 2 to 3 days after the cord stump has sloughed off.

The last step in bathing is washing the hair (a step some suggest doing first). The newborn is swaddled in a dry blanket, leaving only the head exposed, and held in the football hold with the head tilted slightly downward to prevent water from running in the eyes. Water should be brought to the head by a cupped hand. The hair is moistened and lathered with a small amount of mild shampoo. A very soft brush may be used to massage the shampoo over the entire head, including the soft spots. The hair is then rinsed and toweled dry. Oils or lotions are not used on the newborn's head unless there is evidence of cradle cap. Moistening the scaly area with lotion or mineral oil half an hour or more before shampooing softens the crusts or scales and makes it easier to remove them with a soft brush during the shampoo.

TUB BATHS

The baby may be put in a small tub after the cord has fallen off and the circumcision site is healed (approximately 2 weeks) (Figure 30–4 ◆). Newborns usually enjoy a tub bath more than a sponge bath, although some cry during either type.

Only 3 or 4 inches of water is needed in the tub. To prevent slipping, a washcloth is placed in the bottom of the tub or sink. Some parents choose to bring the newborn into the tub with them. The baby's face is washed in the same manner as for a sponge bath. The parent then places the newborn in the tub using the cradle hold and grasping the distal thigh. The neck is supported by the parent's elbow in the cradle position. An alternative hold is to support the newborn's head and neck with the forearm while grasping the distal shoulder and arm.

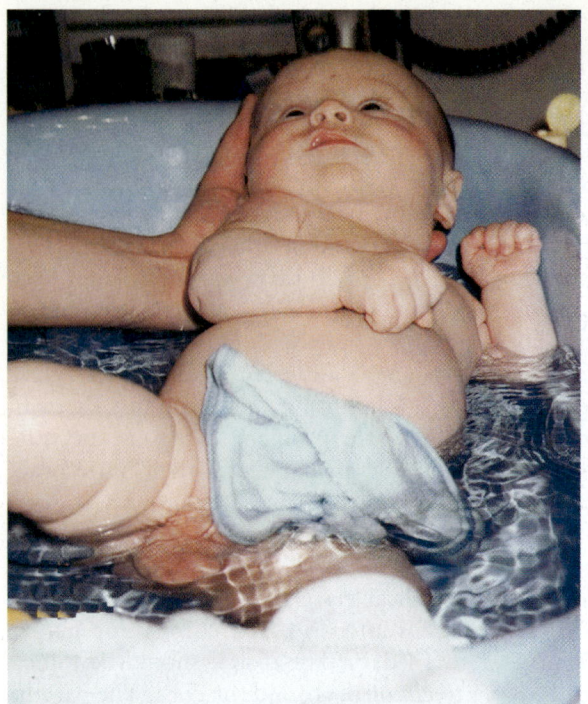

FIGURE 30-4. ◆ When bathing the newborn, it is important to support the head. Wet babies are very slippery.

Because wet newborns are slippery, some parents pull a cotton sock (with holes cut out for the fingers) over the supporting arm to provide a "nonskid" surface. The newborn's body may be washed with a soapy washcloth or hand. To wash the back, the bath giver places his or her noncradling hand on the newborn's chest with the thumb under the newborn's arm closest to the adult. Gently tipping the newborn forward onto the supporting hand frees the cradling arm to wash the back. After the bath, the newborn is lifted out of the tub in the cradle position,

dried well, and wrapped in a dry blanket. The hair is then washed in the same way as for a sponge bath.

Nail Care

The nails of the newborn are seldom cut in the birthing center. During the first days of life, the nails may adhere to the skin of the fingers, and cutting is contraindicated. Within a week the nails separate from the skin and frequently break off. If the nails are long or if the baby is scratching his or her face, the nails may be trimmed. Trimming is most easily done while the infant is asleep. Nails should be cut straight across using blunt-ended cuticle scissors.

Dressing the Newborn

Newborns need to wear a T-shirt, diaper (with a diaper cover or plastic pants if using cloth diapers), and a sleeper. On a fairly cool day, they should be wrapped in a light blanket while being fed. Newborns should be covered with a blanket in air-conditioned buildings. The blanket should be unwrapped or removed when inside a warm building. At home, the temperature determines the amount of clothing the newborn wears. Families who keep their home at 60 to 65°F should dress the infant more warmly than those who maintain a temperature of 70 to 75°F.

Newborns should wear head coverings outdoors to protect their sensitive ears from drafts. A blanket can be wrapped around the baby, leaving one corner free to place over the head while outdoors or in crowds for added protection. Advise families about how easily a newborn's skin can burn in the sun. To prevent sunburn, the newborn should remain shaded, wear a light layer of clothing, or be protected with sunscreen.

Diaper shapes vary (Figure 30–5 ◆). Prefolded and disposable diapers are usually rectangular. Cloth diapers may

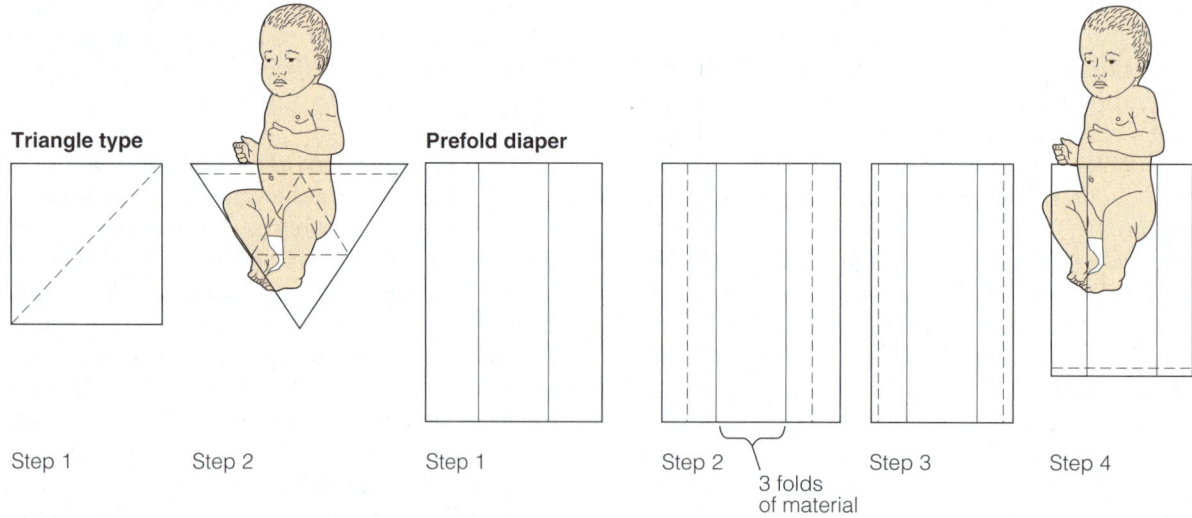

Triangle type — Step 1, Step 2

Prefold diaper — Step 1, Step 2 (3 folds of material), Step 3, Step 4

FIGURE 30-5. ◆ Two basic cloth diaper shapes. Dotted lines indicate folds.

also be triangular or kite folded. Extra material is placed in front for males and toward the back for females to increase absorbency.

Baby clothing may be laundered separately with a mild soap or detergent. Diapers may be presoaked before washing. If the infant develops a rash, it may be necessary for his or her clothing to be rinsed twice to remove soap and residue. Some newborns may not tolerate clothing treated with fabric softeners added to the washer or dryer.

Temperature Assessment

When teaching parents about taking their baby's temperature, provide opportunities for discussion and demonstration. Clarify the times when the family should call their primary health care provider. Discuss the different types of thermometers available for home use. It is important that parents understand the differences and how to select the appropriate one. Although tympanic (ear) thermometers are more expensive, many parents choose them because they are fast and easy to use. Other parents use a digital thermometer. Review the correct procedure for using the chosen thermometer.

Nursing Practice

Health care facilities no longer use glass thermometers because of the risks associated with spilled mercury should one break. Although some parents still have glass thermometers, they are much less common than in the past. Before teaching families about temperature taking, you might find it helpful to visit a local pharmacy and review the types of thermometers available, the costs of the most commonly used methods, and the instructions provided. This will enable you to answer questions accurately when you work with parents or caregivers.

Parents only need to take the newborn's temperature if he or she seems ill. They should call their physician or pediatric nurse practitioner immediately if any signs of illness are present. (See Chapter 26.) Parents should also check with their clinician about over-the-counter medications to be kept in the medicine cabinet.

When parents find their newborn has a fever, they may expect to give an antipyretic such as acetaminophen (Tylenol). They should not give any form of aspirin for an illness that may be viral; use of aspirin in viral illnesses has been linked to Reye syndrome in children. Parents should discuss management of flu, colds, teething, constipation, diarrhea, and other common ailments with their clinician before they occur. When analgesic or antipyretic medication is needed, clinicians often recommend acetaminophen drops.

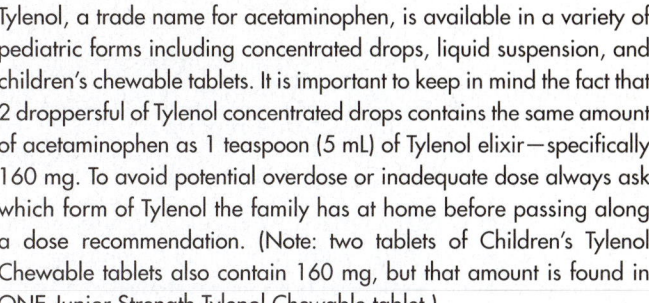

Tylenol, a trade name for acetaminophen, is available in a variety of pediatric forms including concentrated drops, liquid suspension, and children's chewable tablets. It is important to keep in mind the fact that 2 droppersful of Tylenol concentrated drops contains the same amount of acetaminophen as 1 teaspoon (5 mL) of Tylenol elixir—specifically 160 mg. To avoid potential overdose or inadequate dose always ask which form of Tylenol the family has at home before passing along a dose recommendation. (Note: two tablets of Children's Tylenol Chewable tablets also contain 160 mg, but that amount is found in ONE Junior Strength Tylenol Chewable tablet.)

Stools and Urine

The appearance and frequency of a newborn's stools can cause concern for parents. Prepare them by discussing and showing pictures of meconium stools and transitional stools and by describing the difference between breast milk and formula stools. Although each baby develops his or her own stooling patterns, parents can get an idea of what to expect (see Figure 24–8).

- Breastfed newborns may have 6 to 10 small, semiliquid, yellow stools per day by the third or fourth day, when milk production is established, unless the mother is having problems with her milk supply. Once breastfeeding is well established, usually by 1 month, the newborn may have only 1 stool every few days because of the increased digestibility of breast milk, or still may have several daily. Constipation is unlikely in newborns receiving only breast milk. Infrequent stooling in the first few weeks may indicate inadequate milk intake.

- Formula-fed babies may have only one or two stools a day; they are more formed and yellow or yellow-brown.

The parents may also be shown pictures of a constipated stool (small, pelletlike) and diarrhea (loose, green, or perhaps blood tinged). Families need to understand that a green color is common in transitional stools, so that transitional stools are not confused with diarrhea during the first week of a newborn's life. Constipation may indicate that the newborn needs additional fluid. Parents may try offering additional water in an attempt to reverse the constipation.

Babies normally void five to eight times per day. Fewer than six to eight wet diapers a day may indicate that the newborn needs more fluids. Voiding is easy to assess with cloth diapers. Parents who use superabsorbent disposable diapers may have difficulty determining voiding because the surface of the diaper feels dry. The liquid pools inside the filling of the diaper.

Sleep and Activity

The newborn demonstrates several sleep-wake states after the initial periods of reactivity described in Chapter 24. It is not uncommon for a newborn to sleep almost continuously for the first 2 to 3 days following birth, awakening only for feedings every 3 to 4 hours. Some newborns bypass this stage of deep sleep and require only 12 to 16 hours of sleep. The parents need to know that this pattern is normal.

Quiet sleep is characterized by regular breathing and no movement except for sudden body jerks. During this sleep state, normal household noise will not awaken the infant. In the active sleep state, the baby has irregular breathing and fine muscular twitching. The baby may cry out during sleep, but this does not mean he or she is uncomfortable or awake. Unusual noise may awaken the newborn more easily in this state; however, he or she will quickly go back to sleep.

Quiet alert state is a state in which newborns are quietly involved with the environment. They watch a moving mobile, smile, and, as they age, discover and play with their hands and feet. When newborns become uncomfortable due to wet diapers, hunger, or cold, they enter the active awake state and crying state. In these states, parents should identify and eliminate the cause of the crying. Sometimes families are frustrated as they try to identify the external or internal stimuli that are causing the angry, hurt crying. Tell parents that the state may be changed from crying to quiet alert by moving the newborn to a more upright position where he or she can scan and explore. (See Table 30–2.)

Crying

For the newborn, crying is the only way to express needs vocally. Families learn to distinguish different tones and qualities of the newborn's cry. The amount of crying is highly individual. Some cry as little as 15 to 30 minutes in 24 hours, and others cry as long as 2 hours every 24 hours. When crying continues after causes such as discomfort and hunger are eliminated, the newborn may be comforted by swaddling or by rocking and other reassuring activities. There is some indication that newborns who are held more tend to be calmer and cry less when not being held. Some parents are afraid that holding may "spoil" the newborn and need reassurance that this is not the case. Picking babies up when they cry teaches them that adults try to meet their needs and are responsive to them. This helps build a sense of trust in humankind. Excessive crying should be noted and assessed, taking other factors into consideration. After the first 2 or 3 days, newborns settle into individual patterns.

Safety Considerations

Newborns should not have pillows or stuffed animals in the crib while they sleep; these items could cause suffocation. Mattresses should fit snugly in a crib to prevent entrapment and suffocation, and the crib should be inspected regularly to determine whether it is in safe working order. Crib slats should be no more than 2 3/8 inches apart. Encourage parents to attend infant cardiopulmonary resuscitation (CPR) classes, especially if there is a family history of SIDS or the infant requires special care.

Newborn Screening and Immunization Program

Before the newborn and mother are discharged from the hospital, inform the parents about the normal screening tests for newborns and tell them when to return for further tests if needed. Newborn screening tests detect disorders that cause mental retardation, physical handicaps, or death if left undiscovered. Inborn errors of metabolism that can usually be detected from a drop of blood obtained by a heel stick on the second or third day include phenylketonuria (PKU) and congenital hypothyroidism (mandatory screening in all states in the United States), as well as sickle cell disease, galactosemia, and hemocystinuria. Inform parents that a second blood specimen will be required from the newborn after 7 to 14 days; in some states, the second blood specimen is not recommended if the first specimen is obtained 48 hours or longer after birth. Stress that an abnormal test result is not diagnostic. More specific tests must be performed to verify the results.

If additional tests are positive, treatment is begun. Explain to parents that these conditions may be treated by diet or by administration of missing hormones. The inborn conditions cannot be cured, but they can be treated. They are not contagious, but they may be inherited.

Follow-Up Care

Routine well-baby visits should be scheduled with the clinic, pediatric nurse practitioner, or physician. It is helpful to schedule these appointments before the woman leaves the birthing center or hospital.

To help parents care for their newborn at home, some physicians encourage prenatal pediatric visits to establish this contact before the birth. Public health nurses have long been involved in newborn care and parent education. Birthing units are expanding their support for the new family to include one home visit by the nurse who cared for the family in the birthing unit.

The family should be taught all necessary caregiving methods before discharge. A checklist may be helpful to determine whether the teaching has been completed. The mother should have the phone number, address, and any specific instructions from the certified nurse-midwife, nurse practitioner, or physician and the lactation consultant. Having the nursery phone number is also reassuring to a new family. Encourage parents to call with questions.

TABLE 30-2 **Infant State* Chart (Sleep and Awake States)**

			Characteristics of State			
Sleep States	Body Activity	Eye Movement	Facial Movement	Breathing Pattern	Level of Response	Implications for Caregiving
Deep sleep	Nearly still except for occasional startle or twitch	None	Without facial movements except for occasional sucking movement at regular intervals	Smooth and regular	Only very intense and disturbing stimuli will arouse infants.	Caregivers trying to feed infants in deep sleep will probably find the experience frustrating. Infants will be unresponsive, even if caregivers use disturbing stimuli (flicking feet) to arouse infants. Infants may arouse only briefly and then become unresponsive as they return to deep sleep. If caregivers wait until infants move to a higher, more responsive state, feeding or caregiving will be much more pleasant.
Light sleep	Some body movements	Rapid eye movement (REM): fluttering of eyes beneath closed eyelids	May smile and make brief fussy or crying sounds	Irregular	Infants are more responsive to internal and external stimuli. When these stimuli occur, infants may remain in light sleep or move to drowsy state.	Light sleep makes up the highest proportion of newborn sleep and usually precedes awakening. Caregivers who are not aware that the brief fussy or crying sounds made during this state occur normally may think it is time for feeding and may try to feed infants before they are ready to eat.
Awake States						
Drowsy	Activity level variable, with mild startles interspersed from time to time; movements usually smooth	Eyes open and close occasionally; are heavy lidded, with dull glazed appearance	May have some facial movements; often there are none and the face appears still	Irregular	Infants react to sensory stimuli, although responses are delayed. State change after stimulation is frequently noted.	From the drowsy state infants may return to sleep or awaken further. To wake them, caregivers can provide something for infants to see, hear, or suck. This may arouse them to a quiet alert state, a more responsive state. Infants left alone without stimuli may return to a sleep state.
Quiet alert	Minimal	Brightening and widening of eyes	Faces have bright, shining, sparkling looks	Regular	Infants attend most to environment, focusing attention on any stimuli that are present.	Infants in this state provide much pleasure and positive feedback for caregivers. Providing something for infants to see, hear, or suck will often maintain a quiet alert state in the first few hours after birth. Most newborns commonly experience a period of intense alertness before going into a long sleeping period.
Active alert	Much body activity; may have periods of fussiness	Eyes open, with less brightening	Much facial movement; faces not as bright as in alert state	Irregular	Infants are increasingly sensitive to disturbing stimuli (hunger, fatigue, noise, excessive handling).	Caregivers may intervene at this stage to console and to bring infants to a lower state.
Crying	Increased motor activity, with color changes	Eyes may be tightly closed or open	Grimaces	More irregular	Infants are extremely responsive to unpleasant external or internal stimuli.	Crying is the infant's communication signal. It is a response to unpleasant stimuli from the environment or from within infants (fatigue, hunger, discomfort). Crying tells us infants have been reached. Sometimes infants can console themselves and return to lower states. At other times they need help from caregivers.

*State is a group of characteristics that regularly occur together: body activity, eye movements, facial movements, breathing pattern, and level of response to external stimuli (e.g., handling) and internal stimuli (e.g., hunger).

Source: Blackburn, S., & Kang, R. (1991). Early parent-infant relationships (2nd ed., module 3, series 1). In *The first six hours after birth.* White Plains, NY: March of Dimes Birth Defects Foundation. Reprinted with permission of the copyright holder.

Nurses engaged in telephone triage must consider several important strategies to provide optimum care and avoid legal pitfalls. These strategies include (Cady, 1999):

- Develop and follow triage protocols for the most commonly occurring calls.
- Document all triage calls carefully and accurately.
- Initiate timely follow-up contacts. (This may include instructions to the client to call back after a specific period or if the condition does not improve; it may also involve calls from the nurse to the client as a follow-up.)

HOME CARE: THE MOTHER AND FAMILY

The first few days and weeks postpartum bring many changes. The family adjusts to a new member, and siblings become familiar with new roles and responsibilities. During this period the woman must accomplish a variety of physical and developmental tasks, including:

- Restoring her physical condition
- Developing competence in caring for and meeting the needs of her infant
- Establishing a relationship with her new child
- Adapting to altered lifestyles and family structure resulting from the addition of a new member

The nurse can interact with the family following discharge by telephone follow-up, home visit, or a combination. The approach used depends on the mother's needs and preferences and established practices in the community.

Assessment of the Mother and Family

During the first home visit, complete a physical and psychologic assessment. Before doing so, ensure privacy. The physical assessment focuses on the mother's physical adaptation, determined by evaluating vital signs, breasts, abdominal musculature, elimination patterns, reproductive tract, and laboratory values. Talk with the mother about her diet, level of fatigue, ability to rest and sleep, pain management, and signs of postpartum complications. In addition, for breastfeeding mothers, assess the woman's feeding technique and give her information about possible problems that may occur.

The psychologic assessment focuses on attachment, adjustment to the parental role, emotional response to childbirth and parenting, sibling adjustment, and educational needs. Ask specifically about feelings of depression, anger, and the like (see the discussion of postpartum depression in Chapter 23). ⬭ When appropriate, mention available community resources, including public health department follow-up visits. If not already discussed, teaching

about family planning is appropriate at this time, coupled with information about birth control methods.

In ideal situations a family approach with the father or partner and any siblings present provides an opportunity to observe family interactions and gives all family members a chance to ask questions and express concerns. In addition, any questionable family interaction pattern such as one suggestive of abuse or neglect may be evident and further referral could be considered if needed.

If the partner or any siblings of the newborn are not present, it is important to ask the new mother how she believes the family members are adjusting and to seek her perceptions of family dynamics. It is also useful to ask about the role the grandparents play in the family and the support and assistance that they are able and willing to provide. (See "Assessment Guide: Postpartal—First Home Visit and Anticipated Progress at 6 Weeks" on pages 693–695.)

In addition, continue to teach the mother and her family as needed, including descriptions of relevant self-care measures. Discuss infant care and answer questions the family may have. Generally the new mother has a final postpartum examination with her caregiver about 6 weeks after childbirth. However, if the assessment indicates a need, refer the woman to her health care provider for further care before the 6-week check.

BREASTFEEDING ISSUES FOLLOWING DISCHARGE

The mother-baby nurse in the birthing area can offer anticipatory guidance about common breastfeeding issues and provide resources for the woman's use after discharge. Nursing support for breastfeeding mothers can take many forms. Informational support includes written materials, verbal information, demonstration, answering questions, offering tips, providing feedback, and giving nonverbal assistance (such as moving a baby closer to the mother's breast). Encouragement and interpersonal support (such as staying with a breastfeeding woman and supporting the mother's decisions) are also helpful (Gill, 2001). The nurse can also tell the family about various websites that might be helpful. This should include the site for the LaLeche League, an international organization designed to help women breastfeed successfully. ⬭ WEB

Chapter 27 ⬭ provides in-depth discussion of breastfeeding including the physiology of breastfeeding, cultural aspects of the process, hints for getting started, and so forth. ⬭ Because mothers are discharged from the birthing unit before breastfeeding is well established, they are frequently alone when they encounter changes in the breastfeeding process. Many women stop nursing if the situations they encounter seem too hard to handle.

Table 30–3 on page 696 summarizes self-care measures to suggest to a woman with a breastfeeding problem.

Physical Assessment/Normal Findings	Alterations and Possible Causes*	Nursing Responses to Data†
VITAL SIGNS		
Blood pressure: Return to normal prepregnant level.	Elevated blood pressure (anxiety essential hypertension renal disease).	Review history, evaluate normal baseline; refer to physician or CNM if necessary.
Pulse: 60–90 beats/minute (or prepregnant normal rate).	Increased pulse rate (excitement, anxiety, cardiac disorders).	Count pulse for full minute and note irregularities; marked tachycardia or beat irregularities require additional assessment and possible physician or CNM referral.
Respirations: 16–24/minute.	Marked tachypnea or abnormal patterns (respiratory disorders).	Evaluate for respiratory disease, refer to physician or CNM if necessary.
Temperature: 36.2–37.6 °C (98–99.6 °F)	Increased temperature (infection).	Assess for signs and symptoms of infection or disease state.
WEIGHT		
2 days: Possible weight loss of 12–20+ lb.	Minimal weight loss (fluid retention, pregnancy-induced hypertension [PIH]).	Evaluate for fluid retention, edema, deep tendon reflexes, and blood pressure elevation.
6 weeks: Returning to normal prepregnant weight.	Retained weight (excessive caloric intake).	Determine amount of daily exercise. Provide dietary teaching. Refer to dietitian if necessary for additional dietary counseling.
	Extreme weight loss (excessive dieting inadequate caloric intake).	Discuss appropriate diets; refer to dietitian for additional counseling if necessary.
BREASTS		
Nonnursing		
2 days: May have mild tenderness; small amount of milk may be expressed. 6 weeks: Soft with no tenderness; return to prepregnant size.	Some engorgement (incomplete suppression of lactation). Redness; marked tenderness (mastitis). Palpable mass (tumor).	Engorgement may be seen in nonnursing mothers. Advise client to wear a supportive, well-fitted bra, avoid very warm showers, use ice packs for comfort; evaluate for signs and symptoms of mastitis (rare in nonnursing mothers).
Nursing		
Full with prominent nipples, lactation established.	Cracked, fissured nipples (feeding problems). Redness, marked tenderness, or even abscess formation (mastitis). Palpable mass (full milk duct tumor).	Counsel about nipple care. Evaluate client condition, evidence of fever; refer to physician, or certified nurse midwife for initiation of antibiotic therapy, if indicated. Opinion varies as to value of breast examination for nursing mothers; some feel a nursing mother should examine her breasts monthly, after feeding, when breasts are empty; if palpable mass is felt, refer to physician for further evaluation. For breast inflammation instruct the mother to 1. Keep breast empty by frequent feeding. 2. Rest when possible. 3. Take prescribed pain relief med. 4. Force fluids. If symptoms persist for more than 24 hours, instruct her to call her physician or CNM.
	*Possible causes of alterations are placed in parentheses.	**†This column provides guidelines for further assessment and initial nursing interventions.**

(continued)

Physical Assessment/Normal Findings	Alterations and Possible Causes*	Nursing Responses to Data†
ABDOMINAL MUSCULATURE		
2 days: Improved firmness, although "bread-dough" consistency is not unusual, especially in multipara.	Marked relaxation of muscles.	Evaluate exercise level; provide information on appropriate exercise program.
Striae pink and obvious.		
Cesarean incision healing.	Drainage, redness, tenderness, pain, edema (infection).	Evaluate for infection; refer to physician or CNM if necessary.
6 weeks: Muscle tone continues to improve; striae may be beginning to fade, may not achieve a silvery appearance for several more weeks, linea nigra fading.		
ELIMINATION PATTERN		
Urinary Tract		
Return to prepregnant urinary elimination routine.	Urinary incontinence, especially with lifting, coughing, laughing, and so on (urethral trauma, cystocele).	Assess for cystocele; instruct in appropriate muscle tightening exercises; refer to physician or CNM.
	Pain or burning when voiding urgency and/or frequency, pus or white blood cells (WBC) in urine, pathogenic organisms in culture (urinary tract infection).	Evaluate for urinary tract infection; obtain clean-catch urine sample; refer to physician or CNM for treatment if indicated.
Routine urinalysis within normal limits (proteinuria disappeared).	Sugar or ketone in urine—may be some lactose present in urine of breastfeeding mothers (diabetes).	Evaluate diet; assess for signs and symptoms of diabetes; refer to physician or CNM.
Bowel Habits		
2 days: May be some discomfort with defecation, especially if client had severe hemorrhoids or third- or fourth-degree extension.	Severe constipation or pain when defecating (trauma or hemorrhoids).	Discuss dietary patterns; encourage fluid, adequate roughage.
		Continue use of stool softener if necessary to prevent pain associated with straining; continue sitz baths, periods of rest for severe hemorrhoids; assess healing of episiotomy and/or lacerations; severe constipation may require administration of laxatives, stool softeners, and an enema.
6 weeks: Return to normal prepregnancy bowel elimination patterns.	Marked constipation.	See previous discussion.
	Fecal incontinence or constipation (rectocela).	Assess for evidence of rectocele; instruct in muscle-tightening exercises; refer to physician or CNM.
REPRODUCTIVE TRACT		
Lochia		
2 days: Lochia rubra or lochia serosa, scant amounts, fleshy odor.	Excessive amounts (nonfirm uterus), foul odor (infection).	Assess for evidence of infection and/or failure of the uterus to decrease in size; refer to physician or CNM.
6 weeks: No lochia, or return to normal menstruation pattern.	See above.	See above.
Fundus and Perineum		
2 days: Fundus is at least two finger breadths below the umbilicus; uterine muscles still somewhat lax; introitus of vagina lacks tone—gapes when intra-abdominal pressure is increased by coughing or straining.	Uterus not decreasing in size appropriately (infection).	Assess fundus for firmness and/or signs of infection, refer to physician of CNM if indicated.
Episiotomy and/or lacerations healing; no signs of infection.	Evidence of redness, tenderness, poor tissue approximation in eplsiotomy and/or laceration (wound infection).	
6 weeks: Uterus almost returned to prepregnant size, with almost completely restored muscle tone.	Continued flow of lochia, failure to decrease appropriately in size (subinvolution).	Assess for evidence of subinvolution and/or infection; refer to physician for further evaluation and for dilatation and curettage if necessary.

Physical Assessment/Normal Findings	Alterations and Possible Causes*	Nursing Responses to Data†
HEMOGLOBIN AND HEMATOCRIT LEVELS		
6 weeks: Hb 12g/dL. Hct 37% plus or minus 5%.	Hb less than 12g/dL. Hct 32% (anemia).	Assess nutritional status, begin (or continue) supplemental iron for marked anemia (Hb less than or equal to 9g/dL) additional assessment and/or physician or CNM referral may be necessary.
ATTACHMENT		
Bonding process demonstrated by soothing, cuddling, and talking to infant; appropriate feeding techniques; eye-to-eye contact; calling infant by name.	Failure to bond demonstrated by lack of behaviors associated with bonding process, calling infant by nickname that promotes ridicule; inadequate infant weight gain, infant is dirty, hygienic measures are not being maintained, severe diaper rash, failure to obtain adequate supplies to provide infant care (malattachment).	Provide counseling talk with the woman about her feelings regarding the infant; provide support for the caretaking activities that are being performed; refer to public health nurse for continued home visits.
Parent interacts with infant and provides soothing, caretaking activities.	Parent is unable to respond to infant needs (inability to recognize needs; inadequate education and support, fear, family stress).	Provide support for caretaking activities observed; provide information regarding caretaking activities, such as responding to infant cry; methods of wrapping infant; methods of soothing the infant such as swaddling, rocking, increasing stimuli by singing to the infant or decreasing stimuli by putting infant to rest in quiet room; methods of holding the infant; differences in the cry. Identify support system such as friends, neighbors, provide information regarding community resources and support groups.
Parents express feelings of comfort and success with the parent role.	Evidence of stress and anxiety (difficulty moving into or dealing with the parent role).	Provide support and encouragement; provide information regarding progression into parent role and assist parents in talking through their feelings; refer to community resources and support groups.
Woman is in the informal or personal stage of maternal role attainment.	Woman is still greatly influenced by others, has not developed an image or style of her own (woman remains in the anticipatory stage).	Provide role modeling for the woman in working through problem solving with the infant; provide encouragement as she thinks through decisions and develops her sense of problem solving; encourage her to make decisions regarding infant care.
ADJUSTMENT TO PARENTAL ROLE		
Parents are coping with new roles in terms of division of labor, financial status, communication, readjustment of sexual relations, and adjusting to new daily tasks.	Inability to adjust to new roles (immaturity, inadequate education and preparation, ineffective communication patterns, inadequate support, current family crisis).	Provide counseling; refer to parent groups.
EDUCATION		
Mother understands self-care measures	Inadequate knowledge of self-care (inadequate education).	Provide education and counseling.
Parents are knowledgeable regarding infant care.	Inadequate knowledge of infant care (inadequate education).	
Siblings are adjusting to new baby.	Excessive sibling rivalry.	
Parents have a method of contraception.	Birth control method not chosen.	
	*Possible causes of alterations are placed in parentheses.	†This column provides guidelines for further assessment and initial nursing interventions.

TABLE 30-3 Breastfeeding Problems and Remedies

NIPPLES NOT GRASPABLE

Flat or inverted nipples

- Use Hoffman technique to break adhesions.
- Wear milk cups to encourage nipples to protrude.
- Use nipple tug and roll to increase protractility.
- Form the nipple prior to nursing by hand shaping, ice, wearing milk cups a half-hour before feeding.
- As a last resort, use nipple shield for first few minutes of feeding to draw out nipple; then place baby on breast.

Engorged breasts

Treat engorgement by relieving fullness with hand expression of milk prior to nursing and instituting frequent feeding so nipple is more prominent.

Large breasts

- Support breast with opposite hand or use rolled towel under breast to bring nipple to the level of baby's mouth.
- Use C-hold to make nipple accessible to baby.

ENGORGEMENT

Missed or infrequent feedings

- Nurse frequently (every 1 1/2 hours).
- Massage and hand express or pump to empty breasts completely when feedings are missed or when a full feeling develops in breasts and baby is not available or willing to nurse.

Breasts not emptied at feedings

- Nurse long enough to empty breasts (10–15 minutes on each side at each feeding).
- If baby will not nurse long enough to empty breasts, hand express or pump after feeding.

Inadequate letdown

- Use relaxation techniques, massage, and warm or cool compresses before nursing.
- Relax in warm shower with water running from back over shoulders and breasts, hand expressing to relieve fullness.
- If due to anxiety, try to eliminate the source of tension.

Baby sleepy or not eager to nurse

- Use rousing techniques (e.g., hold baby upright, unwrap blanket, change diaper).
- Preexpress milk onto nipple or baby's lips to entice baby.
- Avoid use of bottles of water or formula; these will decrease baby's willingness to suckle.

INADEQUATE LETDOWN

Letdown not well established

- Give the baby ample time at the breast (at least 15 minutes per side) to allow for letdown and complete emptying.
- Nurse in a quiet spot away from distractions.
- Massage breasts before nursing.
- Drink juice, water, tea (no caffeine) before and during nursing.

- Condition letdown by setting up a routine for beginning feedings.
- Use relaxation and breathing techniques.
- Stimulate the nipple manually before nursing.
- Concentrate thought on the baby and milk flow; turn on a faucet so that the sound of running water helps stimulate letdown.
- Use synthetic oxytocin nasal spray several times during a feeding. (This should condition letdown within 24 hours. Then it is no longer needed. Spray must be prescribed by a doctor.

Mother overtired or overextended

- Nap or rest when the baby rests.
- Lie down to nurse.
- Nurse the baby in bed at night.
- Simplify daily chores; set priorities.

Mother tense, pressured

- Identify the causes of tensions and eliminate or minimize them.
- Decrease fatigue.

Mother caught in cycle of little milk, worry, less milk

- Try all the actions mentioned earlier.
- Develop confidence in mothering skills. (A home visit by a counselor may help.)

CRACKED NIPPLES

All causes of sore nipples carried to extreme

- Refer to all actions for sore nipples.
- Consult doctor about using aspirin, acetaminophen (Tylenol), or other painkiller.
- Improve nutritional status, increasing protein, vitamin C, zinc.

Local infection (baby with staph or other organism may have infected mother's nipples)

Refer to physician.

PLUGGED DUCTS

Poor positioning

- Try a variety of positions for complete emptying.

Incomplete emptying of breast

- Nurse at least 10 minutes per side after letdown.
- Alternate nursing positions.
- If baby does not empty breasts, pump or express milk after feedings.

External pressure on breast

- Use larger size bras, insert bra extender, or go braless.
- Use nursing bra instead of pulling up conventional bra to nurse to avoid pressure on ducts.
- Avoid bunching up sweater or nightgown under arm during nursing.

TABLE 30-3 Breastfeeding Problems and Remedies—continued

SORE NIPPLES

Poor positioning

- Alternate nursing positions throughout the day.
- Bring the baby close to nurse so the baby does not pull on the breast.
- Place the nipple and some of the areola in the baby's mouth.
- Check to ensure the baby is put on and off the breast properly.
- Check to ensure the nipple is back far enough in the baby's mouth.
- Hold the baby closely during nursing so the nipple is not constantly being pulled.

Baby chewing or nuzzling onto nipple

- Form the nipple for the baby.
- Set up a pattern of getting the baby onto the breast using the rooting reflex.

Baby nursing on end of nipple

- Ensure the nipple is way back in the baby's mouth by getting the baby properly onto the breast.
- Check for an inverted nipple.
- Check for engorgement.

Baby chewing his or her way off the nipple (nipple being pulled out of baby's mouth at end of feeding)

- Remove the baby from the breast by placing a finger between the baby's gums to ensure suction is broken.
- End feeding when the baby's suckling slows, before he or she has a chance to chew on the nipple.

Baby overly eager to nurse

- Nurse more often.
- Preexpress milk to hasten letdown, avoiding vigorous suckling.

Dry colostrum or milk causing nipple to stick to bra or breast pads

Moisten bra or pads before taking off so as not to remove keratin.

Nipples not allowed to dry

- Remove plastic liners from milk pads.
- Air dry breasts completely after nursing.
- Change milk pads frequently.

Improper use of breast shield

- Use shield only to draw out nipple; then have the baby nurse on the breast.
- Cut tip of shield back bit by bit and eventually discard.

Nipple skin not resistant to stress

- Improve diet, especially adding fresh fruits and vegetables and vitamin supplements.
- Eliminate or decrease use of sugary foods, alcohol, caffeine, cigarettes.
- Check use of cleansing or drying agents.

Natural oils removed or keratin layers broken down by drying agents (soap, alcohol, shampoo, deodorant)

- Eliminate irritants.
- Wash breasts with water only.

Note: From "Breastfeeding Problems and Remedies" (adapted), copyright © 1983, 1990 by Judith Lauwers and Candace Woessner, from Counseling the Nursing Mother, 2nd edition by Judith Lauwers and Candace Woessner. Used by permission of Avery Publishing, a division of Penguin Putnam Inc.

Nipple Soreness

Some discomfort often occurs initially with breastfeeding; it usually peaks between the third and sixth days and then lessens (Riordan & Auerbach, 1999). However, the mother should not switch to bottle-feeding or delay feedings at this point because these measures cause engorgement and more soreness. Discomfort that lasts throughout the feeding or past the first week demands attention.

The baby's position at the breast is a critical factor in nipple soreness. The mother's hand should be off the areola, and the baby should be facing the mother's chest, with ear, shoulder, and hip aligned (see Figure 27–5). To help decrease nipple soreness, encourage the mother to rotate positions when feeding her infant. Changing positions alters the focus of greatest stress and promotes more complete breast emptying.

Nipple soreness may also develop if the infant has faulty sucking habits. If the nipple enters the baby's mouth at an upward angle and rubs against the roof of the mouth, the nipple may have an injured tip that is bruised, scabbed, or blistered (Riordan & Auerbach, 1999). Soreness may also result from continuous negative pressure if the infant falls asleep with the breast in his or her mouth.

Chewed nipples, which result from improper positioning, are cracked or tender at or near the base. In these cases, the baby's jaws close only on the nipple instead of on the areola, the baby's mouth is not opened wide enough, or the infant's mouth has slipped down to the nipple from the areola as a result of engorgement. Soreness on the underside of the nipple is caused by the infant nursing with his or her bottom lip tucked in rather than out, causing a friction burn. In such cases, even vigorous sucking produces little milk because the milk sinuses under the areola are not compressed. This situation results in a frustrated infant and marked soreness for the mother. The problem is overcome by positioning the infant with as much areola as possible in his or her mouth and rotating the baby's positions at the breast.

Nipple soreness is especially pronounced during the first few minutes of a feeding. If the mother is not expecting this discomfort, she may become discouraged and quickly stop. The letdown reflex may take a few minutes to activate, and it may not occur if the mother stops nursing too quickly. The infant is unsatisfied, and the possibility of breast engorgement increases.

Nipple soreness can also result from the vigorous feeding of an overeager infant. In this case the mother may find it helpful to nurse more frequently. The woman can also apply ice to her nipples and areola for a few minutes before feeding to promote nipple erectness and numb the tissue initially. To prevent skin breakdown, after feeding the mother can wash her nipples and areolae with water and allow them to dry well. To promote dryness, the mother may leave her bra flaps down for a few minutes after feeding or expose her nipples to sunlight or ultraviolet light for 30 seconds at first, gradually increasing to 3 minutes. Drying the nipples with a hair dryer on a low heat setting also facilitates drying and promotes healing (Riordan & Auerbach, 1999).

The use of petroleum-based products such as Vaseline, A + D ointment, cocoa butter, and baby oil to lubricate the nipples is discouraged because petroleum interferes with skin respiration and may prolong soreness. Because of the risk of allergic reactions, products such as Massé cream (risk of peanut allergy) and lubricants containing lanolin (risk of wool allergy) are also discouraged. In addition, products that are washed off before breastfeeding should be avoided because washing irritates the nipples (Lauwers & Shinskie, 2000).

Many lactation experts recommend that the mother's own milk be applied to the nipples and allowed to air dry. Breast milk is high in fat, fights infection, and will not irritate the nipples. Moreover, it is readily available at no cost to the mother. In cases of very dry or sore nipples, hypoallergenic medical-grade anhydrous lanolin may be helpful. This product poses a low risk of allergy because the alcohols that contribute to the allergic response have been removed (Lauwers & Shinskie, 2000).

If the woman finds that her bra or clothing rubs against her nipples and adds to her discomfort, she may put shields in her bra. Both Medela Shells and Woolrich Shields relieve friction and promote air circulation. If a woman uses breast pads inside her bra to keep milk from leaking onto her clothes, she should change the pads frequently so the nipples remain dry.

Nipple dermatitis, which causes swollen, reddened, burning nipples, is most commonly caused by thrush or by allergic response to breast cream preparations. If the nipple soreness has a sudden onset and is accompanied by burning or itching, shooting pains through the breast, and a deep pink coloration of the nipple, it may be caused by a thrush infection spread from the infant to the mother. White patches or streaks in the infant's mouth indicate a need for treatment of the mouth and nipple infection. The disease can be treated with a variety of antifungal preparations and does not prevent breastfeeding.

Cracked Nipples

Nipple soreness is often coupled with cracked nipples. When a breastfeeding mother complains of soreness, carefully examine the nipples for fissures or cracks and observe the mother during breastfeeding to see whether the infant is correctly positioned at the breast. If the positioning is correct and cracks exist, interventions are necessary. All the interventions described for sore nipples may be used. It may also help the mother to begin nursing on the breast that is less sore. This approach allows the letdown reflex to occur in the affected breast and permits the infant to more vigorously suck the less tender breast, which decreases trauma to the cracked nipple. With severe cases, the temporary use of a nipple shield for nursing may be appropriate. For the mother's comfort, analgesics may be taken after nursing.

Breast Engorgement

Breast fullness and breast engorgement are not the same. All lactating women experience a transition fullness at first, initially due to venous congestion and later due to accumulating milk. However, this fullness generally lasts only 24 hours, the breasts remain soft enough for the newborn to suckle, and there is no pain. Engorged breasts are hard, painful, and warm and appear taut and shiny.

The infant should nurse for an average of 15 minutes per feeding and should feed at least eight times in 24 hours (Riordan & Auerbach, 1999). If the baby is unable to nurse more frequently, the mother may express some milk manually or with a pump, taking care to avoid traumatizing the breast tissue. Warm or cool compresses before nursing stimulate letdown and soften the breast so that the infant can grasp the areola more easily. Wearing a wellfitting nursing bra 24 hours a day supports the breasts and prevents discomfort.

The use of fresh green cabbage leaves placed inside the bra to treat engorgement is a long-recognized home remedy that has sparked renewed interest. Although the exact action of the cabbage is not understood, it appears to reduce the edema of engorgement. The amount of relief women experience varies. Some women report relief in as little as 30 minutes, whereas other women require more continuous use to perceive an effect. Prolonged use of cabbage can cause the milk to dry up, which may be helpful if sudden weaning is necessary (Lauwers & Shinskie, 2000). Analgesics such as acetaminophen and aspirin, alone or in combination with codeine, are appropriate, especially if taken just before nursing. The pain will be relieved, but the medication will not reach the milk for some time.

Thinking Critically

ASSESSING BREASTFEEDING DIFFICULTIES

Ann calls you from home in tears on her third postpartum day. She states that, although breastfeeding was going well in the hospital, her breasts are now swollen, hard, and very painful, and her baby is refusing to suckle. Ann expresses extreme disappointment that "the breastfeeding didn't work" because she truly believes that breast milk is best for babies and she had enjoyed her breastfeeding experience in the hospital, especially nursing the baby immediately after delivery. But she also states she has not been able to stop crying all day and can no longer tolerate her painful breasts. In addition she says that the baby "seems happier" with the bottle. What would you do? **WEB**

Plugged Ducts

Some mothers experience plugging of one or more ducts, especially in conjunction with or following engorgement. This condition is often referred to as "caked breasts." Manifested as an area of tenderness or lumpiness in an otherwise well woman, plugging may be relieved by heat and massage. Encourage the mother to massage her breasts from her chest wall forward to the nipple while standing in a warm shower or after applying moist heat to the breast (Riordan & Auerbach, 1999). The mother should then nurse her infant, starting on the unaffected breast if the plugged breast is tender. Frequent nursing and varying positions to ensure complete emptying helps prevent the problem.

Breastfeeding and the Working Mother

The best preparation for maintaining lactation after return to work is frequent, unlimited breastfeeding. Even when well planned, the first day back to work may be filled with emotional and physical distress. Anticipatory guidance may ease the transition from maternity leave to work. The earlier the breastfeeding mother returns to work, the more often she will need to pump her breasts to express the breast milk. Because milk production follows the principle of supply and demand, if breasts are not pumped, the milk supply will decrease.

An electric breast pump and double collection system are the best way of expressing milk. However, it is not the only method. Sometimes a mother has a flexible schedule and can return home or have the baby brought to her to nurse at lunch. If this is not possible, the infant may be fed expressed milk. (For proper storage of breast milk, see "Storing Breast Milk" in Chapter 27.) When the mother is absent, the infant can be bottle-fed or spoon-fed. If the baby is 3 months or older, cup feeding is an option. The mother should wait until lactation is well established before introducing the bottle. Most babies adjust to the bottle within 7 to 10 days.

To maintain a milk supply, the working mother must pay special attention to her fluid intake. She can ensure adequate intake by drinking extra fluid at each break and whenever possible during the day. It is also helpful to nurse more on weekends, nurse during the night, eat a nutritionally sound diet, and continue manual expression or pumping when not nursing.

Night nursing presents a dilemma: it may help a working mother maintain her milk supply, but it may also contribute to fatigue. Some women choose to have the infant sleep with them so that breastfeeding is more easily accomplished; other women find it difficult to sleep soundly when the infant is in the same bed. For the mother who works long hours or has a rigid work schedule, the best alternative may be to limit breastfeeding to morning and evening feedings, with supplemental feedings at other times. This choice allows her to maintain a close relationship with the infant and provides some of the unique benefits of breast milk.

Weaning

The decision to wean the baby from the breast may be made for a variety of reasons, including family or cultural pressures, changes in the home situation, or a personal opinion about when weaning should occur. For the woman who is comfortable with breastfeeding and well informed about the process, the appropriate time to wean her infant will become evident if she is sensitive to the child's cues. Often weaning falls between periods of great developmental activity for the child. Thus, weaning commonly occurs at 8 to 9 months, 12 to 14 months, 18 months, 2 years, and 3 years of age. The infant weaned before 12 months should be given iron-fortified infant formula, not cows' milk (American College of Obstetricians and Gynecologists, 2000).

If weaning is timed to respond to the child's cues, and if the mother is comfortable with the timing, it can be accomplished with less difficulty than if the process begins before mother and child are ready emotionally. Nevertheless, weaning is a time of emotional separation for mother and baby; it may be difficult for them to give up the closeness of their nursing sessions. The nurse who is understanding about this possibility can help the mother see that her infant is growing up and plan other comforting, consoling, and play activities to replace breastfeeding. A gradual approach is the easiest and most comforting way to wean the child from breastfeedings.

During weaning, the mother should substitute one cup feeding or bottle-feeding for one breastfeeding session over a few days to a week so that her breasts gradually produce less milk. Eliminating the breastfeedings associated with meals first helps the mother wean the infant more easily. Over a period of several weeks she can substitute more cup feedings or bottle-feedings for breastfeedings. The slow method of weaning prevents breast engorgement, allows infants to alter their eating methods at their own rates, and provides time for psychologic adjustment.

RESUMPTION OF SEXUAL ACTIVITY

Typically, postpartum couples resume sexual intercourse once the episiotomy is healed and the lochial flow has stopped. Because this usually occurs by the end of the third week, prior to the 6-week check, it is important that the woman and her partner have information about what to expect. Inform the couple that, because the vaginal vault is "dry" (hormone poor), some form of lubrication such as K-Y jelly may be necessary during intercourse. The female-superior and side-lying coital positions may be preferable because they allow the woman to control the depth of penile penetration.

Forewarn breastfeeding couples that during orgasm milk may spurt from the nipples due to the release of oxytocin. Some couples find this spurt pleasurable or amusing, but others feel more comfortable if the woman wears a bra during sexual activity. Nursing the baby before lovemaking may reduce the chance of milk release.

Other factors may interfere with satisfactory sexual experiences: the baby's crying may "spoil the mood," the woman's changed body may seem unattractive to her or her partner, maternal sleep deprivation may interfere with desire, and the woman's physiologic response to sexual stimulation may be altered due to hormonal changes. By 3 months postpartum, sexual interest and activity are generally regular in frequency. However, a return to prepregnant levels of sexual activity varies by couple and may take from a few weeks to a year after childbirth.

With anticipatory guidance during the prenatal and postpartum periods, the couple can be forewarned of potential temporary problems. Anticipatory guidance is enhanced if the couple can discuss their feelings and reactions as they are experienced.

Contraception

Information on contraception is often provided as part of discharge teaching. However, the nurse can also be an important resource for the woman and her partner during postpartum follow-up. Couples typically choose to use contraception to control the number of children they will have or to determine the spacing of future children. Whatever the method, consistency of use is essential. Identify the advantages, disadvantages, risks, and contraindications of the various methods to help the couple, or the single mother, make an informed choice. (For a more detailed discussion of contraceptive methods, see Chapter 3.)

Teaching About

RESUMPTION OF SEXUAL ACTIVITY AFTER CHILDBIRTH

- Delay intercourse until no lochia is present because lochia indicates that healing is not yet complete.
- Tenderness of the vagina and perineum may cause discomfort. The partner may test the woman's level of comfort by slipping a lubricated finger inside her vagina. The female-superior and side-lying positions may be preferable because they let the woman control the depth of penetration of the penis.
- Vaginal dryness may occur because the vagina is "hormone poor." It can be avoided by using a water-soluble lubricant.
- Based on the amount of breast engorgement and tenderness present, the partner may need to avoid breast stimulation during foreplay or use a very gentle approach.
- Escape of milk during sexual activity can be minimized by nursing immediately beforehand.
- Fatigue and the new baby's schedule may have a negative impact on the woman's feelings of desire. Napping when the baby sleeps helps decrease fatigue. However, fatigue may be a reality couples need to accept during the early postpartum months.
- Contraception is important even during the early postpartum period. The woman's body needs adequate time to heal and recover from the stress of pregnancy and childbirth. Couples opposed to contraception may choose abstinence at this time.

ADDITIONAL COMMUNITY RESOURCES

Telephone Follow-Up

Telephone follow-up is offered to families prior to discharge, and a mutually agreed upon time is set for the call. Typically the call is made within 3 days after discharge or earlier if desired. To perform effective telephone assessment, the nurse must be able to listen skillfully, ask open-ended questions, and project an attitude of caring. Care provided during a telephone conversation is limited to supportive counseling, teaching, and referral. It is also fairly common for a home care nurse to make a telephone follow-up call to a family a few days after a home visit to provide additional information, address questions or areas of confusion, and make referrals if indicated.

Return Visits

If the mother, family, and physician or certified nurse-midwife have chosen discharge earlier than 48 hours after vaginal birth, in some states, the mother may request a total of three home visits. In such cases the nurse would schedule the first visit about 24 hours after discharge and then space out the other two visits over the next week. In other instances the nurse may schedule additional home visits based on the findings of the first home visit and the follow-up phone call.

Help Lines for Parents

Many communities have established 24-hour help lines for new parents to call when they have questions or need support. In areas where help lines are not available, parents may be directed to call the birthing center. In either case, be sure the family has the number to call.

Postpartum Classes and Support Groups

Postpartum classes are available to help meet the continuing needs of the childbearing family. Classes may focus on topics such as parenting, postpartum exercise, or nutrition, or there may be loosely structured group sessions that address mothers' concerns as they arise. Such classes offer chances for the new mother to socialize, share her concerns, and receive encouragement. Because baby-sitting arrangements may be difficult or expensive, it is desirable to provide child care for newborns and siblings; in some classes infants may remain with mothers.

Many parents today look to the Internet for information and advice. Help them learn criteria that suggest that Internet information is reliable and of high quality, including affiliation with a university medical or nursing school; inclusion of authors' credentials, education, board certification, and affiliations; referencing of information; currency of information; similarity of information when compared with other sources, and easy accessibility (Lamp & Howard, 1999).

CHAPTER HIGHLIGHTS

☞ The overall goal of postpartum home visits is to increase the likelihood of a smooth transition for the new family. The home visit provides opportunities for assessment, teaching, and fostering a caring relationship with new families.

☞ Professional nursing has a role in establishing and maintaining excellence in care for the new family after discharge from the birthing center.

☞ Nurses need to act proactively to maintain their safety when making home visits by exercising reasonable caution and remaining alert to environmental cues.

☞ Nursing goals during home visits include reinforcement of daily newborn care, maintenance of neutral thermal environment, promotion of adequate hydration and nutrition, prevention of complications, promotion of safety, and enhancement of attachment and family knowledge of child care.

☞ Essential care during a home visit includes assessments of the vital signs, weight, overall color, intake and output, umbilical cord and circumcision, newborn nutrition, parent education, and attachment.

☞ The physician or pediatric nurse practitioner should be notified if there is evidence of redness around the umbilicus, bright-red bleeding or puslike drainage near the cord stump, or an unhealed umbilicus.

☞ After a circumcision, the newborn must be observed closely for inability to void and signs of infection.

☞ Signs of illness in newborns include temperature above 38.4 °C (101 °F) or below 36.1 °C (97 °F), more than one episode of forceful vomiting, refusal of two feedings in a row, lethargy, cyanosis with or without a feeding, and absence of breathing for longer than 15 seconds.

☞ Screening for galactosemia, hemocystinuria, hypothyroidism, phenylketonuria, and sickle cell anemia is done on all newborns in the first 1 to 3 days, with a second blood specimen drawn after 7 to 14 days.

☞ Signs of illness in mothers include mastitis, excessive or foul-smelling lochia, failure of the fundus to descend at anticipated rate; temperature of 100.4 °F (38 °C) or above; elevated blood pressure; and tenderness, redness, or pain in the legs.

☞ To prevent sore nipples the nurse can encourage the breastfeeding mother to nurse frequently, to change the infant's position regularly, and to allow her nipples to air dry after breastfeeding.

☞ Sexual intercourse may resume once the episiotomy is healed and lochial flow has stopped. Couples should be forewarned of possible changes. For example, the vagina may be "dry," fatigue may inhibit desire, or the woman's breasts may leak during orgasm.

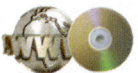 **EXPLORE**MediaLink

NCLEX Review, Case Studies, and other interactive resources for this chapter can be found on the companion website at http://www.prenhall.com/london. Click on "Chapter 30" to select the activities for this chapter.

For animations, more NCLEX review questions, and an audio glossary, access the accompanying CD-ROM in this textbook.

REFERENCES

American Academy of Pediatrics, Committee on Fetus and Newborn. (1995). Hospital stay for healthy term newborns. *Pediatrics, 96*(4, Pt. 1), 788–790.

American College of Obstetricians and Gynecologists. (2000). *Breastfeeding: Maternal and infant aspects* (ACOG Educational Bulletin No. 258). Washington, DC: Author.

Bocar, D. L. (1997). Combining breastfeeding and employment: Increasing success. *Journal of Perinatal and Neonatal Nursing, 11*(2), 23–43.

Bragg, E. J., Rosenn, B. M., Khoury, J. C., Miodovnik, M., & Siddiqi, T. A. (1997). The effect of early discharge after vaginal delivery on neonatal readmission rates. *Obstetrics and Gynecology, 89*(6), 930–933.

Braveman, P., Egerter, S., Pearl, M., Marchi, K., & Miller, C. (1995). Problems associated with early discharge of newborn infants. Early discharge of newborns and mothers: A critical review of the literature. *Pediatrics, 96*(4, Pt. 1), 716–726.

Cady, R. (1999). Telephone triage: Avoiding the pitfalls. American Journal of *Maternal-Child Nursing, 24*(4), 209.

Carpenter, J. A. (1998). Shortening the short stay. *AWHONN Lifelines, 2*(1), 29–34.

Catz, C., Hanson, J. W., Simpson, L., & Yaffe, S. J. (1995). Summary of workshop: Early discharge and neonatal hyperbilirubinemia. *Pediatrics, 96*(4, Pt. 1), 743–745.

Durkin, N., & Wilson, C. (1999). Simple steps to keep yourself safe. *Home Healthcare Nurse, 17*(7), 430–435.

Fishbein, E. G., & Burggraf, E. (1998). Early postpartum discharge: How are mothers managing? *Journal of Obstetric, Gynecologic, and Neonatal Nursing, 27*(2), 142–150.

Gill, S. L. (2001). The little things: Perceptions of breastfeeding support. *Journal of Obstetric, Gynecologic, and Neonatal Nursing, 30*(4), 401–409.

Lamp, J. M., & Howard, P. A. (1999). Guiding parents' use of the Internet for newborn education. *American Journal of Maternal-Child Nursing, 24*, 33–36.

Lauwers, J., & Shinskie, D. (2000). *Counseling the nursing mother: A lactation consultant's guide* (3rd ed.). Boston: Jones & Bartlett.

Locklin, M. P., & Jansson, M. J. (1999). Home visits: Strategies to protect the breastfeeding newborn at risk. *Journal of Obstetric, Gynecologic, and Neonatal Nursing, 28*, 33–40.

Mattson, S. (2000). Providing culturally competent care: Strategies and approaches for perinatal clients. *AWHONN Lifelines, 4*(5), 37–39.

Riordan, J., & Auerbach, K. (1999). *Breastfeeding and human lactation* (2nd ed.). Boston: Jones & Bartlett.

UNIT VI

Care and Needs of Children

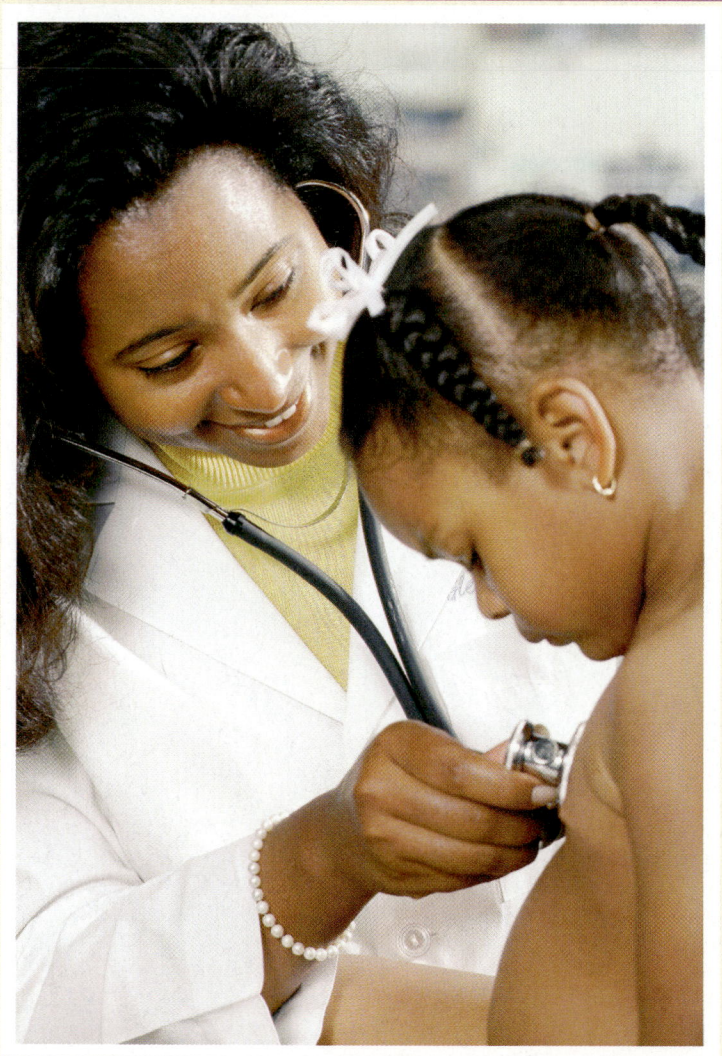

CHAPTER 31

Infant, Child, and Adolescent Nutrition

It is exciting to see Joey progressing into the school setting. Being with children his age will really help him develop in many ways. We're just worried because he needs to get only foods he can chew and swallow so he does not choke. He also needs his tube feedings during school to be sure he gets enough energy to do well.

—MOTHER OF JOEY, 11 YEARS OLD

Key Terms

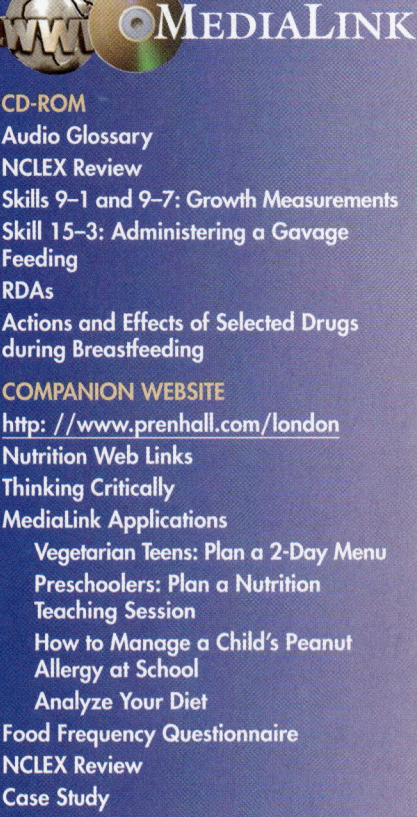

MEDIALINK

CD-ROM
Audio Glossary
NCLEX Review
Skills 9–1 and 9–7: Growth Measurements
Skill 15–3: Administering a Gavage Feeding
RDAs
Actions and Effects of Selected Drugs during Breastfeeding

COMPANION WEBSITE
http://www.prenhall.com/london
Nutrition Web Links
Thinking Critically
MediaLink Applications
  Vegetarian Teens: Plan a 2-Day Menu
  Preschoolers: Plan a Nutrition Teaching Session
  How to Manage a Child's Peanut Allergy at School
  Analyze Your Diet
Food Frequency Questionnaire
NCLEX Review
Case Study

Adequate nutrition is an essential component of growth and development. The child's nutritional status begins before birth and is related to the mother's nutritional state. All children must be assessed for nutritional status, followed by teaching or other interventions to enhance health. Nurses are instrumental in giving parents information about normal nutritional needs of infants and young children. Common techniques to assess nutrition, such as measuring growth and monitoring hematocrit, provide needed information about whether intake of foods is adequate.

Although all children and parents can benefit from information about nutritional needs, some children have additional issues that must be considered. The nurse recognizes the special requirements of children with conditions such as food allergies, cystic fibrosis, cerebral palsy, or diabetes. Nutrition monitoring is provided throughout childhood so that dietary counseling can be integrated with other teaching to promote development. How can the nurse bridge the various settings in which children's nutritional needs are met? These might include home, child care settings, schools, and hospitals. How can the nurse help the family prepare for meeting nutritional needs of a child who has special needs during car or plane travel?

Some children have unique nutritional needs due to their social environments. Parents may not be knowledgeable about child nutritional requirements. Perhaps the family is vegetarian and needs extra help to ensure intake of essential nutrients. If finances are limited, the family may need resources such as food stamps, food banks, or budget planning. The nurse considers the high rate of childhood obesity and common nutritional deficits when applying concepts of health promotion with families. Whatever the nurse's setting, knowledge of nutrition must be integrated within nursing care.

GENERAL CONCEPTS IN NUTRITION

Nutrition refers to taking in food and assimilating it metabolically for use by the body. It is an essential component of life and therefore an important body of knowledge to consider in discussions of child growth and development. The body requires a wide array of intake products, such as carbohydrates, protein, fat, and micronutrients like vitamins and minerals. The need for nutrients is dependent on activity level, state of health and presence of disease or other stress, and age-related requirements.

The **Dietary Reference Intakes (DRIs)** are a set of values established by the Food and Nutrition Board of the Institute of Medicine and the National Academy of Science that can be used to assess and plan intake for individuals of different ages. **WEB** They commonly include four different values that can be considered by nursing, nutrition, and other health personnel. While the DRIs are the approach used in the United States, other countries have developed their own approaches to dietary standards. For example, Canada uses Adequate Intake and Reference Nutrient Intake, whereas the United Kingdom uses Recommended Daily Nutrient Intakes. The aim of these standards is to provide a method to evaluate individual and population diets, and to plan nutrition programs and edu-

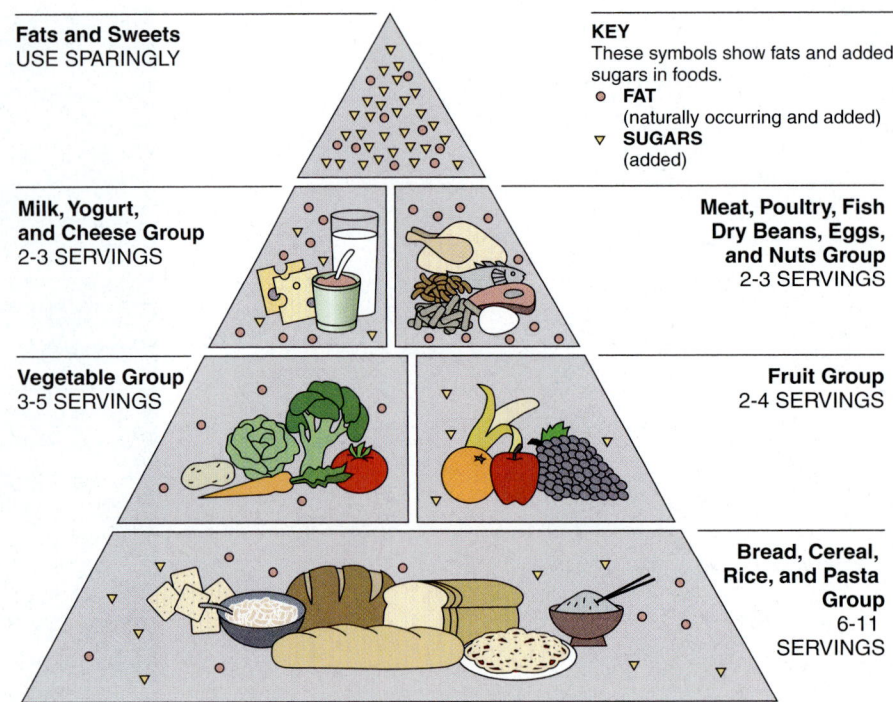

FIGURE 31–1. ◆ The Food Guide Pyramid is used to provide teaching about amounts of foods recommended for daily intake. *Note:* From U.S. Department of Agriculture and U.S. Department of Health and Human.

cation. DRIs are generally specific to males and females in several age categories.

The DRIs provide useful information when evaluating diets, but their use can be time consuming. What "quick check" can provide feedback about the daily diets of children? Learn the Food Guide Pyramid and hang it in schools, clinics, and hospitals. It is a fast way to look at children's intakes for one day and see if they meet most requirements. Instead of calculating amounts of nutrients ingested, the pyramid focuses on categories of foods, which readily reflects the actual intake. The number of servings from various categories stays constant throughout childhood, but the serving sizes increase as the child gets older. See Figure 31–1 ◆ for the Food Guide Pyramid, and consult websites for alternative pyramids for vegetarians and those from various ethnic groups, such as Hispanic and Native American. ⌼ WEB

NUTRITIONAL NEEDS

Infancy

From the first feeding of a few ounces of breast milk to a meal of soft table foods with the family at 1 year of age, the infant demonstrates an amazing growth in ability to ingest and digest a wide variety of foods. Never again will the individual have such a high metabolic rate or high intake requirements in relation to size, or such a change in the types of foods eaten. Infants have an extremely fast rate of growth, since birth weight is usually doubled by about 5 months of age, and tripled by 1 year. Meeting nutritional needs is made difficult by the small size of the infant's stomach and the immaturity of the digestive system. Their great physical activity also necessitates high caloric intake. Nutrient demands for protein and vitamins must be met for the cells of the nervous system and body organs to develop properly.

BREAST- AND BOTTLE-FEEDING

The natural first food is breast milk and its intake should be encouraged for all infants. See Chapter 27 for a discussion of newborn nutrition. ⌼ The American Academy of Pediatrics (AAP) believes that breastfeeding is the best source of nutrition for babies through the first birthday and should be encouraged by health professionals (Committee on Nutrition, 1998). It can be the only food for the first 6 months, and should continue through 12 months of age, with addition of solid foods from 6 to 12 months. Many advantages to breastfeeding are known, including excellent nutritional balance, promotion of gastrointestinal function, fostering immune defense, psychologic benefits, and economic advantage. Although breast milk is the best nutritional source for infants, babies may need some limited supplements.

Providing breastfeeding information and instruction positively influences the number of women who decide to

Teaching About

SUPPLEMENTS FOR BREASTFED BABIES

1. Each baby receives a *vitamin K* injection after birth to promote adequate blood clotting. After that, no further vitamin K is needed since the child manufactures this vitamin in the gut once he or she begins eating.

2. The need for *vitamin D* is not fully established, but 400 IU/day is recommended for infants who are breastfed, live in northern climates and urban settings (especially in winter), are dark skinned, or are kept well covered when outside.

3. *Iron* is not needed unless the infant is not eating food with iron by 4 to 6 months. The baby may need an iron source earlier if the mother was anemic during pregnancy or while breastfeeding.

4. *Fluoride* 0.25 mg is given after 6 months of age if water is not fluoridated to a level of 0.3 parts per million (ppm), or if the baby is not drinking any water.

breastfeed and increases the number of months they choose to continue breastfeeding (Kramer, 2001). Some hospitals have lactation specialists who assist breastfeeding mothers; in others, nurses provide this service. Home visits, phone calls from hospital nursing staff, early visits after the birth to obstetric and pediatric offices, and resources such as La Leche League can provide mothers with needed breastfeeding information and problem-solving suggestions. ⌼ WEB Information is needed so that the mother gets adequate nutritional intake and sufficient rest. Support programs are especially helpful to mothers who have difficulty breastfeeding, feel unsure how it will fit into family and work life, are very young, or have an infant with problems related to feeding. The mother of a hospitalized infant needs special support to continue breastfeeding. The mother should be encouraged to come to the hospital to feed her baby on the same schedule as at home. If the infant cannot breastfeed, the hospital can provide an electric pump so the mother can maintain lactation. Often hospitals provide meals for the mother of a hospitalized baby so that she can maintain good nutrition and quality breast milk while she stays in the hospital with the baby.

Some women decide not to breastfeed or are unable to do so. After several months of breastfeeding, some mothers begin to use supplemental bottles when the infant is away from them. Nurses give these mothers information about formula preparation and feeding. Three types of formula are available—ready to feed, concentrate, and powder. All are nutritionally adequate for infants. The nurse can help parents decide which preparation of formula is best suited for their infant (see Table 31–1). Some infants, such as those with phenylketonuria, other metabolic disorders, or babies with cow milk allergy, require specialized formulas. Breast- or bottle-feeding is discussed at each contact with health professionals to identify potential teaching needs.

Formula Preparation	How Packaged	Advantages	Disadvantages
Ready to feed	Bottles or cans	No preparation needed	Most expensive type of formula
Concentrate	Cans of concentrated liquid	Easy to add equal amounts of formula concentrate and water directly into bottle and shake	Can be incorrectly measured, leading to inadequate or unsafe nutrition for infant; requires access to clean water supply such as city tap water or bottled water; well water may have too high a mineral concentration
Powder	Cans	Least expensive type of formula	Can be incorrectly measured, leading to inadequate or unsafe nutrition for infant; requires shaking to mix thoroughly; requires access to clean water supply such as city tap water or bottled water; well water may have too high a mineral concentration

Nursing Practice

Formula can be mixed with tap water but must be refrigerated once mixed. Formula that the baby does not drink should be discarded after use and not kept for future feedings. This minimizes the chance for bacteria to grow and to cause illness in the baby. When the family lives in older housing, caution them to run tap water for about 2 minutes before using it, and to use only cold water for formula preparation. These practices minimize the chance that lead is leached from the older pipes in the house (see Chapter 46 for further discussion of lead poisoning). If the family has a well, the water should be tested for microorganisms before being used for the baby.

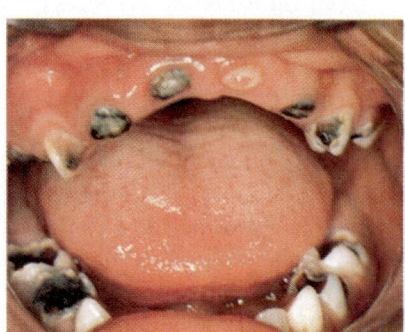

FIGURE 31–2. ◆ Nursing bottle mouth syndrome. This child has had major tooth decay related to sleeping as an infant and toddler while sucking bottles of juice and milk. *Courtesy of Dr. Lezley McIlveen, Department of Dentistry, Children's National Medical Center, Washington, DC.*

During infancy and toddlerhood, nurses should carefully examine the patterns of breast- and bottle-feeding. **Nursing bottle mouth syndrome** can occur when a young child is allowed to nurse or drink from a bottle for long periods, especially when sleeping (Figure 31–2 ◆). The milk, juice, or other fluid pools around the upper anterior teeth, salivary flow decreases, and acid buffering is decreased, resulting in tooth decay. Teach parents to avoid putting the child to bed with a bottle. Encourage pacifier use or a bottle of water instead. Mothers who breastfeed should also be cautioned to limit nursing to specific times so that milk will not pool in the mouth during sleep.

Parents can be taught beginning dental care for the infant, which includes wiping the teeth off daily once they erupt with a piece of moist gauze or a small infant toothbrush. Some pediatric dentists like to see the child for a first dental visit about 1 year of age, whereas others wait until the child is older. Have the parents select and establish contact with a dental provider when the child is nearing the end of infancy.

INTRODUCTION OF SUPPLEMENTAL FOODS

When should other foods be added to the infant's diet? Although some parents add other foods when the infant is only days or weeks old, it is best to take cues from the infant's developmental milestones. The AAP recommends introducing semisolid food at 4 to 6 months (Committee on Nutrition, 1998). At this age the extrusion reflex (or tongue thrust) decreases and the infant can sit well with support. The infant is also developing the ability to appreciate texture and to swallow nonliquid foods, and can indicate desire for food or turn away when full.

The first food added to the infant's diet is usually rice cereal. The advantage of introducing cereal first is that it provides iron at an age when the infant's prenatal iron stores begin to decrease, it seldom causes allergy, and is easy to digest. A tablespoon or two is fed to the infant once or twice daily just before formula- or breastfeeding. The infant may appear to spit out food at first because of normal back-and-forth tongue movement. Parents should not interpret this early feeding behavior as indicating dislike for the food. With a little practice the infant becomes adept at spoon feeding.

Once the infant eats 1/4 cup of cereal twice daily, usually at 6 to 8 months of age, vegetables or fruits can be introduced (Table 31–2). By 8 to 10 months of age, most fruits and vegetables have been introduced and strained meats or other protein (e.g., tofu) can be added to the infant's diet. Finger foods are introduced during the second half of the first year as the infant's palmar and then finger grasp develops and as teeth begin to erupt (Figure 31–3 ◆). Infants enjoy toast, O-shaped cereal, finely sliced meats, cheese and

TABLE 31–2 Introduction of Solid Foods in Infancy

Recommendation	Rationale
Introduce rice cereal at 4–6 months.	Rice cereal is easy to digest, has low allergenic potential, and contains iron.
Introduce fruits or vegetables at 6–8 months.	Fruits and vegetables provide needed vitamins.
Introduce meats at 8–10 months.	Meals are harder to digest, have high protein load, and should not be fed until close to 1 year of age.
Use single-food prepared baby foods rather than combination meals.	Combination meals usually contain more sugar, salt, and fillers.
Introduce one new food at a time, waiting at least 3 days to introduce another.	If a food allergy develops, it will be easy to identify.
Avoid carrots, beets, and spinach before 4 months of age.	Their nitrates can be converted to nitrite by young infants, causing methemoglobinemia.
Infants can be fed mashed portions of table foods such as carrots, rice, and potatoes.	This is a less expensive alternative to jars of commercially prepared baby food; it allows parents of various cultural groups to feed ethnic foods to infants.
Avoid adding sugar, salt, or spices when mixing own baby foods.	Infants need not become accustomed to these flavors; they may get too much sodium from salt or develop gastric distress from some spices.
Avoid honey until at least 1 year of age.	Infants cannot detoxify *Clostridium botulinum* spores sometimes present in honey and can develop botulism.

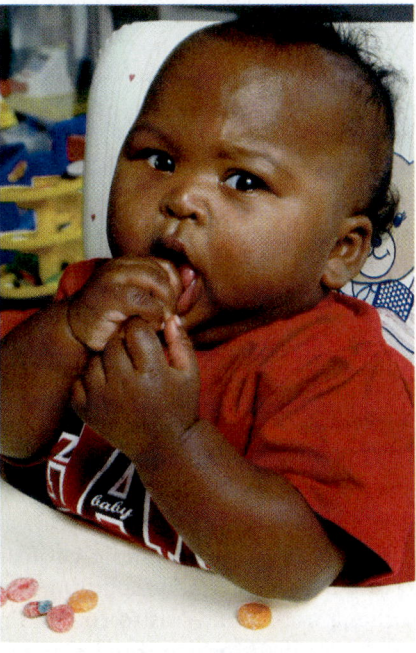

FIGURE 31–3. ◆ The baby who has developed the ability to grasp with thumb and forefinger should receive some foods that can be held in the hand.

Nursing Practice

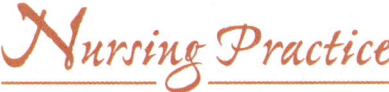

Advise parents to use caution when providing finger foods to the infant. Hard foods and some soft and malleable ones slip easily into the throat and may cause choking. Avoid hot dogs, hard vegetables, candy, and chunks of peanut butter. Infants and other young children should always be supervised while eating. Be sure parents are familiar with techniques for airway obstruction removal and have emergency numbers clearly listed on their phones.

TABLE 31–3 Infant Nutritional Pattern

Birth–1 Month
- Eats every 2–3 hours, breast or bottle
- 2–3 ounces (60–90 mL) per feeding

2–4 Months
- Has coordinated suck-swallow
- Eats every 3–4 hours
- 3–4 ounces (90–120 mL) per feeding

4–6 Months
- Begins baby food, usually rice cereal
- Eats 4 or more times daily
- 4–5 ounces (100–150 mL) per feeding

6–8 Months
- Eats baby food such as rice cereal, fruits, and vegetables
- Eats 4 times daily
- 6–8 ounces (160–225 mL) per feeding

8–10 Months
- Enjoys soft finger foods
- Eats 4 times daily
- 6 ounces (160 mL) per feeding

10–12 Months
- Eats most soft table foods with family
- Uses cup with lid
- Attempts to feed self with spoon though spills often
- Eats 4 times daily
- 6–8 ounces (160–225 mL) per feeding

tofu, and small pieces of cooked, softened vegetables. As food and juice intake increase, formula- or breastfeedings decrease in amount and frequency (Table 31–3).

If breastfeeding is not chosen, or if supplemental feedings are given, only iron-fortified infant formula should be used during the first year of life. Cow's milk (including evaporated milk) can lead to bleeding and anemia (see p. 718), can interfere with absorption of some nutrients, and has a high solute load which immature kidneys can have difficulty excreting. Iron-fortified formula should always be used when the infant under 12 months drinks formula. When breastfed babies are not eating foods with iron by 4 to 6 months, supplemental iron may need to be added. Careful dietary assessment and discussion of intake by the nurse at health visits helps the practitioner decide if supplemental iron is needed. By about 1 year of age, parents should have introduced cups with lids as a method of drinking liquids so that bottles can be slowly withdrawn and replaced by cups. Babies should only be offered cups at meal and snack times so they become accustomed to drinking when thirsty rather than carrying a bottle or cup for much of the day, in order to decrease the chance for dental caries and increased calorie intake.

Parents who want to make baby foods at home can be encouraged and instructed to do so. Some commercially prepared foods have unnecessary additives such as salt, sugar, and food starch, and they may be costly for some families. Parents can easily blend fruits and vegetables the family is eating before adding salt, sugar, or seasoning. Prepared foods should be used promptly and stored in the refrigerator between feedings. Foods can also be placed into ice cube trays and frozen; a cube or two can be defrosted at mealtime. Caution parents not to use honey in foods for infants as it can lead to infant botulism. If foods or fluids are microwaved, they should be shaken, stirred, and checked for temperature so that hot areas in the food do not burn the baby.

Toddlerhood

Why do parents of toddlers frequently become concerned about the small amount of food their children eat? Why do toddlers seem to survive and even thrive with minimal food intake? The toddler often displays the phenomenon of **physiologic anorexia,** caused when the extremely high metabolic demands of infancy slow to keep pace with the more moderate growth rate of toddlerhood. Although it can appear that the toddler eats nothing at times, intake over days or a week is generally sufficient and balanced enough to meet the body's demands for nutrients and energy.

Parents often need knowledge about types of foods that constitute a healthy diet. Some easy to prepare foods are high in salt and other additives, and can lead to exceeding the recommendation of Healthy People 2010 for sodium intake. ⌕ [WEB] Provide alternatives to hot dogs, microwave meals, or fast foods by providing information about easy preparation of sliced meats, cheese, tofu, fruits, and vegetables. Healthy snacks for young children include yogurt, cheese, milk, slices of bread with peanut butter, thinly sliced fruits, and soft vegetables.

Advise parents to offer a variety of nutritious foods several times daily (three meals and two snacks) and let the toddler make choices from the foods offered. Offer foods

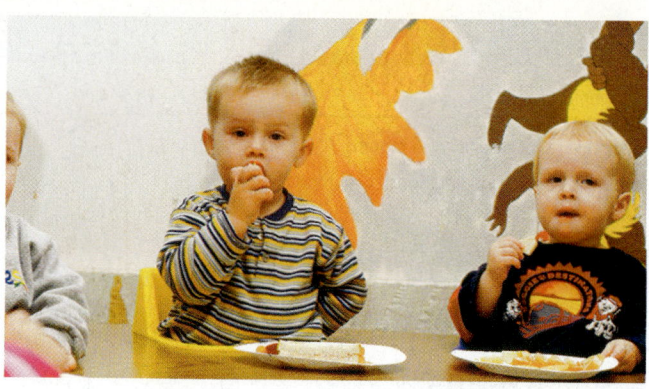

FIGURE 31–4. ◆ Toddlers should sit at a table or in a high chair to eat, to minimize chance of choking and to foster positive eating patterns.

only at mealtimes and have the child sit in a high chair or on a special seat at the table to eat (Figure 31–4 ◆). Small portions are most appealing to the toddler. A general guideline for food quantity at a meal is one tablespoon of each food per year of age. The toddler should drink 16 to 24 oz (1/2 to 3/4 L) of milk daily. Caution parents against giving the toddler more than a quart (one liter) of milk daily, since this interferes with the desire to eat other foods, leading to dietary deficiencies. Recall that the child should not be put to bed with a bottle or allowed to carry a bottle of milk or juice around during the day, due to the risk of nursing bottle mouth syndrome (see previous discussion). In addition, caution parents to limit fruit juice to 4 to 6 ounces daily for children ages 1 to 6 years to decrease the opportunity for overweight, dental caries, and abdominal discomfort (AAP Committee on Nutrition, 2001). Drinking water and eating whole fruits, which provide fiber, is a healthier alternative.

Learning how to eat with others is an important task of toddlerhood. The toddler displays characteristic autonomy or independence during mealtime. Advise parents to provide opportunities for self-feeding of food with fingers and utensils, and to allow some simple choices, such as type of liquid or cup to use. Young children should eat at a table with others, not be allowed to run and play while eating, and eat at specified meal and snack times. Because social skills are developing, the hospitalized toddler may eat better if allowed to have meals with parents or other hospitalized children. See Chapter 34 for further suggestions about management of nutrition in hospitalized children. ⌕

Growth and Development

Toddlers generally eat three meals and two to three snacks daily. Toddlers can drink 2% milk starting at 2 years of age, or "follow-up" formula. Cups are recommended with bottle use discontinued. The child is learning to use utensils but may prefer fingers and still needs small serving sizes.

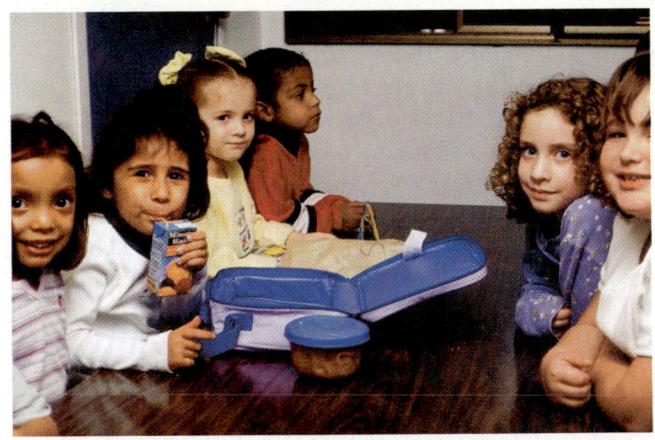

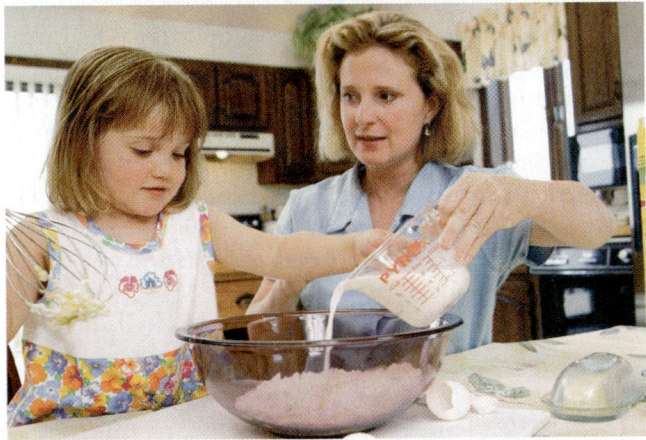

FIGURE 31–5. ◆ Preschoolers learn food habits by eating with others. Engaging them in food preparation enhances knowledge of food and promotes intake at meals.

Preschool

The diet of the preschooler is similar to that of the toddler, but mealtime is now a more social event. Preschoolers like the company of others while they eat, and they enjoy helping with food preparation and table setting (Figure 31–5 ◆). Involving them in these tasks can provide a forum for teaching about nutritious foods and principles of preparation such as the need for refrigeration, safety around stoves, and cleanliness.

Although the rate of growth is slow and steady during the preschool years, the child has periods of **food jags** (eating only a few foods for several days or weeks) and greater or lesser intake. Advise parents to assess food intake over a 1- or 2-week period rather than at each meal to obtain a more accurate impression of total intake. Food jags can be handled by providing the desired food along with other foods to foster choice. The child who chooses not to eat at snacktime or mealtime should not be given other foods in between. The child will become hungry and get accustomed to eating when food is provided. Three meals and two or three snacks daily are the norm. Limit fruit juice to 8 to 12 ounces daily.

The preschool period is a good time to continue encouraging good dental habits. Children can begin to brush their own teeth with parental supervision and help to reach all tooth surfaces. See Chapter 32 for recommended doses of fluoride when the water supply is not fluoridated. ⊂⊃ If the child has not yet visited a dentist, the first dental visit should be scheduled so the child can become accustomed to the routine of dental care.

School-Age Children

The school-age years are a period of gradual growth when energy requirements remain at a steady level, although sometime during these years, most children experience a preadolescent growth spurt. Girls may begin a growth spurt by 10 or 11 years, and boys a year or so later. Nutritional needs increase dramatically with this spurt, with large numbers of calories and increased amounts of other nutrients required. ⊂⊃ [CD]

School-age children are increasingly responsible for preparing snacks, lunches, and even some other meals. These years are a good time to teach children how to choose nutritious foods and plan a well-balanced meal. Because school-age children operate at the concrete level of cognitive thought, nutrition teaching is best presented by using pictures, samples of foods, videotapes, handouts, and hands-on experience.

School-age children often prefer the types of food eaten at home and may be resistant to new food items. A hospitalized child may refuse to eat, slowing the recuperative process. Encourage family members to bring favorite foods from home that meet nutritional requirements. This can be especially helpful when the hospital serves food only from the dominant cultural group. A child accustomed to a diet of rice, tofu, and vegetables may not enjoy a hospital meal of hamburger and fries. By school-age, food has become strongly associated with social interaction, so it is beneficial to have children eat together or to invite family members to take the child off the unit to eat or to bring in food from home and eat with the child. Many hospitals allow children to plan a pizza night or sponsor other events to encourage eating in a social atmosphere.

Most children consume at least one meal daily in school. Although children may bring lunches to school, many participate in the school lunch program, and perhaps the school breakfast program. Become familiar with the policies of school districts in your area for providing foods, snacks, and reduced price food to students in need. How will you plan for Joey to be able to participate in school lunchtime with peers? What types of soft foods are commonly available at school that he might be able to enjoy?

The loss of the first deciduous teeth and the eruption of permanent teeth usually occur at about 6 years, or at the beginning of the school-age period. Of the 32 permanent teeth, 22 to 26 erupt by age 12 years, and the remaining molars follow in the teenage years. See Chapter 33 for the typical sequence of tooth eruption. ⊂⊃ The school-age child should be closely monitored to ensure that brushing and flossing are adequate, that fluoride is taken if the water supply is not fluoridated, that dental care is obtained to provide for examination of teeth and alignment, and that loose teeth are identified before surgery or sports participation.

Adolescence

Most adolescents need well over 2000 calories daily to support the growth spurt, and some adolescent boys require nearly 3000 calories daily. When teenagers are active in a variety of sports, these requirements increase further. Because adolescents prepare much of their own food and often eat with friends, they need to be taught about good nutrition. Developing a diet that includes a large number of calories, meets vitamin and mineral requirements, and is acceptable to the teen may be a challenge. An adolescent who does not like the hospital lunch and reaches for a soft drink and chips may be receptive to juice and pizza, a more nutritious meal. View small improvements positively as they may lead to further changes.

Remember that peer group influence is important, so group sessions in which adolescents eat lunch together can provide a forum for influencing food habits. What other methods might encourage positive nutritional habits among teens?

NUTRITIONAL ASSESSMENT

What is the best indication that the child's nutrition is adequate? Which data-collection methods provide the most accurate information about a child's dietary intake? The nurse plays an important role in assessing the diets of children and in seeking additional evaluation from dietitians and nutritionists in complex situations.

Physical and Behavioral Measurement

GROWTH MEASUREMENT

A common method of evaluating the adequacy of diet is measurement of growth. **Anthropometric measurement** is the term used to refer to assessment of various parts of the body. Anthropometry of young children commonly includes weight, length, and head circumference. Standing height is substituted for length once the child can stand. Head circumference, also known as occipital-frontal circumference (OFC) is measured until about 5 years of age. Additional measurements that may be included in special circumstances include chest circumference, midupper arm circumference, and skinfold measurement at sites such as triceps, abdomen, and subscapular regions. Skills 9–1 through 9–7 in the accompanying CD-ROM and the *Clinical Skills Manual* present techniques for accurate measurement of weight, length, height, and chest and head circumference. ⊂⊃ CD SKILLS

After collecting the measurements, plot them on the appropriate standardized growth curves for weight, length to height, head circumference, and body mass index (see Figure 31–6 ◆). **Body mass index** (BMI) is a calculation based on the child's weight and height, or length, and is calculated as kilograms of weight/m^2 of height. ⊂⊃ CD This is a useful calculation for determining if the child's height and weight are in proportion. Identify on the plots which percentile the child falls in for each measurement. Children normally fall between the 10th and 90th percentiles. A measurement below the 10th percentile, especially for BMI, may indicate undernutrition, whereas one over the 90th percentile can indicate overnutrition. However, it is important to look at the differences between measurements. An infant in the 90th percentile for length, weight, and head circumference is proportional and may be a naturally large baby. On the other hand, a child who is consistently in the 10th percentile for all measurements, but is growing steadily and is at a normal development level, may simply be a small child. Much cultural and individual variation exists in size. See Appendix C and the CD-ROM for standardized growth curves by gender and age for infants, children, and adolescents. Visit our website to find out more about the growth curves. ⊂⊃ WEB CD

Developing Cultural Competence

The revised growth grids now in use were standardized using a cross section of the U.S. population and generally reflect most children. However, children from some other countries or cultures may fall outside of these curves. For example, new immigrants or adoptees may be in lower percentiles, and "catch up" over several months or years. Children of immigrants from developing countries tend to be larger than their parents. Even when small, children should follow normal growth patterns. For example, a child may remain at the 10th or 25th percentile for height, but continues to slowly grow and does not fall to a lower percentile.

Plot measurements on the same growth curve with earlier percentiles for the child. When measurements follow the same percentile over time, growth is generally normal for the child and nutrition is likely adequate. However, a sudden or sustained change in percentile may indicate a chronic disorder, emotional difficulty, or a nutritional intake problem. Further assessment of physical status and dietary intake will be needed.

ADDITIONAL PHYSICAL MEASUREMENT

Many observations from the physical assessment provide clues to nutritional status. Dietary intake can affect every body system, and a combination of certain symptoms may suggest specific nutritional problems. Some common physical manifestations of nutritional status are outlined in Table 31–4.

Weight-for-age percentiles: Boys, birth to 36 months

Age (months)

Laboratory measurements can provide useful information when nutritional status is questionable. Some common studies include hematocrit and hemoglobin, serum glucose and fasting insulin, lipids and lipoproteins, and liver and renal function studies. Adding some further measurements such as chest circumference and skinfolds (measurement of fat at certain body sites such as triceps, scapular, and abdominal areas) may also be useful (Bessler, 1999).

Dietary Intake

The mother's dietary intake during pregnancy may provide information about the child's nutritional state and it can be assessed for pertinent information. Obtain detailed

TABLE 31-4 Indicators of Nutritional Status		
Nutrient Deficiency	Body System	Clinical Manifestation
Protein & Calorie	Growth	Poor growth
	Hair	Dull, scant, loss (alopecia), changed texture, depigmented
	Skin	Depigmented, poor hydration, petechiae
	Nails	Transverse ridging
Minerals	Musculoskeletal	Muscle wasting, weakness

information about the child's dietary intake when there is a potential for nutritional deficiency due to disease, knowledge deficit, or socioeconomic status. After the information is collected, compare the dietary intake to the recommended levels for a child of that age and gender (see Figure 31–1 for Food Guide Pyramid; see the CD-ROM and appendices for Recommended Dietary Allowances [RDAs]). 🔗 CD The 24-hour recall of intake, food frequency questionnaire, and a dietary screening history (see Tables 31–5 and 31–6) provide a good overview of the infant's or child's intake and eating patterns. A food diary provides precise information about the child's food intake.

TWENTY-FOUR-HOUR RECALL OF FOOD INTAKE

The 24-hour diet recall is frequently used to assess the adequacy of the diet. People can generally remember their intake in the past day so results are fairly accurate; it is easy to gather the data and analyze results; only a few minutes are needed. Ask the parent or child to list all foods eaten during the past 24 hours (Figure 31–7 ◆). It is usually helpful to ask for a description of activities in the last day. Then start with the most recent event and move backwards, integrating food intake into the daily schedule. For example, you might begin by saying "You mentioned you got up early to come to the clinic today. What did Sam eat at home before you left? Did he have a snack as you traveled here or after you arrived?" While asking about the foods eaten, inquire specifically about:

- All meals and snacks
- Amounts of each food item consumed (have various size measuring cups, bowls, and plates so accurate amounts can be indicated)
- Types of specific foods used, such as whole milk versus nonfat or 2%, brand names of cereals, specific types of margarine or butter
- Additives used, such as condiments, table salt, spices, milk to mix formula

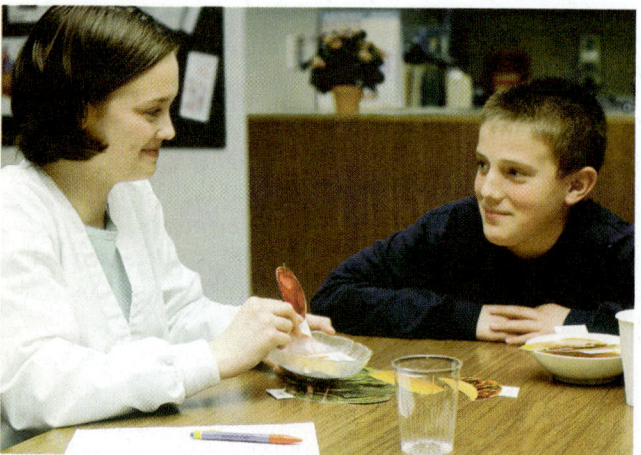

FIGURE 31–7. ◆ The nurse is interviewing a child about foods eaten in the last day. Note the models of food and dishes for accurate assessment of serving sizes.

- Food preparation methods, including adding fats to cook, removal or retention of fats on meats
- Vitamins and supplements, types and doses
- Whether the intake is typical (in situations such as illness or vacation, intake may be different than usual)

Once the 24-hour recall is obtained, analyze the intake. First, do a quick check to compare servings of various food types with the Food Guide Pyramid, as described earlier. Next, do a detailed analysis to compute calories, carbohydrate, protein, and fat intake and compare them to recommended amounts. All major vitamins and minerals are also computed and comparisons made to the DRIs. This computation may be done by hand, using a book of nutrients in common foods, or may be done on the computer. Several computer programs are available, and the federal government has a website that provides intake levels and comparisons to the RDAs. It may be useful to compute a personal 24-hour recall or that of a child in the clinical setting with the Healthy Eating Index. 🔗 WEB

FOOD FREQUENCY QUESTIONNAIRE

Food frequency questionnaires are available that can be easily administered to parents or children. Usually they ask about how often certain types of foods are eaten in a specified period such as a week. Questionnaires can be long and evaluate a total diet, or short to focus on specific items such as fruit and vegetable intake. A short questionnaire about milk intake or fruit and vegetable intake may be helpful before planning a teaching project on nutrition for a class of school-age children. Knowing their usual intake of a food item can provide helpful information for planning the project. See the website for one example of a food frequency questionnaire. 🔗 WEB

DIETARY SCREENING HISTORY

Ask the parent about the infant's or child's eating habits using questions in Tables 31–5 and 31–6. Responses provide information about the family's eating habits and food beliefs beyond that collected on a 24-hour dietary recall or food frequency questionnaire.

FOOD DIARY

Parents are asked to keep a food diary when the child has a nutrition problem or disorder, such as malnutrition, obesity, or type 1 diabetes that requires dietary management. All meals and snacks, with food preparation method and quantities eaten over a 1- to 7-day period, are recorded. Eating patterns change significantly for holidays or family gatherings, so ask parents to select typical days for the food diary or to record specific events affecting food intake. Remind parents of all the places children might have eaten, such as child care center, school, friends' houses, or neighbors. Food diaries can provide a great deal of helpful information, but take time and motivation to complete well (Lee & Nieman, 1996). Be sure instructions are complete and that the form has a place to record amounts, prepara-

TABLE 31-5 Dietary Screening History for Infants
Overview Questions
What was the infant's birth weight?
At what age did the birth weight double and triple?
Was the infant premature?
Does the infant have any feeding problems such as difficulty sucking and swallowing, spitting up, fatigue, or fussiness?
If Infant Is Breastfed
How long does the baby nurse at each breast?
What is the usual schedule for nursing?
Does the baby also take any milk or formula? Amount and frequency? What type?
If Infant Is Fed Other Foods
What formula is used? Is it iron fortified?
How is it prepared?
Do you hold or prop the bottle for feedings?
How much formula is taken at each feeding?
How many bottles are taken each day?
Does the baby take a bottle to bed for naps or nighttime? What is in the bottle?
If Infant Is Formula Fed
At what age did the baby start eating other foods?
Cereal Finger foods
Fruit/juices Meats
Vegetables Other protein sources
Do you use commercial baby food or make your own?
Does the baby eat any table foods?
How often does the baby take solid foods?
How is the baby's appetite?
Do you have any concerns about the baby's feeding habits?
Does the baby take a vitamin supplement?
Have there been any allergic reactions to foods? Which ones?
Does the baby spit up frequently?
Have there been any rashes?
What types of stools does the baby have? Frequency? Consistency?

TABLE 31-6 Dietary Screening History for Children
What foods or beverages does the child dislike?
What types of food or beverage does the child especially like?
What is the child's typical eating schedule? Meals and snacks?
Does the child eat with the family or at separate times?
Where does the child eat each meal?
Who prepares the food for the family?
What method of cooking is used? Baking? Frying? Broiling?
What ethnic foods are commonly eaten?
Does the family eat in a restaurant frequently? What type?
What type of food does the child usually order?
Is the child on a special diet?
Does the child need to be fed, feed himself or herself, need assistance eating, or need any adaptive devices for eating?
What is the child's appetite like?
Does the child take any vitamin supplements (iron, fluoride)?
Does the child have any allergies? What types of symptoms?
What types of regular exercise does the child get?
Are there any concerns about the child's eating habits?

Developing Cultural Competence

Each culture has eating practices that influence dietary intake. It is important to understand the foods commonly eaten by each cultural group and their contribution to the total nutrition of the child.

security is access at all times to enough nourishment for an active, healthy life (Federal Interagency Forum on Child and Family Statistics, 2000). In contrast, **food insecurity** indicates an inability to acquire or consume adequate quality or quantity of foods in socially acceptable ways, or the uncertainty that one will be able to do so (Boyle & Morris, 1999).

The major cause of hunger in children is poverty, and since one in five children is poor, their families may be unable to provide sustainable nutrition at all times (Children's Defense Fund, 2000). Many single-income families have a head of household moving into the workforce, so incomes are often not sufficient to provide for family food needs (see Chapter 1 for a description of Temporary Assistance for Needy Families [TANF]). Families may be ineligible for food assistance programs even though they cannot afford enough food for all their members. Children with special nutritional needs are at particular risk since it may be more costly to buy and prepare formula or foods for a child with allergies, diabetes, or an immune disorder.

Children with insufficient dietary intake are at risk for a wide array of health problems. They may become anemic; have a high rate of infectious disease due to lowered immune response; have slowed developmental maturation, delayed or stunted physical growth, and learning disorders; and be at greater risk of overweight, cardiovascular disease,

tion, events occurring, and where food was eaten. The nurse or parent may need to obtain the school lunch menu and talk with the school lunch personnel to add accurate school intake.

The nurse completes the nutritional assessment indicated for a child, and may consult with or refer the family to a dietitian or nutritionist for additional assessment and teaching.

COMMON NUTRITIONAL CONCERNS

Childhood Hunger

While most Americans live in a "land of plenty," significant numbers of children periodically experience hunger. **Food**

and diabetes in adulthood (Committee on Nutrition, 1998; Hanson, Dahlman-Hoglund, Lundin, et al., 1997; Walter, Olivares, Pizarro, et al., 1997). Subsequently, the national and individual cost of childhood hunger is great.

Nurses are well positioned to evaluate families for food insecurity in a variety of hospital, clinic, school, and home settings. In addition to the assessment of the individual child's nutritional status, further questions can determine families with potential problems. Administer the screening tool to identify risk in families (Table 31–7). Most parents

TABLE 31-7   Food Insecurity Screening

1. Does your household ever run out of money to buy food to make a meal?
2. Do you or members of your household ever eat less than you feel you should because there is not enough money for food?
3. Do you or members of your household ever cut the size of meals or skip meals because there is not enough money for food?
4. Do your children ever eat less than you feel they should because there is not enough money for food?
5. Do you ever cut the size of your children's meals or do they skip meals because there is not enough money for food?
6. Do your children ever say they are hungry because there is not enough food in the house?
7. Do you ever rely on a limited number of foods to feed your children because you are running out of money to buy foods for a meal?
8. Do any of your children ever go to bed hungry because there is not enough money to buy food?

Scoring: 5–8 yes responses = hungry; 1–4 yes responses = risk of hunger. From Washington State Department of Health.

go without food themselves in order to feed their children, so food insecurity may not have directly impacted all children. However, anxiety over providing food can be very stressful for families and diet quality deteriorates as insecurity increases. If families have experienced food insecurity or may be likely to at some time, be sure to provide them with access to community agencies and programs that can help. What resources are available locally to help families with food insecurity?

Overweight and Obesity

After several decades of similar statistics regarding overweight in children, the numbers are now skyrocketing. The current incidence of overweight in the United States has been called an epidemic and is associated with a wide array of health problems, such as the appearance of type 2 diabetes in youth (Troiano & Flegal, 1998). See Chapter 51 for a discussion of diabetes. ◯▭ Overweight can also influence self-image, dietary quality, and amount of physical activity. The Third National Health and Nutrition Examination Survey has found that 11% to 15% of various child and adolescent groups are now overweight (*Healthy People 2010,* 2000). When using the 85th percentile of BMI as indicator of overweight, from 22% to 33% of youth are affected (Troiano, Flegal, Kuczmarski, et al., 1995). Since overweight in childhood and adolescence frequently tracks into adulthood, the implications for health care are obvious.

Many reasons are cited for the increase in overweight children. The number of calories consumed is not increasing. However, children tend to exercise less, particularly in daily life. They infrequently walk or ride bikes, either be-

Teaching About

COMMUNITY RESOURCES FOR FOOD

Food Stamp Program—Eligibility based on household size and income; refer students and those with low incomes, especially when they have young children; education services often available

Child Nutrition Programs—School lunch, breakfast, and milk programs; free and lowered cost meals in schools; assist parents to apply

Special Child Programs—Summer programs, Head Start, child care centers and homeless children programs may provide nutritional support in some communities

Women, Infants, and Children (WIC)—Supplemental foods and nutrition education to pregnant, breastfeeding, and postpartum women and to their young children; assessment of child growth often included

Nutrition Education and Training Program—Nutrition education for teachers and school food service personnel

Community Services—May include food banks, field gleaning, and other programs

Find out what services are available to provide food and nutrition education in your community. Make a list to use in clinical settings with families.

Growth and Development

When a child has one obese parent, chances of the child being overweight are increased. In families with two overweight parents, the incidence of obesity in children increases even more. Finally, the child who has obese parents and is overweight as an adolescent is at very high risk of becoming an obese adult (Whitaker, Wright, Pepe, et al., 1997). Be alert for families with overweight adults and begin prevention early with the children in these families.

Developing Cultural Competence

Overweight is more common among some ethnic and socioeconomic groups. Lack of knowledge about foods and physical activity, limited access to fresh produce and safe places to exercise, and easy access to increasing numbers of fast foods may all constitute risk factors. Lower income, and Hispanic, black, or Native-American ethnic identity are all associated with higher incidence of overweight, especially among women. National goals to eliminate health disparities in income and ethnic groups have been set (*Healthy People 2010,* 2000).

cause of the convenience of driving or due to unsafe neighborhoods. Television viewing is very high among youth and contributes to overweight both from the inactivity associated with it and the pattern of snacking during commercial time. As many as 60% of obese children view excessive television, defined as more than 5 hours daily (Gortmaker, Must, Sobol, et al., 1996). In addition, children may spend time with computer activities and playing video games.

The percentage of calories from fat consumed in the United States is among the highest in the world. Although no more than 30% of calories should come from total dietary fat, and no more than 10% from saturated fat, about 35% of calories consumed in the United States are supplied by fat and 12% by saturated fat (National Cholesterol Education Program, 1991; Krauss, Eckel, Howard, et al., 2001). High levels of dietary fat are associated with higher cholesterol levels and decreased activity. The high rate of dietary fat is related to the large amount of fast food consumed, as fast-food restaurants are convenient and fit well into today's lifestyles. Another factor that contributes to overweight is a pattern of snacking, and there has been an increase in this activity in the last decade. Snacks are often nutrient-poor and calorie-dense (Zizza, Siega-Riz, & Popkin, 2001).

Nurses can help parents and children build good nutritional and exercise habits throughout life, thus decreasing the incidence of overweight and its attendant health risks. Begin with an assessment of growth patterns starting early in life. Address patterns of eating fast foods, meals on the run, and while watching television in early health maintenance visits. Caution parents that television viewing should be limited to a maximum of 2 hours daily, and that television and video games should not be placed in children's bedrooms. Daily exercise routines of at least 30 minutes can be included in most families. Also, teach about the Food Guide Pyramid and its integration into a healthy life. Healthy snacks include fruits, vegetables, grains, and nuts. "Super sizing" fast foods and eating out often should be avoided.

Risks for poor health often cluster together in individuals and families, so be alert for situations in which parents are overweight, and children have elevated blood pressure, exercise infrequently, or are in upper percentiles for weight, BMI, or skinfold. Girls who have menarche before 11 years of age are more often overweight. Being alert for early menarche can help identify overweight girls who need intervention for obesity prevention (Adair & Gordon-Larsen, 2001). Presence of risk factors necessitates further dietary and risk assessment so that a management plan can be implemented. Visit our website for information [WEB] that will be helpful to families in your clinical setting. See resources such as "Helping your overweight child" and "Take charge of your health: a teenager's guide to better health."

Food Safety

Every year in the United States, about 76 million people contract foodborne illnesses. Some are quite mild, while others can be very severe. Children are at greater risk of severe illness and death from food and water due to their immature gastrointestinal and immune systems. The most common pathogens are *Campylobacter, Salmonella, Shigella,* and *Escherichia coli;* infants are at extremely high risk of *Campylobacter, Rotavirus,* and *Salmonella* illness (Morbidity and Mortality Weekly Report [MMWR], 2001a). A former common cause of food-related illness was hepatitis A. Although hepatitis A is still prevalent in some parts of the country, effective management and prevention through immunization has decreased its incidence (see Chapter 46). Worldwide, over 3 million people die of illness related to unsafe drinking water each year, and most of those deaths are among children.

Foodborne illness is relayed by food preparation and storage practices, lack of adequate training of retail employees about foods and hygiene, and increasing amounts and types of foods being imported from other countries. Health personnel should integrate teaching regularly so that families can decrease risks of foodborne illness.

Teaching About

FOODBORNE SAFETY GUIDELINES

Four Key Food Safety Practices:

1. *Clean:* Wash hands and surfaces often.
2. *Separate:* Don't cross-contaminate.
3. *Cook:* Cook to proper temperatures.
4. *Chill:* Refrigerate promptly.

(*Healthy People 2010,* 2000)

Common Dietary Deficiencies

Although children can have deficits in nearly any nutrient, a number of nutrient deficits are more common in childhood. Either limitations in the food supply or patterns of dietary intake cause most deficiencies, and children with certain disease processes, such as metabolic diseases, may have difficulty absorbing or using nutrients ingested (see Chapter 51 for a discussion of inborn errors of metabolism). The nutrient deficiencies of a population are a result of genetic factors and characteristics of the food supply and intake patterns of particular groups.

Developing Cultural Competence

Vitamin A deficiency is common in developing countries. The vitamin is found in liver, dairy products, and fish. Provitamin A sources are yellow and dark green vegetables. The vitamin is fat soluble and stored in the liver. When deficient, children develop night blindness, vision loss, and high rates of infection. Public health efforts have been directed at identifying children with low vitamin A status and providing the vitamin in capsule form or in commonly ingested foods.

IRON

Newborns have a store of iron obtained from their mothers in the uterus, if the maternal nutritional state was satisfactory and the baby is normal gestational age. Breast milk contains little iron but the iron it does contain has high bioavailability. However, by 4 to 6 months of age, the baby's iron stores begin to decrease and a dietary source of iron must be added. Enriched rice cereal is commonly used to meet these initial iron needs. In babies who do not have adequate stores or do not take in enough iron, **anemia,** or a reduction in the number of red blood cells, can result (Figure 31–8 ◆). Feeding cow milk during infancy can also cause anemia by irritating the gut and leading to small but consistent loss of blood from the gastrointestinal tract. When formulas are used, they should be iron fortified to help avoid iron-deficiency anemia.

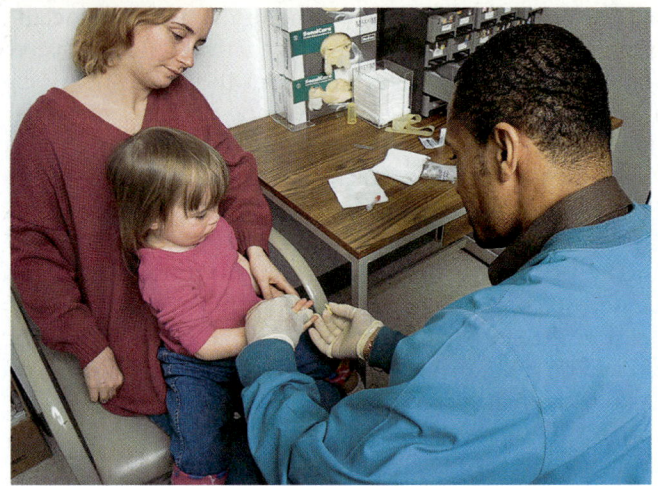

FIGURE 31–8. ◆ Most Head Start centers participate in screening programs to identify children at risk for anemia.

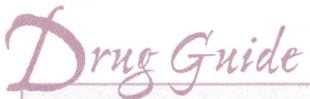

IRON

Overview of Action

Iron is a necessary component of hemoglobin and is therefore essential in the oxygen transfer carried out by red blood cells. It is used in microcytic and hypochromic anemia, which result from iron deficiency. Supplements are frequently used during pregnancy when intake does not meet iron needs, and in infants with decreased iron stores, such as with small-for-gestational-age and premature infants.

Route, Dosage, Frequency

Ferrous Fumarate: 3 mg/kg/day po

Ferrous Gluconate: 8 mg/kg/day po—over 2 years

Ferrous Sulfate: 5 mg/kg/day po

Ferrous Sulfate Dried: 160 mg/day po

Iron Dextran: up to 25 mg/day (under 5 kg weight); up to 50 mg/day (5–10 kg weight); up to 100 mg/day (over 10 kg)—IM, IV

RDAs for Iron

7–12 months: 11 mg

1–3 yr: 7 mg

4–8 yr: 10 mg

9–13 yr: males 8 mg; females 11 mg

14–18 yr: males 8 mg; females 15 mg

Pregnancy: 27 mg

Lactation: 9–10 mg

Nursing Considerations

Administer PO: The mg doses of various forms of iron are not equivalent; rather, the amount of elemental iron in various preparations is important.

Giving with a snack decreases absorption but is often recommended, as GI irritation will be lessened. Accompanying with vitamin C may enhance iron absorption.

Liquid preparations should be given with fluid, such as juice, and by a dropper or straw because they can stain teeth. **IM:** Do not mix with other medications. It is given to the upper outer buttock; therefore, this form is used only in older children. Change needle after drawing up iron. Use long needle and **Z-track** injection technique. Permanent tissue staining can occur if not deep IM. Aspirate after inserting needle and inject slowly. **IV:** Given undiluted. Do not mix with other medications (known to be incompatible with some other medicines) and do not use the multidose bottle (latter only for IM injection). Give at rate slower than 1 mL/minute. Test dose of 25 mg or less given over 5 minutes. If no reaction, remaining dose can be given over 1 to 6 hours. Flush vein after infusion with normal saline.

Assess: Obtain a diet history. Be alert for elements that can decrease iron absorption, such as low-calcium or high-phosphate diet, infection, or decreased GI acid. Watch for signs of deficiency in infants after 4 to 6 months of age when maternal iron stores are depleted (earlier in premature infants). A CBC, including hematocrit, hemoglobin, and reticulocytes, is done to establish iron-deficiency anemia. Before administering parenteral iron, a test dose of 0.5 mL is given.

Monitor: Epinephrine 1:1000 available for parenteral administration. Watch for hypersensitivity. Hemoglobin, hematocrit, other lab studies regularly.

Teaching: Take oral preparation between meals unless GI distress occurs. Teach food sources of iron. Take liquid forms with straw and water to decrease chance of teeth staining. Dairy products, eggs, whole grains, tea, and coffee decrease iron absorption.

Note: From Bindler, R. M., & Howry, L. B. (1997). *Pediatric drugs and nursing implications* (2nd ed.). Upper Saddle River, NJ: Prentice Hall-Health. Adapted.

The other group most commonly deficient in iron is adolescent females, related to loss of blood in menses, metabolic need of the growth spurt, and poor dietary balance due to sporadic dieting. Further discussion of the symptoms and treatment of iron-deficiency anemia can be found in Chapter 44. ⚭ Encourage intake of good iron sources such as meats, eggs, dried fruits, iron-fortified cereal, and iron-fortified baby cereal for infants.

CALCIUM

Calcium is an essential nutrient for bone development during childhood and adolescence. An increased intake of soda pop and fruit juices is related to a decrease in calcium intake, especially among adolescents. During the adolescent growth spurt, almost 40% of the adult bone mass is accumulated (Trahms & Pipes, 1997). Inadequate intake puts the person at risk for osteoporosis later in life since it is not possible to make up for earlier deficits. Although genetic variables account for some of the influence on adult bone mass, increasing calcium intake has been shown to promote bone formation. While the recommended daily intake for adolescents is 1500 mg, the average intake for adolescent males is 1169 mg and for females is only 753 mg (only one half the recommended level) (Food & Nutrition Board, 2001). Encourage foods such as milk and milk products, egg yolks, grains, legumes, nuts, and fruit juice with added calcium.

Adolescents at highest risk for impaired bone development include female athletes and others who diet to a great degree to maintain slimness. Teens who exercise excessively may manifest the "female athlete triad" of excessive thinness, excessive exercise, and amenorrhea. A high rate of fractures and osteomalacia can result, in addition to an extreme risk of osteoporosis in adulthood. Asking about menstrual patterns as well as exercise and diet can be combined with physical measurements of height and weight to obtain pertinent information about the teen athlete. See Chapter 36 for a discussion of the eating disorders anorexia nervosa and bulimia nervosa. ⚭

VITAMIN D

Vitamin D deficiencies are rare since the vitamin can be synthesized in the skin upon exposure to sunlight. However, an increase in cases of vitamin D–deficient rickets has recently been observed. This vitamin is needed to enhance absorption of calcium, so a lack of vitamin D can contribute to calcium deficiency as well. Human milk contains little vitamin D, and if infants are kept wrapped when outside, live in northern climates and rarely get outside in winter months, have extensive sunscreens applied, or are dark in skin color, vitamin D deficiency can result. This has led to a recommendation by the AAP that all breastfed infants receive a 400 IU supplement of vitamin D. Formula-fed babies receive adequate amounts in commercial formulas.

Vitamin D rickets had virtually disappeared from the United States, but several cases have recently been identified. Suggested reasons for the resurgence include failure to provide vitamin D supplementation when breastfeeding is the sole source of intake for over 6 months, use of nonfortified products such as soy milk, and use of sunscreens or covers when infants are outside. Be alert for infants and toddlers with neurologic conditions such as seizures, low height for age, slowness in learning to walk, and malformations (bowing) of spine, legs, and arms. Encourage sunscreen use, but be aware that children who are dark skinned or are kept covered due to religious beliefs may be at higher risk. Be certain that breastfed babies receive vitamin D supplements until other vitamin D sources are added to the diet (MMWR, 2001b).

FOLIC ACID

Epidemiologic evidence has linked increasing maternal folic acid (folate) intake with decreased incidence of neural tube defects such as spina bifida in offspring. More recently, cleft lip and palate incidence has also been found to decrease when folate intake increases, and research is examining the role of folate and B vitamins in prevention of depression. Folate levels are low among adolescents, putting them at particular risk of birth defects when they have babies. The Food and Drug Administration approved fortification of cereals and breads with folate to decrease the population risk of related congenital anomalies. Other good sources of folate include spinach, avocado, green leafy vegetables, beans and peas, liver, and many fruits.

Feeding Disorder of Infancy and Early Childhood (Failure to Thrive)

Feeding disorder of infancy and early childhood, or failure to thrive (FTT), describes a syndrome in which infants or young children fail to eat enough food to be adequately nourished. This disorder accounts for 1% to 5% of pediatric hospitalizations in children under 1 year of age, and many more children are managed in community settings (Maggioni & Lifchitz, 1995).

ETIOLOGY AND PATHOPHYSIOLOGY

The cause of FTT can be organic, as in congenital acquired immunodeficiency (AIDS) (see Chapter 40), inborn errors of metabolism (see Chapter 51), congenital heart defect (see Chapter 43), neurologic disease (see Chapter 49), and esophageal reflux (see Chapter 46). ⚭ However, most cases of FTT are nonorganic in origin. FTT resulting from nonorganic causes is called feeding disorder of infancy or early childhood.

Infants and children whose parents or caretakers suffer from depression, substance abuse, mental retardation, or psychosis are at risk for this disorder. Parents may be socially and emotionally isolated, or may lack knowledge of infant nutritional and nurturing needs. A reciprocal interaction pattern may exist in which the parent does not offer enough food or is not responsive to the infant's hunger cues, and the infant is irritable, not soothed, and does not give clear cues about hunger (Corrales & Utter, 1999).

CLINICAL MANIFESTATIONS

The characteristics of this feeding disorder are persistent failure to eat adequately with no weight gain or with weight loss in a child under 6 years of age, which is not associated with other medical conditions or mental disorders, and is not caused by lack of or unavailability of food (American Psychiatric Association, 2000). Infants with feeding disorder refuse food, may have erratic sleep patterns, are irritable and difficult to soothe, and are often developmentally delayed (see Figure 31–9 ◆).

CLINICAL THERAPY

A thorough history and physical examination are needed to rule out any chronic physical illness. The infant or child may be hospitalized so that health care providers can establish a routine for feeding and sleeping. The goals of treatment are to provide adequate caloric and nutritional intake, promote normal growth and development, and assist parents in developing feeding routines and responding to the infant's cues of physical and psychologic hunger.

Developing Cultural Competence

Each child should maintain a height and weight growth pattern similar to the population standard. Asian-American children may normally be below the fifth percentile on growth charts and not have eating disorder. Suspect an eating disorder when the infant or child falls one standard deviation below his or her own curve and either fails to gain weight or loses weight over several months.

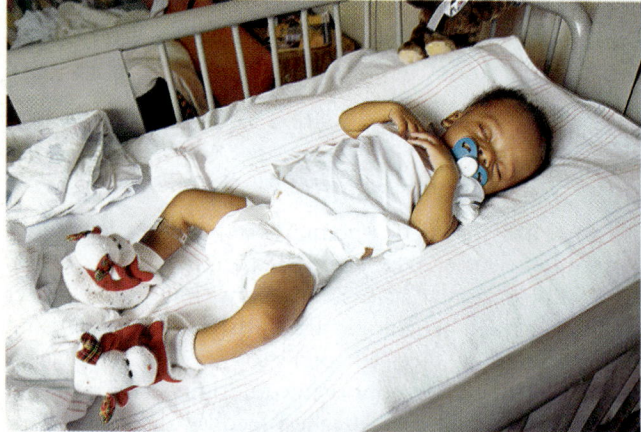

FIGURE 31–9. ◆ Infants with failure to thrive may not look severely malnourished, but they fall well below the expected weight and height norms for their age. This infant, who appears to be about 4 months old, is actually 8 months old. He has been hospitalized for evaluation of failure to thrive.

Nursing Management

Nursing Assessment and Diagnosis

Nursing assessment of the child is essential for establishing the best intervention plan. Accurate weight and height each time any child is seen for health care provides an important record of growth patterns over time. This helps identify the child with an eating disorder. The child's activity level, developmental milestones, and interaction patterns provide important information. When feeding the child, observe how the child indicates hunger or satiety, the ability of the child to be soothed, and general interaction patterns such as eye contact, touch, and "cuddliness."

Ask parents about stresses in their lives; these may prevent appropriate interaction with the child. Asking about the pregnancy and delivery can elicit information about early disturbances in the child-parent relationship. Are there other children in the family and have eating problems occurred with them? Observe the child and parent behaviors while they feed the child; cues given by each person, and interactional modes such as rocking, singing, talking, and body postures are important.

The several nursing diagnoses pertinent for the young child with an eating disorder include:

▶ *Altered nutrition:* less than body requirements related to inability to ingest proper amounts of food

▶ *Altered growth and development* related to inadequate intake

▶ *Altered parenting* related to lack of knowledge about nutritional needs

▶ *Fatigue* related to malnutrition

Planning and Implementation

Nursing care centers on performing a thorough history and physical assessment, observing parent-child interactions during feeding times, and providing necessary teaching to enable parents to respond appropriately to their child's needs. The child is often hospitalized initially and evaluated for physical growth while staff members feed the child. Accurate weights, nutritional assessments, and developmental evaluation should be done to see if the child grows more normally. Additional diagnostic tests may be carried out at this time to rule out organic causes of the poor growth.

Once a diagnosis of nonorganic failure to thrive is confirmed, parents become involved in feeding the child. Observations of feeding and continued careful physical assessments are needed. Carefully record the child's intake at each meal or feeding. Teach parents how to understand and respond to the child's cues of hunger and satiety. Teach them to hold, rock, and touch the infant during feedings, and to establish eye contact with infants and older children.

Upon discharge, referral to an agency that can continue monitoring of the home situation is needed. This provides an opportunity to observe feeding during a home visit and evaluate stresses and behavior patterns among family members. Frequent growth measurement and development must be ensured so the child is adequately nourished. Parents may need referral to community resources to help them manage stressful situations in their lives and to enhance their parenting skills.

Evaluation

Expected outcomes of nursing care include:

▶ Adequate growth and normal development of the infant is achieved.

▶ An improved parent-child relationship is established.

Food Reactions

Food reaction encompasses any adverse reaction to foods or substances ingested in foods. The foods that most commonly cause a reaction are fish, shellfish, nuts, eggs, soy, wheat, corn, strawberries, and cow milk products. Chemical additives, antibiotics, preservatives, and food colorings also can cause food sensitivity reactions.

Allergic reactions are a common cause of food reaction. These IgE-mediated reactions are potentially systemic and characteristically rapid in onset. They may manifest as swelling of the lips, mouth, uvula, or glottis; generalized urticaria; and, in severe reactions, anaphylaxis. Food allergies are the most common cause of anaphylaxis and are more prevalent in children with a family history of allergic reactions to various substances and foods **(atopy).** Children with allergies may experience urticaria of the lips, mouth, and throat when they eat certain foods (Pongracic, 2000). Allergic individuals need to be aware of "hidden" substances in prepared foods. For example, the child allergic to nuts will experience a reaction to a food if nut extracts are used in its preparation.

Delayed hypersensitivity reactions are attributed to digestive products of food and require a thorough diet history over several days to identify the offending food. These reactions are more difficult to diagnose, since the reaction can occur up to 24 hours after ingestion of the food. There may also be biphasic reactions that occur 1 to 30 hours after an initial anaphylaxis. Such reactions can be severe and life threatening.

Food intolerance refers to an abnormal physiologic response to a food and is not IgE-mediated. Examples might include indigestion or flatulence upon eating certain foods, or a sweating reaction to some spices (Burks, 2000).

Cow milk may cause an allergy or food intolerance. In allergy, an IgE-mediated systemic reaction occurs. In intolerance, there is a gastrointestinal response to milk proteins (diarrhea, vomiting, abdominal pain) as a result of lack of the enzyme lactase in the gastrointestinal tract. Infants have difficulty absorbing cow milk and when ingesting it, may have vomiting and watery, blood-streaked, mucoid diarrhea. Even without such overt signs, they may have anemia induced by blood loss not noted by care providers.

Diagnostic tests to identify suspected food allergies include measurement of serum IgE levels, scratch tests, and the **radioallergosorbent test (RAST),** in which radioimmunoassay measures IgE antibodies to specific allergens (see Chapter 40). A diet diary is kept, noting date, type of foods eaten, and reaction, if any. Foods should be eaten singly for several days to determine whether they cause a reaction.

Treatment consists of eliminating the offending foods from the child's diet. Some families will choose to try naturopathic or other treatment modalities.

NURSING MANAGEMENT

Prevention is the first step. Instruct parents of infants to introduce new foods at a rate of not more than one new food every 3 to 5 days. If a sensitivity is noted, the causative food can be easily identified. Discuss any changes in diet or preparation of formula. Reassure parents that the child's symptoms will disappear when the offending foods are removed from the diet.

Be alert for skin, respiratory, and other characteristic manifestations of sensitivity or allergy. Many nurses are involved in administering and measuring skin prick tests for possible allergies.

Nursing care of a child with food allergies is primarily supportive. Help the family identify the offending foods. Explain to parents all tests, use of a food diary, and care of the child should a reaction occur. The child and school may need an EpiPen or other fast treatment for the allergic child. Emphasize the importance of reading food labels for hidden foods that can trigger an allergic reaction (Bock, Munoz-Furlong, & Sampson, 2001). The child with a true food allergy should wear a medical alert bracelet. Be sure that school personnel know about the allergy and know to avoid giving the child the food product. Refer the family to the Food Allergy Network. ⊂‒⊃ **WEB** Recognize that food allergies can be life threatening and plan carefully with the family, child care facilities, schools, and other community contacts to ensure avoidance of food and fast treatment if needed.

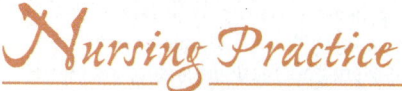

Nursing Practice

Children with food allergies should wear an alert bracelet and carry an emergency medication such as EpiPen. Nurses in schools and offices must instruct families, schoolteachers, and others about the child's allergy and what to do in case of accidental ingestion of the food product.

NUTRITIONAL SUPPORT

Sports Nutrition

Encourage regular physical activity for all children, with at least 30 minutes of activity recommended daily. However, during vigorous or prolonged exercise, or during hot weather, child and adolescent athletes may have special nutritional needs. A well-balanced diet, reflective of the Food Pyramid, is needed. A wide variety of fresh fruits and vegetables, grains, and complex carbohydrates usually provides for adequate caloric intake. When the child is hungry, extra calories should come from the food groups listed here, rather than from increased intake of fat. When the child or teen is very active, sports bars or drinks can provide the additional needed calories in a nutritionally balanced manner. As always, the height, weight, and BMI percentiles are the best assurance that the child is growing adequately over time. Adequate energy to perform the sport as well as be attentive and productive at school and for other activities should also be considered.

Water should be increased during activity both to minimize chance of dehydration and also to maximize performance. About 1 hour before vigorous exercise the child should drink 1 to 2 glasses (8 to 16 ounces) of water, and

should repeat the same amount of fluid just before the exercise begins. Young children may not feel thirsty, and should be encouraged to drink 4 to 6 ounces of fluid every 15 minutes during exercise (Trahms & Pipes, 1997). Water is usually the best replacement, but during extended exercise, sports drinks may be a good alternative for some of the fluid intake. More water is needed after activity. Weight loss of 1 pound indicates a loss of about 1/2 quart of fluid. Be sure the child takes in fluid to replace all losses.

Some common nutrients that may be deficient in all teens, but even more often in the athlete, are calcium and iron. The increased blood volume common in the well-conditioned person necessitates greater intake. Calcium-rich foods such as milk products and dark green vegetables, and iron-rich foods such as meats and grains can guard against deficiencies. Although many adolescents believe that they need extra protein during athletic season, most Americans eat adequate protein to meet even the increased needs of sports. On the other hand, the vegetarian child or adolescent may need help to plan a diet with adequate protein.

Many teens take a wide variety of dietary supplements, believing that they enhance performance during sports. Most of the claims of these products are unproven, and their safety has not usually been investigated, especially in the young. Offer guidance and help the family and teen investigate claims before choosing to use a product. Be sure they know doses, desired effects, and potential side effects of supplements. Be aware that some sports and coaches may encourage small size and dieting. Children and adolescents in activities such as ballet, wrestling, track or running, and horse racing may have health risks associated with inconsistent or poor intake.

Some common amino acid nutritional supplements include creatine, carnitine, and glutamine. Although side effects to these substances are minimal, their possible enhancement of performance is temporary and outcomes of long-term use are unknown. Increasing protein intake to meet needs during high activity is a better alternative. Creatine has been studied more than most supplements; it is made by the body and is present in many protein sources. Supplemental creatine increases the creatine level in muscle and may help to increase performance in short bursts of activity, while not affecting endurance sports. The increase in muscle mass that can occur is actually due to water and is lost quickly when the supplement is discontinued (Johnson, 2001). Some athletes obtain steroids, which can cause serious side effects and can lead to endocrine disturbance and interfere with growth; their use is also illegal in sports. Minerals such as chromium, iron, and calcium are used by some youths. Ask careful and sensitive questions such as "Many athletes take supplements to aid in performance in sports. What supplements do you take or are you considering?" Then provide information to enhance the youth's understanding of nutrition and sports performance. Generally, a balanced diet with adequate carbohydrate, protein, and fat will meet the needs of most athletes and lead to maximal sport performance.

Complementary Care

USE OF DIETARY SUPPLEMENTS IN CHILDREN

The use of complementary and alternative therapies has continued to increase over the last 10 years and this includes the use of dietary supplements in children. Dietary supplements—which include herbs or botanicals, vitamins, minerals, and homeopathic remedies—have been promoted to improve health and prevent illness. Dietary supplements come in many forms and are marketed as capsules, tablets, tinctures, extracts, and tea. Many parents have learned about the use of dietary supplements from magazine and newspaper articles that often claim cures for common childhood conditions. There have been few well-controlled studies using dietary supplements in children. There are some dietary supplements—specifically, herbs—that are considered safe and effective for children and adolescents, such as echinacea (see page 1017 in Chapter 41) and chamomile (see page 1188 in Chapter 46).

Although dietary supplements and pharmaceuticals have similarities such as similar appearance (pills, etc.) and biochemical remedies; they have significant differences as well. Dietary supplements do not have similar regulation in regard to processing, purity, and potency, as does the pharmaceutical industry.

Since dietary supplements are not controlled well for quality or purity, the health care provider is the best advisor to parents and adolescents as to which products to use. Though advertised as "natural," dietary supplements are not always safe to use and may have druglike effects. Parents and children should be urged to use caution if a product claims to be a "miracle cure," and to treat multiple different conditions. Nurses can seek out information on specific dietary substances to help parents and children make informed choices about use.

Health-Related Conditions

Many health conditions influence the child's nutritional state. Conversely, the child's nutritional state can influence the state of health. See "Pathophysiology Illustrated" for examples of some common conditions that influence nutritional needs. These conditions are discussed in various chapters throughout the text. When reading about them, discuss with classmates how to adjust normal nutritional assessment and teaching due to the presence of a health care concern. Which conditions influence absorption of nutrients? Which cause changes in nutritional intake requirements? Some children benefit from special dietary aids, such as eating utensils and cups that are easy to grasp. Therapists can evaluate and make recommendations about devices that can assist the child at meals.

Vegetarianism

Some families choose to eat vegetarian diets and can be helped and encouraged in their endeavors. Several variations in intake occur. **Vegetarians** eat no poultry, meat, or fish. Lacto-ovovegetarians eat eggs and dairy products; lacto-vegetarians eat dairy products. In contrast, **vegans** are strict vegetarians and eat no animal products. When

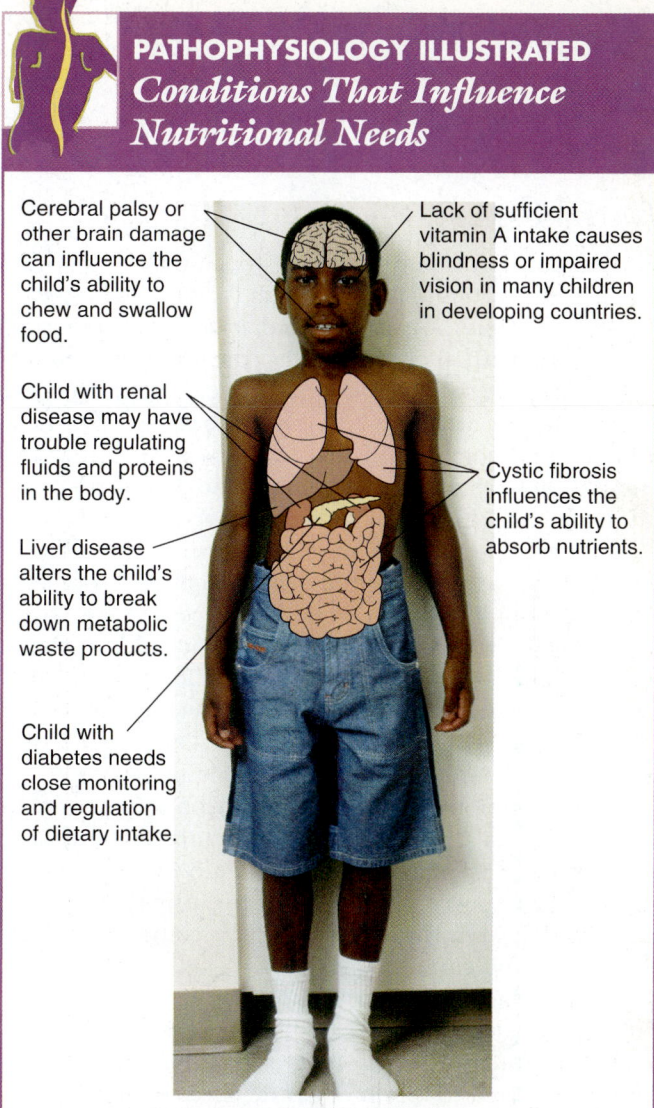

PATHOPHYSIOLOGY ILLUSTRATED
Conditions That Influence Nutritional Needs

Cerebral palsy or other brain damage can influence the child's ability to chew and swallow food.

Child with renal disease may have trouble regulating fluids and proteins in the body.

Liver disease alters the child's ability to break down metabolic waste products.

Child with diabetes needs close monitoring and regulation of dietary intake.

Lack of sufficient vitamin A intake causes blindness or impaired vision in many children in developing countries.

Cystic fibrosis influences the child's ability to absorb nutrients.

Growth and Development

When a pregnant teen follows a vegetarian diet, she needs additional help to encourage adequate nutrition (Rudys-Shapard, 2001). A 24-hour or 2-day diet record helps identify nutritional needs. Consider additional pregnancy needs for protein, iron, and calcium, and note that Vitamin B_{12} is recommended as a supplement. Use the vegetarian Food Guide Pyramid available through the American Dietetic Association. WEB

someone says they are vegetarian, it is best to ask specific questions about what they will and will not eat.

The vegetarian can be very healthy, but may need some additional help to ensure nutritional adequacy. Some common deficiencies include vitamins D and B_{12}, zinc, iron, calories, protein, and fat. Completing a 24-hour diet recall for the pregnant or lactating woman, and for vegetarian children, with analysis for RDAs, can be helpful. Be sure to routinely assess growth and other nutritional measures as well. Provide ideas of various foods to meet nutritional needs and perform other general nutritional teaching. When a vegetarian child is hospitalized, plan with the nutrition department and the child's family to meet intake needs.

Enteral Therapy

Enteral nutrition is a form of nutritional support provided when a child cannot take in enough food orally to sustain health. Since it is the closest form of nutritional support to the natural method of eating, it has the least untoward effects and greatest rate of success. Some children who use enteral therapy are those with cerebral palsy or other neurologic conditions that lead to weakness of the throat and mouth, those with neoplasm or immune dysfunction, and those in acute states of recovery from accidents or illness (see Figure 31–10 ◆). Although a tube can be inserted into the nasal opening and placed through the esophagus into the stomach, a tube surgically placed into the stomach through an abdominal opening, a jejunal or gastric tube, is preferred for long-term use. As long as the child can absorb and use nutrients, enteral therapy can be successful in providing calories and essential nutrients. Commercially prepared formulas are available and specially formulated solutions can be adapted for children with specific dietary needs. The tube and entry site are cared for to prevent infection and skin breakdown. See Chapter 46 for suggestions on management of nursing care during tube feedings plus Skill 15–3 in the accompanying CD-ROM, and the *Clinical Skills Manual*. CD SKILLS

Some of the concerns with enteral feedings relate to the inability to adequately develop hunger/satiety cues in the child, the potential for infection or skin breakdown at the tube site related to action of gastric juice and feedings on the skin, and the need for ongoing care several times daily. Ideally, enteral feedings are temporary and children can begin to take in more foods orally as they grow and develop.

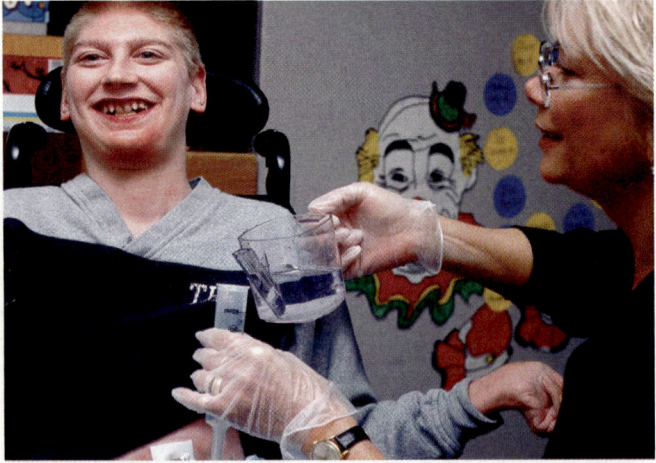

FIGURE 31–10. ◆ This child has returned to school following surgery. Due to cerebral palsy he has difficulty chewing and swallowing food. The school nurse has taught his teacher to safely administer some enteral feedings during school hours.

Total Parenteral Nutrition (TPN)

Parenteral nutrition makes it possible to provide intravenous nutritional support for people who cannot eat or are unable to absorb nutrients from the intestinal tract in a normal manner and are at risk of severe malnutrition (Matarese & Gottschlich, 1998). Examples of children who benefit from this method of nutrition are those with congenital malformation of the gastrointestinal tract, head injury, or severe burns; it may also be used for support after bone marrow transplant, sepsis, or other critical conditions. A catheter is inserted so that a sterile nutrition solution is infused directly into the bloodstream. A central venous catheter is used to promote safe infusion. Fluids usually contain glucose; electrolytes like sodium, potassium, calcium, magnesium, phosphate, and chloride; vitamins; and proteins. Lipid emulsions are another type of TPN used in some children. Meticulous care is needed, whether in the hospital or at home, to ensure safe TPN infusion and treatment. The nurse performs initial assessment, evaluates and monitors ongoing treatment, and administers the solutions in hospital or other settings (Skipper, 1998). See Skill 12–7 for the protocols for TPN management in the *Clinical Skills Manual*. SKILLS

Thinking Critically

THE CHILD WITH SPECIAL NUTRITIONAL NEEDS

Joey was diagnosed with cerebral palsy early in life. He is now 11 years old and has recently been enrolled in school. Part of the health care plan being implemented in the school involves fostering a positive nutritional state. Joey has limited ability to swallow, related to muscle weakness of cerebral palsy, and is therefore unable to ingest enough calories by mouth to ensure his optimal growth and development. Joey had a feeding tube inserted into his stomach at an early age and receives some of his nutrition by this method.

The school nurse has met with Joey's parents and his home health nurse to learn about the amount and type of tube feedings he receives, as well as the texture of oral feedings he can manage. The nurse will plan the feeding schedule at school to facilitate adequate nutrition in that setting. In addition, careful ongoing nutritional assessment will be needed to evaluate if Joey is getting the calories and other nutrients he needs for growth and development. The school nurse is also educating the classroom teachers and other school personnel about Joey's unique nutritional requirements.

- What do the teachers need to know about Joey's nutritional needs during school?
- How will you organize Joey's care if you are the case manager for his integration within the school system?
- How can the nurse help the family prepare for meeting nutritional needs of a child who has special needs like Joey's during travel by car or plane?
- If Joey's family plans to visit another state on a car trip this summer, what will they need to bring with them? (His feeding solution, tubing, and other supplies, and they may need refrigeration to maintain enteral solutions.) WEB

CHAPTER HIGHLIGHTS

☙ Adequate nutritional intake is necessary for the normal growth and development of children.

☙ Children with medical or psychosocial conditions require additional nutritional support.

☙ Dietary intake patterns vary throughout childhood as the child grows, is able to metabolize different types of food, and gains greater gross and fine motor control.

☙ Nutritional assessment is an essential part of nursing care and may involve a number of approaches such as growth measurement and intake records.

☙ Common nutritional concerns in childhood include hunger, overweight, foodborne illness, and dietary deficiencies.

☙ The child with feeding disorder of infancy and childhood requires comprehensive assessment and ongoing management to foster parent-child interaction and adequate nutritional intake.

☙ Children engaging in sports and those who eat vegetarian diets may need guidance to meet nutritional needs.

☙ Alternative feeding methods such as enteral and parenteral feedings are required by some children.

EXPLORE MediaLink

NCLEX Review, Case Studies, and other interactive resources for this chapter can be found on the companion website at http://www.prenhall.com/london. Click on "Chapter 31" to select the activities for this chapter.

For animations, more NCLEX review questions, and an audio glossary, access the accompanying CD-ROM in this textbook.

REFERENCES

Adair, L. S., & Gordon-Larsen, P. (2001). Maturational timing and overweight prevalence in U.S. adolescent girls. *American Journal of Public Health, 91,* 642–644.

American Academy of Pediatrics Committee on Nutrition. (2001). The use and misuse of fruit juice in pediatrics. *Pediatrics, 107,* 1210–1213.

American Psychiatric Association Working Group on Eating Disorders. (2000). Practice guidelines for the treatment of patients with eating disorders. *American Journal of Psychiatry, 157,* 1–39.

Bessler, S. (1999). Nutritional assessment. In P. Q. Samour, K. K. Helm, & C. E. Lang (Eds.), *Handbook of pediatric nutrition* (2nd ed., pp. 17–42). Gaithersburg, MD: Aspen.

Bock, S. A., Munoz-Furlong, A., & Sampson, H. A. (2001). Fatalities due to anaphylactic reactions to foods. *Journal of Allergy and Clinical Immunology, 107,* 191–193.

Boyle, M. A., & Morris, D. H. (1999). *Community nutrition in action* (2nd ed.). Belmont, CA: West/Wadsworth.

Breier, S. J. (2000). Ethics and total parenteral nutrition. *Journal of Intravenous Nursing, 23,* 52–57.

Burks, W. (2000). Diagnosis of allergic reactions to food. *Pediatric Annals, 29,* 744–752.

Children's Defense Fund. (2000). *The state of America's children.* Washington, DC: Author.

Committee on Nutrition. (1998). *Pediatric nutrition handbook* (4th ed.). Elk Grove Village, IL: American Academy of Pediatrics.

Corrales, K. M., & Utter, S. L. (1999). Failure to thrive. In P. Q. Samour, K. K. Helm, & C. E. Lang (Eds.), *Handbook of pediatric nutrition* (2nd ed., pp. 395–412). Gaithersburg, MD: Aspen.

Federal Interagency Forum on Child and Family Statistics. (2000). *America's children: Key national indicators of well-being, 2000.* Washington, DC: Author.

Food and Nutrition Board. (2001). *Dietary reference intakes.* Washington, DC: National Academy Press.

Gortmaker, S. L., Must, A., Sobol, A. M., Peterson, K., Colditz, G. A., & Dietz, W. H. (1996). Television viewing as a cause of increasing obesity among children in the United States. *Archives of Pediatric and Adolescent Medicine, 150,* 356–362.

Gottlieb, B. (2000). *Alternative cures.* Emmaus, PA: Rodale.

Hanson, L. A., Dahlman-Hoglund, A., Lundin, S., Karllson, M., Dahlgren, U., Ahlstedt, S., et al. (1997). Early determinants of immunocompetence. *Nutrition Reviews, 55,* S12–S17.

_____ (2000). *Healthy People 2010.* Washington, DC: U.S. Department of Health and Human Services.

Hensrud, D. D. (1999). Nutrition screening and assessment. *Medical Clinics of North America, 83,* 1525–1546.

Johnson, W. A. (2001). Nutritional supplements: What you need to know. *Contemporary Pediatrics, 18*(7), 63–74.

Kramer, M. S. (2001). Promotion of breastfeeding intervention trial (PROBIT). *Journal of the American Medical Association, 285,* 413–420.

Krauss, R. M., Eckel, R. H., Howard, G., Appel, L. J., Daniels, S. R., Deckelbaum, R. J., et al.

(2001). AHA scientific statement: AHA dietary guideline. *Journal of Nutrition, 131,* 132–146.

Lee, R. D., & Nieman, D. C. (1996). *Nutrition assessment* (2nd ed.). Boston: McGraw-Hill.

Maggioni, A., & Lifchitz, F. (1995). Nutritional management of failure to thrive. *Pediatric Clinics of North America, 42,* 791–810.

Matarese, L. E., & Gottschlich, M. M. (1998). *Contemporary nutrition support practice.* Philadelphia: W.B. Saunders.

McDonough, A. B. (1999). Eating disorders. In P. Q. Samour, K. K. Helm, & C. E. Lang (Eds.), *Handbook of pediatric nutrition* (2nd ed., pp. 191–204). Gaithersburg, MD: Aspen.

MMWR (2001a). Preliminary FoodNet data on the incidence of foodborne illnesses. *Morbidity and Mortality Weekly Report, 50,* 241–246.

MMWR (2001b). Severe malnutrition among young children—Georgia, January 1997–June 1999. *Morbidity and Mortality Weekly Report, 50,* 224–227.

National Cholesterol Education Program. (1991). *Report of the expert panel on blood cholesterol levels in children and adolescents.* Washington, DC: U.S. Department of Health and Human Services.

Neumark-Sztainer, D. (2000). Primary prevention of disordered eating among preadolescent girls. *Journal of the American Dietetic Association, 100,* 1466–1473.

Orbanic, S. (2001). Understanding bulimia. *American Journal of Nursing, 101*(3), 35–41.

Pongracic, J. A. (2000). Is it food allergy? *Contemporary Pediatrics, 17,* 101–112, 117–121.

Rudys-Shapard, R. (2001). Adolescent, pregnant, and vegetarian: A turbulent time for a teen. *Journal of Pediatric Health Care, 15,* 35–40.

Skipper, A. (1998). *Dietitian's handbook of enteral and parenteral nutrition* (2nd ed.). Gaithersburg, MD: Aspen.

Trahms, C. M., & Pipes, P. L. (1997). *Nutrition in infancy and childhood* (6th ed.). New York: WCB/McGraw-Hill.

Troiano, R. P., & Flegal, K. M. (1998). Overweight children and adolescents: Description, epidemiology, and demographics. *Pediatrics, 101* (Suppl. 3), 497–504.

Troiano, R. P., Flegal, K. M., Kuczmarski, R. J., Campbell, S. M., & Johnson, C. L. (1995). Overweight prevalence and trends for children and adolescents. *Archives of Pediatric and Adolescent Medicine, 149,* 1085–1091.

Walter, T., Olivares, M., Pizarro, F., & Munoz, C. (1997). Iron, anemia, and infection. *Nutrition Reviews, 55,* 111–124.

Whitaker, R., Wright, J. A., Pepe, M. S., Seidel, K. D., & Dietz, W. H. (1997). Predicting obesity in young adulthood from childhood and parental obesity. *New England Journal of Medicine, 337,* 869–873.

Zizza, C., Siega-Riz, A. M., & Popkin, B. M. (2001). Significant increase in young children's snacking between 1977–1978 and 1994–1996 represents a cause for concern! *Preventive Medicine, 32,* 303–310.

CHAPTER 32

Growth and Development

We want to help our adopted daughter Irena grow into a normal and special child. She had challenges in her short life in Romania that we can only imagine. We worry about how we can help her grow and develop.

—MOTHER OF IRENA, 2

Key Terms

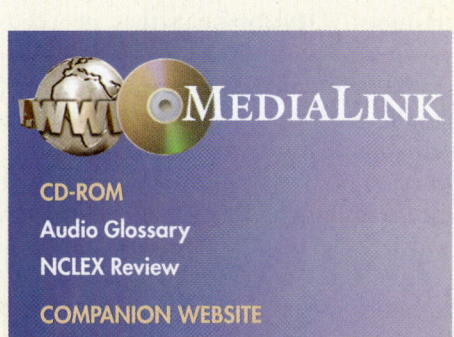

MediaLink

CD-ROM
Audio Glossary
NCLEX Review

COMPANION WEBSITE
http://www.prenhall.com/london
Growth and Development Web Links
Thinking Critically
NCLEX Review
Case Study

Children develop as they interact with their surroundings. They learn skills at different ages, but the order in which they learn them is universal. Development is affected by factors such as nutrition and cultural practices, as well as the social situation in the country or neighborhood. Although each child will develop in a unique manner influenced by genetic makeup, life experiences, and the interaction between these factors, there are certain principles of development that assist parents and the nurse in fostering positive adaptations for the child.

This chapter will cover general principles of growth and development and will explore several theories related to childhood development, as well as their nursing applications. Each age group, from infancy through adolescence, is described in detail. Developmental milestones, physical and cognitive characteristics, health and safety concerns, and communication strategies are presented. This basic information helps guide developmentally appropriate care for children in each age group. These concepts can be applied when caring for all children, including those in special situations like Irena.

PRINCIPLES OF GROWTH AND DEVELOPMENT

It is essential to understand the concepts of growth and development when learning to care for children. **Growth** refers to an increase in physical size. **Development** refers to an increase in capability or function. The quantitative changes in body organ functioning, ability to communicate, and performance of motor skills unfold over time.

Each child displays a unique maturational pattern during the process of development. Although the exact age at which skills emerge differs, the sequence or order of skill performance is uniform among children. Skill development proceeds according to two processes: from the head down and from the center of the body out to the extremities. Development that proceeds from the head downward through the body and toward the feet is called **cephalocaudal development** (Figure 32–1 ◆). For example, at birth, an infant's head is much larger proportionately than the trunk or extremities. Similarly, infants learn to hold up their heads before sitting, and to sit before standing. Skills such as walking that involve the legs and feet develop last in infancy. Development that proceeds from the center of the body outward to the extremities is called **proximodistal development** (see Figure 32–1). For example, infants are first able to control the trunk, then the arms; only later are fine motor movements of the fingers possible.

During the childhood years, extraordinary changes occur in all aspects of development. Physical size, motor skills, cognitive ability, language, sensory ability, and psychosocial patterns all undergo major transformations. Nurses study normal patterns of development so they can perform thorough pediatric assessments and identify children who demonstrate slow or abnormal development. These assessments can guide the nurse in planning interventions for the child and family, such as referring the child for a diagnostic evaluation or rehabilitation, or teaching the parents how to provide adequate stimulation for the child. When development is proceeding normally, the nurse uses his or her knowledge of these normal patterns to plan teaching approaches based on the child's cognitive

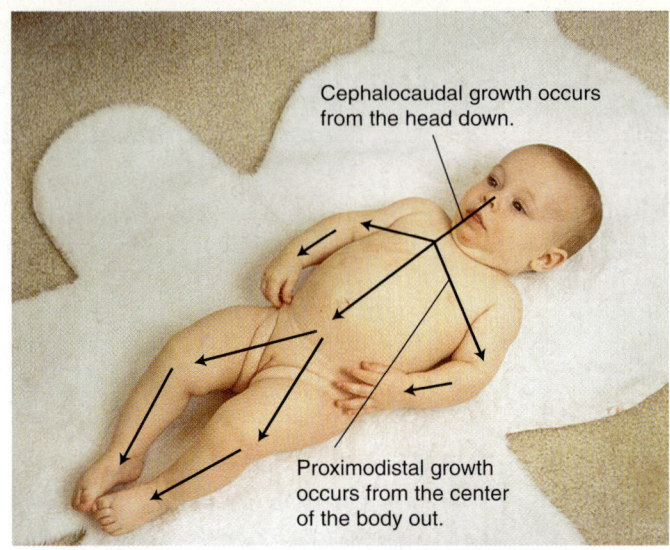

FIGURE 32–1. ◆ In normal *cephalocaudal* growth, the child gains control of the head and neck before the trunk and the limbs. In normal *proximodistal* growth, the child controls arm movements before hand movements. For example, the child reaches for objects before being able to grasp them. Children gain control of their hands before their fingers; that is, they can hold things with the entire hand before they can pick something up with just their fingers.

Cephalocaudal growth occurs from the head down.

Proximodistal growth occurs from the center of the body out.

Growth and Development

One example of children who need careful assessments and nursing interventions to foster development are international adoptees. Nearly 20,000 international adoptions occur annually in the United States, up from less than half that number one decade ago (Jenista, 2000). 🔗 **WEB** While these children can have an array of medical conditions such as infectious diseases, inadequate immunizations, and nutritional disorders, the effects of their early life experiences on development can also be profound. Many international adoptees are small in size, due to poor nutrition of the mother during pregnancy and of the infant after birth, and to growth delay related to emotional issues. The child should be examined closely at the time of adoption for length, weight, and head circumference. Within 6 months of arrival, most children show improvement in growth patterns. If growth does not improve by this time, the child is further assessed for problems such as intestinal parasites, chronic diseases, or other medical problems (Altemeier, 2000; Miller, 2000).

TABLE 32-1 Developmental Age Groups

Infancy—Birth to 12 months. Includes infants or babies up to 1 year of age who require a high level of care in daily activities.

Toddlerhood—1–3 years. Characterized by increased motor ability and independent behavior.

Preschool—3–6 years. The preschooler refines gross and fine motor ability and language skills and often participates in a preschool learning program.

School age—6–12 years. Begins with entry into a school system and is characterized by growing intellectual skills, physical ability, and independence.

Adolescence—12–18 years. Begins with entry into the teen years. Mature cognitive thought, formation of identity, and influence of peers are important characteristics of adolescence.

TABLE 32-2 Common Defense Mechanisms Used by Children

Defense Mechanism	Definition	Example
Regression	Return to an earlier behavior	A previously toilet-trained child becomes incontinent when separated from parents during a hospitalization.
Repression	Involuntary forgetting of uncomfortable situations	An abused child cannot consciously recall episodes of abuse.
Rationalization	An attempt to make unacceptable feelings acceptable	A child explains hitting another because "he took my toy."
Fantasy	A creation of the mind to help deal with unacceptable fear	A hospitalized child who is weak pretends to be Superman.

and language ability, to offer appropriate toys and activities during illness, and to respond therapeutically during interactions with the child.

MAJOR THEORIES OF DEVELOPMENT

Child development is a complex process. Many theorists have attempted to organize their observations of behavior into a description of principles or a set of stages. Each theory focuses on a particular facet of development. Most developmental theorists separate children into age groups by common characteristics (Table 32–1).

Freud's Theory of Psychosexual Development

THEORETICAL FRAMEWORK

Sigmund Freud (1856–1939) was a physician in Vienna, Austria. His work with adults experiencing a variety of nervous disorders led him to develop the approach called psychoanalysis, which explored the driving forces of the unconscious mind. These psychoanalytic techniques led Freud to believe that early childhood experiences form the unconscious motivation for actions in later life. He believed that sexual energy is centered in specific parts of the body at certain ages. Unresolved conflict and unmet needs at a certain stage lead to a fixation of development at that stage (Gemelli, 1996).

Freud viewed the personality as a structure with three parts: the id is the basic sexual energy that is present at birth and drives the individual to seek pleasure; the ego is the realistic part of the person, which develops during infancy and searches for acceptable methods of meeting impulses; and the superego is the moral/ethical system, which develops in childhood and contains a set of values and conscience (Craig, 1999). The ego diverts impulses and protects itself from excess anxiety by use of **defense mechanisms,** including regression to earlier stages and repression or forgetting of painful experiences such as child abuse (Table 32–2).

STAGES

Oral (Birth to 1 Year). The infant derives pleasure largely from the mouth, with sucking and eating as primary desires.

Anal (1 to 3 Years). The young child's pleasure is centered in the anal area, with control over body secretions as a prime force in behavior.

Phallic (3 to 6 Years). Sexual energy becomes centered in the genitalia as the child works out relationships with parents of the same and opposite sexes.

Latency (6 to 12 Years). Sexual energy is at rest in the passage between earlier stages and adolescence.

Genital (12 Years to Adulthood). Mature sexuality is achieved as physical growth is completed and relationships with others occur.

NURSING APPLICATION

Freud emphasized the importance of meeting the needs of each stage in order to move successfully into future developmental stages. The crisis of illness can interfere with normal developmental processes and add challenges for the nurse striving to meet an ill child's needs. For example, the importance of sucking in infancy guides the nurse to provide a pacifier for the infant who cannot have oral fluids. The preschool child's concern about sexuality guides the nurse to provide privacy and clear explanations during any procedures involving the genital area. It may be necessary to teach parents that masturbation by the young child is normal and to help parents deal with it. The adolescent's focus on relationships suggests that the nurse should include questions about significant friends during history taking. Table 32–3 summarizes ways to apply these theoretical concepts to the care of children.

TABLE 32-3 Nursing Applications of Theories of Freud, Erikson, Piaget

Age Group	Developmental Stages	Nursing Applications
Infant (birth to 1 year)	Oral stage (Freud): The baby obtains pleasure and comfort through the mouth.	When a baby is not able to take foods or fluids, offer a pacifier if not contraindicated. After painful procedures, offer a baby a bottle or pacifier or have the mother breastfeed.
	Trust versus mistrust stage (Erikson): The baby establishes a sense of trust when basic needs are met.	Hold the hospitalized baby often. (A) Offer comfort after painful procedures. Meet the baby's needs for food and hygiene. Encourage parents to room in. Manage pain effectively with use of pain medications and other measures.
	Sensorimotor stage (Piaget): The baby learns from movement and sensory input.	Use crib mobiles, manipulative toys, wall murals, and bright colors to provide interesting stimuli and comfort. Use toys to distract the baby during procedures and assessments.
Toddler (1–3 years)	Anal stage (Freud): The child derives gratification from control over body excretions.	Ask about toilet training and the child's rituals and words for elimination during admission history. Continue child's normal patterns of elimination in the hospital. Do not begin toilet training during illness or hospitalization. Accept regression in toileting during illness or hospitalization. Have potty chairs available in hospital and child care centers.
	Autonomy versus shame and doubt stage (Erikson): The child is increasingly independent in many spheres of life.	Allow self-feeding opportunities. Encourage child to remove and put on own clothes, brush teeth, or assist with hygiene. (B) If restraint for a procedure is necessary, proceed quickly, providing explanations and comfort.
	Sensorimotor stage (end); preoperational stage (beginning) (Piaget): The child shows increasing curiosity and explorative behavior. Language skills improve.	Ensure safe surroundings to allow opportunities to manipulate objects. Name objects and give simple explanations.
Preschooler (3–6 years)	Phallic stage (Freud): The child initially identifies with the parent of the opposite sex but by the end of this stage has identifies with the same-sex parent.	Be alert for children who appear more comfortable with male or female nurses, and attempt to accommodate them. Encourage parental involvement in care. Plan for playtime and offer a variety of materials from which to choose.
	Initiative versus guilt stage (Erikson): The child likes to initiate play activities.	Offer medical equipment for play to lessen anxiety about strange objects. (C) Assess children's concerns as expressed through their drawings. Accept the child's choices and expressions of feelings.
	Preoperational stage (Pioget): The child is increasingly verbal but has some limitations in thought processes. Causality is often confused, so the child may feel responsible for causing an illness.	Offer explanations about all procedures and treatments. Clearly explain that the child is not responsible for causing the illness.

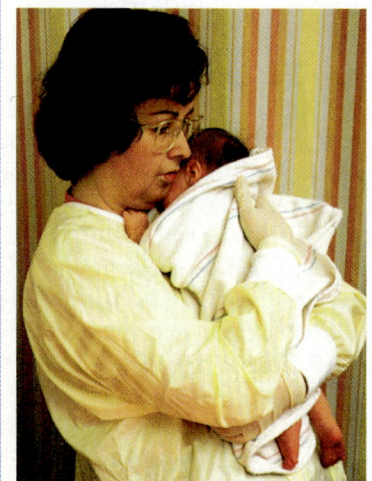

A

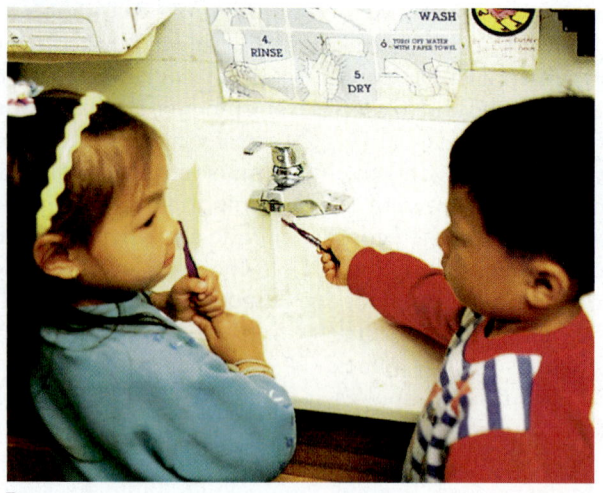

B

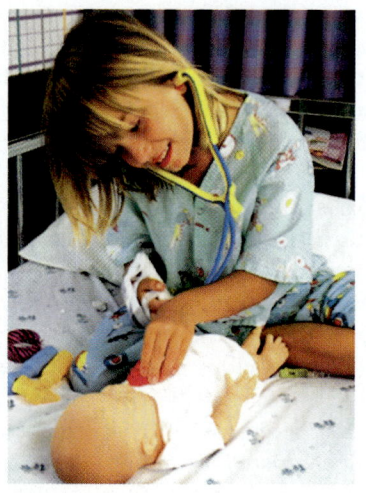

C

Age Group	Developmental Stages	Nursing Applications
School age (6–12 year)	Latency stage (Freud): The child places importance on privacy and understanding the baby.	Provide gowns, covers, and underwear. Knock on door before entering. Explain treatments and procedures.
	Industry versus inferiority stage (Erikson): The child gains a sense of self-worth from involvement in activities.	Encourage the child to continue school work while hospitalized. Encourage child to bring favorite pasttimes to the hospital. (D) Help child adjust to limitations an favorite activities.
	Concrete operational stage (Piaget): The child is capable of mature thought when allowed to manipulate and see objects.	Give clear instructions about details of treatment. Show the child equipment that will be used in treatment.
Adolescent (12–18 years)	Genital stage (Freud): The adolescent's focus is on genital function and relationships.	Ensure access to gynecologic care for adolescent girls. Provide information on sexuality. Ensure privacy during health care. Have brochures and videos available for teaching about sexuality.
	Identity versus role confusion stage (Erikson): The adolescent's search for self-identity leads to independence from parents and reliance on peers.	Provide a separate recreation room for teens who are hospitalized. (E) Take health history and perform examinations without parents present. Introduce adolescent to other teens with same health problem.
	Formal operational stage (Piaget): The adolescent is capable of mature, abstract thought.	Give clear and complete information about health care and treatments. Offer both written and verbal instructions. Continue to provide education about the disease to the adolescent with a chronic illness, as mature thought now leads to greater understanding.

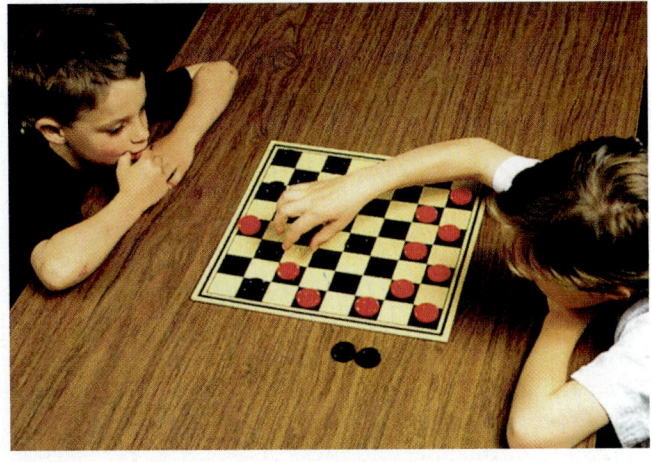

D

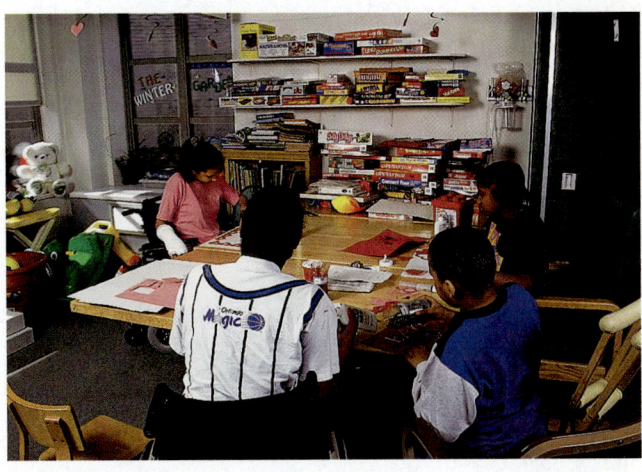

E

Erikson's Theory of Psychosocial Development

THEORETICAL FRAMEWORK

Erik Erikson (1902–1994) studied Freud's theory of psychoanalysis under Freud's daughter, Anna. He later established his own developmental theory which describes psychosocial stages during eight periods of human life. For each stage, Erikson identifies a crisis—that is, a particular challenge that exists for healthy personality development to occur (Erikson, 1963, 1968). The word *crisis* in this context refers to normal maturational social needs rather than to a single critical event. Each developmental crisis has two possible outcomes. When needs are met, the consequence is healthy and the individual moves on to future stages with particular strengths. When needs are not met, an unhealthy outcome occurs that will influence future social relationships.

STAGES

Trust Versus Mistrust (Birth to 1 Year). The task of the first year of life is to establish trust in the people providing care. Trust is fostered by provision of food, clean clothing, touch, and comfort. If basic needs are not met, the infant will eventually learn to mistrust others.

Autonomy Versus Shame and Doubt (1 to 3 Years). The toddler's sense of autonomy or independence is shown by controlling body excretions, saying no when asked to do something, and directing motor activity and play. Children who are consistently criticized for expressions of autonomy or for lack of control—for example, during toilet training—will develop a sense of shame about themselves and doubt in their abilities.

Initiative Versus Guilt (3 to 6 Years). The young child initiates new activities and considers new ideas. This interest in exploring the world creates a child who is involved and busy. Constant criticism, on the other hand, leads to feelings of guilt and a lack of purpose.

Industry Versus Inferiority (6 to 12 Years). The middle years of childhood are characterized by development of new interests and by involvement in activities. The child takes pride in accomplishments in sports, school, home, and community. If the child cannot accomplish what is expected, however, the result will be a sense of inferiority.

Identity Versus Role Confusion (12 to 18 Years). In adolescence, as the body matures and thought processes become more complex, a new sense of identity or self is established. The self, family, peer group, and community are all examined and redefined. The adolescent who is unable to establish a meaningful definition of self will experience confusion in one or more roles of life.

NURSING APPLICATION

Erikson's theory is directly applicable to the nursing care of children. The social situations created by health care in the community provide opportunities for helping caregivers meet children's needs. The child's usual support from family, peers, and others is interrupted by hospitalization. The challenge of hospitalization also adds a situational crisis to the normal developmental crisis a child is experiencing. Although the nurse may meet many of the hospitalized child's needs, continued parental involvement is necessary both during and after hospitalization to ensure progression through expected developmental stages (see Table 32–3).

Piaget's Theory of Cognitive Development

THEORETICAL FRAMEWORK

Jean Piaget (1896–1980) was a Swiss scientist who wrote detailed observations of the behavior of his own and other children. Based on these observations, Piaget formulated a theory of cognitive (or intellectual) development. He believed that the child's view of the world is influenced largely by age and maturational ability. Given nurturing experiences, the child's ability to think matures naturally (Ginsberg & Opper, 1988; Piaget, 1972). The child incorporates new experiences via **assimilation** and changes to deal with these experiences by the process of **accommodation.**

STAGES

Sensorimotor (Birth to 2 Years). Infants learn about the world by input obtained through the senses and by their motor activity. Six substages are characteristic of this stage.

Use of Reflexes (Birth to 1 Month). The infant begins life with a set of reflexes such as sucking, rooting, and grasping. By using these reflexes, the infant receives stimulation via touch, sound, smell, and vision. The reflexes thus pave the way for the first learning to occur.

Primary Circular Reactions (1 to 4 Months). Once the infant responds reflexively, the pleasure gained from that response causes repetition of the behavior. For example, if a toy grasped reflexively makes noise and is interesting to look at, the infant will grasp it again.

Secondary Circular Reactions (4 to 8 Months). Awareness of the environment grows as the infant begins to connect cause and effect. The sounds of bottle preparation will lead to excited behavior. If an object is partially hidden, the infant will attempt to uncover and retrieve it.

Coordination of Secondary Schemes (8 to 12 Months). Intentional behavior is observed as the infant uses learned behavior to obtain objects, create sounds, or engage in other pleasurable activity. **Object permanence** (the knowledge that something continues to exist even when out of sight) begins when the infant remembers where a hidden object is likely to be found; it is no longer "out of sight, out of mind."

Tertiary Circular Reactions (12 to 18 Months). Curiosity, experimentation, and exploration predominate as the toddler tries out actions to learn results. The child turns objects in every direction, places them in the mouth, uses them for banging, and inserts them in containers as he or she explores their qualities and uses.

Mental Combinations (18 to 24 Months). Language provides a new tool for the toddler to use in understanding the world. Language enables the child to think about events and objects before or after they occur. Object permanence is now fully developed as the child actively searches for objects in various locations and out of view.

Preoperational (2 to 7 Years). The young child thinks by using words as symbols, but logic is not well developed. During the preconceptual substage (2 to 4 years), vocabulary and comprehension increase greatly but the child is egocentric (that is, unable to see things from the perspective of another). In the intuitive substage (4 to 7 years), the child relies on transductive reasoning (that is, drawing conclusions from one general fact to another). For example, when a child disobeys a parent and then falls and breaks an arm that day, the child may ascribe the broken arm to bad behavior. Cause-and-effect relationships are often unrealistic or a result of "magical thinking" (the belief that events occur because of thoughts or wishes).

Concrete Operational (7 to 11 Years). Transductive reasoning has given way to a more accurate understanding of cause and effect. The child can reason quite well if concrete objects are used in teaching or experimentation. The concept of conservation (that matter does not change when its form is altered) is learned at this age.

Formal Operational (11 Years to Adulthood). Fully mature intellectual thought has now been attained. The adolescent can think abstractly about objects or concepts and consider different alternatives or outcomes.

NURSING APPLICATION

Piaget's theory is essential to pediatric nursing. The nurse must understand a child's thought processes in order to design stimulating activities and meaningful, appropriate teaching plans. What activities could be planned for a hospitalized child based on his or her expected cognitive level? How can cognitive development be encouraged in a school-age child receiving home health services? Understanding a child's concept of time suggests how far in advance to prepare that child for procedures. Similarly, decisions about offering manipulative toys, reading stories, drawing pictures, or giving the child reading matter to explain health care measures depend on the child's cognitive stage of development (see Table 32–3).

Kohlberg's Theory of Moral Development

THEORETICAL FRAMEWORK

Lawrence Kohlberg (1927–1987) was a German theorist who used Piaget's cognitive theory as a basis for his theory of moral development. He presented stories involving moral dilemmas to children and adults and asked them to solve the dilemmas. Kohlberg then analyzed the motives they expressed when making decisions about the best course to take. Based on the explanations given, Kohlberg established three levels of moral reasoning. Although he provided age guidelines, he stated that they are approximate and that many people never reach the highest (postconventional) stage of development (Santrock, 1999).

STAGES

Preconventional (4 to 7 Years). Decisions are based on the desire to please others and to avoid punishment.

Conventional (7 to 11 Years). Conscience or an internal set of standards becomes important. Rules are important and must be followed to please other people and "be good."

Postconventional (12 Years and Older). The individual has internalized ethical standards on which to base decisions. Social responsibility is recognized. The value in each of two differing moral approaches can be considered and a decision made.

NURSING APPLICATION

Decision making is required in many areas of health care. Children can be assisted to make decisions about health care and to consider alternatives when available. Keep in mind that young children may agree to participate in research simply because they want to comply with adults and appear cooperative. Guidelines for child participation in research are available (see Chapter 1).

Social Learning Theory

THEORETICAL FRAMEWORK

Originally from Canada, psychologist Albert Bandura (1925–) has conducted research at Stanford University for many years. He believes that children learn attitudes, beliefs, customs, and values through their social contacts with adults and other children. Children imitate (or model) the behavior they see; if the behavior is positively reinforced, they tend to repeat it. The external environment and the child's internal processes are key elements in social learning theory (Bandura, 1986, 1997a).

NURSING APPLICATION

The importance of modeling behavior can readily be applied in health care. Children are more likely to cooperate if they see adults or other children performing a task willingly. A frightened child may watch another child perform vision screening or have blood drawn and then decide to allow the procedure to take place. Contact with positive role models is useful when teaching children and adolescents self-care for chronic diseases such as diabetes. Give positive reinforcement for desired performance.

Behaviorism

THEORETICAL FRAMEWORK

John Watson (1878–1958) was an American scientist who applied the research of animal behaviorists like Pavlov and Skinner to children. Pavlov and, later, Skinner worked with animals, presenting a stimulus such as food and pairing it with another stimulus such as a ringing bell. Eventually the animal being fed began to salivate when the bell rang. As Skinner and then Watson began to apply these concepts to children, they showed that behaviors can be elicited by positive reinforcement, such as a food treat, or extinguished by negative reinforcement, such as by scolding or withdrawal of attention. Watson believed that he could make of a child anyone he desired—from a professional to a thief or beggar—simply by reinforcing behavior in certain ways (Santrock, 1999).

NURSING APPLICATION

Behaviorism has been criticized for its simplicity and its denial of the inherent capability of persons to respond willfully to events in the environment. This theory does, however, have some use in health care. When particular behaviors are desired, positive reinforcement can be established to encourage these behaviors. Behavioral techniques are also used to alter behavior of misbehaving children or to teach skills to handicapped children. Parents often use reinforcement in toilet training and other skills learned in childhood.

Ecologic Theory

THEORETICAL FRAMEWORK

You may have noticed that there is controversy among theorists concerning the relative importance of heredity versus environment—or nature versus nurture—in human development. **Nature** refers to the genetic or hereditary capability of an individual. **Nurture** refers to the effects of the environment on a person's performance (Figure 32–2 ◆). ⬭ Piaget believed in the importance of internal cognitive structures that unfold at their appointed times, given any environment that provides basic opportunities. He emphasized the strength of nature. The behaviorist John Watson, on the other hand, believed that behaviors are primarily shaped by environmental responses; he thus stressed the predominance of nurture. Contemporary developmental theories increasingly recognize the interaction of nature and nurture in determining the child's development.

Urie Bronfenbrenner (1917–), a professor at Cornell University, formulated the ecologic theory of development to explain the unique relationship of the child in all of life's

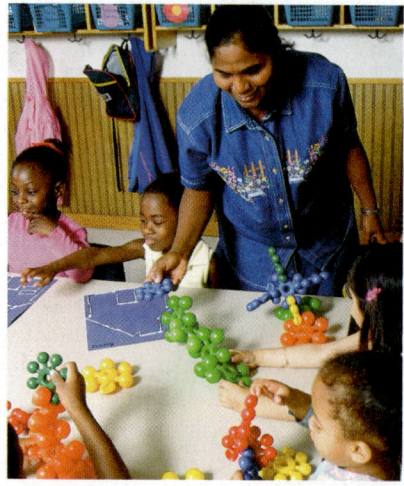

FIGURE 32–2. ◆ Children exposed to pleasant stimulation and who are supported by an adult will develop and refine their skills faster. Group activities such as these provide an environment for both motor skill and psychosocial development. Can you identify which skills are being developed?

settings, from close to remote (Bronfenbrenner, 1986; Bronfenbrenner, McClelland, Ceci, et al., 1996). **Ecologic theory** emphasizes the presence of mutual interactions between the child and these various settings. Neither nature nor nurture is considered of more importance. Bronfenbrenner believes each child brings a unique set of genes—as well as specific attributes such as age, gender, health, and other characteristics—to his or her interactions with the environment. The child then interacts in many settings at different levels or systems (Figure 32–3 ◆).

Levels/Systems

Microsystem. This level is defined as the daily, consistent, close relationships such as home, child care, school, friends, and neighbors. For the child with a chronic illness requiring regular care, the health care providers may even be part of the microsystem. In the ecologic model, the child influences each of these settings in addition to being influenced by them, with reciprocal interactions.

Mesosystem. This level includes relationships of microsystems with one another. For example, two microsystems for most children are the home and the school. The relationships between these microsystems are shown by parents' involvement in their children's school. This involvement, in turn, influences the effects of the home and school settings on the children.

Exosystem. This level is composed of those settings that influence the child even though the child is not in close daily contact with the system. Examples include the parents' jobs and the governing board of the local school district. Although the child may not go to the parents' workplaces, he or she can be influenced by policies related to health care, sick leave, inflexible work hours, overtime, or travel, or even by the mood of the boss (through its impact on the parent). The child's needs may influence a parent to give up a certain job, or to work harder to obtain money for the child's education. Likewise, when a local school board votes to ban certain books or to finance a field trip, the child is influenced by these decisions; the child, in turn, can help establish an atmosphere that will guide future school board decisions.

Macrosystem. This level includes the beliefs, values, and behaviors expressed in the child's environment. Culture is a powerful influence in the macrosystem, as is the political system. For instance, a democratic system creates different beliefs, values, and even eating practices than an anarchic system.

Chronosystem. This final level brings the perspective of time to the previous settings. The time period during which the child grows up influences views of health and illness. For example, the experiences of children with influenza in the 19th versus 20th centuries were quite different.

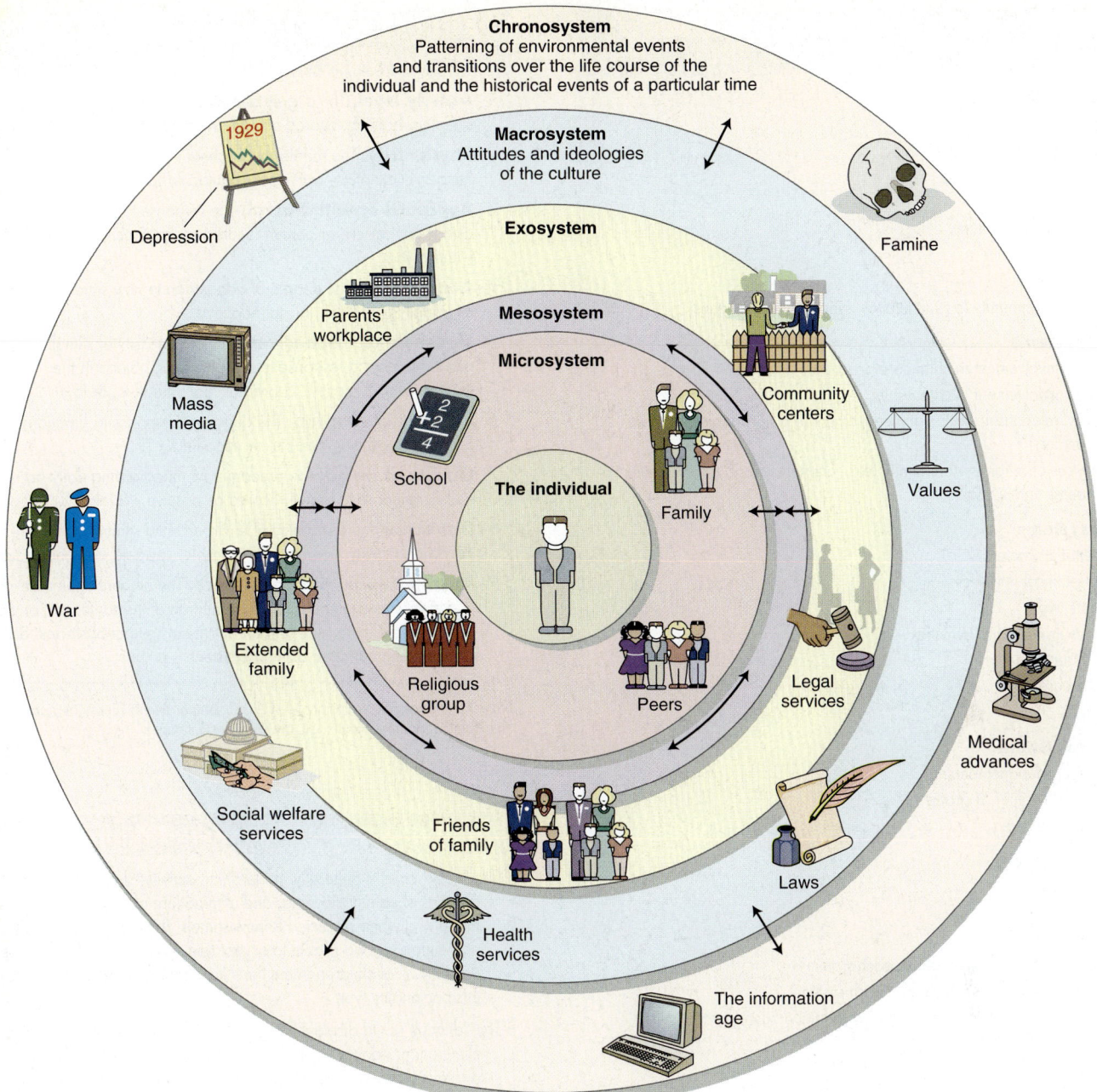

FIGURE 32–3. ◆ Bronfenbrenner's ecologic theory of development views the individual as interacting within five levels or systems.

Note: Redrawn from Santrock, J.W. (2000). *Life span development.* New York, NY: McGraw-Hill. Based on Bronfenbrenner, U. (1979). Contexts of child rearing: Problems and prospects. *American Psychologist, 34,* 844–850, and Bronfenbrenner, U. (1986). Ecology of the family as a context for human development: Research perspectives. *Developmental Psychology, 22,* 723–742.

NURSING APPLICATION

Nurses use ecologic theory when they assess the child's settings to identify influences on development. Table 32–4 provides an assessment tool based on this theory. Interventions are planned to enhance the strengths of the child's settings and to improve on areas that are not supportive.

Temperament Theory

THEORETICAL FRAMEWORK

In contrast to behaviorists such as Watson or maturational theorists such as Piaget, Stella Chess and Alexander Thomas recognize the innate qualities of personality that each individual brings to the events of daily life. They, like

TABLE 32-4   Assessment of Ecologic Systems in Childhood

Microsystem

Parents
Significant others in close contact
Child care arrangements
School
Neighborhood contacts
Clubs
Friends, peers
Religious community (e.g., churches, synagogues, mosques)

Mesosytems

Parents' involvement in child care or school
Parents' involvement in community
Parents' relationship with significant others (e.g., grandparents, care providers)
Influences of religious community (e.g., church, synagogue, mosque) on parents and school

Exosystems

Community centers
Local political influences
Parents' work
Parents' friends and activities
Social services
Health care
Libraries

Macrosystems

Cultural group membership
Beliefs and values of group
Political structure

Chronosystem

Child's age
Parents' ages
Ask yourself:
• How does the child influence each system?
• How is the child influenced by each system?
• Where does this lead you in planning interventions for the child?

TABLE 32-5   Nine Parameters of Personality

1. **Activity level.** The degree of motion during eating, playing, sleeping, bathing. Scored as high, medium, or low.
2. **Rhythmicity.** The regularity of schedule maintained for sleep, hunger, elimination. Scored as regular, variable, or irregular.
3. **Approach or withdrawal.** The response to a new stimulus such as a food, activity, or person. Scored as approachable, variable, or withdrawn.
4. **Adaptability.** The degree of adaptation to new situations. Scored as adaptive, variable, or nonadaptive.
5. **Threshold of responsiveness.** The intensity of stimulation needed to elicit a response to sensory input, objects in the environment, or people. Scored as high, medium, or low.
6. **Intensity of reaction.** The degree of response to situations. Scored as positive, variable, or negative.
7. **Quality of mood.** The predominant mood during daily activity and in response to stimuli. Scored as positive, variable, or negative.
8. **Distractibility.** The ability of environmental stimuli to interfere with the child's activity. Scored as distractible, variable, or nondistractible.
9. **Attention span and persistence.** The amount of time devoted to activities (compared with other children of the same age) and the degree of ability to stick with an activity in spite of obstacles. Scored as persistent, variable, or nonpersistent.

Note: From Chess, S., & Thomas, A. (1996). *Temperament: Theory and practice.* Philadelphia: Brunner/Routledge, div. of Taylor & Francis.

TABLE 32-6   Patterns of Temperament

The "easy" child is generally moderate in activity; shows regularity in patterns of eating, sleeping, and elimination; and is usually positive in mood and when subjected to new stimuli. The easy child adapts to new situations and is able to accept rules and work well with others. About 40% of children in the New York Longitudinal Study displayed this personality type.

The "difficult" child displays irregular schedules for eating, sleeping, and elimination; adapts slowly to new situations and persons; and displays a predominantly negative mood. Intense reactions to the environment are common. About 10% of children in the New York Longitudinal Study displayed this personality type.

The "slow-to-warm-up" child has reactions of mild intensity and slow adaptability to new situations. The child displays initial withdrawal followed by gradual, quiet, and slow interaction with the environment. About 15% of children in the New York Longitudinal Study displayed this personality type.

The remaining 35% of children studied showed some characteristics of each personality type (Chess & Thomas, 1995).

Bronfenbrenner, believe the child is an individual who both influences and is influenced by the environment. However, Chess and Thomas focus on one specific aspect of development—the wide spectrum of behaviors possible in children, identifying nine parameters of response to daily events (Table 32–5). Their theory is based on a research study entitled the *New York Longitudinal Study*, which began with infants in 1956 and has continued into the adulthood of these participating individuals. By careful observations of responses to life events, Chess and Thomas identified characteristics of personality that provide the basis for the study on temperament. Infants generally display clusters of responses, which are classified into three major personality types (Table 32–6). Although most children do not demonstrate all behaviors described for a particular type, they usually show a grouping indicative of one personality type (Chess & Thomas, 1995, 1996).

Recent research demonstrates that personality characteristics displayed during infancy are often consistent with those seen later in life. Predicting future characteristics is not possible, however, because of the complex and dynamic interaction of personality traits and environmental reactions.

Many other researchers have expanded the work of Chess and Thomas, developing assessment tools for temperament types. The concept of "goodness of fit" is an outgrowth of this theory. Goodness of fit refers to whether parents' expectations of their child's behavior are consistent with the child's temperament type. There is a "good fit" when the properties of the environment are in accord with the child's capabilities, characteristics, and style of behavior (Chess & Thomas, 1999). For example, an infant who is very active and reacts strongly to verbal stimuli may be unable to sleep well when placed in a room with older siblings. A child who is slow to warm up may not perform well in the first few months at a new school, much to parents' disappointment. When parents understand a child's temperament characteristics, they are better able to shape the environment to meet the child's needs.

NURSING APPLICATION

The concept of personality type or temperament is a useful one for nurses (Melvin, 1995). Nurses can assess the temperament of young children and alter the environment to meet their needs. This may involve moving a hospitalized child to a single room to ensure adequate rest if the child is easily stimulated, or allowing a shy child time to become accustomed to new surroundings and equipment before beginning procedures or treatments.

Parents are often relieved to learn about temperament characteristics. They learn to appreciate their children's qualities and to adapt the environment to meet the children's needs. A burden of guilt can also be lifted from parents who feel that they are responsible for their child's actions. Teach parents ways of enhancing goodness of fit between the child's personality and the environment (Table 32–7).

INFLUENCES ON DEVELOPMENT

As discussed earlier, both nature and nurture are important in determining individual patterns of development. The interaction of these two forces can explain differences in time frames for acquisition of developmental skills, personality variations between identical twins, and other unique characteristics of individuals. The genetic and environmental factors that contribute to individual differences are explored in more detail next.

Genetics

Each child inherits 23 chromosomes from the mother's egg and 23 from the father's sperm, resulting in a unique individual with 46 chromosomes. Two of these are **sex chromosomes,** and determine the child's gender; the rest are called **autosomal chromosomes,** and govern all remaining characteristics.

Every chromosome carries many genes that determine physical characteristics, intellectual potential, personality type, and other traits. Children are born with the potential for certain features; however, their interaction with the environment influences how and to what extent particular traits are manifested. See Chapter 4 for further discussion of genetic transmission and health-related conditions.

Environmental Influences on Development

PRENATAL INFLUENCES

Some Asian cultures calculate age from the time of conception. This practice acknowledges the profound influence of the prenatal period.

The mother's nutrition and general state of health play a part in pregnancy outcome. Poor nutrition can lead to small infants and infants with compromised neurologic performance, slow development, or impaired immune status with resultant high disease rates. Low maternal stores of iron can result in anemia in the infant (Trahms & Pipes, 1997; UNICEF, 1998). Maternal smoking is associated with low-birth-weight infants. Ingestion of alcoholic beverages, including beer and wine, during pregnancy may lead to fetal alcohol syndrome (Figure 32–4 ◆). Illicit drug

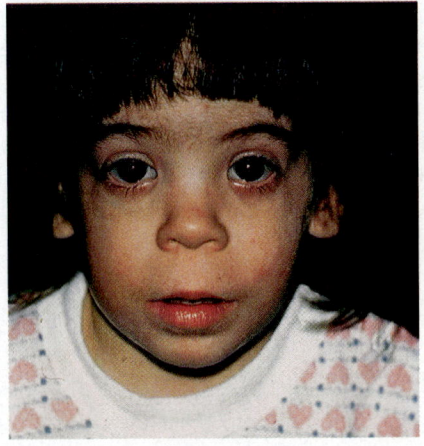

FIGURE 32–4. ◆ Fetal alcohol syndrome. Courtesy of Dr. Sterling Clarren, Seattle, WA. Clarren, S.K., & Smith, D.W. (1978). The fetal alcohol syndrome. *New England Journal of Medicine, 298,* 1063–1067. Copyright 1978, Massachusetts Medical Society. All right reserved.

TABLE 32–7 Ways to Improve Goodness of Fit Between Parents and Child	
Child's Behavior	*Parent's Activity*
Extremely active	Plan periods of active play several times a day. Have restful periods before bedtime to foster sleep.
Shy	Allow time to adapt at own pace to new people and situations.
Easily stimulated	Have quiet room for sleeping as an infant. Have quiet room for homework as a school-age child.
Short attention span	Provide projects that can be completed in a short period. Gradually encourage longer periods at activities.

use by the mother may result in neonatal addiction, convulsions, hyperirritability, poor social responsiveness, and other neurologic disturbances.

Even prescription drugs may adversely affect the fetus. An example is the drug thalidomide, commonly used in Europe to treat nausea during the 1950s. This drug resulted in the birth of infants with limb abnormalities to women who used the drug during pregnancy. Other drugs can cause bleeding, stained teeth, impaired hearing, or other defects in the infant (Briggs, Freeman, & Yaffe, 1998).

Some maternal illnesses are harmful to the developing fetus. An example is rubella (German measles), which is rarely a serious disease for adults but which can cause deafness, vision defects, heart defects, and mental retardation in the fetus if it is acquired by a pregnant woman. A fetus can also acquire diseases such as AIDS/HIV infection or hepatitis B from the mother.

Radiation, chemicals, and other environmental hazards may adversely affect a fetus when the mother is exposed to these influences during her pregnancy. The best outcomes for infants occur when mothers eat well; exercise regularly; seek early prenatal care; refrain from use of drugs, alcohol, tobacco, and excessive caffeine; and follow general principles of good health.

CULTURE

The traditional customs of the many cultural groups represented in North American society influence the development of the children in these groups. Foods commonly eaten vary among people with different cultural backgrounds and influence the incidence of health problems such as cardiovascular disease in these groups. The Native-American practice of carrying infants on boards often delays walking when measured against the norm for walking on some developmental tests. Children who are carried by straddling the mother's hips or back for extended periods have a low incidence of developmental dysplasia of the hip since this keeps their hips in an abducted position. Certain groups are more prone to develop certain diseases due to genetic variations (Table 32–8).

All cultural groups have rules regarding patterns of social interaction. Schedules of language acquisition are determined by the number of languages spoken and the amount of speech in the home. The particular social roles assumed by men and women in the culture affect school activities and ultimately career choices. Attitudes toward

$\mathcal{D}$eveloping Cultural Competence

Cultural differences in childrearing influence personality. For example, Japanese children are taught to respect parents and elders. Gender distinctions are the basis for social behaviors. Girls are praised for maintaining poise, grace, and control; boys for showing determination and strength of will in overcoming obstacles.

TABLE 32-8	Diseases and Conditions More Common among Cultural Groups

African Americans
Sickle cell disease
Hypertension
Stomach and esophageal cancer
Lactose intolerance

Asians/Pacific Islanders
Hypertension
Stomach and liver cancer
Lactose intolerance
Thalassemia

American Indians/ Aleuts/Eskimos
Diabetes
Ear infections
Accidents and suicides
Cirrhosis of the liver
Overweight

Hispanic Americans
Diabetes
Overweight
Lactose intolerance

Jews
Tay-Sachs disease
Niemann-Pick disease
Werdnig-Hoffman disease

Mediterraneans
G6PD deficiency
β-Thalassemia
Familial Mediterranean fever

United Kingdom
Cystic fibrosis
Phenylketonuria
Hereditary amyloidosis
Hyperhomocystinemia

Note: From Jarvis, C. (2000). *Physical examination and health assessment* (3rd ed.). Philadelphia: WB Saunders; and Spector, R. (2000). *Guides to heritage assessment and health traditions.* Upper Saddle River, NJ: Prentice Hall Health. Adapted.

touching and other methods of encouraging developmental skills vary among cultures.

INFANT (BIRTH TO 1 YEAR)

Imagine the experience of tripling body weight in one year, or becoming proficient in understanding fundamental words in a new language and even speaking a few. These and many more accomplishments take place in the first year of life. Starting the year as a mainly reflexive creature, the infant can walk and communicate by the year's end. Never again in life is development so swift.

Physical Growth and Development

The first year of life is one of rapid change for the infant. The birth weight usually doubles by about 5 months and triples by the end of the first year (Figure 32–5 ◆). Height increases by about a foot during this year and body proportion begins to change. Teeth begin to erupt at about 6 months, and by the end of the first year the infant has six to eight deciduous teeth (see Chapter 33). Physical growth is closely associated with type and quality of feeding (see Chapter 31 for a discussion of nutrition in infancy). 🔗

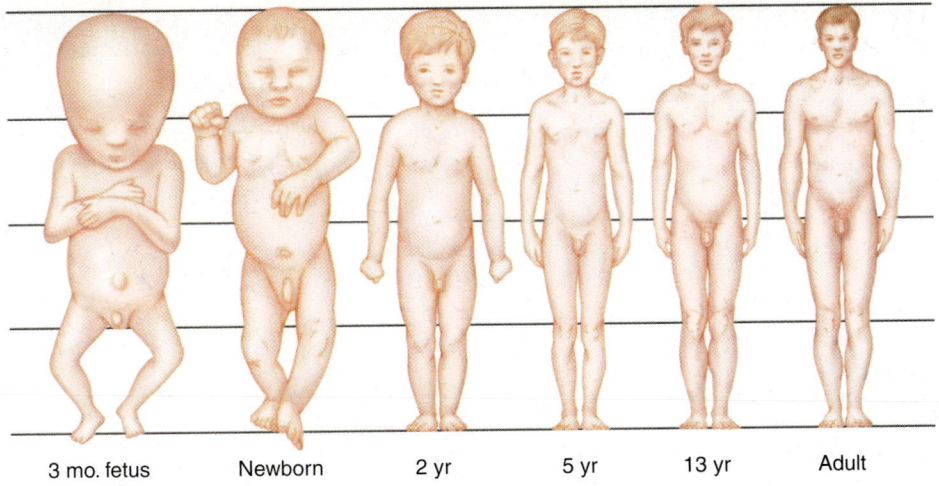

FIGURE 32–5. ◆ Body proportions at various ages.

3 mo. fetus   Newborn   2 yr   5 yr   13 yr   Adult

Growth and Development

Growth charts in use in the United States since 1977 were not based on a wide cross section of the population. A new set of growth charts was issued in 2000 by the Centers for Disease Control and Prevention, based on national cross-sectional survey data from the second and third National Health and Nutritional Examination Survey (NHANES). ⊂▭⊃ **WEB** In addition to previously available percentile charts for height, weight, and head circumference, charts are now available for body mass index so overweight children can more easily be identified. (See Appendix C and the CD-ROM for complete copies of growth grids.) ⊂▭⊃ **CD**

Body organs and systems, although not fully mature at 1 year, function differently than they did at birth. Kidney and liver maturation helps the 1-year-old excrete drugs or other toxic substances more readily than in the first weeks of life. The changing body proportions mirror changes in developing internal organs. Maturation of the nervous system is demonstrated by increased control over body movements, enabling the infant to sit, stand, and walk. Sensory function also increases as the infant begins to discriminate visual images, sounds, and tastes (Table 32–9).

Cognitive Development

The brain continues to increase in complexity during the first year. Most of the growth involves maturation of cells, with only a small increase in number of cells. This growth of the brain is accompanied by development of its functions. One has only to compare the behavior of an infant shortly after birth with that of a 1-year-old to understand the incredible maturation of brain function. The newborn's eyes widen in response to sound; the 1-year-old turns to the sound and recognizes its significance. The 2-month-old cries and coos; the 1-year-old says a few words and understands many more. The 6-week-old grasps a rattle for the first time; the 1-year-old reaches for toys and feeds himself or herself.

The infant's behaviors provide clues about thought processes. Piaget's work outlines the infant's actions in a set of rapidly progressing changes in the first year of life. The infant receives stimulation through sight, sound, and feeling, which the maturing brain interprets. This input from the environment interacts with internal cognitive abilities to enhance cognitive functioning.

Play

An 8-month-old infant is sitting on the floor, grasping blocks and banging them on the floor. When a parent walks by, the infant laughs and waves hands and feet wildly. Physical capabilities enable the infant to move toward and reach out for objects of interest. Cognitive ability is reflected in manipulation of the blocks to create different sounds. Social interaction enhances play. The presence of a parent or other person increases interest in surroundings and teaches the infant different ways to play.

The play of infants begins in a reflexive manner. When an infant moves extremities or grasps objects, the foundations of play are established. The feel and sound of these activities give pleasure to the infant, who gradually performs them purposefully. For example, when a parent places a rattle in the hand of a 6-week-old infant, the infant grasps it reflexively. As the hands move randomly, the rattle makes an enjoyable sound. The infant learns to move the rattle to create the sound and then finally to grasp the rattle at will to play with it.

The next phase of infant play focuses on manipulative behavior. The infant examines toys closely, looking at them, touching them, and placing them in the mouth. The infant learns a great deal about texture, qualities of objects, and all aspects of the surroundings. At the same time,

TABLE 32-9   Growth and Development Milestones During Infancy

Age	Physical Growth	Fine Motor Ability	Gross Motor Ability	Sensory Ability
Birth to 1 month	Gains 5–7 oz (140–200 g)/ week Grows 1.5 cm (½ in) in first month Head circumference increases 1.5 cm (½ in)/ month	Holds hand in fist (A) Draws arms and legs to body when crying	Inborn reflexes such as starte and rooting are predominant activity May lift head briefly if prone (B) Alerts to high-pitched voices Comforts with touch (C)	Prefers to look at faces and black-and-white geometric designs Follows objects in line of vision (D)

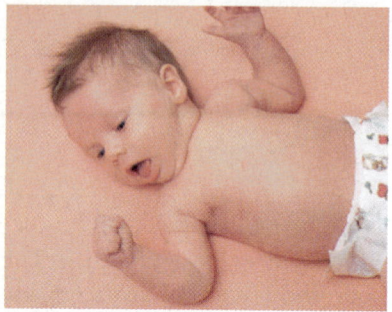

(A) Holds hand in fist

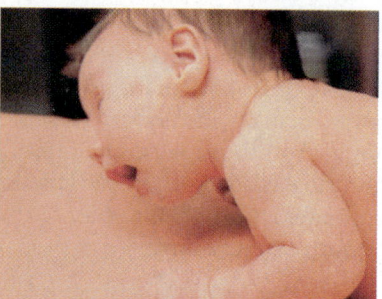

(B) May lift head

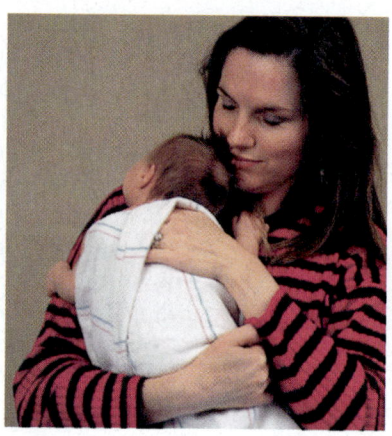

(C) Comforts with touch

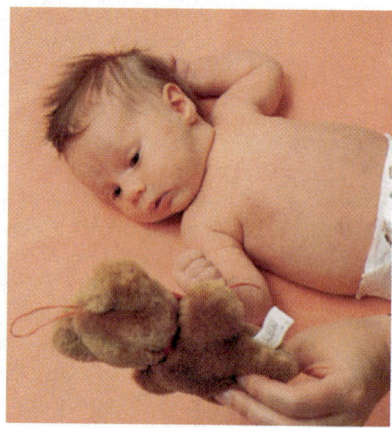

(D) Follows objects

Age	Physical Growth	Fine Motor Ability	Gross Motor Ability	Sensory Ability
2–4 months	Gains 5–7 oz (140–200 g)/ week Grows 1.5 cm (1/2 in)/month Head circumference increases 1.5 cm (1/2 in)/month Posterior fontanel closes Eats 120 mL/kg/24 hr (2 oz/lb/24 hr)	Holds rattle when placed in hand (E) Looks at and plays with own fingers Readily brings objects from hand to mouth	Moro reflex, fauding in strength Can turn from side to back and then return (F) Decrease in head log when pulled to sitting; sits with head held in midline with some bobbing When prone, holds head and supports weight on forearms (G)	Follows objects 180° Turns head to look for voices and sounds

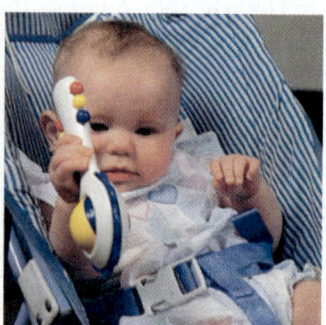

(E) Holds rattle

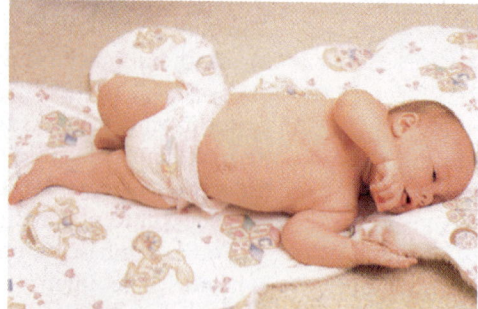

(F) Can turn from side to back

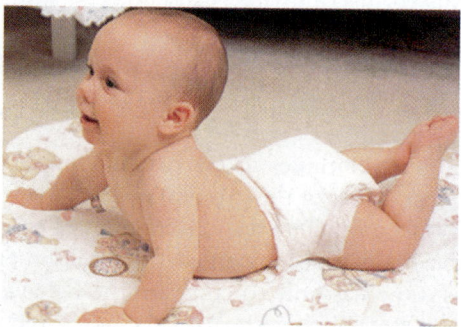

(G) Holds head up and supports weight with arms

TABLE 32-9 **Growth and Development Milestones During Infancy—continued**

Age	Physical Growth	Fine Motor Ability	Gross Motor Ability	Sensory Ability
4–6 months	Gains 5–7 oz (140–200 g)/week Doubles birth weight 5–8 months Grows 1.5 cm (1/2 in), month Head circumference increases 1.5 cm (1/2 in), month Teeth may begin erupting by 6 months Ears 100 mL/kg/24 hr (1 1/2 oz/lb/24 hr)	Grasps rattles and other objects at will: drops them to pick up another offered object (H) Mouths objects Holds feet and pulls to mouth Holds bottle Grasps with whole hand (palmar grasp) Manipulates objects (I)	Head held steady when sitting No head lag when pulled to sitting Turns from abdomen to back by 4 months and then back to abdomen by 6 months When held standing supports much of own weight (J)	Examines complex visual images Watches the course of a falling object Responds readily to sounds

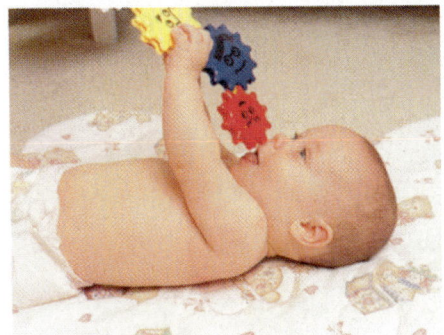

(H) Grasps objects at will

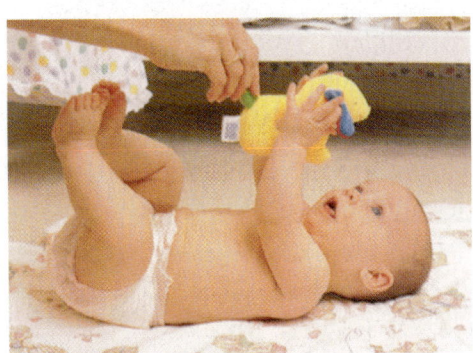

(I) Manipalates objects

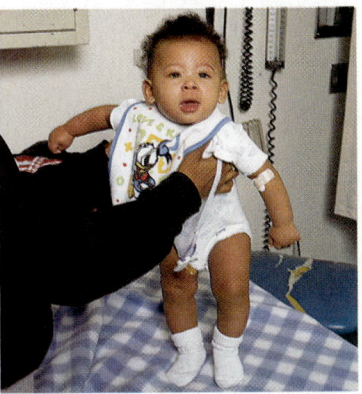

(J) Supports most of weight when held standing

Age	Physical Growth	Fine Motor Ability	Gross Motor Ability	Sensory Ability
6–8 months	Gains 3–5 oz (85–140 g)/week Grows 1 cm (3/8 in)/month Growth rate slower than first 6 months	Bangs two objects held in hands Transfers objects from one hand to the other Beginning pincer grasp at times	Most inborn reflexes extiguished Sits alone steadily without support by 8 months (K) Likes to bounce on legs when held in standing position	Recognizes own name and responds by looking and smiling Enjoys small and complex objects at play

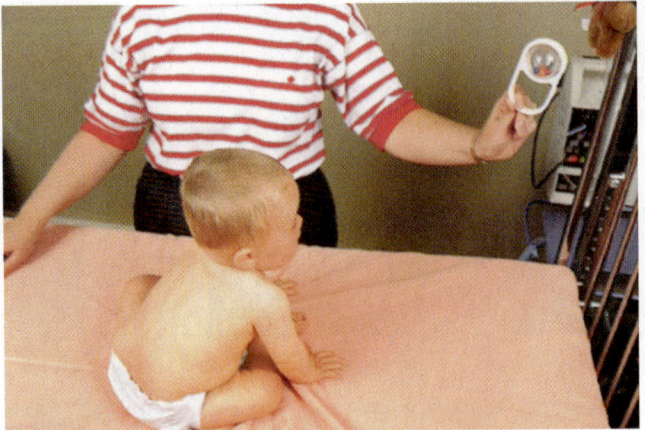

(K) Sits alone without support

(continued)

TABLE 32-9   Growth and Development Milestones During Infancy—continued

Age	Physical Growth	Fine Motor Ability	Gross Motor Ability	Sensory Ability
8–10 months	Gains 3–5 oz (85–140 g) week Grows 1 cm (3/8 in./month)	Picks up small objects (L) Uses pincer grasp well (N)	Crawls or pulls whole body along floor by arms (M) Creeps by using hands and knees to keep trunk off floor Pulls self to standing and sitting by 10 months Recovers balance when sitting	Understands words such as "no" and "cracker" May say one word in addition to "mama" and "dada" Recognizes sound without difficulty

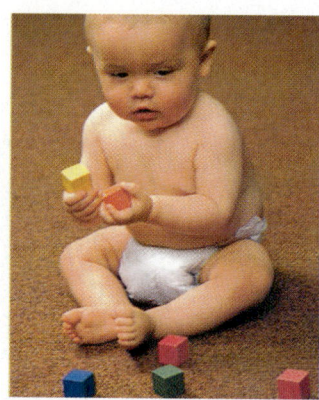

(L) Picks up small objects

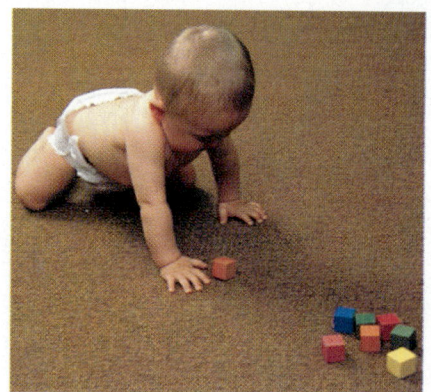

(M) Crawls or pulls body by arms

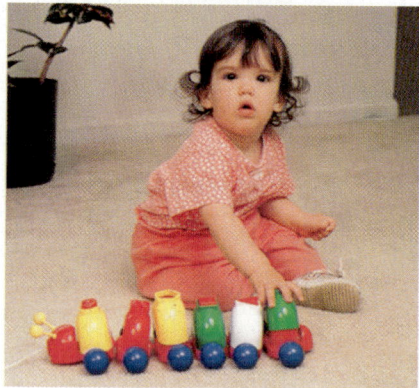

(N) Uses pincer grasp well

Age	Physical Growth	Fine Motor Ability	Gross Motor Ability	Sensory Ability
10–12 months	Gains 3–5 oz (85–140 g)/week Grows 1 cm (3/8 in.)/month Head circumference equals chest circumference Triples birth weight by 1 year	May hold crayon or pencil and make mark on paper Places objects into containers through holes (O)	Stands alone (P) Walks holding onto furniture Sits down from standing (Q)	Plays peek-a-boo and patty cake

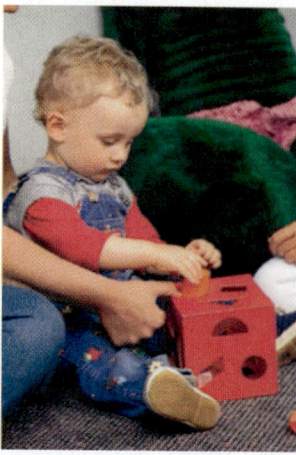

(O) Places objects in container through holes

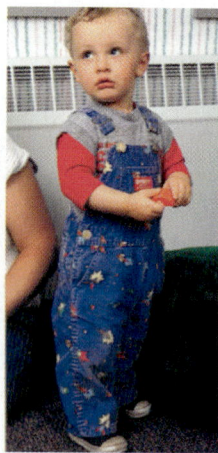

(P) Stands alone

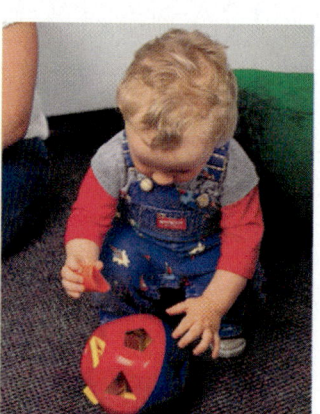

(Q) Sits down from standing

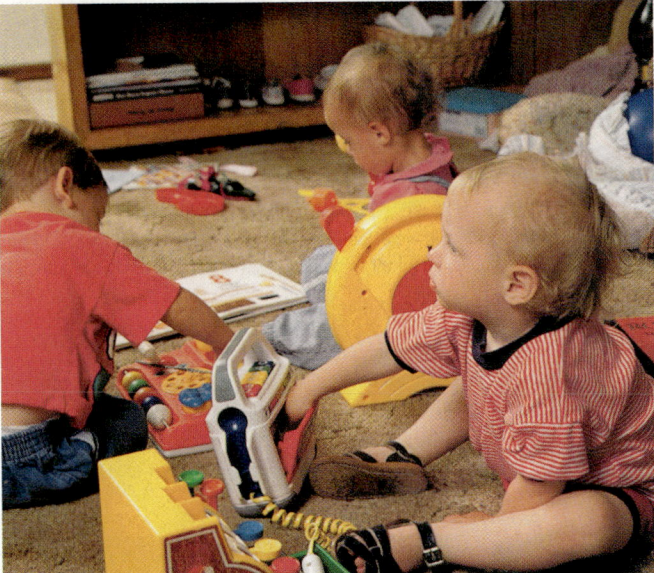

FIGURE 32-6. ◆ Mobility enlarges the sphere of play, allowing the child to seek new toys and spaces and to seek out people for interaction. Which psychosocial, cognitive, and motor skills do you see taking place in this photograph?

TABLE 32-10 Favorite Toys and Activities in Infancy
Birth to 2 months
Mobiles, black-and-white patterns, mirrors
Music boxes, singing, tape players, soft voices
Rocking and cuddling
Moving legs and arms while singing and talking
Varying stimuli—different rooms, sounds, visual images
3–6 months
Rattles
Stuffed animals
Soft toys with contrasting colors
Noise-making objects that are easily grasped
6–12 months
Large blocks
Teething toys
Toys that pop apart and back together
Nesting cups and other objects that fit into one another or stack
Surprise toys such as jack-in-the-box
Social interaction with adults and other children
Games such as peek-a-boo
Soft balls
Push and pull toys

interaction with others becomes an important part of play. The social nature of play is obvious as the infant plays with other children and adults.

Toward the end of the first year the infant's ability to move in space enlarges the sphere of play (Figure 32–6 ◆). Once the infant is crawling or walking, he or she can get to new places, find new toys, discover forgotten objects, or seek out other people for interaction. Play is a reflection of every aspect of development, as well as a method for enhancing learning and maturation (Table 32–10).

Injury Prevention

Injuries are a major cause of death in childhood. The infant is particularly vulnerable to injuries when not adequately supervised. Increasing mobility during the second half of the first year challenges parents to childproof the home and environment. The nurse can provide anticipatory guidance to help prevent unintentional injuries (Table 32–11).

Personality and Temperament

Why does one infant frequently awaken at night crying while another sleeps for 8 to 10 hours undisturbed? Why does one infant smile much of the time and react positively to interactions while another is withdrawn with unfamiliar people and frequently frowns and cries? Such differences in responses to the environment are believed to be inborn characteristics of temperament. Infants are born with a tendency to react in certain ways to noise and to interact differently with people. They may display varying degrees of regularity in activities of eating and sleeping, and manifest

Nursing Practice

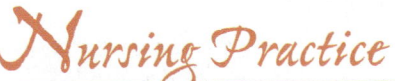

Cognitive and physical development mirror the changing hazards to the health and well-being of children. Injuries are a common cause of death and hospitalization during childhood. See Chapter 1 for statistics about the relationship of injury to morbidity and mortality in childhood. Nurses use **anticipatory guidance,** predicting the upcoming developmental tasks or needs of a child and performing appropriate teaching related to them, to discuss safety hazards and injury prevention for children of various ages with their parents.

Nursing Practice

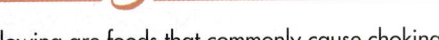

Following are foods that commonly cause choking:

Hot dogs	Ice cubes
Nuts	Grapes
Popcorn	Uncooked vegetable chunks
Hard candy	Lumps of peanut butter

a capacity for concentrating on tasks for different amounts of time.

Nursing assessment identifies personality characteristics of the infant that the nurse can share with the parents. With this information, the parents can appreciate more fully the uniqueness of their infant and design experiences to meet

TABLE 32–11 Injury Prevention in Infancy

Hazard	Developmental Characteristics	Preventive Measures
Falls	Mobility increases in first year of life, progressing from squirming movements to crawling, rolling, and standing	Do not leave infant unsecured in infant seat, even in newborn period. Do not place on high surfaces such as tables or beds unless holding child. (A) Once mobile by crawling, keep doors to stairways closed or use gates. Standing walkers have led to many injuries and are not recommended.
Burns	Infant is dependent on caretakers for environmental control. The second half of the first year is marked by crawling and increased mobility. Objects are explored by touching and placing in mouth.	Check temperature of both water and food liquids for drinking. Cover electrical outlets. Supervise infant so that play with electrical cords cannot occur.
Motor vehicle crashes	Infant is dependent on caretakers for placement in car. On impact with another motor vehicle, an infant held on a lap acts as a torpedo.	Use only approved restraint systems (according to Federal Motor Vehicle Safety Standards) The seat must be used for every trip, even if very short. The seat must be properly buckled to the car's lap belt system. (B)
Drowning	Infant cannot swim and is enable to lift head.	Never leave infant alone in a both of even 2.5 in of water. Supervise when in water even when a life preserver is worn. Flotation devices such as arm inflatables are not certified life preservers.

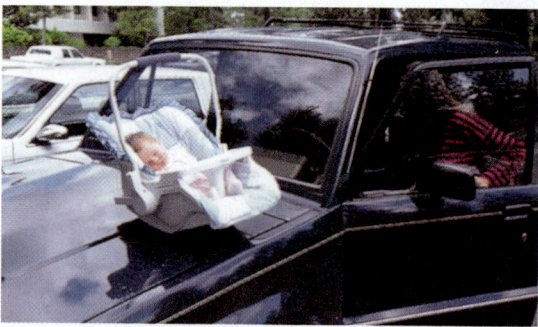

1(A) Never leave infant unsecured or on high surface.

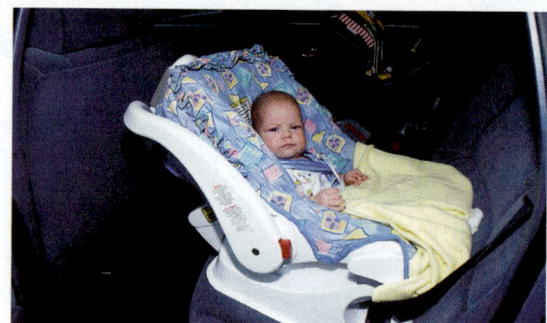

(B) Always use approved restraint system. Place infant in rear-facing seat in backseat of car.

Hazard	Developmental Characteristics	Preventive Measures
Poisoning	Infant is dependent on caretakers to keep harmful substances out of reach. The second half of infancy is marked by exploratory reaching and mouthing objects.	Keep medicines out of reach. Teach proper dosage and administration of medicines to parents. Cleaning products and other harmful substances should not be stored where the infant can reach them. Remove plants from play areas. Have poison control center number by telephone.
Choking	Infant explores objects by placing them in the mouth.(C)	Avoid foods that commonly cause choking. Keep small toys away from infants, especially toys labeled "not intended for use in those under 3 years."
Suffocation	Young infant has minimal head control and may be unable to move it vomiting or having difficulty breathing.	Position infant on back for sleep. Do not place pillows, stuffed toys, or other objects near head. Do not use plastic in crib. Avoid latex balloons. (D)
Strangulation	Infant is able to get head into railings or crib slats but cannot remove it.	Be sure older cribs have slats spaced 6 cm (2 3/8 in) or less apart. The mattress must fit tightly against the crib rails.

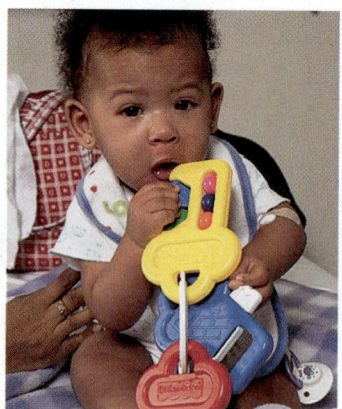

(C) Explores objects with mouth.

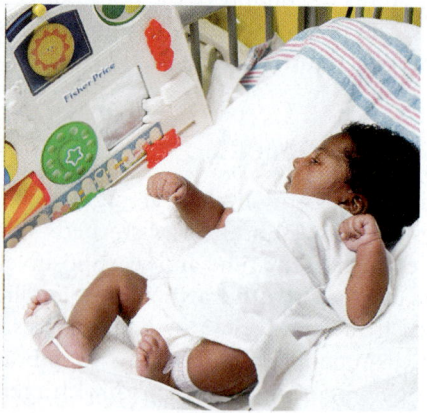

(D) Place infant on back for sleeping, keep toys clear.

the infant's needs. Parents can learn to modify the environment to promote adaptation. For example, an infant who does not adapt easily to new situations may cry, withdraw, or develop another way of coping when adjusting to new people or places. Parents might be advised to use one or two baby-sitters rather than engaging new sitters frequently. If the infant is easily distracted when eating, parents can feed the infant in a quiet setting to encourage a focus on eating. Although the infant's temperament is unchanged, the ability to fit with the environment is enhanced.

Communication

Even at a few weeks of age, infants communicate and engage in two-way interaction. Comfort is expressed by soft sounds, cuddling, and eye contact. The infant displays discomfort by thrashing the extremities, arching the back, and crying vigorously. From these rudimentary skills, communication ability continues to develop until the infant speaks several words at the end of the first year of life (Table 32–12).

Nurses assess communication to identify possible abnormalities or developmental delays. Language ability may be assessed with the Denver II Developmental Test and other specialized language screening tools (see Chapter 35). ⬤▬⬤ Normal infants understand (receptive speech) more words than they can speak (expressive speech). Abnormalities may be caused by a hearing deficit, developmental delay, or lack of verbal stimulation from caretakers. Further assessment may be required to pinpoint the cause of the abnormality.

Nursing interventions focus on providing a stimulating environment. Encourage parents to speak to infants and teach words. Hospital nurses should include the infant's known words when providing care.

TABLE 32–12 Patterns of Infant Communication

Age	Behavior
Birth to 2 months	Coos Babbles Comfort sounds Cries
3–6 months	Vocalizations with play and favorite people Laughs Cries less Squeals and makes pleasure sounds Multisyllabic babbling
6–9 months	Increasing vowel and consonant sounds Links syllables together Speechlike rhythm when "talking" with adult
9–12 months	Understands "no" and other simple commands Says "dada" and "mama" to identify parents Learns one or two other words Receptive speech surpasses expressive speech

Growth and Development

Following are strategies for communicating with the infant:

Hold for feedings.
Hold, rock, and talk to infant often.
Talk and sing frequently during care.
Tell names of objects.
Use high-pitched voice with newborns.
When the infant is upset, swaddle and hold securely.

TODDLER (1 TO 3 YEARS)

Toddlerhood is sometimes called the first adolescence. An infant only months before, the child from 1 to 3 years is now displaying independence and negativism. Pride in newfound accomplishments emerges.

Physical Growth and Development

The rate of growth slows during the second year of life. Parents may become concerned because the child has a limited food intake, and need reassurance that this is normal (see Chapter 31 for further discussion of nutrition in toddlerhood). ⬤▬⬤ By age 2 years, the birth weight has usually quadrupled and the child is about one half of the adult height. Body proportions begin to change, with the legs longer and the head smaller in proportion to body size than during infancy (see Figure 32–5). The toddler has a pot-bellied appearance and stands with feet apart to provide a wide base of support. By approximately 33 months, eruption of deciduous teeth is complete, with 20 teeth present. All parents need anticipatory guidance to meet toddlers needs and some parents, such as those with adopted children or with special health care needs, will need additional guidance.

Gross motor activity develops rapidly (Table 32–13), as the toddler progresses from walking to running, kicking, and riding a Big Wheel tricycle (Figure 32–7◆). As physical

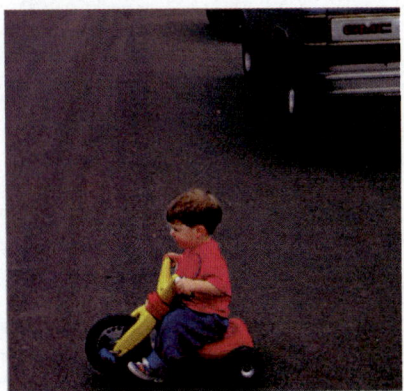

FIGURE 32–7. ◆ This toddler has learned to ride a Big Wheel, which he is doing right into the street. Toddlers must be watched closely to prevent injury.

TABLE 32-13   Growth and Development Milestones During Toddlerhood

Age	Physical Growth	Fine Motor Ability	Gross Motor Ability	Sensory Ability
1–2 years	Gains 227 g (8 oz) or more per month Grows 9–12 cm (3.5–5 in.) during this year Anterior fontanel closes	By end of 2nd year, builds a lower of four blocks (A) Scribbles on paper (B) Can undress self (C) Throws a ball	Runs Walks up and down stairs (E) Likes push and pull toys	Visual acuity 20/50
2–3 years	Gains 1.4–2.3 kg (3–5 lb)/year Grows 5–6.5 cm (2–2.5 in.)/year	Draws a circle and other rudimentary forms Learns to pout Learning to dress self (D)	Jumps Kicks ball (G) Throws ball overhand	

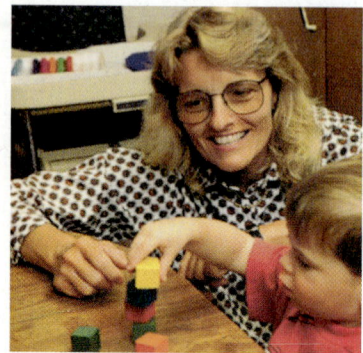

(A) Second year tower of four blocks

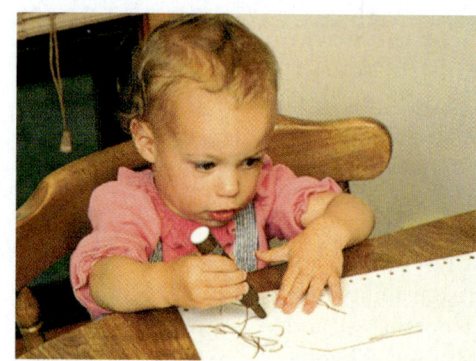

(B) Scribbles on paper

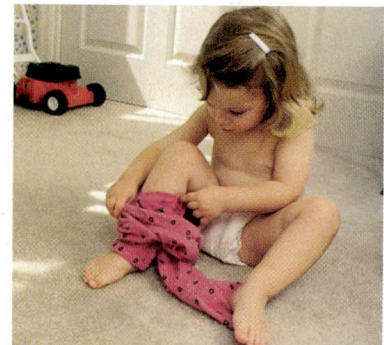

(C) Can undress self

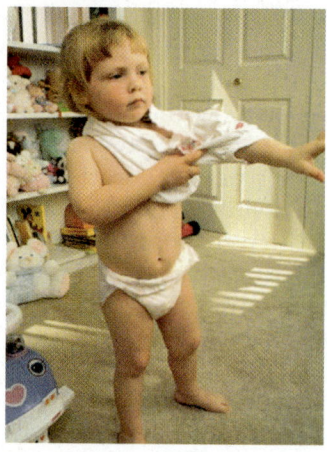

(D) Learning to dress self

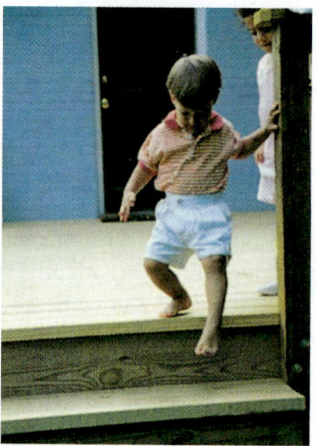

(E) Walks up and down stairs

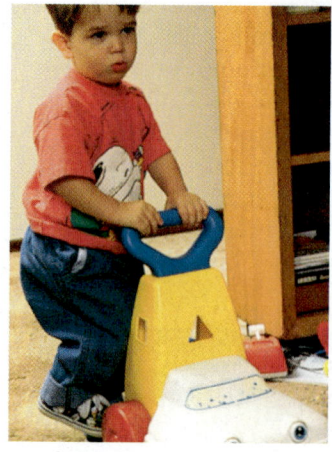

(F) Likes push and pull toys

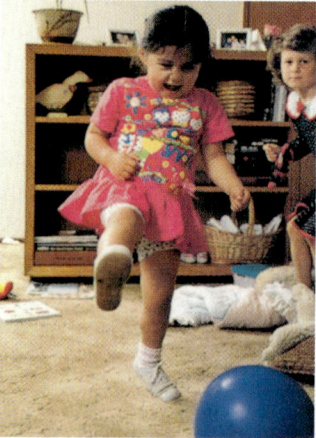

(G) Jumps and kicks ball

Thinking Critically

INTERNATIONAL ADOPTION COUNSELING

Michael and Alyssa had tried for several years to have a biologic child. After an unsuccessful in vitro fertilization, they decided to try to adopt a child. They explored opportunities with adoption agencies, and learned that international adoption would be possible for them. They adopted 2-year-old Irena from Romania several months ago.

Despite thorough investigation of Michael and Alyssa by the adoption agency, they received only scant information about Irena's history. She was given to an orphanage by her mother when she was about 7 months old; the mother stated that the pregnancy and delivery were normal. She was giving the child up because she had two older children to care for and her husband had left home nearly a year before and had not been heard from since. Irena appears small for her age, but is thriving in her new environment. She is learning to say a few English words and is responding appropriately to care and interactions.

How can you work with Michael and Alyssa to ensure special attention to Irena's growth and health care needs? What challenges in her early life may have influenced Irena's physical growth, her ability to interact with others, the timing of developmental milestones, and speech?

What will Irena's cultural needs be as she grows older? How can Michael and Alyssa prepare to tell her about her adoption and background someday? How can they learn about Irena's country of origin? 🔗 **WEB**

TABLE 32-14 Toilet Training

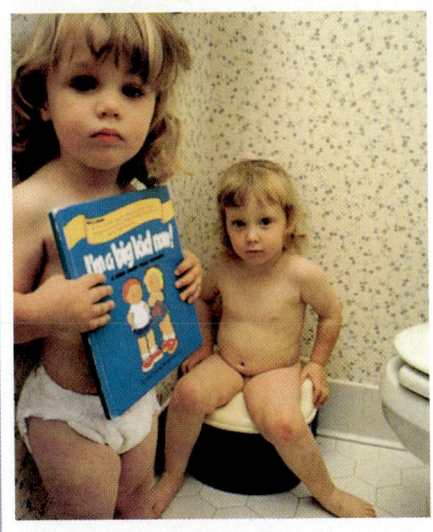

When are children ready to learn toileting? Are parents responsible for the differences in ages at which toilet training is accomplished? Does toilet training provide clues to a child's intellectual ability?

We know that children are not ready for toilet training until several developmental capabilities exist: to stand and walk well, to pull pants up and down, to recognize the need to eliminate and then to be able to wait until in the bathroom. Once this readiness is apparent, the child can be given a small potty chair and the procedure explained.

Children often prefer their own chair on the floor to using the large toilet. The child should be placed on the chair at regular intervals for a few moments and can be given reward or praise for successes. If the child seems not to understand or does not wish to cooperate, it is best to wait a few weeks and then try again. Just as all of development is subject to individual timetables, toilet training occurs with considerable variability from one child to another. Identify for parents the developmental characteristics of their child and encourage them to appreciate without anxiety the unfolding of skills. These timetables are not predictive of future development.

The child who is ill or hospitalized or has other stress often regresses in toilet training activities. It is best to quietly reinstitute attempts at training after the trauma. Potty chairs should be available on pediatric units and toileting habits identified during initial assessment so that regular routines can be followed and the child's usual words for elimination can be used.

---

maturation occurs, the toddler develops the ability to control elimination patterns (Table 32–14).

Cognitive Development

During the toddler years the child moves from the sensorimotor to the preoperational stage of development. The early use of language awakens in the 1-year-old the ability to think about objects or people when they are absent. Object permanence is well developed.

At about 2 years of age, the increasing use of words as symbols enables the toddler to use preoperational thought. Rudimentary problem solving, creative thought, and an understanding of cause-and-effect relationships are now possible.

Play

Many changes in play patterns occur between infancy and toddlerhood. The toddler's motor skills enable him or her to bang pegs into a pounding board with a hammer, for example. The social nature of toddler play is also readily seen. Toddlers find the company of other children pleasurable, even though socially interactive play may not occur. Two toddlers tend to play with similar objects side by side, occasionally trading toys and words. This is called **parallel play.** This playtime with other children helps toddlers develop social skills. Toddlers engage in play activities they

Developing Cultural Competence

In traditional Native-American families, children are allowed to unfold and develop naturally at their own pace. Children thus wean and toilet train themselves with little interference or pressure from parents.

have seen at home, such as pounding with a hammer and talking on the phone. This imitative behavior teaches them new actions and skills.

Physical skills are manifested in play as toddlers push and pull objects, climb in and out and up and down, run, ride a Big Wheel, turn the pages of books, and scribble with a pen. Both gross motor and fine motor abilities are enhanced during this age period.

Cognitive understanding enables the toddler to manipulate objects and learn about their qualities. Stacking blocks and placing rings on a building tower teach spatial relationships and other lessons that provide a foundation for future learning. Various kinds of play objects should be provided for the toddler to meet play needs. These play needs can easily be met whether the child is hospitalized or at home (Table 32–15).

Injury Prevention

By 1 year of age, unintentional injuries are by far the leading cause of death in children (see Chapter 1). Injuries also cause disfigurement and other ongoing health problems. Nurses intervene to care for injured children in the hospital and are responsible for making sure that the hospital environment is free of safety hazards. Nurses are also instrumental in teaching parents how to make the toddler's environment safe (Table 32–16).

Personality and Temperament

The toddler retains most of the temperamental characteristics identified during infancy but may demonstrate some changes. The normal developmental progression of toddlerhood also plays a part in responses. For example, the infant who previously responded positively to stimuli, such as a new baby-sitter, may appear more negative in toddlerhood.

TABLE 32-15 Favorite Toys and Activities in Toddlerhood

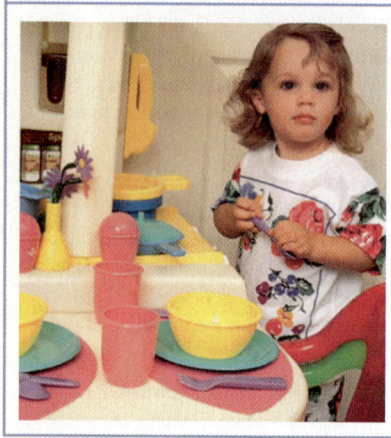

Play Need	Types of Toys and Activities
Facilitate imitative behavior	Play kitchen Grocery carts Pounding board Toy phone
Encourage gross motor activity and provide an outlet for stress	Big Wheel tricycle Soft ball and bat Water and sand Bean bag toss
Foster fine motor skills	Cloth books Large pencil and paper Wooden puzzles
Facilitate cognitive growth	Educational television shows Music Stories and books

TABLE 32-16 Injury Prevention in Toddlerhood

	Hazard	Developmental Characteristics	Preventive Measures
	Falls	Gross motor skills improve. Toddler is able to move chairs to counters and can climb up ladders.	Supervise toddler closely. Provide safe climbing toys. Begin to teach acceptable places for climbing.
	Poisoning	Gross motor skills enable toddler to climb onto chairs and then cabinets. Medicines, cosmetics, and other poisonous substances are easily reached.	Keep medicines and other poisonous materials locked away. Use child resistant containers and cupboard closures. Have poison control center number (1-800-222-1222) by telephone. Keep syrup of ipecac in home (call Poison Control Center before using).
	Burns	Toddler is tall enough to reach stove top. Toddler can walk to fireplace and may reach into fire.	Keep pot handles turned inward on slove. Do not burn fires without close supervision. Use a fire screen.
	Motor vehicle crashes	Toddler may be able to undo seat belt, may resist using car seat, demonstrating characteristic negativism and autonomy.	Insist on safety seat use for all trips. Use approved safety seats only, such as forward-facing convertible seat placed in the car back seat. Toddler is not large enough to use car seat belts.

	Hazard	Developmental Characteristics	Preventive Measures
	Drowning	Toddler can walk onto docks or pool decks. Toddler may stand on or climb seats on boat. Toddler may fall into buckets, toilets, and fish tanks and be unable to get top of body out.	Supervise any child near water. Swimming classes do not protect a toddler from Use child-resistant pool covers. Use approved child life jackets near water and on boats. Empty buckets when not in use.

The increasing independence characteristic of this age is shown by the toddler's use of the word *no*. The parent and child constantly adapt their responses to each other and learn anew how to communicate with each other.

Communication

Because of the phenomenal growth of language skills during the toddler period, adults should communicate frequently with children in this age group. Toddlers imitate words and speech intonations, as well as the social interactions they observe.

At the beginning of toddlerhood, the child may use four to six words in addition to *mama* and *dada*. Receptive speech (the ability to understand words) far outpaces expressive speech. By the end of toddlerhood, however, the 3-year-old has a vocabulary of almost 1000 words and uses short sentences.

Communication occurs in many ways, some of which are nonverbal. Toddler communication includes pointing, pulling an adult over to a room or object, and speaking in expressive jargon. **Expressive jargon** is using unintelligible words with normal speech intonations as if truly communicating in words. Another communication method occurs when the toddler cries, pounds feet, displays a temper tantrum, or uses other means to illustrate dismay. These powerful communication methods can upset parents, who often need suggestions for handling them. It is best to verbalize the feelings shown by the toddler—for example, by saying, "You must be very upset that you cannot have that candy. When you stop crying you can come out of your room"—and then to ignore further negative behavior. The

Teaching About

PROPER CHILD SAFETY USE CHART

	INFANTS	TODDLER	YOUNG CHILDREN
WEIGHT	Birth to 1 year up to 20–22 lbs.	Over 1 year and over 20 lbs.–40 lbs.	Over 40 lbs. Ages 4–8, unless 4'9".
TYPE OF SEAT	Infant only or rear-facing convertible	Convertible/Forward-facing	Belt positioning booster seat
SEAT POSITION	Rear-facing only	Forward-facing	Forward-facing
ALWAYS MAKE SURE:	Children to one year and at least 20 lbs. in rear-facing seats Harness straps at or below shoulder level	Harness traps should be at or above shoulders Most seats require top slot for forward-facing	Belt positioning booster seats must be used with both lap and shoulder belt. Make sure the lap belt fits low and right across the lap/upper thigh area and the shoulder belt fits snug crossing the chest and shoulder to avoid abdominal injuries.
WARNING	All children age 12 and under should ride in the back seat	All children age 12 and under should ride in the back seat	All children age 12 and under should ride in the back seat

Note: From the National Highway Traffic Safety Administration.

Growth and Development

toddler's search for autonomy and independence creates a need for such behavior. Sometimes an upset toddler responds well to holding, rocking, and stroking.

Parents and nurses can promote a toddler's communication by speaking frequently, naming objects, explaining procedures in simple terms, expressing feelings that the toddler seems to be displaying, and encouraging speech. The toddler from a bilingual home is at an optimal age to learn two languages. If the parents do not speak English, the toddler will benefit from a day care experience in which the providers do, so that he or she can learn both languages.

The nurse who understands the communication skills of toddlers is able to assess expressive and receptive language and communicate effectively, thereby promoting positive health care experiences for these children (Table 32–17).

TABLE 32–17 Communicating with a Toddler

Procedures such as drawing blood can be frightening for a toddler. Effective communication minimizes the trauma caused by such procedures:

- Avoid telling toddlers about the procedure too far in advance. They do not have an understanding of time and can become quite anxious.
- Use simple terminology. "We need to get a little blood from your arm. It will help us to find out if you are getting better." If the parent is willing, say, "Your mom will hold your arm still so we can do it quickly."
- Allow the toddler to cry. Acknowledge that it must be frightening and that you understand.
- Perform the procedure in a treatment room so that the toddler's bed and room are a safe haven.
- Be sure the toddler is restrained, with the joints above and below the procedure immobilized.
- Use a Band-Aid to cover up the site. This can reassure the toddler that the body is still intact.
- Allow the toddler to choose a reward such as a sticker after the procedure.
- Praise the toddler for cooperation and acknowledge that you know this was difficult.
- Comfort the toddler by rocking, offering a favorite drink, playing music, and holding. If parents are present, they can offer the comfort needed.

PRESCHOOL CHILD (3 TO 6 YEARS)

The preschool years are a time of new initiative and independence. Most children are in a day care center or school for part of the day and learn a great deal from this social contact. Language skills are well developed, and the child is able to understand and speak clearly. Endless projects characterize the world of busy preschoolers. They may work with play dough to form animals, then cut out and paste paper, then draw and color.

Physical Growth and Development

Preschoolers grow slowly and steadily, with most growth taking place in long bones of the arms and legs. The short, chubby toddler gradually gives way to a slender, long-legged preschooler (Table 32–18).

Physical skills continue to develop (Figure 32–8 ◆). The preschooler runs with ease, holds a bat, and throws balls of various types. Writing ability increases, and the preschooler enjoys drawing and learning to write a few letters.

The preschool period is a good time to encourage good dental habits. Children can begin to brush their own teeth with parental supervision and help to reach all tooth surfaces. Parents should floss children's teeth, give fluoride as ordered if the water supply is not fluoridated (Table 32–19), and schedule the first dental visit

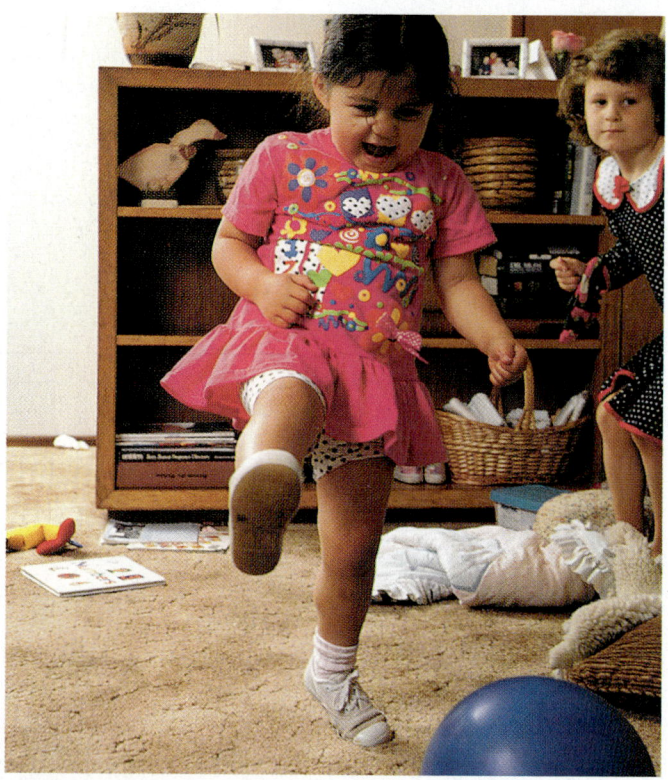

FIGURE 32–8. ◆ Preschoolers continue to develop more advanced skills such as kicking a ball without falling down.

TABLE 32-18 Growth and Development Milestones During Preschool

Physical Growth		Fine Motor Ability

Gains 1.5–2.5 kg (3–5 lb)/year

Grows 4–6 cm (1 1/2–2 1/2 in)/year

Uses scissors (A)

Draws circle, square, cross (B)

Draws at least a six-part person

Enjoys art projects such as pasting, stringing beads, using clay

Learns to tie shoes at end of preschool years (C)

Buttons (D)

Brushes teeth (E)

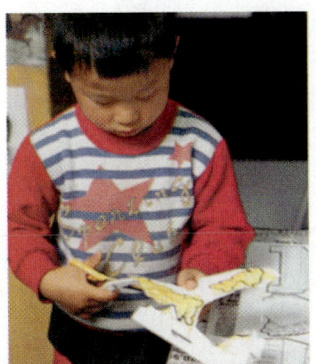

(A) Uses scissors

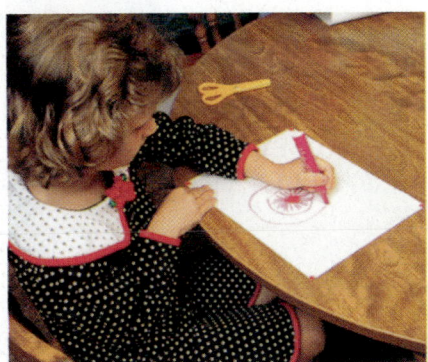

(B) Draws circle, square, cross

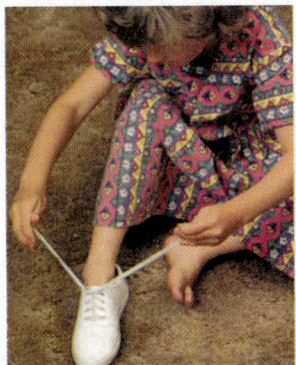

(C) Ties shoes

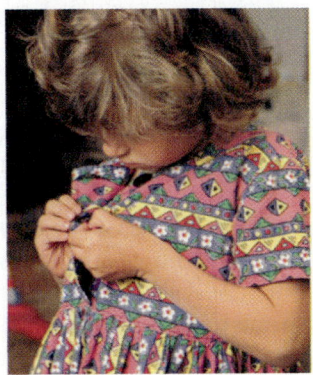

(D) Buttons clothes

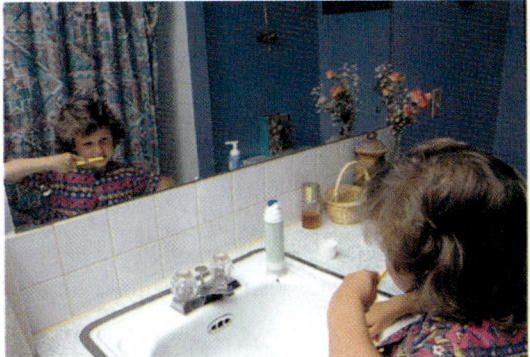

(E) Brushes teeth

Gross Motor Ability
Throws a ball overhand
Climbs well (F)
Rides bicycle (G)

Sensory Ability
Visual acuity continues to improve
Can focus on and learn letters and numbers (H)

Fine Motor Ability
Eats three meals with snacks
Uses spoon, fork, and knife

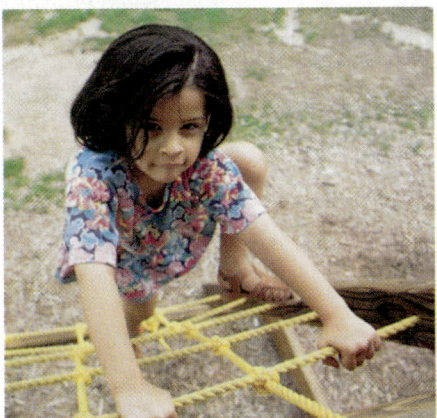

(F) Climbs well

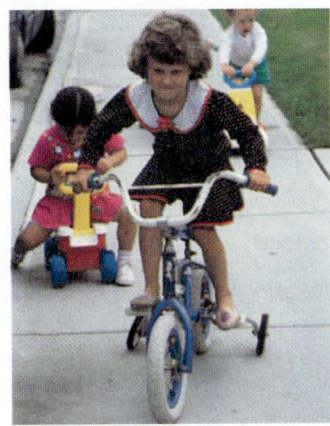

(G) Rides bicycle or bicycle with training wheels

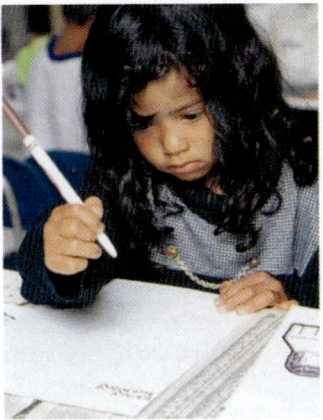

(H) Learns letters and numbers

TABLE 32-19 Recommended Daily Fluoride Dosages

	Amount of Fluoride in Water Supply		
Age	Under 0.3 ppm	0.3–0.6 ppm	Above 0.6 ppm
Under 6 months	0	0	0
6 months to 3 years	0.25 mg	0	0
3–6 years	0.50 mg	0.25 mg	0
6–16 years	1.00 mg	0.50 mg	0
ppm, parts per million.			

Note: Fluoride is available as a liquid to be mixed in a small amount of food or fluid for the infant and toddler and as a chewable tablet for the older child. It acts both systemically to promote strong teeth before they erupt and topically to strengthen tooth surfaces with which it comes in contact. *Note:* From Bindler, R. M., & Howry, L. B. (1997). *Pediatric drugs and nursing implications* (2nd ed., pp. 253–255). Upper Saddle River, NJ: Prentice Hall.

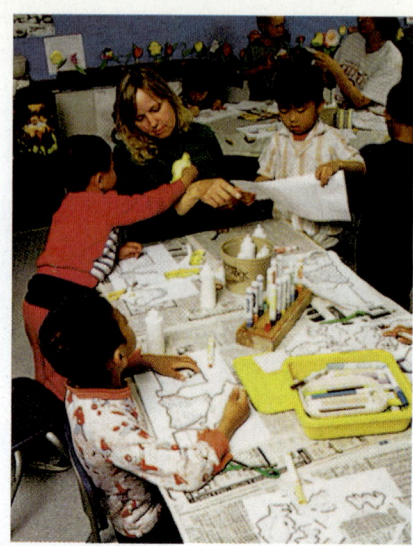

FIGURE 32-9. ◆ These preschoolers are participating in associative play, which means they can interact. One child is cutting out shapes, and the other is gluing them in place. Of course, every job needs a supervisor, who can be seen on the right.

so the child can become accustomed to the routine of periodic dental care.

Cognitive Development

The preschooler exhibits characteristics of preoperational thought. Symbols or words are used to represent objects and people, enabling the young child to think about them. This is a milestone in intellectual development; however, the preschooler still has some limitations in thought (Table 32–20).

Play

The preschooler has begun playing in a new way. Toddlers simply play side by side with friends, each engaging in his or her own activities, but preschoolers interact with others during play. One child cuts out colored paper, for example, while her friend glues it on paper in a design. This new type of interaction is called **associative play** (Figure 32–9 ◆).

In addition to this social dimension of play, other aspects of play also differ. The preschooler enjoys large motor activities such as swinging, riding a tricycle, and throwing a ball. Increasing manual dexterity is demonstrated in greater complexity of drawings and manipulation of blocks and modeling. These changes necessitate planning of playtime to include appropriate activities. Preschool programs and child life departments in hospitals help meet this important need.

Materials provided for play can be simple but should guide activities in which the child engages. Since fine motor activities are popular, paper, pens, scissors, glue, and a variety of other such objects should be available. The child can use them to create important images such as pictures of people, hospital beds, or friends. A collection of dolls, furniture, and clothing can be manipulated to represent parents and children, nurses and physicians, teachers, or

TABLE 32-20 Characteristics of Preoperational Thought

Characteristic	Definition	Example
Egocentrism	Ability to see things only from one's own point of view	The child who cannot understand why parents may need to leave the hospital for work when the child wishes them to be present
Transductive reasoning	Connecting two events in a cause-effect relationship simply because they occur together in time	A child who, awakening after surgery and feeling pain, notices the intravenous infusion and believes that it is causing the pain
Centration	Focusing on only one particular aspect of a situation	The child who is concerned about breathing through on anesthesia mask and will not listen to any other aspects of preoperative teaching
Animism	Giving lifelike qualities to nonliving things	The child who views a monitoring machine as alive because it beeps

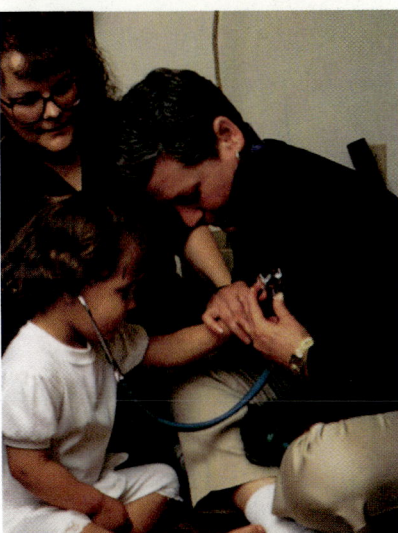

FIGURE 32–10. ◆ Jasmine is participating in dramatic play with a nurse while her mother looks on. In dramatic play the child uses props to play out the drama of human life. It can be an excellent way for a nurse to assess the developmental level of children while talking to them. Notice that the child and the nurse are on the floor of the same level and the atmosphere is informal. Why is it important to be at the same level as the child?

TABLE 32–21 Favorite Toys and Activities in the Preschool Years	
Play Need	*Types of Toys and Activities*
Facilitate associative play	Simple games
	Puzzles
	Nursery rhymes, songs
Promote dramatic play	Dolls and doll clothes
	Play houses and hospitals
	Dress-up clothes
	Puppets
Encourage outlet for stress	Pens, paper
	Glue, scissors
Facilitate cognitive growth	Educational television shows
	Music
	Stories and books

other significant people. Because fantasy life is so powerful at this age, the preschooler readily uses props to engage in **dramatic play,** that is, the living out of the drama of human life (Figure 32–10 ◆).

The nurse can use playtime to assess the preschool child's developmental level, knowledge about health care, and emotions related to health care experiences. Observations about objects chosen for play, content of dramatic play, and pictures drawn can provide important assessment data. The nurse can also use play periods to teach the child about health care procedures and offer an outlet for expression of emotions (Table 32–21).

Injury Prevention

The increasing independence of preschool children puts them at risk of injury. The 3- to 7-year-old group is at high risk of injury from fire, drowning, and motor vehicle and pedestrian accidents (see Chapter 1). Nurses can teach parents preventive measures and can also begin to include preschoolers in safety teaching (Table 32–22).

Personality and Temperament

Characteristics of personality observed in infancy tend to persist over time. The preschooler may need assistance as these characteristics are expressed in the new situations of preschool or nursery school. An excessively active child, for example, will need gentle, consistent handling to adjust to the structure of a classroom. Encourage parents to visit preschool programs to choose the one that would best foster growth in their child. Some preschoolers enjoy the structured learning of a program that focuses on cognitive skills, whereas others are happier and more open to learning in a small group that provides much time for free play. Nurses can help parents to identify their child's personality or temperament characteristics and to find the best environment for growth.

Communication

Language skills blossom during the preschool years. The vocabulary grows to over 2000 words, and children speak in complete sentences of several words and use all parts of speech. They practice these newfound language skills by endlessly talking and asking questions.

The sophisticated speech of preschoolers mirrors the development occurring in their minds and helps them to learn about the world around them. However, this speech can be quite deceptive. Although preschoolers use many words, their grasp of meaning is usually literal and may not match that of adults. These literal interpretations have important implications for health care providers. For example, the preschooler who is told she will be "put to sleep" for surgery may think of a pet recently euthanized; the child who is told that a dye will be injected for a diagnostic test may think he is going to die; mention of "a little stick" in the arm can cause images of tree branches rather than of a simple immunization.

The child may also have difficulty focusing on the content of a conversation. The preschooler is egocentric and may be unable to move from individual thoughts to those the nurse is proposing in a teaching situation.

Concrete visual aids such as pictures of a child undergoing the same procedure or a book to read together enhance teaching by meeting the child's developmental needs. Handling medical equipment such as intravenous bags and stethoscopes increases interest and helps the child to focus. Teaching may have to be done in several short sessions rather than one long session.

TABLE 32-22   **Injury Prevention in the Preschool Years**

	Hazards	Developmental Characteristics	Preventive Measures
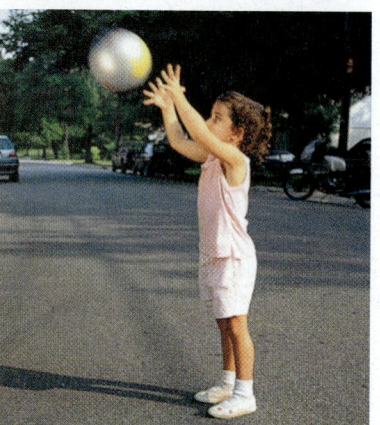	Motor vehicle crashes	Older preschooler independently gets into car and puts on seat belt. Child may forget to belt up or may do so incorrectly.	Verify that child is belted in properly before starting car. Child restraint systems used until child weighs 18 kg (40 lb) and is 100 cm (40 in) tall.
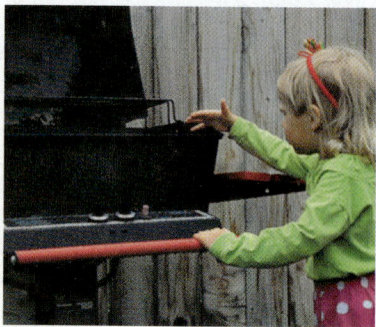	Motor vehicle and pedestrian accidents	Preschooler increasingly plays outside alone or with friends. Preschooler is unable to judge speed of moving car and assumes driver knows that he or she is present.	Teach child never to go into road. A safe, preferably enclosed, play yard is recommended.
	Drowning	Preschooler who has has swimming lessons may choose to go into a lake or pool.	Teach child never to go into water without an adult. Provide supervision when ever child is near water.
	Burns	Preschooler can understand hazards of fire.	Teach child to stop, drop, and roll if clothes are on fire. Practice escapes from home are useful. A visit to a fire station can reinforce learning. Teach child how to call 911.
	Needle sticks in hospitals Electrical injury in hospital	Preschooler can ambulate and is interested in new objects. Preschooler is mobile and may trip over cords and equipment or may choose to examine them.	Keep needles out of reach. Remove immediately after use. Avoid use of electrical cords if possible. Keep equipment out of major traffic areas. Keep beds away from electrical outlets. Monitor child closely.

Growth and Development

Following are strategies for communicating with the preschooler:

Allow time for child to integrate explanations.

Verbalize frequently to the child.

Use drawings and stories to explain care.

Use accurate names for body functions.

Allow choices.

SCHOOL-AGE CHILD (6 TO 12 YEARS)

Errol, 10 years old, arrives home from school shortly after 3 P.M. each day. He immediately calls his friends and goes to visit one of them. They are building models of cars and collecting baseball cards. Endless hours are spent on these projects and on discussions of events at school that day (Figure 32–11◆).

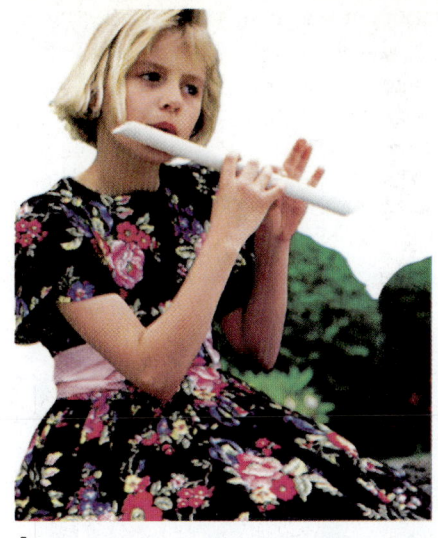

A

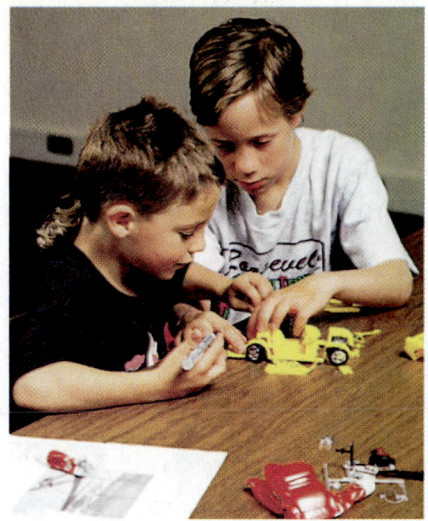

B

FIGURE 32-11. ◆ **A,** School-age children may take part in activities that require practice. This is a consideration when children are hospitalized and unable to practice or perform. Why? **B,** School-age children enjoy spending time with others the same age on projects and discussing the activities of the day. This is an important consideration when they are in an acute care setting. When you are in the clinical setting, look for facilities where this type of interaction is taking place.

Nine-year-old Karen practices soccer two afternoons a week and plays in games each weekend. She also is learning to play the flute and spends her free time at home practicing. Although practice time is not her favorite part of music, Karen enjoys the performances and wants to play well in front of her friends and teacher. Her parents now allow her to ride her bike unaccompanied to the store or to a friend's house.

These two school-age children demonstrate common characteristics of their age group. They are in a stage of industry in which it is important to the child to perform useful work. Meaningful activities take on great importance and are usually carried out in the company of peers. A sense of achievement in these activities is important to develop self-esteem and to prevent a sense of inferiority or poor self-worth.

Physical Growth and Development

School age is the last period in which girls and boys are close in size and body proportions. As the long bones continue to grow, leg length increases (see Figure 32–6). Fat gives

way to muscle, and the child appears leaner. Jaw proportions change as the first deciduous tooth is lost at 6 years and permanent teeth begin to erupt. Body organs and the immune system mature, resulting in fewer illnesses among school-age children. Medications are less likely to cause serious side effects, since they can be metabolized more easily. The urinary system can adjust to changes in fluid status. Physical skills are also refined as children begin to play sports, and fine motor skills are well developed through school activities (Table 32–23 and Figure 32–12 ◆).

Although it is commonly believed that the start of adolescence (age 12 years) heralds a growth spurt, the rapid increases in size commonly occur during school age. Girls may begin a growth spurt by 9 or 10 years and boys a year or so later. Nutritional needs increase dramatically with this spurt.

The loss of the first deciduous teeth and the eruption of permanent teeth usually occur at about age 6, or at the beginning of the school-age period. Of the 30 permanent teeth, 22 to 26 erupt by age 12 and the remaining molars follow during the teenage years. The school-age child should be closely monitored to ensure that brushing and

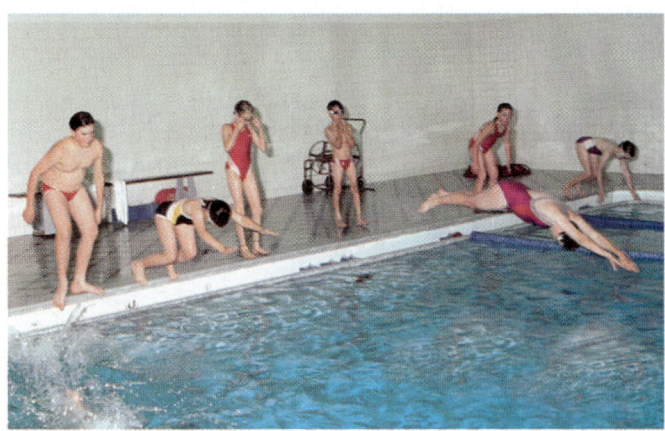

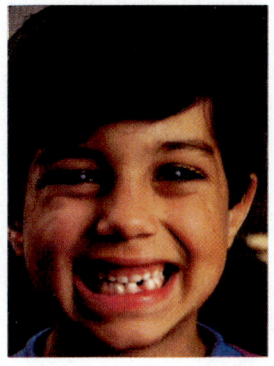

FIGURE 32-12. ◆ School-age girls and boys enjoy participating in sports. They begin to lose fat while developing their muscles, so they appear leaner than at earlier ages. *Inset,* Front teeth are lost around age 6. The family may have rituals associated with the loss of teeth that could affect the child's behavior if he loses a tooth while in the hospital.

TABLE 32–23　Growth and Development Milestones During the School-Age Years

Physical Growth	Fine Motor Ability	Gross Motor Ability	Sensory Ability
Gains 1.4–2.2 kg (3–5 lb), year Grows 4–6 cm (1 1/2–2 1/2 in), year	Enjoys craft projects Plays card and board games	Rides two-wheeler (A) Jumps rope (B) Roller skates or ice skates	Can read Able to concentrate for longer periods on activities by filtering out surrounding sounds (C)

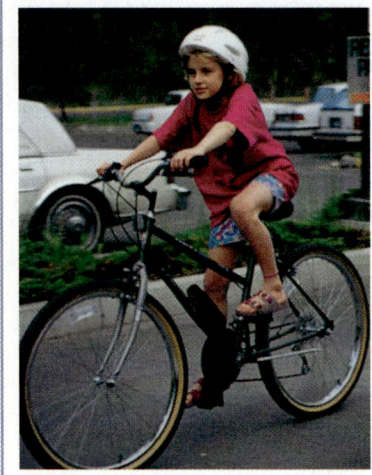

(A) Rides two-wheeler

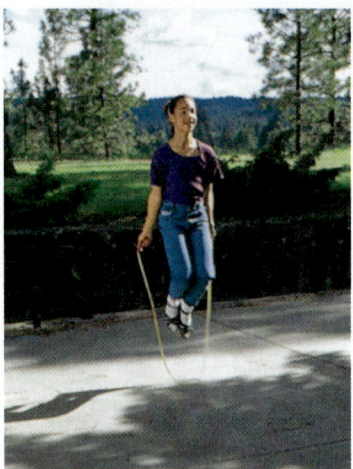

(B) Jumps rope

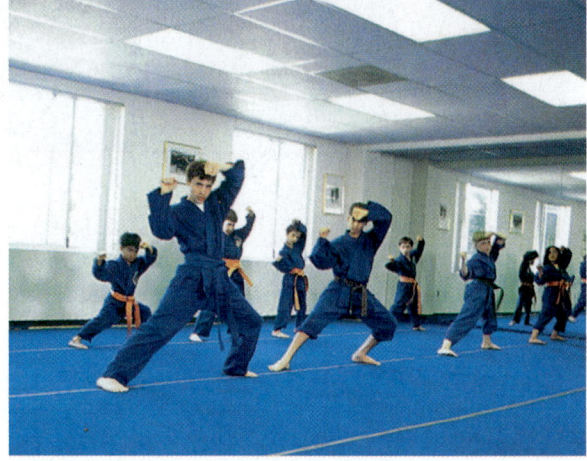

(C) Concentrates an activities for longer periods

flossing are adequate, that fluoride is taken if the water supply is not fluoridated, that dental care is obtained to provide for examination of teeth and alignment, and that loose teeth are identified before surgery or other events that may lead to loss of a tooth.

Cognitive Development

The child enters the stage of concrete operational thought at about 7 years. This stage enables school-age children to consider alternative solutions and solve problems. However, school-age children continue to rely on concrete experiences and materials to form their thought content.

During the school-age years the child learns the concept of **conservation** (that matter is not changed when its form is altered). At earlier ages, a child believes that when water is poured from a short, wide glass into a tall, thin glass, there is more water in the taller glass. The school-age child recognizes that although it may look like the taller glass holds more water, the quantity is the same. The concept of conservation is helpful when the nurse explains medical treatments. The school-age child understands that an incision will heal, that a cast will be removed, and that an arm will look the same as before once the intravenous infusion is removed.

Play

When the preschool teacher tries to organize a game of baseball, both the teacher and the children become frus-

TABLE 32–24　Favorite Play Activities of School-Age Children

Play Need	Types of Activities
Foster gross motor activity	Ball sports Skating Dance lessons Water and snow skiing Biking
Promote sense of industry	Musical instrument Collections (e.g., stamps, miniatures) Hobbies Board and video games
Facilitate cognitive growth	Reading Crafts Word puzzles

trated. Not only are the children physically unable to hold a bat and hit a ball, but they seem to have no understanding of the rules of the game and do not want to wait for their turn at bat. By 6 years of age, however, children have acquired the physical ability to hold the bat properly and may occasionally hit the ball. School-age children also understand that everyone has a role—the pitcher, the catcher, the batter, the outfielders. They cooperate with one another to form a team, are eager to learn the rules of the game, and want to ensure that these rules are followed exactly (Table 32–24).

The characteristics of play exhibited by the school-age child are cooperation with others and the ability to play a part in order to contribute to a unified whole. This type of play is called **cooperative play.** The concrete nature of cognitive thought leads to a reliance on rules to provide structure and security. Children have an increasing desire to spend much of playtime with friends, which demonstrates the social component of play. Play is an extremely important method of learning and living for the school-age child. Active physical play has decreased in recent years as television viewing and playing of computer games have increased, leading to poor nutritional status and other health risks in children. The incidence of children who are overweight (above the 85th percentile) has increased from 15% to 22% in the past three decades (Troiano, Flegel, Kuczmarski, et al., 1995). Nurses can teach healthy snacking habits and the importance of regular daily exercise. Weigh children during each health encounter and perform more detailed dietary history when findings suggest overweight or inadequate nutrition. See Chapter 31 for further discussion of nutrition and physical activity in children.

When a child is hospitalized, the separation from playmates can lead to feelings of sadness and purposelessness. School-age children often feel better when placed in multibed units with other children. Games can be devised even when children are wheelchair bound (Figure 32–13 ◆). Normal, rewarding parts of play should be integrated into care. Friends should be encouraged to visit or call a hospitalized child. Discharge planning for the child who has had a cast or brace applied should address the activities the child can engage in and those the child must avoid. Reinforce the importance of playing games with friends.

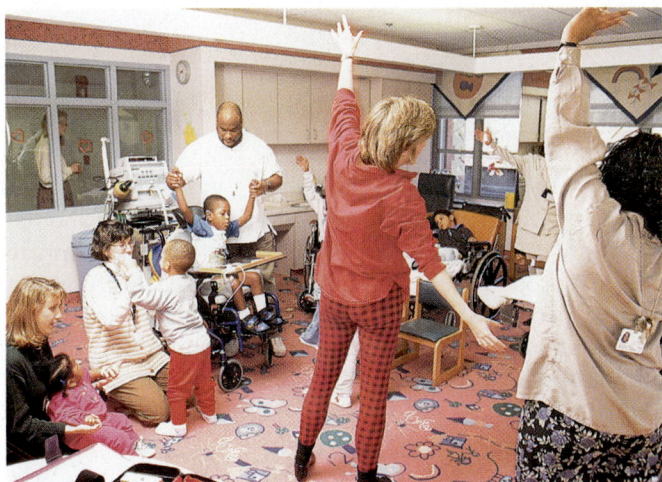

FIGURE 32–13. ◆ The nurse can help the child and family accept and adjust to new circumstances. Encouraging the child in a wheelchair to participate in group activities can help build confidence in physical skills. Good self-esteem, goal attainment, personal satisfaction, and general health are the continued benefits.

Injury Prevention

Because school-age children play in unsupervised settings for longer periods, they are at risk for different types of injuries than younger children (Table 32–25). Motor vehicle crashes are still common, but firearm and burn injuries increase in incidence (See Chapter 1). Safety teaching should be an integral part of each school's curriculum. Anticipatory guidance about violence can easily be integrated into health care visits. This might include questions for parents about how many pushing or shoving fights the child has had in the past year, how the child handles conflict, what types of discipline parents use, and which television shows the child watches. Ask children if they have been touched in a way that makes them "feel bad," how they handle disagreements with friends, and how they spend their time (Stringham, 1998).

Personality and Temperament

The enduring aspects of temperament continue to be manifested during the school years. The child classified as "difficult" at an earlier age may now have trouble in the classroom. Advise parents to provide a quiet setting for homework and to reward the child for concentration. For example, after homework is completed, the child can watch a television show. Creative efforts and alternative methods of learning should be valued. Encourage parents to see their children as individuals who may not all learn in the same way. The "slow-to-warm-up" child may need encouragement to try new activities and to share experiences with others, whereas the "easy" child will readily adapt to new schools, people, and experiences.

Communication

During the school-age years, the child should learn how to correct any lingering pronunciation or grammatical errors. Vocabulary increases, and the child is taught about parts of speech in school. School-age children enjoy writing and can be encouraged to keep a journal of their experiences while in the hospital as a method of dealing with anxiety. It is uncommon for school-age children to understand words as literally as preschoolers do.

Growth and Development

Following are strategies for communicating with the school-age child:

Provide concrete examples of pictures or materials to accompany verbal descriptions.

Assess knowledge before planning teaching.

Allow child to select rewards following procedures.

Teach techniques such as counting or visualization to manage difficult situations.

Include child in discussions and history with parent.

TABLE 32-25 Injury Prevention in the School-Age Years

	Hazard	Developmental Characteristics	Preventive Measures
	Motor vehicle/pedestrian/biking crashes	Child plays outside; may follow ball into road; rides two-wheeler.	Teach child safe outside play, especially near streets. Reinforce use of bike helmet. Teach biking safety rules and provide safe places for riding.
	Firearms	Child may have been shown location of guns; is interested in showing them to friends.	Teach child never to touch guns without parent present. Guns should be kept unloaded and locked away. Guns and ammunition should be stored in different locations. Be sure guns have trigger locks.
	Burns	Child may perform experiments with flames or toxic substances.	Teach child what to do in case of fire or if toxic substances touch skin or eyes. Reinforce teaching about 911.
	Assault	Child may be left alone after school and may walk, bike, or take public transportation alone.	Provide telephone numbers of people to contact in case of an emergency or if child feels lonely. Leave child alone for brief periods initially, and evaluate child's success in managing time. Teach child not to accept rides from or talk to or open doors to strangers. Teach child how to answer the phone.

Sexuality

Although children become aware of sexual differences between genders during preschool years, they deal much more consciously with sexuality during school age. As children mature physically, they need information about their body changes so that they can develop a healthy self-image, and an understanding of the relationships between their bodies and sexuality. Children become interested in sexual issues, and are often exposed to erroneous information on television shows, in magazines, or from friends and siblings. Schools and families need to use opportunities to teach school-age children factual information about sex, as well as fostering healthy concepts of self and others. It is advisable to ask occasional questions about sexual issues to learn how much the child knows and to provide correct information when answers demonstrate confusion. Both friends and the media are common sources of erroneous ideas. Appropriate and inappropriate touch should be discussed, with lists of trusted people who can be approached (teachers, clergy, school counselors, family members, neighbors) to discuss any episodes with which the child feels uncomfortable (Finan, 1997).

ADOLESCENT (12 TO 18 YEARS)

Adolescence is a time of passage signaling the end of childhood and the beginning of adulthood. Although adolescents differ in behaviors and accomplishments, they are in a period of identity formation. If a healthy identity and

TABLE 32–26　Growth and Development Milestones During Adolescence

Physical Growth	Fine Motor Ability	Gross Motor Ability	Sensory Ability
Variation in age of growth spurt During growth spurt, girls gain 7–25 kg (15–55 lb) and grow 2.5–20 cm (2–8 in): boys gain approximately 7–29.5 kg (15–65 lb) and grow 11–30 cm (4 1/2–12 in)	Skills are well developed (A)	New sports activities attempted and muscle development continues (B) Some lack of coordination common during growth spurt	Fully developed

(A) Skills are well developed

(B) New sports activities attempted

sense of self-worth are not developed in this period, role confusion and purposeless struggling will ensue. The adolescents encountered in nursing practice represent various degrees of identity formation, and each will offer unique challenges.

Physical Growth and Development

The physical changes ending in **puberty,** or sexual maturity, begin near the end of the school-age period. The prepubescent period is marked by a growth spurt at an average age of 10 years for girls and 13 years for boys. The increase in height and weight is generally remarkable and is completed in 2 to 3 years (Table 32–26). The growth spurt in girls is accompanied by an increase in breast size and growth of pubic hair. Menstruation occurs last and signals achievement of puberty. In boys the growth spurt is accompanied by growth in size of the penis and testes and by growth of pubic hair. Deepening of the voice and growth of facial hair occur later, at the time of puberty. See Chapter 33 for a description of the pubertal stages.

During adolescence, children grow stronger and more muscular and establish characteristic male and female patterns of fat distribution. The apocrine and eccrine glands mature, leading to increased sweating and a distinct odor to perspiration. All body organs are now fully mature, enabling the adolescent to take adult doses of medications.

The adolescent must adapt to a rapidly changing body for several years. These physical changes and hormonal variations offer challenges to identity formation.

Cognitive Development

Adolescence marks the beginning of Piaget's last stage of cognitive development, the stage of formal operational thought. The adolescent no longer depends on concrete experiences as the basis of thought but develops the ability to reason abstractly. Such concepts as justice, truth, beauty, and power can be understood. The adolescent revels in this newfound ability and spends a great deal of time thinking, reading, and talking about abstract concepts.

The ability to think and act independently leads many adolescents to rebel against parental authority. Through these actions, adolescents seek to establish their own identity and values.

Activities

Maturity leads to new activities. Adolescents may drive, ride buses, or bike independently. They are less dependent on parents for transportation and spend more time with friends. Activities include participation in sports and extracurricular school activities, as well as "hanging out" and attending movies or concerts with friends (Table 32–27). The peer group becomes the focus of activities (Figure 32–14 ◆), regardless of the teen's interests. Peers are important in establishing identity and providing meaning. Although same-sex interactions predominate, boy–girl relationships are more common than at earlier stages. Adolescents thus participate in and learn from social interactions fundamental to adult relationships.

FIGURE 32-14. ◆ Social interaction between children of same and opposite sex is as important inside the acute care setting as it is outside. **A,** Teenagers enjoy playing together. **B,** Emotional relationships form during adolescence.

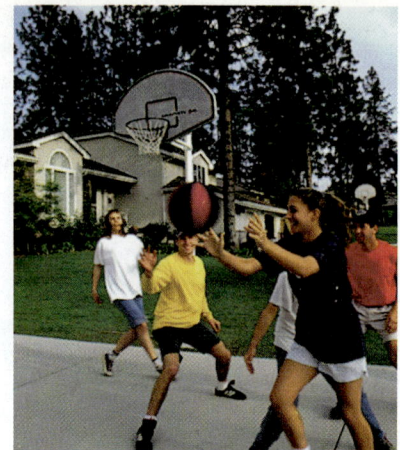

A

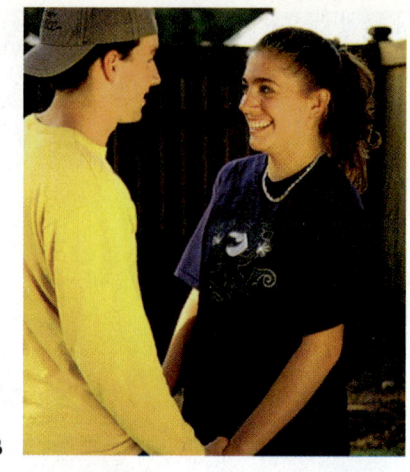

B

TABLE 32-27 in Adolescence	Favorite Activities	
Sports	**Peer Group Activities**
Ball sports	Movies
Gymnastics	Dances
Water and snow skiing	Driving
Swimming	Eating out
School team sports	
	Quiet Activities
School Activities	Reading
Drama	School work
Yearbook	Television and video games
Class officer	Music
Committee participation	

Injury Prevention

Motor vehicle crashes, suicide, and homicide cause 75% of adolescent deaths (see Chapter 1). ⊂⊃ Teenagers have access to potentially harmful objects, such as firearms, motor vehicles, and boats. They often think that no harm can come to them. This encourages adolescents to put themselves at high risk from dangerous behaviors (Table 32–28).

While some types of injuries have decreased in frequency or remained the same in recent years, others have increased. Suicide among adolescents has increased by 300% over the past four decades and is the second leading cause of death from 15 to 19 years (Hayden & Lauer; MMWR, 1995; 2000). The high rate of stress experienced by today's teenagers coupled with easy access to harmful substances and firearms promotes death by suicide (see Chapter 36 for further discussion of suicide and other violent events). ⊂⊃

Nurses can be instrumental in assessing the potential for injury of adolescents seen in practice (see Table 32–28). Teaching about prevention is most successful when young people who have been injured share their experiences with other adolescents. National health objectives to reduce intentional and nonintentional injuries by the year 2010 have been set (Healthy People 2010, 2000). ⊂⊃ WEB

Violence is an increasingly important factor in adolescent injury. Homicide is the number one cause of death for young black males. The environment should be assessed for factors contributing to violence; adolescents at risk should be referred to special programs for violence prevention. By law, nurses must report abuse in homes and schools to law enforcement agencies when they are aware that it may have occurred.

Personality and Temperament

Characteristics of temperament manifested during childhood usually remain stable in the teenage years. For instance, the adolescent who was a calm, scheduled infant and child often demonstrates initiative to regulate study times and other routines. Similarly, the adolescent who was an easily stimulated infant may now have a messy room, a harried schedule with assignments always completed late, and an interest in many activities. It is also common for an adolescent who was an easy child to become more difficult because of the psychologic changes of adolescence and the need to assert independence.

As during the child's earlier ages, the nurse's role may be to inform parents of different personality types and to help them support the teen's uniqueness while providing necessary structure and feedback. Nurses can help parents understand their teen's personality type and work with the adolescent to meet expectations set by teachers and others in authority.

Communication

The adolescent uses and understands all parts of speech. Colloquialisms and slang are commonly used with the peer group. The adolescent often studies a foreign language in school, having the ability to understand and analyze grammar and sentence structure.

The adolescent increasingly leaves the home base and establishes close ties with peers. These relationships become the basis for identity formation. There is generally a period of stress or crisis before a strong identity can

TABLE 32-28 **Injury Prevention in Adolescence**

	Hazard	Developmental Characteristics	Preventive Measures
	Motor vehicle crashes	Adolescents learn to drive, enjoy new independence, and often feel invulnerable.	Insist on driver's education classes. Enforce rules about safe driving. Seat belts should be used for every trip. Discourage drug and alcohol use. Get treatment for teenagers who are known substance abusers.
	Sporting injuries	Adolescents may participate in physically challenging sports such as soccer, gymnastics, or football. They may be allowed to drive motorboats.	Encourage use of protective sporting gear. Teach safe boating practices. Perform teaching related to hazards of drug and alcohol use, especially when using motorized equipment.
	Drowning	Adolescents overestimate endurance when swimming. They take risks diving.	Encourage swimming only with friends. Reinforce rules and teach them about risks.

emerge. The adolescent may try out new roles by learning a new sport or other skills, experimenting with drugs or alcohol, wearing different styles of clothing, or trying other activities. It is important to provide positive role models and a variety of experiences to help the adolescent make wise choices.

The adolescent also has a need to leave the past, to be different, and to change from former patterns to establish his or her own identity. Rules that are repeated constantly and dogmatically will probably be broken in the adolescent's quest for self-identity. This poses difficulties when the adolescent has a health problem, such as diabetes or a heart problem, that requires ongoing care. Introducing the adolescent to other teens who manage the same problem appropriately is usually more successful than telling the adolescent what to do.

Ensure privacy during the taking of health histories or interventions with teens. Even if a parent is present for part of a history or examination, the adolescent should be given the opportunity to relay information or ask questions alone with the health care provider. The adolescent should be given a choice of whether to have a parent present during an examination or while care is provided. Most information shared by an adolescent is confidential. Some states mandate disclosure of certain information to parents, such as an adolescent's desire for an abortion. In these cases, the adolescent should be informed of what will be disclosed to the parent.

Setting up teen rooms (recreation rooms for use only by adolescents) or separate adolescent units in hospitals can provide necessary peer support during hospitalization. Most adolescents are not pleased when placed on a unit or in a room with young children. Choices should be allowed whenever possible. These might include preference for evening or morning bathing, the type of clothes to wear while hospitalized, timing of treatments, and who should be allowed to visit and for how long. Use of contracts with adolescents may increase compliance. Firmness, gentleness, choices, and respect must all be balanced during care of adolescent patients.

Growth and Development

Following are strategies for communicating with the adolescent:

Provide written as well as verbal explanations.

Direct history and explanations to teen alone; then include parent.

Allow for safe exploration of topics by suggesting that teen is similar to other teens. ("Many teens with diabetes have questions about . . . How about you?")

Arrange meetings for discussions with other teens.

Sexuality

With maturation of the body and increased secretion of hormones, the adolescent achieves sexual maturity. This is a complex process involving growing interactions with members of the opposite sex, an interplay of the forces of society and family, and identity formation. The early adolescent progresses from dances and other social events with members of the opposite sex; the late adolescent is mature sexually and may have regular sexual encounters. About half of all high school students in the United States have had intercourse, but only 57% used a condom at their last sexual encounter (Acquavella & Braverman, 1999).

Teenagers need information about their bodies and emerging sexuality. They should understand the interests and forces they experience. Including sex education in school classes and health care encounters is important. Information on how to prevent sexually transmitted diseases is given, with most school districts now providing some teaching on AIDS. Far more common risks to teens, however, are diseases such as gonorrhea and herpes. Health histories should include questions on sexual activity, sexually transmitted diseases, and birth control use and understanding. Most hospitals routinely perform pregnancy screening on adolescent girls before elective procedures.

Adolescents benefit from clear information about sexuality, an opportunity to develop relationships with adolescents in various settings, an open atmosphere at home and school where problems and issues can be discussed, and previous experience in problem solving and self–decision making. Sexual issues should be among topics that adolescents can discuss openly in a variety of settings. Alternatives and support for their decisions should be available.

Some adolescents identify with a sexual minority group such as lesbian, gay, bisexual, or transgendered. They are at particular risk of being stigmatized and harassed by other youth or adults. They are more likely to suffer a variety of problems such as isolation, rejection by significant others, violence, suicide, and taking sexual risks (Stevens & Morgan, 1999, 2001). Nurses are instrumental in helping these youths by providing information for them and their parents, integrating sexual minority content into school sexual curricula, and providing referrals for health and social care when needed. **WEB** See Chapter 36 for further information about the health issues related to homosexuality and other sexual minority practices.

CHAPTER HIGHLIGHTS

- Development unfolds in a predictable pattern, but at different rates dependent on the particular characteristics and experiences of each child.

- Major theories of development encompass the psychosexual (Freud), psychosocial (Erikson), cognitive (Piaget), moral (Kohlberg), social learning (Bandura), and behavioral (Skinner and Watson) components of individuals.

- The ecologic theory of Bronfenbrenner and the temperament theory of Chess and Thomas emphasize the interactions of the individual within the environment.

- Influences on the developmental process include genetic potential and a series of environmental influences unique to each family and individual.

- Infancy spans the time from birth to 1 year, and is marked by rapid physical growth, mastery of basic fine and gross motor skills, and beginning cognitive and language skills.

- Toddlers range in age from 1 to 3 years, and become increasingly mobile and communicative. They master control over excretion and are known for exerting their own opinions and wishes to parents.

- Injury prevention and toilet training are specific parental teaching needs.

- Preschool years range from 3 to 6 and are marked by increasing social skills. Most preschool children attend child care programs and learn to play with other children. Continued mastery of physical skills and language occurs.

- School age spans the years from 6 to 12, when children mature in many areas. They show slow steady growth until reaching puberty between 9 and 12 years, when a growth spurt marks increased height and weight, as well as sexual maturation. School-age children play cooperatively with other children and participate in various school and community activities.

- Adolescence occurs from about 12 years of age through the teen years. Adolescents establish their own identities distinct from parents and other adults. They are mature physically and cognitively. The peer group exerts the major influence at this age.

- The nurse is involved in assessing development at each stage, and in providing anticipatory guidance to families to foster optimal development.

EXPLOREMEDIALINK

NCLEX Review, Case Studies, and other interactive resources for this chapter can be found on the companion website at http://www.prenhall.com/london. Click on "Chapter 32" to select the activities for this chapter.

For animations, more NCLEX review questions, and an audio glossary, access the accompanying CD-ROM in this textbook.

REFERENCES

Acquavella, A., & Braverman, P. (1999). Adolescent gynecology in the office setting. *Pediatric Clinics of North America, 46,* 489–503.

Altemeier, W. A. (2000). Growth charts, low birth weight, and international adoption. *Pediatric Annals, 29,* 204–205.

American Academy of Pediatrics, Committee on Communications. (1995). Children, adolescents and television. *Pediatrics, 96,* 786–787.

Aronson, J. (2000). Medical evaluation and infectious considerations on arrival. *Pediatric Annals, 29,* 218–223.

Bandura, A. (1986). *Social foundations of thought and actions: A social cognitive theory.* Englewood Cliffs, NJ: Prentice Hall.

Bandura, A. (1997a). *Self efficacy in changing societies.* New York: Cambridge University Press.

Bandura, A. (1997b). *Self efficacy: The exercise of control.* New York: WH Freeman.

Baxter, A., & Kahn, J. V. (1996). Effective early intervention for inner-city infants and toddlers: Assessing social supports, needs and stress. *Infant-Toddler Intervention Transdisciplinary Journal, 6,* 197–211.

Board on Children, Youth, and Families, National Research Council and Institute of Medicine. (2001). *From neurons to neighborhoods.* Washington, DC: National Academy Press.

Briggs, G., Freeman, R., & Yaffe, S. (1998). *Drugs in pregnancy and lactation* (5th ed.). Baltimore: Williams & Wilkins.

Bronfenbrenner, U. (1986). Ecology of the family as a context for human development: Research perspectives. *Developmental Psychology, 22,* 723–742.

Bronfenbrenner, U., McClelland, P. D., Ceci, S. J., Moen, P., & Wethington, E. (1996). *The state of Americans.* New York: Free Press.

Chamberlain, L. J. (2001). Children adopted abroad could face life-long psychological problems. *Infectious Diseases in Children, 14*(1), 20.

Centers for Disease Control and Prevention. (2000). *Advance Data, 314,* 1–28.

Chess, S., & Thomas, A. (1995). *Temperament in clinical practice.* New York: Guilford Press.

Chess, S., & Thomas, A. (1996). *Temperament: Theory and practice.* Philadelphia: Brunner/Mazel Publishers.

Chess, S., & Thomas, A. (1999). *Goodness of fit: Clinical applications from infancy through adult life.* Philadelphia: Brunner/Mazel Publishers.

Children's Defense Fund. (2000). *The state of America's children.* Washington, DC: Author.

Craig, G. J. (1999). *Human development.* Upper Saddle River, NJ: Prentice Hall.

Dietz, W. H., Bandini, L. G., Morelli, J. A., Peers, K. F., & Ching, P. L. (1994). Effect of sedentary activities on resting metabolic rate. *American Journal of Clinical Nutrition, 59,* 556–559.

Dowell, D. L. (1998). Effects of television on children: A review of the literature and recommendations for nurse practitioners. *American Journal for Nurse Practitioners, 2*(10), 31–37.

Elkind, D. (1998). *The hurried child: Growing up too fast too soon.* Reading, MA: Perseus Books.

Erikson, E. (1963). *Childhood and society.* New York: W.W. Norton.

Erikson, E. (1968). *Identity: Youth and crisis.* New York: W.W. Norton.

Faber, S. (2000). Behavioral sequelae of orphanage life. *Pediatric Annals, 29,* 242–248.

Federal Interagency Forum on Child and Family Statistics. (2000). *America's children: Key national indicators of well-being.* Washington, DC: U.S. Government Printing Office.

Fields, J., Smith, K., Bass, L. E., & Lugaila, T. (2001). *A child's day: Home, school, and play (selected indicators of child well-being).* Washington, DC: U.S. Department of Commerce.

Finan, S. L. (1997). Promoting healthy sexuality: Guidelines for the school-age child and adolescent. *The Nurse Practitioner, 22,* 62–72.

Friedman, M. M. (1998). *Family nursing (4th ed.).* Stamford, CT: Appleton & Lange.

Gemelli, R. (1996). *Normal child and adolescent development.* Washington, DC: American Psychiatric Press.

Ginsberg, H., & Opper, S. (1988). *Piaget's theory of intellectual development* (3rd ed.). Paramus, NJ: Prentice Hall.

Hayden, D. C., & Lauer, P. (2000). Prevalence of suicide programs in schools and roadblocks to implementation. *Suicide and Life Threatening Behavior, 30,* 239–251.

Healthy People 2010. (2000). *Healthy People 2010 Conference edition.* Washington, DC: United States Department of Health and Human Services.

Jarvis, C. (2000). *Physical examination and health assessment* (3rd ed.). Philadelphia: WB Saunders.

Jenista, J. A. (2000). Preadoption review of medical records. *Pediatric Annals, 29,* 212–215.

Johnson, D. E. (2000). Long-term medical issues in international adoptees. *Pediatric Annals, 29,* 234–241.

Melnyk, B. M., & Alpert-Gillis, L. J. (1997). Coping with marital separation: Smoothing the transition for parents and children. *Journal of Pediatric Health Care, 11,* 165–174.

Melvin, N. (1995). Children's temperament: Intervention for parents. *Journal of Pediatric Nursing, 10,* 152–159.

Miller, L. C. (2000). Initial assessment of growth, development, and the effects of institutionalization in internationally adopted children. *Pediatric Annals, 29,* 224–233.

MMWR. (1995). Suicide among children, adolescents, and young adults—United States, 1980–1992. *Morbidity and Mortality Weekly Report, 44,* 289–291.

MMWR. (2000). Youth risk behavior surveillance—United States 1999. *Morbidity and Mortality Weekly Report, 49,* 1–99.

National Institute of Child Health and Human Development. (1997). The effects of infant child care on infant-mother attachment security. *Child Development, 68,* 860–879.

National Safety Council. (1998). *Child passenger safety.* Washington, DC: Author.

Olds, S., London, M., & Ladewig, P. (2000). *Maternal newborn nursing.* Upper Saddle River, NJ: Prentice Hall.

Piaget, J. (1972). *The child's conception of the world.* Totowa, NJ: Littlefield, Adams Co.

Robinson, T. N. (2001). Intervention to reduce media viewing improves aggressive children's behavior. *Archives of Pediatric and Adolescent Medicine, 155,* 17–23.

Santrock, J. (1999). *Life-span development.* Boston: McGraw-Hill.

Spector, R. (2000). *Guides to heritage assessment and health traditions.* Upper Saddle River, NJ: Prentice Hall Health.

Stein, R. E. K. (1997). *Health care for children.* New York: United Hospital Foundation of New York.

Stevens, P., & Morgan, S. (1999). Health of lesbian, gay, bisexual, and transgender youth. *Journal of Child and Family Nursing, 2,* 237–249.

Stevens, P., & Morgan, S. (2001). Health of lesbian, gay, bisexual, and transgender youth. *Journal of Pediatric Health Care, 15,* 24–34.

Stringham, P. (1998). Violence anticipatory guidance. *Pediatric Clinics of North America, 45,* 439–448.

Thompson, P. (1998). Adolescents from families of divorce: Vulnerability to physiological and psychological disturbances. *Journal of Psychosocial Nursing, 36,* 34–39.

Trahms, C. M., & Pipes, P. L. (1997). *Nutrition in infancy and childhood* (6th ed.). New York: McGraw-Hill.

Troiano, R. P., Flegel, K. M., Kuczmarski, R. J., Campbell, S. M., & Johnson, C. L. (1995). Overweight prevalence and trends for children and adolescents. *Archives of Pediatric and Adolescent Medicine, 149,* 1085–1091.

UNICEF. (1998). The state of the world's children 1998: A UNICEF report. Malnutrition: Causes, consequences, and solutions. *Nutrition Reviews, 56,* 115–123.

Wagner, J. D., Menke, E. M., & Ciccone, J. K. (1995). What is known about the health of rural homeless families. *Public Health Nursing, 12,* 400–408.

Wallerstein, J. S., Corbin, S. B., & Lewis, J. M. (1988). Children of divorce: A ten year study. In E. M. Hetherington & J. B. Arasteh (Eds.), *Impact of divorce, single parenting, and stepparenting on children.* Hillsdale, NJ: Erlbaum Publishers.

Wallerstein, J., & Kelly, J. (1996). *Surviving the breakup.* New York: Harper Collins.

Wallerstein, J., Lewis, J., & Blakeslee, S. (2000). *The unexpected legacy of divorce: A 25 year landmark study.* New York: Hyperion.

Worthington-Roberts, B. S., & Williams, S. R. (1997). *Nutrition in pregnancy and lactation* (6th ed.). Madison, WI: Brown & Benchmark.

CHAPTER 33

Pediatric Assessment

I was scared when we brought Latoya to the hospital. She looked helpless, afraid, and sick. The nurses and doctors took over when we got to the hospital, and I felt better because they seemed to know what to do.

—FATHER OF LATOYA, 6 MONTHS OLD

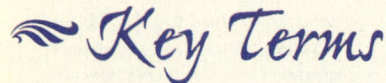

Key Terms

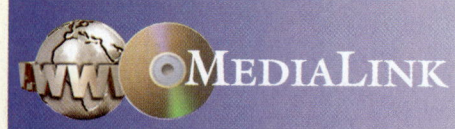

MediaLink

CD-ROM
Audio Glossary
Otoscope Examination Animation
Mouth and Throat Examination Animation
Skills 9–1—9–7: Growth Measurements
Skill 9–10: Blood Pressure
Skills 9–11—9–14: Body Temperature Measurements
Skills 9–17—9–19: Visual Acuity Screening
NCLEX Review

COMPANION WEBSITE
http://www.prenhall.com/london

Pediatric Assessment Web Links
Techniques for Assessing Selected Primitive Reflexes, with Normal Findings and Their Expected Age of Occurrence
Thinking Critically
NCLEX Review
Case Study

Do examination techniques need to vary for children of different ages? How does the nurse encourage infants and toddlers to cooperate with the examination? This chapter answers these questions and provides an overview of pediatric **assessment,** including history taking and examination techniques geared to the unique needs of pediatric patients. Strategies for obtaining the child's history are presented first. The remainder of the chapter then outlines a systematic process for physical examination of the child and guidelines for nutritional assessment.

ANATOMIC AND PHYSIOLOGIC CHARACTERISTICS OF CHILDREN

Children and infants are not only smaller than adults, but also significantly different physiologically. Knowledge of pediatric anatomic and physiologic differences will aid in recognizing normal variations found during the physical examination. It also assists with understanding the different physiologic responses children have to illness and injury. The illustration in "As They Grow" provides an overview of important anatomic and physiologic differences between children and adults.

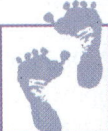

AS THEY GROW ⟆ *Children Are Not Just Small Adults*

Body surface area large for weight, making infants susceptible to hypothermia.

Anterior fontanel and open sutures palpable up to about 18 months. Posterior fontanel closes between 2 and 3 months.

Tongue large relative to small nasal and oral airway passages.

Short, narrow trachea in children under 5 years makes them susceptible to foreign body obstruction.

Until late school age and adolescence, cardiac output is rate dependent not stroke volume dependent, making heart rate more rapid.

Abdomen offers poor protection for the liver and spleen, making them susceptible to trauma.

Until 12 to 18 months of age, kidneys do not concentrate urine effectively and do not exert optimal control over electrolyte secretion and absorption.

Until later school age, proportion of body weight in water is larger, with more water in extracellular spaces. Daily water exchange rate is much higher.

All brain cells present at birth; myelinization and further development of nerve fibers occur during first year.

Head proportionately larger, making child susceptible to head injury.

Higher metabolic rate, higher oxygen needs, higher caloric needs.

Until puberty, percentage of cartilage in ribs is higher, making them more flexible and compliant.

Until about 10 years, there is a faster respiratory rate, fewer and smaller alveoli, and less lung volume. Tidal volume is proportional to weight (7 to 10 ml/kg).

Up to about 4 or 5 years, diaphragm is primary breathing muscle. CO_2 is not effectively expired when child is distressed, making child susceptible to metabolic acidosis.

Until puberty, bones are soft and more easily bent and fractured.

Muscles lack tone, power, and coordination during infancy. Muscles are 25% of weight in infants versus 40% in adults.

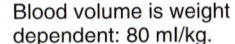

Blood volume is weight dependent: 80 ml/kg.

Children are not just small adults. There are important anatomic and physiologic differences between children and adults that will change based on a child's growth and development.

OBTAINING THE CHILD'S HISTORY
Communication Strategies

What makes communication effective? What does it mean when a parent or caretaker will not look the questioner in the eye? What types of cues indicate that a parent may be withholding historical information?

The health history interview is a very personal conversation with a parent, caretaker, or adolescent during which private concerns and feelings are shared. Try to ensure that this exchange of information with the parent or the child is clearly understood by both parties, that it is an **effective communication.** Effective communication is difficult to accomplish because parents and children often do not correctly interpret what the nurse says, just as the nurse may not understand completely what the parent or child says. People's interpretation of information is based on their life experiences, culture, and education.

STRATEGIES TO BUILD A RAPPORT WITH THE FAMILY

When beginning the history, make sure the parents understand the purpose of the interview and that the information will be used appropriately. To develop rapport, demonstrate interest in and concern for the child and family during the interview. This rapport forms the foundation for the collaborative relationship between the nurse and parent that will provide the best nursing care for the child. The following strategies help to establish rapport with the child's family during the nursing history:

- *Make a self-introduction* (name, title or position, and role in caring for the child). To demonstrate respect, ask all family members present what name they prefer you to use when talking with them.

- *Explain the purpose of the interview* and why the nursing history is different from the information collected by other health professionals. For example, "The nurses will use this information to plan nursing care best suited for your child."

- *Provide privacy* and remove as many distractions as possible during the interview. If the patient's room does not offer privacy, attempt to find a vacant patient room or lounge.

- *Direct the focus of the interview* with open-ended questions. Use close-ended questions or directing statements to clarify information. Open-ended questions are useful to initiate the interview, develop a rapport, and understand the parent's perceptions of the child's problem; for example, "Tell me what problems led to Roberto's admission to the hospital." Close-ended questions are used to obtain detailed information; for example, "How high was Tommy's fever this morning?"

- *Ask one question at a time* so that the parent or child understands what piece of information is desired and so that it is clear which question the parent is

answering. "Does any member of your family have diabetes, heart disease, or sickle cell anemia?" is a multiple question. Ask about each disease separately to ensure the most accurate response.

- *Involve the child in the interview* by asking age-appropriate questions. Young children can be asked "What is your doll's name?" or "Where does it hurt?" Demonstrating an interest in the child initiates development of rapport with both child and parents. Ask older children and teens questions about their illness or injury. Offer them an opportunity to privately discuss their major concerns when their parents are not present.

- *Be honest* with the child when answering questions or when giving information about what will happen. Children need to learn that they can trust their nurse.

- *Choose the language style* best understood by the parent and child. Commonly used phrases can have different meanings to persons in various regions of the country or to different ethnic groups. To improve communication, request frequent feedback from the parents or child to ensure that their interpretation of phrases is accurate.

- *Use an interpreter to improve communication* when not fluent in the family's primary language (Figure 33–1 ◆).

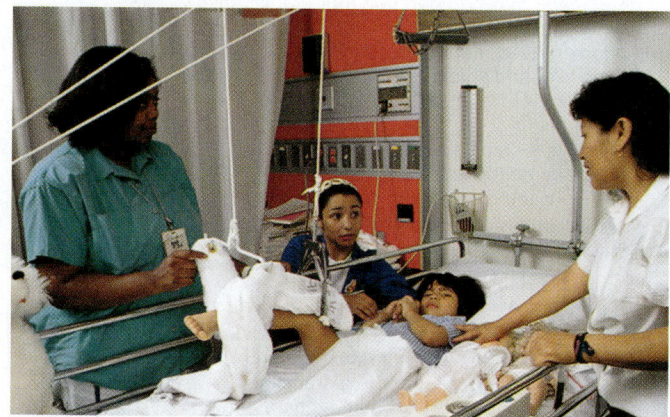

FIGURE 33–1. ◆ Most hospitals have designated interpreters that you should use. If not, find a professional interpreter whom you have identified beforehand and who knows medical terms and the cultural norms of the family. The interpreter *(center)* should be positioned to improve communication. Maintain eye contact with the parent or patient, not the interpreter. To ensure confidentiality of information for parents, avoid using a family member for history taking.

CAREFUL LISTENING

Complete attention is necessary to "hear" and accurately interpret information the parents and child give during the nursing history. Carefully listen to the information provided by the parent, as well as how it is expressed, and observe behavior during the interaction.

- Does the parent hesitate or avoid answering certain questions?

- Pay attention to the parent's attitude or tone of voice when the child's problems are discussed. Determine if it is consistent with the seriousness of the child's problem. The tone of voice can reveal anxiety, anger, or lack of concern.

- Be alert to any underlying themes. For example, the parent who talks about the child's diagnosis, but repeatedly refers to the impact of the illness on the family's finances or on meeting the needs of other family members, is requesting that these issues be addressed.

- Observe the parent's **nonverbal behavior** (posture, gestures, body movements, eye contact, and facial expression) for consistency with the words and tone of voice used. Is the parent interested in and appropriately concerned about the child's condition? Behaviors such as sitting up straight, making eye contact, and appearing apprehensive reflect appropriate concern for the child. Physical withdrawal, failure to make eye contact, or a happy expression could be inconsistent with the child's serious condition.

Developing Cultural Competence

Eye contact with the interviewer may be avoided by many cultural groups (Asian, Native American, and Middle Eastern patients) because it is considered impolite, aggressive, or a sign of disrespect (Spector, 2000).

Subtle nonverbal and verbal cues often indicate that the parent has not provided complete information about the child's problem. Observe for behaviors such as avoiding eye contact, change in voice pitch, or hesitation when responding to a question. Being supportive and asking clarifying questions encourage further description or the expression of information that is difficult for the parent or child to share; for example, "It sounds like that was a very difficult experience. How did Latasha react?"

Encourage parents to share information, even if it is private or sensitive, especially when it influences nursing care planning. Often parents avoid sharing some information because they want to make a good impression, or they do not understand the value of the missing information. If parents hesitate to share information, briefly explain why the question was asked—for example, to make their child's hospital experience more pleasant or to begin planning for the child's discharge and home care.

In some cases the parent becomes too agitated, upset, or angry to continue responding to questions. When the information is not needed immediately, move on to another portion of the history to determine whether the parent is able to respond to other questions. Depending on the emotional status of the parent, it may be more appropriate to collect the remaining historical data later.

Data to Be Collected

Collect and organize the child's health, medical, and personal-social history to plan the child's nursing care. This text uses a modification of the Burns Classification System as the data-collection framework selected (Burns, 1992; Byrnes, 1996). Physiologic, psychosocial, and developmental data are organized to help develop the nursing diagnoses and the nursing care plan. Be alert for nonverbal cues.

PATIENT INFORMATION

Obtain the child's name and nickname, age, sex, and ethnic origin. The child's birth date, race, religion, address, and phone number can be obtained from the admission form. Ask the parent for an emergency contact address and phone number, as well as a work phone number. Record the person providing the patient history and that person's relationship to the patient.

PHYSIOLOGIC DATA

Collect information about the child's health problems and diseases chronologically in a format similar to the traditional medical history.

- The *chief complaint* is the child's primary problem or reason for hospital admission or visit to a health care setting, stated in the parent's or child's exact words.

- The *history of the present illness or injury* is a detailed description of the current health problem. This includes the onset and sequence of events, characteristics of and changes in symptoms over time, influencing factors, and the current status of the problem. Each problem is described separately. Table 33–1 lists the specific data to be collected about each illness and injury.

- The *past history* is a more detailed description of the child's prior health problems. It includes the birth history and all major past illnesses and injuries. A detailed and complete birth history is obtained when the child's present problem may be related to the birth history (Table 33–2). Record the child's age at the time of each illness, injury, related surgery, or hospitalization. Obtain information about each specific diagnosis, treatment, outcomes, complications, or residual problems, and the child's reaction to the event (Table 33–3).

- The *current health status* is a detailed description of the child's typical health status. Obtain information about allergies, current medications, immunization

TABLE 33-1 History of Present Illness or Injury

Characteristic	Defining Variables
Onset	Sudden or gradual, previous episodes, date and time began
Type of symptom	Pain, itching, cough, vomiting, runny nose, diarrhea, rash, etc.
Location	Generalized or localized—anatomically precise
Duration	Continuous or episodic, length of episodes
Severity	Effect on daily activities, e.g., interrupted sleep, decreased appetite, incapacitation
Influencing factors	What relieves or aggravates symptoms, what precipitated the problem, recent exposure to infection or allergen
Past evaluation for the problem	Laboratory studies, physician's office or hospital where done, results of past examinations
Previous and current treatment	Prescribed and over-the-counter drugs used, other measures tried (heat, ice, rest), response to treatments

TABLE 33-2 Birth History

Prenatal

Mother's age, health during pregnancy, prenatal care, weight gained, special diet, expected date of delivery

Details of illnesses, x-ray findings, hospitalizations, medications, complications, and timing during pregnancy

Prior obstetric history

Antenatal—Description of Delivery

Site of delivery (hospital, home, birthing center)

Labor induced or spontaneous

Vaginal or cesarean section, forceps or suction used, vertex or breech position

Single or multiple birth

Condition of Baby at Birth

Weight, Apgar score, cried immediately

Need for incubator, oxygen, suctioning, ventilator

Any abnormalities detected, meconium staining

Postnatal

Difficulties in the nursery—feeding, respiratory difficulties, jaundice, cyanosis, rashes

Length of hospital stay, special nursery, home with mother

Breast- or bottle-fed, weight gained in hospital

Medical care needed in first week—admission to hospital

TABLE 33-3 Past Illnesses and Injuries

Illnesses	Major illnesses including common communicable diseases
Injuries	Major injuries, their mechanism (cause) and severity
Surgery	Specific type, day surgery or hospitalized
Hospitalizations	Reason and length of hospitalization
Transfusions	Circumstances, reactions

TABLE 33-4 Current Health Status

Health Maintenance

Name of primary health care provider; last visit

Name of dentist; last visit

Other health care providers

Allergies

To food, medication, animals, insect bites, environment, etc.

Type of reaction

Immunizations

Types, dates received, unexpected reactions

Safety Measures Used

Car restraint system

Window guards

Medication storage

Sports protective gear

Smoke detectors

Bicycle helmet

Firearm storage

Other

Sociocultural Factors

Environment

Family financial status

Health insurance

Activities and Exercise

Physical mobility

Play and/or sports activities

Limitations and adaptive equipment

Nutrition

Formula-fed or breastfed

When solid foods introduced

Eating and snacking habits

Variety of foods consumed, junk foods eaten

Appetite

Sleep

Length and timing of naps and nighttime sleep

Nightmares or night terrors

Other sleep disturbances

Where the child sleeps

Bedtime rituals

status, activities and exercise, sleep patterns, nutrition, safety measures used, and health maintenance care (Table 33–4).

- The **review of systems** provides a comprehensive overview of the child's health. This is an opportunity to identify additional signs and symptoms associated with the child's admission problem or to identify other problems that have no direct relationship to the child's significant health problem but could be factors complicating nursing care or home care. For example, asking about any urinary problems may reveal that a child still wets the bed at 7 years of age,

TABLE 33-5 Review of Systems

Body Systems	Examples of Problems to Identify
General	General growth pattern, overall health status, ability to keep up with other children or tires easily with feeding or activity, fever, sleep patterns Allergies, type of reaction (hives, rash, respiratory difficulty, swelling, nausea), seasonal or with each exposure
Skin and lymph	Rashes, dry skin, itching, changes in skin color or texture, tendency for bruising, swollen or tender lymph glands
Hair and nails	Hair loss, changes in color or texture, use of dye or chemicals on hair Abnormalities of nail growth or color
Head	Headaches, head injuries
Eyes	Vision problems, squinting, crossed eyes, lazy eye, wears glasses, eye infections, redness, tearing, burning, rubbing, swelling eyelids
Ears	Ear infections, frequent discharge from ears, or tubes in ears Hearing loss (no response to loud noises or questions, inattentiveness, was hearing test ever done?)
Nose and sinuses	Nosebleeds, nasal congestion, colds with runny nose, sinus pain or infections Nasal obstruction, difficulty breathing, snoring at night
Mouth and throat	Mouth breathing, difficulty swallowing, sore throats, strep infections Tooth eruption, cavities, braces Voice change, hoarseness, speech problems
Cardiac and hematologic	Heart murmur, anemia, hypertension, cyanosis, edema, rheumatic fever, chest pain
Chest & respiratory	Trouble breathing, choking episodes, cough, wheezing, cyanosis, exposure to tuberculosis, other infections
Gastrointestinal	Bowel movements, frequency, color, regularity, consistency, discomfort, constipation or diarrhea, abdominal pain, bleeding from rectum, flatulence Nausea or vomiting, appetite
Urinary	Frequency, urgency, dysuria, dribbling, enuresis, strength of urinary stream Toilet trained—age when day and night dryness attained
Reproductive	For pubescent children
Female	Menses onset, amount, duration, frequency, discomfort, problems; vaginal discharge, breast development
Male	Puberty onset, emissions, erections, pain or discharge from penis, swelling or pain in testicles
Both	Sexual activity, use of contraception, sexually transmitted diseases
Musculoskeletal	Weakness, clumsiness, poor coordination, balance, tremors, abnormal gait, painful muscles or joints, swelling or redness of joints, fractures
Neurologic	Seizures, fainting spells, dizziness, numbness, learning problems, attention span, hyperactivity, memory problems

although the admission is for a femur fracture. The nurse would then need to consider how bed-wetting might cause problems with the spica cast. For each problem, obtain the treatment, outcomes, residual problems, and age at time of onset. Data-collection guidelines are given in Table 33–5.

- The *familial and hereditary diseases* summarize the major familial and hereditary diseases in three generations of family members, including the parents, grandparents, aunts, uncles, cousins, child, and siblings. Collect information about the health status of each parent. Record information in either a pedigree or a narrative format. Specific diseases to ask about are listed in Table 33–6.

PSYCHOSOCIAL DATA

Obtain information about family composition to establish a socioeconomic and sociologic context for planning the child's care in the hospital and at home.

- Family composition, including family members living in the home, their relationship to the child, marital status of parents or other family structure, and people helping to care for the child
- Household members employed, family income, and financial resources or agencies used such as health insurance, food stamps, or Temporary Assistance for Needy Families
- Description of the housing and home environment (atmosphere, emotional stresses, family activities); safe play area; use of city or well water; and availability of electricity, heat, and refrigeration

TABLE 33-6 Familial or Hereditary Diseases

Infectious diseases	Tuberculosis, HIV, or hepatitis
Heart disease	Heart defects, myocardial infarctions, hypertension, hyperlipidemia
Allergic disorders	Eczema, hay fever, or asthma
Eye disorders	Glaucoma, cataracts, vision loss
Ear disorders	Hearing loss
Hematologic disorders	Sickle cell anemia, thalassemia, G6PD deficiency, leukemia
Lung disorders	Cystic fibrosis
Cancer	Type, early age of onset
Endocrine disorders	Diabetes mellitus
Mental disorders	Mental retardation, epilepsy, Huntington chorea, psychiatric disorders
Musculoskeletal disorders	Arthritis, muscular dystrophy
Gastrointestinal disorders	Ulcers, colitis, kidney disease
Repeated miscarriages, stillbirths, or sudden childhood deaths	
Learning problems	

- School or child care arrangements; description of the neighborhood, including playgrounds, transportation, and proximity to stores
- Changes in family or lifestyle since last seen; number of times the family has moved; how the child and family members have coped with the changes.

Information about daily routines, psychosocial data, and other living patterns forms the basis for many nursing diagnoses as well as the nursing care plan. Collection of information should focus on issues that have an impact on the quality of daily living, even if some data seem to overlap with disease data (Table 33–7). The psychosocial history for adolescents should focus on critical areas in their lives (home environment, employment and education, activities, drugs, sexual activity/sexuality, suicide and depression, and safety) that may contribute to a less than optimal environment for normal growth and development (Goldenring & Cohen, 1988). Possible screening questions are found in Table 33–8.

DEVELOPMENTAL DATA

Information about the child's motor, cognitive, language, and social development is recorded. Ask the parent about the child's milestones and current fine and gross motor skills. Obtain the age at which the child first used words appropriately and the current words used or language ability. For children in school, ask about academic performance to assess cognitive development. Ask the parent about the child's manner of interaction with other children, family members, and strangers.

TABLE 33–7 Daily Living Patterns

Role Relationships
Family relationships/alterations in family process
Peer relationships
Social interactions: e.g., day care, preschool, school, neighborhood
Communication

Self-Perception/Self-Concept
Personal identity and role identity
Self-esteem
Body image/nonvisible disorder

Coping/Stress Tolerance
Temperament
Coping behaviors
Discipline
Any substance abuse

Values and Beliefs
Religion
Personal values/beliefs

Home Care Provided for Child's Condition
Resources needed/available
Knowledge and skills of parents, other family members
Respite care available

Sensory/Perceptual Problems
Adaptations to daily living for any sensory loss (vision, hearing, cognitive, or motor)

Note: From Burns, C. (1992). A new assessment model and tool for pediatric nurse practitioners. *Journal of Pediatric Health Care, 6,* 73–81. Adapted.

TABLE 33–8 Adolescent Psychosocial Assessment Using the HEADSSS Screening Tool

Home Environment
- With whom do you live?
- Have there been any recent changes in your living situation?
- How are things between your parents (or parent and significant other adult) at home?
- Are your parents employed?

Employment and Education
- Are you currently in school?
- What are your favorite subjects?
- How are your school grades?
- Have you ever been expelled from school or missed a lot of time?
- Do your friends attend school?
- What are your future education or employment plans?

Activities
- What do you do in your spare time?
- What do you do for fun?
- With whom do you spend time?

Drugs
- Have you ever tried street drugs? Alcohol? Steroids? Have you ever smoked or chewed tobacco?
- Are you still using these drugs? Are any of your friends using or selling any drugs?

Sexual Activity/Sexuality
- What is your sexual orientation?
- Are you sexually active?
    At what age did you start having sex?
    How many sexual partners do you have?
    Do you (or your partner) use condoms?
    Do you (or your partner) use contraceptives?
- Have you ever been abused, either physically or sexually?

Suicide/Depression
- Are you ever sad or tearful? Tired or unmotivated?
- Have you ever felt that life is not worth living? Have you ever thought about hurting yourself or tried to hurt yourself? Do you have a suicide plan?

Safety
- Do you use a seat belt or bicycle helmet?
- Do you ever get into dangerous situations where you could be hurt?
- Is there a gun in your home? Have you ever learned about gun safety?

Note: From Goldenring, J. M., & Cohen, E. (1988). Getting into adolescent heads. *Contemporary Pediatrics, 5,* 75–90. © 1988 Thomson Medical Economics. All rights reserved. Adapted with permission.

The developmental data will help when planning nursing care appropriate for the child. Guidelines for a nursing assessment of development can be found in Chapter 32. ⊂⊃

GENERAL APPRAISAL

The examination begins upon first meeting the child, either when admitting the child to the nursing unit or in the patient's room (Figure 33–2 ◆). Measure the infant's weight, length, and head circumference (see Skills 9–1 through 9–7 in the accompanying CD-ROM, as well as the *Clinical Skills Manual*). ⊂⊃ SKILLS CD If the

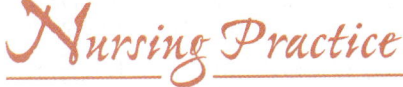
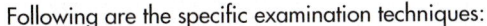

Nursing Practice

Following are the specific examination techniques:

▶ **Inspection.** Purposeful observation of the child's physical features and behaviors. Physical feature characteristics include size, shape, color, movement, position, and location.

▶ **Palpation.** Use of touch to identify characteristics of the skin, internal organs, and masses. Characteristics include texture, moistness, tenderness, temperature, position, shape, consistency, and mobility of masses and organs.

▶ **Auscultation.** Listening to sounds produced by the airway, lungs, stomach, heart, and blood vessels to identify their characteristics. Auscultation is usually performed with a stethoscope to enhance the sounds heard.

▶ **Percussion.** Striking the surface of the body, either directly or indirectly, to set up vibrations that reveal the density of underlying tissues and borders of internal organs.

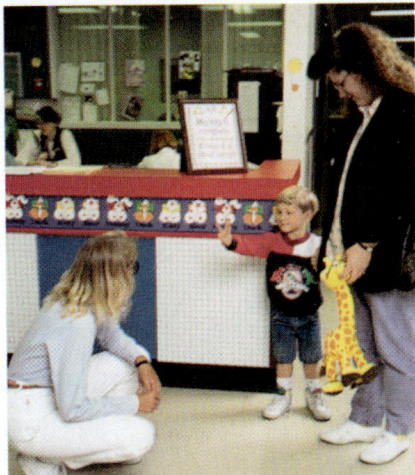

FIGURE 33–2. ◆ Examination of the child begins from the first contact. You should be observing the behavior of the child and parent by using visual cues to make a proper assessment. Does the child appear well nourished? Does the child appear secure with the parent?

child can stand, substitute a standing height measurement for length. Take the child's temperature, heart rate, respiratory rate, and blood pressure (see Skills 9–10 through 9–14). ⊂⊃ SKILLS CD

Observe the child's general appearance and behavior. The child should appear well nourished and well developed. Infants and young children are often fearful and seek reassurance from their parents. The child may resist interacting with the nurse until rapport is established.

Observe the behavior and tone of voice used by the parent when he or she is talking to the child. Is the child encouraged to speak? Is the child appropriately reassured or supported by the parent? The child should feel secure with the parent and perceive permission to interact with the nurse.

ASSESSING SKIN AND HAIR CHARACTERISTICS

Examination of the skin requires good lighting to detect variations in skin color and to identify lesions. Daylight is preferred when available. Rather than inspecting the entire skin surface of the child at one time, examine the skin simultaneously with other body systems as each region of the body is exposed.

Developing Cultural Competence

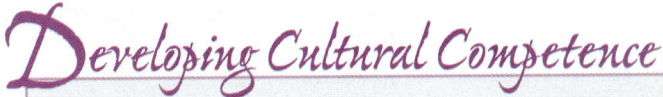

The palms of the hands and soles of the feet are often lighter than the rest of the skin surface in darker skinned children. In addition, their lips may appear slightly bluish.

Inspection of the Skin

Use gloves to inspect the child's skin for color and the presence of imperfections, elevations, or other lesions.

SKIN COLOR

The color of the child's skin usually has an even distribution. Check for color variations—such as increased or decreased pigmentation, pallor, mottling, bruises, erythema, cyanosis, or jaundice—that may be associated with local or generalized conditions. Some variations in skin color are common and normal, such as freckles found in the white population and Mongolian spots found on dark-skinned infants. Bruises are common on the knees, shins, and lower arms as children stumble and fall. Bruises on other parts of the body, especially in various stages of healing, should raise a suspicion of child abuse. See Chapter 25 for more information. ⊂⊃

When a skin color abnormality is suspected, inspect the buccal mucosa and tongue to confirm the color change. This is especially important in darker skinned children

The color of the bruise provides clues to its age (Wilson, 1977).

Color	Age of Bruise
Reddish blue	Up to 48 hours
Brownish blue	2 to 3 days
Brownish green	4 to 7 days
Greenish yellow	7 to 10 days
Yellow-brown	More than 8 days
Normal skin color	2 to 4 weeks

because the mucous membranes are usually pink, regardless of skin color. Press the gums lightly for 1 to 2 seconds. Any residual color, such as that seen in jaundice or cyanosis, is more easily detected in blanched skin. Jaundice may also be noticed in the sclerae of the eyes. Generalized cyanosis is associated with respiratory and cardiac disorders. Jaundice is associated with liver disorders.

Palpation of the Skin

Palpation of the skin provides a sense of its characteristics: temperature, texture, moistness, and resilience or turgor. To evaluate these characteristics, lightly touch or stroke the skin surface. Follow standard precautions by wearing gloves when palpating mucous membranes, open wounds, and lesions. The following list provides details on each of the characteristics of skin palpation:

TEMPERATURE

The child's skin normally feels cool to the touch. A general evaluation of skin temperature can be obtained by placing the wrist or dorsum of the hand against the child's skin. Excessively warm skin may indicate the presence of fever or inflammation, whereas abnormally cool skin may be a sign of shock or cold exposure.

TEXTURE

Children have soft, smooth skin over the entire body. Identify any areas of roughness, thickening, or induration (area of extra firmness with a distinct border). Abnormalities in texture are associated with endocrine disorders, chronic irritation, and inflammation.

MOISTNESS

The child's skin is normally dry to the touch. The skin may feel slightly damp when the child has been exercising or crying. Excessive sweating without exertion is associated with a fever or with an uncorrected congenital heart defect.

RESILIENCE (TURGOR)

The child's skin is taut, elastic, and mobile because of the balanced distribution of intracellular and extracellular fluids. To evaluate skin turgor, pinch a small amount of

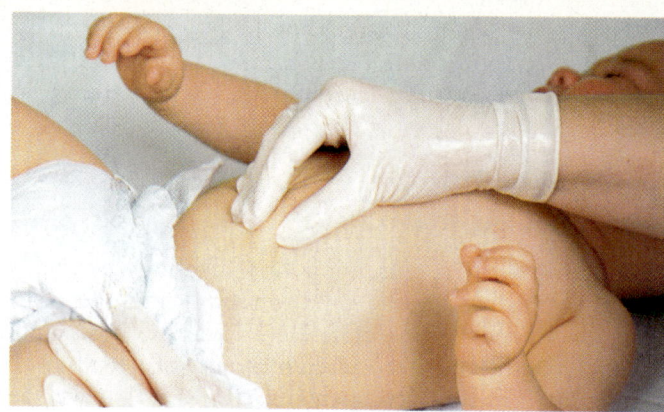

FIGURE 33–3. ◆ Tenting of the skin associated with poor skin turgor. Skin with normal turgor will return to a flat position quickly.

skin on the abdomen between the thumb and forefinger, release the skin, and watch the speed of recoil (Figure 33–3 ◆). Skin with good turgor rapidly returns to its previous contour. Skin with poor turgor tents or stands up rather than resuming its previous contour. Poor skin turgor is commonly associated with dehydration. *Note:* If *edema,* an accumulation of excess fluid in the interstitial spaces, is present, the skin feels doughy or boggy. To test for the degree of edema present, press for 5 seconds against a bone beneath the area of puffy skin, release the pressure, and observe how rapidly the indentation disappears. If the indentation disappears rapidly, the edema is "nonpitting." Slow disappearance of the indentation indicates "pitting" edema, which is commonly associated with kidney or heart disorders.

The degree of dehydration, or weight loss caused by dehydration, can be estimated from the time it takes tented skin to return to its natural contour (Seidel, Ball, Dains, et al., 2003).

Weight Loss from Dehydration	Time to Return to Normal
< 5%	< 2 sec
5% to 8%	2 to 3 sec
9% to 10%	3 to 4 sec
> 10%	> 4 sec

CAPILLARY REFILL AND SMALL-VEIN FILLING TIMES

Two techniques can determine the adequacy of tissue perfusion (oxygen circulating to the tissues). When tissue perfusion is inadequate, immediately assess the child for shock or a physical constriction such as a cast or bandage that is too tight. The capillary refill time is normally less than 2 seconds (Figure 33–4 ◆ A and B). The small-vein filling time is normally less than 4 seconds (Figure 33–4 ◆ C and D).

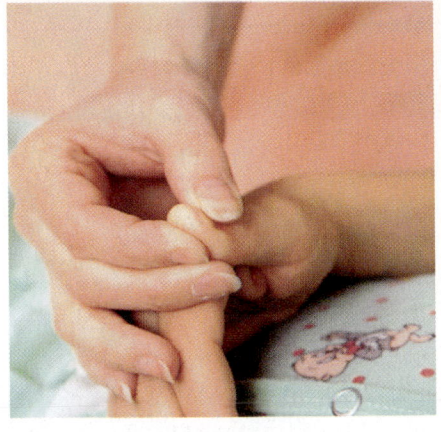

A

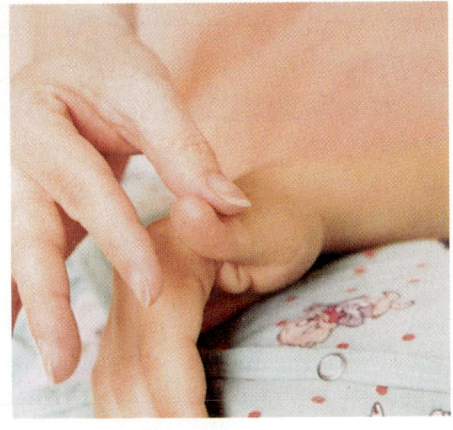

B

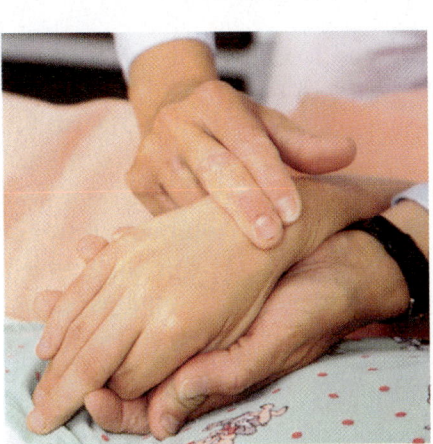

C

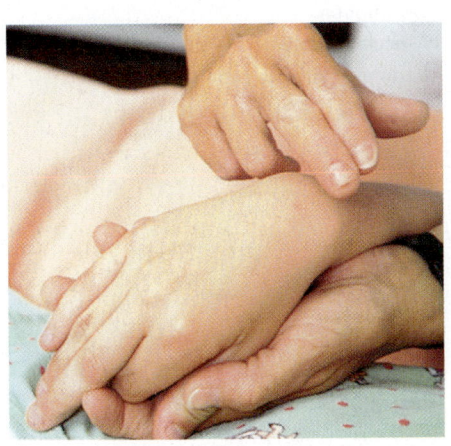

D

FIGURE 33–4. ◆ Capillary refill technique: **A,** Pinch the end of a finger until the skin is blanched. **B,** Quickly release the finger and watch the blood return to the veins. Count the seconds it takes for the color to return or veins to fill. Slow color return or vein filling time could be related to shock or constriction due to a tight bandage or cast. Small vein filling time technique: **C,** Using the index finger, milk a vein on the dorsum of the hand or foot from proximal to distal. **D,** Release your pressure and color should return promptly.

Nursing Practice

Following are common patterns of skin lesions:

Annular:	Circular, begins in center and spreads to periphery
Polycyclic:	Annular lesions running together
Linear:	In a row or stripe
Groups:	Clustered
Gyrate:	Twisted, spiral, coiled

Skin Lesions

Skin lesions usually indicate an abnormal skin condition. Characteristics such as location, size, type of lesion, pattern, and discharge, if present, provide clues about the cause of the condition. Inspect and palpate the isolated or generalized skin color abnormalities, elevations, lesions, or injuries to describe all characteristics present.

Primary lesions (such as macules, papules, and vesicles) are often the skin's initial response to injury or infection. Mongolian spots and freckles are normal findings also classified as primary lesions (see Chapter 25). ⚭ Secondary lesions (such as scars, ulcers, fissures) are the result of irritation, infection, and delayed healing of primary lesions. The illustrations in "Pathophysiology Illustrated" describe common primary lesions.

Inspection of the Hair

Inspect the scalp hair for color, distribution, and cleanliness. The hair shafts should be evenly colored, shiny, and either curly or straight. Variation in hair color not caused by bleaching can be associated with a nutritional deficiency. Normally, hair is distributed evenly over the scalp. Investigate areas of hair loss. Hair loss in a child may result from tight braids or skin lesions such as ringworm (see Chapter 52). ⚭ Notice any unusual hair growth patterns. An unusually low hairline on the neck or forehead may be associated with a congenital disorder such as hypothyroidism.

Children are frequently exposed to head lice. Inspect the individual hair shafts for small nits (lice eggs) that adhere to the hair (Figure 33–5 ◆). None should be present.

Observe the distribution of body hair as other skin surfaces are exposed during examination. Fine hair covers most areas of the body. Body hair in unexpected places should be noted. For example, a tuft of hair at the base of the spine often indicates a spinal defect.

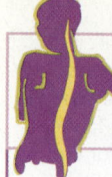
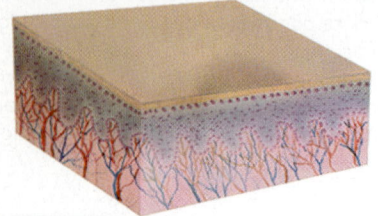

Lesion Name: Macule
Description:
Flat, nonpalpable, diameter <1 cm (½ in)
Example: Freckle, rubella, rubeola, petechiae

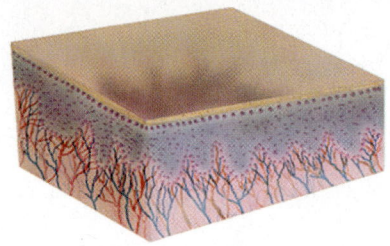

Lesion Name: Patch
Description:
Macule, diameter >1 cm (½ in)
Example: Vitiligo, Mongolian spot

Lesion Name: Papule
Description:
Elevated, firm, diameter <1 cm (½ in)
Example: Warts, pigmented nevi

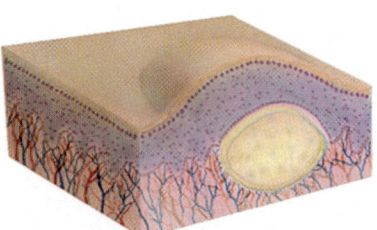

Lesion Name: Nodule
Description:
Elevated, firm, deeper in dermis than papule, diameter 1–2 cm (½ in–1 in)
Example: Erythema nodosum

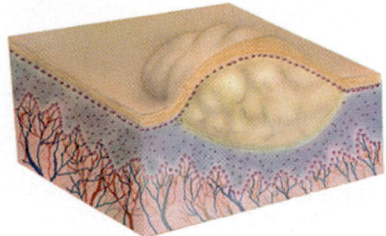

Lesion Name: Tumor
Description:
Elevated, solid, diameter >2 cm (1 in)
Example: Neoplasm, hemangioma

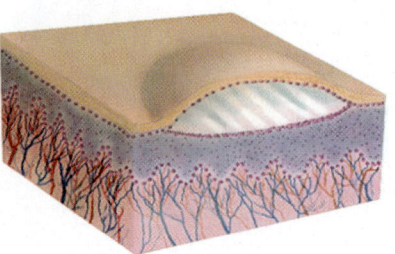

Lesion Name: Vesicle
Description:
Elevated, filled with fluid, diameter <1 cm (½ in)
Example: Early chicken pox, herpes simplex

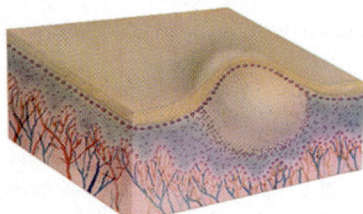

Lesion Name: Pustule
Description:
Vesicle filled with purulent fluid
Example: Impetigo, acne

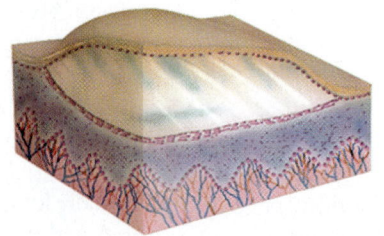

Lesion Name: Bulla
Description:
Vesicle diameter >1 cm (½ in)
Example: Burn blister

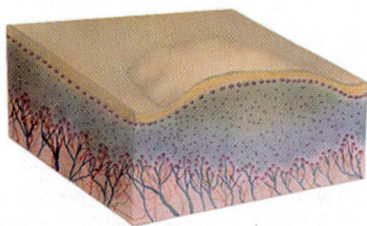

Lesion Name: Wheal
Description:
Irregular elevated solid area of edematous skin
Example: Urticaria, insect bite

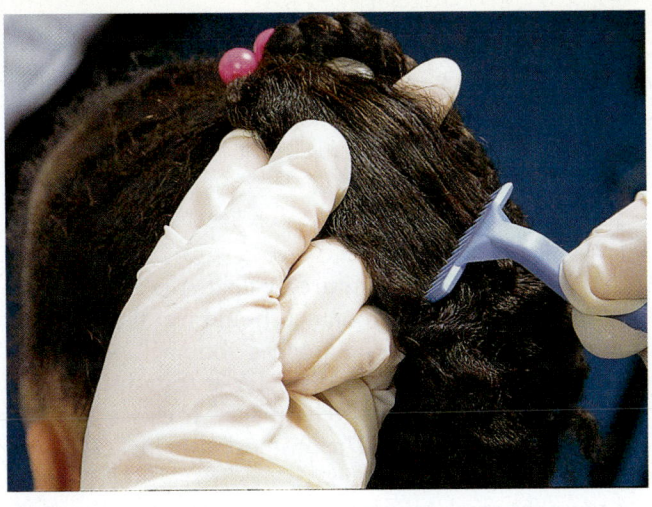

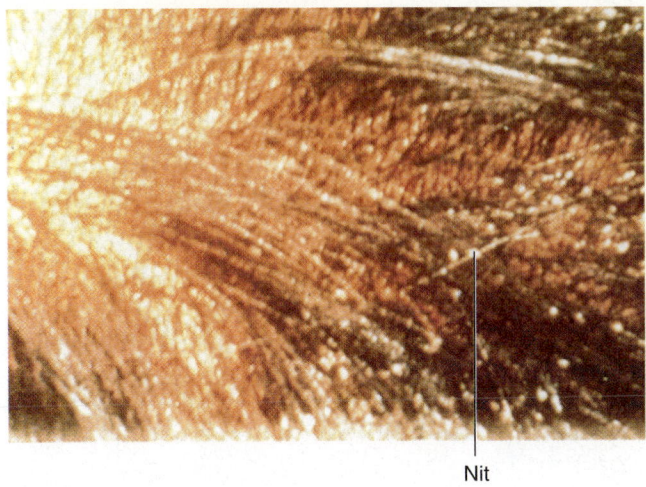

B

Nit

FIGURE 33–5. ◆ **A,** Inspecting for head lice with a fine-tooth comb. **B,** Nits on hair. **B,** *Courtesy of Centers for Disease Control.*

Growth and Development

Pubic hair begins to develop in children between 8 and 12 years of age, and axillary hair develops about 6 months later. Facial hair is noted in boys shortly after axillary hair develops.

It is important to note the age at which pubic and axillary hair develops in the child. Development at an unusually young age is associated with precocious puberty.

Palpation of the Hair

Palpate the hair shafts for texture. Hair should feel soft or silky with fine or thick shafts. Endocrine conditions such as hypothyroidism may result in coarse, brittle hair. Part the hair in various spots over the head to inspect and palpate the scalp for crusting or other lesions. If lesions are present, describe them using the characteristics in "Pathophysiology Illustrated."

ASSESSING THE HEAD FOR SKULL CHARACTERISTICS AND FACIAL FEATURES

What can cause a child's head or face to be asymmetric? How does a normal fontanel feel? What does an unusually large or small head suggest in an infant? What is the ping-pong phenomenon and what does it indicate?

Inspection of the Head and Face

During early childhood the skull's sutures permit expansion for brain growth. Infants and young children normally have a rounded skull with a prominent occipital area. The shape of the head changes during childhood, and the occipital area becomes less prominent. An abnormal skull shape can result from premature closure of the sutures.

Nursing Practice

Children who were low-birth-weight infants often have a flat, elongated skull because the soft skull bones were flattened by the weight of the head early in infancy. Head flattening is also associated with the side- and back-lying sleep positions in infants.

The head circumference of infants and young children is routinely measured until 3 years of age to ensure that adequate growth for brain development has occurred. The *Clinical Skills Manual* ▭▭ **SKILLS** **CD** as well as the CD-ROM describes the proper technique for use of the tape measure. A larger than normal head is associated with hydrocephalus, and a smaller than normal head suggests microcephaly.

Inspect the child's face for symmetry during several facial expressions such as resting, smiling, talking, and crying (Figure 33–6 ◆). Significant asymmetry may result from paralysis of trigeminal or facial nerves (cranial nerves V or VII), in utero positioning, and swelling from infection, allergy, or trauma.

Next inspect the face for unusual facial features such as coarseness, wide eye spacing, or disproportionate size. Tremors, tics, and twitching of facial muscles are often associated with seizures.

Palpation of the Skull

Palpate the skull in infants and young children to assess the sutures and fontanels and to detect soft bones (see "As They Grow").

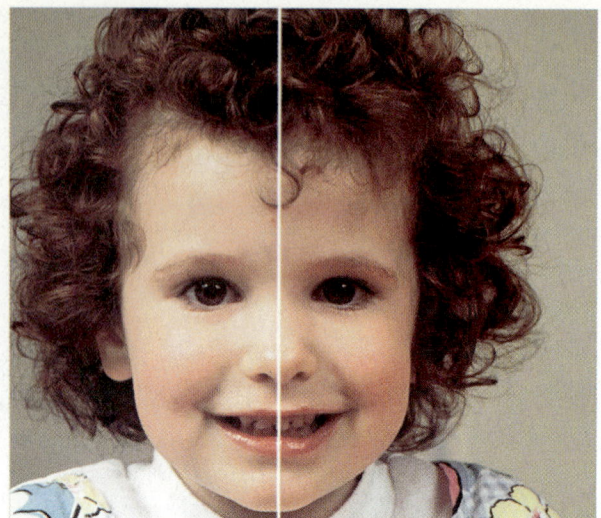

FIGURE 33–6. ◆ Draw on imaginary line down the middle of the face over the nose and compare the features on each side. Significant asymmetry may be caused by paralysis of cranial nerve V or VII, in utero positioning, and swelling from infection, allergy, or trauma.

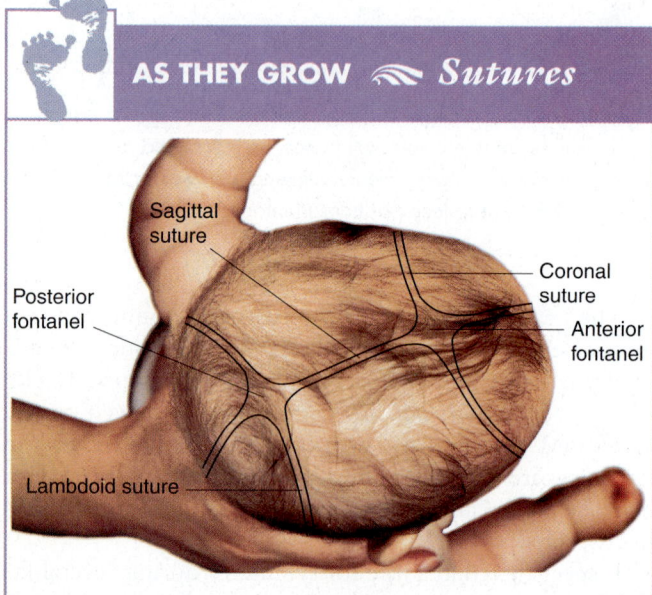

AS THEY GROW ≈ *Sutures*

Sagittal suture

Coronal suture

Posterior fontanel

Anterior fontanel

Lambdoid suture

The sutures are separations between the bones of the skull that have not yet joined. The fontanels are formed at the intersection of these sutures where bone has not yet formed. Fontanels are covered by tough membranous tissue that protects the brain. The posterior fontanel closes between 2 and 3 months. The anterior fontanel and sutures are palpable up to the age of 18 months.

SUTURES

Use your fingerpads to palpate each suture line. The edge of each bone in the suture line can be felt, but normally there is no separation of the two bones. If additional bone edges are felt, it may indicate a skull fracture.

Growth and Development

The suture lines of the skull are seldom palpated after 2 years of age. After that time the sutures rarely split.

FONTANELS

At the intersection of the sutures, palpate the anterior and posterior fontanels. The fontanel should feel flat and firm inside the bony edges. The anterior fontanel is normally smaller than 5 cm (2 in.) in diameter at 6 months of age and then becomes progressively smaller. It closes between 12 and 18 months of age. The posterior fontanel closes between 2 and 3 months of age.

A tense fontanel, bulging above the margin of the skull, is an indication of increased intracranial pressure. A soft fontanel, sunken below the margin of the skull, is associated with dehydration.

Developing Cultural Competence

The head is a sacred part of the body to Southeast Asians. Ask for permission before touching the infant's head to palpate the sutures and fontanels (Spector, 2000). When a Hispanic child is examined, however, not touching the head is considered bad luck.

ASSESSING EYE STRUCTURES, FUNCTION, AND VISION

Inspection of the External Eye Structures

The function of the external and internal eye structures and related cranial nerves makes vision possible. Inspect the external eye structures, including the eyeballs, eyelids, and eye muscles. Test the function of cranial nerves II, III, IV, and VI, which innervate the eye structures (Figure 33–7 ◆). Equipment needed for this examination includes an ophthalmoscope, vision chart, penlight, small toy, and an index card or paper cup.

EYE SIZE AND SPACING

Inspect the eyes and surrounding tissues simultaneously when examining facial features. The eyes should be the same size but not unusually large or small. Observe for eye bulging, which can be identified by retracted eyelids or a sunken appearance. Bulging may be associated with a tumor, and a sunken appearance may reflect dehydration.

Next inspect the eyes to see if they are appropriately distanced from each other. *Hypertelorism*, or widely spaced eyes, can be a normal variation in children.

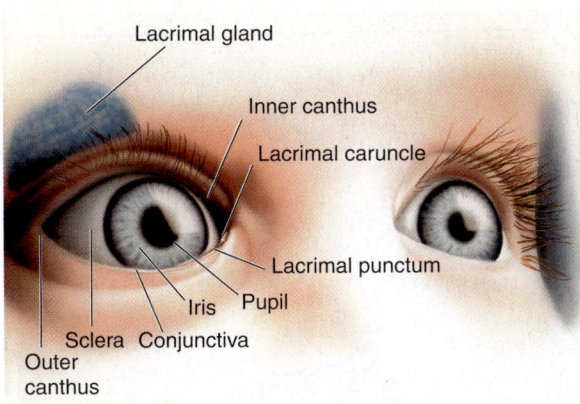

FIGURE 33–7. ◆ External structures of the eye. Notice that the light reflex is at the same location on each eye.

EYELIDS

Inspect the eyelids for color, size, position, mobility, and condition of the eyelashes. Eyelids should be the same color as surrounding facial skin and free of swelling or inflammation along the edges. Sebaceous glands that look like yellow striations are often present near the hair follicles. Eyelashes curl away from the eye to prevent irritation of the conjunctivae.

Inspect the conjunctivae lining the eyelids by pulling down the lower lid and then everting the upper lid. The conjunctivae should be pink and glossy. The lacrimal punctum, the opening for the lacrimal gland on each lid, is located near the medial canthus. No redness or excess tearing should be present.

When the eyes are open, inspect the level at which the upper and lower lids cross the eye. Each lid normally covers part of the iris but not any portion of the pupil. The lids should also close completely over the iris and cornea. Ptosis, drooping of the lid over the pupil, is often associated with injury to the oculomotor nerve, cranial nerve III. Sunset sign, in which the sclera is seen between the upper lid and the iris, may indicate retracted eyelids or hydrocephalus.

Inspect the eyes for the palpebral slant (Figure 33–8 ◆). The eyelids of most people open horizontally. Children of Asian descent often have an extra fold of skin, known as the epicanthal fold, covering all or part of the medial canthus of the eye. An upward or Mongolian slant is a normal finding in Asian children; however, children with Down syndrome also often have a Mongolian slant (Figure 33–9 ◆). A downward or anti-Mongolian slant is seen in some children as a normal variation.

EYE COLOR

Inspect the color of each sclera, iris, and bulbar conjunctiva. The sclera is normally white or ivory in darker skinned

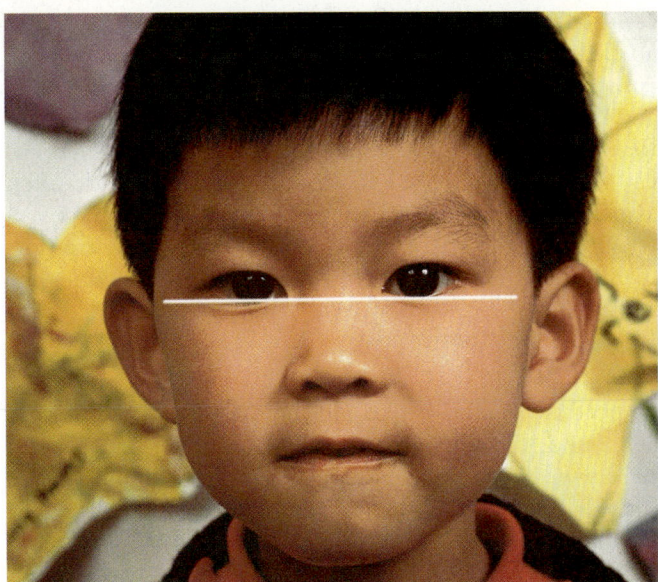

FIGURE 33–8. ◆ Draw an imaginary line across the medial canthi and extend it to each side of the face to identify the slant of the palpebral fissures. When the line crosses the lateral canthi, the palpebral fissures are horizontal and no slant is present. When the lateral canthi fall above the imaginary line, the eyes have an upward or Mongolian slant. A downward or anti-Mongolian slant is present when the lateral canthi fall below the imaginary line. Epicanthal folds are present when an extra fold of skin partially or completely covers the caruncles in the medial canthi. Which type of slant does this child have?

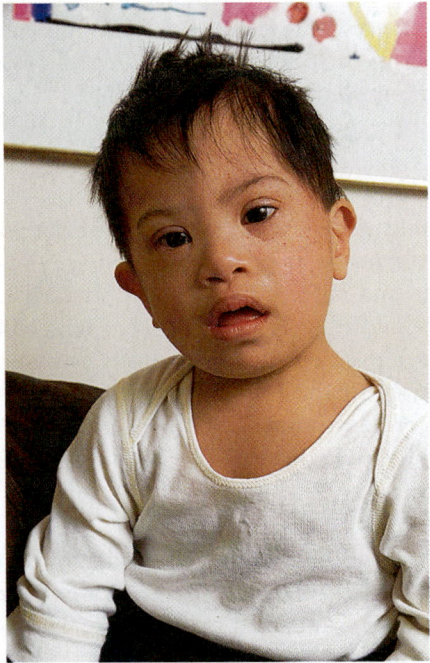

FIGURE 33–9. ◆ The eyes of this boy with Down syndrome show a Mongolian slant.

children. Sclerae of another color suggest the presence of an underlying disease. For example, yellow sclerae indicate jaundice. Typically the iris is blue or light colored at birth and becomes pigmented within 6 months. Inspect the iris for the presence of Brushfield spots, white specks in a linear pattern around the iris circumference, which are often associated with Down syndrome. The bulbar conjunctivae, which cover the sclera to the edge of the cornea, are normally clear. Redness can indicate eyestrain, allergies, or irritation.

PUPILS

Inspect the pupils for size and shape. Normally the pupils are round, clear, and equal in size. Some children have a *coloboma*, a keyhole-shaped pupil caused by a notch in the iris. This sign can indicate that the child has other congenital anomalies.

To test the pupillary response to light, shine a bright light into one eye. A brisk constriction of both the pupil exposed to direct light and the other pupil is a normal finding.

To test pupillary response to accommodation, ask the child to look first at a near object (for example, a toy) and then at a distant object (for example, a picture on the wall). The expected response is pupil constriction with near objects and pupil dilation with distant objects. This procedure tests the optic nerve, cranial nerve II.

Inspection of the Eye Muscles

One of the most common pediatric eye disorders is strabismus, or crossed eyes. This condition is important to detect because, if uncorrected, it can cause vision impairment. Several tests are used to detect a muscle imbalance that can result in strabismus, including the evaluation of extraocular movements, the corneal light reflex, and the cover–uncover test.

EXTRAOCULAR MOVEMENTS

Seat the child at eye level to evaluate the extraocular movements. Hold a toy or penlight 30 cm (12 in.) from the child's eyes and move it through the six cardinal fields of gaze. The child's head may need to be held still until fine motor eye movement develops. Both eyes should move together, tracking the object. This procedure tests the oculomotor, trochlear, and abducens nerves (cranial nerves III, IV, and VI) (Figure 33–10 ◆).

CORNEAL LIGHT REFLEX

To test the corneal light reflex, shine a light on the child's nose, midway between the eyes. Identify the location where the light is reflected on each eye. The light reflection is normally symmetric, at the same spot on each cornea. An asymmetric corneal light reflex indicates strabismus (see Figure 33–7).

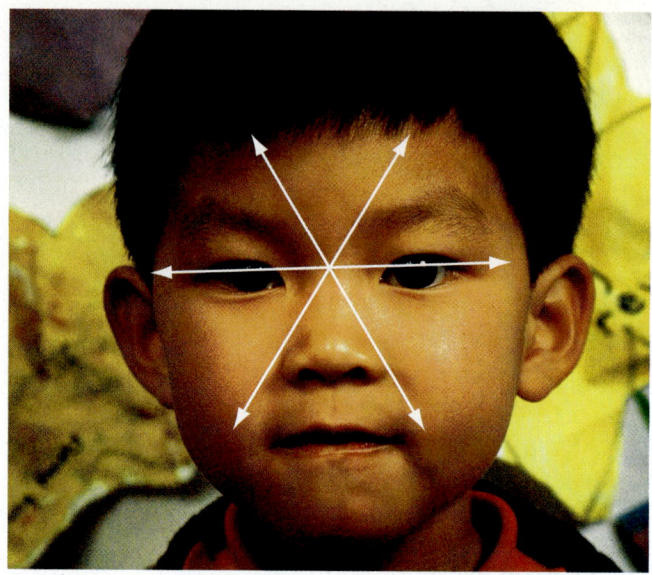

FIGURE 33–10. ◆ Begin the eye muscle examination with inspection of the extraocular movements. Have the child sit at your eye level. Hold a toy or penlight about 30 cm (12 in.) from the child's eyes and move it through the six cardinal fields of gaze. Both eyes should move together, tracking the object. This procedure tests cranial nerves III, IV, and VI.

COVER–UNCOVER TEST

The cover–uncover test can be used only for older, cooperative children. While standing slightly to one side but in a position from which you are still able to see the child's eyes, ask the child to look at a picture on the wall. Cover one of the child's eyes with an index card and simultaneously inspect the uncovered eye for movement as it focuses on the picture. Then remove the card from the covered eye and inspect the eye for movement as it focuses on the picture. Repeat the procedure with the child's other eye covered. Because the eyes work together, no obvious movement of either eye is expected. Eye movement indicates a muscle imbalance.

Vision Assessment

Because vision is such an important sense for learning, assessment is essential to detect any serious problems. Vision is evaluated using an age-appropriate vision test, but no simple method exists. It is possible to assess vision in infants and children by observing their behavior in response to certain maneuvers and during play.

INFANTS AND TODDLERS

When the infant's eyes are open, test the blink reflex by moving your hand quickly toward the infant's eyes. A quick blink is the normal response. Absence of the blink reflex can indicate that the infant is blind.

Growth and Development

Research has discovered that newborns have vision good enough at birth to prefer faces to other patterns and to follow a moving object. The child's visual acuity develops during early childhood (Seidel et al., 2003).

Age	Visual Acuity
3 years	20/50
4 years	20/40
5 years	20/30
6 years	20/20

To test an infant's ability to visually track an object, hold a light or toy about 15 cm (6 in.) from the infant's eyes. When the infant has fixated on or is staring at the object, move it slowly to each side. The infant should follow the object with the eyes and by moving the head.

Once an infant has developed skills to reach for and then pick up objects, observe play behavior to evaluate vision. The ability to easily find and pick up small toys is a good indicator of vision in children under 3 years of age.

STANDARDIZED VISION CHARTS

Standardized vision charts cannot be used to test vision until the child can understand directions and can cooperate, usually at about 3 or 4 years of age. The Snellen E chart and the Picture chart are used to test visual acuity of preschool-age children just as the Snellen Letter chart is used for school-age children and adolescents. Skills 9–17 through 9–19 in the *Clinical Skills Manual,* as well as the accompanying CD-ROM, describes the use of these charts. SKILLS CD

Nursing Practice

A difference in vision of 2 lines or more on the Snellen eye chart between the eyes is an indication for further evaluation.

Inspection of the Internal Eye Structures

The funduscopic examination allows inspection of the structures of the internal eye—the retina, optic disc, arteries and veins, and macula (Figure 33–11 ◆). This examination takes extensive practice because the ophthalmoscope is a complex instrument to master and because the examination is difficult to perform on uncooperative children. Most often it is performed by experienced examiners.

Darken the room so the child's pupils dilate. Explain the procedure to the child to gain his or her cooperation. Have a picture on the wall or have the parent or assistant hold a toy for the child to stare at so that the child's eye will not have to be held open forcibly.

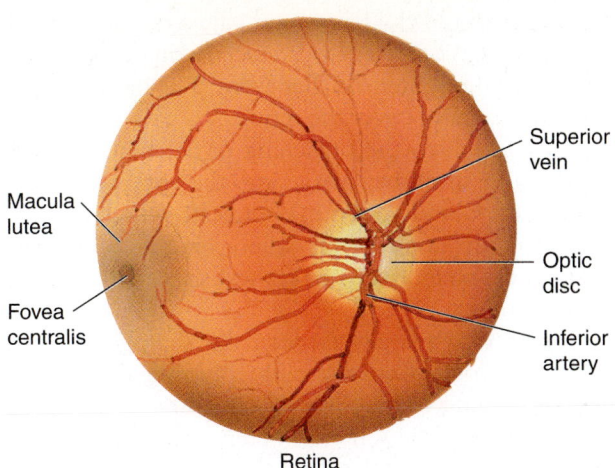

FIGURE 33–11. ◆ Normal fundus.

USING THE OPHTHALMOSCOPE

The ophthalmoscope has a lens-and-mirror system and a bright light for inspecting the structures of the internal eye. Different lens powers are arranged on the rotating disk of the ophthalmic head. This system permits compensation for vision difference between the child and the examiner. The black-numbered plus lenses magnify images, and the red-numbered minus lenses reduce them in a range of powers. The lenses can be changed by turning the disk with the forefinger.

Turn the ophthalmoscope on and set the lens power at 0. Keep a forefinger on the disk to change the lens power as needed. Look through the lens of the ophthalmoscope, stabilizing it by resting the top against an eyebrow and the handle against a cheek. Use your right eye to examine the child's right eye and your left eye to examine the child's left eye. This position is best for visualizing the eye, and it reduces direct exposure to infection. Place a hand on the child's head for stabilization.

Red Reflex. Shine the ophthalmoscope light at the child's eye from a distance of 30 cm (12 in). The first image seen is the red reflex, the red glow of the vascular retina. When the red reflex is seen, the ophthalmoscope is being used correctly and the child's lens is clear. Black spots or opacities within the red reflex are abnormal and may indicate congenital cataracts. If a white reflex is seen rather than a red reflex, a retinoblastoma may be present. The red reflex can also be tested by shining a small flashlight into the eye.

Visualizing the Internal Eye Structures. Slowly move closer to the child. Deeper levels of the vitreous humor are inspected before the pink retina comes into view. The retina is a deeper pink in dark-skinned children. A blood vessel is the first retinal structure usually seen. Continue moving closer to the child's eye and adjust the plus or minus lenses to focus on this blood vessel. Retinal arteries appear smaller and brighter red than veins. The blood vessels branch to spread and cover the retina.

Inspect and follow the branching of the blood vessels toward the nose until they merge into the optic disc. Dark areas along the blood vessels may indicate retinal hemorrhages. Carefully inspect sites where arteries and veins cross. Notches and indentations at these sites are associated with hypertension.

The optic disc margin is normally sharply defined, round, and yellow to creamy pink. Blurring of the disc margins or bulging of the optic disc is a sign of increased intracranial pressure. Use the diameter of the optic disc to identify the location of other landmarks on the retina.

The macula is located approximately 2 disc diameters lateral to the optic disc. To see the macula, ask the child to look at the light. It appears as a yellow dot surrounded by deep pink. The macula is inspected last because the bright light causes the child to blink and look away.

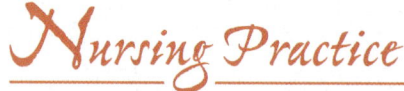

Nursing Practice

Keep the red reflex in view to make sure your head and the ophthalmoscope move as one unit. If you lose the red reflex when moving closer to the child, move back, find the red reflex, and start again.

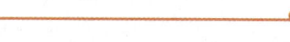

ASSESSING THE EAR STRUCTURES AND HEARING

Inspection of the External Ear Structures

Equipment needed for this examination includes an otoscope, noisemakers (bell, rattle, tissue paper), and a tuning fork 500 to 1000 Hz. The position and characteristics of the pinna, the external ear, are inspected as a continuation of the head and eye examination. The pinna is considered "low set" when the top lies completely below an imaginary line drawn through the medial and lateral canthi of the eye toward the ear. Low-set ears are often associated with congenital renal disorders (Figure 33–12 ◆).

Inspect the pinna for any malformation. The pinna should be completely formed, with an open auditory canal. Next, inspect the tissue around the pinna for abnormalities. A pit or hole in front of the auditory canal may indicate the presence of a sinus. If the pinna protrudes outward, there may be swelling behind the ear, a sign of mastoiditis.

Inspect the external auditory canal for any discharge. A foul-smelling, purulent discharge may indicate the presence of a foreign body or an infection in the external canal. Clear fluid or a blood-tinged discharge may indicate a cerebrospinal fluid leak caused by a basilar skull fracture.

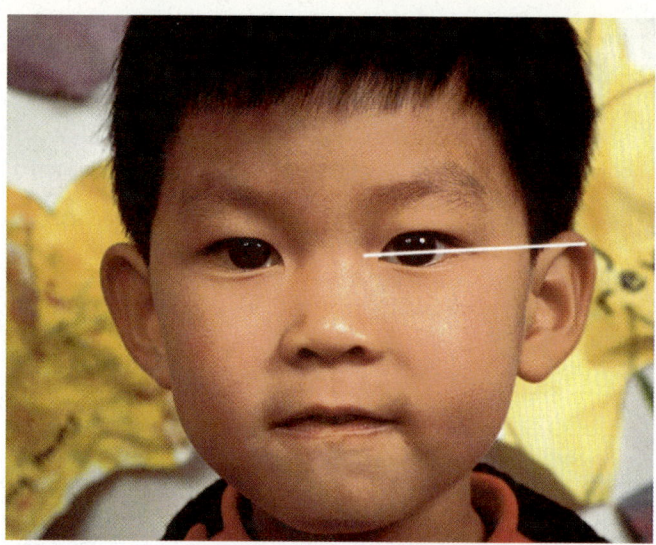

FIGURE 33–12. ◆ To detect the correct placement of the external ears, draw an imaginary line through the medial and lateral canthi of the eye toward the ear. This line normally passes through the upper portion of the pinna. The pinna is considered "low set" when the top lies completely below the imaginary line. Low-set ears are often associated with renal disorders. Is this a normal ear placement? Yes, it is.

Inspection of the Tympanic Membrane

Examination of the tympanic membrane is important in infants and young children because they are prone to otitis media, a middle ear infection. The eustachian tubes are shorter, wider, and more horizontally positioned in infants and young children than in older children and adults. This positioning enables bacteria to move up the eustachian tube from the pharynx, causing an infection.

The otoscope, an instrument with a magnifying lens, bright light, and speculum, is used to examine the internal auditory canal and tympanic membrane. 🔗 [CD] Infants and young children often resist having their ears inspected with the otoscope because of past painful experiences. For that reason it may be wise to delay the otoscopic examination until portions of the assessment requiring cooperation are completed. Use simple explanations to prepare the child. Let the child play with the otoscope or demonstrate how it is used on the parent or a doll. Figure 33–13 ◆ illustrates one method for restraining an uncooperative child. See also Skill 7–3 in the *Clinical Skills Manual.* 🔗 [SKILLS]

USING THE OTOSCOPE

To begin the otoscopic examination, hold the handle of the otoscope in the palm with the thumb pointed toward the base of the handle. 🔗 [CD] If using a pneumatic squeeze bulb, hold it between the index finger and the handle. Choose the largest ear speculum that fits into the auditory canal to form a seal for testing the movement of the tympanic membrane. A large speculum is also less likely to injure the auditory canal if the child moves suddenly.

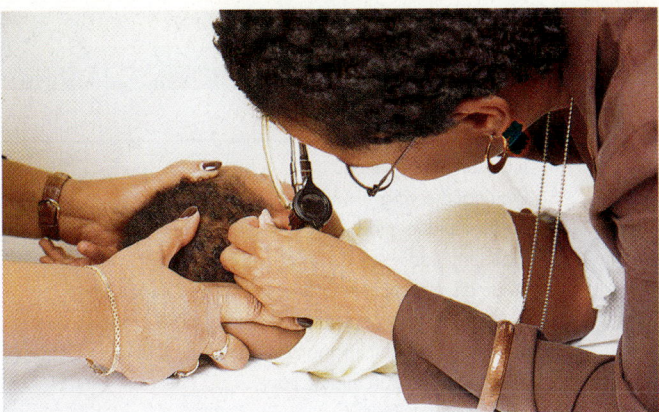

FIGURE 33–13. ◆ To restrain an uncooperative child, place the child prone on the examining table. Have an assistant hold the child's arms next to the head to restrain the child's head movements. Restrain the child's body movements by lying across the child's body. Keep your hands free to hold the otoscope and position the external ear.

Hold the otoscope in the hand closest to the child's face and when the child is cooperative rest the back of that hand against the child's head to stabilize it. Use the other hand to pull the pinna toward the back of the head and either up or down. Pulling the pinna straightens the auditory canal and improves inspection of the tympanic membrane (Figure 33–14 ◆).

Slowly insert the speculum into the auditory canal, inspecting the walls for signs of irritation, discharge, or a foreign body. The walls of the auditory canal are normally pink, and some cerumen is present. Children often put beads, peas, or other small objects into their ears. If the auditory canal is obstructed by cerumen or a foreign body, irrigation can be used to clean the canal.

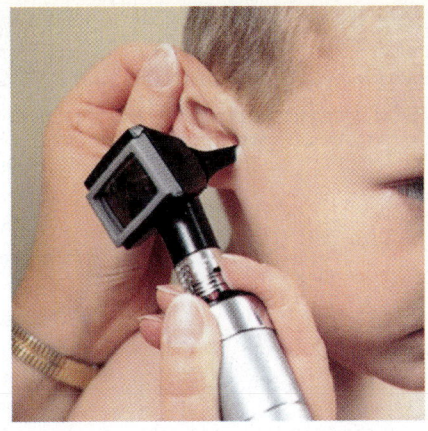

FIGURE 33–14. ◆ To straighten the auditory canal: pull the pinna back and up for children over 3 years of age; pull the pinna down and back for children under 3 years of age.

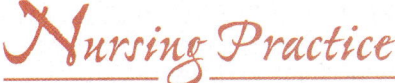

Nursing Practice

Never irrigate the ear canal if any discharge is present. Never use cold water for irrigation.

The tympanic membrane, which separates the outer ear from the middle ear, is usually pearly gray and translucent. It reflects light, and the bones (ossicles) in the middle ear are normally visible. When the pneumatic attachment is squeezed, the tympanic membrane normally moves in and out in response to the positive and negative pressure applied (Figure 33–15 ◆). Table 33–9 lists the abnormal findings of a tympanic membrane examination and their associated conditions.

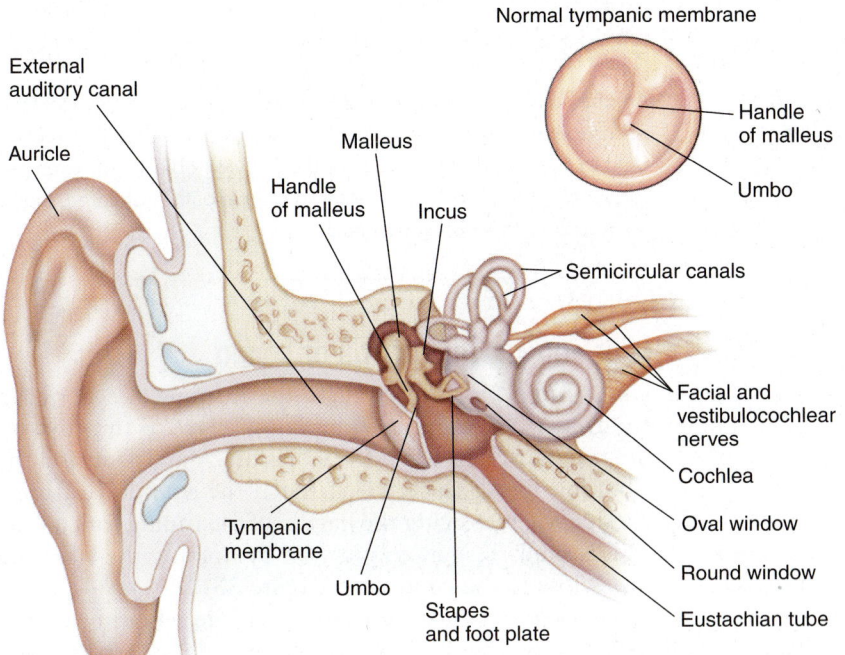

Normal tympanic membrane

External auditory canal

Auricle

Malleus

Handle of malleus

Incus

Handle of malleus

Umbo

Semicircular canals

Facial and vestibulocochlear nerves

Cochlea

Oval window

Round window

Eustachian tube

Tympanic membrane

Umbo

Stapes and foot plate

FIGURE 33–15. ◆ Cross section of the ear. The tympanic membrane normally has a triangular light reflex with the base on the nasal side pointing toward the center. The bony landmarks, the umbo and handle of malleus, are seen through the tympanic membrane.

TABLE 33–9 Unexpected Findings on Examination of the Tympanic Membrane and Their Associated Conditions

Characteristics of Tympanic Membrane	Unexpected Findings	Associated Conditions
Color	Redness	Infection in middle ear
	Slight redness	Prolonged crying
	Amber	Serous fluid in middle ear
	Deep red or blue	Blood in middle ear
Light reflex	Absent	Bulging tympanic membrane, infection in middle ear
	Distorted, loss of triangular shape	Retracted tympanic membrane, serous fluid in middle ear
Bony landmarks	Extra prominent	Retracted tympanic membrane, serous fluid in middle ear
Movement	No motility	Infection or fluid in middle ear
	Excess motility	Healed perforation

Hearing Assessment

Hearing evaluation is important in children of all ages because hearing is essential for normal speech development and learning. With new technology, even newborns can have their hearing screened, and many states require such screening prior to hospital discharge. Often hearing must be evaluated by inspection of the child's responses to various auditory stimuli. Hearing loss may occur at any time during early childhood as the result of birth trauma, frequent otitis media, meningitis, or antibiotics that damage cranial nerve VIII.

Use hearing and speech articulation milestones as an initial hearing screen. Select an age-appropriate method to screen hearing. When a hearing deficiency is suspected as a result of screening, refer the child for audiometry, tympanometry, or evoked response to obtain the most accurate evaluation of hearing. See Skills 9–20 and 9–21 in the *Clinical Skills Manual*. SKILLS

Growth and Development

Indicators of hearing loss in an infant:

• No startle reaction to loud noises
• Does not turn toward sounds by 4 months of age
• Babbles as a young infant but does not keep babbling or develop speech sounds after 6 months of age

Indicators of hearing loss in a young child:

• No speech by 2 years of age
• Speech sounds are not distinct at appropriate ages

INFANTS AND TODDLERS

Select noisemakers with different frequencies, such as a rattle, bell, and tissue paper, that will attract the young child's attention. Ask the parent or an assistant to entertain the infant with a quiet toy, such as a teddy bear. Stand behind the infant, about 2 feet (60 cm) away from the infant's ear but outside the infant's field of vision, and make a soft sound with the noisemaker. Have the parent or assistant observe the child for any of the following responses when the noisemaker is used: widening the eyes, briefly stopping all activity to listen, or turning the head toward the sound. Repeat the test in the other ear and with the other noisemakers.

PRESCHOOL AND OLDER CHILDREN

Use whispered words to evaluate the hearing of children over 3 years of age. Position your head about 12 inches (30 cm) away from the child's ear, but out of the range of vision so the child cannot read your lips. Use words easily recognized by the child, such as Mickey Mouse, hot dog, and Popsicle, and ask the child to repeat the words. Repeat the test with different words in the opposite ear. The child should correctly repeat the whispered words.

Nursing Practice

An alternative procedure is used to assess hearing when the child will not cooperate by repeating whispered words. In a whisper, direct the child to point to different parts of the body or objects, for example, "Show me your eyes" and "Point to your mouth." Children should point to the correct body part each time.

BONE AND AIR CONDUCTION OF SOUND

Use a tuning fork to evaluate the hearing of school-age children who can follow directions. Stroke the tines of the tuning fork to begin the vibration. Avoid touching the vibrating tines, which will dampen the sound. Test bone conduction by placing the handle of the tuning fork on the child's skull. Test air conduction by holding the vibrating tines close to the child's ear (Figure 33–16 ◆).

To perform the *Weber test*, place the vibrating tuning fork on top of the child's skull in the midline. Ask the child

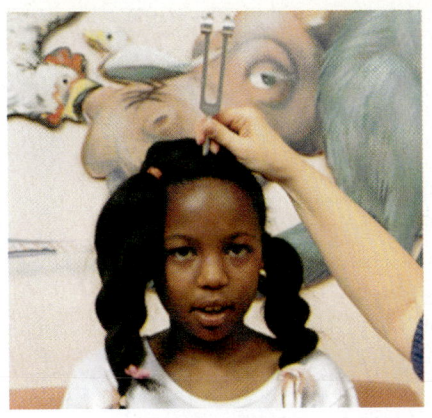 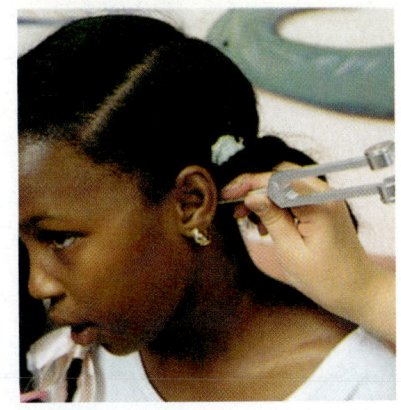 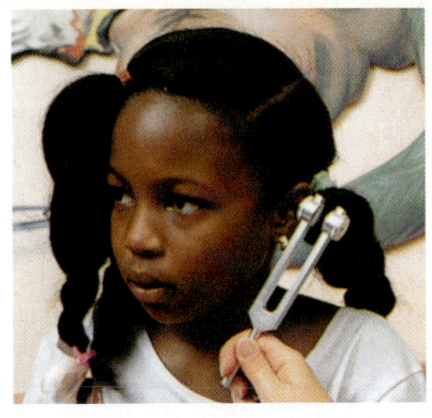

A   **B**   **C**

FIGURE 33–16. ◆ **A,** Weber test. Place vibrating tuning fork on midline of the child's head. **B,** Rinne test, step 1. Place vibrating tuning fork on mastoid process. **C,** Rinne test, step 2. Reposition still vibrating tines between 2.5 and 5 cm (1 and 2 in) from ear.

to say where the sound is heard best, either in both ears equally or in one ear. The sound should be heard equally in both ears.

To perform the *Rinne test,* place the vibrating tuning fork handle on the mastoid process behind an ear. Ask the child to say when the sound is no longer heard. Immediately move the tuning fork, holding the vibrating tines about 2.5 to 5 cm (1 to 2 in) from the same ear. Again, ask the child to indicate when the sound is no longer heard. The child normally hears the air-conducted sound twice as long as the bone-conducted sound. Repeat the Rinne test on the other ear. Table 33–10 provides an interpretation of the Weber and Rinne tests.

ASSESSING THE NOSE AND SINUSES FOR AIRWAY PATENCY AND DISCHARGE

An otoscope with a nasal speculum and a penlight are needed for this examination.

Inspection of the External Nose

Examine the external nose characteristics and placement on the face simultaneously with the facial features. Inspect the external nose for size, shape, symmetry, and midline placement on the face. The nose should be proportional in size to other facial features and positioned in the middle of the face. A flattened nasal bridge is the expected finding in Asian and black children.

The nasolabial folds are normally symmetric. Asymmetry of the nasolabial folds may be associated with injury to the facial nerve (cranial nerve VII). A saddle-shaped nose is associated with congenital defects such as cleft palate.

TABLE 33–10 Interpretation of the Weber and Rinne Tests of Hearing	
Test and Result	*Associated Condition*
Weber Test	
Sound heard equally in both ears	No hearing loss
Sound heard better in one ear (lateralized)	Conductive hearing loss if sound lateralized to deaf ear
Rinne Test	
Sound heard by air conduction twice as long as bone conduction	No hearing loss
Sound heard longer by bone conduction than air conduction	Conductive hearing loss in affected ear
Sound heard longer by air conduction than bone conduction, but less than twice as long	Sensorineural hearing loss in affected ear

Inspect the external nose for unusual characteristics. For example, a crease across the nose between the cartilage and bone is often caused by the allergic child's wiping an itchy nose upward with a hand.

Palpation of the External Nose

When a deformity is noted, gently palpate the nose to detect any pain or break in contour. No tenderness or masses are expected. Pain and a contour deviation are usually the result of trauma.

NASAL PATENCY

The child's airway must be patent to ensure adequate oxygenation. To test for nasal patency, occlude one nostril and observe the child's effort to breathe through the open nostril with the mouth closed. Repeat the procedure with the

Infants under 6 months of age will not automatically open their mouths to breathe when their nose is occluded, such as by mucus.

other nostril. Breathing should be noiseless and effortless. *Nasal flaring,* an effort the child makes to widen the airway, is a sign of respiratory distress and should not be present.

If the child struggles to breathe, a nasal obstruction may be present. Nasal obstruction may be caused by a foreign body, congenital defect, dry mucus, discharge, polyp, or trauma. Newborns may have respiratory distress because of *choanal atresia,* a congenital membranous or bony obstruction between the nose and the nasopharynx. Young children commonly place objects up their nose, and unilateral nasal flaring is a sign of such an obstruction.

Assessment of Smell

The olfactory nerve (cranial nerve I) is rarely tested in preschool children, but it can be tested in school-age children and adolescents. When testing smell, choose scents the child will easily recognize such as orange, chocolate, and mint. When the child's eyes are closed, occlude one nostril and hold the scent under the nose. Ask the child to take a deep sniff and identify the scent. Alternate odors between the nares. The child can normally identify common scents.

Inspection of the Internal Nose

Inspect the internal nose for color of the mucous membranes and the presence of any discharge, swelling, lesions, or other abnormalities. Use a bright light, such as an otoscope light or penlight. For infants and young children, push the tip of the nose upward and shine the light at the end of the nose. The nasal speculum of the otoscope can be used in older children (Figure 33–17 ◆). Avoid touching the septum of the nose with the speculum. Injury to the septum can cause a nosebleed.

MUCOUS MEMBRANES

The mucous membranes should be dark pink and glistening. A film of clear discharge may also be present. Turbinates, if visible, should be the same color as the mucous membranes and have a firm consistency. When the turbinates are pale or bluish gray, the child may have allergies. A *polyp,* a rounded mass projecting from the turbinate, is also associated with allergies.

NASAL SEPTUM

Inspect the nasal septum for alignment, perforations, bleeding, or crusting. The septum should be straight. Crusting will be noted over the site of a nosebleed.

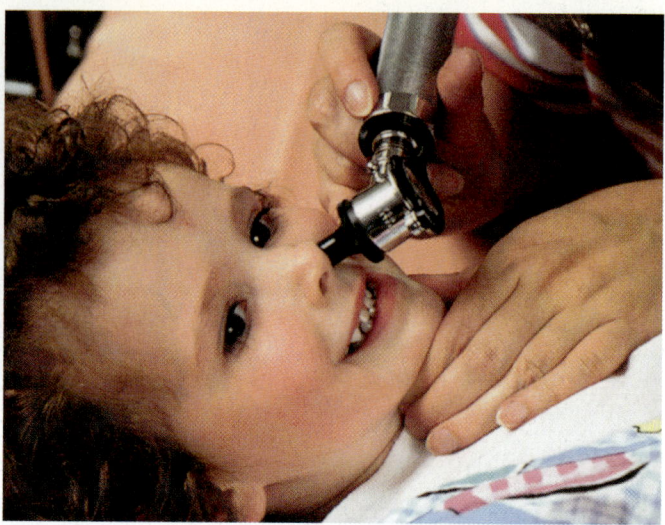

FIGURE 33–17. ◆ Technique for examining nose.

DISCHARGE

Observe for the presence of nasal discharge, noting if the drainage is from one or both nares. Nasal discharge is not a normal finding unless the child is crying. Discharge may be watery, mucoid, purulent, or bloody, depending on the condition present. A foul-smelling discharge in only one nostril is often associated with a foreign body. Table 33–11 lists conditions associated with nasal discharge.

Inspection of the Sinuses

The illustration in "As They Grow" shows how the maxillary and ethmoid sinuses develop during early childhood. Sinus infections can occasionally occur in young children. Suspect a sinus problem when the child has a headache or pain and swelling around one or both eyes.

Inspect the face for any puffiness around one or both eyes. Puffiness and swelling are not normally present. To palpate over the maxillary sinuses, press up under both zygomatic arches with the thumbs. To palpate the ethmoid sinuses, press up against the bone above both eyes with the thumbs. No swelling or tenderness is expected. Tenderness may indicate sinusitis.

TABLE 33-11 Nasal Discharge Characteristics and Associated Conditions	
Discharge Description	Associated Condition
Watery	
Clear, bilateral	Allergy
Serous, unilateral	Spinal fluid from fracture of cribriform plate
Mucoid or purulent	
Bilateral	Upper respiratory infection
Unilateral	Foreign body
Bloody	Nose bleed, trauma

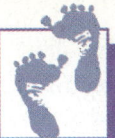
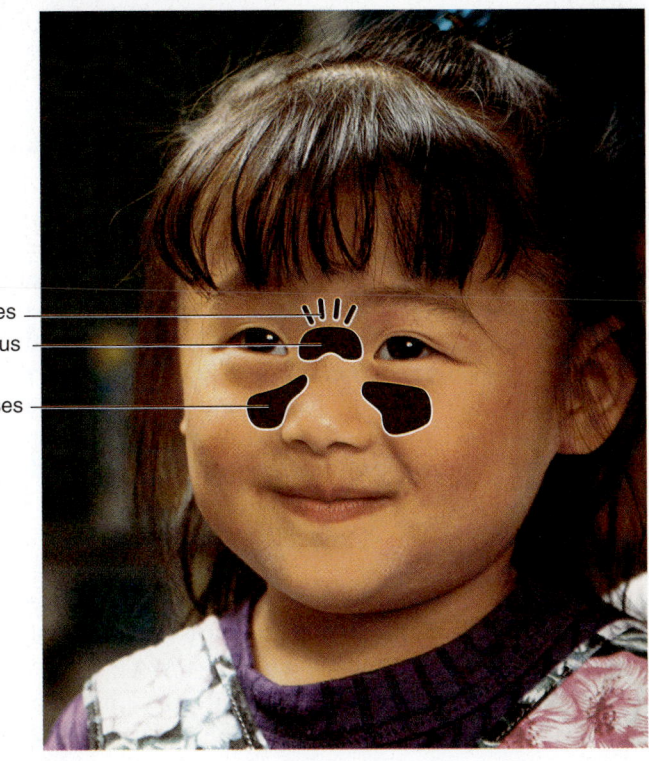

Ethmoid sinuses
Sphenoid sinus
Maxillary sinuses

Sinuses grow and develop during childhood. Maxillary sinuses can be identified in 1-year-old children. Ethmoid sinuses have developed in children by 6 years of age. Sinus problems under 7 years occur infrequently.

ASSESSING THE MOUTH AND THROAT FOR COLOR, FUNCTION, AND SIGNS OF ABNORMAL CONDITIONS

Inspection of the Mouth

Equipment needed to examine the mouth and throat includes a tongue blade and penlight. ⬭ **CD** Young children often need coaxing and simple explanations before they will cooperate with the mouth and throat examination. Most children readily show their teeth. If the child resists by clenching the teeth, they can be gently separated with a tongue blade. Wear gloves when examining the mouth because of contact with mucous membranes (Figure 33–18 ◆).

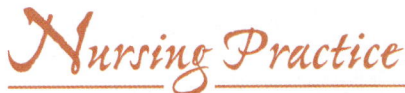

Nursing Practice

Avoid examining the mouth if there are signs of respiratory distress, high fever, drooling, and intense apprehension. These may be signs of epiglottitis. Inspecting the mouth may trigger a total airway obstruction. See Chapter 42 for more information.

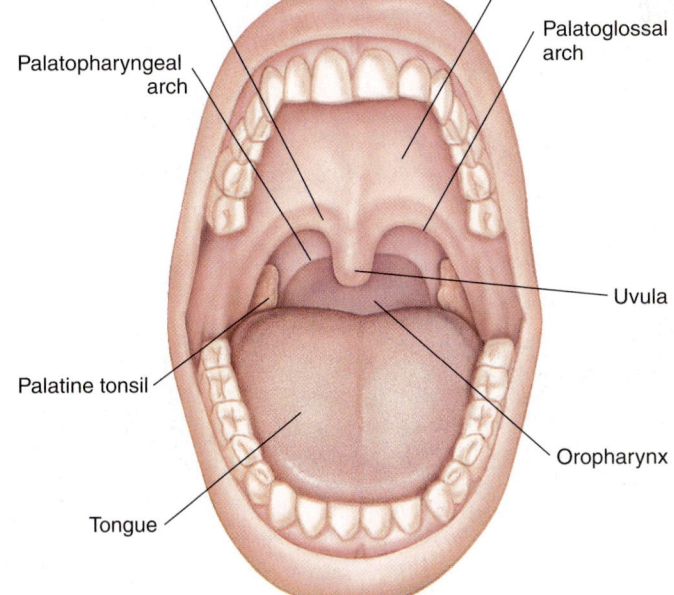

Soft palate
Hard palate
Palatopharyngeal arch
Palatoglossal arch
Palatine tonsil
Uvula
Tongue
Oropharynx

FIGURE 33–18. ◆ The structures of the mouth.

LIPS

Inspect the lips for color, shape, symmetry, moisture, and lesions. The lips are normally symmetric without drying, cracking, or other lesions. Lip color is normally pink in white children and more bluish in darker skinned children. Pale, cyanotic, or cherry-red lips indicate poor tissue perfusion caused by various conditions.

TEETH

Inspect and count the child's teeth. The timing of tooth eruption is often genetically determined, but there is a regular sequence of tooth eruption. Figure 33–19 ◆ presents the typical sequence of tooth eruption for both deciduous and permanent teeth.

Inspect the condition of the teeth, look for loose teeth, and note any spaces where teeth are missing. Compare empty tooth spaces with the child's developmental stage of tooth eruption. Once the permanent teeth have erupted, none should be missing. Teeth are normally white, without a flattened, mottled, or pitted appearance. Discolorations on the crown of a tooth may indicate caries.

MOUTH ODORS

During inspection of the teeth, be alert to any abnormal odors that may indicate problems such as diabetic ketoacidosis, infection, or poor hygiene.

GUMS

Inspect the gums for color and adherence to the teeth. The gums are normally pink, with a stippled or dotted appearance. Use a tongue blade to help visualize the gums around the upper and lower molars. No raised or receding gum areas should be apparent around the teeth. When inflammation, swelling, or bleeding is observed, palpate the gums to detect tenderness. Inflammation and tenderness are associated with infection and poor nutrition.

BUCCAL MUCOSA

Inspect the mucous membrane lining the cheeks for color and moisture. The mucous membrane is usually pink, but patches of hyperpigmentation are commonly seen in darker skinned children. The Stensen duct, the parotid gland opening, is opposite the upper second molar bilaterally. Normally pink, the duct opening becomes red when the child is infected with mumps. Small pink sucking pads can be present in infants. No areas of redness, swelling, or ulcerative lesions should be present.

TONGUE

Inspect the tongue for color, moistness, size, tremors, and lesions. The child's tongue is normally pink and moist, without a coating. The tongue's size permits it to fit easily into

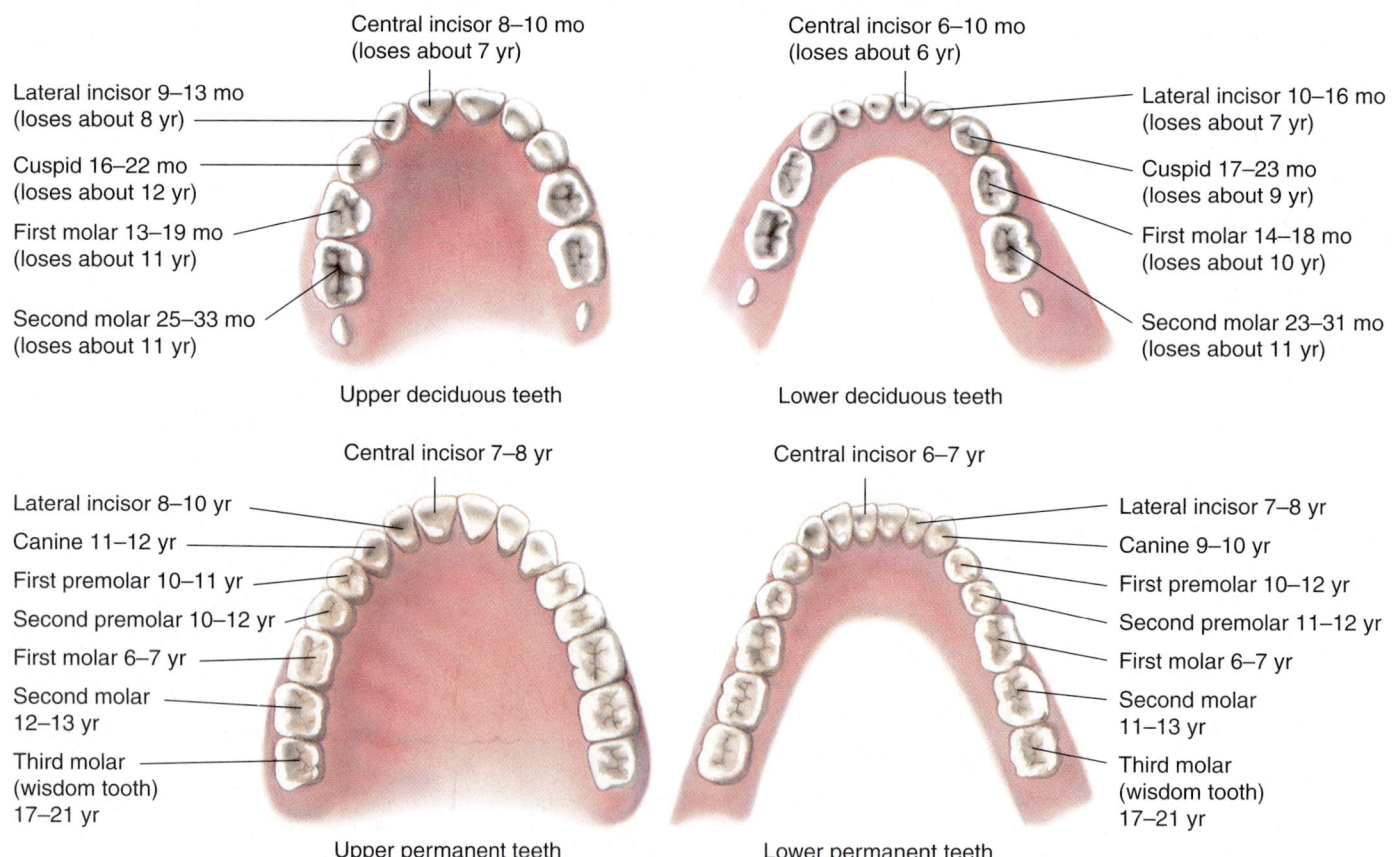

FIGURE 33–19. ◆ Typical sequence of tooth eruption for both deciduous and permanent teeth. Notice that bottom teeth come in first for each kind of tooth: incisors, cuspids, and molars. They are lost in the same pattern.

the mouth. A pattern of gray, irregular borders that form a design (geographic tongue) is often normal, but it may be associated with fever, allergies, or drug reactions. Tremors are abnormal. A white adherent coating on an infant's tongue may be caused by thrush, a *Candida* infection.

Observe the mobility of the tongue. The child should be able to touch the gums above the upper teeth with the tongue. This tongue movement is adequate to enunciate all speech sounds clearly. Ask the child to stick out the tongue and lift it so the underside of the tongue and the floor of the mouth can be inspected for distended veins.

PALATE

Inspect the hard and soft palate to detect any clefts or masses or an unusually high arch. The palate is normally pink, with a dome-shaped arch and no cleft. The uvula hangs freely from the soft palate. Newborns often have Epstein pearls, white papules in the midline of the palate that disappear in a few weeks. A high-arched palate can be associated with sucking difficulties in young infants.

Palpation of the Mouth Structures

Palpate any masses seen in the mouth to determine their characteristics, such as size, shape, firmness, and tenderness. No masses should be found.

TONGUE

To assess the tongue's strength, simultaneously testing the hypoglossal nerve (cranial nerve XII), place the index finger against the child's cheek and ask the child to push against your finger with the tongue. Some pressure against the finger is normally felt.

PALATE

To palpate the palate, insert the little finger, with the fingerpad upward, into the mouth. While the infant sucks against your finger, palpate the entire palate. This procedure also tests the strength of the sucking reflex, innervated by the hypoglossal nerve (cranial nerve XII). No clefts should be palpated.

Inspection of the Throat

Inspect the throat for color, swelling, lesions, and the condition of the tonsils. Ask the child to open the mouth wide and stick out the tongue. Illuminate the throat with a flashlight. Use a tongue blade, if needed, to visualize the posterior pharynx. Moistening the tongue blade may decrease the child's tendency to gag. The throat is normally pink without lesions, drainage, or swelling. Swelling or bulging in the posterior pharynx may be associated with a peritonsillar abscess.

TONSILS

During childhood the tonsils are large in proportion to the size of the pharynx because lymphoid tissue grows fastest in early childhood. The tonsils should be pink without exudate, but *crypts* (fissures) may be present as a result of prior infections.

GAG REFLEX

Use a tongue blade when you are unable to see the posterior pharynx or need to test the gag reflex. Do this at the end of the examination because children dislike the gagging sensation. Prepare the child for what will happen. Ask the child to say "Ah" and watch for the symmetric rising movement of the uvula. This reflex tests the glossopharyngeal and vagal nerves (cranial nerves IX and X). If the uvula does not rise or rises to one side, cranial nerves IX and X may be paralyzed. The epiglottis lies behind the tongue and is normally pink like the rest of the buccal mucosa.

ASSESSING THE NECK FOR CHARACTERISTICS, RANGE OF MOTION, AND LYMPH NODES

Inspection of the Neck

Inspect the neck for size, symmetry, swelling, and any abnormalities. A short neck with skin folds is normal for infants. The neck is normally symmetric. No swelling should be present. Swelling may be caused by local infections such as mumps or a congenital defect. The neck lengthens between 3 and 4 years of age.

Inspect the child's neck for webbing, an extra skin fold on each side of the neck. Webbing is commonly associated with Turner syndrome.

Infants develop head control by 2 months of age. By this age an infant can lift the head up and look around when lying on the stomach. A lack of head control can result from neurologic injury, such as an anoxic episode.

Palpation of the Neck

Face the child and use your fingerpads to simultaneously palpate both sides of the neck for lymph nodes, as well as the trachea and thyroid.

LYMPH NODES

To palpate the lymph nodes, slide your fingerpads gently over the lymph node chains in the head and neck. The sequence for lymph node palpation is as follows: around the ears, under the jaw, the occipital area, and the cervical chain in the neck (Figure 33–20 ◆). Firm, clearly defined, nontender, movable lymph nodes up to 1 cm (1/2 in.) in diameter are common in young children. Enlarged, firm, warm, tender lymph nodes indicate a local infection.

TRACHEA

Palpate the trachea to determine its position and to detect the presence of any masses. The trachea is normally in the

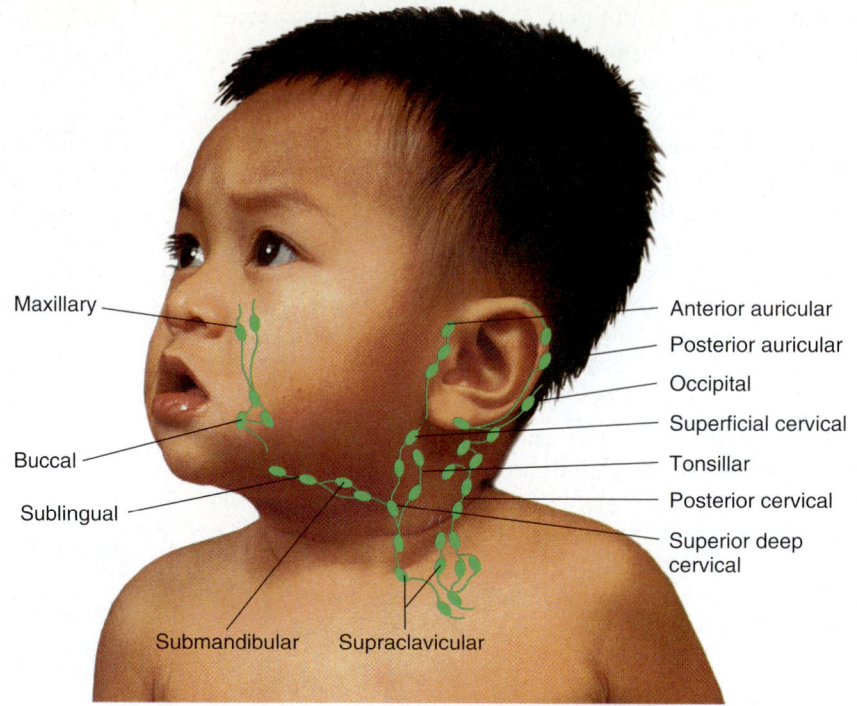

FIGURE 33–20. ◆ The neck is palpated for enlarged lymph nodes around the ears, under the jaw, in the occipital area, and in the cervical chain of the neck.

Maxillary

Buccal

Sublingual

Submandibular

Supraclavicular

Anterior auricular

Posterior auricular

Occipital

Superficial cervical

Tonsillar

Posterior cervical

Superior deep cervical

midline of the neck. It is difficult to palpate in children less than 3 years of age because of their short necks. To palpate the trachea, place your thumb and forefinger on each side of the child's trachea near the chin and slowly slide them down the trachea. Any shift to the right or left of midline may indicate a tumor or a collapsed lung.

THYROID

As the fingers slide over the trachea in the lower neck, attempt to feel the isthmus of the thyroid, a band of glandular tissue crossing over the trachea. The lobes of the thyroid wrap behind the trachea and are normally covered by the sternocleidomastoid muscle. Because of the anatomic position of the thyroid, its lobes are not usually palpable in the child unless they are enlarged.

Range of Motion Assessment

To test the neck's **range of motion,** ask the child to touch the chin to each shoulder and to the chest and then to look at the ceiling. Move a light or toy in all four directions when assessing infants. Children should freely move the neck and head in all four directions without pain.

When the child is unable to move the head voluntarily in all directions, passively move the child's neck through the expected range of motion. Limited horizontal range of motion may be a sign of *torticollis,* persistent head tilting. Torticollis results from a birth injury to the sternocleidomastoid muscle or from unilateral vision or hearing impairment. Pain with flexion of the neck toward the chest (Brudzinski's sign) may indicate meningitis.

ASSESSING THE CHEST FOR SHAPE, MOVEMENT, RESPIRATORY EFFORT, AND LUNG FUNCTION

What terms describe the location of specific sounds heard when auscultating the chest? What does it mean when a child's chest is rounded in shape? What are retractions and what do they indicate? How can normal and adventitious breath sounds be distinguished when auscultating the lungs?

Examination of the chest includes the following procedures: inspecting the size and shape of the chest, palpating chest movement that occurs during respiration, observing the effort of breathing, and auscultating breath sounds. A stethoscope is needed.

Topographic Landmarks of the Chest

The chest skeleton provides most of the landmarks used to describe the location of findings during examination of the chest, lungs, and heart. The intercostal spaces are the horizontal markers. The sternum and spine are the vertical landmarks. When both a horizontal and a vertical landmark are used, the location of findings can be precisely described (Figures 33–21 ◆ and 33–22 ◆). Be sure to indicate whether the finding is on the right or left side of the patient's chest.

Inspection of the Chest

Position the child on the parent's lap or on the examining table with all clothing above the waist removed to inspect

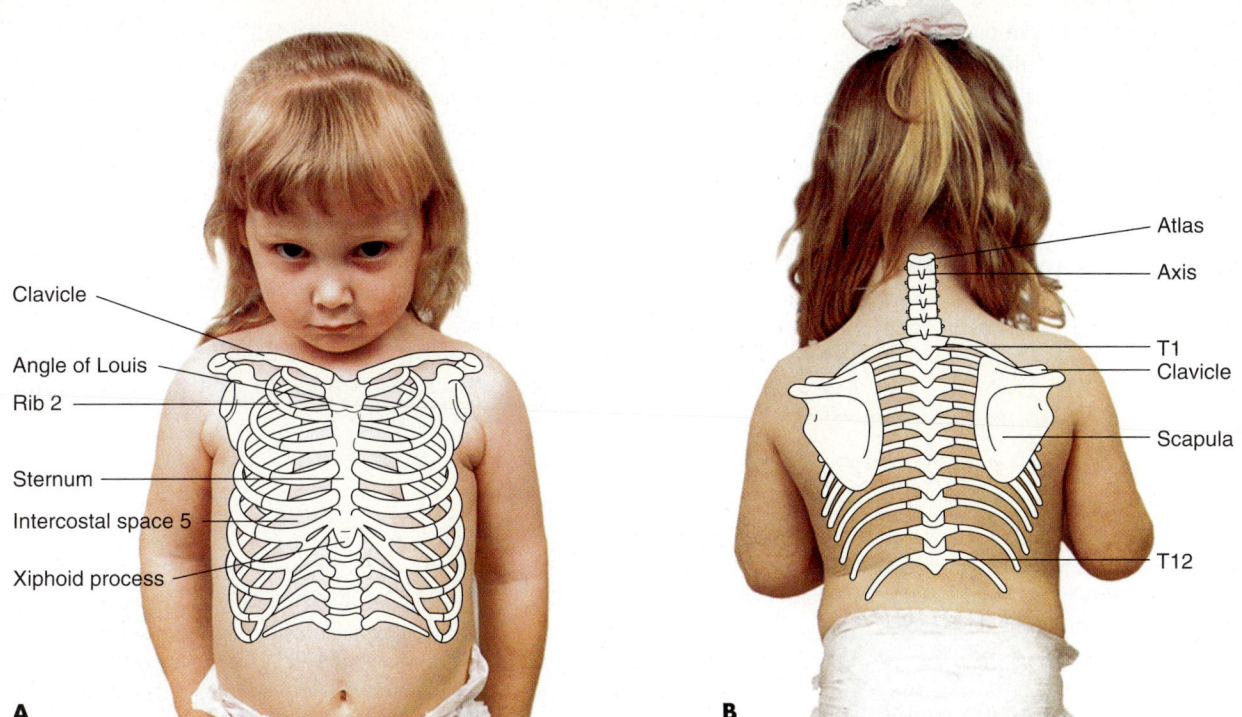

FIGURE 33–21. ◆ Intercostal spaces and ribs are numbered to describe the location of findings. **A,** To determine the rib number on the anterior chest, palpate down from the top of the sternum until a horizontal ridge, the Angle of Louis, is felt. Directly to the right and left of that ridge is the second rib. The second intercostal space is immediately below the second rib. Ribs 3–12 and the corresponding intercostal spaces can be counted as the fingers move toward the abdomen. **B,** To determine the rib number on the posterior chest, find the protruding spinal process of the seventh cervical vertebra at the shoulder level. The next spinal process belongs to the first thoracic vertebra, which attaches to the first rib.

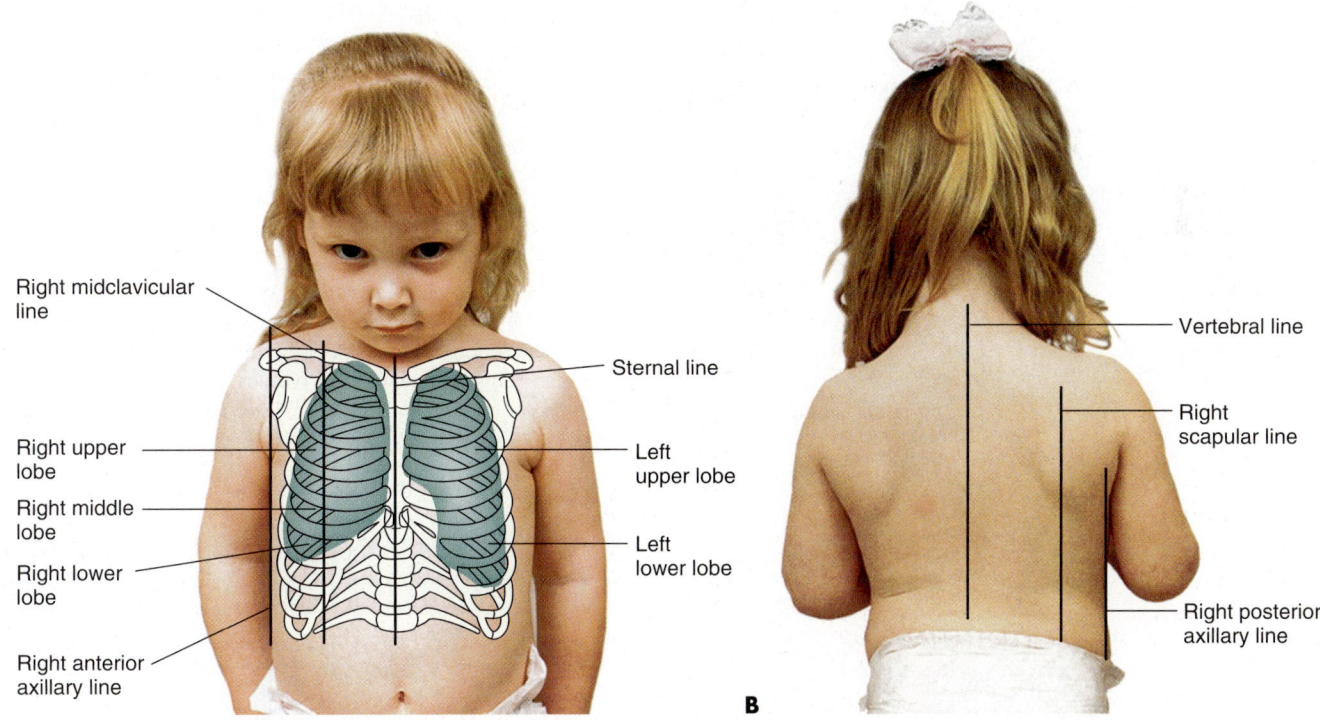

FIGURE 33–22. ◆ The sternum and spine are the vertical landmarks used to describe the anatomic location of findings. The distance between the finding and the center of the sternum (midsternal line) or the spinal line can be measured with a ruler. Imaginary vertical lines, parallel to the midsternal and spinal lines, are used to further describe the location of findings.

the chest. The thoracic muscles and subcutaneous tissue are less developed in children than in adults, so the chest wall is thinner. As a result the rib cage is more prominent.

SIZE AND SHAPE OF THE CHEST

Inspect the chest for any irregularities in shape. A chest is considered rounded when the anteroposterior diameter is approximately equal to the lateral diameter. If a child over 2 years of age has a rounded chest, a chronic obstructive lung condition such as asthma or cystic fibrosis may be present.

Growth and Development

> In infants the chest is rounded with the anteroposterior diameter approximately equal to the lateral diameter. The chest becomes more oval with growth. By 2 years of age the lateral diameter is greater than the anteroposterior diameter.

An abnormal chest shape results from two different structural deformities (Figure 33–23 ◆). If the sternum protrudes, increasing the anteroposterior diameter, pigeon chest (pectus carinatum) may be present. If the lower portion of the sternum is depressed, decreasing the anteroposterior diameter, funnel chest (pectus excavatum) may be present. Scoliosis, curvature of the spine, causes a lateral deviation of the chest. See Chapter 50. ⊂⊐

CHEST MOVEMENT AND RESPIRATORY EFFORT

Inspect for simultaneous chest expansion and abdominal rise. Chest movement is normally symmetric bilaterally, rising with inspiration and falling with expiration. The chest movement of infants and young children is less pronounced than the abdominal movement. The diaphragm is the primary breathing muscle in infants and children under 6 years old. The thoracic muscles are less developed and serve as accessory muscles in cases of respiratory distress. As the thoracic muscles develop, they become primarily responsible for ventilation. On inspiration the chest and abdomen should rise simultaneously. Asymmetric chest rise is associated with a collapsed lung. Retractions, depression of sections of the chest wall with each inspiration, are seen when the accessory muscles are used for breathing in cases of respiratory distress.

Growth and Development

> Infants and children have a faster respiratory rate than adults because of a higher metabolic rate and need for oxygen. Young children are also unable to increase the depth of respirations because not all the alveoli are developed (Hazinski, 1999).

RESPIRATORY RATE

Because young children use the diaphragm as the primary breathing muscle, observe or feel the rise and fall of the abdomen to count the respiratory rate in children under age 6 years (see Skill 9–9 in the *Clinical Skills Manual*). ⊂⊐ SKILLS Table 33–12 gives the normal respiratory rates for each age group. Make every effort to count the respiratory rate when the child is quiet. The respiratory rate rises in response to excitement, fear, respiratory distress, fever, and other conditions that increase oxygen needs.

Nursing Practice

To get the most accurate reading of a newborn's and young infant's respiratory rate, wait until the baby is sleeping or resting quietly. Use the stethoscope to auscultate the rate or place your hand on the abdomen. Count the number of breaths for an entire minute, because newborns and young infants can have irregular respirations.

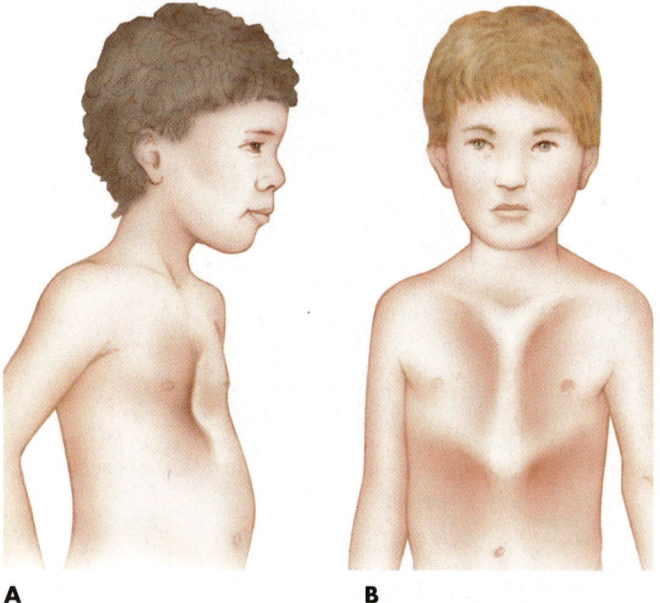

FIGURE 33–23. ◆ Two types of abnormal chest shape. **A,** Funnel chest (pectus excavatum). **B,** Pigeon chest (pectus carinatum).

TABLE 33–12	Normal Respiratory Rate Ranges for Each Age Group
Age	Respiratory Rate per Minute
Newborn	30–60
1 year	20–40
3 years	20–30
6 years	16–22
10 years	16–20
17 years	12–20

A sustained respiratory rate greater than 60 breaths per minute is an important sign in respiratory distress. At that rate, children develop hypoxemia if treatment is not started. The child's airway is very narrow, resulting in higher airway resistance than occurs in adults. When the respiratory rate exceeds 60 breaths per minute, inspired oxygen does not reach the alveoli for gas exchange because air moves no farther than the upper airway (Eichelberger, Ball, Pratsch, et al., 1998).

Palpation of the Chest

Use palpation to evaluate chest movement, respiratory effort, deformities of the chest wall, and tactile fremitus.

CHEST WALL

To palpate the chest motion with respiration, place the palms and outspread fingers on each side of the child's chest. Confirm the bilateral symmetry of chest motion. Use fingerpads to palpate any depressions, bulges, or unusual chest wall shape that might indicate abnormal findings such as tenderness, cysts, other growths, crepitus, or fractures. None should be found. *Crepitus,* a crinkly sensation palpated on the chest surface, is caused by air escaping into the subcutaneous tissues. It often indicates a serious injury to the upper or lower airway. Crepitus may also be felt near a fracture.

TACTILE FREMITUS

Crying and talking produce vibrations, known as *tactile fremitus,* that can be palpated on the chest. Place the palms of your hands on each side of the chest to evaluate the quality and distribution of these vibrations. Ask the child to repeat a series of words or numbers, such as *Mickey Mouse* or *ice cream.* As the child repeats the words, move the hands systematically over the anterior and posterior chest, comparing the quality of findings side to side. The vibration or tingling sensation is normally palpated over the entire chest. Decreased sensations indicate that air is trapped in the lungs, as occurs with asthma. Increased sensations indicate lung consolidation, as occurs with pneumonia.

Auscultation of the Chest

Auscultate the chest with a stethoscope to assess the quality and characteristics of breath sounds, to identify abnormal breath sounds, and to evaluate vocal resonance. Use an infant or pediatric stethoscope when available to help localize any unexpected breath sounds. Use the stethoscope diaphragm because it transmits the high-pitched breath sounds better.

BREATH SOUNDS

Evaluate the quality and characteristics of breath sounds over the entire chest, comparing sounds between the sides. Select a routine sequence for auscultating the entire chest so assessment of all lobes of the lungs will be consistent. Figure 33–24 ◆ shows one suggested chest auscultation

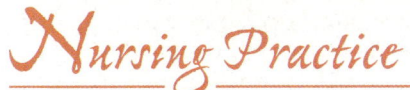

Auscultation of breath sounds is difficult when an infant is crying. First, try to quiet the infant with a pacifier, bottle, or toy. If the infant continues to cry, all is not lost. At the end of each cry the infant takes a deep breath, which you can use to assess breath sounds, vocal resonance, and tactile fremitus. Encourage toddlers and preschoolers to take deep breaths by providing a pinwheel or mobile to blow.

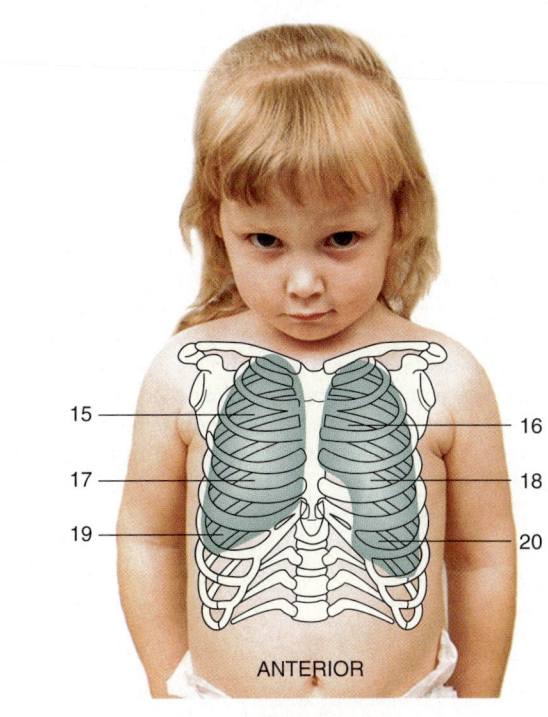

A

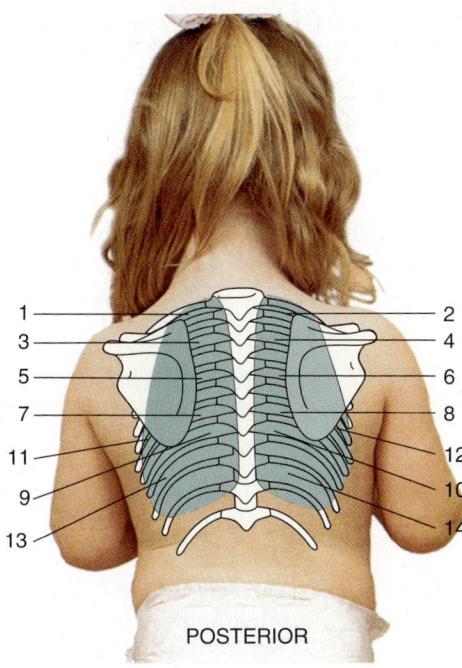

B

FIGURE 33–24. ◆ One example of a sequence for auscultation of the chest.

sequence. Listen to an entire inspiratory and expiratory phase at each spot on the chest before moving to the next site.

Three types of normal breath sounds are usually heard when the chest is auscultated. *Vesicular* breath sounds are low-pitched, swishing, soft, short expiratory sounds. They are usually heard in older children but not in infants and young children. *Bronchovesicular* breath sounds are medium-pitched, hollow, blowing sounds heard equally on inspiration and expiration in all age groups. The location of these sounds on the chest is related to the child's developmental status. *Bronchial/tracheal* breath sounds are hollow and higher pitched than vesicular breath sounds.

Growth and Development

Infants and young children have a thin chest wall because of immature muscle development. The breath sounds of one lung are heard over the entire chest. It takes practice to accurately identify absent or diminished breath sounds in infants and young children. Because the distance between the lungs is greatest at the apices and midaxillary areas in young children, these sites are best for identifying absent or diminished breath sounds. Carefully auscultate, comparing the quality of breath sounds heard bilaterally.

Nursing Practice

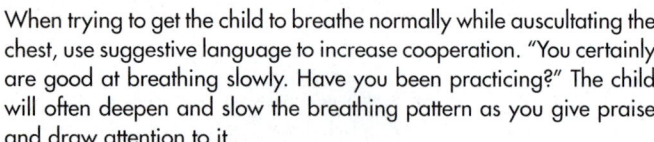

When trying to get the child to breathe normally while auscultating the chest, use suggestive language to increase cooperation. "You certainly are good at breathing slowly. Have you been practicing?" The child will often deepen and slow the breathing pattern as you give praise and draw attention to it.

Breath sounds normally have equal intensity, pitch, and rhythm bilaterally. Absent or diminished breath sounds generally indicate a partial or total obstruction, such as from a foreign body or mucus, that does not permit airflow.

VOCAL RESONANCE

Auscultate the chest to evaluate how well voice sounds are transmitted. Have the child repeat a series of words, either the same as or different from those used for evaluating tactile fremitus. Use the stethoscope to auscultate the chest, comparing the quality of sounds from side to side and over the entire chest. Voice sounds, with words and syllables muffled and indistinct, are normally heard throughout the chest.

If voice sounds are absent or more muffled than usual, an airway obstruction condition such as asthma may be present. When a lung consolidation condition such as pneumonia is present, the vocal resonance quality changes in characteristic ways. These abnormal characteristics are called whispered pectoriloquy, bronchophony, and egophony. *Whispered pectoriloquy* is present when syllables are heard distinctly in a whisper. *Bronchophony* is the increased intensity and clarity of sounds while the words remain indistinct. *Egophony* is the transmission of the "eee" sound as a nasal "ay" sound.

ABNORMAL BREATH SOUNDS

Abnormal breath sounds, also called adventitious sounds, generally indicate disease. Examples of abnormal breath sounds are crackles, rhonchi, and friction rubs. To further assess abnormal breath sounds, the examiner determines their location, the respiratory phase in which they are present, and whether they change or disappear when the child coughs or shifts position. To routinely identify these adventitious sounds takes practice. Table 33–13 describes adventitious sounds.

ABNORMAL VOICE SOUNDS

Observing the quality of the voice and other audible sounds is also important during an examination of the lungs. Examples of these sounds are hoarseness, stridor, and cough. *Stridor* is a noise resulting from air moving through a narrowed trachea and larynx; it is associated with croup. *Wheezing* is a noise resulting from the passage of air through mucus or fluids in a narrowed lower airway; it is associated with asthma. A *cough* is a reflexive clearing of the airway associated with a respiratory infection. *Hoarseness* is associated with inflammation of the larynx.

TABLE 33–13	Description of Selected Adventitious Sounds and Their Cause	
Type	Description	Cause
Fine crackles	High-pitched, discrete, noncontinuous sound heard at end of inspiration (Rub pieces of hair together beside your ear to duplicate the sound.)	Air passing through watery secretions in the smaller airways (alveoli and bronchioles)
Sibilant rhonchi	Musical, squeaking, or hissing noise heard during inspiration or expiration, but generally louder on expiration	Bronchospasm or an anatomic narrowing of the trachea, bronchi, or bronchioles
Sonorous rhonchi	Coarse, low-pitched sound like a snore, heard during inspiration or expiration; may clear with coughing	Air passing through thick secretions that partially obstruct the larger bronchi and trachea

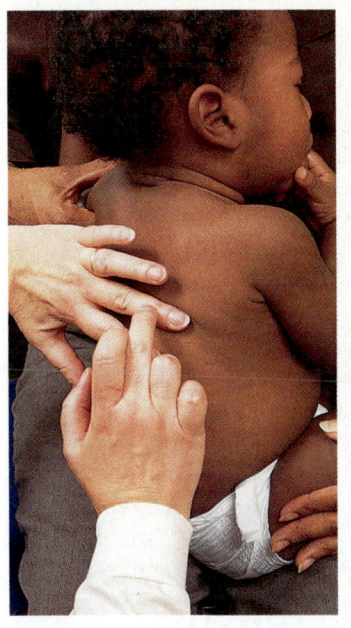
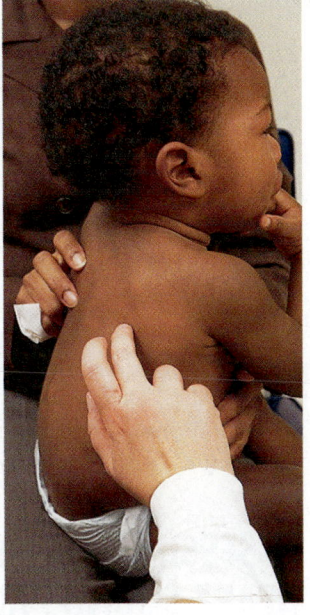

A   **B**

FIGURE 33–25. ◆ **A,** Indirect percussion. Place the middle finger on the child's chest at an intercostal space with the other fingers off of the chest. Tap the finger with a springlike motion with the fingertip of the other hand. **B,** Direct percussion. Tap the infant's chest with the fingertip directly at an intercostal space.

Percussion of the Chest

Percussion is a method sometimes used to assess the resonance of the lungs and the density of underlying organs, such as the heart and liver. Today there is less reliance on percussion to evaluate the lungs because of the frequent use of x-ray examination.

When percussing the anterior and posterior chest, choose a sequence that covers the entire chest and permits comparison bilaterally. The same sequence as that used for auscultation is effective. To perform *indirect percussion*, lay the middle finger of the nondominant hand on the child's chest at an intercostal space. Keep the other fingers off the chest. With a springlike motion, use the fingertip of the other hand to tap the finger in contact with the chest (Figure 33–25A ◆). *Direct percussion* is a technique effective for infants. Tap the chest at an intercostal space with a fingertip to elicit the quality of resonance (Figure 33–25B ◆).

Characteristic patterns of percussion resonance are expected (Figure 33–26 ◆). Characteristic descriptions of sounds heard with percussion of the chest include tympany, flatness, dullness, resonance, and hyperresonance.

ASSESSING THE BREASTS FOR DEVELOPMENT AND MASSES

Inspection of the Breasts

STAGES OF DEVELOPMENT

Inspect the breasts for stage of development. Breast development in girls precedes other pubertal changes. Breast budding, the first stage of pubertal development in girls, normally occurs between 9 and 14 years of age. Breast development before 6 years of age in African Americans and 7 years of age in Caucasians is abnormal (Herman-Giddens, Slora, Wasserman, et al, 1997; Kaplowitz, Oberfield, and the Drug and Therapeutics and Executive Committees of the Lawson Wilkins Pediatric Endocrine Society, 1999). Figure 33–27 ◆ shows normal breast development. A girl's breasts may develop at different rates and appear asymmetric. Boys often have unilateral or bilateral breast enlargement during adolescence. This enlargement can occur as breast buds or actual breast tissue

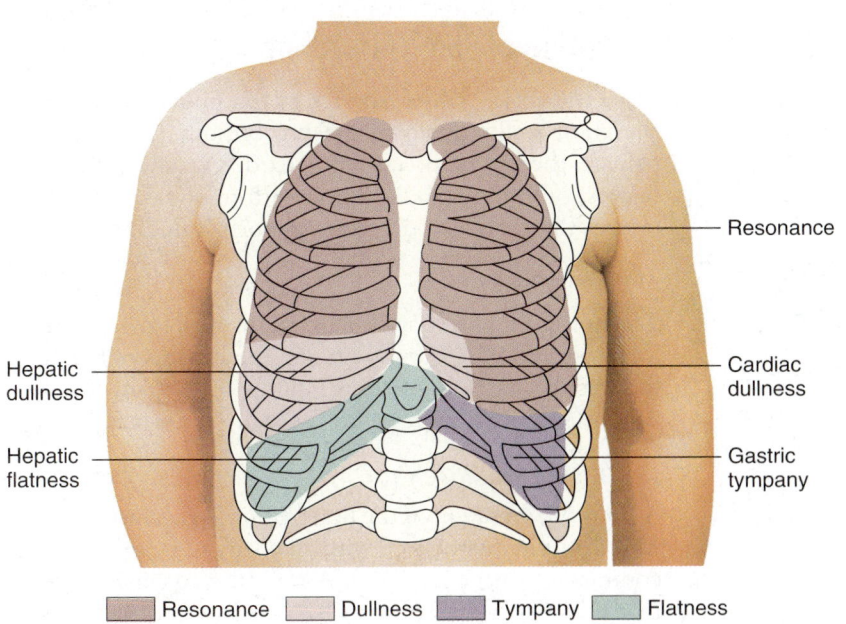

Hepatic dullness
Hepatic flatness
Resonance
Cardiac dullness
Gastric tympany

☐ Resonance   ☐ Dullness   ☐ Tympany   ☐ Flatness

FIGURE 33–26. ◆ Normal resonance patterns expected over the chest. *Tympany* is a loud, high-pitched sound, like a drum. It is usually heard over an air-filled stomach. *Flatness* is a soft, dull sound, like the sound made when percussing your thigh. It is heard over dense muscle and bone. *Dullness* is a moderately loud, thudlike sound. It is heard when percussing over the liver and heart, and at the base of the lungs (at the level of the diaphragm). *Resonance* is a loud, low-pitched, hollow sound, like the sound made when percussing a table. It is heard over the lungs. *Hyperresonance* is a loud, very low-pitched, booming sound. It is usually heard over superinflated lungs. However, because of the thin chest wall in young children, hyperresonance may be a normal finding.

(gynecomastia). It generally disappears without treatment, usually within a year.

Developing Cultural Competence

The age of onset of pubertal changes can vary with race and ethnicity, environmental conditions, geographic location, and nutrition. The mean age for breast development in African-American girls is 8.87 years and for Caucasian girls 9.96 years (Herman-Giddens, Slora, Wasserman, et al. 1997).

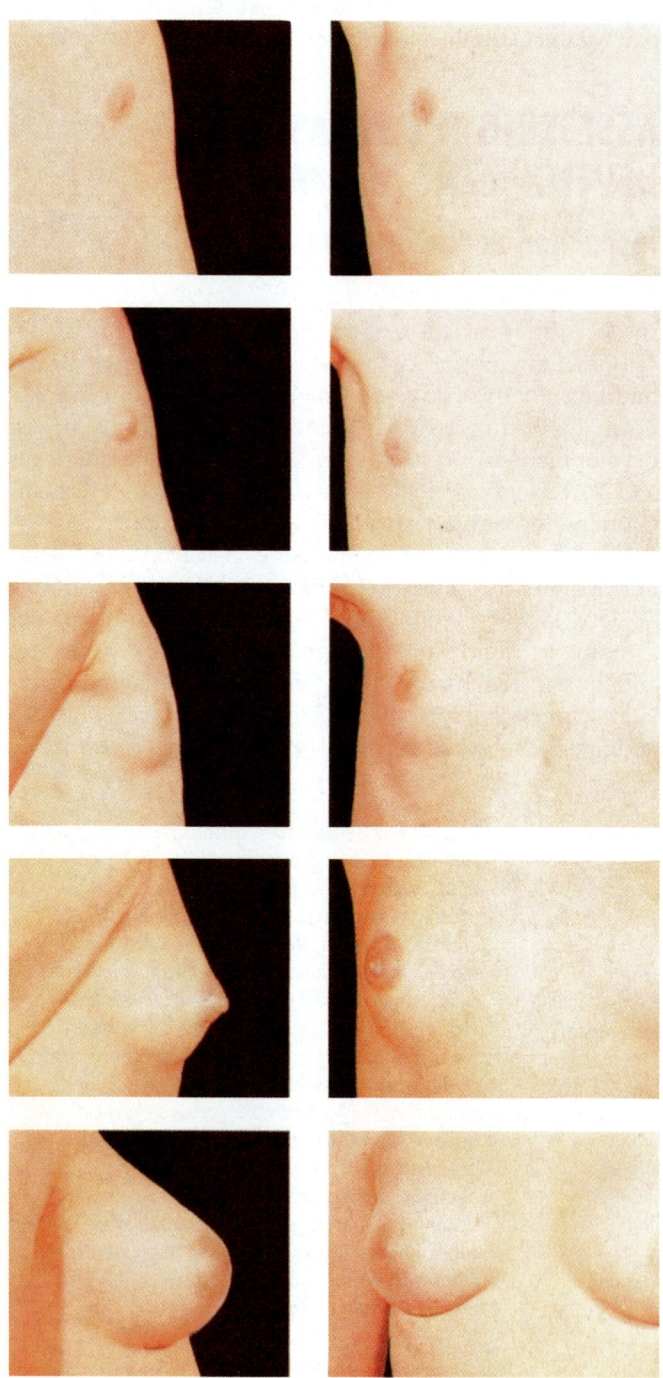

FIGURE 33–27. ◆ Normal stages of breast development.

NIPPLES

The nipples of prepubertal boys and girls are symmetrically located near the midclavicular line at the fourth to sixth ribs. The areola is normally round and more darkly pigmented than the surrounding skin. Inspect the anterior chest for other dark spots that may be *supernumerary nipples*, which are small, undeveloped nipples and areola that may be mistaken for moles. Their presence may be associated with congenital renal or cardiac anomalies.

Palpation of the Breasts

Palpate the developing breasts of adolescent females for abnormal masses or hard nodules. Breast tissue normally feels dense, firm, and elastic.

ASSESSING THE HEART FOR HEART SOUNDS AND FUNCTION

Inspection of the Precordium

A stethoscope and sphygmomanometer is needed to assess the heart. Begin the heart examination by inspecting the *precordium*, or anterior chest. Place the child in a reclining or semi-Fowler's position, either on the parent's lap or on the examining table. Inspect the shape and symmetry of the anterior chest from the front and side views. The rib cage is normally symmetric. Bulging of the left side of the chest wall may indicate an enlarged heart.

Observe for any chest movement associated with the heart's contraction. The *apical impulse,* sometimes called the point of maximum intensity, is located where the left ventricle taps the chest wall during contraction. The apical impulse can normally be seen in thin children. A *heave,* an obvious lifting of the chest wall during contraction, may indicate an enlarged heart.

Palpation of the Precordium

Place the entire palmar surface of the fingers together on the chest wall to palpate the precordium. Systematically palpate the entire precordium to detect any pulsations, heaves, or vibrations. Palpating with minimal pressure increases the chance of detecting abnormal findings.

APICAL IMPULSE

The apical impulse is normally felt as a slight tap against one fingertip. Use the topographic landmarks of the chest to describe its location (see Figures 33–21 and 33–22). Any other sensation palpated is usually abnormal.

ABNORMAL SENSATIONS

A *lift* is the sensation of the heart lifting up against the chest wall. It may be associated with an enlarged heart or a heart contracting with extra force. A *thrill* is a rushing vibration that feels like a cat's purr. It is caused by turbulent blood

Growth and Development

The location of the apical impulse changes as the child's rib cage grows. In children under 7 years old, it is located in the fourth intercostal space just lateral to the left midclavicular line. In children over 7 years old, it is located in the fifth intercostal space at the left midclavicular line.

flow from a defective heart valve and a heart murmur. If present, the thrill is palpated in the right or left second intercostal space. To describe a thrill's location, use the topographic landmarks of the chest (see Figures 33–21 and 33–22) and estimate the diameter of the thrill palpated.

Percussion of the Heart Borders

Percussion of the heart borders is rarely performed during physical examination. The borders of the heart are better identified by x-ray examination. Percussion of the heart should be performed only by an experienced examiner.

Auscultation of the Heart

Auscultation is used to count the apical pulse, to assess the characteristics of the heart sounds, and to detect abnormal heart sounds. Use the bell of the stethoscope to detect these lower pitched sounds.

To assess heart sounds completely, auscultate the heart with the child in both sitting and reclining positions. Differences in heart sounds caused by a change in the child's position or by a change in the position of the heart near the chest wall can then be detected. If differences in heart sounds are detected with a position change, place the child in the left lateral recumbent position and auscultate again.

HEART RATE AND RHYTHM

The apical heart rate can be counted at the site of the apical impulse, (Skill 9–8) [SKILLS] either by palpation or by auscultation. Count the apical rate for 1 minute in infants and in children who have an irregular rhythm. The brachial or radial pulse rate should be the same as the auscultated apical heart rate. Table 33–14 gives normal heart rates in children of different ages.

TABLE 33–14 Normal Heart Rates for Children of Different Ages		
Age	Heart Rate Range (beats/min)	Average Heart Rate (beats/min)
Newborns	100–170	120
Infants to 2 years	80–130	110
2–6 years	70–120	100
6–10 years	70–110	90
10–16 years	60–100	85

Growth and Development

The child's heart rate varies with age, decreasing as the child grows older. The heart rate also increases in response to exercise, excitement, anxiety, and fever. Such stresses increase the child's metabolic rate, creating a simultaneous need for more oxygen. Children respond to the need for more oxygen by increasing their heart rate, a response called sinus tachycardia. They cannot increase their cardiac stroke volume to deliver more oxygen to the tissues as adults do.

Listen carefully to the heart rate rhythm. Children often have a normal cycle of irregular rhythm associated with respiration called sinus arrhythmia. With sinus arrhythmia the child's heart rate is faster on inspiration and slower on expiration. When any rhythm irregularity is detected, ask the child to take a breath and hold it while you listen to the heart rate. The rhythm should become regular during inspiration and expiration. Other rhythm irregularities are abnormal.

DIFFERENTIATION OF HEART SOUNDS

Heart sounds are due to the closure of the valves and vibration or turbulence of blood produced by that valve closure. Two primary sounds, S_1 and S_2, are heard when the chest is auscultated.

S_1, the first heart sound, is produced by closure of the tricuspid and mitral valves when the ventricular contraction begins. The two valves close almost simultaneously, so only one sound is normally heard.

S_2, the second heart sound, is produced by the closure of the aortic and pulmonic valves. Once blood has reached the pulmonic and aortic arteries, the valves close to prevent leakage back into the ventricles during diastole. The timing of the valve closure varies with respirations. Sometimes S_2 is heard as a single sound and at other times as a *split sound*, that is, two sounds heard a fraction of a second apart.

Sound is easily transmitted in liquid, and it travels best in the direction of blood flow. Auscultate heart sounds at specific areas on the chest wall in the direction of blood flow, just beyond the valve (Figure 33–28 ◆). The sounds produced by the heart valves or blood turbulence are heard throughout the chest in thin infants and children. Both S_1 and S_2 can be heard in all listening areas.

Auscultate heart sounds for quality (distinct versus muffled) and intensity (loud versus weak). First, distinguish between S_1 and S_2 in each listening area. Heart sounds are usually distinct and crisp in children because of their thin chest wall. Muffling or indistinct sounds may indicate a heart defect or congestive heart failure. Document the area where heart sounds are heard the best. Table 33–15 and Figure 33–28 review the location where each sound is normally best heard for assessment of quality and intensity.

FIGURE 33–28. ◆ Sound travels in the direction of blood flow. Rather than listen for heart sounds over each heart valve, auscultate heart sounds at specific areas on the chest wall away from the valve itself. These areas are named for the valve producing the sound. *Aortic:* Second right intercostal space near the sternum. *Pulmonic:* Second left intercostal space near the sternum. *Tricuspid:* Fifth right or left intercostal space near the sternum. *Mitral (apical):* In infants—third or fourth intercostal space, just left of the left midclavicular line. In children—fifth intercostal space at the left midclavicular line.

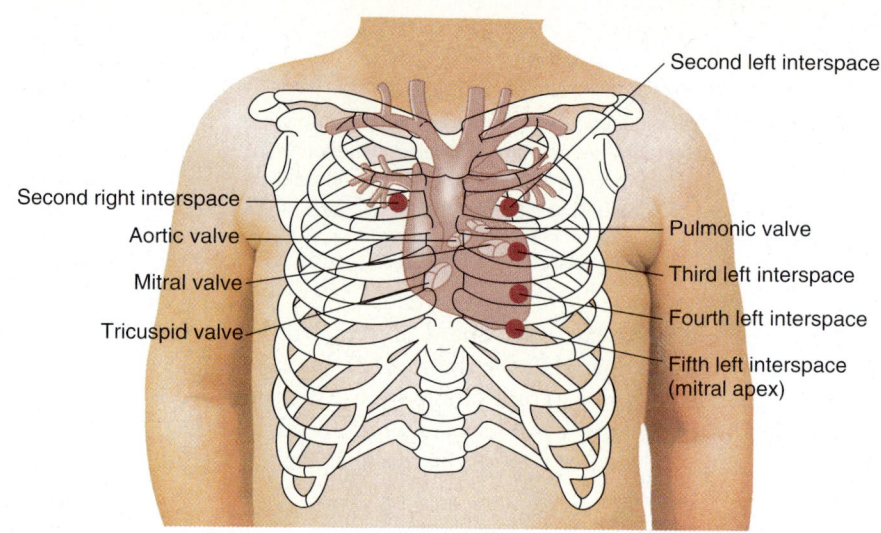

Second left interspace
Second right interspace
Aortic valve
Mitral valve
Tricuspid valve
Pulmonic valve
Third left interspace
Fourth left interspace
Fifth left interspace (mitral apex)

TABLE 33–15 Identification of the Listening Sites for Auscultation of the Quality and Intensity of Heart Sounds

Heart Sound	Locations Best Heard	Where Heard Softly
S_1	Apex of the heart Tricuspid area Mitral area	Base of the heart Aortic area Pulmonic area
S_2	Base of the heart Aortic area Pulmonic area	Apex of the heart Tricuspid area Mitral area
Physiologic splitting	Pulmonic area	
S_3	Mitral area	

Nursing Practice

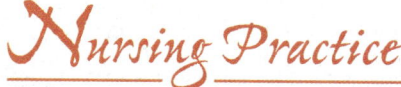

Palpate the carotid pulse when auscultating the heart to distinguish between the two heart sounds. The heart sound heard simultaneously with the pulsation is S_1.

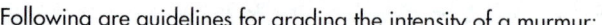

SPLITTING OF THE HEART SOUNDS

After distinguishing the first and second heart sounds, try to detect *physiologic splitting*. The split second heart sound is more apparent during inspiration when the child takes a deep breath. More blood returns to the right ventricle, causing the pulmonic valve to close a fraction of a second later than the aortic valve. To detect physiologic splitting, auscultate over the pulmonic area while the child breathes normally and then while the child takes a deep breath. Splitting is normally more easily detected after a deep breath. The splitting returns to a single sound with regular breathing. If splitting does not vary with respiration, it is called fixed splitting. This is an abnormal finding associated with an atrial septal defect.

THIRD HEART SOUND

A third heart sound, S_3, is occasionally heard in children as a normal finding. S_3 is caused when blood rushes through the mitral valve and splashes into the left ventricle. It is heard in diastole, just after S_2. It is distinguished from a split S_2 because it is louder in the mitral area than in the pulmonic area.

MURMURS

Occasionally abnormal heart sounds are auscultated. These sounds are produced by blood passing through a defective valve, great vessel, or other heart structure.

To hear murmurs in children takes practice. Often, murmurs must be very loud to be detected. For softer murmurs, normal heart sounds must be distinguished before an extra sound is recognized. Once a murmur is detected, define the characteristics of the extra sound.

Murmurs are classified by the following characteristics:

- *Intensity.* How loud is it? Can a thrill also be palpated?

- *Location.* Where is the murmur the loudest? Identify the listening area and precise topographic landmarks. Is the child sitting or lying down?

- *Radiation.* Is the sound transmitted over a larger area of the chest, to the axilla, or to the back?

Nursing Practice

Following are guidelines for grading the intensity of a murmur:

Intensity	Description
Grade I	Barely heard in a quiet room
Grade II	Quiet, but clearly heard
Grade III	Moderately loud, no thrill palpated
Grade IV	Loud, a thrill is usually palpated
Grade V	Very loud, a thrill is easily palpated
Grade VI	Heard without the stethoscope in direct contact with the chest wall

- *Timing.* Is the murmur heard best after S_1 or S_2? Is it heard during the entire phase between S_1 and S_2?
- *Quality.* Describe what the murmur sounds like—for example, machinelike, musical, or blowing.

Completing the Heart Examination

A complete assessment of cardiac function also includes measuring the blood pressure, palpating the pulses, and evaluating signs from other systems.

BLOOD PRESSURE

Assessment of blood pressure is important to detect conditions of hypertension or hypovolemic shock. See Skill 9–10 for the technique for obtaining the blood pressure in children in the *Clinical Skills Manual*, as well as the CD-ROM accompanying this text. SKILLS CD Table 33–16 gives upper limits (95th percentile) of blood pressure readings of children at different ages by selected height percentiles. Persistent readings at or above this level are associated with hypertension.

TABLE 33–16 Upper Limits (95th %) of Systolic and Diastolic Blood Pressure Values for Children of Different Ages by Selected Height Percentiles

BOYS	Systolic BP (mm Hg) by Height Percentile			Diastolic BP (mm Hg) by Height Percentile		
Age in Years	10th	50th	90th	10th	50th	90th
1	99	103	106	54	56	58
2	103	107	110	59	61	63
3	106	109	112	63	65	67
4	108	111	114	68	69	71
5	109	113	116	71	73	75
6	110	114	117	75	76	78
7	111	115	118	77	79	81
8	113	116	119	79	81	83
9	114	118	121	81	82	84
10	116	119	123	82	83	85
11	118	121	125	82	84	86
12	120	124	127	83	85	87
13	122	126	129	83	85	87
14	125	129	132	84	86	87
15	128	132	135	85	86	88
16	131	134	138	86	88	90
17	133	137	140	88	90	92

GIRLS	Systolic BP (mm Hg) by Height Percentile			Diastolic BP (mm Hg) by Height Percentile		
Age in Years	10th	50th	90th	10th	50th	90th
1	102	104	107	56	58	59
2	103	106	108	61	62	64
3	104	107	109	65	66	68
4	106	108	111	68	69	71
5	107	110	112	71	72	74
6	109	111	114	73	74	76
7	111	113	115	75	76	78
8	113	115	117	77	78	79
9	115	117	119	78	79	81
10	117	119	122	79	81	82
11	119	121	124	81	82	83
12	121	123	126	82	83	85
13	123	125	128	83	84	86
14	125	127	129	84	85	87
15	126	128	131	85	86	88
16	127	129	132	85	87	88
17	127	130	132	86	87	88

Note: From Rosner, B., Prineas, R. J., Loggie, J. M. H., & Daniels, S. R. (1993). Blood pressure nomograms for children and adolescents, by height, sex, and age, in the United States. Journal of Pediatrics, 123, 871–886.

PALPATION OF THE PULSES

Palpate the characteristics of the pulses in the extremities to assess the circulation. The technique and sites for palpating the pulse are the same as those used for adults (Figure 33–29 ◆). Evaluate the pulsation for rate, regularity of rhythm, and strength in each extremity and compare your findings bilaterally. The femoral and brachial pulses are the most important pulses to evaluate.

Palpate the femoral arteries and compare their strength with the strength of the brachial pulse. The femoral pulsations are usually stronger than or as strong as the brachial

Growth and Development

Infants have a low systolic blood pressure, and detecting the distal pulses is often difficult. Use the brachial artery in the arms and the popliteal or femoral artery in the legs to evaluate the pulses. The radial and distal tibial pulses are normally palpated easily in older children.

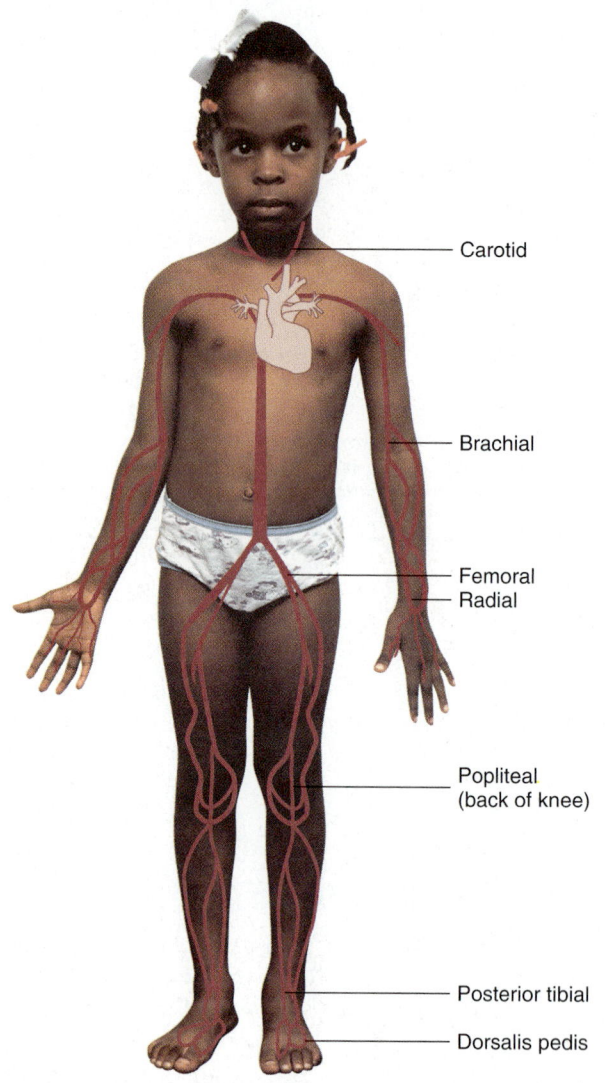

— Carotid

— Brachial

— Femoral
— Radial

— Popliteal
(back of knee)

— Posterior tibial

— Dorsalis pedis

FIGURE 33–29. ◆ The sites used to assess pulses in children.

pulsations. A weaker femoral pulse is associated with coarctation of the aorta.

OTHER SIGNS

To assess the heart and tissue perfusion, consider other signs, including skin color, capillary refill, and respiratory distress. The mucous membranes are usually pink. Cyanosis is most commonly associated with a congenital heart defect in children. Capillary refill is normally less than 2 seconds, indicating good circulation and perfusion of the tissues. Signs of respiratory distress, such as tachypnea, flaring, and retractions, may be associated with the child's attempts to compensate for hypoxemia caused by a congenital heart defect.

ASSESSING THE ABDOMEN FOR SHAPE, BOWEL SOUNDS, AND UNDERLYING ORGANS

Topographic Landmarks of the Abdomen

The location of underlying organs and structures of the abdomen must be considered when the abdomen is examined. The abdomen is commonly divided by imaginary lines into quadrants for the purpose of identifying underlying structures (Figure 33–30 ◆).

Inspection of the Abdomen

Begin the examination of the abdomen by inspecting the shape and contour, condition of the umbilicus and rectus muscle, and abdominal movement. Inspect the child's abdomen from the front and side with good lighting.

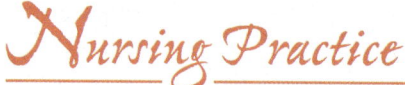

Perform inspection and auscultation before palpation and percussion because touching the abdomen may change the characteristics of bowel sounds.

SHAPE

Inspect the shape of the abdomen to identify an abnormal contour. The child's abdomen is normally symmetric and rounded or flat when the child is supine. A scaphoid or sunken abdomen is abnormal and may indicate dehydration.

UMBILICUS

Observe the newborn's umbilical stump for color, bleeding, odor, and drainage. See Chapter 25 ⬳ for more information. After the stump falls off, inspect the umbilicus for continued drainage which may indicate an infection or a granuloma.

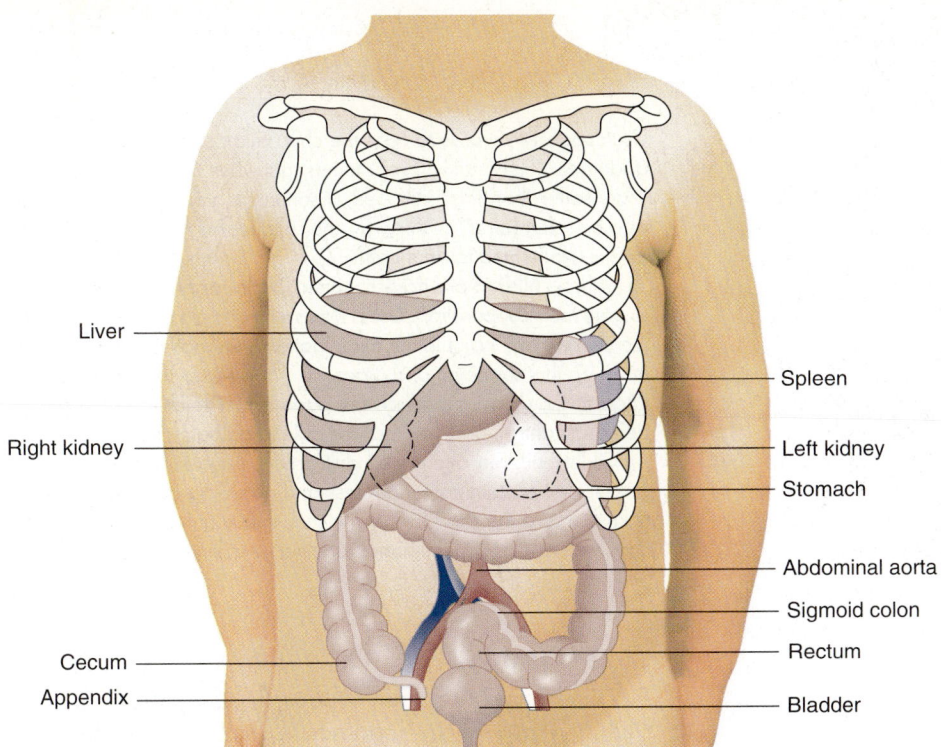

FIGURE 33–30. ◆ Topographic landmarks of the abdomen. The abdomen is commonly divided by imaginary lines into quadrants for the purposes of identifying underlying structures.

Liver

Right kidney

Cecum

Appendix

Spleen

Left kidney

Stomach

Abdominal aorta

Sigmoid colon

Rectum

Bladder

Inspect the umbilicus in older infants and toddlers. Children in these age groups often have an umbilical hernia, a protrusion of abdominal contents through an open umbilical muscle ring.

RECTUS MUSCLE

Inspect the abdominal wall for any depression or bulging at midline above or below the umbilicus, indicating separation of the rectus abdominis muscles. The depression may be up to 5 cm (2 in.) wide. Measure the width of the separation to monitor change over time. As abdominal muscle strength develops, the separation usually becomes less prominent. However, the splitting may persist if congenital muscle weakness is present.

ABDOMINAL MOVEMENT

Infants and children up to 6 years of age breathe with the diaphragm. The abdomen rises with inspiration and falls with expiration, simultaneously with the chest rise and fall. When the abdomen does not rise as expected, peritonitis may be present.

Other abdominal movements such as peristaltic waves are abnormal. *Peristaltic waves* are visible rhythmic contractions of the intestinal wall smooth muscle, which move food through the digestive tract. Their presence generally indicates an intestinal obstruction, such as pyloric stenosis.

Auscultation of the Abdomen

To evaluate bowel sounds, auscultate the abdomen with the diaphragm of the stethoscope. Bowel sounds nor-

mally occur every 10 to 30 seconds. They have a high-pitched, tinkling, metallic quality. Loud gurgling *(borborygmi)* is heard when the child is hungry. Listen in each quadrant long enough to hear at least one bowel sound. Before determining that bowel sounds are absent, auscultate at least 5 minutes. Absence of bowel sounds may indicate peritonitis or a paralytic ileus. Hyperactive bowel sounds may indicate gastroenteritis or a bowel obstruction.

Next auscultate over the abdominal aorta and the renal arteries for a vascular hum or murmur. No murmur should be heard. A murmur may indicate a narrowed or defective artery.

Percussion of the Abdomen

Use indirect percussion to evaluate borders and sizes of abdominal organs and masses. Percussion is performed with the child supine. Choose a sequence to systematically percuss the entire abdomen (Figure 33–31 ◆).

Different tones are expected when the abdomen is percussed, depending on the underlying structures. Organ size can be identified by listening for a percussion tone change at the border of an organ. For example, when you percuss down the chest, the upper edge of the liver is usually detected by a tone change from resonant to dull near the fifth intercostal space at the right midclavicular line. The lower liver edge is usually detected 2 to 3 cm (about 1 in) below the right costal margin in infants and toddlers, but closer to the costal margin in older children.

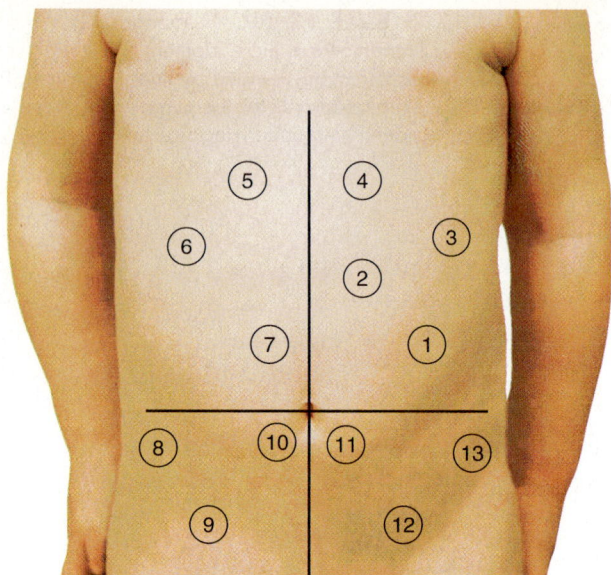

FIGURE 33-31. ◆ Sequence for indirect percussion of the abdomen.

Nursing Practice

Expected pattern of percussion tones over the abdomen: Dullness is found over organs such as the liver, spleen, and full bladder. Tympany is found over the stomach or the intestines when an obstruction is present. Tympany may be found over areas beyond the stomach in infants because of air swallowing. A resonant tone may be heard over other areas.

Palpation of the Abdomen

Both light and deep palpation are used to examine the abdomen's organs and to detect any masses. *Light palpation* evaluates the tenseness of the abdomen (how soft or hard it is), the liver, the presence of any tenderness or masses, and any defects in the abdominal wall. *Deep palpation* detects masses, defines their shape and consistency, and identifies tenderness in the abdomen.

To make the most accurate interpretation, perform the abdominal examination when the child is calm and cooperative. Organs and other masses are more easily palpated when the abdominal wall is relaxed. Infants and toddlers often feel more secure lying supine across both the parent's and the examiner's laps. A bottle, pacifier, or toy may distract the child and improve cooperation for the examination.

To begin palpation, position the child supine with knees flexed. Stand beside the child and place warmed fingertips across the child's abdomen. Palpate with the edge of the fingers, not just the fingerpads, and palpate in a sequence to examine the entire abdomen. Watch the child's face during palpation for a grimace or constriction of the pupils, which indicates pain.

Nursing Practice

Use suggestive words to help the child relax so you can palpate the abdomen. "How soft will your tummy get when my hand feels it? Does it get softer than this? Yes. See, it softens as you breathe out. Will it also be softer here?" In this way, the child learns to relax the abdomen and is challenged to do it better.

When children are ticklish, some special approaches are needed to gain their cooperation. Use a firm touch and do not pretend to tickle the child at any point in the examination. Alternatively, put the child's hand on the abdomen and place your hand over the child's. Let your fingertips slide over to touch the abdomen. The child has a sense of being in control, and you may be able to palpate directly.

Older children often need distraction, especially when there is a question of abdominal tenderness and guarding or when the child is ticklish. Have the child perform a task that requires some concentration, such as pressing the hands together or pulling locked hands apart.

LIGHT PALPATION

For light palpation, use a superficial, gentle touch that slightly depresses the abdomen. Usually the abdomen feels soft and no tenderness is detected. Palpate any bulging along the abdominal wall, especially along the rectus muscle and umbilical ring, which could indicate a hernia. Measure the diameter of the muscle ring, rather than the protrusion, to monitor change over time. The muscle ring normally becomes smaller and closes by 4 years of age. An umbilical hernia that persists beyond this age may need surgical repair.

Liver. Locate and lightly palpate the lower liver edge. Place the fingers in the right midclavicular line at the level of the umbilicus and gently move them toward the costal margin during expiration. As the liver edge descends with inspiration, a flat, narrow ridge is usually felt. Measure the distance of the liver edge from the right costal margin at the right midclavicular line. The liver edge is normally palpated 2 to 3 cm (1 in.) below the right costal margin in infants and toddlers. It may not be palpable in older children. The liver is enlarged when the edge is more than 3 cm (1 in.) below the right costal margin. An enlarged liver may be associated with congestive heart failure or hepatic disease.

DEEP PALPATION

To perform deep palpation, press the fingers of one hand (for small children) or two hands (for older children) more deeply into the abdomen. Because the abdominal muscles are most relaxed when the child takes a deep breath, ask the child to take regular deep breaths when palpating each area of the abdomen.

Spleen. Palpate for the spleen at the left costal margin in the midclavicular line. The spleen tip may be felt when the child takes a deep breath. The spleen is enlarged when it can be easily palpated below the left costal margin.

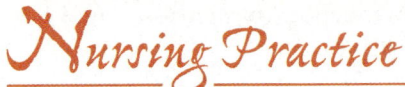

Nursing Practice

If an enlarged kidney or mass is detected, do not continue to palpate the kidney. Pressure on the mass may release cancerous cells.

Kidneys. Palpate for the kidneys deep in the abdomen along each side of the spinal column. The kidneys are difficult to palpate in all children, except newborns, because of the deep layer of abdominal muscles and intestines. If a kidney is actually palpated, an abnormal mass may be present.

Other Masses. Occasionally other masses, both normal and abnormal, can be palpated in the abdomen. A tubular mass commonly palpated in the lower left or right quadrant is often an intestine filled with feces. A distended bladder is often palpated as a firm, central, dome-shaped mass above the symphysis pubis in young children. Any fixed mass that moves laterally, pulsates, or is located along the vertebral column may be a neoplasm.

Assessment of the Inguinal Area

The inguinal area is inspected and palpated during the abdominal examination to detect enlarged lymph nodes or masses. The femoral pulse, a part of the heart examination, may be assessed simultaneously with the abdominal examination.

INSPECTION

Inspect the inguinal area for any change in contour, comparing sides. A small bulging noted over the femoral canal in girls may be associated with a femoral hernia. A bulging in the inguinal area in boys may be associated with an inguinal hernia.

PALPATION

Palpate the inguinal area for lymph nodes and other masses. Small lymph nodes, less than 1 cm (1/2 in.) in diameter, are often present in the inguinal area because of minor injuries on the legs. Any tenderness, heat, or inflammation in these palpated lymph nodes could be associated with a local infection.

ASSESSING THE GENITAL AND PERINEAL AREAS FOR PUBERTAL DEVELOPMENT AND EXTERNAL STRUCTURAL ABNORMALITIES

How is the stage of pubertal development determined in girls and boys? What can a vaginal discharge indicate in a preadolescent girl? Is swelling in a newborn's scrotum normal? Where is the proper location of the urethral meatus on the penis?

Preparation of Children for the Examination

Examination of the genitalia and perineal area can cause stress in children because they sense their privacy has been invaded. To make young children feel more secure, position them on the parent's lap with their legs spread apart. Children can also be positioned on the examining table with their knees flexed and the legs spread apart like a frog.

In younger children the genital and perineal examination is performed immediately after assessment of the abdomen. The genitals and perineum may be examined last in older children and adolescents. Equipment needed for this examination includes gloves, lubricant, and a penlight.

Growth and Development

Preschool-age children are often taught that strangers are not permitted to touch their "private parts." When a child this age actively resists examination of the genital area, ask the parent to tell the child you have permission to look at and touch these parts of the body. Some children develop modesty during the preschool period. Briefly explain what you need to examine and why. Then calmly and efficiently examine the child.

Inspection of the Female Genitalia

Inspect the external genitalia of girls for color, size, and symmetry of the mons pubis, labia, urethra, and vaginal opening (Figure 33–32 ◆). At that time, determine the stage of pubertal maturation. Simultaneously, look for any abnormal findings such as swelling, inflammation, masses, lacerations, or discharge.

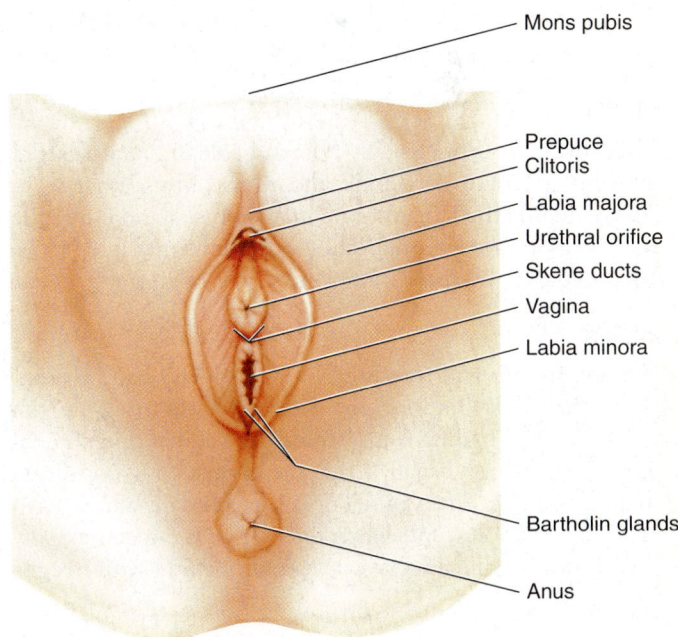

FIGURE 33–32. ◆ Anatomic structures of the female genital and perineal area.

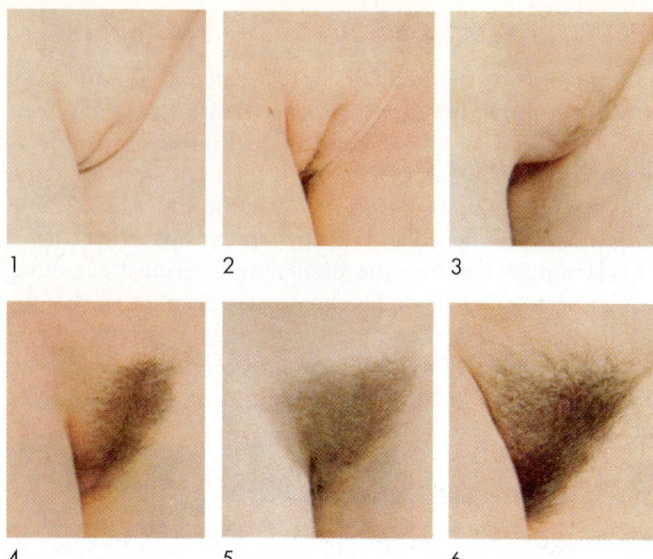

FIGURE 33–33. ◆ The stages of female pubic hair development with sexual maturation. Soft downy hair along the labia majora is an indication that sexual maturation is beginning. Hair grows progressively coarse and curly as development proceeds. From Van Wieringen et al. (1971). *Growth diagrams 1965 Netherlands*, Groningen: Wolters-Noordhof.

MONS PUBIS

Inspect the mons pubis for pubic hair. The presence, amount, and distribution of pubic hair indicates the sexual maturation stage in the girl. Preadolescent girls have no pubic hair. Initial pubic hair is lightly pigmented, sparse, and straight. Pubic hair develops in consistent stages for all girls, but the timing of pubic hair stages is individually determined (Tanner, 1962). Figure 33–33 ◆ illustrates the normal stages of female pubic hair development. Breast development usually precedes pubic hair development. The presence of pubic hair before 8 years of age is unusual.

LABIA

The labia minora are usually thin and pale in preadolescent girls but become dark pink and moist after puberty. In young infants the labia minora may be fused and cover the structures in the vestibule. These adhesions may need to be separated. See Chapter 25 for more information.

HYMEN

Use the thumb and forefinger of one gloved hand to separate the labia minora for viewing structures in the vestibule. The hymen is just inside the vaginal opening. In preadolescents it is usually a thin membrane with a crescent-shaped opening. The vaginal opening is usually about 1 cm (1/2 in.) in adolescents when the hymen is intact. Sexually active adolescents may have a vaginal opening with irregular edges.

URETHRAL AND VAGINAL OPENINGS

Inspect the vestibule for lesions. No lesions or signs of inflammation are expected around the urethral or vaginal opening. Redness and excoriation are often associated with an irritant such as bubble bath.

VAGINAL DISCHARGE

Preadolescent girls do not normally have a vaginal discharge. Adolescents often have a clear discharge without a foul odor. Menses generally begin approximately 2 years after breast bud development. A foul-smelling discharge in preschool-age children may be associated with a foreign body. Various organisms may cause a vaginal infection in older children.

Nursing Practice

Signs of sexual abuse in young children include bruising or swelling of the vulva, foul-smelling vaginal discharge, enlarged opening of the vagina, and rash or sores in the perineal area.

An internal vaginal examination is indicated when abnormal findings such as a vaginal discharge or trauma to the external structures is noted. Only an experienced examiner should perform the vaginal examination of the child.

Palpation of the Female Genitalia

Palpate the vaginal opening with a finger of your free gloved hand. The Bartholin and Skene glands are not usually palpable. Palpation of these glands in preadolescent children indicates enlargement because of an infection such as gonorrhea.

Inspection of the Male Genitalia

Inspect the male genitalia for the structural and pubertal development of the penis, scrotum, and testicles. Place boys in tailor position, seated with their legs crossed in front of them. This position puts pressure on the abdominal wall to push the testicles into the scrotum.

PENIS

Inspect the penis for size, foreskin, hygiene, and position of the urethral meatus. The length of the nonerect penis in the newborn is normally 2 to 3 cm (1 in.). The penis enlarges in length and breadth during puberty. The penis is normally straight. A downward bowing of the penis may be caused by a *chordee*, a fibrous band of tissue associated with hypospadias.

Growth and Development

The foreskin is usually not completely separated from the glans at birth. Separation is normally completed by 3 to 6 years of age. A foreskin opening large enough for a good urinary stream is normal, even when the foreskin does not fully retract.

Nursing Practice

When the boy's foreskin does not easily retract, do not forcefully pull it back. Force may result in torn tissues that heal with adhesions between the foreskin and the glans.

When the penis is circumcised, the glans penis is exposed. To inspect the glans penis of an uncircumcised boy, ask the child or parent to pull the foreskin back. Alternatively, the examiner may retract the foreskin. The foreskin of children over 6 years of age normally retracts easily. If the foreskin is tight and cannot be retracted, phimosis is present.

The glans penis is normally clean and smooth without inflammation or ulceration. The urethral meatus is a slit-shaped opening near the tip of the glans. No discharge should be present. A round, pinpoint urethral meatus may indicate meatal stenosis. Location of the urethral meatus at another site on the penis is abnormal, indicating hypospadias or epispadias. Inspect the urinary stream. The stream is normally strong without dribbling.

SCROTUM

Inspect the scrotum for size, symmetry, presence of the testicles, and any abnormalities. The scrotum is normally loose and pendulous with rugae, or wrinkles. The scrotum of infants often appears large in comparison to the penis. A small, undeveloped scrotum that has no rugae indicates that the testicles are undescended. Enlargement or swelling of the scrotum is abnormal. It may indicate an inguinal hernia, hydrocele, torsion of the spermatic cord, or testicular inflammation. A deep cleft in the scrotum may indicate ambiguous genitalia.

PUBIC HAIR

Inspect the presence, amount, and distribution of pubic hair. Straight, downy pubic hair first develops at the base of the penis. The hair becomes darker, dense, and curly, extending over the pubic area in a diamond pattern by the completion of puberty. The presence of pubic hair before 9 years of age is uncommon. Stages of pubic hair development follow a standard pattern, as illustrated in Figure 33–34 ◆.

Growth and Development

The stage of pubertal maturation is determined by inspecting the amount of pubic hair, size of the penis, and development of the testicles and scrotum. Pubic hair usually appears after the scrotum and testicles start to grow but before the penis begins enlarging (Tanner, 1962).

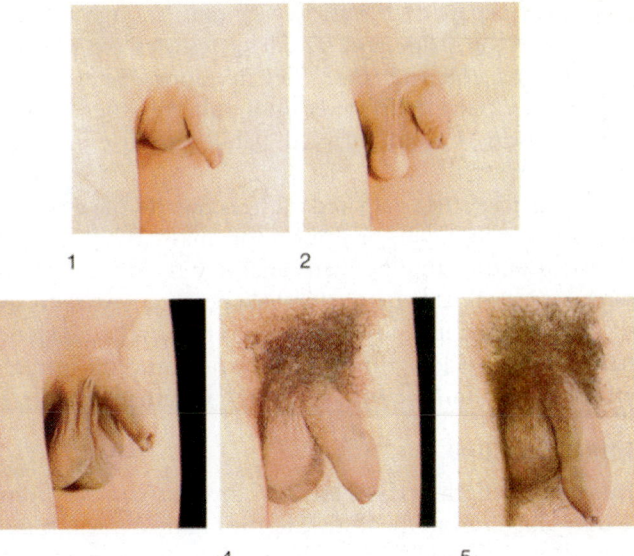

FIGURE 33–34. ◆ The stages of male pubic hair and external genital development with sexual maturation. *From Van Wieringen et al. (1971). Growth diagrams 1965 Netherlands. Groningen: Wolters-Noordhof.*

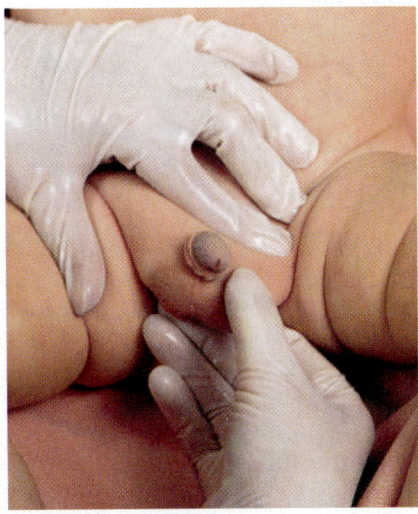

FIGURE 33–35. ◆ Palpating the scrotum for descended testicles and spermatic cords.

Palpation of the Male Genitalia

PENIS

Palpate the shaft of the penis for nodules and masses. None should be present.

TESTICLES

Palpate the scrotum for the presence of the testicles. Make sure your hands are warm to avoid stimulating the cremasteric reflex that causes the testicles to retract. Place your index finger and thumb over both inguinal canals on each side of the penis. This keeps the testicles from retracting into the abdomen (Figure 33–35 ◆).

Gently palpate each testicle with only enough pressure to identify the shape and size. The testicles are normally smooth and equal in size. They are approximately 1 to 1.5 cm (1/2 in.) in diameter until puberty, when they increase in size. A hard, enlarged, painless testicle may indicate a tumor.

If a testicle is not palpated in the scrotum, the examiner palpates the inguinal canal for a soft mass. When the testicle is found in the inguinal canal, try to move it to the scrotum to palpate the size and shape. The testicle is descendable when it can be moved into the scrotum. An undescended testicle is one that does not descend into the scrotum or cannot be palpated in the inguinal canal.

SPERMATIC CORD

Palpate the length of the spermatic cord between the thumb and forefinger from the testicle to the inguinal canal. It normally feels solid and smooth. No tenderness is expected.

ENLARGED SCROTUM

When bulging or swelling of the scrotum is present, palpate the scrotum to identify the characteristics of the mass. Try to determine whether the mass is unilateral or bilateral and attempt to reduce the mass by pushing it back through the external inguinal ring. A mass that decreases may indicate an inguinal hernia. A mass that does not decrease may indicate a hydrocele or an incarcerated hernia.

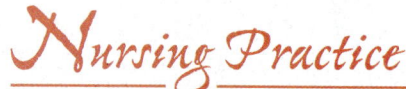

To distinguish between a hydrocele and an incarcerated hernia, place a bright penlight under the scrotum and look for a red glow or transillumination through the scrotum. A hydrocele transilluminates; a hernia does not.

INGUINAL CANAL

Attempt to insert the little finger into the external inguinal canal to determine whether the external inguinal ring is dilated. The inguinal ring is normally too small for the finger to pass into the canal. If the finger passes into the inguinal canal, ask the child to cough. A sensation of abdominal contents coming down to touch the fingertip may indicate an inguinal hernia.

CREMASTERIC REFLEX

Stroke the inner thigh of each leg to stimulate the cremasteric reflex. The testicle and scrotum normally rise on the stroked side. This response indicates intact function of the spinal cord at the T12, L1, and L2 levels.

Inspection of the Anus and Rectum

Inspect the anus for sphincter control and any abnormal findings such as inflammation, fissures, or lesions. The ex-

ternal sphincter is usually closed. Inflammation and scratch marks around the anus may be associated with pinworms. A protrusion from the rectum may be associated with a rectal wall prolapse or a hemorrhoid.

Palpation of the Anus and Rectum

Lightly touching the anal opening should stimulate an anal contraction or "wink." Absence of a contraction may indicate the presence of a lower spinal cord lesion.

PATENCY OF THE ANUS

Passage of meconium by newborns indicates a patent anus. When passage of meconium is delayed, a lubricated catheter can be inserted 1 cm (1/2 in.) into the anus. Resistance in passage of the catheter may indicate an obstruction.

RECTAL EXAMINATION

A rectal examination is not routinely performed on children. It is indicated for symptoms of intra-abdominal, rectal, bowel, or stool abnormalities. Only an experienced examiner should perform a rectal examination.

ASSESSING THE MUSCULOSKELETAL SYSTEM FOR BONE AND JOINT STRUCTURE, MOVEMENT, AND MUSCLE STRENGTH

Inspection of the Bones, Muscles, and Joints

Inspect and compare the arms and then the legs for differences in alignment, contour, skin folds, length, and deformities. The extremities normally have equal length, circumference, and numbers of skin folds bilaterally. Extra skin folds and a larger circumference may indicate a shorter extremity.

Inspect and compare the joints bilaterally for size, discoloration, and ease of voluntary movement. Joints are normally the same color as surrounding skin, with no sign of swelling. Children should voluntarily flex and extend joints during normal activities without pain. Redness, swelling, and pain with movement may indicate injury or infection.

Palpation of the Bones, Muscles, and Joints

Palpate the bones and muscles in each extremity for muscle tone, masses, or tenderness. Muscles normally feel firm, and bony masses are not normally present. Doughy muscles may indicate poor muscle tone. Rigid muscles, or *hypertonia,* may be associated with an active seizure or cerebral palsy. A mass over a long bone may indicate a recent fracture or a bone tumor.

Palpate each joint and surrounding muscles to detect any swelling, masses, heat, or tenderness. None is expected when the joint is palpated. Tenderness, heat, swelling, and redness can result from injury or a chronic joint inflammation such as juvenile rheumatoid arthritis.

Growth and Development

> Palpate the clavicles of the newborn from the sternum to the shoulder. These bones are often fractured during delivery. A mass and crepitus may indicate a fracture.

Range of Motion and Muscle Strength Assessment

ACTIVE RANGE OF MOTION

Observe the child during typical play activities, such as reaching for objects, climbing, and walking, to assess range of motion of all major joints. Children spontaneously move their joints through the full normal range of motion with play activities when no pain is present. Limited range of motion may indicate injury, inflammation of a joint, or a muscle abnormality.

PASSIVE RANGE OF MOTION

When a joint is suspected of having limited active range of motion, perform passive range of motion. Flex and extend, abduct and adduct, or rotate the affected joint cautiously to avoid causing extra pain. Full range of motion without pain is normal. Limitations in movement may indicate injury, inflammation, or malformation. Increased passive range of motion may indicate muscle weakness.

MUSCLE STRENGTH

Observe the child's ability to climb onto an examining table, throw a ball, clap the hands, or move around on the bed. The child's ability to perform age-appropriate play activities indicates good muscle tone and strength. Attainment of age-appropriate motor development is another indicator of good muscle strength (Table 33–17).

To assess the strength of specific muscles in the extremities, engage the child in some games. Compare muscle strength bilaterally to identify muscle weakness. For example, the child squeezes the examiner's fingers tightly with each hand; pushes against and pulls the examiner's hands with his or her hands, lower legs, and feet; and resists extension of a flexed elbow or knee. Children normally have good muscle strength bilaterally. Unilateral muscle weakness may be associated with a nerve injury. Bilateral muscle weakness may result from hypoxemia or a congenital disorder such as Down syndrome.

TABLE 33–17	Selected Gross Motor Milestones for Age
Gross Motor Milestones	Age Attained
Rolls over from prone to supine position	4 months
Sits without support	8 months
Pulls self to standing position	10 months
Walks around room holding onto objects	11 months
Walks alone well	15 months
Kicks ball	24 months
Jumps in place	30 months
Throws ball overhand	36 months

Note: From Frankenburg, W. K., Dodds, J., Archer, P., Shapiro, H., & Bresnick, B. (1992). The Denver II: A major revison and restandardization of the Denver Developmental Screening Test. *Pediatrics, 89,* 91–97. Reproduced with permission from *Pediatrics,* Figure 2, © 1992.

When generalized muscle weakness is suspected in a preschool- or school-age child, ask the child to stand up from the supine position. Children are normally able to rise to a standing position without using their arms as levers. Children who push their body upright using the arms and hands may have generalized muscle weakness, known as a *positive Gowers' sign.* This may indicate muscular dystrophy (see Figure 50–10.)

Posture and Spinal Alignment

POSTURE

Inspect the child's posture when standing from a front, side, and back view. The shoulders and hips are normally level. The head is held erect without a tilt, and the shoulder contour is symmetric. The spine has normal thoracic convex and lumbar concave curves after 6 years of age. Table 33–18 shows normal posture and spinal curvature development.

Growth and Development

> After beginning to walk, young children often have a pot-bellied stance because of a lumbar lordosis. This posture generally disappears by 5 years of age.

SPINAL ALIGNMENT

Assess the school-age child and adolescent for *scoliosis,* a lateral spine curvature. Stand behind the child, observing the height of the shoulders and hips (Figure 33–36 ◆). Ask the child to bend forward slowly at the waist, with arms extended toward the floor. No lateral curve should be present in either position. The ribs normally stay flat bilaterally. The lumbar concave curve should flatten with forward flexion (Figure 33–37 ◆). A lateral curve to the spine or a one-sided rib hump is an indication of scoliosis (see also Chapter 50). ⊂⊃

TABLE 33-18   Normal Development of Posture and Spinal Curves

Infant

2–3 months	6–8 months	10–15 months	Toddler	School-age child

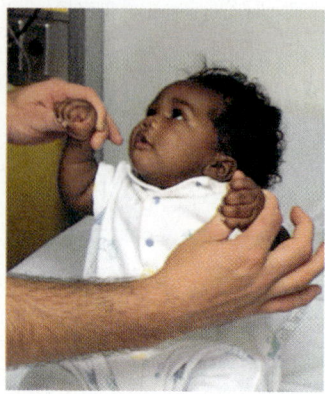 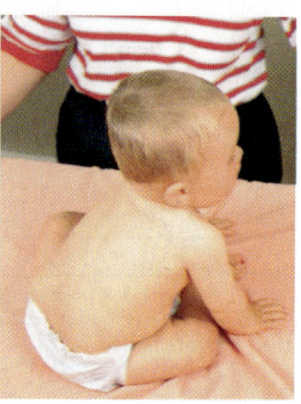 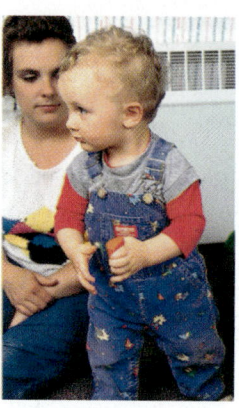 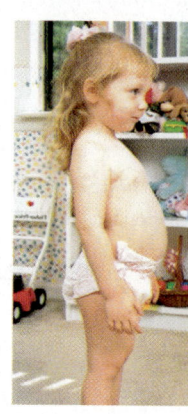 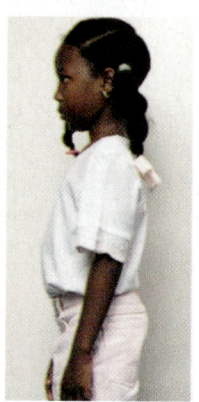

| Holds head erect when held upright; thoracic kyphosis when sitting. | Sits without support; spine is straight. | Walks independently; straight spine. | Protruding abdomen; lumbar lordosis. | Height of shoulders and hips is level; balanced thoracic convex and lumbar concave curves. |

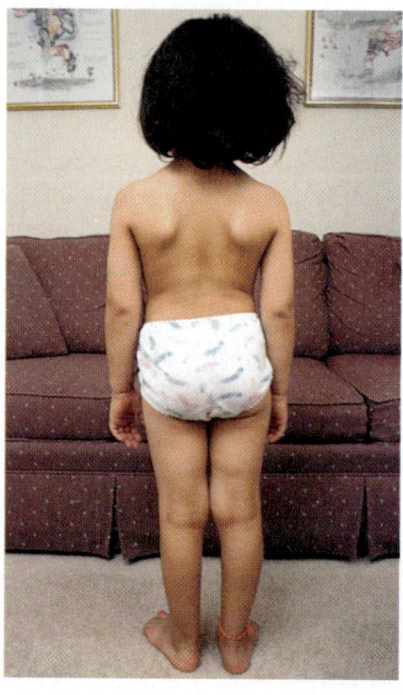

FIGURE 33–36. ◆ Does this child have legs of different lengths or scoliosis? Look at the level of the iliac crests and shoulders to see if they are level. See the more prominent crease at the waist on the right side? This child could have scoliosis.

Inspection of the Upper Extremities

ARMS

The alignment of the arms is normally straight, with a minimal angle at the elbows, where the bones articulate.

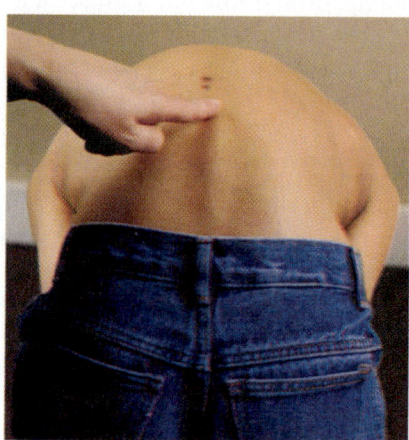

FIGURE 33–37. ◆ Inspection of the spine for scoliosis. Ask the child to slowly bend forward at the waist, with arms extended toward the floor. Run your forefinger down the spinal processes, palpating each vertebra for a change in alignment. A lateral curve to the spine or a one-sided rib hump is an indication of scoliosis.

HANDS

Count the fingers. Extra finger digits (*polydactyly*) or webbed fingers (*syndactyly*) are abnormal. Inspect the creases on the palmar surface of each hand. Multiple creases across the palm are normal. A single crease that crosses the entire palm of the hand, a simian crease, is associated with Down syndrome (Figure 33–38 ◆).

NAILS

Inspect the nails for size, shape, and color. Nails are normally convex, smooth, and pink. *Clubbing,* widening of the nailbed with an increased angle between the proximal nail

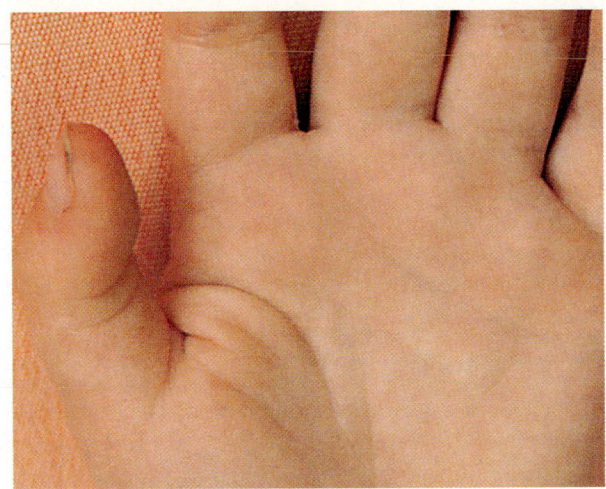

A

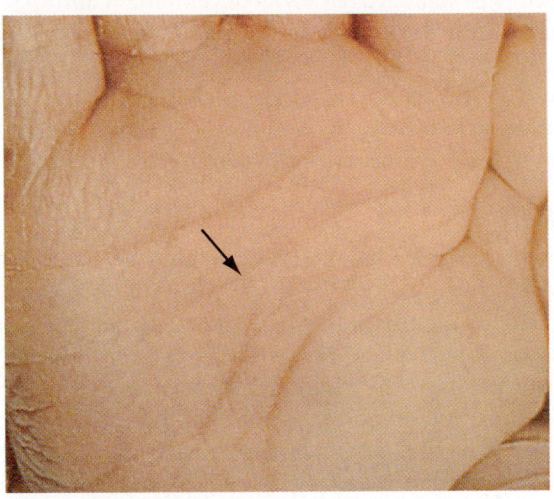

B

FIGURE 33–38. ◆ **A,** Normal palmar creases. **B,** Simian crease associated with Down syndrome. *Source* **B:** From Zitelli, B. J., & Davis, H. W. (Eds.). (1997). Atlas of pediatric physical diagnosis (3rd ed.). St. Louis: Mosby–Year Book.

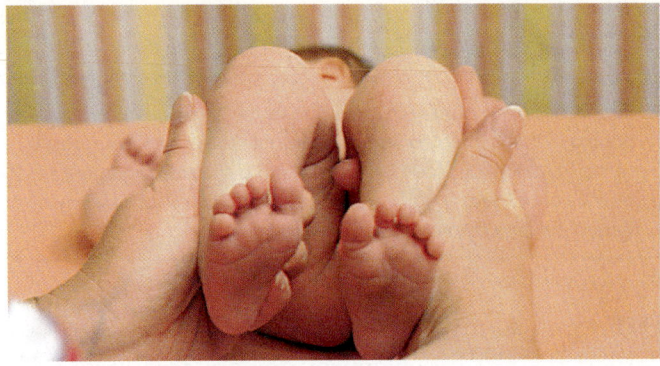

FIGURE 33–39. ◆ Flex the infant's hips and knees so the heels are as close to the buttocks as possible. Place the feet flat on the examining table. The knees are usually the same height. A difference in knee height (Allis sign) is an indicator of hip dislocation (see also Chapter 25). ◖◗ *Courtesy Dee Corbett, RN, Children's National Medical Center, Washington, DC.*

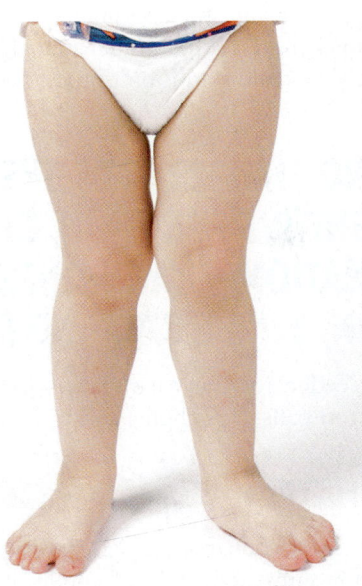

FIGURE 33–40. ◆ To evaluate the child with knock-knees, have the child stand on a firm surface. Measure the distance between the ankles when the child stands with the knees together. The normal distance is not more than 2 in (5 cm) between the ankles.

fold and nail, is abnormal (see Figure 43–6). Clubbing is associated with chronic respiratory and cardiac conditions.

Inspection of the Lower Extremities

HIPS

Assess the hips of newborns and young infants for dislocation or subluxation. First inspect the skin folds on the upper legs. The same number of skin folds should be present on each leg. Uneven skin folds may indicate a hip dislocation or difference in leg length (Allis' sign). Then check for a difference in knee height symmetry (Figure 33–39 ◆). The Ortolani–Barlow maneuver is used to assess an infant's hips for dislocation or subluxation. See Chapter 25 for more information. ◖◗

Ask the child to stand on one leg and then the other. The iliac crests should stay level. If the iliac crest opposite the weight-bearing leg appears lower, the hip bearing weight may be dislocated.

LEGS

Inspect the alignment of the legs. After a child is 4 years of age, the alignment of the long bones is straight, with minimal angle at the knees and feet where the bones articulate. Assess alignment of the lower extremities in infants and toddlers to ensure that normal changes are occurring. To evaluate the toddler with bowlegs, have the child stand on a firm surface. Measure the distance between the knees when the child's ankles are together. No more than 1.5 in (3.5 cm) between the knees is normal. See Figure 33–40 ◆ for assessment of knock-knees.

Growth and Development

Infants are often born with a twisting of the tibia caused by positioning in utero (tibial torsion). The infant's toes turn in as a result of the tibial torsion. Toddlers go through a skeletal alignment sequence of bowlegs (genu varum) and knock-knees (genu valgum) before the legs assume a straight alignment.

FEET

Inspect the feet for alignment, the presence of all toes, and any deformities. The weight-bearing line of the feet is usually in alignment with the legs. Many newborns have a flexible forefoot inversion (metatarsus adductus) that results from uterine positioning. Any fixed deformity is abnormal.

Inspect the feet for the presence of an arch when the child is standing. Children up to 3 years of age normally have a fat pad over the arch, giving the appearance of flat feet. Older children normally have a longitudinal arch. The arch is usually seen when the child stands on tiptoe or is sitting.

ASSESSING THE NERVOUS SYSTEM FOR COGNITIVE FUNCTION, BALANCE, COORDINATION, CRANIAL NERVE FUNCTION, SENSATION, AND REFLEXES

Equipment needed for this examination includes a reflex hammer, cotton balls, a penlight, and tongue blades.

Cognitive Function

Observe the child's behavior, facial expressions, gestures, communication skills, activity level, and level of consciousness to assess cognitive functioning. Match the neurologic examination to the child's stage of development. For example, cognitive function is evaluated much differently in infants than in older children because infants cannot use words to communicate.

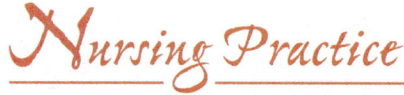

Nursing Practice

The neurologic examination provides an opportunity to develop rapport with the child. Many of the procedures can be presented as games that young children enjoy. You can assess cognitive function by how well the child follows directions for the game. As the assessment proceeds, the child develops trust and is more likely to cooperate with examination of other systems.

BEHAVIOR

The behavior of infants and children during the assessment indicates their alertness. Infants and toddlers are curious but seek the security of the parent, either by clinging or by making frequent eye contact. Older children are often anxious and watch all of the examiner's actions. Lack of interest in assessment or treatment procedures may indicate a serious illness. Excessive activity or an unusually short attention span may be associated with an attention deficit hyperactivity disorder.

COMMUNICATION SKILLS

Speech, language development, and social skills provide good clues to cognitive functioning. Listen to speech articulation and words used, comparing the child's performance with standards of social development and speech articulation for the child's age (Table 33–19). Toddlers can normally follow simple directions such as "Show me your mouth." By 3 years of age the child's speech should be easily understood. Delay in language and social skill development may be associated with mental retardation.

MEMORY

Immediate, recent, and remote memory can be tested in children starting at approximately 4 years of age. To evaluate recent memory, ask the child to remember a special name or object. Then 5 to 10 minutes later during the examination, have the child recall the name or object. To evaluate remote memory, ask the child to repeat his or her address or birth date or a nursery rhyme. By 5 or 6 years of age, children are normally able to recall this information without difficulty.

LEVEL OF CONSCIOUSNESS

When approaching the infant or child, observe his or her level of consciousness and activity, including facial expressions, gestures, and interaction. Children are normally alert, and sleeping children arouse easily. The child who cannot be awakened is unconscious. A lowered level of consciousness may be associated with a number of neuro-

TABLE 33–19 Expected Language Development for Age	
Language Milestones	Age Attained
Understands Mama and Dada	10 months
Says Mama, Dada, 2 other words; imitates animal sounds	12 months
4–6 word vocabulary, points to desired objects	13–15 months
7–20 word vocabulary, points to 5 body parts	18 months
2-word combinations	20 months
3-word sentences, plurals	36 months

Note: From Capute, A. J., Shapiro, B. K., & Palmer, R. B. (1987). Marking the milestones of language development. *Contemporary Pediatrics, 4,* 24–41.

Growth and Development

Test immediate memory by asking the child to repeat a series of words or numbers, such as the names of Disney or Sesame Street characters. Children can remember more words or numbers with age.

Age	Recall Ability
4 years	3 words or numbers
5 years	4 words or numbers
6 years	5 words or numbers

logic conditions such as a head injury, seizure, infection, or brain tumor.

Cerebellar Function

Observe the young child at play to assess coordination and balance. Development of fine motor skills in infants and preschool children provides clues to cerebellar function.

BALANCE

Observe the child's balance during play activities such as walking, standing on one foot, and hopping (Table 33–20). The Romberg procedure can also be used to test balance in children over 3 years of age (Figure 33–41 ◆). Once balance and other motor skills are attained, children do not normally stumble or fall when tested. Poor balance may indicate cerebellar dysfunction or an inner ear disturbance.

COORDINATION

Tests of coordination assess the smoothness and accuracy of movement. Development of fine motor skills can be used to assess coordination in young children (Table 33–21). After 6 years of age the tests for adults (finger-to-nose, finger-to-finger, heel-to-shin, and alternating motion) can be used (Figure 33–42 ◆). The child usually responds enthusiastically when these tests are presented as games. Jerky movements or inaccurate pointing *(past pointing)* indicate poor coordination, which can be associated with delayed development or a cerebellar lesion.

TABLE 33–20 Expected Balance Development for Age

Balance Milestones	Age Attained
Stands without support briefly	12 months
Walks alone well	15 months
Walks backwards	2 years
Balances on 1 foot for 5 seconds	4 years
Hops on 1 foot, heel-toe walking	5 years
Heel-toe walking backwards	6 years

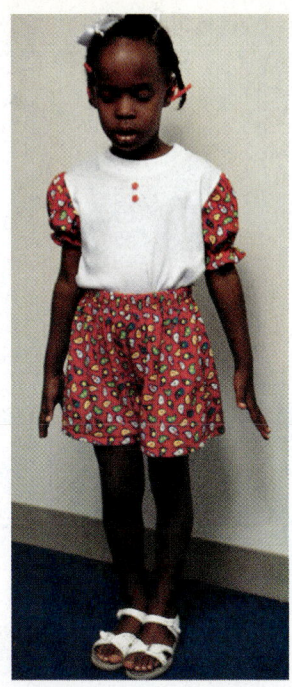

FIGURE 33–41. ◆ Romberg procedure. Ask the child to stand with feet together and eyes closed. Protect the child from falling by standing close. Preschool-age children may extend their arms to maintain balance, but older children can normally stand with their arms at their sides. Leaning or falling to one side is abnormal and indicates poor balance.

TABLE 33–21 Expected Fine Motor Development for Age

Fine Motor Milestones	Age Attained
Transfers objects between hands	7 months
Picks up small objects	10 months
Feeds self with cup and spoon	12 months
Scribbles with crayon or pencil	18 months
Builds 2-block tower	24 months
Builds 4-block tower	30 months
Unfastens front buttons	36 months

Note: From Frankenburg, W. K., Dodds, J., Archer, P., Shapiro, H., & Bresnick, B. (1992). The Denver II: A major revison and restandardization of the Denver Developmental Screening Test. *Pediatrics, 89,* 91–97. Reproduced with permission from *Pediatrics,* Table 2, © 1992.

GAIT

A normal gait requires intact bones and joints, muscle strength, coordination, and balance. Inspect the child when walking from both a front and a rear view. The iliac crests are normally level during walking, and no limp is expected. A limp may indicate injury or joint disease. Staggering or falling may indicate cerebellar ataxia. *Scissoring,* in which the thighs tend to cross forward over each other with each step, may be associated with cerebral palsy or other spastic conditions.

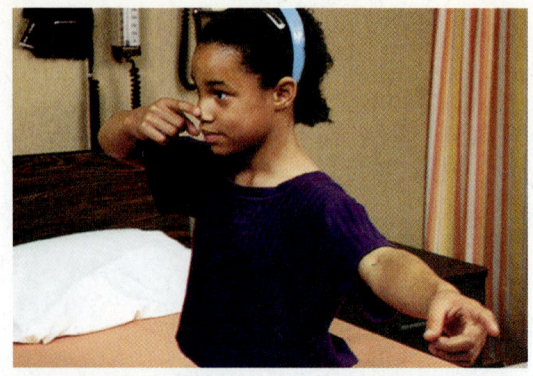

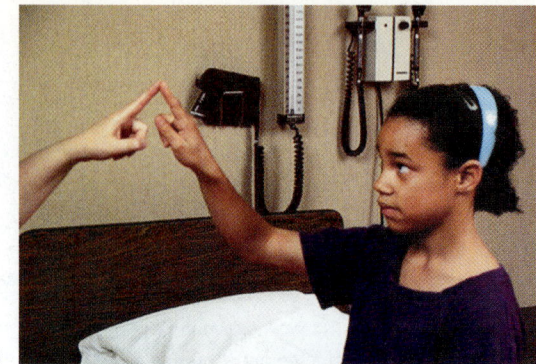

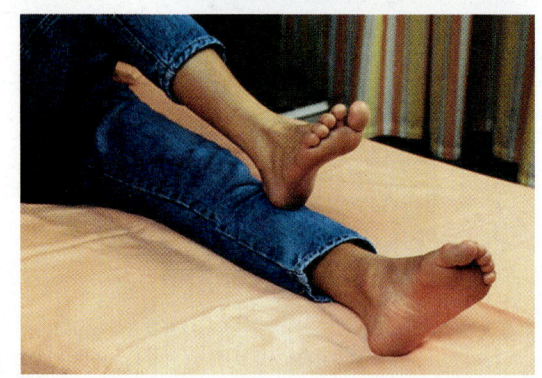

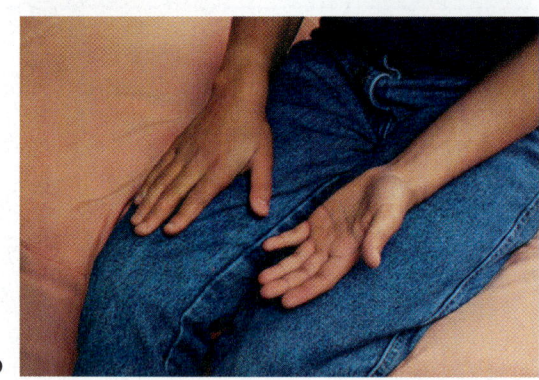

FIGURE 33–42. ◆ Tests of coordination. **A,** *Finger-to-nose test.* Ask the child to close the eyes and touch his or her nose, alternating the index fingers of the hands. **B,** *Finger-to-finger test.* Ask the child to alternately touch his or her nose and your index finger with his or her index finger. Move your hand to several positions within the child's reach to test pointing accuracy. Repeat the test with the child's other hand. **C,** *Heel-to-shin test.* Ask the child to rub his or her leg from the knee to the ankle with the heel of the other foot. Repeat the test with the other foot. This test is normally performed without hesitation or inappropriate placement of the foot. **D,** *Rapid alternating motion test.* Ask the child to rapidly rotate his or her wrist so the palm and dorsum of the hand alternately pat the thigh. Repeat the test with the other hand. Hesitating movements are abnormal. Mirroring movements of the hand not being tested indicate a delay in coordination skill refinement.

Growth and Development

> Gait is related to the motor development of the child. Toddlers beginning to walk have a wide-based gait and limited balance. With practice the toddler's balance improves and the gait develops a narrower base.

Cranial Nerve Function

To assess the cranial nerves in infants and young children, modify the procedures used to assess school-age children and adults (Table 33–22). Abnormalities of cranial nerves may be associated with compression of an individual nerve, head injury, or infections.

Sensory Function

To assess sensory function, compare the responses of both sides of the body to various types of stimulation. Equal responses bilaterally are normal. Loss of sensation may indicate a brain or spinal cord lesion.

SUPERFICIAL TACTILE SENSATION

Stroke the skin on the lower leg or arm with a cotton ball or a finger while the child's eyes are closed. Cooperative children over 2 years of age can normally point to the location touched.

SUPERFICIAL PAIN SENSATION

Break a tongue blade to get a sharp point. After asking the child to close the eyes, touch the child in various places on each arm and leg, alternating the sharp and dull ends of the tongue blade. Children over 4 years of age can normally distinguish between a sharp and dull sensation each time. To improve the child's accuracy with the test, let the child practice telling you the difference between the sharp and dull stimulation.

Nursing Practice

An infant's sensory function is not routinely assessed. Withdrawal responses to painful procedures indicate normal sensory function.

TABLE 33–22	Age-Specific Procedures for Assessment of Cranial Nerves in Infants and Children
Cranial Nerve[a]	Assessment Procedure and Normal Findings[b]
I Olfactory	Infant: Not tested. Child: Not routinely tested. Give familiar odors to child to smell, one naris at a time. *Identifies odors such as orange, peanut butter, and chocolate.*
II Optic	Infant: Shine a bright light in eyes. *A quick blink reflex and dorsal head flexion indicates light perception.* Child: Test vision and visual fields if cooperative. *Visual acuity appropriate for age.*
III Oculomotor IV Trochlear VI Abducens	Infant: Shine a penlight at the eyes and move it side to side. *Focuses on and tracks the light to each side.* Child: Move an object through the six cardinal points of gaze. *Tracks object through all fields of gaze.* All ages: Inspect eyelids for drooping. Inspect pupillary response to light. *Eyelids do not droop and pupils are equal sized and briskly respond to light.*
V Trigeminral	Infant: Stimulate the rooting and sucking reflex. *Turns head toward stimulation at side of mouth and sucking has good strength and pattern.* Child: Observe the child chewing a cracker. Touch forehead and cheeks with cotton ball when eyes are closed. *Bilateral jaw strength is good. Child pushes cotton ball away.*
VII Facial	All ages: Observe facial expressions when crying, smiling, frowning, etc. *Facial features stay symmetric bilaterally.*
VIII Acoustic	Infant: Produce a loud sound near the head. *Blinks in response to sound, moves head toward sound or freezes position.* Child: Use a noisemaker near each ear or whisper words to be repeated. *Turns head toward sound and repeats words correctly.*
IX Glossopharyngeal X Vagus	Infant: Observe swallowing during feeding. *Good swallowing pattern.* All ages: Elicit gag reflex. *Gags with stimulation.*
XI Spinal accessory	Infant: Not tested. Child: Ask child to raise the shoulders and turn the head side to side against resistance. *Good strength in neck and shoulders.*
XII Hypoglossal	Infant: Observe feeding. *Sucking and swallowing are coordinated.* Child: Tell the child to stick out the tongue. Listen to speech. *Tongue is midline with no tremors. Words are clearly articulated.*

[a]Bracketed nerves are tested together.
[b]Italic indicates normal findings.

An inability to identify superficial touch and pain sensation may indicate sensory loss. Identify the extent of sensory loss, such as all areas below the knee. Other sensory function tests (temperature, vibratory, deep pressure pain, and position sense) are performed when sensory loss is found. Refer to other texts for a description of these procedures.

Infant Primitive Reflexes

Evaluate the movement and posture of newborns and young infants by the Moro, ⊂⊃ [WEB] palmar grasp, plantar grasp, placing, stepping, and tonic neck primitive reflexes. These reflexes appear and disappear at expected intervals in the first few months of life as the central nervous system develops. Movements are normally equal bilaterally. An asymmetric response may indicate a serious neurologic problem on the less responsive side. See Chapter 25 for more information. ⊂⊃

Superficial and Deep Tendon Reflexes

Evaluate the superficial and deep tendon reflexes to assess the function of specific segments of the spine.

SUPERFICIAL REFLEXES

Assess superficial reflexes by stroking a specific area of the body. The plantar reflex, testing spine levels L4 to S2, is routinely evaluated in children (Figure 33–43 ◆). Assess the cremasteric reflex in boys (see p. 804). ⊂⊃

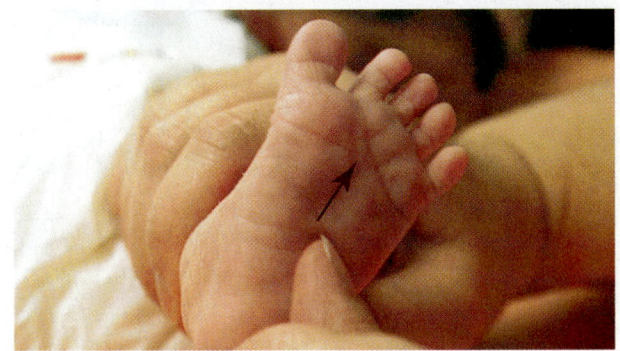

FIGURE 33–43. ◆ To assess the plantar reflex, stroke the bottom of the infant's or child's foot in the direction of the arrow. Watch the toes for plantar flexion or the Babinski response, fanning and dorsiflexion of the big toe. The Babinski response is normal in children under 2 years of age. Plantar flexion, of the toes is the normal response in older children. A Babinski response in children over 2 years of age can indicate neurologic disease.

DEEP TENDON REFLEXES

To assess the deep tendon reflexes, tap a tendon near specific joints with a reflex hammer (or with the index finger for infants), comparing responses bilaterally. The biceps, triceps, brachioradialis, patellar, and Achilles tendons are usually evaluated in children. Inspect for movement in the associated joint and palpate the strength of the expected muscle contraction (Table 33–23). Table 33–24 outlines the numeric scoring of deep tendon reflexes. Responses are normally symmetric bilaterally. The absence of a response is associated with decreased muscle tone and strength. Hyperactive responses are associated with muscle spasticity.

TABLE 33-23	Assessment of Deep Tendon Reflexes and the Spinal Segment Tested with Each	
Deep Tendon Reflex	**Technique and Normal Findings***ᵃ*	**Spine Segment Tested**
Biceps 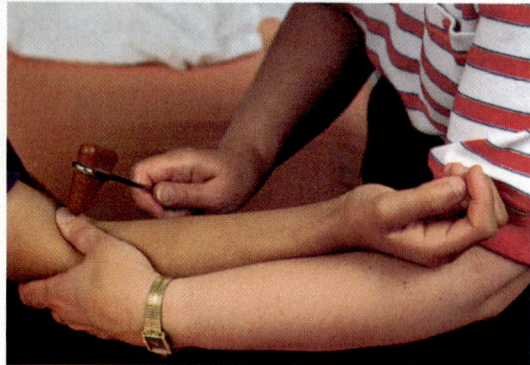	Flex the child's arm at the elbow, and place your thumb over the biceps tendon in the antecubital fossa. Tap your thumb. *Elbow flexes as the biceps muscle contracts.*	C5 and C6
Triceps 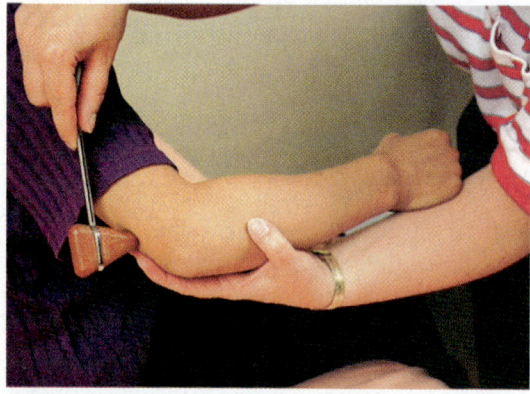	With the child's arm flexed, tap the triceps tendon above the elbow. *Elbow extends as the triceps muscle contracts.*	C6, C7, and C8
Brachioradialis 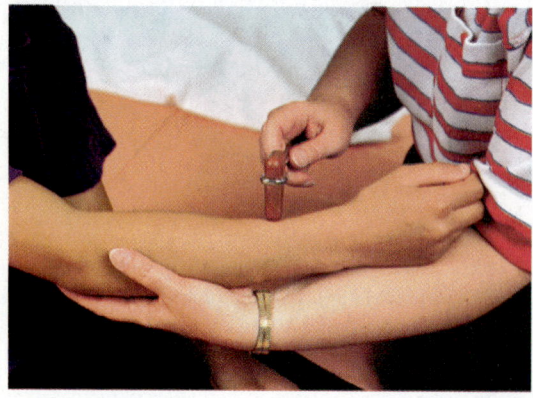	Lay the child's arm with the thumb upright over your arm. Tap the brachioradial tendon 2.5 cm (1 in) above the wrist. *Forearm pronates (palm facing downward) and elbow flexes.*	C5 and C6

TABLE 33-23 Assessment of Deep Tendon Reflexes and the Spinal Segment Tested with Each—continued

Deep Tendon Reflex	Technique and Normal Findings[a]	Spine Segment Tested
Patellar 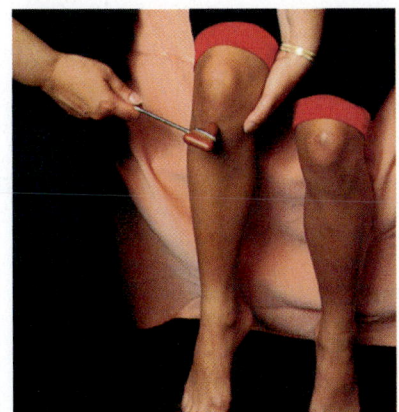	Flex the child's knees, and when the legs are relaxed, tap the patellar tendon just below the knee. *Knee extends (knee jerk) as the quadriceps muscle contracts.*	L2, L3, and L4
Achilles 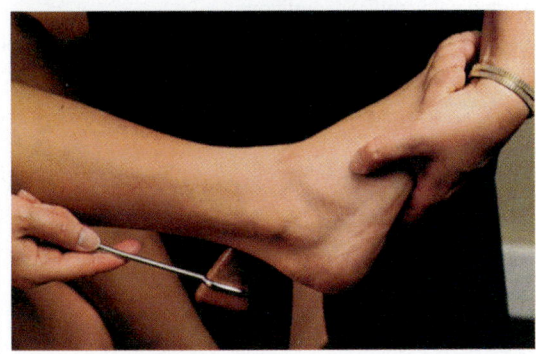	While the child's legs are flexed, support the foot and tap the Achilles' tendon. *Plantar flexion (ankle jerk) as the gastrocnemius muscle contracts.*	S1 and S2

[a]Italics indicate normal findings.

Nursing Practice

The best response to deep tendon reflex testing is achieved when the child is relaxed or distracted. Children often anticipate the knee jerk and either tighten up or exaggerate the response. Making the child focus on another set of muscles may provide a more accurate response. When testing the reflexes on the lower legs, have the child press his or her hands together or try to pull them apart when gripped together.

TABLE 33-24 Numeric Scoring of Deep Tendon Reflex Responses

Grade	Response Interpretation
0	No response
1+	Slow, minimal response
2+	Expected response, active
3+	More active or pronounced than expected
4+	Hyperactive, clonus may be present

Nursing Practice

Be sure to record all findings from the physical assessment legibly, in detail, and in the format approved by your institution.

Thinking Critically

THINKING CRITICALLY: ASSESSING A CHILD WITH BRONCHIOLITIS

Latoya, 6 months old, is brought by her mother and father to the emergency room. She is an emergency admission from the local pediatrician's office with a diagnosis of bronchiolitis. As Latoya's nurse, you are responsible for assessing her condition after she arrives on the pediatric nursing unit.

What historical information do you collect, and what procedures are used to perform a physical examination on a 6-month-old? How do you organize your findings to make sense of them to plan nursing care?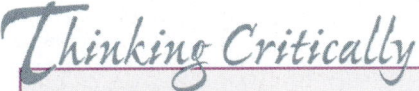

ANALYZING DATA FROM THE PHYSICAL EXAMINATION

Once the physical examination has been completed, group any abnormal findings for each system with those of other systems. Use **clinical judgment** to identify common patterns of physiologic responses associated with medical conditions. Individual abnormal physiologic responses are also the basis of many nursing diagnoses.

CHAPTER HIGHLIGHTS

≈ Establish a rapport with the family and use careful listening techniques to collect historical information about the child's health status.

≈ Historical data to collect includes the chief complaint, history of the present illness or injury, past history, current health status, review of systems, and family history. In addition, collect psychosocial data and developmental data.

≈ The physical examination sequence includes assessment of the following:

- Skin and hair
- Head, eyes, ears, nose, and mouth structures and function
- Neck
- Chest and lungs
- Breasts
- Heart and pulses
- Abdomen
- Inguinal area
- Genitalia and perineal areas
- Musculoskeletal system
- Nervous system

≈ Clinical judgment identifies common patterns of physiologic responses associated with medical conditions.

≈ The physiologic responses and family and child responses to their health condition become the basis for many nursing diagnoses.

EXPLOREMEDIALINK

NCLEX Review, Case Studies, and other interactive resources for this chapter can be found on the companion website at http://www.prenhall.com/london. Click on "Chapter 33" to select the activities for this chapter.

For animations, more NCLEX review questions, and an audio glossary, access the accompanying CD-ROM in this textbook.

REFERENCES

Burns, C. (1992). A new assessment model and tool for pediatric nurse practitioners. *Journal of Pediatric Health Care, 6,* 73–81.

Byrnes, K. (1996). Conducting the pediatric health history: A guide. *Pediatric Nursing, 22,* 135–137.

Eichelberger, M. R., Ball, J. W., Pratsch, G. S., & Clark, J. R. (1998). *Pediatric emergencies: A manual for prehospital care providers* (2nd ed.). Upper Saddle River, NJ: Brady, Prentice Hall.

Goldenring, J. M., & Cohen, E. (1988). Getting into adolescent heads. *Contemporary Pediatrics, 5,* 75–90.

Hazinski, M. F. (1999). *Manual of pediatric critical care* (pp. 289–293). St. Louis, MO: Mosby.

Herman-Giddens, M. E., Slora, E. J., Wasserman, R. C., Bourdony, C. J., Bhapkar, M. V., Koch, G. G. et al. (1997). Secondary sexual characteristics and menses in young girls seen in office practice: A study from the pediatric research in office setting network. *Pediatrics, 99*(4), 505–512.

Kaplowitz, P. B., Oberfield, S. E., and the Drug and Therapeutics and Executive Committees of the Lawson Wilkins Pediatric Endocrine Society. (1999). Reexamination of the age limit for defining when puberty is precocious in girls in the United States: Implications for evaluation and treatment. *Pediatrics, 104*(4), 936–941.

Seidel, H. M., Ball, J. W., Dains, J., & Benedict, G. W. (2003). *Mosby's guide to physical examination* (5th ed.). St. Louis, MO: Mosby.

Spector, R. E. (2000). *Cultural diversity in health and illness* (5th ed.). Upper Saddle River, NJ: Prentice Hall Health.

Tanner, J. M. (1962). *Growth at adolescence* (2nd ed.). Oxford, England: Blackwell Scientific Publications, Inc.

Wilson, E. F. (1977). Estimation of the age of cutaneous contusions in child abuse. *Pediatrics, 60,* 750.

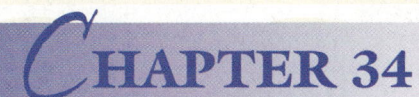

CHAPTER 34

Nursing Considerations for the Hospitalized Child

We live 50 miles from the hospital, and have three other children. We were worried about how we were going to be able to stay with Sabrina. She's only 4, and it's her first time in the hospital. Fortunately, they have beds for parents, so one of us can always be by her side throughout her procedure and recuperation.

—Mother of Sabrina, AGE 4

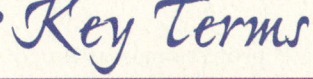 Key Terms

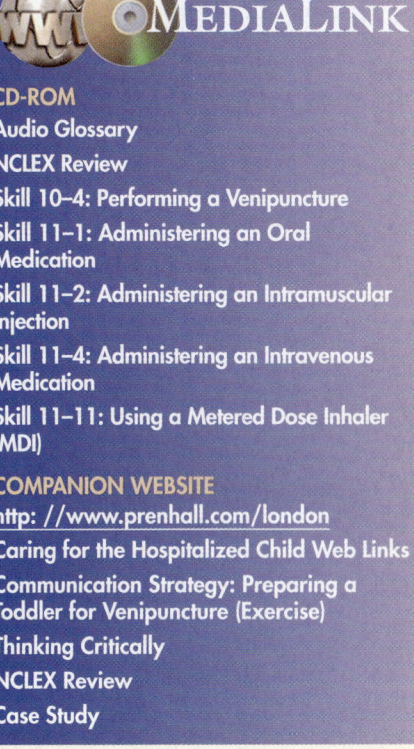

*H*ospitalization, whether it is elective, planned in advance, or the result of an emergency or trauma, is stressful for children of all ages and their families. Today, children are infrequently hospitalized, because most pediatric conditions can be managed within the community. Hospitalized children are usually very ill. They find themselves in an unknown environment, surrounded by strange people and equipment and frightening sights and sounds. They are subjected to unfamiliar procedures, some of which are invasive, and may even have surgery or be in an intensive care unit. For both children and families, routines are disrupted and normal coping strategies are tested.

To minimize the stress of hospitalization, nurses need to provide support to children and their families before, during, and after hospitalization. Through preadmission preparation, children and their families are introduced to the acute care setting. During hospitalization, nurses work collaboratively with parents to use various strategies that promote coping and adaptation, or prepare children for procedures and surgery. Nurses are instrumental in ensuring that the developmental and educational needs of children are met, especially when hospitalization is prolonged. Nurses also work with families to help prepare for discharge or transfer to a long-term care or rehabilitation facility.

EFFECTS OF ILLNESS AND HOSPITALIZATION ON CHILDREN AND FAMILIES

Children's Understanding of Health and Illness

A child is likely to think that yelling at his or her mother caused strep throat. Adolescents may believe that that they never become ill or have an accident. On the other hand, they may fear being in a car crash like that of a friend. Children have limited knowledge about the body and its relation to health and illness. Their understanding is based primarily on their cognitive ability at various developmental stages and on previous experiences with health care professionals.

INFANT

By about 6 months of age, infants have developed an awareness of themselves as separate from their mother or father. They are able to identify primary caretakers and to feel anxious when in contact with strangers. Hospitalization can be a traumatic time for an infant, particularly if the parents are not staying with the child.

Three phases of **separation anxiety** were first identified in young children who were separated from their parents for long periods or permanently and lacked a close relationship with one caretaker after separation (Bowlby,

---

TABLE 34-1   Stages of Separation Anxiety in Young Children

Protest
Screaming, crying
Clinging to parents
Withdrawal from other adults

Despair
Sadness, depression
Withdrawal or compliant behavior
Crying when parents appear

Denial
Lack of protest when parents leave
Appearance of being happy and content with everyone
Close relationships not established
Developmental delay possible

Note: From Bowlby, J. (1960). Separation anxiety. *International Journal of Psychoanalysis, 41,* pp. 89–113. Adapted.

1960). Characteristic behaviors of children in the three phases of separation anxiety are listed in Table 34–1. Hospitalized infants and young children often display some of these behaviors, particularly if parents are unable to remain with the child.

Before the 1970s, health care professionals assumed that the despair and denial manifested by infants and young children after prolonged separation were signs of positive adaptation, since the child in these stages seemed calm and quiet. Infants sometimes protested when their parents visited, and parents were therefore advised not to visit often. However, the protest phase is now viewed as a healthy response to separation from loved ones and as an indication that the infant has meaningful, close relationships. Parents should be encouraged to remain with and provide care to the hospitalized infant, and to visit as often as possible if they cannot remain with the young child.

TODDLER AND PRESCHOOLER

Toddlers and preschoolers are beginning to understand illness but not its cause. Two unrelated events may appear to have a cause-and-effect relationship for young children, who may consider the sun, an animal, bad behavior, or even magic to be the cause of their illness. These children may blame other people, events, or themselves for an illness (Bibace & Walsh, 1981). This is especially true if the other event occurs shortly before the illness.

The child's concept of the body usually is limited to names and locations of some body parts. Although toddlers and preschoolers are not likely to understand how lungs, heart, bones, or other body parts function, they are learning concepts of safety and other health-related issues (Mobley, 1996).

Separation from parents remains the major stressor for the child. When a parent cannot be present, reminders can be left with the child. These might include a piece of cloth saturated with the mother's favorite perfume or father's cologne, an object belonging to the parent, or an audiotape with messages from the parents. Toddlers and preschoolers fear bodily mutilation and change. If, like Sabrina, the child is undergoing an operation, the nurse should explain to the child that surgery will fix the body. The nurse should encourage the parents to be present as much as possible for important rituals such as toileting, carrying out bedtime routines, and singing favorite nursery rhymes.

SCHOOL-AGE CHILD

Older children have a more realistic understanding of the reasons for illness and are able to comprehend explanations. The child's concept of body parts and function is maturing. Concepts of time are well formed, and parents should be encouraged to tell the child when they will return. Parents should also be available for telephone calls to provide support and comfort. Stressful procedures can lead to regression or other behavioral changes. The child relies on parents and others for support and understanding during these events.

Growth and Development

School-age children between the ages of 5 and 8 years believe that the internal body consists of heart and bones. They view the digestive system as having two parts, the mouth and the stomach.

ADOLESCENT

After 11 years of age, adolescents become increasingly aware of the physiologic, psychologic, and behavioral causes of illness and injury. Adolescents are concerned with appearance and perceive an illness or injury in terms of its effect on their body image. Allowing choices in clothing, hair, and music acknowledges the importance of their self-identity (Rosenbaum & Carty, 1996). Privacy and modesty are major concerns of adolescents because their physical characteristics are rapidly changing. Nurses should respect their feelings. Adolescents are in the process of becoming independent of their parents' influence, so control over aspects of their care is important. The peer group is a major influence in their lives, and having recreation and teen lounge facilities available are among their major recommendations. Separation from peers, home, and school are cited as major stressors of hospitalization by adolescents (Gusella, Ward, & Butler, 1998).

Growth and Development

Young adolescents, aged 11 to 13 years, can describe the location and function of major organs such as the brain, nose, eyes, heart, and stomach.

Family Responses to Hospitalization

The illness and hospitalization of a child disrupt a family's usual routines. Sometimes, roles are altered as one parent stays at the hospital while the other parent or siblings take on additional tasks at home. Family members may be anxious and fearful, especially when the outcome is unknown or potentially serious. Watching a child in pain is difficult for a parent. A serious emergency, lengthy illness, chronic condition, poor prognosis, lack of family support, and lack of financial or community services make adjustment more difficult. (See Chapter 37 for a description of nursing support for the child with life-threatening illness or injury.)

Parents report greater satisfaction with their children's care when nurses tailor actions to the family needs and preferences. Positive communication with medical personnel and viewing care as a partnership between parents (as well as other key family members) and clinicians are viewed as predictive of parental satisfaction with their child's hospital care (Marino & Marino, 2000; Conner & Nelson, 1999). Nurses need to see the parents as the ones who know and understand the child best, ask for their participation and partnership in care, and carefully explain all aspects of treatment. Parents need support to lessen their anxiety since those with many fears may not be able to parent children effectively and perform protective, nurturing, and decision-making roles (Melnyk, 2000).

Developing Cultural Competence

For Mexican Americans, family is a strong support. Extended family and godparents (compadres) may want to be with a hospitalized child. Although the father of the child is often the spokesperson, mothers commonly are influential in decisions regarding child health care (Lipson, Dibble, & Minarik, 1996). The nurse should be inclusive of all people the family wishes to have present in the hospital and for explanations about health care.

The siblings of an ill child often receive little attention from the parents. Parents are preoccupied and may not think to take the siblings to visit the child in the hospital. The siblings may fantasize about the illness or injury and the appearance of their brother or sister. Siblings who are not adequately informed about the hospitalized child's condition may fear that the child will be disabled or die, even when this is unlikely. They may feel guilty about fighting with or being mean to their brother or sister in the past and believe that they played a role in causing the illness.

As family roles and routines change, siblings may feel insecure and anxious. Behavioral problems may develop, or school performance may deteriorate. Siblings may feel jealous because the ill brother or sister seems to monopolize the parents' attention. Given support, however, the siblings of an ill child manage well. Chapter 37 describes strategies for working with the siblings of a hospitalized child.

PREPARATION FOR HOSPITALIZATION

Hospitalization may be planned or unexpected. A child may be hospitalized for one of the following reasons:

- The child who has been ill at home gradually or suddenly becomes worse.
- The child needs diagnostic or treatment procedures or requires elective surgery.
- The child who was previously healthy suffers an injury, necessitating unexpected hospitalization.

When hospitalization is planned, both children and their parents have time to prepare for the experience. Assess the family's knowledge and expectations and then provide information about what is likely to happen. A variety of approaches can be used to provide information and allay fears. ⌾ WEB

- Tours of the hospital unit or surgical area are helpful. During tours, allow preschoolers and school-age children to see and touch items with which they will come in contact. The surgical team's attire is less frightening if the child has had a chance to try it on (Figure 34–1 ◆). Medical equipment is not as scary when the child learns what it does and sees how it is used, for example, through demonstration on a doll (Figure 34–2 ◆).
- If a tour is not possible, photographs or a videotape can show the medical setting and procedures.
- Many hospitals offer health fairs to explain health procedures to children. During a tour, while hospitalized, or at home, the child can be exposed to books or films that explain in age-appropriate terms what to expect during various procedures (Table 34–2). Use coloring books and other concrete methods for teaching, as they can help children to cope emotionally with hospitalization (LaMontagne, 2000).

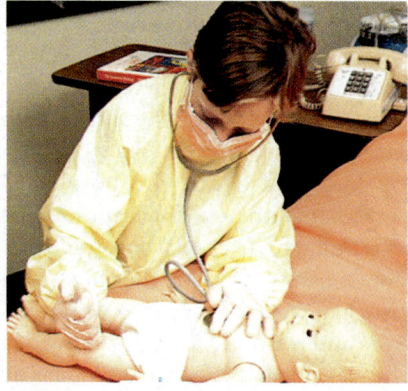

FIGURE 34–1. ◆ Allowing the child to dress up as a doctor or a nurse helps prepare the child for hospitalization. This helps the child adjust to treatment care, and the recovery process. Why? What might the child's concerns be? Can you think of any concerns that could be related to cultural background?

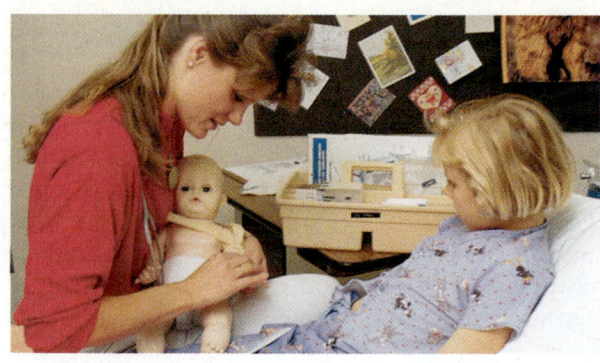

FIGURE 34–2. ◆ The child's anxiety and fear often will be reduced if the nurse explains what is going to happen and demonstrates how the procedure will be done by using a doll. Based on your experience, can you list five things you can do to prepare a school-age child for hospitalization?

TABLE 34–2 Sample Teaching Materials for Children Regarding Hospitalization and Health Care

Videotapes

Clean Intermittent Catheterization	Learner Managed Designs, Inc.
I Have Epilepsy Too.	Epilepsy Foundation
What Do I Tell My Children? How to Help a Child Cope with the Death of a Loved One.	Life Cycle Productions

Books

Barney Is Best. Carlstrom, N. W.	HarperCollins
Barney and Baby Bop Go to the Doctor. Larsen, M.	Lyrick Publishers
The Berenstain Bears Go to the Doctor. Berenstain, S., & Berenstain, B.	Random House
Chris Gets Ear Tubes. Pace, B., & Hutton, K.	Kendall Green Publishers
Curious George Goes to the Hospital. Rey, M., & Rey, H.A.	Houghton Mifflin Company
Cut. McCormick, P., & McCormick, P. (Mental health hospitalization of a teen)	Front Street Publishers
David's Story: A Book about Surgery. Brink, B.	Lerner Publications
Doctors and Nurses: What Do They Do? Green, C.	HarperCollins
The Fall of Freddie the Leaf. Buscaglia, L.	Henry Holt & Co.
Going to the Hospital. Rogers, F., & Judkis, J.	Penguin Putnam Books
The Hospital Book. Howe, J.	Crown Publishers
Let's Talk about Going to the Hospital. Johnston, M.	Rosen Publisher
A Night Without Stars. Howe, J.	Avon
No Measles, No Mumps for Me. Showers, P.	Thomas Y. Crowell
Corduroy Goes to the Doctor. Freeman, D., & McCue, L.	A Golden Book
Rita Goes to the Hospital. Davison, M.	Random Books
Tubes in My Ears: My Trip to the Hospital. Dooley, V., & Katon, M.	Mondo Publishers
A Visit to the Sesame Street Hospital. Hautzig, D.	Random Books
When Molly Was in the Hospital: A Book for Brothers and Sisters of Hospitalized Children. Duncan, D.	Rayve Productions
Why Am I Going to the Hospital? Cilliota, C., & Livingston, C.	Lyle Stuart

TABLE 34-3   Parental Preparation of Children for Hospitalization

- Read stories to the child about the experience.
- Talk about going to the hospital, what it will be like. Talk about coming home.
- Encourage the child to ask questions.
- Encourage the child to draw pictures of what the hospital will be like.
- Visit the hospital unit if possible.
- Let the child touch or see equipment if possible.
- Plan for support via parents' presence, telephone calls, special items of the parents that child can keep during the stay.
- Be honest.

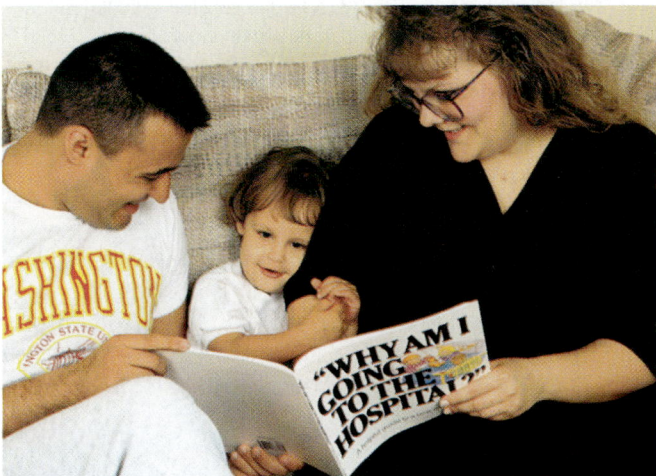

FIGURE 34-3. ◆ Jasmine's parents are taking the time to prepare her for hospitalization by reading a book recommended by the nurse. Such material should be appropriate to the child's age and culture. Why do you think that having the parents read this material to the child is valuable?

Parents can be instrumental in preparing a child for hospitalization by reviewing material presented, being available to answer questions, and by being truthful and supportive (Table 34–3, Figure 34–3 ◆).

Different approaches are useful when adolescents are being prepared for hospitalization. They learn not only from written materials, models, and videotapes, but also from talking with peers who have had similar experiences. Provide a forum for asking questions without parents present.

ADAPTATION TO HOSPITALIZATION

Special Units and Types of Care

Children who are admitted to a hospital may be cared for in one or more of the following units: emergency department, intensive care unit, or short-stay unit. They may require surgical treatment involving preoperative and postoperative care. Children with infectious diseases may require isolation precautions. Other children may need rehabilitative care to achieve or restore maximum potential.

EMERGENCY CARE

When a child is brought to an emergency department, the parents are usually frightened and insecure and may even be in a state of shock. They may demonstrate panic behaviors and need clear directions and frequent repetitions of material (Huckabay & Tilem-Kessler, 1999). The fast pace and critical nature of the unit create an atmosphere in which parents are hesitant to ask questions and are anxious about the outcome. Keep both the child and the family informed about what is being done and when more news may be available. The parents and child should remain together as much as possible. Help parents identify support systems that can help them during this stressful time. It is recommended that parents who wish to remain with a child during even invasive procedures or resuscitation efforts should be allowed to do so. However, further research needs to be performed to study the impact of such presence on family, patients, and health care personnel (Emergency Nurses Association, 1998). Nurses need to ask family members about whether they want to be present in critical situations, and keep them informed about the health care provided.

INTENSIVE CARE

Parents of a child in an intensive care unit are also likely to be anxious, particularly since the child's illness may be severe and the prognosis may be guarded. The unfamiliar equipment may create an atmosphere of fear. Numerous health care professionals come and go, and parents may not know whom to turn to or even what questions to ask. Provide emotional support, explain the purpose of treatments and machines, help parents to hold or touch their child, and provide support and referral to other services if appropriate. (See Chapter 37, and Table 37–1, for a discussion of stressors in parents and children in an intensive care unit and the nursing strategies intended to address these stressors.)

PREOPERATIVE AND POSTOPERATIVE AREAS

Many hospitals now allow parents to be with their child right up until surgery begins and again in the postanesthesia recovery area. Parents often want to support their child before and immediately after a surgical procedure, and their presence may offer reassurance and comfort to the child.

Prepare family members for what will happen and what is expected of them. In some hospitals, only one or two close family members are allowed to see the child. They may need to wear special gowns, shoes, or hats, and they may be restricted to certain areas. Explain special equipment such as intravenous setups and monitoring devices.

SHORT-STAY UNITS

Hospitalizations have generally become short, with minor surgery, diagnostic tests such as radiology studies or cardiac catheterizations, and treatments such as chemotherapy performed in 1 day. The child may be admitted in the morning and go home in the afternoon. In addition, children who have potentially serious illnesses may be placed

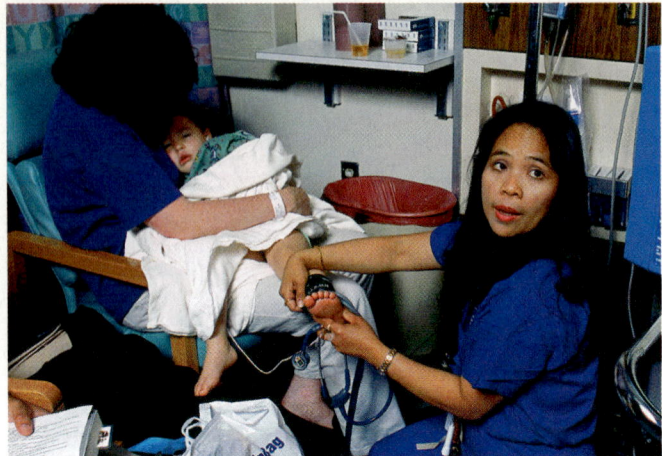

FIGURE 34–4. ◆ The nurse is monitoring a young child who is in a short-stay unit for treatment of dehydration and fever. What support does the mother need?

Thinking Critically

PREPARING CHILDREN FOR HOSPITALIZATION OR SHORT-STAY SURGERY

Six-year-old Kate has had several nosebleeds and fainting spells recently. After examination by her physician and a number of diagnostic studies such as chest x-ray examination, echocardiography, and electrocardiography, coarctation of the aorta is diagnosed. Kate will come in this week for a cardiac catheterization. In 2 weeks, she is scheduled to have open heart surgery.

Kate has had few health problems, and her experiences with health care professionals are limited. Her parents, who are anxious about the heart surgery, are concerned about how their daughter will adapt to hospitalization.

How should you prepare Kate for the cardiac catheterization and for the surgery? How far in advance should teaching take place? What teaching aids are helpful? How can Kate's parents be involved in and reinforce the teaching? What kind of support do her parents, siblings, and friends need during hospitalization? See Table 34–4 for nursing considerations in preparing children for short hospitalizations. ⊂⊃ WEB

on a short-stay or 23-hour unit for monitoring or limited treatment, after which a decision is made to either hospitalize the child for additional treatment or send the child home if improvement occurs (Figure 34–4 ◆). Insurance will often pay for something less than 24 hours so 23-hour or 23–59 (just less than 24) are names of these monitoring units. These short stays are beneficial because they cause minimal disruption of family patterns and are cost effective. Nurses can help parents prepare the child properly for planned admissions, monitor the child during the procedures, encourage family participation in care, and keep families well informed (Table 34–4).

ISOLATION

Children who are placed in isolation may suffer lack of stimulation due to limited contact with other children. Frequent family visits are important and should be encouraged. Family members may be reluctant to wear protective garments either out of fear of using them incorrectly or a belief that they are unnecessary. Be sure the

family understands the reason for isolation and any special procedures. Having contact with and holding the child should be encouraged whenever possible. (Standard precautions are described in the Clinical Skills Manual, as well as the CD-ROM accompanying this text.) ⊂⊃ CD SKILLS

REHABILITATION

Rehabilitation units provide children with ongoing care and support to continue recovery beyond the initial period of illness or injury. These may be separate units within a hospital or independent centers. The objective of **rehabilitation** is to help the child with physical or mental challenges reach his or her fullest potential and to promote achievement of developmentally appropriate skills (Figure 34–5 ◆). Parental involvement is essential.

TABLE 34–4 Nursing Considerations in Preparing Parents and Child for Planned Short-Stay Admission

- Are there special requirements, such as not being permitted food or drink or needing extra fluid intake?
- What time and where must the child appear?
- Are any special forms, insurance numbers, or previous records needed?
- How long will the child stay in the hospital?
- Are parents expected or encouraged to be with the child or stay in the health facility?
- Is there a chance the child may need to remain longer than expected?
- What will the child's condition be for transfer home?
- Will special equipment or care be needed?
- What symptoms can indicate problems?
- Where can the family go or whom can they call in case of problems or questions?

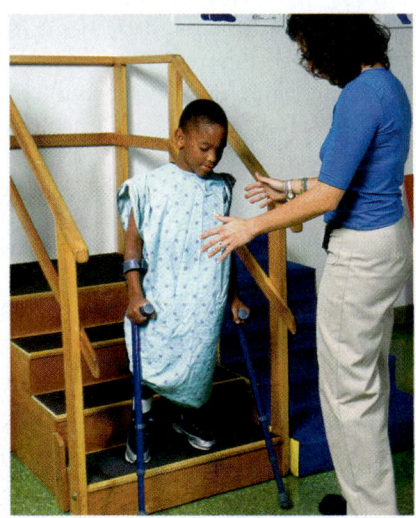

FIGURE 34–5. ◆ Rehabilitation units provide an opportunity for the child to relearn tasks like walking and climbing stairs. They provide an important transition from hospital to home community.

Family Assessment

To develop a plan of care that involves all family members, assess the impact of the child's illness or hospitalization on the family (Table 34–5). Teaching the child and family, providing support, and referring them to community resources are key elements of the plan.

Assess the family's resources frequently. These resources include the coping strategies of family members, financial resources, access to health care, and availability of community services. One family may manage quite well with limited financial support because they have good coping strategies, whereas another family with greater financial resources may have difficulty caring for an ill child. Staying with a hospitalized child can be a financial drain for parents if they must miss work, and perhaps travel to another location and stay away from home.

It is important to assess the family dynamics. Evaluate the quality of communication, methods of handling problems, and sources of strength. Examine how the family has been dealing with the health needs of their child if the child has been hospitalized or required home care in the past. Ask about the roles they want to play in the child's treatment and the roles they would like the nurse to fulfill. Assess cultural beliefs and values. Referrals to family service agencies or other community organizations may be needed. Support groups in the community or agencies that provide medical equipment can also be helpful.

TABLE 34–5   Family Assessment

Family Roles
- What changes will the child's illness create in the family?
- Will household tasks need to be reallocated?
- Will a burden be placed on certain family members?
- Will one parent room in or spend a great deal of time in the hospital?

Knowledge
- What knowledge does the family have about the child's condition and treatment? Do they need further information?
- Is there a need to start discharge planning and teaching early?

Support Systems
- Does the family have medical insurance? What percentage of costs will it cover? Will other financial support be needed?
- Are close friends or family available to provide child care for other children, assist with family tasks, or help in other ways?
- Are there community services such as support groups, camps for children with disabilities, education sessions, or equipment and financial resources to which the nurse can refer the family?

Siblings
- Have they been informed of the ill child's condition and the expected outcome?
- Have they been reassured that they did not cause the illness?
- Do they understand the change in roles and family routines?
- Are they able to visit the ill child?
- Have their teachers been informed of the family stress?
- If the hospitalized child's life is threatened, are the siblings involved in a therapy plan to assist them in dealing with that stress?

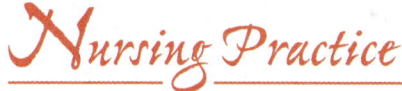 **Developing Cultural Competence**

Many ethnic groups such as Chinese Americans and Mexican Americans use a combination of Western medicine and traditional therapies like home treatments or a traditional healer (curandismo for Mexican Americans). This information may not be shared with nurses or physicians, both out of respect and in fear that they will be told not to use these methods. Recognizing and supporting use of both Western and traditional practices can promote health and provide comfort for children and families.

Child and Family Teaching

Teaching is an essential part of the nurse's role in care of hospitalized children and their parents. Teaching may be informal, as when the nurse provides an explanation during routine care, or structured, as when the nurse plans and implements a formal teaching program. Be sure that explanations or reading materials are at a level the parent can understand. If translators are needed to facilitate understanding, be sure they are available for teaching sessions. Teaching about the behaviors seen in hospitalized children and strategies to deal with these behaviors are helpful for parents. For instance, research has shown that providing information for parents of hospitalized toddlers on the typical behaviors of hospitalized children and on the strategies to assist children leads to less anxiety on the part of the parents and to greater parental involvement and support of the child during the hospitalization (Melnyk, 1995). How can nurses plan to provide such information for parents?

 Nursing Practice

The *American Nurses Association's 1996 Statement on the Scope and Standards of Pediatric Clinical Nursing Practice* mandates teaching as a component of pediatric nursing care.

  Nursing Practice

When children are hospitalized for illness or injury, they are in a vulnerable position. Whereas adults are able to refuse or question treatment, children are often not given those rights. This may be in conflict with the United Nations Convention on the Rights of the Child, which gives children the right to be heard in all matters affecting them. Nurses can carefully examine each situation, being careful not to take for granted that hospitalized children will be unhappy and in pain. We can seek to allow them to speak their wishes and to provide strategies that will best help them during health care (Bricher, 2000).

Teaching directed at children must take into account their developmental level and cognitive abilities. Learning is easier when teaching involves more than one sense (such as hearing, vision, and touch). Teaching directed at parents must be geared to their level of understanding. If English is the parents' second language, a translator may be necessary.

Growth and Development

For children who can hear, touch, see a model or equipment, read, look at pictures, or even smell things like alcohol swabs, learning is more complete. This is particularly important for the school-age child in the stage of concrete operational thought, who must be able to manipulate materials in order to learn.

Timing is a critical factor in teaching. Parents and children are less receptive to teaching when they are preoccupied with other thoughts or activities. Scheduling specific times for teaching sessions may be helpful.

Depending on the information to be presented, teaching may use the cognitive, psychomotor, or affective domains of learning. Teaching that includes all three domains is more effective.

TEACHING PLANS

A teaching plan is a written plan that includes goals and expected outcomes, interventions needed to achieve the specified goals, and a method and time for evaluation of the expected outcomes. The teaching plan may also specify teaching methods and types of materials to be used. Developing a teaching plan helps ensure that all the necessary information is included and makes teaching more efficient.

The child's primary caretaker should participate in the teaching. The primary caretaker is most often a parent but may be a close family member (uncle, aunt, grandparent). The first step in establishing a teaching plan is to assess the child's or parent's knowledge, skills, and feelings by finding the answers to the following questions:

- What does the parent or child know about the health issue?
- What is the cognitive level or ability to learn?
- Is there a desire to learn?
- What previous experiences affect the learning experience, either positively or negatively?
- What resources are available to the parents, child, and nurse to enhance understanding of the health condition?

Teaching About

CARE DURING A SEIZURE

Seizures are characterized as periods of involuntary muscle contractions and relaxations that the child has no control over. Seizures may be caused by high fever, head trauma, birth defects, and other neurologic problems. It is very hard to predict when a seizure is going to occur. Some safety measures can help to prevent injuries to your child during a seizure.

What to do during a seizure

Seizure activity often means that the child is at risk for injury. Here are some safety guidelines to remember when your child has a seizure.

- Remain calm and stay with your child.
- Protect your child from any injury.

  Place your child on the floor when the seizure occurs.

  Remove any dangerous objects from your child's reach, such as furniture, glass, or objects that can fall on the floor. Do not restrain or hold down your child during a seizure.

  If the floor is hard (tile, cement uncarpeted), place a small pillow, sweater, or your hand under your child's head.

  Loosen your child's clothing if it is too tight.

  Turn your child's head to one side to prevent choking. Do not put anything into your child's mouth during a seizure.

- Provide time for your child to recover after the seizure stops. Reassure your child that he or she is okay. Speak softly. Explain what happened. Do not give food or drink until your child has fully recovered from the seizure.

When to call for emergency help

- If your child's seizure continues for more than 5 minutes
- If your child has trouble breathing or does not breath after the seizure
- If your child has one seizure after the other without waking up between each

Everyday safety guidelines

- Have your child wear a safety helmet while riding a bike or skating to reduce the chances of a head injury.
- Keep bathroom and bedroom doors unlocked. It will be easier for you or other family members to get into a room to help.
- If the child prefers a bath rather than a shower, use just a few inches of water in the cub. Supervise the young child during the bath. Be sure someone is at home when a teenager is bathing.
- Your child should always swim with a buddy. If a seizure occurs, it is easier to rescue a child in a pool than a child in a pond or lake.
- Teach your child to hold onto the handrails when using stairs.
- Move glass, furniture, and extra pillows away from the child's bed to reduce the chance of injury during a seizure. Think about placing your child's mattress on the floor. This would keep the child from falling out of bed during a seizure.
- Give antiseizure medicines as prescribed to decrease the number of times your child has a seizure.
- Have your child wear a medical identification bracelet at all times.
- Inform relatives, baby-sitters, and teachers that your child has seizures. Tell them about any special care to be given during a seizure.

Note: From Ball, J. (1998). *Pediatric patient teaching guides* (pp. 1–4). Mosby-YearBook.

- Are there feelings or beliefs that might interfere with the learning process?

The second step involves deciding what knowledge, skill, or change in attitude is desired. Outcome criteria or objectives are established for the parent and child.

- A learning objective for a parent might be: The parent states the importance of checking the child's toes in the casted leg twice daily for temperature, movement, sensations, color, and edema (cognitive domain).
- An objective for a child might be: The child self-catheterizes using correct technique and records the amount of urine in a log (psychomotor domain).
- An objective for an adolescent might be: The adolescent explores methods of managing feelings of loss of control related to diabetes management (affective domain).

Explore possible teaching methods and approaches. A variety of sources, including written materials (books, pamphlets, handouts, and stories), computer software, audiovisual presentations, and others, are available (see Table 34–2). In some settings, audiovisual and computer resources may be limited. Small-group teaching sessions (e.g., for children with recently diagnosed diabetes or cystic fibrosis) may be another option. Gathering two or three parents or children together on a unit to learn and share experiences may be helpful.

For some conditions, standardized teaching plans are available in books and from health care agencies (see page 822 for one example). These plans can serve as a guide in developing an individualized teaching plan.

CHILDREN WITH SPECIAL NEEDS

Children with disabilities may have special learning needs. If they have visual impairment or visual perceptual difficulty, material must be presented in auditory and tactile ways. Children with hearing deficits need visual and tactile presentations. Children with learning disabilities may need more frequent reinforcement and shorter teaching sessions. Evaluate them for comprehension often and adjust teaching as necessary. When psychomotor skill performance is needed, special aids may be necessary so the child can hold a syringe, draw up a liquid, or perform other tasks. Adequate assessment of the child's strengths and disabilities, along with consultation with parents and the child's teachers, can help the nurse plan teaching methods.

Children who have chronic illnesses may have been hospitalized numerous times and have received other health care at home and in the community. They usually have adapted coping mechanisms that help them deal with the chronic illness. Talk to them to see what has helped in the past, provide information about what to expect during this hospitalization, assign staff members familiar to the child when possible, and follow the child's lead in helping them cope (Boyd & Hunsberger, 1998).

Strategies to Promote Coping and Normal Development

During hospitalization, care of the child focuses not only on meeting physiologic needs, but also on meeting psychosocial and developmental needs. Several strategies may help children adapt to the hospital environment, promote effective coping, and provide developmentally appropriate activities. These strategies include child life programs, rooming in, therapeutic play, and therapeutic recreation.

CHILD LIFE PROGRAMS

Many hospitals have child life programs that focus on the psychosocial needs of hospitalized children. Professional child life specialists, paraprofessionals, and volunteers staff these departments. Due to changes in the health care system, more children today are receiving care in outpatient centers, day surgery units, and other community agencies. Pediatric inpatient units are consequently small, and play therapy programs are sometimes curtailed. Nurses need to plan to provide play, whatever the size or services of the unit (DePasquale, 1999). A **child life specialist** plans activities to provide age-appropriate playtime for children either in the child's room or in a playroom. Some activities are designed to assist children in working through feelings about illness. Examples include playing with medical equipment or drawing pictures about hospital treatments. A trusted child life specialist may stay with a child during a particularly frightening procedure such as a venipuncture or bone marrow aspiration. **WEB**

Both the child life department and the nursing staff focus on the emotional needs of hospitalized children. Child life specialists and nurses may formulate a plan together to assist children with particular needs.

ROOMING IN

Rooming in is the practice of having a parent stay in the child's hospital room and care for the hospitalized child. Some hospitals provide cots, others have special built-in beds on pediatric wards, and in some institutions a parent stays in a separate room on the unit. A parent who is rooming in may want to perform all of the child's basic care or help with some of the medical care. Communication between nurse and parent is important so that the parent's desire for involvement is supported.

THERAPEUTIC PLAY

Play is an important part of childhood. The stress of illness and hospitalization increases the value of play. Not only does play facilitate normal development, but play sessions can help the child learn about health care, express anxieties, work through feelings, and achieve a sense of mastery or control over frightening or little-understood situations. In the present era of cost containment, play programs may be minimized in hospitals, so nurses should document the need for and benefits of play. Play that presents an opportunity to deal with the fears and concerns of health experiences is called **therapeutic play.**

Through therapeutic play the child's knowledge of and adaptation to his or her illness or injury can be assessed. Common techniques involve using an outline drawing of the body or stories and asking the child to draw in or talk about what the illness or injury means to him or her (Ramsey, 2000). Alternatively, the child may be asked to draw a picture or make up a story, enabling the nurse to assess fears and other emotions. The Goodenough Draw-A-Person test helps to assess the cognitive level of children between 3 and 13 years of age (Table 34–6). The Gellert Index is another tool that helps to assess the child's knowledge of the body (Table 34–7). In addition to assessment, drawing can be used as a nursing intervention. Show the child on a drawing what will happen during surgery or a treatment. The child's drawings of health care experiences allow him or her to express fears and gain mastery over the situation.

A variety of techniques may be used to promote therapeutic play (Figure 34–6 ◆) (Table 34–8). Specific techniques are chosen to reflect the child's developmental stage.

Toddler. Play is important for toddlers. Through play they explore the environment and learn to identify with significant people in their lives. Play is also an acceptable way for toddlers to release tensions caused by stress or aggressive impulses.

Toddlers should be approached slowly, and the initial approach should be made in their parents' presence, if possible, to decrease feelings of stranger anxiety (wariness of strangers). Playing a variation of peek-a-boo or hide-and-seek using the curtain surrounding the toddler's crib or bed helps promote the realization that objects out of sight, such as parents, do return. Transitional objects, such as a familiar blanket or stuffed animal, can temporarily substitute for the security of parents. The toddler who is re-

---

TABLE 34–6 Goodenough Draw-A-Person Test

- The child is asked to draw a picture of a person and to do so carefully and completely, taking his or her time. It is preferable to have the child take the test alone, away from parents.
- Points are assigned for specific details included in the drawing, for example, 1 point each for the presence of head, legs, arms, trunk, and eyes. Additional points are assigned depending on the complexity of details.
- For every 4 points assigned, another year is added to a baseline age of 3 years. For example, a child who scores 24 points (by including 24 details) would have a total score of 9 years (6 plus 3 baseline years). This number is compared to the child's chronologic age to determine his or her cognitive level.

The Goodenough Test may be obtained from the Psychological Corporation, 555 Academic Court, San Antonio, TX 78204; 1-800-872-1726; www.psychcorp.com

---

TABLE 34–7 Gellert Index of Body Knowledge

Part A

What do you have inside you? Tell me as many things as you can think of that are inside you.

Part B

1. Show me the head. What is in the head? (Tell me all the things that are in the head.)
2. Make a circle showing where and about how big the heart is. What does the heart do? (What is it for?) What would happen if we didn't have a heart?
3. Show me some places where you have bones. (Try for a minimum of five locations.) What do we have bones for? What would happen if we didn't have bones?
4. Make a circle showing where and about how big the stomach is. What does the stomach do? Show me where the food goes after you swallow it. (Sketch in diagram.) And then? (If excretion is not mentioned spontaneously, ask: Does it ever come out anywhere? If the answer is affirmative, ask: Show me where it comes out.)
5. Make a circle showing about where and about how big the ribs are. Why do we have ribs? (What for?) What would happen if we didn't have ribs?
6. Make a circle showing about where and about how big the liver is. What does the liver do? What would happen if we didn't have a liver?
7. What do you think we have a skin for? What would happen if we didn't have a skin?
8. Make a circle showing where and about how big the lungs are. How many lungs are there? What do we have lungs for? What would happen if we didn't have lungs?
9. Do you have any nerves? (If no, ask: Does anybody else? If so, who?) What would happen if we didn't have any nerves?
10. Make a circle showing where and about how big the bladder is. What do we have a bladder for? What would happen if we didn't have a bladder?
11. How come we have bowel movements? (What for?) Where do bowel movements come from? (Probe for derivation from food, stomach, intestines.) Show me on the diagram. What would happen if we didn't have bowel movements? About how often (how many times) should people have bowel movements? About how often do you have bowel movements?

Part C

1. What do you think is the most important part of you? (If you picked one part of you as the most important, which one would you pick?)
2. Are there any parts of you that you could live (get along) without? Which ones?

Note: From Gellert, E. (1962). Children's conceptions of the content and functions of the human body. *Genetic Psychology Monographs, 65,* 293–405. Reprinted with permission of the Helen Dwight Reid Education Foundation. Published by Heldref Publications, 1319 18th St. NW, Washington, DC 20036–1802.

---

strained can be read familiar stories. Repetition of stories promotes a sense of stability in the unfamiliar hospital environment.

A doll is a familiar toy that can be used to re-create a stressful environment, thereby providing an opportunity for the child to express and work through feelings. Other

TABLE 34-8   Therapeutic Play Techniques

Technique	Assessment	Intervention
Stories	Have the child make up a story about a picture. Analyze content and emotional clues in the story. Have children tell a story about an important experience in a group of other children.	Read or make up stories to explain illness, hospitalization, or other specific aspects of health care. Emotions such as fear can be included.
Drawings	Administer Goodenough Draw-A-Person test (see Table 34–6) to evaluate cognitive level. Consider subject matter, size and placement of items in drawings, colors used, presence or absence of physical barriers, and general emotional feeling. Administer Gellert Index (Table 34–7) to learn about the child's knowledge of the body and its functioning before planning teaching.	Use the child's drawings or outlines of the body to explain care, procedures, or conditions. Provide an opportunity for the child to draw pictures of his or her choice or directed topics such as a picture of the child's family or health care encounter. Ask the child: "Tell me about your picture." Be alert to the child's emotions: "This child must be frightened by the big x-ray machine."
Music	Observe types of music chosen and effects of played music on behavior.	Encourage parents and children to bring favorite tapes to the hospital for stress relief. Have tapes playing during tests and procedures. Parents can tape their voices to play for infants and young children during separations. During longer hospitalizations, children can tape messages for siblings or classmates, who are then encouraged to retape their responses. Playtime can include the opportunity to play instruments and sing.
Puppets	The puppets can ask questions of young children, who are often more likely to answer the puppet than a person.	Perform short skits to teach children necessary health care information. Include emotional content when appropriate.
Dramatic play	Provide dolls and medical equipment, and analyze the roles assigned to dolls by the child, the behavior demonstrated by the dolls in the child's play, and the apparent emotions. Dolls with handicaps like those of the child are especially helpful (see Fig. 34–9B).	Provide dolls and equipment for play sessions. To ensure safety, supervise closely when actual equipment is used. Respond to emotions and behavior shown. Use dolls and equipment such as casts, nebulizer, intravenous apparatus and stethoscope to explain care. Use dolls with problems or handicaps similar to those of the child, when available. Provide toys that foster expression of emotion, such as a pounding board and indoor darts.
Pets	Provide pet therapy. Watch the interaction between child and animal.	Respond to emotions the child shows. Facilitate touch and contact with animals.

Additional techniques, such as sand or water play, may be appropriate in specific situations.

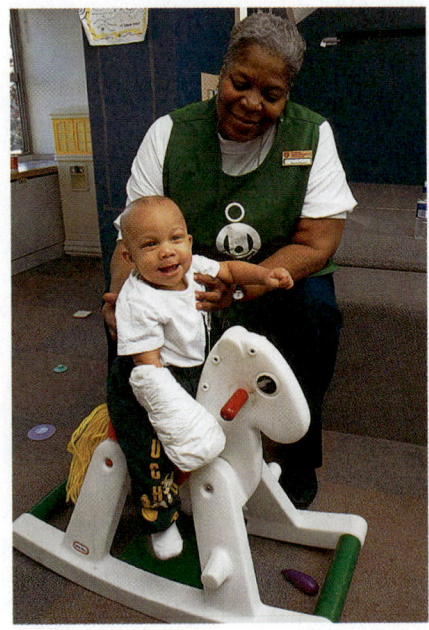 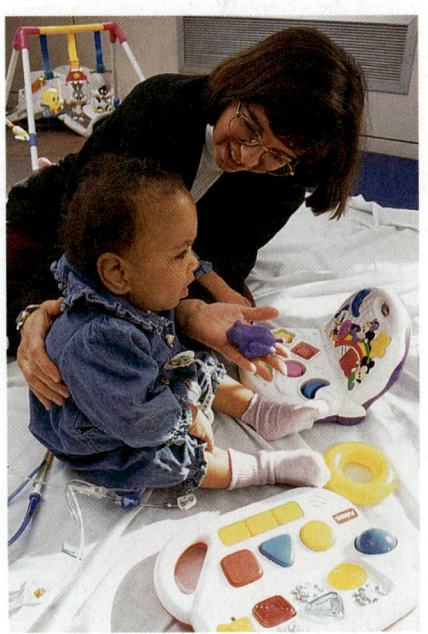

FIGURE 34–6. ◆ **A,** Volunteers such as this foster grandmother can provide stimulation and nurturing to help young children adapt to lengthy hospitalizations. **B,** Child life specialists plan activities for young children in the hospital to facilitate play and stress reduction.

A

B

developmentally appropriate toys for toddlers include familiar objects from home such as measuring cups or spoons, wooden puzzles, building blocks, and push-and-pull toys. Playing with safe hospital equipment (bandages, syringes without needles, and stethoscopes) helps toddlers overcome the anxiety associated with these items. Supervise these play sessions and remove hospital equipment when you leave.

Preschooler. The nurse can intervene to reduce the stress produced by preschoolers' fears through the use of some kinds of play. A simple outline of the body or a doll can be used to address the child's fantasies and fears of bodily harm (Figure 34–7 ◆). Playing with safe hospital equipment may help preschoolers to work through feelings such as aggression (Figure 34–8 ◆).

Preschoolers like crayons and coloring books, puppets, dolls, felt and magnetic boards, play dough, books, and recorded stories (Figure 34–9 ◆). Preschoolers and older children often enjoy pet therapy. Children's hospitals and units can have visits from pets, most commonly dogs, that provide diversion and physical contact (Figure 34–10 ◆). Both preschool and school-age children may enjoy playing with a toy hospital.

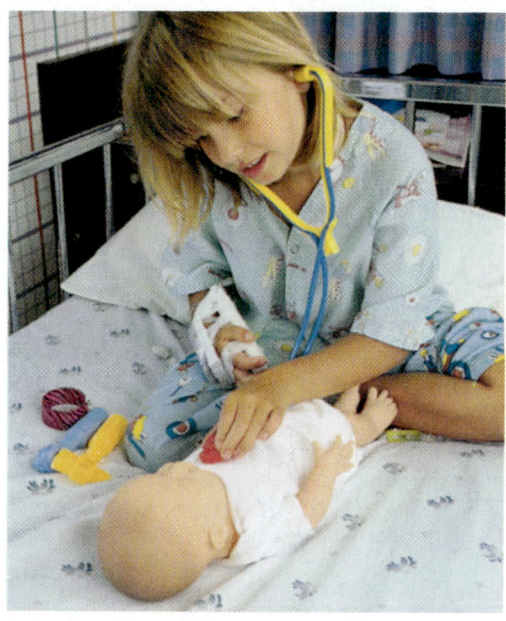
A

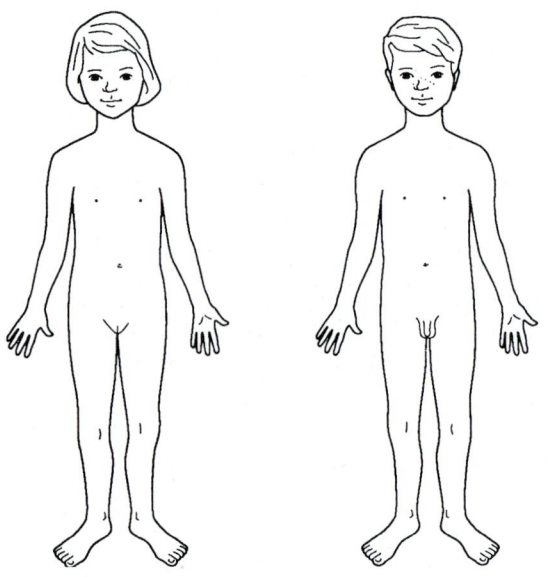

FIGURE 34–7. ◆ The nurse can use a simple gender-specific outline drawing of a child's body to encourage children to draw what they think about their medical problem. Such drawings reveal a child's interpretation, which the nurse can work with to provide appropriate care.

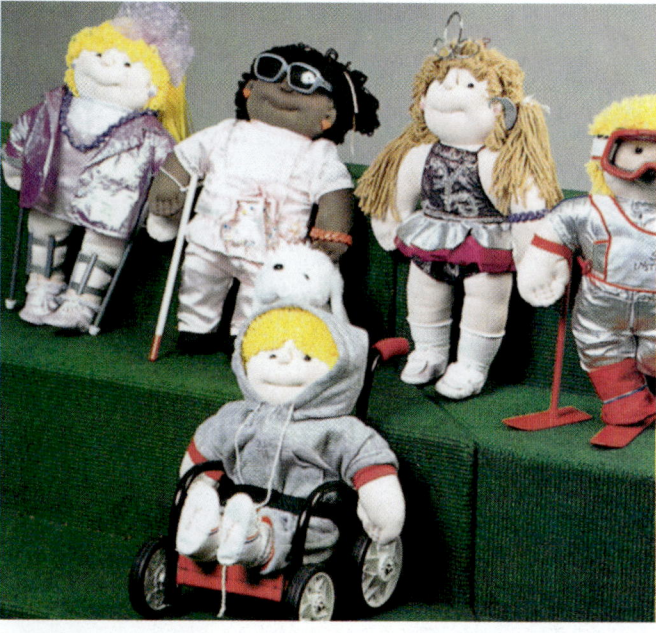
B

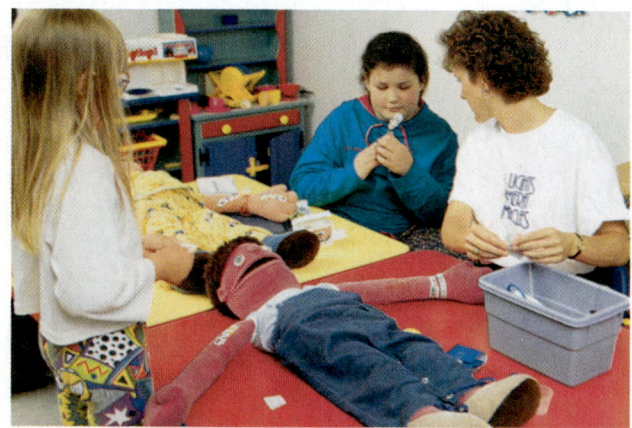

FIGURE 34–8. ◆ A child life specialist works with children being treated for cancer. Special dolls are used to familiarize children with the procedures that they will undergo.

FIGURE 34–9. ◆ **A,** Age-appropriate play will help the child adjust to hospitalization and care. **B,** Having the child play with dolls that have "disabilities" similar to his or her own will help the child adjust. Such play helps the child realize what activities are possible.

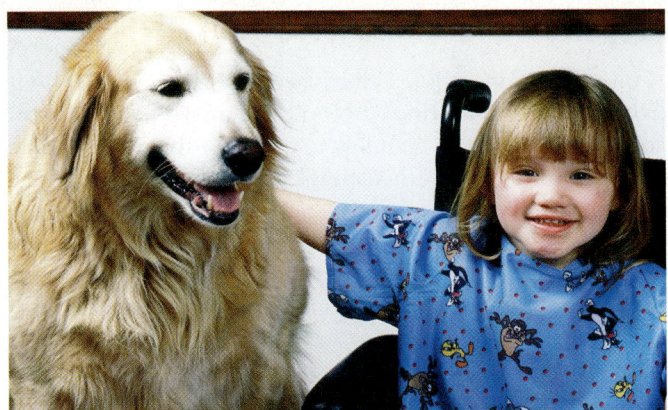

FIGURE 34-10. ◆ Hospitals may have pet therapy from specially trained animals to provide comfort and distraction during health care. Both the child and the dog seem to be smiling.

School-Age Child. Although play begins to lose its importance in the school-age years, the nurse can still use some techniques of therapeutic play to help the hospitalized child deal with stress. School-age children often regress developmentally during hospitalization, demonstrating behaviors characteristic of an earlier state, such as separation anxiety and fear of bodily injury. Outlines of the body and, occasionally, dolls can be used to illustrate the cause and treatment of the child's illness. Use terms for body parts that are suitable for older children. Drawings provide an outlet for expression of fears and anger.

School-age children enjoy collecting and organizing objects and often ask to keep disposable equipment that has been used in their care. They may use these items later to relive the experience with their friends. Games, books, schoolwork, crafts, tape recordings, and computers provide an outlet for aggression and increase self-esteem in the school-age child. The type of play used should promote a sense of mastery and achievement.

Nursing Practice

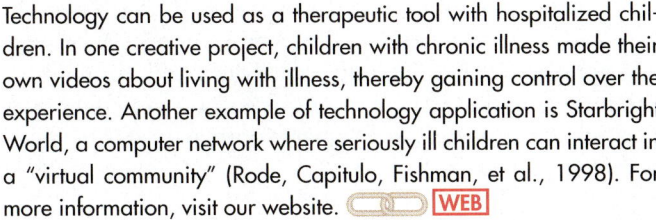

Technology can be used as a therapeutic tool with hospitalized children. In one creative project, children with chronic illness made their own videos about living with illness, thereby gaining control over the experience. Another example of technology application is Starbright World, a computer network where seriously ill children can interact in a "virtual community" (Rode, Capitulo, Fishman, et al., 1998). For more information, visit our website. 🔗 **WEB**

THERAPEUTIC RECREATION

Many of the special play techniques used with younger children are not suitable for adolescents. However, adolescents do need a planned recreation program to help them meet developmental needs during hospitalization. Peers

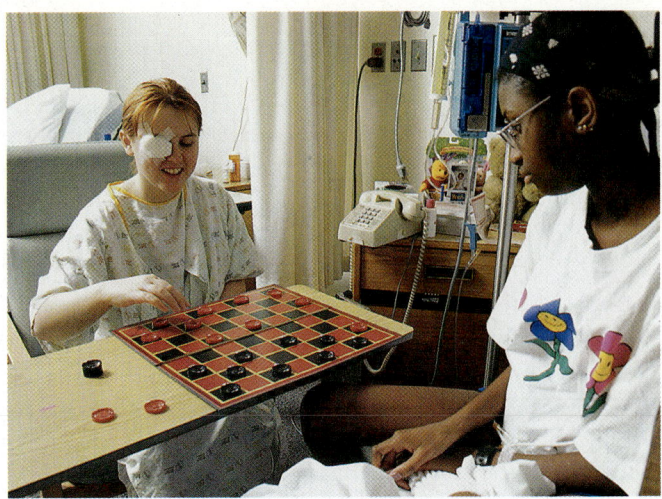

FIGURE 34-11. ◆ Having interaction with other hospitalized adolescents and maintaining contact with friends outside the hospital are very important so that the teenager does not feel isolated and alone. A friendly yet competitive checkers game helps to stimulate these teenagers and allows for self-expression. What are the other benefits?

are important, and the isolation of hospitalization can be difficult. Telephone contact with other teenagers and visits from friends should be encouraged. Interactions with other teenagers at a pizza party, video game, or movie night or during other activities can help adolescents feel normal (Figure 34–11 ◆). Physical activities that provide an outlet for stress are recommended. Even adolescents on bed rest or in wheelchairs can play a modified form of basketball.

The independence of adolescence is interrupted by illness. Give teenagers choices to assist them in regaining control. Giving them options and letting them choose an evening recreational activity can promote their feelings of independence. Passes to leave the hospital for special activities may be possible.

Strategies to Meet Educational Needs

Some hospitalizations are so short that the absence of the child or adolescent from school and peers is of minimal concern. However, if hospitalization is expected to last longer than a few days or if the child's condition will change so that he or she needs special school arrangements, the nurse should assess the effects of hospitalization on the child's education.

When an elective procedure occurs, encourage families to arrange the extended school absence with teachers. The child can then be provided with schoolwork to do in the hospital or at home when well enough. This minimizes educational deficits and future problems for the child. Pencils, paper, comfortable work areas, computers, and quiet work times should be provided. Telephone calls or Internet connections with teachers can be arranged as needed.

The social aspects of school and peers should also be considered. Peers can be encouraged to visit a hospitalized classmate, send cards and letters, call on the phone, or communicate via the Internet. When the child returns to school, the nurse can visit the classroom to inform classmates about the child's medical condition.

The hospital nurse may contact the child's school nurse when special arrangements are necessary. For example, the child who is wearing a large cast or who needs medications or other treatments may offer challenges in a traditional school setting.

The child with chronic health problems or requiring long-term hospitalization has other school-related needs. Hospitals or rehabilitation units may have classrooms, teachers, and facilities to promote learning (Figure 34–12 ◆). Many school districts provide tutors or computer connections for students who are hospitalized or receiving home care for long periods. Teachers can visit children at the hospital or at home. Parents are often pivotal in making arrangements to meet the child's educational needs, since they interact with the child, the school, and the health care team.

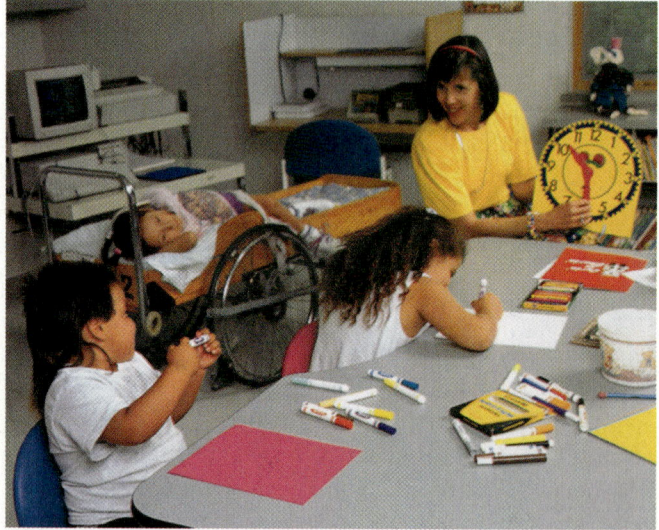

FIGURE 34–12. ◆ Shriners Hospital in Spokane, Washington, has a special classroom and teacher for children undergoing a lengthy hospital stay, enabling them to remain current with their schoolwork. The child who falls behind other students might not fit in when he or she returns to school or might be required to repeat a grade. What are the potential consequences of these situations?

Preparation for Procedures

A number of procedures take place during hospitalization, from collection of urine or blood specimens to spinal taps and surgery. Special techniques can help the child to understand and cope with feelings about these procedures. Never assume that a procedure will not be traumatic for the child. Even providing urine in a specimen cup or undergoing x-ray examination can be frightening if the child does not understand the reason for the procedure or what to expect. Administration of medication can also be frustrating for the child. The nurse should prepare the child for medication administration and adapt techniques from those used with adults so the correct medication is safely given (Table 34–9). See Skills 11–1 through 11–13 in the *Clinical Skills Manual;* Skills 11–1, 11–2, 11–4, and 11–11 can also be found on the CD-ROM that accompanies this text. ⊂⊃ **CD** **SKILLS**

To assess the child's feelings about the procedure, ask the following questions:

- Does the child know the purpose of the procedure?
- Has the child experienced this procedure before? Was the experience painful, frightening, or reassuring?
- What does the child think will happen? Are the child's beliefs accurate?
- Is the procedure painful?
- What techniques does the child use to gain control in challenging situations?
- Will the parents or adult friends be present to provide support?

Preparation may begin a few moments to several days before the procedure, depending on the child's age. Use words that the child understands to describe the procedure and its purpose (see Chapter 32). ⊂⊃ Older children need explanations geared to their cognitive level and previous experiences. They will want to know what is happening, why, and what they can do to cope during the procedure.

Provide written information for adolescents, and schedule time for questions and discussions. Adolescents can make many choices about their own health care. They can be asked such questions as, "Do you want a local or general anesthetic?" or "Do you want your hand numbed for the intravenous start?" Some adolescents want their parents involved in their care, whereas others prefer to minimize the parents' role.

Nursing Practice

When a potentially painful procedure will be occurring, an anesthetic cream or disk, such as EMLA, should be applied from 1 to 2 hours before the planned procedure. This can lessen discomfort and, therefore, fear in the child.

TABLE 34-9 **Variations in Medication Administration to Children**

Route	Developmental Consideration	Techniques
Oral	Children under 5 years cannot generally swallow pills and capsules.	• Medications are usually given in liquid form (elixir, syrup, or suspension). • Sometimes tablets are crushed or capsules are opened and mixed with one spoon of food. Check with pharmacy to be sure this does not inactivate the drug. Never crush enteric-coated or timed-release medicine. • When choosing a vehicle for crushed tablets, use only one spoonful of applesauce, pudding, jelly, or similar food. • Use TB syringe for amounts less than 1 mL to increase accuracy.
	Children may not want to take medicine.	• Position young children upright to avoid choking and aspiration. • Give liquid medicines slowly by oral syringe (for infants) aimed at the inside of the cheek or by medicine cup (for toddler and preschooler) for drinking. • Have the expectation that the medicine will be taken. Let children choose the type of fluid to drink after but do not ask if they will take their medicine now.
Rectal	Colon is small in size.	• For children under 3 years, the nurse's gloved fifth finger is used for insertion. After this age the index finger can usually be used. • Lubricate the tip of the suppository.
Ophthalmic and otic	Young children may be fearful of medicines placed in the eyes or ears.	• Adequate restraint is needed to avoid injury. • The nurse's hand can be stabilized by resting the wrist on the child's head. • Explanations and therapeutic play can be used with children old enough to explain the process of administration. • Have medication at room temperature.
Topical	Skin of infants is thin and fragile.	• Only prescribed doses and medicines appropriate for young children should be used on the skin. • Covering the area or keeping the child's hands occupied may be necessary to ensure adequate contact of medication with the skin.
Intramuscular	Anatomy and physiology of children differs from that of adults.	• Gluteus maximus muscle (dorsal gluteal site) must not be used until the child has been walking for at least 1 year. • Vastus lateralis site is preferred for young children. • Amounts to be administered should be limited to no more than 1 to 2 mL for ventrogluteal site depending on muscle size. • The deltoid muscle is rarely used in young children except for the small amounts injected in some vaccines.
Intravenous	Veins are small and fragile.	• Careful maintenance of sites is needed. • Common infusion sites include hands and feet, although scalp veins are sometimes used in infants.
	Fluid balance is critical.	• Infusion pumps require frequent monitoring. • Syringe pumps are often used when minimal fluid is to be given over an extended period of time. • Central lines are commonly used for long-term intravenous medication therapy.

Developing Cultural Competence

Many American Indian tribes use "smudging," or burning of native plants, as a blessing and purifying of the spirit. This is thought to enhance healing and protect the child. The nurse can provide a safe and facilitative environment for this important ceremony in the hospital.

The procedure should be performed as quickly and efficiently as possible. Parents may wish to be involved or may prefer to be available afterward to comfort the child.

The parents or nurse can be designated to support the child. This may involve gentle touch, talking, singing, reassurance, or a stress-reduction technique.

Procedures on young children are generally performed in a treatment room so the child's own room is viewed as a "safe" and relatively pain-free site. After the procedure the child can be taken back to his or her room for comfort and reassurance. A choice of reward often soothes the young child. An example of a common procedure which children need assistance with during hospitalization is venipuncture (Table 34–10 and Skill 10–4). 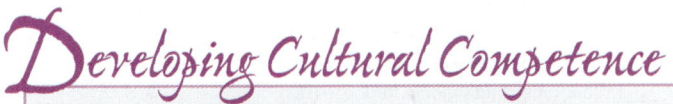 CD SKILLS

TABLE 34–10   Assisting Children Through Procedures

Development Stage	Before Procedure	During Procedure
Infant	None for infant. Explain to parents the procedure, the reason for it, and their role.	Restrain infant securely and gently. Perform procedure quickly. Use touch, voice, pacifier, and bottle as distractions. Have parent hold, rock, and sing to infant after procedure.
Toddler	Give explanation just before procedure, since toddler's concept of time is limited. Explain that child did nothing wrong; the procedure is simply necessary.	Perform in treatment room. Give short explanations and directions in a positive manner. Avoid giving choices when none are available. For example, "We are going to do this now" is better than "Is it okay to do this now?" Allow child to cry or scream. Comfort child after procedure. Give child a choice of favorite drink or special sticker.
Preschool child	Give simple explanations of procedure. Basic drawings may be useful. While providing supervision, allow the child to touch and play with equipment to be used if possible. Since any entry into the body is viewed as a threat, state that the child's body will remain the same, and use adhesive bandages to reassure the child that the body is intact and parts will not "fall out."	Perform in treatment room. Restrain securely. Give short explanations and directions in a positive manner. Encourage control by having the child count to 10 or spell name. Allow child to cry. Give positive feedback for cooperation and getting through procedure. Encourage the child to draw afterward to explore the experience.
School-age child	Clear, thorough explanations are helpful. Use drawings, pictures, books, and contact with equipment. Teach stress reduction techniques such as deep breathing and visualization. Offer a choice of reward after procedure is completed.	Be ready to restrain child if needed. Allow child to remain in position by self if child is able to be still. Explain throughout procedure what is happening. Facilitate use of stress control techniques. Praise cooperative efforts.
Adolescent	Give clear explanations orally and in writing. Teach stress reduction techniques. Explore fear of certain procedures, such as staple removal or venipuncture.	Assist adolescent in self-control. Avoid using restraints. Assist with use of stress control techniques. Explain expected outcome and tell when results of test will be completed.

PREPARATION FOR SURGERY

A child's surgical experience can be elective, planned in advance, or a result of an emergency or trauma. How a child responds to the experience depends on the psychologic and physical preparation he or she receives. See "Nursing Care Plan: The Child Undergoing Surgery" for a summary of the key elements of preoperative and postoperative care.

PREOPERATIVE CARE

Preoperative care of the child includes both psychosocial and physical preparation for surgery.

Psychosocial Preparation.   The goal of preoperative teaching is to reduce the fear associated with the unknown and decrease stress and anxiety associated with surgery. Teaching should be geared to the child's developmental level. If child life teachers are available, they can play an important role in preparing the child for surgery.

If the child will be in an intensive care unit or recovery room after surgery, a visit there before surgery can reduce the fear and anxiety associated with waking up in a strange environment filled with frightening sights, sounds, and smells. The use of tapes, anatomically correct puppets and dolls, drawings, and models is encouraged to teach the child about the surgical procedure. For example, a doll was used as a teaching aid in preparing Sabrina, the preschooler described in the opening quote, for surgery. Playing with stethoscopes, gowns, masks, and syringes without needles also helps the child feel more in control. Reassure children that their parents can accompany them to the operating room floor and will be waiting when they awaken from surgery.

Physical Preparation.   Preoperative procedures and guidelines vary among hospitals and outpatient surgical centers. In ambulatory and acute care settings, preoperative checklists ensure proper physical preparation of patients for surgery. A sample checklist appears in Table 34–11.

TABLE 34–11   Preoperative Checklist

_____ Check that consent forms are witnessed and signed and in the patient's chart.
_____ Be sure the child's name band is in place.
_____ Be sure any allergies are prominently noted in the child's chart.
_____ Remove any prosthetic devices, including orthodontic appliances.
_____ Check the child's mouth for loose teeth.
_____ Remove eyeglasses.
_____ Bathe and cleanse the operative site if ordered.
_____ Put the child in an operating room gown, allowing the child to wear underwear.
_____ Check that all special tests have been completed and the results are in the child's chart.
_____ Have the child void before surgery.
_____ Keep the child NPO (with nothing by mouth) before surgery.
_____ Give the child prescribed medications.
_____ Transport the child safely to the operating room.

GOAL	INTERVENTION	RATIONALE	EXPECTED OUTCOME
Preoperative Care			

1. Knowledge deficit related to preoperative and postoperative events

GOAL	INTERVENTION	RATIONALE	EXPECTED OUTCOME
	NIC Priority Intervention:		*NOC Suggested Outcome:*
	Teaching, preoperative: *Assisting a patient to understand and mentally prepare for surgery and postoperative recovery*		**Knowledge:** *Extent of understanding conveyed about treatment regimen*
The child and family will acquire knowledge related to the operation.	▶ Ask questions of the parent and child about surgery.	▶ Prior knowledge and understanding can be reinforced and used to guide your presentation.	The child and family are able to verbalize details about expected preoperative and postoperative events. They ask questions that demonstrate understanding.
	▶ Teach about preoperative and postoperative events using appropriate developmental methods such as dolls, drawings, stories, and tours.	▶ Developmental level determines the cognitive approach that works best for teaching.	
	▶ Reinforce information the family has received about the purpose of surgery.	▶ The physician may have explained operation.	
	▶ Have the child demonstrate postoperative events that pertain to his or her case such as deep breathing, putting bandage on doll, taping intravenous line on doll, and pressing patient-controlled analgesia button.	▶ Concrete experience promotes learning.	The child demonstrates skills needed in the postoperative period.
	▶ Allow the parents and child to ask questions.	▶ Learners must have opportunity to ask questions.	

2. Anxiety related to change in health status

GOAL	INTERVENTION	RATIONALE	EXPECTED OUTCOME
	NIC Priority Intervention:		*NOC Suggested Outcome:*
	Anxiety reduction: *Minimizing apprehension, dread, foreboding, or uneasiness related to an unidentified source of anticipated danger*		**Coping:** *Actions to manage stressors that tax an individual's resources*
The child and family will show decreased behavior indicating anxiety.	▶ Question the child about expectations of hospitalization and previous experiences.	▶ Previous experiences can influence present anxiety level.	
	▶ Orient the child to the hospital setting, routines, staff, and other patients.	▶ Familiarity with the setting and people can decrease anxiety by removing unknown factors.	
	▶ Institute age-appropriate play and interactions with the child.	▶ Play can increase trust level and decrease anxiety.	
	▶ Explain procedures and prepare for those that might cause trauma. Encourage parents to support the child.	▶ The child is more likely to trust caregivers if they are truthful and if parents are present.	The child and family demonstrate less anxiety. They verbalize understanding and comfort in hospital routines. Parents support the child for traumatic procedures.
	▶ Allow the parents and child to ask questions.	▶ Questioning provides an opportunity to explain the unknown, which decreases anxiety.	

3. Risk for infection and injury related to exposure to nosocomial infection and use of preoperative medication

GOAL	INTERVENTION	RATIONALE	EXPECTED OUTCOME
	NIC Priority Intervention:		*NOC Suggested Outcome: Actions to eliminate or reduce actural, personal, and modifiable health risks*
	Infection control and fall prevention: *Minimizing the acquisition and transmission of infections agents, and instituting special precautions with patient at risk of falling*		
The child will show no signs of infection.	▶ Monitor vital signs at least every 4 hours. Inspect skin and respiratory status each shift.	▶ Increase in vital sign levels, skin lesions, nasal drainage, or adventitious breath sounds can indicate signs of infection in the child.	The child's vital signs and assessment are within normal limits.
The child will remain free of injury.	▶ Report any variations from expected vital signs.	▶ Symptoms are reported so surgery can be canceled if necessary.	
	▶ Keep side rails up after preoperative medication is given. Maintain NPO status when ordered. Transport the child to the operating room safely secured.	▶ Preoperative medication can alter level of consciousness. NPO status prevents aspiration.	The child is transported safely to the operating room.

(continued)

GOAL	INTERVENTION	RATIONALE	EXPECTED OUTCOME

Postoperative Care

4. Impaired skin integrity related to disruption of skin surface

	NIC Priority Intervention		*NOC Suggested Outcome:*
	Wound care: *Prevention of wound complications and promotion of wound healing*		**Wound healing:** *The extent to which cells and tissues have regenerated following intentional closure*
The child will be free of infection.	▶ Monitor vital signs per hospital routine. Record and report changes from baseline.	▶ Changes in vital signs, especially increased temperature and pulse, can indicate infection.	The child shows no signs of infection.
	▶ Monitor surgical dressing and drains every hour.	▶ Excess drainage may indicate infection.	The surgical wound heals without infection.
	▶ Change or reinforce dressings when wet.	▶ Wet dressing can allow organisms to come into contact with surgical wound.	
	▶ Check the intravenous site every 2 hours for redness, swelling, pain, or pallor.	▶ Intravenous lines may become infiltrated or cause thrombophlebitis.	The intravenous line remains patent without signs of infection.
	▶ Teach parents signs of infection before discharge. Teach parents aseptic technique for dressing change and wound care.	▶ Parents report signs of infection and perform home care as needed.	The child continues to demonstrate no signs of infection at home.

5. Risk for constipation related to surgical procedure and anesthetics

	NIC Priority Intervention:		*NOC Suggested Outcome:*
	Constipation management: *Establishment and maintenance of regular bowel elimination*		**Bowel elimination:** *Ability of the gastrointestinal tract to form and evacuate stool effectively*
The child will achieve and maintain normal bowel functioning by the fourth postoperative day.	▶ Auscultate bowel sounds every 4 hours. Offer liquids only when bowel sounds are present. Assess the abdomen for distention.	▶ Restricting fluids avoids distention if peristalsis is not normal.	The child has bowel movement within 2 to 3 days after surgery with normal pattern by the fourth postoperative day.
	▶ Document the character and frequency of bowel movements.	▶ Knowledge of bowel status ensures early identification of constipation.	
	▶ Advance the diet as tolerated.	▶ Fluids and roughage promote normal bowel functioning.	
	▶ Increase activity as ordered and tolerated.	▶ Physical activity promotes peristalsis.	

6. Risk for fluid volume imbalance related to intravenous infusion and NPO status

	NIC Priority Intervention:		*NOC Suggested Outcome:*
	Fluid management		**Fluid balance:** *The child remains in fluid balance with no vomiting in postoperative period.*
The child will achieve and maintain proper circulating volume.	▶ Monitor vital signs per hospital routines.	▶ Changes in vital signs, especially pulse or blood pressure, can indicate fluid imbalance.	
	▶ Record intake and output. Be alert for fluid loss via dressings or watery stools. Evaluate hydration status by skin turgor and mucous membranes.	▶ Intake and output are roughly equivalent. Urinary retention sometimes occurs postoperatively as a result of anesthesia. Fluid status can be assessed by skin and mucous membrane hydration.	
	▶ Monitor laboratory values of hematocrit and hemoglobin.	▶ Increased hematocrit and hemoglobin can indicate hemoconcentration and underhydration. Decreased serum values can indicate hemodilution of overhydration.	
The child will tolerate oral intake when started, with no nausea, vomiting, or dehydration present.	▶ Begin oral intake after assessment of bowel sounds. Record vomiting. Administer antiemetics if indicated.	▶ Vomiting can cause fluid loss.	

GOAL	INTERVENTION	RATIONALE	EXPECTED OUTCOME

7. Impaired gas exchange related to anesthetics and pain

GOAL	INTERVENTION	RATIONALE	EXPECTED OUTCOME
The child will maintain adequate ventilation with no respiratory impairment.	*NIC Priority Intervention:* **Airway management:** *Facilitation of patency of air passages* ▶ Auscultate lungs every 2 hours. Record rate, rhythm, and quality of respiration. Evaluate respiratory rate after analgesics. ▶ Administer oxygen if ordered. ▶ Reposition the child every 2 hours. ▶ Encourage deep breathing and coughing every 2 hours. Use incentive spirometer, pinwheels, or other blow toys appropriate for the development level of the child. ▶ Ensure proper intake and output.	▶ Early identification of respiratory difficulty aids early treatment. Analgesics, especially morphine, may slow respiratory rate. ▶ Oxygen may facilitate breathing status postoperatively. ▶ Repositioning ensures expansion of all lung fields. ▶ All areas of the lungs must be expanded. Mucus is expectorated. ▶ Balanced fluid status ensures liquification of secretions and prevents excess fluid accumulation.	*NOC Suggested Outcome:* **Respiratory Status:** *Ventilation: Movement of air in and out of lungs* The child moves adequate air in and out of lungs.

8. Pain related to surgical procedure

GOAL	INTERVENTION	RATIONALE	EXPECTED OUTCOME
The child will maintain an adequate comfort level.	*NIC Priority Intervention:* **Pain management:** *Alleviation of pain or a reduction in pain to a level of comfort that is acceptable to the patient* ▶ Assess behavioral cues (e.g., crying, movement, guarding). ▶ Use an appropriate pain scale with verbal children ▶ Administer prescribed pain medications on a regular basis. ▶ Use age-appropriate nonpharmacologic methods of pain control (e.g., distraction, repositioning).	▶ Behavior of preverbal children provides clues to pain experience. ▶ Pain scales allow children to quantify the amount of pain (see Chap. 38). ▶ Narcotics and nonnarcotic analgesics alter pain perception. ▶ Nonpharmacologic interventions interfere with pain perception.	*NOC Suggested Outcome:* **Pain control behavior:** *Personal actions to control pain* The child's pain is controlled as demonstrated by a low number on the pain control scale (behavioral or verbal).

9. Risk for impaired skin integrity related to limited mobility after surgery

GOAL	INTERVENTION	RATIONALE	EXPECTED OUTCOME
The child's skin will remain intact.	*NIC Priority Intervention:* **Skin surveillance and pressure management:** *Collection and analysis of patient data to maintain skin integrity and minimizing pressure to body part* ▶ Turn and reposition the child every 2 hours. ▶ Keep linens clean and dry. ▶ Check pressure areas when turning and rub erythemotous areas with lotion. ▶ Get the child up and ambulating when ordered. ▶ Check the incision for drainage, redness, and tactness of staples or stitches every 4–8 hours.	▶ Repositioning takes pressure off the skin and allows increased circulation. ▶ Clean linen decreases the chance of skin breakdown. ▶ Rubbing increases circulation. ▶ Movement decreases pressure on skin. ▶ Early identification of infection or problems with wound healing can ensure fast treatment.	*NOC Suggested Outcome:* **Risk control:** *Actions to eliminate or reduce actual personal and modifiable health threats.* The child develops no pressure areas. The wound heals without complication.

(continued)

GOAL	INTERVENTION	RATIONALE	EXPECTED OUTCOME
10. Anxiety (child and family) related to equipment and surgical outcome			
	NIC Priority Intervention:		*NOC Suggested Outcome:*
	Anxiety reduction: *Minimizing apprehension, dread, foreboding or uneasiness related to an unidentified source of danger*		**Coping:** *Actions to manage stressors that tax an individual's resources*
The child and family will verbalize comfort with postoperative care and outcome.	▶ Explain monitors, drains dressings, intravenous lines, and procedures. ▶ Reassure the child and family that anxiety is of normal response to the stressful event of surgery. ▶ Encourage parental presence and care of the child. ▶ Use touch and other nonverbal and verbal communication with the child and family.	▶ Knowledge of purpose decreases anxiety. ▶ Knowledge of what is expected decreases anxiety. ▶ The child's anxiety decreases with parental presence. ▶ Effective communication reassures child and family.	The child and family demonstrate coping skills to deal with hospitalization.
11. Knowledge Deficit (Child and Family) related to needed home care			
	NIC Priority Intervention:		*NOC Suggested Outcome:*
	Teaching postoperative: *Health system guidance: Facilitating a patient's location and use of appropriate health services.*		**Knowledge:** *Home Care: Extent of understanding conveyed about home care.*
The child and family will verbalize self-care required at home.	▶ Provide oral and written home care instructions regarding surgical wound care, medications, activities, and diet. ▶ Provide a number to call for questions or concerns. Instruct on follow-up visits.	▶ Teaching regarding home care is necessary early in hospitalization. ▶ Parents need to know emergency information and that follow-up care is required.	The child and family demonstrate skills needed for home care following discharge. They verbalize plans for future care.

POSTOPERATIVE CARE

Postoperative care of the child includes both physical and psychologic care. Evaluate the child's level of consciousness, and take vital signs frequently. Observe the surgical site for drainage, and check dressings. Monitor the child's intake and output and provide comfort and pain relief. (See Chapter 38 for details concerning pain management.) Allow parents to visit with the child as soon after surgery as possible and provide culturally competent care (Figure 34–13 ◆). Provide information and support for families that choose to use complementary care. Refer to "Nursing Care Plan: The Child Undergoing Surgery."

PREPARATION FOR LONG-TERM CARE

When ill or injured children require long-term care, they are often transferred from an acute care hospital to a rehabilitation center or other long-term care facility. The rehabilitation phase of the treatment does not begin at the time of discharge from the acute care hospital but, instead, early in the hospitalization phase. The plan of care is instituted in the hospital, interventions and therapies are begun, and plans are made for continued care.

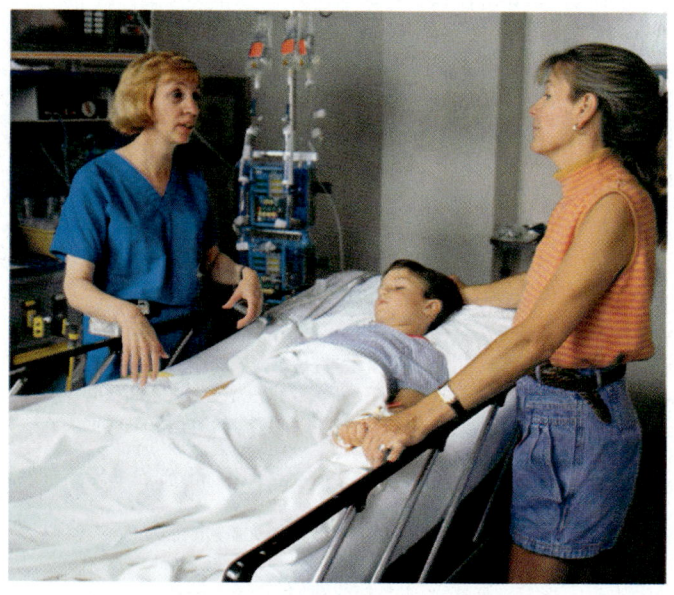

FIGURE 34–13. ◆ This child has just undergone surgery and is in the PICU. Although the child's physical care is immediate and important, remember that both the child and the family have strong psychosocial needs that must be addressed concurrently. It is important to reunite the family as soon as possible after surgery.

Complementary Care

REIKI

Reiki therapy is becoming an increasingly popular complementary modality throughout the United States. Reiki is a treatment modality classified as an energetic healing therapy and shares its foundational principles with other energy-based modalities such as therapeutic touch, polarity therapy, healing touch, and some forms of massage.

Practitioners of Reiki use "laying on of hands" techniques to confer universal life energy to the client for the purpose of healing a wide variety of physical and psychospiritual problems. Although there is great need for further empiric research regarding the efficacy of Reiki, preliminary studies have documented relaxation and decreased pain response during a Reiki treatment. (Nield-Anderson & Ameling, 2001; Olson & Hanson, 1997; Wardell & Engebretson, 2001).

Because Reiki is a noninvasive treatment modality to foster relaxation, it may help children undergoing painful or anxiety-producing procedures. The nurse can help to support parents and children interested in this modality by providing information on the technique, referring to practitioners who perform Reiki, and integrating this therapy with other care provided for the child.

When it becomes apparent that a child will need long-term care, the health care team explores with the family the options and resources available to provide such care:

- Home care with support services such as visiting nurses and physical therapists
- A long-term care facility
- A specialized rehabilitation center that can provide care for an extended period

The family should make the decision about which option will work best, considering the needs of the child, the financial implications, the roles and supports available to the family unit, and the resources available in the community. Guidelines to assist parents in evaluating rehabilitation centers are available from the Brain Injury Association. WEB

Nurses in acute care hospitals frequently coordinate services when transfer to another facility occurs. This involves giving information about the child's history, plan of care, and treatment to the new facility. Forms are available to assist the person responsible for coordinating the transfer. Families will need support and assistance in dealing with the transfer from the acute care setting to another facility.

PREPARATION FOR HOME CARE

Nurses play an important role in preparing the child and family for discharge home; this preparation starts early during the hospitalization. The nurse works with the social service department, home care agencies, and the family to plan for equipment, procedures, and other home care needs. Home care nurses then take over the child's care and assist families to meet the child's health care needs.

Assessing the Child in Preparation for Discharge

Discharge plans should begin early in the child's hospitalization. A health care team, including the physician, nurse, social worker, discharge planner, and family, works together to ensure a smooth transition home. An assessment of the family's ability to manage the child's care and of the appropriateness of the home for providing care should be made (Votroubek & Townsend, 1997).

Children with multisystem problems may require home care involving specialized equipment and personnel. Early planning gives the family time to investigate health insurance benefits, support services in the community, and other needs before discharge.

When a child is to be discharged home, the school district should be contacted and plans for education made. This involves an assessment of the child by the school district and formulation of an **individualized education plan** (IEP). The IEP may include home tutors, specialized services from persons such as physical or speech therapists, or arrangements for transport of the child with a disability to the school and provisions for special medical care as needed. For each child with a chronic disability who is 14 years or older, an **individualized transition plan** focuses on assisting the individual in moving successfully from school into the community (Jackson & Vessey, 2000).

Some common problems that interfere with successful discharge planning include financial concerns, the family's unavailability for teaching and planning, and poor communication and lack of teamwork among involved health care disciplines. Nurses should be alert to these potential problems from the initial contact with the child and family and should take precautions to solve them as soon as possible (Proctor, Morrow-Howell, Kitchen, et al., 1995).

Preparing the Family for Home Care

The family may need to learn physical and rehabilitative procedures for the child's care. Short-term care may be necessary until the child regains full function. In other situations, care may be required throughout the child's life. This may involve measuring vital signs or determining blood glucose levels. For the child requiring complex long-term care, parents may need to learn about intravenous lines, medications, oxygen administration, or ventilators (Figure 34–14 ◆). Parents need to be taught how to use the equipment needed for the child's care and must show that they can use it correctly. They must be able to identify symptoms of distress and report them immediately to the

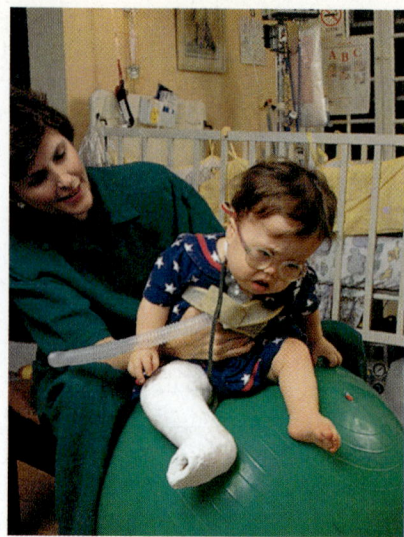

FIGURE 34–14. ◆ This child with chronic medical problems is being cared for at home. Are there any legal implications for the hospital and the nurse associated with the preparation of the child and family for home care?

health care provider. The education provided and the parents' ability to perform care are discussed with a visiting nurse or individual who manages the home care program. Parents should be encouraged to learn cardiopulmonary resuscitation. (Refer to Chapter 35.)

Help parents explore options for respite. If they cannot provide daily care or need a break, they should be able to rely on others for a short period. Some agencies are available to provide respite care. Ongoing assistance may be needed to help families deal with financial, time, and other challenges. Families with the greatest burdens in caring for their children will require the most interventions.

Preparing Parents to Act as Case Managers

The family is an integral part of the plan of care for an ill or hospitalized child. The child with a chronic illness or an injury requiring long-term care will probably require the services of numerous health care personnel or health care agencies. One person needs to be identified as a **case manager** to coordinate health care and to prevent gaps and overlaps. In some hospitals, nurses act as case managers. They may organize a patient care conference while the child with a chronic condition is hospitalized. Management goals are set and decisions are made about which health care provider or agency is responsible for helping the child meet each goal.

Parents can also be case managers. The parent as case manager coordinates medical care, hospital stays, and visits to specialists; meets with school district representatives to plan the individualized education program for the child; finds equipment, personnel, and other services for home care; and manages the child's overall care.

Nurses should strongly encourage parents who want to take over case management to do so. Help them learn the management skills required. Many communities have workshops for parents managing the complex care of their children.

C HAPTER HIGHLIGHTS

☞ Hospitalization is a stressful event for all children and their families, especially when the hospitalization was unplanned and sudden.

☞ Children understand their illnesses and hospitalizations based on cognitive abilities at each developmental stage, and upon previous health care experiences.

☞ Nurses assess the impact of the child's illness or hospitalization on the family unit.

☞ Families are always disrupted by a child's hospitalization, and various approaches can help them understand the process and cope more successfully with this challenge.

☞ When hospitalization is planned, both the child and parents can prepare for the experience. Nurses assist this process by teaching about what to expect.

☞ A teaching plan includes goals and expected outcomes, interventions needed to achieve the specified goals, and a method and time for evaluation of the expected outcomes.

☞ Strategies such as culturally competent care, child life programs, rooming in, therapeutic play, and therapeutic recreation help meet the psychosocial needs of the hospitalized child.

☞ The nurse helps the family plan for the child's long-term health care needs and home care issues. Parents may be trained to act as case managers for the child with long-term needs, or the task may be delegated to a health care provider.

EXPLOREMediaLink

NCLEX Review, Case Studies, and other interactive resources for this chapter can be found on the companion website at http://www.prenhall.com/london. Click on "Chapter 34" to select the activities for this chapter.

For animations, more NCLEX review questions, and an audio glossary, access the accompanying CD-ROM in this textbook.

REFERENCES

Ball, J. W. (1998). *Pediatric patient teaching guides.* St. Louis, MO: Mosby-Yearbook.

Bibace, R., & Walsh, M. (1981). Children's conception of illness. In R. Bibace & M. Walsh (Eds.), *Children's conceptions of health, illness and bodily function.* San Francisco: Jossey-Bass.

Bowlby, J. (1960). Separation anxiety. *International Journal of Psychoanalysis, 41*(2/3), 89–113.

Boyd, J. R., & Hunsberger, M. (1998). Chronically ill children coping with repeated hospitalizations: Their perceptions and suggested interventions. *Journal of Pediatric Nursing, 13,* 330–342.

Bricher, G. (2000). Children in the hospital: Issues of power and vulnerability. *Pediatric Nursing, 26,* 277–282.

Conner, J. M., & Nelson, E. C. (1999). Neonatal intensive care: Satisfaction measured from a parent's perspective. *Pediatrics, 103,* 336–349.

De Pasquale, S. (1999, November). Serious play. *Johns Hopkins Magazine,* 30–36.

Emergency Nurses Association. (1998). *Family presence at the bedside during invasive procedures and/or resuscitation.* Des Plaines, IL: Author.

Gellert, E. (1962). Children's conceptions of the content and functions of the human body. *Genetic Psychology Monographs, 65,* 293–405.

Gusella, J. L., Ward, A. M., & Butler, G. S. (1998). The experience of hospitalized adolescents: How well do we meet their developmental needs? *Children's Health Care, 27,* 131–145.

Huckabay, L. M. D., & Tilem-Kessler, D. (1999). Patterns of parental stress in PICU admission. *Dimensions of Critical Care Nursing, 18*(2), 36–42.

Jackson, P. L., & Vessey, J. A. (2000). *Primary care of the child with a chronic condition* (3rd ed.). St. Louis, MO: Mosby.

LaMontagne, L. L. (2000). Effects of surgery type and attention focus on children's coping. *Nursing Research, 49,* 245–252.

Lipson, J. G., Dibble, S. L., & Minarik, P. A., Eds. (1996). Culture and nursing care: A packet guide. San Fransisco: UCSF Press.

Marino, B. L., & Marino, E. K. (2000). Practice applications of research. Parents' report of children's hospital care: What it means for your practice. *Pediatric Nursing, 26,* 195–198.

Melnyk, B. M. (1995). Parental coping with childhood hospitalization: A theoretical framework to guide research and clinical interventions. *Maternal-Child Nursing Journal, 23,* 123–131.

Melnyk, B. M. (2000). Intervention studies involving parents of hospitalized young children: An analysis of the past and future recommendations. *Journal of Pediatric Nursing, 15,* 4–13.

Mobley, C. E. (1996). Assessment of health knowledge in preschoolers. *Children's Health Care, 25,* 11–18.

Nield-Anderson, L., & Ameling, A. (2001). Reiki. A complementary therapy for nursing practice, *Journal of Psychosocial Nursing and Mental Health Services, 39*(4), 42–49.

Olson, K., & Hanson, J. (1997). Using Reiki to manage pain: A preliminary report. *Cancer Prevention and Control, 1*(2), 108–113.

Proctor, E. K., Morrow-Howell, N., Kitchen, A., & Wang, Y. T. (1995). Pediatric discharge planning: Complications, efficiency, and adequacy. *Social Work in Health Care, 22,* 1–18.

Ramsey, C. A. (2000). Storytelling can be a valuable teaching aid. *Association of Operating Room Nurses Journal, 72,* 497–499.

Rode, D., Capitulo, K. L., Fishman, M., & Holden, G. (1998). The therapeutic use of technology. *American Journal of Nursing, 98*(12), 32–35.

Rosenbaum, J. N., & Carty, L. (1996). The subculture of adolescence: Beliefs about care, health and individuation within Leininger's theory. *Journal of Advanced Nursing, 23,* 741–746.

Votroubek, W. L., & Townsend, J. L. (1997). *Pediatric home care.* Gaithersburg, MD: Aspen Publishers.

Wardell, D. W., & Engebretson, J. (2001). Biological correlates of Reiki touch healing. *Journal Advanced Nursing, 33*(4), 439–445.

CHAPTER 35

Nursing Considerations for the Child in the Community

Sometimes Jessica's asthma attacks really frighten me because she struggles so hard to breathe. She has a lot of trouble with asthma in the summertime with all the heat. I am afraid to let her play outside with her friends for fear that she will have another attack. I would really like to know how to keep Jessica's asthma under control.

—MOTHER OF JESSICA, 8

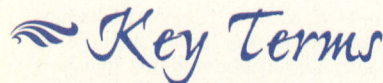

Key Terms

Chronic condition   *850*

Developmental surveillance   *841*

Disability   *850*

Health supervision   *840*

Medical home   *839*

Medically fragile   *858*

Screening tests   *841*

Sensitivity   *841*

Specificity   *841*

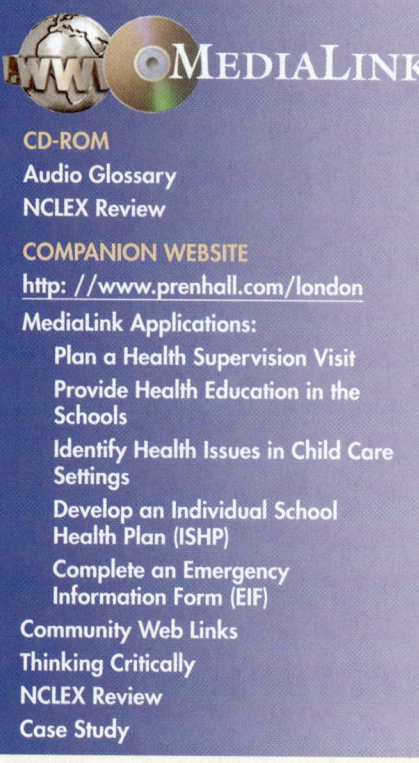

MediaLink

CD-ROM
Audio Glossary
NCLEX Review

COMPANION WEBSITE
http://www.prenhall.com/london

MediaLink Applications:
   Plan a Health Supervision Visit
   Provide Health Education in the Schools
   Identify Health Issues in Child Care Settings
   Develop an Individual School Health Plan (ISHP)
   Complete an Emergency Information Form (EIF)
Community Web Links
Thinking Critically
NCLEX Review
Case Study

Nurses care for children in a wide variety of community settings. Some of these settings include child care centers, schools, camps, physician offices, hospital or public health clinics, homeless shelters, and the home. The range of nursing care varies from monitoring the health and safety of children in child care centers and schools to the provision of acute care to a child at home. Falling within this range are the provision of health supervision or well-child care, care for episodic illnesses and injuries, and assisting families to learn optimal management of their child's chronic conditions. Each of these nursing roles is important in promoting the health of children in the community.

Children receive most of their health care (health supervision and episodic health care for acute illnesses and injuries) in community settings. Depending on the community, health care resources, and age of the child, this care may be provided in any of the settings previously described.

During the past decade, the United States has begun to place a greater emphasis on health promotion and disease and injury prevention (health protection). The purpose is not only to promote optimal well-being and to reduce the pain and suffering of children and families, but also to reduce health care costs. Other patterns of health care delivery are also changing to reduce the costs of health care. Examples of these changes include day surgery in ambulatory surgical centers, newborn discharge after 24 to 48 hours, home care for long-term intravenous antibiotics, and short stay units associated with emergency departments. Health plans and other health care providers continue to explore options to provide safe, high-quality care with fewer hospitalizations or shorter stays when hospitalization is needed. Home care services have developed to support families who now care for more acutely ill children.

This trend in out-of-hospital care is also seen among children with chronic health conditions and advanced disease states. Technologic advances, such as portable medical equipment, now make it possible to provide complex health care services in the home and other community settings (Figure 35–1 ◆). Strategies to support families who provide care to their children in the home have developed. Additionally, federal law mandates that education be provided to all disabled children, and there are no exceptions based on health care status. As a result, schools are now obligated to provide complex health care to children.

Care of children continues to shift rapidly from the hospital to community settings. The nurse working with families in a community setting must use the knowledge of how the larger environment influences the child's health and development and the family's activities. To work effectively in the community the nurse's role includes:

- Making assessments, planning strategies, and implementing and evaluating approaches to care that match

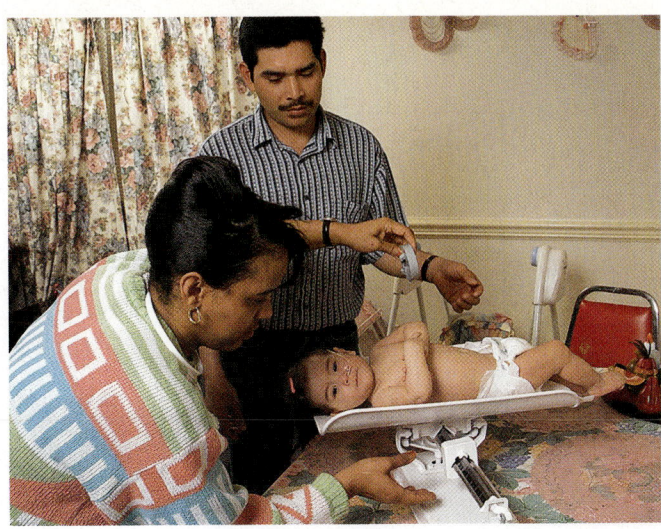

FIGURE 35–1. ◆ Nurses provide both short-term and long-term services to families in the home setting. In some cases, families need support for a short time after the child is discharged from the hospital following an acute illness. In other cases, families need assistance with complex nursing care for the child dependent on technology for survival.

Nursing Practice

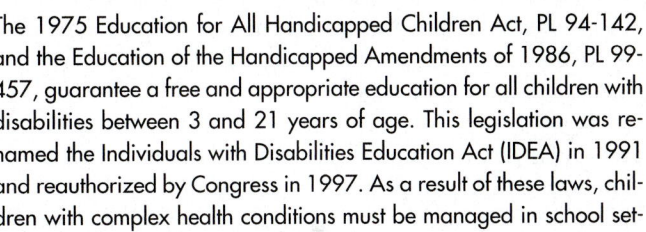

The 1975 Education for All Handicapped Children Act, PL 94-142, and the Education of the Handicapped Amendments of 1986, PL 99-457, guarantee a free and appropriate education for all children with disabilities between 3 and 21 years of age. This legislation was renamed the Individuals with Disabilities Education Act (IDEA) in 1991 and reauthorized by Congress in 1997. As a result of these laws, children with complex health conditions must be managed in school settings in the least restrictive educational environment.

the family's economic and social situation, and available resources.

- Working with others in the community (schools, churches, and other community-based resources) to make assessments, plan strategies, and implement and evaluate approaches addressed to the health care needs of the community's children (Pridham, Broome, & Woodring, 1996).

HEALTH SUPERVISION

How often do children need health supervision visits? What are the elements of a health supervision visit? Why are children screened for health conditions at certain times?

All children need a regular source of health care, a primary care provider or **medical home** that supports the family and child during the important developmental

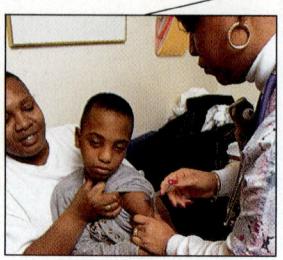 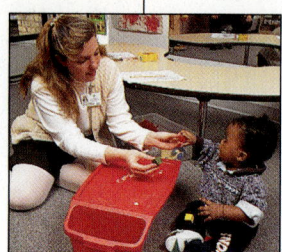 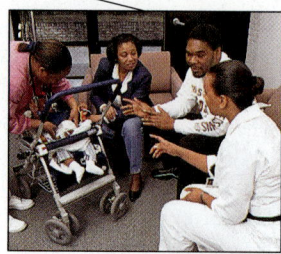

Health supervision

Disease and injury prevention
Screening tests
Immunizations
Safety teaching
Anticipatory guidance

Developmental surveillance
Observation of progress in areas of fine motor, gross motor, language, adaptive skills, and cognition.

Health promotion
Child and family guidance to promote family strengths in areas of healthy lifestyles, social development, coping, and family interactions.

FIGURE 35–2. ◆ Model of pediatric health supervision visits.

years. A medical home includes the following: preventive services, assurance of ambulatory and inpatient care 24 hours a day, continuity of care from infancy through adolescence, appropriate use of subspecialty consultation and referrals, interaction with school and community agencies, and a central record and database containing all pertinent information (Green & Palfrey, 2000). When a family has an established relationship with a primary care provider, comprehensive, family-centered health services can be provided based on the provider's knowledge of the family's strengths and weaknesses.

Health supervision involves services that focus on disease and injury prevention, growth and developmental surveillance, and health promotion at key intervals during the child's life (Figure 35–2 ◆). It is not just a periodic visit for health care services. National guidelines for preventive health services have been developed for infants, children, and adolescents by the U.S. Department of Health and Human Services (DHHS) and the American Medical Association. ⌾ **WEB** Settings for health supervision visits vary widely within a community and include physician offices, community health centers, the home, schools or child care centers, or shelters.

Nursing Practice

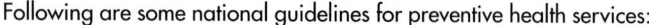

Following are some national guidelines for preventive health services:

▶ *Bright Futures,* Maternal and Child Health Bureau, Health Resources and Services Administration, DHHS

▶ *Put Prevention into Practice,* Office of Disease Prevention and Health Promotion, Public Health Service, DHHS

▶ *Guidelines for Adolescent Preventive Services,* American Medical Association

The health supervision visit must be individualized to the family and child. Every health visit, including an episodic illness visit or maintenance care for a chronic condition, is a potential health promotion visit. A tracking system in the primary care setting helps identify appropriate health supervision activities for each child at every visit. For example, needed immunizations may sometimes be given during a visit for an acute condition if the child has missed a prior health supervision visit. Refer to Chapter 41 for immunization guidelines. ⌾

Nurses play an important role in managing these health supervision visits. Depending on the setting, the nurse may provide all services or support the physician by obtaining an updated health history, screening for diseases and other conditions, conducting a developmental assessment, and providing immunizations, anticipatory guidance, and health education.

Nursing Management

Nursing Assessment and Diagnosis

Nursing assessment of the child and family at each visit for health supervision focuses on the following:

▶ Interviewing the family and child to update the health history, assessing the child's developmental or educational progress, identifying nutritional status and dietary habits, and discussing any concerns the parent or child has (see Chapters 31 and 33). ⌾

▶ Observing the family–child relationships

▶ Conducting developmental surveillance assessments

▶ Performing age-appropriate screening tests (Figure 35–3 ◆)

▶ Performing a physical assessment

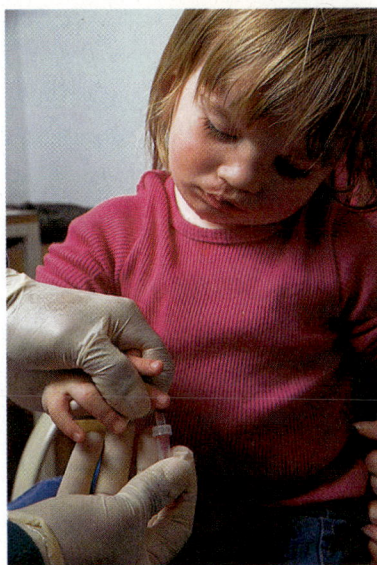

FIGURE 35–3. ◆ This 18-month-old toddler is having a blood screening test to detect iron-deficiency anemia. Children are often screened for adequate levels of iron in the latter stages of infancy and during toddlerhood.

DISEASE AND INJURY PREVENTION

Screening tests detect the presence of a health condition before symptoms are apparent. Once a screening test identifies the existence of a health condition, early intervention can begin, with the goal of reducing the severity or complications of the condition. For example, all newborns are screened within 1 week of birth for at least two genetic diseases, congenital hypothyroidism and phenylketonuria. Appropriate interventions (medication or diet therapy) reduce the chances or severity of mental retardation if either of these conditions is present. (See Chapter 51 for more information about newborn screening.)

Screening tests are administered when children are most likely to develop a condition such as when at high risk for exposure to tuberculosis, or to identify the greatest number of children at highest risk for the condition. Screening tests are also expected to correctly identify children who

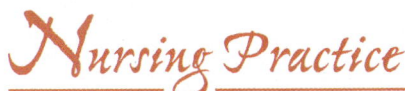

Sensitivity is the proportion of children with a condition who test positive for that condition. Some children who test positive do not have the condition; they are false positives. **Specificity** is the proportion of children who do not have a condition who test negative for that condition. Some children who test negative actually have the condition; they are false negatives.

The best screening tests have both a high sensitivity and high specificity. If a child tests positive on a screening test, additional tests are usually performed to confirm the presence of the condition (Curry & Duby, 1994).

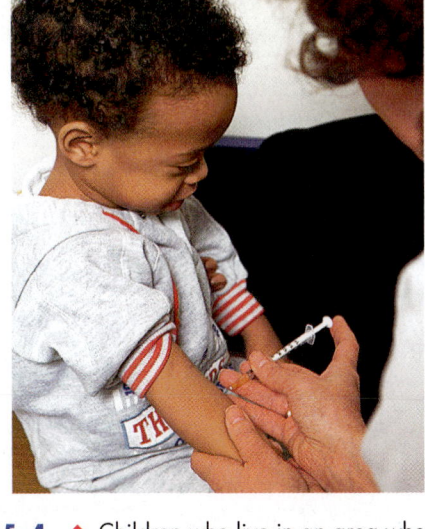

FIGURE 35–4. ◆ Children who live in an area where active tuberculosis has been detected or is epidemic need tuberculosis screening more frequently.

truly have the condition. Some children are at greater risk of contracting certain conditions because of their environment (Figure 35–4 ◆). For example, young children living in housing built before 1960 are screened more frequently for lead poisoning than children who live in newer houses where only lead-free paints have been used. Table 35–1 outlines the recommended screening tests by age for infants, children, and adolescents.

DEVELOPMENTAL SURVEILLANCE

Developmental surveillance is a flexible, continuous process of skilled observations of children's fine and gross motor skills, language, and psychosocial behavior milestones throughout encounters during child health visits. Information may be collected from several sources; for instance, a questionnaire that the parent completes, trigger questions asked during the interview, or observation of the child during the visit. Parents can also be interviewed to identify any developmental concerns they may have about the child. To initiate general health supervision and developmental surveillance, questions such as the following may be used (Deloian, 1997).

▶ Do you have any concerns about Sam's vision and hearing?

▶ What changes have you seen in Hannah's development?

▶ What kind of baby is Jamal?

▶ What do you and Brianna enjoy doing together?

▶ What are Brandon's favorite play activities?

Standardized developmental questionnaires are effective for developmental surveillance of most children, especially when time for health supervision visits is limited. These questionnaires are easy to administer, do not require the child's cooperation, and can be completed by parents

TABLE 35-1   Clinical Preventive Services for Normal-Risk Children, Birth to 18 Years of Age*

Screening Test	Age	Frequency
Newborn screening (PKU, sickle cell hemoglobinopathies, hypothyroidism)	Newborn	Once
Hearing	Newborn, 3 to 8 years, 10 years, 12 years, 15 years, 18 years	Once in each age interval
Head circumference	Birth to 2 years	Periodically
Height and weight	Birth to 18 years	Periodically
Lead	1 year, 2 years	Once at each age
Eye screening	Birth, 3 to 4 years	Once
	5 to 18 years	Periodically
Blood pressure	6 to 12 months	Once
	3 to 18 years	Periodically
Dental	1 to 18 years	Periodically
Alcohol use	11 to 18 years	Periodically

Counseling	Age	Frequency
Development, nutrition, physical activity, safety, unintentional injuries and poisoning, violent behaviors and firearms, STDs and HIV, family planning, tobacco use, drug use	Birth to 18 years	As appropriate for age

* For recommended immunization schedule, see Chapter 41.

Note: From Office of Public Health and Science and Office of Disease Prevention and Promotion. (1998). *Put prevention into practice: Clinician's handbook of preventive services* (2nd ed., Fig. A.2a). Washington, DC: U.S. Department of Health and Human Services, Public Health Services. Adapted.

in the waiting area. Children in need of more extensive developmental surveillance can be identified. See Table 35–2 for a list of commonly used developmental screening questionnaires that have been tested for validity and reliability.

When talking with parents, review physical, social, and communication milestones for infants and young children. Be aware that parents' recall of past developmental milestones is often faulty. The child is often reported to have achieved milestones at ages earlier than actually occurred. When accuracy of developmental milestones is critical, ask to see the child's baby diary or review the past health history at ages closer to the milestone achievement. Past research has

TABLE 35-2   Developmental Surveillance Questionnaires

Questionnaire	Guidelines for Administration
Parents' Evaluation of Developmental Status[a] birth to 8 years	Consists of 10 questions for parents to answer in interview; based on research on parents' concerns. Requires less than 5 minutes to complete. English and Spanish versions are available.
Prescreening Development Questionnaire (PDQ and Revised-PDQ)[b] birth to 6 years	Parents complete one of age-specific forms. Helps identify children who need Denver II assessment. Requires less than 10 minutes to complete. PDQ is available in English, Spanish, and French versions; R-PDQ in English only.
Ages and Stages Questionnaire[c] 04–48 months	Questionnaires for 11 specific ages, with 10–15 items each in areas of fine motor, gross motor, communication, adaptive, personal, and social skills. Parents try each activity with the child. Requires less than 10 minutes to complete. English and Spanish versions are available.
Child Development Inventories[d] 3 to 72 months	Consists of 60 yes-no descriptions for three separate instruments to identify children with developmental difficulties. Requires about 10 minutes to complete.

[a]Frances P. Glascoe, Ellsworth & Vandermeer Press Ltd, 4405 Scenic Drive, Nashville, TN 37204
[b]Denver Developmental Materials, Inc., P.O. Box 6919, Denver, CO 80206-0919
[c]Brookes Publishing Co., P.O. Box 10624, Baltimore, MD 21285-0625
[d]Behavior Science Systems, Box 580274, Minneapolis, MN 55458

indicated that carefully eliciting parents' concerns about their child's development can be as accurate as screening tests in identifying true developmental problems (Glascoe, 1999).

Review school performance for older children and adolescents. Review report cards, school achievement records, and any performance on psychoeducational tests when indicated. Inquire about the child's participation in sports and other activities, as well as noted abilities.

If a developmental delay or abnormality is suspected, a specific developmental screening test is needed to document developmental progress. See Table 35–3 for a list of commonly used developmental screening tests. Some health care providers actually use the Denver II as a developmental chart, like a growth curve to monitor the child's developmental progress (see Figures 35–5 ◆ and 35–6 ◆). Remember: developmental screening tests are not diagnostic tests. They simply help to confirm that most children are progressing along an age-appropriate norm, and they help document suspicions or patterns of developmental problems.

TABLE 35–3	**Developmental Screening Tests for Infants and Young Children**
Screening Test	*Guidelines for Administration*
Denver II[a] birth to 6 years	Consists of observation of the child in four domains: personal–social, fine motor–adaptive, language, and gross motor. Requires 30 minutes to complete. A training video is available.
Bayley Infant Neurodevelopmental Screener (BINS)[b] 3–24 months	Consists of observation of child with 10–13 items for each of six age-specific scales to assess neurologic processes, neurodevelopmental skills, and developmental accomplishments. Requires 10–15 minutes to complete.
McCarthy Scales of Children's Abilities[b] 2.5–8.5 years	Consists of observation of child in domains of motor, verbal, perceptual–performance, quantitative, general cognition, and memory. Requires 45 minutes to complete.
Denver Articulation Screening Exam (DASE)[a] 2.5–6 years	Consists of observation of child's articulation of 30 sound elements and intelligibility. Requires 5 minutes to complete.
Early Language Milestone Scale—2 (ELM)[c] birth to 36 months	Consists of observation of child to assess auditory expressive, auditory receptive, and visual components of speech. Requires 5–10 minutes to complete.

[a]Denver Development Materials, Inc., P.O. Box 6919, Denver, CO 80206-0919
[b]Psychological Corporation, 304 E. 45th Street, New York, NY 10017-3425
[c]PRO-ED, Inc., 8700 Shoal Creek Blvd., Austin, TX 78758-6897

FIGURE 35–5. ◆ Follow all directions for performing the Denver II assessment and for interpreting responses. Develop rapport with the child and approach the assessment as fun. This often helps the child participate more actively during entire Denver II assessment. The 9-month-old boy in this sequence is able to perform the following age-appropriate behaviors: Banging two cubes **A;** playing ball with the examiner **B;** using a thumb-finger grasp **C;** and pulling to stand **D.**

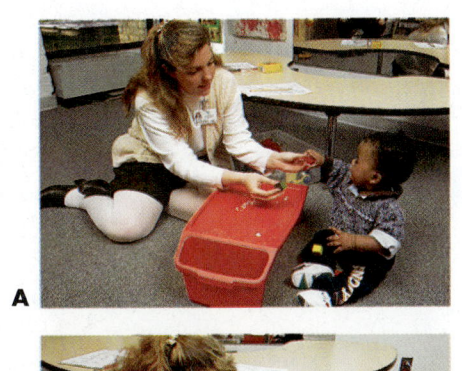
A

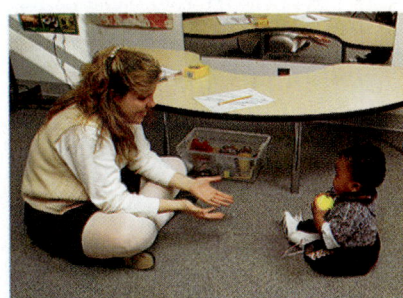
B

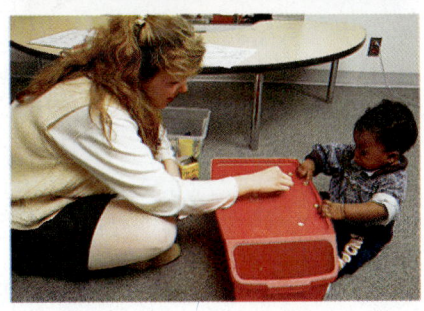
C

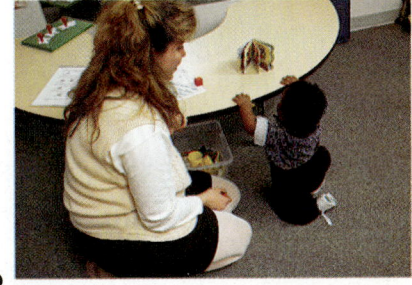
D

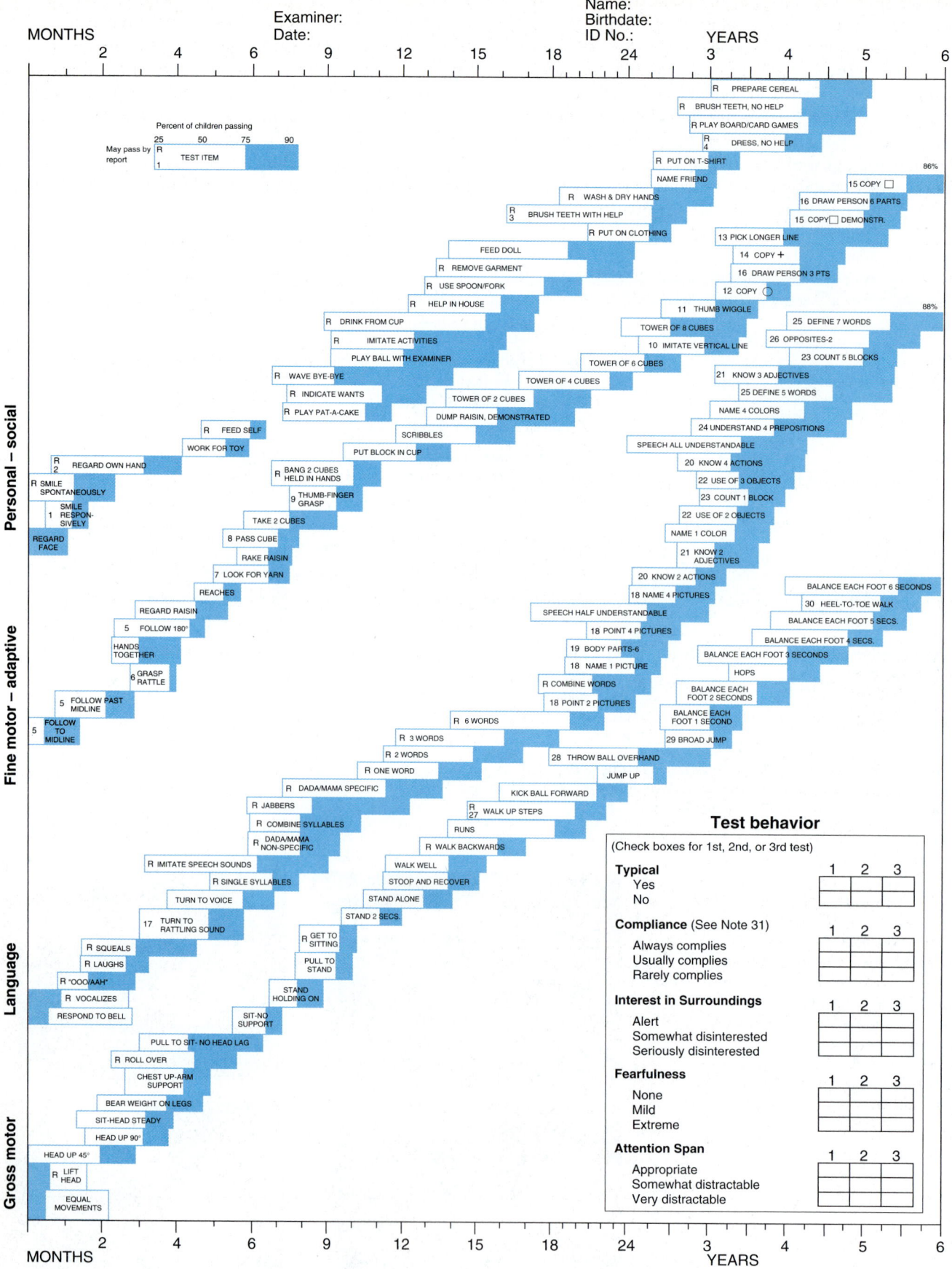

FIGURE 35-6. ◆ Denver II. *Note:* Reproduced with permission from *Pediatrics,* Vol. 89, pages 91–97, Figure 2, © 1992.

1. Try to get child to smile by smiling, talking or waving. Do not touch him/her.
2. Child must stare at hand several seconds.
3. Parent may help guide toothbrush and put toothpaste on brush.
4. Child does not have to be able to tie shoes or button/zip in the back.
5. Move yarn slowly in an arc from one side to the other, about 8" above child's face.
6. Pass if child grasps rattle when it is touched to the backs or tips of fingers.
7. Pass if child tries to see where yarn went. Yarn should be dropped quickly from sight from tester's hand without arm movement.
8. Child must transfer cube from hand to hand without help of body, mouth, or table.
9. Pass if child picks up raisin with any part of thumb and finger.
10. Line can vary only 30 degrees or less from tester's line.
11. Make a fist with thumb pointing upward and wiggle only the thumb. Pass if child imitates and does not move any fingers other than the thumb.

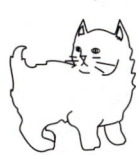 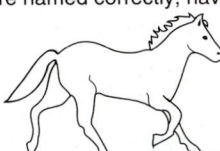 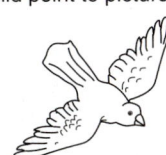 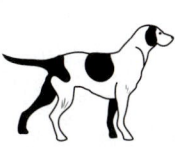

12. Pass any enclosed form. Fail continuous round motions.
13. Which line is longer? (Not bigger.) Turn paper upside down and repeat. (pass 3 of 3 or 5 of 6).
14. Pass any lines crossing near midpoint.
15. Have child copy first. If failed, demonstrate.

When giving items 12, 14, and 15, do not name the forms. Do not demonstrate 12 and 14.

16. When scoring, each pair (2 arms, 2 legs, etc.) counts as one part.
17. Place one cube in cup and shake gently near child's ear, but out of sight. Repeat for other ear.
18. Point to picture and have child name it. (No credit is given for sounds only.)
   If less than 4 pictures are named correctly, have child point to picture as each is named by tester.

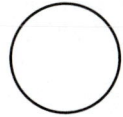  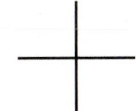  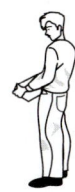

19. Using doll, tell child: Show me the nose, eyes, ears, mouth, hands, feet, tummy, hair. Pass 6 of 8.
20. Using pictures, ask child: Which one flies?... says meow?... talks?... barks?... gallops? Pass 2 of 5, 4 of 5.
21. Ask child: What do you do when you are cold?... tired?... hungry? Pass 2 of 3, 3 of 3.
22. Ask child: What do you do with a cup? What is a chair used for? What is a pencil used for?
   Action words must be included in answers.
23. Pass if child correctly places <u>and</u> says how many blocks are on paper. (1, 5).
24. Tell child: Put block **on** table; **under** table **in front of** me, **behind** me. Pass 4 of 4.
   (Do not help child by pointing, moving head or eyes.)
25. Ask child: What is a ball?... lake?... desk?... house?... banana?... curtain?... fence?... ceiling? Pass if defined in terms of use, shape, what it is made of, or general category (such as banana is fruit, not just yellow). Pass 5 of 8, 7 of 8.
26. Ask child: If a horse is big, a mouse is_____? If fire is hot, ice is_____? If sun shines during the day, the moon shines during the _____? Pass 2 of 3.
27. Child may use wall or rail only, not person. May not crawl.
28. Child must throw ball overhand 3 feet to within arm's reach of tester.
29. Child must perform standing broad jump over width of test sheet (8 1/2 inches).
30. Tell child to walk forward, ⊂⊃⊂⊃⊂⊃⊂⊃ → heel within 1 inch of toe. Tester may demonstrate.
   Child must walk 4 consecutive steps.
31. In the second year, half of normal children are non-compliant.

OBSERVATIONS:

FIGURE 35–6. ◆ Continued. Directions for administration of Denver II.

To perform developmental screening with any of the standardized screening tools, make sure all directions are followed.

- Read directions thoroughly or utilize specific training tools available.
- Calculate the infant's age correctly, especially if premature.
- Attempt to develop rapport with the infant or child to get the best performance.
- In some cases, parents can be asked if a child demonstrates specific skills at home, especially if the child is not cooperative.
- Note the behavior and cooperativeness of the child during the screening process.
- Analyze the findings to make the correct interpretation.

Failure to perform a single item in a single domain does not mean the child has failed the test. The child should be reevaluated at a future visit. Provide parents with guidance on specific methods for stimulating the child. Failure of multiple items within one domain or across multiple domains is of greatest concern. When poor development patterns in one or more domains are revealed, referral for diagnostic developmental assessment is needed.

Examples of nursing diagnoses for an 18-month-old child who is brought by parents for regular health supervision and immunizations may include:

- Altered nutrition: More than body requirements related to lack of basic nutritional knowledge
- Risk for poisoning related to lack of proper precautions with increased mobility to reach and climb
- Health-seeking behaviors related to needed immunizations
- Risk for altered parenting related to mother's plans to return to full-time work

Planning and Implementation

Nursing management for health supervision visits includes providing immunizations, offering anticipatory guidance, educating parents and children about healthy behaviors, carrying out collaborative nurse–family planning for health promotion, and providing referrals for follow-up care. For more information about the recommended schedule for immunizations and the nurse's role in ensuring full immunization status for children, refer to Chapter 41.

Most parents want to know how to contribute to their child's growth and development. Discussions at the conclusion of the health supervision assessments should focus on building family strengths by promoting the development of competence, confidence, and self-esteem in their growing child.

Although some specific interventions are most likely to take place only in a health care facility or physician office, most of the nursing management for health supervision can occur in any setting.

Growth and Development

Community challenges that need to be considered during health supervision visits include:

- Poverty; inadequate housing; limited opportunities for employment; lack of affordable, high-quality child care
- Environmental hazards; unsafe neighborhood; community violence
- Isolation in a rural community; lack of programs for families with special needs; lack of social support; inadequate public services
- Lack of educational programs and social services for adolescent parents; lack of social, educational, cultural, and recreational opportunities
- Lack of access to medical or dental services; inadequate fluoride levels in community water

Parents experiencing more than two of these problems in their community may need extra assistance or guidance to provide a supportive environment for their child that fosters growth and development.

PROVIDE ANTICIPATORY GUIDANCE

Anticipatory guidance provides the family with information on what to expect during the child's current and next stage of development. Topics for each visit should include age-appropriate information about healthy habits, prevention of illness and injury, prevention of poisoning, nutrition, oral health, and sexuality. Health promotion guidance also helps the child and family to develop strategies to support and enhance social development, family relationships, parental health, community interactions, self-responsibility, and school or vocational achievement.

Because the time for each visit is limited, build upon the parent's current knowledge and care practices. Use available time to focus anticipatory guidance, to introduce new information, to reinforce what the family is doing well, and to clear up any poorly understood concepts.

Take advantage of other sources of information in the community to enhance the guidance provided. For example, state and local SAFE KIDS Coalitions help inform families about injury-prevention strategies. School health programs such as the National Fire Prevention Association's "Risk Watch" may educate children about injury prevention, and other school programs may educate students about smoking and drug avoidance. Keep informed about the types of health education provided in different community settings so it is easier to reinforce the concepts already being taught. WEB

ENCOURAGE HEALTH PROMOTION

Often the family needs health education and counseling to promote healthy behaviors in their child. Examples of focused health education and counseling may be information about environmental control to reduce lead exposure; dietary changes to increase iron-rich foods; and reduction of milk intake for weight control or loss strategies. Counseling in the case of the 18-month-old toddler for whom nursing diagnoses were previously stated could focus on child care arrangements and the anticipation and management of potential behavior problems.

Patient education and counseling are most effective when the family understands the relationship between the behavior change needed and the health outcome. The parents and child then work in partnership with the nurse or health care provider and make a commitment to the change or changes needed. Steps in promoting patient education and counseling include:

▶ Working with families to assess barriers to behavior change.

▶ Involving patients in selecting a risk factor to change and the outcome goal.

▶ Gaining commitment from the parents and child to change.

▶ Using a combination of strategies.

▶ Designing a behavior modification program.

▶ Monitoring progress through follow-up contact (Curry & Duby, 1994).

PERFORM HEALTH SUPERVISION INTERVENTIONS

After all of the information from the interviews, physical assessment, and screening tests is collected and analyzed, summarize specific health and developmental achievements for the parents and child. Immunizations are provided as appropriate. (See Chapter 41 for the recommended immunization schedule.) 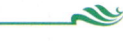 Anticipatory guidance may be offered at various points during the health supervision visit.

When a child is found to be at risk for a health condition, or an actual health problem is detected, follow-up care must be arranged. The child may need to return for another visit to the primary care provider for further evaluation, or referral to another provider may be needed. The nurse needs to learn about all of the available community resources to make appropriate referrals. The range of such services may include:

▶ Hospital and community-based health care specialists from many disciplines (dentists, physicians, physical therapists, speech therapists, nutritionists, social workers)

▶ Community-based programs (child-care centers, developmental stimulation programs, home visitor programs, early intervention programs, mental health centers, diagnostic and evaluation centers, schools, family support centers, food and nutrition referral centers, public health clinics, churches, and other organizations that support families and children)

Evaluation

Expected outcomes of nursing care include:

▶ The child and family collaborate with the health care provider in joint problem solving and decision making regarding the management of the child's condition after appropriate education and counseling.

▶ The child and family prepare for future health supervision visits by identifying questions or concerns they want to discuss.

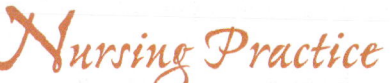

Following is a recommended schedule for health supervision visits from infancy through middle childhood:

Prenatal	6 months	3 years
Newborn	9 months	4 years
First week	1 year	5 years
1 month	15 months	6 years
2 months	18 months	8 years
4 months	2 years	10 years

(Green & Palfrey, 2000)

Health Supervision by Age Group
INFANCY (BIRTH TO 1 YEAR)

Health supervision visits occur frequently during the first year of life because growth and developmental changes are so rapid. Examples of developmental surveillance questions to use during infancy include the following:

• Do you have any specific concerns about Colin's development or behavior?

• How does Taneka communicate what she wants?

• How does Bruce move?

• What do you think Joshua understands?

• How does Tasha act around family members? And other people?

• Tell me about Emily's typical play.

Anticipatory guidance should focus on the infant's stages of rapid growth and development, injury prevention, and nutrition (e.g., adequate amounts of formula or breast milk, when to start solid foods, and avoidance of honey). See Chapters 31 and 32. Make sure the parents recognize their strengths in caring for the infant and other family members.

Health education focuses on issues such as colic, normal sleep patterns, sleep positions, dental hygiene, hand washing, bowel movements, skin and hair care, appropriate dress for weather, safe car transport, and prevention of sun-burn. Teach parents how to recognize signs of early illness in their children, including fever, failure to eat, vomiting, diarrhea, dehydration, unusual irritability or sleepiness, and skin rash.

EARLY CHILDHOOD (1 TO 5 YEARS)

Health supervision visits are needed frequently during early childhood for developmental surveillance, screening for health problems, and immunizations. Examples of developmental surveillance questions to ask during these visits include:

- Do you have any specific concerns about Jawan's development or behavior?
- How does Nicki communicate what she wants?
- What do you think Jerry understands?
- How does Penny get from one place to another?
- How does Kevin act around family members? Around other children?
- How does Lataye react to strangers?
- To what extent does Chris eat independently?
- Tell me about Jodie's typical play.

Anticipatory guidance should focus on promoting growth and development, nutrition, setting limits and discipline, toilet training, injury prevention, family activities, conflict with siblings, child care or play groups, and showing interest in the child's achievements. See Chapters 31 and 32.

Health education should focus on good nutrition; feeding and mealtime strategies; tooth brushing, fluoride supplements (as needed), and dental visits; the child's natural curiosity about genital differences and masturbation; safety approaching dogs; safe car transport; and management of common minor illnesses.

MIDDLE CHILDHOOD (5 TO 10 YEARS)

Health supervision visits occur less frequently during middle childhood as the health of most children is stable, growth has slowed, and screening for health conditions is needed less frequently. Examples of developmental surveillance questions to ask of both the parent and child during visits with children in this age range include:

- Do you have any specific concerns about Shanelle's development or behavior?
- How do you think Ben is performing in school? How is his attendance? Do you have any concerns about his grades?
- Does Shawn seem able to follow the rules at school?
- When Richie plays with other children, can he keep up with them?
- Is Marta proud of her achievements at school? Does she talk with you about what goes on at school? How

do you acknowledge or praise these achievements? Is she in any special classes?

- Have you visited Jorge's classroom? Do you participate in activities at his school? What does the teacher say about him during your parent–teacher conference?

Anticipatory guidance should focus on issues such as growth and development, school entry and educational progress, the growing influence of peers, injury prevention, sports safety, setting reasonable expectations, recognition of achievements, setting limits and discipline, respecting authority, promoting independence, and beginning to have responsibility for chores.

Health education should focus on oral health, nutrition, need for regular physical activity, and teaching the child about personal care and hygiene, preparation for puberty and sexual development, dangers of smoking and smokeless tobacco, and managing anger and resolving conflict. **WEB**

ADOLESCENCE (11 TO 18 YEARS)

Health supervision visits should occur annually during adolescence because of the dramatic changes occurring in physical, social, and emotional development. Adolescents need comprehensive clinical preventive services to deter them from participating in behaviors that jeopardize their health; to detect physical, emotional, and behavioral problems early; and to encourage behaviors that will promote healthy lifestyles (Department of Adolescent Health, 1996). See Table 35–4 for recommended health supervision activities by age.

Developmental surveillance questions should focus on physical, social, and emotional development (Figure 35–7 ◆). The assessment of health behaviors and developmental surveillance become more closely related as the adolescent becomes more heavily influenced by peers. Examples of questions to ask include the following:

- What do you do for fun? What is your favorite activity?
- Who is your best friend? What do you do together? About how many friends do you have? How old are your friends? What do you and your friends do outside of school?
- What are some of the things that worry you? Make you sad? Make you angry? What do you do about these things? Whom do you talk to about them? What do you do when you are really down or depressed? Do these feelings sometimes last more than a week? Have you ever been in trouble at school or with the law? Have you thought about running away? Have you ever thought about hurting yourself or killing yourself?
- What kind of changes have you noticed in your body over the past 6 months? Do you think you are developing pretty much like the rest of your friends? How

TABLE 35-4 Recommended Adolescent Preventive Health Services by Age and Procedure

	Age of Adolescent										
	Early				Middle			Late			
Procedure	11	12	13	14	15	16	17	18	19	20	21
Health guidance											
Parenting[a]			■			■					
Development	■	■	■	■	■	■	■	■	■	■	■
Diet and physical activity	■	■	■	■	■	■	■	■	■	■	■
Healthy lifestyles[b]	■	■	■	■	■	■	■	■	■	■	■
Injury prevention	■	■	■	■	■	■	■	■	■	■	■
Screening history											
Eating disorders	■	■	■	■	■	■	■	■	■	■	■
Sexual activity[c]	■	■	■	■	■	■	■	■	■	■	■
Alcohol and other drug use	■	■	■	■	■	■	■	■	■	■	■
Tobacco use	■	■	■	■	■	■	■	■	■	■	■
Abuse	■	■	■	■	■	■	■	■	■	■	■
School performance	■	■	■	■	■	■	■	■	■	■	■
Depression	■	■	■	■	■	■	■	■	■	■	■
Risk for suicide	■	■	■	■	■	■	■	■	■	■	■
Physical assessment											
Blood pressure	■	■	■	■	■	■	■	■	■	■	■
Body Mass Index	■	■	■	■	■	■	■	■	■	■	■
Comprehensive examination			■			■			■		
Tests											
Cholesterol			1			1			1		
TB			2			2			2		
GC, chlamydia, syphilis, and HPV			3			3			3		
HIV			4			4			4		
Pap smear			5			5			5		
Immunizations											
MMR		■									
Td		■				O					
Hepatitis B		■				6			6		
Hepatitis A			7			7			7		
Varicella			8			8			8		

[a]A parent health guidance visit is recommended during early and middle adolescence.
[b]Includes counseling regarding sexual behavior and avoidance of tobacco, alcohol, and other drug use.
[c]Includes history of unintended pregnancy and STD.

1. Screening test performed once if family history is positive for early cardiovascular disease or hyperlipidemia.
2. Screen if positive for exposure to active TB or lives/works in high-risk situation, e.g., homeless shelter, health care facility.

3. Screen at least annually if sexually active.
4. Screen if high risk for infection.
5. Screen annually if sexually active or if 18 years or older.
6. Vaccinate if high risk for hepatitis B infection.
7. Vaccinate if at risk for hepatitis A infection.
8. Vaccinate if no reliable history of chicken pox.
O. Do not give if administered in last 5 years.

Note: From Department of Adolescent Health (1996). *Guidelines for adolescent preventive services (GAPS).* Chicago: American Medical Association.

do you feel about these changes? Has anyone talked with you about what to expect as your body develops?

- How do you feel about your weight? Are you trying to change your weight? Do you ever fast, vomit, or take laxatives or diet pills to control your weight?
- How are you doing in school?
- What type of responsibilities do you have at home?

- Have you drunk alcohol in the last month? How much? What is the most you have ever had to drink? Have you ever tried other drugs? How often have you taken them in the past month? Do you ever drink and drive? Are you worried about any friends or family members and how much they drink and drive?
- Have you smoked any cigarettes in the last month? Chewed tobacco?

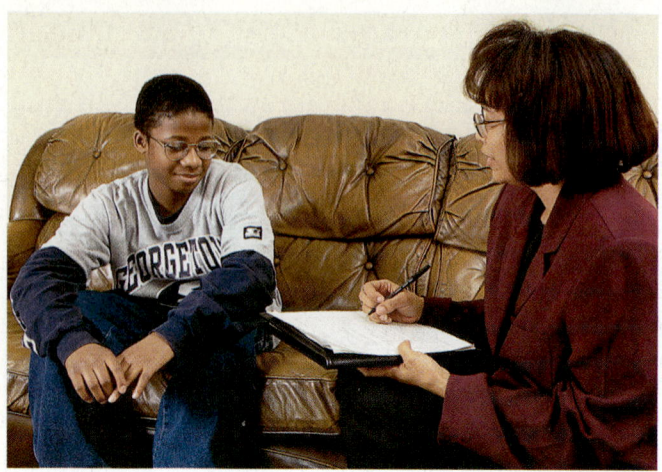

FIGURE 35–7. ◆ With adolescents, in contrast to the earlier developmental stages, developmental surveillance questions should be directed to the child rather than the parent.

- Do your friends pressure you to do things you don't want to do? How do you handle that?
- Have you started dating? Do you date one person or go out as a group? Do you have a steady partner? Are you happy with dating or with this relationship?
- Have you ever been frightened by violent or sexual things someone has said to you? Has anyone ever tried to harm you physically? Has anyone ever touched you in a way you don't like? Forced you to have sex?
- How do you get along with members of your family? What would you like to change about your family if you could?
- Do you own a gun or have access to one?

Anticipatory guidance should focus on future healthy behaviors such as the following: school achievement, identification of talents and interests to pursue, how to deal with stress, use of protective sports gear, use of car safety belts, violence prevention, and use of sun screen to prevent skin cancer. See Chapters 32 and 52. ⌒

Health education should focus on the avoidance of tobacco products, drugs, and alcohol; sexuality and sexual activity options (abstinence, contraception, and safe sex); and good health behaviors including nutrition, oral health, exercise, and sleep. ⌒ **WEB**

HEALTH PROMOTION FOR CHILDREN IN COMMUNITY SETTINGS

What nursing care does the child with a chronic illness need in different community health care settings? How can nurses ease the transition back to school for the child with a chronic condition? How do nurses identify families that need extra support to care for their child at home? Nursing care in all community health care settings (home, school, specialty clinic, primary care office) is focused on minimiz-

ing the impact of the health condition on the child's physical and emotional development and functioning.

Episodic Care for Illnesses and Injuries

During childhood, most children have several episodes of illnesses and injuries that require health care. In most cases, care is provided by the primary health care provider. At other times, the urgency of the condition requires that the child go to an urgent care center or emergency department. The nurse's role in the cases of these episodic health care visits includes the following:

- Collecting health information about the condition
- Performing an assessment
- Assisting the primary care provider with any diagnostic or therapeutic procedures
- Educating the child and family about care of the child at home and how to identify any signs that the health problem is getting more serious

Care of the Child with Special Health Care Needs

Children with a **chronic condition,** a condition that lasts or is expected to last 3 months or more, are also defined as *children with special health care needs*. Many have **disabilities,** impairment in one or more of five categories of function (cognition, communication, motor abilities, social abilities, or patterns of interactions). The overall incidence of children with chronic conditions has not changed much in the last 20 years. The number of years of survival of these children has changed with technology, surgical techniques, and other health care advances (Jackson, 2000). Most children with chronic conditions are cared for in the home without home nursing or other health care services. Children with chronic health conditions need regular health supervision, as well as additional health services to help the child and family manage the condition.

Health promotion, disease prevention, and anticipatory guidance have greater significance for the child with special health care needs. This child already has a condition that places him or her at higher risk for other problems, such as infectious diseases, injury, or developmental delay. The goal is to permit the child to have as normal a childhood as possible.

Growth and Development

"Children with special health care needs are those who have or are at risk for a chronic physical, developmental, behavioral, or emotional condition and who also require health and related services of a type or amount beyond that required by children generally" (McPherson, Arango, Fox, et. al., 1998). Of the 12.6 million U.S. children younger than 18 years, 18% match the definition for children with special health care needs (Newacheck, McManus, Fox, et al., 2000).

The provider of care for children with chronic conditions varies by the type of condition, type of health insurance coverage, preferences of the family, and availability of pediatric specialty resources. Most children with chronic conditions, such as asthma, have a primary care provider. The primary care provider is usually the most knowledgeable about local community resources that may help the child and family. The child is often referred to pediatric specialists, as needed, for a review of the management of the child's health condition, and to make new recommendations according to the child's health status.

A pediatric specialist and advanced practice nurses may collaborate with the primary care provider to coordinate care of the child with chronic conditions, such as spina bifida, cystic fibrosis, or diabetes mellitus. In this manner, the child benefits from the most current health care guidelines and expertise in care for the specific condition. The child and family usually retain a primary care provider, who provides health supervision care and episodic illness care while serving as the child's advocate in the larger health care system. Sometimes a pediatric specialist serves as the child's primary care provider, but it is important to make sure regular health supervision services are not forgotten during the care of acute exacerbations of the chronic condition. Some children with chronic conditions may even require additional health supervision visits for added immunizations, such as meningococcal and influenza vaccines.

Nurses working in hospital specialty clinics and other community settings can help ensure that these children receive the appropriate health supervision services. The nurse in a tertiary care facility needs to identify appropriate resources and to help the family connect with those existing in the child's community. This is a greater challenge if the child and family have traveled a distance to obtain the specialty services. It is often best to make sure the child has a primary care provider in the home community to provide regular care and to help coordinate local community resources.

The role of the nurse in caring for the chronically ill child in a community setting includes providing health supervision, teaching the parents to manage the child's care at home, providing guidelines to promote the child's growth and development, monitoring the child's health status, and referring the family to appropriate community services. Nurses providing care to children with specific chronic conditions need the following knowledge and skills (Jackson, 2000):

- Knowledge of the pathophysiology of the chronic condition and anticipated disease trajectory

- Knowledge of child and family reactions to the stress of the chronic condition

- The ability to work with the family in their efforts to manage the child's normal growth and development

- The ability to provide culturally sensitive care to the child and family experiencing a chronic health condition

- Assessment skills to identify any changes in the child's condition requiring referral or consultation

- The ability to communicate effectively with appropriate health professionals regarding any changes in the child's physical or psychosocial health

- The ability to work collaboratively with other health professionals

- Knowledge of resources (community agencies, tertiary care centers, specialty professionals) appropriate for the child and family with a chronic condition

- The ability to identify a dysfunctional family needing intervention

For example, the recommended care of children with asthma has changed from episodic care for acute asthma attacks with minimal daily management to guidelines for aggressive daily management by the child and family (Figure 35–8 ◆). Recognition of early warning signs of an asthma attack can lead to the initiation of extra medications in an effort to avert a severe attack. (See Chapter 42 for a discussion of asthma management.) ⊂⊃ Refer to "Nursing Care Plan: The Child with Asthma in the Community Setting" for strategies that can be used when working with the child and family to improve asthma management.

Nursing in a School Setting

School nurses work to remove or minimize the health barriers to learning so students can perform academically. Nursing actions for all children focus on the following strategies:

- Reducing infectious disease transmission so school attendance is improved

- Promoting healthy behaviors through health education for many different and diverse audiences

- Providing safe school facilities by inspecting the school environment for hazards

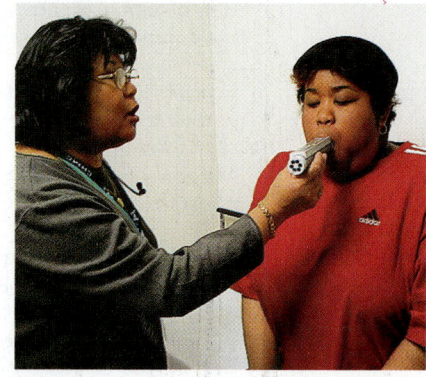

FIGURE 35–8. ◆ Nurses provide patient education to help families learn to recognize the early stages of an asthma attack by using a peak flow meter. The child learns the proper method for taking a deep breath and blowing into the peak flow meter so the best reading is obtained.

GOAL	INTERVENTION	RATIONALE	EXPECTED OUTCOME

1. Family coping: Potential for growth related to increased control of asthma with daily therapeutic care

GOAL	INTERVENTION	RATIONALE	EXPECTED OUTCOME
The child and parents will work in partnership with the nurse to improve the child's asthma management.	*NIC Priority Intervention:* **Family support:** *Promotion of family interests and goals* ▶ Listen to the family's concerns about asthma management and respond with information to correct any misconceptions. ▶ Teach the family skills (assessment, use of equipment, and giving medications) for managing the child's asthma attacks. ▶ Provide telephone consultation to the parents during management of the first few asthma attacks. ▶ Educate the parents about when to call for future medical advice or to seek emergency treatment.	▶ The parents' concerns may not be the same as the nurse's. If the parents' concerns are not addressed, the parents may not comply with recommended care. ▶ Proper use of equipment and appropriate medication dosage will help alleviate asthma symptoms. ▶ Support and reinforcement of learning during an asthma attack will increase the parents' confidence in managing future attacks. ▶ Parents need guidelines for judging the severity of asthma attacks.	*NOC Suggested Outcome:* None developed for this nursing diagnosis The parents express greater confidence in averting and managing their child's asthma attacks.

2. Management of therapeutic regimen, family ineffective related to knowledge deficit

GOAL	INTERVENTION	RATIONALE	EXPECTED OUTCOME
The child and parents will recognize early signs of an asthma attack and begin taking medications.	*NIC Priority Intervention:* **Family involvement:** *Facilitating family participation in the emotional and physical care of the patient* ▶ Teach the child and parents to use a peak flow meter. ▶ Help the child recognize his or her personal best peak flow and range indicating development of asthma symptoms. ▶ Teach the family and child to give medications when the peak flow falls to the yellow range. ▶ Teach the child and family to monitor the child's response to medications with peak flow meter.	▶ The peak flow meter helps quantify changes in respiratory status before symptoms are detected. ▶ Identifying a personal best peak flow helps establish the ranges to be used for future symptom identification. ▶ Giving medications before an asthma attack becomes established may help avert the actual attack. ▶ Monitoring the response gives the family information to determine when home care is inadequate and medical intervention is needed.	*NOC Suggested Outcome:* None developed for this nursing diagnosis The number of asthma attacks requiring medical intervention is reduced.

3. Health maintenance altered, related to lack of school asthma management plan

GOAL	INTERVENTION	RATIONALE	EXPECTED OUTCOME
An individual school health plan (ISHP) will be developed to help control and manage the child's asthma symptoms.	*NIC Priority Intervention:* **Health system guidance:** *Facilitating a patient's location and use of appropriate health services* ▶ Provide the family with educational materials to give to the school nurse and school administrators. ▶ Advocate for all children to have an asthma management plan developed. ▶ Support the family to have a school health plan that includes the physician's written orders customized for the child. ▶ Include in the ISHP participation in regular school/class activities such as field trips and physical education, and what to do if asthma symptoms occur at school. ▶ Help the family to obtain extra equipment and medications that can be provided to the school.	▶ School personnel need the latest information about effective asthma management in school settings. ▶ Establishing a school policy will help all children with asthma receive appropriate care. ▶ The child with severe asthma needs a personalized care plan to be most successful in controlling asthma attacks. ▶ Participation, even with modification or premedication, prior to activities promotes self-esteem and peer relationships. ▶ Schools will provide care, but the families must provide all supplies, equipment, and medications.	*NOC Suggested Outcome:* **Health-promoting behavior:** *Actions to sustain or promote optimal wellness, recovery, and rehabilitation* Implementation of the school health plan reduces the number of school absences for asthma attacks that occur during school hours and increases participation in school activities.

GOAL	INTERVENTION	RATIONALE	EXPECTED OUTCOME
	▶ Work with the parents and school nurse to teach the specific asthma interventions to a designated person in the school nurse's absence.	▶ School nurses often travel between several schools. The school administrator or secretary often serves as the backup care provider.	

4. Self-esteem disturbance (child) related to need to seek special care during school hours

GOAL	INTERVENTION	RATIONALE	EXPECTED OUTCOME
	NIC Priority Intervention: **Self-esteem enhancement:** *Assisting a patient to increase his/her personal judgment of self-worth*		*NOC Suggested Outcome:* **Child development, middle childhood:** *Milestones of physical, cognitive, and psychosocial progression by 8 years of age*
The child's improved control over asthma will increase his or her self-esteem and peer relationships.	▶ Assess the child's peer relationships and opportunities for age-appropriate interactions. ▶ Motivate the child and family to gain increased control of asthma so the child can participate in normal childhood activities. ▶ Identify types of conflict and teasing the child experiences with peers, and teach the child defense tactics to deal with them.	▶ Assessment is important to identify the best strategies to support the child and family. ▶ Motivation may increase compliance with recommended daily asthma control interventions. ▶ If the child is able to gain some control over these situations, his or her self-esteem will be improved.	The child establishes friendships and engages in activities with peers.

- Assessing health status and screening children for health conditions common among school-age children (such as vision and hearing impairments, and scoliosis) (Figure 35–9 ◆)

- Referral and management of acute and chronic health conditions

- Participating as the health specialist on the team developing a child's individual education plan (IEP) and individual school health plan (ISHP)

- Building effective student–family–school–community support systems

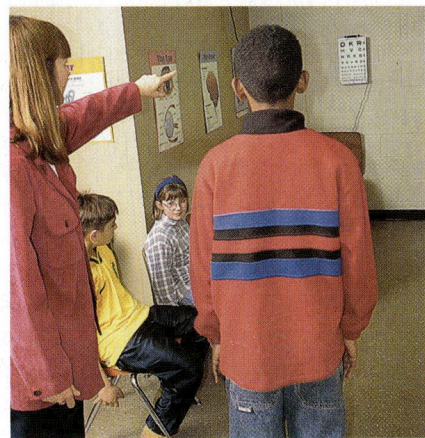

FIGURE 35–9. ◆ The school is often the setting for screening tests of large groups of students at risk for a problem. Screening tests are often organized so all children in a particular grade are assessed, as in this test to detect vision problems.

Table 35–5 presents standards of school nursing care. *Healthy People 2010* includes a specific national objective for the health education of children in school settings to prevent health problems such as unintentional injury, violence, suicide, tobacco use and addiction, alcohol and other drug use, unintended pregnancy, HIV/AIDS, and STD infection, unhealthy dietary patterns, inadequate physical activity, and environmental health. ⊂⊃ **WEB**

Emergency preparedness is important and a plan of managing the emergency care of all students should be developed. Injuries and acute illnesses occur frequently during school hours. School personnel (administrators, secretaries, and health aides in the absence of the school nurse) need to be trained to distinguish between an emergency and an urgent problem that parents should be called to manage. Guidelines for activation of the community's emergency medical services (EMS) should be developed in collaboration with the local EMS agency.

Children with chronic conditions may have special challenges when attending school. An ISHP, developed collaboratively by the parent, child, school nurse, school administrator, and teachers, is a formal mechanism to ensure that the child's health needs are managed in the school setting (Figure 35–10 ◆). The nursing process is the format used for development of the ISHP. In some cases the health plan is integrated into the child's IEP or individual family service plan (IFSP). The information in this plan is treated confidentially, but stored in an easily accessible area for personnel who may have to provide care. The parent provides medications, supplies, and equipment along with the physician's written instructions for care.

TABLE 35–5   Standards of Professional School Nursing Practice

1. The school nurse collects client data.
2. The school nurse analyzes the assessment data in determining nursing diagnoses.
3. The school nurse identifies expected outcomes individualized to the client.
4. The school nurse develops a plan of care/action that specifies interventions to attain expected outcomes.
5. The school nurse implements the interventions identified in the plan of care/action.
6. The school nurse evaluates the client's progress toward attainment of outcomes.
7. The school nurse systematically evaluates the quality and effectiveness of school nursing practice.
8. The school nurse evaluates one's own nursing practice in relation to professional practice standards and relevant statutes, regulations, and policies.
9. The school nurse acquires and maintains current knowledge and competency in school nursing practice.
10. The school nurse interacts with and contributes to the professional development of peers and school personnel as colleagues.
11. The school nurse's decisions and actions on behalf of clients are determined in an ethical manner.
12. The school nurse collaborates with the student, family, school staff, community, and other providers in providing student care.
13. The school nurse promotes use of research findings in school nursing practice.
14. The school nurse considers factors related to safety, effectiveness, and cost when planning and delivering care.
15. The school nurse uses effective written, verbal, and nonverbal communication skills.
16. The school nurse manages school health services.
17. The school nurse assists students, families, school staff, and community to achieve optimal levels of wellness through appropriately designed and delivered health education.

Note: Permission granted for reprint from National Association of School Nurses Inc. (1999). *Standard of professional school nursing practice.* Castle Rock, CO. Adapted.

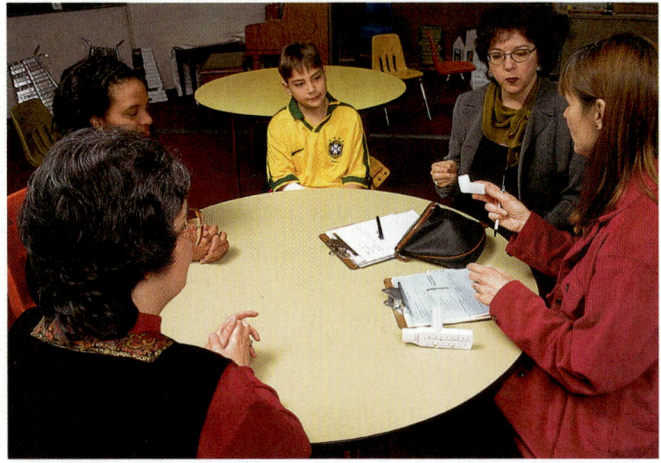

FIGURE 35–10. ◆ Because some children need medications or other therapies during school hours, the parents and child, school nurse, teacher, and school administrators develop a plan to manage the child's condition during school hours. This document is the child's individual school health plan.

Thinking Critically

ASTHMA ATTACKS AT SCHOOL

Carrie, 8 years old, is anxious because her asthma attack is getting worse. Her teacher sees that she is having trouble breathing, so she sends her to the school health office for treatment. Carrie has such severe asthma that a nebulizer is kept at school for her to use. This treatment often relieves Carrie's symptoms and permits her to return to classes. However, in this case, the asthma attack does not respond to the treatment, and the school contacts her mother to come pick her up from school. This means another visit to the emergency department for treatment.

Carrie does not like to miss school or to worry her mother. Her mother wishes there were some way to reduce the number and severity of her asthma attacks.

What are some possible triggers of Carrie's asthma attacks at school? What measures can be taken to control her asthma on a daily basis and reduce the number of attacks? What special arrangements are needed to permit a child to receive care for asthma or another chronic condition while at school? What education does the teacher need to make an assessment and decision for Carrie to go to get her treatment? [WEB]

The ISHP should include directions for the care of the child on the bus, on field trips, and during extracurricular activities. In some cases, school and bus personnel must be trained to care for the child who needs medications or has special equipment, including special precautions when providing care. The school nurse often trains the personnel responsible for providing care.

When a child returns to school following the diagnosis of a chronic condition or a significant change in condition, the child's nurse (in either the hospital or community setting) can help with the child's transition back to the classroom. Contact the school administrators and school nurse. Work with the family to begin preparing teachers and school administrators for the child's special needs. Send educational materials about the child's condition to the school. Often an ISHP must be developed or modified. Work with the child's family and teachers to prepare classmates for the visible changes they will see in the child, such as resulting from an injury. Help them understand more about the child's condition and the importance of having the child get medication before the symptoms worsen.

Nurse's Role in Other Community Settings

In several other settings in the community, the nurse's role may parallel that in a school setting. Promoting health and preventing disease and injury are equally important in child care centers, camps, health department clinics, and disaster or homeless shelters. For example, nurses work with child care center administrators to address infection control issues and to assess the safety of the children's environment. Nurses in camps assess the safety of the children's environment, but also provide nursing care to children with acute illnesses and injuries and plan activities to promote health. Some special camps for children with chronic conditions must have trained personnel to provide needed medical and nursing care while children are participating in recreational activities. Children in health department clinics and shelters need health supervision services as well as linkage with other community resources to promote health.

FAMILY ASSESSMENT

The strength, resilience, coping skills, and resources of a child's family plays a major role in fostering the child's growth and development, as well as managing the child's health problems. When providing care to children in all settings, taking time to assess the family will be helpful when planning and providing nursing care that corresponds to the family's values, resources, and abilities. Collect information about the family's structure, home and community environments, occupation and education, and cultural characteristics. Information about the way the family functions in nurturing its members, problem solving, and communicating may help identify potentially more effective strategies for management of the child's health care. Tables 33–4 and 33–7, in Chapter 33, provide suggestions for information that should be collected for the family assessment.

A chronic illness or disability adds a dimension of developmental risk for an infant, child, or youth. The child and family members can respond with either psychologic or behavioral problems. Families need support to increase their resources and coping behaviors so they can successfully manage the multiple stressors, strains, and hassles of daily living along with the child's chronic condition.

Resilient families bounce back from the stresses and challenges while adapting to successfully manage the child's chronic illness or disability. These families have effective coping behaviors and the ability to acquire and maintain needed resources for managing the demands of the child's condition. Characteristics of a resilient family include (Patterson, 1991):

- Balancing the child's illness with other family needs
- Forming collaborative relationships with health care professionals
- Maintaining a professional relationship rather than a friendship relationship with providers

- Developing competence in communication skills
- Maintaining family flexibility and adapting to changing circumstances
- Maintaining a commitment to the family as a unit
- Attributing positive meaning to the situation
- Maintaining supportive relationships outside the family
- Engaging in active coping efforts with effective and efficient problem-solving abilities

Most families do not naturally develop resilience. Often, nursing support is needed to help family members learn new skills, make adaptations, and gain confidence in their abilities to manage the challenges they face. Nurses need to help families identify their strengths and areas for improvement that will lead to increased resiliency.

Nursing Management

Nursing Assessment and Diagnosis

FAMILY ASSESSMENT TOOLS

Several family assessment tools help measure family coping and functioning. Identification of family strengths and deficits gives nurses information that can be used to support family development—to reinforce family functioning, for family education, for intervention directed to meet special needs, and for referrals to community resources for long-term follow-up.

The Family APGAR is a good initial screening tool that focuses on the family's adaptation, partnership, growth, affection, and resolve (Table 35–6). The five-item questionnaire can be administered quickly. All family members are asked to complete the questionnaire, so the nurse gains a picture of the family's perspective on family functioning. Be more concerned if the majority of responses fall in the "hardly ever" category or responses vary a lot among family members. This may indicate a family that needs much more support to cope with the demands of daily life and management of the child's condition. Discuss the findings with the family members.

The Family Profile (Table 35–7) is another family assessment tool that will be of help when parents are caring for a child with special health care needs in the home. The parents complete this survey of their resources and current use of community services. This assessment may set the stage for the family to become a fully collaborative partner in caring for the child with a serious chronic condition.

HOME ASSESSMENT TOOLS

Assess the home environment to determine factors that promote the child's growth and development. Both assessments help when planning care to promote safety for the child and strategies to promote the child's development.

The Home Observation for Measurement of the Environment (HOME) is an assessment tool that measures the

TABLE 35-6   The Family APGAR Questionnaire

Part I

The following questions have been designed to help us better understand you and your family. You should feel free to ask questions about any item in the questionnaire.

The space for comments should be used when you wish to give additional information or if you wish to discuss the way the question is applied to your family. Please try to answer all questions.

Family is defined as the individual(s) with whom you usually live. If you live alone, your "family" consists of persons with whom you now have the strongest emotional lies.[a]

For each question, check only one box

	Almost always	Some of the time	Hardly ever
I am satisfied that I can turn to my family for help when something is troubling me.	☐	☐	☐
Comments: _____			
I am satisfied with the way my family talks over things with me and shares problems with me.	☐	☐	☐
Comments: _____			
I am satisfied that my family accepts and supports my wishes to take on new activities or directions.	☐	☐	☐
Comments: _____			
I am satisfied with the way my family expresses affection and responds to my emotions, such as anger, sorrow, and love.	☐	☐	☐
Comments: _____			
I am satisfied with the way my family and I share time together.			
Comments: _____			

[a]According to which member of the family is being interviewed the interviewer may substitute for the word "family" either spouse, significant other, parents, or children.
Note: From Smilkstein, G. (1978). The family APGAR: A proposal for a family function test and its use by physicians. *Journal of Family Practice, 6*(6), 1231–1239.

quality and quantity of stimulation and support available to the child in the home environment (Caldwell & Bradley, 1984) (Figure 35–11 ◆). Four age-specific scales are available (birth to 3 years, 3 to 6 years, 6 to 10 years, and 10 to 15 years). Examples of subscales within each age-specific scale include parental responsivity, acceptance of child, the physical environment, learning materials, variety in experience, and parental involvement. Data are collected during an informal, low-stress interview and observation over approximately an hour. The child must be awake during the majority of the interview. Observation of the parent–child interaction is an essential part of the assessment. The intent is to allow family members to act normally.

Several nursing diagnoses may result from the family and home assessment, among them:

▶ *Risk for caregiver role strain* related to child with a newly diagnosed chronic condition and its financial burden

▶ *Impaired social interaction (parents and child)* related to lack of family or respite support for community interaction

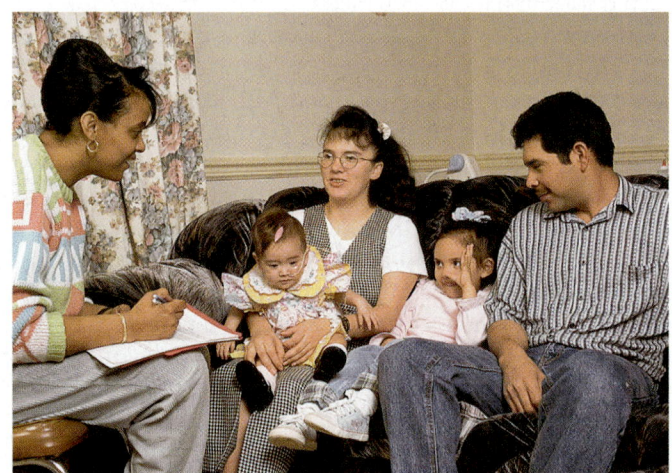

FIGURE 35–11. ◆ A visit to the home when all family members are present provides the best information for completion of an assessment tool such as the Home Observation for Measurement of the Environment (HOME).

TABLE 35-7   Questions from the Family Profile

Family Structure/Roles

Do you want to care for your child at home?

Are you aware of any alternatives to home care?

Who are your child's primary caregivers?

Who are the other members of your household?

Can you identify another person to act as backup caregiver for your child?

Are there others (friends/family members) who can assist you with your child with special needs, with your other children, or with your family obligations?

Medical Management

Have you completed the hospital training in your child's care? If no, what is left to learn?

Has your child's backup caregiver completed training? If no, what is left to learn?

Do you or your backup caregiver need refresher training for anything?

Do you have transportation to medical appointments?

Do you need help in selecting a nursing provider?

Do you need help in selecting a vendor?

Nutrition

How is your child fed? If formula, will you need help to buy/locate the formula?

Have you applied for WIC?

Does your child have a special need for diapers that is greater than the norm?

Education

Will your child be going out to school?

Do you know which school your child will attend?

Has your child been referred for the Infant and Toddler program?

Do you have an IFSP for your child? An IEP?

Do you have a contact person in the school program?

Will your child need adaptive equipment at home?

Parenting/Child Care

What hours/shifts do you think you will need nursing care for your child?

In the event you need to leave home quickly or if you become incapacitated, who will watch your child with special needs? Your other children?

What is your plan for child care in the event of the nurse's absence?

Will you need help in finding child care for your other children?

Do you work outside the home? Any plans for the future?

Do you go to school? Any plans for the future?

Financial Resources

Does your child have medical insurance? Are your other children covered under a family insurance plan?

Do you need more information about or referrals to WIC, SSI, TANF, Food Stamps, housing, respite care?

Do you need help in obtaining everyday supplies for your child?

Do you need a referral for help in obtaining other items for your child, such as furniture, clothing, toys?

Do you need help with budgeting?

Community Resources

Are you involved with any other helping agencies or persons, especially those you would like to include in this planning process?

Do you or other family members belong to a church? Social groups? Clubs? Associations?

Would you like to talk to another parent who has a child with special needs?

Would you like a referral to a support group?

Do you want a referral for counseling? Individual? Marital? Family? Child? Sibling?

Family Life

Do you see your child's homecoming as making a significant change in your lifestyle, and if so, how?

Do you have concerns about your other children?

Can you describe how you see your child in a few months? What are your short-term goals for your child?

Can you describe how you see your child in a few years? What are your long-term goals for your child?

How would you describe your family strengths?

What are your family's needs at this time?

Note: From McCord, B. (1993). *Family profile.* Millersville, MD: Coordinating Center for Home and Community Care.

▶ *Risk for altered parent/child attachment* related to child's dependence on technology

Planning and Implementation

Work to establish a therapeutic relationship with the family. This relationship should be characterized by empathy and trust, as well as the development of mutually identified goals for the child's care. To help families develop resiliency, focus on family competence and strengths. Acknowledge and validate their emotions. Provide information in a clear, timely, and sensitive manner. Ask questions that help direct the family's thinking rather than providing them with all of the answers. Work with families to create solutions until they are able to solve problems independently (Patterson, 1995). Linkage with other families who have faced similar situations may be helpful.

Refer families with moderate or severe dysfunctioning to community resources for social support and counseling as appropriate. Make sure the family has a coordinator of care, especially when a family member seems to be unable to assume the case management role initially. When families seem unable to use referrals and recommendations for identifying and obtaining community assistance, the nurse can help in some additional ways (Taylor & Edwards, 1995):

▶ Call and act as the family's advocate.

▶ Help with role rehearsal.

▶ Provide instructions and support.

▶ Connect the family with a volunteer who can accompany the family to services.

▶ Perform case management services or refer the family for them.

Evaluation

Expected outcomes of nursing care include:

▶ The family assumes the role of case manager or works effectively with an assigned case manager with interventions by nurses and the health care team.

▶ The care needed by the child with a chronic condition is provided by the family according to recommended guidelines.

HOME HEALTH CARE NURSING

Home health care is a component of the continuum of comprehensive health care provided to individuals and families in their home. Many children needing home health care are **medically fragile,** children who need skilled nursing care with or without medical equipment to support vital functions. Only 2% to 5% of these children have chronic conditions serious enough to need regular home health care services (Ahmann, 1996). Home health care services may also be provided for short intervals to help families during their child's acute recovery, such as a child with osteomyelitis receiving home antibiotic infusion therapy. There are two major goals of working with families in the home care setting:

• Promoting or restoring health while attempting to minimize the effects of the disability and illness, including terminal illness

• Promoting child or family self-care capacity in the home

Home care nursing is focused on assisting a family to gain a greater ability to manage the care of a child with a chronic condition more independently. The home is also seen as a much better environment to promote the child's growth and development.

Parents and other care providers without backgrounds in health care are given tremendous responsibilities to provide technology-assisted health care to their child. Technology assistance includes any of the following: ventilators; tracheostomies; suctioning; nasogastric, gastrostomy, or parenteral feeding with feeding pumps; intravenous fluids and medications with intravenous pumps. In some cases,

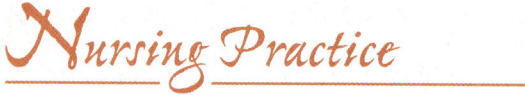

Nursing Practice

Classifications of medically fragile children include:

▶ Children with prolonged dependence on a medical device required to sustain life (mechanical ventilators, intravenous nutrition or drugs, tracheostomy, suctioning, oxygen, or tube feedings)

▶ Children with prolonged dependence on other medical devices that compensate for vital body functions who require daily or near daily nursing care (apnea monitors, renal dialysis, urinary catheters, and colostomies) (Office of Technology Assessment, 1987)

families have created mini–intensive care units in their home. Examples of some serious chronic conditions cared for by families in the home include children with congenital heart defects before corrective surgery, bronchopulmonary dysplasia, and cancer in its terminal stage.

Health care systems (health care providers and insurers) are challenged to simultaneously address the child's illness and developmental needs while providing the support needed by these families so that children do well in their environments. The family also needs help to support the growing child in the school and other peer settings.

To work in the home care setting, nurses need a variety of skills:

• Knowledge and experience in acute care practice with various medical technologies to work with these children. These skills enable nurses to provide direct care, teach the family and child self-care practices, and monitor the child's progress. This may involve collaboration with other health care team members.

• Community assessment skills; an understanding of community resources, financing mechanisms, and multiagency collaboration; and good communication skills (Taylor & Edwards, 1995). Understanding these resources helps nurses to assist families to find the most supportive services to match the child's and family's needs.

• Skill in educating family members to assume care of the child.

Nursing Management

Nursing Assessment and Diagnosis

Assessment in the home is focused on the child being cared for, the family's strengths and coping, and use of community resources.

TRANSITION FROM THE HOSPITAL

For most children, home health care is initiated after an acute hospitalization. The hospital or home care nurse can be responsible for coordinating and linking the transition steps. Clinical care guidelines or case management are methods for promoting a smooth transition. Expected outcomes for the child are documented. The home care nurse works in collaboration with hospital nurses by assessing the following:

▶ Caregiver readiness

▶ Home readiness (safe sleeping arrangements, adequate supplies, ability to meet nutritional and fluid needs, telephone access, heat, electricity, refrigeration, and lack of any communicable diseases in the home). Consider any features of the child's home environment that could cause an acute illness. For example, use of a wood stove or fireplace for heating could cause respiratory distress; renovation of a house built before 1960 could expose the child to lead dust.

Nursing Practice

Assess the home environment for potential hazards related to the child's age, condition, and requirements for technology-assisted care. For example, are extension cords needed to reach electric outlets? The equipment may lose power if someone trips over the cord and disconnects it by mistake.

Nursing diagnoses that could apply as the child transitions from the hospital to home setting include the following:

▶ Ineffective management of therapeutic regimen: Family related to complexity of therapeutic regimen and excessive demands made on the family

▶ Health-seeking behaviors related to information misinterpretation

Planning and Implementation

Nurses help families in the home setting in the following ways (Ahmann, 1996):

▶ Assuring competent care to the child

▶ Providing information about the child's condition and community resources

▶ Assisting families in time management skills and patient care management

▶ Advocating for increased insurance coverage or locating other sources of financial assistance

▶ Identifying appropriate programs in the community such as respite care, therapeutic recreation, or educational opportunities

Developing Cultural Competence

When providing care in the home, recognize potential conflicts between "mainstream" medical care and the family's cultural preferences after carefully listening to the parents' perspectives. Learn and use the family's perspectives of health and disease in discussions and in development of the plan of care (Ahmann, 1996).

Recognize that control belongs to the family in the home care setting. The parents are the employer with the ability to hire and fire. Every interaction is negotiated with the family, or between the family and child if there are differences in what they want. The nurse must be flexible and able to set aside power. House rules for such things as parking, private areas in the home, routines, and discipline of the child must all be followed. Role expectations of the nurse must be clearly understood to reduce stress in the

Nursing Practice

Home care assumes the presence of the child's primary caregiver. Invasive treatments and decisions for provision of emergency care to avoid serious risk to life and limb require informed consent. When the caregiver is not present and the home care nurse provides such care, the home health care agency and the nurse are at significant liability risk (Hogue, 1993).

family. The success of home care is also based upon effective cultural communication.

The range of nursing care activities that may be included in a child's care plan in the home setting include sensory stimulation, routines of daily living, positioning and skin care with gentle handling, respiratory care, nutrition and elimination, medications, and other supportive therapies. A plan for safe evacuation of the home is needed in case of fire. An emergency care plan should be developed for the child that includes an emergency medical history readily available to emergency care providers. The emergency health care provider needs enough information to understand the basics of the child's problem, to prevent delays in disease-specific treatment, and to minimize unnecessary interventions until the child's personal physician can be consulted. The family also needs to notify the emergency medical services agency and the power company that there is a technology-assisted child in the home. Backup generators may be needed if electrical power for life-sustaining equipment is essential. Meeting the child and family before an emergency will help emergency medical technicians be better prepared to care for the child with special health care needs.

Nursing Practice

Special medical problems can develop quickly in a child with severe and complex medical problems. An emergency information form should provide a summary of the child's medical history, baseline physical findings, and important and unique management requirements (American Academy of Pediatrics, 1999).

Evaluation

Expected outcomes of nursing care include:

▶ Care of the child's medical needs are integrated into the family's routines when possible.

▶ The family has an emergency care plan for the child in case of a disaster or weather emergency, or in case the child's condition suddenly worsens.

CHAPTER HIGHLIGHTS

🔊 Care in the community involves health supervision, care for episodic illnesses or injuries, and assisting families to manage their child's chronic health condition.

🔊 Working with the child and family in the community setting requires an understanding of how the larger environment influences the child's health and development and integration of that knowledge into the nursing care plan.

🔊 Health supervision is the provision of services that focus on disease and injury prevention, growth and developmental surveillance, and health promotion at key intervals during the child's life.

🔊 Anticipatory guidance provides the family with information about what to expect during the child's current and future stage of development on topics such as healthy habits; prevention of illness, injury, and poisoning; nutrition; oral health; and sexuality.

🔊 During episodic care for illnesses and injuries the nurse collects health information, assesses the child, assists the primary care provider with diagnostic or therapeutic procedures, and educates the child and family about care of the child at home.

🔊 Caring for the chronically ill child in the community includes health supervision and monitoring the child's health status, teaching the family to manage the child's condition and promote the child's growth and development, and making referrals to community resources.

🔊 An individualized school health plan describes the school-based care of the child with a chronic condition for optimal participation in school and class activities.

🔊 Family assessment tools help nurses identify the family strengths and deficits to support family development and coping.

🔊 Home care nursing focuses on helping the family to gain the ability to manage the child with a chronic condition more independently.

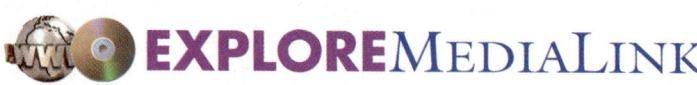

EXPLORE MediaLink

NCLEX Review, Case Studies, and other interactive resources for this chapter can be found on the companion website at http://www.prenhall.com/london. Click on "Chapter 35" to select the activities for this chapter.

For animations, more NCLEX review questions, and an audio glossary, access the accompanying CD-ROM in this textbook.

REFERENCES

Ahmann, E. (1996). *Home care for the high risk infant: A family centered approach* (2nd ed.). Gaithersburg, MD: Aspen Publishers.

American Academy of Pediatrics Committee on Pediatric Emergency Medicine. (1999). Emergency preparedness of children with special health care needs. *Pediatrics, 104*(4), e53.

Caldwell, B. M., & Bradley, R. H. (1984). *The Home Observation for Measurement of the Environment*. Little Rock: University of Arkansas.

Curry, D. M., & Duby, J. C. (1994). Developmental surveillance by pediatric nurses. *Pediatric Nursing, 20*(1), 40–44.

Deloian, B. J. (1997). Screening tests. In J. A. Fox (Ed.), *Primary health care of children* (pp. 148–157). St. Louis, MO: Mosby.

Department of Adolescent Health. (1996). *Guidelines for adolescent preventive services (GAPS)*. Chicago: American Medical Association.

Glascoe, F. P. (1999). Using parents' concerns to detect and address developmental and behavioral problems. *Journal of the Society of Pediatric Nurses, 4*(1), 24–35.

Green, M., & Palfrey, J. S. (2000). *Bright futures: Guidelines for health supervision of infants, children, and adolescents* (2nd ed.). Arlington, VA: National Center for Education in Maternal and Child Health.

Hogue, E. (1993). Care in the absence of primary caregivers. *Pediatric Nursing, 19*(1), 49–50.

Jackson, P. L. (2000). The primary care provider and children with chronic conditions. In P. L. Jackson & J. A. Vessey (Eds.), *Primary care of the child with a chronic condition* (3rd ed., pp. 3–19). St. Louis, MO:Mosby.

McPherson, M., Arango, P., Fox, H., Lauver, C., McManus, M., Newacheck, P. W., et al. (1998). A new definition of children with special health care needs. *Pediatrics, 102*(1), 137–140.

National Association of School Nurses. (1999). *Standards of professional school nursing practice*. Scarborough, ME: Author.

Newacheck, P. A., McManus, M., Fox, H. B., Hung, Y. Y., & Halfon, N. (2000). Access to health care for children with special health care needs. *Pediatrics, 105*(4), 760–766.

Office of Public Health and Science and Office of Disease Prevention and Promotion. (1998). *Put prevention into practice: Clinician's handbook of preventive services* (2nd ed.). Washington, DC: U.S. Department of Health and Human Services, Public Health Services.

Office of Technology Assessment. (1987). *Technology-dependent children: Hospital vs. home care. A technical memorandum*. Washington, DC: Congress of the United States.

Patterson, J. M. (1995). Promoting resilience in families experiencing stress. *Pediatric Clinics of North America, 42*(1), 47–63.

Patterson, J. M. (1991). Family resilience to the challenge of a child's disability. *Pediatric Annals, 20*(9), 491–499.

Pridham, K. F., Broome, M., & Woodring, B. (1996). Education for the nursing of children and their families: Standards and guidelines for prelicensure and early professional education. *Journal of Pediatric Nursing, 11*(5), 273–280.

Taylor, E. H., & Edwards, R. L. (1995). When community resources fail: Assisting the frightened and angry parent. *Pediatric Clinics of North America, 42*(1), 209–216.

CHAPTER 36

Social and Environmental Influences on the Child

A my has always been a challenge. She has already left home a couple of times and lived on the streets. Lately she has been more interested in school and is at home and trying to do well. We want her to succeed and learn the skills she needs in her life. I wish she would not have all of these body piercings, but we don't want to make too big an issue of it as long as she is doing well in school.

—Mother of Amy, 15 YEARS OLD

Key Terms

Adaptation phase *862*
Adjustment phase *862*
Bisexual *876*
Child sexual abuse *881*
Emotional abuse *880*
Emotional neglect *881*
Gay *876*
Homosexuality *876*
Lesbian *876*

Physical abuse *880*
Physical neglect *880*
Resilience *862*
Risk factors *862*
Protective factors *862*
Transgendered *876*
Violence *876*

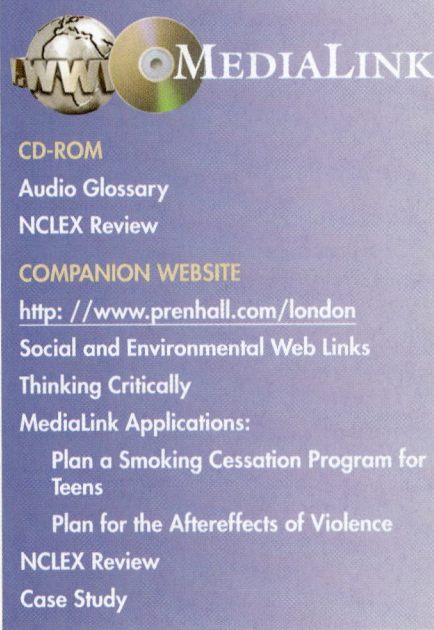

MEDIALINK

CD-ROM
Audio Glossary
NCLEX Review

COMPANION WEBSITE
http://www.prenhall.com/london
Social and Environmental Web Links
Thinking Critically
MediaLink Applications:
   Plan a Smoking Cessation Program for Teens
   Plan for the Aftereffects of Violence
NCLEX Review
Case Study

*M*any of the major causes of mortality and morbidity in children are closely linked with social influences in the child's environment. The social contexts for young children growing up today are different from those of even a decade ago. Examining the social contexts in which children live and grow can provide insights into behavior, and present opportunities for nursing interventions. All nurses must examine the social influences and apply the knowledge gained to plan health care that will benefit youth as they grow into adulthood.

What are the challenges of today's society that children must often face at very young ages? How can nurses help children face these challenges, and emerge healthy and contributing members of society? What roles do nurses play in identifying and using the protective factors and in minimizing the risk factors of youth? This chapter will examine and apply these concepts in a variety of nursing settings.

Examine again the major causes of death for children from 1 year of age through adolescence that are presented in Chapter 1 and on the website. **WEB** Notice that most morbidity is related to preventable causes linked to present-day lifestyles. Car crashes, fires, drowning, and homicides are a few examples of common causes of death in children.

Now examine the major reasons for hospitalization in Chapter 1 and on the website. **WEB** By the time children are 5 years of age, injuries rank as second cause, and by 10 years, mental disorders are the major cause of hospitalization. By the teen years, pregnancy and mental disorders are the most common admitting diagnoses to hospitals. All of these conditions are related, at least in part, to environmental settings. These settings and their influences must be examined in order to understand how to best intervene with children.

BASIC CONCEPTS

In this chapter, two main theories will provide a framework for examining societal influences on children. The ecologic model is discussed in Chapter 32, and should be reviewed now to assist in evaluating the environmental settings that influence children (see Figure 32–3 on page 735). This theory views the child and the environment as interacting forces, with children influencing systems around them, even while they are influenced by these systems (Lackey & Walker, 1998). Close systems providing daily contact are microsystems, but other systems such as parental work and political or cultural environments are also important. Understanding these systems, or the forces in which children function, can provide information that guides care providers. For example, if the parents' employers do not provide health care insurance, their children may not get needed health care such as immunizations, treatment for diseases, and growth monitoring.

Another model that provides a useful framework for understanding the societal influences on child health is the resiliency model. **Resilience** is the ability to function with healthy responses, even with significant stress and adversity (Stewart, Reid, & Mangham, 1997). In this model, the individual or family experiences a crisis that provides a source of stress, and the family interprets or deals with the crisis based on their resources. They may have **protective factors** that provide strength and assistance in dealing with the crisis, and **risk factors** that promote or contribute to health system challenges. Risk and protective factors can be identified in children, in their families, and in their communities. The combination and interplay of all of these factors determines adaptation to the crisis.

Once confronted by a crisis, the child and family first experience the **adjustment phase,** characterized by disorganization and unsuccessful attempts at meeting the crisis. In the **adaptation phase,** the child and family meet the challenge and use resources to deal with the crisis (Malone, 1998). The model and examples are described in Table 36–1. Table 36–2 lists questions that can be helpful as the nurse gathers information from youth or their family members that can be used to maximize resilience in individuals

TABLE 36–1	**Components of Resiliency Model**	
Component	Meaning	Example
A = Crisis event or health challenge	Nature of health care challenge	Parent leaving home
V = Vulnerability; risk factors	Stresses and risks related to dealing with the health challenge	Prior abandonment; financial instability; child's developmental understanding of abandonment
T = Typology	Family methods of functioning	Reliance on extended family; parent alcoholism
B = Protective factors	Strengths for dealing with challenge	Child's desire to succeed in school; positive role modeling of maternal grandparents
C = Appraisal	Family's interpretation of crisis event	Abandonment by loved one; inability to trust others
PS = Problem solving or coping techniques	Skills that help family work toward solution	Use of community resources; acceptance of school and community counselors; child's involvement in classroom activities
X = Response	Positive or negative response to tension created by the health challenge	Remaining parent using counseling available; child identifying with a teacher in school; establishment of sense of mutual interdependence among remaining family members

Note: From Malone, J.A. (1998). The resiliency model of family stress, adjustment, and adaptation. In B. Vaughn–Cole, M.A. Johnson, J.A. Malone, and B.L. Walker. *Family nursing practice.* Philadelphia: W.B. Saunders, p. 52. Adapted.

Questions to determine risk factors:

- Describe the event that occurred and what it has been like for your family.
- What other stressors do you have in your family right now?
- Are there financial worries?
- Are there things you think and worry about late at night?
- Describe your job, your friends.
- What is a typical day like?
- Describe your neighborhood.
- Do you have friends, people to call in emergencies?

Questions to determine protective factors:

- What gives you strength?
- How do you deal with this stress?
- What do you think you do well in your family?
- Who do you call when you need help?
- Do you have a computer? Internet access?
- Are you religious? Spiritual?
- Do you exercise regularly?
- How do you spend free time?

and families. These concepts can be applied to Amy's family as described in the opening quotation. She experienced disruption in family stability. The risk and protective factors interacted with her own personality in ways that resulted in her desire to appear as an independent person, establishing her identity through body art, and finally, a desire to return to school. The National Longitudinal Study of Adolescent Health (ADD) was conducted with over 100,000 adolescents in the United States, and found that parent-family connectedness, school connectedness, a belief in a higher being, and academic success were predictive of youth having lower health risks.

Nurses use concepts of resiliency theory in planning interventions for children and families. Some nursing strategies target risk factors, such as encouraging family behaviors to ensure gun safety by teaching use of gun locks and locked gun cabinets in families with firearms. Others emphasize protective factors, such as suggesting regular exercise to help maintain normal weight and cardiovascular function.

EXTERNAL INFLUENCES ON CHILD HEALTH

Poverty

An important risk factor that influences the health of children is poverty. Conversely, basic financial stability is a protective factor that contributes to the general health and well-being of children. Children who are poor are overrepresented in nearly every health indicator. One in five children is poor, or in a family earning less than $9000 annually for a family of three (Children's Defense Fund, 2000). Children who are poor are more likely to have un-

met health needs, to have difficulty in school, to become teen parents, and to experience multiple health problems. Children are the poorest group in this country and more children are poor now than at any time in our past (Board on Children, Youth, and Families, 2001). Children make up about 38% of the poor in this country and the proportion of poor children in all ethnic groups is increasing (Stein, 1997). [WEB]

Developing Cultural Competence

Ethnic disparities in economic status are present in the United States, with 10% of white children classified as poor, 34% of Hispanic children, and 36% of black children (Federal Interagency Forum on Child and Family Statistics, 2000).

Poverty leads to homelessness for some children. Children comprise one third of the homeless and women represent 20% of the homeless population. Families are the fastest growing group of homeless people. On any night, about 100,000 children are homeless in the United States (Crook, 1998; Menke, 1998). The reasons for homelessness are also common risks for a number of the other challenges to health discussed in this chapter. Homeless people often have poor finances, may have been abused or victims of other violence, and may have mental instability. Children who experience homelessness often have multiple physical and mental health problems, and lack health insurance to provide care for these problems. Teens who have been homeless are more likely to engage in other risky behavior, such as unprotected sex, sex with multiple partners, and substance abuse. They are more likely to need emergency care, to be depressed, and to become pregnant than other teens (Ensign & Santelli, 1998). Health problems related to homelessness, and other family characteristics, continue even after finding a place to live (Vostanis, Grattan, & Cumella, 1998). Complex ongoing care is needed. This may begin in a shelter for the homeless, but should continue while the family obtains a place to live, accesses other community services, gets the children safely enrolled in school, and has financial and mental stability.

Nursing management for families with children that are poor or homeless focuses on identification of poverty, careful assessment of health risks, and linking the family to resources that can assist with stability and health. There is often no way to identify a poor child from appearance and they may hide their status when they are in school or come to a health care facility. Addresses given may not be accurate, or the address of a shelter might be used. Children living at shelters or in cars and on the street usually do not take the school bus but prefer to walk to avoid stigma. Be alert for children who have multiple health problems and repeated infectious diseases. They are often hungry at times, with varying degrees of personal hygiene depending

TABLE 36-3 Common Health Problems and Nursing Management of Poor and Homeless Children

Common Health Problems	Nursing Management
Lack of immunizations	Check immunization records Provide immunizations at schools and in homeless shelters
Common infectious diseases	Facilitate free clinics in shelters, schools, community settings Teach hygiene measures Provide resources for disease management Arrange for medications when needed Provide information about resources for bathing, hygiene
Sleep deficits	Inform parents about respite facilities Arrange for children to have quiet sleep time in school if possible
Vision and hearing deficits	Perform screening for deficits Provide resources for eye glasses, hearing aids, care for ear infections (Service organizations such as Lion's Club are good options)
Nutritional deficits	Perform height and weight checks and nutritional assessment Evaluate family for food security (see Chapter 31) Be sure child is registered for school breakfast and lunch programs if available Assure that children are linked to summer food programs at end of academic year Link to Women, Infants, and Children (WIC) Nutrition Program Inform about resources for meals and field gleaning in the community
Dental care problems	Teach oral hygiene Provide toothbrushes and toothpaste Provide bottled water if child lives in a car or on the street Perform oral assessment Refer to dental programs for people with low incomes
Injuries	Teach basic safety precautions Visit the living situation if possible to assess for safety hazards Teach "street safe" skills Provide helmets, car seats, or other gear needed
Adolescent pregnancy and sexually transmitted diseases	Provide sexuality teaching Inform about access to family planning services Assess for child abuse and prostitution
Mental illness	Assess for depression Evaluate for suicide potential Provide links to services Plan programs to foster self-esteem Arrange for a "Big Brother" or "Big Sister" Refer to extracurricular activities in the school and community Arrange for a school bus stop away from a shelter so other students do not stigmatize the homeless child

on access to laundry and bathing facilities. See Table 36-3 for examples of nursing care needs for homeless children and families.

Stress

The adverse effect of stress on adults is well documented. More recently the impact of stress on children has been recognized. Children manifest stress in a variety of ways, including regressive behavior, interrupted sleep, hyperactive behavior, gastrointestinal symptoms, crying, and withdrawal from normal events. Common stressful events for children include moving to a new home or school, marital difficulties in the family, abuse, and being expected to achieve at an extremely high level in school or sports. The busy pace of today's lifestyles and the media's encouragement of early development in children may put undue stress upon some children (Elkind, 1998). For poor families, commonly reported stressors are related to food, shelter, transportation, medical care, and personal-time needs.

The child experiencing stress has more frequent respiratory and gastrointestinal illnesses and is more likely to be the victim of an injury. The negative long-term effects of stress on body organs and systems suggest that children under stress are more likely to develop illnesses such as strokes, hypertension, and heart attacks later in life.

Nurses help children manage stress by encouraging good coping strategies. With all children, emphasize healthy lifestyles including good nutrition, exercise, and plenty of sleep. The National Heart, Lung and Blood Institute has launched a 5-year program to encourage children to get at least 9 hours of sleep nightly. Encourage parents to provide youth with activities that foster self-esteem, and to avoid unrealistic expectations about performance in sports and other activities. Provide resources to help with food acquisition, shelter, transportation, and medical care for families needing them.

Family Structure

The families into which children are born influence them profoundly. Children are supported in different ways and acquire different world views depending on such factors as whether one or both parents work, how many siblings are present, and whether an extended family is close by. Note variations in family structure such as single parent, homosexual parents, extended family, and stepparents. Societal changes have impacted family life and the needs of children in profound ways. Working parents often raise children with little time for quality relationships and without the financial resources needed for optimum development (Board on Children, Youth, and Families, 2001). All of these factors influence the physical and mental health of children, and can determine their needs for nursing intervention.

First-born children tend to be concerned with achievement and grades, often become leaders, and more commonly obtain advanced degrees. Last-born children more often demonstrate a relaxed approach to school and achievements (Santrock, 1999).

About half of all marriages in the United States end in divorce. Divorce has a profound effect on children, varying with the child's age and cognitive stage. Young children who have limited ability to understand divorce may show such behavioral manifestations as crying, sleep disturbance, regression, and aggressive behavior (Wallerstein, Corbin, & Lewis, 1988; Wallerstein & Kelly, 1996; Wallerstein, Lewis, & Blakeslee, 2000) (see Table 36–4). Older children and adolescents more commonly show inadequate social skills related to cooperation and negotiation, increased aggression, and substance abuse (Thompson, 1998). After divorce, children most often live (about 80% of the time) in a single-parent household with the mother (Friedman, 1998). This can lead to financial strain, decreased health insurance coverage, parental role strain, and other stresses that impact the children. Remarriage, stepparenting, and joint custody arrangements all create additional challenges for families. Nurses can help families recognize the challenges the children are experiencing, cope with their particular needs, and provide resources such as mediation sessions, financial assistance, and support groups (Melnyk & Alpert-Gillis, 1997).

Nurses can complete family diagrams during home visits and in other settings to evaluate the people who are important in a child's life. Identify both the risk factors of the family, such as recent separation, parental stress, and lim-

TABLE 36-4	Effects of Divorce
Age (years)	Behavior
3–5	Fear, anxiety, and dread in daily life events
	Regression
	Searching and questioning
	Self-blame
	Increased aggression
6–8	Extreme sadness
	Fantasies and panic
	Worries about lack of food, money, caretaking
9–12	Intense anger
	Somatic complaints
	Confused self-identity
13–18	Withdrawal from family
	Concern about sex and marriage
	Sense of loss
	Anger

Note: From Wallerstein, J., & Kelly, J. (2000). *Surviving the breakup.* New York: Harper Collins. Adapted.

ited health care coverage, and the family's strengths, such as loving relationships, influential grandparents or other extended family members, and general good health; then use that information in planning care. Nurses can help families experiencing divorce to recognize the challenges the children are facing, help them cope with their particular needs, and provide resources such as mediation sessions, financial assistance, and support groups (Melnyk & Alpert-Gillis, 1997).

School and Child Care

Once a child is 5 or 6 years of age, several hours daily are spent in a school setting. Children develop physical skills through participation in education and sports. Psychosocial stages are met as the child interacts with children and adults and achieves social interaction patterns and pride in accomplishments. The presentation of concepts that challenge thought processes enhances cognitive development.

Although the primary role of schools is educational, they also perform several health-related functions. WEB School health screening programs play an important role in identifying children with such health problems as hearing loss, visual impairment, and scoliosis. Nurses provide assessment, teaching, and clinical management related to some health problems. Some schools have clinics that examine and provide even more complete health care for children. Many schools teach good nutrition, healthful living, safe sexual practices, and other health-related subjects. A school nurse may be present, at least part time, to plan these classes or to work with teachers. Nurses assist school districts in providing plans for emergency health care when needed. With the increase in mainstreaming, school staff now have the responsibility for administering medications, maintaining urinary catheters, and providing respiratory

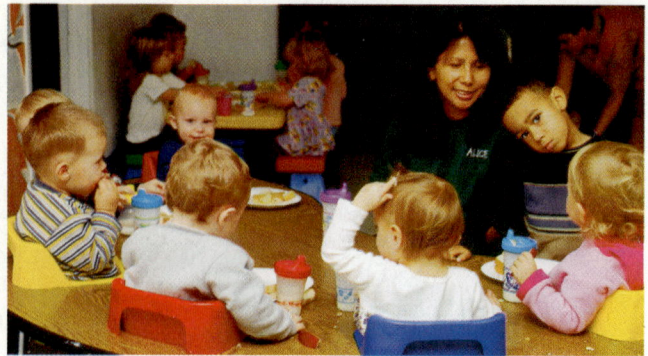

FIGURE 36–1. ◆ Most children will spend time in child care settings. It is important to explore options and find the best fit for the child's needs.

care and other treatments to ensure the child's proper growth and development. See Chapter 35 for a further discussion of school nurse activities. ⊂▭⊃

Some children spend part or nearly all of their days in child care settings (Figure 36–1 ◆). Nearly half of all children are in regular child care by their first birthday (Fields, Smith, Bass, et al., 2001). Although there has been debate about whether child care has a positive or negative impact on children, it appears now that the closeness of the parent-child relationship, the quality of care, and the length of the child care day are important in determining child care effects on children (National Institute of Child Health and Human Development, 1997).

Nursing management involves helping parents to explore types of child care options available and to evaluate programs in their communities (Table 36–5). Care options for young school-age children, either before or after school, can also be shared with parents. When available, recommend early intervention programs with at-risk children, such as the Zero to Three Project and Head Start, which contribute to children's health and welfare. Nurses frequently manage the health programs in early interven-

tion, providing screening, doing health evaluations, and establishing early intervention education plans.

Community

The community in which a child lives may support the child's development or, conversely, expose the child to hazards. Social programs such as Head Start preschools, sports activities, after-school programs, and child abuse treatment centers offer valuable services that improve the experience of growing children. On the other hand, an economically depressed community with scant services and a high homicide rate is unsupportive and hazardous for growing children.

The physical environment is supportive when the child has sidewalks on which to walk to school, open spaces in which to learn and play, and clean air to breathe. Children who must walk to school on unsafe roads, have access to contaminated drinking supplies, or live near polluting manufacturing companies or in crowded housing or old structures are at risk for injuries and health problems such as lead poisoning (see Chapter 46). ⊂▭⊃

Nurses should be aware of the types of neighborhoods in the community. Learn about local resources and hazards. Assessment of every child involves getting information about the community and the health care that the family needs help to obtain. Refer children when appropriate for lead poisoning and for safe programs after school. Teach them about injury prevention specific to their communities.

Culture

The child's cultural group may influence the use of traditional and contemporary health care practices. If the parents or children are recent immigrants, they may still be learning the English language and finding out about health care resources. Even in families that have been in the United States for some time, a combination of approaches to health care is common.

TABLE 36–5	**Types of Child Care**	
Type of Care	Description	Advantage/Disadvantage
In home	Caretaker comes to home of the child	Child can remain at home Little exposure to infectious diseases No need for alternative care when child is ill Limited contact with other children to encourage development Most costly
Family child care	Parent brings child to home of a caretaker	Limited number of children Some exposure to other children and encouragement of development Family type atmosphere Little governmental regulation or examination
Center care a. Private, nonprofit (i.e., church, YMCA) b. Public (i.e., Head Start) c. Private proprietary	Parent brings child to a center where many children receive care	A learning curriculum plan is in place Contact with other children can enhance development Exposure to multiple children increases infectious disease risk

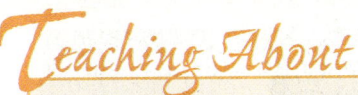

EVALUATION OF CHILD CARE

The nurse can help parents to evaluate child care options and make decisions about placement for their children. Parents should always be welcomed to visit an agency or home child care—this is essential so they can see the routines in action. Some questions they can ask are suggested as follows.

Administration

Is the facility licensed?

Who are the administrators? What is their training and experience?

How many staff are employed? What is their training?

Is there a parent board? What part do they play in administering the center?

Physical Environment, Health, and Safety

What is the neighborhood like? Is transportation to the center convenient?

What is the condition of lighting, heat, cooling, ventilation system, play spaces (inside and out), and the building's general condition?

Is playground equipment safe?

Is there a soft material such as bark, sand, or rubber tiles under climbing equipment?

Is there always supervision for the children?

Are there emergency medical forms and signed forms for field trips?

Who may pick up children? How are they signed in and out?

What is the immunization policy and how are records examined and maintained?

Are criminal background checks of staff done for potential child abuse and other problems?

What is the policy for children with infectious diseases and other illness?

How are foods prepared? Are staff licensed in food handling?

What is the state of general cleanliness?

Who changes diapers? Are recommendations for standard precautions to prevent pathogen transfer followed?

What arrangements and routines are made for naps and quiet times?

Developmental Approaches

Is the curriculum appropriate for different age groups?

Are there materials and plans for gross motor, fine motor, language, and social development?

How much time do children spend in structured time? Free time?

How is discipline handled?

Do the children appear occupied and happy?

What reading materials are available?

What type and quantity of field trips are planned?

What is the educational level and longevity of the child care workers?

Is there a diversity among the children's backgrounds and experiences?

Recent immigrants may experience culture shock, a state of crisis related to the difference in values and lifestyle. This can lead to stress-related symptoms, and create a need for health care intervention. Children whose parents immigrated from another country may feel different from peers and develop conflict with their parents, particularly during adolescence.

All cultural groups have rules about patterns of social interaction. Schedules of language acquisition are determined by the number of languages spoken and the amount of speech in the home. The particular social roles assumed by men and women in the culture affect school activities and ultimately career choices. Attitudes toward touching and other methods of encouraging developmental skills vary among cultures.

Developing Cultural Competence

Cultural differences in childrearing influence personality. For example, Japanese children are taught to respect parents and elders. Gender distinctions are the basis for social behaviors. Girls are praised for maintaining poise, grace, and control; boys for showing determination and strength of will in overcoming obstacles.

Nurses must become aware of common characteristics of the cultural groups they serve so that they can provide culturally competent nursing care. Arrange for translators when needed. Be aware that families often accept and use both traditional and westernized health care, and remain nonjudgmental about traditional healing practices. Provide ethnic foods in health care facilities. Evaluate youth in immigrant families for conflict between family and societal expectations.

LIFESTYLE ACTIVITIES AND THEIR INFLUENCE ON CHILD HEALTH

Many patterns of daily life play a part in determining the length and quality of one's life. The child's use of tobacco products and controlled substances influences both physical and mental health. Patterns of exercise and use of protective gear protect against early disabilities. The use of decorative patterns that can introduce pathogens is an example of a lifestyle pattern that influences mental health, body image, and the body's physical health.

Tobacco Use

Tobacco use is the most preventable cause of adult death in the United States. It leads to 430,000 deaths annually, and will be responsible for the premature death of 5 million of today's youth as they reach adult years (*Healthy People 2010,* 2000). Major health problems linked to tobacco use include cardiovascular disease, cancer, chronic lung disease, low birth weight, and other maternal problems. Even passive smoking or environmental tobacco smoke (ETS) is linked to increased heart disease, blood pressure, and respiratory problems (Werner & Pearson, 1998). Although cigarettes are most common, chewing tobacco, snuff, cigars, and bidis (small, brown, hand-rolled cigarettes) also pose significant health hazards.

Many nurses view tobacco use as an adult issue. Although sale of tobacco products to children and advertisements aimed at this age group are forbidden by federal law, many youths obtain and use tobacco. In fact, the statistics are alarming. At a time when tobacco use by adults has dropped, adolescents are at very high risk of adopting this risky behavior, and their smoking patterns are tracked by the Centers for Disease Control and Prevention, in the annual Youth Risk Behavior Surveillance System. ⬭ WEB About 35% of 12th graders, 26% of 10th graders, and 18% of 8th graders in the United States smoked within the last month. When including children who have ever smoked, the numbers are even larger. About 70% have tried smoking by high school years (MMWR, 2000a). Significant numbers of youth also report using chewing tobacco and cigars in the previous month (*Healthy People 2010*, 2000). It is striking to realize that 3000 youths per day try their first cigarette, and that the major ages for trying tobacco are 9 to 14 years (sixth to ninth grades). Early initiation of smoking is understood as an extremely risky behavior when it is recognized that 82% of current adult smokers began smoking before 18 years of age (MMWR, 2000b). Nicotine is very addictive to youth, with most people becoming addicted to the substance in adolescent years.

Certain characteristics contribute to the likelihood of tobacco use. They include increasing age, male gender, ethnic group, ease of obtaining tobacco products, and smoking among family members. Low socioeconomic group membership, access to tobacco products, low price of products, advertising, and lack of parental involvement in the youths' lives are associated with tobacco use (*Healthy People 2010, 2000*). Girls commonly cite reasons for smoking such as a desire to be slim and to appear mature, whereas boys more often view smoking as a way to be tough and rebellious. Both genders admit that smoking helps them to feel part of a group (Hanson, 1999) (Figure 36–2 ◆).

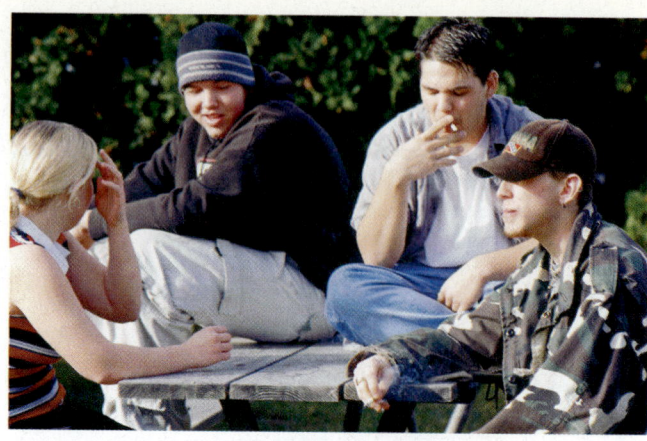

FIGURE 36–2. ◆ About 70% of children have tried smoking by their high school years. Early intervention can begin with discussions about smoking, starting before 9 to 10 years of age.

Several programs have been developed to encourage youth to avoid tobacco use. In addition, smoking cessation programs are available to assist youth who are already regular smokers, and successfully achieve the goals of cessation or decrease in tobacco use (Coleman-Wallace, Lee, Montgomery, et al., 1999). Smoking cessation efforts are more successful in teens who smoke occasionally rather than daily, so keeping occasional smokers from becoming regular smokers is important. Smoking cessation may involve use of peer leadership and support, counseling, and computer instruction. When teens have become regular smokers, nicotine replacement therapy may be needed since they are likely addicted to nicotine (Donovan, 2000; Sergeant, Mott, & Stevens, 1998). Once a teen is identified as a smoker, using a biologic marker such as urine cotinine (a by-product of tobacco) levels can help to identify the frequency of smoking. This information can be used to make suggestions to the teen about the potential outcomes of the behavior and the cessation program which is most likely to be helpful.

Nursing Management

Nursing Assessment and Diagnosis

Nurses are in a unique position to inquire about the incidence of smoking and other tobacco use among youth. Insert questions into all well-child visits, beginning at about 9 to 10 years of age. Inquire about whether family members (especially parents and siblings) smoke or chew, and ask if some of the child's friends have tried smoking. Try to find out the child's knowledge and beliefs about the benefits and risks of tobacco use. As the child gets older, ask more direct and detailed questions. A nonjudgmental approach will be best to obtain a truthful response. School nurses can make observations about numbers of teens smoking and general attitudes about tobacco use. When children come to hospitals and other health facilities for care, use of tobacco should be part of general admission questions.

Developing Cultural Competence

Among youth in the United States, white youth are significantly more likely to smoke than either Hispanic or black peers. About 38.6% of white students report smoking in the previous month, while 32.7% of Hispanic and 19.7% of black students report this behavior (MMWR, 2000). American Indians and Alaska Natives also have high smoking rates, while Asian Americans have low rates (*Healthy People 2010, 2000b*).

Some nursing diagnoses that may apply to youth who smoke or show potential for this behavior include:

▶ *Activity intolerance* related to lowered oxygen supply

▶ *Impaired gas exchange* related to ventilation-perfusion imbalance

▶ *Low self-esteem* related to negative self-appraisal

▶ *Health-seeking behaviors of dangers of tobacco use* related to developmental focus on present

▶ *Altered nutrition, less than body requirements* related to effects of chemical dependence

Planning and Implementation

The roles of nurses in preventing and intervening in youth smoking are to inform youth, identify smokers, and implement programs (Table 36–6). Provide developmentally appropriate information about the hazards of tobacco use in all settings where youth are present. Posters, flyers, and speakers are particularly useful. Addicted teens who share their stories of difficult withdrawal from tobacco, and adults who have had cancer of the lungs or larynx may be effective speakers. Find out where teens obtain tobacco products in the community and where they use the products in order to target these places. 🔗 WEB Offer information on prevention and cessation programs to youths and families in clinics, outpatient surgery centers, community activities, and hospitals. Use opportunities such as adolescent pregnancy and illness to reinforce the hazardous effects of tobacco on the individual and on those around. Speak to young athletes about the effects of tobacco on athletic performance. Show youth the ways this product can interfere with meeting life goals. Role-play how to tell other youth "no" when tobacco is offered. Establish programs that increase the sense of self-esteem without tobacco use. Be sure to include parents in the programs so that they see and acknowledge their role in setting an example about tobacco use, and in providing guidelines for the child. Provide information on the influence of environmental tobacco (secondhand smoke).

Adopt a nonjudgmental attitude when asking questions about smoking so that youth using tobacco can be identified. Ask questions without parents present and assure youth that the information will not be shared. Encourage youth to cut back and to quit use of tobacco products. Offer assistance to them in these efforts.

Work with the schools and school districts to help establish preventive and cessation programs. There should be clear guidelines about school policies regarding smoking on school grounds. Keeping occasional youth smokers from becoming regular users should be a goal in order to avoid nicotine addiction. Find out what positive incentives can be offered to youth who are successful in quitting smoking. Contract with them to achieve their goals.

Evaluation

Expected outcomes of nursing interventions regarding tobacco use are lowered rates of regular use, delayed initiation of use, and success of cessation programs. Use the *Healthy People 2010* (2000). 🔗 WEB objectives as guidelines. They include:

▶ Reduce the proportion of children who are regularly exposed to tobacco smoke at home to 10%.

▶ Increase smoke-free and tobacco-free environments in schools, including all school facilities, property, vehicles, and school events, to 100%.

▶ Eliminate tobacco advertising and promotions that influence adolescents and young adults.

▶ Increase adolescents' disapproval of smoking to 95%.

▶ Reduce tobacco use by adolescents to 21%.

▶ Increase the average age of first use of tobacco products from 12 years to 14 years.

Substance Use

Substance abuse occurs in children and adolescents of all socioeconomic levels and is a growing health problem. It is important to keep in mind that the use of any drug can pose a serious psychologic and physical risk to children and adolescents.

Although a decline in the daily use of marijuana by adolescents has been reported, abuse of other substances, particularly alcohol, cocaine, crack, and heroin, remains high. The Youth Risk Behavior Surveillance of high school seniors reported the following alarming statistics: 81% have had alcohol to drink, 50% had an alcoholic drink in the month prior to being surveyed, 32% engaged in binge drinking of alcohol, and the average age for beginning alcohol and cigarette use was 12 years (MMWR, 2000a). Prevalence increases with advancing age and grade in school, and 47% of children have had their first drink by

---

TABLE 36–6   Nursing Role in Youth Smoking Prevention

Inform
- Hang posters, provide brochures, and facilitate presentations about smoking risks in all settings where youth are present.
- Target smokers with special information about the effects of nicotine on their bodies.

Identify
- Ask questions about smoking and other tobacco use at every health encounter beginning at about 9–10 years of age.
- For users, ask amount and type of tobacco.
- Learn where youth obtain tobacco and be proactive in stopping sales.

Implement
- Encourage youth tobacco users to quit.
- Facilitate referral to cessation programs.
- Arrange positive rewards for youth successful in cessation.

9 years of age (Fetro, Coyle, & Pham, 2001). About 47% of students have used marijuana, 10% have used cocaine, 15% reported inhalant use of glue, paints, or other substances, 9% reported methamphetamine use, and 2% have used heroin (MMWR, 2000a). Synthetic drugs such as phencyclidine (PCP) (commonly called "designer" drugs) mimic other narcotics, stimulants, and hallucinogens and are also dangerous.

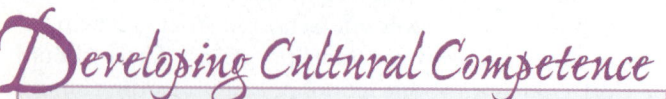
Developing Cultural Competence

In a study of middle school students, Asian students were least likely to drink alcohol (9%), with African Americans next (23%), followed by Hispanics (26%) and whites (29%) (Fetro, Coyle, & Pham, 2001). Nurses can use this information to target groups most at risk of alcohol ingestion, even at these young ages.

Over-the-counter medications are legal, but frequently abused. Easily obtainable at grocery stores and drugstores, these drugs include antihistamines, atropine, bromides, caffeine, ephedrine, pseudoephedrine, phenylpropanolamine, and amphetamine-like substitutes. Volatile inhalants, such as glues, are dangerous substances of abuse, and their use appears to be rising among school-age children and adolescents. **WEB** Anabolic steroids are the drugs of abuse most commonly used by athletes. Some common contemporary drugs and street names are listed in Table 36–7.

ETIOLOGY AND PATHOPHYSIOLOGY

In most cases, substance abuse represents a maladaptive coping response to the stressors of childhood and adolescence. A child may begin using drugs or alcohol to deal with stress because family members or peers do so. Children in families with a history of substance abuse are at higher risk of abusing drugs and alcohol. Other risk factors include rebelliousness, aggressiveness, low self-esteem, dysfunctional parental relationships, lack of adequate support systems, academic underachievement, poor judgment, and poor impulse control.

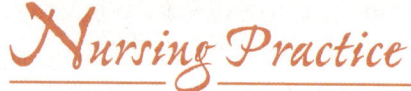
Nursing Practice

Following are common inhalant agents:

Aerosols	**Solvents**
Cooking spray	Nail polish remover
Whipped cream	Paint thinner or cleaner
Spray paint	Lighter fluid
Cosmetic sprays	Degreaser
Adhesives	**Other**
Model glues	Gasoline
Rubber cements	Helium

Note: From Cook (1999). Adapted.

Initial experimentation with alcohol or drugs may be unpleasant. With continued use, however, the adolescent learns to "achieve the high," an illusion of power and well-being. The adolescent wants the high more frequently and actively seeks alcohol or drugs. Tolerance to the substance occurs with continued use, and ever-increasing amounts are required to achieve a pleasurable high. Physical and psychologic dependence ensues as the body's tissues require the substance to function properly. Withdrawal symptoms occur when the child or adolescent is deprived of the substance.

CLINICAL MANIFESTATIONS

Substance abuse in children and adolescents is commonly overlooked and underdiagnosed by health care providers (Pagliaro & Pagliaro, 1996). This is due in part to the wide range of clinical presentations, which vary according to type of drug abused, amount, frequency, time of last use, and severity of drug dependence.

Common physical manifestations include alterations in vital signs, weight loss, chronic fatigue, chronic cough, respiratory congestion, red eyes, and general apathy and malaise. Withdrawal may be shown by anxiety, headache,

---

TABLE 36–7   *Common Contemporary Drugs and Street Names*

Drug	Action	Street Names
Methylenedioxymethamphetamine (MDMA)	Stimulant; appetite suppressant	Ecstasy, XTC, X, Adam, Clarity, Lover's speed
Gamma-hydroxybutyrate (GHB)	CNS depressant	Grievous Bodily Harm, G., Liquid Ecstasy, Georgia Home Boy
Ketamine	Anesthetic	Special K, K, Vitamin K, Cat Valiums
Rohypnol	Amnesia, sedative	Roffies, Rophies, Roche, Forget-me Pill
Methamphetamine	Stimulant	Speed, Ice, Chalk, Meth, Crystal, Crank, Fire, Glass
Lysergic Acid Diethylamide (LSD)	Hallucinogen	Acid, Boomers, Yellow Sunshines

Note: From National Institute on Drug Abuse. (1999). *Some facts about club drugs.* Bethesda, MD: U.S. Department of Health and Human Services. Adapted.

DRUG	POTENTIAL FOR DEPENDENCE	CLINICAL MANIFESTATIONS
Depressants Alcohol, barbiturates (amobarbital, pentobarbital, secobarbital)	*Physical and psychologic:* High; varies somewhat among drugs	*Physical:* Decreased muscle tone and coordination, tremors *Psychologic:* Impaired speech, memory, and judgment, confusion; decreased attention span; emotional lability
Stimulants Amphetamines (e.g., Benzedrine) caffeine, cocaine	*Physical:* Low to moderate *Psychologic:* High; withdrawal from amphetamines and cocaine can lead to severe depression	*Physical:* Dilated pupils, increased pulse and blood pressure, flushing, nausea, loss of appetite, tremors *Psychologic:* Euphoria; increased alertness, agitation, or irritability; hallucinations; insomnia
Opiates Codeine, heroin, meperidine (Demerol), methadone, morphine, opium, oxycodone (Percodan)	*Physical and psychologic:* High; varies somewhat among drugs; withdrawal effects are uncomfortable but rarely life threatening	*Physical:* Analgesia, depressed respirations and muscle tone (may lead to coma or death), nausea, constricted pupils *Psychologic:* Changes in mood (usually euphoria), drowsiness, impaired attention or memory, sense of tranquility
Hallucinogens Lysergic acid diethylamide (LSD), mescaline, phencyclidine (PCP)	*Physical:* None *Psychologic:* Unknown	*Physical:* Lack of coordination, dilated pupils, hypertension, elevated temperature; severe PCP intoxication can result in seizures, respiratory depression, coma, and death *Psychologic:* Visual illusions and hallucinations, altered perceptions of time and space, emotional lability, psychosis
Volatile Inhalants Glues, typing correction fluid, acrylic paints, spot removers, lighter fluid, gasoline, butane	*Physical and psychologic:* Varies with drug used	*Physical:* Impaired coordination, liver damage (in some cases) *Psychologic:* Impaired judgment, delirium
Marijuana	*Physical:* Low *Psychologic:* Usually low; occasionally moderate to high	*Physical:* Tachycardia, reddened conjunctiva, dry mouth, increased appetite *Psychologic:* Initial anxiety followed by euphoria; giddiness; impaired attention, judgment, and memory

tremors, nausea and vomiting, malaise, weakness, insomnia, depressed mood or irritability, and hallucinations. The mental status examination (refer to Chapter 33). ◯◯ may reveal alterations in level of consciousness, impaired attention and concentration, impaired thought processes, delusions, and hallucinations. Low self-esteem, feelings of guilt or worthlessness, and suicidal or homicidal thoughts are also common.

Poor school performance and changes in mood, sleep habits, appetite, dress, and social relationships are nonspecific characteristics of the substance-abusing child.

CLINICAL THERAPY

Multiple psychiatric diagnostic criteria exist for each drug class. Children and adolescents who have other psychosocial disorders commonly use or abuse drugs or alcohol. Treatment should therefore focus not only on the substance use or abuse, but also on the issues underlying the problem. Intervention includes the family as well as the substance-abusing child or adolescent.

The primary goal of treatment is to teach the child and other family members to develop and sustain positive coping patterns, and to support them during this process. Most treatment programs offer inpatient and outpatient services, as well as aftercare programs. These programs usually consist of peer support that focuses on developing a drug- and alcohol-free lifestyle, healthy family relationships, and positive coping skills. Family involvement is strongly encouraged. Hospitalization is required if the physical dependence is significant and withdrawal places the child at risk for complications such as seizures, depression, or suicidal behavior.

Nursing Management
Nursing Assessment and Diagnosis

Nurses may encounter the substance-abusing child or adolescent in the emergency department or outpatient clinic, in schools and other community settings, or during hospitalization for an injury or other acute problem. Nursing assessment includes taking a thorough history from the parents and child, observing the child's behavior, and performing a physical examination. The history should include the age at which drug use began, pattern of use, length of time the drug has been used, amount of drug used, and psychologic state while on drugs. A history of parental drug use and noninvolvement in parenting the child puts the child at higher risk for substance abuse, reflecting the combined effects of genetic and environmental influences. Assessment tools provide useful information. One tool known as PACES collects information about parents and peers, accidents and alcohol or other drug use, cigarette use, emotional problems, and school and sexuality issues (Knight, 1997). Another useful assessment tool, called HEADS, is described in Chapter 35. ⊂◯⊃

PHYSIOLOGIC ASSESSMENT

Look for physical signs and symptoms of substance abuse, including bloodshot eyes, dilated pupils, slurred speech, and weight loss. The adolescent may appear sleepy or restless, or may show signs of clumsiness or inconsistent behavior. Consider all types of substance abuse, including model glue, gasoline, and other sources. Assess for signs of withdrawal as well as current intoxication.

PSYCHOLOGIC ASSESSMENT

Changes in social habits may indicate substance abuse. Parents may report a drop in the school-age child's or adolescent's grades or decreased interest in school activities. The adolescent does not introduce new friends to parents, and has less contact with parents, teachers, and other adults who were previously important. Note the child's current drug use, potential for violence, and motivation to make changes. Assess the degree of family support available.

Teaching About

IDENTIFYING THE YOUTH WHO IS ABUSING SUBSTANCES

Families are often confused about the behavior of adolescents and unsure whether it represents normal development or abuse of substances. Some characteristics of normal development that help to differentiate these occurrences are listed as follows. When concerned about possible substance use the parent can confront the child, or talk with school nurses or counselors.

- Many youth are periodically distant with parents but remain involved with peers in school sports and other activities. Withdrawal from all activities and friends may indicate substance abuse.
- Adolescents often complain about school, but when teachers report the student meets expectations and is consistently performing in the classroom, this is normal behavior.
- Teens may be weepy on occasion when having a difficult time with friends or not performing as desired. Continued, consistent weepiness is more likely to indicate depression or substance abuse.
- Teens like to stay up late and are frequently tired in the morning, whereas abusing teens may "nod off" frequently during the day.
- Many adolescents like to achieve a disheveled look in clothing, but the teen who frequently neglects basic hygiene or does not seem to have the energy to wash and dress may be depressed or be abusing substances.
- All teens get some infections but abusing teens may have reddened eyes, oral sores, and constant respiratory discomfort from "snorting" substances.

Nursing diagnoses for children and adolescents who abuse drugs or alcohol might include the following:

- ▶ *Impaired social interaction* related to altered thought processes
- ▶ *Self-esteem disturbance* related to dysfunctional family and social relationships
- ▶ *Risk for injury* related to altered perceptions and sensorium
- ▶ *Risk for violence: self-directed or directed at others* related to physiologic dependence on drugs, alcohol, and other substances

Planning and Implementation

Care of children and adolescents who abuse drugs, alcohol, and other substances is challenging and often frustrating. Long-term mental health counseling may be necessary to resolve underlying issues and foster lifestyle and behavioral changes.

Prevention is the most desirable intervention. The nurse can play a major role in teaching children and their families about substance abuse. Education should begin in primary school, and continue with intensification during middle and high school years. Nurses also can play a major role in community education. Various prevention programs have been developed by federal and private organizations. Referral to support organizations may be beneficial for the child, parents, and other family members. ⊂◯⊃ **WEB** Self-help groups, available in most communities, include Alcoholics Anonymous, Narcotics Anonymous, Al-Anon, Nar-Anon, and Ala-Teen. Parents may receive support from a group such as Parents Anonymous.

The youth's protective factors can be identified and used in planning appropriate interventions. For example, a child with goals for a future career can be helped to see how substance use will interfere with goal attainment. Identifying a strong role model through a program like Big Brothers or Big Sisters can assist children who lack that strength in their families.

Physical Inactivity

In the past few decades, children have become increasingly inactive physically. This decrease is a reflection of lifestyles in which car travel is valued, computers and televisions are part of daily life, neighborhoods are sometimes unsafe places for play, and schools do not routinely require daily physical education classes (Figure 36–3 ◆). Children and adolescents spend an average of almost 3 hours per day watching television; when video games and computers are included, the total average is 6 1/2 hours daily (Committee on Public Education, 2001; Dowell, 1998). Increasing television time is associated with less physical activity, and poorer sports performance and greater amounts of aggressive behavior (Anderson, Crespo, Bartlett, et al., 1998; Robinson, 2001). Physical inactivity leads to many

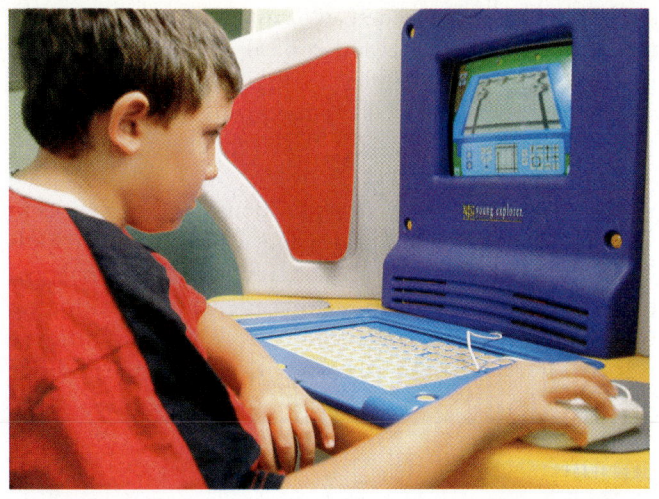
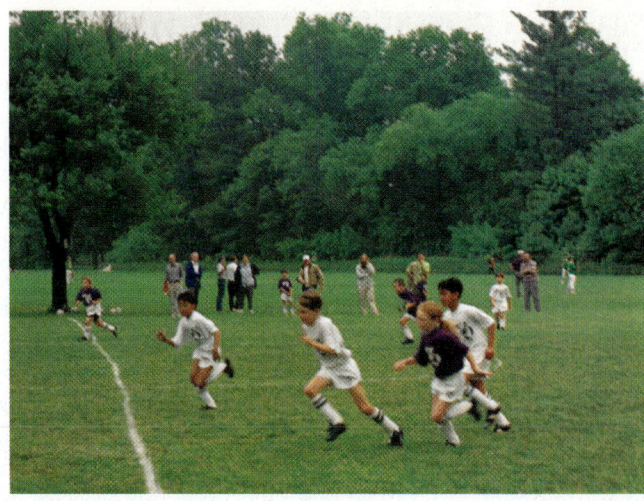

FIGURE 36-3. ◆ Physical inactivity is a growing problem among children, and can contribute to poor health. It is important to balance sedentary activities, such as playing comuter games, with physical and social activities. Sports are an excellent way for children to develop their psychosocial, cognitive, and motor skills. *Soccer photo courtesy of Rebecca Scheirer, Kensington, Maryland.*

health concerns. A primary outcome is overweight or obesity (see Chapter 31). Other outcomes can be an increased rate of type 2 diabetes (see Chapter 51), increased exposure to television/computer game violence and sexual activity at early ages, and early progression of cardiovascular disease (see Chapter 43).

On the other hand, patterns of physical activity established in childhood can increase exercise behaviors in adulthood; contribute to lower rates of low back pain, overweight, osteoporosis, heart disease, diabetes, colon cancer, and high blood pressure; and lead to a more positive self-image.

Although many children demonstrate low levels of physical activity, a profound decrease in vigorous activity is common in grades 9 to 12. Boys who do remain active generally engage in team sports and weight training, whereas girls more commonly enjoy aerobics and dance classes (*Healthy People 2010*, 2000).

Health professionals can integrate assessment of physical activity into all health care, and make recommendations to children and families that will help to increase opportunities for physical activity. Nurses can assess height, weight, and body mass index to look for signs of overweight (see Chapter 31). Children should be asked about how they like to spend free time. Community and school activities should be encouraged and rewarded. Examples include fun runs, walks of benefit causes, aerobics classes, team sports, roadside cleanups, fairs, and carnivals. Help parents and children learn what they can do for physical fitness. **WEB** Work with school physical education personnel to plan activities both in and out of physical education class that promote lifelong exercise routines.

Teaching About

PHYSICAL ACTIVITY GUIDELINES FOR YOUTH

- Engage in moderate physical activity (bike-riding, walking, baseball, rollerblading) at least 30 minutes 5 times weekly.
- Engage in vigorous physical activity that causes sweating and hard breathing (soccer, running, ice hockey) at least 20 minutes 3 times weekly.
- Encourage schools to offer physical education to all students, and have students sign up when this is an elective.
- Encourage walking and bike-riding to friends' homes and stores whenever safe.
- Plan physical activities together as a family.
- Get a pet and plan to walk the pet together daily.
- Limit television and other similar sedentary activities to no more than 2 hours daily.
- On days home, allow the child to watch television for up to 1 hour, and then insist that 1 hour of reading, 1 hour of physical activity, and 1 hour of socializing with others take place before returning to more television.

Complementary Care

YOGA FOR CHILDREN

Yoga has become a very popular practice for adults. Although less common, children can also reap the benefits of this ancient practice through special movements, breathing, and quiet time. Considering how sedentary many children have become, they can benefit from learning about their bodies, how they work, and how to take care of them. Yoga can help the child learn the importance of a balance between activity and calmness. It is easy to learn and can be used by children of every athletic ability, even children with disabilities. Recent research on the use of yoga in children has shown that it can have a calming effect on children 4 to 5 years old and those 12 to 17 years old (Telles, Narendran, Raghuraj, et al., 1997; Telles & Srinivas, 1998). See our website for further information about the use of yoga with children. **WEB**

Injury and Protective Equipment

In the discussion of causes of childhood and adolescent morbidities and mortalities in Chapter 1, unintentional injuries are listed as a common problem. In fact, 72% of all deaths from age 10 years onward result from four causes—motor-vehicle crashes, other unintentional injury, homicide, and suicide (MMWR, 2000a). Chapter 32 discusses the frequent injuries seen in children at different developmental ages, and safety precautions to avoid injuries from car crashes, falls, poisonings, and other developmentally related injuries. Many common injuries are preventable with simple use of protective gear and following of safety guidelines (Figure 36–4 ◆). It is important to consider that 16% of youths rarely or never wear seat belts in automobiles and 38% of those who ride motorcycles do not wear helmets (MMWR, 2000a). Emphasize safe automobile and motorcycle behaviors again in adolescence, with the recognition that risks increase if driving is combined with use of alcohol and controlled substances. Adolescents sometimes engage in practices that put them at particular risk, and nurses should be alert for such activities in their communities. Examples include car surfing (standing on the trunk, hood, or roof of a moving vehicle) (Geiger, Drongowski, & Lenni, 2001) or street racing (racing cars down a street at extremely high speed).

Many children ride bicycles but only about 15% are protected by helmet use, contributing to 23,000 bicycle-related head injuries annually. Bike helmets could prevent up to 88% of serious brain injuries from bicycle crashes (Committee on Injury and Poison Prevention, 2001). Strategies to make helmet use more attractive to children and adolescents are needed. Nurses can play a major role in programs to educate and reward children for helmet use, and can assist families to find affordable helmets. Other risky behaviors that require protective gear include rollerblading, skateboarding, roller hockey, ice hockey, football, soccer, baseball, scooters, and skiing/snowboarding. Nurses can be active in identifying behaviors in youths in specific communities and working with schools and other community groups to establish educational programs. Efforts should also include adequate conditioning for sports, proper treatment of injuries, and prevention of overuse injuries (Committee on Sports Medicine and Fitness, 2001).

Nursing Practice

A recent increase in scooter use led to nearly 28,000 emergency room visits in 2000 for scooter-related injury. Many injuries could be avoided with use of a helmet and knee and elbow pads, riding only on smooth surfaces in areas without cars, and avoiding riding after dark (MMWR, 2000c).

Body Art

Body art in the form of painting, tattooing, and piercing has been used by humans throughout history. In recent years, there has been a resurgence of interest in this decorative art among teens. Many adolescents have multiple body piercings and tattoos and may even resort to performing these decorations on themselves or friends.

From 10% to 25% of adolescents have tattoos, and even more have at least one body piercing (Armstrong & Kelly, 2001). In some states, teens must be 18 years of age or have parental permission to obtain body art, but students often report that it is easy to have an adult present who signs and claims to be a parent. Amy, described at the opening of this chapter and in "Thinking Critically" on page 875, had her piercing done by a friend. In some states, tattoo and body piercing businesses must be licensed and comply with certain regulations, whereas in others there are no regulations. Amy demonstrates some common characteristics of teens who choose to use body art. It may be seen as a way to establish individualism and independence, and helps some teens to feel part of a peer group. Multiple tattoos and piercings are common, as is the case with Amy (Figure 36–5 ◆).

Body art is a common source of infections with skin pathogens, as well as hepatitis B and C. Body piercing is a major method of transmission of hepatitis C, a disease that may not even become manifested until years later. It can be a source of HIV if proper techniques are not followed. Piercings in parts of the body such as the mouth or navel are most prone to bacterial infection and continued redness and irritation.

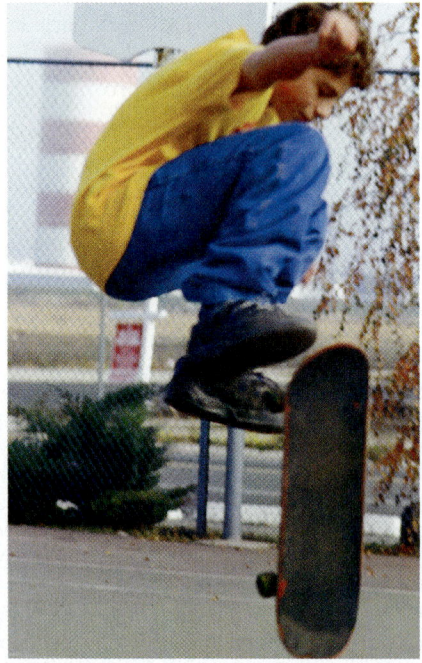

FIGURE 36–4. ◆ What protective gear should children use for skating boarding? How would you convince them to use the protection?

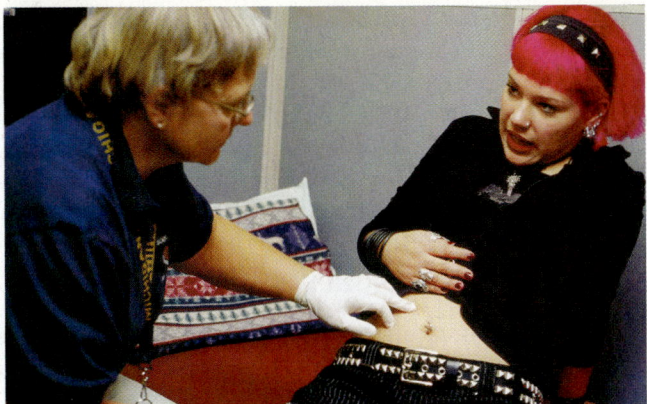

FIGURE 36–5. ◆ Talking openingly with adolescents about their health and teach them to avoid health risks connected with tattoos and piercing. The school nurse is inspecting an adolescent's pierced navel.

Since teens may choose to obtain body art even if parents object and if there are state laws to prohibit or make it difficult, nursing care must focus on providing information for the teen, assessing sites, identifying infections, and referring if needed. Care is almost always provided in community settings such as clinics or schools. Consider asking teens if they are thinking about body art since they often do not seek advice before obtaining the art, and may therefore not get adequate teaching (Montgomery & Parks, 2001).

Thinking Critically

THE ADOLESCENT WITH BODY PIERCINGS

Amy is 15 years old and attends an alternative high school. She recently had an ear piercing and it is sore. She comes to the health room to ask the advice of the school nurse. Upon examination, the area around the piercing is inflamed and mildly edematous. The nurse also learns that Amy recently had her navel pierced. After asking some questions, the nurse learns that Amy's ear was pierced by a friend, using a needle that had been "sterilized" by passing it through a match flame. She has had a slight fever, but otherwise feels fine.

In her home state, adolescents under 18 years of age must have the signature of a parent for body piercings and tattoos, so Amy chose to have the procedure done by a friend. She believes this is safe since her friend has done many piercings on others. She admits that her parents are not very pleased with her body art, but that they allow her to do it as long as she agrees to stay in high school. She had previously run away and spent several weeks living on the streets.

➥ What health care and social needs does Amy have?

➥ How can the nurse support both Amy and her parents?

➥ What physical care does Amy need to treat potential infection at her piercing site?

➥ What systemic infectious diseases is Amy at risk of acquiring due to repeated body piercings with unsterile technique? **WEB**

Teaching About

CARE FOR TATTOOS AND BODY PIERCINGS

Before the Procedure

- Does the studio look clean?
- Visit several studios to make comparisons of techniques, quality, and cleanliness.
- Ask to watch a tattoo or piercing done on someone else.
- What are the artist's sterilization and hygiene practices?
- Is the artist licensed? Trained?
- Look at pictures of completed art and talk with former clients.
- Insist that new, sterile equipment be opened in front of the person to be decorated.
- Consider if this permanent body decoration is desired for a lifetime.
- Consider what the tattoo or piercing will look like in several years.
- Consider the possible side effects of infection, dislike for the art, and allergy to dyes or metals.
- Be sure that hepatitis B vaccination is completed before the procedure.
- Be aware that no immunization is available to protect against the health risks of hepatitis C and HIV.

Care after the Procedure

- Touch the area only after carefully washing your hands.
- Keep the area elevated and use ice for the first 2 days to minimize swelling.
- Avoid contact with another person's body fluids until well healed.
- Turn the piercing jewelry gently several times daily using washed hands.
- Use antibacterial mouthwash or cleaner or ointment as recommended.
- Avoid pressure and rubbing on the site (such as belts on navel piercings).
- Watch carefully for signs of infection and report them to a health care provider:
  - Increased redness
  - Swelling
  - Pain
  - Hot feeling
  - Discharge
- Ask the artist how long healing will take. It varies from 2 months in the mouth or up to 6 or 8 months for a navel.
- Metal is dangerous during some medical procedures such as magnetic resonance imaging (MRI) or during surgery. Be sure to tell doctors and nurses about your piercings when you are hospitalized or receiving medical care, especially if they are in a part of the body not readily visible.
- If you decide to remove a piece of jewelry soon after it is placed, the skin may heal with only a slight scar.

Minority Sexual Practices

Adolescence is a time of identifying emerging sexuality. Most teens establish relationships with members of the opposite sex and learn how to interact in ways guided by their peer group, family, and culture. For some youth, the transition into adult sexuality is more challenging, as they feel emotional and sexual attraction to people of the same sex (**homosexuality**). The term **gay** is often used for homosexual males and **lesbian** for homosexual females. Other youth are **bisexual,** or attracted to both men and women, and some are **transgendered,** or are attracted to dress and act like members of the opposite sex. The initials LGBT are sometimes used to refer collectively to these minority sexuality choices. From 1% to 10% of youth identify as homosexual (Kreiss & Patterson, 1997).

Alternate sexual attractions and practices are not deviant but may be viewed as part of a continuum of sexual expression. No gene, early life experience, or other event causes homosexuality.

LGBT youth are at risk for a variety of problems related to emotional and physical health. These include rejection by family members and peers, verbal harassment, sexual abuse and physical assault, a high rate of suicide, substance abuse, high rate of homelessness, and sexual risks of HIV and other sexually transmitted diseases (Stevens & Morgan, 2001). Their health risks need to be identified and appropriate care provided.

Nurses can provide health care for LGBT youth in a variety of settings. School nurses and clinics can display a sign to demonstrate that they are accepting of persons with minority sexual preferences. Terminology in assessment should be gender-free. Ask "Do you have one or more sexual partners?" rather than "Do you have a boyfriend?" When youth identify as LGBT, provide usual care of all kinds. This includes preventive care such as immunizations, sports assessments, and injury prevention teaching. Be alert that the youth may have additional health challenges. Ask about peer and parental support; refer to support groups if needed. Provide resources when the teen is homeless, depressed, or suicidal (see Chapter 53). Perform testing for sexually transmitted diseases if the teen is having sexual contact and teach preventive measures. Foster a positive sense of self-esteem through encouraging positive activities such as sports, music, and friendships with peers. ⊂⊃ WEB

EFFECTS OF VIOLENCE

Violence is a threatened or actual use of physical force that leads to actual or potential physical or emotional trauma (Hennes, 1998). In the past several years, adults and children alike have been shocked by the violent episodes in schools. Although these incidents had much media coverage, they are just one type of violence that children may be regularly exposed to. Children can be the recipients of violence during child abuse and homicides, and they themselves can perform acts of violence on others. They may be touched by violence when parents are killed in gang conflicts, in terrorist attacks, or in wars. The effects of violence are far-reaching and ongoing; they permeate the victim's entire lifetime. This section explores some types of violence affecting children.

Schools and Communities

At a time when firearm deaths are decreasing overall, unintentional deaths and suicides have increased among children. About 75% of these deaths are committed with firearms found in the home. Forty percent of households with children have guns and in 25% of those homes the firearms are stored loaded or are not secured under lock (Society for Pediatric Nurses, 2000). ⊂⊃ WEB

Nursing Practice

When a group of children is attacked or killed in a school shooting, this tragic occurrence has the attention of the media. Little do many realize that this tragedy is really part of daily life. Nearly 12 children are killed by a firearm every day in the United States, or a classroom full every other day (Children's Defense Fund, 2000). Every 2 hours a child is killed. Nurses must realize and help to intervene in this national tragedy.

Nursing Practice

Nurses in school settings can be aware of the practice of bullying. These behaviors seek to harm or disturb the victim, and include such activities as hitting, verbal abuse, name-calling, threats, or spreading rumors. About 16% of children in a large national survey had suffered bullying, most commonly in grades 6 to 8, and more frequent among males. Children who are socially isolated are more commonly bullied (Nansel, 2001). Nurses can be active in setting up school policies about bullying. Programs should inform students that the behavior is not tolerated, teach what to do when bullying is experienced or witnessed, and set up peer support for those who are victims.

Homicide in children has gained attention in the last several years due to several shootings at schools. Although homicide is an extreme example, there are other types of violence. Children report being threatened verbally and with guns or knives at home, at school, and in their neighborhoods. They may be beaten up or bullied or harassed (Singer et al., 1999). They may view domestic violence in their own homes. They may be subjected to dangerous situations in their neighborhoods or during times of homelessness. About half of youths report experiencing serious threats to their well-being (Pratt & Greydanus, 2000).

Date rape or other sexual violence is reported by up to 15% of teens (Spencer & Bryant, 2000). 🔗 WEB

Risk factors more commonly seen in situations where violence has been committed against children have been identified (see Table 36–8). In addition, children who commit violence more commonly have ready access to firearms, are exposed to violence in the home or community, watch violent media, and have poor self-esteem or depression.

Realizing the impact of violence on and by children, several federal health care initiatives have begun to assist in lowering violence. Some programs have been helpful and incidents of homicides and most other violence have begun to decrease. The most successful programs include individual children, parents, schools, and communities. Health school professionals are instructed to identify signs of violence (Table 36–9). Provide resources for families and children to decrease violence.

Nursing Management

Nursing Assessment and Diagnosis

Nurses are in key positions to identify children at risk of being recipients and victims of violence. The ecologic framework can be used to assess children. Some questions that can be asked are listed in Table 36–9. It is important to detect both the risks that lead to vulnerability and the protective factors that can promote resilience and safety. Adapt questions to each age group and insert them in every health care encounter.

Nursing care for violence is discussed in "Nursing Care Plan: The Child and Violent Behavior." Some additional nursing diagnoses that may be appropriate are:

▶ *Risk for violence: self-directed* related to history of violence

▶ *Chronic low self-esteem* related to history of abuse

▶ *Altered family processes* related to situational crises

▶ *Altered growth and development* related to environmental deficiencies

Planning and Intervention

Nurses intervene with individual children, with families, and in schools and communities to increase safety and decrease violence. Help children and families meet basic needs and access resources to assist with finances, respite care, domestic violence, and other issues. Education is a key element of intervention.

PROVIDING INFORMATION

Teach the family the dangers of firearms and the necessity for use of gun locks, locked cabinets, storing guns unloaded, and storing guns and ammunition in separate places. Suggest alternative activities to minimize child exposure to violence in the media. Inform parents about rating systems for television and other media, and about lockout mechanisms for televisions and computers. Discuss the harmful effects of verbal and physical abuse to the child or other family members and explore alternatives.

Present the school-age child and adolescent with information about bullying and strategies for dealing with it. Provide school and community resources where the child can go if there are threats of any kind. Discuss date rape and violence with all teens and encourage them to report it.

TABLE 36–8 Risk Factors Common in Families with Child Victims of Violence

- History of mental illness, domestic violence, incarceration, or substance abuse in the home
- Family stresses
- Inadequate child care or supervision
- Inadequate family social support
- Use of corporal punishment for the child
- Child abuse
- Access to firearms
- Gang membership in family or neighborhood
- High exposure to media violence
- Child hyperactivity and other developmental behavioral disorders

Note: From Task Force on Violence, American Academy of Pediatrics. (1999). The role of the pediatrician in youth violence prevention in clinical practice and at the community level. *Pediatrics, 103,* 173–181. Adapted.

TABLE 36–9 Assessment Questions to Identify Violence Risk and Protective Factors

Microsystem

- Have you been hurt by your parents or anyone else at home?
- When was the last time you were made fun of or bullied at school? What did you do?
- Have you ever brought a gun or knife or other weapon to school?
- Do you have access to guns and knives at home? At friends' houses?
- What stresses are there in your family now?
- Tell me about school—what you like and don't like.

Mesosystem

- Do your parents attend school meetings? Talk with your teachers?
- Do you participate in any church, synagogue, or mosque services?
- Do you participate in any community activities?

Exosystem

- What stresses do your parents have at work, in their families, with their health or finances?
- Do you feel like your school helps to keep you safe?
- Are there plans for handling violent episodes at your school if they were to occur?
- Do you feel safe in your neighborhood?
- Where would you go or who would you call if you felt unsafe or were hurt and no one was at home?

GOAL	INTERVENTION	RATIONALE	EXPECTED OUTCOME
1. Risk for violence: directed at others related to history of family violence			
	NIC Priority Intervention: **Environmental management: Violence prevention:** *Monitoring and manipulation of the environment to decrease the potential for violent behavior directed toward self, others, or the environment*		*NOC Suggested Outcome:* **Impulse control:** *Ability to restrain compulsive or impulsive behavior in child and others*
The child demonstrates impulse control.	▶ Identify violent behaviors in the child.	▶ Violence in the child usually develops over time.	The child expresses ability to manage problems in acceptable ways.
	▶ Provide a safe place for exploration of feelings by referral to school or other counseling, support groups, and other resources.	▶ The child needs an opportunity to explore feelings and vulnerability.	
	▶ Provide strategies for managing anger, alternative ways for coping with problems.	▶ Coping strategies can be learned from others and can help in dealing with a stressful home situation.	
The child is secure in a safe environment.	▶ Perform thorough assessment of hazards to physical and emotional state in the child's home, neighborhood, and school.	▶ Hazards to physical and emotional health promote violence to and from the child.	The child expresses a sense of physical and emotional safety in daily life.
	▶ Institute actions that will result in removal of child from unsafe situations.	▶ Removal from family, community, or school may be needed to ensure child safety.	
	▶ Use community resources to provide respite care, teaching for families, and safety instruction for the child.	▶ Stress-reduction measures may help to decrease violent behaviors.	
2. Impaired home maintenance management related to insufficient family organization			
	NIC Priority Intervention: **Home maintenance assistance:** *Helping the family to maintain the home as a safe place to live*		*NOC Suggested Outcome:* **Role performance:** *Congruence of an individual's role behavior with role expectations* Family members meet role expectations, contributing to making the home a safe and secure place for the child.
Family members are able to meet role expectations.	▶ Provide information on child's developmental needs.	▶ Parents need to understand the developmental progression of their children.	
	▶ Provide ongoing assessment in the home via home health care visits.	▶ Early identification of hazards can lead to proper interventions to protect against harm to the child.	
	▶ Assist the family in identifying hazards in the environment that can impair the child's growth and development.	▶ Families may need respite care, information about child needs, financial assistance, or other resources to meet the needs of the child.	
	▶ Evaluate ability of adults to provide a safe, secure, nurturing environment.		
3. Hopelessness related to long-term family stress			
	NIC Priority Intervention: **Hope instillation:** *Facilitation of the development of a positive outlook in the given situation*		*NOC Suggested Outcome:* **Hope:** *Presence of internal state of optimism that is personally satisfying and life supporting*
The child will have adequate food and sleep, and express satisfaction with life.	▶ Monitor child's nutritional state and growth and daily patterns.	▶ The child's nutrition, sleep, and other patterns provide clues to the family's ability to perceive hope and provide care for the child.	The child demonstrates normal growth patterns and meets expected developmental outcomes.
	▶ Monitor child's developmental status.		
	▶ Determine adequacy of relationships and support systems.	▶ The child needs close personal relationships in order to grow and learn.	
The family will identify resources to achieve life goals.	▶ Monitor the family's decision-making ability.	▶ Feeling overwhelmed by daily life events leads to an inability to set goals and make decisions to meet the goals.	The family establishes realistic goals for growth and development of its members, and takes steps to meet the goals.
	▶ Provide information on community resources.	▶ Resources can assist the family members in setting and achieving realistic goals.	
	▶ Refer for psychiatric and other services if needed.		
	▶ Assist in goal setting.		

GOAL	INTERVENTION	RATIONALE	EXPECTED OUTCOME
4. Risk for injury related to physical or psychologic conditions in the environment			
	NIC Priority Intervention:		*NOC Suggested Outcome:*
	Safety behavior: *Family actions to minimize risk of physical or emotional trauma*		**Parenting: Social safety:** *Parental actions to avoid social relationships that might cause harm or injury;* **Risk control:** *Actions to eliminate or reduce actual, personal, and modifiable health risks*
Risk for physical and emotional injury to the child is decreased.	▶ Identify physical and psychologic factors that affect child's safety.	▶ Multiple factors in the family can contribute to risk of violence and lack of safety for the child.	
	▶ Assist family to deal with issues such as mental status challenges, fatigue, financial concern, substance abuse, lack of adequate child care resources, and other factors.		The child is not injured in physical or emotional ways in the home or other immediate settings.
	▶ Instruct family on methods of keeping the child safe.	▶ Families need information about the impact of unsafe settings on the child and methods that can decrease risk of injury.	
5. Posttrauma syndrome related to physical or psychosocial abuse			
	NIC Priority Intervention:		*NOC Suggested Outcome:*
	Counseling: *Use of an interactive helping process focusing on the needs, problems, and feelings of the child who is a victim of abuse or other violence*		**Abuse/violence recovery:** *Healing of psychologic and physical wounds of abuse or violence*
The child demonstrates abuse or violence recovery.	▶ Assess the child's affect and behaviors.	▶ Disturbed child behaviors can demonstrate a sense of mistrust and insecurity.	The child identifies feelings related to violent episode(s) and expresses healing of the self.
	▶ Evaluate social interactions and sense of trust in others.	▶ Establishment of close interactions with others demonstrates reestablishment of a sense of trust.	
	▶ Assist the child in identifying feelings and coping strategies by providing counseling, art therapy, and other strategies.	▶ A child who has experienced abuse or other violence needs a therapeutic relationship with a counselor to deal with the trauma, begin to rebuild trust and respect, and learn coping mechanisms.	

Teaching About

RATING SYSTEMS FOR MEDIA

Television Rating	Television MA Categories	Video & Computer	Movies
TV-Y: for all	FV: fantasy violence	E: for everyone	G: general audience
TV-Y7: for older children	L: language	T: for teen	PG: parental guidance suggested
G: general audience	V: violence	M: mature user	PG13: parents strongly cautioned
TV-PG: parental guidance suggested	S: sexual situation	AO: adults only	R: restricted to above 18 years without adult
TV-14: parents strongly cautioned	D: sexual dialogue		NC17: no one under 18 years admitted
TV-MA: mature audience			

Both in schools and community settings, nurses can plan peer mentoring to provide assistance to children at high risk of experiencing violence. Nurses can link and coordinate school and community programs for children to provide for parent involvement and child support. Discuss safety issues, both risks and protective actions, in schools and community groups. Report children at risk. Work to establish extended programs for children so that they are safe after school. Help children learn behaviors that will help them to be safe in their communities and at home. Teach positive problem solving and conflict management techniques to children and parents.

Evaluation

The expected outcomes of nursing care for violence prevention include a decrease in incidents of homicides, firearm injuries, abuse, date rape, and other violence among children. Additional outcomes are establishment of programs to decrease violence and verbalization by all children of what to do if violence occurs, and how to solve problems without becoming violent.

CHILD ABUSE

One of the most common types of violence against children is child abuse. This type of violence can have implications for both the physical and mental health of children, and can influence their health status even long after the abuse has occurred. Awareness of the problem of child abuse is increasing. More cases are being reported; however, these are probably only a small percentage of the total. Approximately 10% to 20% of children between the ages of 3 and 17 years—about 2.8 million children—are physically abused each year (Murry, Baker, & Lewin, 2000).

Physical abuse is only one part of a larger problem. The definition of child abuse has expanded over the past 10 years to include physical neglect, emotional abuse and neglect, verbal abuse, and sexual abuse, as well as physical abuse. Many sexually abused children are under the age of 5 years, some as young as 3 months of age. The average age for sexual molestation is 4 years. The perpetrator is the parent or another person legally responsible who:

- Inflicts or allows another to inflict physical or emotional pain or injury,
- Creates or allows another to create a significant risk of serious physical or emotional pain or injury, or
- Commits or allows another to commit an act of sexual abuse, as defined by law, against the child.

Abuse generally involves an act of commission, that is, actively doing something to a child physically, emotionally, or sexually, such as hitting, belittling, or molesting. Neglect more often involves an act of omission, such as not

TABLE 36–10   Risk Factors for Child Abuse and Neglect
Factors Increasing Risk for Physical Abuse
Poverty
Violence in the family
Prematurity
Unrelated male primary caretaker
Parents who were abused as children
Age less than 3 years
Handicap or condition that requires a great deal of care (e.g., mental retardation, attention deficit hyperactivity disorder)
Parental substance abuse or social isolation
Factors Increasing Risk for Sexual Abuse
Absence of natural father or having a stepfather
Being female
Mother's employment outside the home
Poor relationship with parent
Parental relationship characterized by conflict
Parental substance abuse or social isolation

providing adequate nutrition, emotional contact, or necessary physical care. Because the evidence is often not visible, emotional abuse and neglect are more difficult to identify and prove than physical abuse or neglect. Risk factors for abuse and neglect are listed in Table 36–10.

Physical Abuse

Physical abuse is the deliberate maltreatment of another individual that inflicts pain or injury and may result in permanent or temporary disfigurement or even death. Common methods of physical abuse in children are listed in Table 36–11.

Physical Neglect

Physical neglect is the deliberate withholding of or failure to provide the necessary and available resources to the child. Behaviors constituting physical neglect include failure to provide for the following basic needs: adequate nutrition and hydration, hygiene (e.g., clean diapers and clothes, bathing and toileting facilities), shelter (e.g., warmth in winter), and appropriate health care (e.g., immunizations, dental care, medications, eyeglasses).

Emotional Abuse

Emotional abuse usually involves shaming, ridiculing, embarrassing, or insulting the child. It can also include the destruction of a child's personal property, such as tearing up the child's favorite family photographs or letters or harming, killing, or giving away the child's pet. These actions are frequently used as a means of frightening or controlling the child.

Verbal abuse is a common method of emotional abuse. Words can be a violent and volatile weapon against a child,

TABLE 36-11　Methods of Physical Abuse in Children

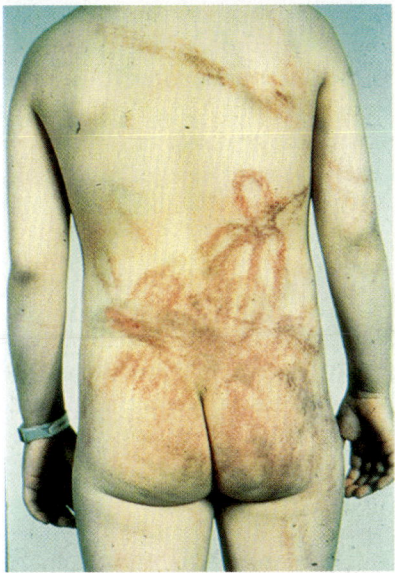

A

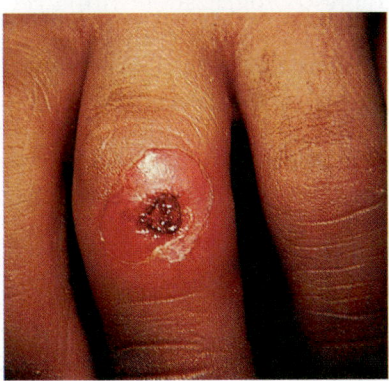

B

Hitting, slapping, kicking, or punching
Whipping with belts, shoes, or electrical cords **(A)**
Inflicting burns with a lit cigarette or lighter **(B)**
Immersing child or body part in scalding water
　(commonly legs, perineal area, hands, or feet; see Fig. 52–14A)
Shaking the child violently ("shaken child" syndrome)
Tying the child to a fence, bed, tree, or other object
Throwing the child against a wall, down stairs, or against a window
Choking or gagging the child
Fracturing the legs, arms, ribs, or skull
Deliberately administering excessive doses of prescribed or
　nonprescribed drugs
Deliberately withholding prescribed medication

Photographs copyright © AAP/Kempe. Used with permission.

eroding the child's fragile sense of self and destroying self-esteem. Common examples of verbal abuse include yelling obscenities at the child, calling the child names, threatening to "put the child away" or to give away or kill the child's pet, telling the child "I wish you were never born" or "You're worthless," and using words to humiliate, shame, or degrade the child.

Emotional Neglect

Emotional neglect is characterized by the caretaker's emotional unavailability to the child. The usual style of interaction is cold and lacking in sensitive personal attention. The child suffers from a lack of nurturance and failure of the parent or caretaker to meet basic dependency needs.

Sexual Abuse

Child sexual abuse is the exploitation of a child for the sexual gratification of an adult. Between 100,000 and 500,000 children in the United States are sexually abused each year. Approximately 75% to 80% of child sexual abusers are immediate family members, other relatives, friends, or neighbors. Male perpetrators make up 92% to 98% of all abusers (Murray, Baker, & Lewin, 2001; Frederickson, 1999). Abusers often threaten to harm or kill the child or another family member if the child discloses the abuse.

Nursing Practice

Following are common forms of sexual abuse:

▸ Oral-genital contact
▸ Fondling and caressing the genitals
▸ Anal intercourse
▸ Sexual intercourse
▸ Rape
▸ Sodomy
▸ Prostitution

ETIOLOGY AND PATHOPHYSIOLOGY

Regardless of the type of abuse, the most common abuser is the child's parent or guardian or the boyfriend of the child's mother. Risk factors associated with abusive behavior in adults include the following:

- Psychopathology, such as drug addiction or alcoholism, low self-esteem, poor impulse control, and other personality disorders

- Poor parenting experiences, such as abuse in the abuser's own childhood, rejection by the abuser's own parent(s), lack of knowledge of alternative methods of discipline, strong belief in or family tradition of harsh discipline, and lack of parental affection

- Marital stressors and problems with partners, such as hostile-dependent, abusive, or nonsupportive relationships, and one-sided decision making

- Environmental stressors, such as legal, financial, medical, or housing problems

- Social isolation, such as few friends and limited use of sitters, family, or other resources

- Inappropriate expectations for the developmental level of the child

CLINICAL MANIFESTATIONS

Clinical manifestations of physical abuse are listed on page. Behaviors inconsistent with developmental stage may be apparent. For example, the toddler or preschool child may be indiscriminately friendly with unfamiliar adults, including health care providers, rather than demonstrating shyness or anxiety. For the infant or young child with "shaken baby syndrome" or "shaken child syndrome," the symptoms are those of central nervous system injury from repeated coup and contrecoup injury (see Chapter 49). ⚭ These may include vomiting, irritability, fatigue, poor feeding, bradycardia, apnea, enlarged fontanel, and seizures. Bruises are usually not present (Castiglia, 2001).

Manifestations of physical neglect include undernourishment (evidenced by constantly feeling hungry, hoarding or stealing food, and being underweight), unclean clothes and body, poor dental health (extensive cavities or generally poor condition of teeth), and inappropriate clothing for the season.

Manifestations of emotional abuse, verbal abuse, and emotional neglect include fear, poor physical growth, and failure to meet appropriate developmental milestones. The child may have difficulty relating to adults, impaired communication skills, and developmental delays. Behavioral manifestations include anxiety, fear, shame, aggression, delinquency, and depression (Frederickson, 1999).

Children who have been sexually abused may exhibit a variety of physical and behavioral signs and symptoms. However, sexual abuse does not always result in apparent injury. Among the many long-term consequences of child sexual abuse are ongoing feelings of shame, guilt, anger, and hostility; decreased self-esteem, which leads to increased self-destructive behavior and risk of suicide; recurrence of victimization experiences; substance abuse; and eating disorders. The results can be long-lasting, with children experiencing posttraumatic stress disorder (PTSD) or substance abuse in adulthood (Walker, Scott, & Koppersmith, 1998). Factors associated with greater psychologic harm to the child include (1) a long period of abuse, (2) use of violent force or threat of violence, (3) abuse involving penetration (intercourse or oral–genital sex), and (4) abuse involving family members, especially the father or stepfather.

CLINICAL THERAPY

Diagnosis of abuse is made on the basis of a careful history and thorough physical examination. X-ray studies may be ordered to identify signs of recurrent abuse (e.g., healed fractures). Some children are admitted directly to the hospital with the diagnosis of suspected abuse or neglect. Less obvious as a victim of abuse is the child admitted with a skull fracture who "fell off a chair."

Neglect, which is more difficult to define and identify, frequently requires hospitalization with a comprehensive medical, social, and psychiatric evaluation. Five basic categories must be considered when attempting to diagnose neglect: (1) medical care neglect (lack of necessary medical care), (2) gross safety neglect (lack of appropriate supervision), (3) physical neglect (lack of food and shelter), (4) emotional neglect, and (5) educational neglect.

All 50 states have extensive, complex statutes about reporting child abuse and neglect. A specialist must be consulted, especially if the child's testimony will be used in court.

CLINICAL MANIFESTATIONS ≈ *Child Abuse*

- Multiple bruises in various stages of healing
- Scald burns with clear lines of demarcation and in a glove or stocking distribution (see Figure 52–14A)
- Rope, belt, or cord marks, usually seen on the mouth, buttocks, back, legs, and arms (see Figure A in Table 36–11)
- Burn scars in various stages of healing

- Multiple fractures in various stages of healing
- Shortness of breath and distress upon being moved, indicating chest contusions and possible rib fractures
- Sedation from overmedication
- Exacerbation of chronic illness (such as diabetes or asthma) because of withholding of medication

---

CLINICAL MANIFESTATIONS ≈ *Sexual Abuse in Children and Adolescents*

- Vaginal discharge
- Bloodstained underpants or diaper
- Genital redness, pain, itching, or bruising
- Difficulty walking or sitting
- Urinary tract infection
- Sexually transmitted disease
- Somatic complaints, such as headaches or stomachaches
- Sleeping problems, such as nightmares or night terrors
- Bed-wetting
- Unwillingness to go to babysitter, family member, neighbor, or other person

- Fear of strangers
- New or excessive sexual curiosity or play
- Constant masturbation
- Curling into fetal position
- Excessively seductive behavior
- Phobias about particular places, people, or things
- Abrupt changes in school performance and attendance
- Changes in eating habits
- Abrupt changes in behavior (especially withdrawal)
- Child or adolescent female acts like a wife or mother

Nursing Practice

Every state has a child abuse law specifying the particular behaviors that define every type of abuse. Any professional who works with children and reasonably suspects that a child has been abused is required to report his or her suspicions to the local agency for child protective services. Reports made in good faith are not liable to countersuits. However, professionals who suspect abuse and do not report it may be held responsible by the courts.

Children do not routinely make false allegations of abuse. If indeed there is reason to believe the allegations are false, a child and adolescent therapist (psychiatrist, psychologist, psychiatric clinical nurse specialist, or social worker) with special expertise should be consulted to determine the truth. Keep in mind that children who withdraw their accusations have often been threatened or coerced into doing so. Because children who have been physically, emotionally, or sexually abused are at risk for major depression, they require skilled care by mental health professionals who are specially trained in this area. Initially the treatment goals include prevention of self-destructive or other dangerous acts. Children must be encouraged to express their fears and feelings in a safe and supportive environment. Equally important is the child's need to build coping skills and self-esteem. The child must be reassured and convinced that he or she is in no way responsible or to blame for what happened.

Individual treatment with art therapy is used initially because it is the least threatening method in the early stages of treatment, it can easily be tailored to meet the child's individual needs, and it prepares the child for other forms of treatment such as family and group therapy (Figure 36–6 ◆). Family or group therapy may be of

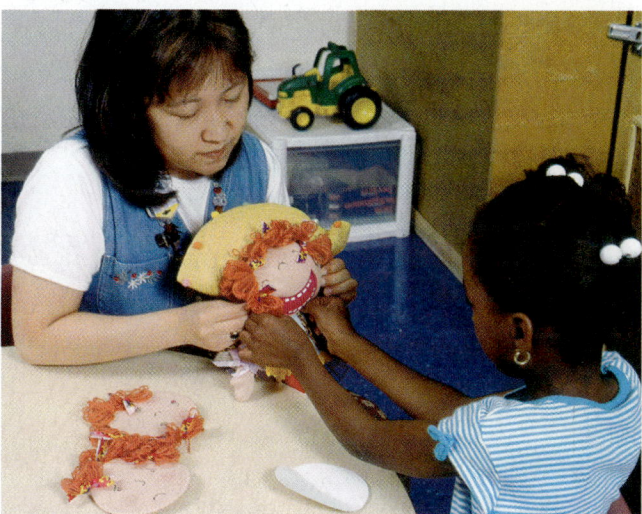

FIGURE 36–6. ◆ Therapeutic strategies with young children involve various methods of communication, such as dramatic play and art.

benefit in exploring the child's concerns and feelings. Anger is common, especially in children who were abused by a trusted adult such as the father or stepfather.

Nursing Management

Nursing Assessment and Diagnosis

Nursing assessment in instances of suspected child abuse or neglect requires a comprehensive history and physical examination, with documentation of findings. Consultation with social service agencies in the community is important if the family is receiving services.

Obtaining the history can be stressful for both the nurse and the parent. Use of therapeutic communication techniques and a quiet, unhurried environment are helpful. Be open, nonjudgmental, and calm. A statement such as "Hello, Mr. S. My name is Joan T. I'm Jonathan's nurse, and will be asking you some questions about his overall health" may be a good start. It is important to differentiate true child abuse from cultural variations that might inaccurately be assumed to indicate abuse (Figures 36–7 ◆ A and B). Obtaining information about abusive and neglectful behaviors requires a trusting relationship with parents, who are often afraid to trust any professional.

Developing Cultural Competence

Traditional treatment practices are sometimes mistaken for signs of physical abuse. The Chinese practice of cupping, which involves heating a bamboo cup and placing it on the skin, is a traditional treatment for headaches or abdominal pain. The Vietnamese practice of caogio (rubbing out the wind), in which a coin or the fingers are forcefully rubbed on the chest, back, or neck, is used to treat minor ailments.

The health history sequence should include (1) parental concerns, (2) general family history, and (3) specific child history. This sequence begins with nonthreatening topics and allows the nurse to demonstrate concern before asking about abuse-related concerns. Obtain details about how injuries occurred. Document the parents' and child's own words verbatim using quotation marks. Compare reports obtained from each family member for lack of consistency and details that change over time.

It is desirable to interview the parent and child separately as well as together. Parent-child interaction during an intensive history-taking session provides an opportunity to observe the child's behavior and the parent's method of handling and responding to the child.

Data gathered during history-taking are particularly important in light of physical findings. Are there discrepancies between the history and physical assessment data? Do the parents give a history of an uncontrollable, inattentive toddler when the nurse observes a child who is attentive

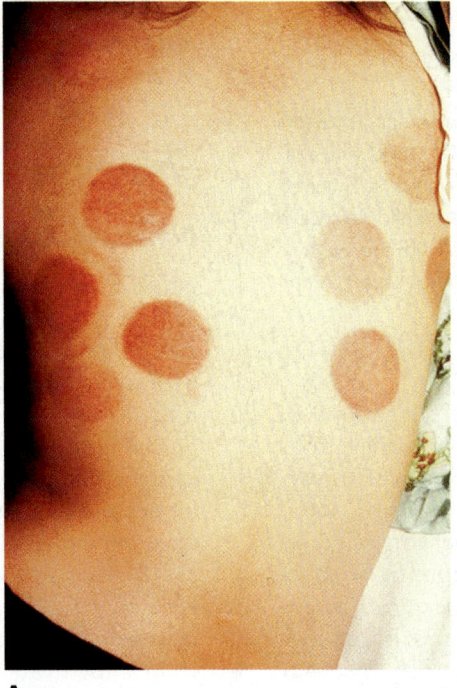
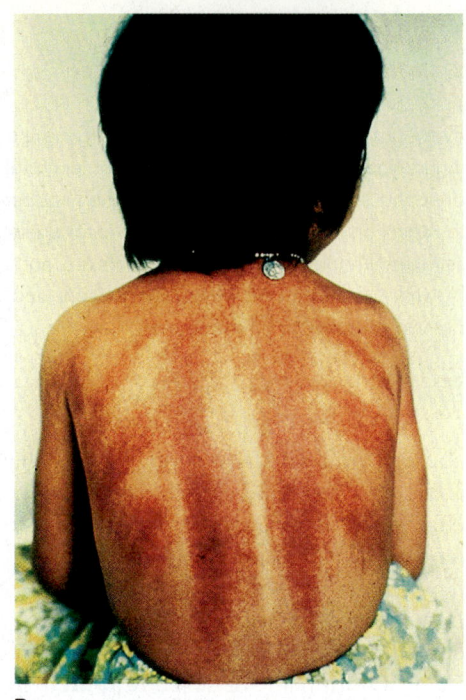

FIGURE 36–7. ◆ It is important to differentiate cultural practices such as cupping (A) and coining (B) from signs of child abuse. Photographs copyright © AAP/Kempe. Used with permission.

A

B

throughout a 15-minute examination? Assess the child's general appearance, including dress and behavior during the assessment. How do the child's affect, behavior, and development compare with those of other children the same age? Be alert for the signs of shaken child syndrome; this most often appears as a subtle neurologic condition. Measure head circumference and perform a neurologic examination (see Chapter 33 ⬭).

Documentation of findings is important in all situations but is essential in cases of suspected child abuse and neglect. Each person who handles a laboratory specimen or other item (e.g., clothing soiled with semen) in cases of suspected child abuse must be identified in the patient's record, and the specimen must never be left unattended. Record physical findings as observed. Use figure diagrams to document skin injuries. Take photographs to document the location, nature, and extent of injuries.

Among the nursing diagnoses that might be appropriate for the physically abused or neglected child are:

- ▶ *Pain* related to inflicted injuries
- ▶ *Impaired skin integrity* related to inflicted injuries
- ▶ *Altered growth and development* related to lack of supportive parenting and environment
- ▶ *Altered nutrition: less than body requirements* related to inadequate caloric intake
- ▶ *Altered health maintenance* related to lack of parental provision of child's essential needs
- ▶ *Fear* related to actual physical harm or repeated risk of injury
- ▶ *Risk for injury* related to physical abuse

- ▶ *Risk for violence (parent)* related to inability to manage anger

Additional diagnoses that might apply to the emotionally abused or neglected child include:

- ▶ *Defensive coping* related to psychologic impairment
- ▶ *Chronic low self-esteem* related to lack of appropriate emotional support from parents
- ▶ *Ineffective family coping: disabling* related to dysfunctional family dynamics and pattern of physical abuse

Diagnoses that might apply to the sexually abused child include the following:

- ▶ *Anxiety* related to potential separation from parent
- ▶ *Rape-trauma syndrome* related to sexual exploitation
- ▶ *Altered role performance* related to domestic violence
- ▶ *Personal identity disturbance* related to disturbance of usual activities of childhood

Planning and Implementation

Nursing care focuses on helping to remove the child from an abusive environment, preventing further injury, providing supportive care, and reinforcing the importance of follow-up care and counseling.

PREVENT FURTHER INJURY

Work with social services and community agencies to assess the child's home environment, individuals living in the home, and the actions surrounding the abuse. Assist in removing the child from the home to temporary custody of the court or foster care of another relative, if indicated. Counsel family members about abuse and refer them for appropriate therapy. **WEB**

PROVIDE SUPPORTIVE CARE

Protect and treat the child's injuries (e.g., fractures, burns). Include parents in the child's treatment plan, and keep them informed about the child's progress. Even if suspected of inflicting injuries to the child, the parent is still the child's primary caretaker. Talk with the parent as you would with any parent. Be supportive of any guilt expressed. Encourage the parent to assist with the child's care. Observe parent–child interactions and document supportive behaviors and the child's response to the parent versus other care providers.

Interacting nonjudgmentally with a parent suspected of abusing his or her child can be difficult. Nurses should talk with a colleague about any anger they feel toward the parents or about the child's injuries or specific actions surrounding the abuse. Use team meetings to develop strategies that enable health care professionals to work with the parents and child.

HOME CARE TEACHING

If there is any question about the child returning to a potentially dangerous situation, support the child's removal from the situation. The child may receive supervised care in the home by court order. Child care, home nursing, and social worker visits may need to be arranged. Parents should be referred to parent effectiveness classes, family therapy, and support groups as necessary. When a neighbor or friend is the abuser, the family may need support and legal advice when a term of incarceration is finished and the perpetrator returns to the community. Some states and communities have sexual offender laws that publicize the presence of an offender on parole within neighborhoods.

Encourage the family to inform other care providers when the child's abuse history may affect a response to care. They should be alert to signs of PTSD so they can seek assistance if the child has continuing problems (see Chapter 53).

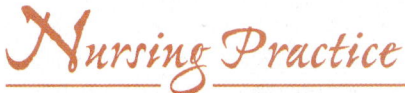

When children have been abused, they are often frightened in new situations. Sexually abused children may resist removing clothes for a physical examination or medical test. They may want to wear undergarments to the surgical suite. They may distrust members of the gender that abused. When aware of a history of abuse, ask the parents or guardians how to best facilitate the child's health care. Be sensitive to fears and allow the child to wear clothing, have a support person present, or whatever may provide a sense of security.

Evaluation

Expected outcomes of nursing care for the child who has been abused or neglected include maintenance of normal growth and development, establishment of a positive sense of self-esteem, provision of parenting information and stress relief for parents, provision of a nurturing environment for the child, and absence of episodes of abuse.

Munchausen Syndrome by Proxy

Munchausen syndrome by proxy is a potentially deadly form of child abuse that involves the fabrication of signs and symptoms of a health condition in a child. Usually it is the mother who creates these fictitious signs in her child (the proxy). The victim is usually under 6 years of age, and commonly under 1 year of age (Paulk, 2001). Frequently the child's symptoms of illness are used to gain entry into the medical system to meet the abuser's own needs.

The issues of abuse are multidimensional. The child is a victim of the feigned illness, repeated hospitalizations, and invasive procedures. Equally disruptive is the deprivation of the child's daily routine caused by the periodic medical crises.

Munchausen syndrome by proxy should be suspected when unexplained, recurrent, or extremely rare conditions occur; illness is unresponsive to treatment; and the history and clinical findings are inconsistent. The most commonly reported signs and symptoms are central nervous system dysfunction, apnea, diarrhea, vomiting, fever, seizures, signs of bleeding (in urine or stool), and rashes. The parent may overdose the child on medications, such as nonprescription drugs and even syrup of ipecac, causing a variety of side effects. The symptoms occur in the presence of the same caretaker and disappear when the child is separated from that caretaker.

The child often appears uncooperative, extremely anxious, fearful, and negative. The caretaker, who in contrast appears very cooperative, competent, and loving, often expresses a desire for the child to recover. The caretaker may even suggest diagnostic procedures to try to determine "what's wrong." Characteristically the caretaker thrives in the health care environment.

The cause of Munchausen syndrome by proxy is often complex and rooted in the caretaker's own abusive or neglectful childhood. The disorder occurs in all socioeconomic classes. Often the perpetrator has some type of health care background, such as nursing or another allied health profession. The abuser is often young, married, and middle socioeconomic class (Paulk, 2001).

A suspicion of Munchausen syndrome by proxy requires a coordinated evaluation by an interdisciplinary team. Members of the team must organize and communicate a strategic plan regarding collection of evidence, confrontation of the abuser, and management of the hospitalized child. The child's safety is the ultimate concern.

The case must also be reported to the appropriate child protective services.

NURSING MANAGEMENT

Take special care to maintain a trusting relationship with the caretaker so that he or she does not become suspicious and leave the hospital. Often the best person on the team to function in the role of "trusted other" is a member of the psychiatric consultation team.

Careful documentation of parent-child interactions, presence or absence of symptoms, and other pertinent observations is essential. The child must be closely monitored. If blood is present in the child's urine, stool, or vomitus, carefully document whether the nurse was present or whether the sample was provided by the parent. Covert video surveillance may be ordered by the hospital when the syndrome is highly suspected in a particular situation. Expert consultants may be needed to ensure legal requirements for investigation are met. When enough evidence is collected to prove Munchausen syndrome by proxy, the physician or another member of the psychiatric team confronts the caretaker.

EATING AND ELIMINATION DISORDERS

A number of eating and elimination disorders affect children and adolescents. The conditions described in this section are clearly linked to the lifestyles common in our country, contributing to an incidence greater than that seen in developing countries or in past decades. The conditions should be examined in light of current stresses, media images, and other environmental forces in order to implement strategies for clinical therapy.

Because food is intricately connected with emotional health, these disorders are often associated with both physiologic and psychologic causes and outcomes. They can create impaired nutritional status, and cause increasing difficulty in family and social relationships for the child or adolescent. The results may be poor nutritional status, depression, isolation and withdrawal, and other self-destructive behaviors.

Eating symbolizes many things. On a basic level, eating represents parental nurturing. The act of being fed or cared for by a parent is the model for all future intimate relationships. For some individuals, however, eating creates anxiety related to a negative association with unpleasant or unsatisfactory parent-child interactions. Elimination, as the outcome of eating, can reflect the same anxieties connected with food intake.

A multidisciplinary team, including a pediatrician, pediatric mental health specialist (psychiatrist, child psycho–logist, clinical nurse specialist, or social worker), family therapist, and nutritionist, assesses the child's physical, developmental, mental health, familial, and nutritional status. Because nutritional deficiencies often accompany eating and elimination disorders, physical assessment focuses on identifying possible associated problems (e.g., anemia). The over-all strengths and weaknesses of the child and family must be evaluated to identify the various factors contributing to the child's inadequate or excessive caloric intake and caloric expenditure. Treatment is then designed to address these factors. Anorexia nervosa and bulimia nervosa, recurrent abdominal pain, irritable bowel syndrome, and encopresis are discussed in the following section. See Chapter 31 for a discussion of eating disorder of infancy and childhood (failure to thrive) and for a discussion of overweight. Other bowel syndromes are discussed in Chapter 46.

ANOREXIA NERVOSA

Anorexia nervosa is a potentially life-threatening eating disorder that occurs primarily in teenage girls and young women, affecting an estimated 5% of young women and 1% of young men in the United States (American Dietetic Association, 2001). The typical patient is white and from a middle- to upper-middle-class family. Age at onset varies, and incidence peaks at 12 to 13 years and again at 17 to 18 years.

Etiology and Pathophysiology

Many causes are now thought to contribute to the onset of anorexia. Cultural overemphasis on thinness may contribute to the overconcern with dieting, body image, and fear of becoming fat experienced by many adolescents. Chemical changes have been found in the brain and blood of anorectic patients, leading to theories about a biologic cause. Often a significant life stress, loss, or change precedes the onset of anorexia. Stress hormones are commonly elevated in anorectics and immune system function may be disturbed (Brambilla, 2001).

Many authorities view family issues as contributory to anorexia. Intrafamilial conflicts and dysfunctional family patterns may occur when parents are overcontrolling and perfectionistic. The adolescent's eating behaviors may be an attempt to exercise independence and resolve internal psychologic conflicts.

The adolescent may engage in lengthy and vigorous exercise (up to 4 hours daily) to prevent weight gain. Laxatives or diuretics may be used to induce weight loss. As the disorder progresses, the adolescent perceives the ever-thinner body as becoming more beautiful. Youth may share weight loss techniques with anorectic friends and search out Internet sites positive about anorexia. The body responds to the abnormal eating behaviors as it would to starvation. Leukopenia, electrolyte imbalance, and hypoglycemia develop as a result of protein–calorie malnutrition. Once the body mass decreases below a critical level, menstruation ceases.

Clinical Manifestations

Anorectic adolescents are characterized by extreme weight loss accompanied by a preoccupation with weight and food,

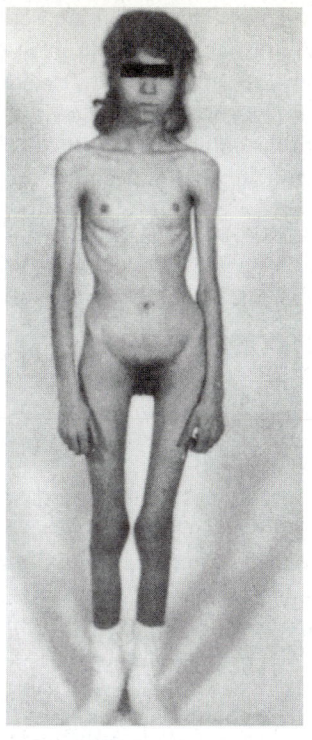
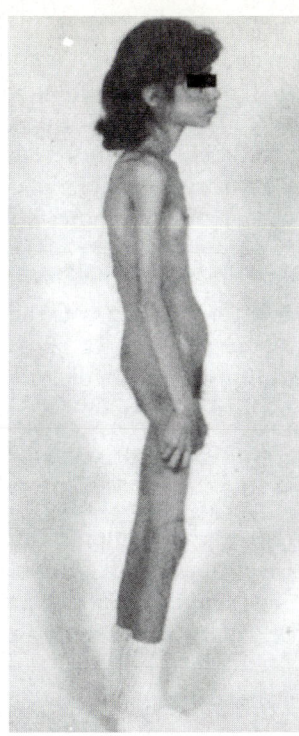

FIGURE 36–8. ◆ Characteristic physical appearance of an adolescent girl with anorexia nervosa. *Note:* From Rawlings, R. P., Williams, S. R., & Beck, C. K. (1992). *Mental-health psychiatric nursing* (3rd ed.), St. Louis, MO: Mosby-Year Book.

excessive compulsive exercising, peculiar patterns of eating and handling food, and distorted body image. They may prepare elaborate meals for others but eat only low-calorie foods. Characteristically the fear of becoming fat does not decrease with continued weight loss. Accompanying signs and symptoms of depression, crying spells, feelings of isolation and loneliness, and suicidal thoughts and feelings are common. The disorder is often associated with mental illness such as obsessive-compulsive disorder, anxiety disorders (see Chapter 53), ⚭ and history of abuse (Herpertz-Dahlmann, Muller, Herpertz, et al., 2001).

Physical findings include cold intolerance, dizziness, constipation, abdominal discomfort, bloating, irregular menses, and malnutrition (Figure 36–8 ◆ A and B). Hypothalamic suppression can lead to disturbances of gynecologic function, osteoporosis, decreased bone density, and fractures (Seidenfeld & Rickert 2001). Lanugo (fine, downy body hair) may be present. Fluid and electrolyte imbalances, especially potassium imbalances, are common. The child or adolescent is usually energetic despite significant weight loss. Extreme weight loss often leads to cardiac arrhythmias (bradycardia).

Clinical Therapy

Diagnosis is based on a comprehensive history, physical examination revealing characteristic clinical manifestations, and the DSM-IV criteria included in Table 36–12.

The goal of treatment is to address the physiologic problems associated with malnutrition, as well as the behavioral and cognitive components of the disorder. A firm focus is placed on reaching a targeted weight with a gradual weight gain of 0.1 to 0.2 kg/day (0.25 to 0.5 lb/day). Enteral feedings or total parenteral nutrition (TPN) may be necessary to replace lost fluid, protein, and nutrients. However, the adolescent often perceives these feedings as a punitive measure.

Individual treatment and family therapy address dysfunctional family patterns and help the family accept and deal with the adolescent as an independent and less than perfect individual. Family involvement is crucial to effect a lasting change in the adolescent.

Long-term outpatient treatment, in either an individual or a group setting, is frequently necessary. Counseling may be continued for 2 to 3 years to ensure that weight gain and self-image are maintained. Antidepressant drugs such as imipramine (Tofranil) or desipramine (Norpramin) may be prescribed for coexisting conditions such as depression, anxiety, or obsessive-compulsive disorders.

Indications for hospitalization include loss of 25% to 30% of body weight, fluid and electrolyte imbalances or arrhythmias, or the need to provide a more intense period of therapy if outpatient treatment fails to produce improvement. Behavior modification techniques are used extensively in combination with counseling and other methods in care of the hospitalized anorectic adolescent.

Nursing Management

Nursing Assessment and Diagnosis

Obtain a thorough individual and family history. Ask about usual eating patterns, daily caloric intake, exercise patterns, and menstrual history. Ask about medication use; include prescription, nonprescription, and herbal products. Is there a family history of eating disorders? Assess for signs of malnutrition. Obtain height and weight measurements, and compare with norms for the general population. Because the anorectic patient often wears layers of clothes when being weighed, attention is needed to obtain an accurate measurement.

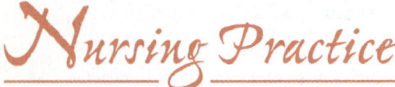

Nursing Practice

In an attempt to lose weight, anorectics and bulimics use products to bring about anorexia, vomiting, and diarrhea. Many herbal products are used for these purposes. One example is ephedra or ma huang. This Chinese herb is used for asthma, coughs, and flu and is present in some weight loss remedies in the United States. It is a chemical source of ephedrine and pseudoephedrine, and in large enough doses can cause increased blood pressure and heart rate, and stimulate the central nervous system (Swerdlow, 2000). Consider that some symptoms seen in those with eating disorders may be related to drugs and herbal products.

Nursing diagnoses for the adolescent with anorexia nervosa might include:

▶ *Altered nutrition: less than body requirements* related to inadequate intake

▶ *Risk for fluid volume deficit* related to inadequate fluid intake or fluid volume loss from overuse of laxatives and diuretics

▶ *Risk for altered body temperature* related to excessive weight loss and absence of subcutaneous fat

▶ *Constipation* related to inadequate food intake and overuse of laxatives

▶ *Body image disturbance* related to distorted perception of body size and shape

▶ *Self-esteem disturbance* related to dysfunctional family dynamics

▶ *Ineffective family coping: compromised or disabling* related to parental tendency to be overcontrolling and perfectionistic

Planning and Implementation

Nursing care centers on meeting nutritional and fluid needs, preventing complications, administering medications, and providing referral to appropriate resources. Specific treatment measures vary depending on physical complications, length and degree of illness, emotional symptoms accompanying the disorder, and family dynamics. Resistance to treatment is common, and nurses who care for anorectic adolescents must deal with their own feelings of frustration and anger.

MEET NUTRITIONAL AND FLUID NEEDS

Monitor nutritional and fluid intake, encourage consumption of food, and observe eating behaviors at mealtime.

Elimination patterns may be altered as a result of increased intake during hospitalization. Monitor for possible problems, including abdominal distention, constipation, or diarrhea. Daily monitoring of serum electrolytes is necessary.

If TPN is administered, watch for complications such as circulatory overload, hyperglycemia, or hypoglycemia. Use strict aseptic technique when changing tubing or dressings.

ADMINISTER MEDICATIONS

Monitor vital signs if the adolescent is receiving antidepressants. Watch for signs of hypertension and tachycardia. Administering medications after meals helps to prevent gastric irritation.

PROVIDE REFERRAL TO APPROPRIATE RESOURCES

Refer parents and other family members to the American Anorexia and Bulimia Association, National Anorectic Aid Society, and National Association of Anorexia Nervosa & Associated Disorders for further information about the disorder and a list of support groups in their area. WEB

Evaluation

Expected outcomes for nursing care include weight gain, maintenance of adequate fluid volume, beginning of positive sense of self-esteem, intake of nutritionally balanced diet, and use of psychologic counseling to understand the disorder.

BULIMIA NERVOSA

Bulimia nervosa is an eating disorder characterized by binge eating (a compulsion to consume large quantities of food in a short period of time). Usually the episodes of bingeing are followed by various methods of weight control (purging), such as self-induced vomiting, large doses of laxatives or diuretics, or a combination of methods. Like anorexia, bulimia affects mainly adolescent girls and young women who are white and in the higher socioeconomic classes. It affects 5% or more of young women. The disorder usually begins in middle to late adolescence, frequently emerging during college.

Etiology and Pathophysiology

Causes of bulimia nervosa are similar to those of anorexia nervosa: sensitivity to social pressure for thinness, body image difficulties, and long-standing dysfunctional family patterns. Families may be chaotic and distant from the girl, rather than overinvolved as with the anorectic. Many bulimic individuals experience depression. It is not clear whether the depression is a cause or a result of the bulimic individual's inability to control the bingeing and purging cycles. A bulimic adolescent often binges after any stressful event.

Bingeing usually occurs in secret for several hours until the individual is stopped by abdominal discomfort, by another person, or by vomiting. At first the episodes of binge eating are pleasurable. Immediately following the binge episode, however, feelings of guilt, shame, anger, depression, and fear of loss of control and weight gain arise. As these feelings intensify, the bulimic adolescent becomes increasingly anxious. This usually initiates the purge behaviors.

Purging eliminates the discomfort from bloating and also prevents weight gain. This relieves the feelings of depression and guilt, but only temporarily. Adolescents with bulimia commonly practice the binge–purge cycle many times a day, losing their ability to respond to normal cues of hunger and satiety.

Clinical Manifestations

Bulimic adolescents, like anorectic ones, are preoccupied with body shape, size, and weight. They may appear overweight or thin and usually report a wide range of average body weight over the years. Physical findings depend on the degree of purging, starvation, dehydration, and electrolyte disturbance. Erosion of tooth enamel, increased dental caries, and gum recession, which result from vomiting of gastric acids, are common findings. The back of a hand can have calloused from inducing vomiting. Abdominal distention is often seen. Esophageal tears and esophagitis may also occur.

Clinical Therapy

A comprehensive history is necessary because most bulimic adolescents appear normal in weight or only slightly underweight. Laboratory evaluation may identify signs of altered electrolyte and hematologic status. The diagnosis is confirmed by the presence of specific DSM-IV criteria (Table 36–13).

TABLE 36–13   DSM-IV Criteria for Bulimia Nervosa

A. Recurrent episodes of binge eating. An episode of binge eating is characterized by both of the following:
1. Eating, in a discrete period of time (e.g., within any 2-hour period), an amount of food that is definitely larger than most people would eat during a similar period of time and under similar circumstances
2. A sense of lack of control over eating during the episode (e.g., a feeling that one cannot stop eating or control what or how much one is eating)
B. Recurrent inappropriate compensatory behavior in order to prevent weight gain, such as self-induced vomiting; misuse of laxatives, diuretics, enemas, or other medications; fasting; or excessive exercise.
C. The binge eating and inappropriate compensatory behaviors both occur, on average, at least twice a week for 3 months.
D. Self-evaluation is unduly influenced by body weight and shape.
E. The disturbance does not occur exclusively during episodes of anorexia nervosa.

Note: From American Psychiatric Association. (2000). *Diagnostic and statistical manual of mental disorders* (4th ed., Text revision). Washington, DC. Copyright © 2000 American Psychiatric Association. Reprinted with permission.

Treatment includes management of physiologic problems, behavior modification, and psychotherapy. Behavior modification focuses on modifying the dysfunctional eating patterns and restoring a normal pattern. Until the episodes of bingeing and purging are under control, feelings of discouragement and hopelessness prevail. Thus, the focus early in treatment is on initiating an immediate behavioral change. Once initial interventions have been successful, group therapy sessions work well for persons with anorexia or bulimia. Specific treatment measures may include:

- Educating the adolescent about good nutrition (including food choice and caloric content)
- Encouraging the adolescent to keep a log or food journal and helping the adolescent make connections between emotional states and stress and the impulse to binge or purge
- Setting up a daily dietary routine of three meals and three snacks a day (using the same foods for each meal and snack every day to change misconceptions about the weight-gaining potential of certain foods and to decrease anxiety about what food must be eaten at the next meal)

Once these initial measures have been taken, the underlying psychosocial issues are explored. The goals of therapy are to provide the bulimic adolescent with adaptive coping skills and to improve self-esteem.

Most bulimic adolescents do not require hospitalization. Serious abnormalities in fluid and electrolyte levels caused by uncontrollable cycles of bingeing and vomiting, accompanied by depression or suicidal activity, indicate the need for hospitalization. The prognosis is good with long-term therapy.

Nursing Management

Nursing Assessment and Diagnosis

Obtain a thorough individual and family history, including daily dietary intake and weight fluctuations. Inquire about problems such as abdominal pain or distention, which may indicate an abnormal eating or elimination pattern. Assess the oral mucosa for signs of damage to tooth enamel caused by purging; examine hands for evidence of vomiting-inducing calloused.

Among the nursing diagnoses that might be appropriate for the adolescent with bulimia nervosa are:

▶ *Altered nutrition: less than or more than body requirements* related to inadequate or excessive intake

▶ *Risk for fluid volume deficit* related to fluid volume loss

▶ *Altered oral mucous membrane* related to chemical effects of vomited gastric acids

- *Health-seeking behaviors (child)* related to health risks of excessive use of laxatives and diuretics
- *Anxiety* related to discomfort with weight and eating patterns
- *Self-esteem disturbance* related to dysfunctional family dynamics
- *Ineffective individual coping* related to life stressors

Planning and Implementation

Nursing care includes monitoring nutritional intake and elimination patterns, preventing complications, and providing appropriate referrals.

During hospitalization the patient keeps a food diary. Be alert to the adolescent who hides, gives away, or discards food from the tray or who exits to use the bathroom after meals. Bulimic adolescents should be with other people for at least a half hour after each meal so that they do not use purging behaviors. Withdrawal from laxatives and diuretics is managed with careful observation for alterations in fluid and electrolyte status. Cardiac monitoring may be necessary if potassium levels are seriously altered. Esophageal tearing or esophagitis is treated to promote mucosal healing. Medications such as antidepressants may be administered. Encourage continuation of group and other therapy sessions.

Refer bulimic adolescents and their families to various organizations for assistance and information about the disorder.

Evaluation

Expected outcomes for nursing care for the adolescent with bulimia include healthy mucous membranes and skin, adequate intake of fluids and food, balanced food intake, maintenance of normal weight, and absence of bingeing and purging.

RECURRENT ABDOMINAL PAIN

Recurrent abdominal pain is a frequent problem among young children and adolescents, particularly girls of school age. Although there may be organic causes such as motility problems, constipation, or inflammatory bowel disease, in most cases an organic cause cannot be found. This disorder is associated with the high-stress lifestyles common in contemporary society and has a strong environmental component. However, parents and health care professionals should not dismiss the child's pain just because the cause is unknown or unidentified (Kaufman, Cromer, Deleiden, et al., 1997).

The pain is generally located in the periumbilical area and occurs on a regular basis. A thorough history and physical examination are necessary to rule out organic causes. Children with recurrent abdominal pain often have little independence and feel controlled by their parents. The history should explore the pressures and stresses in the child's life, the child's temperament or methods of coping, bowel elimination patterns, and history of sexual abuse.

Laboratory studies such as a complete blood count may be ordered to rule out other illness. Gastrointestinal studies may be performed in an outpatient setting. Children are occasionally hospitalized when their condition is severe and not treatable at home.

When no organic cause can be identified, treatment of recurrent abdominal pain focuses on providing outlets for the release of stress within the family and in other settings in the child's life, enhancing the child's coping methods, and promoting dietary changes that encourage regular bowel movements.

Nursing Management

Nursing care includes supporting the child during assessment and diagnostic testing. Teach the child relaxation techniques and methods for coping with stress. Identify what life events are stressors for the child or what he or she worries about. Explore methods for giving more independence to the child in the family. Teach the importance of eating a high-fiber diet and maintaining a regular elimination pattern. The child and family may need explanations to understand the pain, which can be compared to neck pain or a headache as an outcome of stress. Children with continuing or recurrent abdominal pain should be referred to a mental health professional.

IRRITABLE BOWEL SYNDROME

Irritable bowel syndrome occurs in 6% of middle school and 14% of high school students. It is characterized by abdominal pain, with episodes of both diarrhea and constipation. The pain is reduced by defecation. The disorder is believed to be related to recurrent abdominal pain (described earlier) since symptoms and causes are similar, and children with recurrent abdominal pain frequently suffer from irritable bowel syndrome as they get older. Studies have shown that there are sections of disorganized motility in the bowel (Youssef & DiLorenzo, 2001). In contrast with Crohn disease and inflammatory bowel disease (see Chapter 46), irritable bowel syndrome shows no structural or metabolic abnormalities. It is believed that the syndrome is closely related to stress, and that individuals with the abnormality have a heightened autonomic nervous system response to stressful events, leading to hypermotility of sections of the gastrointestinal tract.

Most children with irritable bowel syndrome receive only symptomatic treatment (Fass, Longstreth, Pimentel, et al., 2001). Antispasmodic medicines are sometimes prescribed but may have limited usefulness. Management of stress may be the best solution. Children can be encouraged to exercise, use relaxation techniques, and find other methods of decreasing stress. Ensuring regular bowel movements by eating fresh fruits, vegetables, grains, and fluids can help reduce the pressure in the gastrointestinal tract.

ENCOPRESIS

Encopresis is an abnormal elimination pattern characterized by the recurrent soiling or passage of stool at inappropriate times by a child who should have achieved bowel continence. It occurs in approximately 1% of school-age children. Children with primary encopresis have never achieved bowel control. Children with secondary encopresis have been continent of stool for several months.

Encopresis is usually associated with voluntary or involuntary retention of stool in the lower bowel and rectum, leading to constipation, dilation of the lower bowel, and incompetence of the inner sphincter. The retention of stool is usually a result of being "too busy"; the child puts off going to the bathroom because there are activities occurring and it would be an inconvenience to leave. The retention of stool leads to constipation that is untreated and chronic (Nowicki & Bishop, 1999). Loose stool leaks around the hard feces, and the child becomes unaware of a need to eliminate. Soiling may occur during the day or night. Bowel movements are irregular, painful, small, and hard. The child may be ridiculed by peers because of his or her offensive body odor. This rejection leads to withdrawal and behavioral problems, often resulting in altered school performance and attendance. The child continues to hold stool because the passage has become painful. Parents commonly seek health care, believing that the child has diarrhea or constipation.

The underlying constipation that leads to encopresis may be caused by the stress of environmental changes (birth of a sibling, moving to a new house, attending a new school), issues of anger and control related to bowel training, diet, a full schedule of activities, or a genetic predisposition.

A thorough history, physical examination, and diagnostic studies (possibly including barium enema) are necessary to rule out organic causes and anatomic abnormalities. Examination of mental health and cognitive functioning may be indicated. Information about the child's toilet-training habits and parents' attitudes concerning those habits is obtained. A dietary history, including eating habits and types of foods eaten, is often helpful. Physical examination sometimes reveals a nontender mass in the lower abdomen.

Treatment may include behavior modification techniques, dietary changes, use of lubricants to clear the bowel of impacted stool and encourage normal defecation, and psychotherapy. Behavior modification programs that reward and reinforce appropriate toileting habits can be successful. Dietary changes include incorporating high-fiber foods such as fruits, vegetables, and whole-grain cereals into the diet. Limiting intake of refined and highly processed foods and dairy products also may be helpful. Drugs such as mineral oil, bulk-forming laxatives, and stool softeners are used temporarily to empty the bowel. The child should sit on the toilet for several minutes after morning and evening meals. It takes several months for the bowel to be retrained to respond to sphincter stimulation. Psychotherapy involving the child and family may be indicated in instances of dysfunctional parent-child relationships.

Nursing Management

Prevention of encopresis is a nursing goal. Teach toilet-training techniques to parents, emphasizing the child's developmental readiness (see Chapter 32). Parents should praise the child for successes and avoid punishment and power struggles. Encourage high-fiber diets and regular times for elimination. Daily fiber recommendation is equal to the child's age in years plus 5 to 6 grams, so a 5-year-old child needs 10 to 11 grams of fiber daily. Some high-fiber foods include pears, apples, berries, beans, corn, tomato, potatoes, and whole grains.

Nursing care when a child has encopresis centers on educating the child and parents about the disorder and its treatment and providing emotional support. Explain the treatment plan, including dietary changes and use of laxatives or stool softeners. Reassure the child that he or she has a healthy body and, with treatment, will achieve normal functioning. Follow the child for at least 6 months to be certain new patterns have been established.

CHAPTER HIGHLIGHTS

- Many of the major morbidities and mortalities of childhood and adolescence are related to social and environmental factors.
- The theory of ecologic development provides a framework to use in assessing the interactions of children with factors in their environments.
- The theory of resilience examines children's risk and protective factors to formulate interventions to assist the child dealing with health problems related to social conditions.

- Poverty is a pervasive and important risk factor that influences many health outcomes.
- Tobacco use is high among youths, and the most common time for initiation of tobacco use is middle school years.
- Tobacco prevention and cessation programs are needed throughout the school years.
- Substance abuse of many types occurs in childhood and adolescence and compounds many health risks.

- A major contributor to overweight and other health problems is the lack of physical activity among the young.

- Protective equipment can reduce the number and severity of injuries during risky physical activities.

- Teens need information about body art safety procedures if they choose this method of self-expression.

- Violence can be directed at children, and children can be the perpetrators of violence.

- All families should be regularly assessed for violence and prevention strategies applied when needed.

- The most common eating disorders of adolescence are anorexia and bulimia.

- A combination of behavioral management, counseling, and medication is often used in treatment programs for eating disorders.

EXPLORE MEDIA LINK

NCLEX Review, Case Studies, and other interactive resources for this chapter can be found on the companion website at http://www.prenhall.com/london. Click on "Chapter 36" to select the activities for this chapter.

For animations, more NCLEX review questions, and an audio glossary, access the accompanying CD-ROM in this textbook.

REFERENCES

American Dietetic Association. (2001). Position of the American Dietetic Association. Nutrition intervention in the treatment of anorexia nervosa, bulimia nervosa, and eating disorders not otherwise specified (EDNOS). *Journal of the American Dietetic Association, 101,* 810–819.

Anderson, R. E., Crespo, C. J., Bartlett, S. J., Cheskin, L. J., & Pratt, M. (1998). Relationship of physical activity and television watching with body weight and level of fatness among children: Results from the third National Health and Nutrition Examination Survey. *Journal of the American Medical Association, 279,* 938–942.

Armstrong, M. L. & Kelly, L. (2001). Tattooing, body piercing, and branding are on the rise: Perspectives for school nurses. *Journal of School Nursing 17,* 12–23.

Behrman, R. E. (Ed.). (2000). *The future of children: Unintentional injuries in childhood.* Los Altos, CA: The David and Lucille Packard Foundation.

Board on Children, Youth, and Families, National Research Council and Institute of Medicine. (2001). *From neurons to neighborhoods.* Washington, DC: National Academy Press.

Brambilla, F. (2001). Social stress in anorexia nervosa: A review of immuno-endocrine relationships. *Physiology and Behavior, 73,* 365–369.

Castiglia, P. T. (2001). Shaken baby syndrome. *Journal of Pediatric Health Care, 15,* 78–80.

Children's Defense Fund. (2000). *The state of America's children.* Washington, DC: Author.

Coleman-Wallace, D., Lee, J. W., Montgomery, S., Blix, G., & Wang, D. T. (1999). Evaluation of developmentally appropriate programs for adolescent tobacco cessation. *Journal of School Health, 69,* 314–319.

Committee on Injury and Poison Prevention, American Academy of Pediatrics. (2001). Bicycle helmets. *Pediatrics, 108,* 1030–1032.

Committee on Public Education, American Academy of Pediatrics. (2001). Children, adolescents and television. *Pediatrics, 107,* 423–426.

Committee on Sports Medicine and Fitness, American Academy of Pediatrics. (2001). Risk of injury from baseball and softball in children. *Pediatrics, 107,* 782–784.

Cook, K. R. (1999). Assessment of potential inhalant use by students. *Journal of School Nursing, 15*(20), 20–23.

Crook, W. P. (1998). The new sisters of the road: Homeless women and their children. *Journal of Family Social Work, 3*(4), 49–64.

Donovan, K. A. (2000). Smoking cessation programs for adolescents. *Journal of School Nursing, 16*(4), 36–43.

Dowell, D. L. (1998). Effects of television on children: A review of the literature and recommendations for nurse practitioners. American *Journal for Nurse Practitioners 2*(10), 31–37.

Elkind, D. (1998). *The hurried child: Growing up too fast too soon.* Reading, MA: Perseus Books.

Ensign, J., & Santelli, J. (1998). Health status and service use. *Archives of Pediatric and Adolescent Medicine, 152,* 20–24.

Fass, R., Longstreth, G. F., Pimentel, M., Fullerton, S., Russak, S. M., Chiou, C. F., et al., (2001). Evidence- and consensus-based practice guidelines for the diagnosis of irritable bowel syndrome. *Archives of Internal Medicine, 161,* 2081–2088.

Federal Interagency Forum on Child and Family Statistics. (2000). *America's children: Key national indicators of well-being 2000.* Washington, DC: U.S. Government Printing Office.

Fetro, J. V., Coyle, K. K., & Pham, P. (2001). Health-risk behaviors among middle school students in a large majority-minority school district. *Journal of School Health, 71,* 30–37.

Fields, J., Smith, K., Bass, L. E., & Lugaila, T. (2001). *A child's day: Home, school, and play (selected indicators of child well-being).* Washington, DC: U.S. Department of Commerce.

Frederickson, D. (1999). Maltreatment of children. *Journal of Child and Family Nursing, 2,* 393–401.

Friedman, M. M. (1998). *Family nursing* (4th ed.). Stamford, CT: Appleton & Lange.

Geiger, J. D., Drongowski, R. A., & Lenni, J. L. (2001). Car surfing: An underreported mechanism of serious injury in children and adolescents. *Journal of Pediatric Surgery, 36,* 232–234.

Hanson, M. (1999). Which straw will break the camel's back? *American Journal of Nursing, 99,* 63–69.

_____ (2000). *Healthy People 2010.* Washington, DC: U.S. Department of Health and Human Services.

Hennes, H. (1998). A review of violence statistics among children and adolescents in the United States. *Pediatric Clinics of North America, 45,* 269–280.

Herpertz-Dahlmann, B., Muller, B., Herpertz, S., Heussen, N., Hedebrand, J., & Remschmidt, H. (2001). Prospective 10-year follow-up in adolescent anorexia nervosa—course, outcome, psychiatric comorbidity, and psychosocial adaptation. *Journal of Child Psychology and Psychiatry, 42,* 603–612.

Herrenkohl, T. I., Maguin, E., Hill, K. G., Hawkins, J. D., Abbott, R. D., & Catalano, R. F. (2000). Developmental risk factors for youth violence. *Journal of Adolescent Health, 26,* 176–186.

Kaufman, K. L., Cromer, B., Deleiden, E. L., Zaron-Aqua, A. Aqua, K., Greeley, T., et al. (1997). Recurrent abdominal pain in adolescents: Psychosocial correlates of organic and nonorganic pain. *Children's Health Care, 26,* 15–30.

Knight, J. R. (1997). Adolescent substance use: Screening, assessment, and intervention. *Contemporary Pediatrics, 14,* 45, 51–56, 61–72.

Kreiss, J. L., & Patterson, D. L. (1997). Psychosocial issues in primary care of lesbian, gay, bisexual, and transgender youth. *Journal of Pediatric Health Care, 11,* 266–274.

Lackey, N., & Walker, B. L. (1998). An ecological framework for family nursing practice and research. In B. Vaughan-Cole, M. A. Johnson, J. A. Malone, & B. L. Walker, (Eds.), *Family nursing practice.* (pp. 38–48) Philadelphia: WB Saunders.

Malone, J. A. (1998). The resiliency model of family stress, adjustment, and adaptation. In B. Vaughan-Cole, M. A. Johnson, J. A. Malone, & B. L. Walker, (Eds.), *Family nursing practice* (pp. 49–60). Philadelphia: WB Saunders.

Melnyk, B. M., & Alpert-Gillis, L. J. (1997). Coping with marital separation: Smoothing the transition for parents and children. *Journal of Pediatric Health Care, 11,* 165–174.

Menke, E. M. (1998). The mental health of homeless school-age children. *Journal of Child and Adolescent Psychiatric Nursing, 11,* 87–98.

MMWR. (2000a). Youth risk behavior surveillance—United States, 1999. *Morbidity and Mortality Weekly Report, 49* (SS5).

MMWR. (2000b). Youth tobacco surveillance—United States, 1998–1999. *Morbidity and Mortality Weekly Report, 49* (SS-10), 1–94.

MMWR. (2000c). Unpowered scooter-related injuries—United States, 1998–2000. *Morbidity and Mortality Weekly Report, 49,* 1108–1110.

Montgomery, D. F., & Parks, D. (2001). Tattoos: Counseling the adolescent. *Journal of Pediatric Health Care, 15,* 14–19.

Murry, S. K., Baker, A. W., & Lewin, L. (2000). Screening families with young children for child maltreatment potential. *Pediatric Nursing, 26,* 47–54.

Nansel, T. R. *Journal of the American Medical Association, 285,* 2094–2100.

Nansel, T. R., Overpeck M., Pilla, R. S., Ruan W. J., Simons-Morton, B., & Scheidt, P. (2001) Bullying behaviors among U.S. youth: Prevalence and association with psychosocial adjustment.

National Institute of Child Health and Human Development. (1997). The effects of infant child care on infant-mother attachment security. *Child Development, 68,* 860–879.

National Institute on Drug Abuse. (1999). *Some facts about club drugs.* Bethesda, MD: U.S. Department of Health and Human Services.

Nowicki, M. J., & Bishop, P. R. (1999). Organic causes of constipation in infants and children. *Pediatric Annals, 28,* 293–300.

Pagliaro, A. M., & Pagliaro, L. A. (1996). *Substance abuse among children and adolescents.* New York: John Wiley & Sons.

Paulk, D. (2001). Munchausen syndrome by proxy. *Clinician Reviews, 11*(8), 51–56.

Pratt, H. D., & Greydanus, D. E. (2000). Adolescent violence: Concepts for a new millennium. *Adolescent Medicine, 11,* 103–125.

Robinson, T. N. (2001). Interventions to reduce media viewing improves aggressive children's behavior. *Archives of Pediatric and Adolescent Medicine.*

Santrock, J. (1999). *Life-span development.* Boston: McGraw-Hill.

Sergeant, J. D., Mott, L. A., & Stevens, M. (1998). Predictors of smoking cessation in adolescents. *Archives of Pediatric and Adolescent Medicine, 152,* 388–393.

Seidenfeld, M. E., & Rickert, V. I. (2001). Impact of anorexia, bulimia and obesity on the gynecologic health of adolescents. *American Family Physician, 64,* 445–450.

Singer, M. I., Miller, D. B., Guo, S., Flannery, D. J., Frierson, T., & Slovak, K. (1999). Contributors to violent behavior among elementary and middle school children. *Pediatrics, 104,* 878–884.

Society for Pediatric Nurses, SPN Public Policy Committee. (2000). Gun accidents, suicides increase among children. *SPN News, 9,* 6.

Spencer, G. A., & Bryant, S. A. (2000). Dating violence: A comparison of rural, suburban, and urban teens. *Journal of Adolescent Health, 27,* 302–305.

Stein, R. E. K. (Ed.) (1997). Health care for children. New York: United Hospital Fund of New York.

Stevens, P. E., & Morgan, S. (2001). Health of lesbian, gay, bisexual, and transgender youth. *Journal of Pediatric Health Care, 15,* 24–34.

Stewart, M., Reid, G., & Mangham, C. (1997). Fostering children's resilience. *Journal of Pediatric Nursing, 12,* 21–31.

Swerdlow, J. L. (2000). *Nature's medicine: Plants that heal.* Washington, DC: National Geographic Society.

Task Force on Violence, American Academy of Pediatrics. (1999). The role of the pediatrician in youth violence prevention in clinical practice and at the community level. *Pediatrics, 103,* 173–181.

Telles, S., Narendran, S., Raghuraj, P., Nagarathna, R., & Nagendra, H. R. (1997). Comparisons of changes in autonomic and respiratory parameters of girls after yoga and games at a community home. *Perceptual and Motor Skills, 84*(1), 251–257.

Telles, S., & Srinivas, R. B. (1998). Autonomic and respiratory measures in children with impaired vision following yoga and physical activity programs. *International Journal of Rehabilitation and Health, 4*(2), 117–122.

Thompson, P. (1998). Adolescents from families of divorce: Vulnerability to physiological and psychological disturbances. *Journal of Psychosocial Nursing, 36,* 34–39.

Vostanis, P., Grattan, E., & Cumella, S. (1998). Mental health problems of homeless children and families: A longitudinal study. *British Medical Journal, 346,* 899–902.

Walker, G. C., Scott, P. S., & Koppersmith, G. (1998). The impact of child sexual abuse on addiction severity and analysis of trauma processing. *Journal of Psychosocial Nursing, 36*(3), 10–18.

Wallerstein, J. S., Corbin, S. B., & Lewis, J. M. (1988). Children of divorce: A ten year study. In E. M. Hetherington & J. B. Arasteh (Eds.), *Impact of divorce, single parenting, and stepparenting on children.* Hillsdale, NJ: Erlbaum Publishers.

Wallerstein, J., & Kelly, J. (1996). *Surviving the breakup.* New York: Harper Collins.

Wallerstein, J., Lewis, J., & Blakeslee, S. (2000). *The unexpected legacy of divorce: A 25 year landmark study.* New York: Hyperion.

Werner, R. M., & Pearson, T. A. (1998). What's so passive about passive smoking? *Journal of the American Medical Association, 279,* 157–158.

Youssef, N. N., & DiLorenzo, C. (2001). The role of motility in functional abdominal disorders in children. *Pediatric Annals, 30,* 24–30.

CHAPTER 37

The Child with a Life-Threatening Illness or Injury

I t all happened so fast. We didn't even see the car coming. Next thing I knew, we were in the emergency room talking about abdominal and head injuries. Now we are in the intensive care unit, and I'm worried because Alexa is still unconscious and on a ventilator. It was helpful for the nurse to tell me that even though Alexa couldn't respond it was good to talk to her, because she will probably hear me and be comforted.

—MOTHER OF ALEXA, 6

Key Terms

Coping   896
Death anxiety   909
Death imagery   909
Family crisis   900

Hospice   910
Palliative care   910
Stranger anxiety   896
Support systems   904

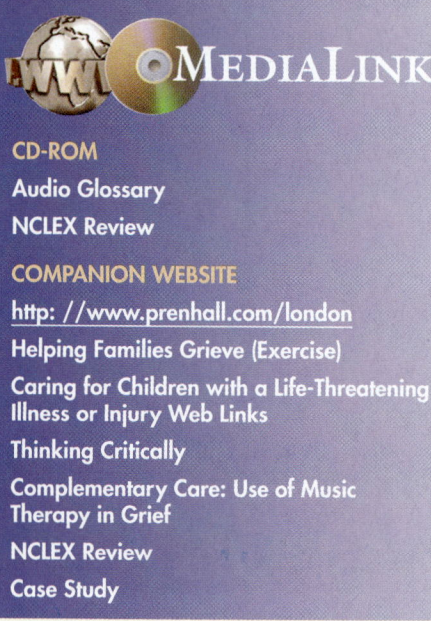

MediaLink

CD-ROM
Audio Glossary
NCLEX Review

COMPANION WEBSITE
http://www.prenhall.com/london
Helping Families Grieve (Exercise)
Caring for Children with a Life-Threatening Illness or Injury Web Links
Thinking Critically
Complementary Care: Use of Music Therapy in Grief
NCLEX Review
Case Study

What do children like Alexa face after admission to the pediatric intensive care unit (PICU)? What nursing strategies can help such critically ill or injured children cope with the experience? What stressors will parents face during the initial period of their child's hospitalization? What interventions could help them in this crisis? What strategies should be used to help siblings understand what has happened to their brother or sister? This chapter will answer these questions and will give guidance about providing supportive care to critically ill and injured children like Alexa and to their families.

The intense emotional and physical demands placed on the critically ill or injured child present a challenge to nurses' attempts to provide developmentally appropriate care. The child's parents and siblings are confronted with a stressful situation. A family-centered model of nursing practice offers a framework for performing interventions that help to minimize stress and enhance coping by parents, siblings, and the ill or injured child.

LIFE-THREATENING ILLNESS OR INJURY

A threat to a child's life may be expected, as in a chronic illness or progressive disabling disease, or unexpected, as in an unintentional injury. How children, parents, and siblings cope with the threat will depend on the anticipated or unanticipated nature of the event and the conditions surrounding the child's admission to the hospital.

When death results from a chronic disease or terminal illness, the child and family have time to adjust to the impending death. Parents can become involved in the child's therapy as integral members of the treatment team. Emergency admission for an acute illness or unintentional injury, on the other hand, brings with it sudden stressors as the child and family are thrust into an unfamiliar environment, confronted with frightening or invasive procedures, and faced with an uncertain outcome.

Nursing care of children and families coping with specific chronic diseases or terminal illnesses such as cancer, cystic fibrosis, or muscular dystrophy is discussed elsewhere in this book. The following discussion focuses on care of children with life-threatening illnesses or injuries and care of the dying child.

CHILD'S EXPERIENCE

Admission to the hospital, emergency department, or PICU is one of the most frightening experiences a child can have. The critically ill child may appear extremely anxious and fearful, or withdrawn, solemn, and preoccupied with his or her physical condition. The illness or injury often brings pain, decreases energy, and changes the child's level of consciousness. Younger children may be unable to understand what is happening to them. The en-

vironment appears overwhelming, fast paced, and frightening. The child's normal sleep patterns can be disrupted because of the lack of day–night patterns in many intensive care units. Being cared for by strangers produces anxiety in the child. The child's limited ability to move intensifies feelings of powerlessness and vulnerability. An increased incidence of posttraumatic stress disorder has been noted in children with life-threatening illnesses and injuries. See Chapter 53.

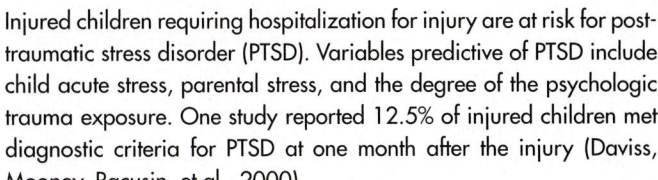
Nursing Practice

Injured children requiring hospitalization for injury are at risk for posttraumatic stress disorder (PTSD). Variables predictive of PTSD include child acute stress, parental stress, and the degree of the psychologic trauma exposure. One study reported 12.5% of injured children met diagnostic criteria for PTSD at one month after the injury (Daviss, Mooney, Racusin, et al., 2000).

Children's responses to stress are influenced by their developmental levels, past experiences, types of illness, coping mechanisms, and available emotional support. Nurses need to take into consideration how the child's developmental level and coping skills will influence his or her ability to deal with the PICU experience. Successful coping can provide the child with the skills to handle difficult situations in the future. WEB

Stressors to the Child

The four most significant stressors for hospitalized children of all ages are (1) separation from parents or the primary caretaker, (2) loss of self-control, autonomy, and privacy, (3) being subjected to multiple painful and invasive procedures, and (4) fear of bodily injury and disfigurement. Table 37–1 highlights key stressors of hospitalization for children at each developmental stage.

In addition to dealing with these stressors, the critically ill child experiences an intense emotional and physical threat to his or her well-being.

An unanticipated admission places the child at emotional risk for several reasons, including the lack of preparation for the experience, the uncertainty and unpredictability of events that follow, the unfamiliarity of the environment, and the heightened anxiety of parents. An admission for exacerbation of a disease such as cystic fibrosis or leukemia can provoke feelings of depression or hopelessness.

INFANT

After 3 months of age, most infants have started to develop a sense of object permanence (the knowledge that an object or person continues to exist when not seen, felt, or heard) and corresponding trust in parents and familiar

TABLE 37-1 Stressors of Hospitalization for Children in Various Developmental Stages

Stages	Responses
Infant	
Separation anxiety	Disrupted sleep/awake cycle
Stranger anxiety	Disrupted feeding routines
Painful, invasive procedures	Excessive irritability
Immobilization	
Sleep deprivation, sensory overload	
Toddler	
Separation anxiety	Frightened if forced to lie supine
Loss of self-control	Associate pain with punishment
Immobilization	Wonder why parents don't rescue them
Painful, invasive procedures	
Bodily injury or mutilation	
Fear of the dark	
Preschooler	
Separation anxiety and fear of abandonment	Difficulty separating reality from fantasy
Loss of self-control	Fear ghosts and monsters
Bodily injury or mutilation	Fear body parts will leak out
Painful, invasive procedures	Withdrawal, projection, aggression, regression
Fear of the dark, ghosts, and monsters	
School-Age Child	
Loss of control	Increased sensitivity to the environment
Loss of privacy and control over body functions	Detailed recall of events to them and other patients
Bodily injury	
Painful, invasive procedures	
Fear of death	
Adolescent	
Loss of control	Denial, regression, withdrawal
Fear of altered body image, disfigurement, disability, and death	Intellectualization, projection, displacement
Separation from peer group	
Loss of privacy and identity	

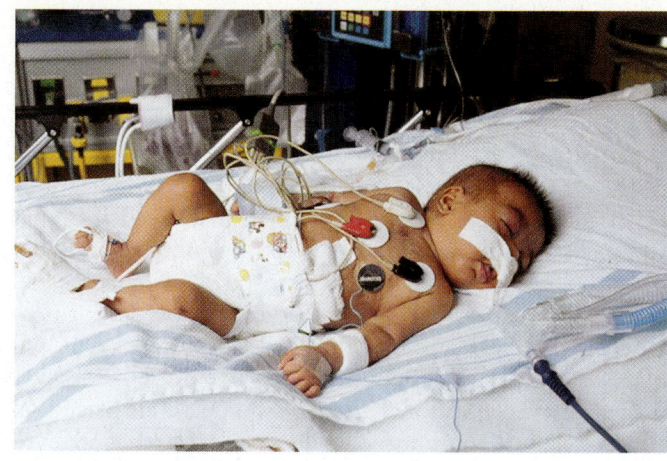

FIGURE 37-1. ◆ Jooti feels pain, hears noises, has her sleep disrupted, and has limited mobility because of all the equipment attached to her.

parents is extremely distressing to toddlers, and they protest vigorously when their parents depart. The toddler often becomes upset when known routines are altered. Having activities limited and being confined is especially threatening to children in this age group. Fear of pain, fear of the dark, and fear of invasive procedures and mutilation are common.

PRESCHOOLER

The greatest stressors to preschoolers are fear of being alone, fear of the dark, fear of abandonment, fear of loss of self-control related to the body and emotions, and fear of bodily injury or mutilation. They may feel guilty about getting sick. Waking up in the PICU and feeling the presence of an endotracheal, nasogastric, or chest tube, along with intravenous, arterial, and urinary catheters, is terrifying to the preschooler.

SCHOOL-AGE CHILD

Major sources of stress for school-age children are loss of control related to body functions, privacy issues, fear of bodily injury, and concerns related to death. School-age children attempt to maintain their composure during painful or invasive procedures but generally still require a great deal of support.

ADOLESCENT

Major stressors to adolescents are separation from the peer group, issues of control and related dependency, privacy, changes in body image, disability, and death. Adolescents often try to maintain rigid self-control when undergoing painful and invasive procedures.

Coping Mechanisms

Coping is cognitive and behavioral responses to manage specific internal and external demands that exceed a per-

caretakers. This makes separation from parents an anxiety-producing experience (see Chapter 34). ⊂⊃ In addition to separation anxiety, infants between 6 and 18 months of age may display **stranger anxiety** (wariness of strangers) when confronted with health care professionals. Other stressors to the infant include painful procedures, immobilization of extremities, and sleep deprivation caused by disruption of normal rhythms and patterns (Figure 37-1 ◆).

TODDLER

Toddlers are the group most at risk for a stressful experience as a result of illness. They lack cognitive ability to understand the reason for hospitalization. Separation from

Thinking Critically

PICU STRESSORS

The PICU receives a call from a community hospital requesting transport for an unstable 12-year-old boy who is in status epilepticus. Jeremiah has a seizure disorder controlled with medications, but several days ago he decided to stop taking his medications. So many seizure medications have been given in the community hospital emergency department to stop Jeremiah's seizures that he is now unconscious and must be intubated to maintain his airway until the medications wear off.

The transport team is in the air within minutes and arrives at the rural community hospital 25 minutes later. They stabilize Jeremiah and receive reports from the medical and nursing teams, meet briefly with his parents, answer a few questions, and are back in the air.

Jeremiah is admitted directly to the PICU, where the unit team has been preparing for his arrival. He is connected to cardiorespiratory and noninvasive blood pressure monitors, while his existing intravenous lines and endotracheal tube are evaluated for patency. Team members quickly complete a head-to-toe assessment. The unit clerk enters Jeremiah's room to say that his parents have arrived in the emergency department and are being escorted to the PICU.

What stressors do children like Jeremiah face after sudden admission to the PICU? What age-specific strategies can you use to help him cope with the experience? What stressors will parents face during the initial period when you work with them? How can you intervene to help them in this crisis? ⚭ WEB

son's resources, enabling the person to solve problems and to respond emotionally. The child may mirror the parents' behaviors and responses, which may help or hinder the child's response to stress. The child's temperament, previous coping experiences, and availability of support systems all combine to influence his or her ability to cope with the current experience.

The nature and severity of the illness and an emergency admission to the hospital stress a child's coping capabilities. Defense mechanisms displayed by children in these situations include regression, or return to an earlier behavior (a common reaction to stress), denial, repression (involuntary forgetting), postponement, and bargaining.

Growth and Development

Coping behavior is influenced by maturation, cognitive development (increased attention span, problem-solving ability, and understanding of cause and effect), and increased impulse control. Young children use more behavioral strategies and ventilate feelings (Ryan-Wenger, 1996).

Nursing Management

Nursing Assessment and Diagnosis

Nursing assessment involves, in addition to physiologic parameters, skilled observation of the child's psychosocial and emotional needs. It is important for the nurse to understand normal psychosocial and cognitive development in order to plan developmentally appropriate interventions. Assessment should include the child's response to illness, the environment, coping strategies, and the need for information and support.

The accompanying "Nursing Care Plan" includes common nursing diagnoses for the child coping with a critical illness or injury. The following nursing diagnoses may also be appropriate:

▶ *Impaired verbal communication* related to the effects of endotracheal intubation and mechanical ventilation

▶ *Impaired social interaction* related to separation from family and friends

▶ *Spiritual distress* related to the crisis of illness or suffering

▶ *Ineffective family coping: compromised,* related to the critical illness of the child

▶ *Impaired physical mobility: Level 2,* related to trauma, musculoskeletal impairment, and pain

▶ *Sleep pattern disturbance* related to circadian asynchrony, excessive stimulation, pain, and anxiety caused by the critical care unit environment

▶ *Diversional activity deficit* related to forced inactivity

▶ *Altered growth and development* related to critical illness or injury, and multiple caretakers

▶ *Body image disturbance* related to loss of body function, severe trauma, or invasive procedures

▶ *Self-esteem: Situational low,* related to hospitalization, or loss of independence and autonomy

▶ *Hopelessness* related to critical illness, deteriorating physical condition, or prolonged activity restrictions creating isolation

▶ *Anticipatory grieving* related to potential loss of body function or impending death of self

Planning and Implementation

Nursing care focuses on promoting a sense of trust, providing education about the illness or injury, preparing the child for procedures, facilitating the use of play, and promoting a sense of control. Children admitted to a PICU are presented with a traumatic experience for which they need support. Nurses play a key role in providing developmentally appropriate support to the child. Nursing interventions are directed at building a trusting relationship, minimizing the stressors experienced by the child, and

GOAL	INTERVENTION	RATIONALE	EXPECTED OUTCOME

1. Anxiety (child) related to separation from parents, foreign environment, strangers as caretakers, invasive procedures

	NIC Priority Intervention:		*NOC Suggested Outcome:*
	Anxiety reduction: *Minimizing apprehension, dread, foreboding, or uneasiness related to an unidentified source of anticipated danger*		**Anxiety control:** *Ability to eliminate or reduce feelings of apprehension and tension from unidentified source*
The child will exhibit or express an increased sense of security.	▶ Encourage parents to remain at the bedside (open visitation) and to participate in the child's care by touching, talking to, reading to, and singing to the child.	▶ Presence of parents is comforting to the child.	The child appears more relaxed and acknowledges parents' presence. Behavioral manifestations of anxiety are absent.
	▶ Talk with the child. Avoid discussions at bedside that the child should not overhear.	▶ The child may overhear and remember, even if unconscious.	
	▶ Offer to arrange a visit from the chaplain or other spiritual support.	▶ Spiritual support often provides comfort and sustenance in a time of crisis.	
	▶ Provide the child with developmentally appropriate explanations when possible. Encourage the child to ask questions and express concerns.	▶ Information reduces anxiety and builds trust.	
	▶ Prepare child in advance for procedures using developmentally appropriate techniques.	▶ Preparation decreases anxiety related to the unknown.	
	▶ Make the child's bedside more personal and familiar by encouraging parents to bring in security objects, family photos, and favorite toys from home.	▶ Security objects decrease foreignness of hospital environment. The child derives comfort from presence of personal items.	
	▶ Involve the child in play appropriate to developmental age (see Chapter 32).	▶ Play provides familiarity, decreases fantasy, and provides motor activity.	
	▶ Provide care using a primary nursing care model.	▶ Consistency in caregivers helps to build the child's trust.	

2. Powerlessness (moderate) related to inability to communicate, and control relinquished to the health care team

	NIC Priority Intervention:		*NOC Suggested Outcome:*
	Self-esteem facilitation: *Encouraging a patient to assume more responsibility for own behavior*		**Health beliefs: Perceived control:** *Personal conviction that one can influence an outcome*
The child or adolescent will have an increased sense of control over the situation.	▶ Provide opportunities for choices when possible.	▶ Such opportunities provide sense of control and autonomy through decision making.	The child or adolescent expresses satisfaction over ability to control some elements of situation.
	▶ Encourage participation in self-care.		
	▶ Prepare the child or adolescent in advance (timing dependent on developmental level) for procedures. Describe the sensations that will be experienced. Allow some choice in timing or method of pain relief.	▶ Information provides anticipatory guidance and a sense of involvement and value to the child.	
	▶ Provide routines for the child both within a 24-hour period and for scheduled care. Tell the child before (timing dependent upon developmental level), repeat explanation of why procedure is necessary, complete procedure in a consistent manner, and offer praise or a special story when completed. When possible, incorporate rituals from home.	▶ Self-control is maintained through rituals.	
	▶ Encourage play as a means of expressing feelings.	▶ Play is a normal activity for children and provides freedom of expression.	

(continued)

GOAL	INTERVENTION	RATIONALE	EXPECTED OUTCOME
	▸ Provide other means of communication to the intubated child (e.g., a word board or finger board). ▸ For the child requiring restraints, use as seldom as possible, provide appropriate explanations, and release at regular intervals. Wrapping IV lines well and using armboards can help maintain lines and avoid restraints.	▸ Maintaining communication provides autonomy and independence for the child. ▸ Release from restraints helps diminish the sense of powerlessness that accompanies their use.	

3. Pain related to injuries, invasive procedures, surgery

GOAL	INTERVENTION	RATIONALE	EXPECTED OUTCOME
	NIC Priority Intervention: **Pain management:** *Alleviation of pain or a reduction in pain to a level of comfort that is acceptable to the patient*		*NOC Suggested Outcome:* **Comfort level:** *Feelings of physical and psychologic ease*
The child will experience reduced pain and improved comfort.	▸ Assess the child's pain: location, intensity, what makes it better or worse. ▸ If appropriate, use pain assessment scale (see Chapter 38). ⌾ ▸ Prepare the child for procedures. Be honest in explanations and use developmentally appropriate language and format. Describe the sensations that the child will feel, smell, taste, or see. Comfort the child after the procedures. Provide rest periods between procedures. ▸ Provide optimal pain relief with prescribed analgesics. Provide comfort measures—position changes, backrubs, etc. Provide diversional activities as appropriate or possible. Incorporate the family in pain relief modality.	▸ Assessment provides baseline information from which a plan of care can be developed. ▸ Use of scale provides continuity and consistency in monitoring of the child's pain. ▸ Information reduces anxiety and fear associated with the unknown and helps the child maintain self-control. ▸ Physiologic and psychologic methods of pain control can be used in combination to maximally improve outcomes.	The child experiences a perceived or actual improvement in comfort level.

promoting coping. Ongoing reassessment of progress in meeting the child's needs is critical. Honesty in all discussions is key to building trust with the child. The accompanying "Nursing Care Plan" summarizes nursing care for the child coping with a life-threatening illness or injury.

PROMOTE A SENSE OF SECURITY

For children of all ages, feeling secure depends on a sense of physical and psychologic safety. A sense of physical security is difficult to attain within the PICU because of the constant barrage of procedures that are part of the child's treatment plan. A sense of psychologic safety is best achieved by the presence of parents. An open visitation policy that enables parents to be at the bedside is optimal. Including parents as partners in the child's care provides comfort and reassurance to the child. Children whose parents have high anxiety levels pick up their parents' emotional cues and become more anxious. Interventions to lower the parents' anxiety may benefit the child (Melnyk & Alpert-Gillis, 1998). Consistency of staff is invaluable in developing familiarity and a trusting relationship with the child.

Personalizing the child's bedside can promote comfort and a sense of security. Pictures from home, a favorite blanket or toy, music tapes, ⌾ WEB or posters can make the environment friendlier and more familiar to the child (Figure 37–2 ◆). Religious or spiritual icons may also provide psychologic support.

PROVIDE EDUCATION ABOUT THE ILLNESS OR INJURY AND PREPARE THE CHILD FOR PROCEDURES

A child's ability to understand the cause of the illness and its therapy depends on his or her cognitive abilities. Help younger children to understand that illness and hospitalization are not a punishment.

Preparation for procedures is important at all ages, even for the unconscious or sedated child. The timing of this preparation depends on the child's cognitive level. Generally, the younger the child, the shorter the interval should be between the time of the teaching and the actual procedure (see Chapter 34) ⌾.

Children often feel and hear even when unconscious, so touch and verbal interchanges are important. Toddlers will

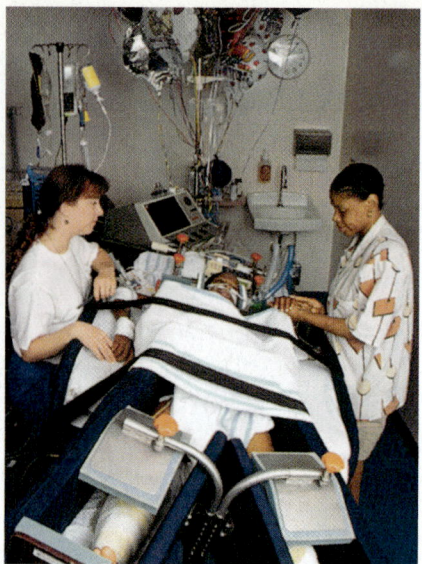

FIGURE 37–2. ◆ By their very nature, PICUs are ominous and sterile. To lessen this effect, it can help to personalize the child's space. Being there with the child and parent, answering questions, or just talking can be a comfort to both.

benefit from being talked to, soothed, and touched during and after the procedure. Provide preschoolers, school-age children, and adolescents with an explanation of the sensations they can expect to experience (temperature, vibrations, sounds, smells, tastes, sight). This information may reduce their stress more than complete details about the procedures (LaMontagne, 1993). In any explanations to the child, avoid medical jargon and use simple language appropriate to the child's developmental level.

FACILITATE THE USE OF PLAY

The use of play is important in alleviating stress and helping children to prepare for procedures. It is also another way for the nurse to assess the child's developmental level. Therapeutic play adds familiarity, diminishes fantasies, provides motor activity, and helps the child develop a sense of mastery (see Chapter 34). Children who are immobilized by tubes and restraints can still feel a sense of accomplishment, for example, by completing a puzzle, even if the nurse points to each piece and responds when the child, through nods and gestures, indicates where it should be placed. Play can help children work through a painful situation, making it more tolerable.

PROMOTE A SENSE OF CONTROL

Children between toddlerhood and adolescence experience a loss of control during a life-threatening illness. This loss of control may be related to the body, emotions, normal routines, or privacy. Nursing interventions should promote a sense of control over these areas.

Give the child choices whenever possible. Even the simple choice of which arm will receive a new intravenous line can help the child feel in control. Scheduling routine activities and treatments at the same time each day adds predictability and lessens anxiety. Limited mobility and the use of restraints, although sometimes necessary, contribute to the child's sense of powerlessness. The Joint Commission on Accreditation of Health Care Organizations requires that hospitals have policies and procedures in place for the use of restraints. If restraints must be used, plan to release them regularly for short periods. Restrain all children as little as possible, and explain the rationale for restraints, emphasizing that they are not a punishment (See Skills 7–1 to 7–6). **SKILLS** Provide diversional activities for the child, for example, by reading stories, playing music, or watching videotapes (see Chapter 34). **WEB**

Enhance the child's coping skills by teaching the child and family a combination of relaxation, visual imagery, or distraction techniques, and comforting self-talk phrases, such as "This will be over soon. If I stay calm, it will be all right. It will be over faster and then I can do something fun." Help the parents become the child's coping coaches.

Evaluation

Expected outcomes of nursing care include:

▶ A trusting relationship is developed with the child and family.

▶ The child's social interactions, coping, and growth and development are promoted through diversional activities.

▶ The child's and family's coping is promoted through education and preparation for procedures.

PARENTS' EXPERIENCE

Families have different reactions and coping mechanisms when challenged. Children who are hospitalized for a critical illness cannot be adequately cared for if their families' needs are not met. Not only will parents find it difficult to support the child if their own needs are not met, but they also can transmit their anxiety to the child, who then becomes even more anxious.

What Makes a Problem a Crisis?

A **family crisis** occurs when a family encounters a problem that seems insurmountable and with which the family cannot cope in its usual ways. The critical care environment and the implications of a life-threatening illness or injury are far removed from the everyday experiences of most families. The unfamiliarity of the environment and the uncertainty and seriousness of the illness or injury create a crisis for the family.

Unexpected illness or injury adds another dimension of stress, since families have little time to prepare for the experience. A sudden admission threatens family integrity, causing enormous stress and separation from loved ones. The interruption of the unique parent-child relationship can be more stressful to parents than the physical PICU environment. Stresses are intensified when divorce, separation, and stepparenting are involved. Other current family stresses such as financial problems, long distance from home to hospital, or another family member with an illness can add to the state of crisis.

Reactions to Life-Threatening Illness or Injury

How do parents react to a threat to their child's life? What parental behaviors might nurses see when a child is critically ill or injured? Parents typically progress through stages that might include shock and disbelief; anger and guilt; deprivation and loss; anticipatory waiting; and readjustment or mourning.

SHOCK AND DISBELIEF

The universal reaction of parents is shock and disbelief. As the familiar is disrupted, parents experience a loss of control, inability to regain their bearings, and feelings of immobility. The hospital environment, emergency department, or PICU may seem unreal. The emotions parents experience initially are intensified by the physical appearance of their child (particularly after traumatic injury); the presence of monitors, tubing, and equipment; and the actual injury or illness (Figure 37–3 ◆). As the mother of a 5-year-old trauma patient said, "I felt distanced, in a daze, in and out of it that first day after the accident."

The stage of shock and disbelief begins in the first few moments after hearing the "news" and can last for days. The shock helps postpone the full impact of the crisis. For most parents, however, the overwhelming sense of shock passes during the first 24 hours. During this period, parents grope for answers and explanations about the illness

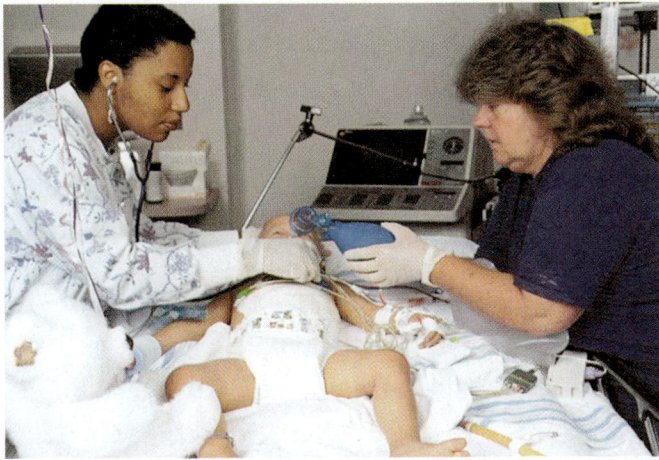

FIGURE 37–3. ◆ Procedures done in the PICU, such as mechanical ventilation, are frightening for parents. Treat the child first, but also remember the needs, fears, and anxieties of the parents and other family members. Anticipating the family's needs and keeping them informed will help them adjust.

or injury. Information must be repeated many times to parents, since in this stage they are often unable to assimilate information easily.

ANGER AND GUILT

Anger and guilt surface as parents become more aware of their child's illness or injury. Their anger may be directed toward themselves, each other, health care providers, or other children or parents, as in the case of a motor vehicle crash involving a group of teenagers. Parents may also be angry with their child. This anger may be a result of injuries the child sustained when breaking known rules such as drinking and driving, playing with matches, or riding a bike without a helmet. Lastly, the anger may not be directed at anyone specifically. Injuries caused by natural disasters such as an earthquake, flood, or hurricane provoke just as much anger as those that result from the actions of people. This may create a challenge to the parents' spiritual beliefs.

Parents typically react to their child's illness or injury with some degree of guilt. This reaction may be magnified in the intensive care environment. The fact that the guilt usually has no basis in real events does not lessen the feeling. A question parents frequently ask at this stage is, "Why not me instead of my child?" Parents' feelings of guilt may have one of two causes:

1. *They may feel responsible for causing the illness or injury.* Statements such as, "If only I hadn't sent him to the store on his bike, this wouldn't have happened," or, from the father of a 2-year-old who nearly drowned, "Maybe if I hadn't been working, he would have been in my care and this wouldn't have happened," reflect feelings of guilt for causing or failing to prevent the injury.

2. *They may feel guilty about not noticing the onset of an illness or disregarding earlier symptoms of an illness.* The mother of a 1-year-old with *Haemophilus influenzae* meningitis repeatedly said, "I shouldn't have waited so long to take her to the doctor!"

DEPRIVATION AND LOSS

As the shock slowly recedes, parents enter a stage of deprivation and loss related to their parental role. Within minutes or hours, parents have gone from the familiar role of being a parent of a healthy child to the unexpected and unfamiliar role of being a parent of a critically ill child. Parents have compared this deprivation and loss to that experienced when a family member dies.

Parents' difficulties and ambivalence in releasing to strangers a part of their responsibility as the child's primary caretakers can threaten their self-esteem and self-control. Moreover, if parents cannot participate in the child's care, they may feel helpless or worthless.

ANTICIPATORY WAITING

Once the child's condition is stabilized and survival seems likely, parents often move into a period of anticipatory waiting. This stage is characterized as "life suspended in time." Parents spend a great deal of time waiting: for test results, for explanations, for their child to become conscious, or for surgery to be over. Parents may fear leaving the area because they may miss an important procedure, physician visit, or decisions or changes in treatment. Lack of mobility decreases the parents' use of typical coping mechanisms, so anxiety and the sense of powerlessness may increase. A pager system has been adopted in some facilities to give parents freedom to take breaks away from the child's bedside, knowing they will be alerted to important events (Ashenberg, Lambert, Maier, et al., 1996).

Parents may have a preoccupation with medical details. During this period, parents may ask questions about the long-term effects of the illness or injury on the child, about the potential for brain damage, or about the need for additional surgeries. Parents may place demands on staff and be frustrated when the child's progress is slow.

READJUSTMENT OR MOURNING

The last stage that parents experience is readjustment or mourning. Readjustment is experienced as the child recovers, improves steadily, and prepares for transfer and discharge. In contrast, parents of the child who dies reenter the cycle of emotions characteristic of grief. Parents also mourn when the child remains seriously ill or unresponsive, when the outcome remains uncertain for an extended period, or when long-term care is required. ⊂⊐ WEB

Table 37–2 lists the most important needs of parents during a child's critical illness or injury.

Nursing Management
Nursing Assessment and Diagnosis

Nurses who work with families of critically ill children have a unique opportunity to help them adapt and to promote family functioning. Begin by assessing the family's reaction to the illness, coping skills, stressors, and needs. This initial assessment provides a baseline of information for developing a care plan and strategies to meet the psychosocial as well as physiologic needs of families.

Several nursing diagnoses may apply to parents who are dealing with their child's critical illness or injury. They include:

▶ *Ineffective denial* related to knowledge deficit of the child's critical condition and uncertain prognosis

▶ *Altered family processes* related to the impact of a critically ill child on the family system

▶ *Parental role conflict* related to the child's critical illness or injury and PICU policies

▶ *Spiritual distress* related to the child's critical illness, suffering, or death

▶ *Disabling ineffective family coping* related to the child's severe or fatal illness

▶ *Family coping: Potential for growth* related to constructive crisis management

▶ *Fatigue* related to extreme stress, sleep deprivation, and crisis

---

TABLE 37–2   Parental Needs During Hospitalization of a Critically Ill or Injured Child

Information (the most important identified need)
- Information and frequent updates about the child's condition. Repeat the information and provide other materials frequently as parents forget or cannot concentrate on details with all their stress.
- Explanations they can understand about the child's condition, equipment being used, and procedures of care.
- Discussion with a physician daily.
- General information about unit policies, team members, phone numbers, etc.

Proximity
- Permission to remain at the bedside.
- Permission to touch and speak with the child.
- Open, flexible visiting hours.

Reestablishment of the parental control
- Recognition as important to the child's recovery.
- Recognition as the decision maker of the child's treatment options.

Participation in the child's care
- Performance of care (bathing, diaper changes, feeding, range of motion exercises, massages, hair care).
- Provision of comfort measures (reading, singing, telling stories, touching, talking).
- Explanation of equipment and procedures to the child to decrease his or her fears.

Confidence in the treatment plan and caregivers
- Continuity in staffing and health care contacts.
- Evidence that staff care about the child.
- Assurance that the child is receiving appropriate treatment and pain management.

Psychologic support
- Acknowledgment that the situation is difficult.
- Help to focus on the positive or unchanged aspects of the child's appearance.
- Rest and nutrition to maintain physical resources necessary for coping.
- Space and privacy as needed.
- Hope—an essential component of coping.
- Choice of other family members to be present.
- Preparation for responses of siblings and the long-term emotional responses of the child patient.

- *Hopelessness* related to the child's deteriorating physiologic condition
- *Caregiver role strain* related to illness severity of the child
- *Anticipatory grieving* related to potential death of the child or loss of body functions

Planning and Implementation

Nursing care focuses on providing information and building trust, promoting parental involvement, providing for physical and emotional needs, facilitating positive staff–parent relationships and communication, and maintaining or strengthening family support systems. Ongoing reassessment provides a measure with which to evaluate the family's ability to manage the crisis. The best way to meet the needs of families, minimize stress, and enhance family coping is to provide care using a family-centered approach (Hazinski, 1999). (See Table 1–1) 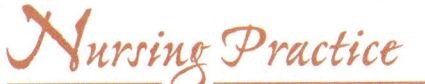 The challenge to nurses is to blend and balance technology with caring.

PROVIDE INFORMATION AND BUILD TRUST

The information given to parents must be provided frequently and accurately. Deliver information on the child's illness, condition, and plan of care in a manner and language readily understandable to parents. Upon admission, parents need to be given an idea of what to expect in the days ahead and prepared for special procedures or major changes in therapy that may become necessary.

Nursing Practice

Explain to the child and parents, in easy-to-understand terms, the purpose of equipment that is being used. Answer alarms quickly. Follow with an explanation of why alarms sound.

Honesty in discussions with parents is extremely important. If parents feel misled or that information is being withheld, a trusting relationship will be impossible. Informed parents, on the other hand, will feel that they are active participants in decision making and care planning for their child. Trust is facilitated when parents believe that the staff truly cares about the child and sees him or her as an individual, special child.

Parents also need a sense of hope regarding their child's illness to help them cope. Focus on the positives as the child progresses through the different phases of the critical illness.

PROMOTE PARENTAL INVOLVEMENT

An important role of nurses is to encourage and strengthen parents in their parenting role. The parents' place when possible is at the bedside—their very presence can comfort the child, minimize fears, and reduce the child's experiences with pain during invasive procedures. They provide continuity and may notice subtle changes that a newly assigned nurse may miss (Giganti, 1998). Parents' needs are best met when they are encouraged to participate in their child's care (Scott, 1998).

If the child is in the PICU, parents need to be prepared before they see their child for the first time. Tell them what tubes and monitors are present and how their child will look and react. Throughout the child's hospitalization, parents will continue to need reassurance and encouragement. Open visitation by parents is important to maintain their parenting role.

PROVIDE FOR PHYSICAL AND EMOTIONAL NEEDS

The experience of having a child with a critical illness drains parents' physical and emotional reserves. Parents often need encouragement to take care of themselves. A statement such as "It is important for you to eat and rest because Alexa is really going to need you when she wakes up" helps parents to realize that becoming exhausted benefits neither them nor the child.

Nursing Practice

Encourage parents to take time for themselves to be alone. Provide parents with a beeper, if possible, to reduce anxiety when they are away from the unit.

Orienting parents to the hospital, as well as to the unit routines, helps them to adapt to their surroundings. Many communities now have a Ronald McDonald house—an inexpensive but warm and supportive environment for parents of ill children. When financial burdens are a consideration, parents may need referrals to family and social service referrals. 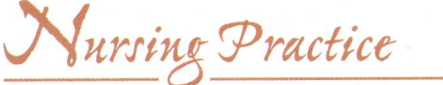 **WEB**

Parents are often at different levels of coping during a crisis. The child's critical illness may foster cohesion between the couple and build a stronger relationship. Unfortunately, the reverse may also be true—differences in styles or levels of coping may foster a sense of isolation, placing a strain on the couple's relationship. Nurses should be alert to family dynamics and refer the family for counseling or therapy, if indicated.

FACILITATE POSITIVE STAFF–PARENT RELATIONSHIPS AND COMMUNICATION

Given the intensity of the parents' experience when their child is critically ill, it is easy to see how problems can arise between staff and parents. Each health care team member must be aware of the child's current status so that parents receive the same information from all staff. Consistency in the message can instill confidence. Provide explanations geared to the parents' level of understanding, using language the parents can understand.

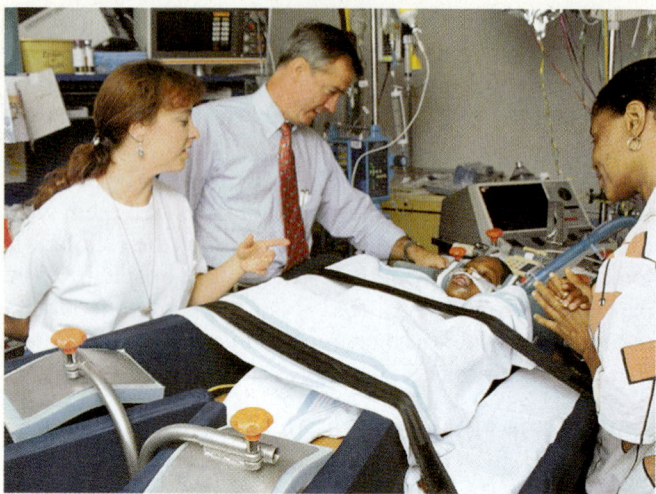

FIGURE 37–4. ◆ In times of crisis, everyone likes to know that someone is in charge and who that person is. The parents should meet and talk with the staff physician in charge and the nurses as often as possible. Parents need to know that someone is responsible, even if different people are providing care.

Parents need to know who has the overall responsibility for the care of their child. They should be introduced to the nurse and physician responsible for the child's care. This is especially important in teaching hospitals that have rotating staff. The staff physician with the overall responsibility should meet with parents as often as necessary to talk about changes in the child's condition or treatment plan and to allow time for parents to ask questions (Figure 37–4 ◆). Encourage parents to keep a daily log or notebook to record information on the child's care, progress, and needs. Family care conferences can be helpful when a large number of team members provide care.

MAINTAIN OR STRENGTHEN FAMILY SUPPORT SYSTEMS

Support systems are the extended network of family, friends, and religious and community contacts that provide nurturance, emotional support, and direct assistance to parents, enabling them to cope with overwhelming problems and crises. Most parents indicate that having family or friends nearby is crucial as a support system.

Parents may need to be reassured that it is all right to ask for help from family, friends, or community services. They may be uncomfortable asking for help, instead attempting to handle multiple responsibilities themselves, often to the point of exhaustion. Some parents are unable to respond to offers of help because it requires too great a mental effort on their part.

Nurses may need to intervene on parents' behalf when they have inappropriate support (Tomlinson & Mitchell, 1992). Parents may be frustrated by people who come to visit unannounced, stay too long, or visit too often, and may find it difficult to tell well-meaning but insensitive friends that they cannot deal with visitors right now. In these situations, offering to serve as a gatekeeper may be helpful.

Families of critically ill or dying children often have emotional needs beyond the support capabilities of the nurse caring for the child. Referrals to family and support services or pastoral care may be beneficial in these instances.

Evaluation

Expected outcomes of nursing care include:

▶ The nurse establishes a trusting relationship and effective communication with the family.

▶ Parents participate in their child's care as much as desired.

▶ Family members receive emotional support and nurturance needed to sustain them through their child's illness.

SIBLINGS' EXPERIENCE WEB

As the parents' focus shifts to the critically ill child, they may need support in dealing with the healthy siblings. Siblings also need care and may feel left out when everyone's attention is focused on the ill child. Siblings of critically ill children may demonstrate behaviors ranging from jealousy or envy to resentment, guilt and hostility, anger, insecurity, regression, and fear. Recognize that siblings may fear becoming ill themselves or believe that they played a role in the child's illness. Siblings often have nightmares about the illness or injury their brother or sister has sustained and about the ill child dying.

Tell siblings about their brother or sister using language and concepts appropriate to their ages and developmental levels. As appropriate, siblings should be allowed to visit. Such a visit should be encouraged if the child could potentially die, to allow the sibling to say good-bye. These visits often help to lift the spirits of the ill child. Because children's fantasies are often worse than reality, unfounded fears may be relieved by a visit.

Preparation for the visit is important. Before the visit, talk with the siblings about what to expect and describe how their brother or sister will look. If the ill child acts, moves, talks, or looks different than usual, provide an explanation beforehand. Describe the hospital environment, including equipment, sounds, and smells. Using a doll, drawing pictures, or showing an actual picture of the child can help prepare the siblings. Table 37–3 summarizes strategies for working with siblings of an ill or injured child.

During the visit, the nurse should demonstrate how to talk to and touch the ill child and encourage the siblings to do the same (Figure 37–5 ◆). After the visit, discuss with siblings what they saw and felt, and answer any questions they may have. When a sibling cannot visit, contact with the ill child can be maintained by sending pictures, drawings, cards, and messages recorded on audiotapes or videotapes (Figure 37–6 ◆).

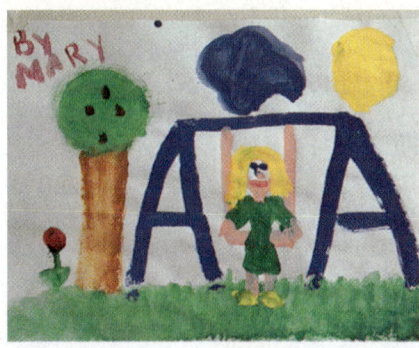
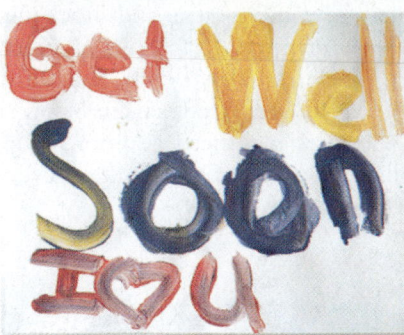

FIGURE 37-6. ◆ It is important that parents and siblings feel comfortable communicating with the seriously ill child. If siblings cannot visit, they should be encouraged to paint or record messages. They need to be able to express themselves and to feel that they are helping.

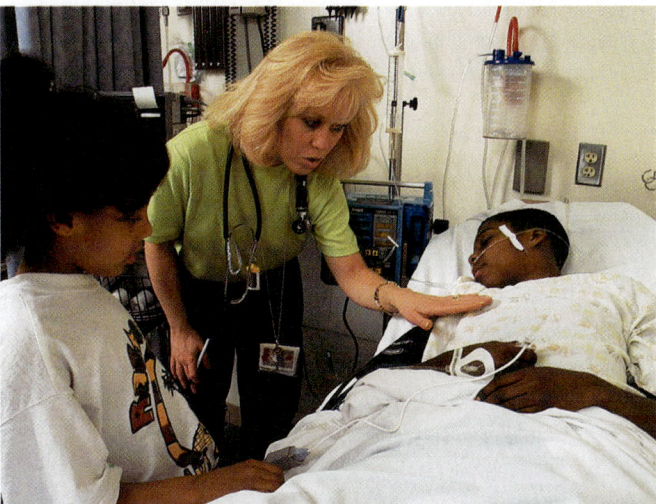

FIGURE 37-5. ◆ During the sibling's visit to the ill child, it is important to talk with the sibling and answer any questions asked in an honest manner at a level the child can understand.

Note: From Anderson, J. E. (1996). Helping parents cope with sudden death. *Contemporary Pediatrics, 13*(12), 42–57. © 1996 Thomson Medical Economics. All rights reserved. Adapted with permission.

If parents are staying at the hospital with the ill child, encourage them to call the siblings at home at a regular time each night. Allowing the siblings at home the opportunity to share their day as well as to receive an update on the ill child provides a feeling of connectedness. The phone call offers siblings a consistent link to the parent as well as the reassurance that they are important and loved.

BEREAVEMENT 〔WEB〕

Parents' Reactions

The death of one's child is probably the most painful experience for a parent. When the loss is sudden and unexpected, the abruptness adds a dimension of shock that may last for 4 to 5 weeks. The goal of the nurse in these situations is to provide comfort and support for the dying child and the family (Table 37–4). Staff education must be built on the premise that grief and mourning are normal, necessary processes.

Grief is painful, individualized, and exhausting. Many factors influence the parents' grief responses, including their perception of the preventability of the illness or injury, the suddenness and other circumstances of the death, the nature of their attachment to the child, previous losses, spiritual or religious orientation, and culture. Suicide produces agonizing anger, guilt, and confusion. The fact that the child ended his or her own life compounds the feelings of guilt.

Although parents progress through distinct stages of grief, the time line and nature of the grief process differ for each individual. The intense pain and shock initially felt by parents gradually give way to feelings of anger, guilt, depression, and loneliness. Very slowly, and with much support, energy returns and parents again begin to enjoy life experiences. Spouses may need additional support when they are at different levels of grieving to prevent a sense of loneliness and isolation.

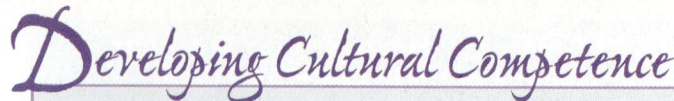

Always ask the parent before cutting a lock of the child's hair. Some cultures and religions, including Native-American groups, forbid it (Nelson, 1995).

The nurse should work closely with the family when the child's death is imminent, since they will remember the experience for the rest of their lives. Prepare the family for changes in the child's appearance and the events to follow. Providing parents with a room in which to be alone with the child ensures privacy at this extremely personal time. Ask the family in a nonjudgmental, supportive manner what is important to them in the last moments or hours of their child's life and what will be important to them in the grief process. Certain religious or cultural practices may

TABLE 37–5	Cultural Traditions in Mourning and After-Death Rites	
Religious Group	Rituals You Might Observe	Organ Donation or Autopsy Beliefs
American Indians	• Beliefs and practices vary widely • Navajo do not touch the deceased or their belongings	
Buddhism	• Last-rite chanting at bedside • Cremation common	Organ donation considered act of mercy, autopsy individual choice
Catholicism	• Sacrament of the sick • Obligated to take ordinary but not extraordinary means to prolong life • Burial usual	Autopsy, organ donation acceptable
Christian Science	• Unlikely to seek medical help to prolong life • Disposal of body and parts decided by family	Individual decides about organ donation
Hinduism	• No restrictions to right-to-die issue • Religious prayers chanted before and after death • Cremation common • Men and women display outward grief • Thread tied around wrist signifies a blessing, do not remove	Autopsy, organ donation acceptable
Islam	• Attempts to shorten life prohibited • Body is washed only by Muslim of same gender	Organ donation acceptable Autopsy only for medical or legal reasons
Jehovah's Witness	• Use of extraordinary means to prolong life is individual choice • Burial determined by family preference	Autopsy if required by law Organ donation forbidden
Judaism	• If death is inevitable, no new procedures needed, but must continue those ongoing • Body ritually washed • Burial as soon as possible, all body parts must be buried together • Seven-day mourning period	Autopsy permitted in certain circumstances, organ donation is complex issue
Mennonite	• Do not believe life must be continued at all cost	Autopsy and organ donation acceptable
Mormonism	• If death inevitable, promote a peaceful and dignified death • Burial in "temple clothes"	Autopsy permitted with permission of next of kin, organ donation is permitted
Protestantism	• Burial or cremation is individual decision	Organ donation, autopsy are individual decisions
Seventh Day Adventist	• Follow ethic of prolonging life • Disposal of body and burial are individual decisions	Autopsy, organ donation acceptable

Note: From Spector, R. E. (2000). *Cultural diversity in health and illness* (5th ed., pp. 137–138, 144–149). Upper Saddle River, NJ: Prentice Hall Health. Adapted.

Questions to use with families whose child has died (Shaefer, 1999):

► I am sorry for your loss. How can I help?
► What are your traditions when an infant or child dies?
► Is there someone I can call for you?
► Has your family ever had this experience before?
► How did they handle it?
► Do you have a funeral service? Is it helpful?

need to be planned. Holding the child is a universal request and should be permitted. Many families find that saying good-bye as a group is helpful. Allowing the family to hold, kiss, and talk to the dying child can help grieving (Nelson, 1995). Encourage parents to continue in their parental role by continuing with caregiving activities such as bathing or dressing the child for the last time. See Table 37–5 for more common mourning and after-death rituals.

After the child's death, allow the family to spend as much time as they need with the child's body. Never rush family members who are saying good-bye to the child. Save all of the child's personal items—especially in the case of an infant, whose parents may have few mementos. A lock of hair, hand or foot prints, the infant's identification band, the child's weight and height, the last clothes or patient gown worn by the child sealed in a plastic bag to retain the child's scent, or a picture of the infant can be sources of comfort and remembrance for families. It may be traumatic to receive the child's possessions, and placing them in a plastic garbage bag is insensitive. When possible, use a special container for this purpose.

Developing Cultural Competence

Many culturally influenced rules and customs surround dying. For instance, the Hmong belief system holds that children will live in eternity in the same state in which they existed at the time of death. Therefore, it is important that the child's body be intact at death.

Parents may need direction about resources available to help with a memorial service or funeral. Information about organ and tissue donation, as well as the need for an autopsy, if required, needs to be discussed. Acknowledge with parents that certain dates—such as the day of the week the child died, the child's birthday, or family holidays—will be difficult and may trigger intense sadness again. Parents may benefit from keeping a journal of their thoughts and memories, or writing letters or poems to or about their child.

Emphasize to parents that although the period surrounding their child's death is difficult, caring for themselves physically and mentally is important. Parents may experience friction due to differing rates and intensity of grief. The nurse can give a list of appropriate support

groups, books, and articles to parents for later use. Parents can be referred to national organizations, such as the Candlelighters Foundation or Compassionate Friends, and to local support groups for bereaved parents or siblings. **WEB** Some institutions have formal follow-up programs for bereaved parents to encourage a healthy progression through the grieving process.

Siblings' Reactions

Siblings experiencing the death of a brother or sister require supportive and compassionate care. In the course of the child's illness the siblings probably will have received less attention from parents. They may fear that they caused their brother or sister to be injured or become ill, or worry that bad thoughts on their part brought on the illness. They need help in adapting to their parents' distraction, grief, and increased protectiveness of them (McIntier, 1995; Schonfeld, 1993). The sibling needs to hear that the parent's grief in no way diminishes the love they have for him or her. Table 37–6 highlights children's understanding of death at different developmental stages and some of the possible behavioral responses.

When talking to the siblings of a dying child, honesty is most important. Provide explanations in language that is developmentally appropriate. Reassure siblings that they did not cause their brother or sister to die and that death was not a punishment for wrongdoing. Allow the siblings to ask questions. Acknowledge the emotions they are feeling, and emphasize that it is all right for them to be sad, angry, frightened, or tearful. Ask how they feel about saying good-bye to the dying child, and provide physical and emotional support. Preparation of the siblings before seeing the dying child involves a brief explanation of what they will see, feel, hear, and smell. Answer questions truthfully. Siblings may have to hear information several times. **WEB**

Growth and Development

Children need to understand the finality of death—that all body functions have stopped. Simple statements that can be told to children include, "Adam's heart will never beat again," "He will never get cold or hungry," and "He will never come home again." These simple statements may need to be repeated several times since young children will test to see if the same answers are given each time (Mahan, 1994).

As appropriate and comfortable, siblings should be permitted to participate in planning the child's memorial or funeral service. The nurse should use the same amount of energy and concern in acknowledging their grief as acknowledging that of adults. Being able to grieve as a family provides siblings with a sense of connectedness to parents and provides security at a vulnerable time. If siblings attend the funeral, prepare them for what to expect and provide a support person. Keep the family together as much as possible.

Understanding of Death	Possible Behaviors
Infant • Lacks understanding of concept of death • May sense caregivers are tense, routines are altered	• May show sadness by turning away from your gaze • Resists cuddling and eats less, crying, clinging • Sleeping more
Toddler • Unable to distinguish fact from fantasy • No understanding of true concept of death • Aware someone is missing—separation anxiety • Unable to distinguish death from temporary separation or abandonment	• Clingy, refuses to let parent out of sight • Stops walking and talking • Shows distress by biting, hitting, tears • Fearfulness • Problems eating and sleeping
Preschooler • Believes death is reversible, temporary • Believes bad thoughts cause death • Believes magical thinking can bring dead person back or can cause death to occur with thoughts • Has beginning experience with death of animals and plants	• May fear going to sleep, has nightmares, afraid of dark • Out-of-control behavior, hyperactivity, tantrums, regression • Problems with bowel and bladder control • Crying spells • Seems morbidly fascinated with death • Asks lots of questions • Displays anger at failure to keep person "alive," breaks toys, aggressive to friends
School-Age Child • Acquires more realistic understanding of death • By 8–10 years, understands that death is permanent and irreversible, and people die from internal and external causes • Believes that death is universal and will happen to him or her • May have exaggerated concerns about death	• May deny sadness by hiding tears and acting more like adults • Difficulty concentrating on school work • Psychosomatic complaints—tummy ache or headache • Acting-out behavior, anger at being abandoned • May try to comfort parents by taking over tasks
Adolescent • Intellectually capable of understanding death • Has a better grasp of association between illness and death • Sense of invincibility conflicts with fear of death • Able to recognize effect of death on others	• Same as school-age child • May have severe depression • Acting-out behavior—risk-taking behavior, delinquency, suicide attempts, promiscuity, pseudo-indifference

Note: From Krulik, T., Holoday, B., & Martinson, I. M. (Eds.). (1987). *The child and family facing life-threatening illness.* Philadelphia: Lippincott; Anderson, J. E. (1996). Helping parents cope with sudden death. *Contemporary Pediatrics, 13,* 42–55; and Grollman, Earl A., Ed., Explaining death to children. Beacon Press: Boston, MA. Adapted.

Growth and Development

Children must also complete a grieving process. This is usually accomplished in three stages (Baker, Sedney, &Gross, 1992).

- Early stage: They understand the death occurred, while using self-protective mechanisms to block the full emotional impact of the loss.
- Middle stage: They accept and rework the loss while experiencing the intense psychologic pain.
- Late stage: They integrate the loss experience into their identity and resume age-appropriate developmental progress.

As with parental bereavement, sibling bereavement is a lifelong process. The nurse should make sure other caregivers and teachers know about the sibling's loss. Let the child express feelings other than sadness, (e.g., guilt and anger). Encourage them to express grief through art, stories, and writing. They may conceal their feelings and suppress their questions to protect their parents (Davies, 1997).

DYING CHILD

Care of the dying child presents one of the greatest challenges to the nurse, requiring the utmost sensitivity and compassion. A child's understanding of death varies according to developmental stages, as described in Table 37–6.

Children as young as 5 years of age can sense when they are seriously ill. A child's awareness of death develops more rapidly when he or she is experiencing the progression of a disease and related medical treatment. Children with life-threatening illnesses often learn about death and their own illness from exposure to other seriously ill and dying children during hospitalization or clinic visits.

Preschool children can see their bodies deteriorate and feel the toxic effects of chemicals during disease progression and treatment. Changes in self-concept occur as they perceive these body changes. They often describe their illness in terms of mutilation to their body. They may realize that they are dying because of these physical changes.

School-age children also have subtle fears about body integrity and anxieties about the seriousness of their illness. This greater preoccupation with illness is considered by many professionals as the child's version of **death anxiety,** a feeling of apprehension or fear of death. Death anxiety occurs in children even though they are unable to conceptualize or describe death at an adult's level of understanding. It can develop from the perception of loneliness associated with a separation from the known world. Children may express death anxiety as a concern with treatments that invade the body or interfere with normal body functions.

Even if children have not been told they are dying, they know their condition is worsening. They are undergoing treatments, not feeling well, and picking up cues from their parents. They usually do not have the same fears about dying that adults do. Some children keep most of their thoughts about death to themselves. If they have not been told that they are dying, they may feel isolated and get the message not to discuss their condition. They may fear that the family members will abandon them emotionally. Children often avoid displaying anger, since they fear desertion more than death. They may also believe that expressing their awareness of death and their fears will place added emotional burdens on family members that could be unbearable to the family. Parents may not recognize the child's death anxiety because of their own fears, concerns, and feelings of helplessness.

Developing Cultural Competence

Depending on the family's cultural and religious beliefs, a chaplain or other health care professional who specializes in working with terminally ill children and families may help reduce a child's spiritual fears and promote peace and comfort among family members.

Waechter's classic study of hospitalized and fatally ill children revealed that children who were given an opportunity to discuss issues related to death openly did not have greater anxiety about death. The permission to discuss any aspect of the illness made the child feel less isolated and alienated from the parents. The child felt that the illness was not too terrible to discuss (Waechter, 1987).

Adolescents have a mature understanding of death, but the normal developmental milestones of adolescence add to their problems in facing a terminal illness. They are struggling to establish their own identity and plans for the future. At a time when body image is extremely important, they may be faced with the possibility of mutilation and disfigurement. Dying teens are often isolated from their peers during a period when peers are the most essential social group. Adolescents with terminal illnesses may be angry because they recognize their loss when the whole world is opening up to them.

Do not expect adolescents to handle feelings in the same way that adults do. Adolescents often avoid expressing anger against the family, seeking to control and direct these feelings elsewhere. They often become angry at

changes in treatment procedures, lack of explanations, and threats to their independence. As death nears, the adolescent may permit comforting and support and may accept care from warm and loving family members, as long as he or she is not treated condescendingly.

Nursing Practice

Some parents ask that their child not be told he or she is dying. Do you abide by their wishes when the child asks you if he or she is dying? Tell the parents that the child asked the question. Offer to set up a meeting with the care team to discuss their fears and concerns about telling their child the truth. Offer words and phrases they can use to talk with their child about his or her death.

Nursing Management

Nurses must make a commitment to children while they are living—to promote growth and development and to foster relationships with family and peers. Help children maintain contact with peers on the hospital unit as long as the child has energy to benefit from the companionship. The comfort of peers reduces the child's feelings of isolation.

Provide opportunities for fantasy play, drawings, and storytelling, without emphasizing or reinforcing death themes. Listen to what children say about themselves and their lives. **Death imagery,** references to death or death-related topics (going away, separation, and funerals), or anticipated experiences with treatment may be themes of their stories. These themes are expected and do not reflect repression or other pathology. See Table 37–7 for strategies for talking with a dying child.

Parents may feel incapable of dealing directly with the child's questions about dying. They may fear that they will

TABLE 37–7 Strategies for Talking to the Dying Child
• Be flexible.
• Recognize that some children communicate best through nonverbal means, i.e., art and music. The child may be willing to talk through a puppet or a stuffed animal.
• Respect the child's need to be alone and the desire to share. Allow communication, but do not force it.
• Be receptive when children initiate a conversation.
• Be specific and literal in explanation of death.
• Acknowledge that a child's life can be complete, even if it is brief. Let dying children know they will always be loved and remembered. Help children find a sense of accomplishment and purpose in the lives they have led.
• Empower children as much as possible in circumstances concerning their deaths. Reassure them of continued love and physical closeness.

Note: From Faulkner, K. W. (1997). Talking about death with a dying child. *American Journal of Nursing, 97*(6), 64–69.

be unable to cope with their own feelings during a frank discussion of the possibility of the child's imminent death. The types of questions that children most frequently ask include the following:

- What will death be like?
- What will happen to me when I die?
- Will I be punished for the bad things I have done?
- When will I be with [person(s) closest to child] again?
- Will my parents be all right?
- Will I experience much pain?

Some parents need help in understanding and answering the child's questions at a developmentally appropriate level for the child. The nurse should provide guidance about appropriate methods and words to use that will support the child. Some parents may prefer that the child's questions be answered honestly by another professional. A professional who has special bereavement counseling training can assist children and families with discussions.

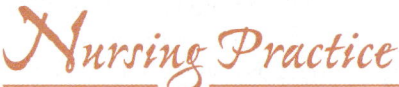
Nursing Practice

The Patient Self-Determination Act of 1990 (PSDA) supports the rights of persons 18 years of age or older in decisions about their medical care and when they should be admitted to a medical facility. Although many adolescents younger than age 18 have the cognitive skills necessary for decision making and are involved in decisions concerning their care, the PSDA limits their legal rights. Creative strategies are needed to develop a model of decision-making rights and responsibilities for adolescents built on the PSDA.

When caring for adolescents, remember that outbursts of anger are common but not personally directed at the nurse. Provide activities to help teens channel their feelings. Continue providing support in spite of their behavior. This approach may encourage teens to accept comforting without losing face. Be available to listen when the teen wants to talk and express feelings and frustrations. Promote friendships with other teens who have similar interests or problems.

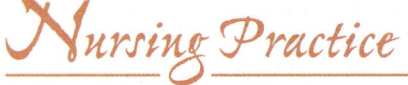
Nursing Practice

The Americans with Disabilities Act of 1990 and the Education for All Handicapped Children Act mandate that all disabled children—including those with terminal illnesses—are entitled to the same education as other students. This has led to policy challenges in the school setting related to hospice care and do-not-resuscitate orders (Ramer-Chrastek, 2000).

The nurse should provide teens with as much independence and control over their situation as possible. Give them a voice in decisions. Answer questions honestly without using a condescending tone.

Palliative care combines active and compassionate therapies intended to comfort and support persons with a short life expectancy. It may be combined with therapies aimed at reducing or curing the illness and treating symptoms more aggressively than hospice care. **Hospice** care helps persons with short life expectancies to live their remaining lives to the fullest—alert, without pain, and with choices and dignity. It does not seek to prolong life. **WEB** Families often delay contact with hospice because it is an admission of death. They may need help to see it as a focus on the time left with the child. Pediatric hospice helps the family to focus on the quality of life by facilitating communication between the child and family. Encourage the family to participate in the child's physical and emotional care. Families need to cry together and to tell each other how much they will miss each other. They need to be assured that the vigil with the child is important so the child does not feel isolated or abandoned as death approaches.

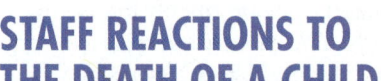
Nursing Practice

Pediatric palliative care is receiving more attention. The American Academy of Pediatrics recently issued care guidelines for children with life-threatening and terminal illnesses. At this time only 1% of children with life-threatening illnesses are receiving hospice care. New federal demonstration programs may help improve end-of-life care for children (Stephenson, 2000).

STAFF REACTIONS TO THE DEATH OF A CHILD

Children are highly valued by society because of their potential future contributions. Children are expected to have a normal life span, and the death of a child is often viewed as a tragedy. Caring for dying children is especially stressful and demanding for health care professionals. Nurses involved in long-term relationships with children experience severe grief when these children die (Davies, Cook, O'Loane, et al., 1996). Nurses often cope by distancing themselves socially from the dying child and family to maintain composure and a professional demeanor. Waechter reported that the total time nurses spent with children decreased as death became more imminent (Davies & Eng, 1993).

Caring for the dying child may be especially difficult for nurses with young children of their own. They tend to identify with the child, making it more likely that they will have difficulty dealing with the death in a professional manner. Nurses may not be able to recognize the dying child's anxiety and fears because of their own personal defenses against their sense of helplessness to alter the course of the child's disease.

Nursing Practice

Nurses who have recognized the inevitability of a child's death experience moral distress with feelings of anger, frustration, sadness, and powerlessness when asked to carry out treatments that cause pain and suffering to the child. Discuss these feelings with members of the care team to determine when curative efforts will stop and the focus of attention will shift to palliative care (Davies, 1996).

Nurses who work with terminally ill children and their families need special preparation to meet the needs of these individuals and to manage personal stress simultaneously. Mentorship with experienced hospice nurses, as well as additional educational experiences, may help promote professional nursing care. Nurses who work with dying children and families must learn to cope effectively with grief and develop empathy, competence, and confidence in their ability to provide more humane and effective nursing care.

Nurses working in emergency departments caring for children who die suddenly or in hospice settings and hospital units that care for terminally ill children need support systems to help balance the stresses of working with dying children. The workplace should acknowledge the stress nurses experience when working with terminally ill children. Support systems may include discussions with peers

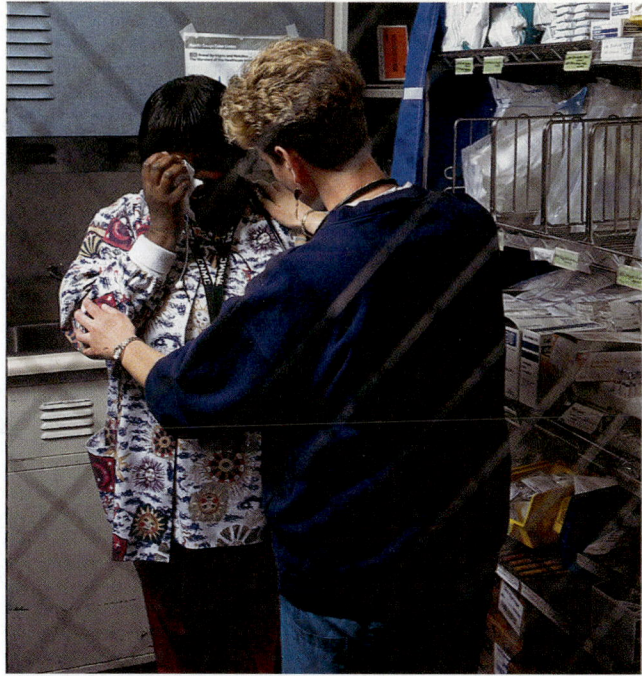

FIGURE 37–7. ◆ Nurses need to express grief in a supportive environment after a child's death. Sharing the sadness and grief or futility of resuscitation efforts with colleagues can often help nurses continue to provide supportive care to the next families who need compassionate care.

or debriefing group sessions with mental health professionals that provide an opportunity to discuss their feelings and concerns (Figure 37–7 ◆). Participating in team decisions regarding the dying child's plan of care (palliative rather than curative) helps many nurses manage their distress.

CHAPTER HIGHLIGHTS

☛ A life-threatening illness or injury places intense emotional and physical demands on the child and family due to the unfamiliar environment of the PICU, frightening or invasive procedures, and an uncertain outcome.

☛ The four most significant stressors for hospitalized children are (1) separation from parents or the primary caretaker, (2) loss of self-control, autonomy, and privacy, (3) being subjected to multiple painful and invasive procedures, and (4) fear of bodily injury and disfigurement.

☛ The child's temperament, previous coping experiences, and having a support system all influence how he or she will cope with the current experience.

☛ When the child is hospitalized, the nurse should work to meet the family members' needs so they can manage their anxiety and support the child.

☛ Parents typically progress through the stages of shock and disbelief; anger and guilt; deprivation and loss; anticipatory waiting; and readjustment or mourning when their child has a life-threatening illness or injury.

☛ The nurse can make sure siblings get information about their critically ill or injured brother or sister and regular messages from the parents to help them control feelings of jealousy, guilt, fear, and insecurity.

☛ Work closely with the family when a child's death is imminent, helping to provide them the support and services most important to them in the last moments or hours of their child's life.

☛ Children with life-threatening illnesses often learn about death and their own illness through exposure to other ill and dying children. Even if they have not been told they are dying, they will know their condition is worsening with extra treatments, feeling ill, and cues from their parents.

☛ Palliative care combines therapies to comfort and support persons with short life expectancy, by providing therapies to improve the quality of remaining life.

☛ Caring for a dying child is difficult, and nurses need special preparation to meet the needs of the child and family while managing their own personal stress.

EXPLOREMediaLink

NCLEX Review, Case Studies, and other interactive resources for this chapter can be found on the companion website at http://www.prenhall.com/london. Click on "Chapter 37" and select the activities for this chapter.

For animations, more NCLEX review questions, and an audio glossary, access the accompanying CD-ROM in this textbook.

REFERENCES

Ashenberg, M. D., Lambert, S. A., Maier, N. P., & McAliley, L. G. (1996). Easing the wait: Development of a pager program for families. *Pediatric Nursing, 22*(2), 103–107.

Baker, J. E., Sedney, M. A., & Gross, E. (1992). Psychological tasks for bereaved children. *American Journal of Orthopsychiatry, 62*(1), 105–116.

Boie, E. T., Moore, G. P., Briummett, C., & Nelson, D. R. (1999). Do parents want to be present during invasive procedures performed on their children in the emergency department? A survey of 400 parents. *Annals of Emergency Medicine, 34*(1), 70–74.

Davies, B. (1997). Commentary on Van Riper's article on sibling bereavement. *Pediatric Nursing, 23*(6), 594–595.

Davies, B., Cook, K., O'Loane, M., Clarke, D., MacKenzie, B., Stutzer, C., et al. (1996). Caring for dying children: Nurses' experiences. *Pediatric Nursing, 22*(6), 500–507.

Davies, B., & Eng, B. (1993). Factors influencing nursing care of children who are terminally ill: A selective review. *Pediatric Nursing, 19*, 9–14.

Daviss, W. B., Mooney, D., Racusin, R., Ford, J. D., Fleischer, A., & McHugo, G. J. (2000). Predicting posttraumatic stress after hospitalization for pediatric injury. *Journal of Ameri-can Academy of Child and Adolescent Psychiatry, 39*(5), 576–583.

Giganti, A. W. (1998). Families in pediatric critical care: The best option. *Pediatric Nursing, 24*(3), 261–265.

Hazinski, M. F. (1999). Psychosocial aspects of pediatric critical care. *In Manual of pediatric critical care* (pp. 14–43). St. Louis, MO: Mosby.

LaMontagne, L. L. (1993). Bolstering personal control in child patients through coping mechanisms. *Pediatric Nursing, 19*(3), 235–237.

Mahan, M. M. (1994). Death of a sibling: Primary care interventions. *Pediatric Nursing, 20*(3), 293–295, 328.

McIntier, T. M., Sr. (1995). Nursing the family when a child dies. *RN, 58*(2), 50–54.

Melnyk, B. M., & Alpert-Gillis, L. J. (1998). The COPE program: A strategy to improve outcomes of critically ill young children and their parents. *Pediatric Nursing, 24*(6), 521–527.

Nelson, L. (1995). When a child dies: Practical, sensitive advice for helping parents through their worst nightmare. *American Journal of Nursing, 95*(3), 61–64.

Ramer-Chrastek, J. (2000). Hospice care for a terminally ill child in the school setting. *Journal of School Nursing, 16*(2), 52–56.

Ryan-Wenger, N. A. (1996). Children, coping, and the stress of illness: A synthesis of research. *Journal of the Society of Pediatric Nurses, 1*(3), 126–138.

Schonfeld, D. J. (1993). Talking with children about death. *Journal of Pediatric Health Care, 7*(6), 269–274.

Scott, L. D. (1998). Perceived needs of parents of critically ill children. *Journal of the Society of Pediatric Nursing, 3*(1), 4–11.

Shaefer, J. (1999, July). *When an infant dies: Cross cultural expressions of grief and loss* (NFIMR Bulletin). Washington, DC: National Fetal and Infant Mortality Review Program.

Stephenson, J. (2000). Palliative and hospice care needed for children with life-threatening conditions. *Journal of the American Medical Association 284*(19), 2437–2438.

Tomlinson, P. S., & Mitchell, K. E. (1992). On the nature of social support for families of critically ill children. *Journal of Pediatric Nursing, 7*(6), 386–394.

Waechter, E. H. (1987). Children's reactions to fatal illness. In T. Krulik, B. Holaday, & I. M. Martinson (Eds.), *The child and family facing life-threatening illness.* Philadelphia: Lippincott.

CHAPTER 38

Pain Assessment and Management in Children

Felicia must be in pain so soon after her surgery. I know I would have pain if it were me. Can she get pain medicine without getting another needle?

—Mother of Felicia, 5

Key Terms

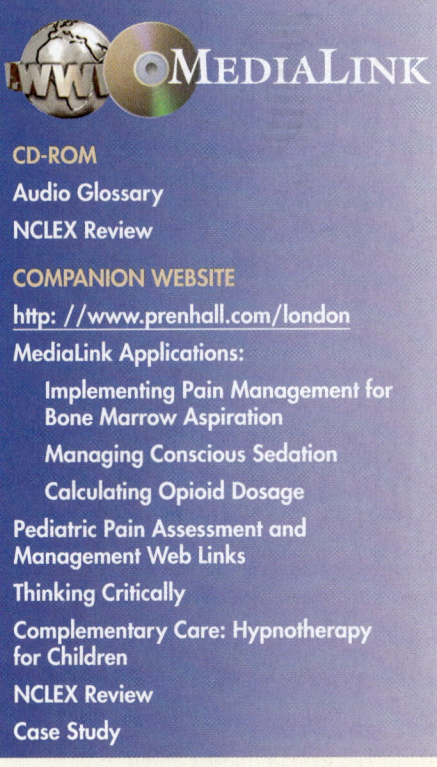

Everyone has his or her own perception of pain. A neurologic response to tissue injury, **pain** is an unpleasant sensory and emotional experience associated with actual or potential tissue damage (see "Pathophysiology Illustrated"). Effective pain management is every child's right.

Nursing Practice

In 2001, the Joint Commission on Accreditation of Healthcare Organizations introduced standards for the assessment and management of pain in patients in accredited hospitals and other health care organizations.

▶ Standard RI.1.2.8 Patients have the right to appropriate assessment and management of pain.

▶ Standard PF.3.4 Patients are educated about pain and managing pain as part of treatment, as appropriate. [WEB]

Pain exists when the patient says it does (McCaffrey & Pasero, 1999). Pain may be either acute or chronic. **Acute pain** is sudden and of short duration; it may be associated with a single event, such as surgery, or an acute exacerbation of a condition such as a sickle cell crisis. **Chronic pain** is persistent, lasting longer than 6 months; it is generally associated with a prolonged disease process such as juvenile rheumatoid arthritis.

OUTDATED BELIEFS ABOUT PAIN IN CHILDREN

In the past, children did not receive adequate treatment for pain. Undertreatment still occurs (Kachoyeanos & Zollok, 1995). Health care professionals once believed that children feel less pain than adults (Table 38–1). In fact, most physicians did not prescribe pain medication for children or ordered it only as needed. This undertreatment was based on the attitudes of health care professionals about pain, the difficulty and complexity of pain assessment in children, and inadequate research.

PATHOPHYSIOLOGY ILLUSTRATED
Pain Perception

Nociceptors (free nerve endings at the site of tissue damage) transmit information by specialized nerve fibers to the spinal cord. Nociceptors are stimulated by mechanical, thermal, and chemical injury. Biochemical mediators (bradykinin, prostaglandin, leukotrienes, and substance P) are produced in response to tissue damage. These substances either activate the pain response or sensitize nerve endings. C fibers slowly transmit dull, burning, diffuse pain as well as chronic pain. A-delta fibers quickly transmit sharp, well-localized pain. After the sensory information reaches the dorsal horn of the spinal cord, the pain signal may be modified depending on the presence of other stimuli, from either the brain or the periphery. The pain signal is then transmitted to the brain through the spinothalamic and reticulospinal nerve pathways, where perception occurs. The spinothalamic and reticulospinal nerve pathways then transmit the pain signal to the brain, where perception occurs. Once the sensation reaches the brain, emotional responses may increase or decrease the intensity of the pain perceived.

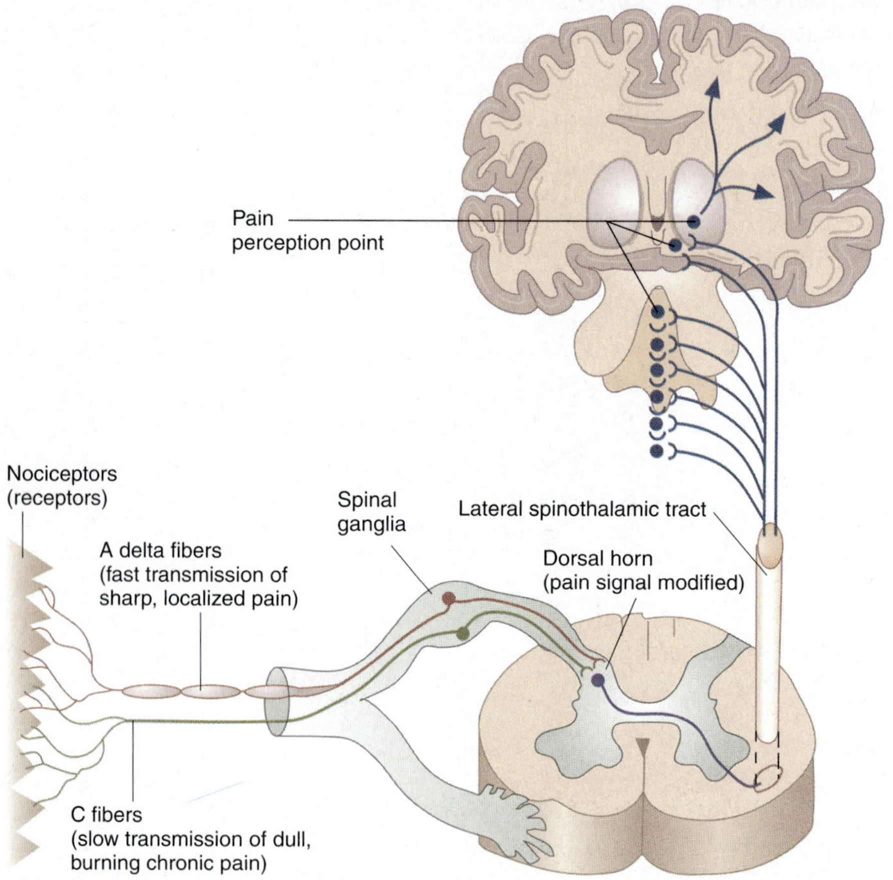

Pain perception point

Nociceptors (receptors)

A delta fibers (fast transmission of sharp, localized pain)

C fibers (slow transmission of dull, burning chronic pain)

Spinal ganglia

Lateral spinothalamic tract

Dorsal horn (pain signal modified)

TABLE 38-1 Outdated Beliefs about Pain and Pain Medication in Children

- Children without obvious physical reasons for pain are not likely to have pain.
- Neonates do not feel pain.
- Children do not feel pain with the same intensity as adults because a child's nervous system is immature.
- Children tolerate discomfort well. They become accustomed to pain after having it for a while.
- Children tell you if they are in pain. They do not need medication unless they appear to be in pain.
- Children are not in pain if they can be distracted or they are sleeping.
- Children recover more quickly than adults from painful experiences such as surgery.
- Parents exaggerate or aggravate their child's pain.
- Children have no memory of pain.
- Narcotics are dangerous for children because they can cause respiratory depression and addiction.
- The best route for giving analgesics is intramuscular.
- After surgery, children should not receive the next analgesic dose until they show obvious signs of pain.
- As-needed medication orders mean that medication should be given as infrequently as possible.

Developing Cultural Competence

The cultural experiences of health care professionals often contribute to their outdated attitudes about pain experienced by children. For example, health care workers may believe that being in pain for a little while is not so bad, that pain helps build character, or that using pain medication is a sign of a weak character.

Research has shown that past beliefs about children's perception of pain were incorrect. Neonates and infants do feel and remember pain. By 6 months of age, children demonstrate anticipatory fear of pain when taken to a location where they once experienced pain (Lutz, 1986). Health care professionals now recognize that children do not complain of pain because they are afraid that the injection to relieve pain will hurt more than the pain already does.

Growth and Development

Even neonates feel pain. Cutaneous sensation is actually present by 20 weeks' gestation. Brain centers necessary for pain perception develop toward the end of gestation. Nerve and biochemical pathways associated with pain transmission are functional at birth, but myelination (further development of the myelin sheath) continues during infancy. Although pain conduction may be slower in neonates, the distance that pain stimuli must travel is much shorter than in adults. Because of their immature nervous systems, young children may actually have a lower pain threshold and pain tolerance. Premature infants may be even more sensitive to pain than full-term infants (Anand & Carr, 1989).

Clinical Manifestations

PHYSIOLOGIC INDICATORS

Acute pain stimulates the adrenergic nervous system and results in physiologic changes, including tachycardia, tachypnea, hypertension, pupil dilation, pallor, and increased perspiration. Changes in these signs demonstrate a complex stress response. As the body adapts physiologically, vital signs return to near normal and perspiration decreases after several minutes. Thus, changes in vital signs are not a reliable indicator of pain in children because they last such a short time.

Chronic pain of long duration permits physiologic adaptation, so normal heart rate, respiratory rate, and blood pressure levels are often seen (Leo & Huether, 1998).

BEHAVIORAL INDICATORS

Children in acute pain behave in many of the same ways as children who show signs of fear and anxiety (Hazinski, 1999; Tesler, Holzemer, & Spreker, 1999). These behaviors include the following:

- Restless and agitated or hyperalert and vigilant
- Short attention span (child is difficult to distract)
- Irritability (child is difficult to comfort)
- Facial grimacing, biting or pursing lips (Figure 38–1 ◆)
- Posturing (guarding a painful joint by avoiding movement), remaining immobile, or protecting the painful area
- Drawing up knees, flexing limbs, massaging affected area
- Anorexia
- Lethargy, remaining quiet, or withdrawal
- Sleep disturbances

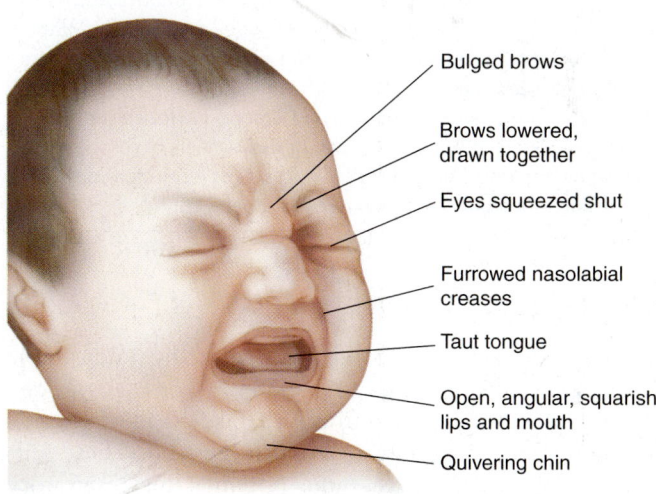

Bulged brows

Brows lowered, drawn together

Eyes squeezed shut

Furrowed nasolabial creases

Taut tongue

Open, angular, squarish lips and mouth

Quivering chin

FIGURE 38–1. ◆ Neonatal characteristic facial responses to pain include bulged brow, eyes squeezed shut, furrowed nasolabial creases, open lips, pursed lips, stretched mouth, taut tongue, and a quivering chin. *Note:* Redrawn from Carlson, K. L., Clement, B. A., & Nash, P. (1996). Neonatal pain: From concept to research questions and the role of the advanced practice nurse. *Journal of Perinatal Neonatal Nursing, 10* (1), 64–71.

Preverbal children may show conflicting signs of pain (increased or decreased vital signs, agitation or withdrawal, grimacing, crying, or anger), making assessment and monitoring pain management more challenging.

Children often suffer additional emotional distress and fear that the discomfort will worsen. Depression and/or aggressive behavior are frequently overlooked as indicators of pain.

Behavioral indicators of chronic pain and pain of long duration include posturing and inactivity to avoid pain, depression, difficulty sleeping, and an inability to concentrate (Shapiro, 1995).

Thinking Critically

DETERMINING WHEN A CHILD IS IN PAIN

Felicia, who is 5 years old, was struck by a car. Six hours ago, she had surgery to repair a liver laceration, but she also has numerous bruises and abrasions on her body. After spending 3 hours in the postanesthesia unit, she was moved to the pediatric inpatient unit. She has an intravenous line in place, as well as a nasogastric tube attached to low suction. Her abdominal dressing is clean and dry.

Felicia's mother is rooming in with her during her hospital stay. Because Felicia is thrashing around, her mother asks the nurse to give her some pain medication. When the nurse enters Felicia's room, she is napping and her facial expression indicates that she is not in pain. When the nurse attempts to straighten her position in bed, she moans. The nurse asks Felicia if she hurts, and she shakes her head no. According to Felicia's chart, she received pain medication just before her transfer from the postanesthesia unit 3 hours ago. Her physician has ordered pain medication every 3 to 4 hours as needed.

How do you know whether Felicia is in pain? Can you expect her to tell you if she feels pain? Is any additional assessment needed to justify giving Felicia more pain medication? What other pain relief measures could reduce or help to control her pain in the first 24 hours?

What is the appropriate dose of IV morphine for Felicia, who weighs 25 kg? What is the timing of assessments of response to pain and potential side effects? What signs of respiratory distress indicate a need for naloxone administration?

Consequences of Pain

Unrelieved pain is stressful and has many undesirable physiologic consequences (Table 38–2). For example, the child with acute postoperative pain takes shallow breaths and suppresses coughing to avoid more pain. These self-protective actions increase the potential for respiratory complications. Unrelieved pain may also delay the return of normal gastric and bowel functions and cause a stress ulcer. Anorexia associated with pain may delay the healing process. The long-term effects of pain on the child's physical or psychologic condition are unknown.

TABLE 38–2 Physiologic Consequences of Unrelieved Pain in Children

Responses to Pain	Potential Physiologic Consequences
Respiratory Changes	
Rapid shallow breathing	Alkalosis
Inadequate lung expansion	Decreased oxygen saturation
Inadequate cough	Retention of secretions
Neurologic Changes	
Increased sympathetic nervous system activity	Tachycardia, change in sleep patterns, increased blood glucose and cortisol levels
Metabolic Changes	
Increased metabolic rate with increased perspiration	Increased fluid and electrolyte losses

Note: From Eland, J. M. (1990). Pain in children. *Nursing Clinics of North America, 25,* 871–884; and Altimier, L., Norwood, S., Dick, M. J., et al. (1994). Postoperative pain management in preverbal children: The prescription and administration of analgesia with and without caudal analgesia. *Journal of Pediatric Nursing, 9*(4), 226–232. Adapted.

PAIN ASSESSMENT

No laboratory tests are routinely used to assess pain. Prolonged, severe pain produces a physiologic stress response that includes the chemical release of catecholamines, cortisol, aldosterone, and other corticosteroids. Insulin secretion also decreases, leading to increased amounts of glucose and severe hyperglycemia (Hazinski, 1999). Existing conditions such as infection, trauma, and anemia can cause the vital sign changes seen with sudden pain.

Nursing Practice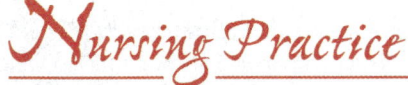

Physiologic symptoms such as nausea, fatigue, dyspnea, bladder and bowel distention, and fever may influence the intensity of pain felt by a child. Fear, anxiety, separation from parents, anger, culture, age, or a previous pain experience may also affect the child's behavior or responses to pain stimuli.

The goal of pain assessment is to provide accurate information about the location and intensity of pain and its effects on the child's functioning. When assessing pain in children, keep the following questions in mind:

- What is happening in tissues that might cause pain? Assume that children who have had surgery, injury, vaso-occlusive episode, or illness are experiencing pain, since these events also cause pain in adults.
- What external factors could be causing pain? For example, is the cast too tight or is the child poorly positioned in bed?

- Are there any indicators of pain, either physiologic or behavioral?
- How is the child responding emotionally?
- How does the child or parent rate the pain?

Pain History

Parents can provide a great deal of information about the child's response to pain, such as the following:

- How the child typically expresses pain, both verbally and behaviorally. Children and parents use similar terms to describe pain. Some examples of words used are *a hurt, owie, boo-boo, stinging, sore, cutting, burning, itching, hot,* and *tight.* Knowing the appropriate word to use makes communicating with the child easier.
- The child's previous experiences with painful situations.
- How the child copes with pain. The child with several past pain experiences may not exhibit the same types of stressful behaviors as the child with few pain experiences.
- The parent's and child's preferences for analgesic use.

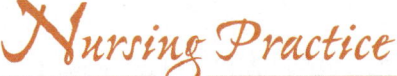

The terms *pain, hurt,* and *ache* have been found to describe pain intensity across cultures. Pain is most intense, hurt is less severe, and ache is least severe (Gaston-Johansson, Albert, Fagan, et al., 1990). The term *tender* or *tenderness* may be confusing for some families in which English is a second language. Tender or tenderness is more commonly associated with caring or romance or with meat rather than soreness or pain.

Older children may be able to give a history of painful procedures. When attempting to obtain information about the child's pain experiences and present level of pain, ask the child and parent similar open-ended questions. Sample questions are given in Table 38–3. Many children modify their pain descriptions depending on the type of questions asked and what they expect will happen as a result of their response.

When help in describing pain is needed, give the child over 6 years of age some words to select from, such as sharp, dull, aching, pounding, cold, hot, burning, throbbing, stinging, tingling, or cutting.

Children with recurrent episodes of pain can be asked to keep a diary or log to describe the characteristics, timing, activities, and potential triggers of their pain, as well as their response to pain treatment measures. This record can help improve pain management.

Cultural Influences on Pain

Children's culture and social learning have a tremendous influence on their expression of pain. Cultural traditions often guide children about self-control, coping, and enlisting the assistance of others (Leo & Huether, 1998). Children learn directly and indirectly from their parents about how to respond to pain. By showing approval and disapproval, parents teach their children how to behave when in pain. This instruction includes the following:

- How much discomfort justifies a complaint

TABLE 38–3 Pediatric Pain History for Children and Parents	
Questions for Children	*Questions for Parents*
Past Pain Experiences	
Tell me what pain is.	What word(s) does your child use to describe pain?
Tell me about the hurt you have had before.	Describe pain experiences your child has previously had.
Do you tell others when you hurt? Who?	Does your child tell you or others when he or she is in pain?
What do you do for yourself when you are hurting?	How do you know when your child is in pain?
What helps the most to take your hurt away?	How does your child usually react to pain?
What do you want others to do for you when you hurt?	What do you do for your child when he or she is in pain?
What don't you want others to do for you when you hurt?	What does your child do to manage pain?
Is there anything special you want me to know about when	What works best to reduce or take away your child's pain?
you hurt? What?	Is there anything special you would like me to know about your child and pain?
Present Pain Experiences	
Where is the pain?	Tell me about the pain your child is having now. Where is it and what does
What does it feel like?	it feel like?
What do you think is causing the pain?	What would you like me to do for your child?
What would you like me to do for you?	

Note: From Hester, N. O., & Barcus, C. S. (1986). Assessment and management of pain in children. *Pediatrics: Nursing Update, 1,* 2–8. Adapted.

- How to express the complaint
- How and when to stop complaining
- Whom to approach for pain relief

For example, boys in the United States are usually encouraged to hide their pain by acting brave and not crying. Girls are often encouraged to express their pain openly. Children also observe other family members in pain and imitate their responses (Abu-Saad, 1984).

Developing Cultural Competence

Some ethnic groups, such as Asian, Anglo-Saxon–Germanic, and Irish, do not openly express pain. People of Italian and Jewish descent are more likely to use both verbal and nonverbal methods to express pain freely. However, children have individualized responses, and younger children have had less time to acquire culturally learned behaviors.

Pain Assessment Scales

A child's responses to and understanding of pain depend on the child's age, stage of development, and other situational factors (McGrath, 1995) (Tables 38–4, 38–5, and 38–6). For example, neonates cannot anticipate pain and may not demonstrate typical behavior associated with a painful response. Young children are unable to give a detailed description of their pain because of their limited vocabulary and pain experiences. Depending on their developmental stage, children use different coping strategies, such as escape, postponement or avoidance, diversion, and imagery, to deal with pain.

TABLE 38–5 Children's Understanding of Pain by Developmental Stage

Developmental Stage	Understanding of Pain
Infants	
< 6 months	No apparent understanding of pain; infants do have memory of pain; neonates exposed to repeated painful experiences in intensive care unit demonstrate memory of pain by holding their breath when approached by care providers
6–12 months	Anticipate a painful event such as an immunization with fear
Toddlers	
1–3 years	Demonstrate a fear of painful situations; use common words for pain such as *owie* and *boo-boo*
Preschoolers	
3–6 years (preoperational)	Pain is a hurt; do not relate pain to illness but may relate pain to an injury; often believe pain is punishment; do not believe an injection takes pain away
School-Age Children	
7–9 years (concrete operations)	Can understand simple relationships between pain and disease but have no clear understanding of the cause of pain; can understand the need for painful procedures to monitor or treat disease; may recognize psychologic pain related to grief and hurt feelings
10–12 years (transitional)	Have a more complex awareness of physical and psychologic pain, such as moral dilemmas and mental pain
Adolescents	
13–18 years (formal operations)	Have a capacity for sophisticated and complex understanding of the causes of physical and mental pain; can relate to the pain experienced by others; pain has both qualitative and quantitative characteristics

TABLE 38–4 Behavioral Responses and Verbal Descriptions of Pain by Children of Different Developmental Stages

Age Group	Behavioral Response	Verbal Description
Infants		
< 6 months	Generalized body movements, chin quivering, facial grimacing, poor feeding	Cries
6–12 months	Reflex withdrawal to stimulus, facial grimacing, disturbed sleep, irritability, restlessness	Cries
Toddlers		
1–3 years	Localized withdrawal, resistance of entire body, aggressive behavior, disturbed sleep	Cries and screams, cannot describe intensity or type of pain
Preschoolers		
3–6 years (preoperational)	Active physical resistance, directed aggressive behavior, strikes out physically and verbally when hurt, low frustration level	Can identify location and intensity of pain, denies pain, may believe his or her pain is obvious to others
School-Age Children		
7–9 years (concrete operations)	Passive resistance, clenches fists, holds body rigidly still, suffers emotional withdrawal, engages in plea bargaining	Can specify location and intensity of pain and describe its physical characteristics
10–12 years (transitional)	May pretend comfort to project bravery, may regress with stress and anxiety	Able to describe intensity and location with more characteristics, able to describe psychologic pain
Adolescents		
13–18 years (formal operations)	Want to behave in a socially acceptable manner (like adults), show a controlled behavioral response	More sophisticated descriptions as experience is gained

TABLE 38–6　Situational Factors Influencing Pain in Children

Cognitive Factors
- Understanding of pain source
- Ability to control what will happen
- Expectations about the quality and strength of pain
- Whether attention is focused on painful event or distractor

Behavioral Factors
- Use of a pain-control strategy
- Response of parents and health care personnel
- Whether or not restrained
- Ability to continue usual activities

Emotional Factors
- Fear
- Anxiety
- Frustration
- Anger
- Depression

Note: From McGrath, P. A. (1995). Pain in the pediatric patient: Practical aspects of assessment. *Pediatric Annals, 24*(3), 126–138. Adapted.

Nursing Practice

Children do not exhibit distress in direct proportion to their pain intensity. Thus, behavioral measures may not match the child's self-report of pain intensity. Older children often appear calm, are expressionless, and limit movement following surgery, but report pain of moderate to severe levels (Tesler et al., 1999).

Various pain scales assess pain in children (see Table 38–7 and Skill 13–1). 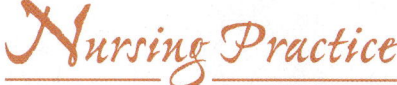 **SKILLS** Physical and behavioral indicators are used to quantify pain in children. Some pain assessment scales rely on the nurse's observation of the child's behavior if the child is nonverbal, for example, the Children's Hospital of Eastern Ontario Pain Scale (CHEOPS) (see Table 38–7) and Neonatal Infant Pain Scale (NIPS) (Table 38–8). These scales can provide only an indirect estimate of pain intensity from the child's behaviors or physical states. Most scales depend on the child's report of pain intensity (Table 38–7). Because adults cannot experience the child's pain, it is not possible to compare the pain felt by children and adults using these assessment tools, even when undergoing the same procedures.

Growth and Development

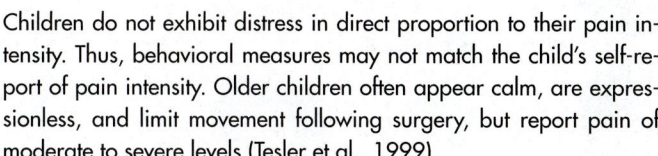

Identify the child's stage of development for readiness to use pain scales.

▶ Assess the child's language skills (ability to use words in sequence, follow simple directions, and answer simple questions).
▶ Ask the child to count his or her fingers or up to 10.
▶ Determine whether the child can understand concepts such as more or less and higher or lower.

Facial scales may be a measure of emotional distress because they reflect the unpleasantness of pain. Comparison of faces pain scales has revealed that those scales with a smiling face as the indicator of no pain resulted in significantly higher pain ratings by children and parents than scales using a neutral expression face as an indicator of no pain (Chambers, Gresbrecht, Craig, et al, 1999).

CLINICAL THERAPY FOR PAIN

Current guidelines for pain management build upon those published by the U.S. government in 1992. The recommendations for pain management include both drug and nondrug measures. Drug interventions include the use of **opioids** and **nonsteroidal anti-inflammatory drugs (NSAIDs).** **WEB**

Opioids

Opioids such as morphine and codeine may be administered by oral, subcutaneous, intramuscular, and intravenous routes. Administration of opioids by an oral route is as effective as by intramuscular and intravenous routes when the drug is given in an **equianalgesic dose** (the amount of drug, whether given by oral or parenteral routes, needed to produce the same analgesic effect) (Table 38–9). Rectal preparations of some opioids are also available. The optimal analgesic dose varies widely among patients in all age groups (American Pain Society, 1999).

Common side effects include sedation, nausea, vomiting, constipation, and itching. Potential complications of opioids include respiratory depression, cardiovascular collapse, and addiction. When the child's condition is unstable, as in trauma or critical illness, the dosage of opioids must be carefully calculated to match the child's cardiorespiratory status, although infants and children are no more likely than adults to develop respiratory depression following administration of a weight-specific dose of narcotics (Holder & Patt, 1995). Addiction is a rare complication in adults treated for painful conditions, and the same holds true for children.

Nursing Practice

Respiratory depression (unresponsiveness and a respiratory rate less than 12 breaths/min in children less than 2 years of age) may progress to respiratory arrest and is the major life-threatening complication of opioid administration. Respiratory depression is most likely to occur when the child is sleeping. This augments the depressant effect on the respiratory center and potential airway obstruction by the tongue (American Pain Society, 1999). Identify the time interval before drug-specific peak respiratory depression occurs, and then carefully monitor the child's vital signs during that period to detect respiratory depression.

TABLE 38-7 **Pain Assessment Scales**

Scale and Age Group	Administration	Use
NIPS		
Preterm and full-term infant to 6 weeks after birth (see Table 38–8)	Observe the neonate's facial expression, cry quality, breathing patterns, arm and leg position, and state of arousal	Useful in measuring pain or pain-elicited distress in infants; overall status of infant and the infant's environment must be factored into the assessment
CHEOPS 1–7 years	Observe the child's cry, facial expression, torso position, leg position, touch-painful area, and verbal complaints; select the numerical score for each category after 5 seconds	Primarily behavioral assessment for postoperative pain or following painful procedures; researchers have no specific score indicating pain in need of medication; in preverbal children scale may measure nonspecific stress rather than only pain.
Eland Color Tool 4–9 years	Child picks a crayon color to represent the most severe pain, then a color for the next most severe pain, until four crayons have been selected; child then colors in an outline of the body to indicate the location of the areas that hurt by level of pain	You need six crayons; black, purple, blue, red, green, and orange; no one color is most often selected by children as representing the most pain; limited reliability and validity of data[a]
Oucher Scale 3–7 years	Child selects a face that best fits his or her level of pain; older child can select a number between 0 and 10	Useful in hospital settings; child must understand concepts of higher/lower and more/less; cultural versions available; tool has been successfully tested for reliability and validity in some age groups[a,b]

A   B   C

(continued)

TABLE 38-7 **Pain Assessment Scales—continued**

Scale and Age Group	Administration	Use
Poker Chip Scale 3–7 years	Child selects the number of chips or checkers that matches level of hurt (1 = a little hurt, 5 = the most hurt)	Useful in hospital settings; child must have number concepts from 1 to 5; you can then obtain a measure of child's perception of pain

A tiny bit of hurt   Little more pain   Still more pain   Most hurt of all

| **Numeric Pain Scale** 9 years–adult | Ask child to rate pain felt on a line with 10 marks (1 = a little pain, 10 = the most pain) | Child must be verbal; easy to carry tool to patient |

0   1   2   3   4   5   6   7   8   9   10

| **Pediatric Pain Questionnaire**[c] | Child selects pain descriptors from checklist, rates current and average pain intensity with visual analog scale and uses own color choices to identify different pain intensities on pain map of body | Parent, child, and adolescent forms exist; parent form provides information about history of pain problem and its management; useful for chronic pain |

[a]Reliability is the extent to which the same score is obtained when an instrument or scale is used either by different persons or by the same person at different times. Validity is the extent to which an instrument or scale measures what it is supposed to measure.

[b]**A,** The Caucasion version of the Oucher, developed and copyrighted by Judith E. Beyer, RN, PhD, 1983. **B,** The African-American version of the Oucher, developed and copyrighted by Mary J. Denyes, RN, PhD, and Antonio M. Villarruel, RN, PhD, 1990. **C,** The Hispanic version of the Oucher, developed and copyrighted by Antonio M. Villarruel, RN, PhD, and Mary J. Denyes, RN, PhD, 1990.

[c]From Varni, J. W., Thompson, K. L., & Hanson V. (1987). The Varni/Thompson pediatric pain questionnaire: Chronic musculoskeletal pain in juvenile rheumatoid arthritis. *Pain, 28*, 27–38.

TABLE 38-8   Neonatal Infant Pain Scale (NIPS)

Characteristic	Scoring Criteria

Facial Expression
0 = Relaxed muscles
1 = Grimace

- Restful face with neutral expression
- Tight facial muscles; furrowed brow, chin, and jaw (Note: At low gestational ages, infants may have no facial expression)

Cry
0 = No cry
1 = Whimper
2 = Vigorous cry

- Quiet, not crying
- Mild moaning, intermittent cry
- Loud screaming, rising, shrill, and continuous (Note: silent cry may be scored if infant is intubated, as indicated by obvious facial movements)

Breathing Patterns
0 = Relaxed

1 = Change in breathing

- Relaxed, usual breathing pattern maintained
- Change in drawing breath; irregular, faster than usual, gagging, or holding breath

Arm Movements
0 = Relaxed/restrained (with soft restraints)
1 = Flexed/extended

- Relaxed, no muscle rigidity, occasional random movements of arms
- Tense, straight arms; rigid; or rapid extension and flexion

Leg Movements
0 = Relaxed/restrained) (with soft restraints
1 = Flexed/extended

- Relaxed, no muscle rigidity, occasional random movements of legs
- Tense, straight legs; rigid; or rapid extension and flexion

State of Arousal
0 = Sleeping/awake

1 = Fussy

- Quiet, peaceful, sleeping; or alert and settled
- Alert and restless or thrashing; fussy

Note: From Lawrence, J., Alcock, D., McGrath, D. P., et al. (1993). The development of a tool to assess neonatal pain. *Neonatal Network, 12*(6), 61.

TABLE 38-9   Opioid Analgesics and Recommended Doses for Children and Adolescents*

Drug	Approximate Equianalgesic Oral Dose	Approximate Equianalgesic Parenteral Dose	Recommended Starting Dose (Adults >50 kg) Oral	Parenteral	Recommended Starting Dose (Children & Adults <50 kg) Oral	Parenteral
Morphine	30 mg	10 mg	15–30 mg q 3–4 hr	10 mg q 3–4 hr	0.3 mg/kg q 3–4 hr	0.1 mg/kg q 3–4 hr
Codeine	130 mg	75 mg IM or Subcutaneous	30–60 mg q 3–4 hr	60 mg q 2 hr	0.5–1 mg q 3–4 hr[a]	NR
Hydromorphone (Dilaudid)	7.5 mg	1.5 mg	4–8 mg q 3–4 hr	1.5 mg q 3–4 hr	0.06 mg/kg q 3–4 hr	0.015 mg/kg q 3–4 hr
Levorphanol (Levo-Dromoran)	4 mg (acute) 1 mg (chronic)	2 mg (acute) 1 mg (chronic)	2–4 mg q 6–8 hr	2 mg q 6–8 hr	0.04 mg/kg q 6–8 hr	0.02 mg/kg q 6–8 hr
Meperidine (Demerol)	300 mg	100 mg	NR	100 mg q 3 hr	NR	0.05–1.5 mg/kg q 2–4 hr
Methadone (Dolophine, others)	20 mg (acute) 2–4 mg (chronic)	10 mg (acute) 2–4 mg (chronic)	5–10 mg q 6–8 hr	10 mg q 6–8 hr	0.2 mg/kg q 6–8 hr	0.1 mg/kg q 6–8 hr
Oxycodone (Roxicodone)	30 mg	NA	5–10 mg q 3–4 hr	NA	0.1–0.2 mg/kg q 3–4 hr[a]	NA
Fentanyl	NA	0.01 mg	5 mcg/kg Lozenge	50–100 mcg q 1–2 hr	5–15 mcg/kg Oralet[b]	1 mcg/kg

NR = Not recommended; NA = Not available
*For all parenteral opioids, start with the low dose and titrate to effective pain control.

[a] Caution: Doses of aspirin and acetaminophen in combination with opioid/NSAID preparation must also be adjusted to the patient's body weight.

[b] The Oralet is not widely used because of nausea and vomiting side effects.

Note: From American Pain Society. (1999). *Principles of analgesic use in the treatment of acute pain and cancer pain* (4th ed., pp. 6–8, 14–15, 20). Glenview, IL: Author; Hazinski, M. F. (1999). Analgesia, sedation, and neuromuscular blockage in pediatric critical care. In M. F. Hazinski, *Manual of pediatric critical care* (pp. 44–72). St. Louis, MO: Mosby; and Acute Pain Management Guideline Panel. (1992). *Acute pain management in infants, children, and adolescents: Operative and medical procedures. Quick reference guide for clinicians* (AHCPR Pub. No. 92–0020). Rockville, MD: Agency for Healthcare Policy and Research, U.S. Public Health Service, Department of Health and Human Services.

Avoid opioid agonists such as nalbuphine (Nubain), pentazocine (Talwin), and butorphanol (Stadol) as first line drugs for pain. These drugs were developed to exert effects on one opioid receptor and antagonize a second receptor. While this mixed agonist/antagonist action may limit potential side effects such as respiratory depression, they have a ceiling to analgesia. They are inappropriate for escalating pain (Hazinski, 1999).

Nonsteroidal Anti-inflammatory Drugs

NSAIDs such as aspirin and acetaminophen, primarily given orally, are effective for the relief of mild to moderate pain and chronic pain. Table 38–10 presents recommended dosages of these drugs. They are most commonly used for bone, inflammatory, and connective tissue conditions. An NSAID may be prescribed in combination with an opioid to increase the effectiveness of the narcotic drug. This combination may ultimately reduce the amount of opioids needed for pain relief.

Drug Administration

Pain from surgery, major trauma, or cancer will be present for predictable periods because of the effects of tissue damage. Pain relief should be provided *around the clock*. Every effort should be made to give the child analgesics without causing more pain. The preferred routes of administration are intravenous, local nerve block, and oral.

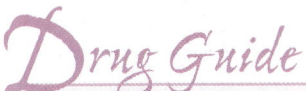

ACETAMINOPHEN

Overview of Action

May interfere with prostaglandin synthesis in the central nervous system to provide analgesia. Acts in the hypothalamus to cause antipyresis. May have a mild anti-inflammatory effect but this is likely not therapeutic. Used in treatment of mild to moderate pain and of fever.

Routes, Dosage, Frequency

Oral or Rectal: 10 to 15 mg/kg every 4 to 6 hours, as needed. Do not exceed 5 doses/day. If not prescribed by health care provider, seek medical advice after 5 doses for either fever or pain.

Contraindications: Previous allergy to the drug and G6PD deficiency. Do not give preparations with aspartame to children with phenylketonuria. Use cautiously in children with hepatic dysfunction, anemia, or renal dysfunction.

Side Effects: Liver damage with overdose.

Nursing Implications

- Assess: Note hepatic and renal function. Assess pain level or actual temperature prior to administration.
- *Administer:* Follow dosage directions carefully for different liquid preparations. Concentration differs between drops and elixir. Plain or chewable tablets may be crushed and given with fluid; avoid giving with high carbohydrate meals, which can decrease drug absorption.
- *Monitor:* Evaluate the response to medication. Periodic renal and hepatic studies may be ordered for patients on long-term therapy.
- *Patient teaching:* Do not give with other over-the-counter medications unless directed by health care provider as they may also contain acetaminophen or aspirin. Consult a physician for dosage in a child younger than 2 to 3 years, if fever or illness persists over 3 days, or if relief is not obtained. Limit child to 5 doses/day. Store out of the child's reach as this medication is a frequent cause of childhood poisoning.

Note: From Bindler, R. M., & Howry, L. B. (1997). *Pediatric drugs and nursing implications* (2nd ed.). Upper Saddle River, NJ: Prentice Hall-Health. Adapted.

TABLE 38-10	NSAIDs and Recommended Doses for Children and Adolescents		
Oral NSAID Peak Action Time	Usual Adult Dose	Usual Pediatric Dose	Comments
Acetaminophen 0.5–2 hr	500–1000 mg q 4–6 hr	10–15 mg/kg q 4–6 hr	Lacks the peripheral anti-inflammatory activity of other NSAIDs; rectal suppository available
Aspirin 1–2 hr	650–975 mg q 4–6 hr	10–15 mg/kg q 4 hr	Do not use in children under 12 years with possible viral illness; may cause gastric upset and bleeding; rectal suppository available
Choline magnesium trisalicylate (Trilisate) 2 hr	1000–1500 mg q 12 hr	25 mg/kg q 12 hr	Does not increase bleeding time like other NSAIDs; also available as oral liquid
Ibuprofen (Motrin, others) 0.5 hr	200–400 mg q 4–6 hr	10 mg/kg q 6–8 hr	Available as oral suspension
Naproxen (Naprosyn) 2–4 hr	500 mg initial dose followed by 250 mg q 6–8 hr	5 mg/kg q 12 hr	Available as oral liquid

Note: From American Pain Society. (1999). *Principles of analgesic use in the treatment of acute pain and cancer pain* (4th ed., pp. 6–8, 14–15, 20). Glenview, IL: Author; Hazinski, M. F. (1999). Analgesia, sedation, and neuromuscular blockage in pediatric critical care. In M. F. Hazinski, *Manual of pediatric critical care* (pp. 44–72). St. Louis, MO: Mosby; and Acute Pain Management Guideline Panel. (1992). *Acute pain management in infants, children, and adolescents: Operative and medical procedures. Quick reference guide for clinicians* (AHCPR Pub. No. 92-0020). Rockville, MD: Agency for Healthcare Policy and Research, U.S. Public Health Service, Department of Health and Human Services.

Continuous-infusion analgesia, which eliminates the peaks and valleys in pain control, is recommended to keep drug levels constant in children with continuous or persistent severe pain. Analgesics may also be given intravenously on a scheduled basis (e.g., every 3 to 4 hours). Delays in giving analgesics on a scheduled basis increase the chances of breakthrough pain and the subsequent anticipation of pain. Giving analgesics on an as-needed basis for acute pain also results in the *loss of pain control*. More medications are often needed to restore pain control than would have been required for continuous infusion analgesia.

Patient-controlled analgesia (PCA) is a method of administering an intravenous or epidural analgesic, such as morphine, using a computerized pump programmed by the health care professional and controlled by the child (Figure 38–2 ◆ and Skill 13–2). [SKILLS] This technique is especially useful for pain control in the first 48 hours after surgery when oral pain management is not possible. PCA is prescribed mostly for children 5 years old and older (Holder & Patt, 1995). Children selected for PCA should be able to push the injection button and should understand that pushing the button will give them medication to relieve pain. Parents are sometimes given responsibility for pushing the injection button for younger children or those with disabilities.

After initial pain control has been achieved with an IV infusion by the nurse, the child presses a button to receive a smaller analgesic dose for episodic pain relief. The PCA monitor can be set up with or without a continuous infusion of opioid drug in addition to the dose administered when the child pushes the button. To prevent overdoses, the PCA computerized pump has safety features that include the ability to set the maximum number of infusions per hour and the maximum amount of drug received in a given time period. A continuous infusion prevents a recurrence of pain during long sleeping periods. Additional pain medication is often ordered as needed to supplement the

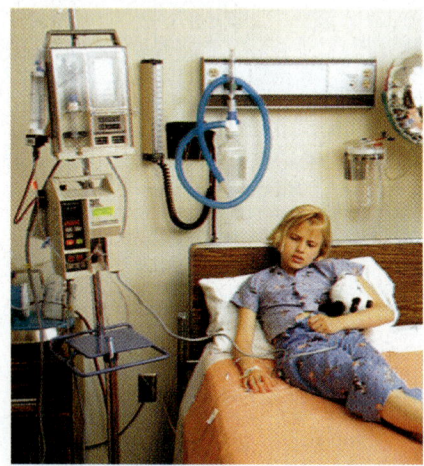

FIGURE 38–2. ◆ By using patient-controlled analgesia, the older child is able to regulate the intake of an intravenous analgesic such as morphine.

Teaching About

PATIENT-CONTROLLED ANALGESIA (PCA)

- What is PCA? Analgesia means pain relief: you get to control the amount of medicine you receive by using the machine.
- The machine gives the medicine by passing it through the tube that is connected to your intravenous line. When you push the button, the machine pumps pain medicine into the intravenous line to make you feel better.
- The machine limits the amount of medicine you can get to what the doctor orders. You can get any amount up to the maximum by pushing the button repeatedly. The push button will not let you make a mistake if you drop it or roll on it.
- Whenever you feel pain, hurt, or discomfort, push the button to get more medicine. You should be the only one to push the button.
- No needles for pain shots are needed as long as the intravenous line is in place.
- The PCA may not relieve all of your pain, but it should make you feel comfortable. Let the nurse know if you think your PCA is not working.
- The PCA will be used until you can take pills or drink liquid pain medicine.

continuous and patient-administered infusion when pain control is not maintained.

Children and adolescents benefit from PCA by receiving continuous pain control and having the ability to control their comfort level with no trauma from injections. Several studies have documented the maintenance of pain relief without an increase in narcotic side effects (Holder & Patt, 1995). Once children can take oral analgesics, PCA is discontinued.

Epidural pain control provides selective analgesia and has become more common for postoperative pain management. A catheter is inserted into either the lumbar or the caudal space. Only minute doses of drugs are needed because of the high concentration achieved at the opioid receptors in the spinal cord's dorsal horn (Holder & Patt, 1995).

Local nerve blocks, such as a popliteal block for anesthesia and analgesia of a lower extremity, are used more frequently for pain control after surgery. A subcutaneous catheter is inserted into the local area for infusion of the analgesia. Pain control is achieved without systemic side effects from the medication.

Nursing Management
Nursing Assessment and Diagnosis

Nurses have an ethical obligation to relieve a child's suffering not only because of the consequences of unrelieved pain but also because appropriate pain management may have benefits such as earlier mobilization, shortened hospital stays, and reduced costs.

Nursing Practice

Most children are unaware of their right to pain relief. Nurses and health care institutions have a duty to prevent and alleviate suffering. Pain management should be an institutional priority with a standard of care. Nurses have an ethical responsibility to monitor implementation of that standard (Kachoyeanos & Zollok, 1995).

To provide effective nursing management of children in pain, anticipate the presence of pain and recognize the child's right to pain control. Assess the child using an appropriate assessment tool (see Tables 38–3 to 38–7). Surgery and trauma can result in multiple sites of pain (incision or laceration, cut or bruised muscles, interrupted blood supply, nasogastric tube placement, insertion sites of intravenous lines). When using pain scales in the assessment of a verbal child, attempt to identify all sites of pain. Then evaluate the intensity of pain at each site.

Examples of nursing diagnoses for children in pain include the following:

▶ *Moderate sharp knee pain* related to injury and orthopedic surgery

▶ *Moderate dull hand chronic pain* related to arthritic joint degeneration

▶ *Anxiety* related to anticipation of pain from an invasive procedure

▶ *Sleep pattern disturbance* related to inadequate pain control

▶ *Ineffective individual management of therapeutic regimen* related to self-management of pain control, and use of nonpharmacologic pain-control measures

▶ *Ineffective breathing pattern: potential for,* related to opioid overdose

▶ *Risk for constipation* related to opioid pain medication and limited activity

Planning and Implementation

Nursing management involves the following actions to increase and maintain patient comfort:

▶ Recognition of pain and formulation of a nursing diagnosis

▶ Pharmacologic intervention

▶ Nonpharmacologic intervention

▶ Monitoring and documenting the effectiveness of pain-control measures to provide optimal comfort

▶ Patient education

The accompanying "Nursing Care Plan" summarizes nursing care for the child with postoperative pain.

PHARMACOLOGIC INTERVENTION

Give analgesics as ordered by the physician, ensuring that the dose is appropriate for the child's weight. When administering an opioid by intravenous infusion or PCA, monitor the flow rate and the site for infiltration. Make sure analgesic antagonists such as naloxone are available should complications develop. Naloxone may be used to treat respiratory depression caused by an opioid drug at a dose and slow infusion rate that does not reverse the pain-control effects of the narcotic. A continuous infusion or repeated doses may be needed for severe overdoses.

Monitor the child's vital signs for complications related to opioids, such as respiratory depression. Clinical signs that predict the development of respiratory depression include sleepiness, small pupils, and shallow breathing. Other vital signs (heart rate and blood pressure) may not change in response to effective analgesia when infection, trauma, or other stressors keep them elevated. Children at particular risk for respiratory depression induced by an opioid are those with an altered level of consciousness, an unstable circulatory status, a history of apnea, or a known airway problem. Check for the presence of other side effects of analgesics, such as sedation, nausea, vomiting, itching, urinary retention, and constipation.

When a regional nerve block is used, the analgesic effect does not recede for several hours after the catheter is removed. Be careful when ambulating a child with a regional nerve block in an extremity. Protect the extremity from injury because the child has reduced feeling in the limb. Monitor the child for tingling of fingers or toes, an indication that the analgesic effect is receding. Begin oral analgesia to maintain pain control.

Evaluate the child's level of pain frequently to determine whether the analgesic eliminated the pain and to identify any increase in pain intensity. Use information collected from the child and parent, as well as from an appropriate pain scale. Dramatic reductions in pain should occur, although not all pain may disappear. Many children sleep after receiving an analgesic. This sleep is not a side effect of the drug or a sign of an overdose, but the result of pain relief. Pain interrupts sleep, and once pain is relieved, the child can sleep comfortably. On the other hand, sleep does not always indicate pain control. A child in pain may fall asleep in exhaustion. Look for other symptoms of pain, such as excess movement or moaning. Be certain to record results of pain-control measures to guide future nursing actions. Use a flowsheet to document assessments and medication administration during the postoperative period.

Become an advocate for children when the dose or type of analgesic ordered is inadequate. **Tolerance** is a decrease in a drug's effect over time or the need for increasing amounts of the drug to produce or maintain the same level of pain relief or sedation effect. This may occur when children with severe pain have been taking opioids or sedatives for several days. Breakthrough pain occurs, and an increase

GOAL	INTERVENTION	RATIONALE	EXPECTED OUTCOME

1. Severe abdominal pain related to surgery and injury

	NIC Priority Intervention:		*NOC Suggested Outcome:*
	Pain management: *Alleviation of pain or a reduction in pain to a level of comfort that is acceptable to the patient*		**Comfort level:** *Feelings of physical and psychologic ease*
The child will report reduced pain.	▶ Give analgesic by a pain-free method.	▶ The child may deny pain to avoid analgesia by painful route.	The child reports reduced pain after administration of analgesia.
	▶ Have the child select a pain scale and rate the amount of pain perceived before and 30–60 minutes after analgesia is given to ensure pain relief.	▶ The child's pain rating is the best indicator of pain. Maintenance of pain control requires less analgesia than treating each acute pain episode.	
	▶ Reposition the child every 2 hr to maintain good body alignment. Provide therapeutic touch or massage.	▶ Anxiety increases perception of pain. New positions decrease muscle cramping and skin pressure.	

2. Sleep pattern disturbance related to inadequate pain control

	NIC Priority Intervention:		*NOC Suggested Outcome:*
	Sleep enhancement: *Facilitation of regular sleep/wake cycles*		**Sleep:** *Extent and pattern of sleep for mental and physical rejuvenation*
The child will experience fewer disruptions of sleep by pain.	▶ Give analgesia by continuous infusion or every 3–4 hr around the clock.	▶ Pain breakthrough occurs even during sleep.	The child's sleep is undisturbed by pain. Child sleeps for age-appropriate number of hours per day.

3. Ineffective individual management of therapeutic regimen related to self-management of pain control and use of nondrug pain-control measures

	NIC Priority Intervention:		*NOC Suggested Outcome:*
	Self-modification assistance: *Reinforcement of self-directed change initiated by the patient to achieve personally important goals*		**Treatment behavior pain control:** *Personal actions to palliate or eliminate pain*
The child and family will effectively use patient-controlled analgesia (PCA) and nondrug pain-control measures.	▶ Teach the child how the PCA works and when to push the button.	▶ The child must know that pushing the PCA button will keep pain under control.	The child's pain rating stays low.
	▶ Teach the family and the child how to use age-appropriate imagery, distraction, relaxation techniques, and other nondrug pain-relief measures.	▶ Nondrug pain-control measures reduce amount of analgesia needed.	The child and family independently use nondrug pain-control measures.
The child and family will use appropriate analgesia after discharge.	▶ Discuss appropriate pain control to use at home after discharge.	▶ The family and child may be anxious about pain management at home.	The family understands pain-relief measures for use at home and knows where to call if help is needed.

4. Risk for ineffective breathing pattern related to opioid overdose

	NIC Priority Intervention:		*NOC Suggested Outcome:*
	Respiratory monitoring: *Collection and analysis of patient data to ensure airway patency and adequate gas exchange*		**Vital signs status:** *Temperature, pulse, respirations, and blood pressure within expected range for the individual*
The child will maintain adequate ventilations.	▶ Verify that correct dose of opioid analgesia is given.	▶ Respiratory depression is a significant complication of opioid analgesia.	There is no episode of respiratory depression associated with analgesia.
	▶ Monitor vital signs and depth of inspirations before analgesic is administered and at time of peak drug action.	▶ Respiratory depression episode must not progress to respiratory arrest. All opioids act on brainstem center which decreases responsiveness to CO_2 tension.	
	▶ Calculate agonist dose ordered by physician to be sure it will reverse respiratory depression, not counteract effect of analgesia.	▶ Valuable time will be saved if agonist is needed for episode of respiratory depression.	

(continued)

GOAL	INTERVENTION	RATIONALE	EXPECTED OUTCOME
5. Constipation related to opioid administration and decreased motility of gastrointestinal tract			
	NIC Priority Intervention:		*NOC Suggested Outcome:*
	Constipation management: *Prevention and alleviation of constipation*		**Bowel elimination:** *Ability of gastrointestinal tract to form and evacuate stool effectively*
The child will have minimal constipation.	▶ Palpate the abdomen, and assess bowel sounds and abdominal distention.	▶ Signs of constipation must be anticipated and identified.	The child has bowel movements at least every 2 days while on opioid pain control.
	▶ Request physician order for stimulating laxative and stool softener.	▶ Opioids increase the transit time of feces and interfere with bile enzymes needed for evacuation.	
	▶ Provide fluids of choice to increase fluid intake when IV fluids are decreased.	▶ Extra fluids will counteract opioid action of increasing the absorption of water from the large intestine.	
	▶ Inform family and child of possible medication-induced constipation.	▶ Parents can become partners in managing fluid intake and monitoring bowel movements.	

in dosage is needed to achieve the previous level of pain relief. Tolerance can be delayed with effective use of pain scales to allow appropriate drug dosing, and often less analgesia is needed. Magnesium may also slow the development of tolerance (Tobias, 2000). Before asking the physician to change the analgesia, review the child's record for documentation that the prescribed drug has been given at the appropriate dose and frequency and that the child's pain relief is ineffective despite the drug administration. After verifying the record, provide the physician with information about the characteristics of the child's pain and ask that the medication be changed. **Withdrawal** is the physical signs and symptoms that occur when a sedative or pain drug is stopped suddenly in a patient who is physically tolerant. Weaning may take 2 to 4 weeks to prevent withdrawal symptoms. See Table 38–11 for signs and symptoms of withdrawal.

Nursing Practice

There is growing consensus that placebo use to assess and manage pain should be avoided, especially without consent. Studies suggest that placebos tend to be used for patients who are disliked, with whom staff have conflicts, or who have failed to respond to standard treatment. Placebo use involves deception. You must respect the patient's right to be informed of treatment (Rushton, 1995).

Oral NSAIDs are generally ordered for less severe pain or chronic pain. These drugs may mask fever. Be alert to the potential complication of gastrointestinal hemorrhage in critically ill children who have increased gastric acids as physiologic stress response to pain.

TABLE 38–11	Signs and Symptoms of Opioid or Sedative Withdrawal
System	*Signs and Symptoms*
Central nervous system	Irritability, increased wakefulness, tremulousness, hyperactive deep tendon reflexes, clonus, inability to concentrate, frequent yawning, sneezing, delirium, hypertonicity, visual or auditory hallucinations
Gastrointestinal system	Feeding intolerance with vomiting, diarrhea, uncoordinated suck and swallow
Sympathetic nervous system	Tachycardia, tachypnea, increased blood pressure, nasal stuffiness, sweating, fever

Note: From Tobias, J. D. (2000). Tolerance, withdrawal, and physical dependency after long term sedation and analgesia of children in the pediatric intensive care unit. *Critical Care Medicine, 28*(6), 2122–2132. Adapted.

NONPHARMACOLOGIC INTERVENTION

Use nonpharmacologic methods of pain control with or without analgesics. One or more of these methods may provide adequate pain relief when the child has low levels of pain. When used with analgesics, nonpharmacologic techniques often increase the effectiveness of the analgesic or reduce the dosage required. When used in association with a medical procedure, remember to use an intervention before, during, and after the procedure. This gives the child a chance to recover, feel mastery, and remember coping (Fanurik, Koh, Schitz, et al., 1997).

Distraction

Distraction involves engaging a child in a wide variety of activities to help him or her focus attention on something other than pain and the anxiety associated with the procedure. Examples of distracting activities are listening to music, singing a song, playing a game, watching television or a video, and focusing on a picture while counting. Select activities that are developmentally appropriate for the child. Children in severe pain cannot be distracted, but do not assume the pain is gone if a child can be distracted.

Teaching About

HELPING A CHILD COPE WITH PAIN

Parents are the single most powerful nonpharmacologic method of pain relief available to children. A parent's presence greatly reduces the anxiety associated with pain and hospitalization (Broome, 2000). Children often feel more secure telling their parents about their pain and anxiety. Parents can help the child to cope with mild or moderate pain using a variety of distraction methods that match the child's developmental stage and individual interests.

- Infants: holding, cuddling, sucking a pacifier
- Preschoolers: engaging in play, watching television or a video
- School-age children: talking about pleasant experiences, playing games, listening to radio, watching television or a video
- Adolescents: having visitors, playing games, watching television, listening to radio or tape player **WEB**

Nursing Practice

Assemble a pain management kit to promote distraction, imagery, and relaxation in children. Items that might be included are magic wands, pinwheels, bubble liquid, a slinky spring toy, a foam ball, party noisemakers, and pop-up books. It may also be helpful to include items for therapeutic play such as syringes, adhesive bandages, alcohol swabs, and other supplies from a medical kit. The pain management kit may be especially helpful for distracting children who are being prepared for surgery or for painful procedures.

Cutaneous Stimulation

Cutaneous stimulation involves gently rubbing the painful area, massaging the skin gently, and holding or rocking the child. Touching provides a stimulus to compete with the pain stimuli transmitted from the peripheral nerves to the spinal cord. These actions may reduce the pain felt by the child.

Swaddling and blanket rolls may calm a distressed neonate by decreasing tactile stimulation and containing gross motor behaviors (Lynn, Ulma, & Spreker, 1999).

Electroanalgesia

Also known as transcutaneous electrical nerve stimulation (TENS), **electroanalgesia** delivers small amounts of electrical stimulation to the skin by electrodes. This stimulation may interfere with the transmission of pain from the peripheral nerves to the spinal cord. TENS may be used for both acute and chronic pain management.

Imagery

Imagery is a cognitive process that encourages the child to focus on and explore a favorite place, event, or funny story unrelated to the pain process. This method is most effective in children over 6 years of age. Ask the child to think about all the sights, sounds, smells, tastes, and feelings that will help him or her to experience the favorite place. Imagery is a form of self-hypnosis, and it is most effective when preceded by a relaxation exercise.

Relaxation Techniques

Relaxation techniques are used to reduce muscle tension. Pain is often aggravated when muscles are tensed. Relaxation methods include rhythmic breathing (repeatedly taking a deep breath and slowly releasing it), alternately tensing and relaxing selected muscle groups for 10 seconds each. Progressively move from specific muscle groups to more central muscles. Relaxation is enhanced if the child is encouraged to focus attention on something pleasant.

Complementary Care

HYPNOTHERAPY FOR CHILDREN

Hypnotherapy is becoming mainstream in Western medicine. It is the most widely studied of the complementary/alternative therapies and is often prescribed as the primary treatment for a variety of childhood problems. Nurses can use hypnotherapeutic language to promote self-efficacy in their patients. Children entering a health care environment are often fearful. Nurses can induce them into a more relaxed state by speaking quietly, as well as asking children to focus on their breathing and to imagine something pleasant—the ingredients of hypnotic induction.

Children have a great capacity to use their imaginations and fantasy worlds for therapeutic gain and are actually more successful than adults in attaining a hypnotic state. Hypnotherapy has been used successfully in children to treat pain, bed-wetting, asthma, stool-withholding, habit disorders, anxiety and fears, migraine headaches, nausea associated with chemotherapy, needle phobias, warts, insomnia, tics, and other problems (Anbar, 2001; Olness & Kohen, 1996; Sugarman, 1996).

Hypnotherapy does not turn one into a quacking duck. It is not a sleep state. Rather, hypnosis is an altered state of awareness within which the individual experiences heightened concentration, a decreased awareness of external stimuli, increased relaxation, and increased suggestibility. Hypnotherapy can be as simple as teaching a child to blow on a pinwheel while getting an injection. This simple form refocuses the child's heightened attention with the goal to diminish the pain and fear of the needle. Hypnotherapy may also be done in a more formal way, where a therapist specially trained in pediatric hypnotherapeutic techniques uses the images and language of the child to induce relaxation and give posthypnotic suggestions. Often, young children have their eyes open during a session. Language such as, "You are the boss of your body and can help make this headache not bother you anymore" is used to help children gain mastery over their physical symptoms. See our website for further information about this modality. **WEB**

Hypnosis

An altered state of consciousness occurs when appropriate suggestions distort perception, memory, and mood in the child. Children who respond to hypnotic suggestions are often more relaxed and experience less pain.

Application of Heat and Cold

Heat application promotes dilation of blood vessels. The increased blood circulation permits the removal of debris of cell breakdown from the site. Heat also promotes muscle relaxation, breaking the pain–spasm–pain cycle. To reduce edema, do not apply heat in the first 24 hours after an injury. The application of cold is believed to slow the ability of pain fibers to transmit pain impulses. Cold also controls pain by decreasing edema and inflammation, and by causing partial or complete anesthesia or numbness of the skin. When cold is applied, assess the skin for redness or signs of irritation. Care should be taken to avoid causing thermal injury. Discontinue cold applications immediately if the skin alternately blanches and reddens afterwards or if blisters or redness do not subside between applications.

DISCHARGE PLANNING AND HOME CARE TEACHING

Children are frequently discharged from the hospital with oral analgesics following surgery, injury, or treatment of acute medical conditions. Parents have the responsibility to provide adequate pain control for their child after day surgery. Because of cultural values, some parents may feel the child should learn to tolerate some amount of pain. Take the time to discuss the importance of pain management and its benefits in promoting the child's healing. Make sure parents know that a sudden increase in pain intensity indicates the development of a complication requiring medical attention.

Provide guidance to help parents assess their child's pain, and for school-age children and adolescents to assess their own pain. Teach parents and children about the dosage and frequency of administration and the side effects of the analgesic ordered. Review nonpharmacologic methods of pain control with parents and children. Encourage children and parents to use the techniques that work best for them.

Children with chronic conditions (arthritis, sickle cell disease) or recurrent painful episodes (headaches, recurrent abdominal pain) often need long-term pain management (Table 38–12). For example, children with severe, long-term pain associated with cancer may be cared for at home with intravenous analgesics. These children are often managed by a home health care team. Educate parents thoroughly about intravenous care and analgesic administration.

Remember that many common health problems (otitis media, pharyngitis, and urinary tract infection) have pain as one of their presenting symptoms. Often the only medication prescribed is an antibiotic to clear the infection. This may leave the child in pain for 48 to 72 hours until

---

TABLE 38–12   Strategies for Chronic Pain Management

- Explain and validate the pain and its causes.
- Define treatment goals, including medications.
- Use distraction, relaxation, self-hypnosis, TENS, and exercise.
- Develop strategies for functional restoration.
- Give guidelines for a gradual increase in activity.
- Have a plan for sudden painful episodes.
- Explore stressors and potential pain triggers.
- Consider whether the child uses manipulatory behaviors for attention or secondary gain.
- Refer to a mental health professional or pain management team as needed.

Note: From Shapiro, B. S. (1995). Treatment of chronic pain in children and adolescents. *Pediatric Annals, 24*(3), 148–156. Adapted.

---

the antibiotic brings the infection under control. Give parents recommendations for pain control and comfort measures during this period.

Evaluation

Expected outcomes of nursing care include:

▶ The child's pain level is assessed frequently and pain management is effective in improving the child's comfort.

▶ The child successfully uses a PCA pump to control acute pain.

▶ Age-appropriate nonpharmacologic methods of pain management enhance the comfort provided by medications.

PAIN ASSOCIATED WITH MEDICAL PROCEDURES

Children undergo a wide variety of painful diagnostic and treatment procedures in the hospital and in outpatient settings. Procedures rated the most painful by children in one study included chest tube insertion, arterial puncture, lumbar puncture, bone marrow aspiration, insertion of a central or peripheral intravenous line, and venipuncture for drawing blood (Wong & Baker, 1988). The anticipation of these procedures causes anxiety and emotional distress that can lead to greater intensity of pain. Children who have experienced severe pain in the past may be unwilling to cooperate with health care personnel.

Clinical Therapy

Procedures such as burn debridement, laceration repair, bone marrow aspiration, and fracture reduction are associated with so much pain and anxiety that children need

TABLE 38-13	Characteristics of Conscious Sedation and Deep Sedation	
Assessment Factors	Conscious Sedation	Deep Sedation
Airway	Able to maintain airway independently and continuously	Unable to maintain airway independently or continuously
Cough and gag reflexes	Reflexes intact	Partial or complete loss of reflexes
Level of consciousness	Easily aroused with verbal or gentle physical stimulation	Not easily aroused, may not respond purposefully to verbal or gentle physical stimulation

Note: From Zimmerman, S. (1993). *Conscious Sedation in the Emergency Medical Trauma Center*. Washington, DC: Children's National Medical Center.

premedication with analgesia and **anxiolysis,** or administration of sedatives. Drugs for sedation include the following:

- Diazepam (Valium)
- Midazolam (Versed)
- Lorazepam (Ativan)
- Ketamine
- Propofol (Diprivan)

A local anesthetic such as lidocaine buffered by sodium bicarbonate is often injected to provide analgesia for emergent invasive procedures. Lidocaine can also be injected subcutaneously in a small area to reduce the pain of deeper needle insertion.

Topical anesthetics can be used to reduce the pain associated with the first needle stick. EMLA (eutetic mixture of local anesthetics) cream, a mixture of lidocaine 2.5% and prilocaine 2.5% in an emulsion, is effective if applied 1 to 2 hours before a needle stick procedure on intact skin (Figure 38–3 ◆). Alternatively, Numby Stuff (2% lidocaine with 1:100,000 epinephrine), can be applied by iontophoresis, electric DC current, to transport the ionizable drugs across intact skin in about 13 minutes (Squire, Kirchoff & Hissong, 2000). ⬭ WEB

Conscious sedation is a light sedation during which the child maintains airway reflexes and responds to verbal stimuli (Table 38–13). It can be used on a cooperative child. With conscious sedation, children have minimal anxiety, less pain, and often no memory of the procedure (Litman, 1995). Analgesia must be given in association with sedation because the sedated child can still feel pain but not communicate its presence. With the combined effects of analgesia and sedatives, the child must be carefully monitored for respiratory depression and **deep sedation,** a controlled state of depressed consciousness or unconsciousness. (See Skills 13–3 and 13–4 for more information.) ⬭ SKILLS

Nursing Management

INCREASE COMFORT DURING PAINFUL PROCEDURES

Help the child cope with a painful procedure by telling the child what sensations to expect and what will happen during the procedure. This reduces stress more effec-

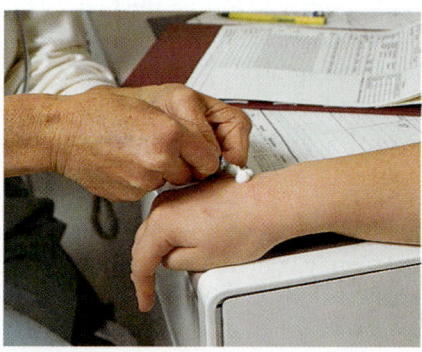

A

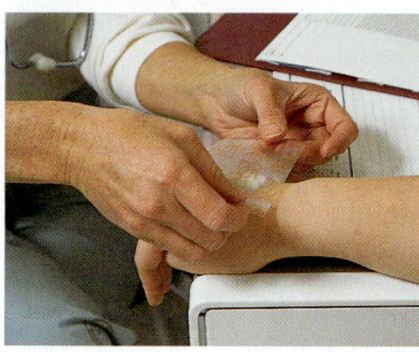

B

FIGURE 38–3. ◆ When painful procedures are planned, use EMLA cream to anesthelize the skin where the painful stick will be made. **A,** Apply a thick layer of cream over intact skin (one half of a 5-g tube). **B,** Cover the cream with a transparent adhesive dressing, sealing all the sides. The cream anesthetizes the dermal surface in 45–60 minutes.

Nursing Practice

Whenever conscious sedation is given, be sure to have the resources available to monitor the child's vital signs and to provide advanced life support if the child should progress to deep sedation. All health care facilities have special protocols for management of children receiving conscious sedation.

In case complications occur, the following equipment should be immediately available: suction apparatus, a bag-valve mask for assisted ventilation with capability of 90% to 100% oxygen delivery, an oxygen supply (5 L/min for more than 60 minutes), and antagonists to sedative medication.

tively than just providing information about the procedure (Broome, 1990). Chapter 34 gives methods for preparing children of different developmental ages for procedures.

Drugs may not be used for quick procedures, such as a dressing change, or an unexpected intravenous insertion, injection, or venipuncture. For a planned injection, intravenous insertion, or venipuncture, EMLA or other local anesthetic medication can be placed on the skin (see Figure 38–3). Nonpharmacologic measures, especially imagery, relaxation techniques, and distraction, may reduce the anxiety associated with the anticipation of the procedure. Teach parents and children to use these interventions before procedures. Help children control their anxiety through therapeutic play.

When pharmacologic pain management is used for a procedure, the nurse's responsibilities include the following:

- Treat anticipated procedure-related pain prophylactically. For example, give an analgesic before a bone marrow aspiration or fracture reduction. Permit time for the drug to become effective.

- Manage preexisting pain before beginning a procedure such as scrubbing a burn.
- Whenever possible, administer drugs by a nonpainful route (oral, transmucosal, intravenous). Avoid intramuscular injections.
- When procedures must be repeated (for example, bone marrow aspirations for children with leukemia), give optimal analgesia for the first procedure to reduce anxiety about future procedures.
- To prevent increased anxiety, avoid delays in performing procedures.
- Document the results of pain management.

When the child receives conscious sedation, monitoring the child's status is important. Nursing assessments include heart and respiratory rates, blood pressure, pulse oximetry, level of consciousness (response to verbal and physical stimulation), and color. Vital signs must be checked every 15 minutes until the child regains full consciousness and level of functioning. If conscious sedation progresses to deep sedation, airway management is essential; check vital signs every 5 minutes.

CHAPTER HIGHLIGHTS

≈ Pain is an unpleasant sensation that is either acute or chronic, perceived in response to tissue damage.

≈ Research has revealed that infants and children feel pain, just as adults do, despite past beliefs to the contrary.

≈ Pain behaviors in children are similar to the behaviors of fearful and anxious children.

≈ Every infant, child, and adolescent has the right to adequate pain control.

≈ The goal of pain assessment is to provide accurate information about the location and intensity of the child's pain and how the child is responding to it.

≈ Learning how the child expresses pain, both verbally and behaviorally, will help the nurse make a better assessment.

≈ Children learn how and when to seek help for pain and how to cope with pain by observing other family members.

≈ Numerous tools have been developed and validated to assess pain in infants and children.

≈ Pharmacologic interventions for pain control include opioids and nonsteroidal anti-inflammatory drugs (NSAIDs).

≈ Opioids are equally as effective when given by mouth, intramuscularly, and intravenously when an equianalgesic dose is used.

≈ Analgesia for continuous or severe pain should be given around the clock to maintain pain control. Patient-controlled analgesia is one method of administering a continuous infusion of an opioid medication and allowing the child to infuse additional small doses for episodic pain.

≈ Epidural and regional nerve blocks are pain-control methods gaining acceptance because they do not have the side effects associated with systemic medications.

≈ Nonpharmacologic methods of pain management include parental presence, distraction, cutaneous stimulation, electroanalgesia, imagery, relaxation techniques, hypnosis, and application of heat and cold.

≈ Parents need education and preparation to provide pain control for children discharged home following surgery and injuries. Children with chronic conditions often need long-term pain management.

≈ Many diagnostic and therapeutic procedures cause pain and anxiety in children. Provide optimal prophylactic pain management to reduce the anxiety associated with future procedures.

≈ Conscious sedation is used to reduce the child's anxiety associated with painful procedures. Analgesia is usually given in association with sedation when the procedure would cause pain or discomfort in an alert child.

EXPLORE MediaLink

NCLEX Review, Case Studies, and other interactive resources for this chapter can be found on the companion website at http://www.prenhall.com/london. Click on "Chapter 38" and select the activities for this chapter.

For animations, more NCLEX review questions, and an audio glossary, access the accompanying CD-ROM in this textbook.

REFERENCES

Abu-Saad, H. (1984). Cultural components of pain: The Asian-American child. *Children's Health Care, 13*, 11–14.

American Pain Society. (1999). *Principles of analgesic use in the treatment of acute pain and cancer pain* (4th ed.). Glenview, IL: Author.

Anand, K. J. S., & Carr, D. B. (1989). The neuroanatomy, neurophysiology, and neurochemistry of pain, stress, and analgesia in newborns and children. *Pediatric Clinics of North America, 36*(4), 795–822.

Anbar, R. (2001). Self-hypnosis for management of chronic dyspnea in pediatric patients. *Pediatrics, 2*, 21.

Broome, M. E. (1990). Preparation of children for painful procedures. *Pediatric Nursing, 16*, 537–541.

Broome, M. E. (2000). Helping parents support their child in pain. *Pediatric Nursing, 26*(3), 315–317.

Chambers, C. T., Gresbrecht, K., Craig, K. D., Bennett, S. M., & Huntsman, E. (1999). A comparison of faces scales for the measurement of pediatric pain: Children's and parent's ratings. *Pain, 83*, 25–35.

Fanurik, D., Koh, J., Schitz, M., & Brown, R. (1997). Pharmacobehavioral intervention: Integrating pharmacologic and behavioral techniques for pediatric procedures. *Children's Health Care, 26*(1), 1–13.

Gaston-Johansson, F., Albert, M., Fagan, E., & Zimmerman, L. (1990). Similarities in pain descriptions of four different ethnic-culture groups. *Journal of Pain and Symptom Management, 5*(2), 94–100.

Hazinski, M. F. (1999). Analgesia, sedation, and neuromuscular blockage in pediatric critical care. In M. F. Hazinski, *Manual of pediatric critical care* (pp. 44–72). St. Louis, MO: Mosby.

Holder, K. A., & Patt, R. B. (1995). Taming the pain monster: Pediatric postoperative pain management. *Pediatric Annals, 24*(3), 164–168.

Joint Commission on the Accreditation of Health Care Organizations. (2001). *Pain standards for 2001.* Oakbrook Terrace, IL: Author.

Kachoyeanos, M. K., & Zollok, M. B. (1995). Ethics in pain management of infants and children. *American Journal of Maternal Child Nursing, 20*, 142–147.

Leo, J., & Huether, S. E. (1998). Pain, temperature regulation, sleep, and sensory function. In K. L. McCance & S. E. Huether (Eds.), *Pathophysiology: The biologic basis for disease in adults and children* (3rd ed., pp. 422–432). St. Louis, MO: Mosby–Year Book.

Litman, R. S. (1995). Recent trends in management of pain during medical procedures in children. *Pediatric Annals, 24*(3), 158–163.

Lutz, W. J. (1986). Helping hospitalized children and their parents cope with painful procedures. *Journal of Pediatric Nursing, 1*, 24–32.

Lynn, A. M., Ulma, G. A., & Spreker, M. (1999). Pain control in very young infants: An update. *Contemporary Pediatrics, 16*(11), 39–66.

McCaffrey, M., & Pasero, C. (1999). *Pain: Clinical manual* (2nd ed.). St. Louis, MO: Mosby.

McGrath, P. A. (1995). Pain in the pediatric patient: Practical aspects of assessment. *Pediatric Annals, 24*(3), 126–138.

Olness, K., & Kohen, D. (1996). *Hypnosis and hypnotherapy with children* (3rd ed.). New York: Guilford Press.

Rushton, C. H. (1995). Placebo pain medication: Ethical and legal issues. *Pediatric Nursing, 21*(2), 166–168.

Shapiro, B. S. (1995). Treatment of chronic pain in children and adolescents. *Pediatric Annals, 24*(3), 148–156.

Squire, S. J., Kirchoff, K. T., & Hissong, K. (2000). Comparing two methods of topical anesthesia used before intravenous cannulation in pediatric patients. *Journal of Pediatric Health Care, 14*(2), 68–72.

Sugarman, L. (1996a). Hypnosis in a primary care practice: Developing skills for the "new morbidities." *Developmental and Behavioral Pediatrics, 17*(5), 300–305.

Sugarman, L. (1996b). Hypnosis: Teaching children self-regulation. *Pediatrics in Review, 17*, 5–11.

Tesler, M. D., Holzemer, W. L., & Spreker, M. (1999). Pain behaviors: Postsurgical responses of children and adolescents. *Journal of Pediatric Nursing, 13*(1), 41–47.

Tobias, J. D. (2000). Tolerance, withdrawal, and physical dependency after long term sedation and analgesia of children in the pediatric intensive care unit. *Critical Care Medicine, 28*(6), 2122–2132.

Wong, D. L., & Baker, C. M. (1988). Pain in children: Comparison of assessment scales. *Pediatric Nursing, 14*, 9–16.

UNIT VII

Caring for Children with Alterations in Health Status

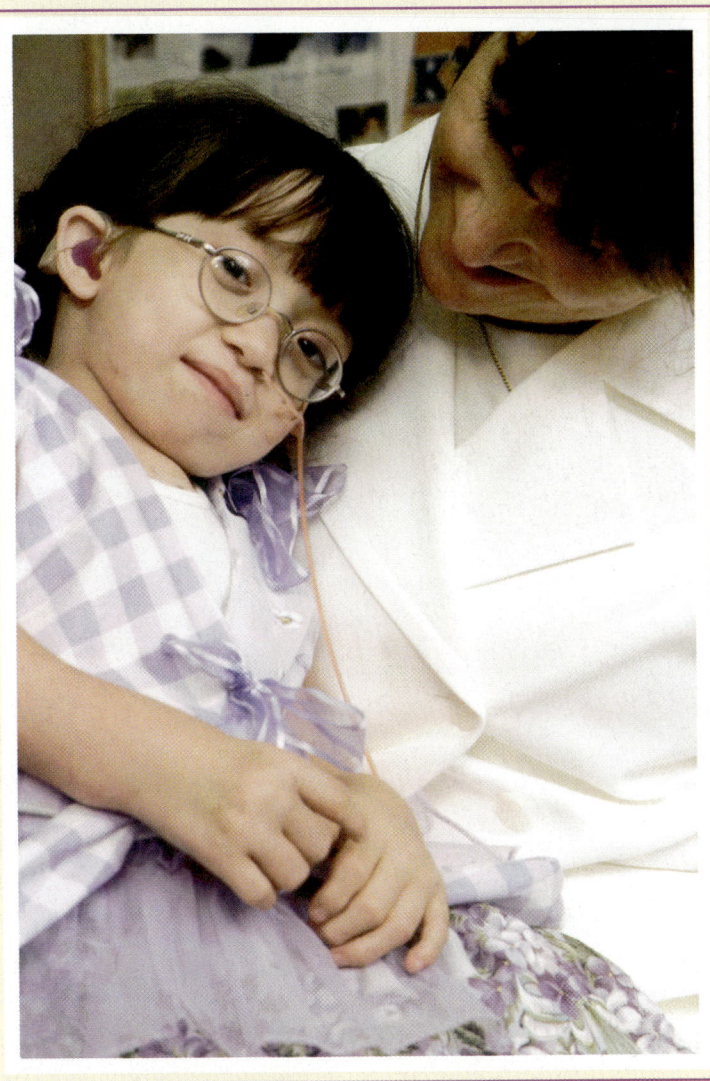

CHAPTER 39

The Child with Alterations in Fluid, Electrolyte, and Acid-Base Balance

Vernon always likes to eat, so when he won't even drink I know he is sick. We just didn't know how sick he was or that he had gotten dehydrated. I wonder if we should have done something else for him at home.

—MOTHER OF VERNON, 18 MONTHS

Key Terms

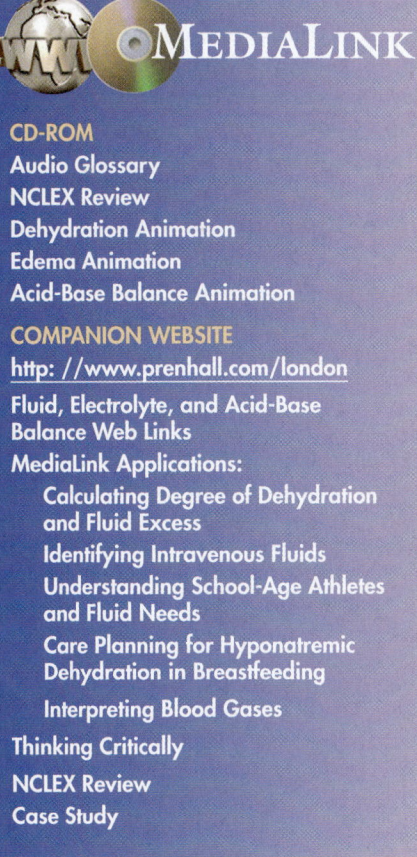

MediaLink

CD-ROM
Audio Glossary
NCLEX Review
Dehydration Animation
Edema Animation
Acid-Base Balance Animation

COMPANION WEBSITE
http://www.prenhall.com/london
Fluid, Electrolyte, and Acid-Base Balance Web Links
MediaLink Applications:
  Calculating Degree of Dehydration and Fluid Excess
  Identifying Intravenous Fluids
  Understanding School-Age Athletes and Fluid Needs
  Care Planning for Hyponatremic Dehydration in Breastfeeding
  Interpreting Blood Gases
Thinking Critically
NCLEX Review
Case Study

A thorough understanding of fluid, electrolyte, and acid-base homeostasis and imbalances is essential when providing nursing care to pediatric patients like Vernon. This chapter presents information about the processes that maintain fluid and electrolyte balance, and describes the common imbalances that may occur in children. It also describes how the body regulates acid-base status and explains the management of acid-base imbalances.

Many health conditions cause changes in body fluids that must be regulated and managed. Sometimes management of fluid status in the home or in a short-term ambulatory facility can prevent more serious illness or hospitalization.

ANATOMY AND PHYSIOLOGY OF PEDIATRIC DIFFERENCES

Infants and young children differ physiologically from adults in ways that make them vulnerable to fluid, electrolyte, and acid-base imbalances.

Fluid in the body is in a dynamic state. In persons of all ages, fluid continuously leaves the body through the skin, in feces and urine, and during respiration. Much of the human body is composed of water. **Body fluid** is body water that has solutes dissolved in it. Some of the solutes are **electrolytes,** or charged particles (ions). Electrolytes such as sodium (Na+), potassium (K+), calcium (Ca++), magnesium (Mg++), chloride (Cl−), and inorganic phosphorus (Pi) ions must be present in the proper concentrations for cells to function effectively.

In people of all ages, body fluid is located in several compartments. The two major fluid compartments contain the **intracellular fluid** (fluid inside the cells) and the **extracellular fluid** (outside the cells). The extracellular fluid is made up of **intravascular fluid** (within the blood vessels) and **interstitial fluid** (between the cells and outside the blood and lymphatic vessels) (Figure 39–1 ◆). Extracellular fluid accounts for about one third of total body water and intracellular fluid for about two thirds (Jospe & Forbes, 1996). The concentrations of electrolytes in the

fluid differ depending on the fluid compartment. For example, extracellular fluid is rich in sodium ions; intracellular fluid, by contrast, is low in sodium ions but rich in potassium ions (Table 39–1).

Fluid moves between the intravascular and interstitial compartments by a process called filtration. Water moves into and out of the cells by the process of osmosis. These processes are discussed later in the chapter.

The percentage of body weight composed of water varies with age. The percentage is highest at birth (and higher in premature than in full-term infants) and decreases with age (Figure 39–2 ◆). Neonates and young infants have a proportionately larger extracellular fluid volume than older children and adults because their brain and skin (both rich in interstitial fluid) occupy a greater proportion of their body weight. Much of our extracellular fluid is exchanged each day (Davenport, 1996). Infants have a high daily fluid requirement with little fluid volume reserve; this makes the infant vulnerable to dehydration. As an infant grows, the proportion of water inside the cells increases.

Infants and children under 2 years of age lose a greater proportion of fluid each day than older children and adults and are thus more dependent on adequate intake. They have a greater amount of skin surface or body surface area (BSA) and thus have greater insensible water losses through the skin. Because of this large BSA, they are also

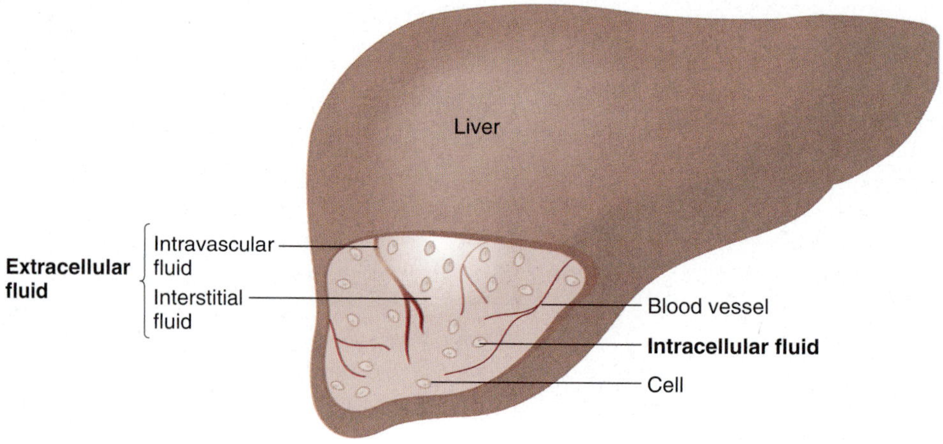

TABLE 39-1 Electrolyte Concentrations in Body Fluid Compartments

Components	Extracellular Fluid (ECF)		Intracellular Fluid (ICF)
	Vascular	Interstitial	
Na+	High	High	Low
K+	Low	Low	High
Ca++	Low	Low	Low (higher than ECF)
Mg++	Low	Low	High
Pi	Low	Low	High
Cl−	High	High	Low
Proteins	High	Low	High

FIGURE 39–1. ◆ The major body fluid compartments. Extracellular fluid is composed mainly of *vascular fluid* (fluid in blood vessels) and *interstitial fluid* (fluid between the cells and outside the blood and lymphatic vessels). Intracellular fluid is that within cells.

Liver

Extracellular fluid — Intravascular fluid — Interstitial fluid

Blood vessel
Intracellular fluid
Cell

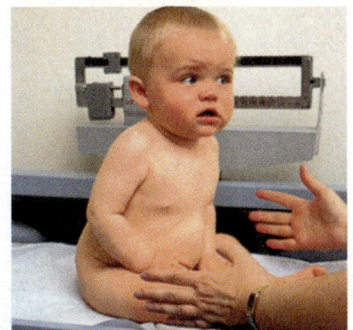
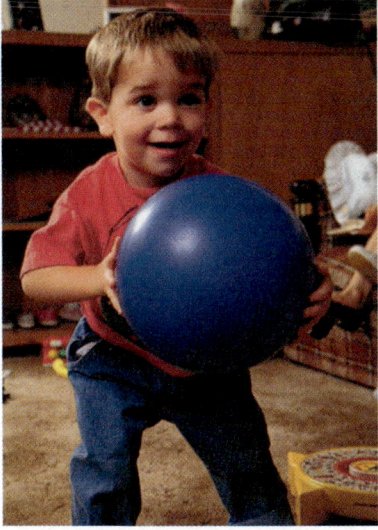
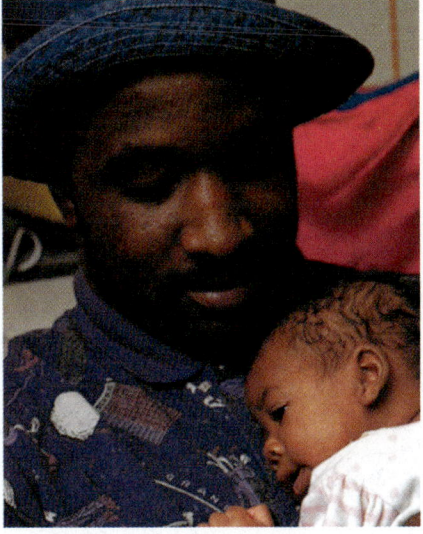
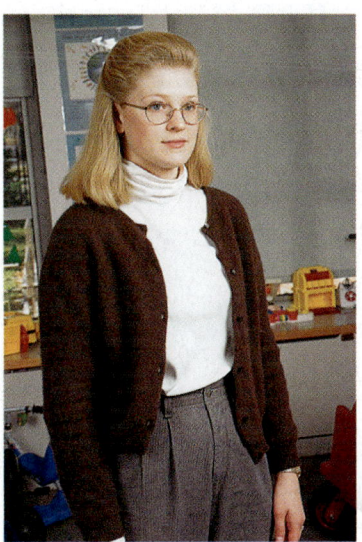

FIGURE 39–2. ◆ The percentage of water in the body varies with age. (ECF = extracellular fluid; ICF = intracellular fluid.)

at greater risk when burned. In addition, respiratory and metabolic rates are high during early childhood, so children have greater water loss from the lungs and greater water demand to fuel the body's metabolic processes (see Figure 39–3 ◆). Due to these factors, the exercising child dehydrates easily and must consume more fluid during physical activity, particularly during hot weather (Committee on Sports Medicine and Fitness, 2000).

When fluid status is compromised, a number of body mechanisms are activated to help restore balance. Several of these mechanisms occur in the kidney. The kidneys conserve water and needed electrolytes while excreting waste products and drug metabolites. In children under 2 years of age, however, the glomeruli, tubules, and nephrons of the kidneys are immature. They are thus unable to conserve or excrete water and solutes effectively (see Chapter 47). ⊂⊃ Because more water is generally excreted, the infant and young child can become dehydrated quickly or develop electrolyte imbalances. In addition, infants have a weaker transport system for ions and bicarbonate, placing them at greater risk for acidosis and acid-base imbalances. Children under 2 years of age also have difficulty regulating electrolytes such as sodium and calcium. Renal response to high solute loads is slower and less developed, with function improving gradually during the first year of life (Hewitt-Taylor, 1999).

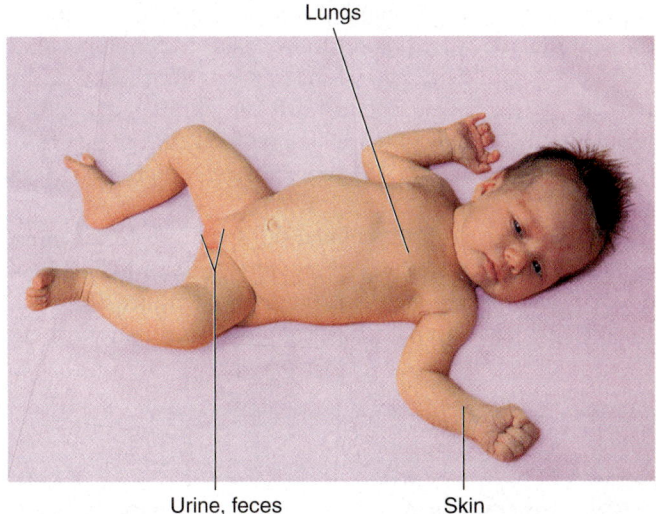

Lungs

Urine, feces   Skin

FIGURE 39–3. ◆ Normal routes of fluid excretion from infants and children.

Finally, in addition to the immaturity of physiologic processes, many health conditions make young children more vulnerable to fluid deficit. Examples include water loss due to phototherapy used to treat newborns with hyperbilirubinemia, water loss with increased respiratory rate during illness, fever, vomiting and diarrhea, and drainage from blood loss or drainage tubes.

❧ FLUID VOLUME IMBALANCES

When fluid excretion and losses are balanced by the proper volume and type of fluid intake, fluid balance will be maintained. If, however, fluid output and intake are not matched, fluid imbalance may occur rapidly. The major types of fluid imbalances are extracellular fluid volume deficit (dehydration), extracellular fluid volume excess, and interstitial fluid volume excess (edema).

EXTRACELLULAR FLUID VOLUME IMBALANCES

Extracellular Fluid Volume Deficit (Dehydration)

Extracellular fluid volume deficit occurs when there is not enough fluid in the extracellular compartment (vascular and interstitial). Because sodium is generally lost along with water, hyponatremia can also be present. (Hyponatremia is described later, on p. 948.) The state of body water deficit is called **dehydration**. ⊂D

ETIOLOGY AND PATHOPHYSIOLOGY

Extracellular fluid volume deficit is usually caused by the loss of sodium-containing fluid from the body. Vomiting, diarrhea, nasogastric suction, hemorrhage, and burns most often cause loss of fluid containing sodium. Vomiting and diarrhea are common manifestations of disease in children throughout the world, and each year up to 5 million children die from dehydration related to diarrhea. In the United States, about 300 to 500 die annually from this problem, about 220,000 are hospitalized, and many more receive outpatient care (Shamir, Zahavi, Abramowich, et al., 1998).

Another cause of extracellular fluid volume deficit in infants is increased water loss in low-birth-weight infants kept under radiant warmers to maintain heat (Figure 39–4 ◆). Less frequently, adrenal insufficiency, accumulation of ex-

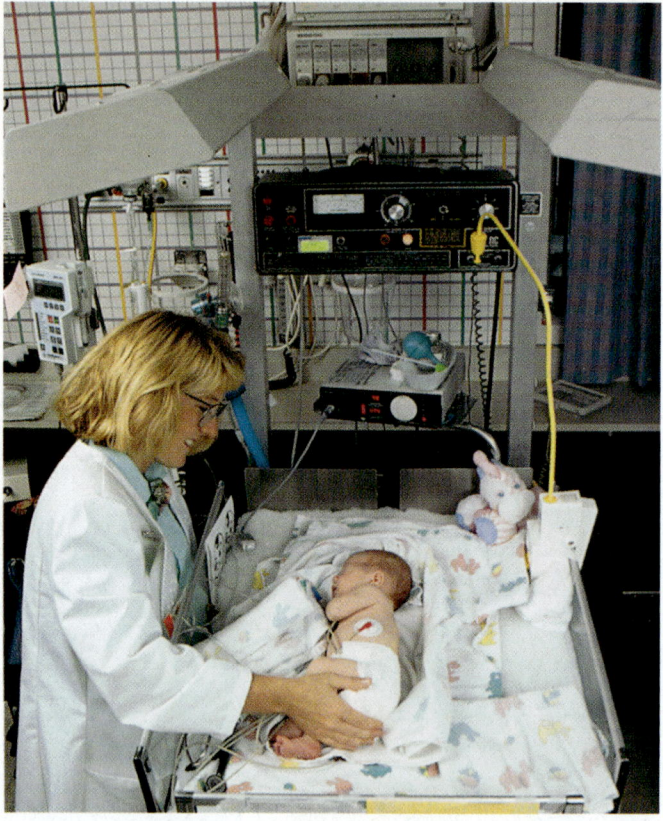

FIGURE 39–4. ◆ Use of an overhead warmer or phototherapy increases insensible fluid excretion through the skin, thus increasing the fluid intake needed.

tracellular fluid in a "third space" such as the peritoneal cavity, and overuse of diuretics may be the cause. The latter etiology is most often seen in bulimic adolescents who are trying to control their weights (see Chapter 36). ⊂D

CLINICAL MANIFESTATIONS

The signs of dehydration relate to the severity or degree of the body water deficit (Table 39–2). They are a result of both the decreased fluid (e.g., diminished turgor and mucous membrane moisture) and the body's response to the fluid deficit (e.g., pulse and blood pressure changes).

CLINICAL MANIFESTATIONS ❧ *Extracellular Fluid Volume Deficit*

SIGNS AND SYMPTOMS	PHYSIOLOGIC BASIS
Weight loss	Decreased fluid volume; 1 L of fluid weighs 1 kg
Postural blood pressure drop (older children)	Inadequate circulating blood volume to offset the force of gravity when in upright position
Increased small vein filling time	Decreased vascular volume
Delayed capillary refill time	Decreased vascular volume
Flat neck veins when supine (older children)	Decreased vascular volume
Dizziness, syncope	Inadequate circulation to brain
Oliguria	Inadequate circulation to kidneys
Thready, rapid pulse	Cardiac reflex response to decreased vascular volume
Sunken fontanel (infants)	Decreased fluid volume
Decreased skin turgor	Decreased interstitial fluid volume

TABLE 39-2   Severity of Clinical Dehydration

	Mild	Moderate	Severe
Percent of body weight lost	Up to 5% (40–50 mL/kg)	6%–9% (60–90 mL/kg)	10% or more (100+/mL/kg)
Level of consciousness	Alert, restless, thirsty	Irritable or lethargic (infants and very young children); alert, thirsty, restless (older children and adolescents)	Lethargic to comatose (infants and young children); often conscious, apprehensive (older children and adolescents)
Blood pressure	Normal	Normal or low; postural hypotension (older children and adolescents)	Low to undetectable
Pulse	Normal	Rapid	Rapid, weak to nonpalpable
Skin turgor	Normal	Poor	Very poor
Mucous membranes	Moist	Dry	Parched
Urine	May appear normal	Decreased output (<1 mL/kg/hr); dark color; increased specific gravity	Very decreased or absent output
Thirst	Slightly increased	Moderately increased	Greatly increased unless lethargic
Fontanel	Normal	Sunken	Sunken
Extremities	Warm; normal capillary refill	Delayed capillary refill (>2 sec)	Cool, discolored; delayed capillary refill (>3–4 sec)
Respirations	Normal	Normal or rapid	Changing rate and pattern

Mild dehydration is hard to detect, because children appear alert and have moist mucous membranes. Infants may be irritable and older children are thirsty. In moderate dehydration, the child is often lethargic and sleepy, but there may be periods of restlessness and irritability, especially in infants. Skin turgor is diminished, mucous membranes appear dry, and urine is dark in color and diminished in amount. Pulse rate is usually increased and blood pressure can be normal or low. Severe dehydration is manifested by increasing lethargy or nonresponsiveness, markedly decreased blood pressure, rapid pulse, poor skin turgor, dry mucous membranes, and markedly decreased or absent urinary output.

Growth and Development

Urine specific gravity may increase in older children who are dehydrated, but children under 2 years of age are not able to concentrate urine effectively. A rising specific gravity may not be seen in the younger dehydrated child.

CLINICAL THERAPY

Medical management depends on accurate identification of the degree of dehydration. In addition to physical signs and symptoms (see Table 39–2), elevated blood urea nitrogen (> 25 mg/dL) and serum bicarbonate (> 17 mEq/L) are useful to identify moderate and severe diarrhea (Eliason & Lewan, 1998; Vega & Avner, 1997). The treatment of extracellular fluid volume deficit is administration of fluid containing sodium, by oral rehydration therapy or by intravenous fluids.

Oral rehydration therapy has been used for years in developing countries without an accessible supply of intravenous fluids. More recently, experts have recognized the benefits of its early use to prevent severe dehydration and to treat mild and moderate dehydration in children in developed countries. The therapy successfully treats the dehydration caused by many gastrointestinal illnesses and prevents hospitalization for many infants and young children (Gavin, Merrick, & Davidson, 1996). It is the treatment of choice for children with diarrhea who have mild to moderate dehydration (Provisional Committee, 1996). Commercially available solutions contain water, carbohydrate (sugar), sodium, potassium, chloride, and lactate. Examples include Pedialyte, Infalyte, Resol, Nutralyte, Hydralyte, and Lytren. Some clinicians allow lactose-free milk, breast milk, or half-strength milk to be given in addition to oral rehydration therapy solution. The WHO/UNICEF solution was developed for use with cholera and is not generally used for diarrhea treatment in the United States, as its sodium and chloride loads are higher than that of other commercial solutions.

Thinking Critically

THE DEHYDRATED CHILD

Vernon is 18 months old. Several days ago he developed vomiting and diarrhea. His parents tried to get him to eat, but he had little appetite. He drank a little water and a few sips of juice, but the next morning he was listless and would not drink anything. The diarrhea continued.

His mother has brought him to the urgent care center. Vernon is irritable on arrival, and his mother reports that he has been alternately irritable and lethargic. His mucous membranes and tongue appear dry, and skin turgor over the abdomen is slightly decreased. His mother notes that Vernon has had only two wet diapers today and says the urine in his diaper was dark in color. She also reports that he weighed 12 kg (26 lb) at the clinic last week. However, when the nurse weighs him, the scale reads only 11 kg (24 1/2 lb). What do Vernon's symptoms suggest? What are his nursing care needs? 🔗 [WEB]

When the child is severely dehydrated, intravenous fluid is given, often accompanied by oral rehydration. The intravenous fluid is often Ringer's lactate followed or accompanied by dilute saline, such as one half or one quarter normal saline. The fluid combination replenishes the extracellular fluid volume and adds solutes to return the body fluid back to normal. The child may be hospitalized or treated with intravenous fluids in a short-stay unit until the dehydration is controlled. Once hydrated, the child resumes an age-appropriate diet (Burkhart, 1999).

Nursing Management

Nursing Assessment and Diagnosis

Weigh the child daily with the same scale and without clothing. Compare to past weights and calculate weight loss. Carefully measure intake and output (see Skill 9–21), 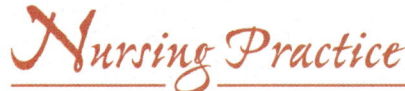 **SKILLS** urine specific gravity, level of consciousness, pulse rate and quality, skin turgor, mucous membrane moisture, quality and rate of respirations, and blood pressure. Compare the blood pressure when the child is supine with the pressure when the child is sitting with legs hanging down or standing. If the child is dehydrated, the sitting or standing blood pressure will be lower than the supine blood pressure, because blood accumulates in the dependent legs. Obtain samples of urine and blood as needed for dehydration evaluation.

Nursing Practice

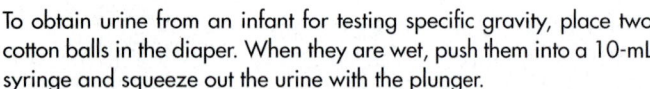

To obtain urine from an infant for testing specific gravity, place two cotton balls in the diaper. When they are wet, push them into a 10-mL syringe and squeeze out the urine with the plunger.

The nursing diagnosis *fluid volume deficit* applies to all children who have an extracellular fluid volume deficit. Other diagnoses depend on the severity of the condition and the age of the child. Several nursing diagnoses that might be appropriate for the mildly to severely dehydrated child are included in the accompanying "Nursing Care Plans." Additional care of the child with dehydration from gastroenteritis can be found in Chapter 46. Nursing diagnoses might include:

▶ *Fluid volume deficit* related to active fluid volume loss or failure of regulatory mechanisms

▶ *Risk for altered peripheral tissue perfusion* related to hypovolemia

▶ *Risk for injury* related to postural hypotension

Planning and Implementation

Nursing care of the dehydrated child focuses on providing oral rehydration fluids, teaching parents oral rehydration methods, and, if necessary, administering intravenous flu-

ids to restore fluid balance. The accompanying "Nursing Care Plans" summarize care of the child with mild to severe dehydration.

PROVIDE ORAL REHYDRATION FLUIDS

In mild or moderate dehydration, oral rehydration fluid is the first intervention. It is given in frequent small amounts; for example, 1 to 3 teaspoons of fluid every 10 to 15 minutes is a useful guideline for starting oral rehydration. For the first 2 to 4 hours of treatment, 50 mL of fluid for each kg of the child's weight should be the target intake (Endsley & Galbraith, 1998; Larson, 2000). Instruct parents to continue to administer 1 teaspoon every 2 to 3 minutes even if the child vomits, as small amounts of the fluid may still be absorbed. Table 39–3 outlines guidelines for oral rehydration therapy.

TEACH PARENTS ORAL REHYDRATION METHODS

Instruct parents about the types of fluids and amounts to be given. Begin teaching with parents of all newborns and reinforce teaching at each well-child visit. Advise parents to continue the child's normal diet in addition to providing the rehydration solution. Cereal, starches, soup, fruits, and vegetables are all allowed. Tell parents to avoid simple sugars, which can worsen diarrhea because of osmotic effects. This includes soft drinks (if used, they should be diluted with equal parts of water), undiluted juice, Jell-O, and sweetened cereal.

Repeated vomiting of large volumes of fluid or a worsening of the child's condition can indicate the need for intravenous therapy. Teach parents when to seek further medical care. If the child's condition worsens or does not improve after 4 hours of oral rehydration therapy, parents should contact a health care professional. Dizziness or lethargy can be manifestations of dehydration.

MONITOR INTRAVENOUS FLUID ADMINISTRATION

The hospitalized child usually requires intravenous fluids. Be sure that the amount of fluid administered corresponds

TABLE 39–3 Oral Rehydration Therapy Guidelines
• Children with diarrhea and no dehydration should be continued on age-appropriate diets.
• For mild dehydration, give 50 mL/kg oral rehydration therapy in 4 hours in addition to replacing fluids lost in stool and emesis. (Measure emesis and give 10 mL/kg of fluid for each diarrheal stool.)
• For moderate dehydration, give 100 mL/kg oral rehydration therapy in 4 hours in addition to replacing fluids lost as described above.
• For severe dehydration, the child is hospitalized and treated with intravenous fluids. When hydrated adequately or concurrently with intravenous rehydration, begin oral rehydration therapy with 50 to 100 mL/kg of fluid in 4 hours and stool replacement as described above.
• When rehydration is complete, resume normal diet.

Note: From Provisional Committee on Quality Improvement, Subcommittee on Acute Gastroenteritis (1996). Practice parameter: The management of acute gastroenteritis in young children. *Pediatrics, 97,* 424–436. Adapted.

with the diagnosed dehydration state of the child (Table 39–4). Usually, about one half of the 24-hour total maintenance and replacement needs are given in the first 6 to 8 hours, with a slower rate infused for the remainder of the 24 hours. During the first 1 to 3 hours, the infusion rate may be highest to rapidly expand the vascular space. Electrolytes, such as potassium, are not usually added until the child has voided a sufficient quantity of urine, in order to avoid hyperkalemia. Rapid infusion of 20 to 30 mL/kg over 1 to 2 hours is sometimes used in outpatient settings, followed by oral fluids. Careful monitoring of intake and output is needed to ensure that the intravenous line

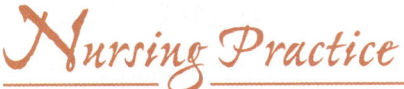

If an oral rehydration solution is too concentrated, it can make diarrhea worse. Juice and cola are very concentrated and should be diluted to half strength if they are given to a child who has diarrhea. Sugar facilitates the absorption of sodium in oral rehydration fluids. Tell parents not to give diet beverages for oral rehydration because they contain no sugar and will not be effectively absorbed.

Encourage parents to keep an oral rehydration solution in liquid or powder form on hand at all times and to use these solutions rather than juice or soda when the child first develops diarrhea (Straughn & English, 1996).

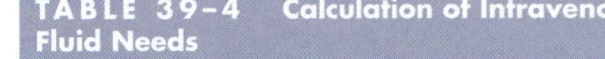

TABLE 39–4   Calculation of Intravenous Fluid Needs

1. First, calculate the maintenance fluid needs of the child, according to the following guideline:

Usual Weight	Maintenance Amount
Up to 10 kg	100 mL/kg/24 hr
11–20 kg	1000 mL + (50 mL/kg for weight above 10 kg)/24 hr
>20 kg	1500 mL + (20 mL/kg for weight above 20 kg)/24 hr

2. Next, calculate replacement fluid for that lost:
Multiply the percentage of body weight loss × 10 × normal weight to obtain the mL/kg/24 hr required.

3. Finally, calculate continued losses and add them to the total of maintenance and replacement needs.

NURSING CARE PLAN   *The Child with Mild or Moderate Dehydration*

GOAL	INTERVENTION	RATIONALE	EXPECTED OUTCOME
1. Ineffective management of therapeutic regimen related to knowledge deficit about diarrhea and vomiting			
	NIC Priority Intervention: **Family Involvement:** *Facilitate family participation in care of the child*		NOC Suggested Outcome: **Effective therapeutic regimen management:**
Parents will describe appropriate home management of fluid replacement for diarrhea and vomiting.	▶ Explain how to replace body fluid with an oral rehydration solution. Encourage parents to keep the solution at home and begin use with the first sign of diarrhea.	▶ Use of an oral rehydration solution can enable successful treatment of vomiting and diarrhea at home.	Parents are successfully able to treat the child's diarrhea and vomiting at home.
	▶ Teach parents to continue the child's normal diet in addition to providing replacement fluids for diarrhea.	▶ Diet plus fluid supplementation leads to faster recovery.	
	▶ Provide verbal and written instructions to parents at each well-child visit.	▶ Parents are provided with a reference for later use.	
2. Knowledge deficit (parent) related to causes of dehydration			
	NIC Priority Intervention: **Teaching:** *Teach causes of dehydration*		NOC Suggested Outcome: **Knowledge:** *Treatment regimen*
Parents will state common causes of childhood dehydration.	▶ Teach parents childhood conditions that commonly lead to dehydration.	▶ If parents recognize situations that can lead to dehydration, they will be more alert to its appearance.	Parents recognize conditions of risk for dehydration in children.
3. Risk for fluid volume deficit related to worsening of child's condition			
	NIC Priority Intervention: **Fluid management:** *Promote fluid balance*		NOC Suggested Outcome: **Fluid balance:** *Balance of water in extra- and intracellular compartments of body*
Parents will seek health care for the child's worsening condition.	▶ Teach parents to seek care when the child's vomiting or diarrhea worsens, or the child's mental alertness changes.	▶ Severe dehydration may occur if milder forms are not successfully treated.	Parents seek prompt attention for the child's worsening condition, preventing the development of severe dehydration.

GOAL	INTERVENTION	RATIONALE	EXPECTED OUTCOME
1. Fluid volume deficit related to excess losses and inadequate intake			
	NIC Priority Intervention:		**NOC Suggested Outcome:**
	Fluid management: *Promote fluid balance*		**Fluid balance:** *Balance of water in extra- and intracellular components of the body*
The child will return to normal hydration status and will not develop hypovolemic shock.	▶ Monitor weight daily. Assess intake and output every shift. Assess heart rate, postural blood pressure, skin turgor, small vein filling time, capillary refill time, fontanel (infant), and urine specific gravity every 4 hours or more frequently as indicated.	▶ Frequent assessment of hydration status facilitates rapid intervention and evaluation of the effectiveness of fluid replacement.	The child has signs of normal hydration.
	▶ Administer intravenous fluids as ordered. Monitor for crackles in dependent portions of the lungs.	▶ Replace fluid lost from the body. Excessive replacement of sodium-containing fluids could cause extracellular fluid volume excess.	
2. Risk for injury related to decreased level of consciousness			
	NIC Priority Intervention:		**NOC Suggested Outcome:**
	Fall prevention: *Institute special precautions*		**Fall prevention:** *Minimize risk factors that precipitate falls*
The child will not experience injury.	▶ Raise the side rails of the bed. Ensure that a small child does not become tangled in bed covers.	▶ Safety measures protect the child.	The child does not fall or suffer other injury.
	▶ Monitor level of consciousness every 2–4 hours or more often as indicated.	▶ Frequent assessment provides evidence of the need for safety interventions and of the effectiveness of therapy.	
	▶ Monitor serum sodium concentration daily or more often.	▶ Elevated serum sodium concentration causes brain cell shrinkage and decreased level of consciousness.	
	▶ Have the child sit before rising from bed and assist to stand slowly.	▶ Slow adjustment to upright posture reduces light-headedness from decreased blood volume.	
3. Activity intolerance related to bedrest immobility			
	NIC Priority Intervention:		**NOC Suggested Outcome:**
	Activity therapy: *Plan activities to meet child's developmental needs*		**Energy conservation:** *Manage energy to sustain activity*
The child will engage in normal activity for age	▶ Plan activities appropriate for the age of the child that can be done in bed.	▶ Activities will provide distraction and promote recovery.	The child engages in normal developmental activities and receives adequate rest.
	▶ Group nursing interventions to provide time for the child to rest.	▶ The child will require more rest than usual.	
	▶ Provide assistance during meals and other activities as needed.	▶ Prevention of overexertion will conserve body fluid and promote healing.	

remains in place until the child is tolerating oral fluids and taking in enough to maintain hydration. When oral fluids are maintained, the child may be discharged and hospitalization avoided (Reid & Bonadio, 1996).

Maintain the intravenous line carefully so fluid infusion can be kept on schedule (see Skill 12–5). ⬡ SKILLS Use a pump to prevent inadvertent, rapid infusion, which can lead to fluid overload and electrolyte imbalance. Play with the toddler and preschool child frequently and use diversionary methods, as necessary, to distract the child from the intravenous line. Monitor the child carefully and implement safety precautions as necessary. Once the child begins to tolerate some oral fluids, substitute oral rehydra-

tion therapy for intravenous fluids; frequent administration of appropriate fluids is needed.

DISCHARGE PLANNING AND HOME CARE TEACHING

Prior to discharge, parents need instructions about types of fluids and amounts to encourage. Teach the signs of dehydration (see Table 39–2) so that if the child does not take in adequate fluids, parents can seek help immediately. Instruct them to begin the child's normal diet once hydration is completed, determined by adequate urinary output and normal behaviors. Review methods of minimizing the child's chance of acquiring gastrointestinal infections (e.g., avoiding contact with other children who are infected; using careful handwashing and dishwashing procedures when another child in the home is sick). During well-child visits, encourage all parents to keep oral rehydration fluids at home in case they are needed; they are available in most grocery stores and pharmacies. Address the needs for increasing fluids in hot weather and when the child is exercising.

Evaluation

Expected outcomes of nursing care for the child with dehydration include:

▶ Balance of water and electrolytes in intracellular and extracellular compartments

▶ Normal urinary output

▶ Adequate fluid intake for maintenance needs

▶ Vital signs within normal limits

Extracellular Fluid Volume Excess

Extracellular fluid volume excess occurs when there is too much fluid in the vascular and interstitial compartment. This imbalance may also be called saline excess or extracellular volume overload. If this disorder occurs by itself (without saline disturbance), the serum sodium concentration is normal. There is simply too much extracellular fluid, even though it has a normal concentration.

Infants and children who develop an extracellular fluid volume excess have a condition that causes them to retain **saline** (sodium and water) or have been given an overload of sodium-containing isotonic intravenous fluid (Figure 39–5 ◆). What conditions cause retention of saline? The hormone aldosterone is secreted by the adrenal cortex. One of its normal functions is to cause the kidneys to retain saline in the body (see "Pathophysiology Illustrated: Aldosterone Effects"). Saline excess can be caused by any condition that results in excessive aldosterone secretion, such as adrenal tumors that secrete aldosterone, congestive heart

failure, liver cirrhosis, and chronic renal failure. Most glucocorticoid medications (such as prednisone) have a mild saline-retaining effect when taken on a long-term basis.

Extracellular fluid volume excess is characterized by sudden weight gain. A gain of 0.5 kg (1 lb) in a day is related to fluid, and represents 500 mL of saline. An overload of fluid in the blood vessels and interstitial spaces can cause clinical manifestations such as bounding pulse, distended neck veins in children (not usually evident in infants), hepatomegaly, dyspnea, orthopnea, and lung crackles. Edema is the sign of overload of the interstitial fluid compartment. In an infant, edema is often generalized (Figure 39–6 ◆). Edema in children with extracellular fluid

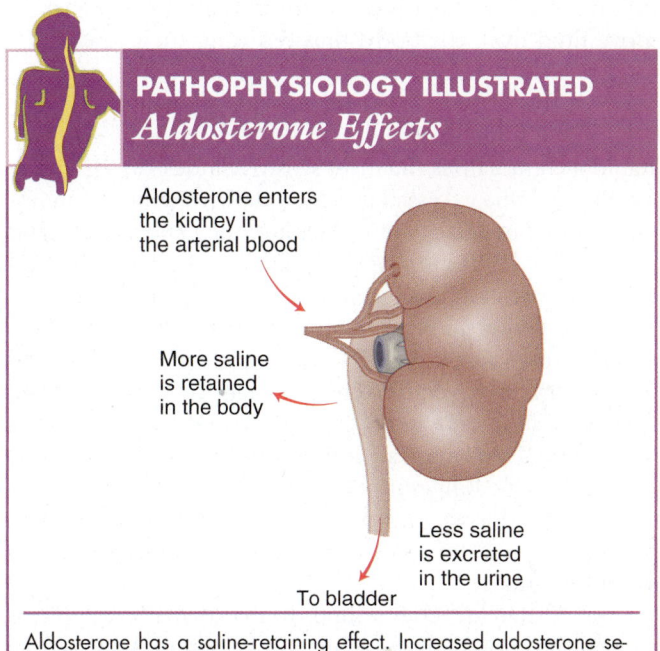

PATHOPHYSIOLOGY ILLUSTRATED
Aldosterone Effects

Aldosterone enters the kidney in the arterial blood

More saline is retained in the body

Less saline is excreted in the urine

To bladder

Aldosterone has a saline-retaining effect. Increased aldosterone secretion can be caused by adrenal tumors or congestive heart failure.

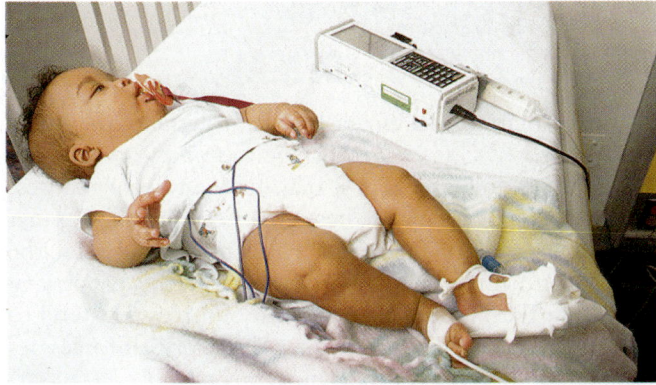

FIGURE 39–5. ◆ If isotonic fluid containing sodium is given too rapidly or in too great an amount, an extracellular fluid volume excess will develop. It is important to monitor fluid intake, excretion, and retention in children.

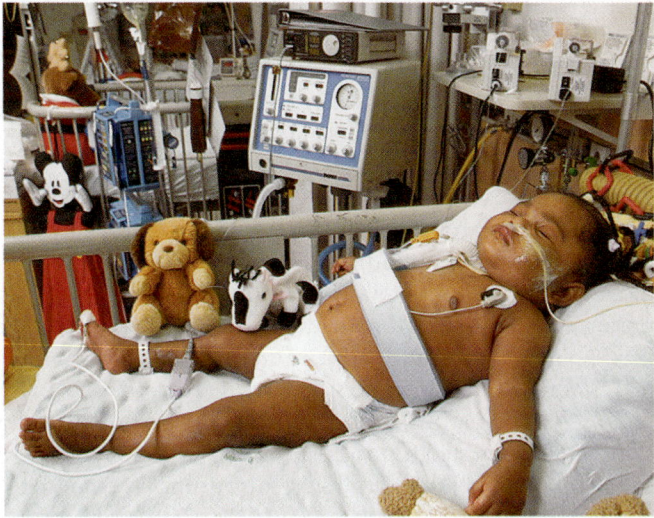

FIGURE 39–6. ◆ This infant with congenital heart disease has signs of generalized edema. Note the fluid retention in the face and abdomen.

volume excess occurs in the dependent parts of the body, that is, in the parts closest to the ground. Thus, edema is evident in sacral areas in a child supine in bed. (Edema that develops from other causes is described in the next section of this chapter.)

Intravenous fluid volume regulation is important, especially in young children. Either inaccurate calculation of needed fluid or inadvertent infusion of excess fluids can cause overload.

The clinical therapy for extracellular fluid volume excess focuses on treating the underlying cause of the disorder. For example, a child who has congestive heart failure is given medications to strengthen the heart's ability to contract. Managing the cause also helps to reduce the extracellular fluid volume excess. Diuretics may be given to remove fluid from the body, thus reducing the extracellular fluid volume directly.

NURSING MANAGEMENT

Rapid weight gain is the most sensitive index of extracellular fluid volume excess. Therefore, daily weighing is an important nursing assessment. Measure the child's intake and output. For babies in diapers, a diaper is weighed dry and then wet, with grams of weight increase equal to urine volume in milliliters. When treatment is successful, output is greater than intake. Assess the character of the pulse and observe for neck vein distention when the child is sitting (usually visible only in older children). Monitor for signs of pulmonary edema (an indication of severe imbalance) by listening to lung sounds in the dependent lung fields (crackles) and assessing for respiratory distress (rapid respiratory rate, use of accessory muscles of respiration). Observe for edema.

A child may develop a fluid overload whenever an isotonic intravenous solution containing sodium, such as normal saline or Ringer's solution, is administered. Therefore, monitor the infusion rate frequently and carefully and use a pump whenever possible to aid in accurate administration (Figure 39–7 ◆). Use only small bags (e.g., 250 or 500 mL) for children, and check pumps frequently.

If an excess of fluid has already developed, administer the medical therapy as prescribed and monitor for any complications of the medical therapy. For example, many diuretics increase potassium excretion in the urine, which may lead to an abnormally low plasma potassium concentration unless potassium intake is increased. (Refer to the discussion of hypokalemia later in this chapter.) It is also important to monitor for the development of extracellular fluid volume deficit as a result of diuretic therapy.

If edema is present, provide careful skin care and protection for edematous areas. Teach parents how to provide skin care and perform position changes at home. See the following section for additional interventions related to edema.

If a child has a long-term condition such as chronic renal failure that predisposes to extracellular fluid volume excess, a dietary sodium restriction may be prescribed (see

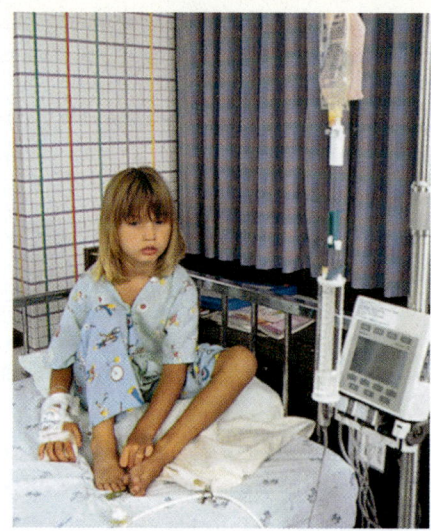

FIGURE 39–7. ◆ The use of a volume control device with an intravenous saline infusion is important to prevent a sudden extracellular fluid volume overload.

Chapter 47 for further detail). ⊂⊃ Teach parents how to manage sodium restriction. Plan low-sodium meals that fit the family's cultural practices. If the child is old enough to participate, incorporate games into the teaching. If a scale is available, teach parents to take and record an accurate daily weight.

Desired outcomes include electrolyte balance, maintenance of intact skin, and dietary intake as prescribed.

Developing Cultural Competence

To adapt teaching about low-sodium diets to the cultural practices of a family, ask them what types of food they usually eat. Help them to choose low-sodium foods from their diets and to avoid high-sodium foods. This approach is more effective than giving the same list of restricted foods to each family.

INTERSTITIAL FLUID VOLUME EXCESS (EDEMA)

Edema is an abnormal increase in the volume of the interstitial fluid. ⊂⊃ CD It may be caused by an extracellular fluid volume excess or it may be due to other causes.

The causes of edema are best understood in the context of normal capillary dynamics. Fluid moves between the vascular and interstitial compartment by the process of **filtration.** Filtration is the net result of forces that tend to move fluid in opposing directions. The strongest forces determine the direction of fluid movement.

At the capillary level, two forces (blood hydrostatic pressure and interstitial osmotic pressure) tend to move fluid from the capillaries into the interstitial fluid, while two other forces (blood colloid osmotic pressure and in-

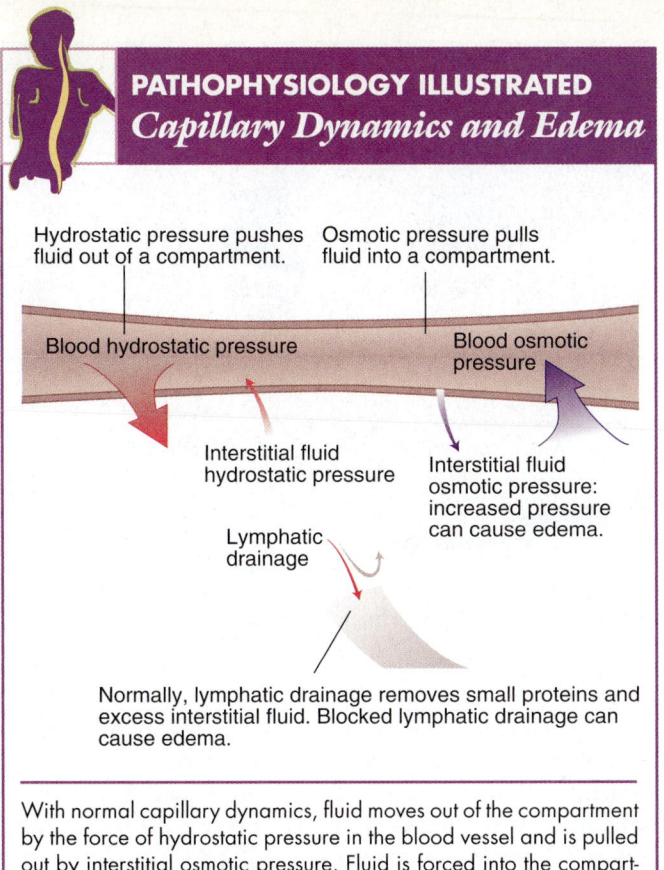

PATHOPHYSIOLOGY ILLUSTRATED
Capillary Dynamics and Edema

Hydrostatic pressure pushes fluid out of a compartment.

Osmotic pressure pulls fluid into a compartment.

Blood hydrostatic pressure

Blood osmotic pressure

Interstitial fluid hydrostatic pressure

Interstitial fluid osmotic pressure: increased pressure can cause edema.

Lymphatic drainage

Normally, lymphatic drainage removes small proteins and excess interstitial fluid. Blocked lymphatic drainage can cause edema.

With normal capillary dynamics, fluid moves out of the compartment by the force of hydrostatic pressure in the blood vessel and is pulled out by interstitial osmotic pressure. Fluid is forced into the compartment by interstitial hydrostatic pressure and pulled in by compartment osmotic pressure. Abnormal capillary dynamics cause edema.

TABLE 39–5 Clinical Conditions That Cause Edema

Edema Due to Increased Blood Hydrostatic Pressure

Increased Capillary Blood Flow
Inflammation
Local infection

Venous Congestion
Extracellular fluid volume excess
Right heart failure
Venous thrombosis
External pressure on vein
Muscle paralysis

Edema Due to Decreased Blood Osmotic Pressure
Increased Albumin Excretion
Nephrotic syndrome (albumin leaks into urine)
Protein-losing enteropathies (excess albumin in feces)

Decreased Albumin Synthesis
Kwashiorkor (low-protein, high-carbohydrate starvation diet provides too few amino acids for liver to make albumin)
Liver cirrhosis (diseased liver unable to make enough albumin)

Edema Due to Increased Interstitial Fluid Osmotic Pressure
Increased Capillary Permeability
Inflammation
Toxins
Hypersensitivity reactions
Burns

Edema Due to Blocked Lymphatic Drainage
Tumors
Goiter
Parasites that obstruct lymph nodes
Surgery that removes lymph nodes

terstitial fluid hydrostatic pressure) tend to move fluid in the opposite direction (from the interstitial fluid into the capillaries). The net result of these forces usually moves fluid from the capillaries into the interstitial compartment at the arterial end of the capillaries and fluid from the interstitial compartment back into the capillaries at the venous end of the capillaries. This process brings oxygen and nutrients to the cells and removes carbon dioxide and other waste products.

Edema occurs if the balance of these four forces is altered so that excess fluid either enters or leaves the interstitial compartment (see "Pathophysiology Illustrated: Capillary Dynamics and Edema"). This may occur through (1) increased blood hydrostatic pressure, (2) decreased blood colloid osmotic pressure, (3) increased interstitial fluid osmotic pressure, or (4) blocked lymphatic drainage. Many clinical conditions are associated with these altered forces (Table 39–5), described in the following list.

1. *Increased blood hydrostatic pressure.* When extracellular fluid volume excess occurs, the increased fluid volume in the vascular compartment congests the veins. The pressure against the sides of the capillary is increased and more fluid then enters the interstitial compartment.

2. *Decreased blood colloid osmotic pressure.* Much of the osmotic pressure that pulls fluid into the capillaries is due to the presence of albumin and other plasma pro-

teins made by the liver. The part of the blood osmotic pressure that is due to plasma proteins is often called **oncotic pressure** or blood colloid osmotic pressure. Any condition that decreases plasma proteins will decrease blood colloid osmotic pressure and cause edema. For example, if a clinical condition causes large amounts of albumin to leak into the urine, the liver will not be able to make albumin fast enough to replace it. As a result, the plasma protein level will fall, decreasing the blood osmotic pressure. Without this pulling force to return fluid to the capillaries, edema will occur. This is the cause of edema in children who have nephrotic syndrome (see Chapter 47).

3. *Increased interstitial fluid osmotic pressure.* Ordinarily, only a few small proteins enter the interstitial fluid, and the interstitial fluid osmotic pressure is small. If the capillary becomes abnormally permeable to proteins, however, the influx of large amounts of proteins into the interstitial fluid causes a dramatic increase in interstitial fluid osmotic pressure. The increased pulling force keeps an abnormal amount of fluid in the interstitial compartment. This mechanism plays an important part in the edema caused by a bee sting or a

sprained ankle. It occurs to a greater extent in burns, leading to swelling at the same time that there is a great loss of fluid volume through the burned skin (see Chapter 52).

4. *Blocked lymphatic drainage.* The lymph vessels normally drain small proteins and excess fluid from the interstitial compartment and return them to the blood vessels. If lymph vessels are blocked, fluid accumulates in the interstitial compartment. This may occur when a tumor blocks lymphatic drainage.

Edema causes localized or generalized swelling, which may cause pain and restrict motion. Edema due to extracellular fluid volume excess or right-sided heart failure usually occurs in the dependent portion of the body. In a child who is walking, dependent edema is observed in the ankles; in a bedfast supine child, it is seen in the sacral area. The skin over an edematous area often appears thin and shiny.

The main focus of clinical therapy for edema is to treat the underlying condition that caused the edema. Such conditions are discussed throughout this book. The edema from inflammation of an injury is initially treated with cold to reduce capillary blood flow and thus reduce blood hydrostatic pressure.

NURSING MANAGEMENT

A child or parent may make comments that alert the nurse to the development of edema. Shoes may become tight by the end of the day (dependent edema); the waistband of pants or a skirt may be "outgrown" suddenly (generalized edema or ascites [accumulation of fluid in the peritoneal cavity]); the eyes may be puffy (periorbital edema); a ring may be too tight; fingers may "feel like sausages." In many cases, visual inspection is sufficient to recognize edema. Observe for pitting edema. To detect changes in the amount of swelling, measure around the edematous part. If the edema is caused by extracellular fluid volume excess, daily measurements of weight and intake and output are a necessary part of the daily assessment. Nursing assessment should also focus on the integrity of the skin, presence of pain, restricted motion, and alterations in the child's body image.

Elevation of an area of localized edema helps to reduce the swelling. The skin over an edematous area needs extra care because it is fragile (Figure 39–8 ◆). Carefully position an infant or child on bed rest and turn frequently to prevent pressure sores. Perform turning carefully to avoid skin abrasion by rubbing against the sheets. Pat the skin dry after cleansing rather than rubbing it. Trim the child's fingernails smooth to prevent scratching. Teach parents skin care for the child at home. Teach older children to inspect their skin carefully to identify areas needing special care.

If restricted mobility is a problem, make specific plans to help the child manage activities. For example, if an edematous finger restricts the motion of a hand, food can be cut into bite-sized portions before the meal is served, so that the child can still eat independently.

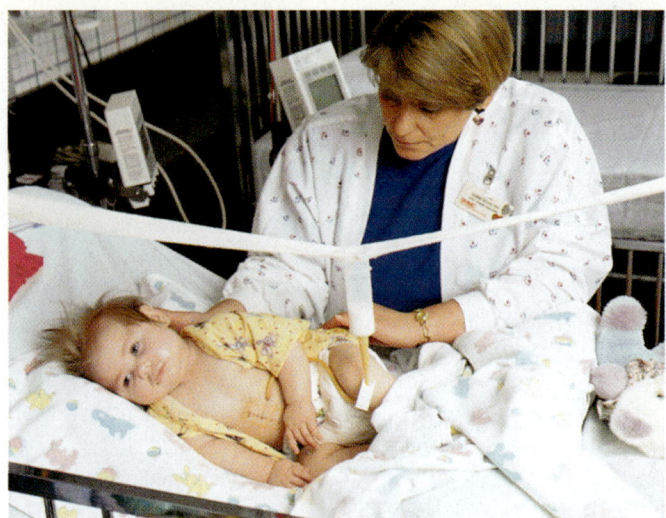

FIGURE 39–8. ◆ Edematous tissue is easily damaged. It must be kept clean and dry and free of pressure.

Discomfort from edema may require creative nursing interventions. Distraction with toys or activities appropriate to the child's developmental level can be useful. Interventions to treat the underlying problem can also reduce the edema and its accompanying discomfort. Interventions for edema should be added to the nursing management of the underlying condition that causes the edema. Administration of the prescribed medical therapy and observation for the complications of therapy are nursing responsibilities.

Discuss with school-age children and adolescents feelings of embarrassment about the edematous appearance. They need to understand the reason for edema and be able to explain it to peers. Arrange for the child to meet other children with similar concerns.

Desired outcomes of care include maintenance of intact skin, normal respiratory sounds and effort, and normal weight patterns.

ELECTROLYTE IMBALANCES

All body fluids contain electrolytes, although the concentration of those electrolytes varies, depending on the type and location of the fluid. When a serum electrolyte value is reported from the laboratory, it provides information about the concentration of that electrolyte in the blood. It may not necessarily reflect the concentration of the electrolyte in other body compartments. Refer to Table 39–1 to see which electrolytes have the highest and lowest concentrations in the blood and other fluid compartments.

Electrolytes are normally gained and lost in relatively equal amounts so the body remains in balance. However, when a child has an abnormal route of loss, such as vomiting, wound drainage, or nasogastric suction, electrolyte balance can be disturbed. Monitoring for signs of imbalance becomes important.

SODIUM IMBALANCES

The serum sodium concentration reflects the **osmolality** of body fluids; that is, their degree of concentration or dilution. It refers to the number of moles of the substance per kilogram of water in the solution. Serum sodium concentration reflects the proportion of water and sodium in the extracellular compartment. When the osmolality of body fluids becomes abnormal, the cells swell or shrink. These cell size changes are due to **osmosis,** the movement of water across a semipermeable membrane into an area of higher particle concentration.

Hypernatremia

Hypernatremia is a condition of increased osmolality of the blood. The body fluids are too concentrated, containing excess sodium relative to water. A serum sodium level above 148 mmol/L in children (146 mmol/L in newborns) is diagnostic of hypernatremia (Table 39–6).

Hypernatremia is caused by conditions that cause the body to lose relatively more water than sodium or to gain relatively more sodium than water (Table 39–7). Special circumstances in which a high solute intake may occur without adequate water include an infant formula that is too concentrated or one that is prepared with salt instead of sugar. A breastfed baby not receiving adequate breast milk who has normal water loss may develop hypernatremic dehydration (Livingstone, Willis, Abdel-Wareth, et al., 2000).

An infant or child who has hypernatremia is generally thirsty. The urine output is small unless the hypernatremia is caused by diabetes insipidus. A decreased level of con-

TABLE 39-7   Causes of Hypernatremia

Loss of Relatively More Water Than Sodium	Gain of Relatively More Sodium Than Water
Diabetes insipidus (not enough antidiuretic hormone)	Inability to communicate thirst
Diarrhea or vomiting without fluid replacement	Limited or no access to water
Excessive sweating without fluid replacement	High solute intake without adequate water (e.g., tube feedings)
High solute intake without adequate water (causes kidneys to excrete water)	Intravenous hypertonic saline

sciousness manifested by confusion, lethargy, or coma results from shrinking of the brain cells. Seizures can occur when hypernatremia occurs rapidly or is severe. Severe hypernatremia can be fatal.

Hypernatremia is treated by intravenous administration of **hypotonic fluid,** or fluid that is more dilute than normal body fluid. This therapy dilutes the body fluids back to normal concentration. If a child is dehydrated, **isotonic fluids** (those with the osmolality of body fluids) may be ordered first to replenish the volume, followed by hypotonic fluid to correct the osmolality. The underlying cause of the disorder is also treated.

NURSING MANAGEMENT

Monitor serum sodium level and measure intake and output and urine specific gravity. Normal specific gravity under 2 years is 1.001 to 1.018; in children over 2 years, 1.01 to 1.03 is the normal range. Specific gravity changes toward normal levels as therapy progresses. Frequently assess responsiveness to monitor the effect of hypernatremia on brain cells. As the concentration of body fluids returns to normal, the child will become more alert and responsive. Watch for rebound hyponatremia while monitoring the fluid replacement. Implement safety interventions such as raised bed rails for protection. Ensure adequate rest and introduce developmentally appropriate activities when the child is alert.

Water deprivation is a form of child neglect or abuse. In neglect, the parents simply do not provide adequate water for the child. A form of child abuse that sometimes includes water deprivation is Munchausen syndrome by proxy (see Chapter 36). A small child who is hospitalized with hypernatremia that does not have a detectable cause may be subject to water deprivation. Assess the child's general condition, developmental tasks, the family dynamics, and the parent's understanding of formula preparation and the child's fluid intake needs.

Teaching can prevent many cases of hypernatremia. Be sure the breastfeeding mother has instruction and resources about lactation before discharge after delivery. If discharged soon after birth, be sure the infant has an appointment to

TABLE 39-6   Normal Serum Values

Blood Component	Values
Sodium	Newborn: 133–146 mmol/L Children: 135–148 mmol/L
Potassium	Premature infants: 4.5–7.2 mmol/L Full-term infants: 3.7–5.2 mmol/L Children: 3.5–5.8 mmol/L
Calcium	Premature infants: 3.5–4.5 mEq/L (1.7–2.3 mmol/L) Full-term infants: 4–5 mEq/L (2–2.5 mmol/L) Children: 4.4–5.3 mEq/L (2.2–2.7 mmol/L)
Magnesium	Children: 1.5–2.4 mg/dL (0.62–0.99 mmol/L)
Arterial pH	Infants: 7.36–7.42 Children: 7.37–7.43 Adolescents: 7.35–7.41
Arterial Pco_2	Infants: 27–41 mm Hg (3.6–5.5 pKa) Children: 32–48 mm Hg (4.3–6.4 pKa)
Arterial Bicarbonate	Infants: 19–24 mmol/L Children: 18–25 mmol/L Adolescents: 23–25 mmol/L

have weight checked within the first few days, and alert the parents to expected output of at least six wet diapers daily. By about 10 days, infants should have regained the birth weight.

When an infant is sick or developing slowly, parents sometimes want to feed the infant more concentrated formula to make him or her stronger. Parents and caregivers of bottle-fed babies should be taught never to give undiluted formula concentrate or evaporated milk. Parents should be cautioned to keep salt out of reach, since eating handfuls of salt has caused hypernatremia. Teach parents to offer extra fluids during hot weather. Teach oral rehydration therapy for use at home during mild vomiting and diarrhea (see p. 940). (see p. 940)

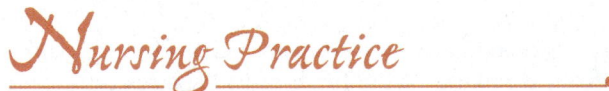

Nursing Practice

Careful teaching about how to mix powdered formula so that it is not too concentrated can help prevent hypernatremia. Pictures are an important teaching tool if the parents are not able to read labels or instructions.

Nurses can prevent hypernatremia in hospitalized infants and children by administering water between tube feedings, keeping water available, and offering it frequently. Offering frequent small amounts and using Popsicles and other creative interventions can increase children's intake.

Desired outcomes of treatment for hypernatremia include balance of electrolytes and fluid in the intracellular and extracellular compartments, and alert level of consciousness.

Hyponatremia

In hyponatremia, the osmolality of the blood is decreased. The body fluids are too dilute, containing excess water relative to sodium. Hyponatremia is the most common sodium imbalance in children (Dabbagh, Ellis, & Gruskin, 1996). A serum sodium level below 135 mmol/L in children (133 mmol/L in newborns) is diagnostic of hyponatremia.

ETIOLOGY AND PATHOPHYSIOLOGY

Hyponatremia is caused by conditions that cause gain of relatively more water than sodium or loss of relatively more sodium than water (Table 39–8). Oral intake of water causes hyponatremia in unusual conditions such as forced fluid intake. More commonly, parents feed an infant only water or dilute formula to save money instead of regular-strength formula or breast milk. Excessive swallowing of swimming pool water by an infant can have the same effect. Infants are vulnerable to the type of hyponatremia caused by water intoxication since they have a poorly developed thirst mechanism and may continue to drink, and then are unable to excrete excess water quickly due to immature kidney function (Fann, 1998).

TABLE 39–8 Causes of Hyponatremia	
Gain of Relatively More Water Than Sodium	Loss of Relatively More Sodium Than Water
Excessive intravenous D5W (5% dextrose in water)	Diarrhea or vomiting with replacement by tap water only instead of fluid containing sodium
Excessive tap water enemas	
Irrigation of body cavities with distilled water	
Excessive antidiuretic hormone	
Forced excessive oral intake of tap water	

CLINICAL MANIFESTATIONS

The child with hyponatremia has a decreased level of consciousness, which results from swelling of brain cells. This can be manifested as anorexia, headache, muscle weakness, decreased deep tendon reflexes, lethargy, confusion, or coma. If hyponatremia arises rapidly or is extreme, seizures may occur. Hyponatremia is a frequent cause of seizures in infants under 6 months of age who have a low body temperature (Farrar, Chande, Fitzpatrick, et al., 1995). Nausea and vomiting also occur in some children. Severe hyponatremia can be fatal.

CLINICAL THERAPY

In most cases, hyponatremia is treated by restricting the intake of water. This therapy allows the kidneys to correct the imbalance by excreting excess water from the body. If a child is having seizures from hyponatremia, intravenous **hypertonic** saline (more concentrated than body fluid) may be administered. Use of this concentrated fluid is a way to rapidly increase body fluid concentration, but it must be monitored carefully because it can easily cause rebound hypernatremia.

Nursing Management

Nursing Assessment and Diagnosis

Monitor serum sodium level and measure intake and output. If an infant with hyponatremia has normal antidiuretic hormone (ADH) levels, and other causes have been ruled out, carefully question parents about proper preparation of formula and feeding practices. A toddler or school-age child may be subjected to forced fluid intake as a form of child abuse. Sensitive interviewing and a caring manner can help identify such problems in a family.

Since hyponatremia is characterized by decreased level of consciousness, frequently assess responsiveness to monitor the response to therapy. The child will become more alert and responsive as the concentration of body fluids returns to normal.

The highest priority nursing diagnosis for hyponatremia addresses the risk for injury related to the child's decreased level of consciousness. The following diagnoses might also apply:

- *Self-care deficit* related to weakness and tiredness
- *Altered health maintenance* related to parental information misinterpretation about infant formula
- *Ineffective breastfeeding* related to inadequate sucking by infant or inadequate milk production

Planning and Implementation

Nurses can prevent hyponatremia in hospitalized children by using normal saline instead of distilled water for irrigations and by avoiding tap water enemas. It is important to help the child comply with prescribed fluid restrictions. WEB Allow the child to choose favorite fluids to drink. Teach parents to replace body fluids lost through diarrhea or vomiting with oral electrolyte solutions (see pp. 939–940).

Evaluation

Expected outcomes of nursing care for hyponatremia include the followng:

- Avoidance of injury
- Balance of fluid and electrolytes
- Establishment of adequate formula and/or breastfeeding intake.

POTASSIUM IMBALANCES

Potassium, an essential electrolyte, performs many necessary functions in the body. Potassium intake in healthy children comes from potassium-rich foods such as fruits and vegetables. Potassium is absorbed easily from the intestine. A normal potassium distribution is important for proper function.

A potassium imbalance arises when the serum potassium concentration rises or falls outside the normal range. Potassium imbalances are caused by alterations in potassium intake, distribution, or excretion; or by loss of potassium through an abnormal route such as burns, emesis, or renal failure.

Most potassium ions in the body are found inside the cells. The sodium-potassium pump in cell membranes moves potassium ions into cells to maintain the high intracellular potassium concentration. Potassium ions can be shifted into or out of cells by various physiologic factors (see "Pathophysiology Illustrated: Potassium Ions"). Potassium is excreted from the body through urine, feces, and sweat. The hormone aldosterone increases potassium excretion in the urine.

Hyperkalemia

Hyperkalemia is an excess of potassium in the blood. It is reflected by a level above 5.8 mmol/L in children or above 5.2 mmol/L in newborns (see Table 39–6).

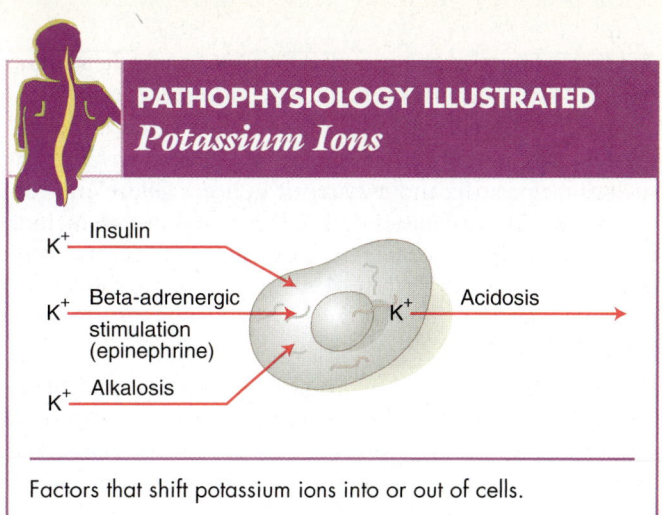

PATHOPHYSIOLOGY ILLUSTRATED
Potassium Ions

K^+ Insulin
K^+ Beta-adrenergic stimulation (epinephrine)
K^+ Alkalosis
K^+ Acidosis

Factors that shift potassium ions into or out of cells.

ETIOLOGY AND PATHOPHYSIOLOGY

Hyperkalemia is caused by conditions that involve increased potassium intake, shift of potassium from cells into the extracellular fluid, and decreased potassium excretion. Increased potassium intake is usually due to intravenous potassium overload. Excessive or too rapid intravenous administration of potassium-containing solutions can occur if potassium requirement is overestimated or if the intravenous infusion runs in too fast.

Blood transfusion is another source of potassium intake that may cause hyperkalemia. Potassium ions leak out of red blood cells that are stored in a blood bank. The longer the blood is stored, the more potassium leaks out of cells and accumulates in the fluid portion of the transfusion. Hyperkalemia from administration of stored blood arises when multiple units are transfused, as when infants receive exchange transfusions or children receive multiple blood transfusions after a serious injury or in surgery.

Shift of potassium from cells into the extracellular fluid occurs when there is massive cell death, as with a crush injury, in sickle cell anemia (hemolytic crisis), or when chemotherapy for a malignancy is rapidly effective. In these situations, the dead cells release their high-potassium contents into the extracellular fluid. Potassium ions also shift out of cells in metabolic acidosis caused by diarrhea and in diabetes mellitus when insulin levels are low.

Decreased potassium excretion occurs with acute or chronic oliguria during renal failure, severe hypovolemia, and conditions that decrease the secretion of aldosterone by the adrenal cortex (lead poisoning, Addison disease, hypoaldosteronism). Several medications can cause hyperkalemia, including some cancer chemotherapy, potassium-sparing diuretics, angiotensin-converting enzyme inhibitors, and nonsteroidal anti-inflammatory analgesics.

CLINICAL MANIFESTATIONS

The clinical manifestations of hyperkalemia are all related to muscle dysfunction since potassium plays a vital role in muscle activity. Hyperactivity of gastrointestinal smooth muscle causes intestinal cramping and diarrhea in some children. The skeletal muscles become weak, beginning typically with leg weakness and ascending. Weakness can progress to flaccid paralysis. The child is often lethargic. Dysfunction of cardiac muscle causes cardiac arrhythmias such as tachycardia and may result in heart failure and cardiac arrest. Abnormalities in the electrocardiogram include a prolonged QRS complex, a peak in T waves, and prolonged PR intervals (White, 1997).

CLINICAL THERAPY

Hyperkalemia is treated by management of the underlying condition that caused the imbalance. If the serum potassium concentration is very high or is causing dangerous cardiac arrhythmias, treatment to decrease the serum potassium level may be ordered. These treatments may remove potassium from the body or drive it from the extracellular fluid into the cells. Potassium is removed from the body by peritoneal dialysis or hemodialysis, by potassium-wasting diuretics, or with a cation exchange resin (Kayexalate) administered orally or rectally. Medical treatments that drive potassium ions into cells are intravenous bicarbonate, intravenous insulin, and glucose.

Nursing Management

Nursing Assessment and Diagnosis

Monitor serum potassium levels with blood draws from intravenous sites. Ongoing assessment of muscle strength is important because the muscle weakness may progress to flaccid paralysis. (This paralysis is reversible on correction of the potassium imbalance.) Diarrhea can occur in infants and children. An older child may complain of intestinal cramping. Monitor the pulse rate carefully.

Growth and Development

> The nursing diagnoses for hyperkalemic children will prompt a nurse to provide safety measures appropriate to the child's developmental level and to assist the child with activities that muscle weakness makes difficult. It is important to provide play and diversional activities that take into account the child's degree of muscle strength as well as the appropriate developmental level.

Nursing diagnoses for a child who has hyperkalemia depend on the severity of the clinical manifestations. The cause of the imbalance may also lead to useful diagnoses that guide teaching for the child and the parents. The following nursing diagnoses may apply:

▶ *Risk for decreased cardiac output* related to cardiac arrhythmias

▶ *Risk for injury* related to muscle weakness

▶ *Self-care deficit: hygiene and dressing* related to neuromuscular impairment

▶ *Anxiety* related to change in health status

▶ *Altered health maintenance* related to parental lack of exposure about potassium intake in chronic renal failure

▶ *Ineffective management of therapeutic regimen* related to complexity of therapy

Planning and Implementation

Nursing care includes measures to prevent hyperkalemia from developing in hospitalized children. If hyperkalemia does develop, care shifts to administering intravenous solutions, monitoring cardiopulmonary status, ensuring safety, promoting adequate nutrition, and preparing the child and family for discharge.

PREVENT HYPERKALEMIA

Any child receiving an intravenous infusion that contains potassium is at risk for hyperkalemia. Check that urine output is normal before administering intravenous potassium solutions. Turn over intravenous solutions to which potassium has been added several times to mix the contents thoroughly before connecting them to the infusion tubing.

Be sure blood or packed red blood cells are fresh, especially for the child receiving multiple transfusions, and for all neonates. Use a cardiac monitor during infusion of these products to watch for arrhythmias.

ADMINISTER INTRAVENOUS SOLUTIONS

Once a child is diagnosed as hyperkalemic, ensure that any infusions with added potassium are stopped. Several infusions may need to be managed, including glucose, bicarbonate, and calcium gluconate. Maintain the infusion at the ordered rate and monitor the child's condition frequently.

MONITOR CARDIOPULMONARY STATUS

Upon diagnosis of hyperkalemia, an electrocardiogram is performed and a cardiac monitor applied. Monitor for any changes in cardiac status and for cardiac arrhythmias. Report abnormal rate and character of pulse as well as shortness of breath.

ENSURE SAFETY

Since the child is weak, raise side rails. Position the child carefully. Assist the child with activities requiring leg muscle strength, such as climbing into bed or pushing up in bed. Encourage quiet activities with frequent rest periods. Document and report any change in muscle weakness.

PROMOTE ADEQUATE NUTRITIONAL INTAKE

Adequate caloric intake is necessary to prevent tissue breakdown and the resultant potassium release from cells. Offer the child nourishing snacks if his or her appetite is decreased. Restrict potassium-rich foods.

DISCHARGE PLANNING AND HOME CARE TEACHING

If the child has chronic renal failure or another condition that decreases aldosterone secretion, teach parents and children to restrict foods high in potassium. Most oral rehydration solutions, including Pedialyte, contain potassium and should not be used to provide fluid for the child. Instruct the family not to use salt substitutes, which commonly contain potassium. Parents should check with the care provider and pharmacist before giving even over-the-counter products to the child, as some of these medications contain potassium. Management of renal failure at home with frequent visits for dialysis and other treatments can be challenging. Refer to Chapter 47 for further suggestions to help parents handle this condition.

Evaluation

Expected outcomes for the child with hyperkalemia include:

▶ Return to a state of fluid and electrolyte balance

▶ Maintenance of safety

▶ Adequate nutritional intake to provide essential potassium

▶ Normal cardiac rate and rhythm

Hypokalemia

Hypokalemia occurs when the serum potassium concentration is too low. Total body potassium may be decreased, normal, or even increased when the serum level is low, depending on the cause of the imbalance. Serum potassium levels below 3.5 mmol/L in children (3.7 mmol/L for newborns) are diagnostic of hypokalemia.

ETIOLOGY AND PATHOPHYSIOLOGY

Hypokalemia is caused by conditions that involve increased potassium excretion, decreased potassium intake, shift of potassium from the extracellular fluid into cells, and loss of potassium by an abnormal route.

Increased potassium excretion is a major cause of hypokalemia in children. In addition to diuretics and other

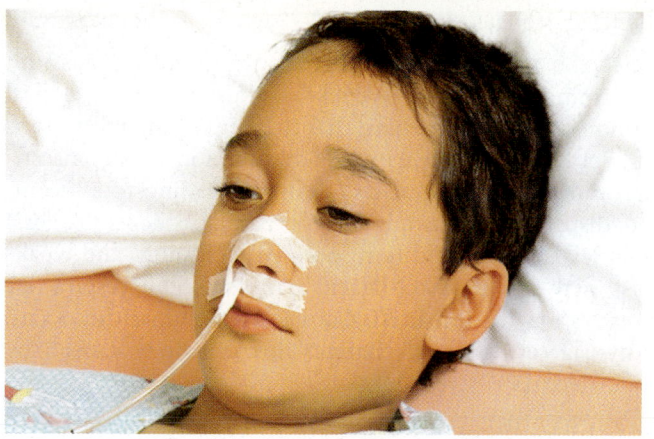

FIGURE 39–9. ◆ Because this child has a nasogastric tube in place that requires suctioning, it is important to monitor his potassium levels.

medications, causes of increased urinary potassium excretion are osmotic diuresis (glucose present in urine), hypomagnesemia, increased aldosterone (hyperaldosteronism, congestive heart failure, nephrotic syndrome, cirrhosis), and increased cortisol (Cushing disease and syndrome). Eating large amounts of black licorice increases renal excretion of potassium. Diarrhea causes potassium to be excreted in the feces.

Decreased potassium intake will lead to hypokalemia slowly, or more rapidly if combined with increased excretion or loss of potassium. Hospitalized children may be placed on NPO status and receive prolonged intravenous therapy without potassium. Adolescents concerned about weight loss or those with anorexia nervosa may embark on diets low in potassium and may take medications that induce diuresis or diarrhea.

Shift of potassium from the extracellular fluid into cells occurs in alkalosis and hypothermia (unintentional or induced for surgery). Hyperalimentation often causes hypersecretion of insulin, which also shifts potassium into cells.

Vomiting is an abnormal route for the loss of potassium; self-induced vomiting in bulimia, for example, can cause hypokalemia. Nasogastric suctioning (Figure 39–9 ◆) and intestinal decompression can cause potassium loss. Hypokalemia can also be caused by several medications (Table 39–9).

TABLE 39–9	Drugs That May Cause Electrolyte Disturbance			
Hyperkalemia	*Hypokalemia*	*Hypocalcemia*	*Hypermagnesemia*	*Hypomagnesemia*
Potassium-containing preparations	Beta-adrenergic agonists	Antacids (if overused)	Magnesium-containing cathartics	Magnesium-wasting diuretics
Cytotoxic agent	Insulin	Laxatives (if overused)	Magnesium antacids	Antineoplastics
Potassium-sparing diuretics	Potassium-wasting diuretics	Oil-based bowel lubricants		Systemic antifungals
Angiotensin-converting enzyme inhibitors	Parenteral penicillins	Anticonvulsants		Aminoglycoside antimicrobials
	Glucocorticoids	Phosphate-containing preparations		Laxatives
	Aminoglycoside antimicrobials	Protein-type plasma expanders during rapid infusion		
	Systemic antifungals			
	Antineoplastics			
	Laxatives			

CLINICAL MANIFESTATIONS

Since the ratio of intracellular to extracellular potassium determines the responsiveness of muscle cells to neural stimuli, it is not surprising that the clinical manifestations of hypokalemia involve muscle dysfunction. Gastrointestinal smooth muscle activity is slowed, leading to abdominal distention, constipation, or paralytic ileus. Skeletal muscles are weak and unresponsive to stimuli, and weakness may progress to flaccid paralysis. The respiratory muscles may be impaired. Cardiac arrhythmias can occur. Polyuria results from changes in the kidney caused by hypokalemia.

CLINICAL THERAPY

Medical management of hypokalemia focuses on replacement of potassium while treating the cause of the imbalance. Potassium replacement may be given intravenously or orally.

Nursing Management

Nursing Assessment and Diagnosis

Monitor serum potassium levels. Observe for muscle weakness, which is frequently detected first in the legs. Parents may report that muscle weakness restricts the child's activities and impairs interactions with peers. Skeletal muscle strength can be difficult to assess if the child is lethargic.

Muscle weakness may affect the respiratory muscles. Assess the child frequently to determine the need for assisted ventilation. Cardiac monitoring is important for continued assessment of hypokalemia-associated arrhythmias.

Assess for diminished bowel sounds. Ask the parents if the child has recently been awakening to use the toilet at night or has begun bed-wetting after previously being dry at night. These may be symptoms of polyuria associated with chronic hypokalemia.

The most important nursing diagnoses in the child with severe hypokalemia relate to cardiac arrhythmias and respiratory muscle weakness. The following nursing diagnoses may apply:

▶ *Risk for decreased cardiac output* related to cardiac arrhythmias

▶ *Ineffective breathing pattern* related to respiratory musculoskeletal impairment

▶ *Risk for injury* related to muscle weakness

▶ *Self-care deficit: hygiene and dressing* related to neuromuscular impairment

▶ *Constipation* related to decreased motility

▶ *Anxiety* related to change in health status

▶ *Health-seeking behaviors (parent)* regarding management of potassium supplements or high-potassium diet

▶ *Ineffective management of therapeutic regimen* related to complexity of potassium therapy

▶ *Health-seeking behaviors (adolescent)* related to information misinterpretation regarding safe weight-loss diet

Planning and Implementation

Nursing care of the child with hypokalemia focuses on ensuring adequate potassium intake, monitoring cardiopulmonary status, promoting normal bowel function, ensuring safety, providing dietary counseling, and preparing the child and family for discharge.

ENSURE ADEQUATE POTASSIUM INTAKE

Since potassium is excreted from the body every day, daily potassium intake is necessary to prevent hypokalemia. A hypokalemic child who is able to eat should be given a high-potassium diet. Teach parents (and the child if old enough) which foods are high in potassium and how to incorporate them into the daily diet (Table 39–10).

Children who have no oral intake for a period of time should receive intravenous fluids that contain potassium. Calculate the dosage to be sure it is accurate. Ensure that the infusion runs on schedule. Sometimes the child will complain of burning along the vein when potassium is infused. The infusion may need to be slowed temporarily to allow it to continue. Check serum potassium to watch for high or low potassium levels. Monitor urine output. An oliguric child can develop hyperkalemia when receiving supplements.

MONITOR CARDIOPULMONARY STATUS

Hypokalemia potentiates digitalis toxicity. A hypokalemic child receiving digitalis needs careful surveillance for digi-

---

TABLE 39–10	Food Sources of Electrolytes			
Potassium-Rich Foods		*Calcium-Rich Foods*		*Magnesium-Rich Foods*
Apricots	Orange juice	Milk	Legumes	Whole-grain cereal
Bananas	Peaches	Cheese	Nuts	Dark green vegetables
Cantaloupe	Potatoes	Yogurt	Figs	Soy
Cherries	Prunes	Pudding	Chicken	Almonds
Dates	Raisins	Egg yolks	Salmon (canned with bones)	Peanut butter
Figs	Strawberries	Grains (cream of wheat, farina, bran muffins)	Tofu	Bananas
Molasses	Tomato juice	Sardines (canned)	Fruit drinks with added calcium	Egg yolk

talis toxicity, which is manifested as anorexia, nausea, vomiting, and bradycardia. Observe for these effects. Take the pulse rate and rhythm regularly. Monitor respirations and ease of breathing to watch for decreased respiratory muscle activity.

Growth and Development

> Bradycardia occurs at a different level for children of various ages. For infants, a pulse rate below 100 is considered bradycardia. For young children, 80 may be the identified number, whereas for adolescents, a pulse below 60 is bradycardia. Look at the child's age and normal pulse range to find changes that indicate bradycardia.

PROMOTE NORMAL BOWEL FUNCTION

Ensure adequate fluids and fiber in the diet. Monitor and record the number of stools and report inadequate stools.

ENSURE SAFETY

Keep side rails up. Assist the child as needed to move into and out of bed. Reposition the child frequently to preserve skin integrity of limbs that are not moved regularly. Perform passive range of motion if the child is not moving. Use supportive pillows to position the child properly.

PROVIDE DIETARY COUNSELING

The adolescent trying to lose weight and not consuming a nutritious diet needs dietary teaching. More intensive treatment will be needed for teens who are anorexic or bulimic (see Chapter 36 for interventions).

DISCHARGE PLANNING AND HOME CARE TEACHING

Teach parents how to give potassium supplements, if prescribed. Liquid or powdered potassium supplements can be mixed with juice or sherbet to improve the bitter taste. The parent should call the mixture "medicine" so that the child does not learn to dislike all juices. Teach the parents signs of hypokalemia and hyperkalemia and whom to call to report these symptoms. These signs must be reported promptly so medications can be adjusted.

Evaluation

Expected outcomes for the child with potassium imbalance include the following:

▶ Normal rate and rhythm of heart and respiratory system

▶ Regular bowel movements

▶ Maintenance of safety

▶ Knowledge of child and family regarding food sources of potassium

CALCIUM IMBALANCES

A normal serum calcium concentration is important for many physiologic functions, including muscle and nerve function, secretion of hormones, bone formation and strength, and clotting of the blood.

Calcium imbalances are caused by alterations in calcium intake, absorption, distribution, or excretion. Calcium absorption requires vitamin D for maximum efficiency and is greatest in the duodenum. Calcium distribution involves calcium entry into and exit from bones and the distribution of different forms of calcium in the plasma. Ionized calcium is the only physiologically active form; additional calcium is bound to protein or ions. Calcium is excreted in urine, feces, and sweat (see "Pathophysiology Illustrated: Calcium Imbalances").

Parathyroid hormone is the major regulator of the plasma calcium concentration. It increases the plasma calcium concentration by increasing calcium absorption, increasing calcium withdrawal from bones, and decreasing calcium excretion in the urine. The plasma calcium concentration has an important influence on cell membrane permeability and influences the threshold potential of

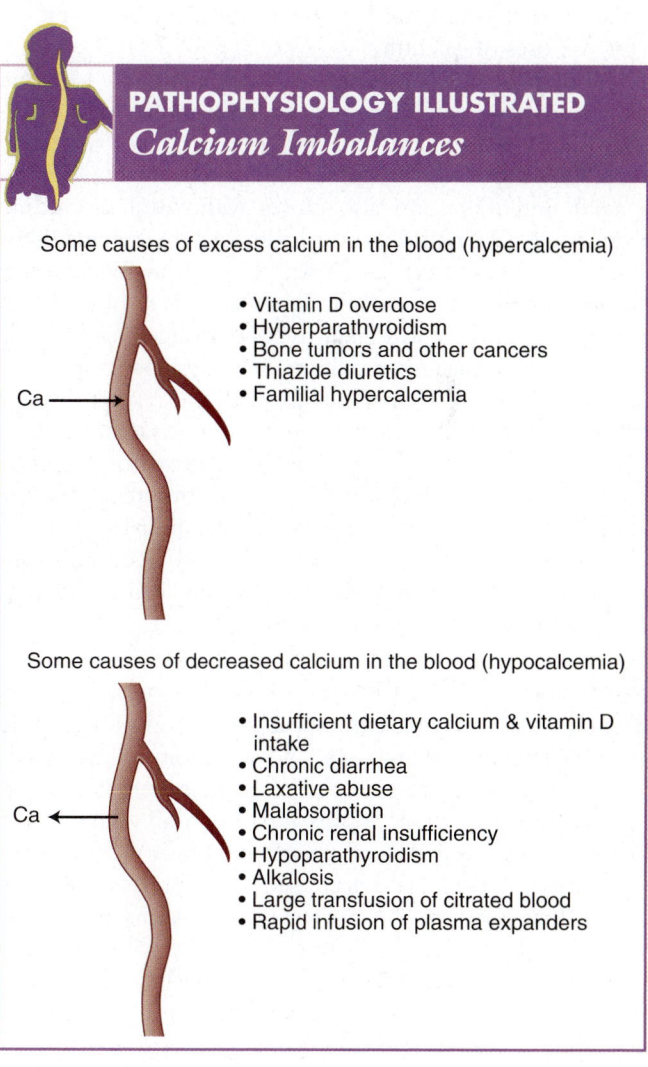

PATHOPHYSIOLOGY ILLUSTRATED
Calcium Imbalances

Some causes of excess calcium in the blood (hypercalcemia)

Ca →

- Vitamin D overdose
- Hyperparathyroidism
- Bone tumors and other cancers
- Thiazide diuretics
- Familial hypercalcemia

Some causes of decreased calcium in the blood (hypocalcemia)

Ca ←

- Insufficient dietary calcium & vitamin D intake
- Chronic diarrhea
- Laxative abuse
- Malabsorption
- Chronic renal insufficiency
- Hypoparathyroidism
- Alkalosis
- Large transfusion of citrated blood
- Rapid infusion of plasma expanders

excitable cells. For this reason, calcium imbalances alter neuromuscular irritability.

Hypercalcemia

Hypercalcemia refers to a plasma excess of calcium (above 5.3 mEq/L [2.7 mmol/L] in children or 5 mEq/L [2.5 mmol/L] in newborns) (see Table 39–6). Because so much calcium is stored in the bones, however, the serum levels of calcium may not reflect body stores.

ETIOLOGY AND PATHOPHYSIOLOGY

Hypercalcemia is caused by conditions that involve increased calcium intake or absorption, shift of calcium from bones into the extracellular fluid, and decreased calcium excretion. Hypercalcemia due to increased calcium intake or absorption may occur if an infant is fed large amounts of chicken liver (source of vitamin A) or is given megadoses of vitamin D or vitamin A, or if a child or adolescent consumes large amounts of calcium-rich foods concurrently with antacids (milk-alkali syndrome). Infants with very low birth weight can develop hypercalcemia if they have inadequate phosphorus intake, as bone phosphorus and calcium will be resorbed. Hypercalcemia may also occur when children receiving total parenteral nutrition are given excessive doses of calcium.

Most cases of hypercalcemia in children are due to a shift of calcium from bones into the extracellular fluid. The excessive amounts of parathyroid hormone produced in hyperparathyroidism cause calcium withdrawal from bones. Prolonged immobilization also causes withdrawal of calcium from bones. Often, the excess calcium ions are excreted in the urine. However, if calcium is withdrawn from bones faster than the kidneys can excrete it, hypercalcemia results. Hypercalcemia also occurs with many types of malignancies such as leukemias. The malignant cells produce substances that circulate in the blood to the bones and cause bone resorption. The calcium from the bones then enters the extracellular fluid, causing hypercalcemia. Bone tumors destroy bone directly, leading to the release of calcium. Familial hypercalcemia and infantile hypercalcemia are rare congenital disorders.

Thiazide diuretics (e.g., thiazide and hydrochlorthiazide) decrease calcium excretion in the urine and may contribute to development of hypercalcemia.

CLINICAL MANIFESTATIONS

Hypercalcemia may have nonspecific symptoms, making diagnosis difficult. Many signs and symptoms of hypercalcemia are manifestations of decreased neuromuscular excitability. Constipation, anorexia, nausea, and vomiting can occur. Fatigue and skeletal muscle weakness predominate. Confusion, lethargy, and decreased attention span are common. Polyuria develops. Severe hypercalcemia may cause cardiac arrhythmias and arrest. Neonates with hypercalcemia have flaccid muscles and exhibit failure to thrive. Hypercalcemia increases sodium and potassium excretion by the kidneys and can lead to polyuria and polydipsia.

CLINICAL THERAPY

Hypercalcemia is treated by increasing fluids and administering the diuretic furosemide (Lasix) to increase excretion of calcium in the urine. Treatment to decrease intestinal absorption of calcium involves effective use of glucocorticoids. Bone resorption can be decreased by administration of glucocorticoids and calcitonin. Phosphate is sometimes given to treat hypercalcemia, but it may cause dangerous precipitation of calcium phosphate salts in body tissues. Dialysis may be used, if necessary.

Nursing Management

Nursing Assessment and Diagnosis

Nursing assessment of a child with hypercalcemia includes monitoring serum calcium levels, level of consciousness, gastrointestinal function, urine volume, specific gravity, cardiac rhythm, and pH. With chronic hypercalcemia, assessment of activity tolerance and developmental level becomes important.

Many nursing diagnoses are appropriate for children who have hypercalcemia. Diagnoses that address cardiac and neuromuscular manifestation are especially important. The following nursing diagnoses may apply:

▶ *Risk for decreased cardiac output* related to cardiac arrest

▶ *Risk for injury* related to decreased level of consciousness

▶ *Risk for injury* related to neuromuscular impairment

▶ *Risk for injury* related to possibility of spontaneous fractures

▶ *Self-care deficit: hygiene and dressing* related to neuromuscular impairment

▶ *Anxiety* related to change in health status

▶ *Constipation* related to decreased motility

▶ *Risk for altered nutrition: less than body requirements* related to anorexia and nausea

▶ *Risk for altered urinary elimination* related to renal calculi

Planning and Intervention

Carefully calculate calcium in total parenteral nutrition and other solutions, administer these solutions with caution, and use cardiac monitoring to prevent hypercalcemia in hospitalized children.

Interventions to increase fluid intake are important for children with hypercalcemia or those who are immobilized. A large fluid intake, appropriate to the child's age, is necessary to keep the urine dilute and to help reduce constipation (a common symptom of hypercalcemia). An acidic urine helps to keep calcium from forming stones. Because urinary tract infections may cause the urine to be alkaline, institute nursing interventions to prevent urinary tract infection. Thiazide diuretics, which decrease calcium excretion, should not be given to the hypercalcemic child. Provide a high-fiber diet to help reduce constipation.

Increasing mobility through assisted weight bearing helps decrease the withdrawal of calcium from bones that is caused by immobility. If the hypercalcemia is caused by withdrawal of calcium from bones, the child is at risk for fractures with minor trauma and must be handled with special care. See Chapter 50 for further discussion of care following fractures and prolonged casting.

Teach parents to avoid giving calcium-rich foods (such as dairy products) and calcium antacids (e.g., Tums) to children with hypercalcemia. Vitamin D supplements should be avoided because they increase calcium absorption from the gastrointestinal tract.

Evaluation

Expected outcomes include the following:

▶ Cardiac pump effectiveness
▶ Safety
▶ Normal bowel excretion
▶ Adequate nutritional status

Hypocalcemia

Hypocalcemia is a serum deficit of calcium (below 4.4 mEq/L [2.2 mmol/L] in children or 4 mEq/L [2 mmol/L] in newborns]). (Remember that serum calcium levels may not reflect body stores of this mineral, as most of the body's calcium is stored in bone.)

ETIOLOGY AND PATHOPHYSIOLOGY

Hypocalcemia is caused by conditions that involve decreased calcium intake or absorption, shift of calcium to a physiologically unavailable form, increased calcium excretion, and loss of calcium by an abnormal route.

Decreased calcium intake or absorption causes hypocalcemia in children with chronic generalized malnutrition, or with a diet low in vitamin D and calcium. Female adolescents trying to lose weight or maintain a low weight often decrease foods that contain calcium and may develop chronic hypocalcemia. They may have premature bone loss and inadequate bone. (See Chapter 31 for further discussion of calcium intake during adolescence.) This deficit cannot be made up later in life, increasing the risk of osteoporosis.

Even with a normal calcium intake, hypocalcemia occurs if the mineral is not absorbed. If a child does not have enough vitamin D, calcium is not absorbed efficiently from the duodenum. Sunlight speeds formation of vitamin D in the skin. Children institutionalized without access to sunlight (e.g., severely developmentally delayed children), those with very dark skin, or children kept well covered when outside may become hypocalcemic because of the lack of vitamin D (see Chapter 31). Uremic syn-

drome is another cause of vitamin D deficiency. It interferes with the kidney's ability to activate vitamin D. High phosphate intake can cause hypocalcemia. Chronic diarrhea and steatorrhea (fatty stools) also reduce calcium absorption from the gastrointestinal tract.

Calcium becomes physiologically unavailable when calcium shifts into bone, or free ionized calcium in plasma binds to proteins or small organic ions in the plasma. Too much calcium shifts into bones in various types of hypoparathyroidism, including DiGeorge syndrome (congenital absence of the parathyroid glands). Hypomagnesemia impairs parathyroid hormone function and may cause hypocalcemia. Some types of neonatal hypocalcemia are associated with delayed parathyroid hormone function or hypomagnesemia. Calcium shifts rapidly into bone when rickets is treated. A high plasma phosphate concentration causes plasma calcium to decrease. Ionized hypocalcemia, due to an increased binding of plasma ionized calcium, occurs very rapidly. The ionized hypocalcemia persists until the alkalosis resolves or the citrate is metabolized by the liver. Children who receive liver transplants are hypocalcemic for several days because of impaired citrate metabolism.

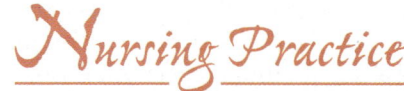

Following are causes of ionized hypocalcemia:

▶ Alkalosis, which causes more calcium to bind to plasma proteins
▶ Citrate in transfused blood products, which binds calcium

Increased calcium excretion occurs in steatorrhea, when calcium secreted into the gastrointestinal fluid binds to the fecal fat in addition to the dietary calcium that is bound in the feces. A similar situation occurs in acute pancreatitis.

Loss of calcium by an abnormal route may contribute to hypocalcemia; calcium is lost through burn or wound drainage or sequestered in acute pancreatitis. Many medications can cause hypocalcemia (see Table 39–9).

CLINICAL MANIFESTATIONS

The signs and symptoms of hypocalcemia are manifestations of increased muscular excitability (tetany). In children they include twitching and cramping, tingling around the mouth or in the fingers, carpal spasm, and pedal spasm. Laryngospasm, seizures, and cardiac arrhythmias are more severe manifestations of hypocalcemia and may be fatal. Hypocalcemia may cause congestive heart failure, especially in neonates.

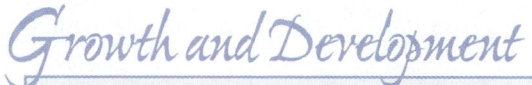

Hypocalcemia in infants is more often seen as tremors, muscle twitches, and brief tonic–clonic seizures.

Although these symptoms are diagnostic of acute calcium deficiency, a more common state in children and adolescents is chronic low intake of calcium. This may be manifested by spontaneous fractures in infants and in adolescents who exercise excessively.

CLINICAL THERAPY

Hypocalcemia is treated by oral or intravenous administration of calcium. The original cause of the imbalance is also treated. If the hypocalcemia is due to hypomagnesemia, the magnesium must be replenished before the calcium replacement can be successful. When the cause is chronic low dietary intake, counseling is needed about high-calcium foods, and perhaps the necessity for vitamin D intake or supplements.

Nursing Management

Nursing Assessment and Diagnosis

Carefully assess growth in the young female who is trying to diet. Whenever an adolescent female is very thin, be sure to ask about excessive sports and other activities, and about regularity of menstrual periods. If periods are irregular or not occurring, collect additional dietary information to help determine whether the girl is lacking in intake of calcium, calories, and other nutrients. These assessments are needed even if serum calcium values are normal. Look for signs of inadequate nutrition such as fat and muscle wasting, dry hair, and cold hands and feet (Johnson, 1994). Assess for muscle cramps, stiffness, and clumsiness; grimacing caused by spasms of facial muscles and twitching of arm muscles; and laryngospasm. Increased neuromuscular excitability may be detected by testing for Trousseau's sign or Chvostek's sign. Many healthy newborns have a positive Chvostek's sign; however, this assessment should be reserved for children over several months of age. Monitor serum calcium levels and perform cardiac monitoring to observe for cardiac arrhythmias.

The effects of increased neuromuscular excitability in the child with hypocalcemia are the basis for several nursing diagnoses. These include:

▶ *Risk for injury* related to potential for fractures

▶ *Risk for injury* related to increased neuromuscular excitability

▶ *Risk for ineffective breathing pattern* related to laryngospasm

▶ *Risk for decreased cardiac output* related to cardiac arrhythmias

▶ *Sensory/perceptual alteration* related to electrolyte imbalance

▶ *Anxiety* related to change in health status

▶ *Health-seeking behaviors* related to misinformation about sources and recommended amounts of calcium intake

Planning and Implementation

To correct calcium deficiency in the hospitalized child, give oral or intravenous calcium as ordered. Monitor for complications of calcium supplementation. Monitor for the side effect of constipation to oral supplements, or for tissue sloughing, elevated serum calcium, or decreased serum phosphate with intravenous supplementation. Calcium is never given intramuscularly because it causes tissue necrosis. A 10% calcium gluconate intravenous solution should be readily available for emergency use in severe hypocalcemia.

Take measures to ensure safety for the child who is hospitalized with hypocalcemia. Seizure precautions may be necessary. Explain the cause of muscle cramps to parents and older children.

Counsel the family about dairy products and nondairy foods rich in calcium (see Table 39–10). For the adolescent female whose weight and menstrual patterns show irregularities, total calories and calcium intake should be increased. Teaching may also be needed about proper calcium intake and its importance both to athletic performance and to prevention of osteoporosis. Encourage three glasses of nonfat milk per day (Snow-Harter, 1994). Teach ways to use milk in the diet. For example, sprinkle nonfat dry milk on cereal and other foods. If the child is lactose-intolerant, emphasize nondairy sources of calcium and advise parents to purchase special milk treated with lactase. This milk is more costly, and inadequate family finances may prevent its use. If a child has a health condition leading to chronic diarrhea, encourage increased intake of calcium-rich foods. Calcium supplements in the form of calcium carbonate tablets may be used.

Evaluation

Expected outcomes of nursing care for hypocalcemia include the following:

▶ Ingestion of recommended dietary allowances for calcium

▶ Absence of discomfort related to calcium imbalance

▶ Freedom from injury

MAGNESIUM IMBALANCES

Magnesium is necessary for enzyme function in cells, acetylcholine release, glycolysis, stimulation of ATPases, and bone formation. Since magnesium is a component of chlorophyll, dark green leafy vegetables are a good dietary source of magnesium. Nuts and grains are also good sources of magnesium. Magnesium is absorbed primarily from the terminal ileum. Magnesium is distributed among the extracellular fluid (small amounts), the cells (larger amounts), and the bones (large amounts). Magnesium excretion occurs in urine, feces, and sweat.

Magnesium imbalances are caused by alterations in magnesium intake, distribution, or excretion; by loss of magnesium through an abnormal route; or by a combination of these factors. The plasma magnesium concentration influences the release of acetylcholine at neuromuscular junctions. Thus, magnesium imbalances are characterized by alterations in neuromuscular irritability.

Hypermagnesemia

Hypermagnesemia occurs when the plasma magnesium con centration is too high (above 2.4 mg/dL [0.99 mmol/L]) (see Table 39–6). Keep in mind that the serum levels measured in the laboratory may not reflect body magnesium stores, because most magnesium in the body is located in the bones and inside the cells.

Hypermagnesemia is caused by conditions that involve increased magnesium intake and decreased magnesium excretion. Impaired renal function leading to decreased magnesium excretion is the most common cause of hypermagnesemia in children. In both oliguric renal failure and adrenal insufficiency, magnesium ions that cannot be excreted in the urine accumulate in the extracellular fluid.

Less frequently, increased magnesium intake may cause hypermagnesemia. Magnesium sulfate (MgSO4) given to treat eclampsia in the mother before delivery causes hypermagnesemia in the newborn. Abnormally high amounts may also be taken in magnesium-containing enemas, laxatives, antacids, and intravenous fluids (see Table 39–9). Aspiration of seawater, as in near-drowning, is an uncommon but potentially serious source of excessive magnesium intake. Children with Addison disease can have abnormally high magnesium levels.

Clinical manifestations of hypermagnesemia include decreased muscle irritability, hypotension, bradycardia, drowsiness, lethargy, and weak or absent deep tendon reflexes. In severe hypermagnesemia, flaccid muscle paralysis, fatal respiratory depression, cardiac arrhythmias, and cardiac arrest occur.

Hypermagnesemia is managed primarily by increasing the urinary excretion of magnesium. This is usually accomplished by increasing fluid intake (except in oliguric renal failure) and by the administration of diuretics. Dialysis may sometimes be necessary.

NURSING MANAGEMENT

Monitor serum magnesium levels. Take the child's blood pressure (to watch for hypotension), heart rate and rhythm (to monitor for bradycardia and cardiac arrhythmias), respiratory rate and depth (to watch for respiratory depression), and deep tendon reflexes (to check muscle tone and paralysis or movement). Keep the side rails of the bed raised. Children with hypermagnesemia or oliguria should not be given magnesium-containing medications or sea salt.

Teach parents of children with chronic renal failure that these children should never be given milk of magnesia, antacids that contain magnesium, or other sources of magnesium. When hypermagnesemia is treated with diuretics, monitor potassium levels to watch for hypokalemia.

Expected outcomes of nursing care include maintenance of electrolyte balance, normal neuromuscular tone, safety, and regular heart rate and rhythm.

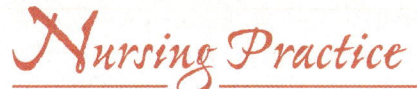

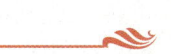

Instruct parents of a child with chronic renal failure to read labels to detect magnesium in antacids and cathartics.

Hypomagnesemia

Hypomagnesemia refers to a plasma magnesium concentration that is too low (below 1.5 to 1.7 mg/dL [0.62 to 0.7 mmol/L]). (Remember that the serum levels of magnesium may not reflect body stores, since most of the magnesium in the body is found in cells and bones.)

Hypomagnesemia is caused by conditions that involve decreased magnesium intake or absorption, shift of magnesium to a physiologically unavailable form, increased magnesium excretion, and loss of magnesium by an abnormal route.

Decreased magnesium intake or absorption can occur if a child who is not eating has prolonged intravenous therapy without magnesium. Chronic malnutrition is another cause of decreased magnesium intake. Magnesium absorption is decreased in chronic diarrhea, short bowel syndrome, malabsorption syndromes, and steatorrhea.

Magnesium may shift to a physiologically unavailable form after transfusion of many units of citrated blood products; magnesium bound to the citrate is not physiologically active. Such transfusions cause prolonged hypomagnesemia in liver transplant patients, who have impaired citrate metabolism. Magnesium shifts rapidly into bones that have been deprived of adequate stores.

Increased magnesium excretion in the urine occurs with diuretic therapy, the diuretic phase of acute renal failure, diabetic ketoacidosis, and hyperaldosteronism. Chronic alcoholism, occasionally seen in adolescents, increases urinary magnesium excretion. Magnesium contained in gastrointestinal secretions is bound to fat and excreted in the stool.

Loss of magnesium by an abnormal route occurs with prolonged nasogastric suction and through sequestration of magnesium in acute pancreatitis. Several medications may cause hypomagnesemia (see Table 39–9).

Hypomagnesemia is characterized by increased neuromuscular excitability (tetany). The clinical manifestations are hyperactive reflexes, skeletal muscle cramps, twitching, tremors, and cardiac arrhythmias. Seizures can occur with severe hypomagnesemia.

Hypomagnesemia is managed by administering magnesium and treating the underlying cause of the imbalance.

NURSING MANAGEMENT

In addition to monitoring serum magnesium levels, nursing assessment of hypomagnesemia includes monitoring deep tendon reflexes, testing for Trousseau's and Chvostek's signs, monitoring cardiac function, and observing for muscle twitching. Children able to talk report muscle cramping. Because magnesium levels are not routinely measured in many settings, request the test for any child who has risk factors and early manifestations of hypomagnesemia. When intramuscular or intravenous magnesium are ordered, administer carefully as directed and monitor vital signs. Electrocardiogram and renal studies may precede drug administration. Have resuscitative drugs and equipment readily available during drug administration.

Teach parents of a child with hypomagnesemia or continuing risk factors such as chronic diarrhea to include magnesium-rich foods in the diet (see Table 39–10). Before administering magnesium supplements, verify that the child's urine output is adequate. Monitor deep tendon reflexes if intravenous magnesium is given, and observe for complications of magnesium supplementation. Oral magnesium may lead to diarrhea, and intravenous magnesium can cause flushing, elevated serum magnesium, cardiac arrhythmias, or decreased deep tendon reflexes.

Expected outcomes are restoration and maintenance of electrolyte balance.

CLINICAL ASSESSMENT OF FLUID AND ELECTROLYTE IMBALANCE

How can a nurse assess children appropriately for fluid and electrolyte imbalance without thinking through the clinical manifestations of every possible disorder one after the other? First, perform a rapid risk factor assessment on each child to see which factors are present (Tables 39–11 and 39–12).

A risk factor assessment may be performed mentally while providing care. Look for factors that alter the intake, retention, and loss of isotonic fluid and water. Use this information to evaluate which fluid imbalance is most likely to occur in a particular child. Next, look for factors that alter electrolyte intake and absorption, distribution between plasma and other electrolyte pools, excretion, and abnormal routes of electrolyte loss. Use this information to evaluate which electrolyte imbalances are most likely to occur in the child. A review of pathophysiology is important to understand the role of the other electrolytes and substances, such as phosphorus, in the body.

TABLE 39–11 Risk Factor Assessment for Fluid Imbalances

Isotonic Fluid (Extracellular Fluid Volume Imbalances)
- Source of increased intake?
- Aldosterone secretion increased or decreased?
- Source of loss from the body?

Water
- Source of increased intake?
- Antidiuretic hormone secretion increased or decreased?
- Source of unusual loss from the body?

TABLE 39–12 Risk Factor Assessment for Electrolyte Imbalances

Electrolyte Intake and Absorption
- Increased?
- Decreased?

Electrolyte Shifts
- From electrolyte pool to plasma?
- From plasma to electrolyte pool?

Electrolyte Excretion
- Increased?
- Decreased?

Electrolyte Loss by Abnormal Route
- Vomiting?
- Diarrhea?
- Nasogastric suction?
- Wound?
- Burn?
- Excessive sweating?

After evaluating possible imbalances for the child, perform a clinical assessment. Assess for fluid imbalances by assessing weight changes, vascular volume, interstitial volume, and cerebral function (Table 39–13). Assess for electrolyte imbalances by assessing serum electrolyte levels, skeletal muscle strength, neuromuscular excitability, gastrointestinal tract function, and cardiac rhythm (Table 39–14). Next, check for other manifestations specific to a particular high-risk imbalance (e.g., polyuria in hypokalemia). Evaluate any serum laboratory values available. This method of risk factor assessment followed by clinical assessment provides a rapid yet thorough approach to assessment for fluid and electrolyte imbalances.

PHYSIOLOGY OF ACID-BASE BALANCE

Normal acid-base balance is necessary for proper function of the cells and the body. The number of hydrogen ions (H+) present in a fluid determines how acidic it is. Increasing the hydrogen ion concentration makes a solution more acidic. Because the hydrogen ion concentration in body fluids is very small, acidity is expressed as **pH** (the negative logarithm of the hydrogen ion concentration) rather than as the hydrogen ion concentration itself. The range of possible pH values is 1 to 14. A pH of 7 is neutral. The lower the pH, the more acidic the solution. A pH above 7 is basic. The higher the pH, the more basic the solution. Body fluids are normally slightly basic.

The pH of body fluids is regulated carefully to provide a suitable environment for cell function. The pH of the blood influences the pH inside the cells. **Acidemia** refers to a decreased blood pH below normal levels, whereas **alkalemia** is an increased blood pH. Normal arterial blood pH ranges are 7.36 to 7.42 for infants, 7.37 to 7.43 for

TABLE 39-13 Summary of Clinical Assessment of Fluid Imbalances

Assessment Category	Specific Assessments	Changes with Fluid Imbalances
Rapid changes in weight	Daily weights	Weight gain—extracellular volume excess Weight loss—extracellular volume deficit; clinical dehydration
Vascular volume	Small vein filling time Capillary refill time Character of pulse	Increased—extracellular volume deficit; clinical dehydration Increased—extracellular volume deficit; clinical dehydration Bounding—extracellular volume excess Thready—extracellular volume deficit; clinical dehydration
	Postural blood pressure measurements Lung sounds in dependent portions Central venous pressure	Postural drop—extracellular volume deficit; clinical dehydration Crackles—extracellular volume excess Increased—extracellular volume excess Decreased—extracellular volume deficit; clinical dehydration
	Tenseness of fontanel (infants)	Bulging—extracellular volume excess Sunken—extracellular volume deficit; clinical dehydration
	Neck vein filling (older children)	Full with upright—extracellular volume excess Flat when supine—extracellular volume deficit; clinical dehydration
Interstitial volume	Skin turgor Presence or absence of edema	Skin tents—extracellular volume deficit; clinical dehydration Edema—extracellular volume excess
Cerebral function	Level of consciousness	Decreased—clinical dehydration

TABLE 39-14 Summary of Clinical Assessment of Electrolyte Imbalances

Assessment Category	Specific Assessments	Changes with Electrolyte Imbalances
Skeletal muscle function	Muscle strength	Weakness, flaccid paralysis—hyperkalemia; hypokalemia
Neuromuscular excitability	Deep tendon reflexes	Depressed—hypercalcemia; hypermagnesemia Hyperactive—hypocalcemia; hypomagnesemia
	Chvostek's sign (not infants) Trousseau's sign Paresthesias Muscle cramping or twitching	Positive—hypocalcemia; hypomagnesemia Positive—hypocalcemia; hypomagnesemia Digital or perioral—hypocalcemia Present—hypocalcemia; hypomagnesemia
Gastrointestinal tract function	Bowel sounds Elimination pattern	Decreased or absent—hypokalemia Constipation—hypokalemia; hypercalcemia Diarrhea—hyperkalemia
Cardiac rhythm	Arrhythmia	Irregular—hyperkalemia; hypokalemia; hypercalcemia; hypocalcemia; hypermagnesemia; hypomagnesemia
	Electrocardiogram	Abnormal—hyperkalemia; hypokalemia; hypercalcemia; hypocalcemia; hypermagnesemia; hypomagnesemia
Cerebral function	Level of consciousness	Decreased—hyponatremia; hypernatremia

children, and 7.35 to 7.41 for adolescents. For the enzymes outside the cells to function optimally, the pH must be in the normal range. If the pH inside the cells becomes too high or too low, then the speed of chemical reactions becomes inappropriate for proper cell function. Cell protein function relies on the correct level of hydrogen ions. Thus, acid-base imbalances result in clinical signs and symptoms, and, in severe cases, they may cause death.

In the course of their normal function, all cells in the body produce acids. Cells produce two kinds of acids: carbonic acid (H_2CO_3) and metabolic (noncarbonic) acids. Carbonic acid is formed from carbon dioxide and water, whereas common metabolic acids are pyruvic, sulfuric, lactic, and hydrochloric acids. These acids are released into the extracellular fluid and must be neutralized or excreted from the body to prevent dangerous accumulation. They can be neutralized to some degree by the buffers in body fluids. The lungs excrete carbonic acid in the form of carbon dioxide and water. Metabolic acids are excreted by the kidneys.

BUFFERS

The maintenance of hydrogen ions within normal range relies heavily on buffers. A **buffer** is a compound that binds hydrogen ions when their concentration rises and releases them when the concentration falls (see "Pathophysiology Illustrated: Buffer Responses to Acid and Base"). Several kinds of buffers are present in the body, such as bicarbonate, protein, hemoglobin, and phosphate. Various body fluids have buffers to meet their special needs

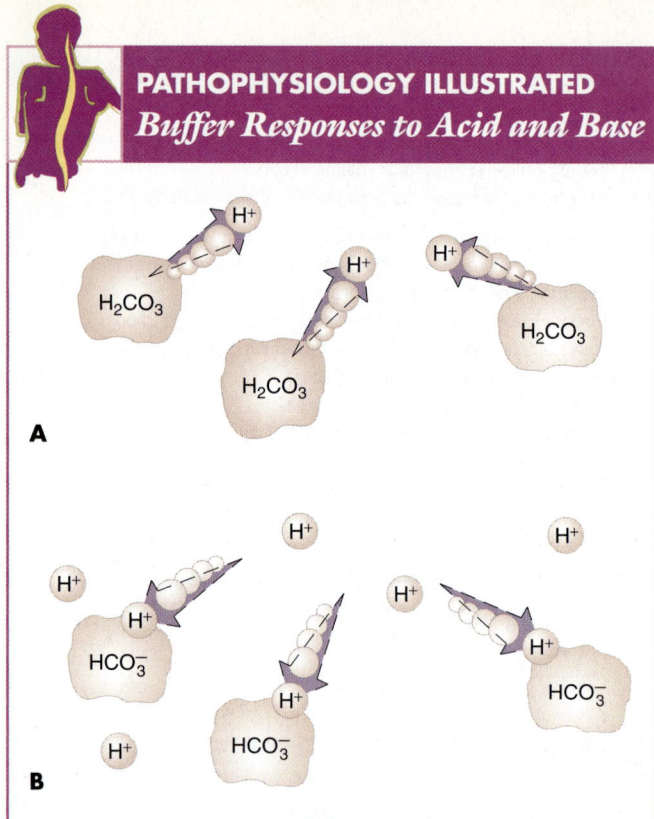

A, How buffers respond to an excess of base. If the blood has too much base, the acid portion of a buffer pair (e.g., H_2CO_3 of the bicarbonate buffer system) releases hydrogen ions (H^+) to help return the pH to normal. **B,** How buffers respond to an excess of acid. If the blood has too much acid, the base portion of a buffer pair (e.g., HCO_3^- of the bicarbonate buffer system) takes up hydrogen ions (H^+) to help return the pH to normal.

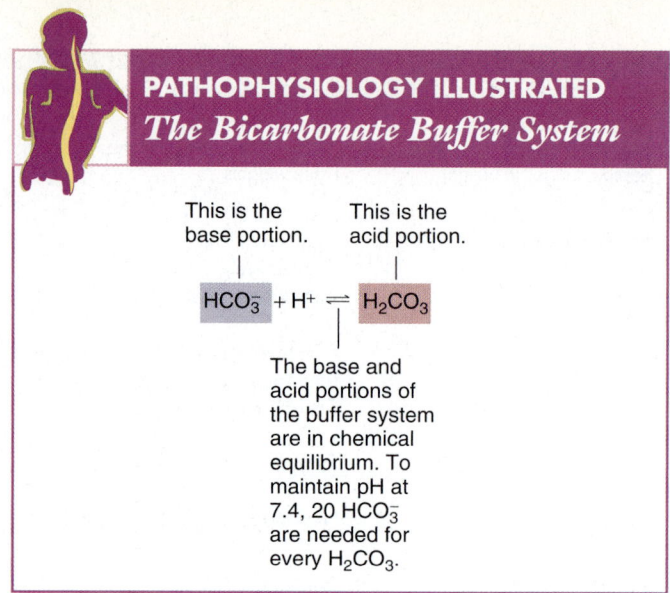

This is the base portion. This is the acid portion.

$$HCO_3^- + H^+ \rightleftharpoons H_2CO_3$$

The base and acid portions of the buffer system are in chemical equilibrium. To maintain pH at 7.4, 20 HCO_3^- are needed for every H_2CO_3.

(Halperin & Goldstein, 1994). The bicarbonate buffer system neutralizes metabolic acids (see "Pathophysiology Illustrated: The Bicarbonate Buffer System"); however, it cannot neutralize carbonic acid.

All buffer systems have limits. For example, if there are too many metabolic acids, the bicarbonate buffers become depleted. The acids then accumulate in the body until they are excreted by the kidneys. Clinically, this is seen as a decreased serum bicarbonate concentration and decreased blood pH.

ROLE OF THE LUNGS

The lungs are responsible for excreting excess carbonic acid from the body. A child breathes out carbon dioxide and water, the components of carbonic acid, with each breath. With faster and deeper breaths, more carbonic acid is excreted. Since carbonic acid is converted in the body to carbon dioxide and water by the enzyme carbonic anhydrase, an indirect laboratory measurement of carbonic acid is P_{CO_2} (see Table 39–6).

Although a child can voluntarily increase or decrease the rate and depth of respirations, they are usually involuntarily controlled. Chemoreceptors in the hypothalamus of the brain and in the aorta and carotid arteries monitor the P_{CO_2} and pH of the blood. These arteries also monitor the P_{O_2} of the blood. The input from the chemoreceptors is combined with other neural input to change breathing according to needs. Rate and depth increase or decrease according to the amount of carbonic acid that needs to be excreted.

If a child has a condition that decreases the excretion of carbonic acid or causes breathing to be too slow or shallow (such as overmedication following surgery), carbonic acid accumulates in the blood. Clinically, this is seen as an increased blood P_{CO_2}. The reverse will also be true.

ROLE OF THE KIDNEYS

The kidneys excrete metabolic acids from the body in two ways. They reabsorb filtered bicarbonate and form bicarbonate when needed to restore balance. Bicarbonate is formed when acids and ammonium combine with extra ions (Hanna, Scheinman, & Chan, 1995). The blood bicarbonate concentration is an indicator of the amount of metabolic acids present, since bicarbonate is used in buffering the acids (see Table 39–6). When the concentration is normal, metabolic acids are present in usual amounts (see "Pathophysiology Illustrated: The Kidneys and Metabolic Acids").

In a healthy child, the result of these renal processes is excretion of metabolic acids and maintenance of blood bicarbonate concentration within normal limits. However, a child whose kidneys are not producing enough urine may be unable to excrete metabolic acids effectively. Accumulation of these acids uses up many of the available bicarbonate buffers, resulting in a decreased serum bicarbonate concentration.

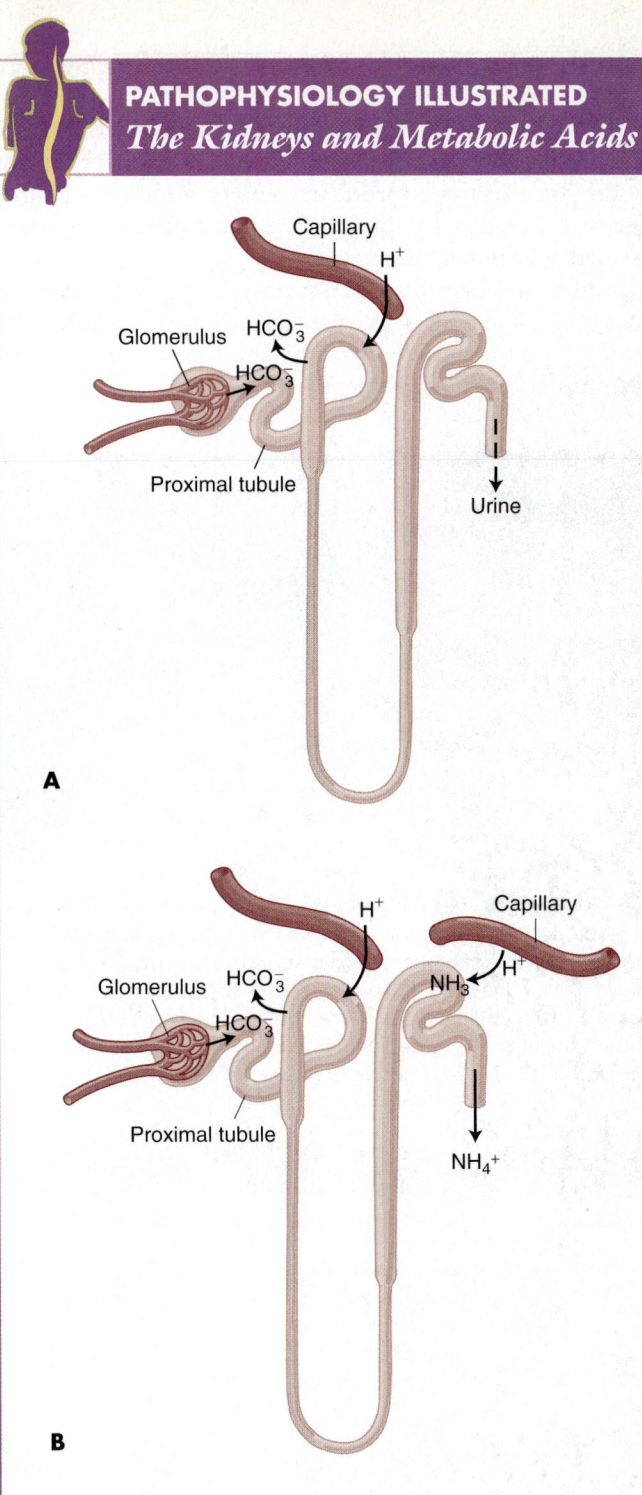

A

B

A, Recycling of bicarbonate by the kidneys. Bicarbonate ions that are in the blood are filtered into the renal tubules at the glomerulus. In the proximal tubules, bicarbonate ions are reabsorbed into the blood at the same time that hydrogen ions are transported from the blood into the renal tubular fluid. **B,** Secretion and buffering of hydrogen ions in the kidneys. If the urine is too acidic, the cells that line the urinary tract could be damaged. To prevent this problem, hydrogen ions secreted into the distal tubules are neutralized by phosphate buffers or bound to ammonia and excreted in the form of ammonium ions.

ROLE OF THE LIVER

The liver also plays a role in maintaining acid-base balance by metabolizing protein, which produces hydrogen ions. It also synthesizes proteins needed to maintain osmotic pressures in the fluid compartments.

ACID-BASE IMBALANCES

There are four acid-base imbalances. Two are the result of processes that cause too much acid in the body and are referred to as **acidosis.** The other two are the result of processes that cause too little acid in the body and are called **alkalosis** (Noble, 1999). An acid-base disorder caused by too much or too little carbonic acid is called a respiratory acid-base imbalance. A disorder caused by too much or too little metabolic acid is called a metabolic acid-base imbalance. CD

Nursing Practice

Acidosis: Relatively too much acid in the body
  Respiratory acidosis: Relatively too much carbonic acid
  Metabolic acidosis: Relatively too much metabolic acid

Alkalosis: Relatively too little acid in the body
  Respiratory alkalosis: Relatively too little carbonic acid
  Metabolic alkalosis: Relatively too little metabolic acid

Arterial blood gas measurements (ABGs) provide a laboratory evaluation of a child's current acid-base status. Table 39–15 provides a method that can help interpret the pH, Pco_2, and bicarbonate concentrations, the most important acid-base measures. End-tidal CO_2 can provide a continuous noninvasive measurement. (Remember that Pco_2 reflects carbonic acid status, and bicarbonate concentration reflects the metabolic acid status.)

RESPIRATORY ACIDOSIS

Respiratory acidosis is caused by the accumulation of carbon dioxide in the blood. Since carbon dioxide and water can be combined into carbonic acid, respiratory acidosis is sometimes called carbonic acid excess. The condition can be acute or chronic. It is controlled by the lungs.

Etiology and Pathophysiology

Any factor that interferes with the ability of the lungs to excrete carbon dioxide can cause respiratory acidosis. These factors may interfere with the gaseous exchange within the lungs, may impair the neuromuscular pump that moves air

TABLE 39-15 How to Interpret Arterial Blood Gas Measurements

Ask the following questions to analyze blood gas results.

1. **What is the pH?** If the pH is normal, the child has no imbalance or has compensated for an imbalance. If the pH is below normal, the child has acidosis. If the pH is above normal, the child has alkalosis.

2. **What is the Pco_2?** If the Pco_2 is normal, the child does not have an acid-base imbalance. If the Pco_2 is above normal, the child has respiratory acidosis. This may be the primary disorder or may be a compensatory response to metabolic alkalosis. Looking at the bicarbonate concentration helps you decide. If the Pco_2 is below normal, the child has respiratory alkalosis. Again, this can be the primary disorder or may be a compensatory response to metabolic acidosis.

3. **What is the bicarbonate concentration?** If the bicarbonate concentration is within normal range, the child does not have a metabolic acid-base imbalance. If the bicarbonate is above normal, the child has metabolic alkalosis. This can be a primary disorder or can be compensatory in respiratory acidosis. When bicarbonate is below normal, the child has metabolic acidosis, either as a direct disorder or as a compensatory response to respiratory alkalosis.

4. **What do the results together tell you?** If the pH is abnormal and either the Pco_2 or bicarbonate concentration is normal, there is an uncompensated acid-base disorder. If all three values are abnormal, the child has a partially compensated disorder and the pH will provide the definitive answer. If Pco_2, pH, and bicarbonate are all decreased, then partially compensated metabolic acidosis is most likely. If pH is normal and Pco_2 and bicarbonate are abnormal, there is a fully compensated acid-base disorder.

5. **What are the child's history and clinical signs?** Does your interpretation fit with what you know about the child's medical condition and with assessments you are making? This last step helps you to integrate laboratory data with the clinical picture to strengthen your nursing care of the child with an acid-base imbalance.

in and out of the lungs, or may depress the respiratory rate (Table 39–16; Figure 39–10 ◆).

As the Pco_2 begins to increase, the pH of the blood begins to decrease. Compensatory mechanisms begin to act in the form of nonbicarbonate buffers, additional hydrogen ion excretion by the kidneys, and formation and decreased bicarbonate excretion by the kidneys. These compensatory mechanisms take several days to become active so the child manifests a changing clinical situation, depending on the underlying cause and the amount of compensation occurring (Table 39–17).

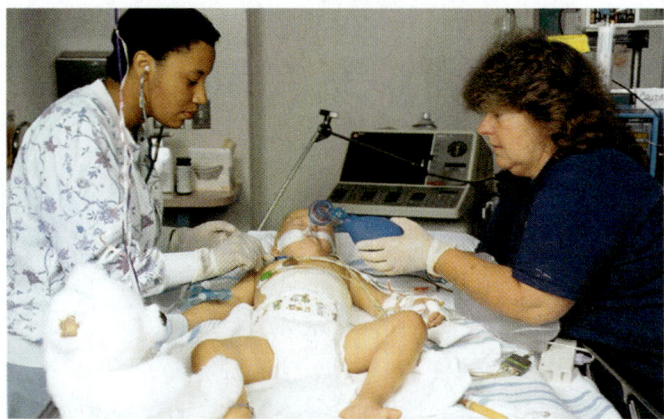

FIGURE 39–10. ◆ This child may develop respiratory acidosis or respiratory alkalosis. If the tidal volume is set too low during mechanical ventilation, carbon dioxide (carbonic acid) will accumulate in the body (respiratory acidosis) because it is not being excreted by the lungs. If the tidal volume is set too high, carbon dioxide will be depleted in the body (respiratory alkalosis) because it is being excreted in great quantities.

TABLE 39-16 Causes of Respiratory Acidosis

Factors Affecting the Lungs	Factors Affecting the Neuromuscular Pump	Factors Affecting Central Control of Respiration
Aspiration	Flail chest	Sedative overdose
Spasm of the airways	Pneumothorax or hemothorax	General anesthesia
Laryngeal edema	Mechanical underventilation	Head injury
Epiglottitis	Hypokalemic muscle weakness	Brain tumor
Croup	High cervical spinal cord injury	Central sleep apnea
Pulmonary edema	Botulism	
Atelectasis	Tetanus	
Severe pneumonia	Kyphoscoliosis	
Cystic fibrosis	Poliomyelitis	
Bronchopulmonary dysplasia	Muscular dystrophy	
Pulmonary embolism	Congenital diaphragmatic hernia	
	Guillain-Barré syndrome	

TABLE 39-17 Laboratory Values in Uncompensated and Compensated Respiratory Acidosis

	Pco_2	pH	HCO_3
Uncompensated	Increased	Decreased	Normal
Partially compensated	Increased	Decreasing but moving toward normal	Increasing
Fully compensated	Increased	Normal	Increased

Clinical Manifestations

Acidosis in the brain cells causes central nervous system depression, manifested by confusion, lethargy, headache, increased intracranial pressure, and even coma (Behrman, Kliegman, & Jenson, 2000). Acute respiratory acidosis can lead to tachycardia and cardiac arrhythmias. The child's arterial blood gases always show an increased Pco_2, the laboratory sign of increased carbonic acid. Serum pH can be decreased or normal.

Clinical Therapy

Treatment of respiratory acidosis requires correction of the underlying cause. For example, treatment may include bronchodilators for bronchospasm, mechanical ventilation for neuromuscular defects, decreasing sedative use, or surgery for kyphoscoliosis.

Nursing Management

Nursing Assessment and Diagnosis

Nursing assessment plays a pivotal role in decisions about interventions for respiratory acidosis. This is especially true in chronic conditions such as cystic fibrosis and kyphoscoliosis. Assess respiratory rate, rhythm, and depth carefully. Take the apical pulse and be alert for tachycardia or arrhythmia. A cardiac monitor may be used. Obtain serial arterial blood gas measurements in acute conditions to evaluate changing status. Assess the level of consciousness and energy. Observe for chronic fatigue, headache, or decreased level of consciousness.

Several nursing diagnoses may apply to the child with respiratory acidosis. The most important addresses the child's risk for injury. Other nursing diagnoses depend on the specific clinical manifestation and the particular cause of the acidosis. Examples include:

▶ *Risk for injury* related to decreased level of consciousness

▶ *Risk for decreased cardiac output* related to cardiac arrhythmias

▶ *Ineffective breathing pattern (hypoventilation)* related to neuromuscular impairment

▶ *Pain (headache)* related to cerebral vasodilation

▶ *Ineffective management of therapeutic regimen* related to complexity of bronchodilator therapy

Planning and Intervention

NURSING CARE IN THE COMMUNITY

Teach children at risk for respiratory acidosis and their parents preventive measures to use at home. For the child with a chronic condition such as cystic fibrosis, muscular dys-

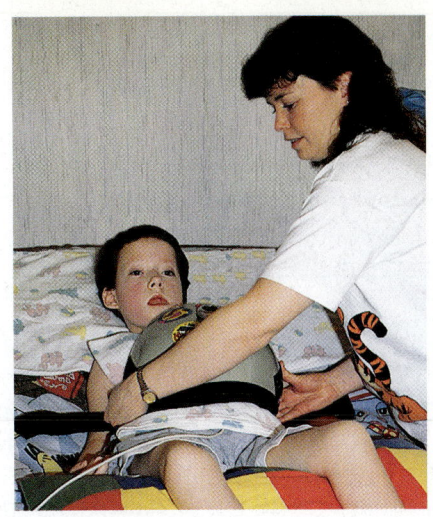

FIGURE 39–11. ◆ This child, who has muscular dystrophy, uses a "turtle" respirator at home to assist with breathing. His parents required instructions from the nurse on use of the respirator. The family has a generator to provide electricity for the respirator during power outages.

trophy, or kyphoscoliosis, demonstrate deep breathing and encourage its use several times each day. Teach the family signs of infection—including fever, increased respiratory secretions, and discomfort with breathing—so these problems can be treated promptly, preventing further respiratory involvement. Position the child to facilitate chest expansion. Teach parents about proper administration of any necessary medications. For example, the child with cystic fibrosis may receive antibiotics to prevent respiratory infections. Teach parents and older children about home respirator use (Figure 39–11 ◆).

Growth and Development

It is usually difficult to get a young child to do deep breathing or to use the "blow bottle" that is often given to older children and adults. To make deep breathing fun, use a pinwheel and have the child turn it during play. Alternatively, give a child a straw and have him or her blow bubbles in a glass of water, or have the child use the straw to blow scraps of paper across the bedside table.

HOSPITAL-BASED NURSING CARE

For the hospitalized child, the focus is on ensuring safety. Keep side rails raised, and turn and position the child frequently. Evaluate mental status and document and report any changes in alertness. When laboratory values of blood pH and Pco_2 are available, evaluate them promptly and report any changes or abnormalities. Administer medications as ordered. Carefully watch the doses of sedatives to avoid further respiratory depression. Provide suctioning and encourage deep breathing.

Evaluation

Expected outcomes of nursing care for the child with respiratory acidosis include the following:

▶ Maintenance of safety

▶ Adequate rate and rhythm of respirations

▶ Management of causative disorders

RESPIRATORY ALKALOSIS

Respiratory alkalosis occurs when the blood contains too little carbon dioxide. It is sometimes called carbonic acid deficit.

Excess carbon dioxide loss is caused by hyperventilation, in which more air than normal is moved into and out of the lungs. Some common causes of hyperventilation are hypoxemia, anxiety, pain, fever, salicylate poisoning, meningitis, and septicemia.

In many cases, respiratory alkalosis lasts for several hours only. Renal compensation does not occur, as these compensatory mechanisms take several days to begin action. An example is the hyperventilation that occurs with acute anxiety. If the condition persists, however, the kidneys will begin to retain more acid and excrete more bicarbonate. Hydrogen ions will be released from body buffers to decrease plasma bicarbonate. While the imbalance continues, cellular function is thus protected by returning pH to normal levels (Table 39–18).

Arterial blood gas measurements show a decreased Pco_2 in respiratory alkalosis. Blood pH is generally elevated. The lack of carbon dioxide causes neuromuscular irritability and paresthesias in the extremities and around the mouth. Muscle cramping and carpal or pedal spasms can occur. The child may be dizzy or confused.

Medical management focuses on correcting the condition that caused the hyperventilation so that the body's compensatory mechanisms can return carbon dioxide levels to normal.

Nursing Management

Assess the child's level of consciousness and ask if the child feels light-headed or has tingling sensations or numbness in the fingers, toes, or around the mouth. Assess the rate and depth of respirations. Monitor the hospitalized child's Po_2 with serial arterial blood gas measurements to evaluate changes in status. Make a careful assessment about the cause of hyperventilation. Did an occurrence cause anxiety for the child? Is the child in pain (see Chapter 38)? Has the child received salicylates in any form? Is the child mechanically ventilated? Is there a central nervous system infection such as meningitis?

Nursing Practice

Check the Po_2 before any therapy for respiratory alkalosis is started, because it is dangerous to stop hyperventilation if oxygenation is poor.

Planning and Implementation

Nursing care for the child with respiratory alkalosis centers on teaching stress management techniques, maintaining pain control, promoting respiratory function, ensuring safety, maintaining fluid status, and providing health supervision and home care.

TEACH STRESS MANAGEMENT TECHNIQUES

When anxiety is the cause of respiratory alkalosis, instruct the child to breathe slowly; demonstrate the rhythm. Use a calm voice, stuffed toys, and supportive reassurance. Teach stress control techniques such as relaxation and imagery for situations that cause anxiety.

MAINTAIN PAIN CONTROL

Use medications, imagery, distraction, positioning, massage, and other techniques to decrease pain and maintain pain management. Chapter 38 describes these and other measures to assist with pain control.

PROMOTE RESPIRATORY FUNCTION

Have the child cough, or suction as needed. Be certain that mechanical ventilation systems are working properly.

ENSURE SAFETY

Provide a safe environment for the child who has a decreased level of consciousness. Be sure the child is supervised when sitting or standing up. Keep bed rails up.

REGULATE FLUID STATUS

Renal compensation to manage ongoing respiratory alkalosis requires adequate urinary output. Regulate fluid intake to ensure urine output unless fluids are restricted due to medical condition.

TABLE 39–18 Laboratory Values in Uncompensated and Compensated Respiratory Alkalosis			
	Pco_2	pH	HCO_3
Uncompensated	Decreased	Increased	Normal
Partially compensated	Decreased	Increased but moving toward normal	Decreasing
Fully compensated	Decreased	Normal	Decreased

Teach parents to keep aspirin and other salicylate products out of reach of children, preferably in a locked medicine box. Instruct parents to keep syrup of ipecac in their homes and how to use it. Provide stickers with the number of the Poison Control Center.

Evaluation

Expected outcomes of nursing care for the child with respiratory alkalosis include the following:

▶ Normal respiratory rate and rhythm
▶ Maintenance of safety
▶ Regulation of fluid status

METABOLIC ACIDOSIS

Metabolic acidosis is a condition in which there is an excess of any acid other than carbonic acid. For this reason, it is sometimes called noncarbonic acid excess.

Etiology and Pathophysiology

Metabolic acidosis is caused by an imbalance in production and excretion of acid or by excess loss of bicarbonate. Excess accumulation occurs by one of two mechanisms. First, a child can eat or drink acids or substances that are converted to acid in the body. Examples include aspirin, boric acid, and antifreeze. Second, cells can make abnormally high amounts of acid that cannot be excreted. This is the case in ketoacidosis of untreated diabetes mellitus, untreated growth hormone deficiency (Glaser, Shirali, Styne, et al., 1998), bladder construction that uses part of the bowel (Mundy, 1999), or the starvation that can occur in anorexia or bulimia. A disorder of excretion occurs in conditions such as oliguric renal failure (Figure 39–12).

The body can lose bicarbonate through the urine or through excessive loss of intestinal fluid. Diarrhea, fistulas, and ileal drainage are all possible sources. Carbonic anhydrase inhibitors can cause loss of excess bicarbonate in the urine.

Below-normal pH of the blood stimulates the chemoreceptors in the brain and arteries and respiratory compensation begins. The child's rate and depth of breathing increase and carbonic acid is removed from the body. The blood pH shifts to a more normal range even though the cause is not corrected. The underlying condition and the degree of compensation alter the clinical laboratory values observed (Table 39–19).

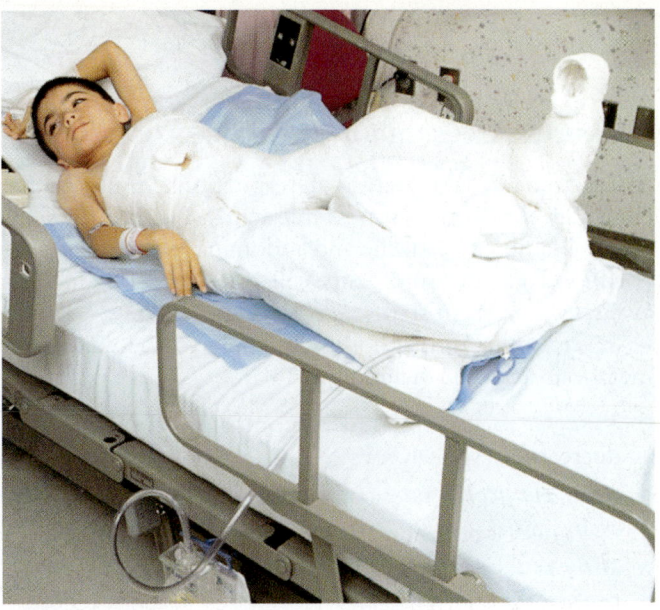

FIGURE 39–12. ◆ With any postoperative or immobilized child, it is important to monitor urine output to detect oliguria. If the kidneys do not produce very much urine, the metabolic acids accumulate in the body and cause metabolic acidosis. Inadequate fluid intake in the postoperative or immobilized child can lead to oliguria and, potentially, metabolic acidosis.

Clinical Manifestations

Laboratory values show decreased blood pH and decreased HCO_3 and Pco_2. An attempt at respiratory compensation causes one of the most important signs of metabolic acidosis, increased rate and depth of respirations (hyperventilation) or **Kussmaul respirations.** Severe acidosis can cause decreased peripheral vascular resistance and resultant cardiac arrhythmias, hypotension, pulmonary edema, and tissue hypoxia. Confusion or drowsiness may result, as well as headache or abdominal pain.

Clinical Therapy

Treatment of metabolic acidosis depends on identification and treatment of the underlying cause. In severe metabolic acidosis, intravenous sodium bicarbonate may be used to increase the pH and to prevent cardiac arrhythmias. This treatment is difficult to manage, because renal excretion can cause excess retention of bicarbonate; therefore, intravenous sodium bicarbonate is used only in severe situations, such as prolonged cardiac arrest.

TABLE 39–19	Laboratory Values in Uncompensated and Compensated Metabolic Acidosis		
	HCO_3	pH	Pco_2
Uncompensated	Decreased	Decreased	Normal
Partially compensated	Decreased	Decreased but moving	Decreasing

Nursing Management

Nursing Assessment and Diagnosis

Assess the rate and depth of respirations. Evaluate the child's level of consciousness frequently. Be alert for signs or complaints of headache and abdominal pain. Serial arterial blood gas measurements will usually be obtained to evaluate changes in status.

Several nursing diagnoses can apply to the child with metabolic acidosis, including:

▶ *Risk for injury* related to confusion/drowsiness or decreased responsiveness

▶ *Risk for decreased cardiac output* related to cardiac arrhythmias

▶ *Altered tissue perfusion: cerebral* related to tissue hypoxia

▶ *Ineffective management of therapeutic regimen* related to complexity of management of diabetes mellitus

Planning and Implementation

Ensure safety, taking into account the child's level of consciousness and alertness. Turn the child and change his or her position to prevent pressure on the skin. Limit the child's activities to decrease cardiac workload.

Position the child to facilitate chest expansion. Provide oral care during rapid respirations since the mouth may become dry.

Monitor intravenous solutions and laboratory values indicating acid-base balance. Report changes promptly.

Once the child is stabilized, provide teaching to compensate for knowledge deficits. Teach parents of young children to keep medications and acids locked up and out of reach to prevent poisoning (Figure 39–13 ◆). This includes medicines with aspirin as well as substances commonly kept in the garage for car maintenance. Teach about home management of diabetes and about early identification and treatment to avoid diabetic ketoacidosis. Expected outcomes of nursing care relate to prevention of acidosis and restoration of normal body balance during disease processes.

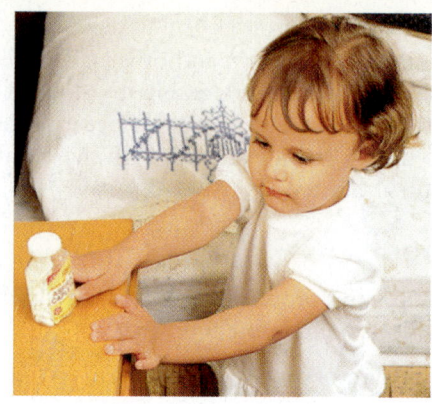

FIGURE 39–13. ◆ Teaching parents to use safety latches on cabinets to keep aspirin away from small children can help prevent one cause of metabolic acidosis.

METABOLIC ALKALOSIS

Metabolic alkalosis occurs when there are too few metabolic acids. It is sometimes called noncarbonic acid deficit.

A gain in bicarbonate or a loss of metabolic acid can cause metabolic alkalosis. Bicarbonate is gained through excessive intake of bicarbonate antacids or baking soda or through metabolism of bicarbonate precursors such as the citrate contained in blood transfusions. Increased renal absorption of bicarbonate can occur in profound hypokalemia, primary hyperaldosteronism, or extreme deficit in extracellular fluid volume. Acid can be lost through severe vomiting, such as that seen in infants with pyloric stenosis, and through continued removal of gastric contents through suction.

When the chemoreceptors in the brain and arteries detect the rising pH of metabolic alkalosis and respirations decrease, the body retains carbonic acid. This carbonic acid can neutralize the bicarbonate and return pH toward normal.

Blood pH, bicarbonate, and P_{CO_2} are usually elevated in metabolic alkalosis (Table 39–20). Hypokalemia often occurs simultaneously (refer to p. 951 to review signs of hypokalemia). Respiratory rate and depth usually decrease. Increased neuromuscular irritability, cramping, paresthesia, tetany, seizures, and excitation can occur. Finally, this state can progress to weakness, confusion, lethargy, and coma.

TABLE 39–20	**Laboratory Values in Uncompensated and Compensated Metabolic Alkalosis**		
	HCO_3	pH	P_{CO_2}
Acute condition; uncompensated	Increased	Increased	Normal
Partially compensated	Increased	Increased but moving toward normal	Increasing
Fully compensated	The need for oxygen drives respirations and limits full compensation for metabolic alkalosis.		

Clinical therapy is directed at treating the underlying cause of the condition. Increasing the extracellular fluid volume with intravenous normal saline facilitates renal excretion of bicarbonate.

Nursing Management

Assess the child's level of consciousness frequently. Alertness may decrease after an initial period of excitement, so regular assessments are needed. Monitor neuromuscular irritability. Observe for nausea and vomiting. Assess the rate and depth of respirations carefully. Obtain serial arterial blood gas measurements as ordered.

Facilitate ease of respirations. Ensure safety by keeping bed rails elevated and by turning the child frequently. Position the child on the side to avoid aspiration of vomitus.

If antacids were the cause of the alkalosis, teach the child and parents about correct use of these medications.

MIXED ACID-BASE IMBALANCES

It is possible for two acid-base imbalances to occur at the same time. For example, a child with cystic fibrosis can develop respiratory acidosis from lung problems and concurrent metabolic alkalosis from vomiting during an illness. Treatment with diuretics may cause concurrent metabolic alkalosis resulting from extracellular volume depletion and hypokalemia in a child with congestive heart failure and chronic respiratory acidosis. In these cases, all underlying causes must be identified and treated. Care of children with mixed acid-base imbalances is often complicated, requiring hospitalization and careful management. Upon discharge, the nurse can teach parents about signs of imbalance that need to be reported and treated in order to prevent further complications. Evaluation of care is based on outcomes of adequate respiratory ventilation and metabolic balance.

CHAPTER HIGHLIGHTS

➤ Young children are at risk for fluid and electrolyte imbalance due to differences in body fluid compartments and regulation systems.

➤ Extracellular fluid volume deficit manifests as dehydration.

➤ Extracellular fluid volume excess is due to an excess of saline in the body.

➤ Interstitial fluid volume excess manifests as edema and weight gain.

➤ Nurses carefully manage fluid status of young children and teach parents prevention and treatment of fluid imbalances caused by gastroenteritis.

➤ The most common electrolyte imbalances involve sodium and potassium.

➤ Normal acid-base balance is necessary for proper function of cells in the body.

➤ The lungs, kidneys, and liver all play a role in maintaining acid-base balance.

➤ Acid-base imbalance can involve alkalosis or acidosis; either can have a respiratory or metabolic origin.

EXPLOREMEDIALINK

NCLEX Review, Case Studies, and other interactive resources for this chapter can be found on the companion website at http://www.prenhall.com/london. Click on "Chapter 39" and select the activities for this chapter.

For animations, more NCLEX review questions, and an audio glossary, access the accompanying CD-ROM in this textbook.

REFERENCES

Aker, J., & O'Sullivan, C. (1998). The selection and administration of perioperative intravenous fluids for the pediatric patient. *Journal of PeriAnesthesia Nursing, 13,* 172–181.

Askin, D. F. (1997a). Interpretation of neonatal blood gases, Part I: Physiology and acid-base homeostasis. *Neonatal Network, 16,* 17–21.

Askin, D. F. (1997b). Interpretation of neonatal blood gases, Part II: Disorders of acid-base balance. *Neonatal Network, 16,* 23–29.

Bar-Or, O. (1996). Water and electrolyte replenishment in the exercising child. *International Journal of Sport Nutrition, 6,* 93–99.

Behrman, R. E., Kliegman, R. M., & Jenson, H. B. (Eds.). (2000). *Nelson textbook of pediatrics* (16th ed.). Philadelphia: WB Saunders.

Burkhart, D. M. (1999). Management of acute gastroenteritis in children. *American Family Physician, 60,* 2555–2563.

Committee on Sports Medicine and Fitness. (2000). Climatic heat stress and the exercising child and adolescent. *Pediatrics, 106,* 158–159.

Davenport, M. (1996). Pediatric fluid balance. *Care of the Chronically Ill Child, 12*(1), 26–28, 30–31.

Dabbagh, S., Ellis, D., & Gruskin, A. B. (1996). In E. K. Motoyama, & P. J. Davis (Eds.). *Smith's Anesthesia for Infants and Children* (6th ed.) p. 105–137. St. Louis: Mosby-Yearbook.

Eliason, B. C., & Lewan, R. B. (1998). Gastroenteritis in children: Principles of diagnosis and treatment. *American Family Physician, 58,* 1769–1776.

Endsley, S., & Galbraith, A. (1998). Are you overlooking oral rehydration therapy in childhood diarrhea? *Postgraduate Medicine, 104,* 159–166, 171.

Fann, B. D. (1998). Fluid and electrolyte balance in the pediatric patient. *Journal of Intravenous Nursing, 21,* 153–159.

Farrar, H. C., Chande, V. T., Fitzpatrick, D. F., & Shema, S. J. (1995). Hyponatremia as the cause of seizures in infants: A retrospective analysis of incidence, severity, and clinical predictors. *Annals of Emergency Medicine, 26,* 42–48.

Gavin, N., Merrick, N., & Davidson, B. (1996). Efficacy of glucose-based oral rehydration therapy. *Pediatrics, 98,* 45–51.

Glaser, N. S., Shirali, A. C., Styne, D. M., & Jones, K. L. (1998). Acid-base homeostasis in children with growth hormone deficiency. *Pediatrics, 102,* 1407–1414.

Halperin, M. L., & Goldstein, M. B. (1994). *Fluid, electrolyte, and acid-base physiology* (2nd ed., pp. 69–144). Philadelphia: Saunders.

Hanna, J. D., Scheinman, J. I., & Chan, J. C. M. (1995). The kidney in acid-base balance. *Pediatric Clinics of North America, 42,* 1365–1396.

Hewitt-Taylor, J. (1999). Children in intensive care: Physiological considerations. *Nursing in Critical Care, 4,* 40–45.

Johnson, M. D. (1994). Disordered eating in active and athletic women. *Clinics in Sports Medicine, 13,* 355–369.

Jospe, N., & Forbes, G. (1996). Fluids and electrolytes—clinical aspects. *Pediatrics in Review, 17,* 395–404.

Larson, C. E. (2000). Safety and efficacy of oral rehydration therapy for the treatment of diarrhea and gastroenteritis in pediatrics. *Pediatric Nursing, 26,* 177–179.

Livingstone, V. H., Willis, C. E., Abdel-Wareth, L. O., Thiessen, P., & Lockitch, G. (2000). Neonatal hypernatremic dehydration associated with breastfeeding malnutrition: A retrospective survey. *Canadian Medical Association Journal, 162,* 647–652.

Mundy, A. R. (1999). Metabolic complications of urinary diversion. *Lancet, 353,* 1813–1814.

Newman, J. (1996). Decision tree and postpartum management for preventing dehydration in the breastfed baby. *Journal of Human Lactation, 12,* 129–135.

Noble, K. A. (1999, June). Putting the puzzle together: Arterial blood gas interpretation. *Advance for Nurses, 28,* 19–22.

Provisional Committee on Quality Improvement, Subcommittee on Acute Gastroenteritis. (1996). Practice parameter: The management of acute gastroenteritis in young children. *Pediatrics, 97,* 424–436.

Reid, S. R., & Bonadio, W. A. (1996). Outpatient rapid intravenous rehydration to correct dehydration and resolve vomiting in children with acute gastroenteritis. *Annals of Emergency Medicine, 28,* 318–323.

Rivera-Brown, A. M., Gutierrez, R., Gutierrez, J. C., Frontera, W. R., & Bar-Or, O. (1999). Drink composition, voluntary drinking, and fluid balance in exercising, trained, heat-acclimatized boys. *Journal of Applied Physiology, 86,* 78–84.

Shamir, R., Zahavi, I., Abramowich, T., Poraz, I., Tal, D., Pollak, S., et al. (1998). Management of acute gastroenteritis in children in Israel. *Pediatrics, 101,* 892–894.

Siberry, G. K., & Iannone, R. (Eds.). (2000). *Harriet Lane Handbook* (15th ed., p. 249). St. Louis, MO: Mosby.

Snow-Harter, C. M. (1994). Bone health and prevention of osteoporosis in active and athletic women. *Clinics in Sports Medicine, 13,* 389–404.

Straughn, A., & English, B. (1996). Oral rehydration therapy. *American Journal of Maternal Child Nursing, 21,* 144–147.

Vega, R. M., & Avner, J. R. (1997). A prospective study of the usefulness of clinical and laboratory parameters for predicting percentage of dehydration in children. *Pediatric Emergency Care 13,* 179–182.

White, V. M. (1997). Hyperkalemia. *American Journal of Nursing, 97*(6), 35.

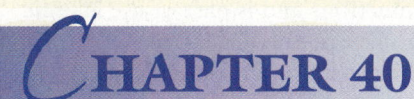

CHAPTER 40

The Child with Alterations in Immune Function

We knew that Raymond might have AIDS—my sister was HIV positive. But we have taken him in as our own child and cared for him. Somehow we thought he would be fine. Now, to get the diagnosis is devastating, especially since my sister is also very ill. We need to learn a lot about how to help him. Can we send him to a preschool next year as we had planned? How will we get money to pay for his medicines? What do we tell other people? How do we get him to eat better? We just don't know where to turn right now.

—Aunt of Raymond, 2 YEARS

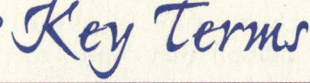

Key Terms

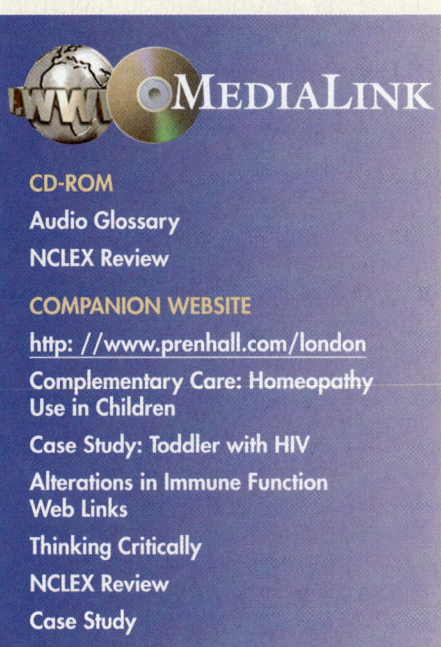

MEDIALINK

CD-ROM

Audio Glossary

NCLEX Review

COMPANION WEBSITE

http://www.prenhall.com/london

Complementary Care: Homeopathy Use in Children

Case Study: Toddler with HIV

Alterations in Immune Function Web Links

Thinking Critically

NCLEX Review

Case Study

*W*hat are the signs and symptoms of immunologic disorders in children? Often they are nonspecific. The immune system is one of the few body systems that regulates, either directly or indirectly, all other body functions. Thus, a problem with the immune system can have multisystem consequences and may be life threatening. Allergic reactions to food or frequent episodes of otitis media may indicate a disorder of immune function. Immune conditions can be mild to severe and life threatening. Congenital abnormalities sometimes signal a defect in cellular immunity. This chapter will examine some of the more common disorders of immune function and discuss nursing care of children who have these diseases and their families.

ANATOMY AND PHYSIOLOGY OF PEDIATRIC DIFFERENCES

The function of the immune system is to recognize any foreign substances within the body—in simple terms, to distinguish "nonself" from "self"—and to eliminate foreign substances as efficiently as possible. Whenever the body recognizes the presence of a substance that it cannot identify as part of itself, the body protects itself through the immune response. Normally, the immune system responds to an invasion of foreign substances, or antigens, in numerous ways. It produces **antibodies,** or proteins that work against **antigens,** the foreign substances that trigger the immune response. There are many types of antibodies, described later in this section. The immune system also produces other types of cells, such as T lymphocytes and natural killer (NK) cells.

Immunity is either natural or acquired. Natural immune defenses are those an infant is born with, such as intact skin, body pH, natural antibodies from the mother, and inflammatory and phagocytic properties. Acquired immunity is composed of humoral (antibody-mediated) and cell-mediated immunity and is not fully developed until a child is about 6 years of age.

Humoral immunity is responsible for destroying bacterial antigens. B lymphocytes, produced in the bone marrow, develop into plasma cells that produce antibodies. Antibodies are a type of protein called **immunoglobulins.** There are five types of immunoglobulins: IgM, IgG, IgA, IgD, and IgE (Table 40–1). IgM, IgG, and IgA act to control a number of body infections, whereas IgE is useful

in combating parasitic infections and is part of the allergic response. The role of IgD is not known.

Antibodies are found in serum, body fluids, and certain tissues. When a child is first exposed to an antigen, the B lymphocyte system begins to produce antibodies that react specifically to that antigen (see "Pathophysiology Illustrated: Primary Immune Response"). It takes approximately 3 days for this process, known as **primary immune response,** to occur. Subsequent encounters with the antigen trigger memory cells, resulting in a **secondary immune response** within 24 hours.

Infants and children have differing amounts of some immunoglobulins. IgG is the only immunoglobulin that crosses the placenta; as a result, a newborn's levels are similar to those of his or her mother. This maternal IgG disappears by 6 to 8 months of age. The infant's IgG then increases gradually until mature levels are reached at 7 to 8 years. IgM levels are low at birth, rise markedly at 1 week of age, and continue to increase until adult levels are reached at about 1 year. IgA and IgE are not present at birth. Manufacture of these immunoglobulins begins by 2 weeks of age; however, normal values are not achieved until 6 to 7 years. It is thus easy to see why children under 6 years of age become ill so often—they do not have a full complement of immunoglobulins.

In contrast, cell-mediated immunity achieves full function early in life. T lymphocytes, produced in the thymus, provide cellular immunity and protect against most viruses, fungi, slowly developing bacterial infections such as tuberculosis, and tumors. In addition, they control the timing of the response in delayed hypersensitivity reactions, such as the purified protein derivative (PPD) test, and they are responsible for the rejection of foreign grafts, such as transplants. For this reason, the blood infused into newborns is generally irradiated to prevent **graft-versus-host disease** (a series of immunologic reactions in response to transplanted cells) from transfused lymphocytes (Stiehm & Ammann, 1997). Specialized types of T lymphocytes include killer T cells, suppressor T cells, and helper T cells. Suppressor T cells inhibit B lymphocytes from differentiating into plasma cells. Helper T cells aid in the proliferation and immunologic function of other cells. T lymphocytes have proteins on their surfaces that can be used to measure the immune activity of these cells. For example, some of the common proteins are CD2, CD3, CD4, CD5, CD7, and CD8.

NK cells (also known as non-B/non-T lymphocytes) originate in the bone marrow and thymus and migrate to the blood and spleen. They play a role in control of viral infection, tumors, and autoimmune disease. Newborns have somewhat lower numbers of NK cells than older children and adults, decreasing their ability to respond to certain antigens.

Complement is a component of blood serum consisting of 11 protein compounds. It is an inactive enzyme that activates in response to antigen–antibody functions, resulting in a generalized inflammatory reaction that kills foreign

TABLE 40–1	**Classes of Immunoglobulins**
IgM	Present in intravascular spaces
IgG	Present in all body fluids
IgA	Present in secretions of gastrointestinal, respiratory, and genitourinary tracts
IgD	Presence and function not yet described
IgE	Present in internal and external body fluids

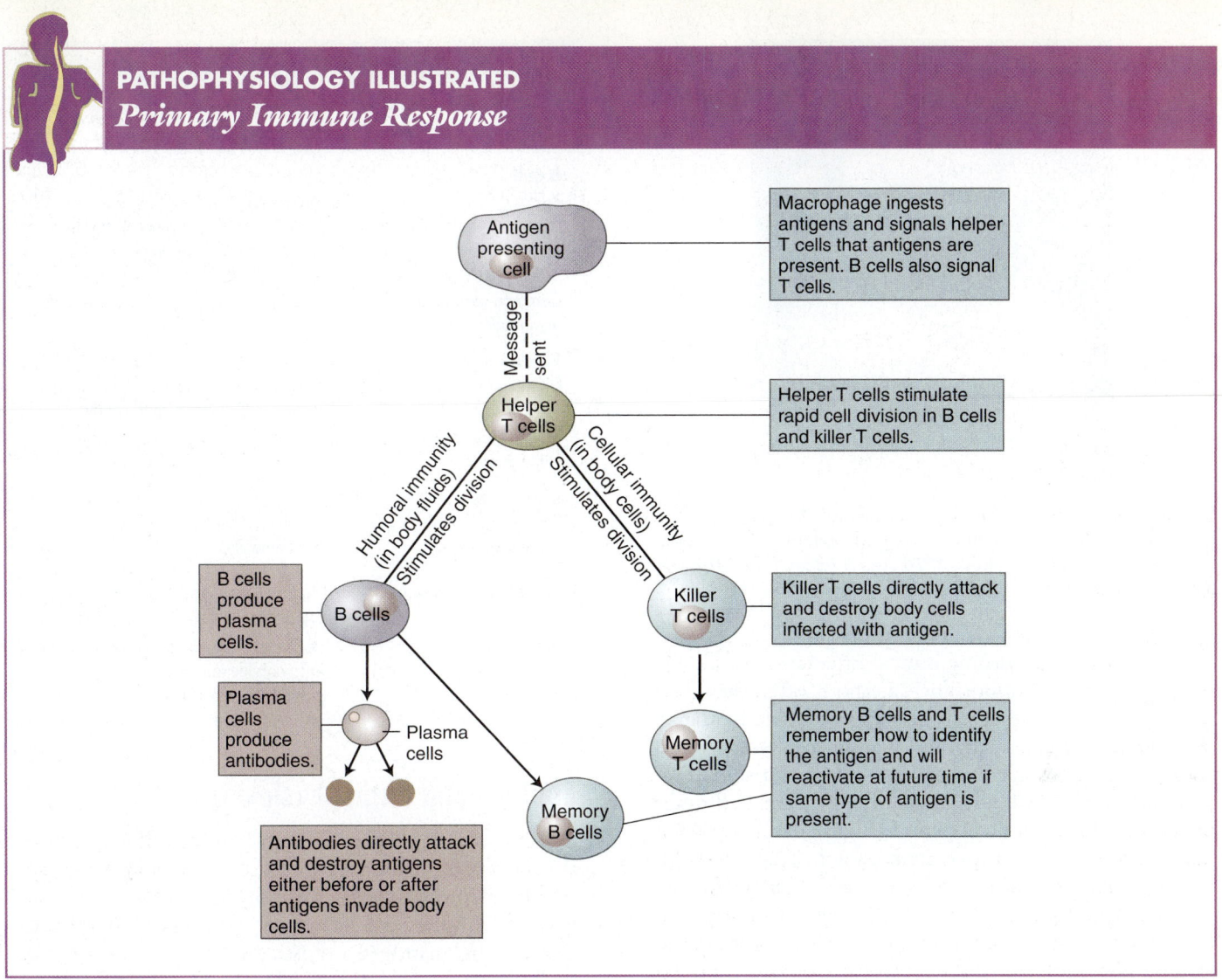

Macrophage ingests antigens and signals helper T cells that antigens are present. B cells also signal T cells.

Helper T cells stimulate rapid cell division in B cells and killer T cells.

Killer T cells directly attack and destroy body cells infected with antigen.

Memory B cells and T cells remember how to identify the antigen and will reactivate at future time if same type of antigen is present.

B cells produce plasma cells.

Plasma cells produce antibodies.

Antibodies directly attack and destroy antigens either before or after antigens invade body cells.

cells. It also plays a role in causing some autoimmune diseases. The levels of some of the complement proteins are lower in newborns than in older children and adults, thus delaying and hampering response to certain infections.

IMMUNODEFICIENCY DISORDERS

Immunodeficiency, a state of decreased responsiveness of the immune system, can occur to varying degrees in response to any number of events. Children with congenital immunodeficiency, or **primary immune deficiency,** are born with a failure of humoral antibody formation (B-cell disorder), a deficient cellular immune system (T-cell disorder), or a combination of both defects. In congenital disorders, the immune deficiency is not caused by another condition. However, immunodeficiency may also be acquired, as in human immunodeficiency virus (HIV) infection. Acquired immunodeficiency is also called **secondary immune deficiency.**

B-CELL AND T-CELL DISORDERS

In B-cell disorders, immunoglobulins may be present in inadequate numbers or nearly absent. X-linked hypogammaglobulinemia, selective IgA deficiency, and common variable immunodeficiency are examples of such disorders. Because newborns are protected from infection by maternal antibodies in the first months after birth, symptoms of B-cell disorders usually become apparent after 3 months of age. Infants with these disorders have frequent recurrent bacterial infections and failure to thrive. With treatment, consisting of intravenous immunoglobulins and antibiotics, most children survive into adulthood. Prognosis depends on the degree of antibody deficiency.

T-cell disorders are characterized by inadequate numbers of T lymphocytes or absence of T-cell functions. Isolated T-cell disorders are rare, usually accompanied by B-cell disorder, and may be associated with congenital abnormalities (as in DiGeorge syndrome) or of unknown

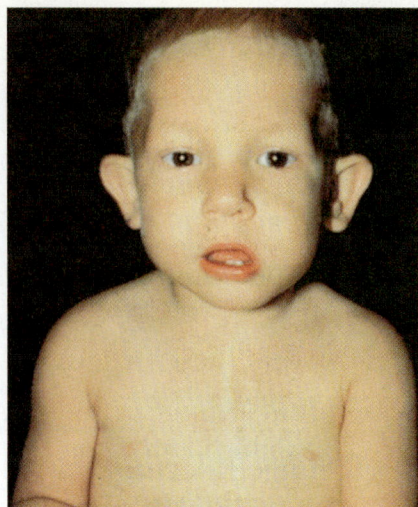

FIGURE 40–1. ◆ This boy has characteristic features of DiGeorge syndrome. Note the low-set and malformed ears. *Note:* From Zitelli, B. J., & Davis, H. W. (Eds.). (1997). *Atlas of Pediatric Physical Diagnosis* 3rd ed., (p. 101, Figure 4–42a). St. Louis, Mosby.

cause. DiGeorge syndrome is most often accompanied by abnormalities in chromosome 22, and is often diagnosed soon after birth. The syndrome is characterized by the absence of parathyroid or thymus glands, resultant hypocalcemia, cardiac defects, low-set ears, hypertelorism (widely set eyes), tetany 48 hours after birth, and viral and fungal infections in the neonatal period (Figure 40–1 ◆). Pneumonia and failure to thrive are common, and T-lymphocyte counts are often <1500/mm³ for CD3 and <1000/mm³ for CD4 cells (Elder, 2000). Children with the disorder are treated with antibiotics for prophylaxis against pneumonia from *Pneumocystis carinii*, oral calcium, thymus transplantation, and HLA-identical bone marrow transplantation. Without thymus transplantation, few children survive beyond 5 years.

Immunodeficiency with hyper-IgM is a T-cell disorder that affects mainly males and causes decreased T-cell function, variable abnormal levels of immunoglobulins, and high titers of some antibodies. It is usually X-linked but is sometimes autosomal. Treatment with intravenous immune globulin (IVIG) therapy is helpful although later malignancies and liver disease can occur (Schwartz, 2000).

Refer to Table 40–2, which compares laboratory values for selected congenital immunodeficiency disorders.

SEVERE COMBINED IMMUNODEFICIENCY DISEASE

Severe combined immunodeficiency disease (SCID) is a congenital condition characterized by absence of both humoral and cellular immunity. SCID occurs in X-linked recessive, autosomal recessive, and sporadic forms. Without appropriate treatment, children born with SCID usually die within the first 2 years of life.

TABLE 40–2 Selected Congenital Immunodeficiency Disorders

Disorders	Laboratory Findings
B cell	
X-linked hypogammaglobulinemia	Reduced IgA, IgM, IgE, IgG (< 100 mg/dL), absence of B cells in peripheral blood, normal T cells
Selective IgA deficiency	IgA < 10 mg/dL
Common variable immunodeficiency	IgA, IgM reduced; IgG < 250 mg/dL
T cell	
DiGeorge syndrome	Lymphopenia; absent T-cell functions, decreased T cells, normal B cells
X-linked immunodeficiency with hyper-IgM	Reduced IgG, IgA; elevated IgM; mutations in T-cell surface proteins
Combined	
Severe combined immunodeficiency syndrome (SCID)	Complete absence of T- and B-cell and NK immunity
Wiskott–Aldrich syndrome	Thrombocytopenia, low platelet volume, nonfunctional B-cells, normal IgG, decreased IgM, increased IgA, increased IgE; inability to respond to polysaccharide antigens

Etiology and Pathophysiology

SCID is caused by genetic mutations of cellular receptors to interleukin. The mutations lead to impaired lymphoid development in children with low T and NK cells. The B lymphocytes may appear normal in number but are defective in performance (Candotti, 2000).

Clinical Manifestations

Symptoms of SCID develop early in life. The neonate often demonstrates a susceptibility to infection by 3 months of age. The disorder is characterized by chronic infection (such as otitis media or pneumonia), failure to completely recover from infection, frequent reinfection, and infection with viruses such as cytomegalovirus and the bacterium *Pneumocystis carinii*. Often the first infection seen is a resistant oral candidiasis. Children are also highly susceptible to serious infections like meningitis, skin or organ infection, osteomyelitis, or sepsis. Failure to thrive is a consequence of persistent illness.

Some infants experience graft-versus-host disease as a result of placental transfer of maternal T lymphocytes. If the child receives foreign tissue, for example, in a blood transfusion, signs such as skin rash, fever, hepatosplenomegaly, and diarrhea may occur.

Clinical Therapy

A marked reduction in lymphocyte counts is indicative of SCID. B and T lymphocytes are generally few in number

TABLE 40-3 Cells Evaluated in Laboratory Studies for Immune Conditions

Test and Type of Cell Evaluated	Action	Implication of Increased or Decreased Levels
White blood cell (WBC) count		
Neutrophil	Phagocytic cell that defends against bacteria	Increased in bacterial infection, inflammatory processes, and some malignancies
Eosinophil	Associated with antigen–antibody reaction	Increased in allergic reaction; decreased in children receiving corticosteroids
Lymphocytes (T, B, non-B/non-T [NK])	Major components of immune system	Increased in many infections; decreased in children with immune deficiency
Immunoglobulins (IgM, IgG, IgA, IgD, IgE)	Many roles in a number of immunologic reactions	Increased in presence of infection or allergic response; decreased in children with immune deficiency

or absent from the peripheral blood and lymphoid tissues. In some cases, the B-lymphocyte count may be elevated, although these cells do not function normally. NK cells are few in number. Immunoglobulin levels are significantly reduced. Refer to Table 40–2 for laboratory findings in SCID. Diagnosis is usually made only after extensive laboratory testing. In addition to a complete blood count, erythrocyte sedimentation rate, and B- and T-cell lymphocyte counts, other studies including IgA, IgG, and IgM antibody titers to immunizations received and neutrophil count may be performed (see Table 40–3).

The goal of medical management is to restore immune function. Thymic hormones have been given to some children with limited success. IVIG may be administered. Bone marrow transplantation offers hope for children with SCID (see Chapter 45). However, the donor must be a histocompatible donor, such as a sibling. The marrow transplantation corrects T-cell function, and new cells appear 3 to 4 months after infusion of the donor marrow. With the identification of the genetic defect for SCID in recent years, gene transfer has been successfully attempted in a small number of children. This experimental therapy will likely be used more often in the future (Candotti, 2000).

Prognosis is poor without aggressive therapy. Some children have survived 10 years after a successful bone marrow transplant.

Nursing Management

Nursing Assessment and Diagnosis

Obtain a thorough history of infections, including age of onset, type of causal organism, frequency, and severity. Take a family history, and find out if the child has had any unusual reactions to vaccines, medications, or foods. Measure the child's height and weight accurately to identify failure to thrive. Look for any evidence of infections involving the skin, subcutaneous tissues, respiratory system, and mucous membranes. Palpate the abdomen for hepatomegaly and the lymph nodes for lymphadenopathy.

Assess family support systems and coping mechanisms when a child is diagnosed with the disorder.

The primary nursing diagnosis for a child with SCID is risk for infection related to immunodeficiency. Other nursing diagnoses may include:

▶ *Risk for altered nutrition: less than body requirements* related to chronic illness

▶ *Risk for impaired skin integrity* related to immunologic deficit

▶ *Risk for caregiver role strain* related to a child with a chronic, life-threatening illness

▶ *Risk for altered growth and development* related to physical disability and chronic illness

Planning and Implementation

Nursing care of the immunodeficient child focuses on preventing infection. However, even with environmental controls, such as keeping children inside special units to maintain a sterile environment, these children are prone to **opportunistic infections** (infections caused by normally nonpathogenic organisms in people who lack normal immunity).

PREVENT SYSTEMIC INFECTION

Frequent and thorough handwashing is important. Always use standard precautions, adding transmission-based precautions when needed. (See the Infection Control Methods chapter in the *Clinical Skills Manual*.) SKILLS Use sterile aseptic technique when caring for all sites where needles, catheters, central lines, endotracheal tubes, pressure-monitoring lines, and peripheral intravenous lines enter the child's body. Food and other items entering the hospital room may need special treatment. The child should have a private room and minimal contact with infectious people.

PROMOTE SKIN INTEGRITY

The skin is the only intact defense that many immunodeficient children have. Provide good skin care, and observe all possible pressure areas closely for signs of breakdown or

TABLE 40-4 Nursing Considerations in the Administration of Intravenous Immune Globulin (IVIG)

Used in treatment of
- Immunodeficiency disease, such as severe combined immunodeficiency and acquired immunodeficiency syndrome (AIDS)
- Antibody deficiency associated with other conditions such as malignancy
- Kawasaki disease

Administration
- IVIG must be administered as stated in the package insert.
- Use separate tubing and do not mix with other medications.
- Start infusion slowly and increase to recommended rate after 30 minutes if no reaction occurs (see below).
- Monitor for hypersensitivity reaction (fever, increased pulse or respiration, decreased blood pressure, chest pain, shaking, chills).
- Schedule immunizations 14 days before or 3 months after IVIG infusion, since immune response will be altered.

Possible adverse reactions
- Headache
- Fever
- Nausea, vomiting
- Arthralgia
- Anaphylaxis

Special types available
- RespiGam (helpful in respiratory syncytial virus)
- CytoGam (enriched with antibodies to cytomegalovirus)

Note: From Lederman, H. M. (1996). IVIG therapy: Separating fact from wishful thinking. *Contemporary Pediatrics, 13,* 75–92. Adapted.

---

infection. Turn the child frequently. Encourage range of motion exercises. Avoid any skin trauma.

MANAGE MEDICATION THERAPY

Many medications used long term in the treatment of children with SCID have numerous side effects. Monitor closely for side effects of antibiotics, such as overgrowth of resistant organisms (e.g., thrush infections in the mouth, *Clostridium difficile* infections of the gastrointestinal tract) and administer IVIG safely (see Table 40–4).

PROVIDE EMOTIONAL SUPPORT AND REFERRAL TO APPROPRIATE SUPPORT GROUPS AND SERVICES

SCID is a life-threatening and devastating disease. Even with aggressive therapy, the prognosis is poor. Evaluate the family's knowledge about the disease. The parents may feel guilt because of the genetic nature of the disease and the difficulties of treatment. Listen closely to their concerns and encourage them to discuss their fears. Refer them to an appropriate support group or counselor if needed. Encourage genetic counseling if the parents plan to have more children.

The family of a child who undergoes bone marrow transplantation requires additional support and referrals. The transplantation procedure involves surgery for both the ill child and the donor, often another child in the fam-

ily. (Refer to the discussion in Chapter 45.) After the infusion of the donor marrow, the ill child will be hospitalized for several months until T-lymphocyte levels are sufficient to provide resistance to infection. During this period, parents may need to rely on social services to help manage the family situation, particularly if the child is hospitalized at a medical center far from the family's home. Assess the family's situation and make appropriate referrals to social services and to support groups. Introduce parents to other families undergoing bone marrow transplantation.

Evaluation

The success of nursing care for the child with SCID is measured by outcomes such as:

▶ Adequate nutritional status as determined by normal growth patterns

▶ Maintenance of intact skin

▶ Adaptive coping by family to demands of a chronic illness

▶ Developmental performance within normal level for age

WISKOTT–ALDRICH SYNDROME

A combined congenital immunodeficiency syndrome, Wiskott–Aldrich syndrome is an X-linked disorder which causes mutation in the WAS gene and changes in WAS protein (Elder, 2000). It is characterized by thrombocytopenia, eczema, hemorrhagic tendencies, and recurrent infections. Thrombocytopenia with bleeding tendencies appears during the neonatal period. Eczema appears by 1 year of age. Infections involve the middle ear and often lead to chronic otitis media. Children are particularly susceptible to infections from herpesviruses and lymphoreticular malignancies, especially of the lymphatic system.

The diagnosis is made in the early neonatal period on the basis of the thrombocytopenia, which leads to petechiae and bleeding (refer to Table 40–2). How and when Wiskott–Aldrich syndrome manifests itself varies, with some children maintaining normal lymphocyte levels for years. Treatment is symptomatic and includes antibiotic prophylaxis together with platelet infusions and sometimes, splenectomy. Without bone marrow transplantation, most children die within the first 5 years of life. Survival beyond adolescence is unusual. Infection, bleeding, or malignancy (leukemia or lymphoma) may be the cause of death (Elder, 2000).

Nursing Management

Nursing care is similar to that for the child with SCID. Refer the parents for genetic counseling to help them understand the transmission of the disease and the probability of having another child with the same disorder. Arrange for psychologic support for parents overwhelmed with guilt from learning that the illness is inherited.

Help the parents and family cope with the knowledge that the child has a chronic and potentially fatal illness. Referral to family counseling may be appropriate. Expected outcomes are return to normal immunologic function or successful coping with a life-threatening illness.

ACQUIRED IMMUNODEFICIENCY SYNDROME

Soon after acquired immunodeficiency syndrome (AIDS) was recognized in homosexual adults and intravenous drug abusers, cases of AIDS were seen in children. Increasing numbers of children infected with HIV have been diagnosed, making HIV infection a leading cause of immune disease in infants and children and a major cause of death in children 1 to 4 years of age. About 7000 children under 5 years are infected, with about 2000 infected children from 5 to 12 years, and about 4000 infected teens. Over 5000 deaths have been reported in children due to AIDS (Centers for Disease Control and Prevention [CDC], 2001).

Most cases of HIV in children—and virtually all new cases—are the result of perinatal transmission. Each year in the United States, approximately 6000 to 7000 infants are born to HIV-infected mothers (Lindegren, Steinberg, & Byers, 2000). **WEB** It is expected and hoped that the number will decrease with new therapies for treating infected women during pregnancy and labor/delivery and their infants after birth. Because of the high rate of transfer from mother to infant, HIV counseling and voluntary testing are encouraged for all pregnant women.

The virus affects multiple systems and eventually destroys the child's immune system (see "Pathophysiology Illustrated: Human Immunodeficiency Virus"). An understanding of the natural history of HIV disease is still evolving, and there are several important differences in the disease progression and clinical manifestations of pediatric and adult HIV infection.

Etiology and Pathophysiology

AIDS is caused by HIV-1. Most children acquire HIV in a form of **vertical transmission** from their mothers transplacentally or during delivery. Transmission can occur during birth from blood, amniotic fluid, and exposure to genital tract secretions, and after birth through breast milk from HIV-positive mothers. However, risk for perinatal transmission has been significantly reduced since mothers identified as infected are now delivered by cesarean, and receive zidovudine (ZDV) during pregnancy (Grosch-Worner, 2000).

HIV has also been transmitted to children through transfusions of infected blood before mandatory screening of blood and blood products was instituted in 1985. Most of these children were infected during treatment of hemophilia.

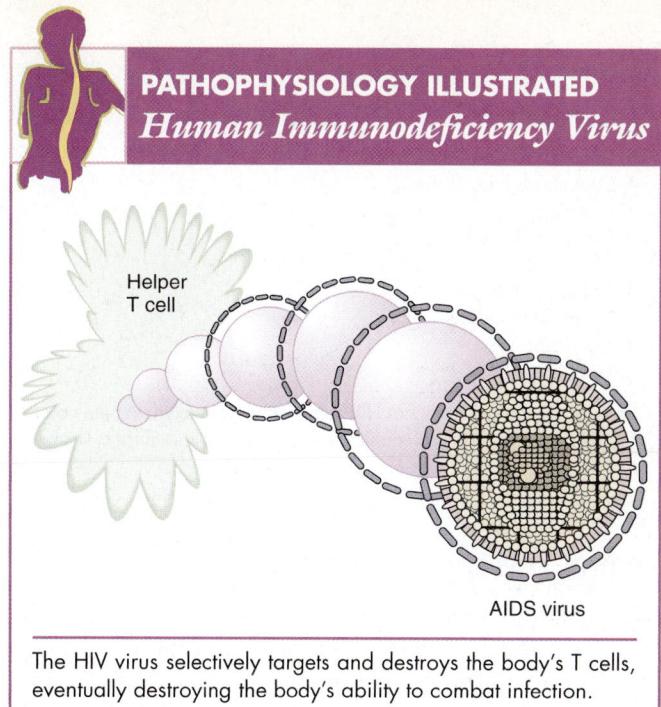

PATHOPHYSIOLOGY ILLUSTRATED
Human Immunodeficiency Virus

The HIV virus selectively targets and destroys the body's T cells, eventually destroying the body's ability to combat infection.

Although 30% of adolescents with AIDS also have hemophilia (with infected blood the expected etiology), adolescents now most commonly acquire the virus through intravenous drug abuse or through unprotected sexual activities.

The HIV virus selectively targets and destroys T cells, thereby decreasing and eventually eliminating cellular immunity. It also affects humoral immunity. Thus, the child is left unprotected against a myriad of bacterial, viral, fungal, and opportunistic infections, which are ultimately fatal. Every organ system can be affected.

Clinical Manifestations

The interval from HIV infection to the onset of overt AIDS is shorter in children than in adults, and shorter in children infected perinatally than in those infected through transfusion. Most children with AIDS have nonspecific findings, including lymphadenopathy, hepatosplenomegaly, nephropathy, oral candidiasis, failure to thrive and weight loss, repeated respiratory infections, diarrhea, chronic eczema and dermatitis, and fever.

Bacterial and opportunistic infections, such as *Streptococcus, Haemophilus influenzae, Salmonella*, and *Pneumocystis carinii* pneumonia (PCP), as well as malignancies such as lymphomas frequently occur as the disease progresses. Children infected with HIV around the time of birth have a higher cancer risk than other children, with the average age of cancer diagnosis at 5 to 6 years (Caselli, 2000). Lymphocytic interstitial pneumonitis is a common manifestation of pediatric AIDS. Frequently, children develop encephalopathy resulting in developmental delay or a deterioration of motor skills and intellectual functioning. Adolescents with HIV infection often are also infected with hepatitis B virus (Rogers, 2000).

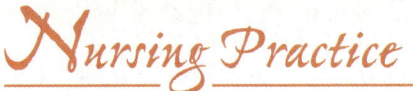

CLINICAL MANIFESTATIONS ❧ HIV

- Chronic, bilateral otitis media
- Oral candidiasis (thrush)
- Pneumocystis carinii pneumonia (PCP)
- Failure to thrive
- Chronic diarrhea
- Hepatosplenomegaly
- Lymphadenopathy
- Skin disorders
- Fever

Be alert for the possibility of HIV infection in infants with some combinations of these clinical manifestations, especially in infants known to be at risk.

Clinical Therapy

Most children with AIDS are diagnosed early in life. Serologic tests for detection of the virus are monitored in infants born to HIV-positive mothers. These tests are performed at birth and repeated at 3 and 6 months. The preferred test is the polymerase chain reaction (PCR); other tests include p24 antigen, or HIV culture (which is not universally available). Any positive result is confirmed by retesting. When the infant has had two negative tests, testing with enzyme-linked immunosorbent assay (ELISA; HIV antibody) should be done at 12, 15, and 18 months. After two consecutive negative results with ELISA, the child is considered free of HIV. In addition, a complete blood count (CBC) and CD4+ T-cell subset is performed at 3 to 6 months. Rapid serologic tests are under study and results are showing promise. Their future use may shorten the diagnosis time and promote better follow-up of potential cases (Nielsen & Bryson, 2000).

The CDC considers children under 13 years of age to be infected if their symptoms meet the CDC criteria for AIDS, if they have HIV in the blood or tissues, or if they have antibodies to HIV. The CDC criteria address two issues: first, the diagnosis of HIV, and second, the clinical classification of children infected with HIV (Table 40–5).

TABLE 40–5 Clinical Staging of Pediatric HIV Infection

Diagnosis of HIV infection in children

- HIV infected (two or more positive tests for HIV or demonstrates AIDS)
- Perinatally exposed (born to a mother known to be infected with HIV)
- Seroconverter (born to a mother known to be infected with HIV but has had two negative HIV tests)

When infected, the child with HIV is classified as

- Category N (not symptomatic)
- Category A (mildly symptomatic)
- Category B (moderately symptomatic)
- Category C (severely symptomatic; multiple, recurrent infection)

Note: From Guidelines for the use of antiretroviral agents in pediatric HIV infection (1998). *Morbidity and Mortality Weekly Report 47,* (RR-4), 1–43.

Two types of tests are commonly used to test for HIV infection. One is enzyme-linked immunosorbent assay (ELISA), and the other is polymerase chain reaction (PCR). Although the PCR has the greatest sensitivity, it is costly (about $175) and identifies some false-positive results. ELISA is less expensive (about $50) but not as sensitive, especially for children under 18 months. For this reason, repeated tests are recommended, especially in the infant who may become HIV-positive after birth to an infected mother. In developing countries where expense prohibits repeated tests, the ELISA is often used with astute clinical observations of the child at risk.

Because of the rapidity of disease progression in perinatally transmitted HIV infection, early identification of infected infants is important to ensure the most effective treatment. HIV-infected mothers should be identified during pregnancy, and their infants should undergo periodic laboratory testing, as described earlier. Regardless of the results of these tests, all infants of infected mothers should start prophylaxis against PCP (a commonly serious or fatal outcome in infants) by the age of 4 to 6 weeks and continue to 12 months, or until two negative HIV tests have been documented (at 1 and 4 months of age). Drugs used for PCP prophylaxis include trimethoprim-sulfamethoxazole (Bactrim or Septra), dapsone, or aerosolized pentamidine. In addition, all infected mothers should receive oral ZDV after the first trimester of pregnancy and intravenous ZDV during labor and delivery; and the newborn should receive 6 weeks of oral ZDV after birth. A CBC with differential is performed at birth, 4 to 6 weeks, and 12 weeks to monitor for drug side effects.

Medical management is supportive, as there is no cure for AIDS. IVIG (see Table 40–4) has been used to prevent bacterial infections in children under the age of 2 years. Treatment involves prompt therapy for bacterial and opportunistic infections. Children between 3 months and 12 years of age are given antiretroviral drugs, including nucleoside reverse transcriptase inhibitors such as ZDV, didanosine (DDI), zalcitabine (DDC), lamivudine (3TC), and stavudine (D4T). (See Table 40–6.) The protease inhibitors (PIs), ritonavir, and nelfinavir have now been approved for use in children over 2 years, and other PIs are now under investigation (Temple, Koranyi, & Nahata, 2001). The PI are most effective in combination with nucleoside reverse transcriptase inhibitors, which slow replication of the virus. Recent drug trials have demonstrated reduction of serum HIV load in perinatally infected infants who were treated with a combination of several antiviral drugs (Luzuriaga, Bryson, Krogstad, et al., 1997). The antineoplastic drug hydroxyurea can be used in combination with nucleoside reverse transcriptase inhibitors (Kline, Calles, Simon, et al., 2000).

TABLE 40-6 Medications Used to Treat HIV

1. **Nucleoside analogues or nucleoside reverse transcriptase inhibitors** (inhibit action of viral reverse transcriptase, an enzyme in the conversion of RNA to DNA)

   Examples: zidovudine, didanosine, zalcitabine, stavudine, lamivudine

2. **Protease inhibitors** (block the function of the enzyme protease needed for viral formation and growth)

   Examples: saquinavir, ritonavir, indinavir, nalfinavir, kaletra (lopinavir/ritonavir combination)

3. **Nonnucleoside reverse transcriptase inhibitors** (bind to viral reverse transcriptase and disrupt the conversion of RNA to DNA)

   Examples: nevirapine, delavirdine

Note: The average cost of annual therapy with a combination of drugs as recommended is about $10,000 (Burpo, 2000). What special financial needs do families have when someone is treated for HIV?

The earlier the child develops AIDS, the poorer the prognosis. However, as treatment improves, more children are living longer with the disease. Younger children are more likely to die of pulmonary diseases or infection, while those who survive past 10 years of age are more likely to die of cardiac disease, wasting syndrome, encephalopathy, and infection with *Mycobacterium avium* complex. The average age for survival of a child after diagnosis of HIV infection is 8 years (Langston, Cooper, Goldfarb, et al., 2001).

Nursing Management
Nursing Assessment and Diagnosis

For infants at risk of HIV infection, obtain the HIV test results of the mother if available. When these are positive, the infant will need to be screened numerous times during infancy for HIV infection, as described in the previous section. Facilitate the screening and explain its necessity to the family.

PHYSIOLOGIC ASSESSMENT

Assessment centers on observation and evaluation of potential sites of infection. Assess breath sounds, respiratory status, arterial blood gases, level of consciousness, and mental status. Report any evidence of lymphocytic interstitial pneumonitis or neurologic abnormalities. Assess the child's height and weight frequently. Observe for signs of failure to thrive and assess for anemia. Look for *Candida* infections in the mouth and the diaper area. Note any developmental delays in motor skills or intellectual functioning, which could result from encephalopathy and poor nutrition, and can signal the progression from HIV infection into AIDS (Pearson, McGrath, Nozyce, et al., 2000). Report them so that the child can receive further medical evaluation.

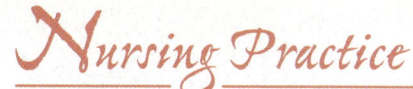

The American Academy of Pediatrics Committee on Pediatric AIDS recommends that school-age children and adolescents with HIV be informed of their diagnosis. Telling the child is difficult for parents and they often avoid doing so. Since parents usually want to be the ones to tell the child, they need help planning how to discuss the issue and ongoing support in the process of communication (Instone, 2000). Nurses can help parents understand the need to discuss the diagnosis with the child, provide information about how to tell the child, and emotionally support them with this difficult task.

PSYCHOSOCIAL ASSESSMENT

Assess family support systems and coping mechanisms, as the stress of caring for a child with AIDS may overwhelm parents. Assess the family's ability to care for the child. If the mother is infected, ask about the extended family's ability to provide daily care and emotional support. Support the family when they decide to inform a school-age child or adolescent of the diagnosis. When assessing an adolescent with AIDS, evaluate the teen's understanding of how AIDS is transmitted and the response to the diagnosis.

"Nursing Care Plan: The Child with Acquired Immunodeficiency Syndrome" includes common nursing diagnoses that may apply to a child hospitalized with AIDS. Other nursing diagnoses may include:

▶ *Diarrhea* related to gastrointestinal infection, malignancy, or drug reactions

▶ *Impaired gas exchange* related to pulmonary disease

▶ *Altered growth and development* related to chronic infection and poor nutrition

▶ *Risk for ineffective family coping: compromised* related to life-threatening illness

Planning and Implementation

The first step in dealing with HIV infection is prevention. Nurses must be active in evaluating test results and instituting measures to prevent vertical transmission of HIV to the infants of infected mothers. Adequate testing, prophylaxis for HIV and PCP, and follow-up visits for evaluation of general health and development for all infants at risk of the disease is advised. Recent guidelines from the American Academy of Pediatrics recommend that pediatricians offer HIV testing and counseling to adolescents who are sexually active or involved in substance abuse (Committee on Pediatric AIDS, 2001). There are also recommendations for including HIV and AIDS education in comprehensive health education for students from kindergarten through 12th grades (Committee on Pediatric AIDS, 1998). Nurses can implement these policies and counsel teens about the dangers and prevention measures for HIV (St. Louis, Levine, Wasserheit, et al., 1998).

GOAL	INTERVENTION	RATIONALE	EXPECTED OUTCOME
1. Risk for infection related to immunosuppression			
Risk factors for infection will be eliminated as evidenced by infection control.	*NIC Priority Intervention:* **Infection control:** *Minimizing the acquisition and transmission of infectious agents* ▸ Assess the child every 2–4 hours for fever; lesions in the mouth; redness, inflammation, soreness, and lesions on the skin or around intravenous lines. ▸ Auscultate for changes in breath sounds every 2 hours. Perform pulmonary toilet (coughing, deep breathing, incentive spirometry) every 2–4 hours. ▸ Enforce strict handwashing. Allow no fresh flowers, fruits, or vegetables in child's room. Screen visitors for colds or recent exposure to varicella. Use blood and body fluid precautions (refer to the *Clinical Skills Manual*). ⬚ **SKILL** Practice strict asepsis for dressing changes and suctioning. ▸ Coordinate patient care assignments to avoid exposing the child to individuals with recent infections or immunizations. ▸ Organize patient care activities to allow for adequate period of rest. ▸ Follow recommendations of CDC and AAP for immunizing immunosuppressed children. Avoid varicella vaccine. Perform annual TB testing.	▸ Fever is one of the few signs of infection in the immunosuppressed child who does not have a sufficient number of white blood cells. ▸ Pneumonia is a likely infection in the child with AIDS. ▸ Control of environmental factors helps prevent infection. ▸ Planning minimizes chances for infection. ▸ Rest periods allow the child to regain energy. ▸ Special recommendations consider the child's decreased immune response and the danger of acquiring disease from certain live virus vaccines.	*NOC Suggested Outcome:* **Risk control:** *Answers to eliminate or reduce actual, personal, and modifiable health threats* The child has no fever and shows no other signs of infection.
2. Altered nutrition: less than body requirements related to loss of appetite and increased absorption of nutrients			
The child will demonstrate adequate nutritional status to meet metabolic needs.	*NIC Priority Intervention:* **Nutrition management:** *Assistance with or provision of a balanced dietary intake of food and fluids* ▸ Encourage frequent small meals to promote nutritional and fluid intake. ▸ Maintain nasogastric tube feeding, if ordered. Hyperalimentation may be necessary to ensure adequate nutrition. ▸ Eliminate unpleasant stimuli and odors from the environment during meals. ▸ Monitor skin turgor every shift. ▸ Involve a nutritionist in planning a diet for the child that includes favorite foods.	▸ Additional nutrition is required to rebuild the immune system. ▸ Unpleasant stimuli decrease the desire for food. ▸ Skin turgor reflects hydration status. ▸ Including favorite foods encourages intake.	*NOC Suggested Outcome:* **Nutritional status:** *Nutrient value: adequacy of nutrients taken into the body* The child eats frequent meals of adequate nutritional content.
3. Risk for impaired skin integrity related to skin infection, immobility, or diarrhea			
The child will have structural intactness and normal physiologic function of skin.	*NIC Priority Intervention:* **Skin surveillance:** *Collection and analysis of patient data to maintain skin integrity* ▸ Observe all pressure areas closely for signs of infection or breakdown. ▸ Keep skin clean and dry. Provide perineal care to minimize irritation from diarrhea.	▸ Skin care is important in the immunocompromised child. The skin may be the only intact defense the child has. ▸ Prevents breaking or cracking of skin.	*NOC Suggested Outcome:* **Risk control:** *Actions to eliminate or reduce actual, personal and modifiable health threats* The child is free of preventable skin breakdown.

GOAL	INTERVENTION	RATIONALE	EXPECTED OUTCOME
4. Risk for altered oral mucous membrane related to infection			
	NIC Priority Intervention:		*NOC Suggested Outcome:*
	Oral health restoration: *Promotion of healing for a patient who has an oral mucosa lesion*		**Tissue integrity** *Structural intactness and normal physiologic function of mucous membranes*
The child will have intact oral mucous membranes.	▶ Inspect mouth for sign of blistering or lesions.	▶ Candidal infection is frequently associated with immunodeficiency.	The child has intact oral mucous membranes.
	▶ Provide mouth care with normal saline solution or lemon–glycerine swabs every 2–4 hours.	▶ Provides comfort and promotes healing.	
5. Pain related to infections			
	NIC Priority Intervention:		*NOC Suggested Outcome:*
	Pain management: *Alleviation of pain or a reduction in pain to level of comfort that is acceptable to the patient*		**Comfort level:** *Feelings of physical and psychologic ease*
The child will be free of pain or experience only mild pain/discomfort.	▶ Observe for signs of pain and discomfort.	▶ Pain relief adds to comfort of the child and family.	The child shows evidence of pain relief.
	▶ Medicate for pain as ordered and document results.		
	▶ Implement general comfort measures (holding, rocking, etc).		
6. Knowledge deficit (parent) related to home care of child with AIDS			
	NIC Priority Intervention:		*NOC Suggested Outcome:*
	Teaching, treatment: *Preparing a patient and family to understand and mentally prepare for a treatment*		**Knowledge, treatment regimen:** *Extent of understanding conveyed about AIDS treatment*
The parent(s) will demonstrate knowledge about home care, measures to prevent infection, and signs and symptoms to report to health care providers.	▶ Explain the importance of optimizing the child's health status and reducing risk of complications through diet, rest, and meticulous personal hygiene. Be sure that parents and other family members understand how AIDS is spread and appropriate precautions.	▶ Knowledge about the disorder and preventive measures is necessary to provide safe and effective home care for the child.	The parent describes appropriate home care and preventive measures for a child with AIDS.
	▶ Discuss with the parents and the child reasons for protective measures.	▶ Knowledge of rationale increases compliance.	
	▶ Inform the family about signs and symptoms of infection that should be reported promptly to the physician or nurse (fever, chills, cough, mild erythema).	▶ Prompt treatment improves outcome.	
7. Caregiver role strain related to anxiety about child's condition and demands of providing care			
	NIC Priority Intervention:		*NOC Suggested Outcome:*
	Caregiver support: *Provision of the necessary information, advocacy, and support to facilitate primary patient care by someone other than a health professional*		**Caregiver emotional health:** *Feelings, attitudes, and emotions of a family care provider while caring for the child over an extended period of time*
The parent(s) will demonstrate emotional health as evidenced by decreased anxiety related to the child's condition and care.	▶ Encourage family members to express fears and concerns regarding the child's prognosis.	▶ Expression of fears helps to decrease anxiety.	The parent states decreased anxiety.
	▶ Advise family about support services or other resources available in the community.	▶ Provides additional support to help family cope with the child's illness and the dying process, when needed.	

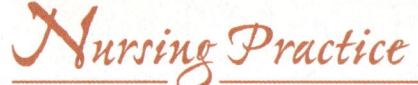

If the child is diagnosed with HIV, close health supervision is needed to ensure medications are taken and examinations are carried out. When HIV progresses to AIDS, nursing care is similar to that of a child with any serious chronic, life-threatening disease. It centers on preventing infection, managing pain, promoting respiratory and other organ function, promoting adequate nutritional intake, and providing emotional support to the parents and child, while promoting the child's growth and development. See "Nursing Care Plan: The Child with Acquired Immunodeficiency Syndrome" for a summary of nursing care.

PREVENT INFECTION

Immunosuppressed children become infected with bacteria as well as other common organisms. Frequent handwashing and limiting the child's exposure to people with upper respiratory or other infections are the best interventions to protect the child with HIV from acquiring other infections (Kaplan, Masur & Holmes, 1997). The child should follow a modified immunization schedule that avoids exposure to live varicella vaccine (Gross & Larkin, 1996). Live measles-mumps-rubella vaccine is used unless the child is severely affected with AIDS, since the risk of serious outcomes for measles disease is great. Tuberculosis is more common in children with AIDS so they should have annual skin tests read by health professionals (Cohen, Chen, Sunkle, et al., 2000). Teach sexually active adolescents the importance of practicing safe sex and the ramifications of high-risk sexual behaviors and intravenous drug abuse.

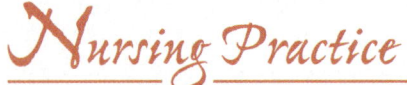
PROMOTE RESPIRATORY FUNCTION

Because many children with AIDS develop pneumonia, encourage the child to cough and deep breathe every 2 to 4 hours. Blowing cotton balls with a straw, blowing bubbles, or other games may engage the interest of a younger child. Reposition infants frequently so all areas of the lungs can aerate. Rest periods to conserve energy and lower the body's demand for oxygen are important.

PROMOTE ADEQUATE NUTRITIONAL INTAKE

Because many children with AIDS have failure to thrive, nutrition is an important part of their care. (See Chapter 31 for information to include in a detailed nutritional assessment.) A nutritionist should be involved in planning an appropriate diet for the child that provides necessary calories, protein, and other nutrients. Vitamins may be especially lacking in the diets of infected children. Antioxidants (vitamin A, vitamin E, zinc, and selenium) enhance general immune system function; children should get recommended levels. Periodic dietary analysis and teaching are needed. Adequate nutrition is sometimes provided by hyperalimentation.

Diarrhea resulting from gastrointestinal infection and lactose intolerance is common in these children and complicates other nutritional disturbances. Antidiarrheal medications may be prescribed, or alternative formulas tried. Keep the child's lips and mouth moist and pay close attention to hydration status. Monitor the skin turgor and urine output, and provide careful perineal skin care to prevent infection.

Frequent *Candida* infections lead to blisters, cracking, and discharge involving the oral mucous membranes. Mouth care with a non-alcohol-based solution such as normal saline or lemon–glycerine swabs should be done every 2 to 4 hours.

PROVIDE EMOTIONAL SUPPORT

The family of the child with AIDS is under great strain. The mother and others in the family may also be infected. Integrate social services and support groups into the care of the child as soon as the diagnosis is made. Spend time talking with the family about their fears and feelings. In many parts of the United States, AIDS still carries a tremendous stigma, and the family may not be able to discuss their feelings outside of the health care environment. Safeguard the family's wishes about the privacy of the diagnosis.

Clarify any misconceptions the older child with AIDS may have about the transmission of the disease. Clearly dis-

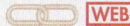

Thinking Critically

THE TODDLER WITH AIDS

Raymond, a 2-year-old child, has had recurrent infections since he was born. After a recent illness with fever, vomiting, and diarrhea, blood tests were done to evaluate his immune function. He was diagnosed with AIDS and admitted to a special unit of the hospital for children with AIDS.

➡ What physical needs does Raymond have at this time?

➡ He manifests failure to thrive, a frequent occurrence with AIDS. How can the nurse and dietitian work together to plan a diet for him to enable him to grow?

➡ What information does Raymond's family need?

➡ What can you do to provide emotional support for them?

➡ What community and Internet resources could be helpful?
 WEB

Nursing Practice

Disclosure of patient information is a breach of confidentiality that may subject you to legal action. Disclosure of confidential information occurs whenever a patient's condition—for example, a diagnosis of AIDS—is discussed inappropriately with any third party.

cuss routes of transmission and the need for safe sexual practices with adolescents. Providing support for adolescents is particularly important, as the dependence which this chronic and terminal disease brings can make it difficult to meet the developmental task of independence. Adolescents may benefit from contact with other infected peers.

DISCHARGE PLANNING

The diagnosis of AIDS is surrounded by strong emotions and fears. Be honest and direct. Education is essential. Explain that there is no evidence that casual contact among family members can spread the infection. For the child hospitalized, identify home care needs well in advance of discharge.

Discuss the family's finances as well as health insurance coverage for the child's care. Assess the family's ability to provide nutritious food, required medications, and a supportive environment. Refer to services as needed to ensure that the child gets quality care after discharge.

Support groups, home health care nursing services, financial assistance, and psychologic counseling are usually needed at some point during the child's illness, and the family should be aware of the availability of such services. Help the family deal with guilt feelings about the child's condition.

NURSING CARE IN THE COMMUNITY

Much of the care of the child with HIV infection or AIDS takes place in the community. Evaluate the family and community support systems and provide resources and referrals

as needed. Many children with HIV infection are placed in foster homes, and these families need careful instruction to manage this multifaceted illness.

School attendance guidelines for children with AIDS by the American Academy of Pediatrics (AAP) and the CDC recommend unrestricted school attendance for children with AIDS or AIDS-related complex as long as their physician approves. Contraindications to school attendance include lack of control of body secretions, biting, and open wounds that cannot be covered. The nurse often prepares the school personnel with training related to care for children with known and unknown cases of HIV. The nurse also may be responsible for providing medicines or other care for the HIV-infected child at school (Gross & Larkin, 1996).

Nursing Practice

Because children with HIV or other bloodborne infections may be enrolled in child care centers, staff in these centers should use standard precautions in handling blood and body fluids. Instruct day care center personnel in use of these precautions. Help child care centers establish procedures to notify all parents when a child with an infectious disease has been at the center. Parents of immunocompromised children can then take any necessary precautions to minimize the chances of their children becoming ill. Parents of HIV-infected children must be very cautious to limit the exposure of their children to infectious diseases.

Help the family alter the home environment to provide standard precautions during care. Make sure the child and family understand that HIV is transmitted through blood, urine, stool, and other body secretions. Teach family members the importance of careful hygiene. Encourage careful handwashing and tell parents to use precautions when handling body fluids. Explain that they should wear gloves when changing diapers; disposing of urine, stool, and emesis; or treating the child's cuts and scrapes. Instruct parents to use a bleach solution for disinfection of objects when necessary and to avoid contact with people with infectious illnesses. Precautions to guard against foodborne illness are particularly important for the HIV-infected child. Parents also need instruction on correct administration and side effects of any medications the child is taking. Giving a child a complicated combination of drugs can be challenging for all families, so use teaching tailored to the particular family and repeatedly evaluate the family's success with medication administration.

Emphasize the importance of promoting the child's development. Perform frequent developmental screening. Teach the parents how to support the child in achieving developmental milestones. Encourage contact with other children and adults, provide for appropriate toys, teach parents how to encourage the child's communication, and praise the family for what the child has already accomplished. Children who manifest decreasing developmental milestones or other neurologic symptoms should be assessed for HIV-induced encephalopathy by the primary care provider. The nurse's record of development will be of great importance in this situation.

The child needs regular health maintenance care, such as child health supervision visits, immunizations, and care for any other health conditions.

Teaching About

FOOD SAFETY

The child with HIV infection is more prone to foodborne disease. Instruct parents to:

1. Use a separate cutting board for meats, and wash it with hot soapy water after use.

2. Wash all utensils with hot soapy water between any uses.

3. Wash and peel fresh fruits and vegetables.

4. Use a disposable cloth or cloth that is washed after each meal to clean dishes. A sponge can harbor organisms and should not be used.

5. Have well water checked for contaminants regularly if that is the source of drinking water.

6. Do not allow the child to eat raw or undercooked meats, fish, eggs, or cookie dough.

7. Bleach solution is the best product for cleaning surfaces in the kitchen.

Nursing Practice

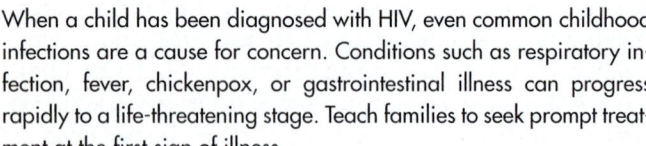

When a child has been diagnosed with HIV, even common childhood infections are a cause for concern. Conditions such as respiratory infection, fever, chickenpox, or gastrointestinal illness can progress rapidly to a life-threatening stage. Teach families to seek prompt treatment at the first sign of illness.

Evaluation

There are many desired outcomes of care for the child with HIV infection or AIDS. These include:

▶ Decreased numbers of cases of pediatric HIV due to vertical transmission from known infected mothers

▶ Prevention of infectious diseases in children with the virus

▶ Adequate respiratory function and perfusion

▶ Nutritional intake to support normal growth patterns and prevent malnutrition

▶ Adequate family coping with the stress of chronic disease

▶ School attendance and support in the educational process

≋ AUTOIMMUNE DISORDERS

An immune system damaged by pathologic changes may react to some of the body's own proteins, resulting in the production of autoantibodies. These pathologic conditions in which the body directs the immune response against itself—identifying "self" as "nonself"—are called autoimmune disorders.

The primary feature of autoimmune disorders is tissue injury caused by a probable immunologic reaction of the host with its own tissues. Structural or functional changes occur as immune cells attack other cells in the body.

The autoimmune disorders are grouped into systemic and organ-specific diseases. Systemic diseases, which largely involve more than one organ, include systemic lupus erythematosus and juvenile rheumatoid arthritis. Organ-specific diseases, which primarily affect a single organ, include insulin-dependent diabetes mellitus (IDDM; see Chapter 51) and thyroiditis. Idiopathic (or immune) thrombocytic purpura is an immune disease affecting blood platelets and clotting and is discussed in Chapter 44.

SYSTEMIC LUPUS ERYTHEMATOSUS

Systemic lupus erythematosus (SLE), a generalized disorder seen mainly in females, is a chronic inflammatory disease of unknown origin that involves many organ systems. SLE is more common in blacks, Hispanics, and Asians than in whites, affecting 4.4 per 100,000 white females from 10 to 20 years of age, 20 per 100,000 black females, 13 per 100,000 Hispanic females, and 31 per 100,000 Asian females (Lehman, 1995). Most cases are diagnosed in the teenage and early adult years. A genetic component is suspected because the disease is often more common in certain families. WEB

Etiology and Pathophysiology

The exact etiology of SLE is unknown. It is believed that an outside environmental agent causes the body to initiate an abnormal immune system response to its own tissues. Antigen–antibody complexes are deposited in the vascular system, leading to widespread inflammation and tissue damage. The tissues most likely to be affected are the small blood vessels, glomeruli, joints, spleen, and heart valves. Because many systems can be affected at the same time, organ damage with subsequent system failure may occur.

Clinical Manifestations

Symptoms depend on the organ involved and the amount of tissue damage that has occurred. Initial symptoms include fever, chills, fatigue, malaise, and weight loss. The most common symptoms are arthritis and skin rash. A butterfly rash on the face, consisting of a pink or red rash over the bridge of the nose extending to the cheeks, is a characteristic finding. Children with SLE may have hemolytic anemia, with a low white blood cell and platelet count; bleeding disorders; hypergammaglobulinemia; and vasculitis.

Clinical Therapy

Blood tests reveal anemia, an elevated blood urea nitrogen (BUN), abnormal plasma proteins, abnormal erythrocyte sedimentation rate (ESR), presence of antinuclear antibodies, and a positive LE (lupus erythematosus) cell reaction, which indicates nonspecific inflammation. The Coombs' test is positive. Urinalysis may reveal proteinuria.

The goals of medical management are to create a remission of symptoms and to prevent complications. Corticosteroids, such as prednisone, are prescribed to control inflammation. Antimalarial preparations, such as hydroxychloroquine and chloroquine, are used to treat symptoms associated with skin lesions and renal and arthritic problems. Although the exact action of these drugs on SLE is not known, they often permit continued remission with a lowered dose of steroids. Nonsteroidal anti-inflammatory drugs (aspirin, ibuprofen, naproxen) are used to relieve muscle and joint pain. Immunosuppressant drugs, such as cyclosporin and methotrexate, have been used to help control SLE. Diet may be restricted if the child has excessive weight gain or fluid retention from steroids and renal damage.

Growth and Development

> The side effects of the corticosteroids, immunosuppressants, and antimalarial drugs used in the treatment of children with SLE are significant and include hair loss, susceptibility to infection, "moon face," retinal damage, and bone loss. These are significant side effects for the adolescent who is commonly concerned about appearance. Teens with SLE may need special teaching, guidance, and support.

Prognosis depends on the severity of the disease. The 5-year survival rate now approaches 80% to 90% because of improved treatment measures (Sack & Fye, 1997).

Nursing Management

Nursing Assessment and Diagnosis

PHYSIOLOGIC ASSESSMENT

A thorough assessment is needed, as symptoms are widespread. Assess for rash, petechiae, cyanosis, skin ulcers, joint deformity, friction rub, edema, and splenomegaly.

PSYCHOSOCIAL ASSESSMENT

Because SLE is a chronic disease that affects primarily adolescents, psychosocial assessment is indicated. Assess family interactions, exploring stressful situations such as divorce

or trauma. Treatment-related restrictions and changes in appearance can lead to withdrawal, depression, and suicidal tendencies.

Several nursing diagnoses may apply to the child with SLE. These include:

▶ *Risk for ineffective management of therapeutic regimen, family,* related to complexity of therapeutic regimen

▶ *Risk for altered tissue perfusion (renal)* related to interrupted blood flow in kidneys

▶ *Risk for impaired skin integrity* related to immunologic deficit

▶ *Risk for activity intolerance* related to chronic disease

▶ *Risk for body image disturbance* related to side effects of medications and skin alterations

▶ *Risk of infection* related to immunosuppressive medications

▶ *Pain* related to joint inflammation and injury

Planning and Implementation

The goals of nursing care are to help the child manage and cope with a chronic disease, and to facilitate a remission.

MAINTAIN FLUID BALANCE

Because most children with SLE have renal involvement, monitor intake and output and frequently evaluate the child's fluid and electrolyte status. Renal dysfunction can manifest itself by edema, muscle cramps, diarrhea, tetany, and convulsions.

PROMOTE SKIN INTEGRITY

The rash on mucous membranes can cause weakening of the tissues, placing the child at increased risk for infection. Encourage good hygienic measures and a mild soap. Recommend that adolescents limit their use of cosmetics. Reinforce the importance of avoiding sunlight as much as possible and the use of sun protection factor (SPF) of 15 or higher at all times when in the sun.

PROMOTE REST AND COMFORT

Because of fatigue and joint pain, the child has little energy reserve during acute episodes of the disease. Encourage frequent rest periods and a nutritious diet to maximize energy stores. A physical therapist can plan a program to encourage mobility and increase muscle strength.

MANAGE SIDE EFFECTS OF MEDICATIONS

Observe for side effects of medications used for treatment, and teach the child and family about these effects. For example, immunosuppressant drugs can promote infection anywhere in the body; and nonsteroidal anti-inflammatory drugs commonly cause gastric distress and bleeding of the gastrointestinal tract. The antimalarial drug hydroxychloroquine can cause serious vision changes; thus, frequent eye examinations are needed.

Adolescents may have an altered body image as a result of rash, alopecia, arthritic changes in the joints, and chronic disease. Referral to a lupus support group, social services, or counseling may be helpful. The American Lupus Society and the Lupus Foundation of America can provide information to help parents and children adjust to the disease. The Arthritis Foundation also publishes a useful pamphlet, *Meeting the Challenge: A Young Person's Guide to Living with Lupus.*

Evaluation

Successful outcomes of nursing care involve management of this chronic disease. Expected outcomes of nursing care include:

▶ Normal intake and output levels, with demonstrated fluid and electrolyte balance

▶ Maintenance of intact skin

▶ A balance of rest and activity to promote development

▶ Medication management

▶ Positive body image

JUVENILE RHEUMATOID ARTHRITIS

Juvenile rheumatoid arthritis (JRA) is an autoimmune inflammatory disease that occurs slightly more often in girls than in boys. It usually occurs in children between 2 and 5 or between 9 and 12 years of age, and it may disappear in adolescence or occasionally continue as a chronic disease.

Etiology and Pathophysiology

The cause of JRA is unknown, but it is thought to have an autoimmune basis. Inflammation begins in the joint and leads to pain and swelling. Scar tissue eventually develops, resulting in limited range of motion. There are three types of JRA: pauciarticular, systemic, and polyarticular.

Clinical Manifestations

JRA may be restricted to a few joints or be systemic with involvement of multiple joints. Symptoms can include fever, rash, lymphadenopathy, splenomegaly, and hepatomegaly. The child may develop a limp or obviously favor one extremity over the other. Pain, stiffness, loss of motion, and swelling occur in the large joints such as the knees. Older children may develop symmetric involvement of the small joints of the hand. The disease is frequently chronic, extending over several years after an initial manifestation with pain and other symptoms.

Clinical Therapy

Diagnosis is made primarily on the basis of the history and assessment findings, in particular, arthritis having an onset before 16 years of age and persisting for at least 6 weeks, with no other identifiable cause (Gottlieb & Ilowite, 2000). There are no specific laboratory tests for the disease. In some children, rheumatoid factor, human leukocyte antigen (HLA) B27, and antinuclear antibody (ANA) tests are positive.

Medical management involves drug therapy, physical therapy, and, when necessary, surgery. The goals of treatment are to relieve pain and prevent contractures. Salicylates (aspirin) or nonsteroidal anti-inflammatory drugs (tolmetin sodium, naproxen, diclofenac, ibuprofen) are prescribed to reduce inflammation. Steroids may be used with children who have moderately active disease. Children who do not respond to aspirin or nonsteroidal anti-inflammatory drugs may be treated with sulfasalazine and methotrexate. Physical therapy increases strength and mobility of joints while protecting them from injury. Surgery is occasionally performed to relieve pain and maintain or improve joint function in children with joint contractures.

Nursing Practice

Infants and children with juvenile rheumatoid arthritis who are receiving aspirin therapy are at risk of developing Reye syndrome if they contract influenza. These children should be immunized with influenza vaccine in the fall of each year.

JRA is generally a chronic disease that has periods of remission and exacerbation. During its course the child may experience pain, impaired mobility, and interference with normal growth and development. Seventy percent of children with JRA have a permanent remission by adulthood. Rarely, the disease is unresponsive to treatment or the child may suffer lasting impairment such as bone and joint changes. Children with early onset have a better prognosis for complete recovery.

Nursing Management

Nursing Assessment and Diagnosis

A careful history is important, as it is sometimes the primary mode of diagnosis. Assess for joint swelling and deformities, fever, nodules under the skin, and enlarged lymph nodes.

Several nursing diagnoses may apply to the child with JRA. They include:

▶ *Activity intolerance* related to chronic pain

- *Impaired physical mobility* related to joint stiffness
- *Anxiety* related to stress of chronic illness
- *Pain* related to joint inflammation
- *Body image disturbance* related to illness

Planning and Implementation

Nursing care focuses on preventing pain, planning measures to enhance development in spite of illness, promoting mobility, encouraging adequate nutrition, and teaching the parents and child about the disease and its management. Most care occurs in the community, including physical therapy, with only occasional hospitalizations during an exacerbation of the disease.

PROMOTE IMPROVED MOBILITY

Physical therapists play an essential role in the child's treatment. The goals of physical therapy are to maintain joint function, strengthen muscles, increase tone, maintain body alignment, and prevent permanent deformities such as contractures. Range of motion exercises, stretching, hydrotherapy, and swimming exercises help to prevent deformities (Figure 40–2 ◆). Encourage the child to perform activities of daily living. Medications may be given to reduce joint swelling and inflammation. Warm compresses to the involved joints are soothing.

ENCOURAGE ADEQUATE NUTRITION

Promote general health by encouraging a well-balanced diet. Children with decreased mobility may have reduced metabolic needs, and excess weight causes additional muscle strain.

NURSING CARE IN THE COMMUNITY

The child with JRA may never, or rarely, be hospitalized. Most care takes place during visits to health care offices, clinics, and physical therapy. Teach parents about the child's condition and prognosis, and answer their questions about the child's treatment. The child may need support to adjust to the diagnosis of a chronic illness. Encourage the child to maintain contact with peers and to attend school whenever possible. Explain to the child and

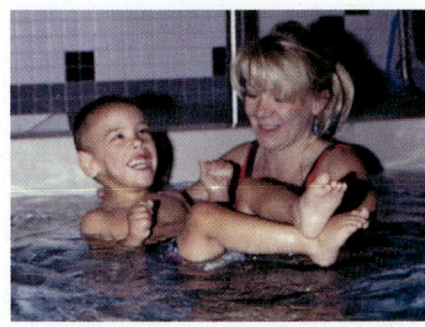

FIGURE 40–2. ◆ The physical therapist uses hydrotherapy to help maintain joint function in a child who has juvenile rheumatoid arthritis.

parents that overexertion may exacerbate the disease. Inform parents about possible complications of JRA, such as altered growth related to early closure of epiphyseal plates, small joint contractures, and synovitis. Refer parents and children to the Arthritis Foundation and the American Juvenile Arthritis Foundation for further information and support.

Evaluation

Desired outcomes for the child with JRA include:

- Maintenance of joint mobility
- Comfort and freedom from pain
- Positive body image
- Avoidance of infection
- Parental understanding and support of the therapeutic process

ALLERGIC REACTIONS

Allergy is one of the major chronic illnesses of children today. Why are some children allergic to cats, for instance, while no one else in the family has allergies? In order to answer this question, the nurse needs a basic understanding of the mechanisms of allergy.

Allergy is an abnormal or altered reaction to an antigen. Antigens responsible for clinical manifestations of allergy are called **allergens.** Allergens can be ingested in food or drugs or injected or absorbed through contact with unbroken skin. Common allergens in children include medications (such as penicillin); animal dander; dust, mites, and mold; plant pollens; and foods (such as nuts, seafood, or egg white). An allergic reaction is an antigen–antibody reaction and can manifest itself as anaphylaxis, atopic disease, serum sickness, or contact dermatitis. Therefore, the symptoms can be mild to severe or life-threatening, and they can be localized or systemic. Characteristic findings in children with allergies are summarized in Table 40–7.

TABLE 40–7 Characteristic Findings in Children with Allergies

Respiratory system: Asthma, rhinitis (seasonal and perennial), serous otitis media, cough, pneumonia, croup, edema of glottis

Gastrointestinal system: Abdominal pain and colic, stomatitis, constipation, diarrhea, bloody stools, geographical tongue, vomiting

Skin: Angioedema, urticaria, eczema, atopic dermatitis, erythema multiforme, purpura, drug and food rashes, contact dermatitis

Nervous system: Headache, tension, fatigue, convulsions, Meniere syndrome, tremor

Eye: Conjunctivitis, cataract, ciliary spasm, iritis

Blood: Thrombocytopenic purpura, hemolytic anemia, leukopenia, agranulocytosis

Musculoskeletal system: Arthralgia, myalgia, rheumatoid arthritis, torticollis

Genitourinary system: Dysuria, vulvovaginitis, enuresis

Miscellaneous: Anaphylactic shock, serum sickness, autoimmune diseases

The **hypersensitivity response,** an overreaction of the immune system, is responsible for allergic reactions. Hypersensitivity reactions have been classified into four types. Type I hypersensitivity reactions are immediate; they occur within seconds or minutes of exposure to the antigen. Symptoms can include a wheal and flare in the skin, edema, spasm of smooth muscle, wheezing, vomiting, diarrhea, or anaphylaxis. The release of chemical substances such as histamine is responsible for the signs and symptoms. The first time a child is exposed to the allergen, there is no reaction. With every exposure thereafter, however, the allergic child may have a reaction to the allergen.

function studies; tests of nasal function; and skin testing. Treatment generally involves avoidance of the allergen, such as substitution of a different drug when the child has a drug allergy. Desensitization may sometimes be used with increasing doses of the allergen administered intradermally in an office where resuscitation is readily available. This treatment is useful for allergy to bees or some pollens. For skin allergies, the allergen is avoided, skin is kept well lubricated, and topical steroids may be used. Oral antihistamines are sometimes used to treat allergy. When exposure to an allergen occurs, medical care may include treatment of anaphylaxis.

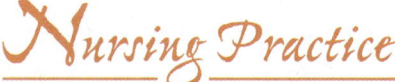

Nursing Practice

Anaphylaxis is an exaggerated hypersensitivity reaction that may manifest with itching; localized or generalized hives on the hands, feet, or mucosa; soft tissue swelling; cough; dyspnea; pallor; sweating; and tachycardia. Severe reactions may lead to respiratory distress or death. Nursing roles involve preventing anaphylactic reactions by teaching families how to minimize exposure and by alerting all health care personnel in hospitals and clinics to the child's allergy. In addition, it is important to know emergency procedures in all facilities such as schools, homes, and hospitals.

Type IV reactions are delayed responses that do not appear until several hours after exposure and require 24 to 72 hours to develop fully. A type IV reaction, which is not confined to any specific tissue, is elicited by relatively complex antigens such as those of bacteria and viruses and by simple antigens such as drugs and metals. Symptoms include contact dermatitis, itching, and blistering.

Assessment of the child with allergy includes a complete physical examination; laboratory, x-ray, and pulmonary

Complementary Care

NETTLE FOR ALLERGIES AND HAY FEVER

Nettle—sometimes called "stinging nettle"—has anti-inflammatory and antihistamine actions and may help to alleviate mild symptoms in children with allergies and hay fever. Although no randomized controlled studies have been done, nettle has generally been felt by herbalists to be safe in children. Nettle should not be given to children under 2 years of age, nor to those with severe allergies (Skidmore-Roth, 2001). This treatment should be used only for *mild* allergies and not when the child's symptoms are serious, or life threatening.

Nursing Management

The child with allergies requires a thorough assessment, including a complete past medical history, family history, personal and social history, and review of symptoms. The history focuses on the following areas:

- What symptoms does the child experience? Encourage the child to describe the difficulty in his or her own words.

CLINICAL MANIFESTATIONS *Types of Hypersensitivity Reactions*

TYPE	ETIOLOGY	CLINICAL MANIFESTATIONS	EXAMPLES
Type I Localized or systemic reactions (anaphylaxis)	Antibodies bind to certain cells, causing release of chemical substances that produce an inflammatory reaction.	Hypotension, wheezing, gastrointestinal or uterine spasm, stridor, urticaria	Extrinsic asthma, hay fever
Type II Tissue-specific reactions	Antibodies cause activation of complement system, which leads to tissue damage.	Variable; may include dyspnea or fever	Transfusion reaction, ABO incompatibility, hemolytic disease of the newborn
Type III Immune-complex reactions	Immune complexes are deposited in tissues, where they activate complement, which results in a generalized inflammatory reaction.	Urticaria, fever, joint pain	Acute glomerulonephritis, serum sickness
Type IV Delayed reactions	Antigens stimulate T cells that release lymphokines, which cause inflammation and tissue damage.	Variable; may include fever, erythema, itching	Contact dermatitis, tuberculin skin test, graft-versus-host disease, allograft rejection

- Are the symptoms continuous or intermittent? What are the frequency and duration of episodes?

- When did the child first begin to experience symptoms? Did the child have eczema or a feeding problem in infancy or childhood? Did the infant have frequent bouts of colic or skin problems when new foods were introduced? Was there a change in symptoms at puberty? Are the symptoms becoming worse or spontaneously improving?

- What known agents in the environment cause difficulties?

- Are there seasonal variations in symptoms? At what time of the day or night do symptoms usually occur?

The nurse may be responsible for performing intradermal skin tests for allergies (Figure 40–3 ◆). Nursing care focuses on treating the symptoms, alleviating the anxiety of the child and parents, and identifying the allergens. Teaching the child and family how to minimize or avoid exposure to allergens is important. Teach parents of children who have had severe reactions to bee or wasp stings how to take precautions and how to provide emergency treatment if the child is stung.

Families may need instructions on allergy-proofing the home. Pets, dust, carpets, fabrics, feather pillows and bedding, and cigarette smoke can all cause allergic reactions. If families are reluctant to give up pets, frequent baths can reduce dander, which is the usual allergen.

When the child has type I reactions to an environmental substance, avoidance of the allergen is most critical. In addition, care providers, families, and school personnel must be able to treat anaphylaxis if exposure to the allergen occurs. Be sure to label the child's chart and bed and apply a red armband to alert others to allergies when the child is hospitalized. School nurses keep records about children's allergies and inform school personnel about the allergies and cautions that need to be followed. See Chapter 31 for more information about food allergies. Nurses must be aware of the resuscitation procedures and equipment in all facilities such as hospital units, offices, child care centers, and schools. ⬭⬭ See Chapter 42 for airway maintenance, and Skill 14–13. ⬭⬭ [SKILLS]

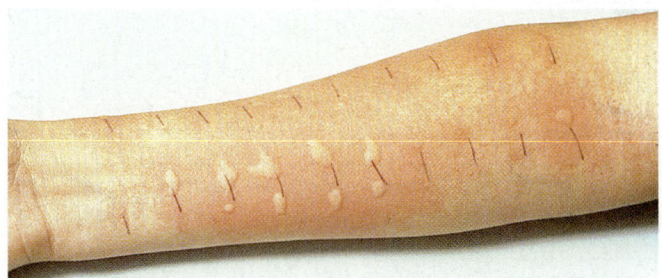

FIGURE 40–3. ◆ Results of intradermal skin testing on the forearm. Injections are given on each side of the markings. Note the positive results marked by induration and erythema in response to certain antigens. From VU/Southern Illinois University/Visuals Unlimited.

Teaching About

REMOVING COMMON ALLERGIES FROM THE HOME

Preventing exposure to the known allergens in the home setting is important. Families can take several measures to minimize contact with allergens. These include:

- Remove household pets.
- Control dust by frequent cleaning.
- Clean with moist cloths and mops to remove dust.
- Use plastic covers on mattresses and pillows.
- Avoid carpeting whenever possible.
- Avoid toys that collect dust (plastic and wood toys are better alternatives than stuffed fabric toys).
- Use high-efficiency air filters.
- Repair homes to prevent entry of water and subsequent molds.
- Consider dehumidification in moist climates.

Nursing Practice

If the child has had a severe or systemic reaction in the past to a bee or wasp sting, ensure that the parents know how to handle an anaphylactic reaction if the child is stung again. Kits with syringes of premeasured adrenaline are available by prescription. Instruct family members how to use the kit. Make sure that the kit is properly stored without exposure to sun or high temperature. Have the family check the expiration date of the adrenaline frequently. The child should wear a medical alert bracelet. A kit should be readily available at school, child care, or other settings, with someone instructed in its use. An allergy specialist should be consulted to determine whether desensitization injections would be helpful for the child.

⬭ LATEX ALLERGY

Latex allergy is common among health care workers, those in other occupations, and patients. About one in five people is sensitive to latex and could develop allergy (Harris, 1997). ⬭⬭ [WEB] Many health care products, such as gloves, drains, catheters, and intravenous ports, contain latex, a sap from the rubber tree. Latex allergy is caused by an IgE-mediated response that develops after repeated exposure to latex. In some cases, intraoperative deaths have occurred when allergic individuals were exposed to latex products during surgery. A reaction to latex products can be manifested as irritant reaction of the skin, type IV of delayed hypersensitivity with redness, inflammation, and blisters on the skin, or type I hypersensitivity, which is immediate and often has systemic manifestations (itchy eyes, asthma, or anaphylaxis).

Nursing Practice

Starting in September 1998, the Food and Drug Association ordered that medical products with latex carry a warning label that reads: "Caution: This product contains natural rubber latex, which may cause allergic reactions." Check on the labels of products in your health care facility to find this label. What products do you expect to need the label?

Children most at risk for latex allergy include those with myelodysplasia and congenital urinary tract anomalies. People who have had repeated surgeries are also at higher risk due to high exposure to latex during surgery. Health care personnel are also at risk for latex allergy because of exposure in the workplace (Table 40–8).

Children and adolescents at high risk should receive allergy testing for latex; the radioallergosorbent test (RAST) is most often used. This test measures circulating IgE antibodies to many allergens, and correlates well with results of allergy skin testing. Health care personnel should use alternative products when caring for people at risk.

When a positive skin test has occurred or when the person has had a reaction to latex, all latex products must be removed from the allergic individual's environment. Alternative products, such as nonlatex gloves and catheters, must be used when providing health care. People allergic to latex should also wear a medical identification bracelet at all times, and should have an epinephrine kit readily

available at home and school. Be alert for any signs of hypersensitivity when the child is receiving health care, and be prepared with drugs and equipment to treat anaphylaxis. This is especially important in operative settings when acute anaphylaxis is often life threatening (Lee & Kim, 1998). Emphasize to parents and children that many everyday products contain latex, including latex balloons and condoms (Table 40–9).

TABLE 40-8 Measures to Protect Against Latex Allergy

Health care personnel are at high risk of developing latex allergy because of intense exposure to products containing latex. An estimated 8% to 12% of health care workers are latex sensitive. You can protect yourself by using the following measures:

- Decrease exposure by using alternative products whenever available (use synthetic rubbers, polyethylene, nitrile, neoprene, vinyl gloves).
- Use powder-free gloves if using latex gloves (the powder has high amounts of latex, which are inhaled).
- Avoid oil-based hand creams and lotions before putting on latex gloves, as these preparations break down the latex.
- When you have symptoms of sensitivity to latex on exposure (rash, hives, nasal congestion, conjunctivitis, cough, or wheeze), contact the Employee Health Department of your facility.
- If severely allergic, avoid all contact and wear a medical identification bracelet.
- Contact the National Institute for Occupational Safety and Health (NIOSH) at 800-346-4647 or the American Nurses Association at 800-637-0323 for more information.

TABLE 40-9   LATEX in the Hospital Environment

Frequently contain Latex	Examples of LATEX-SAFE alternatives/barriers
Adhesives, skin (Smith+Nephew)	Mastisol (Ferndale)
Anesthesia circuits, bags, oxygen masks	Neoprene (Anesthesia Associates, Ohmeda adult), *some* Vital Signs
Bandaids	Active Strip (3M), CURAD Neon, Readi-Bandages, NHP, *some* Airstrip
Blood pressure cuff, tubing (J&J)	Cleen Cuff (Vital Signs), nylon (*some* Trimline)
Bulb syringe	*selected* Davol, Medline, Rusch, Premium, Baxter
Casts: Delta-Lite Podiatry, Orthoflex (J&J)	Scotchcast soft, Delta-Lites, *recent* Conformable (J&J), Caraglas Ultra, liners (Gore)
Catheters, condom	Clear Advantage, ProSys NL, *selected* Coloplast, Rochester, PolyTech (Hollister)
Catheters, indwelling & systems, UDS	*some* Am BioMed, Argyle, Bard, Cook, Dale, Kendall, Lifetech, Mentor, Rochester, Rusch, Vitaid. Adapters & plug (Addto)
Catheters, cardiac, vascular, pulmonary	*some* World Medical, Am BioMed,
Catheters, straight, coude	Mentor, RobNel (Sherwood), Coloplast, *selected* Bard, Rusch catheters
Catheters, feeding	Accumark feeding catheter (Sims Portex)
CPR manikins & Medical training aids	*most* Laerdal products
Dressings: Dyna-flex, butterfly closures (J&J) BDF Elastoplast, Action Wrap, Coban (3M) Lyofoam (Acme), Spandage (Medi-tech), Telfa	Duoderm, Reston foam (3M), Opsite, Venigard, Comfeel, Sorbaview, Telfa (some) Xeroform, PinCare, Bioclusive, Montg'ry strap (J&J), Webril, Metalline, Selopor, Opraflex, Centurion brief, *some* Airstrips, Rainbow Net (Surgilast), VAC

Note: latex in package only: Steri-strip wound closure system, Tegaderm, Tegasorb, Active Strips (3M), Nu-Derm (J&J), CURAD

Note: From the Spina Bifida Association of America. www.sbaa.org.4590 MacArthur Blvd NW Suite 250 Washington DC: 20001-4226. Used with permission.

TABLE 40-9   LATEX in the Hospital Environment—continued

Frequently contain Latex	Examples of LATEX-SAFE alternatives/barriers
Ear Plugs	Grainger (5F767)
Elastic wrap: ACE, Esmarch, Zimmer Dyna-flex, Elastikon (J&J)	E-Cotton, CEB elastic (coNco), Champ (Carolon), Adban Adhesive, X-Mark (Avcor) Co-Flex, PowerFlex (Andover), Comprilan (Jobst), Esmark (DeRoyal, NHP)
Electrode bulbs, pads, grounding	some Baxter, Dantec EMG, Conmed, ValleyLab, Vermont Med, Staodyn, Neotrode
Endotracheal tubes, airways	selected Berman, Mallinckrodt, Polamedco, Portex, Rusch, Sheridan, Shiley
Enemas	BabyLax, Theravac, Bowel Man't Tube (MIC), Pharmaseal set, all Fleet Ready-to-use, cone irrigation set (Convatec), silicone retention cuff tip (Lafayette)
G-tubes, buttons	Silicone (Bard, Flexiflo, MIC, Rusch, Stomate)
Gloves: sterile, clean, surgical, orthodontic	Allergard (J&J), dermaprene (Ansell), N-DEX (Best), Safeskin Nitrile, Neolon, SensiCare, Tru-touch (Maxxim), Nitrex, Tactyl 1,2 (SmartPractice), Duraprene, (Allegiance Healthcare), Elastyren (Hermal, Center Labs), Boston Medical, Masel, Neotech
Incentive deep breathing exerciser	Voldyne 5000 (Sherwood David & Geck), Triflo II
IV access: injection ports, Y-sites, bags, pumps, buretrol ports, PRN adapters, buretrol ports, PRN adapters, needleless systems	**Cover Y-sites and bag ports – do not puncture. Use stopcocks for meds.** Polymer injection caps + burettes + Safsite (Braun), Abbot systems, Walrus, Gemini (IMED), selected Baxter (InterLink), Statlock, Ready Med, ConMed, Clave, Alaris, Hudson, select Sims, IV boards (Avcor), Terumo Pumps: Mach II, ADS 100; Clic-Open (vial top remover – Sepha Pharm.)
OR/Infection Control masks, hats, shoe covers	some by Kimberly Clark, TECNOL; OR & sterile packs (CML, DeRoyal) twill ties
Medication vial stoppers	some AmRegent, Astra, Bedford Labs, Fujisawa, Gensia, Glaxo, Lilly, Roche
Miscellaneous items	Soft-Grip fabric clamp covers (Scanlan), Precision Dynamics I.D. bracelets
Penrose drains	Jackson-Pratt, Zimmer Hemovac
Pulse oximeters, thermometer probes	Nonin oximeters, **selected** Nellcor sensors, Diatec probe covers
Reflex hammers	Cover with plastic bag
Respirators	Advantage (MSA), HEPA-Tech (Uvex), PFR 95 (Tecnol), 3M 1860
Resuscitators, manual	certain Ambu, Armstrong, Laerdal, Puriton Bennett, Vital Blue, Respironics, Rusch
Spacer (for metered dose inhalers)	ACE spacer (Center Labs), OptiHaler (HealthScan)
Stethescope tubing	PVC (some Littman) cover with ScopeCoat or latex-free stockinette (Albahealth)
Suction tubing	PVC (Davol, Laerdal, Mallinckrodt, Superior, Yankauer) Medline, Ballard
Syringes, disposable	Terumo Medical, Abbott PCA Abboject, Norm-Ject (Air-Tite), EpiPen, selected BD syringes, AdvantaJet (Activa)
Tapes: pink, Waterproof (3M), Zonas, Moleskin, cloth, Waterproof (J&J), adhesive felt (Acme)	Dermicel (J&J), Durapore, Microfoam, Micropore, Transpore (3M) Cath-Strip (Genetic Labs), Ice Tape (P.O.Pak), All-Felt (Universal Foot Care)
Tonopen disposable covers (glaucoma tester)	
Tourniquets	Children's Medical, Grafco, VelcroPedic, X-Tourn straps (Avcor), Free-Band (Kent)
Theraband (also strip, tube), Other OT supplies	REP Bands & Cords (OPTP), Exercise putty (Rolyan), new Thera-Band Exercisers plastic tubing-Tygon LR-40
Tubing, sheeting	(Norton), elastic thread, sheets (JPS Elastomerics)
Vascular stockings (Jobst)	Compriform Custom (Jobst)

Latex in the Home and Community

Art supplies: paints, glue, erasers, fabric paints	Elmers (School Glue, Glue-All, GluColors, Carpenters Wood Glue, Sno-Drift paste) FaberCastel erasers, Crayola (**except** stamps, erasers), Liquitex paints, DickBlick Tempera & acrylic paints & soap erasers, Play-Doh
Balloons	Mylar balloons, self-sealing Myloons
Balls: Koosh balls, tennis balls, bowling balls	PVC (Hedstrom Sports Ball), Nerf Foam Balls
Carpet backing, gym floor, basement sealant	Provide barrier–cloth or mat
Chewing gum	Bubblicious, Trident (Warner-Lambert), Wrigley gums (check new products)
Clothes: applique on Tees, elastic on socks, underwear, sneakers, sandals	Cloth-covered elastic, neoprene (Decent Exposures, NOLATEX Industries) Buster Brown elastic-free socks (Vermont Country Store)
Condoms, contraceptive sponges, diaphragm	Polyurethane (Avanti), female condom (Reality), Wideseal Silicone Diaphragms (Milex), Trojan Supra Condom
Crutches: tips, axillary pads, hand grips	Cover with cloth, tape
Dental dams, cups, bands, root canal material orthodontic rubber bands	PURO/M27 intraoral elastics (Midwest Orthodontic), wire springs, sealant (Delton) dams (Meer Dental, Hygenic Corp), John O Butler, Earloop masks (Richmond)
Diapers, Incontinence pads, rubber pants	Huggies, First Quality, Gold Seal, Tranquility, Always, some Attends, Drypers Diapers (not training pants), Confidence (Paper-Pak), Pampers, Luvs

(continued)

TABLE 40-9   LATEX in the Hospital Environment—continued

Frequently contain Latex	Examples of LATEX-SAFE alternatives/barriers
Feeding nipples	Silicone, vinyl (**selected** Gerber, Evenflo, MAM, Ross, Mead Johnson)
Food handled with latex gloves	Synthetic gloves for food handling
NOTE: associated allergies are reported to banana, avocado, chestnut, kiwi and other fruits	
Handles on racquets, tools, bicycles	Vinyl, leather handles, or cover with cloth or tape
Infant toothbrush-massager	Soft bristle brush or cloth, Gerber/NUK
Kitchen cleaning gloves	PVC MYPLEX (Magla), cotton liners (Allerderm)
Miscellaneous items	*some* medical stickers by MediBadge, UAL, Cushie Tushie Potty Seat
Newsprint, ads, coupons, lottery scratch tickets	
Pacifiers	Soothies (Children's Med Ventures), **selected** Binky, Gerber, Infa, Kip, MAM
Rubber bands, bungee cords	Plasti bands
Toys—Stretch Armstrong, old Barbies	Jurassic Park figures (Kenner), 1993 Barbie, Disney dolls (Mattel), many toys by Fisher Price, Little Tikes, Playschool, Discovery, Trolls (Norfin), Silly-putty
Water toys & equipment: beach thongs, masks, bathing suits, caps, scuba gear, goggles	PVC, plastic, nylon, Suits Me Swimwear
Wheelchair cushions, tires	Jay, ROHO cushions, Use leather gloves, Sof Care bed/chair cushions (Gaymar)
Zippered plastic storage bags	Waxed paper, plain plastic bags, Ziploc bags

CHAPTER HIGHLIGHTS

☞ The infant is born with natural immunity from the mother, and develops acquired immunity gradually in the first 6 years of life.

☞ Acquired immunity is humoral (antibody-mediated) and cell mediated.

☞ B cells, T cells, natural killer cells, and complement proteins are the major components of a healthy immune system.

☞ Disorders of the immune system can be due to genetic causes (primary immunodeficiency), or can be acquired (secondary immunodeficiency).

☞ Severe combined immune deficiency (SCID) disease is life threatening and requires careful medical and nursing management.

☞ Human immunodeficiency virus (HIV) can lead to acquired immunodeficiency disease (AIDS); care focuses on prevention of this major viral infection.

☞ A child infected with HIV needs support for nutrition, infection control, and developmental stimulation.

☞ Nurses support families of children with severe immune deficiency with a focus on finances, provision of complex medical care, and emotional support.

☞ Autoimmune disorders such as eczema, juvenile rheumatoid arthritis, and systemic lupus erythematosis occur when the body perceives its own tissue as foreign and mounts a defense against it.

☞ Although progress is slow, the body may return to normal after manifestation of an autoimmune disorder.

☞ A thorough assessment and careful teaching can help the child with allergies to successfully manage reactions.

☞ Allergy to latex products is commonly seen in children, health care workers, and the general population.

EXPLOREMEDIALINK

NCLEX Review, Case Studies, and other interactive resources for this chapter can be found on the companion website at http://www.prenhall.com/london. Click on "Chapter 40" and select the activities for this chapter.

For animations, more NCLEX review questions, and an audio glossary, access the accompanying CD-ROM in this textbook.

REFERENCES

Ammann, A. J., & Stiehm, E. R. (1997). T-cell immunodeficiency disorders. In D. P. Stites, A. I. Terr, & T. G. Parslow (Eds.), *Medical immunology* (pp. 345–351). Stamford, CT: Appleton & Lange.

Burpo, R. H. (2000). Common antiviral agents used in women's and children's care. *Journal of Obstetric, Gynecologic and Neonatal Nursing 29*, 181–200.

Candoti, F. (2000). The potential for therapy of immune disorders with gene therapy. *Pediatric Clinics of North America, 47*, 1389–1408.

Caselli, D. (2000). Human immunodeficiency virus–related cancer in children: Incidence and treatment outcome—Report of the Italian Register. *Journal of Clinical Oncology, 18*, 3854–3861.

Cassileth, B. R. (1998). *The alternative medicine handbook*. New York: W. W. Norton.

Chapman, E. H., Weintraub, R. J., Milburn, M. A., Pirozzi, T. O., & Woo, E. (1999). Homeopathic treatment of mild traumatic brain injury: A randomized, double-blind, placebo-controlled clinical trial. *Journal of Head Trauma Rehabilitation, 14*(6), 521–542.

Cohen, H., Chen, X. C., Sunkle, S., Davis, L., Geromanos, K., Xanthos, G., et al. (2000). Ability of caregivers to read delayed hypersensitivity skin tests in children exposed to and infected by HIV. *Journal of Pediatric Health Care, 14*, 50–55.

Committee on Pediatric AIDS. (1998). Human immunodeficiency virus/ acquired immunodeficiency syndrome education in schools. *Pediatrics, 101*, 933–935.

Committee on Pediatric AIDS and Committee on Adolescence. (2001). Adolescents and human immunodeficiency virus infections: The role of the pediatrician in prevention and intervention. *Pediatrics, 107*, 188–190.

Davenas, E., Beauvais, J., Oberbaum, M., Robinson, B., Miadonna, A., Tedeschi, A., et al. (1988). Human basophil degranulation triggered by very dilute antiserum against IgE. *Nature, 333*, 816–818.

Elder, M. E. (2000). T-cell immunodeficiencies. *Pediatric Clinics of North America, 47*, 1253–1274.

Ferley, J. P., Smirou, D., D'Adhemar, D., & Balducci, F. (1989). A controlled evaluation of a homeopathic preparation in the treatment of influenza-like syndromes. *British Journal of Clinical Pharmacology, 27*, 329–335.

Fisher, P., Greenwood, A., Huskisson, E. C., Turner, P., & Belon, P. (1989). Effect of homeopathic treatment on fibrositis (primary fibromyalgia). *British Medical Journal, 299*, 365–366.

Fugh-Berman, A. (1996). *Alternative medicine: What works*. Tucson, AZ: Odonian Press.

Gottlieb, B. S., & Ilowite, N. T. (2000). Meeting the challenge of rheumatologic diseases in teens. *Contemporary Pediatrics, 17*, 61–98.

Grosch-Worner, I. (2000). An effective and safe protocol involving zidovudine and caesarean section to reduce vertical transmission of HIV-1 infection. *AIDS, 14*, 2903–2911.

Gross, E. J., & Larkin, M. H. (1996). The child with HIV in day care and school. *Nursing Clinics of North America, 31*, 231–242.

Instone, S. L. (2000). Perceptions of children with HIV when not told for so long: Implications for diagnosis disclosure. *Journal of Pediatric Health Care, 14*, 235–243.

Kaplan, J. E., Masur, H., & Holmes, K. K. (1997). 1997 USPHS/IDSA guidelines for the prevention of opportunistic infections in persons infected with human immunodeficiency virus. *Morbidity and Mortality Weekly Report, 46*(RR-12), 1–46.

Kline, M. W., Calles, N. R., Simon, C., & Schwarzwald, H. (2000). Pilot study of hydroxyurea in human immunodeficiency virus infected children receiving didanasine and/or stavudine. *Pediatric Infectious Disease Journal, 19*, 1083–1086.

Langston, C., Cooper, E. R., Goldfarb, J., Easley, K. A., Husak, S., Sunkle, S., et al. (2001). Human immunodeficiency virus-related mortality in infants and children: Data from the pediatric pulmonary and cardiovascular complications of vertically transmitted HIV study. *Pediatrics, 107*, 328–338.

Lee, M. H., & Kim, K. T. (1998). Latex allergy: A relevant issue in the general pediatric population. *Journal of Pediatric Health Care, 12*, 242–246.

Lehman, T. J. A. (1995). A practical guide to systemic lupus erythematosus. *Pediatric Clinics of North America, 42*, 1223–1238.

Linde, K., Clausius, N., Ramirez, G., Melchart, D., Eitel, F., Hedges, L. V., et al. (1997). Are the clinical effects on homoeopathy placebo effects? A meta-analysis of placebo-controlled trials. *Lancet, 350*, 834–843.

Lindegren, M. L., Steinberg, S., & Byers, R. H. (2000). Epidemiology of HIV/AIDS in children. *Pediatric Clinics of North America, 47*, 1–20.

Luzuriaga, K., Bryson, Y., Krogstad, P., Robinson, J., Stechenberg, B., Lamson, M., et al. (1997). Combination treatment with zidovudine, didanosine, and nevirapine in infants with human immunodeficiency virus type infection. *New England Journal of Medicine, 336*, 1343–1344.

Nielsen, K., & Bryson, Y. J. (2000). Diagnosis of HIV infection in children. *Pediatric Clinics of North America, 47*, 39–64.

Pearson, D. A., McGrath, N. M., Nozyce, M., Nichols, S. L., Raskino, C., Brouwers, P., et al. (2000). Predicting HIV progression in children using measures of neuropsychological and neurological functioning. *Pediatrics, 106*(6), (electronic only; full site is http://www.pediatrics.org/cgi/content/full/106/6/e76.

Rogers, A. S. (2000). Serologic examination of hepatitis B infection and immunization in HIV-positive youth and associated risks. *AIDS Patient Care and STDs, 14*, 651–657.

Sack, K. E., & Fye, K. H. (1997). Rheumatic diseases. In D. P. Stites, A. T. Terr, & T. G. Parslow (Eds.), *Medical immunology* (pp. 456–479). Stamford, CT: Appleton & Lange.

Schwartz, S. A. (2000). Intravenous immunoglobulin treatment of immunodeficiency disorders. *Pediatric Clinics of North America, 47*, 1355–1370.

Skidmore-Roth, L. (2001). *Mosby's handbook of herbs and natural supplements*. St. Louis, MO: Mosby.

Spigelblatt, L., Laine-Ammara, G., Pless, I. B., & Guyver, A. (1994). The use of alternative medicine by children. *Pediatrics, 94*(6), 811–814.

St. Louis, M. E., Levine, W. C., Wasserheit, J. N., DeCock, K. M., West, G. R., Holtgrave, D. R., et al. (1998). HIV prevention through early detection and treatment of other sexually transmitted diseases—United States. *Morbidity and Mortality Weekly Report, 47*(RR-12), 1–24.

Stiehm, E. R., & Ammann, A. J. (1997). Combined antibody (B-cell) & cellular (T-cell) immunodeficiency disorders. In D. P. Stites, A. I. Terr, & T. G. Parslow (Eds.), *Medical immunology* (pp. 352–363). Stamford, CT: Appleton & Lange.

Temple, M. E., Koranyi, K., & Nahata, M. C. (2001). The safety and antiviral effect of protease inhibitors in children. *Pharmacotherapy, 21*, 287–294.

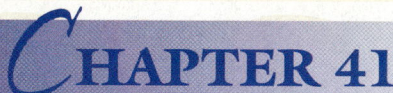
The Child with Infectious and Communicable Diseases

*W*e *came in today because Chang has a fever. I know Lian and Chang need immunizations. Lian will be going to kindergarten in the fall, so it is very important for her to get all of the immunizations she needs now.*

—MOTHER OF LIAN, 5 YEARS OLD AND CHANG, 2 YEARS OLD

~ Key Terms

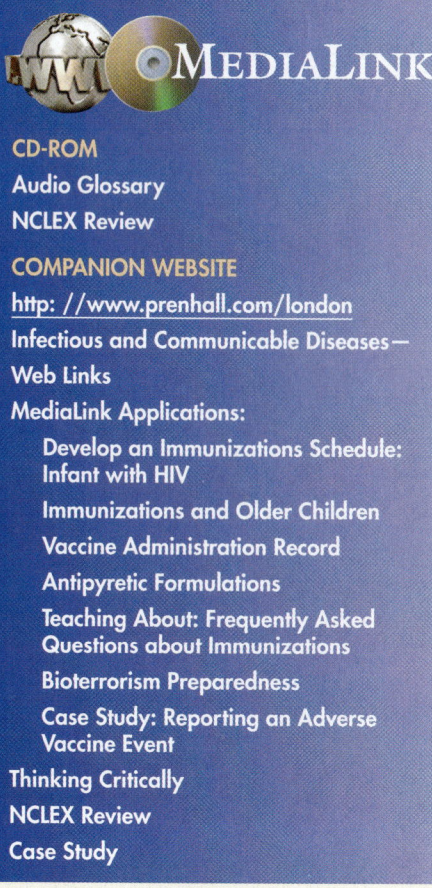

Young children are particularly susceptible to illnesses transmitted among close contacts or through exposure to microorganisms in various settings. Many of these illnesses can be prevented by following the recommended schedule of childhood immunizations. Why are children more vulnerable than adults to infectious and communicable diseases? How are common infectious and communicable diseases recognized, and what is their medical and nursing management? This chapter will answer these questions.

An **infectious disease** is an illness caused by microorganisms commonly communicated from one host (human or otherwise) to another. A **communicable disease** is an illness directly or indirectly transmitted from one person to another. Communicable diseases are a major cause of morbidity in infants and children in the United States, and sometimes result in death.

For a communicable disease to occur, the following need to be present (see "Pathophysiology Illustrated: The Chain of Infection"):

- An infectious agent, or pathogen
- An effective means of transmission
- A susceptible host

An effective chain of transmission for infection requires a suitable habitat, or reservoir, for the pathogen. A reservoir may be living or nonliving, and transmission may be direct or indirect. **Direct transmission** involves physical contact between the source of the infection and the new host. **Indirect transmission** occurs when pathogens survive outside humans before causing infection and disease.

A susceptible host is also necessary for the occurrence of an infectious disease. Young children, whose immune systems are immature and who have not yet developed antibodies to many agents, cannot defend themselves against disease as well as older children. Immunodeficiency and poor health may also increase a child's risk of contracting an infectious disease.

Developing Cultural Competence

In some cultures, infectious diseases are seen as punishment or the result of curses or evil spirits. For example, Native Americans traditionally view illnesses as the result of disharmony or displeasing the spirits. They may not believe in the germ theory of disease causation.

Control of infectious diseases is usually directed at interrupting the chain of transmission or eliminating one or more of the habitats or reservoirs (e.g., spraying insecticide to kill mosquitoes that carry malaria). Isolating an infected individual interferes with disease transmission, and killing the pathogen eliminates the causal agent. Public health authorities monitor patterns of disease occurrence, and health care workers are required to report cases of many infectious diseases to state health officials.

Major public health programs and scientific advances such as safer drinking water, better sanitation, improved standards of living, immunizations, and advanced medical treatment have decreased the occurrence of infectious and communicable diseases. But they remain a significant source of morbidity and mortality in infants and children, especially in developing countries. Special attention is now directed at infectious agents that can become weapons of terrorists and cause disease epidemics. ⬭ **WEB**

SPECIAL VULNERABILITY OF CHILDREN

The capability and function of the immune system, especially of infants, is poorly understood. Infants are particularly vulnerable to infectious diseases for the following reasons:

- Their immune responses are immature.
- Passively acquired maternal antibodies are decreasing.
- Disease protection through immunization is as yet incomplete.

As children grow, they develop immunity through immunization or exposure to the natural disease. As children mature and become more active, they interact more frequently with other children and adults, which increases their exposure to infectious agents (Figure 41–1 ◆). As

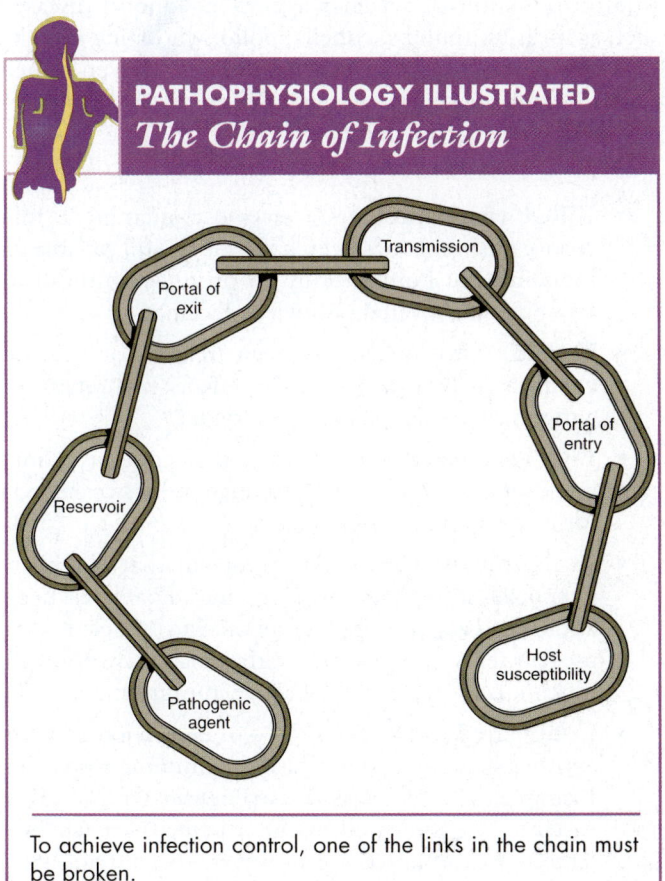

PATHOPHYSIOLOGY ILLUSTRATED
The Chain of Infection

Transmission

Portal of exit

Portal of entry

Reservoir

Host susceptibility

Pathogenic agent

To achieve infection control, one of the links in the chain must be broken.

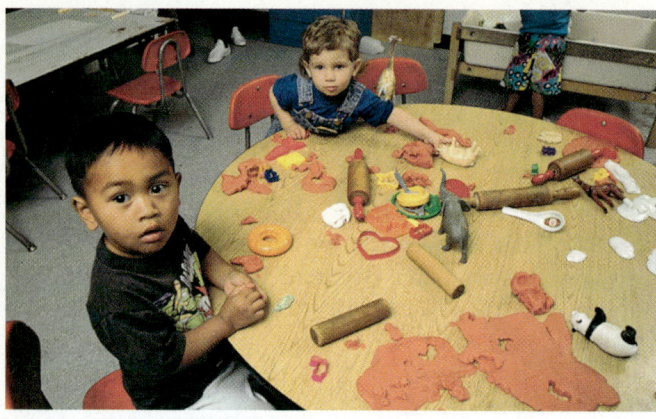

FIGURE 41–1. ◆ Infectious diseases are easily transmitted in settings such as child care centers where children handle common objects.

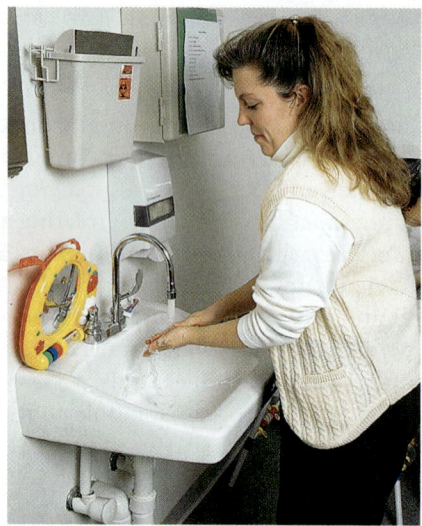

FIGURE 41–2. ◆ Proper handwashing is one of the most effective measures in preventing transmission of microorganisms.

healthy children are exposed to more infections, they develop antibodies naturally. Thus, subsequent infections with the same type of organism may be less severe or avoided. (Refer to "Anatomy and Physiology of Pediatric Differences" in Chapter 40. ◯▭)

The poor hygiene behaviors of young children facilitate transmission of infectious diseases in child care and other close environments. The fecal-oral and respiratory routes are the most common sources of transmission in children. Children usually do not wash their hands after toileting unless they are closely supervised. They put toys and their hands in their mouths, and then rub their nose and eyes. They often are unable to care for a runny nose without help. Diapers may leak stool and provide the fecal exposure to organisms. In addition, the staff in child care centers or other people caring for children may not use proper handwashing techniques (Figure 41–2 ◆). All of these behaviors promote the transmission of infection.

IMMUNIZATION

The development and widespread use of immunizations has been one of the great breakthroughs of modern medicine. Immunization introduces an **antigen** (a foreign substance that triggers an immune system response) into the body, allowing immunity against a disease to develop naturally. The person produces **antibodies,** proteins capable of responding to specific antigens.

To create **active immunity** (in which antibody production is stimulated without causing clinical disease), an antigen is given in the form of a vaccine. However, a child may need antibodies faster than the body can develop them. In this case, **passive immunity** may be induced with antibodies produced in another human or animal host and given to the child. This approach is also used with at-risk children after a single exposure to a disease to prevent the disease from occurring or to reduce its severity. For example, if a child who has never had a tetanus immunization steps on a rusty nail, the child needs immediate protection (passive immunity) from tetanus. Tetanus immune globulin injection is given to combat the tetanus toxin produced by the bacterial spores introduced by the nail. Because passive immunity does not confer lasting immunity, the process of antibody development (active immunity) is then begun by administering a tetanus toxoid vaccine.

Since vaccines were first developed in the late 1800s, many diseases have decreased dramatically in incidence. The introduction of vaccines against childhood diseases such as measles, mumps, rubella, polio, whooping cough, diphtheria, smallpox, *Haemophilus influenzae* type b, hepatitis B, and chickenpox has greatly improved the quality of life for children and adults.

Types of vaccines include the following:

- **Killed virus vaccine.** A vaccine containing a microorganism that has been killed but is still capable of inducing the human body to produce antibodies. Example: inactivated poliovirus vaccine.

- **Toxoid.** A toxin that has been treated (by heat or chemical) to weaken its toxic effects but retain its antigenicity. Example: tetanus toxoid.

- **Live virus vaccine.** A vaccine that contains a microorganism in live but attenuated, or weakened, form. Example: measles vaccine.

- **Recombinant forms.** An organism that has been genetically altered for use in vaccines. Examples: hepatitis B and **acellular pertussis vaccine** (a vaccine that uses proteins from pertussis rather than the whole cell to stimulate the process of active immunity).

- **Conjugated forms.** An altered organism joined with another substance to increase the immune response. Example: The *Haemophilus influenzae* type b (Hib) vaccine is conjugated with a protein-carrier like tetanus toxoid (PRP-T); however, this specific vaccine brand confers no immunity to tetanus.

Improvements in vaccine technology continue to improve the safety and efficacy of immunization against an increasing number of diseases. Today's vaccines are often produced synthetically with recombinant DNA technology or genetic engineering.

Nursing Practice

Thimerosol, a preservative that contains ethyl mercury, is contained in trace elements in some vaccines and immune globulins. Although there is no evidence that the mercury is harmful to children receiving vaccines, some allergic reactions have been reported. Vaccine manufacturers are working to further reduce or eliminate thimerosol from vaccines. At least one brand of each vaccine does not contain thimerosol (Atkinson, 1999).

Vaccines should be administered at specific ages and intervals. Timing for first immunizations is determined by the age at which **transplacental immunity** (passive immunity transferred from mother to infant) decreases or disappears, and the infant or child develops the ability to make antibodies in response to the vaccine. Scientists continue to study the duration of protection from vaccines. Some vaccines do not confer lifelong immunity.

The recommended schedule for immunization is updated annually to reflect new vaccines and the need for repeat immunization. The Advisory Committee on Immunization Practices (ACIP) of the Centers for Disease Control, the American Academy of Pediatrics (AAP), and the American Academy of Family Practitioners (AAFP) collaborate on the recommended schedule. The 2002 recommendations are given in Table 41–1. This schedule applies to immunizations all children should receive, and schedules and recommendations vary for children who begin immunizations later in childhood or need catch-up doses. Other immunization recommendations are made for children who recently received blood products or immunosuppressive agents. **WEB**

Nursing Practice

Two major resources provide more extensive information about immunization schedules and specific vaccines, as well as infectious and communicable diseases. The American Academy of Pediatrics *Red Book: Report of the Committee on Infectious Disease* is updated every few years. The revised immunization schedule is published each January in the American Academy of Pediatrics newsletter and its journal, *Pediatrics*. The Centers for Disease Control maintains a regularly updated website with detailed information about immunizations and infectious and communicable diseases.

Supplemental immunizations for influenza, meningococcal, and pneumococcal infections are recommended for certain children, as noted in Table 41–2.

The effectiveness of vaccines depends on the proper storage of vaccines and the immunization of all susceptible individuals. Lower immunization rates of children are often associated with economic factors, limited access to health care, the lack of primary care at hours convenient for working parents, inadequate education about the importance of immunization, and religious prohibitions. Efforts to administer vaccines and monitor immunization status in children are increasing. For example, managed care organizations require that contracted health care providers comply with the pediatric immunization standards, and patient records are audited to ensure compliance.

Developing Cultural Competence

Vietnamese-American children 3 to 18 years old have lower rates of hepatitis B vaccination than other ethnic groups. This is particularly worrisome as hepatitis B is endemic in those born in Southeast Asia and has a prevalence of 7% to 14% among Vietnamese adults living in the United States. As people with hepatitis B disease can transmit the virus to others and are at increased risk for chronic hepatitis, cirrhosis, and liver cancer, these children should be targeted for special immunization efforts (Jenkins, McPhee, Wong, et al., 2000).

Nursing Practice

Make sure vaccines are stored properly in the refrigerator or freezer. An improperly stored or poorly administered vaccine may be rendered ineffective, thus preventing the child from developing immunity. Read the package inserts of vaccines to determine proper storage conditions. Some vaccines are frozen; others are refrigerated. When reconstituting vaccines, it is important to use the solution provided or follow the manufacturer's directions. Write the date and time on the bottle if it is a multidose vial. Many reconstituted vaccines (e.g., varicella vaccine) have a very short shelf life.

Nursing Management

Nursing Assessment and Diagnosis

Nurses are responsible for reviewing a child's immunization record and determining whether the child needs immunization. **WEB** Inquire about the child's preventive care as well as health problems. Make sure to use the most current guidelines for comparison with the child's record. If the child is behind in appropriate immunizations

TABLE 41-1 Recommended Childhood Immunization Schedule United States, 2002

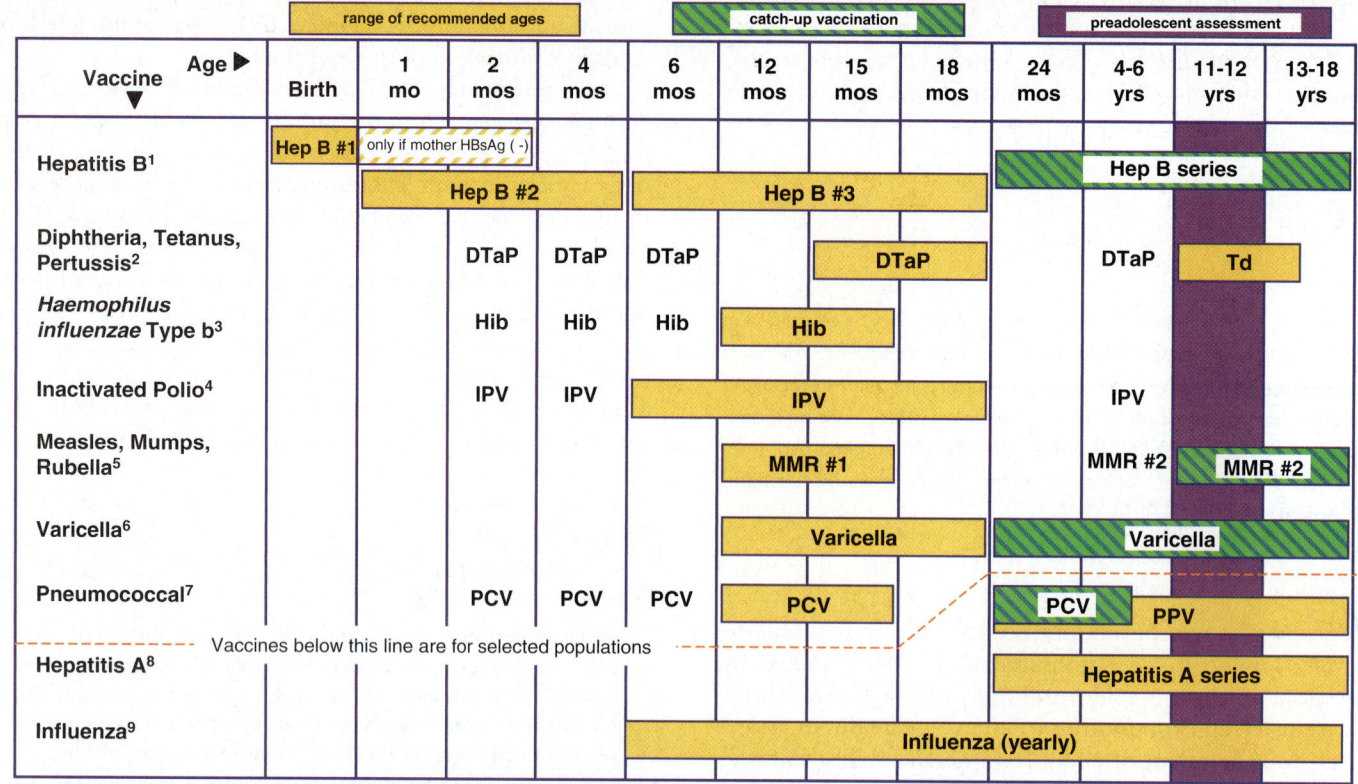

Legend: range of recommended ages | catch-up vaccination | preadolescent assessment

Vaccine ▼ / Age ▶	Birth	1 mo	2 mos	4 mos	6 mos	12 mos	15 mos	18 mos	24 mos	4-6 yrs	11-12 yrs	13-18 yrs
Hepatitis B[1]	Hep B #1	*only if mother HBsAg (-)*									Hep B series	
		Hep B #2			Hep B #3							
Diphtheria, Tetanus, Pertussis[2]			DTaP	DTaP	DTaP		DTaP			DTaP	Td	
Haemophilus influenzae Type b[3]			Hib	Hib	Hib	Hib						
Inactivated Polio[4]			IPV	IPV	IPV					IPV		
Measles, Mumps, Rubella[5]						MMR #1				MMR #2	MMR #2	
Varicella[6]						Varicella					Varicella	
Pneumococcal[7]			PCV	PCV	PCV	PCV			PCV		PPV	
Hepatitis A[8]									Hepatitis A series			
Influenza[9]					Influenza (yearly)							

Vaccines below this line are for selected populations

This schedule indicates the recommended ages for routine administration of currently licensed childhood vaccines, as of December 1, 2001, for children through age 18 years. Any dose not given at the recommended age should be given at any subsequent visit when indicated and feasible. ▨ Indicates age groups that warrant special effort to administer those vaccines not previously given. Additional vaccines may be licensed and recommended during the year. Licensed combination vaccines may be used whenever any components of the combination are indicated and the vaccine's other components are not contraindicated. Providers should consult the manufacturers' package inserts for detailed recommendations.

Approved by the Advisory Committee on Immunization Practices (www.cdc.gov/nip/acip) the American Academy of Pediatrics (www.aap.org), and the American Academy of Family Physicians (www.aafp.org).

1. Hepatitis B vaccine (Hep B). All infants should receive the first dose of hepatitis B vaccine soon after birth and before hospital discharge; the first dose may also be given by age 2 months if the infant's mother is HBsAg-negative. Only monovalent hepatitis B vaccine can be used for the birth dose. Monovalent or combination vaccine containing Hep B may be used to complete the series; four doses of vaccine may be administered if combination vaccine is used. The second dose should be given at least 4 weeks after the first dose, except for Hib-containing vaccine which cannot be administered before age 6 weeks. The third dose should be given at least 16 weeks after the first dose and at least 8 weeks after the second dose. The last dose in the vaccination series (third or fourth dose) should not be administered before age 6 months.

Infants born to HBsAg-positive mothers should receive hepatitis B vaccine and 0.5 mL hepatitis B immune globulin (HBIG) within 12 hours of birth at separate sites. The second dose is recommended at age 1-2 months and the vaccination series should be completed (third or fourth dose) at age 6 months.

Infants born to mothers whose HBsAg status is unknown should receive the first dose of the hepatitis B vaccine series within 12 hours of birth. Maternal blood should be drawn at the time of delivery to determine the mother's HBsAg status; if the HBsAg test is positive, the infant should receive HBIG as soon as possible (no later than age 1 week).

2. Diphtheria and tetanus toxoids and acellular pertussis vaccine (DTaP). The fourth dose of DTaP may be administered as early as age 12 months, provided 6 months have elapsed since the third dose and the child is unlikely to return at age 15-18 months. **Tetanus and diphtheria toxoids (Td)** is recommended at age 11-12 years if at least 5 years have elapsed since the last dose of tetanus and diphtheria toxoid-containing vaccine. Subsequent routine Td boosters are recommended every 10 years.

3. Haemophilus influenzae type b (Hib) conjugate vaccine. Three Hib conjugate vaccines are licensed for infant use. If PRP-OMP (PedvaxHIB® or ComVax®[Merck]) is administered at ages 2 and 4 months, a dose at age 6 months is not required. DTaP/Hib combination products should not be used for primary immunization in infants at age 2, 4 or 6 months, but can be used as boosters following any Hib vaccine.

4. Inactivated poliovirus vaccine (IPV). An all-IPV schedule is recommended for routine childhood poliovirus vaccination in the United States. All children should receive four doses of IPV at age 2 months, 4 months, 6-18 months, and 4-6 years.

5. Measles, mumps, and rubella vaccine (MMR). The second dose of MMR is recommended routinely at age 4-6 years but may be administered during any visit, provided at least 4 weeks have elapsed since the first dose and that both doses are administered beginning at or after age 12 months. Those who have not previously received the second dose should complete the schedule by the visit at age 11-12 years.

6. Varicella vaccine. Varicella vaccine is recommended at any visit at or after age 12 months for susceptible children (i.e. those who lack a reliable history of chickenpox). Susceptible persons aged ≥13 years should receive two doses, given at least 4 weeks apart.

7. Pneumococcal vaccine. The heptavalent **pneumococcal conjugate vaccine (PCV)** is recommended for all children aged 2-23 months and for certain children aged 24-59 months. **Pneumococcal polysaccharide vaccine (PPV)** is recommended in addition to PCV for certain high-risk groups. See MMWR 2000;49(RR-9);1-37.

8. Hepatitis A vaccine. Hepatitis A vaccine is recommended for use in selected states and regions, and for certain high-risk groups; consult your local public health authority. See MMWR 1999;48(RR-12);1-37.

9. Influenza vaccine. Influenza vaccine is recommended annually for children age ≥6 months with certain risk factors (including but not limited to asthma, cardiac disease, sickle cell disease, HIV and diabetes; see MMWR 2001;50(RR-4);1-44), and can be administered to all others wishing to obtain immunity. Children aged ≤12 years should receive vaccine in a dosage appropriate for their age (0.25 mL if age 6-35 months or 0.5 mL if aged ≥3 years). Children aged ≤8 years who are receiving influenza vaccine for the first time should receive two doses separated by at least 4 weeks.

Additional information about vaccines, vaccine supply, and contraindications for immunization, is available at www.cdc.gov/nip or at the National Immunization Hotline, 800-232-2522 (English) or 800-232-0233 (Spanish).

TABLE 41–2 Supplemental Immunizations

Vaccine	Recommendation
Influenza	For children with chronic pulmonary disease, cardiac disease, sickle cell disease or other hemoglobinopathies, diabetes, metabolic disease, human immunodeficiency virus (HIV) infection, or those undergoing immunosuppressive therapy or chronic aspirin therapy (e.g., for rheumatoid arthritis or Kawasaki disease). Administered annually in autumn. Children with no history of influenza illness or vaccine need two doses 1 mo apart.
Meningococcal	For children older than 2 years of age with asplenia. Vaccine duration is 5 years or longer in children older than 4 years at the time of immunization. The vaccine is also suggested for college students. The vaccine should be repeated after 1 year if the child is younger than 4 years at the time of initial immunization.
23-valent Pneumococcal	For children older than 2 years of age with sickle cell disease, asplenia, chronic cardiovascular and pulmonary disorders, nephrotic syndrome, renal failure, HIV infection, cerebrospinal fluid leaks, or those undergoing immunosuppressive therapy. Repeat the immunization after 3–5 years if the child is younger than 10 years and at severe risk for pneumococcal infection.

for age, determine the best combination of vaccines to give at this visit to better protect the child. Also take advantage of opportunities to give needed immunizations to siblings accompanying the family on the visit. A minor illness should not deter immunization.

Health care providers miss many opportunities to immunize children. Children (and siblings present) should have their immunization status assessed during all health care visits, hospitalizations, and in schools. To reduce the number of missed opportunities for full immunization of children, use the following guidelines (American Academy of Pediatrics, 2000).

▶ Several vaccines—diphtheria, tetanus, and acellular pertussis (DTaP); measles, mumps, and rubella (MMR); hepatitis B (HBV); *Haemophilus influenzae* type b (Hib); inactivated polio (IPV); varicella; and heptavalent pneumococcal vaccines—can be given at the same visit.

▶ Two injections can be given in different sites on the same extremity.

▶ Immunizations can be given when the child has a minor illness with or without a low-grade fever, and with antibiotic treatment. Recent exposure to an infectious disease is not a reason to defer a vaccine.

▶ Premature infants need the same immunizations as full-term infants.

▶ Immunizations can be given when there was a local reaction to a prior vaccine or a family member had an adverse response.

True contraindications for a vaccine are an anaphylactic reaction to the vaccine or one of its components and a moderate to severe acute illness. Specific vaccines may have additional contraindications, such as pregnancy and allergy to some components of the vaccine (e.g., neomycin, gelatin, eggs) (see Table 41–3).

Assess the child for potential contraindications to vaccines. Ask about past reactions to vaccines as well as allergy to key vaccine components such as eggs, gelatin, or neomycin. Determine whether female teens could be pregnant.

Ask about recent administration of immune globulin or blood products, which may decrease antibody response to vaccines. Follow guidelines for administration of specific live virus vaccines (e.g., measles, varicella).

The accompanying "Nursing Care Plan" explores three potential nursing diagnoses that may apply to the child needing immunizations. Additional nursing diagnoses may include:

▶ *Ineffective airway clearance* related to an obstructed airway

▶ *Risk for impaired skin integrity* related to vaccine response

▶ *Altered health maintenance* related to cultural beliefs regarding routine immunization

Planning and Implementation

Nursing management focuses on informing parents about immunizations and possible side effects, addressing their fears about possible reactions, obtaining consent, and reporting adverse reactions.

Be a strong advocate for immunization. Being well informed about immunizations, their potential side effects, and recommended schedules assists immunization efforts (see Table 41–3).

Provide written materials about immunizations to the parents or guardian. When teaching about immunizations, explain the risks and benefits of immunization, risks of disease, and common side effects and treatments. Record the child's history carefully, specifying any previous reactions to immunizations, allergies, and immune diseases.

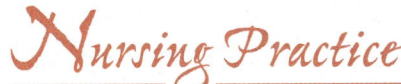

Be prepared for potential vaccine anaphylaxis. Keep epinephrine 1:1000 and resuscitation equipment immediately available. The dose for epinephrine is 0.01 mL/kg per dose and can be repeated every 10 to 20 minutes until symptoms subside or other emergency care interventions are initiated (American Academy of Pediatrics, 2000).

TABLE 41–3 Common Pediatric Immunizations

Immunization Type	Side Effects	Contraindications	Nursing Considerations
Diphtheria and Pertussis Vaccines and Tetanus Toxoid (DTaP) *Route:* Intramuscular *Dosage:* 0.5 mL *Age(s) given:* 2, 4, 6, 15–18 months; 4–6 years (5 doses) *Storage:* Store in body of refrigerator at 2–8 °C (35–46 °F). Do not freeze. *Acel-Imune and Tripedia are licensed for all 5 doses. Infanrix and Certiva are licensed for the first 4 doses (Centers for Disease Control, 2000).	*Common:* Redness, pain, swelling, nodule at injection site; temperature up to 38.3 °C (101 °F); drowsiness, fussiness; anorexia within 2 days of injection. Increase in frequency and magnitude of local reactions with 4th and 5th doses, e.g., entire limb swelling. *Serious:* Anaphylaxis; shock or collapse, fever above 38.8 °C (102 °F); persistent inconsolable crying.	Occurrence of a serious side effect after previous administration of DTaP, such as anaphylaxis. Administration to be delayed for 1 month after immunosuppressive therapy and until moderate to severe febrile illnesses have resolved. Administration of immune serum globulin within last 90 days.	Use same brand for all doses where feasible. Prior to immunization, ask about previous reactions to immunization. DTaP may coincide with or hasten the recognition of a seizure disorder. In children with a history of seizures with or without fever, give acetaminophen at the time of vaccine and then every 4 hours for 24 hours. Shake vaccine before withdrawing. Solution will be cloudy. If it contains clumps that cannot be resuspended, do not use. When required, simultaneous administration of tetanus immune globulin or diphtheria antitoxin should be given in separate sites with a new needle and syringe. Inform parents of the chance of increased reaction to the 4th and 5th doses.
Poliovirus Vaccine Inactivated (IPV) *Route:* Subcutaneous *Dosage:* 0.5 mL *Age(s) given:* 2,4,12–18 months; 4–6 years (4 doses) *Storage:* Store in body of refrigerator at 2–8 °C (35–46 °F). Do not freeze.	*Common:* Swelling and tenderness, irritability, tiredness *Serious:* Anaphylaxis	Hypersensitivity to vaccine components: neomycin, streptomycin, polymyxin B. Anaphylactic response.	Prior to immunization, ask if the child has an allergy to neomycin, streptomycin, or polymyxin B. Clear, colorless suspension. Do not use if it contains particulate matter, becomes cloudy, or changes color. Recommended for use in all vaccine doses.
Measles, Mumps, Rubella Vaccines (MMR) *Route:* Subcutaneous *Dosage:* 0.5 mL *Age(s) given:* 12–15 months; 4–6 years (2 doses) *Storage:* Store in body of refrigerator at 2–8 °C (35–46 °F). When reconstituted, keep refrigerated and away from light; discard if unused within 8 hours. Diluent is stored at room temperature or in refrigerator. Do not freeze.	*Common:* Elevated temperature 1–2 weeks after immunization; redness or pain at injection site; noncontagious rash; joint pain. *Serious:* Anaphylaxis; encephalopathy; thrombocytopenia purpura, chronic arthritis.	Allergy to neomycin or gelatin. Severely impaired immune system due to malignancy, immune deficiency disease, immunosuppressive therapy. MMR vaccine is recommended for those infected with HIV. Wait at least 3 to 11 months after administration of immune serum globulin or blood products (time determined by the type) before giving vaccine. Pregnancy.	Prior to immunization, ask if child has allergy to neomycin or gelatin. Inquire about immunosuppression. Instruct adolescent girls of childbearing age to avoid pregnancy for 3 months after immunization. Give tuberculosis (TB) skin test at same time as MMR or 4–6 weeks later. Reconstituted vaccine is a clear, yellow solution. Give entire contents of vial even if more than 0.5 mL. As college students are at greater risk due to decreasing immunity, make sure they have received a second MMR dose.
Hepatitis B Vaccine (Hep B) *Route:* Intramuscular *Dosage:* Engerix-B: 0.5 mL or Recombivax HB: 0.5 mL *Age(s) given:* Birth–2 months, 1 month after first dose; 6 months after 1st dose *or* Birth–2 months, 1–4 months, 6–18 months (3 doses) *Storage:* Store in body of refrigerator at 2–8 °C (35–46 °F). Do not freeze. Storage out of recommended temperature range decreases potency.	*Common:* Pain or redness at injection site; headache; photophobia; altered liver enzymes. *Serious:* Anaphylaxis.	Prior anaphylaxis, liver abnormalities. Serious allergic reaction to past dose.	Prior to immunization, check status of mother's hepatitis B test and presence of other liver disease. Note: If mother is HBsAg+, vaccine must be given to infant within 12 hours of birth along with hepatitis B immune globulin at the same time in another site with new needle and syringe. Shake vaccine before withdrawing. Solution will appear cloudy. Various formulations (pediatric, adult, dialysis) are available in different strengths. Read package insert carefully to determine the particular formulation's proper dosage for age.

ᵃ Trade names

TABLE 41-3 Common Pediatric Immunizations—continued

Immunization Type	Side Effects	Contraindications	Nursing Considerations
Haemophilus influenza Type B (Hib) _Route:_ Intramuscular _Dosage:_ 0.5 mL _Age(s) given:_ 2, 4, 6, 12–15 months (4 doses for HbOCª [HibTITER] and PRP-Tª [ActHIB or OmniHIB]) or 2,4,12–15 months (3 doses for PRP-OMPª [PedvaxHIB]) _Storage:_ Store in body of refrigerator at 2–8 °C (35–46 °F). Do not freeze. Use or discard reconstituted ActHIB and OmniHIB within 30 minutes. Refrigerate reconstituted PedvaxHIB and discard within 24 hours.	_Common:_ Pain, redness, or swelling at site. _Serious:_ Anaphylaxis (extremely rare).	Prior anaphylactic reaction to this vaccine.	Prior to immunizations, ask if child is immunosuppressed. Solution is clear and colorless. Since schedules for product preparations of different companies vary, it is important to read package inserts carefully. Use the same vaccine preparation for all doses of the primary series if possible. Some preparations combine Hib with DTaP (TriHIBit), DT (VaxemHIB), and Hep B (Comvax).
Heptavalent Pneumococcal Conjugate Vaccine (PCV) _Route:_ Intramuscular _Dosage:_ 0.5 mL _Age(s) given:_ 2,4,6, 12–15 months _Storage:_ Store in body of refrigerator at 2–8 °C (35–46 °F). Do not freeze.	_Common:_ Soreness, swelling, redness at injection site; mild to moderate fever; irritability, drowsiness, restless sleep, decreased appetite, vomiting and diarrhea, rash or hives. _Severe:_ Anaphylaxis.	Hypersensitivity to diphtheria toxoid.	Clear, colorless, or slightly opalescent liquid. In addition to infants this vaccine is a priority for children 2–5 years with sickle cell disease, asplenia, HIV infection, or immunocompromised. The vaccine is also a priority for American Indian and Native Alaskan children 2–5 years because of their increased risk for pneumococcal disease.
Varicella Virus Vaccine _Route:_ Subcutaneous _Dosage:_ 0.5 mL _Age(s) given:_ 12–18 months; or any time up to 12 years of age (1 dose); 13 years or older (2 doses, 4–8 weeks apart) _Storage:_ Frozen at 5 °F or colder. May be stored in refrigerator at 2–8 °C (35–46 °F) up to 72 hours before reconstitution. Once reconstituted, vaccine must be used within 30 minutes or discarded. Do not refreeze. Diluent kept at room temperature.	_Common:_ Pain or redness at injection site; fever up to 38.8 °C (102 °F) in children or up to 37.7 °C (100 °F) in adults; rash at injection site or generalized. _Severe:_ Anaphylaxis.	Allergy to neomycin or gelatin. Immunodeficiency or receiving immunosuppression therapy. Administration of immune serum globulin or blood products in last 3–11 months. Active untreated TB. Pregnancy. Moderate or severe febrile illness.	Prior to immunization, ask if child is immunodeficient or on immunosuppression treatment or has an allergy to neomycin or gelatin. Clear, colorless to pale yellow liquid when reconstituted. Give the entire contents of the vial even if more than 0.5 mL. Instruct adolescent girls of childbearing age to avoid pregnancy for 3 months after immunization.
Hepatitis A, inactivated (Hep A) _Route:_ Intramuscular _Dosage:_ 0.5 mL, 1 mL over 17 years for Vaqtaª, 1 mL over 18 years for Havrixª _Age(s) given:_ 2–18 years, 6–12 months after first dose (2 doses) in areas with increased incidence. _Storage:_ Store in body of refrigerator at 2–8 °C (35–46 °F). Do not freeze; do not use if has been frozen.			Shake well, slightly opaque white suspension. Can be given for postexposure prophylaxis against hepatitis A. Immune globulin and vaccine can be given at the same time in different sites. High incidence areas include the states of Alaska, Arkansas, Arizona, California, Colorado, Idaho, Missouri, Montana, New Mexico, Nevada, Oklahoma, Oregon, South Dakota, Texas, Utah, Washington, and Wyoming. Other high-risk populations to receive vaccine include Native Alaskans and American Indians (Centers for Disease Control, 2001).

GOAL	INTERVENTION	RATIONALE	EXPECTED OUTCOME

1. Risk for infection related to incomplete immunization series

	NIC Priority Interventions: **Immunization Administration**		*NOC Suggested Outcome:* **Risk control**
The child will become adequately protected from disease-preventable illnesses.	▶ Review the child's immunization record for needed vaccines at each health care visit. ▶ Identify all due vaccines that can be provided simultaneously. ▶ Identify potential contraindications to needed vaccines. Review past reactions to vaccines.	▶ Assessment identifies the children who have missed needed immunizations. ▶ Many vaccines can be given at the same visit to more adequately protect the child. This also saves health care trips for families. ▶ Reduces the risk for the child and other caretakers to have adverse reactions to vaccines.	The child is adequately protected from vaccine-preventable illnesses.

2. Knowledge deficit (parent) related to potential side effects of vaccines

	NIC Priority Interventions: **Teaching, prescribed vaccines**		*NOC Suggested Outcome:* **Knowledge:** *Vaccine reactions and comfort measures*
Parents will sign consent for vaccines to be given.	▶ Educate the parents about the need for specific vaccines and the risk if not given. Obtain signed consent before giving vaccines.	▶ Informed consent is required for all treatments.	The parent(s) complete(s) consent form, which is placed in the child's file.
Parents will state the side effects of vaccines given.	▶ Review past reactions to vaccines and describe common potential reactions and why they occur. ▶ Describe serious side effects that should be reported to the health care provider.	▶ Parents should expect common reactions and know they indicate the child's body is building protection to the illness. ▶ Parents need to be prepared for potential serious side effects so they can obtain care if needed.	Parents report all serious side effects to the health care provider.

Parents will manage common side effects of vaccines.	▶ Teach parents general comfort measures for children's common side effects; for example:
	  ▶ Cool pack to tender leg
	  ▶ Acetaminophen for fever and discomfort
	  ▶ Rocking and holding the infant
	  ▶ Gentle movement of affected extremity
		▶ Parents will know how to make the child more comfortable during the 24–48 hours after the vaccine is given.	The child is given comfort measures after vaccine administration.

3. Risk for injury related to vaccine reaction

	NIC Priority Interventions: **Vital sign monitoring**		*NOC Suggested Outcome:* **Risk control**
The child's potential vaccine reactions will be safely managed.	▶ Prepare for life-threatening reactions by having resuscitation drugs and equipment immediately available. ▶ Monitor the child for 15 minutes after the vaccine is given before letting the child go home. ▶ Assess the child for extreme anxiety and injection fearfulness. ▶ Have the fearful child sit or lie down until symptoms of vasovagal response have disappeared. ▶ Report all vaccine-related reactions to the appropriate agency using the standard form.	▶ Anaphylactic reactions must be managed quickly and effectively. ▶ A life-threatening response will usually become apparent within this time frame. ▶ These are potential signs the child may have a vasovagal response to the injection. ▶ The child who faints may sustain a head injury. ▶ Legal requirements for all health care providers.	The child has no reaction, or a severe reaction to a vaccine is managed effectively.

Some parents fear immunization reactions because of stories they have heard. Talk with parents to understand their concerns. Be able to explain the risks and benefits of each immunization. Parents have the right to refuse immunizations for their child on the basis of religious beliefs, but they must sign a waiver noting their decision. If there is a disease outbreak, the nonimmunized child must be kept out of school. Local, city, or state courts decide how to settle any conflicts. WEB

Federal legislation requires consent to be obtained before administering a vaccine. In most institutions it is the nurse's responsibility to inform the parents or the child's legal guardian, supply literature, and obtain written consent before the vaccine is administered. The nurse is required to record the (1) month, day, and year of administration, (2) vaccine given, (3) manufacturer, (4) lot number and expiration date of the immunization given, (5) site and route of administration, and (6) name, title, and address of the person who administers the vaccine. In addition, the nurse ensures that any severe immunization reaction is reported to the National Vaccine Injury Compensation Program (see Skill 7-1). SKILL

Give the appropriate immunizations to the child as efficiently as possible, while providing support to the child (Figure 41–3 ◆). Longer needles (25 mm rather than 16 mm) reduce the rates of local reactions and tenderness in infant immunizations. This may ensure that the vaccine is given intramuscularly rather than subcutaneously (Diggle & Deek, 2000).

Anticipate ways to reduce pain and anxiety associated with immunizations. Do not prolong the process of giving immunizations, and tell the child honestly that the needles will cause some pain. Let the child select the arm or leg for the injection and forms of distraction to promote coping. When finished giving injections, let the parent comfort the child. Provide guidelines for managing expected mild reactions at home. Schedule the child's next appointment for a health supervision visit to complete needed immuniza-

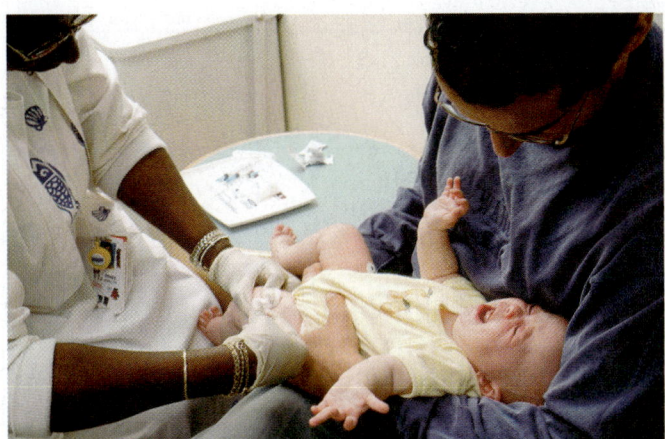

FIGURE 41–3. ◆ Give immunizations quickly and efficiently. Do not prolong the wait and let fear grow. The child will be anxious, especially if more than one injection must be given.

tions. Give parents a record of the child's immunizations, and record the vaccines given in the health care agency's official records.

Certain reactions following immunization are reportable by law to the U.S. Department of Health and Human Services (Table 41–4). Follow guidelines for reporting according to the Vaccine Adverse Event Reporting System. WEB The Vaccine Safety Datalink project continually evaluates vaccine safety on more than 6 million people. Ongoing studies are examining the association of immunizations with diabetes mellitus, and of MMR vaccine with inflammatory bowel disease (American Academy of Pediatrics, 2000).

Evaluation

Expected outcomes of nursing care include:

► Parents are fully informed and give consent for immunizations.
► All immunizations appropriate for the child's age are given at each health visit or to catch up needed immunizations.
► The parents are prepared to manage mild reactions to immunizations at home.

Vaccine	Illness, Disability, Injury, or Condition Covered	Time Period for First Symptom or Manifestation of Onset or of Significant Aggravation after Vaccine Administration—for Compensation
DTaP, P, DT, Td, DTP-Hib, or Tetanus Toxoid; or any other vaccine containing whole cell pertussis bacteria, extracted or partial cell pertussis bacteria, or specific pertussis antigen(s)	Anaphylaxis or anaphylactic shock	0–4 hours
	Encephalopathy (or encephalitis)	72 hours
	Bacterial neuritis	2–28 days
	Any acute complication or sequela (including death) of above events	No limit
	Events described in manufacturer's package insert as contraindications of additional doses of vaccine	Not applicable
Measles, mumps, rubella, or any vaccine containing any of the foregoing as a component needed	Anaphylaxis or anaphylactic shock	0–4 hours
	Encephalopathy (or encephalitis)	5–15 days for measles, mumps, rubella, or any vaccine containing any of the foregoing as a component
	Events described in manufacturer's package insert as contraindications of additional doses of vaccine	Not applicable
Rubella containing vaccines	Chronic arthritis	7–42 days
Measles containing vaccines	Thrombocytopenia purpura	7–30 days
	Vaccine strain measles viral infection in an immunodeficient recipient	0–6 months
Inactivated polio vaccine	Anaphylaxis or anaphylactic shock	0–4 hours
	Any acute complication or sequela (including death) of above events.	No limit
	Events described in manufacturer's package insert as contraindications of additional doses of vaccine	Not applicable
Hepatitis B antigen containing vaccines	Anaphylaxis or anaphylactic shock	0–4 hours
	Any acute complication or sequela (including death) of above events	No limit
	Events described in manufacturer's package insert as contraindications of additional doses of vaccine	Not applicable
Haemophilus influenzae, type B polysaccharide vaccines (unconjugated, PRP vaccines)	Any early-onset Hib disease	0–7 days
	Any acute complication or sequela (including death) of above events	No limit
	Events described in manufacturer's package insert as contraindications of additional doses of vaccine	Not applicable
Haemophilus influenzae, type B polysaccharide conjugate vaccine	No condition specified for compensation	Not applicable
	Events described in manufacturer's package insert as contraindications of additional doses of vaccine	Not applicable
Varicella virus-containing vaccine	No condition specified for compensation	Not applicable
	Events described in manufacturer's package insert as contraindications of additional doses of vaccine	Not applicable

Note: From American Academy of Pediatrics. (2000). *Red Book: Report of the Committee on Infectious Disease* (25th ed.). Elk Grove Village, IL: Author. Adapted.

Thinking Critically

INFECTIOUS AND COMMUNICABLE DISEASES IN CHILDREN ⊂⊃ [WEB]

Infectious and communicable diseases cause acute illnesses. These diseases are caused by bacterial, viral, protozoan, or fungal organisms. As noted earlier, infants and children develop infectious and communicable diseases more frequently than adults do. They develop antibodies as they are exposed to infectious organisms, so they frequently become symptomatic after exposure. The epidemiology, clinical manifestations, treatment, prevention, and nursing care of selected infectious and communicable diseases of childhood are described in detail in Table 41–5.

Clinical Manifestations

The child with an infectious or communicable disease has a cluster of symptoms specific to the disease. Skin rash, poor appetite, malaise, vomiting and/or diarrhea, and body aches are some common signs and symptoms. Fever in a child is often a sign of infectious disease. Why does fever develop in response to certain illnesses and infections? What methods can be used to manage fever in children?

PHYSIOLOGY OF FEVER

The hypothalamus is the control center for the regulation of body temperature and is for that reason frequently compared to a thermostat (see "Pathophysiology Illustrated: Fever"). As blood circulates through the hypothalamus, this brain structure directs body systems to conserve or dissipate heat, depending on the temperature of the blood.

- If body temperature is lower than normal, vasoconstriction is initiated to conserve heat. The adrenal glands produce epinephrine and norepinephrine, which cause an increase in metabolism, more vasoconstriction, and more heat production.
- Shivering or chills may occur, which in turn may increase heat production.

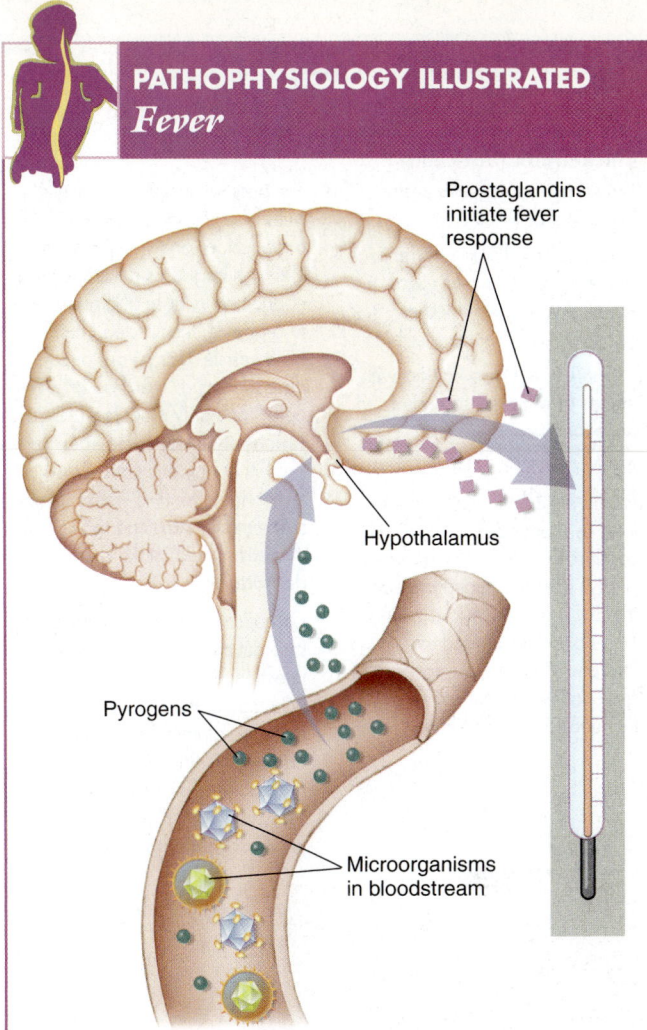

PATHOPHYSIOLOGY ILLUSTRATED
Fever

The hypothalamus functions as the body's thermostat, directing the body to conserve or dissipate heat. When microorganisms invade the body, endogenous pyrogens are released into the bloodstream. These substances travel to the hypothalamus, where they trigger the production and release of prostaglandins, which initiate the fever response. Blood is diverted from the extremities to more central vessels. This helps increase the core body temperature by decreasing heat loss. Shivering increases both metabolic action and heat production. The hypothalamus then maintains the temperature at the new set point.

Nursing Practice

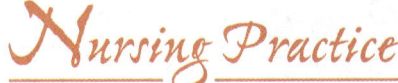

One degree of temperature elevation causes an increase in respiratory rate by four breaths per minute and increases oxygen need by 7%.

- When excess heat is produced, the body's temperature increases. The heart rate and respiratory rate increase.
- Vasodilation occurs and the skin flushes, becoming warm to the touch. As the temperature decreases, the child may start to perspire, and the heart and respiratory rates return to normal.

(text continues on page 1016)

TABLE 41-5   **Selected Infectious and Communicable Diseases in Children**

Disease	Clinical Manifestations	Clinical Therapy	Nursing Management
Chickenpox (Varicella)*+ *Causal agent:* Varicella-zoster, human herpesvirus 3. *Epidemiology:* Peak occurrence is in the late fall, winter, and spring. Maternal antibodies disappear 2–3 months after birth. *Transmission:* Direct contact with lesions or airborne spread of secretions. *Incubation period:* 14–21 days. *Period of communicability:* As long as 5 days before the onset of the rash to a maximum of 6 days after the appearance of the first group of vesicles, when all lesions have crusted over. This period may be prolonged after passive immunization or in immunodeficient children.	The onset of symptoms is acute. Mild fever, malaise, and irritability occur before and with eruption. The rash begins as a macule on an erythematous base and progresses to a papule, then a clear, fluid-filled vesicle. Lesions are often described as a "teardrop on a rose petal" and may erupt for 1–5 days. Lesions of all stages may be present at any one time. Crusts may remain for 1–3 weeks. Lesions in the mouth may lead to decreased fluid intake and dehydration. *Complications:* Complications are rare but can include secondary infection, encephalitis, varicella pneumonia, thrombocytopenia, hepatitis, glomerulonephritis, arthritis, meningitis, and Reye syndrome. This disease may cause very significant illness or death to immunocompromised children.	There is no cure for chickenpox. Medical management is supportive. Oral and IV acyclovir is used for immunocompromised patients. If started within 24 hours will decrease new lesion formation and the total number of lesions, but this is not recommended for healthy children with uncomplicated chickenpox (American Academy of Pediatrics, 2000). *Prognosis:* Most children recover fully. Children who are immunocompromised must be treated aggressively. This includes children on steroids for asthma and other illnesses, and those on long-term salicylate treatment. The disease is more severe when steroids have been given during the incubation period (Twomey, 1998). *Prevention:* Chickenpox is a vaccine-preventable disease. The immunization may be given to susceptible children at any time after 12 months of age. The vaccine may be given within 72 hours after exposure to prevent or significantly modify the disease. Varicella-zoster immune globulin may be given to exposed immunocompromised children with no history of chickenpox or immunization up to 4 days after exposure.	• Use airborne and contact precautions for hospitalized children while they are contagious. • Obtain a varicella immunization history of recent exposure in susceptible children upon admission to the hospital. Place all children exposed to varicella in isolation to protect immunocompromised patients. Nurses caring for the child should have a varicella titer done to be certain of their immune status if they have not had a documented case of chickenpox. • Most children are treated at home. While contagious, isolate them from all susceptible individuals, especially medically fragile children and immunocompromised children or adults, and women early in pregnancy. Notify the school or child care facility of the child's illness. • Give nonaspirin antipyretics to control fever. • Give oral antihistamines for relief of itching. Oatmeal and Aveeno baths are soothing. Caladryl lotion applied in moderation to lesions may also provide relief. • Observe the child closely for drowsiness, meningeal signs, respiratory distress, and dehydration. • Keep the child's fingernails short and clean. Young children may need to wear soft cotton mittens to prevent infections when itching cannot be controlled. • Change bed linens frequently. Linen should be washed in mild soap and rinsed well. • Watch for symptoms of complications. • Disorientation and restlessness may indicate viral encephalitis. • Reassure the child that the lesions are temporary and will go away.

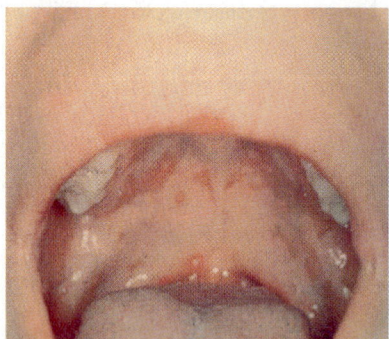

Mouth lesions of chickenpox.
Courtesy of Centers for Disease Control and Prevention, Atlanta, GA.

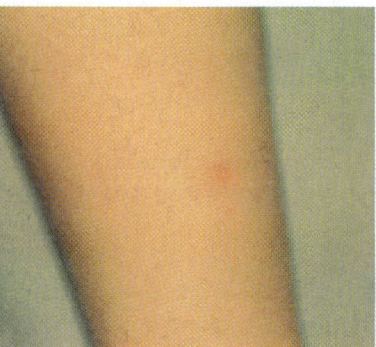

Skin lesions of chickenpox.

𝒩ursing Practice

Chickenpox can be fatal in immunocompromised children. Carefully monitor children undergoing chemotherapy, steroid treatment, or transplant therapy after exposure to the disease. Varicella-zoster immune globulin is usually given as soon as possible after exposure. A chickenpox vaccine is available and recommended for all children who have not had the disease.

*Indicates that a vaccine or antitoxin is available for use in high-risk or as-needed situations.
+Indicates that the disease has a safe and effective vaccine.

Disease	Clinical Manifestations	Clinical Therapy	Nursing Management

Coxsackievirus

Causal agent: Coxsackievirus A16 and enterovirus 71 cause a wide group of acute diseases that range from minor and self-limiting to potentially fatal.

Epidemiology: Occurs worldwide, most commonly in summer and early fall. Sporadic outbreaks are seen, especially among children in out-of-home settings. Illnesses include the common cold; pharyngitis; pneumonia; hand, foot, and mouth disease; and herpangina. Immunity probably occurs after clinical or subclinical infection, but duration of the immunity is unknown.

Transmission: Fecal-oral route; probably respiratory route.

Incubation period: 3–6 days.

Period of communicability: 2 days before rash to 2 days after it disappears.

Each of the coxsackieviruses is responsible for a different set of manifestations.

Herpangina is an acute, self-limiting viral disease characterized by the sudden onset of fever, sore throat, and small, discrete grayish papulovesicular ulcerative pharyngeal lesions that gradually increase in size.

In hand, foot, and mouth disease the lesions are more diffuse and may occur on the buccal surfaces of the cheeks, gums, and sides of the tongue. Papulovesicular lesions occur on the hands and feet and last for 7–10 days. Children may be irritable and have a fever, anorexia, dysphagia, malaise, and a sore throat.

Complications: Enterovirus 71 caused a fatal epidemic in Taiwan in 1998, when 78 deaths resulted from 90,000 cases of hand, foot, and mouth disease (Chang et al., 1999).

There is no specific treatment. An antiviral medication, pleconaril, is being evaluated for use in immunodeficient children (American Academy of Pediatrics, 2000).

Prognosis: Recovery is generally good with supportive care.

Prevention: Avoid contact with infected persons early in the disease.

- Isolate the child while contagious. Use contact precautions if the child is hospitalized.
- Apply topical lotions and give systemic medications as ordered to lessen the pain and relieve the irritation.
- Offer cool drinks and soft, bland foods (no citrus, salty, or spicy foods). Swallowing may be painful.
- Offer warm saline mouth rinses.
- Observe for dehydration.
- Provide reassurance and support to parents.
- Give nonaspirin antipyretics for fever. Keep the child out of school or child care while the child is febrile.

Diphtheria*+

Causal agent: *Corynebacterium diphtheriae,* a bacterium.

Epidemiology: Occurs mostly during colder months in temperate zones in unimmunized, partially immunized, and immunized children with waning immunity. In tropical areas, cases of cutaneous and wound diphtheria occur sporadically. Maternal immunity lasts as long as 6 months after birth. Although there are fewer than 5 cases annually in the U.S., the disease is endemic in areas where immunization is no longer routine, such as Russia.

Transmission: By contact with an infectious patient or carrier's nasal or eye discharge, or skin lesion; or less commonly, indirectly by contact with contaminated articles. Unpasteurized milk has also served as a vehicle.

Incubation period: 2–7 days, sometimes longer.

Period of communicability: Varies but is usually 2–4 weeks or until 4 days after antibiotics were initiated.

Symptoms can be mild or severe with a gradual onset over 1–2 days. Low-grade fever, anorexia, malaise, rhinorrhea with a foul odor, cough, hoarseness, stridor or noisy breathing, cervical lymphadenitis, and pharyngitis may be present. In more severe cases the membranes of the tonsils, pharynx, and larynx are affected. The characteristic membranous lesion is a thick, bluish white to grayish black patch that covers the tonsils. It can spread to cover the soft and hard palates and the posterior portion of the pharynx. Attempts to remove the membrane result in bleeding.

Complications: Produces an endotoxin that causes myocarditis and peripheral neuropathy (diplopia, slurred speech, difficulty swallowing, or paralysis of the palate) or ascending paralysis similar to Guillain-Barré syndrome.

Administration of IV antitoxin and antibiotics within 3 days of onset of symptoms. The child must be tested for sensitivity to horse serum before giving the antitoxin. When diphtheria is suspected, antibiotic therapy (penicillin G or erythromycin) should be initiated without waiting for laboratory results. Removal of membrane may be needed to treat airway obstruction.

Prognosis: With treatment, prognosis is good. If untreated, diphtheria can cause death from airway obstruction.

Prevention: Diphtheria is a vaccine-preventable disease. The immunization series is initiated at 2 months of age and is usually given in combination with tetanus and pertussis. Diphtheria-tetanus (Td) is administered to children over 7 years.

This is a reportable disease.

- Use droplet precautions for pharyngeal disease and contact precautions for cutaneous disease.
- Monitor closely for signs of increasing respiratory distress, as well as cardiac and neurologic complications. Provide humidified oxygen as necessary.
- Have emergency airway equipment available.
- Administer antibiotics. Give no medications containing caffeine or other stimulants.
- Use oral suction gently as necessary.
- Allow children to use mouthwash if desired. Gargling is not permitted because it can irritate the back of the throat.
- Encourage liquids as tolerated. Intravenous fluids may be necessary.
- Provide emotional support to the family.
- Initiate the trace for contacts with the patient to give antibiotics and immunization boosters.

(continued)

Disease	Clinical Manifestations	Clinical Therapy	Nursing Management
Erythema Infectiosum (Fifth Disease) *Causal agent:* Human parvovirus B19. *Epidemiology:* Occurs worldwide, most often in winter and spring. The disease also occurs in epidemics, with peak activity every 6 years. The incidence is highest in children between the ages of 5 and 14 years. *Transmission:* Respiratory secretions and blood. *Incubation period:* 6–14 days. *Period of communicability:* Believed to be the highest before the onset of the disease. Not after rash appears unless in aplastic crisis (Adams & Ware, 1996).	The child first manifests a flulike illness (headache, chills, malaise, nausea, body ache) that lasts 2–3 days; 1 week later, a fiery-red rash appears on the cheeks giving a "slapped face" appearance. The rash is accompanied by circumoral pallor. In 1–4 days a lacelike symmetric, erythematous, maculopapular rash appears on the truck and limbs, spreading proximal to distal. During the third stage, which lasts 1–3 weeks, the rash fades but can reappear if the skin is irritated or exposed to sunlight. The rash may be mildly pruritic. *Complications:* Children with hemolytic conditions may have transient aplastic crisis. The child has flulike symptoms but not rash. Arthritis occurs in 10% of children, lasting 1–6 days after the rash (Cherry, 1999).	There is no specific treatment, and recovery is spontaneous. Children with hemolytic conditions may need blood transfusion if aplastic crisis occurs. *Prognosis:* Fetal infection may occur resulting in spontaneous abortion. *Prevention:* Avoid contact with infected persons early in the disease.	• Children with aplastic crisis are often hospitalized. • Isolation is needed only for children with aplastic crisis or when immunosuppressed. Use contact precautions. • Nonaspirin antipyretics may be given to control fever. • Use soothing oatmeal or Aveeno baths if the rash is pruritic. Antipruritics may also help to relieve itching. • Encourage rest and offer frequent fluids. • Keep children out of direct sunlight if possible. • Provide protective, light, loose clothing if exposure to sunlight cannot be avoided. • Provide quiet diversionary activity. There is no reason to keep the child out of school or day care. • Explain the three stages of rash development to parents.

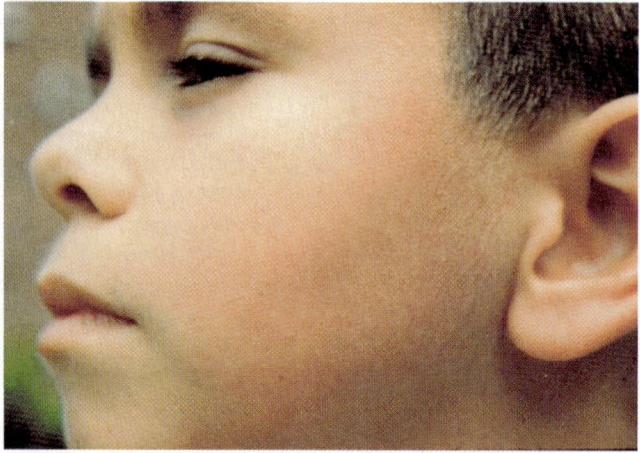 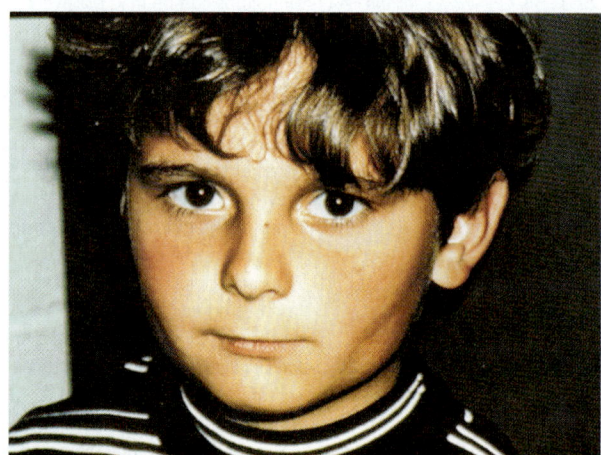

Characteristic facial rash of erythema infectiosum (fifth disease).
Courtesy of Centers for Disease Control and Prevention, Atlanta, GA.

*Indicates that a vaccine or antitoxin is available for use in high-risk or as-needed situations.
⁺Indicates that the disease has a safe and effective vaccine.

Disease	Clinical Manifestations	Clinical Therapy	Nursing Management

Haemophilus Influenzae Type B[+] (H-Influenzae Type B)

Causal agent: Coccobacilli *H. Influenzae* bacteria, which has several serotypes and can be encapsulated or nonencapsulated.

Epidemiology: Occurs most often in the spring and summer. Most commonly affected are infants and young children in child care centers. Low-birth-weight children and children with chronic illnesses also have an increased susceptibility. Invasive disease has decreased 96% in the U.S. from 1987–1995 due to the vaccine (Kaplan, 1999).

Transmission: Direct person-to-person contact or droplet inhalation. The organism is frequently asymptomatically colonized in the respiratory tract.

Incubation period: Unknown.

Period of communicability: 3 days from onset of symptoms.

H. influenzae type B starts with a viral upper respiratory infection. The organism passes through the mucosal barrier to directly invade the bloodstream. It can cause several severe invasive illnesses, including meningitis, epiglottitis, pneumonia, septic arthritis and cellulitis. It is also a cause of sepsis in infants. Other illnesses include sinusitis, otitis media, bronchitis, and pericarditis. Each disease has very specific clinical manifestations.

Complications: Illness caused by *H. influenzae* type B responds to antibiotic therapy. Left untreated, severe sequelae and death, especially in young infants, can occur from conditions such as meningitis, epiglottitis, sinusitis, pneumonitis, and cellulitis.

Treatment consists of antibiotic therapy; however, one third of strains are resistant to ampicillin. Rifampin may be given to unprotected household contacts (not pregnant women), if another child has not completed immunizations, within 1 week after diagnosis. In this case, the infected child also gets rifampin to eliminate nasopharyngeal colonization.

Prognosis: With rapid diagnosis and treatment, the outlook for recovery is good but highly dependent on the disease the organism has caused. When treatment has been delayed, the prognosis for full recovery becomes much more guarded.

Prevention: Immunization is now available for *H. influenzae* type B as part of the recommended childhood immunization series beginning at 2 months of age. Other types of *H. influenzae* are not vaccine-preventable.

- Use droplet precautions until 24 hours after the initiation of antibiotics.
- Antibiotic therapy is administered intravenously for severe infections. Infections such as otitis media can be managed at home with oral antibiotics.
- Children under the age of 4 years who have not been immunized are at increased risk for developing disease from *H. influenzae*. Specific prophylactic measures for susceptible children may be ordered by the physician.
- Administer antipyretics to help the child feel more comfortable.
- Closely monitor IV sites for patency and infiltration.
- Perform nursing care measures specific to the illness.
- Inform family members that rifampin turns urine and other body fluids orange.

Hepatitis A, Hepatitis B, and Hepatitis C See Chapter 46.

Lyme Disease*

Causal agent: *Borrelia burgdorferi*, a spirochete, which is transmitted by ixodid ticks.

Epidemiology: Distribution in the United States correlates highly with the distribution of various tick carriers (vectors). It occurs in 49 states and the District of Columbia. Exposure occurs in any outdoor setting where ticks are endemic. Animals such as dogs and cats can also have the disease. Lyme disease occurs year round, with the highest risk of infection in the summer. Children between 5 and 14 years are at highest risk. Infection does not induce immunity.

Transmission: Tick bite. The tick transmits the infected spirochete when it draws blood. The tick must feed for 36 hours to transmit the disease.

Incubation period: 3–32 days after an infected tick bite. A rash in 48 hours is an allergic reaction or infection, not Lyme disease.

The most typical early symptom is a slowly expanding red rash, called erythema migrans, at the site of the bite, often found on the groin, axilla, or thigh. The rash starts as a flat or raised red area and may progress to partial clearing, or develop blisters or scabs in the center. The rash may look like a bruise in dark-skinned patients. The rash has a "bulls-eye" appearance and is at least 5 cm in diameter. It resolves spontaneously within 4 weeks. Only 50%–75% of patients have the rash (Wade, 2000).

Stage 1 symptoms, lasting 5–21 days, include malaise, fatigue, headache, stiff neck, mild fever, and muscle and joint aches.

Stage 2 (early disseminated) occurs 1–4 months after the bite. The most common symptoms of untreated disease are pain and swelling of the joints, most commonly the knee (Lyme arthritis), facial palsy, meningitis, AV block.

Antibiotics are the treatment of choice. Amoxicillin, cefuroxime axetil, or erythromycin are most often used in children 8 years of age or younger. Doxycycline or tetracycline is given to children over the age of 8 years. A 4-week course of oral medication is given. If no response in 2–4 weeks, IV ceftriaxone, cefotaxime, or penicillin G is needed to prevent progression to later phases (see drug guide for ceftriaxone). Intravenous antibiotics are often required in the later stages of the disease. Relapse can occur.

Prognosis: Lyme disease does not cause acute life-threatening illness, but it may result in significant morbidity, especially when chronic.

- Children with early disease are usually treated at home. Children with progressive symptoms may be hospitalized. Use standard precautions.
- Educate parents about the need for the long course of medications, informing them that the spirochete can go dormant.
- Tell parents to have the child avoid sun exposure when taking doxycycline. Nonaspirin analgesics and antipyretics may provide relief of mild fevers, headaches, and muscle and joint aches.
- Children with Lyme disease may tire easily. Promote rest and avoid vigorous activities that may be difficult.
- Educate parents and children about the disease and early recognition of the symptoms. Teach them to safely remove ticks.

(continued)

Disease	Clinical Manifestations	Clinical Therapy	Nursing Management
Lyme Disease*—continued	Stage 3 (late disseminated) occurs months later and includes problems such as Lyme arthritis and central nervous system changes. These may become chronic problems. *Complications:* Left untreated, Lyme disease can cause significant neurologic deficits, including arm and leg weakness, Bell's palsy, encephalopathy, meningitis, severe headaches, and cognitive and behavioral changes as well as chronic arthritis, and disorders of the peripheral nerves. The spriochete can cross the placental barrier and infect the fetus (Wade, 2000).	*Prevention:* A vaccine, LYMErix, is approved for high-risk patients 15–70 years. Some clinical trials in younger children appear promising. Avoid areas that are heavily tick infested, and wear protective clothing. Check for ticks (especially hidden in hair) after every outing. Check pets because they can carry home ticks that are then transferred to the child. Remove ticks as soon as possible. There is no acquired immunity.	• To remove a tick, grasp it gently but firmly with fine-point tweezers where the mouth parts are attached. Pull gently—avoid squeezing of the tick's body—until it releases. Clean the area with soap and water. If any tick parts are left under the skin, take the child to a health care provider for removal. Tell them to mark the date of tick bite on the calendar and monitor the child's health for flulike symptoms over the next 2 weeks. Encourage them to seek medical attention promptly if symptoms develop. • Provide emotional support.

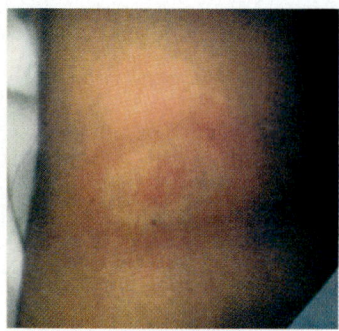 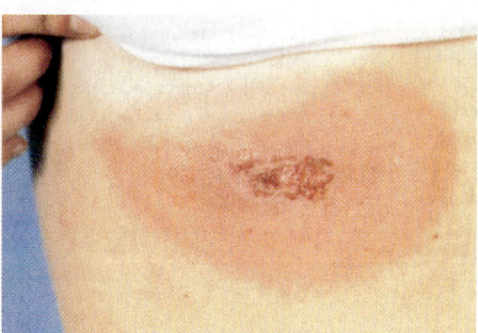

The appearance of the erythema migrons rash may vary in early Lyme disease.
From Pfizer Central Research. (1989). *Lyme disease.* Groton, CT: Author.

Nursing Practice

Patients are sometimes denied health insurance coverage for oral and IV medications for long courses of treatment for Lyme disease. Connecticut passed legislation in 1999 requiring insurers to cover treatment. Other states are considering such legislation (Healy, 2000).

Malaria *Causal agent: Plasmodium*, 4 species (*P. falciparum, P. vivax, P. ovale, P. malariae*). *Epidemiology:* Occurs in tropical and subtropical regions on 4 continents (Africa, Americas, Asia, and Oceania). The disease is acquired during travel to an endemic area. *Transmission:* The bite of an infected female Anopheles mosquito during a nocturnal blood meal permits the parasite to enter the human bloodstream. The parasite passes to the liver and infects hepatic cells. During an asymptomatic 5- to 16-day cycle, the parasite transforms to become a merozoite. The merozoites are released and infect the red blood cells.	Nonspecific signs such as myalgia, malaise, headache, abdominal pain, back pain, diarrhea, nausea, and vomiting are common. Spiking fever occurs at the time red blood cells rupture, becoming a classical cyclic pattern every 48–72 hours. Periods of symptomatic improvement are sometimes seen between spells.	The patient is hospitalized to receive fluid replacement, antipyretics, and anemia management. In severe disease with greater than 5% parasitemia, intensive care and IV treatment is needed. The blood is regularly monitored for parasite density. Quinine sulfate and tetracycline are used for chloroquine-resistant *P. falciparum*. Hypoglycemia may result from quinine treatment. Sulfadoxine-pyremethamine rather than tetracycline is used for children under 8 years of age. Mefloquine is used for chloroquine-sensitive organisms. Primaquine will cause severe anemia if given to individuals with G6PD disorder (Barat & Zucker, 1999).	• Use standard precautions for the hospitalized patient. • Maintain fluid intake. Monitor intake and output. • Monitor blood glucose level and be prepared to respond to sudden hypoglycemia. • Observe for signs of increasing illness severity such as confusion, seizures, and shock. Be prepared to protect the patient from injury and provide emergency support with airways and oxygen supplementation until the child can be transferred to intensive care. • Monitor the hematocrit and hemoglobin levels. • Administer antipyretics to control the fever and promote comfort.

*Indicates that a vaccine or antitoxin is available for use in high-risk or as-needed situations.
⁺Indicates that the disease has a safe and effective vaccine.

Disease	Clinical Manifestations	Clinical Therapy	Nursing Management
Malaria—continued *Period of communicability:* Not communicable except by blood or blood product transfusion, or the transplantation of organs from an infected person.	*Complications:* When more than 5% of red blood cells are infected, severe anemia is seen; seizures and cerebral malaria (increased intracranial pressure, confusion, stupor, coma, and sometimes death) are most common in children. Pulmonary edema, respiratory failure, renal failure, spontaneous bleeding, and shock are seen in older children and adolescents. Children with asplenia are at high risk for death. Causes 1–2 million deaths worldwide annually.	*Prevention:* Minimize contact with mosquitoes, use DEET insect repellent, screened rooms, DEET-treated mosquito netting, and cover the body with clothing when traveling in endemic regions. Antimalarial chemoprophylaxis (mefloquine) should be used 1 week before arrival, weekly during travel, and 4 weeks after leaving the risk area. Doxycycline is sometimes used as an alternate chemoprophylaxis, but must be taken daily.	• Educate families traveling to endemic areas about the importance of antimalarial chemoprophylaxis. Explain the need to take the medication correctly despite the common side effects of nausea and vomiting. Discuss the need to protect children during nocturnal feeding times of mosquitoes with protective clothing, mosquito repellent, and mosquito netting around the bed.
Measles (Rubeola)** *Causal agent: Morbillivirus,* a member of the paramyxovirus group. *Epidemiology:* Occurrence peaks in the late winter and early spring. In developed countries, measles occurs mostly in outbreaks among children. The outbreaks are largely the result of lack of immunization or possibly declining immunity. Many cases are imported from countries without routine immunization. Maternal immunity is active in the infant until the age of approximately 12–15 months. Vaccination induces lifelong immunity. In developing countries, measles remains largely an endemic problem and is a significant cause of infant and child morbidity and mortality. *Transmission:* Airborne, respiratory droplets, and contact with infected persons. *Incubation period:* about 8–12 days. *Period of communicability:* Begins during the prodromal phase and ends about 2–4 days after the rash appears.	Children are quite ill in the 3- to 5-day prodromal phase, with symptoms including high fever, conjunctivitis, coryza, cough, anorexia, and malaise. Small, irregular, bluish white spots on a red background, called Koplik's spots, appear on the buccal mucosa about 2 days before and after the onset of the rash. The characteristic red, blotchy, maculopapular rash that becomes confluent usually appears 2–4 days after onset of prodromal phase. The rash begins on the face and spreads to the trunk and extremities. Symptoms gradually subside in 4–7 days. Other symptoms include anorexia, malaise, fatigue, and generalized lymphadenopathy. *Complications:* Diarrhea, otitis media, bronchopneumonia, bronchitis, laryngotracheobronchitis, and encephalitis. Complications and sequelae occur most often in children who are malnourished, medically fragile, and immunosuppressed. The younger the child, the greater the risk for complications.	There is no cure for measles. Treatment is supportive. Antibiotics are used for bacterial secondary infections. *Prognosis:* Recovery is generally good with supportive care. *Prevention:* Measles is a vaccine-preventable disease. The measles vaccine is available alone (M), in combination with the rubella vaccine (MR), or in combination with the rubella and mumps vaccines (MMR). Immune globulin, administered up to 6 days after exposure, may be helpful in preventing the disease in susceptible persons (immunocompromised children, infants less than 1 year of age, pregnant women). All health care workers should have documented immunity. This is a reportable disease.	• If the child is hospitalized, maintain airborne precautions during the contagious period (5 days after the rash appears). • Use a cool-mist vaporizer to help clear respiratory passages. • Suction nose and oral cavity very gently as necessary. • Give nonaspirin antipyretics for fever and antipruritics for itching. • Assess lungs carefully, especially in young children, in whom pneumonias are a common complication. • Antitussives may be ordered to control coughing. • Keep lights dim, and cover windows if the child has photophobia. • Elevate the head of the bed. Keep the room cool with good air circulation. Provide light, nonirritating blankets. • Keep skin clean and dry. No soaps should be used. • Maintain fluid intake. Offer cool liquids frequently in small amounts. Blended, pureed, and mashed foods are most easily tolerated. • Maintain bed rest. Visitors should be immune to measles. • Provide diversions such as music, stories, and favorite toys.

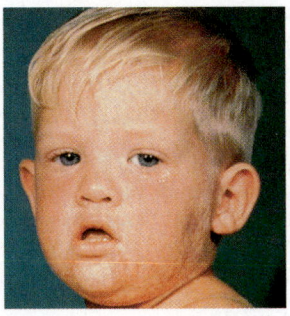
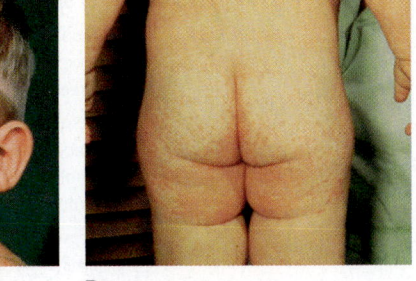
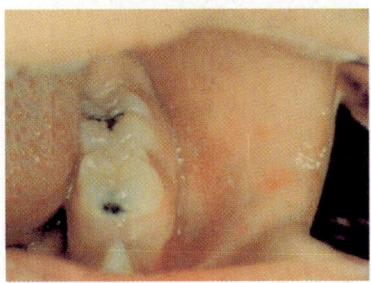

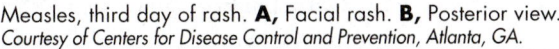

A   **B**

Measles, third day of rash. **A,** Facial rash. **B,** Posterior view.
Courtesy of Centers for Disease Control and Prevention, Atlanta, GA.

Koplik spots on oral mucosa, fifth day of rash.
Courtesy of Centers for Disease Control and Prevention, Atlanta, GA.

(continued)

Disease	Clinical Manifestations	Clinical Therapy	Nursing Management
Mononucleosis *Causal agent:* Epstein-Barr virus (EBV), a member of the herpesvirus group. *Epidemiology:* Occurs worldwide. In developing countries, the disease occurs in young children and may be asymptomatic or mild. In developed countries, the disease is more common in older children and adolescents. *Transmission:* Direct contact with infected oropharyngeal and genital tract secretions. EBV can also be transmitted by blood transfusion. *Incubation period:* 30–50 days. *Period of communicability:* Virus is shed for up to 18 months after the clinical course of the disease.	In very young children, mononucleosis may cause irritability, but be otherwise asymptomatic. A maculopapular rash may be seen in a few cases. In other children, the disease is characterized by malaise, headache, anorexia, abdominal pain, fatigue, and fever for 2–3 days, followed by lymphadenopathy and a sore throat. Hepatosplenomegaly may occur. Pain from swelling of the tonsils and lymph nodes may be significant. The syndrome typically lasts 2–3 weeks and is self-limited. *Complications:* Rare side effects include central nervous system symptoms such as encephalitis, aseptic meningitis, and Guillain-Barré syndrome. Splenic rupture, respiratory failure, and hematologic complications such as thrombocytopenia can also occur. In immunodeficient children, fatal infections or lymphomas can develop.	There is no specific treatment. Corticosteroids may be used to control tonsillar swelling and pain when there is impending airway obstruction. Antibiotics (penicillin or erythromycin) are used for secondary infections. A rash may develop with antibiotic treatment (Sullivan, 1999). *Prognosis:* After recovery, the virus remains latent in the lymphoid system. It can be reactivated during periods of immunosuppression. The child will be a virus carrier for life. *Prevention:* No known prevention.	• Children are usually treated at home. Standard precautions should be used. • Give antipyretics and analgesics for fever and sore throat. Offer warm salt water for gargling. Offer soft foods and encourage fluids. • Maintain bed rest. • Give adolescents a sense of responsibility by involving them in decisions about care whenever possible. Be sure to include parents and adolescents in discussions. • Reassure adolescents who may be worried about keeping up with schoolwork that they can return to school when the fever is gone and swallowing is normal. • Teens should avoid kissing until the fever has been gone several days. • Contact sports should be avoided until the liver and spleen are normal, usually in about 4 weeks.
Mumps (Parotitis)⁺ *Causal agent:* A paramyxovirus. *Epidemiology:* Occurs worldwide in unvaccinated children, most often in winter and spring. Infection and vaccination induce lifelong immunity. Maternal antibodies begin to disappear in infants at the age of 12–15 months. *Transmission:* Saliva droplets and direct contact. *Incubation period:* 12–25 days. *Period of communicability:* 7 days before parotid swelling until 9 days after swelling subsides.	Malaise; low-grade fever; and earache, headache, pain with chewing, decreased appetite and activity; followed by bilateral or unilateral parotid gland swelling. Swelling peaks around the third day. Meningeal signs (stiff neck, headache, photophobia) occur in about 15% of patients. *Complications:* Orchitis (inflammation of the epididymis, pain on testicular palpation, and scrotal swelling—most often unilateral) may occur in postpubertal males; sterility is relatively rare (Taber & Demmler, 1999a). Oorphoritis, pancreatitis, aseptic meningoencephalitis, and unilateral permanent deafness are sometimes seen.	There is no specific treatment. Therapy is supportive, focused on symptom relief. *Prognosis:* Mumps is usually self-limiting. *Prevention:* Mumps is a vaccine-preventable disease. The vaccine is usually administered in combination with measles and rubella vaccines (MMR) at 12–15 months of age and again at either 4–6 years or 11–12 years. This is a reportable disease.	• Children are generally uncomfortable but are rarely very ill. They are usually cared for at home. • Use droplet precautions for hospitalized children while contagious. Avoid exposure to immunocompromised individuals or susceptible persons. • Keep children out of school or child care until all symptoms subside. Encourage diversional activities. • Give nonaspirin analgesics and antipyretics to control fever and pain. Give steroids if ordered. Encourage fluid intake. Swallowing and chewing may be painful. Offer soft and blended foods. Avoid foods and beverages that increase salivary flow (citrus, spices, and candies) because they cause pain. • Talking may be painful. Provide a bell or other attention-getting device. • Apply warm or cool compresses, whichever is preferred, to the parotid area. • Be alert for signs of complications. Headache, stiff neck, vomiting, and photophobia may indicate meningeal irritation. • Provide scrotal supports if testicular swelling occurs. • Reassure children who may be upset about the facial swelling that it will go away.

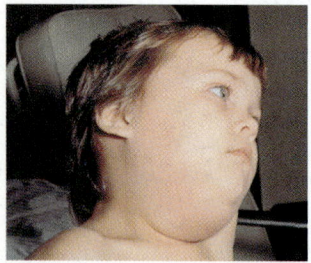 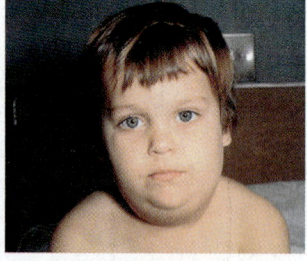

A   **B**

This child has mumps with diffuse lymphedema of the neck.
A, Side view. **B,** Front view. *Courtesy Centers for Disease Control and Prevention, Atlanta, GA.*

Disease	Clinical Manifestations	Clinical Therapy	Nursing Management
Pertussis (Whooping Cough)[+] *Causal agent:* Bordella pertussis *Epidemiology:* Occurs worldwide. Predominantly a childhood disease that is most common in children under 6 months of age. Epidemic cycles occur every 2–5 years. Pertussis also occurs in health care workers or adults who may have weakened or incomplete immunity. Adults may become only mildly ill but can spread the disease to unimmunized children. *Transmission:* Respiratory droplets and direct contact with discharge from the respiratory membranes. *Incubation period:* 7–21 days (commonly 7–10 days). *Period of communicability:* Begins approximately 1 week after exposure. Pertussis is communicable for 5–7 days after the initiation of antibiotic therapy. The disease is most contagious before the paroxysmal cough stage.	The onset is insidious. The disease begins with a runny nose, followed by an irregular, nonproductive cough. The cough becomes more severe at night and changes into spasms of paroxysmal coughing followed by inspiration, stridor, or "whooping." (Young infants do not manifest the "whooping.") The whoop sound results from forceful inhalation and a narrowed glottis. Sucking on a bottle may trigger the coughing spell. May be accompanied by flushing, cyanosis, vomiting, profuse drainage from the nose, eyes, and mouth. Dehydration may result from decreased oral intake. Paroxysmal coughing may last 1–4 weeks or more. *Complications:* Pneumonia, atelectasis, otitis media, and seizures.	Treatment consists of antibiotics (erythromycin and other macrolides), corticosteroids, if ordered, and supportive care. *Prognosis:* The disease is most severe in infants under 1 year of age, and most deaths occur in this age group. *Prevention:* Pertussis is a vaccine-preventable disease. Active immunization should be given in early infancy. Health care professionals who are in close contact with infected children before diagnosis may need antibiotics to prevent transmission. This is a reportable disease.	• Use droplet precautions until 5–7 days after the initiation of antibiotics. Most hospitalized cases occur in children under the age of 5 years. • Closely monitor respirations and oxygen saturation. The smaller the child, the greater the risk for respiratory distress and apnea. • Remain with the child during coughing spells, when hypoxic and apneic episodes are most likely. Give oxygen if ordered. Have emergency equipment available. • Provide humidification. Gentle suctioning may be necessary. • Give nonaspirin antipyretics as needed for fever. • Encourage frequent rest periods. • Allow the child to eat desired foods. • Encourage the child to take fluids. The child may need IV hydration if oral intake is not tolerated. • Provide emotional support to parents. • Teach parents to watch for signs of respiratory failure and dehydration if the child is managed at home.
Pneumococcal infection[+] *Causative agent: Streptococcus pneumoniae,* a gram-positive diplococcus. *Epidemiology:* The organism is found in the pharynx of healthy people. Outbreaks occur in the winter and spring when people are more crowded in physical settings. In temperate climates, 6 serotypes account for most of the infections found in children. The disease is more common in African Americans, American Indians, and Native Alaskans. It occurs most commonly in the 6-month to 2-year age group. Of particular concern is the development of strains that are resistant to penicillin and other antibiotics. *Transmission:* Respiratory secretions, and droplets. Upper respiratory infections help the spread. *Incubation period:* 1–3 days. *Period of communicability:* Unknown. Probably less than 24 hours after initiation of effective antibiotic therapy.	The signs and symptoms are related to the focal area of infection. The organism causes otitis media, sinusitis, pharyngitis, laryngotracheobronchitis, pneumonia, meningitis, and bacteremia. In otitis media, upper respiratory infection, fever, ear pain, and decreased appetite are seen. In bacteremia, there is unexplained fever and no localized infection site. In pneumonia, fever, chills, chest pain, dyspnea, malaise, and a productive cough are seen. In meningitis, inconsolable crying, increased irritability, lethargy, refusal to eat, nausea, vomiting, diarrhea, myalgia, photophobia, and seizures are seen. *Complications:* This organism is one of the leading causes of morbidity and mortality. It causes 85% of bacteremia, is the leading cause of meningitis, and is responsible for 40% of acute otitis media (Rennels, 1999). Other complications include septic arthritis, osteomyelitis, endocarditis, and brain abscess.	Penicillin is given for penicillin-sensitive strains, but up to 48% of infections are penicillin resistant. Macrolide antibiotics are used for mild disease if the child is allergic to penicillin. Penicillin-resistant strains are treated with third-generation cephalosporins (cefotaxime or ceftriaxone). Vancomycin and rifampen are used in combination when strains are resistant to antibiotics listed above (American Academy of Pediatrics, 2000). Symptomatic care is also provided. *Prevention:* Many serotypes are preventable with immunization. Active immunization should begin in infancy with the 7-valent vaccine (Prevnar). In studies testing the efficacy of the vaccine, the new pneumococcal conjugate vaccine resulted in significant reduction in pneumonia, meningitis, bacteremia, and otitis media (Rennels, Edwards, & Keyserling, 1998). A 23-valent vaccine is available for older children at high risk of pneumococcal disease.	• If the child is hospitalized, maintain standard precautions. • Provide nonaspirin antipyretics for control of fever and comfort. • Encourage fluids, and monitor intake and output. • Monitor vital signs and consciousness level to identify signs of worsening condition. • Educate parents about the need for the vaccine, as the unimmunized child could become infected with another serotype. • Many children with mild disease are treated at home. Educate parents about signs indicating a need to seek additional medical care, the need for proper medication administration, and comfort measures for the child.

(continued)

Disease	Clinical Manifestations	Clinical Therapy	Nursing Management
Poliomyelitis[+] *Causal agent:* There are three serotypes of poliovirus. *Epidemiology:* Occurs worldwide. Polio primarily affects children, although some of the cases involve transmission to immunocompromised or non-polio-protected adults caring for infants who had received live polio virus vaccine. The disease can be mild or severe. The vaccine induces lifelong immunity. The live poliovirus vaccine was associated with paralytic disease and is no longer recommended for routine immunization in the U.S. *Transmission:* Primarily by the fecal-oral route, possibly respiratory. *Incubation period:* Usually 7–10 days (range 3–36 days). *Period of communicability:* Unknown. Infectious for up to several weeks before symptoms develop. The virus is shed in pharyngeal secretions for a few days and in the stool for several weeks.	Affects the central nervous system. Less severe infections may be limited to fever and stiffness in the neck and back, headache, vomiting, and sore throat. In other cases, fever, headache, stiff neck, Kernig's or Brudzinski's sign, decreased deep tendon reflexes, and progressive weakness occur. There may be respiratory difficulties, and an increased respiratory rate that may interfere with the ability to talk because frequent pauses are needed. Onset of paralysis may be sudden, in hours, or gradual over 3–5 days. Paralysis results from damage to neurons. *Complications:* Permanent motor paralysis, respiratory arrest, myocardial failure, aseptic meningitis, and postpolio syndrome.	Treatment is supportive. No chemotherapeutic agents that directly kill the polio virus are available. *Prognosis:* Respiratory complication is life-threatening and involves 5%–10% of all cases. Respiratory paralysis may lead to death. *Prevention:* Poliomyelitis is a vaccine-preventable disease. Children should be immunized with the inactivated poliovirus vaccine (IPV) according to the recommended schedule. This is a reportable disease.	• Use standard and droplet precautions in the hospital and keep the child on strict bed rest. • Observe closely for respiratory paralysis (ineffective cough, talking with frequent pauses, shallow and rapid respiratory rate). Have emergency equipment at bedside. Assist ventilations as needed until mechanical ventilation is set up. • Administer sedatives and nonaspirin analgesics as ordered to allow for rest and comfort. Hot packs may relieve discomfort. • Encourage fluids. • Position the child to promote body alignment. • Perform range of motion exercises to prevent contractures after the acute phase. • Provide emotional support. • Patients are alert and aware. Tell them what is happening to them. • Long-term orthopedic (physical therapy) support may be needed by some children.
Rabies (Hydrophobia)* *Causal agent:* Rhabdoviridae, two types (urban, in dogs; wild, in wildlife). *Epidemiology:* Occurs worldwide. Urban rabies is generally controlled by vaccination of domestic animals susceptible to the infection, especially dogs and cats. Rabies can occur in many wild animals, particularly bats, foxes, skunks, and raccoons. *Transmission:* Infected saliva from bite of rabid animal. Virus enters the wound and travels along the nerves from point of entry to the brain where it multiplies and migrates along the efferent nerves to the salivary glands.	Children may be free of symptoms during the long incubation period. Initial acute symptoms include pain or paresthesia at the site of exposure along with headache, fever, loss of appetite, and malaise. Painful contractures in the muscles used for swallowing lead to hydrophobia (50% of patients), a reflex contraction at the sight of liquid. Neurologic symptoms such as hallucinations, disorientation, periods of excitability (mania) and quiet, and seizures later occur. Some patients may have confusion with or without agitation with progression to stupor and coma. Symptoms last about 2 weeks.	Immediately wash animal bites thoroughly with soap and water and irrigate well. Suturing should be avoided if possible. Human rabies immune globulin (HRIG) and human diploid cell rabies vaccine (HDCV) should be given to all persons bitten by animals that may be rabid. Half of the HRIG is infiltrated around the wound and the remainder is given IM. HRIG and HDCV can be delayed 48 hours if testing of the animal's brain is done (Phelps, 1997). The vaccine is of no value once rabies symptoms are present. *Prognosis:* If symptoms develop, no drug improves the prognosis.	• Administer RIG and HDCV as ordered. Assist family with obtaining help to find and quarantine the animal for observation. • Provide emotional support to the family while reinforcing the urgency for the vaccine and the need for a series of injections. • Inform parents and the child about the side effects of the vaccine—irritation at the injection site, itching, headache, muscle aches, nausea, and dizziness. • If the child acquires rabies, he or she will be hospitalized.

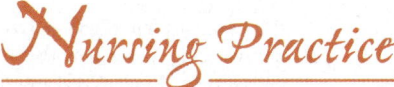

Nursing Practice

Any animal suspected of having rabies should be quarantined, if possible (Phelps, 1997). Rabies is diagnosed on the basis of history and clinical symptoms. The importance of history cannot be underestimated. Diagnosis is usually confirmed by fluorescent antibody staining of the dead animal's brain tissue.

*Indicates that a vaccine or antitoxin is available for use in high-risk or as-needed situations.
[+]Indicates that the disease has a safe and effective vaccine.

Disease	Clinical Manifestations	Clinical Therapy	Nursing Management
Rabies (Hydrophobia)*–continued *Incubation period:* Highly variable (3–7 weeks); average 6 weeks. This period depends on the amount of virus in the saliva, how close to the brain or major nerves the bite occurred, and how deeply the saliva penetrated the skin.	*Complications:* Usually results in death.	*Prevention:* Postexposure prophylaxis with HRIG and HDCV should be given as soon as possible after exposure. HDCV is repeated on days 3, 7, 14, and 28 after the bite (5 doses). The HDCV series may be stopped if the animal is found free of rabies. Expert advice on the administration of these vaccines is available from state and local health officials. Prevention also includes immunizing all domestic animals against rabies. Teach children to avoid contact with all unknown animals, dead or alive.	• Institute standard and contact precautions. The virus is transmitted primarily in the saliva and cerebrospinal fluid. • Make the child as comfortable as possible. • Keep liquids out of sight of the hydrophobic child. • Use caution in the late stages of the disease when children are usually combative. Various medications, paralyzing agents, and sedatives may be used to provide relief. Coma and death occur after an exhaustive period of excitement and agitation that may last for days. • Provide emotional support to the family of the dying child.
Rocky Mountain Spotted Fever (Tickborne Typhus Fever, Sao Paulo Typhus) *Causal agent: Rickettsia rickettsii,* a bacterium that is transmitted by infected ticks. *Epidemiology:* Rocky Mountain spotted fever (RMSF) occurs in most of the U.S., southwestern Canada, and Mexico. In the U.S., cases are most prevalent in the southeastern region. Nearly half of all cases occur in Oklahoma, North Carolina, South Carolina, and Tennessee. Generally occurs between April and September. Most infections occur in children who are less than 15 years of age. Infection induces immunity. *Transmission:* Transmitted by bites of ticks, principally dog ticks. There is no evidence of person-to-person transmission. *Incubation period:* 2–8 days (most commonly 7 days) after bite of an infected tick.	RMSF is a multisystem disease that can be mild, moderate, or severe. Onset may be gradual or rapid. Children may be very ill. Sudden onset is characterized by a moderate to high fever (40 °C) that ordinarily lasts for 2–3 weeks, significant malaise, deep muscle pain, persistent headache, chills, and conjunctival injection. The characteristic rash, which usually appears between the third and fifth days, starts on the extremities, including the palms and soles, and moves to the trunk. Initially the rash is maculopapular and blanches with pressure. It later becomes petechial and more defined; it is rarely pruritic. The child may have splenomegaly, hepatomegaly, and jaundice. *Complications:* In severe cases bleeding from disseminated intravascular coagulation (DIC) can be significant. Gastrointestinal symptoms often occur early in the disease. Pulmonary complications, especially pneumonitis, are common and can become life threatening. Central nervous system involvement can cause significant encephalitis and overall severe neurologic dysfunction. Cardiac and renal complications can also occur, leading to shock in severe cases.	Treatment consists of antibiotics, such as chloramphenicol and doxycycline. *Prognosis:* Without early recognition and treatment, morbidity is significant and mortality in children is 4%–7% (Feigin & Bloom, 1999). If the rash occurs late or not at all, the disease is likely to be more severe. *Prevention:* Avoid heavily tick-infested areas, and wear protective clothing. Check for ticks and if found remove promptly. Infected ticks must be attached and feeding for 4–6 hours to transmit the disease. Seek medical attention promptly for a child who has been bitten and becomes symptomatic.	• Use standard precautions. • Children may require prolonged hospitalization, including monitoring in the intensive care unit. • Have hemodynamic monitoring equipment and emergency supplies readily available. • Administer antibiotics as ordered. • Observe for any abnormal bleeding. • Make the child as comfortable as possible. If the child is unconscious, support the extremities and keep the eyes closed and lubricated. • Provide quiet diversional activities. • Provide emotional support, and keep parents informed about the child's condition.

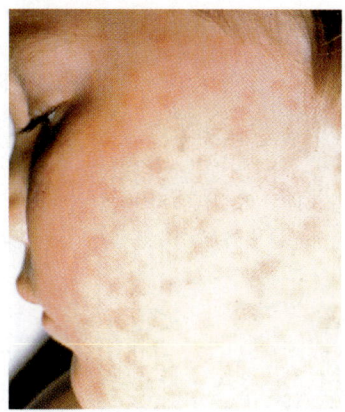

Rash of Rocky Mountain spotted fever.

(continued)

Disease	Clinical Manifestations	Clinical Therapy	Nursing Management
Roseola (Exanthem Subitum) *Causal agent:* Herpesvirus type 6. *Epidemiology:* Occurs worldwide, primarily in children 6–24 months of age during the spring and summer months. Maternal antibodies are present in infants at birth. *Transmission:* Unknown. A latent virus is probably shed by a caregiver in saliva. *Incubation period:* Appears to be 5–15 days. *Period of communicability:* Unknown. Probably infectious but person-to-person spread is not reported.	Sudden, high fever up to 40.5 °C (105 °F) for 3–8 days, during which the child does not appear toxic (normal appetite and behavior). The fever phase is followed by a characteristic pale pink, discrete, maculopapular rash, which starts on the trunk and spreads to the face, neck, and extremities. The rash can last for 1–2 days. The child's appetite is normal. *Complications:* Children may have febrile seizures.	Roseola is self-limiting, and there is no treatment other than supportive care. *Prognosis:* Roseola is benign in most cases.	• Children are rarely hospitalized, but if they are, use standard precautions. • Give nonaspirin antipyretics to control fever. • Observe closely for any seizure activity, especially during the acute febrile periods. • Encourage fluids. • Reassure parents that the rash will disappear in a few days.
Rubella (German Measles)[+] *Causal agent:* An RNA virus, member of the family Togaviridae, genus *Rubivirus*. *Epidemiology:* Occurs worldwide and is most prevalent in the winter and spring. Children are susceptible after loss of transplacentally acquired maternal antibodies about 6–9 months after birth. Natural infection or vaccination induces lifelong immunity. Most cases occur in adults older than 20 years. Congenital rubella syndrome is most likely the result of lack of immunization rather than vaccine failure. Rates of congenital rubella syndrome have increased since 1989 because 25% of postpubertal women lack antibody to rubella virus (Taber & Demmler, 1999b). *Transmission:* Droplet spread, direct contact with infected persons, or contact with articles soiled by nasal secretions. *Incubation period:* 14–21 days (most commonly 16–18 days). *Period of communicability:* From about 7 days before until about 4 days after the onset of the rash. Infants with congenital rubella may shed the virus for months after birth and should not be exposed or cared for by persons who are not immune to the disease.	Rubella is generally a mild disease with a characteristic pink, nonconfluent, maculopapular rash. The rash appears on the face, progresses to the neck, trunk, and legs, and disappears in the same order. Prodromal symptoms occur 1–5 days before the rash and include low-grade fever, headache, malaise, coryza, sore throat, and anorexia. Forschheimer spots (discrete, erythematous pinpoint or larger lesions on the soft palate) are seen during the prodromal phase. Generalized lymphadenopathy involving the postauricular, suboccipital, and posterior cervical areas is common up to 7 days before the rash. *Complications:* Complications are rare, but include arthritis in adolescents, encephalitis, and congenital rubella syndrome.	Treatment is supportive. Rubella is generally self-limiting in children. *Prognosis:* Disease is usually mild and benign. Major risk is for fetus if the mother is infected in the first trimester. Abortion, stillbirth, or fetal death are common (10% die after birth). Many other anomalies may be present, such as intrauterine growth retardation, and cardiac, ear, and eye deficits. *Prevention:* Rubella is a vaccine-preventable disease. It is important that females of childbearing age be immunized because of the severe complications rubella poses to the fetus during the first trimester. All health care workers should have documented immunity.	• Children are usually treated at home and rarely require hospitalization. They should not attend school or day care while contagious, and they should be isolated from pregnant women. School and child care facilities should be notified of the child's illness. • Maintain droplet precautions for contagious children. Maintain contact precautions for infants with congenital rubella syndrome until 1 year of age (American Academy of Pediatrics, 2000). • Give nonaspirin analgesics and antipyretics for any pain and fever. • Allow children to choose what they would like to eat and drink. Encourage fluids. • Provide quiet activities.

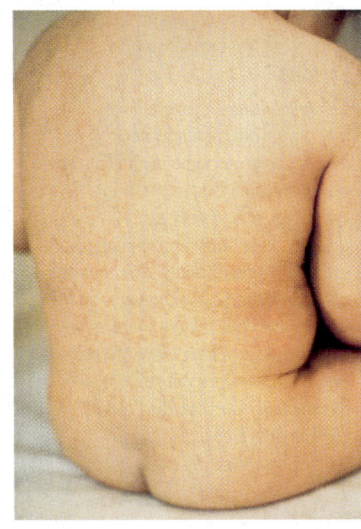

Discrete maculopapular erythematous rash of rubella.

Disease	Clinical Manifestations	Clinical Therapy	Nursing Management
Streptococcus *Causal agent:* Group A streptococci (GAS). *Epidemiology:* The illness is caused by various M-protein groups of group A alpha- and beta-hemolytic streptococci. In recent years severe infections have appeared, in some cases threatening life and limb. Different strains are associated with pharyngeal and pyodermal infections. Pharyngeal infections tend to occur more in late fall, winter, and spring. Pyodermal infections tend to occur in warmer seasons because of the association with minor skin trauma and insect bites. *Transmission:* Airborne respiratory droplets, and direct contact. *Incubation period:* Pharyngeal: usually 2–5 days; Pyodermal: usually 7–10 days. *Period of communicability:* Four weeks in untreated pharyngeal infections. The child is most contagious during the acute stage of the illness.	*Pharyngeal:* Onset is abrupt, with a sore throat, dysphagia, malaise, high fever, chills, headache, abdominal pain, anorexia, and vomiting. A beefy red pharynx with exudate (strep throat), and tender cervical nodes is seen. Palatal petechia may be seen. A characteristic erythematous rash associated with scarlet fever appears in some cases 12–48 hours after onset of symptoms, starting on the neck and spreading to the trunk and extremities. In 3–4 days, the rash begins to fade and the tips of the toes and fingers begin to peel. The classic strawberry tongue is seen on day 4–5. *Pyodermal:* Lesions (impetigo) are honey-colored crusts at the site of open lesions. *Complications:* If untreated, retropharyngeal abscess, cervical lymphadenitis, acute rheumatic fever, acute glomerulonephritis, toxic shock syndrome, bacteremia, and necrotizing fasciitis or myositis can occur.	Prompt antibiotic treatment is effective. Penicillin is the drug of choice. Erythromycin is used if the child is allergic to penicillin. The fever decreases after treatment is begun. Uncomplicated impetigo is treated with bacitracin or mupirocin ointment. Invasive strains causing necrotizing fasciitis or myositis need surgical intervention (exploration and debridement of dead tissue). Clindamycin may be needed for toxic shock syndrome and necrotizing fasciitis (McMillan & Feigin, 1999). *Prognosis:* Recovery is usually good with antibiotic therapy; 10%–20% of school-age children become chronic carriers. *Prevention:* None.	• Children with uncomplicated streptococcal infections are usually cared for at home. Promote bed rest during the febrile stage. Give nonaspirin antipyretics to control fever. Teach parents important signs of a worsening condition. • For pharyngeal infections, offer warm salt water for gargling; a soft diet and nonacidic beverages. Encourage fluids. Provide cool, clear liquids. Swallowing may be difficult. • Explain to parents the importance of the child's taking antibiotics for the full number of days prescribed. • Encourage other family members with sore throats to have throat cultures taken. • For impetigo, teach the parents to wash the skin, remove crusts, and apply antibiotic ointment. If the child is hospitalized, maintain droplet precautions for pharyngeal infections and contact precautions for skin lesions for 24 hours after beginning antibiotics. Monitor vital signs, especially temperature. Administer antibiotics as ordered. • If the child develops invasive streptococcal infection, use standard precautions. The child with toxic shock syndrome needs intensive care to manage shock and fluid and electrolyte imbalances.

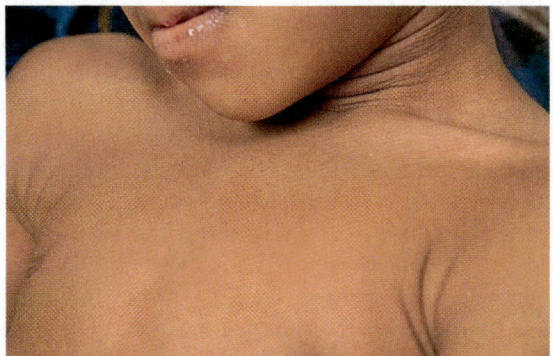

Skin Rash of scarlet fever.

*Indicates that a vaccine or antitoxin is available for use in high-risk or as-needed situations.
⁺ Indicates that the disease has a safe and effective vaccine.

Disease	Clinical Manifestations	Clinical Therapy	Nursing Management
Tetanus *Causal agent: Clostridium tetani* or tetanus bacillus. *Epidemiology:* The bacillus is common and exists as a spore in soil, dust, and animal excretions. The organism produces an endotoxin that affects the central nervous system. *Transmission:* The organism is transmitted to humans through wounds in the skin from contact with contaminated soil or implements. Newborns can acquire tetanus via the umbilical cord if they are born in an unclean area or if a contaminated implement is used to cut the cord. *Incubation period:* 3 days–3 weeks (average 8 days). *Period of communicability:* Not communicable to other individuals except through skin wounds.	Stiffness of the neck and jaw, with painful facial spasms and difficulty swallowing over a few days. Noise or sudden movement may stimulate spasms. Localized prolonged and painful muscle contraction may occur at the site of the wound. There is eventual rigidity of the abdomen and trunk. There is difficulty swallowing the increased oral secretions. Newborns have difficulty with sucking, progressing to an inability to suck, irritability, and nuchal rigidity. *Complications:* Laryngospasm, respiratory distress, death.	Tetanus immune globulin is given to unimmunized persons as soon as possible. Tetanus toxoid is given at the same time in a separate site. Medications are provided to treat muscle spasms. Intensive care is provided with cardiorespiratory monitoring, assisted ventilation, IV metronidazole or penicillin G, nutrition, and supportive care. Survival beyond 4 days indicates an increased chance of recovery. Paroxysms become less frequent and complete recovery may take weeks. *Prognosis:* 30% mortality; much higher in newborns. Intensive care has improved mortality. *Prevention:* Tetanus immunizations are routinely given. They must be updated every 10 years, or, if a potentially contaminated wound occurs, in 5 years. Proper surgical debridement of wounds decreases the chance of infection.	• Prevent disease by checking immunization records and administering immunizations as necessary. • Give immune globulin to unimmunized persons. • Assist with wound debridement. • The child with tetanus is hospitalized. Use standard precautions. • Monitor the child's condition. Handle as little as possible. Reduce stimulation by placing child in a quiet, darkened room. • Offer skin and respiratory care. The child may need an endotracheal tube, suctioning, and supplemental oxygen for airway support. • Provide feedings via total parenteral nutrition or feeding tube. • Maintain hydration with IV fluids and electrolytes. • Try to reduce the child's anxiety, as mental status may be unaffected. • Prepare the family for a possible poor prognosis.
Tuberculosis See Chapter 42.			

Endogenous pyrogens (interleukins, interferons, and tumor necrosis factor) are released by macrophages in response to an invasive organism. These pyrogens travel through the circulatory system to the hypothalamus, where they trigger the production of prostaglandins. Prostaglandins are believed to raise the body's thermoregulatory set point, causing fever (Cimpella, Goldman, & Khine, 2000).

Clinical Therapy

Diagnostic tests include cultures from sites where the infection may potentially be located (skin, pharynx, blood, urine, feces, cerebrospinal fluid, etc.). In some cases, x-rays or special imaging may be used to identify localized infection in an organ, such as the lungs.

For many infectious and communicable diseases, management is supportive. (See Skills 9–11—9–14 on the accompanying CD-ROM, as well as the *Clinical Skills Manual*). **SKILL** An elevated temperature can be a beneficial physiologic response, helping to eradicate organisms that thrive at lower body temperatures, and mobilizing the immune response. It may also enhance the effect of antibiotics. In addition, fever decreases the plasma iron concentration, which may limit the growth of microorganisms

(Cimpella et al., 2000). Fever is not inherently harmful until it reaches 41 °C (105.9 °F). For this reason, medical management may include postponing treatment of low-grade fevers under 38.9 °C (102 °F) to promote the body's natural defenses against an infection. If not managed, elevated temperatures can result in febrile seizures, which usually have no long-term sequelae. Thus, fevers greater than 38.9 °C (102 °F) should be treated, especially if associated with discomfort. Persistent temperatures of 38.3 to 38.5 °C (101 to 101.5 °F) may also benefit from antipyretic treatment. Acetaminophen and ibuprofen are the preferred antipyretics for children. Aspirin is no longer recommended for children because of its association with Reye syndrome. Antipyretics reduce fever by inhibiting prostaglandin synthesis, thus lowering the body's temperature set point.

Antibiotics are often another component of clinical therapy for infectious diseases. Before the introduction of antibiotics, children were often unable to fight infection and died as the result of overwhelming sepsis; antibiotics have decreased morbidity and mortality from infections among children. However, strains of bacteria have developed resistance to many antibiotics. Children with chronic illnesses such as cystic fibrosis, sickle cell disease, and AIDS are particularly susceptible to infection by drug-resistant pathogens.

Complementary Care

HERBAL THERAPIES FOR THE COMMON COLD

Parents often turn to herbal therapies to alleviate discomfort, especially when over-the-counter medications do not alleviate symptoms. Various forms of children's herbal remedies exist, including glycerine extracts, syrups, capsules, and chewable tablets. Tinctures are generally not recommended for children due to the high alcohol content and objectionable taste. Use of herbal supplements should be limited to children over 1 year of age (and in some cases, to children over 2, as shown below). Patients of all ages should limit use of the following herbs to 14 days unless otherwise noted.

- **Echinacea** *(E. purpurea, E. spp.)*—The most popular herbal remedy for upper respiratory infections on the common market is echinacea root. Echinacea is generally considered safe for children over 2 years old and appropriate for decreasing the frequency and severity of the common cold (Romm, 2000; Skidmore-Roth, 2001). Herbal practitioners recommend using echinacea immediately at the first signs of a cold, giving four doses per day for 3 days. If acute symptoms develop, practition-

ers recommend that TID dosage be continued throughout symptomatic period and for 2 days following. Echinacea has been found to limit severity of symptoms of the common viral cold (Schoneberger, 1992). Although some disagreement exists, most practitioners adhere to the belief that echinacea root is contraindicated for patients with autoimmune disorders.

- **Astragalus** *(A. membranaceus)*—Generally used preventively. In traditional Chinese medicine (TCM), practitioners advise cooking astragalus roots in soup during cold and flu season. Antiviral and immunostimulatory effects have been shown to reduce severity and length of symptoms for acute treatment of common cold (McGuffin, 1997; Murray & Pizzorno, 1998).

- **Elderberry** *(Sambucus nigra)*—Elderberry syrup has been shown to inhibit Type A and B influenza viruses in vitro (Zakay-Rones, 1995) and to reduce frequency and duration of influenza in adults and children (McGuffin, 1997; Mumcuoglu, 1995). The syrup is pleasant tasting, and is available in a sugar-free form.

Complementary Care

AYURVEDIC TREATMENT OF THE COMMON COLD

Ayurveda is an ancient system of natural and medical healing that originated in India. *Ayur* means "life" and *veda* means "science." It includes a wide range of modalities, including the use of diet, herbs, massage, exercise, music therapy, aromatherapy, meditation, and yoga, among others. According to Ayurveda, everything in nature, including the body, is composed of five elements: space, fire, air, water, and earth. Ayurvedic practitioners group these five elements into three categories, or doshas: vata (space and air); pitta (fire and water); and kapha (earth and water). Practitioners believe that disease is caused by an excess of one or more of these elements. Someone with a cold, for example, might be found to have an excess of kapha (Gottlieb, 2000).

Ayurveda states that, from birth to around mid-teenage years, children generally have a more watery constitution (kapha). Ayurveda says that this is the reason children are prone to colds, sinus problems, and lung fluid problems. The treatments in Ayurvedic medicine are aimed at restoring balance by decreasing excessive elements and increasing the others. An example is the commonly used herbal tea ginger (fire) for healing colds. Ayurvedic practitioners would also advise a diet that avoids mucus-increasing foods, such as dairy products. **Note that ginger is contraindicated in children with fevers** (Skidmore-Roth, 2001). Yoga would also most likely be "prescribed" by an Ayurvedic practitioner for many childhood illnesses, including a cold. Specific yoga postures are targeted toward healing particular organs and organ systems.

Nursing Management

Nursing Assessment and Diagnosis

Assess the child's hydration status and fluid intake, vital signs, comfort level, and appetite. Observe for seizures and for a **toxic appearance** (lethargy, poor perfusion, hypoventilation or hyperventilation, and cyanosis). The child with a fever may be irritable and restless, sleep fitfully, and have nonspecific muscular pain. Identify children who may be at higher risk for a serious illness in association with a fever, in particular (Thomas, 1995):

- Children having a toxic appearance
- Children less than 28 days of age with a temperature over 38 °C (100.4 °F)

- Children less than 4 years of age with a temperature over 41 °C (105.8 °F)
- Children with conditions such as a ventriculoperitoneal shunt, congenital heart disease, asplenia, and sickle cell anemia

Observe the child for other signs of infection, such as a rash, nausea and vomiting, and/or diarrhea, as well as generalized symptoms of a poor appetite and malaise.

The following nursing diagnoses may be appropriate for children with infectious and communicable diseases:

- *Hyperthermia* related to infectious disease process
- *Risk for fluid volume deficit* related to hypermetabolic state
- *Impaired skin integrity* related to hyperthermia and self-mutilation of skin lesions

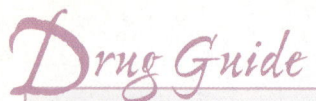

CEFTRIAXONE SODIUM (ROCEPHIN)

Overview of Action

Semisynthetic cephalosporin that acts by inhibiting mucopeptide synthesis in bacterial cell wall, causing osmotic instability. More active against wide range of gram-negative bacteria, such as *Neisseria gonorrhoeae, Haemophilus influenzae, Shigella, Enterobacter aerogenes, Escherichia coli, Klebsiella,* and *Pseudomonas aeruginosa.* Also active against some gram-positive strains (e.g., *Staphylococcus aureus, Staphylococcus pyogenes, Streptococcus pneumoniae*). Used to treat infections of lower respiratory tract, skin, intra-abdominal area, genitourinary tract (uncomplicated gonorrhea, pelvic inflammatory disease), bones, joints, and septicemia and meningitis.

Routes, Dosage, Frequency

IM, IV

- Neonates: 50 mg/kg/day as single dose
- Infants, children: 50 to 75 mg/kg/day in equally divided doses every 12 hours (dosage not to exceed 2 g/day)
- Meningitis: Neonates to 12 years: Loading dose: 75 to 100 mg/kg once, then 100 mg/kg/day in equally divided doses every 12 hours
- Skin and skin structure infections: Less than 12 years: Loading dose: 50 to 75 mg/kg once daily or in equally divided doses twice daily (not to exceed 2 g)
- Prophylaxis for infants of mothers with peripartum gonococcal infections: Single dose 50 mg/kg IM or IV given at birth (125 mg maximum dose)

Contraindications: Hypersensitivity to the drug or cephalosporins, neonates with hyperbilirubinemia. Use with caution if allergic to penicillin and other drugs, or if impaired renal or hepatic function.

Side Effects: Diarrhea, rash, pruritis, hypersensitivity, pain and induration at injection site.

Nursing Implications

- Assess: Determine if previous allergic reaction to ceftriaxone, penicillins, or cephalosporins. Obtain cultures and sensitivity before treatment, but treatment can start before results are obtained.
- Administer: **IM:** Reconstitute with either sterile or bacteriostatic water, saline, 5% dextrose, or 1% lidocaine hydrochloride (without epinephrine) for injection. Solution will be light yellow to amber. Injection is painful. Give into deep muscle appropriate for age and development; adequately restrain child, rotate and record sites. Do not use bacteriostatic water with benzyl alcohol for reconstitution in neonates. **IV:** Reconstitute according to package insert with compatible IV fluid. Intermittent infusion is given over 10 to 30 minutes in recommended concentrations of 10 to 40 mg/ml; compatible with D5W, D10W, D5W/0.5% NS, D5W/NS. Do not premix with other aminoglycosides and other bacteriostatic agents. Use of large vein with small-bore needle may reduce local IV reactions. Has 3.6 mEq sodium/1 Gram of drug.
- Monitor: Check IM site for induration. Observe IV site for vein irritation and extravasation, and change peripheral site every 48 to 72 hours. Monitor child for hypersensitivity and side effects, especially if renal or hepatic impairment is present, or if on long-term therapy periodically. Monitor CBC, prothrombin time, and hepatic and renal function levels. Watch for symptoms of superinfection or diarrhea (may indicate pseudomembranous colitis), check for fever and report. Yogurt (4 oz) daily may maintain normal intestinal flora. Watch for symptoms of bleeding due to possible prolonged bleeding time especially in malnutrition, children on anticoagulants, and other susceptible patients. If given for group A beta-hemolytic streptococcal infections, a 10-day therapy course is needed to reduce risk of rheumatic fever and glomerulonephritis. Usual therapy course is 4 to 14 days, or 2 days after symptoms subside.
- Patient teaching: Cold compresses for 24 hours after IM injection. Heat to injection site after 24 hours for local pain management.

Note: From Bindler, R. M., & Howry, L. B. (1997). *Pediatric drugs and nursing implications* (2nd ed.). Upper Saddle River NJ: Prentice Hall-Health. Adapted.

▶ *Altered oral mucous membranes* related to infectious disease process

▶ *Fluid volume deficit* related to repeated episodes of vomiting and diarrhea

▶ *Ineffective management of therapeutic regimen (family)* related to complexity of therapeutic regimen

Planning and Implementation

Most children with infectious diseases are cared for at home; however, children may be evaluated in various health care settings.

Nursing care of children with infectious diseases in health care settings focuses on preventing the spread of infection. Isolate children with suspicious rashes from other children. When possible, hard surfaces in the examining room where the child was seen should be wiped down with antiseptic solution before another child uses the room. Linens are disposed of in appropriately marked linen bags.

Nursing care for treatment of fever includes administering antipyretics, removing unnecessary clothing, and encouraging increased fluid intake. Tepid baths or sponging may be ordered when the child's temperature is greater than 40 °C (104 °F) while waiting for the antipyretic to work. Use water that is about 26.6 °C (80 °F).

Children are often admitted to the hospital for treatment of severe infections. In addition, countless numbers of **nosocomial** (hospital-acquired) **infections** occur each year. The fecal–oral and respiratory routes are the most common sources of infections in children. All items with which the infected child comes into contact are considered contaminated (linens, toys, medical equipment, etc.).

GUIDELINES FOR EVALUATING AND TREATING FEVER IN CHILDREN

Call your health care provider immediately if:

- The child is under 2 months old or has a fever over 40.1 °C (104.2 °F).
- The child is crying inconsolably or whimpering.
- The child cries when moved or otherwise touched by the parent or other family members.
- The child is difficult to awaken.
- The child's neck is stiff.
- There are any purple spots present on the skin.
- Breathing is difficult and no better after the nose is cleared.
- The child is drooling saliva and is unable to swallow anything.
- The child has a convulsion.
- The child acts or looks very sick.

Call your health care provider within 24 hours if:

- The child is 2 to 4 months old (unless fever occurs within 48 hours of a DTaP shot and the infant has no other serious symptoms).
- The fever is higher than 40.1 °C (104.2 °F) (especially if the child is under 3 years old).
- The child complains of burning or pain with urination.
- The fever has been present more than 24 hours without an obvious cause or location of infection.
- The fever went away for more than 24 hours and then returned.
- The fever has been present for more than 72 hours.

Treating the fever

- Use acetaminophen or ibuprofen to lower a fever.
- Use the correct dose of the medication—drops and syrups do not have the same concentration.
- Ibuprofen lasts 1 to 2 hours longer than acetaminophen, so it may be given less often.
- Remove all but a light layer of the child's clothing to help lower the temperature.

Note: From Hay, W. W., Jr., Groothuis, J. R., Hayward, A. R., & Lewin, M. J. (Eds.). (2001). *Current pediatric diagnosis and treatment* (15th ed.). New York: McGraw-Hill. Adapted.

Transmission-based precautions, including isolation, must be implemented to reduce exposure of other children and staff to the infectious agent. Follow the facility's standard precautions and transmission-based precautions to reduce the spread of infectious diseases to staff and other patients. Bring any questions and concerns to the hospital's infection control nurse. (See the Infection Control chapter in the *Clinical Skills Manual* for more detailed information).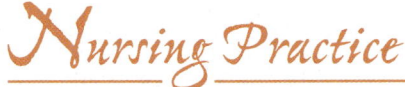

Involve the parents by allowing them to assist with their child's care. Nursing care also includes treating infection, administering antibiotics on schedule, monitoring antibiotic blood levels if indicated to ensure appropriate results, and educating parents.

Nursing Practice

A study comparing methods of fever reduction in febrile children with temperatures of more than 38.9 °C (102 °F) found no significant differences in temperature reduction over a 2-hour period when the child was given acetaminophen alone or with a 15-minute tepid sponge bath. However, the children who were given sponge baths had significantly higher discomfort scores (Sharber, 1997).

NURSING CARE IN THE COMMUNITY

Teach parents to care for their child at home. This includes how and when to give antipyretics and antibiotics if ordered, appropriate foods and beverages to provide, and care of rashes and other topical symptoms. Parents often fear fevers and need information and reassurance. Help them to recognize the signs of the child's worsening condition in association with the child's specific disease.

Correct any misconceptions parents and child care workers may have about the occurrence or cause of the infectious disease in their child. The parents and other providers may feel that they have exposed the child to certain germs or bacteria. Teach them that infection control will reduce exposure of other children and family members to the infectious disease. Specific infection-control measures include the following:

▶ Good handwashing is one of the best ways to decrease the spread of infection.

Developing Cultural Competence

Many Latino and Asian cultures subscribe to the hot and cold theory of disease causation. Fever, a hot condition, is treated by giving the patient cold substances (foods or medicines). "Hot" and "cold" do not refer to temperature but to categories. Cold foods include vegetables, fruits, and fish. Cold medicines include orange flower water, linden, and sage. Ask parents how they think the illness should be treated. Encourage them to use that treatment as long as it seems safe. Teach them additional Western medicine treatments they can use.

- Disinfect hard surfaces such as those touched by the child with a cold, diaper-changing areas, diaper pails, and cribs.
- Tell children not to kiss pets on the mouth.
- Remove toys that the child has mouthed and disinfect them before other children play with them.
- Make sure all children in the house are fully immunized.

Evaluation

Expected outcomes of nursing care include:

- Opportunities for spread of infection are minimized between patients and family members.
- The child's fever is effectively managed with antipyretics.

CHAPTER HIGHLIGHTS

✎ Infectious and communicable diseases remain a significant source of morbidity and mortality in children, especially in developing countries.

✎ Infants are especially vulnerable to infectious diseases because their immune system is immature, their passively acquired maternal antibodies are decreasing, and disease protection through immunization is not yet complete.

✎ For a child to acquire a communicable disease, an infectious agent or pathogen, an effective means of transmission, and a susceptible host need to be present.

✎ Major public health efforts that have decreased the occurrence of infectious and communicable diseases include safer drinking water, better sanitation, improved standards of living, increased immunization, and advanced medical treatment.

✎ Vaccines must be given at specific ages and intervals. Immunization timing is related to decreasing maternal antibody protection, the child's developing ability to make antibodies in response to a vaccine, and whether or not the vaccine provides lifelong immunity.

✎ Vaccines must be stored properly and administered appropriately to ensure their effectiveness.

✎ The National Childhood Vaccine Injury Act of 1986 provides compensation if a link between immunization and a serious adverse effect is found. The Vaccine Adverse Event Reporting System has been established to track serious vaccine reactions.

✎ Infectious and communicable diseases are caused by bacterial, viral, protozoan, or fungal organisms.

✎ Fever is often a sign of infectious disease in children. The hypothalamus functions as the body's thermostat, directing the body to conserve or dissipate heat. When microorganisms invade the body, endogenous pyrogens are released into the bloodstream. These substances travel to the hypothalamus, where they trigger the production and release of prostaglandins, which initiate the fever response.

✎ The child with a toxic or septic appearance has the following signs: lethargy, poor perfusion, tachypnea or bradypnea, and pallor or cyanosis.

✎ Infection-control measures caregivers can take include the following: using good handwashing techniques, disinfecting hard surfaces touched by the child, telling children not to kiss pets, disinfecting toys the child has mouthed before letting other children play with them, and making sure all children are fully immunized.

EXPLOREMEDIALINK

NCLEX Review, Case Studies, and other interactive resources for this chapter can be found on the companion website at http://www.prenhall.com/london. Click on "Chapter 41" to select the activities for this chapter.

For animations, more NCLEX review questions, and an audio glossary, access the accompanying CD-ROM in this textbook.

REFERENCES

Adams, D. M., & Ware, R. E. (1996). Parvovirus B19: How much should you worry? *Contemporary Pediatrics, 13*(4), 85–96.

American Academy of Pediatrics Committee on Infectious Disease. (2000). *Red book: Report of the Committee on Infectious Disease* (25th ed). Elk Grove Village, IL: Author.

Atkinson, W. L. (1999). Thimerosol. *Needle Tips and the Hepatitis B Coalition News, 9*(2), 1, 15.

Barat, L. M., & Zucker, J. R. (1999). Malaria. In J. A. McMillan, C. D. DeAngelis, R. D. Feigin, & J. B. Warshaw (Eds.), *Oski's pediatrics: Principles & practice* (3rd ed., pp. 1177–1184). Philadelphia: Lippincott, Williams & Wilkins.

Centers for Disease Control Advisory Committee on Immunization Practices. (2000). Use of diphtheria toxoid-tetanus toxoid-acellular pertussis vaccine in a 5-dose series. *Morbidity and Mortality Weekly Reports, 49*(RR-13); 1–7.

Centers for Disease Control Advisory Committee on Immunization Practices. (2001). Recommended childhood immunization schedule—United States, 2001, *Morbidity and Mortality Weekly Report, 50*(01); 7–10, 19.

Chang, L. Y., Lin, T. Y., Hsu, K. H., Huang, Y. C., Lin, K. L., Hsueh, C., et al. (1999). Clinical features and risk factors of pulmonary edema after enterovirus 71–related hand, foot, and mouth disease. *Lancet, 354*(9191), 1682–1686.

Cherry, J. D. (1999). Parvoviruses. In J. A. McMillan, C. D. DeAngelis, R. D. Feigin, & J. B. Warshaw (Eds.), *Oski's pediatrics: Principles & practice* (3rd ed., pp. 1098–1100). Philadelphia: Lippincott, Williams & Wilkins.

Cimpella, L. B., Goldman, D. L., & Khine, H. (2000). Fever pathophysiology. *Clinical Pediatric Emergency Medicine, 1*(2), 84–93.

Diggle, L., & Deek, J. (2000). Effect of needle length on incidence of local reactions to routine immunizations in infants aged 4 months: Randomized control trial. *British Medical Journal, 321*(7266), 931–933.

Feigin, R. D., & Bloom, M. L. (1999). Rickettsial disease. In J. A. McMillan, C. D. DeAngelis,

R. D. Feigin, & J. B. Warshaw (Eds.), *Oski's pediatrics: Principles & practice* (3rd ed., pp. 898–902). Philadelphia: Lippincott, Williams & Wilkins.

Gottlieb, B. (2000). *Alternative cures.* Emmaus, PA: Rodale Press.

Grimm, W., & Muller, H. H. (1999). A randomized controlled trial of the effect of fluid extract of *Echinacea purpurea* on the incidence and severity of colds and respiratory infections. *American Journal of Medicine, 106*(2), 138–143.

Healy, T. L. (2000). The impact of Lyme disease on school children. *Journal of School Nursing, 16*(2), 12–18.

Jenkins, C. N. H., McPhee, S. J., Wong, C., Nguyen, T., & Euler, G. L. (2000). Hepatitis B immunization coverage among Vietnamese-American children 3 to 18 years old. *Pediatrics, 106*(6), 1–8.

Kaplan, S. L. (1999). Haemophilis influenzae. In J. A. McMillan, C. D. DeAngelis, R. D. Feigin, & J. B. Warshaw (Eds.), *Oski's pediatrics: Principles & practice* (3rd ed., pp. 969–973). Philadelphia: Lippincott, Williams & Wilkins.

McGuffin, M., Hobbs, C., Upton, R., & Goldberg, A. (1997). *Botanical safety handbook.* Boca Raton, FL: CRC Press.

McMillan, J. A., & Feigin, R. D. (1999). Group A streptococcal infections. In J. A. McMillan, C. D. DeAngelis, R. D. Feigin, & J. B. Warshaw (Eds.), *Oski's pediatrics: Principles and practice* (3rd ed., pp. 1012–1017), Philadelphia: Lippincott, Williams & Wilkins.

Mumcuoglu, *Sambucus Nigra* L. (1995). *Black elderberry extract: A breakthrough in the treatment of influenza.* Skokie, IL: RSS Publishing.

Murray, M., & Pizzorno, J. (1998). *Encyclopedia of natural medicine.* Roseville, CA: Prima Publishing.

Phelps, R. (1997). Rabies: Confronting the continuing threat. *Contemporary Pediatrics, 14*(7), 137–150.

Rennels, M. B. (1999). Resistant pneumococcal disease: Treatment and prevention. *Contemporary Pediatrics* (Suppl. 3), 4–10.

Rennels, M. B., Edwards, K. M., & Keyserling, H. L. (1998). Safety and immunogenicity of heptavalent pneumococcal vaccine conjugated to CRM in United States infants. *Pediatrics, 101*(4), 604–611.

Romm, A. (2000). Better Nutrition's 2000 guide to children's supplements. *Better Nutrition, 62*(10), 38–43.

Schoneberger, D. (1992). The influence of immune-stimulating effects of pressed juice from *Echinacea purpurea* on the course and severity of colds: Results of a double-blind study. *Forum Immunology, 8,* 2–12.

Sharber, J. (1997). The efficacy of tepid sponge bathing to reduce fever in young children. *American Journal of Emergency Medicine, 15*(2), 211–213.

Skidmore-Roth, L. (2001). *Mosby's handbook of herbs and natural supplements.* St. Louis, MO: Mosby.

Sullivan, J. L. (1999). Epstein-Barr virus infection in children. In J. A. McMillan, C. D. DeAngelis, R. D. Feigin, & J. B. Warshaw (Eds.), *Oski's pediatrics: Principles & practice* (3rd ed., pp. 1107–1110). Philadelphia: Lippincott, Williams & Wilkins.

Taber, L. H., & Demmler, G. J. (1999a). Mumps. In J. A. McMillan, C. D. DeAngelis, R. D. Feigin, & J. B. Warshaw (Eds.), *Oski's pediatrics: Principles & practice* (3rd ed., pp. 1141–1142). Philadelphia: Lippincott, Williams & Wilkins.

Taber, L. H., & Demmler, G. J. (1999b). Rubella (German measles). In J. A. McMillan, C. D. DeAngelis, R. D. Feigin, & J. B. Warshaw (Eds.), *Oski's pediatrics: Principles & practice* (3rd ed., pp. 1134–1137). Philadelphia: Lippincott, Williams & Wilkins.

Thomas, D. O. (1995). Fever in children: Friend or foe? *RN, 58*(4), 42–47.

Twomey, J. (1998). Varicella exposure in a child at risk of being immunosuppressed. *Pediatric Nursing, 23*(5), 459–464.

Wade, C. F. (2000). Keeping Lyme disease at bay: An integrated approach to prevention. *American Journal of Nursing, 100*(7), 26–31.

Zakay-Rones, Z. Varsano, N., Zlotnick, M., Manor, O., Regev, L., Schlesinger, M. et al. (1995). Inhibition of several strains of influenza virus *in vitro* and reduction of symptoms by an elderberry extract during an outbreak of influenza B Panama. *Journal of Alternative and Complementary Medicine, 1*(4), 361–369.

CHAPTER 42

The Child with Alterations in Respiratory Function

Emily gets sick so much faster than my other children. I guess the bronchopulmonary dysplasia and her tracheostomy make her more susceptible to infections. I really get concerned because she struggles so hard to breathe when she gets all these extra secretions. I have learned to suction and change her tracheostomy, but I am afraid that one day she will completely obstruct her airway. I just hope I remember all the things I have been taught if that happens, and that the emergency medical personnel come quickly.

—FATHER OF EMILY, 8 MONTHS

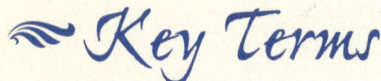

Key Terms

Adventitious *1023*

Airway resistance *1023*

Alveolar hypoventilation *1030*

Apnea *1026*

Dysphagia *1034*

Dysphonia *1034*

Dyspnea *1030*

Hypercapnia *1029*

Hypoxemia *1029*

Hypoxia *1030*

Laryngospasm *1032*

Paradoxical breathing *1023*

Periodic breathing *1026*

Retractions *1024*

Stridor *1031*

Tachypnea *1030*

Trigger *1035*

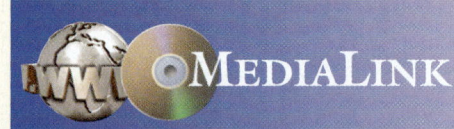

MediaLink

CD-ROM

Audio Glossary

NCLEX Review

Skill 11-11: Using a Metered Dose Inhaler

Skill 14-2: Oxygen Saturation: Pulse Oximetry

Skill 14-5: Peak Expiratory Flow Meter

Skill 14-9: Tracheostomy Care

Skill 14-20: Performing Chest Physiotherapy/Postural Drainage

COMPANION WEBSITE

http://www.prenhall.com/london

Nursing Care Plan: The Child with Bronchiolitis

Respiratory Web Links

Thinking Critically

Teaching Plan: Metered Dose Inhaler

NCLEX Review

Case Study

This chapter explores several special factors in the child's respiratory system that create ongoing threats to respiratory function and overall health. Most respiratory problems in children produce mild symptoms, last a short time, and can be managed at home. Nevertheless, acute respiratory problems are the most common cause of illness requiring hospitalization in infants and children under 15 years of age (Health Resources and Services Administration, 2000).

Pediatric respiratory conditions may occur as a primary problem or as a complication of nonrespiratory conditions and may be life threatening or have long-term implications. Nurses must learn to assess the child's current respiratory status quickly, monitor progress, and anticipate potential complications (Table 42–1).

Respiratory problems may result from structural problems, functional problems, or a combination of both. Structural problems involve alterations in the size and shape of parts of the respiratory tract. Functional problems involve alterations in gas exchange and threats to this normal process from irritants (such as large particles and chemicals) or invaders (such as viruses or bacteria). Alterations in other organ systems, especially the immune and neurologic systems, may also threaten respiratory function. When reading this chapter, keep the distinction between structural and functional problems in mind to help distinguish between what is normal and what is abnormal about the child's maturing respiratory system. Refer to Chapter 48 for information on upper respiratory tract infections.

ANATOMY AND PHYSIOLOGY OF PEDIATRIC DIFFERENCES

The child's respiratory tract constantly grows and changes until about 12 years of age. The young child's neck is shorter than an adult's, resulting in airway structures that are closer together.

Upper Airway Differences

The child's airway is shorter and narrower than an adult's. These differences create a greater potential for obstruction (see "As They Grow: Airway Development"). The infant's airway is approximately 4 mm in diameter, about the width of a drinking straw, in contrast to the adult's airway diameter of 20 mm. The upper airway primarily increases in length rather than diameter during the first 5 years of life. The diameter of a child's trachea closely approximates the diameter of the child's little finger. This "rule of finger" can be used for quick assessment of airway size.

The child's narrower airway causes an increase in **airway resistance,** the effort or force needed to move oxygen through the trachea to the lungs. As air moves from the child's nares down the trachea to the distal airways (alveoli), it must flow through a relatively small area. Friction and increasing resistance are generated as air passes through the airway. Airway resistance in infancy is 15 times greater than in adults (Webster & Huether, 1998). When edema and swelling occur in response to a virus, bacterium, or other irritant, the airway is further narrowed, increasing airway resistance even more. The trachea in a child is higher and at a different angle than the adult's (see "As They Grow: Trachea Position").

Physiologically the upper airway is the port for inspiration of oxygen and expiration of carbon dioxide. Infants, children, and adults can breathe through either the nose or the mouth. Until 4 weeks of age, newborns are obligatory nose breathers. The coordination of mouth breathing is controlled by maturing neurologic pathways; thus, young infants do not automatically open the mouth to breathe when the nose is obstructed. The only time a newborn breathes through the mouth is when he or she is crying. Nasal patency in newborns is therefore essential for such activities as breathing and eating.

TABLE 42–1   Assessment Guidelines for a Child in Respiratory Distress[a]

Quality of Respirations
- Inspect the rate, depth, and ease of respirations.
- Identify the signs of respiratory distress: tachypnea (abnormally rapid rate of respirations), retractions, nasal flaring, inspiratory stridor, expiratory grunting.
- Note lack of simultaneous chest and abdominal rise with inspiration **(paradoxical breathing).**
- Auscultate breath sounds: bilateral, diminished or absent, **adventitious** (sounds that are not normally heard, such as wheezes, crackles, rhonchi).

Quality of Pulse
- Assess the rate and rhythm: tachycardia may indicate hypoxia.
- Compare pulse sites (apical to brachial) for strength and rate.

Color
- Observe overall color: with respiratory distress, color progresses from pallor to mottled to cyanosis; central cyanosis is a late sign of respiratory distress.
- Compare peripheral and central color: assess capillary refill and nailbed color and inspect mucous membranes; central cyanosis in mucous membranes is more ominous.
- Note whether crying improves or worsens color.

Cough
- Quality: note whether dry (nonproductive), wet (productive, mucousy), brassy (noisy, musical), croupy (barking, seal-like).
- Effort: note whether forceful or weak; weak cough may indicate an airway obstruction or fatigue from prolonged respiratory effort (not valid in neonates).

Behavior Change
- Note level of consciousness: alert or lethargic.
- Restlessness and irritability are associated with hypoxia.
- Watch for abrupt behavior changes (restlessness, irritability) and lowered level of consciousness, which indicate increasing hypoxia.

Signs of Dehydration
- Inspect for dry mucous membranes, lack of tears, poor skin turgor, and decreased urine output, which indicate that fluid needs are not being met.

[a]Refer to Chapter 33 for the actual techniques of assessment mentioned in this table.

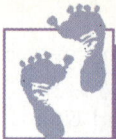
Smaller nasopharynx, easily occluded during infection.

Lymph tissue (tonsils, adenoids) grows rapidly in early childhood; atrophies after age 12.

Smaller nares, easily occluded.

Small oral cavity and large tongue increase risk of obstruction.

Long, floppy epiglottis vulnerable to swelling with resulting obstruction.

Larynx and glottis are higher in neck, increasing risk of aspiration.

Because thyroid, cricoid, and tracheal cartilages are immature, they may easily collapse when neck is flexed.

Because fewer muscles are functional in airway, it is less able to compensate for edema, spasm, and trauma.

The large amounts of soft tissue and loosely anchored mucous membranes lining the airway increase risk of edema and obstruction.

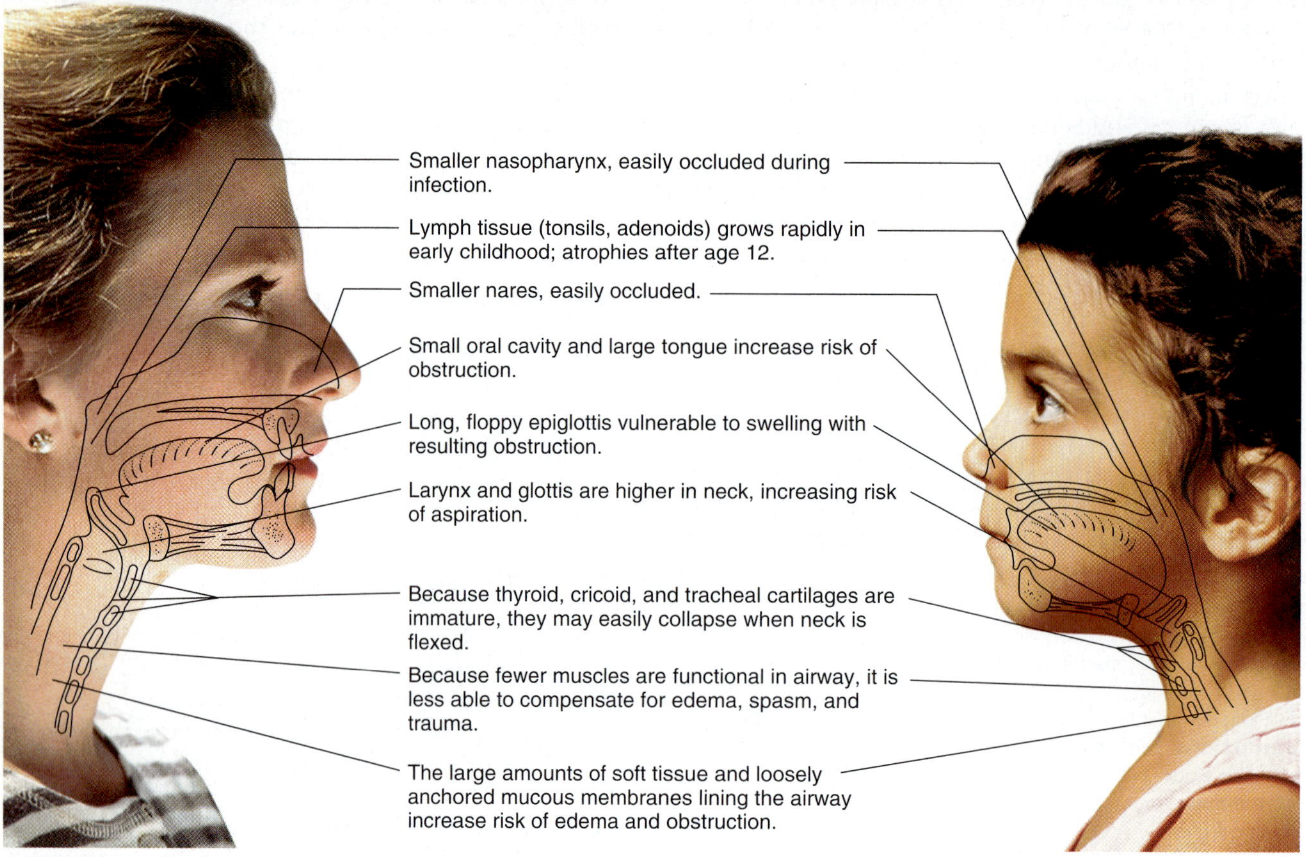

It is easy to see that a child's airway is smaller and less developed than an adult's airway, but why is this important? An upper respiratory tract infection, allergic reaction, positioning of the head and neck during sleep, and the small objects children play with can have serious consequences in the child.

Lower Airway Differences

The child's lower airway is also constantly growing. The developing alveoli change size and shape, and their numbers increase until respiratory maturity is attained at 12 years of age. This alveolar growth increases the area available for gas exchange. At birth the distal (peripheral) bronchioles that extend to the alveoli are narrow and fewer in number than in an adult. The child's overall growth can be correlated to the increased branching of the peripheral bronchioles as the alveoli continue to multiply. The taller the child, the greater the lung surface area.

The bronchi and bronchioles are lined with smooth muscle. The newborn does not have enough smooth muscle bundles to help trap airway invaders. By 5 months of age, however, a baby has enough muscles to react to irritants by bronchospasm and muscle contraction. Smooth muscle development is complete and comparable to that of an adult by 1 year of age (Webster & Huether, 1998).

The lungs, which have no muscles of their own, rely on the diaphragm and intercostal muscles to power respiration.

Growth and Development

At birth the lung tissue contains only 25 million alveoli, which are not fully developed. The number of alveoli increases to 300 million by 8 years of age, after which these structures begin increasing in size and complexity until puberty (Webster & Huether, 1998).

Children up to 6 years of age are primarily diaphragmatic breathers. Because the intercostal muscles are immature and the ribs are primarily cartilage and very flexible, their efficiency in assisting ventilation is reduced. The chest wall is so flexible that the negative pressure created by the downward movement of the diaphragm draws in air, but in cases of respiratory distress causes the chest wall to be drawn inward, causing **retractions.** By 6 years of age, the child begins to use the intercostal muscles more effectively for breathing (see "Pathophysiology Illustrated: Retraction Sites").

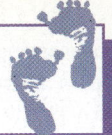
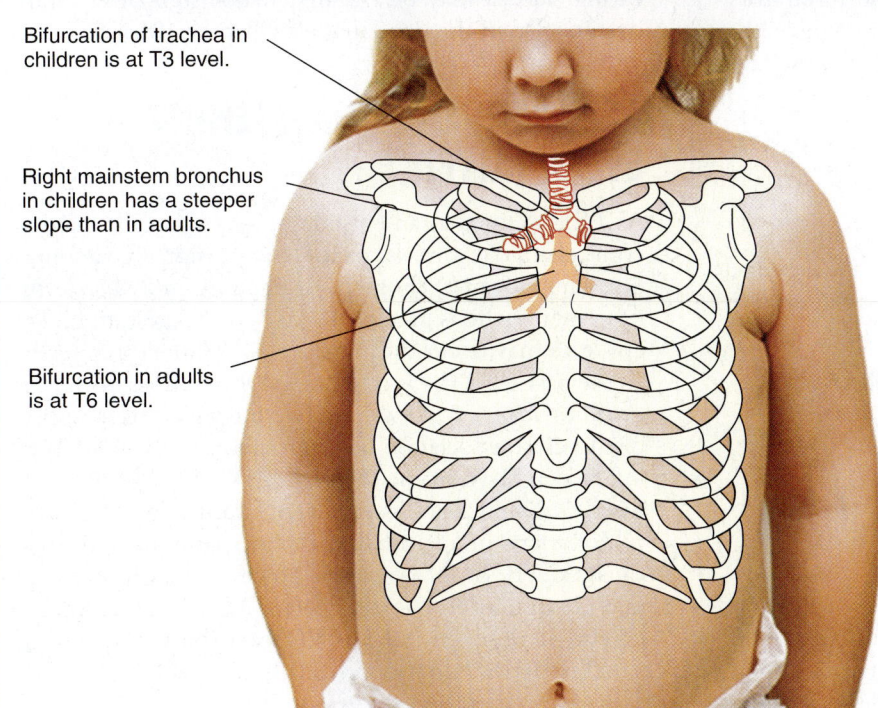

Bifurcation of trachea in children is at T3 level.

Right mainstem bronchus in children has a steeper slope than in adults.

Bifurcation in adults is at T6 level.

In children, the trachea is shorter and the angle of the right bronchus at bifurcation is more acute than in the adult. When you are resuscitating or suctioning, you must allow for the differences. Do you think that this difference is significant in respiratory infection? Why?

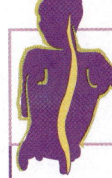

PATHOPHYSIOLOGY ILLUSTRATED
Retraction Sites

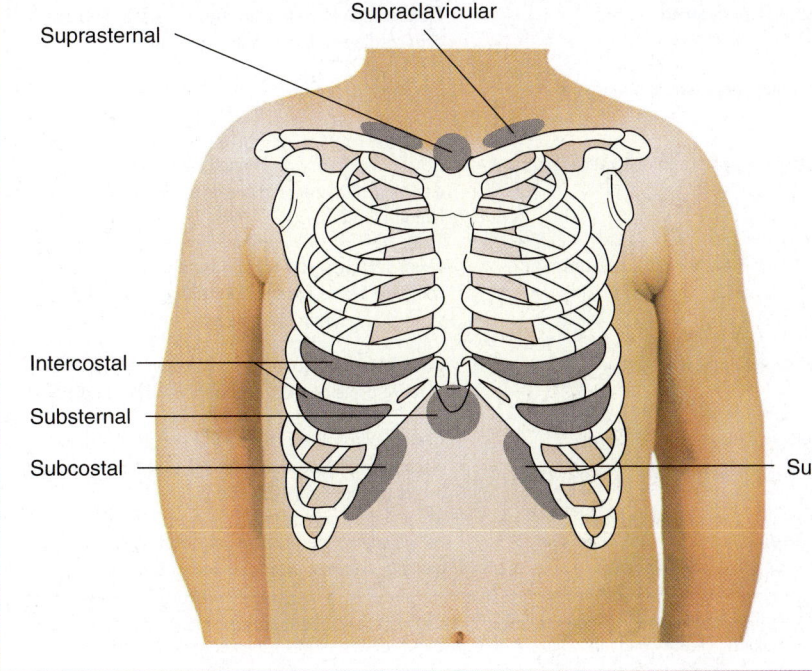

Suprasternal

Supraclavicular

Intercostal

Substernal

Subcostal

Subcostal

Retractions may occur in the very young infant in the suprasternal area. In the older infant and child, retractions occur when the airway is severely obstructed, as in croup. The depth and location of retractions is associated with the severity of respiratory distress. Isolated intercostal retractions indicate mild distress. Subcostal, suprasternal, and supraclavicular retractions indicate moderate distress. These retractions accompanied by use of accessory muscles indicate severe distress.

URGENT RESPIRATORY THREATS

From the moment a child is born, airway integrity is threatened because of the immaturity of the respiratory muscles and neurologic system. Learn to recognize the early signs of respiratory compromise to enable quick intervention to assist the infant in distress.

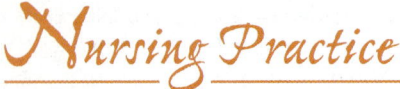

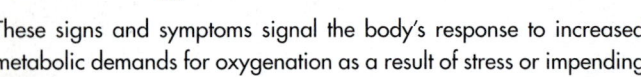

These signs and symptoms signal the body's response to increased metabolic demands for oxygenation as a result of stress or impending illness:

▸ Increasing restlessness, irritability, unexplained sudden confusion
▸ Rapid heart rate accompanied by rapid respiratory rate

APNEA

Infants normally breathe with an irregular rhythm and may have pauses of up to 20 seconds between breaths. This **periodic breathing** should not be confused with apnea.

Apnea, by definition, is cessation of respiration lasting longer than 20 seconds, or any pause in respiration associated with cyanosis, marked pallor, hypotonia, or bradycardia. Apnea may be the first major sign of respiratory dysfunction in the neonate (see Chapter 28).

APPARENT LIFE-THREATENING EVENT (ALTE)

ALTE is defined as an episode of apnea accompanied by a color change (cyanosis, pallor, or occasionally ruddiness), limp muscle tone, choking, or gagging in a near-term or term infant who is greater than 37 weeks' gestation. These episodes may occur during sleep, wakefulness, or feeding. In the past, ALTE was often called *near-miss sudden infant death* or *aborted crib death*. These terms erroneously implied a close association between such episodes and sudden infant death syndrome (SIDS). SIDS should not be confused with apnea and is discussed later in this chapter.

A variety of identifiable diseases and conditions can cause ALTE. In 50% of cases, however, no cause is identified (Loughlin & Carroll, 1999). ALTE can frighten the parent or observer, who often fears the infant has died. Emergency resuscitation is usually required.

CLINICAL MANIFESTATIONS ~ *Causes of Apparent Life-Threatening Events*

CAUSE	CLINICAL MANIFESTATIONS	DIAGNOSTIC TESTS
Functional or structural airway problem or immaturity	Apnea of 20 sec or longer; accompanied by bradycardia or cyanosis	Cardiorespiratory monitoring, sleep study, pneumogram, sepsis workup
Aspiration as a result of dysfunctional swallowing or gastroesophageal reflux	Choking, coughing, cyanosis, vomiting	Barium swallow, esophageal pH probe
Cardiac problems	Tachycardia, tachypnea, dyspnea	Cardiorespiratory monitoring, electrocardiogram, echocardiogram, arterial blood gases
Drug toxicity or poisoning; maternal history of ingestion	Central nervous system depression, hypotonia	Serum magnesium level, toxicity screen
Environmental, thermoregulation problem	Lethargy, tachypnea, hypothermia or hyperthermia	Cardiorespiratory and temperature monitoring, environmental temperature level (ambient air temperature)
Impaired oxygenation, respiratory disease (pulmonary edema, atelectasis, pneumonia)	Cyanosis, tachypnea, respiratory distress, anemia, choking, coughing	Oximetry, chest radiograph, arterial blood gases, complete blood count, upper airway evaluation, sleep study, serum electrolytes
Acute infection (sepsis, meningitis, necrotizing enterocolitis)	Feeding intolerance, lethargy, temperature instability	Complete blood count, cultures when appropriate, C-reactive protein, chest and abdominal radiographs
Intracranial pathology (intraventricular hemorrhage, ventricular dilation, central nervous system anomalies, meningitis)	Abnormal neurologic examination, seizures	Cranial ultrasound, computed tomography scan, electroencephalogram, magnetic resonance imaging, cerebrospinal fluid evaluation
Metabolic disorders	Jitteriness, poor feeding, lethargy, central nervous system depression or irritability, hypotonia	Serum electrolytes (potassium, sodium, chloride), glucose, calcium, arterial blood gases

Note: From Theobald, K., Botwinski, C., Albanna, S., & McWilliam, P. (2000). Apnea of prematurity: Diagnosis, implications for care, and pharmacologic management. *Neonatal Network, 19*(6), 17–24; and Eichenwald, E., & Stark, A. (1992). Apnea of prematurity: Etiology and management. *Tufts University School of Medicine Reports on Neonatal Respiratory Diseases, 2*(1), 1–11. Adapted.

Nursing Management

After ALTE, infants are usually admitted to the hospital for evaluation and cardiorespiratory monitoring. Nursing care includes collecting a detailed history of the event, observing and monitoring cardiorespiratory status, providing supportive care to the infant and family, and anticipating the need for emergency resuscitation and for the diagnostic process.

MONITOR CARDIORESPIRATORY STATUS

Cardiorespiratory monitoring records heart rate and respiratory rate while the infant is awake and asleep. Transcutaneous PO_2 (oxygen saturation or oximetry) monitoring provides a noninvasive continuous evaluation of the infant's oxygenation status. An SaO_2 less than 95% indicates hypoxemia. (See Skills 14-2–14-4.) 🔗 **SKILLS** **CD**

PROVIDE EMOTIONAL SUPPORT

Establishing rapport and open communication with the parents is essential for creating a sense of trust. To obtain further information about the episode, use open-ended questions and active listening skills. Do not give parents the impression that their parenting skills are being judged or questioned. Parents are fearful and anxious about the infant's prognosis. Explanations of tests and treatment help to decrease their anxiety and increase their understanding of the situation.

During hospitalization the infant should be held and cuddled to provide a sense of security and well-being. Encouraging parents' participation in the infant's care helps to meet these needs and promotes family bonding. Often parents are afraid to touch the infant because they might disconnect the monitoring cable. Wrapping the cable inside the infant's blanket helps secure the wires, increasing parents' feelings of confidence in handling the infant.

PROVIDE TACTILE STIMULATION

Tactile stimulation, such as rubbing the infant's back or feet, often is enough to halt an apneic episode. Continuous stimulation from an oscillating waterbed reduces the frequency of apneic episodes in some infants (Theobald, Botwinski, Albanna, et al., 2000). Both methods of stimulation remind the infant to take a breath.

ADMINISTER MEDICATIONS

Methylxanthines (aminophylline, caffeine) or doxapram may be administered to stimulate the respiratory center in the brain. Caffeine is preferred because it enhances diaphragmatic contraction and has a longer action time, fewer side effects, and more stable plasma concentration. Infants have immature hepatic and renal systems, so the rate and efficiency of drug absorption and excretion are affected. Monitor serum drug levels frequently because the metabolism and distribution of the drug can be unpredictable.

ANTICIPATE EMERGENCY RESUSCITATION

Because the infant who has had ALTE continues to be at risk for cardiopulmonary arrest, keep emergency resuscitation equipment and drugs readily accessible at all times.

Teaching About

HOME CARE INSTRUCTIONS FOR THE INFANT REQUIRING APNEA MONITORING

Apnea Equipment
- Understand monitor type, lead wires, placement of skin electrodes or chest belt, battery power, manual for troubleshooting.

Emergency Preparation
- Notify telephone company, electric company, local rescue squad, local emergency department (establishes priority status).
- Post phone numbers of rescue squad, physician, equipment company, power company, emergency number, cardiopulmonary resuscitation (CPR) guidelines, other important numbers (neighbor, parents' work numbers) in at least two places in the home; have at least one added extension phone.
- Keep the apnea monitor battery fully charged.

Safety Precautions
- Place monitor on firm surface; keep away from other appliances (television, microwave oven) and water.
- Ensure that alarms are audible from all locations.
- Double-check that monitor is on before going to bed.
- Thread cable and wires through lower end of infant's clothes.
- Ensure integrity of leads, monitor cable, and power cord (replace if frayed).

Routine Care
- Understand reasons for apnea monitor and frequency of use.
- Be able to attach and detach infant chest leads and belt.
- Evaluate skin for irritation or breakdown from electrode placement and give skin care (no oils or lotion; move patches correctly).

Emergency Care
- Develop plan for respiratory failure and power failure.
- Demonstrate CPR and back blows and chest thrusts for airway obstruction.
- Understand how to respond to alarms for apnea, bradycardia, or loose lead.

Apnea Alarm
- Observe infant's respiratory movement.
- If respiration is absent or infant is lethargic, stimulate by calling name and gently touching, proceeding to vigorous touch if needed.
- If no response, proceed with CPR.

Bradycardia Alarm
- Stimulate infant; infant should respond quickly.

Loose Lead
- Check electrode patch. Is it loose? Dirty? Belt loose?
- Check wires from electrode or monitor cable.
- Check power supply. Is battery low? Power failure? Monitor malfunctioning?

DISCHARGE PLANNING AND HOME CARE TEACHING

Identify and address home care needs well in advance of discharge. Teach parents how to operate an apnea monitor, what to do when the infant has an apneic episode, and how to perform cardiopulmonary resuscitation (CPR) and choking-prevention techniques (see Skill 14-13). **SKILLS**

SUDDEN INFANT DEATH SYNDROME (SIDS)

SIDS has been defined as the sudden death of an infant under 1 year of age that remains unexplained after a complete autopsy, a death scene investigation, and review of the history. It remains a leading cause of death in infants between 1 month and 1 year of age, with 90% of cases occurring before 6 months of age (American Academy of Pediatrics [AAP] Committee on Child Abuse and Neglect, 2001). SIDS occurs rarely in infants younger than 2 weeks. It is currently unpredictable and unpreventable. The first symptom is cardiopulmonary arrest.

SIDS is referred to as a "syndrome" because of the many and varied autopsy and clinical findings that characterize most infants who die of the disorder. The autopsy typically does not identify a disease process that caused the death. Clinical findings include evidence of a struggle or change in position and the presence of frothy, blood-tinged secretions from the mouth and nares. SIDS occurs more often in the fall and winter and during sleep. Most deaths are unobserved. Typically parents find the infant dead in the crib in the morning and report having heard no cries or disturbances during the night. A mild respiratory illness often precedes the death.

The current thinking about the etiology of SIDS is that an abnormality of the arcuate nucleus of the brainstem causes a delayed development of arousal, cardiorespiratory control, or cardiovascular control (Panigrahy, Filiano, Sleeper, et al. 1997). Other proposed causes include *H. pylori* gastrointestinal infection, and a cardiac dysrhythmia called long QT syndrome. Several infant, maternal, and familial factors appear to place infants at risk for SIDS (Table 42–2). SIDS has not been found to be associated with newborn apnea or immunizations for diphtheria, tetanus, and pertussis (DTP). Child abuse or homicide may be associated with 1% to 5% of SIDS cases (AAP Committee on Child Abuse and Neglect, 2001).

Nursing Management

The sudden, unexpected nature of the infant's death is confirmed in the emergency department. The nurse's role is to be empathetic and provide support during one of the greatest crises a family must face. The focus is on supporting the family during the acute grieving period (Table 42–3).

Reassure the parents that they are not responsible for the infant's death and help them contact other family members and mobilize support. Older children may need

TABLE 42–2 Risk Factors for Sudden Infant Death Syndrome (SIDS)

Infant
- Prematurity
- Low birth weight
- Twin or triplet birth
- Race (in decreasing order of frequency): most common in Native-American infants, followed by African-American, Hispanic, white, and Asian infants
- Gender: more common in males than females
- Age: most common in infants between 2 and 4 months of age
- Time of year: more prevalent in winter months
- Exposure to passive smoke
- History of cyanosis, respiratory distress, irritability, and poor feeding in the nursery
- Sleeping prone

Maternal and Familial
- Maternal age less than 20 years
- History of smoking and illicit drug use (increases incidence 10 times)
- Anemia
- Multiple pregnancies, with short intervals between births
- History of sibling with SIDS (increases incidence four to five times)
- Low socioeconomic status; crowding
- Poor prenatal care, low weight gain

Nursing Practice

Guidelines for the support of families experiencing SIDS should include baptism services, religious support, grief counseling, assistance with funeral arrangements, and counseling on cessation of breast-feeding and sibling reactions.

reassurance that SIDS will not happen to them (see Chapter 37). They may also believe that bad thoughts or wishes about their baby brother or sister caused the death. Support groups can help parents, siblings, and other family members express these fears and work through their feelings about the infant's death. The SIDS Alliance and SHARE are organizations that can help families locate a support group in their area. **WEB**

Nurses can play an important role in educating the public about the link between SIDS and infant positioning during sleep. The AAP recommends that infants be placed on their back to sleep. The dramatic decrease in SIDS deaths, from 67% of postneonatal deaths in 1993 to 28% in 1998, is believed to be related the success of educational campaigns about infant sleep position. Recent findings indicate that infants placed to sleep on their stomach who typically sleep on their backs have an increased incidence of SIDS. This is believed to be a factor in the rising incidence of SIDS in child care settings (Cote, Gerez, Brouillette, et al., 2000; Moon, Patel, & Shaefer, 2000). Place hospitalized infants to sleep in supine position rather than side-lying or prone.

TABLE 42–3 Supportive Care for the Family of an Infant with Sudden Infant Death Syndrome (SIDS)

Nursing Interventions	Rationale
1. Provide parents with a private area and a support person who reinforces that the infant's death was not their fault.	1. Parents need to be able to express their grief in their own way and hear that they are not being blamed for the infant's death.
2. Prepare the family for the viewing of the infant. Describe how the infant will look and feel.	2. You can say "Paul's [use the infant's name] skin will feel cool. He will be very still and his eyes will be closed." They probably know this, but a gentle explanation demonstrates empathy. Explain that pooling of blood on the dependent areas will look like bruises.
3. Allow parents to hold, touch, and rock the infant if desired.	3. Viewing the infant allows parents a chance to say good-bye. Before bringing the infant to parents, wrap in a clean blanket, comb the hair, wash the face, swab the mouth clean, and apply Vaseline to lips.
4. Reinforce the physician's explanation about the need for an autopsy.	4. An autopsy is required for all unexplained deaths. You can say to parents, "It is the only way we can be sure of what caused your baby's death."
5. Answer parents' questions and provide them with sources for further information. Provide literature and a name of the local contact for a SIDS support group, as well as for the national foundation.	5. Parents may not be able to take in all of your answers. Many emergency departments and pediatric units have a social worker who provides ongoing contact with the family. Provide names of resource people and phone numbers for SIDS support groups.
6. Advise parents that surviving siblings may benefit from psychologic support.	6. Siblings often require emotional support in the weeks and months after the death. Social workers can help the family obtain counseling and support for all members.
7. Provide parents with a lock of hair, footprints, and handprints, if they desire.	7. Personal items can be placed in a memory book. This reaffirms the child's existence for many parents.

RESPIRATORY FAILURE

Respiratory failure occurs when the body can no longer maintain effective gas exchange. An inflammatory response and alveolar capillary damage lead to respiratory failure. Other body systems may also contribute directly or indirectly to an increased workload, causing the respiratory system to fail. The clinical manifestations of respiratory failure are signs of respiratory distress: **hypoxemia** (lower than normal blood oxygen level) and **hypercapnia** (an excess of carbon dioxide in the blood). Arterial blood gas levels indicative of respiratory failure are a PO_2 level less than 50 mm Hg and a PCO_2 level greater than 50 mm Hg. See Appendix **B** for expected laboratory values by age.

CLINICAL MANIFESTATIONS ~ *Respiratory Failure and Imminent Respiratory Arrest*

PHYSIOLOGIC CAUSE	CLINICAL MANIFESTATIONS
Respiratory failure These signs occur because the child is trying to compensate for oxygen deficit and airway blockage. Oxygen supply is inadequate; behavior and vital signs reflect compensation and beginning hypoxia.	*Initial signs* Restlessness Tachypnea Tachycardia Diaphoresis
The child tries to use accessory muscles to assist oxygen intake; hypoxia persists and efforts now waste more oxygen than is obtained.	*Early decompensation* Nasal flaring Retractions Grunting Wheezing Anxiety and irritability Mood changes Headache Hypertension Confusion
Imminent respiratory arrest These signs occur because oxygen deficit is overwhelming and beyond spontaneous recovery. Cerebral oxygenation is dramatically affected; central nervous system changes are ominous.	*Severe hypoxia* Dyspnea Bradycardia Cyanosis Stupor and coma

The physiologic process that ends in respiratory failure begins with **alveolar hypoventilation.** Alveolar hypoventilation occurs when any of these factors exist: (1) oxygen need exceeds actual oxygen intake, (2) the airway is partially occluded, or (3) the transfer of oxygen and carbon dioxide in the alveoli is disrupted. This disruption may occur either because of a malfunction of respiratory center stimulation (the alveoli do not receive the message to diffuse) or because the alveolar membrane is defective (a structural problem).

Alveolar hypoventilation results in hypoxemia and hypercapnia. When the blood levels of oxygen and carbon dioxide reach abnormal levels, **hypoxia** (lower than normal oxygen in the tissues) occurs and respiratory failure begins. Signs of impending respiratory failure include irritability, lethargy, cyanosis, and increased respiratory effort such as **dyspnea** (difficulty breathing), **tachypnea** (increased respiratory rate), nasal flaring, and intercostal retractions. Grunting slows the expiratory flow and increases the lung volume and alveolar pressures. This is a sign of severe disease and suggests the onset of respiratory failure (Margolis & Gadomski, 1998). Report any signs of respiratory failure immediately.

Nursing Management

Early recognition of impending respiratory failure is the most important aspect of care for a child with any signs of respiratory compromise. Immediately place a child who has even a slight degree of respiratory distress in an upright position (by elevating the head of the bed). Assess respiratory quality and rate, followed by apical pulse rate and temperature. Oxygen saturation and end-tidal CO_2 monitoring are also helpful. Keep oxygen administration equipment and respiratory emergency equipment at the child's bedside. Ensure that an order for oxygen is obtained or that oxygen is administered. Monitor the child for changes in vital signs, respiratory status, and level of responsiveness. Be prepared to assist ventilations if respiratory status deteriorates. (See Skills 9-8–9-14.) [SKILLS]

USING ARTIFICIAL AIRWAYS

Respiratory problems that do not respond to oxygen therapy, medications, or position changes require the insertion of an artificial airway. As the child's level of responsiveness deteriorates, the ability to keep the airway open decreases.

Thinking Critically

OXYGEN DELIVERY DEVICES

Oxygen delivery devices are selected to match the concentration of oxygen needed by the child. In respiratory failure, a higher concentration of oxygen is needed to reverse the hypoxemia. Which oxygen delivery device should be used? Are there any contraindications to oxygen use in a child who is hypoxic? [WEB]

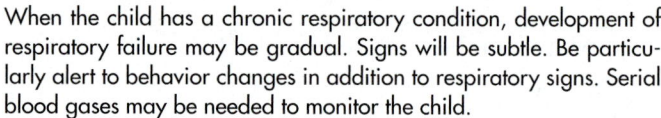 *Nursing Practice*

When the child has a chronic respiratory condition, development of respiratory failure may be gradual. Signs will be subtle. Be particularly alert to behavior changes in addition to respiratory signs. Serial blood gases may be needed to monitor the child.

Endotracheal intubation is a short-term, emergency measure to stabilize the airway by placing a tube in the trachea. The tube must be protected and stabilized to prevent its displacement. (See Skills 14-8 and 14-9.) [SKILLS] [CD] A tracheostomy is the creation of a surgical opening into the trachea through the anterior neck at the cricoid cartilage. Surgeons prefer to perform this procedure in the operating room; however, a tracheostomy may also be performed in an emergency department or other setting when immediate intervention is needed. These children usually require admission to the intensive care unit (ICU) for monitoring and ventilatory support.

Because endotracheal and tracheostomy tubes prevent vocal cord vibration, intubated children cannot cry or talk. Infants and young children often express initial frustration when they realize they cannot communicate verbally. They often develop other noise-making behaviors, such as striking the mattress to gain attention. When time permits, teach the parents and child what to expect before insertion of the endotracheal or tracheostomy tube. A communication board can be used with older children.

Many children are discharged from the hospital and cared for at home for an extended period with a tracheostomy tube in place. It is essential to teach parents how to maintain the airway, clean the tracheostomy site, and change the tube. A home health care nurse can provide follow-up care and support for the child and family. (See Skill 14-10.) [SKILLS]

REACTIVE AIRWAY DISORDERS

Reactive airway disorders occur when airway tissue reacts to invasion by a virus, bacterium, allergen, or irritant. These invaders cause airway tissue to respond with inflammation, edema, increased mucus production, and bronchospasm. Reactive airway disorders are reversible, usually self-limiting, and generally responsive to supportive therapies. They occur in either upper or lower airways and include croup syndromes, asthma, and bronchiolitis.

CROUP SYNDROMES

Croup is a term applied to a broad classification of upper airway illnesses that result from swelling of the epiglottis and larynx. The swelling usually extends into the trachea and bronchi. Included under the classification of croup syndromes are viral syndromes, such as spasmodic laryngitis (spasmodic croup), laryngotracheitis, and laryngotracheobronchitis (LTB), and bacterial syndromes, such as bacterial tracheitis and epiglottitis (see "Pathophysiology Illustrated: Airway Changes with Croup" and Table 42–4).

LTB, epiglottitis, and bacterial tracheitis are referred to as the "big three" of pediatric respiratory illness because they affect the greatest number of children across all age groups in both sexes. The initial symptoms of all three conditions include inspiratory **stridor** (a high-pitched, musical sound that is created by narrowing of the airway), a "seal-like" barking cough, and hoarseness. LTB is the most common disorder, but epiglottitis and bacterial tracheitis are more serious.

Laryngitis and laryngotracheitis are mild illnesses that can be managed at home. LTB is the most serious type of viral croup, frequently necessitating an emergency department visit for infants and children under 6 years of age.

Laryngotracheobronchitis

Although the term *croup* is applied to several viral and bacterial syndromes, it is most often used to refer to LTB, a viral invasion of the upper airway that extends throughout the larynx, trachea, and bronchi. Table 42–4 compares LTB and other croup syndromes.

ETIOLOGY AND PATHOPHYSIOLOGY

Acute viral LTB is most common in children 3 months to 4 years of age but can occur up to 8 years of age. Boys are affected more often than girls. LTB is of greatest concern

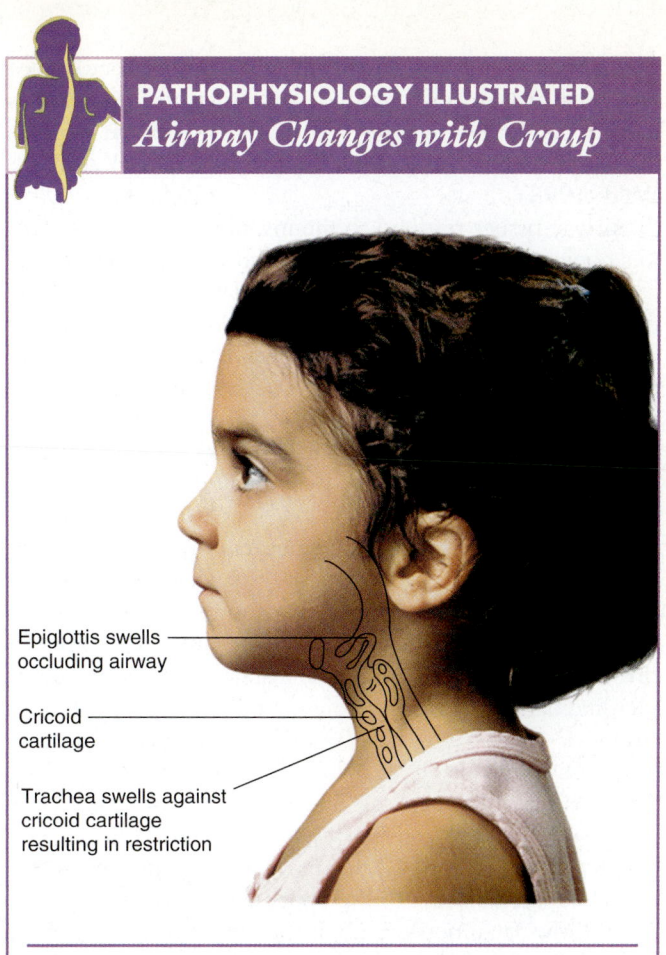

PATHOPHYSIOLOGY ILLUSTRATED
Airway Changes with Croup

Epiglottis swells occluding airway

Cricoid cartilage

Trachea swells against cricoid cartilage resulting in restriction

There are two important changes in the upper airway in croup: the epiglottis swells, thereby occluding the airway, and the trachea swells against the cricoid cartilage, causing restriction.

TABLE 42–4	Summary of Croup Syndromes				
	Viral Syndromes			*Bacterial Syndromes*	
	Acute Spasmodic Laryngitis (Spasmodic Croup)	*Laryngotracheitis*	*Laryngotracheobronchitis*	*Bacterial Tracheitis*	*Epiglottitis (Supraglottitis)*
Severity	Least serious	Most common[a]	Most serious; progresses if untreated	Guarded; requires close observation	Most life threatening (medical emergency)[a]
Age affected	3 months to 3 years	3 months to 8 years	3 months to 8 years	1 month to 13 years[a]	2 years to 8 years
Onset	Abrupt onset; peaks at night, resolves by morning (recurs)[a]	Gradual onset; starts as URI, progresses to moderate respiratory difficulty	Gradual onset; starts as URI, progresses to symptoms of respiratory distress	Progressive from URI (1–2 days)	Progresses rapidly (hours)[a]
Clinical manifestations	Afebrile; mild respiratory distress; barking-seal cough	*Early:* mild fever [<39 °C (102.2 °F)]; hoarseness; barking-seal, brassy, croupy cough; rhinorrhea; sore throat; stridor (inspiratory); apprehension *Progressing to* labored respirations	*Early:* mild fever [<39 °C (102.2 °F)]; barking-seal, brassy, croupy cough; rhinorrhea; sore throat; stridor (inspiratory); apprehension; restless/irritable *Progressing to* retractions (progressive); increasing stridor; cyanosis	High fever [>39 °C (102.2 °F)]; URI appears as viral croupy cough; croup initially; stridor (tracheal); purulent secretions	High fever [>39 °C (102.2 °F)]; URI; intense sore throat; dysphagia[a]; drooling[a]; increased pulse and respiratory rate; prefers upright position (tripod position with chin thrust)[a]
Etiology	Unknown; suspect viral with allergic/emotional influences	Parainfluenza, types I and II, RSV, or influenza	Parainfluenza, types I and II, RSV, or influenza	*Staphylococcus*	*Haemophilus influenzae*

[a]Classic parameter or key point (distinguishes condition).

in infants and children under the age of 6 years, because of potential airway obstruction. The causative organism is usually parainfluenza virus type I, II, or III, that appears during winter months in clustered outbreaks (Kaditis & Wald, 1998).

Airway tissues respond to the invading virus by producing copious, tenacious secretions and swelling, which increase the child's respiratory distress. The laryngeal inflammation causes the airway diameter to narrow in the subglottic area, the narrowest part of the airway. Even small amounts of mucus or edema can quickly obstruct the airway (see "Pathophysiology Illustrated: Airway Changes with Croup"). Both the large and small airways can be affected.

CLINICAL MANIFESTATIONS

Most children brought to the emergency department with LTB have been ill for a couple of days with upper respiratory symptoms. These symptoms progress to a cough and hoarseness. Fever may or may not be present. Common presenting signs are tachypnea, inspiratory stridor, and a seal-like barking cough.

CLINICAL THERAPY

Diagnosis is often made by clinical signs. Pulse oximetry is used to detect hypoxemia (see Skill 14-2). 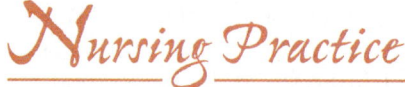 If the diagnosis of LTB is in question, anteroposterior (AP) and lateral x-rays of the upper airway are taken; these may show symmetric subglottic narrowing called a "steeple sign." Throat cultures and visual inspection of the inner mouth and throat are contraindicated in children with LTB and epiglottitis. These procedures can cause **laryngospasms** (spasmodic vibrations that close the larynx) as a result of the child's anxiety or of probing this reactive and already compromised area.

Medical management consists of maintaining and improving respiratory effort with humidification, medications, and supplemental oxygen when the saturated oxygen level is less than 92% (see Table 42–5).

Children with a good response to medications are often sent home from the emergency department after an obser-

vation period. Children with moderate to severe symptoms after medications are admitted for further observation and treatment. Airway obstruction is a potential complication of LTB. The child may require intubation and transfer to the ICU to maintain airway patency if obstruction is imminent. Most children, however, respond positively to the medications and oxygen therapy and are discharged within 48 to 72 hours.

Nursing Management

Nursing Assessment and Diagnosis

The initial and ongoing physical assessment of the child with LTB focuses on adequacy of respiratory functioning. Close monitoring is required to identify changes in airway patency. Continuously monitor the child in the emergency department observation area or the ICU. When the child's condition stabilizes, monitoring can be less frequent (Tables 42–6 and 42–7).

Nursing Practice

Observe the child continuously for inability to swallow, absence of voice sounds, increasing degree of respiratory distress, and acute onset of drooling (an ominous sign of supraglottic obstruction). If any of these signs occur, get medical assistance immediately. The quieter the child, the greater the cause for concern.

Pay particular attention to the child's respiratory effort, breath sounds, and responsiveness. Physical exhaustion can diminish the intensity of retractions and stridor. As the child uses the remaining energy reserve to maintain ventilation, breath sounds may actually diminish. Noisy breathing (audible airway congestion, coarse breath sounds) in this situation verifies adequate energy stores. Responsiveness decreases as hypoxemia increases.

TABLE 42–5	**Medications Used for Symptomatic Treatment of Laryngotracheobronchitis**	
Medication	*Action/Indication*	*Nursing Considerations*
Beta-agonists and beta-adrenergics (e.g., albuterol, racemic epinephrine): aerosolized through face mask	Rapid-acting bronchodilator, decreases bronchial and tracheal secretions and mucosal edema, used to decrease symptoms of moderate to severe respiratory distress; and constriction of subglottic mucosa and submucosal capillaries	Provides only temporary relief; improvement in 30 minutes which lasts about 2 hours, it gives time for the steroid to work; the child may experience tachycardia (160–200 beats/min) and hypertension; dizziness, headache, and nausea may necessitate stopping medication; reduces the need for artificial airway
Corticosteroids (e.g., dexamethasone): IM, PO, nebulized budesonide	Anti-inflammatory, used to decrease edema; has a long half-life of 36–54 hours	The child may experience cardiovascular symptoms (hypertension): requires close observation for individual response; children less frequently need emergency airways; stridor resolves faster

TABLE 42-6 Nursing Assessment of Child with a Reactive Airway Disorder

Nursing Action	Rationale
Assess heart rate and respiratory rate	Tachypnea and tachycardia indicate increasing respiratory effort
Check position of the child (sitting? prone? supine?)	Upright or semi-Fowler's promotes airway patency; the child's change to a more upright position may signal increased distress
Assess overall quality of respiratory effort: Determine inspiratory and expiratory breath sounds, ability to speak, and presence of stridor, cough, retractions, nasal flaring, cyanosis	Reflects overall adequacy of airway and respiratory function
Initiate croup score (Table 42–7) and continue scoring every 2–4 hours or more frequently if distress increases; initiate nursing actions appropriate for croup score	Provides consistent and objective assessment data with quantitative score for future comparison
Attach cardiorespiratory monitor and pulse oximeter	Provides continuous assessment data as part of ongoing physiologic monitoring

TABLE 42-7 Croup Scale to Identify the Severity of Croup

	Severity Score			
Signs	0	1	2	3
Stridor	None	Mild	Moderate at rest	Severe, on inspiration + expiration
Retractions	None	Mild	Suprasternal, intercostal	Severe, may see sternal retractions
Color	Normal	–	–	Dusky or cyanotic
Breath sounds	Normal	Mildly decreased	Moderately decreased	Markedly decreased
Level of consciousness	Normal	Restless when disturbed	Anxious, agitated	Lethargic

Scoring: To quantify the severity of croup, add up the individual scores for each of the sign categories. A score between 0 and 15 is possible. The rating of mild, moderate, and severe is as follows: 4–5 is mild, 6–8 is moderate, > 8 or any sign in the severe category is severe.

Note: From Davis, H. W., Gartner, J. C., Galvis, A. G., Michaels, R. H., & Mestad, P. H. (1981). Acute upper airway obstruction: Croup and epiglottitis. *Pediatric Clinics of North America, 28*(4), 859–880. Modified.

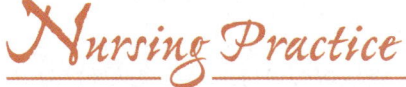

Nursing Practice

Infants and preverbal toddlers with laryngotracheobronchitis require constant supervision to monitor respiratory status. A means of communication (sign language or simple word cues) must be established so the older child can alert nursing staff to respiratory difficulty.

The following nursing diagnoses might be appropriate for the child with acute LTB:

▶ *Ineffective breathing pattern* related to tracheobronchial obstruction, decreased energy, and fatigue

▶ *Risk for fluid volume deficit* related to inadequate fluid intake prior to admission

▶ *Fear (child)* related to unfamiliar surroundings, procedures, and separation from support system

Planning and Implementation

Skillful nursing care can greatly help children with LTB and their families cope with the symptoms of the illness. Nursing care focuses on maintaining airway patency, promoting fluid balance, reducing stress, and teaching the family how to care for the child at home.

MAINTAIN AIRWAY PATENCY

Supplemental oxygen with humidity may be needed for hypoxemia. High-humidity mist tents are rarely used, as studies have not demonstrated any improvement in symptoms. Allow the child to assume a comfortable position. Be immediately available to attend to the child's respiratory needs. The child should be roomed near the nurses' station and emergency resuscitation equipment kept at the bedside.

MEET FLUID AND NUTRITIONAL NEEDS

The illness preceding the emergency department visit may have compromised the child's fluid status. Recognizing fluid deficit and monitoring the child's hydration and nutritional status are essential. Fluids promote liquification of secretions and provide calories for energy and metabolism.

Children with laryngotracheobronchitis usually prefer cool, noncarbonated, nonacidic drinks such as apple juice or fruit-flavored drinks. Remember that gelatin, ice, and fruit-flavored ice pops are also fluids. Oral rehydration fluids may also be used. Encourage parents to participate in gaining the child's cooperation in taking oral fluids. An intravenous infusion may be necessary to rehydrate the child, maintain fluid balance, or provide emergency access. Observe the child closely for difficulty in swallowing, which may be an early sign of epiglottitis or bacterial tracheitis.

During the child's observation period, take every opportunity to assess the parents' knowledge of symptoms of LTB and discuss actions to take if symptoms recur. For example, instruct parents to call the child's physician if:

▶ Mild symptoms do not improve after 1 hour of humidity and cool air treatment.

▶ The child's breathing is rapid and labored.

Evaluation

Expected outcomes of nursing care include:

▶ The child responds to medications with decreased respiratory distress.

▶ The child's fear and anxiety is managed with family support and explanations about care.

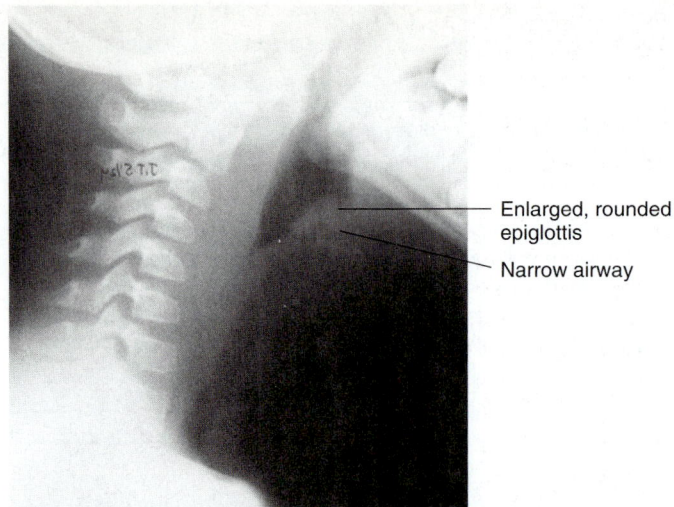

Enlarged, rounded epiglottis

Narrow airway

FIGURE 42–1. ◆ The phrase "thumb sign" has been used to describe this enlargement of the epiglottis. Recall the trachea's usual "little finger" size. Do you see the stiff, enlarged "thumb" above it in this lateral neck x-ray?

Epiglottitis (Supraglottitis)

Epiglottitis (also known as supraglottitis) is an inflammation of the epiglottis, the long narrow structure that closes off the glottis during swallowing (see "Pathophysiology Illustrated: Airway Changes with Croup"). Because edema in this area can rapidly (within minutes or hours) obstruct the airway by occluding the trachea, epiglottitis is considered a potentially life-threatening condition. (Table 42–4 compares epiglottitis and other croup syndromes.)

Epiglottitis is caused by bacterial invasion of the soft tissue of the larynx by streptococcus and staphylococcus, and by *Haemophilus influenzae* type B (Hib) in unimmunized children. The resulting inflammation and edema in the tissues and surrounding the epiglottis lead to airway obstruction. Fortunately, since Hib vaccination has become widespread, the number of cases of epiglottitis has decreased significantly.

Characteristically, a previously healthy child suddenly becomes very ill. The child initially develops a high fever (greater than 39 °C [102.2 °F]), with a sore throat, **dysphonia** (muffled, hoarse, or absent voice sounds), and **dysphagia** (difficulty in swallowing). As the larynx becomes obstructed, inspiratory stridor and respiratory distress develop. The child resists normal swallowing of saliva because of intense throat pain and swelling, resulting in drooling. To fully open the airway and improve air intake, the child sits up and leans forward with the jaw thrust forward in the classic "sniffing" or tripod posture and refuses to lie down.

Diagnosis is often based on a lateral neck x-ray (Figure 42–1), which reveals a narrowed airway and an enlarged, rounded epiglottis, seen as a mass at the base of the tongue. A blood culture may be taken after the child is stabilized. Laryngospasm and airway obstruction can occur as a result of the severe irritation and hypersensitivity of the airway muscles. For this reason, *visual inspection of the mouth and throat is contraindicated in children with suspected epiglottitis until immediate intubation or tracheostomy can be performed* (Eichelberger, Ball, Pratsch, et al., 1998).

Immediate clinical therapy usually involves insertion of an endotracheal tube to maintain the airway. Antibiotics effective for gram-positive organisms and *H. influenzae* are given until blood culture sensitivities are available. Antipyretics (acetaminophen, ibuprofen) may be useful in managing fever and sore throat pain.

NURSING MANAGEMENT

Nursing management consists of airway management, drug therapy, hydration, and emotional and psychosocial support of the child and parents. Until the endotracheal tube is removed, the child is usually managed in the ICU to ensure continual observation. (See Skills 14-1 and 14-10.) SKILLS

Until the child is intubated, allow the child to sit upright or to assume a comfortable position to maintain the airway and breathe more easily. Supplemental humidified oxygen may be used initially to reverse hypoxemia. Observe the child's respiratory and airway status closely and often. Provide a quiet environment with as little stress as possible to decrease anxiety and crying. Crying stimulates the airway, increases oxygen consumption, and can precipitate laryngospasm; the calmer the child, the better the respiratory function (Eichelberger et al., 1998).

Administer antibiotics to treat the infection and provide fluids to provide hydration. Because the child was febrile with a sore throat before admission, fluid intake may have been compromised.

The loss of voice, or even the inability to create sounds, can be frightening to a child. The unfamiliar hospital environment and strange equipment can create stress for child and parent alike. Reassure the parents that the child's voice loss is temporary and explain the need for the various pieces of equipment.

Most children show rapid improvement once cool mist and oxygen, antibiotics, and fluid therapy are started. The endotracheal tube can usually be removed within 24 to 36 hours (Hazinski, 1999). Home care may involve completing the course of antibiotics. Parents need instructions on proper administration and potential problems of drug therapy.

Bacterial Tracheitis

Bacterial tracheitis is a secondary infection of the upper trachea after viral laryngotracheitis that is most often caused by group A streptococcus or *Haemophilus influenzae*. The disorder starts with croupy cough and stridor but progresses to include a high fever (greater than 39 °C [102.2 °F]), which persists for several days (Bank & Krug, 1995). (Table 42–4 compares bacterial tracheitis and other croup syndromes.)

Because of the similarity of symptoms, bacterial tracheitis is often misdiagnosed initially as LTB. Instead of improving with therapy, however, the child's condition becomes worse. Children generally prefer lying flat to sitting up. This seems to be a position of comfort that allows the child to conserve energy. Diagnosis is often made by blood cultures after the child is found unresponsive to usual LTB management. Antibiotics are given for a full 10-day course. Most children need a secured artificial airway and ventilatory support.

NURSING MANAGEMENT

Nursing management involves the following:

- Careful airway assessment and support
- Airway maintenance (artificial airway assistance is often required because of the thick tracheal secretions that pool high in the upper airway)
- Suctioning as needed (mechanical suction enables easier removal of secretions and helps maintain a patent airway)
- Administration of humidified oxygen
- Administration of antibiotics
- Preparation for resuscitation

The earlier section on epiglottitis discusses other nursing care interventions that may also be appropriate for the child with bacterial tracheitis.

ASTHMA

Asthma (also called bronchial asthma) is a chronic inflammatory disorder of the airway with airway obstruction that can be partially or completely reversed, and increased airway responsiveness to stimuli (Kieckhefer & Ratcliffe, 2000). It affects about 5 million children in the United States. Affected children have about 10 days of school absenteeism and 20 days of restricted activity per year (Sydnor-Greenberg & Dokken, 2000). Most children with asthma experience their first symptoms before the age of 5 years. Asthma occurs more frequently in boys than girls until the teen years, when the incidence equalizes (Kieckhefer & Ratcliffe, 2000). WEB

Passive smoke exposure (secondhand smoke) contributes significantly to the development of respiratory problems in children. It has been linked specifically to an increase in asthma symptoms, emergency department visits, and hospital admissions in children of parents who smoke. It is believed to be responsible for thousands of new cases of asthma in children each year. In addition, children exposed to tobacco smoke in utero have a higher rate of asthma. The increased number of women smokers may be contributing to the increased rates of asthma (Gilliland, YU-Fen, & Peters, 2001).

Asthma is a chronic condition with acute exacerbations or persistent symptoms. Children require continuous coordinated care to control sudden symptoms and minimize long-term airway changes. Although unusual in the past, severe persistent asthma is more common now. Mortality from asthma in children rose 31% between 1980 and 1987, and continues to rise (National Asthma Education and Prevention Program, 1997). How does this chronic condition pose a threat to children?

Etiology and Pathophysiology

The respiratory difficulties of an asthma attack result from inflammation that contributes to airway obstruction (Richman, 1997). The inflammation causes the normal protective mechanisms of the lungs (mucus formation, mucosal swelling, and airway muscle contraction) to react excessively in response to a stimulus.

The stimulus, more correctly termed a **trigger,** that initiates an asthmatic episode can be inflammatory or noninflammatory. Triggers increase the frequency and severity of smooth muscle contraction, and airway responsiveness is enhanced through inflammatory mechanisms. During the acute reaction, an antigen binds to the specific immunoglobulin E surface on the mast cell, and histamine is released along with intercellular chemical mediators, resulting in bronchospasm. Inflammation peaks in 12 to 24 hours (Kieckhefer & Ratcliffe, 2000). Asthmatic triggers include exercise, viral or bacterial agents, allergens (mold, dust, or pollen), food additives, pollutants, weather changes (humidity and temperature), and emotions. The reactive airway responses to stimuli are present *before* the trigger initiates the physiologic sequence that results in an asthma attack.

Airway narrowing results from airway swelling and production of copious amounts of mucus. Mucus clogs small airways, trapping air below the plugs (see "Pathophysiology Illustrated: Asthma"). The airways swell, creating muscle spasms that often become uncontrolled in the large airways. With time, repeated episodes of bronchospasm,

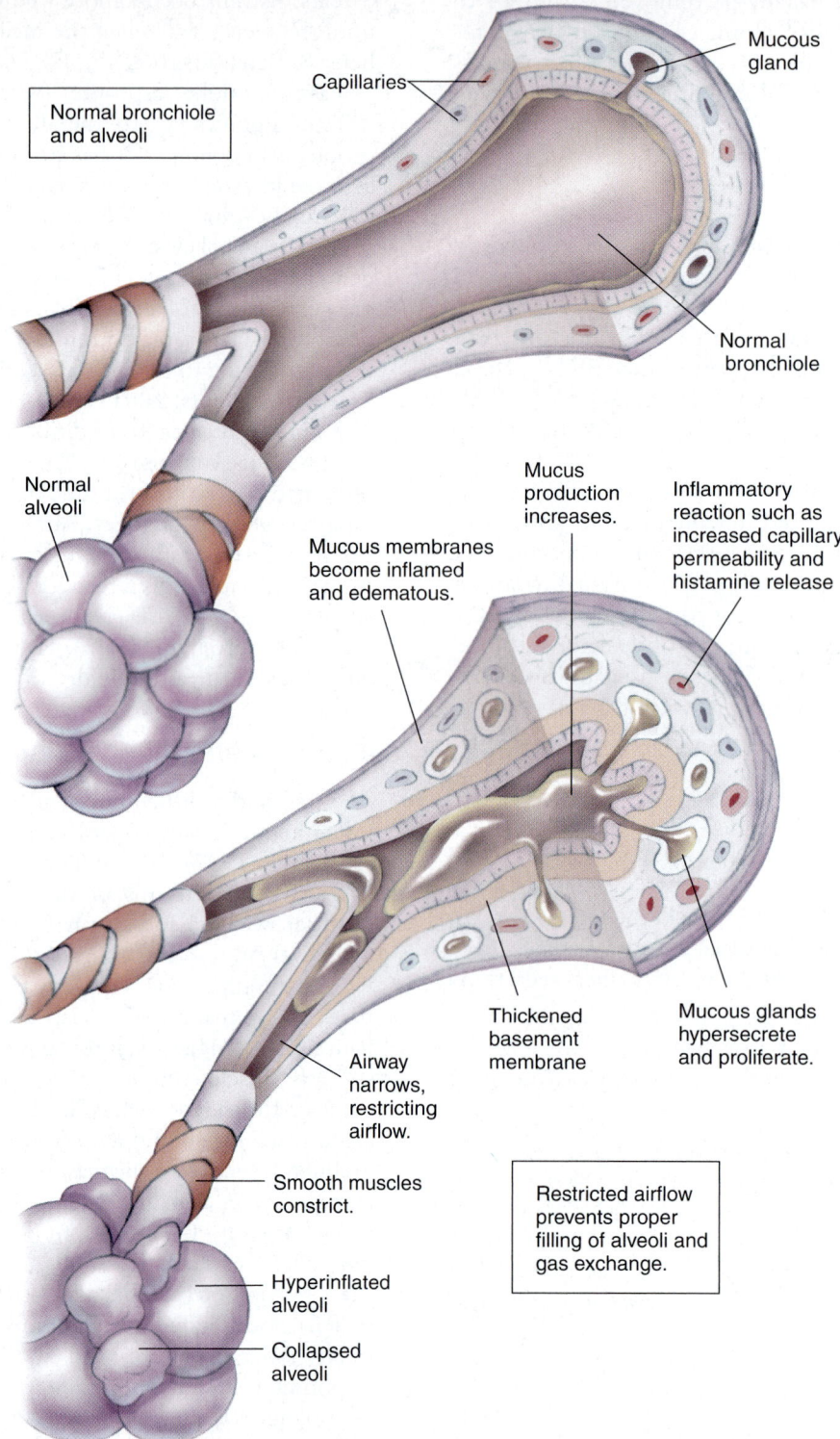

Normal bronchiole and alveoli

Capillaries

Mucous gland

Normal bronchiole

Normal alveoli

Mucous membranes become inflamed and edematous.

Mucus production increases.

Inflammatory reaction such as increased capillary permeability and histamine release

Thickened basement membrane

Mucous glands hypersecrete and proliferate.

Airway narrows, restricting airflow.

Smooth muscles constrict.

Restricted airflow prevents proper filling of alveoli and gas exchange.

Hyperinflated alveoli

Collapsed alveoli

Some asthma triggers are exercise, infection, and allergies. Shown is how asthma obstructs airflow through constriction and narrowing of the airway, along with increased production of mucus.

mucosal edema, and mucus plugging can damage the respiratory cells that line the airway. This process leaves the airway chronically irritated and scarred and results in air trapping, called hyperinflation.

The psychologic sequence of events during an asthmatic episode starts with moderate anxiety as the episode begins. The anxiety becomes severe as the episode intensifies. Severe anxiety, in turn, intensifies physical responses and symptoms, and a vicious cycle is established. Recognizing and addressing the child's fear and panic are essential for reestablishing normal respirations.

Clinical Manifestations

Asthma is characterized by airway inflammation, airway obstruction or narrowing, and airway hyperreactivity. The sudden appearance of breathing difficulty is often referred to as an asthma "attack" or "episode." The infant or child who has had episodes of frequent coughing or frequent respiratory infections (especially pneumonia or bronchitis) should also be evaluated for asthma. The cough is the warning signal that the child's airway is very sensitive to stimuli; it may be the only sign in "silent" asthma.

During an acute attack, respirations are rapid and labored and the child often appears tired because of the ongoing exertion of breathing. Nasal flaring and intercostal retractions may be visible. The child exhibits a productive cough and expiratory wheezing, use of accessory muscles, decreased air movement, and respiratory fatigue. The resulting hypoxia, as well as the cumulative effect of previously administered medications, contributes to behaviors ranging from wide-eyed agitation to lethargic irritability.

In children who have repeated acute exacerbations, a barrel chest and the use of accessory muscles of respiration are common findings (see "Pathophysiology Illustrated: Barrel Chest," p. 1047).

Clinical Therapy

The diagnosis of asthma has four key elements: symptoms of episodic airflow obstruction; partial reversibility of bronchospasm with bronchodilator treatment; exclusion of alternate diagnosis; and confirmation by spirometry of measurement of peak expiratory flow variability (see Skill 14-5). **SKILLS** **CD** A spirometer measures the forced expiration of air within 25 to 75 seconds to assess the severity of airway obstruction. Because the test requires children to cooperate and follow instructions, it is usually administered to children over 4 or 5 years of age. Findings determine the extent of airway restriction and assist in selecting the appropriate treatment. (See Tables 42–8 and 42–9.) Skin testing may be used to identify allergens (asthma triggers).

Medical management includes medications, support of parents and child, and education. Pharmacologic treatment attempts to promote optimal respiratory function. Anti-inflammatory medications should begin early in the course

TABLE 42–8 Assessing Peak Expiratory Flow Rate (PEFR)

Zone	PEFR (Best or Predicted for Age)	Action
Green	80%–100%	Continue regular management plan.
Yellow	50%–80%	Implement action plan provided by physician.
Red	< 50%	**Medical Alert:** Implement action plan predetermined by physician. Call provider if PEFR does not return to yellow or green zone.

The child's personal best is determined after reviewing the recorded PEFRs measured two to four times a day for 2 to 3 weeks. The child should be optimally treated with medications during the day so the best reading is obtained (Richman, 1997).

TABLE 42–9 Revised Asthma Severity Classification

Classification (Steps)	Description	Clinical Therapy
Step 1: Mild intermittent	Brief exacerbations with symptoms no more often than twice a week. Nighttime symptoms less than twice a week. PEFR ≥ 80% of predicted with variability < 20%.	Quick relief bronchodilator as needed. If needed more than twice a week, move to next level.
Step 2: Mild persistent	Exacerbations more than twice a week, but less than once a day. May affect activity. PEFR ≥ 80% of predicted.	Daily anti-inflammatory medication. Quick relief bronchodilator as needed.
Step 3: Moderate persistent	Daily symptoms. Daily use of inhaled short-acting beta-agonist. Exacerbations at least twice a week that may last for days; nighttime symptoms more than once per week. Affects activity. PEFR > 60% but < 80% of predicted with variability > 30%.	Daily anti-inflammatory medication, medium dose. Bronchodilator as needed up to three times a day.
Step 4: Severe persistent	Continuous symptoms, limited physical activity. Frequent exacerbations and frequent nighttime symptoms. PEFR ≤ 60% of predicted with variability > 30%.	Daily anti-inflammatory medication, high dose. Systemic corticosteroid. Bronchodilator as needed for symptoms up to three times a day.

Note: From National Asthma Education and Prevention Program. (1997). Expert Panel Report II: Guidelines for the diagnosis and management of asthma (NIH Publication No. 97–4051, pp. 45–48). Bethesda, MD: National Institutes of Health.

TABLE 42-10 Medications Used to Treat Asthma

Medication	Action/Indication	Nursing Considerations
Bronchodilators Beta$_2$-agonists (short-acting and long-acting) Albuterol, metaproterenal, terbutaline, or salmeterol: SQ, PO, aerosol Methylxanthines Theophylline (related to caffeine): PO	Relax smooth muscle in airway, resulting in rapid bronchodilation within 5–10 minutes; drugs of choice for acute or daily therapy (inhaled route); used for nocturnal symptoms and exercise-induced bronchospasm. Relax muscle bundles that constrict airways; dilate airway; provide continuous airway relaxation; sustained release for prevention of nocturnal symptoms.	Have some side effects (tachycardia, nervousness, nausea and vomiting, headaches), but these are usually dose-related; repetitive or excessive use can mask increasing airway inflammation and hyperresponsiveness. Used later in the treatment course for moderate to severe symptoms. Used for long-term control, so continuous administration needed; works best when a specific amount is maintained in the bloodstream (therapeutic serum level, 10–20 µg/L); requires serum level checks and dose adjustment; have many and varied side effects (including tachycardia, dysrhythmias, restlessness, tremors, seizures, insomnia, hypotension, severe headaches, vomiting, and diarrhea).
Anti-inflammatory Agents Cromolyn sodium: aerosol only Nedocromil: aerosol only Corticosteroids: IV, PO, or aerosol Beclomethasone, triamcinolone, prednisone	Preventive medications, best taken daily to stop chemicals associated with producing asthma; controls seasonal, allergic, and exercise-induced asthma; may be used for unavoidable allergen exposure. Effectively reduce mucosal edema in airways; usually combined with other asthma medications for prompt control.	Less effective in older children; prophylactic medications, once wheezing starts, these medications are ineffective. Short courses of IV corticosteroids used to gain control and speed resolution of moderate to severe asthma. Side effects (such as abnormalities in glucose metabolism, increased appetite, fluid retention, weight gain, moon face, mood alteration, and hypertension) may be severe if used long term; if used daily, lowest therapeutic dose should be given; growth suppression possible with long-term use.
Leukotriene Modifiers Montelukast: PO	Steroid-sparing adjunct for exercise-induced asthma to prevent bronchospasm. Alternate therapy to low doses of inhaled corticosteroids. Improves pulmonary function, but less well than corticosteroids; enhances effect of corticosteroids and may permit lowering of dosage.	Increased risk of diarrhea, laryngitis, pharyngitis, nausea, otitis, sinusitis, give at bedtime once a day, easier for compliance. Infrequent adverse effects of mild headache and gastrointestinal disturbances.
Other Hyposensitization (allergy shots), SQ	Series of injections that can reduce sensitivity to unavoidable allergens (e.g., environmental organisms—mold, pollen); gradual dose increase over time (called a "buildup") increases the child's tolerance to allergic substances; has been of help in some children.	Use is controversial; some question about actual effect.

to prevent irreversible changes in the asthmatic airway (Steinbach, 2000) (see Table 42–10). See "Clinical Pathway: Stages of Inpatient Care for Children with Severe Asthma."

In children as young as 4 to 5 years, a peak expiratory flow meter can assist in the management of asthma by helping to identify when obstruction occurs (Kieckhefer & Ratcliffe, 2000). This device measures the child's ability to push air forcefully out of the lungs. Medication administration can be based on peak expiratory flow rate (PEFR) readings and the effectiveness of treatment confirmed by improved PEFR numbers.

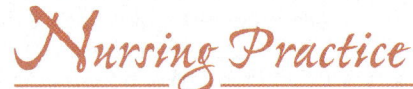

Spacers with valves are often used with metered dose inhalers (MDI) for children who cannot coordinate inspiration with medication release. The spacer captures the aerosol released by the MDI in a reservoir for the child to breathe in over a couple of minutes. This provides a benefit similar to nebulizer treatment, but it takes less time and is less expensive (Steinbach, 2000).

Category	Continuous Nebulizer Treatments	Frequent Nebulizer Treatments	Transition to Discharge, Nebulizer Treatmentss every 4–6 hr
Outcomes	Patient will: • Evidence stabilization of vital signs. • Exhibit patent airway; experience resolution of acute respiratory distress. • Verbalize understanding and demonstrate cooperation with respiratory therapy. • Have oral intake equal to fluid maintenance needs. • Demonstrate proficiency with peak flow meter. Family verbalizes feelings about illness. Family displays effective coping. Family understands plan of care for hospitalization. Family verbalizes beginning understanding of asthma and ongoing care and treatments.	Patient will: • Evidence stable vital signs and be afebrile. • Exhibit unlabored respirations and patent airway. • Tolerate full diet. • Tolerate age-appropriate activity without evidence of respiratory distress, weakness, or exhaustion. • Have moist mucous membranes. • Verbalize understanding and demonstrate cooperation with respiratory therapy. Family exhibits effective coping mechanisms.	Patient is afebrile with stable vital signs. Patient exhibits a patent airway and unlabored respirations with activity. Patient's respiratory rate and status has returned to baseline. Patient tolerates activity without evidence of respiratory distress, weakness, or exhaustion. Patient's mucous membranes are moist. Family verbalizes/demonstrates home care instructions, including strategies to reduce exposure to infectious illnesses and respiratory irritants. Family exhibits willingness to make lifestyle changes and cope with effects of chronic illness. Family demonstrates/verbalizes ability to cope with ongoing stressors. Family verbalizes beginning understanding of home care instruction including trigger agents, signs and symptoms of impending attack, and appropriate actions.
Assessments	Vital signs q 1–2 hr and prn. Continuous O_2 saturation monitoring. Cardiorespiratory monitoring while on continuous nebulizer treatments. Potassium level 12 hr after on continuous nebulizer treatments, then q 12 hr. Assess respiratory status q 1–2 hr and prn. Monitor carefully for changes in respiratory rate, skin color, retractions, and/or flaring. Strict intake and output. Urine specific gravity q 8hr. Humidification as ordered. Position patient in semi-Fowler's or high Fowler's position. Oxygen as ordered to maintain O_2 saturation ≥ 95%. Provide quiet, restful environment. Assess cognitive/developmental level.	Vital signs q 4 hr and prn. Assess respiratory status q 4 hr and prn. Monitor carefully for changes in respiratory rate, skin color, retractions, and/or flaring. Discontinue cardiorespiratory monitor. Strict intake and output. Urine specific gravity q 8hr. Humidification as ordered. Position patient in semi-Fowler's or high Fowler's position. Continue O_2 saturation while on oxygen. Wean oxygen, keeping O_2 saturation at ≥ 92%. Provide quiet, restful environment.	Vital signs q 8 hr and prn. O_2 saturation q 4 hr if patient is on oxygen. Continue weaning oxygen if O_2 saturation ≥ 92%. Assess respiratory status q 8 hr and prn. Monitor carefully for changes in respiratory rate, skin color, retractions, and/or flaring. Provide quiet, restful environment.
Knowledge	Initiate teaching regarding ongoing care, including procedures, treatments, and medications. Initiate patient and family teaching about asthma, its treatments, peak flow meter use, trigger agents, avoidance of respiratory infections and irritants, and early signs and symptoms of infections. Evaluate understanding of teaching. Provide information at developmental/cognitive level.	Reinforce earlier teaching about ongoing care. Reinforce teaching about asthma and treatments. Renew detailed teaching with family and patient about home care including medications, respiratory therapy, activity, trigger agents, avoidance of respiratory infections and irritants, early signs and symptoms of impending attack, and follow-up care. Evaluate understanding of teaching.	Reinforce earlier teaching about ongoing care. Complete discharge teaching to include diet, follow-up care, signs and symptoms to report, follow-up physician visit, activity, and medications: name, purpose, dose, frequency, route, dietary interactions, and side effects. Provide family/patient with written discharge instructions. Refer unmet teaching needs to outpatient services. Evaluate understanding of teaching. Refer knowledge deficits to community resources.

(continued)

Category	Continuous Nebulizer Treatments	Frequent Nebulizer Treatments	Transition to Discharge, Nebulizer Treatmentss every 4–6 hr
Psychosocial	Orient patient to setting. Provide age-appropriate communication and support. Encourage verbalization of concerns. Encourage family to participate in care. Reassure patient and family of ongoing surveillance of patient status and responses to therapy.	Provide age-appropriate communication and support. Encourage verbalization of concerns. Encourage family to participate in care. Reassure patient and family of ongoing surveillance of patient status and responses to therapy.	Provide age-appropriate communication and support. Encourage verbalization of concerns. Provide ongoing support and encouragement to family.
Diet	Clear liquids as tolerated. Avoid cold fluids and foods. Encourage fluid intake.	Age-appropriate diet as tolerated, providing small, frequent, nutritious feedings. Avoid cold fluids and foods. Encourage fluid intake.	Age-appropriate diet as tolerated, providing small, frequent, nutritious feedings. Avoid cold fluids and foods. Encourage fluid intake.
Activity	Assess safety needs and provide adequate precautions. Encourage age- and status-appropriate diversional activities. Balance activity with planned rest periods.	Maintain safety precautions. Balance activity with planned rest periods. Increase activity as tolerated. Encourage age- and status-appropriate diversional activities.	Maintain safety precautions. Balance activity with planned rest periods. Encourage age- and status-appropriate diversional activities. Activity as tolerated.
Medications	IV fluids only if unable to take oral fluids to equal maintenance. Oral steroids as ordered. Ipratropium as ordered. Continuous albuterol nebulizer treatments until respiratory distress decreases. Give oral potassium if K level is less than 3.5. Tylenol as ordered for temperature over 38.3 °C (101 °F).	Oral steroids as ordered. Albuterol nebulizer treatments q 2 hr. Tylenol as ordered for temperature over 38.3 °C (101 °F).	Oral steroids as ordered. Albuterol nebulizer treatment q 4–6 hr. Start or restart home therapy. Observe patient for reaction to new medications, if applicable. Patient sent home with inhaler.
Transfer/ discharge plans	Continue to review progress toward discharge goals. Review discharge plans.	Continue to review progress toward discharge goals. Determine need for home respiratory therapy and outpatient teaching for breathing exercises. Finalize discharge plans. Make appropriate referrals.	Finalize plans for home care if needed. Make appropriate referrals. Complete discharge teaching.

Most children with acute exacerbations respond to aggressive management in the emergency department. Children who do not respond or who are already being managed at home on corticosteroids have a greater chance of being admitted. Some children need mechanical ventilation. Support of the parents and child should focus on helping them to cope with and understand the diagnosis and the need for daily management to promote near-normal respiratory function while the child continues to grow and develop normally.

Nursing Management

Nursing Assessment and Diagnosis

The nurse usually encounters the child and family in the emergency department or nursing unit. In these settings, acute care has become necessary because the child's level of respiratory compromise cannot be managed at home. What needs to be done first? What is the nurse's role during an acute asthmatic episode?

PHYSIOLOGIC ASSESSMENT

Identify the child's current respiratory status first by assessing the airway, breathing, and circulation (see "Clinical Manifestations of Asthma in Children by Severity of Acute Exacerbations" on page 1042). If the child is moving air or talking, assess the quality of breathing. Is the child wheezing? Is stridor present? Are retractions visible (see "Pathophysiology Illustrated: Retraction Sites" on p. 1025)? ▭ What is the respiratory rate? What is the quality of breath sounds? Observe the child's color and assess the heart rate. Obtain oxygen saturation via pulse oximeter. Only move on to other symptoms after finding

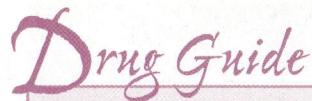

Drug Guide

ALBUTEROL

Overview of Action A synthetic sympathomimetic amine that appears to act on β-adrenergic receptors, resulting in bronchodilation; it seems to have greatest effect on bronchial, uterine, and vascular muscles. Used for relief of reversible obstructive bronchospasms of asthma, bronchitis, and cystic fibrosis.

Routes, Dosage, Frequency
Oral

- **2 to 6 years:** Initial: 0.1 mg/kg/day in divided doses (syrup) (maximum dosage 2 mg 3 times daily); if child fails to respond, gradually increase 0.2 mg/kg/day in 3 divided doses (maximum dosage 4 mg 3 times per day)
- **6 to 14 years:** 2 mg 3 to 4 times per day (may be increased to maximum of 24 mg/day cautiously, in stepwise increments)
- **Over 14 years:** 2 to 4 mg 3 to 4 times per day; extended-release tablets: 4 to 8 mg every 12 hours

Inhalation: Oral inhalation for relief of acute bronchospasms or prevention of asthma symptoms

- **Over 4 years:** 1 to 2 inhalations (90 μg/inhalation) every 4 to 6 hours. If second inhalation is prescribed, manufacturer recommends 1 minute elapse between inhalations; however, some clinicians believe 10 to 20 minutes should elapse before second inhalation.

Inhalation capsules via Rotahaler: for exercise-induced bronchospasms

- **Over 4 years:** 200 μg via oral inhaler 15 minutes before exercise

Nebulizer: Manufacturer does not recommend use of nebulization in those under 12 years; however, some clinicians recommend:

- **Under 5 years:** 1.25 to 2.5 mg every 4 to 6 hours as necessary
- **Over 5 years:** 2.5 to 5 mg every 4 to 6 hours as necessary
- **Over 12 years:** 2.5 mg 3 to 4 times a day

Contraindications: Hypersensitivity to drug or its ingredients. Use cautiously in children with diabetes mellitus, hypertension, hyperthyroidism, cardiovascular disorders.

Side Effects: Excitement, nervousness, hyperactivity, tremors, dizziness, tachycardia, palpitations, hypertension or hypotension, peripheral vasodilation, irritation of nose and throat.

Nursing Implications

Assessment: Assess the respiratory status and obtain baseline pulse. **Administer: For oral:** Plain tablets can be crushed and mixed with small amounts of food or fluids. Do not crush coated tablets. Side effects are more common with oral form. **Inhalation:** Shake container well. If second inhalation is prescribed, manufacturer recommends that 1 minute elapse between doses. **Nebulizer:** Follow agency policy for operation of IPPB apparatus. Follow package insert directions for solution dilution. If solution is discolored, do not use. Do not remove nebulization capsules from the original package until just prior to use.

Monitor: Monitor pulse (cardiovascular effects may occur), respiratory response to medication. Maintain hydration for weight. Do not use other sympathomimetic agents with this drug; it increases risk of cardiovascular symptoms. If long-term therapy has been prescribed, periodically monitor serum potassium.

Patient teaching: Teach the proper use and care of the inhaler. Have child demonstrate inhaler use. Emphasize that inhaler should not be used more frequently than prescribed, and to contact physician if symptoms worsen.

Note: From Bindler, R. M., & Howry, L. B. (1997). *Pediatric drugs and nursing implications* (2nd ed.). Upper Saddle River, NJ: Prentice Hall-Health. Adapted.

---

no life-threatening respiratory distress. Assess PEFR, skin turgor, intake and output, and specific gravity. Because asthma can be a symptom of another illness, perform a head-to-toe assessment to identify other associated problems (Tables 42–1 and 42–6). (See Skills 9-1–9-21.)

SKILLS CD

PSYCHOSOCIAL ASSESSMENT

Is the child anxious? Crying? (See Table 42–11.) In an older child whose asthma was previously diagnosed, have the asthmatic episode and hospitalization created guilt about doing something the child thinks he or she should have avoided or about forgetting to take medication? Look for clues to hidden stress and self-blaming.

Common nursing diagnoses for the child experiencing an acute asthmatic episode include the following:

▶ *Ineffective airway clearance* related to airway compromise, copious mucus secretions, and coughing

TABLE 42–11 Psychosocial Assessment of the Child with an Acute Respiratory Illness

Child

- Assess for indications of anxiety or fear that may have an impact on respiratory status.
- For young children, ask about security objects (such as a blanket or doll), the child's reaction to strangers, and reaction to absence of parents.
- For older children, ask whether this is the first hospital stay and what previous illness and hospital experiences have meant to the child.

Parents

- Assess parents' reactions: Are they anxious? Fearful? Verbal or quiet? Asking appropriate questions?
- Observe for nonverbal cues. Often parents have financial worries (cost of hospital stay, lost work and wages) and personal worries (siblings at home who are ill) that they may not readily share with staff.

ASSESSMENT CRITERIA	MILD	MODERATE	SEVERE
PEFR[a]	70%–90% predicted or personal best	50%–70% predicted or personal best	< 50% predicted or personal best
Respiratory rate, resting or sleeping	Normal to 30% increase above the mean	30%–50% increase above mean	Increase over 50% above mean
Alertness	Normal	Normal	May be decreased
Dyspnea[b]	Absent or mild; speaks in complete sentences	Moderate; speaks in phrases or partial sentences; infant's cry softer and shorter; has difficulty sucking and feeding	Severe; speaks only in single words or short phrases; infant's cry softer and shorter; stops sucking and feeding
Pulsus paradoxus[c]	< 10 mm Hg	10–20 mm Hg	20–40 mm Hg
Accessory muscle use	No intercostal to mild retractions	Moderate intercostal retractions with tracheosternal retractions; use of sternocleidomastoid muscles; chest hyperinflation	Severe intercostal retractions, tracheosternal retractions with nasal flaring during inspiration; chest hyperinflation
Color	Good	Pale	Possibly cyanotic
Auscultation	End-expiratory wheeze only	Wheeze during entire expiration and inspiration	Breath sounds becoming inaudible
Oxygen saturation	> 95%	90%–95%	< 90%
PCO$_2$	< 35	< 40	> 40

Note: Within each category, the presence of several parameters, but not necessarily all, indicates the general classification of the exacerbation.
[a]For children 5 years of age or older.
[b]Parents' or physicians' impression of degree of children's breathlessness.
[c]Pulsus paradoxus does not correlate with phase of respiration in small children.
Note: From National Asthma Education and Prevention Program. (1994). *Acute exacerbations of asthma: Care in a hospital-based emergency department* (p. 13). Bethesda, MD: National Heart, Lung, and Blood Institute, National Institutes of Health.

▶ *Impaired gas exchange* related to airway obstruction, possible additional respiratory illness, and poor response to medication

▶ *Anxiety/fear (child or parents)* related to change in health status, difficulty breathing

▶ *Ineffective management of therapeutic regimen (family)* related to acute and daily medical management of chronic disease

Planning and Implementation

Pharmacologic and supportive therapies are used to reverse the airway obstruction and promote respiratory function. Nursing interventions center on maintaining airway patency, meeting fluid needs, promoting rest and stress reduction for the child and parents, supporting the family's participation in care, and giving the family information that lets them manage the child's acute asthmatic episodes and ongoing needs.

MAINTAIN AIRWAY PATENCY

If the child is exhibiting breathing difficulty, supplemental oxygen is required. Oxygen is best administered by nasal cannula or face mask. Humidified oxygen should be used to prevent drying and thickening of mucus secretions. Place the child in a sitting (semi-Fowler's) or upright position to promote and ease respiratory effort. Evaluate the effectiveness of positioning and oxygen administration by transcutaneous oxygen monitoring (pulse oximeter) and by observing for improved respiratory status. (See Skill 14-1.) 🔗 **SKILLS**

The respiratory distress and need for supplemental oxygen can be stressful for parents and child alike (Figure 42–2 ◆). Encouraging the parents' presence can be reassuring for the child. Keep the parents informed of proce-

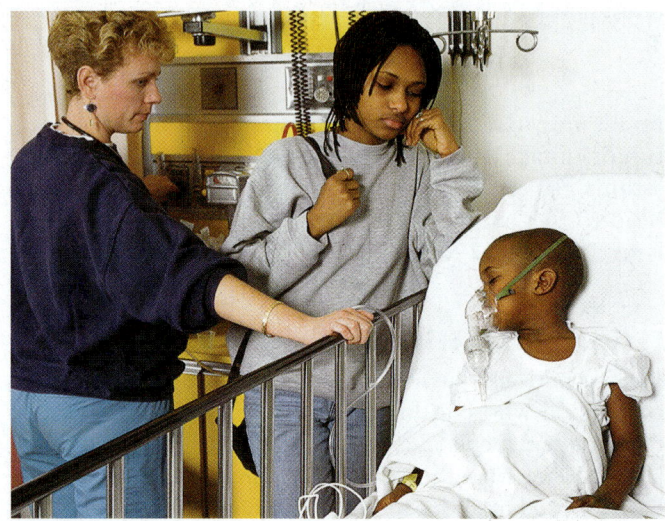

FIGURE 42–2. ◆ Acute exacerbations of asthma may require management in the emergency department. The child is placed in a semisitting position to facilitate respiratory effort. Providing support to both the child and parent is an important part of nursing care during these acute episodes. This mother is exhausted after a sleepless night of caring for her son.

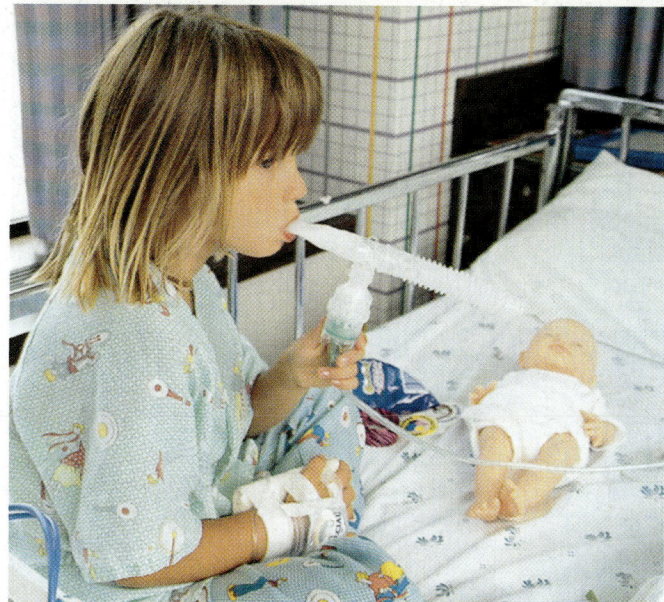

FIGURE 42–3. ◆ Medications given by aerosol therapy allow children the freedom to play and entertain themselves.

dures and results, and get their input when developing the treatment plan.

Many medications are given by the aerosol route (Figure 42–3 ◆). The advantages of aerosol are that the medication acts quickly, enabling the pulmonary blood vessels to absorb the inhaled medication, systemic effects are minimized, and the inhaled droplets provide the added benefit of moisture. Because the medication is quickly absorbed, continuous aerosol treatments may be implemented. Monitor the child for side effects. The frequency of vital sign assessment is related to the severity of symptoms. (See Skill 11-10.) ⊂⊃ SKILLS

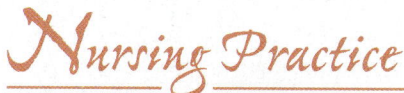

Nursing Practice

To help toddlers learn to use a peak flow meter, have them practice by blowing into party favors (i.e., noisemakers). To teach the use of a metered-dose inhaler, let the child learn to breathe in slowly with straws.

MEET FLUID NEEDS

Fluid therapy is often necessary to restore and maintain adequate fluid balance. Adequate hydration is essential to thin and break up trapped mucus plugs in the narrowed airways. An adequate oral intake may not be possible with the child's compromised respiratory status. An intravenous infusion may be needed, and this route also may be used for administering medications and providing glucose. Overhydration must be avoided to prevent pulmonary edema in severe asthma attacks.

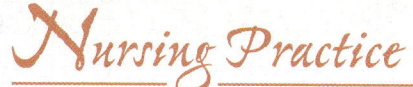
Nursing Practice

Iced beverages precipitate bronchospasms in some children with asthma. It is safest to offer the asthmatic child room temperature or slightly cooled fluids without ice.

As respiratory difficulty diminishes, offer oral fluids slowly. Monitor intake and output and assess specific gravity frequently to evaluate the child's hydration status. Involving parents in feeding can help gain the child's cooperation in taking oral fluids. Determine the child's fluid preferences and give choices where possible.

PROMOTE REST AND STRESS REDUCTION

The child who has had an acute asthmatic episode is usually very tired when admitted to the nursing unit. Labored breathing and low oxygen status have left the child exhausted. Put the child in a quiet, private room if possible, to promote relaxation and rest. Avoid repeatedly disturbing the child by grouping tasks.

SUPPORT FAMILY PARTICIPATION

The parents may stay with the child, but may be exhausted after hours of their child's respiratory distress. Give parents the option of assisting with the child's treatments, rather than expecting them to do it in addition to comforting the child. Provide frequent updates about the child's condition and encourage the parents to take breaks as needed.

Length of hospitalization depends on the child's response to therapy. Any underlying or accompanying health problem, such as preexisting lung disease or pneumonia, can complicate and extend the child's hospital stay. Communicate with the family of the hospitalized child at least once a day about the child's condition.

DISCHARGE PLANNING AND HOME CARE TEACHING

Parents need a thorough understanding of asthma—how to prevent attacks and treatment to maintain the child's health and avoid unnecessary hospitalization. When possible, educate parents when they are rested. Provide a written treatment plan about how to manage asthma on a daily basis and in a crisis (see Skill 11-11). ⊂⊃ SKILLS CD *Pediatric Asthma: Promoting Best Practice* is a good resource for families available from the American Academy of Asthma, Allergy, and Immunology. ⊂⊃ WEB Through printed educational materials and referral to a local support group, parents gain additional knowledge and confidence that enable them to help their child lead a normal life (National Asthma Education and Prevention Program, 1997) (Figure 42–4 ◆). Special summer camps for asthmatic children are available.

Discharge planning for the asthmatic child focuses on increasing the family's knowledge about the disease,

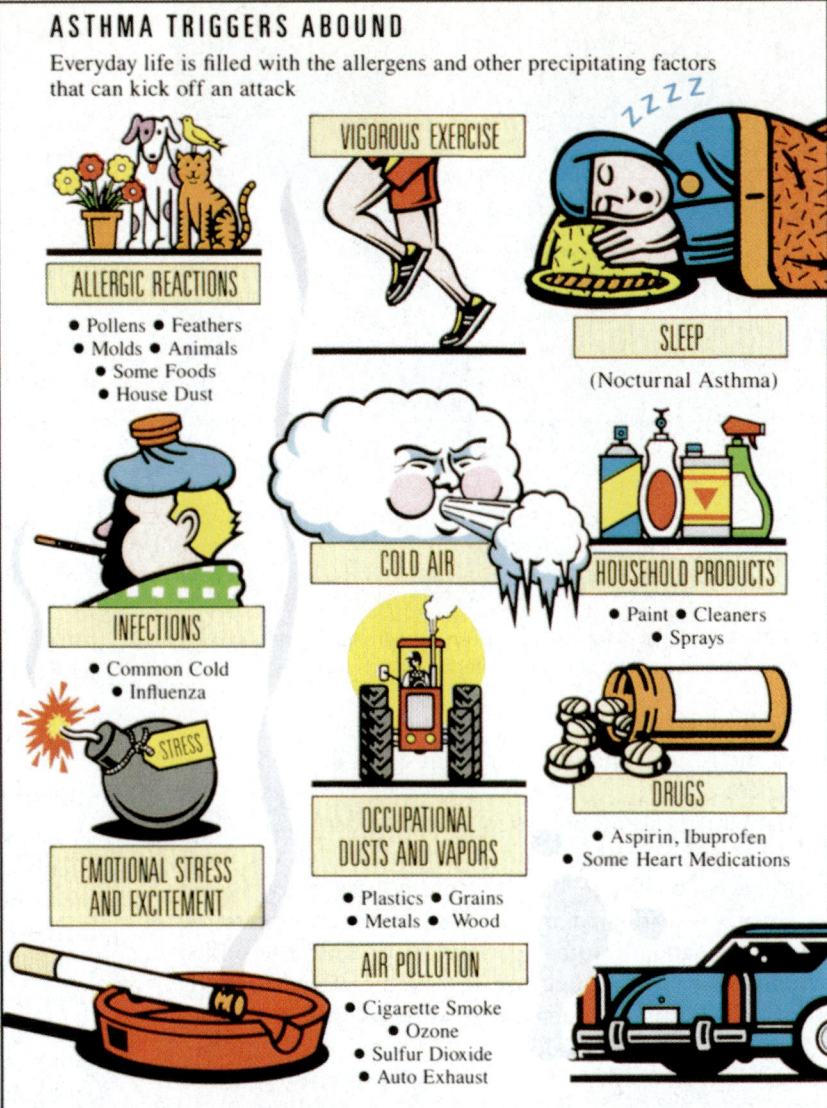

ASTHMA TRIGGERS ABOUND

Everyday life is filled with the allergens and other precipitating factors that can kick off an attack

VIGOROUS EXERCISE

SLEEP
(Nocturnal Asthma)

ALLERGIC REACTIONS
- Pollens • Feathers
- Molds • Animals
- Some Foods
- House Dust

COLD AIR

HOUSEHOLD PRODUCTS
- Paint • Cleaners
- Sprays

INFECTIONS
- Common Cold
- Influenza

STRESS

DRUGS
- Aspirin, Ibuprofen
- Some Heart Medications

EMOTIONAL STRESS AND EXCITEMENT

OCCUPATIONAL DUSTS AND VAPORS
- Plastics • Grains
- Metals • Wood

AIR POLLUTION
- Cigarette Smoke
- Ozone
- Sulfur Dioxide
- Auto Exhaust

FIGURE 42–4. ◆ This educational piece from the American Lung Association explains what triggers an asthma attack. The required lifestyle changes for the child and family will be significant, so be sensitive to the family's situation and needs. Culture sometimes plays a significant part in exposure to lifestyle triggers. Note: Reprinted with permission. © 2002 American Lung Association. For more information on how you can support to fight lung disease, the third leading cause of death in the U.S., please contact The American Lung Association at 1-800-LUNG-USA or log on to the website at www.lungusa.com.

medication therapy, and the need for follow-up care according to guidelines of the National Asthma Education and Prevention Program. The required lifestyle changes may be difficult for the child and parents. The need to modify the home by removing a loved pet, for example, may create stress. The nurse can play a role in keeping lines of communication open and can facilitate discussion and clarification of ways to prevent asthmatic episodes. Teach the family how to measure peak expiratory flow and necessary medications to manage asthma attacks early on. Reassure the family that most children with asthma can lead a normal life with some modifications.

NURSING CARE IN THE COMMUNITY

Nurses provide care to children with asthma in pediatricians' offices, specialty asthma clinics, schools, and summer camps. Once the stress of the acute episode has passed, opportunities exist to provide more extensive education (Figure 42–5 ◆).

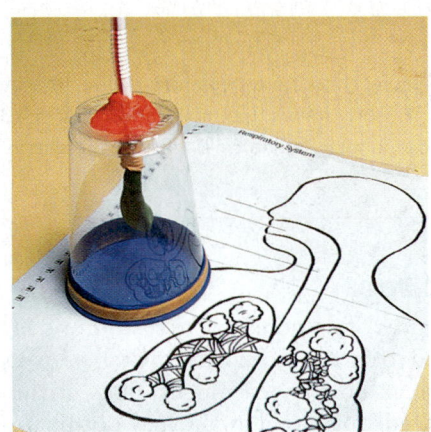

FIGURE 42–5. ◆ School-age children can be taught how the lung functions using simple activities such as this project, in which a "lung" is made using a plastic cup, a straw, and balloons. This activity illustrates how the lung takes in air, expanding and contracting during breathing.

TABLE 42–12	Markers of Good Asthma Control

- Prevents chronic and troublesome symptoms of cough, wheeze, difficulty breathing and chest tightness
- Maintains normal or near-normal pulmonary function
- Maintains normal activity levels including physical exercise
- Prevents recurrent exacerbations and minimizes the need for urgent care or hospitalization
- Provides optimal pharmacotherapy with minimal or no adverse effects
- Meets patient's and family's expectations of asthma care and maintains their satisfaction with care.

Note: From the National Asthma Education and Prevention Program (1997).

If the child has severe asthma and uses high doses of aerosol or oral glucocorticoids to control asthma attacks, monitor the child's growth every 6 months as the disease and medications may affect overall growth. Review the family's daily plan for monitoring the child's respiratory status. Evaluate the child's technique for PEFR and the parent's ability to identify the timing and type of stepped-up care needed to manage worsening symptoms. The goal is to bring asthma attacks under control with stepped-up care before a significant episode occurs. This can be achieved only with daily monitoring (Table 42–12).

Environmental control is an important part of asthma management. When possible, pets should not be kept in the home (and never in the child's bedroom). Cockroaches and dust mites should be eliminated or controlled. Smoke from cigarettes, wood stoves, and fireplaces all have the potential to trigger an asthma attack.

Help the child learn the signs of early respiratory distress so that treatment can be obtained before signs get more serious. Parents should communicate with school personnel regarding the child's condition, and have an individual school health plan developed to ensure that medications are given as needed, even in preparation for exercise. Make sure the child has a supply of medications at school or child care as well as at home. For a young school-age child, make sure the child's teacher can help recognize respiratory distress and reduce the child's fear of going to the nurse for rescue medications.

Refer to "Nursing Care Plan: The Child with Asthma in the Community Setting" in Chapter 35 for additional information.

Teaching About

HOME CARE INSTRUCTIONS FOR THE CHILD WITH ASTHMA

Identify parents' knowledge about the condition:

1. Review why asthma occurs and assess parents' understanding of the physiologic process. Ask:
   - Do you understand what happens in your child's lungs during an asthma attack?
   - Do you know the early warning signs of an asthma episode in your child?
   - What are your child's symptoms and how does he or she respond to them? Does your child use the peak expiratory flow meter to evaluate symptoms?
2. Identify asthma triggers and assess parents' understanding of how to prevent, avoid, or minimize their effect in a timely manner. Ask:
   - Do you know your child's personal asthma triggers? (Suggest that the parents and child keep a notebook to track episodes so they can learn more about these triggers.)
   - What steps can you take to minimize or eliminate your child's exposure (quitting smoking, environmental control, etc.)?

Set up a schedule for parents to learn asthma management. Ask:

- Do you know when and where to seek emergency medical help?
- What actions can you take before seeking medical assistance?

Review parents' understanding of medication therapy:

- Provide information about medications: name, type of drug, dose, method of administration, expected effect, possible side effects.
- Evaluate the child's technique for the use of an inhaler and peak flow meter.

Address associated issues:

- Do parents know how to store and properly transport medications?
- What are the financial considerations of medication cost and lifestyle changes?
- Has the child's school or teacher been notified? What arrangements have been made for the child's use of medications at school?
- Has a medical identification bracelet or medallion been obtained for the child to facilitate assistance when away from home?

Identify need for follow-up care:

- Do parents know when to see a physician? When drug levels need to be checked?
- Does child need to see an allergist?
- Do the child or parents have special emotional needs?
- Would a self-help group or camp experience be helpful for the child?

Evaluation

Expected outcomes of nursing care include:

▶ The child recognizes asthma symptoms and uses rescue medications before severe respiratory distress occurs.

▶ The child and family implement a daily treatment plan for asthma and reduce the number of asthma attacks the child has.

▶ The child with a serious asthma attack responds to oxygen, fluids, and medication therapy, avoiding hospital admission.

STATUS ASTHMATICUS

Status asthmaticus is unrelenting, severe respiratory distress and bronchospasm in an asthmatic child, which persists despite pharmacologic and supportive interventions. Without immediate intervention the child with status asthmaticus may die. The child is placed in an ICU and may require endotracheal intubation with assisted ventilation. The section on respiratory failure earlier in the chapter gives additional information on the nurse's role in providing emergency respiratory care.

 LOWER AIRWAY DISORDERS

The lower airway, or bronchial tree, lies below the trachea and includes the bronchi, bronchioles, and alveoli. Lower airway disorders occur because a structural or functional problem interferes with the lungs' ability to complete the respiratory cycle. Lower airway disorders include neonatal respiratory distress syndrome, bronchopulmonary dysplasia, bronchitis, bronchiolitis, pneumonia, tuberculosis, and cystic fibrosis.

BRONCHOPULMONARY DYSPLASIA

Bronchopulmonary dysplasia (BPD) is the most chronic and serious respiratory disorder that begins during infancy. The infant has an acute lung injury in which an abnormal radiograph is found and oxygen is required at 36 weeks' postconceptional age. Premature infants are affected more often than full-term infants, and morbidity is greater in

Complementary Care

ALTERNATIVES IN TREATING CHILDREN WITH ASTHMA

Complementary and alternative therapies, especially herbal remedies, are used worldwide to treat asthma; many have been shown to be effective. Herbal remedies (including dietary supplements and botanicals) have the least amount of studies to support their use in children. However, other therapies such as lifestyle therapies and mind-body therapies have been shown to be effective in children (Kemper & Lester, 1999).

"Self-Regulating Therapies": Relaxation, Self-Hypnosis, Breathing Exercises, and Guided Imagery: Since asthma is an inflammatory process and involves the autonomic nervous system, an emotional component to asthma symptoms has been recognized. Anxiety from triggers or from the symptoms of asthma may exacerbate the condition.

Over the last 20 years there have been numerous studies regarding the use of "self-regulating" therapies for asthma. They have shown to help with decreasing medication use, decreasing health care visits, improving pulmonary function, and improving quality of life. Self-hypnosis, relaxation, breathing exercises, and guided imagery in children have all been successful in decreasing medication use, improving pulmonary function, and improving a sense of well-being in children with asthma (Anbar, 2001; Kohen and Wynne, 1997; Vedanthan, Kesavalu, Murthy, et al., 1998).

Massage Therapy: Another traditional therapy that has been studied in children is massage. Children whose parents gave them a nightly massage at bedtime had improved pulmonary function. It is not known whether long-term benefits would result from chronic or intermittent massage, but this is a safe modality that can be recommended to all families with children with asthma (Field, Henteleff, Hernandez-Reif, et al., 1998).

Exercise: Although exercise is a frequent trigger of asthma symptoms in the majority of patients, the benefits of routine exercise on asthma symptoms have been documented in both children and adults (Markowitz, 2000; Milgrom & Taussig, 1999; van Veldhoven, Vermeer, Bogaard, et al., 2001). There is no real benefit of one type of exercise over another, although swimming has been routinely recommended (Stricker, 2000). The improvement in cardiovascular fitness along with self-esteem are added benefits that come from routine exercise.

Dietary Therapies: The use of diet in treating asthma is common and many families think that "allergies" to certain foods play a significant role in their child's illness. There are few studies in children to show the benefit of a nondairy diet or elimination of particular grains or food groups. However, there is more data to support that being obese in itself leads to an increase in asthma problems in childhood; weight reduction improves asthma symptoms. Epidemiologic studies in adults have also demonstrated less asthma in populations that have a more vegetarian diet, a diet with fewer polyunsaturated fats (vegetable oils), and a diet rich in omega-3 fatty acids (especially fish oils such as sardines, herring, and mackerel). Lycopene, a natural antioxidant in vegetables such as tomatoes, has been found to reduce exercise-induced asthma (Neuman, Nahum, & Ben-Amotz 2000). These are recommendations that may, in addition to conventional medications (and their proper use) and environmental control, be demonstrated to improve a child's asthma so that less school is missed, sleep disruption is reduced, and lung function is improved.

males than in females. The incidence is increasing due to advances in medical technology that permit very-low-birth-weight infants to survive (Daigle & Cloutier, 1997).

BPD is a direct result of the treatment provided to premature and term infants with such conditions as RDS, congenital heart disease, meconium aspiration, patent ductus arteriosus, and fluid overload and edema in newborns (see Chapter 28). The sequence of events is an immature lung leading to respiratory failure requiring mechanical ventilation resulting in barotrauma, oxygen toxicity, inflammation, cellular damage, and death. Fibrosis and edema of the bronchioles along with smooth muscle hypertrophy follows (Harvey, 2000). Potential long-term outcomes of BPD include developmental delays, growth retardation, continuing airway obstruction, and persistent airway hyperactivity.

The infant with BPD has persistent signs of respiratory distress: tachypnea, wheezing, crackles, irritability, nasal flaring, grunting, retractions, pulmonary edema, and failure to thrive. Cyanosis may be seen in severe cases. Normal activities, such as feeding, can create increased oxygen demands that are difficult for the compromised infant to meet.

The chest x-ray is the best indicator of lung changes and is the key to medical diagnosis. There may be cystic changes or fine lacy densities with or without hyperinflation (Harvey, 2000). The air trapping persists and in time causes the chest to assume a barrel shape (see "Pathophysiology Illustrated: Barrel Chest"). Medical management focuses on symptomatic treatment that supports respiratory function

TABLE 42–13	Medications Used to Treat Bronchopulmonary Dysplasia
Medication	Action/Indication
Bronchodilators (beta2-adrenergics, anticholinergics, theophylline, albuterol nebulizer)	Decreases airway resistance; increases expiratory flow in small airways; stimulates mucous clearance; different drugs work together for best response
Anti-inflammatory agents (corticosteroids, inhaled cromolyn, becholmethasone)	Reduces pulmonary edema and inflammation in small airways; enhances effect of bronchodilators; helps decrease the need for other drugs and oxygen; for moderate disease only
Diuretics (furosemide, chlorothiazide, spironolactone)	Helps remove excess fluid from lungs; decreases pulmonary resistance and increases pulmonary compliance; may cause electrolyte imbalances
Potassium chloride	Prevents electrolyte imbalances associated with diuretics
Antibiotics	Low-dose prophylactic therapy to prevent severe illness; specific treatment for identified organisms
RSV immune globulin	Prevents respiratory syncytial virus

and on good nutrition, which helps to accelerate lung maturity. Supplemental oxygen with humidity is used to keep the SaO_2 more than 90% to 92% even during sleep and feeding. Chest physiotherapy and medications (diuretics, bronchodilators, anti-inflammatories, and inhaled corticosteroids) are also used (see Table 42–13). With improvement and adequate weight gain, the child is weaned off of oxygen, diuretics, and bronchodilators. Long-term sequelae include asthma and respiratory infections with frequent rehospitalization rates.

Nursing Management

Nursing management focuses on promoting respiratory function and preparing the family for home care needs. Nursing assessment includes close monitoring of respirations, pulse, color, behavior changes, and vital signs. The infant with chronic BPD may become acutely ill at any time.

Thinking Critically

INFANT WITH BPD

Emily, an 8-month-old infant with bronchopulmonary dysplasia, is cared for at home by her mother. She has a tracheostomy and receives humidification. Emily has frequent infections and episodes of respiratory distress that require hospitalization. When she develops a fever, more secretions than usual collect in the trachea. Suctioning is needed to ease Emily's breathing. What signs indicate that Emily needs to be suctioned? How do you select the correctly sized suction catheter? How do you suction Emily without causing hypoxia? When is it necessary to change Emily's tracheostomy tube? WEB

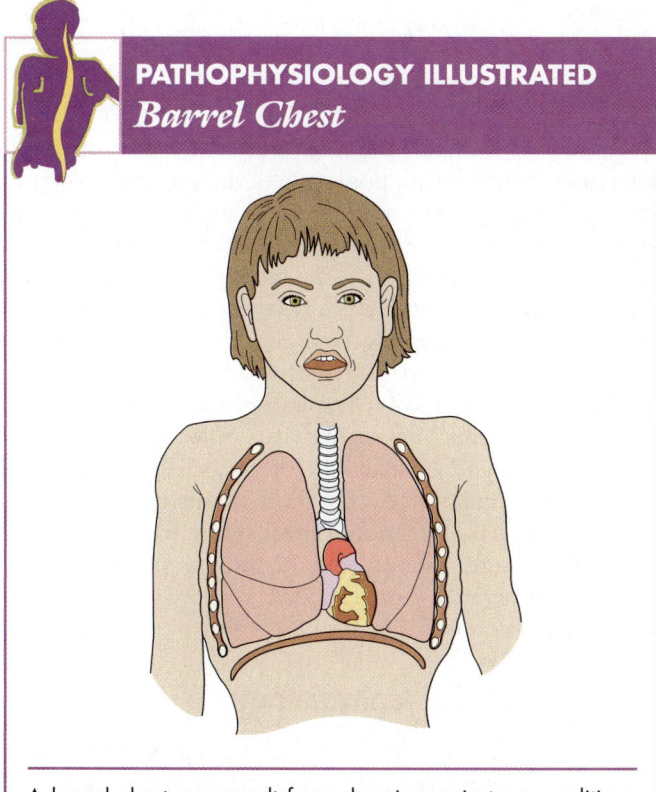

PATHOPHYSIOLOGY ILLUSTRATED
Barrel Chest

A barrel chest may result from chronic respiratory conditions such as bronchopulmonary dysplasia or asthma, in which air trapping or hyperinflation of the alveoli occur.

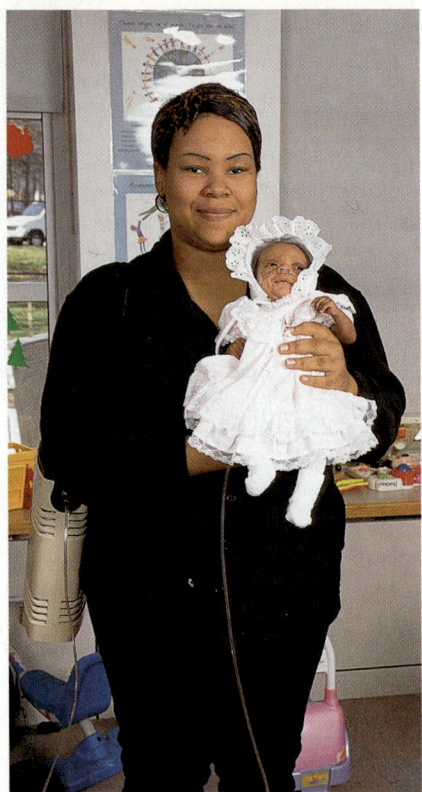

FIGURE 42–6. ◆ Many children with BPD are cared for at home, with the support of a home care program to monitor the family's ability to provide airway management, oxygen, and ventilator support. This premature infant girl, who is now 4 months old but weighs only about 5 pounds, requires respiratory support, which is provided by a portable oxygen tank.

Once home, many infants need ventilation therapy, oxygen respiratory support, and drug therapy (Figure 42–6 ◆). Frequent rehospitalization may be necessary because, although the lungs may function adequately, they remain vulnerable throughout childhood to common respiratory illnesses. Infants with BPD do not have the same respiratory reserve as healthy infants, and they can become very ill very quickly. Nutritional requirements to support growth must be balanced with fluid restrictions. A formula supplemented with carbohydrates and medium chain triglycerides may be given to promote weight gain. Some children need nasogastric or gastrostomy tube feedings to get adequate nutrition when cyanosis is noted with feeding. Electrolytes must be monitored monthly.

It is important to provide for the infant's normal development through rest, nutrition, stimulation, and family support. Including parents in the infant's care early on promotes bonding and prepares them for home care responsibilities. Some families require home nursing assistance. Carefully plan and coordinate referrals for needed respiratory supplies, medications, an early intervention program, and follow-up care well in advance of the infant's discharge date. ◯▭ WEB

BRONCHITIS

Acute bronchitis, inflammation of the trachea and bronchi, rarely occurs in childhood as an isolated problem. The bronchi can be affected simultaneously with adjacent respiratory structures during a respiratory illness. Bronchitis occurs most often in children under 4 years of age, usually following a mild upper respiratory tract problem (D'Auria, 1997). Bronchitis is caused most often by a virus but may also result from invasion of bacteria or in response to an allergen or irritant.

The classic symptom of bronchitis is a coarse, hacking cough, which increases in severity at night. Children with bronchitis look tired and report that they feel awful. The chest and ribs may be sore because of the deep and frequent coughing. There is often a deep, rattling quality to breathing. Some children have audible wheezing that can be heard without a stethoscope. Treatment is palliative unless a secondary bacterial infection occurs.

Nursing Management

Nursing management includes supporting respiratory function through rest, humidification, hydration, and symptomatic treatment. Refer to the sections on asthma and pneumonia for detailed information on treatment measures.

Home care should emphasize the self-limiting nature of the disorder. Advise parents who smoke that quitting or refraining from smoking in the child's presence may benefit the child.

BRONCHIOLITIS

Bronchiolitis is one of the most frequent causes of hospitalization in infants and poses one of the greatest threats to the respiratory system of infants and small children (Webster & Huether, 1998). Although some infants and children have mild symptoms easily managed at home, others become acutely ill with severe respiratory distress that can become a life-threatening emergency. What makes bronchiolitis such a potential threat?

Bronchiolitis is a lower respiratory tract illness that occurs when an infecting agent (virus or bacterium) causes inflammation and obstruction of the small airways, the bronchioles. Infection occurs most frequently in toddlers and preschoolers. Infection is most severe in infants under 6 months of age. Infants under 2 months of age are particularly vulnerable, and they are routinely hospitalized when bronchiolitis is diagnosed.

Etiology and Pathophysiology

Viral, bacterial, and mycoplasmal organisms may cause bronchiolitis; however, infection with respiratory syncytial virus (RSV) is the most common cause.

RSV occurs in annual epidemics from October to March. Nearly all children have been infected with RSV by

2 years of age, and reinfection (via siblings or close family contacts) throughout life is common (National Respiratory and Enteric Virus Surveillance System, 2000). RSV is transmitted through direct or close contact with respiratory secretions of infected individuals. Viruses, acting as parasites, are able to invade the mucosal cells that line the small bronchi and bronchioles. The invaded cells die when the virus bursts from inside the cell to invade adjacent cells. The resulting cell debris clogs and obstructs the bronchioles and irritates the airway. In response, the airway lining swells and produces excessive mucus. Despite this protective effort by the bronchioles, the actual effect is partial airway obstruction and bronchospasms.

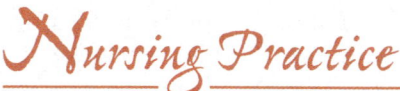

Respiratory syncytial virus (RSV) is the most common cause of lower respiratory tract infections in infants and children. RSV causes severe or fatal illness in infants with conditions such as congenital heart disease, bronchopulmonary dysplasia (BPD), prematurity, and immunosuppression. Health care workers should follow principles of good handwashing, as the virus is easily transmitted and can survive on the hands for 1 hour.

The cycle is repeated throughout both lungs as the airway cells are invaded by the virus. The partially obstructed airways allow air in, but the mucus and airway swelling block expulsion of the air. This creates the wheezing and crackles in the airways. Air trapped below the obstruction also interferes with normal gas exchange. The child with RSV is therefore at risk for respiratory failure as the oxygen level decreases and the carbon dioxide level increases. Apnea and pulmonary edema may occur.

As the airflow continues to decrease, breath sounds diminish. Thus the noisier the lungs, the better, as this indicates that the child is still able to move air in and out of the lungs.

Clinical Manifestations

The infant or child with bronchiolitis may have been ill with upper respiratory symptoms such as nasal stuffiness, cough (not usually noted in infants), and fever (less than 39 °C [102.2 °F]) for a few days. As the illness progresses and the lower respiratory tract becomes involved, symptoms increase and include wheezing, a deeper, more frequent cough, and more labored breathing. Respirations are rapid, shallow, and accompanied by nasal flaring and retractions (signs of severe distress). Parents report that the infant or child is acting more ill—appearing sicker, less playful, and less interested in eating. Infants, especially, may refuse to feed or may spit up what they do eat along with thick, clear mucus.

Clinical Therapy

The history and physical examination provide the data needed to diagnose bronchiolitis. Chest x-rays show nonspecific findings of inflammation.

Viral cultures or antigen testing of an immunofluorescent stain of respiratory secretions obtained by either a nasal swab in special culture medium or a nasopharyngeal wash confirm the presence of RSV (see Skills 10-13 and 10-14). SKILLS Children who test positive for RSV are isolated, roomed together, or placed on the same ward to minimize the spread of the virus to other hospitalized children. Medical management is frequently supportive, especially when the causative agent is unknown and the condition is mild to moderate in severity (Table 42–14). The child may be intubated and ventilated for apnea or respiratory failure.

TABLE 42-14   Clinical Therapy for Bronchiolitis

Clinical Therapy	Rationale
Cardiorespiratory monitor and pulse oximetry	Enable provider to follow course and assess need for specific therapies.
Humidified oxygen therapy via hood or face tent, tent, or nasal cannula	Delivery method determined by desired concentration of oxygen, degree of moisture, and child's response.
Intubation and assisted ventilation	Used when the child becomes too fatigued to breathe effectively.
Hydration via intravenous or oral fluids	Provider must consider insensible fluid loss, decreased intake, the child's current electrolyte and hydration status, and risk for pulmonary edema.
Aerosol medications	Bronchodilators, steroids, and beta-antagonists act directly on inflamed and obstructed airways; bronchodilators help prevent apnea episodes in premature infants; ribavirin (RSV antiviral agent) reduces the severity of the illness, improves oxygenation, and decreases inflammatory injury.
Pulmonary hygiene (postural drainage and chest physiotherapy)	Helps to further loosen trapped mucus.
Systemic medications	Symptomatic treatment may include antipyretics (acetaminophen or ibuprofen preferred; no antibiotics are given unless evidence of secondary bacterial infection [e.g., otitis media] is present).
High-Risk Infant or Child[a]	
RespiGam (RSV immune globulin) IV	Give for 5 consecutive months during RSV season to high-risk children. May prevent RSV bronchiolitis.
Palivizumab IM	Both are very expensive, but less than hospitalization.

[a]Defined as a child with congenital heart disease, bronchopulmonary dysplasia, chronic lung problems, or cystic fibrosis or who is premature or severely ill and less than 6 weeks old.

Ribavirin is the only antiviral drug available for treatment. Studies have not confirmed its effectiveness, so it is reserved for life-threatening cases (Margo & Shaughnessy, 1998).

There is evidence that bronchiolitis in infancy may increase the chances of childhood wheezing and asthma. It also may be a major risk factor for chronic obstructive pulmonary disease later in life (Webster & Huether, 1998).

Nursing Management

Nursing Assessment and Diagnosis

PHYSIOLOGIC ASSESSMENT

Assess airway and respiratory function carefully. Good observation skills are important to ensure timely interventions for worsening respiratory symptoms and prevention of respiratory distress (see Table 42–1 and "Clinical Manifestations" on page 1029). A decreased oxygen saturation level is the best indicator of the severity of the disease. See the Nursing Care Plan: The Child with Bronchiolitis on the Companion Website. WEB

PSYCHOSOCIAL ASSESSMENT

Observe children and their parents for signs of fear and anxiety (see Table 42–11). The unfamiliar hospital environment and procedures can increase stress. Parents' questions, as well as their nonverbal cues, help direct nursing interventions during admission and throughout hospitalization.

DEVELOPMENTAL ASSESSMENT

Observe for signs of stranger and separation anxieties, which are common in the age group most often hospitalized for bronchiolitis (infants and small children). Involving parents in procedures and care, when appropriate, can promote emotional security.

Common nursing diagnoses for the child with bronchiolitis include:

▶ *Ineffective breathing pattern* related to increased work of breathing and decreased energy (fatigue)

▶ *Activity intolerance* related to imbalance between oxygen supply and demand

▶ *Risk for fluid volume deficit* related to inability to meet fluid needs and increased metabolic demands (insensible loss, fever, thickened or increased respiratory secretions)

▶ *Anxiety (child and parent)* related to acute illness, hospitalization, uncertain course of illness and treatment, and home care needs

Planning and Implementation

Nursing management focuses on maintaining respiratory function, supporting overall physiologic function and hydration, reducing the child's and family's anxiety, and preparing the family for home care.

MAINTAIN RESPIRATORY FUNCTION

Close monitoring is essential to evaluate the child's improvement or to spot early signs of deterioration. Administer oxygen and pulmonary care therapies. High humidity and supplemental oxygen may be provided with a mist tent if the child requires only moisture and minimal oxygen. If more concentrated oxygen is required, it can be given via nasal cannula, hood, or tent. Use pulse oximetry to evaluate oxygenation.

Patent nares are important to promote oxygen intake. A bulb syringe is a helpful tool that can quickly and easily clear the nasal passages. Elevate the head of the bed to ease the work of breathing and drain mucus from the upper airways. Pulmonary hygiene and nebulized medications are usually administered by a respiratory therapist. Maintenance of a nebulizer for medications may be needed.

SUPPORT PHYSIOLOGIC FUNCTION

Grouping nursing tasks promotes the child's physiologic function by decreasing stress and promoting rest. Rest is a key to improving the child's breathing and overall health. Medications may be administered to control temperature and promote comfort as needed. An intravenous infusion may be ordered to rehydrate and maintain fluid balance until the child is capable of taking sufficient oral fluids.

REDUCE ANXIETY

The need for hospitalization and assistive therapies creates anxiety and fear in the child and parents. An important part of nursing care is anticipating, recognizing, and acting to decrease the child's and parents' anxiety. Provide parents with thorough explanations and daily updates, and encourage their participation in the child's care.

The presence of parents and their ability to calm the infant or child can be helpful in the child's recovery. The parents may themselves be frightened by the child's continued respiratory difficulty and the assistive equipment at the bedside. Reassure them that holding or touching the child will not dislodge wires or tubing.

If the child has been ill for a few days before admission, the parents are likely to be tired. Acknowledging parents' physical and emotional needs creates a spirit of caring and enhances communication between staff and family. Encourage the parents to take turns at the child's bedside and to take breaks for meals and rest.

DISCHARGE PLANNING AND HOME CARE TEACHING

Children are discharged once they show sufficient stability in maintaining adequate oxygenation (as evidenced by easing of respiratory effort, decreased mucus production, and absence of coughing). In most children, symptoms abate within 24 to 72 hours; however, resolution of all symptoms may take weeks. The same supportive therapies implemented in the hospital may be needed at home:

DISCHARGE TEACHING FOR BRONCHIOLITIS

Advise parents to call the physician if:

- Respiratory symptoms interfere with sleep or eating.
- Breathing is rapid or difficult.
- Symptoms persist in a child who is less than 1 year old, has heart or lung disease, or was premature and had lung disease after birth.
- The child acts sicker—appears tired, less playful, and less interested in food (parents just "feel" the child is not improving).

▶ Use of the bulb syringe to suction the nares of an infant under 1 year of age (see Skill 14-15) **SKILLS**

▶ Fluid intake to thin respiratory secretions (making them easier to clear) and provide glucose for energy (since the child's appetite may not return to normal for several days)

▶ Rest

Children can usually recognize their own activity limits. However, parents should encourage active toddlers to nap and take rest periods. Teach the parents proper administration of medications. Acetaminophen may be prescribed for persistent low-grade fevers and general discomfort. Advise parents that RSV infection can recur; therefore, they need to know how to recognize symptoms and when to call the physician.

Evaluation

Expected outcomes of nursing care for the child with bronchiolitis include:

▶ The child returns to respiratory baseline within 48 to 72 hours.

▶ Child's hydration status is maintained during acute phase of illness.

▶ Parents and child show decreasing anxiety and decreasing fear as symptoms improve and as child and parents feel more secure in hospital environment.

PNEUMONIA

Pneumonia is an inflammation or infection of the bronchioles and alveolar spaces of the lungs. It occurs most often in infants and young children. Pneumonia in children often resolves much sooner than in adults. The key is early recognition, enabling the child to be managed at home rather than in the hospital.

Pneumonia may be viral, mycoplasmal, or bacterial in origin. Common organisms causing pneumonia include RSV, parainfluenza virus, adenovirus, enterovirus, and pneumococcus. Immunosuppressed children are susceptible to many other bacterial, parasitic, or fungal infections.

Regardless of the causative agent, symptoms include elevated temperature, rhonchi, crackles, wheezes, cough, dyspnea, tachypnea, restlessness, and decreased breath sounds if consolidation exists.

What physiologic process occurs to precipitate the symptoms? Bacterial and viral invaders act differently within the lungs. Bacterial invaders circulate through the bloodstream to the lungs, where they damage cells. Bacteria tend to be distributed evenly throughout one or more lobes of a single lung, a pattern termed *unilateral lobar pneumonia*. Viral or mycoplasma invaders, on the other hand, are parasites of cells. Viruses frequently enter from the upper respiratory tract, infiltrating the alveoli nearest the bronchi of one or both lungs. There they invade the cells, replicate, and burst out forcefully, killing the cells and sending out cell debris. They rapidly invade adjacent areas, distributing themselves in a scattered, patchy pattern referred to as bronchopneumonia. The end result of bacterial, viral, or mycoplasma invasion is exudate resulting from cell death, which fills the alveolar spaces, pooling and clumping in dependent areas of the lung to create areas of consolidation.

Diagnosis is made by chest x-ray, which shows an abnormal density of tissue, such as a lobar consolidation. There is no clinical way to differentiate bacterial and viral cause. The child's age, severity of symptoms, and presence of an underlying lung, cardiac, or immunodeficiency disease can create varying responses.

Clinical management for all types of pneumonia includes symptomatic therapy (pain and fever control) and supportive care through airway management, fluids, and rest. Mycoplasma and other bacterial pneumonias are treated with organism-sensitive antibiotics; viral pneumonias usually improve without antibiotics. Some children need oxygen and anti-inflammatory medications.

Nursing Management

Nursing care incorporates supportive measures and medical therapies as appropriate. Nursing measures used to manage the child with bronchiolitis are generally applicable to the child with pneumonia.

In addition to ongoing respiratory assessment and supportive therapies (pulmonary care, antibiotics, hydration), the child may need relief from pain when coughing and deep breathing. Teach the child and parent how to splint the chest, by hugging a small pillow, teddy bear, or doll, to make coughing less painful. Pain medication (acetaminophen or ibuprofen) can provide the added benefits of temperature control and may aid in sleep. Hospitalization is reserved for seriously ill children.

The goal of nursing care is to restore optimal respiratory function. Address discharge planning early in the hospital stay. Medications, especially antibiotics, must be taken at prescribed intervals and for the full course. Teach parents the proper administration of drugs and any side effects. Follow-up may include a chest x-ray to see if the lungs are clear. Symptoms of pneumonia usually disappear long before the lungs are completely healed. Some children continue to have worsening reactive airway problems or abnormal results on pulmonary function tests. Most children, however, recover uneventfully.

Preventive measures against pneumonia are limited. An immunization against pneumococcal bacteria is recommended for children over 2 years of age who are immunosuppressed or have chronic diseases. (See Chapter 41.) ⊂⊃

TUBERCULOSIS

Tuberculosis (TB) is caused by the organism *Mycobacterium tuberculosis,* which is transmitted through the air in infectious particles called droplet nuclei. Since 1988, the incidence of TB has been on the rise, particularly among immigrants, minorities, and children younger than 15 years (Brashers & Davey, 1998). An estimated 15 million people are infected in the United States, creating a large reservoir for infection in children. The risk of developing TB is greatest during the first 2 years of life (American Thoracic Society, 2000). Adults with active laryngeal or pulmonary TB may transmit the disease to children.

By coughing, sneezing, speaking, or singing, a person with active TB sends out tiny droplets of moisture that remain in the air. If these droplets are inhaled, the bacillus is small enough to travel directly to the alveoli. Frequently, however, the organism is trapped in the upper airway, preventing infection. Pulmonary infection occurs only when the bacillus reaches the alveoli.

Once the organism reaches the alveoli, an immune response is initiated to combat the invader. The immune system sends macrophages to surround and wall off the bacillus in small hard capsules, called tubercles. There the bacillus can remain dormant (inactive) indefinitely or can progress to active TB. In young children, the disease develops as an immediate complication of the primary infection. Children with HIV infection or immunosuppression may have more rapidly progressive disease. If the tubercle extends into a blood vessel, the bacillus may spread through the bloodstream to affect the liver, spleen, bone marrow, or meninges (tubercular meningitis). This systemic form of TB (meningeal or miliary tuberculosis) may lead to serious illness or death. Miliary tuberculosis is not, however, transmissible; only active pulmonary TB has the potential to infect another individual.

Clinical manifestations of TB in infants include a persistent cough, weight loss or failure to gain weight, and fever. Wheezing and decreased breath sounds may be present. Older children may be asymptomatic.

Several tests may be required to confirm the diagnosis (Table 42–15). Medical management focuses on diagnosis and treatment of active TB with antitubercular drug therapy. Drugs to treat TB include isoniazid, rifampicin, pyrazinamide, ethambutol, and streptomycin. Challenges to treat-

TABLE 42–15	Diagnostic Tests for Tuberculosis
Test	Indication
Mantoux test (intradermal injection of purified protein derivative [PPD])	Confirms infection with the TB organism (3–12 weeks after exposure)
Chest x-ray examination (anteroposterior and lateral views)	Confirms presence of pulmonary tuberculosis (small, seedlike opacities may be visible)
Blood cultures for *Mycobacterium tuberculosis*	Proves diagnosis; defines specific drug sensitivity
Gastric washings (early morning after overnight fast; 3 consecutive days)	Confirms pulmonary tuberculosis (active form of tuberculosis). Used in children under 12 years because they do not produce sputum.
Sputum cultures (expectorated or from bronchoscopic examination)	Confirms active pulmonary tuberculosis
Pleural biopsy for culture and tissue examination	Taken when pleural effusion is present
Lumbar puncture	Confirms meningeal tuberculosis (inactive form of tuberculosis)

ment have occurred with the development of multidrug-resistant TB. Up to 90% of cases are resistant to certain drugs (Brashers & Davey, 1998). Tuberculosis is a major public health problem and must be promptly reported to local health departments.

In suspected cases of tuberculosis, the child, immediate family, and supposed carrier should be skin tested for TB. Intradermal testing using purified protein derivative (PPD, the Mantoux test) is considered the most accurate test. A control skin test verifies the response status of the immune system. High-risk children who should receive a TB skin test include those with a TB contact, travel to a TB endemic area, contact with adults at high risk or TB, and positive HIV status (Ozuah, Ozuah, Stein, et al., 2001).)

Nursing Management

Nursing care centers on administering medications and providing supportive care. Teach parents about the disease process, medications, possible side effects, and the importance of long-term therapy (e.g., that drug therapy may last for 6 to 12 months). Most children with TB can lead essentially normal lives. Emphasize the importance of taking medications as prescribed on an empty stomach, and ensuring proper nutrition and rest to promote normal growth and development.

The discussion of pneumonia earlier in this chapter and the discussion of tubercular meningitis in Chapter 49 give other nursing care measures appropriate for the child with TB. ⊂⊃

CYSTIC FIBROSIS

Cystic fibrosis is a common inherited autosomal recessive disorder of the exocrine glands that results in physiologic alterations in the respiratory, gastrointestinal, integumentary, musculoskeletal, and reproductive systems. The disorder occurs predominantly in white children, but other populations are also affected. Incidence varies by race—1:3200 in whites, 1:15,000 in blacks, 1:31,000 in Asian Americans (Rosenstein & Cutting, 1998). Gender is not a factor in incidence (Figure 42–7). The median life span for individuals with cystic fibrosis is 30 years.

Etiology and Pathophysiology

A gene isolated on the long arm of chromosome 7 directs the function of the cystic fibrosis transmembrane conductance regulator (CFTR). With a defective CFTR, the exocrine and epithelial cells have defective chloride-ion transport. This results in an abnormal accumulation of viscous, dehydrated mucus that affects the respiratory, gastrointestinal, and genitourinary systems. Inflammation and lung changes are present as early as 4 weeks of age. Ultimately, all body organs with mucous ducts become obstructed and damaged (McMullen, 2000).

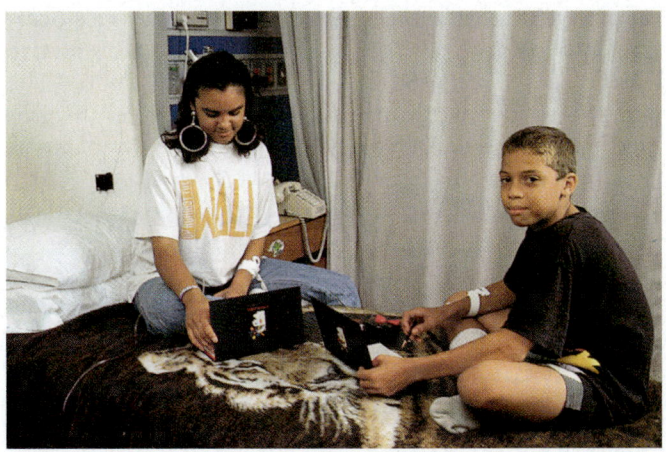

FIGURE 42–7. ◆ Cystic fibrosis is an inherited autosomal recessive disorder of the exocrine glands, so it is not uncommon to see siblings with it such as this brother and sister.

Because of the blocked pancreatic ducts and resulting pancreatic damage, the natural enzymes necessary to digest fats and proteins are not secreted and essential nutrients are excreted in the stool. Stools of the child with cystic fibrosis characteristically are frothy (bulky and large quantity), smell foul, contain fat (are greasy), and float.

The classic cough occurs because the lungs are always filled with mucus, which the respiratory cilia cannot clear. This causes air to become trapped in the small airways, resulting in atelectasis (pulmonary collapse). Secondary respiratory infections occur because secretions provide an environment conducive to bacterial growth. This is a major cause of morbidity and mortality.

Nearly all males who have cystic fibrosis are sterile because of blockage or absence of the vas deferens. Females have difficulty conceiving because increased mucus secretions in the reproductive tract interfere with the passage of sperm (McMullen, 2000).

Metabolic function is altered as a result of the imbalances created by excessive electrolyte loss through perspiration, saliva, and mucus secretion. The "salty taste" of the skin is the result of sodium chloride that makes its way through skin pores to the skin surface.

Clinical Manifestations

The primary symptom of cystic fibrosis is the production of thick, sticky mucus. One of the earliest signs in the newborn is meconium ileus, a small bowel obstruction that occurs during the first few days of life. In infants and toddlers, fecal impaction and intussusception ("telescoping" of the bowel) may be the first signs of the disorder. Steatorrhea (fatty stool) is one of the characteristic signs of cystic fibrosis. The sticky, thick stool is thought to create the initial obstruction. Intestinal peristalsis (controlled by the autonomic nervous system) is also adversely affected. Rectal prolapse, resulting from the large, bulky, difficult-to-pass stools, may occur (Figure 42–8 ◆).

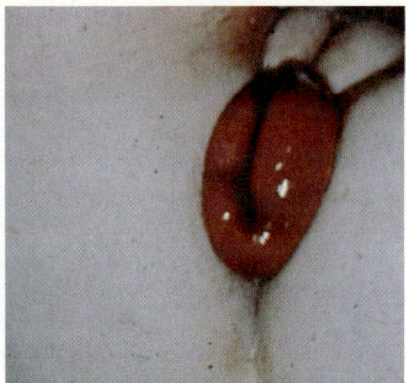

FIGURE 42–8. ◆ Rectal prolapse.

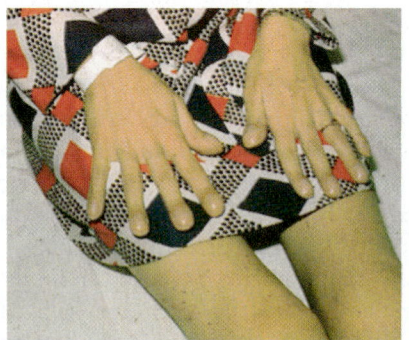

FIGURE 42–9. ◆ Digital clubbing.

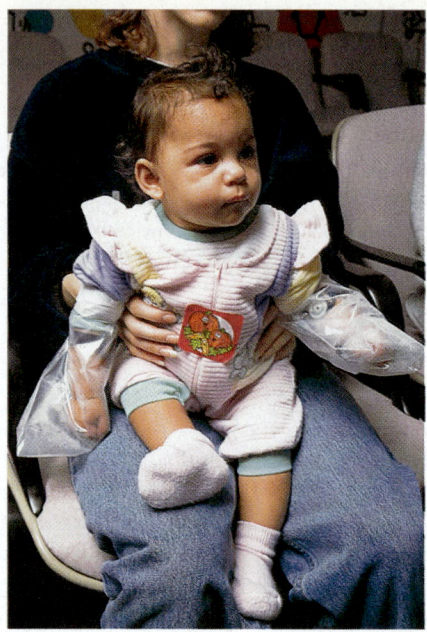

FIGURE 42–10. ◆ This 6-month-old girl is being evaluated for cystic fibrosis using the sweat test.

Other signs and symptoms include a chronic moist, productive cough and frequent respiratory infections. Most children have difficulty maintaining and gaining weight despite a voracious appetite. Infants and children may have a delayed bone age, short stature, and delayed onset of puberty. Clubbing of the tips of the fingers and toes occurs as the disease progresses (Figure 42–9 ◆).

Clinical Therapy

Cystic fibrosis is usually diagnosed in infancy or early childhood with one of three major presentations: newborn meconium ileus, malabsorption or failure to thrive, or chronic recurrent respiratory infections. Some children with a milder form of the disease, however, may reach the teen or young adult years before symptoms appear. The mean age at diagnosis is 4.8 years (Farrell, Kosorok, Rock, et al., 2001).

Cystic fibrosis is diagnosed definitively by a positive sweat test and the presence of classic symptoms or a positive family history (McMullen, 2000). A chloride concentration of 50 to 60 mEq/L is suspicious. If the chloride concentration is >60 mEq/L, it is diagnostic with other signs. Genetic testing of the child's DNA along with blood immunoreactive trypsinogen can be used for newborn screening (Farrell et al., 2001). The sweat test may be performed at the child's bedside or on an outpatient basis. The parents should be present to hold and reassure the in-

fant or small child (Figure 42–10 ◆). Tell them that the test will indicate whether the child has cystic fibrosis and that a second test may be ordered to confirm the diagnosis. Pulmonary function tests are performed on children older than 6 years.

Clinical therapy focuses on maintaining respiratory function, managing infection, promoting optimal nutrition and exercise, and preventing gastrointestinal blockage (Table 42–16). Newly diagnosed children will have no or minimal symptoms and near-normal lung function if aggressively treated. Pulmonary function declines 2% to 4% per year even with aggressive treatment (Varlotta, 1998).

Improvements in medical management and optimal nutrition now enable many children with cystic fibrosis to survive well into adulthood. Lung transplantation is occasionally performed, and approximately 50% of cases survive for the first 5 years (Stubblefield & Murray, 2000). The disease is ultimately terminal, however, because of the progressive multisystem changes and the difficulty of long-term infection management.

Care of the child with previously diagnosed cystic fibrosis is the focus of the following discussion.

Nursing Management

Nursing Assessment and Diagnosis

PHYSIOLOGIC ASSESSMENT

Physical assessment of the child focuses on adequacy of respiratory function. The child with cystic fibrosis usually is admitted with symptoms of an upper respiratory infection. Obtain a set of baseline vital signs, including temper-

TABLE 42-16   Clinical Therapy for Cystic Fibrosis

Clinical Therapy	Rationale
Respiratory Therapy	
Aerosol bronchodilators	Opens large and small airways; use before chest physiotherapy; and with symptoms
Aerosol DNAse	Loosens, liquefies, and thins pulmonary secretions; decreases risk of developing pulmonary infections requiring parenteral treatment in some patients (McMullen, 2000)
Anti-inflammatory agents: steroids, high-dose ibuprofen	Reduces inflammatory response to chronic infection; short courses to decrease side effects of steroids; decreases progression of lung damage in preadolescents with mild disease
Chest physiotherapy for all lung segments (bilateral percussion-vibration and forceful coughing)	Mobilizes secretions to bronchi for expectoration; performed twice a day
Infection Management (Most Susceptible to *H. influenzae, S. aureus,* and *Pseudomonas aeruginosa* bacteria, *Burkholderia cepacia,* and Viral Agents)	
Antibiotics (oral, IV, aerosol routes)	Treatment based on sputum-culture results; may need higher than normal doses to be effective
Nutritional Needs	
Pancreatic enzyme supplements (Cotazym-S, Pancrease, Viokase) taken with meals and snacks	Assists in digestion of nutrients and decreasing fat and bulk; given prior to food ingestion
Diet supplies well-balanced food with 120%–150% of RDA recommended calories and 200% of RDA recommended protein, and moderate fat; nutritional counseling necessary	Promotes essential nutrient balance for health, growth, and weight maintenance; considers child, food, and cultural-socioeconomic issues
Multivitamins and vitamin E in water-soluble form; vitamins A, D, and K given when deficient; iron	Cystic fibrosis interferes with vitamin production; supplements are required in water-soluble form for better absorption supplementation (vitamins A, D, E, and K are naturally fat soluble); iron deficiency results from malabsorption syndrome

ature, pulse, respirations, and blood pressure, along with a weight measurement, on admission. Observe the child's physical appearance, noting overall body proportions and any changes characteristic of long-term cystic fibrosis.

PSYCHOSOCIAL ASSESSMENT

The emotional stress of this chronic disease may not be readily apparent on admission, particularly if the child's symptoms are mild and not imminently life threatening. Ongoing observation of the child's and parents' behavior helps direct nursing interventions throughout hospitalization (see Table 42–11). Parents may feel guilt as carriers of the disease. Siblings may also show signs of difficulty in dealing with the illness. Link the family to support groups.

Ask parents how the child's illness has affected day-to-day functioning and how they have adapted to the child's plan of care. What have parents told the child and siblings about the disease? What kind of questions have the child and siblings asked about cystic fibrosis, and how have parents answered them? Has the child ever asked about his or her life expectancy? If not, what would parents say if asked?

DEVELOPMENTAL ASSESSMENT

Growth and development may be altered by the chronic nature of the disease. Children with cystic fibrosis may be growth retarded. Compare the child's height and weight to age norms and observe the adolescent for the appearance of secondary sex characteristics, which are often delayed. School-age children and adolescents often are embarrassed at being viewed as different from playmates and peers. Ask how the child and adolescent feel about the need for a special diet, medications, and limitations.

Common nursing diagnoses for the child with cystic fibrosis include the following:

▶ *Ineffective airway clearance* related to thick mucus in lungs

▶ *Risk for infection* related to the presence of mucous secretions conducive to bacterial growth

▶ *Altered nutrition: less than body requirements* related to inability to digest nutrients

▶ *Parental role conflict* related to interruptions in family life due to the home care regimen

Planning and Implementation

Nursing management involves supporting the child and family initially, when the diagnosis is made, during subsequent hospitalizations, and during visits to specialty and primary health care providers. The nurse's role begins with implementing specific medical therapies and providing nursing care to meet the child's physiologic and psychosocial needs. Respiratory therapy, medications, and diet must be coordinated to promote optimal body function. Psychosocial support and reinforcement of the child's daily care needs are important in preparation for home care.

Children with cystic fibrosis require periodic hospitalization when a severe infection occurs or for a pulmonary and nutritional "tune-up". Respect the parents' experiences as the child's primary care provider and include them in the child's routine care as much as possible. However, parents may view the hospital stay as a break from the rigorous daily pulmonary routine at home and need support in taking advantage of some "down" time. The family often becomes proficient at providing physical care to the child, but the nurse should take the opportunity provided during rehospitalization to review basic and new information about respiratory care, medications, and nutrition. Keeping lines of communication open and validating parents' understanding of their child's disease and care needs are important steps in preparing the family to cope with this chronic health challenge.

PROVIDE RESPIRATORY THERAPY

Chest physiotherapy is usually performed one to three times per day before meals to clear secretions from the lungs, as coughing may stimulate vomiting (Figure 42–11 ◆). Parents and other family members can learn to help with these necessary treatments. Pulmonary care may involve aerosol treatments and antibiotics when indicated (see Table 42–13). (See Skill 14-20.) ⟨⊃ SKILLS CD

ADMINISTER MEDICATIONS AND MEET NUTRITIONAL NEEDS

Special medications and dietary modification can ease digestive problems (see Table 42–16). Pancreatic enzyme supplements come in powder sprinkles and capsule form and are taken orally with all meals and large snacks. The amount needed is individualized based on the child's nutritional needs and digestive response to these supplements. The goal is to achieve near-normal, well-formed stools and adequate weight gain.

Some fat-soluble vitamins (A, D, E, and K) are not completely absorbed from food; therefore, they must be taken in water-soluble form. Multivitamins taken twice daily usually are sufficient to prevent deficiency. The diet should be well-balanced, with an emphasis on high caloric value. Respiratory complications necessitate additional energy expenditure, and some children require special nutritional supplements, and sometimes supplemental nasogastric or gastrostomy feedings, to gain and maintain weight.

Fats and salt are both necessary in the diet. Balanced with pancreatic enzyme supplements, moderate fat intake adds an important source of extra fuel.

PROVIDE ANTICIPATORY GUIDANCE

Help the parents and child learn what they must do to maintain health after discharge. Emotional support is essential because the diagnosis of this disorder creates anxiety and fear in both the parents and the child. They need assistance with emotional and psychosocial issues relating to discipline, body image (stooling and odor), frequent rehospitalization, the potential fatal nature of the illness, the child's feeling of being different from friends, and overall financial, social, and family concerns. Because the disorder is inherited, families may have more than one child with cystic fibrosis. Parents may have unspoken feelings of anger and guilt, blaming themselves for their children's condition.

DISCHARGE PLANNING AND HOME CARE TEACHING

A family already overwhelmed by the diagnosis may not immediately recognize the financial burden of medications, supplies, and medical follow-up. Because of the chronicity of cystic fibrosis, home care is as important as care of the child in the hospital. Initially, parents need assistance in obtaining necessary equipment. If the family requires financial assistance, refer them to the appropriate social services. Home care of the child with cystic fibrosis is expensive and can be draining on the family's finances.

Parents need to learn chest physiotherapy, which the child needs as often as three or four times a day. Arranging for a visiting nurse and a respiratory therapist to visit the family frequently can provide reassurance and relief to the family. Managing the child's nutritional needs is important and takes time and energy.

Parents need to learn how to mix enzymes for young children, what vitamins need to be given daily, and what foods should be avoided or eliminated because of the

FIGURE 42–11. ◆ Postural drainage can be achieved by clapping with a cupped hand on the chest wall over the segment to be drained to create vibrations that are transmitted to the bronchi to dislodge secretions. **A,** If the obstruction is in the posterior apical segment of the lung, the nurse can do this with the child sitting up. **B,** If the obstruction is in the left posterior segment, the child should be lying on the right side. Several other positions can be used depending on the location of the obstruction.

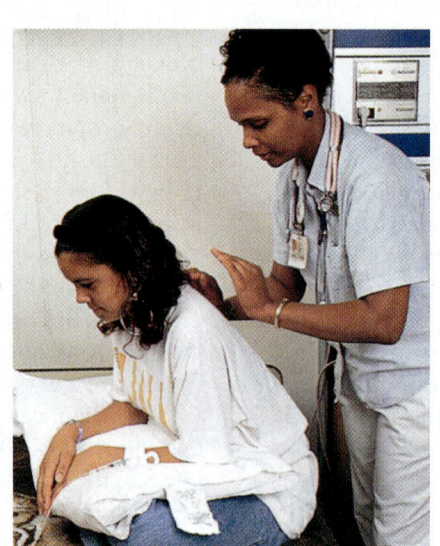

A

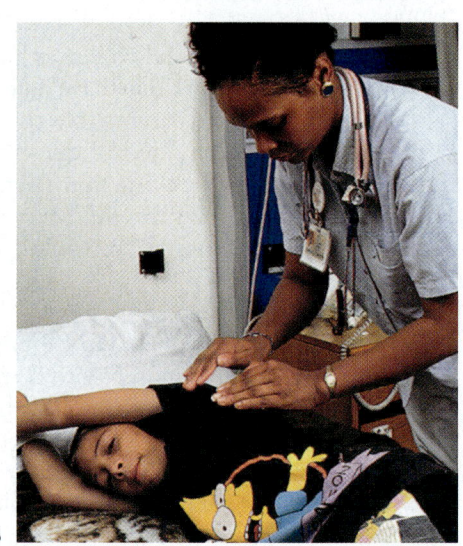

B

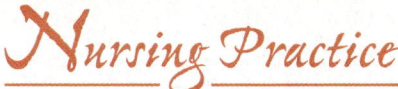

Nursing Practice

Parents often have a difficult time getting the child with cystic fibrosis to eat the extra calories needed for optimal nutrition, setting the stage for a potential mealtime battleground. To be successful, parents need guidance about managing mealtime behaviors in addition to guidelines for preparing nutritional calorie-dense foods. Increase calorie intake by adding fats and high-calorie snacks between meals and before bed. Extra intervention may be needed when the child's weight is 85% to 90% of ideal weight for height (Wilson & Pencharz, 1998).

child's digestive problems. Make a referral to a nutritionist either before or at the time of discharge.

Cystic fibrosis affects all family members and disrupts activities of daily living for everyone. It is important to refer families to family counseling and group therapy with families of other children with cystic fibrosis if indicated. The Cystic Fibrosis Foundation is a source for information on current advances in cystic fibrosis. **WEB** Local chapter activities also provide emotional support for parents and children.

NURSING CARE IN THE COMMUNITY

Nurses may encounter the child with cystic fibrosis in any of the following settings: clinics specializing in the disease, pediatricians' offices, and schools. The primary goal is to keep the disease under control by promoting optimal nutrition and assisting the family to reduce the incidence of infection. Nurses may also provide home care to the child with cystic fibrosis following hospitalization for an acute exacerbation or provide hospice care.

Assessment

Assess the child's respiratory status. Inquire about the frequency and character of the child's cough and characteristics of the sputum. Compare this information with the child's baseline. Changes in the cough may be more important than its presence or absence. Auscultate the chest for breath sounds, crackles, and wheezes. Note any cyanosis or clubbing of the extremities. Obtain oxygen saturation and spirometry readings if changes in respiratory status are suspected.

Evaluate the child's growth, plotting the weight and height on a growth curve. Determine whether the child is maintaining an appropriate growth pattern. Inquire about the child's appetite and dietary intake. How are nutritional supplements, pancreatic enzymes, and vitamins used?

Assess the child's stooling pattern. Identify whether the child has problems with abdominal pain or bloating, and whether these problems can be related to eating, stooling, or other activities. Palpate the abdomen for liver size, fecal masses, and evidence of pain.

Inquire about the family's and child's emotional and psychosocial responses to managing the illness. These issues are very important when the child is going through major developmental stages.

Management

Review the child's use of bronchodilators and airway clearance techniques. To prevent a change in pulmonary status from progressing, short-term changes in care may be recommended. These may include intravenous and aerosol medications and antibiotics, an increase in the number of times chest physiotherapy is performed daily, and changes in dietary management. Help the family select the best time to fit the additional treatment into their schedule.

Malnutrition is a major problem for children with cystic fibrosis. Parents often need to plan meals and snacks for the young child to ensure that adequate calories are consumed. Nutritional supplements may be suggested when growth is not adequate. Arrange for a consultation with a nutritionist if the family would benefit from new strategies to help meet the child's nutritional needs. Children with adequate nutrition have a longer life expectancy.

Children with cystic fibrosis lose more than normal amounts of salt in their sweat. This loss can become intensified during hot weather, strenuous exercise, and fever. Parents should allow the child to add extra salt to food and should permit some salty snacks (pretzels with salt, pickles, carbonated soda). During periods of increased sweating, the child should be encouraged to drink more fluids and increase salt intake. Teach parents to recognize early symptoms of salt depletion, including fatigue, weakness, abdominal pain, and vomiting, and to contact the child's health care provider if these symptoms occur.

Talk with the child and family to identify any assistance needed with emotional and psychosocial issues. Depending on the child's developmental stage, issues related to discipline, body image (stooling and odor), or the child's feeling of being different from friends may be major concerns. The family may also have overall financial, social, and family management concerns that can be discussed.

Adolescents with cystic fibrosis need special assistance in coping with their disorder. Help them identify normal adolescent changes versus those related to cystic fibrosis. Plan transitional care as they take on more responsibility for self-care and decision making, as well as preparing for a job that fits their energy level. Adolescents should also have a supportive grief process as they recognize how their remaining life will be different from their peers (Muscari, 1998).

Evaluation

Expected outcomes of nursing care include:

▶ The child and family develop proficiency in providing the daily pulmonary care and reducing the incidence of respiratory infections.

▶ The child and family develop a schedule and routine for daily pulmonary care that fits into family and school activities.

▶ The child consumes adequate calories and pancreatic enzymes to support growth and to stay within desirable weight ranges.

Airway compromise after an unintentional injury can cause death if not managed quickly and effectively. Why are children so vulnerable to changes in respiratory function after accidental injury?

The small size of the child's airway makes it vulnerable to obstruction. The tongue, small amounts of blood, mucus, or foreign debris or swelling in the respiratory tract or adjacent neck tissue may block the airway and lead to hypoxia and respiratory failure. If the child's neck is flexed or hyperextended, the soft laryngeal cartilage may compress and obstruct the airway.

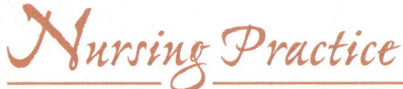
Nursing Practice

Never allow a child's neck to hyperextend (bend completely backward) or hyperflex (bend completely forward). Hyperextension flattens the trachea because there is no firm cartilage to provide structural support. Hyperflexion can kink and compress the trachea. Both maneuvers obstruct rather than open the airway.

Infants and young children rely on the diaphragm for air movement. They are abdominal (or "belly") breathers. Excessive crying and anxiety deplete metabolic reserves. External ventilatory support and vigorous crying may impede diaphragm function if the stomach becomes distended with air. Because the child's metabolic rate is about double that of an adult, the child has a greater need for oxygen. Respiratory distress, anxiety, and even fever can dramatically add to the child's oxygen demand.

AIRWAY OBSTRUCTION

Airway obstruction exists when air passage in the respiratory tract and lungs is slowed or blocked. If the blockage occurs above the trachea, inspiration is more affected. If the blockage occurs below the trachea, expiration is more affected. Earlier sections dealt with structural and functional problems that may lead to airway obstruction. This section addresses two common conditions of airway obstruction in children that result from unintentional injury: foreign body aspiration and near-drowning.

Foreign-Body Aspiration

Foreign-body aspiration is the inhalation of any object (solid or liquid, food or nonfood) into the respiratory tract. Aspiration occurs most often during feeding and reaching activities, while crawling, or during playtime in children aged 6 months to 4 years. However, aspiration may occur in children of any age.

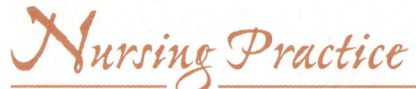
Nursing Practice

Foreign-body aspiration is a major health problem for infants and young toddlers because of their increasing mobility and tendency to place small objects in the mouth.

ETIOLOGY AND PATHOPHYSIOLOGY

In infants over 6 months of age and in children, any number of small objects that make their way into the child's mouth may cause aspiration. Foods such as nuts, popcorn, or small pieces of raw vegetables or hot dog; small, loose toy parts such as small wheels and bells; or household objects and substances such as beads, safety pins, coins, buttons, latex balloon pieces, and colorful liquids (mouthwash, perfume) in enticing packages (screw top bottles) are frequent causes of airway obstruction.

The severity of the obstruction depends on the size and composition of the object or substance and its location within the respiratory tract. Most aspirated foreign bodies (AFBs) usually cause bronchial, not tracheal, obstruction. An object lodged high in the airway above the vocal cords is frequently coughed out easily or with some assistance (such as use of chest thrusts and back blows or the abdominal thrust). An object lodged in the trachea is a life-threatening situation. (See Skill 14-14). **SKILLS**

Coughing, choking, gagging, dysphonia, and wheezing may be brief or may persist for several hours if the object drops below the trachea into one of the mainstem bronchi. The right lung is the most common site of lower airway aspiration because of the sloped angle of its bronchus (see "As They Grow: Trachea Position" on p. 1025). Objects may migrate from higher to lower airway locations. An object may also move back up to the trachea, creating extreme respiratory difficulty. If oxygen is depleted for an extended time, brain damage may occur.

CLINICAL MANIFESTATIONS

Children are usually brought to the hospital after a sudden episode of coughing. Discovery of an open container with small objects may prompt parents to seek medical assistance for the child. The child may have spasmodic coughing, respiratory distress, or gagging. If the child cannot say the "P" in words like *Pluto* or *Peter Pan,* the foreign body has noticeably diminished expiratory effort. Sudden respiratory distress in the absence of fever or other symptoms of illness strongly suggests foreign-body aspiration (Hazinski, 1999).

CLINICAL THERAPY

Clinical therapy focuses on taking a careful history to determine whether aspiration has indeed occurred. Choking associated with feeding or crawling on the floor is usually a confirming event. The physical examination often reveals decreased breath sounds, stridor, and respiratory distress in

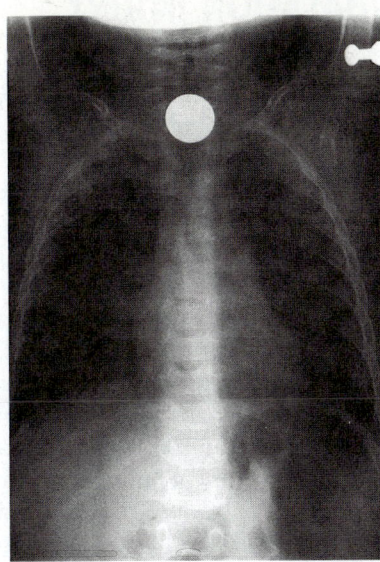

FIGURE 42–12. ◆ An aspirated foreign body (coin) is clearly visible in the child's trachea on this chest x-ray. *Courtesy of Rockwood Clinic, Spokane, WA.*

the child without a witnessed aspiration. A special radiograph, called a forced expiratory film, may be ordered. This shows local hyperinflation (air trapping) and a mediastinal shift away from the affected side (Hazinski, 1999). Sometimes, when the object aspirated is radiopaque, it can be seen on an x-ray film (Figure 42–12 ◆). Fluoroscopy and fiberoptic bronchoscopy may be used to identify, locate, and extract the AFB.

The child with an AFB that is removed is usually stabilized in the emergency department and observed for a few hours. Depending on the type of object and degree of obstruction, surgical removal of the object and hospitalization may be required.

Nursing Management

Nursing Assessment and Diagnosis

PHYSIOLOGIC ASSESSMENT

If the object remains lodged, observe the child for increasing signs of respiratory distress, especially vital signs and audible wheezing on auscultation. Note changes in breath sounds, from noisy to decreasing to absent, on the affected side. This can indicate that the object is moving and blocking a mainstem bronchus.

PSYCHOSOCIAL ASSESSMENT

The unexpected and acute nature of the event creates anxiety for both parents and child. The child and parents also may be experiencing a variety of other emotions—fear, anger, or guilt. Assess coping and level of stress. Providing a quiet environment and encouraging the presence of the parents can help reduce the child's fear and anxiety.

DEVELOPMENTAL ASSESSMENT

As the child's condition stabilizes, observe how well the child's abilities match the parents' understanding of age-appropriate behaviors. Providing anticipatory teaching or reinforcing information about developmental characteristics (see Chapter 32) ⚬▭ helps parents to anticipate safety hazards in the future.

Common nursing diagnoses for a child with an AFB include:

▶ *Ineffective airway clearance* related to foreign object trauma (previously removed or coughed out object)
▶ *Inability to sustain spontaneous ventilations* related to foreign object and respiratory muscle fatigue
▶ *Fear/anxiety (parent or child)* related to uncertainty of prognosis, unfamiliar surroundings and procedures

Planning and Implementation

The first 12 hours after aspiration are critical; promptly document and report any subtle changes in the child's respiratory status during this period. Explain procedures to the child and family and provide emotional support. Be prepared to perform back blows and chest thrusts for an infant or abdominal thrusts for the child with complete obstruction. (See Skill 14-13.) ⚬▭

DISCHARGE PLANNING AND HOME CARE TEACHING

Discharge planning centers on anticipatory guidance about childproofing the home (see Chapter 32) ⚬▭ and encouraging the parents to learn CPR, choking-prevention techniques, and back blows, chest thrusts, or abdominal thrusts.

Evaluation

Expected outcomes of nursing care include:

▶ The child regains the ability to ventilate spontaneously after removal of the foreign body.
▶ No future incidents of aspiration of a foreign body occur because of the parent's prevention efforts.

NEAR-DROWNING

Near-drowning incidents and death by drowning are most prevalent in children under 5 years of age. In this age group, drowning is a leading cause of death resulting from injury (Murphy, 2000). Groups at high risk include toddlers, teenage boys, and children with seizure disorders. Children with seizure disorders may experience sudden and uncontrollable loss of body position that places them at risk without warning.

Near-drowning is defined as resuscitation and survival for 24 hours following a submersion injury. Near-drowning may result in complete recovery, severe brain injury, or variable neurologic deficits. A key feature influencing survival is initiation of immediate resuscitation, followed, it is hoped, by spontaneous respiratory effort by the child within 5 minutes after removal from the water. The mouth is cleaned of foreign matter, but time should not be wasted trying to remove water from the lungs. The sooner the child is ventilated, the better the chance of survival with normal neurologic potential. Emergency transport to a hospital should occur as soon as possible, even if the child begins spontaneous breathing.

Nursing Practice

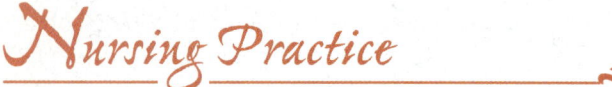

Toddlers have large heads, which makes them top heavy, and an unsteady gait that compromises body control and speed of movement. When propelled into a body of water, they may be unable to escape. Teenage boys may engage in risky behavior around or in a body of water, placing themselves or others at risk.

Most drownings occur in the child's home pool or at the residence of a neighbor, friend, or relative. Usually the child is playing, is not wearing a swimsuit, and is briefly unsupervised before the immersion. Other common drowning sites for young children include bathtubs, hot tubs, toilets, and even large water-filled buckets. A child can drown in as little water as it takes to cover the nose and mouth. In most immersion cases, hypoxemia begins within seconds and irreversible nervous system cell changes begin within 4 to 6 minutes (refer to Chapter 49). Hypoxemia is the most important consequence of near-drowning. Supportive care for any progression of pathology related to cerebral edema and aspiration of water is key. Damage to the airways from loss of surface-active material can lead to capillary leakage, pulmonary edema, and acute respiratory distress syndrome (Hazinski, 1999).

Nursing Management

Nursing management focuses on observation and support of cardiopulmonary and central nervous system function. Oxygen and mechanical ventilation with positive end expiratory pressure will be needed if acute respiratory distress develops. Frequent neurologic monitoring with the Glasgow Coma Scale and assessment of vital signs provide valuable baseline information. (See Chapter 49.) A chest x-ray may be ordered to establish baseline information about lung expansion and pulmonary integrity. Pulse oximetry will be ordered to provide ongoing data about the child's oxygenation status. Document any change in respiratory status and notify the physician promptly. (See Skill 9-15.) **SKILLS**

The child and family need support to work through the feelings surrounding the near-drowning incident, the unexpected hospitalization, and an uncertain prognosis that may mean the child will not return to normal functioning. Prevention is the key to avoiding a similar mishap in the future.

SMOKE-INHALATION INJURY

Exposure to fire conditions sets up dramatic responses in the respiratory tract of children. In every age group, inhalation injury significantly increases the child's chance of death (Allshouse & Eichelberger, 1993).

The severity of the smoke-inhalation injury is influenced by the type of material burned and whether the child was found in an open or closed space. The composition of materials determines how easily they ignite, how fast they burn, and how much heat they release. These factors influence the production of smoke and toxic gases. Smoke, a product of the burning process that is composed of gases and particles, is generated in varying volumes and density. The type and concentration of toxic gases, which are usually invisible, affect the severity of pulmonary damage. The duration of exposure to the smoke produced and any toxic gases contribute significantly to the child's prognosis.

Exposure to extreme heat, common in house fires, leads to surface injury and upper airway damage. The upper airway normally removes heat from inhaled gases, sparing the lower airway from thermal damage. However, this action results in marked edema, placing the small child at particular risk for airway obstruction. Edema develops rapidly over a few hours and may lead to acute respiratory distress syndrome. Burns of the face and neck, singed nasal hairs, soot around the mouth or nose, and hoarseness with stridor or voice change all indicate inhalation injury.

Carbon monoxide (CO) is a clear, colorless, odorless gas present in all fire conditions as the fire consumes oxygen. The CO molecule binds more firmly to hemoglobin than does oxygen. As a result, it replaces oxygen in circulation and rapidly produces hypoxia in the child. The longer the exposure to CO, the greater the hypoxia. The brain receives inadequate oxygen, resulting in confusion. This accounts for the inability of fire victims to escape as confusion progresses to loss of consciousness. The process can be rapidly reversed, however, by timely administration of 100% oxygen (Schweich & Zempsky, 1999).

Damage to the lower airway most often results from chemicals or toxic gas inhalation. Soot is carried deep into the lungs, where it combines with water in the lungs to deposit acid-producing chemicals on the lung tissue. These acids burn the tissue, causing loss of cilia, loss of surfactant, and edema. Tissue destruction, edema, and disruption of gas exchange produce the initial insult to the lungs and potential airway obstruction. Days later, the damaged tissue sloughs off, obstructing the airways. Because the cilia that normally help remove debris have been destroyed, the lungs become a breeding ground for microorganisms. Pneumonia becomes a major health concern. The damaged alveoli heal by scar tissue formation. This can greatly reduce future lung function.

Nursing Management

Most children who survive smoke-inhalation injury are admitted for close observation, airway management, and ventilatory support, if indicated. Respiratory assessment and pulmonary therapy are usually required to reestablish adequate oxygenation and respiratory function.

BLUNT CHEST TRAUMA

Blunt trauma is a common injury in children, especially associated with motor vehicle crashes (Pieper, 2000). Chest injuries may not be obvious and can be extremely difficult to evaluate.

After sustaining severe blunt trauma, most children die from lack of oxygen caused by poor airway and ventilatory control. A child's elastic, pliable chest wall and thin abdominal muscles provide minimal protection to underlying organs. This elasticity often spares bone but not the underlying organs. A rib fracture in children under 12 years old indicates trauma of significant force. The energy from blunt trauma is transferred directly from an external force to the internal organs, often causing a pulmonary contusion or pneumothorax.

PULMONARY CONTUSION

A pulmonary contusion is defined as bruising damage to the tissues of the lung. This causes bleeding into the alveoli, which may lead to capillary rupture in the air sacs. Pulmonary edema develops in the lower airways as blood and fluid from damaged tissues accumulate. Lower airway obstruction and atelectasis may result in impaired gas exchange, acute respiratory distress, and respiratory failure (Hazinski, 1999).

Pulmonary contusion occurs in up to 76% of children with nonpenetrating chest trauma. Initially the child may appear asymptomatic. Respiratory distress often develops over several hours, so careful observation is required during the first 12 hours after the injury to detect decreased perfusion related to ventilatory impairment.

Nursing Management

Nursing care centers on providing necessary physiologic support, such as oxygen therapy, positioning, positive pressure ventilation, oxygen, and comfort measures. The child's level of consciousness is an excellent indicator of respiratory function. Agitation and lethargy can signal increasing hypoxia. When monitoring the status of a child who has a pulmonary contusion, do not rely on the child's color as an indicator of adequate oxygenation. Cyanosis in children is often a late indicator of respiratory distress. Observe for hemoptysis (fresh blood in the emesis), dyspnea, decreased breath sounds, wheezes, crackles, and a transient temperature elevation.

Inspect the thorax for symmetric chest wall movement and equal presence of breath sounds in both lungs. The child may initially appear well but requires careful and thorough monitoring to detect signs of deterioration.

Children with significant injuries are cared for in the ICU. Some children require ventilator support as the pulmonary tissues heal.

PNEUMOTHORAX

A pneumothorax occurs when air collects between the pleural layers, causing the lung to collapse. If blood collects in the pleural space, it is called a *hemothorax,* and if blood and air collect, it is called a *pneumohemothorax.* A pneumothorax is one of the more common thoracic injuries in pediatric trauma patients.

There are three types of pneumothorax: open, closed, and tension. An open pneumothorax, sometimes referred to as a sucking chest wound, results from any penetrating injury that exposes the pleural space to atmospheric pressure, thereby collapsing the lung.

A closed pneumothorax is sometimes caused by blunt chest trauma with no evidence of rib fracture (see "Pathophysiology Illustrated: Pneumothorax"). The chest may be compressed against a closed glottis, causing a sudden increase in pressure within the thoracic cavity. The child spontaneously holds his or her breath when the thorax is struck, accounting for the involuntary closing of the glottis. The pressure increase is transferred to the alveoli, causing them to burst. A single burst alveolus may be able to seal itself off, but with the destruction of many alveoli the lung collapses. Breath sounds are decreased or absent on the injured side, and the child is in respiratory distress. A thoracostomy is performed and a chest tube inserted. A closed drainage system is attached to help remove the air and reinflate the lung by reestablishing negative pressure.

A tension pneumothorax is a life-threatening emergency that results when the internal pressure from a closed pneumothorax is not vented and continues to build, compressing the chest contents and collapsing the lung. Air leaks into the chest cavity during inhalation but is trapped from escape during exhalation. Venous return to the heart is impaired as the trachea, heart, vena cava, and esophagus are compressed toward the unaffected lung when the mediastinum shifts, leading to decreased cardiac output. Signs of tension pneumothorax include increasing respiratory distress, decreased breath sounds, and paradoxical breathing.

Nursing Management

Nursing management focuses on airway management and maintaining lung inflation. The child arrives on the nursing unit with a chest tube and drainage system in place. Continued close observation for respiratory distress is essential. Carefully monitor vital signs. Complications include hemothorax (if the thoracostomy and chest tube are improperly placed), lung tissue injury, and scarring from poor tube placement (especially if the tube is placed too near the breast in girls).

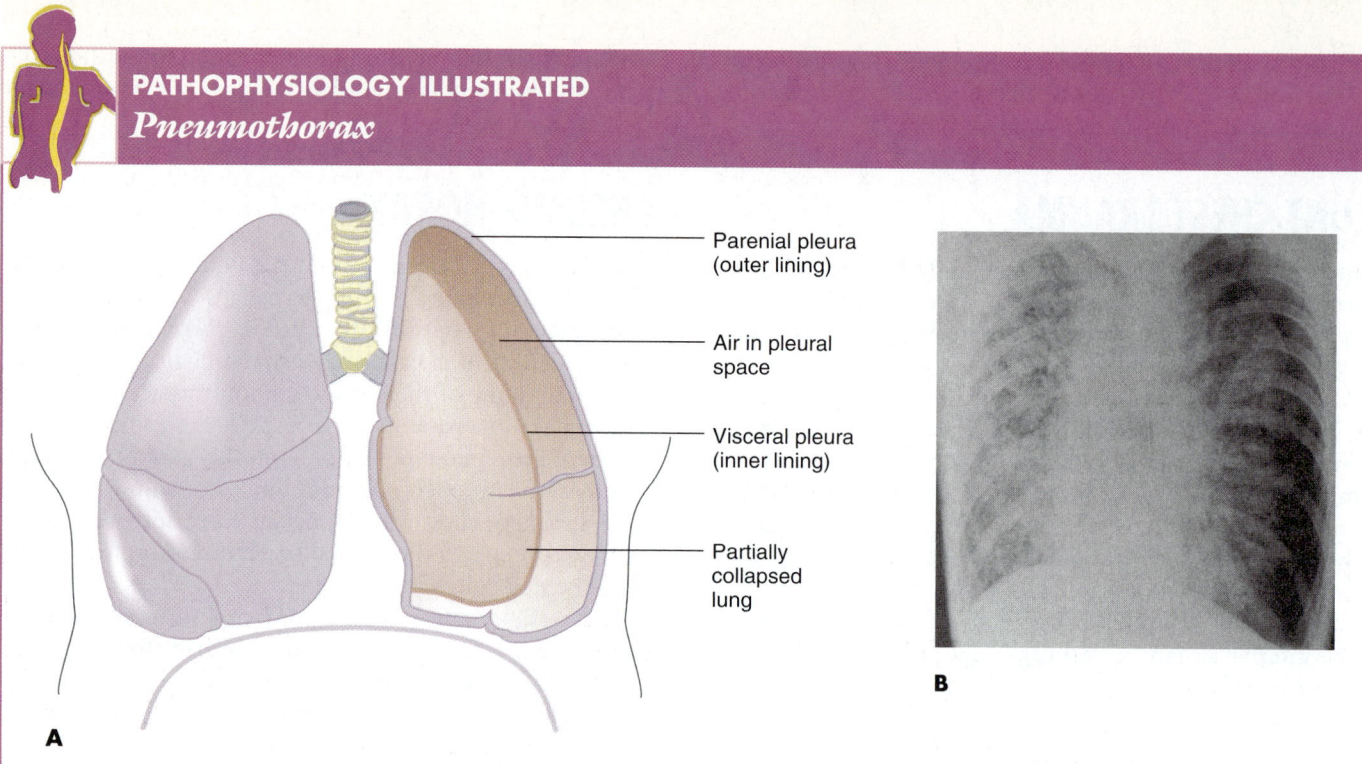

Parenial pleura
(outer lining)

Air in pleural
space

Visceral pleura
(inner lining)

Partially
collapsed
lung

A

B

A, A pneumothorax is air in the pleural space that causes a lung to collapse. Whether the air results from an open injury or from bursting of alveoli due to a blunt injury, it is important to focus on airway management and maintain lung inflation. **B,** Pneumothorax (right lung). **B,** Note: From Fleisher, G. R., Ludwig, S. (1993). *Textbook of Pediatric Emergency Medicine*, 3rd ed., Fig. 89.10A, p. 398. Philadelphia: Lippincott.

*C*HAPTER HIGHLIGHTS

➣ Acute respiratory problems are the most common cause of illness requiring hospitalization in infants and children less than 15 years of age.

➣ The child's airway is shorter and narrower than an adult's. These differences create a greater potential for obstruction. The lungs have no muscles of their own, so the diaphragm and intercostal muscles power respiration.

➣ Apnea, by definition, is cessation of respiration lasting longer than 20 seconds, or any pause in respiration associated with cyanosis, marked pallor, hypotonia, or bradycardia.

➣ Sudden infant death syndrome (SIDS), a leading cause of death in infants, is the sudden death of an infant under 1 year of age that remains unexplained after a complete autopsy, a death scene investigation, and review of the history.

➣ Signs of impending respiratory failure in infants and children include irritability, lethargy, cyanosis, and increased respiratory effort such as dyspnea (difficulty breathing), tachypnea (increased respiratory rate), nasal flaring, and intercostal retractions.

➣ Laryngotracheobronchitis (LTB) is a croup syndrome viral illness with signs of an upper respiratory illness, hoarseness, tachypnea, inspiratory stridor, and a seal-like barking cough. Fever may or may not be present.

➣ Epiglottitis is caused by bacterial invasion of the soft tissue of the larynx causing inflammation and edema of the tissues and the epiglot-

tis that can result in life-threatening airway obstruction. Fortunately, the number of cases of epiglottitis has decreased significantly because of the Hib vaccine.

➣ Asthma affects about 5 million children in the United States and, for each of those children, results in about 10 days of school absenteeism and 20 days of restricted activity per year.

➣ Bronchopulmonary dysplasia (BPD) is often a consequence of neonatal respiratory distress syndrome, congenital heart disease, meconium aspiration, and fluid overload and edema in the newborn. It is associated with respiratory infections requiring frequent hospitalization.

➣ Although many bacterial and mycoplasmal organisms may cause bronchiolitis, infection with respiratory syncytial virus (RSV) is the most common cause.

➣ Symptoms of pneumonia in infants and children include elevated temperature, rhonchi, crackles, wheezes, cough, dyspnea, tachypnea, restlessness, and if consolidation exists, decreased breath sounds.

➣ Clinical manifestations of tuberculosis in infants include a persistent cough, weight loss or failure to gain weight, and fever. Wheezing and decreased breath sounds may be present. Older children may be asymptomatic.

➣ In cystic fibrosis, defective chloride-ion transport across the exocrine and epithelial cells results in an abnormal accumulation of viscous, dehydrated mucus that affects the respiratory, gastrointestinal, and genitourinary systems.

- Foreign body aspiration is most often caused by small objects that make their way into the child's mouth, such as foods, small toy parts, or household objects like beads, safety pins, coins, or buttons.

- A child can drown in as little water as it takes to cover the nose and mouth. Most drownings occur in the child's home pool or at the residence of a neighbor, friend, or relative. Other common drowning sites for young children include bathtubs, hot tubs, toilets, and even large water-filled buckets.

- Signs of smoke inhalation injury in children include burns of the face and neck, singed nasal hairs, soot around the mouth or nose, and hoarseness with stridor or voice change.

- Pulmonary contusion occurs in most children with nonpenetrating chest trauma. Although the child may appear initially asymptomatic, respiratory distress often develops in a few hours.

- A pneumothorax may become life threatening if internal pressure from a closed pneumothorax is not vented. Air leaking into the chest cavity during inspiration cannot escape during expiration, increasing compression. Venous blood return to the heart is impaired as the mediastinum shifts toward the unaffected lung.

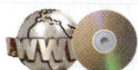

EXPLOREMEDIALINK

NCLEX Review, Case Studies, and other interactive resources for this chapter can be found on the companion website at http://www.prenhall.com/london. Click on "Chapter 42" and select the activities for this chapter.

For animations, more NCLEX review questions, and an audio glossary, access the accompanying CD-ROM in this textbook.

REFERENCES

Allshouse, M. J., & Eichelberger, M. R. (1993). Patterns of thoracic injury. In M. R. Eichelberger (Ed.), *Pediatric trauma: Prevention, acute care, rehabilitation* (pp. 437–448). St. Louis, MO: Mosby.

American Academy of Pediatrics Committee on Child Abuse and Neglect. (2001). Distinguishing sudden infant death syndrome from child abuse fatalities. *Pediatrics, 107*(2), 437–441.

American Thoracic Society and Centers for Disease Control and Prevention. (2000). Diagnostic standards and classification of tuberculosis in adults and children. *American Journal of Respiratory and Critical Care Medicine, 161,* 1376–1395.

Anbar, R. D. (2001, February). Self-hypnosis for management of chronic dyspnea in pediatric patients. *Pediatrics, 107*(2), E21.

Bank, D. E., & Krug, S. E. (1995). New approaches to upper airway disease. *Emergency Medical Clinics of North America, 13*(2), 473–487.

Brashers, V. L., & Davey, S. S. (1998). Alterations in pulmonary function. In K. L. McCance & S. E. Huether (Eds.), *Pathophysiology: The biologic basis for disease in adults and children* (3rd ed., pp. 1158–1200). St. Louis, MO: Mosby.

Cote, A., Gerez, T., Brouillette, R. T., & Laplante, S. (2000). Circumstances leading to a change to prone sleeping in sudden infant death syndrome victims. *Pediatrics, 106*(6), 1–5.

Daigle, K. L., & Cloutier, M. M. (1997). Office management of bronchopulmonary dysplasia. *Comprehensive Therapy, 23*(10), 656–663.

D'Auria, J. P. (1997). Respiratory system. In J. A. Fox (Ed.), *Primary health care of children* (pp. 415–418). St. Louis, MO: Mosby.

Eichelberger, M. R., Ball, J. W., Pratsch, G. S., & Clark, J. R. (1998). *Pediatric emergencies* (2nd ed.). Englewood Cliffs, NJ: Brady.

Farrell, P. M., Kosorok, M. R., Rock, M. J., Laxova, A., Zeng, L., Lai, H. C. et al. (2001). Early diagnosis of cystic fibrosis through neonatal screening prevents severe malnutrition and improves long term growth. *Pediatrics, 107*(1), 1–13.

Field, T., Henteleff, T., Hernandez-Reif, M., Martinez, E., Mavanda, K., Kuhn, C., et al. (1998). Children with asthma have improved pulmonary functions after massage therapy. *Journal of Pediatrics, 132*(5), 854–858.

Gilliland, F. D., YU-Fen, L., & Peters, J. M. (2001). Effects of maternal smoking during pregnancy and environmental tobacco smoke on asthmatic and wheezing in children. *American Journal of Respiratory and Critical Care Medicine, 163,* 429–436.

Gross, I. (1999). Respiratory distress syndrome. In J. A. McMillan, C. D. DeAngelis, R. D. Feigin, & J. B. Warshaw *Oski's pediatrics: Principles and practice* (3rd ed., pp. 254–258). Philadelphia: Lippincott, Williams & Wilkins.

Harvey, K. (2000). Bronchopulmonary dysplasia. In P. L. Jackson & J. A. Vessey (Eds.), *Primary care of the child with a chronic condition* (3rd ed., pp. 242–265). St. Louis, MO: Mosby.

Hazinski, M. F. (1999). *Manual of pediatric critical care.* St. Louis, MO: Mosby.

Health Resources and Services Administration's Maternal and Child Health Bureau. (2000). *Child health USA 2000.* Washington, DC: Government Printing Office.

Kaditis, A. G., & Wald, E. R. (1998). Viral croup: Current diagnosis and treatment. *Pediatric Infectious Disease Journal, 17*(9), 827–834.

Kemper, K. J., & Lester, M. R. (1999). Alternative asthma therapies: An evidence-based review. *Contemporary Pediatrics, 16,* 162–195.

Kieckhefer, G., & Ratcliffe, M. (2000). Asthma. In P. L. Jackson & J. A. Vessey (Eds.), *Primary care of the child with a chronic condition* (3rd ed., pp. 164–190). St. Louis, MO: Mosby.

Kohen, D. P., & Wynne, E. (1997). Applying hypnosis in a preschool family asthma education program: Uses of storytelling, imagery and relaxation. *American Journal of Clinical Hypnosis, 39,* 169–181.

Loughlin, G. M., & Carroll, J. L. (1999). Apparent life-threatening events. In J. A. McMillan, C. D. DeAngelis, R. D. Feigin & J. B. Warshaw *Oski's pediatrics: Principles and practice* (3rd ed., pp. 589–596). Philadelphia: Lippincott, Williams & Wilkins.

Margo, K., & Shaughnessy, A. (1998). Antiviral drugs in healthy children. *American Family Physician, 57*(5), 1073–1077.

Margolis, P., & Gadomski, A., (1998). Does this infant have pneumonia? *Journal of the American Medical Association, 279*(4), 308–313.

Markowitz, G. (2000, April). Don't be sidelined. Managing exercise-induced asthma in children. *Advanced Nurse Practitioner, 8*(4), 77–80.

McMullen, A. H. (2000). Cystic fibrosis. In P. L. Jackson & J. A. Vessey (Eds.), *Primary care of the child with a chronic condition* (3rd ed., pp. 401–425). St. Louis, MO: Mosby.

Merelle, M. E., Lees, C. M., Nagelkerke, A. F., & Dezateux, C. (2000). Newborn screening for cystic fibrosis. *The Cochrane Library, 4,* 1–19.

Milgrom, H., & Taussig, L. M. (1999, September). Keeping children with exercise-induced asthma active. *Pediatrics, 104*(3), e38.

Moon, R. Y., Patel, K. M., & Shaefer, S. J. M. (2000). Sudden infant death syndrome in child care settings. *Pediatrics, 106*(2), 295–300.

Murphy, S. A. (2000). *Deaths: Final data for 1998. National Vital Statistics Reports, 48*(11). Hyattsville, MD: National Center for Health Statistics.

Muscari, M. E. (1998). Coping with chronic illness. *American Journal of Nursing, 98*(9), 20–22.

National Asthma Education and Prevention Program. (1997). *Expert Panel Report II: Guide-*

lines for diagnosis and management of asthma (NIH Publication No. 97-4051). Bethesda, MD: National Institutes of Health.

National Respiratory and Enteric Virus Surveillance System. (2000). Respiratory syncytial virus activity—U.S., 1999–2000 season. *Morbidity and Mortality Weekly Report, 49*(48), 1091–1093.

Neuman, I., Nahum, H., & Ben-Amotz, A. (2000, December). Reduction of exercise-induced asthma oxidative stress by lycopene, a natural antioxidant. *Allergy, 55*(12), 1184–1189.

Ozuah, P. O., Ozuah, T. P., Stein, R. E. K., Burton, W., & Mulvihill, M. (2001). Evaluation of risk assessment questionnaire used to target tuberculin skin testing in children. *Journal of the American Medical Association, 285*(4), 451–453.

Panigrahy, A., Filiano, J. J., Sleeper, L. A., Mandell, F., Valdes-Depena, M., Krous, H. F., et al. (1997). Decreased kainite binding in the arcuate nucleus of the sudden infant death syndrome. *Journal of Neuropathology and Experimental Neurology, 56*(11), 1253–1261.

Pieper, P. (2000). Pediatric trauma. In B. V. Wise, C. McKenna, G. Garvin, & B. J. Harmon (Eds.), *Nursing care of the general pediatric surgical patient* (pp. 459–479). Gaithersburg, MD: Aspen.

Richman, E. (1997). Asthma diagnosis and management: New severity classifications and therapy alternatives. *Clinician Reviews, 7*(8), 76–112.

Rosenstein, B. J., & Cutting, G. R. (1998). The diagnosis of cystic fibrosis: A consensus statement. *Journal of Pediatrics, 132*(4), 589–595.

Rubin, R. (2001, April 2). Cystic fibrosis carrier testing gains support. *USA Today,* p. 5D.

Schweich, P. J., & Zempsky, W. T. (1999). Emergent issues. In J. A. McMillan, C. D. DeAngelis, R. D. Feigin & J. B. Warshaw *Oski's pediatrics: Principles and practice* (3rd ed., pp. 584–585). Philadelphia: Lippincott, Williams & Wilkins.

Steinbach, S. F. (2000). Four controversies in pediatric asthma care. *Contemporary Pediatrics, 17*(10), 150–172.

Stowe, C. D., & Jacobs, R. F. (1999). Treatment of tuberculosis infection and disease in children: The North American perspective. *Pediatric Drugs, 1*(4), 299–312.

Stricker, P. R. (2000). Swimming: A case-based approach to exercise-induced asthma and rotator cuff tendonitis. *Pediatric Annals, 29*(3), 166–70.

Stubblefield, C., & Murray, R. L. (2000). Making the transition: Pediatric lung transplantation. *Journal of Pediatric Health Care, 14*(6), 280–287.

Sydnor-Greenberg, N., & Dokken, D. (2000). Communicating information at diagnosis: Helping families and children manage asthma. *Journal of Child and Family Nursing, 3*(4), 290–295.

Theobald, K., Botwinski, C., Albanna, S., & McWilliam, P. (2000). Apnea of prematurity: Diagnosis, implications for care, and pharma-cologic management. *Neonatal Network, 19*(6), 17–24.

Tooley, W. H. (1996). Hyaline membrane disease. In A. M. Rudolph, J. I. E. Hoffman, & C. D. Rudolph (Eds.), *Rudolph's pediatrics* (20th ed., pp. 1598–1605). Stamford, CT: Appleton & Lange.

van Veldhoven, N. H., Vermeer, A., Bogaard, J. M., Hessels, M. G., Wijnroks, L., Colland, V. T., et al. (2001, August). Children with asthma and physical exercise: Effects of an exercise programme. *Clinical Rehabilitation, 15*(4), 360–370.

Varlotta, L. (1998). Management and care of the newly diagnosed patient with cystic fibrosis. *Current Opinion in Pulmonary Medicine, 4,* 311–318.

Vedanthan, P. K., Kesavalu, L. K., Murthy, K. C., Duvall, K., Hall, M. J., Baker, S., et al. (1998). Clinical study of yoga techniques in university students with asthma: A controlled study. *Allergy and Asthma Proceedings, 19*(1), 3–9.

Webster, H., & Huether, S. E. (1998). Alterations in pulmonary function in children. In K. L. McCance & S. E. Huether (Eds.), *Pathophysiology: The biologic basis for disease in adults and children* (3rd ed., pp. 1201–1220). St. Louis, MO: Mosby.

Wilson, D. C., & Pencharz, P. P. (1998). Nutrition and cystic fibrosis. *Nutrition, 14*(10), 792–795.

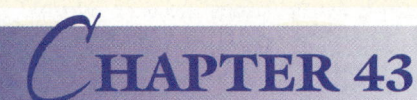

CHAPTER 43

The Child with Alterations in Cardiovascular Function

Brandy got sick so fast. Look how hard she is working to breathe. She gets tired before she can finish her formula. We didn't expect her to have to have heart surgery when she was still so small. We were told her chances for successful surgery would improve if she grew some more. I just want her to get stronger and have the chance to grow up to be like other kids.

—MOTHER OF BRANDY, 1 MONTH

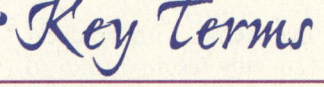

Key Terms

Compliance   *1066*
Desaturated blood   *1066*
Digitalization   *1067*
Hemodynamics   *1074*
Palliative procedure   *1085*

Polycythemia   *1066*
Preload   *1087*
Shunt   *1077*
Syncope   *1078*

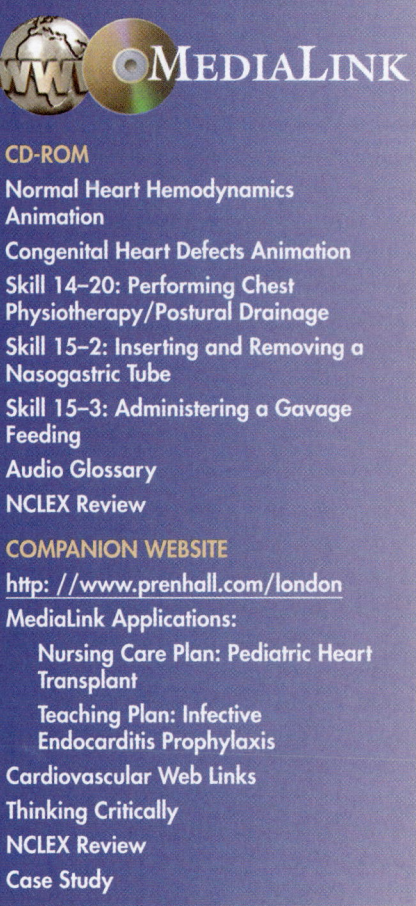

MEDIALINK

CD-ROM
Normal Heart Hemodynamics Animation
Congenital Heart Defects Animation
Skill 14–20: Performing Chest Physiotherapy/Postural Drainage
Skill 15–2: Inserting and Removing a Nasogastric Tube
Skill 15–3: Administering a Gavage Feeding
Audio Glossary
NCLEX Review

COMPANION WEBSITE
http://www.prenhall.com/london
MediaLink Applications:
   Nursing Care Plan: Pediatric Heart Transplant
   Teaching Plan: Infective Endocarditis Prophylaxis
Cardiovascular Web Links
Thinking Critically
NCLEX Review
Case Study

Alterations in cardiovascular function may be a result of a congenital defect, acquired infection, or injury. Congenital heart disease is the leading cause of death, excluding prematurity, during the first year of life (Kohr & Sims, 1998). At least 35 types of heart defects are recognized (American Heart Association, 2001). Congenital heart defects occur in approximately 1% of all live births and often require surgical correction (Hoffman, 1995). Rapid advances in the treatment of congenital heart defects allow children to have surgery at younger ages. As a result, nursing care required to identify and manage responses of infants and children with heart disease has become more challenging. [WEB]

ANATOMY AND PHYSIOLOGY OF PEDIATRIC DIFFERENCES

The transition from fetal to pulmonary circulation is described in Chapter 28. Systemic vascular resistance increases after the umbilical cord is cut. The increased blood and pressure in the left side of the heart stimulates the closure of the foramen ovale. The ductus arteriosus normally constricts and closes within 10 to 15 hours after birth in response to higher oxygen saturation levels. The ventricles are equal in size at birth, but by 2 months of age the left ventricle is twice as large as the right ventricle. The higher systemic vascular pressures force the left ventricle to develop quickly. [CD]

Infants have a greater risk of heart failure than older children because the immature heart is more sensitive to volume or pressure overload. During infancy the muscle fibers of the heart are less developed and less organized, resulting in limited functional capacity. Less **compliance** (amount of distention or expansion the ventricles can achieve to increase stroke volume) of the heart muscle means that the stroke volume (cardiac output) cannot increase substantially. The heart muscle fibers develop during early childhood and by 9 years of age, the weight of the heart has increased by 6 times (Kohr & Sims, 1998).

Oxygenation

Oxygen bound to hemoglobin is transported to the tissues by the systemic circulation. Hematocrit and hemoglobin concentrations appropriate for the child's age are necessary for adequate oxygen transport (see Chapter 44). The oxygen arterial saturation is the amount of oxygen that can potentially be delivered to the tissues. **Desaturated blood** results when oxygenated and unoxygenated blood mix because of a congenital heart defect. Cyanosis, which indicates hypoxemia (lower than normal amounts of oxygen in the blood), results when 5 or more grams of unoxygenated hemoglobin are present per 100 mL of blood (Park, 1996). A pulse oximeter provides a noninvasive arterial oxygen saturation level. A reading of 95% to 98% is normal in children. The following values indicate hypoxemia:

- Mild hypoxemia: 90% to 95%
- Moderate hypoxemia: 85% to 90%
- Severe hypoxemia: < 85%

The child's bone marrow responds to chronic hypoxemia by producing more red blood cells to increase the amount of hemoglobin available for oxygenation. This increase is known as **polycythemia.** A hematocrit value of 50% or higher is common in children with cyanotic heart defects. Extreme polycythemia, a hemoglobin concentration greater than 20 g/dL and a hematocrit greater than 55% to 60%, is dangerous. Blood viscosity is increased, and the child is at risk for a thromboembolism (Park, 1996).

Cardiac Functioning

Oxygen requirements are high for the first 8 weeks of life. Normally the newborn's heart rate increases to provide adequate oxygen transport. The infant has little cardiac output reserve capacity until oxygen requirements begin to decrease. Cardiac output depends almost completely on heart rate until the heart muscle is fully developed at 5 years of age. Weight-specific cardiac output decreases during childhood. During stress, exercise, fever, or respiratory distress, infants and children have tachycardia, which increases their cardiac output.

Children respond to severe hypoxemia with bradycardia. Cardiac arrest in children generally results from prolonged hypoxemia related to respiratory failure or shock rather than from a primary cardiac insult as in adults. Bradycardia is therefore a significant warning sign of cardiac arrest. Appropriate management of hypoxemia reverses bradycardia and prevents cardiac arrest.

CONGESTIVE HEART FAILURE

Congestive heart failure is a disorder of circulation in which cardiac output is inadequate to support the body's circulatory and metabolic needs. It may result from a congenital heart defect that causes increased pulmonary blood flow or obstruction to the blood outflow tract, from problems with heart contractility, or from pathologic conditions that require high cardiac output, such as severe anemia, acidosis, or respiratory disease.

Etiology and Pathophysiology

Congenital heart defects [CD] are the most common cause of congestive heart failure in children (Wolfe, Boucek, Schaffer, et al., 1997). Some defects allow blood to flow from the left side of the heart to the right so that extra blood must be pumped to the pulmonary system rather than through the aorta when the left ventricle contracts. This overloads the pulmonary system, and if prolonged can lead to pulmonary artery hypertension, an often irreversible condition leading to life-threatening pulmonary vascular resistance (see p. 1088). Obstructive congenital defects (i.e., abnormally small pulmonary vessels) restrict the flow of blood so the heart hypertrophies to work harder to force blood through these structures. This increases cardiac output initially, but eventually the hypertrophied muscle becomes ineffective (Balaguru, Artman, & Auslender, 2000). Initially one side of the heart may fail, but eventually failure is bilateral.

When cardiac output remains insufficient, the body's organs and tissues do not receive adequate oxygen. The kidneys respond to the lowered circulating volume by activating the renin-angiotensin mechanism to retain salt and water. A sympathetic response increases the heart rate and heart muscle contractility. Both responses increase cardiac output to the vital organs. Without intervention, the compensatory mechanisms increase their intensity, demanding more effort from the compromised heart. This results in progressive systemic edema and pulmonary congestion.

Clinical Manifestations

Congestive heart failure often develops subtly, and symptoms may not be recognized at first. The infant tires easily, especially during feeding. Weight loss or lack of normal weight gain, diaphoresis, irritability, and frequent infections may be evident. Older children may have exercise intolerance, dyspnea, abdominal pain or distention, and peripheral edema.

As the disease progresses, symptoms such as tachypnea, tachycardia, pallor or cyanosis, nasal flaring, grunting, retractions, cough, or crackles may occur. Generalized fluid volume overload is seen more commonly in toddlers and older children. Periorbital and facial edema and hepatomegaly are signs of fluid volume excess. Jugular vein distention is seen in older children.

Cardiomegaly occurs as the heart attempts to maintain cardiac output. Cyanosis, weak peripheral pulses, cool extremities, hypotension, and heart murmur are precursors of cardiogenic shock, which can occur if congestive heart failure is not adequately treated. (Cardiogenic shock is discussed later in this chapter.)

Clinical Therapy

Diagnosis is based primarily on clinical manifestations such as tachycardia, respiratory distress, and crackles. A chest x-ray study reveals cardiac enlargement and venous congestion or signs of pulmonary edema. Echocardiography may be performed to diagnose specific cardiac defects or dysfunction. An electrocardiogram may show tachycardia, bradycardia, or ventricular hypertrophy.

The goals of medical management are to make the heart work more efficiently and to remove excess fluid, thus improving systemic circulation without flooding the pulmonary system. Inotropic medicines and afterload-reducing agents (angiotensin-converting enzyme inhibitors) are sometimes used to lessen the workload of the heart and help it to work more efficiently (Balaguru et al., 2000). Digoxin is the drug most commonly used to improve the heart's ability to contract and therefore increase its output. Occasionally a higher than normal dose is given initially, followed by a lower maintenance dose. This process, called **digitalization,** speeds the child's response to the drug. β-blockers are used in some cases to reduce the effects of catecholamines on heart rate and contractility (O'Laughlin, 1999).

Nursing Practice

Digoxin and digitoxin are both digitalis preparations but are not the same drug. Digoxin is the drug of choice in pediatrics. Digitoxin is 10 times more powerful than digoxin, and is rarely used in children. Read labels carefully and double-check doses to ensure that you give the child the right dose of the right drug.

Diuretics, such as furosemide, chlorothiazide, and spironolactone, are given to promote fluid excretion (Table 43–1). Furosemide is the most commonly used medication during hospitalization; thiazides are commonly used to maintain diuresis at home. Because most diuretics (except for spironolactone) cause potassium loss, serum potassium levels are monitored and potassium supplements may be ordered. Vasodilating drugs may be given to reduce pulmonary and systemic vasoconstriction and to decrease the work of the heart.

CLINICAL MANIFESTATIONS ≈ *Congestive Heart Failure*	
CAUSE	**CLINICAL MANIFESTATION**
Pulmonary venous congestion	Tachypnea, wheezing, crackles, retractions, cough, grunting, nasal flaring, feeding difficulties, irritability, tiring with play
Systemic venous congestion	Hepatomegaly, ascites, peripheral edema
Impaired cardiac output	Tachycardia, diminished pulses, hypotension, capillary refill time > 2 seconds, pallor, cool extremities, oliguria
High metabolic rate	Failure to thrive or slow weight gain

TABLE 43–1	Drugs Used in Treatment of Congestive Heart Failure
Drug	Action
Digoxin	Increases myocardial contractility
Furosemide	Rapid diuresis
Thiazides	Maintenance diuresis
Chlorothiazide (suspension)	
Hydrochlorthiazide (tablets)	
Spironolactone	Maintenance diuresis (potassium-sparing)
ACEi (angiotensin-converting enzyme inhibitor)	Promotes vascular relaxation and reduced peripheral vascular resistance
Propranolol	Increases contractility

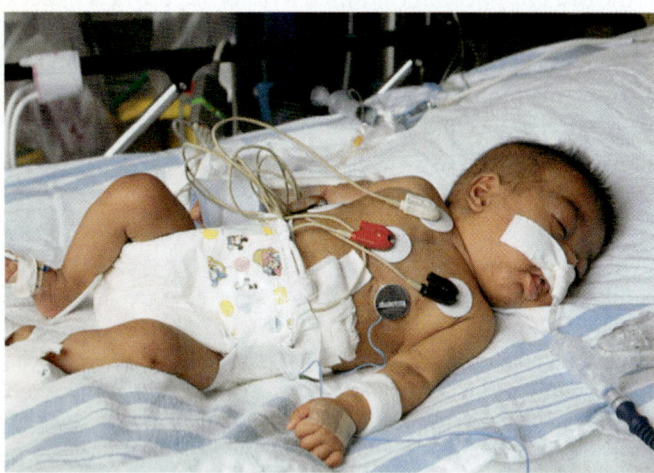

FIGURE 43–1. ◆ Jooti is receiving intravenous fluids and oxygen. Her condition is being continuously monitored for congestive heart failure.

Surgery or interventional catheterization to correct a congenital heart defect may become the treatment of choice. Cardiac transplantation may be performed for children with end-stage cardiomyopathy or complex congenital heart defects such as hypoplastic left heart syndrome.

Other medical therapy is supportive. Airway management, ventilatory support, rest, and fluid and dietary management are also part of the treatment plan. Oxygen may be ordered (Figure 43–1 ◆). Most children improve rapidly after medication is administered.

Nursing Management

Nursing Assessment and Diagnosis

PHYSIOLOGIC ASSESSMENT

As diagnosis of congestive heart failure depends primarily on physical symptoms, nursing observations are important. Assess the child's behavioral patterns (e.g., playfulness, irritability), cardiac function, respiratory function, and fluid status. Use the age-specific heart and respiratory rates in Tables 33–12 and 33–14 to identify tachycardia and tachypnea. ⚬▭ Obtain a detailed history of the onset of symptoms from the parents, as congestive heart failure often develops slowly.

PSYCHOSOCIAL ASSESSMENT

Take a history of the child's previous hospitalizations and assess the family's knowledge about the child's condition. Families of children with congestive heart failure are anxious and fear the potentially serious outcome of the problem and the need to provide ongoing care. Assess the family's anxiety level and coping strategies. Evaluate the family's economic status. Medication is crucial to treatment, and a family's inability to afford or obtain the necessary medications jeopardizes the child's outcome.

The family is often overprotective and reluctant to leave the child with other caregivers. Find out if a knowledgeable person who can safely administer medications and watch the child is available for respite care.

DEVELOPMENTAL ASSESSMENT

Since fatigue limits the activities of the child with congestive heart failure, the child does not have the opportunity to practice the skills needed to attain normal developmental milestones. Assess development with a tool such as the Denver II (see Chapter 35). ⚬▭ In addition, parents can provide information about the attainment of expected developmental milestones such as sitting, manipulating objects, standing, or walking. When congestive heart failure is well controlled, the child's energy level increases and developmental skills often improve. In infants and toddlers, assessments every 2 to 3 months are useful to observe development and evaluate disease management.

Parents may limit the child's contact with other children because of frequent infections and exercise intolerance. Ask parents about contact and play with other children and a typical day's activity schedule.

Several nursing diagnoses that may apply to the child with congestive heart failure can be found in the accompanying "Nursing Care Plans." The primary nursing diagnosis is decreased cardiac output related to cardiac anomaly.

Planning and Implementation

Nursing care for the child with congestive heart failure focuses on administering and monitoring effects of medications, maintaining adequate oxygenation and myocardial function, promoting rest, fostering development, providing adequate nutrition, and providing emotional support to the child and family. (See "Nursing Care Plan: The Child Hospitalized with Congestive Heart Failure.")

ADMINISTER AND MONITOR PRESCRIBED MEDICATIONS

Children with congestive heart failure usually receive digoxin and furosemide. These medications are potent and must be administered correctly.

GOAL	INTERVENTION	RATIONALE	EXPECTED OUTCOME

1. Decreased cardiac output related to cardiac anomaly (VSD)

	NIC Priority Intervention:		*NOC Suggested Outcome:*
	Hemodynamic regulation: *Optimization of heart rate, preload, afterload, and contractility*		**Cardiac pump effectiveness:** *Extent to which blood is ejected from the left ventricle per minute to support systemic perfusion pressure*
The child's cardiac output will be sufficient to meet the body's metabolic demands.	▸ Administer digoxin as ordered.	▸ Digoxin increases contractility of the heart and force of contraction.	The child's cardiac output is sufficient as indicated by increased energy, adequate feeding intake, and decreased edema.
	▸ Take apical pulse and listen to heart sounds regularly, especially before each dose of digoxin. Record apical pulse with each recorded dose of digoxin.	▸ Digoxin may cause bradycardia. Pulse and heart sounds provide information about heart functioning.	
	▸ Use cardiac monitor if ordered.	▸ Monitor notes tachycardia and arrhythmias.	
	▸ Prevent injury by monitoring for digoxin side effects and serum potassium level.	▸ Digoxin is a potent drug with serious side effects. Hypokalemia increases risk of digoxin toxicity.	The child maintains normal serum levels of potassium and therapeutic levels of digoxin.
	▸ Provide for rest periods each hour.	▸ Rest decreases need for high cardiac output.	The child rests hourly and has adequate energy to eat and play.
The child will manifest adequate oxygenation.	▸ Place child in semi-Fowler's position.	▸ Position facilitates lung expansion.	
	▸ Evaluate respiratory rate and sounds. Take pulse oximetry readings to determine oxygen saturation.	▸ Absence of tachypnea and adventitious sounds and oxygen saturation above 95% indicate ease of respiration.	The child has normal respiratory rate for age with no evidence of adventitious sounds or diaphoresis.
	▸ Provide oxygen and humidification if ordered. Observe for diaphoresis, a sign of increased respiratory effort.	▸ Supplemental oxygen decreases tachypnea, and humidification moistens secretions to keep airway clear.	

2. Fluid volume excess related to heart failure

	NIC Priority Intervention:		*NOC Suggested Outcome:*
	Fluid management: *Promotion of fluid balance and prevention of complications resulting from abnormal or undesired fluid levels*		**Fluid balance:** *Balance of water in the intracellular and extracellular compartments of the body*
The child's urinary output will remain within normal levels. Intake and output will be balanced.	▸ Measure intake and output carefully. Weigh diapers to obtain output of young child.	▸ Adequate output is a good indicator of renal perfusion.	The child's intake and output are proportional, and electrolyte levels remain within normal ranges.
	▸ Maintain fluid-restricted diet if ordered.	▸ Fluid restriction is sometimes used to decrease cardiac load.	
	▸ Administer diuretics as ordered.	▸ Diuretics mobilize fluids and facilitate excretion.	
	▸ Monitor electrolytes.	▸ Electrolyte imbalance is common when fluids are restricted and diuretics are given.	
	▸ Weigh daily. Measure abdominal girth daily if present. Observe for peripheral edema.	▸ Evaluations demonstrate effectiveness of treatment.	

3. Risk for impaired skin integrity related to altered fluid status.

	NIC Priority Intervention:		*NOC Suggested Outcome:*
	Pressure management: *Minimizing pressure to body parts*		**Risk control:** *Actions to eliminate or reduce actual, personal, and modifiable health threats*
The child's peripheral and central edema will decrease.	▸ Provide skin care for edematous body parts and elevate extremities.	▸ Edematous skin injures easily. Elevation promotes return of fluid from extremities.	The child has no skin breakdown after edema resolves.
	▸ Change child's position frequently.	▸ Position change promotes circulation to skin over pressure points.	
	▸ Inspect skin frequently for redness and skin breakdown over pressure points.	▸ Inspection identifies earliest stages of skin breakdown.	

(continued)

GOAL	INTERVENTION	RATIONALE	EXPECTED OUTCOME
4. Altered nutrition: less than body requirements related to high metabolic needs and rapid tiring while feeding			
	NIC Priority Intervention:		*NOC Suggested Outcome:*
	Nutrition management: *Assistance with or provision of a balanced dietary intake of food and fluids*		**Nutrition status:** *Extent to which nutrients are available to meet metabolic needs*
The infant or child will demonstrate normal weight gain for age.	▸ Hold infant at 45-degree angle for feeding.	▸ Position facilitates breathing while eating.	The infant or child gains recommended weight according to growth grids. All dietary requirements are met, and mealtimes are pleasant.
	▸ Record intake carefully.	▸ Evaluation of intake indicates whether caloric and other nutritional needs are met.	
	▸ Weigh child daily.	▸ Weight indicates growth (in absence of edematous symptoms of congestive heart failure).	
	▸ Give frequent small meals with rest periods in between. Give high-calorie snacks.	▸ Digesting small meals requires less energy. High-calorie snacks provide calories efficiently.	
	▸ Use soothing approaches such as holding infants for feeding and having parents eat with older child.	▸ Restful approach facilitates intake with minimum cardiac work.	
5. Ineffective family coping, compromised, related to unknown nature of child's disease			
	NIC Priority Intervention:		*NOC Suggested Outcome:* Not yet developed
	Family involvement: *Facilitating family participation in the emotional and physical care of the patient*		
Parents will express lessened anxiety as hospitalization proceeds.	▸ Encourage parents to room-in or stay with child. Explain procedures and treatment. Involve parents in care as much as possible. Have parents plan child's play periods.	▸ Involvement in child's care lessens parental anxiety and fear of unknown.	Parents participate in developing and implementing the treatment plan and providing care to the child.
	▸ At discharge, provide clear instructions and information about what to do in an emergency, and whom and where to call with questions.	▸ Having resources available provides feelings of security.	
	▸ Allow parents to verbalize questions, concerns, and feelings. Refer parents to support groups or other resources as needed.	▸ Emotional support is needed to lessen anxiety.	

Measure intake and output carefully (see Skill 9–21). SKILLS Weigh the infant's diapers before and after changing (1 g = 1 mL urine). Observe for changes in peripheral edema and circulation. Weigh the child at the same time each day because fluid volume varies throughout the day (see Skill 9–3). If ascites is present, take serial abdominal measurements to monitor changes (see Skill 9–7). SKILLS CD Turn the child frequently, and provide skin care when edema is present (see Figure 39–8).

MAINTAIN OXYGENATION AND MYOCARDIAL FUNCTION

Oxygen therapy may be ordered. Make sure that tubing is patent, the oxygen flow rate is correct, the oxygen delivery device is working properly, and humidification is provided. Keep the child calm and quiet. Position the child in a semi-Fowler's or 45-degree angle position to promote maximum oxygenation.

PROMOTE REST

Group assessments and interventions together to ensure that the child has some uninterrupted rest each hour. Feedings should last no more than 20 to 30 minutes. Frequent small feedings generally work best, with burping after every half ounce of intake to minimize vomiting. Rocking is restful for infants. Encourage older children to engage in quiet activities such as playing board games or watching television.

FOSTER DEVELOPMENT

Encourage parents to play with the child, using toys to stimulate eye–hand coordination and fine motor movements. Such toys include rattles, blocks, and stuffed animals for infants and books, paper and pencil, and dolls for older children. Encourage sitting, standing, or walking for short periods with adequate rest afterward to promote the

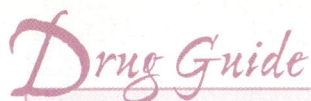

DIGOXIN

Action

Digoxin acts on the heart to increase myocardial contractility and automaticity, to reduce excitability and conduction velocity, and to prolong the refractory period. It inhibits activity of an enzyme that transports sodium across cell membranes, thus, sodium may be retained and potassium lost from the myocardium. Digoxin is used in the treatment of congestive heart failure and for ventricular rate control in atrial flutter and atrial fibrillation.

Routes, Dosage, Frequency

Dosage varies by age and whether giving a digitalizing or maintenance dose.

Tablets and Elixir

Digitalizing dose:

- Premature neonates: 20 to 35 μg/kg in 2 or more doses
- Neonates: 25 to 35 μg/kg in 2 or more doses
- 1 to 24 months: 35 to 60 μg/kg in 2 or more doses
- 2 to 5 years: 30 to 40 μg/kg in 2 or more doses
- 5 to 10 years: 20 to 35 μg/kg in 2 or more doses
- Over 10 years: 10 to 15 μg/kg in 2 or more doses

Maintenance dose:

- Premature neonates: 20% to 30% of digitalizing dose given daily
- Neonates, infants, children: 25% to 35% of digitalizing dose given daily
- 10 years and over: 125 to 250 μg/day

Alternate for maintenance dose: elixir may be calculated as 17 μg/kg given in divided doses.

Capsules

Digitalizing dose:

- 2 to 5 years: 25 to 35 μg/kg in 2 or more doses
- 5 to10 years: 15 to 30 μg/kg in 2 or more doses
- Over 10 years: 8 to 12 μg/kg/day in 2 or more doses

Maintenance dose:

- Children 25% to 35% of digitalizing dose in 2 to 3 daily doses
- 10 years and over: 125 to 250 μg/day

Intravenous

Digitalizing dose:

- Premature neonate: 15 to 25 μg/kg in 3 or more doses
- Neonate: 20 to 30 μg/kg in 3 or more doses
- 1 to 24 months: 30 to 50 μg/kg in 3 or more doses
- 2 to 5 years: 25 to 35 μg/kg in 3 or more doses
- 5 to 10 years: 15 to 30 μg/kg in 3 or more doses
- Over 10 years: 8 to 12 μg/kg in 3 or more doses

Maintenance dose:

- Premature neonates: 20% to 30% of digitalizing dose in 2 to 3 daily doses
- Neonates, infants, children: 25% to 35% of digitalizing dose in 2 to 3 daily doses
- 10 years and over: 25% to 35% of digitalizing dose given once daily

Doses are reduced in renal dysfunction, especially if creatinine clearance is under 10 mL/minute.

Nursing Management

Assessment: Before giving digitalizing dose, establish baseline vital signs and ECG. Check serum electrolytes, hepatic and renal function. Assess hydration status, and hydrate if hypovolemic.

Administration: Digoxin is given intravenously or orally in extremely small doses. Carefully measure and verify the doses. Digitalizing or loading doses are divided, with about half given initially and a quarter dose at 4 to 8 hours intravenously or at 6 to 8 hours orally.

PO: Give at same times daily with or without food to ensure equivalent bioavailability. Food will slow absorption, but it does not decrease total absorption. Use the provided calibrated dropper for the elixir. Be certain to administer digoxin, *not digitoxin*, tablets.

IV: Dilute dose with at least four times the volume, using sterile water, 5% dextrose, or saline, and administer over at least 5 minutes. Use immediately after dilution. Do not mix with other medications. Patients are changed from IV to PO form as soon as possible.

Monitor

- Before giving any dose take apical pulse for 1 minute. If bradycardia is detected (< 100 beats/min for infants and toddlers, < 80 beats/min in older children, or < 60 beats/min in adolescents, or below a guideline noted in the physician's order), call for a physician's advice before administering the drug.
- Monitor ECG during IV dose. The dosage is carefully individualized, and the drug has a low therapeutic index; so monitoring is critical.
- Monitor hepatic and renal functions. Dosage will be reduced if creatinine clearance is 50 mL/minute or less. Check serum electrolytes, particularly potassium, calcium, and magnesium; closely monitor those also on diuretics.
- Digoxin overdose is more common when potassium levels are low, so check serum potassium levels when a potassium-depleting diuretic is given. Serum potassium of 3.5 mmol/L or less may be a contraindication to digoxin administration; clarify this possible contraindication with the child's physician. If a child taking digoxin orally is NPO or vomiting, seek a physician's order regarding the course of action; the drug must not be omitted.
- Observe the child carefully for digoxin toxicity. Early signs include tachycardia in young children and nausea, vomiting, anorexia, dizziness, headache, weakness, fatigue, arrhythmia, or bradycardia in older children.
- Serum digoxin levels are taken 6 to 8 hours after a dose. A therapeutic serum level ranges from 1.1 to 1.7 ng/mL. Levels below 0.5 ng/mL are ineffective, and those over 2 ng/mL can lead to toxicity.
- If routes of administration are changed, absorption of digoxin may be altered, so careful monitoring of intake and output is required.
- Generally, tablets and elixir dosages will need to be decreased by 20% to 25% when changing to IV or capsule preparations.

Note: From Bindler, R. M., & Howry, L. B. (1997). *Pediatric drugs and nursing implications* (2nd ed.). Upper Saddle River, NJ: Prentice Hall-Health.

development of large muscles. Singing, talking, and playing music facilitate cognitive and language skills.

PROVIDE ADEQUATE NUTRITION

Teach parents about feeding techniques. Encourage the mother who chooses to breastfeed the infant. The antibodies in breast milk reduce infections, and the milk is naturally low in sodium. However, the sucking involved in breast- or bottle-feeding may cause dyspnea that forces the infant to rest frequently during feeding.

Infants should be burped frequently to permit rest and prevent vomiting. They may need small frequent feedings and longer feeding periods. Positioning the baby in an infant seat at a 45-degree angle decreases venous return to the heart and decreases its metabolic demand. This is a favorable position for feeding and other activities (Kohr & Sims, 1998).

Make sure parents understand that changes in feeding habits (decreased intake, vomiting, sleeping through feedings, increased perspiration with feedings) may indicate deteriorating cardiac status. The American Heart Association publishes the booklet *Feeding Infants with Congenital Heart Disease* for parents. ⊂⊃ WEB

The infant needs adequate nutrition to support growth. It is not unusual for infants with heart problems to develop failure to thrive as the result of feeding difficulties. (See Chapter 31.) ⊂⊃ When infants have significant dyspnea with feeding, special feeding techniques are needed. Some infants need a higher caloric formula (24 to 30 calories per ounce) to obtain adequate nutrition. Other infants require nutritional supplementation by nasogastric or gastrostomy tube (Figure 43–2 ◆). Parents are often advised to give the infant a chance to feed normally for a specific

period. The remainder of the formula is then given by nasogastric or gastrostomy tube. (See Skills 15–2 and 15-3) ⊂⊃ SKILLS CD

PROVIDE EMOTIONAL SUPPORT

When a child is hospitalized with congestive heart failure, the family is often anxious about his or her condition. Give parents a chance to express concerns about their child's condition. Explain the child's treatment regimen, and make sure family members understand the child's need for nutrition and rest. Answering questions about the child's prognosis and the ultimate outcome can be reassuring. Give family members information, and relay questions to the physician. Talking to other parents of children with cardiac conditions may be a source of emotional support. Refer parents to the appropriate support groups.

DISCHARGE PLANNING AND HOME CARE TEACHING

Identify and address home care needs well in advance of discharge. Show parents how to feed the child to maximize nutritional intake. While the child is hospitalized, teach the family about the administration of medications and signs of a worsening condition. Tell them to watch for symptoms such as increased feeding difficulty, irritability, lethargy, breathing difficulty, and puffiness around the eyes or extremities, which indicate that congestive heart failure is worsening. Parents are frequently taught to take the child's pulse and to report any significant change to the physician. An increase in pulse rate can signal congestive heart failure, and a decrease can indicate digoxin toxicity.

Demonstrate administration of drugs, and then supervise while the parents measure and administer medications. Teach parents about the toxic effects of digoxin and other drugs. Advise them to notify the physician immediately if any of these side effects occur. Because digoxin is a potential poison, encourage parents to keep it locked up at home and away from children. In case of accidental ingestion, immediate medical care is needed. Be sure parents keep the poison control number on all phones.

NURSING CARE IN THE COMMUNITY

"Nursing Care Plan: The Child with Congestive Heart Failure Being Cared for at Home" outlines home care. Parents play a critical role in the care of the child with heart disease by facilitating normal development and limiting the incidence of congestive heart failure.

Evaluate family resources so that adequate child or respite care can be arranged if needed. Show the family how to assess the child's energy level, and how to observe for feeding problems and edema. Observe medication administration and correct any errors. Watch the child feeding and make suggestions as necessary.

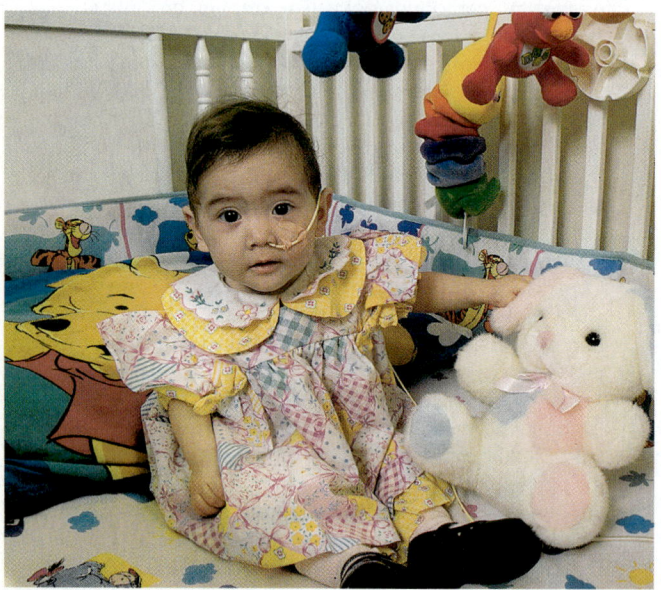

FIGURE 43–2. ◆ Infants with cardiac conditions often require supplemental feedings to provide sufficient nutrients for growth and development. The parents of this infant girl have been taught how to give her nasogastric feedings at home.

Evaluation

Expected outcomes of nursing care can be found in the "Nursing Care Plans."

GOAL	INTERVENTION	RATIONALE	EXPECTED OUTCOME
1. Altered growth and development related to effects of physical disability			
	NIC Priority Intervention: **Developmental enhancement:** *Teaching parents to facilitate optimal gross motor, fine motor, language, cognitive, social, and emotional growth of preschool children*		NOC Suggested Outcome: **Child development** (2 years): *Milestones of physical, cognitive, and psychosocial progression by 2 years of age*
The child will meet developmental milestones for age group.	▸ Perform baseline developmental assessment. ▸ Plan for short play periods after rest. ▸ Introduce age-appropriate toys and activities such as rattles and blocks for infants and art projects for older children. ▸ Plan for interactions with healthy children.	▸ Assessment provides comparison for later assessments and basis for planning specific games, toys, and activities. ▸ Short play periods maintain energy and facilitate play. ▸ Play activities facilitate learning and mastery of developmental tasks. ▸ Social skills are learned through contact with others.	The child displays normal language, fine motor, and gross motor activity.
2. Ineffective management of therapeutic regimen (family) related to complexity of therapeutic regimen			
	NIC Priority Intervention: **Family involvement:** *Facilitating family participation in the emotional and physical care of the patient*		NOC Suggested Outcome: Not yet developed
Parents will demonstrate correct administration of medications. Parents will state side effects of medications and symptoms of congestive heart failure.	▸ Demonstrate administration of digoxin, diuretics, and other medications. Have parents administer them under supervision of nurse. ▸ Describe side effects of medications. Give parents handouts with telephone number to call to ask questions or report side effects. ▸ Describe subtle onset of congestive heart failure and its symptoms (increasing weakness, exhaustion, irritability, difficulty feeding, cough or difficult respirations, edema).	▸ Demonstration with return demonstration is an excellent method of learning psychomotor skills. ▸ If side effects are understood, serious complications can be avoided. ▸ Parents can evaluate child regularly and note subtle changes requiring medical management.	Parents report that child continues to demonstrate improvement and adequate cardiac output with absence of congestive heart failure.
3. Altered nutrition: less than body requirements related to chronic illness and tiring while feeding			
	NIC Priority Intervention: **Weight gain assistance:** *Facilitation of body weight gain*		NOC Suggested Outcome: **Nutritional status: Food and fluid intake:** *Amount of food and fluid taken into the body over a 24-hour period*
The infant or child will demonstrate normal weight gain for age.	▸ Teach parents methods to promote food intake related to positioning, size of feedings, food choices. ▸ Observe feeding during home visit.	▸ Positioning, frequency of feedings, size of feedings, and use of high-caloric foods can enhance nutritional intake. ▸ Feedback can assist parents in integrating positive feeding techniques.	The infant or child shows normal weight gain. Parents report and demonstrate successful feedings of child.
4. Activity intolerance (child) related to poor cardiac output			
	NIC Priority Intervention: **Energy management:** *Regulating energy use to treat or prevent fatigue and optimize function*		NOC Suggested Outcome: **Energy conservation:** *Extent of active management of energy to initiate or sustain activity*
The child will perform all necessary activities of daily living without undue tiring.	▸ Help parents alternate activities and rest throughout the child's day. ▸ Have parents limit child's exposure to persons with contagious disease. ▸ Help family plan quiet surroundings to provide for child's rest.	▸ Activities to promote development must be alternated with rest due to decreased cardiac output. ▸ When the child is ill and tired, the immune system can be compromised. ▸ Home setting may need to be altered to promote rest.	The child performs necessary activities and rests frequently each day.

(continued)

GOAL	INTERVENTION	RATIONALE	EXPECTED OUTCOME
5. Caregiver role strain (parent) related to 24-hour responsibility for child's care			
	NIC Priority Intervention: **Caregiver support:** *Provision of the necessary information, advocacy, and support to facilitate primary patient care by someone other than a health care professional*		*NOC Suggested Outcome:* **Caregiver endurance potential:** *Factors that promote family care provider continuance over an extended period of time*
Parents will express ability to meet own needs.	▶ Assess family and community supports. Provide information related to respite care. ▶ Encourage parents to seek activities to meet personal needs.	▶ Variable family and community supports are available. ▶ Parents need time to meet own personal needs in order to successfully care for child.	Parents report some time away from the child and report renewal in caring for the child.

〰 CONGENITAL HEART DISEASE

Congenital heart disease refers to a defect in the heart or great vessels, or persistence of a fetal structure after birth. Congenital heart defects occur in an estimated 1% of live births (American Heart Association, 2001). In spontaneously aborted and stillborn fetuses the incidence is much higher. People with congenital heart disease are living longer. Between 1979 and 1997, deaths from heart defects declined by 39.4% (Boneva, Botto, Moore, et al., 2001). This is attributed to diagnostic advances, surgical technique refinements, and intensive care.

Congenital heart defects develop during the early weeks of pregnancy. They are usually the result of a combined or interactive effect of genetic and environmental factors, such as:

- Fetal exposure to drugs such as phenytoin and lithium
- Maternal viral infections such as rubella
- Maternal metabolic disorders such as phenylketonuria and diabetes mellitus
- Maternal complications of pregnancy such as increased age and antepartal bleeding
- Genetic factors (family recurrence patterns)
- Chromosomal abnormalities such as Turner syndrome, Noonan syndrome, Marfan syndrome, DiGeorge syndrome, cri du chat syndrome, Down syndrome, and trisomy syndromes 13, 15, 18, and 21 (Kohr & Sims, 1998). The prevalence of heart defects in children with Down syndrome is about 40% (Lewin, 2000).

Chromosome 22q11 is one of the most frequent genetic sites associated with development of cardiovascular defects such as truncus arteriosus, tetralogy of Fallot, and pulmonary atresia (Lewin, 2000). Because of this genetic component, the incidence of congenital heart defects is expected to slowly rise as people with some of these defects

survive and have children of their own. A child often has more than one defect at the same time. Depending on the type of defect, signs and symptoms may be present at birth or develop later.

Nursing Practice

Evidence is emerging that the use of multivitamins by women at the time of conception may reduce the risk of certain defects (transposition of the great vessels, tetralogy of Fallot, and truncus arteriosus) (Botto, Khoury, Mulinare, et al., 1996).

Congenital heart defects 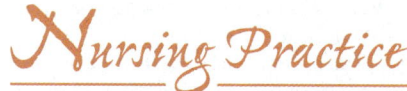 are generally divided into two categories, cyanotic and acyanotic, based on the hallmark sign of cyanosis. However, a child with an acyanotic defect may show clinical signs of cyanosis. The pathophysiology of a heart defect is related to **hemodynamics,** the pressures generated by blood and the pathways blood takes through the heart and pulmonary system. In some cases the blood flow to the pulmonary system is increased, leading to congestive heart failure.

ACYANOTIC DEFECTS

Most children with congenital heart defects have acyanotic conditions. There are two types of acyanotic defects: nonobstructive lesions, which do not interfere with the flow of blood, and obstructive lesions, which block the outflow of blood from the heart. Nonobstructive defects include patent ductus arteriosus (PDA), atrial septal defect (ASD), atrioventricular canal (endocardial cushion defect), and ventricular septal defect (VSD). Obstructive defects include pulmonic stenosis (PS), aortic stenosis (AS), and coarctation of the aorta. Tables 43–2 and 43–3 summarize the pathophysiology, clinical manifestations, and clinical therapy for these defects.

Patent Ductus Arteriosus (PDA)

PDA is a common congenital defect caused by persistent fetal circulation that accounts for 9% to 12% of all congenital heart defects (Driscoll, 1999). When pulmonary circulation is established and systemic vascular resistance increases at birth, pressures in the aorta become greater than in the pulmonary arteries. Blood is then shunted from the aorta to the pulmonary arteries, increasing circulation to the pulmonary system.

Clinical Manifestations

Dyspnea; tachypnea; full, bounding pulses; and poor development occur. Infant is at risk for frequent respiratory infections and infective endocarditis. With a large PDA, right-sided congestive heart failure, intercostal retractions, hepatomegaly, and growth failure are also seen. A continuous systolic murmur is auscultated, and a thrill may be palpated in the pulmonic area.

Clinical Therapy

When murmur is detected, diagnosis is confirmed by chest x-ray study, electrocardiogram (ECG), and echocardiogram. Chest x-ray film and ECG show left ventricular hypertrophy. PDA can be visualized, and left-to-right shunt can be measured on echocardiogram.

Surgical ligation of PDA is the treatment of choice. Intravenous indomethacin often stimulates closure of the ductus arteriosus in premature infants. Transcatheter closure by obstructive device is sometimes attempted in children over 18 months of age.

PROGNOSIS: If PDA is not treated, the child's life span is shortened because pulmonary hypertension and vascular obstructive disease develop.

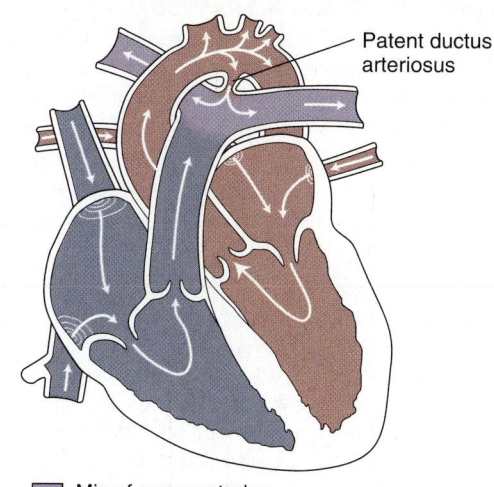

Patent ductus arteriosus

Mix of oxygenated and unoxygenated blood

Atrial Septal Defect (ASD)

ASD is an opening at any point in the atrial septum that permits left-to-right shunting of blood, and increased pulmonary blood flow. The opening may be small, as when the foramen ovale fails to close, or large, as when the septum is completely absent. Of children with congenital heart defects, 6% to 10% have an ASD (Driscoll, 1999).

Clinical Manifestations

Infants and young children usually have no symptoms. Small and moderate-sized ASDs are usually not diagnosed until preschool years or later. Congestive heart failure, easy tiring, and poor growth occur with a large ASD. A soft systolic murmur is usually heard in the pulmonic area with wide splitting of S_2.

Clinical Therapy

Diagnosis is made by echocardiogram that identifies right ventricular overload and shunt size. Chest x-ray film and ECG reveal little information unless ASD is large and excessive shunting is present.

Surgery to close or patch ASD is performed to prevent pulmonary vascular obstructive disease. Some ASDs may be closed by transcatheter device (septal occluder) during cardiac catheterization.

PROGNOSIS: Many people with uncorrected small and moderate-sized ASDs have lived to middle age without symptoms. Atrial arrhythmias are common late complications.

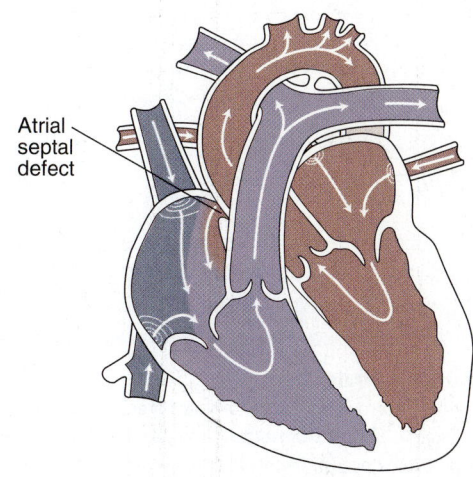

Atrial septal defect

Atrioventricular Canal (Endocardial Cushion Defect)

Atrioventricular (AV) canal refers to a combination of defects in the atrial and ventricular septa and portions of tricuspid and mitral valves. Of children with congenital heart defects, 4% to 5% have a total or partial AV canal (Driscoll, 1999). This defect is associated with Down syndrome. Endocardial cushions are fetal growth centers for mitral and tricuspid valves and AV septum. The most complex AV canal malformation results in one AV valve and large septal defects between both atria and ventricles.

Clinical Manifestations

Severity of symptoms depends on amount of mitral regurgitation. Infants have congestive heart failure, tachypnea, tachycardia, poor growth, and repeated respiratory failure, as well as systolic murmur, which is loudest at the left lower sternal border.

Clinical Therapy

On chest x-ray film, the heart appears large and pulmonary vascular markings are present. Echocardiogram reveals septal defects and details of valvular malformation. Cardiac catheterization is performed to evaluate pulmonary hypertension and pulmonary resistance.

Surgery is performed during infancy to prevent pulmonary vascular disease. Patches are placed over septal defects, and valve tissue is used to form functioning valves. Occasionally the mitral valve is replaced. Oxygen may be required until surgery.

PROGNOSIS: Information on long-term survival following successful surgery is lacking. Arrhythmias and mitral valve insufficiency occur postoperatively. There is no difference in short-term survival rates between infants with and without Down syndrome.

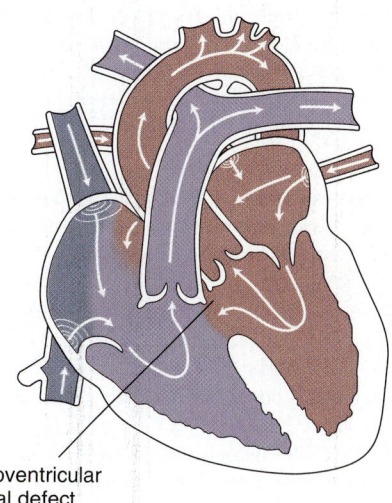

Atrioventricular canal defect

(continued)

Ventricular Septal Defect (VSD)

An opening in the ventricular septum results in increased pulmonary blood flow. Blood is shunted from the left ventricle directly across the open septum into the pulmonary artery. This most common congenital heart defect occurs in approximately 20% of all children with congenital heart disease (Driscoll, 1999).

Clinical Manifestations

Only 15% of VSDs are large enough to cause symptoms, such as tachypnea, dyspnea, poor growth, congestive heart failure, and pulmonary hypertension. Systolic murmur is auscultated in the lower left sternal border.

Clinical Therapy

Chest x-ray film and ECG reveal few findings in cases of small VSDs. Larger VSDs with shunting are associated with an enlarged heart and pulmonary vascular markings on chest x-ray film and left ventricular hypertrophy on ECG. Echocardiogram establishes diagnosis if shunting is present. Cardiac catheterization is used only in preparation for surgery.

Most small VSDs close spontaneously. Treatment is conservative when no signs of congestive heart failure or pulmonary hypertension are present. Surgical patching of VSD during infancy is performed when poor growth is evident. Closure of VSD by transcatheter device (i.e., Rashkind device) during cardiac catheterization may be attempted for some defects. Prophylaxis for infective endocarditis is required.

PROGNOSIS: Highest risk associated with surgical repair is in the first few months of life. Children respond well to surgery and experience substantial "catch-up" growth. Malignant tachyarrhythmias and heart block are a possible complication.

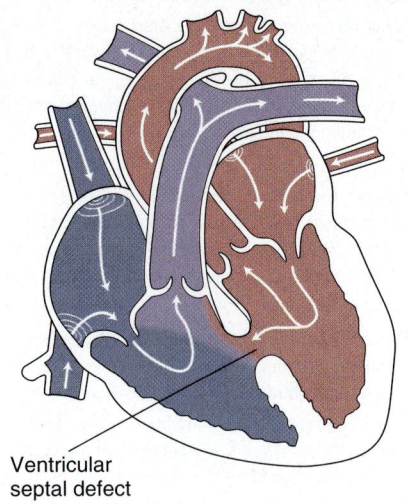

Ventricular septal defect

Pulmonic Stenosis

Stenosis (narrowing of valve or valve area) can be above valve, below valve, or at valve. Stenosis obstructs blood flow into pulmonary artery, increasing preload. Right ventricular hypertrophy occurs. Pulmonic stenosis is the second most frequent congenital heart defect, accounting for 8% to 12% of all cases.

Clinical Manifestation

Children with mild stenosis may have no symptoms and grow normally. In moderate stenosis, dyspnea and fatigue occur on exertion. Signs of heart failure are rare but may result from chronic pressure overload. A systolic murmur with a fixed split S_2 and thrill may be found in the pulmonic listening area. Heart failure and chest pain on exertion may occur in severe cases.

Clinical Therapy

Diagnosis is usually made at birth after auscultation of murmur. The chest x-ray film may show heart enlargement, and the ECG may demonstrate right ventricular hypertrophy. Echocardiogram provides information about the pressure gradient across the valve and size of valve ring.

Dilation by balloon valvuloplasty, performed during cardiac catheterization, has been widely successful for treatment of simple pulmonic stenosis. Surgical valvotomy may still be used, especially when other defects such as VSD are present. Surgical resection may be needed for narrowing above the valve area. Pulmonary regurgitation may result, but is not a significant problem.

PROGNOSIS: Pulmonic stenosis does not typically increase in severity. Lifelong infective endocarditis prophylaxis is necessary.

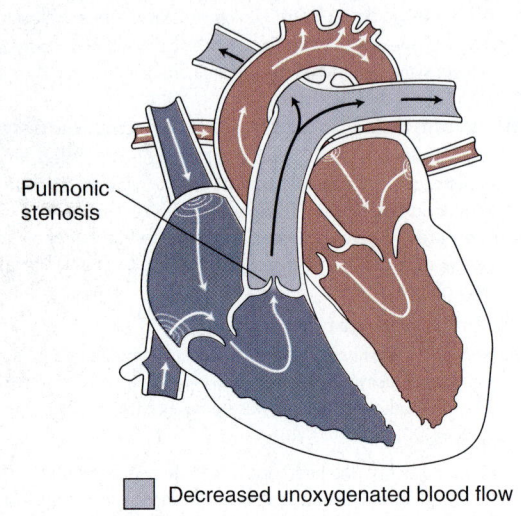

Pulmonic stenosis

▨ Decreased unoxygenated blood flow

(continued)

Aortic Stenosis

Narrowing of the aortic valve obstructs blood flow to systemic circulation. Aortic stenosis accounts for 3% to 6% of all cases of congenital heart defects (Fedderly, 1999). This defect is often associated with a bicuspid rather than a normal tricuspid valve. Stenosis is usually progressive during childhood.

Clinical Manifestations

Most infants and young children are asymptomatic and grow and develop normally. The blood pressure is normal, but there is often a narrow pulse pressure. Occasionally the child complains of chest pain after exercise, but exercise intolerance is uncommon. Peripheral pulses may be weak. Fainting and dizziness are serious signs that require intervention. Congestive heart failure develops in symptomatic infants. A systolic heart murmur and thrill in the aortic listening area are usually detected in routine physical examination in the school-age child or adolescent.

Clinical Therapy

Chest x-ray film and ECG are usually normal in mild cases. An echocardiogram reveals the number of the valve cusps, pressure gradient across the valve, and size of the aorta. Stress testing may be used in asymptomatic children to determine the amount of obstruction present with exercise.

The aortic valve may be successfully dilated by balloon valvuloplasty during cardiac catheterization. Surgical valvuloplasty may also be performed. Aortic valve replacement is performed when stenosis is severe or if significant regurgitation results from other interventions. Surgical treatment is palliative rather than curative.

PROGNOSIS: Chest pain, syncope, and sudden death can occur in symptomatic children, particularly during vigorous exercise. Stenosis is usually progressive during childhood as the valve calcifies. Valve replacement may ultimately be necessary. Lifelong infective endocarditis prophylaxis is required.

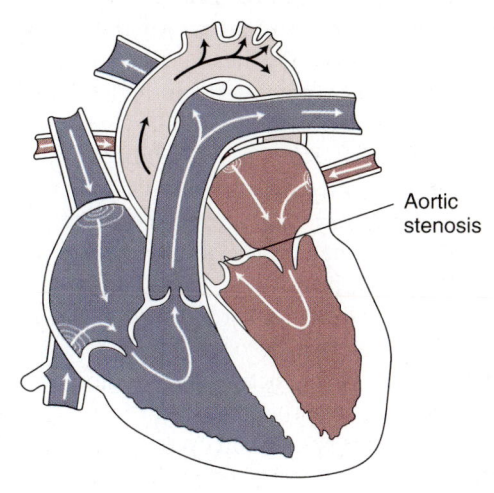

Aortic stenosis

Coarctation of the Aorta

Narrowing or constriction in the descending aorta, often near the ductus arteriosus, obstructs systemic blood outflow. This defect is common, occurring in 5% to 8% of all children with congenital heart disease (Fedderly, 1999).

Clinical Manifestations

Many children are asymptomatic and grow normally, but constriction is progressive; 20% to 30% of children develop congestive heart failure by 3 months of age. Reduction in blood flow through the descending aorta causes lower blood pressure in the legs and higher blood pressure in the arms, neck, and head. Brachial and radial pulses are full, but femoral pulses are weak or absent. Older children may complain of weakness and pain in the legs after exercise.

Clinical Therapy

ECG shows left ventricular hypertrophy. Chest x-ray film may reveal enlargement and pulmonary venous congestion, and indentation of the descending aorta. Rib notching (change in the smooth contour of the rib, apparent on x-ray) is rarely seen before 10 years of age. Magnetic resonance imaging shows coarctation.

Balloon dilation during cardiac catheterization provides both initial and recoarctation relief. Surgical resection and anastomosis are palliative, since coarctation may recur. The subclavian artery can be used as a patch in the infant. Repair in the first year of life is preferred to decrease exposure to hypertension.

PROGNOSIS: Post-coarctectomy syndrome (abdominal pain and distention) occurs in 20% of patients (Walters, 2000). Persistent hypertension in adulthood is common. Infective endocarditis prophylaxis is needed.

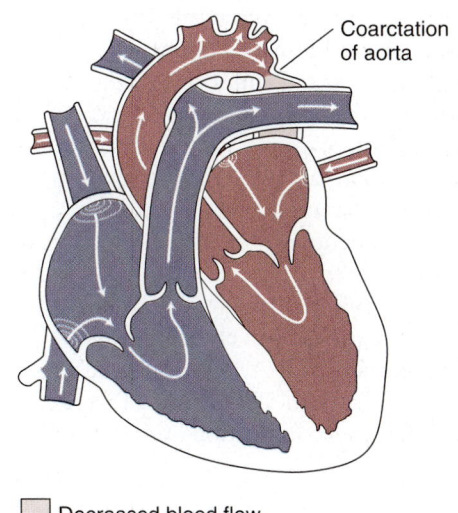

Coarctation of aorta

☐ Decreased blood flow

Etiology and Pathophysiology

Beginning at birth the left side of the heart normally generates higher pressures than the right side in response to increasing systemic vascular resistance and decreasing pulmonary vascular resistance. Children with nonobstructive defects such as openings in the septal wall have a left-to-right **shunt** (movement of blood between heart chambers through an abnormal opening). Oxygenated blood mixes with unoxygenated blood, and the extra blood volume overloads the pulmonary system, causing congestive heart failure. Pulmonary artery hypertension occurs if chronic volume overload of the pulmonary arteries is not corrected.

Clinical Manifestations

The child with a nonobstructive acyanotic heart defect may be asymptomatic except for a heart murmur. The most important consequence of these defects is volume overload. Congestive heart failure may develop if the amount of blood passing from the left to the right side of the heart overloads the pulmonary system (Nouri, 1997). If this occurs, the child has hepatomegaly, dyspnea, tachypnea, intercostal retractions, poor growth, and frequent respiratory infections. The more severe and complex the heart defect, the sooner symptoms of congestive heart failure appear.

The child with an obstructive acyanotic heart defect also has a heart murmur. See Chapter 33 for assessment of murmurs. 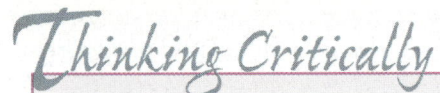 Obstructive defects cause pressure overload and hypertrophy of the closest ventricle. Although some children experience fatigue and exercise intolerance because they cannot increase cardiac output, many children are asymptomatic and grow normally. Signs and symptoms of congenital heart disease in older children include exercise intolerance, chest pain, arrhythmias, syncope, and sudden death.

Older children with congenital heart disease may have additional symptoms. Exercise-induced dizziness and **syncope** (transient loss of consciousness and muscle tone) are serious signs indicating a need for medical evaluation.

Clinical Therapy

A heart murmur is often the first indication of an acyanotic defect. A loud murmur indicates higher pressures of blood flowing across the shunt or through the narrowed valve or vessel. Once the heart murmur is discovered, a chest x-ray study, electrocardiography, and echocardiography are performed. See Table 43–4 to review tests used for the diagnosis of congenital heart disease.

The selection of treatment for acyanotic defects depends on the severity of symptoms and whether the condition is imminently life threatening. Surgical correction is the treatment of choice for most acyanotic defects. Table 43–5 lists the types of surgical procedures performed on children with congenital heart defects. Conservative treatment, such as waiting until the child is symptomatic or

THE INFANT WITH VSD

Brandy, who is 1 month old, was diagnosed with a ventricular septal defect (VSD) at birth. Her parents were just beginning to accept that she had a heart defect that might require surgical repair when signs of respiratory distress and difficulty in feeding developed.

Brandy's mother had been alerted to watch for these signs as a possible indication of congestive heart failure. Brandy was quickly hospitalized so her congestive heart failure could be treated with digoxin, furosemide (Lasix), and potassium. Over the next 2 days she lost the weight she had gained due to fluid retention.

Corrective surgery was performed to place a patch over the septal opening. Brandy was cared for in the intensive care unit before being transferred to another unit.

➡ *Why did Brandy develop congestive heart failure?*

➡ *Why was corrective surgery performed so soon?*

➡ *Is Brandy at risk to develop congestive heart failure after having had corrective surgery?*

➡ *What teaching and support do Brandy's parents need to care for her at home after the heart surgery?* WEB

older, may be selected initially. For example, a VSD may close spontaneously or the child's growth may increase the probability of surgical success. Surgical correction of defects that cause pulmonary hypertension is performed in infancy to prevent irreversible pulmonary vascular disease.

Surgery often completely repairs the acyanotic defect. Unless complications develop before surgery, the child should make a complete recovery without limitations. The major complication of acyanotic heart defects is pulmonary hypertension.

Cardiac catheterization, an invasive procedure previously used exclusively for diagnosis of some congenital heart defects, is now more often performed as a therapeutic procedure. Recently developed techniques using balloons and other transcatheter devices permit treatment of many acyanotic heart defects during cardiac catheterization.

Potential complications of cardiac catheterization include perforation of the pulmonary artery, allergic reaction

TABLE 43–4	Diagnostic Tests Used in Children with Congenital Heart Disease
Diagnostic Test	*Purpose*
Chest x-ray study	Reveals size and contour of the heart and characteristics of pulmonary vascular markings
Electrocardiogram (ECG)	Records quality of major electrical activity in the heart, identifies arrhythmias
Echocardiogram	Identifies heart's structures, the pattern of movement, hemodynamics, and the presence of defects
Cardiac catheterization	Allows precise measurement of oxygen saturation, cardiac output, and pressures in each chamber and heart vessel; also identifies anatomic alterations
Holter monitor	Allows 24–48 hour ECG recording
Exercise testing	Enables ECG recording with controlled increase in activity to identify significant cardiac compensation or inadequate cardiac output
Hyperoxia test	Measures differences in arterial blood gas level when child is on room air and on 100% oxygen

TABLE 43-5   Surgical Procedures for Congenital Heart Defects

Procedure	Purpose	Therapeutic Use
Angioplasty	Dilatation of coarctation of aorta during cardiac catheterization.	Palliative
Fontan	Creation of conduit between right atrium (inferior vena cava) and pulmonary artery to increase pulmonary blood flow—total right heart bypass.	Corrective or palliative
Glenn	Superior vena cava connected to right pulmonary artery along with closure of aortopulmonary shunt. Systemic venous blood is sent to the lungs directly without ventricular pumping.	Palliative
Jartene (arterial switch)	Aorta and pulmonary arteries are transected and reanastomosed to opposite stumps, coronary arteries are moved to new aorta area.	Corrective
Modified Blalock-Taussig shunt	Creation of aortopulmonary conduit to increase pulmonary blood flow.	Palliative
Mustard or Senning	Baffling blood in atria to reestablish a proper blood flow in transposition of great vessels.	Corrective
Norwood	Creation of conduit between aorta and pulmonary artery to increase blood flow to aorta.	Palliative or corrective
Patent ductus arteriosus closure	Closure of ductus arteriosus by surgery or an umbrella device during cardiac catheterization.	Corrective
Pulmonary artery banding	Placement of constricting band around pulmonary artery to reduce pulmonary blood flow.	Palliative
Rashkind—Balloon atrial septostomy	Creation of larger defect between atria to increase blood mixing, performed during cardiac catheterization.	Palliative
Rastelli	Pulmonary arteries removed from truncus and conduit is placed (or a connection is made) between the right ventricle and pulmonary artery.	Corrective
Transcatheter closure	Closure of a septal defect by a septal occluder or Rashkind device during cardiac catheterization.	Corrective
Transplant	Replacement of diseased heart with donor heart.	Corrective
Valvuloplasty	Repair of valve to relieve stenosis by balloon dilatation during cardiac catheterization or surgery.	Palliative or corrective

to the contrast media, arrhythmias, hypotension, stroke, vascular compromise in the leg, and bleeding.

Nursing Care of the Child Undergoing a Cardiac Catheterization

Prepare the child for cardiac catheterization with age-appropriate information. A tour of the catheterization laboratory may reduce the child's fears about the large equipment. Because the child will be sedated but arousable for the procedure, explain the sensations that he or she will experience.

Cardiac catheterization is often an outpatient procedure, but some children will be admitted for observation. The child is NPO for several hours, except for medications, and arrives at the catheterization laboratory 1 to 2 hours before the procedure. Before entering the laboratory, the child is asked to void and is given an oral sedative.

Nursing Management

Nursing Assessment and Diagnosis

Before the procedure, assess the child's vital signs, hematocrit and hemoglobin concentrations, and strength of pedal pulses for comparison with postcatheterization assessments.

For several hours after the procedure, monitor the child for potential complications such as arrhythmia, bleeding, hematoma development, thrombus formation, and infection. No bleeding should occur at the catheterization site. Assess vital signs, neurovascular status of the lower extremities, and the pressure dressing over the catheterization site every 15 minutes for 1 hour and then every 30 minutes for 1 hour. The child's temperature, heart rate, respiratory rate, and blood pressure should remain stable. Monitor intake and output because the contrast medium may cause diuresis. The child's intake and output should be balanced. Pedal pulses, capillary refill, sensation, warmth, and color of the lower extremities should match the precatheterization assessment.

The following nursing diagnoses may apply to the child who undergoes cardiac catheterization:

▶ *Fear* related to separation from support system in a stressful situation

▶ *Risk for fluid volume deficit* related to inadequate fluid intake due to NPO status and diuretic effect of contrast medium

▶ *Altered tissue perfusion (cardiopulmonary)* related to mechanical reduction of arterial and venous blood flow

▶ *Risk for decreased cardiac output* related to ventricular restriction (obstruction by balloon catheter)

Planning and Implementation

Nursing care during a cardiac catheterization focuses on monitoring the child's vital signs, reassuring the child, and providing emergency care if necessary. After the catheters and guidewires are removed at the end of the procedure, direct pressure must be applied for 15 minutes. A pressure dressing is then placed over the site for 6 hours.

The child is kept on bed rest for 6 hours to decrease the risk for bleeding from the catheter insertion site. Activity is then limited for 24 hours. Provide quiet diversional activities to keep the child occupied.

Encourage the child to drink small amounts of clear liquids initially, and then progress to other fluids and food as the child tolerates them. Maintaining hydration is important because the contrast medium used during the procedure has a diuretic effect. Monitor intake and output.

DISCHARGE PLANNING AND HOME CARE TEACHING

Children are routinely discharged several hours after the cardiac catheterization. Teach the parents to watch the child for signs of complications and make sure they know when to notify the physician.

Teaching About

> **HOME CARE AFTER CARDIAC CATHETERIZATION**
>
> Check for signs of complications several times in the first 24 hours after catheterization:
>
> - Fever
> - Bleeding or a bruise increasing in size at the catheterization site
> - Foot on side of catheterization site is cooler than other foot
> - Loss of feeling in foot on side of catheterization
>
> Notify physician immediately if any of these signs are noted within the first 24 hours after the catheterization.
> Encourage fluids to help flush the dye out of the body.
> Permit quiet play such as games, puzzles, and videos for first 24 hours after procedure.

Children whose heart defect is corrected by cardiac catheterization have the same risks for infective endocarditis as children with surgical correction. Use the information in Table 43–6, later in this chapter, to teach parents about infective endocarditis prophylaxis.

Evaluation

Expected outcomes of nursing care include:

- Any potential complications (thrombosis or hemorrhage) following cardiac catheterization are rapidly identified and cared for.
- The child maintains fluid balance.

Nursing Care of the Child Undergoing Surgery for an Acyanotic Defect

Children with acyanotic heart defects are hospitalized either because of complications, such as congestive heart failure, or for surgery. Refer to the earlier discussion of nursing management of congestive heart failure for care of children with this condition.

Nursing Management

Nursing Assessment and Diagnosis

Assess parents' ability to cope with the diagnosis of their child's congenital heart defect. Initially parents may be in shock and feel guilty and anxious. The child often looks healthy and has few symptoms.

Parents need a chance to express their feelings and to begin learning to cope with their child's illness. They need special support if their infant has a life-threatening heart defect. Members of the cardiology team, including nurses, must provide counseling for the family. Counseling information may include the following:

- General information about the congenital heart disease, including a description of the heart's anatomy and physiology and the defect
- Specific information about the multiple interactive factors associated with congenital heart disease; this information can often help reduce parents' guilt about the child's defect
- Sample case histories with good and poor prognoses
- Overview of the child's prognosis and timing of medical and surgical interventions

Parents may need genetic counseling if planning a future pregnancy. Parents are at higher risk of having a child with a congenital heart defect if any of the following factors are present: family history of congenital heart disease, maternal age greater than 35 years, coexisting maternal disease (diabetes mellitus, collagen vascular disease, phenylketonuria), and exposure to teratogens or rubella infection (Stumpflen, Stumpflen, Wimmer, et al., 1996). Fetal echocardiography can identify structural heart defects as early as 18 to 20 weeks of gestation.

Parents may need support for their anxiety about an uncertain outcome of surgery. **WEB** Some parents may be concerned that signing a consent for surgery is like signing the child's death warrant. The American Heart Association publishes a booklet, *If Your Child Has a Congenital Heart Defect,* that can be used for education.

Following surgical correction of the heart defect, the child is usually cared for in an intensive care unit until stable. The child may be intubated and ventilated for a few hours. In the immediate postoperative period, assess the child's vital signs, level of consciousness, pain level, heart functioning, and arrhythmias. Monitor intake and output. Monitor for hemorrhage, adequate ventilation and tissue perfusion, and acid–base and electrolyte imbalances.

After the child's return to the general nursing unit, nursing assessment focuses on signs of surgical complications such as infection, arrhythmias, and impaired tissue perfusion. Monitor the child's temperature, and inspect the surgical incision site. Fever, excessive incisional pain, spreading erythema around the incision, and wound drainage beginning 3 to 4 days postoperatively may be early signs of infection. Assess the respiratory system for breath sounds, respiratory effort, and signs of distress that may indicate pneumonia or fluid in the pleural space.

Because the child may no longer be on a cardiac monitor, auscultation of the apical pulse to detect an irregular heart rate or bradycardia is essential. Either condition indicates reduced cardiac output that requires intervention. To assess for impaired tissue perfusion, check capillary refill, extremity warmth, pedal pulses, level of consciousness, and urine output. Reduced urine output is a sign of decreased cardiac output. Continue to assess the child's pain.

Examples of nursing diagnoses associated with acyanotic heart defects and their complications include:

▶ *Fluid volume excess* related to heart failure and pulmonary vasculature overload

▶ *Decreased cardiac output* related to ventricular restriction and an obstructed outflow tract

▶ *Ineffective breathing pattern* related to respiratory muscle fatigue

▶ *Ineffective infant feeding pattern* related to shortness of breath and fatigue

▶ *Fatigue* related to chronic pulmonary vasculature overload

▶ *Altered family processes* related to crisis of child's serious illness

Planning and Implementation

Children are often managed at home until surgery is scheduled. Nursing care following surgery focuses on promoting the child's recuperation. Provide pain management for several days postoperatively. Follow the guidelines given in Chapter 38. ⬭ Avoid pulling on the child's arms to prevent stress on the sternum and pain.

Encourage the child to perform spirometry exercises regularly to promote full lung expansion. Chest physiotherapy may be performed in children under 3 years of age. Inspect the child's incision regularly and cleanse it with hydrogen peroxide if ordered (Figure 43–3 ◆). (See Skill 14–20) ⬭ **SKILLS** **CD**

Administer antibiotics as ordered. Intravenous lines are often converted to heparin or saline locks to continue antibiotic administration once the child's oral intake is normal. Although oral fluids are rarely limited, intake and output should be assessed carefully.

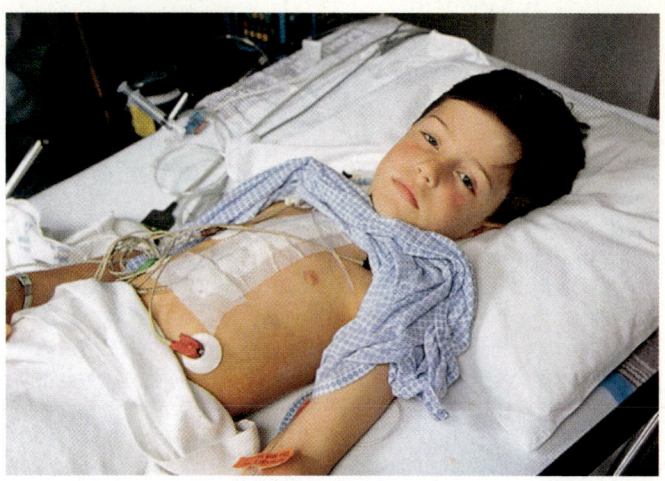

FIGURE 43–3. ◆ A child with atrial septal defect repair. Surgery is performed with this type of defect to prevent pulmonary vascular obstructive disease.

Teaching About

> **HOME CARE OF CHILDREN WITH CONGENITAL HEART DEFECTS BEFORE SURGERY**
>
> **Routine Health Care**
> Provide well-child care and all immunizations, including influenza vaccine.
> Provide preventive dental care with fluoride treatment.
>
> **Administration of Medications**
> Give medications safely with a dosage schedule that fits the family's routine.
>
> **Signs of Illness**
> Notify physician if the child has the following signs: fever, vomiting, diarrhea, or is feeding poorly. Avoid dehydration.
>
> **Activity**
> Allow the child to set his or her own activity level. Children with congenital heart defects usually do not overexert themselves.

Note: From Stinson, J., & McKeever, P. (1995). Mother's information needs related to caring for infants at home following cardiac surgery. *Journal of Pediatric Nursing, 10*(1), 48–57. Modified.

Encourage the child to increase activity gradually with longer periods out of bed every day. Provide opportunities for therapeutic play so the child can better manage the stresses associated with pain and frightening procedures.

DISCHARGE PLANNING AND HOME CARE TEACHING

Infants and children may be discharged from the hospital within a few days of surgery. Parents need discharge teaching in preparation for continuing care of the child at home.

Reassure parents by telling them that the child with a repaired cardiac defect should have no further cardiovascular problems. Encourage them to allow the child to live a normal and active life.

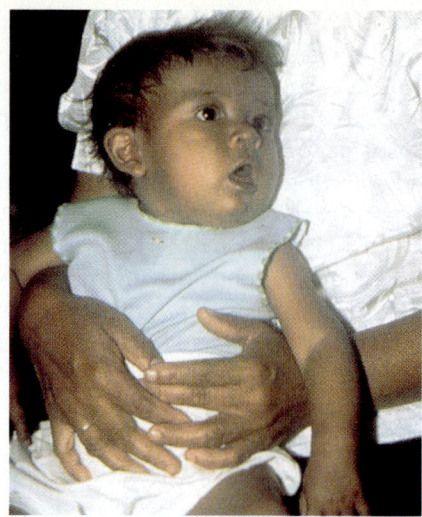

FIGURE 43–4. ◆ This infant has a cyanotic heart defect.

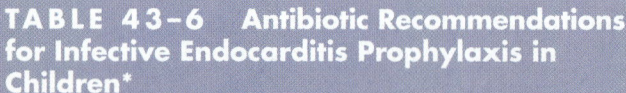

Teaching About

CARE OF THE CHILD AFTER CARDIAC SURGERY

- Allow the child to increase activity gradually as tolerated. Report increased fatigue or decreased activity tolerance to the physician.
- Report any signs of wound infection, fever, flulike symptoms, or an increased respiratory rate or respiratory distress to the physician.
- Allow the child to return to school in approximately 3 weeks. Physical activities such as rough play, bike riding, or climbing should be postponed for 6 weeks until the incision has healed completely.
- Report any unexplained fever or illness during the first 2 months following surgery as the child is at higher risk for infective endocarditis during that time. Antibiotics should be given for dental and surgical procedures.

TABLE 43–6 Antibiotic Recommendations for Infective Endocarditis Prophylaxis in Children*
For Dental, Oral, or Upper Respiratory Tract Procedures
Amoxicillin
For Children Allergic to Penicillin
Clindamycin, cephalexin, cefadroxil, azithromycin, clarithromycin
For Genitourinary and Gastrointestinal Procedures
Ampicillin, gentamicin, amoxicillin
For Children Allergic to Penicillin
Vancomycin, gentamicin

*One large dose is given 1 hour before the procedures. In high-risk patients, a smaller dose may be given 6 hours after the procedure. *Note:* From Dajani, A. S., Taubert, K. A., Wilson, W., Bolger, A. F., Bayer, A., et al. (1997). Prevention of bacterial endocarditis: Recommendations of the American Heart Association. *Journal of the American Medical Association, 277*(22), 1794–1801. Modified.

Children are at risk for infective endocarditis, especially within the first 6 months after surgery. The child should receive prophylactic antibiotics according to the American Heart Association recommendations (Table 43–6). Any unexplained fever or malaise in the 2 months following repair or after dental work may be a sign of infection. The child should be examined for petechiae and splenomegaly. Blood cultures, blood cell count, and urinalysis should be performed.

Evaluation

Examples of expected outcomes of nursing care include:

▶ The child's pain is effectively managed.

▶ Full lung expansion is maintained with spirometry exercises or chest physiotherapy.

▶ The child's incision heals without infection.

CYANOTIC DEFECTS

Cyanotic heart disease is generally caused by a valvular or vascular malformation. The most common malformations are tetralogy of Fallot and transposition of the great vessels (Figure 43–4 ◆). Table 43–7 summarizes clinical manifestations, diagnostic tests, and medical management for these defects.

Other less common congenital heart defects include hypoplastic left heart syndrome, tricuspid atresia, pulmonary atresia, truncus arteriosus, and total anomalous pulmonary venous return (Table 43–8). Not all of these defects cause cyanosis.

Etiology and Pathophysiology

Cyanotic defects are generally caused by a malformation or combination of defects that prevents adequate oxygenation of the blood. When the defect is associated with decreased pulmonary blood flow, pressures from obstructed blood in the right side of the heart exceed those in the left. Unoxygenated blood is shunted to the left side of the heart. Oxygenated blood destined for the systemic circulation is diluted, resulting in chronic hypoxemia and cyanosis.

When children with cyanosis rise in the morning, they may experience an abrupt decrease in systemic resistance and pulmonary blood flow. A hypercyanotic spell may be triggered by this decrease when combined with a sudden increase in cardiac output and venous return caused by crying, feeding, exercise, warm bath, and straining with defecation. The partial pressure of oxygen (PO_2) is lowered, and the partial pressure of carbon dioxide (PCO_2) rises. The hypoxemia becomes progressively worse as the respiratory center in the brain overreacts, increasing the respiratory effort. The additional respiratory effort further increases the cardiac output and contributes to a life-threatening decline unless rapid intervention is successful.

TABLE 43-7 **Cyanotic Heart Defects**

Tetralogy of Fallot

Combination of four defects: pulmonic stenosis, right ventricular hypertrophy, ventricular septal defect (VSD), and overriding of aorta. Some children have a fifth defect: open foramen ovale or atrial septal defect (ASD). About 10% of children with congenital heart defects have tetralogy of Fallot (Fyler, 1992). This defect is characterized by elevated pressures in right side of heart, causing right-to-left shunt.

Clinical Manifestations

As ductus arteriosus closes, the infant becomes hypoxic and cyanotic. The degree of pulmonary stenosis determines severity of symptoms. Polycythemia, hypoxic spells, metabolic acidosis, poor growth, clubbing, and exercise intolerance may develop. Infants have a systolic murmur heard in the pulmonic area that is transmitted to the suprasternal notch.

Clinical Therapy

Chest x-ray film shows a boot-shaped heart due to the large right ventricle with decreased pulmonary vascular markings. Electrocardiogram (ECG) shows right ventricular hypertrophy. Echocardiogram demonstrates VSD, obstruction of pulmonary outflow, and overriding aorta. Cardiac catheterization is required before surgical correction to completely identify the location of all anatomic structures and any additional defects.

Hypercyanotic spells are managed according to guidelines given in the section on nursing management of cyanotic defects. Monitoring the child for metabolic acidosis or prolonged unconsciousness is critical. A total repair is performed before 6 months of age when the infant has a hypercyanotic spell. Corrective surgery may be attempted in asymptomatic children by 6 months of age.

PROGNOSIS: Not all children are cured by surgery, but most have improved quality of life and longevity. Arrhythmias and right ventricular dysfunction may be residual problems (Waldman & Wernly, 1999). Lifelong infective endocarditis prophylaxis is required.

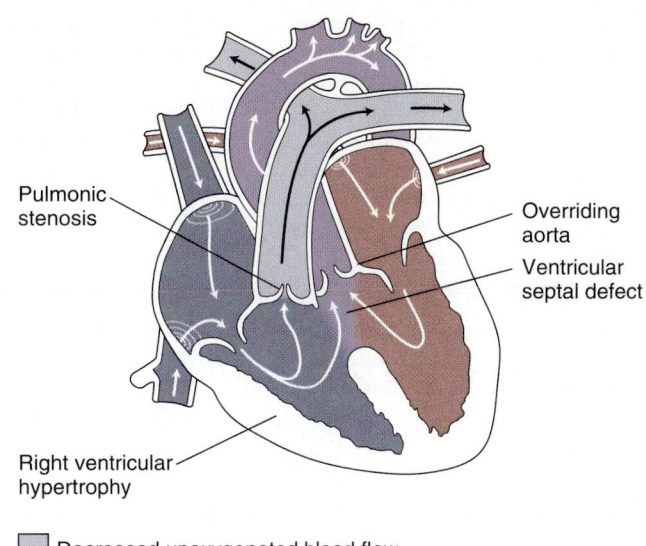

Pulmonic stenosis

Overriding aorta

Ventricular septal defect

Right ventricular hypertrophy

■ Decreased unoxygenated blood flow

■ Mixed oxygenated and unoxygenated blood

Transposition of the Great Arteries (TGA)

Pulmonary artery is the outflow for the left ventricle, and aorta is the outflow for the right ventricle. This condition is life threatening at birth, and survival initially depends on open ductus arteriosus and foramen ovale. This condition occurs in about 5% of children with congenital heart disease (Grifka, 1999). ASD or VSD may also be present with TGA.

Clinical Manifestations

Cyanosis, apparent soon after birth, progresses to hypoxia and acidosis. Cyanosis does not improve with oxygen administration. However, cyanosis may be less apparent when a large VSD is also present. Congestive heart failure may develop over days or weeks. Tachypnea (60 respirations/min) is often present without retractions or other signs of dyspnea. Infants take a long time to feed and need frequent rest periods because of rapid respiratory rate and fatigue. Growth failure may be evident as early as 2 weeks of age if corrective surgery is not performed.

Clinical Therapy

Chest x-ray study may reveal a classic egg-shaped heart on a string (narrow superior mediastinum). Diagnosis is made by echocardiogram when position of arteries arising from ventricles is visible.

Prostaglandin E_1 is initially ordered to maintain a patent ductus arteriosus until a palliative procedure such as balloon atrial septostomy can be performed. Corrective surgery (arterial switch) is usually performed before 1 week of age. Balloon atrial septostomy may be performed during cardiac catheterization in newborns as a first stage. This may also be corrected surgically.

PROGNOSIS: Survival without surgery is impossible. Arrhythmias, right ventricular failure, and sudden death are long-term complications (8 to 15 years) after the Mustard procedure, so the Mustard or Rastelli procedure are performed only when significant pulmonary valve stenosis is present (Grifka, 1999). Infective endocarditis prophylaxis may be necessary.

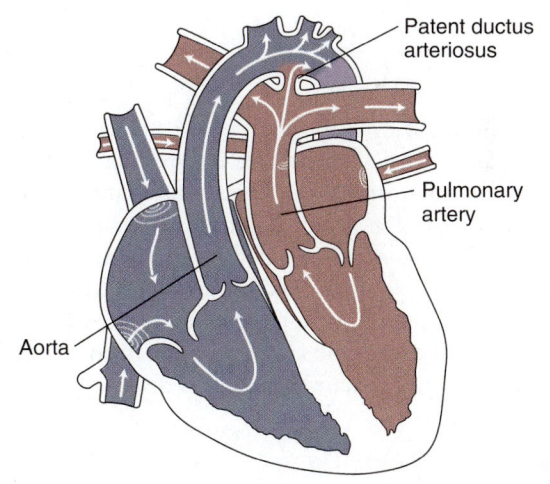

Patent ductus arteriosus

Pulmonary artery

Aorta

TABLE 43-8 Less Common Congenital Heart Defects

Condition	Clinical Manifestations	Clinical Therapy
Hypoplastic Left Heart Syndrome Absence or stenosis of mitral and aortic valves associated with an abnormally small left ventricle and aortic arch. Signs are initiated with closure of ductus arteriosus. Largest contributor of infant deaths due to congenital heart disease (Petrini, Damus, & Johnston, 1998). Possible genetic predisposition to the condition.	Signs include tachypnea, retractions, decreased peripheral pulses, poor peripheral perfusion, pulmonary edema, and congestive heart failure eventually leading to shock, acidosis, and death.	Echocardiogram is used for initial diagnosis. May be diagnosed prenatally in the first trimester. Prostaglandin E$_1$ given to maintain patent ductus arteriosus. Supplemental oxygen avoided. Surgery is done in 3 stages—Norwood procedure first, Glenn procedure next, and Fontan last. A heart transplant may also be performed. The survival rate is improving. May have failure of single ventricle over time.
Tricuspid Atresia/Pulmonary Atresia Absence of tricuspid or pulmonary valve. A ventricular septal defect (VSD) or transposition of the great arteries (TGA) is also often present.	Early cyanosis, dyspnea, congestive heart failure, pulmonary edema, hepatomegaly, acidosis, hypoxic spells, clubbing, polycythemia, and growth delays occur. Continuous murmur is heard in aortic area.	Chest x-ray study and echocardiogram are used for initial diagnosis. Prostaglandin E$_1$ is given to maintain patent ductus arteriosus. Digoxin and diuretics are also used. Palliative surgery (Rashkind procedure) increases pulmonary blood flow. The modified Fontan procedure results in improved survival.
Truncus Arteriosus A single large vessel empties both ventricles. VSD is usually present.	Cyanosis develops soon after birth. Severe congestive heart failure, dyspnea, retractions, fatigue, poor feeding, polycythemia, clubbing, increased pulse pressure, bounding peripheral pulses, increased respiratory infections, and cardiomegaly also occur.	Chest x-ray study and echocardiogram give initial diagnosis. Cardiac catheterization is done before surgery. Rastelli procedure is performed to close VSD and create a passage to pulmonary arteries. Digoxin and diuretics are given. Repeated surgery is necessary to enlarge pulmonary artery conduit. Survival is improved, but truncal valve stenosis and regurgitation result. Long-term prognosis is unknown.
Total Anomalous Pulmonary Venous Return Pulmonary veins empty into right atrium or veins leading to the right atrium.	Increased right ventricular impulse may occur. With severe pulmonary overload, tachycardia, dyspnea, pulmonary edema, retractions, cyanosis, hepatomegaly, poor feedings, irritability, and failure to thrive are seen.	Chest x-ray study, echocardiogram, and cardiac catheterization are used for diagnosis. Prostaglandin E$_1$ is given to maintain patent ductus arteriosus. Surgery to reconnect or baffle the pulmonary veins to the left atrium is performed. Survivors have lived more than 20 years after correction.

Children with cyanotic defects are at increased risk for thromboembolism. The chronic hypoxemia leads to polycythemia in an attempt to increase the hemoglobin available to carry oxygen. Brain abscesses are more common in children with cyanotic heart defects. Bacteria in the blood returning from the systemic circulation are usually filtered out by the capillaries in the lungs. However, when unoxygenated blood enters the systemic circulation through the right-to-left shunt, bacteria can travel directly to the brain.

Clinical Manifestations

Cyanosis often occurs when the ductus arteriosus closes, causing hypoxemia. Signs and symptoms of chronic hypoxemia include fatigue, clubbing of the fingers and toes, exertional dyspnea, and delayed developmental milestones. Because infants tire easily with feeding, they receive fewer calories, and do not grow normally. Congestive heart failure develops in some children.

The skin may have a ruddy or mottled appearance before cyanosis is observed. When pulmonary circulation is impaired, hemoglobin may not become reoxygenated. The

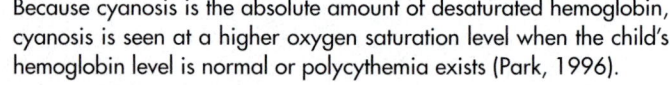

Because cyanosis is the absolute amount of desaturated hemoglobin, cyanosis is seen at a higher oxygen saturation level when the child's hemoglobin level is normal or polycythemia exists (Park, 1996).

Hemoglobin Level	Oxygen Saturation Level
6 g% (anemia)	45% to 50%
15 g% (normal)	75% to 80%
20 g% (polycythemia)	80% to 85%

appearance of cyanosis is related to the hemoglobin level and the oxygen saturation level.

Hypercyanotic (hypoxic) spells, the most significant problem to develop in infants and toddlers with heart defects, usually appear between 2 months and 2 years of age. Hypercyanotic spells can develop suddenly. Signs include:

- Increased rate and depth of respirations

- Increased cyanosis

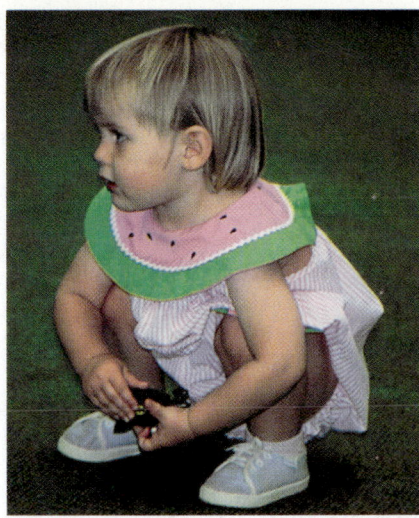

FIGURE 43–5. ◆ A child with a cyanotic heart defect squats (assumes a knee—chest position) to relieve cyanotic spells.

- Increased heart rate
- Pallor and poor tissue perfusion
- Agitation or irritability progressing to lethargy and decreased responsiveness without treatment

Children with uncorrected cyanotic heart disease often squat to relieve dyspnea (Figure 43–5 ◆). The knee–chest position reduces the cardiac output by decreasing the venous return from the lower extremities and by increasing the systemic vascular resistance.

Clinical Therapy

A systolic heart murmur may be apparent after cyanosis develops. A chest x-ray study, electrocardiogram, and echocardiogram are obtained. Usually the echocardiogram clearly shows the defect, shunt, and heart pressures. Cardiac catheterization is often used to obtain detailed anatomic information before surgery.

Early management of cyanotic heart defects is important to prevent secondary damage to the heart, lungs, and brain, including the adverse effects of hypoxemia on the child's cognitive and psychomotor development. For this reason, corrective surgery is being performed at younger ages, often in infancy. Recent studies comparing cognitive performance of school-age children with heart defects revealed that most preschool and school-age children have normal IQ scores. Some children with complex lesions (transposition of great arteries and hypoplastic left heart syndrome) seem to have an increased risk for neurodevelopmental problems (Mahle & Wernovsky, 2001).

A **palliative procedure** may be performed to preserve life in children with potentially lethal heart defects and complications (see Table 43–5). With some defects, corrective surgery can be postponed with a palliative procedure. This gives the infant an opportunity to grow and improves the success of corrective surgery.

If closure of the ductus arteriosus causes life-threatening cyanosis in newborns, prostaglandin E_1 (PGE_1) is prescribed to maintain or reopen the ductus arteriosus. These infants depend on a PDA for survival or improvement in pulmonary or systemic blood flow due to an obstructive defect. Treatment with PGE_1 provides time for the newborn to be transferred to a cardiac center for diagnostic evaluation and surgical intervention. Response time to PGE_1 varies depending on the type of defect.

The child's hemoglobin level and hematocrit values must be monitored to ensure that the blood does not become too viscous. Polycythemia may be managed by red blood cell pheresis if the blood viscosity becomes too high. Also monitor the child for anemia, as these children do not tolerate the lower hemoglobin and oxygen-carrying capacity.

Hypercyanotic spells become life threatening if not treated immediately. The child becomes progressively more hypoxic and limp, loses consciousness, is likely to have a seizure or cerebrovascular accident, and may die. To decrease the pulmonary vascular resistance, the initial treatment involves calming the child, giving oxygen, and administering morphine and propranolol intravenously. Packed red blood cells may be administered to improve oxygen delivery to the tissues when the child is anemic. Postpone all unpleasant procedures. To increase the systemic vascular resistance, the child is placed in knee–chest position and given intravenous fluids to expand circulatory volume. Dopamine or phenylephrine (Neosynephrine) are also given. Once a hypercyanotic spell has occurred, immediate palliative or corrective surgery is often scheduled. Oral propranolol is administered to decrease the frequency of hypercyanotic spells because of its action to minimize spasms of the pulmonary outflow tract (DeBoer, 1996).

Antibiotic prophylaxis for infective endocarditis is needed before and after surgical correction for all cyanotic conditions. See Table 43–6 for a list of recommended antibiotics.

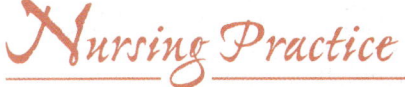

Nursing Practice

Crying may improve cyanosis caused by lung disease or disorders of the central nervous system. In children with cyanotic heart disease, crying usually makes cyanosis worse.

Nursing Management

Nursing Assessment and Diagnosis

The cardiovascular status of infants receiving PGE_1 therapy needs careful monitoring. Assess vital signs, heart rhythm, skin color, peripheral pulses, and capillary refill time (see Skills 9–8—9–14). 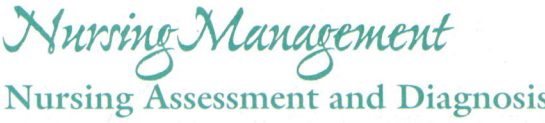 Observe for improvement in vital signs and color as the oxygen saturation increases and

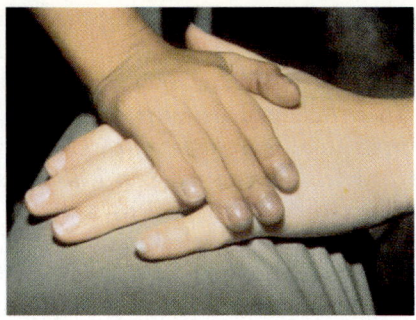

FIGURE 43–6. ◆ Clubbing of the fingers is one manifestation of a cyanotic defect in an older child.

acidosis decreases following the initial treatment. In addition, watch for tachycardia, tachypnea, crackles, frothy secretions, low urine output, and edema, because these infants are at risk for congestive heart failure.

The child needs careful observation for signs of increased cyanosis in the morning or at other high-risk times. Watch for neurologic signs of thromboembolitic complications from polycythemia such as headache, dizziness, excessive irritability, and paralysis. Older children with cyanotic defects may have clubbing of the fingers (Figure 43–6 ◆). Among the nursing diagnoses that might apply to a child with cyanotic heart disease are:

▶ *Risk for infection* related to unfiltered bacteria in the blood and sites of blood shunting that promote bacterial growth

▶ *Pain* related to palliative or corrective surgery

▶ *Risk for caregiver role strain* related to care of a child with chronic illness

▶ *Activity intolerance* related to cyanosis and dyspnea on exertion

▶ *Altered growth and development* related to congenital anomaly and hypoxemia

▶ *Risk for ineffective management of therapeutic regimen* related to complexity of therapeutic regimen: assessment and management of cyanotic spells, which are unpredictable events

Planning and Implementation

Children with tetralogy of Fallot are often managed at home until surgery is scheduled. Home care involves reducing parental anxiety, providing adequate nutrition, helping parents recognize signs of illness, and formulating a plan for emergency treatment. Nursing care of the hospitalized child focuses on monitoring PGE_1 therapy (for newborns only; used until palliative surgery is performed), treating hypercyanotic spells, and providing postsurgical care.

HOME CARE OF THE CHILD BEFORE SURGERY

Parents are usually anxious because of the need to wait before surgery can be performed. They often fear that the

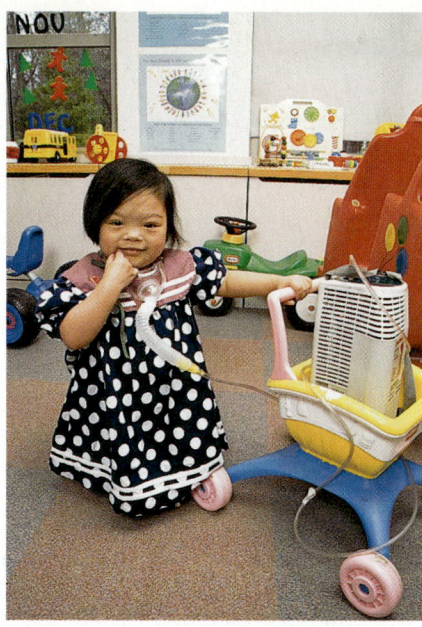

FIGURE 43–7. ◆ By pushing her oxygen cannister in a toy shopping cart, this toddler is able to move around in her environment. This strategy meets both her physiologic need for supplemental oxygen and her developmental need for independence.

infant will not survive until surgery or that they will be unable to manage any problems the infant may have. Give parents information and teach them how to care for the child at home. Some infants have such special home care needs that home health nursing and other community services are required. Many of these children require supplemental oxygen and nutrition, either for emergencies or for regular use (Figure 43–7 ◆).

Cyanosis with or without congestive heart failure often results in delayed gross motor skills. Developmental specialists can help parents set realistic developmental goals for the child. Make referrals to community-based early-intervention programs to promote the child's development.

Encourage parents to treat the infant as normally as possible. Children with mild cyanotic lesions do not need to adjust activity. The child with moderate to severe disease should be able to tolerate crying for a few minutes without difficulty. Prolonged crying should not be permitted because it causes fatigue and further hypoxia.

Vomiting and diarrhea may lead to dehydration, and parents must notify the physician whenever the infant or child has these symptoms. Dehydration is a particular risk in children with polycythemia because the blood can become even more viscous. Fever and dehydration may increase cyanosis. The systemic vascular resistance is decreased, resulting in a further decrease in blood flow to the pulmonary system. Aggressive management with antipyretic medication and fluid volume replacement is necessary (DeBoer, 1996).

Teach parents to observe the child for signs of infective endocarditis, including low-grade fever, fatigue, and malaise. They need to notify the physician if these symptoms occur within 2 months of surgery or a high-risk procedure. Parents must learn to request antibiotic prophylaxis for the child (see Table 43–6). Children also need preventive dental care to reduce the risk of endocarditis.

Parents may want to make an emergency plan in case the infant develops acute problems such as a hypercyanotic spell or respiratory distress. They should learn cardiopulmonary resuscitation. Ask parents to notify the local rescue squad about the infant's problem. Prepare a card or brief history form with information about the child's condition, medications, and necessary emergency care and the physician's name for parents to keep at home (American Academy of Pediatrics, 1999). When an acute problem occurs, this form gives important information to the emergency medical technicians and emergency department staff.

Although parents may travel with cyanotic children, they should not take these children to areas of high altitude without consulting with the physician first. The child may need supplemental oxygen when traveling on an airplane.

CARE OF THE INFANT AND CHILD UNDERGOING SURGERY

Monitor and carefully maintain the central, umbilical, or peripheral intravenous lines in the infant receiving continuous infusion of PGE_1. Observe the infant for cutaneous vasodilation, bradycardia, tachycardia, hypotension, seizure activity, fever, and apnea, common side effects of prostaglandin treatment. Have intubation equipment and a bag and mask at the bedside in case apnea occurs. Have intravenous fluids available to control hypotension.

If a cyanotic spell occurs, immediately place the child in the knee–chest position and administer oxygen. Administer morphine as ordered. Immediately notify the physician for further orders if these procedures are ineffective and the spell continues. Avoid any unpleasant or anxiety-provoking procedures.

Nursing Practice

Teach parents of infants with cyanotic heart defects to provide initial care for a hypercyanotic spell. Calm and reassure the infant while simultaneously positioning him or her in knee-chest position with the infant facing your chest. Place one arm under the knees and fold the legs upward toward the infant's chest. Use the other arm to support the infant's back. Then seek emergency care for the infant.

Children are admitted to the intensive care unit following surgery. Refer to the section on nursing assessment in the discussion of nursing care of the child undergoing surgery on page 1080. Postoperative bleeding is a potential risk in children with polycythemia because bleeding times are prolonged and platelet counts are low. Monitor chest tube output carefully for bright red blood or excessive volume. Bright red blood in the chest tube is a signif-

icant sign of hemorrhage. Fluids and diuretics maintain **preload** (the volume of blood in the ventricle at the end of diastole that stretches the heart muscle before contraction) in the right ventricle, whereas inotropic drugs support cardiac output. Children are transferred to the general nursing unit once heart function has stabilized.

Monitor the heart functioning of children following surgery. Assess vital signs, skin color, perfusion of the skin by capillary refill, and distal pulses. A sudden sustained increase in pulse and respirations and a decrease in peripheral perfusion may be early signs of hemorrhage. Monitoring fluid intake and output following surgery is critical. Note any signs of respiratory distress that may indicate the development of a pneumothorax or congestive heart failure.

Evaluation

Examples of expected nursing care outcomes include:

▶ The parents recognize a hypercyanotic spell, initiate emergency treatment, and get the child to medical care immediately.

▶ The parents manage fever and medical illnesses to prevent dehydration and potential hypercyanotic spells.

▶ The child attains expected developmental progress in gross motor, fine motor, and language skills.

HEART TRANSPLANTATION

In 1999, 307 pediatric heart transplantations were performed. Conditions associated with transplantation include the following by age group (Odim, Laks, Burch, et al., 2000):

• Infants—primarily congenital heart disease, such as hypoplastic left heart syndrome and other complex defects

• Children 1 to 10 years—cardiomyopathy (> 50%), congenital heart disease (40%)

• Adolescents—cardiomyopathy (65%), congenital heart disease (25%)

With improved immunosuppressive protocols and surgical techniques, survival rates are increasing (75% at 1 year and 65% at 5 years) (Boucek, 2000).

Infection and rejection are the major causes of mortality and morbidity. The immunosuppression regimen usually includes cyclosporin A, azathioprine, and corticosteroids. Signs of organ rejection include the following (Duitsman, Suddaby, & Masterson, 1999):

• Increasing resting heart rate, arrhythmias, bradycardia

• Presence of a third heart sound

• Cool and mottled extremities

• Inspiratory crackles, diaphoresis, tachypnea, pulmonary edema

- Hepatosplenomegaly
- Oliguria

Bacterial, fungal, and viral (i.e., cytomegalovirus) infections cause the most problems; however, some common childhood illnesses (acute otitis, colds) may be well tolerated.

After recovery from surgery, children may have near-normal exercise capabilities, normal heart function, and return to school and other activities. Immunosuppressive medications will be continued long term and can cause a variety of physical side effects such as hair growth, gum hyperplasia, weight gain, moon face, acne, and rashes. Children and adolescents may need support to develop positive self-esteem.

Depending upon the age at time of transplant, the child may not have had all immunizations (see Chapter 41). Live virus vaccines are often not given to immunosuppressed children. Help parents arrange for schools and child care centers to provide early notification of cases of measles, mumps, rubella, and chickenpox. Preventive treatment for the child can be provided as necessary. Handwashing and other methods to reduce the spread of infection should be encouraged both at home and at school.

Organ rejection is a major concern of families. Provide education for the parents and child to recognize the signs and to seek treatment promptly.

PULMONARY ARTERY HYPERTENSION

Pulmonary artery hypertension is a complication of many congenital heart defects, as well as pulmonary conditions. In some children with congenital heart defects, excessive pulmonary blood flow over time causes pulmonary vascular changes to decrease the blood flow. Inflammation, hypertrophy of pulmonary vessels, and fibrosis develop. Pulmonary venous hypertension develops. The increased pressure leads to a right-to-left shunt and right heart function is impaired. The condition may become life threatening (Barst, 1999).

Hypoxemia results from pulmonary hypertension, and the infant displays tachypnea, cyanosis, retractions, and fatigue. Feeding is difficult, and weight loss with fluid and electrolyte imbalance is likely. Older children have exertional dyspnea, chest pain, and syncope.

Clinical therapy involves surgery to correct an obstructive lesion or close a defect. Therapy for pulmonary artery hypertension related to noncardiac conditions involves bronchodilators, antibiotics, corticosteroids, and low-flow oxygen. No cure is available, but these measures can prolong life (Barst, 1999).

Nursing care focuses on promoting rest for oxygen conservation, monitoring fluid intake and output carefully, and administering medications and oxygen. Airplane travel may be possible with supplemental oxygen. Exercise should be tailored to avoid dyspnea. Give parents needed support and information about their child.

ACQUIRED HEART DISEASES

RHEUMATIC FEVER

Rheumatic fever is an inflammatory disorder of connective tissue that follows an initial infection by some strains of group A beta-hemolytic streptococci. This disorder causes changes in the heart, joints, brain, and skin tissues. Although not common, the disorder has occurred more frequently since the 1980s, probably because of a virulent strain of group A streptococcal infections (Steeg, Walsh, & Glickstein, 2000). The exact cause of the disorder is unknown. Possible causes include an autoimmune response in a genetically predisposed child (Steeg, 2000).

One to 3 weeks after an untreated streptococcal infection, the hallmark signs of rheumatic fever may occur. Aschoff's bodies (hemorrhagic bullous lesions) develop in the connective tissue of the heart. Endocarditis may lead to permanent mitral or aortic heart valve damage. The child's joints become inflamed and painful (migratory polyarthritis), although this condition improves in several weeks. Subcutaneous nodules may be palpable near joints. A skin rash called erythema marginatum, with pink macules and blanching in the middle of the lesions, is frequently seen. Spiking fever often occurs. A condition known as Sydenham chorea (St. Vitus dance), which is characterized by aimless movements of the extremities and facial grimacing, may be seen if the central nervous system is involved. Mild anemia may also occur.

Diagnosis is based on clinical signs (Jones criteria; Table 43–9) and laboratory testing for antistreptolysin-O (ASO). An elevated ASO antibody titer indicates a recent streptococcal infection.

TABLE 43–9 Guidelines for Diagnosis of Initial Attack of Rheumatic Fever (Jones Criteria, updated 1992)*	
Major Manifestations	*Minor Manifestations*
Carditis	**Clinical findings**
Polyarthritis	Arthralgia
Chorea	Fever
Erythema marginatum	**Laboratory findings**
Subcutaneous nodules	Elevated acute-phase reactants
	Erythrocyte sedimentation rate
	C-reactive protein
	Prolonged PR interval

Supporting evidence of antecedent group A streptococcal infection: (1) positive throat culture or rapid streptococcal antigen test; (2) elevated or rising streptococcal antibody titer.

*If supported by evidence of preceding group A streptococcal infection, the presence of two major manifestations or one major and two minor manifestations indicates a high probability of acute rheumatic fever.

Note: Data from Special Writing Group of the Committee on Rheumatic Fever, Endocarditis, and Kawasaki Disease of the Council on Cardiovascular Disease in the Young of the American Heart Association. (1992). Guidelines for the diagnosis of rheumatic fever. Jones Criteria, 1992 update. *Journal of the American Medical Association, 268*(15), 2069–2073.

Clinical therapy includes antibiotics (penicillin, sulfadiazine, or erythromycin) to eradicate the streptococcal infection. Aspirin may be given to control joint inflammation and reduce fever. Children should be monitored carefully by echocardiogram for potential heart involvement. Steroids may be used for severe carditis with congestive heart failure. Most children recover fully.

Nursing Management

The most important role of the nurse is prevention of rheumatic fever. Nurses in clinics, offices, and schools need to ensure that all children with possible streptococcal infections have a throat culture taken. Even if the sore throat is mild, a culture is needed if family members or other contacts have had a streptococcal infection. Emphasize to the family the importance of giving the entire 10-day course of antibiotics when a culture is positive.

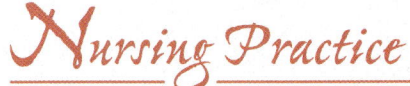
Nursing Practice

Often, the sore throat that precedes the child's illness is mild and goes untreated. Carefully evaluate pharyngitis, especially when cases of group A streptococcal infection have been identified in the family or community.

In a case of severe rheumatic fever, the child is hospitalized. Nursing care focuses on assessing the child's condition, promoting recovery, and ensuring compliance with the treatment regimen.

During the acute inflammatory phase, take the child's temperature at least every 4 hours and monitor vital signs. The child is on bed rest while monitoring for the onset of carditis, and for 4 weeks if carditis develops. Auscultate the child's heart and note any unusual sounds. Observe the child for changes in skin, joints, or behavior. Be sure family members have throat cultures done to identify possible asymptomatic streptococcal carriers.

Administer antibiotics and aspirin as ordered. The child is usually lethargic and often has joint pain. Aspirin often relieves pain dramatically after a few doses. Position and handle the child's joints carefully. Provide quiet activities, as the child is often confined to bed. Encourage visits or telephone calls from family members and friends. For the child with chorea, provide emotional support; the purposeless involuntary movements that can last for 5 to 15 weeks can be disturbing. Encourage the family to participate in the child's hospital care.

During the recovery phase, the child is generally cared for at home. Activities may be limited, especially if heart damage is suspected. Help parents plan quiet activities, such as playing board games, working with computers, or reading, and arrange rest periods after the child returns to school. Reassure the child and parents that the effects of chorea will eventually subside.

On discharge, a daily oral low-dose antibiotic is prescribed or a monthly long-acting antibiotic injection is given. Make sure the child and parents understand the importance of taking prescribed medication until adulthood to prevent future infection and possible heart damage from recurrent rheumatic fever. Stress the importance of telling future health care providers, including dentists and surgeons, about the child's rheumatic fever history so prophylactic antibiotics can be given to prevent infective endocarditis during invasive procedures.

Make sure the parents understand that the child's future sore throats may be streptococcal and that a throat culture should be taken even when the child is taking daily antibiotics. The child may need additional antibiotics for the infection. Emphasize the importance of follow-up care to prevent new infections and to monitor heart function.

INFECTIVE ENDOCARDITIS

Infective endocarditis is an inflammation of the lining, valves, and arterial vessels of the heart caused by bacterial, enterococci, and fungal infections. Children who have a congenital heart defect, rheumatic heart disease, or a central venous catheter or who have had heart surgery are at risk for infective endocarditis. Infections may occur after the causal organism enters the bloodstream during dental work or surgery and lodge on damaged or abnormal endocardial tissue. It is a significant cause of morbidity and mortality in children with complex heart defects treated with prosthetic aortopulmonary shunts and in immunocompromised children with long-term central venous catheter use (Brook, 1999).

Symptoms can be mild and develop slowly, or they can be severe and develop rapidly. Common symptoms are fever (often with elevations in the afternoon), fatigue, joint and muscle aches, headache, and nausea and vomiting. Signs may include a new or changing murmur, congestive heart failure, dyspnea, hematuria, petechia, and splenomegaly (Brook, 1999).

Infective endocarditis is diagnosed primarily by blood culture; however, urine and cerebrospinal fluid also may be cultured. Elevated erythrocyte sedimentation rate, anemia, elevated C-reactive protein level, increased white blood cell count, alterations in the electrocardiogram, and changes in heart sounds and murmurs are indicators of the condition. Echocardiography may be used to identify vegetation or infective lesions in the heart.

Clinical therapy consists of administering antibiotics such as penicillin G, ampicillin, vancomycin, nafcillin, or gentamicin. Intravenous administration is preferred, with therapy continuing for 2 to 8 weeks until the infective organism is eradicated. Serum levels of antibiotics are monitored to maintain a therapeutic range. Occasionally surgery is necessary to drain an abscess or because of heart valve failure. If congestive heart failure occurs, bed rest and medications such as digoxin and furosemide are prescribed.

Nursing Management

Nursing care focuses on assessing the child's condition, administering medications, and teaching the parents about the child's care. Take the child's vital signs and assess gastrointestinal discomfort. Administer medications as ordered and monitor serum antibiotic levels. Monitor for side effects of antibiotics and for infiltration or extravasation at the infusion site. Keep invasive procedures to a minimum. Use careful aseptic technique in performing venipunctures, urinary catheterizations, and other procedures.

The child is often lethargic and on bed rest. Encourage parents to assist with the child's care and plan quiet age-appropriate activities. Home infusion antibiotic therapy may be ordered so that care can be provided on an outpatient basis. At discharge, arrange home health nursing and instruct parents about care needed for the child's recuperation. Reinforce the need for follow-up visits. Explain the importance of telling physicians and dentists about the child's history of endocarditis so that they will take care to prevent infection before invasive procedures.

CARDIAC ARRHYTHMIAS

Cardiac arrhythmias (abnormal rhythms) are not uncommon in children. These include tachyarrhythmias (sinus tachycardia) and bradyarrhythmias (sinus bradycardia) that occur with acute conditions and resolve once the condition is treated. Less common arrhythmias are often associated with congenital heart disease, including atrial fibrillation, atrial flutter, ventricular fibrillation, and heart block.

Supraventricular Tachycardia

Supraventricular tachycardia (SVT), the most common pathologic tachycardia, is the abrupt onset of a rapid, regular heart rate, often too fast to count. Neonates and young children may be predisposed to the condition because of a congenital heart defect or Wolff-Parkinson-White syndrome. Short periods of arrhythmia (several seconds), which may be caused by paroxysmal atrial tachycardia, are rarely dangerous. However, prolonged episodes of continuous SVT for more than 24 hours may lead to congestive heart failure. Cardiac output is affected because diastolic filling cannot occur with such a rapid heart rate.

Recurrent attacks are common. Prolonged episodes of SVT are life threatening and can progress to congestive heart failure or cardiogenic shock if untreated.

Growth and Development

> The presenting heart rate in infants with supraventricular tachycardia (SVT) may be up to 260 beats/min. In older children, a heart rate between 150 and 240 beats/min may be seen. A heart rate of 230 beats/min is seen in 60% of children under 18 years of age (Robinson, Anisman, & Eshaghpour, 1996).

Early signs in infants include poor feeding, irritability, and pallor. Older children may have episodes of altered consciousness (dizziness or syncope).

Electrocardiography, including a 24-hour rhythm recording, confirms the diagnosis. Vagal stimulation such as applying ice or iced saline solution to the face may reduce the heart rate. An older child can perform the Valsalva maneuver (holding the breath and straining, or blowing forcefully on the thumb) to increase intrathoracic and venous pressures and thus slow the heart rate. Adenosine or amiodarone are the recommended emergency medications when vagal stimulation does not work. Cardioversion may be used for life-threatening episodes if other treatments are not effective. Digoxin and propranolol may be given to reduce the frequency of episodes (Starr & Freitas-Nichols, 2000). Radio-frequency catheter ablation is used with much success in chronic cyclic tachycardia to obliterate the accessory pathway (Case, 1999).

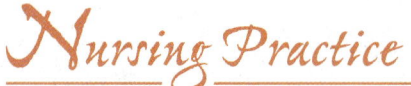

Nursing Practice

The child with SVT should avoid subsequent use of cardiac stimulant drugs such as decongestants. These drugs might trigger another episode of SVT.

Long QT Syndrome

Long QT syndrome is a rhythm disturbance of autosomal dominant and autosomal recessive inheritance that puts children at risk for ventricular fibrillation and sudden death. It may also result from electrolyte abnormalities, malnutrition associated with anorexia and bulimia, myocarditis, and central nervous system trauma (Berul, 2000). It is thought to be associated with some cases of sudden infant death syndrome.

The arrhythmia commonly occurs without warning and often results in death. It may be triggered by exercise or emotional stress, but in some cases has occurred during rest. Early signs include a fast heart rate (too fast to count), irritability, lethargy, poor feeding, poor perfusion (cool pale skin, increased capillary refill time), decreased responsiveness, and decreased blood pressure.

If the child is resuscitated or evaluated because of early signs, the arrhythmia is commonly detected by electrocardiogram. The disorder is treated by beta-adrenergic blockade, antiarrhythmic agents, and often a pacemaker (Lewin, 2000).

NURSING MANAGEMENT

Nursing care of children with SVT or Long QT Syndrome focuses on assessing the child's condition, administering medications, and providing emotional support to the child and parents. Children are treated in the emergency department or intensive care unit. The child is placed on a cardiac monitor, and frequent assessment is critical. Report continued abnormal rates or rhythms to the physician. Carefully observe and record changes in level of consciousness, color, weakness, irritability, and feeding pattern. Administer medications as ordered. Have emergency drugs and resuscitation equipment available at the bedside. Provide for rest and adequate nutrition.

Episodes of arrhythmia are frightening for both the child and parents. Carefully explain the treatment plan and home care. Teach parents to take the child's apical pulse. Make sure parents are trained in cardiopulmonary resuscitation. Provide telephone numbers of emergency medical facilities and help parents plan how to seek emergency care. Emphasize that medications help prevent or reduce the frequency of the episodes.

⤳ VASCULAR DISEASES

KAWASAKI DISEASE

Kawasaki disease, also known as mucocutaneous lymph node syndrome, is an acute systemic inflammatory illness. Although this disorder is most common in Asian children, it is seen in all races. The disorder occurs primarily in children under 5 years of age. In the United States, Kawasaki disease is the most common cause of acquired heart disease in children. The etiology of Kawasaki disease is unknown, but the primary cause is thought to be infectious in genetically predisposed children. It does not appear to be spread by person-to-person contact, but there is often a preceding upper respiratory tract infection.

There are three stages of the disease: acute, subacute, and convalescent. The acute stage is characterized by fever, conjunctival hyperemia, red throat, swollen hands and feet, rash on the trunk, enlargement of the cervical lymph nodes, diarrhea, and hepatic dysfunction (Figure 43–8 ◆). The subacute stage is characterized by cracking lips and fissures, desquamation of the skin on the tips of the fingers and toes, joint pain, cardiac disease, and thrombocytosis. In the convalescent stage, 6 to 8 weeks after disease onset, the child appears normal but may have lingering signs of inflammation.

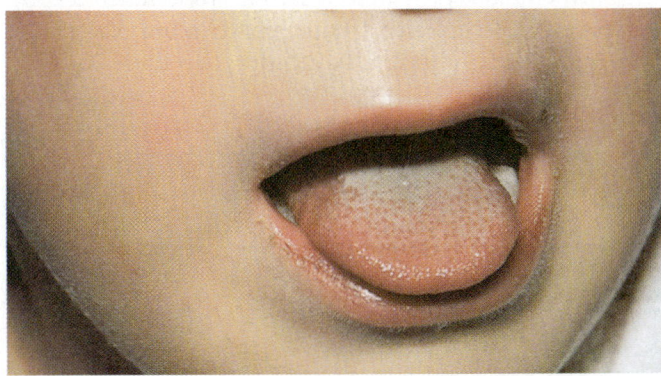

FIGURE 43–8. ◆ This child shows many of the signs of the acute stage of Kawasaki disease.

TABLE 43–10	Diagnostic Criteria for Kawasaki Disease

Kawasaki disease is diagnosed when a high spiking fever over 39 °C (102.2 °F) for 5 days or longer is present along with four of the following five criteria:

- Bilateral conjunctivitis without exudate, typically with distinctly visible vessels early in the disease
- Intense erythema of the buccal and pharyngeal surfaces with dry, swollen, cracked, and fissuring lips and a strawberry tongue
- Dermatitis of the extremities, intense palmar and plantar erythema, induration of the hands and feet, and then desquamation after 2 or more weeks of symptoms
- Dermatitis of the trunk with an erythematous maculopapular rash
- Acute cervical lymphadenopathy, frequently unilateral, with a node over 1.5 cm in diameter found early in the disease and an illness not explained by another disease process.

Note: From Rowley, A. H., & Shulman, S. T. (1999). Kawasaki syndrome. *Pediatric Clinics of North America, 46*(2), 313–329. Modified.

Diagnosis is based on clinical signs using the criteria given in Table 43–10. Blood studies show some abnormalities such as elevated erythrocyte sedimentation rate, elevated white blood cell count, mild anemia, thrombocytosis, elevated platelet count, and elevated C-reactive protein level. An echocardiogram may reveal some heart changes.

Clinical therapy for Kawasaki disease involves aspirin and immune globulin. High doses of aspirin (80 to 100 mg/kg/day) are given while the fever is high. The dose is decreased to 10 mg/kg/day or less once the fever has dropped. Aspirin is taken until the platelet count is normal and may be continued on a long-term basis if cardiac abnormalities occur. High doses of immune globulin and of aspirin given early in the disease have been shown to reduce the incidence of coronary artery lesions and aneurysms, and to decrease fever and inflammatory signs (Rowley & Shulman, 1999).

Children are usually hospitalized as long as fever persists. Most children recover fully. Careful monitoring for cardiac disease continues for several weeks or months. Cardiac involvement is the most serious complication. Aneurysms and early atherosclerosis lead to arrhythmias, congestive heart failure, coronary stenosis, myocardial infarction, and, potentially, death.

Nursing Management

Nursing care focuses on promoting comfort, monitoring for early signs of complications or disease progression, and supporting the family.

Assessment is important in identifying signs of Kawasaki disease, as the acute phase of this disorder is commonly confused with other diseases. The nurse in the community must be alert to early signs and symptoms. When the child is hospitalized, take the temperature every 4 hours and before each dose of aspirin. Carefully assess the extremities for edema, redness, and desquamation every 8 hours.

Examine the eyes for conjunctivitis and the mucous membranes for inflammation. Monitor the child's dietary and fluid intake and weigh the child daily. Carefully assess heart sounds and rhythm.

Administer aspirin and immune globulin as ordered. Monitor for side effects of aspirin such as bleeding and gastrointestinal upset. Administer intravenous immune globulin as a blood product, carefully regulating the infusion rate to run slowly according to the physician's orders, and watching for any reactions to the infusion. The infusion rate should not be over 1 mL/min. If symptoms of reaction occur, stop the infusion immediately (see Chapter 40).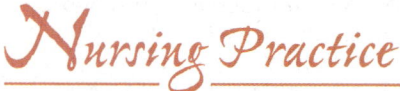

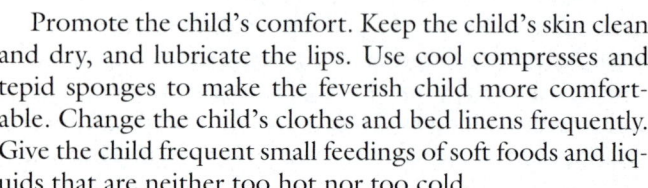

Nursing Practice

Inform the parents of a child with Kawasaki disease to postpone any scheduled immunizations for 5 months after immune globulin administration, as immune response to the vaccine may not be fully effective (Rowley & Shulman, 1999).

Promote the child's comfort. Keep the child's skin clean and dry, and lubricate the lips. Use cool compresses and tepid sponges to make the feverish child more comfortable. Change the child's clothes and bed linens frequently. Give the child frequent small feedings of soft foods and liquids that are neither too hot nor too cold.

Use passive range of motion exercises to facilitate joint movement. Because the child with Kawasaki disease is often lethargic and irritable, plan rest periods and quiet age-appropriate activities. Encourage the parents to participate in their child's care. This comforts and reassures the child. Give the parents information about the disease and the child's treatment.

Before the child is discharged, teach the parents to administer aspirin as ordered and to watch for side effects. Advise the parents that the child may need to avoid contact sports or other activities that could cause bleeding. Have them take the child's temperature daily and report any fever above 37.8 °C (100 °F) to the physician. Emphasize the need for follow-up care to monitor for cardiac complications.

HYPERLIPIDEMIA

Hyperlipidemia is a condition of excessive fat in the blood that may eventually lead to atherosclerosis. Although children do not usually die of atherosclerotic heart disease, coronary heart disease, the major cause of death in the United States, begins in childhood and progresses through the adult years (Giddings, 1999). It is important to identify children who have a genetic history or lifestyle that makes them more susceptible to future coronary heart disease. Risk factors for hyperlipidemia include the following: family history of coronary heart disease before age 55, cigarette smoking, hypertension, diabetes, lack of exercise, high total and saturated fat intake, and overweight.

Some children have hereditary disorders of lipid metabolism characterized by high levels of total cholesterol, low-density lipoprotein, or triglycerides, or by low levels of high-density lipoprotein (Winter, House, & Schatz, 1999). Children with familial hypercholesterolemia, for example, have cholesterol levels as high as 600 to 1000 mg/dL, resulting in lipid deposits in their corneas and tendons. As the excessive fat circulates, it causes changes in blood vessels. More commonly, children have milder lipid abnormalities that arise from a combination of heredity and lifestyle factors. The fatty streaks that appear in childhood become fibrous plaques in adolescence. These atherosclerotic plaques continue to grow in adulthood and may cause hemorrhage, thrombi, and occlusion of vessels (Williams & Bollella, 1995).

A blood test identifies hyperlipidemia. Cholesterol, including total cholesterol (TC) and high-density lipoprotein cholesterol (HDL-C), and triglycerides are measured. The low-density lipoprotein cholesterol (LDL-C) level is calculated using an equation based on the triglyceride, HDL, and total cholesterol levels. All children who have a family history of cardiovascular disease before age 55 years (parents or grandparents) or who have a parent with elevated total serum cholesterol (240 mg/dL) should be screened (Winter et al., 1999). Some clinicians choose to screen all children, especially those with an unknown family history, during childhood or sometime after the age of 2 years. This helps identify children who have no risk factors but demonstrate hyperlipidemia (Purath, Lansinger, & Ragheb, 1995). Based on total cholesterol value, children are placed in a low-, moderate-, or high-risk category (See Table 43–11).

TABLE 43–11	Recommended Lipid/Lipoprotein Levels for Children		
Lipid/Lipoprotein	Recommended Level	Borderline High Level	High Level
Total cholesterol	< 170 mg/dL	170–200 mg/dL	> 200 mg/dL
LDL-C	< 110 mg/dL	110–130 mg/dL	> 130 mg/dL
Triglyceride	< 100 mg/dL	< 100 mg/dL	> 130 mg/dL
HDL-C	> 35 mg/dL	—	—

Note: From the National Cholesterol Education Program Coordinating Committee. (1991). *Report of the expert panel on blood cholesterol levels in children and adolescents.* Washington, DC: U.S. Department of Health and Human Services. Adapted.

TABLE 43–12   Recommended Nutrient Intake in Children and Adolescents with Hyperlipidemia

Nutrient	Recommended Intake
Saturated fatty acid	Less than 10% of calories
Total fat	No more than 30% of calories
Polyunsaturated fat	Up to 10% of calories
Monounsaturated fat	10–15% of calories
Cholesterol	Less than 300 mg/day

Note: From the National Cholesterol Education Program Coordinating Committee. (1991). *Report of the expert panel on blood cholesterol levels in children and adolescents.* Washington, DC: U.S. Department of Health and Human Services; and Kris-Etherton, P., Daniels, S. R., Eckel, R. H., et. al. (2001). AHA scientific statement: Summary of the scientific conference on dietary fatty acids and cardiovascular health. Conference summary of the Nutrition Committee of the American Heart Association. *Journal of Nutrition, 131*(4), 1322–6. Modified.

The LDL cholesterol level is examined carefully in children with elevated total cholesterol (200 mg/dL). LDL cholesterol should be less than 110 mg/dL. High HDL and low LDL cholesterol levels provide protection against heart disease.

Hyperlipidemia in most children can be managed by dietary modifications, exercise, and other changes in lifestyle. The child's diet is carefully analyzed and changes are made to satisfy the dietary guidelines given in Table 43–12. If the child continues to have high serum lipid levels, a lipid specialist should be consulted. Cholestyramine or colestipol, which bind bile acid in the intestine; niacin; or some of the statin drugs are occasionally prescribed for children over 10 years of age.

Long-term studies of the effect of childhood lipid levels on life span have not yet been concluded. It is hoped that careful monitoring and management of lipid levels in childhood will decrease the incidence of cardiovascular disease. A long-term study evaluating the safety and efficacy of a cholesterol-lowering diet in children with elevated LDL-C revealed that dietary fat modification can be achieved and sustained in actively growing children. LDL-C levels can be improved without adverse effects on the child's growth and maturational development (Obarzanek, Kimm, Barton, et al., 2001).

Nursing Management

Nursing care focuses on identifying children at risk for hyperlipidemia, providing education about diet and exercise, and monitoring eating patterns. Identification and management of hyperlipidemia takes place in a variety of community agencies. Office and clinic nurses identify children who need to have serum lipid measured. Nurses in schools provide education on ways to reduce risk factors (Howard, Bindler, Synoground, et al., 1996). The child's history of exercise patterns, weight percentile, and dietary intake provides important information. Obtain information on familial heart disease, hypertension, diabetes, and smoking to determine risk factors. Although a screening for total cholesterol level does not require fasting, the child needs to fast for 12 hours before blood is drawn for a complete lipid evaluation.

Work with nutritionists to provide dietary teaching and monitor family eating patterns. Emphasize the importance of exercise in keeping the heart and blood vessels free from atherosclerotic changes. Help the child select an aerobic activity such as running, biking, swimming, soccer, hiking, fast walking, aerobic dancing, and rollerblading. Encourage participation at least five times weekly for 30 minutes each time.

Discourage smoking by the child or the parents. Secondhand smoke may affect blood pressure and plaque formation, and thus increase the risk for the development of cardiovascular disease (Giddings, 1999).

Include the entire family in the treatment plan, as changing eating and exercise patterns is difficult for a single family member. The family of a child with hyperlipidemia requires continual teaching and reinforcement. Periodically perform nutrition assessments and evaluation of family diet.

HYPERTENSION

Hypertension is present in 1% to 3% of children (Porto, 2000). Most cases have unknown cause, labeled as primary or essential hypertension (Hohn, 1997). Some underlying conditions such as kidney disease or heart defects may cause secondary hypertension. A genetic predisposition to hypertension may be manifested in some children by high normal or slightly elevated blood pressures. Mildly elevated blood pressure in children and adolescents may precede adult hypertension (National High Blood Pressure Education Program, 1996). High blood pressure in adolescents is correlated with obesity and high serum lipid level (Bartosh & Aronson, 1999). All children with blood pressures in the 90th percentile for age are significantly more likely to develop hypertension as adults (Bartosh & Aronson, 1999).

Developing Cultural Competence

African-American children may be particularly susceptible to increased blood pressure caused by dietary intake of sodium. Encouraging these children to follow a low-salt diet is important. Increasing intake of low-fat dairy products and fruits can contribute to blood pressure control.

The child with an elevated blood pressure should have blood chemistry (BUN, creatinine, glucose, and electrolytes), urinalysis, and urine culture tests done to detect secondary causes of hypertension. Serum lipid studies should be performed to determine whether hyperlipidemia exists. Nonpharmacologic measures for reduction of blood pressure include dietary counseling for obesity, low-sodium and high-potassium diet, increased physical exercise, adequate calcium and dietary fiber with less than 10% of calories from saturated fats, three to five daily fruit servings, discontinuation of smoking, alcohol, and drugs, and behavioral modification (Hohn, 1997). Medications are used for children with persistent, severe hypertension.

Nursing Management

Take a complete history for the child with borderline hypertension and no other associated diseases. Are parents or siblings hypertensive? Is the child obese? How many servings of fruits does the child eat daily? What is the daily number of dairy product servings? What is the child's daily salt intake? What are the child's daily exercise routines? Take the child's blood pressure regularly to monitor changes (see Skill 9–10). ⬭ SKILLS CD Compare readings to normal blood pressure for age and gender (see Table 33–16). ⬭

Teach both the child and the parents how to improve the diet and develop exercise routines. Emphasize the importance of avoiding smoking. Teaching that involves the entire family is usually the most effective. Instruct the family on correct administration of prescribed medications when used.

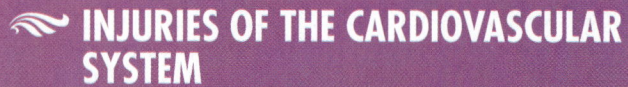

⌇ INJURIES OF THE CARDIOVASCULAR SYSTEM

SHOCK

Shock is an acute, complex state of circulatory dysfunction resulting in failure to deliver sufficient oxygen and other nutrients to meet cell and tissue demands. It can be caused by a variety of conditions such as hemorrhage, dehydration, sepsis, obstruction of blood flow, and cardiac pump failure.

Hypovolemic Shock

Hypovolemic shock is a clinical state of inadequate tissue and organ perfusion resulting from the movement of blood or plasma out of the intravascular compartment (see "Pathophysiology Illustrated: Hypovolemic Shock"). The blood or plasma in the vascular space may be decreased because of hemorrhage or fluid movement into the interstitial spaces.

ETIOLOGY AND PATHOPHYSIOLOGY

Major causes of decreased intravascular blood volume include:

- Hemorrhage from significant injury
- Plasma loss from burns, nephrotic syndrome, and sepsis
- Fluid and electrolyte loss associated with dehydration, diabetic ketoacidosis, and diabetes insipidus
- Vasodilating drugs

Shock results in inadequate delivery of oxygen and nutrients to cells and accumulation of toxic wastes in the capillaries. The reduction in circulating blood volume causes a decrease in cardiac output and mean arterial pressure. Cellular hypoxia and acidosis develop simultaneously. The accumulation of toxins and inadequate tissue oxygenation cause cellular damage.

The child's body attempts to compensate by the following measures:

- The heart rate and myocardial contractility increase to improve cardiac output.
- The respiratory rate increases to improve oxygenation and decrease waste accumulation in the cells.
- The hydrostatic pressure falls, permitting fluid to shift into the vascular space and increasing the circulating blood volume.
- The peripheral vasculature constricts to maintain the systemic vascular resistance as long as possible.

The child can compensate until 20% to 25% of volume loss occurs, and then life-threatening hypotension results.

CLINICAL MANIFESTATIONS

Signs of early hypovolemic shock in children are nonspecific but need to be recognized before hypotension occurs. Signs that the child is compensating for a decreased blood volume are tachycardia, usually sustained at a rate greater than 130 beats per minute; increased respiratory effort; delayed capillary refill (> 2 seconds); weak peripheral pulses; pallor; and cold extremities (signs of decreased perfusion). Although the child's body attempts to compensate by preserving circulation to vital organs, urine output decreases when renal blood flow drops. In cases of dehydration, dry mucous membranes and poor skin turgor are also present.

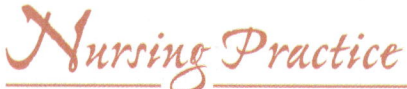

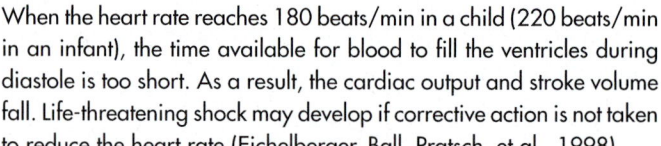

When the heart rate reaches 180 beats/min in a child (220 beats/min in an infant), the time available for blood to fill the ventricles during diastole is too short. As a result, the cardiac output and stroke volume fall. Life-threatening shock may develop if corrective action is not taken to reduce the heart rate (Eichelberger, Ball, Pratsch, et al., 1998).

If treatment is not begun in the early stages of hypovolemic shock, the condition progresses until the child can no longer compensate. At that time the systolic blood pressure drops and the pulse pressure decreases. Reduced cerebral blood flow ultimately results in a decreased level of consciousness. If shock is not reversed, the condition progresses to cardiopulmonary failure. "Clinical Manifestations of Hypovolemic Shock" compares the signs associated with early, uncompensated, and profound shock.

PATHOPHYSIOLOGY ILLUSTRATED
Hypovolemic Shock

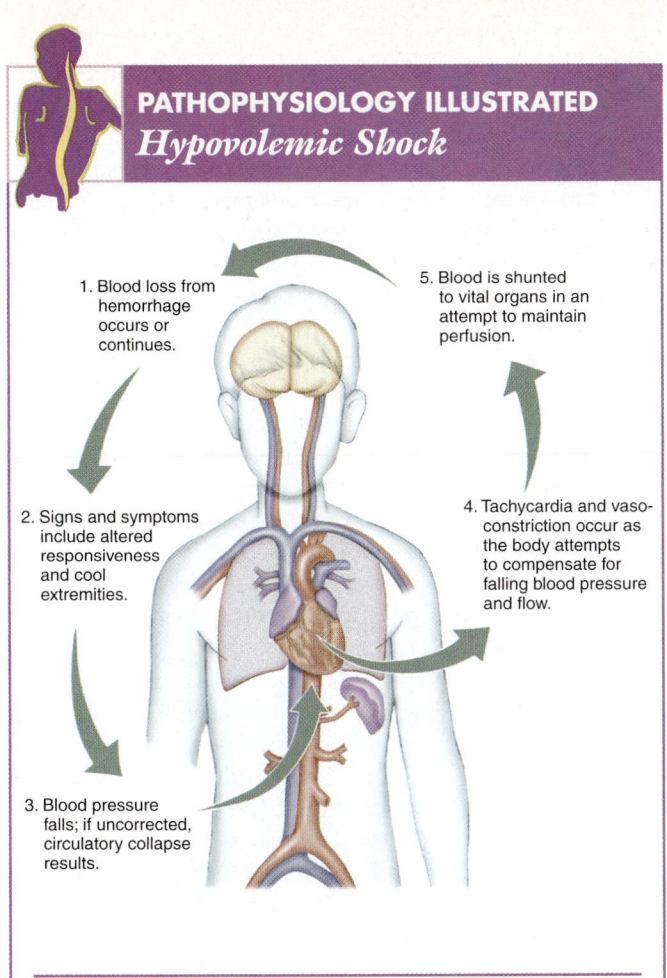

1. Blood loss from hemorrhage occurs or continues.

2. Signs and symptoms include altered responsiveness and cool extremities.

3. Blood pressure falls; if uncorrected, circulatory collapse results.

4. Tachycardia and vaso-constriction occur as the body attempts to compensate for falling blood pressure and flow.

5. Blood is shunted to vital organs in an attempt to maintain perfusion.

If hemorrhage reduces the circulating blood volume sufficiently, vasoconstriction occurs, shifting blood to maintain the perfusion of vital organs. When the blood loss exceeds 20% to 25%, the child's body can no longer compensate and hypovolemic shock ensues.

CLINICAL THERAPY

No laboratory values can be used to evaluate the volume deficit rapidly enough to diagnose hypovolemic shock. The child is examined for characteristic signs to confirm the diagnosis. Laboratory tests commonly performed after hypovolemic shock is diagnosed include hematocrit and hemoglobin, arterial blood gases, serum electrolytes, glucose, osmolality, blood urea nitrogen, and urinalysis.

Emergency care focuses on improving tissue perfusion. An open airway is established, oxygen is administered, and ventilation is assisted if necessary. Bleeding is controlled, and an intravenous or intraosseous line is started to provide large volumes of crystalloid fluids (Ringer's lactate).

Ringer's lactate solution is the preferred fluid for initial resuscitation. A fluid volume of 20 mL/kg is administered rapidly over 5 minutes. The same amount of fluid is given in 5 minutes if the child's physiologic condition does not improve after fluid is first administered. Signs that a child is responding to fluid resuscitation include improved color, improved responsiveness, lower heart rate, and faster capillary refill time. If no improvement is seen after the second fluid bolus, blood or albumin is usually ordered.

Once the child's physiologic condition is stabilized, the cause of the hypovolemic shock becomes the focus of examination and treatment.

Nursing Management
Nursing Assessment and Diagnosis

Ask the parent (or child, if appropriate) about possible injuries or the duration and severity of acute illnesses. If no external bleeding is evident, determine whether an injury may be causing internal bleeding. For example, the liver and spleen are highly vascular organs that have little protection from direct blunt forces. Significant bleeding from injury to one of these organs can cause hypovolemic shock without evidence of bleeding. An acute illness such as

CLINICAL MANIFESTATIONS ～ Hypovolemic Shock

SYSTEM	EARLY SHOCK	UNCOMPENSATED SHOCK	PROFOUND SHOCK
Cardiac	Tachycardia, weak distal pulses	Tachycardia, absent distal pulses, decreasing systolic blood pressure	Frank hypotension, bradycardia, weak central pulses
Neurologic	Normal, anxious, irritable, or combative behavior	Confusion, lethargy, decreased pain response	Comatose state
Skin	Mottled appearance; capillary refill time > 2 seconds; cool, clammy extremities	Cyanosis, capillary refill time > 3 seconds, cold extremities	Pale, cold skin
Renal	Decreased urine output, increased specific gravity	Oliguria, increased specific gravity	No urine output

Note: From Waisman, H., & Eichelberger, M. R. (1993). Hypovolemic shock. In M. R. Eichelberger (Ed.), Pediatric trauma: Prevention, acute care, rehabilitation (p. 182). St. Louis, MO: Mosby-Yearbook. Modified.

gastroenteritis with prolonged vomiting and diarrhea can also result in dehydration and hypovolemic shock.

If external bleeding is apparent, determine the amount of blood lost. Although children lose the same amount of blood from a laceration as adults, the total volume of blood lost is proportional to their weight.

Growth and Development

> The child's total blood volume varies by weight. The child has approximately 80 mL of blood for every kilogram of body weight.
>
> - Newborn: 3 kg × 80 mL = 240 mL (1 cup)
> - 5-year-old child: 25 kg × 80 mL = 2000 mL (2 quarts)
> - 13-year-old child: 50 kg × 80 mL = 4000 mL (1 gallon)

When an injured child is admitted to the hospital for a problem such as a liver or spleen laceration, assess the child's circulatory status frequently. Current medical treatment for these injuries is conservative. Surgeons give the liver or spleen a chance to heal spontaneously rather than perform immediate surgery to control bleeding and repair the laceration. Even if the child's circulatory condition was stabilized during emergency care, shock can develop again if bleeding continues.

Frequently assess the child's heart rate, respiratory rate, blood pressure, capillary refill time, level of consciousness with the Glasgow Coma Scale (see Chapter 49), color, and skin temperature to identify any changes that indicate improvement or deterioration in the child's condition. Monitor urine output and specific gravity hourly. Signs of the child's improved status include:

- A decrease in heart rate, respiratory rate, and capillary refill time
- An increase in systolic blood pressure and urine output
- Improved color, level of consciousness, and skin temperature
- Regaining of lost weight

Several nursing diagnoses may apply to the child with hypovolemic shock. They include:

- *Decreased cardiac output* related to hypovolemia
- *Fluid volume deficit* related to active fluid volume loss
- *Altered tissue perfusion (cardiopulmonary, renal, and cerebral)* related to impaired transport of oxygen across alveolar and capillary membrane
- *Ineffective airway clearance* related to altered level of consciousness
- *Ineffective family coping: compromised* related to life-threatening condition of the child

Planning and Implementation

Nurses in the emergency department and intensive care unit participate in the resuscitation of the child in hypov-

olemic shock. Assist with the child's assessment and the establishment of intravenous access. Calculate and prepare the amount of intravenous fluid needed for administration according to the child's weight (20 mL/kg). Ensure rapid fluid administration by intravenous push or pressure bag. Monitor the child's physiologic response to the fluid bolus within 5 minutes. Prepare a second and third fluid bolus.

Use warmed intravenous fluids for resuscitation because hypothermia may interfere with the child's response to treatment. Keep the child covered or use heat lamps to reduce body-heat loss.

When packed red blood cells are administered, verify that the correct blood has been obtained for the child. Change the intravenous fluid to normal saline solution to prevent clotting during blood administration. Assess the child carefully for a transfusion reaction (see Chapter 44). Monitor the child's physiologic circulatory responses for improvement or deterioration in status. Notify the physician of any deterioration.

Provide support to the child and family during the acute phase of treatment. Parents and children with hypovolemic shock resulting from injury are usually apprehensive. The child may be fearful because of the sudden hospitalization or agitated because of an altered level of consciousness. Determine the causes of the child's anxiety. The parents often fear for the child's life in cases of injury. Update the parents about the child's condition frequently. Explain the care being provided and how it helps the child. Listen to their concerns and correct any misconceptions.

Evaluation

Examples of expected nursing care outcomes include:

- The child receives adequate fluid resuscitation to prevent progression to uncompensated shock.
- The family copes with the stress of the child's injury.

Distributive Shock

Distributive (septic) shock is an abnormal pooling of blood in the extremities that may be caused by anaphylaxis, sepsis, or spinal cord injury. Immunodeficient children are at high risk for septic shock. The blood accumulates in the extremities because of vasodilation and capillary permeability. Less blood is returned to the heart, so preload drops and cardiac output falls.

Septic shock begins as an infection and progresses to sepsis. Once a bacterial toxin enters the circulatory system, the body's inflammatory processes go out of control. White blood cells multiply throughout the body and macrophages produce cytokines, which dilate the blood vessels and increase permeability. Congestion occurs in some tissue beds, and bacteria may be trapped and multiply unchecked. Systemic and pulmonary edema develop as organ ischemia occurs (Hazinski, 1999) (see "Pathophysiology Illustrated: Septic Shock").

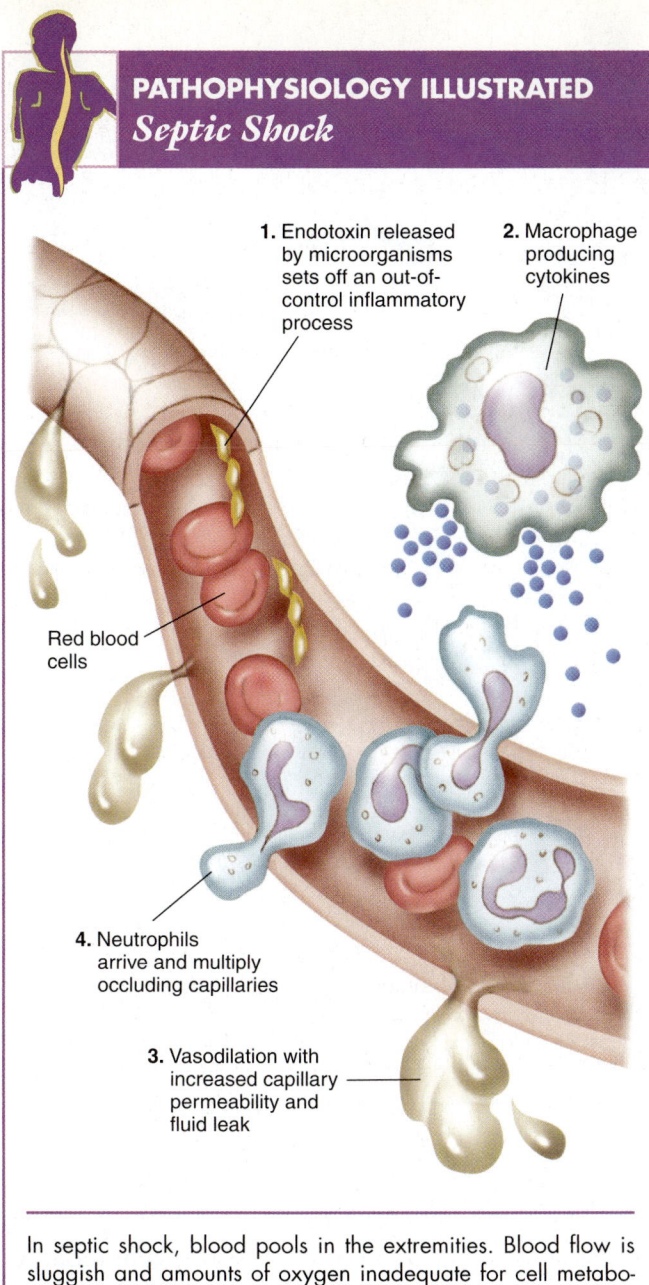

1. Endotoxin released by microorganisms sets off an out-of-control inflammatory process

2. Macrophage producing cytokines

Red blood cells

4. Neutrophils arrive and multiply occluding capillaries

3. Vasodilation with increased capillary permeability and fluid leak

In septic shock, blood pools in the extremities. Blood flow is sluggish and amounts of oxygen inadequate for cell metabolism are received by the tissues.

Septic shock has two phases: hyperdynamic and hypodynamic. During the hyperdynamic phase, the child has a fever, tachycardia, tachypnea, warm extremities, bounding pulses, and brisk capillary refill. Perfusion appears adequate; however, because of infection and fever, oxygen demand in the tissues is much higher and perfusion is really inadequate.

Cardiac output is high but systemic vascular resistance is low, leading to an uneven flow and pooling in the extremities. Blood moves sluggishly, and anaerobic metabolism and lactic acidosis occur in tissue beds where oxygen no longer circulates. As the syndrome progresses, the hypodynamic phase develops. Cardiac output is low, and systemic vascular resistance is high. Blood has already pooled in the extremities. During the hypodynamic phase the child is cool, hypotensive, pale, and oliguric. Blood is shunted away from the kidneys, muscles, and skin to the heart and brain. Multisystem organ failure occurs if treatment does not improve regional perfusion.

Treatment for septic shock is begun even before the diagnosis is confirmed. Fluid resuscitation is used in early septic shock to stabilize the circulation and ensure adequate tissue perfusion. Antibiotics effective against the suspected organism are given. Vasopressors are given during the hypodynamic phase. Morbidity and mortality are high even when treatment is initiated early. Complications include disseminated intravascular coagulation and adult respiratory distress syndrome.

Obstructive Shock

Obstructive shock occurs when a blockage of the main bloodstream interferes with tissue perfusion (see "Pathophysiology Illustrated: Mediastinal Shift"). Causes in children include compression of the vena cava, pericardial tamponade, pulmonary embolism, tension pneumothorax, pleural effusion, and congenital heart defects with outflow obstruction (e.g., coarctation of the aorta). Management is focused on treatment of the underlying condition.

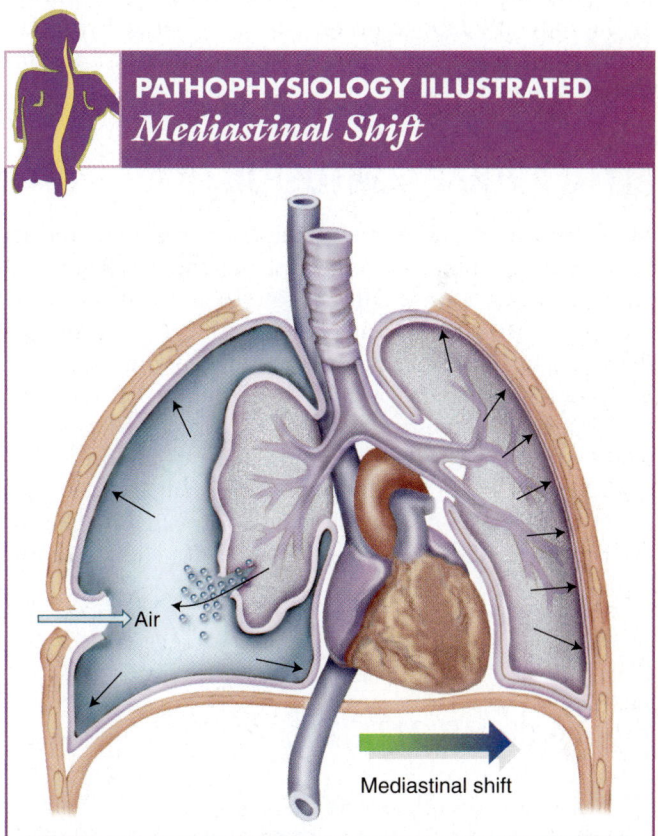

Air

Mediastinal shift

Obstructive shock can occur when a tension pneumothorax obstructs blood flow to and from the heart. Here, the great vessels are compressed during the mediastinal shift.

Cardiogenic Shock

Cardiogenic shock is an abnormality of myocardial function in which the heart fails to maintain adequate cardiac output and tissue perfusion (see "Pathophysiology Illustrated: Cardiogenic Shock"). Causes of cardiogenic shock in children may include congestive heart failure, congenital heart disease, cardiomyopathy, and arrhythmias such as bradycardia and supraventricular tachycardia. Cardiogenic shock may also be an end stage for other acute and chronic conditions such as sepsis, prolonged shock, asphyxia, hypoglycemia, and muscular dystrophy. Heart failure may result from obstructed outflow in congenital heart defects such as severe coarctation of the aorta and hypoplastic left heart syndrome.

Clinically, cardiogenic shock resembles hypovolemic shock with low cardiac output. Tachycardia, tachypnea, decreased oxygen saturation, hypotension, diminished peripheral pulses, and cool, pale extremities are common signs. The child becomes disoriented and restless as the compensatory mechanisms fail. Increased systemic vascular resistance puts more stress on the failing heart. Each contraction causes more blood to accumulate in the heart and pulmonary vessels, eventually leading to congestive heart failure, metabolic acidosis, and circulatory collapse.

The goals of medical treatment are rapid restoration of myocardial function with adequate ventilation, resolution of the initial metabolic insult, correction of arrhythmias, fluid management, and administration of diuretics and inotropic drugs.

MYOCARDIAL CONTUSION

Myocardial contusion, a rare injury in children, results from a strong, blunt force against the chest wall that injures the heart muscle. Blood flow to areas of the heart muscle is disrupted, or myocardial cells are directly destroyed. This potentially life-threatening condition is often associated with a motor vehicle–related injury. It most often occurs in adolescents who have struck the steering wheel of a motor vehicle during a crash or children who have been struck in the chest with a baseball.

A myocardial contusion should be suspected in cases of injury to the anterior chest. The child has chest discomfort because of fractured ribs or chest wall contusion. An electrocardiogram reveals arrhythmias or signs of myocardial infarct. An echocardiogram may show an abnormality in heart wall movement. Cardiac isoenzyme concentrations are elevated. Because of the risk of sudden arrhythmias, the child is admitted to the intensive care unit for cardiac monitoring.

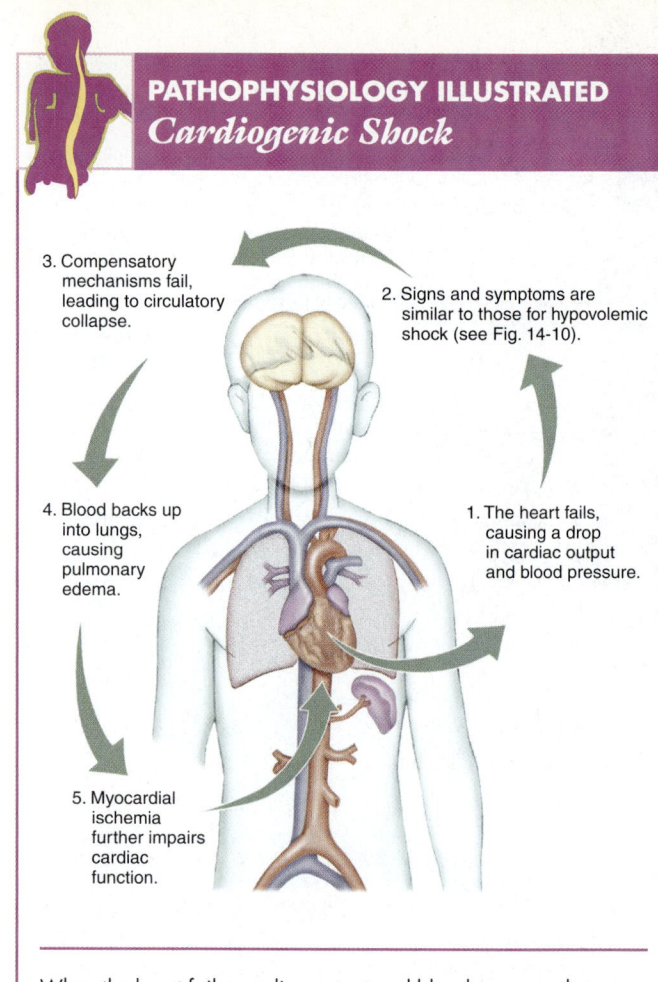

PATHOPHYSIOLOGY ILLUSTRATED
Cardiogenic Shock

3. Compensatory mechanisms fail, leading to circulatory collapse.

2. Signs and symptoms are similar to those for hypovolemic shock (see Fig. 14-10).

4. Blood backs up into lungs, causing pulmonary edema.

1. The heart fails, causing a drop in cardiac output and blood pressure.

5. Myocardial ischemia further impairs cardiac function.

When the heart fails, cardiac output and blood pressure decrease. Blood backs up into the lungs, causing pulmonary edema. Inadequate amounts of oxygen reach the myocardium, further impairing the heart's pumping action. The result is cardiogenic shock.

CHAPTER HIGHLIGHTS

☞ Infants are at risk of heart failure because their immature heart is more sensitive to volume or pressure overload. The heart muscle fibers are less developed and the ventricles have less compliance so that stroke volume cannot increase substantially.

☞ Cardiac output depends almost completely on heart rate until the heart muscle is fully developed at 5 years of age.

☞ Congenital heart defects are the most common cause of congestive heart failure in infants and children.

☞ Signs of congestive heart failure may include tachypnea, tachycardia, pallor or cyanosis, nasal flaring, grunting, retractions, cough, crackles, periorbital and facial edema, jugular vein distention, and hepatomegaly.

- Congenital heart defects develop during the early weeks of pregnancy and are usually the result of a combined or interactive effect of genetic and environmental factors.

- In nonobstructive acyanotic heart defects a left-to-right shunt allows extra blood volume to overload the pulmonary system and potentially cause congestive heart failure.

- An obstructive defect (i.e., aortic or pulmonic stenosis) causes pressure overload and hypertrophy of the closest ventricle.

- Cardiac catheterization provides a way to evaluate hemodynamics and pressure gradients within the heart, and to noninvasively correct some heart defects.

- The child with a cyanotic heart defect may have life-threatening hypercyanotic spells requiring emergency treatment. Palliative or corrective surgery is often performed soon afterwards to prevent other life-threatening attacks.

- Heart transplantation is performed in infants and children for complex heart defects or in children for cardiomyopathy.

- Pulmonary artery hypertension is a life-threatening complication of congenital heart disease with excessive pulmonary blood flow. Irreversible pulmonary vascular changes include inflammation, hypertrophy of pulmonary vessels, and fibrosis.

- Rheumatic fever is an inflammatory connective tissue disease following a streptococcal infection that may affect the heart, joints, skin, or central nervous system.

- Children who have a congenital heart defect, rheumatic heart disease, or a central venous catheter or who have had heart surgery are at risk for infective endocarditis.

- Two potentially life-threatening cardiac arrhythmias are supraventricular tachycardias and long QT syndrome.

- Kawasaki disease is the most common cause of acquired heart disease in children in the United States.

- Some children have familial or lifestyle-related hyperlipidemia that causes undesirable levels of cholesterol or triglycerides. These children should have dietary intervention to reduce the risk of coronary artery disease as adults.

- All children with blood pressures in the 90th percentile for age are significantly more likely to develop hypertension as adults.

- Shock is an acute, complex state of circulatory dysfunction resulting in failure to deliver sufficient oxygen and other nutrients to meet cell and tissue demands.

- Signs that a child is in compensated hypovolemic shock include tachycardia, increased respiratory effort, delayed capillary refill, weak peripheral pulses, pallor, and cold extremities.

- Distributive shock is an abnormal pooling of blood in the extremities that may be caused by anaphylaxis, sepsis, or spinal cord injury.

- Myocardial contusion results from a strong, blunt force against the chest wall that injures the heart muscle, and may cause an arrhythmia.

EXPLOREMediaLink

NCLEX Review, Case Studies, and other interactive resources for this chapter can be found on the companion website at http://www.prenhall.com/london. Click on "Chapter 43" and select the activities for this chapter.

For animations, more NCLEX review questions, and an audio glossary, access the accompanying CD-ROM in this textbook.

References

American Academy of Pediatrics Committee on Pediatric Emergency Medicine. (1999). Emergency preparedness of children with special health care needs. *Pediatrics, 104*(4), e53.

American Heart Association. (2001). *Incidence of congenital heart defects.* WEB

Balaguru, D., Artman, M., & Auslender, M. (2000). Management of heart failure in children. *Current Problems in Pediatrics, 30*(1), 1–36.

Barst, R. J. (1999). Recent advances in the treatment of pediatric pulmonary artery hypertension. *Pediatric Clinics of North America, 46*(2), 331–345.

Bartosh, S. M., & Aronson, A. J. (1999). Childhood hypertension: An update on etiology, diagnosis, and treatment. *Pediatric Clinics of North America, 46*(2), 235–252.

Berul, C. I. (2000). Cardiac evaluation in the young athlete. *Pediatric Annals, 29*(3), 162–165.

Boneva, R. S., Botto, L. D., Moore, C. A., Yang, Q., Correa, A., & Erickson, J. D. (2001). Mortality associated with congenital heart defects in the United States: Trends and racial disparities, 1979–1997, *Circulation, 103*(19), 2376–2381.

Botto, L. D., Khoury, M. J., Mulinare, J., & Erickson, J. D. (1996). Periconceptional multivitamin use and the occurrence of contruncal heart defects: Results from a population-based, case-control study. *Pediatrics, 98*(5), 911–917.

Boucek, M. M. (2000). *Issues in pediatric heart transplantation.* WEB

Brook, M. M. (1999). Pediatric bacterial endocarditis: Treatment and prophylaxis. *Pediatric Clinics of North America, 46*(2), 275–287.

Case, C. L. (1999). Diagnosis and treatment of pediatric arrhythmias. *Pediatric Clinics of North America, 46*(2), 347–354.

Dajani, A. S., Taubert, K. A., Wilson, W., Bolger, A. F., Bayer, A., Ferrieri, P., et.al. (1997). Prevention of bacterial endocarditis: Recommendations of the American Heart Association. *Journal of the American Medical Association, 277*(22), 1794–1801.

DeBoer, S. (1996). The care of the blue baby: Emergency department management of tetralogy of Fallot. *Journal of Emergency Nursing, 22*(2), 73–76.

Driscoll, D. J. (1999). Left-to-right shunt lesions. *Pediatric Clinics of North America, 46*(2), 355–368.

Duitsman, D. M., Suddaby, E. C., & Masterson, G. (1999). Unique considerations for the pediatric heart transplant recipient: The role of the school nurse. *Journal of School Nursing, 15*(3), 10–13.

Eichelberger, M. R., Ball, J. W., Pratsch, G. S., & Clark, J. R. (1998). *Pediatric emergencies* (2nd ed.). Englewood Cliffs, NJ: Brady.

Fedderly, R. T. (1999). Left ventricular outflow obstruction. *Pediatric Clinics of North America, 46*(2), 369–384.

Giddings, S. (1999). Preventive pediatric cardiology: Tobacco, cholesterol, obesity, and physical activity. *Pediatric Clinics of North America, 46*(2), 253–262.

Grifka, R. G. (1999). Cyanotic congenital heart disease with increased pulmonary blood flow. *Pediatric Clinics of North America, 46*(2), 405–425.

Hazinski, M. F. (1999). *Manual of pediatric critical care* (pp. 130–160). St. Louis, MO: Mosby.

Hoffman, J. I. E. (1995). Incidence of congenital heart disease: I. Postnatal incidence. *Pediatric Cardiology, 16*(3), 103–113.

Hohn, A. R. (1997). Diagnosis and management of hypertension in childhood. *Pediatric Annals, 26*(2), 105–110.

Howard, J. K., Bindler, R. M., Synoground, G., & Van Gemert, F. C. (1996). A cardiovascular risk reduction program for the classroom. *Journal of School Nursing, 12*(4), 5–11.

Kohr, L. M., & Sims, S. L. (1998). Alterations in cardiovascular function in children. In K. L. McCance & S. E. Huether (Eds.), *Pathophysiology: The biologic basis for disease in adults and children* (3rd ed., pp. 1093–1130). St. Louis, MO: Mosby.

Kris-Etherton, P., Daniels, S. R., Eckel, R. H., Engler, M., Howard, B. V., Krauss, R. M., et al. (2001). AHA scientific statement: Summary of the Scientific Conference on dietary fatty acids and cardiovascular health. Conference summary of the Nutrition Committee of the American Heart Association. *Journal of Nutrition, 131*(4), 1322–6.

Lewin, M. B. (2000). The genetic basis of congenital heart disease. *Pediatric Annals, 29*(8), 469–480.

Mahle, W. T., & Wernovsky, G. (2001). Long-term developmental outcome of children with complex congenital heart disease. *Clinics in Perinatology, 28*(1), 235–247.

National High Blood Pressure Education Program Working Group on Hypertension Control in Children and Adolescents. (1996). Update on the 1987 task force report on high blood pressure in children and adolescents: A working group report from the National High Blood Pressure Education Program. *Pediatrics, 98*(4), 649–658.

Nouri, S. (1997). Congenital heart defects: Cyanotic and acyanotic. *Pediatric Annals, 26*(2), 94–98.

Obarzanek, E., Kimm, S. Y. S., Barton, B. A., Van Horn, L., Kwiterovich, P. O., Simons-Morton, D. G., et al. (2001). Long-term safety and efficacy of a cholesterol-lowering diet in children with elevated low-density lipoprotein cholesterol: Seven-year results of the dietary intervention study in children (DISC). *Pediatrics, 107*(2), 256–264.

Odim, J., Laks, H., Burch, C., Komanapalli, C., & Alejos, J. C. (2000). Transplantation for congenital heart disease. *Advances in Cardiac Surgery, 12,* 59–76.

O'Laughlin, M. P. (1999). Congestive heart failure in children. *Pediatric Clinics of North America, 46*(2), 263–273.

Park, M. K. (1996). *Pediatric cardiology for practitioners* (3rd ed.). St. Louis, MO: Mosby–Year Book.

Petrini, J., Damus, K., & Johnston, R. B., Jr. (1998, September 25). Trends in infant mortality attributable to birth defects—United States, 1980–1995. *Morbidity and Mortality Weekly Report, 47,* 773–778.

Porto, I. (2000). Hypertensive emergencies in children. *Journal of Pediatric Health Care, 14*(6), 312–317.

Purath, J., Lansinger, T., & Ragheb, C. (1995). Cardiac risk evaluation for elementary school children. *Public Health Nursing, 12*(3), 189–195.

Robinson, B., Anisman, P., & Eshaghpour, E. (1996). Is that fast heart beat dangerous (and what should you do about it)? *Contemporary Pediatrics, 13*(9), 52–85.

Rowley, A. H., & Shulman, S. T. (1999). Kawasaki syndrome. *Pediatric Clinics of North America, 46*(2), 313–329.

Starr, N. B., & Freitas-Nichols, J. (2000). Cardiac arrythmias in children. *Journal of Pediatric Health Care, 14*(3), 127–129.

Steeg, C. N., Walsh, C. A., & Glickstein, J. S. (2000). Rheumatic fever: No cause for complaisance. *Contemporary Pediatrics, 17*(1), 128–141.

Stinson, J., & McKeever, P. (1995). Mother's information needs related to caring for infants at home following cardiac surgery. *Journal of Pediatric Nursing, 10*(1), 48–57.

Stumpflen, I., Stumpflen, A., Wimmer, M., & Bernaschek, G. (1996, September 28). Effects of detailed fetal echocardiography as part of routine prenatal ultrasonographic screening on detection of congenital heart disease. *Lancet, 348,* 854–857.

Waldman, J. D., & Wernly, J. A. (1999). Cyanotic congenital heart disease with decreased pulmonary blood flow in children. *Pediatric Clinics of North America, 46*(2), 385–404.

Walters, H. L. (2000). Congenital cardiac surgical strategies and outcomes: HEARTS. *Pediatric Annals, 29*(8), 489–498.

Williams, C. L., & Bollella, M. (1995). Guideline for screening, evaluating, and treating children with hypercholesterolemia. *Journal of Pediatric Health Care, 9*(4), 153–161.

Winter, W. E., House, D. V., & Schatz, D. (1999). Measuring and managing lipid levels. *Contemporary Pediatrics, 16*(5), 96–105.

Wolfe, R. R., Boucek, M., Schaffer, M. S., & Wiggins, J. W. (1997). Cardiovascular diseases. In W. W. Hay, J. R. Groothius, A. R. Hayward, & M. J. Levin (Eds.), *Current pediatric diagnosis and treatment* (13th ed., pp. 474–536). Stamford, CT: Appleton & Lange.

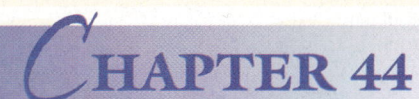

CHAPTER 44

The Child with Alterations in Hematologic Function

Having a child with sickle cell disease is very difficult for us. We know this is a genetic disease, and we feel responsible for Michael's pain. We also never seem to expect the bad times when they come. He'll be doing well and we almost forget. . .then he gets sick or doesn't drink enough and we're in the hospital again. His older sister has started talking about how she worries that sometime she'll have a child with sickle cell disease and we don't know what to tell her.

—FATHER OF MICHAEL, 12 YEARS OLD

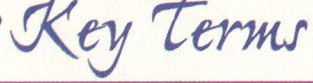

Key Terms

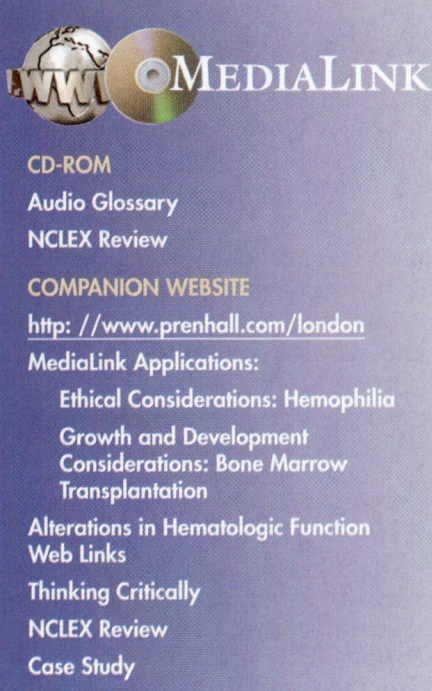

MediaLink

CD-ROM

Audio Glossary

NCLEX Review

COMPANION WEBSITE

http://www.prenhall.com/london

MediaLink Applications:

Ethical Considerations: Hemophilia

Growth and Development Considerations: Bone Marrow Transplantation

Alterations in Hematologic Function Web Links

Thinking Critically

NCLEX Review

Case Study

The hematologic system is one of a few body systems that regulate, directly or indirectly, all other body functions. Because blood is involved in the function of all tissues and organs, changes in the blood may result in altered functioning of many body organs and structures. A tendency toward easy bruising is a characteristic sign of many bleeding disorders. Other signs include nosebleeds, pallor, frequent infections, and lethargy. This chapter discusses the most common disorders of the blood and blood-forming organs in children. (See Chapter 45 for a discussion of leukemia.)

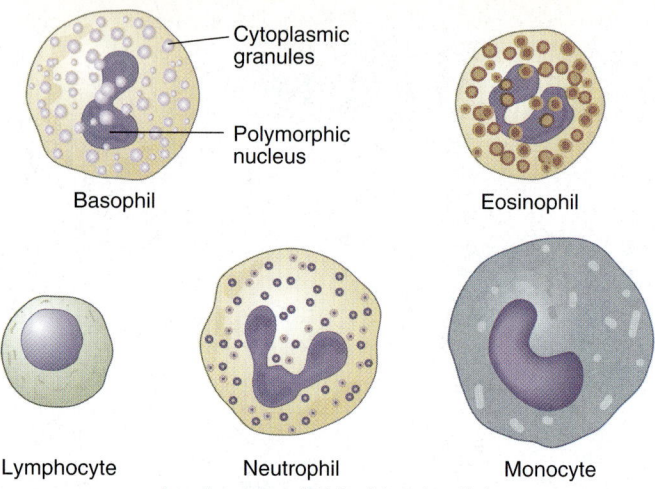

Leukocytes (white blood cells)

ANATOMY AND PHYSIOLOGY OF PEDIATRIC DIFFERENCES

Blood has two components: a fluid portion called plasma and a cellular portion known as the formed elements of the blood. The cellular elements are red blood cells (erythrocytes), white blood cells (leukocytes), and platelets (thrombocytes) (Figure 44–1 ◆). Table 44–1 gives normal values for these blood components in children.

The fetus produces red blood cells by the second week of gestation, with white blood cell and platelet production beginning at 8 weeks. Most of this early production occurs in the liver; however, by 20 to 24 weeks' gestation, liver production decreases as bone marrow production begins to predominate (Ohls & Christensen, 2000).

At birth, **hematopoiesis,** or blood cell production, occurs in the marrow of almost every bone. The flat bones, such as the sternum, ribs, pelvic and shoulder girdles, vertebrae, and hips, retain most of their hematopoietic activity throughout life.

Red Blood Cells

Red blood cells, or erythrocytes, are the most abundant of the cellular elements of blood. They are formed through the process of **erythropoiesis.** The primary function of red blood cells is to transport oxygen from the lungs to the tissues. They also help to carry carbon dioxide back to the lungs. Hemoglobin, a red pigment composed of protein and iron, is essential to this function.

Polycythemia is an above-average increase in the number of red cells in the blood. Any condition that causes the

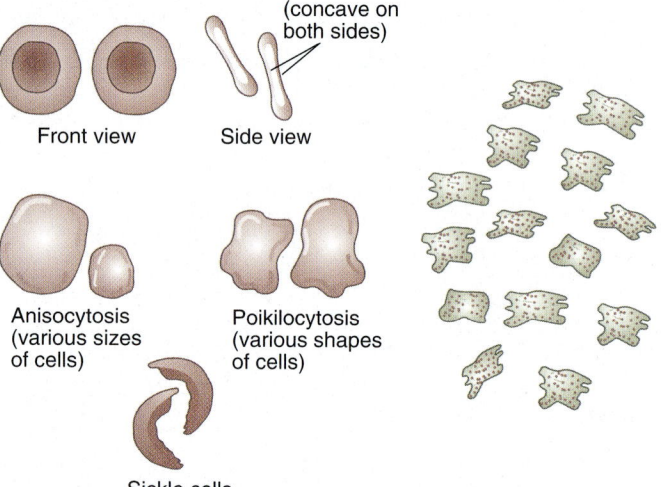

Erythrocytes (red blood cells)   Platelets

FIGURE 44–1. ◆ Types of blood cells.

quantity of oxygen transported to the tissues to decrease ordinarily increases the rate of red blood cell production. When a child becomes anemic after a hemorrhage, for instance, the bone marrow immediately begins to produce large quantities of red cells. **Anemia** is a reduction in the number of red blood cells; the various types of anemia will be discussed in the following section.

TABLE 44–1	Normal Blood Values in Children			
	Newborn	2 Years	12 Years	18 Years
Red blood cells (RBCs) (values × 10⁶/μL)	3.4–5.5	4.0–4.9	4.0–5.3	3.8–5.4
Hematocrit (Hct) (%)	37.4–56.1	31.7–37.7	34.0–43.9	33.0–46.2
Hemoglobin (Hgb) (g/dL)	12.7–18.6	10.5–12.7	14.8–13.6	10.7–15.7
White blood cells (WBCs) (values × 10³/μL)	6.8–14.3	5.3–11.5	4.5–10.1	4.4–10.2
Platelets (values × 10³/μL)	164–351	204–405	165–335	143–326

Note: From Soldin, S. J., Brugnara, C., & Hicks, J. M. (1999). *Pediatric reference ranges* (3rd ed.). Washington, DC: AACC Press. Adapted.

At birth, the newborn has a naturally occurring elevation in red blood cells (RBCs) due to a high level of erythropoietin, which stimulates red cell production (see Table 44–1). Once the newborn begins breathing air and the oxygen level in the blood increases, this production slows. Levels of RBCs fall until about 2 to 3 months of age, and then begin increasing. Adult levels are reached during adolescence. Teenage males have RBC levels slightly higher than teenage females (see Appendix B) (Lane, Nuss, & Ambruso, 1999).

White Blood Cells

White blood cells, or leukocytes, are the mobile units of the body's protective system. They are formed in bone marrow and lymph tissue. The white blood cell count is highest at birth, although levels vary greatly among infants. By 1 week of age, white blood cell values stabilize. Throughout childhood, there is a very slow decrease in white blood cell count (Boxer, 2000).

There are five types of white blood cells, each with a distinct function (Table 44–2). A differential blood count indicates the percentages of the different types of white cells in the blood and is sometimes useful in identifying the cause of an illness. For example, infections cause an increase in neutrophils; and allergies are related to an increase in eosinophils. The role of lymphocytes is discussed with AIDS in Chapter 40. A decrease in the number of white blood cells is called **leukopenia,** and can be caused by immune or bone marrow disorders.

Platelets

Platelets, or thrombocytes, are cell fragments that can form hemostatic plugs to stop bleeding. They are synthesized from components in the red bone marrow and are stored in the spleen. Platelet levels in newborns are lower than in older children and adults. Levels of many clotting factors, particularly those requiring vitamin K for activation, are also lower in infants. For this reason, all newborns receive a prophylactic injection of vitamin K at birth. Values of platelets and other coagulation products soon reach normal childhood levels (Montgomery & Scott, 2000). A deficiency of platelets can lead to bleeding disorder and is termed **thrombocytopenia.**

TABLE 44–2	White Blood Cells and Their Functions
Type	Function
Neutrophils	Phagocytosis
Eosinophils	Allergic reactions
Basophils	Inflammatory reactions
Monocytes (macrophages)	Phagocytosis, antigen processing
Lymphocytes	Humoral immunity (B cell), cellular immunity (T cell)

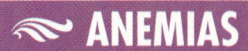

ANEMIAS

Anemia is defined as a reduction in the number of RBCs, the quantity of hemoglobin, and the volume of packed red cells to below-normal levels. It can be caused by loss or destruction of existing RBCs or by an impaired or decreased rate of red cell production. Anemia also can be a clinical manifestation of an underlying disorder, such as lead poisoning or hypersplenism (a syndrome characterized by splenomegaly and blood cell deficiencies). The major types of anemia seen in children include iron-deficiency anemia, beta-thalassemia, aplastic anemia, normocytic anemia, and sickle cell anemia.

IRON-DEFICIENCY ANEMIA

Iron-deficiency anemia is the most common type and the most common nutritional deficiency in children. It can occur because of blood loss, or as a result of increased internal demands (rapid growth) for blood production, or due to poor nutritional intake. See Chapter 31 for a discussion of iron-deficiency anemia due to deficits in nutritional intake.

Developing Cultural Competence

A number of genetic abnormalities of red blood cells rare in the United States are found among Southeast Asian immigrants. Many of these conditions can be confused with iron deficiency; however, most do not cause serious illness. If you work with these cultural groups, seek out more specific information about such conditions (Glader & Look, 1996).

Rapidly growing adolescents whose diets are high in fat and low in vitamins and minerals are particularly susceptible to iron-deficiency anemia. Infants who do not take in adequate solid foods after 6 months of age and are fed only breast milk or formula that is not fortified with iron are also at risk because neonatal iron stores have been depleted by this time and their iron needs are not being met. Similarly, if the mother's nutritional status during pregnancy was inadequate, or the infant was born prematurely or as part of a multiple birth, insufficient iron may have been stored in the latter part of pregnancy, placing the infant at higher risk for anemia in the first months of life.

Chronic blood loss is always a potential cause of iron-deficiency anemia. The infant who has had bleeding in the neonatal period, the child who loses blood as a result of conditions such as hemophilia or parasitic gastrointestinal illness, and the adolescent girl who has **menorrhagia** (heavy menstrual bleeding) may all be at risk of anemia.

Clinical manifestations depend on the severity of the anemia. Pallor, fatigue, and irritability are characteristic findings. With prolonged anemia, nailbed deformities,

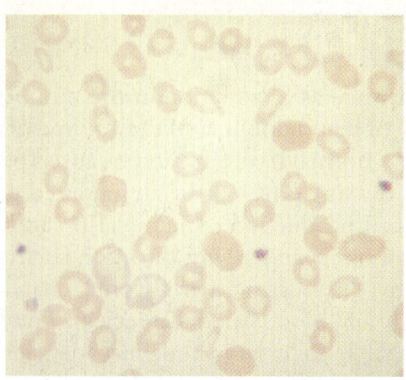

FIGURE 44–2. ◆ In iron-deficiency anemia, red blood cells appear hypochromic as a result of decreased hemoglobin synthesis. *Courtesy of Dr. Ed Wong, Laboratory Medicine, Children's National Medical Center, Washington, DC.*

growth retardation, developmental delay, tachycardia, and systolic heart murmur can occur.

Diagnosis is made on the basis of laboratory studies, including hemoglobin level, mean corpuscular volume, microscopic analysis (Figure 44–2 ◆), and serum iron-binding capacity. The RBCs are microcytic (small) in size and hypochromic (pale) in appearance (Cook, 2000). A diet history and analysis can provide information about food intake; see Chapter 31 for guidelines about diet history. ⊂▭⊃

Treatment involves correction of the iron deficiency with oral elemental iron preparations and a diet high in iron. Because oral iron preparations cause several side effects such as constipation and gastrointestinal discomfort, the child may receive iron supplements (to restore blood levels of iron) while the iron content of the diet is increased above the recommended dietary allowances (RDAs). Oral supplements can then be tapered off once the child's food intake can supply the needed iron. If the anemia is a result of bleeding, the cause is identified and treated to prevent future excess blood loss.

Nursing Management

The child with iron-deficiency anemia is usually not hospitalized unless he or she has another serious illness. Nursing care focuses on screening for the disorder and educating the parents and child about the causes of iron-deficiency anemia, dietary management, and the importance of complying with the medication regimen.

Screening for anemia is recommended at 9 months of age and again at adolescence (see Chapter 35) ⊂▭⊃ (American Academy of Pediatrics, 2000). A hematocrit or hemoglobin level is obtained. More detailed tests are performed if the blood test is abnormal. Children at high risk for nutritional deficiencies, such as those in low-income groups and WIC programs, may require additional tests. Nurses screen most children in Head Start annually. In addition, children showing signs of anemia should be screened. Take height and weight measurements at each health care visit, plot them on growth charts, and compare to percentiles obtained at previous visits. Slow downward trends in percentiles are of concern and require further nutritional analysis (see Chapter 31). ⊂▭⊃ Do developmental screening tests to assess for developmental delays (see Chapter 35). ⊂▭⊃

Developing Cultural Competence

According to traditional Chinese beliefs, a person who does not feel well is lacking in chi (inner energy) and blood. Chinese Americans who follow traditional practices may be hesitant to have blood drawn for laboratory studies for fear of causing bodily weakness.

Dietary management is the preferred long-term treatment for iron-deficiency anemia. Teach the family and child about foods rich in iron. The infant's diet should include iron-fortified formula and baby cereals. Older infants and toddlers can eat finger foods such as thinly sliced meats. Adolescents can be encouraged to eat foods with a high iron content, such as hamburgers and dried fruits.

Oral iron preparations are given to correct anemia (see Drug Guide, Chapter 31). ⊂▭⊃ Teach the child and family that the liquid iron preparation should be taken through a straw because it stains the teeth. Instruct about side effects such as black stools, constipation, and a foul aftertaste. Emphasize the importance of drinking fluids and eating foods high in dietary fiber to minimize these side effects. The medicine should be stored safely to avoid accidental poisoning. Expected outcomes of care are intake of recommended levels of iron and return to normal hematocrit level.

NORMOCYTIC ANEMIA

In normocytic anemia, the RBCs, although decreased in number, are of normal size with a pale center (Cook, 2000). This type of anemia may occur as a result of hemorrhage, disease-induced inflammation, disseminated intravascular coagulation (DIC; see the discussion later in this chapter), G6PD deficiency, hemolytic–uremic syndrome (see Chapter 47), ⊂▭⊃ or several other conditions. When one of these conditions exists in a child diagnosed with anemia, the infectious or inflammatory condition should be suspected as the cause of the identified anemia and treated first. The anemia will often then correct itself over time (Abshire, 1996). Some infectious and inflammatory causes of anemia are listed in Table 44–3.

Clinical manifestations are similar to those seen in iron-deficiency anemia, with the possible occurrence of he-

TABLE 44-3 Infectious and Inflammatory Causes of Anemia

Infections	Inflammations
Haemophilus influenzae type b	Arthritis
HIV/AIDS	Cancers
Orbital cellulitis	Chronic heart or liver disease
Meningitis	
Septic arthritis	

TABLE 44-4 Sickle Cell Disorders

Sickle Cell Trait (Hgb SA)
Most common form of sickle cell disease in the United States
Heterozygous condition (child has one sickle cell hemoglobin gene and one normal hemoglobin gene)
Child is carrier of sickle cell anemia and rarely has symptoms of the disease

Sickle Cell Anemia (Hgb SS)
Homozygous condition (child has two sickle hemoglobin genes)
Child is subject to sickle cell crises

Sickle Cell Syndromes
Sickle cell–Hgb C disease (Hgb SC)
Second most frequent form of sickle cell disease in African Americans
Different from sickle cell anemia only in that the sickle cell assumes a C shape instead of an S shape
Sickle Cell–β-Thalassemia Disease (Hgb SB)
Rarely occurs
Combination of sickle cell trait and thalassemia trait most often seen in people of Mediterranean descent

patomegaly and splenomegaly, as well. The etiology of normocytic anemia associated with chronic inflammation or infection is related to increased RBC destruction, decreased iron release from storage sites, and ineffective bone marrow response (Lane et al., 1999). In hemorrhage, anemia is a direct result of loss of blood.

Treatment of normocytic anemia depends on the underlying cause. When the anemia is associated with inflammation or infection, the underlying condition is treated. For anemia caused by renal failure, recombinant human erythropoietin is administered. When hemorrhage is the underlying cause, the source of the bleeding is identified and treated. In acute emergencies, blood products are infused to make up for some of the losses.

Nursing management of normocytic anemia depends on the cause of the decreased RBCs. Children with inflammatory or infectious diseases require careful assessment and management of medication and other treatment regimens. Administer blood products and other intravenous fluids as ordered to restore blood volume. Use follow-up and home visits to assess hematocrit, hemoglobin, and dietary intake. (Refer to the discussion later in this chapter for management of DIC; to Chapter 46 for management of intestinal infections; and to Chapter 47 for management of hemolytic–uremic syndrome).

SICKLE CELL ANEMIA

Sickle cell anemia is a hereditary **hemoglobinopathy,** in which normal hemoglobin is partly or completely replaced with abnormal hemoglobin S (Hgb S) (Table 44–4). Sickle cell anemia occurs primarily in blacks, although occasionally it affects people of Mediterranean descent. Sickle cell anemia occurs in about 1 in 375 black infants born in the United States, and 1 in 12 blacks have sickle cell trait (i.e., they carry one gene for the disease) (Jakubik & Thompson, 2000). **WEB**

Etiology and Pathophysiology

Sickle cell anemia is an autosomal recessive disorder. If both parents have the trait, with each pregnancy the risk of having a child with the disease is 25%. (See Chapter 4 for a discussion of recessive gene transmission.)

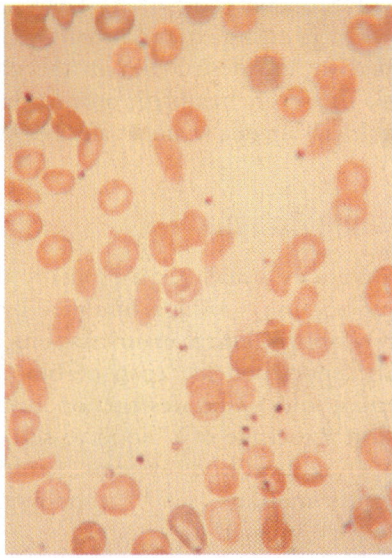

FIGURE 44–3. ◆ Many of these red blood cells show an elongated crescent shape characteristic of sickle cell anemia. Courtesy of Dr. Ed Wong, Laboratory Medicine, Children's National Medical Center, Washington, DC.

In sickle cell anemia, the hemoglobin in the RBC acquires an elongated crescent or sickle shape (Figure 44–3 ◆). The rigid sickled cells obstruct capillary blood flow. Microscopic obstructions lead to engorgement and tissue ischemia. This local tissue hypoxia causes further sickling and ultimately large infarctions. Damaged tissues in organs throughout the body become scarred, resulting in impaired function. For example, children with sickle cell anemia can suffer from splenic sequestration when blood is trapped in the spleen, a life-threatening complication.

Many children must undergo splenectomy in early childhood, leading to severely compromised immunity. Infection rate is high due to impaired immunity, and bacterial infections are the leading cause of death in young children with sickle cell disease. Strokes occur in 5% to 10% of children with sickle cell disease and can lead to developmental delay, mental retardation, and other neurologic outcomes (Hendricks-Ferguson & Nelson, 1999).

Sickling may be triggered by fever and emotional or physical stress. Precipitating factors for sickle cell crisis include increased blood viscosity (such as from a low fluid intake or fever) and hypoxia or low oxygen tension. Potential causes of hypoxia or low oxygen tension include high altitudes, poorly pressurized airplanes, hypoventilation, vasoconstriction when cold, or an emotionally stressful event. Any condition that increases the body's need for oxygen or alters the transport of oxygen (such as infection, trauma, or dehydration) may result in sickle cell crisis.

Sickled cells can resume a normal shape when rehydrated and reoxygenated. The membrane of these cells becomes more fragile, however, and cell life is shortened to 10 to 20 days rather than the usual 120 days. In response, bone marrow spaces enlarge to produce more RBCs. Continuous formation and destruction of the child's RBCs contributes to the severe hemolytic anemia that is characteristic of sickle cell anemia (Lane et al., 1999).

Clinical Manifestations

Affected children are usually asymptomatic until 4 to 6 months of age because sickling is inhibited by high levels of fetal hemoglobin. Clinical manifestations are directly related to the shortened life span of blood cells (hemolytic anemia) and tissue destruction resulting from **vaso-occlusion** (blockage of a blood vessel). Pathologic changes happen in most body systems, resulting in multiple signs and symptoms (see "Pathophysiology Illustrated: Sickle Cell Anemia").

Illness results from recurrent vaso-occlusive events that involve painful crises and chronic organ damage (Odesina, 2001). Sickle cell crises are acute exacerbations of the disease that vary markedly in severity and frequency. Table 44–5 outlines the most common types of crises affecting children with sickle cell disease. These crises may occur individually or in combination.

Children with sickle cell trait rarely have such crises. However, because they have some abnormal hemoglobin, they may develop symptoms of the disease under conditions of abnormally low oxygen such as flying in an unpressurized airplane over 7000 feet, or during anesthesia. The most common symptoms experienced by those with sickle cell trait are splenic infarction and hematuria. However, most persons who carry the trait never have symptoms, even with low oxygen concentrations.

TABLE 44-5	**Types of Sickle Cell Crises**

Vaso-occlusive Crises (Thrombotic)
Most common type of crisis; painful
Caused by stasis of blood with clumping of cells in the microcirculation, ischemia, and infarction
Signs include fever, pain, tissue engorgement

Splenic Sequestration
Life-threatening crisis; death can occur within hours
Caused by pooling of blood in the spleen
Signs include profound anemia, hypovolemia, and shock

Aplastic Crises
Diminished production and increased destruction of red blood cells
Triggered by viral infection or depletion of folic acid
Signs include profound anemia, pallor

Clinical Therapy

The initial diagnosis of sickle cell anemia in newborns is often made by testing cord blood using hemoglobin electrophoresis. The sickle-turbidity test (Sickledex) may be used for quick screening in children over 6 months of age, once the fetal hemoglobin levels have fallen. Hemoglobin electrophoresis verifies positive Sickledex test results. Newborns are screened hemoglobinopathies in 43 states (Zimmerman, Ware, & Kinney, 1997). It is recommended that all newborns be screened, because sickle cell disease can occur in several groups in addition to blacks, such as Mediterranean, South American, Arabian, and East Indian. A child's heritage cannot be predicted from appearance or name alone.

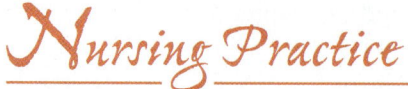

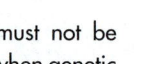

Information about genetic testing is confidential and must not be shared with people other than those tested. In the 1970s, when genetic testing for sickle cell disease and trait first became available, blacks who had the trait for sickle cell disease experienced discrimination in jobs and insurance.

No cure for sickle cell anemia exists. Supportive care is aimed at the prevention and treatment of sickling episodes. Preventing exposure to infections and maintaining normal hydration are important steps in avoiding crises. Aggressive treatment of infection with antibiotics and use of daily prophylactic penicillin in children from 2 months to 5 years of age is effective (Davis, Schoendorf, Gergen, et al., 1997). The reticulocyte count is monitored regularly to make sure that the bone marrow is still functioning.

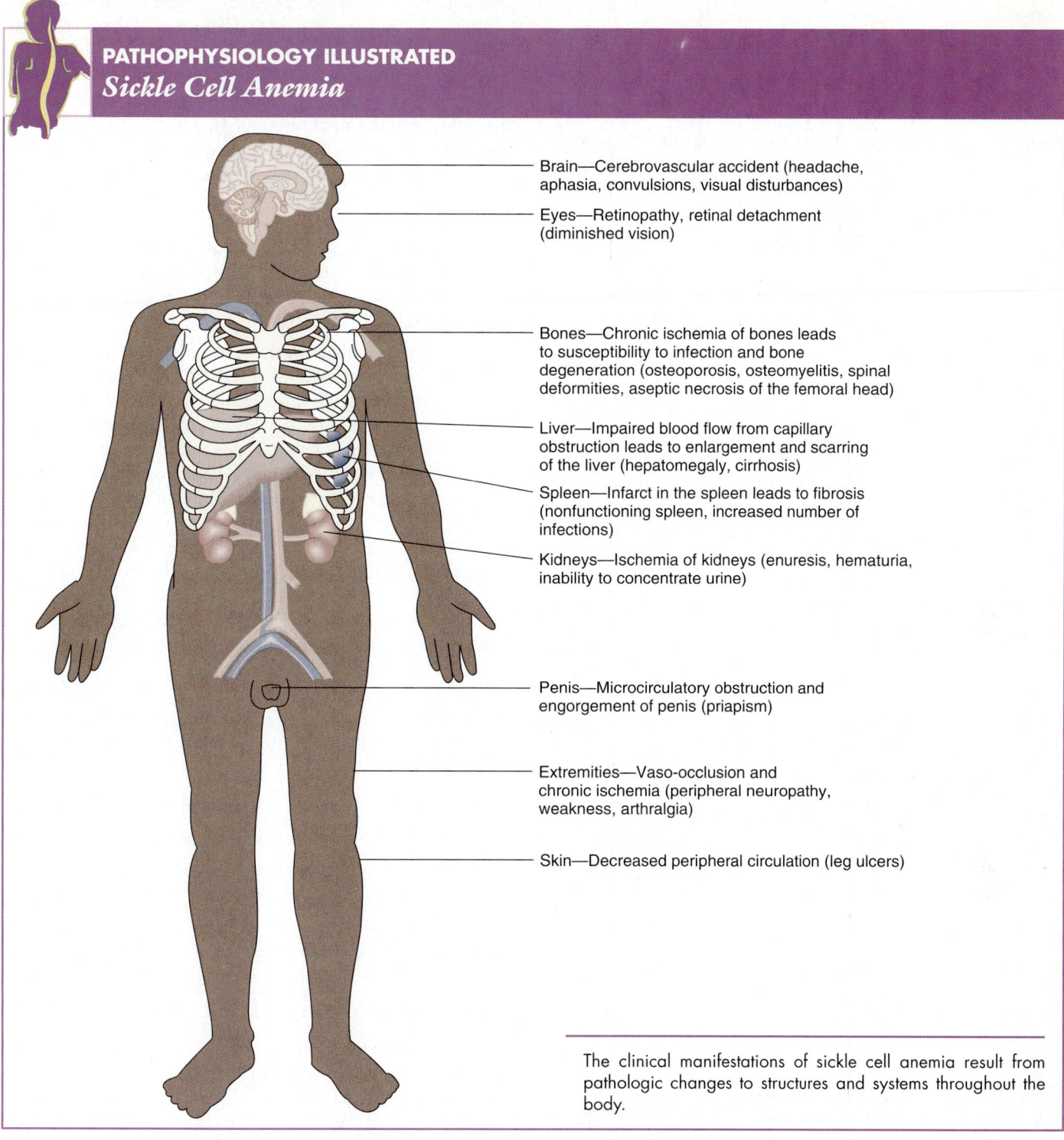

PATHOPHYSIOLOGY ILLUSTRATED
Sickle Cell Anemia

Brain—Cerebrovascular accident (headache, aphasia, convulsions, visual disturbances)

Eyes—Retinopathy, retinal detachment (diminished vision)

Bones—Chronic ischemia of bones leads to susceptibility to infection and bone degeneration (osteoporosis, osteomyelitis, spinal deformities, aseptic necrosis of the femoral head)

Liver—Impaired blood flow from capillary obstruction leads to enlargement and scarring of the liver (hepatomegaly, cirrhosis)

Spleen—Infarct in the spleen leads to fibrosis (nonfunctioning spleen, increased number of infections)

Kidneys—Ischemia of kidneys (enuresis, hematuria, inability to concentrate urine)

Penis—Microcirculatory obstruction and engorgement of penis (priapism)

Extremities—Vaso-occlusion and chronic ischemia (peripheral neuropathy, weakness, arthralgia)

Skin—Decreased peripheral circulation (leg ulcers)

The clinical manifestations of sickle cell anemia result from pathologic changes to structures and systems throughout the body.

Treatment of crises involves hydration, oxygen, pain management, and bed rest to reduce energy expenditure. Cultures (blood, urine, and throat) are taken to identify sources of infection. Other therapeutic measures include blood transfusions to treat the anemia and to make the sickled blood less viscous. In children who have had strokes from the disease, periodic transfusions (about every 3 to 4 weeks) can reduce the incidence of future strokes (National Heart, Lung, and Blood Institute, 1997). If given early in the crisis, blood transfusions may sometimes relieve the ischemia in major organs and body parts (spleen, lung, kidney, brain, and penis) caused by the vaso-occlusion. Antibiotics treat acute infection and are sometimes used as a prophylactic measure. Treatment with hydroxyurea has been helpful in adults, and is now sometimes used in children. This cytotoxic drug decreases production of abnormal blood cells and leads to less pain (Day & Wynn, 2000). (See Skill 12-6.) 🔗 **SKILLS**

It is important for all health facilities to have current guidelines for transfusion protocols. Become familiar with the policies and procedures where you work. For example, does the child's blood type and patient identification need to be checked by two nurses before starting the infusion? See the *Clinical Skills Manual* for further information on blood transfusions. 🔗 SKILLS

Children who have suffered a cerebrovascular accident (stroke) as a complication of the disease may be treated with blood transfusions on a regular basis. However, frequent transfusions may result in an overload of iron in the body. The iron is stored in tissues and organs (**hemosiderosis**) because the body has no way of excreting it. For this reason, an iron-chelating drug such as deferoxamine may be given along with vitamin C to promote iron excretion.

Neonatal screening, early intervention, prophylactic antibiotics, and parent education have allowed children with sickle cell disease to live into adulthood. Prognosis depends on the severity of the child's disease; children with more frequent exacerbations and hospitalization have poorer prognoses.

Nursing Management

Nursing Assessment and Diagnosis

The nurse may be involved in sickle cell gene testing to identify carriers and children who have the disease. Once a child is diagnosed with the disease, a comprehensive physical assessment is essential because sickle cell anemia can affect any body system.

Thinking Critically

SICKLE CELL ANEMIA

Michael is a 12-year-old black child with sickle cell disease who is admitted to the hospital with severe abdominal pain. Which organ is likely filled with sickled cells and causing his pain? Michael is receiving oxygen by nasal cannula; why would he need this? 🔗 WEB

PHYSIOLOGIC ASSESSMENT

In children who are known to have sickle cell anemia, take a detailed history from the parents or child about past crises, precipitating events, medical treatment, and home

management. Measure the child's height and weight accurately and compare to past measurements, since failure to thrive is common. Ask about chronic or acute pain that the child is experiencing. Pain may occur in nearly any body part, but most commonly manifests as headache, extremity pain, or abdominal discomfort. The ill child with sickle cell disease should receive a careful multisystem assessment. Fever is an emergency necessitating prompt treatment (Zimmerman et al., 1997).

When the child is in crisis, assess pain and note the presence of any signs of inflammation or infection. Carefully monitor the child for signs of shock (see Chapter 43). 🔗

PSYCHOSOCIAL ASSESSMENT

The family of a child with sickle cell disease requires a thorough psychosocial assessment. If the child is newly diagnosed with the disorder, the family needs assistance to deal with feelings related to the serious, life-threatening nature of the disease. Assess parents' understanding of the disease transmission and ask whether genetic counseling has been obtained. Determine whether the family has adequate health care coverage to pay for the child's medical expenses. Ask older children about their knowledge of the disease, and explore their feelings related to the management of a chronic condition. When siblings or other family members are carriers, periodic counseling is needed so they can understand implications for dating, marriage, and having children.

Several nursing diagnoses that might apply to the child with sickle cell anemia are presented in the accompanying "Nursing Care Plan." Other nursing diagnoses might include:

▶ *Caregiver role strain* related to illness chronicity

▶ *Risk for altered parenting* related to having a child with a physical illness

▶ *Altered growth and development* related to effects of physical disability

▶ *Impaired physical mobility* related to pain

Planning and Implementation

The accompanying "Nursing Care Plan" summarizes nursing care for the child with sickle cell anemia. Nursing management for the child in crisis focuses on increasing tissue perfusion, promoting hydration, controlling pain, preventing infection, ensuring adequate nutrition, preventing complications, and providing emotional support to the child and family.

INCREASE TISSUE PERFUSION

Administer blood transfusions and oxygen as ordered. To prevent hemolysis, the intravenous fluid used before and after a blood transfusion must be saline rather than D5W. In small children, the blood is usually infused without saline

GOAL	INTERVENTION	RATIONALE	EXPECTED OUTCOME
1. Risk for altered peripheral tissue perfusion related to affinity of hemoglobin for oxygen			
	NIC Priority Intervention: **Circulation care:** *Promotion of arterial and venous circulation*		*NOC Suggested Outcome:* **Tissue perfusion, peripheral:** *Extent to which blood flows through the small vessels of the extremities and maintains tissue function*
The child will show few signs and symptoms of tissue hypoxia.	▸ Instruct child to avoid physical exertion, emotional stress, low-oxygen environments (e.g., airplanes, high altitudes); and known sources of infection.	▸ Decreased activity and exposure reduce body's need for oxygen.	The child has no shortness of breath and shows no signs of hypoxia.
Repeated cerebrovascular accidents will be avoided.	▸ Administer blood transfusions as ordered.	▸ Packed cells increase number of red blood cells available to carry oxygen to tissue cells. Transfusions promote circulation.	
	▸ Perform several caregiving activities together whenever possible. ▸ Give oxygen as ordered.	▸ Grouping activities allows for optimum rest. ▸ High concentration of oxygen in alveoli increases diffusion of gas across membranes.	
	▸ Administer and teach the family to administer prophylactic transfusions for the child who has had a cerebrovascular accident.	▸ Lowers potential for a future cerebrovascular accident.	The child does not suffer a cerebrovascular accident.
2. Risk for fluid volume deficit related to inadequate fluid intake			
	NIC Priority Intervention: **Fluid management:** *Promotion of electrolyte balance and prevention of complications resulting from abnormal or undesired fluid levels*		*NOC Suggested Outcome:* **Hydration:** *Amount of water in the intracellular and extracellular compartments of the body*
The child will maintain or be restored to adequate hydration.	▸ Calculate the child's daily fluid requirements. Monitor the child's usual fluid consumption and make necessary adjustments. Encourage the child to take fluids. Observe for signs dehydration. ▸ Record intake and output.	▸ Optimizing fluid intake ensures that the child gets needed fluid. Dehydration exacerbates crises. ▸ Recording enables you to monitor daily fluid intake and spacing throughout the day.	The child shows signs of adequate hydration.
3. Pain related to chromic physical disability			
	NIC Priority Intervention: **Pain management:** *Alleviation of pain or a reduction in pain to a level of comfort acceptable to the patient*		*NOC Suggested Outcome:* **Comfort level:** *Feelings of physical and psychologic ease*
The child will verbalize that pain is controlled.	▸ Administer analgesics, such as morphine or hydromorphine (Dilaudid), as ordered. Continuous intravenous infusion is used for the duration of a painful crisis. ▸ Position carefully.	▸ Pain of sickle cell crises is excruciating. ▸ Joints and extremities can be extremely painful.	The child is pain-free or pain control is significantly improved.
4. Risk for infection related to chronic disease and splenic malfunction			
	NIC Priority Intervention: **Infectious control:** *Minimizing the acquisition and transmission of infectious agents*		*NOC Suggested Outcome:* **Risk control:** *Actions to eliminate or reduce actual, personal, and modifiable health threats*
The child will not develop infection.	▸ Ensure adequate nutrition by providing high-calorie high-protein diet. Make sure that the child's immunizations are up to date. Report any signs of infection to physician immediately. ▸ Isolate the child from possible sources of infection. Instruct parents about signs of infection and encourage them to seek prompt healthcare.	▸ Chronically ill children are at greater risk of infection. ▸ Restriction of persons with infection decreases the child's contact with infectious agents. Prompt care for infection reduces the chance of sickle cell crisis.	The child is free of infection.

(continued)

GOAL	INTERVENTION	RATIONALE	EXPECTED OUTCOME
5. Knowledge deficit (child and parents) related to lack of exposure about cause and treatment of sickle cell anemia			
The child and family will verbalize understanding of risk factors for sickle cell crises and how to minimize them.	*NIC Priority Intervention:* **Teaching disease process:** *Assisting the patient to understand information related to a specific disease process* ▶ Review basics of sickle cell disease. Teach the child and family about signs and symptoms of crises. ▶ Arrange for genetic counseling and testing for sickle cell trait for family members if desired.	▶ Knowledge of disease helps ensure compliance with treatment regimen and adherence to preventive measures. ▶ Questions and concerns regarding future pregnancies can be allayed through knowledge of disease and transmission.	*NOC Suggested Outcome:* **Knowledge:** *Extent of understanding conveyed about sickle cell disease* The child and parent can verbalize precipitating events of crises.

because the child cannot manage the extra volume. Monitor for transfusion reactions (see "Clinical Manifestations of Blood Transfusion Reactions"). Encourage the child to rest. Work with the child and family to avoid emotional stress. Any activities that increase cellular metabolism also result in tissue hypoxia. Schedule caregiving activities and play to allow for optimal rest.

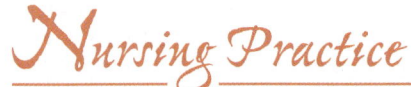

When giving a transfusion, never infuse cold blood since it may increase sickling. Use a blood-warming coil to bring blood to room temperature.

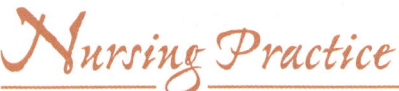

Blood reactions can occur as soon as the blood transfusion begins. Administer the first 20 mL of blood slowly and observe the child carefully for a reaction. Repeatedly assess the child according to hospital policy.

PROMOTE HYDRATION

The child with sickle cell anemia is adversely affected by dehydration. Calculate the child's fluid maintenance requirements (minimum daily fluid intake) (see Chapter 39) 〇⊃ and monitor the child's oral fluid intake. Administer intravenous fluids as ordered. Adjust oral intake as necessary to keep the child well hydrated.

Growth and Development

To encourage fluid intake in a small child:

- Use a favorite cup or glass.
- Use straws.
- Take advantage of times the child is thirsty, such as on awakening or after play.
- Leave a cup within easy reach of the child.
- Offer frozen juice pops, crushed ice drinks, and flavored ice chips.

CONTROL PAIN

Give prescribed analgesics around the clock during crises. If patient-controlled analgesia is used, be sure that the constant infusions run as ordered and that the parent or child understands the use of bolus infusions, when needed (see Chapter 38). Help the child assume a comfortable position. Avoid putting stress on painful joints.

CLINICAL MANIFESTATIONS 〜 *Blood Transfusion Reactions*

TYPE OF REACTION	ETIOLOGY	CLINICAL MANIFESTATIONS	CLINICAL THERAPY
Allergic reaction Hemolytic reaction	Immune response Mismatched blood, history of multiple transfusions	Urticaria, itching, respiratory distress Fever, chills, hematuria, headache, chest pain; can progress to shock	Stop the transfusion; call physician; give antihistamines as ordered; monitor vital signs; maintain intravenous infusion of normal saline; keep intravenous line open; check urine for hematuria

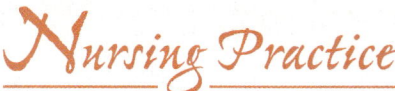

Use neither hot nor cold compresses for pain management in the child with sickle cell anemia. Ischemic tissue is fragile and has reduced sensation, increasing the risk of burn injury. Cold compresses promote sickling.

PREVENT INFECTION

Infection makes the child more susceptible to a crisis, and the crisis, in turn, increases susceptibility to infection. Teach the parents how to administer antibiotics for prophylaxis or treatment of infection. Be sure they have the finances and other resources to obtain and give daily antibiotics. Because infections are particularly virulent in these children, tell parents to get immediate care when the child is ill. Encourage the pneumococcal vaccine in all infants and children with the disease. The *Haemophilus influenzae* type b (Hib) vaccine series should be started by 2 months of age and continued at recommended ages to prevent another common source of infection.

ENSURE ADEQUATE NUTRITION

Emphasize the importance of adequate nutrition to promote growth. Encourage the child to eat a high-protein, high-calorie diet. Emphasize the importance of folic acid supplements as ordered.

PREVENT COMPLICATIONS OF CRISES

Poor growth and delayed maturation are frequently observed, so measure growth and evaluate developmental skills. Watch for signs of increasing anemia, infection, and shock (mental status change, pallor, vital sign changes). Assess the child's neurologic status for evidence of altered cerebral function. If ordered, assess for an enlarged spleen by gentle palpation. Administer blood transfusions and watch the child for any adverse reaction.

PROVIDE EMOTIONAL SUPPORT

Sickle cell anemia is a chronic disease accompanied by life-threatening episodic crises. Family members often need support to help them deal with their feelings about the diagnosis and its implications. Explore resources in the home and community to see if parents will be able to administer medications and fluids and to provide adequate nutrition. Assess their knowledge of signs of infection and of sickle cell crisis and when to seek medical care for the child. Refer the parents for genetic counseling, particularly if they plan to have more children. Encourage adolescents and young adults in the family to receive genetic counseling and testing, as well. Referrals to support groups and contact with others with the disease can be helpful.

HOME CARE CONSIDERATIONS FOR THE CHILD WITH SICKLE CELL ANEMIA

Follow recommended schedules for well-child care visits.

Be sure the child is up-to-date with immunizations, including hepatitis B, annual influenza, pneumococcal vaccine, and tuberculosis skin test.

Special testing, such as heart and eye examinations, may be needed periodically to check for sequelae of the disease.

Special medications, such as antibiotics, may be needed; pain relief medicine and blood transfusions may be administered.

Dehydration is dangerous. Be sure the child gets extra fluids in hot weather, when ill, during physical activity, and during travel.

As the child develops, provide information about the disease and encourage self-care. Be sure the school personnel understand the child's diagnosis and any care required during school hours.

Contact your health care provider if the child has a high fever, a common illness that lasts more than one day, seizures, change in behavior, severe pain, abnormal skin color or breathing pattern, or any other symptoms that concern you.

DISCHARGE PLANNING AND HOME CARE TEACHING

Identify and address home care needs well in advance of discharge. Give parents information about sickle cell disease and the child's treatment. Even parents of a child previously diagnosed with the disorder may benefit from information about the disease process and its management. Explain the basic effect of tissue hypoxia and the effects of sickling on circulation. Refer parents to support groups such as the National Association of Sickle Cell Disease for further information. **WEB**

Teach parents to look for signs of dehydration, such as dry mucous membranes, weight loss, and sunken fontanels in infants. Give specific instructions about how many ounces of liquid the child needs to drink each day. Emphasize that increased fluid intake is needed to replace the fluids lost from overheating or exposure to hot weather. Make sure both the child and family understand the triggers and precipitating factors for sickle cell crises. Encourage them to avoid situations that cause crises. Instruct the child and parents about signs and symptoms of crises that should be reported to their health care provider (see Table 44–5).

Provide the family with careful instructions about infusion therapy. When regular blood infusions are used, the resulting iron overload is damaging to body organs. These children need infusion of deferoxamine (Desferal) for iron overload. The medication is usually given by subcutaneous or intravenous routes over 8 to 10 hours. Prompt recognition of side effects and careful management of the lengthy infusion process are important. The child needs to be monitored for skin reactions and allergic responses. Have parents demonstrate the infusion technique and state what to do in case of reactions. Pain management is needed during infusion as the site may be tender and uncomfortable (Odesina, 2001).

Tell parents that it is important to inform all treating physicians and dentists of the child's medical condition. The child should also wear medical identification (e.g., medical identification bracelet). Special precautions are necessary when the child undergoes surgery of any kind, as hypoxia resulting from anesthesia is a major surgical risk.

Family members need ongoing support to deal with the stress of having a child with a chronic condition. Provide resources, respite care for parents, and information as needed for siblings.

Encourage older children with sickle cell anemia to participate in activities with other children between crises but to avoid strenuous physical exertion and contact sports. Play and social interactions that promote learning and development are important.

Evaluation

Expected outcomes of nursing care for the child with sickle cell anemia include:

▶ Management of pain to facilitate comfort level

▶ Maintenance of adequate hydration state to prevent cell sickling

▶ Absence of side effects of disease in respiratory system, central nervous system, and body organs

▶ Maintenance of normal immune status and prevention of infection

▶ Prompt recognition and treatment of complications of the disease

▶ Maintenance of normal growth and development for the child

▶ Provision of necessary services and resources for the parents and other family members

▶ Knowledge of disease and treatment by family

β-THALASSEMIA

The thalassemias are a group of inherited blood disorders of hemoglobin synthesis characterized by anemia that can be mild or severe. β-thalassemia, also known as Cooley anemia, is the most common type. These disorders most often occur in people of Mediterranean descent but are also found among Middle Eastern, Asian, and African populations (Cook, 2000; Lane et al., 1999). If both parents carry the abnormal gene, with each pregnancy there is a 25% chance of passing the disorder on to the child.

There are three types of β-thalassemia: thalassemia minor, or thalassemia trait (produces mild anemia); thalassemia intermedia (produces severe anemia); and thalassemia major (produces anemia requiring transfusion). Clinical

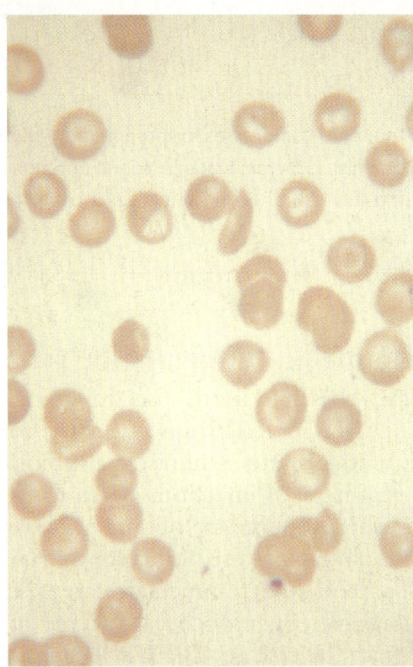

FIGURE 44–4. ◆ Red blood cell appearance in β-thalassemia. What characteristic abnormalities can be seen on this microscopic view? Courtesy of Dr. Ed Wong, Laboratory Medicine, Children's National Medical Center, Washington, DC.

manifestations of β-thalassemia are caused by the defective synthesis of hemoglobin, structurally impaired RBCs (Figure 44–4 ◆), and the shortened life span of the RBCs. β-thalassemia can be detected early in infancy. The infant with β-thalassemia manifests pallor, failure to thrive, hepatosplenomegaly, and severe anemia (hemoglobin <6 g/dL). Diagnosis is made by hemoglobin electrophoresis, which shows a decreased production of one of the globin chains in hemoglobin. Characteristic erythrocyte cell changes often can be recognized in infants by 6 weeks of age.

Treatment is supportive. The goal of medical management is to maintain normal hemoglobin levels. Blood transfusion is the conventional therapy used to treat children with severe disease. Since iron overload is a side effect of this treatment, children may need to receive an iron-chelating drug such as deferoxamine, which binds excess iron so it can be excreted by the kidneys. Other potential complications of long-term transfusion therapy are transfusion reactions and alloimmunization (antibody formation). Bone marrow transplantation may be offered as an alternative therapy for children newly diagnosed with the disorder.

Nursing Management

Nursing care focuses on observing for complications of transfusion therapy, providing emotional support, and referring the family for genetic counseling. Transfusions of packed cells are often given and careful evaluation for transfusion reactions is needed (see "Clinical Manifestations of Blood Transfusion Reactions" on page 1110).

BODY ORGAN	CLINICAL MANIFESTATIONS
Red Blood Cells (Anemia)	Hypochromic and microcytic changes Folic acid deficiency Frequent epistaxis
Skeletal Changes	Osteoporosis Delayed growth Susceptibility to pathologic fractures Facial deformities: enlarged head, prominent forehead due to frontal and parietal bossing, prominent cheek bones, broadened and depressed bridge of nose, enlarged maxilla with protruding front teeth, eyes with mongolian slant and epicanthal fold
Heart	Chronic congestive heart failure Myocardial fibrosis Murmurs
Liver/Gallbladder	Hepatomegaly Hepatic insufficiency
Spleen	Splenomegaly
Endocrine System	Delayed sexual maturation Fibrotic pancreas, resulting in diabetes mellitus
Skin	Darkening of skin

Teach parents the technique for subcutaneous infusion of deferoxamine if that route is to be used for therapy at home. Give parents information about thalassemia and its treatment, and encourage them to obtain genetic counseling. Provide emotional support and encourage parents to take an active role in the child's treatment regimen.

Compliance with transfusion therapy often becomes an issue as children reach adolescence. Offering the adolescent treatment options, such as when to undergo transfusion, can help improve compliance. Adolescents with β-thalassemia and parents of newly diagnosed children can be referred to the Thalassemia Action Group, a national organization for patients, or to the Cooley's Anemia Foundation. ⬤ WEB Expected outcomes of nursing care include maintenance of normal hemoglobin and hematocrit, safe transfusion of blood products, maintenance of recommended body iron levels, and family understanding about the genetic transmission of the disease.

APLASTIC ANEMIA

Aplastic anemia is a deficiency of the blood cells that results from failure of the bone marrow to produce adequate numbers of circulating blood cells. The condition may be congenital or acquired.

Congenital aplastic anemia (Fanconi anemia) is a rare autosomal recessive syndrome consisting of multiple congenital anomalies. Symptoms can include **purpura** (bleeding into the tissues), **petechiae** (pinpoint lesions), bleeding, fatigue, and pallor. Laboratory findings include neutropenia or anemia and thrombocytopenia (low platelet count) that progresses to **pancytopenia** (decreased number of blood cell components).

Children with congenital aplastic anemia are at risk for developing malignancies such as acute nonlymphocytic leukemia (Pizzo & D'Andrea, 2000). The treatment of choice is bone marrow transplantation. However, the prognosis is poor, and death usually results from overwhelming infection, hemorrhage, or malignancy.

Acquired aplastic anemia in children is either idiopathic or occurs from a drug reaction. It can develop after exposure to ionizing radiation or insecticides or after ingestion of drugs such as sulfonamides, chloramphenicol, quinacrine, benzene solvents in model airplane glue, or lead. This type of anemia can also be a result of an infectious process such as viral hepatitis or mononucleosis.

Symptoms are related to the degree of bone marrow failure and can include petechiae, purpura, bleeding, pallor, weakness, tachycardia, and fatigue. Diagnosis is made by blood studies, which reveal leukopenia (low white blood cell count) with marked neutropenia, thrombocytopenia, and pancytopenia; and by bone marrow aspiration, which reveals yellow, fatty bone marrow instead of red bone marrow.

Supportive treatment includes transfusions of packed cells and/or platelets. Immunosuppressive drug therapy is effective for many children. The treatment of choice is bone marrow transplantation from a compatible sibling or family member donor.

Nursing Management

Nursing care is similar to that for the child with leukemia (see Chapter 45). ⊂⊃ Nursing actions focus on preventing bleeding, administering and monitoring blood transfusions, preventing infection, encouraging mobility as tolerated, educating the parents and child about the disorder, and providing emotional support. Families need support in dealing with a child who has a life-threatening disease. Refer them to support groups for counseling, if indicated, and to social services. ⊂⊃ [WEB] Expected outcomes of nursing care include maintenance of normal levels of white and red blood cells and platelets to support body functions.

⌇ CLOTTING DISORDERS

HEMOPHILIA

Hemophilia refers to a group of hereditary bleeding disorders that result from a deficiency in specific clotting factors. Hemophilia A, or classic hemophilia, is caused by a deficiency of factor VIII in the blood and accounts for 80% of persons with hemophilia. About 1 in 5000 male babies has hemophilia A (DiMichele, 1996). Hemophilia B, known as Christmas disease, is caused by a deficiency of factor IX. Of people with hemophilia, 15% have hemophilia B.

Etiology and Pathophysiology

Hemophilia is an X-linked recessive trait, which manifests almost exclusively as affected males and carrier females. A daughter who inherits the trait from her father has a 50% chance at each pregnancy of transmitting it to her sons (see Chapter 4 for a description of genetic transmission). ⊂⊃ However, as many as one third of hemophiliacs have no family members with a history of clotting disorders. In these cases, the disorder is caused by a new mutation. The degree of bleeding is related to the amount of clotting factor and the severity of the injury.

Clinical Manifestations

Hemophilia is manifested in different children by bleeding tendencies that range from mild to moderate or severe. Children with hemophilia often do not manifest symptoms until after 6 months of age as they become more mobile and incur injuries and bleeding from falls or from tooth eruption. Spontaneous bleeding, **hemarthrosis** (bleeding into a joint space), and deep tissue hemorrhage occur. Affected children frequently experience bleeding into the joint spaces of the knees, ankles, and elbows. Bleeding into joint spaces or bursae causes the child to have limited motion because of pain, tenderness, and swelling. Bone changes, contractures, and disabling deformities can result from immobility and from the effects of blood in the joint structures.

Children may have bleeding after circumcision, easy bruising (**ecchymosis,**) nosebleeds, hematuria, and bleeding after tooth extraction, minor trauma, or minor surgical procedures. Large subcutaneous and intramuscular hemorrhages sometimes occur. Bleeding into the tissues of the neck, mouth, or chest is particularly serious because of the potential for airway obstruction. Retroperitoneal and intracranial bleeding may also occur and can be life threatening (Stover, 2000).

Females who carry the trait for hemophilia do not usually manifest symptoms of the disease. However, they may have prolonged bleeding during dental work, surgery, or trauma.

Clinical Therapy

Affected people and carriers can be diagnosed before birth through chorionic villus sampling or amniocentesis. Genes for clotting factors VIII and IX are located near the terminal long arm of the X chromosome (Montgomery & Scott, 2000). Genetic testing of family members is increasingly being used to identify carriers. Diagnosis can also be made on the basis of the history, physical examination, and laboratory data. Laboratory tests show low levels of factor VIII or IX, and prolonged activated partial prothrombin time (APPT). Prothrombin time (PT), thrombin time (TT), fibrinogen, and platelet count are normal.

The goal of medical management is to control bleeding by replacing the missing clotting factor. Replacement therapy is indicated when the child experiences a mild or major hemorrhage or faces a life-threatening situation. Prompt, adequate treatment is needed to prevent serious bleeding episodes and their sequelae (Stover, 2000). A synthetic drug effective against mild hemophilia is desmopressin acetate (DDAVP). An analogue of vasopressin, DDAVP is administered intravenously and causes a two- to fourfold increase in factor VIII activity.

The outlook for children with hemophilia has been greatly improved by the availability of transfusion therapy. Transfusions started at home and early interventions prevent many disease complications. In the past, many children with factor VIII deficiency died in the first 5 years of life. Today, children with moderate or mild hemophilia can lead normal lives. Gene therapy is being explored for treatment of hemophilia. One approach is to infuse carrier organisms into the body where they would act on target cells to promote manufacture of deficient clotting factor. These research approaches offer the promise of new treatment options in the future (White, 2001).

Nursing Management

Nursing Assessment and Diagnosis

PHYSIOLOGIC ASSESSMENT

Obtain a complete medical history from the parents or child. In particular, ask about previous episodes of bleeding and the occurrence of hemophilia or any other bleeding disorders in family members. The history of bleeding will vary, depending on the severity of the disease.

Assess the child for any joint pain, swelling, or permanent deformity, particularly around the knees, elbows, ankles, and shoulders. Note the presence of hematuria and mild flank pain. Conduct a neurologic assessment, as the risk for intracranial hemorrhage and bleeding can lead to peripheral neuropathies.

Screen the adolescent with hemophilia for HIV. Present testing methods make transmission of HIV to individuals with hemophilia very unusual. However, before universal testing of the blood supply began in 1985, significant numbers of hemophiliacs acquired HIV from infusions (see Chapter 40).

PSYCHOLOGIC ASSESSMENT

It is difficult for families to manage care of the hemophiliac child, especially if the disease is severe. Assess the family's coping mechanisms and support systems. Ask whether the family's health insurance covers the child's medical expenses; the factor concentrates and infusion equipment are costly. Find out if the parents have respite care that lets them take time for themselves while knowing that the child is cared for safely. Assess older children's understanding of the disease and their adaptation to it.

DEVELOPMENTAL ASSESSMENT

Because the child with hemophilia may have physical activity restrictions, physical skills may be delayed. Perform frequent developmental assessments, being particularly attentive to fine and gross motor skills.

The most important nursing diagnosis for the child with hemophilia is risk for injury related to bleeding disorder. Some of the other nursing diagnoses that might apply include:

▶ *Pain* related to bleeding episodes
▶ *Impaired physical mobility* related to joint stiffness or contractures
▶ *Impaired home maintenance management* related to challenges of hemophilia
▶ *Altered family processes* related to family role shift required to care for a child with a chronic illness
▶ *Altered growth and development* related to effects of physical disability

Planning and Implementation

Nursing care focuses on preventing and controlling bleeding episodes, limiting joint involvement and managing pain, and providing emotional support. Both short-term interventions and long-term management are necessary.

PREVENT AND CONTROL BLEEDING EPISODES

Bleeding problems are rare in infants with hemophilia. As children learn to walk and develop other motor skills,

however, they often fall and suffer cuts and bruises. The risk of injury can be reduced by emphasizing to parents the need for close supervision and a safe environment. Parents should encourage children to play with safe, age-appropriate toys.

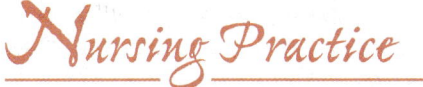

Take the following precautions when caring for children with bleeding disorders:

▶ Avoid taking temperatures rectally or giving suppositories.
▶ Check blood pressure by cuff as infrequently as possible.
▶ Avoid intramuscular or subcutaneous injections.
▶ Use only paper or silk tape for dressings.
▶ When indicated, perform mouth care every 3 hours with a glycerin swab.
▶ Except for factor replacement therapy, avoid all venipunctures.
▶ Use a peripheral fingerstick to obtain blood samples.
▶ Do not give aspirin.

If dental surgery or tooth extraction is necessary, it is performed in a controlled environment by experienced staff. Use of a dental irrigation device is often recommended if the child has excess bleeding from gums. Advise adolescents to shave only with an electric razor.

Control any superficial bleeding by applying pressure to the area for at least 15 minutes. Immobilize and elevate the affected area, and apply ice packs to promote vasoconstriction.

If significant bleeding does occur, offer supportive measures and assist with factor replacement therapy. Carefully monitor the child's condition for any side effects when factor replacement therapy is administered.

LIMIT JOINT INVOLVEMENT AND MANAGE PAIN

During bleeding episodes, hemarthrosis is managed by elevating and immobilizing the joint and applying ice packs. Administer analgesics as ordered. Once bleeding has been controlled, range of motion exercises strengthen muscles and joints and prevent flexion contractures. Physical therapy may be needed. Because excessive weight can place an added stress on joints, encourage the child to maintain an appropriate weight.

PROVIDE EMOTIONAL SUPPORT

The needs of families with hemophiliac children are best met through a comprehensive team approach. Refer the parents for genetic counseling as soon as possible after diagnosis. It is important to identify family members who carry the trait, as they may suffer excessive bleeding during surgery.

Encourage the parents to verbalize their feelings. Be understanding and sensitive to their needs. Teach the parents about hemophilia and explain how the disorder affects both the child and other family members. Refer the parents and child to organizations such as the National Hemophilia Foundation for further information. **WEB**

DISCHARGE PLANNING AND HOME CARE TEACHING

The child may be hospitalized briefly during the first manifestation of bleeding or diagnosis and management. After that, most care takes place in the home. Identify and address home care needs well in advance of discharge. Advise parents to have the child wear a medical identification bracelet. Explain the cause of bleeding so both the child and parents understand the disease process. Teach the child and family how to identify internal bleeding. Signs and symptoms such as joint pain, abdominal pain, and obvious bleeding are indicators for immediate factor infusion. Make sure the child and parents know what situations could cause bleeding to occur. Teach parents to give acetaminophen instead of aspirin to relieve pain.

Instruct the parents and the child, when appropriate, to prepare and administer factor concentrate. If infusion of the missing factor is scheduled regularly, bleeding episodes can be controlled or avoided. Have the parents demonstrate the procedure and make sure they can administer the product correctly. The parents need to be familiar with properties of the factor concentrate to prepare the mixture correctly.

The child will need an individualized school health plan (see Chapter 35). Members of the school staff should be instructed in management of emergencies, and infusion equipment should be readily available. Identify key school personnel and teach them to provide competent and prompt care for the hemophiliac child.

Help the family and school plan an appropriate schedule of activities without overprotecting the child. Children with hemophilia should not engage in contact sports such as football and soccer, which may result in injury and trauma. Instead, encourage sports such as swimming, hiking, and bicycling.

Explain how the parents can coordinate their child's care with a number of health professionals. Provide ongoing case management, assisting the family to take on this task if able.

Growth and Development

Encourage adolescents with hemophilia to participate in leisure activities such as computer games, reading clubs, and crafts. They should use knee pads, elbow pads, and helmets when participating in any physical sports. Activities important to development can be encouraged when coaches, teachers, and others know how to treat bleeding episodes.

Hemophilia is not only a debilitating disorder for the child. It also can be financially draining for the family. Frequent outpatient visits, emergency department visits, hospital admissions, and the cost of factor concentrate can exhaust a family's resources. If indicated, refer families to appropriate social services (e.g., the state's maternal and child health program for children with special health care needs) and organizations such as the National Hemophilia Foundation. Sharing experiences with other families of children with hemophilia can provide support.

Evaluation

Expected outcomes of nursing care include:

▶ Prevention of injury to the child

▶ Management of pain to promote comfort level

▶ Promotion of normal growth and development

▶ Adequate knowledge of child and family for disease management, including recognition of bleeding and prompt initiation of infusions

VON WILLEBRAND DISEASE

Like hemophilia, von Willebrand disease is a hereditary bleeding disorder. There are about 20 different disorders involving a deficiency of von Willebrand factor, a plasma protein and the carrier for clotting factor VIII; it plays a necessary role in platelet adhesion (McDaniel, 2000). The most common form of the disorder is transmitted as an autosomal dominant trait, and it can occur in both males and females. The gene for the disease is located on chromosome 12.

The characteristic manifestations are easy bruising and epistaxis. Children with von Willebrand disease frequently have gingival bleeding and increased bleeding with lacerations or during surgery. Affected teenage girls may have menorrhagia (increased menstrual bleeding).

Diagnosis of von Willebrand disease is made after laboratory studies reveal decreased von Willebrand factor levels, von Willebrand factor antigen levels, and factor VIII activity; reduced platelet agglutination; prolonged bleeding time; and prolonged or normal activated partial thromboplastin time (APPT). Treatment is similar to that for the child with hemophilia and involves infusion of von Willebrand protein concentrate. For bleeding episodes or prior to surgery, DDAVP is infused. Locally administered medications such as aminocaproic acid are sometimes used to manage bleeding in the mucous membranes.

Nursing Management

Teach parents about the disorder and instruct them not to give the child any aspirin or other drugs that can cause bleeding or inhibit platelet function. Teach management of bleeding episodes and intravenous infusion techniques, as for hemophilia. The prognosis is good, and children with von Willebrand disease usually have a normal life expectancy. Expected outcomes of nursing care include prompt management of bleeding and prevention of disease complications.

DISSEMINATED INTRAVASCULAR COAGULATION

Disseminated intravascular coagulation (DIC) is a life-threatening, acquired pathologic process in which the clotting system is abnormally activated, resulting in widespread clot formation in the small vessels throughout the body. Excess thrombin is generated, followed by deposition of fibrin strands in body tissues. These changes cause tissue hypoxia, resulting in eventual tissue necrosis. The circulating fibrin fragments later begin to interfere with platelet aggregation and other aspects of the clotting mechanism, resulting in bleeding or hemorrhage.

DIC is a complication of other serious illnesses in infants and children, such as hypoxia, shock, cancer, and viruses. Symptoms can include diffuse bleeding manifested by hematuria, petechiae, or purpura; an injection site that continues to ooze; circulatory collapse; and major vessel thrombosis (Lane, et al., 1999). The prothrombin time and partial thromboplastin time are prolonged, platelet count and fibrinogen levels are increased, and levels of fibrin–fibrinogen split products are high.

Medical management is supportive and includes identification and treatment of the underlying disorder; replacement of depleted coagulation factors, fibrinogen, and platelets; and anticoagulant therapy (heparin).

Nursing Management

DIC is a complex disorder managed by a critical care team. Nursing care focuses on assessing the bleeding, preventing further injury, and administering prescribed therapies. Observe for petechiae, ecchymoses, and oozing every 1 to 2 hours. Be sure to check dependent areas, as blood pools in these areas. Intravenous sites are particularly prone to oozing and should be assessed every 15 minutes. Examine stool for the presence of blood, and measure blood loss as accurately as possible. Measure intake and output.

Because all body systems can be involved, careful, continuous assessment of all systems is needed. Institute bleeding control precautions, monitor prescribed therapy (transfusion, anticoagulant therapy), and report any signs of complications. Desired outcomes of nursing care are management of bleeding and adequate function of all body systems. Adequate family support in this life-threatening situation is a focus of nursing care.

IDIOPATHIC THROMBOCYTOPENIC PURPURA

Idiopathic thrombocytopenic purpura (ITP), also known as autoimmune thrombocytopenic purpura, is a disorder characterized by increased destruction of platelets, even though platelet production in the bone marrow is normal. When the rate of platelet destruction exceeds the rate of platelet production, the number of circulating platelets decreases and blood clotting slows.

ITP is the most common bleeding disorder in children. It occurs most frequently in children 2 to 10 years of age and usually follows a viral infection such as measles, chickenpox, or rubella, as part of an inappropriate immune response (Bolton-Maggs, 2000). Symptoms include multiple ecchymoses and petechiae. Diagnosis is made by history and through physical and laboratory findings, which show a decreased platelet count and antiplatelet antibodies in the peripheral blood. Treatment includes administering corticosteroids and intravenous immunoglobulins. For children who do not respond to drug therapy over a period of 6 months to 1 year, splenectomy may be the treatment of choice. Spontaneous remission is seen in 90% of children with ITP.

Nursing Management

Nursing care focuses on controlling and reducing the number of bleeding episodes. Preventive measures are similar to those for the child with hemophilia. Teach parents to use acetaminophen, rather than aspirin, to control pain. Provide emotional support. Expected outcomes of care are prevention of bleeding and restoration of normal coagulation patterns.

MENINGOCOCCEMIA

Meningococcemia is the most severe disease process that follows infection with *Neisseria meningitidis* or, occasionally, other microorganisms such as *H. influenzae* or *Streptococcus pneumoniae*. The disorder is thought to be an immune response to the endotoxins of the organism.

Onset is sudden: A respiratory infection is followed by high fever, petechial rash, massive skin and mucosal hemorrhage, hypotension, disseminated intravascular coagulation, and shock (Herf, Nichols, Fruh, et al., 1998). The child, usually under 2 years of age, is critically ill and demonstrates multisystem disease. Symptoms can progress to a critical level within 12 to 48 hours of onset. Commonly the skin turns pink and then black as the tissues are damaged by reduced oxygen delivery. Limbs may need to be amputated as a result of impaired circulation.

Treatment consists of antibiotics, removal from sources of infection, and multisystem shock management (Refer to Chapter 43 for a description of distributive shock). Prompt administration of antibiotics to the child who manifests fever with purpura can decrease the severity of outcome. Depending on the child's condition, total parenteral nutrition, sedation and pain relief, dialysis, or amputation may be required. Close contacts of the child should receive prophylactic antibiotics.

Nursing Management

Nursing care of the child with meningococcemia is complex. Treatment must begin quickly and the child generally has a lengthy hospitalization in a pediatric intensive care unit (Hoag-Apel, 1997). Perform thorough assessments of all body systems. Administer intravenous infusions when ordered to ensure correct and timely administration of antibiotics and other therapies. Measure urinary output to evaluate kidney function. Meticulous skin care is necessary to preserve the integrity of tissues. Take care to prevent further infections. Nutritional support in the form of total parenteral nutrition is common. The family needs support to deal with the changing critical nature of the child's illness and the possibility that death or permanent, severe deformities will result. When the child improves, continuing comprehensive care in the hospital and then in the community is needed to manage complex issues related to growth, development, nutrition, amputations, and prosthetics. Expected outcomes of nursing care include prevention of further infection, maintenance of body systems during acute phase of illness, and positive adjustment to amputations and deformities resulting from the disease.

BONE MARROW TRANSPLANTATION

Bone marrow transplantation is a treatment used for diseases such as severe combined immunodeficiency disease, severe and unresponsive aplastic anemia, and leukemia (see Chapter 45 for a description of the related treatment of stem cell transplantation).

There are three types of bone marrow transplant: autologous, isogeneic (or syngeneic), and allogeneic. In autologous transplantation, the child's own marrow is taken, stored, and reinfused after the child has received chemotherapy. In isogeneic transplantation, the marrow is taken from an identical twin. In allogeneic transplantation, the donor, usually a sibling, has a compatible human leukocyte antigen (HLA). When no relative is found to match the child, a histocompatible donor may be sought from the National Bone Marrow Registry.

The transplantation procedure begins with chemotherapy and, sometimes, total body irradiation directed at destroying circulating blood cells and the diseased bone marrow in the ill child. Following this treatment, the child is transfused with the donor marrow. If the transplantation is successful, the donor marrow implants itself in the bone and begins to grow. Healthy bone marrow, capable of making blood cells, is the result.

The chemotherapy program for destruction of bone marrow takes 4 to 12 days. During this time, the child is cared for in strict isolation in a special unit that provides a germ-free environment (Figure 44–5 ◆). Side effects of chemotherapy provide challenges for care in addition to those of preventing infection (see Chapter 45). The child is without any immunity for a minimum of 10

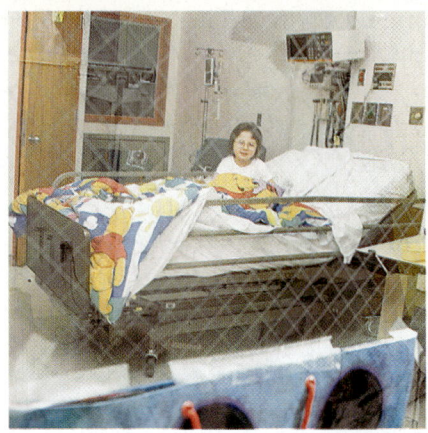

FIGURE 44–5. ◆ The child undergoing bone marrow transplantation is hospitalized in a special unit while receiving chemotherapy before the transfusion. The child remains in the unit for several weeks afterward until the new marrow produces enough cells to maintain immunity.

days after transplantation. It takes 2 to 4 weeks for the donor cells to begin proliferation and maturation. Medications to stimulate the production of red and white blood cells are administered during this period.

Once the bone marrow begins to produce new cells, graft-versus-host disease (rejection) is the major threat. Refer to Chapter 40 for a discussion of graft-versus-host disease.

Monitor for this multisystem disorder by assessing the skin, mucous membranes, gastrointestinal function, respiratory function, cardiac function, and hydration status. Because graft-versus-host disease may occur at any time, even after the child returns home, frequent thorough assessments are necessary after discharge.

Supportive care after the transplantation procedure focuses on preventing infection, controlling bleeding, maintaining adequate nutrition and hydration, monitoring for signs of rejection, and providing psychosocial support. The treatment is lengthy, the child is often critically ill, and parents may have traveled to a medical center many miles from home for the procedure. Ask parents about other family members and how they are managing. Provide information about inexpensive housing available near the medical center, such as in a Ronald McDonald house. Encourage parents to discuss their feelings with other parents of children receiving bone marrow transplantation. Organizations such as the Bone Marrow Transplant Family Support Network can serve as resources for families. WEB

Growth and Development

Hospitalizations of children undergoing bone marrow transplantation are usually lengthy. Evaluate the child's age and developmental stage and establish developmental goals to be met during the hospitalization. Implement nursing plans to meet the child's developmental needs and encourage further growth.

When the child is ready for discharge, be sure the family is prepared to administer medications, recognize signs of graft-versus-host disease, provide adequate nutrition for the child, and perform other necessary care. Arrange for follow-up visits and provide the names of local health care contact people who can offer support and provide information. The child may need tutors or other educational assistance to promote integration back into the school setting. The major expected outcome of nursing care is the proper activity of bone marrow in the child with resulting normal levels and function of blood cells. Other outcomes are provision of family support, ongoing care and education for the child, adequate nutrition, and prevention of infection.

CHAPTER HIGHLIGHTS

≈ Erythrocytes (red cells) are a major component of the blood and transport oxygen from the lungs to body tissues.

≈ Polycythemia is an increase in the number of red blood cells, and anemia is characterized by a decrease in red blood cell number. Leukocytes (white cells) are important in the cell's defenses against disease.

≈ Thrombocytes (platelets) are necessary for normal clotting of blood.

≈ The major anemias of childhood include iron-deficiency anemia, thalassemia, aplastic anemia, normocytic anemia, and sickle cell anemia.

≈ Sickle cell anemia is a genetic disease in which an abnormal shape, or sickling of red blood cells, prevents the normal flow of blood.

≈ Major complications of sickle cell anemia include pain, strokes, retinopathy, enlarged liver and spleen, urinary complications, poor peripheral blood flow, and osteoporosis.

≈ Nurses help families deal with chronic diseases such as sickle cell anemia by providing information about the disorder and resources that can provide assistance, monitoring child growth and development, instituting preventive care, and managing exacerbations of the disease.

≈ Thalassemia is also a genetic disease of red blood cells, and causes defective synthesis of hemoglobin.

≈ Treatment of thalassemia frequently involves regular blood transfusions; bone marrow transplantation is used in severe cases.

≈ Aplastic anemia is a deficiency of all blood cells related to poor bone marrow function; it can be congenital or acquired after exposure to certain drugs or harmful environmental toxins.

≈ Hemophilia is a genetic bleeding disorder; hemophilia A is most common and causes a decrease in clotting factor VIII.

≈ The goal of hemophilia treatment is to control bleeding by preventive care and replacement of the missing factor.

≈ Major nursing concerns for the child with hemophilia include managing bleeding episodes, controlling pain during bleeds, minimizing physical immobility, supporting the family in learning management of this chronic disease, and explaining genetic implications of the disease.

≈ Disseminated intravascular coagulation is a serious condition in which clotting mechanisms are disturbed, leading to extensive clotting and tissue damage.

≈ Idiopathic thrombocytopenic purpura causes destruction of platelets and most frequently follows a childhood viral disease.

≈ Management of idiopathic thrombocytopenic purpura includes corticosteroids and immunoglobulins since the disease is considered to be autoimmune in nature.

≈ Occasionally, infection with organisms such as *Neisseria meningitidis* or *Streptococcus pneumoniae* is followed by a severe systemic disease known as meningococcemia.

≈ Meningococcemia is manifested by sudden high fever, rash, skin and mucosal hemorrhage, and shock; prompt treatment with antibiotics is needed.

≈ Bone marrow transplantation is a useful treatment in some diseases of the hematologic system and some cancers; it involves infusion of bone marrow from a donor into the blood where it circulates, implants into the bone marrow, and begins making new blood cells.

≈ Nursing care before and after bone marrow transfusions includes infection prevention, careful physical assessment, administration of medications, and providing support for the family.

EXPLORE MEDIALINK

NCLEX Review, Case Studies, and other interactive resources for this chapter can be found on the companion website at http://www.prenhall.com/london. Click on "Chapter 44" and select the activities for this chapter.

For animations, more NCLEX review questions, and an audio glossary, access the accompanying CD-ROM in this textbook.

REFERENCES

Abshire, T. C. (1996). The anemia of inflammation: A common cause of childhood anemia. *Pediatric Clinics of North America, 43*(3), 623–638.

American Academy of Pediatrics. (2000). *Guidelines for health supervision III.* Elk Grove Village, IL: American Academy of Pediatrics.

Bolton-Maggs, P. H. B. (2000). Idiopathic thrombocytopenic purpura. *Archives of Disease in Childhood, 83,* 220–223.

Boxer, L. A. (2000). Leukopenia. In R. E. Behrman, R. M. Kliegman, & H. B. Jenson (Eds.), *Nelson textbook of pediatrics* (16th ed, pp. 621–626). Philadelphia: WB Saunders.

Cook, L. S. (2000). A simple case of anemia: Pathophysiology of a common symptom. *Journal of Intravenous Nursing, 23,* 271–281.

Davis, H., Schoendorf, K. C., Gergen, P. J., & Moore, R. M. (1997). National trends in the mortality of children with sickle cell disease,

1968 through 1992. *American Journal of Public Health, 87*(8), 1317–1322.

Day, S. W., & Wynn, L. W. (2000). Sickle cell pain & hydroxyurea. *American Journal of Nursing, 100,* 32–38.

DiMichele, D. (1996). Hemophilia 1996: New approach to an old disease. *Pediatric Clinics of North America, 43*(3), 709–736.

Glader, B. E., & Look, K. A. (1996). Hematologic disorders in children from Southeast Asia. *Pediatric Clinics of North America, 43*(3), 665–682.

Hendricks-Ferguson, V. L., & Nelson, M. (1999). Update of the health care management needs of infants with sickle cell disease. *Journal of Pediatric Health Care, 13,* 217–222.

Herf, C., Nichols, J., Fruh, S., Holloway, B., & Anderson, C. U. (1998). Meningococcal disease: Recognition, treatment, and prevention. *Nurse Practitioner, 23*(8), 33–36, 39–40.

Hoag-Apel, C. (1997). Meningococcal disease. *American Journal of Nursing, 97,* 33.

Jakubik, L. D., & Thompson, M. (2000). Care of the child with sickle cell disease: Acute complications. *Pediatric Nursing, 26,* 373–380.

Jarvinen, O., Lehesjoki, A., Lindlof, M., Uutela, A., & Kaariainen, H. (2000). Carrier testing of children for two x-linked diseases: A retrospective study of comprehension of the test results and social and psychological significance of the testing. *Pediatrics, 106,* 1460–1465.

Lane, P. A., Nuss, R., & Ambruso, D. R. (1999). Hematologic disorders. In W. W. Hay, A. R. Hayward, M. J. Levin, & J. M. Sondheimer (Eds.), *Current pediatric diagnosis and treatment* (14th ed., pp. 723–773). Stamford, CT: Appleton & Lange.

McDaniel, P. (2000). Focus on factors. *Journal of Intravenous Nursing, 23,* 282–289.

Mentzer, W. C., & Cowan, M. J. (2000). Bone marrow transplantation for beta-thalassemia: The University of California San Francisco experience. *Journal of Pediatric Hematology and Oncology, 22,* 598–601.

Merenstein, G. B., Kaplan, D. W., & Rosenberg, A. A. (1997). *Handbook of pediatrics* (18th ed., pp. 986–989). Stamford, CA: Appleton & Lange.

Montgomery, R. R., & Scott, J. P. (2000). Hemorrhagic and thrombotic diseases. In R. E. Behrman, R. M. Kliegman, & H. B. Jenson (Eds.), *Nelson textbook of pediatrics* (16th ed., pp. 1504–1515). Philadelphia: WB Saunders.

National Heart, Lung, and Blood Institute. (1997). *Periodic transfusions lower stroke risk in children with sickle cell anemia.* Washington, DC: U.S. National Library of Medicine.

Northington, L. (2000). Chronic sorrow in caregivers of school age children with sickle cell disease: A grounded theory approach. *Issues in Comprehensive Pediatric Nursing, 23,* 141–154.

Odesina, V. (2001). Intravenous support for the patient in sickle cell crisis. *Journal of Intravenous Nursing, 24,* 32–37.

Ohls, R. K., & Christensen, R. D. (2000). The hematopoietic system. In R. E. Behrman, R. M. Kliegman, & H. B. Jenson (Eds.), *Nelson textbook of pediatrics* (16th ed., pp. 1456–1460). Philadelphia: WB Saunders.

Pizzo, A. P. & D'Andrea, A. D. (2000). The pancytopenias. In R. E. Behrman, R. M. Kliegman, & H. B. Jenson (Eds.), *Nelson textbook of pediatrics* (16th ed., pp. 1495–1498). Philadelphia: WB Saunders.

Reed, W., Walters, M., & Lubin, B. H. (2000). Collection of sibling donor cord blood for children with thalassemia. *Journal of Pediatric Hematology and Oncology, 22,* 602–604.

Stover, B. (2000). Training the client in self-management of hemophilia. *Journal of Intravenous Nursing, 23,* 304–309.

White, G. C. (2001). Gene therapy in hemophilia: Clinical trials update. *Thrombosis and Haemostasis, 86,* 172–177.

Zimmerman, S., Ware, R., & Kinney, T. (1997). Gaining ground in the fight against sickle cell disease. *Contemporary Pediatrics, 14*(10), 154–177.

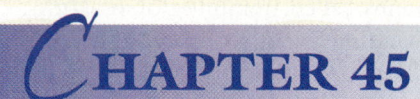

CHAPTER 45

The Child with Alterations in Cellular Growth

Rasheed was just diagnosed with leukemia seven months ago, but already, he has been in the hospital five times. This time he had enterocolitis, an infection of the intestines. But he has done really well and is determined to fight the disease. It is his will and strength that help us all to be strong and to know that he will do well after his treatment is finished.

—MOTHER OF RASHEED, 12 YEARS OLD

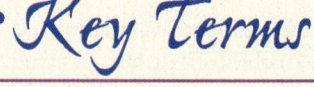

Key Terms

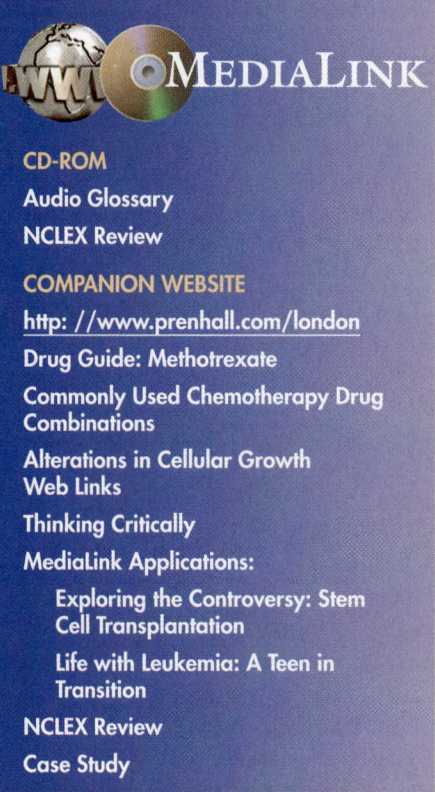

MEDIALINK

CD-ROM
Audio Glossary
NCLEX Review

COMPANION WEBSITE
http://www.prenhall.com/london
Drug Guide: Methotrexate
Commonly Used Chemotherapy Drug Combinations
Alterations in Cellular Growth Web Links
Thinking Critically
MediaLink Applications:
Exploring the Controversy: Stem Cell Transplantation
Life with Leukemia: A Teen in Transition
NCLEX Review
Case Study

Why do children develop different types of cancers than adults? Cancer in adults is often the result of dietary practices or habits such as smoking. Some adult-onset cancers are the result of oncogenic responses to stimuli—that is, responses that stimulate cancerous changes in cells. Other cancers that occur in adults result from prolonged exposure to toxins such as coal dust and asbestos. Some cancers are known to be related to genetic causes. In adults, prevention through general lifestyle changes is a major focus of interventions. However, in children, cancer is usually embryonic (occurring during development of the fetus) or oncogenic in origin. Thus, lifestyle changes that begin in childhood have little effect on the incidence of childhood cancer, although they may help reduce the incidence of later cancer or other diseases. Occasionally, an environmental exposure is linked to the incidence of cancer in children.

Abnormal cellular growth can occur in any area of the body. Why are some growths called cancer and others not? Changes in cellular growth within the body are called **neoplasms** (meaning new growth). A neoplasm is further classified as benign or malignant. **Benign** means that a growth does not endanger life or health. **Malignant** means that progressive growth of the tumor will, if not checked by treatment, result in spread to other sites in the body (**metastasis**), ending in death. The common term for this type of cellular growth is cancer.

ANATOMY AND PHYSIOLOGY OF PEDIATRIC DIFFERENCES

The major physiologic difference between adults and children that affects cellular growth involves the immune system and how well it defends the body. The rate of cell growth in children also can play a role in the rapid progression of some childhood cancers. The continuing presence of fetal cells in small children is related to some cancers.

The immune system defends the body against foreign organisms and substances through two responses: nonspecific and specific. In a nonspecific response the components of the immune system attack a variety of targets. Nonspecific components include phagocytic (cell-destroying) cells such as mononuclear leukocytes, polymorphonuclear (PMN) leukocytes, natural killer (NK) cells, and complements (noncellular proteins) that work together to destroy invading cells and substances. During the first month of a child's life the nonspecific response is immature, so phagocytic cells have little ability to move toward cancer cells and fulfill their function. The nonspecific response is also impaired in premature and small-for-gestational-age (SGA) infants.

In a specific response, T lymphocytes and immunoglobulin (Ig) attack only one type of invader. The specific response capability also is immature in infants. B-cell production of various proteins called immunoglobins (IgM, IgG, and IgA) is below adult levels, so that the infant is vulnerable to bacterial and viral infections. (For a discussion of immune function, see Chapter 40.)

In children, many cells are growing quickly; this fast growth can lead to the proliferation of cancerous as well as normal cells.

CHILDHOOD CANCER

The care of children who have cancer is a challenging specialty in pediatric nursing. For several years, the child undergoes aggressive treatments that may be life threatening and cause temporary illness. Often the prognosis is quite hopeful; at other times, a terminal result may be expected. The child is cared for at home with outpatient visits for treatment and occasional hospitalization when needed. The periods of hospitalization are times of intense physical vulnerability for the child and intense emotional vulnerability for both the child and the family. To monitor the child closely, nurses need a sound knowledge of physiologic and psychologic responses, medical interventions, and nursing care. Effective communication skills are necessary to support the child and family and promote realistic hope.

Incidence

During 2001, in the United States, cancer was diagnosed in approximately 8600 children. In children under 15 years of age, cancer is the leading cause of disease-related death. In 2001, about 1500 U.S. children died of cancer, one third of these from leukemia (American Cancer Society, 2001). Mortality rates have declined by over 60% since 1960, and the rates continue to improve. Children treated in the 1980s and 1990s have had significantly lower mortality rates than those treated in the 1960s and 1970s. Mortality rates are higher for females than males, for those diagnosed before 5 years of age, and for children with central nervous system tumor or leukemia. The cause of death for most children is recurrence of the primary cancer (Moller, Garwicz, Barlow, et al. 2001). The most common forms of childhood cancers among children in different age groups are shown in Figure 45–1 ◆.

Etiology and Pathophysiology

Alterations in cellular growth occur in response to external and internal stimuli. Neoplasms are caused by one or a combination of three factors: (1) external stimuli that cause genetic mutations, (2) immune system and gene abnormalities, and (3) chromosomal abnormalities.

EXTERNAL STIMULI

External stimuli may affect the child's general health and cause mutations in body cells. **Carcinogens** are chemicals or industrial processes that, when combined with genetic

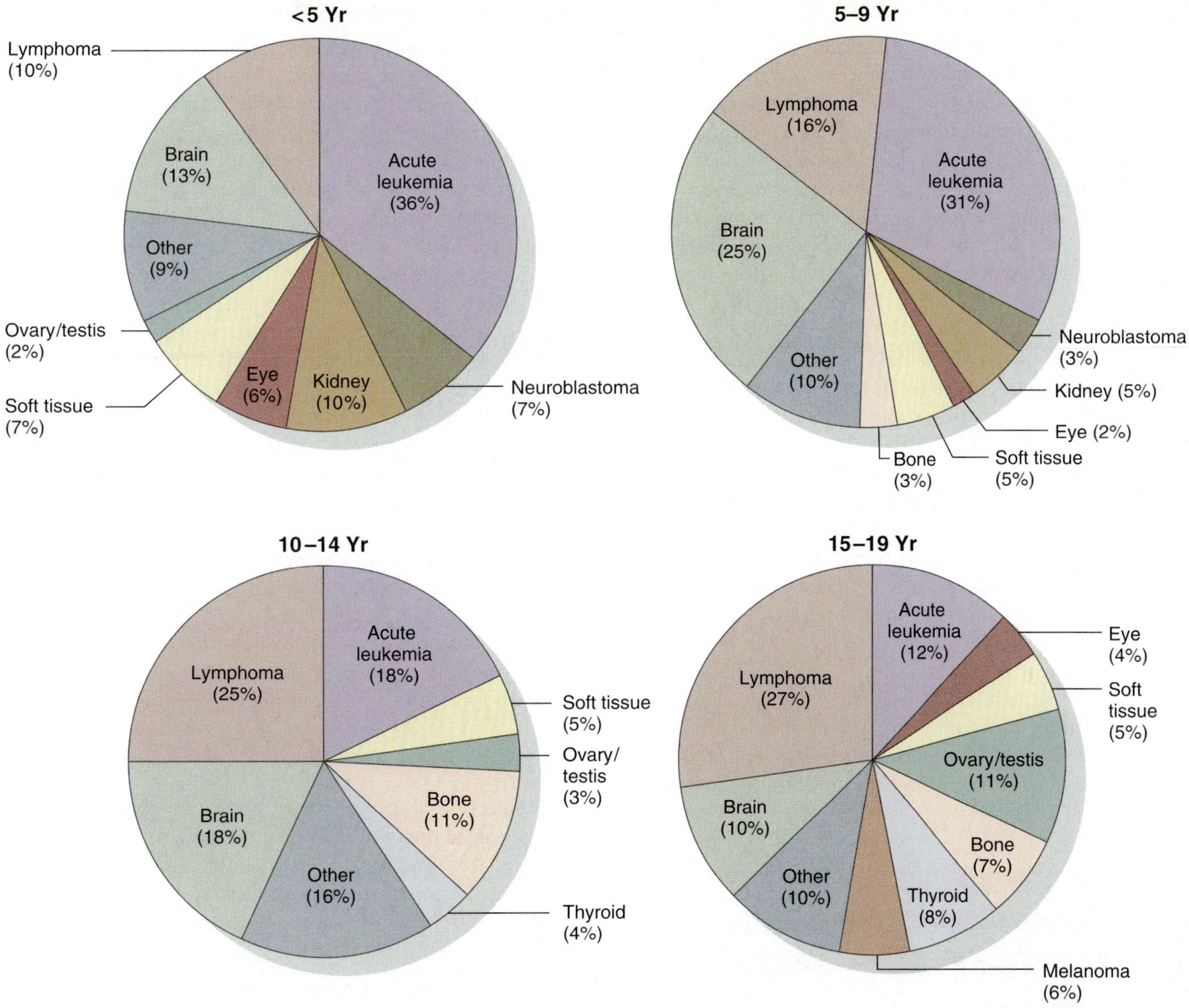

<5 Yr

Lymphoma (10%)
Brain (13%)
Other (9%)
Ovary/testis (2%)
Soft tissue (7%)
Eye (6%)
Kidney (10%)
Neuroblastoma (7%)
Acute leukemia (36%)

5–9 Yr

Lymphoma (16%)
Acute leukemia (31%)
Brain (25%)
Other (10%)
Bone (3%)
Soft tissue (5%)
Eye (2%)
Kidney (5%)
Neuroblastoma (3%)

10–14 Yr

Lymphoma (25%)
Acute leukemia (18%)
Soft tissue (5%)
Ovary/testis (3%)
Bone (11%)
Thyroid (4%)
Other (16%)
Brain (18%)

15–19 Yr

Lymphoma (27%)
Acute leukemia (12%)
Eye (4%)
Soft tissue (5%)
Ovary/testis (11%)
Bone (7%)
Thyroid (8%)
Melanoma (6%)
Other (10%)
Brain (10%)

FIGURE 45–1. ◆ Percentage of primary tumors by site of origin for different age groups. *Note:* From Crist, W. M. (2000). Neoplastic diseases and tumors. In R. E. Behrman, R. M. Kliegman, & H. B. Jenson (Eds.), *Nelson textbook of pediatrics* (16th ed., p. 1531). Philadelphia: Saunders.

traits and in interaction with one another, result in cancer. Several carcinogens cause cancers that are diagnosed during childhood. Others cause cancers that begin in childhood but are not identified until adulthood. Some chemicals suspected of causing childhood cancer include diethylstilbestrol (maternal use of therapeutic estrogen hormones), anabolic androgenic steroids, alkylating chemotherapy agents, and immunosuppressants used for organ transplantation. Radiation exposure has been known to cause cancers such as leukemia and thyroid tumors in children exposed to excessive radiation during diagnostic medical procedures and to atomic bombs. Secondary cancers can result when the child is treated for a primary cancer with high doses of radiation. Excessive exposure to ultraviolet radiation from the sun predisposes children to development of skin cancer in adulthood.

Nursing Practice

Many parents ask what they can do to decrease the incidence of cancer in children as they grow into adulthood. The three major teaching areas to address are:

1. Have children increase intake of fruits and vegetables. Most children do not eat enough of these foods and increased intake is associated with lower rates of many cancers.
2. Protect skin with sunscreen. Early excessive exposure to sun and having been sunburned increase the chance of skin cancers in adulthood.
3. Discourage smoking among children and be sure children are not exposed to environmental tobacco smoke. This will decrease the future chance of developing lung cancer.

IMMUNE SYSTEM AND GENE ABNORMALITIES

One critical function of a normal immune system is immune surveillance, in which phagocytic cells circulate throughout the body, detecting and destroying abnormal and cancerous cells. Children with congenital immune deficiencies, such as Wiskott–Aldrich syndrome, in which immune surveillance may fail, are at high risk for cancer. A form of non-Hodgkin lymphoma develops in some children treated with immune system–suppressing drugs. Children with AIDS may be at higher risk of certain types of cancer, such as lymphoma, Kaposi sarcoma, and leiomyosarcoma (Biggar, Frisch, & Goedert, 2000).

Viruses and other substances may alter the immune system, thereby allowing cancer to occur (see "Pathophysiology Illustrated: Proto-oncogene Alteration"). Their action is based on changing certain genes that normally regulate cellular growth and development (called **proto-oncogenes**) to related genes that allow unregulated cell division and cancerous growth (called **oncogenes**). Among the cancers thought to be linked to virus action and the change of proto-oncogenes to oncogenes are certain leukemias, rhabdomyosarcoma, Burkitt lymphoma, and some forms of Hodgkin disease.

Tumor suppressor genes counteract the effect of oncogenes, keeping cellular growth within normal limits. When tumor suppressor genes are missing, unstemmed cellular growth can occur. These genes are commonly missing in children with retinoblastoma and Wilms' tumor.

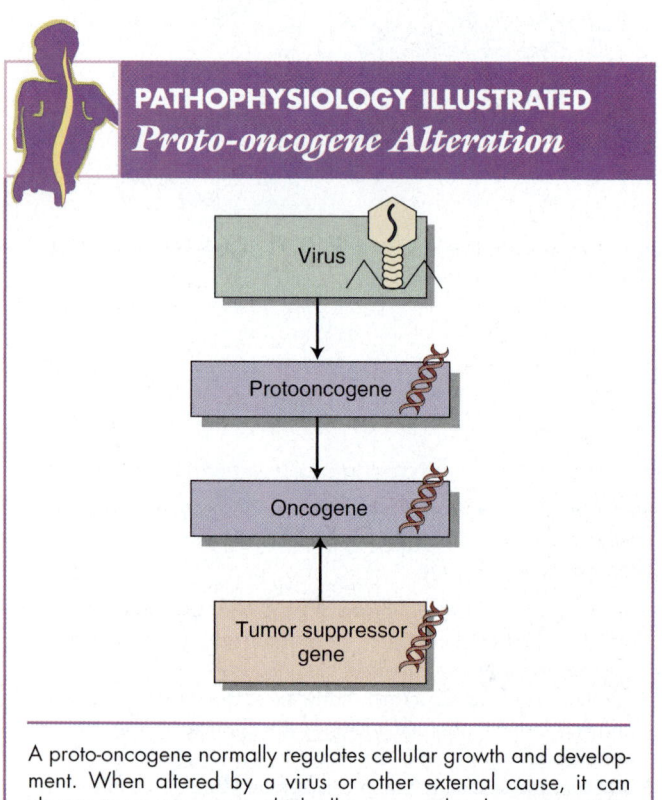

PATHOPHYSIOLOGY ILLUSTRATED
Proto-oncogene Alteration

A proto-oncogene normally regulates cellular growth and development. When altered by a virus or other external cause, it can change to an oncogene, which allows unregulated genetic activity and tumor growth. Tumor-suppressor genes regulate the effects of oncogenes to decrease wildly proliferating cellular growth.

CHROMOSOMAL ABNORMALITIES

Normal chromosomes undergo change as a part of the genetic process. Most changes are not harmful. However, some result in chromosomal abnormalities such as hyperploidy (more than the normal number of chromosomes), deletion, translocation, and breakage.

Some chromosomal abnormalities have been linked to an increased incidence of cancer. Children with Down syndrome have a 200 times higher incidence of leukemia than nonaffected children. Children missing a band of genetic material on chromosome 13 often have retinoblastoma. Similarly, a Wilms' tumor often develops in children missing part of the genetic material from chromosome 11.

Regardless of the location of abnormal cellular growth, the pathophysiologic process is similar. The altered cell begins to multiply as directed by the altered genetic structure of its DNA and the absence or inactivation of tumor suppressor genes. Each new cell transmits the new or altered pattern to the next generation. As the abnormal cells replicate, the neoplastic mass grows. Normal cells usually die as the increased metabolic rate of the neoplastic cells depletes available nutrition. The altered DNA in the tumor cells may also cause the abnormal cells to invade adjoining tissue. Through continued growth the mass expands until it enters and disrupts a major vessel or a vital organ.

Clinical Manifestations

Each type of childhood cancer signals its presence differently. Because many of the presenting signs and symptoms of cancer are typical of common childhood illnesses, diagnosis may be delayed. In some cases, no symptoms are noted until the cancer is advanced. Some of the common presenting symptoms of cancer follow.

- *Pain* may be the result of a neoplasm either directly or indirectly affecting nerve receptors through obstruction, inflammation, tissue damage, stretching of visceral tissue, or invasion of susceptible tissue.

- *Cachexia* is a syndrome characterized by anorexia, weight loss, anemia, asthenia (weakness), and early satiety (feeling of being full).

- *Anemia* may be experienced during times of chronic bleeding or iron deficiency. In chronic illness the body uses iron poorly. Anemia is also present in cancers of the bone marrow when the number of red blood cells (RBCs) is reduced, in part because of the presence of large numbers of other bone marrow products. Treatment of cancer often promotes further anemia.

- *Infection* is usually a result of an altered or immature immune system. In addition, infection occurs when bone marrow cancers inhibit maturation of normal immune system cells. Infection may also occur in children treated with corticosteroids. Because their immune response is altered, the normal signs of infection may not appear.

- *Bruising* can occur if the bone marrow cannot produce enough platelets and bleeding occurs after minor trauma.

Clinical Therapy

The most common diagnostic tests performed on children with cancer are complete blood counts, bone marrow aspiration, lumbar puncture (Table 45–1), peripheral blood studies, radiographic examination, magnetic resonance imaging (MRI), computed tomography (CT; Figure 45–2 ◆), ultrasound, and biopsy.

Nursing Practice

Any child who has an implanted metallic object in his or her body should not undergo MRI scanning because of the strong magnetic field generated. Metallic objects include orthodontic braces, metal dental bridgework, surgical clips or plates, and orthopedic rods. Remove all jewelry and clothes with metal snaps from the child before the test.

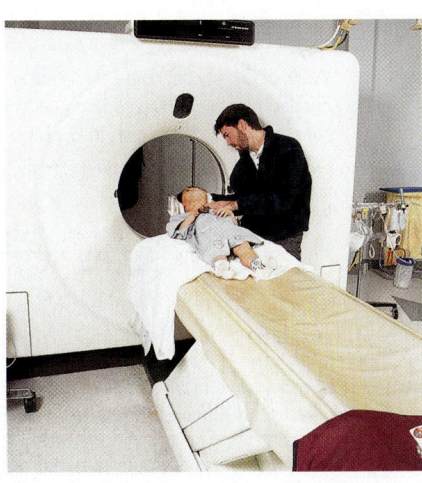

FIGURE 45–2. ◆ Computed tomography (CT) can be a frightening procedure for children. This 2-year-old boy is comforted by his father before the procedure.

Cancer is treated with one or a combination of therapies: surgery, chemotherapy, radiation, biotherapy, and bone marrow transplantation. Many families also choose to use some type of complementary therapy, in addition to traditional medical approaches. The choice of treatment is determined by the type of cancer, its location, and the degree of metastasis (spread to other sites in the body).

Teaching About

CANCER THERAPY

Most parents are not aware of the effects of cancer treatment and how they can help children through this experience. Depending on the stage and type of treatment, there are several ways to help:

- Children in radiation and chemotherapy are fatigued. Provide extra rest periods with shorter activity periods between them.
- Have a bag ready in case the child develops a complication and needs to be taken to stay in the hospital for a few days. Several hospital stays of a few days are normal during treatment.
- When concerned about a symptom in the child, ask the care provider. Parents are often key in identifying problems early.
- Parents are usually concerned about central line care but feel more comfortable after a few days of caring for the line.
- Children may not feel hungry so when they are ready to eat intake should be nutritious.
- Remember that the child is still at the normal developmental age. Treat them appropriately for their age, not as if they are older or younger.
- Try to maintain contact with the child's peer group and family members.
- Seek information from other parents and resources on cancer care.

Remind parents to get time away and relax so that they have enough energy and are better able to deal with the child's therapy.

TABLE 45–1	**Selected Diagnostic Tests for Childhood Cancer**		
Test	*Purpose*	*Normal Laboratory Values*	*Diagnostic Values*
Bone marrow aspiration	Examines bone marrow	<5% blast cells (immature)	>25% blast cells in acute lymphoblastic leukemia, most with hypercellular marrow
Lumbar puncture	Examines cerebrospinal fluid	Cell count (μL) Polymorphonuclear leukocytes 0 Monocytes 0–5 RBCs 0–5	Presence of malignant cells indicates central nervous system involvement
Complete blood count and differential	Examines cellular components of blood	WBC <10,000/μL Platelets 150,000–400,000/μL Hemoglobin 12–16 g/dL	WBC >10,000/μL Platelets 20,000–100,000/μL Hemoglobin 7–10 g/dL

The goal of treatment may be curative, supportive, or palliative. Curative treatment rids the child's body of the cancer. Supportive treatment includes transfusions, pain management, antibiotics, and other interventions to assist the body's defenses and increase the child's comfort. Palliative treatment is designed to make the child as comfortable as possible when no curative treatment is possible (see Chapter 37 for a detailed discussion of palliative care for children). Whatever combination of treatment is used, families have many questions and need resources for information.

SURGERY

Surgery is used to remove or debulk (reduce the size of) a solid tumor. An example of a cancer that is commonly treated with surgery is a Wilms' tumor. Surgery may also determine the stage and type of cancer.

CHEMOTHERAPY

Chemotherapy is the administration of specific drugs that kill both normal and cancerous cells. The administration of various chemotherapeutic drugs is timed to achieve the greatest cellular destruction. The cell's cycle of replication determines the schedule (see "Pathophysiology Illustrated: Chemotherapy Drug Action"). Several chemotherapeutic drugs are administered simultaneously to maximize their lethal impact on cells at all stages of activity (see Table 45–2). Whereas DNA in a normal cell can repair itself after chemotherapy, the DNA in a neoplastic cell cannot. The particular chemotherapy treatment protocol used is based on research into different types of cancer cells. A **protocol** is a plan of action for chemotherapy based on the type of cancer, its stage, and the particular cell type (Figure 45–3 ◆).

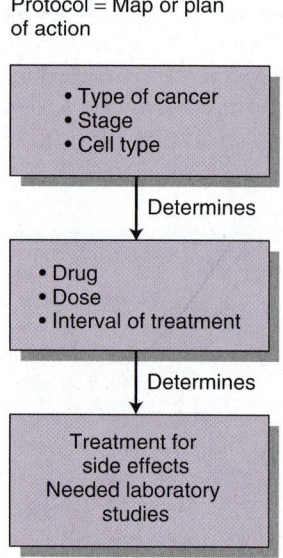

FIGURE 45–3. ◆ Chemotherapy protocol. A protocol is a map or plan of action that directs therapy by identifying the drug and its accompanying treatment.

Other drugs used in the treatment of children with cancer include colony-stimulating factors, antiemetics, and nutritional supplements. Colony-stimulating factors are hormonelike glycoproteins that enhance blood cell production and counteract the myelosuppressive effects of

TABLE 45–2 Medications for Chemotherapy and Their Actions	
Cell cycle specific agents (active in specific phases of the cell cycle) (see "Pathophysiology Illustrated: Chemotherapy Drug Action")	
Antimetabolites	Work at synthesis phase; interfere with function of nucleic acid, inhibiting DNA or RNA synthesis 5-Azacytidine 5-Fluorouracil 6-Mercaptopurine 6-Thioguanine Cytosine arabinoside Methotrexate
Vinca alkaloids	Work at mitosis phase; bind with cell proteins to inhibit nucleic acid and protein synthesis Etoposide Teniposide Vinblastine Vincristine
Miscellaneous	Work at G1 phase; cause depletion of asparagine, needed by cancer cells, and cause lysis of lymphoid cells; make cells in G phase vulnerable to other agents; interfere with prosynthesis L-Asparaginase Prednisone
Miscellaneous	Work at G2 phase; bind cellular proteins to cause metaphase arrest Bleomycin Etoposide
Cell cycle nonspecific agents (active in all stages of the cell cycle) (see "Pathophysiology Illustrated: Chemotherapy Drug Action")	
Alkylating agents	Substitute an alkyl group for a hydrogen atom, leading to DNA replication Cyclophosphamide Cisplatin Busulfan Chlorambucil Thiotepa Mechlorethamine
Antibiotics	Interfere with nucleic acid, inhibiting DNA or RNA synthesis Doxorubicin Mitomycin-C Dactinomycin Bleomycin Daunorubicin
Nitrosureas	Cause breakage in DNA; cross blood–brain barrier Carmustine Lomustine
Miscellaneous	Affect DNA and RNA synthesis Dacarbazine Procarbazine

Nucleus

G₂	Premitotic	→ Prophase
M	Mitotic	→ Metaphase
G₀	Resting	→ Anaphase
G₁	Postmitotic	→ Telophase
S	Synthesis	

Interphase (G₁, G₂, S)

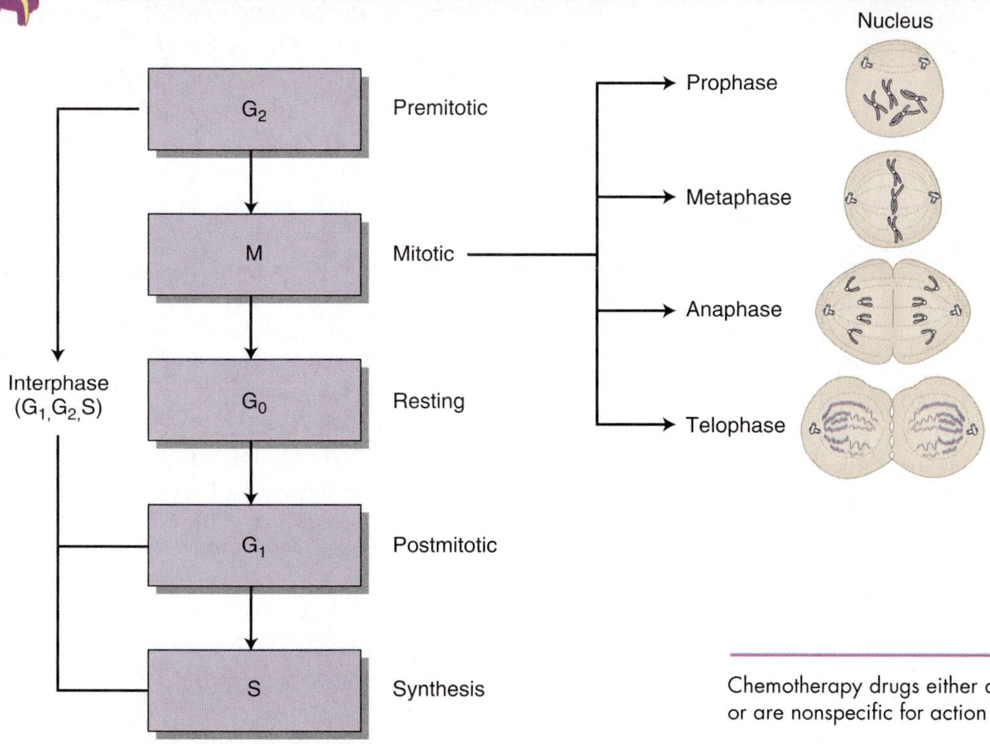

Chemotherapy drugs either act at specific parts of the cell cycle or are nonspecific for action (act throughout all cell phases).

chemotherapy drugs. For example, erythropoietin is produced in the kidney, and a recombinant form (epoetin) is available which can be used to treat anemia of cancer, thereby decreasing the number of transfusions needed (Agency for Healthcare Research and Quality, 2001a). Filgrastim (Neupogen) is a drug that stimulates neutrophil production. Antiemetics treat the nausea and vomiting that are common side effects of therapy. Nutritional supplements help maintain nutritional status.

RADIATION

Radiation therapy involves unstable isotopes that release varying levels of energy to cause breaks in the DNA molecule and thereby destroy cells. Radiation has been used as a treatment method since the early 1900s, shortly after its discovery. It is often used for the local and regional control of cancer, and in combination with surgery and chemotherapy.

Nursing Practice

Nurses who care for a child receiving implant radiation or who work in a radiation department need to wear a dosimeter film badge at all times to measure their radiation exposure.

The area to be irradiated (treatment field) includes the tumor site and sometimes other involved areas, such as lymph glands. The goal is to irradiate the tumor but not healthy adjacent tissue. The total dose of radiation is divided (or fractionated) and given over several weeks. A common course of radiation treatment might be once daily 4 or 5 days per week for a period of 2 to 6 weeks.

Tumors highly sensitive to radiation include Hodgkin disease, Wilms' tumor, retinoblastoma, and rhabdomyosarcoma. Tumors that have a low sensitivity to radiation, such as osteosarcoma and soft tissue sarcomas, require higher doses of radiation.

BIOTHERAPY

Biotherapy is the use of biologic response modifiers, such as interleukins, interferons, or radiolabeled monoclonal antibodies, to treat cancer (Bertolone, 1997). There are three major classes of biologic response modifiers: (1) agents that restore, augment, or modulate the host's immunologic mechanisms, (2) agents that have direct antitumor activity, and (3) agents that have other biologic effects. The actions of many of these agents are not completely understood, and some agents have more than one effect. For example, interferon has both antiviral and antiproliferative effects on some malignant cells. Interferon and tumor necrosis factor are undergoing clinical trials to study their effectiveness and to develop protocols for their safe use against selected cancers.

BONE MARROW AND BLOOD STEM CELL TRANSPLANTATION

Bone marrow transplantation is used to treat leukemia, neuroblastoma, and some noncancerous conditions, such as aplastic anemia. The goal of therapy is to administer a lethal dose of chemotherapy and radiation that will kill the cancer, and then to resupply the body with bone marrow stem cells either from the child's own marrow previously removed and stored (autologous transplant) or from a compatible donor (allogenic transplant).

Bone marrow transplantation has become the treatment of choice when a relapse occurs while the child is receiving another form of cancer therapy. First, a histocompatible donor must be located. The child then receives intensive chemotherapy, often followed by total body irradiation. This treatment kills all circulating blood cells and bone marrow contents, and begins 7 to 10 days before the transplant (Alcoser & Burchett, 1999). Following this treatment, the child is intravenously transfused with the donor bone marrow. New blood cells usually form within 6 to 8 weeks. (See Chapter 44 for a description of care for the child undergoing bone marrow transplantation.) The child's rights and needs must be carefully considered since the procedure requires long-term and life-threatening care.

Stem cells that become established in the host child's bone marrow can also be obtained from newborn cord blood. For some children this has become a better option than waiting for a matching bone marrow donor. Cord blood can be easily collected at birth from a sibling of the ill child, since histocompatible matches often occur in siblings, or cord blood banks may offer a match. The cord blood is then infused into the child undergoing treatment and the same mechanism occurs as in bone marrow transplantation—the stem cells implant into the child's bone marrow and produce normal blood cells over about 2 to 6 weeks. Advantages of cord blood are that, unlike bone marrow collection, it is not painful for the donor and does not require anesthesia; it is possible to easily collect samples from many ethnic groups that are underrepresented in bone marrow donor registries; graft versus host disease after treatment is less prevalent; and storage of cord blood for use later in life is possible (Chang, 1998; Crooks, Lill, Feig, et al., 1997). A variety of federally funded and private blood banks are available to store and provide cord blood. WEB

COMPLEMENTARY THERAPIES

Many families use **complementary therapies** in treatment of a child's cancer. These approaches to care are also referred to as alternative or unconventional, and may involve nutritional supplements, taking herbs, touch therapy, and mind/body interventions. Very little research has been done on complementary therapies, although up to 80% of children have used at least one such therapeutic approach (Kelly, Jacobsen, Kennedy, et al., 2000). Health care providers should be aware of these practices, inquire in a non-judgmental manner about the therapies, and attempt to learn about specific therapies and practices. WEB Although some herbs and nutritional products such as St. John's Wort may decrease serum concentration of chemotherapeutic agents, or some may act as hormones in the body, most are not known to negatively impact contemporary medical treatment, and the families should be assisted in seeking information and supported in use of their chosen therapies (Chase, 2000; Dean, 2000). Eating fruits and vegetables is associated with lower cancer incidence in adults, and some foods such as garlic and oranges may slow cancer growth or enhance medical chemotherapy (Swerdlow, 2000). Some people use some herbal supplements to treat cancer; these include cat's claw (bark of a tree root), mistletoe, and shark cartilage. The Food and Drug Administration has allowed testing of the efficacy of some herbal treatments for cancer (Kemper & Longwood Herbal Task Force, 1999). Several cancer drugs such as vincristine and paclitaxel are obtained from plant products. Some herbs can decrease nausea and vomiting, and others can boost the immune system's function (Kemper & Longwood Herbal Task Force, 1999).

Developing Cultural Competence

Traditional Chinese view cancer as a result of weak or toxic blood, which allows pollutants to accumulate and become toxic. A variety of plant products and acupuncture are used to detoxify the blood, and good nutrition helps it to rebuild. Some common foods used in various cultures to prevent and treat cancer include carrots, garlic, green tea, cabbage, citrus fruits, ginger root, and willow bark (Swerdlow, 2000).

PALLIATIVE CARE

In spite of modern medicinal practices and complementary therapies, some children do not survive childhood cancer. In these cases the focus of health care is to provide comfort and emotional support for the child and family. Too often, health care providers feel uncomfortable when a child is expected to die and may withdraw from close contact with the child or family, fail to provide adequate comfort measures, and leave the family without access to needed resources. When recognition of prognosis is delayed, children suffer more and palliative care is less integrated (Wolfe, Klar, Grier, et al., 2000). Some symptoms for which children are commonly undertreated include pain, dyspnea, nutrition, elimination, and fatigue (Wolfe, Grier, Klar, et al., 2000). On the other hand, the care provided for the dying child can be enhanced by a palliative care team; an integrated plan of care; collaboration between families, primary care provider, and other practitioners; and a focus on the child's developmental level and family needs (Chaffee, 2001; Hilden, Emanuel, Fairelogh, et al., 2001). See Chapter 37 for a detailed description of palliative care for children with terminal disease.

ONCOLOGIC EMERGENCIES

Oncologic emergencies can be organized into three groups: metabolic, hematologic, and those involving space-occupying lesions.

Metabolic Emergencies. Metabolic emergencies result from the lysis (dissolving or decomposing) of tumor cells, a process called tumor lysis syndrome. This cell destruction releases high levels of uric acid, potassium, phosphates, and calcium into the blood and can lower serum sodium levels. It is seen most commonly in children with Burkitt's lymphoma and acute lymphocytic leukemia (Kelly & Lange, 1997). Table 45–3 presents laboratory tests and management of tumor lysis syndrome.

A second type of metabolic emergency is septic shock. During periods of immune suppression the child is vulnerable to overwhelming infection, resulting in circulatory failure, inadequate tissue perfusion, and hypotension. Septic shock can be fatal (see Chapter 43 for a description of septic shock). Factors contributing to massive infection include inadequate neutrophil production, abnormal granulocytes (not able to be actively phagocytic), erosions through normal barriers such as blood vessels and mucous membranes, and altered bone marrow production caused by chemotherapy and some forms of radiation. Such infections may manifest with hyperthermia or hypothermia, tachycardia, tachypnea, hypotension, mental changes, and peripheral cyanosis and coolness, and must be vigorously treated with antimicrobial therapy and hydration management.

A third type of metabolic emergency occurs when treatment destroys large amounts of bone, resulting in hypercalcemia (elevated calcium in the serum). Hypercalcemia is most common in children with acute lymphocytic leukemia and rhabdomyosarcoma. Treatment includes hydration and adequate oral phosphate supplement.

Hematologic Emergencies. Hematologic emergencies result from bone marrow suppression or infiltration of brain and respiratory tissue with high numbers of leukemic blast cells (hyperleukocytosis). Bone marrow suppression results in anemia and thrombocytopenia with resultant hemorrhage. Gastrointestinal and central nervous system bleeding (strokes) are common.

Treatment involves infusion of packed RBCs for anemia; and platelet transfusion, vitamin K, and fresh frozen plasma for thrombocytopenia and hemorrhage. Hyperleukocytosis is treated by hydration, bicarbonate infusion, and allopurinol (Kelly & Lang, 1997).

Space-Occupying Lesions. Extensive tumor growth may result in spinal cord compression, increased intracranial pressure, brain herniation, seizures, massive hepatomegaly, and superior vena cava syndrome (obstruction of the superior vena cava by tumor). These emergencies are often caused by neuroblastoma, medulloblastoma, astrocytoma, Hodgkin disease, or lymphoma. After biopsy of the mass, treatment involves radiation therapy, chemotherapy, and corticosteroids.

Nursing Management

Nursing Assessment and Diagnosis

PHYSIOLOGIC ASSESSMENT

Physiologic assessment focuses on identifying the signs and symptoms of cancer and ongoing assessment of the side effects of treatment (see the discussion of side effects following under "Planning and Implementation"). Assessment of children with the most significant types of childhood cancers is presented later in the chapter.

A thorough physical assessment of all systems is needed to help identify the presence and extent of cancer (see Chapter 33). Carefully measure height and weight, and compare with prior findings for the child. Observe gait and coordination, as well as any changes in mental status. Evaluate pain, nutritional intake, fatigue, infections, bruising, shortness of breath, and elimination problems. Periodic laboratory studies will be performed. (See Skills 9-1–9-21.) SKILLS CD

PSYCHOSOCIAL ASSESSMENT

Assessment of body image, stress and coping abilities, knowledge of the condition and cognitive level, support systems, and developmental level provides data that helps determine the appropriate nursing interventions for the child with cancer and the family.

TABLE 45–3 Tumor Lysis Syndrome
Laboratory Evaluation
CBC
Serum sodium, potassium, chloride, bicarbonate, calcium, phosphorus, uric acid, BUN, creatinine, magnesium
Urinalysis
ECG if potassium is > 7 mEq/L
Management
Hydration to maintain urine specific gravity < 1.010
Alkalinization with drugs and intravenous fluids to keep urine pH between 7 and 7.5
Diuretics
Phosphate reduction with aluminum hydroxide

Growth and Development

Children of different ages experience differing threats to body image as a result of cancer treatment. A preschool girl may be most upset at hair loss, since she now looks like a boy. A school-age child has the most difficult time with changes that interfere with the developmental task of industry. Amputation, which decreases the child's ability to participate in activities such as sports, dancing, and school work, can be a major challenge during the school-age years. Teenagers are often most worried about changes like hair loss and cushingoid features, which cause them to look different from peers.

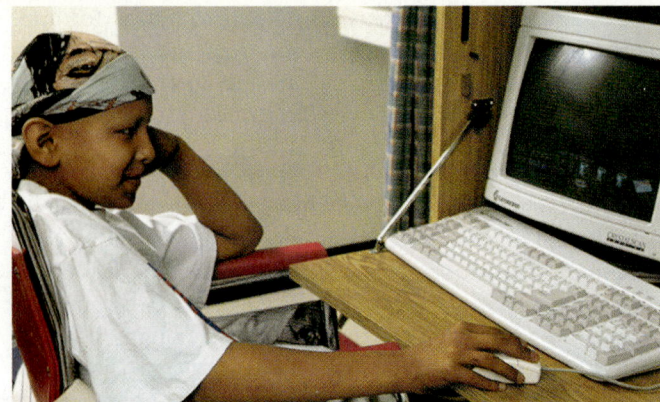

FIGURE 45–4. ◆ One of the most common threats to a child's body image at any age is hair loss induced by chemotherapy. Use of hats can improve self-concept.

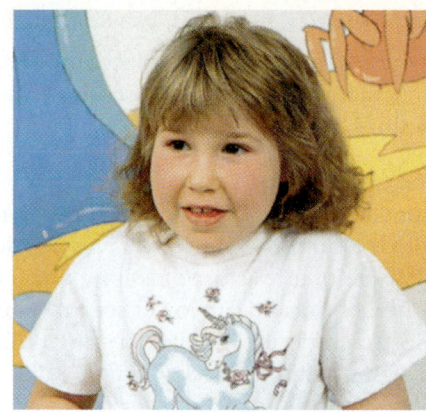

FIGURE 45–5. ◆ The child with cushingoid changes frequently has a rounded face and prominent cheeks.

Body Image

Hair loss, surgical scars, and cushingoid changes are three common treatment-induced threats to body image. Most children being treated for cancer experience hair loss (Figure 45–4 ◆). Children who have cranial surgery lose hair as part of the surgical preparation. Chemotherapy frequently results in some degree of hair loss. The speed of hair loss is unique to the child and can be as rapid as overnight or slower, with hair left on the pillow and in the hairbrush.

Nursing Practice

For many parents, especially of daughters, the loss of the child's hair can be devastating. Ask the parents and the child what the loss is like for them. Prepare them for the fact that it can be rapid or slow. Find out how they will plan to cope. Some children want the hair cut very short so its loss will not be as traumatic. Offer resources for wigs, hats, or other ideas. Put them in touch with children who have lost hair and with those who have now regrown it.

A second challenge to the child's body image is surgery. The scars of cranial and neck surgery are obvious, as are amputation and limb salvaging. Abdominal surgery for lymphoma is more easily concealed but is still a threat to the child's body image.

A third source of altered body image is the cushingoid features such as round and flushed face, prominent cheeks, double chin, and generalized obesity (Figure 45–5 ◆) that result from the use of corticosteroids. As the child's weight increases, stretch marks similar to those of pregnancy may occur. These stretch marks often remain after the corticosteroids are decreased.

Body image disturbances occur when a child cannot integrate changes and continues to cling to old images despite their inconsistency with reality. Common means for assessing body image are drawings, colored pictures cut out by the child to form a collage, discussion, and observation. See Chapter 33 for further discussion of these and other assessment techniques that can be used with children. ⌾

Stress and Coping

The diagnosis of cancer is a major stressor for both the child and the family. Although each child's prognosis and each family's coping mechanisms are unique, most families deal with the diagnosis in a manner similar to that of other families who have a child with a life-threatening illness (see Chapter 37). ⌾ Assess the family (and child if old enough) for their understanding and acceptance of the diagnosis. Find out if the family has told the child about the diagnosis and if they need assistance in deciding how to do this (Ishibashi, 2001). Assess the level of anxiety during health care visits and scheduled treatments (Figure 45–6 ◆). Evaluate the family's methods of coping, such as the ability to integrate relaxing and meaningful activities into family life, the use of support systems in the community and extended family, and the ability to alter expectations to take into account the child's health status. Concurrent stressors increase the difficulty of coping with childhood cancer. Evaluate the family for stressors such as illness or death of an-

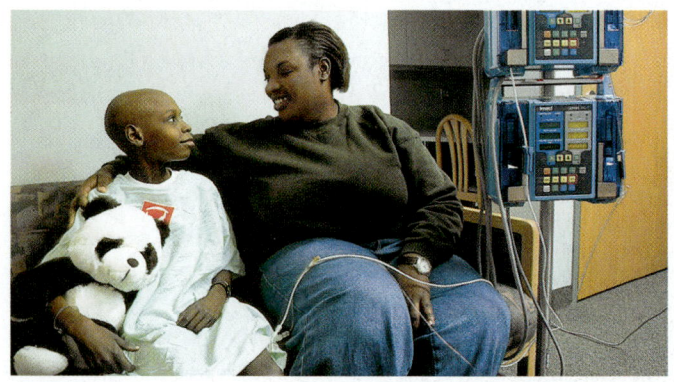

FIGURE 45–6. ◆ The child with cancer depends on parents and family members to provide support. Nurses can assist families to draw upon their strengths to help the child.

other family member, occupational changes, financial problems, relocation, and change in vacation plans.

Knowledge

Anxious people tend to narrow their scope of attention and may read unintended messages into the behaviors of health care personnel. Anxiety also limits a person's ability to retain information.

Assess the child's knowledge of cancer and its treatment throughout the treatment period. As the child matures cognitively, reevaluate knowledge. Cancer and its treatment are complex topics and parents are exposed to information in various forms, including written material, news reports, and Internet websites and resources. Evaluate their knowledge and give them a chance to ask questions.

Support Systems

Cancer treatment generally occurs over a long time. The extended family is crucial in providing necessary support to the child, parents, and siblings. Identify key people in the family. They may be the parents, grandparents, or aunts and uncles. Thoroughly assess the coping strategies the family uses to meet the various challenges posed by the child's illness. This information helps to predict the success of interventions, such as home care with intravenous medications, and to decide when referrals for other supportive therapies are needed.

Assess family resources to identify support systems available to help the family during crises and if a child is expected to die. Extended supports include friends, jobs, insurance coverage, religious affiliations, cultural support systems, and the school system. Parents commonly lose contact with close friends after the diagnosis of cancer in a child. This is an additional stressor for the family. Jobs are often a source of support because coworkers may have gone through the same experience. It may also be comforting for a parent to return to a job where he or she can feel a sense of security in tangible accomplishments. However, jobs can also be a source of stress if employers are unsympathetic to the demands of the child's hospitalization and clinic or office visits. The nurse caring for a child and family in the palliative care phase can best support family members by helping them to view the child's unique characteristics, conveying care and concern for the family, and continuing to have close contact with the dying child (James & Johnson, 1997). Religious affiliations can be an important source of support. Evaluate whether such affiliations are meaningful for the family and, if so, plan for visits from the appropriate clergy. In some cultures, spiritual leaders are an important part of the family's support.

The return to school may pose difficulties for the child with cancer or it may be a source of support to be connected again to peers. The child is encouraged to go to school, even if only for half a day per week, to stay connected to peers. Evaluate the school's ability to accept a medically vulnerable child into the classroom. Assess whether the other children and teachers have been prepared for the appearance and needs of the child with can-

cer. Help the teacher devise a plan to prepare the children, and offer to visit the classroom to explain what the child with cancer is experiencing. Arrangements can be made for tutors to help the child keep up with schoolwork if he or she cannot attend school.

DEVELOPMENTAL ASSESSMENT

Developmental assessment of children should be performed regularly during treatment for cancer. Assessment of the child's physical and neurologic development helps determine the progress made during treatment and provides a baseline for evaluating the long-term effects of treatment. Children under 6 years of age who have cancer should receive regular developmental assessment with a standardized tool such as the Denver Screening Test (see Chapter 35). Performance in school and social activities with friends provides important information about expected developmental milestones in older children. If the parents have signed up for a clinical trial (research) treatment for the child, the child should also give verbal or written assent when he or she has the cognitive maturity to do so.

Children who have received cranial radiation and intrathecal chemotherapy need regular scholastic evaluations. Impaired neurocognitive performance may be a long-term effect of treatment and appropriate interventions should be planned in these cases (Challinor, Miaskowski, Moore, et al., 2000).

Children with cancer have a variety of common psychologic and physiologic problems, regardless of their specific type of cancer. They and their families are dealing with a complex illness that influences their lives for years. The impact of this experience extends into all areas of function.

The accompanying "Nursing Care Plans" include several diagnoses that may be appropriate for the child with cancer who is receiving care in the hospital or at home. Among the many other diagnoses that may be appropriate for a child with cancer are the following:

▶ *Diarrhea* related to radiation therapy and toxins

▶ *Altered urinary elimination* related to chemotherapy

▶ *Altered oral mucous membrane* related to chemotherapy and radiation therapy

▶ *Impaired skin integrity* related to altered nutritional state, effects of medication, radiation, and immobilization

▶ *Ineffective individual coping* related to situational crisis of chronic and acute illness

▶ *Sleep pattern disturbance* related to biochemical agents, anxiety, and unfamiliar surroundings

▶ *Diversional activity deficit* related to frequent lengthy treatments

▶ *Body image disturbance* related to chronic illness and treatments

▶ *Impaired home maintenance management* related to challenges of cancer

▶ *Anticipatory grieving* related to actual or potential loss

GOAL	INTERVENTION	RATIONALE	EXPECTED OUTCOME
1. Pain related to tissue injury			
	NIC Priority Intervention:		*NOC Suggested Outcome:*
	Pain management: *Alleviation or reduction in pain to a level of comfort acceptable to patient*		**Comfort level:** *Feelings of physical and psychologic ease*
The child will report reduced pain that is manageable.	▶ Give analgesics as ordered. ▶ Teach relaxation techniques, deep breathing and distraction.	▶ Adequate medications can reduce pain. ▶ Nonpharmacologic methods work with the medication to reduce pain.	The child experiences pain reduced to the level that allows child to interact appropriately and gain rest.
2. Sleep pattern disturbance related to lack of sleep privacy			
	NIC Priority Intervention:		*NOC Suggested Outcome:*
	Sleep enhancement: *Facilitation of regular sleep/wake cycles*		**Rest:** *Extent and pattern of diminished activity for mental and physical rejuvenation*
The child will sleep for hours appropriate to age. The child will report feeling rested.	▶ Alter the environment to allow designated rest periods. ▶ Plan care to reduce frequency of interruptions during normal rest and sleep times.	▶ A quiet environment encourages relaxation needed for resting. ▶ Reduced interruptions allow continuous sleep and rest.	The child rests and sleeps for an age-appropriate amount of time per day.
3. Altered nutrition: less than body requirements related to inability to ingest or digest food or absorb nutrients			
	NIC Priority Intervention:		*NOC Suggested Outcome:*
	Nutrition management: *Assistance with and provision of a balanced dietary intake*		**Nutritional status:** *Extent to which nutrients are available to meet metabolic needs*
The child will maintain adequate nutritional intake.	▶ Offer small feedings. Encourage favorite foods. Refer to dietitian for special meals. Weigh daily.	▶ Measures can increase caloric intake. Taste changes and mouth sores alter desire for food.	The child maintains admission weight.
The child will experience reduced effects of chemotherapy (i.e., nausea and vomiting).	▶ Teach the child distraction and relaxation techniques. Give antiemetics according to orders.	▶ Pharmacologic and nonpharmacologic methods are effective in helping to reduce nausea.	The child has minimal side effects of nausea and vomiting.
4. Constipation related to change in usual foods and eating patterns			
	NIC Priority Intervention:		*NOC Suggested Outcome:*
	Constipation management: *Prevention and alleviation of constipation*		**Bowel elimination:** *The ability of the gastrointestinal tract to form and evacuate stool effectively*
The child will reestablish normal bowel pattern.	▶ Record all output by size and description. Administer stool softeners. Test stool for guaiac. Report changes in stool to physician. Encourage adequate fluid intake.	▶ Chemotherapy or tumor may create constipation, diarrhea, or blood in stool.	The child has normal bowel pattern.
5. Fluid volume excess or deficit related to medications			
	NIC Priority Intervention:		*NOC Suggested Outcome:*
	Fluid management: *Promotion of fluid balance and prevention of complications resulting from abnormal fluid levels*		**Fluid balance:** *Balance of water in the intracellular and extracellular compartments of the body*
The child will be adequately hydrated.	▶ Record all intake. Monitor intravenous rate and solution as appropriate.	▶ Some drugs (e.g., cyclophosphamide) necessitate a high level of fluid intake to prevent complications.	The child demonstrates adequate hydration. Mucous membranes are hydrated.
	▶ Test specific gravity of urine daily.	▶ Renal function may be affected by chemotherapy.	Specific gravity remains within normal range.

(continued)

GOAL	INTERVENTION	RATIONALE	EXPECTED OUTCOME

6. Risk for infection related to immunosuppression, invasive procedures, malnutrition, or pharmaceutical agents

	NOC Suggested Outcome:		NOC Suggested Outcome:
	Infection protection: *Prevention and early detection of infection in patient at risk*		**Risk control:** *Actions to eliminate or reduce health threats*
The child will remain free of infection.	▶ Wash hands often. Maintain in isolation if needed.	▶ Handwashing is effective in killing organisms.	The child remains infection free.
The child will return to normal, uninfected state.	▶ Monitor temperature. Report elevation to physician.	▶ Elevated temperature is a sign of infection.	The child with an infection is effectively treated.
	▶ Administer intravenous antibiotics as ordered. Monitor temperature. Use cooling mattress as ordered. Report elevations over 38 °C (101 °F) to physician.	▶ Multiple antibiotics are needed to deal with bacterial and fungal infections during neutropenia. Blood cultures may be taken to identify organism.	

7. Ineffective individual coping related to situational crisis

	NIC Priority Intervention:		NOC Suggested Outcome:
	Coping enhancement: *Assisting a patient to adapt to stressors which interfere with meeting life demands and roles*		**Coping:** *Actions to manage stressors that tax an individual's resources*
The child will demonstrate normal adaptive coping methods.	▶ Encourage drawings and other therapeutic play for expression of feelings. Allow for expression of angry feelings, such as hitting dolls and throwing sponge balls. Discuss how to behave during treatments.	▶ Expression of feelings helps identify avoidance coping for further intervention. Play is a normal way for child to express self and ideas. Misinterpretations can be corrected. Knowledge of appropriate and helpful behaviors supports self-esteem.	The child continues to use usual coping strategies expected for developmental stage.

8. Altered health maintenance related to complex treatment, and lack of resources

	NOC Suggested Outcome:		NOC Suggested Outcome:
	Health system guidance: *Facilitating use of health services*		**Knowledge: Health behaviors:** *Extent of understanding conveyed about promotion and protection of health*
The child will state understanding of treatments and procedures.	▶ Use age-appropriate teaching methods. Content areas include child's cancer, medications (actions and side effects), how to deal with body changes, and how to deal with response of others to those changes. Correct misinterpretations. Anticipate upcoming events and teach the child and family about them.	▶ Education helps by increasing understanding, removing fantasy, and clarifying fears. Education promotes the use of new learning in all areas of life.	The child demonstrates age-appropriate knowledge of the cancer, its treatments, and medications.
			The child has age-appropriate understanding of how to deal with changes in the body.

Planning and Implementation

The nursing care of children newly diagnosed with cancer and their families includes immediate physiologic and psychologic support, along with anticipatory guidance about imminent and future medical interventions. Assist and support the family in making decisions about types of treatment that are appropriate for their child.

Nursing care of the hospitalized child with cancer and the child receiving ongoing therapy at home is summarized in the accompanying "Nursing Care Plans." These care plans are designed for the child who is beyond the cancer diagnosis phase and is receiving chemotherapy.

Physiologic care of the hospitalized child focuses on providing support during treatment. This includes ensuring optimal nutritional intake, administering medications, managing the multiple side effects of chemotherapy and radiation, ensuring adequate hydration, preventing infection, and managing pain during diagnostic procedures and treatment.

ENSURE OPTIMAL NUTRITIONAL INTAKE

The high metabolic rate of cancer growth depletes the child's nutritional stores. Added to this is the catabolic effect of chemotherapy and radiation on normal cells, necessitating additional cellular replacement. The child needs

GOAL	INTERVENTION	RATIONALE	EXPECTED OUTCOME

1. Risk for infection related to immunosuppression, chemotherapy, and presence of invasive lines

	NIC Priority Intervention:		*NOC Suggested Outcome:*
	Infection protection: *Prevention and early detection of infection in child at risk*		**Risk control:** *Actions to eliminate or reduce health risks*
The child will remain infection free.	▶ Educate the child and parents about meaning of blood counts.	▶ Knowledgeable parents and child can protect themselves.	The child remains infection free.
	▶ Encourage parents/family members to use masks when they are ill.	▶ Masks help decrease airborne infection if used properly.	All exposures are reported to physician immediately.
	▶ Encourage good handwashing at all times.	▶ Handwashing is best prevention.	
	▶ Advise the child's teacher to tell parents if the child is exposed to communicable illness at school.	▶ Exposure can be reported to physician for possible use of acyclovir or admission for treatment.	
	▶ Clean vascular access site and inject heparin per protocol. Observe for signs of infection. Report infection to physician.	▶ Use of heparin maintains an open access route by preventing clotting.	

2. Altered nutrition: less than body requirements related to inability to ingest or digest adequate quantities of food or absorb adequate nutrients

	NIC Priority Intervention:		*NOC Suggested Outcome:*
	Nutrition management: *Assistance with and provision of a balanced dietary intake*		**Nutritional status:** *Extent to which nutrients are available to meet metabolic needs*
The child will maintain adequate nutritional intake.	▶ Encourage small and frequent high-calorie meals. Encourage small bites of a variety of foods.	▶ Measures to increase caloric intake. Taste changes and favorite foods may no longer be preferred.	The child maintains normal weight for height.
	▶ Promote good oral hygiene and use of nonalcohol mouthwashes.	▶ Mouth sores interrupt eating. Alcohol stings open sores.	
	▶ Teach home parenteral nutrition if ordered.	▶ Parenteral nutritional support may be used to enhance intake.	

3. Ineffective management of therapeutic regimen related to complex therapy

	NIC Priority Intervention:		*NOC Suggested Outcome:*
	Family involvement: *Facilitating family participation in the emotional and physical care of the child*		**Care management:** *Family ability to manage complex therapy*
The child will comply with oral medication regimen.	▶ Educate parents and child about the importance of taking medication as prescribed.	▶ Understanding can assist parents and child in placing importance on medication intake.	The child takes all medications according to prescription.
	▶ Set up calendar with dates, times, and medications clearly labeled.	▶ Visual reminders can help them recall instructions.	
	▶ Reward the child for taking medications.	▶ Reinforcing desired behaviors through rewards is effective with children.	

4. Altered growth and development related to serious illness

	NIC Priority Intervention:		*NOC Suggested Outcome:*
	Developmental enhancement: *Facilitating patient's caregivers to promote optimal growth and development of child*		**Child growth and development:** *Normal increase in body size and developmental skills*
The child will demonstrate normal physical, emotional, and cognitive development.	▶ Encourage play appropriate to age.	▶ Normal activities support self-esteem and self-knowledge.	The child continues to develop physically, emotionally, and cognitively at a normal pace.
	▶ Encourage the child to attend school.	▶ School is the work of the child and promotes cognitive and social growth.	
	▶ Encourage seeing peers when unable to attend school.	▶ Peer contacts help the child in normal developmental tasks.	
	▶ Work with teachers to support reentry to school. Use puppets, videotape, and discussion with classmates.	▶ Classmates need to understand what has happened to their friend without asking the child directly.	

GOAL	INTERVENTION	RATIONALE	EXPECTED OUTCOME
5. Fatigue related to disease state			
	NIC Priority Intervention:		*NOC Suggested Outcome:*
	Energy management: *Regulating energy use to prevent fatigue and optimize function*		**Energy conservation:** *Extent of management of energy to initiate and sustain activity*
The child will maintain energy levels necessary for normal activities.	▸ Problem-solve ways to save energy for play and school. ▸ Plan with child for quiet activities during low-energy times.	▸ The child and parents are assisted to see school and play as important. ▸ Child is empowered to select and plan own activities.	The child plans use of time effectively to maintain energy for school and play. The child conserves energy during times of increased fatigue.
7. Altered family processes related to situational crisis			
	NIC Priority Intervention:		*NOC Suggested Outcome:*
	Family process maintenance: *Minimization of family process disruption events*		**Family process:** *Extent of maintenance of family support system*
The child and family will demonstrate healthy adaptation.	▸ Encourage open communication. ▸ Suggest that all family members develop support networks. ▸ Parents should be proactive with siblings about their feelings and needs. ▸ Encourage attendance of all family members at oncology camps.	▸ Open discussion allows problem solving and ego support. ▸ Networks expand support systems. ▸ Siblings feel valued and problems are confronted early. ▸ Oncology camps promote open discussion between peers for further support and fun.	Parents report better communication between themselves and the children. Family members report an increase in friends with whom they can share feelings. Family reports attending oncology camp and describes benefit of sharing with other families in same situation.

increased nutritional intake at a time when nausea and vomiting are occurring as drug side effects, and when decreased activity and general health status result in diminished appetite. This often leads to extreme concern on the part of parents, and they may focus excessive attention on the child's intake.

Administer antiemetic drugs to lessen nausea from chemotherapy. Offer frequent, small meals. It may be helpful to offer the child's favorite foods at times when nausea and vomiting are decreased. Ask the family what treatments they use to decrease the child's nausea and vomiting. Perform 24-hour dietary recalls to assess the child's intake, and evaluate height and weight regularly. Special nutritional products may be given orally, nasogastric or nasoduodenal tube feedings may be given, or total parenteral nutrition may be necessary.

Teaching About

NUTRITION AND THE CHILD WITH CANCER

Because of the effects of cancer and chemotherapy or other treatment, the child often has a poor appetite. Mucosal sores lead to difficulty chewing and swallowing. Parents can enhance the nutritional intake of the child in a variety of ways:

- Provide frequent small feedings rather than three meals daily.
- Integrate the child's favorite foods into daily menus.
- Have nutritious snacks available for times when the child feels like eating.
- Sprinkle dried milk on top of cereals and other foods.
- Smooth, soft foods are usually preferred. Milkshakes with added peanut butter, puddings, and soft casseroles may be well tolerated. Try a variety of liquid protein-calorie supplements to find those the child likes.
- Avoid making food an area for disagreement. Do not force foods but rather, make them readily available.

- If the child is vomiting due to therapy, do not encourage food at that time. The child may develop food aversions to foods that are vomited.
- Administer antiemetics as ordered during therapy since they can prevent nausea and vomiting.
- Report weight loss and increased fatigue.
- Bring the child in for scheduled health visits so growth, development, and effects of therapy can be monitored.
- Some children need a temporary feeding tube to ensure adequate nutrition. Feedings at night can often increase intake and promote health. Occasionally a central line is inserted to provide total parenteral nutrition.
- Supplements and tube feedings will usually be covered by insurance if the provider writes an order for them.

ADMINISTER MEDICATIONS

One of the most important interventions of the oncology nurse is administering medications safely. Most chemotherapeutic drugs are prescribed and calculated as dose per meter squared (dose/m²), with m² calculated from the child's height and weight. (See Skills 11-1–11-13.)

SKILLS **CD**

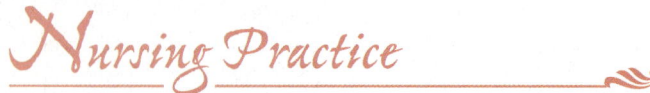

Nursing Practice

Health care professionals who have contact with chemotherapy drugs must follow careful guidelines. The Occupational Safety and Health Administration (OSHA) publishes an instruction manual entitled *Controlling Occupational Exposure to Hazardous Drugs,* which outlines general guidelines, protective equipment, and procedures (OSHA Instruction TED 1–0.15, Office of Science and Technology Assessment, Washington, DC, 1999).

A number of chemotherapeutic drugs are commonly used in combinations. **WEB** These drugs are prepared with special techniques under laminar flow devices to minimize potential toxic effects on health care providers. Gloves and other hazardous drug protocols are used. Care must be taken to avoid **extravasation** of intravenous drugs (leakage into the soft tissue around the infusion site), as permanent tissue damage can result.

In addition to chemotherapy drugs, the nurse administers other medications, such as antiemetics to control nausea, vitamin supplements, and antibiotics. Ask parents about complementary therapy and medications they are obtaining from other sources and using at home. All medications must be safely administered and the child should be monitored for side effects. **Polypharmacy** (the use of several drugs at one time to treat multiple health conditions) can lead to multiple side effects and can challenge the body's ability to metabolize and excrete drugs.

MANAGE TREATMENT SIDE EFFECTS

All cancer treatments affect some normal body cells as well as cancer cells, causing a wide variety of side effects. A frequent occurrence is **myelosuppression,** or suppression of blood cell production in the bone marrow. Be alert for signs of a decreased white blood cell count, such as infections. Take the child's temperature, isolate the child from others with infections, and perform serum laboratory studies as ordered. A colony-stimulating factor for white cell production may be administered, if necessary. Leucovorin is a form of folic acid given during methotrexate chemotherapy to protect normal cells from the destructive effects of methotrexate.

Protect the child from bruises and be alert for signs of bleeding such as petechiae, an effect of decreased platelets. When **thrombocytopenia** (decreased platelets) occurs, minimize needle sticks and other intrusive procedures. Be ready to deal with nosebleeds and watch for bleeding gums. Report any bleeding episodes to the physician.

Inadequate RBC production can result in anemia. Encourage the child to eat iron-rich foods and administer nutritional supplements, as needed.

Chemotherapy affects all rapidly growing cells in the body, but especially those of the mucous membranes. Provide good oral hygiene with a soft toothbrush, foam wand, or water irrigation device. Report oral breakdown promptly. Be alert for blood in vomitus and stool, which can indicate bleeding in the gastrointestinal tract. Evaluate the effects of hair loss on the child.

Radiation can cause burns to the skin. Examine the skin daily during hospitalization or weekly when making home visits. Leave the marks on the skin that outline the radiation target area. Avoid use of lotions, powders, and soaps on the target skin area. Some children may need to be anesthetized to ensure correct positioning for radiation; postanesthesia care will then be needed.

ENSURE ADEQUATE HYDRATION

Hydration management can be a challenge as the child may not be thirsty but is excreting large numbers of cell fragments and other substances as a result of treatment. Offer frequent small amounts of fluid. Include frozen ice pops or other fluid-containing foods such as Jell-O. Measure intake and output. To ensure adequate excretion, a number of chemotherapy drugs are given with intravenous fluids. It is important to administer fluids as ordered and ensure that the recommended urinary output excretion rate is maintained after drug administration.

PREVENT INFECTION

Children with cancer have an altered immune system, both from the disease and from the effects of immunosuppressant drugs, and must be kept away from persons with known infections. Teach parents to avoid taking the child to places that attract large gatherings of people, such as department stores, once the child returns home. Emphasize the need to report any exposure to contagious diseases, especially chickenpox. Some drugs may mask signs of infection, so be alert for any signs of mild infection. Fever, malaise, and mild respiratory infection must all be reported promptly. Follow recommendations for the immunization of children with cancer as published by the Centers for Disease Control and Prevention and the American Academy of Pediatrics. **WEB** Usually, no immunizations are given to the child until 6 months after he or she has stopped receiving chemotherapy.

MANAGE PAIN

The child with cancer may experience pain from the disease itself and from the medical interventions, such as lumbar puncture, bone marrow aspiration, and frequent intravenous infusions and blood draws. Use all possible pain management techniques to keep the child comfortable,

SIDE EFFECT	CLINICAL MANIFESTATIONS	CLINICAL THERAPY
Bone marrow suppression	Evidence of suppression usually appears 7–10 days after administration of chemotherapy; recovery is usually complete within 3–4 weeks.	Blood transfusions are administered when anemia is severe (Hgb < 7 g/dL) or platelets are very low. Some institutions use a low-microbial diet to decrease the possibility that infectious organisms will colonize the intestine. Septra is used for *Pneumocystis carinii* pneumonia prophylaxis; nystatin and oral vancomycin for antifungal and antibacterial prophylaxis. Instruct the family and child about the importance of protecting the body from bruising during periods of mild to moderate thrombocytopenia (platelet count < 5000/mm^3). Careful handwashing is essential. Encourage use of masks if family or staff have nasopharyngeal infections.
Nausea and vomiting	Symptoms may occur immediately or 5–6 hours after administration of chemotherapy and may last 48 hours.	Antiemetics, such as ondansetron, Kytril, Reglan, and Benadryl are used to treat this side effect. Teach relaxation techniques, hypnosis, and systematic desensitization (a hypnotic process that progressively reduces reactions to objects that cause strong emotional or physical responses) to help to decrease the child's symptoms. Encourage mild exercise and change of diet (eating only easily digestible foods) 12 hours before chemotherapy.
Anorexia and weight loss	May occur at any time.	Hyperalimentation is necessary if dietary changes are unsuccessful in halting the child's weight loss. Pay careful attention to changes in taste that affect food preferences. Referral to a dietician may be helpful to achieve successful modification of the child's diet.
Mouth sores	The oral mucositis resulting from chemotherapy usually occurs within 3–4 days and is often a contributing factor in anorexia.	Antifungal agents, such as nystatin or clotrimazole, lessen the possibility of candidal infection. Promote good oral hygiene, use soft foam wand or water irrigation to clean teeth; commercial mouthwashes are not recommended because they contain alcohol and increase drying of the oral cavity.
Constipation	Can occur at any time in treatment but becomes more common as therapy progresses and dietary intake and physical activity decrease.	Stool softeners and laxatives are used to treat this side effect. Advise parents to increase fluids and fibrous foods in the child's diet.
Pain	Pain can occur at any time and is best understood by subjective explanations of the child.	Acetaminophen, morphine, steroids, nonsteroidal anti-inflammatory drugs, and antidepressants may be used to manage pain. Careful pain assessment is important; the location of the pain may provide a clue to its cause, for example, metastasis to the skull, infiltration of joints, or damage to soft tissue; pain associated with chemotherapy may also be related to oral mucositis, myalgia, or tumor embolization; painful polyneuropathy can follow treatment with vincristine or cisplatin. Acetaminophen for pain can mask the presence of fever, which signals infection; careful and complete physical assessment is needed to identify infection. Pharmacologic, nonhypnotic (deep breathing, self-control), and hypnotic methods of pain control may be used; the nonpharmacologic methods often prove helpful to children with pain from multiple etiologies.

(See Skills 13-1–13-4) SKILLS as this encourages cooperation throughout the long treatment period. (See Chapter 38 for suggestions on methods of pain management.)

Management of cancer pain has been the subject of an evidence-based practice report by the Agency for Healthcare Research and Quality. The agency concluded that there is a lack of adequate studies on pain management, and there is limited application of existing work. These factors limit effective pain management in many patients with cancer (Agency for Healthcare Research and Quality, 2001b). Nurses must examine research on effective pain management for children and integrate findings into practice. WEB

Conscious sedation (see Chapter 38) may be used for some procedures. Administer sedation as ordered for young children who are undergoing radiation. Coordinate other painful or intrusive tests so they can be done while the child is sedated for radiation.

Topical anesthetics such as EMLA cream may be used to numb the skin before an intravenous start, lumbar puncture, or bone marrow aspiration. Whenever possible, include the parents in comforting the child after painful procedures.

PROVIDE PSYCHOSOCIAL SUPPORT

A diagnosis of cancer brings with it many emotions for the family. Initially parents experience shock and anger. They need basic information about the disease and the purpose of the tests that will be performed. Instructions often need to be repeated as parents may not process information the first time it is presented due to their increased stress levels. Help the parents plan how and when to tell the child the diagnosis. What the child needs to know is based on his or her developmental level and understanding.

Once the family has progressed from their initial state of shock about the diagnosis, they need to learn more about the disease. They may be interested in the pathophysiology, treatment, and expected outcome or the prognosis. Clarify their understanding of these areas and ask what questions they have. Provide verbal explanations and written material. Parents may talk with friends, purchase books, or search the Internet for information. Find out where they are getting information and provide additional resources when appropriate. Correct misconceptions and misinformation.

The family needs many strategies to deal with the challenge of long-term treatment for cancer. As the child experiences remissions and exacerbations or complications, the family feels alternately hopeful and discouraged. Identify the family's support systems and intervene as needed to enhance these systems. Facilitate contact with extended family members who might be of help, religious or spiritual connections, social service agencies, and other resources such as Internet and parent support groups. Assist parents who are concerned about job obligations and financial concerns. Help the parents to identify sources of

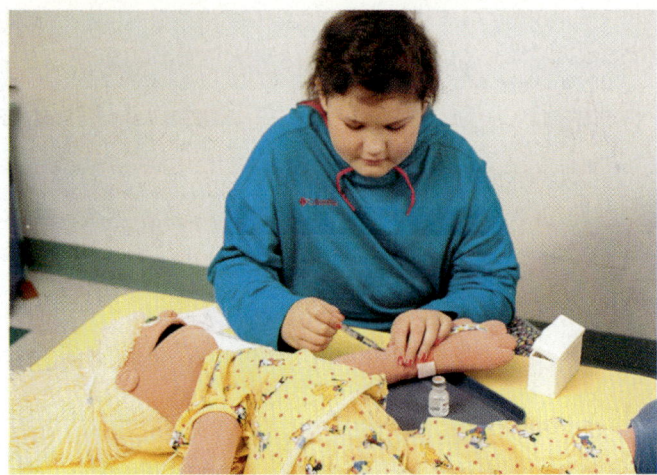

FIGURE 45–7. ◆ A child in a pediatric oncology clinic giving injections to a doll. This type of play therapy helps the child deal with fear and thus lowering her stress level.

financial assistance, respite from child care, and time for themselves (Mercer & Ritchie, 1997).

The child undergoing treatment for cancer needs support appropriate to his or her developmental stage and cognitive level. (See Chapters 32 and 34 for developmental levels and effective support strategies for children of different ages.) Younger children primarily need support during painful procedures and separation from parents. Older children need intervention strategies to help work through feelings about treatments (Figure 45–7 ◆). A major developmental task of adolescence is to attain independence and control, but cancer often interferes with adolescents' ability to achieve this task. Therefore, plan nursing strategies that empower adolescents as much as possible. Introduce them to other teens with similar diagnoses and allow them to make decisions and choices independent of parents when possible (Enskar, Carlsson, Golsater, et al., 1997).

Growth and Development

An adolescent can decide which type of medication port would be best (e.g., an implantable port under the skin or a venous access device with tubing outside the body). Making this choice enables the teen to feel more in control of the disease and treatment.

Talk with the child's teachers before the return to school after treatment to explain the child's condition. Arrange for tutors if necessary to assist the child with school work during hospitalization and home care. Explore the option of summer camp for children with cancer. The Make-a-Wish Foundation strives to make dreams come true for ill children by sponsoring them for a desired activity or outing. Refer the child to this foundation if appropriate.

The siblings of a child who has cancer can be stressed by the changes in the family. They may grieve over the ill brother or sister and may feel sad and depressed. They also can experience anger, guilt, or resentment and may have a lack of knowledge about the disease and treatment. Inquire about siblings and ask what they know about the child's condition. Find out who is caring for siblings and whether their teachers have been informed about the family situation. Include siblings in care when possible. Invite them to visit and to participate both during hospitalization and at home care visits. They can be involved in play therapy sessions and recreational activities with the ill child. Ask the parents if the siblings are demonstrating symptoms such as depression, behavioral changes, or decrease in school performance and suggest interventions as appropriate. They may benefit from speaking with a school counselor or can be referred to a support group for siblings of children with cancer. Some cancer summer camps welcome siblings as well as children with cancer.

The family of a child with cancer is faced with a life-threatening illness. Refer to Chapter 37 for strategies to assist the family in coping with this stressor. For some types of cancer, the child may experience a remission with treatment, but a recurrence of disease later as cancer cells grow again. The family may become angry or depressed about the relapse. Repeated treatments challenge the family's support systems. Waiting for the outcome of diagnostic tests can be an especially challenging time. Provide information as soon as possible. If the child's illness progresses, refer the family to hospice to help them care for the terminally ill child and work through the grieving process. Explore cancer support groups and information, and share this information with families.

DISCHARGE PLANNING AND HOME CARE TEACHING

Preparation for home care centers on creating a normal environment while supporting the child's physiologic and psychosocial responses to the cancer and treatments. Education is the primary focus of discharge planning. Teach the parents how to ensure adequate nutritional intake, to be alert for signs of infection, to protect the child from exposure to communicable diseases during times of neutropenia, to administer medications at home, as well as methods to handle vomiting and pain. Help the parents and child deal with any obstacles to normal development and functioning. Teach the parents and family about symptoms that need to be treated immediately.

Home management of a vascular access device or central line (see Chapter 12 in the *Clinical Skills Manual*), SKILLS such as a Broviac catheter, initially challenges parents (Figure 45–8 ◆). An implanted port may be used; it allows the child freedom to swim and engage in other activities. Parents will need information about whatever device the child has received. Demonstrate details about cleaning the site, instilling heparin in the line or reservoir, and other needed care. After teaching the parents, observe them performing the procedure before the child is discharged.

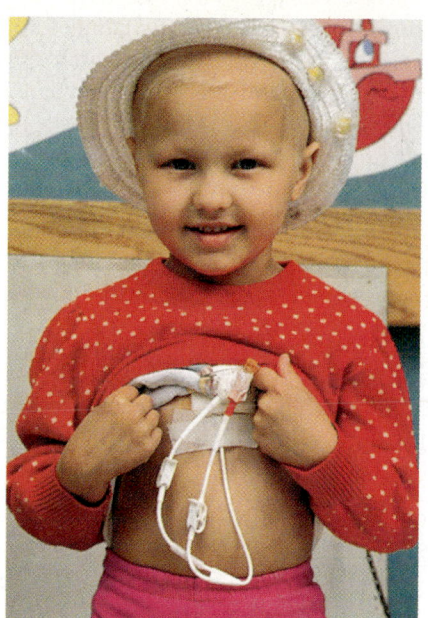

FIGURE 45–8. ◆ A vascular access device allows chemotherapeutic agents to be administered without the need for repeated "sticks" to the child.

Teaching About

REPORTABLE EVENTS FOR CHILDREN RECEIVING CHEMOTHERAPY

Report the following events to your child's oncologist if they occur while the child is receiving chemotherapy:

- Temperature above 38 °C (101 °F)
- Any bleeding, such as nosebleeds, blood in stool or urine, petechiae, bruising
- Pain or discomfort with urination or defecation
- Sores in the mouth
- Vomiting or diarrhea
- Persistent pain anywhere, including headache
- Signs of infection, such as cough, fever, runny nose, tugging at ears
- Signs of infection in central lines, such as redness, drainage, or tenderness
- Exposure to communicable diseases, especially varicella (chickenpox)

Inform dentists and other health care providers that the child is receiving chemotherapy prior to procedures. Prophylactic antibiotics should be given before and after dental care.

Note: From Bindler, R. M., & Howry, L. B. (1997). *Pediatric drugs and nursing implications* (2nd ed.). Upper Saddle River, NJ: Prentice Hall-Health. Adapted.

Emphasize the need for the child and family to have fun and be as normal as possible. Play distracts the child and is essential in reducing fears. Children, parents, and siblings often benefit from participation in cancer support groups and cancer summer camps. These activities create additional support systems, build the child's self-esteem, and enhance coping skills through role modeling.

Make home visits to evaluate the family's strengths and needs. Be sure that the family has adequate support from hospice and other end-of-life services when the child's condition is terminal.

Evaluation

Expected outcomes of nursing care for the child with cancer relate to the specific disease, treatments, and responses. Some examples of outcomes include:

▶ Adequate intake to promote normal growth
▶ Hydration that supports body processes and ensures drug and cancer cell product elimination
▶ Prompt identification and treatment to minimize treatment side effects
▶ Management of pain to a level of comfort satisfactory to child and family
▶ Family use of resources to provide necessary support during hospitalizations and treatments
▶ Knowledge of management of treatment regimens
▶ Acceptance of prognosis and support of all family members

BRAIN TUMORS

Central nervous system or brain tumors are the most commonly occurring solid tumors in children and the second most common malignancy, after leukemia (Baker, 1998; Smith, Freidlia, Ries, et al., 1998). Each year approximately 1500 children under the age of 15 years are diagnosed with tumors of the brain and central nervous system, accounting for one in five childhood cancers (Conway, Asuncion, & DaRosso, 1999).

Etiology and Pathophysiology

Brain tumors in children usually occur below the roof of the cerebellum and involve the cerebellum, midbrain, and brainstem (see "Pathophysiology Illustrated: Brain Tumors"). In contrast, brain tumors in adults are usually located above the areas between the cerebrum and cerebellum.

The most common brain tumors in children are medulloblastoma, cerebral and cerebellar astrocytoma, ependymoma, and gliomas of the cerebrum or brainstem. Less common are supratentorial embryonal tumors and craniopharyngioma.

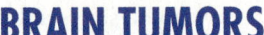

PATHOPHYSIOLOGY ILLUSTRATED
Brain Tumors

- Supratentorial tumors (cerebral astrocytoma, ependymoma, optic nerve gliomas)
- Tentorial notch tumors (pineal region tumors, hypothalamic glioma)
- Tentorial tumors
- Infratentorial tumors (brainstem gliomas, medulloblastoma, cerebellar astrocytoma, ependymoma)
- Foramen magnum tumors

- Supratentorial tumors
- Tentorial notch tumors
- Tentorial tumors
- Infratentorial tumors
- Foramen magnum tumors

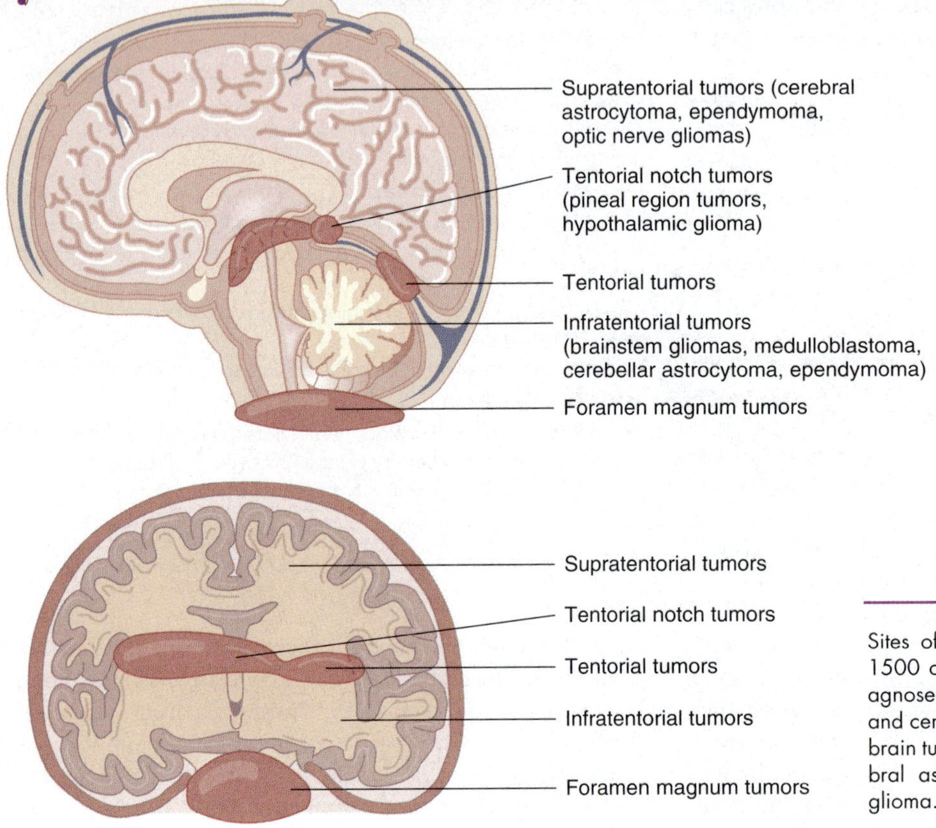

Sites of brain tumors in children. Approximately 1500 children under the age of 15 years are diagnosed annually as having tumors of the brain and central nervous system. The four most common brain tumors in children are medulloblastoma, cerebral astrocytoma, ependymoma, and brainstem glioma.

TUMOR	ETIOLOGY	CLINICAL MANIFESTATIONS	CLINICAL THERAPY
Medulloblastoma	External layer of cerebellum	Headache, vomiting, ataxia	Surgery; chemotherapy with lomustine, vincristine, prednisone, cisplatin, radiation
Astrocytoma	Glial cells, supratentorial or infratentorial	Seizures, visual disturbances, increased intracranial pressure; vomiting	Surgery, chemotherapy with vincristine, dactinomycin; radiation
Ependymoma	Fourth ventricle, posterior fossa	Hydrocephalus	Surgery, radiation
Brainstem glioma	Pons	Cranial nerve (VI + VII) tract signs, nystagmus, ataxia, motor symptoms	Surgery, radiation

Clinical Manifestations

Brain tumors in children can be manifested by behavioral and nervous system changes that occur either rapidly or more slowly and subtly. Some common symptoms include headache, nausea, vomiting, dizziness, change in vision or hearing, fatigue, and nonspecific signs. Nonspecific signs include slight behavior change, decreased school performance, or slight incoordination. See "Clinical Manifestations: Brain Tumors" for common manifestations of certain types of tumors. 🔗

Medulloblastomas are brain tumors in the external layer of the cerebellum. They account for 20% of childhood brain tumors, and commonly occur in children aged 5 to 6 years. Astrocytomas arise from glial cells and can be either above or below the area between the cerebrum and cerebellum. They account for 40% of childhood brain tumors (Kun, 1997). Ependymomas commonly occur in the fourth ventricle of the posterior fossa and comprise 8% of childhood brain tumors. Brainstem gliomas are located in the pons and typically spread into the surrounding tissue. They account for 15% of childhood brain tumors (Conway et al., 1999). Cerebral gliomas are another common cancer type in children.

Nursing Practice

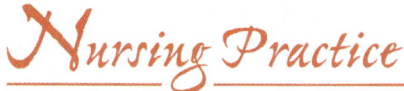

The following drugs are used to treat brain tumors:

Cyclophosphamide   VP-16
Ifosfamide   Cisplatin
Lomustine   Carboplatin
Vincristine

Clinical Therapy

Brain tumors are commonly diagnosed with CT, MRI, myelography, and angiography. Neurophysiologic tests (electroencephalography and brainstem evoked potentials) are used to assess sensory pathway integrity and disease- or drug-related sensory dysfunction. Other tests that may be performed are tumor markers and cerebrospinal fluid cytology. Lumbar puncture identifies abnormal cells in the cerebrospinal fluid. Bone marrow aspiration identifies any extracranial primary neoplastic growth, since cancers in other sites can metastasize to the brain.

Treatment depends on the type of brain tumor. Surgery is common. It may be performed to obtain a biopsy specimen, to debulk (reduce the tumor by partial removal) or excise the tumor, or to treat any hydrocephalus that may be present. During surgery, radiology images allow the neurosurgeon to see computerized images of the brain while at the same time stimulating nerves to determine their functioning. These techniques provide rapid feedback to the neurosurgeon. Laser surgery, which has delicate precise control and accuracy, is used when tumors are close to sensitive neural or vascular structures.

Use of radiation after surgery and chemotherapy has improved the survival of children with medulloblastoma and ependymoma. High-dose chemotherapy is often used, and this modality has improved the survival of children with central nervous system tumors (Conway et al., 1999). Low-dose chemotherapy can shrink and help manage some tumors. Intrathecal administration of chemotherapy is useful in some cases. However, the blood–brain barrier reduces the effectiveness of chemotherapy for children with brain tumors. For example, when methotrexate is administered intrathecally (in the spinal canal), only a small amount crosses normal brain capillaries. Radiation is not used in children under 3 years because of resultant damage to brain cells. Bone marrow and stem cell transplantation is increasingly used.

Complications of treatment for children with brain tumors are significant. They include severe infections (associated with high-dose chemotherapy), seizure activity, sensorimotor defects, hydrocephalus, and growth problems. Care is taken to treat infections early and aggressively. If a cerebrospinal shunt is used, infection or blockage can occur (see Chapter 49 for further discussion of cerebrospinal shunts in children). 🔗 Anticonvulsants are commonly given prophylactically after surgery. Endocrine problems, such as growth hormone changes, hypothyroidism, and panhypopituitarism, may occur when the tumor is in the hypothalamic–pituitary area (Vernon-Levett & Geller,

1997). Treatment may also lead to impaired cognitive function and emotional or behavioral problems in some children. Memory deficits and selective attention deficits are the most common problems.

Diabetes insipidus is a special consideration in children with midline brain tumors, such as those that compress the hypothalamus, pituitary stalk, or posterior pituitary gland. Manifestations of diabetes insipidus include voiding of large amounts of dilute urine with a specific gravity of less than 1.005 (see Chapter 47). ⊂⊃

Nursing Management

Nursing Assessment and Diagnosis

The focus of physiologic assessment of the child with a brain tumor is determined by its presentation (Table 45–4). Presenting signs can be categorized as follows:

▶ *Nonspecific signs* related to increasing intracranial pressure

▶ *Secondary signs* related to displacement of intracranial structures

▶ *Focal signs* suggesting direct involvement of the brain and cranial nerves

Thorough neurologic examination before surgery is essential to provide a record of baseline functioning. The neurologic examination also allows the evaluation of the child's changing physiologic status before surgery. Ask if the child has manifested slow changes over time or has had quickly developing symptoms. Measurement of head circumference and assessment of the anterior fontanel are necessary in children under the age of 18 months.

Perform developmental screening on young children using the Denver II or other developmental test (see Chapter 35). ⊂⊃ Ask about the child's social interactions, school performance, and any behavior changes that have occurred.

Several nursing diagnoses can be identified for the child with a brain tumor, depending on the type and location of the tumor. Some common examples are:

▶ *Altered nutrition: less than body requirements* related to loss of appetite

▶ *Impaired physical mobility* related to tumor pressure on coordination centers

▶ *Altered growth and development* related to effects of disability

▶ *Impaired memory* related to neurologic disturbance

▶ *Pain* related to physical injury

Planning and Implementation

The child with a brain tumor requires multidisciplinary care by, among others, a neurologist, neurosurgeon, pediatrician, dietitian, and social worker. Other specialists are also often needed. The nurse can act as a case manager to coordinate the complex care needed by the child.

For the nursing care of children immediately following surgery, refer to Chapter 34. ⊂⊃ In addition, close monitoring of neurologic status is needed postoperatively (refer to Chapter 49). ⊂⊃ Be especially alert for signs of increased intracranial pressure and infection. Observe for seizure activity. Administer drugs such as antibiotics and anticonvulsants as ordered.

Signs and symptoms of diabetes insipidus may occur following brain surgery (see Chapter 47 for a description of diabetes insipidus). ⊂⊃ Nursing care includes hourly measurement of intake and output, measurement of serum sodium levels every 4 to 6 hours, accurate fluid replacement, and frequent assessment of neurologic status. An indwelling urinary catheter is useful for accurate measurement of urinary output. Both abnormally high or low urinary output can indicate problems and should be promptly reported.

DISCHARGE PLANNING AND HOME CARE TEACHING

Teach the parents to watch for an increase in voiding of dilute urine. Be sure they can recognize the signs of infection and changes in the child's neurologic status. Once the child is ready for discharge, chemotherapy or radiation may begin; tell parents the reason and potential side effects of these treatments. Help the family get any special equipment they may need to care for the child at home, such as a wheelchair, bed rails, or dressings. The American Cancer Society is a potential resource for assistance with these needs.

Children with brain tumors, especially those who have received radiation, often have some permanent sequelae. They may have slowed development, incoordination, learning disabilities, or other effects. These sequelae are most common in children who are 3 years of age or younger at the time of radiation therapy. Perform accurate height and weight measures at each health care visit. Assess developmental milestones. Ask about progress in school and any special services that might be needed. Perform thorough neurologic assessments. Support the family as they learn to deal with unknown or changed expectations for the child's performance (Freeman, O'Dell, & Meola, 2000).

TABLE 45–4 Physiologic Assessment of Brain Tumors	
Clinical Manifestations	Assessment
Nonspecific signs: headache, morning vomiting, somnolence, irritability	Level of consciousness, pupil response, pupil shape and size
Secondary signs: disturbances of cranial nerves; other signs depend on site of tumor	All cranial nerves
Focal signs: truncal ataxia (midline brain tumors), general nystagmus, head tilting	Motor ability, head positions when watching television or looking at people (double vision, sixth cranial nerve involvement)

Evaluation

Expected outcomes of nursing care for the child with a brain tumor depend on the site of tumor, clinical therapy, and medical outcome. Some outcomes might include:

▶ Adequate nutritional intake to support growth and prevent malnutrition

▶ Maintenance of a safe environment

▶ Physical mobility allowed by developmental level and alterations of disease

▶ Provision of an environment to meet normal developmental milestones within capability of the child

▶ Management of pain to comfort level

▶ Parental understanding of diagnosis and treatment plan

NEUROBLASTOMA

Neuroblastoma is the solid tumor most commonly occurring outside the cranium of children. It is responsible for 8% of childhood cancers and 15% of cancer deaths in children. The average age at onset is 22 months. Prognosis varies, depending on the staging of the tumor (Table 45–5) and the age of the child, with more favorable outcomes in infants under 1 year of age (Castleberry, 1997).

Neuroblastoma is commonly a smooth, hard, nontender mass that can occur anywhere along the sympathetic nervous system chain. A frequent location is the abdomen,

although other sites are the adrenal, thoracic, and cervical areas. It is usually diagnosed in children under 5 years of age, with the median age at diagnosis being 2 years.

Etiology and Pathophysiology

Neuroblastoma originates in primitive neurocrest cells that form the adrenal medulla, paraganglia, and sympathetic nervous system of the cervical sympathetic chain and the thoracic chain. A majority of neuroblastomas develop in the adrenal medulla or peritoneal sympathetic ganglia. Other develop in the thorax and elsewhere along the sympathetic chain. Lymph node metastasis is common.

The cause of neuroblastoma is unknown. Theories center on the possible effects of environmental factors such as prenatal drug exposure from the mother and disturbed cellular nerve growth factors. Oncogenes are present in neuroblastoma cells in a DNA sequence known as N-myc. High levels of the N-myc oncogene are associated with rapid disease progression and a poorer prognosis. Tumors in infants are commonly treatable, with poorer prognosis in older children (McManus & Gilchrist, 2000)

Clinical Manifestations

The location of the mass determines the symptoms. A retroperitoneal mass causes altered bowel and bladder function; characteristic signs are weight loss, abdominal fullness, irritability, fatigue, and fever. Dyspnea or infection may occur when the tumor is mediastinal. Neck and facial edema may result from vena cava syndrome if the tumor is mediastinal and large. Malaise, fever, and a limp can occur if there has been metastasis to the bone (Castleberry, 1997).

Clinical Therapy

The International Neuroblastoma Staging System (INSS) recommends different diagnostic and laboratory evaluations for diagnosis of the primary disease and of metastases. Biopsy of the tumor is used for initial diagnosis. Metastases are diagnosed by bone marrow biopsy, radiolabeled scanning, x-ray, CT, and MRI.

Vanillylmandelic acid (VMA) and homovanillic acid (HVA) are byproducts of adrenal hormones and their levels are usually elevated in the urine and blood (see Appendix B and the CD for normal values). They are used initially to diagnose the disease and later to follow its progress. Areas of necrosis and calcification are readily identifiable with radiologic tests. These tests also help in the staging of the disease by identifying metastases.

Routine blood cell counts may reveal anemia and thrombocytopenia. There is no classic white blood cell (WBC) response, although thrombocytopenia may occur in association with disseminated intravascular coagulation. **Leukocytosis** (higher than normal leukocyte count) and **leukopenia** (lower than normal leukocyte count) have been observed with bone marrow involvement.

TABLE 45–5	International Neuroblastoma Staging System
Stage	**Description**
1	Localized tumor confined to the area of origin; complete gross excision, with or without microscopic residual disease; identifiable ipsilateral and contralateral lymph nodes negative microscopically
2A	Unilateral tumor with incomplete gross excision; identifiable ipsilateral and contralateral lymph nodes negative microscopically
2B	Unilateral tumor with complete or incomplete gross excision; with positive ipsilateral regional lymph nodes; identifiable contralateral lymph nodes negative microscopically
3	Tumor infiltrating across the midline with or without regional lymph node involvement; or unilateral tumor with contralateral regional lymph node involvement; or midline tumor with bilateral regional lymph node involvement
4	Dissemination of tumor to distant lymph nodes, bone, bone marrow, liver, and/or other organs (except as defined in stage 4S)
4S	Localized primary tumor as defined for stage 1 or 2 with dissemination limited to liver, skin, and/or bone marrow

Note: From Castleberry, R. P. (1997). Biology and treatment of neuroblastoma. *Pediatric Clinics of North America, 44,* 919–938. Adapted.

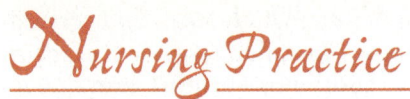

Nursing Practice

The following drugs are used to treat neuroblastoma:

Cyclophosphamide	Teniposide
Doxorubicin	Etoposide
Cisplatin	Carboplatin
Ifosfamide	

The stage of the tumor (see Table 45–5) determines the treatment protocol. Surgical excision of the mass is performed, followed by chemotherapy with a combination of drugs. Radiation is occasionally used. Bone marrow transplantation may be performed for advanced disease. Neuroblastoma is most responsive to treatment in children under 1 year of age.

Nursing Management

Nursing Assessment and Diagnosis

Assess the presenting site of the tumor, such as the neck or abdomen, by observation and inspection. Palpation is contraindicated. Carefully document related functioning, such as bowel and bladder function. Take vital signs to watch for elevated temperature and vital sign changes caused by a thoracic mass. Observe gait and coordination. Take weight and height and compare to earlier percentiles for the child. Specific assessments during treatment will depend on the treatment methods used (refer to the earlier discussions of chemotherapy and radiation treatment). Psychosocial assessment and emotional assessment of the family are needed.

A variety of nursing diagnoses may be appropriate for the child with neuroblastoma, depending on the location and extent of the presenting disease. Some common diagnoses might include:

▶ *Impaired gas exchange* related to ventilation-perfusion imbalance

▶ *Impaired physical mobility* related to neuromuscular impairment

▶ *Sensory/perceptual alteration (visual)* related to altered sensory perception

▶ *Pain* related to tumor pressure and injury

▶ *Anticipatory grieving (family)* related to potential loss of significant person

Planning and Implementation

The nursing management of the child with neuroblastoma can encompass the three phases of medical treatment: chemotherapy, surgery, and radiation. Specific postsurgical care depends on the size and site of the tumor. Normal postoperative care includes providing fluid support and respiratory care and preventing infection.

Nursing care during the chemotherapy phase includes minimizing side effects, preventing infection, teaching parents about the medications their child is receiving, and monitoring physical and emotional growth and development of the young child. When radiation is part of the treatment, use common nursing measures described earlier in the chapter.

Topics for parent and family teaching and discharge planning are presented in "Teaching About: The Child with a Neuroblastoma." Ongoing support and connection to resources to assist in management of the child's treatment at home will be needed. When the prognosis is poor, parents may appreciate referrals to hospice, to other parents who have experienced similar child illnesses, and to other community resources. See Chapter 37 for additional nursing care for end of life. ⊂▭⊃

Teaching About

THE CHILD WITH A NEUROBLASTOMA

Surgery Phase
- Teach the parents to observe for signs of infection at the wound site and to take the child's temperature, if necessary.
- Advise parents to note bowel movements and report a lack of one for 3 days to the physician.
- Continue with progression to a regular diet.

Chemotherapy Phase
- The child frequently has a central line placed early in the chemotherapy phase. The central line greatly reduces the emotional trauma associated with chemotherapy and blood tests.
    Teach the child how to help the parents with cleaning of the central line.
    Teach the child how to protect the central line.
    Teach the parents how to clean and dress the site of the central line.
    Have the parents practice central line care with a model and then on the child before discharge to increase the parents' confidence.
    Give the parents written and illustrated information about care of a central line.
    Arrange for home care dressing supplies before discharge.
- Give the parents detailed chemotherapy information.
- Refer the family to the American Cancer Society for coloring books for children receiving chemotherapy.

Evaluation

Expected outcomes of nursing care for the child with neuroblastoma include:

▶ Respiratory exchange to support daily activities

▶ Physical mobility to level possible considering developmental age

- Management of sensory/perceptual alterations to provide for safety and sensory input
- Management of pain to level of comfort
- Acceptance and integration of diagnosis into lives of family members

WILMS' TUMOR (NEPHROBLASTOMA)

Nephroblastoma, an intrarenal tumor that is called Wilms' tumor, is a common abdominal tumor of childhood and accounts for 6% to 7% of all childhood tumors (Anderson, 2000). Each year the incidence is 8.1 cases per million children. Wilms' tumor occurs most frequently between 2 and 5 years of age, but may also occur in adolescents and adults.

Etiology and Pathophysiology

Wilms' tumor is associated with several congenital anomalies: aniridia (absence of the iris), hemihypertrophy (abnormal growth of one half of the body or a body structure), genitourinary anomalies, nevi, and hamartomas (benign, nodulelike growths). This connection suggests a genetic link. However, most children with Wilms' tumor have no other abnormalities. A tumor suppressor gene has been identified that acts to promote normal kidney development. This gene and others may be missing in children with Wilms' tumor (Anderson, 2000).

Clinical Manifestations

Wilms' tumor is usually an asymptomatic, firm, lobulated mass located to one side of the midline in the abdomen. Often a parent discovers the mass during the child's bath. Hypertension caused by increased renin activity related to renal damage is reported in 25% of cases. Hematuria is sometimes present. Bilateral Wilms' tumors occur in 5% to 10% of cases (Anderson, 2000).

Clinical Therapy

The diagnosis of Wilms' tumor is based on an ultrasound study of the abdomen and an intravenous pyelogram. CT scanning or MRI of the lungs, liver, spleen, and brain may be performed to identify any metastasis. This information is used in staging the tumor (Table 45–6). A complete blood count is obtained, as well as BUN and creatinine levels. Liver function tests are performed.

Treatment is multifaceted. Surgery is performed to remove the affected kidney, to examine the opposite kidney, and to look for other sites of metastasis. Chemotherapy or radiation therapy, alone or in combination, is sometimes used before surgery to reduce the size of the tumor. Radiation and/or chemotherapy may also follow surgery. Children whose tumors are almost completely excised and who have a favorable prognosis do not require irradiation of the tumor bed.

TABLE 45–6 National Wilms' Tumor Study Staging System

Stage	Description
I	The tumor is limited to the kidney and completely excised. The surface of the renal capsule is intact. The tumor is not ruptured before or during removal. No residual tumor is apparent beyond the margins of the excision.
II	The tumor extends beyond the kidney but is completely excised. Regional extension of the tumor is present, i.e., penetration through the outer surface of the renal capsule into the perirenal soft tissues. Vessels outside the kidney substance are infiltrated or contain tumor thrombus. Biopsy may have been performed on the tumor, or local spillage of tumor confined to the flank has occurred. No residual tumor is apparent at or beyond the margin of excision.
III	Residual nonhematogenous tumor is confined to the abdomen. Any of the following may occur: Lymph nodes on biopsy are found to be involved in the hilus, the periaortic chains, or beyond. Diffuse peritoneal contamination by the tumor has occurred, such as by spillage of tumor beyond the flank before or during surgery, or by tumor growth that has penetrated through the peritoneal surface. Implants are found on peritoneal surfaces. The tumor extends beyond the surgical margins either microscopically or grossly. The tumor is not completely resectable because of local infiltration into vital structures.
IV	Hematogenous metastasis: deposits are present beyond stage III, e.g., lung, liver, bone, and/or brain.
V	Bilateral renal involvement is present at diagnosis. An attempt should be made to stage each side according to the above criteria on the basis of extent of disease before biopsy.

Note: From Green, D. M., Grigoriev, Y. A., Nan, B., Takashima, J. R., Norkool, P. A., D'Angio, G. J., et al. (2001). Congestive heart failure after treatment for Wilms' tumor: A report from the National Wilms' Tumor study group. *Journal of Clinical Oncology, 19,* 1926–1934. Adapted.

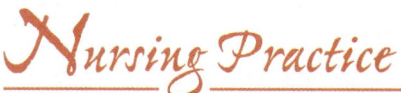

Nursing Practice

The following drugs are used to treat Wilms' tumor:

Vincristine
Actinomycin D
Doxorubicin
Cyclophosphamide

Long-term complications of treatment include liver damage, portal hypertension, and mild cirrhosis, which may occur in children treated for right-sided Wilms' tumor. Radiation damage (such as thinning or weakening) of the skeleton, pelvis, and thorax has been reported. Kyphosis and scoliosis may occur from irradiation of vertebral bodies and the pelvis. Glomerular damage to the remaining kidney may also occur. Second malignancies in the original radiation field have occurred with orthovoltage radiation, but recent changes in radiation therapy have reduced this risk.

Nursing Management

Nursing Assessment and Diagnosis

Perform a thorough baseline assessment of the child. Do not palpate the abdomen because of the potential for spreading the cancerous cells. Monitor the child's blood pressure carefully as hypertension is a common finding that may require treatment.

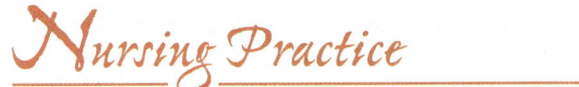

Nursing Practice

If you feel a mass during palpation of a child's abdomen, stop palpating immediately and report the finding to the physician. Never palpate the liver or abdomen of a child with Wilms' tumor as this could cause a piece of the tumor to dislodge. Place a sign on the child's bed and in the chart alerting health providers not to palpate the abdomen.

Nursing diagnoses for a child with Wilms' tumor will differ depending on the phase of treatment. Some common nursing diagnoses might include:

▶ *Risk for infection* related to inadequate defenses

▶ *Altered urinary elimination* related to anatomic obstruction

▶ *Altered cardiopulmonary tissue perfusion* related to hypertension caused by mechanical reduction of blood flow

▶ *Risk for caregiver role strain* related to child's illness severity

▶ *Risk for impaired home maintenance management* related to child's disease

Planning and Implementation

Nursing management can be divided into two phases: the postrenal surgery phase and the chemotherapy phase. (See Chapter 34 for general care of the child after surgery.) Drawings and special teaching dolls with removable kidneys can be used to teach young children about the surgery. Although chemotherapy may occur at two different times, before and after surgery, nursing management considerations remain the same.

Nursing care during the postrenal surgery phase focuses on pain management and close monitoring of fluid levels. A large incision is necessary to remove the kidney, and the resultant postoperative shift of organs and fluid in the abdominal cavity may create discomfort for the child. Fre-

quently reposition the child and use noninvasive and pharmacologic pain interventions to improve the child's comfort. Gentle handling is important. Monitor fluids closely following surgery to prevent hypovolemia and to assess the shift of fluids out of the third space and out of the body. Assess daily weight, intake and output (I&O), and urine specific gravity. Monitor the function of the remaining kidney. Take blood pressure frequently to watch for signs of shock and to assess the functioning of the remaining kidney.

During the chemotherapy phase, monitor the child for side effects of drugs, the potential for infection from the central line site, and the function of the remaining kidney. Advise parents about home care needs, administration of medications, and monitoring for drug side effects and ongoing needs for health monitoring. A long-term complication in children who received doxorubicin treatment is congestive heart failure, so ongoing periodic health care evaluations are needed.

Evaluation

Desired outcomes for nursing care of the child with nephroblastoma include balanced I&O, normal vital signs, recovery from surgery, and successful family management of postsurgical care and ongoing treatments.

BONE TUMORS

Osteosarcoma

Osteosarcoma is a rare, malignant bone tumor that occurs predominantly in adolescent boys. Its peak incidence is during the rapid growth years. The tumor is usually located at the metaphysis of the distal femur, proximal tibia, or proximal humerus (Meyers & Gorlick, 1997).

ETIOLOGY AND PATHOPHYSIOLOGY

Bone tissue produced by osteosarcoma never matures into compact bone. Although the cause of osteosarcoma is unknown, radiation exposure (either environmental or treatment related) is associated with its development. Survivors of retinoblastoma have a greatly increased incidence of osteosarcoma. An abnormality of gene p53 has been noted in some cases of this cancer, leading to oncogene malformations and possibly to an absence of tumor suppressor genes (Meyers & Gorlick, 1997).

CLINICAL MANIFESTATIONS

The common initial symptoms are pain and swelling. The pain can be referred to the hip or back, which can delay diagnosis. Pulmonary metastasis occurs in 20% of cases.

CLINICAL THERAPY

Diagnosis is made through radiographic tests (radiographic studies of the affected area, bone scan, CT, or MRI scans of involved bone), blood test for serum alkaline phosphatase (level may be elevated), and tumor biopsy (to confirm the diagnosis). Arteriography may be performed if limb-sparing surgery is contemplated.

Treatment involves both surgery and chemotherapy. The surgery is either a limb-sparing procedure or limb amputation. In limb-sparing procedures the tumor is removed and an internal prosthesis is inserted. A limb-sparing procedure is possible if bone growth has taken place and a neurobundle (area where several nerves converge) is not involved in the tumor. If these two criteria are not met, limb amputation is necessary. Aggressive chemotherapy following surgery has improved the survival rate. At the time of diagnosis, most children have metastases (even though they may not be identifiable), so chemotherapy is needed. Chemotherapy may be started before surgery, especially when limb-sparing surgery is performed.

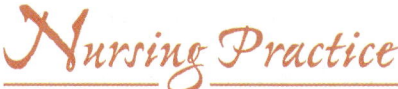

The following drugs are used to treat osteosarcoma:

Methotrexate	Bleomycin
Doxorubicin	Dactinomycin
Cisplatin	Ifosfamide
Cyclophosphamide	

Research is testing the benefit of drugs to stimulate the immune system in the treatment for osteosarcoma. In addition, muramyl-tripeptide (MTP), a derivative of the tuberculosis vaccine BCG, is showing promise in reducing the risk of recurrence (Meyers & Gorlick, 1997).

Ewing's Sarcoma

Ewing's sarcoma is a malignant, small, round cell tumor usually involving the diaphyseal (shaft) portion of the long bones. The most common sites are the femur, pelvis, tibia, fibula, ribs, humerus, scapula, and clavicle, but any bone may be involved. Ewing's sarcoma occurs in 2 children per million, is most common in whites and Hispanics, and is rare in black and Asian-American children. The incidence is highest in children between the ages of 10 and 20 years (Grier, 1997).

Although full mechanisms have not been described, abnormalities on chromosomes 11 and 22 have been identified in children with Ewing's sarcoma. A translocation of genetic material is apparent. In addition, these tumors express a proto-oncogene, c-myc.

The symptoms are similar to those of osteosarcoma and may include pain, swelling, fever, an elevated WBC count, and elevated erythrocyte sedimentation rate. A tumor biopsy is necessary for diagnosis. Diagnostic tests are the same as those for osteosarcoma.

Initial treatment for Ewing's sarcoma is chemotherapy to reduce the tumor, followed by surgical removal of the entire bone or intensive high-dose irradiation of the entire bone. Surgery is preferred because of the possibility of a secondary cancer from radiation. Chemotherapy is always used after initial treatment, as nondetectable metastases are nearly always present (Grier, 1997).

Nursing Practice

The following drugs are used to treat Ewing's sarcoma:

Vincristine	Ifosfamide
Cyclophosphamide	Etoposide
Dactinomycin	Adriamycin
Doxorubicin	

Nursing Management

Nursing Assessment and Diagnosis

Physiologic assessment of the child with a bone tumor includes assessment of the site before surgery. Assess the child's pain or discomfort, mobility, and gait. Take careful vital signs, especially noting temperature and respirations. Psychologic assessments of the child and family are needed, especially if amputation is planned. Loss of a limb causes body image disturbances, particularly with school-age children and adolescents. Assess the child's understanding of the treatment and of care after surgery. Find out what support systems are available for assistance.

Observe the wound postoperatively for infection and hemorrhage. Assess circulation above and below the operative site. If edema is found, elevate the limb. If a limb salvage procedure is performed, the child's extremity will remain, but it will not function as before because muscle insertion sites and mass have been removed with the tumor during surgery. Detailed charting of the condition of the surgical site and limb function is important.

If the limb has been amputated, assess the child for the following signs indicating a disturbed body image:

▶ Refusal to look at or touch the altered or missing body part

▶ Preoccupation with loss or change

▶ Feelings of shame or embarrassment, either verbalized or demonstrated

▶ Distorted perception of normal body (easily seen in the child's drawings of the body)

▶ Fears of rejection or unwanted attention from others

▶ Overexposure or hiding of the affected body part

▶ Actual or perceived change in the structure and function of the body or body parts

Psychosocial assessment of the child and family is discussed in more detail earlier in the chapter under "Childhood Cancer" (see pp. 1129–1131).

Nursing diagnoses for the child with a bone tumor are based on the treatment and needs of each child. Among the nursing diagnoses that might be appropriate are:

- *Risk for infection* related to amputation
- *Impaired skin integrity* related to mechanical forces of prosthesis
- *Impaired physical mobility* related to musculoskeletal impairment
- *Impaired adjustment* related to disability and lifestyle change
- *Body image disturbance* related to treatment and injury
- *Pain* related to physical injury of tissues

Planning and Implementation

Care of the child after surgery involves general postoperative care (see Chapter 34). The child who has had an amputation has special needs regarding skin care and rehabilitation. Inspect the tissue at the surgical site, using sterile technique, and turn the child at least every 2 hours. The site needs to heal completely before chemotherapy can begin and a prosthesis can be made.

Discuss insurance and other financial arrangements with the parents, as prosthetics can be costly. Referral to a Shriners Hospital is an option for some families.

Implement plans to help the child deal with body image disturbance. Plan for a visit from another child who is well adjusted to a prosthesis. Help the child gradually learn how to care for the stump. Slow progress may be made as the child first looks briefly, then for longer periods, and finally is willing to touch the stump. Show the child how it is possible to continue with sports such as baseball, skiing, or biking with a prosthesis. A discussion group with others can be very useful for adolescents. Plan with the child how to tell friends about the surgery and what issues he or she may face upon return to school. Make plans for elevator access if needed and emergency evacuation procedures. Some children or adolescents may need referral for counseling to assist in dealing with body image disturbance.

The child will receive physical rehabilitation while hospitalized and after discharge. When the child is discharged, explain to the family the importance of bringing the child for outpatient chemotherapy and physical rehabilitation visits. Special arrangements may be needed at the child's school to accommodate a wheelchair, crutches, or ambulation with a new prosthesis. Call or visit the school to see whether there are buttons to open doors, wide doorways to facilitate passage, and any limitations of the building. Contact school personnel to plan the child's return.

Evaluation

Expected outcomes of nursing care for the child with a bone tumor focus on the treatments required and adaptation to changes in lifestyle. Examples include:

- Healed surgical site with no signs of infection
- Adaptation to changes in mobility status
- Successful adjustment to changes required in school settings
- Maintenance of healthy skin
- Positive body image
- Management of pain to comfort level
- Successful integration of continuing medical therapy

LEUKEMIA

Leukemia is among the most commonly diagnosed pediatric malignancies; an increase of acute leukemia in children has occurred in the last decade, perhaps due to improved early diagnosis (Friebert & Shurin, 1998). A cancer of the blood-forming organs, leukemia is characterized by a proliferation of abnormal WBCs in the body. Several types of leukemia are differentiated, depending on the blood cells affected. The main types are acute lymphoblastic leukemia, acute myelogenous leukemia, and the rare chronic leukemias of childhood.

The most common type of childhood leukemia is acute lymphoblastic leukemia (ALL), which accounts for 25% of all childhood cancer and 75% of leukemias in children. The peak age at onset is 2 to 4 years (Landier, 2001). ALL is more common in whites and in boys (Friebert & Shurin, 1998). Acute myelogenous leukemia (AML) affects all ethnic groups equally, and there is no peak age at onset (Golub, Weinstein, & Grier, 1997). Because chronic leukemias such as chronic myelocytic, chronic myelomonocytic, and chronic lymphocytic leukemia are rare in children, the following discussion will focus on ALL and AML.

Etiology and Pathophysiology

The causes of leukemia are not well understood. Genetic factors are believed to play a role in some types of the disease. For instance, children with chromosomal defects such as Down syndrome have an increased incidence of ALL, and chromosomal abnormalities are present in most children with ALL (Friebert & Shurin, 1998). Ionizing radiation and chemical agents such as treatment with chemotherapy for other cancers are thought to play some role in the development of AML. Children with immune deficiency states, such as ataxia-telangiectasia, congenital hypogammaglobulinemia, and Wiskott–Aldrich syndrome have an increased risk of ALL. Some investigators theorize that exposure to infectious agents can predispose children to leukemia (Kinlen & Balkwill, 2001).

Leukemia occurs when the stem cells in the bone marrow produce immature WBCs that cannot function normally. These cells proliferate rapidly by cloning instead of normal mitosis, causing the bone marrow to fill with abnormal WBCs. The abnormal cells then spill out into the circulatory system where they steadily replace the normally functioning WBCs. As this occurs, the protective lymphocytic functions such as cellular and humeral immunity are reduced, leaving the body vulnerable to infections.

The malignant WBCs rapidly fill the bone marrow, replacing stem cells that produce erythrocytes (RBCs) and other blood products such as platelets, thereby decreasing the amount of these products in circulation. The stem cells are replaced by leukemic clones, eventually resulting in anemia. Children with leukemia commonly experience abnormal bleeding because of the reduced amounts of platelets.

Clinical Manifestations

Children with ALL and AML usually have fever, pallor, overt signs of bleeding, lethargy, malaise, anorexia, and large joint or bone pain. Petechiae, frank bleeding, and joint pain are cardinal signs of bone marrow failure. Enlargement of the liver and spleen (hepatosplenomegaly) and changes in the lymph nodes (lymphadenopathy) are common. If the leukemia has infiltrated the central nervous system (entered it by means of the circulatory or lymphoid system), the child will have signs such as headache, vomiting, papilledema, and sixth cranial nerve palsy (inability to move the eye laterally). These findings are caused by the leukemic cells massing and putting pressure on nerves. The testicles, spinal cord, and bone marrow are common sites for infiltration. The leukemic cells in the testicle become a mass that causes the testicle to enlarge, often painlessly.

Clinical Therapy

Diagnosis is based initially on blood counts and bone marrow aspiration. Blood counts reveal anemia, thrombocytopenia, and neutropenia. Bone marrow aspiration reveals immature and abnormal lymphoblasts and hypercellular marrow. Bone marrow aspiration is the differential test. Neutropenia, thrombocytopenia, and anemia are commonly noted. Other abnormal laboratory findings include elevated serum uric acid and elevated calcium, potassium, and phosphorus levels. New laboratory studies such as rapid flow cytometric assay are making the detection of even very small numbers of leukemic cells possible, so that treatment can improve prognosis in children with minimal residual disease.

Treatment of ALL involves radiation and chemotherapy. Radiation is used for central nervous system prophylaxis and involvement and for testicular involvement. Chemotherapy is organized into four phases: (1) induction, (2) consolidation, (3) delayed intensification, and (4) maintenance of remission. Additional drugs may be used for treatment of central nervous system involvement. Maintenance therapy may continue for 2 to 3 years, causing decreased resistance to infection for this prolonged period (Kanarek, 1998). Treatment of AML involves use of a wide variety of drugs during the induction and consolidation phases.

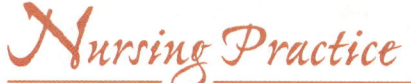 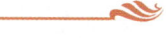

The following drugs are used to treat acute lymphoblastic leukemia:

Induction phase

Prednisone   L-asparaginase

Vincristine   Daunorubicin

Central nervous system prophylaxis

Intrathecal methotrexate

Consolidation phase

L-asparaginase   Doxorubicin

Delayed intensification

Vincristine   Cyclophosphamide

Ara-C

Maintenance phase

6-mercaptopurine or 6-thioguanine

Methotrexate

 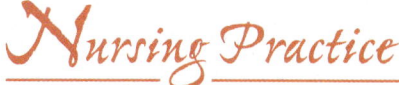 

The following drugs are used to treat acute myelogenous leukemia:

Induction phase

Daunorubicin   Mitoxantrone

Doxorubicin   Cytarabine

Consolidation phase

Etoposide   Teniposide

Maximum cell death occurs during the induction phase. The cells that remain after this period are more resistant to treatment. After 3 to 4 weeks, when a remission has occurred, central nervous system prophylaxis begins. Drugs are used in combination with cranial irradiation. During the consolidation phase, chemotherapy with l-asparaginase and doxorubicin is administered. Delayed intensification uses additional drugs to target the leukemic cells that have survived. Treatment during the maintenance phase is aimed at destroying the remaining leukemic cells. Combinations of active drugs are used to prevent resistance. Occasionally other drugs are added to the regimen, such as vincristine, prednisone, cyclophosphamide, intravenous methotrexate (see "Drug Guide" on the Companion Website), [WEB] cytosine arabinoside, or anthracyclines.

The prognosis for children with leukemia is much improved with current therapy. However, several risk factors affect the long-term outcome. The most favorable findings are:

- Age at onset between 2 and 10 years
- Initial hemoglobin level less than 10 g/dL

- Low initial WBC count
- Lack of B- or T-cell antigens
- Absence of extramedullary (outside bone marrow or spinal cord) involvement
- Rapid response to chemotherapy

The most important factor is the initial leukocyte count. The higher the leukocyte count (over 50,000/mm3) at diagnosis, the worse the prognosis. For children in the low-risk group, the probability of prolonged survival is as high as 90%. Infants under 12 months of age have a poor prognosis. Treatment methods and duration are adjusted for each child, depending on that child's risk factors. More aggressive treatment is undertaken for those in the higher risk groups.

Nursing Practice
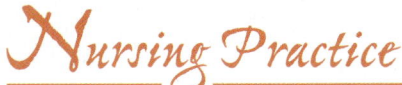

Following are the laboratory values in leukemia:

Usual	*Common Values in Leukemia*
Leukocytes	
<10,000/mm^3	>10,000/mm^3
Platelets	
150,000–400,000/mm^3	20,000–100,000/mm^3
Hemoglobin	
12–16g/dL	7–11g/dL

Approximately 10% of children have a relapse within a year after completing treatment. Treatment for relapse consists of additional chemotherapy drugs. The prognosis is best if the relapse occurs late after the initial diagnosis and after the initial treatment is completed. Bone marrow transplantation is a treatment option for the child who has a relapse with ALL or who is in remission from AML. Chemotherapy itself can create numerous complications, affecting all body organs. Central nervous system toxicity, damage to organs such as pituitary, liver, kidneys, heart, and lungs, and secondary malignancies sometimes occur.

Nursing Management

Nursing Assessment and Diagnosis

A thorough physical assessment is important to ensure prompt identification of problems without injuring the child who has deficient coagulation and immune function. Perform assessments every 8 hours or more often depending on the chemotherapy regimen. Observe carefully for bruising and other new sites of bleeding. Once chemotherapy has begun, closely monitor renal functioning through specific gravity, I&O, and daily weight measurement.

Monitor dietary intake, nausea, vomiting, and constipation. Observe for mucosal sores in the mouth. A central line is usually in place for intravenous infusion of medications, so carefully assess the line for proper functioning and for signs of infection (see Skill 12-8). **SKILLS** Ask the parents about any behavioral changes. Central nervous system infiltration can affect the child's level of consciousness, causing irritability, vomiting, and lethargy. However, chemotherapeutic drugs and antiemetics can also induce these nonspecific signs. Frequent venipunctures, bone marrow aspirations, and spinal taps require pain assessment, and an evaluation of the level of knowledge and coping skills of child and family.

Leukemia causes many changes in the body, and confirmation of the disease is difficult for families to face. Among the many nursing diagnoses that might be appropriate for the child with leukemia are:

- ▶ *Altered nutrition: less than body requirements* related to inability to ingest food
- ▶ *Risk for infection* related to altered immune system functioning
- ▶ *Risk for injury* related to bleeding
- ▶ *Activity intolerance* related to generalized weakness
- ▶ *Pain* related to chemotherapy and disease process
- ▶ *Anxiety (child and parent)* related to change in health status

Planning and Implementation

Bone marrow suppression may necessitate transmission-based precautions. **SKILLS** Instruct parents in the prevention of infection. Care of mouth sores and other side effects of chemotherapy is presented in "Nursing Care Plan: Hospital Care of the Child with Cancer," earlier in this chapter.

Special attention to renal function is needed when the child receives cyclophosphamide. Gross hematuria is a side effect of this drug. Hydration with intravenous fluids to attain a specific gravity of less than 1.010 prevents or reduces the severity of hematuria. To achieve this specific gravity, the child receives intravenous fluids at 1 1/2 times maintenance volume for at least 6 to 8 hours before and at least 1 1/2 hours after administration of the drug. Careful monitoring of I&O is required to record the intravenous fluids and assess kidney functioning. Monitor specific gravity every 8 hours, as well as before and during administration of the drug, and when the intravenous fluids are reduced to maintenance volume levels. Daily weight measurements are important to assist in planning adequate hydration during chemotherapy, as well as to measure nutritional status.

Many children are treated in an oncology clinic, staying in the hospital only on the day of intravenous drug administration, and receiving oral medications at home. Careful teaching for the family is needed to ensure safe drug administration and identification of symptoms requiring care.

Nurses play a key role in the long-term multidisciplinary treatment of children with leukemia. The impact of a diagnosis of leukemia and the long-term nature of treatment can severely stress the coping abilities of both the child and the family. Ongoing psychosocial assessment and emotional support are essential (see the general discussion of psychosocial assessment in the section titled "Childhood Cancer" on pp. 1129–1131). Referral to support groups and social services may be beneficial. Help the family explore alternative therapies such as relaxation, imagery, and nutritional support that may aid the child. Be alert for any interactions that could occur between alternative therapies and the medical regimen.

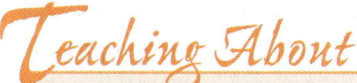

CHEMOTHERAPY FOR LEUKEMIA

Physical Care

- Have rest periods each day.
- Avoid exposure to people with illnesses.
- Drink generous amounts of water.
- Eat a healthy diet, using frequent, small, and nutritious meals to obtain enough nutrients.
- Take medicines prescribed to decrease nausea.
- Maintain good oral hygiene with soft toothbrush and water pick.
- Avoid sun exposure and check skin each day for any signs of bruises, pressure areas, cuts, or scratches.
- Allow time for and eat foods to promote bowel elimination.
- Report any signs of infection, changes in condition, or other concerns.

Emotional Care

- Be prepared for loss of hair with plans for hats, wigs, or other alternatives.
- Continue contact with friends via phone, Internet, and in person when possible.
- Try relaxation techniques to aid in sleep and management of treatments.
- Talk with clergy, teachers, parents, counselors, friends, or other supportive people about the experience of having leukemia.
- Keep a journal to record feelings and experiences.

Evaluation

Expected outcomes for nursing care of the child with leukemia include:

▶ Prevention of infection

▶ Adequate hydration

▶ Normal urinary output

▶ Blood values within normal limits

▶ Successful family adaptation to parenting a child with chronic illness

▶ Adequate parental knowledge related to disease process

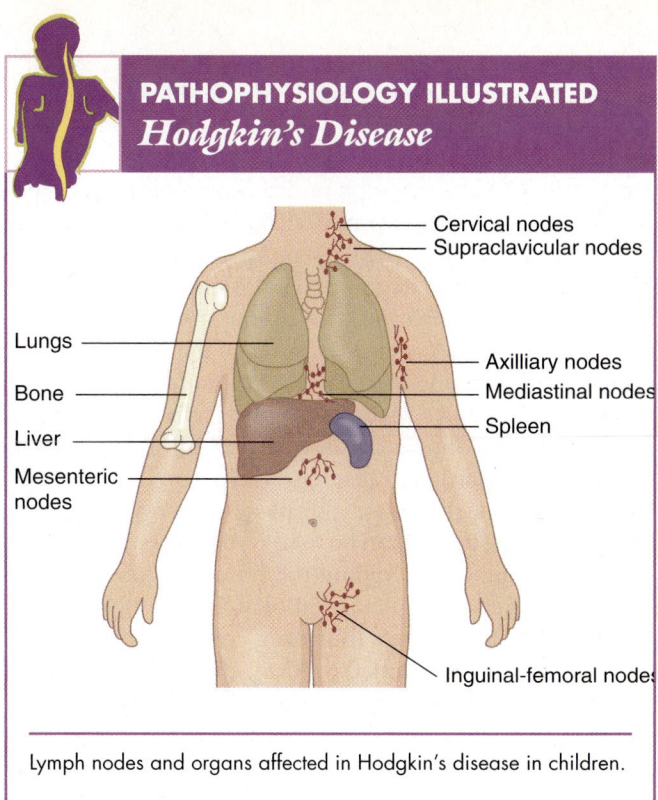

PATHOPHYSIOLOGY ILLUSTRATED
Hodgkin's Disease

Cervical nodes
Supraclavicular nodes
Axilliary nodes
Mediastinal nodes
Spleen
Inguinal-femoral nodes
Lungs
Bone
Liver
Mesenteric nodes

Lymph nodes and organs affected in Hodgkin's disease in children.

SOFT TISSUE TUMORS

Hodgkin's Disease

Hodgkin's disease is a disorder of the lymphoid system. It usually arises in a single lymph node or an anatomic group of lymph nodes (see "Pathophysiology Illustrated: Hodgkin's Disease"). There are approximately 3 cases per 100,000 people, with the peak occurrence in adolescent boys. Hodgkin's disease has a childhood form but is rare in those under 14 years. Most cases involve a young adult form that affects those between 15 and 35 years of age, and an older adult form, usually seen in persons over 55 years of age (Thompson, 1999).

ETIOLOGY AND PATHOPHYSIOLOGY

Hodgkin's disease occurs in clusters and has been reported in families. This suggests a possible genetic link as well as an infectious agent or environmental hazard. Some potential infectious agents may be herpes virus, cytomegalovirus, and Epstein-Barr virus.

CLINICAL MANIFESTATIONS

The main symptom of Hodgkin's disease is nontender, firm lymphadenopathy, usually in the supraclavicular and cervical nodes but occasionally in the mediastinal area. A mediastinal growth can cause respiratory difficulty because of pressure on the trachea or bronchi. Fever, night sweats, and weight loss occur in one third of children with Hodgkin's disease and are associated with a more aggressive form of the disease. The leukocyte count and erythrocyte sedimentation rate (ESR) may be elevated.

CLINICAL THERAPY

Diagnosis is based on lymph node biopsy; Reed-Sternberg cells (large cells with two nucleoli) are present. Staging is done using the Ann Arbor staging classification (Table 45–7). The basis for staging is data obtained from the history, physical examination, chest x-ray study (for metastasis), chest CT scan, CT or MRI scans of the retroperitoneal nodes, lymphangiogram, laboratory studies (complete blood count, ESR, serum copper level, liver function tests), and a radionuclide scan with gallium. Bone marrow biopsy, bone scan, or a staging laparotomy may be performed if advanced disease is suspected. Increasingly, minimally invasive surgery can be used to biopsy or remove the spleen for diagnosis, avoiding the potential complications of major surgery (Kleinhaus & Boley, 1999).

Chemotherapy using a four-drug combination has been found to be the most effective drug treatment. Radiation is commonly added, with low doses for children who are still growing, and larger doses for those who are physically mature or those whose disease is more advanced at diagnosis. The 5-year survival rate is approximately 80% to 90%, depending on the stage of the disease at diagnosis.

Nursing Practice

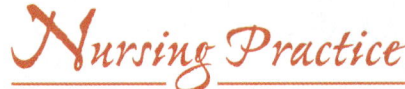

The following drugs are used to treat Hodgkin's disease:

MOPP (mechlorethamine, Oncovin [vincristine], procarbazine, prednisone)

COPP (cyclophosphamide, Oncovin, procarbazine, prednisone)

COMP (cyclophosphamide, Oncovin, methotrexate, prednisone)

OPPA (Oncovin, procarbazine, prednisone, Adriamycin)

ABVD (Adriamycin, bleomycin, vinblastine, dacarbazine)

TABLE 45–7   Ann Arbor Staging System for Hodgkin's Disease

Stage	Description
I	Disease within a single lymph node region
IE	Disease within a single extralymphatic organ
II	Disease within two or more lymph node regions on same side of diaphragm
IIE	Disease within extralymphatic organ, and of one or more lymph node regions on same side of diaphragm
III	Disease of lymph node regions on both sides of diaphragm
IIIE	Disease of lymph node regions on both sides of the diaphragm with involvement of extralymphatic organ
IIIS	As in III, plus disease within spleen
IIISE	As in III, plus disease in extralymphatic organs and spleen
IV	Disseminated disease within one or more lymphatic organs with or without lymph node involvement

Bone marrow transplantation is a treatment option in children with advanced disease or relapse.

Non-Hodgkin's Lymphoma

Non-Hodgkin's lymphoma includes all lymphomas that are not classified as Hodgkin's disease (about 60% of pediatric lymphomas). There are three types of pediatric non-Hodgkin's lymphoma: (1) lymphoblastic lymphoma (30% to 40%), (2) small noncleaved cell (Burkitt's) lymphoma (40% to 50%), and (3) large cell lymphoma ($\le$ 15%) (Derengowski, 1999). Lymphomas of all types are the third most common group of malignancies in children, following leukemia and brain tumors (Shad & Magrath, 1997). Non-Hodgkin's lymphomas are malignant tumors of lymphoreticular (internal framework of the lymph system) origin. The peak incidence for lymphomas occurs between the ages of 7 and 11 years, and they are three times more common in boys than in girls.

Fifty percent of non-Hodgkin's lymphomas are caused by T-cell abnormalities. These abnormal T cells are diffuse, highly malignant, and very aggressive; they do not mature. T-cell lymphomas produced by these cells often occur in children with congenital or acquired immunodeficiency states, chronic immune stimulation, or autoimmune disease. Some lymphomas are observed with B-cell abnormalities. The incidence of lymphomas shows geographic variability. For example, a high incidence of Burkitt lymphoma is found in equatorial Africa, where it causes 50% of childhood cancer. Incidence in Hispanic children is higher than in whites, and blacks have the lowest incidence (Wilkinson, Fleming, MacKinnon, et al., 2001).

Nursing Practice

The following drugs are used to treat non-Hodgkin's lymphoma:

Cyclophosphamide	ARA-C
Ifosfamide	VM-26
Prednisone	Adriamycin
Methotrexate	Vincristine

Children with non-Hodgkin's lymphoma frequently present with fever and weight loss. The lymph glands are usually enlarged or nodular, with the most frequent sites being the cervical, axillary, inguinal, and femoral nodes. However, the disease may be diffuse, without nodular glands. The anterior mediastinum is the primary site for T-cell lymphomas. Tumors that occur in this area may compress the airway (causing breathing difficulty) or superior vena cava (leading to swelling of the face, neck, or arms), and can cause pain. Jaw involvement is common in Burkitt lymphoma.

Tissue biopsy confirms the diagnosis. There are several staging systems that relate to the tumor mass and extension to other body areas. Because 80% of children with non-Hodgkin's lymphoma have systemic disease, the treatment is aggressive chemotherapy similar to that used for ALL. The induction phase of chemotherapy results in a 90% remission rate. Treatment also includes localized radiation and surgery to remove the tumor mass. Between 50% and 75% of children with non-Hodgkin's lymphoma have a good outcome. Children with localized diseases have a more favorable prognosis.

Rhabdomyosarcoma

Rhabdomyosarcoma is a soft tissue cancer common in children. It occurs most often in the muscles around the eyes (extraorbital), in the neck, and less commonly in the abdomen and genitourinary tract. Among children under 15 years of age, rhabdomyosarcoma occurs more often in whites than in blacks or Asians (Wexler & Helman, 1997). Most cases are diagnosed in children under 5 years of age.

Tumors close to the eye produce swelling, ptosis, visual disturbances, and eye movement abnormalities (Figure 45–9 ◆). When the tumor occurs in the genitourinary tract, the result can be obstruction, hematuria, dysuria, vaginal discharge, and a protruding vaginal mass. Rhabdomyosarcoma occurring in the abdomen may be asymptomatic. There is rapid metastasis to the lungs, bones, bone marrow, and distant lymph nodes.

Diagnosis is confirmed by CT, MRI, bone marrow aspiration, and biopsy. A useful biologic marker, desmin, allows differentiation of rhabdomyosarcoma from other round cell tumors. Because 20% of children have metastatic disease at the time of diagnosis, chest and lung CT scans are performed.

Treatment includes surgical removal of the tumor followed by wide-field radiation and chemotherapy with a combination of drugs. Prognosis depends on the site, staging (Table 45–8), and histologic findings. Children with stage II or IV disease or abdominal tumors have a poor prognosis.

TABLE 45–8	Classification of Rhabdomyosarcoma

Group	Description
I	Localized, completely resected disease
II	Total gross resection with regional microscopic spread
III	Incomplete gross resection or biopsy
IV	Distant metastatic disease present

Note: From Wexler, L. H., & Helma, L. J. (1997). Rhabdomyosarcoma and the undifferentiated sarcomas. In P. A. Pizzo & D. G. Poplack (Eds.), *Principles and practices of pediatric oncology* (3rd ed., p. 808). Philadelphia: Lippincott-Raven.

Nursing Practice

The following drugs are used to treat rhabdomyosarcoma:

Dactinomycin	Cisplatin
Cyclophosphamide	Etoposide
Vincristine	Dacarbazine
Doxorubicin	

Retinoblastoma

Retinoblastoma is an intraocular malignancy of the retina. It may be bilateral (20% to 30%) or unilateral. In 40% of children, the disease is inherited by an autosomal dominant gene (Donaldson, Egbert, Newsham, et al., 1997).

The first sign of retinoblastoma is a white pupil, termed leukokoria or cat's-eye reflex (Figure 45–10 ◆). Other symptoms may include a fixed strabismus (a constant deviation of one eye from the other), orbital inflammation, glaucoma, and heterochromia (irises of different colors).

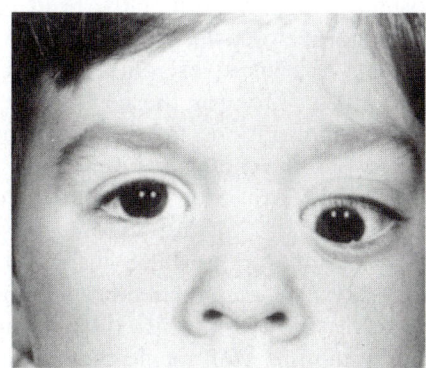

FIGURE 45–9. ◆ Rhabdomyosarcoma is characterized by ptosis and swelling. *Note:* From Vaughan, D., Asbury, T., & Riordan-Eva, P. (1995). *General ophthalmology* (14th ed.). Norwalk, CT: Appleton & Lange.

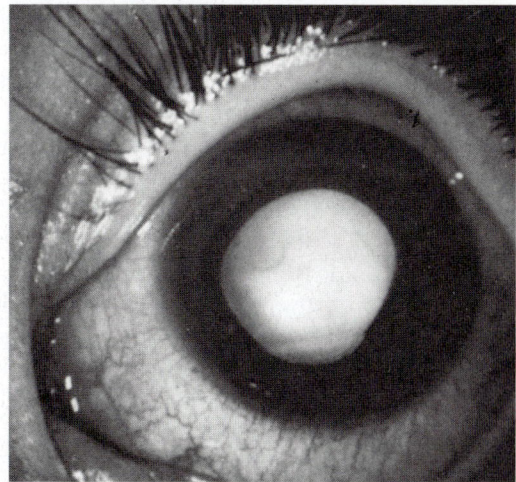

FIGURE 45–10. ◆ Retinoblastoma is characterized by leukokoria, a white reflection in the pupil. *Note:* From Hathaway, W. E., Hay, W. W., Jr., Groothuis, J. R., & Paisley, J. W. (1993). *Current pediatric diagnosis and treatment* (11th ed.). New York: McGraw-Hill Companies.

Retinoblastoma is usually diagnosed when the child is between 1 and 2 years of age. The overall tumor-free survival rate is 90%, 5 to 10 years after diagnosis. Diagnostic tests include full ocular examination and CT or MRI scans of the eye orbit. All children with a family history of retinoblastoma should be examined by an ophthalmologist after birth and on a regular basis to aid in early diagnosis. Tumors are classified according to a staging system, from a very small localized tumor (group I) to tumors involving more than half the retina and with seeding into the vitreous (group V).

Treatment for retinoblastoma may include removal of the eye. Other surgical treatments involve cyrotherapy or photocoagulation (argon laser therapy). Radiation is nearly always used, either as the sole treatment or before surgery to shrink the tumor. Chemotherapy is occasionally used but is generally ineffective as the drugs often fail to penetrate sufficiently into the eye. Multiple therapies are more commonly used in children with bilateral retinoblastoma. Children with retinoblastoma are at increased risk of developing a secondary tumor, including another retinoblastoma or a sarcoma, most commonly osteogenic sarcoma. However, most young children who have been treated for the disease have good health and normal mental abilities several years after treatment. Over 90% of children with small unilateral tumors survive. Increased size and invasion by a tumor decrease success of treatment. The most common sequela of retinoblastoma is decrease in visual acuity (Ross, Lipper, Abramson, et al., 2001).

Nursing Management

Nursing Assessment and Diagnosis

PHYSIOLOGIC ASSESSMENT

Physiologic assessment of the child with a soft tissue tumor, such as Hodgkin's disease, non-Hodgkin's lymphoma, rhabdomyosarcoma, and other lymphomas, focuses on the child's general condition. Accurate height and weight measurements are essential to provide a baseline against which to measure the child's growth during treatment, as well as for calculation of chemotherapeutic drug dosages.

Observe the area of the tumor, such as the face, neck, and abdomen, and describe any changes. Monitor respiratory status if the tumor is in the face or neck. Report any changes in respiratory pattern to the physician. Avoid palpation of any tumor site or enlarged area; injudicious palpation and manipulation of a tumor site can influence metastasis. Notify the physician of a change in any lymph node or any other area of the body.

Gastrointestinal and genitourinary function can be altered by the presence of a tumor and by treatment such as chemotherapy and radiation. Careful monitoring of the child's I & O measurement is essential. Abdominal tumors may affect defecation, so charting of all bowel movements

is important. Explain to the family and child why keeping accurate records is necessary.

Observe wounds closely for lack of healing as a result of chemotherapy or radiation. Examine the mouth and extremities for wounds or ulcers. Nutritional changes caused by treatment will affect the body's ability to support healthy cells and heal wounds.

A thorough eye examination is warranted for any child who has a family history of retinoblastoma or has undergone treatment for a prior tumor. Assess color and position of the iris, eye movements, cover–uncover test, and other eye tests described in Chapter 33. Ask whether the child has been evaluated by an ophthalmologist.

PSYCHOSOCIAL ASSESSMENT

Assessment of the family's psychosocial status and coping mechanisms is an essential component of nursing care. Refer to the general discussion of psychosocial assessment under "Childhood Cancer," earlier in this chapter. Assessment of body image is needed when the child has a soft tissue tumor affecting appearance of the head and neck.

The location and type of soft tissue tumor determine the specific nursing diagnoses for a particular child. Common nursing diagnoses might include:

▶ *Altered tissue perfusion (peripheral)* related to interruption of blood flow

▶ *Ineffective breathing pattern* related to effect of tumor deformity on neck or chest wall

▶ *Impaired swallowing* related to acquired anatomic defect

▶ *Altered growth and development* related to effects of treatment

▶ *Body image disturbance* related to illness and treatment

▶ *Sensory/perceptual alteration (visual)* related to illness

Planning and Implementation

Nursing management of children with soft tissue tumors varies depending on the specific tumor. Children with lymphoma affecting the mediastinum may need respiratory support. Position the child so that the head is elevated. Administer chemotherapy drugs as ordered, maintaining adequate fluids to facilitate excretion of the resultant breakdown products. Monitor the central line used for chemotherapy administration, and teach parents care of the central line when the child is at home.

For the child with a rhabdomyosarcoma involving the bladder, monitor urinary output carefully. Report hematuria and painful urination. Monitor the changes that occur during therapy. For example, in children with eye tumors, observe for a decrease in ptosis, which may indicate successful treatment. Administer pain medications as needed and use distraction and other techniques to decrease the child's discomfort. Emphasize to parents the need for follow-up CT and MRI scans after completion of treatment.

When the child with retinoblastoma undergoes removal of the eye, the parents and child will need detailed instructions on postsurgical care. Demonstrate to the parents care of the socket and use of a conformer to maintain the eye socket shape. When healing is complete and the child receives a prosthetic eye, instruct parents about its insertion and care. The child can gradually be taught to take over this care when old enough. Encourage periodic health care visits to monitor for signs of a tumor in the other eye. Interventions to encourage normal developmental milestones are adapted if sensory alteration has resulted.

Pay attention to the body changes of the cancer and its treatment. Children and adolescents may need suggestions to deal with hair loss, disfigurement, and living with serious illness. Referral to other children and teens with similar concerns may be helpful. Parents of all children need help to encourage normal development in the child with cancer.

The child with a soft tissue tumor often receives chemotherapy or radiation, or sometimes both modalities. Nursing management during chemotherapy and radiation is discussed earlier in this chapter in the general sections on these treatment measures (beginning on 1125–1127) and in "Nursing Care Plan: Hospital Care of the Child with Cancer." Generally, the family needs help to adjust to the diagnosis of a life-threatening disease and to the care of the ill child. Refer to Chapter 34 for a description of postsurgical care. Consult Chapter 48 for strategies to assist the child and family if the child has a visual impairment resulting from a retinoblastoma. Topics for parent and family teaching and discharge planning are similar to those previously presented. Referral resources to support the families of children with these types of cancer can be found at our companion website.

Evaluation

The following expected outcomes of nursing care for the child with a soft tissue tumor are examples that illustrate the varied tumor presentations.

▶ Successful management of treatment side effects

Teaching About

THE CHILD WITH A SOFT TISSUE TUMOR

- Teach the family about the chemotherapy drugs and their side effects.
- Teach about the care of venous access devices surgically placed.
- Provide written and illustrated information about the chemotherapy protocol(s).
- Provide radiation and surgery education specific to the tumor treatment.
- Refer the family to nutrition resources such as dietitians to improve the child's nutritional status.

▶ Healed surgical site with no signs of infection

▶ Adaptation to sensory loss

▶ Growth and development to maximum potential

▶ Anticipatory grieving by parents in cases of terminal disease

IMPACT OF CANCER SURVIVAL

Over the past two to three decades, treatment for childhood cancers has been increasingly successful. About 1 in 1000 young adults is a survivor of childhood cancer. The success of new modalities and treatment combinations has, however, created special health care needs for many survivors (see Figures 45–11A, B, and C).

Surgery can have many results. Body organs may be removed and manipulated, leading to adhesions, intestinal obstruction, visual impairment, neurologic disruption, and even sterility. Removal of the spleen can lead to serious infections. Amputation creates a need for prosthetic devices and physical rehabilitation.

Radiation has several long-term effects. It can impair the growth of bones and teeth, leading to conditions such as scoliosis, leg length discrepancy, or poor dental health. Cardiotoxicity and pulmonary toxicity can result from mediastinal radiation. Delayed puberty and sterility can result from radiation effects to the cranium and spinal regions. Neural damage can occur. Secondary cancers, most commonly solid tumors, occur in some survivors.

Chemotherapy can cause a wide variety of effects, both during its administration and for years afterward. Cardiomyopathy can occur with some drugs, especially the anthracyclines. Pulmonary toxicity and renal complications can develop. Neurologic effects of some drugs can lead to hearing loss (e.g., cisplatin and ifosfamide), cataracts, and paraplegia (e.g., intrathecal methotrexate for leukemia). Learning disabilities and change in intelligence quotient (IQ) occur in some children (Blatt, Copeland, & Bleyer, 1997). Although radiation is responsible for most secondary tumors, some chemotherapy drugs have also been implicated.

The diagnosis, treatment, and risk of recurrence are significant stressors for the child with cancer. See Chapter 37 for a discussion of the stresses that are experienced by families when a child has a life-threatening illness. Families may find it difficult to obtain full insurance coverage for the child who has had a prior cancer. Employment can be a potential problem for cancer survivors if employers have concerns about the earlier cancer diagnosis (Monaco, Fiduccia, & Smith, 1997). Most people with cancer report fear of recurrence of the disease, which is a stressor. On the other hand, hopefulness and the sense of having an added purpose in life can be positive outcomes for many cancer survivors.

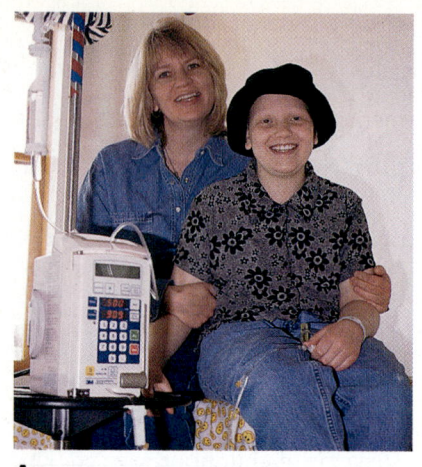
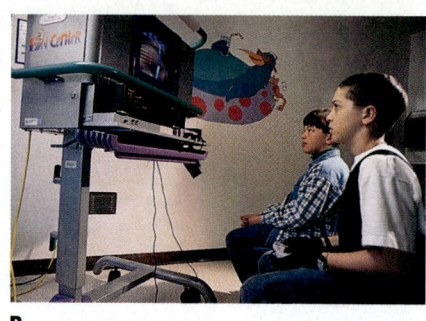
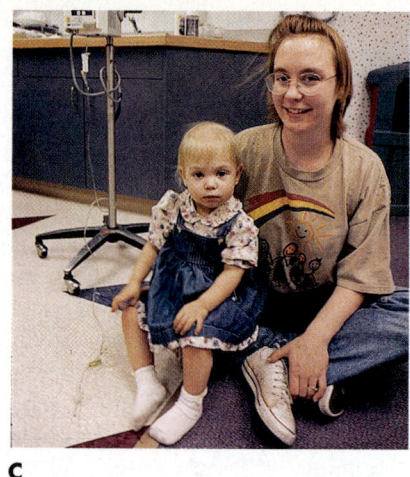

FIGURE 45–11. ◆ Survivors of childhood cancer. **A,** Nicole, 11 years old, is undergoing chemotherapy for Ewing sarcoma. Her mother emphasizes, "It's our faith that has gotten us through this. The hardest part is how busy you are coming to treatments all the time. Nicole's younger brother sometimes feels neglected." **B,** According to Jesse, who is 10 years old and waiting for a bone marrow transplant, "The thing that has helped me the most [in dealing with acute lymph oblastic leukemia] is all the mail I got from my friends." His mother adds, "We're just really positive and think that everything will turn out all right." **C,** Cassie, 19 months old, has been diagnosed with neuroblastoma. At this age, it is hard for her to understand what is happening. Her mother has stayed with her each time she has come to the hospital, which has helped Cassie adjust to therapy. Her caregivers are confident that she will respond well to her treatment.

Nurses are involved with families when a diagnosis of cancer is made, during the therapy process, and in the years that follow. For a child who survives cancer, ongoing care is essential. Evaluate the child regularly with thorough physical, psychosocial, developmental, and cognitive assessments. Carefully monitor all body systems (e.g., cardiovascular; respiratory; musculoskeletal; eye, ear, nose, and throat; genitourinary). Record height and weight and general growth patterns. Ask about the child's interactions with peers and performance at school. Be alert for signs and symptoms that could indicate a secondary tumor. Ask the parents about insurance coverage and other financial difficulties with ongoing care.

Plan care to help the family manage any long-term effects of cancer treatment. This may involve physical rehabilitation, support related to visual impairment, or treatment for cardiac or musculoskeletal abnormalities. Provide resources for information and support. Facilitate periodic evaluations in a health care agency so that serious outcomes of treatment can be identified early.

*C*HAPTER HIGHLIGHTS

- Cancer is a leading cause of illness and death among children.

- In spite of improvement in mortality and prevalence rates from childhood cancer, the incidence of some types of cancer, such as brain tumors and leukemia, continues to rise.

- Cancer may be caused by chromosomal alterations or genetic messages, environmental carcinogens, or infectious processes. Often a combination of factors seems to be present.

- Cancer treatments include surgery, chemotherapy, radiation, biotherapy, and alternative therapies. Palliative care is needed when the prognosis is poor.

- Oncologic emergencies are life-threatening conditions caused by cancer or its treatment.

- Main types of oncologic emergencies are metabolic, hematologic, or space-occupying.

- Key signs of childhood cancer are pain, cachexia, anemia, infection, and bruising.

- A protocol is a plan of action for chemotherapy that is based on the type of cancer, its stage, and the particular cell type.

- Nursing assessment for children with cancer involves detailed physical data, as well as psychologic factors and developmental achievements.

- Common physical nursing interventions for children with cancer involve nutrition, medication administration, hydration, infection prevention, pain management, and measures to decrease side effects of treatment. Families require ongoing psychosocial support, information, and referral to diverse resources when caring for a child with cancer.

- Common brain tumors in children include medulloblastoma, astrocytoma, ependymoma, and gliomas.

- Headache, vomiting, ataxia, seizures, increased intracranial pressure, hydrocephalus, and sensory disturbances are the major clinical manifestations of brain tumors.

- Neuroblastoma is a tumor located along the sympathetic nervous system chain.

- Nephroblastoma (Wilms' tumor) is an intrarenal tumor; when suspected the abdomen should not be palpated.

- Common bone tumors in childhood are osteosarcoma and Ewing's sarcoma; both are most common among adolescents.

- Leukemia is a common childhood malignancy, with the major types being acute lymphoblastic leukemia and acute myelogenous leukemia.

- A variety of soft tissue tumors are seen in children and adolescents; they include Hodgkin's disease, non-Hodgkin's lymphoma, rhabdomyosarcoma, and retinoblastoma.

- While the number of children who are long-term survivors continues to grow, some of these children experience lasting effects such as cognitive or behavioral problems, recurrent or secondary cancers, or discrimination.

- Nurses are in a key position to assist families during a diagnosis for cancer, while therapy is carried out, in adjustment to school and other life tasks, and in providing palliative care for children who do not survive.

EXPLORE MediaLink

NCLEX Review, Case Studies, and other interactive resources for this chapter can be found on the companion website at http://www.prenhall.com/london. Click on "Chapter 45" and select the activities for this chapter.

For animations, more NCLEX review questions, and an audio glossary, access the accompanying CD-ROM in this textbook.

REFERENCES

Agency for Healthcare Research and Quality. (2001a). *Uses of epoetin for anemia in oncology* (Evidence Report/Technology Assessment No. 30). Washington, DC: U.S. Department of Health and Human Services.

Agency for Healthcare Research and Quality. (2001b). *Management of cancer pain,* (Evidence Report/Technology Assessment No. 35). Washington, DC: U.S. Department of Health and Human Services.

Alcoser, P. W., & Burchett, S. (1999). Bone marrow transplantation. *American Journal of Nursing, 99,* 26–31.

American Cancer Society. (2001). *Statistics.* www.cancer.org.

Anderson, P. M. (2000). Neoplasms of the kidney. In R. E. Behrman, R. M. Kliegman, & H. B. Jenson (Eds.), *Nelson textbook of pediatrics* (16th ed., pp. 1554–1556). Philadelphia: WB Saunders.

Baker, B. (1998). CNS tumors now most common cancer in children. *Pediatric News, 32*(7), 12.

Bertolone, K. (1997). Pediatric oncology: Past, present, and new modalities of treatment. *Journal of Intravenous Nursing, 20,* 136–140.

Biggar, R. J., Frisch, M., & Goedert, J. J. (2000). Risk of cancer in children with AIDS. *Journal of the American Medical Association, 284,* 205–209.

Bindler, R. M., & Howry, L. B. (1997). *Pediatric drugs and nursing implications* (2nd ed., pp. 579–580, 587). Stamford, CT: Appleton & Lange.

Blatt, J., Copeland, D. R., & Bleyer, W. A. (1997). Late effects of childhood cancer and its treatment. In P. A. Pizzo & D. G. Poplack (Eds.), *Principles and practice of pediatric oncology* (3rd ed., pp. 1301–1330). Philadelphia: Lippincott-Raven.

Castleberry, R. P. (1997). Biology and treatment of neuroblastoma. *Pediatric Clinics of North America, 44,* 919–938.

Chaffee, S. (2001). Pediatric palliative care. *Primary Care, 28,* 365–370.

Challinor, J., Miaskowski, C., Moore, I., Slaughter, R., & Franck, L. (2000). Review of research studies that evaluated the impact of treatment for childhood cancers on neurorecognition and behavioral and social competence: Nursing implications. *Journal of the Society for Pediatric Nurses, 5,* 57–74.

Chang, C. C. (1998). Cord blood stem cell transplantation. *Clinician Reviews, 8,* 67–83.

Chase, S. (2000). St. John's Wort: Not so safe. *RN, 63,* 114.

Conway, E. E., Asuncion, A., & DaRosso, R. (1999). Diagnosing and managing brain tumors: The pediatrician's role. *Contemporary Pediatrics, 16,* 84–97.

Coustan-Smith, E., Sancho, J., Hancock, M. L., Boyett, J. M., Behm, F. G., Raimondi, S. C., et al. (2000). Clinical importance of minimal residual disease in childhood acute lymphoblastic leukemia. *Blood, 96,* 2691–2696.

Crooks, G. M., Lill, J., Feig, S., & Parkman, R. (1997). Cord blood—new source of stem cells for transplants. *Contemporary Pediatrics, 14,* 25–26, 30, 34–36, 41.

Dean, R. (2000). Alternative therapies may cause interactions in oncology patients. American College of Clinical Pharmacology meeting, September 2000. Reported by Reuters. http://pediatrics.medscape.com/reuters/prof/2000/09/09.19/2000091prof003.html. Retrieved from world wide web 9/25/2000.

Derengowski, S. (1999, June). Pediatric non-Hodgkin's lymphoma. *Advance for Nurses, 14,* 26–28.

Donaldson, S. S., Egbert, P. R., Newsham, Il, & Cavenee, W. K. (1997). Retinoblastoma. In P. A. Pizzo & D. G. Poplack (Eds.), *Principles and practice of pediatric oncology* (3rd ed., pp. 699–716). Philadelphia: Lippincott-Raven.

Enskar, K., Carlsson, M., Golsater, M., & Hamrin, E. (1997). Symptom distress and life situation in adolescents with cancer. *Cancer Nursing, 20,* 23–33.

Freeman, K., O'Dell, C., & Meola, C. (2000). Issues in families of children with brain tumors. *Oncology Nursing Forum, 27,* 843–848.

Friebert, S. E., & Shurin, S. B. (1998). ALL: Diagnosis and outlook. *Contemporary Pediatrics, 15,* 118–119, 123–124, 127–128, 131–132, 134, 136.

Golub, T. R., Weinstein, H. J., & Grier, H. E. (1997). Acute myelogenous leukemia. In P. A. Pizzo & D. G. Poplack (Eds.), *Principles and practice of pediatric oncology* (3rd ed., pp. 463–482). Philadelphia: Lippincott-Raven.

Green, D. M., Grigoriev, Y. A., Nan, B., Takashima, J. R., Norkool, P. A., D'Angio, G. J., et al. (2001). Congestive heart failure after treatment for Wilms' tumor: A report from the National Wilms' Tumor study group. *Journal of Clinical Oncology, 19,* 1926–1934.

Grier, H. E. (1997). The Ewing family of tumors: Ewing's sarcoma and primitive neuroectodermal tumors. *Pediatric Clinics of North America, 44,* 991–1004.

Hilden, J. M., Emanuel, E. J., Fairclogh, D. L., Link, M. P., Foley, K. M., Clarridge, B. C., et al. (2001). Attitudes and practices among pediatric oncologists regarding end-of-life care: Results of the 1998 American Society of Clinical Oncology survey. *Journal of Clinical Oncology, 19,* 205–212.

Ishibashi, A. (2001). The needs of children and adolescents with cancer for information and social support. *Cancer Nursing, 24,* 61–67.

James, L., & Johnson, B. (1997). The needs of parents of pediatric oncology patients during the palliative care phase. *Journal of Pediatric Oncology Nursing, 14,* 83–95.

Kanarek, R. C. (1998). Facing the challenge of childhood leukemia. *American Journal of Nursing, 98,* 42–50.

Kelly, K. M., & Lange, B. (1997). Oncologic emergencies. *Pediatric Clinics of North America, 44,* 809–830.

Kelly, K. M., Jacobsen, J. S., Kennedy, D. D., Braudt, S. M., Mallick, M., & Weiner, M. A. (2000). Use of unconventional therapies by children at an urban medical center. *Journal of Pediatric Hematology/Oncology, 22,* 412–416.

Kemper, K. J., & Longwood Herbal Task Force. (1999). Shark cartilage, cat's claw, and other complementary cancer therapies. *Contemporary Pediatrics, 16,* 101–102, 105–106, 112, 115, 117–118, 121, 125–126.

Kinlen, L. J., & Balkwill, A. (2001).Infective cause of childhood leukemia and wartime population mixing in Orkney and Shetland, UK. *Lancet, 357,* 858.

Kleinhaus, S., & Boley, S. J. (1999). The latest news about minimally invasive surgery. *Contemporary Pediatrics, 16,* 125–134.

Kun, L. E. (1997). Brain tumors: Challenges and directions. *Pediatric Clinics of North America, 44,* 907–918.

Landier, W. (2001). Childhood acute lymphoblastic leukemia: Current perspectives. *Oncology Nursing Forum, 28,* 823–833.

McManus, J., & Gilchrist, G. S. (2000). Neuroblastoma. In R. E. Behrman, R. M. Kliegman, & H. B. Jenson (Eds.), *Nelson textbook of pediatrics* (16th ed., pp. 1552–1554). Philadelphia: WB Saunders.

Mercer, M., & Ritchie, J. A. (1997). Home community care: Parents' perspectives. *Journal of Pediatric Nursing, 12,* 133–141.

Meyers, P. A., & Gorlick, R. (1997). Osteosarcoma. *Pediatric Clinics of North America, 44,* 973–990.

Moller, T. R., Garwicz, S., Barlow, L., Falck Winther, J., Glattre, E., Olafsdotti, G., et al. (2001). Decreasing late mortality among five-year survivors of cancer in childhood and adolescence: A population-based study in the Nordic countries. *Journal of Clinical Oncology, 19,* 3161–3181.

Monaco, G. P., Fiduccia, D., & Smith, G. (1997). Legal and societal issues facing survivors of childhood cancer. *Pediatric Clinics of North America, 44,* 1043–1058.

Ross, G., Lipper, E. G., Abramson, D., & Preiser, L. (2001). The development of young children with retinoblastoma. *Archives of Pediatric and Adolescent Medicine, 155,* 80–83.

Shad, A., & Magrath, L. J. (1997). Non-Hodgkin's lymphoma. *Pediatric Clinics of North America, 44,* 863–890.

Smith, M. A., Freidlin, B., Ries, L. A., & Simon, R. (1998). Trends in reported incidence of primary malignant brain tumor in children in the United States. *Journal of the National Cancer Institute, 90,* 1269–1277.

Swerdlow, J. L. (2000). *Nature's medicine: Plants that heal.* Washington, DC: National Geographic Society.

Thompson, K. A. (1999). Detecting Hodgkin's disease. *American Journal of Nursing, 99,* 61–64.

Vernon-Levett, P., & Geller, M. (1997). Posterior fossa tumors in children: A case study. *AACN Critical Issues, 8,* 214–226.

Wexler, L. H., & Helman, L. J. (1997). Rhabdomyosarcoma and the undifferentiated sarcomas. In P. A. Pizzo & D. G. Poplack (Eds.), *Principles and practice of pediatric oncology* (3rd ed., pp. 799–830). Philadelphia: Lippincott-Raven.

Wilkinson, J. D., Fleming, L. E., MacKinnon, J., Voti, L., Wohler-Torres, B., Peace, S., et al. (2001). Lymphoma and lymphoid leukemia incidence in Florida children: Ethnic and racial distribution.*Cancer, 91,* 1402–1408.

Wolfe, J., Grier, H. E., & Klar, N. (2000). Symptoms and suffering at the end of life in children with cancer. *New England Journal of Medicine, 342,* 326–333.

Wolfe, J., Klar, N., Grier, H. E., Duncan, J., Salem-Schatz, S., Emanuel, E. J., et al. (2000). Understanding of prognosis among parents of children who died of cancer. *Journal of the American Medical Association, 284,* 2469–2475.

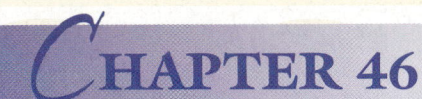

CHAPTER 46

The Child with Alterations in Gastrointestinal Function

I was so worried when Jerome was born. He had no anal opening and his esophagus did not lead to his stomach. Now that he's had several surgeries, he is growing and doing pretty well, and I'm so happy to see him starting to smile. I can't wait until he is able to eat on his own instead of having tube feedings.

—MOTHER OF JEROME, 8 MONTHS OLD

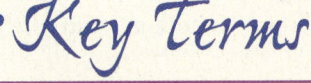

Key Terms

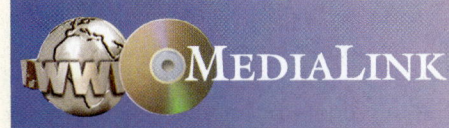

CD-ROM
Skill 12-7: Total Parenteral Nutrition
Skill 15-3: Administering a Gavage Feeding
Skill 16-3: Changing the Dressing for an Infant with an Ostomy
Skill 16-4: Changing an Ostomy Pouch for an Infant or Child
Insider's View: Effects of Lead in the Body—Animation
Audio Glossary
NCLEX Review

COMPANION WEBSITE
http://www.prenhall.com/london
Alterations in Gastrointestinal Function—Web Links
Thinking Critically
Complementary Care: Chamomile for Digestive Disorders
Complementary Care: Therapies for Pediatric Constipation
MediaLink Applications:
 Care of the Child with Cleft Palate
 Evaluating the Home for Poisons
 Managing Emesis in Pediatric Conditions
NCLEX Review
Case Study

What causes structural defects of the gastrointestinal tract such as the esophageal atresia and imperforate anus experienced by Jerome? What special care do children with gastrointestinal abnormalities need to promote growth and development during treatment for anomalies? This chapter discusses the care of infants who have structural defects and those with other common disorders of gastrointestinal functioning.

Through the gastrointestinal (GI) tract, a child ingests and absorbs the foods and fluids necessary to sustain life and promote growth. Most GI disturbances produce short-term symptoms that interfere with nutrition and fluid balance only briefly. Some disorders or severe defects lead to complications that prevent optimal nutrition and adequate growth. This chapter explores some common GI disorders in children. (See Chapter 39 for a discussion of specific fluid imbalances that may accompany GI disorders.) 🔗

GI disorders can result from a congenital defect, acquired disease, infection, or injury. Structural problems may occur when development is altered or ceases in the first trimester of gestation. Because various parts of the GI system are developing at this point in gestation, it is not unusual for infants to have more than one structural defect of the GI system. This was the case with Jerome in the opening vignette. Infections can cause an increase or decrease in motility and prevent proper absorption of nutrients. Interruption or destruction of the GI system can also result from trauma or ingestion of caustic substances. While reading this chapter, remember that any interruption or alteration in the GI system decreases the body's ability to obtain nutrients, thus impairing growth.

ANATOMY AND PHYSIOLOGY OF PEDIATRIC DIFFERENCES

Although the fetus makes sucking and swallowing movements in utero and ingests amniotic fluid, the GI system is immature at birth. The processes of absorption and excretion do not begin until after birth because the placenta provides nutrients and removes waste. Sucking is a primitive reflex that occurs whenever the lips or cheeks are stroked. The infant does not have voluntary control over swallowing until about 6 weeks of age.

The stomach capacity of the newborn is quite small, and intestinal motility (**peristalsis**) is greater than in older children. These characteristics explain the newborn's need for small, frequent feedings and the increased frequency and liquid consistency of bowel movements. Because of the relaxed cardiac sphincter, infants frequently regurgitate small amounts of feedings.

Digestion takes place in the duodenum. Infants have a deficiency of several enzymes: amylase (which digests carbohydrates), lipase (which enhances fat absorption), and trypsin (which catabolizes protein into polypeptides and

Growth and Development

Stomach capacity increases throughout early childhood:

Age	Capacity (mL)
Newborn	10 to 20
1 week	30 to 90
2 to 3 weeks	75 to 100
1 month	90 to 150
3 months	150 to 200
1 year	210 to 360
2 years	500

some amino acids). Enzymes are usually not present in sufficient quantities to aid digestion until 4 to 6 months of age. Thus, abdominal distention from gas is common.

Liver function is also immature. After the first few weeks of life the liver is able to conjugate bilirubin and excrete bile. The processes of **gluconeogenesis** (formation of glycogen from noncarbohydrates), plasma protein and ketone formation, vitamin storage, and **deamination** (removal of amino group from amino compound) remain immature during the first year of life.

By the second year of life, digestive processes are fairly complete. Stomach capacity increases to accommodate a three-meals-per-day feeding schedule. At about the same time, myelination of the spinal cord becomes complete and voluntary control over excretory functions can be achieved.

〰 STRUCTURAL DEFECTS

Structural defects can involve one or more areas of the GI tract. These defects occur when growth and development of fetal structures are interrupted during the first trimester. This can leave the structure incomplete, resulting in atresia (absence or closure of a normal body orifice), malposition, nonclosure, or other abnormalities.

CLEFT LIP AND CLEFT PALATE

Cleft lip and cleft palate are two distinct facial defects that can occur singly or in combination (Figure 46–1 ◆). Incomplete fusion of the lip occurs in approximately 1 in 700 births (Mitchell & Wood, 2000). It is more common in Native Americans and Asians than in whites, and less common in blacks. Incomplete fusion of the palate occurs in approximately 1 in 2000 births (Balasubrahmanyam, Scherer, Martin, et al., 1998). Each defect can vary in severity.

Etiology and Pathophysiology

Cleft lip with or without cleft palate results when the maxillary processes fail to fuse with the elevations on the frontal prominence during the sixth week of gestation. Normally

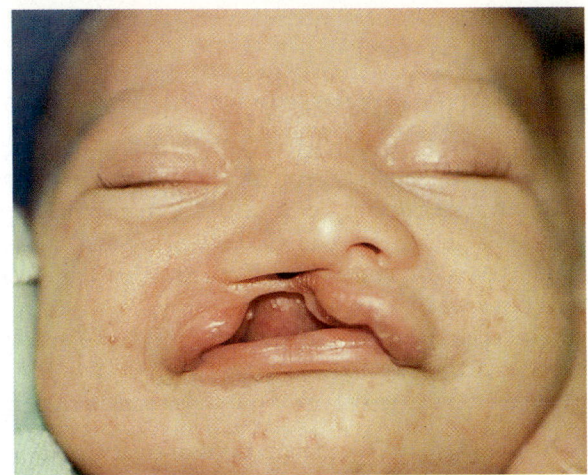

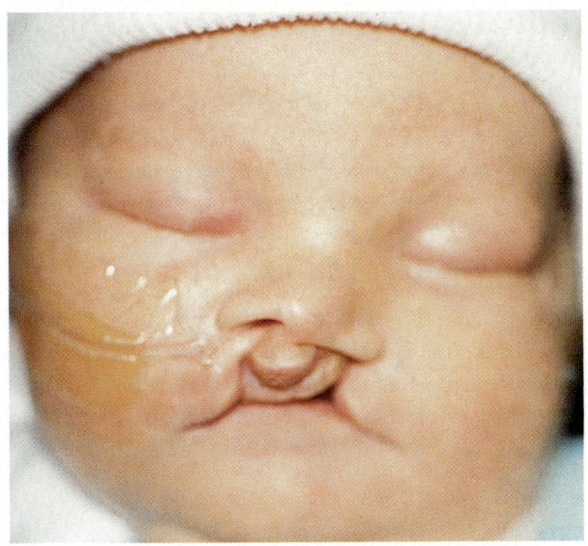

FIGURE 46–1. ◆ **A,** Unilateral cleft lip. **B,** Bilateral cleft lip.
Courtesy of Dr. Elizabeth Peterson, Spokane, WA.

union of the upper lip is complete by the seventh week. Fusion of the secondary palate occurs between 5 and 12 weeks of gestation. Failure of the tongue to move downward at the correct time prevents the palatine processes from fusing.

The intrauterine development of the hard and soft palates is completed in the first trimester. It is during this time that other major organ systems develop. Congenital defects such as tracheoesophageal fistula, omphalocele, trisomy 13, and skeletal dysplasias are associated with cleft lip and palate defects in 20% to 30% of cases. There is an increased incidence in families with a prior history of cleft lip or palate. The cause is believed to be multifactorial, involving a combination of environmental and genetic influences. When fortification of cereals and breads with folate began in the United States in 1996 as a measure to decrease neural tube defects, the incidence of orofacial clefts also decreased. This may suggest that folate plays a role in formation of maxillary processes in the fetus (Wong, Eskes, Kuihpers-Jagtman, et al., 1999).

Clinical Manifestations

Cleft lip may be seen on ultrasound by 13 to 16 weeks' gestation (Mitchell & Wood, 2000). A cleft that involves the lip is apparent at birth. It may be a simple dimple in the vermilion border of the lip or a complete separation extending to the floor of the nose. The defect may be unilateral or bilateral and may occur alone or in combination with a cleft palate defect. Varying degrees of nasal deformity may also be present.

Cleft palate defects are less obvious when they occur without a cleft lip and may not be detected at birth. Clefts of the hard palate form a continuous opening between the mouth and nasal cavity and may be unilateral or bilateral, involving just the soft palate or both the soft and hard palate.

Clinical Therapy

Cleft lip and palate are usually diagnosed at birth or during the newborn assessment. Medical management requires the combined efforts of a multidisciplinary team. Because speech, hearing, and dentition may be affected, coordinated care by specialists in plastic surgery, hearing, speech, and dentistry is necessary.

The cleft lip is usually repaired by about 2 to 3 months of age (Figure 46–2 ◆). The lip is sutured together, and a Logan bow or other stabilizing device or dressing is put in place to prevent tension on the suture line. After surgery, the infant's elbows are restrained to prevent flexion (see Skill 7-6). ⊂▭ **SKILLS** To prevent injury to the suture line, the child is medicated to minimize crying.

Early closure of the lip enables the infant to form a better seal around the nipple for feeding. The sucking motion strengthens the muscles necessary for speech. Special feeding devices such as longer nipples with enlarged holes are available to help meet the infant's nutritional needs before surgical correction.

Developing Cultural Competence

In many developing countries, infants do not have access to surgery for correction of cleft lip and palate. They may grow into childhood and adulthood with these abnormalities. Medical teams from the United States, Canada, and other countries sometimes travel to developing nations for short medical missions, performing surgery on the children and teaching local doctors surgical techniques.

Timing of the cleft palate repair is controversial and depends on the size and severity of the cleft. Most surgeons perform closure operations when the infant is about 18 months old. This protects the formation of tooth buds and allows the infant to develop more normal speech patterns.

Infants with cleft lip and cleft palate are prone to recurrent otitis media, which can lead to tympanic membrane scarring and hearing loss. Antibiotics are prescribed to

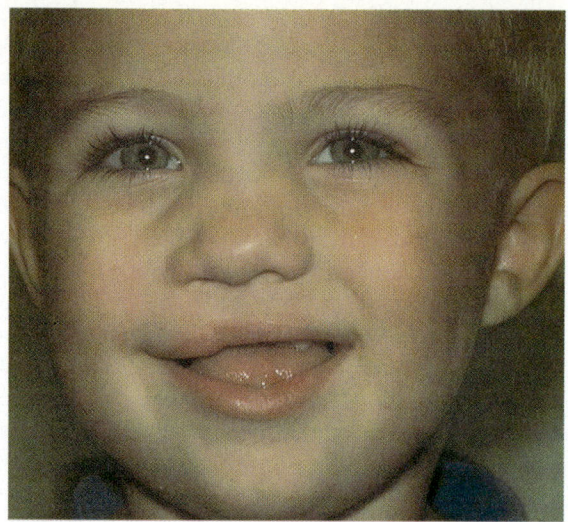

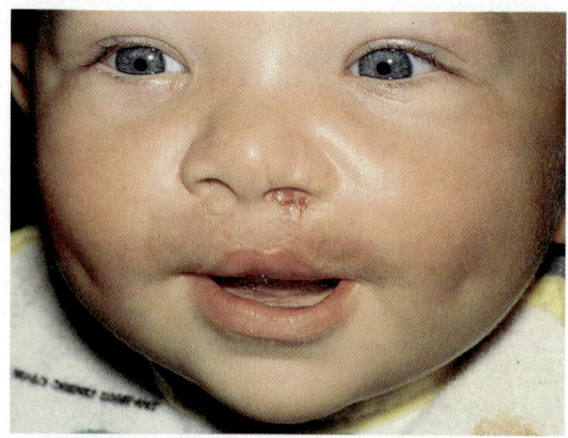

FIGURE 46–2. ◆ **A,** Repaired unilateral cleft lip (see Fig. 46–1A). **B,** Repaired bilateral cleft lip (see Fig. 46–1B). *Courtesy of Dr. Elizabeth Peterson, Spokane, WA.*

treat any infections that might lead to an ear infection. Because infants with chronic otitis media often have difficulty hearing, speech patterns may be altered. These infants require early, continuous intervention to prevent complications. (Refer to Chapter 48 for care of the child with chronic otitis media.) ⌾▭ The child who has had cleft palate repair requires orthodontic care. Early visits permit assessment of tooth eruption and the need for future orthodontic work.

Nursing Management

Nursing Assessment and Diagnosis

PHYSIOLOGIC ASSESSMENT

A cleft lip defect is observable at birth. A cleft palate defect is usually noted during the newborn assessment by palpation of the hard palate with the finger. A description of the location and extent of the defect helps the nurse determine the correct method of feeding. Thorough and complete

physical assessment is needed since additional defects are sometimes present.

PSYCHOSOCIAL ASSESSMENT

Assessment of the family's reactions is an integral part of the overall nursing assessment. Physical deformities, especially of the face, can be devastating to parents. A poorly corrected defect can lead to low self-esteem in the older child. Assess the child's developmental level and social interactions with peers.

The accompanying "Nursing Care Plan" lists common nursing diagnoses for the infant with a cleft lip and/or palate. Other diagnoses that might be appropriate include:

▶ *Anxiety (parent)* related to situational crisis and threat to self-concept

▶ *Ineffective infant feeding pattern* related to anatomic abnormality

▶ *Risk for caregiver role strain* related to complexity of caregiving tasks

▶ *Risk for impaired home maintenance management* related to infant's defect(s) and inadequate family support

Planning and Implementation

Nursing care involves providing emotional support, performing postsurgical care, helping parents coordinate care and maintain a healthy home environment, and making appropriate referrals. See "Nursing Care Plan: The Infant with a Cleft Lip and/or Palate" for a summary of nursing care.

PROVIDE EMOTIONAL SUPPORT

Parents may need assistance to view their infant as a whole person, rather than focusing solely on the physical defect. Promote parent–infant bonding by explaining the nature of the structural defect and the procedure for correction. Interact and speak to the infant in the parents' presence and point out positive attributes such as alertness, soft skin, or active movements. Self-blame is common among parents. Parents can also be referred to the American Cleft Palate Association for information ⌾▭ WEB about the disorder. Some plastic surgeons have photos of children before and after correction to show parents; this may reassure parents that their child can have a "normal" appearance (Uhrich & Mackin, 2001).

Parental anxiety is usual when children undergo surgery, and it is heightened when the surgery involves an infant. To minimize anxiety, give clear, concise explanations to parents. Allow sufficient time for parents to ask questions. Encourage parents to hold and cuddle the infant before surgery.

PROVIDE POSTOPERATIVE CARE

Provide general postoperative care for the infant. (See "Nursing Care Plan: The Infant with a Cleft Lip and/or Palate" in this chapter and "Nursing Care Plan: The Child

GOAL	INTERVENTION	RATIONALE	EXPECTED OUTCOME
Preoperative Care			

1. Risk for aspiration (breast milk, formula, or mucus) related to anatomic defect

GOAL	INTERVENTION	RATIONALE	EXPECTED OUTCOME
	NIC Priority Intervention:		*NOC Suggested Outcome:*
	Aspiration precautions: *Prevention or minimization of risk factors in the patient at risk of aspiration*		**Airway maintenance:** *Toleration of enteral feedings without aspiration*
The infant will have no episodes of gagging or aspiration.	▶ Assess respiratory status and monitor vital signs at least every 2 hours.	▶ Allows for early identification of problems.	The infant exhibits no signs of respiratory distress.
	▶ Position on side after feedings.	▶ Prevents aspiration of feedings.	
	▶ Feed slowly and use adaptive equipment as needed.	▶ Facilitates intake while minimizing risk of aspiration.	
	▶ Burp frequently (after every 15–30 mL of fluid).	▶ Helps to prevent regurgitation and aspiration.	
	▶ Position upright for feedings.	▶ Minimizes passage of feedings through cleft.	
	▶ Keep suction equipment and bulb syringe at bedside.	▶ Suctioning may be necessary to remove milk or mucus.	

2. Ineffective family coping related to birth of a child with a defect

GOAL	INTERVENTION	RATIONALE	EXPECTED OUTCOME
	NIC Priority Intervention:		*NOC Suggested Outcome:*
	Family Involvement: *Facilitating family participation in the emotional and physical care of the child*		**Positive coping:** *Extent of coping mechanisms and ability to perform child's physical and emotional care* Parents hold, comfort, and show concern for the infant.
Parents will begin bonding process with the infant.	▶ Help parents to hold the infant and facilitate feeding process.	▶ Contact is essential for bonding.	
	▶ Point out positive attributes of infant (hair, eyes, alertness, etc).	▶ Helps parents see the child as a whole, rather than concentrating on the defect.	
	▶ Explain surgical procedure and expected outcome. Show pictures of other children's cleft lip repair.	▶ Eliminating unknown factors helps to decrease anxiety.	
The family's coping ability will be maximized. Parents will verbalize the nature and sequelae of the defect.	▶ Assess parents' knowledge of the defect, their degree of anxiety and level of discomfort, and the interpersonal relationships among family members.	▶ Helps to determine the appropriate timing and amount of information to be given regarding the child's defect.	The family demonstrates improved coping ability before discharge.
	▶ Explore the reactions of extended family members.	▶ Extended family is an important source of support for most parents of a newborn. Family members can often help promote acceptance and compliance with the treatment plan.	Parents receive necessary support to care for their infant.
	▶ Support open visitation.	▶ Allows parents to continue the bonding process.	
	▶ Encourage parents to participate in caretaking activities (holding, diapering, feeding).	▶ Participation in infant care decreases anxiety and provides parents with a sense of purpose.	
	▶ Provide information about the etiology of cleft lip and palate defects and the special needs of these infants. Encourage questions.	▶ Concrete information allows parents time to understand the defect and reduces guilt.	
	▶ Refer to parent support groups.	▶ Support groups allow parents to express their feelings and concerns, to find people with concerns similar to their own, and to seek additional information.	

3. Altered nutrition: less than body requirements related to the infant's inability to ingest nutrients

GOAL	INTERVENTION	RATIONALE	EXPECTED OUTCOME
	NIC Priority Intervention:		*NOC Suggested Outcome:*
	Nutrition management: *Provision of a balanced dietary intake of foods and fluids*		**Nutrition status:** *Amount of food and fluid taken into the body over a 24-hour period* The infant maintains adequate nutritional intake and gains weight appropriately.
The infant will gain weight steadily.	▶ Assess fluid and calorie intake daily. Assess weight daily (same scale, same time, with infant completely undressed).	▶ Provides an objective measurement of whether the infant is receiving sufficient caloric intake to promote growth. Using the same scale and procedure when weighing the infant provides for comparability between daily weights.	

(continued)

GOAL	INTERVENTION	RATIONALE	EXPECTED OUTCOME

Preoperative Care—continued

3. Altered nutrition: less than body requirements related to the infant's inability to ingest nutrients—continued

	▶ Observe for any respiratory impairment.	▶ Any symptoms of respiratory compromise will interfere with the infant's ability to suck. Feedings should be initiated only if there are no signs of respiratory distress.	
	▶ Provide 100–150 cal/kg/day and 100–130 ml/kg/day of feedings and fluid. If the infant needs an increased number of calories to grow, referral to a nutritionist should be made. Formulas with higher calorie concentrations per ounce are available without increasing total fluids.	▶ Provides optimal calories and fluids for growth and hydration.	
	▶ Facilitate breastfeeding.	▶ Breast milk is recommended as the best food for an infant. The process of breastfeeding helps to promote bonding between mother and infant.	Successful breastfeeding is achieved if desired.
	▶ Hold the infant in a semisitting position.	▶ Makes swallowing easier and reduces the amount of fluid return from the nose.	
	▶ Give the mother information on breastfeeding the infant with a cleft lip and/or palate such as plugging the cleft lip and eliciting a letdown reflex before nursing.	▶ Information and specific suggestions may encourage the mother to persist with breastfeeding.	
	▶ Contact the La Leche League for the name of a support person.	▶ The La Leche League promotes breastfeeding for all infants. It can provide support people with experience who will aid the mother.	
	▶ If the mother is unable to breastfeed (or prefers not to), initiate bottle-feeding: Hold infant in an upright or semisitting position for feeding.	▶ Facilitates swallowing and minimizes the amount of fluid return from the nose.	Feeding provides necessary nutrients and is a positive experience for parents and infant.
	▶ Place nipple against the inside cheek toward the back of the tongue. May need to use a premature nipple (slightly longer and softer than regular nipple with a larger opening) or a Brecht feeder (an oval bottle with a long, soft nipple).	▶ Use of longer, softer nipples makes it easier for the infant to suck. A Brecht feeder decreases the amount of pressure in the bottle and makes the formula flow more easily.	
	▶ Feed small amounts slowly.	▶ Small amounts and slow feeding do not tire the infant as quickly as do larger amounts given at a faster rate. They also decrease the calories used during feeding.	
	▶ Burp frequently, after 15–30 mL of formula has been given.	▶ Frequent burping prevents the accumulation of air in the stomach, which can cause regurgitation or vomiting.	
	▶ Initiate nasogastric feedings if the infant is unable to ingest sufficient calories by mouth.	▶ Adequate nutrition must be maintained. Use of a feeding tube allows the infant who has difficulty with oral feeding to receive adequate nutrition for growth.	

Postoperative Care

1. Risk for infection related to location of surgical procedure

GOAL	INTERVENTION	RATIONALE	EXPECTED OUTCOME
	NIC Priority Intervention:		*NOC Suggested Outcome:*
The infant's mucosal tissue will heal without infection.	**Infection control:** *Minimizing the acquisition and transmission of infectious agents*		**Risk control:** *Actions to eliminate or reduce actual, personal, or modifiable health risks*
	▶ Assess vital signs every 2 hours.	▶ Elevated temperature may indicate infection.	The infant remains free of infection in the oral cavity. Tissues remain intact and pink.
	▶ Assess oral cavity every 2 hours or as needed for tenderness, reddened areas, lesions, or presence of secretions.	▶ Aids in identifying infection.	
	▶ Cleanse suture line with normal saline or sterile water if ordered.	▶ Helps decrease the presence of bacteria.	Healing process progresses without adverse events in postoperative period.
	▶ Cleanse the cleft areas by giving 5–15 mL of water after each feeding.	▶ Prevents accumulation of carbohydrates, which encourage bacterial growth.	

GOAL	INTERVENTION	RATIONALE	EXPECTED OUTCOME

Postoperative Care—continued

	▶ If a crust has formed, use a cotton swab to apply a half-strength peroxide solution.	▶ Helps loosen the crust, aiding in removal.	
	▶ Apply antibiotic cream to suture line as ordered.	▶ Counteracts the growth of bacteria.	
	▶ Use careful handwashing and sterile technique when working with suture line.	▶ Prevents the spread of microorganisms from other sources.	

2. Ineffective breathing pattern related to surgical correction of defect

	NIC Priority Intervention:		*NOC Suggested Outcome:*
	Airway management: *Facilitation of patency of air passages*		**Vital signs status:** *Temperature, pulse, respiration, and blood pressure within expected range for the infant/child*
The infant will maintain an effective breathing pattern.	▶ Assess respiratory status and monitor vital signs at least every 2 hours.	▶ Allows for early identification of problems.	The infant shows no signs of respiratory infection or compromise.
	▶ Apply a cardiorespiratory monitor.	▶ Enables early detection of abnormal respirations, facilitating prompt intervention.	
	▶ Keep suction equipment and bulb syringe at bedside. Gently suction oropharynx and nasopharynx as needed.	▶ Gentle suctioning will keep the airway clear. Suctioning that is too vigorous can irritate the mucosa.	
	▶ Provide cool mist for first 24 hours postoperatively if ordered.	▶ Moisturizes secretions to reduce pooling in lungs. Moisturizes oral cavity.	
	▶ Reposition every 2 hours.	▶ Ensures expansion of all lung fields.	

3. Impaired tissue integrity related to mechanical factors

	NIC Priority Intervention:		*NOC Suggested Outcome:*
	Wound care: *Prevention of wound complications and promotion of wound healing*		**Wound healing:** *The extent to which cells and tissues have regenerated following intentional closure*
Lip and/or palate will heal with minimal scarring or disruption.	▶ Position the infant with cleft lip repair on side or back only.	▶ Prone position could cause rubbing on suture line.	Lip/palate heals without complications.
	▶ Use soft elbow restraints. Remove every 2 hours and replace. Do not leave the infant unattended when restraints are removed.	▶ Prevents the infant's hands from rubbing surgical site. Regular removal allows for skin and neurovascular checks.	
	▶ Maintain metal bar (Logan bow) or Steri-Strips placed over cleft lip repair.	▶ Maintaining suture line will minimize scarring.	
	▶ Avoid metal utensils or straws after cleft palate repair.	▶ These devices may disrupt suture line.	
	▶ Keep the infant well medicated for pain in initial postoperative period. Have parents hold and comfort the infant.	▶ Good pain management minimizes crying, which can cause stress on suture line. Increases bonding and soothes the child to decrease crying.	
	▶ Provide developmentally appropriate activities (i.e., mobiles, music).	▶ Soothes and keeps the infant calm.	

4. Knowledge deficit (parent) related to lack of exposure and unfamiliarity with resources

	NIC Priority Intervention:		*NOC Suggested Outcome:*
	Teaching, disease process: *Assisting the patient to understand information related to cleft lip/palate*		**Knowledge:** *Extent of understanding conveyed about cleft lip/palate treatment*
Before discharge, parents will verbalize home care methods for care of the infant with cleft lip and palate defect.	▶ Explain care and treatment (both short-term and long-term). Discuss potential complications.	▶ Assists the family to deal with the physical and psychosocial aspects of a child with a congenital defect.	Parents accurately describe and demonstrate feeding techniques to facilitate optimal growth of the infant; describe interventions if respiratory distress occurs; and take the written instructions home with them on discharge.
	▶ Demonstrate feeding techniques and alternatives. Allow parents to demonstrate before discharge.	▶ Provides visual instructions. Redemonstration confirms learning.	
	▶ Provide written instructions for follow-up care arrangements.	▶ Written instructions reinforce verbal instruction and provide a reference after discharge.	
	▶ Introduce the parents (if possible) to a primary care provider in the setting where the infant will receive follow-up care after discharge.	▶ Continuity of care is important. Since the infant will require long-term follow-up, a contact with the new provider is helpful.	

(continued)

GOAL	INTERVENTION	RATIONALE	EXPECTED OUTCOME
Postoperative Care			
5. Altered nutrition: less than body requirements related to inability to ingest nutrients			
The infant will receive adequate nutritional intake.	NIC Priority Intervention: **Nutrition management:** *Promotion of a balanced dietary intake of foods and fluids* ▶ Maintain intravenous infusion as ordered. ▶ Begin with clear liquids, then give half-strength formula or breast milk as ordered. ▶ Use Asepto syringe or dropper in side of mouth. ▶ Do not allow pacifiers. ▶ Give high-calorie soft foods after cleft palate repair.	▶ Provides fluid when NPO. ▶ Ensures adequate fluids and nutrients. ▶ Avoids suture line and resultant accumulation of formula in that area. ▶ Sucking can disrupt suture line. ▶ Rough foods, utensils, and straws could disrupt the surgical site.	NOC Suggested Outcome: **Nutritional status:** *Extent to which nutrients are available to meet metabolic needs* The infant receives adequate nutritional intake. Infant resumes usual feeding patterns and gains weight appropriately.

Undergoing Surgery" in Chapter 34.) ⊂▭⊃ Assess vital signs frequently and maintain the infant's airway. Measure intake and output. When oral fluids with clear liquids are started, they are usually given through a dropper or an Asepto syringe. Position the infant in a sitting position for the feedings to avoid aspiration. The infant then progresses to half-strength formula or breast milk. After each feeding, clean the suture line with water or normal saline to avoid accumulation of feedings.

It is important to maintain the suture line to ensure healing. Position the infant in a supine or a side-lying position to avoid rubbing the suture line on the bedding. Keep elbows in soft restraints. Maintain the metal device or Steri-Strips placed over the incision. Place antibiotic cream on the incision site as ordered. Medicate the infant regularly to control pain and to minimize crying and stress on the suture line. After cleft palate surgery, avoid the use of metal utensils or straws, which may disrupt the surgical site.

Growth and Development

An infant who has had a cleft lip repair needs stimulation to provide distraction. This approach will minimize crying, which can damage the suture line. Soft, colorful toys, mobiles, and other visual objects are helpful. Music also can be used to soothe the infant.

NURSING CARE IN THE COMMUNITY

Identify and address home care needs well in advance of discharge. Discuss all aspects of the infant's care with the parents throughout hospitalization and after surgery. Involve parents in the infant's care to increase their comfort level before discharge and to promote bonding. Teach them feeding techniques, how to recognize signs of infection, how to position the infant, and how to care for the suture line. Breastfeeding is usually possible with some assistance from a lactation specialist, even if the mother pumps her breasts and milk is fed by a special nurser. Some infants may need a device placed in the mouth to enable them to establish suction. Several companies make special nursers that may be helpful for children with cleft lip or palate.

Management, especially in the first few months of life, involves many different health care professionals. In addition to hospital, clinic, and home health nurses, members of the health care team often include specialists such as the surgeon, speech specialist, geneticist, dentist, prosthodontist, audiologist, social worker, and pediatrician (Balasubrahmanyam, et al., 1998). The parents are the best coordinators of the child's care. Encourage them to keep a diary listing the professionals with whom they talk and the content of the discussions.

Discuss with the parents the financial implications of long-term care. Private insurance does not always cover all the costs of care necessary for the child. Refer parents to social services familiar with programs and financial aid for which the parents and child may be eligible. Relief of financial worries enables parents to concentrate on caring for the child.

Teach parents how to care for the child after discharge. If the child has siblings, emphasize that they will need preparation to accept the child. Sibling rivalry can be heightened when one child receives more attention at the home. Remind parents of the importance of setting limits and of spending time with each child. Determine whether additional family supports are necessary. Provide parents with information on support groups, physicians, social workers, Internet resources, and local services that can help maintain family continuity.

Discuss ways to prevent the infant from touching the suture line. Teach parents how to bundle an infant in a blanket with arms tucked inside the blanket. A front-sling baby carrier may also be used to immobilize the arms. Front-sling carriers provide the additional benefits of comforting the infant through contact with the parent and of holding the infant upright, which aids in optimal positioning after feedings.

After surgical repair, parents need to be taught how to feed the infant and identify signs of complications (fever, vomiting, respiratory distress). Referral to a home health care agency for support may be helpful. Encourage follow-up visits with health care professionals. The child may need further evaluation of speech development, ear infections, or a recommendation for plastic surgery.

Evaluation

Expected outcomes of nursing care in the preoperative period include:

▶ Absence of respiratory distress and maintenance of normal respirations

▶ Positive parent-infant bonding

▶ Parental expression of support and comfort by family and community

▶ Maintenance of normal weight by infant

▶ Parental knowledge of defect, its correction, and infant needs

Expected outcomes of postoperative nursing care include:

▶ Absence of infection

▶ Clean healing of surgical area

▶ Absence of respiratory distress

▶ Effective pain management

▶ Fluid and electrolyte balance and adequate weight gain

▶ Parental description of infant care and feeding

ESOPHAGEAL ATRESIA AND TRACHEOESOPHAGEAL FISTULA

Esophageal atresia is a malformation that results from failure of the esophagus to develop as a continuous tube during the fourth and fifth weeks of gestation. Esophageal atresia with tracheoesophageal fistula occurs in 1 in 3000 to 4500 births. About 30% of the infants are premature (Herbst, 2000).

In esophageal atresia, the foregut fails to lengthen, separate, and fuse into two parallel tubes (the esophagus and trachea) during fetal development. Instead the esophagus may end in a blind pouch or develop as a pouch connected to the trachea by a fistula (tracheoesophageal fistula) (see "Pathophysiology Illustrated: Esophageal Atresia and

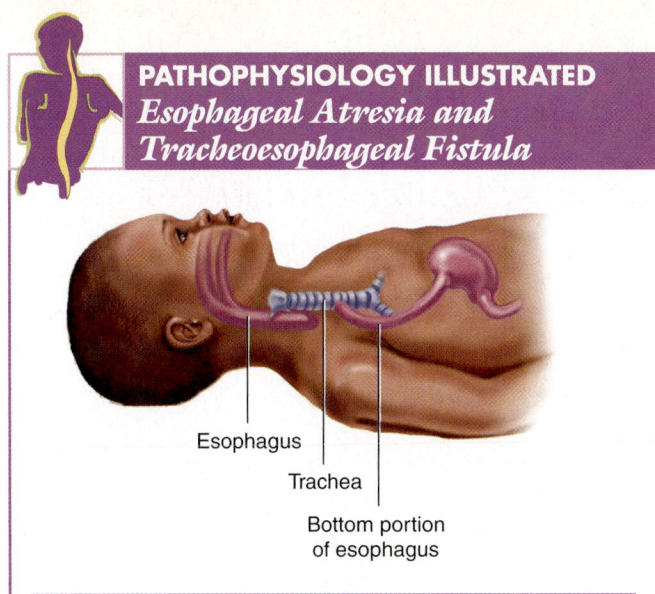

PATHOPHYSIOLOGY ILLUSTRATED
Esophageal Atresia and Tracheoesophageal Fistula

Esophagus

Trachea

Bottom portion of esophagus

In the most common type of esophageal atresia and tracheoesophageal fistula, the upper segment of the esophagus ends in a blind pouch connected to the trachea; a fistula connects the lower segment to the trachea.

Tracheoesophageal Fistula"). Esophageal atresia is often associated with a maternal history of polyhydramnios. Associated anomalies may occur, including congenital heart defects, gastrointestinal or urinary tract anomalies, and musculoskeletal abnormalities. Jerome, described at the beginning of the chapter, had esophageal atresia as well as an imperforate anus.

Symptoms in the newborn include excessive salivation and drooling, often accompanied by cyanosis, choking, coughing, and sneezing. During feeding, the infant returns fluid through the nose and mouth. Aspiration places the infant at risk for pneumonia. Depending on the type of defect, the abdomen may become distended because of air trapping.

Diagnosis is usually confirmed by attempting to pass a 5 or 8 French nasogastric tube into the stomach. In most cases, the tube meets resistance and can be advanced only minimally. Specific defects and associated anomalies are determined by x-ray examination. Echocardiogram and abdominal ultrasound are performed. Careful examination of the lungs is needed. A delay in diagnosis can be fatal because ingested fluid or secretions may enter the lungs.

A tube is inserted to suction the upper pouch. Intravenous antibiotics and fluids are begun. Surgery is performed as soon as possible. Surgical correction may be accomplished in several stages. The first stage usually involves ligation of the fistula and insertion of a gastrostomy tube. In the second stage, the two ends of the esophagus are reconnected, if possible. When surgical closure (anastomosis) is not possible, a gastrostomy tube must remain in place for use in feeding. Potential postoperative complications include gastroesophageal reflux, aspiration, and stricture formation. The prognosis is usually good with surgery.

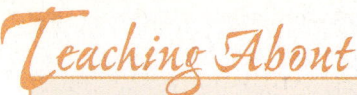

HOME CARE INSTRUCTIONS FOR THE CHILD REQUIRING GASTROSTOMY TUBE FEEDINGS AND CARE

Equipment

Prepared, prescribed feeding; enteral feeding pump; long-nosed syringe

Procedure

1. Wash hands.
2. Warm prescribed formula to room temperature.
3. Pour formula to run through the feeding bag.
4. Allow formula to run through the tubing to remove air. Close clamp.
5. Attach syringe to the end of the gastrostomy tube. Unclamp the gastrostomy tube.
6. Pull plunger back until resistance is felt. Check amount of formula in syringe. If more than half of the prescribed amount is withdrawn, refer to the section on problem solving (below). If less than the prescribed amount is withdrawn, push the formula gently back through the syringe.
7. Instill water through the tube.
8. Attach the feeding bag to the gastrostomy tube. Infuse at the prescribed rate.
9. Burp or bubble the infant throughout the feeding.
10. After feeding, flush the gastrostomy tube with water and clamp the tube.
11. Position the infant prone or side lying for 1/2 to 1 hour after feedings.

Psychosocial Needs

Hold and rock the infant or child during feedings.

Give a pacifier to an infant or a bottle or cup to a child to meet developmental needs.

Medication Administration

Use liquid medication whenever possible.

Crush only uncoated tablets.

Crush tablets to a fine powder and mix with water or juice.

Flush tubing before and after medication administration.

Stoma Care

Wash the area around the stoma twice a day with soap and water.

Use half-strength hydrogen peroxide to remove any crusting.

Look for signs of infection, such as redness, swelling, and discharge.

Notify the physician if any signs of infection or leakage are present.

Problem Solving

Problem	Cause	Action
Formula will not flow	Blocked tube (clamped, foreign material, viscous formula)	Check clamp. Reposition.
		Pull back on syringe. Instill water. Milk tube. Notify physician.
	Pump malfunction	Check pump. Call company.
		Give feeding by gravity.
Large volume of undigested formula removed before feeding	Delayed absorption	Reinfuse remaining formula. If more than half of feeding, subtract from amount given in the next feeding.
		Do not discard the residual.
Constipation	Decreased free fluids	Check for last bowel movement.
		Notify physician.
		Give water and juice between feedings as tolerated. Report bowel problems or hard stools to physician.
Diarrhea	Hyperosmolar formula	Dilute formula.
	Rapid rate of flow	Feed at a slower rate.
	Cold formula	Warm formula to room temperature before feeding.
	Bacterial contamination	Treat with antibiotics.
Dislodged tube	Inadequate stabilization	Bring child for emergency care
Skin irritation	Formula leakage	Skin care; barrier if needed

Note: From Borkowski, S. (1998). Pediatric stomas, tubes, and appliances. *Pediatric Clinics of North America, 45,* 1419–1435; and Young, C., & White, S. (1992). Preparing patients for tube feeding at home. *American Journal of Nursing, 92,* 46–53.

Nursing Management

Esophageal atresia is a surgical emergency. Preoperatively the infant requires close observation and intervention to maintain a patent airway. Suction should be readily available to remove any secretions that accumulate in the nasopharyngeal airway. Place the infant with the head of the bed slightly lowered to minimize aspiration of secretions into the trachea. Use continuous or low intermittent suction to remove secretions from the blind pouch. To confirm correct placement of the tube, aspiration of stomach contents and pH testing are required. Withhold oral fluids, and maintain the infant with intravenous fluids administered through an umbilical artery catheter.

After surgery, maintain gastrostomy drainage, and administer intravenous fluids and antibiotics. Total parenteral nutrition may be needed until gastrostomy or oral feedings are tolerated.

The parents require emotional support throughout the infant's hospitalization. Clearly explain all procedures. Encourage parents to bond with the infant by stroking and talking to the infant. Eliciting questions and allowing parents to participate in the infant's care, especially feeding (when permitted), can facilitate bonding and help to prepare parents for care of the infant after discharge.

Once enteral feedings have been established, the infant may be discharged from the hospital with a gastrostomy tube in place (Figure 46–3 ◆ and Skill 15-3). **SKILLS** **CD** Teach the parents about gastrostomy tube care and feeding, signs of infection, and how to prevent postoperative complications.

The outcomes of nursing care will depend on the extent of the defect and correction. Examples include:

- Adequate intake of fluids to promote hydration and growth
- Absence of respiratory distress

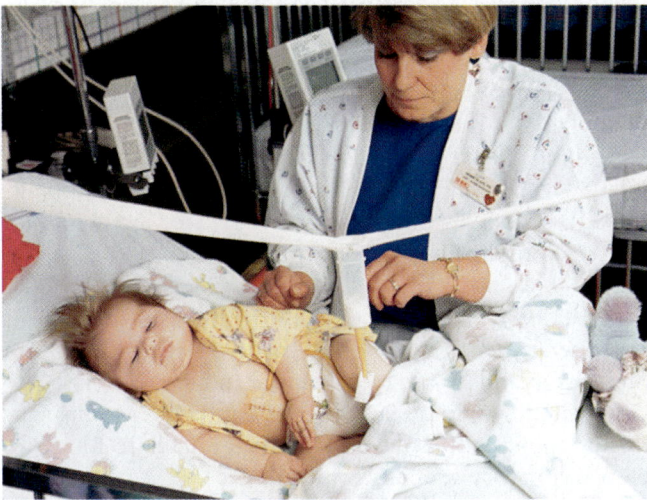

FIGURE 46–3. ◆ A gastrostomy tube is used to feed the child with a gastrointestinal disorder such as esophageal atresia.

- Positive parent-infant bonding
- Absence of infection
- Parental use of support and information resources regarding the condition

PYLORIC STENOSIS

Pyloric stenosis is a hypertrophic obstruction of the circular muscle of the pyloric canal. It is a common problem that most often affects first-born male infants.

Etiology and Pathophysiology

The exact cause of pyloric stenosis is unknown, although frequently there is a family history of the disorder. It is relatively common, with about 3 cases in 100 births (Irish, Pearl, Caty, et al., 1998). Hypertrophy of the circular pylorus muscle results in stenosis of the passage between the stomach and the duodenum, partially obstructing the lumen of the stomach (see "Pathophysiology Illustrated: Pyloric Stenosis"). The lumen becomes inflamed and edematous, which narrows the opening until the obstruction becomes complete. At this time vomiting becomes more forceful. As the obstruction progresses, the infant becomes dehydrated and electrolytes are depleted, resulting in metabolic imbalances.

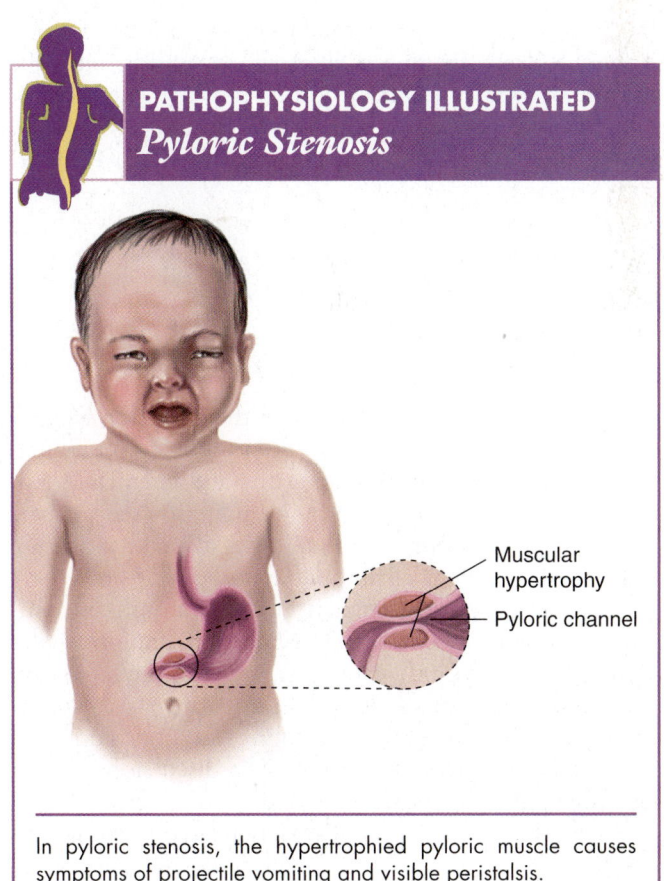

PATHOPHYSIOLOGY ILLUSTRATED
Pyloric Stenosis

Muscular hypertrophy
Pyloric channel

In pyloric stenosis, the hypertrophied pyloric muscle causes symptoms of projectile vomiting and visible peristalsis.

Clinical Manifestations

Symptoms usually become evident 2 to 4 weeks after birth, although onset may vary. Initially the infant appears well or regurgitates slightly after feedings. The parents may describe the infant as a "good eater" who vomits occasionally. As the obstruction progresses, the vomiting becomes projectile. In **projectile vomiting,** the contents of the stomach may be ejected up to 3 feet from the infant. The vomitus is nonbilious and may become blood tinged because of repeated irritation to the esophagus. The infant is always hungry, appears irritable, fails to gain weight, and has fewer and smaller stools. Dehydration, alkalosis, and hyperbilirubinemia can occur.

Clinical Therapy

On physical examination, visible peristaltic waves across the abdomen and an olive-sized mass in the left upper quadrant are often found. A sonogram is usually performed to confirm the diagnosis, and an upper GI series may be performed as well. Blood tests determine the degree of dehydration, electrolyte imbalance, and anemia (see Chapter 39). ⌐⊃

Surgical correction is the treatment of choice. Preoperatively the infant's condition is stabilized with intravenous fluids and electrolytes. A nasogastric tube is inserted to decompress the stomach. Surgery is performed as soon as possible after the infant's condition is stabilized. During surgery the circular muscle fibers are released to allow the passage of food and fluid (pyloromyotomy). The prognosis is good. The infant is usually taking fluids in 12 to 24 hours, and discharged on a regular diet by 36 to 48 hours after surgery.

Nursing Management

Nursing Assessment and Diagnosis

Observe the infant's abdomen for the presence of peristaltic waves. Bowel sounds are hyperactive on auscultation. Auscultate before palpating the abdomen since palpation can cause a change in bowel patterns (see Chapter 33). ⌐⊃ Palpation reveals an olive-shaped mass in the right upper quadrant of the abdomen.

Assess skin turgor, fontanels, urinary output, and mucous membranes to determine whether hydration is adequate. Measure vomitus and describe vomiting episodes. Be alert for signs of an electrolyte imbalance, particularly low levels of serum chloride, sodium, and potassium, and an elevated pH. (See Chapter 39 for a discussion of these electrolyte imbalances.) ⌐⊃

Assess the parents' level of anxiety related to the child's condition.

Among the nursing diagnoses that might be appropriate for the child with pyloric stenosis are:

▶ *Fluid volume deficit* related to active fluid volume loss
▶ *Altered nutrition: less than body requirements* related to vomiting and inability to ingest nutrients
▶ *Sleep pattern disturbance* related to discomfort
▶ *Altered family processes* related to health status of family member

Planning and Implementation

Nursing care centers on meeting the infant's fluid and electrolyte needs, minimizing weight loss, promoting rest and comfort, preventing infection, and providing supportive care for parents.

MEET FLUID AND ELECTROLYTE NEEDS

Because projectile vomiting will continue until the obstruction is relieved surgically, withhold oral feedings. Administer intravenous fluid therapy to correct fluid and electrolyte imbalances and to maintain adequate hydration. Because gastric fluid is high in potassium, hypokalemia can result (see Chapter 39 for a discussion of this electrolyte imbalance and the signs of its occurrence). ⌐⊃ Monitor intake and output (including vomitus) and urine specific gravity. Inform parents that all diapers will be weighed to measure the infant's output of urine and stool.

MINIMIZE WEIGHT LOSS

The infant loses weight because of frequent vomiting. Monitor weight daily both preoperatively and postoperatively. Begin small, frequent feedings of clear liquids within 4 to 6 hours postoperatively. If clear liquids are tolerated, advance the infant to formula or breast milk feedings.

PROMOTE REST AND COMFORT

During the preoperative period the infant is hungry and cries often. Swaddle the infant to maintain warmth and provide comfort. Encourage the parents to hold and cuddle the infant. Provide a pacifier to meet the infant's need to suck.

Postoperatively the infant is uncomfortable because of the surgical incision. Instruct parents to avoid pressure on the incision. When diapering the infant, slide the diaper gently under the buttocks rather than lifting the legs. Swaddling, rocking, and use of a pacifier help to relax the infant. Acetaminophen or other analgesics can be administered to relieve discomfort as ordered. (See Chapter 38 for a discussion of pain management.) ⌐⊃

PREVENT INFECTION

Postoperatively the incision is covered with collodion or Steri-Strips and should be kept clean and dry. Check the incision site for redness, swelling, or discharge. Monitor the infant's temperature every 4 hours. Auscultate lungs for clear respiratory sounds.

PROVIDE SUPPORTIVE CARE

The need for hospitalization and surgery creates anxiety for parents. Encourage them to participate in the infant's care and to discuss their fears and concerns. Provide simple and clear explanations about the infant's condition and care. Advise parents that occasional vomiting after surgery may occur.

DISCHARGE PLANNING AND HOME CARE TEACHING

Instruct parents to observe the incision for redness, swelling, or discharge and to notify the physician immediately if these occur or if the infant's temperature is higher than 38.5 °C (101 °F). To reduce the possibility of infec-

tion, advise parents to fold the infant's diaper so that it does not touch the incision.

Evaluation

Expected outcomes of care include pain control, intake of recommended fluid and food with absence of vomiting, and manifestation of normal growth patterns. See "Clinical Pathway: Pyloric Stenosis."

CLINICAL PATHWAY ～ *Pyloric Stenosis*

Category	Immediate Postoperative Period	Transition to Discharge	Discharge to Home Care
Daily outcomes	Client will: • have stable vital signs and be alert and responsive • have lungs clear to auscultation • have unlabored respirations and maintain oxygen saturation above 95% • have a clean, dry dressing • recover from anesthesia • have moist mucous membranes • have a urine specific gravity = 1.005–1.020 • demonstrate pain control Family displays effective coping with ongoing stressors Family verbalizes beginning understanding of expected postoperative course	Client will: • have stable vital signs and be alert and responsive • have lungs clear to auscultation • have unlabored respirations and maintain oxygen saturation above 95% • have a clean, dry wound with edges well-approximated, healing by first intention • tolerate ordered diet without vomiting • have moist mucous membranes • have a urine specific gravity = 1.005–1.020 Family demonstrates understanding of home care Instructions Family displays effective coping with ongoing stressors	Client is afebrile, has stable vital signs, and is alert and oriented Client has lungs clear to auscultation and unlabored respirations with an O_2 saturation >95% Client has clean, dry wound with edges well-approximated Client has moist mucous membranes and urine specific gravity = 1.005–1.020 Family successfully plans for and transfers child home Client tolerates ordered diet without vomiting Family exhibits ability to cope with ongoing stressors
Assessments, tests, and treatments	Electrolytes Urine specific gravity q8hr Weight Vital signs and O_2 saturation and wound drainage assessment q15min × 4; q30min × 4; q1hr × 24 and prn Assess respiratory status q2–4hr and prn Level of consciousness Change position frequently Assess abdomen and bowel sounds q2–4hr Oxygen as ordered Strict intake and output Record and report vomiting Monitor temperature and provide warming measures as indicated Provide ongoing emotional support to family	Weight Urine specific gravity q8hr Vital signs, O_2 saturation, and dressing and wound drainage assessment q2–4hr and prn Assess respiratory status q4hr and prn Change position frequently Assess abdomen and bowel sounds q4hr Dressing change and wound assessment BID and prn Strict intake and output Observe responses to feeding and feeding technique Record and report vomiting Monitor temperature and provide warming or cooling measures as indicated	Weight Vital signs, O_2 saturation, and dressing and wound drainage assessment upon discharge Assess respiratory status Change position frequently Assess wound and apply dry sterile dressing every day and prn Assess abdomen and bowel sounds upon discharge Observe responses to feeding and feeding technique Record and report vomiting Monitor temperature and return for health care if needed
Knowledge deficit	Orient family to room and surroundings Provide simple, brief instructions Encourage family involvement in care Review specific postoperative care: turning, intravenous, pain management Evaluate understanding of teaching	Review plan of care Begin discharge teaching regarding wound care/dressing change and diet Review written discharge instructions with family Continue to encourage family participation in care Observe and coach family members regarding feeding Evaluate understanding of teaching	Complete discharge teaching to include wound care, diet, follow-up care and appointment, signs and symptoms to report, activity, and medication: name, purpose, dose, frequency, route, food interactions, and side effects Provide family with written discharge instructions regarding home care Evaluate understanding of teaching Provide telephone number/resource for questions

(continued)

Category	Immediate Postoperative Period	Transition to Discharge	Discharge to Home Care
Psychosocial	Assess anxiety related to surgery Encourage verbalization of concerns Assess coping status of family Provide emotional support to client and family Cuddle prn and encourage parents to cuddle child	Assess level of anxiety Encourage verbalization of concerns Assess coping status of family Provide emotional support to client and family Provide information and ongoing encouragement	Assess level of anxiety Encourage verbalization of concerns Assess coping status of family Provide emotional support to client and family Provide information and ongoing encouragement
Diet	NPO until feeding ordered	When fully awake, begin progressive diet as ordered Continue progressing diet as ordered Position on right side with head up after feedings Burp before feedings and frequently during feedings	Diet as ordered Position on right side with head up after feedings Burp before feedings and frequently during feedings Pacifier between meals if desired
Activity	Assess safety needs and provide adequate precautions	Maintain safety precautions	Maintain safety precautions
Medications	IV fluids Analgesics as ordered	Maintain IV line as ordered Analgesics as ordered	Analgesics as ordered D/C IV line
Transfer/discharge plans	Establish discharge objectives with family Determine discharge needs Assess support system Begin home care instructions	Review progress toward discharge goals Make appropriate referrals Finalize discharge plans	Complete discharge instructions Ensure safe transfer home

Note: From Beyea, S. C. (1996). *Critical pathways for collaborative nursing care.* Upper Saddle River, NJ: Prentice Hall-Health. Modified.

GASTROESOPHAGEAL REFLUX

Gastroesophageal reflux, the return of gastric contents into the esophagus, is the result of relaxation of the lower esophageal sphincter. It may occur at any time and is not necessarily related to having a full stomach.

Some "spitting up" after feedings is considered normal in newborn infants, because of the weak cardiac sphincter of the stomach. However, regurgitation that continues and increases in frequency, resulting in delayed growth, may be called "reflux disease," and requires further investigation. Gastroesophageal reflux is more common in premature infants and in children with neurologic impairments. It often resolves without surgical intervention by 12 to 18 months of age (Berube, 1997).

Children with gastroesophageal reflux are frequently hungry and irritable. They eat often but still lose weight. They have a history of vomiting and frequent upper respiratory infections. Reflux of stomach contents can lead to aspiration, resulting in frequent bouts of pneumonia, reactive airway disease, color changes during feeding, apnea, or hematemesis (Levy, 2001).

Diagnosis is confirmed by a thorough history of the child's feeding patterns and by diagnostic evaluation using contrast upper GI series, upper GI endoscopy, pH probe monitoring (insertion of a small catheter into the esophagus through the nose that is left in place for 18 to 24 hours to measure pH and thus determine number of reflux episodes), or gastroesophageal scintigraphy (radionuclide scanning to evaluate gastric emptying) (Murray & Christie, 2000).

Treatment depends on the severity of the condition. Mild cases may require only a modification of feeding habits, and usually resolve by 12 to 18 months (Murray & Christie, 2000). One to six teaspoons of rice cereal can be added to each ounce of formula in the infant's bottle to thicken feedings. Fatty foods and citrus juices are avoided. Medications (cholinergics, antacids, and histamine antagonists) may be prescribed to reduce the amount of stomach acid and lessen the child's discomfort (see Table 46–1). The child should be positioned with the upper body raised 30 degrees after feedings.

Treatment for severe cases may include surgery to create a valve mechanism by wrapping the greater curvature of the stomach (fundus) around the distal esophagus (Nissen fundoplication). A gastrostomy tube is usually inserted during surgery and left in place for 6 weeks. Both infants with mild conditions and those undergoing surgical correction usually have decreased incidence of reflux. **WEB** They may have episodes of mild reflux throughout life and may occasionally require medication for treatment.

TABLE 46-1 Medications Used to Treat Gastroesophageal Reflux

Drug	Action
Antacid (aluminum hydroxide, aluminum carbonate)	Neutralizes refluxed material and decreases resultant discomfort
Mucosal protectant	Forms a barrier on ulcers to protect them from pepsin and bile
Histamine blocker Ranitidine Cimetidine	Decreases gastric acid production
Metoclopramide	Increases esophageal motility and tone
Cisapride	Increases esophageal motility and tone
Acetaminophen	Controls pain

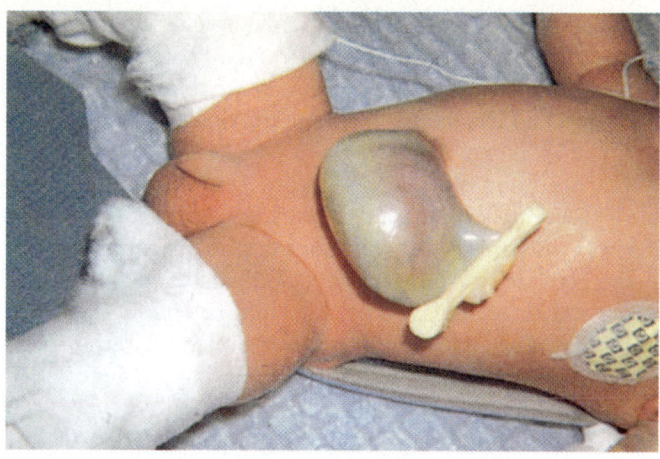

FIGURE 46-4. ◆ In omphalocele, the size of the sack depends on the extent of the protrusion of abdominal contents through the umbilical cord. *Note:* From Rudolph, A. M., Hoffman, J. I. E., & Rudolph, C. D. (Eds.). (1991). *Rudolph's pediatrics* (19th ed., p. 1040). Stamford, CT: Appleton & Lange.

Nursing Management

Nursing management focuses on obtaining a thorough history of the child's feeding patterns. Observe vomiting episodes and document amount, color, and consistency of emesis.

Monitor the infant's weight daily and plot on a growth chart to note progress. Observe for any signs of respiratory distress, and keep the infant's nose and mouth clear of vomitus.

Adequate nutrition must be maintained. Infants receiving oral feedings should be given small, frequent feedings. Elevate the head of the bed to prevent aspiration if vomiting should occur. If the child has difficulty maintaining this position, a Tracy harness or reflux board may be used. The harness, which is pinned to the mattress, supports the infant in an upright position. If the child has a gastrostomy tube, it is important to maintain skin integrity around the stoma site. Secure the tube so the infant cannot dislodge or pull on it, and check daily to be sure the length is the same, indicating correct placement.

Discharge planning focuses on instructing parents in how to feed and position the infant, as well as providing comfort and emotional support. Encourage parents to hold and cuddle the infant during all feedings. Providing the infant with a pacifier helps to meet nonnutritive sucking needs. Teach parents how to suction the nose and mouth if vomiting occurs. Discourage use of infant seats since they usually increase intra-abdominal pressure and worsen reflux symptoms.

OMPHALOCELE

Omphaloceles are congenital malformations in which intra-abdominal contents herniate through the umbilical cord (Figure 46-4 ◆). They result when the abdominal contents, such as intestines and liver, fail to return to the abdomen when the abdominal wall begins to close by the tenth week of gestation. The protrusion is covered by a translucent sac (peritoneum) into which the umbilical cord inserts. Omphalocele is often associated with other congenital anomalies such as cardiac defects; genitourinary anomalies; trisomy 13, 18, or 21; craniofacial abnormalities; and diaphragmatic abnormalities (Brown, Irish, Rice, et al., 1998). Omphalocele with intestinal contents in the sac occurs in 1 in 5000 births, while those involving liver and intestines occur in 1 in 10,000 births (Stoll & Kliegman, 2000).

The size of the sac varies depending on the extent of the protrusion. Rupture of the sac results in evisceration of the abdominal contents. Treatment involves protecting the sac from injury, providing fluids and warmth, and surgical repair to replace the abdominal contents and close the abdominal wall. For smaller defects, primary closure is accomplished with one surgery. If the defect is severe, surgical correction may be performed in several steps. If an omphalocele occurs without associated defects, the child usually recovers from the surgery without incident and leads a normal life.

Nursing Management

Be alert for signs of associated congenital anomalies. (Refer to the discussions of tracheoesophageal fistula earlier in this chapter; to genitourinary anomalies in Chapter 47; and to congenital heart defects in Chapter 43.) ⊂⊃

Immediately after birth, cover the sac with sterile gauze soaked in normal saline solution to prevent drying of the abdominal contents. Place a layer of plastic wrap over the gauze to provide additional protection against heat and moisture loss. Monitor vital signs every 2 to 4 hours, paying close attention to temperature, as the infant can lose heat through the sac. The child should be in a warmer or isolette for maintenance of temperature control. Inspect the area for signs of infection.

Because the infant is NPO preoperatively, maintain fluid and electrolyte with intravenous fluids. Postoperative care includes measures to control pain, prevent infection, maintain fluid and electrolyte balance, and ensure adequate nutritional intake.

Throughout the infant's hospitalization, parents need clear, accurate explanations about the infant's condition. To help the parents deal with the crisis of an acutely ill newborn, provide emotional support and encourage parents to express their feelings. When the child has multiple anomalies, parents need ongoing support for the lengthy treatment, numerous hospitalizations, and management of nutritional intake.

Expected outcomes of nursing care depend on the severity of defect and its correction. Some examples include maintenance of normal vital signs, prompt identification of additional problems, healing of surgical site without signs of infection, pain control, proper intake of fluids, and establishment of an intake to support growth patterns.

INTUSSUSCEPTION

Intussusception occurs when one portion of the intestine prolapses and then invaginates or telescopes into another. It is one of the most frequent causes of intestinal obstruction during infancy, with an incidence of 1 to 4 in 1000 births. Most cases occur in boys between the ages of 3 months and 6 years (Wylie, 2000).

The most common site of intussusception is the ileocecal valve. Telescoping of the intestine obstructs the passage of stool. The walls of the intestine rub together, causing inflammation, edema, and decreased blood flow. This can lead to necrosis, perforation, hemorrhage, and peritonitis.

The onset is usually abrupt. A previously healthy infant or child suddenly experiences acute abdominal pain with vomiting and passage of brown stool. There may be periods of comfort between acute episodes of pain. As the condition worsens, painful episodes increase. The stools become red and resemble currant jelly because of the mix of blood and mucus. A palpable mass may be present in the upper right quadrant or mid-upper abdomen.

Diagnosis is made on the basis of the history and confirmed by radiographs and ultrasound of the abdomen; barium enema may be used (Orenstein, 2000). In some cases the hydrostatic pressure from the barium moves the bowel back into place. Oxygen, saline, and aqueous contrast material may also be used to reduce the intussusception. If these treatments are ineffective, surgical intervention to reduce the invaginated bowel and remove any necrotic tissue is necessary. Surgery usually corrects the problem.

Nursing Management

Nursing management focuses on maintaining or restoring fluid and electrolyte balance. Intravenous fluids are started immediately. Serum electrolyte monitoring is essential to correct imbalances.

Postoperative care focuses on monitoring for early signs of infection, managing the child's pain, and maintaining nasogastric tube patency. Assess vital signs, check for abdominal distention, and listen for bowel sounds every 4 hours. After normal bowel function returns, begin clear liquid feedings. Feedings are advanced to half-strength milk and other foods as the infant or child tolerates it.

Discharge usually occurs shortly after the infant or child begins taking full feedings. Instruct parents to watch for infection and to call the physician if symptoms recur, a fever develops, or appetite decreases.

HIRSCHSPRUNG DISEASE

Hirschsprung disease, also known as congenital aganglionic megacolon, is a congenital anomaly in which inadequate motility causes mechanical obstruction of the intestine. The absence of autonomic parasympathetic ganglion cells in the colon prevents peristalsis at that portion of the intestine, resulting in the accumulation of intestinal contents and abdominal distention. Hirschsprung disease is more common in boys (4:1) and can occur in combination with congenital heart defects, Down syndrome, and some other syndromes such as Smith-Lemli-Opitz syndrome and Waardenburg syndrome. It can be acute or chronic and occurs in 1 in 5000 births (Nowicki & Bishop, 1999). A family history is involved in about 10% of cases; a proto-oncogene and other genetic causes have been identified (Pearl, Irish, Caty, et al., 1998). In contrast, another disorder known as chronic intestinal pseudo-obstruction (pseudo-Hirschsprung) is very rare and affects small bowel motility (Barr, 2000).

Clinical manifestations of Hirschsprung disease vary depending on the child's age at onset. In newborns, symptoms include failure to pass meconium, refusal to suck, abdominal distention, and bile-stained emesis. If Hirschsprung disease is not treated, the condition can lead to complete obstruction, respiratory distress, and shock.

In the older child, symptoms may include failure to gain weight and delayed growth. The child may have a history of abdominal distention, severe constipation alternating with **diarrhea** (frequent, watery stools), and vomiting. The stool may be normal size or have a ribbonlike appearance.

Diagnosis is made on the basis of the history, bowel patterns, anorectal manometry (reaction of the anal sphincter to distention of the rectum), radiographic contrast studies, and rectal biopsy for presence or absence of ganglion cells (Pearl et al., 1998). The rectum is small in size on palpation and does not contain stool.

Treatment in infancy involves surgical removal of the aganglionic bowel. In severe cases or in ill infants, a temporary colostomy is created. Closure of the colostomy and reanastomosis are performed at a later point (Pearl et al., 1998).

For the child with a milder defect, management may involve dietary modification, stool softeners, and isotonic irrigations to prevent impaction until the child is toilet trained.

The return of normal bowel function depends on the amount of bowel involved. Some fecal incontinence and constipation may persist following surgery. A serious complication is enterocolitis (inflammation of the intestines), which occurs in 20% to 60% of children after surgery (Pearl et al., 1998). Symptoms of enterocolitis include GI bleeding and diarrhea. Enterocolitis can occur before or after surgery, resulting in ischemia and ulceration of the bowel wall. Treatment may include total parenteral nutrition and a lactose-free diet.

Nursing Management

Nursing assessment in the newborn period includes careful observation for the passage of meconium. Because newborns are often discharged within 24 hours of birth, tell parents to notify the physician if no stool is passed or the abdomen becomes distended. When the disease is diagnosed later in infancy or in childhood, take a thorough history of weight gain, nutritional intake, and bowel habits.

Nursing management consists of carefully monitoring fluid and electrolyte balance and maintaining nutrition. Teach parents how to ensure regular bowel movements. Daily rectal irrigations with normal saline solution are necessary to promote adequate elimination and prevent obstruction. Teach parents how to prevent skin breakdown in the rectal area by changing diapers frequently, cleansing the area carefully, and applying protective ointment at each diaper change.

If surgical correction is necessary, nursing care includes monitoring for infection, managing pain, maintaining hydration, measuring abdominal circumference to detect any distention, and providing support to the child and family. Parents need instruction in ostomy care if the child has a colostomy (refer to the discussion later in this chapter). Provide appropriate referrals to an ostomy support group and enterostomal nurse specialist when indicated. Teach parents to be alert for and immediately report signs of complications. These include diarrhea and pelvic abscess from leakage of intestinal contents at the surgical site (characterized by fever and pain). Children occasionally develop constipation, and parents may need guidance to adapt the diet and fluid intake to manage this complication. Because some children develop malabsorption, be alert for signs of poor growth or malnutrition.

Expected outcomes of nursing care include prompt identification of obstruction, maintenance of normal bowel patterns, adequate hydration, and maintenance of clear skin.

ANORECTAL MALFORMATIONS

Malformations of the anus and rectum are common congenital anomalies. Minor anomalies occur in 1 in 4000 to 5000 births. They are often associated with anomalies of the urinary tract, esophagus, and duodenum (Brown et al., 1998). Table 46–2 describes the most common anorectal anomalies.

TABLE 46-2	Management of Anorectal Malformations	
Condition	Management
Males	
Cutaneous fistula Anal stenosis Anal membrane	No colostomy required

Rectourethral fistula
    Bulbar
    Prostatic
Rectovesical fistula
Anorectal agenesis without fistula
Rectal atresia
	Colostomy required

Females	
Cutaneous perineal fistula	No colostomy required
Vestibular fistula Vaginal fistula Anorectal agenesis without fistula Rectal atresia Persistent cloaca	Colostomy required

Note: From Warner, B. W. (1996). Classification of congenital disorders of the anorectum. In A. M. Rudolph et al., *Rudolph's pediatrics* (29th ed., p. 1112). Stamford, CT: Appleton & Lange.

Diagnosis is usually made at birth or during the newborn assessment of anorectal structures and rectal patency. Failure to pass meconium may indicate a malformation high in the colon. Stool in the urine indicates a fistula between the colon and urinary tract. Ribbonlike stools may occur with some malformations. Ultrasound and lower GI radiographic studies confirm the diagnosis and demonstrate the extent of the anomaly. Higher defects are often less apparent at birth and involve more complicated treatment (Hendren, 1998).

Medical management depends on the extent of the malformation. Some stenosed anal openings can be treated with dilation alone. An imperforate anal membrane is excised surgically, followed by daily manual dilations. More severe defects require reconstructive surgery. A temporary colostomy is sometimes performed to rest the bowel after reconstruction. The colostomy is generally closed between the age of 6 months and 1 year.

Nursing Management

During the initial newborn assessment, inspect the perineal area for a poorly developed anal dimple or sacral anomalies. Lubricate a rectal thermometer and insert it a short distance into the rectum to determine patency. Observation and recording of passage of meconium are essential.

Once the diagnosis has been made, intravenous fluids are initiated and a nasogastric tube is inserted to decompress the stomach. Monitor the child's intake and output and cardiorespiratory functioning. Provide emotional support to the parents and give them information about the upcoming surgery.

Postoperative care centers on preventing infection and respiratory complications from surgery, as well as maintaining hydration. Observe the incision for signs of infection, and provide careful wound care. Assess vital signs at least every 4 hours. Once the child's condition is stable, clear fluid oral intake is allowed, advancing to half- and full-strength formula or breast milk as tolerated. The infant will have a colostomy after surgery, and careful skin care around the stoma is essential to prevent breakdown of the fragile area. Colostomy care was a particular focus of nursing management for Jerome, described at the beginning of this chapter.

DISCHARGE PLANNING AND HOME CARE TEACHING

Infants are increasingly discharged shortly after birth, so parents need clear instructions about normal newborn stools and what abnormalities to report.

After surgery, teach parents how to take the infant's temperature using the axillary route (see Skill 9-13). SKILLS CD Have them demonstrate the proper technique before discharge. Explain the signs and symptoms of infection. Discuss feeding regimens and bowel habits necessary to maintain adequate nutrition for growth and development. Advise parents that children with anorectal malformations may have difficulty achieving bowel control. Patience in toilet training is important. When the child reaches an age appropriate for toilet training, encourage the family to speak with a health care provider to discuss the child's progress.

If a colostomy is performed, teach parents how to care for the ostomy site (see discussion of ostomies later in this chapter). Reassure parents that the colostomy will be closed in the future, and help them plan for that hospitalization. Discuss follow-up care and long-term management. Arrange follow-up visits and home care visits to evaluate the child's ostomy site and monitor growth.

Expected outcomes of nursing care include adequate fluid intake, normal bowel patterns, parental knowledge of ostomy or other treatment protocols, and eventual success with toilet training.

❧ HERNIAS

A **hernia** is the protrusion or projection of an organ or a part of an organ through the muscle wall of the cavity that normally contains it. This protrusion may result from the failure of normal openings to close during fetal development or from weakness in the supporting musculature. When intra-abdominal pressure increases (as when the infant cries or strains to pass stool), the weakened area separates, causing a protrusion of underlying organs. Inguinal hernias are the most common type of hernia occurring in children (see Chapter 47). Other hernias that occur frequently in children are diaphragmatic and umbilical.

DIAPHRAGMATIC HERNIA

In a diaphragmatic hernia, abdominal contents protrude into the thoracic cavity through an opening in the diaphragm. Sites of herniation include the substernal space, posterolateral region, and the esophageal hiatus. The posterolateral site (foramen of Bochdalek) is the most common location. The cause is a delay or failure in closure of the pleuroperitoneal musculature. The overall incidence of diaphragmatic hernia is 1 in 5000 live births, and 1 in 2000 stillbirths (Hartman, 2000). Associated anomalies, particularly cardiac defects, occur in some infants.

A diaphragmatic hernia is a life-threatening condition. Severe respiratory distress occurs shortly after birth. As the infant cries, abdominal organs extend into the thorax, decreasing the size of the thoracic cavity. The infant becomes dyspneic and cyanotic. Characteristic findings include a barrel-shaped chest and sunken abdomen.

Some cases of congenital diaphragmatic hernia are diagnosed in utero by ultrasound. Chest x-ray examination confirms postnatal diagnosis. Immediate respiratory support is essential. The infant is positioned with the head and thorax higher than the abdomen to facilitate downward movement of abdominal organs. A nasogastric tube is inserted to decompress the stomach. Ventilator support is necessary to manage respiratory compromise. Intravenous fluids are administered through an umbilical artery catheter.

Once the infant's condition is stabilized, the defect is corrected surgically. Extracorporeal membrane oxygenation (ECMO) may be used to provide cardiopulmonary bypass to rest the lungs. The prognosis is poor. Only 50% of infants survive, with death usually resulting from pulmonary hypoplasia. Even after surgery the infant may do well initially and then manifest severe respiratory decompensation.

Nursing Management

The infant with a diaphragmatic hernia is admitted to the neonatal intensive care unit (NICU) and requires continuous monitoring. Preoperative management centers on providing supportive care to the infant and parents. Note the infant's vital signs every 30 minutes on the cardiorespiratory monitor. Observe for worsening of respiratory compromise. Maintain intravenous fluid administration. Promote decreased stimulation to keep the infant calm and thus maintain low abdominal pressure. Keep parents informed about the infant's condition, and provide emotional support both before and after surgery.

Postoperative care includes positioning the infant on the affected side to facilitate expansion of the lung on the unaffected side, observing closely for signs of infection, maintaining respiratory support, and carefully monitoring fluid and electrolyte balance.

Before discharge, instruct parents in wound care, prevention of infection, and feeding techniques.

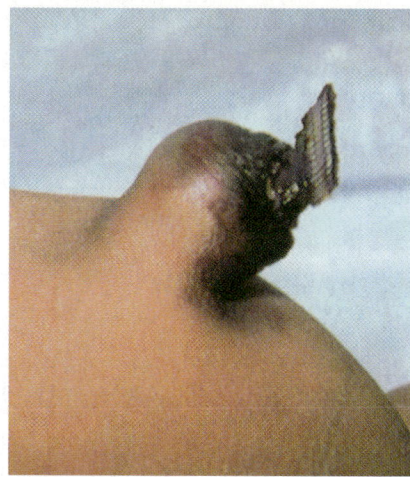

FIGURE 46–5. ◆ The umbilical hernia of the newborn usually closes as the muscles strengthen in later infancy and childhood. *Note:* From Zitelli, B., & Davis, H. (Eds.). (1994). *Atlas of pediatric physical diagnosis* (2nd ed.). London: Mosby-Wolfe Publishing.

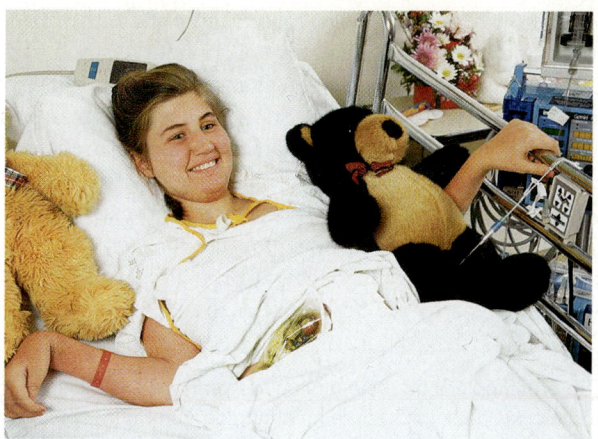

FIGURE 46–6. ◆ Nursing strategies to address altered perceptions of body image and increased feelings of dependence are important when working with adolescents who have ostomies. Support groups or a visit from another teenager who has had an ostomy can facilitate positive coping, as demonstrated by this teenage girl.

UMBILICAL HERNIA

An umbilical hernia results from a weak or imperfectly closed umbilical ring (Figure 46–5 ◆). The condition is often associated with diastasis recti (lateral separation of the abdominal muscles). It is more common in black children, in girls, and in low-birth-weight infants (O'Donnell, Glick, & Caty, 1998).

The hernia appears as a soft swelling covered by skin. The herniated area protrudes with coughing, crying, or straining during a bowel movement. It is easily reduced by pushing the bowel back through the fibrous ring. The size of the defect may vary among individuals. Contents of the hernia include omentum or portions of the small intestine.

Most defects resolve spontaneously by 3 to 4 years of age. Surgery is indicated in cases of strangulation (closure of the umbilical ring around a portion of the bowel, preventing it from moving back into the abdomen), increased protrusion of the hernia after the age of 2 years, or little or no improvement in a large defect after the age of 4 years.

Nursing management is generally supportive. Instruct parents not to apply tape, straps, or coins to reduce the hernia. This can cause strangulation of the hernia, necessitating immediate surgery. If surgery is required, it is usually performed in a short-stay unit. Postoperatively, teach parents how to care for the surgical site, to watch for bleeding, and to recognize signs of infection. Reinforce the importance of returning for follow-up evaluation.

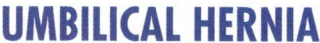 OSTOMIES

An intestinal **ostomy** is an opening, or **stoma,** into the small or large intestine that diverts fecal matter, providing an outlet when a distal surgical anastomosis, obstruction, or nonfunctioning structure prevents normal elimination. Depending on the integrity and function of anatomic structures, the ostomy may be temporary or permanent. Infants and small children with necrotizing enterocolitis, Hirschsprung disease, volvulus, or intussusception may require a temporary colostomy or ileostomy. Ostomies may also be indicated for children with inflammatory bowel disease, intestinal tumors, or abdominal trauma.

An ostomy may be elective or a surgical emergency. In all cases it affects a child's lifestyle, alters body image, causes anxiety, and increases the risk for alterations in physiologic processes (electrolyte imbalance, increased nutritional requirements). For adolescents, it may also result in dependence at a time when autonomy is a major developmental need (Figure 46–6 ◆).

In assessing the family and child approaching ostomy surgery, it is important to determine their ability to understand and accept the physical changes that will occur. Parents may feel guilt and anger about the ostomy surgery when the child has a genetically transmitted disease, is injured, or has developed an obstruction from necrosis of the bowel. Encourage the parents and child to express their feelings, and correct any misunderstandings. Parents and older children may be referred for counseling and to support groups to help them deal with their feelings. Adolescents often benefit from a visit with an adolescent ostomate (someone who has an ostomy) who can answer questions about living with an ostomy.

PREOPERATIVE CARE

Preoperative education focuses on educating the child and family and preparing them for postoperative management.

Discuss how the appliance will look, and explain the purpose of the pouch in developmentally appropriate terms. Encourage the parents and child to touch and manipulate all equipment. A younger child can be shown how to place a pouch on a doll. Older children can practice placing a pouch on their skin. These measures help relieve anxiety by providing information and increasing familiarity with the appliance.

Growth and Development

> The preschooler has some manual dexterity and can help with some parts of the procedure for changing an ostomy appliance and cleaning the stoma. Teach the child using a doll or stuffed animal. Many school-age children are able to care for their ostomy independently. Teach them how to avoid leakage around the bag, which could be embarrassing. Adolescents are generally totally independent in their self-care of ostomies. However, they may need support to deal with the fact that they are different from their peers.

In addition to discussion of the appliance, preoperative education should include discussion of pain control and measures that will be used to prevent postoperative complications (turning, coughing, and breathing deeply). Gear the instructions to the child's developmental level. Encourage parental participation to promote compliance.

POSTOPERATIVE CARE

Postoperative care of a child with an ostomy is similar to that for any child who undergoes abdominal surgery. (See the earlier discussion of nursing management for appendicitis and "Nursing Care Plan: The Child Undergoing Surgery" in Chapter 34.) Management of the stoma may be done by an "ostomy nurse" or other nurses. Major interventions involve ensuring proper function of the stoma, identifying complications, and instituting daily stoma care. Assess the stoma, quality and amount of fecal matter, skin condition, and adherence of the pouch. Evaluate for the most common complications, which are prolapse, retraction, stenosis, and skin breakdown around the stoma (Borkowski, 1998). Evaluate the family's understanding and their ability to care for the ostomy.

Identify and address home care needs well in advance of discharge. Instructions include skin care, care of the stoma, appliance removal and application, and frequency of appliance changes (see Skills 16-3–16-4). **SKILLS** **CD** Begin teaching immediately after surgery with responsibility for care transferred gradually to the parents and child as they are ready. Discuss diet, activity level, hygiene, clothing, equipment, and financial considerations. Arrange for home visits to check periodically on the home management program.

Parents and children can be referred to the United Ostomy Association **WEB** or a local ostomy group for information and support. Make referrals to social service, counseling, and a home health agency, if appropriate.

Expected outcomes of nursing care include successful adjustment to the ostomy, thorough evacuation of the bowel, absence of infection and other complications, intact skin, and formation of a positive self-image in the child.

Nursing Practice
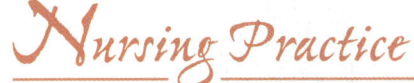

Avoid adhesive enhancers on the skin of newborns and premature infants. Their skin layers are so thin that removal of the appliance can strip off the skin. Remember also that adhesive contains latex and its constant use is not advised due to risk of latex allergy development (see Chapter 40).

⚋ INFLAMMATORY DISORDERS

Inflammatory disorders are reactions of specific tissues of the GI tract to trauma caused by injuries, foreign bodies, chemicals, microorganisms, or surgery. These disorders may be acute or chronic and may involve various segments of the GI tract.

APPENDICITIS

Appendicitis is an inflammation of the vermiform appendix, the small sac near the end of the cecum. The condition occurs most often in adolescent boys (10 to 19 years of age) (Hamilton, Rao, Wagner, et al., 1998). It is rarely seen before 2 years of age.

Etiology and Pathophysiology

Appendicitis almost always results from an obstruction in the appendiceal lumen. It can be caused by a fecalith (hard fecal mass), parasitic infestations, stenosis, hyperplasia of lymphoid tissue, or a tumor. Continued secretion of mucus following acute obstruction of the lumen increases pressure, causing ischemia, cellular death, and ulceration.

The appendix may perforate or rupture, resulting in fecal and bacterial contamination of the peritoneum. Peritonitis spreads quickly and if untreated can result in small bowel obstruction, electrolyte imbalances, septicemia, and hypovolemic shock.

Clinical Manifestations

At onset, symptoms include periumbilical cramps, abdominal tenderness, and fever (Pena, Taylor, & Lund, 1999). In adolescent and young adult females, symptoms must be differentiated from those associated with ovulation (mittelschmerz), ruptured ectopic pregnancy, and pelvic inflammatory disease. As the inflammation progresses, pain

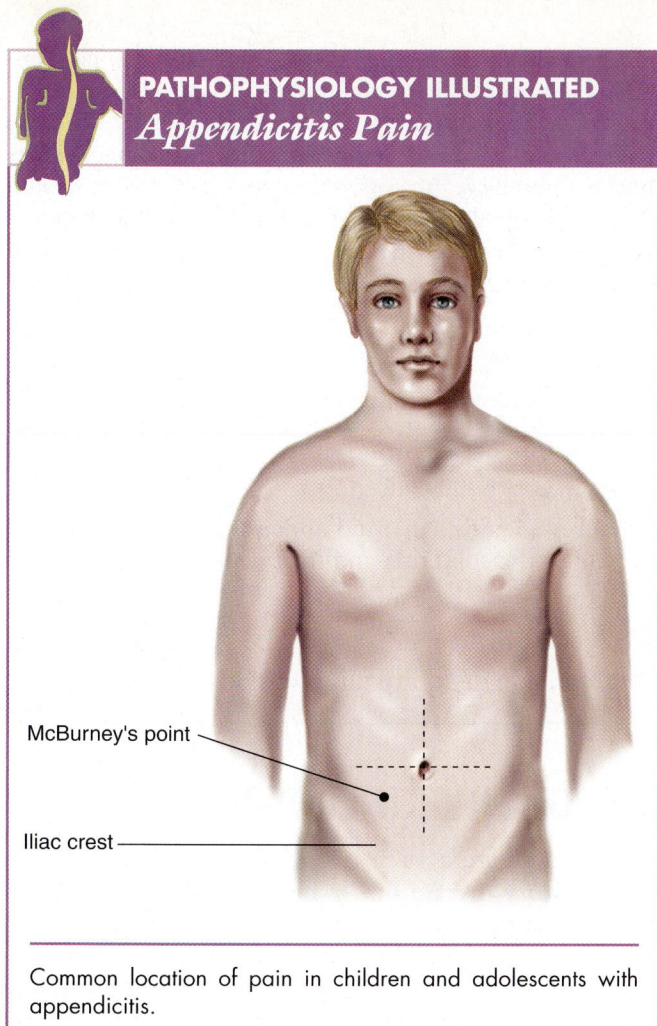

McBurney's point

Iliac crest

Common location of pain in children and adolescents with appendicitis.

An elevated white blood cell count (above 15,000/mm³) may occur. This leukocytosis occurs less often in young children than in teenagers. A history of abdominal pain, presence of a fecalith in the right lower abdomen on x-ray, and abdominal ultrasound help to confirm the diagnosis. Focused appendiceal computerized tomography (FACT) is a new technique that shows success in diagnosing the condition (Rao, Rhea, Novelline, et al., 1998).

Treatment involves immediate surgical removal (appendectomy). Preoperatively the child is kept NPO. Intravenous fluids, electrolytes, and antibiotics are administered. A nasogastric tube may be inserted before or after surgery. Postoperatively the child has an abdominal incision, and intravenous antibiotics are administered to prevent infection. If the appendix has ruptured before surgery, a Penrose drain is inserted and the wound may not be completely sutured. Wound irrigations may be needed to help cleanse the peritoneum. Recovery is usually complete following uncomplicated removal of the appendix.

Nursing Management

Nursing Assessment and Diagnosis

PHYSIOLOGIC ASSESSMENT

A detailed assessment of the child's pain is necessary to differentiate appendicitis from other illnesses (see Chapter 38). Ask the child to point to the painful area and to describe the pain. Recognize that localizing the pain may be difficult for young children. Note onset, location, and intensity of pain; precipitating factors; and relief measures tried. During abdominal assessment, palpate last to avoid causing additional pain. Assess vital signs to determine baseline values, and monitor every 4 hours thereafter.

PSYCHOSOCIAL ASSESSMENT

Because appendicitis usually occurs in school-age children and adolescents, assessment of the child's coping skills is important. Adolescents, because of their preoccupation with body image, may be concerned about the surgical scar. Assess the parents' and child's anxiety about the sudden hospitalization and need for emergency surgery.

Among the nursing diagnoses that might be appropriate for the child with appendicitis are:

▶ *Pain* related to inflammation and surgery
▶ *Risk for fluid volume deficit* related to fluid volume loss and inadequate fluid volume intake
▶ *Anxiety/fear* related to physical condition
▶ *Risk for infection* related to bowel trauma
▶ *Risk for ineffective airway clearance* related to retained secretions
▶ *Anxiety (parent and child)* related to child's change in health status

in the right lower abdomen becomes constant. Pain is often most intense halfway between the anterior superior iliac crest and the umbilicus (see "Pathophysiology Illustrated: Appendicitis"). In 30% of children, however, the appendix is in a different location, so the pain may occur elsewhere. Symptoms progress to include guarding, rigidity, and rebound tenderness following palpation over the right lower quadrant (Hamilton et al., 1998). If the appendix ruptures, there is usually fever, sudden relief from abdominal pain, guarding and distention of the abdomen, rapid breathing, pallor, chills, and irritability.

Vomiting, diarrhea, or constipation may be present. As appendicitis progresses, the child remains motionless, usually in a side-lying position with knees flexed. Sudden relief of pain usually means that the appendix has ruptured.

Clinical Therapy

Diagnosis of appendicitis in young children can be difficult because their pain may be less localized and their symptoms more diffuse than in the older child. Continuing evaluations over several hours are often needed to establish the diagnosis.

Planning and Intervention

Nursing management focuses on promoting comfort, maintaining hydration, providing emotional support, supporting respiratory function, providing care of the surgical site, and monitoring for symptoms of infection.

PROMOTE COMFORT

A side-lying position with knees bent is usually the most comfortable. Administer analgesics as ordered, and note relief from pain. Manage postoperative pain in a similar manner. The child should be placed in a semi-Fowler or side-lying position on the right side. If the appendix has ruptured, lying on the right side helps the peritoneal cavity drain. Administer pain medication as ordered. Avoid a heating pad, which increases inflammation.

MAINTAIN HYDRATION

Assess fluid volume status every 2 hours. Assess skin turgor, eyes, and mucous membranes for signs of dehydration. Monitor intake and output, and assess vital signs. An intravenous infusion is initiated preoperatively and continued until bowel function returns after surgery. Once bowel sounds return, offer water in small amounts and then other clear fluids.

PROVIDE EMOTIONAL SUPPORT

For many children, this may be their first hospitalization and their first experience with health care personnel beyond their usual provider. The nurse must elicit a history, perform a physical examination, coordinate diagnostic tests, and prepare the child for surgery in a short period of time. Emotional support is essential for both child and parents. Good preoperative education can reduce anxiety. Answer any questions the child or parents may have. In the postoperative period, phone calls from friends or family members may be helpful.

SUPPORT RESPIRATORY FUNCTION

General anesthesia during surgery compromises respiratory function. It is important for the child to turn, cough, and breathe deeply to prevent atelectasis. Encourage the child to splint the incision area with a pillow during coughing to decrease pain.

RECOGNIZE SYMPTOMS OF INFECTION

Assess vital signs and observe the abdominal incision every 4 hours for redness, edema, or drainage. If a drain is present, assess drainage for color, consistency, and amount. After the initial dressing has been changed, perform dressing changes frequently and keep the incision area clean and dry. Administer antibiotics as prescribed.

DISCHARGE PLANNING AND HOME CARE TEACHING

The child is discharged once bowel function returns and he or she has a bowel movement. Give parents instructions on reestablishing a nutritious diet slowly and as tolerated.

Teach parents to recognize the signs and symptoms of infection and to seek early treatment.

Normal activities can be resumed fairly quickly, but the child should avoid strenuous activities and contact sports in the immediate postoperative period. Parents should check with the child's physician before allowing the child to resume sports activities. Home tutoring may be needed for a short time so the child can keep up with schoolwork.

Evaluation

Expected outcomes of nursing care include:

▶ Successful management of pain
▶ Absence of bodily infection
▶ Expressed knowledge and understanding by parent and child of the condition and treatment
▶ Clear respiratory sounds
▶ Adequate hydration
▶ Restoration of normal nutritional intake

NECROTIZING ENTEROCOLITIS

Necrotizing enterocolitis is a potentially life-threatening inflammatory disease of the intestinal tract that occurs primarily in premature infants. It affects from 1% to 8% of infants in the NICU, and has up to a 40% mortality rate (Pearl et al., 1998). It can be caused by several factors, among them intestinal ischemia, bacterial or viral infection (a result of the premature infant's decreased immune response and greater risk for infection), and immaturity of the gut (a result of the premature infant's decreased amount of gastric acid and proteolytic enzymes and underdeveloped protective intestinal mucin layer). The disease occurs most often in the terminal ileum and colon.

The infant may initially show signs of feeding intolerance (increased gastric residuals, vomiting, irritability, and abdominal distention). These signs are caused by inflammation and dilation of the bowel and accumulation of gas in the intestine. Bloody diarrhea may be present because of the hemorrhagic bowel. Signs of sepsis usually follow, and the infant's condition rapidly deteriorates.

Diagnosis is made on the basis of characteristic clinical findings and the presence of free peritoneal gas, dilated bowel loops, bowel distention, and bowel wall thickening on abdominal x-rays. Necrotizing enterocolitis requires prompt intervention. Management begins with discontinuation of all enteral feedings. An orogastric tube is inserted to prevent gastric distention, and intravenous fluids are started. Total parenteral nutrition may be initiated through a central line. Antibiotics are administered prophylactically or to treat sepsis. Perforation or necrosis of the bowel necessitates surgical resection of the bowel. An ileostomy or colostomy may sometimes be performed.

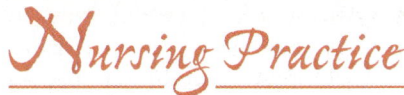

Nursing Practice

Signs of sepsis include:

- ▶ Hypothermia or hyperthermia
- ▶ Jaundice
- ▶ Respiratory distress
- ▶ Hepatomegaly
- ▶ Abdominal distention
- ▶ Anorexia
- ▶ Vomiting
- ▶ Lethargy

All cases of necrotizing enterocolitis are treated with strict enteric precautions to prevent the spread of infection to other premature infants on the unit. Early aggressive enteral formula feedings of premature infants is avoided because of the increased incidence of the disease in these cases. Human milk has been shown to protect against the disease; thus, breastfeeding or feeding the mother's expressed milk is the feeding method of choice for premature infants.

Long-term complications of necrotizing enterocolitis include short bowel syndrome, strictures, **cholestasis,** impaired nutrition and growth, and delayed developmental performance.

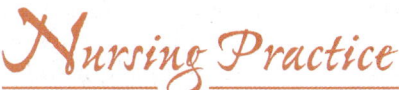

Nursing Practice

Cholestasis is a disruption of bile flow. This is the most common problem in survivors of necrotizing enterocolitis. It is a complication of total parenteral nutrition (TPN) and commonly occurs 2 weeks after TPN therapy has been initiated. It is characterized by an elevated bilirubin (>2 mg/dL), hepatomegaly, and elevated serum transaminase.

Nursing Management

Nursing care centers on prevention and early detection of necrotizing enterocolitis to minimize bowel loss, and providing postoperative care. Watch for feeding intolerance by aspirating gastric residual (if the infant is receiving enteral feedings). Enteral feedings should slowly progress, by no more than 20 mL/kg/day (Committee on Nutrition, American Academy of Pediatrics, 1998). Measure abdominal circumference in the premature or high-risk infant every 4 to 8 hours. Even minimal changes in circumference can indicate necrotizing enterocolitis; report them to the physician.

Maintaining fluid and electrolyte balance is essential. Provide comfort by holding and cuddling an infant who is NPO, and offer a pacifier to meet nonnutritive sucking needs. Careful assessment for infection and maintenance of skin integrity are essential. Gradually reestablish feedings once bowel function returns.

Parents need emotional support and reassurance and help in bonding with their infant. They are coping with the birth of a critically ill infant. Because the symptoms of necrotizing enterocolitis do not appear until approximately 5 to 7 days after feedings are begun, parents may not be prepared for the infant's decline. The recovery of a premature infant is slow and can be complicated. Give clear explanations and encourage parents to ask questions and express their fears and concerns. If the infant's condition worsens, offer support for the parents of a dying child (see Chapter 37).

Once the child is discharged, frequent follow-up is needed. Encourage regular health care visits. Schedule home visits to help the family manage health care and normal developmental issues. If total parenteral nutrition is administered at home, the parents need to know how to administer it correctly and how to care for the central line. Carefully assess oral and enteral nutritional intake. Monitor the child's growth and compare it to previous findings. Several medications are likely to be used, and correct administration techniques must be reinforced. The infant requires regular and thorough physical assessments to identify any complications. Parents need to learn care of the ostomy if the child has one in place. Assess developmental progress by regular use of a test such as the Denver II (see Chapter 35).

Expected outcomes of nursing care for the child with necrotizing enterocolitis include successful treatment of infection, absence of signs of sepsis, management of fluid and electrolyte status, and provision of adequate nutrition. If surgery is performed, complete healing without infection or other complication is desired. If the infant is not successfully treated, support and comfort for the parents is a necessary outcome. When the child survives, long-term outcomes include normal developmental progression and nutrition to support growth.

MECKEL'S DIVERTICULUM

Meckel's diverticulum results when the omphalomesenteric duct, which connects the midgut to the yolk sac during embryonic development, fails to atrophy. Instead, an outpouching of the ileum remains, usually located near the ileocecal valve. The pouch contains gastric or pancreatic tissue, which secretes acid, causing irritation and ulceration. Meckel's diverticulum is the most common GI malformation and cause of lower GI bleeding in children; it occurs in 2% of the population, although many people are asymptomatic and do not know they have the disorder (Pearl et al., 1998).

Clinical manifestations usually appear by 2 years of age. The most common sign is painless dark or bright red rectal bleeding, which results from the obstruction or ulceration. Often blood is passed without stool. Abdominal pain is uncommon, but when it occurs, it may resemble the pain of appendicitis. The child may have symptoms of intussusception, incarcerated hernia, volvulus, or intestinal obstruction. If untreated, diverticulitis may progress to perforation and peritonitis.

Diagnosis is based on the history. Contrast studies are usually not helpful because the diverticulum is often too small to visualize and may not fill with barium. Radionuclide imaging and scanning can usually detect the gastric tissue, confirming the diagnosis.

Treatment is surgical excision of the diverticulum and removal of any involved bowel. The prognosis is good following surgical excision.

Nursing Management

Preoperatively an intravenous infusion is initiated to correct fluid and electrolyte imbalances. Monitor intake and output. Observe for rectal bleeding, and test stools for **occult blood** (blood that is present in small quantities and is measurable only by laboratory testing). Keep the child on bed rest. Assess vital signs every 2 hours, and monitor for signs of shock. Postoperative care is similar to that for an infant or child undergoing abdominal surgery. (See the earlier discussion of postsurgical nursing management of appendicitis and "Nursing Care Plan: The Child Undergoing Surgery" in Chapter 34.)

At discharge, parents need instructions on caring for the surgical site, preventing infection, providing an adequate diet, and administering prescribed medications.

INFLAMMATORY BOWEL DISEASE
Crohn's Disease and Ulcerative Colitis

Inflammatory bowel disease encompasses two distinct chronic disorders, Crohn's disease and ulcerative colitis, that have similar symptoms and treatment. Both diseases involve faulty regulation of the immune response of the intestinal mucosa in genetically predisposed people who have a genetic trigger (Gokhale, 2001). Inflammatory bowel disease differs from irritable bowel syndrome, which is discussed in the section on feeding and elimination disorders in Chapter 36.

Crohn's disease is a chronic, inflammatory process. It can occur randomly throughout the GI tract, with the ileum, colon, and rectum the most common sites. A distinct feature of Crohn's disease is the development of enteric fistulas between loops of bowel or nearby organs. Mucosal ulcers begin in small locations, and then grow in size and depth into the mucosal wall. Submucosal inflammation can be severe. The etiology is unknown. There is strong evidence to support a genetic association. Crohn's disease is more common in whites and three to six times more prevalent in individuals of Jewish descent. It most often develops between 15 and 25 years of age, and has been increasing in incidence (Gokhale, 2001).

The onset of Crohn's disease is subtle. Crampy abdominal pain is usually reported first, followed by diarrhea. Other symptoms include fever, anorexia, growth failure or weight loss, general malaise, and joint pain. Diagnosis is based on laboratory evaluation (anemia is common; an elevated erythrocyte sedimentation rate, hypoalbuminemia, and thrombocytosis are other possible findings), diffuse abdominal tenderness, and radiologic and biopsy examinations.

Ulcerative colitis is a chronic recurrent disease of the colon and rectal mucosa of unknown etiology. Inflammation is limited to the mucosa and can involve the entire length of the bowel with varying degrees of inflammation, ulceration, hemorrhage, and edema. Emotional and other psychosocial factors may influence the presentation and course of the disease. It is more prevalent among persons of Jewish heritage. The disease develops before 20 years of age with peak onset at about 12 years.

The first symptom of ulcerative colitis is usually diarrhea. Lower abdominal pain and cramping are present before and during a bowel movement and are relieved by the passage of stool and flatus. The stool is often mixed with blood and mucus. Weight loss or delayed growth, nutritional deficiencies, and arthralgias often occur as effects of the disease.

Diagnosis centers on evaluating the cause and identifying the extent of involved bowel and differentiating an infectious process (organisms such as *Shigella* and *Salmonella*) from ulcerative colitis. Endoscopy with biopsy is helpful to determine the extent and severity of the inflammatory process. Laboratory and bone age studies help to identify related nutritional, growth, and blood abnormalities.

Crohn's disease and ulcerative colitis have periods of remission and exacerbation. Treatment for both diseases

CLINICAL MANIFESTATIONS ～ *Ulcerative Colitis and Crohn's Disease*

	ULCERATIVE COLITIS	CROHN'S DISEASE
Type of lesions	Continuous, superficial involvement	Segmental, transmural (through the wall) involvement
Clinical manifestations		
Anal or perianal lesions	Rare	Common
Anorexia	Mild to moderate	Can be severe
Diarrhea	Often severe	Moderate
Growth retardation	Mild	Significant
Pain	Present	Common
Rectal bleeding	Present	Absent
Weight loss	Moderate	Severe
Risk of cancer	Slightly increased	Greatly increased

includes pharmacologic interventions (antibiotic, anti-inflammatory, immunosuppressive, and antidiarrheal medications), nutrition therapy, and, in severe cases, surgery. Corticosteroids are given orally and as enemas to children with more severe disease. For children with milder disease, sulfasalazine decreases the number of relapses.

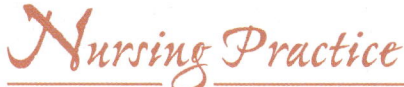

Nursing Practice

The following drugs are used in the treatment of inflammatory bowel disease:

Aminosalicylates	Immunosuppressants
Sulfasalazine	6-Mercaptopurine (6-MP)
Mesalamine	Azathioprine
Olsalazine	Cyclosporine
Balsalazide	Methotrexate
	Tacrolimus (FK-506)
Corticosteroids	
Prednisone	Antibacterial
Methylprednisone	Metronidazole
Hydrocortisone enema	Ciprofloxacin

A nutritionist is part of the team treating the child. The goal of nutrition therapy is to provide adequate caloric intake and nutrients necessary for growth. Vitamin, iron, zinc, and folic acid supplementation is frequently required. Total parenteral nutrition (TPN) is often given to treat nutritional deficiencies and malnutrition, which accompany inflammatory bowel disease (see Skill 12–7). **SKILLS** **CD** A high-protein, high-carbohydrate, low-fiber diet with normal amounts of fat is recommended.

If other treatment measures fail to reduce inflammation, surgery is generally indicated. A temporary colostomy or ileostomy is performed to allow the bowel to rest. In Crohn's disease, however, ulcerations tend to recur elsewhere in the GI tract. Research is being done to see if intravenous infusion of antitumor necrosis factor antibody is successful in treating the disorder (Gokhale, 2001). In ulcerative colitis, removal of the diseased bowel provides a permanent cure.

NURSING MANAGEMENT

Nursing management occurs mainly in the community and home and focuses on helping the child and family adjust to the emotional impact of a chronic disease, administering medications and diet therapy, monitoring nutritional status, and providing appropriate referrals. Provide emotional support and counseling to help the child adjust to feeling "different" from peers. Inability to compete with peers and frequent absences from school can affect the child's self-esteem. Have the parents contact the school district to arrange for tutoring in case extended absences from school become necessary. Encourage the child who is not attending school regularly to maintain contact with friends through telephone calls, cards, and visits.

Growth and Development

Providing adequate stress reduction may be helpful in control of inflammatory bowel disease. Teach young children relaxation techniques, such as deep breathing, progressive tensing and relaxing of muscles, and visualization of favorite places. Encourage busy school-age children and teens to have quiet and restful times each day, in addition to physical activity periods.

If the child is unable to eat or the intake of calories is insufficient to meet basic nutritional and metabolic needs, TPN is ordered (see Skill 12-7). **SKILLS** **CD** If the child is able to eat, parents need instructions about dietary needs. Frequently measure growth and assess nutrition.

Teaching About

DIET INSTRUCTIONS FOR INFLAMMATORY BOWEL DISEASE

- Several small feedings are usually better tolerated than three meals daily.
- Limiting fiber intake can help to decrease intestine motility and inflammation. Peel fruits and avoid large quantities of whole grains and nuts.
- If the child is not eating well, offer high-calorie meals. If lactose intolerance is not a problem for the particular child, cream soups, milkshakes, puddings, and custards can be offered.
- Liquid dietary supplements may be helpful to ensure protein and caloric requirements are met.
- Watch for foods that cause intestinal problems for the individual child, and avoid them in the future.
- Avoid having mealtime become a reason for family strife. Seek help of nurses and dietitians if needed.

Body image is a major concern for children and adolescents with inflammatory bowel disease. Corticosteroid therapy causes growth retardation and delayed sexual maturation. Encourage the child to discuss feelings about these side effects. If a permanent colostomy or ileostomy is required, help the child and family understand the need for surgical treatment. (See the discussion of ostomies earlier in this chapter.) Introduce the child and family to other children who have stomas.

Teach parents about medication administration and diet therapy. Reinforce to both the parents and child the importance of adhering to a strict medication regimen. Emphasize that medications should be continued even when the child is asymptomatic. Discuss the side effects of the drugs and what to do if any of these symptoms occur. When the child is taking systemic corticosteroids, immunizations are generally delayed until after the medication is discontinued.

Parents also need instructions for TPN and care of a central venous catheter, including dressing changes, sterile and nonsterile techniques, signs of infection, how to handle infusion pumps and tubing, and how to measure the child's intake and output. Assist parents in obtaining equipment and supplies necessary for the child's care. Have parents demonstrate their mastery of care for the central venous catheter and their understanding of TPN techniques during home visits and appointments for health care.

Refer parents to social services, the visiting nurse association, and home health care agencies, if they are not receiving any of these services. For information about inflammatory bowel disease, refer families to the Crohn's and Colitis Foundation.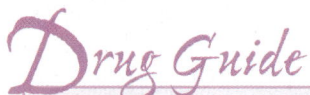

Expected outcomes of nursing care for the child with inflammatory bowel disease include:

- Normal growth and development
- Absence of gastrointestinal distress
- Successful management of medications without demonstration of side effects
- Freedom from infection due to TPN line
- Establishment of positive body image
- Integration of stress-lowering practices into daily life

PEPTIC ULCER

A peptic ulcer is an erosion of the mucosal tissue in the lower end of the esophagus, in the stomach (usually along the lesser curvature), or in the duodenum. Boys are more likely to have peptic ulcers than girls. Peptic ulcers are much less common in children than in adults.

Ulcers are classified as primary or secondary, depending on their etiology. Primary peptic ulcers occur in healthy children. Secondary (stress) ulcers occur in children with a preexisting illness or injury (often a burn) and in children receiving medications such as salicylates, corticosteroids, and nonsteroidal anti-inflammatory drugs. Diet usually is not a major factor in the development of peptic ulcers in children, although caffeine and alcohol consumption in adolescents may exacerbate the disease. It is now known that ulcers in both adults and children are often caused by *Helicobacter pylori*, a gram-negative rod (Herbst, 2000). This organism is transmitted by the fecal–oral or oral–oral routes. Infections often occur in several members of a family, especially when the family's water supply is contaminated.

Clinical manifestations vary according to the age of the child and location of the ulcer. The most common symptom is abdominal pain (burning) associated with an empty stomach, which may awaken the child at night. Vomiting and pain after meals, anemia, occult blood in stools, and abdominal distention may also be present.

Diagnosis is based on the history and radiologic studies. *H. pylori* can be diagnosed by culture of the organism taken via gastroscopy, and by measuring urea in the urine and on the breath, since the organism hydrolyzes urea. The goals of medical management are to relieve discomfort and promote healing. When *H. pylori* is the causative agent, antimicrobial agents such as bismuth salts, tetracycline, and metronidazole combination are given. Other drug combinations, such as a combination of antacids in liquid form (Maalox, Mylanta) and histamine antagonists (ranitidine, cimetidine, and famotidine), are also used. Antibody titers are measured several times over 6 months to evaluate the effectiveness of therapy. The prognosis is usually good with early intervention.

Drug Guide

RANITIDINE

Overview of Action

Ranitidine inhibits histamine action at the H2 receptor sites of parietal cells, prohibiting basal and nocturnal secretion of gastric acid. It also suppresses the gastric acid secretion caused by food, insulin, amino acids, and pentagastrin. It is used for treatment of active GI hemorrhage or peptic ulcer disease, hypersecretory syndrome, and gastroesophageal reflux.

Routes, Dosage, Frequency

Modify dosage for renal impairment.

- **PO:** 2 to 4 mg/kg/day in equally divided doses every 12 hours
- **IM, IV:** Newborns: 1 to 2 mg/kg/day in equally divided doses every 6 to 8 hours; Infants and Children: 4 to 5 mg/kg/day in equally divided doses every 8 to 12 hours; Adolescents and Adults: 50 mg every 6 to 8 hours (maximum daily dosage 400 mg or 6 mg/kg)

Nursing Implications

Assess: Assess amount and location of abdominal pain.

Administer: PO: Unaffected by food, usually given with or after meals. Syrup contains alcohol; peppermint flavored. Tablets can be crushed, mixed with small amounts of food and fluid. Effervescent preparations must be diluted in 80 to 240 mL just prior to ingestion.

IM: Do not use if discolored or has precipitate. Injection may cause burning. **IV:** For those over 12 years old: each 50 mg of drug must be diluted with at least 20 mL of 0.9% sodium chloride, 5% dextrose, or other compatible IV solutions; infuse slowly over at least 5 minutes maximum concentration 2.5 mg/mL. Rapid administration may cause bradycardia, tachycardia, or premature ventricular contractions. For intermittent infusion, dilution is 50 mg/100 mL (5 to 7 mL/min) infused over 15 to 20 min; continuous infusion over 24 hours preferred. Compatible with D5W, D10W, NS, LR.

Monitor: Assess for side effects. Side effects include malaise, dizziness, and vertigo; cardiac arrhythmia; constipation or diarrhea; hepatitis. Monitor blood counts, renal and hepatic function during therapy.

Contraindications and Precautions: The drug is contraindicated in those with prior hypersensitivity to the drug. It is discontinued if liver abnormalities occur, and the dosage is lowered in renal disease.

Note: From Bindler, R. M., & Howry, L. B. (1997). *Pediatric drugs and nursing implications* (2nd ed.). Upper Saddle River, NJ: Prentice Hall-Health. Adapted.

Nursing Management

Nurses may identify children with peptic ulcer disease by looking for the symptoms and noting family history of *H. pylori* infection. Nursing care centers on interventions to promote adequate nutritional intake, promote healing, and prevent recurrences. Provide a nutritionally sound, age-appropriate diet. Omit foods only if they exacerbate the disorder.

Antibiotics must be given as scheduled. Emphasize the importance of continuing drug therapy. The family needs encouragement to continue the medications as ordered and to return for follow-up visits. Children who attend school may prefer to take antacids in the form of tablets, which are easier to carry than liquid preparations. A permission form to take medications at school needs to be filled out by the prescriber. Parents should check with the child's physician before giving any additional medication. Caution parents to avoid aspirin products, which irritate the gastric mucosa. If an antipyretic or pain medication is needed, acetaminophen should be given. Advise parents to read medication labels if they are unsure of product contents.

Because psychologic stress can contribute to peptic ulcer disease, help the parents and child identify sources of stress in the child's life. Assess coping mechanisms and provide referral for psychologic counseling, if appropriate. Teach relaxation techniques and recommend community classes on yoga or other stress reduction.

☙ DISORDERS OF MOTILITY

Fluids are produced in large quantities as part of normal GI functioning. As food passes through the intestines, fluids are reabsorbed and moderately soft stool is formed and evacuated. In disorders such as diarrhea and constipation, fluid production is altered, causing either more or less fluid to be reabsorbed. This can severely alter the characteristics of the stool. Reabsorption of too little water produces diarrhea and can lead to fluid and electrolyte alterations. Reabsorption of too much fluid can cause constipation, which if untreated can lead to bowel obstruction.

GASTROENTERITIS (ACUTE DIARRHEA)

Gastroenteritis is an inflammation of the stomach and intestines that may be accompanied by vomiting and diarrhea. It can affect any part of the GI tract. Diarrhea is a common problem in children. It may be an acute problem, caused by viral, bacterial, or parasitic infections, or a chronic problem. Children under age 5 years average approximately two episodes of gastroenteritis each year (Burkhart, 1999). Infants and small children with gastroenteritis or diarrhea can quickly become dehydrated and are at risk for hypovolemic shock if fluid and electrolyte losses are not replaced (see Chapter 39). 🔗

TABLE 46-3 Causes of Diarrhea in Children

Etiology	Bowel Manifestations
Emotional stress (anxiety, fatigue)	Increased motility
Intestinal infection (bacteria [*E. coli, Salmonella, Shigella*], viral [human rotavirus, enteric adenovirus], fungal overgrowth)	Inflammation of mucosa; increased mucus secretion in colon
Food sensitivity (gluten, cow's milk)	Decreased digestion of food
Food intolerance (lactose, introduction of new foods, overfeeding)	Increased motility; increased mucus secretion in colon
Medications (iron, antibiotics)	Irritation and suprainfection
Colon disease (colitis, necrotizing enterocolitis, enterocolitis)	Inflammation and ulceration of intestinal walls; reduced absorption of fluid; increased intestinal motility
Surgical alterations (short bowel syndrome)	Reduced size of colon; decreased absorption surface

Etiology and Pathophysiology

Diarrhea in children can have many different causes (Table 46–3). The specific etiology is not always identified. The common mechanism is a decrease in the absorptive capacity of the bowel through inflammation, decrease in surface area for absorption, or alteration of parasympathetic innervation. Children in child care centers and those living in substandard housing with improper sanitation are at increased risk.

Clinical Manifestations

Diarrhea may be mild, moderate, or severe. In mild diarrhea, stools are slightly increased in number and have a more liquid consistency. In moderate diarrhea the child has several loose or watery stools. Other symptoms include irritability, anorexia, nausea, and vomiting. Moderate diarrhea is usually self-limiting, resolving without treatment within 1 or 2 days. In severe diarrhea, watery stools are continuous. The child exhibits symptoms of fluid and electrolyte imbalance (see Chapter 39), 🔗 has cramping, and is extremely irritable and difficult to console.

Clinical Therapy

Diagnosis is based on the history, physical examination, and laboratory findings. A thorough history may help identify the cause. Ask parents about recent exposure to illnesses, use of antibiotics, travel, food and formula preparation, food sensitivities or allergies, and whether the child attends day care. Physical examination provides a guide to the severity of dehydration (see Chapter 39). 🔗 The stool can be examined for the presence of ova, parasites, infectious organisms, viruses, fat, and undigested sugars. Laboratory evaluation of serum and urine helps identify electrolyte imbalances and other deficiencies (Murphy, 1998).

DEHYDRATION	CLINICAL THERAPY
None	Feed age-appropriate diet of breast milk or regular formula, complex carbohydrates, and meats (especially chicken) Oral rehydration of 10 mL/kg/stool for ongoing losses
Mild (3%–5%)	Oral rehydration with 50 mL/kg for 4–6 hours or until rehydrated 10 mL/kg/stool for ongoing losses and replacement of estimated emesis volume After rehydration, feed age-appropriate diet
Moderate (6%–9%)	100 mL/kg plus replacement of continuing losses during a 4-hour period Reassess ongoing losses every hour and replace volume for volume After rehydration, feed age-appropriate diet
Severe (≥10%)	True emergency which causes shock or near-shock condition Bolus intravenous therapy with normal saline or Ringer's lactate, 20–40 mL/kg/hr Begin oral rehydration solution when level of consciousness improves After rehydration, feed age-appropriate diet

Note: From Provisional Committee on Quality Improvement, Subcommittee on Acute Gastroenteritis (1996). Practice parameter: the management of acute gastroenteritis in young children. *Pediatrics, 97,* 424–436. Adapted.

Medical management depends on the severity of the diarrhea and fluid and electrolyte imbalances. The goal of treatment is to correct the fluid and electrolyte imbalances. For mild to moderate dehydration the child is rehydrated with oral rehydration therapy (see Chapter 39). ⊂⊃ This may be accomplished at home or in the short-stay observation unit in a hospital with solutions such as Pedialyte, Ricelyte, or Lytren. Carbonated and very sugary beverages should not be given. Fermentation of sugar in the GI tract causes increased gas, abdominal distention, and an increased frequency of diarrhea.

For severe dehydration, rehydration is accomplished by intravenous infusion with a solution chosen to correct the specific imbalances. Isotonic fluid such as normal saline with glucose or Ringer's lactate are commonly used solutions (see Chapter 39 for further information about solutions to correct dehydration). ⊂⊃ As soon as possible, clear liquids are introduced and then the child progresses to a regular diet. Foods generally are not withheld for more than 1 to 2 days (Eliason & Lewan, 1998).

If the diarrhea is caused by bacteria or parasites, antimicrobial therapy may be prescribed. Antiemetics and antidiarrheals are generally not used in young children since they can mask the signs and symptoms of more serious illness.

Nursing Management

Nursing Assessment and Diagnosis

The nurse may encounter the child and family in the emergency department, urgent care center, clinic, or office. The child may be cared for over several hours at a clinic or urgent care center so that dehydration is treated with intravenous infusion and/or oral rehydration, and then sent home with instructions for parents to care for the child. If the child is hospitalized, it is important to assess onset, frequency, color, amount, and consistency of stools. If the child is also vomiting, monitor the amount and type of vomitus. Initial and ongoing physical assessment of the child focuses on observing for signs and symptoms of dehydration, which reflect underlying fluid and electrolyte status. Evaluate urinary output and specific gravity. Weigh the infant or child on admission and daily thereafter. Monitor vital signs every 2 to 4 hours. A febrile child has increased water loss, contributing to the dehydration. Assess skin integrity, especially in the perineal and rectal areas, and note any breakdown or rashes. Avoid commercial baby wipes, which can promote additional skin irritation and breakdown.

"Nursing Care Plan: The Child with Gastroenteritis" lists common nursing diagnoses. Other diagnoses that might also be appropriate include:

▶ *Anxiety (child and parent)* related to change in health status

▶ *Sleep pattern disturbance* related to pain

▶ *Altered nutrition: less than body requirements* related to inability to ingest sufficient nutrients

Planning and Implementation

Nursing care focuses on providing emotional support, promoting rest and comfort, and ensuring adequate nutrition. See "Nursing Care Plan: The Child with Gastroenteritis" for a summary of nursing care.

PROVIDE EMOTIONAL SUPPORT

The child may have been ill for several days or become suddenly ill a short time before seeking health care. The child and parents are usually anxious, so it is important to allow them to talk and ask questions. The child may require blood tests to help direct rehydration therapy. Using ther-

GOAL	INTERVENTION	RATIONALE	EXPECTED OUTCOME

1. Diarrhea related to infectious process

	NIC Priority Intervention:		*NOC Suggested Outcome:*
	Diarrhea management: *Prevention and alleviation of diarrhea*		**Fluid and electrolyte balance:** *Balance of water and electrolytes in the intracellular and extracellular compartments of the body*
The child's bowel function will be restored to normal.	▸ Obtain baseline vital signs and monitor every 2–4 hours.	▸ Fluid and electrolyte imbalances can alter vital body functions.	The child's bowel function returns to normal.
	▸ Observe stools for amount, color, consistency, odor, and frequency.	▸ Aids in the diagnosis and in monitoring the child's status.	
	▸ Test stools for occult blood.	▸ Frequent defecation and some infectious organisms can cause bleeding.	
	▸ Monitor results of stool culture and sample for ova and parasites.	▸ Rapid notification of the physician will facilitate treatment.	
	▸ Wash hands well before and after contact with the child.	▸ Helps prevent transmission of microorganisms.	
	▸ Isolate the child until the cause of the diarrhea is determined.	▸ Prevents exposure of other patients and staff.	
	▸ Assist the child with toileting and hygiene.	▸ The child may be weak, incontinent, physically impaired, or anxious and require assistance to use the bathroom.	
	▸ Administer prescribed oral rehydration and intravenous solutions.	▸ Provides necessary fluids and nutrients.	
	▸ Notify the physician if diarrhea persists, stool characteristics change, or other symptoms of dehydration electrolyte imbalance occur	▸ Ensures early intervention.	

2. Fluid volume deficit related to active fluid volume loss

	NIC Priority Intervention:		*NOC Suggested Outcome:*
	Fluid monitoring: *Collection and analysis of patient data to regulate fluid balance*		**Fluid and electrolyte balance:** *Balance of water and electrolytes in the intracellular and extracellular compartments of the body*
The child will remain hydrated and will begin to drink fluids within 24 hours of admission.	▸ Monitor intake and output. Be sure to document time of each voiding.	▸ Will determine if output exceeds input. Long periods of time without urine output can be an early indicator of poor renal function. A child should produce 1 mL of urine/kg/hr.	The child has normal fluid and electrolyte balance as indicated by laboratory evaluation and physical examination.
	▸ Compare admission weight to preadmission weight. Assess weight daily.	▸ The degree of dehydration can be determined by the percentage of weight loss. Daily weights aid in determining progress toward rehydration.	
	▸ Assess level of consciousness, skin turgor, mucous membranes, skin color and temperature, capillary refill, eyes, and fontanels every 4 hours.	▸ Will determine degree of hydration and adequacy of interventions.	
	▸ Assess for vomiting.	▸ Vomiting frequently accompanies diarrhea and contributes to the child's fluid loss.	
	▸ Provide oral fluid and electrolyte replacement solution if able to tolerate.	▸ Less invasive than IV fluids. Provides for replacement of essential fluids and electrolytes.	
	▸ Provide and maintain IV replacement therapy, as ordered.	▸ Use of IV replacement is based on the degree of dehydration, ongoing losses, insensible water losses, and electrolyte results.	

3. Risk for impaired skin integrity related to altered fluid status

	NIC Priority Intervention:		*NOC Suggested Outcome:*
	Skin surveillance: *Collection and analysis of patient data to maintain skin integrity*		**Tissue integrity:** *Structural intactness and normal physiologic function of skin*
The child will remain free of skin breakdown and rashes.	▸ Assess skin of perineum and rectum for signs of skin breakdown or irritation.	▸ Early assessment and intervention can prevent worsening of the condition.	The child's perianal and rectal tissue remains pink and intact.
	▸ Provide prevention or restorative care for infants as follows:		

(continued)

GOAL	INTERVENTION	RATIONALE	EXPECTED OUTCOME
Preventive care:	▶ Change diapers every 2 hours or as needed.	▶ Minimizes skin contact with chemical irritants from stool and urine.	
	▶ Use cloth diapers rather than disposable.	▶ Minimizes the mechanical and chemical irritation from disposables.	
	▶ Wash diaper area after each soiling.	▶ Removes traces of stool if present.	
	▶ Apply A & D ointment.	▶ Provides a barrier and protects intact or reddened skin from becoming excoriated.	
Restorative care:	▶ Place the infant prone and leave the buttocks open to air.	▶ Promotes air circulation to the area.	
	▶ Notify the physician if the skin is severely broken or peeling or if a rash is present.	▶ Additional measures may be needed to ensure skin healing.	
	▶ For toddlers and older children: Tub bathe at least daily (if condition allows) in tepid water. Pat the area dry.	▶ Helps loosen any fecal matter without scrubbing, which can cause additional irritation to the skin.	
	▶ Discourage the wearing of underwear if possible.	▶ Allows air to circulate and prevents accumulation of moisture.	
	▶ Apply A & D ointment at least four times daily.	▶ Provides a barrier and protects intact or reddened skin from becoming excoriated.	

apeutic play techniques, such as allowing the child to manipulate equipment, can reduce anxiety (see Chapter 34). To promote trust, be honest if a procedure will hurt. Encourage the child to express anger, fear, and pain.

PROMOTE REST AND COMFORT

Most children with gastroenteritis are quite ill and awaken frequently with periods of vomiting and diarrhea. Provide a quiet, restful environment. Darken the room and keep interruptions to a minimum. To reduce the child's anxiety, encourage parents to room-in. Place the child's favorite toys and comfort objects within reach. Keep the child's mouth moistened with a glycerine swab, a wet washcloth, or an occasional ice chip.

ENSURE ADEQUATE NUTRITION

Offer liquids throughout the illness, even if an intravenous infusion is in place. Follow guidelines for oral rehydration therapy in Chapter 39. Find out what fluids the family uses at home. If tolerated, the CRAM diet can be started. This includes complex carbohydrates such as cereals and toast, rice, and milk. Infants are breastfed or given formula. After about 1 week, the child should be consuming a normal diet for age.

DISCHARGE PLANNING AND CARE IN THE COMMUNITY

Discharge teaching should begin on arrival at the health care facility. Teach family members that handwashing is the most important measure that can be taken to prevent the spread of gastroenteritis. Tell parents what to expect as the child's GI system returns to normal. Teach the parents about the symptoms of dehydration and what to do if diarrhea recurs. Be sure that parents understand the recom-

mended diet progression. Emphasize the necessity of good hygiene practices to prevent the spread of microorganisms that can cause gastroenteritis. If the child attends child care, have the parent inform the care center about the infection so the staff can be alerted to watch for other cases and can take steps to prevent the spread of infection.

Complementary Care

CHAMOMILE FOR DIGESTIVE DISORDERS

Chamomile has been used for digestive disorders such as vomiting, colic, diarrhea, and flatulence, as well as parasitic infections. In human and animal studies, chamomile has shown efficacy as an anti-inflammatory and antispasmodic (DerMarderosian, 2000; Lucassen, Assendelft, Gubbels, et al., 1998; O'Hara, Kiefer, Farrell, et al., 1998). See the website for further information on chamomile. **WEB**

Evaluation

Expected outcomes of nursing care for the child with gastroenteritis include:

▶ Correction of dehydration

▶ Adequate nutritional intake

▶ Return to normal bowel function

▶ Parental description of signs of dehydration

▶ Parental knowledge of importance of handwashing in decreasing transmission of infectious agents

▶ Maintenance of intact skin

CONSTIPATION

Constipation is characterized by a decrease in the frequency or passage of stools; the formation of hard, dry stools; or the oozing of liquid stool past a collection of hard, dry stool. Because stooling patterns vary among children, identification of an abnormal pattern is sometimes difficult. Infants usually have several bowel movements a day. For a young child, one bowel movement a day may be normal. As the child grows, however, three to four bowel movements a week may be a normal pattern.

Constipation may be caused by an underlying disease, diet, or psychologic factor. It may result from defects in filling, or more commonly emptying, of the rectum. Pathologic causes of defective filling include ineffective colonic propulsive activity, caused by hypothyroidism or use of medication, and obstruction, caused by a structural anomaly (stricture or stenosis) or by an aganglionic segment (Hirschsprung disease). If the rectum fails to fill, stasis leads to excessive drying of the stools. Emptying of the rectum depends on the defecation reflex. Lesions of the spinal cord, weakness of the abdominal muscles, and local lesions blocking sphincter relaxation all may impede attempts to defecate.

Constipation during infancy is rare and is most often caused by mismanagement of diet. The transition from formula to cow's milk may cause a transient constipation because the bowel must adjust to the increased protein content of cow's milk. Constipation in young infants can usually be corrected by increasing the amount of fluids or adding 2 oz. of pear of apple juice to daily intake. In older infants, increasing the intake of cereals, fruits, and vegetables in the diet should correct the problem.

Constipation occurs most frequently in the toddler and preschool age groups. This increased incidence is often associated with learning to control body functions. Many children do not like the sensations of a bowel movement and may begin withholding stool, which accumulates in and dilates the rectum until the next urge to defecate. The increasingly hard and painful bowel movement reinforces the child's behavior, and a pattern develops (Castiglia, 2001). See Chapter 36 for a discussion of encopresis.

Removing constipating foods (bananas, rice, and cheese) from the child's diet often decreases the constipation. Increasing the child's intake of high-fiber foods (whole grain breads, raw fruits and vegetables) and increasing fluids also promote defecation.

The school-age child may become constipated because time for toileting is limited. Busy school-age children may delay going to the bathroom. Children may also be hesitant to use an unfamiliar bathroom. Encouragement from parents and relaxation of bathroom privileges at school promote regularity and return of usual bowel patterns within a short time.

Diagnosis is based on a thorough history and physical examination. When constipation occurs along with growth failure, vomiting, or abdominal pain, further investigation is necessary to rule out other disorders. Dietary management is the treatment of choice for constipation that has no underlying pathologic cause. A single glycerin suppository or enema may be needed to remove hard stool, followed by dietary and fluid management.

Constipation may follow surgery, especially in children who are immobilized, such as by traction or a body cast. Stool softeners and a diet high in roughage and fluids prevent and treat constipation. Many families use herbal or other plant remedies to treat constipation.

Complementary Care

FLAXSEED AND PSYLLIUM IN THE TREATMENT OF CONSTIPATION

Flaxseed is an age-old botanical treatment for constipation. The seeds bind with water and swell to form a demulcent gel in the intestines, thus softening the stools and increasing the bowel content. The increased stool content causes stretching in the bowel wall creating peristalsis and stool evacuation. The protective oils of the flaxseed also are healing for the intestinal lining and therefore are helpful for colons damaged by irritable bowel syndrome and gastritis (Blumenthal, Goldberg, & Brinckmann, 2000.)

Psyllium seeds are another botanical remedy for constipation. Much like flaxseed, psyllium is a stool softener. The German Commission E approved black psyllium seed for chronic constipation and irritable bowel syndrome especially when a soft stool is the goal of therapy (Blumenthal et al., 2000.) See our website for further information, including other complementary therapies such as movement therapies and massage for the treatment of constipation. ⊂⊃ WEB

Nursing Management

Take a diet history and obtain a description of bowel patterns from parents. Ask what the family does to treat constipation. Assessment of the child's food likes and dislikes may provide a clue to the cause of constipation. Nursing care focuses on teaching parents what constitutes normal bowel patterns in children and the importance of diet in maintaining normal bowel patterns. Regular bowel habits are encouraged by placing the child on the toilet 30 minutes after a meal or around the time defecation usually occurs. Providing positive reinforcement during toilet training helps prevent a withholding pattern.

Teach parents dietary measures to promote regularity of bowel movements. Children can be given a high-fiber diet that includes fruits and vegetables. Cut-up fresh fruits, dried fruits, and fruit juice can be offered as snacks. A glycerine suppository can be used periodically. This is a natural stimulant and lubricant of the bowel. Caution parents to avoid frequent use of laxatives, stool softeners, and enemas, since overuse can cause bowel dependency. Herbal stimulant laxatives are discouraged for children less than 12 years, whereas other intestinal motility aids are not generally harmful. Find out more about any herbs the family commonly uses. ⊂⊃ WEB

Complementary Care

CULTURAL USE OF HERBAL LAXATIVES

Herbal stimulant laxatives are used by some cultures as complementary therapies. The following are not recommended for use in children under 12 years:

- Aloe
- Buckthorn bark
- Cascara sagrada bark
- Senna leaf or pod
- Coffee
- Tea
- Cola nut
- Maté (yerba maté)
- Ma huang

≈ INTESTINAL PARASITIC DISORDERS

Intestinal parasitic disorders occur most frequently in tropical regions. Outbreaks take place where water is not treated, food is incorrectly prepared, or people live in crowded conditions with poor sanitation. In the United States, outbreaks of diseases caused by protozoa or helminths (worms) are increasing. Young children, especially those in day care, are most at risk of infection. Young children often lack good hygiene practices and are likely to put objects and their hands into their mouths. (See "Clinical Manifestations: Common Intestinal Parasitic Disorders.")

CLINICAL MANIFESTATIONS ≈ *Common Intestinal Parasitic Disorders*

PARASITIC INFECTION	TRANSMISSION, LIFE CYCLE, PATHOGENESIS	CLINICAL MANIFESTATIONS	CLINICAL THERAPY	COMMENTS
Giardiasis Organism: protozoan *Giardia lamblia*	Transmission is through person-to-person contact, unfiltered water, improperly prepared infected food, and contact with animals. Cysts are ingested and passed into the duodenum and proximal jejunum, where they begin actively feeding. They are excreted in the stool.	May be asymptomatic. *Infants:* diarrhea, vomiting, anorexia, failure to thrive *Older children:* abdominal cramps; intermittent loose, foul-smelling, watery, pale, and greasy stools	Available medications include furazolidone and quinacrine. Furazolidone has fewer side effects than quinacrine but is more expensive. Metronidazole is also effective but is not licensed in the United States for treatment of giardiasis.	Most common intestinal parasitic organism in the United States. Infection may resolve spontaneously in 4–6 weeks without treatment. Parents or caregivers should wear gloves when handling diapers or stool of parasite-infected infant or child.
Enterobiasis (Pinworm) Organism: nematode *Enterobius vermicularis*	Transmission is from discharged eggs inhaled or carried from hand to mouth. Eggs hatch in the upper intestine and mature in 15–28 days. Larvae then migrate to the cecum. After mating, the female migrates out of the anus and lays up to 17,000 eggs. Movement of worms causes intense itching. Scratching deposits eggs on the hands and under the nails.	Intense perianal itching, irritability, restlessness, and short attention span; in females, can migrate to the vagina and urethra to cause infection. Itching intensifies at night when the female comes to the anal opening to lay eggs.	Available medications include mebendazole, pyrantel pamoate, and piperazine citrate. The child and all household members should be treated at the same time. Treatment may be repeated in 2–3 weeks.	Most common helminthic infection in United States. Transmission is increased in crowded conditions such as housing developments, schools, and day care centers.

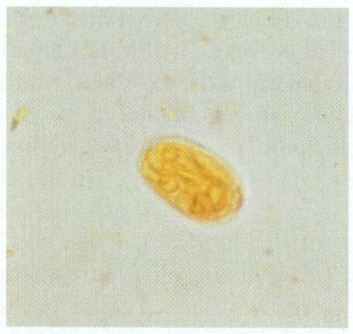

Giardia lamblia

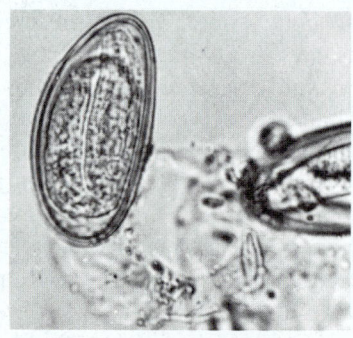

Pinworm

Giardia lamblia courtesy of the Centers for Disease Control and Prevention, Atlanta, GA. Pinworm, roundworm, hookworm, and threadworm from Rudolph, A. W., Hoffman, I.I.E., and Rudolph, C. D. (1996). *Rudolph's pediatrics* (20th ed.) Stamford, CT: Appleton & Lange.

PARASITIC INFECTION	TRANSMISSION, LIFE CYCLE, PATHOGENESIS	CLINICAL MANIFESTATIONS	CLINICAL THERAPY	COMMENTS
Ascariasis (Roundworm) Organism: nematode *Ascaris lumbricoides*	Transmission is from discharged eggs carried from hand to mouth. Adult lays eggs in small intestine. Eggs are excreted in stool, where they incubate for 2–3 weeks. Swallowed eggs hatch in the small intestine. Larvae may penetrate intestinal villi, entering the portal vein and liver, then moving to the lung. Larvae that ascend to upper respiratory tract are swallowed and proceed to the small intestine, where they repeat the cycle.	Mild infection may be asymptomatic. Severe infection may result in intestinal obstruction, peritonitis, obstructive jaundice, and lung involvement.	Available anthelmintic medications include mebendazole, pyrantel pamoate, or piperazine citrate. Stools should be examined 2 weeks after treatment and monthly for 3 months. Family members and contacts of the child should be treated if indicated. If the child has intestinal obstruction, treatment may include administering piperazine through a nasogastric tube and duodenal suction. Obstructing worms sometimes have to be surgically removed.	Most common in warm climates. Primarily affects children 1–4 years of age.
Hookworm disease Organism: nematode *Necator americanus*	Transmission is through direct contact with infected soil containing larvae. Worms live in the small intestine and feed on villi, causing bleeding. Eggs are deposited in the bowel and excreted in feces. Eggs hatch in damp shaded soil. Larvae attach to and penetrate the skin then enter the bloodstream, migrating to the lungs. Larvae then migrate to the upper respiratory passages and are swallowed.	In healthy individuals mild infection seldom causes problems. More severe infection may result in anemia and malnutrition. Presence of larvae on the skin may cause burning and itching, followed by redness and papular eruption.	Available medications include mebendazole and pyrantel pamoate. Stools should be examined 2 weeks after treatment and monthly for 3 months. Family members and contacts of the child should be treated if indicated.	Children should wear shoes when outdoors, although other unprotected areas of the skin may still come in contact with larvae.

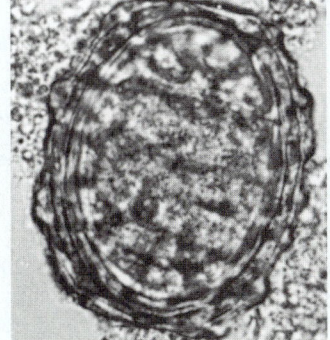

Roundworm

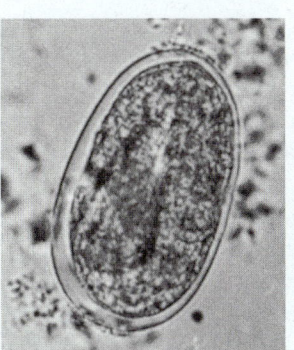

Hookworm

(continued)

PARASITIC INFECTION	TRANSMISSION, LIFE CYCLE, PATHOGENESIS	CLINICAL MANIFESTATIONS	CLINICAL THERAPY	COMMENTS
Strongyloidiasis (Threadworm) Organism: nematode *Strongyloides stercoralis*	Transmission is from the ingestion of discharged larvae in the soil. Life cycle is similar to that of the hookworm, except the threadworm does not attach to the intestinal mucosa and feeding larvae (rather than eggs) may be deposited in the soil.	Mild infection may be asymptomatic. Severe infection may result in abdominal pain and distention, nausea, vomiting, and diarrhea. Stools may be large and pale, with mucus. Severe infection may lead to a nutritional deficiency.	Available medications include thiabendazole or mebendazole. Treatment may need to be repeated if symptoms recur after treatment. Family members and contacts of the child should be examined and treated if indicated.	Most common in older children and adolescents.

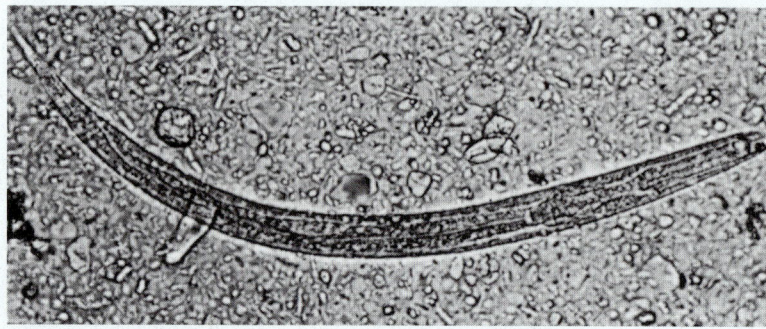

Threadworm

Visceral larva migrans (toxocariasis) Organism: nematode *Toxocara canis* or *T. catis,* commonly found in dogs and cats	Transmission is through the ingestion of eggs in the soil. Ingested eggs hatch in the intestine. Mobile larvae then migrate to the liver and eventually to all major organs (including the brain). Once migration is complete, they encapsulate in dense fibrous tissue.	Most cases are asymptomatic. Affected children may have a low-grade fever and recurrent upper airway diseases. Severe symptoms include hepatomegaly, pulmonary infiltration, and neurologic disturbances. In all cases there is a hypereosinophilia of the blood.	There is no specific treatment. Corticosteroids have been used in severe cases. Thiabendazole has been recommended but efficacy is not established (infection usually resolves spontaneously).	Most common in toddlers. Deworm household pets monthly if indicated. Keep children away from areas contaminated with animal droppings.

In addition, previously uncommon parasites are emerging in the United States. The possibility of enteric infection should always be considered in children with continuing diarrhea or other intestinal symptoms (Cowden & Hotez, 2001).

Another common cause of young child infection is exposure to pets and wildlife. Pets should be checked for parasites and dewormed regularly. Public policies for cleanup of pet fecal material in parks can also decrease contamination. Sand and play boxes should be kept covered when not in use and children should be taught good handwashing after exposure to their pets and not to approach or touch unfamiliar or wild animals (Kazacos, 2000).

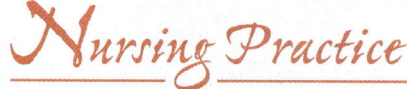

Nursing Practice

The following drugs are used in the treatment of intestinal protozoan infections:

Diloxanide furoate
Furazolidone
Iodoquinol
Mebendazole
Metronidazole
Paromomycin

Piperazine citrate
Pyrantel pamoate
Tetracycline
Thiabendazole
Trimethoprim/sulfamethoxazole

Laboratory examination of stool specimens identifies the causative organism (protozoa, worms, larvae, or ova). Treatment usually involves an anthelmintic. Nursing care centers on preventive teaching. Emphasize the importance of good hygiene practices, especially careful handwashing, after toileting and when handling food. Instruct parents to give prescribed medications as directed even if the child's condition seems to be improved.

FEEDING DISORDERS

Feeding problems that interfere with a child's ability to ingest or tolerate formulas and foods usually become apparent during the first year of life. To prevent complications of poor nutrition, feeding methods or diet may need to be altered. The following discussion focuses on the common disorders of colic and rumination. See Chapter 31 for a discussion of food allergy and sensitivity and of feeding disorder of infancy and childhood (failure to thrive). Chapter 36 has a discussion of the eating disorders anorexia nervosa and bulimia.

COLIC

Colic is a feeding disorder characterized by paroxysmal abdominal pain of intestinal origin and severe crying. It usually occurs in infants under 3 months of age. The etiology of colic is unknown. Proposed causes include feeding too rapidly and swallowing large amounts of air.

Characteristically the infant cries loudly and continuously, often for several hours. The infant's face may become flushed. The abdomen is distended and tense. Often the infant draws up the legs and clenches the hands. Episodes occur at the same time each day, usually in the late afternoon or early evening. Crying may stop only when the child is completely exhausted or after passage of flatus or stool. Carrying the child in the upright position is often helpful.

The symptoms initially may resemble intestinal obstruction or peritoneal infection. These conditions must be ruled out along with sensitivity to formula. Treatment is supportive. Usually by 3 months of age the severity and frequency of symptoms decrease.

Nursing Practice

Vomiting and feeding disorders can occur throughout childhood as well as in infancy. In older children, a pattern of **chronic vomiting** (low-grade nearly daily emesis) or **cyclic vomiting** (repeated severe vomiting of an episodic nature) can occur. These patterns differ from vomiting seen in colic or gastroesophageal reflux. Chronic vomiting is most often associated with peptic ulcer or irritable bowel, and cyclic vomiting is indicative of a syndrome known as abdominal migraine. Continuous vomiting of any nature should be evaluated (Li, 1996).

Nursing Management

Nursing care requires a thorough history of the infant's diet and daily schedule and the events surrounding episodes of colicky behavior. Assess the infant's feeding patterns and diet including type, frequency, and amount of feeding (if breastfeeding, maternal diet history) and frequency of burping. Assess episodes of colic for onset, duration, and characteristics of cry. What measures are used to relieve crying? How effective are they? When possible, observe the feeding method. Parents of infants with colic are often tired and frustrated. They require frequent reassurance that they are not to blame for the infant's condition. Suggest ways of alleviating some of the infant's symptoms and discomfort.

Teaching About

SUGGESTIONS FOR ALLEVIATING COLIC

Provide Rhythmic Movement
Front-carrying sling carriers
Infant swing (battery-operated swing provides continuous motion)
Car ride

Alternate Positions
Swaddle infant in a soft, stretchy blanket with knees flexed up against abdomen or with legs straight
Place infant prone on parent's arm, supporting the body with one hand under the abdomen and cradling the head in the crook of the other arm

Reduce Environmental Stimuli
Respond to crying
Provide quiet, soothing music
Prevent sudden loud noises
Avoid smoking

Provide Various Tactile Stimuli
Offer a pacifier
Provide a warm bath
Massage abdomen

Alter Intake
Feed smaller amount and burp frequently
Use a bottle with a collapsible bag to prevent sucking air
Breastfeeding mothers: eliminate milk products and spicy or gas-producing foods
Hold upright for ½ hour after feeding

RUMINATION

Rumination is a rare and serious form of chronic regurgitation that may lead to malnutrition and growth failure in infancy. Chewing movements and mouthing of fingers often precede or accompany regurgitation. Close observation may reveal the infant actively initiating gagging with the tongue and fingers.

Rumination is most often associated with poor maternal–infant bonding. This kind of behavior is seen in infants deprived of tactile, visual, or auditory stimuli for long periods. The infant substitutes repetitive self-stimulation for the lack of appropriate external stimulation. (See the discussion of failure to thrive in Chapter 31.)

Diagnostic evaluation focuses on ruling out an organic cause and determining the degree and type of nutritional deficiencies. Treatment involves correcting the nutritional deficits and developing normal feeding patterns. Medical and nursing staff and social services are often involved in helping parents meet the infant's nutritional and psychologic needs (see Chapter 31).

Nursing Management

Nursing care focuses on establishing a warm, caring relationship with the infant and the parents. Making eye contact with the infant, providing food regularly, and stimulating the infant through all the senses are ways to break the pattern of rumination.

Parents need to be included in the infant's care. Discuss proper nutrition and demonstrate feeding techniques and interactions that promote development. Determine the parents' support needs and make a referral to social service agencies as appropriate. A parent preoccupied with financial or other problems is less likely to attend to an infant's needs, resulting in continuation or recurrence of the pattern of rumination.

≈ DISORDERS OF MALABSORPTION

Malabsorption occurs when a child cannot digest or absorb nutrients in the diet. Disorders of malabsorption include celiac disease, lactose intolerance, and short bowel syndrome. Cystic fibrosis, a common cause of malabsorption, is discussed in Chapter 42.

CELIAC DISEASE

Celiac disease, or gluten-sensitive enteropathy, is a chronic malabsorption syndrome that is more common in Caucasian, European children and is uncommon in African-American or Asian children. It is also more common among members of the same family, so a genetic factor may play a role in etiology (Connon, 1999). About 1% to 4% of children with Down syndrome have celiac disease (Nehring & Vessey, 2000). Current research is directed at locating the potential genetic abnormalities that occur in celiac disease, and using knowledge of genetics to carry out antibody titer level diagnostic testing (Hoffenberg, Bao, Eisenbarth, et al., 2000). The disease is characterized by an intolerance for gluten, a protein found in wheat, barley, rye, and oats. Inability to digest glutenin and gliadin (pro-

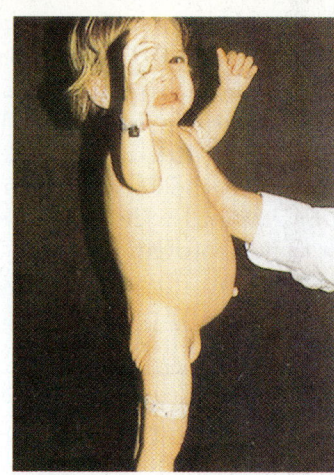

FIGURE 46–7. ◆ The child with celiac disease commonly shows failure to grow and wasting of extremities. The abdomen can appear large due to intestinal bloating and malnutrition. Note: From Zitelli, B. J., & Davis, H. W. (Eds.). (1997). *Atlas of Pediatric Physical Diagnosis,* 3rd ed. (page 294, Figure 10–15a). St. Louis: Mosby.

tein fractions) results in the accumulation of the amino acid glutamine, which is toxic to mucosal cells in the intestine. Damage to the villi ultimately impairs the absorptive process in the small intestine.

In the early stages, celiac disease affects fat absorption, resulting in excretion of large quantities of fat in the stools (steatorrhea). Stools are greasy, foul smelling, frothy, and excessive. As changes in the villi continue, the absorption of protein, carbohydrates, calcium, iron, folate, and vitamins A, D, E, K, and B_{12} becomes impaired.

Symptoms usually occur when solid foods containing gluten are introduced to the child's diet (in the first 2 years of life), although celiac disease is sometimes first diagnosed in adulthood (Connon, 1999). The child exhibits chronic diarrhea, vomiting, irritability, and failure to grow (Figure 46–7 ◆). If diagnosis is delayed, the child begins to show evidence of protein deficiency (wasted musculature, abdominal distention), delayed dentition, and changes in bone density.

Diagnosis is confirmed through measurement of fecal fat content, jejunal biopsy, and improvement with removal of gluten products from the diet. Blood screening tests are more often being used successfully for diagnosis. Serum antigliadin antibody (AGA) and reticulin antibody levels are elevated. Symptoms usually improve within a few days to weeks. The intestinal villi return to normal in about 6 months. Growth should improve steadily, and height and weight should reach normal range within 1 year. Vitamin supplementation may be needed for a time if the child has become malnourished.

Nursing Management

Nursing care focuses on supporting the parents in maintaining a gluten-free diet for the child. Thoroughly explain the disease process to the parents. Emphasize the necessity of following a gluten-free diet. Help parents understand that celiac disease requires lifelong dietary modifications that should not be discontinued when the child is symptom free. Discontinuation of the diet places the child at risk for growth retardation and the development of GI cancers in adulthood. All children with celiac disease should be seen by a dietitian several times during childhood. Nutritional assessment and continued teaching to maintain a gluten-free diet take place at these visits. Dietary management is made difficult by hidden gluten in many prepared foods, such as chocolate candy, prepared meats, ice cream, soups, condiments, and food starch.

An infant or toddler's diet is easily monitored at home. When the child enters school, however, ensuring adherence to dietary restrictions becomes more difficult. In addition to easily identified gluten-based foods, such as bread, cake, doughnuts, cookies, and crackers, the child must also avoid processed foods that contain gluten as a filler. School-age children and adolescents are often tempted to eat these foods, especially when among peers. Emphasize the need for compliance while meeting the child's developmental needs.

The child's special dietary needs can place a financial burden on the family. Parents need to purchase prepared rice or corn flour products or make their own bread and bakery products. Advise parents that getting a dietary prescription enables them to deduct the cost of these ingredients and commercially prepared products as a medical expense.

Because the entire family must adapt to the diet, parents and siblings need support and management skills (Huff, 1997). For information and support, refer parents and children to several organizations, including the American Celiac Society, the Celiac Sprue Association/United States of America, and the Gluten Intolerance Group. Written materials are also available from Children's Memorial Hospital in Chicago. ⬭ **WEB**

Expected outcomes of nursing care include:

- Maintenance of normal dietary patterns
- Adequate absorption of essential nutrients as demonstrated by normal growth patterns and absence of deficiency symptoms
- Child and family knowledge of sources of dietary gluten

LACTOSE INTOLERANCE

Lactose intolerance is the inability to digest lactose, a disaccharide found in milk and other dairy products. It results from a congenital or acquired deficiency of the enzyme lactase. Congenital lactase deficiency of infancy is rare. See Chapter 31 for a general discussion of food intolerance.

⬭ Abdominal pain, flatulence, and diarrhea occur shortly after birth when the infant is unable to hydrolyze lactose. The prevalence of secondary (acquired) lactase deficiency is highest (approximately 100%) among Asian and Native-American children and affects approximately 70% of blacks after the age of 3 years. Diarrhea develops rapidly after the child ingests milk and milk products. Some children can tolerate small ingestions of lactose but have symptoms when larger amounts are consumed. Incidence of lactose intolerance increases with advancing age throughout childhood.

Diagnosis is based on a thorough history and a hydrogen breath test, which measures the amount of hydrogen left after fermentation of unabsorbed carbohydrates. A lactose-free diet may eliminate the symptoms, confirming the diagnosis. Treatment for infants includes switching to a soy-based formula. For older children, eliminating lactose-containing foods is recommended. Enzyme tablets such as LactAid can be added to milk or sprinkled on foods to aid digestion.

Nursing Management

Nursing care is primarily supportive. Carefully explain dietary modifications to parents and discuss alternate sources of calcium (see Chapter 39). ⬭ Discuss the need for supplementation of calcium and vitamin D to prevent deficiencies. Teach families how to read food labels to find hidden sources of lactose. For example, milk solids may be found in breads, cakes, candies, salad dressings, margarine, and processed food. Suggest lactase tablets for children who want to eat some dairy products.

SHORT BOWEL SYNDROME

Short bowel syndrome is a decreased ability to digest and absorb a regular diet because of a shortened intestine. Loss of intestine may result from extensive bowel resection for treatment of necrotizing enterocolitis or inflammatory disorders or from a congenital bowel anomaly such as intestinal malrotation, gastroschisis, or atresia.

The extent and location of the involved bowel determine the severity of the disorder. Because specific types of absorption occur primarily in certain parts of the bowel, the section lost determines which vitamins and other nutrients are inadequate. During the first 3 months after bowel resection, watery diarrhea is common. In the transition period, the remaining bowel usually increases its absorptive surface area and partially compensates for the absent intestine. At first, the infant or young child requires nutritional support to provide sufficient nutrients for growth and development. A combination of total parenteral nutrition via central line and oral fluids may be required. Once the bowel begins to recover, enteral feedings may be started. Careful management of enteral feedings includes a high-fat, low-carbohydrate diet with added stimulants for mucosal growth hormones (gastrin, insulin, enteroglucagon, and growth hormone). Careful management of nucleotide, glutamine, polyamine, and fatty acid components in enteral feedings can also encourage growth of normal intestinal mucosa (Committee on Nutrition, American Academy of Pediatrics, 1998).

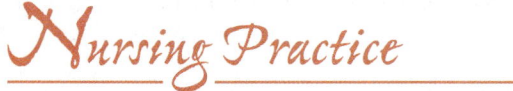

Nursing Practice

The section of the intestine that is resected will determine the vitamin and nutrient deficiencies of the child with short bowel syndrome. When the ileum is resected, bile salts, fluids, and electrolyte absorption decrease so diarrhea can result. Loss of ileum also leads to steatorrhea and fat-soluble vitamins. When the colon is resected, fluid and electrolyte management is impaired. Resection of the jejunum is compensated for effectively by the remaining bowel (Jakubik, Colfer, & Grossman, 2000).

Nursing Management

Nursing care focuses on meeting the child's nutritional and fluid needs and teaching parents how to care for the child at home. Establishing an adequate nutritional intake and bowel pattern is a lengthy process. TPN is provided initially until a feeding regimen can be established. Oral and enteral feedings are instituted gradually to allow the bowel time to compensate. Provide support to the family and child throughout this period. Teach parents how to prepare and administer total parenteral feedings and care for the central line (see Skill 12-7). **SKILLS** **CD** Once enteral or tube feedings are begun, teach management of the feeding pump and care of the feeding tube. Ensure regular bowel function and maintain skin integrity. Arrange home visits to monitor the child's growth and development, care of the central line and tube feeding site, and any side effects such as fluid and electrolyte imbalance and diarrhea.

❧ HEPATIC DISORDERS

The liver is one of the most vital organs in the body. Its essential functions include blood storage and filtration; secretion of bile and bilirubin; metabolism of fat, protein, and carbohydrates; synthesis of blood-clotting components; detoxification of hormones, drugs, and other substances; and storage of glycogen, iron, fat-soluble vitamins, and vitamin B_{12}. Thus any inflammatory, obstructive, or degenerative disorder that affects liver function can be life threatening. The following discussion focuses on three common liver disorders in children: biliary atresia, viral hepatitis, and cirrhosis.

BILIARY ATRESIA

Biliary atresia is the pathologic closure or absence of bile ducts outside the liver. It is the most common pediatric liver disease necessitating transplantation and the most common cause of infant jaundice (Brown et al., 1998; Cox, 2000).

Initially the newborn is asymptomatic. Jaundice may not be detected until 2 to 3 weeks after birth. At that point bilirubin levels increase, accompanied by abdominal distention and hepatomegaly (see Appendix B + the CD-ROM for bilirubin levels and other liver function tests). **CD** As the disease progresses, splenomegaly occurs. The infant experiences easy bruising, prolonged bleeding time, and intense itching. Stools have puttylike consistency and are white or clay colored because of the absence of bile pigments. Excretion of bilirubin and bile salts results in tea-colored urine. Failure to thrive and malnutrition occur as the destructive changes of the disease progress.

The cause of biliary atresia is unknown. Absence or blockage of the extrahepatic bile ducts results in blocked bile flow from the liver to the duodenum. This altered bile flow soon causes inflammation and fibrotic changes in the liver. In addition to blockage, the disease can also be caused by hepatocellular dysfunction (Brown et al., 1998). Lack of bile acids also interferes with digestion of fat and absorption of fat-soluble vitamins A, D, E, and K, resulting in steatorrhea and nutritional deficiencies. Without treatment the disease is fatal.

Diagnosis is based on the history, physical examination, and laboratory evaluation. Laboratory findings reveal elevated bilirubin levels, elevated serum aminotransferase and alkaline phosphatase values, prolonged prothrombin time, and increased ammonia levels. Ultrasound rules out other causes, and a liver biopsy is performed. Because liver damage develops rapidly in infants with biliary atresia, early diagnosis is essential.

Treatment involves surgery to attempt correction of the obstruction (hepatoportoenterostomy) and supportive care. In the hepatoportoenterostomy (Kasai procedure), a segment of the intestine is anastomosed to the porta hepatis. In most children this is a palliative treatment to promote bile drainage, maintain as much hepatic function as possible, and prevent the complications of liver failure. Supportive treatment is directed at managing the bleeding tendencies by administering oral vitamin K; preventing rickets through vitamin D supplementation; controlling itching and irritability with cholestyramine and antihistamines; and promoting adequate nutrition.

Although the hepatoportoenterostomy improves the prognosis, complications of liver disease continue to develop; liver transplantation is eventually needed. Advances in transplantation surgery now make it possible to perform partial liver transplants from living donor resections. This enables transplantation to be performed when the child is in optimal health, rather than waiting until an appropriate-size cadaver liver is available, and allows for donations from close family members who are often good tissue matches.

These advances, along with the development of cyclosporine and other immunosuppressants, have improved the first-year survival rate for children receiving liver transplantation to between 75% and 85% (SPLIT Research Group, 2001).

Nursing Management

Nursing care in the initial stages of biliary atresia is the same as that for any healthy newborn. As symptoms develop, the focus of nursing care becomes long-term management and support.

Diagnosis of this potentially fatal disorder can be devastating to parents. Provide emotional support and offer frequent explanations of tests during the initial diagnostic evaluation. As the disease progresses, the infant becomes irritable because of intense itching and the accumulation of toxins. Tepid baths may help to relieve itching and provide comfort. Dry skin by patting rather than rubbing to avoid further skin irritation. Promote rest by grouping nursing activities while the infant is awake. Care following a hepatoportoenterostomy is similar to that for a child undergoing abdominal surgery. (See the earlier discussion of postsurgical nursing management for appendicitis and "Nursing Care Plan: The Child Undergoing Surgery" in Chapter 34. Posttransplant care includes immunosuppressant drugs and close monitoring for vascular complications (see Table 46–4).

Discharge planning focuses on teaching parents how to care for the child's skin, provide for nutritional needs, administer medications, and monitor for increasing symptoms of liver disease. When the child has received a transplant, teach parents how to identify signs of rejection (nausea, vomiting, fever, and jaundice), as well as the administration and side effects of immunosuppressant medications. Refer parents to support groups, clergy, or social services if indicated. They will need ongoing visits from a home health care nurse to help them manage the child's complex care. The main expected outcomes of nursing care are the parent's ability to cope with the child's health status and to provide the necessary care. The child is expected to function at maximum potential considering the extent of disease.

VIRAL HEPATITIS

Hepatitis is an inflammation of the liver caused by a viral infection. It may be acute or chronic. Acute hepatitis is rapid in onset and if untreated may develop into chronic hepatitis. The most frequently diagnosed causative organisms are hepatitis A virus (HAV), hepatitis B virus (HBV), hepatitis C virus (HCV), hepatitis D virus (HDV), and hepatitis E virus (HEV). An estimated 136,000 cases of hepatitis occur annually in the United States, and one third of these are in children. WEB Most cases are types A and B (Table 46–5).

Etiology and Pathophysiology

Hepatitis A is the most common form of acute viral hepatitis. It is highly contagious and traditionally has been called infectious hepatitis. Infection occurs primarily through the fecal–oral route. Transmission is by direct person-to-person spread or through ingestion of contaminated water or food (particularly shellfish). Hepatitis A frequently occurs in children in child care settings where hygiene practices are poor. Food handlers can spread hepatitis A if not aware of their infection; it is a common cause of foodborne illness. The virus can live on surfaces for one month. Because the virus is transmitted in the early stages of the disease when individuals are often asymptomatic or only mildly ill, large numbers of people may be exposed before the diagnosis is confirmed (Table 46–6). Although a mild disease in many people, it may cause severe liver damage (Shovein, Damazo, & Hyams, 2000).

Hepatitis B, known traditionally as serum hepatitis, is a serious disease. Transmission is usually by the parenteral route through the exchange of blood or any body secretion or fluid. Other common transmission routes include sexual activity and transmission from mother to fetus in utero. Adolescents who use intravenous drugs and have unprotected sexual intercourse are at risk for contracting hepatitis B. Major sources for the spread of HBV are healthy chronic carriers. All body fluids of infected individuals are potentially contaminated with the virus.

The hepatitis C virus is transmitted primarily through blood and blood products, and blood banks now test for this virus. Infected children have commonly had repeated transfusions (as in sickle cell disease or hemophilia). Intravenous drug use, body piercing, and multiple sexual

---

TABLE 46–4 Problems Encountered in Pediatric Liver Transplant

- **Lack of donors.** This problem is being solved by increasing use of split liver transplants when a partial transplant is provided by a family member, alleviating the need to wait for cadaver donations.
- **Immunosuppression.** Immunosuppressive therapies have been tested less in children than in adults and increased research is needed.
- **Morbidity and mortality of treatment.** Many of the drugs used after transplant have side effects of renal toxicity, malignancy, and other serious sequelae. The effects can be magnified in children who have decades of exposure to these drugs.
- **Recurrent and new diseases.** Diseases that may be caused by immunosuppression can occur, such as those caused by infectious agents. Other liver diseases such as cirrhosis and nonspecific hepatitis are seen in some children.
- **Influences on growth and development.** Drugs, liver disease, emotional strain, and disturbed nutritional intake and metabolism may all influence the growth, cognitive function, and developmental variation of children. Attention and consistent screening of development and family adaptation are needed.

Note: From McDiarnid, S. V. (2000). Liver transplantation. The pediatric challenge. *Clinical Liver Disease, 4,* 879–927.

TABLE 46-5 Comparison of Hepatitis Types

Type	Incubation	% Icteric	% Who Become Chronic Carriers	Clinical Features
Hepatitis A				
Children < 5 years	4 weeks (10–50 days)	< 5	0	More acute onset; frequently subclinical in young children
Adults		50–75		
Hepatitis B				
Infants	1–6 months	< 5	> 90	Extrahepatic manifestations more common
Adults		20–60	5–10	
Hepatitis C				
All ages	6–7 weeks	20–30	≥ 60	Frequently anicteric; predisposes to hepatocellular carcinoma
Hepatitis D				
Coinfection with HBV	2–8 weeks		< 5	Most common viral cause of fulminant hepatitis
Superinfection of HBV carrier			> 80	
Hepatitis E				
All ages	2–9 weeks	~10	0	Severe in pregnant women; high mortality and fetal loss

Note: From Holst, B., & Ritter, D. (2001). Managing viral hepatitis. *Clinician Reviews, 11,* 51–62. Adapted.

TABLE 46-6 Transmission, Immunization, and Prophylaxis for Hepatitis

Type	Primary Transmission	Immunization Available	Prophylaxis
Hepatitis A	Fecal–oral	Yes	Immune serum globulin Hepatitis A vaccine
Hepatitis B	Blood products Intravenous drug use In utero Sexual activity	Yes	Hepatitis B immune globulin Hepatitis B vaccine
Hepatitis C	Blood products Sexual activity Intravenous drug use	No	None
Hepatitis D	Blood products Intravenous drug use In utero Sexual activity	No	Hepatitis B vaccine
Hepatitis E	Fecal–oral	No	None

Note: From Holst, B., & Ritter, D. (2001). Managing viral hepatitis. *Clinician Reviews, 11,* 51–62. Adapted.

partners are also risk factors. Infected mothers may infect their children before birth or during breastfeeding (Estrada, 2000; National Institute on Drug Abuse, 2000).

Hepatitis D (delta virus) is a defective virus that can gain entry to a human only in connection with hepatitis B. This virus is suspected when someone diagnosed with hepatitis B has diminishing liver function, increasing jaundice, and deteriorating mental status.

Hepatitis E infection is primarily transmitted through contaminated water and is most common in developing countries. Outbreaks may occur in flooding and rainy seasons. A related infection transferred primarily through blood transfusion is hepatitis G (Holst & Ritter, 2001).

The liver's response to injury by the viruses that cause hepatitis is similar (see "Pathophysiology Illustrated: Viral Hepatitis"). Initially, invasion of the parenchymal cells by the virus results in local degeneration and necrosis. Subsequent infiltration of the parenchyma by lymphocytes, macrophages, plasma cells, eosinophils, and neutrophils causes inflammation that blocks biliary drainage into the intestine. Impaired bile excretion causes a buildup of bile in the blood, urine, and skin (jaundice). Structural changes in the parenchymal cells account for other altered liver functions. Regeneration of parenchymal cells occurs within 3 months, and most children recover completely.

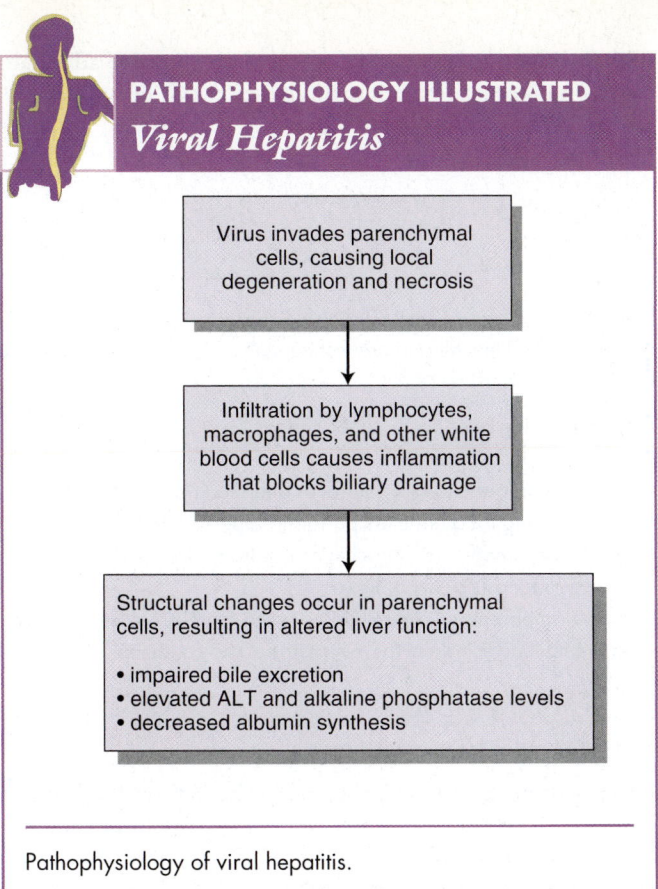

PATHOPHYSIOLOGY ILLUSTRATED
Viral Hepatitis

Virus invades parenchymal cells, causing local degeneration and necrosis

↓

Infiltration by lymphocytes, macrophages, and other white blood cells causes inflammation that blocks biliary drainage

↓

Structural changes occur in parenchymal cells, resulting in altered liver function:

- impaired bile excretion
- elevated ALT and alkaline phosphatase levels
- decreased albumin synthesis

Pathophysiology of viral hepatitis.

In some children, however, a progressive and total destruction of the hepatic parenchyma known as acute fulminating hepatitis develops. Children with this form of the disease usually die of liver failure within 2 weeks of onset unless they receive a liver transplant. Another complication, chronic active hepatitis, may lead to scarring of the liver and progressive deterioration of liver function. The prognosis depends on the degree of liver involvement. In some people, especially those who develop chronic hepatitis, liver cancers and cirrhosis can develop.

Clinical Manifestations

Acute hepatitis infection is characterized by two phases, the anicteric (absence of jaundice) phase and the icteric (jaundice) phase. The anicteric phase usually lasts 5 to 7 days. Signs and symptoms include nausea, vomiting, anorexia, malaise, fatigue, right upper quadrant pain, hepatosplenomegaly, and fever (see Table 46–5). The child becomes irritable, looks ill, and requires rest. In the icteric phase, signs and symptoms include darkening of urine, clay-colored stools, and the characteristic yellowing of the skin and sclera. Many children with hepatitis do not have jaundice, leading to difficulty in disease diagnosis and management. As the jaundice worsens, the child begins to feel better. This phase lasts approximately 4 weeks. Complete recovery with return of normal liver function and laboratory values may take 1 to 3 months.

In some cases, hepatitis becomes chronic. A person with chronic hepatitis carries the virus, can transfer it to others, and may develop serious liver disease after several years.

Clinical Therapy

Diagnosis is often made on the basis of a thorough history and physical examination. A history of exposure to persons with the disease is significant. Physical examination reveals a tender, enlarged liver, abdominal pain, and flulike symptoms. Laboratory evaluation includes serologic testing (to detect the presence of antigens and antibodies to HAV, HBV, HCV, or HDV) and liver function studies. Although a test for HEV has been developed, it is not available in developing countries, so diagnosis is usually based on the history.

The three goals of medical management are early detection to prevent complications, support and monitoring during the acute phase of the disease, and prevention of the spread of the disease. Early diagnosis is essential to follow the course of the illness and identify potential complications. Management includes bed rest during the flulike phase. If prothrombin times are increased, vitamin K is administered.

The spread of viral infections can be interrupted by elimination of the virus from the infected population, institution of proper hygiene, and passive or active immunization. To date, no antiviral agent has been developed to combat the hepatitis viruses. Prevention depends on breaking the cycle of infection. Active immunization for hepatitis A, a two-dose series, is recommended for all people at risk of acquiring and transmitting the disease and for children and child care workers in certain states with endemic disease (see Chapter 41). People at risk include child care staff and food handlers (Centers for Disease Control and Prevention [CDC], 1999). Immunization for hepatitis B, a three-dose series, is recommended for all children and at-risk adults. The first dose is given within 12 hours of birth to the infant born of an infected mother (refer to the discussion of immunization in Chapter 41).

Passive immunity to HAV can be achieved with standard pooled immune globulin. It must be administered within 2 weeks of exposure. Passive immunity to HBV can be achieved with hepatitis B immune globulin (HBIG). Used for one-time exposure and for infants of infected mothers, it is given within 12 hours of birth.

Nursing Management

Nursing Assessment and Diagnosis

The nurse usually encounters the child and family in an outpatient setting. In addition to observing the child for characteristic signs of hepatitis (jaundiced skin and sclera), assess for abdominal pain, anorexia, nausea and vomiting, malaise, and arthralgia. Also get a history of the child's contacts over the past 45 days for HAV and up to 180 days for HBV. For an infant, the hepatitis history of the mother and other family members is important.

Common nursing diagnoses for the child with acute hepatitis might include:

▶ *Risk for altered nutrition: less than body requirements* related to chronic illness

▶ *Fatigue* related to disease state

▶ *Risk for diversional activity deficit* related to forced inactivity

▶ *Risk for body image disturbance (older child)* related to jaundice

▶ *Anxiety (parent and child)* related to threat to health status

▶ *Pain* related to liver injury

Planning and Implementation

Nursing care involves home and community considerations, as children are seldom admitted to the hospital for hepatitis treatment. The hospitalized child is placed in isolation. Prevention of the diseases is integrated into all health care by discussion of immunization and universal precautions. When hepatitis cases have occurred in the family or community, parents need additional detailed information about health precautions and infection-control measures. In addition, teach parents the importance of checking with health professionals before administering any medications (even nonprescription medicines), maintaining adequate nutrition, promoting rest and comfort, and providing diversional activities.

PREVENT SPREAD OF INFECTION

Teach the parents and the child infection-control measures to help prevent transmission of the virus. For parents, reinforce good hygiene practices, such as washing hands before and after toileting and proper disposal of soiled diapers. Siblings of a child with hepatitis B who have not already been immunized with the hepatitis B vaccine should be vaccinated immediately. Contacts of the child with hepatitis A should receive immune serum globulin and the first immunization in the hepatitis A series. Rifampin may be given in some cases. All health providers should receive the hepatitis B immunization series and use standard precautions at all times with everyone in health care. **SKILLS**

MAINTAIN ADEQUATE NUTRITION

Initially, encourage the child to eat favorite foods. Once the anorexia and nausea have resolved, a high-protein, high-carbohydrate, low-fat diet is recommended. Increased protein helps maintain protein stores and prevent

muscle wasting. Increased carbohydrates ensure adequate caloric intake and prevent protein depletion. Low-fat foods lessen stomach distention. Offer the child small, frequent feedings.

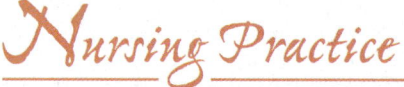

Nurses in child care centers can provide assessment of the center's procedures and teaching to prevent hepatitis A transmission. Help the center to set standards about:

▸ Handwashing after each diaper change
▸ Proper disposal of diapers
▸ Cleaning diaper-changing surfaces after each diaper change
▸ Never having food handlers perform diaper changes
▸ Instructing parents to keep children at home for at least 2 weeks after a diagnosis of hepatitis A
▸ Informing parents of other children when there is a case of hepatitis A and teaching them the symptoms of the condition

PROMOTE REST AND COMFORT

Bed rest is necessary only if the child has severe fatigue and malaise. However, most children voluntarily limit their activities during the initial phase of the disease. Keep the child quiet and comfortable. Offer comfort items such as favorite toys, blankets, and pillows.

PROVIDE DIVERSIONAL ACTIVITIES

Hospitalized children with hepatitis are kept in isolation. Nonhospitalized children with hepatitis do not need to be isolated, but they should be kept at home for 2 weeks following the onset of symptoms. Parents who cannot take time off from work may need to arrange home sitters to stay with the child. Offer suggestions for diversional activities during this period. Young children can be given a new toy or favorite activities. Older children and adolescents can be given board games, puzzles, books or magazines, movies, or video games. Phone calls and short visits from friends help school-age children and adolescents maintain contact with peers.

Expected outcomes of nursing care for hepatitis include the following:

▶ Prevention of new cases of the disease

▶ Full immunization coverage at recommended ages

▶ Restoration to normal liver function

▶ Reestablishment of nutritional intake to support growth

▶ Return to full energy and activity level

▶ Developmental progression during and after the disease

▶ Control of pain to level of comfort

▶ Absence of chronic liver disease

ETIOLOGY	CLINICAL MANIFESTATIONS	CLINICAL THERAPY
Fluid and electrolyte imbalance	Ascites	Restrict sodium, protein, and fluids. Administer diuretics (e.g., furosemide [Lasix]). Administer intravenous albumin.
Liver dysfunction	Hepatic encephalopathy	Restrict protein. Administer lactulose to control increased ammonia levels. Administer antibiotics. Correct any imbalances that can lead to coma (fluid and electrolyte imbalance).
Esophageal varices	Hemorrhage	Administer blood and blood products. Replace fluid and electrolytes. Administer vitamin B complex and vitamin K.
		Insert Sengstaken-Blakemore tube in cases of severe bleeding.

CIRRHOSIS

Cirrhosis is a degenerative disease process that results in fibrotic changes and fatty infiltration in the liver. It can occur in children of any age as the end stage of several disorders. The diffuse destruction and regeneration of the hepatic parenchymal cells result in an increase in fibrous connective tissue and disorganization of the liver structure. The balance between destruction and regeneration determines the specific clinical presentation.

Clinical manifestations of cirrhosis vary. When the disease process results from obstruction, as in biliary atresia, jaundice is an initial sign that intensifies with progression of the disease. In other diseases that cause cirrhosis, jaundice may be a late sign, intermittent, or absent. Steatorrhea is frequently present and can lead to rickets, hemorrhage, and failure to gain weight. Anemia can occur as a result of chronic blood loss from the GI tract. Pruritus is common, particularly in children with biliary malformations. Clubbing of the digits and cyanosis are other common findings. Severe end-stage complications signaling hepatic failure can occur at any time and with little warning.

Diagnostic evaluation is based on the child's history of infection or disease with liver involvement. Physical examination may reveal jaundice, skin changes, ascites, and hemodynamic changes. Laboratory evaluation reveals abnormal liver function tests. A liver biopsy may help determine the extent of the parenchymal damage.

Medical management focuses on treating the child's symptoms and achieving optimal nutritional status and growth. See "Clinical Manifestations of Cirrhosis Complications" for a summary of treatment. Liver transplantation is the most common treatment for biliary atresia and metabolic disorders and is the only treatment for end-stage liver disease.

Nursing Management

Nursing care focuses on monitoring physiologic and psychosocial changes to identify early signs of end-stage hepatic failure. Monitor vital signs every 2 to 4 hours. Measure weight daily to assess for fluid retention. Close monitoring of electrolytes and liver function test results helps determine the need for fluid replacement therapy.

Careful administration of medications and monitoring for side effects are necessary because drug metabolism is altered in liver disorders. If ascites is present, provide a low-sodium, low-protein diet and restrict fluids. Remove all water pitchers, glasses, and straws to minimize the child's desire to drink.

Parents of a child with cirrhosis are coping with a life-threatening disorder, and their anxiety and stress are high. The child may be awaiting a liver transplantation that represents the only hope for recovery. Support parents and encourage them to talk about their fears and concerns (see Chapter 37). ⊂⊃ Encourage parents to participate in the child's care. Referral to a support group or counseling may be beneficial.

∼ INJURIES TO THE GASTROINTESTINAL SYSTEM

ABDOMINAL TRAUMA

Abdominal injuries may be caused by blunt or penetrating trauma. The kind of injury determines the extent of organ damage. Low-velocity trauma, which may occur when a child strikes the handlebars of a bicycle, usually injures a single organ.

High-velocity blunt trauma, which may occur in motor vehicle crashes, usually results in multiple-organ involvement. Solid organs such as the liver and spleen are more vulnerable to injury than hollow organs such as the stomach, intestines, and bladder.

Motor vehicle crashes are the most common and also the most preventable unintentional injury in children (National Safety Council, 2000). On impact, small children held on a parent's lap or improperly restrained in a safety seat can easily become airborne, striking objects or being thrown from the car. When older children involved in severe crashes are wearing only lap belts, injury to the hollow organs may result. Bicycles are another cause of abdominal injuries in children. Such injuries commonly occur when the child strikes the handlebars during a fall or sudden stop or is struck by a car. Child abuse is another major cause of abdominal trauma.

Suspected abdominal trauma in a child necessitates a thorough history and physical examination. The description of the event should be compared with the child's signs and symptoms. Clinical manifestations of abdominal injury include pain, abdominal distention, muscle guarding, decreased or absent bowel sounds, nausea and vomiting, hypotension, and shock. See Chapter 33 for techniques of abdominal assessment.

A sonogram or a CT scan assesses for internal bleeding and air in the abdomen. CT scans are also used to locate areas of internal trauma. Peritoneal lavage may be performed by inserting a catheter into the abdominal cavity, instilling saline or lactated Ringer's solution, and draining and analyzing the fluid. Baseline laboratory studies, including blood type and crossmatch, are done. A urinary catheter may be inserted to check for blood and bladder rupture.

A liver or spleen injury is treated in the ICU; the focus is on preventing or managing hemorrhage and monitoring for signs of shock. An intravenous infusion is started for fluid maintenance and to provide access for blood products. The child is kept NPO. A nasogastric tube is inserted. Blood transfusions and pharmacologic management treat blood loss. Use of analgesics is minimized to avoid masking symptoms. Serial hematocrit levels are monitored during this period. Healing of the liver and spleen usually occurs without further intervention.

Exploratory laparotomy resects hollow organ injuries or repairs liver or spleen lacerations when bleeding is not controlled. The spleen is salvaged to help maintain immune function. The child is usually discharged within 5 to 7 days. No strenuous activity is allowed for 6 to 8 weeks. The prognosis is generally good.

Nursing Management

Nursing care includes initial and ongoing assessments of the child's condition. Monitor vital signs every hour as warranted. Measurement of abdominal circumference, intake and output monitoring, serial hematocrits, and auscultation of bowel sounds are also performed hourly. Notify the physician of any changes.

The child and parents are usually fearful and anxious when the child is admitted to the hospital. If the injury was preventable, parents feel guilt or anger. Provide emotional support and avoid judgmental comments or statements that assign blame.

Once the child's condition is stabilized, the focus of nursing care shifts to preventive teaching. Teach parents safety measures to prevent future injuries and give them written materials, when available, to use as a reference when they return home.

Discuss the use of car safety restraint devices for riding in an automobile (see Chapter 32). If the child's injury was the result of a bicycle fall or crash, discuss the importance of the proper bicycle size and teach bike safety measures such as use of a helmet and proper use of hand signals (see Chapter 32). Have the child practice safe biking habits at a bike rodeo sponsored by a local affiliate of the National SAFE KIDS Campaign. WEB

POISONING

Poisoning is a common cause of death and injury in children between 1 and 4 years of age. About 1.5 million poisonings occur annually in the United States (Powers, 2000). Young children are at risk for poisoning because they characteristically explore their environments (see Chapter 32). Infants and toddlers commonly place objects in their mouths. Some household items are nontoxic and cause little harm. However, items that contain caustic agents or toxic chemicals can cause irreversible damage or death.

The Poison Prevention Packaging Act of 1970 mandates child-protective devices for all potentially toxic substances, such as household cleansers and medications. However, children still ingest many of them; analgesics and hydrocarbons remain the two most common causes of poisoning deaths (Powers, 2000). Many other items commonly found in the home are less obvious sources of toxins. The leaves, stems, or flowers of many common household and garden plants are poisonous. Examples include Boston ivy, poinsettia, philodendron, lily-of-the-valley, daffodil (bulbs), azalea, and rhododendron. Nail care products, mothballs, weed and bug killers, and rodent killers are other potential hazards (Emery & Singer, 1998). See "Clinical Manifestations: Commonly Ingested Toxic Agents" for treatments for several commonly ingested household toxins.

Most poisonings occur in the home (see Chapter 32). While 75% of poisons are ingested, other routes of contamination include dermal, inhalation, and ocular (Litovitz, Klein-Schwartz, White, et al., 2001). Parents who suspect that their child has ingested a poison should immediately call the Poison Control Center (PCC). The PCC will advise parents about treatment to begin at home, and if the child needs treatment in the emergency department. If the child has vomited, the vomitus should be brought to the emergency department. With older children, the possibility of intentional ingestion needs to be considered.

In the emergency department the child's vital signs and level of consciousness are assessed and specific information about the poison is obtained from the parent. The goal of treatment is to prevent further absorption of the poison and to reverse or eliminate its effects. Management focuses on stabilizing the child's condition, identifying the toxic substance, reversing any undesirable effects, and eliminat-

TYPE	SOURCES	CLINICAL MANIFESTATIONS	CLINICAL THERAPY
Corrosives (strong acids and alkaline products that cause chemical burns of mucosal surfaces)	Batteries, household cleaners, Clinitest tablets, denture cleaners, bleach, toilet bowl cleaners	Severe burning pain in mouth, throat, or stomach; swelling of mucous membranes; edema of lips, tongue, and pharynx (respiratory obstruction); violent vomiting; hemoptysis; drooling; inability to clear secretions; signs of shock, anxiety, and agitation	*Do not induce vomiting!* Dilute toxin with water to prevent further damage. Give activated charcoal.
Hydrocarbons (organic compounds that contain carbon and hydrogen; most are distillates of petroleum)	Gasoline, kerosene, furniture polish, lighter fluid, paint thinners	Gagging, choking, coughing, nausea, vomiting, alteration in sensorium (lethargy), weakness, respiratory symptoms of pulmonary involvement, tachypnea, cyanosis, retractions, grunting	*Do not induce vomiting!* (Aspiration of hydrocarbons places child at high risk for pneumonia.) Use gastric lavage if severe central nervous system and respiratory impairment are present. Use of activated charcoal is controversial. Provide supportive care. Decontaminate skin by removing clothing and cleansing skin.
Acetaminophen	Many over-the-counter products	Nausea, vomiting, sweating, pallor, hepatic involvement (pain in upper right quadrant, jaundice, confusion, stupor, coagulation abnormalities)	Induce vomiting or perform gastric lavage, depending on amount ingested. Administer charcoal or NAC (concentrated form of Mucomyst), which binds with the metabolite, preventing absorption and protecting the liver.
Salicylate	Products containing aspirin	Nausea, disorientation, vomiting, dehydration, diaphoresis, hyperpnea, hyperpyrexia, bleeding tendencies, oliguria, tinnitus, convulsions, coma	Depends on amount ingested. Induce vomiting. Administer intravenous sodium bicarbonate, fluids, and vitamin K.
Mercury	Broken thermometers, chemicals, paints, pesticides, fungicides	Tremors, memory loss, insomnia, weight loss, diarrhea, anorexia, gingivitis	Similar to that for lead poisoning (see text discussion).
Iron	Multiple vitamin supplements	Vomiting, hematemesis, diarrhea, bloody stools, abdominal pain, metabolic acidosis, shock, seizures, coma	Induce vomiting. Administer intravenous fluids and sodium bicarbonate. Desferoxamine chelation therapy.

ing the substance from the child's body. Table 46–7 summarizes emergency management for poisoning.

Nursing Management

Once immediate care has been provided, the focus of nursing care shifts to providing emotional support and preventing recurrence.

PROVIDE EMOTIONAL SUPPORT

Wait until the child is out of immediate danger before questioning parents in detail about the incident. Encourage parents to express anger, guilt, or fear about the incident.

PREVENT RECURRENCE

Discuss with parents the need to supervise infants and young children at all times. Ask parents how medicines and cleaning agents are stored and whether the house contains any plants. Teach proper methods of childproofing the home. Instruct parents to keep two bottles of syrup of ipecac available for each child in the home and to be fa-

miliar with its use and proper dosage. They must contact the PCC before administering this medication at home. Suggest ways to prevent recurrence of poisoning.

Teaching About

AVOIDING CHILDHOOD POISONING

- Put PCC phone number by every phone in the house.
- Place household cleaners, medications, vitamins, and other potentially poisonous substances out of the reach of children or in locked cabinets. Use warning stickers such as Mr. Yuk on all containers.
- Buy products with childproof caps.
- Store products in their original containers. Never place household cleansers or other products in food or beverage containers.
- Remove all house plants from the child's play areas.
- Use caution when visiting other settings that are not childproofed (e.g., grandparents' homes). Remember that visitors may have pills in their purses or pockets that are easily accessible.

TABLE 46–7   Emergency Management for Poisoning

1. Stabilize the child. Assess ABCs (airway, breathing, circulation). Provide ventilatory and oxygen support.
2. Perform a rapid physical examination, start an IV infusion, draw blood for toxicology screen, and apply a cardiac monitor.
3. Obtain a history of the ingestion, including substance ingested, where child was found, by whom, position, when, how long unsupervised, history of depression or suicide, allergies, and any other medical problems.
4. Reverse or eliminate the toxic substance using the appropriate method:

Syrup of ipecac

The use of ipecac is no longer widely promoted since it may not remove all poison and can be harmful in some situations. Activated charcoal is used instead for many types of poisons (West, 1997).

- Assess level of consciousness before administering. Recommended doses are:
  6–12 months: 10 mL; do not repeat
  1–12 years: 15 mL; may repeat one time if vomiting does not occur
  Over 12 years: 30 mL; may repeat one time if vomiting does not occur
- Administer clear fluids, 10–20 mL/kg, after giving ipecac.

Apomorphine

- Assess level of consciousness before administering.
- Given IM or SQ; has rapid onset.
- Give plenty of oral fluids.

Gastric lavage

- Insert a gastric tube through the mouth (use the largest size possible for the size of the child).
- Instill and aspirate normal saline solution until the return is clear. Considered a less effective method of removing ingested substances from the stomach than vomiting. Reserved for children with central nervous system depression, diminished or absent gag reflex, or unwillingness to cooperate with other measures.
- *Contraindicated* in children who have ingested alkaline corrosive substances, since insertion of the tube might cause esophageal perforation. Used in children who have ingested acids to decrease continued damage and potential perforation of stomach and intestines.

Activated charcoal

- Given to absorb and remove any remaining particles of toxic substances.
- Give a commercial preparation of activated charcoal orally or through a gastric tube. It is available as a ready-to-drink solution in an opaque container. Use a covered cup and straw when giving orally, to prevent the child from seeing the black liquid and to minimize spillage. Give activated charcoal only after the child has stopped vomiting, since aspiration of charcoal is damaging to lung tissue.

Cathartics

- Hasten excretion of a toxic substance and minimize absorption. The most commonly used cathartic is magnesium sulfate.

Antidotes and antagonists

There are a few of these agents. The most common is Narcan, for opiate ingestion.

5. Other measures will depend on the child's condition, the nature of the ingested substance, and the time since ingestion. May include diuresis, fluid loading, cooling or warming measures, anticonvulsive measures, antiarrhythmic therapy, hemodialysis, or exchange transfusions.
6. Remember always to treat the child first, not the poison. Maintain airway, breathing, and circulation.

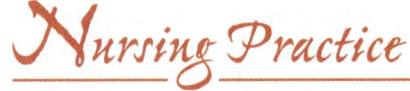 *Nursing Practice*

The toll-free number for the American Association of Poison Control Centers (AAPCC) is 1-800-222-1222. This number can be accessed from anywhere in the United States and Puerto Rico and the caller will be connected to the nearest PCC.

LEAD POISONING

Lead poisoning has been successfully prevented in many areas of the United States, with a substantial decline in lead levels from the mid-1970s. The average serum lead level for children is now 0.6 µg/dL, down from 15 µg/dL in 1976. About 7.6% of children (1.5 million) have levels above the recommended level of <10 µg/dL. Many of these children are poor, and live in older houses in inner cities (CDC, 2000). Even children with levels below 10 µg/dL may experience cognitive defects due to lead exposure. Lead in paint is the most common source of lead exposure for preschool children. Children are also exposed to lead when they ingest contaminated food, water, and soil or when they inhale dust contaminated with lead. Some major sources of lead include lead-based paint, soil and dust, food grown in contaminated soil, drinking water from lead-lined pipes or teapots, lead dust on parents' clothing from occupations like some artwork or construction, and air near smelters and battery-manufacturing plants.

Children are at greater risk for lead poisoning because they absorb and retain more lead in proportion to their weight than adults do. Lead is particularly harmful to children under the age of 7 years.

Lead interferes with normal cell function, primarily of the nervous system, blood cells, and kidneys, and adversely affects the metabolism of vitamin D and calcium.   Clinical manifestations depend on the degree of toxicity. Neurologic effects include decreased IQ scores, cognitive deficits, impaired hearing, and growth delays. Impaired mental function can occur with blood levels even lower than 10 µg/dL. Lead ingestion by a woman during pregnancy can result in fetal malformations, reduced birth weight, and premature birth. Severe lead poisoning, which can result in encephalopathy, coma, and death, is now rare.

Once in the body, lead accumulates in the blood, soft tissues (kidney, bone marrow, liver, and brain), bones, and teeth. Lead absorbed by the bones and teeth is released slowly. Thus, exposure to even small doses, over time, can result in dangerously high levels of lead in the body.

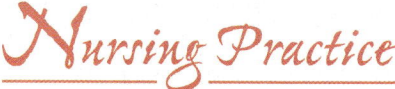

Mercury is another heavy metal that can produce similar effects in the body to those seen in lead poisoning. Recent mercury levels measured in the National Health and Nutrition Examination Survey found that about 10% of women of childbearing age have had more mercury exposure than is recommended. The major source of mercury begins with pollution from power plants, waste incinerators, and industrial processes. Mercury is emitted into the air and falls to waters where it is ingested by fish. In most states, women of childbearing age and young children are warned to limit consumption of fish. Other sources of potential mercury contamination such as mercury thermometers should be eliminated (CDC, 2001).

The CDC now recommends screening children at high risk, with reduced screening for those at low risk (CDC 1997; Harvey, 1997). In addition, all children enrolled in Medicaid should be tested, with follow-up management and care (Advisory Committee on Childhood Lead Poisoning, 2000). A blood lead (Pb-B) level is the most useful screening and diagnostic test for lead exposure.

A Pb-B below 10 μg/dL is considered acceptable, although it may still not screen out all children with impaired development due to lead. An environmental history should be obtained for children with Pb-B levels between 10 and 19 μg/dL to identify removable sources of lead. Follow-up testing is required. Children with Pb-B levels between 20 and 69 μg/dL require a full medical evaluation, including a detailed environmental and behavioral history,

physical examination, and tests for iron deficiency. Interventions to remove sources of lead from the child's environment are necessary. For levels above 25 μg/dL, chelation therapy is also administered. Children with Pb-B levels greater than 70 μg/dL are critically ill from lead poisoning and require immediate chelation therapy and interventions to provide a lead-free environment.

Chelation therapy involves the administration of an agent that binds with lead, increasing its rate of excretion from the body. Calcium disodium ethylenediaminetetraacetate (CaNa$_2$ EDTA), dimercaprol (BAL), d-penicillamine, or succimer (DMSA) may be used. Children with Pb-B levels between 25 and 69 μg/dL receive CaNa$_2$ EDTA for 5 to 7 days, followed by a rest period and then a second chelation treatment. Children with Pb-B levels greater than 70 μg/dL are given both BAL and CaNa$_2$ EDTA, followed by a rest period and a second chelation treatment using CaNa$_2$ EDTA alone. Long-term follow-up of children receiving chelation therapy is essential. The child should never be discharged unless a lead-free home environment has been ensured.

Nursing Management

Nursing care centers on screening, education, and follow-up. Nurses often work with state and local health officials to plan screening for children at high risk of lead exposure. Ask parents about the child's development and eating habits and be alert for risk of lead exposure. Educate parents about sources of lead in the environment and techniques to reduce exposure. Emphasize the importance of housekeeping interventions to reduce exposure to lead dust. These interventions include damp mopping of hard surfaces, floors, window sills, and baseboards; washing the child's hands and face before meals; and frequent washing of toys and pacifiers.

CLINICAL MANIFESTATIONS ～ *Lead Poisoning*

MILD TOXICITY (10–15 μg/dL)	MODERATE TOXICITY (25–69 μg/dL)	SEVERE TOXICITY (>70 μg/dL)
Myalgia or paresthesia	Arthralgia	Paresis or paralysis
Mild fatigue	General fatigue	Encephalopathy (may lead abruptly to seizures, changes in consciousness, coma, and death)
Irritability	Difficulty concentrating	Lead line (blue-black) on gingival tissue
Lethargy		
Occasional abdominal discomfort	Muscular exhaustibility	Colic (intermittent, severe abdominal cramps)
	Tremor	
	Headache	
	Diffuse abdominal pain	
	Vomiting	
	Weight loss	
	Constipation	
	Anemia	

Note: From Agency for Toxic Substances and Disease Registry. (1990). *Lead toxicity, Case studies in environmental medicine* (p. 11). Atlanta: Author. Adapted.

Developing Cultural Competence

Traditional medicines and cosmetics may contain large amounts of lead. Examples include azarcon and greta, preparations that are used by Mexican Americans to treat empacho, a coliclike illness; chifong tokuwan, pay-loo-ah, ghasard, bali goli, and kandu, used by some Asian communities; and alkohl, kohl, surma, saoott, and cebagin, used by some Middle Eastern communities.

Teach parents the importance of including foods high in iron and calcium in the child's diet to counteract losses of these minerals associated with lead exposure. The child should eat meals at regular intervals, since lead is absorbed more readily on an empty stomach.

Be sure that parents understand the importance of follow-up testing of lead levels. If the child is developmentally delayed, refer the family to an infant stimulation or child development program. Referral to social services and either a visiting nurse or home health care nurse may also be appropriate.

Expected outcomes of nursing care for the child with lead or other poisoning include:

- Normal growth and development, including cognition
- Adequate nutritional intake
- Removal of lead or other poisons from the child's environment
- Expressed understanding by family of measures to establish a safe environment for the child

CHAPTER HIGHLIGHTS

- A variety of structural defects caused by fetal development alterations can affect the gastrointestinal system of infants.

- Cleft lip and palate are structural defects that often involve care by a team of providers, such as plastic surgeon, pediatrician, nurse, audiologist, speech therapist, and orthodontist.

- A variety of defects of the esophagus can manifest as mild to life-threatening problems in newborns.

- Pyloric stenosis is a common cause of projectile vomiting in newborns.

- Children with gastroesophageal reflux are irritable due to lack of food and discomfort when feeding.

- Anatomic malformations of the intestines include omphalocele, Hirschsprung disease, and anorectal disorders.

- Hernias can be present in the diaphragmatic area, umbilicus, or inguinal canal.

- The most common inflammatory disorder of the gastrointestinal tract is appendicitis.

- Necrotizing enterocolitis is a potentially life-threatening inflammatory disease of the intestines seen primarily in premature infants after enteral feedings are begun.

- Common inflammatory bowel diseases affecting primarily adolescent and young adult age groups are Crohn's disease and ulcerative colitis.

- Peptic ulcer may be primary (often caused by *H. pylori*) or secondary, in situations of stress, trauma, or other disease.

- Several intestinal problems of childhood necessitate temporary or permanent ostomy placement.

- Acute vomiting and diarrhea (gastroenteritis) is a common disease that threatens the fluid and electrolyte status of young children.

- A variety of parasitic disorders are seen in children, and preventive methods can minimize their spread.

- Feeding disorders such as colic and rumination may require teaching and other nursing interventions.

- Celiac disease is a malabsorption disorder caused by gluten sensitivity.

- Short bowel syndrome occurs when surgery to treat an intestinal disease removes significant sections of the bowel.

- Biliary atresia and hepatitis are the most common liver diseases in young children.

- Abdominal trauma most often occurs to children during car and other crashes.

- Children accidentally ingest a number of medicines, plants, pesticides, and other household products. Nurses teach parents how to avoid these poisonings and how to contact the Poison Control Center in case of accidental exposure.

EXPLORE MediaLink

NCLEX Review, Case Studies, and other interactive resources for this chapter can be found on the companion website at http://www.prenhall.com/london. Click on "Chapter 46" to select the activities for this chapter.

For animations, more NCLEX review questions, and an audio glossary, access the accompanying CD-ROM in this textbook.

REFERENCES

Advisory Committee on Childhood Lead Poisoning Prevention. (2000). Recommendations for blood lead screening of young children enrolled in Medicaid: Targeting a group at high risk. *Morbidity and Mortality Weekly Report, 49* (RR14), 1–13.

Balasubrahmanyam, G., Scherer, N. J., Martin, J. A., & Michal, M. L. (1998). Cleft lip and palate: Keys to successful management. *Contemporary Pediatrics, 15,* 133–153.

Barr, J. M. B. (2000). Chronic intestinal pseudo-obstruction: Pediatric case presentations and review of the literature. *Journal of the Society of Pediatric Nurses, 5,* 175–182.

Berube, M. (1997). Gastroesophageal reflux. *Journal of the Society of Pediatric Nurses, 2,* 43–46.

Blumenthal, M., Goldberg, A. & Brinckmann, J. (2000). *Herbal medicine, expanded commission E monographs.* Newton, MA: Integrative Medicine Communications.

Borkowski, S. (1998). Pediatric stomas, tubes, and appliances. *Pediatric Clinics of North America, 45,* 1419–1436.

Brown, R. L., Irish, M. S., Rice, H. E., Caty, M. G., & Glick, P. L. (1998). Care of the surgical intensive care nursery graduate: The primary care pediatrician's perspective. *Pediatric Clinics of North America, 45,* 1327–1352.

Burkhart, D. M. (1999). Management of acute gastroenteritis in children. *American Family Physician, 60,* 2555–2566.

Castiglia, P. T. (2001). Constipation in children. *Journal of Pediatric Health Care, 15,* 200–202.

Centers for Disease Control and Prevention. (1997). *Screening young children for lead poisoning: Guidance for state and local public health officials.* Atlanta: Author.

Centers for Disease Control and Prevention. (1999). Prevention of hepatitis A through active or passive immunization: Recommendations of the ACIP. *Morbidity and Mortality Weekly Report, 48* (RR12), 1–37.

Centers for Disease Control and Prevention. (2000). Blood lead levels in young children— United States and selected states, 1996–1999. *Morbidity and Mortality Weekly Report, 49,* 1133–1137.

Centers for Disease Control and Prevention. (2001). Blood and hair mercury levels in young children and women of childbearing age—United States, 1999. *Morbidity and Mortality Weekly Report, 50,* 140–143.

Committee on Nutrition, American Academy of Pediatrics. (1998). *Pediatric nutrition handbook.* Elk Grove Village, IL: American Academy of Pediatrics.

Connon, J. J. (1999). Celiac disease. In M. E. Shils, J. A. Olson, J. Shike, & A. C Ross (Eds.), *Modern nutrition in health and disease* (9th ed., pp. 1163–1168). Baltimore: Williams & Wilkins.

Cowden, J. D., & Hotez, P. J. (2001). A field guide to emerging enteric protozoa. *Contemporary Pediatrics, 18,* 440–447.

Cox, K. L. (2000). Liver transplantation. In R. E. Behrman, R. M. Kliegman, & H. B. Jenson (Eds.), *Nelson textbook of pediatrics* (16th ed., pp. 1227–1229). Philadelphia: Saunders.

DerMarderosian, A. (Ed.). (2000). *Chamomile. The review of natural products: Facts and comparisons* [Monograph]. St. Louis, MO: Wolters Kluwer Co.

Eliason, B. C., & Lewan, R. B. (1998). Gastroenteritis in children: Principles of diagnosis and treatment. *American Family Physician, 58,* 1769–1776.

Emery, D., & Singer, J. I. (1998). Highly toxic ingestions for toddlers: When a pill can kill. *Emergency Medicine Reports, 3,* 111–122.

Estrada, B. (2000). Breast-feeding and vertical transmission of hepatitis C. *Infectious Medicine, 17,* 526–528.

Gokhale, R. (2001). Chronic abdominal pain: Inflammatory bowel disease and eosinophilic gastroenteropathy. *Pediatric Annals, 30,* 49–55.

Hamilton, J., Rao, P. M., Wagner, J. M., & Miller, D. (1998). Appendicitis: Unmasking the great masquerader. *Patient Care Nurse Practitioner, 1*(5), 11–27.

Hartman, G. E. (2000). Diaphragmatic hernia. In R. E. Behrman, R. M. Kliegman, & H. B. Jenson (Eds.), *Nelson textbook of pediatrics* (16th ed., pp. 1231–1234). Philadelphia: Saunders.

Harvey, B. (1997). New lead screening guidelines from the Centers for Disease Control and Prevention: How will they affect pediatricians? *Pediatrics, 100,* 384–388.

Hendren, W. H. (1998). Pediatric rectal and perianal problems. *Pediatric Clinics of North America, 45,* 1353–1372.

Herbst, J. J. (2000). The esophagus: Ulcer disease. In R. E. Behrman, R. M. Kliegman, & H. B. Jenson (Eds.), *Nelson textbook of pediatrics* (16th ed., pp. 1121–1128, 1147–1150). Philadelphia: Saunders.

Hoffenberg, E. J., Bao, F., Eisenbarth, G. S., Uhlhom, C., Haas, J. E., Sokol, R. J., et al. (2000). Transglutaminase antibodies in children with a genetic risk for celiac disease. *Journal of Pediatrics, 137,* 356–366.

Holst, B., & Ritter, D. (2001). Managing viral hepatitis. *Clinician Reviews, 11,* 51–62.

Huff, C. (1997). Celiac disease: Helping families adapt. *Gastroenterology Nursing, 20,* 79–81.

Irish, M. S., Pearl, R. H., Caty, M. G., & Glick, P. L. (1998). The approach to common abdominal diagnoses in infants and children. *Pediatric Clinics of North America, 45,* 729–773.

Jakubik, L. D., Colfer, A., & Grossman, M. B. (2000). Pediatric short bowel syndrome: Pathophysiology, nursing care, and management issues. *Journal of the Society of Pediatric Nurses, 5,* 111–121.

Kazacos, K. R. (2000). Protecting children from helminthic zoonoses. *Contemporary Pediatrics* (Suppl.), 1–24.

Levy, J. (2001). Gastroesophageal reflux and other causes of abdominal pain. *Pediatric Annals, 30,* 42–47.

Li, B. U. K. (1996). Cyclic vomiting: New understanding of an old disorder. *Contemporary Pediatrics, 13,* 48–62.

Litovitz, T. L., Klein-Schwartz, W., White, S., Cobaugh, D. J., Youniss, J., Omslaer, J. C., et al. (2001). 2000 annual report of the American Association of Poison Control Centers Toxic Exposure Surveillance System. *American Journal of Emergency Medicine, 19,* 337–395.

Lucassen, P. L., Assendelft, W. J., & Gubbels, J. W. (1998). Review: Some behavioral interventions, drugs, and dietary changes reduce infantile colic. *British Medical Journal, 316,* 1563–1569.

McDiarnid, S. V. (2000). Liver transplantation. The pediatric challenge. *Clinical Liver Disease, 4,* 879–927.

Mitchell, J. C., & Wood, R. J. (2000). Management of cleft lip and palate in primary care. *Journal of Pediatric Health Care, 14,* 13–19.

Murphy, M. S. (1998). Guidelines for managing acute gastroenteritis based on a systematic review of published research. *Archives of Disease in Childhood, 79,* 279–288.

Murray, K. F., & Christie, D. L. (2000). Vomiting in infancy: When should you worry. *Contemporary Pediatrics, 17,* 81–115.

National Institute on Drug Abuse. (2000). *Hepatitis C. Community drug alert bulletin* (NIH Publication No. 00–4663). Bethesda: National Institutes of Health.

National Safety Council. (2000). *Injury facts.* Itasca, IL: Author.

Nehring, W. M., & Vessey, J. A. (2000). Down syndrome. In P. L. Jackson & J. A. Vessey (Eds.), *Primary care of the child with a chronic condition* (pp. 445–474). St. Louis, MO: Mosby.

Nowicki, M. J., & Bishop, P. R. (1999). Organic causes of constipation in infants and children. *Pediatric Annals, 28,* 293–300.

O'Donnell, K. A., Glick, P. L., & Caty, M. G. (1998). Pediatric umbilical problems. *Pediatric Clinics of North America, 45,* 791–812.

O'Hara, M., Kiefer, D., Farrell, K., & Kemper, K. (1998). A review of 12 commonly used medicinal herbs. *Archives of Family Medicine, 7,* 523–536.

Orenstein, J. (2000). Update on intussusception. *Contemporary Pediatrics, 17,* 180–191.

Pearl, R. H., Irish, M. S., Caty, M. G., & Glick, P. L. (1998). The approach to common abdominal diagnoses in infants and children: Part II. *Pediatric Clinics of North America, 45,* 1287–1326.

Pena, B. M. G., Taylor, G. A., & Lund, D. P. (1999). Appendicitis revisited: New insights into an age-old problem. *Contemporary Pediatrics, 16,* 122–133.

Powers, K. S. (2000). Diagnosis and management of common toxic ingestions and inhalations. *Pediatric Annals, 29,* 330–343.

Rao, P. M., Rhea, J. J., Novelline, R. A., Mostatavi, A. A., & McCabe, C. J. (1998). Effect of computed tomography of the appendix. *New England Journal of Medicine, 338,* 141–146.

Shovein, J. T., Damazo, R. J., & Hyams, I. (2000). Hepatitis A: How benign is it? *American Journal of Nursing, 100,* 43–48.

Snyder, J. (1997, July). Feeding during diarrhea: New AAP guidelines and innovations in oral rehydration solutions. *Contemporary Pediatrics Reporter, 6.*

SPLIT Research Group. (2001). Studies of pediatric liver transplantation (SPLIT): Year 2000 outcomes. *Transplantation, 72,* 463–476.

Stoll, B. J., & Kliegman, R. M. (2000). Digestive system disorders. In R. E. Behrman, R. M. Kliegman, & H. B. Jenson (Eds.), *Nelson textbook of pediatrics* (16th ed., pp. 510–518). Philadelphia: Saunders.

Uhrich, K. S., & Mackin, A. L. (2001). Cleft lip and palate. *American Journal of Nursing, 101,* 24AA–FF.

Warner, B. W. (1996). Classification of congenital disorders of the anorectum. In A. M. Rudolph, J. I. E. Hoffman, & C. D. Rudolph (Eds.), *Rudolph's pediatrics* (29th ed., p. 1112). Stamford, CT: Appleton & Lange.

West, L. (1997). Innovative approaches to the administration of activated charcoal in pediatric toxic ingestions. *Pediatric Nursing, 23,* 616–619.

Westerdahl, J. (1999). Botanicals in pediatrics. In P. Q. Samour, K. K. Helm, & C. E. Lang (Eds.), *Handbook of pediatric nutrition* (2nd ed., pp. 589–600). Gaithersburg, MD: Aspen Publishers.

Wong, W. Y., Eskes, T. K., Kuihpers-Jagtman, A. M., Spauwen, P. H., Steegers, E. A., Thomas, C. M., et al. (1999). Nonsyndromic orofacial clefts: Association with maternal hyperhomocysteinemia. *Teratology, 60,* 253–257.

Wylie, R. (2000). Ileus, adhesions, intussusception, and closed loop obstructions. In R. E. Behrman, R. M. Kliegman, & H. B. Jenson (Eds.), *Nelson textbook of pediatrics* (16th ed., pp. 1141–1144). Philadelphia: Saunders.

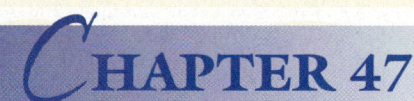

CHAPTER 47

The Child with Alterations in Genitourinary Function

Planning Terrell's day can be a challenge, because his treatment often interferes with his activities. We all hope that Terrell receives a kidney transplant soon so his growth will improve and he will not have to miss school during treatment.

—AUNT OF TERRELL, 5 YEARS OLD

Key Terms

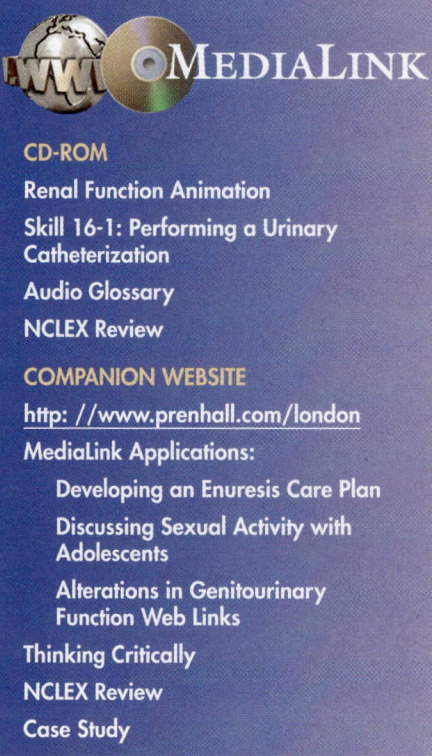

MEDIALINK

CD-ROM

Renal Function Animation

Skill 16-1: Performing a Urinary Catheterization

Audio Glossary

NCLEX Review

COMPANION WEBSITE

http://www.prenhall.com/london

MediaLink Applications:

Developing an Enuresis Care Plan

Discussing Sexual Activity with Adolescents

Alterations in Genitourinary Function Web Links

Thinking Critically

NCLEX Review

Case Study

Many infections, structural disorders, and disease processes alter genitourinary function. Because the kidneys and other urinary system organs perform several essential body functions, including removing waste products and maintaining fluid and electrolyte balance, disorders that affect these organs pose a significant threat to the health of children.

Although the reproductive system is functionally immature until puberty, uncorrected structural defects and sexually transmitted diseases can have both psychologic and physiologic implications for the developing child.

ANATOMY AND PHYSIOLOGY OF PEDIATRIC DIFFERENCES

The genitourinary system is made up of the urinary and reproductive organs. The urinary system—kidneys, ureters, bladder, and urethra (Figure 47–1 ◆)—excretes wastes and maintains acid-base and fluid and electrolyte balance. The reproductive system consists of internal and external organs that at maturity promote the conception and healthy development of a fetus.

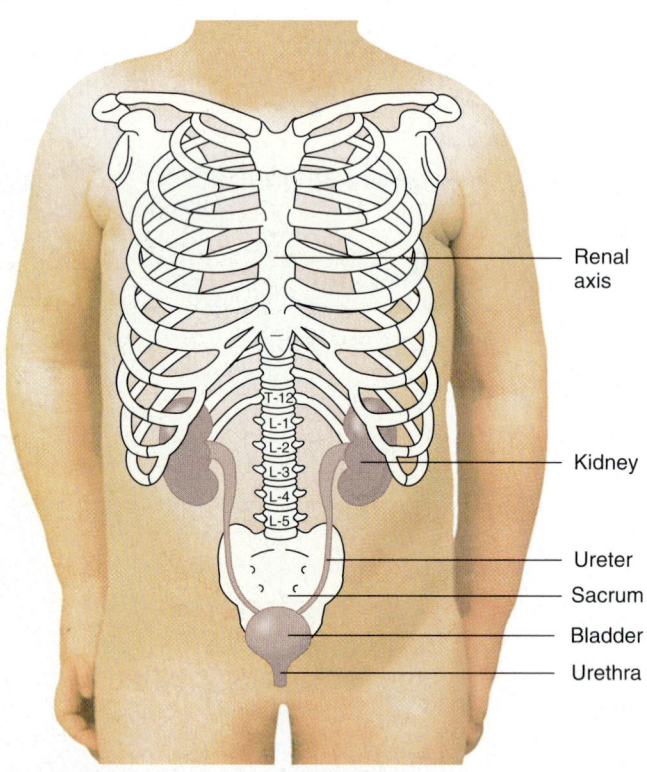

FIGURE 47–1. ◆ The kidneys are located between the twelfth thoracic (T12) and third lumbar (L3) vertebrae.

Urinary System

All of the nephrons that will make up the mature kidney are present at birth. The kidneys grow and the tubular system matures gradually during childhood, reaching full size by adolescence. Most renal growth occurs during the first 5 years of life. This increase in size is due primarily to enlargement of the nephrons. The efficiency of the kidney also increases with age. During the first 2 years of life, the kidneys are less efficient at regulating electrolyte and acid-base balance (see Chapter 39) ⊂⊃ and eliminating some drugs from the body. After the age of 2 years, the kidneys' efficiency increases markedly.

Growth and Development

Urinary output per kilogram of body weight decreases as the child ages because the kidney becomes more efficient at concentrating urine. Expected output:

Infants	2 mL/kg/hr
Children	0.5 to 1 mL/kg/hr
Adolescents	40 to 80 mL/hr

Bladder capacity increases with age from 20 to 50 mL at birth to 700 mL in adulthood. A child's bladder capacity (in ounces) can be estimated by adding 2 to the child's age (e.g., a 4-year-old has a bladder capacity of 6 ounces). Stimulation of "stretch receptors" within the bladder wall initiates urination. Simultaneous contraction of the detrusor muscle of the bladder and relaxation of the internal and external sphincters result in emptying of the bladder. Children less than 2 years of age cannot maintain bladder control because of insufficient nerve development.

Normal renal function requires the following: unimpaired renal blood flow, adequate glomerular ultrafiltration, normal tubular function, and unobstructed urine flow. ⊂⊃ CD

Reproductive System

The reproductive system in children is functionally immature until puberty. Throughout childhood the genitalia (with the exception of the clitoris in girls) enlarge gradually. The hormonal changes of puberty accelerate anatomic and functional development (see Chapter 33 and Figures 33–32 and 33–33). ⊂⊃ In girls, the mons pubis becomes more prominent and hair begins to grow. The vagina lengthens, and the epithelial layers thicken. The uterus and ovaries enlarge, and the musculature and vascularization of the uterus also increase. In boys, downy hair begins to appear at the base of the penis, and the scrotum becomes increasingly pendulous. The penis grows longer and wider.

BLADDER EXSTROPHY

Bladder exstrophy is a rare defect in which the posterior bladder wall extrudes through the lower abdominal wall (Figure 47–2 ◆). Failure of the abdominal wall to close during fetal development results in eversion and protuberance of the bladder wall and a wide separation of the rectus muscles and the symphysis pubis. The upper urinary tract is usually normal. The defect occurs in approximately 1 in every 400,000 live births and is more common in boys than girls by a ratio of 3 to 1 (Ben-Chaim, Docimo, Jeffs, et al., 1996). The bladder mucosa appears as a mass of bright red tissue, and urine continually leaks from an open urethra. Females have a bifid clitoris. Males have a short, stubby penis, and the glans is flattened with dorsal chordee and a ventral prepuce. Epispadias and bilateral inguinal hernias are also common.

Treatment is surgical reconstruction, which is performed in several stages. The initial stage (bladder closure) is usually completed within 24 to 48 hours after birth. Epispadias repair and closure of the symphysis pubis are often performed at the same time. Surgery to reconstruct the bladder neck and reimplant the ureters is performed when the child is 2 to 3 years of age. The goals of surgical reconstruction are (1) bladder and abdominal wall closure; (2) urinary continence, with preservation of renal function; (3) creation of functional and normal-appearing genitalia; and (4) improvement of sexual functioning. Some

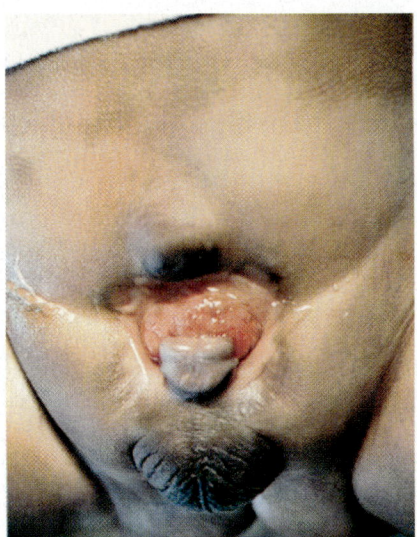

FIGURE 47–2. ◆ This child has bladder exstrophy, noted by extrusion of the posterior bladder wall through the lower abdominal wall.

children require permanent urinary diversion because a functional bladder cannot be reconstructed. In some patients with a very small or bifid penis, gender reassignment may be considered.

Because the bladder epithelium is abnormal, it is prone to neoplasms. Yearly cystoscopy after the age of 20 years is recommended to evaluate for possible malignancies (Feeg & Harbin, 1991).

Nursing Management

Preoperative nursing care centers on preventing infection and trauma to the exposed bladder. The bladder mucosa is covered in sterile plastic wrap to prevent trauma and irritation, and the surrounding area is cleaned daily and protected from leaking urine with a skin sealant.

Postoperatively the wound and pelvis are immobilized to facilitate healing. Internal and external immobilization techniques are used for pelvic closure (see Chapter 50). Avoid abduction of the infant's legs. Nursing care includes maintaining proper alignment, monitoring peripheral circulation, and providing meticulous wound and skin care.

Monitor renal function by assessing the adequacy of urine output and blood and urine chemistries. Observe for any signs of obstruction in the drainage tubes such as increased intensity of bladder spasms, decreased urine output, or urine or blood draining from the urethral meatus. Promote comfort and give antibiotics as ordered.

Parents need emotional support to help them cope with the disfiguring nature of the infant's defect and the uncertainty of complete repair. To promote parent–infant bonding, encourage parents to participate in all aspects of the infant's care, including bathing, feeding, and wound care. Discharge teaching should include instructions about dressing changes and diapering and the need to immediately report any signs of infection or change in renal function. Emphasize the need for routine follow-up visits after surgery to assess urinary function and to ensure that the next stages of surgery for continence control are performed at the appropriate time in the child's development. However, these children do not always achieve continence. Parents need help to promote the child's self-esteem and self-confidence with sexual identity and function. Psychologic counseling may help the child during adolescence.

HYPOSPADIAS AND EPISPADIAS

Hypospadias and epispadias are congenital anomalies involving the location of the urethral meatus in males (Figure 47–3 ◆). Both defects result when the urethral folds fail to fuse completely over the urethral groove. The reported incidence of hypospadias of 1 in every 300 male births is increasing, possibly due to environmental elements or genetic factors (Paulozzi, Erickson, & Jackson, 1997).

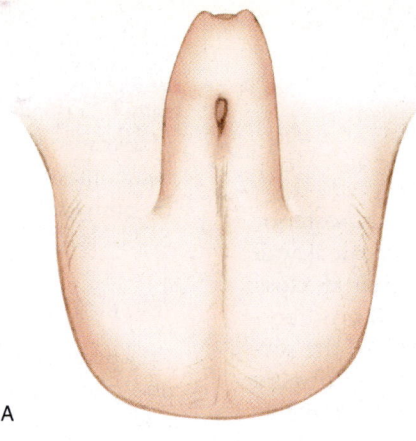

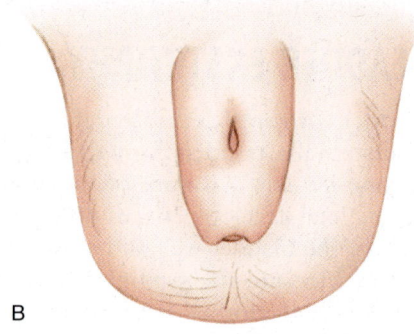

FIGURE 47–3. ◆ Hypospadias and epispadias. **A,** In hypospadias the urethral canal is open on the ventral surface of the penis. **B,** In epispadias the canal is open on the dorsal surface.

A

B

With hypospadias, the urethral meatus can be located anywhere along the course of the anterior urethra on the ventral surface of the penile shaft, from the perineum to the tip of the glans. Most cases are mild, with the meatus slightly off center from the tip of the penis; in severe cases, the meatus is located on the scrotum. Hypospadias often occurs in conjunction with congenital chordee, a fibrous line of tissue that results in ventral curvature of the penile shaft and undescended testes.

In epispadias, the meatal opening is located on the dorsal surface of the penile shaft. Epispadias often occurs in conjunction with exstrophy of the bladder.

Diagnosis is made prenatally by ultrasound or by examination at birth. The infant should not be circumcised because the dorsal foreskin tissue will be used for surgical repair. The defects are corrected surgically, usually during the first year of life, to minimize psychologic effects when the child is older. Surgery is usually performed in a single operation, often as an outpatient procedure. The goals of surgical repair are (1) placement of the urethral meatus at the end of the glans penis with satisfactory caliber and configuration for a urinary stream (enabling the child to void in a standing position) and (2) release of chordee to straighten the penis (enabling future sexual function).

A caudal nerve block is often used for postoperative pain relief. Muscle relaxants may be prescribed to relieve bladder spasms.

Nursing Management

It is important to address parents' concerns at the time of birth. Preoperative teaching can relieve some of their anxiety about the future appearance and functioning of the penis.

Postoperative care focuses on protecting the surgical site from injury. The infant or child returns from surgery with the penis wrapped in a simple dressing, and sometimes a urethral **stent** (a device used to maintain patency of the urethral canal) is placed to keep the new urethral canal open. Plan care to ensure that the stent does not get removed. Refer to the hospital's policy for the appropriate use of physical restraints in this situation.

Encourage fluid intake to maintain adequate urinary output and patency of the stent. Accurate documentation of intake and output is essential. Notify the physician if there is no urine drainage for 1 hour as this may indicate kinks in the system or obstruction by sediment. Pain may be associated with bladder spasms. Anticholinergic medications such as oxybutynin or hyoscyamine may be prescribed. Acetaminophen may also be given for pain. Antibiotics are often prescribed until the urinary stent falls out.

Patients are often discharged the day of surgery. Discharge teaching should include instructions for parents about care of the reconstructed area, double diapering to protect the stent, fluid intake, medication administration, and signs and symptoms of infection (see "Teaching About Caring for the Child after Hypospadias and Epispadias Repair" and Skill 16-2 in the *Clinical Skills Manual*). **SKILLS** Tell parents that they need to take the child to the physician's office for dressing removal about 4 days after surgery.

OBSTRUCTIVE UROPATHY

Obstructive uropathy refers to structural or functional abnormalities of the urinary system that interfere with urine flow. The pressure caused by urine backup compromises kidney function and often causes **hydronephrosis** (accumulation of urine in the renal pelvis as a result of obstructed outflow). Physiologic changes that may occur as a result of hydronephrosis include:

- Cessation of glomerular filtration when the pressure in the kidney pelvis equals the filtration pressure in the glomerular capillaries. In response, the blood pressure increases as the body attempts to increase the glomerular filtration pressure.

- Metabolic acidosis, which results when the distal nephrons' ability to secrete hydrogen ions is impaired.

- Impairment of the kidney's ability to concentrate urine, resulting in polydipsia and polyuria.

- Obstruction resulting in urinary stasis, which promotes the growth of bacteria.

CARING FOR THE CHILD AFTER HYPOSPADIAS AND EPISPADIAS REPAIR

- Use double-diapering to protect the stent (the small tube that drains the urine). See Skill 16-2. **SKILLS**
- Restrict the infant or toddler from activities (e.g., playing on riding toys) that put pressure on the surgical site. Avoid holding the infant or child straddled on the hip. Limit the child's activity for 2 weeks.
- Encourage the infant or toddler to drink fluids to ensure adequate hydration. Provide fluids in a pleasant environment or using a special cup. Offer fruit juice, fruit-flavored ice pops, fruit-flavored juices, flavored ice cubes, and gelatin.
- Be sure to give the complete course of prescribed antibiotics to avoid infection.
- Watch for signs of infection: fever, swelling, redness, pain, strong-smelling urine, or change in flow of the urinary stream.
- The urine will be blood tinged for several days. Call the physician if urine is seen leaking from any area other than the penis.

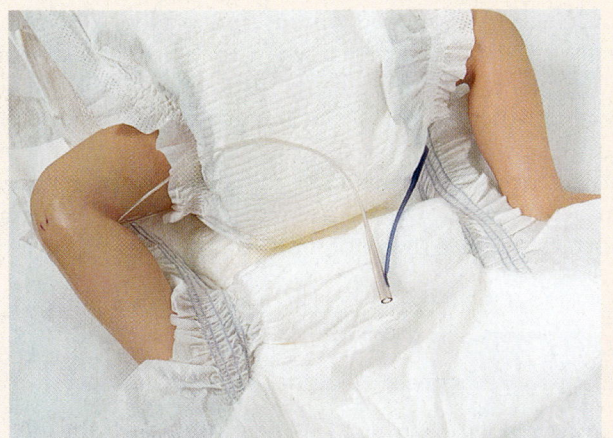

A double diapering technique protects the urinary stent after surgery for hypospadias or epispadias repair. The inner diaper collects stool; the outer diaper, urine.

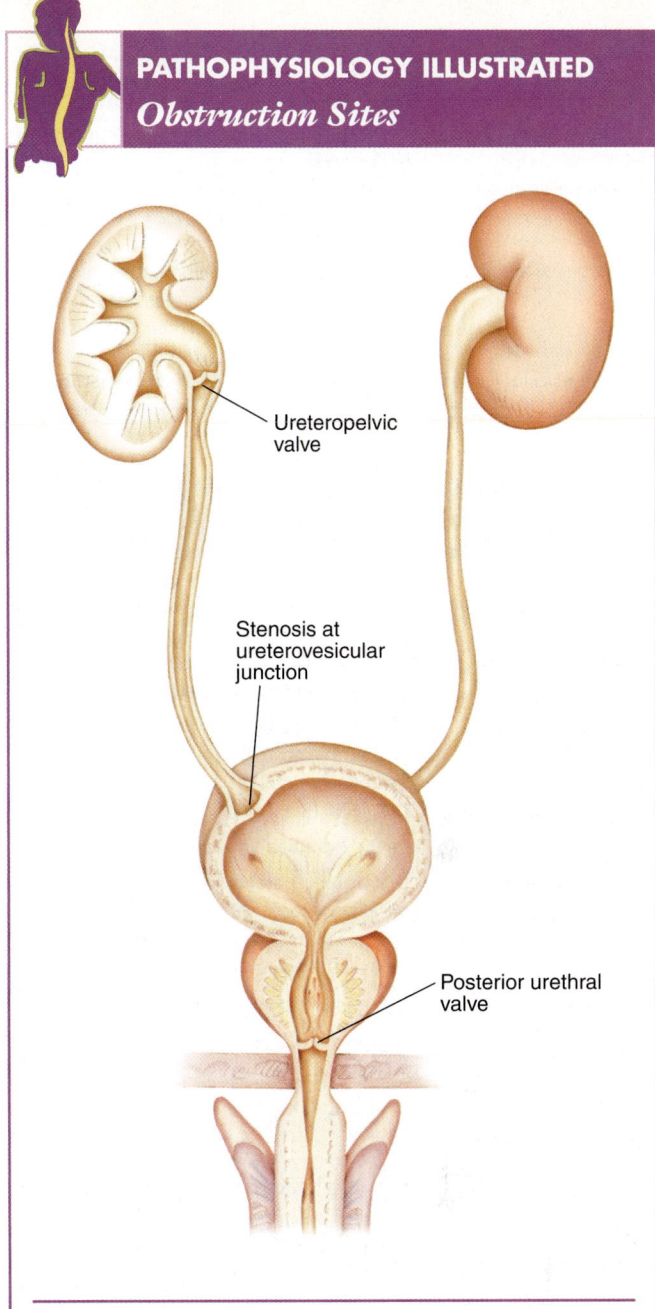

PATHOPHYSIOLOGY ILLUSTRATED
Obstruction Sites

Ureteropelvic valve

Stenosis at ureterovesicular junction

Posterior urethral valve

The common sites of obstruction in the upper and lower urinary tract. Why would damage from posterior urethral valves potentially be worse than other obstructions? Upper urinary tract infections are often unilateral. Renal failure is most likely to occur when both kidneys are affected by hydronephrosis.

- Restriction of urinary outflow, which causes progressive renal damage if left untreated. As a consequence, the growth of the kidneys may be arrested, or renal failure may occur.

Obstructive uropathy may be caused by several congenital lesions such as ureteropelvic junction (UPJ) obstruction, posterior urethral valves (PUVs), and stenosis at the ureterovesicular junction (see "Pathophysiology Illustrated: Obstruction Sites"). The UPJ is the most common site of obstruction of the upper urinary tract in infants and children. PUVs (abnormal folds of mucosa in the male urethra) are the most common cause of anatomic bladder outlet obstruction, occurring in approximately 1 in 5000 to 8000 live male births.

Prune-belly syndrome, also known as Eagle–Barrett syndrome, is another cause of hydronephrosis. In this congenital defect the abdominal musculature fails to develop. The skin covering the abdominal wall is thin and resembles a wrinkled prune. Other characteristics include urinary tract anomalies, poor ureteral peristalsis, enlarged bladder, high risk for recurrent urinary tract infection, and bilateral cryptorchidism. Prune-belly syndrome occurs predominantly in males (95%), with an incidence of 1 in 29,000 to 40,000 births (Becker & Avner, 1995).

OBSTRUCTIVE LESION	CLINICAL MANIFESTATIONS
Ureteropelvic junction obstruction	In infants: abdominal mass (enlarged kidney), hypertension, urinary tract infection In children: hematuria, pain, intermittent nausea and vomiting
Posterior urethral valves	In infants: abdominal mass (enlarged kidney), distended bladder, poor urinary stream, urinary tract infection, sepsis, low specific gravity, polyuria, increased creatinine level, failure to thrive In children: urinary frequency and incontinence
Ureterovesicular junction obstruction	Urinary tract infection (recurrent or chronic), hematuria, pain, abdominal mass (enlarged kidney), enuresis

TABLE 47–1   Diagnostic Tests for Urinary System Conditions

Test	Use
Voiding cystourethrogram	Shows bladder structure and function, urethral anatomy, bladder masses. Detects vesicoureteral reflux.
Renal ultrasound	Identifies large renal scars, renal anomalies, obstruction, abscesses, masses, and hydronephrosis.
Diuretic renogram	Identifies lesions that become symptomatic during increased urine flow.
Radionucleotide scan	Detects renal parenchymal lesions, renal atrophy, or scars. Differentiates between hydronephrosis caused by obstructive lesions, reflux, or a cyst.
Renal cortical scintigraphy	Documents pyelonephritis and renal scarring.
Serum creatinine	Evaluates kidney function.

Other conditions that can lead to hydronephrosis include myelomeningocele and neoplasms. Clinical manifestations vary, depending on the cause and location of the obstruction.

Early diagnosis and treatment prevent kidney damage and deterioration of renal function. Prenatal ultrasound may detect hydronephrosis, but milder obstructions may not become apparent until later in infancy or childhood. Table 47–1 lists diagnostic tests commonly used to identify urinary tract conditions.

The goals of surgical correction or diversion are to lower the pressure within the collecting system, which prevents parenchymal damage, and to prevent stasis, which decreases the risk of infection. Surgical correction may necessitate **pyeloplasty** (removal of an obstructed segment of the ureter and reimplantation into the renal pelvis) or valve repair or reconstruction, depending on the cause of the obstruction. Urinary incontinence resulting from sphincter weakness is a common problem after surgery.

Nursing Management

Preoperative nursing care focuses on preparing the parents and child for the procedure and addressing parents' concerns about the postsurgical outcome. Give parents a chance to discuss concerns about how the disorder will affect the child's long-term renal functioning.

Postoperative care involves monitoring vital signs and intake and output and observing for signs of urine retention, such as decreased output and bladder distention. Many children are discharged with stents or catheters. Teach parents how to change dressings, double diaper, care for catheters, assess pain and give analgesics, and recognize signs of possible obstruction or infection. Parents should encourage the child to participate in age-appropriate activities. However, children should avoid contact sports because of their potential to injure the bladder.

≈ URINARY TRACT INFECTION

A urinary tract infection (UTI) may be bacterial, viral, or fungal; it occurs in the urinary tract. Cystitis is a lower UTI that involves the urethra or bladder. Pyelonephritis is an upper UTI that involves the ureters, renal pelvis, and renal parenchyma. UTIs can be acute or chronic (the latter either recurrent or persistent).

UTIs are the second most common infections in children. What accounts for the high incidence of these infections? Among newborns and young infants, most infections occur in boys. They are usually associated with structural defects having a higher incidence in males (e.g., obstructive uropathy), which predispose the infant to infection. A higher rate of UTIs also occurs among uncircumcised infants (Anderson & Anderson, 1999). Among older infants and children, the incidence of UTIs is higher in girls. This is attributed to the shorter female urethra (2 cm [1 in] in young girls) and its proximity to the anus and vagina, which increases the risk of contamination by fecal bacteria.

Etiology and Pathophysiology

Many first UTIs are caused by *Escherichia coli*, a common gram-negative enteric bacterium. Other causative organisms include *Staphylococcus, Klebsiella, Proteus, Pseudomonas, Enterobacter,* and *Enterococcus.*

Urinary stasis enhances the risk of UTI. Stasis may be caused by abnormal anatomic structures or abnormal function (e.g., neurogenic bladder, common in children with myelomeningocele). Infrequent voiding, which is common in school-age children, also increases the risk of UTI. Children normally void five to six times a day. Some children, however, develop the habit of urinating only once or twice a day, which results in incomplete emptying of the bladder and urinary stasis. Other factors associated with increased risk of UTI include an irritated perineum, constipation, masturbation, sexual abuse, and sexually active adolescent females.

Another cause of UTI is **vesicoureteral reflux,** the backflow of urine from the bladder into the ureters during voiding. This prevents complete emptying of the bladder and creates a reservoir for bacterial growth. Vesicoureteral reflux can also result from a structural anomaly in which the ureters insert in an abnormal position into the bladder.

Renal scarring can result from hydronephrosis or pyelonephritis due to the inflammatory and ischemic effects of the infection. Scars have been associated with hypertension, proteinuria, and kidney failure. The risk of kidney damage increases in the following instances:

- Child less than 1 year of age
- Delay in diagnosis and effective antibacterial treatment for an upper UTI
- Anatomic or neurologic obstruction
- Recurrent episodes of upper UTIs

Clinical Manifestations

Symptoms depend not only on the location of the infection, but also on the age of the child. Symptoms in the newborn period tend to be nonspecific—unexplained fever, failure to thrive, poor feeding, vomiting and diarrhea, strong-smelling urine, and irritability. Any child under 2 years of age with a fever of unknown origin should be tested for a UTI. Not until the toddler years, are the more "classic" symptoms of lower UTI seen as listed in the clinical manifestations table. About 40% of UTIs are asymptomatic.

Clinical Therapy

A urine specimen is examined for the presence of bacteria. A dipstick leukocyte esterase test identifies white blood cells and pyuria. A nitrite dipstick detects bacteria. Using both dipsticks increases the sensitivity (88%) and specificity (93%) for diagnosing a UTI (Shaw & Gorelick, 1999). Diagnosis is confirmed with a urine culture collected by midstream clean-catch void, sterile catheterization, or suprapubic aspiration (see Skills 10-7 and 10-8). **SKILLS** Urine collection bags used on infants are reliable only when no pathogens are found as sterility of the specimen cannot be guaranteed. The diagnosis of infection is made from the number of colony-forming units (between 10^3 to 10^5) depending upon the method of urine collection (Shaw & Gorelick, 1999). Antibiotic sensitivity for the specific organisms cultured is then determined.

Radiologic studies are often performed to detect structural abnormalities and renal scarring. The most common tests performed are a renal ultrasound soon after the diagnosis and a voiding cystourethrogram (VCUG) after the infection has cleared. Renal cortical scintigraphy has become the most commonly used imaging study to detect pyelonephritis and renal scarring (Hellerstein, 2000).

Antibiotic therapy is begun as soon as urine samples have been collected. The antibiotic is changed if necessary after culture sensitivity is determined. Follow-up cultures should be obtained 48 to 72 hours after drug therapy has started, at which time the urine should be sterile. Follow-up urine cultures should then be obtained monthly for 3 months, every 3 months for 6 months, and then annually. Subsequent infections may be asymptomatic. For children with vesicoureteral reflux or recurrent infections, a long-term, suppressive dose of an antibiotic may be ordered for prophylaxis. Children with renal scarring should have their blood pressure monitored.

CLINICAL MANIFESTATIONS ≈ *Urinary Tract Infection Clinical Manifestations and Therapy*

TYPE OF UTI	CLINICAL MANIFESTATIONS	CLINICAL THERAPY
Lower UTI—cystitis	Frequency, dysuria, urgency, enuresis, strong smelling urine	5- to 7-day course of trimethoprim or sulfamethoxazole or antibiotic matching organism sensitivity, encourage fluids, analgesic such as acetaminophen or pyridium
Upper UTI—pyelonephritis	High fever, chills, abdominal pain, flank pain, persistent vomiting, moderate to severe dehydration	Rehydration, antipyretics, IV antibiotics initially then transitioned to oral antibiotics matching organism sensitivity for a total of 7 to 10 days

Children who appear ill and cannot tolerate oral antibiotics are often hospitalized because they need rehydration and parenteral antibiotic treatment. Infants may develop permanent kidney damage or generalized sepsis if the UTI is not treated aggressively. If a structural defect is identified, surgical correction may be necessary to prevent recurrent infections that could lead to renal damage.

Nursing Management

Nursing Assessment and Diagnosis

PHYSIOLOGIC ASSESSMENT

Take a history of urinary symptoms. Assess the infant for toxic (very ill) appearance, fever, and oral fluid intake. Measure the child's height and weight and plot on a growth curve to identify any change in growth pattern associated with a chronic illness. Take the infant's or child's blood pressure. Palpate the abdomen and suprapubic and costovertebral areas for masses, tenderness, and distention. Observe the urinary stream if possible and perform a urinalysis, including specific gravity. Proper collection of the urine specimen is essential. Get a clean-catch urine specimen if the child is able to cooperate. If not, get a catheterized sample (see Skills 10-7 and 10-8). **SKILLS** An early morning urine specimen is preferred because the urine is more concentrated.

PSYCHOSOCIAL ASSESSMENT

Sexually active adolescents may deny having symptoms because they fear disclosing their sexual activity to their parents. Careful questioning may be necessary to elicit these concerns. Be open and approachable and give the patient and family the chance to address their concerns.

Common nursing diagnoses for the child with a UTI include:

▶ *Altered urinary elimination* related to recurrent urinary tract infections
▶ *Risk for altered growth* related to chronic infection and renal damage
▶ *Urinary retention* related to infrequent voiding habits or vesicoureteral reflux
▶ *Risk for ineffective management of therapeutic regimen* related to lack of knowledge of preventive measures (adequate fluid intake, proper hygiene, signs and prophylactic antibiotics)
▶ *Risk for fluid volume deficit* related to fever and inadequate intake

Planning and Implementation

Nursing care for the hospitalized child with a complicated UTI centers on administering prescribed medications, promoting rehydration, assessing renal function, and teaching parents and older children how to minimize the risk of future infection.

Administer antibiotics and antipyretics as prescribed to maintain therapeutic drug levels and reduce fever. Encourage fluid intake to dilute the urine and flush the bladder. Document intake and output. Assess renal function by comparing the child's output to the expected measure of 1 mL/kg/hr and weigh the child daily.

Frequent voiding minimizes urinary stasis. Postvoid catheterization may be needed to determine the amount of residual urine left after urinating (see Skill 16-1). **SKILLS** **CD** Palpate or percuss the bladder after voiding to evaluate bladder emptying.

Because bladder training is such an important milestone for young children, any disorder that affects voiding may have developmental implications. A toddler who has been toilet trained may regress and require diapers temporarily due to incontinence related to the UTI. Reassure parents that this is normal and emphasize that they should offer the toddler support rather than disapproval. A preschooler may perceive the infection as punishment for an imagined wrong such as masturbation. Provide support and reassurance that the child is not being punished for any actions.

NURSING CARE IN THE COMMUNITY

Children with UTIs are usually cared for at home. Teach parents the importance of giving antibiotics as prescribed and assist them to develop an effective schedule. Emphasize that antibiotics must be taken for the full course and that they may be continued even after the infection has cleared to prevent a recurrence. Teach prevention through proper hygiene and avoidance of risk behaviors.

Give parents specific guidelines for oral fluid intake. Make sure the amount of fluids recommended for a 24–hour period equals the maintenance fluids needed plus additional fluids required because of fever and diuresis to flush out pathogens. (See Chapter 39.) Suggest that the parents avoid giving the child caffeinated and carbonated beverages as these may potentially irritate the bladder mucosa (Miller, 1996).

Teaching About

PREVENTION OF URINARY TRACT INFECTIONS

- Teach proper perineal hygiene. Girls should always wipe the perineum from front to back after voiding.
- Encourage the child to drink plenty of fluids and avoid long periods of "holding urine."
- Caution against tight underwear; children should wear cotton rather than nylon underwear.
- Encourage the child to void more frequently and to fully empty the bladder.
- Discourage bubble baths and hot tubs, which can irritate the urethra.
- Instruct sexually active adolescent girls to void before and after sexual intercourse to prevent urinary stasis and flush out bacteria introduced during intercourse.

Encourage the child to void more frequently even after the infection has cleared. A wristwatch with an alarm may be a helpful reminder. The child with a neurogenic bladder needs to have clean intermittent catheterization performed several times a day to reduce urinary stasis and the potential for UTI.

Teach parents the signs and symptoms of recurrent infection and to seek care promptly.

Evaluation

Expected outcomes of nursing care include:

▶ The child increases fluid intake and number of times voiding each day.

▶ Future UTIs are prevented.

ENURESIS

Enuresis is repeated involuntary voiding by a child old enough that bladder control is expected, usually about 5 to 6 years of age. (See Table 47–2 for bladder control milestones.) Enuresis can occur either at night (nocturnal, 50% of cases), during the day (diurnal, 10% of cases), or both night and day (40% of cases) (Kelleher, 1997). Nocturnal enuresis occurs more often in boys than in girls, with 3.5:1 ratio, whereas diurnal enuresis is more common in girls. Enuresis can be primary, intermittent, **WEB** or secondary. In primary enuresis the child has never had a dry night. It is thought to be due to a maturational delay and small functional bladder, not stress or a psychologic cause. In intermittent enuresis the child has occasional nights or periods of dryness. With secondary enuresis a child who has been reliably dry for 6 to 12 months begins bed-wetting. It is associated with stress, infections, and sleep disorders.

TABLE 47–2	Milestones in the Development of Bladder Control
Age	Developmental Milestone
1 1/2 years	Child passes urine at regular intervals.
2 years	Child announces when he or she is voiding.
2 1/2 years	Child makes known need to void; can hold urine.
3 years	Child goes to the bathroom by himself or herself; holds urge if preoccupied with play.
2 1/2–3 1/2 years	Child achieves nighttime control.
4 years	Child shows great interest in going to bathrooms when away from home (shopping centers, movies).
5 years	Child voids approximately 7 times a day; prefers privacy; is able to initiate emptying of bladder at any degree of fullness.

Growth and Development

An estimated 15% to 20% of children who are partially toilet trained will continue to have wetting episodes after 5 years of age. An estimated 5% of 10-year-olds and 2% of 12- to 14-year-olds continue to have nocturnal enuresis (Issenman, Filmer, & Gorski, 1999).

Enuresis may result from neurologic or congenital structural disorders, illness, or stress. Nocturnal enuresis occurs frequently in children whose parents have a history of bed-wetting. There is a 77% risk if both parents had enuresis, a 44% risk if one parent had enuresis, and a 15% risk if neither parent had enuresis (Tobias, 2000). In most children with primary enuresis, the bladder has a smaller functional capacity, and neuromuscular maturation of the inhibitory fibers is delayed. Minor abnormalities of the bladder neck and urethra are also associated with enuresis. Some children are believed to have mild developmental delays. Often children with nocturnal enuresis are harder to arouse and may fail to respond to full bladder signals. In some children, unstable bladder contractions may occur during sleep resulting in enuresis. The majority of cases (95%) are not associated with structural or neurologic pathology.

Diabetes mellitus or renal insufficiency should be ruled out in children with both enuresis and polyuria or oliguria. The child's lower spine is examined for fistulas, sacral dimples, or tufts of hair that could be signs of occult spina bifida. Prolonged hospitalization, family stressors, and preoccupation with school concerns also have been associated with secondary enuresis. Children with diurnal enuresis may have frequency, urgency, constant dribbling, and involuntary loss of control after voiding.

A thorough history can help identify potential causes of enuresis (Table 47–3). Asking about the child's elimination patterns and developmental milestones and the parents' methods of toilet training can provide essential information (see Table 32–16). Enuretic children often have a history of constipation. Rectal pressure on the posterior bladder wall stimulates the bladder to empty. Laboratory evaluation includes urinalysis and urine culture. Renal studies such as ultrasound and VCUG are done in cases of secondary enuresis.

A multitreatment approach is usually most effective. Fluid restriction, bladder training, and enuresis alarms are common approaches (Table 47–4). A spontaneous cure happens in 15% of children each year, regardless of intervention or lack of intervention. Approximately one third of children with nocturnal enuresis are treated with medications. Imipramine, a tricyclic antidepressant, is often used but requires close monitoring because of its effects on mood and sleep-arousal patterns and the associated danger of overdoses. Desmopressin, given as a nasal spray, has an antidiuretic effect but is not used long term because of its

TABLE 47-3 Questions to Ask When Taking an Enuresis History

Family History

Is there a family history of renal or urinary structural abnormalities?

Is there a family history of bed-wetting?

Family Management

How serious is the problem for the family?

What happens when the child wets? (Who gets up and changes sheets?)

How is the child treated? Is the child punished or blamed for wetting?

What remedies have been tried?

Toilet Training

Did the child have a difficult time with toilet training?

What method of toilet training did you use? When was toilet training initiated?

What are the child's current voiding and stooling patterns?

How long is the child's longest dry period, and when does it occur?

Does the child have a history of constipation or encopresis?

Stressors

How is the child doing in school?

Are any new or chronic stressors present in the child's life?

How does the problem interfere with play and other activities?

Risk Factors

Diabetes

• Does the child void often or have urgency?

• Is the child frequently thirsty?

Urinary Tract Infection

• Does the child experience burning on urination?

• Has the child had a urinary tract infection before?

TABLE 47-4 Treatment Approaches for Enuresis

Approach	Description
Fluid restriction	Fluid intake is limited in the evening and before the child goes to bed.
Bladder exercises	The child drinks a large amount and then holds urine as long as he or she can. The child practices stopping voiding midstream. Exercises should continue for at least 6 months.
Timed voiding	The child with diurnal enuresis is instructed to void every 2 hours and to use a double voiding pattern; this trains the bladder to empty completely and avoid overdistention.
Enuresis alarms	A detector strip is attached to the child's pants. The alarm sounds a buzzer that alerts the child when wetting occurs, so the child can get up and finish voiding in the bathroom. This works best for children over 7 years old, and takes 3 to 4 months for success.
Reward system	Set realistic goals for the child and reinforce dry days or nights with stars and stickers on a chart.
Medications	Imipramine is prescribed nightly for 2 to 4 months and then tapered over several months to reduce the rate of relapse. It is effective in 50% to 70% of children. Desmopressin is prescribed to children with nocturnal enuresis for special events such as camp or sleepovers. Oxybutynin is used for diurnal enuresis to relieve urgency and frequency from bladder irritability.

expense. It is usually reserved for times when the child is away from home for a short period (e.g., sleepovers or camp). Relapse often occurs when medications are stopped. It may be a good idea for the child to avoid foods believed to contribute to enuresis, such as those containing caffeine, milk, chocolate, and citrus (Tobias, 2000).

Nursing Management

Teach the child and parents about the physiologic development of bladder control and causes and treatment of enuresis. Explore feelings of guilt or blame. Make sure the parents are aware that the child cannot control the wetting. Psychosocial support is an essential part of care since stress is an important cause of secondary enuresis. Provide emotional support to the parents and child, and encourage the child's participation in the treatment plan. Refer the child for counseling or therapy if appropriate.

Assess the parents' and child's motivation and readiness for interventions. Before parents buy an enuresis alarm, suggest they use an alarm clock in the child's room for several nights to see if the child will arouse. Find out whether the child shares a room with others who will be disturbed by the alarm. Ask if the child and parents are willing to per-

sist with an enuresis alarm, as it may take months to work. Evaluation of nursing care includes families choosing the intervention best for them, and an increase in the number of dry nights.

RENAL DISORDERS

NEPHROTIC SYNDROME

Nephrotic syndrome refers not to a specific disease, but rather to a clinical state characterized by edema, massive proteinuria, hypoalbuminemia, hypoproteinemia, hyperlipidemia, and altered immunity. Nephrotic syndrome is classified as congenital, primary, or secondary. Congenital nephrotic (CNF) syndrome, an autosomal recessive disorder, is extremely rare. The CNF gene is localized on the long arm of chromosome 19 (19q 13.1) (Goodyer & Kashtan, 1998). Primary nephrotic syndrome results from a disease that affects only the kidney, such as glomerulonephritis. Secondary nephrotic syndrome results from a disease with multisystem effects, such as diabetes, lupus, or sickle cell anemia.

Approximately 80% of children with nephrotic syndrome have a type of primary disease called minimal change nephrotic syndrome (MCNS). MCNS usually occurs in children between the ages of 2 and 7 years, with an incidence of 3 per 100,000 children, and is approximately twice as common in boys as in girls (Gilman & Mooney, 1998). MCNS derives its name from the normal or only minimally changed appearance of the glomeruli on light microscopic evaluation. Because MCNS is the most common form of nephrotic syndrome, it is the focus of the following discussion.

Etiology and Pathophysiology

The cause of primary MCNS is unknown, but an immune system role is strongly suspected. The mechanism of increased glomerular permeability is unknown as the glomeruli appear normal. Normally, only a minute amount of protein is present in the urine. In MCNS, however, increased permeability of the glomerular membrane permits large, negatively charged molecules such as albumin to pass through the membrane and be excreted in the urine. Proteinuria results in decreased oncotic pressure and edema, because fluid remains in the interstitial spaces instead of being pulled back into the vascular compartment. Loss of protein in the urine, as well as insufficient albumin production by the liver and a decreased albumin concentration as a result of salt and water retention by the kidney contribute to hypoalbuminemia.

Because the kidney reabsorbs salt and water, edema develops. Immunoglobulins are lost, resulting in altered immunity. The liver, stimulated perhaps by hypoalbuminemia or decreased osmotic pressure, responds by increasing synthesis of lipoprotein (cholesterol), resulting in hyperlipidemia.

Clinical Manifestations

In most children, edema develops gradually over several weeks. Children may have a history of periorbital edema on waking that resolves during the day as fluid shifts to the abdomen and lower extremities. Other signs include weight gain greater than expected based upon previous growth pattern, snug fit of clothing and shoes, pallor, hypertension, irritability, anorexia, hematuria, decreased urine output, and nonspecific malaise (Gilman & Mooney, 1998). The child's urine may be frothy or foamy. Parents often do not seek medical treatment until generalized edema develops on the child's extremities, abdomen, or genitals (Figure 47–4 ◆). Respiratory distress from pleural effusion may occur in some cases.

Massive edema resulting in a dramatic weight gain and abdominal pain, with or without vomiting, may occur, depending on the amount of albumin lost and the amount of sodium ingested. The child becomes malnourished as a result of protein loss in the urine. The skin is pale and shiny with prominent veins, and the hair becomes more brittle.

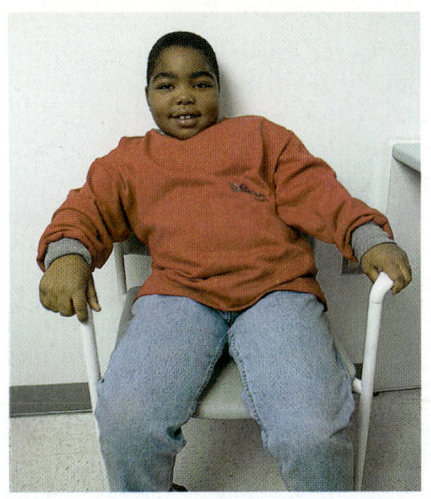

FIGURE 47–4. ◆ This boy has generalized edema, a characteristic finding in nephrotic syndrome.

Clinical Therapy

Diagnosis is based on the history, physical examination, characteristic symptoms, and laboratory findings. Serum albumin and other blood studies may be ordered. Edema begins to develop in children when the serum albumin concentration falls below 20 g/L (Tune & Mendoza, 1997). Urinalysis reveals massive proteinuria (50 mg/kg/day), the primary indicator of nephrotic syndrome. Microscopic hematuria may also be present. The serum creatinine or BUN are increased in some cases.

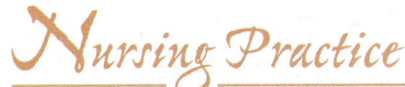

A protein-to-creatinine (PR/CR) ratio of the first morning void is used to estimate protein excretion in children because of the challenges in obtaining 24-hour urines. A ratio of > 0.2 is found in children over 2 years with MCNS.

Children may be hospitalized when severe edema or a major infection is present, but usually get treatment as outpatients. Clinical therapy focuses on decreasing proteinuria, relieving edema, managing associated symptoms, improving nutrition, and preventing infection. A corticosteroid (such as prednisone), the drug of choice, is prescribed to decrease proteinuria. In most children, urine protein levels fall to trace or negative values within 2 to 3 weeks of the start of therapy. Children who respond successfully to therapy continue to take corticosteroids daily for 6 weeks, and then 6 weeks of alternate-day treatment. The relapse rate has been improved with this protocol (Tune & Mendoza, 1997).

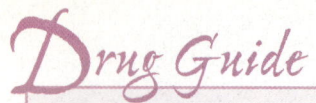

PREDNISONE

Overview of Action

Natural or synthetic, intermediate-acting glucocorticoid that has strong anti-inflammatory, immunosuppressant, and metabolic actions. Treats diseases such as renal, connective tissue, dermatologic, allergy, acute leukemia, and respiratory distress syndrome.

Routes, Dosage, Frequency

PO:

- 0.14 to 2 mg/kg/day or 40 to 60 mg/m²/day in equally divided doses 4 times a day
- Nephrosis: 2 mg/kg/dose 3 to 4 times per day until urine is protein free for 5 days or for 28-day course (maximum of 80 mg/day). For persistent proteinuria may increase to 4 mg/kg/dose every other day for additional 28 days. Maintenance: 2 mg/kg/dose every other day for 28 days. To discontinue: taper over 4 to 6 weeks.
- Asthma: Acute: 0.5 to 1 mg/kg/day for 3 to 5 days (maximum of 20 to 40 mg/day). Severe: 5 to 10 mg/day or 10 to 30 mg every other day, taper to aerosol corticosteroids.

Note: dosage is determined by severity of condition and child's response.

Contraindications: Hypersensitivity to the drug, immunizations with live virus vaccines, HIV infection, varicella, and systemic fungal infection.

Side Effects: Usually dependent upon dosage and duration of treatment, but includes possible growth suppression, hypertension, congestive heart failure, psychotic behavior, increased appetite, impaired wound healing, and Cushing state.

Nursing Implications

- *Assess:* Obtain baseline weight and height; before long-term therapy, obtain ECG, chest and spinal x-rays, glucose tolerance tests, evaluation of HPA-axis function, and blood pressure therapy.

- *Administer:* Dosage is based on child's response to drug and severity of condition rather than strictly on weight or body surface. PO: Take with food or milk to reduce gastrointestinal irritation. Tablets can be crushed and mixed with small amounts of food or fluid. Tablets are very bitter. If child is able to swallow capsules, they can be placed in a gelatin capsule. Follow with fluids to cleanse child's palate. Best to give daily dosage before 9 A.M. It suppresses adrenal cortex less, which may reduce risk of HPA-axis suppression. Alternate-day therapy is recommended to reduce growth-retarding effects.

- *Monitor:* Carefully assess child's response to drug to determine need for dosage adjustments. Observe for side effects, especially hypocalcemia, signs of adrenal insufficiency, symptoms of infection, or worsening of condition. Monitor blood pressure and daily weights; report any sudden weight gain to the physician. With long-term usage, monitor serum electrolytes and height. Encourage well-balanced diet low in sodium, and encourage good hygiene and dental care (possible oral fungal infections). Tonometry (eye) examinations every 6 weeks. To discontinue the medication, reduce the dose gradually, especially after long-term use, so it does not cause acute life-threatening adrenal insufficiency. After discontinuation of short-term therapy (up to 5 days) with high dosage, adrenal recovery may occur within 1 week. After prolonged high-dose therapy, complete recovery of adrenal function may take up to 1 year.

- *Patient Teaching:* Do not alter dose or stop medication abruptly as it could cause serious side effects or even death. Gradual tapering of dosage is necessary. Increasing the amount of medication will not speed the healing process. Monitor signs and symptoms of medication reactions; report these and symptoms of adrenal insufficiency or worsening of condition to physician. Obtain daily weights; report any sudden weight gain to physician. Stress importance of close medical supervision and follow-up. Get regular ophthalmologic examinations if on long-term therapy. Caution not to receive skin tests or immunizations. Inform any health care provider, including dentists, surgeons, or emergency care personnel, that child is on medication. Child should carry medical identification card. Observe for symptoms of infection. Do not use over-the-counter medications without contacting health care provider.

Note: From Bindler, R. M., & Howry, L. B. (1997). *Pediatric drugs and nursing implications* (2nd ed.). Upper Saddle River, NJ: Prentice Hall-Health. Adapted.

Approximately 85% of children experience complete remission with corticosteroid therapy. Relapses commonly happen with a respiratory infection or live virus immunizations; however, relapses become less frequent or stop during puberty (Gilman & Mooney, 1998). Children who have a relapse after drug therapy is discontinued get repeat therapy. Alkylating agents such as chlorambucil and cyclophosphamide have been effective in children with frequently recurring nephrotic syndrome, but they have serious side effects, including carcinogenesis and 15% to 20% risk of sterility in males (Tune & Mendoza, 1997). If steroid therapy is ineffective, a renal biopsy is performed to identify other causes for the child's symptoms.

To reduce massive edema, intravenous administration of albumin or oral diuretics may be ordered. Since diuretics can precipitate hypovolemia, hyponatremia, and hypokalemia, electrolyte levels should be carefully monitored. An angiotensin-converting enzyme (ACE) inhibitor may be used to decrease protein excretion. Broad-spectrum antibiotics treat any infections.

A normal diet for the child's age is recommended. No attempt should be made either to restrict or to increase protein intake. A high protein intake increases urinary protein loss and could accelerate the development of renal failure. A low protein diet may lead to protein deficiency. A "no added salt" diet is recommended during corticosteroid treatment.

Nursing Management

Nursing Assessment and Diagnoses

PHYSIOLOGIC ASSESSMENT

Careful assessment of the child's hydration status and edema is essential. Monitor intake and output and vital signs and record these findings accurately. Carefully assess for respiratory distress associated with pleural effusion (see Chapter 42). Test urine for proteinuria and specific gravity at least once each shift.

PSYCHOSOCIAL ASSESSMENT

Children and parents are often fearful or anxious on admission. Because edema often develops gradually, parents may feel guilty if they did not seek medical attention immediately. School-age children with generalized edema are often concerned about their appearance. Careful questioning may be necessary to elicit these concerns. The child hospitalized for a recurrence of nephrotic syndrome may be frustrated or depressed. Assess individual and family coping mechanisms, support systems, and level of stress.

Common nursing diagnoses for the child with MCNS include:

- *Risk for infection* related to immunosuppressive therapy
- *Risk for impaired skin integrity* related to edema, lowered resistance to infection and injury, immobility, and malnutrition
- *Fluid volume excess* related to renal dysfunction and sodium retention
- *Altered nutrition: less than body requirements* related to loss of appetite and protein loss in urine
- *Fatigue* related to fluid and electrolyte imbalance, albumin loss, altered nutrition, and renal failure
- *Diversional activity deficit* related to fatigue, immobility, and social isolation

Planning and Implementation

Nursing care is mainly supportive and focuses on administering medications, preventing infection, preventing skin breakdown, meeting nutritional and fluid needs, promoting rest, and providing emotional support to the parents and child.

ADMINISTER MEDICATIONS

It is important to give prescribed medications at the scheduled times. Watch for side effects of corticosteroids such as moon face, increased appetite, increased hair growth, abdominal distention, and mood swings. If the child is receiving albumin intravenously, monitor closely for hypertension or signs of volume overload caused by fluid shifts. If diuretics are used, observe for shock. The child may need to have albumin infused simultaneously with diuretics.

PREVENT INFECTION

Children with MCNS are at risk for infection because of the loss of immunoglobulins in the urine, other alterations of the immune system associated with renal failure, and corticosteroid therapy. Careful handwashing is important. Use standard precautions. Strict aseptic technique is essential during invasive procedures. Monitor the child's white blood cell count when cytotoxic drugs are given because of bone marrow suppression. Monitor vital signs carefully to detect early signs of infection that may be masked by corticosteroid therapy. Decrease the child's social contacts during immunosuppressive treatment, and caution parents and children to avoid exposure to people with respiratory infections and communicable diseases. Emphasize the importance of avoiding shopping malls, sporting arenas, grocery stores, game stores, and other public areas where the risk of exposure to such infections is increased.

PREVENT SKIN BREAKDOWN

Meticulous skin care is essential to prevent skin breakdown and potential infection. Assess the skin repeatedly, turn the child frequently, and use therapeutic mattresses (e.g., egg crate, airflow) to help prevent skin breakdown. Keep the skin clean and dry.

MEET NUTRITIONAL AND FLUID NEEDS

Keep the child's food preferences in mind when planning menus. Encourage the child to eat by presenting attractive meals with small portions. Mealtimes should center on pleasurable socialization. Encourage the child to eat meals with other children on the unit. Fluids are not usually restricted.

Carefully monitor intake and output. Weigh the child daily using the same scale, and measure abdominal girth to monitor changes in edema and ascites (see Figure 39–8). Monitor vital signs every 4 hours to watch for signs of respiratory distress, hypertension, or circulatory overload.

PROMOTE REST

Provide opportunities for quiet play as tolerated, such as drawing, playing board games, listening to tapes, and watching videos. Adjust the child's daily schedule to allow rest periods after activities. Signs of fatigue may include irritability, mood swings, or withdrawal. Tell the parents and child about the importance of rest. Limiting visitors during the acute phase of the illness may be necessary. Telephone contacts may be encouraged as an alternative to visitors. To provide a sense of control, encourage the child to set his or her own limits on activity.

PROVIDE EMOTIONAL SUPPORT

Parents and children often need support to cope with this chronic disease. Thoroughly explain the child's disease and treatment regimen to parents. Parental anxiety in combination with the hospitalization may interfere with the child's independence. Help parents promote the child's independence by allowing the child to choose from the menu or to select the daily activity schedule. This gives the child some sense of control.

Children with MCNS may have a distorted body image because of sudden weight gain and edema. They may refuse to look in the mirror, refuse to participate in care, and take less interest in their appearance. Encourage children to express their feelings. Help them maintain a normal appearance by promoting normal grooming routines. Encourage children to wear their own pajamas rather than hospital gowns. Scarves or hats may be used to lessen the child's edematous appearance.

DISCHARGE PLANNING AND HOME CARE TEACHING

Explain the disease process, prognosis, and treatment plan to parents and school-age children. Make sure parents know how to administer medications and can identify potential side effects. Inform parents about restricting fluid intake until the edema resolves. Instruct parents about the need to monitor urine daily for protein, and have them keep a diary to record results. Monitoring the child's weight each week may help identify early stages of fluid retention. This helps parents to spot a relapse before edema occurs.

Tutoring may be required for a short period after discharge. However, encourage parents to allow the child to return to normal activities once the acute episode has resolved. Emphasize the importance of avoiding contact with people with infectious diseases, because of the child's reduced immunity. Reinforce to parents that it is important to follow the "no added salt" diet as long as the child is receiving corticosteroid therapy or shows signs of MCNS. Warn them that steroids stimulate appetite, so they need to control the child's food intake and weight gain. No live immunizations should be given to the child who is relapsing or taking corticosteroid therapy. Withhold immunizations until 6 months after the completion of corticosteroid therapy. Although immunizations may trigger a relapse, pneumococcal vaccine and other immunizations are important to protect the child from serious preventable infections.

Most children do well with corticosteroid therapy; however, relapses are common. Even children with frequent relapses usually have a spontaneous resolution of MCNS before 30 years of age.

Evaluation

Expected outcomes of nursing care include:

▸ The child responds to corticosteroid therapy.
▸ Dietary guidelines of no added salt are followed and food intake is controlled during corticosteroid therapy.
▸ Relapses are identified by parents before edema occurs.
▸ The child receives the additional recommended immunizations.

A discussion of Wilms' tumor can be found in Chapter 45.

RENAL FAILURE

Renal failure, which may be acute or chronic, occurs when the kidney is unable to excrete wastes and concentrate urine. Acute renal failure occurs suddenly (over days or weeks) and may be reversible, whereas in chronic renal failure, kidney function diminishes gradually and permanently over months or years.

Both types of renal failure are characterized by **azotemia** (accumulation of nitrogenous wastes in the blood) and sometimes **oliguria** (urine output less than 0.5 to 1 mL/kg/hr), indicating the kidney's inability to excrete metabolic waste products. The degree of renal impairment is estimated by the degree of azotemia and the increase in serum creatinine level. **Uremia** occurs when there is an excess of urea and other nitrogenous waste products in the blood.

Acute Renal Failure

Acute renal failure (ARF), in which kidney function abruptly diminishes, is characterized by a rapid rise in the BUN level. The kidneys are also unable to regulate extracellular fluid volume, sodium balance, and acid-base homeostasis. ARF occurs most frequently in neonates who are critically ill with asphyxia, shock, and sepsis. It can also be a postoperative complication of cardiac surgery or may result from drug toxicity.

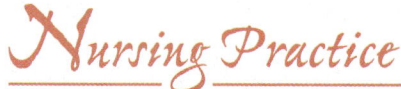

The following factors by age group increase the risk of acute renal failure:

Infants
▸ Critically ill neonate
▸ Obstructive uropathy
▸ Dehydration
▸ Hemolytic-uremic syndrome

Toddler
▸ Poisoning (e.g., acetaminophen, mushrooms)

School-Age Child and Adolescent
▸ Trauma

ETIOLOGY AND PATHOPHYSIOLOGY

ARF may be caused by prerenal, postrenal, or intrinsic factors. Prerenal ARF is a result of decreased perfusion to an otherwise normal kidney in association with a systemic condition. Hypovolemia (hemorrhage or dehydration), septic shock, or cardiac failure may precipitate prerenal ARF. This is the most common type of ARF in infants and young children.

Intrinsic ARF results from primary damage to the parenchymal cells of the kidneys. Damage can be caused by infection, diseases such as hemolytic-uremic syndrome or acute glomerulonephritis, cortical necrosis, nephrotoxic drugs, or accidental ingestion of drugs or poisons. The structure most susceptible to damage is the kidney tubule. Injury to the tubule resulting in acute tubular necrosis is the most frequent cause of intrinsic renal failure in children.

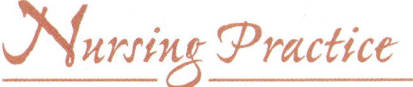

Nephrotoxic drugs include the following:

▶ Antimicrobials: aminoglycosides, cephalosporins, tetracycline, sulfonamides
▶ Radiographic contrast media with iodine
▶ Heavy metals: lead, barium, iron
▶ Nonsteroidal anti-inflammatory drugs: indomethacin, aspirin

Postrenal ARF is caused by obstruction of the urinary flow from both kidneys, such as occurs in posterior urethral valves or a neurogenic bladder. Children may have oliguria, or normal or increased urine output. Renal failure without oliguria usually indicates a less severe renal injury. Children who recover from ARF may have residual kidney damage and compromised renal function.

CLINICAL MANIFESTATIONS

Characteristically, a healthy child suddenly becomes ill with nonspecific symptoms, including nausea, vomiting, lethargy, edema, gross hematuria, oliguria, and hypertension (Vogt, 1997). These symptoms are a result of electrolyte imbalances, uremia, and fluid overload. The child appears pale and lethargic. See the clinical manifestations tables for more information.

Hyperkalemia is the most life-threatening electrolyte disorder associated with ARF. An increase in serum potassium

CLINICAL MANIFESTATIONS ∽ *Acute Versus Chronic Renal Failure*

TYPE OF RENAL FAILURE	CLINICAL MANIFESTATIONS
Acute renal failure	Gross hematuria, headache, edema, severe hypertension, lethargy, nausea and vomiting, oliguria
Chronic renal failure	Fatigue, malaise, poor appetite, prolonged unexplained nausea and vomiting, failure to thrive, poor school performance, secondary enuresis, chronic anemia, hypertension, and unusual bone disease (fractures with minimal trauma, rickets, valgus deformity)

Note: From Vogt, B. A. (1997). Identifying kidney disease: Simple steps can make a difference. *Contemporary Pediatrics, 14*(3), 115–119.

CLINICAL MANIFESTATIONS ∽ *Electrolyte Imbalances in Acute Renal Failure*

ELECTROLYTE IMBALANCE AND CAUSE	CLINICAL MANIFESTATIONS
Hyperkalemia Results from inability to adequately excrete potassium derived from diet and catabolized cells. In metabolic acidosis, potassium also moves from intracellular fluid to extracellular fluid.	• Peaked T waves, widening of QRS waves on ECG. • Dysrhythmias: ventricular dysrhythmias, heart block, ventricular fibrillation, cardiac arrest • Diarrhea • Muscle weakness
Hyponatremia In the acute oliguric phase, hyponatremia is related to the accumulation of fluid in excess of solute.	• Change in level of consciousness • Muscle cramps • Anorexia • Abdominal reflexes, depressed deep tendon reflexes • Cheyne-Stokes respirations • Seizures
Hypocalcemia Phosphate retention (hyperphosphatemia) depresses the serum calcium concentration. Calcium is deposited in injured cells. Hyperkalemia and metabolic acidosis may mask the common clinical manifestations of severe hypocalcemia.	• Muscle tingling • Changes in muscle tone • Seizures • Muscle cramps and twitching • Positive Chvostek sign (contraction of facial muscles after tapping facial nerve just anterior to parotid gland)

Note: From Chan, J. C. M, Alon, U., & Oken, D. E. (1992). Acute renal failure. In C. M. Edelman, Jr. (Ed.), *Pediatric kidney disease* (2nd ed., pp. 1923–1940). Boston: Little, Brown. Adapted.

adversely affects the electrical conductivity within the heart. Hyponatremia affects central nervous system function, resulting in symptoms that range from fatigue to seizures. Edema occurs as a result of sodium and water retention. (Refer to Chapter 39 for a discussion of these fluid and electrolyte alterations.) 🔗 Children with ARF are also more susceptible to infection because of depressed immune functioning.

CLINICAL THERAPY

Diagnosis of renal failure is based primarily on urinalysis and blood chemistry results, including BUN, serum crea-tinine, sodium, potassium, and calcium levels (Table 47–5). The kidneys are normal in size and no signs of osteodystrophy are found on x-ray. Various imaging studies to assess kidney size, renal blood flow, and renal perfusion and function may be performed to determine whether the child has ARF or chronic renal failure.

Treatment depends on the underlying cause of the renal failure. The goal is to minimize or prevent permanent renal damage while maintaining fluid and electrolyte balance and managing complications. Eliminate all potential sources of potassium intake until hyperkalemia is controlled (see Chapter 39). 🔗 Initial emergency treatment of children with fluid depletion focuses on fluid replacement at 20 mL/kg of saline or lactated Ringer's solution given rapidly or over 5 to 10 minutes to ensure renal perfusion. Albumin may also be administered when blood loss is the cause of circulatory depletion. If oliguria persists after restoration of adequate fluid volume, intrinsic renal damage is suspected. Children with fluid overload, like those with pulmonary edema, need diuretic therapy, and dialysis if they respond poorly to diuretics.

Fluid requirements are calculated to maintain zero water balance. Intake should equal output. Nutrition must be maintained with extra carbohydrate intake during the catabolic state. Antibiotics are prescribed for infection. Nephrotoxic antibiotics such as aminoglycosides are avoided.

Some children whose ARF is unresponsive to management require dialysis to correct severe electrolyte imbalances, manage fluid overload, and cleanse the blood of waste products. The clinical situation and age of the child determines whether hemodialysis or peritoneal dialysis is used. Refer to "Renal Replacement Therapy" later in this chapter.

Prognosis depends on the cause of ARF. When renal failure results from drug toxicity or dehydration, the prognosis is generally good. However, ARF that results from diseases such as hemolytic-uremic syndrome or acute glomerulonephritis may be associated with residual kidney damage (see Table 47–6).

TABLE 47–5 Diagnostic Tests for Renal Failure

Test	Normal Values	Findings in ARF
Urinalysis		
pH	4.5–8	Lowered
Osmolarity	50–1400 mosm/L	> 500 prerenal
		< 350 intrinsic
Specific gravity	1.001–1.030	High: prerenal ARF
		Low: intrinsic ARF
		Normal: postrenal ARF
Protein	Negative	Positive
Blood Chemistry		
Potassium	3.5–5.8 mmol/L	Elevated
Sodium	135–148 mmol/L	Normal, low, or high, depends solely on the amount of water in the body
Calcium	2.2–2.7 mmol/L	Low
Phosphorus	1.23–2 mmol/L	High
Urea nitrogen	3.5–7.1 mmol/L	Increased
Creatinine	0.2–0.9 mmol/L	Increased
pH	7.38–7.42	Low acidic

ARF: acute renal failure

TABLE 47–6 Medications Used to Treat Complications of Acute Renal Failure

Complication	Medication	Action or Indication	Nursing Implications
Hyperkalemia (> 5.8 mmol/L)	Kayexalate	Exchanges sodium for potassium	May require up to 4 hours to take effect.
	Calcium gluconate 10%	Counteracts potassium-induced increased myocardial irritability	Monitor for ECG changes. Intravenous infiltration may result in tissue necrosis.
	Albuterol	Shifts potassium to the cells	Give by aerosol.
	Sodium bicarbonate	Helps correct metabolic acidosis by exchanging hydrogen for potassium	*Do not mix with calcium.* Complications include fluid overload, hypertension, and tetany.
Hypocalcemia (< 2.2 mmol/L)	Calcium gluconate 10%	Used in presence of tetany; provides ionized calcium to restore nervous tissue function to control serum phosphorus	Administer slowly to prevent bradycardia. Monitor for ECG changes.
Malignant hypertension (blood pressure > 95% for age)	Sodium nitroprusside, nitroglycerin	Relaxes smooth muscle in peripheral arterioles	Administer by continuous intravenous infusion; fall in blood pressure is seen within 10–20 minutes.

Nursing Management

Nursing Assessment and Diagnoses

A complete history and physical examination are necessary to identify progression of symptoms and possible causes for renal failure.

PHYSIOLOGIC ASSESSMENT

Assess vital signs, level of consciousness, and other neurologic indicators to help identify clinical signs of electrolyte imbalance (see "Causes and Clinical Manifestations of Electrolyte Imbalances in Acute Renal Failure" on page 1223). Measure the child's weight on admission to provide a baseline for evaluating changes in fluid status. Monitor urinalysis, urine culture, and blood chemistry studies. Inspect urine for color (Figure 47–5 ◆). Cloudy urine may indicate infection; tea-colored urine suggests hematuria. Assess urine specific gravity and intake and output.

PSYCHOSOCIAL ASSESSMENT

The unexpected and acute nature of the child's hospitalization creates anxiety for both parents and child. Assess for feelings of anger, guilt, or fear associated with the hospitalization. Such feelings are likely if ARF developed as a result of dehydration, a preventable injury, or poisoning. Assess coping mechanisms, family support systems, and level of stress.

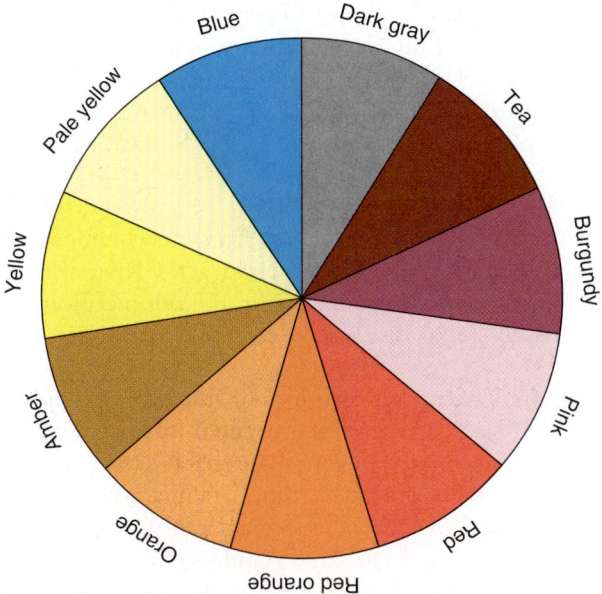

FIGURE 47–5. ◆ A color wheel, such as the one shown here, can be used as a guide in standardizing descriptions of urine color. Normal urine is pale yellow. Changes in urine color can indicate the following alterations: *yellow*—concentrated urine; *amber*—bile in urine; *orange*—alkaline or concentrated urine; *red-orange*—acid pH, medications; *red*—blood; menses; *pink*—dilute blood; *burgundy*—laxatives; *tea*—melanin, hematuria; *dark gray*—medications, dyes; *blues*—dyes, medications. *Note:* From Cooper, C. (1993). What color is that urine specimen? *American Journal of Nursing, 93,* 37 Copyright © 1993 Connie Cooper, R.N., M.S.N.; graphics by Mike O'Grady, R.N., M.S.N.

Several nursing diagnoses may apply to the child with ARF, including:

- ▶ *Altered renal tissue perfusion* related to hypovolemia, sepsis, or drug toxicity
- ▶ *Fluid volume excess* related to renal dysfunction and sodium retention
- ▶ *Altered nutrition: less than body requirements* related to anorexia, nausea, vomiting, and catabolic state
- ▶ *Risk for infection* related to invasive procedures and monitoring equipment, and diminished immune functioning
- ▶ *Ineffective family coping (compromised)* related to sudden hospitalization and uncertain prognosis of child

Planning and Implementation

Nursing care focuses on preventing complications, maintaining fluid balance, administering medications, meeting nutritional needs, preventing infection, and providing emotional support to the child and parents.

PREVENT COMPLICATIONS

Complications are best prevented by ensuring compliance with the treatment plan. Careful monitoring of vital signs, intake and output, serum electrolytes, and level of consciousness can alert the nurse to changes that indicate potential complications. For example, if the serum sodium concentration rises and weight falls, insufficient fluids are being administered. If the serum sodium level falls and the weight increases, excessive fluids are being administered.

MAINTAIN FLUID BALANCE

Estimate the child's fluid status by monitoring weight (on the same scale), intake and output, and blood pressure two or three times a day. Also monitor serum chemistry values, especially for sodium. The aim of maintaining fluid balance is to achieve a stable serum sodium concentration and a decrease in body weight by 0.5% to 1% a day.

If the child has oliguria, limit fluid intake, including parenteral nutrition, to replacement of insensible fluid loss from the lungs, skin, and gastrointestinal tract (about one third the daily maintenance requirements in afebrile children). The child with **renal insufficiency** (i.e., as the kidneys' ability to conserve sodium and concentrate the urine decreases) is at greater risk for fluid loss with illness. If the child is febrile, fluid administration is increased by 12% for each centigrade degree of temperature elevation. In cases of acute gastrointestinal illness, children are at greater risk for dehydration.

ADMINISTER MEDICATIONS

Because the kidney's ability to excrete drugs is impaired in ARF, dosages of all medications should be adjusted. The actual dosage of the drug can be reduced or the time interval between doses can be increased. Check drug levels to monitor for drug toxicity. Know the signs of drug toxicity for each medication the child is receiving.

MEET NUTRITIONAL NEEDS

Children are at risk for malnutrition because of their high metabolic rate. Parenteral or enteral feeding may be used initially to minimize protein catabolism. The diet is tailored to the individual child's need for calories, carbohydrates, fats, and amino acids or protein hydrolysates. Depending on the degree of renal failure, sodium, potassium, and phosphorus may be restricted. Initiate oral feeding as soon as the child can tolerate it.

PREVENT INFECTION

The child with ARF is extremely susceptible to nosocomial infections because of altered nutritional status, compromised immunity, and numerous invasive procedures. Thorough handwashing and standard precautions are imperative to decrease the risk of infection. Use sterile technique for all invasive procedures and when caring for lines. Drainage from catheter sites should be cultured to check for the presence of infectious organisms. Assess vital signs and lung sounds frequently.

PROVIDE EMOTIONAL SUPPORT

The sudden onset of ARF presents parents with an unexpected threat to their child's life. Both the child and the parents experience anxiety because of the unexpected hospitalization and the uncertainty of the prognosis. Parents often feel guilty, regardless of the cause of renal failure. This guilt is intensified when renal failure is a result of dehydration or poisoning. Encourage parents to verbalize their fears and help them work through feelings of guilt. Explain procedures and treatment measures to decrease anxiety. Encouraging parents and older siblings to participate in the child's care can increase their sense of control.

DISCHARGE PLANNING AND HOME CARE TEACHING

Encourage parental involvement early in the child's hospitalization. Be sure parents understand the importance of administering medications correctly. Teach family members proper technique for measuring blood pressure so they can monitor the child's hypertension, if ordered. Have them demonstrate how to take the blood pressure.

Diet counseling is a key component of discharge planning and is usually performed by a renal dietitian. Depending on the degree of renal failure, the child's diet may include restrictions on protein, water, sodium, potassium, and phosphorus. The parents should be given written guidelines listing appropriate food choices to assist in menu planning. Ethnic and cultural preferences should be considered in listing menu options.

Continued monitoring of renal function during follow-up examinations is critical as deterioration may occur over time. Referral to support groups can be helpful for both parents and children. The National Kidney Foundation is a source of numerous publications. **WEB**

Evaluation

Expected outcomes of nursing care include:

▶ The child's fluid status is balanced with edema-associated weight loss.

▶ Nutritional needs are met.

▶ The child acquires no secondary infections.

Chronic Renal Failure

Chronic renal failure (CRF) is a progressive, irreversible reduction in kidney function. CRF is rare in children, occurring in 0.6 to 1.6 per million (Saborio, Hahn, Hisano, et al., 1998). Blacks have a higher rate of end-stage renal disease than whites by a ratio of 2.7:1 (Balinsky, 2000).

ETIOLOGY AND PATHOPHYSIOLOGY

In children, CRF usually results from developmental abnormalities of the kidney or urinary tract. CRF may also be caused by hemolytic-uremic syndrome, glomerulonephritis, or other renal diseases. (See discussions later in the chapter.)

The gradual, progressive loss of functioning nephrons ultimately results in **end-stage renal disease (ESRD)**. ESRD is characterized by minimal renal function (less than 5% of normal), uremic syndrome, anemia, and abnormal blood values. In ESRD, the kidneys can no longer maintain homeostasis and the child requires dialysis.

The kidneys excrete excess acid in the body and regulate the body's fluid and electrolyte balance. Renal failure upsets this fluid and electrolyte balance. As renal failure progresses, metabolic acidosis occurs because the kidneys cannot excrete the acids that build up in the body. Retention of excessive sodium and water is a common cause of the elevated blood pressure associated with CRF. Insufficient calcium loss, phosphorus retention, and elevated parathyroid hormone levels lead to uremic bone disease. The kidneys also produce erythropoietin (the growth factor responsible for the production and maturation of red cells); lack of erythropoietin and progressive renal disease are the underlying causes of the anemia of CRF.

CLINICAL MANIFESTATIONS

Children with CRF frequently have no symptoms initially, as the following progression occurs:

- Early renal failure with glomerular filtration rate (GFR) of 50% to 75% of normal; few or no clinical signs,
- Chronic renal insufficiency with GFR of 25% of normal and some clinical signs,
- Chronic renal failure with GFR of 10% to 15% of normal with more clinical signs, and
- ESRD with GFR of less than 10% of normal. Clinical signs require treatment with dialysis or renal transplantation (Taylor, 1996).

In the early stages, the child may appear pale and complain of headache, nausea, and fatigue. Decreased mental alertness and ability to concentrate may be seen. The child may have anemia leading to tachycardia, tachypnea, and dyspnea on exertion. As the disease progresses, the child loses his or her appetite and has complications of renal impairment, including hypertension, pulmonary edema, growth retardation, **osteodystrophy** (defective mineralization of bone caused by renal failure and chronic hyperphosphatemia), delayed fine and gross motor development, and delayed sexual maturation. See the contrast with signs of acute renal failure on page 1223.

Growth retardation is caused by disturbances in the metabolism of calcium, phosphorus, and vitamin D; decreased caloric intake; and metabolic acidosis. Osteodystrophy increases the child's risk for spontaneous fractures, rickets, and valgus deformity of the legs.

In ESRD, the most advanced form of CRF, renal failure adversely affects all body systems. As the severity of the clinical and biochemical disturbances resulting from progressive renal deterioration increases, uremic symptoms develop. Signs and symptoms of uremic syndrome include nausea and vomiting, progressive anemia, anorexia, dyspnea, malaise, uremic frost (urea crystals deposited on the skin), unpleasant (uremic) breath odor, headache, progressive confusion, tremors, pulmonary edema, and congestive heart failure.

CLINICAL THERAPY

Laboratory evaluation, including serum electrolyte, phosphate, BUN, and creatinine levels and pH, is used to confirm the diagnosis of CRF. A urine sample is collected for culture, and a 24-hour urine sample is obtained to quantify creatinine and protein excretion. From the 24-hour urine creatinine and serum creatinine levels, it is possible to calculate the remaining glomerular filtration rate. Laboratory values vary depending on the child's size and muscle mass. Age-specific normal ranges for laboratory values must be used. Tests to identify renal diseases

that could be causing the renal failure are also performed if necessary. A renal biopsy is the best method for establishing or confirming the diagnosis, predicting the prognosis, and directing treatment (Taylor, 1996).

The goals of treatment are to slow the progression of renal disease and to prevent complications. Conservative treatment includes a combination of dietary, fluid, and electrolyte management, and control of hypertension. If that fails and the child progresses to ESRD, dialysis is initiated.

Dietary management focuses on maximizing caloric intake for growth while limiting demands on the kidneys and minimizing fluid and electrolyte disturbances. Tube feedings or parenteral nutrition may be required to achieve optimal protein intake, especially in children under 1 year of age. When CRF is present, optimal protein intake for infants is 2 to 2.5 g/kg/day; for older children it is 1.5 to 2 g/kg/day.

Sodium bicarbonate (Bicitra) treats metabolic acidosis. Restricting sodium to as little as 2 g/day may be necessary if the child is hypertensive or edematous. As renal failure progresses, potassium and phosphate restrictions become necessary. Calcium-based phosphate binders may be prescribed to remove the excess phosphate.

Diuretics reduce the edema associated with renal failure. Antihypertensives (calcium channel blockers or ACE inhibitors) reduce blood pressure and prevent the progression of renal disease. As in ARF, medication dosages are adjusted because of the reduced glomerular filtration rate. Supplementation of vitamins (pyridoxine and folic acid) and minerals (iron and calcium) is usually necessary to offset dietary deficiencies. Ergocalciferol and calcitriol (vitamin D) increase calcium absorption and treat renal osteodystrophy. Ascorbic acid is administered to enhance iron absorption. Erythropoietin is given to stimulate increased production of red blood cells, improve energy tolerance and school performance, and reduce the need for transfusions. Human growth hormone is given during the course of renal failure, until ESRD occurs, to increase muscle mass and total body weight gain.

Children who progress to ESRD require renal replacement therapy (see the following discussion). The timetable for dialysis or renal transplantation is different from that of adults; earlier initiation can prevent some complications of ESRD. Rather than use the absolute BUN or serum creatinine as the guide, nonspecific signs such as uremic syndrome, poorly controlled hypertension, renal osteodystrophy, failure of head circumference measurement to increase normally, developmental delay, and poor growth are used in determining when to initiate therapy. (Refer to "Renal Replacement Therapy" later in this chapter.)

CRF is irreversible. However, the course of the disease is variable. Some children progress quickly to renal failure, necessitating dialysis. Other children are managed with a combination of medication and diet therapy for some time before significant renal impairment occurs. Frequent modifications in the treatment plan are often necessary to address the child's changing status.

Nursing Management

Nursing Assessment and Diagnoses

PHYSIOLOGIC ASSESSMENT

The initial and ongoing assessment of the child focuses on identifying complications of renal failure. Observe for signs of edema, poor growth and development, osteodystrophy, and anemia. Assess vital signs to help identify electrolyte alterations (see page 1223).

PSYCHOSOCIAL ASSESSMENT

As renal disease progresses, the number of stressors on the child and family increases. Denial and disbelief are commonly the first reactions. A thorough family assessment can help to identify particular needs of the child and family (see Table 35–7). The development of ESRD is particularly challenging during adolescence. Noncompliance with treatments can endanger the adolescent's life.

Nursing diagnoses for the child with CRF are similar to those previously listed for ARF. Additional diagnoses might include:

▶ *Altered growth* related to decreased protein and caloric intake and loss of protein in dialysate

▶ *Impaired social isolation* related to hemodialysis schedule during school hours

▶ *Activity intolerance* related to renal disease, anemia, and fatigue

▶ *Ineffective management of therapeutic regimen* related to complexity of care plan and economic difficulties

▶ *Body image disturbance* related to short stature and visible external catheter for dialysis

Planning and Implementation

HOSPITAL-BASED CARE

Children with CRF are usually hospitalized for initial diagnostic evaluation, to initiate dialysis treatment, to monitor problems that develop in the treatment plan, or to treat infection or another concurrent problem. Nursing care for the hospitalized child with CRF focuses on monitoring for side effects of medications, preventing infection, meeting nutritional needs, and providing emotional support and anticipatory teaching.

MONITOR FOR SIDE EFFECTS OF MEDICATIONS

Watch for signs of electrolyte imbalance such as weakness, muscle cramps, dizziness, headache, and nausea and vomiting in children taking diuretics. Supervise the child's activities closely to prevent falls resulting from dizziness, especially at the beginning of diuretic therapy. If antihypertensive medications such as hydralazine are being administered, monitor the child's weight to detect excessive gain resulting from water and sodium retention.

PREVENT INFECTION

The child with CRF is extremely susceptible to infections. Be alert for signs of infection, such as elevated temperature; cloudy, strong-smelling urine; dysuria; changes in respiratory pattern; or productive cough. Emphasize to the child and family the importance of good handwashing practices. Make sure the child receives influenza, 23-valent pneumococcal, and meningococcal vaccines in addition to usual childhood immunizations.

MEET NUTRITIONAL NEEDS

Maintaining adequate nutritional intake in a child with CRF who has dietary restrictions is challenging. Provide small, frequent feedings and present meals attractively to encourage the child to eat.

PROVIDE EMOTIONAL SUPPORT

Progressive CRF requires a total lifestyle change for the child and family. The parents and child need opportunities to express and work through their feelings related to the disease, prognosis, and treatment restrictions. Help children express their feelings through drawings or therapeutic play.

The need for ongoing dialysis treatments and the wait for a suitable donor kidney are stressful for both parents and child. Identify effective coping methods and family support systems to promote treatment compliance. The National Kidney Foundation and local support groups for kidney disease can give the family information or additional support. **WEB**

DISCHARGE PLANNING AND HOME CARE TEACHING

Parents need to understand the necessity of long-term treatments and follow-up care. Help the family develop a schedule for medication administration that fits with their routine. Emphasize the importance of consistency in administration times. Teach parents how to recognize side effects and complications.

Make appropriate referrals to the local visiting nurse association and to home care nursing agencies. Home care nurses help the parents care for the child receiving dialysis and provide necessary support and reassurance. Parents of children receiving dialysis at home should be taught how to perform the treatment and how to identify complications (Table 47–7). Strict aseptic technique is necessary to prevent infection at the catheter site.

NURSING CARE IN THE COMMUNITY

Children with CRF require frequent outpatient visits to monitor the progression of signs and symptoms, and to evaluate the effectiveness of current treatments.

When assessing the child, compare height, weight, and head circumference to age-specific norms to identify growth retardation and to plot progress. Assess developmental progress using the Denver II or another screening tool (see Chapter 35). Assess the adolescent for signs of delayed sexual maturation and, in girls, amenorrhea. Blood and urine tests are performed to monitor renal function. Radiographs of the bones are taken at 6-month intervals to assess changes caused by osteodystrophy.

Promote good dentition and oral hygiene. Regular dental visits are important to reduce infections. Make sure the family understands the need for antibiotic prophylaxis before certain invasive procedures, including dental care (see Table 43–8). If possible, all immunizations should be provided before renal transplantation, as long-term immunosuppressive therapy will then be prescribed. Live vaccines should not be given to the child taking immunosuppressive agents.

Review any dietary restrictions with parents. Provide sample menus for meal planning to help parents incorporate dietary changes into daily meals. A renal dietitian usually helps the child make food selections and restrict fluids and sodium as necessary, taking into account the child's likes and dislikes and cultural background. High caloric supplements may be needed because of anorexia. School-age children may not understand the consequences of noncompliance with dietary restrictions and may perceive these restrictions as punishment. Adolescents often resent the dietary restrictions and ongoing dialysis treatments, which pose a threat to their independence and evolving sense of self. Noncooperation, depression, and hostility are common responses. Discuss possible behavioral responses to dietary restrictions and limitations imposed by the treatment plan.

Growth and Development

> Adequate protein intake helps improve the child's growth and height velocity. Recommendations are as follows:
>
> | | |
> |---|---|
> | < 3 years | 2.5 to 3 g/kg/day |
> | 3 to puberty | 2 to 2.5 g/kg/day |
> | puberty | 2 g/kg/day |
> | postpubertal | 1.5 g/kg/day (Warady et al., 1999) |

School-age children and adolescents are often embarrassed about being seen as different from peers. Ask the child how he or she feels about the need to follow a special diet, take medications, and undergo dialysis treatments. To minimize the psychologic consequences of coping with a chronic disease, encourage parents to promote the child's participation in age-appropriate activities. Attendance at school and contacts with peers promote normal growth and development. Work to promote the child's self-worth and a healthy self-esteem. Prepare the child for peer conflict. Encourage adolescents to participate in a program that helps them transition to adult health services and job skill training.

Give the parents timely information about the disease process, dialysis treatments, and issues related to renal transplantation, as the child's renal impairment progresses.

Evaluation

Expected outcomes of nursing care include:

▶ The child is fully immunized with childhood and additional vaccines.

▶ The child's fluid status is maintained.

▶ The child eats foods that meet nutritional needs while adhering to dietary restrictions.

Renal Replacement Therapy

Renal replacement therapy is the treatment for renal failure and includes both dialysis and renal transplantation. In 2000, 5300 children between birth and 19 years of age received some form of renal replacement therapy, and 1602 children (200 of them less than 2 years old) received regular dialysis. Approximately 41% of children managed at home with ESRD receive peritoneal dialysis and 59% receive hemodialysis (United States Renal Data System, 2000). Dialysis treatment can cost more than $50,000 per year.

PERITONEAL DIALYSIS

Peritoneal dialysis is the preferred form of dialysis for small children because it continuously removes fluids and waste products. The resulting continuous steady state of dialysis clearance decreases the toxic effects of waste products on the child's developing body. Dietary and fluid restrictions are less severe. The timing of the treatment can be set to minimize the interruption of school, play, or other social events.

Two types of peritoneal dialysis are commonly used: continuous ambulatory peritoneal dialysis and automated peritoneal dialysis. Buretrols or graduated cylinders are used to monitor the volume of fluid exchanged.

- Continuous ambulatory peritoneal dialysis uses gravity to instill prefilled bags of **dialysate** (dialysis solution) into the peritoneal cavity four or five times a day. The fluid remains in the cavity for 4 to 8 hours. An attached bag is folded under the child's clothes, permitting normal activity. After the allotted time, the dialysate is drained by hanging the bag lower than the pelvis. The repeated connections and disconnections with this method are time consuming for the child and family and increase the risk of infection.

- Automated peritoneal dialysis uses an automatic cycler to instill and drain the dialysate about five times over a 10-hour period, usually overnight. With this method, only one connection and disconnection is needed per day, which reduces demands on the family as well as the risk of infection. This is the preferred peritoneal dialysis method because it delivers more dialysate (Warady, Alexander, Watkins, et al., 1999).

In children receiving peritoneal dialysis for ARF, a percutaneously placed catheter can be used for a few weeks. In children with CRF, a catheter is placed surgically for long-term use.

The primary complications of peritoneal dialysis are peritonitis and abdominal hernia (see Table 47–7). Signs and symptoms of peritonitis associated with peritoneal dialysis include fever, vomiting, diarrhea, abdominal pain, tenderness, and cloudy dialysate. Patients average one episode of peritonitis per year (Evans, Greenbaum, & Ettenger, 1995).

Teach the family to perform peritoneal dialysis and to use sterile technique when performing dialysis and when doing catheter care. Peritoneal dialysis is time consuming, and family members must be committed to managing this procedure daily. Help the family develop home routines that minimize disruptions to daily family life. For additional information, refer to "Nursing Care Plan: The Child Receiving Home Peritoneal Dialysis."

TABLE 47–7   Complications of Peritoneal Dialysis

Complication	Cause
Peritonitis Cloudy dialysate, abdominal pain, tenderness, leukocytosis, fever (neonatal hypothermia), constipation	*Staphylococcus aureus, Staphylococcus* epidermidis, fungal infections, gram-negative rods (risk is proportional to duration of dialysis and inversely proportional to age)
Pain During inflow	Too rapid a rate of infusion, too large a volume of dialysate, encasement of catheter in a false passage, extremes in temperature of dialysate
During outflow at end of emptying	Omentum entering catheter at end of outflow
Leakage Fluid around catheter, edema of penis or scrotum secondary to leakage into abdominal subcutaneous tissue, fluid leakage to pleural spaces through diaphragm	Overfilling of abdomen, catheter that has migrated from peritoneal cavity
Respiratory symptoms Shortness of breath, decreased breath sounds in lower lobes, inadequate chest expansion	Abdominal fullness that compromises diaphragm movement, hole in diaphragm allowing dialysate into chest cavity

NURSING CARE PLAN 〰 *The Child Receiving Home Peritoneal Dialysis*

GOAL	INTERVENTION	RATIONALE	EXPECTED OUTCOME
1. Altered nutrition: less than body requirements related to poor appetite, feeling of fullness after a small amount, and loss of protein in dialysate			
	NIC Priority Intervention: **Nutrition management:** *Assistance with or provision of a balanced dietary intake of foods and fluids*		*NOC Suggested Outcome:* **Nutrition status:** *Food and fluid intake. Amount of food and fluid taken into the body over a 24-hour period.*
The child will obtain adequate nutrients each day.	▶ With a nutritionist, develop a diet plan to identify the amounts of essential nutrients needed.	▶ Parents need concrete guidelines for food preparation.	The child's intake is adequate for an expected growth pattern to be maintained.
	▶ Provide small, frequent meals of needed nutrients.	▶ The child will feel full with smaller amounts of food because of the dialysate.	
	▶ Make mealtimes pleasant and avoid battles over the child's intake.	▶ The child will be more inclined to eat if there is less stress.	
	▶ Provide supplements by tube feeding if adequate oral intake is not possible.	▶ Adequate nutrition is important for growth and development, and must be supported if oral intake is inadequate.	
2. Risk for infection related to daily invasive procedure			
	NIC Priority Intervention: **Infection control:** *Minimizing the acquisition and transmission of infectious agents*		*NOC Suggested Outcome:* **Risk control:** *Actions to eliminate or reduce actual personal, and modifiable health threats*
The child will not develop peritonitis.	▶ Use aseptic technique for connection and disconnection of catheters.	▶ Aseptic technique reduces chance of introducing bacteria into the abdomen.	The child does not develop peritonitis.
	▶ Perform daily catheter site care.	▶ Skin around the catheter site will have fewer organisms that could potentially cause infection.	
If peritonitis occurs, it will be treated appropriately.	▶ Observe for signs of infection (fever, abdominal pain, cloudy dialysate).	▶ Early identification of infection will reduce complications.	Hospitalization will not be needed for peritonitis due to early identification and prompt treatment.
	▶ Report signs of infection to physician immediately.	▶ Rapid intervention may reduce need for hospitalization.	

GOAL	INTERVENTION	RATIONALE	EXPECTED OUTCOME

3. Caregiver role strain related to daily dialysis treatments

	NIC Priority Intervention:		*NOC Suggested Outcome:*
	Caregiver support: *Provision of necessary information, advocacy, and support to facilitate primary patient care by someone other than a health care professional*		**Caregiver performance:** *Direct care: Provision by family care provider of appropriate personal and health care for a family member or significant other*
The family copes with daily demands for the child's dialysis treatments.	▶ Discuss the importance of daily, consistent dialysis treatments for the child's overall health status.	▶ If parents understand the need for consistent dialysis treatments, they are more likely to comply.	The family complies with daily dialysis treatment guidelines.
	▶ Collaborate with the family to identify strategies that could reduce the impact of dialysis on the family's life.	▶ When the family participates in planning care, compliance is more likely.	
	▶ Refer the family to local support groups for emotional support, treatment strategies, and respite care.	▶ Support groups may help the family develop effective coping strategies.	

4. Body image disturbance related to small size and perception of being and looking different

	NIC Priority Intervention:		*NOC Suggested Outcome:*
	Body image enhancement: *Improving a patient's conscious and unconscious perceptions and attitudes toward his/her body*		**Psychosocial adjustment:** *Life change: Psychosocial adaptation of an individual to a life change*
The child will develop a sense of self-worth and self-esteem.	▶ Identify and emphasize strengths the child has (e.g., interaction style, skills, or cognitive abilities) despite being smaller than peers.	▶ Perception of personal strengths should increase self-esteem.	The child effectively interacts with peers and participates in age-appropriate activities.
	▶ Assist the child and family to identify popular clothing styles that hide the dialysate bag and catheter.	▶ Clothing that conforms to current styles, but still hides dialysate, will help the child feel less different from peers.	
	▶ Increase the child's participation in self-care as appropriate for developmental age.	▶ Ability to perform self-care increases the child's sense of control.	
	▶ Promote participation in safe activities with peers.	▶ Social interaction with peers helps reinforce similarities with others.	
	▶ Encourage the child to participate in support groups with other children receiving dialysis when possible.	▶ Interactions with other affected children provide a chance to express feelings and frustrations, and to develop successful coping strategies.	

5. Altered health maintenance related to chronic condition

	NIC Priority Intervention:		*NOC Suggested Outcome:*
	Health system guidance: *Facilitating a patient's location and use of appropriate health services*		**Health-seeking behaviors:** *Actions to promote optimal wellness, recovery, and rehabilitation.*
The child's routine health maintenance visits will be integrated with the management of the chronic condition.	▶ If a renal specialty team is not conveniently located and providing general health care, make sure the child has a primary care provider working in collaboration with the renal them.	▶ A source of health maintenance and acute minor illness care is important, especially if the family lives a distance from the tertiary care center.	The child is fully immunized at appropriate intervals and the family has a source of regular care in the community.
	▶ Assess the child regularly for growth and developmental progress and signs that the chronic condition is being managed effectively.	▶ Routine assessments will allow potential complications to be identified earlier.	
	▶ Provide immunizations as recommended for the child with a chronic condition.	▶ Immunizations may reduce the risk of potentially life-threatening infections in a child at high risk.	
	▶ Provide anticipatory guidance related to safety, developmental progress, appropriate physical activities, and behavior management.	▶ Information will help the family support the child's health status and promote development.	

HEMODIALYSIS

Hemodialysis is used in the critical care setting, and for those children with CRF when peritoneal dialysis is not possible for technical reasons or when the family is unable to safely provide it. Hemodialysis for children is offered in a special center. Infants as small as 4 kg (8.8 lb) can be hemodialyzed with current technology. Treatment is usually performed three times a week, with each session lasting approximately 3 to 4 hours.

In emergency hemodialysis and for infants, a double-lumen cannula is inserted into a large vein (e.g., the femoral, jugular, or subclavian vein). Children over 20 kg (44 lb) often have an artificial blood vessel, an arteriovenous shunt or fistula, created. Blood is pumped out of the body and through a dialyzer, where waste products and extra fluids diffuse out across a semipermeable membrane. Dialysate is pumped in the direction opposite blood flow to promote waste extraction. Differences in osmolarity and concentration between the child's blood and the dialysate alter the intravascular electrolyte concentration and reduce the intravascular volume (Figure 47–6 ◆).

Hemodialysis is more efficient than peritoneal dialysis but requires close monitoring for symptoms related to hypotension or rapid changes in fluid and electrolyte balance. Uncommonly, a disequilibrium syndrome may occur during or soon after the dialysis procedure is initiated. Other complications include access thrombosis and infection. Heparin is used to achieve an active clotting time of 150%, which reduces the risk of thrombosis.

Nursing management focuses on care of the child during dialysis and teaching the child and family about the administration of heparin and the control of bleeding from minor trauma. Carefully monitor fluid balance in the child undergoing hemodialysis. Check vital signs and blood pressure every half hour. Monitor oral intake and urinary output every half hour when the child is on the dialysis equipment. Weigh the child before and after the dialysis to determine any fluid imbalances that must be adjusted in the next hemodialysis session.

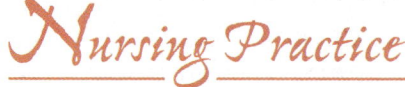

Monitor the child receiving hemodialysis for complications that can occur suddenly.

▶ Hypotension—sudden nausea and vomiting, abdominal cramping, tachycardia, and dizziness
▶ Rapid fluid and electrolyte exchange—muscle cramping, nausea and vomiting, and dizziness
▶ Dysequilibrium syndrome—restlessness, headache, nausea and vomiting, blurred vision, muscle twitching, and altered level of consciousness

Because dietary limitations are needed more often with hemodialysis than with peritoneal dialysis, make sure the family knows how to plan and provide for the child's daily nutritional needs. Review ways to reduce the risk of infection, including the daily care of the catheter site. Encourage showering rather than tub baths. Activities such as swimming may be discouraged.

RENAL TRANSPLANTATION

Renal transplantation provides the only alternative to long-term dialysis for children with ESRD. It can normalize physiology and may let children grow normally. Because delaying transplantation has adverse effects on growth and development, children are given some priority over adults awaiting transplantation. For a transplant to be successful,

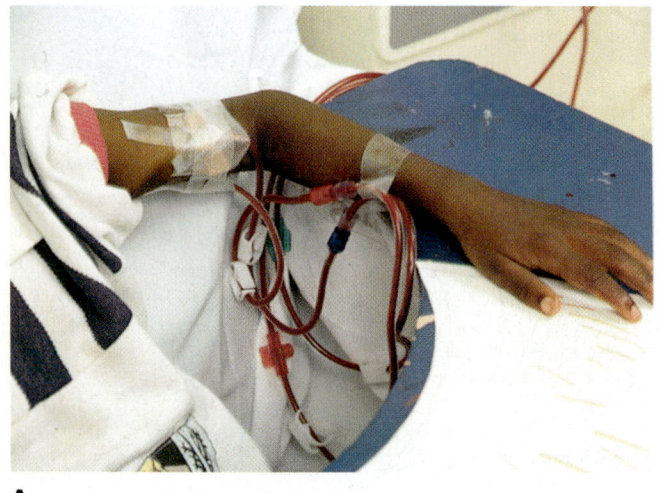

A

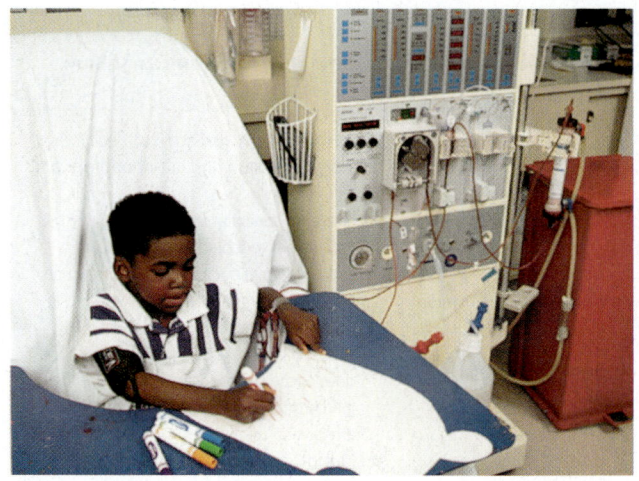

B

FIGURE 47–6. ◆ This child is undergoing hemodialysis. **A,** A surgically implanted vascular graft is being used here. One needle is placed in the arterialized end of the graft (red tubing), and one needle is placed in the venous end (blue tubing) for blood return. **B,** The child is able to draw or perform other quiet activities during dialysis treatment. Note that the child's blood pressure is monitored carefully throughout the treatment.

the donor and recipient must have ABO compatibility. A human leukocyte antigen (HLA) system match also improves survival of the graft. A living relative donor kidney has a higher survival rate than a cadaver kidney.

After transplantation, the child must take immunosuppressive medications such as corticosteroids, azathioprine, cyclosporine, and antilymphocyte antibodies to suppress rejection. Immunosuppression regimens use various combinations and sequences of these drugs to reduce the incidence of acute and chronic rejection. Signs of rejection include fever, increased BUN and serum creatinine levels, pain and tenderness over the abdomen, irritability, and weight gain.

Complications of immunosuppression therapy include opportunistic infection, lymphomas and skin cancer, and hypertension. Noncompliance with management is highest among families with instability, adolescents, females, and children and youth with low self-esteem (Bereket & Fine, 1995). Some primary kidney diseases, such as glomerulonephritis and hemolytic-uremic syndrome, can also recur in the transplanted kidney.

Nursing management includes teaching parents about the transplantation process before it occurs to help prepare them for the experience. Discuss all aspects of the child's care that will have an impact on the family's life, including follow-up appointments, medications, and general health promotion. Teach parents about the signs of acute rejection and infection, including when and how to notify the child's physician if immediate care is required.

POLYCYSTIC KIDNEY DISEASE

Polycystic kidney disease (PKD) is a genetic disorder that has autosomal recessive and autosomal dominant forms. Liver abnormalities are associated with both forms of the disease. They each have a spectrum of severity and may be detected in the fetus or become apparent during infancy or childhood. The incidence of the autosomal recessive form is 1 per 10,000 to 40,000, and is most often detected in fetuses and infants (Barratt, Avner, & Harmon, 1999). The autosomal dominant form is the most common inherited kidney disease, with a prevalence of 1 per 1000 patients (Barratt et al., 1999). The most common PKD results from mutations on the PKD1 locus on chromosome 16 (Goodyer & Kashtan, 1998).

In PKD, cellular hyperplasia of the collecting ducts causes them to dilate. Fluid secreted into these ducts enables cyst sacs to form. Initially, cysts are usually less than 2 mm in size and do not obstruct urinary flow. As the child grows, however, the cysts become larger and fibrosis occurs. Tubular atrophy may occur in some children, whereas others have minimal changes in renal function. Polycystic kidney disease is also associated with liver abnormalities that progress to fibrosis, portal hypertension, and biliary infection, which gets more severe with age.

Newborns with polycystic kidney disease may have enlarged kidneys, detected at birth. Those with the most severe form of the disease die shortly after birth of pulmonary hypoplasia. Clinical manifestations in infants and children include hypertension, hematuria, frequent urination, poor growth, urinary tract infections, and proteinuria. Polyuria and polydipsia develop with progressive renal insufficiency. As uremia develops, infants and children develop renal osteodystrophy and progressive developmental delay and growth failure.

Sonogram or renal biopsy confirms the diagnosis. The disease is often diagnosed on prenatal ultrasound. If identified, other family members should be screened for subclinical cases of the disease. Liver function tests are usually normal.

Treatment is supportive. Medications such as diuretics are prescribed for hypertension. Antibiotics treat urinary tract infection. Erythropoietin is prescribed to prevent and treat anemia. Growth hormones may be used in some children to promote growth. Renal osteodystrophy is treated to suppress the parathyroid hormone. Chronic renal failure is managed as described earlier. Surgery is performed for portal hypertension. Renal dialysis or a transplant prolong survival. However, liver problems may continue to complicate the child's health, even when the renal condition is well controlled.

Nursing Management

Nursing care is the same as that for the child with renal insufficiency and chronic renal failure. Observe the child for signs of progressive renal impairment. Make sure the family schedules follow-up appointments to assess growth, developmental progress, and the effectiveness of the treatment plan. Family teaching for home management focuses on medications, diet adequate in protein and calories to support growth, management of acute gastrointestinal illnesses, and care for the child with progressive renal insufficiency and a liver disorder.

HEMOLYTIC-UREMIC SYNDROME

Hemolytic-uremic syndrome (HUS) is a relatively rare, acute renal disease that occurs most often in children under 4 years. The syndrome has a classic triad of signs: (1) hemolytic anemia, (2) thrombocytopenia, and (3) ARF. It is an important cause of CRF.

The development of HUS is often linked to enterohemorrhagic *Escherichia coli* strain 0157:H7, which produces a toxin that attaches to the kidneys and other organs. Hamburger is the vector in more than half of cases. The toxin damages the lining of the glomerular arterioles, causing the endothelial cells to swell. In response, clotting mechanisms deposit fibrin in the renal arterioles and capillaries. This partial occlusion damages the red blood cells, resulting in hemolysis and subsequent anemia. Platelet agglutination occurs in areas of vascular endothelial damage, causing thrombocytopenia. ARF develops as a consequence of blood clotting in the arterioles as well as the toxic effect of hemolyzed red blood cells on renal tubular cells, leading to acute tubular necrosis. Autosomal recessive and autosomal dominant forms of HUS also exist, accounting for less than 5% of cases (Varade, 2000).

An episode of mild gastroenteritis with diarrhea, upper respiratory infection, or UTI precedes the development of HUS by 1 to 2 weeks. Signs and symptoms of HUS are described below. The child may also have hyperkalemia and metabolic acidosis as a result of renal failure. A peripheral blood smear with fragments of red blood cells, fibrin split products, and a decreased platelet count ($<140,000/$ $\mu L[mm^3]$) confirms the diagnosis.

Treatment focuses on the complications of ARF and includes fluid restrictions, antihypertensive medications, and a high-calorie, high-carbohydrate diet that is low in protein, sodium, potassium, and phosphorus. A recent study showed that antibiotic treatment of the child exposed to *E. coli* 0157:H7 increases the risk of HUS due to the release of toxins and alteration of the intestinal flora (Wong, Jelacic, Habeeb, et al., 2000). Treatment of diarrhea with antimotility medications is contraindicated because they increase the risk of toxic megacolon or progression from hemorrhagic colitis to HUS (Varade, 2000).

Enteral nutritional support is sometimes needed. (Refer to the earlier discussion of ARF.) About 60% of children need dialysis; peritoneal dialysis is preferred unless the child has severe colitis and abdominal tenderness. It generally takes about 8 days to recover normal renal function (Varade, 2000). Some children may develop chronic renal failure. Transfusions of fresh packed red blood cells may be ordered to treat severe anemia. Platelets are given if the child is bleeding or if surgery is needed. Transfusions should be administered carefully to prevent hypertension caused by hypervolemia. Mortality from HUS is now less than 5%.

Nursing Management

Nursing care is the same as that for the child with ARF, described earlier. Careful monitoring of neurologic signs, laboratory values, and fluid and electrolyte balance is essential. Observe the child carefully for signs of progressive renal impairment. Discharge planning focuses on teaching parents about medications and dietary and fluid restrictions. Follow-up visits are necessary to evaluate the effectiveness of the treatment plan. Teach parents that HUS can be largely prevented by cooking of ground beef to 155 °F throughout, meaning no more rare hamburgers. Teach them to wash hands carefully when handling raw ground meats, and to make sure utensils touching raw meat do not come into contact with cooked meats.

ACUTE POSTINFECTIOUS GLOMERULONEPHRITIS

Glomerulonephritis is an inflammation of the glomeruli of the kidneys. In children, it is most often a response to a group A beta-hemolytic streptococcal infection of the skin or pharynx. It is also caused by other organisms, including *Staphylococcus, Pneumococcus,* and coxsackieviruses. The incidence of acute postinfectious glomerulonephritis (APIGN) is highest in children who are 5 to 8 years of age,

---

CLINICAL MANIFESTATIONS ~ *Hemolytic-Uremic Syndrome*

STAGE	CLINICAL MANIFESTATIONS
Prodromal stage (1–7 days)	Upper respiratory illness Abdominal pain with nausea, vomiting, and bloody diarrhea Pallor Fever and irritability Lymphadenopathy Skin rash Edema Severe gastroenteritis with bloody diarrhea in 90% of cases
Acute stage	Hemolytic anemia Hypertension Purpura Neurologic involvement (irritability, seizures, lethargy, stupor, coma, cerebral edema) Hematuria and proteinuria Oliguria or anuria Edema and ascites

and the disorder is more common in boys than in girls. Early antibiotic therapy for streptococcal infection does not seem to prevent the development of APIGN.

Etiology and Pathophysiology

The child with APIGN usually becomes ill after a nephritogenic strain of group A beta-hemolytic streptococcal infection of the upper respiratory tract or the skin. Often the child becomes ill with strep throat, recovers, and then develops signs of APIGN after 8 to 14 days.

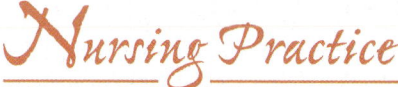

Encourage prompt treatment of streptococcal infections with a full course of antibiotics to prevent APIGN when possible. Ensure that children with possible streptococcal infections, such as a severe or continuing sore throat, are seen by a health care provider.

Glomerular damage occurs as a result of an immune complex reaction that localizes on the glomerular capillary wall. Antibody–antigen complexes become lodged in the glomeruli, leading to inflammation and obstruction. Dam-age to the glomerular membrane allows red blood cells and red cell casts to be excreted. Sodium and water are retained, expanding the intravascular and interstitial compartments and resulting in the characteristic finding of edema (see "Pathophysiology Illustrated: Glomerulonephritis").

Clinical Manifestations

Onset is usually abrupt. Microscopic hematuria is present in nearly all cases, and gross hematuria, resulting in tea-colored urine, is found in up to 50% of cases. Mild periorbital edema occurs early, but edema may become more severe if fluid intake is not restricted during the acute stage. Most hospitalized children become hypertensive. As the disease progresses, the child becomes lethargic and feverish and may complain of abdominal pain, headache, and costovertebral tenderness (related to stretching of the renal capsule from edema).

Clinical Therapy

Blood tests may reveal elevated BUN and creatinine concentrations. The erythrocyte sedimentation rate is increased in the acute phase, and serum lipid levels are increased in about 40% of cases. An elevated antistreptolysin O (ASO) titer reflects the presence of antibodies from a

---

PATHOPHYSIOLOGY ILLUSTRATED
Acute Postinfectious Glomerulonephritis

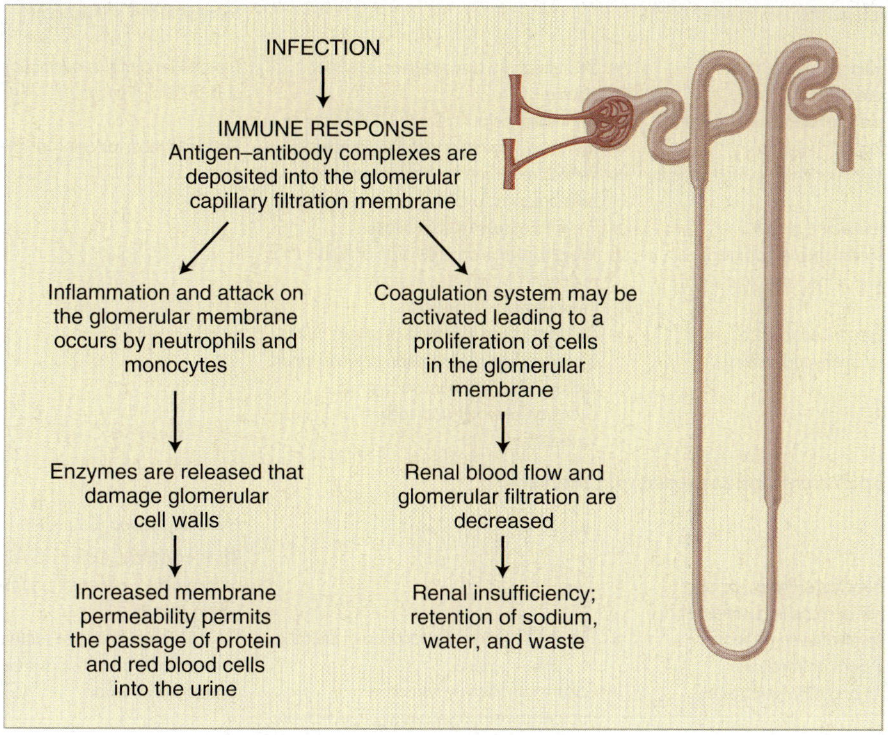

INFECTION
↓
IMMUNE RESPONSE
Antigen–antibody complexes are deposited into the glomerular capillary filtration membrane

Inflammation and attack on the glomerular membrane occurs by neutrophils and monocytes
↓
Enzymes are released that damage glomerular cell walls
↓
Increased membrane permeability permits the passage of protein and red blood cells into the urine

Coagulation system may be activated leading to a proliferation of cells in the glomerular membrane
↓
Renal blood flow and glomerular filtration are decreased
↓
Renal insufficiency; retention of sodium, water, and waste

recent streptococcal respiratory infection, but the ASO level associated with a recent skin infection is low. The anti-DNAse B titer is helpful for detecting antibodies associated with recent skin infections. Up to 90% of children have reduced serum C3. Urinalysis reveals an acid pH, hematuria, proteinuria (trace to 2 +), reddish brown color due to red blood cells, and white blood cells. Anemia is common in the acute phase, usually because extracellular fluid dilutes the serum. The hemoglobin level and hematocrit value may decrease during the late phase as a result of hematuria. The white blood cell count may be normal or slightly elevated.

Treatment focuses on relief of symptoms and supportive therapy. Bed rest is a key component of the treatment plan during the acute phase. Hypertension can be managed with a combination of an antihypertensive medication (such as hydralazine [Apresoline]) and a diuretic (such as furosemide [Lasix]). Mild to moderate hypertension should be treated with fluid and salt restriction. A course of antibiotics may be given to ensure eradication of the infectious agent.

Fluid requirements are determined by careful monitoring of urinary output, weight, blood pressure, and serum electrolytes. Initially, only insensible losses are replaced until the status of renal function is known. The severity of edema determines the degree of dietary restriction. Sodium and potassium intake are restricted. With severe azotemia, protein intake may have to be limited.

The prognosis for over 95% of children with APIGN is good. Most children recover completely within a few weeks. Recurrences are unusual. Rarely, some children do develop chronic glomerulonephritis.

Nursing Management

Nursing Assessment and Diagnoses

Assess edema, which may be periorbital or dependent and shifts as the child's position is changed. Assess for circulatory congestion (crackles, dyspnea, and cough). Monitor blood pressure, which can rise as high as 200/120 mm Hg. With severe hypertension, assess for signs of central nervous system problems (headache, blurred vision, vomiting, decreased level of consciousness, confusion, and convulsions).

Refer to "Nursing Care Plan: The Child with Acute Postinfectious Glomerulonephritis" for several nursing diagnoses that may apply to the child with APIGN.

NURSING CARE PLAN ∼ *The Child With Acute Postinfectious Glomerulonephritis*

GOAL	INTERVENTION	RATIONALE	EXPECTED OUTCOME
1. Fluid volume excess related to decreased glomerular filtration and increased sodium retention			
	NIC Priority Intervention: **Fluid management:** *Promotion of fluid balance and prevention of complications resulting from abnormal or undesired fluid levels*		*NOC Suggested Outcome:* **Fluid balance:** *Balance of water in the intracellular and extracellular compartments of the body*
The child will regain normal fluid balance.	▶ Assess for edema (periorbital or dependent areas). ▶ Calculate fluid intake and plan amounts to offer throughout the day. ▶ Limit foods with moderate to high sodium content. ▶ Document intake and output. ▶ Perform daily weight measurement on the same scale at the same time of day. ▶ Administer prescribed medications (diuretics and antihypertensives).	▶ Sodium and water retention leads to edema. ▶ An intake/output ratio of 1:1 reflects normal hydration and kidney function. ▶ Further reduction in sodium intake will help balance fluid and sodium retention. ▶ Prevents excessive fluid intake. ▶ Weight gain is an early sign of fluid retention. Weight loss indicates improvement in condition. ▶ Diuretics cause excretion of excess fluid by preventing reabsorption of water and sodium. Antihypertensives increase excretion of water and sodium and cause vasodilation.	The child maintains normal urine output of 0.5–1 mL/kg/hr. The child receives appropriate fluid each day.
2. Risk for infection related to renal impairment and corticosteroid therapy			
	NIC Priority Intervention: **Infection protection:** *Prevention and early detection of infection in a patient at risk* ▶ Assess temperature every 4 hours. Observe for signs of infection. ▶ Obtain throat and other cultures as ordered.	▶ The child is at risk for secondary infection. ▶ Culture can identify causative microorganism in secondary infection or presence of residual streptococcal infection.	*NOC Suggested Outcome:* **Risk control:** *Actions to eliminate or reduce actual personal and modifiable health threats.* The child's temperature remains within normal limits and child is free of secondary infection.
The child will be infection-free.			

Planning and Implementation

As with other renal disorders, care of the child with APIGN requires careful monitoring of vital signs and fluid–electrolyte balance to evaluate renal functioning and identify complications. Bed rest is required during the acute phase. Immediate emergency care is needed for severe hypertension with cerebral dysfunction; diazoxide or hydralazine is administered intravenously. Nursing care focuses on monitoring fluid status, preventing infection, preventing skin breakdown, meeting nutritional needs, and providing emotional support to the child and family.

NURSING CARE PLAN ～ *The Child Acute Postinfectious Glomerulonephritis—continued*

GOAL	INTERVENTION	RATIONALE	EXPECTED OUTCOME
3. Risk for impaired skin integrity related to tissue edema			
	NIC Priority Intervention: **Pressure management:** *Minimizing pressure to body parts*		*NOC Suggested Outcome:* **Risk control:** *Actions to eliminate or reduce actual personal and modifiable health threats.*
The child will be free of skin breakdown.	▶ Assess skin for breakdown secondary to edema and bed rest. ▶ Encourage position changes every 1–2 hours. Provide skin care. Use a therapeutic mattress.	▶ Ensures early identification and implementation of preventive measures. ▶ Prolonged pressure leads to skin breakdown.	The child has unimpaired skin integrity.
4. Altered nutrition: less than body requirements related to loss of appetite			
	NIC Priority Intervention: **Nutrition management:** *Assistance with or provision of balanced dietary intake of foods and fluids*		*NOC Suggested Outcome:* **Food and fluid intake:** *Amount of food and fluid taken into the body over a 24-hour period*
The child will maintain adequate caloric intake.	▶ Maintain meal schedule similar to that at home. Serve food in age-appropriate servings. Assess for food likes and dislikes. Provide favorite foods, as possible.	▶ Normal routine and preferred food choices help to encourage the child to eat.	Child maintains weight and tolerates daily intake that meets nutritional requirements.
5. Activity intolerance related to fluid and electrolyte imbalance, infectious process, and altered nutrition			
	NIC Priority Intervention: **Energy management:** *Regulating energy use to treat or prevent fatigue and optimize function*		*NOC Suggested Outcome:* **Energy conservation:** *Extent of active management of energy to initiate and sustain activity*
The child will progress in activity tolerance without excess fatigue as the disease process improves.	▶ Maintain bed rest during acute stage. Encourage gradual activity increase as the condition improves. ▶ Provide for quiet play according to the developmental stage of the child (e.g., coloring books, music, videotapes, television).	▶ Rest decreases the production of waste materials, which place increased stress on the kidneys. ▶ Quiet activities minimize energy expenditures and stress on the kidneys.	The child avoids fatigue and exhibits the ability to tolerate activity for longer periods.
6. Effective management of therapeutic regimen (parents) related to child's medication schedule and treatment regimen after discharge			
	NIC Priority Intervention: **Anticipatory guidance:** *Preparation of patient for an anticipated developmental and/or situational crisis*		*NOC Suggested Outcome:* **Compliance behavior:** *Actions taken on the basis of professional advice to promote wellness, recovery, and rehabilitation*
The parents will state knowledge of the child's treatment regimen after discharge.	▶ Assess parents' understanding of need for compliance with medication schedule. ▶ Describe best schedule for giving medications to match child's and family's routines. ▶ Inform parents about potential side effects of prescribed medications and signs and symptoms of complications.	▶ Diuretics and antihypertensives are central to treatment plan. ▶ Improves compliance. ▶ Allows early intervention to prevent side effects.	The parents administer medications as prescribed.

MONITOR FLUID STATUS

Monitor vital signs, fluid and electrolyte status, and intake and output. Hypovolemia can occur as a result of fluid shifting from vascular to interstitial spaces despite the outward clinical signs of excess fluid retention. Monitor the degree of ascites by measuring abdominal girth. Document urine specific gravity.

PREVENT INFECTION

Impaired renal function puts the child at risk for infection. Monitor for signs of infection, including fever, increased malaise, and an elevated white blood cell count. Instruct the family in good handwashing technique. Limit visitors, and screen for upper respiratory infections.

PREVENT SKIN BREAKDOWN

Dependent areas or areas prone to pressure are vulnerable to skin breakdown. Turn the child frequently. Pad bony prominences or susceptible areas with sheepskin, or protect skin with a transparent dressing. Make sure the child's bed is free of crumbs or sharp toys. Keep sheets tight and free of wrinkles.

MEET NUTRITIONAL NEEDS

A team approach (including the nurse, renal dietitian, parents, and child) is often needed to meet the child's nutritional needs. In most cases the child follows a "no added salt" and low-protein diet. Anorexia presents the greatest challenge to meeting daily nutritional requirements during the acute phase of the disease. To increase the child's appetite, encourage parents to bring the child's favorite foods from home, serve foods in age-appropriate quantities, and allow the child to eat with other children or with family members.

PROVIDE EMOTIONAL SUPPORT

Parents of a child with APIGN commonly feel guilty. Parents may blame themselves for not responding more quickly to the child's initial symptoms or may believe they could have prevented the development of glomerular damage. Discuss the etiology of the disease and the child's treatment, and correct any misconceptions. Emphasize that APIGN develops in only a few children with streptococcal infection.

DISCHARGE PLANNING AND HOME CARE TEACHING

Children are hospitalized for a few days, but it may take 3 weeks for hypertension and gross hematuria to resolve and longer for the disorder to resolve completely. Discharge planning focuses on teaching parents about the child's medication regimen, potential side effects of medications, dietary restrictions, and signs and symptoms of complications. Teach parents how to take the child's blood pressure and how to test urine for albumin, if ordered. Have them demonstrate these procedures. Emphasize that it is important to avoid exposing the child to people with upper respiratory tract infections. Recommend family

screening for streptococcal infection if this is found to be the cause of the child's APIGN. Advise parents to allow the child to return to his or her normal routine and activities after discharge, with periods allowed for rest.

Evaluation

Expected outcomes of nursing care are listed on the nursing care plan.

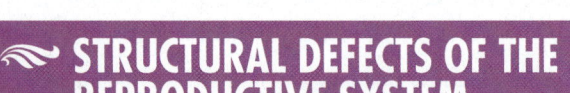

PHIMOSIS

In phimosis, the foreskin over the glans penis cannot be pulled back, due to adhesions or infection. Circumcision, surgical removal of the foreskin, is often performed during the newborn period to prevent phimosis, for ease of proper male hygiene, and to prevent UTIs, balanitis (inflammation of the glans penis), and penile cancer (see Chapter 26). Approximately 12% of males who are not circumcised as newborns eventually need the surgery (Williamson, 1997). Betamethasone cream 0.05% applied twice daily for a month to the glans is an effective alternative to surgery (Van Howe, 1998).

CRYPTORCHIDISM

Cryptorchidism (undescended testes) occurs when one or both testes fail to descend through the inguinal canal into the scrotum. Normally, the testes descend during the seventh to ninth month of gestation.

Cryptorchidism may be the result of a testosterone deficiency, an absent or defective testis, or a structural problem such as a narrow inguinal canal, short spermatic cord, or adhesions. The disorder occurs in 3% to 4% of term male infants and in approximately 30% of premature infants (Fonkalsrud, 1996). The higher temperature in the abdomen than in the scrotum results in morphologic change to the testis, beginning after the second birthday. Lower sperm counts are the ultimate result. Complications of uncorrected cryptorchidism include infertility, malignancy or torsion of the undescended testis, atrophy, and the psychologic effects of "empty" scrotum.

Cryptorchidism is usually detected during the newborn examination when palpation of the scrotum fails to reveal one or both testes. It is not unusual for boys with cryptorchidism to have an inguinal hernia as well. In 75% of cases, the testes descend spontaneously by 3 months of age. If descent does not occur within the first year, human chorionic gonadotropin may be prescribed to detect the presence of nonpalpable testes. An orchiopexy is performed at 1 year of age before further damage to the testes occurs. An incision is made at the location of the testis, either in the abdomen or in the inguinal area. Blood vessels are disentangled to allow the testis to reach into the lower scrotum. A second incision is made in the scrotum at the point where the testis is stitched to the inside wall to keep it in place. If the testis is defective or undeveloped, it may be removed surgically to decrease the risk of later malignancies and a prosthesis may be placed in the scrotum. The goals of surgery are repair of any hernia, enhanced fertility, and psychologic benefit. The orchiopexy also makes it easier to examine the testis for tumors. The risk of testicular cancer is 35 to 50 times greater in men with a history of cryptorchidism (Ferrer & McKenna, 2000).

Nursing Management

Preoperative nursing care includes preparing the parents and child for the procedure and addressing parents' concerns about the postsurgical outcome. Orchiopexy is often performed as an outpatient procedure. If the child is hospitalized, postoperative nursing care focuses on maintaining comfort and preventing infection. Encourage bed rest, and monitor voiding. Apply ice to the surgical area, and administer prescribed analgesics to relieve pain.

Discharge instructions should include demonstration of proper incision care. The diaper area should be cleaned well with each diaper change to decrease chances of infection. Teach parents to identify signs of infection such as redness, warmth, swelling, and discharge. All vigorous activity should be restricted for 2 weeks following surgery to promote healing and prevent injury.

INGUINAL HERNIA AND HYDROCELE

An inguinal hernia is a painless inguinal or scrotal swelling of variable size. A hydrocele is a fluid-filled mass in the scrotum. A hernia is found in 1% to 5% of infants, more commonly in boys than girls by a 4:1 ratio. Inguinal hernias occur more commonly in premature infants.

During fetal development, a peritoneal sac precedes the testicle's descent to the scrotum. The lower sac enfolds the testis to become the tunica vaginalis, and the upper sac atrophies before birth. Fluid may become trapped in the tunica vaginalis and cause the hydrocele. When the tunica vaginalis does not atrophy, an abdominal structure may move into it.

Diagnosis is made by physical examination at birth or in early infancy. Palpation of the scrotum reveals a round, smooth, nontender mass. Transillumination helps determine whether the mass is a hernia or hydrocele (see Chapter 33). Swelling associated with a hernia may become more apparent with straining. Some hernias reduce in size during sleep.

Outpatient surgery is performed at an early age (usually after 3 months of age to reduce anesthesia risks) to avoid incarceration, which is a medical emergency. A nerve

block may be given in the operating room to reduce postoperative pain. The prognosis is generally excellent. Most hydroceles without inguinal hernia resolve spontaneously as the fluid reabsorbs by the time an infant is 1 to 2 years of age.

Nursing Practice

Inguinal hernias can become incarcerated when a bit of bowel becomes trapped in the inguinal opening. The child has a sudden painful swelling in the groin, increased irritability, vomiting, and abdominal distention. A bowel obstruction is seen on x-ray. Efforts are made to reduce the hernia before surgery by placing the child in the Trendelenburg position and applying firm manual pressure on the affected side. The child needs surgery within 24 to 48 hours.

Nursing care for hydrocele and inguinal hernia includes explaining the disorder and its treatment and providing preoperative and postoperative teaching and care. Inform parents that the scrotum may be edematous and may appear bruised after surgery. Incision care involves careful cleaning of the diaper area. The incision is covered with a protective sealant rather than a dressing.

TESTICULAR TORSION

Testicular torsion is an emergency condition in which the testis suddenly rotates on its spermatic cord, cutting off its blood supply. The arteries and veins in the spermatic cord become twisted and interrupt the blood supply, leading to vascular engorgement and ischemia. The incidence is highest at puberty; however, the condition may occur at any time between 3 and 20 years of age. Often the testicles are positioned horizontally in the scrotum, a congenital anomaly known as a bell clapper deformity, which predisposes the boy to this condition.

Manifestations include severe pain and erythema in the scrotum, nausea and vomiting, abdominal pain, and scrotal swelling that is not relieved by rest or scrotal support. The cremasteric reflex is absent. Symptoms generally start when the child is sleeping or inactive, but they can occur after trauma, sexual activity, or exercise. The testis is positioned higher in the scrotum than the unaffected testis because of the shortened vascular pedicle. A testicular scan or sonogram may be performed, if necessary to confirm the diagnosis.

Torsion must be reduced within 6 hours to save the testis. Manual reduction with an analgesic is sometimes attempted, but emergency surgery is more common. During surgery, the testis is untwisted and stitched to the side of the scrotum in the correct position. The procedure is usually performed bilaterally to prevent future torsion in the other testis.

Nursing management involves psychologic support for the child and family related to the need for emergency surgery and concern about the child's future fertility.

Reassure parents that as only one testis is usually involved, fertility should not be affected. The child often goes home within a few hours of surgery; thus, the child and family need to be taught about proper care of the incision and pain management. Explain to parents that the child should not lift heavy objects for 4 weeks or participate in strenuous activity for 2 weeks after surgery to promote healing. Teach the adolescent testicular self-examination. See Chapter 3 for more information on sexually transmitted infections.

CHAPTER HIGHLIGHTS

- Bladder capacity increases with growth, from 20 to 50 mL in newborns to 700 mL in adults.

- Structural defects of the urinary system, including bladder exstrophy, hypospadias and epispadias, and obstructive uropathy, generally require surgical treatment.

- Urinary tract infections are the second most common infection in children. Symptoms vary by the age of the child. Children who do not receive aggressive treatment may develop permanent kidney damage or sepsis.

- Nocturnal enuresis often occurs in children whose parents have a history of enuresis. A structural or neurologic cause is identified in very few children.

- Minimal change nephrotic syndrome is characterized by edema that develops over several weeks, weight gain, hypertension, irritability, hematuria, malaise, anorexia, and foamy or frothy urine.

- Acute renal failure occurs when kidney function diminishes abruptly and is often reversible. It may occur as a complication of cardiac surgery or drug toxicity. It is also seen in critically ill neonates with asphyxia, sepsis, or shock.

- Chronic renal failure is progressive, irreversible reduced function of the kidneys, eventually resulting in end-stage renal disease. It often results from developmental abnormalities of the kidneys or urinary tract.

- Children with end-stage renal disease are treated with hemodialysis, peritoneal dialysis, or renal transplant.

- Polycystic kidney disease is a genetic disorder with both autosomal recessive and autosomal dominant forms that leads to chronic renal failure. It may be detected prenatally or in young children.

- Hemolytic-uremic syndrome is often associated with ingestion of *E. coli* strain 0157:H7, which produces a toxin that attacks the kidneys. The child develops hemolytic anemia, thrombocytopenia, and acute renal failure that can progress to chronic renal failure.

- Acute postinfectious glomerulonephritis results from a beta-hemolytic group A streptococcal infection of the respiratory tract or skin. Most children's kidney function recovers completely.

- Structural defects of the male reproductive system include phimosis, cryptorchidism, inguinal hernia and hydrocele, and testicular torsion.

EXPLORE MediaLink

NCLEX Review, Case Studies, and other interactive resources for this chapter can be found on the companion website at http://www.prenhall.com/london. Click on "Chapter 47" and select the activities for this chapter.

For animations, more NCLEX review questions, and an audio glossary, access the accompanying CD-ROM in this textbook.

REFERENCES

American Academy of Pediatrics. (2000). *The red book: Report of the Committee on Infectious Disease* (25th ed.). Elk Grove Village, IL: Author.

Anderson, J. E., & Anderson, K. A. (1999). What to tell parents about circumcision. *Contemporary Pediatrics, 16*(2), 87–102.

Balinsky, W. (2000). Pediatric end-stage renal disease: Incidence, management, and prevention. *Journal of Pediatric Health Care, 14*(6), 304–308.

Barratt, T. M., Avner, E. D., & Harmon, W. E. (1999). *Pediatric nephrology* (4th ed.). Philadelphia: Lippincott, Williams & Wilkins.

Becker, N., & Avner, E. D. (1995). Congenital neuropathies and uropathies. *Pediatric Clinics of North America, 42*(6), 1319–1341.

Ben-Chaim, J., Docimo, S. G., Jeffs, R. D., & Gearhart, J. P. (1996). Bladder exstrophy from childhood to adult life. *Journal of the Royal Society of Medicine, 89*(1), 39P–46P.

Bereket, G., & Fine, R. N. (1995). Pediatric renal transplantation. *Pediatric Clinics of North America, 42*(6), 1603–1628.

Evans, E. D., Greenbaum, L. A., & Ettenger, R. B. (1995). Principles of renal replacement therapy in children. *Pediatric Clinics of North America, 42*(6), 1579–1602.

Ferrer, F. A., & McKenna, P. H. (2000). Current approaches to the undescended testicle. *Contemporary Pediatrics, 17*(1), 106–111.

Fonkalsrud, E. W. (1996). Current management of the undescended testis. *Seminars in Pediatric Surgery, 5*(1), 2–7.

Furth, S. L., Garg, P. P., Neu, A. M., Hwang, W., Fivush, B. A., & Powe, N. R. (2000). Racial differences in access to the kidney transplant waiting list for children and adolescents with end-stage renal disease. *Pediatrics, 106*(4), 756–761.

Gilman, C. M., & Mooney, K. H. (1998). Alterations in renal and urinary tract function in children. In K. L. McCance & S. E. Huether (Eds.), *Pathophysiology: The biologic basis for disease in adults and children* (3rd ed., pp. 1273–1287). St. Louis, MO: Mosby.

Goodyer, P., & Kashtan, C. (1998). The genetic basis of pediatric renal disease. *Seminars in Nephrology, 18*(3), 244–255.

Hellerstein, S. (2000). Long term consequences of urinary tract infections. *Current Opinion in Pediatrics, 12*, 125–128.

Issenman, R. M., Filmer, R. B., & Gorski, P. A. (1999). A review of bowel and bladder control development in children: How gastrointestinal and urologic conditions relate to problems in toilet training. *Pediatrics, 103*(6), 1346–1352.

Kelleher, R. E. (1997). Daytime and night time wetting in children: A review of management. *Journal of the Society of Pediatric Nurses, 2*(2), 73–82.

Miller, K. L. (1996). Urinary tract infections: Children are not small adults. *Pediatric Nursing, 22*(6), 473–480, 544.

Miller, K. M. (1999). Testicular torsion. *American Journal of Nursing, 99*(6), 33.

Paulozzi, L. J., Erickson, J. D., & Jackson, R. J. (1997). Hypospadias trends in two U.S. surveillance systems. *Pediatrics, 100*(5), 831–834.

Saborio, P., Hahn, S., Hisano, S., Lotta, K., Scheinman, J. I., & Chan, J. C. M. (1998). Chronic renal failure: An overview from a pediatric perspective. *Nephron, 80,* 134–148.

Shaw, K. N., & Gorelick, M. H. (1999). Urinary tract infection in the pediatric patient. *Pediatric Clinics of North America, 46*(6), 1111–1123.

Taylor, J. H. (1996). End stage renal disease in children: Diagnosis, management, and interventions. *Pediatric Nursing, 22*(6), 481–490.

Tobias, N. E. (2000). Management of nocturnal enuresis. *Nursing Clinics of North America, 35*(1), 37–60.

Tune, B. M., & Mendoza, S. A. (1997). Treatment of idiopathic nephritic syndrome: Regimens and outcomes in children and adults. *Journal of the American Society of Nephrology, 8*(5), 824–832.

United States Renal Data System. (2000). *2000 annual data report: Atlas of end-stage renal disease in the United States.* Minneapolis, MN: USRDS Coordinating Center.

Van Howe, R. S. (1998). Cost-effective treatment of phimosis. *Pediatrics, 102*(4), e43.

Varade, W. S. (2000). Hemolytic uremic syndrome: Reducing the risks. *Contemporary Pediatrics, 17*(9), 54–64.

Vogt, B. A. (1997). Identifying kidney disease: Simple steps can make a difference. *Contemporary Pediatrics, 14*(3), 115–127.

Warady, B. A., Alexander, S. R., Watkins, S., Kohout, E., & Harmon, W. E. (1999). Optimal care of the pediatric end-stage renal disease patient on dialysis. *American Journal of Kidney Diseases, 33*(3), 567–583.

Williamson, M. L. (1997). Circumcision anesthesia: A study of nursing implications for dorsal penile nerve blocks. *Pediatric Nursing, 23*(1), 59–63.

Wong, C. S., Jelacic, S., Habeeb, R. L., Watkins, S. L., & Tarr, P. I. (2000). The risk of HUS after antibiotic treatment of *Escherichia coli* 0157:H7 infection. *New England Journal of Medicine, 342*(26), 1930–1936.

CHAPTER 48

The Child with Alterations in Eye, Ear, Nose, and Throat Function

The early intervention program that Raeanne attended to help her deal with her visual impairment really helped her to prepare for preschool. We learned a lot too about how to help her. We are still really nervous about her starting at preschool and being with a lot of other children. We want it to go well for her.

—MOTHER OF RAEANNE, 3 YEARS OLD

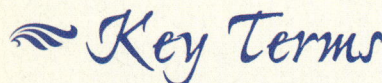

Key Terms

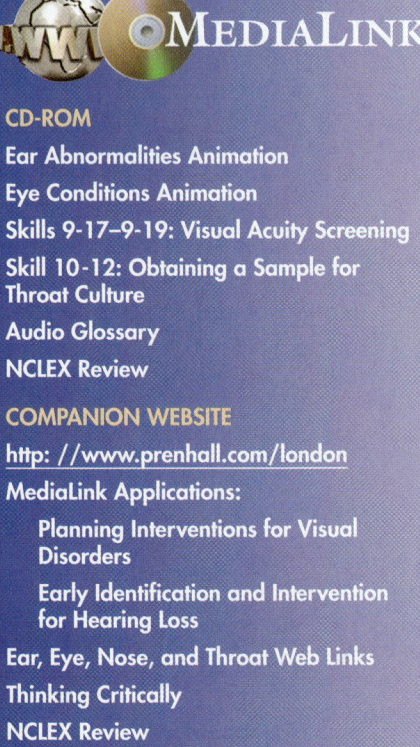

MEDIALINK

CD-ROM

Ear Abnormalities Animation

Eye Conditions Animation

Skills 9-17–9-19: Visual Acuity Screening

Skill 10-12: Obtaining a Sample for Throat Culture

Audio Glossary

NCLEX Review

COMPANION WEBSITE

http://www.prenhall.com/london

MediaLink Applications:

    Planning Interventions for Visual Disorders

    Early Identification and Intervention for Hearing Loss

Ear, Eye, Nose, and Throat Web Links

Thinking Critically

NCLEX Review

Case Study

*H*ow are conditions of the eye, ear, nose, and throat related? Which conditions have the potential to affect a child's growth, development, and behavior? In what settings do children with eye, ear, nose, and throat conditions receive care? How can parents be helped to foster development in their children when they have a visual or hearing disorder?

Because the eye, ear, nose, and throat are connected, a malformation, infection, or other condition in one of these structures may affect them all. Intact sensory structures enable children to reach developmental milestones; thus alterations, especially to the eye and ear, may delay a child's development. Most children with eye, ear, nose, and throat disorders are treated at home or in the community rather than in the hospital.

ANATOMY AND PHYSIOLOGY OF PEDIATRIC DIFFERENCES

Eye

How are the eyes of children different from those of adults? Chapter 33 provides a detailed discussion of the assessment of the eyes and **visual acuity,** the ability to discriminate letters or other objects. ⬭ The eyes of neonates differ from the eyes of adults in several ways. Visual acuity in neonates ranges between 20/100 and 20/400. The lens is more spherical and cannot accommodate to both near and far objects, which means that the neonate sees best at a distance of about 8 inches (20 cm). Since the optic nerve is not yet completely myelinated, the ability to distinguish color and other details is decreased. If the infant is preterm, especially less than 32 weeks' gestation, retinal vascularization, particularly in the periphery of the retina, may be incomplete. The rectus muscles that control binocular vision may be somewhat uncoordinated at birth. The eyes should be aligned and movement coordinated by the age of 3 months.

The eyeball of the infant and young child occupies a larger portion of the orbit than in the adult. Since the eyeball is relatively unprotected laterally, it is more easily injured. The sclera of the neonate is thin and translucent with a bluish tinge, and the iris is blue or gray. Eye color changes during the first 6 months of life. Infants produce tears to nourish and oxygenate the outer layers of the cornea. Parents do not see tears when a young infant cries because the infant's lacrimal system drains them efficiently into the nasal cavity.

As infants grow, their eyes mature and their vision improves. By the age of 2 or 3 years, most children have a visual acuity of 20/50, and by the age of 6 or 7 years, it is 20/20. Visual acuity is measured using standardized letter or picture charts. (See Chapter 33.) ⬭ **Vision** refers to the complex process of acquiring meaning from what is seen, involving the eye, brain, and related neuro-

logic and physiologic structures. Development interacts with a child's maturing physiologic system to bring increasing meaning to objects in sight (Table 48–1).

Ear

Why do infants and young children have more ear problems than adults? The eustachian tube, which connects the nasopharynx to the middle ear, is proportionately shorter, wider, and more horizontal in infants than in older children or adults (see "As They Grow"). During sucking, yawning, and other movements, the tube opens for milliseconds, allowing free passage of air between the nasopharynx and the middle ear.

The external ear canal is small at birth, although the internal ear and middle ear are relatively large. As a result, the tympanic membrane is close to the surface and can be easily injured.

Nose and Throat

Up to the age of 6 months, infants breathe primarily through the nose and not through the mouth. Edema and nasal discharge may interfere with adequate air intake and feeding. Mucosal swelling and exudate may block the small nasal passages of young children.

The palatine tonsils, visible on oral examination, are located on each side of the oropharynx. The method for examining a child's throat is discussed in Chapter 33. ⬭ Although tonsils vary in size considerably during childhood, they are normally large, especially in school-age children. The nasopharyngeal tonsils (adenoids) lie in the

TABLE 48–1 Visually Related Developmental Milestones

Age	Milestone
Term neonate	Demonstrates alertness to visual stimulus presented 8–12 in (20–30 cm) from eyes
1 month	Follows an object 60 degrees horizontally and 30 degrees vertically; blinks at an approaching object
2 months	Follows a person from 6 ft (2 m) away; smiles in response to a face; raises head 30 degrees from prone
3 months	Tracks an object through 180 degrees; regards own hand; begins visual-motor coordination
4–5 months	Social smile; reaches for a cube 12 in (30 cm) away; notices a raisin 12 in (30 cm) away
7–8 months	Picks up a raisin by raking
8–9 months	Pokes at holes in a peg board; neat pincer grasp; crawling
12–14 months	Stacks blocks; places a peg in a round hole; stands and walks

Note: From Scheiner, A. P. (1996). Vision problems: Impairment to blindness. In A. M. Rudolph, J. I. E. Hoffman, & C. D. Rudolph (Eds.), *Rudolph's pediatrics* (20th ed., p. 167). Stamford, CT: Appleton & Lange.

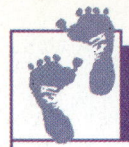
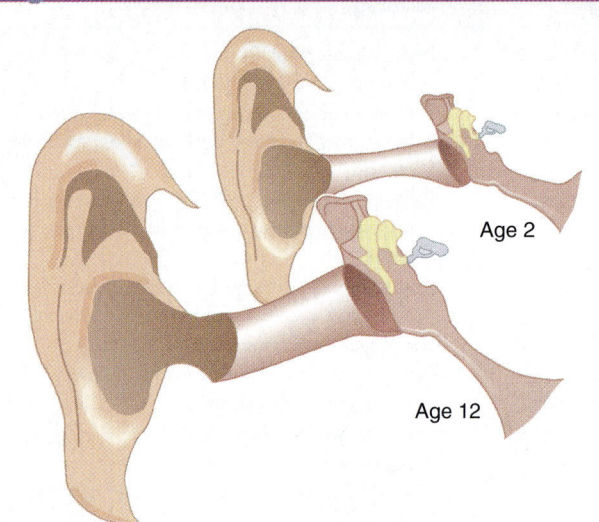

Position of eustachian tube is at less of an angle in the young child, resulting in decreased drainage. (more horizontal)

Age 2

End of eustachian tube in nasal pharynx opens during sucking.

Age 12

Eustachian tube equalizes air pressure between the middle ear and the outside environment and allows for drainage of secretions from middle ear mucosa.

Of the three anatomic differences in the eustachian tube between adults and small children (shorter, wider, more horizontal), which do you think could cause more problems for the child and why?

posterior wall of the nasopharynx, just above the oropharynx. In children, the adenoids may become enlarged, harboring bacteria and interfering with breathing.

～ DISORDERS OF THE EYE

INFECTIOUS CONJUNCTIVITIS

Conjunctivitis is an inflammation of the conjunctiva, the clear membrane that lines the inside of the lid and sclera. Bacteria, viruses, allergies, trauma, or irritants cause the conjunctiva to become swollen and red with a yellow or white discharge (Figure 48–1 ◆).

Conjunctivitis in an infant under 30 days of age is called ophthalmia neonatorum. These infections are usually acquired from the mother during vaginal delivery as a result of contact with infected vaginal discharge containing organisms such as *Chlamydia trachomatis* and *Neisseria gonorrhoeae*. See Chapter 26 for information on prophylactic eye treatment. ⬯ For the infection caused by herpesvirus, prompt and vigorous treatment is needed to prevent eye injury or blindness, which can occur in children with recurrent herpesvirus infections as a result of antibody reaction to the viral antigen. Infants with herpesvirus infections of the eye are treated with intravenous acyclovir as well as topical drops. Newborns occasionally get chemical conjunctivitis in response to prophylactic eye treatment. This may be a cause when the conjunctivitis develops within 24 to 48 hours after instillation of the medication (Alcorn, 2001).

In infants who have frequent tearing and "mattering" (eyelid discharge that has formed a crust) on awakening, a plugged lacrimal duct may mimic conjunctivitis. Treat-

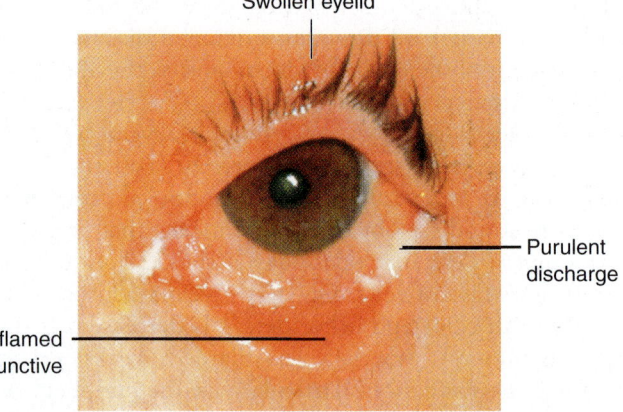

Swollen eyelid

Purulent discharge

Inflamed conjunctive

FIGURE 48–1. ◆ Acute conjunctivitis. The major difference between bacterial and viral conjunctivitis is that bacterial conjunctivitis has a purulent discharge that may result in crusting whereas the discharge from viral conjunctivitis is serous (watery). Allergic conjunctivitis produces watery to thick drainage and is characterized by itching. Note: From Newell, F. W. (1996). *Ophthalmology: Principles and concepts* (8th ed.). St. Louis, MO: Mosby-Year Book, Adapted.

ment involves massaging the tear duct every 4 hours when the infant is awake. Lacrimal ducts that remain plugged after the age of 1 year may have to be opened surgically.

Older children with conjunctivitis complain of itching or burning, mild photophobia, and a feeling of scratching under the lids. Parents may notice increased tearing or a mucoid or mucopurulent discharge, redness and swelling of the conjunctiva, a pink sclera, and crusty eyelids, especially in the morning. There is no change in vision. Common infectious organisms in older children include *Haemophilus influenzae, Streptococcus pneumoniae,* and *Staphylococcus aureus* (Wagner, 2000). A viral cause is also possible, with adenoviruses the most common organism. Viral conjunctivitis is more often bilateral than unilateral.

When conjunctivitis is caused by an allergy, the child complains of intense itching. Eyes are red with watery discharge, and can also be puffy and swollen.

Antibiotic eye medication is prescribed in droplet or ointment form if a bacterial infection is suspected. Amoxicillin and erythromycin are common choices. When gonococcal conjunctivitis occurs in newborns, ceftriaxone is recommended since the disease is resistant to penicillin. Careful total evaluation of the newborn is also performed to watch for other signs of infection.

Instructions for instilling eye medication are provided in the skills manual (see Skill 11-5). 🔗 SKILLS Viral conjunctivitis may be treated with comfort measures such as cleaning drainage away with a warm clean cloth, and avoiding bright lights and reading. Ophthalmic antibiotics may sometimes be given to prevent bacterial invasion due to frequent rubbing of the eyes. If an allergen is believed to be the cause, antihistamines administered orally or ophthalmically may be prescribed. Topical steroids and vasoconstrictors may also be used (Alcorn, 2001).

Nursing Management

Nurses routinely instill antibiotics into the eyes of newborns after birth. Perform a careful examination so that any cases of ophthalmia neonatorum can be referred promptly to an ophthalmologist. Women infected with gonococcus or chlamydia should be identified so their babies can receive attention and medication at birth to prevent infection (Brocklehurst & Rooney, 2000). Babies born at home should have ocular examinations soon after birth.

Teaching About

INSTILLING EYE MEDICATIONS

It can be challenging to safely instill eye medication into young children. Give parents the following suggestions:

- Wash your hands well.
- Be sure the medicine is warmed at least to room temperature.
- Remove any drainage from the eye with a clean or sterile moist, warm cloth or gauze.
- Wash your hands again.
- Have the child lying on the back with eyes closed.
- Gently pull the lower lid down to form a small pocket.
- Apply a thin string (for ointment) or drops of the medicine.
- Allow the eyelid to return to normal position.
- Have the child keep the eye closed for several seconds.
- Help prevent spread of the infection by keeping the child's hands clean.

Enhance comfort by keeping the head elevated to decrease swelling and avoiding exposure to bright light.

In suspected conjunctivitis, gentle pressure for several seconds with a gloved index finger placed next to the inner corner of the eye may cause a discharge of mucopurulent drainage. Since infectious conjunctivitis is extremely contagious, tell parents that children should not return to child care or school until they have been taking an antibiotic for 24 hours. Teach parents the importance of careful handwashing and the avoidance of shared towels. Tell parents that children should not rub their eyes. Mittens may help prevent infants from rubbing their eyes. Toddlers may be distracted by activities that keep their hands busy. Teach parents the proper techniques for instilling eye medications. For children with allergies, alert parents to signs of infection so if the child gets an eye infection, they will seek prompt treatment.

PERIORBITAL CELLULITIS

Periorbital cellulitis is an infection of the eyelid and surrounding tissues, usually caused by bacteria (Figure 48–2 ◆). Children present with swollen, tender, red or purple eyelids; restricted, painful movement of the area around the eye; and fever. Periorbital cellulitis should be treated promptly to prevent the spread of the infection to the posterior orbit. Management includes hospitalization for intravenous antibiotics and the application of hot packs. Children usually respond favorably within 48 to 72 hours.

VISUAL DISORDERS

Vision, the complex process of acquiring meaning from what is seen, depends on many factors. The eyes must move quickly and in a coordinated manner. (See Chapter 33 for discussion of eye movement assessment.) 🔗 They must function together for clear, single vision to occur. If this ability, called **binocularity,** is not present (perhaps due to strabismus or amblyopia), the child cannot make sense of the images the brain receives. Normally, the objects seen are integrated with other senses through eye–hand coordination, and with the brain through visual

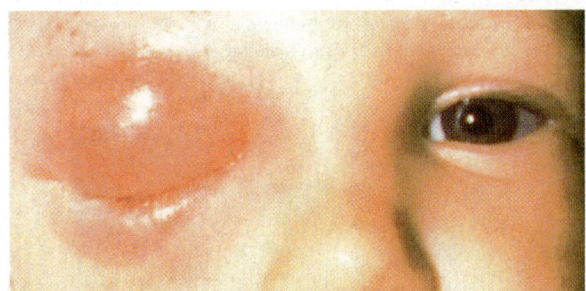

FIGURE 48–2. ◆ Periorbital cellulitis is an infection of the eyelid and surrounding tissues, not the eye itself. It is a serious bacterial infection that can spread to the optic nerve if not treated promptly with intravenous antibiotics. Note: From Malinow, I., & Powell, K. R. (1993). Periorbital cellulitis. *Pediatric Annals, 22*(4), 241–246.

imagery and discrimination of objects seen. Although visual acuity is essential, the child's movements, mental processes, and other senses all interact to give meaning to objects that are viewed. Vision therefore influences learning and school performance.

Visual disturbances must be diagnosed and treated promptly to prevent impairment or loss of visual acuity (Altemeier, 2000). Most children undergo a simple test for visual acuity during health care visits as soon as they can cooperate with the examiner. Once in school, children's visual acuity is screened every 2 to 3 years during the elementary years. Nurses often organize vision screening programs for children. Table 48–2 provides a series of questions that can be used to identify visual disturbances in children. A child who does not pass vision screening is referred to an ophthalmologist or optometrist for more detailed examination of near and far vision, eye structure and movement, and color discrimination.

Some of the common visual disorders in children are: 🔗 CD

- *Hyperopia* (farsightedness): Light rays focus posterior to the retina, resulting in an inability to focus on nearby objects. All children have some degree of hyperopia until 9 to 10 years of age. However, their eyes can accommodate sufficiently to enable them to see near objects clearly. Blurring of vision occurs only in children with excessive hyperopia, or a difference in accommodation between the two eyes. Amblyopia, or a weakening of the poorer eye, can occur in these children if treatment is not obtained.

- *Myopia* (nearsightedness): Light rays focus anterior to the retina, resulting in an inability to see far-off objects. Although children of any age can manifest myopia, it most commonly develops at about 8 years

---

TABLE 48–2   Assessment Questions for Identifying Visual Disturbances in Children

Young Child
Ask the parents:
Does your child follow you with his or her eyes as you come into a room?
Are other objects followed with ease?
Do both eyes work together or does one seem to wander off?
At what age did your baby sit, stand, walk?
Does your child have any difficulty picking up objects?

School-Age Child
Ask the parents:
Does your child like to look at pictures and read?
Does your child hold toys or books close, or sit very close to the television?
Does your child squint or rub the eyes?
Is he or she at grade level in all subjects?
Has your child demonstrated any learning difficulties?
Does he or she use a computer, watch television, or play computer games?
Does your child play sports and games at the same level of ability as peers?

---

of age. The child may complain of headaches and often squints to improve distance vision.

- *Astigmatism:* Light rays are refracted differently depending on their place of entry to the eye. The curvature of the cornea or lens is not uniformly spherical, causing blurred images. The child with astigmatism often holds pages very close to the face to obtain the best visual image. (DeRespinis, 2001)

For the description and management of four disorders that can significantly affect vision—strabismus, amblyopia, cataracts, and glaucoma—see "Clinical Manifestations: Visual Disorders".

CLINICAL MANIFESTATIONS 〰 *Visual Disorders*

ETIOLOGY	CLINICAL MANIFESTATIONS	CLINICAL THERAPY
Strabismus Can be congenital or acquired. Most common types: Esotropia: inward deviation of eyes ("crossed eyes") Exotropia: outward deviation of eyes ("wall-eyes")	Eyes appear misaligned to observer. May occur only when child is tired. Symptoms include: squinting and frowning when reading; closing one eye to see; having trouble picking up objects; dizziness and headache. Corneal light reflex and cover–uncover tests confirm diagnosis.	Occlusion therapy (patching the fixating or good eye to force use of the weak eye) Compensatory lenses Surgery of the rectus muscles to correct muscle imbalance. Eye drops to cause blurring of the good eye. Prisms Vision therapy (eye exercises) If treatment is begun before 24 months of age, amblyopia (reduced vision in one or both eyes) may be prevented.

Strabismus

Note: Reprinted from Paediatrics, 2e, Thomas & Harvey, p. 130, 1997, by permission of the publisher Churchill Livingtstone.

ETIOLOGY	CLINICAL MANIFESTATIONS	CLINICAL THERAPY
Amblyopia ("lazy eye") Reduced vision in one or both eyes Amblyopia can result from anything which causes visual deprivation to one eye. The most common causes are untreated strabismus, with the child "tuning out" the image in deviating eye, congenital cataract or visual differences between eyes.	Symptoms are the same as for strabismus. Vision testing can be used to diagnose condition.	Compensatory lenses Occlusion therapy Occasionally vision therapy (eye exercises) is used in an attempt to improve the weaker eye. Treatment is discontinued when visual acuity no longer improves; 20/20 acuity rarely attained. Treatment is most successful if done by 5–6 years of age.
Cataracts Occur when all or part of lens of eye becomes opaque, which prevents refraction of light rays onto retina Congenital cataract. From Vaughan, D., Asbury, T. & Riordan-Eva, P. (1992). *General ophthalmology* (13th ed., p. 172). New York: The McGraw-Hill Companies, Inc.	Can affect one or both eyes and may be congenital or acquired Clouding of lens indicates presence of cataract; however, cataracts are not always visible to naked eye. Symptoms include: distorted red reflex; symptoms of vision loss (see strabismus).	Specific treatment depends on whether one or both eyes are affected, extent of clouding, and presence of other ocular abnormalities. Surgical removal of lens and corrective lenses; contact lenses frequently used; results of surgery are good; surgery before the age of 2 months is associated with the best results; visual acuity in 55% of children is 20/40 or better. Lens implant may be used. Eye protectors and restraints are used postoperatively to prevent injury; antibiotic or steroid drops may be used for several weeks; treatment for amblyopia may be necessary.
Glaucoma Increased intraocular pressure damages eye and impairs visual function; ciliary body of eye produces aqueous fluid that flows between iris and lens into anterior chamber; if enough fluid accumulates, blindness results. May be congenital or acquired and affect one or both eyes Congenital glaucoma. From Vaughan, D., Asbury, T. & Riordan-Eva, P. (1992). *General ophthalmology* (13th ed., p. 172). New York: The McGraw-Hill Companies, Inc.	Symptoms of congenital glaucoma include: learning, corneal clouding, eyelid spasms, and progressive enlargement of eye; photophobia (extreme sensitivity to light). Symptoms of acquired glaucoma include: constant bumping into objects in child's periphery (painless visual field loss); seeing halos around objects. Diagnosis is made using tonometer, which measures intraocular pressure.	Surgery to reduce intraocular pressure is treatment of choice, since medications used to combat glaucoma in adults are not effective in children. Compensatory lenses used following surgery Treatment is not always successful, especially if the child has congenital glaucoma, so parents' feelings regarding care of a visually handicapped child should be explored.

Note: From Altemeier, 2000; Bacal & Wilson, 2000; Slaur, 2000.

Compensatory lenses are prescribed for most visual disorders. A significant difference in visual acuity between the eyes is often a result of amblyopia or strabismus, and further treatment may be needed. The visual acuity of a child with compensatory lenses should be reevaluated every 1 to 2 years. More frequent visits to an eye specialist are needed when a child is being treated for amblyopia or strabismus.

Color Blindness

Color blindness is an X-linked recessive disorder found in 8% of white and 4% of black males and almost never in females. The most common form affects the ability to distinguish between the colors red and green, but there are other variations. Preschool boys are tested for color blindness in some clinics to identify those with the disorder. Color blindness is not treatable and management focuses on issues of safety (e.g., problems in distinguishing between red and green traffic signals) and techniques to improve discrimination of colors in the affected color groups.

RETINOPATHY OF PREMATURITY

Retinopathy of prematurity (ROP) occurs when immature blood vessels in the retina constrict and become necrotic. This condition, which may occur in infants of low birth weight or of short gestation, can heal completely or lead to mild myopia or retinal detachment and blindness.

Etiology and Pathophysiology

Retinopathy of prematurity results from injury to the developing capillaries of the retina. Oxygen therapy is associated with the development of retinopathy of prematurity (Figure 48–3 ◆), but other factors such as respiratory dis-

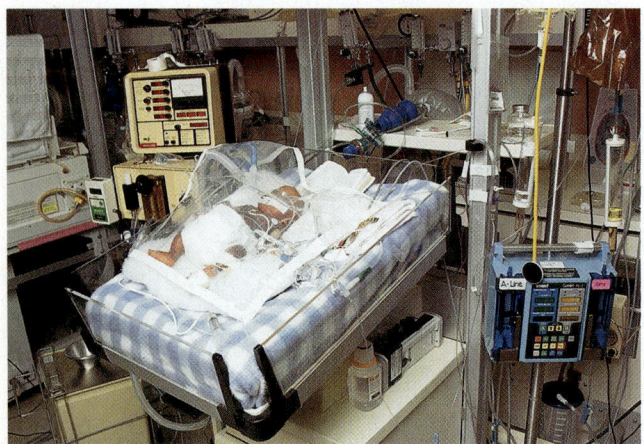

FIGURE 48–3. ◆ This premature infant in the neonatal intensive care unit is receiving artificial ventilation—a risk factor for retinopathy of prematurity. The infant will need careful management of oxygen exposure and periodic eye examinations.

tress, artificial ventilation, apnea, bradycardia, heart disease, multiple blood transfusions, infection, hypoxia, hypercarbia, acidosis, shock, and sepsis have also been linked with the disorder. It is most common in infants born before 28 weeks of gestation and weighing under 1600 g (3 lb, 8 oz) at birth.

The retina is normally vascularized by about 8 months' gestation. For the premature infant, however, this process must continue after birth and the environmental and other conditions listed in the preceding paragraph appear to affect its course. Arteriole constriction, followed by vascular proliferation of abnormal vessels, occurs. In most cases, the abnormal vessels gradually regress and normal vascularization occurs. Sometimes, however, the abnormal vascularization continues into the vitreous cavity, causing abnormalities of the retina, optic disc, and macula. It is not known why the disease progresses in some cases, but progression is directly linked to lower birth weight, greater prematurity, and duration (not necessarily concentration) of oxygen therapy. Raeanne, the child described in the scenario at the beginning of this chapter, developed retinopathy of prematurity after receiving oxygen therapy to aid her underdeveloped lungs.

Although the developing capillaries are lost, in up to 90% of cases there is some degree of revascularization later. The degree of visual loss, varying from slight to total, is determined by the degree of revascularization.

Clinical Manifestations

Retinopathy of prematurity is characterized by progressive changes in the retinal blood vessels, and in severe disease, by retinal detachment. Premature and low-birth-weight infants at risk for the disease are given frequent ocular examinations to ensure early detection of these changes. For infants who do not receive ophthalmologic examinations, resulting visual impairment may be detected only later in infancy when the child progresses slowly in meeting developmental milestones, fails to reach for objects, and does not follow objects or faces with the eyes. When visual impairment is present, the child usually manifests myopia. Total loss of vision can occur in the child who suffers a retinal detachment.

Clinical Therapy

Diagnosis is made by ophthalmologic examination. A classification system is used to describe the location, extent, and severity of the disease (American Academy of Pediatrics, 2001). All infants at risk, particularly those under 2000 g (4 lb, 3 oz) at birth or born before 33 weeks of gestation, are assessed frequently by an ophthalmologist experienced with the condition. The disease does not manifest itself before 4 to 6 weeks after birth, so it is important that the infant receive regular eye examinations until the risk is discounted. If the infant shows signs of disease, eye examinations continue every 1 to 2 weeks. Involvement of blood vessels in the periphery of the retina rarely leads to visual impairment. With involvement in other areas of the retina, visual problems are more common.

Treatment of infants with severe retinopathy of prematurity involves using cryotherapy or laser therapy to stop progression of the disease process. Other surgical procedures such as a scleral buckle procedure and vitrectomy have been used in retinal detachments. Prompt treatment of accompanying problems such as strabismus, amblyopia, and myopia can promote maximal development.

Nursing Management

Nursing Assessment and Diagnosis

Assessment of the infant at risk for retinopathy of prematurity begins at birth by identifying infants who may require oxygen therapy. Look for risk factors such as prematurity and low birth weight. Assess the infant's breathing efforts and report any changes. Be certain the ventilation equipment is properly set to deliver the correct amount of oxygen (see Skill 14-12). ⊂▭⊃ **SKILLS** Note the cumulative risks in a particular case and suggest the need for a referral to an ophthalmologist, as necessary.

"Nursing Care Plan: The Child with a Visual Impairment Secondary to Retinopathy of Prematurity" outlines several nursing diagnoses. Other nursing diagnoses may be appropriate for an infant with the potential to develop retinopathy of prematurity or a child with resulting visual impairment. They include:

▶ *Sensory/perceptual alteration (visual)* related to altered transmission of impulses

▶ *Impaired gas exchange* related to ventilation-perfusion imbalance

▶ *Alteration in growth and development* related to effects of visual impairment

▶ *Altered family processes* related to a child with a visual impairment

---

NURSING CARE PLAN ～ *The Child with a Visual Impairment Secondary to Retinopathy of Prematurity*			
GOAL	**INTERVENTION**	**RATIONALE**	**EXPECTED OUTCOME**
1. Sensory/perceptual alteration related to altered reception, transmission, and integration resulting from retinopathy of prematurity			
	NIC Priority Intervention: **Visual deficit enhancement:** *Assistance in accepting and learning alternate methods for living with diminished vision*		*NOC Suggested Outcome:* **Developmental progression:** *Compensate for sensory deficits by maximizing use of impaired senses*
The child will receive adequate sensory input	▶ Provide kinesthetic, tactile, and auditory stimulation during play and in daily care (e.g., talking and playing). Provide music while bathing an infant using bells and other noises on each side of infant. Verbally describe to a child all actions being carried out by adult.	▶ Because visual sensory input is not present, the child needs input from all other senses to compensate and provide adequate sensory stimulation.	The child demonstrates minimal signs of sensory deprivation.
2. Risk for injury related to impaired vision			
	NIC Priority Intervention: **Fall prevention:** *Instituting special precautions with patients at risk for injury*		*NOC Suggested Outcome:* **Risk control:** *Actions to eliminate or reduce modifiable health threats* The child will experience no injuries.
The child will be protected from safety hazards that can lead to injury.	▶ Evaluate environment for potential safety hazards based on age of child and degree of impairment. Be particularly alert to objects that give visual cues to their dangers (e.g., stoves, fireplaces, candles). Eliminate safety hazards and protect the child from exposure. Take the child on a tour of new rooms, explaining safety hazards (e.g., schools, hotel room, hospital room).	▶ The child may be at risk for injury related both to developmental stage and inability to visualize hazards.	

(continued)

GOAL	INTERVENTION	RATIONALE	EXPECTED OUTCOME
3. Risk for altered growth and development related to impaired vision			
	NIC Priority Intervention: **Developmental enhancement:** *Facilitating or teaching parents/caregivers to facilitate optimal growth and development of children*		*NOC Suggested Outcome:* **Child growth and development:** *Milestones of developmental progression*
The child has experiences necessary to faster normal growth and development.	▶ Help parents plan early, regular social activities with other children.	▶ The visually impaired child benefits developmentally from contact with other children.	The child demonstrates normal growth and development milestones.
	▶ Provide opportunities and encourage self-feeding activities.	▶ To obtain adequate nutrients, the child needs to feel comfortable feeding self.	
	▶ Provide an environment rich in sensory input.	▶ Sensory input is needed for normal development to occur.	
	▶ Assess growth and development during regular examinations to identify the child's strengths and needs.	▶ Regular examinations aid in early identification of growth problems or developmental delays, so that appropriate interventions can be planned.	
4. Risk for ineffective family coping related to child is prolonged disability from sensory impairment			
	NIC Priority Intervention: **Family mobilization:** *Utilization of family strengths to influence child's health positively*		*NOC Suggested Outcome:* **Positive coping:** *Extent to which family can mobilize resources to deal with the child's needs*
The family identifies methods for coping with their visually impaired child.	▶ Provide explanation of visual impairment as appropriate.	▶ The parents may feel guilt about the child's visual impairment, which can be allayed by knowledge of the cause.	The family successfully copes with the experience of having a visually impaired child.
	▶ Refer parents to organizations, early intervention programs, and other parents of visually impaired children.	▶ The parents will receive needed information and support from others.	
	▶ Assist parents to plan for meeting developmental, educational, and safety needs of their visually impaired child. Offer resources for changing home environment to assist visually impaired child.	▶ The child may require an enhanced environment in order to foster developmental progress.	

Planning and Implementation

The nurse plays an important role in preventing retinopathy of prematurity. Encourage early and regular prenatal care to prevent unnecessary premature births. Administer oxygen only to newborns who need it, and in the amount specified by the physician. Ensure that the proper ventilatory settings are used. Shield newborns from excessive exposure to light, since that may decrease susceptibility to retinopathy of prematurity. Be alert for infants with multiple risk factors and refer them, when appropriate, for ophthalmologic examination. Parents of infants at risk for retinopathy of prematurity require information about the disorder, as well as support, as the long-term effects on the child's vision are often identified only after subsequent examinations as the child grows.

The accompanying "Nursing Care Plan" summarizes care for the child with a visual impairment resulting from retinopathy of prematurity. The nurse is instrumental in case management for such children. Reinforce to parents the importance of follow-up eye examinations. Teach methods of stimulating development for the visually impaired child (refer to the next section).

Evaluation

Expected outcomes of nursing care for the child with retinopathy of prematurity include:

▶ Early identification of visual impairment

▶ Normal developmental milestone achievement

▶ Positive management of child's visual condition by the family

TABLE 48–3 Common Causes of Visual Impairment in Children	
Congenital or Hereditary	**Acquired**
Cataracts	Injury to eye or head
Glaucoma	Infections
Tay–Sachs disease	Rubella
Marfan syndrome	Measles
Down syndrome	Chickenpox
Fetal alcohol syndrome	Brain tumor
Prenatal infections (maternal infection)	Retinopathy of prematurity
Rubella	Cerebral palsy
Toxoplasmosis	
Herpes simplex	
Retinoblastoma	

TABLE 48–4 Signs of Visual Impairment	
Infants	**Toddlers and Older Children**
May be unable to follow lights or objects	May rub, shut, or cover eyes
Do not make eye contact	Tilt or thrust head forward
Have a dull, vacant stare	Blink frequently
Do not imitate facial expressions	Hold objects close
	Bump into objects
	Squint

VISUAL IMPAIRMENT

Visual impairment accounts for 11% of chronic medical conditions in children. Legal blindness (defined as visual acuity of 20/200 or worse in the corrected eye or significantly reduced visual fields) occurs in 1 per 35,000 children. About 1 in 500 children has partial vision. About half of the children who are blind or have partial vision have other disabilities as well. One in 25 preschoolers and 1 in 4 school-age children have a vision problem that requires corrections (Burns, Brady, Dunn, et al., 2000).

Many conditions discussed earlier in this chapter lead to temporary or permanent visual impairment. Infants who are premature; whose mothers were infected prenatally with rubella, toxoplasmosis, or other viruses; and who have certain congenital and hereditary conditions have a high risk of visual problems (Table 48–3). Fetal alcohol syndrome (FAS) is a major cause of visual disturbance; 90% of children with FAS have eye abnormalities.

Growth and Development

Infants with visual impairment use kinesthesia, touch, and language to socialize. They appreciate and use touch more than other children and respond to verbal explanations when others use nonverbal communication. Vision affects both fine and gross motor skills, so skills such as hand-to-mouth coordination and walking may be delayed in children who are visually impaired.

The signs of visual impairment depend on the cause and degree of the problem and the age of the child (Table 48–4). The child's eyes may appear crossed or watery, and the lids may be crusty. Verbal children may complain of itching, dizziness, headache, or blurred, double, or poor vision.

Clinical therapy depends on the child's condition and may include surgery, medication, and supportive aids. In the case of a disorder that results in permanent visual impairment, an interdisciplinary team of specialists works with the child and family. Nurses have an important role in this team to ensure developmental progression for the child and ongoing support for the family.

Nursing Management

Nursing Assessment and Diagnosis

Prevent visual deficits by teaching safety in activities that can injure the eye. For example, be sure that children are not allowed to play with laser pointers since young children are at great risk of retinal damage from these pointers due to a slower blink and gaze aversion response.

Vision screening facilitates early detection and treatment of conditions that can lead to vision loss. Visual testing can be done at any age, including immediately after birth. Developmental milestones that require vision, such as following bright lights, reaching for objects, or looking at pictures in a book, can be used to assess vision. For children over the age of 3 years, visual acuity is most frequently measured by means of an age-appropriate acuity test (see Skills 9-17–9-19). SKILLS CD Vision screening should begin at 3 years of age and take place during annual health care visits. Most states mandate school screening of vision. (See Chapter 33.) The photo screener, a device that can be used to take a photo of the child's eyes, is useful for infants, toddlers, and preschoolers. The photo can be used to diagnose refraction errors, eye opacities, and misalignment (Gomez & Davis, 2001). Visual fields and the ability to discriminate colors are tested at school age, when children can cooperate.

Children who are visually impaired may lag in development of cognitive and other skills. Sighted children learn the word *cup* using four senses—sight, touch, hearing, and taste—to obtain the information necessary to connect words with the objects they represent. In contrast, children with visual impairments rely on only three senses—touch, hearing, and taste. They learn concepts through differences in sounds, textures, and shapes.

Many visual disorders are linked with conditions that influence development. Thus, a child with cerebral palsy or fetal alcohol syndrome should be assessed frequently to identify a visual disorder, as well as to evaluate normal developmental milestones.

Nursing diagnoses for the child with impaired vision might include:

▶ *Sensory/perceptual alteration (visual)* related to altered sensory perception

▶ *Risk for injury* related to poor vision

▶ *Risk for altered growth and development* related to visual impairment

▶ *Risk for ineffective family coping* related to demands of a child with a sensory impairment

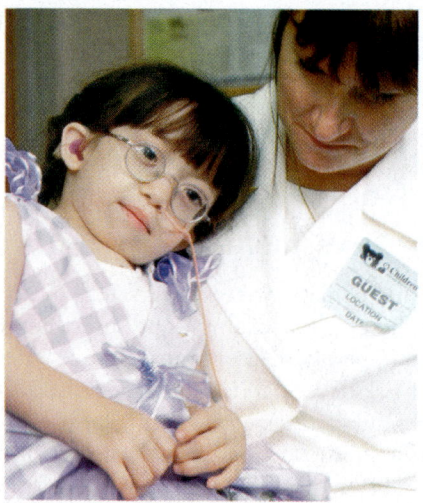

FIGURE 48–4. ◆ This child needs ongoing developmental assessment and a comprehensive individual education plan. As is true with many children, she has several health care needs. Note that she is receiving tube feedings.

ENHANCING DEVELOPMENT OF THE VISUALLY IMPAIRED CHILD

- Encourage a toddler or preschooler who is visually impaired to look at pictures in well-lit settings. Have a school-age child read large-print books. Computers designed for the visually impaired are also available. The Optacon (a device that raises print so it can be felt by the child) and View Scan (which magnifies print) improve reading ability.
- Expose the infant and child to everyday sounds.
- Encourage the infant to use the sense of touch to explore people and objects. Have the parents purchase toys with sound and texture in mind. Directional concepts can be taught using games. Responding to the infant's and child's vocalizations encourages the use of speech.
- Teach specific techniques for toileting, dressing, bathing, eating, and safety.
- When the child becomes mobile, furniture and other objects in the environment should be kept in the same positions so the child can safely move around independently. Extra care must be taken to prevent injuries when a child does not see.
- Emphasize the child's abilities. Adolescents can use seeing-eye dogs or a white cane to function independently.
- Encourage the child to function independently within normal developmental parameters.
- If the child goes to a hospital or another strange environment, orient the child to the placement of objects and do not rearrange them.
- Teach those around the child to:
  - Announce their presence to the child when approaching.
  - Walk slightly ahead of the child so he or she can sense their movements.
  - Let the child hold the seeing person's arm rather than the reverse.
  - Identify the contents of meals and encourage the child to feed self.

Planning and Implementation

Nursing care for a child with a visual impairment focuses on encouraging the child's use of all senses, promoting socialization, helping parents to meet the child's developmental and educational needs, and providing emotional support to parents. Refer the parents to an early intervention program as soon as the diagnosis is made. Nearly all care occurs in community and home settings.

ENCOURAGE USE OF ALL SENSES

Children who are partially sighted or blind use other senses to a great extent. Encouraging the use of the eyes as much as possible is important even if a child has poor vision (Figure 48–4 ◆).

PROMOTE SOCIALIZATION

The child's interactions and socializations should be as normal as possible (similar to those of sighted children of the same age and development).

▶ Stroke, rock, and hug infants and children who are visually impaired. Sing and talk to them. These infants do not make eye contact and have rather blank expressions.

▶ Call the child's name and speak before touching the child. Tell the child when the nurse and others are leaving the room. Describe locations of foods on the plate and tray to orient the child.

▶ Teach parents to read body language and vocalization as expressions of emotion. Facial expressions give a great deal of information, but infants and children with poor vision do not have the ability to learn by visual imitation. Show parents how to use tactile means to teach appropriate facial expressions. For example, a touch on the arm can be soft and stroking to indicate a smile, but firmer to indicate dismay or frown.

▶ Describe procedures such as blood pressure, ear examination, or cast application so the child knows what they will feel like. Let the child touch the equipment.

▶ Explain to parents that discipline and rewards for children with poor vision should be the same as those for other children in the family. The child should be given age-appropriate tasks.

▶ Encourage contact with peers as the child grows older. Teach the child to look directly at persons who are talking to him or her. Play, sports, and other activities can be modified to give the visually impaired child the same social experiences as a sighted child.

NURSING CARE IN THE COMMUNITY

Public laws require that each state provide educational and related services for children with disabilities (see Chapter 1). Parents and professionals should develop an individual education plan (as discussed in Chapter 35) that maximizes the child's learning ability. If possible, the child with a vision problem should attend child care and preschool with children who have normal visual acuity. What nursing actions are needed to help a child with a visual impairment adjust to child care or school?

▶ Provide parents with information about educational options before their child reaches school age. Education should take place in a setting that allows the child to have contact with other children and to participate in social activities.

▶ The child may be mainstreamed with a tutor, be partially mainstreamed in a resource room, attend special classes, or be tutored at home. If the child is to attend public school, suggest to parents that they contact the school well before enrollment to ensure that school personnel understand the child's disability.

▶ Make sure that equipment such as large-print books, braille materials, audio equipment, or an Optacon (described in "Teaching About" on page 1252) is available. Ensure that frequent eye examinations are performed and assist with proper use and care of prescribed glasses or contact lenses, as necessary. Clean glasses daily with warm water and dry with a clean, soft cloth. Follow family directions for cleaning contact lenses.

▶ Familiarize the child with the new environment.

PROVIDE EMOTIONAL SUPPORT

The family often needs help to understand the child's abilities and disabilities. Support them as they learn about their child's visual problems, tell friends and family, and then adjust to supporting the child.

▶ Encourage habilitation as soon as realistically possible. Make the adjustment easier by providing information about the child's specific type of visual impairment, available community services, and groups or associations for children with similar vision conditions. Suggest resources to families of children with visual disorders.

▶ Be supportive and listen to the family's concerns about the child's visual deficit.

▶ Make sure the parents meet their own physical and emotional needs so they are better able to care for and provide support to their child.

Growth and Development

Children with visual impairment may take longer to master self-help skills such as feeding and dressing.

Evaluation

Expected outcomes of nursing care for the child with a visual impairment include:

▶ Prevention of injury

▶ Growth and development to maximum potential

▶ Establishment of successful individualized education plan

INJURIES OF THE EYE

In the United States eye injuries are common in boys 11 to 15 years of age and in all children aged 9 to 11 years (Coody, Banks, Yetman, et al., 1997). Foreign bodies, blunt and sharp objects, chemical and thermal burns, physical irritants, and abuse may cause eye trauma. Recreational activities such as sports and projectile toys are common causes. Older children may be injured by chemicals in school science laboratories.

TABLE 48-5   Emergency Treatment of Eye Injuries

Injury	Treatment
Subconjunctival hemorrhage (caused by coughing, mild trauma, or increased physical activity)	Usually heals spontaneously; child should see ophthalmologist if most of sclera is covered or if condition does not clear up in 1–2 weeks
Periorbital ecchymosis ("black eye")	Apply ice to eye area (both eyes) for 5–15 minutes every hour for the first 1–2 days after injury (even if only one eye is affected, both eyes may discolor); then apply warm compresses
Foreign body on conjunctiva	Do not let child rub eye; remove material on surface of eye by closing upper lid over lower lid, irrigating or everting upper lid, visualizing material, and removing it with slightly damp handkerchief; patch eye and transport child to emergency department if foreign body cannot be removed
Corneal abrasion	Superficial corneal abrasions are diagnosed by touching sterile fluorescein strip to lower conjunctiva; dye remains where corneal epithelial cells are disrupted; most corneal abrasions heal spontaneously or antibiotic ointment may be prescribed and eyes patched in some children
Burns (alkaline burns readily penetrate cornea and are more serious than acid burns)	For child with chemical burn, irrigate eye for 15–30 minutes; transport child to emergency department, where irrigation should continue (see *Skills Manual*); pupils are dilated to reduce pain and prevent adhesions; after irrigation is complete, eyes are patched and antibiotics are prescribed
Penetrating & perforating injuries	Obtain medical assistance immediately; never try to remove an object that has penetrated the child's eye; such objects should be removed by an ophthalmologist; prevent the child from rubbing injured eye; cover both eyes with shield before transportation to emergency department
Eye injuries caused by severe blows to head and eye (blunt trauma can seriously injure all eye structures, including orbit, which can be fractured)	Transport immediately to ophthalmologist's office or emergency department for evaluation and treatment

Some injuries can be treated at home, but many require emergency care or hospitalization. If a tetanus booster has not been given in the last 5 years, the child is reimmunized. A careful history of the injury is taken, assessment of the eye is performed, and visual acuity is measured. Table 48–5 summarizes emergency treatment of common eye injuries. Nurses should teach children and parents methods to prevent eye injuries. Chemicals and objects such as scissors and knives should be placed out of reach. Protective eye wear is recommended, especially for children who participate in athletics and have poor vision or only one functional eye.

❧ DISORDERS OF THE EAR

OTITIS MEDIA

Otitis media, or inflammation of the middle ear, is sometimes accompanied by infection. 🔗 CD This condition is one of the most common childhood illnesses. Between 75% and 95% of all children have at least one episode by 6 years of age, with peak incidence at 2 years (Hoberman & Paradise, 2000). Otitis media occurs more frequently among boys and in children who attend child care centers. It is most common during winter.

Etiology and Pathophysiology

The specific cause of otitis media is unknown, but it appears to be related to eustachian tube dysfunction. Often an upper respiratory infection precedes otitis media. This infection causes the mucous membranes of the eustachian tube to become edematous. As a result, air that normally flows to the middle ear is blocked, and the air in the middle ear is reabsorbed into the bloodstream. Fluid is pulled from the mucosal lining into the former air space, providing a medium for the rapid growth of pathogens. The tympanic membrane and fluid behind it become infected. The most common causative organisms are *Streptococcus pneumoniae, Haemophilus influenzae,* and *Moraxella catarrhalis* (Dowell, Butler, Geibink, et al., 1999).

Growth and Development

Fluid accumulation in the middle ear prevents the efficient transmission of sound and can result in hearing loss over time, potentially delaying speech and language development. These delays may manifest as cognitive deficits or behavior problems. Motor development has been found to be impaired in children with chronic ear infections.

Conditions such as enlarged adenoids or edema from allergic rhinitis can also obstruct the eustachian tube and lead to otitis media. Since children with certain facial malformations (cleft palate) and genetic conditions (Down syndrome) usually have compromised eustachian tubes, these children are more vulnerable to otitis media. Children who live in crowded conditions, those exposed to cigarette smoke, and those who attend child care with multiple children are at higher risk. Breastfeeding protects against otitis media (Dowell et al., 2000)

Clinical Manifestations

Otitis media is categorized according to symptoms and the length of time the condition has been present. Pulling at the ear is a sign of ear pain (Figure 48–5 ◆). Diarrhea, vomiting, and fever are typical of otitis media. Irritability and "acting out" may be signs of a related hearing impairment. Some children with otitis media are asymptomatic; therefore, an ear examination should be performed at every health care visit (see Chapter 33). ⟮CD⟯ A red, bulging, nonmobile tympanic membrane is a sign of otitis media (Figure 48–6 ◆). If fluid lines and air bubbles are visible, the child has otitis media with effusion (Figure 48–7 ◆).

Bulging tympanic membrane

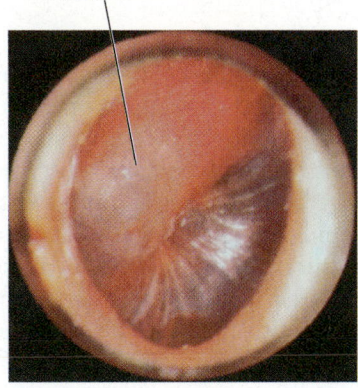

FIGURE 48–6. ◆ Acute otitis media is characterized by pain and a red, bulging, nonmobile tympanic membrane. Note: From Malasanos, L., Barkauskas, V., & Stoltenberg-Allen, K. (1990). *Health assessment* (4th ed., Plate 2). St. Louis, MO: Mosby-Year Book. Courtesy of Richard A. Buckingham, M. D., Clinical Professor, Otolaryngology, University of Illinois College of Medicine at Chicago.

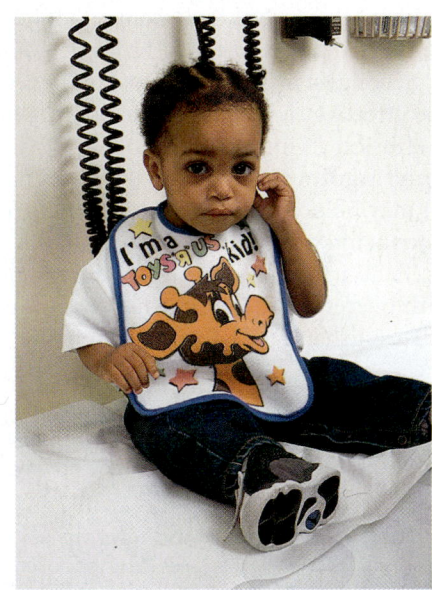

FIGURE 48–5. ◆ This young child is pulling at the ear and acting fussy, two important signs of otitis media. Ask the parents about presence of fever and night awakenings, additional signs that are often observed in children with this condition.

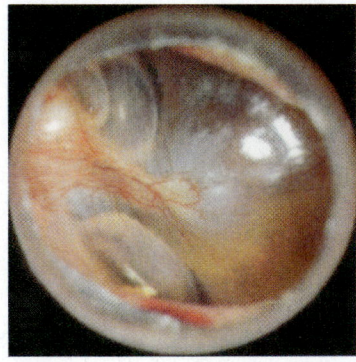

FIGURE 48–7. ◆ Otitis media with effusion is noted on otoscopy by fluid line or air bubbles. Note: From Malasanos, L., Barkauskas, V., & Stoltenberg-Allen, K. (1990). *Health assessment* (4th ed., Plate 2). St Louis, MO: Mosby-Year Book. Courtesy of Richard A. Buckingham, M. D., Clinical Professor, Otolaryngology, University of Illinois College of Medicine of Chicago.

CLINICAL MANIFESTATIONS ∼ *Otitis Media*

TYPE	DURATION	CLINICAL MANIFESTATIONS
Acute otitis media (AOM)	Rapid onset; 1–3 weeks duration	Tympanic membrane (TM) red, retracted or bulging, and painful; ear pulling; fever; hearing loss caused by presence of fluid; possible spontaneous TM rupture resulting in fluid drainage and reduction of pain
Recurrent otitis media (ROM)	Similar onset and duration to AOM, but repeated episodes in succession (three in 6 months or four in 12 months)	Similar to those of AOM
Otitis media with effusion (OME)	May precede or follow any stage of otitis media	Ear popping; feeling of pressure in middle ear; pain; hearing loss; TM retracted; fluid line or bubbles via otoscopy; symptoms of acute infection are absent
Chronic otitis media (COM)	Slow onset and persistence of 3 months of more	TM thick, immobile, retracted; if TM perforated, drainage from ear; tympanogram abnormal; hearing loss

Clinical Therapy

Diagnosis is based on otoscopic examination. Redness, inflammation, or bulging of the tympanic membrane is usually present. The trained clinician can perform pneumatic otoscopy in which positive air pressure in the external canal is used to measure the movement of the tympanic membrane. Special gradient acoustic reflectometry (SGAR) measures the condition of the middle ear by introducing a sound and measuring the tympanic membrane response (Hoberman & Paradise, 2000). A "flat" tympanogram is also suggestive of otitis media. (The tympanogram is described in the next section, on hearing impairment.)

Acute and recurrent otitis media have traditionally been treated with antibiotic therapy for 10 to 14 days. The choice of antibiotic depended on the probable organism, ease of administration, cost, previous effectiveness, and any history of allergies. First-line therapy is amoxicillin. Amoxicillin with clavulanate or cefuroxime axetil are second-line drugs, and ceftriaxone is used if other drugs are not successful (Dowell et al., 1999).

Concern has developed about the increasing appearance of drug-resistant microbials as causative agents in otitis media. These organisms may explain the increase in otitis media observed in the last decade (Carlson & Fall, 1998).

Since the specific pathogen is not usually known, wide-spectrum antibiotics are used and microbial overgrowth may result. To learn if antibiotic treatment was essential, use of medication has been delayed in some cases, and children improved without drugs. Many clinicians now believe that a more cautious approach is warranted, with treatment delayed for 3 days to see if the child improves, as long as the child does not appear extremely ill (Little, Gould, Williamson, et al., 2001). Dosing with medication when needed for 5 or 7 days, rather than the traditional 10 days, is also becoming more common. A one-dose injection is sometimes given rather than more extended therapy (Agency for Healthcare Research and Quality, 2001).

Chronic otitis media with effusion and recurrent otitis media may result in sensorineural or conductive hearing loss and cochlear damage, so treatment and follow-up with audiology are essential (Roddey & Hoover, 2000).

Neither decongestants nor antihistamines have been shown to be effective in the treatment of otitis media with or without effusion. If infection recurs inspite of antibiotic treatment, **myringotomy** (surgical incision of the tympanic membrane) may be performed and **tympanostomy tubes** (pressure equalizing tubes) inserted to drain fluid from the middle ear. Tube insertion is generally recommended for children with bilateral middle ear effusion and hearing deficiency of greater than 20 decibels (dB) for over 3 months.

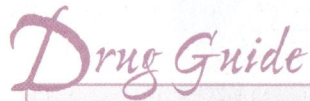

AMOXICILLIN

Overview of Action

Bactericidal action inhibits cell-wall synthesis, a broader spectrum of activities than penicillin G. Effective on some gram-positive and gram-negative organisms, such as *Haemophilus influenzae, Escherichia coli, Proteus mirabilis, Neisseria gonorrhoeae,* meningococci, enterococci, and *Salmonella.* Used to treat infections of the ear, upper respiratory tract, GU system, skin, and soft tissue and as a prophylaxis against bacterial endocarditis. Topical forms may be used for eye infections.

Routes, Dosage, Frequency
PO

- **Under 20 kg:** 20 to 40 mg/kg/day in equally divided doses every 6 to 12 hours
- **Over 20 kg:** 250 to 500 mg every 8 hours (maximum dose 2 to 3 g)

For prophylaxis against bacterial endocarditis in susceptible children who are undergoing procedures:

Child: 50 mg/kg given 1 hour prior to procedure and 25 mg/kg 6 hours later

Adolescents: 3 g 1 hour before procedure and 1.5 g 6 hours later

Nursing Implications

Assess: Assess previous allergy to this drug, penicillins, cephalosporins, other drugs, asthma, or family history of allergies. Obtain culture and sensitivity before treatment when ordered, but can start treatment before results.

Administer PO: Stable in gastric acid, give without regard to meals. Shake suspension well. Capsules may be taken apart or tablets crushed; mixed in small amount of food or fluid. Chewable tablets should be chewed thoroughly or crushed and followed with fluids.

Side Effects: Nausea, vomiting, diarrhea, pruritus, urticaria, anaphylaxis.

Monitor: Monitor child for hypersensitivity (especially within first 20 minutes following dose), rash (onset and characteristics), and side effects. Monitor blood counts, renal and hepatic function with prolonged or high-dose therapy or with premature infants and neonates. Maintain fluid intake. Watch for signs of superinfection; diarrhea (may indicate pseudomembranous colitis, which can occur while on drug or 4 to 6 weeks after drug is discontinued). If given for β-hemolytic streptococcal infection, 10-day course is needed to prevent risk of acute rheumatic fever or glomerulonephritis. If ampicillin rash occurs, it usually subsides in 6 to 14 days; however, rash can become severe, requiring drug discontinuance. Rash then usually resolves in 1 to 7 days.

Teaching: Child must take the medicine for the recommended time. If a revisit is scheduled, such as one for evaluation of treatment success in otitis media, parents are encouraged to keep this appointment. Report diarrhea, nausea, rash, or other side effects. Report if the child seems to have continued symptoms of infection (fever, irritability, pain, discharge from infected site, fatigue, or lethargy).

Note: From Bindler, R. M., & Howry, L. B. (1997). *Pediatric drugs and nursing implications* (2nd ed.). Upper Saddle River, NJ: Prentice Hall-Health. Adapted.

Enlarged and infected adenoids may be removed at the same time (Paradise, Feldman, Campbell, et al., 2001). Alternatively, a tympanostomy may be done to extract middle ear fluid for culture and sensitivity so that antimicrobial therapy can be directed at the cause of infection.

Nursing Management

Nursing Assessment and Diagnosis

Assess the tympanic membrane for color, transparency, mobility, presence of landmarks, and light reflex. Ask the parents whether the child has had a fever, been fussy, or been pulling at the ears. Observe for signs of impaired hearing.

Several nursing diagnoses that may apply are included in "Nursing Care Plan: The Child with Otitis Media." Additional nursing diagnoses might include:

▶ *Risk for altered body temperature: hyperthermia* related to infectious process
▶ *Fatigue (child and parent)* related to sleep deprivation
▶ *Sensory/perceptual alteration (auditory)* related to chronic ear infections and altered sensory reception

Planning and Implementation

Most children with otitis media are not hospitalized; therefore, nursing management centers on care of the child in the home. The child having tympanostomy tubes inserted is generally treated in a day surgery setting. Occasionally, children admitted to the hospital for other problems have a concurrent ear infection. The accompanying "Nursing Care Plan" summarizes nursing care for the child with otitis media.

Emphasize preventive measures. Exposure to second-hand smoke in the home increases the incidence of otitis media in children, so encourage parents who smoke to avoid smoking near the child or in the home. If young children are in child care with fewer than 10 children, incidence decreases. Breastfeeding provides some protection from the disease. Placing babies to sleep with a pacifier may increase incidence and should be avoided in the infant with prior infections (Niemela, Pihakari, Pokka, et al., 2000). Many cases of otitis media are related to microbials such as *Haemophilus influenzae* and *Pneumococcal pneumoniae*, so immunization against these pathogens (see Chapter 41) ⊂⊃ can be effective preventive measures.

NURSING CARE PLAN 〰 *The Child with Otitis Media*

GOAL	INTERVENTION	RATIONALE	EXPECTED OUTCOME
1. Pain related to inflammation and pressure on tympanic membrane			
	NIC Priority Intervention:		NOC Suggested Outcome:
	Pain management: *Alleviation or reduction in pain to a level of comfort acceptable to patient and family*		**Pain level:** *Amount of reported or demonstrated pain*
The child or parent will indicate absence of pain.	▶ Give analgesic such as acetaminophen. Use analgesic eardrops.	▶ Analgesics alter perception or response to pain.	Verbal child states that pain is relieved. Nonverbal child has improved disposition and comfort.
	▶ Have the child sit up, raise head on pillows, or lie on unaffected ear.	▶ Elevation decreases pressure from fluid.	
	▶ Apply heating pad or warm hot water bottle	▶ Heat increases blood supply and reduces discomfort.	
	▶ Have the child chew gum or blow on balloon to relieve pressure in ear.	▶ Attempts to open the eustachian tube may help aerate the middle ear.	
2. Infection related to presence of pathogens			
	NIC Priority Intervention:		NOC Suggested Outcome:
	Infection control: *Minimizing the acquisition and transmission of infectious agents*		**Risk control:** *Actions to eliminate or reduce health threats*
The child will be free of infection.	▶ Encourage breastfeeding of infants.	▶ Breastfeeding affords natural immunity to infectious agents.	The child's temperature is normal, symptoms have disappeared, and tympanic membrane shows no signs of infection.
	▶ Instruct the parents to administer antibiotics exactly as directed and to complete prescribed course of medication.	▶ Taking antibiotics as prescribed minimizes chance for overgrowth of pathogens.	
	▶ Telephone the parents 2 or 3 days after initial examination.	▶ If symptoms have not improved in 36 hours, treatment should be evaluated.	
	▶ Examine ear 3 or 4 days after completion of antibiotic treatment, or if symptoms worsen in child on symptomatic treatment.	▶ Checkup determines whether treatment is effective.	

(continued)

GOAL	INTERVENTION	RATIONALE	EXPECTED OUTCOME
3. Risk for caregiver role strain related to chronic disease			
	NIC Priority Intervention:		NOC Suggested Outcome:
	Caregiver support: *Provision of necessary support, information, and advocacy to facilitate care by parents*		**Caregiver performance:** *Provision by family care provider of health care for child*
The parents will manage the child's condition with minimal stress.	▶ Determine the parents' ability to manage condition. Provide frequent information and feedback.	▶ Many parents can treat children at home. Knowledge of condition allows parents to make informed decisions and to manage condition effectively.	The parents express confidence about treating the child and state that stress is reduced.
	▶ Encourage parental input in managing care.	▶ Active participation increases confidence and ability to manage condition.	
	▶ Listen carefully to parental expressions of frustration and fatigue and try to understand parents' feelings.	▶ Reacting empathically encourages parents to communicate.	
4. Knowledge deficit related to unfamiliarity with information of infection in children			
	NIC Priority Intervention:		NOC Suggested Outcome:
	Infection control: *Minimizing the acquisition and transmission of infectious agents*		**Knowledge:** *Extent of understanding conveyed about infectious disease prevention*
The parents will state understanding of preventive measures.	▶ Teach family members to cover mouths and noses when sneezing or coughing and to wash hands frequently. Have parents isolate sick children.	▶ Good hygiene prevents spread of pathogens.	Parents express understanding of measures to lead to fewer infections.
	▶ Encourage optimal nutrition, rest, and exercise.	▶ Physical well-being helps the body fight disease.	
	▶ Position bottle-fed infants upright when feeding. Do not prop bottles.	▶ Elevated position prevents injection of milk and pathogens into the eustachian tube.	
	▶ Eliminate allergens and upper respiratory irritants such as tobacco, smoke, and dust.	▶ Fewer irritants and allergens may decrease susceptibility to respiratory infections. Secondhand smoke contributes to higher incidence of otitis media.	
5. Risk for altered growth and development related to hearing loss			
	NIC Priority Intervention:		NOC Suggested Outcome:
	Developmental enhancement: *Facilitating optimal growth and development of the child*		**Growth and development:** *Milestones of developmental progression*
The child will have normal hearing.	▶ Assess hearing ability frequently.	▶ Monitoring detects hearing loss early.	The child's general health and hearing improve, and incidence of condition decreases.
The child will have normal motor and language development.	▶ Assess motor and language development at each health care visit.	▶ Early detection of developmental delays can lead to appropriate intervention.	The child has language and motor development within norms for age group.

Chronic otitis media can create many problems for the family. The child's waking at night with ear pain results in lack of sleep and parental fatigue. Parents often become frustrated and disillusioned by the health care system's inability to cure the child and may fear a permanent hearing impairment. Reassure parents that as the child grows older, the recurrent infections eventually cease. Teach them that asking for courses of antibiotics for every infection may not be the best treatment. Make sure parents of children with tympanostomy tubes know how to care for the child and what symptoms to report.

Evaluation

Expected outcomes of nursing care for the child with otitis media include:

▶ Return to normal sleep and feeding patterns

▶ Maintenance of normal hearing

▶ Effective pain and temperature management

▶ Understanding of treatment regimen by parents

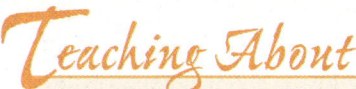

Teaching About

CARE OF THE CHILD WITH TYMPANOTOMY TUBES

After Surgery

Encourage the child to drink generous amounts of fluids.

Reestablish a regular diet as tolerated.

Give pain medication (acetaminophen) as ordered for discomfort and at bedtime.

Place drops in child's ears if instructed.

Restrict the child to quiet activities.

Following Postoperative Period

Follow the physician's instructions regarding swimming and water (some caution against swimming and other activities that might get water in ears; others do not).

Ear plugs can be used to prevent water from getting into ears.

Be alert for tubes becoming dislodged and falling out and alert physician (they usually fall out within 1 year).

Report purulent discharge from the ear, which may indicate a new ear infection. Contact the care provider.

Complementary Care

ACUPUNCTURE

Acupuncture is the complementary therapy most frequently recommended by physicians (Lee, Highfield, Berde, et al., 1999), and some physicians are educated in acupuncture treatment. Acupuncture is a treatment modality that is part of traditional Chinese medicine (TCM). It is based on the circulation of life-energy, or "chi." In acupuncture, sterile needles are inserted into specific points on the body in order to control the flow of chi, and to correct an imbalance that may be creating symptoms. Some practitioners will also use a variety of non-needle techniques to stimulate acupuncture points, such as magnets, massage, and electrical stimulation, among others (Lee et al., 1999). Conditions for which pediatric patients and their families frequently seek acupuncture treatment include otitis media, headaches, pain, and nausea.

Acupuncture is now provided as a treatment option in approximately one third of pediatric pain treatment programs at academic medical centers in North America (Kemper, 2001; Lee et al., 1999). Most families pay for acupuncture services out-of-pocket, but third-party payment is offered by some insurance carriers. Recent studies suggest that certain children readily accept acupuncture as a potential treatment option (Kemper, 2001; Kemper & Sarah, 2000).

HEARING IMPAIRMENT

Approximately 1 million children in the United States have some form of hearing impairment. Hearing impairment is expressed in terms of **decibels** (dB), which are units of loudness, and rated according to severity (Table 48–6).

TABLE 48-6	Severity of Hearing Loss
Type of Loss	**Hearing Ability**
Slight/mild	Some speech sounds are difficult to perceive, particularly unvoiced consonant sounds
Moderate	Most normal conversational speech sounds are missed
Severe	Speech sounds cannot be heard at a normal conversational level
Profound	No speech sounds can be heard; considered legally deaf
Deaf	No sound at all can be heard

Children who have only a mild hearing loss (35 to 40 dB) may miss 50% of everyday conversation and are considered at high risk for school failure. Children with a hearing loss of more than 90 dB are considered legally deaf. From 2 to 6 children per 1000 have a hearing loss (Bachman & Arvedson, 1998).

Etiology and Pathophysiology

About 50% of hearing loss is genetically caused, usually with a recessive inheritance pattern. Another 25% is due to environmental causes around the time of birth; the remainder is due to unknown causes. Infants and children at risk for hearing loss include those with a family history of hearing loss, recurrent otitis media, congenital perinatal infections such as rubella or herpes, anatomic malformations involving the head or neck, low birth weight (less than 1500 g [3 lb, 4 oz]), hyperbilirubinemia, bacterial meningitis, severe asphyxia at birth, and prolonged mechanical ventilation, and those who have received ototoxic medications (Bachman & Arvedson, 1998). Parents should be aware of excessive noise at home and at school. Teenagers who use earphones at high volumes or attend many rock concerts are at risk for hearing loss (Figure 48–8 ◆). Other noise hazards include firecrackers, guns, power tools, and farm equipment (Niskar, Kieszak, Holmes, et al., 2001).

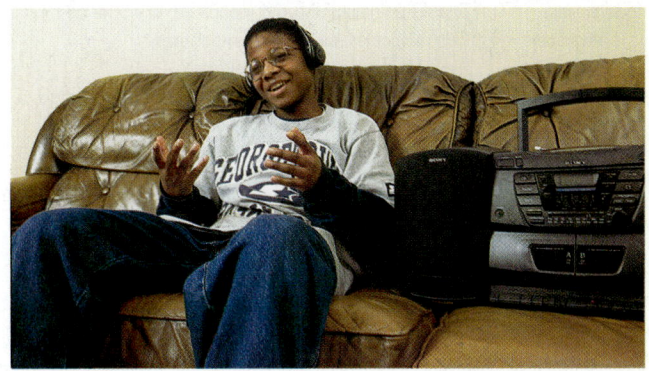

FIGURE 48–8. ◆ Listening to loud music with headphones or at rock concerts is a frequent cause of hearing loss among teenagers and young adults. This adolescent needs to be informed about the possible outcomes of this activity.

Clinical Manifestations

Hearing disorders can be classified according to the location of the deficit. **Conductive hearing loss** occurs when conditions in the external auditory canal or tympanic membrane prevent sound from reaching the middle ear. Common causes include impacted cerumen, the most frequent reason for conductive loss; outer ear infection ("swimmer's ear"); trauma; or a foreign body. Conductive loss also occurs if the tympanic membrane does not fully vibrate, as in otitis media. The loss of acuity may be gradual or rapid and results in diminished hearing in all ranges.

Sensorineural hearing loss occurs when the hair cells in the cochlea or along the auditory nerve (cranial nerve VIII) are damaged. This leads to permanent hearing loss. Conditions leading to this type of hearing loss may be congenital (maternal rubella), genetic (Tay–Sachs disease), or acquired (from ototoxic drugs or loud noise). In sensorineural hearing loss, high-frequency sounds are most affected.

A **mixed hearing loss** indicates a hearing loss having a combination of conductive and sensorineural causes.

Hearing is both an innate and a learned behavior. Infants and children who are hearing impaired exhibit a range of behaviors, depending on their age and the severity of the deficit. Infants who hear normally respond to sound in both obvious and subtle ways that do not occur in those who are hearing impaired (Table 48–7). As children mature, their hearing impairments affect their language skills. Hearing loss is often manifested as a cognitive deficit, a behavioral problem, or both.

TABLE 48–7	**Behaviors Suggestive of Hearing Impairment**
Age	Behavior
Infant	Has a diminished or absent startle reflex to loud sound
	Does not awaken when environment is very noisy
	Awakens only to touch
	Does not turn head to sound at 3–4 months
	Does not localize sound at 6–10 months
	Babbles little or not at all
Toddler and preschooler	Speaks unintelligibly, in a monotone, or not at all
	Communicates needs through gestures
	Appears developmentally delayed
	Appears emotionally immature, yells inappropriately
	Does not respond to doorbell or telephone
	Appears more interested in objects than people and prefers to play alone
	Focuses on facial expressions rather than verbal communications
School-age child and adolescent	Asks to have statements repeated
	Answers questions inappropriately, except when able to view speaker's face
	Daydreams and is inattentive
	Performs poorly at school or is truant
	Has speech abnormalities or speaks in a monotone
	Sits close to or turns television or radio up loudly
	Prefers to play alone

Clinical Therapy

Early identification of hearing loss is a key element in successful treatment. Detection of hearing loss in infants is important to ensure optimal development. Universal screening of all infants and children is recommended with rescreening and monitoring of those at risk (American Academy of Pediatrics, 1999; Hayes, 1999). Observations of response to noise in all newborns should be accompanied by more sophisticated testing such as auditory brainstem response or transient evoked otoacoustic emissions in those at high risk of deficits (White & Maxon, 1999).

Growth and Development

Infants and young children respond automatically with a blink or the startle reflex to unexpected or loud noises. As they mature, they localize the sound source, then understand speech, and then communicate verbally.

Nursing Practice

Although it is recommended that infants with significant hearing loss be identified by 3 months of age and receive treatment by 6 months, most children with hearing deficits are not identified until later in childhood. Early intervention is crucial for maximizing the child's ability to use any hearing present and to learn communication methods. Development is profoundly impacted by difficulty in communication. Nurses need to test all newborns and infants for signs of hearing disorders and refer as needed. Parents often are the first to notice a problem with hearing, so ask for their observations of the infant's hearing during each visit (Garganta & Seashore, 2000).

An otoscopic examination with a tympanogram can be performed on an older infant to determine conductive hearing loss. The **tympanogram** is a test that provides a graph of the ability of the middle ear to transmit sound. An airtight probe is inserted into the external ear canal and a tone is emitted. The probe measures the pressure, which is plotted on a graph. A "flat" tympanogram suggests conductive hearing loss. **Audiography** can be used with cooperative children over 3 years of age. Sounds of various frequencies and intensities are presented to the child through earphones, and the child is instructed to raise his or her hand when the sound is heard. Audiography cannot detect hearing loss caused by middle ear effusion but can indicate sensorineural loss.

The hearing of preschool and school-age children is tested by asking them to repeat whispered words. Hearing of school-age children and adolescents also is assessed with the Weber and Rinne tests (see Chapter 33).

If a hearing loss is uncorrectable, a multidisciplinary team composed of pediatrician, audiologist, otolaryngolo-

TABLE 48-8 Communication Techniques for Children Who Are Hearing Impaired

Technique	Description
Cued speech	Supplement to lipreading; eight hand shapes represent groups of consonant sounds and four positions about the face represent groups of vowel sounds; based on the sounds the letters make, not the letters themselves; child can "see-hear" every spoken syllable a hearing person hears
Oral approach	Uses only spoken language for face-to-face communication; avoids use of formal signs; uses hearing aids and residual hearing
Total communication	Uses speech and sign, fingerspelling, lipreading, and residual hearing simultaneously; child selects communication technique depending on the situation

Note: From Schwartz, S. (1996). *Choices in deafness: A parent's guide* (2nd ed.). Rockville, MD: Woodbine House. Reprinted with permission. For publications related to hearing-impaired children, contact Woodbine House. ⬭ **WEB**

gist, speech–language pathologist, nurse, teacher, and social worker should help the child and family adapt to the disability (Brookhouse, Beauchaine, & Osberger, 1999). If the deficit is due to recurrent ear infections, tympanostomy tube insertion may improve hearing.

A hearing aid may be prescribed for a conductive loss. A sensorineural loss is more difficult to treat, but cochlear implants and bone conduction hearing aids have been used in some children. Cochlear implants are increasingly being used in children and have restored hearing in some who are profoundly deaf (Cheng, Rubin, Powe, et al., 2000).

For children with uncorrectable hearing loss, several approaches are used to enhance communication (Table 48–8). Children with hearing impairment may receive speech therapy and instructions in lipreading, signing, cuing, and fingerspelling.

Nursing Management

Nursing Assessment and Diagnosis

Nurses conduct newborn hearing tests soon after birth and make observations of the infant's responses to sound. As the child grows, assess hearing at every well-child visit. The best judges of hearing are parents; ask them if they have any concerns about their child's hearing. An infant's reaction to rattles, bells, or handclapping (about 12 in [30 cm] from the ear) is an important observation. Evaluate language milestones when examining the older infant and child. Language development is a major area of focus in deaf children. Deaf infants begin to babble at about 5 to 6 months of age, the same age as hearing infants. However, this babbling ceases several months later in the hearing-impaired child.

School nurses use audiometers to evaluate hearing during screening programs in schools, and refer children who do not pass the screening test (see Skills 9-20 and 9-21). ⬭ **SKILLS**

Measures to promote speech and communication development as well as safety are implemented.

Common nursing diagnoses for the child with impaired hearing include:

▶ *Sensory/perceptual alteration (auditory)* related to altered sensory perception

▶ *Risk for impaired verbal communication* related to hearing loss

▶ *Risk for altered growth and development* related to communication impairment

▶ *Risk for ineffective family coping* related to caring for a child with a hearing impairment

Planning and Implementation

Nurses can encourage prevention of hearing loss from exposure to loud noises such as loud music and power and farm equipment. Music should be turned down and ear protection worn for other activities. Newborn screening, developmental assessment, and childhood hearing screening facilitate identification of hearing loss in infants and children. Infants should be tested for hearing loss by 3 months of age and in cases of loss, intervention should begin before 6 months of age (Joint Committee on Infant Hearing, 2000).

Nursing care of the child with a hearing impairment focuses on facilitating the child's ability to receive spoken language and to send information, helping parents meet the child's schooling needs, and providing emotional support to parents. Refer the parents to an early intervention program as soon as the diagnosis of hearing impairment is made, in order to foster the child's development. If a cochlear implant is planned, the child needs surgical care and follow-up to monitor results and integrate sound gradually into the child's life (Slattery & Fayad, 1999).

FACILITATE ABILITY TO RECEIVE SPOKEN LANGUAGE

Be aware of how the child compensates for hearing loss and use these strategies in communication.

▶ If hearing loss is mild or temporary or if the child reads lips, first obtain the child's visual attention by lightly touching the child or saying the child's name.

▶ Position your face 3 to 6 ft (1 to 2 m) from the child's face and make sure that the child's eyes are focused on your face and lips. Make sure the room is well lit, with no backlighting. Speak at a normal rate and tone, and use facial expressions that show caring or concern. If the child does not understand, rephrase the information in shorter, simpler sentences. Use specific, concrete explanations, and give the child time to comprehend. Watch for subtle signs of misinterpretations and give consistent and immediate feedback since only 30% of the English language is visible on the lips.

▶ Be familiar with the different types of hearing aids. Hearing aids, which are microphones that amplify all sounds, can be worn in or behind the ear, in the frame of glasses, or on the body with a wire attached to the ear. Place the hearing aid in the ear with the volume off, then slowly turn up to half volume. Adjust as needed. When talking to a child with a hearing aid, speak slowly within 6 to 18 inches (15 to 45 cm) from the microphone using a normal conversational tone. Talk to the child even if the child is not looking at you. Make sure the batteries are fresh for the best reception. Since all sound is amplified, reduce background noise as much as possible. Clean the hearing aid daily with a damp cloth. Change the batteries as needed, usually about once a week. The child's growth necessitates a new fitting, usually about once annually.

Acoustic feedback, an audible whistling sound that cannot always be heard by the child, is one of the most common problems with hearing aids. To eliminate this sound, readjust the hearing aid to make sure that it is inserted properly and that no hair or ear wax is caught between the ear mold and canal. Turning down the volume may also help.

A remote microphone system is another type of device designed to improve hearing. This is often used in the classroom situation because it eliminates background noise. The speaker wears a transmitter that picks up the voice and transmits it to a receiver worn by the child.

FACILITATE ABILITY TO SEND INFORMATION

Maintain the child's hearing aid in proper condition. Many children with impaired hearing communicate using speech, which is enhanced through speech therapy. In addition, they are taught to sign, fingerspell, or use cued speech (Figure 48–9 ◆). Articulation may be difficult, and understanding what the child is trying to say may be frustrating for both the nurse and the child. Taking time to listen carefully is important.

Take measures to promote speech and communication development as well as safety. Ask the parents to explain the child's communication techniques and to help interpret words. Have younger children point to pictures. Use assisted technologies such as a computer or picture board as well as drawings or gestures if necessary. This is especially helpful for communicating feelings of pain and hunger during hospitalization. If the child signs or fingerspells, make sure that you understand the signs for important functions. Give older children a pad of paper and pencil to write requests. People other than parents should be able to understand what the child is trying to communicate. Have an interpreter available if the child uses American Sign Language. Learn some common signs to communicate simple words or phrases. Orient the child carefully to new settings such as the hospital room or a new school.

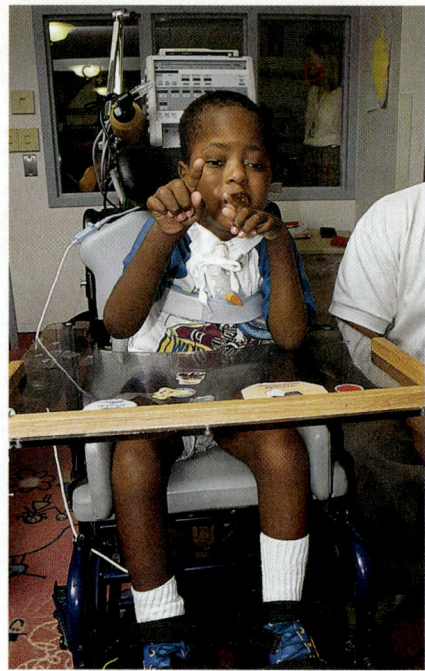

FIGURE 48–9. ◆ This child with a hearing impairment and tracheostomy is communicating by means of American Sign Language.

HELP PARENTS TO MEET CHILD'S EDUCATIONAL NEEDS

Public laws apply to the education of children who are hearing impaired (see Chapter 1). ⬯ After diagnosis, the parents and professionals together agree on an individual education plan (see discussion in Chapter 35). ⬯ Day care and preschool are recommended for children with hearing problems.

▶ Give parents information about adjustments that may have to be made for the hearing-impaired child who attends public school. By sitting at the front of the classroom, the child can hear and see more clearly. The teacher should always face the child when speaking, and background noise should be reduced.

▶ Tell parents that children who are hearing impaired have the same intelligence quotient (IQ) distribution as children without hearing impairment. However, communication and learning can be difficult, and extra support is needed.

▶ Children with hearing impairment should reach their intellectual potential, although development in certain areas may take place more slowly than it does in non-hearing-impaired children.

PROVIDE EMOTIONAL SUPPORT

By recognizing the effects of the diagnosis on the family, the nurse can help the family deal with their reaction to the child's hearing loss. Supporting healthy coping is an important intervention to help the parents carry on with their lives.

- Help the parents understand the child's disability and its effect on speech and language development. Provide accurate information about their concerns. Work jointly with other health care professionals and social service workers if necessary.
- Tell the family about the community services available for medical, nursing, psychologic, and financial assistance. ⬭ WEB

Evaluation

Expected outcomes of nursing care for a child with hearing impairment include:

- Successful establishment of communication method
- Growth and development to maximum potential
- Establishment of successful individualized education plan
- Positive family coping

INJURIES OF THE EAR

Ear injuries of many types commonly occur in children. Lacerations, infections, and hematomas may occur in the external ear structures, especially the pinna. Children may place foreign objects in the ear, and insects may enter the ear canal. Rupture of the tympanic membrane may result from head injuries, blows to the ear, or insertion of objects into the ear canal. Caution children and parents not to place anything into the ear, including cotton swabs for cleaning.

See Table 48–9 for information on the emergency treatment of ear injuries. Any injury resulting in earache, decreased hearing, persistent bleeding, or other discharge should be seen by a physician.

➤ DISORDERS OF THE NOSE, THROAT, AND MOUTH

EPISTAXIS

Epistaxis, or nosebleed, is common in school-age children, especially boys. Kiesselbach's plexus, an area of plentiful veins located in the anterior nares, is the most common source of bleeding. The most common cause is irritation from nosepicking, foreign bodies, or low humidity. Other causes include forceful coughing, allergies, or infections resulting in congestion of the nasal mucosa. Bleeding from the posterior septum is more serious and may be life threatening. Hospitalization may be necessary. Posterior nosebleeds have a variety of causes, some of which may indicate systemic disease (i.e., bleeding disorder) or injury.

Children with nosebleeds are sometimes brought to the emergency department by a parent who has been unable to stop the flow of blood within a few minutes. Both parent and child may be frightened. Ask the parent briefly about any history of nosebleeds and other contributing factors, including medications. Take the child's pulse and blood pressure to assess for excessive blood loss. Carefully examine the nasal mucosa by asking the child to blow any clots out gently, if possible. Suctioning may be necessary.

Observing the flow may help determine whether the blood is coming from an anterior or a posterior location. A nosebleed confined to one side of the nose is almost always anterior, but posterior bleeding can flow on one or both sides. If blood cannot be seen, the child may be swallowing it and may become nauseated. Suspect posterior bleeding in children who have sustained blunt trauma or in other children at high risk.

TABLE 48-9	Emergency Treatment of Ear Injuries
Injury	Treatment
Pinna	
Minor cuts or abrasions	Wash thoroughly with soap and water and rinse well; leave exposed to air if possible or apply adhesive bandage; monitor for infection.
Hematomas	Needle aspiration should be performed and pressure dressing applied; undrained hematomas may become fibrotic; "cauliflower ear" deformity may develop.
Cellulitis or abscesses	Apply moist heat intermittently; make sure that prescribed antibiotic is taken; minor surgery may be performed for an abscess.
Deep lacerations	Apply pressure to stop bleeding; transport to physician's office or emergency department for suturing.
Ear Canal	
Foreign bodies	Have child lie on back and turn head over edge of bed, with affected side down; wiggle earlobe and have child shake head; foreign object may fall out as result of gravity; if object remains in ear, call physician; do not try to remove foreign body with tweezers since this may push the object further into the ear.
Insects	Shine flashlights into ear to try to attract insect; instilling a few drops of mineral oil, olive oil, or alcohol kills insect, and irrigating ear canal gently may remove dead insect. See Skill 11-8. ⬭ SKILLS
Tympanic Membrane	
Ruptures	Call physician if child has persistent ear pain after blow, blast injury, or insertion of foreign object; cover external ear loosely with piece of sterile cotton or gauze; if tympanic membrane has been ruptured, systemic antibiotics are prescribed.

The child with anterior bleeding should sit upright quietly. The head should be tilted forward to prevent blood from trickling down the throat, which can lead to vomiting. The nares should be squeezed just below the nasal bone and held for 10 to 15 minutes while the child breathes through the mouth. If the bleeding does not stop, a cotton ball or swab soaked with Neo-Synephrine, epinephrine, thrombin, or lidocaine may be inserted into the affected nostril to promote topical vasoconstriction or anesthesia. Once the bleeding has stopped, the nostril may have to be cauterized with silver nitrate or electrocautery. If the bleeding cannot be stopped, absorbable packing may be used.

Posterior bleeding must also be stopped by packing, and the child must be monitored carefully. Arterial ligation is occasionally needed. Repeated or severe nosebleeds need further evaluation (Newland & Rich, 1998).

Nursing Management

Assess the child's hematocrit or hemoglobin if significant bleeding has occurred. Take a complete history and do a physical examination of children with frequent epistaxis to rule out systemic disease.

Teaching About

PREVENTION AND HOME MANAGEMENT OF EPISTAXIS

Prevention
- Humidify the child's room, especially during the winter.
- Discourage the child from picking or rubbing the nose or inserting foreign objects in the nose.
- Instruct the child to blow the nose gently and release sneezes through the mouth.

Home Management
- Keep the child calm.
- Sit the child upright with head tilted slightly forward so blood does not run down the throat.
- Press a roll of cotton under the upper lip to compress the labial artery.
- Apply steady pressure to both nostrils just below the nasal bone with the thumb and forefinger for 15 to 20 minutes. Time by the clock.
- Apply an ice pack or cold compress to the bridge of the nose or the back of the neck.
- Call health care provider if the bleeding does not stop.
- Avoid further bleeds by sleeping with the head elevated on pillows, avoiding hot showers and drinks, and avoiding aspirin or other noncoagulant drugs during the first few days after a nosebleed.

Note: From Newland, J. A., & Rich, E. (1998). Epistaxis. *American Journal of Nursing, 98*, 16HHH. Adapted.

After the nosebleed has stopped, the child is more vulnerable to recurrent bleeding and should avoid bending over, stooping, strenuous exercise, hot drinks, and hot baths or showers for the next 3 to 4 days. Sleeping with the head elevated on two or three pillows and humidifying the air with a vaporizer may also prevent a recurrence. Give parents suggestions for prevention and home management of epistaxis.

NASOPHARYNGITIS

Nasopharyngitis, also known as the "common cold," causes inflammation and infection of the nose and throat and is probably the most common illness of infancy and childhood. More than 200 viruses and numerous bacteria can cause this condition. The most common viruses include rhinovirus and coronavirus, and the most frequently occurring bacterium is group A *Streptococcus*. The organisms incubate in 1 to 3 days, and the infection is communicable several hours before symptoms develop and for 1 to 2 days after they begin. Symptoms may last 4 to 10 days or longer. The pathogens are believed to spread when the infected person touches the hand of an uninfected person, who then touches his or her mouth or nose, resulting in self-inoculation.

A red nasal mucosa with clear nasal discharge and an infected throat with enlarged tonsils may be apparent in children with nasopharyngitis. Vesicles may be present on the soft palate and in the pharynx. Accompanying symptoms may vary, depending on the child's age (Table 48–10).

Between episodes of nasopharyngitis, the child should be asymptomatic. If a child continues to have upper respiratory infections, an underlying condition such as allergy, asthma, or polyps should be ruled out.

TABLE 48–10	Nasopharyngitis
Infants Younger Than 3 Months of Age	
Lethargy	Feeding poorly
Irritability	Fever (may be absent)
Infants 3 Months of Age or Older	
Fever	Anorexia
Vomiting	Irritability
Diarrhea	Restlessness
Sneezing	
Older Children	
Dry, irritated nose and throat	
Chills, fever	
Generalized muscle aches	
Headache	
Malaise	
Anorexia	
Thin nasal discharge, which may later become thick and purulent	
Possible sneezing	

Nursing Management

For infants who cannot breathe through the mouth, normal saline nose drops can be administered every 3 to 4 hours, especially before feeding (see Skill 11-9). ⊂⊃ **SKILLS** For infants over 9 months of age, nasal stuffiness can be treated with either normal saline nose drops or a decongestant such as phenylephrine (0.125% to 0.25%, depending on the child's age). Older children can use nasal sprays.

Although nose drops and sprays are more effective than systemic decongestants, they should not be used for more than 4 or 5 days or more often than recommended. Antihistamines may be helpful for children with allergic rhinitis or profuse nasal drainage. Long-acting nasal sprays and medications with several ingredients are not recommended.

Room humidification may help prevent drying of nasal secretions. Antipyretics such as acetaminophen reduce fever and make the child more comfortable. Aspirin is not recommended because of its association with Reye syndrome (refer to Chapter 49). ⊂⊃

Children should avoid strenuous physical activity and engage in quiet play such as reading, listening to music or stories, or watching television or videotapes. Children should not be forced to eat. Encourage the intake of favorite fluids to liquify secretions. Tell parents that no medicine or vaccine can prevent the common cold, but eliminating contact with infected persons can reduce the spread of infection. Proper handwashing and disposal of tissues helps to decrease the spread of the infection.

Developing Cultural Competence

Many Hispanic and Asian cultural groups believe in the "hot and cold theory" of disease, in which health problems are viewed as the result of imbalance. For example, Mexican Americans traditionally treat a "cold disease" such as an earache or common cold with "hot" substances. Ask families if they prefer to eat certain foods during an illness. Incorporating such preferences can help the child to get better and increase the confidence of the family in health care providers.

SINUSITIS

Sinusitis is an inflammation of one or more of the paranasal sinuses. These sinuses, which have respiratory epithelium and are continuous with the respiratory tract, include the maxillary, ethmoid, frontal, and sphenoid sinuses. The sinuses may become infected with bacteria following a viral upper respiratory infection. In most cases, the child's history reveals a cold for several days, followed by improvement in the cold symptoms but an increase in purulent nasal drainage. There is accompanying facial pain, headache, and fever. Chronic sinusitis may occur in children with uncontrolled allergies and asthma.

Although most physicians treat suspected sinusitis with antibiotics, many cases clear spontaneously without treatment. Amoxicillin is the first choice for therapy; amoxicillin/clavulanate and cephalosporins are also sometimes used (Sinus and Allergy Health Partnership, 2000; Batieha, Kakish, Mahafza, et al., 2000).

Tell parents whose child has persistent and purulent nasal drainage to have the child seen by a health care provider, particularly if the drainage is accompanied by facial pain, headache, and fever. Teach parents the correct administration of antibiotics (i.e., to take for the full course) if prescribed, and the use of saline nose drops if needed for comfort. Infants may need to have the nose cleared with nose drops and a bulb syringe prior to feedings (see Skill 14-15). ⊂⊃ **SKILLS** Antipyretics can be given for fever and to relieve pain.

PHARYNGITIS

Acute pharyngitis is an infection that primarily affects the pharynx, including the tonsils (Figure 48–10 ◆). It is seen most frequently in children 4 to 7 years of age and is rare in children less than 1 year of age. Approximately 80% of these infections are caused by viruses; the rest are caused by bacteria. Bacterial pharyngitis is commonly known as "strep throat," since it is most often caused by group A beta-hemolytic streptococcus (GABHS). Viral pharyngitis is caused by a large number of enteroviruses.

The major complaint is a sore throat. See "Clinical Manifestations of Viral Pharyngitis and Strep Throat." Children with symptoms of strep throat who have minimal throat redness and pain, exudate, mild lymphadenopathy, and a low-grade fever, and who have been exposed to someone who has pharyngitis should have a throat culture. The classic signs of purulent drainage and white patches are not present in all cases of strep throat. A child who finds swallowing difficult or extremely painful, who drools, or who exhibits signs of dehydration or respiratory distress should be seen by a physician immediately. These signs

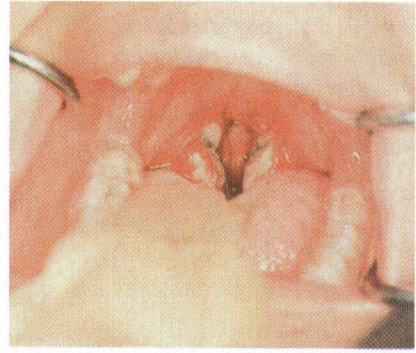

FIGURE 48–10. ◆ Acute pharyngitis primarily affects the pharynx but often involves the tonsils, as in this child. Note: From Malasanos, L., Barkauskas, V., & Stoltenberg-Allen, K. (1990). *Health assessment* (4th ed., Plate 2). St. Louis, MO: Mosby-Year Book. Courtesy of Edward L. Applebaum, M. D., Chicago, IL.

VIRAL PHARYNGITIS	STREP THROAT
Nasal congestion	Tonsillar exudate[b]
Mild sore throat	Painful cervical lymphadenopathy[b]
Conjunctivitis	Abdominal pain
Cough	Vomiting
Hoarseness	Severe sore throat
Mild pharyngeal redness	Headache
Minimal tonsillar exudate	Fever >38.3 °C (101 °F)
Mildly tender anterior cervical lymphadenopathy	Petechial mottling of soft palate
Fever <38.3 °C (101 °F)	

a = Children 6 months to 3 years of age may have streptococcus with symptoms that resemble those of viral pharyngitis. Children with scarlet fever have the symptoms of strep throat plus a sandpaper-textured erythematous generalized rash and pallor of the lips.

b = Classic signs of strep throat

could be indicators of serious conditions such as epiglottitis, peritonsillar or retropharyngeal abscess, or diphtheria.

The diagnosis of strep throat is made by throat culture, using the rapid or traditional strep tests (see Skill 10-12). 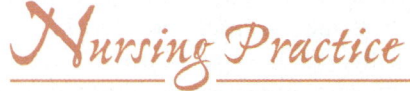 SKILLS CD Results of the rapid strep test may be available within minutes; those for the traditional test are available in 24 to 48 hours. Early signs of strep throat should be treated with oral penicillin for 10 days or by long-acting penicillin given in one injection immediately, even before the result of the culture is available. If the child is allergic to penicillin, erythromycin is given. Acute symptoms should resolve within 24 hours of therapy, at which time the child is no longer contagious. For viral pharyngitis, symptomatic treatment alone is used.

Nursing Practice

Throat cultures must be properly performed for accurate diagnosis. Swab a sterile cotton-tip applicator across the tonsils, posterior edge of the soft palate, and uvula. Ask cooperative children to put their hands under their buttocks, open their mouth, and laugh or pant like a dog. Quickly swab the throat. You can place uncooperative and young children on their backs with their hands next to their heads and have a parent or an assistant hold them. Depress the tongue gently with a tongue blade and swab the throat.

Nursing Management

Nursing care focuses on symptomatic relief. Acetaminophen reduces throat pain and generalized fever. Cool, nonacidic fluids and soft foods, ice chips, or frozen juice pops given frequently in small amounts facilitate swallowing and prevent dehydration. Humidification, chewing gum, and gargling with warm salt water (1 teaspoon [5 g]

salt to 8 oz [250 mL] water) soothe an irritated throat. Alternatively, the salt water can be placed in a spray bottle and sprayed gently toward the throat. Commercial throat sprays or throat lozenges are not generally more effective than these home remedies. Encourage the child to rest, to conserve energy and promote recovery.

Teach parents the importance of completing the 10–day course of antibiotics if prescribed for bacterial pharyngitis. Reinforce to parents the importance of treating streptococcal infections, as untreated infections may lead to rheumatic fever, cervical adenitis, sinusitis, glomerulonephritis, or meningitis.

TONSILLITIS

Tonsillitis is an infection or inflammation (hypertrophy) of the palatine tonsils. Although most children with pharyngitis may have infected tonsils, they do not necessarily have tonsillitis.

Etiology and Pathophysiology

Like pharyngitis, tonsillitis may be caused by a virus or bacterium. The primary site of infection is the tonsils.

Clinical Manifestations

Symptoms suggestive of tonsillitis include frequent throat infections with breathing and swallowing difficulties; persistent redness of the anterior pillars; and enlargement of the cervical lymph nodes. If children breathe through their mouths continuously, the mucous membranes may become dry and irritated.

Clinical Therapy

Diagnosis is made on the basis of visual inspection and clinical manifestations. Symptomatic treatment for tonsillitis is the same as for pharyngitis. Surgical removal of tonsils (tonsillectomy) is often recommended when children have recurrent throat infections (about three per year for 3 years), chronic tonsillitis, obstructive sleep apnea, or malformations causing nasal speech or a facial growth abnormality. If the child is under 3 years of age, the surgery is postponed if possible because it may stimulate growth of other lymphoid tissue in the nasopharynx. If the pharyngeal tonsils (adenoids) are enlarged, as suggested by mouth breathing, cough, impaired taste and smell, a muffled quality to the voice, and chronic otitis media, they may be removed at the same time.

Nursing Management

Nursing Assessment and Diagnosis

Assess the throat carefully during each physical examination. Observe for tonsils that are simply large (a common finding in childhood) and those that are inflamed. Look for the degree of redness and presence of any exudate. Ask if the child has pain or difficulty swallowing. Ask about the history of past tonsillar infections and the length of time of the present discomfort.

If surgery is indicated, take a complete history of the child preoperatively. Monitor vital signs and observe for respiratory distress, hemorrhage, and dehydration postoperatively.

Several nursing diagnoses may apply to the child with tonsillitis. They include:

▶ *Pain* related to inflammation of the pharynx

▶ *Risk for fluid volume deficit* related to inadequate intake

▶ *Risk for ineffective breathing pattern* related to obstruction by enlarged tonsils

▶ *Impaired swallowing* related to inflammation and pain

▶ *Health-seeking behaviors (parents)* related to home care following discharge

Planning and Implementation

The nurse provides general supportive care and, if medication is prescribed, encourages completion of the full course of treatment. The nursing management of children with tonsillitis is similar to that of children with pharyngitis (see earlier discussion).

If surgery is indicated, help the parents prepare their child for a short-term surgical procedure with a possible overnight stay in the hospital (see Chapter 34). Children should be free of sore throat, fever, or upper respiratory infection for at least 1 week before surgery. They should not be given aspirin or ibuprofen for 2 weeks before surgery, since these medications can increase bleeding. Check if any herbal medications are taken and report them to the physician and anesthesiologist since some may interfere with anesthetic drugs used in surgery.

DISCHARGE PLANNING AND HOME CARE TEACHING

Discharge planning includes teaching parents about pain management, fluid and nutrition intake, activity restrictions, and possible complications in the postoperative period. Most children have a sore throat for 7 to 10 days after tonsillectomy. Advise parents how to relieve the child's throat pain.

Children may experience ear pain, especially when swallowing, between 4 and 8 days after tonsillectomy. Advise parents that this pain is referred from the tonsillar area and does not indicate an ear infection.

Emphasize to parents the importance of adequate fluid intake. Children should be given any liquid they prefer for the first week, except citrus juices, which may produce a burning sensation in the throat. Soft foods such as gelatin, applesauce, frozen juice pops, and mashed potatoes can be added as tolerated.

Teaching About

CARE AFTER TONSILLECTOMY

After tonsillectomy the parent can take measures to increase the child's comfort.

- Have the child drink adequate cool fluids or chew gum, as this reduces spasms in the muscles surrounding the throat.
- Give acetaminophen elixir, as ordered.
- Apply an ice collar around the child's neck.
- Have the child gargle with a solution of 1/2 teaspoon (2.5 g) each of baking soda and salt in a glass of water.
- Have the child rinse the mouth well with viscous lidocaine and then swallow the solution.

Teaching About

COMPLICATIONS OF TONSILLECTOMY AND ADENOIDECTOMY

Bleeding

- To prevent bleeding, aspirin or ibuprofen should not be given for pain for the first postoperative week. Use acetaminophen instead.
- Bleeding is most likely to occur within the first 24 hours or 7 to 10 days after the tonsillectomy, when the scar is forming. Report any trickle of bright red blood to the physician immediately.

Infection

- The back of the throat will look white and have an odor for the first 7 to 8 days after the surgery. The child may also have a low-grade fever. These are not signs of infection.
- For temperatures over 38.3 °C (101 °F), acetaminophen may be used.
- Call the physician if the child develops a fever above 38.8 °C (102 °F).

Pain

- Administer acetaminophen as ordered.
- Offer frequent small amounts of cool liquids. Avoid citrus juice.
- Provide for rest and quiet activities for several days.

Children do not need to be confined to bed, but they should avoid vigorous exercise for the first week after surgery. Advise parents that the child may return to school approximately 10 days after tonsillectomy.

Any surgery carries the risk of postoperative complications. Teach parents the normal signs of healing in the postoperative period, as well as signs of complications. See "Clinical Pathway: Tonsillectomy and Adenoidectomy."

Category	Immediate Perioperative Period	Discharge to Home Care
Daily outcomes	Parent/client verbalizes understanding of preoperative teaching including IV fluids, antiemetics, ice pack to neck, activity, and pain management Parent/client displays effective coping Validate informed consent	Client has a patent airway and has minimal drainage in the throat Client has stable vital signs and is alert and responsive Client remains free of signs/symptoms of hemorrhage and hemoglobin and hematocrit remains within normal limits Client manages pain with ordered medications Parent/client verbalizes/demonstrates home care instructions Client tolerates liquids without complaints of severe pain or vomiting
Assessments, tests and treatments	*Preoperative:* CBC Urinalysis PTT Baseline physical assessment with a focus on respiratory status Anesthesia consult Assess cognitive/developmental level *Postoperative:* Position on side until fully awake; then Fowler's position Level of consciousness Vital signs and O_2 saturation, neurovascular assessment, and bleeding assessment q15min × 4; q30min × 4; q1hr × 4 and then q4hr and prn Assess lung sounds q1–2hr and prn Discourage coughing or clearing of throat Monitor for frequent swallowing Ice pack to neck Monitor intake and output; encourage voiding prior to discharge Offer/administer analgesics on schedule as ordered Assess pain and effectiveness of pain medications	Perform complete discharge assessment
Knowledge deficit	Orient to room and surroundings Include family in teaching Provide simple, brief instructions Review preoperative preparation, Including hospital and surgical routines Emphasize probability of the presence of old blood in the nose, between the teeth, and in emesis Reinforce preoperative teaching Evaluate understanding of teaching Provide information at developmental/cognitive level	Review plan of care as well as diet and activity restrictions Complete discharge teaching regarding postoperative assessments, follow-up care, signs and symptoms to report, medications, and diet Explain to client to avoid coughing or clearing throat and to avoid gargling Review the importance of reporting any signs or symptoms of bleeding during the postoperative period up to 10 days following surgery Evaluate understanding of teaching
Psychosocial	Assess anxiety related to pending surgery Assess fears of the unknown related to surgery Encourage verbalization of concerns Provide emotional support to client and family Minimize external stimuli (e.g., noise, movement) Reassure child that he/she will be able to talk	Assess level of anxiety Encourage verbalization of concerns Provide emotional support to client and family Provide information and encouragement to client and family
Diet	*Preoperative:* NPO Baseline nutritional assessment *Postoperative:* Advance to clear liquid to full liquid following surgery; offer cool fluids Encourage large sips of fluids No straws No citrus juices	Advance to regular diet as tolerated

Note: From Beyea, S. C. (1996). Critical pathways for collaborative nursing care. Upper Saddle River: Prentice Hall-Health. Modified.

Category	Immediate Perioperative Period	Discharge to Home Care
Activity	As desired until premedicated for surgery In bed with rails up once premediated Progress from bed rest to dangling on side of bed to walking postoperatively as tolerated	Provide safety precautions Encourage bed rest for first 24 hours, then advance as tolerated to normal activity
Medications	Preoperative mediations, postoperative analgesics, and antibiotics as ordered	Analgesics as ordered Antibiotics if ordered NO ASPIRIN
Transfer/discharge plans	Assess discharge plans and support system	Probable discharge within 6 hours of surgery Complete discharge home care teaching when fully awake and oriented and before discharge Provide a written copy of discharge instructions Provide telephone number of other resource for questions

Note: From Beyea, S.C. (1996). Critical pathways for collaborative nursing care. Upper Saddle River: Printice Hall-Health. Modified.

Evaluation

Expected outcomes of nursing care for the child with tonsillitis include:

▶ Adequate intake of food and fluids

▶ Management of pain and fever

▶ Healing without impairment following tonsillectomy

〜 MOUTH AND DENTAL EMERGENCIES

Children may have trauma to the mouth and teeth during sporting activities and during other injuries. About 10% of children experience some dental trauma (Diangelis & Bakland, 1998). Nurses inform parents of proper treatment for injuries and may provide emergency treatment in schools and other community settings. Injury prevention includes use of protective gear during sports. See Chapter 45 for a discussion of oral care during treatment for cancer, and see Chapter 36 for a discussion of protective sporting gear and of body piercing which may include the oral cavity.

Since the mouth has a profuse blood supply, bleeding may be extensive for even minor injuries. It is best to use clean cloths to absorb the blood and prevent choking on it, and get the child to an emergency facility to have the lesion carefully examined.

Dental injuries may involve fracture of a tooth, luxation (partial extrusion), or avulsion (complete removal). The child should be transported immediately to an emergency facility. If the child is otherwise stable, an emergency dental visit is the best choice. When avulsion has occurred, fast care can improve chances that a permanent tooth can be reimplanted and kept alive. Chances of tooth survival are best when reimplanted within 30 minutes (Rudy, 2001). Nurses can perform care or teach parents what to do in case of dental emergency. Referral to dental resources may be needed. Families with financial constraints may lack dental care and resources. Seek resources in the local community for families in need of dental assistance.

Teaching About

CARE OF A TOOTH AVULSION

When a tooth is removed during an injury, prompt treatment may improve the chance that it can be reimplanted. If the child's condition is stable, try to reimplant the tooth and then transfer to an emergency dental facility.

• Handle the tooth only by the crown (its top).

• Gently rinse the tooth in a bowl of tap water. Do NOT place it under running water.

• Insert into the socket.

• Have the child provide gentle pressure by biting a piece of gauze or a tea bag.

If the child is unstable or has other injuries, enlist emergency medical transportation (call 911). In this case the tooth is transported with the child.

• Place the tooth in milk, saline, saliva, or water. If a dental aid kit is available it may contain a transport liquid called Hank's Balanced Salt Solution.

Note: From Rudy, C. A. (2001). Dental trauma. *School Nurse News, 18*(1), 33–35. Adapted.

CHAPTER HIGHLIGHTS

☞ Health conditions affecting the eyes and ears are common in childhood, partially due to anatomic differences in structure.

☞ Disorders of the eye and ear can lead to developmental delay and communication disorders.

☞ Conjunctivitis can occur throughout childhood, and be caused by bacteria, viruses, and allergy.

☞ Conjunctivitis in the newborn, ophthalmia neonatorum, can be acquired during birth from the mother, and can provide a serious health threat.

☞ Children manifest a wide array of visual disorders such as hyperopia, myopia, and astigmatism.

☞ Conditions that can have serious effects on vision are strabismus, amblyopia, cataracts, and glaucoma.

☞ Retinopathy of prematurity is an iatrogenically caused visual disorder.

☞ Nurses commonly screen vision of children in schools and health facilities to identify those with visual impairment.

☞ Interventions for the child with visual impairment center on providing input through other senses to maximize child development.

☞ Otitis media is the most common childhood health condition, and has increased in incidence in the past decade.

☞ Overgrowth of resistant organisms has made treatment of otitis media difficult.

☞ Treatment may begin with up to 3 days of monitoring, followed by antibiotic therapy if the child's condition worsens.

☞ Newborns should be screened for response to sounds, and those at high risk of hearing impairment should get careful monitoring in early childhood.

☞ Hearing loss may be conductive, sensorineural, or mixed.

☞ Nurses plan interventions to maximize development and communication in the child with a hearing impairment.

☞ Common disorders of the nose and throat in children include epistaxis, nasopharyngitis, pharyngitis, and tonsillitis.

EXPLORE MediaLink

NCLEX Review, Case Studies, and other interactive resources for this chapter can be found on the companion website at http://www.prenhall.com/london. Click on "Chapter 48" and select the activities for this chapter.

For animations, more NCLEX review questions, and an audio glossary, access the accompanying CD-ROM in this textbook.

REFERENCES

Agency for Healthcare Research and Quality. (2001). *Management of acute otitis media* (AHRQ Pub. No. 00-E010). Rockville, MD: Author.

Alcorn, D. M. (2001, March). Red eye: When to treat and when to refer. *Infectious Diseases in Children, 3*–8.

Altemeier, W. A. (2000). Preschool vision screening: The importance of the two-line difference. *Pediatric Annals, 29,* 264–267.

American Academy of Pediatrics, Section on Ophthalmology. (2001). Screening examination of premature infants for retinopathy of prematurity. *Pediatrics, 108,* 809–811.

American Academy of Pediatrics, Task Force on Newborn and Infant Hearing. (1999). Newborn and infant hearing loss: Detection and intervention. *Pediatrics, 103,* 527–530.

Bacal, D. A., & Wilson, M. C. (2000). Strabismus: Getting it straight. *Contemporary Pediatrics, 17,* 49–60.

Bachman, K. R., & Arvedson, J. C. (1998). Early identification and intervention for children who are hearing impaired. *Pediatrics in Review, 19,* 155–165.

Brocklehurst, P., & Rooney, G. (2000). Interventions for treating genital *Chlamydia trachomatis* infection in pregnancy. *Cochrane Database Systematic Review 2000, (2),* CD000054.

Brookhouse, P. E., Beauchaine, K. L., & Osberger, M. J. (1999). Management of the child with sensorineural hearing loss: Medical, surgical, hearing aids, cochlear implants. *Pediatric Clinics of North America, 46,* 121–142.

Burns, C. E., Brady, M. A., Dunn, A. M., & Starr, N. B. (2000). *Pediatric primary care* (2nd ed.). Philadelphia: WB Saunders.

Carlson, L. H., & Fall, P. A. (1998). Otitis media: An update. *Journal of Pediatric Health Care, 12,* 313–319.

Cheng, A. K., Rubin, H. R., Powe, N. R., Mellon, N. K., Francis, H. W., & Niparko, J. K. (2000). Cost-utility of the cochlear implant in children. *Journal of the American Medical Association, 284,* 850–856.

Coody, D., Banks, J. M., Yetman, R. J., & Musgrove, K. (1997). Eye trauma in children: Epidemiology, management, and prevention. *Journal of Pediatric Health Care, 11,* 182–188.

DeRespinis, P. A. (2001). Eyeglasses: Why and when do children need them? *Pediatric Annals, 30,* 455–461.

Diangelis, A. J., & Bakland, L. K. (1998). Traumatic dental injuries: Current treatment concepts. *Journal of the American Dental Association, 129,* 1401–1414.

Dowell, S. F., Butler, J. C., Geibink, G. S., & Drug-Resistant *Streptococcal pneumoniae* Thera-

peutic Working Group. (1999). Acute otitis media: Management and surveillance in an era of pneumococcal resistance. *Pediatric Infectious Disease Journal, 18,* 1–9.

Garganta, C., & Seashore, M. R. (2000). Universal screening for congenital hearing loss. *Pediatric Annals, 29,* 302–308.

Gomez, S., & Davis, R. L. (2001). Photoscreening—A viable method for referral. *School Nurse News, 18*(1), 18–20.

Hayes, D. (1999). State programs for universal newborn hearing screening. *Pediatric Clinics of North America, 46,* 89–94.

Hoberman, A., & Paradise, J. L. (2000). Acute otitis media: Diagnosis and management in the year 2000. *Pediatric Annals, 29,* 609–620.

Joint Committee on Infant Hearing (2000). Joint committee on infant hearing 2000 position statement: Principles and guidelines for early hearing detection and intervention programs. *Pediatrics 106,* 798–817.

Kakish, K. S., Mahafza, T., Batieha, A., Ekteish, F., & Daoud, A. (2000). Clinical sinusitis in children attending primary care centers. *Pediatric Infectious Disease Journal, 19,* 1071–1074.

Kemper, K. J. (2001). Complementary and alternative medicine for children: Does it work? *Archives of Disease in Childhood, 84*(1), 6–9.

Kemper, K. J., & Sarah, R. (2000). On pins and needles? Pediatric pain patients' experience with acupuncture. *Pediatrics, 105,* 941–947.

Lee, A. C., Highfield, E. S., Berde, C. B., & Kemper, K. J. (1999). Survey of acupuncturists: Practice characteristics and pediatric care. *Western Journal of Medicine, 171*(3), 153–157.

Little, P., Gould, C., Williamson, I., Moore, M., Warner, G., & Dunleavey, J. (2001). Pragmatic randomized controlled trial of two prescribing strategies for childhood acute otitis media. *British Medical Journal, 322,* 336–342.

Newland, J. A., & Rich, E. (1998). Epistaxis. *American Journal of Nursing, 98,* 16HHH.

Niemela, M., Pihakari, O., Pokka, T., Uhari, M., & Uhari, M. (2000). Pacifier as a risk factor for acute otitis media: A randomized, controlled trial of parental counseling. *Pediatrics, 106,* 483–488.

Niskar, A. S., Kieszak, S. M., Holmes, A. E., Esteban, E., Rubin, C., & Brody, D. J. (2001). Estimated prevalence of noise-induced hearing threshold shifts among children 6 to 19 years of age: The third national health and nutrition examination survey, 1988–1994, United States. *Pediatrics, 108,* 40–43.

Paradise, J. L., Feldman, H. M., Campbell, T. F., Dollaghan, C. A., Colburn, D. K., Bernard, B. S., et al. (2001). Effect of early or delayed insertion of tympanostomy tubes for persistent otitis media on developmental outcome at the age of 3 years. *New England Journal of Medicine, 344,* 1170–1187.

Roddey, O. F., & Hoover, H. A. (2000). Otitis media with effusion in children: A pediatric office perspective. *Pediatric Annals, 29,* 623–629.

Rudy, C. A. (2001). Dental trauma. *School Nurse News, 18(1),* 33–35.

Scheiner, A. P. (1996). Vision problems: Impairment to blindness. In A. M. Rudolph, J. I. E. Hoffman, & C. D. Rudolph (Eds.), *Rudolph's pediatrics* (20th ed., p. 167). Stamford, CT: Appleton & Lange.

Sinus and Allergy Health Partnership. (2000). Antimicrobial treatment guidelines for acute bacterial rhinosinusitis. *Otolaryngology and Head and Neck Surgery, 123,* 5–31.

Slattery, W. H., & Fayad, J. N. (1999). Cochlear implants in children with sensorineural inner ear hearing loss. *Pediatric Annals, 28,* 359–363.

Starr, N. B. (2000). Vision therapy for learning disabilities and dyslexia. *Journal of Pediatric Health Care, 14,* 32–33.

Wagner, R. S. (2000). Management of conjunctivitis. *Contemporary Pediatrics Supplement 2000,* 3–14.

White, K. R., & Maxon, A. B. (1999). *Early identification of hearing loss: Implementing universal newborn hearing screening programs.* Rockville, MD: U.S. Department of Health & Human Services, Maternal & Child Health Bureau.

CHAPTER 49

The Child with Alterations in Neurologic Function

It's so hard to watch your child experience a head injury and lie in a coma. All we can do is be here every day for Antwan. We keep talking to him and trying to get him to respond to us. We keep hoping that he will fully recover.

—MOTHER OF ANTWAN, 7 YEARS OLD

Key Terms

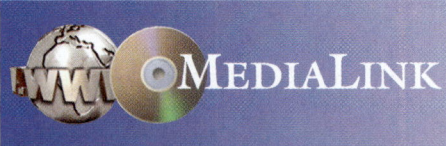

MediaLink

CD-ROM

Skill 14–2: Oxygen Saturation: Pulse Oximetry

Skill 14–20: Performing Chest Physiotherapy/Postural Drainage

Skill 15–2: Inserting and Removing a Nasogastric Tube

Skill 16–1: Performing a Urinary Catheterization

Audio Glossary

NCLEX Review

COMPANION WEBSITE

http://www.prenhall.com/london

Complementary Care: Music Therapy for Special Needs Children

Neurology Web Links

Thinking Critically

MediaLink Applications:

   Soothing Newborns with Neonatal Abstinence Syndrome

   Assess a Child with a Concussion for Return to Competitive Play

NCLEX Review

Case Study

ANATOMY AND PHYSIOLOGY OF PEDIATRIC DIFFERENCES

Knowledge of the anatomy of the nervous system makes neurologic symptoms easier to understand. The brain, spinal cord, and nerves are the major structures of the nervous system (Figure 49–1 ◆). The spinal cord transmits impulses to and from the brain, conveying sensory information and relaying impulses that stimulate motor responses. Because the nervous system helps control and coordinate many body functions, alterations in neurologic function can have widespread effects on the body's metabolism.

Central nervous system (CNS) defects account for approximately one third of all apparent congenital malformations in live infants, and 90% of these are neural tube defects (Farley & Mooney, 1998). CNS defects are responsible for 40% of infant deaths in the first year of life (Farley & Dunleavy, 2000).

At birth, the nervous system is complete but immature. The infant is born with all the nerve cells he or she will have throughout life. However, the number of glial cells and dendrites, which enable receipt of nerve impulses, continues to increase until approximately 4 years of age. Myelination, which increases the speed and accuracy of nerve impulses, is also incomplete at birth. The myelination process accounts for the progressive acquisition of fine and gross motor skills and coordination during early childhood. This development proceeds in a cephalocaudal direction.

The anatomic and physiologic differences between the nervous systems of children and adults help explain why children and adults have different neurologic problems (Table 49–1). For example, the skeletal structures of the skull and vertebrae protect the brain and spinal cord. In infants, however, the cranial bones and vertebrae are not completely ossified. The infant's brain and spinal cord are thus at greater risk for injury from trauma.

TABLE 49–1 Summary of Anatomic and Physiologic Differences Between Children and Adults

Difference in Children	Significance
Top heavy; head is large in proportion to body; neck muscles not well developed	Prone to head injuries with falls; neck may not be able to support large head
Thin cranial bones that are not well developed; unfused sutures	Prone to fracture
Highly vascular brain; subarachnoid space small; dura firmly attached but can strip away from pericranium	Brain prone to hemorrhage; there is less cerebrospinal fluid to cushion the brain
Excessive spinal mobility; muscles, joint capsules, and ligaments of cervical spine immature	Greater risk for high cervical spine injury at C1–C2 level
Wedge-shaped, cartilaginous vertebral bodies; ossification of vertebral bodies incomplete	Greater risk for compression fractures of vertebrae with falls

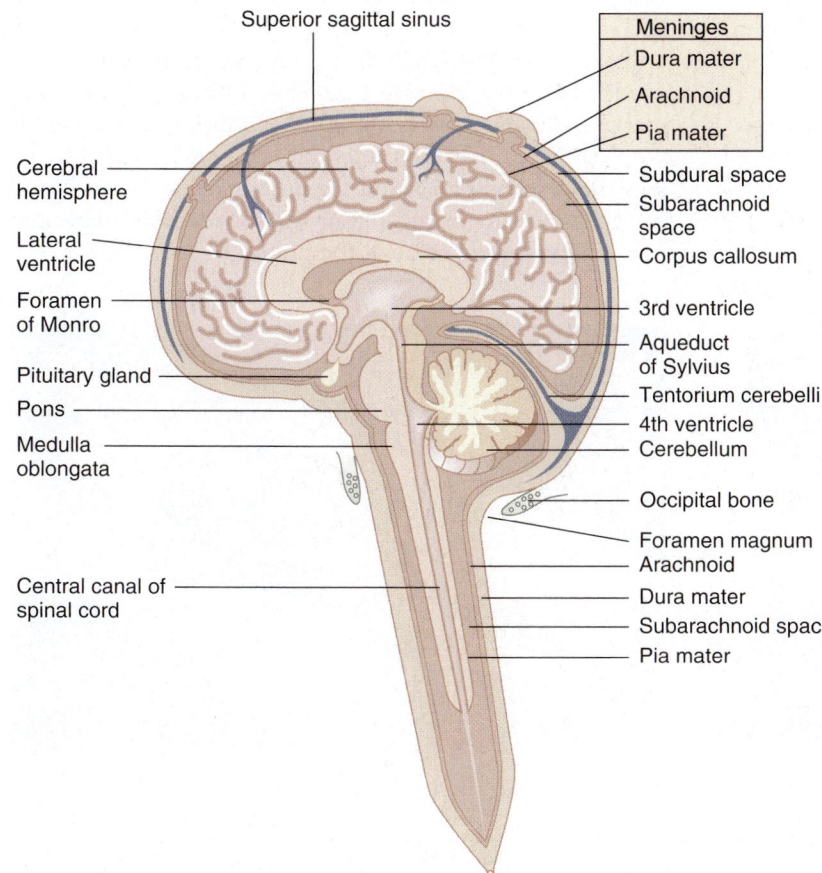

FIGURE 49–1. ◆ Transverse section of the brain and spinal cord. Knowledge of the anatomy of the brain is helpful in understanding the symptoms of neurologic dysfunction.

✎ ALTERED STATES OF CONSCIOUSNESS

Level of consciousness (LOC) is perhaps the most important indicator of neurologic dysfunction. Consciousness, the responsiveness of the mind to sensory stimuli, has two components: *alertness,* or the ability to react to stimuli, and *cognitive power,* or the ability to process the data and respond either verbally or physically. Unconsciousness, on the other hand, is depressed cerebral function, or the inability of the brain to respond to stimuli.

Levels of deterioration can be further categorized as:

- *Confusion:* disorientation to time, place, or person. The child may seem alert. Answers to simple questions may be correct, but responses to complex ones may be inaccurate.
- *Delirium:* state characterized by confusion, fear, agitation, hyperactivity, or anxiety.
- *Obtunded:* limited response to the environment; the child falls asleep unless given verbal or tactile stimulation.
- *Stupor:* response to vigorous stimulation only; the child returns to the unresponsive state when the stimulus is removed. For example, the child may react to a needle stick but not respond to a milder stimulus such as touching the skin.
- *Coma:* severely diminished response; the child cannot be aroused even by painful stimuli.

Etiology and Pathophysiology

Many conditions may alter the level of consciousness, including the following: trauma, hypoxia, infection, poisoning, seizures, endocrine or metabolic disturbances, electrolyte or acid-base imbalance, CNS pathology, and a congenital structural defect. Any of these pathologic processes can also cause increased **intracranial pressure** (force exerted by brain tissue, cerebrospinal fluid, and blood within the cranial vault). Discovering the cause of the decreased level of consciousness is essential so that immediate treatment can begin, to prevent possible secondary effects of the illness or injury.

Clinical Manifestations

Decline in a child's level of consciousness often follows a sequential pattern of deterioration. A child may first appear awake and alert, and may respond appropriately. Initial changes may be subtle: a slight disorientation to time, place, and person. The child may become restless or fussy, and actions that normally calm or soothe the child only increase irritability. As responsiveness decreases, the child may become drowsy but still respond to loud verbal commands and withdraw from painful stimuli. Keeping the child awake is sometimes difficult. Then response to pain progresses from purposeful to nonpurposeful. The child may exhibit decorticate or decerebrate **posturing,** the abnormal positions assumed after injury or damage to the brain (Figure 49–2 ◆).

Clinical manifestations of increased intracranial pressure are provided in Table 49–2.

Clinical Therapy

Clinical therapy focuses on early diagnosis, intervention, and prevention of complications. A thorough history is taken to identify a potential cause of altered consciousness, such as a recent head trauma, an infection, or a poisoning.

Laboratory tests include a complete blood cell count, blood chemistry, clotting factors, and blood culture; toxicology assessments of both blood and urine; and urinalysis with culture. A lumbar puncture may be performed to assess the cerebrospinal fluid for protein, glucose, or blood cells. An electroencephalogram (EEG) identifies damaged or nonfunctioning areas of the brain.

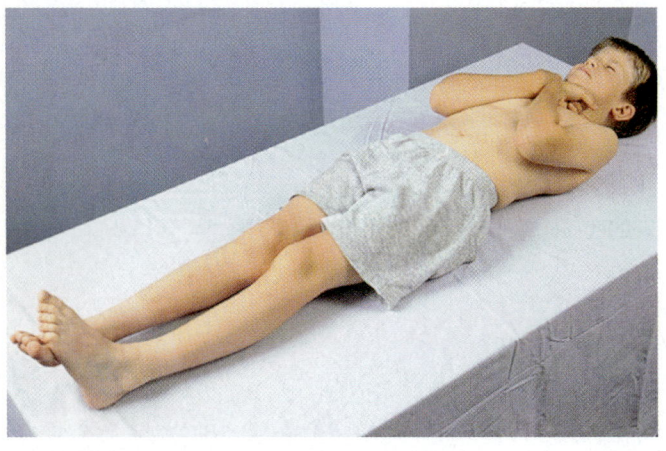

A

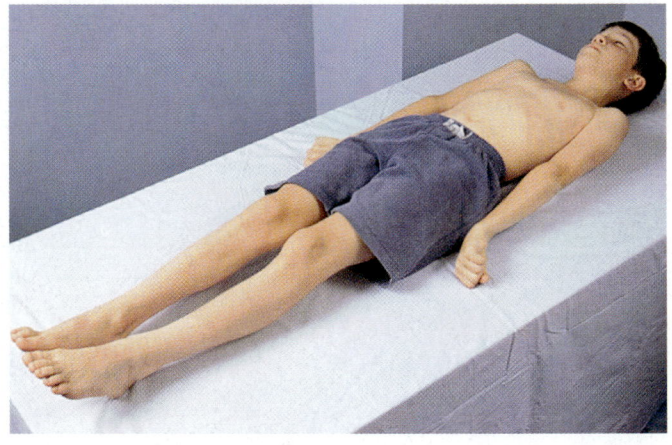

B

FIGURE 49–2. ◆ **A,** Decorticate posturing, characterized by rigid flexion, is associated with lesions above the brainstem in the corticospinal tracts. **B,** Decerebrate posturing, distinguished by rigid extension, is associated with lesions of the brainstem.

TABLE 49-2 Signs of Increased Intracranial Pressure

Early Signs

Headache
Visual disturbances, diplopia
Nausea and vomiting
Dizziness or vertigo
Slight change in vital signs
Pupils not as reactive or equal
Sunsetting eyes
Seizures
Slight change in level of consciousness

Infant has above signs plus:
Bulging fontanel
Wide sutures, increased head circumference
Dilated scalp veins
High-pitched, catlike cry

Late Signs

Significant decrease in level of consciousness
Cushing's triad
• Increased systolic blood pressure and widened pulse pressure
• Brachycardia
• Irregular respirations
Fixed and dilated pupils

---

ment or deterioration in the child's condition. Pediatric criteria take into account the child's developmental age for each category of the test (Table 49–3).

The child is treated with oxygen and assisted ventilation is provided when gas exchange is inadequate. Any metabolic, acid-base, or electrolyte imbalances are corrected. Antibiotics are initiated for suspected infection.

Growth and Development

Following are developmentally appropriate cues in the Glasgow Coma Scale assessment:

• Eye opening. Note whether eye opening is spontaneous or occurs in response to stimuli.

• Verbal response. Crying in an infant is a positive response. The 2-year-old child who says "no" to each command is also responding in an age-appropriate way.

• Motor response. Motor score is probably the most critical aspect of this test, since the child cannot control reflexes. A fearful toddler may refuse to open his or her eyes or talk to strangers, but the child's reflexes should automatically respond to appropriate stimuli. Ask the child to reach for a finger puppet or doll rather than your hand. This makes the child feel less threatened, and the toy can be a reward.

Computed tomography (CT) or magnetic resonance imaging (MRI) is used to detect any lesions, structural abnormalities, vascular malformations, or edema. Skull x-ray studies are used to detect fractures or bony malformations.

The Glasgow Coma Scale quantifies the level of consciousness, thus enabling future comparison of improve-

Efforts are made to maintain the **cerebral perfusion pressure** (the amount of pressure needed to ensure that adequate oxygen and nutrients will be delivered to the brain). In cases of hypovolemia, intravenous fluids are given. In cases of poor perfusion and fluid overload, dopamine or dobutamine is administered. If the intracranial

TABLE 49-3 Glasgow Coma Scale for Assessment of Coma in Infants and Children

Category	Score	Infant and Young Child Criteria	Older Child and Adult Criteria
Eye opening	4	Spontaneous opening	Spontaneous
	3	To loud noise	To verbal stimuli
	2	To pain	To pain
	1	No response	No response
Verbal response	5	Smiles, coos, cries to appropriate stimuli	Oriented to time, place, and person; uses appropriate words and phrases
	4	Irritable; cries	Confused
	3	Inappropriate crying	Inappropriate words or verbal response
	2	Grunts, moans	Incomprehensible words
	1	No response	No response
Motor response	6	Spontaneous movement	Obeys commands
	5	Withdraws to touch	Localizes pain
	4	Withdraws to pain	Withdraws to pain
	3	Abnormal flexion (decorticate)	Flexion to pain (decorticate)
	2	Abnormal extension (decerebrate)	Extention to pain (decerebrate)
	1	No response	No response

Add the score from each category to get the total. The maximum score is 15, indicating the best level of neurologic functioning. The minimum is 3, indicating total neurologic unresponsiveness.

Note: From Teasdale, G., & Jennett, B. (1974). Assessment of coma and impaired consciousness. *Lancet, 2,* 81–84; and James, H. E. (1986). Neurologic evaluation and support in the child with acute brain insult. *Pediatric Annals, 15*(1), 17.

pressure is markedly increased and results from the accumulation of cerebrospinal fluid because of obstruction, a ventricular tap can be performed to decrease the pressure, relieving a life-threatening condition that can lead to coma.

Nursing Management

Nursing Assessment and Diagnosis

Initially assess the child's physiologic status, focusing on the child's responsiveness to the environment or stimuli, ability to maintain the airway, vital signs, and breathing patterns. Use the Glasgow Coma Scale to assess the child at specified intervals (see Skill 9-15). 🔗 SKILLS

Assess the child's cranial nerves (see Table 33–24). The child's responses may differ significantly when stress and anxiety are reduced. Encourage the parents to take part in the examination to reduce the child's anxiety. In the unconscious child, cranial nerve assessment and interpretation are more challenging (see Table 49–4).

Assess the child's respiratory effort and color. Monitor pulse oximetry or arterial blood gas measurements. Adequate air exchange to keep oxygen and carbon dioxide levels within normal ranges is critical to reduce the risk of increased intracranial pressure. If the child cannot maintain an adequate respiratory effort, mechanical ventilation will be necessary.

Among the nursing diagnoses that might be appropriate for the child with an altered level of consciousness or increased intracranial pressure are:

▶ *Ineffective breathing pattern* related to neuromuscular dysfunction associated with increased intracranial pressure

▶ *Risk for aspiration* related to decreased level of consciousness

▶ *Risk for impaired skin integrity* related to decreased level of consciousness and impaired mobility

▶ *Impaired verbal communication* related to physiologic condition of decreased level of consciousness

▶ *Altered family processes* related to care of a child with an acquired disability

Planning and Implementation

HOSPITAL-BASED NURSING CARE

Nursing care of the child with altered consciousness or increased intracranial pressure focuses on maintaining airway patency, monitoring neurologic status, performing routine care, providing sensory stimulation, and providing emotional support to parents.

Make sure the child's airway is clear at all times. If the child is having difficulty swallowing secretions or does not have a gag reflex, intubation or a tracheostomy is performed. Frequent suctioning may be required (see Skill 14-17). 🔗 SKILLS Keep suction apparatus with catheters, oxygen, resuscitation bag and mask, and extra tracheostomy tubes (if applicable) at the bedside. Perform pulse oximetry or arterial blood gas analysis at regular intervals to ensure that gas exchange is adequate. Mechanical ventilation may be required.

Perform routine neurologic checks. Evaluate pupil size and reactivity, eye movements, and motor function (Figure 49–3 ◆). Monitor vital signs. Increased systolic blood pressure, a wide pulse pressure, and bradycardia indicate increased intracranial pressure. Observe for other signs of increased intracranial pressure listed in Table 49–2. If seizures occur, raise the side rails to protect the child from injury.

Perform routine nursing care. If the corneal reflex is absent, place artificial tears in the eyes and cover them with gauze, taping over so they remain closed. Perform routine mouth care by brushing the teeth and using glycerine swabs.

Provide adequate nutrition. Initially nutrients may be supplied intravenously. A nasogastric or gastrostomy tube may be inserted if the child remains unconscious or is not alert enough to take food by mouth (see Skill 15-2). 🔗 SKILLS CD

TABLE 49–4	Assessment of Cranial Nerves in the Unconsious Child	
Cranial Nerves	Reflex	Assessment Procedure and Normal Findings[a]
II, III	Pupillary	Shine a light source in eye. *Rapid, concentrically constricting pupils indicate intact cranial nerves, II, III.*
II, IV, VI	Oculocephalic	Should be performed with eyes held open (doll's eyes) and head turned from side to side. *Eyes gazing straight up or logging slightly behind head motion indicate intact cranial nerves.* Precaution: Cervical spine injury must be ruled out before this assessment is performed.
III, VIII	Oculovestibular	Place the head in a midline and slightly elevated position. Inject ice water into ear canal. *Eyes deviating toward the irrigated ear indicate intact cranial nerves III, VIII.* Precautions: Cervical spine injury must be ruled out before this assessment is performed. Tympanic membrane must be intact; otherwise brain may be filled with bacteria-laden fluid. Note: This assessment is usually performed by a physician.
V, VII	Corneal	Cornea is gently swabbed with sterile cotton swab. *A blink indicates intact cranial nerves V, VII.*
IX, X	Gag	Pharynx is irritated with tongue depressor or cotton swab. *Gagging response indicates intact cranial nerves IX, X.*

[a]Italic indicates normal findings.

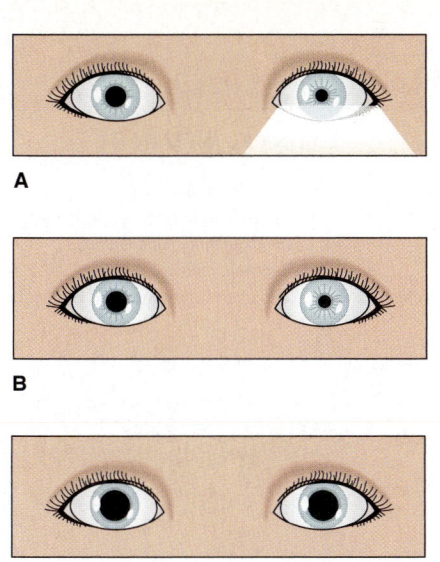

A

B

C

FIGURE 49–3. ◆ Pupil findings in various neurologic conditions with altered consciousness. **A,** A unilateral dilated and reactive pupil is associated with an intracranial mass. **B,** A fixed and dilated pupil may be a sign of impending brainstem herniation. **C,** Bilateral fixed and dilated pupils are associated with brainstem herniation from increased intracranial pressure.

TABLE 49–5 Care of the Immobile Child
• Help keep body in proper alignment with splints or rolls made of towels or blankets.
• Perform passive or gentle range of motion exercises three or four times per day according to physician's orders.
• Maintain skin integrity:
• Change position every 2 hours.
• Place child on foam or egg-crate mattress or sheepskin covering.
• Massage child gently using lotion.

Prevent complications associated with immobility (muscle atrophy, contractures, and skin breakdown) as described in Table 49–5. Support physical therapy efforts with extra passive range of motion exercises.

Provide sensory stimulation. Because the child with a severely altered level of consciousness may still be able to hear, talking to him or her may be beneficial. Listening to music or tapes of family members talking or reading can soothe a child who has an altered level of consciousness when family members cannot be present. Explain all procedures and actions.

When the child becomes more alert, orient the child to time, place, and person, depending on his or her age and level of understanding. Encourage parents to bring objects or toys from home to make the environment more familiar and promote a feeling of security.

Provide emotional support to the child and family. Explain the child's condition in simple terms. Encourage parents to take part in the child's care and therapy as much as possible. If the child's normal functioning has been permanently impaired, refer the family to the appropriate psychologic and social services for emotional support. (See Chapter 37 for more information about helping families cope with a child's life-threatening illness.) Give family members chances to express their feelings.

DISCHARGE PLANNING AND HOME CARE TEACHING

The child's transition from the hospital to home, a long-term care facility, or inpatient rehabilitation center must be planned well in advance of discharge. Identify a case manager or social worker who can help plan the child's long-term care needs, including home health nursing, adaptation of the home, and the purchase of special equipment.

NURSING CARE IN THE COMMUNITY

Home care nurses play a vital role in the care of the child with an acquired neurologic dysfunction and prolonged altered consciousness. Teach the family how to care for the child with severe neurologic dysfunction and to perform routine procedures such as maintaining the airway, skin care, feeding, positioning, exercises, and stimulation. Regular follow-up visits are needed to assess the child's progress and to modify the treatment plan.

The child also needs to be linked with community rehabilitation services through an early intervention program or school-based program. The home health nurse or case manager should help the family have an individual education plan developed for the child (see Chapter 35).

Evaluation

Expected outcomes of nursing care include the following:

▶ The child's airway is maintained and the cerebral perfusion pressure is maintained to oxygenate the brain.

▶ The family provides appropriate care to the child with prolonged altered consciousness to promote minimal long-term disabilities.

HEADACHES

Children commonly experience headaches. They may be the cause of school absence, decreased extracurricular activity, and poor academic achievement. Up to 82% of children experience a headache by late adolescence (O'Hara & Koch, 1998).

Headaches have both benign (migraine, inflammatory, and tension) and structural causes. See "Causes and Clinical Manifestations of Headaches." Migraine headaches are the most common benign headaches in children, estimated to occur in 5% of children. Most children are affected by 9 years of age. Migraines may be triggered by stress; foods containing nitrates, glutamate, caffeine, tyramine, and salt; menses; oral contraceptives; fatigue; and hunger. Another family member often has similar headaches, so there may be a genetic predisposition.

TYPE OF HEADACHE AND CAUSE	CLINICAL MANIFESTATIONS	CLINICAL THERAPY
Migraine—vascular	• Unilateral or bilateral pulsatile throbbing pain lasting for hours or days • Nausea and vomiting • Photophobia • Visual or motor aura several minutes before headache starts • Recurrent abdominal pain • Increased pain with activity • Relief with sleep	• Food elimination trial • Medications to abort migraine (ergot, isometheptene, supatriptan) • Analgesic medication • Relaxation techniques and biofeedback
Tension—muscular contraction	• Dull, achy pain in band around head, in neck and shoulders that may last for days • Intermittent or constant pain with fluctuations in degree of pain • Nausea, no vomiting • Sensitive to light or sound • Pain not aggravated by physical activity	• Relaxation techniques • Analgesic and anti-inflammatory medications • Ice pack • Rest
Inflammatory—sinusitis or dental abscess	• Frontal pain or tenderness over affected sinus • Fever	• Analgesic, antipyretic, and anti-inflammatory medications • Antibiotic medications • Cold or heat application
Structural—space-occupying lesion, hemorrhage, increased intracranial pressure	• Pain that awakens child in morning • Pain worse in morning, with coughing, sneezing, or straining • Morning vomiting, no nausea • Worsening pain with increasing frequency, abnormal neurologic signs within 2–6 months of headache onset (i.e., double vision, papilledema)	• Surgery • Analgesic medications

Clinical therapy involves taking a detailed history of the headache characteristics, onset, warning signs, duration, severity, and associated symptoms. The child is assessed for neurologic signs such as altered consciousness, abnormal cranial nerves, papilledema, and motor or sensory deficits. Radiologic studies (CT scan or MRI) are used only if a structural problem is suspected. Treatment includes relaxation techniques, analgesics, and anti-inflammatory medications. Food elimination diet trials are often used to identify foods that trigger headaches. Medications to abort migraines (ergot or isometheptene) are used in children old enough to identify an aura, or warning. Adolescents may use sumatriptan in oral or nasal spray form to abort migraines. Beta-blockers may be used prophylactically if headaches significantly interfere with usual activities.

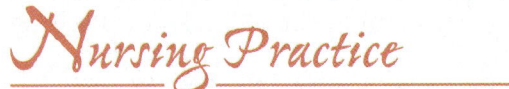

Nursing Practice

An **aura** is a sensation (visual, auditory, taste, or motor) that warns of an impending migraine headache or epileptic seizure. Before migraine headaches, children may report seeing spots or a shimmery film that gets larger and affects their vision. In the case of the migraine, the child has time to take medications in an effort to abort the headache. In epilepsy, the child may have time to avoid injury by getting to the floor.

Nursing management involves assessing the child for potential neurologic signs associated with headaches and assisting the child and family to identify strategies for relieving the headaches. Help the family and child implement the food elimination trial and gradually add foods to identify offending chemical triggers. Make sure the child learns to take the prescribed medications appropriately. Teach the child relaxation techniques (breathing control training, mental imagery, progressive relaxation, and biofeedback) to manage stress and the pain associated with the headaches. **WEB**

~ SEIZURE DISORDERS

Seizures are periods of abnormal electrical discharges in the brain that cause involuntary movement, and behavior and sensory alterations. They are a common neurologic disorder in children. Approximately 2% to 4% of children have one or more seizures during childhood from a variety of causes, most often during infancy. Infants are susceptible to developing epilepsy in the first year of life with an incidence of 1 per 1000. The incidence decreases with age. Approximately 20% of all epilepsy cases develop by 5 years of age (Farley & McEwan, 2000). Epilepsy is a chronic disorder characterized by recurrent, unprovoked seizures secondary to a CNS disorder. One in 100 people has epilepsy (Valente, 2000).

Etiology and Pathophysiology

Seizures are believed to be the result of abnormal electrical discharges of brain neurons. These cells can be triggered by either environmental or physiologic stimuli such as emotional stress, anxiety, fatigue, infection, or metabolic disturbances. The most common causes in children are CNS infection and head trauma.

Some seizures are idiopathic, or not provoked by known stimuli. Genetic factors may lower the seizure threshold by making brain cells more vulnerable to abnormal electrical discharges. Acquired seizures may be caused by underlying pathologic conditions such as trauma, infection, hypoglycemia, endocrine dysfunction, toxins, tumors, or lesions that may be manifested at any time. See "Clinical Manifestations: Seizures."

CLINICAL MANIFESTATIONS ∿ *Seizures*

TYPE OF SEIZURE AND CAUSE	CLINICAL MANIFESTATIONS
Partial Seizures ***Complex partial seizures*** (psychomotor seizures) Lesions, cysts, or tumors Perinatal trauma Focal sclerosis, i.e., scarring of the mediotemporal lobe from prolonged febrile seizures Vascular anomalies, i.e., arteriovenous malformations Head trauma	*Onset:* 3 years of age to adolescence Consciousness is impaired immediately or gradually after a simple partial onset; lasts 5–10 seconds up to 1–2 minutes; postseizure confusion Aura frequently present, unusual taste or odor Feelings of anxiety, fear or déjà vu (sensation that event occurred before) Abdominal pain Staring into space, mental confusion Posturing **Automatisms**—lip smacking, lip chewing, sucking
Simple partial seizures (focal seizures) Focal damage (e.g., with cerebral palsy) Tumors or lesions Arteriovenous malformation Brain abscesses	*Onset:* any age No loss of consciousness; lasts 5–10 seconds; no postseizure confusion No aura Motor responses may involve one extremity, part of extremity, or ipsilateral extremities with eyes and head turning in opposite direction Sensory responses involve paresthesias (decreased sensation or tingling); auditory, olfactory, or visual sensations; autonomic (sweating, papillary dilation) or psychic symptoms Motor and sensory involvement may be combined Jacksonian march (rare in children): tonic contractions of either fingers of one hand, toes of one foot, or one side of face become clonic or tonic-clonic movements; activity then "marches" up to adjacent muscles of either affected extremity or same side of body (such as face)
Generalized Seizures ***Tonic-clonic seizures*** (grand mal seizures) Cerebral damage from perinatal trauma, head trauma, tumors, structural lesions, metabolic and neuromuscular degenerative disorders Genetic link Many are idiopathic	*Onset:* any age, rare before 6 months of age, strong familial incidence Abrupt onset seizure, 1–2 minute loss of consciousness, postseizure confusion (few minutes to hours) May or may not have aura Falls to ground when all muscles contract Eyes roll upward or deviate to one side with pupils dilated Abdominal or chest wall rigidity with leg, head, and neck extended, and arms flexed or contracted Cry or grunt as air is forced out when diaphragm and chest muscles contract Urinary or bowel incontinence as muscles become flaccid during clonic phase Characterized by sleepiness, difficulty in arousal; hypertension; diaphoresis; headache, nausea, vomiting; poor coordination, decreased muscle tone; confusion, amnesia; slurred speech; visual disturbances; combativeness
Absence seizures (petit mal, or lapse seizures) Hyperventilation Genetic predisposition	*Onset:* age 4–5 years with remission in adolescence More prevalent in females May go on to develop other generalized seizures Brief loss of consciousness, usually lasts 5–10 seconds, rarely exceeds 30 seconds, no postseizure confusion, lethargy, or sleepiness Frequent attacks (50–100 per day), may cluster No aura Abrupt cessation of current activity Staring; episodes may be confused with daydreaming or inattentiveness Rolling of eyes, eye blinking, ptosis or fluttering of eyelids Slight increase or loss of muscle tone (head may droop, handheld objects may be dropped) Amnesia

(continued)

TYPE OF SEIZURE AND CAUSE	CLINICAL MANIFESTATIONS
Myoclonic seizures Progressive or degenerative encephalopathy	*Onset:* as early as 2 years, but more prevalent in school-age child or adolescent No loss of consciousness, child recovers in seconds, no postictal period Attacks occur most often upon falling asleep or awakening Quick involuntary muscle jerks, may appear to drop or throw object; head, extremity, or body contractions, may be limited to one body part or whole body
Infantile spasms (myoclonic epilepsy of infancy, salaam seizures) Prenatal and perinatal encephalopathy Metabolic disorder Tuberous sclerosis Microcephaly	*Onset:* begin at age 3 months and resolve by 2 years Positive history of gestational difficulties, developmental delays or other neurologic abnormalities Possible loss of consciousness Several seizures can occur throughout the day Episodes usually occur when infant is falling asleep or awakening Dropping of head, flexion of neck, extension of arms, and flexion of legs; sudden flexion or extension of trunk (or both) Eye rolling, either upward or downward Crying, pallor, or cyanosis Regression in development and irritability
Akinetic or atonic seizures (drop attacks) Gray matter degenerative diseases and subacute seizures Sclerosing panencephalitis Many are idiopathic	*Onset:* first seen at 2 years, disappear by 6 years Momentary loss of consciousness Falls to ground with sudden loss of postural tone, inability to break fall

Partial, or **focal,** seizures are caused by abnormal electrical activity in one hemisphere or a specific area of the cerebral cortex, most often the temporal, frontal, or parietal lobes. The symptoms depend on the region of the cortex affected.

In contrast, generalized seizures are the result of diffuse electrical activity that begins in both hemispheres of the brain simultaneously and spreads throughout the cortex into the brainstem. As a result, movements and spasms displayed by the child are bilateral and symmetric.

The length of a seizure, especially of a generalized seizure, is important because the airway may be compromised during the tonic phase. The basal metabolic rate rises during the peak of seizure activity. This change, in turn, increases the demand for oxygen and glucose. During a seizure the child may become pale or cyanotic as a result of hypoxia or hypoglycemia.

Febrile seizures occur in connection with a sudden rise in temperature in association with an acute illness. No evidence of intracranial infection or other defined cause is found. They are usually seen between 3 months and 5 years with a peak incidence between 18 to 24 months of age. There is often a family history of febrile seizures. In addition, children who have one febrile seizure have a 30% to 50% greater chance of having future seizures (Sagraves, 1999). The lower convulsive threshold of infants may explain this type of seizure.

Clinical Manifestations

The symptoms of a seizure depend on the type and duration of the seizure. Seizures are classified into two types: *partial (focal) seizures* and *generalized seizures* of nonfocal origin. The specific characteristics of the various types of partial and generalized seizures are presented on page 1279. The initial manifestations of the **tonic** phase of a generalized seizure are unconsciousness and continuous muscular contraction. The tonic phase is followed by the **clonic** phase, characterized by alternating muscular contraction and relaxation. During the **postictal period** following seizure activity the level of consciousness is decreased. The length of the postictal period varies among children. An olfactory or visual aura providing an early warning sign of a seizure occurs only in partial seizures (Vendanarayan, 1999).

Febrile seizures—generalized seizures that usually occur in children as the result of rapid temperature rise above 39 °C (102 °F)—involve generalized tonic–clonic movements that last less than 15 minutes.

Clinical Therapy

After the child's first seizure, it is essential that a thorough history be taken from the parent, primary caretaker, or witnesses to the event. Table 49–6 lists the questions that should be asked. Details such as the description and length of the seizure, presence or absence of an aura, and whether or not the child lost consciousness should be noted. This information is used to identify the type of seizure according to the International Classification of Epileptic Seizures. 🔗 WEB

A complete physical and neurologic examination is performed. Based on the physical findings and history, diagnostic tests are ordered. Laboratory tests include a

TABLE 49-6 Questions to Ask About Seizures

- Did the child complain of not feeling well or feeling "funny" just before the seizure?
- Did the child complain of headache, nausea, muscle pain? Did the child vomit?
- Did the child suffer any trauma before the seizure?
- Did the child get into any medications or poisons before the seizure?
- Was the child sick or feverish before the seizure?
- What movements of the arms and legs were seen? On one side of the body or in one extremity only?
- Was the child's vision normal?
- Were the pupils dilated or the eyes deviated to one side?
- Was the child aware of surroundings? Could the child respond to questions?
- Was the child incontinent of urine or stool?
- How long did the episode last? When did the child begin to wake up?
- Was the child lethargic, weak, or uncoordinated upon arousal?
- Was the child injured during the convulsion?
- Did the child's color change (pale, red, blue)?

TABLE 49-7 Management of Status Epilepticus

- Maintain a patent airway. Muscle rigidity may compromise the airway.
- Perform a jaw thrust maneuver if the airway is obstructed.
- Keep suction equipment at the bedside in case secretions are excessive.
- Give oxygen by mask, as increased metabolic demands deplete oxygen stores.
- Monitor vital signs and circulation with pulse oximeter and cardiorespiratory monitor.
- Assess neurologic level.
- Establish an intravenous line to administer any necessary fluids or medications.
- Administer glucose if the child is hypoglycemic; the physical stress of the seizure may result in declining glucose levels.
- Insert a nasogastric tube.
- Protect the child from injury.
- Manage thermoregulation.
- Administer benzodiazepines such as diazepam, lorazepam, or midazolam. If there is no response, the dose may be repeated. Phenytoin or phenobarbital may be necessary if seizure activity continues. Cumulative doses of drugs may produce apnea, so be prepared to assist ventilations.

TABLE 49-8 Anticonvulsants Used to Treat Seizure Disorders

Emergency Medications	First Line Medications	Second Line Medications
Diazepam	Carbamazepine	Clonazepam
	Ethosuximide	Felbamate
	Phenobarbital	Gabapentin
	Phenytoin	Lamotrigine
	Primidone	Tiagabine
	Valproic Acid	Topiramate

complete blood cell count, blood chemistry, urine culture, and lumbar puncture. If the child is taking any anticonvulsants, blood levels of the medication should be monitored. An EEG may be performed. A lead level, toxicology screening, and radiologic tests such as CT scanning or MRI and angiography may be performed to identify a cerebral lesion.

Many convulsions are self-limiting and require no emergency intervention. Children with febrile seizures may be treated with an anticonvulsant for the remainder of the presenting febrile illness. However, long-term anticonvulsants are not generally used. Instead, parents are taught to lower fevers by using antipyretics and keeping the child cool with light clothing, and to prepare for future seizures.

Any generalized seizure lasting longer than 10 minutes needs to be monitored for electrolytes, glucose, blood gases, increasing fever, and abnormal blood pressure. Anticonvulsants are given intravenously or rectally. Monitor for continued motor activity and the potential for status epilepticus (a continuous seizure that lasts for more than 30 minutes or a series of seizures during which consciousness is not regained). Motor activity may become less apparent after anticonvulsants are given, even though the child is still unconscious (Altemeier, 1999). The postictal period ranges from 30 minutes to 2 hours. Management of the child in status epilepticus is described in Table 49-7.

Most seizure disorders are treated with anticonvulsants. A single medication (monotherapy) is preferred for seizure control to minimize the side effects. Monotherapy works for 80% of children with new onset epilepsy (Valente, 2000). See Table 49-8 for first and second line medications used. Serum drug levels are monitored to achieve therapeutic levels or when toxicity is possible. Therapeutic ranges of medications may be exceeded to control seizures

when tolerated by the child. Medication dosage adjustments are often needed as the child grows. Approximately 25% to 30% of children have refractory or **intractable seizures,** seizures that continue to occur even with optimal medical management (Danielpour & Peacock, 2000). These children are often treated with multiple anticonvulsants. Surgery may occasionally be performed to remove a tumor, lesion, or portion of the brain that has been identified as causing the seizures.

A ketogenic diet is occasionally used for children under the age of 8 years with myoclonic and absence seizures. This diet involves a high intake of fat and low intake of carbohydrates and protein. This high-fat diet causes a mild state of starvation, resulting in ketosis as the body uses fat for metabolism. A mild state of dehydration is maintained so the level of ketones in the circulation is not diluted. Ketosis is believed to slow the electrical impulses that cause seizures. Medium-chain triglycerides may be given as a supplement to increase the acidosis. Family motivation must be high to maintain the diet for 2 to 3 years and to

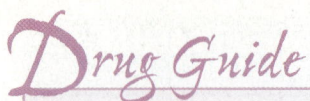

Drug Guide

PHENYTOIN

Overview of Action

Controls seizure propagation by modifying the activities of sodium, potassium, and calcium ions and prevents seizure discharge from seizure foci. Used for control of tonic-clonic (generalized) and partial seizures with complex symptomatology (psychomotor), as well as seizures caused by factors other than epilepsy. May be used in status epilepticus, particulary in combination with diazepam.

Routes, Dosage, Frequency

PO: For seizures

- 5 mg/kg or 250 mg/m^2/day in 2 to 3 doses initially; adjusted as needed; not to exceed 300mg/day.
- Maintenance dose is usually 4 to 8 mg/kg/day or 200 mg/day.
- A loading dose in several doses over 24 hours may be used to reach therapeutic serum levels more quickly. The lower maintenance dose is then used. The loading dose in infants is 8 to 20 mg/kg, followed by 4 to 8 mg/kg/day. The loading dose in children is 10 to 20 mg/kg followed by 8 to 15 mg/kg/day (under 9 years) or 4 to 8 mg/kg/day (over 9 years).

IM: Rarely used, temporary use when patients unable to take PO form. Reduce usual oral dose by half and give IM. Because of the potential slow drug release from IM storage locations, one half of the PO dose is used for 1 week when returning to PO administration.

IV: Status epilepticus: 250 mg/m^2 or 10 to 15 mg/kg, not to exceed 20 mg/kg/day.

Contraindications:
Hypersensitivity to the drug, sinus bradycardia, heart block. Use with caution in respiratory depression and congestive heart failure, especially IV form. Previous exfoliative, purpuric, or bullous rash with therapy. Do not use preparation containing sodium bisulfite in children with sulfite allergy.

Side Effects:
Confusion, drowsiness during early therapy, dizziness, headache, anorexia, decreased taste, weight loss, hirsutism, anemia, thrombocytopenia, leukopenia, pancytopenia, hyperglycemia, gingival hyperplasia, osteomalacia.

Nursing Implications

Assess: Baseline CBC, liver function tests, and urinalysis are done. Serum levels of drug may be monitored. **IV:** Take vital signs before administration; watch for irritation and necroses, which can occur even without filtration.

Administer: Give the PO form with food or fluid to prevent gastric irritation. If given by feeding tube, dilute the solution with sterile water, D5W, or normal saline and flush tube with at least 20 mL after administration to avoid adherence to feeding tube. Have emergency drugs and equipment available if given IV.

Monitor: CBC, liver function tests, and urinalysis are done monthly. Observe for side effects, especially gingival hyperplasia and rashes. Observe for and record seizure activity, neuropathy, and mental changes.

Patient Teaching: The child should use good dental hygiene to reduce the severity of dental hyperplasia. A medical alert band indicating seizures and phenytoin medication use should be worn. Avoid alcohol and other central nervous system depressants, including those in over-the-counter medications. Mental alertness may be altered with this medication, so driving cars or other mechanical equipment should be avoided.

Note: From Bindler, R. M., & Howry, L. B. (1997). *Pediatric drugs and nursing implications* (2nd ed.). Upper Saddle River, NJ: Prentice Hall-Health. Adapted.

---

frequently monitor the child's urine ketone values (Katyal, Koehler, McGhee, et al., 2000).

A trial of medication withdrawal is attempted for some types of seizures (such as absence) during adolescence as some children have spontaneous remissions.

Nursing Management

Nursing Assessment and Diagnosis

Assess and monitor the child's physiologic status. During the postictal period, monitor the child's vital signs, perform neurologic checks, and keep the environment safe. Once the child is stable, a more definitive assessment can be made. Level of consciousness is one of the most important indicators of neurologic function. Remember that the child's lack of response may be the result of the postictal state.

Collect and analyze historical information about the seizure activity, clustering, aura, description of motor activity or changes in muscle tone, automatisms, and any

changes in development or school performance to help determine the type of seizures the child has.

Common nursing diagnoses for the child with a seizure disorder include:

- ▶ *Ineffective breathing pattern* related to neuromuscular dysfunction during the tonic phase of a seizure
- ▶ *Ineffective airway clearance* related to inability to control secretions during seizure
- ▶ *Risk for trauma* related to seizure activity
- ▶ *Chronic low self-esteem* related to refractory seizures and loss of bowel and bladder control during seizure activity
- ▶ *Risk for anxiety* related to unpredictable nature of seizure disorder
- ▶ *Ineffective management of therapeutic regimen (individual)* related to poor compliance with pharmacologic management of seizures
- ▶ *Altered family processes* related to care of a child with a chronic disorder

Planning and Implementation

Nursing care focuses on maintaining airway patency, ensuring safety, administering medications, and providing emotional support. Both acute care and long-term management are involved.

MAINTAIN AIRWAY PATENCY

Be sure that nothing is placed in the child's mouth during a seizure; loose teeth may be knocked out and aspirated. Monitor the child to ensure adequate oxygenation: the child's color should be pink, the heart rate at a normal or slightly above normal rate for age, and the pulse oximetry reading greater than 95%. Oxygen is usually given at levels below 95% (see Skill 14-2). SKILLS CD

ENSURE SAFETY

Protect the child from self-harm during violent seizures (Figure 49–4 ◆). If the child is in bed, the side rails should be padded to prevent injury. Children who have frequent,

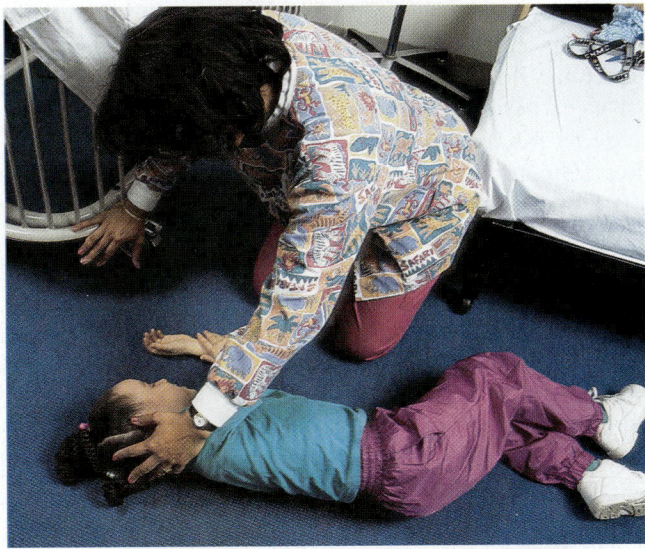

FIGURE 49–4. ◆ A child who has a seizure when standing should be gently assisted to the floor and placed in a side-lying position. Clear the area of any objects that might cause harm to the child.

recurrent seizures should wear helmets to protect their heads in case they fall. All children with seizure disorders should wear some form of medical identification (e.g., a Medic-Alert bracelet).

ADMINISTER MEDICATIONS

Take special precautions when administering intravenous medications for the acute management of seizures. Give these medications very slowly to minimize the risk of respiratory or circulatory collapse.

Medications for the management of chronic seizures are given orally. Crushing pills and mixing them in a teaspoonful of applesauce, pudding, or other soft food make them more palatable and easier for the child to swallow.

When a child is NPO due to illness or on the day of surgery, seizure medications are usually given with a swallow of water. Check with the prescriber for clear orders in such cases.

PROVIDE EMOTIONAL SUPPORT

The loss of control of body movements and possible loss of consciousness make seizures frightening and difficult to accept for the child, parents, and other family members.

Parents often feel guilty about the child's seizure disorder and compensate by not disciplining or restricting the child appropriately. Stress the need to treat the child as normally as possible. Refer the child and family to support groups and counseling services if indicated.

DISCHARGE PLANNING AND HOME CARE TEACHING

Encourage parents to express their fears and anxieties. Answer their questions honestly, and refer them to organizations such as the Epilepsy Foundation of America, where they can get more information about the child's disorder. Be sure parents know how to administer medications and keep the child safe. Discuss with them whom to call with questions and when to return for follow-up. WEB

NURSING CARE IN THE COMMUNITY

Educate the child and parents about medication regimens. Explain the purpose of each drug, its schedule for administration, and the importance of giving all doses. Teaching the older child to take medications without parental intervention gives the child a feeling of control. Provide information about the side effects of medications ordered, and alert parents to the signs of toxic reactions or undermedication. Regular dental care is important because of the effect of certain anticonvulsants on the gingiva. Explain the importance of follow-up visits to health care providers so the effectiveness of the child's medications can be monitored.

Teach families about safety guidelines for the child. Families of children with severe seizure disorders need to develop an emergency care plan so that emergency personnel know about their needs for care in advance (see Chapter 35).

SAFETY FOR THE CHILD WITH A SEIZURE DISORDER

Children with epilepsy have more injuries of all sorts, including burns and falls. Children are at increased risk for death due to drowning.

Planning for safety includes the following:

- Do not leave the child alone in the bathtub.
- Children who bathe alone should use the shower.
- A buddy and lifeguard should always be present when the child swims.
- A life vest should always be worn when boating.
- The child should not play or stand around open flames or outdoor grills.
- The child should avoid areas where fall risks are increased.

Assist the family to develop an individual school health plan so the child can receive medications during school hours, if necessary. Teachers and school administrators should know what to do if the child has a seizure and what information to report about the seizure. Encourage participation in sports when good supervision is provided.

The child may be afraid of having a seizure in front of friends. Reassure the child and family that taking medications regularly should control seizures. Children need to be able to explain to peers what a seizure is and what to do if they are present when one occurs. Summer camps for children with seizures can be a safe and comfortable place for the child to enjoy outdoor activities. Tell parents to boost the child's self-image by emphasizing what the child can do, rather than focusing on contraindicated activities. Depending on state laws, most adolescents can drive after they have been seizure-free for at least 2 years.

Teach parents of children with recurrent febrile seizures how to give antipyretics and the proper dose. Antipyretic doses need to be updated as the child grows. Parents need to know that antipyretics and anticonvulsants may not prevent a future febrile seizure associated with an acute illness. The potential toxicity of an anticonvulsant in a child with febrile seizures often outweighs the risk of the seizures, and parents can be reassured that complications from febrile seizures are rare.

Evaluation

Expected outcomes of nursing management include the following:

▶ The child is not injured when seizures occur because safety measures are used.

▶ The child's self-esteem is enhanced through participation in well-supervised sports and activities.

≈ INFECTIOUS DISEASES

BACTERIAL MENINGITIS

Meningitis, an inflammation of the meninges, can be caused by either bacterial or viral agents. Bacterial meningitis is more virulent than viral meningitis and is sometimes fatal. Children under 1 year of age are at greatest risk for bacterial meningitis. Seventy percent of all cases appear before 5 years of age (Farley & Mooney, 1998).

Etiology and Pathophysiology

Meningitis may occur secondary to other infections such as otitis media, sinusitis, pharyngitis, cellulitis, pneumonia, or septic arthritis; head trauma; or a neurosurgical procedure. Most cases are caused by three organisms: *Haemophilus influenzae* type b, *Neisseria meningitidis,* and *Streptococcus pneumoniae* (Farley & Mooney, 1998). The number of cases of bacterial meningitis caused by *Streptococcus pneumoniae* is expected to decline as more infants and children are immunized with the new heptovalent pneumococcal conjugate vaccine (see Chapter 41).

In many cases, bacteremia spreads the infectious agent to the CNS (see "Pathophysiology Illustrated: Central Nervous System Infection"). An inflammatory response follows. White blood cells accumulate, covering the surface of the brain with a thick, white, purulent exudate. The brain then becomes hyperemic and edematous. If the infection spreads to the ventricles, they can become obstructed and impede the flow of cerebrospinal fluid, causing hydrocephalus.

Clinical Manifestations

Symptoms are variable and depend on the child's age, the pathogen, and the length of the illness before diagnosis. Onset may be sudden or the illness may develop over about a 1-week period. Symptoms in the young infant may include fever, change in feeding pattern, vomiting, or diarrhea. The anterior fontanel may be bulging or flat. The infant may be alert, restless, lethargic, or irritable. Rocking or cuddling, which normally calms a fussy infant, only irritates the infant with meningitis.

Older children are usually febrile; can be irritable, lethargic, or confused; have vomiting; and complain of muscle or joint pain. A hemorrhagic rash, first appearing as petechiae and changing to purpura or large necrotic patches, may be seen in meningococcal meningitis. The child displays other symptoms consistent with meningeal irritation: headache (most often frontal), photophobia, esotropia, and nuchal rigidity (resistance to neck flexion). The child is comfortable only in an opisthotonic position (hyperextension of the head and neck to relieve discomfort; Figure 49–5 ◆). The child may have a positive Kernig or Brudzinski sign, or both, on examination (Figures 49–6 ◆ and 49–7 ◆).

Pathogens lead to exudate
and swelling in subarachnoid space

Arachnoid

Pia mater

Pia mater   Arachnoid

Choroid plexus produces
the cerebrospinal fluid

Pathogens are circulated throughout
the brain and spinal cord by the
cerebrospinal fluid

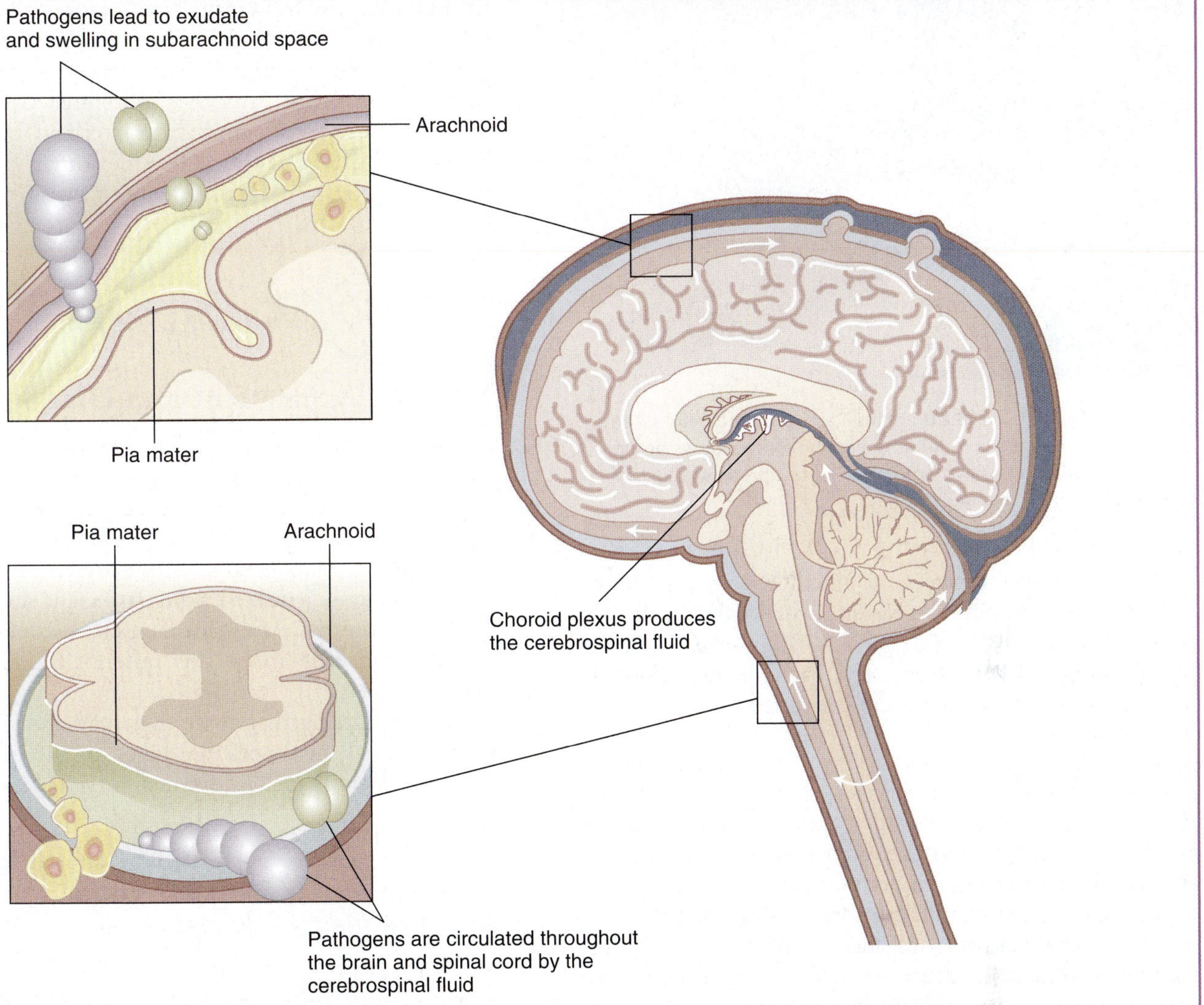

After bacteria reach the central nervous system, the pia mater, the arachnoid, and the cerebrospinal fluid–filled subarachnoid space become infected. The cerebrospinal fluid then circulates the pathogens throughout the brain and spinal cord.

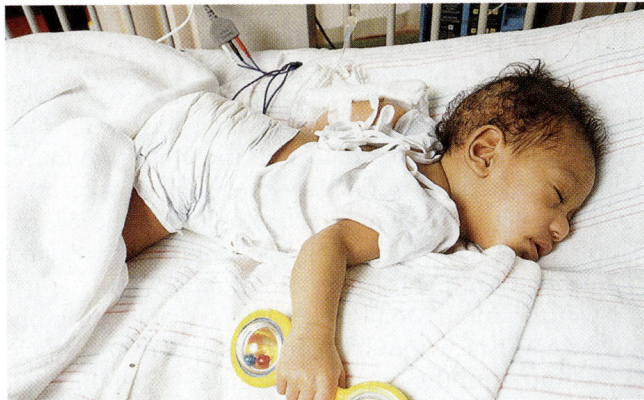

FIGURE 49-5. ◆ The child with bacterial meningitis assumes an opisthotonic position, with the neck and the head hyperextended, to relieve discomfort.

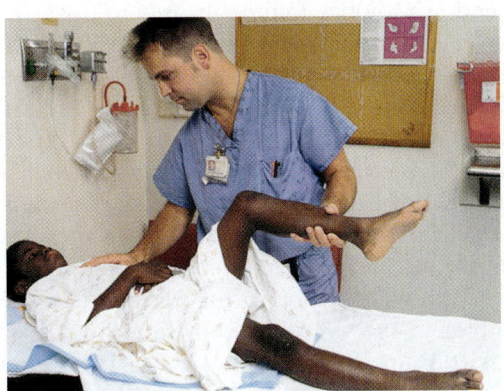

FIGURE 49-6. ◆ To test for Kernig sign, raise the child's leg with the knee flexed. Then extend the child's leg at the knee. If any resistance is noted or pain is felt, the result is a positive Kernig sign. This is a common finding in meningitis.

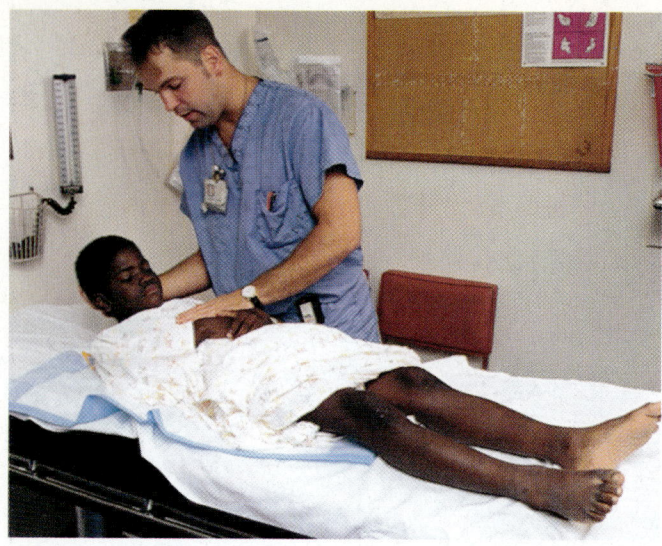

FIGURE 49–7. ◆ To test Brudzinski sign, flex the child's head while in a supine position. If this action makes the knees or hips flex involuntarily, a positive Brudzinski sign is present. This is a common finding in meningitis.

Symptoms can progress to include seizures, apnea, cerebral edema, subdural effusion, hydrocephalus, disseminated intravascular coagulation (DIC), shock, and increased intracranial pressure. The bacteria may also colonize within a joint, causing septic arthritis.

Clinical Therapy

Diagnosis is based on the history, clinical presentation, and laboratory findings. A thorough history should be taken and a physical examination performed.

Laboratory tests include a complete blood count, blood cultures, serum electrolytes and osmolality, and clotting factors. A lumbar puncture is performed to evaluate the cerebrospinal fluid for number of white blood cells and protein and glucose levels. A Gram stain and culture are done on the cerebrospinal fluid.

Antibiotics are administered as soon as diagnostic tests are obtained. Antibiotics commonly used to treat bacterial meningitis include ampicillin, aminoglycosides, cefotaxime, ceftriaxone, and penicillin G. Antibiotics are often changed once culture and sensitivity results are known, especially as many organisms have resistance to certain antibiotics. These medications are administered intravenously for 7 to 21 days, depending on the organism and the child's clinical response. Depending on the causative organism, the disease may need to be reported to the local health department, and contacts may need to take prophylactic antibiotics, such as rifampin or ciprofloxacin. Corticosteroids (dexamethasone) are given as an adjunct to children over 6 weeks of age to reduce the risk of severe neurologic sequelae such as sensorineural hearing loss (Leake & Perkins, 2000). In some cases, anticonvulsants and antipyretics are given.

Some infants and children who have had bacterial meningitis suffer neurologic damage despite early, aggressive management. The most common sequelae involve cranial nerves, especially the eighth, resulting in hearing loss. In addition, children may have seizures, hydrocephalus, subdural effusion, syndrome of insufficient antidiuretic hormone, developmental delay, learning problems, and behavior problems. Another potential complication is meningococcal septicemia, characterized by high fever, hypotension, DIC, and multisystem organ failure (Harrison, 2001). See the discussion about meningococcemia in Chapter 44. ⌒

Nursing Management

Nursing Assessment and Diagnosis

Assess the child's physiologic status, including vital signs and level of consciousness. Measure head circumference often in infants because of the potential for hydrocephalus. Be alert for signs of a change in the child's condition and response to treatment. Monitor the child's ability to control secretions and to drink sufficient fluids. Monitor intake and output. Assess for any sensory deficits. Identify parents' concerns about this potentially life-threatening condition.

Several nursing diagnoses that may apply to the child with bacterial meningitis are given in the accompanying "Nursing Care Plan." Additional nursing diagnoses might include:

▶ *Risk for aspiration* related to altered level of consciousness and poor secretion control

▶ *Risk for fluid volume deficit* related to poor oral fluid intake

▶ *Anticipatory grieving (parent)* related to the child's potentially life-threatening condition

▶ *Caregiver role strain* related to a hospitalized child and other family responsibilities

Planning and Implementation

The "Nursing Care Plan" summarizes care for the child with bacterial meningitis. Nursing care begins with emergency treatment and continues as the child's condition stabilizes. Monitor respiratory and neurologic status, maintain hydration, administer medications, and prevent complications. Promote the child's comfort with reduced stimulation (dim lights, quiet room) and by placing in a side-lying position. Monitor the child's response to antibiotic therapy. Isolate the child and use standard and droplet precautions until the causative organism is identified and effective treatment is under way.

Maintenance and replacement fluids are usually given to children with bacterial meningitis. However, it is impor-

GOAL	INTERVENTION	RATIONALE	EXPECTED OUTCOME

1. Inability to sustain spontaneous ventilation related to level of consciousness

	NIC Priority Intervention:		*NOC Suggested Outcome:*
	Respiratory monitoring: *Collection and analysis of patient data to assure airway patency and adequate gas exchange*		**Vital sign status:** *Pulse, respiration, and blood pressure are within expected range for age*
The child's respiratory failure does not progress to respiratory arrest.	▶ Place the child on a cardiorespiratory monitor with a 20-second alarm.	▶ The alarm on the monitor alerts staff that the child is having bradycardia or an apneic spell.	The child's respiratory failure is easily managed with prompt assessment and treatment.
	▶ Have resuscitation equipment, including oxygen, resuscitation bag with mask, and suction apparatus, at the bedside.	▶ Equipment should be at the bedside in case of respiratory arrest. Bag-valve-mask ventilation is recommended as the child's respiratory secretions contain bacteria.	
	▶ Stimulate the child if apneic; if no response, begin manual ventilations and call for emergency resuscitation.	▶ Stimulation may encourage spontaneous respirations; if not, ventilation is necessary. Calling for emergency resuscitation ensures help in managing the child in a timely manner.	
	▶ Monitor heart rate and perform compressions if necessary.	▶ The apneic child may have bradycardia resulting from cardiac hypoxia.	

2. Risk for injury related to infection of cerebrospinal fluid and potential sequelae

	NIC Priority Intervention:		*NOC Suggested Outcome:*
	Complication monitoring: *Evaluation of fever, shock, and consciousness responses to bacterial infection of the meninges*		**Risk control:** *Actions to eliminate or reduce actual personal and modifiable health threats*
The child will suffer minimal CNS injury secondary to infection.	▶ Administer prescribed antibiotics and corticosteroids as scheduled.	▶ Antibiotics help eradicate the pathogen and prevent cerebral edema. Corticosteroids diminish inflammatory response and reduce the chance of neurologic sequelae.	The child's condition improves significantly within 48–72 hours (fever decreases and no signs of neurologic sequelae are detected).
	▶ Note return of fever, nuchal rigidity, or irritability. Monitor vital signs, assess for signs of increased intracranial pressure, measure head circumference once or twice daily, note changes in responsiveness. Notify the physician immediately if any signs are detected.	▶ Watching for common sequelae such as subdural effusions or septic arthritis ensures prompt treatment.	
The child will not develop cerebral edema as a result of water retention.	▶ Monitor for syndrome of inappropriate antidiuretic hormone secretion (SIADH) and watch for signs of increased intracranial pressure (ICP).	▶ SIADH can be either avoided or quickly managed if recognized early.	Cerebral edema does not develop. If SIADH or increased ICP occurs, the condition is treated promptly so effects are minimal.
	▶ Perform strict intake and output measurements. Determine urine specific gravity. Check electrolytes and osmolality of both serum and urine. Weigh the child daily. Restrict fluids and give sodium chloride as ordered.	▶ Low urine output with a high specific gravity is a sign of fluid retention and SIADH. The child is maintained with lower fluids and provided sodium supplements to reduce the possibility for cerebral edema.	
The child will be free of injury resulting from DIC.	▶ Be aware of needle sticks that continue to bleed and lesions that continue to ooze. Monitor clotting times.	▶ Prompt recognition leads to management of the coagulopathy.	The child does not sustain injury from DIC.
	▶ Administer blood products, vitamin K, or heparin as ordered.	▶ Prompt recognition allows for early initial treatment of DIC. The child may bleed to death if treatment is delayed.	
The child will be free of injury secondary to shock.	▶ Monitor vital signs including pulse, respirations, and blood pressure. Note perfusion (capillary refill, central versus proximal pulses). Check level of consciousness. Note urine output.	▶ Monitoring allows for prompt diagnosis of shock based on clinical signs.	The child recovers from shock quickly with no complications. Prompt management of shock can enhance the child's recovery, since it prevents complications associated with poor perfusion (tissue acidosis and ischemia).
	▶ Begin fluid resuscitation as ordered.	▶ Intravenous fluid bolus may improve perfusion.	
	▶ Administer inotropes if ordered.	▶ Inotropes enhance perfusion when response to fluid challenge is minimal.	

(continued)

GOAL	INTERVENTION	RATIONALE	EXPECTED OUTCOME
3. Impaired social interaction related to decreased level of consciousness, hospitalization, and isolation			
	NIC Priority Intervention: **Socialization enhancement:** *Facilitation of the child's ability to interact with others*		*NOC Suggested Outcome:* **Role performance:** *Congruence of the child's role behavior with role expectations*
The child's social interaction will be near normal despite isolation.	▶ Educate parents and other visitors to use proper infection control techniques. ▶ Encourage parents to help with daily activities such as feeding and bathing.	▶ Family members help fulfill the emotional and social needs of the ill and contagious child. ▶ Parental involvement in the child's care provides the child with a sense of security and emotional well-being. Parents have a sense of control and a feeling that they are doing something to enhance the child's recovery.	The child's social and developmental needs are met by family members despite the child's illness and hospitalization.
	▶ Have age-appropriate games and toys in the room. Play with the child. When the child is feeling better, encourage watching television/videotape or listening to the radio/audiotape.	▶ Providing the child with toys and games as well as sensory stimulation helps the child achieve a sense of well-being.	
The child with any degree of hearing loss will be identified.	▶ Arrange for hearing assessment prior to discharge.	▶ Hearing loss is a common complication. Early intervention is needed to promote growth and development.	The child with identified hearing loss is referred to appropriate specialist or program for intervention.
4. Pain related to meningeal irritation			
	NIC Priority Intervention: **Pain management:** *Alleviation of pain or reduction in pain to a level of comfort acceptable to patient*		*NOC Suggested Outcome:* **Comfort level:** *Feelings of physical and psychologic ease*
The child will be as comfortable as possible.	▶ Minimize tactile stimulation. ▶ Allow the child to assume a comfortable position.	▶ Sensory stimulation increases discomfort. ▶ The child determines the most comfortable position. Opisthotonic position, with the head and neck hyper-extended, may be the most comfortable.	The child is calm and expresses increased comfort.
	▶ Keep the lights dim.	▶ Dim lights reduce the discomfort from photophobia.	
	▶ Maintain a quiet environment. Keep doors closed.	▶ Noise can disturb the child.	
5. Risk for infection (family and close contacts) related to pathogens in the cerebrospinal fluid			
	NIC Priority Intervention: **Infection control:** *Minimizing the acquisition and transmission of infectious agents*		*NOC Suggested Outcome:* **Risk control:** *Actions to eliminate an actual health threat*
Caretakers or family members will have no apparent evidence of infection.	▶ Explain rationale and dose schedule for taking rifampin or ciprofloxacin.	▶ Rifampin and ciprofloxacin provide prophylaxis for many bacterial pathogens responsible for meningitis.	Family members and other close contacts verbalize schedule for rifampin or ciprofloxacin therapy.

tant to monitor the serum sodium concentration and urine specific gravity because these children are at risk for the syndrome of insufficient antidiuretic hormone (SIADH; see Chapter 47). ⊂⊃ Fluids are restricted. Sodium chloride, potassium, and acetate or lactate are administered intravenously to balance sodium excretion.

Respond to parents' concerns about their child's condition, explaining all measures to reduce the child's discomfort and treat the illness. Identify ways parents can help meet the child's comfort needs. Parents may also need help figuring out how to meet the needs of other children at home while spending time with the hospitalized child.

DISCHARGE PLANNING AND HOME CARE TEACHING

Identify and address home care needs well in advance of discharge. Follow-up visits are important to monitor for complications and sequelae. Help parents deal with any physical requirements resulting from the child's illness and any emotional, social, and financial repercussions of the child's condition. Teach parents what to do if the child has a seizure. Remember that gastrointestinal bleeding is a potential complication of corticosteroid use. Teach parents to monitor the child on long-term corticosteroids for signs of intestinal discomfort and for blood in the stools.

Infants and toddlers with neurologic sequelae should be referred to an early intervention program. If the child has had a hearing loss, referral to an otolaryngologist and speech and language specialist should be made. Encourage early identification of other neurologic sequelae, such as learning problems. Children with hearing, learning, or attention disorders need individual education plans (see Chapter 35), and parents may need help planning for the child's special educational needs. Refer parents to the appropriate social service agencies for support and assistance.

Adolescents entering college should be encouraged to get the meningococcal vaccine to prevent meningococcal meningitis.

Evaluation

Expected outcomes of nursing care are provided in the "Nursing Care Plan."

VIRAL (ASEPTIC) MENINGITIS

Viral meningitis is an inflammatory response of the meninges characterized by an increased number of blood cells and protein in the cerebrospinal fluid. In the United States, an enterovirus is often the cause of aseptic meningitis (Cherry, 1999).

Generally, the child with aseptic meningitis does seem as ill as the child with bacterial meningitis. The child may be irritable or lethargic and usually has a fever. Other symptoms include general malaise, headache, photophobia, gastrointestinal distress, upper respiratory symptoms, and a maculopapular rash. The child may also show signs of meningeal irritation such as stiff neck, back pain, and positive Kernig and Brudzinski signs (see Figures 49–6 and 49–7). The infant may have a tense anterior fontanel. Seizures are rare. Symptoms usually resolve spontaneously within 3 to 10 days.

The child with fever and meningeal signs is hospitalized. Blood, urine, and cerebrospinal fluid analyses are performed. Until the diagnosis of aseptic meningitis is confirmed, the child is treated aggressively, as if he or she has bacterial meningitis.

Nursing Management

Initial nursing care focuses on providing supportive care as described for the child with bacterial meningitis. Give acetaminophen as ordered to reduce fever, headache, and muscle or joint pain. Keep the room dark and quiet (to decrease stimuli and meningeal irritation), give fluids either intravenously or orally, and promote comfort with proper positioning.

The child and family need information about the disease. Explain medical and nursing procedures in terms that the child and family can understand. Keep parents informed about the child's progress. Once the diagnosis of viral meningitis is made, immediately begin discharge planning and teaching for home care. Explain that recovery may take several weeks but that complete recovery is expected.

ENCEPHALITIS

Encephalitis is an inflammation of the brain usually caused by a viral infection. Inflammation of the meninges is also common (Moe & Seay, 1997).

Viruses are believed to cause most cases of encephalitis. Herpes simplex type I is the most common cause after the newborn period, and is associated with a high mortality rate. Other viruses causing encephalitis include enteroviruses (poliovirus, echovirus, and coxsackievirus), adenoviruses and herpesviruses, arboviruses, measles, mumps, rubella, rabies, and hepatitis B.

Signs and symptoms depend on the causative organism and the location of the infection within the brain. An acute onset of a febrile illness with neurologic signs is the classic manifestation of encephalitis. Initially the child may have a severe headache, fever, signs of an upper respiratory infection, and nausea or vomiting. Meningeal irritation signs such as nuchal rigidity, photophobia, and positive Kernig and Brudzinski signs are uncommon. Other neurologic signs vary. The child may be disoriented or confused, with behavioral or personality changes. Speech disturbances; motor dysfunction such as hemiparesis, ataxia, or weakness; cranial nerve deficits; or alterations in reflex response may be present. Focal or generalized seizures may occur, alternating with periods of screaming, hallucinating, and moving in a bizarre fashion. The child's level of consciousness may deteriorate from stupor to coma.

Diagnosis is based on history and laboratory findings. Information about recent immunizations, insect bites, or travel to areas where vectors are present should be obtained. Cerebrospinal fluid analysis, blood serologic tests, and nasopharyngeal and stool specimens are evaluated to identify viral pathogens. A CT scan, MRI, and EEG may also be performed. The nucleic acid detection test is used to assay for herpes DNA in the spinal fluid. Brain biopsy may be performed to diagnose herpes simplex and parasitic infections.

The child with encephalitis is at risk for seizures, respiratory failure, and increased intracranial pressure and should be cared for in an intensive care unit. Treatment is both pharmacologic and supportive. The child with a suspected bacterial infection should be treated with antibiotics until bacterial pathogens have been ruled out.

Children with encephalitis have many permanent neurologic sequelae. Although some children recover completely, many more are left with intellectual, motor, visual, or auditory deficits. The cardiovascular system, lungs, or liver may also be affected. Generally, the younger the child, the more serious the illness and the more severe the residual effects.

Nursing Management

Nursing care focuses on monitoring cardiorespiratory function, preventing complications resulting from immobility, reorienting the child, and teaching the parents about the child's condition.

Monitor the child's cardiorespiratory function. Check the child's airway and ability to handle secretions. Monitor respiratory status by observing color, pulse oximetry readings, and arterial blood gas values. Observe cardiopulmonary status by monitoring heart rate, blood pressure, capillary refill time, and urine output. Provide seizure precautions, and have appropriate equipment for managing seizures at the bedside (see Skill 14-20). **SKILLS** **CD**

Prevent complications resulting from immobility as described in Table 49–5. Maintain skin integrity. Proper positioning with frequent turning is important. When indicated by the physician, perform chest physiotherapy to prevent pneumonia.

The child whose level of consciousness begins to improve may at first be confused and disoriented and may have residual effects of the disease. Orient the child to the hospital environment. Have the family help to reorient the child by bringing favorite stuffed animals or music from home. Engage in therapeutic play (refer to Chapter 34 for techniques). Give the child age-appropriate toys to encourage a return to normal behavior.

Give the parents information about their child's condition and prognosis. If the child receives physical, occupational, or speech therapy, explain the treatment regimen to the parents.

DISCHARGE PLANNING AND HOME CARE TEACHING

Encourage parents to take an active role in the child's physical and emotional care in the hospital, and give them written instructions about home care. Encourage the parents to learn specific physical, occupational, and speech therapies so they can work with their child at home between home care visits. Refer parents to home care, social services, family counseling, and support groups. Plan follow-up visits so the child can be evaluated for neurologic sequelae.

REYE SYNDROME

Reye syndrome is an acute **encephalopathy,** a cerebral dysfunction caused by a toxic, injury, inflammatory, or anoxic insult that may result in permanent tissue damage, although the dysfunction may improve over time. In Reye syndrome the encephalopathy is parainfectious, and it also affects the liver, causing hepatic dysfunction. It is characterized by cerebral edema and an enlarged, fatty, poorly functioning liver.

The etiology of Reye syndrome is unclear. The disorder usually develops after a mild viral illness, such as varicella or influenza. It has also been associated with aspirin use. Since most parents give children acetaminophen rather than aspirin for flulike symptoms and varicella, Reye syndrome has become rare, but the mortality rate for children who develop the condition is high.

Nursing Practice

Make sure all parents know not to give aspirin when the child has a viral illness such as chickenpox or influenza because aspirin is associated with the development of Reye syndrome. Instruct parents to check all over-the-counter medicines for the presence of aspirin compounds. Emphasize the importance of obtaining health care whenever a child's condition worsens at the end of a viral illness.

Reye syndrome begins with nausea and vomiting, mental status changes, seizures, and progressive unresponsiveness (Ressler & Nelson, 2000). The condition has five stages, as described in Table 49–9. The condition is most severe in younger children.

The diagnosis of Reye syndrome is based on an abrupt change in the child's level of consciousness and diagnostic laboratory tests. The child has often progressed to coma or stage III by the time of diagnosis. Liver enzyme levels (aspartate aminotransferase [AST] or alanine aminotransferase [ALT]) are elevated to twice their normal levels, ammonia levels are elevated, blood glucose levels are below normal, and prothrombin time is prolonged. A liver biopsy is sometimes performed to confirm the diagnosis (by showing small droplet fat deposits).

The child with Reye syndrome should be placed in a pediatric intensive care unit because of the potential for rapid deterioration. The goal of medical management is to provide supportive treatment and to prevent the secondary effects of cerebral edema and metabolic injury. As-

TABLE 49–9	Stages of Reye Syndrome
Stage	Clinical Manifestations
I	Vomiting; lethargy; appropriate responses to verbal commands; purposeful responses to pain; brisk pupillary reaction
II	Combativeness; stupor; inappropriate language; confusion; anxiety, fear; purposeful and nonpurposeful responses to pain; sluggish pupillary reaction; conjugate deviation with oculocephalic reflex; hyperactive reflexes; progresses to coma but interrupted by periods of screaming and ranting
III	Coma; decorticate rigidity; conjugate deviation with diminished oculocephalic reflex; sluggish pupillary reaction; decorticate posturing
IV	Coma with brainstem dysfunction; decerebrate rigidity; inconsistent or absent oculocephalic reflex; loss of corneal reflex; sluggish pupillary reaction; decerebrate posturing
V	Coma with seizures; flaccidity; loss of deep tendon reflexes; respiratory arrest

sisted ventilation is often needed once the child is comatose. The child is monitored for signs of increased intracranial pressure, which can be secondary to cerebral edema. Hypoglycemia is treated with intravenous glucose, and electrolytes, blood chemistry, and blood pH are monitored.

Nursing Management

Nursing care focuses on monitoring the child's physical status, providing emotional support, and teaching parents about disease prevention.

Check the child's respiratory and neurologic status frequently, and note any signs of improvement or deterioration. Orient the child who awakens from coma. Refer to the discussion of nursing management of altered states of consciousness at the beginning of this chapter for specific nursing interventions. Look for changes in laboratory values that indicate acidosis, an elevation of ammonia levels, or hypoglycemia. Monitor the child's intake and output. Correct imbalances by administering fluids, electrolytes, or medications as ordered. Prevent complications associated with immobility.

Provide emotional support to the parents, who may feel guilty because they did not seek medical attention sooner. Keep them informed about the child's condition, and prepare them for potential deterioration. Explain treatments to help reduce anxiety. Encourage the parents to participate in the child's care whenever possible.

Once the child is discharged, monitoring is needed to observe for sequelae of the illness. Developmental and neurologic deficits may occur and are more severe in children under 2 years of age. Arrange for home nursing visits during the recovery period so that developmental and neurologic status monitoring can be assessed. Be sure the parents know about community resources that can help them deal with the child's recovery.

GUILLAIN-BARRÉ SYNDROME (POSTINFECTIOUS POLYNEURITIS)

Guillain-Barré syndrome is an acute inflammatory demyelinating polyneuropathy. This condition may lead to deteriorating motor function and paralysis that progresses in an ascending pattern. It is the most common cause of acute flaccid paralysis in infants and children (Jones, 2000). Guillain-Barré syndrome is caused by an immune response to an infectious organism, usually from a gastrointestinal or respiratory illness 2 to 3 weeks prior to onset. It has also been associated with immunizations and cytomegalovirus.

Infants have an onset of rapidly progressive severe hypotonia, possible respiratory distress, and feeding difficulties. Older children have rapidly progressive symmetric weakness and muscle pain with varying degrees of distal paresthesia and numbness in the legs. This weakness spreads to the upper extremities, trunk, chest, neck, face, and head. Deep tendon reflexes may be diminished or absent. The child may develop acute ataxia. Respiratory effort may be inadequate for proper ventilation. Facial paresis and difficulty swallowing follow. Cranial nerves may be affected, causing Bell's palsy, for example. A dysfunctional autonomic nervous system may cause such symptoms as hypertension, postural hypertension, sinus tachycardia or bradycardia, excessive diaphoresis, urinary and bowel incontinence, and facial flushing.

Diagnostic criteria of Guillain-Barré syndrome include (1) progressive motor weakness (minimal weakness of the legs to total paralysis of all extremities), and (2) areflexia of varying degrees. Two tests are diagnostic. Lumbar puncture obtains cerebrospinal fluid; increased protein levels (80 to 200 mg/dL) with fewer than 50 lymphocytes per cubic millimeter indicate the condition (Jones, 2000). Electroconduction tests such as electromyography are also used. An abnormal pattern of nerve conduction indicates Guillain-Barré syndrome.

Clinical therapy for Guillain-Barré syndrome is plasmapheresis or intravenous immune globulin if the child cannot ambulate. Guidelines for administration of intravenous immune globulin can be found in Chapter 40. Responses to intravenous immune globulin are dramatic, often within days. If the child can ambulate, physical therapy and supportive care are provided. The condition is rarely fatal.

Nursing Management

Nursing care focuses on monitoring respiratory status, meeting nutritional needs, managing autonomic nervous system dysfunction, preventing complications associated with immobility, providing emotional support, and teaching the parents how to care for the child after discharge.

MONITOR RESPIRATORY STATUS

Monitor the child's respiratory status closely, especially in the early phase of illness. Look for such signs as dyspnea, inability to handle secretions, inadequate respiratory effort, and color changes that may indicate the need for endotracheal intubation and mechanical ventilation.

MANAGE AUTONOMIC NERVOUS SYSTEM DYSFUNCTION

Monitor the child's vital signs closely for episodes of tachycardia, bradycardia, and hypotension. Blood pressure fluctuations and autonomic instability are linked to fatal cardiac arrythmias (Jones, 2000). Observe frequently for decreased responsiveness. Intervene promptly if these or other signs of autonomic nervous system dysfunction are noted.

MEET NUTRITIONAL NEEDS

Assess whether the child is having difficulty swallowing. If the child has no gag reflex, maintain nutritional needs with intravenous supplements or nasogastric tube feedings.

PREVENT COMPLICATIONS

Prevent complications associated with immobility (see Table 49–5). Ensure good postural alignment, and turn the child every 2 hours. Maintaining skin integrity is also important.

Evaluate the child's muscle tone, strength, and symmetry. When the child's condition begins to improve, recovery of lost strength is the priority. Active exercise is emphasized in physical therapy. Encourage family members to participate in the child's care, especially during the recovery phase. They can help with the activities of daily living and reinforce what the child has learned in physical therapy.

PROVIDE EMOTIONAL SUPPORT

Explain the progression of Guillain-Barré syndrome to the parents during the initial stages. Witnessing a rapid deterioration in their child's physical status can be frightening; therefore, preparation is essential to reduce their anxieties. Be honest when discussing recovery and prognosis for the child.

Have parents bring in favorite toys, dolls, or books to make the child feel more secure. Playing with or reading to the child can be comforting.

DISCHARGE PLANNING AND HOME CARE TEACHING

Identify and address home care needs well in advance of discharge. Support the parents as they prepare for the child's return home. Provide referral to home care nurses who can manage all aspects of treatment, rehabilitation, and follow-up. Refer the parents to social workers, who can help with financial arrangements and school considerations.

NURSING CARE IN THE COMMUNITY

Help the child to adjust to any residual effects of Guillain-Barré syndrome. Help the child practice exercises learned in physical therapy sessions, and encourage the child to perform activities of daily living, such as brushing the teeth or combing the hair. Refer the child to outpatient rehabilitation programs to promote recovery.

To promote a positive self-image, praise any effort the child makes to be self-sufficient. The child may be frustrated and angry. Allow the child to express these feelings in an appropriate way, either during play or in conversation.

⁓ STRUCTURAL DEFECTS

HYDROCEPHALUS

Hydrocephalus is the body's response to an imbalance between the production and absorption of cerebrospinal fluid. The condition is often congenital, but may be related to prematurity. The incidence is 3 to 4 per 1000 births. A recessive X-linked genetic hydrocephalus accounts for a small number of cases (Jackson & Harvey, 2000). Hydrocephalus can develop in older children as a complication of illness or trauma.

Etiology and Pathophysiology

Hydrocephalus may be either communicating or noncommunicating, and congenital or acquired. Communicating hydrocephalus is the blockage of flow or absorption of cerebrospinal fluid in the subarachnoid space and the arachnoid villi. It can be acquired from postinfectious meningitis or intraventricular hemorrhage; be congenital; or be of unknown etiology.

Noncommunicating hydrocephalus is responsible for most cases in children. It results from a blockage in the ventricular system that prevents cerebrospinal fluid from entering the subarachnoid space (see "Pathophysiology Illustrated: Hydrocephalus"). This obstruction can be caused by infection, hemorrhage, tumor, or structural deformity. Congenital structural defects such as the Arnold-Chiari II malformation (found in most children with myelomeningocele) and the Dandy-Walker syndrome block the flow of cerebrospinal fluid (Jackson & Harvey, 2000).

Clinical Manifestations

The signs and symptoms of hydrocephalus vary with the age of the child (see "Clinical Manifestations: Hydrocephalus"). The predominant manifestation of the condition in infants is rapid head growth (Figure 49–8 ◆). Older children show signs of increased intracranial pressure (see Table 49–2).

Clinical Therapy

The diagnosis of hydrocephalus in infants is based on clinical manifestations. In the hospital setting, daily measurements of the infant's head circumference are critical in any infant at risk of developing hydrocephalus. In older children, signs of increased intracranial pressure are noted.

CT scanning and MRI diagnose hydrocephalus, and in some cases reveal the anatomic cause. In the infant whose

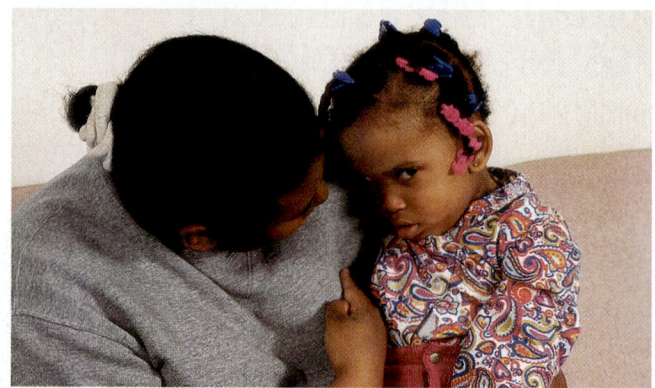

FIGURE 49–8. ◆ In communicating hydrocephalus, an excessive amount of cerebrospinal fluid accumulates in the subarachnoid space, producing the characteristic head enlargement seen here. Note the downward deviation of the eyes so that the lower half of the iris is hidden by the lower eyelid. This finding occurs in severe hydrocephalus.

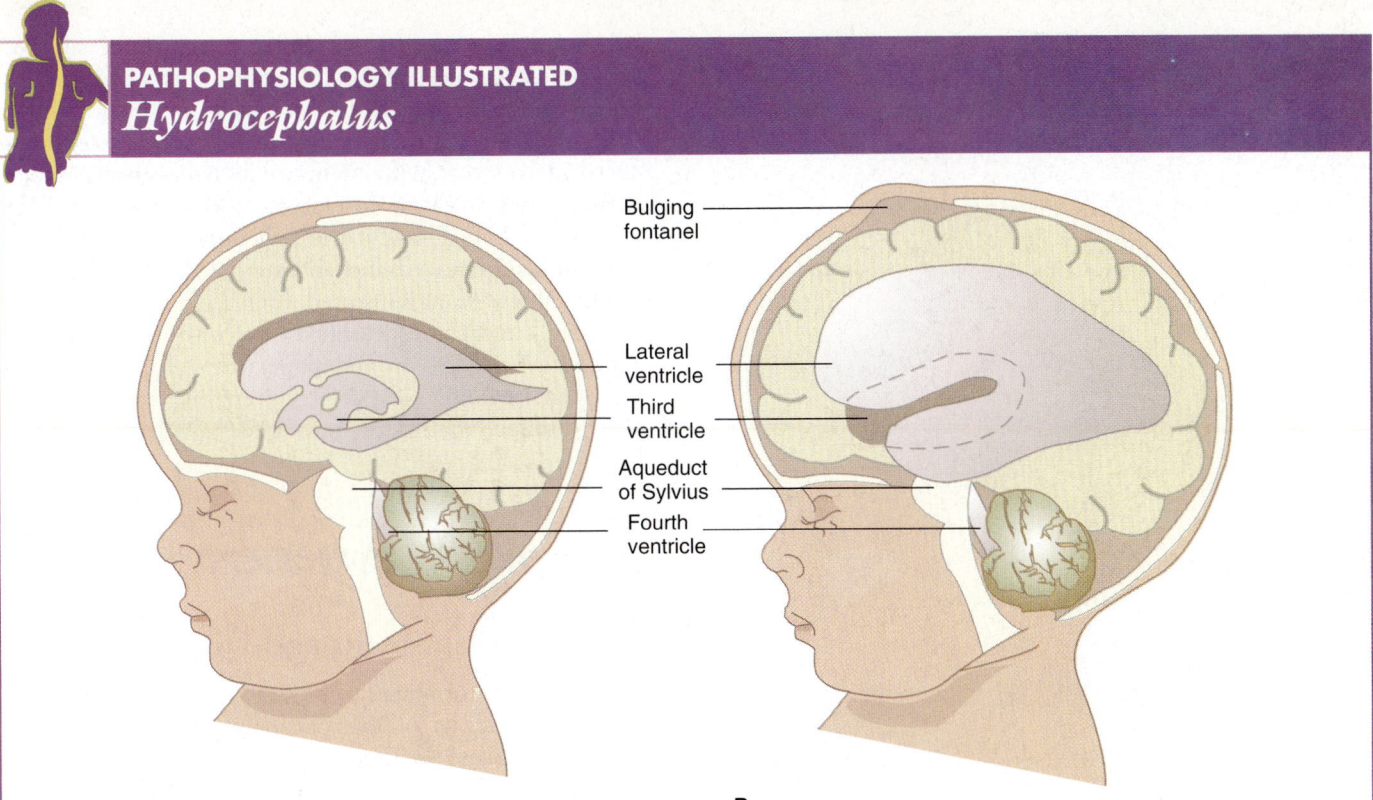

Bulging fontanel

Lateral ventricle

Third ventricle

Aqueduct of Sylvius

Fourth ventricle

A

B

A, Normal size of ventricle. **B,** Enlarged ventricles, characteristic of hydrocephalus.

CLINICAL MANIFESTATIONS ∼ *Hydrocephalus*

CAUSES	CLINICAL MANIFESTATIONS
Congenital Structural Defect in Infancy 　Dandy-Walker syndrome 　Arnold-Chiari II malformation	Early signs 　Rapid head growth 　Tense, bulging fontanel, split sutures 　Bossing (protrusion) of frontal area 　Prominent scalp veins 　Translucent skin 　Increased tone or hyperreflexia 　Irritability or lethargy, poor feeding 　Decline in level of consciousness Late signs 　Shrill, high-pitched cry 　Difficulty swallowing or feeding 　Macewen's or "cracked-pot" sign 　Sunsetting eyes (sclera visible above iris), sixth cranial nerve palsy 　Vomiting 　Cardiopulmonary depression (severe cases)
Acquired Hydrocephalus in Older Child 　Postinfectious 　Tumor 　Hemorrhage	No head enlargement Headache upon arising with vomiting Fussiness, sleepiness, confusion, or apathy Personality change, loss of interest in daily activities Poor judgment or verbal incoherence Ataxia, spasticity, or other alterations in motor development Visual defects secondary to pressure on second, third, and sixth cranial nerves Signs of increased intracranial pressure

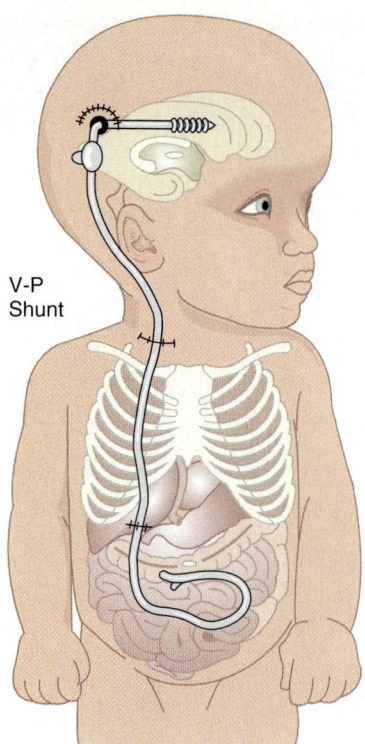

FIGURE 49–9. ◆ A ventriculoperitoneal shunt, commonly used to treat children with hydrocephalus, is usually placed at 3–4 months of age.

V-P Shunt

fontanel is still open, ultrasonography or echoencephalography may be used to confirm the diagnosis.

Clinical therapy for hydrocephalus involves removing the obstruction (e.g., surgical removal of a tumor) or creating a new cerebrospinal fluid (CSF) pathway to divert excess CSF. A catheter or shunt is placed in the ventricle and passes the CSF to the peritoneal cavity, atrium of the heart, or the pleural spaces. Ventriculoperitoneal shunts (Figure 49–9 ◆) are commonly used. Shunt systems consist of four parts: a ventricular catheter, a pumping chamber or reservoir, a one-way pressure valve, and a distal catheter. Initial shunt placement is usually performed early in infancy, with replacement two to four times as the child grows. Researchers in neuroendoscopy are developing techniques to create a new pathway for CSF to flow between the ventricles and spinal cord in people with obstructive hydrocephalus. The new endoscopy procedure may be used in some patients in the future to avoid shunt placement (Jackson & Harvey, 2000).

Mechanical complications may include blockage at either the proximal or the distal end of the catheter, kinking of the tubing, or valve breakdown. Infants or children with shunt failure show signs and symptoms of recurrent hydrocephalus and increased intracranial pressure. Shunt failure and ventricular size are confirmed by CT scanning or MRI. Shunt materials and systems continue to be refined in an attempt to reduce mechanical problems.

The most serious complication is shunt infection, which may occur at any time but is most prevalent in the first 2 months after placement. The most important signs of shunt infection are changes in responsiveness and irritability after fever is controlled. Other signs include low-grade fever, malaise, headache, and nausea. The infection rate is 4% to 12% per year, with infants under 6 months having the highest rates (Jackson & Harvey, 2000). Antibiotics are usually prescribed, but if the infection is overwhelming, the shunt is removed and an external drainage device is placed. A new shunt is inserted when the infection resolves.

Some children, especially those with ventriculoatrial shunts, are placed on the same prophylactic antibiotic treatment regimen used for children with cardiac anomalies to reduce the risk of shunt infections (refer to Chapter 43). 🔗

Nursing Management

Nursing Assessment and Diagnosis

It is important for nurses to become familiar with the clinical manifestations of hydrocephalus to ensure prompt identification and treatment of children with this condition. Measure head circumference of all infants at each well-child visit to detect the condition at an early stage.

Assess the child with a ventriculoperitoneal shunt for signs and symptoms of shunt failure and infection. Measure the infant's head circumference daily when shunt failure is suspected (see Skill 9-5). 🔗 **SKILLS** Report any abnormalities to the physician immediately.

Nursing diagnoses that might be appropriate for the child with hydrocephalus include:

▶ *Risk for infection* related to presence of shunt

▶ *Impaired physical mobility (level 2)* related to decreased muscle mass to lift the increased weight of head

▶ *Risk for caregiver role strain* related to care of a child with a chronic condition or life-threatening illness

▶ *Anxiety (parent)* related to repeated surgeries and life-threatening illness

▶ *Risk for injury* related to potential shunt failure

Planning and Implementation

HOSPITAL-BASED NURSING CARE

Nursing care focuses on providing preoperative and postoperative care and providing emotional support.

Provide preoperative care. Measure the child's head circumference daily and watch for signs of increased intracranial pressure (see Table 49–2). Measure fluid intake and output as ordered. Carefully assess respiratory status. Provide good skin care.

Position the child carefully; do not stretch or strain the neck muscles, since they must support the large head. Holding the child may be difficult because of the additional weight of the head. Reduce the chances for skin breakdown by placing sheepskin or a lamb's wool blanket under the head. Prevent any other complications associated with immobility (see Table 49–5).

Attend to the child's special nutritional needs. Because the infant is prone to vomiting, frequent small feedings with frequent burping are beneficial.

After surgery the child is usually placed in a flat position to prevent rapid CSF drainage. The head of the bed is elevated gradually. Take vital signs every 2 to 4 hours. Monitor the child carefully for any signs of shunt malfunction, increased intracranial pressure, or infection.

Support the parents and explain the child's condition and all procedures to be performed. Encourage parents and family to help with the child's care in the hospital when appropriate. Be sympathetic and understanding, and allow parents to express their concerns. If hydrocephalus occurs during early infancy, the parents will be anxious about the impact of the chronic condition and subsequent surgical procedures. If hydrocephalus is secondary to neoplasm, however, the parents' anxieties are compounded by their child's life-threatening illness. Assure parents that most children with shunts lead normal lives, attending school and interacting with others no differently from their peers.

DISCHARGE PLANNING AND HOME CARE TEACHING

Identify and address home care needs well in advance of discharge. Teach parents how to care for a child with a shunt. Make parents and other family members aware of the signs and symptoms of both shunt failure (signs of increased intracranial pressure) and infection (changes in responsiveness, irritability, malaise, headache, nausea, and low-grade fever). Give them the telephone numbers of the pediatrician and the neurosurgeon, and make sure that they understand that they should contact a physician immediately if they suspect a problem. Inform them that the shunt may need to be replaced one or more times in childhood as the child grows. Arrange appropriate home care referrals. Refer families to the appropriate psychologic and social services, such as the Hydrocephalus Association. 🔗 WEB

NURSING CARE IN THE COMMUNITY

Infants and children need frequent monitoring to ensure proper shunt functioning. Head circumference is measured at each visit to monitor growth. Assess the child for visual problems and cognitive, speech, and motor developmental delays. Refer the child and family to an early intervention program to promote developmental progress. School-age children may need to have an individual education plan developed (see Chapter 35). 🔗 Intellectual functioning outcomes may be associated with the cause of the hydrocephalus. For example, children with uncomplicated congenital causes do better than those with brain injury, infection, or intraventricular hemorrhage causes. About 70% of hydrocephalic children function below the normal IQ range (Jackson & Harvey, 2000).

Encourage parents seeking child care for their infant to use a setting with fewer children to decrease exposure to infection. Review the signs of shunt failure and infection with parents at each visit and make sure they have a plan to manage the emergency of a shunt failure.

Teach parents to protect the infant from injury. Infants with poor head control due to an enlarged head should not be placed in forward-facing car safety seats, regardless of their age. For these children, this position increases the risk of cervical spine injury and death in a car crash. As the child grows, encourage parents to avoid becoming overprotective and to allow the child to develop normally. Participation in sports with a high potential for head and abdominal impact should be discouraged.

Evaluation

Expected outcomes of nursing care include the following:

▶ The child develops adequate neck muscle control to interact with the environment.

▶ Shunt infections and malfunctions are identified by the parents and medical attention is sought quickly.

▶ Potential for growth and development is maximized by care and a stimulating environment.

SPINA BIFIDA

Spina bifida, a congenital neural tube defect that affects the head and spinal column, is the most common developmental disorder of the CNS. It is a malformation of the neural tube that can occur anywhere along the spine. Another less common neural tube defect is anencephaly, an exposed or absent brain. Spina bifida occurs in about 1 per 2000 births in the United States each year but varies by region of the country (Northrup & Volcik, 2000).

Developing Cultural Competence

The incidence of spina bifida varies with ethnicity and geographic location in the United States. Hispanic people, especially those in Texas, have the highest rate. The incidence in other ethnic groups in descending order are Caucasians, African Americans, and Asian Americans (Northrup, 2000).

The cause of spina bifida is unknown, although environmental factors such as chemicals, medications (e.g., valproic acid used for seizures), and maternal health conditions (insulin-dependent diabetes mellitus, gestational diabetes, folic acid deficiency, and maternal obesity) have been implicated. The increased incidence of the condition in families indicates a possible genetic influence. Mandatory fortification of all enriched grain products with folate has reduced the prevalence of neural tube defects by 19%.

Educational efforts to increase folic acid supplementation to women of childbearing age has led to fewer cases of spina bifida (Honein, Paulozzi, Matthew, et al., 2001).

There are several different types of spina bifida (see "Pathophysiology Illustrated: Types of Spina Bifida"). A saclike protrusion on the infant's back indicates meningocele or myelomeningocele (see Figure 49–10 ◆). The clinical manifestations seen depend on the location of the defect: the higher the defect, the greater the neurologic dysfunction. The lower extremities may be completely paralyzed with anesthesia of the skin, or there may be varying degrees of immobility with orthopedic problems of the hips, knees, and feet. Bowel and bladder sphincters may be affected. Renal involvement may occur secondary to neurologic impairment and urinary retention. Hydrocephalus is usually present in children with myelomeningocele because of the Arnold-Chiari II malformation, in which there is downward displacement of the cerebellum, brainstem, and fourth ventricle. Because these structures control respiration and the protective reflexes, as well as house the cranial nerves, the displacement can have varying effects such as sudden death, respiratory difficulty, swallowing difficulties, and the need for assisted ventilation. Signs and symptoms may occur at any time, and this is the leading cause of death for children with spina bifida. The range of potential problems for the child with spina bifida is listed in "Clinical Manifestations: Spina Bifida."

Diagnosis is usually made prenatally, but after birth the lesion is examined and the neurologic status is evaluated. Radiologic imaging by CT scan, MRI, and flat films of the spinal column can pinpoint the bony defect. Surgery to

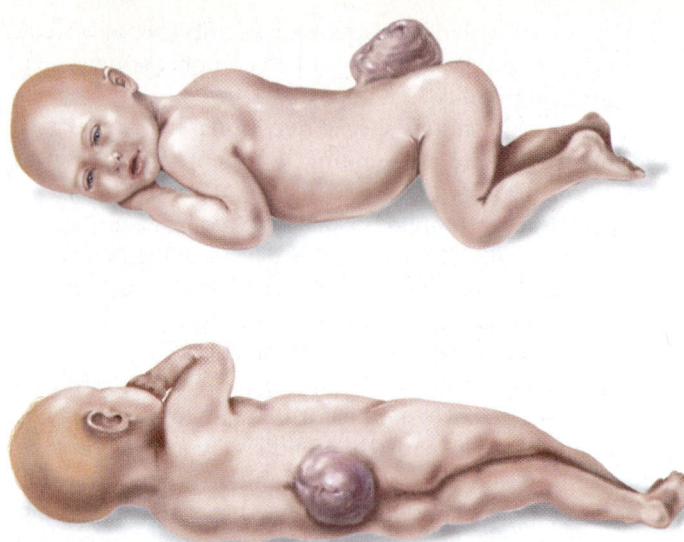

FIGURE 49–10. ◆ Lumbosacral myelomeningocele is caused by a neural tube defect that results in incomplete closure of the vertebral column. As shown here, the meninges (and sometimes the spinal cord) protrude as a saclike structure.

close and repair the lesion usually occurs within 24 to 48 hours of the infant's birth to reduce infection. In some cases, uteromyelomeningocele repairs are performed. Early outcomes for carefully selected infants for this procedure show decreased shunting for hydrocephalus and resolution of the Arnold-Chiari II malformation (Sutton, Adzick, Belaniuk, et al., 1999).

CLINICAL MANIFESTATIONS ≈ *Spina Bifida*

CAUSE	CLINICAL MANIFESTATIONS
Interruption of the spinal cord at site of the spinal defect	Paralysis of legs Scoliosis or kyphosis Incontinence of urine and feces, constipation Anesthesia of skin
Muscle imbalance	Hip abnormalities, hip dysplasia Foot deformities, e.g., clubfoot

Arnold-Chiari II malformation	Hydrocephalus
	Infants:
	    Difficulty swallowing
	    Apnea, respiratory difficulty, inspiratory stridor
	    Weak or poor cry
	    Sustained arching of head
	Older children:
	    Stiffness or spasticity of arms and hands
	    Loss of feeling or sensation

Brain and spinal cord abnormalities	Learning problems, attention deficit disorder Problems with perceptual motor skills Memory and organization problems Problems with numerical reasoning

Note: From Northrup, H., & Volcik, K. A. (2000). Spinal bifida and other neural tube defects. *Current Problems in Pediatrics, 30*(10), 417–431. Adapted.

PATHOPHYSIOLOGY ILLUSTRATED
Types of Spina Bifida

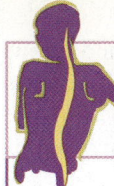

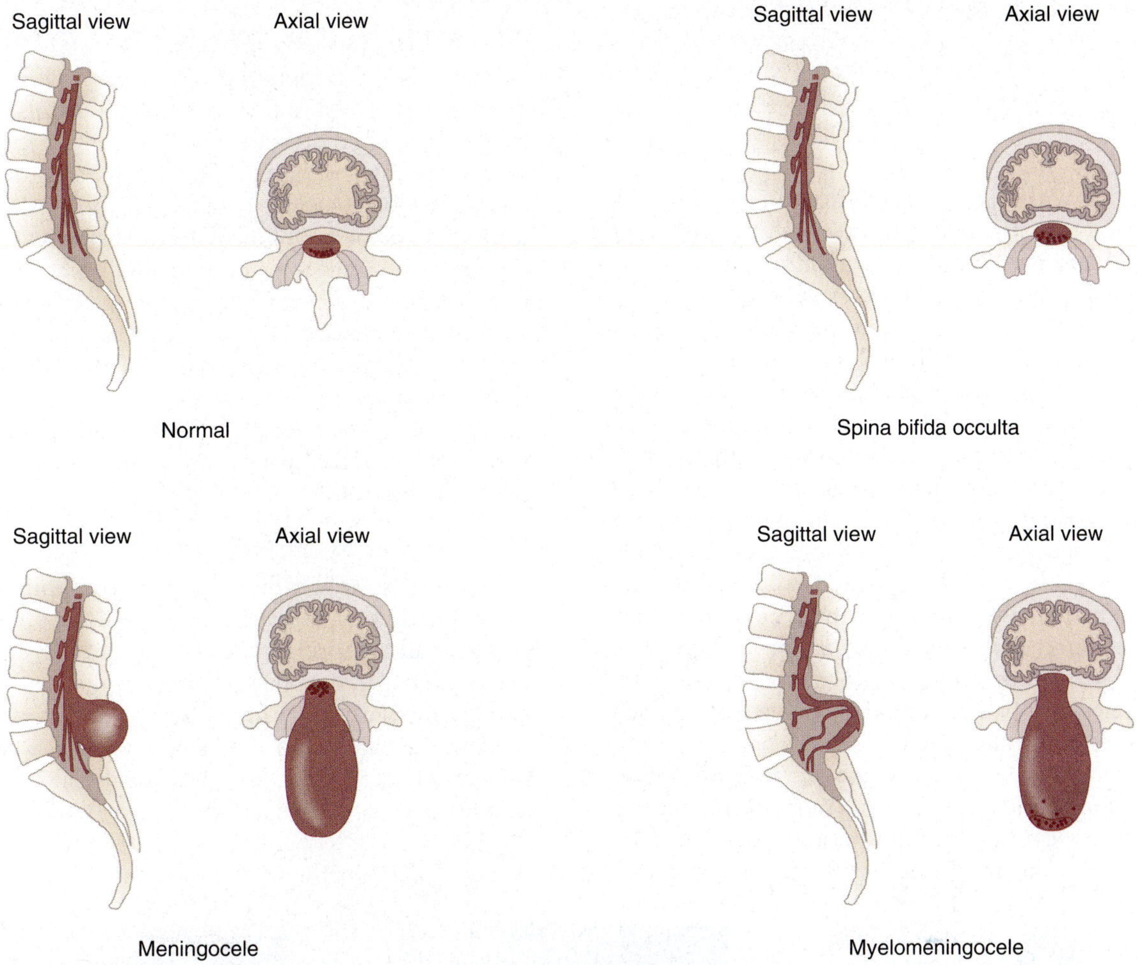
Sagittal view
Axial view
Normal
Sagittal view
Axial view
Spina bifida occulta
Sagittal view
Axial view
Meningocele
Sagittal view
Axial view
Myelomeningocele

Spina bifida occulta	Failure of posterior vertebral arches to fuse, most commonly at fifth lumbar or first sacral vertebrae; spinal cord and meninges entirely within vertebral canal; condition usually not visible externally; tuft of hair, a dermoid cyst, or hemangioma may be found over the site; mildest form
Spina bifida cystica	Defect in closure of posterior vertebral arch with protrusion through bony spine
Meningocele	Saclike protrusion through bony defect containing meninges and cerebrospinal fluid; sac covering defect may be translucent or membranous; spinal cord and spinal root in normal position
Myelomeningocele	Saclike herniation through bony defect holding meninges, cerebrospinal fluid, as well as a portion of spinal cord or nerve roots; fluid leakage may also occur; lesion poorly covered with imperfect tissue; handicap 99% of time; more common than meningocele

Prognosis depends on the type of defect, the level of the lesion, and other complicating factors. Children need multiple surgeries and invasive procedures. A team of physicians, nurses, and therapists from the neurosurgery, orthopedic, urology, and physical medicine departments work with the child and family to form a comprehensive care plan.

Nursing Management

HOSPITAL-BASED NURSING CARE

Nursing care focuses on providing preoperative and postoperative care, promoting mobility, and providing emotional support.

Growth and Development

Treat older children according to their intellectual level, not their motor development. Encourage them to take responsibility for self-care, and recognize their need to control their body functions. Promote interaction with peers in the hospital and participation in activities. If children are hospitalized for an extended time, arrange schooling.

Cover the sac with a sterile saline dressing to protect its integrity. Place the infant in a prone position with hips slightly flexed and legs abducted to minimize tension on the sac. Maintain this position using towel rolls placed between the knees. Assess the infant regularly for motor deficits as well as bladder and bowel involvement.

The infant is difficult to handle before surgery. Feed the infant with the head turned to one side until surgery has been performed. Comfort the infant before surgery with tactile stimulation such as touching, patting, and cuddling.

Following surgery, monitor the infant's vital signs carefully. Watch closely for symptoms of infection, especially meningitis. If a ventriculoperitoneal shunt was placed, watch for hydrocephalus, increased intracranial pressure, or infection. Inspect the surgical site for CSF leakage. The infant should be placed in the prone or side-lying position, or in some cases may be held upright. Splints may be used to maintain extremity alignment.

Promote mobility by beginning gentle range of motion exercises as soon as possible to prevent muscle contractures and atrophy. Use extreme caution because these children have brittle bones and are subject to idiopathic fractures.

Support the parents by keeping them informed about their child's status. Allow them to express their frustrations and anger. As soon as parents are able to cope with the child's condition, encourage them to become involved in the child's care in the hospital.

DISCHARGE PLANNING AND HOME CARE TEACHING

Identify and address home care needs well in advance of discharge. Make sure family members understand how to care for the child at home. Help them get special devices such as splints, wedges, and rolls, if needed, to prevent complications. Instruct parents how to position, handle, feed, and perform range of motion exercises. Teach them the signs and symptoms of increased intracranial pressure, hydrocephalus, shunt infection or malfunction, and urinary tract infection. Arrange home care nursing, if necessary. The home care nurse reinforces the skills learned in the hospital setting and coordinates the numerous health care professionals working with the child and family. Refer parents to resource groups such as the Spina Bifida Association of America. 🔗 WEB

NURSING CARE IN THE COMMUNITY

To reduce complications and promote optimal development, children with spina bifida need comprehensive care planned and coordinated by a knowledgeable team of health care professionals. This care may be provided in partnership with the primary care physician.

Promote safety and independent mobility with proper use of braces, walkers, crutches, canes, and in some cases custom-designed wheelchairs and car safety seats (Figure 49–11 ◆). For other safety guidelines, see "Teaching About: Safety for the Child with Spina Bifida."

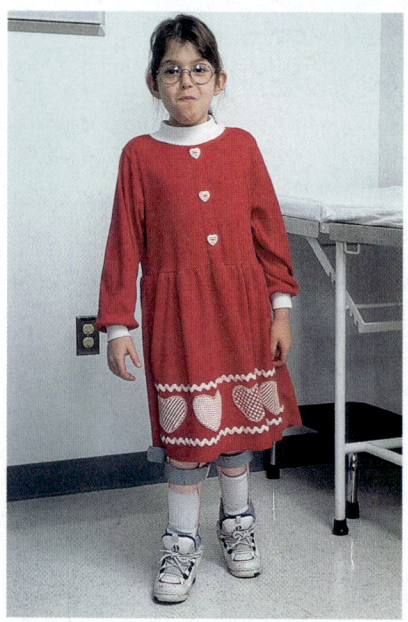
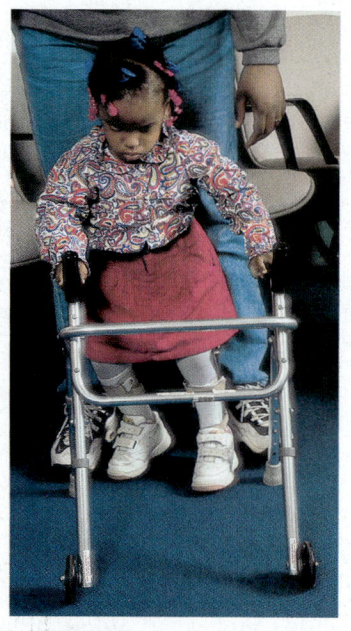
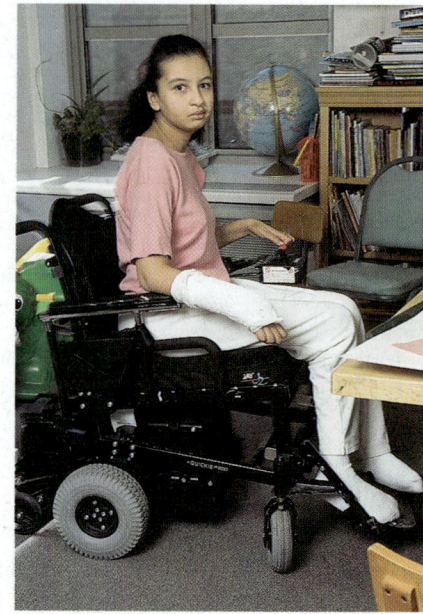

A   **B**   **C**

FIGURE 49–11. ◆ Help determine the best assistive device for the child to gain the most independence for mobilizing and to promote development. The child may change devices in different settings to promote optimal independence. **A** and **B,** Braces and walkers may be best for young children to promote an upright posture that encourages a normal interaction with the environment. **C,** A motorized wheelchair can assist the child with a significant neurologic impairment to achieve independence and mobility.

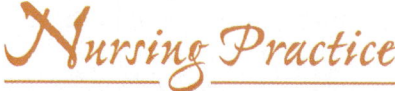

Teaching About

SAFETY FOR THE CHILD WITH SPINA BIFIDA

Due to the loss of sensation in the lower extremities, injuries to the skin are not noticed by the child.

- Each day, check all skin surfaces and pressure points associated with sitting, braces, shoes, etc., for abrasions, scrapes, reddened areas, and other lesions.
- Keep all skin surfaces clean and dry.
- Use a gel-filled cushion and teach the child to shift position when in the wheelchair to avoid pressure sores.
- Avoid burns to the lower extremities by checking the temperature of bath water and car safety seats in a hot car.
- Take latex precautions as the child is at high risk for latex allergy. Inform all health care providers about the child's latex allergy.
- Use safe ambulation techniques with walkers, canes, and crutches.

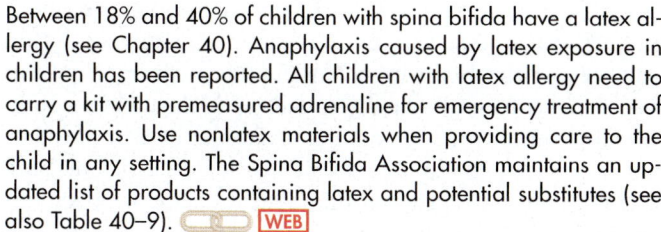

Between 18% and 40% of children with spina bifida have a latex allergy (see Chapter 40). Anaphylaxis caused by latex exposure in children has been reported. All children with latex allergy need to carry a kit with premeasured adrenaline for emergency treatment of anaphylaxis. Use nonlatex materials when providing care to the child in any setting. The Spina Bifida Association maintains an updated list of products containing latex and potential substitutes (see also Table 40–9). **WEB**

Parents may need to learn how to catheterize the child and then at an appropriate age teach the child intermittent self-catheterization to prevent urinary tract infections and other renal complications. Good nutrition planning is important to prevent obesity and to reduce constipation and complications such as fecal impaction. Surgery to create a channel between the skin and bowel (Malone antegrade continence enema) is sometimes performed. Children need to be taught to assume greater responsibility for self-care as they get older.

Parents are faced with the long-term financial issues of caring for the child who needs regular new adaptive equipment to match growth, as well as other medical supplies. At least 75% of children born with spina bifida generally survive to at least the early adult years (Bowman, McLone, Grant, et al., 2001). Parents thus need to learn how to act as the child's case manager, or to work effectively with another person in this role.

CRANIOSYNOSTOSIS

Craniosynostosis is the premature closing of the cranial sutures during the first 18 months of life. This condition occurs in up to 1 in 2000 births (Renier, Lajeunie, Arnaud, et al., 2000). Most children have no family history of the condition, although 15% have autosomal dominant inherited syndromes such as Alpert syndrome and Crouzon syndrome (Robinson, 1999).

The cause of craniosynostosis is unknown. Closure of the sutures usually takes place at predetermined times during the child's development. Problems arise if one or more sutures close early. Bone growth continues in a direction parallel to the suture line, which leads to compensatory overgrowth at normal suture lines and the classic skull deformities associated with craniosynostosis (Figure 49–12 ◆). Positional plagiocephaly, a totally flat occiput, is seen increasingly in healthy infants because they are put to sleep on their back to prevent sudden infant death syndrome. Since the infant's sleep position does not change, the weight of the head sometimes flattens the skull. A helmet device that corrects the deformation from positional plagiocephaly has been approved by the Food and Drug Administration. It is worn for 3 to 4 hours a day and it generally improves the head shape in 3 to 4 months.

Diagnosis is made by clinical appearance. Palpation of the skull reveals a bony ridge along a suture. Skull x-ray films, CT scan, and MRI confirm the diagnosis. The hands and feet should be carefully examined to detect any skeletal defect that could be associated with a syndrome (Renier et al., 2000).

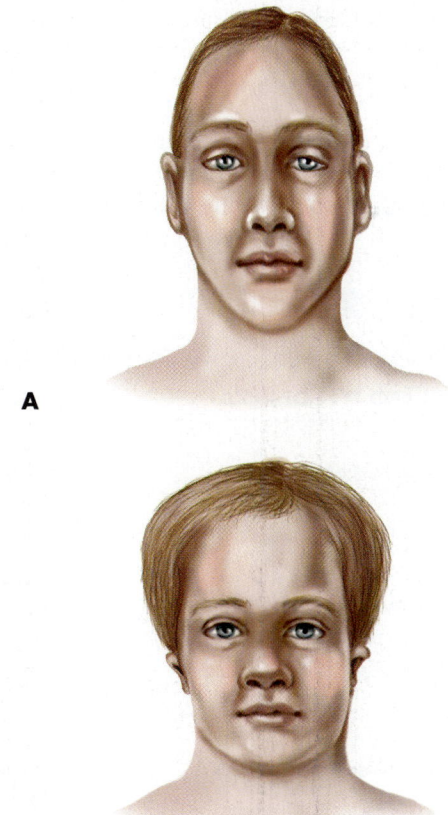

A

B

FIGURE 49–12. ◆ In craniosynostosis, the head shape is dependent upon which sutures are involved. Examples of different head shapes include those shown in **A** and **B.**

Reconstructive surgery, the most common form of treatment, is performed to protect mental development and vision. Many children need multiple procedures. Children having surgery before 1 year of age have a better outcome. After surgery, it is important for the incision to remain dry and intact. The nurse should also observe the child for symptoms of increased intracranial pressure (see Table 49–2).

Explain to parents that surgery will improve the child's appearance. Assure them that most children with craniosynostosis are healthy, and that their brains develop normally.

For information on neonatal substance abuse see Chapter 28.

CEREBRAL PALSY

Cerebral palsy is a nonprogressive motor and posture dysfunction that occurs secondary to CNS insults of congenital, hypoxic, ischemic, or traumatic origin, occurring in the prenatal, perinatal, or postnatal (up to 2 years) periods. Cerebral palsy is the most common chronic disorder of childhood, occurring in an estimated 1.4 to 3 per 1000 births (Nehring, 2000). Four types of motor dysfunction are seen with cerebral palsy—spastic, dyskinetic, ataxic, and mixed—related to the location of brain insult (see "Clinical Manifestations of Cerebral Palsy by Type of Insult").

Etiology and Pathophysiology

Most cerebral palsy cases are believed to be caused by intrauterine insults or structural abnormalities of the CNS (Nelson & Grether, 1999). During gestation, insufficient nutrients and oxygen can cause damage to the developing brain of the fetus. Very premature infants are at high risk because of their immature central nervous systems and the measures taken at birth to promote their survival. The survival of more premature infants has led to higher numbers of anoxic episodes. The incidence of cerebral palsy has not decreased, and the incidence of spastic diplegia has increased with technology improvements (Nelson & Grether, 1999). Injury at birth may be due to direct trauma to the brain or to asphyxia resulting from cord collapse, strangulation, or meconium aspiration. Asphyxia accounts for a small proportion of cerebral palsy cases. Neonatal sepsis and hyperbilirubinemia place the child at higher risk. In young children, CNS infection and head trauma are the major sources of acquired brain injury and subsequent motor dysfunction.

Clinical Manifestations

Cerebral palsy is characterized by abnormal muscle tone and lack of coordination with spasticity found in the majority of cases (Table 49–10). Children have a variety of symptoms depending on their ages. See table below for clinical manifestations by type of central nervous system injury. There is wide variability in symptoms depending on the area of the brain involved and the degree of anoxia. Children with cerebral palsy usually are delayed in meeting developmental milestones. For example, at 6 months of age, they may be unable to sit up, have persistent back arching, and have little spontaneous movement. They frequently have other problems, including visual defects such as strabismus, nystagmus, or refractory errors; hearing loss; language delay; speech impediment; seizures; or mental retardation.

CLINICAL MANIFESTATIONS ～ Cerebral Palsy by Type of Insult

CLASSIFICATION AND TYPE OF INSULT	CLINICAL MANIFESTATIONS
Spastic Cerebral cortex or pyramidal tract injury	Persistent hypertonia, rigidity Exaggerated deep tendon reflexes Persistent primitive reflexes Leads to contractures and abnormal curvature of the spine
Dyskinetic Extrapyramidal, basal ganglia injury	Impairment of voluntary muscle control Bizarre twisting movements Tremors, difficulty with fine and purposeful motor movements Exaggerated posturing Inconsistent muscle tone
Ataxic Cerebellar (extrapyramidal) injury	Lack of balance and position sense Hypotonia in infancy Muscle instability and gait disturbances
Mixed Injuries to multiple areas	Unique compensatory movements and posture to maintain control over specific neuromotor deficits Combination of characteristics from other types

TABLE 49–10 Clinical Characteristics of Cerebral Palsy

Clinical Characteristics	Definitions
Hypotonia	Floppiness, increased range of motion of joints, diminished reflex response
Hypertonia	
Rigidity	Tense, tight muscles
Spasticity	Uncoordinated, awkward, stiff movements; scissoring or crossing of the legs; exaggerated reflex reactions
Athetosis	Constant involuntary writhing motions that are more severe distally
Ataxia	Irregularity in muscle coordination or action
Hemiplegia	Involvement of one side of the body with the upper extremities being more dysfunctional than the lower extremities
Diplegia	Involvement of all extremities, but the lower extremities are more affected than the upper, usually spastic
Quadriplegia	Involvement of all extremities with the arms in flexion and legs in extension

Clinical Therapy

Diagnosis is usually based on clinical findings. Generally, cerebral palsy is difficult to diagnose in the early months of life as it must be distinguished from other neurologic conditions and signs may be subtle. Suspicious findings include an infant who is small for age; has a history of prematurity, low Apgar score (0–3 at 5 minutes), or inflammatory, traumatic, or anoxic event; and also demonstrates abnormal positions and developmental delays (DeLuca, 1996). It is not uncommon for children who are delayed in meeting developmental milestones or who have neuromuscular abnormalities at 1 year of age to show gradual improvement in function. In some cases, signs of dysfunction disappear entirely with physical maturation.

Clinical therapy focuses on helping the child develop to his or her maximum level of independence. Referrals are made for physical, occupational, and speech therapy, as well as special education to improve motor function and ability. Surgical interventions may be required to improve function by balancing muscle power and stabilizing uncontrollable joints. The Achille's tendon may be lengthened to increase range of motion in the ankle, which allows the heel to touch the floor and thus improves ambulation. The hamstrings may be released to correct knee flexion contractures. Other procedures may be performed to improve hip adduction or correct the natural position of the foot. Physical therapy and occupational therapy promote optimal independent functioning.

Medications are given to control seizures, to control spasms (skeletal muscle relaxants, baclofen, and benzodiazepines), and to minimize gastrointestinal side effects (cimetidine or ranitidine). Baclofen is administered by intrathecal pump to decrease muscle tone and vasospasms when oral administration is ineffective or causes side effects (Wiens, 1998).

The prognosis for infants and children with cerebral palsy depends on the level of physical involvement and on the presence of intellectual, visual, or hearing deficits. Many children with hemiplegia or ataxia show some improvement with maturation and are able to ambulate. Others need assistance with mobility and activities of daily living. They are usually cared for in their homes, but some receive care in long-term care facilities.

Nursing Management

Nursing Assessment and Diagnosis

Be alert for children whose histories indicate an increased risk for cerebral palsy. Assess all children at each health care visit for developmental delays. Note any orthopedic, visual, auditory, or intellectual deficits. Assess for newborn reflexes, which may persist beyond the normal age in a child with cerebral palsy. Record dietary intake as well as height and weight percentiles for children suspected to have or diagnosed with the condition.

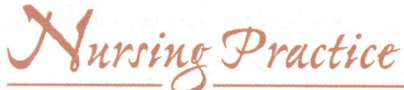

Evaluate all infants who show symptoms of developmental delays, feeding difficulties caused by poor sucking, or abnormalities of muscle tone. Two simple screening assessments are:

 Place a clean diaper on the infant's face. The normal child will use two hands to remove it, but the infant with cerebral palsy will either use one hand or not remove the cloth at all.

▶ Turn the infant's head to one side. A persistent asymmetric tonic neck reflex (beyond 6 months of age) indicates a pathologic condition. Suspect cerebral palsy in any infant who has persistent primitive reflexes.

Nursing diagnoses for the child with cerebral palsy vary, depending on the type of cerebral palsy, the particular child's symptoms and age, and the family situation. "Nursing Care Plan: The Child with Cerebral Palsy" includes several diagnoses that might be appropriate. Additional nursing diagnoses might include:

▶ *Constipation* related to low intake of fiber and fluids and insufficient physical activity

▶ *Impaired tissue integrity* related to decreased physical mobility and limited self-care ability

GOAL	INTERVENTION	RATIONALE	EXPECTED OUTCOME

1. Impaired physical mobility related to decreased muscle strength and control

	NIC Priority Intervention:		*NOC Suggested Outcome:*
	Exercise therapy, joint mobility: *Use of active and passive body movement to maintain joint flexibility*		**Joint movement—active:** *Range of motion of joints with self-limited movement*
The child will attain maximum physical abilities possible.	▶ Perform development assessment and record age of achievement of milestones (e.g., reaching for objects, sitting).	▶ Delayed development milestones are common with cerebral palsy. Once the child achieves one milestone, interventions are revised to assist in the next skill necessary.	The child reaches maximum physical mobility and all developmental milestones.
	▶ Plan activities to use gross and fine motor skills (e.g., holding pen or eating utensils, toys positioned to encourage reaching and rolling over).	▶ Many activities of daily living and play activities promote physical development.	
	▶ Allow time for the child to complete activities.	▶ The child may perform tasks more slowly than most children.	
	▶ Perform range of motion exercises every 4 hours for the child unable to move body parts. Position the child to promote tendon stretching (e.g., foot plantar flexion instead of dorsiflexion, legs extended instead of flexed at knees and hips).	▶ Promotes mobility and increased circulation, and decreases the risk of contractures.	
	▶ Arrange for and encourage parents to keep appointments with a rehabilitation therapist.	▶ A regular and frequently reevaluated rehabilitation program assists in promoting development.	
	▶ Teach the family to maintain appropriate brace wear.	▶ Adaptive devices are often necessary to maximize physical mobility.	

2. Sensory/perceptual alteration: visual or auditory related to cerebral damage

	NIC Priority Intervention:		*NOC Suggested Outcome:*
	Communication enhancement: Visual deficit or auditory deficit: *Assistance with accepting or learning alternative methods for living with diminished vision or hearing*		**Body image:** *Positive perception of own appearance and body functioning*
The child will receive and benefit from varied forms of sensory and perceptual input.	▶ Facilitate eye and auditory examinations by specialist. Promote the use of adaptive devices (glasses, contact lenses, hearing aids), and encourage recommended return visits to specialists.	▶ Adaptive devices often enhance sensory input. These devices need frequent changes as the child grows.	The child receives adequate sensory/perceptual input to maximize developmental outcome.
	▶ Maximize the use of intact senses (e.g., verbally describe the surroundings to a child with poor vision, allow touching of objects, provide visual materials to enhance learning in the child with impaired hearing, use computers to promote communication).	▶ Other senses can compensate for those that are impaired.	

3. Altered nutrition: less than body requirements related to difficulty in chewing and swallowing and high metabolic needs

	NIC Priority Intervention:		*NOC Suggested Outcome:*
	Weight gain assistance: *Facilitation of body weight gain*		**Nutritional status:** *Extent to which nutrients are available to meet metabolic needs*
The child will receive nutrients needed for normal growth.	▶ Monitor height and weight and plot on a growth grid. Perform hydration status assessment.	▶ Insufficient intake can lead to impaired growth and dehydration.	The child shows normal growth patterns for height, weight, and other physical parameters.

GOAL	INTERVENTION	RATIONALE	EXPECTED OUTCOME
	▶ Teach the family techniques to promote caloric and nutrient intake: ▶ Position the child upright for feedings. ▶ Place foods far back in the mouth to overcome tongue thrust. ▶ Use soft and blended foods. ▶ Allow extra time and quiet environment for meals. ▶ Perform frequent respiratory assessment. Teach the family to avoid aspiration pneumonia. Teach care of gastrostomy and tube feeding technique as appropriate.	▶ Special techniques can facilitate food intake. ▶ Aspiration pneumonia is a risk for the child with poor swallowing. Special feeding techniques may be needed.	

4. Ineffective management of therapeutic regimen: family related to excessive demands made on family with child's complex care needs

	NIC Priority Intervention:		*NOC Suggested Outcome:*
	Family process maintenance: *Minimization of family process disruption effects*		Not yet developed
The family will adapt to growth and development needs of the child with cerebral palsy.	▶ Allow chances for parents to verbalize the impact of cerebral palsy on the family. Refer to other parents and support groups. ▶ Explore community services for rehabilitation, respite care, child care, and other needs and refer family as appropriate. ▶ During home and office visits, review the child's achievements and praise the family for care provided. ▶ Teach the family skills needed to manage the child's care (e.g., medication administration, physical rehabilitation, seizure management). ▶ Teach case management techniques. ▶ Involve siblings in the care for the child with cerebral palsy. Review for parents the needs of all children in the family.	▶ The family needs a chance to explore the emotional and social impact of the child's care so they can integrate and grow from the experience. ▶ Diverse services are available and will be needed due to the multiple impacts of cerebral palsy on the child. ▶ The child's achievements are positive reinforcement of the family's efforts. ▶ Complex skills must be learned before they can be performed efficiently. ▶ The child requires care by many specialists. Many parents become case managers to coordinate care. ▶ Siblings of the child with cerebral palsy may feel left out because of the care provided. Special efforts contribute to meeting the developmental needs of all family members.	The family continues its development and provides support for all of its members.

5. Diversional activity deficit (child) related to poor social skills

	NIC Priority Intervention:		*NOC Suggested Outcome:*
	Recreation therapy: *Purposeful use of recreation to promote relaxation and enhancement of social skills*		**Play participation:** *Use of activities as needed for enjoyment, entertainment, and development by children*
The child engages in activities that maximize growth and development.	▶ Refer the family to early childhood stimulation programs. Encourage contact with other children. When hospitalized, place the child in a room with other children whenever possible. ▶ Work with the local school to develop an individual education plan that allows the child contact with other children and a variety of activities. ▶ Investigate recreational programs for children with disabilities and share information with the parents.	▶ The child needs a variety of activities and contact with other children and adults to maximize development. ▶ Public schools must provide an individual education plan. Parents may need help to interact effectively with the school system. ▶ Recreational programs for children with disabilities may promote social experiences and physical activity.	The child engages in activities to maximize development.

- *Impaired verbal communication* related to hearing and/or speech impairment
- *Impaired home maintenance management* related to child's developmental disability and inadequate support system
- *Altered growth and development* related to lack of muscle strength or limited social interaction

Planning and Implementation

The accompanying "Nursing Care Plan" summarizes care for the child with cerebral palsy. Since the condition can range from mild to severe and have a range of manifestations, interventions need to be adapted to the particular child and family. Nursing care focuses on providing adequate nutrition, maintaining skin integrity, promoting physical mobility, promoting safety, promoting growth and development, teaching parents how to care for the child, and providing emotional support.

PROVIDE ADEQUATE NUTRITION

Children with cerebral palsy require high-calorie diets or supplements to the diet because of feeding difficulties associated with spasticity. Many children have difficulty chewing and swallowing. Give the child small amounts of soft foods at a time. Utensils with large, padded handles may be easier for the child to use.

MAINTAIN SKIN INTEGRITY

Take special care to protect the bony prominences from skin breakdown. See Table 49–5 for specific nursing interventions.

Maintain the child's proper body alignment at all times. Support the child with pillows, towels, and bolsters whether the child is in bed or in a chair. Support the head and body of a floppy infant. A spastic child with scissored, extended legs or an athetoid child who writhes constantly is difficult to carry and transport.

PROMOTE PHYSICAL MOBILITY

Range of motion exercises are essential to maintain joint flexibility and to prevent contractures. Consult with the physical therapists who work with the child and help with recommended exercises. Teach parents to position the child to foster flexion rather than extension so that the child can more easily interact with the environment (for example, by bringing objects closer to the face). Encourage parents to bring the child's adaptive appliances (customized wheelchairs, braces) to the hospital to prevent deterioration during hospitalizations. Refer parents to the appropriate resources for help getting adaptive devices (Figure 49–13 ◆).

PROMOTE SAFETY

Teach parents the importance of using safety belts with children in strollers and wheelchairs (see Skill 8-3). ⌾

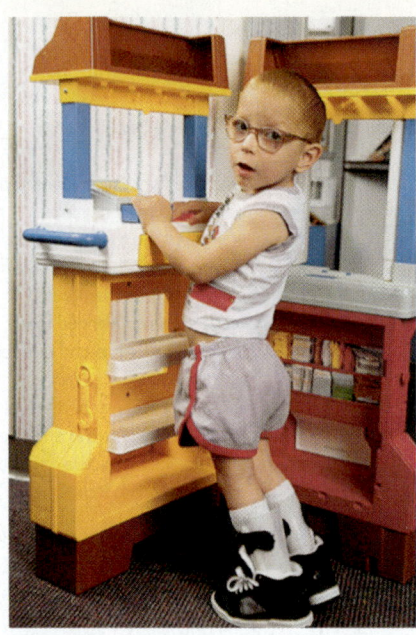

FIGURE 49–13. ◆ A child with cerebral palsy has abnormal muscle tone and lack of physical coordination.

SKILLS A child with chronic seizures should wear a helmet to protect against further injury.

PROMOTE GROWTH AND DEVELOPMENT

Remember that many children with cerebral palsy are physically but not intellectually disabled. Use terminology appropriate for the child's developmental level. Help the child develop a positive self-image to ensure emotional health and social growth. Children with a hearing impairment may need referral to learn American Sign Language or other communication methods.

Provide audio and visual activities for the child who is quadriplegic. Encourage the use of a computer to interact with peers, participate in educational programs, and locate resources for adaptation to the disability. Television, videotapes, and music are good diversions. Encourage the child who is paraplegic to use his or her arms and hands in interactive games. Children can use special hand controls or pointers to use the computer or play video games and other adaptive devices to manipulate the television or radio.

FOSTER PARENTAL KNOWLEDGE

Teach parents about the disorder and arrange sessions to teach them about all of the child's special needs. Teach administration, desired effects, and side effects of medications prescribed for seizures. Make sure parents are aware of the need for dental care for children taking anticonvulsants.

PROVIDE EMOTIONAL SUPPORT

Refer parents to individual and family counseling if appropriate. Listen to the parents' concerns and encourage them to express their feelings and ask questions. Explain what they can expect from future treatment. Work with other health care professionals to help families adjust to this chronic disease.

NURSING CARE IN THE COMMUNITY

Children with cerebral palsy need continuous support in the community. A case manager such as the parent or nurse is likely needed to coordinate care. As they grow, these children need new adaptive devices, ongoing developmental assessment and care planning, and possibly surgery. Although the brain lesion does not change, it manifests itself in different ways as the child grows. For example, once the child begins to walk, the extensor tone may cause Achilles' cord tightening. Braces may decrease deformities, but surgery may eventually be needed, perhaps to loosen tight tendons in the knees or hips (Dzienkowski, Smith, Dillow, et al., 1996). Speech therapy may be needed, as well as new glasses and eye examinations as the child grows. The child may need an individual education plan to maximize learning potential (see Chapter 35). Other parents of children with cerebral palsy can provide needed support. **Assistive technology,** any item, piece of equipment, or product system modified or customized for use to improve or maintain functional capabilities of individuals with disabilities, helps the child be as independent as possible.

Early intervention programs can help parents learn to meet their child's special needs, including physical, occupational, and speech therapy, as well as educational needs. Parents may need financial assistance to provide the care that the child needs and to obtain appliances such as braces, wheelchairs, or adaptive utensils. Technology offers many new strategies to promote communication and self-care by these children. The nurse can be instrumental in helping parents meet the needs of the child with cerebral palsy in preschools, schools, offices, clinics, and other settings. In addition, the nurse makes referrals as appropriate to early intervention programs, support groups, and organizations such as the United Cerebral Palsy Association and Shriners Hospitals. Recreational activities may be identified through the National Association of Sports for Cerebral Palsy. **WEB**

Transition programs assist the family and adolescent with cerebral palsy develop plans for adult living. The young adult (18 to 21 years) may be able to move into a group home or live independently if desired. Vocational training options can be explored. Nurses in hospital programs may coordinate transition into smaller communities and settings and help the family access available resources.

Evaluation

Expected outcomes of nursing care for the child with cerebral palsy are provided on the "Nursing Care Plan."

◆ INJURIES OF THE NEUROLOGIC SYSTEM

TRAUMATIC BRAIN INJURY

A traumatic brain injury can be defined as any trauma involving the scalp, cranial bones, or structures within the skull resulting from force or penetration. Traumatic brain injuries are the most common injuries in childhood, with approximately 200,000 children hospitalized each year and 5000 deaths. Approximately 30,000 children and adolescents under 19 years of age develop a permanent disability from a moderate or severe injury, such as epilepsy, cognitive impairment, learning problems, and behavioral or emotional problems (Rosman, 1999).

Children are prone to skull fractures, often resulting in hematomas and brain injury. They may suffer from the secondary effects of trauma, such as diffuse cerebral edema, malignant brain edema, and increased intracranial pressure.

Young children with moderate and severe traumatic brain injury are at risk for long-term cognitive deficits. Most recovery occurs in the first 12 months postinjury. With fewer well-established skills and knowledge and the slowed processing of information and attention impairment after the brain injury, the child has more challenges when developing cognitive and social competence (Anderson, Catroppa, Morse, et al., 2000).

Etiology and Pathophysiology

Falls are a major cause of unintentional head injuries in young children. Infants fall from dressing tables, beds, and sofas and also tumble down stairs, especially in walkers (American Academy of Pediatrics, 2001). Child abuse, including shaken baby syndrome, accounts for a large number of traumatic brain injuries in children under 1 year old. Toddlers and preschool-age children lack good judgment, and they may run out into the street without looking where they are going, or they may lean out of windows and fall. School-age children may be injured in motor vehicle crashes, either as passengers or as pedestrians, and they may also be injured in bicycle, rollerblading, scooter, or skateboard mishaps. Adolescents are frequently the drivers in motor vehicle crashes; often alcohol or drugs are involved. Teenagers are also injured in sports-related accidents (see Chapter 36).

Brain injuries can be categorized as either primary or secondary. Primary injuries occur at the time of the insult when the initial cellular damage takes place. These injuries result from either a direct blow to the head (coup injury) or from acceleration-deceleration movement of the brain within the skull (contrecoup injury; see "Pathophysiology Illustrated: Brain Injury"). At the time of impact, arterial and intracranial pressures increase, and apnea and loss of consciousness occur.

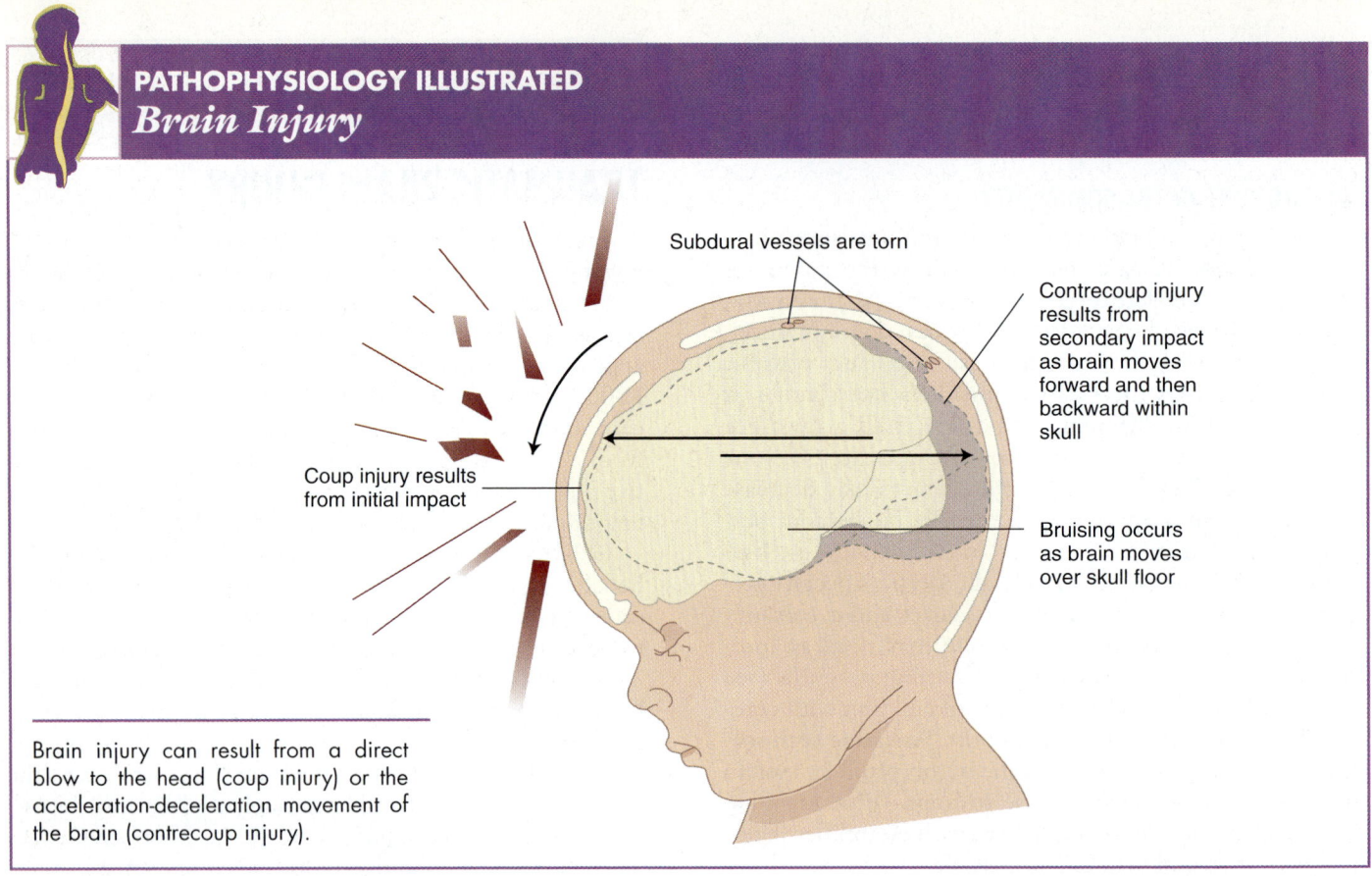

Subdural vessels are torn

Contrecoup injury results from secondary impact as brain moves forward and then backward within skull

Coup injury results from initial impact

Bruising occurs as brain moves over skull floor

Brain injury can result from a direct blow to the head (coup injury) or the acceleration-deceleration movement of the brain (contrecoup injury).

The secondary phase of head trauma is a biochemical and cellular response to the initial insult, and it can be manifested immediately or over hours, days, or weeks. Damage usually results from destruction of brain tissue secondary to hypoxia, hypotension, edema, change in the blood–brain barrier, or hemorrhage (Rosman, 1999). The result is increased intracranial pressure.

Clinical Manifestations

The signs and symptoms of head injuries in children depend on the pathologic features and severity of the injury. The child with a mild head injury may remain conscious or have brief loss of consciousness. The child with a moderate head injury loses consciousness for 5 to 10 minutes. Following mild and moderate head injuries, children may have amnesia about the event, headache, nausea, and vomiting. A child with a severe head injury is usually unconscious for more than 10 minutes and may rapidly show signs of increased intracranial pressure. Unconsciousness may result from increased intracranial pressure, edema, hemorrhage, or parenchymal damage to both cerebral cortices or the brainstem. Posttraumatic seizures are common. Retinal hemorrhages are seen in 65% to 90% of children with inflicted traumatic brain injury (Schutzman & Greenes, 2001).

Vital signs are important indicators of head injury. Changes in respiratory effort or periods of apnea can occur secondary to shock, injury to the spinal cord above C4, or damage to or pressure on the medulla. Heart rate and blood pressure are indices of brainstem function. Tachycardia can be a sign of blood loss, shock, hypoxia, anxiety, or pain. **Cushing's triad,** associated with increased intracranial pressure or compromised blood flow to the brainstem, is characterized by hypertension, increased systolic pressure with wide pulse pressure, bradycardia, and irregular respirations. Refer to the earlier discussion of altered states of consciousness for more information about increased intracranial pressure.

Reflexes may be hyporesponsive, hyperresponsive, or nonexistent. The child may assume a decorticate, decerebrate, **areflexic** (no response to verbal, sensory, or pain stimulation), or flaccid posture (see Figure 49–2).

Clinical Therapy

Identifying the severity of a brain injury involves history, observation, examination, and diagnostic testing. Ask questions about how the injury occurred, the child's initial responses and current responses, any loss of consciousness, and the child's memory of the event.

Neurologic evaluation with the pediatric Glasgow Coma Scale is performed frequently to detect changes in the child's condition (see Table 49–3). Cranial nerves are assessed (see Table 49–4). See Chapter 33 and the earlier discussion in this chapter of altered states of consciousness for further details.

Laboratory tests include a complete blood cell count, blood chemistry, toxicology screening, and urinalysis.

Radiologic examination identifies the specific injury. Skull films detect fractures. A CT scan detects fractures, hematomas, lacerations, or contusions. An MRI scan may be performed to visualize subtle damage or injury. A fracture indicates a more serious injury. Many children with brain injuries have multiple other injuries. Even though cervical spine injuries are rare, all children with a brain injury should have a potential cervical spine injury ruled out by radiologic examination.

The initial management of a child with a brain injury is based on the child's physiologic status. The airway must be clear and stable, and hypoxia must be prevented. If indicated, the child is intubated, sedated, and chemically paralyzed.

Perfusion of the brain must be maintained to ensure that it gets adequate oxygen and nutrients. Shock is treated aggressively with fluid boluses. Keep the head of the bed flat until adequate cerebral perfusion pressure is ensured. Inotropes may be used to ensure perfusion if the child has **cerebral edema** (the increase in intracellular and extracellular fluid in the brain that results from anoxia, vasodilation, or vascular stasis).

Increased intracranial pressure must be controlled. Hypoxia and hypercapnia have disastrous effects on cerebral function, as they can cause vasodilation and increased intracranial pressure. Effective assisted ventilation with 100% oxygen at the child's normal respiratory rate is used in the first 24 hours after injury; however, hyperventilation may be used in subsequent days (Rosman, 1999). If there is no cervical spine injury, the head of the bed is elevated up to 30 degrees. The child's head is kept in the midline to promote venous (jugular) drainage. Hip flexion is avoided. Acetaminophen can be given for pain. The child's body temperature is kept within normal limits. The environment is kept as quiet as possible. Fluids may be restricted only after the child is hemodynamically stable. Diuretics such as mannitol or furosemide may be given to shrink brain volume. A urinary catheter is inserted to monitor output, and electrolytes should be checked frequently.

Invasive procedures may be necessary to reduce increased intracranial pressure. Bur holes may be made or more extensive surgery may be performed to evacuate a lesion or hematoma. A ventricular catheter may be placed to drain CSF and to monitor pressure.

Aggressive support continues until the child regains consciousness and rehabilitation can be initiated. Reliable predictions of outcome in the child who has suffered a severe brain injury cannot be made until 6 to 12 months postinjury.

Nursing Management

Nursing Assessment and Diagnosis

Assess the child's neurologic status frequently. Evaluate the child's level of consciousness continually using the pediatric Glasgow Coma Scale (see Table 49–3). Monitor vital signs closely. Changes in these signs may indicate hypoxia, decreased perfusion, shock, or increased intracranial pressure. When the child has a decreased level of consciousness shortly after a head injury, consider if a posttraumatic seizure occurred and if the child is still in the postictal state. Compare the child's neurologic status to his or her previous state, noting improvement, stability, or deterioration. The cause of any deterioration must be quickly determined and appropriate interventions taken.

Nursing diagnoses that might be appropriate for the child with a head injury include:

▶ *Altered cerebral tissue perfusion* related to hypoventilation, hypovolemia, and/or reduction of arterial blood flow to the brain due to increased intracranial pressure

▶ *Risk for aspiration* related to decreased level of consciousness

▶ *Caregiver role strain* related to 24-hour care responsibility of a child with neurologic complications

▶ *Altered family processes* related to shift in health status of child

▶ *Altered growth and development* related to serious brain injury

Planning and Implementation

HOSPITAL-BASED NURSING CARE

Nursing care focuses on maintaining cardiopulmonary function, preventing complications, promoting recovery, and providing emotional support. Nursing management is based on prevention of secondary injury and return to an optimal level of function.

Thinking Critically

Antwan, 7 years old, was injured when he was struck by a car and thrown several feet into the air. He was unconscious upon admission to the emergency department and showed some signs of increased intracranial pressure (dilated and fixed pupils). He was treated for shock, and his neurologic status and vital signs were frequently assessed. The initial evaluation revealed that Antwan had sustained several contusions of the brain, but no skull fracture. He was intubated and medicated to manage the increased intracranial pressure.

Antwan's intracranial pressure has now stabilized, but he still has not totally regained consciousness. He is restless and agitated, and unable to follow directions. His parents stay at his bedside and provide auditory and tactile stimulation, hoping he will eventually respond. Physical therapy has been initiated to prevent contractures and to maintain function. Long-term rehabilitation will be needed to help Antwan and his family achieve the best outcome possible after this injury.

What is the role of the nurse in acute care of the brain-injured child? What support does the family need to contribute to the child's care? How would you work with other health care professionals to coordinate care during the acute care phase? How would you help plan the long-term care for a child such as Antwan? 🔗 **WEB**

Maintain cardiopulmonary function. In the moderately injured child, observe breathing patterns and check color and level of consciousness. Check the pulse oximeter. Report any sign of decreased oxygenation to the physician immediately.

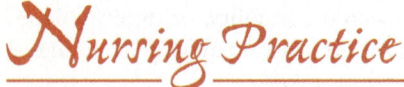

Prevent complications by padding the side rails of the bed to protect the child if a seizure occurs. Keep equipment for suction and ventilation at the bedside. Position the child properly, maintain a quiet environment, and control body temperature. Administer medications as ordered. Check intracranial monitors or surgical sites if invasive measures have been taken. Report any signs and symptoms of increased intracranial pressure (see Table 49–2) to the physician immediately.

Promote recovery and prevent physical deformities. Physical, occupational, and speech therapy should begin in the hospital. Work with these therapists to reinforce exercises and help teach parents the techniques so they can work with the child in the hospital and at home. The nurse can reinforce what has been done during these sessions, noting positive changes. Using toys, books, music, or games, provide stimulation based on the child's age and ability. Encourage parents to bring in favorite toys, stuffed animals, and tape recordings of the child's favorite music or of family members talking.

Provide emotional support to the family in collaboration with the social workers, physicians, psychologists, rehabilitation therapists, and members of the clergy caring for the child and family. All can help the family adjust to having a child with a new disability.

DISCHARGE PLANNING AND HOME CARE TEACHING

Identify and address home care needs well in advance of discharge. Children with significant injuries benefit from inpatient or outpatient rehabilitation to promote optimal achievement of function. A case manager may be needed to coordinate services and resources during rehabilitation.

Give parents information about caring for children with head injuries at home and possible behaviors to expect from the child. For children with disabilities, determine what adaptations are needed in the home to care for the child, such as a wheelchair, walker, braces, or special bed. Social work and home health agencies can often help the parents make special arrangements.

Even though the child looks normal within days of a mild or moderate head injury, brain healing takes up to 6 weeks. Make sure parents and teachers know that typical behavior during this period may include any of the following behaviors: tiring easily, memory loss or forgetfulness, easy distractibility, difficulty concentrating, difficulty following directions, irritability or short temper, and needing help starting and finishing tasks. Educational assessment should be initiated if recovery takes longer than 6 weeks.

NURSING CARE IN THE COMMUNITY

Arrange for home care nursing and follow-up care, if necessary. The home care nurse can take over the case management for the disabled child and make sure the environment is safe. Many children with head injuries are disabled enough to qualify for Social Security Supplemental Security Income (SSI) benefits or the state program for children with special health care needs. Public Law 104-166, the Traumatic Brain Injury Act, was enacted by Congress in 1996 to prevent head injuries and to minimize the severity of dysfunction as a result of head injury by providing funding to states to identify mechanisms to improve access to services (United States Congress, 1996). Find out whether any services are available through a state program funded by this act.

Parents of children with mild or moderate injuries need to be prepared for typical behavior after a head injury, until full recovery has occurred. If the child returns to school, help prepare the teachers, school administrators, and other children for how their classmate is "different." Such sensitivity training makes reintegrating the child into the classroom easier.

The child or adolescent facing long-term rehabilitation needs support to adjust to the disability and to find the strength to maximize his or her abilities. Identify recreational opportunities for the child with disabilities to promote exercise and self-esteem. The adolescent may need to gain vocational skills and learn to live independently. Refer parents to the Brain Injury Association for further information. WEB

Evaluation

Examples of expected outcomes of nursing care for the child with traumatic brain injury include the following:

▶ Cerebral perfusion pressure is maintained at an adequate rate to sustain oxygenation of the brain.

▶ Muscle function is maintained and physical deformities are prevented with range of motion exercises and splinting during the recovery stages of the brain injury.

▶ Parents are supported through the child's acute recovery phase and learn to provide care the child will need at home.

SPECIFIC HEAD INJURIES

Scalp Injuries

Injuries to the scalp, which can be caused by falls, blunt trauma, or penetration of a foreign body, are usually benign. Although bleeding may be extensive, hypovolemia or shock is uncommon unless the patient is an infant.

Lacerations should be irrigated with copious amounts of sterile normal saline solution and inspected for bony fragments or depressions, CSF leakage with a dural tear, or debris. If the injury is simple, the laceration can be sutured and the child discharged from the emergency department. If not, a neurosurgeon should be consulted.

Concussion

A concussion can involve transient impairment of consciousness that usually results from blunt head trauma. It is secondary to stretching, compression, or shearing of nerve fibers. There is usually no gross structural damage or focal injury. The child has an alteration in mental status (e.g., amnesia, dizziness, memory or orientation impairment, unsteady gait), but not necessarily loss of consciousness. Concussions are categorized by three levels of severity (Table 49–11).

Treatment is supportive. Children are observed in the emergency department for several hours before being sent home with instructions to the parents to watch them closely for decreased responsiveness. Any child who is unconscious for more than 5 minutes or has amnesia of the event may be admitted to the hospital or observed in a short-stay unit to rule out other injury.

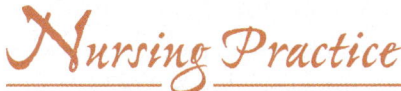

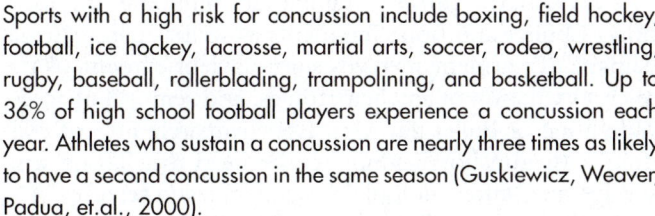

Sports with a high risk for concussion include boxing, field hockey, football, ice hockey, lacrosse, martial arts, soccer, rodeo, wrestling, rugby, baseball, rollerblading, trampolining, and basketball. Up to 36% of high school football players experience a concussion each year. Athletes who sustain a concussion are nearly three times as likely to have a second concussion in the same season (Guskiewicz, Weaver, Padua, et.al., 2000).

TABLE 49-11 Levels of Concussion Severity
Grade 1
Transient confusion, no loss of consciousness, and a duration of mental status abnormalities of less than 15 minutes.
Grade 2
Transient confusion, no loss of consciousness, and a duration of mental status abnormalities of 15 minutes or longer.
Grade 3
Loss of consciousness, either brief (seconds) or prolonged (minutes or longer).

Note: From the Quality Standards Subcommittee, American Academy of Neurology. (1997). Practice parameters: The management of concussion in sports. *Neurology, 48,* 581–585. Adapted.

Pediatric concussive syndrome, which is believed to be caused by an injury to the brainstem, is seen in children who are less than 3 years old. Toddlers seem stunned at the time of injury, but they do not lose consciousness. Later, however, these children become pale, clammy, and lethargic, and they may vomit. They are usually brought to the hospital for treatment when these symptoms appear. These children may be placed in a short-stay unit for observation and usually recover within 24 hours.

Postconcussive syndrome, which is common in both children and adults, may occur anytime after the initial head injury. Signs and symptoms can include headache, dizziness or vertigo, fatigue, irritability, photophobia, subtle changes in personality, poor concentration, poor memory, and ataxia. Treatment is supportive. Symptoms usually disappear within several weeks but may last up to 6 months. Parents and teachers should be told to expect altered behavior in the child and encouraged to help the child maintain self-esteem.

Young athletes suffering a second concussion before complete recovery from the first develop *"second impact" syndrome.* This syndrome results in acute brain swelling, neurologic or cognitive deficits, and sometimes death from the cumulative effect of these concussions. Recommendations should be followed for the management of sports-related concussions to reduce the risk of disability and death. Removal from sports participation ranges from 1 week to the entire season, depending on the severity of concussion and neurologic symptoms (Guskiewicz, Weaver, Padua, et al., 2000).

Skull Fractures

A fracture to any of the eight cranial bones is caused by a considerable force to the head. Any area of the skull with swelling or a hematoma should be evaluated for possible fracture. Diagnosis is made by visual inspection, palpation, radiologic study, or CT scan. Treatment should always include neurosurgical consultation.

Management of skull fractures depends on the type and extent of the injury (Table 49–12).

Cerebral Contusion

A cerebral contusion, or the bruising of brain tissue, is secondary to blunt trauma and can occur with either coup or contrecoup injuries (see "Pathophysiology Illustrated: Brain Injury"). Such injuries are rare in children less than 1 year of age. The temporal or frontal sections of the skull are the most common sites of this injury, which involves damage to the parenchyma with tears in vessels or tissue, pulping, and subsequent areas of necrosis or infarction.

The child may have focal symptoms depending on the area of injury. Altered levels of consciousness range from confusion and disorientation to being obtunded. A CT scan is used for diagnosis.

TABLE 49–12 Skull Fractures

Injury	Clinical Therapy
Linear Fracture Results from impact to large area of the skull. Usually no symptoms. May have overlying hematoma or soft tissue swelling.	If fracture is on temporal bone or crosses sagittal suture line a CT scan is performed to detect potential epidural hematoma. Consider the possibility of inflicted injury.
Depressed Fracture Break in skull itself or an area shattered into many fragments. Pieces of bone may be depressed into brain tissue with hematoma forming on top.	Plain radiographic film or CT scan. Surgery to elevate bone fragments when depression is greater than 5 mm. Tetanus prophylaxis is given as needed. Many are associated with intracranial injury and posttraumatic epilepsy.
Compound Fracture Combination of a full thickness scalp laceration and depressed skull fracture with the bone exposed. Are considered penetrating fractures if the dura is torn.	Visual diagnosis along with radiographic studies. Surgical debridement, a search for foreign bodies, and copious irrigation are performed. Parenteral antibiotics and tetanus prophylaxis are provided as needed.
Basilar Fracture Fracture at the base of the skull that may involve the frontal, ethmoid, sphenoid, temporal, or occipital bones. A dural tear may be present.	Diagnosis is confirmed by signs of blood behind the tympanic membranes, CSF leakage from the nose or ears, periorbital ecchymosis (raccoon eyes) or bruising of the mastoid (Battle sign). Radiographic imaging locates the fracture site. Antibiotics may be prescribed. Surgical repair of the site of the CSF leak is performed if the leak persists after 7–10 days. Transient or permanent cranial nerve injuries occur (e.g., hearing loss).

Note: From Rosman, N. P. (1999). Acute head trauma. In J. A., McMillan, C. D., DeAngelis, R. D., Feigin, & J. B. Warshaw (Eds.), *Oski's pediatrics: Principles and practice* (3rd ed., pp. 603–617). Philadelphia: Lippincott, Williams, & Wilkins. Adapted.

Treatment involves hospitalization for observation and to rule out other injuries. Surgical treatment is rarely necessary.

Sequelae are focal and specific to the area of the brain that was injured. For example, an injury to the left temporal area may affect speech.

Intracranial Hematomas

Intracranial hematomas are space-occupying lesions that expand rapidly or slowly, depending on whether they are arterial or venous in origin. They must be located quickly. Some lesions require evacuation as soon as possible to minimize the secondary effects of the injury. Table 49–13 describes types of intracranial hematomas and their treatment.

Subarachnoid hemorrhages, associated with severe head injuries such as intracranial hematomas or contusions, result from laceration of arteries or veins in the subarachnoid space. Symptoms include decreased level of consciousness, ipsilateral pupil dilation, diplopia, hemiparesis, nausea and vomiting, nuchal rigidity, and headache.

Diagnosis is confirmed by CT scan. There is no specific treatment, and the clinical course depends on associated injuries.

Penetrating Injuries

Gunshot wounds to the head can damage tissue, bone, and vessels. Low-velocity bullets enter but do not exit the skull; instead they ricochet within the cranial vault, destroying brain tissue and vessels. Although the child may be con-

scious just after the injury, the level of consciousness quickly deteriorates because of the edema surrounding the penetration tract. High-velocity bullets, on the other hand, cause immediate, severe damage on impact. See Chapter 36 for a discussion of violence in childhood.

CT evaluates gunshot trauma and pinpoints the location of bullet and bone fragments as well as parenchymal damage. Treatment involves surgical debridement of the tract, evacuation of any hematomas, and removal of accessible bone or bullet particles. Approximately 50% of children with gunshot wounds to the head die. Those who survive may suffer multiple focal deficits and seizures.

Impalement injuries frequently occur in children in association with lawn darts or dog bites. All objects must be left in place and removed in the operating room by a neurosurgeon. The child with an impalement injury is at high risk for focal injury and infection. After surgery, children with this type of injury are managed as with other postoperative head injuries, with attention focused on level of consciousness, increased intracranial pressure, and infection control.

SPINAL CORD INJURY

Less than 5% of spinal cord injuries occur in children under 16 years of age annually (Massagli, 2000). Many children with these injuries die within the first hour of trauma or during the first 3 months after trauma.

Motor vehicle crashes are the leading cause of spinal cord injuries, either pedestrian-vehicular, bicycle-vehicular,

TABLE 49-13 Intracranial Hematomas

Type of Hematoma	Diagnosis and Management

Subdural Hematoma
Result of severe head trauma such as falls, assaults, motor vehicle crashes, or shaken child syndrome
Occurs most frequently in children less than 1 year old
Caused by laceration of the bridging veins; clot forms and presses directly on brain, leading to damage from two sources: original contusion and hematoma, usually venous
Symptoms (may not appear until 48–72 hours after the injury) include:
    Change in level of consciousness (confusion, agitation, or lethargy)
    Nausea or vomiting
    Headache
    Retinal hemorrhages in both eyes
    Pupil on side of injury may be fixed and dilated
    Seizures
    Fever
	Diagnosis confirmed by CT scan
	Treatment is usually surgical; subdural taps may be necessary after surgery to give the brain room to expand
	More than half of children with subdural hematomas die; those who survive have 75% chance of developing seizures
	
	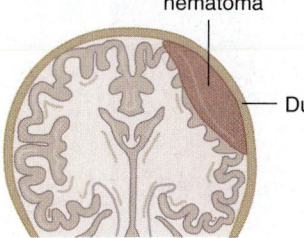
	Bleeding occurs between dura and brain

Epidural Hematoma
Rare in children and almost never occurs in children less than 4 years of age
Results from blunt trauma (most often falls), motor vehicle crashes, assaults, or baseball to temporal area
Temporal and parietal areas are most common sites.
May be associated with linear skull fracture
May be fatal if bleeding is arterial
Symptoms include:
    Brief loss of consciousness followed by lucid period and rapid deterioration
    Sleepiness or lethargy
    Headache
    Full fontanel
    Paresis of cranial nerves III and VI
    Papilledema
    Fixed and dilated pupil
    Signs of increased intracranial pressure
	Diagnosis confirmed by CT scan
	Treatment involves immediate surgical intervention; craniotomy is performed followed by evacuation of the hematoma
	Prognosis is good, although 25% of children have seizures
	
	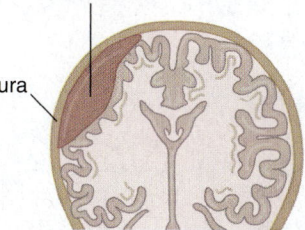
	Bleeding occurs between dura and skull

Intracerebral Hematoma Result of deep contusion or intracerebral laceration (secondary to foreign body or bony penetration or impalement) Causes diffuse bleeding in parenchyma; there may be a hematoma with associated small areas of bleeding	Diagnosis confirmed by CT scan Surgical treatment not indicated Neurologic effects depend on size and location of lesion and whether bleeding can be controlled; hemiplegia or visual loss may result 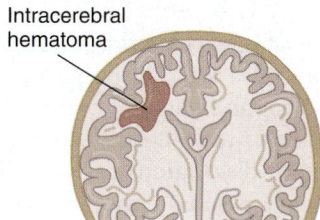 Bleeding occurs within cerebrum

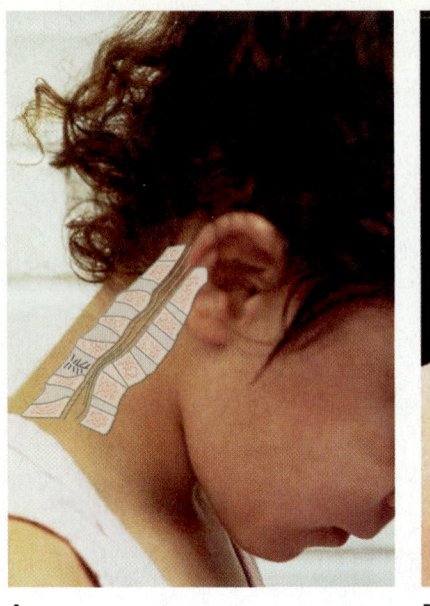
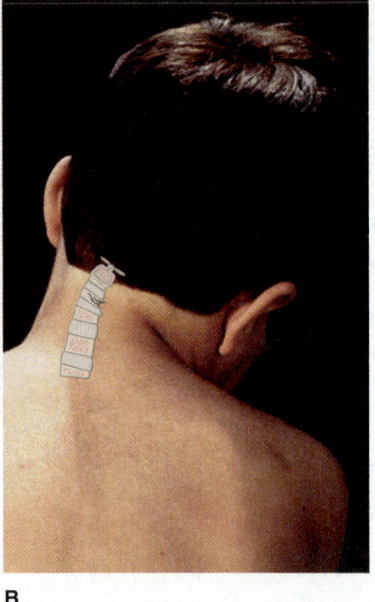
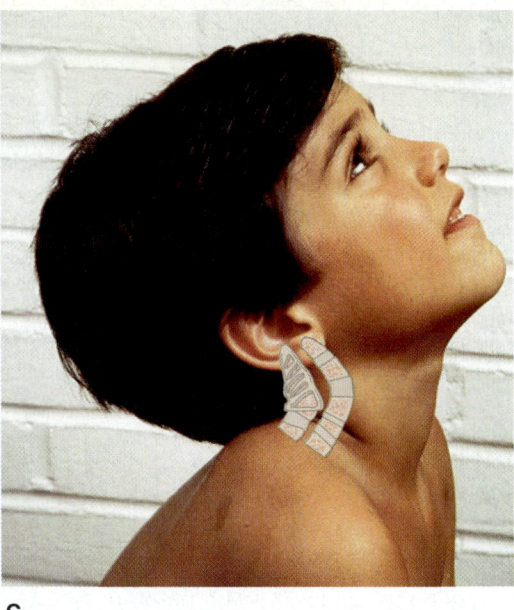

A **B** **C**

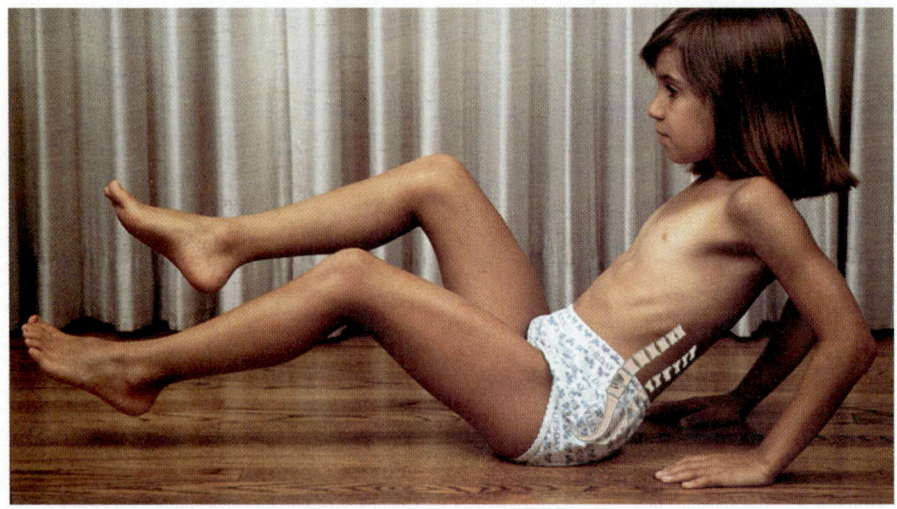

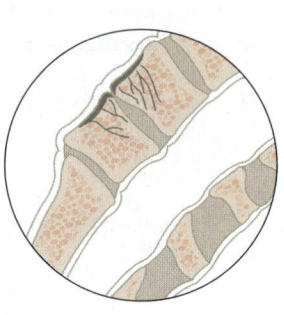

D

FIGURE 49–14. ◆ Mechanics of injury to the spinal cord. **A,** Hyperflexion. **B,** Lateral flexion, **C,** Extension. **D,** Compression.

passenger, or driver-related. Other causes of spinal injuries, especially in toddlers and young children, include falls and child abuse. Recreation or sports-related trauma accounts for more injuries as children grow older. Penetrating injuries such as stab and gunshot wounds are becoming more prevalent.

The mechanism of injury determines the type of lesion that occurs (Figure 49–14 ◆). Hyperflexion injuries produce tears or avulsions and fractures of vertebral bodies, as well as subluxation and dislocation. Lateral flexion (rotation) may cause joint dislocations or unstable spinal fractures. Extension may result in the so-called hangman's fracture, ligament tears, avulsion fractures of vertebral bodies, as well as central or posterior spinal cord syndrome. Compression injuries cause anterior cord syndrome.

Growth and Development

The vertebrae are incompletely ossified in children under 9 years. The facet joints are more shallow and horizontal. The young child's head is relatively large compared to the strength of the neck muscles. The fulcrum is at the C2 to C3 level so injuries are more likely to occur at the C1 to C3 level under 9 years and at the C4 to C6 level for children 9 to 15 years (Massagli, 2000).

Spinal cord injuries are classified as complete or incomplete. Complete lesions are irreversible and involve a loss of sensory, motor, and autonomic function below the level of the injury. Incomplete lesions involve varying degrees of sensory, motor, and autonomic function below the level of injury.

Children are prone to specific kinds of spinal cord injuries because of the extreme mobility and flexibility of their spinal column. Table 49–14 describes the spinal cord injuries most common in children.

The higher the level of spinal cord injury, the more severe the neurologic damage. The child is often a victim of multiple trauma and may display signs of hypovolemic shock resulting from other injuries, increased intracranial pressure, or respiratory depression. Children can also experience neurogenic or spinal shock (see Chapter 43).

At the time of injury, the child is flaccid and areflexic below the lesion and responds only to stimuli above the level of the injury. Priapism may be present. Muscle spasticity below the lesion occurs later. Respiration may be compromised due to paralysis of the diaphragm.

Diagnosis is made by observation, neurologic examination, and x-ray studies. X-ray studies include lateral cervical spine and anteroposterior and lateral views of the thoracic and lumbosacral spine. In addition, CT scanning, MRI, fluoroscopy, or myelography may be performed. Many children have spinal cord injury without radiographic abnormality (SCIWORA) accounting for 15% to 25% of all pediatric spinal cord trauma (Massagli, 2000). SCIWORA occurs when initial films or CT scans show no bony deformity and the child is believed to be free of injury. Profound or progressive paralysis is found either immediately or within 48 hours. An MRI can detect the injury.

Spinal injuries are managed aggressively. The child with a spinal cord injury may be placed in skeletal traction or a halo device. Further surgical management of the injury may be necessary. Debridement and decompression should be accomplished within the first 8 hours after penetrating injury. A fusion using bone from another part of the body may be performed to stabilize the spinal cord. If more drastic measures are necessary, an internal fixation device may be required.

To further decrease neurologic sequelae, methylprednisolone is administered in high doses to children with motor deficits. Administration must be started within 8 hours of the injury.

Complications of spinal cord injury include:

- Scoliosis if injury occurs before the skeleton is mature
- Impaired respiratory function due to a paralyzed diaphragm or diminished vital capacity
- Hip instability due to poor acetabular development
- Pathologic fractures of the long bones due to immobilization hypercalcemia
- Pressure sores
- Deep vein thrombosis
- Autonomic dysreflexia (hypertension, bradycardia, severe headaches, pallor below and flushing above the level of the cord lesion, and seizures)

An interdisciplinary approach is required to manage the rehabilitation and long-term care needs of the child and family.

Nursing Management

HOSPITAL-BASED NURSING CARE

Nursing care focuses on monitoring vital signs, meeting nutritional needs, maintaining skin integrity, promoting independent functioning, encouraging therapeutic play, providing emotional support, and promoting rehabilitation.

Monitor vital signs and be alert for any changes, especially those that may signify increased intracranial pressure (see Table 49–2) or autonomic dysreflexia. Monitor the child's respiratory status. Some children with cervical lesions have tracheostomies to help maintain airway patency; others with very high lesions need ventilators. Keep proper emergency equipment at the bedside at all times.

Ensure adequate nutrition. A child with complete paralysis may require a gastrostomy tube.

Prevent skin breakdown (see Table 49–5). Observe surgical sites for signs of infection or inflammation. Perform good skin care at the insertion of the external fixation device (see Table 50–5 on page 1346).

Promote independent functioning by reinforcing the exercises and skills learned in physical and occupational therapy. Use supports, boots, footboards, splints, and braces as recommended by the therapists to prevent contractures (Figure 49–15 ◆). If hand mobility is limited, explore options for independence. Encourage the child to be as independent as possible in a wheelchair. An important mobility goal is to achieve wheelchair transfer and to perform self-care. Identify adaptive equipment that make these goals possible.

Bowel and bladder control may be difficult. Intermittent catheterizations may be necessary (see Skill 16-1). SKILLS CD Bowel training involves a diet high in fiber and the use of stool softeners.

Therapeutic play appropriate for the child's developmental level is an important part of the healing process.

TABLE 49–14 Spinal Cord Injuries in Children

Cervical Region
- Site of 75% of spinal injuries in children through 8 years and 60% between 8 and 14 years
- Highest incidence above C3 segment
- Many of these injuries are fatal

Thoracolumbar Region
- Second most common area of injury; probably a result of improperly placed lap belts
- Most injuries occur at the L2 to L4 levels

Thoracic Region
- Site of 20% of spinal injuries usually between 8 and 14 years

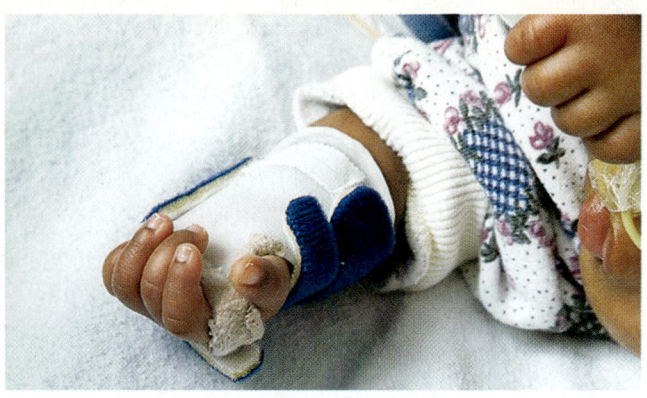

FIGURE 49–15. ◆ Splints are often used to prevent contractures, thus maintaining optimal functioning of the child's hands or feet.

Provide as many normal activities for the child as possible, but do not give the child tasks that he or she will have difficulty completing. Child life teachers or tutors can help the child keep up with schoolwork.

Television, videotapes, and music can offer diversion for prolonged hospitalization. Paraplegic children can learn to use their arms and hands to play interactive games. Devices can also be adapted so that the child can play video games or manipulate the television or radio.

Support the child emotionally. Encourage the child to meet small, short-term goals, including those that involve self-care. Encourage the child to express fears and frustrations.

Be compassionate and understanding. Encourage siblings to visit, answer their questions honestly, and help them to discuss their feelings. Involve the parents and siblings in the child's care as much as possible. When appropriate, encourage them to help with activities of daily living.

DISCHARGE PLANNING AND HOME CARE TEACHING

Many children are discharged to inpatient rehabilitation facilities. Help arrange the child's transfer from the hospital to the rehabilitation facility. Work closely with the child, parents, and other members of the health care team concerning placement. Identify and address home care needs, reintegration into educational programs, and safety issues well in advance of discharge from the rehabilitation facility. Refer families to social services, family counseling, and support groups if indicated. ▭▭ **WEB**

The young child's ultimate functioning will be related to cognitive development, the amount of upper body strength, and the family's expectations (Massagli, 2000).

HYPOXIC-ISCHEMIC BRAIN INJURY (DROWNING AND NEAR-DROWNING)

Drowning is defined as death within 24 hours of a submersion incident. Near-drowning is survival for at least 24 hours after submersion. Over 90% of drownings occur in fresh water such as ponds and residential swimming pools (Zuckerman & Conway, 2000). Drowning is the second leading cause of injury-related deaths in children. Most pediatric victims are very young (under age 4 years) or in their teen years. Boys are five times more likely than girls to die from drowning.

Growth and Development

Between 40% and 50% of children injured in drowning incidents are under 4 years of age, with peak incidence between ages 1 and 2 years. The majority (55%) of infant drownings are in bathtubs. The most common drowning locations for children 1 to 4 years old are artificial pools (56%) and other bodies of fresh water (26%). Among older children, 63% of drownings occur in natural bodies of fresh water (Brenner, Trumble, Smith, et al., 2001).

There are two types of drowning. Wet drowning, which occurs more frequently, is the result of aspiration of fluid into the lungs. Dry drowning, seen in 10% of cases, is due to hypoxemia resulting from laryngospasm, with small or insignificant amounts of liquid aspirated.

The events preceding drowning follow a sequential pattern. The child trapped in water panics, struggles, tries to move using swimming motions, and holds his or her breath. Then the child swallows a small amount of fluid, vomits, and aspirates the vomitus. This leads to a brief period of laryngospasm, which lasts no more than 2 minutes. Because of the increasing panic and hypoxia, the child swallows more liquid. Then either the child goes into profound laryngospasm, becomes severely hypoxic, has a seizure, and dies (dry drowning), or the child becomes unconscious, the laryngospasm relaxes as reflexes are lost, and the child passively aspirates even greater amounts of water into the airway and stomach (wet drowning).

Anoxia is the major insult associated with drowning. Anoxia leads to cerebral edema and increased intracranial pressure. Little can be done to resuscitate the brain, but with aggressive cardiopulmonary resuscitation, more severely brain-injured children are surviving in a permanent vegetative state. Aspiration leads to impaired gas exchange and ultimately affects pulmonary, cardiac, cerebral, and renal functions. See Chapter 42 for a brief discussion of the effects of drowning on the respiratory system. ▭▭

Prognosis and outcome are highly individual. Anoxic brain injury is the leading cause of mortality. Predictors of good outcome are submersion less than 5 minutes and cardiopulmonary resuscitation for less than 10 minutes (Zuckerman & Conway, 2000).

The child who has been immersed exhibits a wide variety of signs and symptoms depending on the length of time underwater, the temperature of the water, the response to the episode, and the initial treatment performed at the scene. Children submerged for short periods have few symptoms and recover without complication. The child with a longer submersion can experience the following symptoms: decreased level of consciousness ranging from stupor to total unresponsiveness, cerebral edema, increased intracranial pressure, seizures, respiratory acidosis, irregular respirations, apnea, and gastric distention.

Medical intervention begins at the scene of the drowning with immediate ventilation and compressions, when indicated. The sooner the treatment is started, the better the child's prognosis. All near-drowning victims should be admitted to the hospital for at least 24 hours or observed in a short-stay observation unit for several hours, even when asymptomatic. Many life-threatening complications, including respiratory distress and cerebral edema, may not become evident for at least 12 hours after the incident.

Nursing Management

Nursing care of the child who survives a near-drowning focuses on monitoring the child's cardiopulmonary status and providing emotional support.

Monitor the child's respiratory status, cardiopulmonary function, and neurologic status. Administer prescribed medications and position the child properly. Other nursing interventions, especially for the comatose child, can be found in the earlier discussion of altered states of consciousness.

Provide emotional support to the family. Be nonjudgmental and provide a forum for parents to express their feelings. Reassure parents who exhibit guilt reactions that their child is receiving all possible medical treatment. Parents may be faced with an unknown prognosis. Encourage them to seek assistance from social workers, members of the clergy, close friends, and relatives. Arrange for appropriate referrals.

Identify and address home care needs well in advance of discharge. Assist with arrangements for the child with minor deficits. Help the parents decide whether the comatose child will go home or to a long-term facility.

Drowning can be prevented by education, legislation, and changes in the environment. Pool owners should erect climb-proof 5-foot fences around all four sides of the pool. Local ordinances may require such fences. Adolescents should learn the dangers of mixing alcohol and swimming. Five-and 10-gallon buckets should be kept empty when not in use. Emphasize the importance of closely supervising children when near or in the water, whether at pools, at the beach, or in the bathtub.

CHAPTER HIGHLIGHTS

🙢 Altered level of consciousness is caused by trauma, infection, poisoning, seizures, or any other process that affects the central nervous system. Cerebral perfusion pressure (the amount of pressure needed to ensure that adequate oxygen and nutrients will be delivered to the brain) is decreased with hypovolemia and increased intracranial pressure.

🙢 More than 80% of children have had a headache by late adolescence, and migraine is the most common type of benign headache in children.

🙢 Monitor any child with a generalized seizure lasting longer than 10 minutes for electrolytes, glucose, blood gases, increasing fever, and abnormal blood pressure to identify any conditions that can be treated and reduce the risk of significant CNS injury.

🙢 Neurologic damage from bacterial meningitis often occurs in infants and young children despite early, aggressive management. The most common sequelae involve cranial nerves, especially the eighth resulting in hearing loss, seizures, and developmental delay.

🙢 Viral (aseptic) meningitis is not as virulent as bacterial meningitis, and the child with aseptic meningitis appears less ill than the child with bacterial meningitis.

🙢 Encephalitis is usually caused by a virus, often herpes simplex I. It has a high mortality rate.

🙢 Reye syndrome is an encephalopathy with a high mortality rate that is associated with aspirin use for a mild viral illness. Since most parents give children acetaminophen rather than aspirin for flulike symptoms and varicella, Reye syndrome has become rare.

🙢 Guillain-Barré syndrome is the most common cause of flaccid paralysis in infants and children. It is caused by an immune response to an infectious organism, usually from a gastrointestinal or respiratory illness 2 to 3 weeks prior to onset.

🙢 Hydrocephalus is caused by the blockage of flow or absorption of cerebrospinal fluid in the subarachnoid space and the arachnoid villi, or by blockage in the ventricular system. It can be associated with a congenital condition or acquired from meningitis or intraventricular hemorrhage, tumor, or structural deformity.

🙢 Spina bifida, a congenital neural tube defect, is the most common developmental disorder of the central nervous system. Its prevalence is decreasing due to the fortification of all enriched grain products with folate.

🙢 Positional plagiocephaly, a totally flat occiput, is seen increasingly because of the "Back to Sleep" campaign for sudden infant death syndrome.

🙢 Most cases of cerebral palsy are characterized by spasticity and a lack of coordination. The majority of cases are believed to be caused by intrauterine insults, such as infection, or structural abnormalities of the central nervous system.

🙢 Traumatic brain injuries are the most common injuries during childhood. They result from falls, motor vehicle crashes, sports injuries, and child abuse.

🙢 Spinal cord injuries, although relatively rare in children, are often associated with the extreme mobility and flexibility of the spinal column. The cervical and lumbar regions are the locations most commonly affected.

🙢 Children who have the best outcomes following a near-drowning include those submerged less than 5 minutes and those who need cardiopulmonary resuscitation for less than 10 minutes.

![EXPLORE Media Link logo]

EXPLOREMediaLink

NCLEX Review, Case Studies, and other interactive resources for this chapter can be found on the companion website at http://www.prenhall.com/london. Click on "Chapter 49" and select the activities for this chapter.

For animations, more NCLEX review questions, and an audio glossary, access the accompanying CD-ROM in this textbook.

REFERENCES

Altmeier, W. A. (1999). Status epilepticus. *Pediatric Annals, 28*(4), 206–208.

American Academy of Pediatrics Committee on Injury and Poison Prevention. (2001). Injuries associated with infant walkers. *Pediatrics, 108*(3), 790–792.

Anderson, V., Catroppa, C., Morse, S., Haritou, F., & Rosenfeld, J. (2000). Recovery of intellectual ability following traumatic brain injury in childhood: Impact of injury severity and age at injury. *Pediatric Neurosurgery, 32*(6), 282–290.

Bowman, R. M., McLone, D. G., Grant, J. A., Tomita, T., & Ito, J. A. (2001). Spina bifida outcome: A 25 year perspective. *Pediatric Neurosurgery, 34*(3), 114–120.

Brenner, R. A., Trumble, A. C., Smith, G. S., Kessler, E. P., & Overpeck, M. D. (2001). Where children drown, United States, 1995. *Pediatrics, 108*(1), 85–89.

Bruce, M. G., Rosenstein, N. E., Capparella, K. A., Shutt, K. A., Perkins, B. A., & Collins, M. Risk for meningococcal disease in college students. *Journal of the American Medical Association, 286*, 688–693.

Cherry, J. D. (1999). Nonpolio enteroviruses. In J. A. McMillan, C. D. DeAngelis, R. D. Feigin, & J. B. Warshaw (Eds.), *Oski's pediatrics: Principles and practice* (3rd ed., pp. 1102–1107). Philadelphia: Lippincott, Williams, & Wilkins.

Danielpour, M., & Peacock, W. J. (2000). Epilepsy surgery in children. *Clinical Neurosurgery, 47*, 400–421.

DeLuca, P. A. (1996). The musculoskeletal management of children with cerebral palsy. *Pediatric Clinics of North America, 43*(5), 1135–1150.

Dzienkowski, R. C., Smith, K. K., Dillow, K. A., & Yucha, C. B. (1996). Cerebral palsy: A comprehensive review. *Nurse Practitioner, 21*(2), 45–59.

Fadiman, A. (1997). *The spirit catches you and you fall down.* New York: Farrar, Strauss, Giroux.

Farley, J. A., & Dunleavy, M. J. (2000). Myelodysplasia. In P. L. Jackson & J. A. Vessey (Eds.), *Primary care of the child with a chronic condition* (3rd ed., pp. 658–675). St. Louis, MO: Mosby.

Farley, J. A., & McEwan, M. (2000). Epilepsy. In P. L. Jackson & J. A. Vessey (Eds.), *Primary care of the child with a chronic condition* (3rd ed., pp. 475–494). St. Louis, MO: Mosby.

Farley, J. A., & Mooney, K. H. (1998). Alterations in neurologic function in children. In

K. L. McCance & S. E. Huether (Eds.), *Pathophysiology: The biologic basis for disease in adults and children* (3rd ed., pp. 591–624). St. Louis, MO: Mosby.

Guskiewicz, K. M., Weaver, N. L., Padua, D. A., & Garrett, W. E. (2000). Epidemiology of concussion in collegiate and high school football players. *American Journal of Sports Medicine, 28*(5), 643–650.

Harrison, L. H. (2001, May). Meningococcal infection in adolescents and young adults. *Contemporary Pediatrics* (Spring Supp), 4–15.

Honein, M. A., Paulozzi, L. J., Matthews, T. J., Erickson, J. D., & Wong, L. Y. (2001). Impact of folic acid fortification of the U.S. food supply on the occurrence of neural tube defects. *Journal of the American Medical Association, 285*(23), 2981–2986.

Jackson, P. L., & Harvey, J. (2000). Hydrocephalus. In P. L. Jackson & J. A. Vessey (Eds.), *Primary care of the child with a chronic condition* (3rd ed., pp. 560–582). St. Louis, MO: Mosby.

Jones, H. R. (2000). Guillain-Barre syndrome: Perspectives with infants and children. *Seminars in Pediatric Neurology, 7*(2), 91–102.

Katyal, N. G., Koehler, A. N., McGhee, B., Foley, C. M., & Crumrine, P. K. (2000). The ketogenic diet in refractory epilepsy: The experience of Children's Hospital of Pittsburgh. *Clinical Pediatrics, 39*(3), 153–159.

Leake, J. A. D., & Perkins, B. (2000). Meningococcal disease: Challenges in prevention and management. *Infections in Medicine, 17*(5), 364–377.

Massagli, T. L. (2000). Medical and rehabilitation issues in the care of children with spinal cord injury. *Physical Medicine and Rehabilitation Clinics of North America, 11*(1), 169–182.

Moe, P. G., & Seay, A. R. (1997). Neurologic and muscular disorders. In W. W. Hay, J. R. Groothius, A. R. Hayward, & M. J. Levin (eds.), *Current pediatric diagnosis and treatment* (13th ed., pp. 686–689). Stamford, CT: Appleton & Lange.

Nehring, W. M. (2000). Cerebral palsy. In P. L. Jackson & J. A. Vessey (eds.), *Primary care of the child with a chronic condition* (3rd ed., pp. 305–330). St. Louis, MO: Mosby.

Nelson, K. B., & Grether, J. K. (1999). Causes of cerebral palsy. *Current Opinion in Pediatrics, 11*(6), 487–491.

Northrup, H., & Volcik, K. A. (2000). Spina bifida and other neural tube defects. *Current Problems in Pediatrics, 30*(10), 317–331.

O'Hara, J., & Koch, T. K. (1998). Heading off headaches. *Contemporary Pediatrics, 15*(3), 97–116.

Renier, D., Lajeunie, E., Arnaud, E., & Marchac, D. (2000). Management of craniosynostosis. *Children's Nervous System, 16*, 645–658.

Ressler, J. A., & Nelson, M. (2000). Central nervous system infections in the pediatric population. *Neuroimaging Clinics of North America, 10*(2), 427–443.

Robinson, T. M. S. (1999). Perinatal substance abuse. Working with neonates and families. *Neonatal Network, 18*(2), 68–70.

Rosman, N. P. (1999). Acute head trauma. In J. A. McMillan, C. D. DeAngelis, R. D. Feigin, & J. B. Warshaw (Eds.), *Oski's pediatrics: Principles and practice* (3rd ed., pp. 603–617). Philadelphia: Lippincott, Williams, & Wilkins.

Sagraves, R. (1999). Febrile seizures—Treatment and prevention or not? *Journal of Pediatric Health Care, 13*(2), 79–83.

Schutzman, S. A., & Greenes, D. S. (2001). Pediatric minor head trauma. *Annals of Emergency Medicine, 27*(1), 65–74.

Spector, R. E. (2000). *Cultural diversity in health and illness* (5th ed., p. 71). Upper Saddle River, NJ: Prentice Hall Health.

Sutton, L., Adzick, N. S., Belaniuk, L. T., Johnson, M. P., Crombleholme, T. M., & Flake, A. W. (1999). Improvement of hindbrain herniation demonstrated by serial fetal magnetic resonance imaging following fetal surgery for myelomeningocele. *Journal of the American Medical Association, 282*(19), 1826–1831.

United States Congress. (1996). Traumatic brain injury act of 1996. *Congressional Record, 142* (July 29, 1996), 110 STAT, 1445–1449.

Valente, L. R. (2000). Seizures and epilepsy: Optimizing patient management. *Clinician Reviews, 10*(3), 79–104.

Vendanarayan, V. V. (1999). Diagnosis of epilepsy in children. *Pediatric Annals, 28*(4), 218–224.

Weins, H. D. (1998). Spasticity in children with cerebral palsy: A retrospective review of effects of intrathecal baclofen. *Issues in Comprehensive Pediatric Nursing, 21*, 49–61.

Zuckerman, G. B., & Conway, E. E. (2000). Drowning and near-drowning: A pediatric epidemic. *Pediatric Annals, 29*(6), 360–366.

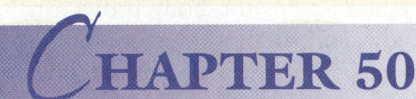

CHAPTER 50

The Child with Alterations in Musculoskeletal Function

When I got the call that Douglass was in the emergency room I was so scared. I guess we're lucky it was just a broken leg. I don't know what to do now, though—he broke his leg on a friend's trampoline. Should he go back to his friend's house? Should I tell him not to use the trampoline? It's hard to decide. And I never had a cast. What do you need to do with it?

—MOTHER OF DOUGLASS, 12 YEARS OLD

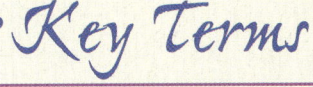

Key Terms

Chondrolysis   *1329*
Compartment syndrome   *1344*
Dislocation   *1324*
Dysplasia   *1324*
Equinus   *1321*
Ossification   *1319*

Osteotomy   *1323*
Pseudohypertrophy   *1339*
Sprain   *1319*
Subluxation   *1324*
Varus   *1321*

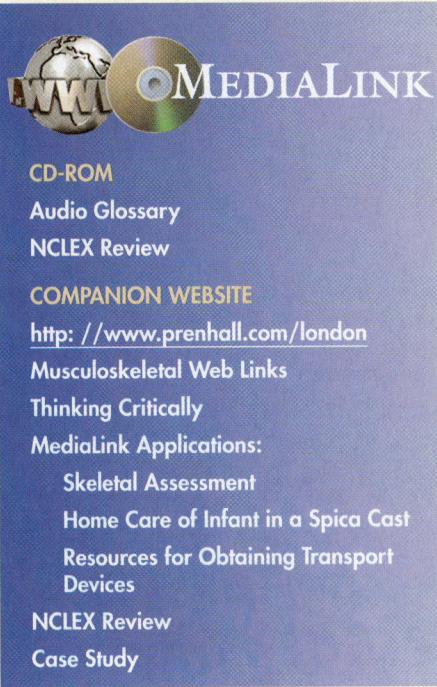

MEDIALINK

CD-ROM
Audio Glossary
NCLEX Review

COMPANION WEBSITE
http://www.prenhall.com/london
Musculoskeletal Web Links
Thinking Critically
MediaLink Applications:
   Skeletal Assessment
   Home Care of Infant in a Spica Cast
   Resources for Obtaining Transport Devices
NCLEX Review
Case Study

What concerns do parents and children have when a child has musculoskeletal conditions? Will the child need any special adaptations in the home and school? Can musculoskeletal injuries be prevented? The information in this chapter will answer these questions, and enable nurses to provide effective care for children who have musculoskeletal disorders.

The musculoskeletal system helps the body protect its vital organs, support weight, control motion, store minerals, and supply red blood cells. Bones provide a rigid framework for the body, muscles provide for active movement, and tendons and ligaments hold the bones and muscles together. Alterations in musculoskeletal functioning, therefore, can have a significant impact on a child's growth and development.

TABLE 50–1   Musculoskeletal Positions

Varus
An abnormal position of a limb that involves bending inward toward the midline of the body

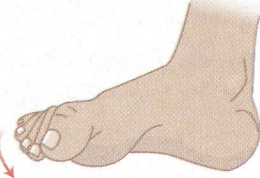

Valgus
An abnormal position of a limb that involves bending outward away from the midline of the body

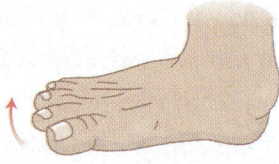

Adduction
Lateral movement of limbs toward the midline of the body

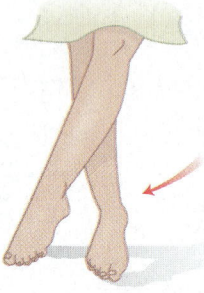

Abduction
Lateral movement of limbs away from the midline of the body

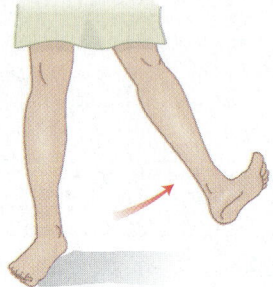

Inversion
Turning inward, usually more than normal

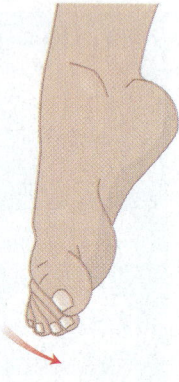

Eversion
Turning outward

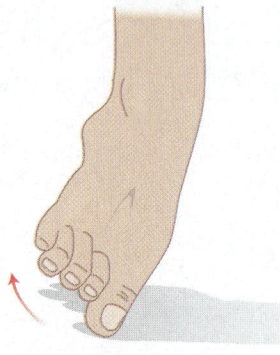

Supination
Lying on the back or placing the hand so the palm faces upward

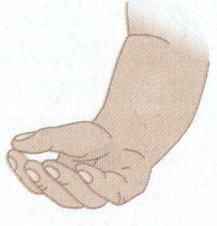

Pronation
Lying on the stomach or placing the hand so the palm faces downward

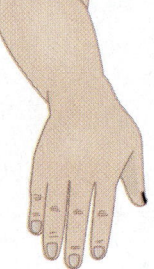

Musculoskeletal disorders may be congenital, such as clubfoot, or acquired, such as osteomyelitis. They may require short- or long-term management, and may be treated on an outpatient basis or require hospitalization. Many musculoskeletal disorders require surgical correction, casting, or braces.

Table 50–1 reviews several terms that will be used throughout this chapter in describing the positioning of a child's limbs.

ANATOMY AND PHYSIOLOGY OF PEDIATRIC DIFFERENCES

Bones

The bones of children and those of adults differ in several ways. Although primary centers of **ossification** (bone formation) are nearly complete at birth, a fibrous membrane still exists between the cranial bones (fontanels) (see "As They Grow: Sutures" on page 776). The posterior fontanel closes between 2 and 3 months of age. The anterior fontanel does not close until approximately 18 months of age, allowing for growth of the brain and skull. In addition, the ends of the long bones (epiphyses) remain cartilaginous (Figure 50–1 ◆). Long bone growth continues until approximately age 20, when skeletal maturation is complete.

Secondary ossification occurs as the long bones grow. Cartilage cells at the epiphyses are replaced by osteoblasts

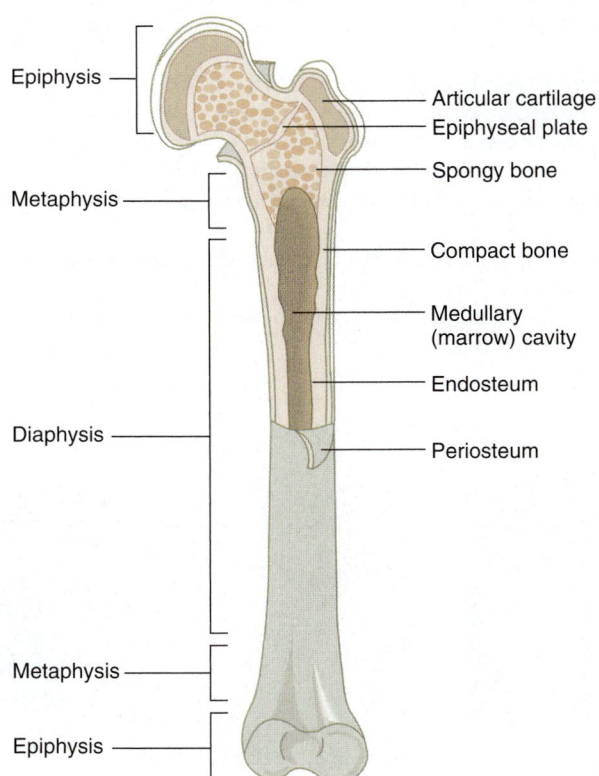

Epiphysis

Articular cartilage
Epiphyseal plate

Metaphysis

Spongy bone

Compact bone

Medullary (marrow) cavity

Endosteum

Diaphysis

Periosteum

Metaphysis

Epiphysis

FIGURE 50–1. ◆ The parts of long bones.

(immature bone cells), resulting in the deposition of calcium. Calcium intake during childhood and adolescence is essential to provide adequate bone density that will prevent osteoporosis and fractures in adulthood. See Chapter 31 for a discussion of inadequate calcium intake during school age and adolescence. Because growth takes place at the epiphyseal plates, injuries to this portion of a long bone are of particular concern in young children.

The long bones of children are porous and less dense than those of adults. For this reason, children's bones can bend, buckle, or break as a result of a simple fall. In addition to the structural differences between the bones of children and adults, there are also functional differences in the skeletal system of children (see "As They Grow: Children Are Not Just Small Adults" on page 765). Before birth, the thoracic and sacral regions of the spine are convex curves. As the infant learns to hold up the head, the cervical region becomes concave. When the child learns to stand, the lumbar region also becomes concave. Failure of the spine to assume these final curves results in an abnormal curvature of the spine (kyphosis or lordosis). The rapid bone growth of childhood facilitates healing after fractures, but may also lead to "growing pains," as muscles are pulled when bones grow quickly (Muscari, 1998).

Muscles, Tendons, and Ligaments

The muscular system, unlike the skeletal system, is almost completely formed at birth. As a child grows, muscles do not increase in number, but rather in length and circumference. Until puberty, both ligaments and tendons are stronger than bone. When these structural differences are not recognized, a childhood fracture is sometimes mistaken for a sprain. A **sprain** is a tearing of ligaments, the structural support connecting bones, usually caused when a joint is twisted or otherwise traumatized. Tendons, which connect bones to muscles, grow in length and fibrous tissue as mechanical pressure is placed on them.

⟿ DISORDERS OF THE FEET AND LEGS

METATARSUS ADDUCTUS

Metatarsus adductus, the most common congenital foot deformity, is characterized by an inward turning of the forefoot at the tarsometatarsal joints (Figure 50–2 ◆). Often referred to as "intoeing," metatarsus adductus affects male and female infants equally and occurs in approximately 1 in 1000 births, with more common incidence among siblings. This condition is most likely caused by both intrauterine positioning and genetic factors (Ryan, 2001). Metatarsus adductus is differentiated from other causes of intoeing, such as internal tibial torsion (more common in children 12 to 18 months and learning to walk), and femoral anteversion (seen more often in preschool-age children).

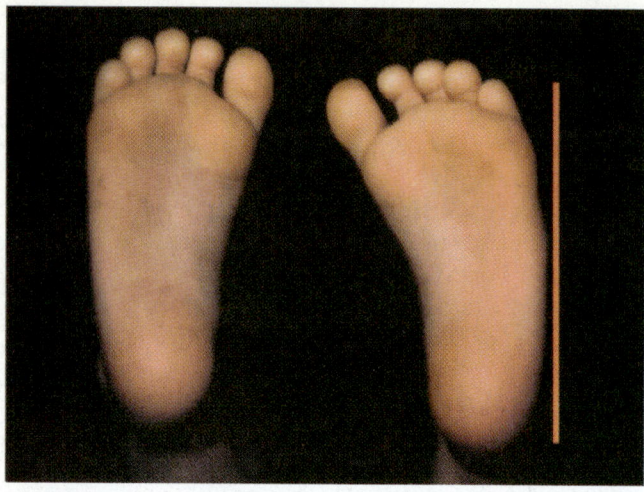

FIGURE 50-2. ◆ Metatarsus adductus is characterized by convexity (curvature) of the lateral border of the foot, as shown by the red line. *Note:* From Staheli, L. T. (1992). *Fundamentals of pediatric orthopedics* (p. 5.7). New York: Roven Press.

Treatment depends on the degree of foot flexibility. If the foot can be readily maneuvered past the neutral position, simple exercises may correct the problem. Most cases resolve spontaneously by the time the infant is about 3 months of age. Serial casting is the treatment of choice for curvature angles greater than 15 degrees, or in cases that do not improve. The infant's feet are placed in a position as close to neutral as possible and are held secure with casts. Casts are changed weekly until the desired correction is achieved. Braces and orthopedic shoes may also be used to maintain correction after casting (Mankin & Zimbler, 1997).

Nursing Management

Reassure parents that the child's condition can be corrected. If the child's deformity is mild, teach parents simple stretching exercises to perform at each diaper change. The foot is held securely by the heel and the forefoot is moved outward from the body with the other hand. The position is maintained for 5 seconds, and repeated 5 times

TABLE 50-2   Nursing Care of the Child in a Cast

- A plaster cast takes anywhere from 24 to 48 hours to dry. When handling the wet cast, be gentle and use the palms of your hands, as fingertips can indent plaster and create pressure areas.
- After the cast is applied, elevate the extremity on a pillow above the level of the heart. Elevation helps reduce swelling and increases venous return.
- If the cast is applied after surgery, there may be drainage or bleeding through the cast material. Circle the stain and note the date and time on the cast to provide a way to assess the amount of fluid lost.
- Assess the distal pulses, and check the fingers and toes for color, warmth, capillary refill, and edema. Assess sensation as well as movement. Any deviation from normal may indicate nerve damage or decreased blood supply.
- During the first 24 hours, check the casted extremity every 15–30 minutes for 2 hours, then every 1–2 hours thereafter. The skin should be warm. It should blanch when slight pressure is applied and then return to its normal color within 3 seconds (A). For the next 2 days, assess the casted extremity at least every 4 hours.
- Check the edges of the cast for roughness or crumbling. If necessary, pull the inner stockinette over the edge of the cast and tape in place.

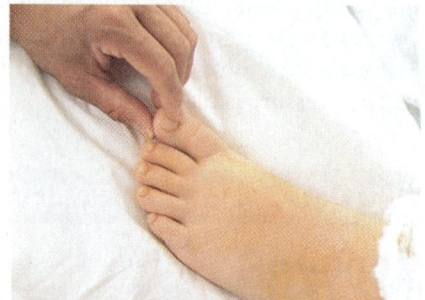

A

- The rough edges of the cast may also be alleviated by "petaling." This is done by securing adhesive tape to the inside of the cast and pulling it over the edge, covering the jagged or broken pieces of plaster, and securing it to the outer surface of the cast (B, C, D). Moleskin may be used on the cast as well.
- Keep the cast as clean and dry as possible. Cover the cast with a plastic bag or plastic wrap when the child bathes or showers.
- The skin under the cast may itch; however, do not use powders or lotions near the edges or under the cast as they can cause skin irritation.
- Be sure that children do not put small objects between the casts and their extremities; that can cause skin irritation as well as neurovascular compromise.

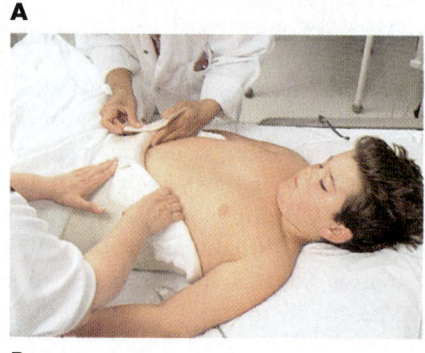

B

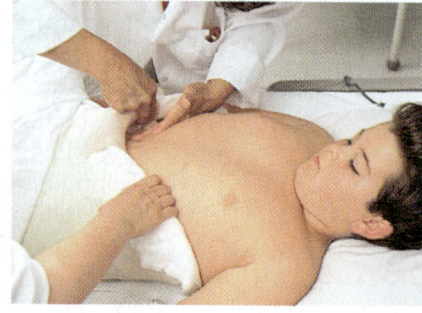

C

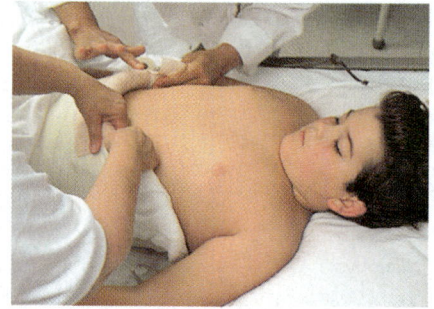

D

CARE OF THE CHILD WITH A CAST

Skin Care

- Check the skin around the cast edges for irritation, rubbing, or blistering. The skin should be clean and dry.
- You may cleanse the skin just under the cast edges and between the toes or fingers with a cotton-tipped applicator and rubbing alcohol. Avoid using lotions, oils, and powders near the cast as they may cause caking.
- Avoid poking sharp objects down inside the cast as this may result in sores.

Cast Care

- Keep the cast dry. Protect plaster with a cast shoe, thick sock, or sling.
- Allow a new, wet cast to air-dry for 24 hours.
- You may walk on a leg cast only if your physician has given you permission to do so.

Be Alert for Possible Complications

- Toes or fingers should be pink, not blue or white.
- Skin should be warm and the tips of the toes should blanch when pinched.
- Raise the casted arm or leg above heart level and rest it on pillows to prevent or reduce any swelling.

Notify Your Health Care Provider If Any of the Following Occur

- Unusual odor beneath the cast
- Tingling
- Burning or numbness in the casted arm or leg
- Drainage through the cast
- Swelling or inability to move the fingers or toes
- Slippage of the cast
- Cast cracked, soft, or loose
- Sudden unexplained fever
- Unusual fussiness or irritability in an infant or child
- Fingers or toes that are blue or white
- Pain that is not relieved by any comfort measures (i.e., repositioning or pain medication)

Courtesy of Shriners Hospital for Children, Spokane, WA.

at each diaper change. If casting is necessary, provide cast care as outlined in Table 50–2 and teach parents how to care for the child in a cast at home (see Skill 17-1). [SKILLS] If metatarsus adductus persists into childhood without correction, the challenge is to find shoes that accommodate the unusual shape of the foot.

CLUBFOOT

Clubfoot is a congenital abnormality in which the foot is twisted out of its normal position. It occurs in approximately 1 to 3 in 1000 births and affects boys nearly twice as often as girls (Fernbach, 1998).

Etiology and Pathophysiology

The exact cause of clubfoot is unknown; however, several possible etiologies have been proposed. Some authorities believe abnormal intrauterine positioning causes the deformity. Others suspect neuromuscular or vascular problems as causes. Yet other experts believe there is a genetic component, either at the chromosomal level or by the arrest of normal fetal development. A positive family history increases the chance of the deformity (Blakeslee, 1997).

Clinical Manifestations

A true clubfoot (talipes equinovarus) involves three areas of deformity: the midfoot is directed downward (**equinus**), the hindfoot turns inward (**varus**), and the forefoot curls toward the heel (adduction) and turns upward in partial supination. Most children have this combination of findings. The foot is small with a shortened Achilles' tendon. Muscles in the lower leg are atrophied, but leg lengths are generally normal. Clubfoot is bilateral in 50% of cases (see "Pathophysiology Illustrated: Clubfoot"). Clubhand is a rare occurrence that has similar characteristics to the foot deformity.

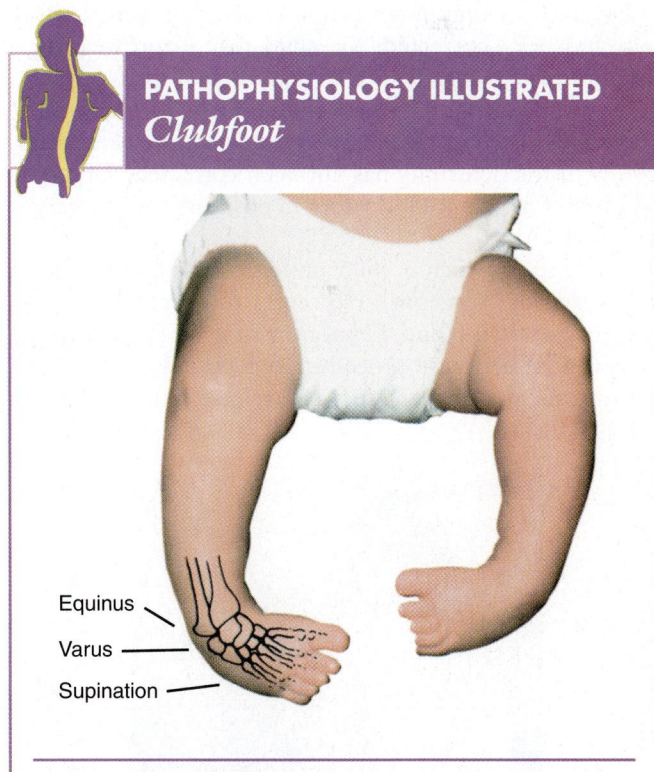

PATHOPHYSIOLOGY ILLUSTRATED
Clubfoot

Equinus
Varus
Supination

Bilateral clubfoot deformity. Parents of a child with clubfoot will have many questions. Can the condition be treated? Will the child be able to walk normally after surgery? Will they need help caring for the infant? How much will surgery and other care cost? Will any subsequent children have a clubfoot?

Note: From Staheli, L. T. (1992). *Fundamentals of pediatric orthopedics* (p. 5.10). New York: Raven Press. Modified.

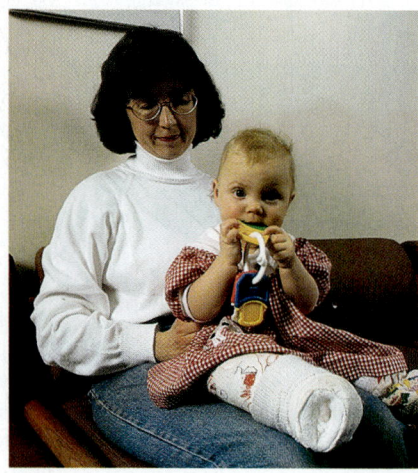

Developing Cultural Competence

The incidence of talipes equinovarus (clubfoot) varies among ethnic groups. The condition is least common in Asian groups and Caucasians, with a higher incidence in groups from the Middle East, South Africa, and Mexico. It is most common in Polynesian groups (Blakeslee, 1997).

Clinical Therapy

Diagnosis is made at birth on the basis of visual inspection. Radiographs are used to confirm the severity of the condition.

Early treatment is essential to achieve successful correction and reduce the chance of complications. Serial casting is the treatment of choice. Casting should begin as soon as possible after birth. Timing is critical because the short bones of the foot, which are primarily cartilaginous at birth, begin to ossify shortly thereafter. The foot is manipulated to achieve maximum correction first of the varus deformity and then of the equinus deformity. A long leg cast holds the foot in the desired position (Figure 50–3 ◆). The cast is changed every 1 to 2 weeks. This regimen of manipulation and casting continues for approximately 8 to 12 weeks until maximum correction is achieved. If the deformity has been corrected, the child may begin wearing a splint or reverse last (shaped so that the foot turns outward away from the body instead of the normal inward turn) corrective shoes to maintain the correction (Fernbach, 1998). If the deformity has not been corrected, surgery is required. Casting holds the foot in position until surgery is performed.

The age at which a child undergoes clubfoot surgery varies among surgeons. However, most children have surgery between 3 and 12 months of age. The one-stage posteromedial release procedure, which involves realignment of the bones of the foot and release of the constrict-ing soft tissue, is most common. The foot is held in the proper position by one or more stainless steel pins. A cast is then applied with the knee flexed to prevent damage to the pin and to discourage weight bearing. Casting continues for 6 to 12 weeks. The child may then need to wear a brace or corrective shoes, depending on the severity of the deformity and the surgeon's preference.

More severe cases or those not corrected in infancy may require more than one surgery to correct the foot.

Nursing Management

Nursing Assessment and Diagnosis

Nursing assessment, which begins at birth and continues throughout the child's subsequent outpatient casting visits and hospitalization for surgery, includes taking a genetic and birth history, performing a physical examination (including position and appearance of the foot), and assessing the child's motor development and family's coping mechanisms. Because parents will need to bring the child for frequent cast changes, ask about transportation and other arrangements needed for these visits.

Among the nursing diagnoses that might apply to the child with a clubfoot deformity are:

▶ *Impaired physical mobility* related to prescribed movement restriction of cast

▶ *Risk for impaired skin integrity* related to cast

▶ *Altered parenting* related to birth of a child with a physical defect

▶ *Health-seeking behaviors (parent)* related to need for information about deformity, treatment, and home care

Planning and Implementation

Nursing management involves providing emotional support, educating the family about home care of the child in a cast and the importance of keeping appointments at the outpatient facility for cast changes, preparation of the family for the child's hospitalization if surgery is to occur, and providing postsurgical care.

PROVIDE EMOTIONAL SUPPORT

Clubfoot affects both the child and the family. The child's foot deformity is upsetting to parents, and they need emotional support to allay their fears. Helping parents understand the condition and its treatment is essential.

Promote bonding by encouraging parents to hold and cuddle the child and to take an active role in the child's care. Explain that, with treatment, the child will grow and develop normally.

PROVIDE CAST AND BRACE CARE

Routine cast care is outlined in Table 50–2. After serial casting is complete, or after surgery, the child may progress to

FIGURE 50–3. ◆ This girl has a long leg cast, which was applied after surgery to correct her clubfoot deformity.

wearing a brace or special shoe for 6 to 12 months. Braces should fit snugly but should not interfere with neurovascular function. Before the child begins to wear a brace, check the skin for any areas of redness or breakdown. Give parents guidelines for brace wear. Emphasize that proper skin care is essential. If skin redness develops, arrange to have the fit of the brace evaluated and modified if necessary.

Teaching About

GUIDELINES FOR BRACE WEAR

- Braces should be as comfortable as possible and the child should have adequate mobility while wearing the brace.
- Begin wearing the brace for periods of 1 to 2 hours and then progress to 2 to 4 hours.
- Check the skin at 1- to 2-hour intervals initially, then lengthening to every 4 hours once skin has been clear for several days. If redness is apparent, leave the brace off and allow the skin to clear. If breakdown has occurred, the brace cannot be replaced until healing is complete. (See Chapter 52 for a discussion of pressure ulcers.)
- Always have the child wear a clean white sock, T-shirt, or other thin white liner beneath the brace. Be sure the liner is wrinkle-free under the brace. Avoid using powders or lotions that can cause skin to break down. Toughen any sensitive areas using alcohol wipes.
- Reapply the brace when the skin returns to its normal color.
- Return to the physician or orthotic specialist if discomfort or red areas persist or if the brace needs adjustment or repair or is outgrown.
- Check the brace daily for rough edges.

PROVIDE POSTSURGICAL CARE

Routine postoperative care after surgical correction includes neurovascular status checks every 2 hours for the first 24 hours and observing for any swelling around the cast edges (see Table 50–2). Apply ice bags to the foot, and keep the ankle and foot elevated on a pillow for 24 hours. This promotes healing and helps with venous return. Check for drainage or bleeding. Administer pain medication routinely for 24 to 48 hours. Popliteal or epidural blocks may be placed during surgery and used in the immediate postsurgical period for pain control (see Skill 13-4). SKILLS Monitor these blocks for effectiveness and any undesired effects (see Chapter 38 for detailed instructions on pain management).

DISCHARGE PLANNING AND HOME CARE TEACHING

Give parents written instructions for care of the child with a cast (see page 1321). In addition, assist them in the following ways:

- Demonstrate the use of a sponge bath to protect the cast from water breakdown.
- Discuss options for clothing that accommodate a cast, for example, one-piece snap suits or sweatpants.

- Discuss potential safety hazards that may result from awkward positioning. Be sure the child is properly situated in a car safety seat for the trip home.
- Provide resources for strollers and other equipment that will support the cast so it does not hang down during the baby's activities.
- Suggest that parents try to place toys within the child's reach, since the movements of a child in a cast may be slowed.

Evaluation

Expected outcomes of nursing care include maintenance of skin integrity, recovery without complications after surgery, normal developmental progression of the child, and demonstrated parental knowledge of care of braces or casts, as needed.

GENU VARUM AND GENU VALGUM

Genu varum (bowlegs) is a deformity in which the knees are widely separated and the lower legs are turned inward (varus). In genu valgum (knock-knees), the knees are close together and the lower legs are directed outward (valgus).

At certain stages of a child's development, the appearance of bowlegs or knock-knees is normal. Until 2 to 3 years of age, the knees are normally bowed, showing varus alignment, and by 4 to 5 years, some knock-knee or valgus alignment is common (Mankin & Zimbler, 1997). However, the persistence of knock-knees beyond the age of 4 to 5 years necessitates further evaluation. The most common pathologic causes of bowed legs are Blount disease (disruption of tibial growth plate) and rickets (see Chapter 31). Chapter 33 discusses the assessment of bowlegs and knock-knees in children.

Braces are often used to correct mild deformities that could worsen as the child grows. Braces for bowlegs are worn at night; those for knock-knees both day and night. Duration of brace wear is determined by the severity of the deformity, which is usually evaluated by radiographs. If the deformity continues to worsen, surgery is necessary. An **osteotomy** (cutting of the bone) is performed and the tibiofemoral angle surgically corrected. The child is then placed in a cast for approximately 6 to 10 weeks, or until completely healed.

Nursing Management

Reassure parents that bowlegs and knock-knees are usually a normal part of a child's growth and development. These conditions often resolve on their own and need no treatment other than monitoring.

Nursing care focuses on educating the parents and child about the condition and its treatment. Give the child and family guidelines for brace wear and maintenance (see "Teaching About: Guidlines for Brace Wear").

✎ DISORDERS OF THE HIP

DEVELOPMENTAL DYSPLASIA OF THE HIP

Developmental dysplasia of the hip (DDH) refers to a variety of conditions in which the femoral head and the acetabulum are improperly aligned. These conditions include hip instability, **dislocation** (displacement of the bone from its normal articulation with the joint), **subluxation** (in this instance, a partial dislocation), and acetabular **dysplasia** (abnormal cellular or structural development) (American Academy of Pediatrics, 2000). In the past, DDH was referred to as congenital dislocated hip (CDH). The revised name of the disorder emphasizes that many cases of dislocation, subluxation, and dysplasia occur well after the neonatal period and involve more than a simple dislocation.

One in 100 newborns has hip instability, while dislocation occurs in 1 to 2 in 1000 births, and the condition affects girls four times as often as boys. It is unilateral in 80% of affected children, and the left hip is affected three times as often as the right (American Academy of Pediatrics, 2000).

Etiology and Pathophysiology

Although the exact cause of DDH is unknown, genetic factors appear to play a role. DDH is 20 to 50 times more common in first-degree relatives of an infant with the condition than in the general population. If one child of a set of identical twins has DDH, the other twin is affected 30% to 40% of the time.

Prenatal conditions may affect the development of DDH. The left hip is involved more often than the right hip as a result of intrauterine positioning of the left side of the fetus against the mother's sacrum. Maternal estrogen may cause laxity of the hip joint and capsule, leading to joint instability, especially in females who respond to these estrogen levels. DDH is more common in infants born in the breech position. Cultural factors may also be associated with DDH.

✎ Developing Cultural Competence

Infants positioned on cradle boards or traditionally swaddled, as in some Native-American cultures, have a high incidence of developmental dysplasia of the hip (DDH). Among cultures in which mothers carry infants on their hips or backs with the infants' legs abducted—as in Korean, Chinese, and some African groups—the incidence of DDH is low (Novacheck, 1996).

Clinical Manifestations

Common signs and symptoms of DDH include limited abduction of the affected hip, asymmetry of the gluteal and thigh fat folds, and telescoping or pistoning of the thigh

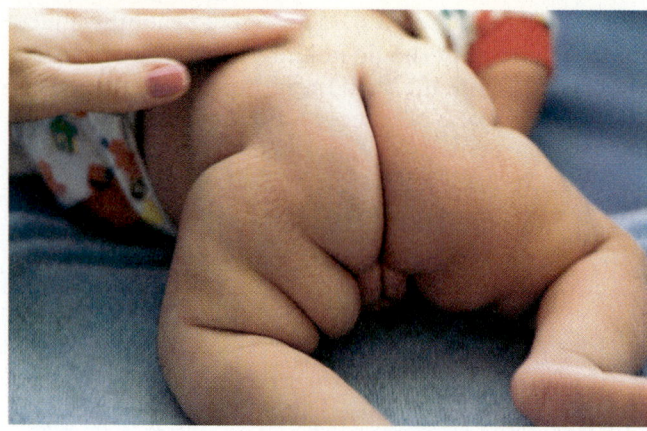

FIGURE 50–4. ◆ The asymmetry of the gluteal and thigh fat folds is easy to see in this child with developmental dysplasia of the hip.

(Figure 50–4 ◆). The older child with untreated DDH walks with a significant limp, which results from telescoping of the femoral head into the pelvis. The longer the disorder goes untreated, the more pronounced the clinical manifestations become, and the worse the prognosis.

Clinical Therapy

Physical examination reveals Allis' sign (one knee lower than the other when the knees are flexed) and positive Ortolani and Barlow maneuvers in babies under 8 to 12 weeks. Refer to Chapter 33 for a discussion of the assessment of hip dysplasia in newborns and infants. ⟨⊃ Radiographs are generally not reliable until approximately 4 months of age because the pelvis in a newborn is still primarily cartilaginous. Before 4 months of age, ultrasonography may be useful for diagnosis. After that age, radiographs are used for diagnosis.

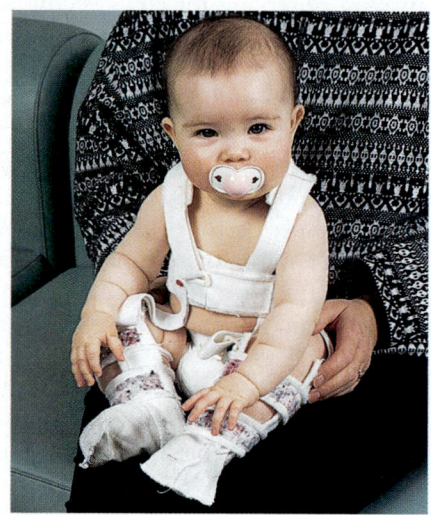

FIGURE 50–5. ◆ The most common treatment for DDH in a child under 3 months of age is a Pavlik harness. A shirt should be worn under the harness to prevent skin irritation. (It was omitted for clarity in this photograph.)

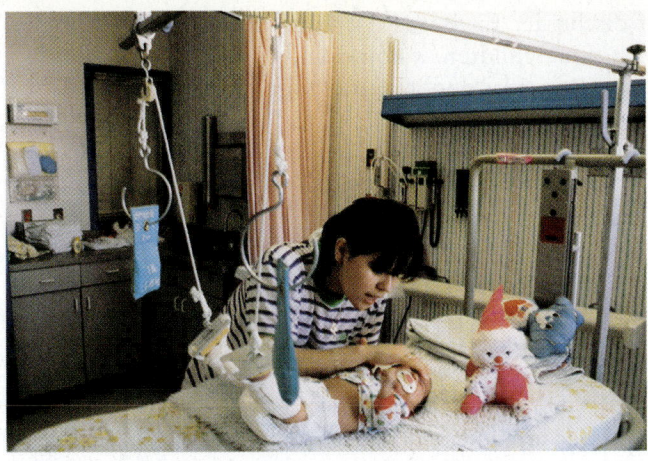

FIGURE 50–6. ◆ For infants older than 3 months of age, skin traction is commonly used for treatment of DDH.

Treatment plans vary according to the child's age. For infants younger than 3 months of age, the Pavlik harness is the most commonly used method for hip reduction (Figure 50–5 ◆). The Pavlik harness is a dynamic splint—that is, a splint that allows movement. It ensures hip flexion and abduction and does not allow hip extension or adduction. For infants older than 3 months of age, skin traction is used (Figure 50–6 ◆). Correct positioning, which involves relocating the femoral head into the acetabulum while gently stretching the restrictive soft tissue, is essential. Surgery and a spica cast may be necessary. In children over 18 months of age, surgery and casting are usually necessary and bracing may also be required.

Early screening, detection, and treatment enable most affected children to attain normal hip function.

Nursing Management

Nursing Assessment and Diagnosis

Assessment for DDH begins at delivery and continues through all well-child checkups. The family history or birth data may indicate a high-risk infant. Instructions for performing the physical examination to assess the infant for DDH are given in Chapter 33. ⊂⊃ Further assessments are determined by the treatment provided. Assess the skin of the child in traction or a cast. Include respiratory and circulatory assessments when the child is immobilized. Ongoing assessment of the child's growth and development is needed. Weigh the casted child once the cast is dry so a baseline casted weight can be used for comparison while the cast remains in place.

Several nursing diagnoses may apply to the child with DDH. They include:

▶ *Impaired physical mobility* related to prescribed movement restriction (Pavlik harness, traction, spica cast, brace)

▶ *Risk for impaired skin integrity* related to irritation from harness straps or skin traction

▶ *Risk for altered urinary elimination or constipation* related to immobility caused by treatment

▶ *Risk for altered nutrition* related to decreased appetite

▶ *Risk for altered growth and development* related to limited mobility and potential decreased exposure to stimulation

▶ *Health-seeking behaviors (parent)* related to need for information about disease process and treatment

Planning and Implementation

The infant with DDH is often cared for at home and in outpatient facilities. If surgery is performed the child is hospitalized for surgery and the immediate postoperative period. Nursing care varies according to the medical treatment and the child's age. Management includes maintaining traction, if ordered; providing cast care; preventing complications resulting from immobility; promoting normal growth and development; and teaching parents how to care for a child in a cast, traction, or a Pavlik harness at home. Because treatment may interfere with the child's normal movement, the treatment plan should take into consideration the age and developmental stage of the child.

MAINTAIN TRACTION

Bryant skin traction is the most common form of traction used in the treatment of DDH. (Types of traction are discussed later in the chapter and presented in Table 50–4). Check the traction apparatus frequently to ensure proper alignment and healing. Traction may also be used in the home. The family needs careful instruction in how to care for the child in traction. In addition, a nurse needs to make several home visits to set up the traction apparatus and monitor the child's progress after discharge (see Table 50–5 later in the chapter). The apparatus should be set up so that nuts and bolts are tight, knots are secure, weights are hanging free, and lines are straight (see Skill 17-3). ⊂⊃ **SKILLS**

PROVIDE CAST CARE

The principles of routine cast care presented in Table 50–2 apply to the care of spica casts. Special techniques should be used to help keep the cast clean and dry in children who are not toilet trained. Female and male urinals can be used for older children. Use a plastic lining to protect the cast edges during elimination for older children and use a small disposable diaper to cover the perineum in babies, tucking edges beneath the cast. Be sure to change the diaper frequently to prevent soiling of the cast.

PREVENT COMPLICATIONS RESULTING FROM IMMOBILITY

Immobilization from traction or a cast can cause alterations in physiologic functioning. To prevent complications:

▶ Assess breathing patterns and lung sounds frequently for congestion or respiratory compromise.

- Perform skin and neurovascular assessments approximately every 2 hours.

- Use adequate padding and skin wrapping to avoid placing pressure on the popliteal space. Such pressure could lead to nerve damage.

- For the child in a cast, change the child's position every 2 to 3 hours while awake to help avoid areas of pressure and promote increased circulation. The child can be placed either prone or supine or positioned on the floor and supported with pillows.

- Help prevent skin irritation and breakdown in the child with a cast. Use moleskin to protect from rough edges. Place tape around the perineal opening of the cast to prevent soiling.

- Increase fluids and fiber in the child's diet, as a change in bowel or bladder status is commonly associated with immobility.

- If permitted by physician orders, release the child from traction for meals and daily care. The time out of traction should not exceed 1 hour per day. Encourage parents to hold and cuddle the child at this time to promote comfort and bonding.

PROMOTE NORMAL GROWTH AND DEVELOPMENT

Engage the child in activities that stimulate the upper extremities and all five senses. Provide stimulating toys such as stacking blocks, brightly colored mobiles, soft balls, or musical toys. Position toys within the child's reach and interact with the child as much as possible.

DISCHARGE PLANNING AND HOME CARE TEACHING

Teach parents how to care for a child in traction or a spica cast at home. Family members' active participation in the child's daily care during hospitalization gradually increases their confidence in their ability to provide care once home. Identify and address home care needs well in advance of discharge. Before discharge, be sure the parents have:

- Information about general cast care (see page 1321), positioning, bathing, toileting, and age-appropriate diversional activities.

- Safety teaching to minimize chance of injury to a casted child.

- Instruction about types of toys that are age-appropriate and measures to prevent them from being placed into cast (a t-shirt should be placed over the cast covering its edges).

- Appropriate referrals for periodic assessment by a visiting nurse or home health nurse.

- Family resources to care for the child.

Before discharge, have parents demonstrate how to dress and feed a child in a spica cast. Ensure that safe travel arrangements have been made for the day of discharge. Help parents get an appropriate car safety seat in advance

of discharge. Encourage parents to let the child interact with other children at home, and to provide the child in a cast with similar opportunities for play and social activities.

Teaching About

TRANSPORTING THE CHILD WITH ORTHOPEDIC DEVICES

The American Academy of Pediatrics (1999) has established guidelines for transporting children with special health care needs.

- Riding in the rear seat is preferable.

- If the front seat must be used, the front passenger airbag should be disconnected.

- Use only car seat transport systems approved for use with special needs children. 🔗 WEB

- Install and use seats as instructed.

- Move a child from a wheelchair or other special device to the vehicle safety seat whenever this is reasonable.

- Pieces of medical equipment required during transportation (such as monitors or oxygen) or that are being transported with the child (such as wheelchair or walker) should be secured to the floor of the vehicle.

- If the child is transported by school bus, follow state and federal recommendations for school bus transportation of children with special needs.

NURSING CARE IN THE COMMUNITY

Have parents of an infant in a Pavlik harness demonstrate proper application of the harness and care of the infant in the harness. Teach family members about daily care (bathing, dressing, and feeding) of the infant. Ideally, the harness is worn 23 hours per day and is removed only for skin checks and bathing. The hips and buttocks should be supported carefully when the infant is out of the harness. Demonstrate how to feed the infant in an upright position to maintain abduction and how to change a diaper without removing the harness. Double diapering may be recommended to support the hips.

Instruct the parents of an infant with a harness or a child in a cast to look for any reddened or irritated areas near the harness or cast edges and to check toes frequently for proper circulation. Frequent repositioning reduces the risk of pressure sores or circulatory compromise. The infant should wear an undershirt and socks under the harness to prevent rubbing of the skin.

Safety precautions are important as the child will not have normal mobility. Parents will need to use a specially designed car seat that accommodates the child with abducted hips (see "Teaching About: Transporting the Child with Orthopedic Devices"). Strollers and cribs should provide sufficient room to protect the legs from injury and to prevent hip adduction.

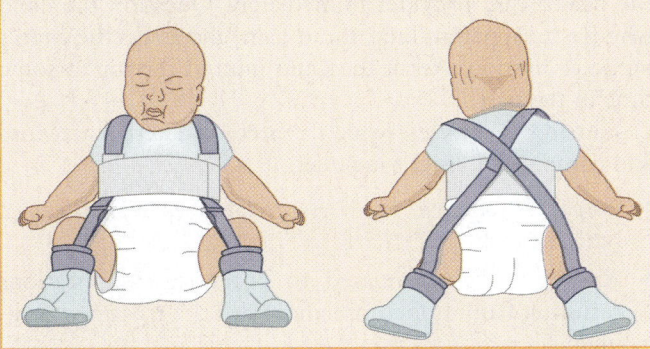

Teaching About

GUIDELINES FOR PAVLIK HARNESS APPLICATION

1. Position the chest halter at nipple line and fasten with Velcro.
2. Position the legs and feet in the stirrups, being sure the hips are flexed and abducted. Fasten with Velcro.
3. Connect the chest halter and leg straps in front.
4. Connect the chest halter and leg straps in back.

All the straps are marked at the first fitting with indelible ink so they can be reattached easily after the harness is rinsed and dried.

Evaluation

Expected outcomes for nursing care of the child with developmental dysplasia of the hip include:

▶ Maintenance of skin integrity
▶ Absence of symptoms of immobility
▶ Knowledge by parents about the condition, treatment, and necessary home care
▶ Maintenance of a safe environment for the child

LEGG-CALVÉ-PERTHES DISEASE

Legg-Calvé-Perthes disease is a self-limiting condition characterized by avascular necrosis of the femoral head. The disease occurs in approximately 1 in 12,000 children and affects boys four times more often than girls. It usually occurs between the ages of 2 and 12 years, with a peak incidence between 4 and 8 years. The disease is bilateral in 10% of cases (Roy, 1999).

Etiology and Pathophysiology

The necrosis associated with Legg-Calvé-Perthes disease results from an interruption of the blood supply to the femoral epiphysis. How and why this occurs is not completely understood, but several predisposing factors have been identified. The incidence of Legg-Calvé-Perthes disease is up to 20% higher in families with a history of the disease than in the general population, which suggests that genetic factors may play a role. In one quarter of the cases, onset of the disease is preceded by a mild traumatic injury. Trauma may cause a subchondral fracture and resultant synovitis, which in turn causes pressure that occludes the blood supply. Children with Legg-Calvé-Perthes disease often have delayed skeletal maturation, increased thyroid levels, and low somatomedin C (insulin-like growth factor). It is more common in those with low birth weight, increased parental age, and exposure to environmental tobacco smoke (Roy, 1999).

Developing Cultural Competence

Legg-Calvé-Perthes disease is most common among white and Chinese children. It is less common among blacks and Native Americans.

Clinical Manifestations

Legg-Calvé-Perthes disease progresses through four distinct stages after the original insult (usually unknown) occurs, over a period of 1 to 4 years. Early symptoms of Legg-Calvé-Perthes disease include a mild pain in the hip or anterior thigh and a limp, which are aggravated by increased activity and relieved by rest. The child favors the affected hip and limits hip movement to avoid discomfort (Davids, 1998).

CLINICAL MANIFESTATIONS ～ *Legg-Calvé-Perthes Disease*

STAGE	CLINICAL MANIFESTATIONS
Prenecrosis	An insult causes loss of blood supply to the femoral head.
I—Necrosis	Avascular stage (3–6 months); the child is asymptomatic, bone radiographs are normal, and the head of the femur is structurally intact but avascular.
II—Revascularization	Period of 1–4 years characterized by pain and limitation of movement. Bone radiographs show new bone deposition and dead bone resorption. Fracture and deformity of the head of the femur can occur.
III—Bone healing	Reossification takes place; pain decreases.
IV—Remodeling	The disease process is over, pain is absent, and improvement in joint function occurs.

As the disease progresses, range of motion becomes limited and weakness and muscle wasting develop. The affected thigh is 2 to 3 cm smaller than the unaffected thigh. Over time, prolonged hip irritability may produce muscle spasms.

Clinical Therapy

Because the child's initial symptoms are so mild, parents often do not seek medical attention until symptoms have been present for several months. Diagnosis is made using standard anteroposterior and frog-leg radiographs. As noted on page 1327, radiographs taken early in the course of the disease may be normal or show vague widening of the cartilage space. Bone scans and magnetic resonance imaging (MRI) may show the disease process earlier than radiographs. Laboratory studies of the blood, such as white blood cell count, help to rule out inflammatory synovitis of the hip.

Medical management and prognosis depend on the degree of femoral involvement. Early detection is important. The desired outcome is a pain-free hip that functions properly. To promote healing and prevent deformity, the femoral head must be contained within the hip socket until ossification is complete. This can happen only if the hips remain in an abducted position. At the beginning of treatment, traction can be used to maintain the hips in an abducted and internally rotated position. Once abduction is accomplished, treatment consists of Petrie (leg abduction) casting, or surgical soft tissue releases such as adductor tenotomy, followed by bracing. Toronto (Figure 50–7 ◆) and Scottish-Rite braces are most commonly used. Prognosis is good if the femoral head can be contained long enough for proper healing to occur. Severe disease may be treated by surgery to release adductor muscles, treat the acetabulum or femur, and restore range of motion. Children with untreated disease or those diagnosed late in the

disease process occasionally develop osteoarthritis and hip dysfunction later in life (Roy, 1999).

Nursing Management

Nursing Assessment and Diagnosis

Suspect Legg-Calvé-Perthes disease in any child, especially a boy aged 2 to 12 years, who complains of hip discomfort accompanied by a limp. The school nurse may be the first person to observe the child with symptoms of Legg-Calvé-Perthes disease. The child may complain of pain and have to rest during physical education classes. Refer the child to the health care provider immediately. Question the child who has an apparent limp about pain, and assess the child's range of motion. Ask if the child injured the hip at some time in the past.

Nursing diagnoses, which center on altered activities and compliance, might include:

▶ *Impaired physical mobility* related to restriction of brace or cast

▶ *Risk for injury* related to potential complications resulting from noncompliance with the treatment regimen

▶ *Risk for noncompliance* related to duration of treatment

▶ *Diversional activity deficit* related to forced inactivity

▶ *Potential body image disturbance* related to brace

Planning and Implementation

Children with Legg-Calvé-Perthes disease often receive all of their treatment at home. Helping the child and family comply with the prescribed treatment plan may be challenging, because children develop the disease at an age when they are usually very active. The child, who may have little pain, often finds immobilization difficult.

PROMOTE NORMAL GROWTH AND DEVELOPMENT

Give parents suggestions to help redirect the child's energy within the limitations in mobility imposed by treatment. A return to school promotes a feeling of normalcy. Coordinate the return to school by facilitating the child's use of elevator or ramp as needed in that setting. Activities that involve peers also help the child achieve developmental milestones. Help the child adjust to wearing a brace.

Growth and Development

Legg-Calvé-Perthes disease primarily affects boys with an average age of 6 years. These school-age children are industrious and independent. Suggest activities that redirect energy and promote normal development. These may include horseback riding, which promotes hip abduction; swimming to increase mobility; handcrafts to promote fine motor skills; and computer activities to stimulate cognitive development.

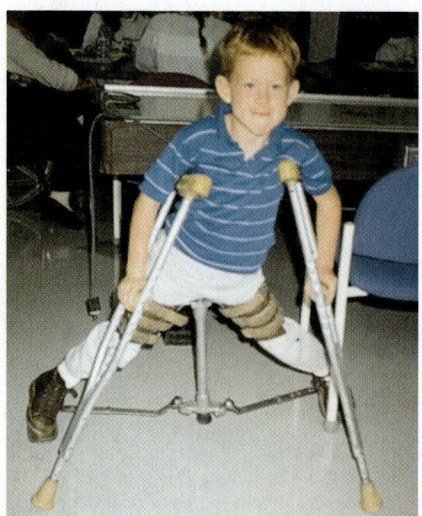

FIGURE 50–7. ◆ Although the Toronto brace may seem formidable for a child to wear, you can see by this photograph that, as usual, children adapt quite well to it.

NURSING CARE IN THE COMMUNITY

Both the child and the family should be aware that treatment generally takes more than 2 years. Emphasize the importance of following the treatment plan to ensure adequate hip containment and proper healing. Teach the family how to care for a child in traction and how to check the child's skin for breakdown (see Table 50–5). Follow-up visits should be arranged at regular intervals, in addition to home care visits during the period of traction.

Evaluation

Expected outcomes of nursing care are elimination of hip pain and discomfort, normal development during the period of immobilization, and parent and child knowledge of treatment regimen.

SLIPPED CAPITAL FEMORAL EPIPHYSIS

Slipped capital femoral epiphysis (SCFE) occurs when the femoral head is displaced from the femoral neck. This condition is commonly seen during the adolescent growth spurt, between the ages of 8 to 16 years. Boys are more often affected than girls (Theophilopoulos & Barrett, 1998).

Etiology and Pathophysiology

The cause of SCFE is unknown. Predisposing factors include obesity, a recent growth spurt, and endocrine disorders such as hypothyroidism and hypogonadism. There may be a genetic predisposition to the development of the disorder.

Slippage of the femoral head occurs at the proximal epiphyseal plate, and the femur displaces from the epiphysis (see "Pathophysiology Illustrated: Slipped Epiphysis"). Slippage is usually gradual (chronic), but may also result from acute trauma. The synovial membrane becomes inflamed, edematous, and painful. If untreated, callous formation occurs, resulting in a deformed hip with limited range of motion.

Clinical Manifestations

Symptoms include limp, pain, and loss of hip motion. The condition is categorized as acute (sudden onset with less than 3 weeks' duration), chronic (longer than 3 weeks' duration), or acute-on-chronic (an additional slippage in a child with a chronic condition), depending on the onset and severity of symptoms. The child with an acute slip has sudden, severe pain and cannot bear weight. An acute slip may be associated with traumatic injury.

A chronic slip presents with persistent hip pain, which is generally aching or mild and can be referred to the thigh, knee, or both. A limp and decreased range of motion may also occur.

When the child has had a chronic slip and then sustains a traumatic incident that causes further slippage of the

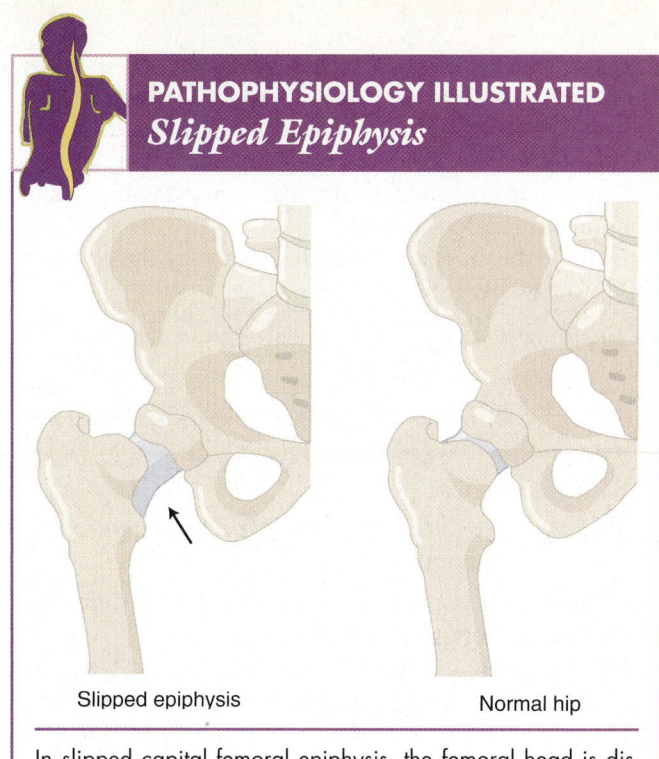

PATHOPHYSIOLOGY ILLUSTRATED
Slipped Epiphysis

Slipped epiphysis   Normal hip

In slipped capital femoral epiphysis, the femoral head is displaced from the femoral neck at the proximal epiphyseal plate.

femoral head, an acute-on-chronic slip is said to have occurred. The child experiences sudden, severe pain.

Clinical Therapy

A complete history provides information about risk factors and the development of the condition. Radiographs confirm the diagnosis. A bone scan may also be performed.

The goal of medical management is to stabilize the femoral head while keeping displacement to a minimum and retaining as much hip function as possible. Surgical treatment is usually necessary; this involves fixation of the epiphysis with screws or pins. If treated early, a single screw into the hip in an outpatient procedure is sufficient for stabilization; in more advanced cases surgery becomes more complicated (Shaw, Gerardi, & Hennrikus, 1998). Medical treatment, which is occasionally used, includes a regimen of no weight bearing, bed rest, a spica cast, and Buck or Russell traction (see Table 50–4).

Prognosis is related to the severity of the deformity and the occurrence of complications, such as avascular necrosis of the femoral head or **chondrolysis** (the breaking down and absorption of cartilage).

Nursing Management

Nursing Assessment and Diagnosis

The child usually presents with hip pain or referred pain to the groin, thigh, or knee, and limited mobility. A thorough history is needed to assess for injury as a cause. Assess the child's range of motion, pain, and limp, if apparent. Refer the child for treatment immediately if SCFE is suspected. This condition is considered to be an emergency, and it is essential that the child be treated immediately to keep weight off the affected joint.

Among the nursing diagnoses that may apply to the child with SCFE are:

▶ *Impaired physical mobility* related to treatment

▶ *Pain* related to hip injury

▶ *Risk for body image disturbance* related to treatment

▶ *Risk for altered growth and development* related to mobility restrictions

▶ *Risk for altered nutrition: more than body requirements* related to immobility

▶ *Altered tissue perfusion: peripheral* related to traction, casting, and other treatments

▶ *Health-seeking behaviors (child and parent)* related to disease process and treatment

Planning and Implementation

Nursing management involves caring for the child in traction or after surgery, administering medications and other pain-control interventions, maintaining mobility within the limits imposed by treatment, providing adequate nutrition, educating the child and family about the disorder, providing emotional support, and promoting compliance with the treatment plan.

ENCOURAGE APPROPRIATE NUTRITIONAL INTAKE

A growing adolescent needs increased amounts of proteins, carbohydrates, and calcium to promote skeletal healing. Provide written instructions about nutritional requirements to promote bone healing and maintain an ideal body weight. If a child is overweight, encourage weight loss by decreasing the percentage of fat in the diet. Weight loss decreases pressure on the femoral epiphysis and can also lead to a more positive self-image.

PROVIDE EMOTIONAL SUPPORT

Because the onset of SCFE is usually unexpected, the child and family may find themselves facing surgery with little warning. Explain the treatment plan simply and thoroughly. Reassure the child and family that with proper compliance, treatment should be successful.

DISCHARGE PLANNING AND HOME CARE TEACHING

Help the family plan for return to school. If attendance is not possible for a time due to traction or surgery, arrange for tutors and computer communication with school as needed. Follow-up visits are necessary until the child's epiphyseal plates close. It is not uncommon for SCFE to

occur in the other hip. Make sure the child and family are aware of symptoms such as decreased range of motion or pain that could indicate onset of the disorder in the other hip. Tell parents to contact their health care provider immediately if these symptoms occur.

Evaluation

Expected outcomes of nursing care for the child with SCFE include maintenance of normal weight and recommended nutritional intake, absence of complications of immobility, successful adaptation to school following treatment, and family recognition of need for ongoing monitoring for complications.

⮕ DISORDERS OF THE SPINE

SCOLIOSIS

Scoliosis is a lateral S- or C-shaped curvature of the spine that is often associated with a rotational deformity of the spine and ribs. Many people exhibit some degree of spinal curvature; curvatures of more than 10 degrees are considered abnormal. Curves are either structural or compensatory, as the spine curves to compensate for a structural deformity along its length. Idiopathic scoliosis occurs most often in girls, especially during the growth spurt between the ages of 10 and 13 years. Early onset of idiopathic scoliosis occurs before 10 years of age and comprises 15% of cases (Kautz & Skaggs, 1998).

Etiology and Pathophysiology

The cause of scoliosis is complex. Structural scoliosis may be congenital, idiopathic, or acquired (associated with neuromuscular disorders such as muscular dystrophy or myelodysplasia, or secondary to spinal cord injuries).

In idiopathic structural scoliosis (the most common type), the spine for unknown reasons begins to curve laterally, with vertebral rotation. The most common curve is a right thoracic and left lumbar deformity. As the curve progresses, structural changes occur. The ribs on the concave side (inside of the curve) are forced closer together, while the ribs on the convex side separate widely, causing narrowing of the thoracic cage and formation of the rib hump. The lateral curvature affects the vertebral structure. Disk spaces are narrowed on the concave side and spread wider on the convex side, resulting in an asymmetric vertebral canal (Figure 50–8 ◆).

Scoliosis can also occur in congenital diseases involving the spinal structure and in the musculoskeletal changes seen in conditions such as myelomeningocele, cerebral palsy (see Chapter 49), or muscular dystrophy. It can also be acquired after injury to the spinal cord.

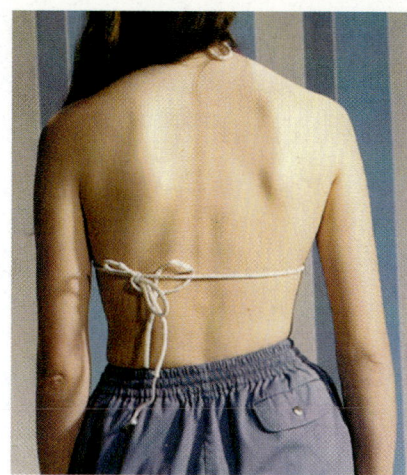

FIGURE 50–8. ◆ A child may have varying degrees of scoliosis. For mild forms, treatment will focus on strengthening and stretching. Moderate forms will require bracing. Severe forms may necessitate surgery and fusion. Clothes that fit at an angle, such as this teenage girl's shorts, and anatomic asymmetry of the back provide clues for early detection.

Clinical Manifestations

The classic signs of scoliosis include truncal asymmetry, uneven shoulders and hips, a one-sided rib hump, and a prominent scapula. The child does not complain of pain or discomfort.

Clinical Therapy

Generally, observation and radiographic examination diagnose scoliosis. Additional diagnostic studies include MRI, computed tomography (CT), and bone scanning, which are used occasionally to assess the degree of curvature. Moiré photography using a special screen and a point light source documents asymmetry of the spine and other bony landmarks.

The goal of medical management is to limit or stop progression of the curvature. Early detection is essential to successful treatment. Adequate treatment and follow-up maximize the child's chances for proper spinal alignment. The treatment regimen chosen depends on the degree and progression of the curvature and the reaction of the child and family to medical management.

Treatment of children with mild scoliosis (curvatures of 10 to 20 degrees) consists of exercises to improve posture and muscle tone and to maintain, or possibly increase, flexibility of the spine. Emphasis is placed on bending strength toward the outside of the curve while stretching the inside of the curve. These exercises are not a cure, however, and the child should be evaluated by a physician at 3–month intervals, with radiographic evaluation every 6 months.

Medical management of moderate scoliosis (curvatures of 20 to 40 degrees) includes bracing with either a Boston or Milwaukee brace. The goal of wearing a brace is to maintain the existing spinal curvature with no increase. Brace wear begins immediately after diagnosis. To achieve maximum effectiveness, the brace should be worn 23 hours per day. Brace treatment is lengthy and requires a high degree of compliance, which can be difficult for adolescents, for whom body image or sports involvement is often important.

Electrical stimulation is used occasionally as an alternative treatment. An electric current stimulates the back muscles to contract, thus helping to correct the spinal curvature. This treatment, performed at night, eliminates the need for bracing. There is controversy about the usefulness of this therapy.

Children with severe scoliosis (curvatures of 40 degrees or more) require surgery, which involves spinal fusion. The majority of spinal fusions are performed using instrumentation with Luque wires or Coutrel-Dubosset (CD) instrumentation. These treatments stabilize the spine well during surgery, may be accompanied by bone grafting to the spine, and require no long-term therapy (Killian, Mayberry, & Wilkinson, 1999). Following surgery with wires or instrumentation, the child is on bed rest during a recovery period and then is generally fitted with anteroposterior plastic shells that are worn for several months to provide stability for the spine.

Nursing Management

Nursing Assessment and Diagnosis

School nurses often screen children for scoliosis, generally in the fifth and seventh grades. Several states mandate this screening. When abnormalities are noted, refer the child to an orthopedic center for further evaluation. Children should be examined every 6 to 9 months thereafter. If scoliosis is detected, the child's brothers and sisters should be examined and observed closely. Chapter 33 discusses screening children for scoliosis.

Once scoliosis has been identified, the focus becomes education and follow-up. Any child with scoliosis should have a comprehensive neurologic, cardiac, and respiratory examination, since the rib cage deformity can influence the functioning of these systems.

The following nursing diagnoses may apply to the child with scoliosis who is not having surgery:

▶ *Risk for noncompliance with exercise program* related to duration and intensity of exercise

▶ *Impaired physical mobility* related to brace

▶ *Risk for impaired skin integrity* related to brace

▶ *Health-seeking behaviors (child and parent)* related to unfamiliarity with disease process

Common nursing diagnoses can be found in "Nursing Care Plan: The Child Undergoing Surgery for Scoliosis."

GOAL	INTERVENTION	RATIONALE	EXPECTED OUTCOME

1. Knowledge deficit (child and parents) related to lack of information about surgery

	NIC Priority Intervention:		*NOC Suggested Outcome:*
	Teaching disease process and preoperative: *Assisting the patient to understand information and mentally prepare for surgery and postoperative recovery*		**Knowledge:** *Extent of understanding conveyed about scoliosis treatment*
The child and parents will verbalize understanding of the disease, its treatment, and the surgical procedure.	▶ Teach the child and family about the course of the disease, its signs and symptoms, and treatment. Provide appropriate handouts. Encourage the child and parents to ask questions.	▶ Understanding and involvement increase motivation and compliance while reducing fear.	The child and family accurately verbalize knowledge about the disease and its treatment. The child and family ask appropriate questions about postoperative care.
	▶ Begin preoperative teaching at the time of admission. Orient the child to hospital and postoperative procedures. Before surgery, have the child demonstrate log-rolling, range of motion exercises, and the use of an incentive spirometer. Discuss pain management.	▶ Preoperative teaching and familiarity with hospital procedures reduces the stress related to surgery and postoperative complications.	

2. Ineffective breathing pattern related to hypoventilation syndrome

	NIC Priority Intervention:		*NOC Suggested Outcome:*
	Airway management and respiratory monitoring: *Facilitation of patency of air passages and analysis of patient data*		**Respiratory status ventilation:** *Movement of air in and out of the lungs*
The child will show no signs of respiratory compromise.	▶ Monitor respiratory status, especially after the administration of analgesics. Apply pulse oximeter.	▶ Evaluation of the child's respiratory condition anticipates and avoids complications. Analgesics such as morphine may increase or potentiate respiratory compromise.	The child has normal respiratory patterns.
	▶ Administer oxygen if ordered.	▶ Oxygen increases peripheral oxygen saturation to 95%–100%.	
	▶ Have the child use an incentive spirometer.	▶ Spirometry increases lung expansion and aeration of the alveoli.	
	▶ Monitor intake and output.	▶ Good hydration promotes loose secretions and helps prevent infection.	
	▶ Reposition the child at least every 2 hours.	▶ Repositioning ensures inflation of the lung fields.	

3. Risk for injury related to neurovascular deficit secondary to instrumentation

	NIC Priority Intervention:		*NOC Suggested Outcome:*
	Injury prevention: *Instituting special precautions with patient at risk*		**Risk control:** *Actions to eliminate or reduce modifiable health risks*
The child's neurovascular system will remain intact as evidenced by circulation, sensation, and motor checks.	▶ Monitor the child's color, circulation, capillary refill, warmth, sensation, and motion in all extremities. Perform neurovascular checks every 2 hours for the first 24 hours and then every 4 hours for the next 48 hours. Record presence of pedal and tistal libial pulses every hour for 48 hours. Report changes and abnormal findings immediately.	▶ When the spinal column is manipulated during surgery, altered neurovascular status, thrombus formation, and paralysis are possible complications. Postoperative risks include loss of bowel or bladder control, weakness or paralysis, and impaired vision or sensation.	The child exhibits only temporary alteration (pale skin, faint pulse, and edema occur but then resolve within the initial postoperative phase). The child returns to the preoperative baseline state by discharge.
The child will feel no numbness or tingling.	▶ Have the child wear antiembolism stockings until ambulatory. The stockings may be removed for 1 hour 2–3 times daily.	▶ Antiembolism stockings prevent blood clots and promote venous return. Thrombus formation is a postoperative risk.	

GOAL	INTERVENTION	RATIONALE	EXPECTED OUTCOME
	▶ Check for any pain, swelling, or a positive Homans' sign in the legs. Record any evidence of edema. ▶ Monitor input and output. ▶ Encourage and assist the child with range of motion exercises, both passive and active.	▶ Swelling may indicate a tight dressing and tissue damage. A positive Homans' sign and pain may indicate thrombus formation. ▶ Abnormalities may indicate a fluid shift problem. ▶ Activity promotes mobility and reduces risk of thrombus formation.	

4. Pain related to spinal fusion with instrumentation

GOAL	INTERVENTION	RATIONALE	EXPECTED OUTCOME
	NIC Priority Intervention: **Pain management:** *Alleviation of pain or a reduction of pain to a level of comfort acceptable to the patient*		*NOC Suggested Outcome:* **Pain level:** *Amount of reported or demonstrated pain*
The child will verbalize an adequate level of comfort or show absence of pain behavior within 1 hour of a specific nursing intervention.	▶ Assess the level of pain and initiate pain management strategies as soon as possible. Use patient-controlled analgesia if ordered. ▶ Administer pain medication around-the-clock to help ensure pain relief, especially during the first 48 hours. Monitor epidural blocks and patient-controlled analgesia or other methods used for pain control. ▶ Use nonpharmacologic pain manage-ment techniques, such as imagery, relaxation, touch, music, application of heat and cold, and reduced environ-mental stimulation to supplement medi-cations (see Chapter 38). 🔗 ▶ Document pain assessment, interventions, and the child's reactions. ▶ Reassure the child that some discomfort is expected and that a variety of measures can be tried to reduce discomfort.	▶ Adequate pain management allows for faster healing and a more cooperative patient. Patient-controlled analgesics may be effective. ▶ Medicating around-the-clock helps to maintain comfort. Monitoring ensures patient safety. ▶ Alternative treatments also interrupt the pain stimulus and provide relief. Nonpharmacologic methods can be an effective adjunct to pain management. ▶ Proper documentation guides the selection of the most effective means of pain control. ▶ Realistic expectations decrease anxiety and give the child a sense of control.	The child experiences pain relief early in the postoperative period.

5. Impaired physical mobility related to movement restrictions and pain

GOAL	INTERVENTION	RATIONALE	EXPECTED OUTCOME
	NIC Priority Intervention: **Positioning and ambulation:** *Moving the patient to provide comfort and promote healing, assist with walking*		*NOC Suggested Outcome:* **Ambulation:** *Ability to walk from place to place*
The child will maintain proper body alignment and progress with activity as ordered by the physician. If no anteroposterior shell bracing is required, the child will have active mobility by the third to fifth postoperative day.	▶ Reposition the child every 2 hours using the log-roll technique. Support the back, feet, and knees with pillows. ▶ Have the child do passive and active range of motion exercises every 2 hours for 48 hours and then every 4 hours while awake. Have the child dangle his or her legs at the bedside by the second to fourth postoperative day. Begin ambulation by the third to fifth postoperative day. Note any complaints of dizziness, pallor, etc. Proceed slowly.	▶ Proper positioning prevents twisting or turning the spine. ▶ Exercises help maintain strength, circulation, and muscle tone. If the spine is stable and the physician has ordered no external support, the child may progress to full ambulation as tolerated. If the spine is not stable, great care must be taken until external supportive devices are used.	The child is as mobile as appropriate for condition with 3–5 days after surgery.

(continued)

GOAL	INTERVENTION	RATIONALE	EXPECTED OUTCOME
6. Risk for body image disturbance related to treatment			
	NIC Priority Intervention:		*NOC Suggested Outcome:*
	Body image enhancement: *Improving conscious and unconscious perceptions toward the body*		**Body image:** *Positive perception of own appearance and body*
The child will verbalize feelings about body image and self-esteem in relation to the disease and its treatment. The child will be informed about available support services and use them as needed.	▶ Encourage independence in daily activities within allowable limits. Use positive reinforcements. Encourage the child to participate in community activities, if possible. Involve the child in scoliosis support groups.	▶ Involvement in activities demonstrates that a "normal" life is realistic.	The child has a positive self-image and is involved in community activities or support groups.
	▶ Provide contact with a peer resource person who has undergone treatment for scoliosis.	▶ Peers are an effective means of support.	
7. Risk for knowledge deficit (child and parent) related to lack of information about home care			
	NIC Priority Intervention:		*NOC Suggested Outcome:*
	Teaching: prescribed treatment: *Preparing family to understand and perform prescribed treatment*		**Knowledge:** *Extent of understanding conveyed about postoperative treatment and follow-up care*
The child and family will verbalize reduced anxiety about home care. The child will demonstrate knowledge of self-care and permitted activities.	▶ Teach cast or brace care as appropriate (see pp. 1321 and 1323). Provide oral and written instructions and a list of activity limitations. Have the child and family demonstrate adequate knowledge.	▶ Providing education decreases anxiety and increases compliance with treatment plan. Demonstration reinforces the learning process.	The child and family demonstrate home care and implementation of discharge teaching.
	▶ Arrange for follow-up appointments as ordered by the physician. Encourage the child and family to notify the nurse or physician if they have any questions or concerns.	▶ Follow-up visits help the nurse and physician evaluate the effectiveness of the treatment plan and patient compliance.	

Planning and Implementation

An important aspect of nursing care is patient education. Patient compliance is critical to the success of treatment. Children and their families need to understand the condition and the stages of treatment. This is particularly true for adolescents undergoing treatment for scoliosis. Children or adolescents facing surgery require education, reassurance, and support. The accompanying "Nursing Care Plan" summarizes nursing care for the child undergoing surgery for scoliosis.

PROMOTE COMPLIANCE WITH THE TREATMENT PLAN

Provide instructions about exercises that will help to decrease the severity of the spinal curvature. Demonstrate the exercises, and explain their purpose (i.e., to strengthen back muscles). Help the child adjust to wearing a brace. Adolescents, in particular, may be reluctant to wear an external device such as a brace. To promote a sense of control, allow the adolescent to choose when to exercise and when to be out of the brace, within the treatment guidelines. Provide reassurance and encouragement and promote interaction with peers. Suggesting that the adoles-

cent work with a peer support person who is being treated for scoliosis or has had the condition in the past may be beneficial. Provide information about fashionable clothing that can be worn with the brace and facilitate visits to department stores that will help the teen shop for clothing.

DISCHARGE PLANNING AND HOME CARE TEACHING

Identify and address home care needs well in advance of discharge after spinal surgery. The child will need to learn to adapt to a new set of body mechanics. Show the child how to do simple tasks without bending or twisting the torso. Have the child demonstrate the ability to perform activities of daily living before discharge from the hospital.

Activities for the child who has had spinal surgery are commonly limited for a period of time. The child can usually walk and perform physical activity such as gentle swimming, but lifting heavy loads, bending or twisting at the waist, or engaging in activities such as skiing, rollerblading, bicycle riding, and many other sports may not be allowed. Restrictions usually should be followed for 6 to 8 months, depending on the type of surgery and the surgeon. Emphasize to both the child and the family the importance of compliance. Give written discharge instructions to the child and family. Follow-up visits are important. The child should be examined 4 to 6 weeks after discharge, then every 3 to 4 months for 1 year, and every 1 to 2 years thereafter. The metal hardware in the back necessitates that after surgery the teen must carry a written physician explanation since they will set off metal detectors at airports.

Several organizations provide information and assistance to families of children with scoliosis. **WEB** Make referrals as appropriate.

Evaluation

Expected outcomes of nursing care for the child with scoliosis treated by brace are maintenance of intact skin and compliance with prescribed therapy. Expected outcomes after surgical correction are listed on the accompanying "Nursing Care Plan."

TORTICOLLIS, KYPHOSIS, AND LORDOSIS

Torticollis is tilt of the head caused by rotation of the cervical spine. Stretching exercises or surgical lengthening of the sternocleidomastoid muscle are usual treatments. Kyphosis (hunchback) and lordosis (swayback) are two other types of spinal curvature that may occur in children. Nurses can perform thorough musculoskeletal assessments of children (see Chapter 33) and refer any children with abnormalities for further evaluation. Clinical therapy depends on the cause and degree of the curvature, and the age of the child at onset. Refer to "Clinical Manifestations: Kyphosis and Lordosis".

DISORDERS OF THE BONES AND JOINTS

OSTEOMYELITIS

Osteomyelitis is an infection of the bone, most often one of the long bones of the lower extremity. It may be acute or chronic and may spread into surrounding tissues. Although osteomyelitis may occur at any age, it is most common in children between the ages of 1 and 12 years. Boys are affected two to three times as often as girls, primarily because they have a greater incidence of trauma (Carek, Dickerson, & Sack, 2001).

Etiology and Pathophysiology

Osteomyelitis is caused by a microorganism, usually bacterial but possibly viral or fungal. *Staphylococcus aureus* is the most common causative pathogen, followed by *Escherichia coli*, group B streptococci, *Streptococcus aureus, Streptococcus pyogenes,* and *Haemophilus influenzae.* Common sources of infection are an upper respiratory infection, trauma to the bone, and surgery.

The infecting organism spreads through the bloodstream or through a penetrating injury to the bone, where

		DIAGNOSTIC TESTS	
CLINICAL MANIFESTATIONS *Kyphosis and Lordosis*			
CONDITION	**CLINICAL MANIFESTATIONS**	**AND CLINICAL THERAPY**	**NURSING MANAGEMENT**
Kyphosis Excessive convex curvature of the cervical thoracic spine	Visible hunchback or rounded shoulders; shortness of breath or fatigue; abdominal creases and tight hamstrings in severe cases	*Diagnostic tests:* Spinal curvature is assessed by having the child bend 90 degrees at the waist and looking at the scapular area from side. Diagnosis is confirmed by radiograph. *Clinical therapy:* Exercises are prescribed for mild condition; bracing is commonly used; surgery is performed in severe cases.	Provide support. Encourage exercises and diligent brace wear. Help the child to deal with the psychologic stress of altered body image.
Lordosis Excessive concave curvature of the lumbar spine with an angle of more than 60 degrees; most common in prepubescent girls and African Americans	Presence of swayback; prominent buttocks; hip flexion contractures; tight hamstrings	*Diagnostic tests:* Spinal curvature is assessed by looking at the standing child from the side. Lumbar lordosis is confirmed by visualizing the spine on standing, lateral radiograph. *Clinical therapy:* Treatment focuses on exercises and postural awareness. Bracing and surgery are rarely prescribed.	Provide support. Reassure the child and family that the condition is often outgrown as the child matures. Encourage physical conditioning exercises and follow-up examinations on a yearly basis.

it becomes established. Most infections in children begin in the metaphysis (see Figure 50–1), which has a sluggish blood supply. Eventually the infection may penetrate the bone cortex and periosteum. Inflammation and abscess formation can interrupt the blood supply to the underlying bone, affect the surrounding soft tissue, and, if the infection is left untreated, lead to necrosis.

Clinical Manifestations

Symptoms include pain and tenderness with swelling, decreased mobility of the infected joint, and fever. Redness over the area may occur. The onset of acute osteomyelitis is generally rapid, and is therefore sometimes misdiagnosed as a sports injury (Shaw, Gerardi, & Hennrikus, 1998).

Clinical Therapy

A history suggestive of osteomyelitis includes an upper respiratory infection or blunt trauma followed by pain at the area of a growth plate. Laboratory evaluation shows leukocytosis and an elevated erythrocyte sedimentation rate (ESR) and C-reactive protein (Carek, Dickerson, & Sack, 2001; Theophilopoulos & Barrett, 1998). The degree of ESR elevation is directly related to the severity of the infection. Radiographs and bone scans may identify the area of involvement. A needle aspiration of the site or a blood culture can confirm the diagnosis and provide a culture of the causative organism.

Medical management begins with the intravenous administration of a broad-spectrum antibiotic, even before culture results are available. Once the culture results are obtained, the antibiotic may be altered. Oral antibiotics are given once an adequate response has occurred. However, extended intravenous home therapy may be used. Antibiotic therapy continues for about 6 weeks. When an adequate response is not obtained within 2 to 3 days, the area may be aspirated again, or surgically drained. Intravenous fluids may be administered to ensure adequate hydration. In children with extensive orthopedic surgery, or in those with immunosuppression, a short course of prophylactic antibiotic may be administered after surgery (De Baun, 1998).

Prompt diagnosis and treatment usually completely resolve the infection. The prognosis is related to the initiation of therapy—the earlier treatment begins, the better the outcome. Long-term unfavorable outcomes include disruption of the growth plate, which can interrupt growth and damage the joints from septic arthritis.

Growth and Development

Osteomyelitis in a newborn is of great concern, as before 18 months of age the blood vessels cross the growth plates. This creates a higher risk of epiphyseal involvement with resultant limb length discrepancy.

Nursing Management

Nursing Assessment and Diagnosis

A thorough history, including information about the onset of symptoms and a history of recent infections or puncture wounds, is essential. Assess the affected area for signs of redness, swelling, pain, and decreased range of motion. When osteomyelitis is possible, all cultures of blood or wound must be taken before antibiotic therapy is started.

Among the nursing diagnoses that may apply to the child with osteomyelitis are:

▶ *Pain* related to biologic injury

▶ *Impaired physical mobility* related to discomfort

▶ *Risk for sepsis* related to spread of infection

▶ *Risk for altered nutrition: less than body requirements* related to loss of appetite

▶ *Risk for noncompliance* related to duration of antibiotic therapy

▶ *Health-seeking behaviors (child and parent)* related to need for information about disease process

Planning and Implementation

Nursing management focuses on administering antibiotics, protecting the child from spread of the infection, and encouraging a well-balanced diet. Use standard precautions, with transmission-based precautions for any drainage from the site of infection.

ADMINISTER FLUIDS AND MEDICATIONS

Administer intravenous fluids as ordered to maintain the child's hydration status. Antibiotics are administered intravenously at first, then orally. Monitor the intravenous site and provide care for the central line, if one is used (see Skill 12-8). SKILLS In the early stages of the infection, analgesics are prescribed to relieve the associated pain and joint tenderness.

PROTECT FROM THE SPREAD OF INFECTION

Strict aseptic technique and transmission-based precautions should be used during all dressing changes. Children and family members should avoid direct contact with any dressings or drainage. Teach good hygiene practices, including handwashing, to maintain infection control. Take vital signs and evaluate the child frequently for symptoms indicating the spread of infection (e.g., increasing pain, difficulty breathing, increased pulse rate, fever).

ENCOURAGE A WELL-BALANCED DIET

Educate both the child and the parents about healthy dietary choices that promote healing. A high-protein diet and extra vitamin C will contribute to this process. Encourage increased fluid intake to provide adequate hydration and circulation.

DISCHARGE PLANNING AND HOME CARE TEACHING

Emphasize the importance of completing the full course of antibiotic therapy, especially for children who have had an abscess or lesion surgically drained. Explain that failure to follow the prescribed antibiotic therapy may result in chronic infection. Provide suggestions for the family if the child will be immobilized at home.

Nursing Practice

If the child needs to remain home for a period of time during treatment for osteomyelitis, help the family plan for completion of school tasks.

▶ Contact the school and ask that work be sent home.
▶ Arrange for a tutor if needed.
▶ Facilitate computer communication between child, teacher, and other students.
▶ Help the family plan for help at home to monitor the child when they need to be at work or performing other tasks.
▶ Refer families to financial resources as appropriate for the services the child needs.
▶ Suggest activities that the child can do at home that foster developmental progress.

Evaluation

Expected outcomes of nursing care for the child with osteomyelitis include:

▶ Absence of signs of infection or sepsis
▶ Completion of prescribed course of antibiotics
▶ Prevention of infection in contacts
▶ Adequate intake of fluids and nutrients
▶ Absence of pain
▶ Return to normal activities of daily living

SKELETAL TUBERCULOSIS AND SEPTIC ARTHRITIS

Skeletal tuberculosis (Figure 50–9) and septic arthritis are two infections that, although infrequent, may affect children and adolescents. See "Clinical Manifestations and Treatment of Skeletal Tuberculosis and Septic Arthritis."

OSTEOGENESIS IMPERFECTA

Osteogenesis imperfecta, also known as brittle bone disease, is a connective tissue disorder that primarily affects the bones. Children with this condition have fragile bones that are more likely to fracture. The major type of osteogenesis imperfecta occurs in 1 in 30,000 live births and affects boys

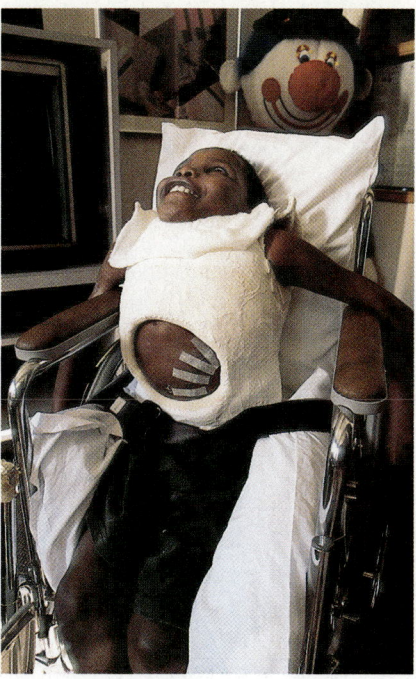

FIGURE 50–9. This boy from Kenya had surgery to correct severe kyphosis and scoliosis, caused by tuberculosis of the spine. A Risser cast has been applied to maintain stability of the spine and thoracic cage during healing. Notice the area cut out of the cast to allow for auscultation of the abdomen, as well as to facilitate the child's comfort and adequate intake of food.

and girls equally. Clinical manifestations include multiple and frequent fractures; blue sclerae; thin, soft skin; increased joint flexibility; enlargement of the anterior fontanel; weak muscles; soft, pliable, brittle bones; and short stature. Conductive hearing loss can occur by adolescence or young adulthood (Paterson, Monk, & McAllion, 2001).

The underlying disorder is a biochemical defect in the production of collagen. The disease is genetically transmitted, generally in an autosomal dominant inheritance pattern, although some types are transmitted in a recessive pattern.

The disease is classified into four types. In type I disease, the most common form, children have fragile bones, blue sclerae, weakened tooth dentin, and hearing loss that manifests in adolescence. In type II disease, the ribs and skeleton are extensively involved; most children with this form of the disease die in utero or shortly after birth. Type III disease is identified in the newborn period or in infancy when the child sustains numerous fractures and manifests blue sclera. Severe bone fragility and kyphoscoliosis are observed. Most children with type III disease die in childhood as a result of cardiorespiratory failure. Type IV disease is characterized by fractures without other symptoms of the disease. Bowing of the legs and other structural deformities can occur; however, the incidence of fractures decreases beginning in puberty.

Improved knowledge about the genetic transmission of this disease means that some cases of osteogenesis imperfecta can be identified before birth using ultrasound or

CONDITION	CLINICAL MANIFESTATIONS	DIAGNOSTIC TEST AND CLINICAL THERAPY	NURSING MANAGEMENT
Skeletal Tuberculosis Rare microbacterial infection that can be very destructive. The spine is the most frequent site of infection (Pott's disease), with joints and other sites sometimes affected.	Depending on the site, pain, limp, severe muscle spasms, kyphosis, muscle atrophy, "doughy" swelling of joints, decreased joint motion, changes in reflexes, low-grade fever	*Diagnostic tests:* Diagnostic studies include tuberculosis skin test, complete blood count, synovial fluid analysis, and radiographs of affected limb or joint. *Clinical therapy:* Antibiotic therapy (using a combination of drugs) for 6–9 months is the treatment of choice. The affected site is immobilized. Disease may become resistant to these drugs, and additional drug therapy may be necessary.	Educate the child and family about the disorder and stress the importance of complying with long-term antibiotic therapy. Test all members of the family for tuberculosis. Report the disease to the local health department. Facilitate the immobilization and physical therapy of the child at home.
Septic Arthritis Joint infection of the synovial space most often caused by *Haemophilus influenzae*, *Staphylococcus*, and *Streptococcus*. The most common site of infection is the knee, followed by the hip, ankle, and elbow.	Fever, pain and local inflammation, joint tenderness, swelling, loss of spontaneous movement	*Diagnostic tests:* Diagnosis is made based on joint aspiration findings. Radiographic changes may not be evident until later in the disease process. *Clinical therapy:* This is a medical emergency requiring prompt treatment to avoid permanent disability. Treatment involves joint aspiration, open drainage, and irrigation, followed by intravenous antibiotic therapy for 3–4 weeks and then oral antibiotics. If the full course of antibiotic treatment is not completed, the child risks recurrent infection and further degeneration of the infected joint.	Educate the child and family about the disorder and emphasize the importance of proper antibiotic therapy. Carefully position the painful joint.

collagen analysis of chorionic villus cells. In many cases, however, diagnosis of osteogenesis imperfecta is made only when the child has a delay in walking or sustains a fracture. Radiographic evaluation may detect old as well as new fractures. This may lead to an erroneous diagnosis of child abuse.

There is no cure for osteogenesis imperfecta. Medical management consists primarily of fracture care and prevention of deformities. The goal is to maximize the child's independence and mobility while minimizing the risk of fractures. Treatment includes physical therapy; casting, bracing, or splinting; surgical stabilization, nutritional management with high vitamin D and calcium, and biphosphonate medication such as pamidronate (Gonzalez, Pavia, Ros, et al., 2001). Bone marrow transplant has been used successfully in some children with severe osteogenesis imperfecta and is under further research (Horwitz, Prockop, Gordon, et al., 2001).

Nursing Management

Nursing care is primarily supportive and focuses on educating the parents and child about the disease and its treatment. The family may have been suspected of child abuse before the disease was diagnosed; explain the similar presenting symptoms of these cases.

To prevent fractures, children with osteogenesis imperfecta must be handled gently. Support the trunk and extremities using a blanket whenever moving the child. Such tasks as bathing and diapering may cause fractures and should be performed carefully. Never pull the legs upward during diaper changes, but slip a hand gently under the hips to raise them.

Emphasize the importance of maintaining normal patterns of growth and development. Help toddlers explore and interact safely in their environment. Socialization is essential during the school-age and adolescent years. Encourage exercise, such as swimming, to improve muscle tone and prevent obesity. Adaptive equipment and motorized wheelchairs promote independent functioning. Maintenance of function can depend on proper rehabilitation services. Arrange and manage such services for the family.

The Osteogenesis Imperfecta Foundation provides information about the disease and can put families in touch with others who have the disease. Parents should receive genetic counseling.

❧ MUSCULAR DYSTROPHIES

The muscular dystrophies are a group of inherited diseases characterized by muscle fiber degeneration and muscle

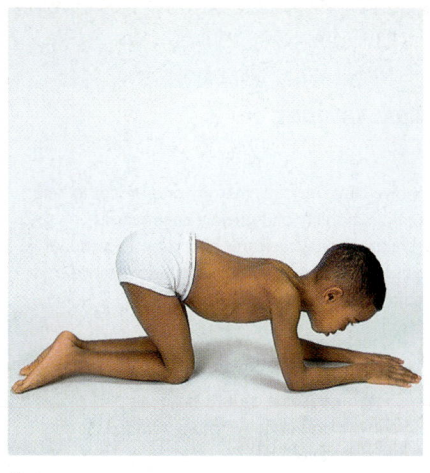

A

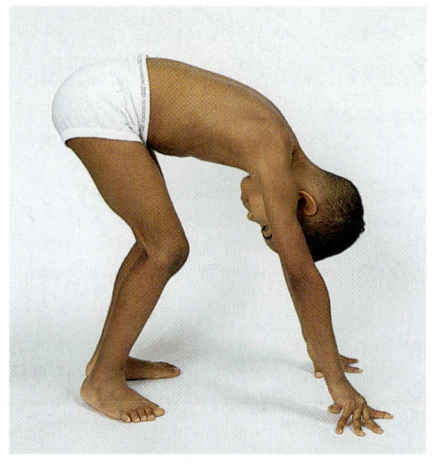

B

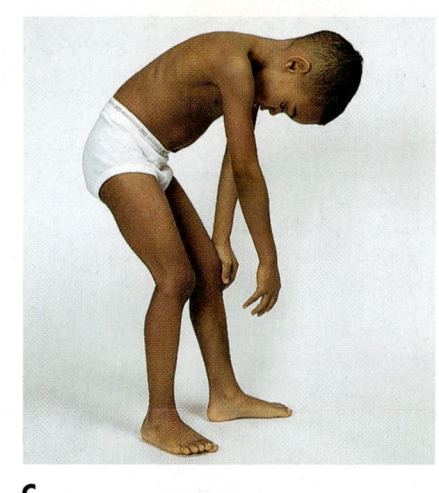

C

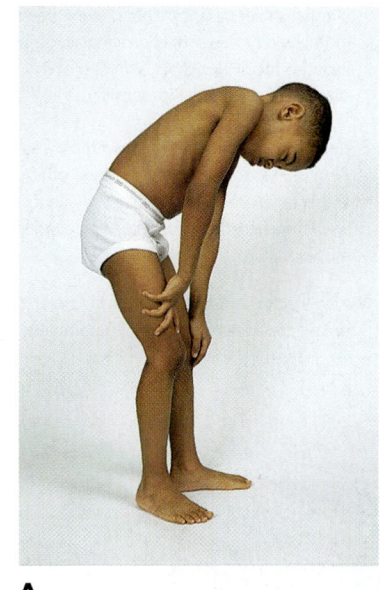

A

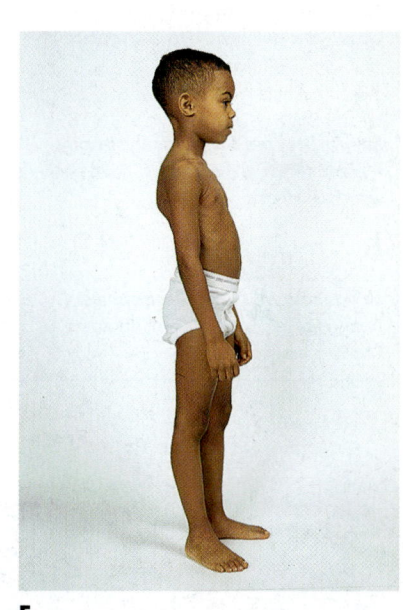

E

FIGURE 50–10. ◆ Since the leg muscles of children with muscular dystrophy are weak, these children must perform the Gowers' maneuver to raise themselves to a standing position. **A** and **B,** The child first maneuvers to a position supported by arms and legs. **C,** The child next pushes off the floor and rests one hand on the knee. **D** and **E,** The child then pushes himself upright.

wasting. These disorders can begin early or late in life, and onset can be at birth or gradual.

Many kinds of muscular dystrophies affect children and adults (see page 1340). ⊂▭⊃ The most common form of childhood muscular dystrophy is Duchenne muscular dystrophy (pseudohypertrophic), which occurs in 1 in 3500 live male births. **Pseudohypertrophy** refers to enlargement of the muscles as a result of their infiltration with fatty tissue. The gene for Duchenne muscular dystrophy was identified in 1987; it is carried in the Xp21.2 region of the chromosome and is either absent or deleted in affected children.

Diagnosis and classification are most often based on clinical signs and the pattern of muscle involvement. Children with muscular dystrophy have generalized muscle weakness. They compensate for weak lower extremities by using the upper extremity muscles to raise themselves to a standing position (Gower's maneuver) (Figure 50–10 ◆).

Biochemical examinations such as serum enzyme assay, muscle biopsy, and electromyography confirm the diagnosis. Serum creatine kinase (CK) is elevated early in the disease. Muscle biopsy can measure dystrophin, the muscle protein that is deficient in muscular dystrophy.

There is no effective treatment for childhood muscular dystrophy. Research is being directed at several techniques to repair mutations by gene therapy (Takeda & Miyagoe-Suzuki, 2001). Progressive weakness and muscle deformity result in chronic disability (Figure 50–11 ◆). The goal of medical management is to provide support and prevent complications such as infection or spinal deformities (Figure 50–12 ◆). The team approach to managing the child with muscular dystrophy ensures a comprehensive management plan. Team members should include physicians (pediatrician, orthopedic surgeon, neurologist), nurses, physical and occupational therapists, a nutritionist, and a social worker.

TYPE OF DYSTROPHY	CLINICAL MANIFESTATIONS	CLINICAL THERAPY
Duchenne Muscular Dystrophy X-linked recessive disorder seen in boys (on Xp21 gene); however, 30%–50% of affected children have no family history Onset: within the first 3–4 years of life	Delayed walking; frequent falls; easily tired when walking, running, or climbing stairs; toe walking, hypertrophied calves; waddling gait; lordosis; positive Gower's maneuver; mental retardation frequently seen	Supportive care; physical therapy and braces to help maintain mobility and prevent contractures Most children are wheelchair bound by 12 years of age; death usually occurs during adolescence from respiratory or cardiac failure
Becker Muscular Dystrophy X-linked recessive disorder Onset: usually after 5 years	Symptoms are similar to those of Duchenne muscular dystrophy, but milder and delayed; child is mobile until late teens; normal intelligence; congestive heart failure; contractures	Supportive care, same as for Duchenne muscular dystrophy Slow progression (same as for Duchenne muscular dystrophy); death usually occurs from the third to the fifth decade of life
Facioscapulohumeral Muscular Dystrophy Autosomal dominant disorder (on 4q35 chromosome) Onset: later childhood and adolescence	Face, shoulder girdle, lower limbs affected; unable to raise arms over head; lordosis; cannot close eyes, whistle, smile, or drink from a straw because of inability to move face; characteristic appearance includes facial weakness, winging of the scapula, thin arms, well-developed forearms	Physical therapy Slow progression; confined to wheelchair as older adult, but usually attains normal life span
Emery-Dreifuss Muscular Dystrophy X-linked recessive disorder (on Xq28 gene) Onset: childhood	Early onset of contractures followed by weakness; Achilles' tendon, elbow, and spine affected; muscle weakness in upper body follows, with lower body weakness occurring later; cardiac conduction defect may occur	Physical therapy Surgery Pacemaker insertion
Congenital Muscular Dystrophies Autosomal recessive group of disorders Onset: present at birth	Muscle weaknesses present at birth; motor development delay; contractures and joint deformities; hypotonia	Correction of skeletal deformity (orthosis or surgery) Usually nonprogressive

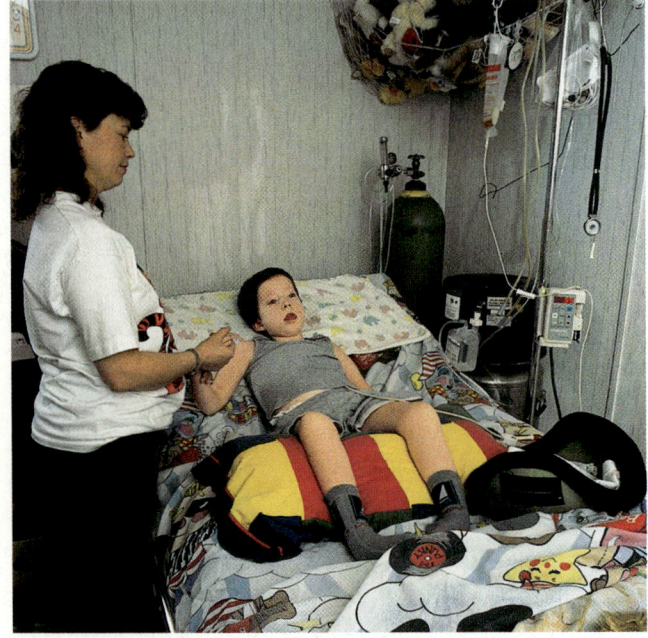

FIGURE 50–11. ◆ This young boy with muscular dystrophy needs to receive tube feedings and home nursing care. He attends school when possible and is able to use an adapted computer.

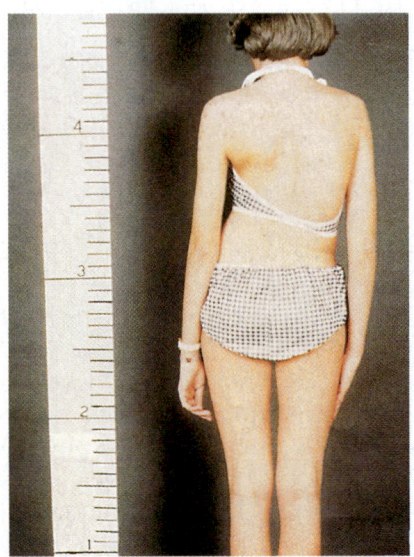

FIGURE 50–12. ◆ Spinal deviation with spinal muscular atrophy. *Note:* From Zitelli, B. J., & Davis, H. W. (Eds.). (1997). *Atlas of Pediatric physical diagnosis,* 3rd ed. (page 658, Figure 21–71). St Louis: Mosby.

Nursing Management

Nursing care focuses on promoting independence and mobility and providing psychosocial support that helps the child and family deal with this progressive, incapacitating disease.

Monitor cardiac and respiratory functioning frequently. Administer oxygen or respiratory therapy as ordered. Perform periodic developmental assessments, and give parents suggestions for encouraging the child's development. Meet with teachers to evaluate the child's learning needs and functioning in the classroom.

Encourage the child to be independent for as long as possible. Concentrate on what the child can accomplish and do not ask the child to complete tasks that may prove frustrating. Reading books to the child, listening to tapes, and watching television offer the child stimulation during hospitalization. Exercise as tolerated contributes to muscle strength. Physical therapy helps the child ambulate and prevents joint contractures. It is important to provide good back support and posture by keeping the child's body in alignment when confined to a wheelchair.

Parents may feel guilty and hopeless. Encourage parents to express their feelings. Genetic counseling is recommended for the entire family, and it is especially important to identify women who are carriers of one of the X-linked disorders. Siblings may feel neglected because their brother or sister is receiving so much attention. They may be concerned that they will develop the disease. Encourage the parents to involve siblings in the child's care to reassure them of their importance.

Refer family members to resource and support groups such as the Muscular Dystrophy Association. 🔗 **WEB**

≋ INJURIES TO THE MUSCULOSKELETAL SYSTEM

Musculoskeletal injuries are classified according to the mechanism, the location, and the force of the injury. Strains, sprains, dislocations, and fractures are the most common musculoskeletal injuries in children. Distinguishing among these injuries is often difficult. See "Clinical Manifestations of Strains, Sprains, and Dislocations." A detailed discussion of fractures follows.

FRACTURES

A fracture is a break in a bone that occurs when more stress is placed on the bone than the bone can withstand. Fractures may occur at any age; they are frequent in children because their bones are less dense and more porous than those of adults (see "Pathophysiology Illustrated: Classification and Types of Fractures").

CLINICAL MANIFESTATIONS ≋ *Strains, Sprains, and Dislocations*

CONDITION	CLINICAL MANIFESTATIONS	CLINICAL THERAPY
Strain • Stretching or tearing of either a muscle or a tendon, usually from overuse (example: back strain resulting from improper or overly heavy lifting).	• Vary according to the type and severity of the strain. Pain can be acute or chronic.	• Rest and support of the injured part until the muscle or tendon heals and normal activity can occur.
Sprain • Stretching or tearing of a ligament, usually caused by falls, sports injuries, or motor vehicle crashes.	• Edema, joint immobility, and pain.	• For the first 24–36 hours: **R**est **I**ce **C**ompression **E**levation • After the first 24–36 hours, mobility is gradually increased.
Dislocation • Complete displacement of an articular joint surface, usually associated with falls, sports injuries, or motor vehicle crashes. Although almost any joint may be dislocated, most dislocations occur in the shoulder, knee, and hip.	• Pain and tenderness, swelling and obvious deformity, and instability of the joint.	• Varies according to the site and severity of the injury, and consists of: Shoulder: Open or closed reduction followed by the application of a sling. Knee: Closed reduction with gentle traction, then immobilization with a splint. Hip (posterior): Immediate closed reduction or possibly open reduction, traction, or hip spica cast. Hip (anterior): Immediate closed reduction, extension traction, and hip spica cast.

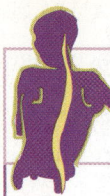

CLASSIFICATION	TYPE

Complete (transverse) fracture

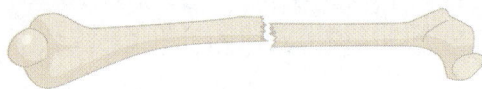

Break across entire section of a bone at a right angle to the bone shaft resulting in two or more fragments

Spiral fracture

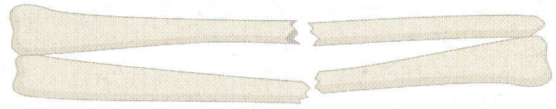

Associated with twisting force; fracture coils around the bone

Open fracture

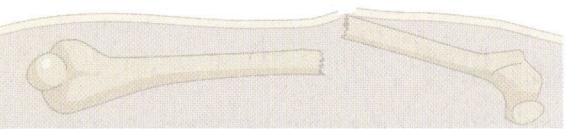

Broken bone protrudes through the skin leaving a path to the fracture site; high risk of infection exists

Closed fracture

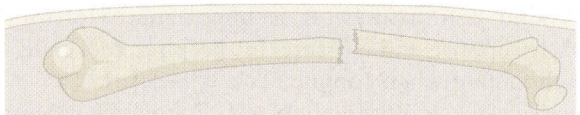

Broken bone does not protrude through the skin

Greenstick fracture

Caused by compression force; often seen in young children

Comminuted fracture

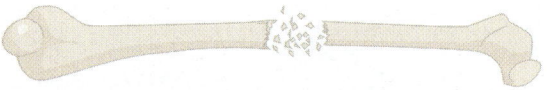

Associated with high impact forces; bone breaks into three or more segments

Additional types of fractures include: *incomplete,* in which the break occurs in only one side of the cortex; *oblique,* in which the fracture slants across the long axis of the bone; *compression,* in which two bones are jammed together (usually occurs in spinal area); and *compacted,* in which one bone fragment is wedged into another.

Etiology and Pathophysiology

Fractures in children may result from direct trauma to a bone (falls, sports injuries, abuse, motor vehicle crashes) or bone diseases that result in weakening of the bone (osteogenesis imperfecta). Trauma may be caused by an acute injury, or direct and forceful impact, or by overuse such as in chronic and repetitive activities (O'Connor, 1998).

Clinical Manifestations

Signs and symptoms of fractures vary depending on the location, type, and nature of the causative injury. Fractures are generally characterized by pain, abnormal positioning, edema, immobility or decreased range of motion, ecchymosis, guarding, and crepitus. Childhood fractures most often involve the clavicle, tibia, ulna, and femur, with dis-

tal forearm fractures the most common type. Douglass, described in the opening vignette, had a fracture of his tibia. Fractures to the pelvis are often associated with motor vehicle crashes. Epiphyseal (growth plate) injuries are common in children. These injuries are described using the Salter-Harris classification system (Figure 50–13 ◆).

Growth and Development

Stress fractures are becoming more common in adolescents who limit their intake of calories and calcium in an attempt to remain lean for sports such as distance running or gymnastics. These fractures may present with chronic pain that changes in intensity. Be alert to this possibility when teenagers' diets and athletic activities place them at risk.

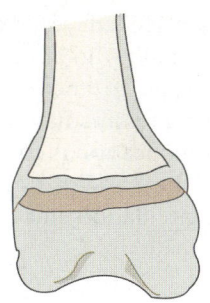

Type I
Common
Growth plate undisturbed
Growth disturbances rare

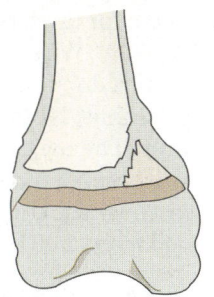

Type II
Most common
Growth disturbances rare

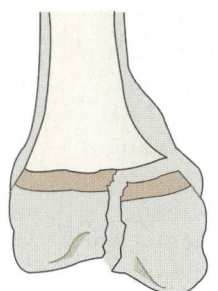

Type III
Less common
Serious threat to growth
   and joint

FIGURE 50-13. ◆ The Salter-Harris classification system is based on the angle of the fracture in relation to the epiphysis.

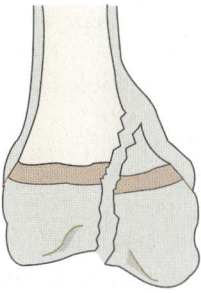

Type IV
Serious threat to growth

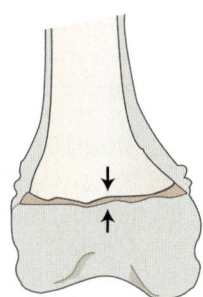

Type V
Rare
Crush injury causes cell death in growth plate,
   resulting in arrested growth and limited
   bone length
If growth plate is partially destroyed, angular
   deformities may result

Growth and Development

The risk of bone fractures in adolescent females who drink carbonated beverages is three times higher than in those who do not drink these beverages. It is thought that the high phosphorus content of carbonated beverages fosters bone loss and that these beverages displace milk, a major calcium source, in the diet (Wyshak, 2000).

Clinical Therapy

Radiographs are useful for determining the exact location and type of the fracture. Medical management consists of two basic steps: (1) reduction to realign displaced or fragmented bones, and (2) immobilization so that healing can take place.

A closed reduction aligns the bone by manual manipulation or traction. Conscious sedation or pain management may be used during closed reduction. An open reduction requires surgical alignment of the bone, often using pins, plates, wires, or screws. For open fractures, surgery must also be performed for debridement, to remove dead tissue and clean the wound. Casting is the most common external method of immobilization. Casts may be placed on ex-

TABLE 50-3	**Complications of Fracture Reduction**
Complication	*Clinical Therapy*
Infection Acute (may occur with open fractures) Chronic (osteomyelitis)	Debridement, drainage, culture, and treatment with antibiotics
Neurovascular injury resulting from physical nerve damage	Nerve repair
Vascular injury	Vascular repair, amputation, tendon lengthening
Malunion (undesired healed alignment of bone) or delayed union	Corrective osteotomy; prolonged immobilization
Nonunion	Surgical intervention; internal fixation
Leg length discrepancy	Shoe lift

tremities (short or long leg or arm cast), on the upper body to immobilize the spine, or from chest to legs to stabilize pelvis or hips (spica cast). Leg casts may be walking or nonwalking casts. Cast material is either plaster or a synthetic fabric. Other external methods of stabilization include traction and splinting (see Table 50–4 for types of traction). Pins may be inserted to stabilize the fracture, and can be used with or without casts or traction. A child with multiple fractures following a car crash or other trauma may need a combination of treatments (Frye & Luterman, 1999).

Healing of fractures is influenced by factors including age, size of the involved bone, and fracture site. Fractures heal in less time in children than in adults. Immobilization is essential for the bone healing process. If a fracture is properly reduced, complications should be minimal (Table 50–3). Fractures involving the epiphyseal growth plate must be treated properly to minimize the chance for limb length discrepancy, joint incongruity, and angular deformities.

Nursing Management

Nursing Assessment and Diagnosis

When dealing with an injured child, be alert to the signs and symptoms of fractures before moving the child. When in doubt about the type of injury, apply a splint to immobilize the joints above and below the injury. Try to identify the cause of the injury by asking the child, parents, or other family members what happened. Evaluate pain, swelling, and any abnormal positioning of the injured area. When a child is admitted to the emergency department or hospital, nursing assessment includes the extent of the injury, the degree of pain, and the child's vital signs (respiratory status, pulse, blood pressure).

Several nursing diagnoses may apply to the child with a fracture. They include:

▶ *Pain* related to injury

▶ *Risk for impaired skin integrity* related to treatment

▶ *Risk for infection* related to open fracture or trauma

▶ *Impaired physical mobility* related to treatment

▶ *Health-seeking behaviors* related to need for information about treatment and expected outcome

Planning and Implementation

Nurses may be in community settings when children experience a fracture, and need to provide emergency care and arrange for transport. Inform emergency personnel of the assessment data to provide for safe care. In addition, be aware that repeated fractures in the same child can be a sign of other health care conditions. Young children may have osteogenesis imperfecta, an older child may be experimenting with risky behavior, and child abuse may have occurred if there are several fractures in various states of healing or if the parental explanation does not match the clinical presentation. Nursing care focuses on care of the child before and after fracture reduction, encouraging mobility as ordered, maintaining skin integrity, preventing infection, and teaching the parents and child how to care for the fracture. If conscious sedation or pain blocks are

used, nursing care for these procedures is needed (see Skill 13-3). **SKILLS** When caring for a child who has undergone fracture reduction, it is important to know the signs of complications. Notify the physician immediately if these signs occur. The major serious complication is **compartment syndrome,** or a condition of increased pressure in a limited space which compromises circulation and tissue function (Harvey, 2001).

MAINTAIN PROPER ALIGNMENT

Immobilization maintains proper alignment of the fracture. Casts and traction are methods used for immobilizing an injured child. Cast care guidelines are included in Table 50–2, earlier in this chapter.

Different types of traction are used, depending on the location and type of fracture (Table 50–4). Nursing care for the child in traction is described in Table 50–5.

MONITOR NEUROVASCULAR STATUS

Neurovascular assessment is used for early detection of compartment syndrome (see Skill 9-16). **SKILLS** Compartment syndrome may occur with a crush injury or when a fracture is reduced. The swelling of inflammation reduces blood flow to the affected area, and casting causes further constriction of blood flow. Douglass had a splint applied for several days, with casting later, to allow swelling to decrease and to minimize risk for compartment syndrome. Monitor the child's sensation to touch, temperature, movement, strength of the pulse, and capillary refill time in the extremity distal to the injury. Monitor every 15 minutes after the cast is applied for at least 2 hours and then every 1 to 2 hours, depending on the facility's policy and the child's condition. Keep the cast elevated above heart level to minimize edema.

PROMOTE MOBILITY

The amount of mobility the child is allowed is ordered by the physician; restrictions depend on the extent and site of the fracture. Fractures of the hip or pelvis may involve body casts; wheeled carts make mobility possible. Children with leg fractures can sometimes bear weight on the cast, but if they cannot, they move around with crutches, walkers, or wheelchairs (see Skill 17-2). **SKILLS**

DISCHARGE PLANNING AND HOME CARE TEACHING

Most fractures can be easily managed at home. Activities are generally limited for approximately 8 weeks. Teach the parents and child cast care, activity restrictions, and how to identify problems that should be reported (see p. 1321). Help parents to identify any modifications that may be needed at home and school. The child who has to manage steps at home or school may need special training with crutches or a temporary ramp. Refer parents to home health nurses or home teaching services if indicated. Provide pertinent teaching to prevent future injuries. Reinforce need for protective gear for many sports (see Chapter 36).

TABLE 50-4   Types of Traction

Skin Traction

Pull is applied to the skin surface, which puts traction directly on the bones and muscles. Traction is attached to the skin with adhesive materials or straps, or foam boots, belts, or halters.

Dunlop Traction (can be either skeletal or skin)

Used for fracture of the humerus. The flexed arm is suspended horizontally with straps placed on both the upper and lower portions for pull from both sides.

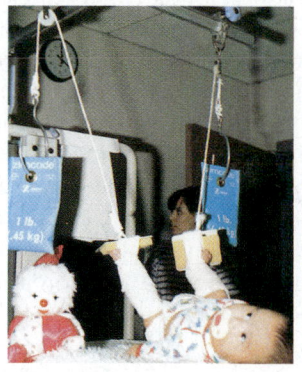

A

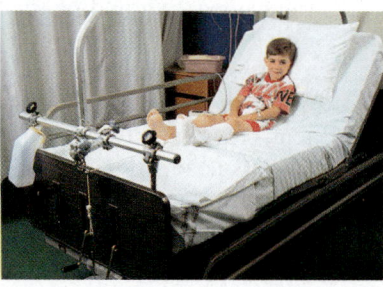

B

Bryant Traction (A)

Used specifically for the child under 3 years of age and weighing less than 35 pounds (17.5 kg), who has developmental dysplasia of the hip or a fractured femur. This bilateral traction is applied to the child's legs and kept in place by wrapping the legs from foot to thigh with elastic bandages. The hips are flexed at a 90-degree angle, with knees extended. This position is maintained by attaching the traction appliance to weights and pulleys suspended above the crib. The buttocks do not rest on the mattress, but are slightly elevated off the bed.

Buck Traction (B)

Used for knee immobilization; to correct contractures or deformities; or for short-term immobilization of a fracture. It keeps the leg in an extended position, without hip flexion. Traction is applied to the extremity in one direction (straight line) with a single pulley system.

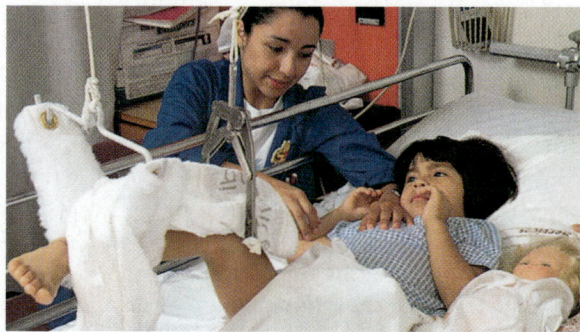

D

90–90 Traction (D)

Used for fractures of the femur or tibia. A skeletal pin or wire is surgically placed through the distal part of the femur, while the lower part of the extremity is in a boot cast. Traction ropes and pulleys are applied at the pin site and on the boot cast to maintain the flexion of both the hip and knee at 90 degrees. This traction can also be used for treatment of an upper extremity fracture.

Skeletal Traction

Pull is directly applied to the bone by pins, wires, tongs, or other apparatus that have been surgically placed through the distal end of the bone.

Skeletal Cervical Traction

Used for cervical spine injuries to reduce fractures and dislocations. Crutchfield, Gardner-Wells, or Vinke tongs are placed in the skull with bur holes. Weights are attached to the apparatus with a rope and pulley system to the hyperextended head.

Halo Traction

Used to immobilize the head and neck after cervical injury or dislocation. Also used for positioning and immobilization after cervical injury.

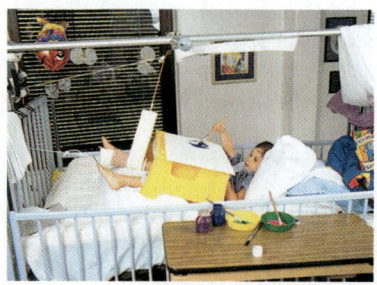

C

Russell Traction (C)

Used for fractures of the femur and lower leg. Traction is placed on the lower leg while the knee is suspended in a padded sling. The slightly flexed hips and knees are immobilized. One force is applied by a double pulley to the foot and another force is applied upward using a sling under the knee and an overhead pulley.

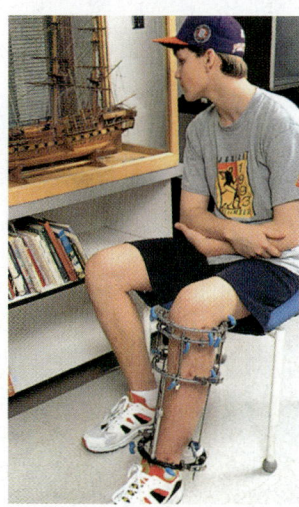

E

External Fixators (E)

These devices can be used in the treatment of simple fractures, both open and closed; complex fractures with extensive soft tissue involvement; correction of bony or soft tissue deformities; pseudoarthroses; and limb length discrepancy. They are attached to the extremity by percutaneous transfixing of pins or wires to the bone. When used to lengthen an extremity, the device can be "distracted" or turned as ordered by the surgeon for a very small amount several times daily. This separates the bone and allows new growth, gradually lengthening the extremity.

TABLE 50-5 Care of the Child with Traction or External Fixator

1. Assess the child in traction by first checking the equipment. Make sure that the equipment is in the proper position. Observe both the body appliance and the attached weights and pulleys. Make certain that the child's body is in proper alignment.

2. Assess the skin under the straps and pin insertion sites for any signs of redness, edema, or skin breakdown.

3. Assess the extremity by checking neurovascular status frequently (check warmth, color, distal pulses, capillary refill time, movement, sensation).

4. Provide pin care when ordered using sterile technique. Clean the area surrounding the pin with cotton-tipped applicators saturated with normal saline or half-strength hydrogen peroxide. Clean the area again with sterile water or more saline. Apply an antibacterial ointment, if ordered, using another cotton-tipped applicator.

5. When the traction equipment can be removed, skin care should be performed every 4 hours.

6. Place a sheepskin pad under the child's extremity if orders permit.

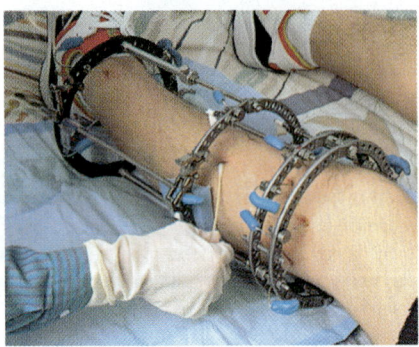

CLINICAL MANIFESTATIONS
Compartment Syndrome

Clinical manifestations begin about 30 minutes after tissue ischemia starts. Major manifestations are:

- Paresthesia (tingling, burning, loss of 2-point discrimination)
- Pain (unrelieved by medication, characterized by crying in the young child)
- Pressure (skin is tense, cast appears tight)
- Pallor* (pale, gray or white skin tone)
- Paralysis* (weakness or inability to move extremity)
- Pulselessness* (weak or absent pulse)

* = late sign

Check extremities for:

- Color
- Temperature
- Capillary refill
- Peripheral pulses
- Edema
- Sensation
- Motor ability
- Pain

Document results and report changes or abnormal results immediately.

Note: From Kunkler, C. E. (1999). Neurovascular assessment. Orthopaedic Nursing, 18(3), 63–71; and Harvey, C. (2001). Compartment syndrome: When it is least expected. Orthopaedic Nursing, 20(3), 15–26. Adapted.

AMPUTATIONS

Amputation—the complete absence of a body extremity—can be either congenital or acquired. Approximately two thirds of amputations in children are congenital and one third are acquired. Congenital amputations can be caused by constrictive amniotic bands, drugs, or irradiation. Acquired amputations are generally associated with trauma or the result of a disease or disorder.

The child with an absent limb should be fitted with a prosthesis as soon as feasible. This fosters a positive body image, independence, and self-confidence and also ensures that motor skills develop as normally as possible. The prosthetic device should be reevaluated as the child progresses physically and developmentally. Children with traumatic amputations may need frequent stump reconstructions because as children grow, so do their bones, and the skin tends to adhere to the bone. Bone may need to be cut and soft tissue added to keep the stump rounded. Joint fusions or stump lengthenings may also be needed to allow the effective use of a prosthesis.

Nursing Management

Nursing care focuses on providing emotional support regarding altered body image, managing pain, maintaining skin integrity, and encouraging maximal independent functioning.

Recovering from the loss of a limb is one of the most difficult challenges facing a child. Emphasize what the child can do rather than what he or she cannot do. Good listening skills are important.

The child who has had surgery or a traumatic injury experiences pain. Many techniques discussed in Chapter 38 are useful interventions. After surgery, an epidural may be the treatment of choice. Oral analgesics are used during the period of adaptation to a prosthesis if the stump is tender. Children may have "phantom" limb pain in the lost extremity although this phenomenon is less common in children than adults (Ray, 2000).

The child usually begins wearing the prosthetic device for 1- to 2-hour intervals. Check the skin for any redness or breakdown. If redness or breakdown develops, leave the prosthesis off and allow the skin to clear before reapplying. Have the prosthesis adjusted if necessary, and increase wearing time as tolerated by the child.

Children with amputated limbs quickly learn how to accommodate to the prosthetic device. Use physical therapy programs specifically designed to help the child perform activities of daily living.

DISCHARGE PLANNING AND HOME CARE TEACHING

Answer any questions the family has about how to care for the prosthetic device and how to perform skin checks. Encourage parents to allow the child to participate in physically and emotionally challenging peer activities. Sporting activities that enable the child to participate using modified equipment are a good way to build self-confidence and motivation. For example, ski centers may offer programs that teach children with physical disabilities how to ski, or Special Olympics is motivating for some children. ⊂⊃ **WEB** Assess the need for counseling and offer referrals as appropriate.

Thinking Critically

THE CHILD WEARING A CAST

Douglass was admitted to the clinic today for application of a short leg cast. He broke his leg nearly a week ago when he was on a trampoline with three friends, trying to see who could jump the highest. Douglass slipped and his leg hit the frame on the side. His friends helped him off the trampoline and found someone to transport Douglass to the emergency room. They then reached his mother by phone, who rushed to the hospital when she heard the news.

His mother states that he is now 12 years old and in middle school. He has been going to a friend's house nearly every day after school and spending time on activities such as the trampoline and rollerblading, as well as watching television and playing video games. She felt this was safer than him being at home alone during her work hours, but is now starting to wonder about whether to allow Douglass to engage in activities with his friend.

A splint has provided support for several days and has allowed the swelling to decrease before today's cast application. Douglass has been non–weight bearing on his leg and has been using crutches. He returned to school yesterday for part of the day and found it was hard to get to all of his classes.

- What concerns will Douglass have once his cast is in place?
- What teaching should you provide to help him keep the cast intact and to ensure his safety?
- What signs or symptoms might indicate infection or loss of circulation and need to be reported immediately?
- Will any special adaptations be needed in his home and school?
- Is there any way his injury could have been avoided? What teaching does he need now to avoid further injuries? ⊂⊃ **WEB**

*C*HAPTER HIGHLIGHTS

➷ Children may develop musculoskeletal conditions as a result of congenital conditions, developmental variations, or trauma.

➷ Talipes equinovarus (clubfoot) is a common unilateral or bilateral variation in newborns that is treated by casting, traction, and/or surgery.

➷ Genu varum and genu valgum are normal variations at certain times in development that may need treatment if they persist.

➷ The nurse may identify developmental dysplasia of the hip (DDH) during newborn assessments and needs to refer the child for care to a specialist.

➷ Mild DDH may be treated by a harness, whereas more severe cases may require surgery for the child to walk normally.

➷ Legg-Calvé-Perthes is a disease most commonly seen in school-age boys; it causes necrosis of the femoral head.

➷ Slipped capital femoral epiphysis is treated by casting, traction, or more commonly surgery with pinning, to stabilize the epiphysis.

➷ Scoliosis is a lateral curvature of the spine; nurses commonly screen adolescents to identify the disorder.

➷ Osteomyelitis most commonly follows another infection and requires prompt treatment to prevent sepsis and serious injury to the bone.

➷ The child with osteogenesis imperfecta (brittle bone disease) requires careful handling by the nurse and parents to prevent fractures while fostering developmental progress.

➷ Muscular dystrophies are inherited diseases characterized by muscle wasting and degeneration.

➷ Children can experience a variety of fractures due to sports, car crashes, and other injury.

➷ Cast and traction care are common interventions for fractures; nursing interventions minimize problem development from these treatments.

EXPLOREMEDIALINK

NCLEX Review, Case Studies, and other interactive resources for this chapter can be found on the companion website at http://www.prenhall.com/london. Click on "Chapter 50" and select the activities for this chapter.

For animations, more NCLEX review questions, and an audio glossary, access the accompanying CD-ROM in this textbook.

REFERENCES

American Academy of Pediatrics, Committee on Injury and Poison Prevention. (1999). Transporting children with special health care needs. *Pediatrics, 104,* 988–992.

American Academy of Pediatrics, Committee on Quality Improvement and Subcommittee on Developmental Dysplasia of the Hip. (2000). *Pediatrics, 105,* 896–905.

Blakeslee, T. J. (1997). Congenital talipes equinovarus (clubfoot). *Clinics in Podiatric Medicine and Surgery, 14,* 9–55.

Carek, P. J., Dickerson, L. M., & Sack, J. L. (2001). Diagnosis and management of osteomyelitis. *American Family Physician, 63,* 2413–2420.

Davids, J. R. (1998). Limping. In L. T. Staheli (Ed.), *Pediatric orthopedic secrets* (pp. 195–199). Philadelphia: Hanley & Belfus.

DeBaun, B. J. (1998). Prevention of infection in the orthopedic surgery patient. *Nursing Clinics of North America, 33,* 671–684.

Fernbach, S. A. (1998). Common orthopedic problems of the newborn. *Nursing Clinics of North America, 33,* 583–596.

Frye, K. E., & Luterman, A. (1999). Burns and fractures. *Orthopaedic Nursing, 18*(1), 30–35.

Gonzalez, E., Pavia, C., Ros, J., Villaronga, M., Valls, C., & Exxcola, J. (2001). Efficacy of low dose schedule pamidronate infusion in children with osteogenesis imperfecta. *Journal of Pediatric Endocrinology and Metabolism, 14,* 529–533.

Harvey, C. (2001). Compartment syndrome: When it is least expected. *Orthopaedic Nursing 20*(3), 15–26.

Horwitz, E. M., Prockop, D. J., Gordon, P. L., Koo, W. W., Fitzpatrick, L. A., Neel, M. D., et al. (2001). Clinical responses to bone marrow transplantation in children with severe osteogenesis imperfecta. *Blood, 97,* 1227–1231.

Kautz, S. M., & Skaggs, D. L. (1998). Getting an angle on spinal deformities. *Contemporary Pediatrics, 15,* 111–128.

Killian, J. T., Mayberry, S., & Wilkinson, L. (1999). Current concepts in adolescent idiopathic scoliosis. *Pediatric Annals, 28,* 755–761.

Kunkler, C. E. (1999). Neurovascular assessment. *Orthopaedic Nursing, 18*(3), 63–71.

Mankin, K. P., & Zimbler, S. (1997). Gait and leg alignment: What's normal and what's not. *Contemporary Pediatrics, 14,* 41–70.

Muscari, M. E. (1998). Preventing sports injuries. *American Journal of Nursing, 98,* 58–60.

Novacheck, T. F. (1996). Developmental dysplasia of the hip. *Pediatric Clinics of North America, 43,* 829–848.

O'Connor, D. L. (1998). Preventing sports injuries in kids. *Patient Care Nurse Practitioner, 1*(4), 24–36.

Paterson, C. R., Monk, E. A., & McAllion, S. J. (2001). How common is hearing impairment in osteogenesis imperfecta? *Journal of Laryngology and Otolaryngology, 115,* 280–282.

Ray, R. L. (2000). Complications of lower extremity amputations. *Topics in Emergency Medicine, 22*(3), 35–43.

Roy, D. R. (1999). Current concept in Legg-Calve-Perthes disease. *Pediatric Annals, 28,* 748–754.

Ryan, D. J. (2001). Intoeing: A developmental norm. *Orthopaedic Nursing, 20*(2), 13–18.

Shaw, B. A., Gerardi, J. A., & Hennrikus, W. L. (1998). Avoiding the pitfalls of orthopedic disorders. *Contemporary Pediatrics, 15,* 122–135.

Takeda, S., & Miyagoe-Suzuki, Y. (2001). Gene therapy for muscular dystrophies: Current status and future prospects. *Biodrugs, 15,* 635–644.

Theophilopoulos, E. P., & Barrett, D. J. (1998). Get a grip on the pediatric hip. *Contemporary Pediatrics 15,* 43–65.

Wyshak, G. (2000). Teenaged girls, carbonated beverage consumption, and bone fractures. *Archives of Pediatrics and Adolescent Medicine, 154,* 610–613.

CHAPTER 51

The Child with Alterations in Endocrine Function

I am really worried about how Anthony is going to learn to manage all these aspects of diabetes care. Learning to check his blood sugar is pretty easy compared to counting calories and figuring out how much insulin to take and when to take it. I hope we have some time to get into a routine with his diabetes management before he gets sick. We have to work hard to keep the diabetes under control.

—MOTHER OF ANTHONY, 12 YEARS OLD

Key Terms

Acanthosis nigricans   *1375*

Bone age   *1352*

Euthyroid   *1356*

Glucagon   *1374*

Glycosuria   *1363*

Goiter   *1356*

Hormones   *1350*

Hyperinsulinemia   *1375*

Inborn errors of metabolism   *1350*

Insulin resistance   *1374*

Karyotype   *1360*

Polydipsia   *1354*

Polyphagia   *1364*

Polyuria   *1353*

Pseudohermaphroditism   *1360*

Puberty   *1350*

Thyrotoxicosis   *1358*

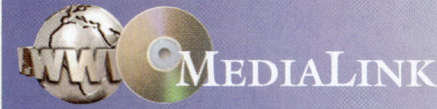

MEDIALINK

CD-ROM

Hormone Regulation and Secretion Animation

Audio Glossary

NCLEX Review

COMPANION WEBSITE

http://www.prenhall.com/london

MediaLink Applications:

Identify Strategies to Help Girls Understand Early Pubertal Development

Develop a Plan: Child with Type 1 Diabetes Returning to Elementary School

Develop a Peer Strategy: Child with Inborn Errors of Metabolism and Diet

Endocrine Web Links

Thinking Critically

NCLEX Review

Case Study

The endocrine system controls the cellular activity that regulates growth and body metabolism through the release of hormones. **Hormones** are chemical messengers secreted by various glands that exert controlling effects on the cells of the body. Overlapping with all body systems, the general functions of the endocrine system include the following:

- Differentiation of the reproductive and central nervous systems in the fetus
- Regulation of the pace of growth and development in concert with the central nervous system throughout childhood and adolescence
- Coordination of the male and female reproductive systems, enabling sexual reproduction
- Maintenance of an optimal level of hormones for body functioning
- Maintenance of homeostasis, a healthy internal environment, in the presence of a constantly changing external environment

Inborn errors of metabolism—inherited biochemical abnormalities of the urea cycle and amino acid and organic acid metabolism—often have a significant impact on the endocrine system's ability to support growth and development. Some chromosomal abnormalities also result in disturbances in growth and sexual development.

Endocrine disturbances result in alterations in metabolism, growth and development, and behavior that may have significant implications for children. If not diagnosed and treated early, these conditions can result in delays in growth and development, mental retardation, and, occasionally, death. However, treatment, which usually consists of supplementation of missing hormones, adjustment of hormone levels, or dietary measures, allows most children to live a normal life.

ANATOMY AND PHYSIOLOGY OF PEDIATRIC DIFFERENCES

The hypothalamic-pituitary axis produces a number of releasing and inhibiting hormones that regulate the function of many endocrine glands, including the thyroid, adrenal, and male and female reproductive glands. In addition, hormones originating from this axis regulate growth. Other endocrine glands include the parathyroid glands, and islets of Langerhans in the pancreas (Figure 51–1 ◆). All of these glands secrete hormones into the bloodstream, which carries them to target organs or tissues. Most hormones exert their influence through interaction with receptors in the target cells of specific tissues (Table 51–1).

The regulation of hormone secretion occurs through a negative feedback mechanism that functions to maintain an optimal internal environment in the body. 🔗 CD

Negative feedback occurs when an endocrine gland or secretory tissue receives a message that the target cells have received an adequate amount of hormone. In response, further secretion is inhibited. Secretion is resumed only when the secretory tissue receives another message indicating that levels of the hormone are low.

The endocrine system is responsible for sexual differentiation during fetal development and for stimulating growth and development during childhood and adolescence. This includes stimulating development of the reproductive system in both sexes.

Puberty (sexual maturation, lasting 2 to 3 years) occurs when the gonads secrete increased amounts of the sex hormones estrogen and testosterone. At the average age of 10 years in girls and 11 years in boys, the hypothalamus produces increased amounts of gonadotropin-releasing hormone. This hormone stimulates the anterior pituitary gland to increase the production of luteinizing hormone (LH) and follicle-stimulating hormone (FSH). These hormones in turn stimulate the gonads to secrete more sex hormones (Figure 51–2 ◆), resulting in the development of primary and secondary sex characteristics.

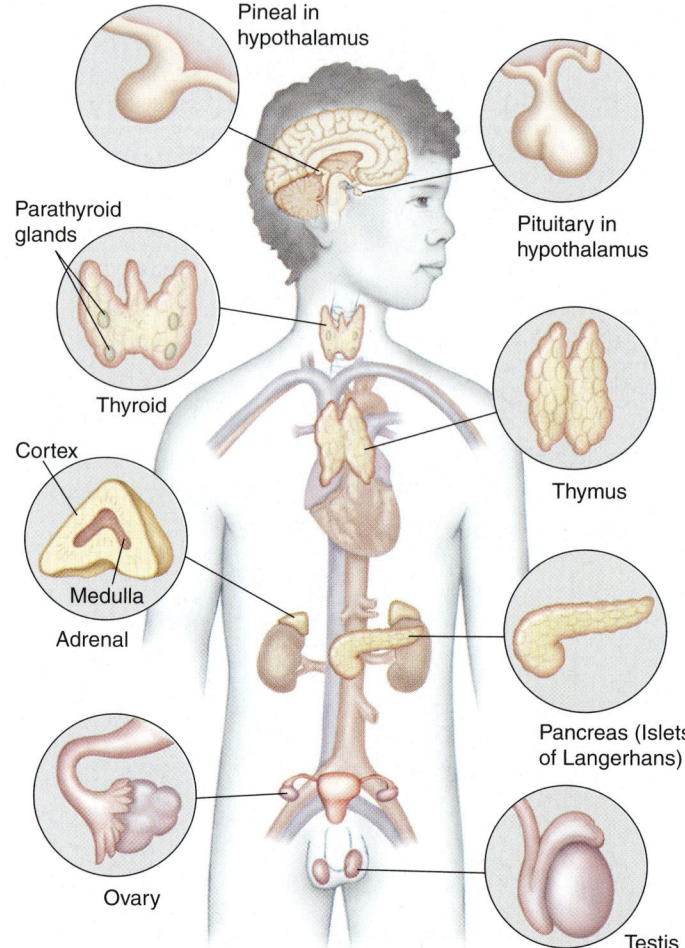

FIGURE 51–1. ◆ Major organs and glands of the endocrine system.

TABLE 51-1 Endocrine Glands and Their Functions

Gland/Hormone	Function
Anterior Pituitary	
Growth hormone	Stimulates growth of all body tissues
Thyroid-stimulating hormone (TSH)	Stimulates thyroid hormone secretion
Adrenocorticotropic hormone (ACTH)	Stimulates secretion of glucocorticoids and androgens
Follicle-stimulating hormone (FSH)	Stimulates secretion of estrogen; supports follicle development in ovaries
Luteinizing hormone (LH) and Interstitial cell-stimulating hormone (ICSH) (Male analogue)	Stimulates secretion of androgens in males and progesterone in females
Prolactin-releasing hormone	Stimulates secretion of prolactin that stimulates the secretion of milk during lactation
Melanocyte-stimulating hormone (MSH)	Stimulates skin pigmentation
Posterior Pituitary	
Antidiuretic hormone (ADH)	Stimulates permeability of distal renal tubules and collecting ducts
Oxytocin	Stimulates uterine contractions and breast milk letdown reflex
Beta endorphins	May regulate body temperature, food and water intake
Thyroid	
Thyroxine (T4) and triiodothyronine (T3)	Regulates metabolic rate of all cells, body heat production; protein, fat, and carbohydrate catabolism in all cells
Thyrocalcitonin	Stimulates bone ossification and development
Parathyroid	
Parathyroid hormone	Regulates serum calcium levels and excretion of phosphorus
Adrenal	
Aldosterone	Conserves sodium and excretion of potassium
Androgens	Stimulates bone development and secondary sexual characteristics
Cortisol	Stimulates anti-inflammatory reactions, protects from stress
Epinephrine	Activates sympathetic nervous system; stimulates increase in blood pressure and blood glucose levels
Pancreas (Islets of Langerhans)	
Insulin	Facilitates cellular glucose utilization
Glucagon	Increases blood glucose
Somatostatin	Stimulates inhibition of insulin and glucagon secretion; may prevent excess insulin secretion
Ovaries	
Estrogen	Stimulates development of breasts and ova
Progesterone	Stimulates breast glandular development; acts to maintain pregnancy
Testes	
Testosterone	Stimulates production of sperm, development of secondary sexual characteristics, and closure of epiphysis

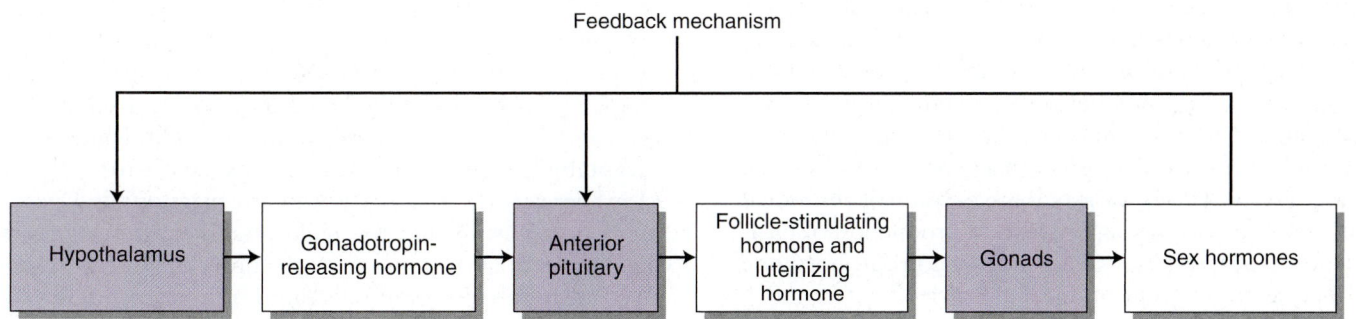

FIGURE 51-2. ◆ Feedback mechanism in hormonal stimulation of the gonads during puberty.

✍ DISORDERS OF PITUITARY FUNCTION

GROWTH HORMONE DEFICIENCY (HYPOPITUITARISM)

Growth hormone deficiency (GHD) is a disorder caused by decreased activity of the pituitary gland. Because most children with this disorder secrete inadequate amounts of growth hormone, the term *growth hormone deficiency* is often preferred to *hypopituitarism*. As many as 10,000 school-age children have GHD (Shulman & Bercu, 1998).

The release of growth hormone from the anterior pituitary gland is controlled by the hypothalamus, which secretes releasing and inhibitory factors. Growth hormone stimulates linear growth and bone mineral density, as well as the growth of all body tissues. It also stimulates the synthesis of proteins in the liver, among them the somatomedins or insulin-like growth factors (IGFs), which promote glucose use by the cells and cell proliferation.

Infection, infarction of the pituitary gland (related to sickle cell disease), central nervous system disease, tumors of the pituitary gland or hypothalamus (primarily craniopharyngiomas and gliomas), other brain tumors, cranial irradiation, brain trauma, and psychosocial deprivation may cause GHD by interfering with the production or release of growth hormone. Dominant or recessive inheritance or a genetic mutation may cause deficiency of growth hormone or abnormalities of hormone receptors (Finegold, 1997).

Children with GHD have normal birth weights and lengths. By the age of 1 year, however, they are below the third percentile on the growth chart. They characteristically grow at a rate of less than 5 cm (2 in) per year. Other characteristic findings in infants include hypoglycemic seizures, hyponatremia, neonatal jaundice, pale optic discs, micropenis, and undescended testicles. Children with GHD tend to be overweight and to have youthful facial features, higher pitched voices, delayed dentition, "ripply" abdominal fat, decreased muscle mass, delayed skeletal maturation, delayed sexual maturation, and hypoglycemia.

Any child whose height is 2 to 3 standard deviations below the mean height for age or whose measurement is falling off the normal growth chart should be evaluated for short stature (Table 51–2). Major causes of short stature include GHD, familial short stature, hypothyroidism, Turner syndrome, constitutional growth delay, chronic renal failure, Cushing syndrome, inborn error of metabolism, and severe cardiac, pulmonary, or gastrointestinal disease. Psychosocial dwarfism is a syndrome of emotional deprivation that causes suppression of production of pituitary hormones, resulting in adrenocorticotropic hormone (ACTH) and growth hormone deficiencies.

A child whose screening tests reveal low levels of IGF-1 requires further evaluation by a pediatric endocrinologist. A

TABLE 51–2 Diagnostic Tests for Short Stature

Test	Purpose Related to Short Stature
IGF-1 and IGFBP-3	Excludes GHD if normal
Radiographic views of the sella turcica (site of the pituitary gland)	Demonstrates size of the sella turcica or a tumor
Karyotype (girls)	Detects Turner syndrome (see page 1377) 🔗
Thyroid function studies	Detects hypothyroidism (see page 1355) 🔗
Urine creatinine, pH, specific gravity, urea nitrogen, electrolytes	Detects chronic renal failure (see Chapter 47) 🔗
Bone age	Identifies other potential causes of delayed growth
Complete blood count and erythrocyte sedimentation rate	Screens for inflammatory bowel disease with anemia
Antigliadin antibodies	Screens for celiac disease

Note: From D'Ercole, A. J., & Underwood, L. (1996). Anterior pituitary gland and hypothalamus. In A. M. Rudolph, J. I. E. Hoffman, & C. D. Rudolph (Eds.), *Rudolph's pediatrics* (20th ed., p. 1692). Stamford, CT: Appleton & Lange. Modified.

careful history, physical examination, assessment of pubertal development and unusual facies, and radiologic studies are necessary to identify possible causes of short stature. A radiograph of the bones of the wrist is used to evaluate the stage of bone ossification, and thus the **bone age** of the child. Using standardized norms for bone ossification, it can be determined if the child's chronologic and bone ages match. A significantly delayed (less than the child's age) or advanced (greater than the child's age) bone age indicates the possibility of a systemic chronic disease or hormone abnormality. Provocative growth hormone testing, in which various medications (arginine, clonidine, glucagon, insulin, L-dopa) are administered to stimulate release of growth hormone, is the definitive diagnostic test in most children.

Treatment depends on the cause of the deficiency. Brain tumors must be treated effectively before growth hormone therapy can be considered. See Chapter 45. 🔗 Approved indications for growth hormone therapy include GHD and growth retardation due to chronic renal failure, Turner syndrome, small for gestational age, Russell-Silver syndrome, and Prader-Willi syndrome. Most children receive subcutaneous injections 3 to 7 times a week, and have increased growth velocity for 1 year, followed by more normal growth velocity. Close monitoring of growth and endocrinology visits every 3 to 4 months are needed. Replacement therapy continues until the child achieves an acceptable height or growth velocity drops to < 2 cm (1 in) per year (Willhaus, 1999). Early diagnosis and treatment help ensure that the child attains maximum adult height potential. In some cases the onset of puberty is delayed with gonadotropin-releasing hormone analogues to provide more time for growth hormone therapy to stimulate growth.

The increased availability of synthetic growth hormone has raised legal and ethical questions about its use for short children who are not growth hormone deficient. The medication is expensive (up to $15,000 per year), the injections are invasive, and its long-term effects, such as actually increasing adult height, are still being investigated.

Nursing Management

Nursing care consists of monitoring growth, teaching the child and family about the disorder and its treatment, and providing emotional support. Carefully measure the child's height and weight and plot them on a growth chart (see Appendix C and Skills 9–1—9–7). ⊂⊃ SKILLS CD

Teach the parents and child about the growth hormone replacement therapy and how to give injections. Provide the parents with ideas about how to minimize the trauma to the child receiving regular injections. Give parents educational resources, such as information from the Magic Foundation, Human Growth Foundation, and the Short Stature Foundation. Since replacement therapy is expensive and may not be covered by insurance, parents may need financial assistance that is sometimes available from the growth hormone manufacturers. ⊂⊃ WEB

Children with GHD, especially those due to tumors and trauma from radiation or surgery, may have academic problems because of acquired learning disabilities. Before the child enters or returns to school, a comprehensive evaluation should be performed to identify potential problems.

The best results occur when treatment is begun at an early age, before the psychologic effects of short stature become apparent. People often treat short children on the basis of their size rather than their age, and such children experience social prejudice about height. Teasing is a common problem. The teenage years may be particularly stressful because of adolescents' characteristic preoccupation with body image.

Encourage parents and teachers to treat the child in an age-appropriate manner. The child should dress in clothing that reflects chronologic age. Emphasize the child's strengths, support independence, and encourage participation in age-appropriate activities to aid in the development of a positive self-image. Suggest that the child take part in sports in which ability does not depend on size (e.g., swimming, gymnastics, wrestling, ice skating, and martial arts). Identifying positive role models, short people who accomplish their goals, also promotes a positive image. Refer the child for counseling if appropriate.

HYPERPITUITARISM

Hyperpituitarism, a disorder in which excessive secretion of growth hormone increases the growth rate, is rare in children. Oversecretion of growth hormone is usually caused by a pituitary adenoma. If combined with precocious puberty, a tumor of the hypothalamus may be pres-

ent. Affected children can grow to 7 or 8 feet in height when oversecretion occurs before closure of the epiphyseal plates. If the disorder occurs after closure of the epiphyseal plates, acromegaly occurs.

Because tall stature is valued in our society, assessment of children (particularly boys) with accelerated growth is often delayed. Any child whose predicted height exceeds that consistent with parental height should be evaluated for possible growth problems and underlying pathologic conditions.

A complete history is obtained, and physical examination and laboratory testing are performed. Increased levels of IGF-1 establish the diagnosis of hyperpituitarism. A bone age is done, and a bone scan is usually obtained to determine whether the epiphyseal plates have begun to fuse. Radiologic studies are used to detect a tumor. Thorough evaluation is required to differentiate hyperpituitarism from familial tall stature.

Treatment depends on the cause of the excessive growth and may involve surgical removal of a tumor, radiation therapy, radioactive implants, or high doses of sex steroids given to close the epiphyseal plates. The child may need pituitary hormone replacement following surgery.

Nursing Management

Tall stature, like short stature, can be stressful for children. Tall children are often treated as if they are older than their chronologic age. Tall adolescents may have problems with self-image, and girls in particular may worry about their appearance.

Nursing care focuses on teaching the parents and child about the disorder and its treatment, providing emotional support, and, if surgery is required, providing preoperative and postoperative teaching and care (see Chapter 34). ⊂⊃

DIABETES INSIPIDUS

Diabetes insipidus, a rare disorder of the posterior pituitary gland, may begin at any age. Two forms of diabetes insipidus occur in children: true (or central) antidiuretic hormone (ADH) deficiency and familial nephrogenic diabetes insipidus, in which the renal collecting tubules are unable to respond to the ADH that is present.

True ADH deficiency in children is usually familial or idiopathic. Secondary causes include central nervous system trauma, infection, tumor, hypoxic brain damage, vascular anomalies, or infiltrative diseases like leukemia. Most cases of nephrogenic diabetes insipidus are familial, with either an X-linked or an autosomal recessive form. It may also result from drug toxicity or recurrent infection.

ADH facilitates concentration of the urine by stimulating reabsorption of water from the distal tubule of the kidney. When ADH is inadequate, the tubules do not resorb, leading to **polyuria** (passage of a large volume of urine in a given period).

CAUSE	CLINICAL MANIFESTATIONS	CLINICAL THERAPY
True Diabetes Insipidus ADH deficiency Familial or idiopathic	Polyuria, polydipsia Nocturia, enuresis Thirsty at night, irritable if fluids withheld Constipation, fever, dehydration	Desmopressin acetate
Nephrogenic Diabetes Insipidus Familial, decreased responsiveness of kidneys to ADH	Polyuria, polydipsia Hypernatremia in neonatal period Dehydration, fever, vomiting Mental status changes	Diuretics High fluid intake Salt and protein restricted diet

Polyuria and **polydipsia** (excessive thirst) are the cardinal signs of diabetes insipidus above. See "Clinical Manifestations: Diabetes Insipidus." Although the onset of symptoms is usually sudden, diagnosis is often delayed. Children who can quench their thirst may not complain to parents about symptoms. The child may be obese due to an excessive intake of high-caloric fluids.

In all forms of diabetes insipidus, the urine cannot be concentrated, no matter how dehydrated the child becomes. Dehydration usually precipitates diagnosis. Serum sodium concentration and osmolality increase rapidly to pathologic levels. Often an unconscious child is admitted to the emergency department with dehydration and hypernatremia.

Serum electrolytes and both serum and urine osmolalities are tested. Diagnosis is confirmed by measuring the plasma arginine vasopressin (AVP) level before and during a fluid deprivation test, which is usually conducted in the hospital or in a carefully controlled outpatient setting for up to 7 hours. Urine osmolality, urine specific gravity, serum sodium, and serum osmolality are monitored hourly. The specific gravity will remain less than 1.010 even after dehydration. A dose of aqueous vasopressin is given after several hours. A decreased urine output and increased urine concentration confirm the diagnosis.

Nursing Practice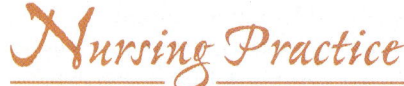

During the fluid deprivation test, advise parents that the child will be frustrated and irritable from thirst. No one should drink in front of the child during the testing period. Monitor the child's vital signs and intake and output carefully. The test is stopped if the child loses 3% to 5% of body weight and develops a fever and hypotension (Dveirin & Tunnessen, 2000).

Treatment of true ADH deficiency consists of the subcutaneous, intranasal, or oral desmopressin acetate (DDAVP) with an effect lasting 8 to 12 hours. DDAVP reduces urinary output, enabling the child to live a more normal life with a decrease in thirst, urinary output, and nocturia. The dose of DDAVP must be titered so the child receives adequate caloric intake for growth and development. Because DDAVP does not control nephrogenic diabetes insipidus, these children are treated with diuretics, a high fluid intake, and a salt- and protein-restricted diet. The child's sodium and potassium levels must be carefully monitored to prevent hypernatremia and hypokalemia (see Chapter 39).

Nursing Management

Nursing care centers on administering medications and teaching parents how to manage the condition and recognize signs of altered fluid status. Parent education is of primary importance. Administration of synthetic vasopressin (DDAVP) in small doses by intranasal insufflation (blowing the medication into the nasal cavity) in infants and young children often results in inconsistent absorption. If too large a dose is given, the child may swallow the medication, resulting in lack of absorption.

Help parents monitor fluid intake after DDAVP treatment is begun. Infants usually need fluid intake even during the night. Many infants have coexisting brain damage and decreased thirst and need nasogastric or gastrostomy feeding to maintain adequate hydration and nutrition. When the child has compensated for the condition with an excessive fluid intake, he or she must learn about the diminished need for fluids. The child will not be able to excrete the excess water load with DDAVP treatment.

Teach parents to recognize signs of inadequate fluid intake (see Chapter 39) and to adjust the child's fluid intake to prevent dehydration. When the child with nephrogenic diabetes insipidus has an acute illness, the child's physician should be notified immediately because the increased metabolic activity may cause dehydration and hypernatremia that can cause mental retardation, seizures, and cerebral calcification. Additional fluids are needed to prevent dehydration (Kirchlechner, Koller, Seidl, et al., 1999).

Parents may need help managing the child's care. Arrangements for a visiting nurse, a home health nurse, or respite care may be needed.

PRECOCIOUS PUBERTY

Puberty normally occurs between 8 and 13 years of age in girls and between 9 1/2 and 14 years of age in boys. Precocious puberty is defined as the appearance of any secondary sexual characteristics before 8 years of age in girls and 9 years of age in boys.

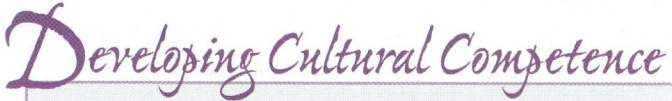

A national study of the age at which pubertal development begins in girls has revealed an earlier average age of puberty than described in texts. African-American girls begin puberty between 8 and 9 years of age. Caucasian girls begin puberty by 10 years of age (Herman-Giddens, Slora, Wasserman, et al, 1997).

Early secretion of the normal hormones responsible for pubertal changes usually is not associated with abnormalities. However, a benign hypothalamic tumor may be present. Other causes include brain injury, brain tumor, postinfectious encephalitis or meningitis, congenital adrenal hyperplasia, tumors of the ovary, adrenal gland, or testicle, and exogenous sources or androgens (i.e., anabolic steroids). Children with precocious puberty have an advanced bone age (premature skeletal maturation) and may appear unusually tall for their age. Their growth ceases prematurely, however, as the hormones stimulate closure of the epiphyseal plates, resulting in short stature.

When the cause of the condition cannot be treated, the child's development may be monitored for 6 to 12 months to see how quickly pubertal changes are occurring. If development is stalled or slow, no treatment is initiated. If pubertal changes occur rapidly, a gonadotropin-releasing hormone analogue is used to stop the development of secondary sexual characteristics, bone age progression, and rapid growth. This extends the time for pubertal growth. In some cases growth hormone is given to increase the ultimate height of the child (Kohn, Julius, & Blethen, 1999).

Nursing Management

Nursing care centers on teaching the child and parents about the condition and its treatment and providing emotional support. Inform the child in age-appropriate terms that physiologic changes are normal but occurring at an earlier than usual age. Reassure the child that friends will go through the same stages of development eventually. Remember that the child's social, cognitive, and emotional development matches his or her age, even though the physical development is advanced.

Children with precocious puberty become self-conscious as body changes occur. Parents should be advised to dress the child in a manner appropriate to his or her chronologic age, even though the child may look older. Looser cloth-ing may help hide some of the body changes that are occurring. Provide privacy during examinations. Encourage the child to express his or her feelings about the changes. The child may need to practice role-playing as a coping mechanism to manage teasing by other children. Parents should be advised that they may need to discuss issues of sexuality with the child at an earlier age than normal. Refer the child for counseling if appropriate.

≈ DISORDERS OF THYROID FUNCTION

HYPOTHYROIDISM

Hypothyroidism is a disorder in which levels of active thyroid hormones are decreased. It may be congenital or acquired. Congenital hypothyroidism occurs in approximately 1 in 4000 live births and is twice as common in girls as in boys. It is less prevalent in African-American infants but more frequent in infants of Far Eastern and Hispanic origin (1 in 2000 births). It also occurs more commonly in children with Down syndrome. Acquired hypothyroidism has an estimated prevalence of 1 in 500,000 school-age children, and is more common in girls than in boys (Donohoue, 1999).

Etiology and Pathophysiology

Thyroid hormones are important for growth and development and for metabolizing nutrients and energy. When these hormones are not available to stimulate other hormones or specific target cells, growth is delayed and mental retardation develops.

Congenital hypothyroidism is usually caused by a spontaneous gene mutation, an autosomal recessive genetic transmission of an enzyme deficiency, hypoplasia or aplasia of the thyroid gland, failure of the central nervous system–thyroid feedback mechanism to develop, or iodine deficiency. Mental retardation is irreversible if the disorder is not treated.

Acquired hypothyroidism can be idiopathic or result from autoimmune thyroiditis (Hashimoto thyroiditis), late-onset thyroid dysfunction, isolated thyroid-stimulating hormone (TSH) deficiency due to pituitary or hypothalamic dysfunction, or exposure to drugs or substances such as lithium that interfere with thyroid hormone synthesis.

Clinical Manifestations

Infants with congenital hypothyroidism have few clinical signs of the disorder in the first weeks of life. In untreated infants the characteristic cretinoid features (thickened protuberant tongue, thick lips, dull appearance) appear during the first few months of life. Other signs include prolonged neonatal jaundice, hypotonia, macroglossia, respiratory distress, bradycardia, decreased pulse pressure, cool extremities, mottling, umbilical hernia, a posterior fontanel larger than 1 cm in diameter, difficulty feeding, lethargy, constipation, and a hoarse cry.

Children with acquired hypothyroidism have many of the same signs as adults: decreased appetite, dry, cool skin, thinning hair or hair loss, depressed deep tendon reflexes, bradycardia, constipation, sensitivity to cold temperatures, abnormal menses, and a **goiter** (a nontender enlarged thyroid gland). Manifestations unique to children include change in past normal growth patterns with a weight increase, decreased height velocity, delayed bone and dental age, muscle hypertrophy with muscle weakness, and delayed or precocious puberty.

Clinical Therapy

Congenital hypothyroidism is usually detected during newborn screening of thyroxine (T_4) and TSH levels, which is mandatory in all 50 states. An elevated TSH level indicates that the disease originated in the thyroid, not the pituitary. Two tests are frequently performed so that the disorder is identified, before the newborn leaves the hospital and at the first health care visit at 1 to 2 weeks of age. Rapid response from the laboratory testing the samples is important to reduce the time to diagnosis and the effects of hypothyroidism on the infant's development.

If the T_4 level is below normal and the TSH level is increased, the synthetic thyroid hormone levothyroxine (Synthroid) is prescribed. The dose is increased gradually as the child grows to ensure a **euthyroid** (normal thyroid) state. A pediatric endocrinologist monitors treatment. Periodic evaluation of T_4 and TSH serum levels, bone age, and growth parameters is necessary to assess for signs of excess or inadequate thyroid hormone.

Antithyroid antibodies are measured in children with a goiter and suspected Hashimoto thyroiditis, as increased titers of antithyroglobin and antimicrosomal antibodies are often found.

To ensure an adequate growth rate and prevent mental retardation, the hormone must be taken throughout life. Children with congenital hypothyroidism that is diagnosed before 3 months of age have the best prognosis for optimal mental development. Treated children with the most severe form of congenital hypothyroidism lose 6 to 15 IQ points, while the less severely affected children have an IQ similar to their siblings (Van Vliet, 2001). Children with acquired hypothyroidism usually have normal growth following a period of catch-up growth. Many adolescents with Hashimoto thyroiditis have a spontaneous remission.

Nursing Management

Nursing Assessment and Diagnosis

Routine neonatal screening is performed before discharge from the hospital and is often repeated at the infant's first health visit to evaluate levels of circulating thy-

roid hormones. Sometimes nurses make home visits a few days after discharge to assess the health of the mother and infant. Neonatal screening may be performed at that visit (see Skill 10–2). **SKILLS**

Peform serial measurement and recording of height and weight at each follow-up visit. The child is assessed for signs of inadequate growth to determine if the dose of thyroid hormone needs to be adjusted and to monitor compliance with medication.

Among the nursing diagnoses that might be appropriate for the child with hypothyroidism are:

▶ *Altered nutrition: less than body requirements* related to loss of appetite

▶ *Hypothermia* related to decreased basal metabolic rate

▶ *Constipation* related to decreased bowel motility

▶ *Fatigue* related to altered body chemistry

▶ *Altered health maintenance* related to lack of understanding about the treatment regimen

Planning and Implementation

Nursing care focuses on teaching the parents and child about the disorder and its treatment and monitoring the child's growth rate. When the cause is genetic, make a referral for genetic counseling. Explain how to administer thyroid hormone (e.g., tablets can be crushed and mixed in a small amount of formula or applesauce). Advise parents that the child may experience temporary sleep disturbances or behavioral changes in response to therapy. Teach the parents how to assess for an increased pulse rate, which could indicate the presence of too much thyroid hormone, and advise them to report problems such as fatigue, which could indicate an improper drug dose that needs to be adjusted.

Caution parents to dress the child appropriately for the season to prevent hypothermia. Modify the child's diet by increasing the amount of fruits and bulk if constipation is a problem.

Reassure the family that the child will develop normally with hormone replacement therapy. Reinforce the importance of follow-up visits to assess growth rate and response to therapy and to regulate drug dosages as the child grows. Periodic assessments of educational achievement are needed. Even with good control, adolescents have persistent visual-spatial deficits, and memory and attention problems. Those with more severe disease or who take longer to get to euthyroid status have the poorest academic achievement and more behavior problems (Rovet & Erlich, 2000). Parents should be informed that therapy will be lifelong and is needed to promote the child's mental development.

Evaluation

Expected outcomes of nursing care of the child with hypothyroidism include:

- The child maintains adequate growth of height and weight, following a percentile curve throughout childhood.
- The child's diet contains adequate fruits and bulk to prevent constipation.
- The child's cognitive develop is appropriate for age.

HYPERTHYROIDISM

Hyperthyroidism occurs when thyroid hormone levels are increased. It is rare in children and adolescents with a rate of 8 cases per 1 million children (Castiglia, 1997). It is most common in adolescent girls and is almost always due to Graves disease.

Etiology and Pathophysiology

Graves disease is an autoimmune disorder in which the body produces antibodies that attack the cells of the thyroid gland. It has a high familial incidence. Immunoglobulins produced by the B lymphocytes stimulate oversecretion of thyroid hormones, resulting in the clinical symptoms. Signs and symptoms are caused by hyperactivity of the sympathetic nervous system.

Other more unusual forms of hyperthyroidism result from thyroiditis and thyroid hormone–producing tumors, including thyroid adenomas and carcinomas, and pituitary adenomas. Congenital hyperthyroidism can occur in infants of mothers with Graves disease because of transplacental transfer of immunoglobulins.

Clinical Manifestations

Characteristic findings include an enlarged, nontender thyroid gland (goiter), prominent or bulging eyes (exophthalmos) (Figure 51–3), eyelid lag, tachycardia, nervousness, restlessness or irritability, increased appetite with weight loss, emotional lability, heat intolerance, increased sweating, insomnia, tremor, and muscle weakness. The thyroid gland may be slightly enlarged or grow to three to four times its normal size, feel warm, soft, and fleshy, and have an auditory bruit on auscultation. The disorder often presents in the preschool years, but with an increased incidence in adolescence. Onset is subtle, and the condition often goes unrecognized for 1 to 2 years.

Children with Graves disease usually have behavioral problems and declining performance in school. They become easily frustrated in the classroom and overheated and fatigued during physical education class. It is difficult for them to relax or sleep. These symptoms usually prompt parents to seek medical treatment for them. Other symptoms include an increased appetite with weight loss, tremors, and tachycardia. Exophthalmos is less pronounced in children than in adults.

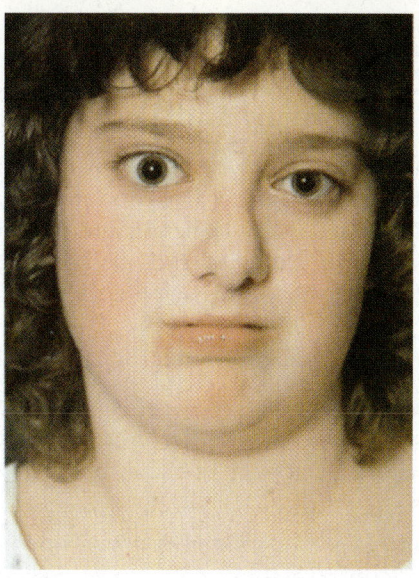

FIGURE 51–3. ◆ Exophthalmos and an enlarged thyroid in an adolescent with Graves disease. *Note:* From Zitelli, B., & Davis, H. (Eds.). (1997). *Atlas of pediatric physical diagnosis* (3rd ed., p 271). St Louis, MO: Mosby-Wolfe.

Clinical Therapy

Diagnostic studies include laboratory evaluation of serum TSH, T_3 (triiodothyronine), and T_4 levels, and a thyroid scan. Blood studies are also performed to detect autoantibodies specific for the various thyroid disorders.

The goal of clinical therapy is to inhibit excessive secretion of thyroid hormones. Treatment may include antithyroid drug therapy, radiation therapy, or surgery. Drug therapy is most often the initial treatment, but compliance is often a problem because of drug side effects. Methimazole (Tapazole) and propylthiouracil (PTU) are given to inhibit thyroid hormone secretion. PTU therapy can cause temporary side effects, including skin rashes, urticaria, and lymphadenopathy. If fever or sore throat develops, a health care professional should evaluate the child to rule out granulocytopenia. Treatment continues for 18 months to 2 years or until the thyroid decreases in size. Symptoms usually improve within weeks of starting treatment. Approximately 25% of children have a remission of symptoms every 2 years (Castiglia, 1997).

If drug therapy is ineffective, radiation therapy using radioactive iodine (131I) is the next treatment choice. Current data do not indicate a relationship between radioactive iodine and cancer or leukemia. It also does not appear to increase the risk of birth defects in future offspring in those treated (Castiglia, 1997). Thyroidectomy is the third alternative; however, destruction or removal of the thyroid gland often results in permanent hypothyroidism, necessitating hormone replacement therapy.

Nursing Management

Nursing Assessment and Diagnosis

Assess the child's vital signs, as blood pressure and pulse may be elevated. Keep a record of food intake. Accurate measurement and recording of height and weight are important to establish baselines and identify patterns of growth. Observe the child's behavior, activity, and level of fatigue.

Common nursing diagnoses for the child with hyperthyroidism include:

▶ *Ineffective thermoregulation (elevated)* related to illness and excessive activity of the sympathetic nervous system

▶ *Altered nutrition: less than body requirements* related to high metabolic needs

▶ *Body image disturbance* related to changes caused by illness (prominent eyes, excessive perspiration, and tremors)

▶ *Fatigue* related to disease state and sleep deprivation

▶ *Self-esteem disturbance* related to chronic illness and declining school performance

Planning and Implementation

Nursing care focuses on teaching the child and parents about the disorder and its treatment, promoting rest, providing emotional support, and, if the child needs surgery, providing preoperative and postoperative teaching and care. Promote increased caloric intake by providing five or six moderate meals per day. Encourage the child and family to express their feelings and concerns about the disorder. Pointing out even slight improvements in the child's condition increases compliance with therapy.

Children with hyperthyroidism are easily fatigued. Rest periods should be scheduled at school and home and physical activities kept to a minimum until symptoms resolve. Encourage parents to provide a cool environment and allow the child to wear fewer clothes until symptoms subside.

Children who have partial or total removal of the thyroid gland receive antithyroid drugs, such as iodine, for approximately 2 weeks before surgery. Teach the child and parents about drug therapy and instruct parents to watch for side effects of antithyroid drugs, including fever, urticaria, and lymphadenopathy. Provide preoperative teaching (see Chapter 34). Young children, in particular, may be fearful about having their throat "cut."

Postoperatively, observe for life-threatening signs of hypercalcemia and severe **thyrotoxicosis** or thyroid "storm" when thyroid hormone is suddenly released into the bloodstream during surgery. The child experiences fever, diaphoresis, and tachycardia, progressing to shock and, if untreated, death. Treatment includes antithyroid drugs and propranolol. Monitor the child's surgical site. Assess the child for bleeding, hoarseness, and difficulty breathing, which may be signs of inflammation.

Teach the family about the need for lifelong thyroid hormone replacement if radiation or surgery is performed. The child should wear a medical alert bracelet. Make sure the child is monitored regularly to ensure that the T_4 level is adequate to sustain growth.

Evaluation

Expected outcomes of nursing care for the child with hyperthyroidism include:

▶ The child regains lost weight and then follows the previously established growth curve because the T_4 level remains appropriate.

▶ Any difficulty breathing, bleeding, or hoarseness as a result of thyroid surgery are rapidly managed and controlled.

See Chapter 39 for parathyroid conditions.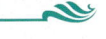

❧ DISORDERS OF ADRENAL FUNCTION

CUSHING SYNDROME

Cushing syndrome, also called adrenocortical hyperfunction, is characterized by a group of symptoms resulting from excess levels of glucocorticoids (especially cortisol) in the bloodstream. It is uncommon in children and the true incidence is unknown. During infancy and childhood, most cases of Cushing syndrome are due to malignant adrenal tumor. After 8 years of age more than half of the cases are due to secretion of ACTH by a pituitary adenoma causing cortisol secretion. Another cause is hyperplasia of one or both adrenal glands. The increased secretion of cortisol alters metabolism.

The initial sign in most children is gradual excessive weight gain and growth retardation. It generally takes up to 5 years for the child to develop the characteristic "cushingoid" appearance, which includes a moon face (chubby cheeks and a double chin) and fat pads over the shoulders and back (buffalo hump). The most common reasons for cushingoid features in children are excessive doses of corticosteroids and prolonged use of corticosteroids as treatment for other diseases. Corticosteroids suppress adrenal function when given long term. These children do not have Cushing syndrome. See "Clinical Manifestations: Cushing Syndrome."  Other signs include mental changes and delayed puberty.

Diagnosis is based on characteristic physical findings and laboratory values, including reduced serum levels of potassium and phosphorus; elevated serum calcium and sodium concentrations; increased 24-hour urinary levels of

CLINICAL MANIFESTATIONS *Cushing Syndrome*

CAUSE	CLINICAL MANIFESTATIONS
Catabolism of protein	Muscle weakness and wasting, capillary weakness and bruising, growth failure with delayed bone age, fatigue
Decreased absorption of calcium from the intestines	Demineralization of bones, osteoporosis
Increased appetite	Weight gain primarily on the trunk, striae on the abdomen, buttocks, thighs
Salt-retention	Increased blood volume and hypertension

free cortisol, and 17-hydroxycorticosteroid (17-OHCs); and loss of diurnal rhythm in serum cortisol (usually elevated at night). The child has chronic hyperglycemia and an elevated glycosylated hemoglobin concentration. See Appendix B for lab values.

The adrenal suppression test is used for the initial screening of children with suspected adrenocortical hyperfunction. If this test reveals that adrenal cortisol output is not suppressed overnight after a dose of dexamethasone, further diagnostic testing is necessary to determine the cause of hypercortisolism. Computed tomography (CT) and magnetic resonance imaging (MRI) detect tumors in the adrenal and pituitary glands.

Surgical removal is the current treatment of choice for adrenal tumors or pituitary adenomas. Cortisol replacement is required when both adrenal glands are removed. The prognosis for children with malignant adrenal tumors is poor.

Nursing Management

The nurse usually encounters a child with Cushing syndrome when the child is hospitalized for diagnostic evaluation or surgery. Nursing assessment includes monitoring the child's vital signs and fluid and nutritional status, and assessing muscle strength and endurance during hospital play activities.

Teach the child and family about the disorder and its treatment, and, for children undergoing surgery, provide preoperative and postoperative teaching and care. Answer any questions the child and family may have and explain all laboratory and diagnostic tests. Explain to parents that the child's cushingoid appearance is reversible with treatment. Provide nutritional guidance or refer the child and parents to a nutritionist to promote maintenance of an appropriate weight.

Preoperative and postoperative teaching and care are similar to those for the child undergoing surgery (see Chapter 34). Refer to Chapter 45 for general nursing care of the child with cancer.

For children who need cortisol replacement therapy because both adrenal glands were surgically removed, administering the drug early in the morning or every other day causes fewer symptoms than daily administration and mim-

ics the normal diurnal pattern of cortisol secretion. Cortisol replacement in the postoperative period must be explained carefully to parents. Hydrocortisone (Cortef, Solu-Cortef, cortisone acetate) comes in liquid, tablet, or injectable form. Teach parents how and when to administer the injectable form, usually when the child is vomiting or has diarrhea, or cannot take the oral medication. The oral preparations of cortisone have a bitter taste and can cause gastric irritation. Giving the dose at mealtimes and using antacids between meals helps reduce these side effects.

Nursing Practice

Signs of acute adrenal insufficiency may include increased irritability, headache, confusion, restlessness, nausea and vomiting, diarrhea, abdominal pain, dehydration, fever, loss of appetite, and lethargy. If untreated, the child will go into shock. In newborns, the symptoms include failure to thrive, weakness, vomiting, and dehydration. Hyponatremia and hyperkalemia are key signs.

Teach parents to be alert to signs of acute adrenal insufficiency during the withdrawal of corticosteroid therapy, and to inform all health care providers of the child's condition and medication. The child should wear a medical alert bracelet at all times.

CONGENITAL ADRENAL HYPERPLASIA

Congenital adrenal hyperplasia, sometimes called adrenogenital syndrome, adrenocortical hyperplasia, or congenital adrenogenital hyperplasia, is an autosomal recessive disorder that causes a deficiency of one of the enzymes necessary for the synthesis of cortisol and aldosterone. **WEB**. The defective gene CYP21 is located on the short arm of chromosome 6. It occurs in 1 in 10,000 to 16,000 live births, and males and females are affected equally. The incidence is highest in Native Alaskans (American Academy of Pediatrics, 2000). Of the two classic forms of the disorder, 75% are salt-losing, caused by the blockage of aldosterone production, and 25% are non-salt-losing, or simple virilization.

Etiology and Pathophysiology

More than 80% of children with congenital adrenal hyperplasia have partial or complete 21-hydroxylase enzyme deficiency in which deficient aldosterone synthesis leads to excessive renal excretion of salt (salt losing). This form has an autosomal recessive inheritance pattern. About 10% of children have 11-hydroxylase deficiency. The remainder have deficiencies involving five other enzymes. In its most severe form the disorder can be life threatening. In all forms, increased secretion of ACTH occurs in response to diminished cortisol levels.

During fetal development the lack of cortisol triggers the pituitary to continue secretion of ACTH. This in turn stimulates overproduction of the adrenal androgens. Female virilization of the external genitalia begins in week 10 of gestation. If untreated, the overproduction of androgens results in accelerated height, early closure of the epiphyseal plates, and premature sexual development with both pubic and axillary hair.

Approximately 65% to 75% of children have a disturbance in mineralocorticoid regulation that can lead to acute adrenal insufficiency with any serious illness or injury (Therrell, Berenbaum, Manter-Kapanke, et al., 1998).

Clinical Manifestations

Congenital adrenal hyperplasia is the most common cause of **pseudohermaphroditism** (ambiguous genitalia) in newborn girls. Virilization begins in utero. The female infant is born with an enlarged clitoris and labial fusions (Figure 51–4 ◆). Severely virilized females may be mistaken for males with cryptorchidism, hypospadias, or micropenis. The male infant may look normal at birth or may have a slightly enlarged penis and hyperpigmented scrotum. The boy may have an adult-sized penis by

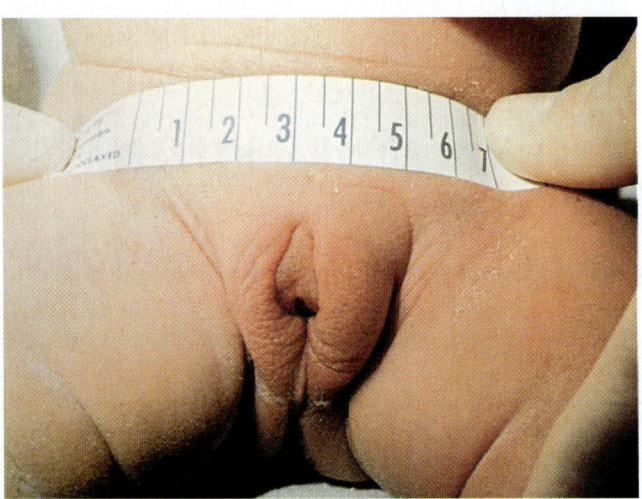

FIGURE 51–4. ◆ Newborn girl with ambiguous genitalia. Courtesy of Patrick C. Walsh, MD.

school age, but the testes are appropriately sized for age. Partial enzyme deficiency produces less obvious symptoms. Precocious puberty and tall stature for age may be noted later. Due to early epiphyseal fusion, adults have short stature.

Recurrent vomiting, dehydration, metabolic acidosis, hypotension, and hypoglycemia are characteristic signs of the salt-wasting form of the disorder. Hypertension with hypokalemic alkalosis is alternately found in children with 11-hydroxylase deficiency.

Clinical Therapy

Diagnosis in infants and children is usually confirmed by laboratory evaluation of serum 17-hydroxyprogesterone (17-OHP) level. Routine newborn screening for congenital adrenal hyperplasia is performed in 19 states (American Academy of Pediatrics, 2001). Prenatal screening is available. In instances of ambiguous genitalia, a **karyotype** (a microscopic chromosome study in which the 46 chromosomes of the child are lined up in pairs from largest to smallest to detect errors in chromosome number, shape, and size) determines the infant's gender. Ultrasonography may be used to visualize pelvic structures.

In the salt-wasting form of the disorder the child may have hyponatremia, hyperkalemia, a high urine sodium level, and low serum and urinary aldosterone levels. Serum concentrations of testosterone in girls and androstenedione in boys and girls are elevated in affected infants. Elevated ACTH with measurement of serum cortisol and 17-OHP levels are necessary to confirm the diagnosis (American Academy of Pediatrics, 2000). Diagnosis may be delayed in the non-salt-losing form until 3 to 7 years.

The goal of treatment is to suppress adrenal secretion of androgens by replacing deficient hormones. This is accomplished by the lifelong use of oral glucocorticoids (dexamethasone or hydrocortisone). The glucocorticoid replacement reduces secretion of ACTH which had overstimulated the adrenal cortex. As a result, excessive adrenal androgen production is suppressed. The dose is individualized by monitoring growth parameters, bone age, and hormone levels. If the infant has the salt-wasting form of the disorder, salt is added to the infant's formula and a mineralocorticoid (Florinef) is given to replace the missing hormone. Hormone dosage must be doubled or tripled during acute illnesses or injury and for surgery. Injectable hydrocortisone is used for severe stress. A combination of flutamide and testolactone along with a reduced dose of glucocorticoids have shown promise in efforts to reduce excess androgen production that control the accelerated growth and slow bone maturation (Merke & Culter, 1997)

Reconstructive surgery of the enlarged clitoris is often performed on girls during the first year of life. Vaginal reconstruction is performed later.

Nursing Management

Nursing Assessment and Diagnosis

Assess the infant and child for signs of dehydration, electrolyte imbalance, and shock in the salt-wasting form of the disease (see Skill 9–22). ⚭ **SKILLS** Monitor vital signs and assess peripheral perfusion (capillary refill, distal pulses, color and temperature of the extremities) frequently to detect early changes in condition.

Assess the parents' emotional response to a child with ambiguous genitalia and a chronic condition. Explore their values and beliefs regarding gender roles and sexuality while awaiting results of the karyotype.

Nursing diagnoses for the child with congenital adrenal hyperplasia might include:

▶ *Risk for altered parenting* related to a child with undetermined gender identity

▶ *Caregiver role strain* related to care of a child with a chronic, potentially life-threatening condition

▶ *Risk for fluid volume deficit* related to failure of regulatory mechanisms and excess excretion of salt by the kidneys

▶ *Risk for altered growth* related to premature development of secondary sex characteristics and accelerated growth

Planning and Implementation

Nursing care of the newborn with congenital adrenal hyperplasia focuses on teaching parents about the disorder and its treatment, providing emotional support, and preoperative and postoperative teaching for parents of infants undergoing reconstructive surgery. Because of the risk for adrenal insufficiency, the child will most likely be hospitalized for surgery rather than having outpatient surgery. The administration of glucocorticoids and mineralocorticoids must be carefully controlled.

It is often difficult for parents to accept that their infant, whose genitalia look male, is really female. With medication and surgery the genitalia assume a female appearance and all organs necessary for future childbearing are usually functional. Several surgeries may be performed before 2 years of age and then during adolescence to dilate the vagina.

Nurses can assist parents in educating the child's siblings, grandparents, other family members, and child care workers about the condition. In the newborn nursery the infant should be referred to as "your beautiful infant," not "your son" or "your daughter," until gender identity is confirmed.

Inform parents that genetic counseling should be provided for the child during adolescence. Parents considering a future pregnancy should also be informed that prenatal testing may detect congenital adrenal hyperplasia in the fetus. Refer the family for counseling if indicated.

NURSING CARE IN THE COMMUNITY

Teach parents about the special problems that develop in the salt-wasting form of the disease during acute illness. Explain the medication regimen and help the family develop an emergency care plan. The child should wear a medical alert bracelet. Teach parents how to administer intramuscular injections of hydrocortisone. Make sure the parents have an emergency kit of injectable hydrocortisone at home and at school to be used when the child is vomiting or has diarrhea. It should be carried wherever the child goes. If injectable hydrocortisone is not available, the child needs urgent treatment in an emergency department. The child may become dehydrated quickly and need intravenous fluid and electrolyte replacement in addition to higher doses of hydrocortisone.

Evaluation

Expected outcomes of nursing care for congenital adrenal hyperplasia include:

▶ Parents learn to give glucocorticoids appropriately when the child is ill and prevent episodes of adrenal crisis.

▶ Families effectively cope with the virilized appearance of the child's genitalia and bond with the child.

ADRENAL INSUFFICIENCY (ADDISON DISEASE)

Adrenal insufficiency, also known as Addison disease, is a rare disorder in childhood characterized by a deficiency of glucocorticoids (cortisone) and mineralocorticoids (aldosterone). It may be acquired after trauma; with tuberculosis, AIDS, or fungal infections that destroy the adrenal glands; or as the result of an autoimmune process.

Adrenal insufficiency usually develops slowly as the adrenal glands deteriorate. The early signs may not be noticed but include weakness with fatigue; anorexia and salt craving; poor weight gain or weight loss; hyperpigmentation at pressure points, lip borders and gingival margins, nipples, palms and soles, body creases, and scarred areas of the body; generalized bronzing of the skin or freckling without tan lines even in winter months; abdominal pain; nausea and vomiting; and diarrhea. Symptomatic hypoglycemia may also be present. If the child experiences a stressful period (illness, injury, or surgery), acute adrenal insufficiency may occur. Signs of an adrenal crisis include weakness, fever, abdominal pain, hypoglycemia with seizures, hypotension, dehydration, and shock.

Serum cortisol and urinary 17-hydroxycorticoid levels are measured in the early morning. Low levels are associated with adrenal insufficiency. The ACTH stimulation test is used to detect adrenal gland reserve. Electrolyte values generally reveal low serum sodium, elevated serum potassium, and low fasting blood glucose levels. CT may be used to visualize the adrenal glands.

Treatment involves replacement of the deficient hormones. Oral hydrocortisone is given in the lowest therapeutic dose to control symptoms and promote normal growth. Fludrocortisone acetate (Florinef) replaces the missing mineralocorticoid in children with aldosterone deficiency. Adrenal crisis is treated by fluid and electrolyte resuscitation, treatment of the precipitating illness or injury, adequate doses of glucocorticoid, and maintenance doses of mineralocorticoid.

Nursing Management

Nursing management focuses on educating the child and parents about the disorder, providing emotional support, and caring for the child during acute episodes. See the earlier discussion of congenital adrenal hyperplasia for further detail.

PHEOCHROMOCYTOMA

Pheochromocytoma is a tumor of the adrenal gland, but it may be extra-adrenal with no anatomic connection. In most cases these tumors are benign and curable. They can occur in a familial pattern (autosomal dominant trait) with a 3:2 male to female ratio. The incidence is 1 to 500,000 children, and most tumors are diagnosed in children between the ages of 6 and 14 years (Reddy, O'Neill, Holcomb, et al., 2000).

Clinical manifestations include labile hypertension with a systolic reading that may reach 250 mm Hg, tachycardia, arrhythmias, palpitations, profuse sweating with cool extremities, flushing, headache, abdominal pain, nausea and vomiting, weight loss, visual disturbances, weakness, polydipsia, and polyuria. The classic triad of signs includes new onset hypertension, new or worsening diabetes mellitus, and hypertensive crisis. Because release of catecholamines (norepinephrine and epinephrine) from the tumor is not continuous, these symptoms occur intermittently. Attacks may occur daily or monthly. In some cases the condition may be silent until a stressor such as surgery causes a hypertensive crisis.

Diagnosis is based on 24-hour urine studies to detect the presence of urinary catecholamines and vanilmandelic acid (VMA) levels, and CT, MRI, and ultrasound studies to locate the tumor (see Appendix B). ⚭ The treatment of choice is surgical removal of the tumor; however, the procedure is dangerous and may result in pheochromocytoma crisis, manifested by seizures, shock, altered level of consciousness, disseminated intravascular coagulation, rhabdomyolysis (skeletal muscle destruction), and acute renal failure. Alpha- and beta-adrenergic blocking agents to control hypertension and catecholamine release are given for 10 to 14 days before surgery. Plasma catecholamines are used to measure the effectiveness of the

preoperative adrenergic blockade. Postoperatively, for several days, a 24-hour urine collection is measured for catecholamines to determine if all tumor sites were removed. With successful removal of all tumor sites, the prognosis is generally good. Follow-up is important to assess for recurrence.

Nursing Management

Nursing care is mainly supportive. Provide preoperative and postoperative teaching and care (see Chapter 34). ⚭ Preoperatively, monitor vital signs and observe for signs of complications associated with pheochromocytoma crisis. Administer antihypertensives and watch for any signs of hyperglycemia (see page 1374). ⚭ Postoperatively, the child may be managed initially in an intensive care unit. Monitor blood pressure, and observe for neurologic signs, respiratory distress, and signs of shock. Lifelong follow-up care with screening for hypertension and increased urinary catecholamine levels is required as symptoms recur in up to 20% of patients 2 to 7 years after surgery (Reddy et al., 2000).

⚭ DISORDERS OF PANCREATIC FUNCTION

DIABETES MELLITUS

Diabetes mellitus, the most common metabolic disease in children, is a disorder of carbohydrate, protein, and fat metabolism. There are two main types of diabetes. Most children have immune-mediated type 1 diabetes, formerly called insulin-dependent diabetes mellitus or juvenile diabetes. However, a disturbingly large number of children are being diagnosed with type 2 diabetes, formerly called noninsulin-dependent diabetes.

About 1.5 million children and adolescents in the United States have diabetes, 70% to 85% with type 1 and up to 30% with type 2 (Selekman, Scofield, & Swenson-Brousell, 1999). The national prevalence for diabetes of all types in 12- to 19-year-olds is 4.1 per 1000 adolescents (American Diabetes Association, 2000).

Type 1 Diabetes

Most children with diabetes have immune-mediated type 1. The annual incidence of type 1 diabetes is 18 per 100,000 children under 20 years old. The peak age of onset is 10 to 12 years in girls and 12 to 14 years in boys (Boland & Grey, 2000).

ETIOLOGY AND PATHOPHYSIOLOGY

Type 1 diabetes is thought to be caused by a genetic component, environmental influences, and an autoimmune response. Type 1 diabetes has strong familial tendencies but does not show any specific pattern of inheritance. The long arm of chromosome 14 at the 14q24 locus is the type 1 diabetes-11 marker. This is a polygenic multifactorial pattern of inheritance since 18 different chromosomes show linkage to type 1 diabetes (Rennert & Francis, 1999). Inheritance of the DR3 and DR4 markers on the human leukocyte antigen (HLA) complex on chromosome 6 increases the likelihood of developing type 1 diabetes. If the child inherits one marker, the child's risk is 3 to 5 times higher. If both markers are inherited, the child's risk is 10 to 20 times higher (Selekman et al., 1999). Approximately 5% of children with type 1 diabetes have a first- or second-degree relative with the type 1 diabetes (American Diabetes Association, 2000). The child inherits a susceptibility to the disease rather than the disease itself.

Insulin helps transport glucose into the cells so that the body can use it as an energy source. It also prevents the outflow of glucose from the liver to the general circulation. Environmental factors such as enteroviruses or toxins are believed to lead to an autoimmune destruction of the beta cells in the Islets of Langerhans (Figure 51–5 ◆). Antigens are generated that lead to production of antibodies that indicate ongoing destruction of the islet cells. As the destruction continues, the child develops glucose intolerance. The preclinical stage may last up to 13 years as the autoimmune process begins early in life (Silverstein & Rosenbloom, 2000). Lack of insulin results in a rise in blood glucose level and a decrease in the glucose level inside the cells. When the renal threshold for glucose (160 mg/dL) is exceeded, **glycosuria** (abnormal amount of glucose in the urine) occurs. Up to 1000 calories per day can be lost in the urine.

When glucose is unavailable to the cells for metabolism, free fatty acids provide an alternate source of energy. The liver metabolizes them at an increased rate, producing acetyl coenzyme A (CoA). The by-products of acetyl CoA metabolism (ketone bodies) accumulate in the body, resulting in a state of metabolic acidosis, or ketoacidosis. (Refer to Chapter 39 ⊙ for discussion of metabolic acidosis.)

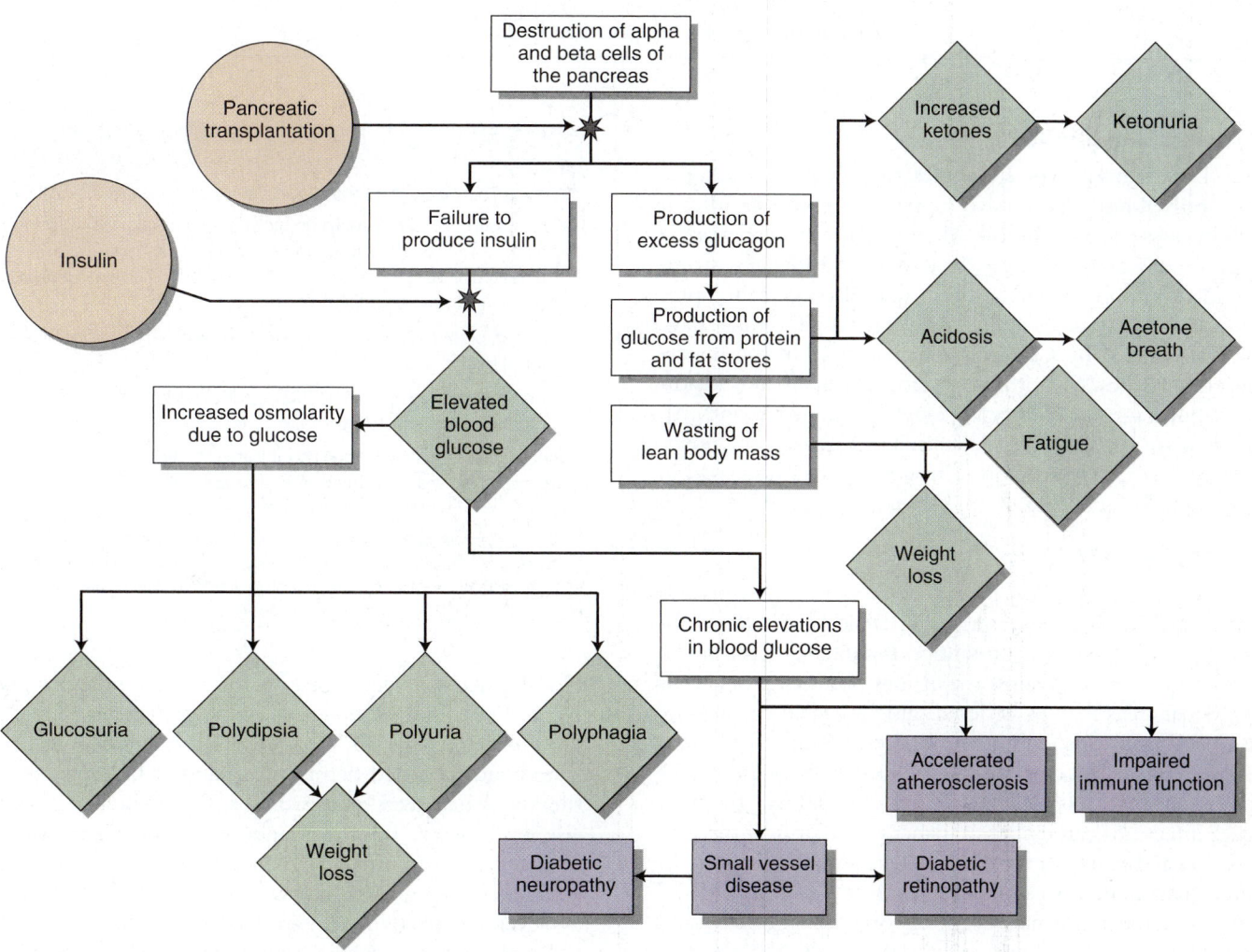

FIGURE 51–5. ◆ Pathophysiology of diabetes mellitus. *Note:* From Black, J. M., & Matassarian-Jocobs, E. (1997). *Medical-surgical nursing: Clinical management for continuity of care* (5th ed., p. 1958). Philadelphia: Saunders. Adapted.

CLINICAL MANIFESTATIONS ❧ *Diabetes by Type*

CAUSE	CLINICAL MANIFESTATIONS	CLINICAL THERAPY
Type 1—immune mediated, insulin deficiency due to pancreatic beta cell destruction	Polyuria, polydipsia Recent weight loss, but may be overweight Ketoacidosis on initial presentation in 30% to 40% of cases, at continued risk for ketoacidosis Short duration of symptoms Ketosis Initial period of decreased insulin requirement, then need insulin for survival	Blood glucose monitoring Insulin Dietary management, balancing carbohydrate intake to insulin Exercise
Type 2—insulin resistance with relative insulin secretory defect	Obese, little or no weight loss, or may have significant weight loss Acanthosis nigricans Long duration of symptoms Polyuria, polydipsia, may be mild or absent Glycosuria without ketonuria in 33% of cases on initial presentation Ketoacidosis on initial presentation in 5% to 25% of cases Lipid disorders Hypertension Androgen-mediated problems such as acne, hirsutism, menstrual disturbances, polycystic ovary disease Excessive weight gain and fatigue due to insulin resistance	Diet with decreased calories and low-fat foods Decrease sedentary activity time or increase routine physical activity Blood glucose monitoring Oral medication (metformin) to improve insulin sensitivity

CLINICAL MANIFESTATIONS

The classic signs of type 1 diabetes are polyuria, polydipsia, and **polyphagia** (excessive appetite) with significant weight loss. See "Clinical Manifestations: Diabetes by Type." Unexplained fatigue or lethargy, headaches, stomachaches, and occasional enuresis may also occur in a previously toilet-trained child. Adolescent girls may have vaginitis caused by *Candida*, which thrives in the hyperglycemic tissues. Symptoms develop gradually and insidiously but have usually been present less than a month. In severe cases diabetic ketoacidosis (DKA), a type of metabolic acidosis, may develop. This condition is discussed in more detail on p. 1373. ⊂⊃

CLINICAL THERAPY

Diagnosis is based on the presence of classic symptoms and plasma glucose levels as described in Table 51–3. Other laboratory tests for known autoantibodies that can indicate an autoimmune attack against the insulin-producing beta cells of the pancreas may be ordered: glutamic acid decarboxylase (GAD-65), insulin autoantibodies, and islet cell cytoplasmic autoantibodies. A careful history is necessary to rule out a stress-related illness, corticosteroid use, fracture, acute infection, cystic fibrosis, pancreatitis, or liver disease.

Clinical therapy for type 1 diabetes combines insulin, dietary management to support growth and maintain blood glucose at near normal levels, an exercise regimen, and physiologic support. The goal of initial insulin therapy is to lower blood glucose levels and eliminate ketones. Blood glucose levels are then further lowered until stabilized. Long-term insulin therapy is calculated to maintain a

TABLE 51–3 Criteria for the Diagnosis of All Types of Diabetes Mellitus

- Symptoms of diabetes (polyuria, polydipsia, unexplained weight loss for type 1, or acanthosis nigricans and obesity for type 2) *plus* plasma glucose concentration ≥ 200 mg/dL (11.1 mmol/L) taken at any time of day regardless of time of last meal.
- Fasting plasma glucose ≥126 mg/dL (7 mmol/L), no caloric intake for at least 8 hours.
- Two-hour plasma glucose ≥ 200 mg/dL (11.1 mmol/L) during an oral glucose tolerance test.

Repeat the testing on a second day if there is no unequivocal hyperglycemia with acute metabolic decompensation.

Note: Reprinted with permission from the Expert Committee on the Diagnosis and Classification of Diabetes Mellitus. (1999). Report of the expert committee on the diagnosis and classification of diabetes mellitus. *Diabetes Care, 22* (Suppl. 1), S5–S19. © 1999 American Diabetes Association.

blood glucose level as close to the normal range as possible and to minimize episodes of hyperglycemia and hypoglycemia (see page 1374). ⊂⊃ Blood glucose levels are tested and recorded before meals and at bedtime. Insulin therapy is balanced by the child's dietary intake and exercise level. Stress, infection, and illness may either increase or decrease insulin needs. In addition, insulin doses must be adjusted for growth and at puberty.

Several forms of insulin are available (Table 51–4). Multiple approaches to insulin therapy for children and adolescents are available, and an approach that works for the child and family should be selected. In children, conventional insulin therapy is commonly used, requiring 2 to 3

TABLE 51-4 Insulin Action (Subcutaneous Route)

Type	Onset	Peak	Duration
Rapid Acting			
Lispro/Humalog	5–15 min	1 hr	~4 hr
Short Acting			
Regular	1/2–1 hr	2–4 hr	6–8 hr
Intermediate Acting			
NPH	1–2 hr	6–12 hr	18–26 hr
Lente	1–2 hr	6–12 hr	24–26 hr
Long Acting			
Ultralente	4–8 hr	10–20 hr	16–24 hr
Lantus/insulin glargine		none/slight	24 hr

injections a day. One example of conventional insulin therapy consists of daily administration of a combination of a short-acting (regular) insulin and an intermediate-acting (NPH or Lente) or long-acting insulin (Ultralente) before breakfast and before the evening meal (Figure 51–6 ◆). Older children and adolescents often use a regimen of tighter control that includes two injections a day of intermediate or long-acting insulin and an injection of rapid-acting insulin with each meal to match carbohydrate intake. Rapid-acting insulin (Lispro) therapy may also be used to achieve tight glucose control for the following reasons: a decreased number of nocturnal hypoglycemic episodes, meal coverage for toddlers who have unpredictable food consumption, and flexibility for adolescents concerned about weight gain who do not want to eat a mid-morning snack.

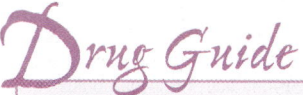

Drug Guide

INSULIN

Overview of Action

Insulin is an endogenous hormone, secreted by the beta cells of the pancreas, that facilitates the transport of glucose to body tissues. Other physiologic functions of insulin include (1) stimulation of glycogen synthesis by the liver; (2) inhibition of lipolysis, the breakdown of triglycerides to fatty acids and glycerol; and (3) stimulation of protein synthesis by facilitating storage of ingested amino acids. It is used as a replacement for physiologic production of endogenous insulin in type 1 diabetes and as an IV diagnostic tool to evaluate pituitary growth hormone. Insulin human injection is derived by enzyme modification of pork pancreas or from microbial synthesis.

Routes, Dosage, Frequency

Insulin is usually provided in a concentration of 100 units/mL. Diluted insulin prepared by a pharmacist may be used for infants and toddlers who require a small insulin dosage. Doses are individualized. Factors such as stress, activity, dietary intake, and status of health cause variations in the insulin dose. The following recommendations can be used for initiating therapy:

SC, IM, IV (Regular = Fast acting): Diabetic ketoacidosis (DKA): IV: 0.1 U/kg bolus, then 0.1 U/kg/hour or SC: 0.25 to 2 U/kg/dose; may repeat every 4 to 6 hours depending on glucose levels, degree of acidosis, and patient's clinical condition.

SC (Lente or NPH = intermediate-acting): Maintenance: 0.5 U/kg in early A.M.; additional regular insulin 0.25 U/kg in the afternoon, depending on urine results. Dose of the long-acting insulin should be increased in the morning if additional doses of regular insulin were needed in previous 24 hours or reduced if urine glucose is negative for two consecutive mornings. Adolescents

in growth spurts may require 1 to 1.5 U/kg/day. Newly diagnosed children with DKA should receive half-doses because they may be very sensitive to insulin. Adjust dosage in renal dysfunction.

Side Effects: Skin reactions such as hives, wheal, induration, or hypertrophy; hypoglycemia; allergic reaction.

Nursing Implications

Assessment: Assess for symptoms of hypergylcemia or hypoglycemia, including urine and blood glucose levels. History of events leading to onset of symptoms, time, and amount of last insulin dosage, illness, exercise, stress, or dietary intake. Assess child's level of growth and development, attitude, and understanding of disease and treatment, and family dynamics and interactions. If newly diagnosed, assess diabetic family and child's level of acceptance, willingness to learn, and ability to grasp large amount of information.

Administer: Use only insulin ordered and carefully read label to prevent giving incorrect insulin. Do not switch brands, strengths, type, species, or purity because it may affect dosage adjustment. First dose of insulin is given early A.M. about 30 minutes before breakfast. Rotate sites using SC tissue of upper arms, thighs, upper buttocks, and stomach.

Monitor: Monitor for symptoms of hypoglycemia, hypergylcemia, and Somogyi reactions, as well as for presence of glycosuria. Identify peak action times for insulin used, as that is when hypoglycemia is most likely to occur. Be aware that hypoglycemic attacks associated with Ultralente insulin are most likely to occur during the night or early morning. Plan for snacks and meal times accordingly. Observe child for clammy skin and restlessness. Give child sucrose or glucose PO and check blood level immediately. Monitor blood glucose levels several times daily.

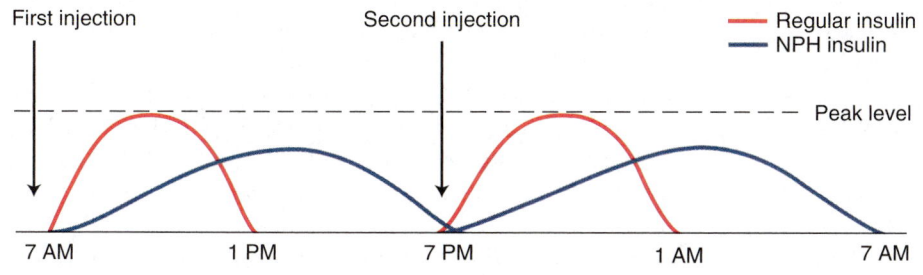

FIGURE 51–6. ◆ Conventional therapy. Insulin levels vary over a 24-hour period in relation to injections and mealtimes.

Thinking Critically

MANAGING ADOLESCENT DIABETES

Anthony, 12 years old, has just been diagnosed with diabetes mellitus. His parents took him to their family physician after Anthony complained of being constantly thirsty and hungry for over a week. Despite this he lost 5 pounds. They note that he had a viral illness about 1 month ago but seemed to recover from it. His mother says that Anthony seemed lethargic for several days.

Anthony and his family must now learn to manage his diabetes using a combination of diet, exercise, and insulin therapy. Monitoring his blood glucose level is important in determining how much insulin he will need every day. Anthony and his mother will need to learn to schedule his meals and snacks, and to have appropriate amounts of protein, fat, and carbohydrates at each meal, and to count carbohydrates. Anthony's meals and activity will need to be coordinated with the insulin doses. Anthony and his parents will need to watch closely for signs of hypoglycemia.

➡ *What causes diabetes?*

➡ *What potential problems need prompt treatment?*

➡ *What does Anthony need to monitor for when he gets sick?*

➡ *Intensive therapy will be a goal of Anthony's treatment—how can you help Anthony and his family decide if this should be accomplished with insulin injections or an insulin pump?*

➡ *What are some strategies to help an adolescent actively participate in his disease management and maintain optimal control?* 🔗 **WEB**

TABLE 51–5 Advantages and Disadvantages of an External Insulin Infusion Pump

Advantages	Disadvantages
• Delivers a continuous infusion of insulin to match the basal rate needed plus an insulin bolus at mealtime	• Requires highly motivated child and supportive parents and health care professionals
• Helps maintain blood glucose control between meals	• Requires willingness to live connected to a device (can be disconnected for short periods by removing or clamping the catheter; however, DKA can occur within hours of interruption of insulin flow)
• Improves growth in children	
• Reduces number of injections	
• Allows child to eat with less regard to a schedule	• The site must be changed every 2–4 days, at least 1 inch from the last site
• Reduces number of injection sites, so variation in absorption decreases	• Necessitates more time and energy to monitor blood glucose levels, dietary intake, and insulin bolus calculation
• More closely simulates normal pancreatic function	• Involves changing syringe, catheter, and skin setup every 2–3 days
• Frequency of severe hypoglycemia has been decreased	• Infections can occur at the injection site
• More flexible lifestyle is permitted	• Weight gain is common when blood glucose control improves

Note: From Saudek, C. D. (1997). Novel forms of insulin delivery. *Endocrinology and Metabolism Clinics of North America, 26*(3), 599–610; and Maniatis, A. K., Klingensmith, G. J., Slover, R. H., Mowry, C. J., & Chase, H. P. (2001). Continuous subcutaneous insulin infusion therapy for children and adolescents: An option for routine diabetes care. *Pediatrics, 107*(2), 351–356. Adapted.

The American Diabetes Association recommends that all adolescents use the intensive therapy regimen with 3 or more insulin injections a day or a continuous subcutaneous insulin infusion (CSII) by an insulin pump. Research revealed that the risk for developing retinopathy, microalbuminuria, albuminuria, and clinical neuropathy was significantly lower with this treatment regimen over more conventional regimens. Advantages and disadvantages of an insulin pump are outlined in Table 51–5. Adolescents taking frequent insulin injections during the day may also use an easy-to-carry, pen-shaped device that contains an insulin-filled cartridge.

Intensive therapy for type 1 diabetes includes:

- Monitoring blood glucose four times a day and once a week at 3 A.M.
- Monitoring dietary intake
- Varying the insulin dose to fit the carbohydrates eaten at each meal or snack if doing carbohydrate counting
- Anticipating exercise in the routine

Laboratory evaluation of hemoglobin A_{1c} (HbA_{1c}) to measure glycosylated hemoglobin should be performed every 3 months. It provides an objective measurement of glycemic control because it represents the amount of glucose irreversibly attached to the hemoglobin molecule over an extended period (the life span of the red blood cell, approximately 120 days). The HbA_{1c} is below 6.2% for individuals without diabetes, and the goal for children with diabetes is 7.5% to 9.3% depending upon age and physician preferences. It is also important to determine if the HbA_{1c} matches recorded blood sugars.

Physical activity is associated with increased insulin sensitivity. Regular exercise and fitness improve metabolic control with a lower insulin dose. Blood lipid levels are also positively affected. However, the child must have an adequate caloric intake to prevent hypoglycemia. Excessive exercise associated with sports requires careful planning and management.

Many new developments for diabetes management are being evaluated. An implantable insulin infusion pump with a glucose-sensing device that can work for years without being accessed is now being used experimentally. FDA approval has not yet been sought (Saudek, 1997). Studies of the effectiveness of inhaled insulin for administration before meals also are being conducted. The goal is to find alternative methods of intensive insulin control without increasing injections. Noninvasive or continuous glucose monitoring techniques are being investigated and have been approved by the FDA for adults (Silverstein & Rosenbloom, 2000).

Complications of type 1 diabetes (retinopathy, heart disease, renal failure, and peripheral vascular disease) result from long-term hyperglycemic effects on the blood vessels. Without careful management, diabetic children may develop renal failure and loss of vision in adulthood. Intensive therapy is expected to reduce the risk for or delay the development of these complications. Risk may be further reduced if the adolescent does not begin smoking and if the blood pressure is controlled.

Nursing Management

Nursing Assessment and Diagnosis

PHYSIOLOGIC ASSESSMENT

Children are generally admitted to the hospital at the time of diagnosis. Assess the child's physiologic status, focusing on vital signs and level of consciousness. Assess hydration by checking mucous membranes, skin turgor, and urine output. Blood initially is collected hourly to monitor blood gases, glucose, and electrolytes. Once the child is stable, assess dietary and caloric intake and the ability of the child or family to manage care.

PSYCHOSOCIAL ASSESSMENT

Parents may feel guilty at the time of diagnosis if they waited to seek care until the child began to experience symptoms of DKA. Assess coping mechanisms, ability to manage the disease, and educational needs of both the child and parents. Examples of questions to use in assessing the family's strengths and limitations in the child's disease management include:

▶ Do both parents or the single parent work? What hours?

▶ Who else is involved in the child's care?

▶ What is the child's usual daily schedule? Does the schedule vary on the weekend or any other days of the week?

▶ Does the child have health insurance? What coverage exists for diabetes education, treatment, and home management?

▶ Does the child have any cognitive, behavioral, motor, or visual problems coexisting with this condition?

▶ What other family stressors coexist with the diagnosis?

DEVELOPMENTAL ASSESSMENT

Assess the child's developmental level, particularly fine motor skills and cognitive level. The child will need to learn how to obtain and read a blood glucose sample and how to draw up and administer insulin (see Skill 10–3). **SKILLS** Children can usually perform some of these tasks with supervision by 6 to 8 years of age. Self-management is the eventual goal, and the child's responsibilities are gradually increased.

Adolescents perceive type 1 diabetes as a disability and often deny having the disease so they can be like their peers when eating and exercising. Talk with the adolescent to evaluate motivation to manage diet, the exercise regimen, blood glucose testing, and insulin therapy. Although the adolescent is cognitively able to manage self-care, the desire to be like peers often interferes with compliance.

Several diagnoses that may apply to the child newly diagnosed with type 1 diabetes are provided in the accompanying "Nursing Care Plans." Additional diagnoses that may be appropriate include the following:

▶ *Risk for fluid volume deficit* related to active fluid loss associated with hyperglycemia

▶ *Ineffective breathing pattern* related to neuromuscular dysfunction associated with metabolic acidosis

▶ *Ineffective denial* related to inability to admit impact of disease on lifestyle

Planning and Implementation

Nursing care focuses on teaching the child and parents about the disease and its management, managing dietary intake, providing emotional support, and planning strategies for daily management in the community. Refer to the accompanying "Nursing Care Plans," which summarize nursing care for the child who is hospitalized with newly diagnosed type 1 diabetes, and the child who is receiving care in the community. Some hospitals have developed clinical pathways to streamline and standardize diabetes care.

PROVIDE EDUCATION

The nurse is an important member of the management team (physician, nurse, nutritionist, and social worker) and is usually responsible for educating the child and family. A diabetic nurse educator in the clinic setting often does this teaching, since children may be hospitalized only briefly following diagnosis.

The timing and amount of information provided are especially important in the first days following diagnosis. Both the child and parents are very tired, and they are often in a state of shock and disbelief. Information presented during this period needs to be repeated. Use this time to assess learning needs and to answer the family's questions. Initial teaching focuses on the survival skills necessary for home management (insulin administration, blood glucose testing, record keeping, dietary management, and the recognition and treatment of both hypoglycemia and hyperglycemia).

Explain the goals of insulin therapy. Teach the child and parents how to administer insulin and perform blood glucose tests (Figure 51–7 ◆). Rotating the injection sites is

GOAL	INTERVENTION	RATIONALE	EXPECTED OUTCOME
1. Health-seeking behaviors (child and parents) related to lack of exposure to diabetic management in the newly diagnosed child			
	NIC Priority Intervention:		*NOC Suggested Outcome:*
	Individual teaching: *Planning, implementation, and evaluating a teaching program designed to address a patient's particular need*		**Knowledge:** *Extent of understanding conveyed about treatment regimen*
The child and parents will acquire survival skills for home management.	▶ Assess the child's developmental level and select an educational approach and self-care activities to match. ▶ Teach blood glucose monitoring, drawing up and injecting insulin, urine testing for ketones, record keeping, survival food guidelines, and when to call the doctor. ▶ Use demonstration/return demonstration until the child and family are comfortable with procedures.	▶ Learning goals for the child must match knowledge and skill expectations appropriate for developmental stage. ▶ Diabetic management survival skills are needed for initial home management until more extensive education can be completed that permits more independent management. ▶ Evaluation permits positive reinforcement and guidance for modification of techniques.	The child and parents demonstrate proper technique for blood glucose monitoring, urine testing for ketones, drawing up insulin doses and injection, and record keeping.
The child and parents will recognize signs and symptoms of hypoglycemia and hyperglycemia.	▶ Teach signs and symptoms of hypoglycemic and hyperglycemic reactions. ▶ Teach child to test blood glucose when feeling different than usual, and record the reading and symptoms felt.	▶ Recognition of and treatment of poor glucose control will prevent progression of symptoms. ▶ Permits child to learn his/her specific symptoms of hyper- and hypoglycemia.	The child and family can describe symptoms of hypoglycemia and hyperglycemia.
2. Risk for injury related to periods of hypoglycemia and diabetic ketoacidosis			
	NIC Priority Intervention:		*NOC Suggested Outcome:*
	Hypoglycemia monitoring: *Instituting special precautions with patient at risk for injury*		**Risk control:** *Actions to eliminate or reduce actual, personal, and modifiable health threats*
The child will experience few episodes of hypoglycemia during hospitalization.	▶ Assess the child at least every 2 hours for signs of hypoglycemia. If signs are present, check blood glucose to verify and administer source of quick sugar. ▶ When the child is NPO for a special procedure, verify with physician when food, fluids, and insulin are to be given, or if an intravenous infusion with dextrose is to be given. ▶ Have glucose paste or 50% dextrose solution readily available.	▶ Hypoglycemia commonly occurs during hospitalization because of change in diet, lack of food intake, or illness. ▶ Giving insulin without food intake can lead to hypoglycemia. Intravenous dextrose and insulin can be used when the child must be NPO. ▶ Dextrose is used for emergency intravenous treatment of severe hypoglycemia. Glucose paste is used for oral treatment.	The child and staff manage episodes of hypoglycemia without a crisis developing.
The child's condition is treated slowly to gradually reverse hyperglycemia and ketoacidosis and to prevent cerebral edema.	▶ Assess the child's mental status for improvement or deterioration. ▶ Check blood glucose and urine ketones frequently to confirm reduction in blood glucose level and ketosis, to identify the insulin dose for administration. ▶ Monitor and control IV fluid intake. Measure output. ▶ Have insulin doses checked by a second nurse.	▶ Improvement in mental status may indicate successful treatment. Deterioration may indicate onset of cerebral edema. ▶ Frequent blood glucose and ketone level determination helps assess progress in treating ketoacidosis. ▶ The child with ketoacidosis will be dehydrated. IV fluid intake needs to be carefully controlled to prevent cerebral edema. ▶ Doses are frequently small, and the possibility of error is great.	The child's hyperglycemia and ketoacidosis resolves without additional complications.
The child and parents will demonstrate emergency management of hypoglycemia.	▶ Identify sources of glucose to give in case of hypoglycemic reaction. Tell the child and parent to carry glucose tablets or paste with them at all times.	▶ Access to sources of glucose and its rapid administration are important for emergency care.	The child and family can identify several glucose sources for emergencies. The child and family have a source of glucose with them at each visit.

GOAL	INTERVENTION	RATIONALE	EXPECTED OUTCOME
2. Risk for injury related to periods of hypoglycemia and diabetic ketoacidosis—continued			
The child and parents will demonstrate management of sick days.	▶ Teach the child and family to test blood glucose and urine for ketones with acute symptoms and notify the physician.	▶ When the child is ill, hyperglycemia needs special management to prevent progression to ketoacidosis.	The child's hyperglycemic episodes do not progress to ketoacidosis.
3. Risk for altered nutrition: less than body requirements related to glycosuria			
	NIC Priority Intervention:		*NOC Suggested Outcome:*
	Nutrition management: *Assistance with or provision of a balanced dietary intake of foods and fluids*		**Nutritional status:** *Extent to which nutrients are available to meet metabolic needs*
The child will eat a well-balanced diet and maintain normal height and weight proportions.	▶ Encourage and serve meals and snacks with consistent carbohydrates at the same time each day.	▶ Keeps blood glucose levels stable during initial disease management stages.	The child regains weight lost and demonstrates normal growth and stable blood glucose levels.
	▶ Provide a calorie nonrestricted diet.	▶ Enables weight lost during onset of diabetes to be regained.	
The child and parents will state understanding of dietary management of diabetes mellitus.	▶ Make an appointment with a nutritionist who can assess the child's favorite foods and promote their integration into the child's diet. Reinforce the dietary information taught.	▶ The nutritionist can develop dietary recommendations that fit the specific needs of the child and include favorite foods, thereby increasing compliance with the diet.	The child and parents describe nutritional needs of the child and select the dietary management best suited to the family's and child's eating habits.
	▶ Provide sample menus and food exchanges, or teach the use of carbohydrate counting.	▶ Assists the family and adolescent with diet planning.	

GOAL	INTERVENTION	RATIONALE	EXPECTED OUTCOME
1. Risk for altered nutrition: less than body requirements related to chronic illness (diabetes mellitus)			
	NIC Priority Intervention:		*NOC Suggested Outcome:*
	Weight management: *Assistance with or provision of a balanced dietary intake of foods and fluids*		**Nutritional status: Nutrient value:** *Adequacy of nutrients taken into body*
The child will eat a well-balanced diet that maintains weight proportional to height.	▶ Assess height and weight regularly and plot on growth chart.	▶ Assesses change in body mass index to identify potential weight problem early.	Diet records indicate meals and snacks have the appropriate distribution of carbohydrates, protein, and fats, and daily caloric intake goals are met.
	▶ Make an appointment with a nutritionist who can assess the child's favorite foods and integrate them into a diet plan that controls caloric intake. Encourage the child to keep a food diary.	▶ Inclusion of child's favorite foods helps child adapt to changes in diet.	
2. Altered family processes related to management of a chronic disease			
	NIC Priority Intervention:		*NOC Suggested Outcome:* To be developed
	Family process maintenance: *Minimization of family process disruption effects*		
The child and family will manage the dietary modifications, exercise, blood glucose monitoring, and medications regimen.	▶ Assess the family's lifestyle and attempt to fit the child's care needs into the family's schedule.	▶ Fitting the care to the family's lifestyle promotes compliance with regimen.	The child and family make minimal changes in usual lifestyle while managing the type 1 diabetes.
	▶ Discuss the family's routines for special occasions and vacations. Identify ways to modify the child's management for these occasions.	▶ It is important for the child to participate in special events with the family and peers as a normal child to promote psychologic development.	

(continued)

GOAL	INTERVENTION	RATIONALE	EXPECTED OUTCOME

3. Ineffective coping (individual) related to inadequate level of confidence in ability to cope

	NIC Priority Intervention:		*NOC Suggested Outcome:*
	Coping enhancement: *Assisting a patient to adapt to perceived stressors, changes, or threats which interfere with meeting life demands and roles*		**Coping:** *Actions to manage stressors that tax an individual's resources*
The child will demonstrate enhanced coping skills.	▶ Ask how the child has solved problems in the past. Review possible problems the child may encounter. Together evaluate the effectiveness of solutions. Suggest other solutions to consider.	▶ Children's success in mastering maturational conflicts and daily psychosocial problems will influence their pattern of coping.	The child demonstrates enhanced coping skills and expresses positive attitude toward self. The child displays warmth and affection toward family.
The child will develop positive self-esteem.	▶ Role-play ways to talk about diabetes with friends and teachers. Encourage the child to express feelings about diabetes to those he or she trusts. ▶ Encourage the child to attend diabetes camp. ▶ Encourage the child to continue previous social activities and hobbies.	▶ Sharing information about the condition helps others understand changes in lifestyle needed by the child. Expressing feelings decreases anxiety. ▶ Learning and support networks developed at camp can promote self-esteem. ▶ Increased social interaction, especially in group sessions, improves self-esteem.	

4. Health-seeking behaviors (child) related to learning self-management of chronic disorder

	NIC Priority Intervention:		*NOC Suggested Outcome:*
	Self-modification assistance: *Reinforcement of self-directed change initiated by the patient to achieve personally important goals*		**Health promotion:** *Actions to sustain or increase wellness*
The child will develop independent ability to manage diabetes care.	▶ Allow the child to perform as many self-care procedures as possible at each developmental stage. ▶ Encourage the child to make decisions regarding care. Review decisions and discuss possible alternative solutions. Role-play possible scenarios. ▶ Encourage parents to stay involved even when the adolescent takes primary responsibility for care. ▶ Provide 24-hour access to physician or diabetes nurse educator. Encourage the child to seek help early.	▶ Normal growth and development are ensured if the child is encouraged to participate in care from the beginning. ▶ Feelings of trust are developed when children sense that their decisions are respected or at least considered by others. ▶ The child's diabetic control is likely to be better when the parents continue to show interest and supervise care. ▶ The child needs to overcome concerns about calling for guidance, and thus maintain better control.	The child is able to perform as many diabetic care techniques as possible for age.

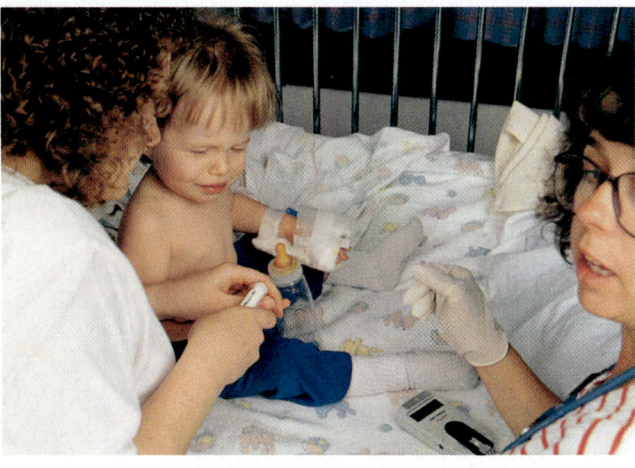
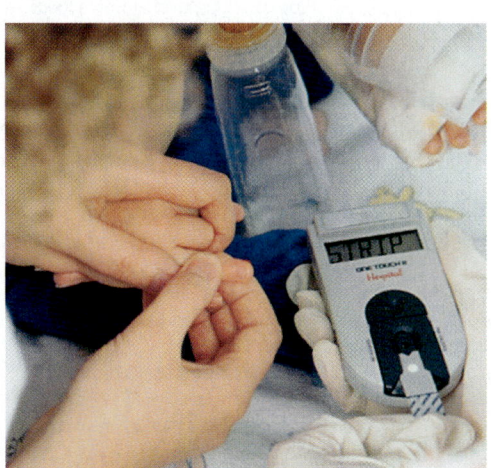

FIGURE 51–7. ◆ This mother is being taught how to test her child's blood glucose level.

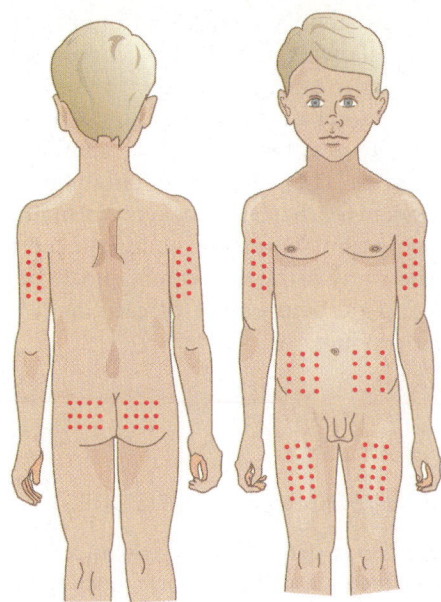

FIGURE 51–8. ◆ Insulin injection sites. Give all morning insulin in one site (e.g., arms) and all evening insulin in another (e.g., legs) because of different rates of absorption from these sites. Space injections about 1/2 inch (1.25 cm) apart.

important to decrease the chances of hypertrophy (Figure 51–8 ◆). The absorption rate of insulin varies by the site used. Encourage the child to give the morning injections in one body area (e.g., an arm) and the evening injections in another (e.g., the thigh). An understanding of the different types of insulin and their actions is essential.

Once the child and parents demonstrate understanding of this information, teach guidelines for managing episodes of hyperglycemia during acute illness and using a sliding scale. A sliding scale indicates specific insulin dosages appropriate for a particular blood glucose level. The family also needs to learn "sick day" care guidelines to prevent diabetic ketoacidosis.

Caution parents to check the blood glucose level of a toddler who is extremely sleepy or irritable, as these can be signs of either hypoglycemia or hyperglycemia.

MANAGE DIETARY INTAKE

The preferred diet for children with type 1 diabetes is a low-saturated-fat, low-sodium diet. The total amount of carbohydrates consumed is more important than whether they are simple or complex. A variety of carbohydrates should be eaten. The child needs adequate calories to reach or maintain a desirable body weight. Usually at the time of diagnosis the child needs to regain lost weight, so calorie limitation is not recommended.

For conventional treatment, dietary intake should include three meals per day, eaten at consistent intervals, plus a midafternoon carbohydrate snack and a bedtime snack high in protein. Some children need a morning snack depending upon the time of the morning insulin dose, how much breakfast is eaten, and the scheduled lunchtime. Although the child with diabetes is not restricted from eating any food, certain foods need to be balanced by extra insulin. A nutritionist can help the family integrate preferred ethnic foods into the child's diet. The recommended distribution of total calories by food group for children with type 1 diabetes is 50% to 55% carbohydrates, 20% to 25% protein, and 25% to 30% fat (Kaufman & Halvorson, 1999). A consistent intake of carbohydrates at each meal and snack is needed. The American Diabetes Association's exchange lists facilitate dietary management by suggesting portions and types of foods and noting allowed substitutions.

Many adolescents find that carbohydrate counting for dietary management gives them more flexibility in disease management. One carbohydrate choice equals 15 grams of carbohydrate. They then determine the number of units of insulin needed to cover the grams of carbohydrates eaten.

PROVIDE EMOTIONAL SUPPORT

The diagnosis of type 1 diabetes often comes as a shock to the family. If there is a familial history, parents may feel guilty about having caused the disease. The diagnosis of a chronic disease that requires daily management can be difficult to accept. Give parents information about diabetes education programs, put them in touch with other parents of diabetic children, and help them to learn the role they can play in managing the disease.

Support for the child depends on age and developmental stage. Encourage the child to express feelings about the disease and its management. The adolescent may benefit from contact with other adolescents who have diabetes.

DISCHARGE PLANNING AND HOME CARE TEACHING

Home care needs should be identified and addressed before discharge. Initial survival skills described earlier are taught with the plans for ongoing outpatient education.

Make every effort to incorporate the diabetic regimen (insulin administration, diet, blood glucose monitoring, and exercise) into the family's present lifestyle. The fewer changes the family has to make, the greater the chance of compliance.

Testing strips for blood glucose meters cost between $0.50 and $1.00 each. Learn about the allowable expenses covered by the child's health insurance. Try to work within those guidelines to reduce the family's out-of-pocket expenses.

Provide written materials and refer parents to books and other materials they can use in teaching the child about diabetes. The Juvenile Diabetic Research Foundation and the American Diabetes Association are good sources of information. ⌐⌐ WEB

NURSING CARE IN THE COMMUNITY

During follow-up visits, ask the child or parents about signs indicating problems of diabetic control. Questions to ask that could help identify problems in diabetic control include:

▶ Is the child hungry at meals? Between meals?

▶ How much fluid is the child drinking?

▶ Has the child been going to the bathroom frequently or had episodes of bed-wetting?

▶ Does the child have dry skin?

▶ Are there sores on the feet? Do scratches or scrapes take a long time to heal?

▶ Has the child had any skin infections?

▶ Doess the child have changes in mood (depression, unexplained sadness, irritability) or energy level from day to day or throughout the day?

▶ Have there been any changes in vision?

Record growth measurements and vital signs in the child's chart. Review the child's typical dietary intake and exercise regimens. Assess the child's sexual development using Tanner staging guidelines (see Chapter 33). Puberty may be delayed if diabetic control is inadequate.

Education is ongoing, especially for children who develop diabetes at a young age. As they grow and assume more responsibility for their care, remember that they need to learn more about the pathophysiology of the disease and the rationale for its management.

Continually work with the child to help him or her assume responsibility for self-care, and with parents to promote the child's self-care (Figure 51–9 ◆). The child's developmental stage and cognitive level influence his or her readiness to take on responsibility for self-care. Summer camps and other programs for diabetic children are often helpful in providing education and support.

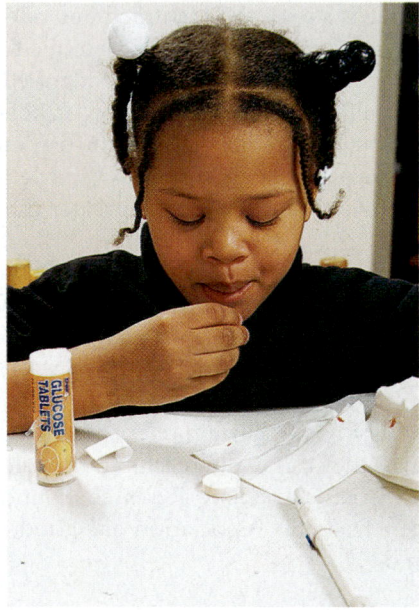

FIGURE 51–9. ◆ This girl is old enough to understand the need to take glucose tablets or another form of a rapidly absorbed sugar when her blood glucose level is low.

The preschool child's need for autonomy and control can be met by allowing the child to choose snacks or to pick which finger to stick for glucose testing and by helping parents to gather necessary supplies. School-age children can learn to test blood glucose, administer insulin, and keep records. They should be taught how to select foods appropriate for dietary management and how to plan an exercise program. School-age children need to learn to recognize the signs of hypoglycemia and hyperglycemia, and understand the importance of carrying a rapidly absorbed sugar product.

Teaching About

TREATING HYPOGLYCEMIC EPISODES

- If the child shows signs of hypoglycemia (pallor, sweating, tremors, dizziness, numb lips or mouth, confusion, irritability, altered mental status), test the blood glucose level.

- Assist the child to do the test as skills needed to get an accurate reading deteriorate with altered mental status.

- If the blood glucose reading is ≤ 70 mg/dL, give glucose rapidly. Use one of the following:
  - 1/2 cup orange juice
  - 3/4 cup of sugar-sweetened beverage
  - 1 small box raisins
  - 3 to 4 glucose tablets

- Wait 15 minutes and recheck the blood glucose level. Repeat the glucose if it is still ≤ 70/mg/dL. Recheck the blood glucose level in another 15 minutes.

- Once blood sugar has returned to at least 80 mg/dL, give a more substantial snack such as cheese and crackers if the next meal will be more than 30 minutes later or an activity or exercise is planned.

- If the child is unconscious, administer IM or SQ glucagon.

Adolescents should take on total responsibility for self-care; however, they benefit from the ongoing supervision by the family. Although they understand explanations about the potential complications of diabetes, they are present-time oriented and may rebel against the daily regimentation of insulin injections and dietary management. Successful self-care depends in part on the adolescent's adjustment to the chronic nature of the disease and feelings of being different from peers.

Children with type 1 diabetes often learn manipulative behaviors, using their disease to obtain something they want. Teach parents to be alert to signs of manipulation, such as helpless, demanding, or whining behaviors, and any evidence of poor coping. Food may become a battleground for toddlers who are picky eaters, but must eat enough for the insulin dose. Referral for counseling may be appropriate for some families.

The child with type 1 diabetes may develop circulatory and neurologic changes over time. Emphasize the importance of good foot care from an early age, for example, wearing clean cotton socks; changing socks and shoes when they are damp; washing, drying, and powdering feet; and keeping toenails short.

Explain to parents that the child should wear some type of medical alert identification. Help them have an individual school health plan developed (see Chapter 35) to ensure that school administrators and teachers can identify the signs of hypoglycemia or hyperglycemia and provide emergency management.

Evaluation

Expected outcomes of nursing care for children with type 1 diabetes can be found in the "Nursing Care Plans."

Diabetic Ketoacidosis

Diabetic ketoacidosis (DKA) is the common and potentially life-threatening condition that occurs in children with type 1 diabetes when the body must burn fat for energy because no insulin is available to metabolize glucose.

Potential causes of DKA include incorrect or missed insulin doses or administration just under the skin, an illness, trauma, or surgery. Most have no clinical evidence of infection (Flood & Chiang, 2001). Insulin deficiency is accompanied by a compensatory increase in hormones (epinephrine, norepinephrine, cortisol, growth hormone, and glucagon) leading to failure to deliver enough glucose to the cells. The muscle cells break down protein into amino acids that are then converted to glucose by the liver, leading to hyperglycemia. The adipose tissue releases fatty acids that are transformed by the liver into ketone bodies. Their accumulation leads to ketoacidosis. The hyperglycemia causes an osmotic diuresis resulting in dehydration, acidosis, and hyperosmolality. Altered consciousness occurs as symptoms progress (Hafeez & Vuguin, 2000).

Characteristic signs of DKA include dehydration, weight loss, tachycardia, flushed ears and cheeks, Kussmaul respirations, acetone breath, altered level of consciousness, and hypotension. The disorder may progress to electrolyte disturbances, arrhythmias, and shock. Children complain of abdominal or chest pain, begin to vomit, have labored breathing, and can slowly slip into a semiconscious state. Hyperglycemia, glycosuria, and ketonuria are also present.

DKA is present with the following findings: blood glucose level greater than 300 mg/dL, ketones in the serum, acidosis (pH less than or equal to 7.3 and bicarbonate less than 15 mEq/L), glycosuria, and ketonuria. Electrolyte disorders also occur (hyperkalemia, hyperchloremia, hyponatremia, hypophosphatemia, hypocalcemia, and hypomagnesemia). Diabetic coma occurs when the serum osmolality exceeds 350 mOsm/kg. Normal serum osmolality is 275 to 295 mOsm/kg. Cerebral edema is a life-threatening complication thought to be related to hyperosmolality.

The child with ketoacidosis is usually hospitalized. Medical management includes intravenous fluids and electrolytes for dehydration and acidosis. Insulin is given by continuous infusion pump to decrease the serum glucose level at a rate not to exceed 100 mg/dL/hr. Faster reduction of hyperglycemia and serum osmolality may be related to the development of cerebral edema. Mannitol is kept on standby for treatment of neurologic deterioration. Bicarbonate is no longer used for treatment of DKA as it places the child at risk for increased central nervous system acidosis and hyperosmolality.

Cerebral edema occurs in about 3% of children with DKA, but it accounts for 30% of DKA deaths and 20% of the overall childhood diabetes mortality (Felner & White, 2001). See Chapter 49 for information about cerebral edema.

NURSING MANAGEMENT

Continuously monitor the child's vital signs, respiratory status, perfusion, and mental status. Frequently monitor the electrolytes and acid-base status, and the blood glucose levels and urine ketone levels. Monitor intake and output.

Give intravenous fluids in boluses of 10 to 20 mL/kg per hour if the child is in shock. Give enough fluids to reverse the fluid deficit. Replace electrolytes as needed. The insulin infusion must be carefully maintained to control the gradual reduction in hyperglycemia. Wean the child off of intravenous insulin when clinically stable.

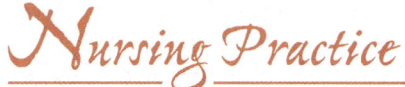

Insulin binds to IV tubing. Let 50 to 100 mL run through new IV tubing to saturate all the binding sites. This assures that the full dose of insulin reaches the child from the outset.

PREVENTING DKA

Call the child's health care provider if the child has the following signs (Kaufman & Halvorson, 1999):

- Vomiting more than two times or for longer than 4 hours
- More than five diarrheal stools
- Sick and cannot eat
- Change in mental status
- Temperature over 101 °F (38.4 °C)
- Blood glucose > 350 mg/dL on two separate readings, or > 200 mg/dL and moderate to large ketones
- Large ketones are present, acetone breath
- There is evidence of a bacterial infection
- The patient has trouble breathing

The prevention of future episodes of DKA is important. The parents and child need to learn strategies to keep hyperglycemic episodes from progressing to DKA. For example, the child's urine should be tested for ketones if three or four consecutive blood glucose readings are higher than 200 mg/dL, or if the child is sick. If the child has a high blood glucose and moderate or large amounts of ketones, treatment with extra insulin and fluids can be initiated. This monitoring is especially important when the child has significant stressors such as an illness. Insulin is needed even when the child is not eating to counter the hormones secreted in response to the stressor.

Hypoglycemia

Hypoglycemia can develop within minutes in children with type 1 diabetes mellitus. The symptoms outlined below may occur when blood glucose levels suddenly drop. Children are at risk of hypoglycemia due to their rapid growth rates and unpredictable eating habits and physical activity. Common causes include an error in insulin dosage, errors in injection technique, inadequate calories because of missed meals, or exercise without a corresponding increase in caloric intake.

Hypoglycemia can be diagnosed on the basis of the sudden onset of signs and symptoms. A blood glucose reading should be taken to confirm the diagnosis, since signs of hyperglycemia and hypoglycemia may be difficult to distinguish. Give glucose immediately in the form of a carbohydrate-containing snack or drink, sugar gel like Cakemate, glucose tablets, or glucose paste. Do not use cake frosting or candy bars for treatment of hypoglycemia. The fat in the frosting and candy prevents the sugar from working quickly. Hard candy takes too long to dissolve to provide rapid treatment for hypoglycemia. In the hospital, administer an intravenous infusion of dextrose to prevent progression of symptoms. If the child becomes unconscious, sugar gel or glucose paste can be squeezed onto the gums.

NURSING MANAGEMENT

Teach parents and children to recognize the signs of hypoglycemia and take appropriate action. Teach parents to give an intramuscular or subcutaneous dose of **glucagon** (a hormone produced by the pancreas that helps release stored glucose from the liver) for severe cases of hypoglycemia. Reinforce the importance of balancing dietary intake, insulin, and exercise every day.

Complementary Care

CHROMIUM FOR DIABETES

Chromium, an essential trace mineral that is required for proper metabolic functioning, may be helpful in treating diabetes, especially if nutritional deficiencies exist (Skidmore-Roth, 2001). It is available in capsule or tablet form, and it is also found in such dietary sources as brewer's yeast and molasses. A recent study showed beneficial antioxidant effects in adults with type 2 diabetes when chromium was combined with zinc, a mineral (Anderson, Roussel, Zouari, et al., 2001).

Type 2 Diabetes

Type 2 diabetes is a disease associated with **insulin resistance** (an alteration of the insulin receptor that signals the presence of insulin in the interior of cells), and it may be connected with an insulin secretory defect in the pancreas.

CLINICAL MANIFESTATIONS ~ *Hypoglycemia and Hyperglycemia*

CAUSE	CLINICAL MANIFESTATIONS	CLINICAL THERAPY
Hypoglycemia • Insulin dose too high for food eaten • Insulin injection into muscle • Too much exercise for insulin dose • Too long between meals/snacks • Too few carbohydrates eaten • Illness, stress	Rapid onset Irritability, nervousness, tremors, shaky feeling, difficulty concentrating or speaking, behavior change, confusion, repeating something over and over Unconsciousness, seizure, shallow breathing, tachycardia Pallor, sweating Moist mucous membranes, hunger Headache, dizziness, blurred vision, double vision, photophobia Numb lips or mouth	If conscious, give 15 grams of carbohydrate. Wait 15 minutes and recheck blood glucose level. Give another 15 grams of carbohydrate if ≤ 70 mg/dL. Recheck the blood glucose level in 15 minutes. If unconscious, give glucagon by injection.
Hyperglycemia • Insulin dose too low for food eaten • Illness or injury, stress • Too many carbohydrates eaten • Meals/snacks too close together • Insulin injected just under skin or injected into hypertrophied areas • Decreased activity	Gradual onset Lethargy, sleepiness, slowed responses, or confusion Deep, rapid breathing Flushed skin, dry skin Dry mucous membranes, thirst, hunger, dehydration Weakness, fatigue Headache, abdominal pain, nausea, vomiting Blurred vision Shock	Additional insulin given at usual injection time. Sliding scale insulin doses for specific blood glucose levels when ill or injured. Extra injections if hyperglycemia and moderate to large ketones. Increased fluids.

Type 2 diabetes was formerly called noninsulin-dependent diabetes. Risk factors include obesity, low physical exercise, and type 2 diabetes in a first-degree relative. Between 74% and 100% of children with type 2 diabetes have a first- or second-degree relative with the same type of diabetes (American Diabetes Association, 2000). The peak age of onset in children is at the time of puberty, and females are affected more than males with a 1.7:1 ratio (Pinhas-Hamiel & Zeitler, 2001).

The increasing number of children being diagnosed with type 2 diabetes has caused significant concern in the health care community. Up to 45% of children with a new diagnosis of diabetes have type 2. The increasing rate of obesity among children is thought to be a contributing factor (American Diabetes Association, 2000). The true incidence in children is unknown as many children are undiagnosed.

Developing Cultural Competence

Children of African-American, American-Indian, Hispanic, and Asian origin are at greater risk for developing type 2 diabetes (American Diabetes Association, 2000). The disease in children appears to be following the same racial and ethnic distribution as found in adults (Brosnan, Upchurch, & Schreiner, 2001). Particularly affected are members of some American-Indian tribes that historically had a high level of exercise and had hunter-gatherer types of diet. In some groups, such as the Pima Indians of the Southwest, the majority have diabetes and face complications from the disease.

ETIOLOGY AND PATHOPHYSIOLOGY

Type 2 diabetes is a complex metabolic disorder in which the child has insulin resistance, which prevents insulin from transferring glucose into the cells. With the weight, the visceral fat produces a cytokine hormone (tumor necrosis factor) that desensitizes the insulin receptor to insulin. The pancreatic cells produce more insulin in an attempt to facilitate glucose transfer and overcome the insulin resistance. This results in **hyperinsulinemia** (elevated insulin levels in the blood). The child maintains a balance between hyperinsulinemia and insulin resistance and a normal glycemic state. As insulin resistance worsens, the islet of Langerhans beta cells fail in their ability to hypersecrete insulin. This leads to impaired glucose tolerance and overt diabetes develops. The growth hormone secretion may have a role during puberty in promoting insulin resistance.

CLINICAL MANIFESTATIONS

Signs and symptoms of type 2 diabetes upon initial presentation are very different from type 1. **Acanthosis nigricans,** hyperpigmentation and thickening of the skin with velvety irregularities in the skin folds of the neck, axillae, elbows, knees, groin, and abdomen, is a common finding associated with chronic hyperinsulinemia (see Fig-

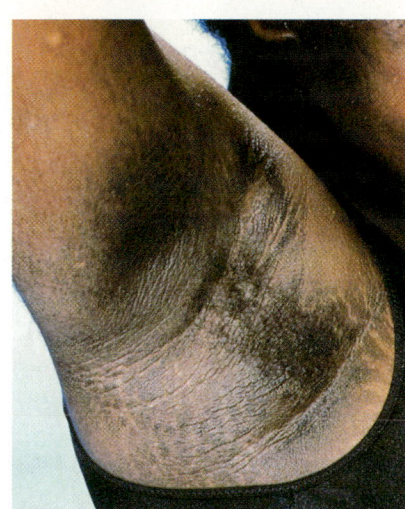

FIGURE 51–10. ◆ Acanthosis nigricans. Courtesy of Audrey Austin, M. D., Children's National Medical Center, Washington, D.C.

ure 51–10 ◆) The child is usually obese, usually with truncal (or central) adiposity. The child may present in diabetic ketoacidosis. Other clinical manifestations can be found on page 1364.

CLINICAL THERAPY

Obesity and the presence of acanthosis nigricans on physical exam are clues to the diagnosis. Blood glucose levels ≥ 200 mg/dL without fasting, or a fasting glucose ≥ 126 mg/dL are diagnostic of diabetes. Urine is tested and ketones are found in about 50% of children. Islet cell autoantibodies, insulin levels, glutamic acid decarboxylase autoantibody test (GAD-65), and fasting C-peptid level are used to differentiate between type 1 and type 2 diabetes. The child with type 2 diabetes has higher insulin and fasting C-peptid levels than the child with type 1 diabetes. Islet cell and GAD-65 autoantibodies will not be present. A fasting lipid profile is obtained since dyslipidemia (primarily elevated LDL-C and triglycerides) is usually present. Elevated fasting insulin levels are present (see Appendix B).

The goal of clinical therapy is normal physical and emotional development, control of hypo- and hyperglycemia, and minimization of long-term complications. To accomplish this, the child needs to have gradual sustained weight loss, metabolic control of blood glucose levels, exercise, and emotional support. Oral medication is used when diet and exercise efforts are inadequate to control hyperglycemia. Metformin enhances insulin sensitivity, slows the gastrointestinal absorption of glucose, and reduces the hepatic and renal glucose production. It can be used when there is normal liver and kidney function and no ketosis. If additional medication is needed, sulfonylurea may be used. The adolescent may ultimately need insulin for glycemic control.

If the child presents in ketoacidosis, insulin is initially used to reverse the metabolic decompensation. Insulin may not be required after the metabolic deterioration is resolved.

Nursing Management

Nursing Assessment and Diagnosis

Because the child does not often have an acute onset, assess any child with a BMI greater than 85th percentile for age and sex for signs of insulin resistance (acanthosis nigricans, hypertension, and dyslipidemia). Family history of diabetes in an overweight child is a reason to begin screening for the condition. Once the child has been diagnosed, monitor the child's blood glucose levels and blood pressure. Assess the child's diet and activity patterns to determine appropriate changes for disease management. Consider evaluating the siblings for diabetes. Nursing diagnoses that may apply to the child with type 2 diabetes include:

▶ *Altered nutrition, more than body requirements* related to obesity in one or both parents and ethnic and cultural norms

▶ *Activity intolerance* related to sedentary lifestyle

▶ *Fatigue* related to disease state (insulin resistance)

▶ *Ineffective management of therapeutic regimen, family and individual* related to family conflict over changing eating patterns

▶ *Self-esteem disturbance* related to situational crisis associated with diagnosis of new onset chronic illness

Planning and Implementation

The child with type 2 diabetes may be hospitalized at the time of diagnosis because of ketoacidosis. However, the nurse in an inpatient setting is more likely to encounter this child when hospitalized for another condition or during visits for health care in clinics or schools. Nursing care focuses on managing the child's blood glucose levels and hypertension during the hospitalization, assessing growth and dietary intake, evaluating goals for weight loss and exercise programs, and reviewing the child's knowledge about diabetes and strategies for management at home.

NURSING CARE IN THE COMMUNITY

Since the child is initially diagnosed and managed on an outpatient basis, nursing care focuses on teaching the child and parents about the disease and its management, managing dietary intake, providing emotional support, and planning strategies for daily management in the community.

Educate the child and family about the disease and lifestyle changes required for effective management of the condition. Focus on the need to increase activity with routine exercise of at least 30 to 60 minutes daily and by decreasing sedentary activity time, such as computer and television viewing time to no more than 2 hours daily. Customize the activity strategy for each child with motivation to develop a regular routine.

Work with the family to decrease high-calorie and high-fat foods with a diet plan sensitive to the family's re-sources and ethnic preferences. Limit fast food to once weekly and have snacks with natural products like fruits and vegetables. Assess the child's height, weight, and BMI on each visit, and plot on the appropriate growth curve for age and sex on each visit. A gradual sustained weight loss or decrease in BMI is the goal. If the child is going through a growth height spurt, maintenance of weight rather than weight loss is the goal. Make sure the child takes a multivitamin daily because of dietary restrictions. Encourage the entire family to make dietary changes, especially since other family members are also at risk for the condition.

Teach the child and family to perform home blood glucose testing to monitor glycemic control. This will let the child and family know that efforts to manage the disease are successful. Take HbA_{1c} levels at each visit to determine the average blood glucose level for the past 3 months. A HbA_{1c} level of 7% is the goal. When dietary control and exercise are not successful in reducing blood glucose levels, teach the child and family about the prescribed oral medication.

Give the child and family chances to talk about the impact of the disease on their lives. Identify resources for information about strategies that have worked for other families. Identify local support groups and peer groups for the family and child.

Make sure the child gets annual evaluations for potential complications of diabetes. The tests to be performed include blood for lipid levels, blood pressure, liver and renal function, urine for albumin, an eye exam for retinopathy, and a neurologic exam of the extremities for neuropathies. The child with type 2 diabetes has the same risk for developing long-term vascular complications as the child with type 1 diabetes when hyperglycemia is poorly controlled.

Evaluation

Examples of expected outcomes of nursing care include:

▶ The child decreases sedentary activity time to under 2 hours a day.

▶ The child's daily intake of fruits and vegetables increases to 5 to 8 daily and total fat intake decreases to less than 30% of total calories.

▶ The child's body mass index slowly and consistently decreases.

⚕ DISORDERS OF GONADAL FUNCTION

GYNECOMASTIA

Gynecomastia is the presence of unilateral or bilateral enlarged breast tissue in males. It is a common finding during adolescence and is sometimes confused with subcutaneous fat pads in obese boys. Gynecomastia occurs when the ratio of estrogen to testosterone is greater than the usual male ratio. It is also associated with drugs that increase the circulating concentration of prolactin such as marijuana and tricyclic antidepressants (Wilson, 1999). The amount of breast tissue varies among boys. The condition usually disappears in 1 to 2 years.

Nursing care focuses on reassuring the boy and his parents that gynecomastia is common and transient. Because of the body image concerns common during adolescence, embarrassment is a frequent problem. Alerting the teen's teachers may be necessary if teasing becomes a problem.

AMENORRHEA

Amenorrhea, or lack of menstruation, may be primary or secondary. Criteria for primary amenorrhea include:

- Absence of menarche by age 14 in association with no growth or development of secondary sexual characteristics
- Absence of menses by age 16 when secondary sexual characteristics and growth are present
- Absence of menarche 2 years after completing breast development and peak height velocity (Prose, Ford, & Lovely, 1998).

Secondary amenorrhea is the cessation of menstrual periods 6 months or 3 cycles after menstruation has begun; it is characterized by an absence of spontaneous bleeding for at least 120 days. Pregnancy is the most common cause of secondary amenorrhea in adolescents. It is common for adolescents to have irregular menstrual cycles and duration of the menstrual period for 1 to 2 years after menarche. A large number of cycles are anovulatory for the first 2 years after menarche.

Primary amenorrhea is most often caused by structural defects of the reproductive system; chromosomal abnormalities (such as Turner syndrome); or hypothalamic or pituitary tumors, thyroid dysfunction, or polycystic ovary disease. No underlying pathologic condition is found in some adolescents. Primary or secondary amenorrhea may be found in competitive athletes.

A thorough history, physical examination, and laboratory evaluation are required to determine the cause of amenorrhea. The history focuses on asking questions about recent excessive weight loss or gain; excessive physical activity or sports training; chronic illness; use of illegal drugs, birth control pills, or phenothiazines; emotional problems; and age of the mother at menarche. The physical examination focuses on evaluating the adolescent's stage of sexual development and assessing for hirsutism (see Chapter 33). A vaginal exam is performed to determine vaginal patency and if the vaginal mucosa is estrogenized. A pregnancy test is performed. A bone age and hormone levels are evaluated (estrogen, LH, FSH, and prolactin).

Treatment of amenorrhea depends on the specific cause. The most common approach is to give birth control pills containing both estrogen and progesterone. Athletic teenagers are encouraged to eat a well-balanced, high-calorie diet. Calcium supplements may be ordered. Estrogen with progesterone in low doses may be prescribed for athletes to reduce the risk for osteoporosis. Nursing management centers on patient education and emotional support. The goal is to maintain normal growth and development.

See Chapter 3 for information on dysmenorrhea.

≈ DISORDERS RELATED TO SEX CHROMOSOME ABNORMALITIES

TURNER SYNDROME

Turner syndrome is the most common sex chromosome abnormality in females. Affected girls have a missing or abnormal X chromosome. It occurs in approximately 1 in 1500 to 2500 live female births (Prose et al., 1998). The cause of the chromosomal error is unknown.

Characteristic clinical findings include significant short stature (less than 5th percentile); undeveloped ovaries; a short, webbed neck with a low posterior hairline; cubitus valgus (increased angle at the elbow); broad chest with widely spaced nipples; lymphedema; hyperconvex fingernails; dark, pigmented nevi; delayed puberty; amenorrhea; and infertility (Figure 51–11 ◆). Few girls have all of these features. Pubertal development occurs spontaneously, but delayed, in up to 30% of affected girls (Ranke & Saenger 2001).

Among the conditions that may be associated with Turner syndrome are congenital heart disease; coarctation of aorta; structural abnormalities of the kidney; congenital lymphedema; hypothyroidism or Hashimoto thyroiditis; chronic or recurrent otitis media; ptosis, myopia, or amblyopia (lazy eye); inflammatory bowel disease; idiopathic hypertension; and scoliosis (Sanger, 1996).

Growth usually proceeds at a normal rate for the first 2 to 3 years of life and then slows. Breast tissue, which begins to bud at about 10 to 12 years, fails to develop fully. Only in rare instances does a girl with Turner syndrome menstruate spontaneously or become able to conceive. Without treatment, final height is approximately 4 feet 8 inches.

Growth and Development

Girls competing in sports such as gymnastics, ballet, and long-distance running need to maintain a low weight and a perfect body type. The inadequate nutrition and strenuous activity may cause hypothalamic dysfunction and a low estrogen level. This results in amenorrhea (Prose et al., 1998). This, in turn, may increase the girl's risk of fractures and osteoporosis in young adulthood. See Chapter 31.

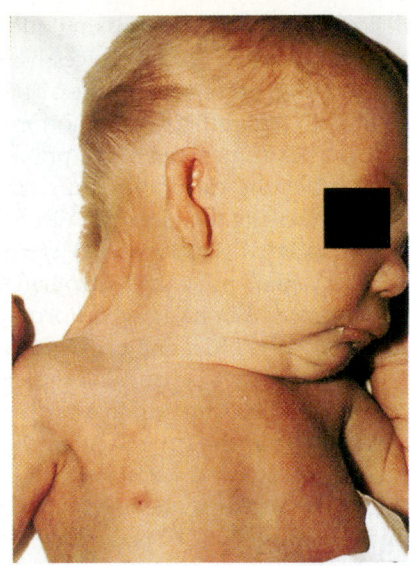

FIGURE 51–11. ◆ What characteristic physical manifestations of Turner syndrome can you identify in this girl? Note: From Zitelli, B. J., & Davis, H. W. (Eds.). (1997). *Atlas of Pediatric Physical Diagnosis*, 3rd ed., (p. 14, Fig. 1–19a). St. Louis: Mosby.

Characteristic physical findings may alert health care providers to suspect Turner syndrome. Some infants, however, have few of these characteristics. In some instances diagnosis is made only when short stature and delayed puberty become apparent in the teenage years. The condition is diagnosed definitively by a karyotype, which reveals the classic 45,XO chromosome pattern or 46,XX pattern with one misshapen X chromosome. WEB

Treatment involves carefully monitoring the child's growth. A growth chart made especially for girls with Turner syndrome is available. Growth hormone therapy may be prescribed to promote growth during childhood (Ranke & Saenger, 2001). Low-dose estrogen therapy is usually begun at about 15 years of age, with dosage increases over the next 2 to 3 years. Waiting until 15 years gives the girl the opportunity to achieve her maximum height before hormones cause the growth plates to close. This treatment produces pubertal changes such as breast development and pubic hair. Progesterone is added to the estrogen therapy to initiate menstrual periods.

Nursing Management

The lack of growth and sexual development associated with Turner syndrome presents problems not only for physical growth but also for psychosocial development. The girl's perception of her body and how she differs from peers affects self-image, self-consciousness, and self-esteem.

In the United States, cultural values place importance on attaining normal to tall stature. Short children tend to be treated according to their size rather than their age. Emphasis is also placed on sexual maturity. Television, advertisements, and movies encourage adolescents to dress

and behave in a sexually mature manner. Girls with Turner syndrome are often self-conscious and easily embarrassed and suffer from low self-esteem. Even though their intelligence is generally normal, they have a higher incidence of learning problems because of visual–spatial deficits that affect performance on mathematical and manual dexterity tasks (Ranke & Saenger, 2001).

The nurse can be instrumental in helping the child adapt to the condition and gain self-esteem. Be an active listener and reinforce abilities and skills that the girl exhibits. Encourage parents to provide support. The Turner Syndrome Society can provide additional information about the disorder for parents and adolescents. WEB

KLINEFELTER SYNDROME

Klinefelter syndrome is a genetic condition that occurs in boys who have an extra X chromosome (usually 47,XXY). It occurs in approximately 1 in 500 male births (Lewanda & Jabs, 1999). It is the single most common cause of hypogonadism (decreased secretory activity of the gonad) and infertility in males.

Most infants appear normal at birth. The condition is usually diagnosed during the school-age years when the boy's behavior becomes a problem in the classroom. Boys with Klinefelter syndrome may have emotional problems because of delayed language development and auditory processing problems that are frustrating to the child. Intelligence quotient (IQ) scores are often 10 to 15 points below those of unaffected siblings, and IQs below 80 are not uncommon. Boys with Klinefelter syndrome are tall and thin, with overly long arms and legs. The arm span to height ratio is normal. The onset of puberty may be delayed with an abnormal progression. Testicular size is decreased at all ages. Less facial and body hair may develop. Gynecomastia is a characteristic finding.

Chromosomal analysis revealing one or more extra X chromosomes confirms the diagnosis. The goal of treatment is to stimulate masculinization and the development of secondary sex characteristics when adolescence is delayed. Testosterone replacement is begun when the boy is 11 or 12 years of age. Depo-Testosterone is given by intramuscular injection every 3 to 4 weeks to maintain serum testosterone levels within the normal range. The dose is increased gradually until an adult dose is reached between 15 and 17 years of age; however, this does not improve fertility. Gynecomastia does not typically disappear with hormone treatment. Cosmetic surgery may be needed if breast size is distressing.

Nursing Management

Nursing care consists of educating the parents and child about the syndrome, evaluating the child's and family's coping mechanisms, assisting with school problems, and reinforcing the child's strengths. Encourage parents to channel their son's energy into areas that will provide opportunities for success and productive experiences. Emphasize the importance of rewarding the boy's successes in school, sports, or hobbies. Make genetic counseling available to adolescents, if indicated, because sexual functioning and fertility may be impaired.

INBORN ERRORS OF METABOLISM

Inborn errors of metabolism are inherited biochemical abnormalities of the urea cycle, amino acid, and organic acid metabolism. Individually they are rare disorders; however, as a group they are a significant health problem in infancy.

The biochemical defect usually causes an abnormal chemical by-product to accumulate in the blood, urine, or tissues or results in a decreased amount of normal enzymes. Most disorders are associated with protein intolerance, and symptoms develop shortly after formula or breast milk feedings are begun.

Clinical manifestations usually occur within days or weeks of birth. Signs and symptoms may include lethargy and poor feeding, persistent vomiting, abnormal muscle tone and seizures, apnea and tachycardia, and an unusual urine or body odor (musty, sweet odor of maple syrup or burnt sugar, or cheesy or sweaty feet).

In many states, neonatal screening is used to detect several of these conditions before symptoms develop. Four million newborns are screened each year for metabolic disorders (e.g., phenylketonuria), hematologic disorders (e.g., sickle cell anemia), and endocrinopathies (e.g., hypothyroidism) (Centers for Disease Control and Prevention, 2001).

Nursing Practice

Neonatal screening for hypothyroidism and phenylketonuria is mandated by state law in all 50 states. When a state law exists, signed informed consent of the parents is not required. All states but South Dakota permit parents to refuse screening for religious or personal reasons. If parents refuse the test, obtain a signature of "informed dissent" to include in the child's medical record (American Academy of Pediatrics, 2001).

However, most inborn errors of metabolism are not detected until signs and symptoms are present. Initial laboratory tests include measurement of serum glucose, electrolytes, blood gases, and serum ammonia. Test results make it possible to classify the disorder by the presence of hypoglycemia, metabolic acidosis, hyperammonemia, or liver dysfunction. Further diagnostic laboratory tests are then performed.

Treatment, when available, focuses on replacing or reducing the amount of the substance causing the biochemical abnormality.

Three of the more common inborn errors of metabolism, phenylketonuria, maple syrup urine disease, and galactosemia, are presented here. Congenital hypothyroidism and congenital adrenal hyperplasia, also considered inborn errors of metabolism, were discussed earlier in this chapter.

PHENYLKETONURIA

Phenylketonuria (PKU) is an autosomal recessive inherited disorder of amino acid metabolism that affects the body's use of protein. It is caused by a mutation of the phenylalanine hydroxylase gene. The incidence is 1 in 10,000 live births per year, with great ethnic variability (Yule, 2000).

Developing Cultural Competence

Phenylketonuria is rare in African, Jewish, and Japanese populations. It is more commonly found in isolated communities with numerous intermarriages between families over several generations.

Children with PKU have a deficiency of the liver enzyme phenylalanine hydroxylase that normally breaks down the essential amino acid phenylalanine into tyrosine. As a result, phenylalanine accumulates in the blood, causing a musty or mousey body and urine odor, irritability, vomiting, hyperactivity, seizures, and an eczema-like rash. Persistence of elevated phenylalanine leads to disruption of cellular processes of myelination and protein synthesis, and results in a seizure disorder and untreatable mental retardation.

Infants appear normal at birth. Screening for PKU is required by state law in all 50 states. For best results the newborn should have begun formula or breast milk feeding before specimen collection. Early hospital discharge places newborns at risk for false negative screening tests if screened within 24 hours of birth. Screening needs to occur no sooner than 48 hours after birth, or the test should be repeated at 1 to 2 weeks of age. If the test shows elevated levels of plasma phenylalanine, a repeat test is performed. If the second test is positive, the family is referred to an outpatient treatment center.

PKU is treated using special formulas (e.g., Lofenalac, Minafen, and Albumaid XP) and a diet low in phenylalanine to keep plasma phenylalanine levels between 2 and 6 mg/dL. The diet must also meet the child's needs for optimal growth. High-protein foods (meats and dairy products) and aspartame are avoided because they contain large amounts of phenylalanine. Elemental medical foods (modified protein hydrosylates in which the phenylalanine has been removed) are used instead. The low-phenylalanine diet should be maintained throughout life. If dietary control is lost before 6 years of age, there is a significant impact on IQ (Yule, 2000). If adults go off the diet, there is no change in their IQ, but they may perform less well on tasks requiring attention and processing speed (Phenylketonuria: Screening and Management: National Institutes of Health, 2000). The low phenylalanine diet is especially important for adolescent females and women prior to conception and during pregnancy to prevent congenital anomalies (low birth weight, mental retardation, microcephaly) in the fetus.

Nursing Management

Nursing care is mainly supportive and focuses on teaching parents about the disorder and its management. Measure serum levels of phenylalanine periodically throughout life.

The low-phenylalanine diet is a rigid, strict diet that excludes many foods. Parents and children need a great deal of support to promote compliance. The formula and elemental medical food costs are relatively high. Usually only the formula is reimbursed by insurance. Like children with diabetes mellitus, children with PKU may rebel against the dietary limitations in an effort to be like their peers. For this reason the low-phenylalanine diet may be discontinued during the late school-age years or adolescence. If the child has problems concentrating or sitting still, resuming the low-phenylalanine diet may improve behavior and cognitive functioning.

Refer parents of an affected child who are considering a future pregnancy and adolescents with the disorder for genetic counseling.

GALACTOSEMIA

Galactosemia, a disorder of carbohydrate metabolism, has an autosomal recessive inheritance pattern. It occurs in 1 in 70,000 live births (Kirschner, Kolb, Pandit, et al., 2000).

Galactosemia results from a deficiency of the liver enzyme galactose 1-phosphate uridyltransferase (GALT), one of three enzymes needed to convert galactose to glucose. The lack of enzyme leads to an accumulation of galactose metabolites in the eyes, liver, kidney, and brain, rapidly damaging the organs and causing life-threatening problems. Children become susceptible to gram negative sepsis.

Early signs include feeding problems, failure to gain weight due to vomiting followed by diarrhea, hypoglycemia, and an enlarged liver. Later signs include mental retardation, jaundice, ascites, sepsis, lethargy, seizures, hypotonia, cataracts, and coma. Babies may die within 1 month of birth without treatment, usually due to sepsis.

Routine newborn screening for galactosemia is performed in 44 states and the District of Columbia (Kirschner et al., 2000). (See Skill 10–2.) SKILLS Infants in other states are identified once they become symptomatic. The diagnosis is based upon history, physical ex-

amination, and laboratory tests (galactose, SGOT, and SGPT are abnormally high). Urines are checked for reducing substances (the Clinitest is positive and the Clinistix is negative). Infants with galactosemia are placed on a lactose- or galactose-free formula (e.g., Nutramigen, a meat-based or soybean formula), which remains the child's milk substitute for life. Improvement in the infant's condition is generally seen within 24 hours. A galactose-free diet (no milk or cheese products, including foods with dry milk products) is prescribed when the infant is ready for solids. In spite of compliance with the diet, complications (learning disabilities, speech defects, ovarian failure, and neurologic syndromes) develop in many children.

Nursing management focuses on educating the parents and child about the disorder and required diet, assessing coping abilities, and providing emotional support. Refer the family to a nutritionist for diet counseling. Families must learn to screen foods for added milk solids and to avoid medications, such as antibiotics, that have lactose fillers. Calcium supplementation may be needed. Advise parents that several galactose-free cheeses are sold commercially. Because the disorder is inherited, refer the family for genetic counseling.

MAPLE SYRUP URINE DISEASE

Maple syrup urine disease (MSUD), a disorder of amino acid metabolism, has an autosomal recessive inheritance pattern. It is rare—found in 1 in 225,000 live births—but has a high incidence in some Pennsylvania Mennonites (1 in 380 live births) (Robinson & Drumm, 2001).

In MSUD, three essential amino acids (leucine, isoleucine, and valine) cannot be broken down because of absent or defective enzyme branched chain alpha-ketoacid dehydrogenase. This results in alpha ketoacidosis. All three amino acids are essential to form normal structures such as the hair, skin, and muscle. Leucine has the potential to build up in the brain and cause cerebral edema, progressive neurologic impairment, and death.

Within 3 to 7 days of life, the newborn develops symptoms of poor appetite, lethargy, vomiting, variable muscle tone, irritability, seizures, high-pitched cry, and a sweet smell. Not all states require newborn screening for this condition. Diagnosis is made with laboratory tests of the urine for positive ketones and blood tests for elevated leucine, isoleucine, and valine. Specially designed medical formulas and foods rich in amino acids, calories, vitamins, minerals, and other nutrients are prescribed. These special medical foods have the three amino acids removed. The child needs special low-protein foods that are adequate for growth with enough calories to support twice the child's basal metabolic rate. Daily urine testing is required to determine if ketones are being excreted, an indication that the body is in a catabolic state.

Nursing care includes educating the family about the disorder and special dietary requirements. The parents need to learn how to mix the child's special formula with natural protein source, amino acid supplements, and water. The child needs formula even when ill; provide a sick day plan to prevent ketoacidosis. The child should be permitted moderate exercise only to prevent increases in leucine levels. Help families identify sources of information or support groups who can share recipes and tips for managing the child's condition. ⟬⟭ [WEB]

When the child starts child care or school, it is important for teachers and other care providers to know foods the child should avoid and a list of snacks for special occasions. The child should have formula and other supplements available to ensure a steady intake of calories during the day. An individual school health plan should be developed with the school nurse so that teachers and other school personnel are informed.

CHAPTER HIGHLIGHTS

🙢 Puberty is the process of sexual maturation that occurs when the gonads secrete increased amounts of the sex hormones estrogen and testosterone, resulting in the development of primary and secondary sex characteristics.

🙢 Children with hypopituitarism have short stature as a result of growth hormone deficiency. Treatment with growth hormone early in life enables these children to have near normal heights.

🙢 An excessive secretion of growth hormone or hyperpituitarism may cause children to grow 7 or 8 feet in height when it occurs before the epiphyseal plates close.

🙢 In diabetes insipidus, the urine cannot be concentrated, no matter how dehydrated the child becomes. Diagnosis rarely occurs until the child experiences hypernatremic dehydration.

🙢 Precocious puberty is the appearance of any secondary sexual characteristics before 8 years of age in girls and 9 years of age in boys. If no treatment is provided the hormones will stimulate closure of the epiphyseal plates and the child will have short stature as an adult.

🙢 Untreated or ineffectively treated congenital hypothyroidism results in impaired growth and mental retardation.

🙢 Signs of hyperthyroidism include an enlarged, nontender thyroid gland (goiter), prominent eyes, eyelid lag, tachycardia, nervousness, restlessness or irritability, increased appetite with weight loss, emotional lability, heat intolerance, increased sweating, insomnia, tremor, and muscle weakness.

🙢 During infancy and childhood, most cases of Cushing syndrome are due to malignant adrenal tumor. It generally takes up to 5 years for the child to develop the characteristic "cushingoid" appearance.

🙢 Congenital adrenal hyperplasia has two forms, salt-losing or simple virilization. Approximately 65% to 75% of children have a disturbance in mineralocorticoid regulation that can lead to acute adrenal insufficiency with any serious illness or injury.

🙢 Adrenal insufficiency, though rare in children, is characterized by weakness with fatigue; anorexia and salt craving; poor weight gain or weight loss; hyperpigmentation at pressure points; generalized bronzing of the skin; abdominal pain; nausea and vomiting; and diarrhea.

🙢 Pheochromocytoma is a benign tumor of the adrenal gland that causes labile hypertension and intermittent signs associated with epinephrine and norepinephrine secretion.

🙢 The American Diabetes Association recommends that all adolescents with type 1 diabetes mellitus use an intensive therapy regimen with 3 or more insulin injections a day or a continuous subcutaneous insulin infusion (CSII) by an insulin pump.

🙢 Treatment of the child with diabetic ketoacidosis includes intravenous fluids and electrolytes for dehydration and acidosis. Insulin is given by continuous infusion pump to decrease the serum glucose level slowly but steadily to prevent cerebral edema.

🙢 Common causes of hypoglycemia in children with type 1 diabetes include an error in insulin dosage, errors in injection technique, inadequate calories because of missed meals, or exercise without a corresponding increase in caloric intake.

🙢 Type 2 diabetes mellitus is a new epidemic among children and adolescents that results from insulin resistance. Children most commonly affected are obese and the majority have family members with the same type of diabetes.

🙢 Secondary amenorrhea is the cessation of spontaneous bleeding for at least 120 days that occurs 6 months or 3 cycles after menarche.

🙢 Turner syndrome is diagnosed definitively by a karyotype, which reveals the classic 45,XO chromosome pattern or 46,XX pattern with one misshapen X chromosome.

🙢 Signs of Klinefelter syndrome include gynecomastia, delayed onset of puberty with an abnormal progression, decreased testicular size, and less facial and body hair than normal.

🙢 Children with phenylketonuria (PKU) have a deficiency of the liver enzyme phenylalanine hydroxylase that normally breaks down the essential amino acid phenylalanine into tyrosine. It is treated with special formula and engineered foods.

🙢 Galactosemia results from a deficiency of a liver enzyme needed to convert galactose to glucose. This leads to an accumulation of galactose metabolites in the eyes, liver, kidney, and brain, rapidly damaging the organs and causing life-threatening problems.

🙢 Maple syrup urine disease is a rare inherited enzyme deficiency that results in ketoacidosis unless special formula, engineered foods, and extra calories are eaten.

EXPLOREMEDIALINK

NCLEX Review, Case Studies, and other interactive resources for this chapter can be found on the companion website at http://www.prenhall.com/london. Click on "Chapter 51" to select the activities for this chapter.

For animations, more NCLEX review questions, and an audio glossary, access the accompanying CD-ROM in this textbook.

REFERENCES

American Academy of Pediatrics Committee on Bioethics. (2001). Ethical issues with genetic testing in pediatrics. *Pediatrics, 107*(6), 1451–1455.

American Academy of Pediatrics Section on Endocrinology and Committee on Genetics. (2000). Technical report: Congenital adrenal hyperplasia. *Pediatrics, 106*(6), 1511–1518.

American Diabetes Association. (2000). Type 2 diabetes in children and adolescents. *Diabetes Care, 23*(3), 381–389.

Anderson, R. A., Roussel, A. M., Zouari, N., Mahjoub, S., Matheau, J. M., & Kerkeni, A. (2001). Potential antioxidant effects of zinc and chromium supplementation in people with type 2 diabetes mellitus. *Journal of the American College of Nutrition, 20*(3), 212–218.

Boland, E. A., & Grey, M. (2000). Diabetes mellitus (type 1). In P. L. Jackson & J. A. Vessey (Eds.), *Primary care of the child with a chronic condition* (3rd ed., pp. 426–444). St. Louis, MO: Mosby.

Brosnan, C. A., Upchurch, S., & Schreiner, B. (2001). Type 2 diabetes in children and adolescents: An emerging disease. *Journal of Pediatric Health Care, 15*(4), 187–193.

Castiglia, P. T. (1997). Hyperthyroidism. *Journal of Pediatric Health Care, 11*(5), 227–229.

Centers for Disease Control and Prevention. (2001). Using tandem mass spectrometry for metabolic disease screening among newborns: A report of a work group. *Morbidity and Mortality Weekly Report 50*(RR-31), 1–34.

Donohoue, P. A. (1999). The thyroid. In J. A. McMillan, C. D. DeAngelis, R. D. Feigin, & J. B. Warshaw (Eds.), *Oski's pediatrics: Principles and practice* (3rd ed., pp. 1803–1812). Philadelphia: Lippincott Williams & Wilkins.

Dveirin, K., & Tunnessen, W. W. (2000). A 14-month-old with polyuria and polydipsia: Searching for buried treasure. *Contemporary Pediatrics, 17*(10), 23–30.

Expert Committee on the Diagnosis and Classification of Diabetes Mellitus. (1999). Report of the expert committee on the diagnosis and classification of diabetes mellitus. *Diabetes Care, 22* (Suppl. 1), S5–S19.

Felner, E. I., & White, P. C. (2001). Improving management of diabetic ketoacidosis in children. *Pediatrics, 108*(3), 735–740.

Finegold, D. (1997). Endocrinology. In B. J. Zitelli & H. W. Davis (Eds.), *Atlas of pediatric physical diagnosis* (3rd ed., p. 270). St. Louis, MO: Mosby–Wolfe.

Flood, R. G., & Chiang, V. W. (2001). Rate and prediction of infection in children with diabetic ketoacidosis. *Journal of Emergency Medicine, 19*(4), 270–273.

Hafeez, W., & Vuguin, P. (2000). Managing diabetic ketoacidosis: A delicate balance. *Contemporary Pediatrics, 17*(6), 72–83.

Herman-Giddens, M. E., Slora, E. J., Wasserman, R. C., Bourdony, C. J., Bhapkar, M. V., Koch, G. G., et al. (1997). Secondary sexual characteristics and menses in young girls seen in office practice: A study from the pediatric research in office settings network. *Pediatrics, 99*(4), 505–512.

Kaufman, F. R., & Halvorson, M. (1999a). New trends in managing type 1 diabetes. *Contemporary Pediatrics, 16*(10), 112–123.

Kaufman, F. R., & Halvorson, M. (1999b). The treatment and prevention of diabetic ketoacidosis in children and adolescents with type 1 diabetes. *Pediatric Annals, 28*(9), 576–582.

Kirchlechner, V., Koller, D. Y., Seidl, R., & Waldhauser, F. (1999). Treatment of nephrogenic diabetes insipidus with hydrochlorothiazide and amiloride. *Archives of Diseases in Children, 80*, 548–552.

Kirschner, C., Kolb, A., Pandit, S., & Tunnessen, W. W. (2000). A 4-week-old with poor weight gain and jaundice: A diagnosis in space. *Contemporary Pediatrics, 17*(11), 27–33.

Kohn, B., Julius, J. R., & Blethen, S. L. (1999). Combined use of growth hormone and gonadotropin-releasing hormone analogues: The National Cooperative Growth Study experience. *Pediatrics, 104*(4, pt. 2), 1014–1017.

Lewanda, A. F., & Jabs, E. W. (1999). Dysmorphology: Genetic syndromes and associations. In J. A. McMillan, C. D. DeAngelis, R. D. Feigin, & J. B. Warshaw (Eds.), *Oski's pediatrics: Principles and practice* (3rd ed., p. 2231). Philadelphia: Lippincott Williams & Wilkins.

Merke, D. P., & Cutler, G. B. (1997). New approaches to the treatment of congenital adrenal hyperplasia. *Journal of the American Medical Association, 277*(13), 1073–1076.

Phenylketonuria: Screening and management, NIH Consensus statement. (2000, Oct. 16–18), 17(3), 1–33.

Pinhas-Hamiel, O., & Zeitler, P. (2001). Type 2 diabetes: Not just for grownups anymore. *Contemporary Pediatrics, 18*(1), 102–125.

Prose, C. C., Ford, C. A., & Lovely, L. P. (1998). Evaluating amenorrhea: The pediatrician's role. *Contemporary Pediatrics, 15*(10), 83–110.

Ranke, W. B., & Saenger, P. (2001, July 28). Turner's syndrome. *Lancet, 358*, 309–314.

Reddy, V. S., O'Neill, J. A., Holcomb, G. W., Neblett, W. W., Pietsch, J. B., & Morgan, W. M. (2000). Twenty-five year surgical experience with pheochromocytoma in children. *American Surgeon, 66*(12), 1085–1091.

Rennert, O. M., & Francis, G. L. (1999). Update on the genetics and pathophysiology of type 1 diabetes. *Pediatric Annals, 28*(9), 570–575.

Robinson, D., & Drumm, L. (2001). Maple syrup urine disease: A standard of nursing care. *Pediatric Nursing, 27*(3), 255–264, 270.

Rovet, J. F., & Ehrlich, R. (2000). Psychoeducational outcome in children with early-treated congenital hypothyroidism. *Pediatrics, 105*(3), 515–522.

Sanger, P. (1996). Turner's syndrome. *Current Concepts, 335*(2), 1749–1754.

Saudek, C. D. (1997). Novel forms of insulin delivery. *Endocrinology and Metabolism Clinics of North America, 26*(3), 599–610.

Selekman, J., Scofield, S., & Swenson-Brousell, C. (1999). Diabetes update in the pediatric population. *Pediatric Nursing, 25*(6), 666–669.

Shulman, D. I., & Bercu, B. B. (1998). Growth hormone therapy: An update. *Contemporary Pediatrics, 15*(8), 95–110.

Silverstein, J. H., & Rosenbloom, A. L. (2000). New developments in type 1 (insulin dependent) diabetes. *Clinical Pediatrics, 39*(5), 257–266.

Skidmore-Roth, L. (2001). *Mosby's handbook of herbs and natural supplements.* St. Louis, MO: Mosby.

Therrell, B. L., Berenbaum, S. A., Manter-Kapanke, V., Simmank, J., Korman, K., Prentice, L., et al. (1998). Results of screening 1.9 million Texas newborns for 21-hydroxylase-deficient congenital adrenal hyperplasia. *Pediatrics, 101*(4), 583–590.

Van Vliet, G. (2001, July 14). Treatment of congenital hypothyroidism. *Lancet, 358*, 86–87.

Willhaus, J. (1999). Growth hormone therapy and children with idiopathic short stature: A viable option? *Pediatric Nursing, 25*(6), 662–665.

Wilson, M. D. (1999). Breast problems. In J. A. McMillan, C. D. DeAngelis, R. D. Feigin, & J. B. Warshaw (Eds.), *Oski's pediatrics: Principles and practice* (3rd ed., pp. 536–539). Philadelphia: Lippincott Williams & Wilkins.

Yule, K. S. (2000). Phenylketonuria. In P. L. Jackson & J. A. Vessey (Eds.), *Primary care of the child with a chronic condition* (3rd ed., pp. 706–731). St. Louis, MO: Mosby.

CHAPTER 52

The Child with Alterations in Skin Integrity

I didn't know that soup could cause such a bad injury. The hardest thing for me to deal with is all the pain Sherray has with each dressing change.

—Mother of Sherray, 6 years old

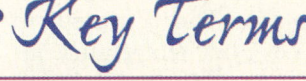

Key Terms

Atopy   *1390*

Autografting   *1406*

Circumferential   *1403*

Debridement   *1385*

Dermatophytoses   *1399*

Eschar   *1405*

Escharotomy   *1405*

Intertriginous   *1388*

Lichenification   *1385*

Melanin   *1412*

Phototoxic   *1395*

Xerosis   *1390*

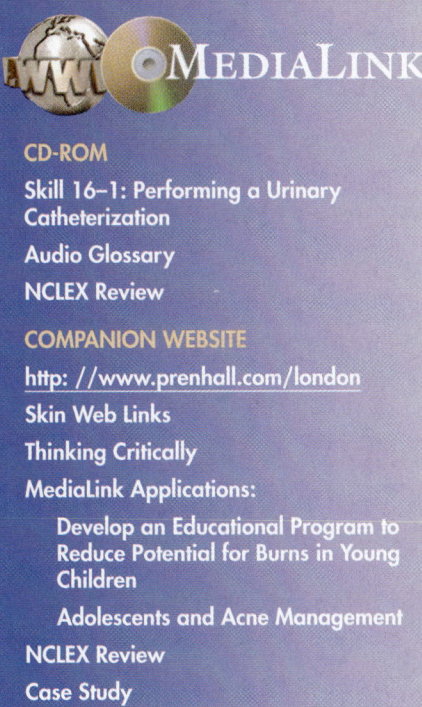

MediaLink

CD-ROM

Skill 16–1: Performing a Urinary Catheterization

Audio Glossary

NCLEX Review

COMPANION WEBSITE

http://www.prenhall.com/london

Skin Web Links

Thinking Critically

MediaLink Applications:

Develop an Educational Program to Reduce Potential for Burns in Young Children

Adolescents and Acne Management

NCLEX Review

Case Study

$\mathcal{T}$he skin is the largest organ in the body. It performs several essential functions, among them perception, protection, temperature regulation, vitamin D synthesis, and excretion. The skin protects underlying tissues from invasion by microorganisms and from trauma. The nerves in the skin enable the perception of pain, heat, and cold.

The body regulates its temperature by dilation or constriction of blood vessels and sweat glands that act under the control of the central nervous system. The skin also supplements the body's intake of vitamin D by synthesizing this vitamin from ultraviolet light. The sweat glands secrete a solution of water, electrolytes, and urea, thus helping to rid the body of toxins.

Nurses who work in outpatient clinics, schools, emergency departments, and pediatric units of hospitals frequently see skin disorders. Many are not unique to children, but children are at greater risk for some skin conditions.

ANATOMY AND PHYSIOLOGY OF PEDIATRIC DIFFERENCES

The skin has three distinct layers: the epidermis, the dermis, and the subcutaneous fatty layer that separates the skin from the underlying tissue (Figure 52–1 ◆). Within the

dermis are nerves, muscles, connective tissue, hair follicles, sebaceous and sweat glands, lymph channels, and blood vessels.

The infant's skin is thin, with little underlying subcutaneous fat. Because of this the infant loses heat more rapidly, has greater difficulty regulating body temperature, and becomes more easily chilled than an older child or an adult. The thinner skin also leads to increased absorption of harmful chemical substances. The infant's skin contains more water than an adult's and has loosely attached cells. As the infant grows, the skin toughens and becomes less hydrated, making it less susceptible to bacteria.

The accessory structures of the skin (hair, sebaceous glands, eccrine glands, and apocrine glands) are present at birth. Like other body structures, however, they are still immature.

Sebaceous glands function at birth, although somewhat immaturely. They vary in size and appear all over the body except on the hands and soles of the feet. Sebum, a lipid substance produced and secreted into the hair follicle or directly onto the skin, lubricates the skin and hair.

Eccrine glands, located in the dermis, open onto the skin surface. They secrete an odorless, watery fluid, primarily in response to emotional stress. They also respond to changes in body temperature. As body temperature in-

FIGURE 52–1. ◆ Layers of the skin with accessory structures.

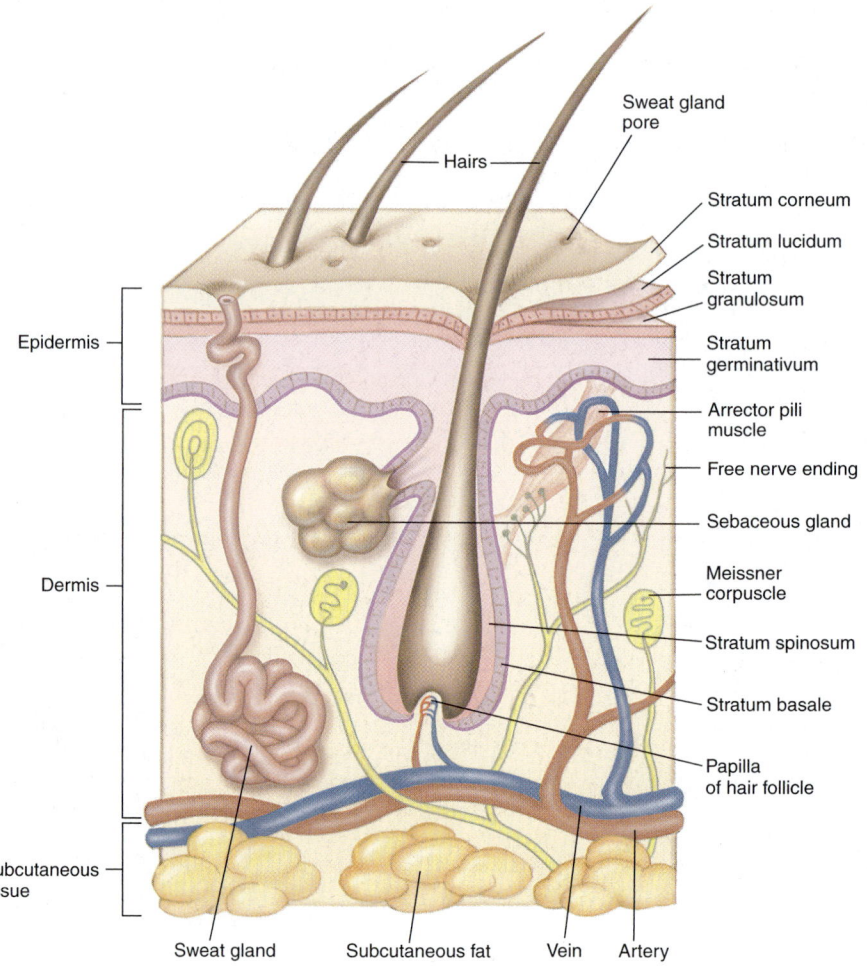

creases, the glands increase production of sweat; its evaporation cools the body. Because the eccrine sweat glands usually are not fully functional until middle childhood, infants and young children cannot regulate temperature as effectively as older children and adults.

Apocrine glands, located mainly in the axillary and genital areas, do not function until puberty. Decomposition of the fluid secreted by these glands leads to body odor. Their biologic function, however, is unknown.

SKIN LESIONS

Skin lesions vary in size, shape, color, and texture characteristics. The two major types of skin lesions are primary lesions and secondary lesions. Primary lesions arise from previously healthy skin and include macules, patches, papules, nodules, tumors, vesicles, pustules, bullae, and wheals (see "Pathophysiology Illustrated" on page 774). Secondary lesions result from changes in primary lesions. They include crusts, scales, **lichenification** (thickening of the skin), scars, keloids, excoriation, fissures, erosion, and ulcers (Table 52–1). It is important for the nurse to be able to identify and describe the primary and secondary skin lesions and understand their underlying cause and treatment.

WOUND HEALING

Wound healing occurs in three overlapping phases: inflammation, reconstruction, and maturation (see "Pathophysiology Illustrated: Phases of Wound Healing") (Rote, 1998; Valencia, Falabella, & Schachner, 2001).

Inflammation, the initial response at the injury site, lasts approximately 3 to 5 days. This phase prepares the injury site for the repair process. The blood coagulates as platelets, red blood cells, and fibrin gather to form a clot. This seals the wound, preventing bacterial invasion and joining the wound edges. Vasodilation, which occurs shortly after injury, allows leukocytes to travel to the injury site, where they ingest bacteria and debris.

Reconstruction or reepithelialization, the second phase, may last from 5 days to 4 weeks, depending on the extent of the injury. Capillary budding to reestablish the blood flow and natural **debridement** (enzyme action to clean the lesion and dissolve the clot or scab) occur. The wound contracts. Fibroblasts multiply, producing collagen and granulation tissue to fill the wound to skin level. A fine layer of epithelial cells forms over the site.

Maturation or remodeling, the third phase, involves continued collagen production for scar production. Although the scar gradually strengthens and devascularizes, it will never be as strong as normal skin. Maturation can take months to years, depending on the extent of the injury.

Complementary Care

COMPLEMENTARY THERAPIES FOR SKIN LESIONS

Condition	Complementary Therapy	Use
Poison ivy	Aloe, calendula, oatmeal (topical)	Relief from itching
Atopic dermatitis	Evening primrose oil (oral)	Decreases excoriations and lichenification
		Decreases need for antihistamines for itching
Accelerated wound healing, burns, abrasions	Aloe vera gel (topical)	Antimicrobial effects, bacteriostatic, bacteriocidal
Skin inflammation	Chamomile (topical)	Wound drying, antimicrobial properties
Acne	5% Tea tree oil (topical)	Antibiotic, decreases open and closed comedones

Note: From Gardner, P., Coles, D., & Kemper, K. J. (2001). The skinny on herbal remedies for dermatologic disorders. *Contemporary Pediatrics, 18*(7), 103–114. Adapted.

TABLE 52–1   Common Secondary Skin Lesions and Associated Conditions

Lesion Name	Description	Example
Crust	Dried residue of serum, pus, or blood	Impetigo
Scale	Thin flake of exfoliated epidermis	Dandruff, psoriasis
Lichenification	Thickening of skin with increased visibility of normal skin furrows	Eczema (atopic dermatitis)
Scar	Replacement of destroyed tissue with fibrous tissue	Healed surgical incision
Keloid	Overdevelopment or hypertrophy of scar that extends beyond wound edges and above skin line due to excess collagen	Healed skin area following traumatic injury
Excoriation	Abrasion or scratch mark	Scratched insect bite
Fissure	Linear crack in skin	Tinea pedis (athlete's foot)
Erosion	Loss of superficial epidermis; moist but does not bleed	Ruptured chickenpox vesicle
Ulcer	Deeper loss of skin surface; bleeding or scarring may ensue	Chancre

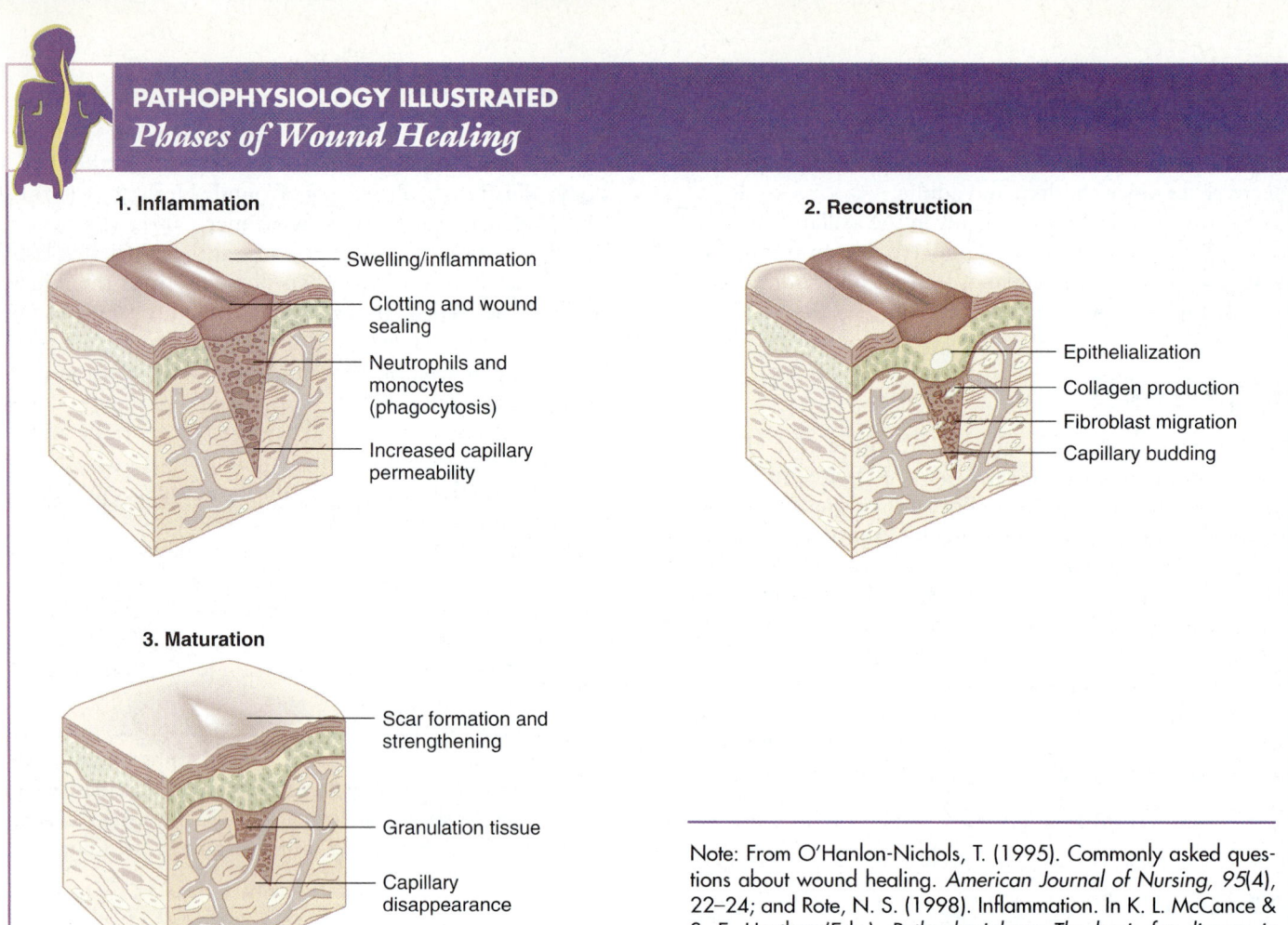

1. Inflammation

Swelling/inflammation
Clotting and wound sealing
Neutrophils and monocytes (phagocytosis)
Increased capillary permeability

2. Reconstruction

Epithelialization
Collagen production
Fibroblast migration
Capillary budding

3. Maturation

Scar formation and strengthening
Granulation tissue
Capillary disappearance

Note: From O'Hanlon-Nichols, T. (1995). Commonly asked questions about wound healing. *American Journal of Nursing, 95*(4), 22–24; and Rote, N. S. (1998). Inflammation. In K. L. McCance & S. E. Huether (Eds.), *Pathophysiology: The basis for disease in adults and children* (3rd ed., pp. 205–236.). St. Louis; MO: Mosby. Adapted.

≈ DERMATITIS

Many skin inflammations occur in early childhood. Most are easily treated and do not have long-term consequences. Dermatitis is a condition in which the skin changes in response to external stimuli. The four most common types of dermatitis in infants, children, and adolescents are contact dermatitis, diaper dermatitis, seborrheic dermatitis, and eczema (atopic dermatitis). It is important to understand that these skin disorders bring emotional problems for the family and child. Be sympathetic and remember that the family and child can see the skin condition and need to be reassured that the child is not infectious.

CONTACT DERMATITIS

Contact dermatitis is an inflammation of the skin that occurs in response to direct contact with an allergen or irritant. Up to 35% of the infant population is affected, most commonly between 9 and 12 months of age (Kazaks & Lane, 2000).

At least 20% of children are at risk for allergic contact dermatitis (Weston & Bruckner, 2000). Generally, repeated exposures or a long-term exposure are required to cause the immune response and the dermatitis. An irritant does not require an immune response. Common allergens include poison ivy, poison oak, lanolin, neomycin, rubber, chemicals in shoe leather, and nickel. Common irritants include soaps, detergents, fabric softeners, bleaches, lotions, urine, and stool. Children may have both irritant and allergic reactions to latex, found in many types of hospital equipment and supplies, as well as in products in the home and community (see Chapter 40).

The rash of allergic contact dermatitis is characterized by erythematous papules with oozing, crusting, pruritis, and edema, and it is usually limited to the area of contact. Symptoms of allergic contact dermatitis can develop within 12 to 72 hours after contact, and can last up to 3 to 4 weeks without treatment. In contrast, irritant contact dermatitis is a discrete area of redness that corresponds to the exposure location. The rash usually develops within a few hours of contact, peaks within 24 hours, and quickly resolves with removal of the irritant.

TABLE 52–2 Distribution of Lesions by Type of Allergen	
Distribution of Lesion	Allergen
Linear	Plant exposure
Ear lobes, neck	Nickel
Dorsal aspects of toes and feet	Rubber or leather chemical in shoes
Face, eyelids	Cosmetics
Subumbilical	Snaps on pants

Note: From Weston, W. L., & Bruckner, A. (2000). Allergic contact dermatitis. *Pediatric Clinics of North America, 47*(4), 897–907. Adapted.

Photodermatitis can result when the child has contact with citrus rinds and juice or fig leaves followed by sun exposure. The child develops erythema and blistering at the site of the exposure that then becomes hyperpigmented. The hyperpigmentation fades over time (Friedlander, 1998).

Sweating and friction enhance the absorption of the allergen or irritant. The distribution of the lesions provides clues about the source and identity of the allergen. See Table 52–2. Treatment involves removing the offending agent (e.g., clothes, plant, soap). Calamine lotion or hydrocortisone cream or ointment can be applied to the affected skin. Cool compresses with aluminum acetate (Burow's solution) promote drying. Colloidal oatmeal soaks relieve itching. Antihistamines may be given for a sedative effect when the child is too irritable to sleep. Reactions to poison ivy covering more than 10% of the body surface area require treatment with oral corticosteroids. See Chapter 47 for information about prednisone. ⊂⊃

Nursing Management

Patient education for home care management focuses on ways to avoid the offending agent and on care of the skin. Advise parents to wash all clothes before the first wearing and to rinse clothes an extra time to remove all the soap. Mild soap should be used to clean the skin. When oatmeal soaks are used, caution parents that the tub will be slippery, and to pat the child dry to leave the oatmeal film in place. Familiarize parents with the symptoms of infection in the affected area (i.e., increased redness, oozing, fever) and tell them when to return for follow-up care.

DIAPER DERMATITIS

Diaper dermatitis, one of the most common causes of irritant contact dermatitis, occurs in approximately one third of young children, usually in a mild form. It is most common in infants from 4 to 12 months of age. Breastfed babies' stools have a lower pH, and this helps reduce their incidence of diaper rash (Kazaks & Lane, 2000).

Diaper dermatitis is a primary reaction to urine, feces, moisture, or friction. Urine and feces interact to cause der-

Teaching About

EXPOSURE TO POISON IVY OR POISON OAK

- React quickly after contact. Wash off sap with soap and water and scrub under the nails.
- Do not rub fingers against broken skin or in eyes.
- Avoid hugging a pet exposed to poison ivy until after it has been bathed.
- Launder clothing worn during exposure, and wash hands after handling exposed clothing.
- Wear vinyl gloves to handle plants (cloth and rubber gloves allow sap to penetrate).
- Search the yard and remove all plants. Do not burn plants removed. A person with a sensitivity may inhale the smoke and develop airway inflammation.

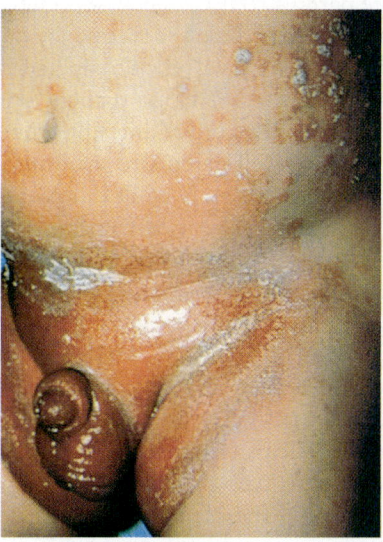

FIGURE 52–2. ◆ Diaper dermatitis. Courtesy of the Centers for Disease Control, Atlanta, GA.

matitis. The urine increases the wetness and pH of the skin, increasing abrasion and its permeability to irritants and microbes. Fecal organisms provide more irritants. *Candida albicans,* a secondary infection, is a common complication of diaper dermatitis or antibiotic therapy for another condition. It is frequently the underlying cause of severe diaper rash. Diaper candidiasis often occurs simultaneously with oral candidiasis (see later discussion).

The rash is characterized by erythema, edema, vesicles, papules, and scaling that appear in areas in direct contact with the diaper. Usually the perineum, genitals, and buttocks are affected, and the skin folds are spared. In severe cases, the infant develops a rash that is fiery red, raised, and confluent. Pustules with tenderness can also be present (Figure 52–2 ◆).

Mild diaper dermatitis is treated with a barrier or protective sealant such as zinc oxide, Desitin, or Balmex. Treatment for moderate or severe diaper dermatitis involves application of low potency (0.25% or 0.5%) hydrocortisone cream with each diaper change for 5 to 7 days and good basic hygiene. The cream must be applied before any protective sealant is used. Diaper candidiasis is treated with alternating applications of 1% hydrocortisone cream and antifungal creams (nystatin) applied to the affected areas at diaper change. An oral antifungal agent may be given to clear the candidiasis from the intestines. Fluorinated topical corticosteroids should not be used because of the higher rate of absorption through damaged skin.

Nursing Management

Severe diaper dermatitis can be a major source of stress for parents who must deal with a child in constant discomfort. Instruct parents to change the diaper as soon as the infant is wet, or at least every 2 hours during the day and once during the night.

Encourage parents to use superabsorbent disposable diapers, which tend to reduce the frequency and severity of diaper dermatitis. When wet, these diapers form a gel that keeps the skin drier than cloth diapers. However, this should not be an excuse for waiting until the diaper is saturated to change it. Tell parents to avoid using tight diapers and waterproof pants. A & D ointment, zinc oxide, Desitin, and Balmex can be used to protect the skin from urine and stool.

Advise parents to wash the perianal area with warm water and a mild soap (such as Dove or Tone) or a cleanser not needing water (Aquanil HC lotion or Cetaphil) only after a bowel movement. If baby wipes are preferred, advise parents to use those without alcohol. Cornstarch or zeaSORB powder helps to decrease friction and moisture, but it is important to keep these powders away from the infant's face. Exposing the diaper area to air helps aid healing; for example, parents could allow the child to go without a diaper while lying on an absorbent pad or cloth. Watch for signs of infection since the skin is damaged and can allow infectious organisms to grow. If this occurs, additional treatment will be needed.

SEBORRHEIC DERMATITIS

Seborrheic dermatitis is a recurrent inflammatory skin condition caused by an overgrowth of *Pityrosporum* yeast, commonly found in areas of sebaceous gland activity (Armsmeier & Paller, 1997). The condition is influenced by hormones and associated with an oily complexion. The rash is found over the areas of the body where the sebaceous glands are most plentiful: scalp (cradle cap), forehead, and postauricular and periorbital areas. It may also occur on the skin of the eyelids, inguinal area, or nasolabial folds. The condition is frequently seen in infants up to 3 months of age and adolescents.

Common symptoms are pruritus and a mildly erythematous, adherent, waxy scaling of the scalp (or "dandruff").

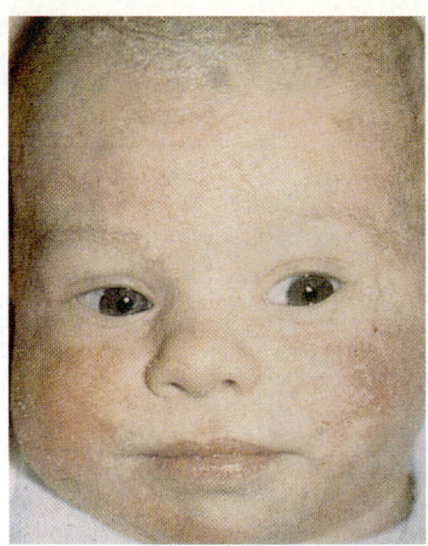

FIGURE 52-3. ◆ Seborrheic dermatitis.

Yellow-red patches with greasy scaling may be present, typically on the scalp and nasolabial folds on the face, behind the ears, on the upper chest, and sometimes on the **intertriginous** (skin folds of the neck, axillae, antecubital fossa) areas (Figure 52-3 ◆).

Treatment for seborrheic dermatitis consists of daily shampooing with a medicated shampoo (e.g., Selsun or Head and Shoulders). An emollient is left on the scalp for about 20 minutes to soften the crusts. The scales are removed by brushing with the fingertips or with a baby hairbrush. The hair is then rinsed thoroughly. Lesions on the body can be treated with shampoos containing selenium sulfide or salicylic acid. Use baby shampoo to wash lesions on the eyelids and eyelashes. Treatments are continued for several days after the lesions disappear. Topical corticosteriods are used to treat seborrhea that is not on the scalp.

Nursing Management

Seborrheic dermatitis in newborns can often be prevented with proper scalp hygiene. Teach new parents to wash the infant's hair regularly with each bath. Reassure parents that gentle cleansing will not harm the infant's "soft spot." Demonstrate bathing to show them the proper technique, if necessary. Follow-up is seldom necessary, as the condition resolves with treatment. Advise adolescents that emotional distress may trigger future flare-ups and to initiate treatment promptly when symptoms begin.

DRUG REACTIONS

Adverse reactions to over-the-counter or prescription medications are relatively common. Children with drug allergies usually have reactions after ingestion (e.g., aspirin, antibiotics, sedatives), injection (e.g., penicillin), or direct skin contact with medications. Drug sensitivities may result from variations in an individual's ability to tolerate a particular drug or concentration of a drug or from allergic responses. (See Chapter 40 for a description of allergic reactions.)

Sensitivity reactions to a drug not previously administered may take up to 7 days to develop. If the child has been sensitized to a drug, the reaction is almost immediate. The most common reactions in children are erythematous macules and papules or urticaria, which may be pruritic. Drugs most likely to cause maculopapular eruptions, urticaria, and pruritis include the following: amoxicillin, ampicillin, cephalosporins, erythromycin, penicillin G, semisynthetic penicillins, sulfamethoxazole, and trimethoprim (Vanderhooft, 1998). Some drug reactions can be life threatening. Be alert to the possibility of serious drug reactions that may become a medical emergency.

The treatment of choice for most drug sensitivity reactions is discontinuation of the causative drug. In some cases, a drug may be continued when the child has a sensitivity reaction because it is the best treatment choice. Supportive measures should be taken to decrease the intensity of the reaction. An antihistamine may be used to block the release of histamine, which causes the rash. Topical corticosteroids, cool compresses, and baths may also be prescribed for pruritis.

Nursing Management

Teach parents to be alert for the signs of drug sensitivity reactions. Obtain a careful history of the child's past reactions to medications before starting new therapies. If a reaction occurs, discontinue the medication until the physician is notified. Children with a true drug allergy (having a past serious systemic reaction) should never be treated with that drug again. Prominently mark the child's records so that all allergies are easily identified. The child should wear a medical alert bracelet.

CLINICAL MANIFESTATIONS ∼ *Drug Reactions*

TYPE OF REACTION	CLINICAL MANIFESTATIONS	CLINICAL THERAPY
Allergic drug reaction	Erythematous macules and papules Pruritus Urticaria, move from one part of body to another	Remove offending drug Topical antipruritics Oral antihistamines Lubricate skin when scaly Systemic corticosteroids if no response to other treatment
Stevens-Johnson syndrome (erythema multiform major) Hypersensitivity reaction to the drug or reaction to an infectious agent	Target lesions coalesce to form large areas of erythema and bullae Fever, malaise Headache, muscle aches, joint pain Itching Cough, coryza, sore throat Vomiting and diarrhea	Remove offending drug Balance intake and output Gentle debridement of crusts Oral antihistamines Topical antipruritics Nutritional support Ophthalmic consultation Corticosteroid use is controversial—may delay wound healing and increase risk of secondary infection or sepsis
Toxic epidermal necrolysis Potential life-threatening hypersensitivity reaction to NSAIDS, sulfa, antibiotics, and anticonvulsants	Rash like Stevens-Johnson syndrome Appearance of tender skin, then bullae or erosions occur over more than 20% of body surface area Full-thickness epidermis peels off in sheets	May be cared for in a burn center, see page 1403 Debridement of blisters may or may not be performed Gentle cleaning with saline or Burow's solution (aluminum acetate) compresses Topical antibiotic ointment Sterile nonadherent dressings Wounds may be covered with biosynthetic dressing Intensive nutritional support Ophthalmic consultation No corticosteroids No creams with sulfa as this may be cause of original toxicity
Erythema multiform Hypersensitivity reaction to anticonvulsants, penicillins, salicylates, and sulfa antibiotics	Fixed annular erythematous papules and placques Target lesions with dusky centers, may become bullae Edema	Remove offending drug Oral antihistamines Topical antipruritics Use of corticosteroids is controversial

Note: From Vanderhooft, S. L. (1998). Is the rash really an adverse drug reaction? *Contemporary Pediatrics, 15*(5), 118–137; and Valencia, I. C., Falabela, A. F., & Schachner, L. A. (2001). New developments in wound care for infants and children. *Pediatric Annals, 30*(4), 211–218. Adapted.

ECZEMA (ATOPIC DERMATITIS)

Eczema, also called atopic dermatitis, is a chronic, superficial inflammatory skin disorder characterized by intense pruritus. The condition affects infants, children, and adolescents. It is common, and is believed to affect 10% of children. Up to 75% of children who develop the condition do so during the first 6 months of life, and most of the remainder who have the condition develop it by 5 years of age (Nicol, 2000). An increasing prevalence has been noted in developed countries that also exhibit an increased rate of asthma, demonstrating the allergic tendency for this condition (Raimer, 2000).

Etiology and Pathophysiology

The etiology of eczema is unknown, but the disorder tends to occur in children with hereditary allergic tendencies (**atopy.**) If one parent has allergies (e.g., hay fever, asthma, or contact dermatitis), the child has a 60% greater chance of having allergies. This increases to 80% if both parents have allergies (Nicol, 2000). A family history of asthma or hay fever frequently predisposes a child to eczema. Infantile eczema is more likely to be food induced when the condition is severe (Hebert, Rakes, Loach, et al., 1997). Several factors exacerbate the condition: triggers (house mites, animal dander, pollens), food allergies, irritants (soaps, detergents, chemicals, solvents, abrasive clothing), hormonal changes, and emotional stress. Increased IgE levels are found in 80% to 85% of patients (Nicol, 2000). See Chapter 40 for a discussion of IgE.

Children with eczema have **xerosis,** generally dry skin that is more likely to crack and fissure. The barrier function of the skin is impaired leading to increased water loss from the epidermis and decreased elasticity. When the skin is chronically dry, irritants have a greater chance to penetrate, and the child is more susceptible to infection.

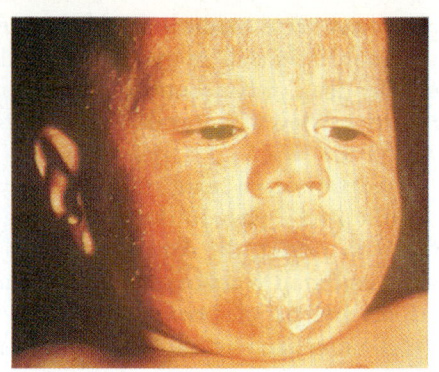

FIGURE 52–4. ◆ Chronic eczema.

Clinical Manifestations

Acute eczema is characterized by pruritus and erythematous patches with vesicles, exudate, and crusts (Figure 52–4 ◆). Subacute eczema is characterized by scaling with erythema and excoriation. There are often postinflammatory pigment changes. Symptoms of chronic eczema are pruritus, dryness, scaling, and lichenification (thickening of the skin with increased visibility of normal skin furrows). Inflammation usually occurs on the face, upper arms, back, upper thighs, and back of the hands and feet.

Eczema occurs in three forms: infantile (ages 2 months to 2 years), childhood (ages 2 years to puberty), and adolescent.

Clinical Therapy

Eczema is more likely than other types of dermatitis to have a generalized distribution with no known exposure to an allergen. Eczema is distinguished from other forms of dermatitis by its history and clinical manifestations. No laboratory tests are diagnostic. Diagnostic criteria for eczema include an itching skin condition with three of these factors:

CLINICAL MANIFESTATIONS ⪡ *Eczema*

TYPE	CLINICAL MANIFESTATIONS	OUTCOME
Infantile (2 months to 2 years)	Exudative, crusty, papulovesicular, and erythematous lesions on cheeks, scalp, forehead, neck, trunk, and extensor surfaces of extremities Intensely pruritic Lichenification after the child can scratch at about 2 months of age	50% of cases resolve by age 2 to 3 years
Childhood (2 years to puberty)	Erythematous, dry, scaly, well-circumscribed, papular, more thickened and lichenified lesions on flexor surfaces of extremities, neck, and retroauricular folds	Subacute and chronic 75% of cases have no recurrence after adolescence
Adolescent (puberty and onward)	Much the same as childhood eczema Large plaques thickened and lichenified on face, neck, back, hands, feet, and upper arms	May recur often as it is more often a chronic inflammation

- History of flexural dermatitis (knees, ankles, neck, or cheeks) if less than 4 years old
- History of asthma or hay fever in a child, or in a first-degree relative if less than 4 years old
- History of dry skin in past year
- Skin rash occurring before 2 years of age
- Visible flexural dermatitis; dermatitis on cheeks, forehead, and outer limbs if less than 4 years old (Raimer, 2000)

As there is no cure, the goals of treatment are to hydrate and lubricate the skin, reduce pruritus, minimize inflammatory changes, and try to determine what triggers flare-ups. The cardinal principle of topical therapy for oozing or weeping is "wet on wet." If lesions are weeping, wet compresses (cotton cloths) soaked in aluminum acetate solution sometimes are used. Applying occlusive topical ointment after bathing traps moisture, provides lubrication, and prevents drying of the skin. Moisturizing ointments and creams to use for eczema include Eucerin cream, Aquaphor ointment, Vanicream, Cetaphil cream, SBR-Lipocream, and white petrolatum. Moisturizing ointments and creams should be applied 3 to 4 times a day or whenever the skin feels dry.

Topical corticosteroids reduce inflammation. Ointments are preferred over creams because of their occlusive effect, which ensures a stronger barrier and absorption into the skin. Hydrocortisone 1% to 2.5% or triamcinolone 0.1% is usually the drug of choice. Newer corticosteroid ointments such as fluticasone propionate bind better with the glucocorticoid receptor, maximizing the ointment's penetration and its anti-inflammatory properties. They also have fewer adverse effects (Nicol, 2000). Corticosteroids are used two times daily for 2 weeks and must be applied before the skin moisturizer is used. Lower potency ointments are used for thinner skin areas, such as the face and skin folds. A more potent ointment is used for flare-ups, with tapering to lower potency as the dermatitis improves. When the dermatitis resolves, only moisturizers are used. Steroids are not used on healthy skin. Oral corticosteroids may be used for an acute exacerbation; however, there is often a rebound effect (i.e., after the medication is discontinued, the rash returns). Systemic antibiotics are given only if the child has a superimposed infection.

Antihistamine agents such as hydroxyzine (Vistaril and Atarax) can be given to relieve itching at night. Nonsedating antihistamine agents have a limited effect on itching. Methods to reduce pruritus include environmental controls, such as humidification in the winter and air conditioning in the summer. A humidifier counteracts dryness of the surrounding air, minimizing loss of skin moisture. Air conditioning limits unnecessary sweating that can exacerbate inflamed areas.

Because food allergies are common in infants under 2 years of age, a food elimination test may be suggested for infants and young children with moderate to severe eczema needing daily treatment. Milk, wheat, eggs, soy products, citrus, and peanuts are the foods most often withheld for 2 or more weeks to determine if any change in skin condition occurs. Foods withheld are then introduced one at a time to determine which ones are the allergens. A RAST (radioallergosorbent) test is sometimes used to exclude allergens (see Chapter 40).

Nursing Management

Nursing Assessment and Diagnosis

Take a thorough history, including any family history of allergy, environmental or dietary factors, and past exacerbations. Note distribution and type of lesions.

Common nursing diagnoses that may be appropriate for the child with eczema include:

▶ *Impaired tissue integrity* related to chemical irritants and mechanical factors (abrasive clothing)
▶ *Sleep deprivation* related to prolonged physical discomfort (itching)
▶ *Risk for infection* related to breaks in skin barrier
▶ *Self-esteem disturbance* related to chronic illness and peer reaction to visible skin lesions
▶ *Ineffective management of therapeutic regimen (families)* related to excessive demands made on the family to keep the condition under control

Planning and Implementation

Nursing management focuses on education and emotional support. Although it has no "cure," eczema can be controlled. Advise parents that the lesions are not contagious and will not result in scarring. Help parents and adolescents deal with the frustration of the acute flare-ups of the condition by reinforcing that remissions do occur with good home care.

Teach parents or adolescents to avoid using harsh or perfumed soaps. Use a mild soap (e.g., Dove or Tone), but only where the skin is dirty. Washing clean skin with soap only dries it out. Use wet wraps for severely affected skin to give moisture back to the skin. Hot water can exacerbate the condition and increase itching. Recommend tepid baths and patting dry or air-drying afterward. Moisturizers should be applied within 3 minutes of exiting the bath to help retain moisture, once or twice daily. Wool clothing should be avoided because it can increase skin irritation and pruritus. Encourage loose cotton clothing.

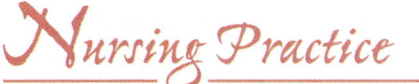

Nursing Practice

Wet occlusive dressings increase penetration of corticosteroid ointments, and also help decrease itching. Apply the topical ointment and then wrap the child in a wet towel for 10 minutes, then reapply the topical ointment followed by an emollient (Raimer, 2000).

Teach parents and adolescents how to apply topical ointments or creams. Topical corticosteroids should not be used in the periorbital area; posterior cataracts are a side effect. Instruct parents to place clean cotton gloves or socks over the infant or young child's hands and to keep the child's fingernails cut short to decrease scratching and reduce the chance of secondary infection.

Complementary Care

MASSAGE THERAPY FOR ATOPIC DERMATITIS

A study of the effectiveness of massage in treating eczema showed a benefit for the child and parent. Daily massage of the child for 20 minutes over 1 month resulted in improvements in redness, scaling, lichenification, excoriation, and pruritus. The child's activity level and disposition also improved. Parents doing the massage reported decreased anxiety (Schachner, Field, Hernandez-Ruif, et al., 1998).

Eczema produces visible changes that can affect a child's self-confidence and self-esteem. Children need to be educated about the disorder and its treatment. Emphasize the importance of following the treatment plan to promote healing of existing lesions and to reduce the risk of secondary infections. Eczema that is difficult to manage is more stressful and has a more profound effect on the child's and family's quality of life than diabetes mellitus (Su, Kemp, & Varigos, 1997).

Once the condition is under control, counsel the parents about how to introduce a food that was previously eliminated when an allergen cause of eczema was suspected (see Chapter 40). ⊂⊃ Emphasize that increased itching within hours of eating a food may be associated with the eczema flare-up. Teach parents how to control the skin inflammation that results, as described earlier. Once a specific food allergy has been identified, refer the parents to a nutritionist for counseling about alternative food options that will fulfill daily nutritional requirements. Tell parents that food allergies can change, so foods connected with eczema can sometimes be safely eaten later in life. Different food sensitivities may also develop. Refer the family to the Food Allergy Network. ⊂⊃ WEB

Evaluation

Expected outcomes of nursing care include the following:

▶ Control of the child's eczema is maintained and no infection occurs.

▶ Parents identify triggers of the child's eczema and avoid or eliminate them.

▶ The child's sleep is minimally disturbed by itching.

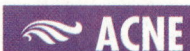

ACNE

Acne is an inflammatory disorder of the sebaceous hair follicles on the face and trunk. It is the most common skin disorder in the pediatric population. It is triggered by the increased androgen production of puberty and the overproduction of sebum. The prevalence in adolescents aged 12 to 15 years is estimated to approach 85% (Sidbury & Paller, 2000). The condition is often more severe in the winter. Acne may also occur in neonates in response to maternal androgen hormones. This form of acne usually develops between 2 and 4 weeks of age and resolves by 4 to 6 months of age.

Etiology and Pathophysiology

Acne is caused by the interaction of several factors: an overgrowth of residential bacteria on the skin, increased sebum production, and abnormal follicular shedding of skin cells that are more adherent than normal. The extra sebum caused by androgen secretion mixes with the shed skin cells and causes them to clump together. The keratin and sebum that usually flow to the skin surface are obstructed in the follicular canal, causing comedones (whiteheads and blackheads). The sebum behind the comedo is an ideal environment for the anerobic *Propionibacterium acnes*, and this bacterium metabolizes the sebum, causing an inflammatory reaction. When the inflammatory reaction is close to the surface, a papule or pustule develops. If the inflammatory reaction is deeper, a larger papule or nodule develops. Although acne follows familial trends, hard data to define a pattern of inheritance are not conclusive. Medications associated with the appearance of acne lesions include corticosteroids, barbiturates, phenytoin, lithium, isoniazid, and cyclosporin.

Clinical Manifestations

There are three main types of acne: comedomal (characterized by open and closed comedones), papulopustular (characterized by papules and pustules) (Figure 52–5 ◆), and cystic (characterized by nodules and cysts). Lesions occur most often on the face, upper chest, shoulders, and back.

Clinical Therapy

Diagnosis is based upon the examination of the skin. The severity of skin lesions is graded, and treatment is customized to the severity level. See Table 52–3.

Treatment depends on the type of lesion. Most adolescent acne is treated with topical and oral medications, alone or in combination. The goal of treatment is to suppress lesions until the condition is outgrown, thus preventing infection and scarring, and minimizing psychologic distress. Increasing numbers of cases of bacterial resistance

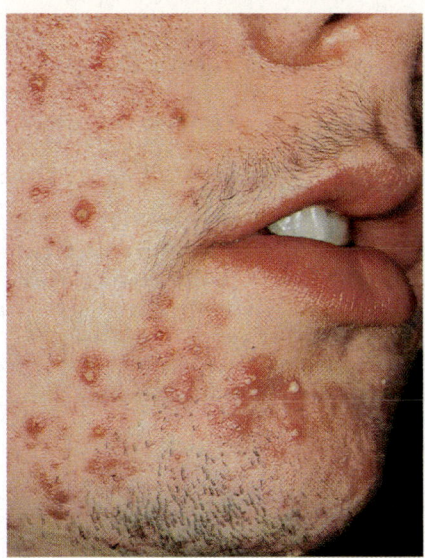

FIGURE 52–5. ◆ Pustular acne can have a significant effect on an adolescent's self-esteem. *Note:* From Habif, T. P. (1990). *Clinical dermatology: A color guide to diagnosis and therapy* (2nd ed., p. 113). St. Louis, MO: Mosby-Year Book.

TABLE 52–3	Treatment Protocols for Acne
Appearance	*Treatment*
Grade I Comedonal acne (comedones only)	Tretinoin (Retin-A) 0.025% cream daily, in the evening, salicylic acid, adapalene, tazarotene
Grade II Papulopustular acne (red papules, pustules)	2.5% benzoyl peroxide gel, Tretinoin (Retin-A) in evening, topical clindamycin and erythromycin, topical tetracycline, azaleic acid cream twice a day
Grade III Cystic acne (red papules, many pustules, cysts)	Tretinoin (Retin-A) and benzoyl peroxide twice a day, with oral antibiotics (tetracycline, minocycline, or doxycycline)
Grade IV Pustulocystic nodular (severe, resistant to other treatment)	Isotretinoin (Accutane)

Note: From Sidbury, R., & Paller, A. S. (2000). The diagnosis and management of acne. *Pediatric Annals, 29*(1), 17–24. Adapted.

to antibiotics have been noted. A recurrence or flare-up of acne after it has been controlled may indicate that the bacteria have developed resistance to the antibiotic.

Gels and liquids are prescribed to dry the skin, and dryness and scaling are typical after several days of treatment. The condition may appear to worsen for the first 1 to 3 weeks of treatment (Sidbury, 2000).

Isotretinoin (Accutane) is reserved for the most serious cases of acne because of its teratogenicity. Patients started

on isotretinoin need two negative pregnancy tests and a monthly pregnancy test. A one-month supply is provided to promote compliance with testing. In addition, two forms of contraception must be used when taking isotretinoin (Buck, 2001). A recent study examining the association between isotretinoin (Accutane) and mental health problems found no increased risk for depression, suicide, or other psychologic problems (Jick, Kremers, & Vasilakis-Scaramozza, 2000).

Oral contraceptives with norgestimate and ethinyl estradiol are FDA approved for the treatment of acne (Sidbury & Paller, 2000).

Nursing Management

Nursing Assessment and Diagnosis

Physical assessment should include documentation regarding distribution, type, and severity of acne lesions. Assess the adolescent's and parents' knowledge about the cause and treatment of acne. Also explore the amount of emotional distress the acne is causing the adolescent.

Common nursing diagnoses are presented in "Nursing Care Plan: The Adolescent with Acne."

Planning and Implementation

Nursing care for the adolescent with acne is summarized in the accompanying "Nursing Care Plan." Nursing management focuses on educating the child and parents about acne and its treatment. Advise adolescents not to touch the affected areas and to avoid picking or squeezing the lesions. Remind them that the inflammation occurs with the rupture of lesions below the skin surface, which picking and squeezing may cause. In addition, advise them to avoid using any cleansing products that have a greasy base, to shampoo hair regularly (to treat seborrhea that can accompany acne), to expect flare-ups despite treatment, and to eat a well-balanced diet.

Teaching About

CARING FOR ACNE

- Avoid picking and squeezing pimples.
- Avoid hats or gear that can cause friction and occlusion of the skin.
- Greasy foods may leave a residual oil on the face and hands that can be occlusive.
- Avoid touching the face.
- Limit the use of pomades or petrolatum-based hair products.
- Use noncomedonic sunscreen and emollients for the skin.
- Use oil-free or water-based makeup.
- Use sunscreen even on cloudy days.

GOAL	INTERVENTION	RATIONALE	EXPECTED OUTCOME
1. Management of therapeutic regimen: individual, effective			
	NIC Priority Intervention: **Anticipatory guidance:** *Preparation of patient for an anticipated developmental and/or situational crisis*		*NOC Suggested Outcome:* **Symptom control behavior:** *Personal actions to minimize perceived adverse changes in physical and emotional functioning*
The adolescent will verbalize proper hygiene, nutrition, and treatment of acne.	▶ Teach good skin care: 　▶ Wash skin with mild soap and water twice a day. 　▶ Do not use astringents. 　▶ Avoid vigorous scrubbing. ▶ Praise good habits. ▶ Advise the adolescent to wash hair with antiseborrheic shampoo, avoid oil-based cosmetics or lotions. ▶ Encourage a balanced diet, adequate fluids, exercise, and adequate rest. ▶ Encourage the adolescent to keep a diary of health and diet habits.	▶ Good hygiene and appropriate skin care reduce surface oils and bacteria, which intensify inflammatory reactions. ▶ Positive reinforcement encourages continued effort. ▶ Treats seborrhea, which frequently accompanies acne. Oil-based preparations can obstruct sebaceous glands, exacerbating acne. ▶ Adequate nutrients, water, and exercise promote healthy skin. ▶ A record may help identify associations with flare-ups that can be avoided in the future.	The adolescent exhibits good hygiene habits.
The adolescent will verbalize understanding of treatment regimen.	▶ Educate the adolescent about medications (action, side effects, dosage, method of application). ▶ Encourage application of tretinoin at night. Encourage use of nonoil sunscreens of at least SPF 15. ▶ Educate the adolescent about time needed for response and importance of daily compliance.	▶ Proper application of medication enhances healing of lesions. ▶ Helps reduce sensitivity to sun and avoid sunburn. ▶ May take up to 3 months for significant improvement to occur. The adolescent needs a reason to continue with the care plan.	The adolescent implements the treatment regimen as outlined, resulting in a noticeable reduction in lesions.
2. Body image disturbance related to biophysical factors (visible facial lesions)			
	NIC Priority Intervention: **Body image enhancement:** *Improving a patient's conscious and unconscious perceptions and attitudes toward his/her body*		*NOC Suggested Outcome:* **Self-esteem:** *Personal judgment of self-worth*
The adolescent will demonstrate increased self-confidence and self-esteem.	▶ Establish a rapport with the adolescent. ▶ Provide education about the condition and therapy modalities. ▶ Encourage the adolescent to be responsible for treatment and follow-up, and give positive reinforcement. ▶ Encourage the adolescent to become involved with school activities and peers.	▶ A trusting relationship promotes verbalization of concerns and fears. ▶ Providing information better enables the adolescent to take control of the condition. ▶ Responsibility reinforces sense of self-esteem. ▶ Involvement in activities helps enhance self-esteem and allows the adolescent to explore new experiences and friendships.	The adolescent freely discusses concerns and fears. The adolescent demonstrates active involvement in own care. The adolescent shows increased confidence, as demonstrated by involvement in extracurricular activities.

Tell adolescents to wash the face no more than two to three times a day with a mild soap, then wait about 20 to 30 minutes before applying tretinoin (Retin-A), if prescribed. Topical medications should be spread in a thin film over the skin, according to directions. Emphasize that treatment is often long term. Significant improvement may not be seen until at least 6 to 12 weeks after the start of treatment.

Correct misconceptions about dietary causes. Although no food has been found to cause acne or an increase in severity of lesions, good nutrition is important. Teach parents and children that increased sweating, as well as heat and humidity, may exacerbate acne. Emotional stress may increase adrenal androgen production, resulting in increased sebum production and acne flare-ups.

Caution patients using tretinoin that this medication is **phototoxic** (a rapid nonimmunologic reaction of the skin when exposed to sunlight), resulting in sunburn with even minimal exposure. Teach correct procedures for taking other prescribed drugs, such as tetracycline and isotretinoin (Accutane), and discuss possible side effects. Emphasize the importance of return visits to the adolescent's health care provider to monitor medication side effects. WEB

Psychologic support is an important aspect of care. Because adolescents are preoccupied with their body image and peer relationships, they often find having acne embarrassing. Encourage them to express their feelings and refer for counseling, if necessary.

Evaluation

Expected outcomes of nursing care can be found in "Nursing Care Plan: The Adolescent with Acne."

INFECTIOUS DISORDERS

IMPETIGO

Impetigo is a highly contagious, superficial (epidermal) infection caused by streptococci, staphylococci, or both. The most common sites are the face, around the mouth, the hands, the neck, and the extremities. It is the most common bacterial skin condition in children and accounts for nearly 10% of all skin problems (Darmstadt, 1997).

Minor skin abrasions, lacerations, insect bites, burns, and dermatitis provide the portal for the infectious agent commonly present in the environment. *Group A beta-hemolytic streptococcus* and *Staphylococcus aureus* are usually responsible. This infection occurs more commonly in children who are in close physical contact with others, such as in child care settings, or who have poor hygiene.

Clinical manifestations include a lesion, pruritus, and regional lymphadenopathy. There is little erythema. The lesion begins as a vesicle or pustule surrounded by edema

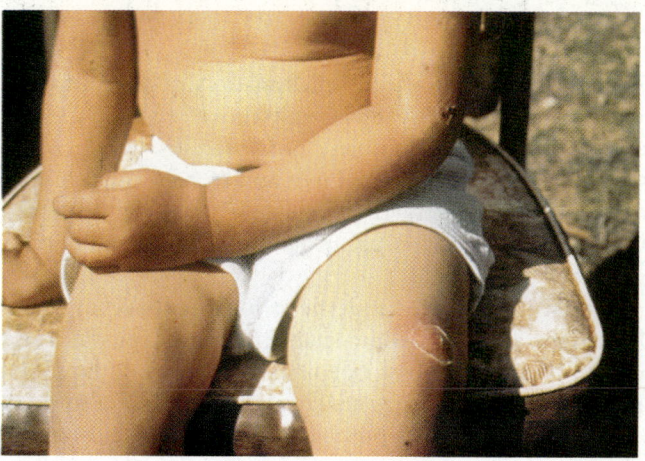

FIGURE 52–6. ◆ Characteristic lesions of impetigo. Courtesy of the Centers for Disease Control, Atlanta, GA.

and redness, usually at a site that has been injured. This progresses to an exudative and crusting stage. The initially serous vesicular fluid becomes cloudy, and the vesicle ruptures, leaving a honey-colored crust covering an ulcerated base (Figure 52–6 ◆). Common sites include the intertriginous areas, skinfolds such as in the neck, axillae, or diaper area. The rash may spread to the face and extremities by self-innoculation. Bullous impetigo, in which the vesicles enlarge into bullae with straw-colored fluid and then rupture, is less common. A moist, erythematous erosion with a collar of skin around the erosion is seen in this localized scalded skin syndrome.

Impetigo is diagnosed by a Gram stain and bacterial culture. Local treatment involves removal of the crusts and application of a topical antibiotic. Crusts are soaked in warm water and gently scrubbed off with an antiseptic soap. A topical bactericidal ointment (such as bacitracin, or mupirocin) is applied for 5 to 7 days. If there is no response to topical antibiotics, a systemic antibiotic (e.g., dicloxacillin or erythromycin) may be needed. The infection is communicable for 48 hours after antibiotic ointment treatment is begun.

If the child has a history of recurrent impetigo, determine if a person in contact with the child is a nasal carrier of *Staphylococcus aureus*. The carrier can be effectively treated with topical mupirocin ointment applied to the nares four times daily (Mancini, 2000).

Nursing Management

Advise parents that they must continue oral or topical medications for the full number of days prescribed. Tell the parents to observe all close contacts and family members for lesions. Caution them that an infected child should not share towels or toiletries with others and that all linens and clothing used by the child should be washed separately with detergent in hot water. Fingernails should be kept short and clean to prevent spreading infection by scratching. Inform the child's child care center about the infection, so staff can sanitize toys and surfaces.

FOLLICULITIS

Folliculitis is a superficial inflammation of the pilosebaceous follicle caused by infection, trauma, or irritation. The causative organism is usually *Staphylococcus aureus*. The condition is common in children and teenagers because of increased sweat production. Folliculitis may be associated with *Pseudomonas* exposure in a poorly chlorinated pool or hot tub.

Symptoms include tenderness, localized swelling, and the formation of tiny dome-shaped, yellowish pustules and red papules at follicular openings with surrounding erythema. Individual lesions may become deeper and form an abscess (furuncle). Lesions are usually seen in clusters on the face, scalp, trunk, and extremities. Ruptured lesions heal with hyperpigmentation and no scarring.

Treatment of inflamed follicles consists of washing the affected area with a topical antibiotic cleanser and water, followed by application of hot compresses for 20 minutes, four times a day. Complications are rare. If lesions do not resolve within a week, the child may need systemic antibiotics (e.g., cephalexin or dicloxacillin) and, if the infection is deep, incision and drainage.

Nursing Management

Nursing management focuses on educating the parents and child about prevention. Advise children to shower daily and shortly after exercise, to cleanse with an antibacterial soap, and to wear loose cotton clothing.

CELLULITIS

Cellulitis is an acute inflammation of the dermis and underlying connective tissue characterized by red or lilac, tender, warm, edematous skin that may have an ill-defined, nonelevated border. The condition usually occurs on the face and extremities as a result of trauma or a compromised skin barrier.

Etiology and Pathophysiology

Children with cellulitis often have a history of trauma, impetigo, folliculitis, or recent otitis media. Common causative organisms are *Staphylococcus aureus, Streptococcus pneumoniae, Haemophilus influenzae,* and beta-hemolytic and group A *streptococcus*. The condition may also result from a nearby abscess or sinusitis. Onset is usually rapid.

Clinical Manifestations

Children with cellulitis have a rapid onset and they appear ill. Classic signs and symptoms include erythema, edema of the face or infected limb, warmth, and tenderness around the infected site (Figure 52–7 ◆). Other symptoms include fever, chills, malaise, and enlargement and tenderness of regional lymph nodes. In some cases, a rapidly progressive lesion may result in septicemia.

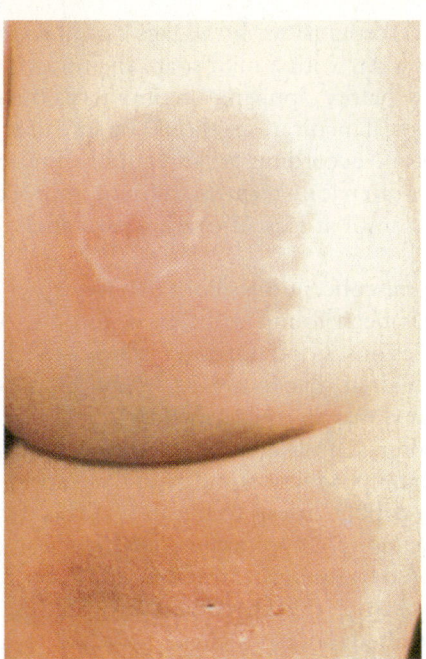

FIGURE 52–7. ◆ Characteristic appearance of cellulitis. *Note:* From Ben-Amitai, D., & Ashkenazi, S. (1993). Common bacterial skin infections in children. *Pediatric Annals, 22*(4), 226. Photograph courtesy of Dr. Aryeh Metzker.

Clinical Therapy

Blood studies may show an increase in white blood cells. Cultures are taken by needle aspiration, if possible, to identify the causative organisms. Blood cultures are taken if the child has a toxic (very ill) appearance (see Skill 10–5). **SKILLS** If the face is involved, antibiotic therapy is administered to avoid serious complications. (Periorbital cellulitis is discussed in Chapter 48.)

Children with cellulitis on the trunk, limbs, or perianal area may be treated on an outpatient basis with oral antibiotics. Recovery begins within 48 hours, but therapy should continue for at least 10 days.

Children with severe cases or a large affected surface area are hospitalized to prevent sepsis. They receive systemic antibiotics and analgesics. Untreated cellulitis or cellulitis that does not respond to treatment can lead to osteomyelitis, arthritis, or serious systemic infection.

Nursing Management

Nursing Assessment and Diagnosis

Assessment centers on recognition of infection, documentation of location and related symptoms, and monitoring of vital signs.

Among the nursing diagnoses that may be appropriate for the child with cellulitis are:

▶ *Impaired skin integrity* related to mechanical factors (injury, the inflammatory process, and presence of infection)

- *Pain* related to injury agents (swelling and inflammation of the skin)
- *Parental role conflict* related to home care needs of child with special needs

Planning and Implementation

Because of the risk of sepsis, manage cellulitis carefully. Administer prescribed antibiotics. Supportive care includes warm compresses to the affected area four times daily, elevation of the affected limb, and bed rest. Outpatient follow-up is crucial.

Advise parents about possible complications, such as abscess formation. Instruct parents of children treated at home to contact their health care provider if the child has any of the following signs:

- Spread of the infected area in the 24- to 48-hour period after the start of treatment
- Temperature over 38.3 °C (101 °F)
- Increased lethargy

Reinforce to parents the importance of compliance with the treatment regimen and the seriousness of the possible complications.

Evaluation

Expected outcomes of nursing care include pain control, compliance with administration of antibiotics, and resolution of the infection without progression to systemic infection.

PEDICULOSIS CAPITIS (LICE)

Pediculosis capitis is an infestation of the hair and scalp with lice. Head lice live and reproduce only on humans and are transmitted by direct hair-to-hair contact or indirect contact such as sharing of hair accessories, brushes, hats, towels, and bedding. Lice do not fly or jump, but they can crawl quickly. The female louse lays her eggs (nits) on the hair shaft, close to the scalp (see Figure 33–5). The incubation period is 8 to 10 days. Children between 3 and 10 years of age are most often affected.

Infestation occurs among children of all socioeconomic levels. Parents or teachers may be the first to notice lice, or health care providers may spot them during routine examination (see Chapter 33). Outbreaks occur periodically among preschool and school-age children, particularly those in day care and elementary school.

Clinical manifestations include intense pruritus and complaints of "dandruff" that sticks to the hair (actually the nits) and "bugs" in the hair. Nits look like silvery white 1-mm teardrops adhering to one side of the hair shaft. Secondary effects of scratching include inflammation, pustules, and bacterial infection. Nits are found most commonly behind the ears and at the base of the head. Lice move quickly away from light and are not commonly seen. Posterior cervical nodes are frequently palpable.

Treatment involves a pediculicide shampoo, such as pyrethrum with an enzymatic lice egg remover, or an ovicidal rinse, such as permethrin (Nix). Permethrin resistance has been reported, but a 5% concentration is effective. An alternate therapy is malathion (Ovide); however, it is flammable, smells bad, and costs more. Lindane shampoo is not recommended because of lice resistance and toxicity (Angel, Nigro, & Levy, 2000).

Permethrin cream rinse is applied to washed and towel-dried hair. The preparation is applied, left in place for 10 minutes, and then rinsed. The hair is towel dried, and the nits are removed with a fine-toothed comb. Distilled white vinegar or an over-the-counter formic acid solution helps loosen the nit's bond to the hair shaft. A second treatment is needed in 7 days.

Nursing Management

Carefully assess children who have been exposed to head lice (see Chapter 33). To avoid potential reinfestation of other children, change gloves frequently when assessing several children in a classroom setting.

Infestation with lice can be upsetting for both the child and family. Emphasize to the family that anyone can get lice. Thorough interventions and education are essential for effective treatment. **WEB** All contacts of the child should be examined for infestation and should be treated as necessary. Tell parents that children infested with lice should not return to day care or school until after the first pediculicide treatment is completed. Teach the child not to share clothing, headwear, or combs.

Explain to parents that the shampoo and rinses prescribed are pesticides and must be used as directed. Keep these products out of the eyes and mouth of the child during their use. When combing the hair to remove nits, a creme rinse or oil may make combing easier. Comb 1–inch sections from the scalp outward and pin these out of the way when done. All nits should be removed. Put the child under a bright light and use distractions such as a video to keep the child entertained during the procedure.

Although lice can survive for only about 3 days away from a human host, shed nits may hatch 8 to 10 days later. For this reason, the child's bedding and clothing should be changed daily, laundered in hot water with detergent, and dried in a hot dryer for 20 minutes. Nonessential bedding and clothing can be stored in a tightly sealed bag for 2 to 3 weeks and then washed. Hair accessories, brushes, and combs should be discarded or soaked in hot soapy water (54.4 °C [130 °F]). Vacuum furniture and carpets and treat them with a hot iron when possible. Use of an insecticide in the home to kill the lice on carpets, furniture, and other items with which young children and pets come into contact is not recommended. Seal toys and other personal items that cannot be washed or dry cleaned in a plastic bag for 2 weeks.

SCABIES

Scabies is a highly contagious infestation caused by the mite *Sarcoptes scabiei*. It is spread by skin-to-skin contact. Children of all ages and both sexes can be affected. The highest prevalence is in children under 2 years of age (Angel et al., 2000).

The female mite burrows into the outer layer of the epidermis (stratum corneum) to lay her eggs, leaving a trail of debris and feces. The larvae hatch in approximately 2 to 4 days and proceed toward the surface of the skin. The cycle is repeated 14 to 17 days later. Hypersensitivity to the ova and mite feces causes irritation and intense pruritus approximately 1 month after infestation. Nodules, which can persist for weeks after effective treatment, develop as a granulomatous response to the dead mite antigens and feces. Because the mite usually takes at least 45 minutes to burrow into the skin, transient contact is unlikely to cause infestation.

Symptoms include a rash with various types of lesions, severe pruritus that worsens at night, and restlessness. Lesions are usually located in the webs of the fingers, in the intergluteal folds, around the axillae, or on the palms, wrists, head, neck, legs, buttocks, chest, abdomen, and waist (Figure 52–8 ◆). In infants the palms, insteps of the feet, and scalp and face can be affected. Lesions appear as linear, threadlike, grayish burrows 1 to 10 cm in length, which may end in a pinpoint vesicle. The lesion may have been obliterated by the child's scratching and secondary infection.

Diagnosis is confirmed by examination under the microscope of scrapings from a burrow, which reveals ac-

tively moving mites, fecal pellets, eggs, or nits. Treatment involves application of a scabicide, such as 5% permethrin lotion, over the entire body from the chin down. Lindane is no longer recommended for full-body application in infants and young children because of toxicity (Angel et al., 2000). Apply scabicide only to the scalp and forehead of infants. The lotion can be applied to the face of older children if lesions are present. Precipitated sulfur in petrolatum for three successive nights is used to treat scabies in infants under 2 months of age who should not be exposed to the more toxic scabicide lotions (Metry & Hebert, 2000). It is malodorous and messy and stains the bedding and clothing, so parents do not like using it.

Application of 5% permethrin lotion or malathion (Ovide) is preceded by a warm soap and water bath. Skin must be cool and dry before the lotion is applied. The lotion is left in place for 8 to 12 hours (overnight) before washing it off. A second treatment is used one week later. All members of the household and child care contacts should be treated at the same time, even if they have no symptoms. Itching may persist for 1 to 2 weeks after treatment. An oral antihistamine (e.g., Benadryl, Atarax) may be prescribed to help relieve itching.

Nursing Management

Advise parents that scabies is transmitted by close contact and is very contagious. All clothing, bedding, and pillowcases used by the child should be changed daily, washed with hot water, and ironed before reuse. Nonwashable toys and other items should be sealed in plastic bags for 5 to 7 days.

Family members who are not infected should avoid touching the affected child until after treatment is completed. If they do, they should wash their hands well. Inform the parents about signs of secondary infections and that itching and nodules may persist for weeks after effective treatment.

Scabies, like pediculosis, can be embarrassing or upsetting for the child and family. Educate the child and parents about the condition, its spread, and treatment measures to prevent recurrence.

FUNGAL INFECTIONS

Oral Candidiasis (Thrush)

Oral candidiasis (moniliasis or thrush) is a fungal infection that occurs as an acute condition in newborns (usually acquired during birth from the vaginal canal of an infected mother) and a chronic condition in young children who:

- Have an immune disorder
- Regularly use a corticosteroid inhaler
- Are receiving antibiotics, which have disturbed the normal flora, allowing the growth of the fungus

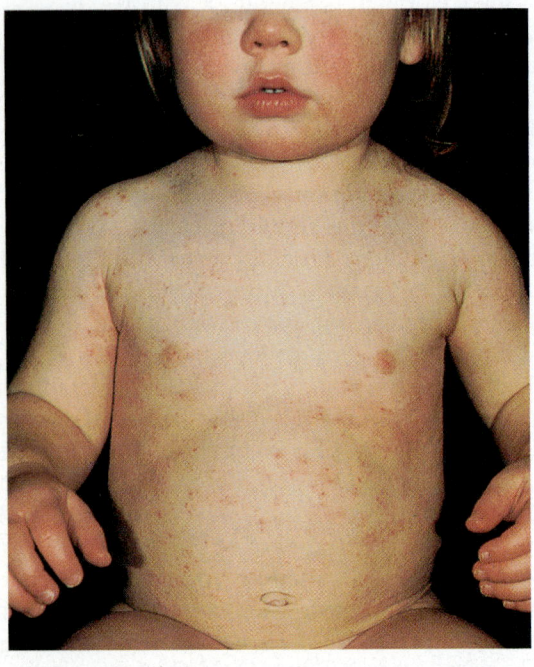

FIGURE 52–8. ◆ Diffuse scabies in an infant. The lesions are most numerous around the axillae, chest, and abdomen. *Note:* From Habif, T. P. (1990). *Clinical dermatology: A color guide to diagnosis and therapy* (2nd ed., p. 298). St. Louis, MO: Mosby-Year Book.

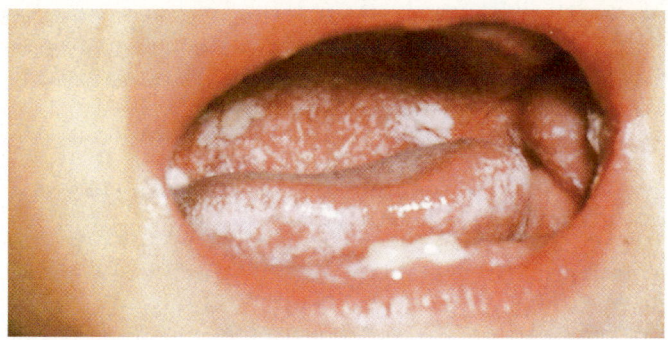

FIGURE 52–9. ◆ Thrush, an acute pseudomembranous form of oral candidiasis, is a common fungal infection in infants and children. Note: From Zitelli, B. J., & Davis, H. W. (Eds.). (1997). *Atlas of pediatric physical diagnosis*, 3rd ed., (p. 104, Fig. 4–50a). St. Louis: Mosby.

Thrush is characterized by white patches that look like coagulated milk on the oral mucosa and may bleed when removed (Figure 52–9 ◆). Milk residue can be removed from the oral mucosa with gentle swabbing. With candidiasis, however, attempts at gentle removal are unsuccessful. The infant may refuse to nurse or feed because of discomfort and pain. The infant may also have diaper dermatitis superinfection with candidiasis. Fever is usually not present.

Treatment involves oral nystatin suspension, which is applied to the mouth and tongue after feedings. For infants, parents should use a swab to apply the suspension to the buccal mucosa and tongue surfaces, allowing the infant to swallow the remaining suspension. They should tell older children to swish the solution around in the mouth before swallowing it.

If infection is severe, occurs in the esophagus, or invades other body systems, oral fluconazole or intravenous amphotericin B may be prescribed.

NURSING MANAGEMENT

To prevent a reinfection, educate parents about sterilizing bottle nipples and pacifiers. A commercial antiseptic spray may be used on toys that cannot be autoclaved, but follow directions carefully so the child does not ingest any harmful residue. Teach parents and older children with asthma to rinse the mouth well with water after using a corticosteroid inhaler to prevent candidiasis. If they use a spacer, they should also rinse it with water after use.

Dermatophytoses (Ringworm)

Dermatophytoses are fungal infections that affect the skin, hair, or nails. Children of all ages may be affected. Dermatophytoses may be spread from person to person or from animal to person. The most common infections are tinea capitis, tinea corporis, tinea cruris, and tinea pedis. See "Clinical Manifestations: Tinea Infections."

Diagnosis is confirmed through microscopic examination of the hair and scale scrapings using a potassium hydroxide (KOH) wet mount to reveal rows and chains of spores within the hair shaft. A fungal culture can also be taken from a scalp lesion by rubbing a cotton-tipped applicator across the scalp and placing it in a throat culture tube. A Wood's lamp is also useful in identifying some forms of tinea that fluoresce under ultraviolet light. However, *Trichophyton tonsurans,* the most common cause of tinea capitis, does not fluoresce with a Wood's lamp (McDonald & Smith, 1998). An oral antifungal agent (e.g., griseofulvin) is usually prescribed for tinea capitis, but resistance is developing. Other drugs not yet approved for use in children include itraconazole, fluconazole, and terbinafine (American Academy of Pediatrics, 2000).

NURSING MANAGEMENT

Assess all members of the family and household pets for fungal lesions. Advise parents to give oral griseofulvin with fatty foods such as whole milk or peanut butter to enhance absorption. The medications must be used for the entire prescribed period, even if the lesions are gone, to prevent recurrence of the infection. Teach parents and older children or teenagers that fungi are found in soil and animals and are transmitted through direct contact.

Since person-to-person transmission is common, it is best to avoid personal contact with hair and sharing hair accessories, brushes, and hats. In some cases, there may be an asymptomatic carrier in the family, in which case everyone should be treated. For children with tinea cruris, encourage loose-fitting undergarments to promote dryness. With tinea pedis, feet should be kept clean and dry and nails clipped short. Discourage occlusive footwear or nylon socks, which trap moisture.

Parents of children with tinea capitis should be told that hair regrowth is slow and may take 6 to 12 months. In some cases hair loss is permanent, which can be particularly stressful for older children or adolescents. Provide emotional support.

✎ INJURIES TO THE SKIN

PRESSURE ULCERS

More and more children with disabilities are cared for in hospital, community, and home care settings. Many are at risk for skin breakdown and pressure ulcers. Children at greatest risk are those with limited mobility, sensory deficits, or the inability to change positions (Table 52–4).

TABLE 52–4   Sites and Potential Causes of Pressure Ulcers

Sites	Potential Causes
Occipital region of scalp	Inability to lift head
Sacrum and buttocks	Confinement to bed or wheelchair
Legs and feet	Leg braces
Spine and neck	Scoliosis brace
Knees and elbows	Rubbing against bed sheet

SITE AND INCIDENCE	CLINICAL MANIFESTATIONS	CLINICAL THERAPY
Tinea capitus (scalp) Usually prepubertal children between 1 and 10 years	Circumscribed hair loss Broken hairs; black, dotted stubbed appearance where weakened hair has broken off Diffuse fine scaling Many scaly pustular bald areas with indistinct margins Mild itching Boggy nodules with superficial pustules as an allergic response to fungus Suboccipital or posterior cervical nodes	Griseofulvin orally for 8 to 12 weeks Selenium sulfide shampoo 2 to 3 times weekly, leave on for 10 minutes before rinsing
Tinea corporis (trunk) Children and adolescents	One or several circular erythematous patches, may be scaly or erythematous throughout Slightly raised borders with a clearing center	Topical cream (e.g., clotrimazole, miconazole, tolnaftate, naftifine, or terbinafine) twice a day for 4 weeks Wash with selenium sulfide shampoo
Tinea cruris ("jock itch") (inner thighs, inguinal creases) Rare before adolescence	Scaly, erythematous eruption symmetric bilaterally Possibly elevated lesions, possible papules or vesicles	Same as for tinea corporis
Tinea pedis ("athlete's foot") (feet and toes)	Vesicles or erosions on instep or between toes (fissures, red scaly) Peeling maceration and fissures in lateral toe web spaces Dry scaly patches or plaques with mild erythema on plantar and lateral surfaces of foot Itching	Same as for tinea corporis and cruris Keep feet dry with absorbent talc Allow to air dry Use 100% cotton socks, change twice daily

Tinea capitis

Tinea corporis

Photographs of tinea capitis and tinea corporis courtesy of the Centers for Disease Control and Prevention, Atlanta, GA.

Etiology and Pathophysiology

Soft tissues may be compressed between a bony prominence and another surface. Tissue ischemia occurs when high pressure is maintained over a short period of time or low pressure is maintained over a prolonged time. The cells are deprived of oxygen and nutrients, and metabolic waste products accumulate, injuring the soft tissue. Without appropriate intervention, the injury progresses rapidly and a pressure ulcer forms. Various factors place the child at greater risk for skin breakdown, including prolonged pressure, decreased mobility and activity, decreased sensory perception of pressure-related discomfort or injury, increased exposure to moisture, incontinence of urine and feces, friction and shearing forces, poor nutritional status,

an extended pediatric intensive care stay, and impaired tissue perfusion and oxygenation requiring ventilator support (Loman, 2000).

Clinical Manifestations

The earliest sign of skin damage is an area of redness that does not go away within 30 minutes of removing the pressure or skin irritant. In the next stage the skin looks rubbed or raw (superficial or partial thickness injury), similar to an abrasion or blister. Without intervention, the skin damage extends through the epidermis and dermis (full-thickness injury) and an ulcer forms. Injury deepens to underlying tissue (muscles, bone, or connective tissue) unless treated (see "Pathophysiology Illus-

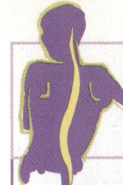
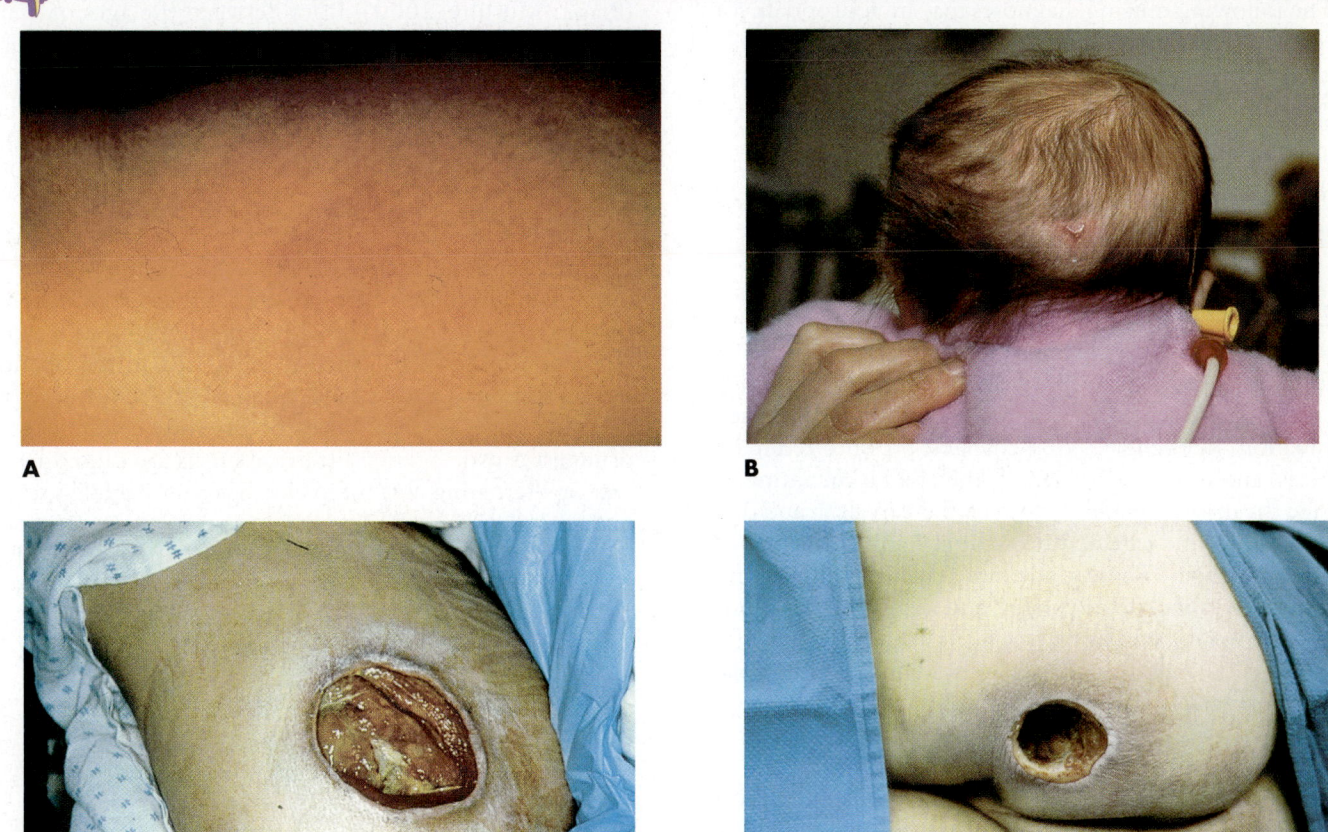

A, Stage 1, nonblanchable erythema of intact skin. **B,** Stage 2, blister or abrasion, partial thickness loss with damage through epidermis, dermis, or both. **C,** Stage 3, full thickness loss with exposure of subcutaneous tissue. **D,** Stage 4, full thickness loss that extends to muscle, bone, or supporting tissues. Courtesy of Sandra Quigley, Children's Hospital, Boston, MA.

trated: The Four Stages of Pressure Ulcer Formation") (Ball, 1998; Quigley & Curley, 1996).

Clinical Therapy

Initial treatment for early stages of skin damage involves removing pressure from the affected site until the skin has healed. Children who use leg braces for alignment and mobility are often put in wheelchairs. Children who use wheelchairs are often put on bed rest on a pressure-reducing surface. Frequent repositioning is needed. A transparent film may be applied to affected red skin to minimize friction. Pressure ulcers are treated with various dressings, such as hydrocolloids, gels or hydrogels, and calcium alginates (Quigley & Curley, 1996).

Nursing Management

Nursing Assessment and Diagnosis

Carefully inspect the dependent skin surfaces of all infants and children confined to bed at least three times in each 24-hour period. Evaluate the risk for skin damage based on factors that can contribute to skin breakdown.

Growth and Development

The site of greatest pressure in infants and young children is the occiput. Older children have increased pressure on the sacral and occipital areas.

Identify the size (diameter and depth) and character of the skin lesion. Note any signs of infection, the appearance of wound edges, and the type of tissue at the wound base. Describe drainage amount, color, and type.

The following nursing diagnoses may be appropriate for the child at risk for pressure sores:

▶ *Risk for impaired skin integrity* related to inability to shift position
▶ *Risk for injury* related to sensory/perceptual alterations
▶ *Impaired physical mobility* related to decreased muscle strength and control

Planning and Implementation

Develop protocols for pressure ulcer prevention so that children at high risk are identified and receive appropriate interventions. Such interventions may include increased ambulation, frequent position changes, pressure-reducing surfaces, and moisture barriers. If the child is incontinent, change the diaper frequently to keep the skin clean and dry.

Provide wound care and dressing changes according to agency guidelines. These guidelines may include irrigating the site with saline, debridement, and a dressing appropriate for the wound condition (see Skills 10–10 and 10–11). SKILLS Avoid using tape to hold dressings in place unless a protective skin barrier is used.

NURSING CARE IN THE COMMUNITY

Teach parents of children with impaired mobility and diminished pain sensation to inspect the braces and skin under the braces every day for signs of irritation (redness or blisters). Take the braces off and help the child to use a mirror with a long handle to inspect skin on the bottom and sides of the feet, behind the knees, and on the lower legs. Check all edges of the braces for roughness or breakage that can pinch or scrape the skin. If any sign of skin irritation is seen and redness does not go away within 30 minutes, do not put the brace back on until the skin heals. Inform the child's physician so that treatment can be started immediately. To prevent braces from rubbing on bare skin, have the child wear cotton socks under the braces. To avoid irritation of the foot, the child should wear shoes large enough to accommodate the brace and the foot. Advise parents to return to a prosthetist regularly for refitting as the child grows.

Children who use a wheelchair are at risk for skin breakdown on the buttocks and lower back because of the pressure from sitting for hours. A wheelchair cushion can distribute and shift the child's weight when sitting in the chair. The child needs to change position often to relieve the pressure on the skin. Teach the child to do wheelchair push-ups or to shift the weight by leaning to the side or forward for several minutes every 10 to 15 minutes. Make sure the child wears a safety belt when sitting in the wheelchair. Teach school personnel about the child's recommended protocol so they can provide opportunities in school to change positions and reinforce the routine.

BURNS

Burns are the second leading cause of injury deaths (after motor vehicle crashes) in children between 5 and 14 years of age (Murphy, 2000). Boys between the ages of 1 and 4 years are twice as likely as girls to be burned. The national average age of pediatric burn patients is 32 months. In 1997, 83,000 children were hospitalized for burns (Hernandez-Reif, Field, Largie, et al., 2001). About 440,000 children are treated for burns each year (Stewart, 2000). WEB

There are four main types of burns: thermal, chemical, electrical, and radioactive. Thermal burns, the most common in children, result from flames, scalds (such as coffee or grease), or contact with hot objects (such as a wood stove or curling iron). Sherray, described in the opening quote, sustained a scald burn when a bowl of hot soup fell onto her leg. Chemical burns occur when children touch or ingest caustic agents. Electrical burns are caused by direct or alternating current in electrical wires, appliances, or high-voltage wires. Radiation burns result from exposure to radioactive substances or sunlight. About 10% of all burns in children are due to child abuse (Rodgers, 2000). See Chapter 36 for a description of child abuse.

Etiology and Pathophysiology

Children at different developmental stages are at risk for different types of burns.

- Infants are most often injured by thermal burns (scalding liquids, house fires) (Figure 52–10 ◆).
- Toddlers are at risk for thermal burns (pulling hot liquids or grease onto themselves), electrical burns (biting electrical cords) (Figure 52–11 ◆), contact burns, and chemical burns (ingesting cleaning agents and other substances) associated with exploring the environment.

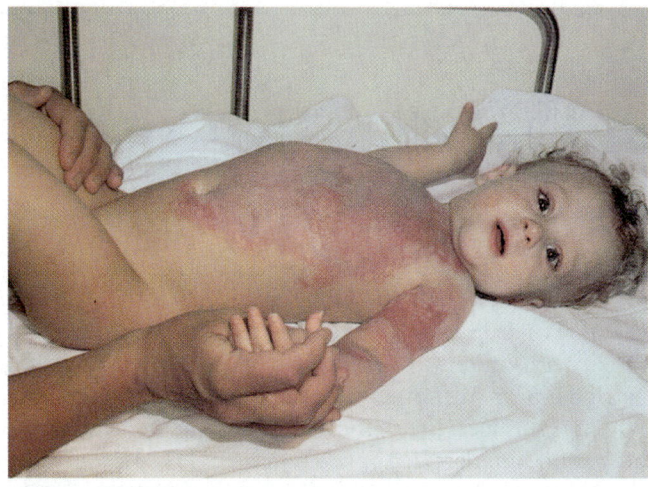

FIGURE 52–10. ◆ Thermal (scald) burns are the most common burn injury in infancy.

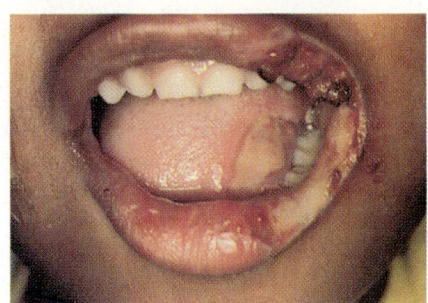

FIGURE 52-11. ◆ Electrical burn caused by biting on electrical cord. *Courtesy Dr. Lezley McIveen, Department of Dentistry, Children's National Medical Center, Washington, DC.*

- Preschool-age children are most often injured by scalding or contact with hot appliances (curling irons, ovens).
- School-age children are at risk for thermal burns (playing with matches, fireworks), electrical burns (climbing high-voltage towers, climbing trees, and contact with electrical wires), and chemical burns (combustion experiments) associated with their curiosity and interest in experimentation.
- Adolescents also experience thermal, chemical, and electrical burns.

Immediately after the burn, intense vasoconstriction occurs in response to substances released by the injured cells. Then vasodilation and capillary permeability allow plasma to seep into the wound. Ischemia due to vasoconstriction may increase the depth of the burn injury. The child loses increased water and heat through the injured epidermis. The child's metabolic rate and need for calories increase in the attempt to maintain body temperature.

Clinical Manifestations

Burns are classified by depth. Burn depth may be defined as partial thickness or full thickness. Partial-thickness burns, in which the injured tissue can regenerate and heal, may be either first- or second-degree. Full-thickness burns, in which the injured tissue cannot regenerate, are also known as third-degree burns. The depth of the burn depends upon the temperature and duration of the heat application, and on the ability of tissues to dissipate the transferred energy. See "Pathophysiology Illustrated: Classification of Burns" (on page 1404) for clinical manifestations by burn depth.

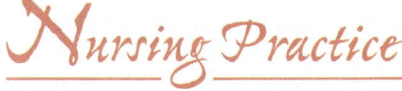

A full-thickness burn can occur in adults after only 2 seconds' immersion in water with a temperature of 65 °C (149 °F). The amount of time for a burn to occur increases to 10 minutes when water temperature is 50 °C (122 °F). Because infants and children have more sensitive skin, they need less time to receive a serious burn (Stewart, 2000).

Signs of infection include purulent drainage, focal areas of necrosis, edema, erythema, discoloration of wound margins, and conversion from partial-thickness to full-thickness injury depth (Rogers, 2000).

Clinical Therapy

ASSESSMENT OF BURN SEVERITY

Burn severity is determined by the depth of the burn injury, percentage of body surface area (BSA) affected, and involvement of specific body parts (Table 52-5). A Lund and Browder chart with BSA distributions for various body parts at different ages is used to calculate the area affected by the burn injury (Figure 52-12 ◆). The palm of a child's hand is 1% of his or her body surface area and can be used to make a quick estimate of the burn size. Once the affected BSA is calculated, the burn can be classified as minor, moderate, or major. Children with moderate and major burns require hospitalization, and those with major burns will usually be transferred to a burn center.

The involvement of specific body parts or specific burn distributions increases the burn severity, regardless of the percentage of BSA affected. Burns to the face, hands, feet, or perineal area are treated as major injuries because of the potential for functional impairment. **Circumferential** burns (injury completely surrounding the thorax or an extremity), anterior chest burns, and smoke inhalation are also classified as major burns.

INITIAL TREATMENT

The first step is to stop the burning process by removing jewelry and clothing. Moist soaks or ice (if small surface area affected) are used to stop the burning process and to relieve pain. A tetanus vaccine booster is given if more than 5 years have passed since the last vaccine, or when the child has not completed the full vaccine series.

TREATMENT OF MAJOR BURNS

The goals of treatment include: decrease burn fluid losses, prevent infection, control pain, and salvage all viable tissue.

TABLE 52-5	Classification of Burn Severity
Minor	Partial thickness < 10% BSA Full thickness < 2% BSA
Moderate	Partial thickness of 10%–20% BSA Full thickness 3%–10% BSA
Major	Partial thickness of > 20% BSA Full thickness of >10% BSA Burns involving face, eyes, ears, hands, feet, and perineum Electrical burns, inhalation injury, other injuries, and preexisting chronic conditions

Note: From Stewart, C. (2000). Emergency care of pediatric burns. *Pediatric Emergency Medicine Reports, 5*(10), 101–112. Adapted.

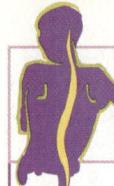
Superficial Partial Thickness (first degree)

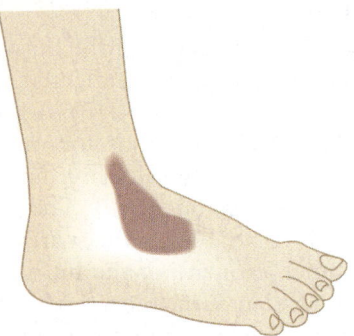

Damages only outer layer of skin; burn is painful and red; heals in a few days (e.g., sunburn)

Erythema, blanches on pressure, no bullae, peeling after a few days due to premature cell death

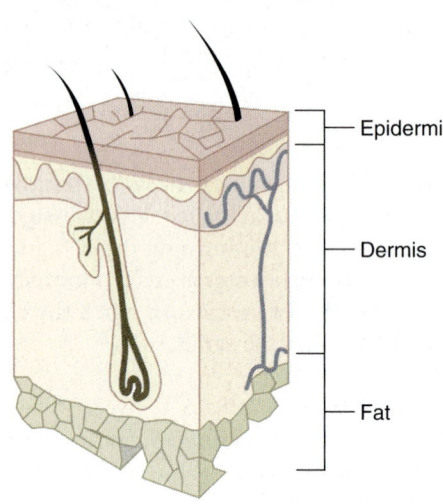

— Epidermis

— Dermis

— Fat

Partial Thickness (second degree)

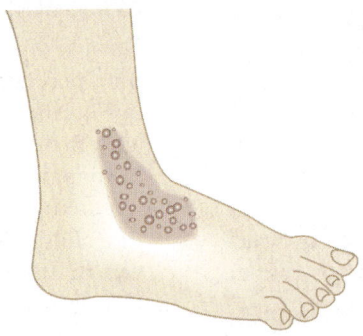

Involves epidermis and upper layers of dermis; may have sparing of sweat glands and sebaceous glands; heals in 10–14 days

Blisters or bullae, erythema, blanches on pressure, pain and sensitivity to cold air, minimal scar formation

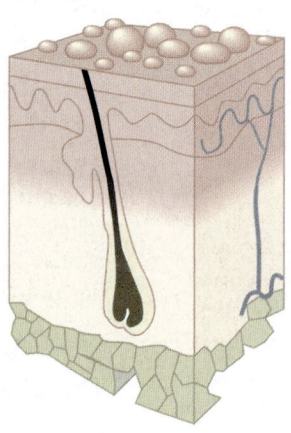

Full Thickness (third degree)

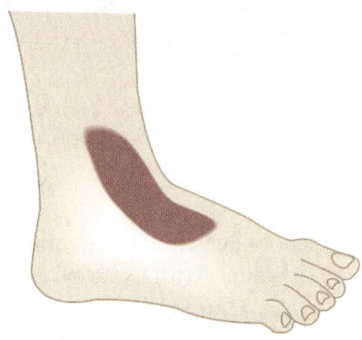

Involves all of epidermis and dermis; may also involve underlying tissue; nerve endings usually destroyed; requires skin grafting

Skin may appear brown, black, deep cherry red, white to gray, waxy or translucent; usually no pain, injured area may appear sunken

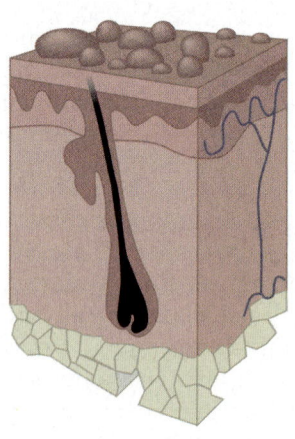

Fluid replacement is necessary to prevent hypovolemic shock in cases of major burn injury. Fluid shifts from the vasculature to the interstitial spaces (third spacing) occur soon after the burn, with the most dramatic occurring within the first 8 to 12 hours after injury. Fluid replacement for the first 24 hours after the injury is based on a fluid volume formula calculated from the child's body weight, affected BSA, and normal maintenance needs. Several formulas exist for this calculation. Lactated Ringer's or normal saline solutions are the preferred fluids. Hypotonic intravenous solutions such as D5W increase the risk of hyponatremia and subsequent cerebral edema and seizures (Stewart, 2000). Half of the total volume calculated for the 24-hour period is infused over the first 8 hours, and the remainder is distributed evenly over the next 16 hours. Resuscitation efforts also focus on maintaining the child's temperature because heat is lost rapidly through burned skin. Vascular integrity is usually restored after the first 24 hours.

Fever is a normal, expected outcome of any significant thermal injury, but it is not always a sign of infection. Treatment may include analgesics, ice packs, cooling blankets, or cool hydrotherapy sessions. Infection, however, is a frequent complication, and can cause a partial-thickness burn to convert to a full-thickness burn (Rodgers, 2000).

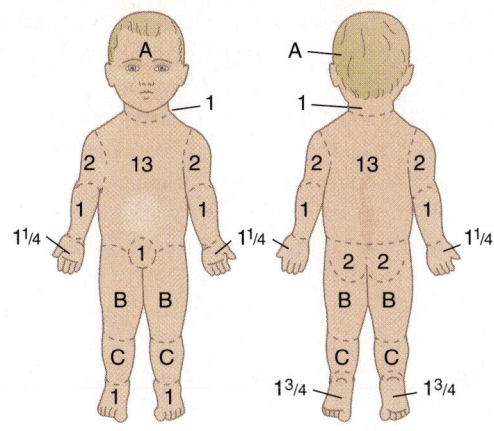

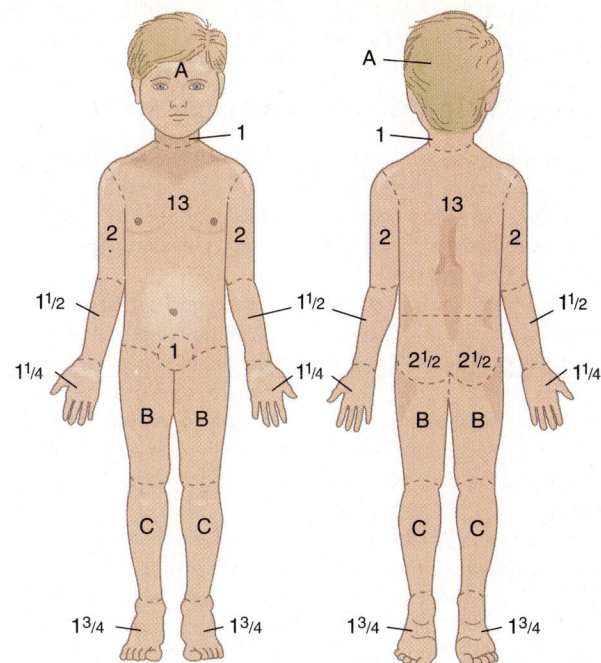

Relative Percentages of Areas Affected by Growth

Area	Age in years					
	0	1	5	10	11	Adult
A = $1/2$ of head	$9^{1/2}$	$8^{1/2}$	$6^{1/2}$	$5^{1/2}$	$4^{1/2}$	$3^{1/2}$
B = $1/2$ of one thigh	$2^{3/4}$	$3^{1/4}$	4	$4^{1/2}$	$4^{1/2}$	$4^{3/4}$
C = $1/2$ of one lower leg	$2^{1/2}$	$2^{1/2}$	$2^{3/4}$	3	$3^{1/4}$	$3^{1/2}$

FIGURE 52–12. ◆ Lund and Browder chart for determining percentage of body surface areas in pediatric burn injuries. Note: From Artz, C. P., & Moncrief, J. A. (1969). *The treatment of burns* (2nd ed.). Philadelphia: Saunders. Adapted.

Enteral feedings are often begun within 6 hours of the burn injury to support the child's increased nutritional requirements, which result from the increased metabolic rate needed to support healing and the body's stress response to injury (Herndon & Spies, 2001). Burned children often need nearly twice the basal metabolic caloric requirements and nearly 2 g/kg body weight of protein (Smith, 2000).

Aggressive pain management with intravenous opioids is needed as all procedures cause pain. In addition, the burns cause a significant emotional overlay that increases the perception of pain. See Chapter 38 for a discussion of pain management. ⚭ Cimetidine or other H₂ blockers may be ordered to prevent a burn stress ulcer.

Special consideration is needed when burns involve certain areas of the body:

- Deep partial-thickness and full-thickness burns develop **eschar** (the tough leathery scab that forms over severely burned areas) with no elasticity. When the burn is circumferential, blood flow can become restricted due to edema and cause tissue hypoxia. An **escharotomy** (incision into the constricting tissue) may be necessary to restore peripheral circulation.

Nursing Practice

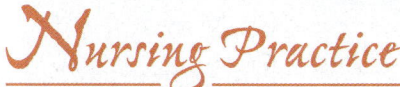

Assess for increases in cyanosis, deep tissue pain, and capillary refill time, and a decreased pulse distal to a circumferential burn. If you detect these signs, notify the physician immediately.

- Facial burns usually cause significant edema. Care must be taken to ensure airway patency. For burns to the eye, an ophthalmologist should be consulted to assess damage and prescribe treatment. If the lips are burned, an infant may be unable to suck.

- Burns of the hands require careful management to maintain function. Special splinting and physical therapy are usually necessary.

- Perineal burns are at higher risk for infection because of frequent contamination with urine and stool. Frequent dressing changes are required. A urinary catheter is usually inserted but is removed once hydration status is stable to minimize the risk of urinary tract infection.

WOUND MANAGEMENT

Burn wound care has several goals: (1) to speed wound debridement, (2) to protect granulation tissue and new grafts, (3) to conserve body heat and fluids, and (4) to control scarring and prevent scar contracture. Several treatment regimens help achieve these goals.

The entire body is bathed to initiate debridement (removal of dead tissue to speed the healing process). Conscious sedation and anesthesiology support may be ordered for pain management during debridement. Intact blisters provide a natural, pain-free, sterile dressing. If blisters break open, the tissue should be carefully cut away. After initial cleansing, antibacterial agents, such as Silvadene, are applied to prevent bacterial infection and dressings are added to cover the burned area (see Skill 11–12). ⚭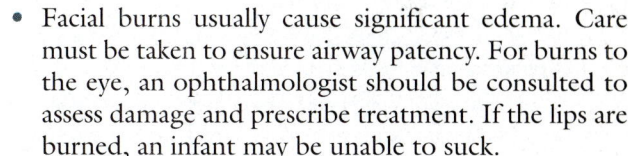

Thinking Critically

THE CHILD WITH A PARTIAL-THICKNESS BURN

Sherray, 6 years old, was admitted to the hospital with a deep partial-thickness burn after dropping a bowl of soup on her leg. By her second day in the hospital, it is clear that Sherray's burn is not full thickness and that no skin grafting is needed. She will be discharged the next day.

Sherray's treatment includes a bath with wound debridement and dressing changes twice a day. Although pain medication is provided, the debridement and dressing changes cause a lot of anxiety and pain. Sherray needs a high-protein, high-calorie diet to promote wound healing. She has a hard time extending her leg and walking because movement stretches the burned skin, so she needs assistance to get out of bed and participate in child life activities.

Sherray's mother is rooming in, and remains at her side during the dressing changes. Her greatest concern right now is to help Sherray deal with the burn injury and to reduce the chance of infection. Over the next couple of days, Sherray's mother will take more responsibility for the dressing changes in anticipation of continuing her daughter's care at home.

➥ *What signs of infection must you watch for?*

➥ *What is the procedure Sherray's mother will need to use to provide care to the wound at home?*

➥ *What are some suggestions for pain management during wound care that could be used at home?*

➥ *What suggestions can you make to help Sherray extend and use her leg, despite the pain movement causes?*

➥ *What are some foods that Sherray's mother can prepare at home to provide the high-protein and high-calorie diet needed for healing?* 🔗 WEB

Dressing changes are performed once or twice daily. These changes are often very painful. When an old dressing is removed, a layer of eschar is also debrided.

Hydrotherapy (whirlpool) baths are given before debridement to loosen eschar. Hydrotherapy is performed twice daily to increase vasodilation and circulation and to speed healing. As a rule, tap water is used for debridement. Gentle washing is necessary to protect new epithelial cells. Granulation tissue forms as a result of daily debridement. Superficial second-degree burns reepithelialize within 3 weeks.

Skin grafting is necessary with any deep second- or third-degree burn. Often a temporary skin substitute is used to cover a second-degree burn until it heals, or to cover a deep second- and third-degree burn until **autografting** (use of healthy skin taken from a nonburned area of the child's body). The graft is placed after the wound is debrided in the operating room to reveal healthy, bleeding tissue.

Trans-Cyte is a temporary skin substitute approved by the Food and Drug Administration that is bioengineered from newborn foreskin tissue. It forms a protective barrier over the wound surface to decrease infection risk and to protect against fluid loss. Research conducted in children indicates that it promotes healing more rapidly than silvadene, decreases infection risk, avoids painful burn dressings, and reduces length of hospital stay (Figure 52–13 ◆) (Lukish, Eichelberger, Newman, et al., 2001; Wiebelhaus & Hansen, 2001). It is applied with a surgical adhesive or staples and covered with a bulky dressing or pressure dressing.

An autograft is permanent. The donor site (where the autograft was harvested) is a new wound, causing pain and requiring close monitoring for signs of infection. A temporary skin substitute may cover that wound until it heals.

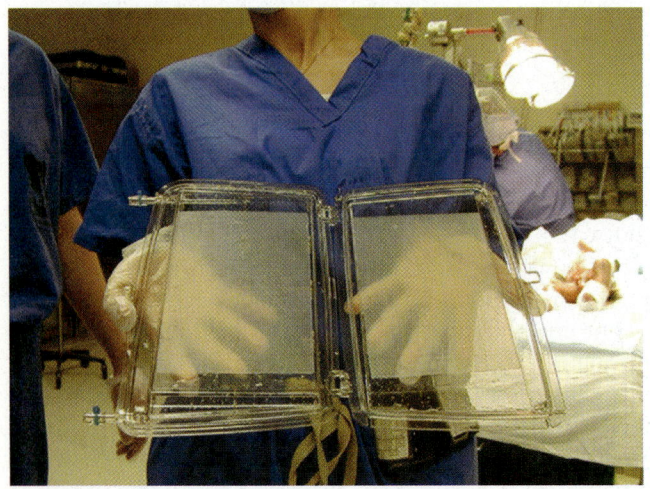 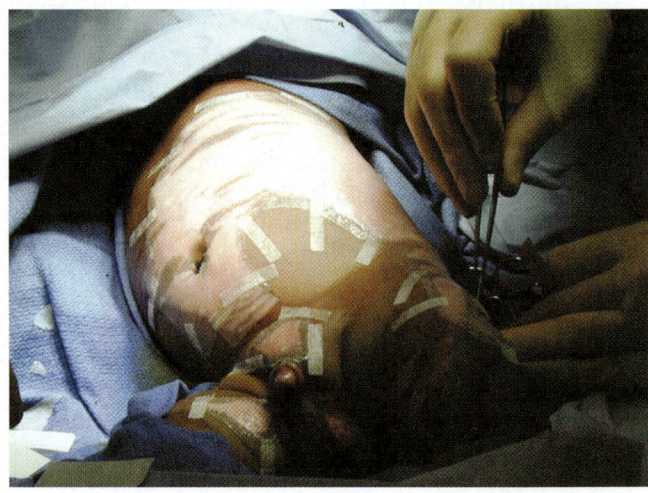

FIGURE 52–13. ◆ **A,** Trans-Cyte, a temporary skin substitute, prior to application. **B,** Application of Trans-Cyte after debridement of a scald burn. Courtesy of Martin R. Eichelberger, M.D., Children's National Medical Center, Washington, D.C.

Nursing Management

Nursing Assessment and Diagnosis

Emergency assessment is based on the ABCs of basic life support (airway, breathing, and circulation). Assess airway patency, especially when there are signs of smoke inhalation or burns to the face and neck. Assess the child for other potential injuries when the mechanism of injury also includes a fall or explosion. Identify signs of respiratory distress and any potential bleeding source. A weak, thready pulse, tachycardia, and pallor are important signs of early shock that may provide clues to an internal injury.

Find out about the type of burn (e.g., thermal, electrical, chemical), and take a complete history. When taking a burn history, carefully document type of injury, time of injury, people present at the time of the injury, first aid administered, and history of other unusual injuries or emergency department visits. Thorough documentation is essential to rule out child abuse. Be alert to signs of abuse such as glove and stocking burns, burns that spare flexor surfaces, contact burns from cigarettes or irons, and zebra burn lines from contact with a hot grate (Figure 52–14 ◆). Child neglect can be a factor in the burn of an inadequately supervised child. If a burn injury was preventable, parents may be emotionally stressed by guilt. Be careful to avoid sounding accusatory when questioning parents about the injury.

Physical assessment should be thorough, including frequent monitoring of vital signs, pain control, and daily weight measurement. Perform a head-to-toe assessment at the beginning of every shift followed by system-specific assessments, depending on clinical findings and changes in the child's status. Be alert to signs of infection such as purulent drainage and edematous, red, or discolored wound margins.

Assess the child's concerns over appearance and the stress of hospitalization. Determine if the child has memories or nightmares about the burn and arrange psychologic support as needed.

Common nursing diagnoses for the child with a major burn injury are included in the accompanying "Nursing Care Plan." Additional nursing diagnoses for the child with a major burn might include:

▶ *Impaired physical mobility* related to movement prescriptions (limb immobilization) and pain

▶ *Body image disturbance* related to burn injury

▶ *Anxiety* related to situational crisis and threat of death or disfigurement

Planning and Implementation

Nursing care focuses on performing burn care, preventing complications, and providing emotional support. Care of the burned child involves various treatments designed to promote healing and prevent complications. These include dressing changes, hydrotherapy, antibiotic therapy, analgesic support, physical therapy, play therapy, and possibly skin grafting.

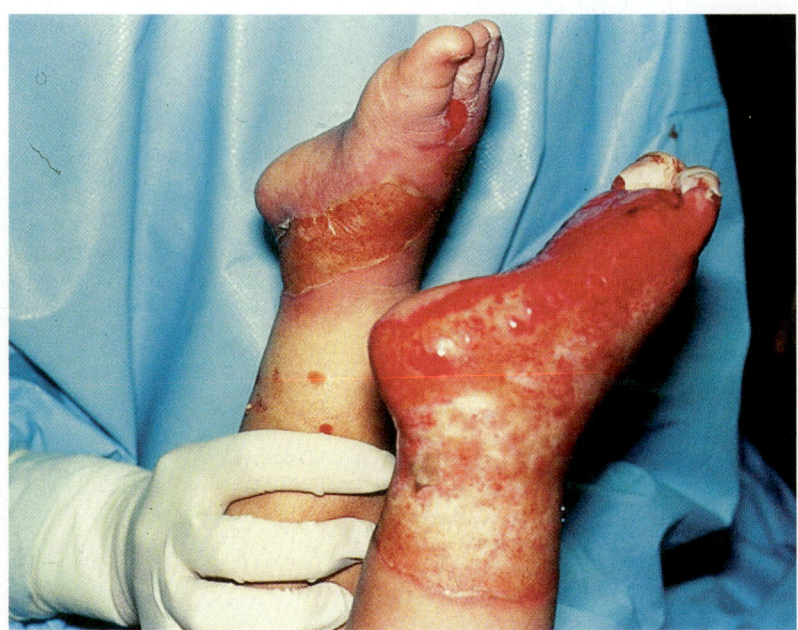
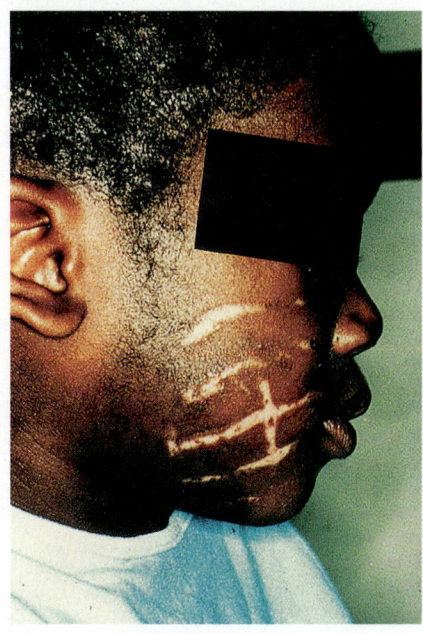

FIGURE 52–14. ◆ Burn injuries associated with child abuse. **A,** Burns of the hands or feet that are distributed like gloves or stockings. **B,** Zebra burns from a grate. *Courtesy of American Academy of Pediatrics, Elk Grove Village, IL, and the Kempe Children's Center, Denver, CO.*

GOAL	INTERVENTION	RATIONALE	EXPECTED OUTCOME
1. Pain related to physical injury agents			
	NIC Priority Intervention:		*NOC Suggested Outcome:*
	Pain management: *Alleviation of pain or a reduction in pain to a level of comfort that is acceptable to the patient*		**Comfort level:** *Feelings of physical and psychologic ease*
The child will verbalize adequate relief from pain and will be able to perform activities of daily living (ADLs).	▶ Assess the level of pain frequently using pain scales (see Chapter 38). 🔗	▶ Pain scale provides objective measurement. Pain is always present, but changes in location and intensity may indicate complications.	The child verbalizes adequate relief from pain and is able to perform ADLs.
	▶ Cover burns as much as possible.	▶ Temperature changes or movement of air causes pain.	
	▶ Change the child's position frequently. Perform range of motion exercises.	▶ Reduces joint stiffness and prevents contractures.	
	▶ Encourage verbalization about pain.	▶ Provides outlet for emotions and helps the child cope.	
	▶ Provide diversional activities.	▶ Helps lessen focus on pain.	
	▶ Promote uninterrupted sleep with use of medications.	▶ Sleep deprivation can increase pain perception.	
	▶ Use analgesics before all dressing changes and burn care.	▶ Helps to reduce pain and decreases anxiety for subsequent dressing changes.	
2. Risk for infection related to trauma and destruction of skin barrier			
	NIC Priority Intervention:		*NOC Suggested Outcome:*
	Infection protection: *Prevention and early detection of infection in a patient at risk*		**Risk control:** *Actions to eliminate or reduce actual, personal, and modifiable health threats*
The child will be free of infection during healing process.	▶ Take vital signs frequently.	▶ Increased temperature is an early sign of infection.	The child either stays free of secondary infection, or has infection diagnosed and treated early.
	▶ Use standard precautions (gown, gloves, mask) when wounds of a major burn are exposed. Limit visitors (no one with an upper respiratory infection or other contagious disease).	▶ Reduces risk of wound contamination.	
	▶ Clip hair around burns.	▶ Hair harbors bacteria.	
	▶ Keep biosynthetic burn dressing dry.	▶ Helps reduce the number of bacteria introduced to the burned site.	
	▶ Do not place the IV in any burned area.	▶ Reduces risk of wound contamination.	
	▶ Administer oral or IV antibiotics for diagnosed infections as prescribed.	▶ Antibiotics administered as prescribed help to clear the infection quickly.	
3. Risk for fluid volume imbalance related to loss of fluids through wounds and to subsequent excess fluid intake			
The child will maintain adequate urine output.	*NIC Priority Intervention:* To be developed		*NOC Suggested Outcome:* To be developed
	▶ Monitor vital signs, central venous pressure, capillary refill time, pulses.	▶ The child is initially at risk for hypovolemic shock and needs fluid resuscitation (see Chapter 39). 🔗	The child maintains normal urine output and burn site edema is not excessive.
	▶ Administer IV and oral fluids as ordered.	▶ Careful calculation of fluid needs and ensuring proper intake helps keep the child properly hydrated.	
	▶ Estimate insensible fluid losses.	▶ Losses are increased during the first 72 hours after burn injury; may need replacement. Plasma is lost through burn site because of capillary damage.	
	▶ Monitor intake and output.	▶ The child is at risk for fluid overload during hydration, and for edema in the tissues at the burn site.	
	▶ Weigh child daily.	▶ Significant weight loss or gain can help determine fluid imbalances.	
	▶ Insert urinary catheter.	▶ Helps maintain accurate output measurement during critical care stage.	
	▶ Monitor for hyponatremia and hypercalcemia (see Chapter 39). 🔗	▶ Sodium is lost with burn fluid and potassium is lost from damaged cells, causing electrolyte imbalances.	

GOAL	INTERVENTION	RATIONALE	EXPECTED OUTCOME

4. Altered peripheral tissue perfusion related to mechanical reduction of venous and/or arterial blood flow (edema) of circumferential burns

	NIC Priority Intervention:		NOC Suggested Outcomes:
	Circulatory care: *Promotion of arterial and venous circulation*		**Tissue perfusion (peripheral):** *Extent to which blood flows through the small vessels of the extremities and maintains tissue function*
The child will maintain adequate perfusion in burned extremities.	▶ Elevate extremities. Check distal pulse hourly. Notify the physician of decreased or absent pulses.	▶ Elevation helps to reduce dependent edema by promoting venous return. Dependent edema can constrict peripheral circulation.	The child has no episodes of poor perfusion in the burned extremity.
	▶ Check eschar.	▶ Eschar can constrict peripheral circulation in edematous extremity.	

5. Ineffective breathing pattern related to respiratory muscle fatigue due to smoke inhalation and airway edema

	NIC Priority Intervention:		NOC Suggested Outcomes:
	Respiratory monitoring: *Collection and analysis of patient data to ensure airway patency and adequate gas exchange*		**Vital signs status:** *Temperature, pulse, respiration, and blood pressure within expected range for the individual.*
The child will maintain or demonstrate improvement in breathing pattern.	▶ Closely monitor quality of respirations, breath sounds, mucus secretions, pulse oximetry.	▶ Excess fluid replacement can cause pulmonary edema; toxins from burning products can cause airway inflammation.	The child has regular and unlabored breathing pattern.
	▶ Provide thorough pulmonary care.	▶ Pulmonary care assists in removal of secretions to prevent infection.	
	▶ Elevate head of bed. Keep intubation tube at bedside.	▶ Dyspnea, nasal flaring, air hunger (respiratory distress) may develop.	
	▶ Administer corticosteroids, as prescribed.	▶ Reduces airway edema.	

6. Impaired physical mobility related to joint stiffness due to burns

	NIC Priority Intervention:		NOC Suggested Outcome:
	Exercise therapy, joint mobility: *Use of active or passive body movement to maintain or restore joint flexibility*		**Joint movement (active):** *Range of motion of joints with self-initiated movement*
The child will maintain maximum range of motion.	▶ Arrange physical and occupational therapy twice daily for stretching and range of motion exercises. Splint as ordered. Encourage independent ADLs.	▶ Good positioning, range of motion exercises, and alignment prevent contractures.	The child maintains maximum range of motion without contactures.

7. Altered nutrition: less than body requirements related to high metabolic needs

	NIC Priority Intervention:		NOC Suggested Outcome:
	Nutrition management: *Assistance with or provision of balanced dietary intake of foods and fluids*		**Nutritional status:** *Extent to which nutrients are available to meet metabolic needs*
The child will maintain weight and demonstrate adequate serum albumin and hydration.	▶ Provide an opportunity to choose meals. Offer a variety of foods. Provide snacks.	▶ Encourages intake. General malaise and anorexia lead to poor healing.	The child maintains weight, adequate hydration, normal serum albumin.
	▶ Encourage the child to have meals with other children.	▶ Socialization improves intake.	
	▶ Provide a multivitamin supplement.		
	▶ Substitute milk and juices for water.	▶ Vitamin C aids zinc absorption; zinc aids in healing.	
	▶ Provide nasogastric feedings as needed.	▶ A child with a burn greater than 10% of BSA cannot usually meet nutrition requirements without assistance.	
	▶ Weigh the child daily.	▶ Provides objective evaluation.	

(continued)

GOAL	INTERVENTION	RATIONALE	EXPECTED OUTCOME
8. Anxiety (child) related to threat to or change in health status			
	NIC Priority Intervention:		*NOC Suggested Outcome:*
	Anxiety reduction: *Minimizing apprehension, dread, foreboding, or uneasiness related to an unidentified source of anticipated danger*		**Coping:** *Actions to manage stressors that tax an individual's resources*
The child will verbalize reduced anxiety.	▸ Provide continuity of care providers.	▸ Helps to build a trusting relationship.	The child expresses and shows signs of reduced anxiety.
	▸ Encourage parents to stay with the child; calls from home; pictures from classmates.	▸ Familiar surroundings, people, and items encourage relaxation.	
	▸ Group tasks and activities.	▸ Reduces overstimulation and encourages rest.	
9. Anxiety (parent) related to situational crisis			
	NIC Priority Intervention:		*NOC Suggested Outcome:*
	Anxiety reduction: *Minimizing apprehension, dread, foreboding, or uneasiness related to an unidentified source of anticipated danger*		**Anxiety control:** *Ability to eliminate or reduce feelings of apprehension and tension from an unidentified source*
Parents will verbalize decreased anxiety.	▸ Provide educational materials about healing, grafting, dressing changes, and course of action.	▸ Knowledge reduces anxiety.	Parents state decreased anxiety.
	▸ Be flexible when teaching parents about wound care.	▸ Adults learn in many different ways.	
	▸ Refer to social services or parent support group.	▸ Allows for venting of fears and guilt feelings, and provides exchange of ideas on dealing with hospitalization and long-term care.	

Begin pain management as soon as possible. Soak charred clothing off with sterile saline and clip any hair within 2 inches of the burn to keep it out of the burn site. Cleanse the burn with mild soap and water and remove any foreign matter. If a chemical is the burning agent, remove the clothing and wash with lots of water. Elevate burned extremities. See "Nursing Care Plan: The Child with a Major Burn Injury."

Severe morbidity is likely with major burns. Significant scarring may occur regardless of autografting. Contractures and loss of function are also possible. Inadequate fluid replacement may lead to irreversible renal damage or cardiac damage, necessitating close follow-up unrelated to the actual burn injury. Monitor intake and output closely. A urinary catheter may be inserted to enable close monitoring of urine output (see Skill 16–1). SKILLS CD

Children with major burns require comprehensive follow-up, sometimes involving repeated hospitalizations for surgery to release burn contractures, perform new grafting, or provide scar revision.

PREVENT COMPLICATIONS

Severe complications of burns include infections, pneumonia, and renal failure, as well as possible irreversible loss of function of the burned area. The health care team's goal is to prevent complications. Parents need to be involved in their child's care and to learn how to change dressings, assess for infection and dehydration (see Chapter 39), and perform range of motion exercises to aid in the child's recovery.

WOUND CARE

When a synthetic skin cover such as Trans-Cyte is used, protect the area from moisture and ointments, as these interfere with adherence. Since Trans-Cyte is transparent, the site can be monitored for signs of infection and wound healing. Assess the skin covering for air bubbles or fluid, and aspirate or drain as ordered. If the covering is used over a joint, a splint will be used to prevent movement. When the burn heals, the synthetic skin covering loosens, permitting it to be trimmed.

PROVIDE EMOTIONAL SUPPORT

Burned children have received a profound insult to their body and their self-image. Fear and anxiety about disfigurement and scarring are common, especially among adolescents. The shock and pain of the injury cause increased stress, as do the unfamiliar surroundings and presence of health care providers.

An attitude of genuine interest and concern is essential. Orient the child to his or her surroundings frequently and give ample preparation for procedures, when possible. Continuity of care providers is important in developing a trusting relationship with the child. Encourage the child to voice concerns, and show understanding and support.

Play therapy is encouraged for children, even if they can only observe initially. Play therapy serves several purposes for the child with a major burn:

▶ It provides an outlet for frustration, independence, and creativity.

▶ It promotes activities that challenge range of motion.

▶ It normalizes the child's daily routine.

▶ It encourages the child, who sees the progress other children make day by day.

Families are at risk for emotional stress. Forewarn them about the expected edema and the resulting gross changes in the child's body. Parents often feel guilty and responsible for the child's injury. Help parents focus on recovery rather than past actions. Fear usually results from lack of knowledge about the severity of the burn and the child's status, especially in the early stages of burn care and admission to the hospital ICU. Include the family in the child's care whenever possible. The family needs information and frequent updates. This promotes trust between the family and the health care team.

Autografting procedures enable the child to recover from major burns, but the operation leaves visible scarring. Psychologic support is therefore essential to the child's recovery. Social workers, chaplains, art therapists, child life specialists, and play therapists are all trained to help the child and family deal with the stressors of recovery. Make appropriate referrals to ensure that the child and family receive necessary services.

DISCHARGE PLANNING AND HOME CARE TEACHING

Identify and address home care needs well in advance of discharge. Thorough assessment is necessary to identify the family's needs related to the child's discharge home or to a rehabilitation facility. Discharge planning may include instructing parents in nutrition and diet needs, safety in the home, burn wound care, and range of motion exercises to prevent contractures.

Provide support and encouragement to parents as they learn how to care for the burned child. Many parents find it difficult to perform dressing change procedures they know will inflict pain to their child. Provide pain medication for dressing changes, and outline specific guidelines so that parents and health care team members have the same focus. Parents should first observe care being performed and then provide repeat demonstrations until competent.

NURSING CARE IN THE COMMUNITY

Care of the child with a burn requires long-term therapy and rehabilitation. Nurses in clinic and home care settings continue the care provided during hospitalization. Long-term care commonly occurs in the home, with frequent visits to health care professionals. In some cases, children regularly return to the hospital clinic for dressing changes. Children with extensive burns or with burns in locations where scarring may limit function must often wear an elasticized (Jobst) garment, and sometimes a face mask if the face was burned. The Jobst garment may present a threat to the child's body image, but it is an important way to decrease scarring. Scarring may also be managed through drug injections or surgery (i.e., revision, grafting, or Z-plasty). Help families understand the need for the special garments and masks and how to clean and care for them.

Continued physical therapy and occupational therapy are often needed to increase strength and dexterity in performing activities of daily living (ADLs) and to prevent contractures. Emphasize returning to normal ADLs as soon as possible. This includes returning to school as soon as health permits. Some children have home tutors for a while to decrease their risk of exposure to infection.

School reentry is often a traumatic experience, especially for older children and adolescents, because of the fear of rejection, decreased self-esteem, and impaired body image. The child's primary nurse, social worker, and child life specialist may visit the school of a child with a burn injury before the child returns to school—bringing photographs of the child, pressure garments, or other items—to desensitize the class and allow them to explore their feelings about the child's burn injury. Several communities offer support groups for families and children with burn injuries. Referral to these groups may be beneficial. ⊂▭⊃ **WEB**

MANAGEMENT OF MINOR BURNS

Many children with minor burns are cared for at home after an initial visit to the emergency department or urgent care clinic. For superficial burns covering a small area, use moist soaks or ice to stop the burning process and to relieve pain. Any open blisters are debrided, and a thin layer of silver sulfadiazine is applied over the burn. Do not place this medication close to the eyes or mouth. The burn is then covered with one or two layers of gauze. Burn dressings should be changed twice daily. This involves cleaning the burn and reapplying antibiotic cream.

Teaching About

CARING FOR MINOR BURNS

- Place burn under cool, running water to stop the burning process and to help reduce pain.
- Do not use ice as it can cause more damage to the injured skin.
- Remove all clothing and jewelry from the burned area.
- Apply a topical antibiotic such as Neosporin to the burned area on the face.

Tell parents to increase the child's fluid intake to compensate for loss of fluid through damaged skin. A high-calorie, high-protein diet is necessary to meet the increased nutritional requirements of healing. Acetaminophen (Tylenol) with codeine is often given, especially before dressing changes. Infection is a common complication. The child should be seen within 48 hours of treatment to monitor progress. Reinforce to parents the importance of follow-up appointments.

Moisturizing creams can be used after healing to relieve residual drying. The healed skin is very sensitive to sunburn, so cover the area or use a sunscreen. Sunscreen also helps prevent hyperpigmentation after burn healing.

SUNBURN

Sunburn is a burn injury to the outer layer of skin caused by excess sun exposure, or sun exposure after taking phototoxic drugs (acne medication, chlorpheniramine, diphenylhydramine, sulfonamides, tetracycline) (Laughlin-Richard, 2000). It occurs more often in fair-skinned children, who have less **melanin** (skin pigment) to protect their skin against these harmful rays. Repeated sunburns during childhood correlate strongly with malignant melanoma in adulthood. Melanoma is the most common cancer in women between 25 and 29 years (Schachner, 2000). Avoiding sunburn during childhood is believed to be more important than protecting skin during adulthood.

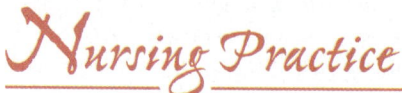 *Nursing Practice*

An estimated 80% of a person's lifetime exposure to sunburns occurs before 21 years of age, while the epidermis is relatively thin. Melanin is also present in low levels during infancy and childhood (Laughlin-Richard, 2000). For these reasons, children should use a sunscreen with an SPF of 15 or higher during all outdoor activities.

Erythema and skin tenderness usually develop between 30 minutes and 4 hours after exposure to sunlight. Increased vasodilation and vascular permeability result in the extravasation of fluid to the tissues and white blood cell migration to the damaged skin. The erythema peaks at 24 hours. Prolonged exposure can result in edema, vesiculation, bullae, or ulceration. Systemic complaints include malaise, insomnia (because of skin tenderness), fatigue, headaches, and chilling (because of rapid heat loss).

Treatment is generally supportive. Pain can be relieved by cool compresses followed by a topical corticosteroid. Children with severe sunburn may need nonsteroidal anti-inflammatory drugs for pain relief and to reduce inflammation. See Chapter 38.

Nursing Management

Educate parents and children about preventing sunburn. Advise them that repeated sunburns may lead to permanent skin damage and skin cancer. Recommend to parents that children use sunscreens of at least SPF 15, reapplied

several times daily, wear protective clothing, and limit the amount of time they spend in the sun. Children should also wear sunglasses with 99% ultraviolet blockage. WEB

Teaching About

PREVENTING SUNBURN

- Keep children out of direct sunlight as much as possible, especially the mid-day sun. Avoid scheduling outdoor activities during the hours of maximum exposure (10 A.M. to 2 P.M.).
- When outdoors, minimize exposed areas by wearing hats and long-sleeved, closely woven cotton clothing and pants; wear T-shirts while swimming. Special sun protection clothing is now available from some manufacturers.
- Be aware that water, concrete, and sand reflect sunlight and increase exposure up to 90% by reflecting up to 85% of the ultraviolet rays.
- Use sunscreen (preferably 30 SPF). For optimal protection, apply as thickly as directed to all exposed areas 30 to 45 minutes before sun exposure. Reapply every 2 hours as needed, or sooner if swimming, toweling off, or perspiring heavily.
- Use a waterproof sunscreen when swimming; this provides protection in water for approximately 60 to 80 minutes. Then reapply. Avoid getting waterproof sunscreen in the eyes because it causes severe pain and a chemical burn. Call the poison control center immediately for guidance.
- Avoid using sunscreens in infants less than 6 months of age because they may absorb the chemicals through their skin.
- Remember that a child can be burned even on a cloudy day. Up to 80% of ultraviolet rays can penetrate the cloud cover.
- If the child is taking any medications, check with your health care practitioner before exposure (some medications cause hypersensitivity to sunlight).

HYPOTHERMIA

Hypothermia is a condition in which the core body temperature falls below 35 °C (95 °F). This occurs when the heat produced by the body is less than the heat lost. Hypothermia is a life-threatening emergency.

Hypothermia is associated with near-drowning episodes because body heat is lost quickly in water, as compared with air. Children are at greater risk for hypothermia because of their thinner skin, limited subcutaneous fat, and high surface area to body mass ratio. As the body temperature falls, the body tries to conserve the core temperature at the expense of the extremities. Increased muscle tone and an increased metabolic rate occur. Shivering is the body's attempt to rewarm the blood before it returns to the core of the body. Other causes of hypothermia include exposure to a cold environment, ingestion of alcohol or barbiturates, trauma or a brain disorder that interferes with temperature regulation, and overwhelming sepsis (Eichelberger, Ball, Pratsch, et al., 1998).

Symptoms of mild hypothermia include slurred speech, incoordination, poor judgment, and shivering. Symptoms of moderate hypothermia include depressed respirations, slow pulse, low blood pressure, pale or cyanotic color, shivering, dilated pupils, and confusion. Profound hypothermia (body temperature below 29 °C [84 °F]) may result in absence of respirations and pulse, ventricular arrhythmia, dilated pupils, and loss of consciousness.

Clinical therapy focuses on resuscitation, if necessary, and gradual rewarming of the body. The child who has been immersed in cold water for a long time (up to 30 to 45 minutes) should receive CPR until the body temperature returns to normal because of the diving reflex, a cardiovascular system response triggered by immersion of the face and nose in cold water, in which the heart rate decreases and blood flow is decreased to all body areas except the brain, thus conserving oxygen and preserving vital organs. Assess body temperature with a rectal thermometer. For mild hypothermia (temperature above 35 °C [95 °F]), external heat lamps, immersion in warm water, and an electric blanket may be all that are necessary. More aggressive techniques are required for profound hypothermia. These may include humidified, warm oxygen; warmed intravenous fluids; hemodialysis; or application of warmth to core circulation areas (axilla, groin, and posterior neck).

If a child becomes hypothermic during an outing such as a camping trip, a warm person should get into a sleeping bag (or under the blankets) next to the child. This action will warm the child and prevent further heat loss. First aid for hypothermia includes moving the child to a dry area and removing any wet clothing. Replace with warm, dry clothing, and encourage the child to drink a warm, high-calorie liquid, if able.

Nursing Management

Monitor vital signs and urine output during rewarming. Prevention is geared toward educating parents to layer children's clothing in cold climates, recognize signs of hypothermia, decrease time of exposure to cold, and know how to treat mild hypothermia. Teach school-age children and adolescents who go on camping and hunting trips how to recognize and manage hypothermia in themselves and others. Teach preventive techniques such as avoiding riding snowmobiles or walking on ice that is not known to be deep enough to support the weight.

FROSTBITE

Frostbite is an extreme form of hypothermia that results from overexposure to extremely low temperatures. The hands, feet, cheeks, nose, and ears are at high risk for frostbite. Skin cells have a high concentration of water. Ice crystallizes in the tissues, resulting in cellular dehydration and ischemic damage.

Clinical manifestations depend on the severity of the cellular damage. The skin at first appears pale and is numb.

Rapid rewarming causes a flush and the sensation of tingling, burning, or prickling in the affected area. The erythema and mild swelling develop into bullae. The extent of injury usually is not initially apparent.

If frostbite is suspected, loosen all constricting clothing and remove any wet clothes. Obtain health care as soon as possible. Rewarming is done slowly to decrease the chance of cellular damage. Immerse the affected part for 10 to 15 minutes in water warmed to between 38 and 40 °C (100.4 and 104 °F). Analgesics may be given to manage pain. Elevate the affected part, if possible, to improve venous return. Encourage the child to drink warm fluids. This will help to warm the child slowly. Because the frostbitten area is numb, extreme caution is needed to protect it from any trauma.

Lengthy treatment and amputation are sometimes necessary when tissues are permanently damaged.

Nursing Management

As with hypothermia, the goal of management is prevention. Teach parents to layer children's clothing for warmth and to pack extra blankets and clothing if cold temperatures are expected during outdoor activities. Teach adolescents how to avoid frostbite during hunting and other cold weather expeditions. Wet clothing should be changed quickly. Early care is instrumental in minimizing permanent injury. Severe frostbite requires hospitalization, with fluid management, dressing changes, antibiotic therapy, and careful attention to diet.

BITES

Animal Bites

Each year 5 million people are bitten by animals in the United States. Dog bites account for 80% of animal bites treated in the United States. [WEB] Other animals that may bite include cats, birds, turtles, and wild animals such as bats, squirrels, and raccoons. Children, especially those less than 8 years old, are at higher risk for animal bites, and boys are bitten more than twice as often as girls (Bernardo, Gardner, O'Connor, et al., 2000). Most dogs are known by the child.

Assessment includes noting the location and number of puncture wounds, abrasions, lacerations, and crushing injuries, redness or swelling at entry sites, redness extending out from site (possible cellulitis), and any drainage related to the bite. Check for nerve, muscle, tendon, or vascular damage. Carefully document findings. Head and neck bites require radiographic examination to rule out any associated injury, such as trauma to the airway or breathing structures or a depressed skull fracture.

To decrease infection, initial treatment involves high-pressure wound irrigation with large quantities of sterile saline or lactated Ringer's solution rather than scrubbing. A 19-gauge needle on a 60-cc syringe may be used. Any devitalized tissue is debrided. Some children may need conscious sedation. A clean pressure dressing is applied, and the affected part is elevated to reduce bleeding. Small wounds may be closed with adhesive strips rather than suturing because of the potential for infection. Severe bites sometimes require surgical closure or reconstruction. Wounds over joints should be immobilized and elevated. Puncture wounds should not be irrigated or sutured.

Dog bites tend to be crushing, rather than clean, sharp lacerations. The major complication of bites is infection. Antibiotics and early treatment can greatly decrease this sequela. Dog bites should be reported to the police, and the dog should be observed for 10 days for signs of rabies. Cat bites are also dangerous because they tend to be puncture wounds and are therefore associated with a higher rate of infection, cellulitis, and abscesses.

Bites by wild animals in areas with endemic rabies require rabies prophylaxis. Human rabies immune globulin (HRIG) or human diploid cell rabies (HDCV) vaccine should be given to all children bitten by wild animals in which rabies cannot be excluded, as well as to children bitten by domestic animals (cats and dogs) suspected or proven to be rabid. See Chapter 41 for a description of rabies treatment. ⊂⊃

Check the child's immunization record to determine whether a tetanus booster is necessary. Instruct parents about how to care for the wound.

Human Bites

Human bites are more common than most people realize. They usually occur in toddlers and young children. Because the mouth harbors many bacteria, infection is fairly common. Assess the risk for hepatitis B and HIV infection. Antibiotics may be prescribed to prevent systemic complications. Initial treatment includes irrigating with sterile saline and debridement. Instruct parents about how to care for the wound. Follow-up is important to watch for infection.

NURSING MANAGEMENT

If a child is bitten by an animal, take a complete and accurate history that includes the following information: extent of the injury, circumstances surrounding the attack, present location of the animal, and attempts to assess the animal's health.

Educate parents about preventing animal and human bites and the importance of teaching children appropriate behavior around other children and animals. When these bites occur in a child care or school setting, inform parents about the human bite so they can discuss potential risks and follow up with a health care provider.

As children with bites are often cared for at home, teach the parents about the normal healing process, proper wound care, and the signs and symptoms of infection.

Children who receive traumatic animal bites often experience significant psychologic trauma. They may develop a fear of strange animals and a decreased capacity to enjoy household pets. Counseling and follow-up may be necessary to evaluate such concerns.

Teaching About

PREVENTING ANIMAL BITES

- Teach children the following rules:
  —Avoid all unfamiliar animals and report them to a parent.
  —Avoid contact with all wild animals.
  —Do not touch an animal when it is eating, sleeping, or nursing.
  —Never overexcite an animal, even in play. No roughhouse or games that stimulate aggressive behavior.
  —Never tease or throw objects at an animal.
  —Never put your face close to an animal. Seek permission before hugging or petting an animal.
    –If approached by a dog, stay calm, stand still, talk softly, and back away slowly until the dog loses interest; don't run.
    –If attacked, be a tree or a log and protect the face.
- If an animal is sick or acting strangely, notify the health department.
- Never leave a young child alone with an animal.
- Do not buy a pet unless you are confident of your child's ability to respect it.
- Spay or neuter the pet to reduce aggression.

Insect Bites and Stings

Insect bites and stings occur frequently in children and usually are not a cause for concern. Exceptions include bites or stings by insects that carry parasites or communicable diseases (ticks, mosquitos), those of venomous insects (spiders), and those that produce an allergic reaction. About 4% of the population is sensitized to bee stings (Herman & Skokan, 1999). (For a discussion of Lyme disease and Rocky Mountain spotted fever, see Chapter 41.) ⊂⊃

Reactions to mosquito and flea bites can be localized or systemic. Local reactions include discrete, red papules and edema at the bite site, as well as itching, burning, pain, and hives. Local inflammation results from injected foreign protein or chemicals. Most bites produce minimal discomfort. Systemic reactions can include wheezing, urticaria, laryngeal edema, and shock.

Treatment is usually supportive and focuses on relieving itching and reducing inflammation. Pruritus is treated with cold compresses or ice applied to the site and an antihistamine. In children sensitized to insect bites, pruritic wheals and bullae tend to develop with repeat exposure. In rare cases, exposure can lead to an anaphylactic reaction. If large wheals, swelling of extremities, or respiratory difficulty occurs, emergency medical treatment is needed.

Bees and fire ants (Hymenoptera) inject a hemolytic, neurotoxic venom that causes a histaminelike response. Fire ants bite repeatedly in a small area. A black center is seen at the point of the bite along with pustules and local swelling. Reactions to either bee stings or fire ant bites may be local inflammation or a systemic allergic response (wheezing, urticaria, diarrhea, vomiting, and dizziness). In some cases an anaphylactic response occurs. Antihistamines may be used to treat local reactions. A dash of meat tenderizer (papain powder) and a drop of water massaged into the skin for 5 minutes quickly relieves the pain of most insect bites and stings. Ice is also effective. For systemic reactions, treat with glucocorticoids and antihistamines or intravenous or subcutaneous 1:1000 epinephrine solution. Desensitization for the Hymenoptera group should also be considered when the child has a systemic reaction.

Nursing Practice

Remove a bee stinger as soon as possible, but do not use tweezers or squeeze the venom sack. This pushes more venom into the skin. Use a straight edge, such as a piece of cardboard, to pull the stinger out in a scraping motion.

Black widow spider bites are characterized by a stinging sensation at the time of the bite followed by swelling, redness, and pain at the site. Red fang marks can be seen in a target lesion. Systemic symptoms can occur 15 minutes to 2 hours after the bite and include dizziness, fever, regional lymph node tenderness, severe abdominal pain (abdominal muscle rigidity), and weakness. Profuse sweating, vomiting, hypertension, and tachycardia may also be seen. Muscle cramps begin near the bite and can involve all skeletal muscles. If large doses of venom are absorbed, the bite may lead to paralysis and death. A neurotoxin produced by the spider is responsible for the symptoms. The black widow spider can be recognized by the red and orange hourglass-shaped markings on its underside. It usually bites in self-defense and avoids light areas. Treatment involves cleansing the wound, elevating the extremity, and immediately applying ice packs. Sedatives, analgesics, or muscle relaxants may be prescribed. Intravenous calcium gluconate may be given for muscle spasms. Antivenom (produced in horse serum) is used only in severe or high-risk cases because of the risk for anaphylaxis (Metry & Hebert, 2000). Hydrocortisone may decrease the inflammatory response. Symptoms generally peak in 3 to 12 hours and diminish within 72 hours.

The brown recluse spider bite is characterized by a sharp pain resembling a sting. Most bites are mild and cause only minimal edema and mild erythema. Severe bites can become necrotic over 48 to 72 hours in 10% of cases (Metry & Hebert, 2000). The child experiences mild to severe pain and tenderness. Within 3 to 4 days a purple, star-shaped area forms at the site with a white ischemic halo and outer ring of erythema, progressing to black eschar that is sloughed off. The wound usually heals with a scar in 6 to 8 weeks. Severe progressive reactions may include associated fever, chills, restlessness, malaise, joint pain, and nau-

sea and vomiting. The child may also have intravascular hemolysis with a severe reaction that results in anemia. The brown recluse spider is recognized by the fiddle-shaped marking on its head. It is usually unaggressive and bites only when provoked. Treatment involves prophylactic antibiotics, analgesics, application of cool compresses to the site, and corticosteroids for inflammation. In some cases a skin graft is needed.

NURSING MANAGEMENT

The goal of nursing care is prevention. Become familiar with the harmful insects in your area, so you can identify them and recognize their effects. Children should be taught to avoid spiders and other biting or stinging insects. Many commercial repellents (OFF, Cutter's, Deep Woods OFF) are available. Most products contain DEET (diethyltoluamide) and are effective against many insects including mosquitos, fleas, ticks, and chiggers. Use insect repellent containing DEET in concentrations less than 10% for children. If combined with sunscreen the effectiveness of the sunscreen is reduced by a third or half, so use sunscreen with an SPF of 30 (Metry & Hebert, 2000). However, caution parents to avoid overuse of products containing DEET, especially with infants and small children. Cases of toxic encephalopathy have been reported following repeated use on children's bedding and clothing (Metry & Hebert, 2000). DEET does not repel stinging insects.

Warn parents against using heavily perfumed shampoos, powders, soaps, or lotions, or dressing children in bright clothing when outdoors, as these may attract insects. Household pets may be a source of fleas or ticks. Encourage frequent inspection of pets and preventive treatments against fleas and ticks before pets are allowed prolonged contact with children. When a known allergy to Hymenoptera has occurred, the child should wear a medical alert identification and carry an emergency kit with epinephrine. Desensitization injections may be given. Teach parents and school personnel how to administer epinephrine.

Snake Bites

Venomous snakes are found in most areas of the country. During warm months, snakes are active and likely to bite if disturbed. Fortunately, many bites are dry, delivering no venom. Fatalities are rare. Rattlesnake, copperhead, and cottonmouth venom affects the blood coagulation system (Bond & Burkhart, 1998). Coral snake venom causes neuromuscular paralysis.

Puncture marks, white wheal, and severe pain appear at the site of the bite. Erythema and edema rapidly develop and extend from the site. Numbness may occur. Systemic signs include dizziness, nausea and vomiting, sweating and chills, weakness, hematemesis, and bleeding from the nose, intestines, or bladder. Numbness of the tongue and perioral areas may develop. Intracranial hemorrhage may be fatal. Clinical therapy involves immobilization of the extremity and a cold compress to slow the spread of the venom. Excision of the bite is no longer recommended. Laboratory studies include complete blood count, platelet count, coagulation studies, electrolytes, and renal function. Specific antivenom is quickly administered, but because antivenom contains a horse serum base, a skin test may be performed first to detect hypersensitivity. A tetanus booster is given if vaccination status is unknown or the tetanus series is incomplete.

NURSING MANAGEMENT

Nursing care involves assessing the child for initial and progressive signs of envenomation. First aid involves immobilizing the extremity, keeping it in a dependent position to slow the spread of venom, and cold compresses. Remove any jewelry from the injured extremity. Keep the child quiet and calm to slow the circulation. Help the child identify the snake from pictures of snakes common to the area; however, keep in mind that other venomous snakes may be kept as exotic pets.

Administer the antivenom intravenously. Help locate additional antivenom if the hospital does not have an adequate supply. Monitor the child for progressive signs of envenomation, and for hypersensitivity responses to antivenom. Provide emotional support to the child and family.

Teach children and their family to avoid future snakebites.

CONTUSIONS

Contusions are soft tissue injuries that have a variety of causes. Often it is difficult to assess whether an injury has caused underlying tissue damage. An injury does not have to break the skin to result in internal damage. Radiographic examination may be necessary to rule out broken bones or further tissue damage. Signs and symptoms that indicate a need for treatment include swelling that does not subside within 72 hours, intense pain, inability to move the injured part, and infection.

Elevate the injured extremity and apply ice as soon as possible after injury. This can reduce inflammation and swelling in the area.

FOREIGN BODIES

Many skin injuries result from penetration of foreign particles. Common substances include gravel from abrasions, bee stingers, and splinters. Treatment of superficial foreign bodies involves irrigating the wound to try to forcibly dislodge the debris. A deeply embedded foreign body is best removed under medical supervision to avoid permanent injury or scarring.

CHAPTER HIGHLIGHTS

≈ The skin has several essential functions: perception of pain, heat, and cold; protection from invasion by microorganisms and trauma; temperature regulation; vitamin D synthesis; and excretion.

≈ Wound healing has three phases—inflammation, reconstruction, and maturation.

≈ Contact dermatitis is an inflammation of the skin that occurs in response to direct contact with an allergen causing an immune response or irritant without an immune response.

≈ Superabsorbent disposable diapers reduce the frequency and severity of diaper dermatitis because wetness forms a gel, keeping the skin drier than cloth diapers.

≈ Seborrheic dermatitis is an inflammatory skin condition due to an overgrowth of *Pityrosporum* yeast in areas of sebaceous gland activity. It is commonly found on the scalp, forehead, and postauricular and periorbital areas.

≈ Treatment of atopic dermatitis involves hydration and lubrication of the skin with moisturizing ointments. Inflammation is treated with wet compresses and corticosteroid ointments.

≈ The acne medications tretinoin and isotretinoin are phototoxic. Avoidance of sun exposure or the use of sunscreen is important to prevent a significant sunburn.

≈ The classic impetigo lesion begins as a vesicle surrounded by edema and redness. The vesicle fluid turns cloudy and ruptures, leaving a honey-colored crust on an ulcerated base.

≈ Folliculitis, a superficial inflammation of the pilosebaceous follicle, may be associated with *Pseudomonas* exposure in a poorly chlorinated pool or hot tub.

≈ Children with cellulitis appear ill with fever, chills, malaise, and enlarged lymph nodes. The infected site is erythematous, warm, and tender.

≈ Treatment for lice includes a pediculicide shampoo, distilled white vinegar to loosen the nits' bonds to the hair shafts, and combing the hair with a fine-toothed comb to remove all the nits. A second treatment is needed in 7 days.

≈ Scabies lesions appear as linear, threadlike, grayish burrows 1 to 10 cm in length that may end in a pinpoint vesicle. Often the child's scratching and secondary infection change the appearance of the lesions.

≈ Children using oral inhalers with corticosteroids are at risk for thrush (oral candidiasis). Rinsing the mouth well with water after using the inhaler helps to prevent thrush.

≈ Treatment for tinea capitus involves 8 to 12 weeks of oral griseofulvin. Giving this medication with fatty foods such as whole milk or peanut butter enhances its absorption.

≈ Children at greatest risk for pressure ulcers are those with limited mobility, sensory deficits, or the inability to change positions.

≈ Of the four main types of burns (thermal, chemical, electrical, and radioactive), thermal burns are most common in children. They occur through exposure to flames or scalds and contact with a hot object.

- Repeated sunburns during childhood increase the risk for developing malignant melanoma in early adulthood.
- Children are at greater risk for hypothermia because of their thinner skin, limited subcutaneous fat, and high surface area to body mass ratio.
- Frostbite occurs when ice crystallizes in the tissues, causing cellular dehydration and ischemic damage.
- Dog bites account for 80% of animal bites treated in the United States. Boys less than 8 years old are at greater risk for animal bites. Most children know the dog that bites them.
- Insects and spiders with venomous bites include bees, fire ants, black widow spiders, and brown recluse spiders.
- Venomous snakes living in the wild in the United States include rattlesnakes, copperheads, cottonmouths, and coral snakes.

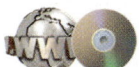 **EXPLORE**MEDIA**LINK**

NCLEX Review, Case Studies, and other interactive resources for this chapter can be found on the companion website at http://www.prenhall.com/london. Click on "Chapter 52" and select the activities for this chapter.

For animations, more NCLEX review questions, and an audio glossary, access the accompanying CD-ROM in this textbook.

REFERENCES

American Academy of Pediatrics Committee on Infectious Disease. (2000). *Red Book, Report of the Committee on Infectious Disease* (25th ed.). Elk Grove Village, IL: Author.

Angel, T. A., Nigro, J., & Levy, M. L. (2000). Infestations in the pediatric patient. *Pediatric Clinics of North America, 47*(4), 921–935.

Armsmeier, S. L., & Paller, A. S. (1997). Getting to the bottom of diaper dermatitis. *Contemporary Pediatrics, 14*(11), 115–129.

Ball, J. W. (1998). *Mosby's pediatric patient teaching guides.* St. Louis, MO: Mosby.

Bernardo, L. M., Gardner, M. J., O'Connor, J., & Amon, N. (2000). Dog bites in children treated in a pediatric emergency department. *Journal of Society of Pediatric Nurses, 5*(2), 87–95.

Bond, R. G., & Burkhart, K. K. (1997). Thrombocytopenia following timber rattlesnake envenomation. *Annals of Emergency Medicine, 30*(1), 40–44.

Buck, M. L. (2001). Isotretinoin: Improving patient education and reducing risk. *Pediatric Pharmacology, 7*(7), 1–6.

Darmstadt, G. L. (1997). A guide to superficial strep and staph skin infections. *Contemporary Pediatrics, 14*(5), 95–116.

Eichelberger, M. R., Ball, J. W., Pratsch, G. L., & Clark, J. R. (1998). *Pediatric emergencies* (2nd ed., p. 182). Upper Saddle River, NJ: Prentice-Hall.

Friedlander, S. F. (1998). Contact dermatitis. *Pediatrics in Review, 19*(5), 166–170.

Gardner, P., Coles, D., & Kemper, K. J. (2001). The skinny on herbal remedies for dermatologic disorders. *Contemporary Pediatrics, 18*(7), 103–114.

Hebert, P. W., Rakes, G. P., Loach, T. C., & Murphy, D. D. (1997). Recognizing the young atopic child. *Contemporary Pediatrics, 14*(4), 131–139.

Herman, B. E., & Skokan, E. G. (1999). Bites that poison: A tale of spiders, snakes, and scorpions. *Contemporary Pediatrics, 16*(8), 41–65.

Hernandez-Reif, M., Field, T., Largie, S., Hart, S., Redezepi, M., Nierenberg, B., et al. (2001).

Children's distress during burn treatment reduced by massage therapy. *Journal of Burn Care Rehabilitation, 22*(2), 191–195.

Herndon, D. N., & Spies, M. (2001). Modern burn care. *Seminars in Pediatric Surgery, 10*(1), 28–31.

Jick, S. S., Kremers, H. M., & Vasilakis-Scarmoza, C. (2000). Isotretinoin use and risk of depression, psychotic symptoms, suicide, and attempted suicide. *Archives of Dermatology, 136*(10), 1231–1236.

Kazaks, E. L., & Lane, A. T. (2000). Diaper dermatitis. *Pediatric Clinics of North America, 47*(4), 909–919.

Laughlin-Richard, N. (2000). Sun exposure and skin cancer prevention in children and adolescents. *Journal of School Nursing, 16*(2), 20–26.

Loman, D. G. (2000). Assessment of skin breakdown risk in children. *Journal of Child and Family Nursing, 3*(3), 234–238.

Lukish, J. R., Eichelberger, M. R., Newman, K. D., Pao, M., Nobuhara, K., Keating, M., et al. (2001). The use of a bioactive skin substitute decreases length of stay for pediatric burn patients. *Journal of Pediatric Surgery, 36*(8), 1118–1121.

Mancini, A. J. (2000). Acne vulgaris: A treatment update. *Contemporary Pediatrics, 17*(12), 122–133.

McDonald, L. L., & Smith, M. L. (1998). Diagnostic dilemmas in pediatric/adolescent dermatology: Scaly scalp. *Journal of Pediatric Health Care, 12*(2), 80–84.

Metry, D. W., & Hebert, A. A. (2000). Insect and arachnid stings, bites, infestations, and repellents. *Pediatric Annals, 29*(1), 39–48.

Murphy, S. A. (2000). Deaths: Final data for 1998. *National Vital Statistics Reports, 48*(11). Hyattsville, MD: National Center for Health Statistics.

Nicol, N. H. (2000). Managing atopic dermatitis in children and adults. *Nurse Practitioner, 25*(4), 54–76.

Quigley, S. M., & Curley, M. A. Q. (1996). Skin integrity in the pediatric population: Preventing and managing pressure ulcers. *Journal of the Society of Pediatric Nurses, 1*(1), 7–18.

Raimer, S. S. (2000). Managing pediatric atopic dermatitis. *Clinical Pediatrics, 39*(1), 1–14.

Rodgers, G. L. (2000). Reducing the toll of childhood burns. *Contemporary Pediatrics, 17*(4), 152–173.

Rote, N. S. (1998). Inflammation. In K. L. McCance & S. E. Huether (Eds.), *Pathophysiology: The biologic basis for disease in adults and children* (3rd ed., pp. 205–236). St. Louis, MO: Mosby.

Schachner, L. A. (2000 May). Sun protection in three ways. *Contemporary Pediatrics,* (Suppl.), 8–11.

Schachner, L., Field, T., Hernandez-Ruif, M., Duarte, A. M., & Krasnegor, J. (1998). Atopic dermatitis symptoms decreased in children following massage therapy. *Pediatric Dermatology, 15*(5), 390–395.

Sidbury, R., & Paller, A. S. (2000). The diagnosis and management of acne. *Pediatric Annals, 29*(1), 17–24.

Smith, M. L. (2000). Pediatric burns: Management of thermal, electrical, and chemical burns and burn-like dermatologic conditions. *Pediatric Annals, 29*(6), 367–378.

Stewart, C. (2000). Emergency care of pediatric burns. *Pediatric Emergency Medicine Reports, 5*(10), 101–112.

Su, J. C., Kemp, A. S., Varigos, G. A., & Nolan, T. M. (1997). Atopic eczema: Its impact on the family and financial cost. *Archives of Diseases in Children, 76*(2), 159–162.

Valencia, I. C., Falabella, A. F., & Schachner, L. A. (2001). New developments in wound care for infants and children. *Pediatric Annals, 30*(4), 211–218.

Vanderhooft, S. L. (1998). Is the rash really a drug reaction? *Contemporary Pediatrics, 15*(5), 118–137.

Weston, W. L., & Bruckner, A. (2000). Allergic contact dermatitis. *Pediatric Clinics of North America, 47*(4), 897–907.

Wiebelhaus, P., & Hansen, S. L. (2001). Another choice for burn victims. *RN, 64*(9), 34–37.

CHAPTER 53

The Child with Alterations in Mental Health Function

*W*e've been so worried about Cassandra. After being in the car crash, she has become so frightened of everything. She wakes up at night screaming and has lost interest in school and friends. We hope that her work with the therapist will help to decrease her fears and get her involved in all of her activities again.

—MOTHER OF CASSANDRA, 9 YEARS OLD

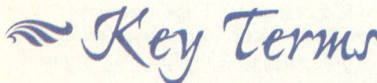

Key Terms

Adaptive functioning   *1429*
Affect   *1433*
Agoraphobia   *1438*
Behavior modification   *1420*
Cognitive therapy   *1420*
Echolalia   *1423*

Evidence-based practice   *1419*
Pervasive developmental disorders   *1423*
Play therapy   *1420*
Stereotypy   *1423*

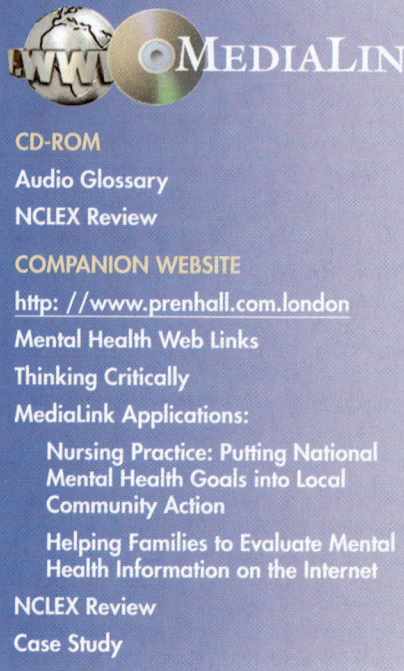

MediaLink

CD-ROM
Audio Glossary
NCLEX Review

COMPANION WEBSITE
http://www.prenhall.com.london
Mental Health Web Links
Thinking Critically
MediaLink Applications:

Nursing Practice: Putting National Mental Health Goals into Local Community Action

Helping Families to Evaluate Mental Health Information on the Internet

NCLEX Review

Case Study

$\mathcal{T}$his chapter will provide the knowledge and tools needed to provide appropriate care for children with alterations in mental health. Because much of this care is provided by psychiatric–mental health specialists, the nurse's role often centers on identification, support of the therapy, teaching, and referral.

Some mental health conditions in children originate from a genetic or physiologic cause. Examples include mental retardation and childhood schizophrenia. Often the environments in which children live influence their characteristics and contributes to dysfunctions such as anxiety, depression, and posttraumatic stress disorder.

Most mental health conditions are treated in community settings, and nurses in these settings play an active role in the treatment and support of the child and family. Nurses may function as case managers, assisting a family to deal with all areas of the child's care. Occasionally a child is hospitalized for treatment of a significant mental health disruption, or a child hospitalized for another health problem requires continued mental health services.

PSYCHOTHERAPEUTIC MANAGEMENT OF CHILDREN AND ADOLESCENTS

Mental health is foundational to a sense of personal well-being. However, 10% of children in the United States suffer from mental illness severe enough to impair functioning, and only 50% of those children receive any mental health services. Further, some of the services received are not comprehensive or multidisciplinary, leading to unmet mental health needs (Navon, Nelson, Pageno, et al., 2001). In other cases, the interventions used are not supported by theory and research.

The Surgeon General is leading an initiative to examine mental health in the United States and has identified a series of goals and steps toward improving mental health care for children (Department of Health and Human Services, 2000). From the ages of 10 to 21 years, mental health issues are among the top two leading causes of hospitalization in all age groups (see Chapter 1). 🔗 This high rate of hospitalization suggests that children are not receiving mental health services early, when outpatient care is appropriate and prognosis is best. In order to confront this childhood mental health crisis, the Surgeon General's agenda includes promoting mental health as an essential part of child health, integrating mental health services into all health services provided to children, engaging families and youth in planning for mental health care, and developing and enhancing the infrastructure to support child and youth mental health services (Department of Health and Human Services, 2000). See Table 53–1 for a list of the goals established in the Surgeon General's report. 🔗 WEB

TABLE 53-1 Goals of the Surgeon General's National Action Agenda for Children's Mental Health

1. Promote public awareness of children's mental health issues and reduce stigma associated with mental illness.
2. Continue to develop, disseminate, and implement scientifically proven prevention and treatment services in the field of children's mental health.
3. Improve the assessment and recognition of mental health needs in children.
4. Eliminate racial/ethnic and socioeconomic disparities in access to mental health care.
5. Improve the infrastructure for children's mental health services, including support for scientifically proven interventions across professions.
6. Increase access to and coordination of quality mental health care services.
7. Train frontline providers to recognize and manage mental health issues, and educate mental health providers in scientifically proven prevention and treatment services.
8. Monitor the access to and coordination of quality mental health care services.

Note: From Department of Health and Human Services, 2000.

The primary treatment goal for children and adolescents with psychosocial disorders is to assist the child and family to achieve and maintain an optimal level of functioning through interventions designed to reduce the impact of stressors. Therapeutic interventions and communication are based on the principle that feelings motivate behaviors. Parents and others close to the child often fall into the habit of reacting to the child's behaviors rather than trying to find out what feelings may be precipitating the undesirable actions. While behaviors may be considered in treatment, feelings and life experiences are often explored to provide insight and to lead to behavior change. Medication may be used to enhance and support other therapy, or may be the major therapeutic measure.

When possible, mental health interventions should be founded on **evidence-based practice,** or a body of scientific knowledge. Such research knowledge is scant in pediatric mental health services, but is increasing due to health care research in this area. Nurses can include evidence-based practice and outcome measurement in mental health care whenever possible (Hoagwood, Burns, Kiser, et al., 2001).

Treatment Modes

Three basic treatment modes are used: individual, family, and group therapy. The choice of treatment mode must take into account the child's age and developmental stage. Most therapists use several intervention strategies simultaneously. Different strategies are more or less effective and appropriate for children and adolescents in various stages of development. A thorough understanding of developmental needs, expectations, and abilities is therefore essential for mental health professionals.

INDIVIDUAL THERAPY

Individual therapy involves only the child and the therapist. Treatment of specific emotional problems or disorders may involve various techniques such as play therapy, psychodrama, art therapy, and **cognitive therapy** (a technique used to help a person recognize automatic negative thinking). Individual therapy may be short term (four to six sessions) or long term (lasting for several years).

FAMILY THERAPY

Family therapy involves the exploration of a particular emotional problem and its manifestations among the family members. Family therapy is based on the idea that the emotional symptoms or problems of an individual are an expression of emotional symptoms or problems in the family. The focus is on the relationships among the family members, not the psychologic conflict within each individual member.

GROUP THERAPY

Group therapy involves an ongoing or limited number of sessions in which several individuals participate. The emphasis is on the interpersonal styles of relating to one another in the group. Group therapy is particularly effective with adolescents because of the importance of the peer group at this age. An advantage of group therapy is that stimuli and feedback come from multiple sources (the group members) instead of just one person (the therapist).

Therapeutic Strategies

PLAY THERAPY

Play is often called the language or work of the child. From a developmental perspective, children progressively learn to express feelings and needs through action, fantasy, and finally language. The special quality of play buffers children against the pressures and demands of daily life. Play helps children master developmental stages by strengthening physical and neurologic processes. Play also assists in cognitive learning, setting the stage for problem solving and creativity.

Play therapy is a technique that reveals problems on a fantasy level through the use of toys, dolls, clay, art, and other creative objects. It is often used with preschool and school-age children who are experiencing anxiety, stress, and other specific nonpsychotic mental disorders. Play therapy encourages the child to act out feelings such as anger, hostility, sadness, and fear. It also gives the therapist a chance to help the child understand, on a conscious or unconscious level, his or her own responses and behavior in a safe, supportive environment. This type of therapy was used for Cassandra, described in the opening quotation, who needed to gain some control over a frightening environment by acting out fears and trying solutions during play with a therapist. Play therapy is different from therapeutic play, which may be used with hospitalized children (see Chapter 34). Only a specialist is qualified to provide play therapy for mental health disorders.

ART THERAPY

Children who may be apprehensive about playing can sometimes be encouraged to participate in art therapy, using brief drawing exercises. This technique is appropriate for children of all ages, including adolescents. The drawings can help the therapist gain information about the child, the family, and the interactions between the child and family. However, children's drawings should never be the only basis for a definitive diagnosis.

When used in conjunction with a thorough history and appropriate psychologic testing information, art therapy can guide the child's treatment. These drawing exercises provide an opportunity to help in the healing process. The therapist can assist the child to release feelings of anger, pain, or fear onto paper, where they can be examined objectively. (Figures 53–1 ♦ to 53–4 ♦ present several examples of this technique.)

BEHAVIOR AND COGNITIVE THERAPY

Behavior modification is a therapeutic technique that uses stimulus and response conditioning to alter inappropriate behaviors. It reinforces desirable behaviors, helping the child to replace maladaptive behaviors with more appropriate ones. This technique is based on the assumption

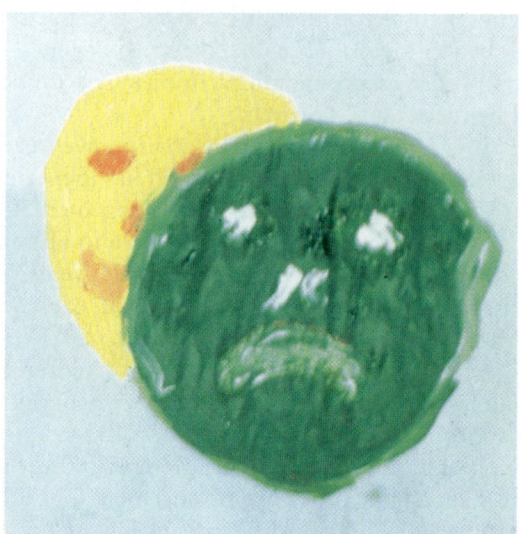

FIGURE 53–1. ♦ "Me." Drawn by a 14-year-old girl with major depression, anxiety, and school phobia who had experienced multiple losses over several years. Her mother had severe chronic lung problems and diabetes, and the girl had stopped attending school for fear that something would happen to her mother. This drawing represents the girl's obvious feelings of sadness and depression but also indicates a glimmer of hope (represented by the yellow mask coming from behind the dark mask of depression).

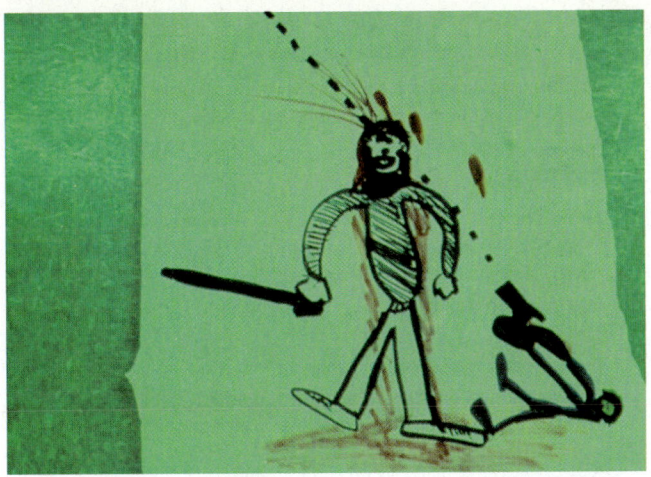

FIGURE 53–2. ◆ "Self-Portrait." Drawn by a 15-year-old boy who was admitted through the emergency department after a failed suicide attempt by hanging. He had a psychiatric diagnosis of depression and polysubstance abuse (including inhalants and alcohol) and insisted that he was a member of a satanic cult in his hometown. Most of his drawings depicted a preoccupation with violence and suicide. The boy said that he always felt a "darkness" like a shadow that followed him around and wanted him dead. His family history was significant for depression and suicide on both his mother's and his father's side. His father also had a lengthy history of polysubstance abuse and alcoholism. The boy was discharged to a long-term residential treatment facility for adolescents.

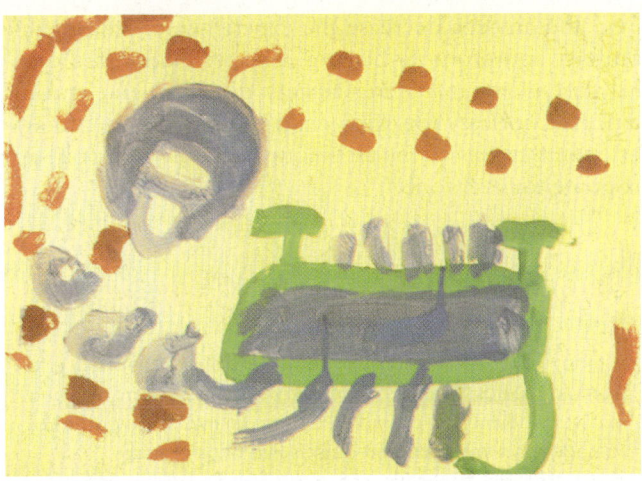

FIGURE 53–4. ◆ "A Family Activity." By the same boy who drew Figure 53–3. This drawing depicts a recurring incident of physical and emotional abuse by his mother's live-in boyfriend. It shows the family bathtub with feces and blood smeared on the floors and walls. The boy reported that when either he or his 3-year-old brother had a toileting accident the boyfriend would make them go into the bathroom and stand in the bathtub while he smeared the feces on the walls. He would then hit the children and make them clean up the mess. The boy had previously been removed from the mother's custody for neglect. He was transferred from the medical-surgical area to the inpatient children's psychiatric unit, where he received a diagnosis of depression, overanxious disorder, and child abuse (physical and emotional). Charges were filed against the mother's boyfriend and custody of both children was temporarily revoked.

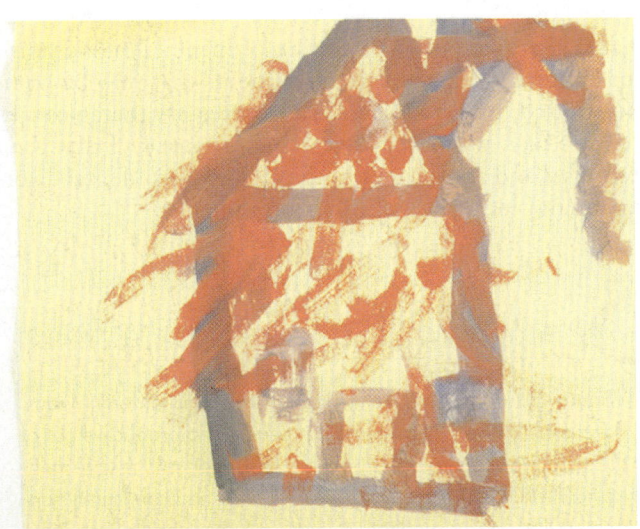

FIGURE 53–3. ◆ "An Activity." Drawn by an 8-year-old boy who was initially admitted to the medical-surgical floor of a pediatric hospital for dehydration resulting from vomiting and diarrhea. Psychiatric evaluation was ordered for extreme anxiety. These drawings, completed during the initial interview, led to further investigation, which revealed that the child had started a house fire in which his grandmother (his primary caretaker at the time) was killed. The family's home and all their belongings were lost. No one had known that the child had set the fire. Further sessions indicated that he had been setting neighborhood garage fires and watching them burn from a distance.

that any learned behavior can be unlearned. Thus, if parents, nurses, teachers, and other adults consistently reinforce desirable behaviors, the child will eventually alter or discontinue undesirable behaviors.

Behavior modification may include (1) removing the child from the home to a more structured environment, such as a hospital, for a brief time, and (2) teaching the parents, teachers, and other appropriate adults to be agents of behavioral change. Several ongoing sessions may be required with the adults involved, using role play and other techniques. Consistency is the most important principle in the success of behavior modification.

Cognitive therapy teaches thinking patterns to change reactions to situations that cause anxiety or other undesirable conditions. The child is taught how his or her brain and body are working; this understanding assists the child in having control over the experience. Often a combination of cognitive and behavioral approaches is useful in treating children.

VISUALIZATION AND GUIDED IMAGERY

The techniques of visualization and guided imagery begin with specific directions for progressive relaxation according to the child's ability. This form of therapy uses the child's own imagination and positive thinking to reduce stress and anxiety, decrease the experience of pain or discomfort, and promote healing. The techniques are especially useful for managing anxiety disorders and chronic pain. It is not easy for every child to use his or her imagination in this way, so the technique may not work or be appropriate for everyone.

Developing Cultural Competence

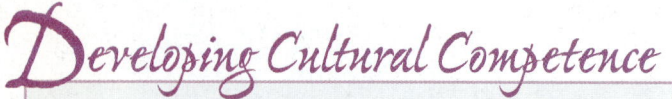

In many cultures, care of the "spirit" is believed necessary to promote mental health. An identity with one's community and spiritual wholeness is promoted by storytelling, singing, rites of passage, and use of certain objects like bags of herbs.

HYPNOSIS

Hypnosis involves varying degrees of suggestibility and deep relaxation effects. This technique is useful for children and adolescents because they can usually be hypnotized more easily than adults. Hypnosis is especially helpful in treating physical symptoms with a psychologic component, anxiety, and phobias. It is also useful in managing severe physical symptoms or discomfort (pain or nausea) associated with a physiologic disorder or its treatment (e.g., cancer or juvenile rheumatoid arthritis). Refer to "Complementary Care: Hypnotherapy for Children" in Chapter 38, page 928.

Nurse's Role

Although many mental health disorders are managed effectively with therapy and/or medication on an outpatient basis, some necessitate admission to an inpatient psychiatric setting. The nurse may encounter the child with a mental health disorder during hospitalization for a concurrent physiologic problem, or in a variety of community settings. If a child is hospitalized for a concurrent problem, assess the child's current level of functioning in relation to the mental health disorder.

Nursing assessment also focuses on identifying medications being taken, common abnormal behaviors (what triggers them, what reduces them), family interactions, and routines to maintain appropriate behaviors (Table 53–2). Then consider how to support the child within the hospital environment.

Nursing care includes carrying out the prescribed treatment plan and administering psychotropic medications. Evaluate the child's medication regimen for administration schedule, dosage, side effects, and effectiveness. Inform the therapist of the child's hospitalization if the child has been hospitalized for a concurrent condition, and consult with the therapist about appropriate approaches for the child. Provide supportive care for the child and family. Continuation of family involvement is critical. The nurse frequently is the liaison between the family and the therapist in making follow-up arrangements at the time of dis-

---

TABLE 53–2 Mental Health Assessment

Gather information about the child's mental health by asking questions and making observations. Some components to include are:

- Appearance
  - Clothing appropriate for age, setting, and developmental level
  - Facial expression and response to you
  - Body size and posture
  - Interactions with parents or others
  - Interest in surroundings
- Behavior
  - Level of consciousness and interaction with surroundings
  - Recent reported changes in behavior (i.e., sleep, eating patterns, communication with others, school performance, friendships, risky activities)
  - Problem behaviors identified by child or parent
  - Events associated with problem behaviors
- Development
  - Results of developmental testing
  - Progression of skills reported by family
  - Unusual capabilities or deficits
  - Progression in school and extracurricular activities
- Life Events
  - Recent stress or trauma
  - Changes in family structure
  - Chronic health conditions in family members
- History
  - Prenatal events or birth trauma
  - Diagnosed mental health disorder in child or other family members
  - Neurologic injuries or diseases

---

charge. Be aware of the meaning of mental illness in various cultural groups and the treatments that may be commonly used. Integrate these complementary therapies into the care plan whenever safe. Families must feel that their responses and approaches to the child with a mental disorder are not judged by health professionals.

Developing Cultural Competence

Various cultural groups define mental health in different ways. For most it is a sense of well-being, peace, and productive use of the mind. Various therapies are used to support and restore mental health. They may include healers, family and community support, relaxation or meditation, teas and other herbal products, and exorcism. Find out how individuals and groups define mental health and how they believe health is maintained. Be alert to learn if mental disorders are viewed as a negative stigma or are openly accepted and discussed.

The nurse in the community assesses how a child with a mental health disorder is functioning in each microsystem (see Chapter 32), such as home, day care, school, and with friends. Assess risk and protective factors of the child and family (see Chapter 36). 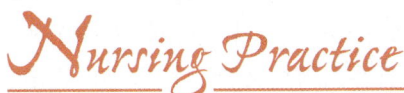 Evaluate involvement in therapy sessions and ability to manage prescribed pharmacologic interventions.

(see Chapter 36)

≈ DEVELOPMENTAL AND BEHAVIORAL DISORDERS

AUTISTIC SPECTRUM DISORDER

Pervasive developmental disorders (PDDs) begin in early childhood and are characterized by impaired social interactions and communication, with restricted interests, activities, and behaviors (Baird, Charman, Cox, et al., 2001). Autism or autistic spectrum disorder (ASD) is the most common of the PDDs. (Rett syndrome and Asperger syndrome are two examples of nonautistic PDDs.) Autistic disorder is a complex childhood disorder that involves abnormalities in behavior, social interactions, and communication. The essential features typically become apparent by the time a child is 3 years of age. For every 1000 births, 1 to 2 children are found to have autistic disorder, and an increasing incidence has been noted in the last few years (American Academy of Pediatrics [AAP], 2001a). The disorder occurs four times more often in boys than in girls.

𝒩urnsing 𝒫ractice

Rett syndrome is a pervasive developmental disorder similar in some ways to autistic disorder. Rett syndrome, however, occurs only in girls. The child usually appears normal until 6 to 18 months of age. Symptoms of increasing ataxia, hand-wringing, intermittent hyperventilation, dementia, and growth retardation then progress until the child requires total care.

𝒩urnsing 𝒫ractice

Asperger syndrome is manifested by impaired social interaction and repetitive behavior. Pitch, tone, and other characteristics of speech may be abnormal. However, cognition and language skills are usually normal for age.

Etiology and Pathophysiology

The cause of autistic disorder is unknown. Genetic transmission, immune responses, and neuroanatomy are all being investigated as causes (Williams, Dalrymple, & Neal, 2000). Neurotransmitters such as dopamine, serotonin,

and opioids are abnormal in some children and a focus of present research (Cade & Tidwell, 2001). Congenital rubella syndrome and tuberous sclerosis can lead to autism (AAP, 2001a). Recent studies have demonstrated that there is no link between the measles-mumps-rubella (MMR) vaccine and autism (Dales, Hammer, & Smith, 2001). Autistic children are frequently cognitively impaired, but can demonstrate a wide range of intellectual ability and functioning.

Clinical Manifestations

Autistic children may manifest disturbances in the rate or sequence of development. A primary finding is impairment in social interactions. Autistic children are unable to relate to people or to respond to social and emotional cues. In addition, they engage in **stereotypy,** or rigid and obsessive behavior. Characteristically these repetitive behaviors in affected children include head banging, twirling in circles, biting themselves, and flapping their hands or arms. Frequently a child's behavior is self-stimulating or self-destructive. Responses to sensory stimuli are frequently abnormal and include an extreme aversion to touch, loud noises, and bright lights. Emotional lability is common.

Difficulties or delays in speech and language are common and are often the first symptoms that lead to diagnosis. Abnormal communication patterns include both verbal and nonverbal communication. Autistic children may eventually learn to talk, in some cases well, but their speech is likely to show certain abnormalities: use of *you* in place of *I;* **echolalia** (a compulsive parroting of what is heard); repeating questions rather than answering them; and fascination with rhythmic, repetitive songs and verses.

About 75% of children with ASD are mentally retarded (Koenig, 1998). Although 25% have microcephaly, most children have normal appearance. Cognitive impairment may become apparent early in life by slow developmental progression, particularly in social skills.

Clinical Therapy

Diagnosis is based on the presence of specific criteria, as described in the American Psychiatric Association's *Diagnostic and Statistical Manual of Mental Disorders,* 4th edition (DSM-IV), outlined in Table 53–3. Additional testing is done to rule out other causes of the child's behavior. Tests may include neuroimaging (CT scan or MRI), lead screening, DNA analysis, and electroencephalogram. See Chapters 4 and 20 for further descriptions related to the neurologic system.

Early intervention helps maximize the child's potential and establish helpful support for parents. Treatment focuses on behavior management to reward appropriate behaviors, foster positive or adaptive coping skills, and facilitate effective communication. The goals of treatment are to reduce rigidity or stereotypy (repetitive, obsessive, machine-like movements) and other maladaptive behaviors.

TABLE 53-3 DSM-IV-TR Diagnostic Criteria for Autistic Disorder

A. A total of six or more items from 1, 2, and 3, with at least two from 1, and one each from 2 and 3:

  1. Qualitative impairment in social interaction, as manifested by at least two of the following:

    a. Marked impairment in the use of multiple nonverbal behaviors such as eye-to-eye gaze, facial expression, body posture, and gestures to regulate social interaction

    b. Failure to develop peer relationships appropriate to developmental level

    c. A lack of spontaneous seeking to share enjoyment, interests, or achievements with other people

    d. Lack of social or emotional reciprocity

  2. Qualitative impairments in communication as manifested by at least one of the following:

    a. Delay in, or total lack of, the development of spoken language (not accompanied by an attempt to compensate through alternative modes of communication such as gesture or mime)

    b. In individuals with adequate speech, marked impairment in the ability to initiate or sustain a conversation with others

    c. Stereotyped and repetitive use of language or idiosyncratic language

    d. Lack of varied, spontaneous make-believe play or social imitative play appropriate to developmental level

  3. Restricted repetitive and stereotyped patterns of behavior, interests, and activities, as manifested by at least one of the following:

    a. Encompassing preoccupation with one or more stereotyped and restricted patterns of interest that is abnormal either in intensity or in focus

    b. Apparently inflexible adherence to specific, nonfunctional routines or rituals

    c. Stereotyped and repetitive motor mannerisms (e.g., hand or finger flapping or twisting, or complex whole-body movements)

    d. Persistent preoccupation with parts of objects

B. Delays or abnormal functioning in at least one of the following areas, with onset prior to age 3 years: (1) social interaction, (2) language as used in social communication, or (3) symbolic or imaginative play.

C. The disturbance is not better accounted for by Rett Syndrome or Childhood Disintegrative Disorder.

Note: From American Psychiatric Association. (2000). *Diagnostic and statistical manual of mental disorders* Text Revision (4th ed.). Washington, DC: Author. Copyright © 2000 American Psychiatric Association.

Often the child must be physically restrained from aggressive or self-destructive behaviors. Some parents choose to use complementary therapies such as vitamin supplements and dimethylglycine. Foods such as sugar, aspartame, milk products, and wheat are sometimes eliminated from the diet. Some families use medicines such as secretin (a pancreatic hormone) and antacids (Hyman & Levy, 2000).

The overall prognosis for autistic children to become functioning members of society is guarded. The extent of adequate adjustment varies greatly. Successful adjustment is more likely for children with higher IQs, adequate speech, and access to specialized programs.

Nursing Management

Nursing Assessment and Diagnosis

The nurse may encounter the autistic child when parents seek care for a suspected hearing impairment, speech difficulty, or developmental delay. Early and frequent developmental screening of all children can help in referral for thorough assessment and identification of cases. Parents may report abnormal interaction such as lack of eye contact, disinterest in cuddling, minimal facial responsiveness, and failure to talk. Initial assessment focuses on language development, response to others, and hearing acuity (see Chapters 33 and 48). Specialized screening tests for autism are available online and are being evaluated for their usefulness.

When a child with a diagnosis of autistic disorder is hospitalized for a concurrent problem, obtain a history from the parents about the child's routines, rituals, and likes and dislikes, as well as ways to promote interaction and cooperation. Autistic children may carry a special toy or object that they play with during times of stress. Ask parents about these objects and their use.

Ask about the child's behaviors and observe them on admission. Obtain a history of acute and chronic illnesses and injuries. Ask about eating patterns and food restrictions. Inquire about complementary and alternative medicine treatments in a nonjudgmental and supportive manner.

Nursing diagnoses must be tailored to fit the individual needs of the child. Examples of nursing diagnoses that might be appropriate for autistic children include the following:

▶ *Impaired verbal communication* related to psychologic condition

▶ *Impaired social interaction* related to developmental disability

▶ *Altered thought processes* related to mental disorder

▶ *Risk for injury* related to cognitive impairment

▶ *Risk for caregiver role strain* related to chronicity and demands of child's condition

▶ *Ineffective family coping: compromised or disabling* related to having a child with prolonged disability

Planning and Implementation

Nursing care focuses on stabilizing environmental stimuli, providing supportive care, enhancing communication, maintaining a safe environment, giving the parents anticipatory guidance, and providing emotional support.

STABILIZE ENVIRONMENTAL STIMULI

Autistic children interpret and respond to the environment differently from other individuals. Sounds that are not distressing to the average person may be interpreted by autistic children as louder, more frightening, and overwhelming. The child needs to be oriented to new settings such as a classroom or the hospital room and may adjust best to a small classroom or a hospital room with only one other child. Encourage parents to bring the child's favorite objects from home, and try to keep these objects in the same places, because the child does not cope well with changes in the environment.

PROVIDE SUPPORTIVE CARE

Developing a trusting relationship with the autistic child is often difficult. Adjust communication techniques and teaching to the child's developmental level. Ask parents about the child's usual home routines, and maintain these routines as much as possible. Because self-care abilities are often limited, the child may need help meeting basic needs. School programs and individual education plans (see Chapter 35) 🔗 can help the child learn self-care skills. When possible, schedule daily care and routine procedures at consistent times to maintain predictability. Encourage parents to remain with the hospitalized child and to participate in daily care planning. Parents are integral parts of the treatment team when the child's learning goals are established in early intervention or school programs. Identify rituals for naptime and bedtime, and maintain them to promote rest and sleep. Establish patterns that help the child eat nutritious foods at mealtimes.

ENHANCE COMMUNICATION

Since children with autism have impaired communication, nursing care focuses on using and improving communication with the child (Cade & Tidwell, 2001). Use speech when possible. When the child responds well to visual cues, pictures, computers, and other visual aids may form an important part of interactions. Some children use sign language.

MAINTAIN A SAFE ENVIRONMENT

Monitor autistic children at all times, including bathtime and bedtime. Close supervision is needed to ensure that the child does not obtain any harmful objects or engage in dangerous behaviors. Bicycle helmets and mittens are sometimes used to protect autistic children so that they can safely participate in activities.

PROVIDE ANTICIPATORY GUIDANCE

Approximately half of all children with autistic disorder require lifelong supervision and support. This is especially true if the disorder is accompanied by mental retardation. Some children may grow up to lead independent lives, although they will have social limitations with impaired interpersonal relationships. Encourage parents to promote the child's development through behavior modification and specialized educational programs. The overall goal is to provide the child with the guidance, education, and support necessary for optimal functioning.

NURSING CARE IN THE COMMUNITY

Families of autistic children need a great deal of support to cope with the challenges of caring for the autistic child. Help the family identify resources for child care, such as special toddler programs and preschools. The child will need an individual education plan. The parent or primary caretaker often has a hard time getting respite care and may need assistance to find suitable resources. Siblings of the autistic child may need help explaining the disorder to their friends or teachers. Family support programs are available in some states to provide assistance to parents.

Offer the family genetic counseling. Parents need information on the need for immunizations since they may have heard about a potential connection between immunization and the disorder. Encourage parents to have the child immunized on the recommended schedule. Parents may have questions about where to find information on complementary and alternative therapies.

Local support groups for parents of autistic children are available in most areas. Parents can also be referred to the Autism Society of America for information. 🔗

Evaluation

Expected outcomes of nursing care for the child with autism include:

▶ Management of behavioral symptoms
▶ Maximization of self-care
▶ Maintenance of safe environment
▶ Consistent developmental progression
▶ Successful communication strategies

ATTENTION DEFICIT DISORDER AND ATTENTION DEFICIT HYPERACTIVITY DISORDER

Attention deficit disorder (ADD) is a variation in central nervous system processing characterized by developmentally inappropriate behaviors involving inattention. When hyperactivity and impulsivity accompany inattention, the disorder is called attention deficit hyperactivity disorder (ADHD). ADHD is the more common condition and affects approximately 5% of all children, boys more commonly than girls (Hunt, Paguin, & Payton, 2001).

Etiology and Pathophysiology

Although a variety of physical and neurologic disorders are associated with ADHD, children with identifiable causes represent a small proportion of this population. Examples of known associations include exposure to high levels of lead in childhood and prenatal exposure to alcohol. There may be a deficit in the catecholamines dopamine and norepinephrine in some children, lowering the threshold for stimuli input. Probably there are many types of attention deficit, resulting from several different mechanisms. Genetic factors may be important, as well as family dynamics and environmental characteristics. Although ADHD occurs more commonly within families, a single gene has not been located and a specific mechanism of genetic transmission is not known. It is believed that a genetic predisposition interacts with the child's environment, so that both factors contribute to the appearance of the condition. Some children with the condition have additional problems such as aggressive behaviors, learning disabilities, and motor disorders (Blondis, 1999; Fletcher, Shaywitz, & Shaywitz, 1999).

Clinical Manifestations

Children with ADD and ADHD have problems related to decreased attention span, impulsiveness, and/or increased motor activity. Symptoms can range from mild to severe. The disorders often coexist with various developmental learning disabilities. The child has difficulty completing tasks, fidgets constantly, is frequently loud, and interrupts others. Sleep disturbances are common. Because of these behaviors, the child often has difficulty developing and maintaining social relationships and may be shunned or teased by other children. This only increases the anxiety of the already compromised child, whose behavior is set on a downward-spiraling course.

Typically, girls with ADHD show less aggression and impulsiveness than boys, but far more anxiety, mood swings, social withdrawal, rejection, and cognitive and language problems. Girls tend to be older at the time of diagnosis. Children are frequently diagnosed with the disorder soon after beginning school, with its demands for attentive behavior (AAP, 2000).

Clinical Therapy

Children are usually brought for evaluation when behaviors escalate to the point of interfering with the daily functioning of teachers or parents. When children have learning disabilities or anxiety disorders, the problem is commonly misdiagnosed as ADHD without further evaluation of the child's symptoms. Therefore, obtaining an accurate diagnosis by a pediatric mental health specialist is important (AAP, 2000).

Specific diagnostic criteria (Table 53–4) must be applied to all children with the potential diagnosis. Behaviors both at home and school or child care must be evaluated, since abnormal patterns in two settings are needed for diagnosis. Based on the findings, desired outcomes are established for the child's performance and management of the disorder.

Treatment is established to meet the desired behavioral outcomes, and includes a combination of approaches, such as environmental changes, behavior therapy, and pharmacotherapy (AAP, 2001b). It is expected that treatment will be long term.

TABLE 53–4 DSM-IV-TR Diagnostic Criteria for Attention Deficit Hyperactivity Disorder

A. Either 1 or 2:
  1. **Inattention:** Six (or more) of the following symptoms of inattention have persisted for at least 6 months to a degree that is maladaptive and inconsistent with developmental level:
     a. Often fails to give close attention to details or makes careless mistakes in schoolwork, work, and other activities
     b. Often has difficulty sustaining attention in tasks or play activities
     c. Often does not seem to listen when spoken to directly
     d. Often does not follow through on instructions and fails to finish schoolwork, chores, or duties in the workplace (not due to oppositional behavior or failure to understand instructions)
     e. Often has difficulty organizing tasks and activities
     f. Often avoids, dislikes, or is reluctant to engage in tasks that require sustained mental effort (such as schoolwork or homework)
     g. Often loses things necessary for tasks or activities (e.g., toys, school assignments, pencils, books, or tools)
     h. Is often easily distracted by extraneous stimuli
     i. Is often forgetful in daily activities
  2. **Hyperactivity-impulsivity:** Six (or more) of the following symptoms of hyperactivity-impulsivity have persisted for at least 6 months to a degree that is maladaptive and inconsistent with developmental level:
     Hyperactivity
     a. Often fidgets with hands or feet or squirms in seat
     b. Often leaves seat in classroom or in other situations in which remaining seated is expected
     c. Often runs about or climbs excessively in situations in which it is inappropriate (in adolescents or adults, may be limited to subjective feelings of restlessness)
     d. Often has difficulty playing or engaging in leisure activities quietly
     e. Is often "on the go" or often acts as if "driven by a motor"
     f. Often talks excessively
     Impulsivity
     g. Often blurts out answers before questions have been completed
     h. Often has difficulty awaiting turn
     i. Often interrupts or intrudes on others (e.g., butts into conversations or games)
B. Some hyperactive-impulsive or inattentive symptoms that caused impairment were present before age 7 years.
C. Some impairment from the symptoms is present in two or more settings (e.g., at school [or work] and at home).
D. There must be clear evidence of clinically significant impairment in social, academic, or occupational functioning.
E. The symptoms do not occur exclusively during the course of a Pervasive Developmental Disorder, Schizophrenia, or other Psychotic Disorder and are not better accounted for by another mental disorder (e.g., Mood Disorder, Anxiety Disorder, Dissociative Disorder, or a Personality Disorder).

Note: From American Psychiatric Association. 2000. *Diagnostic and statistical manual of mental disorders* Text Revision (4th ed.). Washington, DC: Author. Copyright © 2000 American Psychiatric Association.

Children often benefit from environmental changes. Decreasing stimulation—for example, by turning off television, keeping the environment quiet, and maintaining an orderly and clutter-free desk or study area without distraction—may help the child to stay focused on the task at hand. Another relatively simple change is appropriate classroom placement, preferably in a small class with a teacher who can provide close supervision and a structured daily routine. Consistent limits and expectations should be set for the child. Children living in chaotic homes and communities may function better if the environment can be simplified. When aggressive behaviors occur, therapeutic approaches such as play and group therapy may be useful.

Behavior therapy involves rewarding the child for desired behaviors and applying consequences for undesirable behaviors. Children may be rewarded by praise or earn points toward a movie or other desired outing for staying seated during meals or quietly listening in a classroom.

Children with moderate to severe ADHD are treated with pharmacotherapy. Methylphenidate (Ritalin, Concerta) is most often prescribed. Usually a favorable response (a decrease in impulsive behaviors and an increase in the ability to sit still and attend to an activity for at least 15 minutes) is seen in the first 10 days of treatment and frequently with the first few doses. Other medications that may be used include dextroamphetamine (Dexedrine or Adderall), the tricyclic antidepressants desipramine and imipramine, and the antidepressant bupropion (Wellbutrin) (AAP, 2001b).

In addition to drug therapy, a variety of other treatments have been attempted for ADHD, and are commonly used by families. Chiropractic manipulation, biofeedback, visual or auditory therapy, and dietary interventions are examples of common complementary or alternative therapies. Some dietary interventions include elimination of dietary components, such as highly processed foods, sugar, aspartame, or yeast. Other therapies include supplements, such as iron, magnesium, zinc, and vitamin B_6. Herbs such as Pycnogenol, melatonin, and *Ginkgo biloba* are sometimes used (Arnold, Pinkham, & Votolato, 2000; Baumgaertel, 1999).

Complementary Care

ESSENTIAL FATTY ACIDS FOR ADHD
Essential fatty acids (EFAs) have been studied for their beneficial effects on ADHD, specifically omega-3 and omega-6 fatty acids, (Burgess, Stevens, Zhang, et al., 2000; Kidd, 2000). Because the body does not manufacture EFAs, they must be obtained from the diet. Sources of omega-3 and omega-6 fatty acids include evening primrose oil, flaxseed oil, borage oil, and oils from cold-water fish such as cod and salmon.

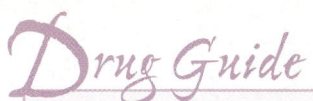

Drug Guide

METHYLPHENIDATE HYDROCHLORIDE (RITALIN)

Overview of Action

Methylphenidate hydrochloride (Ritalin) is a derivative of peridine that acts like an amphetamine. It causes CNS and respiratory stimulation and has some sympathomimetic activity. It may work by enhancing catecholamine effects in the reticular activating system, thereby affecting the cortex to improve attention span and the task performance. It may also prevent flooding of sensory impulses into the cortex so that they enter in a more integrated manner. It is used to treat children with attention deficit hyperactivity disorder and adults with narcolepsy.

Routes, Dosage, Frequency

PO: For children 6 years or over: 5 mg before breakfast and lunch initially, increased in 5- to 10-mg increments weekly as needed or 0.25 mg/kg/day in 2 doses initially, increased by doubling weekly as needed; not to exceed 2 mg/kg/day or 60 mg/day. A sustained-release form is available so that children can take one pill in the morning and do not have to take more at school in the middle of the day.

Side Effects: Insomnia, nervousness and agitation, anorexia and weight loss

Contraindications: Tic syndromes, allergy to the drug, children under 6 years

Nursing Implications

Measure height and weight and plot on growth grid. Take baseline vital signs. Do CBC and platelet count. Take history of previous drug therapy and reactions.

- *Administer:* Schedule II drug under Federal Controlled Substance Act. Do not give tablets late in afternoon or evening because doing so may interrupt sleep. Extended–release tablets are given once daily in early morning and should not be crushed or chewed.

- *Monitor:* Patient is seen in office for regular visits, when vital signs, height, weight, and CBC and platelet counts are done. Observe for signs of bleeding and bruising. Question parents and teachers about child's behavior and ability to concentrate and perform tasks. If drug is to be effective, behavior change occurs within 1 month. Some drug-free holidays are recommended; monitor for behavior changes at these times.

- *Patient Teaching:* Take drug as directed. Do not withdraw quickly; tapering is recommended under supervision of prescriber. Measure child's weight weekly and report weight loss. Report signs of bleeding, fever, sore throat, bruising. Report changes in child's ability to concentrate and general behavior.

Note: From Bindler, R. M., & Howry, L. B. (1997). *Pediatric drugs and nursing implications* (2nd ed.). Upper Saddle River, NJ: Prentice Hall-Health. Adapted.

Although ADHD was once thought to be a disorder of childhood that gradually improved with age, it is now believed that symptoms continue into adulthood and that careful management in childhood helps lessen problems of social functioning later in life.

Nursing Management

Nursing Assessment and Diagnosis

Nurses may encounter the child with ADHD in the hospital when parents bring the child for treatment of an injury (e.g., fracture) or other problem. Explore the parent's report of the child's attention span in detail. Usually within a few minutes in an unstructured setting or waiting area, the child with ADHD becomes restless and searches for distraction. Gather information about the child's activity level and impulsiveness. Be alert for information that reveals a serious problem, such as hurting animals or other children. Find out about distractibility, attention deficit in activities of daily living, characteristic ways of reacting, and the extent of impulsiveness when the child is receiving medication. Find out how the family manages at home. Ask about a family history of the disorder, as that is a common finding among children with ADHD.

Examples of nursing diagnoses that might be appropriate for a child with ADHD include the following:

▶ *Impaired verbal communication* related to altered perceptions

▶ *Impaired social interaction* related to chronic episodes of impulsive behavior

▶ *Chronic low self-esteem* related to behaviors associated with ADHD

▶ *Risk for injury* related to high level of impulsiveness and excitability

▶ *Risk for caregiver role strain* related to management of child with unpredictable moods and high energy

Planning and Implementation

Nursing care of the hospitalized child with ADHD focuses on administering medications, managing the child's environment, implementing behavioral management plans, providing emotional support to the child and family, promoting self-esteem, and ensuring ongoing care.

ADMINISTER MEDICATIONS

Methylphenidate and other medications increase the child's attention span and decrease distractibility. Be alert for the common side effects of these medications, including anorexia, insomnia, and tachycardia. Administering medication early in the day helps to alleviate insomnia. Anorexia can be managed by giving medication at mealtimes. Careful monitoring of weight, height, and blood pressure is necessary.

MINIMIZE ENVIRONMENTAL DISTRACTIONS

The child may need an environment with minimal distractions. When hospitalized, this may mean a room with only one other child. Keep potentially harmful equipment out of reach. Monitor and limit television and video game time. Use shades to darken the room at nap- or bedtime, and minimize noise. Teach parents to minimize distractions at home during periods when the child needs to concentrate; for example, when doing schoolwork. Visits to areas such as shopping malls and playgrounds may need to be limited. Plenty of daily exercise and minimal use of television/video games may help the child concentrate when needed for school work.

IMPLEMENT BEHAVIORAL MANAGEMENT PLANS

Behavior modification programs can help reduce specific impulsive behaviors. An example is setting up a reward program for the child who has taken medication as ordered or completed a homework assignment. The rewards may be daily as well as weekly or monthly, depending on the child's age. (For example, one completed homework assignment might be rewarded with 30 minutes of basketball or a bike ride; assignments completed for a week might be rewarded with an activity of the child's choice on the weekend.)

If punishment is necessary, the behavior should be corrected while simultaneously supporting the child as a person. Punishment is generally withdrawal of a privilege, and should follow the offense quickly as the child may not otherwise connect the punishment with the behavior.

PROVIDE EMOTIONAL SUPPORT

Children with ADHD offer a special challenge to parents, teachers, and health care providers. Parents must cope simultaneously with managing the difficult needs and demands of a hard-to-handle child, obtaining appropriate evaluation and treatment, and understanding and accepting the diagnosis, even when the child exhibits different behaviors with different people. Family support is essential. Educate both the parents and the child about the importance of appropriate expectations and consequences of behaviors. Teach skills that will help as the child grows older: making lists of tasks to accomplish; having routines for eating, sleeping, recreation, and school work; minimizing stimuli in the environment when completing work; asking teachers and friends to identify when behavior is inappropriate.

PROMOTE SELF-ESTEEM

Help the child understand the disorder at an appropriate developmental level, and facilitate a trusting relationship with health care providers. Assist the child with social skills through role-play, playing in small groups, and modeling. Promote the child's self-esteem by pointing out the positive aspects of behavior and treating instances of negative behavior as learning opportunities. Help the child to develop ego strengths (the consciousness to be able to screen outside stimuli and control internal demands), which will result in better impulse control and thus increase self-esteem over time.

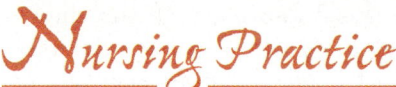

Nursing Practice

Many families who have a child with ADHD or another mental health disorder are embarrassed and feel shame because of the diagnosis. This may be especially true in certain cultures, such as some Asian groups, and in highly structured and highly achieving families. When taking histories from family members, it is best to be sensitive to the stigma some may feel. Ask questions in a private setting and ask about the family's feelings about a mental health disorder. Provide information in a nonjudgmental manner and if appropriate provide support from other families with similar experiences.

NURSING CARE IN THE COMMUNITY

Most children with ADHD are not hospitalized. Only occasionally will a child be hospitalized when needing care for another condition. Parents need support to understand the diagnosis and to learn how to manage the child. Emphasize the importance of a stable environment, at home as well as at school. At home the child may have difficulty staying on task. Parents need to consider age and developmental appropriateness of tasks, give clear and simple instructions, and provide frequent reminders to ensure completion. Routines in the evening can promote good sleep patterns.

The nurse can serve as a liaison to teachers and school personnel, or as the case manager for the child. An individual education plan may be needed (see Chapter 35), with clear expected outcomes stated for the child's behaviors. Special classrooms or periods of instruction free from the distractions of the entire class may enable the child to improve school performance. Parents may have difficulty understanding the need for these approaches because the child often tests with above-average intelligence. Reinforce the importance of providing a structured environment free from unnecessary external stimuli. Be sure that parents understand behavioral approaches that will help the child, how to administer prescribed medications, and the importance of returning for health care visits to monitor for side effects. Medication should be locked safely away at home to keep it away from other children and prevent illegal use of this controlled substance. An individual school health plan may be needed for medication management.

Parents may have heard about ADHD in the media and often have many questions about its cause and management. Providing information about complementary and alternative treatments is a nursing role.

As the child grows older, explain the disorder and teach about techniques that will assist in dealing with problems. Emphasize the importance of doing homework or other tasks requiring concentration in a quiet environment without background noise from a television or radio. Encourage children with ADHD to write down instructions from teachers and to use checklists to help them accomplish specific tasks.

Evaluation

Expected outcomes of nursing care for the child with ADD or ADHD include:

▶ Understanding of disorder by parents and child
▶ Management of medication administration
▶ Increase in attentiveness and decrease in hyperactivity, impulsivity, and sleep disturbances
▶ Formation of positive self-image in the child

MENTAL RETARDATION

Mental retardation is defined as significantly subaverage general intellectual functioning (IQ below 70 to 75), as well as impairments in **adaptive functioning** (the ability to meet the standards expected for a cultural group). The mentally retarded child has adaptive deficits in at least two areas such as communication, self-care, home living, social/interpersonal skills, use of community resources, self-direction, functional academic skills, work, leisure, health, or safety. A low IQ score by itself does not necessarily correlate with an impaired ability to carry out adaptive skills. The IQ score and the level of adaptive skills together determine the degree of severity of mental retardation.

Etiology and Pathophysiology

Mild retardation occurs in 3 to 6 per 1000 people, and mental retardation affects about 3% of the population (Baralle, 2001). The causes of mental retardation can be grouped into three general categories: prenatal errors in the development of the central nervous system, prenatal or postnatal changes in the person's biologic environment, and external forces leading to central nervous system damage. In each instance, the precipitating factor changes the form, function, and adaptation of the central nervous system. Table 53–5 provides examples of common causes of mental retardation for each category.

TABLE 53-5 Common Causes of Mental Retardation	
Prenatal Conditions	**External Forces**
Down syndrome	Traumatic brain injury
Fragile X syndrome	(e.g., accident)
Fetal alcohol syndrome	Poison ingestion
Maternal infection (e.g.,	(acute or chronic)
rubella, cytomegalovirus)	Hypoxia/anoxic insult
Biologic Environment	Infection (e.g., meningitis)
Inborn errors of metabolism (e.g.,	Environmental deprivation
phenylketonuria, hypothyroidism)	

Three common causes of retardation from the prenatal category are Down syndrome, fragile X, and fetal alcohol syndrome. About 1 in 1000 infants, or 4000 infants each year, are born with *Down syndrome* in the United States (Zickler, Morrow, & Bull, 1998). It is caused by an extra chromosome so the child has 47 rather than 46 chromosomes (see discussion of genetic transmission in Chapter 32). ⊂⊃ The most common chromosome affected is 21 so that the child often has "trisomy 21," or three instead of two number 21 chromosomes. In addition to mental retardation and physical signs, the child with Down syndrome is at higher risk of developing some other conditions such as cardiac defects, hearing loss, thyroid disease, and leukemia (Van Riper & Cohen, 2001).

Fragile X is caused by a single recessive gene abnormality on the X chromosome. A premutation to the X chromosome may occur in males or females. When a father or mother give the faulty X chromosome to a daughter, it may remain as a premutation or may change into a true mutation. The daughter has two X chromosomes and therefore does not manifest this recessive disorder. However, she can give the mutated X chromosome to her son who becomes affected with fragile X. The mutation of fragile X is on gene FMRP-1, which instructs cells to make a protein necessary for normal brain development (Bailey, Roberts, Mirrett, et al., 2001).

Fetal alcohol syndrome (FAS) is caused by the effect of ethyl alcohol on the developing fetus. Alcohol ingestion by the pregnant woman can influence development of many body organs and effects can range from mild to severe.

Developing Cultural Competence

Fetal alcohol syndrome is more common in groups with higher intake of alcohol. Since some Native-American tribes have a high rate of alcoholism, the federal government and some tribes have joined together to lower that risk among this ethnic group. On some reservations, such as the Yakama Nation in Washington State, alcoholic beverages are not sold and educational programs are in place.

Chapter 51 discusses phenylketonuria and hypothyroidism, two common biochemical causes of mental retardation. ⊂⊃ Other causes involve traumatic brain injury and infections of the central nervous system (see Chapter 49). ⊂⊃ Mental retardation is more common in children born prematurely.

Clinical Manifestations

Mild mental retardation was originally described as an intelligence quotient (IQ) between 50 to 70, moderate retardation with IQ of 35 to 50, severe retardation for IQ 20 to 35, and profound retardation below 20. However, although an IQ below 70 is generally considered indicative of retardation, the functional assessment of the child is now considered a more accurate identification of children's performance and needs. Children who are mentally retarded manifest delays in all areas of development, including motor movement, language, and adaptive behavior. They usually achieve developmental milestones more slowly than the average child. These developmental delays may be the first indication to parents and care providers of the child's condition.

Mental retardation is sometimes accompanied by sensory impairment, speech problems, motor and orthopedic disabilities, and seizure disorders. Of children with mental retardation, 10% to 30% manifest one of these other disorders. Table 53–6 lists several physical characteristics associated with Down syndrome, fragile X syndrome, and fetal alcohol syndrome.

TABLE 53–6 *Characteristics Associated with Three Common Types of Mental Retardation*

Down Syndrome (see Figures 33–9 and 33–38) ⊂⊃
Small head (microcephaly)
Flattened forehead
Wide, short neck
Epicanthal eye folds
White spots on eye iris (Brushfield spots)
Congenital cataracts
Flat nose
Small, low-set ears
Protruding tongue
Short broad hands
Simian line on palm
Wide space between first and second toes
Hearing loss
Increased incidence of diabetes, congenital heart defect, and leukemia
Hypotonia

Fragile X Syndrome
Long face
Prominent jaw
Large ears
Frequent otitis media
Large testicles
Epicanthal eye folds
Strabismus
High arched palate
Scoliosis
Pliable joints

Fetal Alcohol Syndrome (see Figure 32–4) ⊂⊃
Flat midface
Low nasal bridge
Long philtrum with narrow upper lip
Short upturned nose
Poor coordination
Failure to thrive
Skeletal and joint abnormalities
Hearing loss

TABLE 53-7 DSM-IV-TR Diagnostic Criteria for Mental Retardation

A. Significantly subaverage intellectual functioning: an IQ of approximately 70 or below on an individually administered IQ test (for infants, a clinical judgment of significantly subaverage intellectual functioning)

B. Concurrent deficits or impairments in present adaptive functioning (i.e., the person's effectiveness in meeting the standards expected for his or her age by his or her cultural group) in at least two of the following areas: communication, self-care, home living, social/interpersonal skills, use of community resources, self-direction, functional academic skills, work, leisure, health, and safety

C. The onset is before age 18 years

Note: From American Psychiatric Association (2000). *Diagnostic and statistical manual of mental disorders* Text Revision (4th ed.). Washington, DC: Author. Copyright © 2000 American Psychiatric Association.

Clinical Therapy

Mental retardation is diagnosed and initial treatment is planned in a multistep process, and by involving a multidisciplinary team (Frederic & Williams, 1998). The team may include a developmental specialist, physician, nurse, teacher, language therapist, occupational therapist, and physical rehabilitation specialist. See Table 53–7 for a description of the DSM-IV-TR diagnostic criteria for mental retardation. Diagnosis begins with a comprehensive history and evaluation of the child's physical characteristics, developmental level, and intellectual and adaptive functioning. Laboratory tests such as chromosome analysis, blood enzyme levels, lead levels, or cranial imaging provide valuable information in some circumstances.

Developmental screening using a test such as the Denver II (see Chapter 35) can help identify children at risk. Intellectual and adaptive functioning are tested when mental retardation is suspected. A neurologic examination may indicate asymmetry of movement or strength, irritability or lethargy, or abnormal pitch to an infant's cry. Because mental retardation may be accompanied by physical abnormalities, it is important to observe the child for facial symmetry, distance between the eyes, level of the ears, hair growth, and palmar creases. These abnormalities may be clues to other health problems.

Based on the results of the evaluation, a multidisciplinary team plans the support needed to maximize the child's potential for development. Management focuses on early intervention to improve the degree of adaptive functioning. Associated physical, emotional, and behavioral problems are treated simultaneously. Depending on the child's condition, special education programs and physical or occupational therapy may be necessary (Figure 53–5 ◆). The child may require supportive care and assistance with activities of daily living. The plans for intervention need to change as the child grows and the family situation alters.

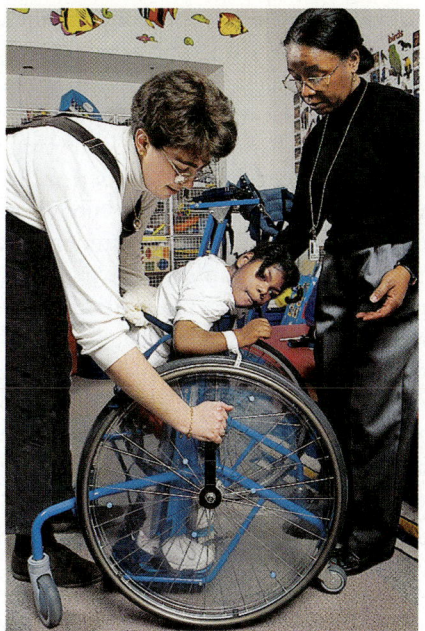

A

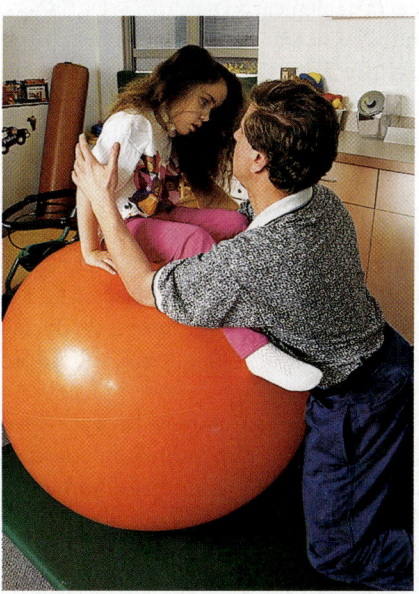

B

FIGURE 53–5. ◆ Physical therapy is an important component of medical management for many children who are mentally retarded. **A,** This girl, who is severely retarded and uses a wheelchair, is being positioned in a mobile prone stander, which enables her to interact in a different manner with her therapists and the environment. **B,** Physical therapists also provide outpatient care in the community to children with varying degrees of disability.

Nursing Management

Nursing Assessment and Diagnosis

Nurses can help to identify children with mental retardation through history taking, observation, and developmental screening during early childhood. The history should provide information about the mental and adaptive functioning of birth parents and other family members, as mental retardation may cluster in some families, and conditions such as fragile X syndrome are genetic. The pregnancy and birth history can provide important information about the mother's alcohol and drug use during pregnancy. Be alert for a history of difficult pregnancy and problems during delivery. When genetic conditions in the family predispose family members to mental retardation, assess the child carefully. Children from deprived environments or those at risk because of environmental factors such as lead poisoning (see Chapter 46) ⬯ are more likely to manifest mental retardation.

Many mentally retarded children are not diagnosed until they reach school age, particularly if the condition is mild or moderate. Early intervention, however, can help to enhance the child's functioning later. During home visits, during clinic appointments, in child care centers, and during hospitalization, be alert for signs such as developmental delays, multiple (more than three) physical anomalies associated with a specific condition (see Table 53–6), or neurologic alterations. Developmental assessment should be part of each health care visit.

Once the diagnosis of mental retardation has been made, assess the adaptive functioning of the child and family. Perform a functional assessment of the child, including toileting, dressing, and feeding skills. Assess the child's language, sensory, and psychomotor functioning. Assess the home and community for safety hazards. Observe how the family is managing with the child. Ask about family activities that can include the child, and community and school attitudes and support. Assess the availability of services such as groups for parents and special education opportunities for children. Evaluate the coping skills of family members.

Several nursing diagnoses may be appropriate for the mentally retarded child, depending on the degree, cause, and outcome of the child's condition. Some of these diagnoses relate to impairments in adaptive functioning; others relate to the impact on the family. Examples include:

▶ *Altered growth and development* related to neonatal disease or condition

▶ *Altered nutrition: less than body requirements* related to inability to ingest sufficient food

▶ *Self-care deficit: dressing, toileting, bathing* related to developmental disability

▶ *Impaired verbal communication* related to developmental disability

▶ *Risk for injury* related to lack of understanding of environmental hazards

▶ *Ineffective family coping: compromised* related to the child's developmental variations

Planning and Implementation

Nearly all mentally retarded children are cared for in the community. However, they may have conditions that require periodic hospitalization or frequent health care visits.

Wherever nursing care occurs, it focuses on providing emotional support and information to family members, assisting the child with adaptive functioning, and fostering parental management of the child's activities. Whenever possible, the nurse uses preventive teaching to lower the risk of mental retardation. For example, nurses can integrate teaching into care for all women about the importance of avoiding all alcohol during any times when they might become pregnant. This helps prevent fetal alcohol syndrome, especially in early pregnancy when women may not know they are pregnant.

PROVIDE EMOTIONAL SUPPORT AND INFORMATION

Family members need empathy and support both at the time of diagnosis and in the ensuing years. Parents may be in an acute or chronic state of grief over the loss of the perfect child. Encourage them to verbalize their feelings. Introducing them to parents of other mentally retarded children may help and support them as they learn how to manage the child's needs. Discuss the availability of respite care to provide parents with a break from caretaking. Other family members such as grandparents and siblings may also feel grief or guilt and should be given an opportunity to talk about their feelings.

Parents need honest information and answers to their questions about the child's condition. Reinforce information provided by genetic counselors and other health care professionals. Parents need to know about community resources designed to assist children with mental retardation. The Education for All Handicapped Children Act, PL 94-142, provides free appropriate education to all handicapped children between 2 and 21 years of age. States and local communities may provide early intervention services for infants and toddlers with disabilities. Examples of programs include the Zero to Three project early intervention programs, special education preschools and schools, county health services, and respite care, among others. Refer parents to Internet sources if that may be helpful, and help them interpret information they find and analyze its strengths and limitations. ⬯ WEB

MAINTAIN A SAFE ENVIRONMENT

The child with mental retardation requires close supervision because he or she may not understand common hazards. Ensure safety in the hospital. Assist parents to provide safety at home and school, and teach the child necessary skills such as pedestrian safety. Consider both physical and emotional safety. The mentally retarded child may be indiscriminately trusting and sometimes is at risk for physical or sexual abuse.

PROVIDE ASSISTANCE WITH ADAPTIVE FUNCTIONING

Encourage parents' efforts to maximize the child's areas of strength and identify needs related to adaptive behaviors. Refer them to resources to help with the child's impaired areas of adaptive functioning, such as communication, self-care, or social skills. During hospitalization, support parents' efforts to maintain the child's skills in toileting, dressing, and self-care by planning interventions to use the skills being taught at home.

NURSING CARE IN THE COMMUNITY

The child with mental retardation needs ongoing care throughout childhood; interventions must be adapted as the child develops and the family's needs evolve. Parents often act as case managers for the child's care. Assist parents as necessary to acquire the skills required to coordinate the child's plan of care. Evaluate the child's needs regularly and help parents with the treatment plan as necessary. Assist with plans for education and for services such as physical or speech therapy. Most children with mental retardation have an individual education plan designed to meet their specific learning needs. Parents, nurses, and others such as teachers and language therapists are part of the team that establishes the child's individual education plan. Promote optimal development and socialization. As the child reaches adolescence, education is directed toward a vocation, issues of sexuality, and the goal of independent living, when appropriate. Transition classes for adolescents with mental retardation can teach self-care skills that may enable some to live in group homes or other community settings. Parents need help planning for the child's future and their own retirement.

Specific guidelines for care are available for the child with Down syndrome. These guidelines suggest times for evaluation of hearing, growth, cardiac function, and other areas designed for early identification and treatment of associated disorders (Van Riper & Cohen, 2001). There are growth grids for children with Down syndrome, and specific topics to suggest for anticipatory guidance during health care visits (AAP, 2001c). ⬤ WEB

Evaluation

The expected outcomes of nursing care depend on the child's needs and developmental level. Early in the diagnostic phase, desired outcomes may involve the family's understanding of the diagnosis and the child's special needs. Later outcomes may focus on the child's communication of self-help skills. Outcomes related to cognitive performance and adaptive skills may be developed during childhood.

SCHIZOPHRENIA

Schizophrenia is a psychotic disorder that is relatively rare in young children and adolescents, although it can occur in children as young as 5 years of age. The prevalence of schizophrenia increases after puberty and reaches adult levels by late adolescence. About 1 in 10,000 children develops schizophrenia (Lambert, 2001).

The cause of schizophrenia is unknown, but genetic predisposition or a neurovirus during pregnancy may play a role (Lambert, 2001). The brain is altered in the disease, with progressively enlarged ventricles, and nervous system arousal. Impaired glucose metabolism is often present. The disorder most often manifests between 15 and 20 years of age. Onset is usually slow with increasing intensity. Most often the child demonstrates restlessness, poor appetite, and social withdrawal over several weeks to months. Behavioral problems, slowed development, and minor neurologic symptoms may occur.

The clinical manifestations of schizophrenia are the same in children as in adults. Characteristic behaviors include social withdrawal, impaired social relationships, flat **affect** (outward appearance of feeling or emotion), regression, loose associations (thought characterized by speech in which ideas shift from one subject to another that is unrelated), poor judgment and problem-solving, anxiety, delusions, and hallucinations. Motor abnormalities may include rocking and arm flapping.

During adolescence, acute schizophrenia can occur suddenly while the teenager is making plans to leave home and family to attend college, marry, or work in another area. Onset of symptoms may be triggered by an important loss (death of a significant other, parent, child, or friend).

Clinical therapy for childhood schizophrenia is multifaceted, including individual psychotherapy, family therapy, and various psychotropic medications (antipsychotics such as haloperidol [Haldol], antianxiety agents such as lorazepam [Ativan], antidepressants such as imipramine [Tofranil], and newer antipsychotics such as clozapine, olanzapine, and risperidone). Drugs are only moderately effective at controlling hallucinations and delusions, responses vary considerably, and children may have different responses than adults. Side effects determine what drugs are used and for how long. Antipsychotic medication is continued for at least 4 to 6 weeks before effectiveness can be determined. Medications often must be continued for several months or years after recovery from an acute schizophrenic episode, although medication-free trials may be tried in children who have not shown symptoms for 6 to 12 months (American Academy of Child & Adolescent Psychiatry, 2001).

Often, episodes of acute schizophrenia require inpatient hospitalization on a psychiatric unit for thorough diagnosis and beginning management. Treatment may include an intensive school-based program in a structured, supervised setting with specially trained professionals. The goal of initial treatment is to reduce or control psychotic episodes and provide a safe, structured environment for the child or adolescent, enabling the child to live each day at an optimal level of functioning. Outpatient care is provided in the community following initial diagnosis and establishment of treatment regimen.

Most children require long-term treatment, including intermittent periods of hospitalization. Children or adolescents whose symptoms are difficult to control and who present a safety risk to themselves or others may require long-term residential treatment. Earlier age at diagnosis and delay in treatment lead to poorer prognosis.

Nursing Management

The nurse may encounter the child or adolescent with schizophrenia during hospitalization for an acute episode, for treatment of another problem, or while working with the individual in the community. Nursing care centers on providing for physical safety and psychologic care, and normal growth and development for the child.

Family education and involvement in the treatment plan are essential. The family is taught to monitor the child's symptoms and progression. Educating the child and parents about the risk of recurrence and methods to alleviate side effects of prescribed medications may increase compliance with the treatment plan. The nurse assesses the child for common medication side effects. For example, when excess weight is a potential side effect, frequent growth measurements are made. Neurologic assessment and laboratory studies may be needed with some medications. Extrapyramidal side effects such as dystonia, Parkinson-like movement, and akathisia may occur with some drugs.

Help the family establish educational plans and integration within the school system. The nurse communicates with school personnel in order to ensure understanding of the child's condition and ongoing management of the individual education plan.

MOOD DISORDERS

DEPRESSION

Depression is psychologic distress that can range from mild to severe. Only in recent years has depression in children been recognized as a clinical condition. Many children referred to child guidance centers and mental health professionals because of behavioral difficulties or poor achievement actually suffer from depression. The incidence of major depression is estimated to be about 5% in prepubertal children and about 10% to 20% in adolescents (Castiglia, 2000; Moldenhauer & Melnyk, 1999). Before puberty, depression is more common in boys than girls. Incidence of depressive symptoms and disorders increases with age, as does the female:male ratio.

Etiology and Pathophysiology

Many theories have been proposed to explain the cause of depression in children and adolescents. Depression may be biologic in origin or a result of learned helplessness, cognitive distortion, social skills deficit, or family dysfunction. Childhood depression sometimes occurs secondary to parental depression because the parental depression deprives the child of effective parenting. Abuse and neglect predispose children to depression, especially very young children. In about half of all children with depression, at least one other psychiatric diagnosis is made; these include conditions such as ADHD, anxiety disorder, or another

personality disorder. Depressive disorders may contribute to other mental illness such as disturbed relationships, substance abuse, and suicide (Lyon & Morgan-Judge, 2000).

Clinical Manifestations

Characteristic findings of major depression in children and adolescents include declining school performance; withdrawal from social activities; sleep disturbance (either too much or too little); appetite disturbance (too much or too little); multiple somatic complaints, especially headaches and stomachaches; decreased energy; difficulty concentrating and making decisions; low self-esteem; and feelings of hopelessness. There is much variation among children in the symptoms displayed, and they often have some but not all of the major criteria (Williamson, Birmaher, Brent, et al., 2000).

Growth and Development

Symptoms of depression in children vary according to their developmental levels. Infants may fail to eat and grow, toddlers can show regressive behaviors in toileting and other activities, and school children may show a decrease in academic performance, increased or decreased activity, somatic complaints, and loss of friends. The adolescent can have a wide array of symptoms such as anxiety, decreased social contact, poor school performance, lack of prior involvement in activities, poor self-care, difficulty with parents and teachers, or focus on violence.

Clinical Therapy

Initial assessment is performed by a child psychologist or child psychiatrist. A variety of scales and techniques are used; however, very little guidance is available about evaluating children under 6 years of age. Examples of useful tools are the Children's Depression Inventory and the Revised Children's Manifest Anxiety Scale.

Treatment may include psychotherapy in combination with psychotropic medication. Often a combination of individual, family, and group therapy provides the greatest benefits for young children and adolescents. Involving parents and other family members in the treatment plan is essential. Group therapy is effective for adolescents because of the importance of peer group relationships during the teenage years. Cognitive therapy may be used with adolescents, and play therapy with younger children (see discussion of play therapy earlier in this chapter).

Antidepressant medications, most commonly the selective serotonin reuptake inhibitors (SSRIs), imipramine (Tofranil), desipramine (Norpramin), and amitriptyline (Elavil), may be prescribed (see Table 53–8). The SSRIs act to block reuptake of serotonin in the synapse, so that serotonin (which influences mood) levels increase. Although the SSRIs are generally considered safer than

TABLE 53-8	Selective Serotonin Reuptake Inhibitor (SSRI) Drugs Used to Treat Depression		
Medication	Pediatric Dose	Adolescent Dose	Selected Side Effects
Fluoxetine (Prozac)	5–40 mg qd	10–60 mg qd	Restlessness, headaches, akathisia
Sertraline (Zoloft)	25–125 mg qd	50–200 mg qd	Dry mouth, gastric upset
Paroxetine (Paxil)	5–40 mg qd	20–40 mg pd	Dry mouth, weight gain
Fluvoxamine (Luvox)	25–125 mg bid	200–300 mg qd	Dry mouth, gastric upset
Citalopram (Celexa)	Little data available	20–40 mg qd	Dry mouth, nausea, sleep disturbance

Note: From Labellarte, Walkup, & Riddle, 1998; Lyon & Morgan-Judge, 2000. Adapted.

some other antidepressants, their use in children has been limited, so side effects must be monitored. The major serious side effect is serotonin syndrome. This condition is characterized by agitation, muscle twitching, gastric upset, chills, fever, confusion, and dizziness. Generally the child is started with a low dose and it is increased slowly to minimize chance of side effects.

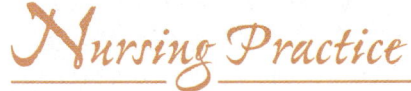
Nursing Practice

Serotonin syndrome, the serious and life-threatening side effect of SSRIs, is caused by overstimulation of serotonin receptors. It is more likely to develop when the child or adolescent is also taking St. John's Wort, other antidepressants, alcohol, diet pills, or drugs such as ecstasy and LSD (Lyon & Morgan-Judge, 2000). Be certain to ask questions in a nonjudgmental way about intake of any alternative therapies, other medications, or substance use to identify those most at risk.

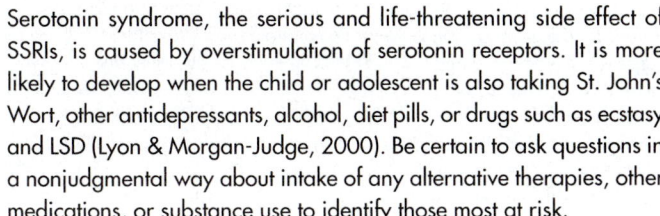
Nursing Management

Nursing Assessment and Diagnosis

Take a thorough history and physical examination, including observation of behavior, at the time of admission. Assess the child for common risk factors for depression (Table 53–9).

Several nursing diagnoses that might be appropriate for the child or adolescent hospitalized with depression are

TABLE 53-9 Risk Factors for Depression and Anxiety in Children and Adolescents
Parental neglect, abuse, or loss
Stressful social relationships
Academic pressures and underachievement
Dysfunctional family relationships
Family history of depression, suicide, substance abuse, alcoholism, or other psychopathology
Chronic illness and frequent hospitalization

included in the accompanying "Nursing Care Plan." Other diagnoses might include:

▶ *Altered nutrition: more than body requirements* related to eating in response to internal cues other than hunger

▶ *Powerlessness* related to sense of helplessness

▶ *Low self-esteem* related to negative self-evaluation

Planning and Implementation

Nursing care of the child or adolescent hospitalized for depression includes administering medications and other therapy, and providing supportive care. Monitor vital signs of youth receiving antidepressant medications. Watch for common side effects of the agent(s) used. Carefully monitor for serious side effects of SSRIs and be aware that lower doses are used at initiation with doses increasing slowly to desired level. Monitor cardiovascular status, including hypertension and tachycardia, observe motor movement, and record dietary intake. Help parents to evaluate inpatient settings to be certain the care provided will best meet the needs of the child or adolescent. Refer to "Nursing Care Plan: The Child or Adolescent Hospitalized with Depression" for specific nursing interventions.

DISCHARGE PLANNING AND HOME CARE TEACHING

When the child has been hospitalized and is returning home, teach parents to recognize signs and symptoms of worsening depression. Also teach them dosages and side effects of any prescribed medications. Refer the family to appropriate health care professionals and to support groups for family members dealing with depression. WEB

NURSING CARE IN THE COMMUNITY

Most children with depression are cared for in the community. Maintain regular contact with the family through their health care visits to outpatient agencies and by making home visits. Monitor the child's affect, activity, and food intake. School teachers and counselors often are aware of the child's ability to perform in the school setting. Have the family schedule after-school care so young children are not left at home alone for extended periods. Assist the family in finding support for financial and emotional needs related to managing the child's depression.

GOAL	INTERVENTION	RATIONALE	EXPECTED OUTCOME
1. Hopelessness related to long-term stress			
	NIC Priority Intervention: **Hope instillation:** *Facilitation of the development of a positive outlook*		*NOC Suggested Outcome:* **Hope:** *Presence of internal state of optimism that is personally satisfying and life supporting.*
The child or adolescent will discuss feelings of hopelessness.	▶ Encourage open expression of feelings. Explore hopeless, sad, or lonely feelings. Point out the connection between feelings and behavior. Assess the child or adolescent to identify the precipitating event when feelings of sadness arose. ▶ Encourage the child or adolescent to take part in self-care and unit activities. Use routines to establish feelings of control. ▶ Medicate as ordered and document results.	▶ Expressing feelings may help to relieve sadness, loneliness, despair, and hopelessness. An accepting and nonjudgmental attitude must be maintained regarding any feelings expressed by the child. ▶ An active role in self-care and treatment helps the child or adolescent to feel more in control. ▶ Antidepressants modify mood to a more hopeful outlook.	By discharge, the child or adolescent expresses an interest in the future
2. Ineffective individual coping related to inadequate social support or disturbance in pattern of appraisal of threaten			
	NIC Priority Intervention: **Coping enhancement:** *Assisting a patient to adapt to perceived stressors, changes, or threats which interfere with meeting life demands and roles*		*NOC Suggested Outcome:* **Coping:** *Actions to manage stressors that tax an individual's resources*
The child or adolescent will use effective coping skills.	▶ Teach positive, effective coping strategies such as guided imagery and relaxation. Assist the child or adolescent to focus on strengths rather than weaknesses. ▶ Assist the child or adolescent to identify friends, family members, and others who are positive and supportive.	▶ Therapeutic techniques can help the child or adolescent to replace negative thoughts and images with more positive and effective beliefs and images. These interventions foster resilience. ▶ Helps the child or adolescent to become aware that people can be caring and supportive (thus validating self-esteem).	The child or adolescent verbalizes and demonstrates ability to cope appropriately for his or her age.
3. Impaired social interaction related to self-concept disturbance			
	NIC Priority Intervention: **Socialization enhancement:** *Facilitation of ability to interact with others*		*NOC Suggested Outcome:* **Social interaction skills:** *An individual's use of effective interaction behaviors*
The child or adolescent will participate in and initiate activities and conversation.	▶ Assist the child or adolescent to identify topics and activities of interest. ▶ Encourage interaction with peers and staff. ▶ Facilitate visits from family and friends. ▶ Provide guidance to family regarding interaction that promotes self-esteem.	▶ The more the child or adolescent focuses on areas of interest, the less he or she will focus on internal anxiety and depression. ▶ Each positive interaction reinforces feelings of success. Each success reinforces the desire for future social interaction. ▶ Reinforces positive and rewarding relationships. ▶ The family's existing interaction style is often negative.	By discharge, the child or adolescent initiates conversation and activities with staff and peers.
4. Altered nutrition: less than body requirements related to loss of appetite secondary to depression			
	NIC Priority Intervention: **Nutrition management:** *Assistance with or provision of a balanced dietary intake of foods and fluids*		*NOC Suggested Outcome:* **Nutritional status:** *Amount of food and fluid taken into the body over a 24-hour period*
The child or adolescent's daily intake will be adequate to maintain optimal nutritional status.	▶ Offer nutritious finger foods, sandwiches, and high-calorie liquid supplements frequently throughout the day. ▶ Offer easy-to-carry drinks that are high in vitamins, minerals, and calories. ▶ Encourage daily vigorous physical activity of at least 30 minutes.	▶ Convenient easy-to-eat foods encourage the child or adolescent to eat and maintain nutritional status. ▶ These are a convenient method for meeting hydration and electrolyte needs. ▶ Physical activity stimulates appetite.	The child or adolescent's daily intake will be adequate to maintain optimal nutritional status by discharge.

Teaching About

Major expected outcomes for nursing care of the child with depression are found on the accompanying "Nursing Care Plan."

BIPOLAR DISORDER (MANIC-DEPRESSION)

Bipolar disorder is a mental illness in which extreme changes in affect and energy are manifested. Moods most often alter between mania and depression. Children often present with irritability or hyperactivity. About 1.5% of the total population suffers from bipolar illness, although diagnosis and accurate numbers are difficult to obtain due to the frequency of accompanying additional mental illness (St. Dennis & Synoground, 1998). About 10% to 20% of individuals with bipolar illness commit suicide. The average age for children to demonstrate bipolar disorder is 11 years. Children may show mainly depressive symptoms, and then develop mania in adolescence, or may have episodes of both mania and depression in the same day (Jellinek & Snyder, 1998).

The manic phase of bipolar illness is characterized by hyperactivity and high energy, irritability, aggression, and sometimes hallucinations. In the depressive phase, the child is sad, has alterations in sleep and eating patterns, and is socially withdrawn, similar to any depressive illness.

Diagnosis and treatment of bipolar disorder should be performed by mental health specialists. Use of alcohol or illegal drugs should be ruled out as a cause of symptoms, even in children. Since the manic phase is often manifested by hyperactivity, the child may incorrectly be treated with stimulants (see discussion of ADHD earlier in this chapter), and the disease can be worsened. The treatment of bipolar disease involves a variety of drugs used to stabilize mood. Nurses are instrumental in identifying children with the disorder, providing information to families, and monitoring the drugs and psychotherapy for the child.

❧ ANXIETY AND RELATED DISORDERS

GENERALIZED ANXIETY

Anxiety is a subjective feeling of uncertainty and helplessness, usually accompanied by central nervous system signs, including restlessness, trembling, perspiration, and rapid pulse. Anxiety is second to only substance abuse (see Chapter 36) in incidence for mental disorders and is a common mental disorder among children (Smoller, Finn, & White, 2000). Anxiety disorders are strongly linked to familial and genetic factors.

Separation anxiety disorder is characterized by an extreme state of uneasiness when in unfamiliar surroundings and often by refusal to visit friends' homes or attend school for at least 2 weeks. Approximately 75% of children with separation anxiety disorder refuse to attend school (see the school phobia discussion that follows). This disorder occurs in approximately 4% to 5% of children and in twice as many girls as boys (Masi, Mucci, & Millepiedi, 2001).

Growth and Development

The separation anxiety commonly experienced by a 2-year-old differs from the psychiatric disorder in age appropriateness, duration, and severity. Separation anxiety disorder affects children of preschool age or older, lasts for at least 2 weeks, and is characterized by excessive anxiety. In contrast, the separation anxiety experienced by the 2-year-old involves a single episode of separation from a familiar caretaker and is a characteristic response in toddlers.

Children with separation anxiety disorder tend to be perfectionistic, overly compliant, and eager to please. They appear to cling to the parent or caretaker. They may use physical complaints such as headaches, abdominal pain, nausea, and vomiting in an attempt to avoid being away from the parent. Depression frequently accompanies separation anxiety disorder. The resulting avoidant behaviors can interfere with personal growth and development, academic achievement, and social functioning.

Anxiety disorders are best treated by behavioral, family, and individual therapy. For children with significant or long-lasting impairment in functioning, drugs such as the SSRIs or other antidepressants may be tried.

Nursing care centers on educating parents about the disorder and management techniques. Encourage attendance at therapy sessions. Children with separation anxiety disorder benefit from a predictable routine and environment. Advise children in advance of any expected changes in routine. Help parents plan consistent and reassuring contacts for the child after school and during activities. Instruct about medication administration and side effects if this therapy is used.

Thinking Critically

POSTTRAUMATIC STRESS DISORDER

Cassandra is a 9-year-old girl who has recently become fearful about attending school and has awakened crying at night. She is in the third grade at a school she has attended for 2 years. A few weeks ago she was in a car crash as her mother drove her to school. She received only minor injuries and returned to school the next day. However, her mother believes that Cassandra's behavior has been worsening since the car crash. She spoke with the school nurse who is aware of no trauma at school, but did learn from the teacher that Cassandra has not been paying attention in class recently. Cassandra cannot explain why she does not want to go to school, only that her stomach aches or some other part of her body hurts.

Cassandra visited her pediatrician who ruled out any physical cause for her complaints, and referred her to a child psychologist. The psychologist has scheduled several sessions with Cassandra to help her learn to verbalize her fears and learn strategies to deal with them. She uses dolls in an attempt to help Cassandra act out her fears and gain some understanding. The psychologist communicates Cassandra's progress to you, the school nurse.

➡ *How can you ensure Cassandra's attendance at school?*

➡ *What does the teacher need to know to support Cassandra in the classroom?*

➡ *What is your role as liaison between the psychologist, family, and school personnel?*

➡ *Parents often feel guilty when a child experiences a mental health disorder. What type of information and support do Cassandra's parents need?* 🔗 WEB

PANIC

Panic disorder is the presence of recurrent, unexpected panic attacks. Panic attacks are periods of intense fear and discomfort in the absence of real danger. The risk of panic disorder ranges from 1.5% to 3.5% of the population (Smoller et al., 2000), with adolescence a common age for the onset of symptoms. The risk of panic disorder is 20 times more likely when there is a family history of the disorder (American Psychiatric Association, 2000).

Examples of the physical symptoms experienced are palpitations, sweating, chills, hot flashes, shaking, shortness of breath, choking, chest pain, nausea, and dizziness. The person describes feelings of danger or doom. Some people may have accompanying agoraphobia. **Agoraphobia** is an anxiety of being in places or situations from which escape may be difficult or embarrassing, or in which help may not be available. The attacks may be continuous or episodic, but generally are chronic.

Similar to anxiety, treatment may involve individual and family therapy, with use of medication in some cases. Nurses can help identify the disorder, refer for evaluation, and provide care in the community so that the child attends therapy sessions and takes medication as ordered (Carson, 2000).

OBSESSIVE-COMPULSIVE DISORDER

People with obsessive-compulsive disorder may be mildly or severely affected. One in about 200 children is affected, and there may be associated conditions such as tic disorders or attention deficit-hyperactivity (Leonard, Freeman, Barcia, et al., 2001). Affected children have recurrent ritualistic thoughts or actions; these obsessions or compulsions interfere with daily life. Examples of behaviors and concerns are obsessions about dirt or germs, worries about harm, and sexual thoughts. Common behaviors are excessive handwashing, counting objects, and hoarding substances. These practices may take one hour or more of time each day.

The basal ganglia of the brain are affected and a genetic link is observed. Post-streptococcal autoimmune disorder may be a cause in some cases. Treatment may involve cognitive-behavioral therapy, where the feared occurrence is presented and the person learns that no harm will occur. Medications, particularly SSRIs, are effective in most children. Nurses can identify cases and refer for psychiatric evaluation. Families need instruction about medications and potential side effects.

Nursing Practice

A connection has been observed between neuropsychiatric abnormalities and people who have acute rheumatic fever (a disease caused by *Streptococcus*). Some types of obsessive/compulsive and tic disorders may worsen after infection with infections such as strep throat; this connection has been called Pediatric Autoimmune Neuropsychiatric Disorders Associated with Streptococcus (PANDAS). Current federal research is investigating the treatment of PANDAS with plasma exchange treatments and with antibiotics (Kaplan, 2000).

SCHOOL PHOBIA

School phobia (also called school avoidance or school refusal) is a persistent, irrational, or excessive fear of attending school. The child may fear being harmed or losing control. School phobia is common in children between 5 and 12 years of age, but can occur in children up to 16 years. The child's avoidance of school is often a manifestation of fear of leaving the parent or primary caretaker. Children commonly report that teachers and peers "pick on" them. Somatic complaints are similar to those in children with separation anxiety disorder. Characteristically, symptoms are present only on school days and not on weekends or holidays.

Treatment includes the family and child, and establishes firm limits for behavioral expectations and consequences. Antidepressant medications may sometimes be needed to help the child feel comfortable. The longer a child is out of school, the greater the likelihood that a chronic, treatment-resistant condition will result. Referral for psychiatric evaluation is indicated for persistent symptoms.

POSTTRAUMATIC STRESS DISORDER

Posttraumatic stress victims have experienced or witnessed a life-threatening event with death or severe injury (Meltzer-Brody, Hidalgo, Connor, et al., 2000). Although accurate statistics are not available on children, about 1% to 2% of children are probably affected, with increasing numbers as more children are exposed to war and other violence (Kessler, 2000). The child or adolescent with the disorder has feelings of fear, terror, and helplessness, and may relive the event frequently in thought and nightmares. The child may become emotionally numb in a subconscious attempt to protect the self, but may have a persistently increased state of arousal (Kent, Sullivan, & Rauch, 2000). Examples of events associated with posttraumatic stress include sexual or other child abuse, rape, car crash, fire, witnessing violence, and having experience in war. The events that occurred in the United States on September 11, 2001, are potential causes of posttraumatic stress in children who either had a family member involved, lived near the events, or in some other way were profoundly affected. Cassandra, described in the opening quotation of this chapter, was experiencing posttraumatic stress disorder (PTSD) due to a frightening car crash as she was driven to school. She was too young to describe her feelings verbally to her mother or school personnel; however, she manifested the sleep abnormalities and other complaints common in the disorder (Figure 53–6). Even children of Holocaust victims experience PTSD, leading mental health professionals to believe that PTSD can be transmitted from parent to child (Yehud, Hallig, & Grossman, 2001). There is a relatively high incidence of PTSD among incarcerated youth (Lamberg, 2001).

The disorder involves both a traumatic event and the child's reaction to this event. It is believed that brain changes occur in trauma, leading to neurobiologic alterations that cause dysfunction of memory. Female gender, having other psychiatric disorders, a family history of psychiatric illness, and severe or lengthy trauma are all risk factors. The incidence ranges from 1% to 9% (Meltzer-Brody et al., 2000).

A variety of antidepressants and SSRIs are used for pharmacologic treatment. Counseling and other mechanisms of

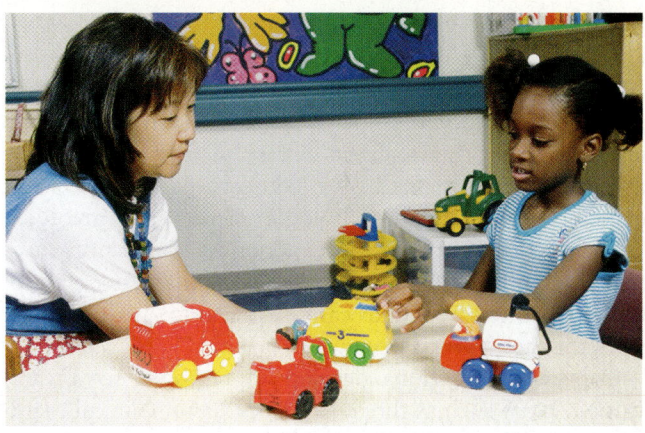

FIGURE 53–6. ◆ The psychologist uses play therapy to help Cassandra reenact her car crash. This helps her gain some control over the event so that it is not so frightening.

care can help the victim deal with the events. Cassandra saw a clinical psychologist who used play therapy to help her communicate her fears related to a car crash. Once the fears are clearly communicated, they often lose their power over the person, so that normal behaviors can resume. Nurses often help identify PTSD victims so that they can get care. Mental health nurses may conduct group therapy sessions. All nurses should recognize that they are at risk for the disorder when their jobs present them with frequent traumatic events. They should seek assistance from counselors and use various resources to deal with the trauma.

Teaching About

TALKING WITH CHILDREN ABOUT TRAUMATIC EVENTS

Whether a child or adolescent experiences trauma from a car crash, abuse, or environmental event, parents can help to decrease the effects of the stress and prevent the appearance of PTSD. Some suggestions for parents include:

- Be sure children feel free to ask parents, teachers, or others about the events and their feelings.
- Assure children that their feelings are normal and may return over time.
- Be honest and open in responses, without overloading children with more details than they need.
- Be prepared to repeat answers and discuss the same topics many times.
- Get help from counselors who can suggest how to talk with the child.
- Use communication methods appropriate at various ages, such as reading books, doing art projects, or drawing.
- Show children that they are loved by spending time and planning activities with them.
- Limit the television and other media time where the child is exposed to violence and traumatic events.
- Restore a sense of normal routines into the child's life.
- Be alert for increasing signs of distress and seek care from a professional if they occur.

CONVERSION REACTION

Conversion reaction is a disorder in which a disturbance or loss of sensory, motor, or other physical functions suggests neurologic or other somatic disease. The disturbance or loss cannot be explained by any known pathophysiologic mechanism. Instead, psychologic factors are involved. About 3% of the population experiences conversion reactions at some time (American Psychiatric Association, 2000). Adolescence and early adulthood are common times for the onset to occur.

Conversion reactions develop in response to a catastrophic event such as threat or loss or harm. Clinical manifestations include altered sensations, such as blindness or deafness; paralysis or ataxia, including inability to stand or walk and loss of ability to speak (aphonia); involuntary movements, such as pseudoepileptic convulsions; and constant complaints of pain with no physical basis (psychogenic pain). Children under 10 years usually present with gait abnormalities or seizures. The onset of conversion symptoms is usually dramatic and sudden. Symptoms often appear to be neurologic, but on careful examination obvious discrepancies are found. The person is usually calm about the symptoms even though they are serious. Often the child or family members appear indifferent or unconcerned over what health care providers consider an overwhelming physical disability.

Children suspected of having a conversion reaction require a complete physical and neurologic evaluation to rule out any possible physiologic basis for the symptoms. Individual and family therapy is usually necessary to identify the source of the psychologic conflict, pain, or need resulting in the conversion symptoms.

≈ SUICIDE

Suicide is the third leading cause of death in adolescents between 15 and 19 years of age. Over the past 40 years, teenage suicide has nearly tripled (Fish, 2000; National Strategy for Suicide Prevention, 2001). Suicide accounts for about 16% of deaths in teens. Nine percent of teens and 1% of prepubertal children have attempted suicide (Jellinek & Snyder, 1998).

Developing Cultural Competence

Some ethnic groups have a high rate of suicide. For example, Native Americans have a rate of suicide 1.5 times the national average. Many youth in this group are suicide victims, so it is a major cause of death in Native-American youth. The historic pain experienced by this ethnic group and lack of opportunities for many youth may be some of the reasons for a high suicide rate. Healthy People 2010 goals focus on eliminating health disparities such as this by finding the causes, setting up prevention programs, and providing more support and opportunities for native populations.

Boys die as a result of suicide four times more often than girls. This statistic is reversed for suicide attempts, perhaps because boys use lethal methods such as guns, hanging, and jumping more often than girls, who use drug overdose and wrist cutting. Boys attempt suicide more often when depressed or in a challenging social situation, whereas girls more commonly attempt suicide as an impulsive act when in an unstable situation. It is not unusual for health care professionals and parents to label suicide attempts by children and adolescents "accidents." Up to half of childhood suicides may be recorded as accidents; suicide data for children under age 10 years are not maintained. Adults may have difficulty believing that young children, in particular, would have any reason to want to end their lives. Because of this, many children brought to the emergency department with indications of a suicide attempt are often classified as unintentional injury victims and released without arrangements for appropriate follow-up care.

Many risk factors for suicide exist in children and adolescents (Table 53–10). The most common precursor to adolescent suicide is depression (see earlier discussion). Common signs or symptoms of an underlying depression that could lead to suicide include boredom, restlessness, problems with concentration, irritability, lethargy, intentional misbehavior, preoccupation with one's own body or health, and excessive dependence on or isolation from others (especially adults or caregivers).

The child or adolescent at high risk for suicide may be admitted to a psychiatric unit for care or cared for in a community mental health facility. Treatment may include individual, group, or family therapy. Negotiating a "no suicide" contract is one method that may be used with a suicidal youth. In the contract, the child agrees not to attempt suicide during a specified time period. When a suicide attempt is made, the child or adolescent may be hospitalized for 24 hours, kept in a short-term monitoring unit, or sent home under close observation to ensure adequate assessment and monitoring. It is important to provide crisis intervention at the time of suicide attempt to minimize the opportunity for repeat attempts and begin a therapeutic treatment plan.

TABLE 53–10   Risk Factors for Suicide in Children and Adolescents
School problems
Pregnancy
Drug use or abuse
Problems with a romantic relationship
Feelings of anxiety
History of chronic family problems
Chronic illness
Physical, emotional, or sexual abuse
History of suicide in a family member
History of depression
Chronic low self-esteem

Nursing Management

The major nursing role is in prevention of suicide. Take all suicide threats seriously. Most suicides are committed with firearms present in the home. Ask at each health care visit if the family has firearms. Encourage parents to keep guns unloaded, with ammunition and firearms locked in separate locations. Be sure that children and adolescents do not have access to the keys for the locked firearms. Never underestimate the resourcefulness or abilities of a suicidal child or adolescent, regardless of age, IQ, or physical abilities.

Education in all school settings is appropriate to teach children about resources that can help them if they need it and to identify peers at risk. Be alert for children and adolescents at risk for suicide in any setting. Assess children and adolescents in schools, outpatient settings, and emergency rooms for the possibility of suicidal behavior. Report threats of suicide and depressive behavior. When a child or adolescent persists in threatening suicide after establishment of a "no suicide" contract, hospitalization is necessary to ensure safety. Recognize that when a child or adolescent has committed suicide, friends of the victim may be at increased risk. Teach students to report to teachers, nurses, or counselors about friends who have threatened suicide or seem depressed or display behaviors different from usual. Nurses often plan with mental health specialists to implement suicide prevention programs in schools and communities. Provide supportive services to family and friends whenever suicide occurs.

Nursing care centers on taking appropriate precautions to ensure the child's safety. Monitor both the child and the hospital environment for any object that could be used for self-harm. Remove all potentially harmful objects, such as shoestrings, belts, pantyhose, and hair ribbons. Keep all personal care items (including toothbrush and shampoo) locked at the nursing station and monitor them constantly when used by the child.

Children or adolescents considered at high risk for suicidal behaviors are attended by a nursing staff member at all times, including while using the bathroom and sleeping. It may be necessary for the child to dress in a plain hospital gown, be kept in a visually monitored seclusion room, or (if seriously impaired and self-abusive) be medicated for restraint for a period of time. Restraints are used only when ordered by the physician and interdisciplinary team caring for the youth. Physical restraint is only a short-term approach to provide immediate safety if necessary. Chemical (medication) restraint may need to be used to prevent self-injury by the suicidal person. See page 1437 for information to help families consider when choosing care for their suicidal child. 🔗

Hospitalization continues as long as the child's behavior is self-destructive. Children are referred for intensive individual and family therapy. Encourage parents to keep follow-up clinic appointments, to watch for self-destructive behaviors, and to administer any prescribed medications according to the treatment schedule. Arrange home visits and other community resources for families. 🔗

〰 TIC DISORDERS AND TOURETTE SYNDROME

Tics are sudden, rapid, recurrent, nonrhythmic, and brief motor movements or vocalizations. They may involve movement of the head or upper body, blinking of eyes, or a variety of verbal noises. They may be worse during periods of stress or tiredness. Severe motor tics accompanied by verbal utterances are known as Tourette syndrome. The syndrome is often accompanied by other diagnoses such as attention deficit and learning disabilities (Kurlan, McDermott, Deeley, et al., 2001). Many children have mild motor tics at some time which gradually disappear with no intervention. When the tics are severe or last over one year, they are considered chronic and may require attention from a mental health provider. This disorder is believed to be caused by dopamine abnormalities in the brain and can be successfully treated by haloperidol or other psychotropic medications. Children with Tourette syndrome may initially be incorrectly diagnosed with ADHD due to the increased motor activity. If they are medicated with a drug such as methylphenidate (Ritalin), their behaviors will worsen. Nursing care involves supporting parents and encouraging normal developmental progression for the child. Carefully monitor symptoms after medication is begun. Minimize stress and teach relaxation techniques.

*C*HAPTER HIGHLIGHTS

〰 Major treatment modes for children with mental health disorders include individual therapy, family therapy, and group therapy.

〰 Therapeutic strategies for treatment of children and adolescents with mental health disorders include play therapy, art therapy, behavior therapy, visualization, and hypnosis.

〰 Families often attempt to treat mental health conditions with alternative and complementary therapy; nurses can provide information to assist families in evaluating the results of these therapies.

〰 Nurses are involved in conducting mental health assessments, preventing disorders when possible, participating in intervention to treat disorders, and evaluating success of treatments.

- Autistic spectrum disorder is the major type of pervasive developmental disorder, and is manifested by abnormal behavior, social interaction, and communication.

- Attention deficit disorder (ADD) and attention deficit hyperactivity disorder (ADHD) are characterized by developmentally inappropriate behaviors involving inattention, and sometimes hyperactivity.

- ADD and ADHD must be diagnosed using recommended criteria and are commonly treated with a combination of behavioral, environmental, and medication therapy.

- Mental retardation is a subaverage intellectual and adaptive functioning, and is caused by chromosomal, genetic, or environmental factors.

- Nurses identify children with possible mental retardation by carefully evaluating development.

- A multidisciplinary team plans the care for children with mental retardation and periodically evaluates the child's progress and the family's needs.

- Schizophrenia is a psychotic disorder manifested by social withdrawal, delusions, and hallucinations.

- Mood disorders in childhood and adolescents are commonly manifested as depression or manic-depression (bipolar disorder).

- Several anxiety disorders occur in children and adolescents, most notably anxiety, panic, obsessive-compulsive disorder, and school phobia.

- Behavioral therapy and selective serotonin reuptake inhibitors (SSRIs) are used to treat anxiety disorders.

- Posttraumatic stress disorder may occur as victims relive the terror of traumatic events.

- Suicide is a frequent cause of death among youth.

- Nurses have a key role in identifying youth at risk of suicide, instituting suicide prevention programs, and counseling family and friends of suicide victims.

- Children may experience tic disorders which impair development and social interactions; medications are helpful in treatment of these disorders.

- Nurses play a vital role in maintaining the mental health of children, identifying children at risk of mental health disorders, and providing care or referring families for mental health services.

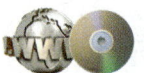

EXPLOREMEDIALINK

NCLEX Review, Case Studies, and other interactive resources for this chapter can be found on the companion website at http://www.prenhall.com/london. Click on "Chapter 53" and select the activities for this chapter.

For animations, more NCLEX review questions, and an audio glossary, access the accompanying CD-ROM in this textbook.

REFERENCES

American Academy of Child and Adolescent Psychiatry. (2001). The practice parameter for the assessment and treatment of children and adolescents with schizophrenia. *Journal of the American Academy of Child & Adolescent Psychiatry, 40(7)*, 4S–23S.

American Academy of Pediatrics, Committee on Quality Improvement, Subcommittee on Attention-Deficit / Hyperactivity Disorder. (2000). Diagnosis and evaluation of the child with attention-deficit/hyperactivity disorder. *Pediatrics, 105*, 1158–1170.

American Academy of Pediatrics. (2001a). Diagnosis and management of autistic spectrum disorder. *Pediatrics, 107*, 1221–1226.

American Academy of Pediatrics, Committee on Quality Improvement, Subcommittee on Attention-Deficit / Hyperactivity Disorder. (2001b). Clinical practice guideline: Treatment of the school-aged child with attention-deficit/hyperactivity disorder. *Pediatrics, 108*, 1033–1044.

American Academy of Pediatrics, Committee on Genetics. (2001c). Health supervision for children with Down syndrome. *Pediatrics, 107*, 442–449.

American Psychiatric Association. (2000). *Diagnostic and statistical manual of mental disorders* (4th ed.): text revision (DSM-IV-TR). Washington, DC: Author.

Arnold, L. E., Pinkham, S. M., & Votolato, N. (2000). Does zinc moderate essential fatty acid and amphetamine treatment of attention-deficit/hyperactivity disorder? *Journal of Adolescent Psychopharmacology, 10(2)*, 111–117.

Bailey, D. B., Roberts, J. E., Mirrett, P., & Hatton, D. D. (2001). Identifying infants and toddlers with fragile X syndrome: Issues and recommendations. *Infants and Young Children, 14*, 24–33.

Baird, G., Charman, T., Cox, A., Baron-Cohen, S., Swettenham, J., Wheelwright, S., et al. (2001). Screening and surveillance for autism and pervasive developmental disorders. *Archives of Disease in Childhood, 84*, 468–475.

Baralle, D. (2001). Chromosomal aberrations, subtelomeric defects, and mental retardation. *Lancet, 358*, 7–8.

Baumgqertel, A. (1999). Alternative and controversial treatments for attention-deficit/hyperactivity disorder. *Pediatric Clinics of North America, 46*, 977–992.

Blondis, T. A. (1999). Motor disorders and attention-deficit/hyperactivity disorder. *Pediatric Clinics of North America, 46*, 899–914.

Bryden, K. E., Carrey, N. J., & Kutcher, S. P. (2001). Update and recommendations for the use of antipsychotics in early-onset psychosis. *Journal of Child and Adolescent Psycho-pharmacology, 11*, 113–130.

Burgess, J. R., Stevens, L., Zhang, W., & Peck, L. (2000). Long-chain polyunsaturated fatty acids in children with attention-deficit hyperactivity disorder. *American Journal of Clinical Nutrition, 71(1)*, 327–330.

Cade, M., & Tidwell, S. (2001). Autism and the school nurse. *Journal of School Health, 71*, 96–100.

Carson, V. B. (2000). *Mental health nursing* (2nd ed.). Philadelphia: WB Saunders.

Castiglia, P. T. (2000). Depression in children. *Journal of Pediatric Health Care, 14*, 73–75.

Dales, L., Hammer, S. J., & Smith, N. J. (2001). Time trends in autism and in MMR immunization coverage in California. *Journal of the American Medical Association, 285*, 1183.

Department of Health and Human Services. (2000). *Report of the Surgeon General's conference on children's mental health: A national action agenda.* Washington, DC: U.S. Department of Health and Human Services.

Diagnostic and Statistical Manual of Mental Disorders, Fourth Edition, Text Revision. Washington, D.C., American Psychiatric Association, 2000.

Fish, K. B. (2000). Suicide awareness at the elementary school level. *Journal of Psychosocial Nursing, 38*, 20–23.

Fletcher, J. M., Shaywitz, S. E., & Shaywitz, B. A. (1999). Comorbidity of learning and attention disorders: Separate but equal. *Pediatric Clinics of North America, 46*, 885–898.

Frederic, D. W., & Williams, S. L. (1998). New definition of mental retardation for the American Association of Mental Retardation. *Image, 30*, 53–56.

Hoagwood, K., Burns, B. J., Kiser, L., Rindeisen, H., & Schoenwald, S. K. (2001). Evidence-based practice in child and adolescent mental health services. *Psychiatric Services, 52,* 1179–1189.

Hunt, R. D., Paguin, A., & Payton, K. (2001). An update on assessment and treatment of complex attention-deficit hyperactivity disorder. *Pediatric Annals, 30,* 162–172.

Hyman, S. L., & Levy, S. E. (2000). Autistic spectrum disorders: When traditional medicine is not enough. *Contemporary Pediatrics, 17,* 101–116.

Jellinek, M. S., & Snyder, J. B. (1998). Depression and suicide in children and adolescents. *Pediatrics in Review, 19,* 255–263.

Kaplan, E. L. (2000). PANDAS? Or PAND? Or both? Or neither? *Contemporary Pediatrics, 17,* 81–96.

Kent, J. M., Sullivan, G. M., & Rauch, S. L. (2000). The neurobiology of fear: Relevance to panic disorder and posttraumatic stress disorder. *Psychiatric Annals, 30,* 733–742.

Kessler, R. C. (2000). Posttraumatic stress disorder. *Journal of Clinical Psychiatry, 61*(Suppl. 15), 4–12.

Kidd, P. M. (2000). Attention deficit/hyperactivity disorder (ADHD) in children: Rationale for its integrative management. *Alternative Medicine Review, 5*(5), 402–428.

Koenig, K. (1998). Pervasive developmental disorders: Diagnosis, intervention and education. *American Journal for Nurse Practitioners, 2*(8), 15–28.

Kurlan, R., McDermott, M. P., Deeley, C., Como, P. G., Brower, C., Eapen, S., et al. (2001). Prevalence of tics in school children and adolescents associated with placement in special education. *Neurology, 57,* 1383–1388.

Labellarte, M. J., Walkup, J. T., & Riddle, M. A. (1998). The new antidepressants: Selective serotonin reuptake inhibitors. *Pediatric Clinics of North America, 45,* 1137–1155.

Lamberg, L. (2001). Psychiatrists explore the legacy of traumatic stress in early life. *Journal of the American Medical Association, 286,* 523–526.

Lambert, L. T. (2001). Identification and management of schizophrenia in childhood. *Journal of Child and Adolescent Psychiatric Nursing, 14,* 73–80.

Leonard, H. L., Freeman, J., Barcia, A., Garvey, M., Snider, L., & Swedo, S. E. (2001). Obsessive-compulsive disorder and related conditions. *Pediatric Annals, 30,* 154–160.

Lyon, D. E., & Morgan-Judge, T. (2000). Childhood depressive disorders. *Journal of School Nursing, 16*(3), 29–31.

Masi, G., Mucci, M., & Millepiedi, S. (2001). Separation anxiety disorder in children and adolescents: Epidemiology, diagnosis and management. *CNS Drugs, 15,* 93–104.

Meltzer-Brody, S., Hidalgo, R., Connor, K. M., & Davidson, J. R. T. (2000). Posttraumatic stress disorder: Prevalence, health care use and costs, and pharmacologic considerations. *Psychiatric Annals, 30,* 722–730.

Moldenhauer, Z., & Melnyk, B. M. (1999). Use of antidepressants in the treatment of child and adolescent depression: Are they effective? *Pediatric Nursing, 25,* 643–645.

National Strategy for Suicide Prevention. (2001). www.mentalhealth.org/suicideprevention. Retrieved November 5, 2001 from the world wide web.

Navon, M., Nelson, D., Pagano, M., & Murphy, M. (2001). Use of the pediatric symptom checklist in strategies to improve preventive

behavioral health care. *Psychiatric Services, 52,* 800–804.

Rohde, P., Seeley, J. R., & Mace, D. E. (1997). Correlates of suicidal behavior in a juvenile detention center. *Suicide and Life-Threatening Behavior, 27,* 164–175.

Smoller, J. W., Finn, C., & White, C. (2000). The genetics of anxiety disorders: An overview. *Psychiatry Annals, 30,* 745–753.

St. Dennis, C., & Synoground, G. (1998). Medications for early onset bipolar illness: New drug update. *Journal of School Nursing, 14*(5), 29–41.

Van Riper, M., & Cohen, W. I. (2001). Caring for children with Down syndrome and their families. *Journal of Pediatric Health Care, 15,* 123–131.

Williams, P. G., Dalrymple, N., & Neal, J. (2000). Eating habits of children with autism. *Pediatric Nursing, 26,* 259–264.

Williamson, D. E., Birmaher, B., Brent, D. A., Bolach, L., Dahl, R. E., & Ryan, N. D. (2000). Atypical symptoms of depression in a sample of depressed child and adolescent outpatients. *Journal of the American Academy of Child and Adolescent Psychiatry, 39,* 1253–1259.

Yehud, R., Hallig, S. L., & Grossman, R. (2001). Childhood trauma and risk for PTSD: Relationship to intergenerational effects of trauma, parental PTSD, and cortisol excretion. *Developmental Psychopathology, 13,* 733–753.

Zickler, C. F., Morrow, J. D., & Bull, M. J. (1998). Infants with Down syndrome: A look at temperament. *Journal of Pediatric Health Care, 12,* 111–117.

Appendices

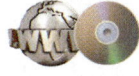

Please note: Additional maternal-newborn and pediatric resources can be found on the accompanying CD-ROM and Companion Website. ⊂▭⊃ [CD] [WEB]

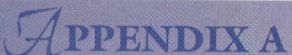

Selected Maternal-Newborn Laboratory Values*

NORMAL MATERNAL LABORATORY VALUES

Test	Nonpregnant Values	Pregnant Values
Hematocrit	37%–47%	32%–42%
Hemoglobin	12–16 g/dL**	10–14 g/dL**
Platelets	150,000–350,000/mm³	Significant increase 3–5 days after birth (predisposes to thrombosis)
Partial thromboplastin time (PTT)	12–14 seconds	Slight decrease in pregnancy and again in labor (placental site clotting)
Fibrinogen	250 mg/dL	400 mg/dL
Serum glucose		
··Fasting	70–80 mg/dL	65 mg/dL
··2-hour postprandial	60–110 mg/dL	Less than 140 mg/dL
Total protein	6.7–8.3 g/dL	5.5–7.5 g/dL
White blood cell total	4500–10,000/mm³	5000–15,000/mm³
Polymorphonuclear cells	54%–62%	60%–85%
Lymphocytes	38%–46%	15%–40%

** At sea level

NORMAL TERM NEONATAL CORD BLOOD LABORATORY VALUES

Test	Normal Values
Hematocrit	43%–63%*
Hemoglobin	14–20 g/dL
Platelets	150,000–350,000/mm³
Reticulocyte	3%–7%
White blood cell total	10,000–30,000/mm³
White blood cell differential	
··Polymorphonuclear (segs)	40%–80%
··Lymphocytes	20%–40%
··Monocytes	3%–10%
Serum glucose	45–96 mg/dL*
Serum electrolytes	
··Sodium	126–166 mEq/L*
··Potassium	5.6–120 mEq/L*
··Chloride	98–110 mEq/L*
··Carbon dioxide	13–29 mmo l/L
··Bicarbonate	18–23 mEq/L
··Calcium	8.2–11.1 mg/dL
Total protein	4.8–7.3 g/dL

Note: From Fanaroff, A. A., & Martin, R. J. (Eds.). (2002). *Neonatal-perinatal medicine* (7th ed.). St. Louis, MO: Mosby. Adapted.

* All laboratory values are approximate. Consult your local laboratory for guidelines as to normal values.

** at sea level

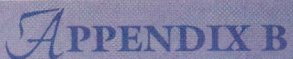

Selected Normal Pediatric Laboratory Values

All laboratory values listed are approximate. Consult your local laboratory for guidelines as to normal values for the specific testing procedures used. This appendix can also be found on the accompanying CD-ROM.

NORMAL VALUES: BLOOD

Albumin (S)[1]

Newborn:	2.6–3.6 g/dL
1–3 years:	3.4–4.2 g/dL
4–6 years:	3.5–5.2 g/dL
7–9 years:	3.7–5.6 g/dL
10–19 years:	3.7–5.6 g/dL

Aldolase (S)[1]

10–24 months:	3.4–11.8 U/L
2–7 years:	1.2–8.8 U/L
Adults:	1.7–4.9 U/L

Aldosterone (S)[1]

6–9 years:	1–24 ng/dL
10–11 years:	2–15 ng/dL
12–14 years:	1–22 ng/dL
15–17 years:	1–32 ng/dL

Alkaline Phosphatase (S)[2]

Values in IU/L at 37°C (98.6°F) using *p*-nitrophenol phosphate buffered with AMP (kinetic).

Age	Males	Females
Newborns (1–3 days)	95–368	95–368
2–24 months	115–460	115–460
2–5 years	115–391	115–391
6–7 years	115–460	115–460
8–9 years	115–345	115–345
10–11 years	115–336	115–437
12–13 years	127–403	92–336
14–15 years	79–446	78–212
16–18 years	58–331	35–124
Adults	41–137	39–118

a₁Antitrysin (S)[1]

Newborn:	143–440 mg/dL
1–3 years:	147–244 mg/dL
4–9 years:	160–245 mg/dL
10–13 years:	166–267 mg/dL
14–19 years:	152–317 mg/dL

Note: Modified from:
[1]Soldin, S.J., Brugnara, C., & Hicks, J.M. (1999). *Pediatric reference ranges* (3rd ed.). Washington, DC: AACC Press.
[2]Hay, W.W., Hayward, A.R., Levin, M.J., Sondheimer, J.M. (2000). *Current pediatric diagnosis and treatment* (15th ed.). New York: Lange Medical Books/McGraw Hill.

Ammonia (P)[1]

Newborns:	<50 mmol/L
Thereafter:	0–35 mmol/L

Base Excess (B)[1]

Newborn:	–10 to –2 mmol/L
Infant:	–7 to –1 mmol/L
Child:	–4 to +2 mmol/L
Thereafter:	–3 to +3 mmol/L

Bicarbonate, Actual (P)[2]

Calculated from pH and $PaCO_2$

Newborns:	17.2–23.6 mmol/L
2 months–2 years:	19–24 mmol/L
Children:	18–25 mmol/L
Adult males:	20.1–28.9 mmol/L
Adult females:	18.4–28.8 mmol/L

Bilirubin, Conjugated (S)[1]

Neonates:	<10 μmol/L
Neonate:	<2 μmol/L
Preterm (1–6 days):	<10 μmol/L

Bleeding Time (Simplate)[2]

2–9 min.

Blood Volume[2]

Premature infants: 98 mL/kg	
At 1 year:	86 mL/kg (range, 69–112 mL/kg)
Older children:	70 mL/kg (range, 51–86 mL/kg)

Calcium (S)[2]

Premature infants (first week):	3.5–4.5 mEq/L (1.7–2.3 mmol/L)
Full-term infants (first week):	4.0–5.0 mEq/L (2.0–2.5 mmol/L)
Thereafter:	4.4–5.3 mEq/L (2.2–2.7 mmol/L)

Carbon Dioxide, Partial Pressure (PCO_2) (B)[1]

Newborn:	27–40 mmHg	(3.6–5.5 kPa)
Infant:	27–41 mmHg	(3.6–5.5 kPa)
Children:	32–48 mmHg	(4.3–6.4 kPa)

Carbon Dioxide, Total (P)[1]

Cord blood:	13–29 mmol/L
<1 year:	17–31 mmol/L
Adults:	24–30 mmol/L

Chloride (S, P)[1]

<1 year:	96–111 mmol/L
1–17 years:	102–112 mmol/L
Adults:	100–108 mmol/L

Cholesterol, High-Density Lipoprotein (S)[1]

1–9 years:	35–82 mg/dL	(0.91–2.12 mmol/L)
10–13 years:	36–84 mg/dL	(0.93–2.17 mmol/L)
14–19 years:	35–65 mg/dL	(0.91–1.68 mmol/L)

Cholesterol, Low-Density Lipoprotein (S)[1]

5–9 years:	63–140 mg/dL	(1.63–3.63 mmol/L)
10–14 years:	64–136 mg/dL	(1.66–3.52 mmol/L)
15–19 years:	59–137 mg/dL	(1.53–3.55 mmol/L)

Cholesterol, Total (S, P)[1]

1–3 years:	44–181 mg/dL	(1.15–4.70 mmol/L)
4–6 years:	108–187 mg/dL	(2.80–4.80 mmol/L)
7–9 years:	112–247 mg/dL	(2.90–6.40 mmol/L)
10–13 years:	125–244 mg/dL	(3.25–6.30 mmol/L)
14–19 years:	106–224 mg/dL	(2.75–5.80 mmol/L)

Complement (S)[2]

C3:	96–195 mg/dL
C4:	15–20 mg/dL

Creatine Kinase (S, P)[2]

Newborns (1–3 days):	40–474 IU/L at 37°C (98.6°F)
Adult males:	30–210 IU/L at 37°C (98°F)
Adult females:	20–128 IU/L at 37°C (98.6°F)

Creatine (S, P)[2]

Values in mg/dL (μmol/L)

Age	Males	Females
1–3 days[a]	0.2–1.0 (17.7–88.4)	0.2–1.0 (17.7–88.4)
1 year	0.2–0.6 (17.7–53.0)	0.2–0.5 (17.7–44.2)
2–3 years	0.2–0.7 (17.7–61.9)	0.3–0.6 (26.5–53.0)
4–7 years	0.2–0.8 (17.7–70.7)	0.2–0.7 (17.7–61.9)
8–10 years	0.3–0.9 (26.5–79.6)	0.3–0.8 (26.5–70.7)
11–12 years	0.3–1.0 (26.5–88.4)	0.3–0.9 (26.5–79.6)
13–17 years	0.3–1.2 (26.5–106.1)	0.3–1.1 (26.5–97.2)
18–20 years	0.5–1.3 (44.2–115.0)	0.3–1.1 (26.5–97.2)

[a] Values may be higher in premature newborns.

Creatinine Clearance[2]

Values show great variability and depend on specificity of analytical methods used.

Newborns (1 day):	5–50 mL/min/1.73 m² (mean, 18 mL/min/1.73 m²)
Newborns (6 days):	15–90 mL/min/1.73 m² (mean, 36 mL/min/1.73 m²)
Adult males:	85–125 mL/min/1.73 m²
Adult females:	75–115 mL/min/1.73 m²

C-Reactive Protien (S)[1]

Cord blood:	10–350 μg/L
Adult:	68–8,200 μg/L

Fasting Insulin Level[3]

1.8–24.6 mU/L

Fibrinogen (P)[2]

200–500 mg/dL (5.9–14.7 μmol/L)

Galactose (S, P)[2]

1.1–2.1 mg/dL (0.06–0.12 mmol/L)

Galactose 1-Phosphate (RBC)

Normal: 1 mg/dL of packed erythrocyte lysate; slightly higher in cord blood
Infants with congenital galactosemia on a milk-free diet: <2 mg/dL
Infants with congenital galactosemia taking milk: 9–20 mg/dL

Galactose 1-Phosphate Uridyl Transferase (RBC)[2]

Normal:	308–475 mIU/g of hemoglobin
Heterozygous for Duarte variant:	225–308 mIU/g of hemoglobin
Homozygous for Duarte variant:	142–225 mIU/g of hemoglobin
Heterozygous for congenital galactosemia:	142–225 mIU/g of hemoglobin
Homozygous for congenital galactosemia:	<8 mIU/g of hemoglobin

Glucose (S, P)[2]

Premature infants:	20–80 mg/dL (1.11–4.44 mmol/L)
Full-term infants:	30–100 mg/dL (1.67–5.56 mmol/L)
Children and adults (fasting):	60–105 mg/dL (3.33–5.88 mmol/L)

Glucose 6-Phosphate Dehydrogenase (RBC)[2]

150–215 units/dL

Glucose Tolerance Test Results in Serum [a][2]

	GLUCOSE		INSULIN	
TIME	mg/dL	mmol/L	μU/mL	pmol/L
Fasting	59–96	3.11–5.33	5–40	36–287
30 min	91–185	5.05–10.27	36–110	258–789
60 min	66–164	3.66–9.10	22–124	158–890
90 min	68–148	3.77–8.22	17–105	122–753
2 hr	66–122	3.66–6.77	6–84	43–603
3 hr	47–99	2.61–5.49	2–46	14–330
4 hr	61–93	3.39–5.16	3–32	21–230
5 hr	63–86	3.50–4.77	5–37	36–265

[a] Normal levels based on results in 13 normal children given glucose, 1.75 g/kg orally in one dose, after 2 weeks on a high-carbohydrate diet.

Glycosylated Hemoglobin (Hemoglobin A₁) (B)[1]

Normal:	4–7% of total hemoglobin
Diabetic patients in good control of their condition:	8–10%
Diabetic patients in poor control:	8–18%
Pregnant Women:	5%–8%
Values tend to vary with testing technique.	

[a] Note: These values reflect total Hemoglobin A_1 levels. When Hemoglobin A_{1c} is computed, values are usually 2–4% lower.

Growth Hormone (S)[2]

After infancy (fasting specimen): 0–5 ng/mL

In response to natural and artificial provocation (e.g., sleep, arginine, insulin, hypoglycemia): >8 ng/mL

During the newborn period (fasting specimen): GH levels are high (15–40 ng/mL) and responses to provocation variable

Hematocrit (B)[1]

Age	Males (%)	Females (%)
Newborns	43.4–56.1	37.4–55.9
6 months–2 years	30.9–37.0	31.2–37.2
2–6 years	31.7–37.7	32.0–37.1
6–12 years	32.7–39.3	33.0–39.6
12–18 years	34.8–43.9	34.0–40.7
>18 years	33.4–46.2	33.0–41.0

Hemoglobin (B)[1]

Age	Males (g/dL)	Females (g/dL)
Newborns	14.7–18.6	12.7–18.3
6 months–2 years	10.3–12.4	10.4–12.4
2–6 years	10.5–12.7	10.7–12.7
6–12 years	11.0–13.3	10.9–13.3
12–18 years	11.5–14.8	11.2–13.6
>18 years	10.9–15.7	10.7–13.5

Hemoglobin A$_{1C}$

See Glycosylated Hemoglobin.

Hemoglobin Electrophoresis (B)[2]

A$_1$ hemoglobin:	96%–98.5% of total hemoglobin
A$_2$ hemoglobin:	1.5%–4% of total hemoglobin

Hemoglobin, Fetal (B)[2]

At birth:	50%–85% of total hemoglobin
At 1 year:	<15% of total hemoglobin
Up to 2 years:	≤5% of total hemoglobin
Thereafter:	<2% of total hemoglobin

Immunoglobulins (S)[1]

Age	IgG (mg/dL)	IgA (mg/dL)	IgM (mg/dL)
1–30 days	221–1031	1–19	12–117
1–6 months	195–794	1–59	9–212
7–12 months	184–974	9–107	4–216
1–3 years	507–1407	18–171	63–298
4–6 years	571–1550	47–231	64–298
7–9 years	589–1717	41–252	49–270
10–12 years	705–1871	61–269	58–340
13–15 years	709–1907	42–304	57–361
16–18 years	632–2108	89–322	59–360

Immunoglobulin D (S)[1]

Newborn:	0 mg/dL
Thereafter:	0–8 mg/dL

Immunoglobulin E (S, P)[1]

0–12 months	<1 KIU/L
1–3 years	<90 KIU/L
4–10 years	<193 KIU/L
11–18 years	<398 KIU/L

Iron (S, P)[2]

Newborns:	20–157 µg/dL (3.6–28.1 µmol/L)
6 weeks–3 years:	20–115 µg/dL (3.6–20.6 µmol/L)
3–9 years:	20–141 µg/dL (3.6–25.2 µmol/L)
9–14 years:	21–151 µg/dL (3.8–27 µmol/L)
14–16 years:	20–181 µg/dL (3.6–32.4 µmol/L)
Adults:	44–196 µg/dL (7.2–31.3 µmol/L)

Iron-Binding Capacity (S, P)[2]

Newborns:	59–175 µg/dL (10.6–31.3 µmol/L)
Children and adults:	275–458 µg/dL (45–72 µmol/L)

Lactate Dehydrogenase (LDH) (S, P)[2]

Values using lactate substrate (kinetic).

1–3 days:	40–348 IU/L at 37°C (98.6°F)
1 month–5 years:	150–360 IU/L at 37°C (98.6°F)
5–8 years:	150–300 IU/L at 37°C (98.6°F)
8–12 years:	130–300 IU/L at 37°C (98.6°F)
12–14 years:	130–280 IU/L at 37°C (98.6°F)
14–16 years:	130–230 IU/L at 37°C (98.6°F)
Adult males:	70–178 IU/L at 37°C (98.6°F)
Adult females:	42–166 IU/L at 37°C (98.6°F)

Lead (B)[1]

0–15 years   <10 µg/dL (<0.48 µmol/L)

Magnesium (P)[1]

Values in mg/dL (mmol/L)

Age	Males	Females
1–30 days	1.7–2.4 (0.70–0.99)	1.7–2.5 (0.70–1.03)
31–365 days	1.6–2.5 (0.66–1.03)	1.9–2.4 (0.78–0.99)
1–3 years	1.7–2.4 (0.70–0.99)	1.7–2.4 (0.70–0.99)
4–9 years	1.7–2.4 (0.70–0.99)	1.6–2.3 (0.66–0.95)
10–15 years	1.6–2.2 (0.66–0.91)	1.6–2.2 (0.66–0.91)
16–18 years	1.5–2.2 (0.62–0.91)	1.5–2.2 (0.62–0.91)

Osmolality (S)[1]

Birth–1 month:	275–305 mOsm/kg
Adults:	282–300 mOsm/kg

Oxygen, Partial Pressure (PO$_2$) (B)[1]

Birth:	8–24 mmHg	1.1–3.2 kPa
>1 hour:	55–80 mmHg	7.3–10.6 kPa
>1 day:	83–108 mmHg	11.0–14.4 kPa

Oxygen Saturation (B)[1]

Newborns:	85%–90%
Thereafter:	95%–99%

Partial Thromboplastin Time (P)[2]

Children:	42–54 sec

PH (B)[1]

0–6 months	7.18–7.50
6–12 months	7.27–7.49

Phenylalanine (S, P)[2]

0.7–3.5 mg/dL (0.04–0.21 mmol/L)

Phosphorus, Inorganic (S, P)[2]

Newborns:	5.0–7.8 mg/dL (1.61–2.52 mmol/L)
1 year:	3.8–6.2 mg/dL (1.23–2.0 mmol/L)
10 years:	3.6–5.6 mg/dL (1.16–1.81 mmol/L)
Adults:	3.1–5.1 mg/dL (1.0–1.65 mmol/L)

Platelet Count (RBC)[1]

Value $\times 10^3/\mu$L. (μL = mm³)

Age	Males	Females
Newborns	164–351	234–346
1–2 months	275–567	295–615
2–6 months	275–566	288–598
6 months–2 years	219–452	229–465
2–6 years	204–405	204–402
6–12 years	194–364	183–369
12–18 years	165–332	185–335
>18 years	143–320	171–326

Potassium (S, P)[2]

Premature infants:	4.5–7.2 mmol/L
Full-term infants:	3.7–5.2 mmol/L
Children:	3.5–5.8 mmol/L
Adults:	3.5–5.5 mmol/L

Proteins in Serum[a][2]

Age	Total Protein	α_1-Globulin	α_2-Globulin
At birth	4.6–7.0	0.1–0.3	0.2–0.3
3 months	4.5–6.5	0.1–0.3	0.3–0.7
1 year	5.4–7.5	0.1–0.3	0.5–1.1
>4 years	5.9–8.0	0.1–0.3	0.4–0.8

Age	β-Globulin	λ-Globulin
At birth	0.3–0.6	0.6–1.2
3 months	0.3–0.7	0.2–0.7
1 year	0.4–1.0	0.2–0.9
>4 years	0.5–1.0	0.4–1.3

[a]Values are for cellulose acetate electrophoresis and are in g/dL. SI conversion factor: g/dL $\times$ 10 = g/L.

Prothrombin Time (P)[2]

Children:	11–15 sec

Protoporphyrin, "Free" (FEP, ZPP) (B)[2]

Values for free erythrocyte protoporphyrin (FEP) and zinc protoporphyrin (ZPP) are 1.2–2.7 μg/g of hemoglobin.

Red Blood Cell Count (B)[1]

Values $\times 10^6/\mu$L. (μL = mm³)

Age	Males	Females
Newborns–6 months	4.2–5.5	3.4–5.4
6 months–2 years	4.1–5.0	4.1–4.9
2–12 years	4.0–4.9	4.0–4.9
12–18 years	4.2–5.3	4.0–4.9
>18 years	3.8–5.4	3.8–4.8

Sedimentation Rate (Micro) (B)[2]

<2 years:	1–5 mm/hr
>2 years:	1–8 mm/hr

Sodium (P)[1]

Newborns:	133–146 mmol/L
Children and adults:	135–148 mmol/L

Thrombin Time (P)[2]

Children:	12–16 sec

Thyroid-stimulating Hormone (TSH) (P, S)[1]

Values in mU/L.

Age	Males	Females
1–30 days	0.52–16.00	0.72–13.10
1 month–5 years	0.55–7.10	0.46–8.10
6–18 years	0.37–6.00	0.36–5.80

Thyroxine (T4) (S, P)[1]

Values in μg/dL (nmol/L).

Age	Males	Females
1–30 days	5.9–21.5 (76–276)	6.3–21.5 (81–276)
1–12 months	6.4–13.9 (82–179)	4.9–13.7 (63–176)
1–3 years	7.0–13.1 (90–169)	7.1–14.1 (91–180)
4–6 years	6.1–12.6 (79–162)	7.2–14.0 (93–180)
7–12 years	6.7–13.4 (86–172)	6.1–12.1 (79–156)
13–15 years	4.8–11.5 (62–148)	5.8–11.2 (75–144)
16–18 years	5.9–11.5 (76–148)	5.2–13.2 (67–170)

Thyroxine, "Free" (Free T4) (S, P)[1]

Newborns:	0.80–2.78 ng/dL (10–36 pmol/L)
1–12 months:	0.76–2.00 ng/dL (10–26 pmol/L)
1–5 years:	0.90–1.72 ng/dL (12–22 pmol/L)
6–10 years:	0.81–1.68 ng/dL (10–22 pmol/L)
11–15 years:	0.79–1.57 ng/dL (10–20 pmol/L)
16–18 years:	0.83–1.53 ng/dL (11–20 pmol/L)

Thyroxine-binding Globulin (TBG) (P)1

1–12 months:	16.2–32.9 mg/L
1–3 years:	16.4–33.8 mg/L
4–6 years:	16.6–30.8 mg/L
7–12 years:	15.0–29.2 mg/L
13–18 years:	13.4–28.7 mg/L

Triglycerides (S)[1]

Values in mg/dL (mmol/L)

Age	Males	Females
1–3 years	27–125 (0.31–1.41)	27–125 (0.31–1.41)
4–6 years	32–116 (0.36–1.31)	32–116 (0.36–1.31)
7–9 years	28–129 (0.32–1.46)	28–129 (0.32–1.46)
10–11 years	24–137 (0.27–1.55)	39–140 (0.44–1.58)
12–13 years	24–145 (0.27–1.64)	37–130 (0.42–1.47)
14–15 years	34–165 (0.38–1.86)	38–135 (0.43–1.52)
16–19 years	34–140 (0.38–1.58)	37–140 (0.42–1.58)

Triiodothyronine (T3) (S, P)[1]

1–30 days	15–210 ng/dL
1–12 months	50–275 ng/dL
1–5 years	80–258 ng/dL
6–10 years	96–232 ng/dL
11–15 years	73–211 ng/dL
16–18 years	69–201 ng/dL

Urea Clearance[2]

Premature infants:	3.5–17.3 mL/min/1.73 m^2
Newborns:	8.7–33 mL/min/1.73 m^2
2–12 months:	40–95 mL/min/1.73 m^2
=2 years:	>52 mL/min/1.73 m^2

Urea Nitrogen (P)[1]

1–3 years	5–17 mg/dL (1.8–6.0 mmol/L)
4–13 years	7–17 mg/dL (2.5–6.0 mmol/L)
14–19 years	8–21 mg/dL (2.9–7.5 mmol/L)

Uric Acid (S, P)[2]

Males:
0–14 years:	2–7 mg/dL (119–416 μmol/L)
>14 years:	3–8 mg/dL (178–476 μmol/L)

Females:
All ages:	2–7 mg/dL (119–416 μmol/L)

White Blood Cell Count (B)[1]

Values $\times 10^3$/μmL. (μL = mm^3)

Age	Males	Females
Newborns	6.8–13.3	8.0–14.3
6 months–2 years	6.2–14.5	6.4–15.0
2–6 years	5.3–11.5	5.3–11.5
6–12 years	4.5–10.5	4.7–10.3
12–18 years	4.5–10.0	4.8–10.1
>18 years	4.4–10.2	4.9–10.0

NORMAL VALUES: URINE

Addis Count[2]

Red cells (12-hr specimen):	<1 million
White cells (12-hr specimen):	<2 million
Casts (12-hr specimen):	<10,000
Protein (12-hr specimen):	<55 mg

Albumin[2]

First month:	1–100 mg/L
Second month:	0.2–34 mg/L
2–12 months:	0.5–19 mg/L

Ammonia[2]

2–12 months:	4–20 mEq/min/m^2
1–16 years:	6–16 mEq/min/m^2

Calcium[2]

4–12 years:	4–8 mEq/L (2–4 mmol/L)

Catecholamines (Norepinephrine, Epinephrine)[2]

Values in μg/24 hr (nmol/24 hr).

AGE	TOTAL CATE-CHOLAMINES	NOREPI-NEPHRINE	EPINEPHRINE
<1 year	20	5.4–15.9 (32–94)	0.1–4.3 (0.5–23.5)
1–5 years	40	8.1–30.8 (48–182)	0.8–9.1 (4.4–49.7)
6–15 years	80	19.0–71.1 (112–421)	1.3–10.5 (7.1–57.3)
>15 years	100	34.4–87.0 (203–514)	3.5–13.2 (19.1–72.1)

Chloride[2]

Infants:	1.7–8.5 mmol/24 hr
Children:	17–34 mmol/24 hr
Adults:	140–240 mmol/24 hr

Corticosteroids (17-Hydroxycorticosteroids)[1]

0–2 years:	2–4 mg/24 hr (5.5–11 mmol)
2–6 years:	3–6 mg/24 hr (8.3–16.6 mmol)
6–10 years:	6–8 mg/24 hr (16.6–22.1 mmol)
10–14 years:	8–10 mg/24 hr (22.1–27.6 mmol)

Creatine[2]

18–58 mg/L (1.37–4.42 mmol/L)

Creatinine[2]

Newborns:	7–10 mg/kg/24 hr
Children:	20–30 mg/kg/24 hr
Adult males:	21–26 mg/kg/24 hr
Adult females:	16–22 mg/kg/24 hr

Growth Hormone[1]

2.2–13.3 years (Tanner 1):	0.4–6.3 ng/24 hr (0.9–12.3 ng/g creatinine)
10.3–14.6 years (Tanner 2):	0.8–12.0 ng/24 hr (1.0–14.1 ng/g creatinine)
11.5–15.3 years (Tanner 3):	1.7–20.4 ng/24 hr (1.9–17.0 ng/g creatinine)
12.7–17.1 years (Tanner 4):	1.5–18.2 ng/24 hr (1.3–14.4 ng/g creatinine)
13.5–19.9 years (Tanner 5):	1.2–14.5 ng/24 hr (0.8–11.0 ng/g creatinine)

Homovanillic Acid[2]

Children:	3–16 μg/mg of creatinine
Adults:	2–4 μg/mg of creatinine

Mucopolysaccharides[2]

Acid mucopolysaccharide screen should yield negative results. Positive results after dialysis of the urine should be followed up with a thin-layer chromatogram for evaluation of the acid mucopolysaccharide excretion pattern.

Osmolality[2]

Infants:	50–600 mosm/L
Older children:	50–1400 mosm/L

Phosphorus, Tubular Reabsorption

78%–97%.

Porphyrins[2]

δ-Aminolevulinic acid:	0–7 mg/24 hr (0–53.4 μmol/24 hr)
Porphobilinogen:	0–2 mg/24 hr (0–8.8 μmol/24 hr)
Coproporphyrin:	0–160 mg/24 hr (0–244 μmol/24 hr)
Uroporphyrin:	0–26 mg/24 hr (0–31 μmol/24 hr)

Potassium[2]

26–123 mmol/L

Sodium[2]

Infants: 0.3–3.5 mmol/24 hr (6–10 mmol/m[2])
Children and adults: 5.6–17 mmol/24 hr

Specific Gravity

1.010–1.030

Urobilinogen[2]

<3 mg/24 hr (<5.1 μmol/24 hr)

Vanillymandelic Acid (VMA)

Because of the difficulty in obtaining an accurately timed 24-hour collection, values based on microgram per milligram of creatinine are the most reliable indications of VMA excretion in young children.

1–12 months:	1–35 μg/mg of creatinine (31–135 mg/kg/24 hr)
1–2 years:	1–30 μg/mg of creatinine
2–5 years:	1–15 μg/mg of creatinine
5–10 years:	1–14 μg/mg of creatinine
10–15 years:	1–10 μg/mg of creatinine (1–7 mg/24 hr; 5–35 mmol/24hr)
Adults:	1–7 μg/mg of creatinine (1–7 mg/24 hr; 5–35 mmol/24 hr)

NORMAL VALUES: FECES

Fat, Total[2]

2–6 months:	0.3–1.3 g/d
6 months–1 year:	<4 g/d
Children:	<3 g/d
Adolescents:	<5 g/d
Adults:	<7 g/d

NORMAL VALUES: SWEAT

Electrolytes[2]

Normal:	<40 mmol/L for both sodium and chloride.
Patients with cystic fibrosis:	>60 mmol/L for both sodium and chloride.

NORMAL VALUES: CEREBROSPINAL FLUID

Protein[1]

Newborns:	40–120 mg/dL
<1 month:	20–80 mg/dL
>1 month:	15–45 mg/dL

Glucose[1]

All ages: 60%–80% of blood glucose

Physical Growth Charts

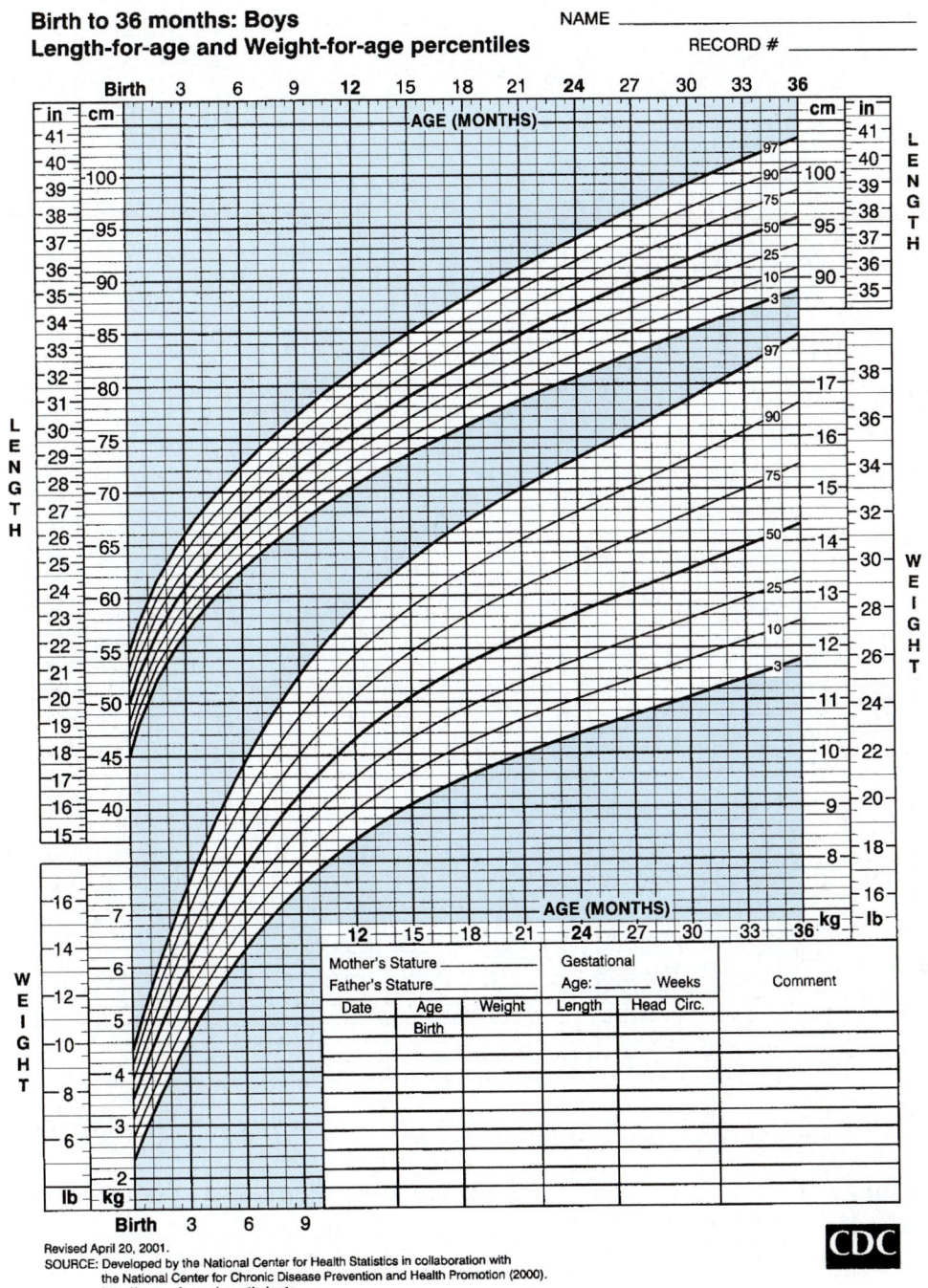

Birth to 36 months: Boys
Length-for-age and Weight-for-age percentiles

NAME _____

RECORD # _____

Revised April 20, 2001.
SOURCE: Developed by the National Center for Health Statistics in collaboration with
the National Center for Chronic Disease Prevention and Health Promotion (2000).
http://www.cdc.gov/growthcharts

FIGURE C-1. ◆ Physical growth percentiles for length and weight—boys: birth to 36 months.
From CDC, 2001. www.cdc.gov/growthcharts

Birth to 36 months: Boys
Head circumference-for-age and
Weight-for-length percentiles

NAME _____

RECORD # _____

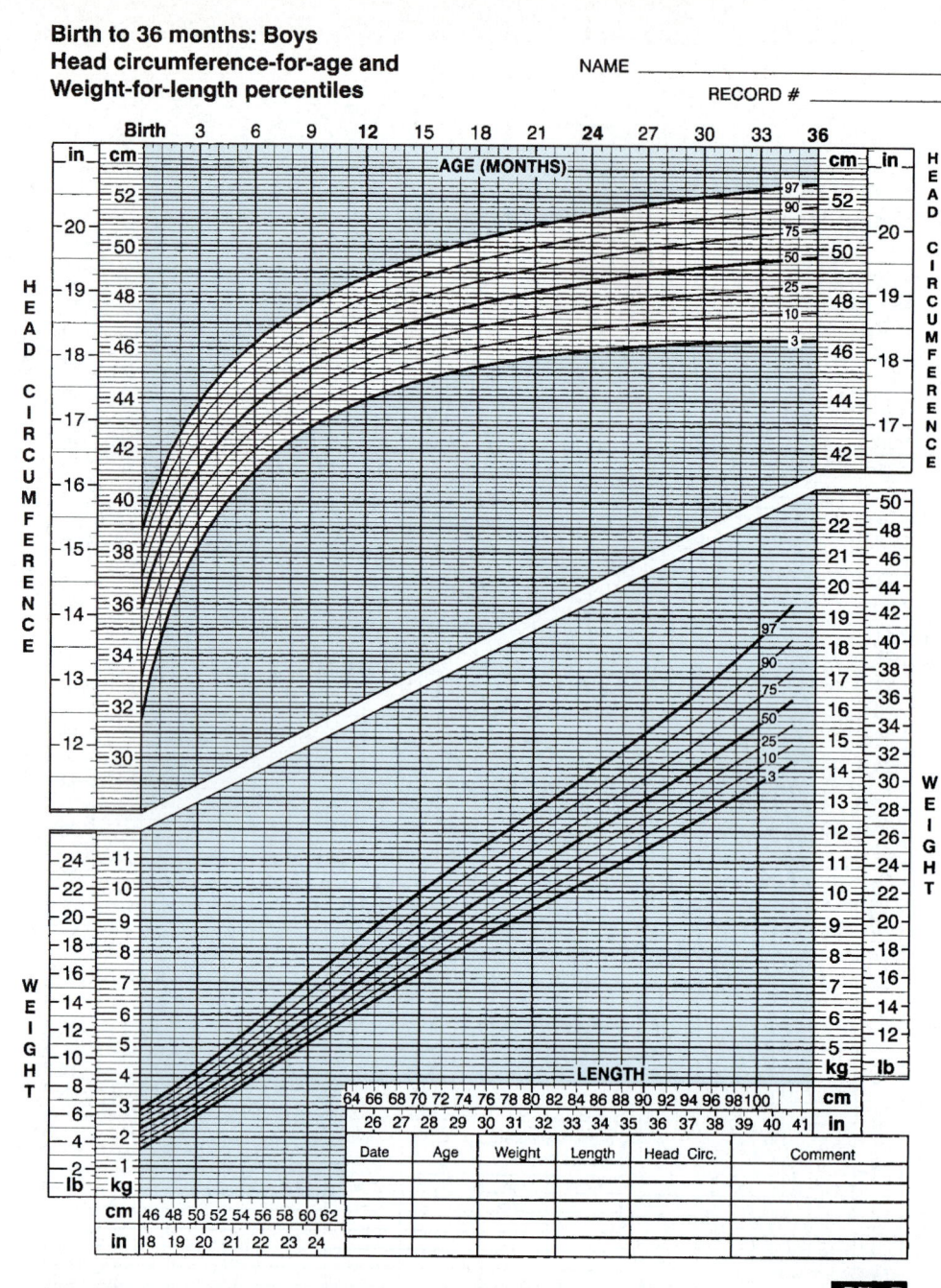

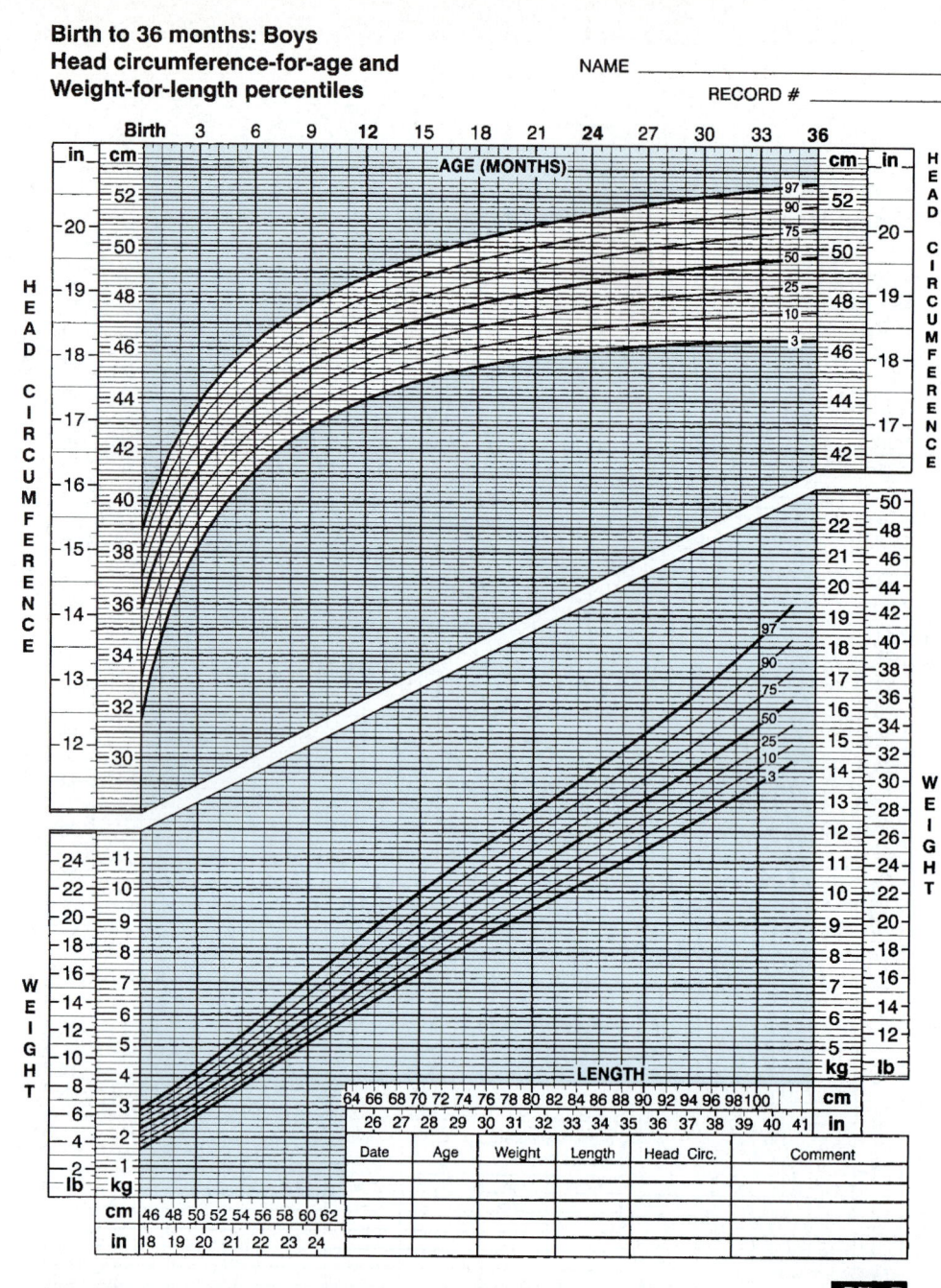

SOURCE: Developed by the National Center for Health Statistics in collaboration with
the National Center for Chronic Disease Prevention and Health Promotion (2000).
http://www.cdc.gov/growthcharts

CDC

FIGURE C–2. ◆ Physical growth percentiles for head circumference, weight for length—boys: birth to 36 months.
From CDC, 2001. www.cdc.gov/growthcharts

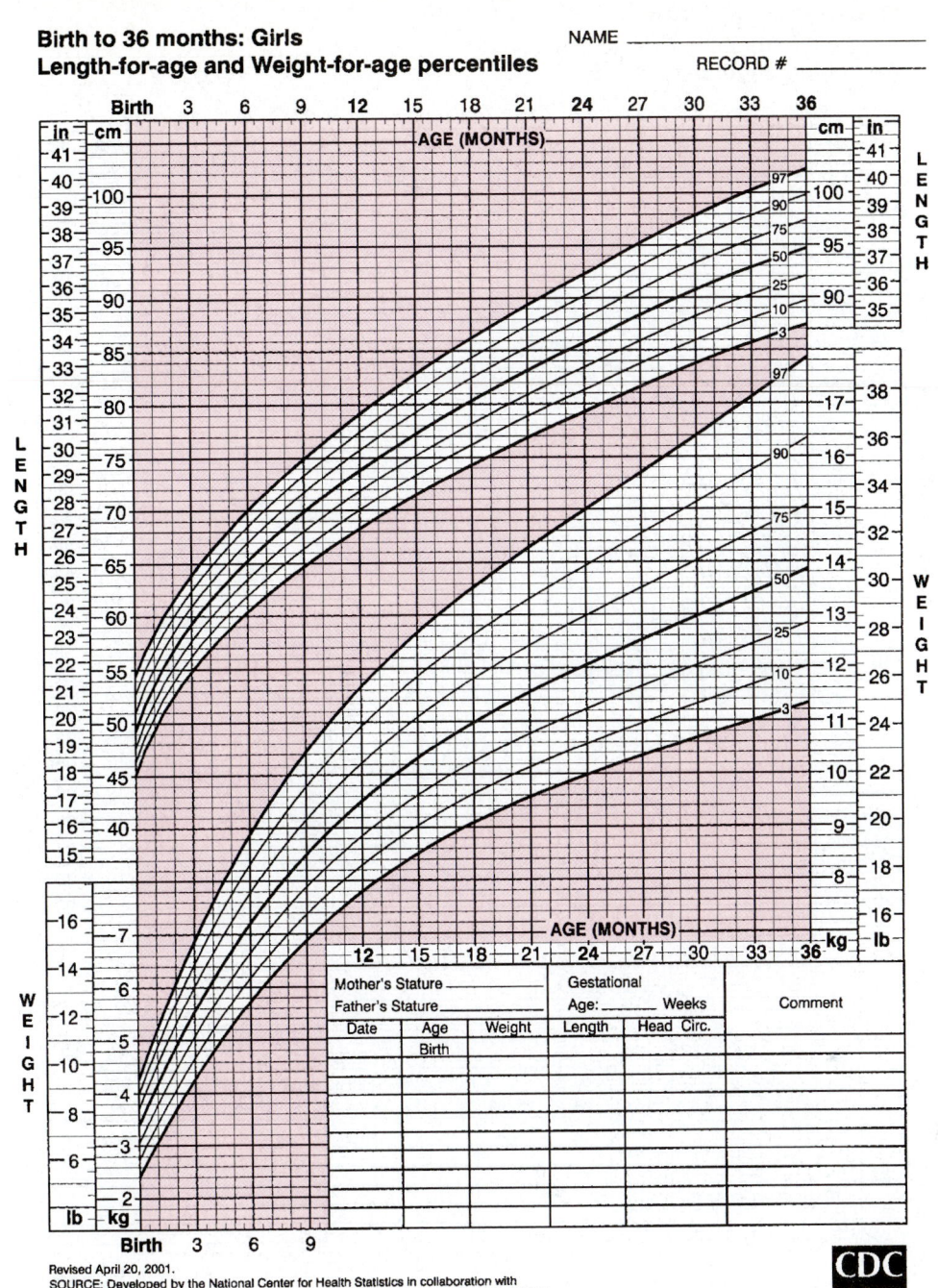

Birth to 36 months: Girls
Length-for-age and Weight-for-age percentiles

NAME _____

RECORD # _____

Revised April 20, 2001.
SOURCE: Developed by the National Center for Health Statistics in collaboration with
the National Center for Chronic Disease Prevention and Health Promotion (2000).
http://www.cdc.gov/growthcharts

FIGURE C-3. ◆ Physical growth percentiles for length and weight—girls: birth to 36 months.

From CDC, 2001. www.cdc.gov/growthcharts

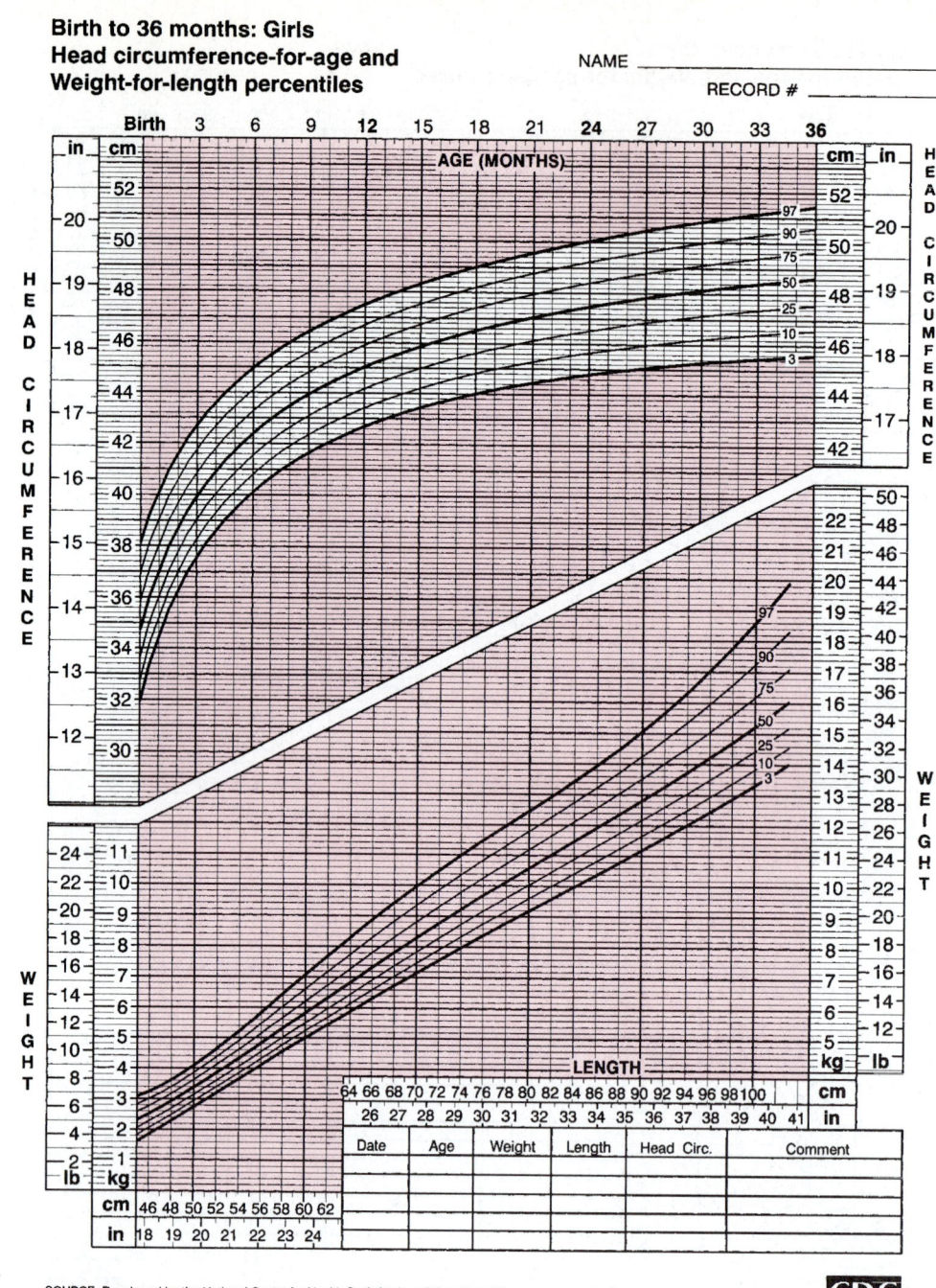

Birth to 36 months: Girls
Head circumference-for-age and
Weight-for-length percentiles

NAME _____

RECORD # _____

SOURCE: Developed by the National Center for Health Statistics in collaboration with
the National Center for Chronic Disease Prevention and Health Promotion (2000).
http://www.cdc.gov/growthcharts

FIGURE C-4. ◆ Physical growth percentiles for head circumference, weight for length—girls: birth to 36 months.
From CDC, 2001. www.cdc.gov/growthcharts

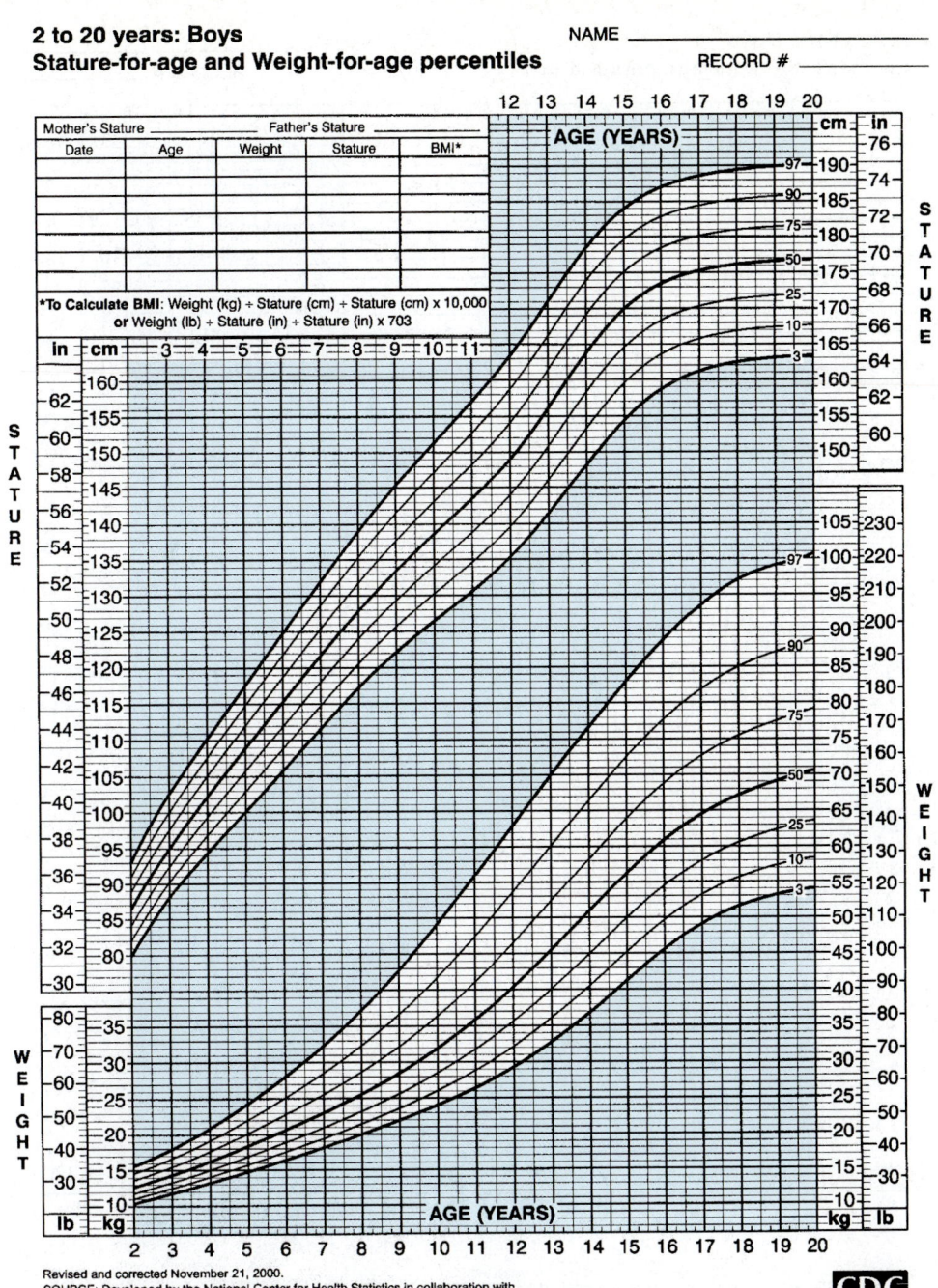

2 to 20 years: Boys
Stature-for-age and Weight-for-age percentiles

NAME _____

RECORD # _____

Revised and corrected November 21, 2000.
SOURCE: Developed by the National Center for Health Statistics in collaboration with
the National Center for Chronic Disease Prevention and Health Promotion (2000).
http://www.cdc.gov/growthcharts

FIGURE C–5. ◆ Physical growth percentiles for stature and weight according to age—boys: 2 to 20 years.
From CDC, 2001. www.cdc.gov/growthcharts

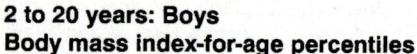

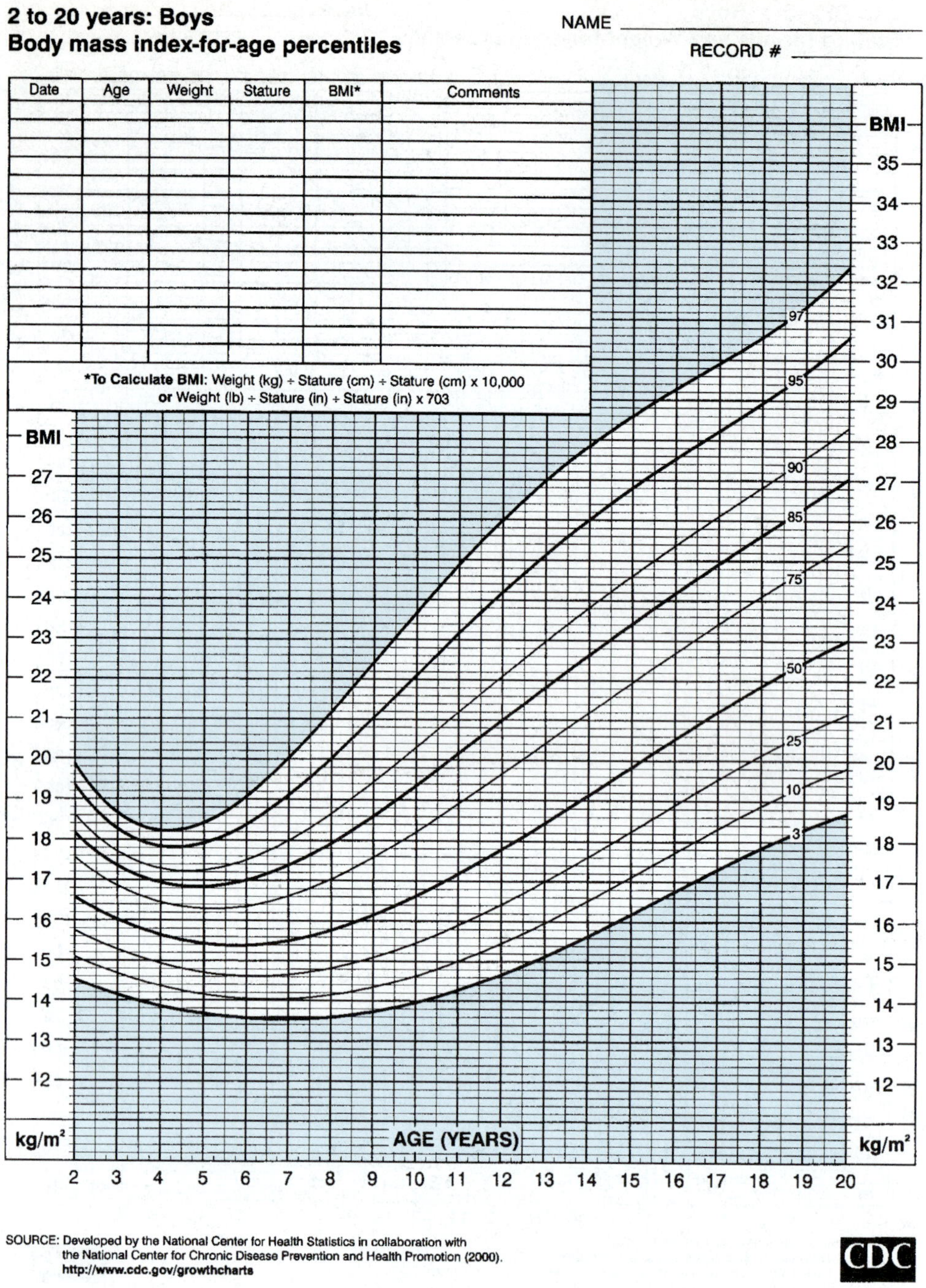
2 to 20 years: Boys
Body mass index-for-age percentiles
NAME
RECORD #
Date
Age
Weight
Stature
BMI*
Comments
*To Calculate BMI: Weight (kg) ÷ Stature (cm) ÷ Stature (cm) x 10,000
or Weight (lb) ÷ Stature (in) ÷ Stature (in) x 703
BMI
kg/m²
AGE (YEARS)
97
95
90
85
75
50
25
10
3
2 3 4 5 6 7 8 9 10 11 12 13 14 15 16 17 18 19 20
12 13 14 15 16 17 18 19 20 21 22 23 24 25 26 27 28 29 30 31 32 33 34 35
SOURCE: Developed by the National Center for Health Statistics in collaboration with
the National Center for Chronic Disease Prevention and Health Promotion (2000).
http://www.cdc.gov/growthcharts
CDC

FIGURE C–6. ◆ Physical growth percentiles for body mass index according to age—boys: 2 to 20 years. From CDC, 2001. www.cdc.gov/growthcharts

Weight-for-stature percentiles: Boys

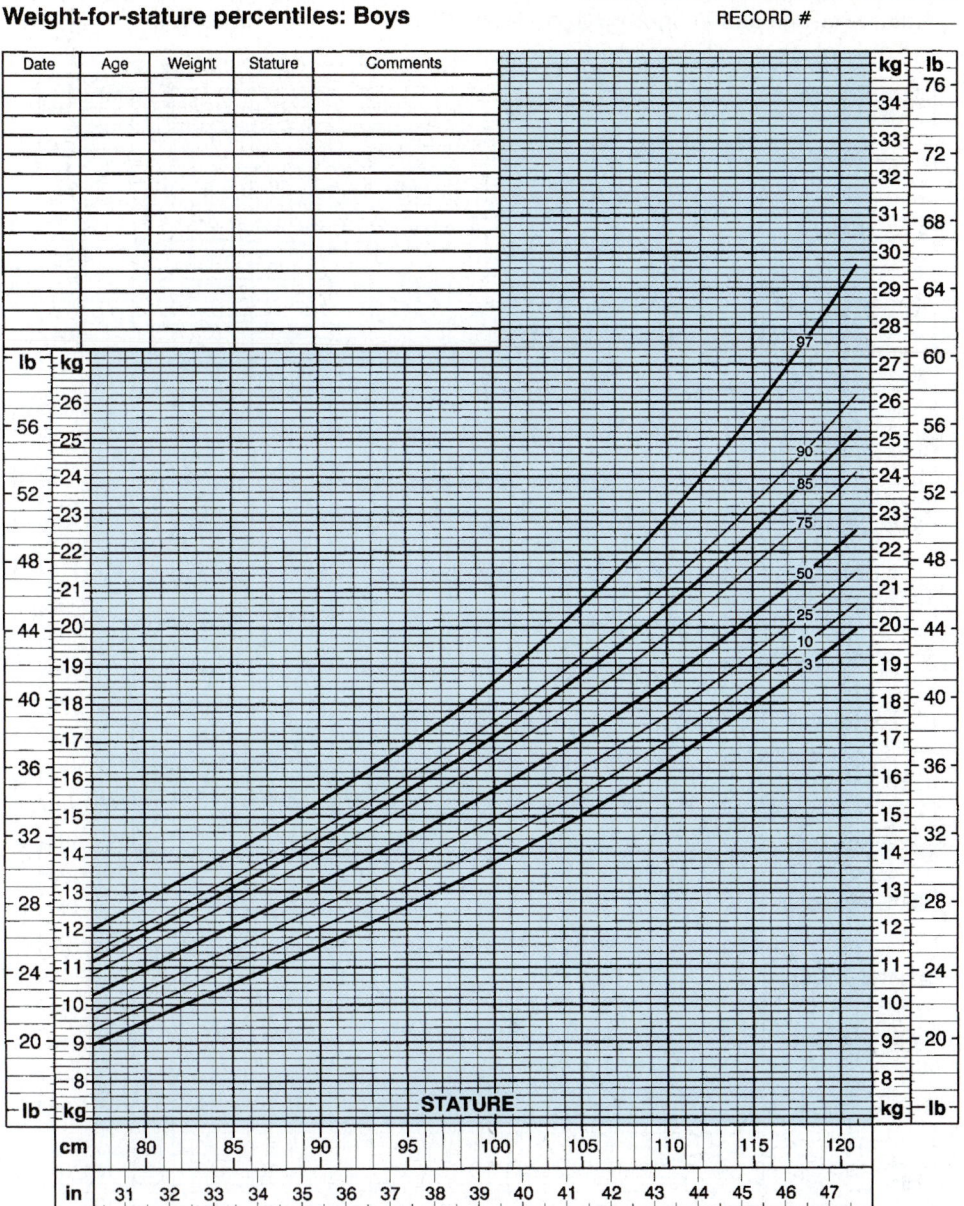

Date	Age	Weight	Stature	Comments

SOURCE: Developed by the National Center for Health Statistics in collaboration with
the National Center for Chronic Disease Prevention and Health Promotion (2000).
http://www.cdc.gov/growthcharts

CDC

FIGURE C–7. ◆ Physical growth percentiles for weight for stature—boys: 2 to 20 years.
From CDC, 2001. www.cdc.gov/growthcharts

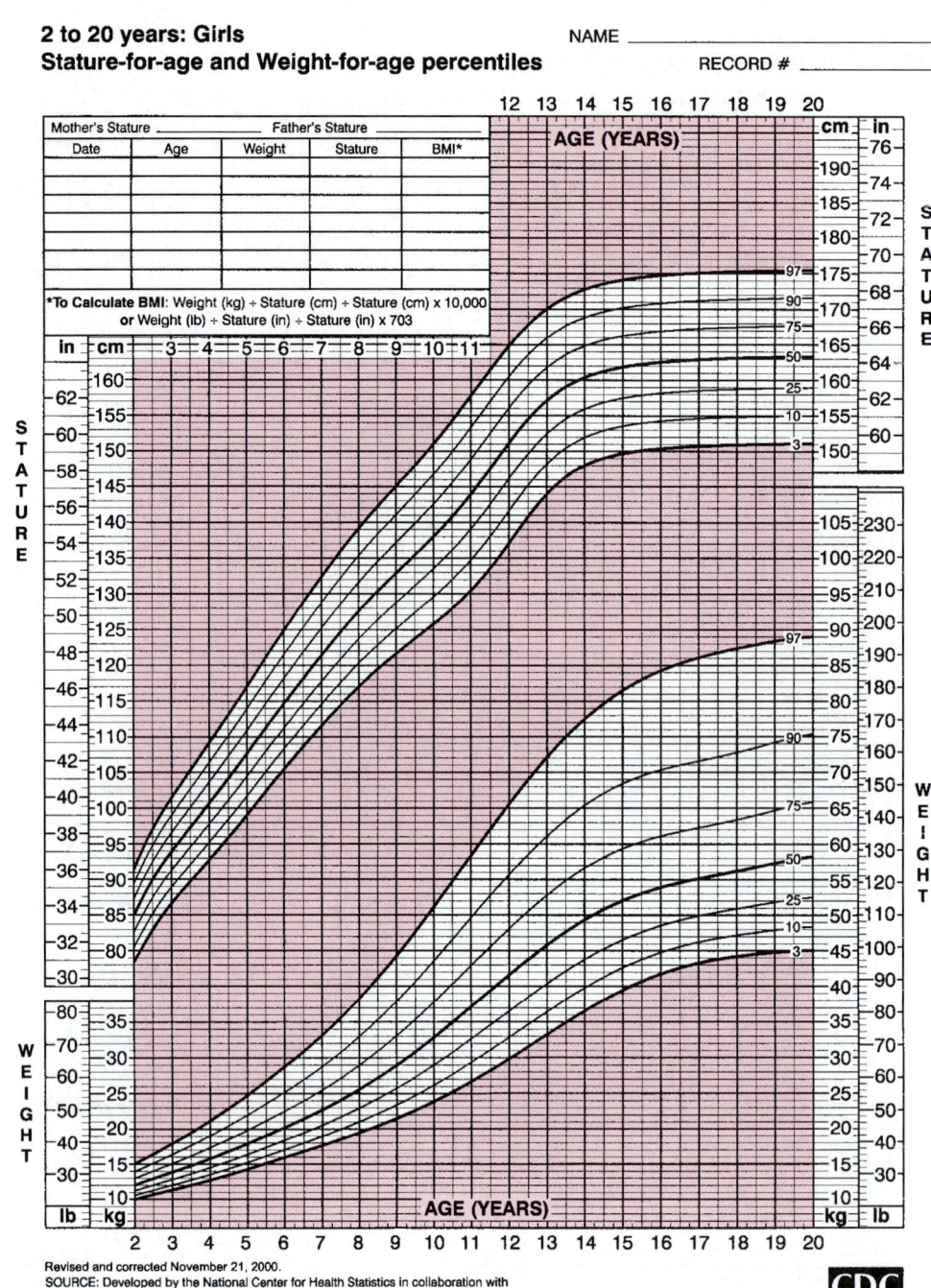

2 to 20 years: Girls
Stature-for-age and Weight-for-age percentiles

NAME _____

RECORD # _____

*To Calculate BMI: Weight (kg) ÷ Stature (cm) ÷ Stature (cm) x 10,000
or Weight (lb) ÷ Stature (in) ÷ Stature (in) x 703

Revised and corrected November 21, 2000.
SOURCE: Developed by the National Center for Health Statistics in collaboration with
the National Center for Chronic Disease Prevention and Health Promotion (2000).
http://www.cdc.gov/growthcharts

FIGURE C–8. ◆ Physical growth percentiles for stature and weight according to age—girls: 2 to 20 years.
From CDC, 2001. www.cdc.gov/growthcharts

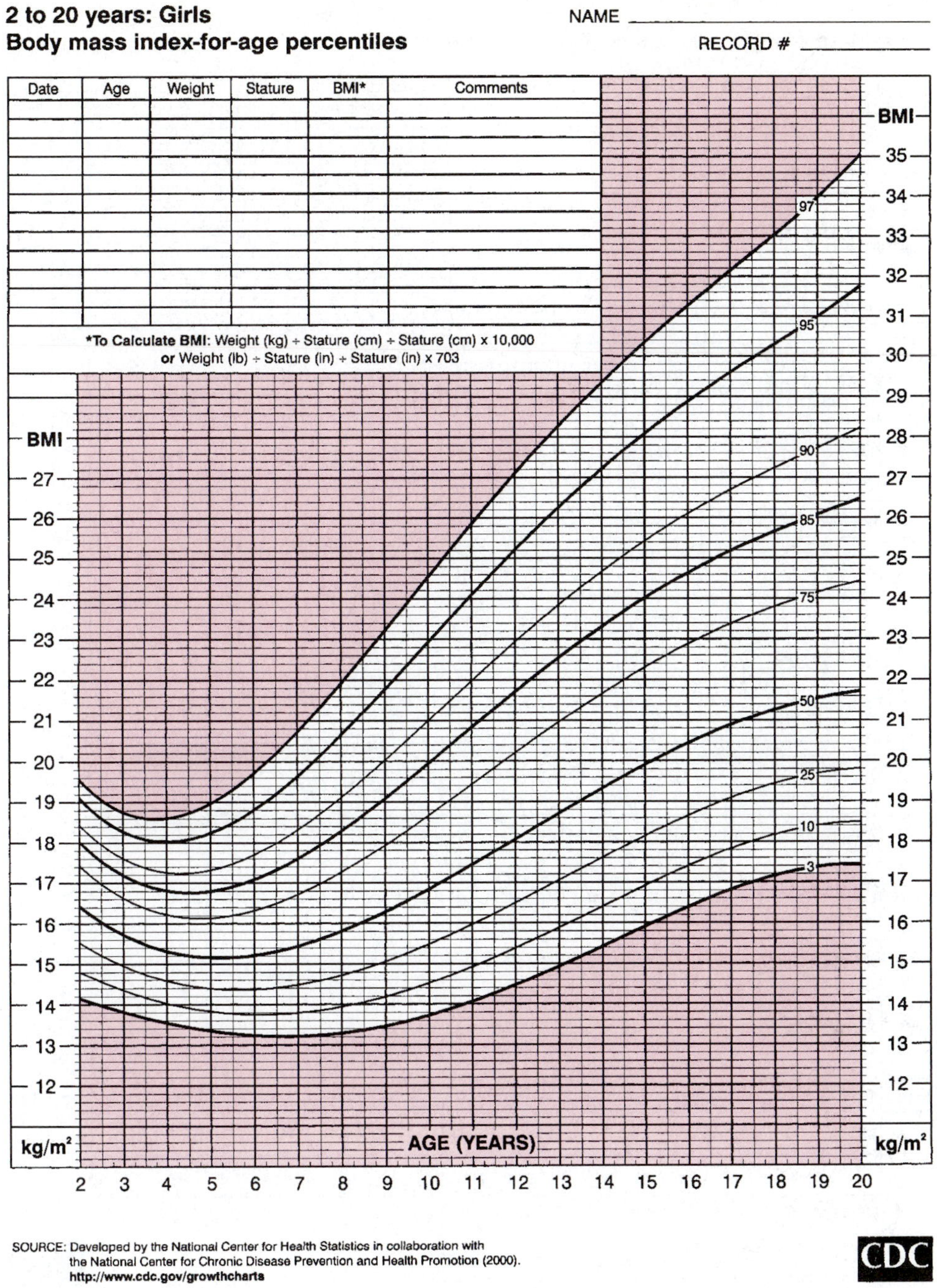
2 to 20 years: Girls
Body mass index-for-age percentiles
NAME
RECORD #
Date
Age
Weight
Stature
BMI*
Comments
*To Calculate BMI: Weight (kg) ÷ Stature (cm) ÷ Stature (cm) x 10,000
or Weight (lb) ÷ Stature (in) ÷ Stature (in) x 703
BMI
35
34
33
32
31
30
29
28
27
26
25
24
23
22
21
20
19
18
17
16
15
14
13
12
kg/m²
97
95
90
85
75
50
25
10
3
AGE (YEARS)
2 3 4 5 6 7 8 9 10 11 12 13 14 15 16 17 18 19 20
SOURCE: Developed by the National Center for Health Statistics in collaboration with
the National Center for Chronic Disease Prevention and Health Promotion (2000).
http://www.cdc.gov/growthcharts
CDC

FIGURE C–9. ◆ Physical growth percentiles for body mass index according to age—girls: 2 to 20 years. From CDC, 2001. www.cdc.gov/growthcharts

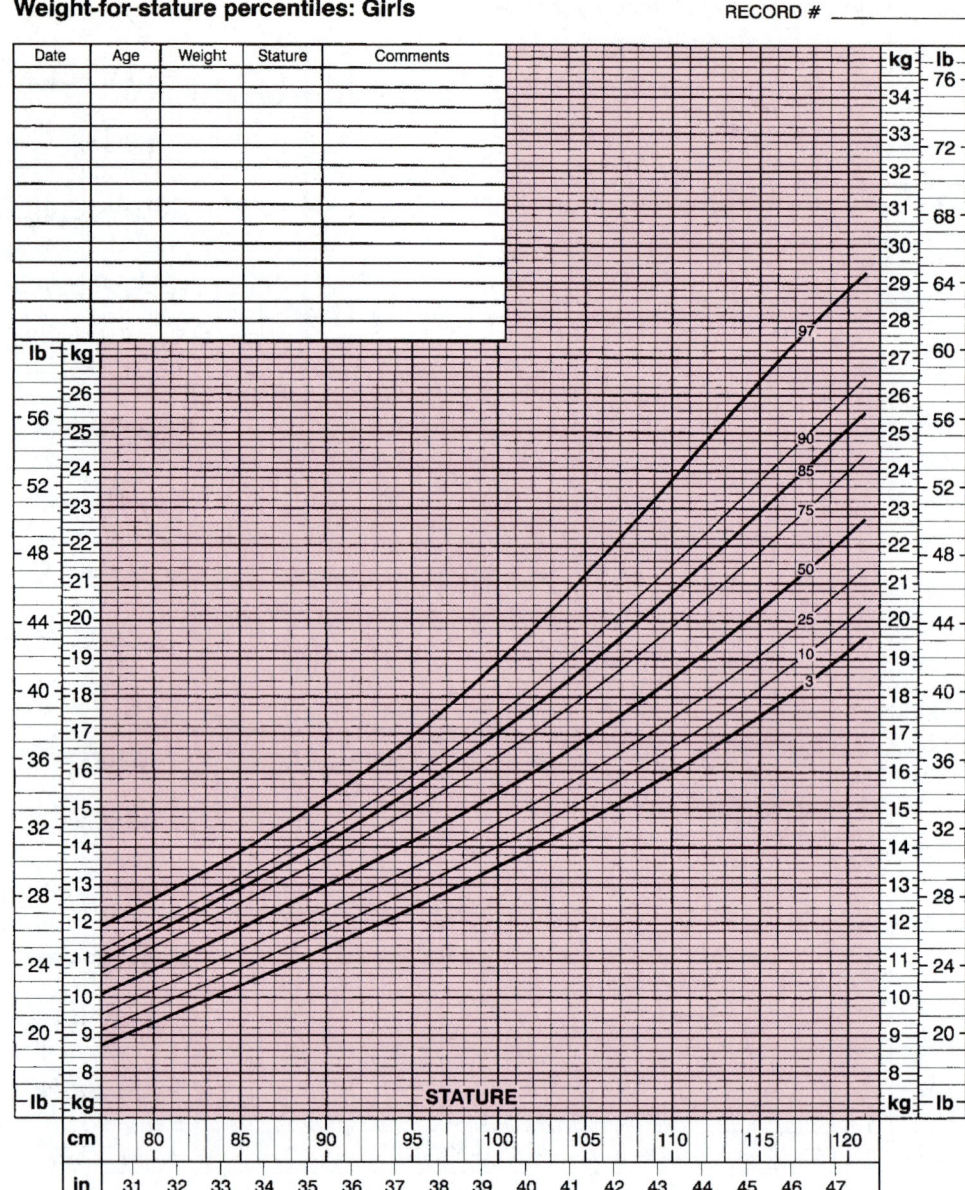

Weight-for-stature percentiles: Girls

Date	Age	Weight	Stature	Comments

SOURCE: Developed by the National Center for Health Statistics in collaboration with
the National Center for Chronic Disease Prevention and Health Promotion (2000).
http://www.cdc.gov/growthcharts

CDC

FIGURE C–10. ◆ Physical growth percentiles for weight for stature—girls: 2 to 20 years.
From CDC, 2001. www.cdc.gov/growthcharts

Conversions and Equivalents

TEMPERATURE CONVERSION

(Fahrenheit temperature − 32) × 5/9 = Centigrade temperature

(Centigrade temperature × 9/5) + 32 = Fahrenheit temperature

SELECTED CONVERSION TO METRIC MEASURES

Known Value	Multiply by	To find
inches	2.54	centimeters
ounces	28	grams
pounds	454	grams
pounds	0.45	kilograms

SELECTED CONVERSION FROM METRIC MEASURES

Known Value	Multiply by	To find
centimeters	0.4	inches
grams	0.035	ounces
grams	0.0022	pounds
kilograms	2.2	pounds

CONVERSION OF POUNDS AND OUNCES TO GRAMS

Pounds	Ounces															
S	0	1	2	3	4	5	6	7	8	9	10	11	12	13	14	15
0	–	28	57	85	113	142	170	198	227	255	283	312	340	369	397	425
1	454	482	510	539	567	595	624	652	680	709	737	765	794	822	850	879
2	907	936	964	992	1021	1049	1077	1106	1134	1162	1191	1219	1247	1276	1304	1332
3	1361	1389	1417	1446	1474	1503	1531	1559	1588	1616	1644	1673	1701	1729	1758	1786
4	1814	1843	1871	1899	1928	1956	1984	2013	2041	2070	2098	2126	2155	2183	2211	2240
5	2268	2296	2325	2353	2381	2410	2438	2466	2495	2523	2551	2580	2608	2637	2665	2693
6	2722	2750	2778	2807	2835	2863	2892	2920	2948	2977	3005	3033	3062	3090	3118	3147
7	3175	3203	3232	3260	3289	3317	3345	3374	3402	3430	3459	3487	3515	3544	3572	3600
8	3629	3657	3685	3714	3742	3770	3799	3827	3856	3884	3912	3941	3969	3997	4026	4054
9	4082	4111	4139	4167	4196	4224	4252	4281	4309	4337	4366	4394	4423	4451	4479	4508
10	4536	4564	4593	4621	4649	4678	4706	4734	4763	4791	4819	4848	4876	4904	4933	4961
11	4990	5018	5046	5075	5103	5131	5160	5188	5216	5245	5273	5301	5330	5358	5386	5415
12	5443	5471	5500	5528	5557	5585	5613	5642	5670	5698	5727	5755	5783	5812	5840	5868
13	5897	5925	5953	5982	6010	6038	6067	6095	6123	6152	6180	6209	6237	6265	6294	6322
14	6350	6379	6407	6435	6464	6492	6520	6549	6577	6605	6634	6662	6690	6719	6747	6776
15	6804	6832	6860	6889	6917	6945	6973	7002	7030	7059	7087	7115	7144	7172	7201	7228
16	7257	7286	7313	7342	7371	7399	7427	7456	7484	7512	7541	7569	7597	7626	7654	7682
17	7711	7739	7768	7796	7824	7853	7881	7909	7938	7966	7994	8023	8051	8079	8108	8136
18	8165	8192	8221	8249	8278	8306	8335	8363	8391	8420	8448	8476	8504	8533	8561	8590
19	8618	8646	8675	8703	8731	8760	8788	8816	8845	8873	8902	8930	8958	8987	9015	9043
20	9072	9100	9128	9157	9185	9213	9242	9270	9298	9327	9355	9383	9412	9440	9469	9497
21	9525	9554	9582	9610	9639	9667	9695	9724	9752	9780	9809	9837	9865	9894	9922	9950
22	9979	10007	10036	10064	10092	10120	10149	10177	10206	10234	10262	10291	10319	10347	10376	10404

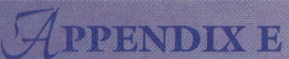

Actions and Effects of Selected Drugs during Breastfeeding*

ANTICOAGULANTS
Coumarin derivatives (warfarin, dicumarol): Relatively safe to use; only small amount in breast milk; check PTT
Heparin: Does not cross into breast milk; check PTT

ANTICONVULSANTS
Phenytoin (Dilantin), phenobarbital: Generally considered safe; if high doses of phenobarbital are ingested, may cause drowsiness; short-acting phenobarbiturates (secobarbital) preferred, because they appear in lower concentration in milk
Magnesium sulfate: Lactogenesis may be delayed

ANTIDEPRESSANTS
SSRI class (Fluoxetin, Fluvoxamine) Effect on newborn unknown current concern.

ANTIHISTAMINES
Diphenhydramine (Benadryl), pheniramine (Dimetane), Claritin, Allegra: May cause decreased milk supply; infant may become drowsy or irritable

ANTIMETABOLITES
Unknown, probably long-term anti-DNA effect on the infant; potentially very toxic

ANTIMICROBIALS
Aminoglycosides: May cause ototoxicity or nephrotoxicity if given for more than 2 weeks
Ampicillin: Skin rash, candidiasis; diarrhea
Azithromycin: No risk to newborn
Chloramphenicol: Possible bone marrow suppression; too low a dose for Gray syndrome; refusal of breast
Methacycline: Possible inhibition of bone growth; may cause discoloration of the teeth; use should be avoided
Metronidazole (Flagyl): Possible neurologic disorders or blood dyscrasias; delay breastfeeding for 12 hours after dose
Penicillin: Possible allergic response; candidiasis
Quinolones (synthetic antibiotics): Can cause arthropathies
Sulfonamides: May cause hyperbilirubinemia; use contraindicated until infant over 1 week old
Tetracycline: Long-term use and large doses should be avoided; may cause tooth staining or inhibition of bone growth

ANTITHYROIDS
Thiouracil: Contraindicated during lactation; may cause goiter or agranulocytosis

BARBITURATES
Propylthiouracil: Safe; monitor infant thyroid function
Phenothiazines: May produce sedation

BRONCHODILATORS
Aminophylline: May cause insomnia or irritability in the infant
Ephedrine, cromolyn (Intal): Relatively safe

CAFFEINE
Excessive consumption may cause jitteriness or wakefulness

CARDIOVASCULAR
Methyldopa: Increase in milk volume
Propranolol (Inderal): May cause hypoglycemia; possibility of other blocking effects, especially if infant has renal or liver dysfunction
Quinidine: May cause arrhythmias in infant
Reserpine (Serpasil): Nasal stuffiness, lethargy, or diarrhea in infant

CORTICOSTEROIDS
Adrenal suppression may occur with long-term administration of doses greater than 10 mg/day

DIURETICS
Furosemide (Lasix): Not excreted in breast milk
Thiazide diuretics (Esidrix, Hydrodiuril, Oretic): Safe but can cause dehydration, reduce milk production

HEAVY METALS
Gold: Potentially toxic; gold salts—compatible with nursing
Lead: Excreted in breast milk; high maternal levels can effect neuropsychologic development
Mercury: Excreted in the milk and hazardous to infant

HORMONES
Androgens: Suppress lactation
Thyroid hormones: May mask hypothyroidism

LAXATIVES
Peri-Colaces Ducolax: Relatively safe
Milk of magnesia, metamucil: Relatively safe

NARCOTIC ANALGESICS
Codeine: Accumulation may lead to neonatal depression
Meperidine: May lead to neonatal depression
Morphine: Long-term use may cause newborn addiction

NONNARCOTIC ANALGESICS, NSAIDS

Acetaminophen (Tylenol): Relatively safe for short-term analgesia

Ibuprofen (Motrin): Safe

Propoxyphene (Darvon): May cause sleepiness and poor nursing in infant

Salicylates (aspirin): Safe after first week of life; monitor protime

ORAL CONTRACEPTIVES

Combined estrogen/progestin pills: Significantly decrease milk supply; may alter milk composition; may cause gynecomastia in male infants

Progestin only (DMPA, Norplant): Safe if started after lactation is established

RADIOACTIVE MATERIALS FOR TESTING

Gallium citrate (^{67}*G): Insignificant amount excreted in breast milk; no nursing for 2 weeks*

Iodine: Contraindicated; may affect infant's thyroid gland

^{125}*I:* Discontinue nursing for 48 hours

^{131}*I:* Nursing should be discontinued until excretion is no longer significant; nursing may be resumed after 10 days

Technetium-99m: Discontinue nursing for 3 days (half-life = 6 hours)

SEDATIVES/TRANQUILIZERS

Diazepam (Valium): May accumulate to high levels; may increase neonatal jaundice; may cause lethargy and weight loss

Lithium: Contraindicated; may cause neonatal flaccidity and hypotonia

SUBSTANCE ABUSE

Alcohol: Potential motor developmental delay; mild sedative effect

Amphetamines: Controversial; may cause irritability, poor sleeping pattern

Cocaine, crack: Extreme irritability, tachycardia, vomiting, apnea

Marijuana: Drowsiness

Heroin: Tremors, restlessness, vomiting, poor feeding

Nicotine (smoking): Shock, vomiting, diarrhea, decreased milk production

*Based on data from Riordan, J., & Auerbach, K. J. (1999). *Breastfeeding and human lactation* (2nd ed., pp. 163–220). Boston: Jones & Bartlett. Briggs, G. G., Freeman, R. K., & Yaffe, S. J. (2002). *Drugs in pregnancy and lactation* (6th ed.). Baltimore: Williams & Wilkins. Hale, T. (2000). *Medications and mothers' milk.* (9th ed.). Amarillo, Tx.: Pharmasoft Publishing; Committee on Drugs, American Academy of Pediatrics. (1994). The transfer of drugs and other chemicals into human milk. *Pediatrics, 93,* 137–150.

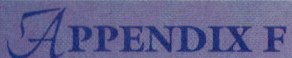

Common Abbreviations in Maternal-Newborn and Women's Health Nursing

AC	Abdominal circumference		**FAD**	Fetal activity diary
accel	Acceleration of fetal heart rate		**FAE**	Fetal alcohol effects
AFI	Amniotic fluid index		**FAS**	Fetal alcohol syndrome
AFP	Alpha-fetoprotein		**FBD**	Fibrocystic breast disease
AFV	Amniotic fluid volume		**FBM**	Fetal breathing movements
AGA	Average for gestational age		**FBS**	Fetal blood sample *or* Fasting blood sugar test
AI	Amnioinfusion		**FHR**	Fetal heart rate
AMOL	Active management of labor		**FHT**	Fetal heart tones
AROM	Artificial rupture of membranes		**FL**	Femur length
ART	Artificial reproductive technology		**FMR**	Fetal movement record
			FPG	Fasting plasma glucose test
BAT	Brown adipose tissue (brown fat)		**FSH**	Follicle-stimulating hormone
BBT	Basal body temperature		**FSHRH**	Follicle-stimulating hormone–releasing hormone
BL	Baseline (fetal heart rate baseline)			
BOW	Bag of waters			
BPD	Biparietal diameter *or* Bronchopulmonary dysplasia		**G or grav**	Gravida
			GDM	Gestational diabetes mellitus
BPP	Biophysical profile		**GIFT**	Gamete intrafallopian transfer
BSE	Breast self-examination		**GnRF**	Gonadotropin-releasing factor
			GnRH	Gonadotropin-releasing hormone
CC	Chest circumference *or* Cord compression		**GTD**	Gestational trophoblastic disease
C–H	Crown-to-heel length		**GTPAL**	Gravida, term, preterm, abortion, living children; a system of recording maternity history
CID	Cytomegalic inclusion disease			
CMV	Cytomegalovirus			
CNM	Certified nurse-midwife			
CNS	Clinical nurse specialist		**HA**	Head-abdominal ratio
CPAP	Continuous positive airway pressure		**HAI**	Hemagglutination-inhibition test
CPD	Cephalopelvic disproportion *or* Citrate-phosphate-dextrose		**HC**	Head compression
			hCG	Human chorionic gonadotropin
CRL	Crown-rump length		**hCS**	Human chorionic somatomammotropin (same as hPL)
C/S	Cesarean section (or C-section)			
CST	Contraction stress test		**HMD**	Hyaline membrane disease
CVA	Costovertebral angle		**hMG**	Human menopausal gonadotropin
CVS	Chorionic villus sampling		**hPL**	Human placental lactogen
			HPV	Human papilloma virus
D&C	Dilatation and curettage		**HRT**	Hormone replacement therapy
decels	Deceleration of fetal heart rate		**HSV**	Herpes simplex virus
DFMR	Daily fetal movement response			
dil	Dilatation		**IDM**	Infant of a diabetic mother
DTR	Deep tendon reflexes		**IPG**	Impedance phlebography
			ISAM	Infant of a substance abusing mother
ECMO	Extracorporal membrane oxygenator		**IU**	International units
EDB	Estimated date of birth		**IUD**	Intrauterine device
EDC	Estimated date of confinement		**IUFD**	Intrauterine fetal death
EFM	Electronic fetal monitoring		**IUGR**	Intrauterine growth restriction
EFW	Estimated fetal weight		**IVF**	In vitro fertilization
EIA	Enzyme immunoassay			
ELF	Elective low forceps		**LADA**	Left-acromion-dorsal-anterior
ELISA	Enzyme-linked immunosorbent assay		**LADP**	Left-acromion-dorsal-posterior
EP	Ectopic pregnancy		**LBW**	Low birth weight
epis	Episiotomy		**LDR**	Labor, delivery, and recovery room

LGA	Large for gestational age	**PMS**	Premenstrual syndrome
LH	Luteinizing hormone	**PPHN**	Persistent pulmonary hypertension
LHRH	Luteinizing hormone–releasing hormone	**Premie**	Premature infant
LMA	Left-mentum-anterior	**primip**	Primipara
LML	Left mediolateral (episiotomy)	**PROM**	Premature rupture of membranes
LMP	Last menstrual period *or* Left-mentum-posterior	**PUBS**	Percutaneous umbilical blood sampling
LMT	Left-mentum-transverse	**RADA**	Right-acromion-dorsal-anterior
LOA	Left-occiput-anterior	**RADP**	Right-acromion-dorsal-posterior
LOF	Low outlet forceps	**RDS**	Respiratory distress syndrome
LOP	Left-occiput-posterior	**REM**	Rapid eye movements
LOT	Left-occiput-transverse	**RIA**	Radioimmunoassay
L/S	Lecithin/sphingomyelin ratio	**RMA**	Right-mentum-anterior
LSA	Left-sacrum-anterior	**RMP**	Right-mentum-posterior
LSP	Left-sacrum-posterior	**RMT**	Right-mentum-transverse
LST	Left-sacrum-transverse	**ROA**	Right-occiput-anterior
		ROM	Rupture of membranes
MAS	Meconium aspiration syndrome	**ROP**	Right-occiput-posterior *or* Retinopathy of prematurity
mec	Meconium		
mec st	Meconium stain	**ROT**	Right-occiput-transverse
ML	Midline (episiotomy)	**RRA**	Radioreceptor assay
MSAFP	Maternal serum alpha-fetoprotein	**RSA**	Right-sacrum-anterior
multip	Multipara	**RSP**	Right-sacrum-posterior
		RST	Right-sacrum-transverse
NGU	Nongonococcal urethritis		
NP	Nurse practitioner	**SET**	Surrogate embryo transfer
NSCST	Nipple stimulation contraction stress test	**SGA**	Small for gestational age
NST	Nonstress test *or* Nonshivering thermogenesis	**SIDS**	Sudden infant death syndrome
NTE	Neutral thermal environment	**SMB**	Submentobregmatic diameter
NSVD	Normal sterile vaginal delivery	**SOB**	Suboccipitobregmatic diameter
NTD	Neural tube defects	**SPA**	Sperm penetration assay
		SROM	Spontaneous rupture of membranes
OA	Occiput anterior	**STI**	Sexually transmitted infection
OC	Oral contraceptives	**SVE**	Sterile vaginal exam
OCT	Oxytocin challenge test		
OF	Occipitofrontal diameter of fetal head	**TC**	Thoracic circumference
OFC	Occipitofrontal circumference	**TCM**	Transcutaneous monitoring
OGTT	Oral glucose tolerance test	**TDI**	Therapeutic donor insemination
OM	Occipitomental (diameter)	**TET**	Tubal embryo transfer
OP	Occiput posterior	**TOL**	Trail of labor
		TORCH	Toxoplasmosis, rubella, cytomegalovirus, herpesvirus hominis type 2
p	Para		
Pap smear	Papanicolaou smear	**TSS**	Toxic shock syndrome
PDA	Patent ductus arteriosus	**ū**	Umbilicus
PEEP	Positive end-expiratory pressure	**UA**	Uterine activity
PG	Phosphatidylglycerol *or* Prostaglandin	**UAC**	Umbilical artery catheter
PID	Pelvic inflammatory disease		
PIH	Pregnancy-induced hypertension	**VBAC**	Vaginal birth after cesarean
Pit	Pitocin	**VVC**	Vulvovaginal Candidiasis
PKU	Phenylketonuria		

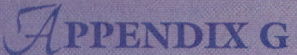

Common Abbreviations in Nursing Care of Children

ACTH	Adrenocorticotropic hormone	**H&H**	Hematocrit and hemoglobin
ADD	Attention deficit disorder	**H-Flu**	*Haemophilus influenzae*
ADH	Antidiuretic hormone	**HIB**	*Haemophilus influenzae* immunization
ADHD	Attention deficit hyperactivity disorder	**HIV**	Human immunodeficiency virus
AFB	Aspirated foreign body	**HOME**	Home Observation for Measurement of the Environment
AI	Adequate intake		
ALL	Acute lymphocytic leukemia	**HUS**	Hemolytic uremic syndrome
ALTE	Apparent life-threatening event	**Hz**	Hertz
AML	Acute myelogenous leukemia		
AOP	Apnea of prematurity	**IEP**	Individualized Education Plan
APIGN	Acute postinfectious glomerulonephritis	**IGF**	Insulinlike growth factor
ARF	Acute renal failure	**ISHP**	Individualized School Health Plan
AS	Aortic stenosis	**IVIG**	Intravenous immunoglobulin
ASD	Atrial septal defect	**IPV**	Inactivated poliovirus vaccine
ASO	Antistreptolysin-O	**IVP**	Intravenous pyelogram
BMI	Body mass index	**JRA**	Juvenile rheumatoid arthritis
BPD	Bronchopulmonary dysplasia		
BSA	Body surface area	**LOC**	Level of consciousness
		LTB	Laryngotracheobronchitis
CBC	Complete blood count		
CF	Cystic fibrosis	**MCNS**	Minimal change nephrotic syndrome
CHD	Congenital heart defect *or* congenital heart disease	**MDI**	Metered dose inhaler
		MMR	Measles, mumps, rubella immunization
CHF	Congestive heart failure	**MR**	Mental retardation
CHIP	Child health insurance program	**MRI**	Magnetic resonance imaging
COA	Coarctation of aorta		
CP	Cerebral palsy	**NEC**	Necrotizing enterocolitis
CRF	Chronic renal failure	**NSAIDs**	Nonsteroidal anti-inflammatory drugs
CSHCN	Children with special health care needs		
CT	Computerized tomography	**OFC**	Occipital frontal circumference
dB	Decibel	**PCA**	Patient controlled analgesia
DDH	Development displasia hip	**PDA**	Patent ductus arteriosis
DDAVP	Desmopressin acetate	**PEFR**	Peak expiratory flow rate
DKA	Diabetic ketoacidosis	**PGE$_1$**	Prostaglandin E$_1$
DPT	Diphtheria, pertussis and tetanus immunization, *or* Demerol, phenergan and thorazine (for conscious sedation)	**PICU**	Pediatric intensive care unit
		PKU	Phenylketonuria
		PPD	Purified protein derivative (TB test)
DRI	Dietary Reference Intake	**PS**	Pulmonic stenosis
DSM	Diagnostic and Statistical Manual of Mental Disorders		
		RAST	Radioallergosorbent test
DTRs	Deep tendon reflexes	**RBC**	Red blood cell
		RDA	Recommended dietary allowance
EAR	Estimated average requirement	**RDS**	Respiratory distress syndrome
EEG	Electroencephalogram	**RSV**	Respiratory syncytial virus
EMLA	Eutectic mixture of local anesthetics		
ESRD	End stage renal disease	**S$_1$**	First heart sound
		S$_2$	Second heart sound
FTT	Failure to Thrive	**SBE**	Subacute bacterial endocarditis
		SCID	Severe combined immunodeficiency disease
GC	Gonorrhea		
GCS	Glasgow coma scale *or* Glasgow coma score	**SIDS**	Sudden infant death syndrome

STI	Sexually transmitted infection	UA	Urinalysis
SVT	Supraventricular tachycardia	UI	Upper intake
		UTI	Urinary tract infection
TANF	Temporary Assistance for Needy Families		
TB	Tuberculosis	VSD	Ventricular septal defect
TEF	Tracheoesophageal fistula		
TGA	Transposition of the great arteries	WBC	White blood cell
TPN	Total parenteral nutrition	WIC	Women, Infant and Children Nutrition Program
TSH	Thyroid stimulating hormone		
Tx	Traction		

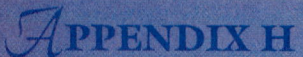

Family Assessment

FAMILY STRUCTURE

- Do you want to care for your child at home?
- Are you aware of any alternatives to home care?
- Who are your child's primary caregivers?
- Who are the other members of your household?
- Can you identify another person to act as backup caregiver for your child?
- Are there others (friends/family members) who can assist you with your child with special needs, with your other children, or with your family's obligations?

MEDICAL MANAGEMENT

- Have you completed the hospital training in your child's care? If no, what is left to learn?
- Has your child's backup caregiver completed training? If no, what is left to learn?
- Do you or your backup caregiver need refresher training for anything?
- Do you have transportation to medical appointments?
- Do you need help in selecting a nursing provider?
- Do you need help in selecting a vendor?

NUTRITION

- How is your child fed?
- If formula, will you need help to buy/locate the formula?
- Have you applied for WIC?
- Does your child have a special need for diapers that is greater than the norm?

PARENTING/CHILD CARE

- During what hours/shifts do you think you will need nursing for your child?
- In the event you need to leave home quickly or if you become incapacitated, who will watch your child with special needs? Who will watch your other children?
- What is your plan for child care in the event of the nurse's absence?
- Will you need help in finding day care for your other children?

- Do you work outside the home? Any plans for the future?
- Do you go to school? Any plans for the future?

FINANCIAL RESOURCES

- Does your child have medical insurance? Are your other children covered under a family insurance plan?
- Do you need more information about or referrals to WIC, SSI, TANF, Food Stamps, Housing, Respite Care?
- Do you need help in obtaining everyday supplies for your child?
- Do you need a referral for help in obtaining other items for your child, such as furniture, clothing, toys?
- Do you need help with budgeting?

COMMUNITY RESOURCES

- Are you involved with any other helping agencies or persons, especially those you would like to include in this planning process?
- Do you or other family members belong to a religious group? Social groups? Clubs? Associations?
- Would you like to talk to another parent who has a child with special needs?
- Would you like a referral to a support group?
- Do you want a referral for counseling? Individual? Marital? Family? Child? Sibling?

FAMILY LIFE

- Do you see your child's homecoming as making a significant change in your lifestyle, and if so, how?
- Do you have concerns about your other children?
- Can you describe how you see your child in a few months? What are your short-term goals for your child?
- Can you describe how you see your child in a few years? What are your long-term goals for your child?
- How would you describe your family strengths?
- What are your family's needs at this time?

Key: WIC = Woman, Infant, Children Nutritional Program; IFSP = Individualized Family Service Plan; IEP = Individualized Education Plan; TANF = Temporary Assistance for Needy Families
From McCord, B. (1993). *Family Profile*. Millersville, MD: Coordinating Center for Home and Community Care.

Guidelines for Working with Deaf Clients and Interpreters

1. First, remember that it requires trust on the part of the client to allow nonsigning caregivers and an interpreter into her life.

2. It is important to use a registered interpreter. Medical interpreters are registered with the Registry of Interpreters for the Deaf. Although family members and friends may offer to interpret, it is best to use registered medical interpreters because they are required to translate the clients' and nurses' words accurately without adding in any other opinion.

3. Greet the client and family with a handshake and body posture that indicates welcome. You may point to your name tag and use the American Sign Language (ASL) alphabet cards to spell out your name. The client may wish to select cards to indicate her name. It is especially important as you work together to make the effort to provide a greeting as you would with speaking clients; greetings help develop rapport.

4. Once the interpreter is present, continue to look at the client and speak directly to her. There will be a temptation to look at the interpreter, and it will help to remember that you are speaking to the client.

5. Avoid phrasing your words as if you are talking to the interpreter (eg, "Can you tell her . . . ?"). Instead, phrase your questions as you do with speaking clients (eg, "I'm going to ask you some questions now.").

6. Depend on the deaf client to ask questions.

7. Look at the client's face for signs of difficulty in understanding. Deaf clients have a behavior of "gesturing" that involves shaking their heads as if to indicate "yes" even when they do not understand. If the client is nodding "yes," ask her to repeat the directions you have just given.

8. Be as direct as possible. Keep to what you want to know or what you want to convey. Speak in short sentences, using nontechnical words. Avoid colloquial or slang words. Be sure to explain what you want to do before you do it. For instance, tell her you want to start an IV and explain the equipment. Then, with her permission, start the IV.

9. Be aware that deaf clients may have difficulty understanding when to take medications. It will be helpful to associate taking medications or completing some treatment or activity with meals. (For instance, while showing her the two capsules she is to take when she goes home, tell her to take the two capsules at breakfast and another two capsules at bedtime.) Avoid saying "take two capsules at 8:00 A.M., 2:00 P.M., and 12:00 A.M."

10. The difference in interpreting time may also affect obtaining a history. It is best to begin with a specific event in the past and work forward.

WHAT TO DO UNTIL THE INTERPRETER ARRIVES

1. Role-play as much as possible.

2. Demonstrate what you want the client to do or what you want to do.

3. Be resourceful.

4. Remember that some deaf clients can read lips. Some may read written language, but use care in assuming the client understands.

WHAT TO DO TO PREPARE FOR WORKING WITH A DEAF CLIENT

1. Contact local agencies that work with deaf clients to see what resources are available. Ask about classes in ASL. Being able to use some basic signs will be very helpful while waiting for an interpreter to arrive.

2. Read to learn more about the deaf culture. Contact your local agency or the National Information Center on Deafness, Silver Springs, Maryland, to get suggestions on books you might read.

3. Investigate your health facility. What is available to assist you? Look for videos used for teaching in the maternal-child unit and note if they have captions. Remember that many deaf clients do not read written language, so it will be important to review the content of the video with an interpreter present.

Prepared with the kind assistance of Mr. Gerald Dement, Interpreter Coordinator, Pikes Peak Center on Deafness, Colorado Springs, Colorado.

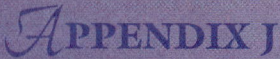

Recommended Dietary Allowances for Childhood and Adolescence

RECOMMENDED DIETARY ALLOWANCES

	AGE	VITAMIN A (μg/d)	VITAMIN D (μg/d)	VITAMIN E (mg/d α-tocopherol)	VITAMIN K (μg/d)	VITAMIN C (mg/d)	THIAMIN (mg/d)	RIBOFLAVIN (mg/d)	NIACIN (mg/d)
Infants	0–6 months	400*	5*	4*	2.0*	40*	0.2*	0.3*	~0.2*
	7–12 months	500*	5*	5*	2.5*	50*	0.3*	0.4*	~0.4*
Children	1–3 years	300	5*	6	30*	15	0.5	0.5	6
	4–8 years	400	5*	7	55*	25	0.6	0.6	8
Males	9–13 years	600	5*	11	60*	45	0.9	0.9	12
	14–18 years	900	5*	15	75*	75	1.2	1.3	16
Females	9–13 years	600	5*	11	60*	45	0.9	0.9	12
	14–18 years	700	5*	15	75*	65	1.0	1.0	14

*Values are Adequate Intakes (AI) rather than Recommended Dietary Allowances (RDAs). All other values on chart are RDAs. See Chapter 3 for a discussion of nutrient requirements.

Note: All data from Institute of Medicine. (1997–2001). *Dietary reference intakes.* Washington DC: National Academy Press. Available also at http://www.nas.edu/iom

VITAMIN B$_6$ (mg/d)	FOLATE (μg/d)	VITAMIN B$_{12}$ (μg/d)	CALCIUM (mg/d)	PHOSPHORUS (mg/d)	MAGNESIUM (mg/d)	IRON (mg/d)	ZINC (mg/d)	IODINE (μg/d)	SELENIUM (μg/d)
0.1*	65*	0.4*	210*	100*	30*	0.27*	2.0*	110*	15*
0.3*	80*	0.5*	270*	275*	75*	11	3	130*	20*
0.5	150	0.9	500*	460	80	7	3	90	20
0.6	200	1.2	800*	500	130	10	5	90	30
1.0	300	1.8	1300*	1250	240	8	8	120	40
1.3	400	2.4	1300*	1250	240	11	11	150	55
1.0	300	1.8	1300*	1250	410	8	8	120	40
1.2	400	2.4	1300*	1250	360	15	9	150	55

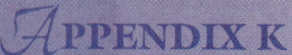

APPENDIX K

Recommended Dietary Allowances for Females, Pregnancy, and Lactation

RECOMMENDED DIETARY ALLOWANCES

	Age	Vitamin A (µg/d)	Vitamin D (µg/d)	Vitamin E (mg/d α-tocopherol)	Vitamin K (µg/d)	Vitamin C (mg/d)	Thiamin (mg/d)	Riboflavin (mg/d)	Niacin (mg/d)	Vitamin B₆ (mg/d)	Folate (µg/d)	Vitamin B₁₂ (µg/d)	Calcium (mg/d)	Phosphorus (mg/d)	Magnesium (mg/d)	Iron (mg/d)	Zinc (mg/d)	Iodine (µg/d)	Selenium (µg/d)
Females	9–13 y	600	5*	11	60*	45	0.9	0.9	12	1.0	300	1.8	1,300*	1,250	240	8	8	120	40
	14–18 y	700	5*	15	75*	65	1.0	1.0	14	1.2	400	2.4	1,300*	1,250	360	15	9	150	55
	19–30 y	700	5*	15	90*	75	1.1	1.1	14	1.3	400	2.4	1,000*	700	310	18	8	150	55
	31–50 y	700	5*	15	90*	75	1.1	1.1	14	1.3	400	2.4	1,000*	700	320	18	8	150	55
	50–70 y	700	10*	15	90*	75	1.1	1.1	14	1.5	400	2.4	1,200*	700	320	8	8	150	55
	>70 y	700	15*	15	90*	75	1.1	1.1	14	1.5	400	2.4	1,200*	700	320	8	8	150	55
Pregnancy	≤18 y	750	5*	15	75*	80	1.4	1.4	18	1.9	600	2.6	1,300*	1,250	400	27	12	220	60
	19–30 y	770	5*	15	90*	85	1.4	1.4	18	1.9	600	2.6	1,000*	700	350	27	11	220	60
	31–50 y	770	5*	15	90*	85	1.4	1.4	18	1.9	600	2.6	1,000*	700	360	27	11	220	60
Lactation	≤18 y	1200	5*	19	75*	115	1.4	1.6	17	2.0	500	2.8	1,300*	1,250	360	10	13	290	70
	19–30 y	1300	5*	19	90*	120	1.4	1.6	17	2.0	500	2.8	1,000*	700	310	9	12	290	70
	31–50 y	1300	5*	19	90*	120	1.4	1.6	17	2.0	500	2.8	1,000*	700	320	9	12	290	70

*Values are Adequate Intakes (AI) rather than Recommended Dietary Allowances (RDAs). All other values on chart are RDAs.

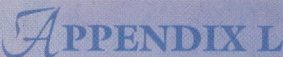

Standards for Maternal-Newborn and Child Health Nursing

PROFESSIONAL PRACTICE STANDARDS IN THE CARE OF WOMEN AND NEWBORNS

Standards of Care for Nurses in the Care of Women and Newborns include:

- Collecting health data.
- Analyzing the assessment data in determining diagnoses.
- Identifying expected outcomes individualized to the woman or newborn.
- Developing a plan of care that prescribes interventions to attain expected outcome.
- Implementing the interventions identified in the plan of care.
- Evaluating the patient's progress toward outcomes.

Standards of Professional Performance in the Care of Women and Newborns include:

- Systematically evaluates the quality and effectiveness of nursing practice.
- Evaluating his/her own nursing practice in relation to professional practice standards and relevant statutes and regulations.
- Acquiring and maintaining current knowledge in nursing practice.
- Contributing to the professional development of peers, colleagues, and others.
- Making nursing decisions and actions on behalf of patients that are determined in an ethical manner.
- Collaborating with the patient, significant others, and health care providers in providing patient care.
- Using research findings in practice.
- Considering factors related to safety, effectiveness, and cost in planning and delivering patient care.
- Contributing to the environment of care delivery within the practice setting.
- Being professionally and legally accountable for his/her practice.

Source: From Association of Women's Health, Obstetric & Neonatal Nurses. (1998). *Standards & Guidelines for Professional Nursing Practice in the Care of Women and Newborns.* (5th ed.). Washington, DC: AWHONN ©

PROFESSIONAL PRACTICE STANDARDS FOR PEDIATRIC CLINICAL NURSING PRACTICE

Standards of Care for the Pediatric Nursing include

- Collecting health data.
- Analyzing the assessment data in determining diagnoses.
- Implementing the interventions identified in the plan of care.
- Evaluating the child's and family's progress toward attainment of outcomes.

Standards of Performance for the Pediatric Nurse include

- Systematically evaluating the quality and effectiveness of pediatric nursing practice.
- Evaluating his or her own nursing practice in relation to professional practice standards and relevant statutes and regulations.
- Acquiring and maintaining current knowledge in pediatric nursing practice.
- Contributing to the professional development of peers, colleagues, and others.
- Making decisions and taking action on behalf of children and their families that are determined in an ethical manner.
- Collaborating with the child, family, and health care providers in providing patient care.
- Using research findings in practice.
- Considering factors related to safety, effectiveness, and cost in planning and delivering care.

Note: From American Nurses Association & the Society of Pediatric Nurses. (1996). *Statement on the scope and standards of pediatric clinical nursing practice.* (MCH-17). Washington, DC: American Nurses Publishing. © 1996 American Nurses Publishing, American Nurses Foundation/ American Nurses Association, 600 Maryland Ave SW, Suite 100W, Washington, DC 20024-2571.

West Nomogram-Body Surface Area

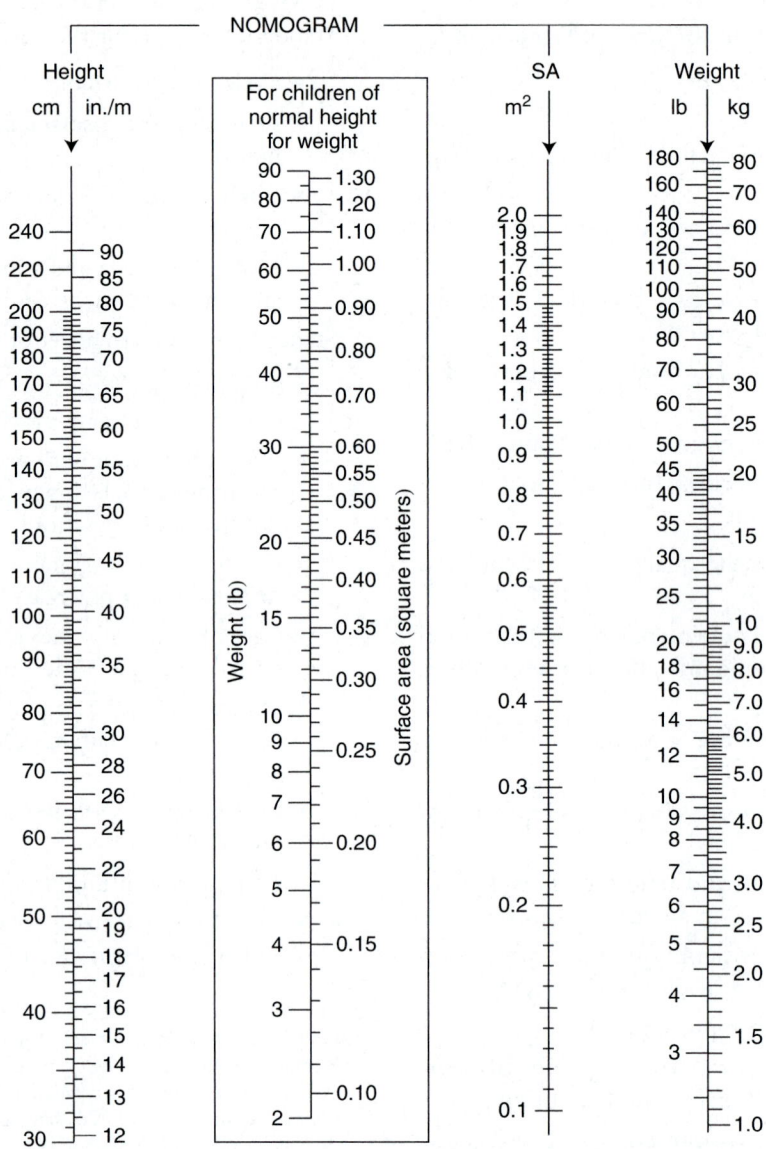

Note: Nomogram modified from data of E. Boyd by C.D. West; from Behrman, R.E., Kliegman, R.M., & Jenson, H.B. (eds.). (2000). Nelson textbook of pediatrics (16th ed.). Philadelphia: W.B. Saunders.

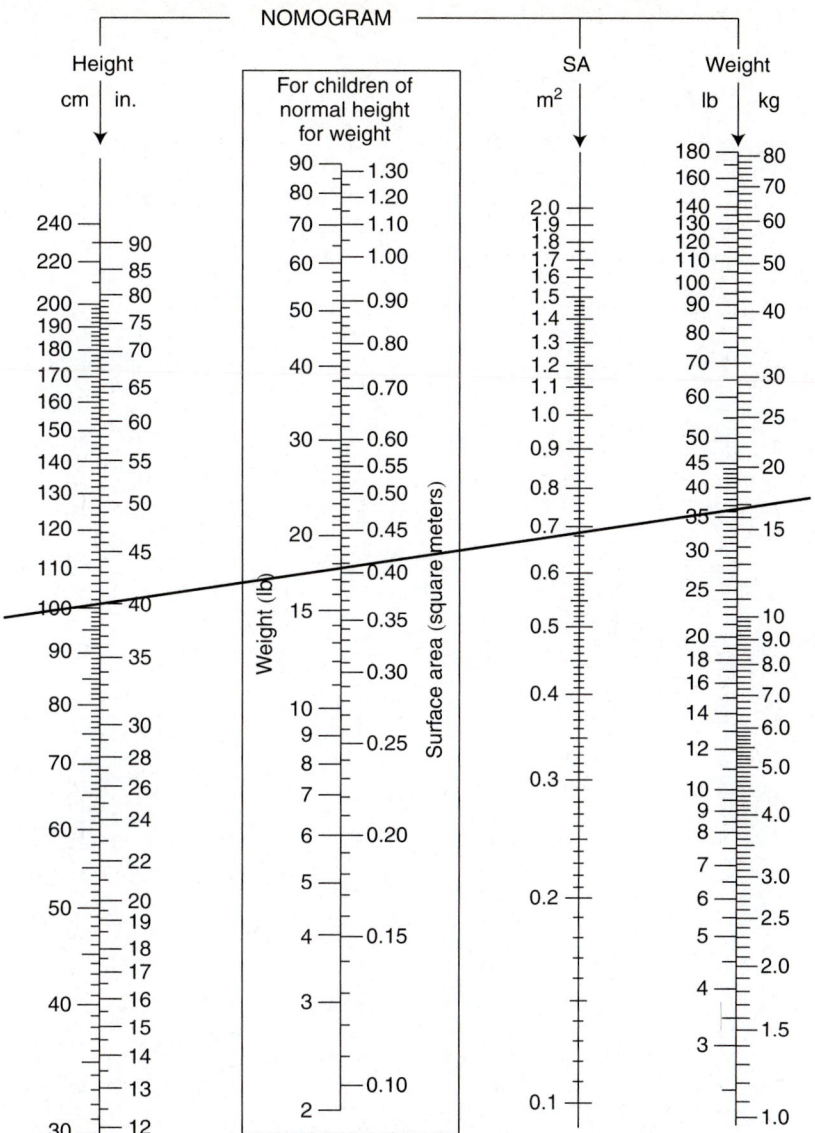

Pediatric doses of medications are generally based on body surface area (BSA) or weight. To calculate a child's BSA, draw a straight line from the height (in the left-hand column) to the weight (in the right-hand column). The point at which the line intersects the surface area (SA) column is the BSA (measured in square meters [m²]). If the child is of roughly normal proportion, BSA can be calculated from the weight alone (in the enclosed area).

Credits

ART CREDITS

Chapter 2 2-4: Wendy Hiller Gee/Biomed Arts Associates. 2-6: Wendy Hiller Gee/Biomed Arts Associates. 2-8: Wendy Hiller Gee/Biomed Arts Associates. 2-9: Wendy Hiller Gee/Biomed Arts Associates. 2-14: Wendy Hiller Gee/Biomed Arts Associates.

Chapter 20 20-2A-B: Wendy Hiller Gee/Biomed Arts Associates.

Chapter 28 Artwork within Pathophysiology Illustrated: Cardiac Defects of Early Newborn Period: Courtesy of Ross Laboratories, Columbus, OH.

PHOTOGRAPHY CREDITS

Chapter 3 3-10: Courtesy of Centers for Disease Control and Prevention. 3-11: Courtesy of Centers for Disease Control and Prevention.

Chapter 4 4-3B: Courtesy of Lovena L. Porter.

Chapter 5 5-8: Courtesy of Marcia London, RNC, MSN, NNP. 5-9: Courtesy of Marcia London, RNC, MSN, NNP. 5-13: © Petit Format/Nestle/Science Source/Photo Researchers, Inc. 5-14: © Petit Format/Nestle/Science Source/Photo Researchers, Inc.

Chapter 8 8-2: © Elena Dorfman. 8-4: © Elena Dorfman.

Chapter 9 9-4: © Jenny Thomas Photography. 9-5: © Elena Dorfman. 9-7: © Elena Dorfman. 9-8A-D: © Elena Dorfman.

Chapter 10 10-2: © Elena Dorfman. 10-3: © Jenny Thomas Photography.

Chapter 11 11-3: © Elena Dorfman.

Chapter 12 12-1: © Jenny Thomas Photography.

Chapter 13 13-2: © Elena Dorfman.

Chapter 14 14-1: © Elena Dorfman. 14-2: © Elena Dorfman.

Chapter 15 15-12: © 2002 Stella Johnson.

Chapter 16 16-1: © 2002 Stella Johnson.

Chapter 17 17-1: © Elena Dorfman. 17-2: © Elena Dorfman. 17-3: © Elena Dorfman. 17-4: © Suzanne Arms. 17-5A: © Elena Dorfman. 17-5B: © 2002 Stella Johnson. 17-6: © 2002 Stella Johnson. 17-8: © Elena Dorfman. 17-10: © Suzanne Arms.

Chapter 21 21-3: © 2002 Stella Johnson. 21-7: © Elena Dorfman.

Chapter 22 22-2: © 2002 Stella Johnson.

Chapter 24 24-10: © Elena Dorfman.

Chapter 25 25-4C: © Suzanne Arms. 25-5C: © Suzanne Arms. 25-6B: © Suzanne Arms. 25-13: © Elena Dorfman. 25-16: © Elena Dorfman. 25-28: © 2002 Stella Johnson. 25-31A-B: © Elena Dorfman. 25-32: © Elena Dorfman. 25-35B: © 2002 Stella Johnson. 25-36: © 2002 Stella Johnson. 25-37: © 2002 Stella Johnson. 25-38: © 2002 Stella Johnson. 25-39: © 2002 Stella Johnson.

Chapter 26 26-1: © 2002 Stella Johnson. 26-2: © Elena Dorfman. 26-8: © 2002 Stella Johnson. 26-9: © 2002 Stella Johnson.

Chapter 27 27-1: © 2002 Stella Johnson. 27-3: © 2002 Stella Johnson. 27-4B: © 2002 Stella Johnson. 27-7: © 2002 Stella Johnson. 27-8: © Jenny Thomas Photography.

Chapter 28 28-4: © 2002 Stella Johnson. 28-7: © 2002 Stella Johnson.

Chapter 29 29-1: © 2002 Stella Johnson. 29-5: © 2002 Stella Johnson. 29-7: © Elena Dorfman. 29-9: © 2002 Stella Johnson. 29–10: © 2002 Stella Johnson. 29-13: © 2002 Stella Johnson.

Chapter 30 30-1: © Kathy Kieliszewski. 30-4: © Kathy Kieliszewski.

All photographs/illustrations not credited on page, adjacent to the piece, or credited above, were photographed/rendered on assignment and are property of Pearson Education/Prentice Hall Health. These include illustrations and photographs supplied by the following illustrators and photographers.

ILLUSTRATORS

Shirley Bortoli, Barbara Cousins, Nea Hanscomb, Left Coast Group, Kristin Mount, Precision Graphics, Robert Voights.

PHOTOGRAPHERS

Kathleen Cameron, Annie Dowie, Beth Elkin, Alain McLaughlin, Richard Tauber.

CONTENT CREDIT

Appendix B: The fasting insulin level value is from Barone, M.A. (1999). Laboratory values. In J.A. McMillan, C.D. DeAngelis, R.D. Feigin, & J.B. Warshaw. *Oski's pediatrics: Principles and practice* (3rd ed., pp. 2216–2225). Philadelphia: Lippincott Williams & Wilkins.

Index

*Page numbers in bold indicate tables and figures.

F

Face
  newborns, 543
  pediatric assessment,
    775–776
Face presentation, 313, 401–402,
  403
Facilitated transport, 120
Failure to thrive (FTT), 719–721
Faintness, 189
Fallopian tubes, 29–30
False labor, 148, 320, 321
False pelvis, 32
Family
  adolescent pregnancy and,
    211–215
  asthma, 1043
  at-risk newborns, 672–679
  caesarian birth education for,
    138
  care of, 183
  cesarean birth and, 438–441
  first stage of labor, 360
  home care, 692, 693–695,
    835–836
  home visit, 684
  hospitalization and, 817, 821
  postpartal risks, 483
  prenatal education for,
    136–138
  psychologic response to
    pregnancy, 150–155
  teaching, 821–823
Family adaptation, 214
Family assessment
  community, 855–858
  hospitalization, 821
Family-centered childbirth, 5
Family-centered maternal-child
  care, 5–8
Family crisis, 900–901
Family profile, **857**
Family structure, 865
Family therapy, 1420
Family wellness, promotion of,
  475–476
Fantasy, **729**
Farsightedness, 1246
Fat, 222
Father
  care of, 183
  psychologic response to
    pregnancy, 153–154
  See also Parents
Father-infant interactions, 452.
  See also Attachment
Fatigue, 186
Fat-soluble vitamins, 223–224
Fear, 394–395
Feeding
  breast milk, 587–589 (*see
    also* Breastfeeding)
  cultural considerations,
    593–594
  formula, 589–591
  home care, 686
  patterns, 591–592
  promotion of, 592–593

See also Bottle-feeding;
  Formula feeding
Feeding disorder of infancy and
  early childhood, 719–721
Feeding disorders, 1193–1194
Feet, 808
  disorders, 1319–1323
  newborns, 549–550
Female condoms, 49–50, **51**
Female genitals, 23–25, 532, 548
  inspection of, 801–802
  palpation of, 802
Female hormones, effects of,
  34–36
Female partner abuse, 61–63
Female reproductive cycle (FRC),
  34–38
Female reproductive system, 23
  breasts, 34
  external genitals, 23–25
  internal organs, 25–34
Ferning capacity, 86–87
Fertility awareness, 48–49, **83**
Fertilization, process of, 112–114
Fetal acoustic stimulation test
  (FAST), 299
Fetal activity
  maternal assessment of, 294
  monitoring, 191, **192**
Fetal alcohol syndrome (FAS),
  200, 236, 633, 1430
Fetal assessment, intrapartal,
  341–352
Fetal attitude, 312, **313**
Fetal blood sampling, 352
Fetal bradycardia, 347
Fetal breathing movements, 507
Fetal circulation, **510**
Fetal circulatory system, 121, **122**
Fetal death, 10
Fetal development, 121–129,
  173–174
Fetal distress, 408–409
Fetal fibronectin (fFN), 269
Fetal head, 311–312
Fetal heartbeat, 150, 173
Fetal heart rate (FHR)
  auscultation of, 343–344
  electronic monitoring of,
    344–352
  tracing, 396
Fetal lie, 312
Fetal lung development, 507
Fetal malposition. *See* Malposition
Fetal malpresentation. *See*
  Malpresentation
Fetal maturity, 429
Fetal movement, 150
Fetal movement record (FMR),
  191, **192**
Fetal-neonatal risks/implications
  abruption placentae, 412–413
  cephalopelvic disproportion,
    422
  diabetes mellitus, 240
  forceps-assisted birth, 436
  herpes simplex virus, 286–287
  hydramnios, 420

multiple gestation, 406
oligohydramnios, 421
placenta previa, 413–414
preeclampsia-eclampsia, 274
prolapsed umbilical cord, 419
Rh sensitization, 280
rubella, 285
toxoplasmosis, 285
Fetal-newborn transitional physiology, 510–511
Fetal outline, 149
Fetal position, 315, **316**, 341, 343
Fetal presentation, 312–313,
  314, 341, 343
Fetal scalp blood sampling, 352
Fetal sensation, 329
Fetal stage, 126–128
Fetal status, 293
  amniotic fluid analysis,
    302–303
  biophysical profile, 299–300
  chorionic villus sampling, 304
  contraction stress test,
    300–302
  Doppler blood flow studies,
    296–297
  fetal acoustic stimulation test
    and vibroacoustic stimula-
    tion test, 299
  maternal assessment, 294
  nonstress test, 297–299
  percutaneous umbilical blood
    sampling, 304
  ultrasound, 294–296
Fetal tachycardia, 346
Fetus
  cardinal movements, 323, 325
  diabetes mellitus, 241
  labor and, 311–314, 329
  Rh sensitization, 282
  visualization of, 150
Fever, 1003, 1016, 1019
Fibroadenoma, 66
Fibrocystic breast disease, 65–66
Filtration, 944
Fimbriae, 29
Fimbria ovarica, 29
Fine motor development, **809**
First feeding, 573–574, 591
First stage (of labor), 322–323
  assessment guide, 335–339
  nursing management during,
    359–370
First trimester
  discomforts of, 183–186
  father's psychologic response
    to, 153
  mother's psychologic
    response to, 152
Flatulence, 187
Flaxseed, 1189
Flexion, 323
Fluids, 225
  acute postinfectious
    glomerulonephritis, 1238
  acute renal failure, 1225
  anorexia nervosa, 888
  asthma, 1043

laryngotracheobronchitis,
  1033
nephrotic syndrome, 1221
osteomyelitis, 1336
preterm newborns, 619, 622
pyloric stenosis, 1170
respiratory alkalosis, 964
systemic lupus erythema-
  tosus, 983
Fluid volume imbalances
  anatomy and physiology of,
    936–937
  clinical assessment, 958
  edema, 944–946
  extracellular, 938–944
Fluoride, **752**
Focal seizures, 1280
Folic acid, 224, 719
Folic acid deficiency anemia, **247**
Follicle-stimulating hormone
  (FSH), 23, 85
Follicular phase, 37
Folliculitis, 1396
Follow-up care, for newborns,
  690, 692
Fontanelles, 312, 542, 776
Food diary, 714–715
Food frequency questionnaire,
  714
Food groups, vegetarian, **226**
Food Guide Pyramid, **221, 706**
Food insecurity, 715
Food insecurity screening, **716**
Food jags, 711
Food reactions, 721–722
Food safety, 717, 982
Food security, 715
Food Stamp Program, 716
Foot disorders, 1319–1323. *See
  also* Feet
Footling breech, 313
Foramen ovale, 121
Forceps marks, 540
Forceps, 436
Forceps-assisted birth, 436–437
Forces of labor, 317
Foreign bodies, 1416
Foreign-body aspiration, 1058
Foremilk, 587
Foreskin, 39
Formal operational stage, 733
Formula feeding, 589–591
  education for, 601–603
  nutritional needs and,
    707–708
Fornix, 26
Fourchette, 24
Fourth stage (of labor), 326
  complications, 422
  nursing management during,
    373–378
Fractures, 1309, **1310,**
  1341–1344, **1345, 1346**
Fragile X syndrome, 99, 1430
Frank breech, 313
Frequency, 317
Freud, Sigmund, 729, **730–731**
Frontal suture, 312

SINGLE PC LICENSE AGREEMENT AND LIMITED WARRANTY

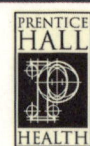
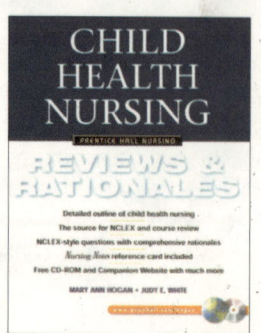
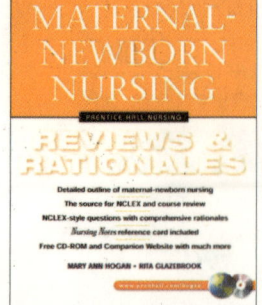
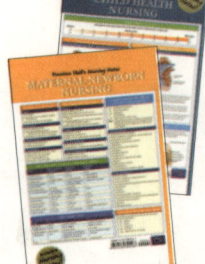